KU-728-252

OXFORD TEXTBOOK OF MEDICINE

OXFORD MEDICAL PUBLICATIONS

OXFORD TEXTBOOK OF MEDICINE

THIRD EDITION

VOLUME 1
Sections 1–10 and Index

Edited by

D. J. Weatherall

Regius Professor of Medicine, University of Oxford;
Honorary Director, Institute of Molecular Medicine, Oxford

J. G. G. Ledingham

Clinical Professor and May Reader in Medicine,
Nuffield Department of Clinical Medicine, University of Oxford

D. A. Warrell

Professor of Tropical Medicine and Infectious Diseases,
Nuffield Department of Clinical Medicine, University of Oxford

Oxford New York Tokyo
OXFORD UNIVERSITY PRESS
1996

Oxford University Press, Walton Street, Oxford OX2 6DP
Oxford New York
Athens Auckland Bangkok Bombay
Calcutta Cape Town Dar es Salaam Delhi
Florence Hong Kong Istanbul Karachi
Kuala Lumpur Madras Madrid Melbourne
Mexico City Nairobi Paris Singapore
Taipei Tokyo Toronto
and associated companies in
Berlin Ibadan

Oxford is a trade mark of Oxford University Press

Published in the United States
by Oxford University Press Inc., New York

First published 1983
Second edition 1987
Third edition 1996

A catalogue record for this book is available from the British Library

Library of Congress Cataloging in Publication Data
(Data Available)

ISBN 0 19 262140 8 (Three volume set)
ISBN 0 19 262706 6 (vol 1)
ISBN 0 19 262707 4 (vol 2)
ISBN 0 19 262708 2 (vol 3)
Available as a three volume set only

Typeset by University Graphics Inc, New Jersey, USA
Printed in the United States of America

Preface to the Third Edition

As the third edition of the *Oxford Textbook of Medicine* begins to see the light of day, medical textbooks are having a bad press in Great Britain. The stimulus to the recent resurgence of the age-old argument about the educational value, or lack of it, of textbooks was a presentation to a House of Lords Select Committee that suggested that many patients are losing their lives because doctors rely on information obtained from outdated texts and clinical teaching based on archaic practice.

In the preface to the first edition of the *Textbook* we discussed the late Professor Mitchell's similarly jaundiced views on the value of medical textbooks. He had suggested that they were likely to suffer the same fate as dinosaurs in that their very weight would preclude survival (it is not just the medical sciences that need constant revision; this view of the reason for the extinction of the dinosaurs may also have to be modified!). He went on to say that textbooks were already out of date before they were published, and hence, as well as being a health hazard due to their weight, were of limited educational value to their readers. However, having had a few more years to ponder further on Professor Mitchell's forecasts, we remain largely unrepentant.

A number of factors have combined greatly to increase the complexity of medical practice over the relatively short timespan since this *Textbook* was first published. There has been a major revolution in the basic biological sciences that has enormous implications for clinical practice in the future. In the richer countries the mean age of the population has risen dramatically and hence the pattern of disease has become much more complex and multifactorial. The populations of the developing countries continue to expand and, if anything, malnutrition and infectious disease present an even more frightening problem than they did fifteen years ago. And the remarkable achievements of the basic biomedical sciences combined with the inability of the richer countries to contain the costs of health care, and the poorer ones to provide it, are raising many new ethical problems for doctors.

Set against this complex and rapidly changing scene what should be the objective of a textbook of medicine? Clearly, no student or practitioner can own a library of monographs and journals that covers the whole of internal medicine. One important function is to provide a sound basic account of the many disorders that comprise internal medicine and thus give the background to more recent advances that are best sought in specialist journals. Furthermore, as well as the greater complexity of the diseases of the richer countries, the increasing ease of international travel and the movements of massive refugee populations round the world mean that internal medicine today is truly global; diseases that once were restricted to tropical climates or particular countries can turn up in hospitals or consulting rooms anywhere in the world. It is clear, therefore, that some basic textbooks that give students and doctors a 'way in' to the literature on the bulk of the diseases that they are likely to encounter, common or rare, are still required. With this background in mind we have added a number of new chapters and topics to this edition and have had many of the previous ones completely rewritten. We have expanded some of the background chapters on the basic sciences, particularly for students and doctors in countries in which access to current literature in these fields is limited. We have introduced new sections on medical ethics, clinical trials and evidence-based medicine, forensic medicine, and related topics that are an important part of the modern medical scene. As in previous editions, we have attempted to provide a global view of internal medicine rather than describe it as it is seen in day-to-day practice in the richer industrialized countries. And because of the increasing evidence of the clinical value of the management of cancer by specialists in the field we have included a new section on clinical oncology as a background to the descriptions of malignant disease in individual sections.

We are well aware that parts of this book will rapidly date and hence it is important that students and practitioners continue to augment their reading with up-to-date journals, and refresh themselves by regular visits to postgraduate meetings. Information systems and related technology are rapidly changing the face of communication in medicine and readers should avail themselves of every opportunity of learning the complexities and potentials of this rapidly evolving branch of practice.

As before we are particularly grateful to those of our colleagues who helped in the planning of particular sections: Dr J.A. Vale (poisoning by drugs and chemicals); Dr E. Hodgson and Professor J.M. Harrington (occupational and environmental health and safety); Dr R.W.E. Watts (metabolic disorders); Professor Alan McGregor (endocrine disorders); Professor C. Redman (medical disorders of pregnancy); Dr Derek Jewell, Dr Margaret Bassendine, and Professor Sir Leslie Turnberg (gastroenterology); Professor Stuart Cobbe (cardiovascular disorders); Drs Julian Hopkin and Donald Lane (respiratory medicine); Professor M.W. Adler (sexually-transmitted diseases and sexual health); Professor Paul Dieppe (rheumatology); Professors John Goldman and Sam Machin (disorders of the blood); Drs J. Strang, I. Glass, and M. Farrell (alcohol and drug-related problems); Professor J. Newsom-Davis (neurology and disorders of voluntary muscle). The section on Psychiatry was organized and edited by Professor Michael Gelder.

We wish to thank Dr Irene Butcher who has edited this edition of the *Textbook*; her forbearance with its editors, some of its more errant authors, and Oxford University Press has, at times, bordered on the saintly. We also thank Mrs Pam Herridge for invaluable editorial work. Finally, we are particularly grateful to our personal secretaries who have stayed the course with us through yet another phase of this saga, Mrs Janet Watt, Mrs Maureen Stacey, and Miss Eunice Berry.

Oxford
April 1995

D.J. WEATHERALL
J.G.G. LEDINGHAM
D.A. WARRELL

Dose schedules are being continually revised and new side-effects recognized. Oxford University Press makes no representation, express or implied, that the drug dosages in this book are correct. For these reasons the reader is strongly urged to consult the drug company's printed instructions before administering any of the drugs recommended in this book.

Summary of Contents

Volume 1

Volume 2

Volume 3

Contents

Volume 1

Volume 2

Volume 3

Contributors

P. AABY
Senior Researcher, Statens Seruminstitut, Copenhagen, Denmark
7.10.2 Measles

J.P. ACKERS
Senior Lecturer, Department of Medical Parasitology, London School of Hygiene and Tropical Medicine, London, UK
7.13.13 Trichomoniasis

A.A. ADISH
% McGill Community Health Project, Addis Ababa, Ethiopia
8.5.5(h) Podoconiosis (non-filarial endemic elephantiasis of the lower legs)

M.W. ADLER
Professor of Genito-Urinary Medicine, Academic Department of Genito-Urinary Medicine, University College London Medical School, UK
21.1 Sexually transmitted diseases and sexual health

D. ADU
Consultant Nephrologist, Queen Elizabeth Hospital, Birmingham, UK
20.4.2 Idiopathic glomerulonephritis
20.5.2 Infections and associated nephropathies

M.P. ALPERS
Director, Papua New Guinea Institute of Medical Research, Goroka, Papua New Guinea
24.7.5 Kuru

P.D. ANDERSON
Consultant, World Health Organization Regional Office for Europe, Copenhagen, Denmark
28.2.1 Alcohol and drug-related problems: screening and brief intervention

H. ANNETT
Head, Health Department, Secretariat de Son Altesse l'Aga Khan, Aiglemont, Gouvieux, France
3.4 Health care in developing countries

J.K. ARONSON
Clinical Reader in Clinical Pharmacology, University of Oxford; Honorary Consultant Physician, Anglia and Oxfordshire Health Authority, Oxford, UK
9 Principles of clinical pharmacology and drug therapy

A.W. ASSCHER
Principal, St George's Hospital Medical School, University of London, UK
20.9.4 Balkan (endemic) nephropathy and irradiation nephritis

TAR-CHING AW
Senior Lecturer in Occupational Medicine, Institute of Occupational Health, University of Birmingham, UK
8.3.6 Poisoning from metals
8.5.5(k) Environmental factors and disease: vibration

J.G. AYRES
Consultant Respiratory Physician, Heartlands Hospital, Birmingham, UK
8.5.5(l) Environmental factors and disease: air pollution

R.R. BAILEY
Nephrologist, Christchurch Hospital, New Zealand
20.8.1 Urinary tract infection
20.8.2 Vesicoureteric reflux and reflux nephropathy

M.J. BAINES
Consultant Physician, St Christopher's Hospice, London, UK
32 Terminal illness

E.L. BAKER
Centers for Disease Control and Prevention, Atlanta, Georgia, USA
8.5.3(d) The main occupational diseases: neurological disorders

L.R.I. BAKER
Consultant Physician and Nephrologist, St Bartholomew's Hospital, London, UK
20.10 Urinary-tract obstruction
20.15 Genitourinary tuberculosis

J.E. BANATVALA
Professor of Clinical Virology, United Medical and Dental Schools of Guy's and St Thomas's Hospital, St Thomas's Campus, London, UK
13.12.1 Viral infections in pregnancy

C.R.M. BANGHAM
Consultant Virologist, John Radcliffe Hospital, Oxford, UK
7.10.31 HTLV-I and -II associated diseases

SIR ROGER BANNISTER
Honorary Consultant Neurologist, The National Hospital for Neurology and Neurosurgery, London, and Oxford Regional and District Health Authority, UK
24.3.7 The autonomic nervous system

K.M. BANNISTER
Senior Consultant, Renal Unit and Department of Nuclear Medicine, Royal Adelaide Hospital, South Australia
20.1 Clinical physiology of the kidney: tests of renal function and structure

D. BARLOW
Consultant Physician, Department of Genitourinary Medicine, St Thomas's Hospital, London, UK
7.11.6 Neisseria gonorrhoeae

A.J. BARRETT
Chief, Bone Marrow Transplant Unit, National Heart, Lung, and Blood Institute, National Institutes of Health, Bethesda, Maryland, USA
22.3.3 Acute myeloblastic leukaemia

C. BASS

Consultant in Liaison Psychiatry, John Radcliffe Hospital, Oxford, UK

27.3.1 Psychological factors and the presentation and course of illness

M.F. BASSENDINE

Professor of Hepatology, Department of Medicine, The Medical School, University of Newcastle; Consultant Physician, Freeman Hospital, Newcastle upon Tyne, UK

14.27.2 Primary biliary cirrhosis

P.J. BAXTER

Consultant Occupational Physician, University of Cambridge and Addenbrooke's Hospital, Cambridge, UK

8.5.5(m) Environmental factors and disease: environmental disasters

M.A.H. BAYLES

Senior Specialist and Senior Lecturer, Department of Dermatology, King Edward VIII Hospital and Medical School, University of Natal, Durban, South Africa

7.12.3 Chromoblastomycosis

P.H. BAYLIS

Professor of Experimental Medicine, University of Newcastle upon Tyne; Consultant Physician, Royal Victoria Infirmary, Newcastle upon Tyne, UK

12.3 The posterior pituitary

20.2.1 Water and sodium homeostasis and their disorders

J.I. BELL

Nuffield Professor of Clinical Medicine, John Radcliffe Hospital, University of Oxford; Consultant Physician in General Medicine, Oxford Radcliffe NHS Trust, UK

5.2 Immune mechanisms of disease

11.11 Diabetes mellitus

E.J. BELL*

Regional Virus Laboratory, Ruchill Hospital, Glasgow, UK

7.10.13 Enteroviruses

M.K. BENSON

Consultant Chest Physician, Osler Chest Unit, The Churchill Hospital, Oxford, UK

17.11 Pleural disease

17.13.2 Pleural tumours

17.13.3 Mediastinal tumours and cysts

V. BERAL

Director, Imperial Cancer Research Fund's Cancer Epidemiology Unit, Oxford, UK

21.8 Cervical cancer and other cancers caused by sexually transmitted infections

R.J. BERRY

Director, Westlakes Research Institute, Moor Row, Cumbria, UK

8.5.5(i) Environmental factors and disease: radiation

* It is with regret that we report the deaths of those authors marked with an asterisk. Although their deaths occurred between the appearance of the second edition and preparation of the third edition, much of their contribution to the former has been incorporated into this edition, with appropriate updating from their coauthors.

P.C.L. BEVERLEY

Professor of Tumour Immunology and Staff Member of the Imperial Cancer Research Fund, University College London Medical School, UK

6.4 Tumour immunology

C.M. BLACK

Professor of Rheumatology, Royal Free Hospital and School of Medicine, University of London, UK

18.11.1 Connective tissue disorders and vasculitis—introduction

18.11.4 Systemic sclerosis

S.R. BLOOM

Professor of Endocrinology, Royal Postgraduate Medical School, Hammersmith Hospital, London, UK

12.10 Non-diabetic pancreatic endocrine disorders and multiple endocrine neoplasia

14.8 Hormones and the gastrointestinal tract

L.D. BLUMHARDT

Professor of Clinical Neurology, University of Nottingham; Consultant Neurologist, University Hospital, Queen's Medical Centre, Nottingham, UK

24.4.2 Syncope

N.A. BOON

Consultant Cardiologist, Royal Infirmary of Edinburgh, UK

15.14.2 HIV-related heart muscle disease

15.28.3 Coarctation of the aorta as a cause of secondary hypertension in the adult

R.T. BOOTH

Professor of Safety and Health, Health and Safety Unit, Aston University, Birmingham, UK

8.5.4 Occupational safety

I.C.G. BOWLER

Consultant Microbiologist, Oxford Regional Public Health Laboratory, John Radcliffe Hospital, Oxford, UK

7.9 Nosocomial infection

D. BRADLEY

Professor of Tropical Hygiene, London School of Hygiene and Tropical Medicine, University of London, UK

7.13.2 Malaria

R.D. BRADLEY

Emeritus Professor of Intensive Care Medicine, St Thomas's Hospital, London, UK

16 Intensive care

D.P. BRENTON

Reader in Inherited Metabolic Diseases, Department of Medicine, University of College London School of Medicine, UK

11.3 Inborn errors of amino acid and organic acid metabolism

R.P. BRETTLE

Consultant Physician and Part-time Senior Lecturer, Regional Infectious Disease Unit, City Hospital, Edinburgh, UK

28.3.1 Complications of drug use, particularly injecting drug use

V. BROADBENT
Consultant Paediatric Oncologist, Addenbrooke's Hospital, Cambridge, UK
22.5.6 The histiocytoses

M. BROWN
Professor of Clinical Pharmacology, University of Cambridge; Honorary Consultant Physician, Addenbrooke's Hospital, Cambridge, UK
15.28.2 Phaeochromocytoma

A.D.M. BRYCESON
Consultant Physician, Hospital for Tropical Diseases, London
7.13.12 Leishmaniasis

C. BUNCH
Medical Director, Oxford Radcliffe Hospital NHS Trust, John Radcliffe Hospital, Oxford, UK
22.5.2 Introduction to the lymphoproliferative disorders
22.5.3 The lymphomas
22.8.2 Marrow transplantation

DANAI BUNNAG
Professor Emeritus, Clinical Tropical Medicine, Mahidol University, Bangkok, Thailand
7.16.2 Liver fluke diseases of humans

W. BURGDORFER
Scientist Emeritus, Laboratory of Vectors and Pathogens, National Institutes of Health, Rocky Mountain Laboratories, Hamilton, Montana, USA
7.11.30 Lyme disease

A.K. BURROUGHS
Consultant Physician and Hepatologist, Liver Transplantation and Hepato-biliary Medicine, Royal Free Hospital, London, UK
14.29 Cirrhosis, portal hypertension, and ascites

T. BUTLER
Professor of Internal Medicine and of Microbiology and Immunology, Texas Technical University, Health Sciences Center; Attending Physician, University Medical Center, Lubbock, USA
7.11.6 Plague

A.E. BUTTERWORTH
Medical Research Council External Scientific Staff and Honorary Professor of Medical Parasitology, Department of Pathology, University of Cambridge, UK
7.16.1 Schistosomiasis

F.I. CAIRD
Formerly David Cargill Professor of Geriatric Medicine, University of Glasgow, UK
31 Medicine in old age

J.S. CAMERON
Professor of Renal Medicine, United Medical and Dental Schools, Guy's Campus, London, UK
20.3 Common presentations of renal disease
20.5.6 Rheumatological disorders and the kidney
20.9.2 Gout, purines, and interstitial nephritis

D.M. CAMPBELL
Senior Lecturer in Obstetrics and Gynaecology and Reproductive Physiology, University of Aberdeen, UK
13.11 Nutrition in pregnancy

M.J. CARDOSA
Lecturer, School of Pharmaceutical Sciences, Universiti Sains Malaysia, Penang, Malaysia
7.10.20 Dengue haemorrhagic fever

D.J.S. CARMICHAEL
Consultant Nephrologist, Southend Health Care NHS Trust, Essex, UK
20.14 Drugs and the kidney

J. CARMICHAEL
J.B. Cochrane Professor of Clinical Oncology, University of Nottingham, UK
6.8. New approaches to cancer therapy

C.C.J. CARPENTER
Professor of Medicine, Brown University, Providence, Rhode Island, USA
7.11.11 Cholera

R.W. CARRELL
Professor of Haematology, University of Cambridge, Addenbrooke's Hospital, Cambridge, UK
11.15 α_1-Antitrypsin deficiency

D.P. CASEMORE
Clinical Scientist, PHLS Cryptosporidium Reference Unit, Glan Clwyd District General Hospital, Bodelwyddan, Clwyd, UK
7.13.5 Cryptosporidium and cryptosporidiosis
7.13.6 Cyclospora

A. CASSELS
Independent Health Systems Development Consultant, Chilham, Canterbury, Kent, UK
3.4 Health care in developing countries

D. CATOVSKY
Professor of Haematology, Institute of Cancer Research and Royal Marsden Hospital, London, UK
22.3.2 The classification of leukaemia
22.3.6 Chronic lymphocytic leukaemia and other leukaemias of mature B and T cells
22.3.7 Myelodysplastic syndromes

D.A. CHAMBERLAIN
Consultant Cardiologist, Royal Sussex County Hospital, Brighton: Senior Visiting Research Fellow, University of Sussex, UK
15.6.2 Digitalis

H.M. CHAPEL
Consultant Immunologist and Senior Clinical Lecturer, John Radcliffe Hospital, Oxford, UK
5.4 Complement and disease

L.E. CHAPMAN
Supervising Medical Epidemiologist, Division of Viral and Rickettsial Diseases, National Center for Infectious Diseases, Center for Disease Control, Atlanta, Georgia, USA
7.10.5 Human infections caused by simian herpesviruses

R.W. CHAPMAN
Consultant Gastroenterologist, John Radcliffe Hospital, Oxford, UK
14.27.3 Primary sclerosing cholangitis

SEUNG-YULL CHO
Professor of Parasitology, College of Medicine, Chung-Ang University, Seoul, Korea
7.15.4 Diphyllobothriasis and sparganosis

A.B. CHRISTIE*
Honorary Consultant, Fazakerley Hospital, Liverpool, UK
7.10.11 Mumps: epidemic parotitis
7.11.1 Diphtheria
7.11.18 Anthrax

M.L. CLARK
Senior Lecturer, St Bartholomew's Hospital Medical College, London, UK
14.16 Tumours of the gastrointestinal tract

A.R. CLARKSON
Associate Professor of Medicine, University of Adelaide; Director, Renal Unit, Royal Adelaide Hospital, Australia
20.4.1 IgA nephropathy, Henoch-Schönlein purpura, and thin membrane nephropathy

SIR CECIL CLOTHIER
Formerly Parliamentary Commissioner for Administration and Health Service Commissioner for England and Wales, and Scotland
1 On being a patient

A.J.S. COATS
Senior Lecturer and Honorary Consultant Cardiologist, Royal Brompton Hospital, London, UK
15.5 The syndrome of heart failure

S.M. COBBE
Professor of Medical Cardiology, University of Glasgow, Glasgow Royal Infirmary, UK
15.8.1 Cardiac arrhythmias

J. COHEN
Professor of Infectious Diseases and Bacteriology, Royal Postgraduate Medical School, Hammersmith Hospital, London, UK
7.19.3 Infection in the immunocompromised host

R.D. COHEN
Professor of Medicine, The London Hospital Medical College, University of London, UK
11.14 Disturbances of acid-base homeostasis
20.19.1 The renal tubular acidoses

* It is with regret that we report the deaths of those authors marked with an asterisk. Although their deaths occurred between the appearance of the second edition and preparation of the third edition, much of their contribution to the former has been incorporated into this edition, with appropriate updating from their coauthors.

J. COLLINGE
Wellcome Senior Research Fellow in the Clinical Sciences and Honorary Consultant in Neurology and Molecular Genetics, St Mary's Hospital Medical School, Imperial College London, UK
24.7.4 Prion diseases

R. COLLINS
British Heart Foundation Research Fellow and Co-ordinator, Clinical Trial Service Unit, Nuffield Department of Clinical Medicine, University of Oxford, UK
2.4 Large-scale randomized evidence: trials and overviews

G. COLMAN
Formerly Consultant Microbiologist, Division of Hospital Infection, Central Public Health Laboratory, Colindale, London, UK
7.11.2 Pathogenic streptococci

D.A.S. COMPSTON
Professor of Neurology, University of Cambridge, UK
24.9 Demyelinating disorders of the central nervous system

C.P. CONLON
Consultant Physician, Infectious Diseases Unit, Nuffield Department of Medicine, John Radcliffe Hospital, Oxford, UK
7.8 Travel and expedition medicine
7.10.29 HIV infection and AIDS
14.18 Gastrointestinal infections

M. CONTRERAS
Chief Executive and Medical Director, North London Blood Transfusion Centre, London, UK
22.4.13 Acquired haemolytic anaemia

M.R. COOPER
Formerly Commonwealth Bureau of Animal Health, Central Veterinary Laboratory, Addlestone, Surrey, UK
8.4.2 Poisonous plants and fungi

J. COUVREUR
Associate Professor of Paediatrics, Hôpital Trousseau, Paris, France
7.13.4 Toxoplasmosis

P.J. COWEN
Medical Research Council Clinical Scientist, University Department of Psychiatry, Littlemore Hospital, Oxford, UK
27.4.1 Psychopharmacology in medical practice

T.M. COX
Professor of Medicine, University of Cambridge, and Honorary Consultant Physician, Addenbrooke's Hospital, Cambridge, UK
11.2.1 Glycogen storage diseases
11.2.2 Inborn errors of fructose metabolism
11.2.3 Disorders of galactose metabolism
14.9.5 Disaccharidase deficiency

W.I. CRANSTON
Emeritus Professor of Medicine, United Medical and Dental Schools, St Thomas's Hospital, London, UK
8.5.5(b) Environmental factors and disease: drug-induced increases of body temperature

D.H. CRAWFORD
Professor of Microbiology, London School of Hygiene and Tropical Medicine, UK
7.10.4 The Epstein–Barr virus

P. CREAMER
Senior Registrar in Rheumatology, Bristol Royal Infirmary, UK
18.3 Rheumatology: use and abuse of investigations

I.B. CROME
Consultant Psychiatrist, Keele, Staffordshire, UK
28.1.2 Assessing substance use and misuse
28.1.3 Diagnoses and classifications: substance problems and dependence—what is the difference?
28.3.2 The management of substance-related problems in a general ward

D.W.M. CROOK
Consultant Microbiologist, Public Health Laboratory, John Radcliffe Hospital, Oxford, UK
7.9 Nosocomial infection
15.17 Infective endocarditis
15.21 Cardiovascular syphilis
17.6.3 Microbiological methods in the diagnosis of respiratory infections
24.15.1 Bacterial meningitis

G.W. CSONKA
Consultant Physician in Genitourinary Medicine (retired), Charing Cross Hospital, London, UK
7.11.34 Syphilis

J. CUNNINGHAM
Consultant Physician and Honorary Senior Lecturer in Nephrology, Royal London Hospital and Medical College, London, UK
20.19 Renal tubular disorders

SIR JOHN DACIE
Emeritus Professor of Haematology, Royal Postgraduate Medical School, University of London, UK
22.3.12 Paroxysmal nocturnal haemoglobinuria

D.A.B. DANCE
Director/Consultant Microbiologist, Public Health Laboratory, Derifford Hospital, Plymouth, Devon, UK
7.11.15 Melioidosis and glanders

J.H. DARGIE
Consultant Cardiologist, Western Infirmary, Glasgow, UK
15.6.3 Vasodilators

J.H. DARK
Consultant Cardiothoracic Surgeon, Freeman Hospital, Newcastle upon Tyne, UK
15.7 Cardiac transplantation

P.G. DAVEY
Reader in Clinical Pharmacology and Infectious Diseases, Ninewells Hospital and Medical School, Dundee, UK
7.6 Antimicrobial chemotherapy

M.J. DAVIES
BHF Professor of Cardiovascular Pathology, St George's Hospital Medical School, University of London, UK
15.10.2 The pathology of ischaemic heart disease

S.W. DAVIES
Consultant Cardiologist, The Royal Brompton Hospital, London, UK
15.3.1 Breathlessness
15.3.4 Fatigue

P.D.O DAVIES
Consultant Respiratory Physician, Cardiothoracic Centre and Aintree Hospital NHS Trust, Liverpool, UK
7.11.22 Tuberculosis
7.11.24 Disease caused by environmental bacteria

A.M. DAVISON
Consultant Renal Physician, St James's University Hospital, Leeds, UK
20.5.4 Renal manifestations of malignant disease
20.5.5 Sarcoid and the kidney

P.T. DAWES
Consultant Rheumatologist, Staffordshire Rheumatology Centre; Senior Lecturer, University of Keele, Staffordshire, UK
18.2 Rheumatology: clinical presentation and diagnosis

K. DAWKINS
Consultant Cardiologist and Clinical Services Manager, Wessex Cardiothoracic Centre, Southampton General Hospital, UK
15.4.7 Exercise testing

D.P. DE BONO
British Heart Foundation Professor of Cardiology, University of Leicester Medical School, UK
15.10.5 Coronary angioplasty

M. DE SWIET
Consultant Physician, Queen Charlotte's Hospital for Women and University College Hospital, London and Northwick Park Hospital, Harrow, Middlesex, UK
13.5 Thromboembolism in pregnancy
13.6 Chest diseases in pregnancy

D.M. DENISON
Professor and Director, Lung Function Unit, Royal Bromptom Hospital, London, UK
8.5.5(e) Environmental factors and disease: aerospace medicine
8.5.5(f) Environmental factors and disease: diving medicine

J. DENT
Gastroenterology Unit, Royal Adelaide Hospital, South Australia
14.2.1 Dysphagia and other symptoms in oesophageal disease
14.6 Diseases of the oesophagus

R. DICK
Consultant Radiologist, Royal Free Hospital Trust, London, UK
14.20.1 Computed tomography and magnetic resonance imaging of the liver and pancreas

P. DIEPPE
ARC Professor of Rheumatology, Bristol University, UK
18.1 Rheumatology: introduction
18.3 Rheumatology: use and abuse of investigations

M. DOHERTY
Reader in Rheumatology, University of Nottingham Medical School, Rheumatology Unit, City Hospital, Nottingham, UK
18.7 Crystal-related arthropathies

SIR RICHARD DOLL
Honorary Consultant, Imperial Cancer Research Fund, Radcliffe Infirmary, Oxford, UK
6.2. Epidemiology of cancer

M. DONAGHY
Clinical Reader in Neurology, University of Oxford; Consultant Neurologist, Radcliffe Infirmary, Oxford, UK
24.1 Neurology: introduction
24.16 The motor neurone diseases

S. DOVER
Senior Registrar in Medicine and Gastroenterology, Fazakerley Hospital, Liverpool, UK
11.5 Porphyrin metabolism and the porphyrias

R.H. DOWLING
Professor of Gastroenterology, United Medical Schools of St Thomas's and Guy's Hospitals, Guy's Campus, London, UK
14.9.3 Small-bowel bacterial overgrowth

R.M. DU BOIS
Consultant Physician, Royal Brompton Hospital and Honorary Senior Lecturer, National Heart and Lung Institute, London, UK
17.10.1 Alveolar and interstitial disease: introduction
17.10.2 Cryptogenic fibrosing alveolitis

C.R.K. DUDLEY
Consultant Nephrologist, The Richard Bright Renal Unit, Southmead Hospital, Bristol, UK
15.12 Cholesterol embolism

B.O.L. DUKE
River Blindness Foundation, Lancaster, UK
7.14.1 General principles of filarial infections and diseases

M.S. DUNNILL
Fellow of Merton College, Sometime Consultant Histopathologist, John Radcliffe Hospital, Oxford, UK
17.6.5 Histopathology and cytology in diagnosis of lung disease

G.R. DUNSTAN
Professor Emeritus of Moral and Social Theology, University of London; Honorary Research Fellow, University of Exeter, UK
2.2. Medical ethics

D.T. DURACK
Consulting Professor of Medicine, Duke University Medical Center, Durham, North Carolina, USA
7.19.1 Fever of unknown origin

S.R. DURHAM
Senior Lecturer and Honorary Consultant Physician, Royal Brompton Hospital, London, UK
17.8.1 Allergic rhinitis ('hay fever')

B.G.M. DURIE
Division of Hematology/Oncology, Department of Medicine, Cedars-Sinai Medical Center, Los Angeles, California, USA
22.5.5 Myeloma and other paraproteinaemias

P.N. DURRINGTON
Reader in Medicine, University of Manchester Department of Medicine, Manchester Royal Infirmary, Chester, UK
11.6 Lipid and lipoprotein disorders

G.M. DUSHEIKO
Reader in Medicine, Royal Free Hospital and School of Medicine, London, UK
14.33 Hepatic granulomas

C.J. EASTMOND
Consultant Physician, Department of Rheumatology, Aberdeen Royal Infirmary, UK
18.5 Seronegative spondarthropathies

S. EBER
Professor of Paediatrics, Universitäts-Kinderklinik, Göttingen, Germany
22.4.10 Genetic disorders of the red cell membrane

A.L.W.F. EDDLESTON
Professor of Liver Immunology and Dean of Clinical Medicine, King's College School of Medicine and Dentistry, London, UK
14.27.1 Autoimmune hepatitis

C.R.W. EDWARDS
Professor of Clinical Medicine, University of Edinburgh, UK
12.7.1 Adrenocortical diseases

G. EDWARDS
Emeritus Professor of Addiction Behaviour, National Addiction Centre, University of London, UK
28.1.1 Drug problems as every doctor's business

A.M. EL NAHAS
Consultant Renal Physician, Sheffield Kidney Institute, Northern General Hospital, Shefffield, UK
20.17.1 Chronic renal failure

M. ELIA
Head of Clinical Nutrition Group, MRC, Dunn Clinical Nutrition Centre; Honorary Consultant Physician, Addenbrooke's Hospital, Cambridge, UK
10.6 Special nutritional problems and the use of enteral and parenteral nutrition

M. ELIAKIM
Professor of Internal Medicine; Chairman, Department of Medicine, Bikur Cholim Hospital, Jerusalem, Israel
11.13.2 Recurrent polyserositis (familial Mediterranean fever, periodic disease)

E. ELIAS
Consultant Physician, Liver Unit, Queen Elizabeth Hospital, Birmingham, UK
14.25 Jaundice

C.M. ELLIOTT
Dean of Trinity Hall, Cambridge, UK
3.1 The diseases of gods: some newer threats to health

B.T. EMMERSON
Professor of Medicine, University of Queensland and Consultant Physician, Princess Alexandra Hospital, Brisbane, Australia
20.13 Toxic nephropathy

SIR ANTHONY EPSTEIN
Professor Emeritus of Pathology, University of Bristol; Fellow of Wolfson College, Oxford, UK
7.10.4 The Epstein–Barr virus

S.J. EYKYN

Reader (Honorary Consultant) in Clinical Microbiology, United Medical and Dental Schools, St Thomas's Hospital, London, UK
7.11.4 Staphylococci
7.11.4 Anaerobic bacteria

E.A. FAGAN

Senior Lecturer in Medicine, Royal Free Hospital School of Medicine and University College London Medical School, London
13.13 Liver and gastrointestinal disease in pregnancy

C.G. FAIRBURN

Wellcome Trust Senior Lecturer, Department of Psychiatry, University of Oxford, UK
10.4 Eating disorders
27.2.7 Psychiatric disorders as they concern the physician: eating disorders

M. FARRELL

Senior Lecturer/Consultant Psychiatrist, National Addiction Centre, the Maudsley Hospital, London, UK
28.1.2 Assessing substance use and misuse
28.2.2 Harm reduction
28.3.2 The management of substance-related problems in a general ward
28.3.8 Caring for the HIV-positive drug user

M.J.G. FARTHING

Professor of Gastroenterology and Honorary Consultant Physician, St Bartholomew's Hospital, London, UK
14.9.9 Malabsorption in the tropics

M.F. FIELD

Associate Professor of Medicine, University of Sydney, Concord Hospital, New South Wales, Australia
20.1 Clinical physiology of the kidney: tests of renal function and structure

J.D. FIRTH

Wellcome Fellow, Honorary Consultant Physician, Oxford, UK
15.3.3 Oedema
20.16 Acute renal failure

S. FISHER-HOCH

Department of Pathology, Aga Khan Hospital Medical School, Karachi, Pakistan
7.10.22 Arenaviruses

R.A. FISHMAN

Professor of Neurology, University of California, San Francisco, USA
24.2.6 Lumbar puncture

E. FITZSIMONS

Consultant and Senior Lecturer in Haematology, Monklands Hospital, Airdrie and Western Infirmary, Glasgow, UK
11.5 Porphyrin metabolism and the porphyrias

A.F. FLEMING

Professor of Haematology at Baragwanath Hospital, Soweto School of Pathology of the South African Institute for Medical Research and the University of the Witwatersrand, Soweto, South Africa
22.4.3 Anaemia as a world health problem

E.W.L. FLETCHER

Consultant Radiologist, John Radcliffe Hospital, Oxford, UK
14.3.2 Methods for investigation of gastrointestinal diseases: radiology

D. FLISER

Physician, Department of Internal Medicine, Division of Nephrology, University of Heidelberg, Germany
20.5.1 Diabetic nephropathy

P. FOËX

Nuffield Professor of Anaesthetics, University of Oxford, Radcliffe Infirmary, Oxford, UK
17.10.20 Adult respiratory distress syndrome

J.C. FORFAR

Consultant Physician, John Radcliffe Hospital, Oxford, UK
13.4 Heart disease in pregnancy
15.6.4 Catecholamines and the sympathetic nervous system

I. FOULDS

Senior Lecturer, Occupational Dermatology, Institute of Occupational Health, University of Birmingham, UK
8.5.3(a) Occupational dermatology

G.H. FOWLER

Reader in General Practice, University of Oxford; Honorary Director, Imperial Cancer Research Fund General Practice Research Group, Oxford, UK
3.3 Primary care

A.J. FREW

Senior Lecturer in Medicine, University Medicine, University of Southampton, UK
17.9.1(a) Asthma: basic mechanisms and pathophysiology

P. FRITH

Consultant Medical Ophthalmologist, University College Hospitals, London, UK
26 The eye in general medicine

H.R. GAMSU

Professor of Neonatology, King's College Hospital School of Medicine and Dentistry, University of London, UK
13.12.2 Bacterial, fungal, and protozoal infections in pregnancy and the newborn

D. GARDNER-MEDWIN

Consultant Paediatric Neurologist, Newcastle General Hospital, Newcastle upon Tyne, UK
24.18 Developmental abnormalities of the nervous system

C. GARRARD

Consultant Physician in Intensive Care, John Radcliffe Hospital, Oxford, UK
17.10.20 Adult respiratory distress syndrome
17.14.3(a) Acute respiratory failure: intensive care

J.S. GARROW

Professor of Human Nutrition, St Bartholomew's Hospital Medical College, University of London, UK
10.5 Obesity

D.H. GATH
Clinical Reader in Psychiatry, University Department of Psychiatry, Warneford Hospital, Oxford, UK
27.2.8 Affective disorders

K.C. GATTER
University Lecturer in Pathology, Department of Cellular Science, John Radcliffe Hospital, Oxford, UK
22.5.2 Introduction to the lymphoproliferative disorders
22.5.3 The lymphomas

M.G. Gelder
Handley Professor of Psychiatry, University of Oxford, UK
27.1 Psychiatry in medicine: introduction
27.2.1 Reactions to stressful events
27.2.2 Anxiety and obsessional disorders
27.2.3 Psychiatric conditions with physical complaints
27.2.4 Dissociative disorder
27.2.5 Malingering and factitious disorders
27.2.6 Personality and its disorders
27.2.9 Schizophrenia
27.4.2 Psychological treatment in medical practice

C. GERADA
Principal in General Practice, Hurley Clinic, Kennington, London, UK
28.3.6 The pregnancy drug abuser

A.H. GHODSE
Professor of Psychiatry and Director, Centre for Addiction Studies, St George's Hospital Medical School, University of London, UK
28.3.5 Drug misusers and addicts in accident and emergency

C.J. GIBSON
Professor of Respiratory Medicine, University of Newcastle upon Tyne and Consultant Physician, Freeman Hospital, Newcastle upon Tyne, UK
17.10.19 Drug-induced lung disease

D.G. GIBSON
Consultant Cardiologist, Royal Brompton Hospital, London, UK
15.18 Valve disease
15.20 Pericardial disease

A.M. GILES
Medical Laboratory Scientific Officer, Department of Clinical Biochemistry, John Radcliffe Hospital, Oxford, UK
33 Reference intervals for biochemical data

F.J. GILES
Assistant Professor, University of California at Los Angeles; Director, Myeloma Research and Treatment Center, Bone Marrow Transplantation Unit, Cedars-Sinai Medical Center, Los Angeles, California, USA
22.5.5 Myeloma and other paraproteinaemias

C.F. GILKS
Senior Lecturer and Consultant Physician, Liverpool School of Tropical Medicine, Liverpool, UK
7.10.30 Human immunodeficiency virus in the developing world

M.D.G. GILLMER
Honorary Lecturer, Nuffield Department of Obstetrics and Gynaecology, University of Oxford and Consultant Obstetrician and Gynaecologist, John Radcliffe Hospital, Oxford, UK
13.8 Diabetes in pregnancy

D.J. GIRLING
Clinical Coordinator, MRC Cancer Trials Office, Cambridge, UK
7.11.22 Tuberculosis
7.11.24 Disease caused by environmental mycobacteria

R. GOKAL
Consultant Nephrologist and Honarary Lecturer, Manchester Royal Infirmary, UK
20.17.2 Replacement therapy by dialysis

M.J. GOLDACRE
Consultant in Public Health Medicine, Anglia and Oxford Regional Health Authority, and Honorary Senior Clinical Lecturer in Public Health, University of Oxford, UK
3.2 Health and sickness in the community

M.H.N GOLDEN
Professor of Medicine (Nutrition), University of Aberdeen, UK
10.3 Severe malnutrition

S.J. GOLDING
Lecturer in Radiology, University of Oxford, UK
6.5 Medical imaging in oncology

J. GOLDMAN
Professor of Leukaemia Biology, Royal Postgraduate Medical School, Hammersmith Hospital, London, UK
22.3.5 Chronic myeloid leukaemia

S. GORDON
Glaxo Professor of Cellular Pathology, Sir William Dunn School of Pathology, University of Oxford, UK
4.2.3 The mononuclear phagocyte system and tissue homeostasis

E.C. GORDON-SMITH
Professor of Haematology, St George's Hospital Medical School, University of London, UK
22.3.11 Aplastic anaemia and other causes of bone marrow failure
22.4.11 Haemolysis due to red-cell enzyme deficiencies
22.4.13 Acquired haemolytic anaemia

M. GOSSOP
Head of Research, Drug Dependence Unit, National Addiction Centre, The Maudsley Hospital, London, UK
28.3.7 Management of pain in the drug abuser

J.M. GRANGE
Reader in Clinical Microbiology, National Heart and Lung Institute, University of London, UK
7.11.22 Tuberculosis
7.11.24 Disease caused by environmental mycobacteria

R. GRAY
Senior Research Fellow, Clinical Trial Service Unit, Nuffield Department of Clinical Medicine, University of Oxford, UK
2.4 Large-scale randomized evidence: trials and overviews

D.W.R. GRAY
Reader in Transplantation and Consultant Surgeon, Nuffield Department of Surgery, University of Oxford, UK
20.17.3 Renal transplantation

J.R. GRAYBILL
Professor of Medicine, University of Texas Health Science Center, San Antonio, USA
7.12.2 Coccidioidomycosis

M.F. GREAVES
Professor of Cell Biology and Director, Leukaemia Research Fund Centre at the Institute for Cancer Research, London, UK
22.3.1 Cell and molecular biology of leukaemia

M. GREAVES
Reader in Haematology, Central Sheffield University Hospital, UK
22.6.7 Thrombotic disease

B.M. GREENWOOD
Director, MRC Laboratories, Fajara, The Gambia
7.3 The host's response to infection
7.11.3 Pneumococcal infection
7.11.5 Meningococcal infection

R.J. GREENWOOD
Consultant Neurologist, St Bartholomew's and The National Hospitals for Neurology and Neurosurgery, London, UK
24.15.5 Neurosyphilis

B. GRIBBIN
Consultant Cardiologist, The John Radcliffe Hospital, Oxford, UK
15.17 Infective endocarditis
15.21 Cardiovascular syphilis

J. GRIMLEY EVANS
Professor of Clinical Geratology, University of Oxford, UK
31 Medicine in old age

N.R. GRIST
Emeritus Professor of Infectious Diseases, University of Glasgow; formerly Consultant Virologist, Head of Regional Virus Laboratory, Ruchill, Glasgow, UK
7.10.13 Enteroviruses

D.I. GROVE
Director of Clinical Microbiology and Infectious Diseases, The Queen Elizabeth Hospital, Woodville, South Australia
7.14.5 Nematode infections of lesser importance

D.J. GRUNDY
Consultant in Spinal Injuries, The Duke of Cornwall Spinal Treatment Centre, Salisbury District Hospital, UK
24.3.10 Spinal cord injury and the management of paraplegia

J.-P. GRÜNFELD
Professor of Nephrology, Necker Medical School, University René Descartes, Necker Hospital, Paris, France
20.5.3 Amyloid, myeloma, light chain deposition disease, fibrillary glomerulonephritis and cryoglobulinaemia
20.7 Clinical aspects of inherited renal disorders

W.J. GULLICK
Principal Scientist, Imperial Cancer Research Fund, Hammersmith Hospital, London, UK
6.3 Growth factors and oncogenes

H.H. GUNSON
Medical Director, National Blood Authority, Manchester, UK
22.8.1 Blood transfusion

M.R. HAENEY
Consultant Immunologist, Salford General Hospitals Trust, Salford, UK
14.4 Immune disorders of the gastrointestinal tract

A.M. HALLIDAY
Formerly Consultant in Clinical Neurophysiology, National Hospital for Neurology and Neurosurgery, London; Member of the External Staff of the Medical Research Council, UK
24.2.3 Evoked potentials

P.J. HAMMOND
Senior Registrar, St James's University Hospital, Leeds, West Yorkshire, UK
12.10 Non-diabetic pancreatic endocrine disorders and multiple endocrine neoplasia
14.8 Hormones and the gastrointestinal tract

D.M. HANSELL
Consultant Radiologist, Royal Brompton Hospital, London, UK
17.6.1 Thoracic imaging

A.E. HARDING
Professor of Clinical Neurology, Institute of Neurology; Consultant Neurologist, National Hospital for Neurology and Neurosurgery, London, UK
25.9 Mitochondrial myopathies and encephalomyopathies

KHUNYING TRANAKCHIT HARINASUTA
Professor of Tropical Medicine and Consultant, Faculty of Tropical Medicine, Mahidol University, Bangkok, Thailand
7.16.4 Intestinal trematodiasis

J.M. HARRINGTON
Professor of Occupational Health, University of Birmingham, UK
8.5.1 Occupational and environmental health and safety: general introduction
8.5.2 The investigation of occupational disease
8.5.3 The main occupational diseases. (b) Occupational cancer. (e) Cardiovascular system. (f) Genitourinary system

A.L. HARRIS
Imperial Cancer Research Fund Professor of Clinical Oncology, University of Oxford, ICRF Clinical Oncology Unit, Churchill Hospital, Oxford, UK
6.8 New approaches to cancer therapy
13.15 Malignant disease in pregnancy

SIR HENRY HARRIS
Regius Professor of Medicine Emeritus, University of Oxford
6.1 General characteristics of neoplasia

M.J.G. HARRISON
Professor in Clinical Neurology, University College London Medical School; Consultant Neurologist, Middlesex Hospital and the National Hospital, London, UK
24.4.4 Coma
24.21 Neurological complications of systemic diseases

C. HASLETT

Professor of Respiratory Medicine, Edinburgh University and Honorary Consultant Physician, Royal Infirmary, Edinburgh, UK
17.3.1 Non-immune defence mechanisms of the lung
17.3.2 Inflammation and the lung

I. HASLOCK

Consultant Rheumatologist, South Tees Acute Hospitals Trust; Visiting Professor of Clinical Bio-engineering, University of Durham, UK
18.8 Back pain and periarticular disease

D.A. HAWKINS

Consultant Physician in Genitourinary Medicine, Chelsea and Westminster Hospital, London, UK
28.2.3(b) Physical complications of drug abuse

K.E. HAWTON

Consultant Psychiatrist, University Department of Psychiatry, Warneford Hospital, Oxford, UK
27.3.4 Sexual problems associated with physical illness

R.J. HAY

Mary Dunhill Professor of Cutaneous Medicine, United Medical and Dental Schools, Guy's Hospital, London, UK
7.11.28 Nocardiosis
7.12.1 Fungal infections

B. HAZLEMAN

Consultant Rheumatologist, Addenbrooke's Hospital, Cambridge, UK
18.10 Miscellaneous conditions

A.H. HENDERSON

Professor of Cardiology, University of Wales College of Medicine, Cardiff, UK
15.3.2 Chest pain

D.J. HENDRICK

Consultant Physician and Honorary Senior Lecturer, Newcastle General Hospital, University of Newcastle upon Tyne, UK
17.10.8 Lymphocytic infiltrations of the lung
17.10.9 Extrinsic allergic alveolitis
17.10.12 Pulmonary alveolar proteinosis
17.10.13 Pulmonary amyloidosis
17.10.14 Lipoid (lipid) pneumonia
17.10.15 Pulmonary alveolar microlithiasis
17.10.21 Lung disorders in genetic syndromes

M.F. HEYWORTH

Associate Professor of Medicine, University of California; Staff Physician, Veterans Affairs Medical Center, San Francisco, USA
7.13.8 Giardiasis, balantidiasis, isosporiasis, and microsporidiosis

TRAN TINH HIEN

Clinical Research Unit, Centre for Tropical Diseases (Cho Quan Hospital), Ho Chi Minh City, Vietnam
7.11.1 Diphtheria

T.W. HIGENBOTTAM

Consultant Physician and Respiratory Physiologist, Papworth and Addenbrooke's Hospitals, Cambridge, UK
17.14.4 Lung and heart-lung transplantation

S.L. HILLIER

Research Associate Professor of Obstetrics and Gynecology, University of Washington, Seattle, USA
21.4 Vaginal discharge

D. HILTON-JONES

Consultant Neurologist, Radcliffe Infirmary, Oxford, and Milton Keynes General Hospital, UK
25.8 Metabolic and endocrine myopathies

T.D.R. HOCKADAY

Honorary Consultant Physician, Radcliffe Infirmary, Oxford, UK
11.11 Diabetes mellitus

J.R. HODGES

University Lecturer and Consultant Neurologist, University of Cambridge Clinical School, Addenbrooke's Hospital, Cambridge, UK
24.7.1 Dementia: introduction
24.7.3 Pick's disease (focal lobar atrophy)

H.J.F. HODGSON

Professor of Gastroenterology, Royal Postgraduate Medical School, London, UK
14.9.6 Whipple's disease
14.9.7 Short gut syndrome

E.S. HODGSON

Occupational Health Physician and Lecturer in Occupational Health, University of Oxford: Honorary Consultant Occupational Physician, Radcliffe Hospital, Oxford, UK
8.5.1 Occupational and environmental health and safety: general introduction
8.5.2 The investigation of occupational medicine
8.5.3 The main occupational diseases: (g) Gastrointestinal tract; (h) The haematopoietic system; (i) Infections

A.V. HOFFBRAND

Professor of Haematology, Royal Free Hospital, London, UK
22.4.6 Megaloblastic anaemia and miscellaneous deficiency anaemias

S.T. HOLGATE

MRC Clinical Professor of Immunopharmacology, Southampton General Hospital, UK
17.9.1(a) Asthma: basic mechanisms and pathophysiology

P. HOLLOWAY

Clinical Lecturer and Senior Registrar, Department of Clinical Biochemistry, John Radcliffe Hospital, Oxford, UK
33 Reference intervals for biochemical data

J.M. HOPKIN

Consultant Physician, John Radcliffe Hospital, UK
7.12.5 Pneumocystis carinii
17.1 Respiratory medicine: introduction
17.7.1 Upper respiratory tract infection
17.7.3 Suppurative pulmonary and pleural infections
17.7.4 Chronic specific infections
17.7.5 Respiratory infection in the immunosuppressed
17.10.3 Bronchiolitis obliterans
17.10.5 Pulmonary vasculitis and granulomatosis
17.10.17 Toxic gases and fumes
17.10.18 Radiation pneumonitis

A.P. HOPKINS

Director of the Research Unit, Royal College of Physicians: Consultant Neurologist, Royal Hospital NHS Trust, London, UK
24.4.1 Epilepsy in later childhood and adult life

J.A.C. HOPKIRK
Consultant Physician, King Edward VII Hospital, Midhurst, West Sussex, UK
8.5.5(e) Environmental factors and disease: aerospace medicine

A. HORWICH
Professor of Radiotherapy, Institute of Cancer Research, London University; Consultant in Clinical Oncology, Royal Marsden Hospital, London, UK
6.7 Role of radiotherapy in the treatment of cancer

I.A. HUGHES
Professor of Paediatrics, University of Cambridge, UK
12.7.3 Congenital adrenal hyperplasia

B.J. HUNT
Consultant/Honorary Senior Lecturer in Haematology, St Thomas's Hospital; Honorary Senior Lecturer in Cardiothoracic Surgery at The National Heart and Lung Hospital, London, UK
22.6.6 Acquired coagulation disorders

C.W. HUTTON
Consultant Rheumatologist, Mount Gould Hospital, Plymouth, UK
18.6 Osteoarthritis

C.W. IMRIE
Honorary Senior Lecturer, University of Glasgow; Consultant Surgeon, Royal Infirmary, Glasgow, UK
14.23.1 Acute pancreatitis

M. IRVING
Professor of Surgery, Hope Hospital (University of Manchester School of Medicine), Salford, UK
14.19 The peritoneum, omentum, and appendix

D. ISAACS
Head of Department of Immunology and Infectious Diseases, Royal Alexandra Hospital for Children, Sydney: Associate Professor, University of Sydney, Australia
7.7 Immunization
7.10.1 Respiratory tract viruses

P.G. ISAACSON
Professor of Morbid Anatomy, University College London Medical School, London, UK
14.9.8 Enteropathy-associated T-cell lymphoma

D.A. ISENBERG
Professor of Rheumatology, Bloomsbury Rheumatology Unit, The Middlesex Hospital, London, UK
18.11.3 Systemic lupus erythematosus and related disorders

I. ISHERWOOD
Emeritus Professor of Diagnostic Radiology, University of Manchester, UK
24.2.1. Principles of neuroradiology

K. ISHIKAWA
Director, Department of Internal Medicine, Higashi Nagahara Hospital, Osaka, Japan
15.13 Takayasu's disease

C.A. ISON
Lecturer in Medical Microbiology, St Mary's Hospital Medical School, London, UK
7.11.6 Neisseria gonorrhoeae

A. JACKSON
Senior Lecturer in Neuroradiology, University of Manchester, UK
24.2.1 Principles of neuroradiology

H.S. JACOBS
Professor of Reproductive Endocrinology, University College London Medical School; Consultant Physician, The Middlesex Hospital, London, UK
12.8.1 The ovary
12.8.3 The breast

R.J. JACOBY
Clinical Reader in Old Age Psychiatry, University of Oxford, UK
27.2.11 Mental disorders of old age

O.F.W. JAMES
Professor of Geriatric Medicine, University of Newcastle upon Tyne, UK
14.28 Alcoholic liver disease

W.P.T. JAMES
Professor and Director, Rowett Research Institute, Aberdeen, UK
10.1 Nutrition: introduction

J.L. JAMESON
C.F. Kettering Professor of Medicine, Northwestern University School of Medicine, Chicago, Illinois, USA
12.1 Principles of hormone action

B. JENNETT
Emeritus Professor of Neurosurgery, Institute of Neurological Science, Glasgow, UK
24.4.5 Brain death and the vegetative state

D.P. JEWELL
Consultant Physician, John Radcliffe Hospital; Clinical Lecturer, University of Oxford, UK
14.1 Gastroenterology: introduction
14.2.2 Vomiting
14.2.3 Abdominal pain
14.2.6 Gastrointestinal bleeding
14.3.1 Endoscopy
14.9.4 Coeliac disease
14.10 Crohn's disease
14.11 Ulcerative colitis
14.36 Miscellaneous disorders of the gastrointestinal tract and liver

A.R. JOHNS
Senior Lecturer, Division of Psychiatry of Addictive Behaviour, St George's Hospital Medical School, University of London, UK
28.3.4 Management of withdrawal syndromes

A.M. JOHNSON
Reader in Epidemiology, Academic Department of Genito-urinary Medicine, University College London Medical School, UK
21.2 Sexual behavior

A.W. JOHNSON
Formerly Commonwealth Bureau of Animal Health, Central Veterinary Laboratory, Addlestone, Surrey, UK
8.4.2 Poisonous animals and plants

P.J. JOHNSON
Institute of Liver Studies, King's College School of Medicine and Dentistry, London, UK
14.27.1 Autoimmune hepatitis

E.A. JONES
Chief of Hepatology, Department of Gastrointestinal and Liver Diseases, Academic Medical Centre, Amsterdam, The Netherlands
14.30 Hepatocellular failure

M. JOY
Consultant Cardiologist, St Peter's District General Hospital, Chertsey, Surrey, UK
15.10.7 Vocational aspects of coronary artery disease

R.W. JUBB
Consultant Rheumatologist, Selly Oak Hospital, Birmingham, UK
8.5.3(c) The main occupational diseases: musculoskeletal disorders

B.E. JUEL-JENSEN
Honorary Consultant Physician, Nuffield Department of Clinical Medicine, John Radcliffe, Hospital, Oxford, UK
7.10.2 Herpes simplex virus infections
7.10.3 Varicella-zoster virus infections: chickenpox and zoster
7.10.9 Orf
7.10.10 Molluscum contagiosum

J.A. KANIS
Professor in Human Metabolism and Clinical Biochemistry, University of Sheffield Medical School, UK
12.6 Disorders of calcium metabolism
20.18 Renal bone disease

TOMISAKU KAWASAKI
Director, Japan Kawasaki Disease Research Center, Tokyo, Japan
18.11.10 Kawasaki disease

W.R. KEATINGE
Professor of Physiology, Queen Mary and Westfield College, University of London
8.5.5 Environmental factors and disease: (a) heat; (c) Cold, drowning, and seasonal mortality

P.G.E. KENNEDY
Burton Professor of Neurology, University of Glasgow, UK
24.15.2 Acute viral infections of the central nervous system
24.15.3 Neurological manifestations of infections with human immunodeficiency virus type 1

S. KESHAV
Research Fellow, Sir William Dunn School of Pathology, University of Oxford, UK
4.2.4 Cytokines

M. KETTLEWELL
Consultant Surgeon, Oxford Radcliffe Trust; Fellow, Green College, Oxford, UK
14.14 Colonic diverticular disease

M. KING
Honorary Research Fellow, University of Leeds, UK
3.1 The diseases of gods: some newer threats to health

M.M. KLIKS
President and Director of Research, CTS Foundation, Honolulu, Hawaii, USA
7.14.3 Guinea-worm disease: human dracunculiasis

B. KNIGHT
Professor of Forensic Pathology, University of Wales College of Medicine, Cardiff, Wales, UK
29 Forensic medicine

R. KNIGHT
Associate Professor of Parasitology, Department of Medical Microbiology, Faculty of Medicine, Unity of Nairobi, Kenya
7.13.1 Amoebiasis
7.14.4 Strongyloidiasis, hookworm, and other gut cestodes
7.15.1 Gut cestodes

J.B. KURTZ
Consultant Virologist, John Radcliffe Hospital, Oxford, UK
7.11.36 Legionellosis and legionnaires' disease

H.P. LAMBERT
Emeritus Professor of Microbial Diseases, St George's Hospital Medical School, London; Visiting Professor, London School of Hygiene and Tropical Medicine, UK
7.1 Clinical approach to the patient with suspected infection

D.J. LANE
Consultant Chest Physician, Oxford Radcliffe Hospital, The Churchill, Oxford
17.1 Respiratory medicine: introduction
17.5 The clinical presentation of chest diseases
17.9.2 Cystic fibrosis
17.9.1(b) Asthma: clinical features and management
17.10.5 Pulmonary vasculitis and granulomatosis
17.10.6 Pulmonary haemorrhagic disorders
17.10.7 Pulmonary eosinophilia

H.E. LARSON
Consultant in Infectious Disease and General Medicine, Southborough, Massachusetts, USA
7.11.21 Botulism, gas gangrene, and clostridial gastrointestinal infections

N.F. LAWTON
Consultant Neurologist, Wessex Neurological Centre, Southampton General Hospital; Honorary Senior Lecturer, University of Southampton, UK
24.13 Benign intracranial hypertension

J.G.G. LEDINGHAM
May Reader in Medicine and Honorary Consultant Physician, John Radcliffe Hospital, Oxford, UK
13.3 Renal disease in pregnancy
15.3.3 Oedema
15.6.1 Diuretics
15.26 Pulmonary embolism
15.28.1 Renal and renovascular hypertension
15.29 Lymphoedema
20.20.2 Idiopathic oedema of women
20.20.3 Disorders of potassium metabolism
24.17.1 The POEMS syndrome

J.W. LeDUC
Medical Officer, Division of Communicable Diseases, World Health Organization, Geneva, Switzerland
7.10.21 Bunyaviridae

T. LEHNER
Head of Division of Immunology, United Medical and Dental Schools of Guy's and St Thomas's Hospital, Guy's Hospital, London
14.5 The mouth and salivary glands
18.11.8 Behçet's disease

G.G. LENNOX
Senior Lecturer in Clinical Neurology, University of Nottingham Medical School, UK
13.10 Neurological disease in pregnancy

E.A. LETSKY
Consultant Haematologist, Queen Charlotte's and Chelsea Hospitals, London, UK
13.9 Blood disorders in pregnancy

S.M. LEWIS
Emeritus Reader in Haematology, University of London; Senior Research Fellow, Department of Haematology, Royal Postgraduate Medical School, London, UK
22.5.4 The spleen and its disorders

D.C. LINCH
Professor of Haematology, University College London, UK
22.2.2 Stem-cell disorders

C.C. LINNEMANN JR.
Professor, Departments of Medicine and Pathology and Laboratory Medicine, University of Cincinnati, Ohio, USA
7.11.14 Bordetella

D. LIPKIN
Consultant Cardiologist, The Royal Free Hospital, London, UK
15.3.1 Breathlessness
15.3.4 Fatigue

W.A. LISHMAN
Emeritus Professor of Neuropsychiatry, Institute of Psychiatry, London, UK
27.3.3 Specific conditions giving rise to mental disorder

A. LLANOS-CUENTAS
Professor of Medicine and Public Health, Universidad Peruana Cayetano Heredia; Senior Research Assistant at Instituto de Medicina Tropical 'Alexander von Humboldt', Lima, Peru
7.11.45 Bartonellosis

C.M. LOCKWOOD
Wellcome Reader in the School of Clinical Medicine, Addenbrooke's Hospital, Cambridge, UK
18.11.3 Small-vessel vasculitis

S. LOGAN
Senior Lecturer in Paediatric Epidemiology, Institute of Child Health, London, UK
7.10.18 Rubella

D.A. LOMAS
Lecturer in Medicine/Honorary Consultant Respiratory Physician, University of Cambridge, UK
11.5.α_1-Antitypsin deficiency

M.S. LOSOWSKY
Professor of Medicine and Dean of the Faculty of Medicine, University of Leeds, UK
14.9.2 Investigation and differential diagnosis of malabsorption

P.F. LUDMAN
Senior Registrar in Cardiology, Papworth Hospital NHS Trust, Papworth Everard, Cambridgeshire, UK
15.4.5 Magnetic resonance and computed X-ray tomography

S.E. LUX
Professor of Pediatrics, Harvard Medical School; Chief, Division of Hematology/Oncology, Children's Hospital, Boston, Massachusetts, USA
22.4.10 Genetic disorders of the red-cell membrane

L. LUZZATTO
Professor of Haematology, Royal Postgraduate Medical School, Hammersmith Hospital, London, UK
22.3.12 Paroxysmal nocturnal haemoglobinuria
22.4.12 Glucose 6-phosphate dehydrogenase (G6PD) deficiency

D.C.W. MABEY
Professor of Communicable Diseases, London School of Hygiene and Tropical Medicine, UK
7.11.42 Chlamydial infections

J.T. MacFARLANE
Consultant Physician in General and Respiratory Medicine, City Hospital, Nottingham; Clinical Teacher, University of Nottingham, UK
7.11.36 Legionellosis and legionnaires' disease
17.7.2 Acute lower respiratory tract infections

B.B. MacGILLIVRAY
Physician in charge, Department of Clinical Neurophysiology, Royal Free Hospital; Consultant in Clinical Neurophysiology, National Hospitals for Neurology and Neurosurgery, London, UK
24.2.2 Electroencephalography

S.J. MACHIN
Professor of Haematology, University College London, UK
22.6.2 Introduction to disorders of haemostasis and coagulation
22.6.3 Purpura

D.W.R. MacKENZIE
Visiting Professor of Medical Mycology, London School of Hygiene and Tropical Medicine, UK
7.12.1 Fungal infections (mycoses)

I.J. MACKIE
Non-Clinical Lecturer in Haematology, University College London, UK
22.6.1 The biology of haemostasis and thrombosis
22.6.2 Introduction to disorders of haemostasis and coagulation

C.R. MADELEY
Professor of Clinical Virology, University of Newcastle upon Tyne, UK
7.10.14 Viruses in diarrhoea and vomiting

A. MADEN
Senior Lecturer in Forensic Psychiatry, The Institute of Psychiatry, London, UK
28.3.9 The needs of the alcohol/drug user in custody

M.M. MADKOUR
Consultant Physician, Military Hospital, Riyadh, Saudi Arabia
7.11.19 Brucellosis

C. MAGUIÑA-VARGAS
Professor of Medicine, Cayetano Heredia Peruvian University; Physician, Instituto Nacional de Salud; President, Instituto de Medicina Tropical 'Alexander von Humboldt', Lima, Peru
7.11.45 Bartonellosis

J.I. MANN
Professor in Human Nutrition and Medicine, University of Otago, Dunedin, New Zealand
10.7 Diseases of overnourished societies and the need for dietary change
15.10.1 Ischaemic heart disease: epidemiology and prevention

M.G. MARMOT
Professor of Epidemiology and Public Health, University College London, UK
15.10.1 Ischaemic heart disease; epidemiology and prevention

T.J. MARRIE
Professor of Medicine and Associate Professor of Microbiology, Dalhousie University; Active Staff Physician, Victoria General Hospital, Halifax, Nova Scotia, Canada
7.11.39 Coxiella burnetti infections (Q fever)

T.C. MARRS
Senior Medical Officer, Department of Health, London, UK
8.3.7 Poisoning by conflict

P.D. MARSDEN
Professor of Medicine, University of Brasilia, Brazil
7.13.11 American trypanosomiasis

C.D. MARSDEN
Professor and Head of Neurology, Institute of Neurology and the National Hospital for Neurology and Neurosurgery, London, UK
24.4.3 Narcolepsy and related sleep disorders
24.10 Movement disorders
24.19 Metabolic and deficiency disorders of the nervous system
24.20 Neurological disorders due to physical agents

V.J. MARTLEW
Chief Executive and Medical Director, National Blood Service: Mersey and North Wales, Liverpool, UK
22.8.1 Blood transfusion

A.D. MASON
Chief, Laboratory Division, US Army Institute of Surgical Research, Fort Sam Houston, Texas, USA
8.5.5(g) Environmental factors and disease: lightning and electric shock

W.B. MATTHEWS
Professor Emeritus of Clinical Neurology, University of Oxford, UK
24.3.2 The motor and sensory systems, midbrain, and brain-stem
24.3.9 Spinal cord

R.S. MAURICE-WILLIAMS
Consultant Neurosurgeon, The Royal Free Hospital, London, UK
24.3.11 Disorders of the spinal nerve roots

R.L. MAYNARD
Senior Medical Officer, Department of Health, UK
8.3.7 Poisoning in conflict

R.T. MAYON-WHITE
Consultant in Communicable Disease Control, Oxfordshire Health Authority, Oxford, UK
7.4 Epidemiology and public health

R.A. MAYOU
Clinical Reader in Psychiatry and Honorary Consultant, Warneford Hospital, Oxford, UK
27.2.10 Organic (cognitive) mental disorders
27.3.2 Emotional reactions in the bereaved and dying
27.4.3 Psychiatric emergencies

E. McCLOY
Medical Adviser to the Civil Service; Director, Civil Service Occupational Health Service, Edinburgh, UK
8.5.3 The main occupational diseases: reproductive system

K.E.L. McCOLL
Professor of Gastroenterology, University Department of Medicine and Therapeutics, Western Infirmary, Glasgow, UK
11.5 Porphyrin metabolism and the porphyrias

J.B. McCORMICK
Center for Bacterial and Mycotic Diseases, Centers for Disease Control, Atlanta, Georgia, USA
7.10.22 Arenaviruses

A.M. McGREGOR
Professor of Medicine, King's College School of Medicine, London, UK
12.4 The thyroid gland and disorders of thyroid function
13.7 Endocrine disease in pregnancy

N. McINTYRE
Professor of Medicine, Royal Free Hospital School of Medicine, London, UK
14.29 Cirrhosis, portal hypertension, and ascites

W.J. McKENNA
Professor of Cardiac Medicine, St George's Hospital Medical School, London, UK
15.14.1 The cardiomyopathies, myocarditis, and specific heart muscle disorders

A.J. McMICHAEL
MRC Clinical Research Professor of Immunology, Nuffield Department of Medicine, Institute of Molecular Medicine, Oxford, UK
5.1. Principles of immunology

A. McMILLAN
Consultant Physician, Department of Genito-urinary Medicine, Edinburgh Royal Infirmary, UK
21.6 Infections and other medical problems in homosexual men

T.W. MEADE
Director of MRC Epidemiology and Medical Care Unit and Professor of Epidemiology, Medical College of St Bartholomew's Hospital, London, UK
15.9.3 Haemostatic variables in ischaemic heart disease

A. MEHEUS
Professor of Epidemiology and Community Medicine, University of Antwerp, Belgium
21.1 Sexually transmitted diseases and sexual health

T.J. MEREDITH

Professor of Medicine and Pathology, School of Medicine, Vanderbilt University and Director, Center for Clinical Toxicology, Vanderbilt University Medical Center, Nashville, Tennessee, USA
8.1.1 Poisoning: introduction and epidemiology
8.1.2 Poisoning: clinical and metabolic features and general principles of management
8.2.1 Poisoning caused by analgesic drugs
8.2.2 Poisoning from antidepressants, hypnotics, antihistamines, anticonvulsants, and antiparkinsonian drugs
8.2.3 Poisoning from cardiovascular drugs
8.2.4 Poisoning caused by respiratory drugs
8.2.5 Poisoning caused by drugs acting on the gastrointestinal system
8.2.6 Poisoning by haematinics and vitamins
8.2.7 Poisoning by endocrine drugs
8.2.8 Poisoning from antimicrobials
8.2.10 Poisoning from drugs of abuse
8.2.11 Poisoning due to miscellaneous drugs
8.3.1 Poisoning from household products
8.3.2 Poisoning by alcohols and glycols
8.3.3 Poisoning by hydrocarbons and chlorofluorocarbons
8.3.4 Poisoning by inhalational agents
8.3.5 Poisoning due to corrosive substances

K.R. MILLS

University Lecturer and Consultant in Clinical Neurophysiology, The Radcliffe Infirmary, Oxford, UK
24.2.4 Investigation of central motor pathways: magnetic brain stimulation

A. MINDEL

Professor of Sexual Health Medicine, Universities of Sydney and New South Wales, Sydney, Australia
21.3 Genital herpes

S.A. MISBAH

Consultant Immunologist, Leeds General Infirmary; Senior Clinical Lecturer in Immunology, University of Leeds, UK
18.11.10 Cryoglobulinaemia

J.J. MISIEWICZ

Consultant Physician and Joint Director, Department of Gastroenterology and Nutrition, Central Middlesex Hospital, London, UK
14.7 Peptic ulceration

T.P. MONATH

Chief, Virology Division, USAMRIDD, Fort Detrick, Frederick, Maryland, USA
7.10.19 Flaviviruses

M.R. MOORE

Professor of Medicine, National Research Centre for Environmental Toxicology, University of Queensland, Australia
11.5 Porphyrin metabolism and the porphyrias

H.G. MORGAN

Professor of Mental Health, University of Bristol, Avon, UK
27.2.12 The patient who has attempted suicide

P.J. MORRIS

Nuffield Professor of Surgery and Director of the Oxford Transplant Centre, University of Oxford, John Radcliffe Hospital, Oxford, UK
5.5 Principles of transplantation immunology
15.11 Peripheral arterial disease

W.L. MORRISON

Consultant Cardiologist, Cardiothoracic Centre, Liverpool, UK
15.3.6 Cardiac cachexia

N.J.McC. MORTENSEN

Consultant Surgeon and Clinical Reader in Colorectal Surgery, John Radcliffe Hospital, Oxford, UK
14.14 Colonic diverticular disease

A.G. MOWAT

Honorary Senior Clinical Lecturer in Rheumatology, Oxford University; Consultant Rheumatologist, Nuffield Orthopaedic Centre, Oxford, UK
18.11.7 Polymyalgia rheumatica and giant-cell arteritis

J. MOXHAM

Professor of Thoracic Medicine, King's College Hospital, London, UK
17.14.1 Respiratory failure: definition and causes
17.14.3(b) Chronic respiratory failure

E.R. MOXON

Action Research Professor of Paediatrics, University of Oxford, UK
7.7 Immunization
7.11.12 Haemophilus influenzae

M.F. MUERS

Consultant Physician, Respiratory Unit, Regional Cardiothoracic Centre, Killingbeck Hospital, Leeds, UK
17.6.4 Diagnostic bronchoscopy and tissue biopsy

P.A. MURPHY

Professor of Medicine, Johns Hopkins University School of Medicine, Baltimore, Maryland, USA
7.5 Physiological changes in infected patients
7.19.2 Septicaemia

I.M. MURRAY-LYON

Consultant Gastroenterologist, Charing Cross Hospital, London, UK
14.32 Liver tumours

D.G. NATHAN

Robert A. Stranahan Professor of Pediatrics, Harvard Medical School, Boston, Massachusetts, USA
22.2.1 Stem cells and haematopoiesis

G. NEALE

Consultant Physician, Addenbrooke's Hospital, Cambridge, UK
14.17 Vascular and collagen disorders

G.H. NEILD

Professor of Nephrology, Institute of Urology and Nephrology, University College London Medical School, UK
20.6 Haemolytic uraemic syndrome

J. NEUBERGER

Consultant Physician, Queen Elizabeth Hospital, Birmingham, UK
14.34 Drugs and liver damage
14.35 The liver in systemic disease

J.M. NEUTZE

Chairman, Department of Cardiology, Green Lane Hospital, Auckland, New Zealand
15.16 The cardiac aspects of rheumatic fever

C.I. NEWBOLD

University Lecturer, University of Oxford, UK
7.13.2 Malaria

A.J. NEWMAN TAYLOR

Professor of Occupational and Environmental Medicine, National Heart and Lung Institute and Consultant Physician, Royal Brompton Hospital, London, UK
17.9.13 Occupational asthma

J. NEWSOM-DAVIS

Professor of Clinical Neurology, University of Oxford, Radcliffe Infirmary, Oxford, UK
24.1 Neurology: introduction
24.3.8 Respiratory problems in neurological disease
25.7 Disorders of neuromuscular transmission

S. NIGHTINGALE

Consultant Neurologist, Midland Centre for Neurosurgery and Neurology, West Midlands, UK
7.10.31 HTLV-I and -II associated diseases

SUCHITRA NIMMANNITYA

Consultant Paediatrician, Children's Hospital, Bangkok, Thailand
7.10.20 Dengue haemorrhagic fever

D.J. NOLAN

Consultant Radiologist, John Radcliffe Hospital, Oxford, UK
14.3.2 Methods for investigation of gastrointestinal disease: radiology

G. NUKI

Professor of Rheumatology, Department of Medicine, University of Edinburgh; Consultant Rheumatologist, Western General Hospital and Royal Infirmary of Edinburgh, UK
11.5 Disorders of purine and pyrimidine metabolism

R.E. O'HEHIR

Academic Head of Allergy and Clinical Immunology, St Mary's Hospital Medical School, London, UK
5.2 Immune mechanisms of disease

J.D. ORIEL

Formerly Consultant Physician in Genito-Urinary Medicine, University College Hospital, London, UK
21.7 Genital warts

D. OVERBOSCH

Consultant Physician, Department of Internal Medicine and Imported Tropical Medicine, Red Cross Hospital, The Hague, The Netherlands
7.15.3 Cysticercosis

S.M. OXBURY

Consultant Clinical Neuropsychologist, Radcliffe Infirmary, Oxford, UK
24.3.1 Disturbances of higher cerebral function

J.M. OXBURY

Consultant Neurologist, Radcliffe Infirmary, Oxford, UK
24.3.1 Disturbances of higher cerebral function

S. PARISH

Senior Research Fellow, Clinical Trial Service Unit, Nuffield Department of Clinical Medicine, University of Oxford, UK
2.4 Large-scale randomized evidence: trials and overviews

J.R. PATTISON

Professor of Medical Microbiology, University College London Medical School, UK
7.10.25 Parvoviruses

J. PAUL

Senior Registrar, Public Health Laboratory, John Radcliffe Hospital, Oxford, UK
7.11.46 'Newer' and lesser known bacteria causing infection in humans
7.17 Non-venomous arthropods

J. PAYAN

Consultant in Clinical Neurophysiology to Guy's and King's College Hospitals and the Hospital for Sick Children, London, UK
24.2.5 Electrophysiological investigation of the peripheral nervous system

I. PEAKE

Professor of Molecular Medicine, University of Sheffield, UK
22.6.4 The pathogenesis of genetic disorders of coagulation

J.M.S. PEARCE

Honorary Consultant Neurologist, Hull Royal Infirmary, Hull, UK
24.11 Headache

A.D. PEARSON

Senior Lecturer in Microbiology and Public Health Medicine; Clinical Director, Infection Control Department, St Thomas's Hospital, London, UK
7.11.17(a) Tularaemia (b) Pasteurellosis. (c) Yersiniosis

P.E. PELLETT

Chief, Herpesvirus Section, Centers for Disease Control and Prevention, Atlanta, Georgia, USA
7.10.7 Human herpesvirus 6

M.E. PEMBREY

Professor of Paediatric Genetics, Institute of Child Health, University of London, UK
4.3 Genetic factors in disease

M.B. PEPYS

Professor of Immunological Medicine, Royal Postgraduate Medical School, Hammersmith Hospital, London, UK
11.13.1 Amyloidosis
11.13.3 The acute phase response and C-reactive protein

S. PEREIRA

Research Fellow in Gastroenterology, United Medical Schools of St Thomas's and Guy's Hospitals, Guy's Campus, London, UK
14.9.3 Small-bowel bacterial overgrowth

B.A. PERKINS

Medical Epidemiologist, Childhood and Respiratory Diseases Branch, Centers for Disease Control and Prevention, Atlanta, Georgia, USA
7.11.41 Cat scratch disease, bacillary angiomatosis, and trench fever

P.L. PERRINE

Professor of Epidemiology, School of Public and Community Medicine, University of Washington, Seattle, USA
7.11.33 Non-venereal treponemes: yaws, endemic syphilis, and pinta
7.11.43 Lymphogranuloma venereum

C.J. PETERS

Chief, Special Pathogens Branch, Centers for Disease Control and Prevention, Atlanta, Georgia, USA
7.10.5 Human infections caused by simian herpesviruses

T.J. PETERS

Professor of Clinical Biochemistry, King's College; Consultant Physician and Chemical Pathologist, King's College Hospital, London, UK
28.2.3(a) Physical complications of alcohol misuse

R. PETO

Professor of Medical Statistics and Epidemiology, ICRF Cancer Studies Unit, Radcliffe Infirmary, Oxford, UK
2.4 Large-scale randomized evidence: trials and overviews
6.2 Epidemiology of cancer

T.E.A. PETO

Consultant Physician, Infectious Diseases, John Radcliffe Hospital, Oxford, UK
7.10.2 Herpes simplex virus infections
7.10.3 Varicella-zoster infections: chickenpox and zoster
7.10.9 Orf
7.10.10 Molluscum contagiosum
7.10.29 HIV infection and AIDS
17.6.3 Microbiological methods in the diagnosis of respiratory infections

R.K.H. PETTY

Lecturer in Neurology and Neurovirology, Institute of Neurological Sciences, University of Glasgow, UK
24.15.3 Neurological manifestations of infection with human immunodeficiency virus type 1

P.A. PHILIP

Senior Registrar in Medical Oncology, ICRF Clinical Oncology Unit, Churchill Hospital, Oxford, UK
13.15 Malignant disease in pregnancy

PRIDA PHUAPRADIT

Professor of Neurology, Division of Neurology, Department of Medicine, Ramathibodi Hospital, Mahidol University, Bangkok, Thailand
24.15 Bacterial meningitis

M.J. PIPPARD

Professor of Haematology, Ninewells Hospital and Medical School, University of Dundee, UK
22.4.4 Iron metabolism and its disorders

J.M. POLAK

Professor of Endocrine Pathology, Royal Postgraduate Medical School, Hammersmith Hospital, London, UK
14.8 Hormones and the gastrointestinal tract

P.A. POOLE-WILSON

Professor of Cardiology, National Heart and Lung Institute; Honorary Physician, Royal Brompton Hospital, London, UK
15.1 Cardiovascular disease: physiological considerations: biochemistry and cellular physiology of heart muscle
15.5 The treatment of heart failure

J.S. PORTERFIELD

Formerly Reader in Bacteriology, Sir William Dunn School of Pathology, University of Oxford, UK
7.10.21 Bunyaviridae

R.E. POUNDER

Professor of Medicine, Royal Free Hospital School of Medicine, University of London, UK
14.7 Peptic ulceration

M.A. PREECE

Professor of Child Health and Growth, Institute of Child Health, University of London, UK
12.9.2 Normal growth and its disorders

E.W. PRICE*

Research Fellow, Department of Clinical and Tropical Medicine, London School of Hygiene and Tropical Medicine, London, UK
8.5.5(h) Podoconiosis (non-filarial endemic elephantiasis of the lower legs)

J.S. PRICHARD

Professor of Medicine, St James's Hospital, Dublin, Eire
15.22.7 The pulmonary circulation in health and disease
15.23 Pulmonary oedema
15.24 Pulmonary hypertension
15.25 Cor pulmonale

N.B. PRIDE

Professor of Respiratory Medicine, Royal Postgraduate Medical School, Hammersmith Hospital, London, UK
17.6.2 Tests of ventilatory mechanics
17.9.4 Chronic obstructive pulmonary disease

J. PRITCHARD

Senior Lecturer in Paediatric Oncology, Institute of Child Health and Consultant, Hospital for Sick Children, Great Ormond Street, London, UK
22.5.6 The histiocytoses

A.T. PROUDFOOT

Consultant Physician, Royal Infirmary of Edinburgh NHS Trust; Director, Scottish, Poisons Information Bureau, Edinburgh, UK
8.1 Poisoning: introduction and epidemiology
8.1.2 Poisoning: clinical and metabolic features and general principles of management
8.2.1 Poisoning caused by analgesic drugs
8.2.2 Poisoning from antidepressants, hypnotics, antihistamines, anticonvulsants, and antiparkinsonian drugs
8.2.3 Poisoning from cardiovascular drugs
8.2.4 Poisoning caused by respiratory drugs
8.2.5 Poisoning caused by drugs acting on the gastrointestinal system
8.2.6 Poisoning by haematinics and vitamins
8.2.7 Poisoning by endocrine drugs
8.2.8 Poisoning from antimicrobials
8.2.10 Poisoning from drugs of abuse
8.2.11 Poisoning due to miscellaneous drugs
8.3.1 Poisoning from household products
8.3.2 Poisoning by alcohols and glycols
8.3.3 Poisoning from hydrocarbons and chlorofluorocarbons
8.3.4 Poisoning by inhalational agents
8.3.5 Poisoning due to corrosive substances
8.3.8 Pesticides

* It is with regret that we report the deaths of those authors marked with an asterisk. Although their deaths occurred between the appearance of the second edition and preparation of the third edition, much of their contribution to the former has been incorporated into this edition, with appropriate updating from their coauthors.

B.A. PRUITT
Commander and Director, US Army Institute of Surgical Research, Fort Sam Houston, Texas, USA
8.5.5(g) Environmental factors and disease: lightning and electric shock

SWANGJAI PUNGPAK
Associate Professor of Clinical Tropical Medicine, Mahidol University, Bangkok, Thailand
7.16.2 Liver fluke diseases in man

SOMPONE PUNYAGUPTA
President and Chairman, Department of Medicine, Vichaiyut Hospital, Bangkok, Thailand
7.14.8 Angiostrongyliasis

C.D. PUSEY
Reader in Renal Medicine, Royal Postgraduate Medical School, Hammersmith Hospital, London, UK
20.4.3 Rapidly progressive glomerulonephritis and antiglomerular basement membrane disease

N.P. QUINN
Reader in Clinical Neurology, Institute of Neurology, London, UK
24.3.3 Subcortical structures—the cerebellum, thalamus, and basal ganglia

A.J. RADFORD
Professor of Primary Health Care, Flinders University of South Australia
7.15.1 Hydatid disease
7.17 Non-venomous arthropods

PRAYONG RADOMYOS
Associate Professor of Parasitology, Bangkok School of Tropical Medicine, Faculty of Tropical Medicine, Mahidol University, Bangkok, Thailand
7.16.4 Intestinal trematodiasis

A.E.G. RAINE
Professor of Renal Medicine, St Bartholomew's Hospital Medical College, London, UK
15.6.1 Diuretics
15.28.1 Renal and renovascular hypertension
20.11 Hypertension: its effects on the kidney

A.C. RANKIN
Senior Lecturer in Medical Cardiology, Glasgow Royal Infirmary, UK
15.8.1 Cardiac arrhythmias

P.J. RATCLIFFE
University Lecturer and Honorary Consultant Physician, Nuffield Department of Medicine, Oxford, UK
20.17.3 Renal transplantation

C.W.G. REDMAN
Professor of Obstetric Medicine, Nuffield Department of Obstetrics and Gynaecology, John Radcliffe Hospital, Oxford, UK
13.2 Hypertension in pregnancy
13.3 Renal disease in pregnancy

A.J. REES
Regius Professor of Medicine, University of Aberdeen; Honorary Consultant Physician, Aberdeen Royal Hospitals, UK
20.4.3 Rapidly progressive glomerulonephritis and antiglomerular basement membrane disease

D. RENNIE
Professor of Medicine, Institute for Health Policy Studies, University of California, San Francisco, USA
8.5.5(d) Environmental factors and disease: diseases of high terrestrial altitudes

J. RICHENS
Clinical Lecturer, University College London Medical School, UK
7.11.8 Typhoid and paratyphoid fevers
7.11.9 Rhinoscleroma
7.11.45 Donovanosis (granuloma inguinale)

B.K. RIMA
Professor of Molecular Biology, School of Biology and Biochemistry, The Queen's University of Belfast, UK
7.10.11 Mumps: epidemic parotitis

E. RITZ
Professor of Medicine and Head of the Division of Nephrology, Ruperto Carola University of Heidelberg, Germany
20.5.1 Diabetic nephropathy

I.A.G. ROBERTS
Senior Lecturer and Honorary Consultant in Haematology, Royal Postgraduate Medical School, Hammersmith Hospital, London, UK
22.3.4 Acute lymphoblastic leukaemia

A.R. RONALD
Associate Dean, Research University of Manitoba; Director of Infectious Diseases, St Boniface Hospital, Winnipeg, Canada
7.11.13 Haemophilus ducreyi and chancroid

R.J.M. ROSS
Senior Lecturer in Endocrinology, Northern General Hospital, Sheffield, UK
12.9.3 Puberty

R.W. ROSS RUSSELL
Consultant Physician, St Thomas's Hospital, National Hospital of Neurology and Neurosurgery, and Moorfields Eye Hospital, London, UK
24.3.4 Visual pathways

M.N. ROSSOR
Consultant Neurologist, National Hospital for Neurology and Neurosurgery and St Mary's Hospital, London, UK
24.7.2 Alzheimer's disease

D.J. ROWLANDS
Consultant Cardiologist, Royal Infirmary, Manchester, UK
15.4.2 The electrocardiogram
15.4.4 Nuclear techniques

M.B. RUBENS
Consultant Radiologist, Royal Brompton Hospital, London and Honorary Senior Lecturer, National Heart and Lung Institute, University of London, UK
15.4.1 Chest radiography in heart disease

P.C. RUBIN
Professor of Therapeutics, University of Nottingham; Consultant Physician, University Hospital, Birmingham, UK
13.16 Prescribing in pregnancy

P. RUDGE
Consultant Neurologist, National Hospital for Neurology and Neurosurgery, London, UK
24.3.5 The eighth cranial nerve

T.K. RUEBUSH
Chief, Malaria Section, Division of Parasitic Diseases, Centers for Disease Control and Prevention, Atlanta, Georgia, USA
7.13.3 Babesia

R.C.G. RUSSELL
Consultant Surgeon, The Middlesex Hospital, London, UK
14.23.3 Tumours of the pancreas

T.J. RYAN
Clinical Professor of Dermatology, Oxford Radcliffe Trust, UK
23 Diseases of the skin

D.L. SACKETT
Professor of Clinical Epidemiology and Director, Centre for Evidence-Based Medicine, University of Oxford, UK
2.3 Evaluation of clinical method

P.J. SANSONETTI
Professeur à l'Institut Pasteur, Chef de l'Unite de Pathogenie Microbienne Moleculaire and INSERM U389, Institut Pasteur, Paris, France
7.2.1 Introduction to the diversity of bacterial pathogens
7.2.2 Molecular taxonomy of bacterial pathogens

M.O. SAVAGE
Reader in Paediatric Endocrinology, St Bartholomew's Hospital, London, UK
12.9.1 Normal and abnormal sexual differentiation
12.9.3 Puberty

G.F. SAVIDGE
Director, Haemophilia Reference Centre, St Thomas's Hospital, London, UK
22.6.5 Clinical features and management of the hereditary disorders of haemostasis

J.W. SCADDING
Consultant Neurologist, The National Hospital for Neurology and Neurosurgery, London, UK
24.5 Pain: pathophysiology and treatment

K.P. SCHAAL
Professor and Director, Institutes of Medical Microbiology and Immunology, University of Bonn, Germany
7.11.27 Actinomycoses

R.B.H. SCHUTGENS
Associate Professor and Clinical Chemist, Department of Paediatrics, University of Amsterdam, The Netherlands
11.9 Peroxisomal disorders

T.G. SCHWAN
Acting Head, Arthropod-borne Diseases Section, Laboratory of Vectors and Pathogens, National Institutes of Health, Rocky Mountain Laboratories, Hamilton, Montana, USA
7.11.30 Lyme disease

J. SCHWEBKE
Assistant Professor of Medicine, University of Alabama at Birmingham, USA
21.4 Vaginal discharge

J. SCOTT
Professor of Medicine, Royal Postgraduate Medical School, Hammersmith Hospital, London, UK
15.9.1 The pathogenesis of atherosclerosis

D.G.I. SCOTT
Consultant Rheumatologist, Norfolk and Norwich Health Care Trust, UK
18.11.1 Connective tissue diseases: introduction

A. SEATON
Professor of Environmental and Occupational Medicine, University of Aberdeen Medical School, UK
17.10.16 Pneumoconioses

A.W. SEGAL
Charles Dent Professor of Medicine, The Rayne Institute, University College London Medical School, UK
22.5.1 Leucocytes in health and disease

M.H. SEIFERT
Consultant Rheumatologist and Honorary Clinical Senior Lecturer in Medicine, St Mary's Hospital Medical School, London, UK
18.9 Septic arthritis

G.R. SERJEANT
Director, MRC Laboratories (Jamaica), University of the West Indies, Kingston, Jamaica
20.5.7 Renal manifestations of systemic disease: sickle-cell disease

C.A. SEYMOUR
Professor of Clinical Biochemistry and Metabolism and Honorary Consultant Physician, St George's Hospital Medical School, University of London, UK
11.7 Trace metal disorders
14.22 Hereditary disease of the liver and pancreas

K.V. SHAH
Professor of Immunology and Infectious Diseases, Johns Hopkins University School of Hygiene and Public Health, Baltimore, Maryland, USA
7.10.24 Papovaviruses

M. SHARPE
Clinical Tutor in Psychiatry, Oxford University, UK
7.19.4 Chronic fatigue syndrome (postviral fatigue syndrome and myalgic encephalomyelitis)

R.J. SHAW
Senior Lecturer and Consultant Physician in Respiratory Medicine, St Mary's Hospital Medical School, London, UK
17.10.4 The lung in collagen–vascular diseases
17.10.11 Pulmonary histiocytosis X (eosinophilic granuloma of the lung) and lymphangiomatosis
17.10.21 Lung disorders in genetic syndromes

M.C. SHEPPARD
Professor of Medicine, University of Birmingham, UK
12.5 Thyroid cancer

J.M. SHNEERSON
Director, Respiratory Support and Sleep Centre, Papworth Hospital, Cambridge, UK
17.12 Disorders of the thoracic cage and diaphragm

M. SIEBELS
Department of Internal Medicine, Division of Nephrology, University of Heidelberg, Germany
20.5.1 Diabetic nephropathy

C.A. SIEFF
Associate Professor in Pediatrics, Harvard Medical School and Dana Farber Cancer Institute; Senior Associate in Medicine, Children's Hospital, Boston, Massachusetts, USA
22.2.1 Stem cells and haematopoiesis

H.A. SIMMONDS
Senior Lecturer, Purine Research Laboratory, United Medical Schools of Guy's and St Thomas's Hospitals, London Bridge, UK
20.9.2 Gout, purines, and interstitial nephritis

I.A. SIMPSON
Consultant Cardiologist, Southampton General Hospital, UK
15.4.3 Doppler echocardiography

D.I.H. SIMPSON
Professor of Microbiology, Department of Microbiology and Immunology, Queen's University of Belfast, UK
7.10.17 Alphaviruses
7.10.23 Filoviruses: Marburg and Ebola fevers

V. SITPRIJA
Professor and Chairman, Department of Medicine, Chulalongkorn University; Director of Queen Saovabha Memorial Institute, Thai Red Cross, Bangkok, Thailand
7.11.32 Leptospirosis

M.B. SKIRROW
Honorary Emeritus Consultant Microbiologist, Public Health Laboratory, Gloucester Royal Hospital, UK
7.11.7 Enterobacteria and miscellaneous enteropathogenic and food-poisoning bacteria

P. SLEIGHT
Field Marshal Alexander Professor Emeritus of Cardiovascular Medicine, John Radcliffe Hospital, Oxford, UK
15.10.4 Myocardial infarction

R. SMITH
Consultant Physician and Consultant in Metabolic Medicine, John Radcliffe Hospital and Nuffield Orthopaedic Centre, Oxford, UK
10.1 Nutrition: introduction
10.2 Nutrition: biochemical background
11.6 Metabolic effects of accidental injury and surgery
19 Disorders of the skeleton

G.L. SMITH
Reader in Bacteriology, Sir William Dunn School of Pathology, University of Oxford, UK
7.10.8 Poxviruses

D.H. SMITH
Senior Lecturer and Honorary Consultant Physician in Tropical Medicine; Head of Division of Tropical Medicine, Liverpool School of Tropical Medicine, UK
7.13.10 Human African trypanosomiasis

M.L. SNAITH
Senior Lecturer in Rheumatic Diseases, Section of Rheumatology, University of Sheffield Medical School, UK
18.11.3 Systemic lupus erythematosus and related disorders

J. SOMERVILLE
Consultant Physician for Congenital Diseases, Cardiology Directorate, Royal Brompton Hospital, London, UK
15.15 Congenital heart disease in adolescents and adults

R.L. SOUHAMI
Kathleen Ferrier Professor of Clinical Oncology, University College London Medical School, UK
6.6 Cancer: clinical features and management

B.A. SOUTHGATE
Senior Lecturer in Tropical Disease Epidemiology, London School of Hygiene and Tropical Medicine, University of London, UK
7.14.2 Lymphatic filariasis

S.G. SPIRO
Consultant Physician, University College Hospitals London Trust, UK
17.13.1(a) Lung cancer. (b) Pulmonary metastases

C.J.F. SPRY
B.H.F. Professor of Cardiovascular Immunology, St George's Hospital Medical School, University of London, UK
15.4.3 The hypereosinophilic syndrome and the heart
22.5.7 The white cells and lymphoproliferative disorders: the hypereosinophilic syndrome

A. SPURGEON
Lecturer in Occupational Health Psychology, Institute of Occupational Health, University of Birmingham, UK
8.5.3(k) The main occupational disorders: neuropsychological disorders

S. STAGNO
Katharine Reynolds Ireland Professor and Chairman, Department of Pediatrics, University of Alabama, Birmingham, USA
7.10.6 Cytomegalovirus

J.C. STEVENSON
Director, Wynn Institute for Metabolic Research; Honorary Senior Lecturer, National Heart and Lung Institute, University of London; Honorary Consultant Physician, Royal Brompton Hospital, London, UK
13.17 Benefits and risks of hormone therapy

J.A. STEWART
Chief, Clinical Virology Section, Centers for Disease Control and Prevention, Atlanta, Georgia, USA
7.10.7 Human herpesvirus 6

J.H. STEWART
Professor in Medicine and Associate Dean, Western Clinical School, University of Sydney, Australia
20.9.1 Kidney disease from analgesics and non-steroidal anti-inflammatory drugs

R.A. STOCKLEY
Reader in Respiratory Medicine, Queen Elizabeth Hospital, Edgbaston, Birmingham, UK
17.9.3 Bronchiectasis
17.9.4 Chronic obstructive pulmonary disease

J.R. STRADLING

Consultant Physician, Oxford Radcliffe Trust (Churchill), Oxford, UK
17.2.2 The upper respiratory tract
17.8.2 Upper airways obstruction
17.14.2 Sleep-related disorders of breathing

J. STRANG

Professor and Director, Addiction Research Unit, National Addiction Centre, The Maudsley/Institute of Psychiatry, London, UK
28 Alcohol and drug-related problems: introduction
28.1.2 Assessing substance use and misuse
28.2.2 Harm reduction
28.3.2 The management of substance-related problems in a general ward
28.3.3 Drugs and the law
28.3.8 Caring for the HIV-positive drug user

P.R. STUDDY

Consultant Physician, Harefield Hospital NHS Trust and Mount Vernon and Watford Hospitals Trust, Hertfordshire, UK
17.10.10 Sarcoidosis

P.H. SUGDEN

Reader in Biochemistry, Department of Cardiac Medicine, National Heart and Lung Institute, University of London, UK
15.1 Cardiovascular disease: physiological considerations: biochemistry and cellular physiology of heart muscle

J.A. SUMMERFIELD

Professor of Experimental Medicine, St Mary's Hospital Medical School, Imperial College London, UK
14.21 Congenital disorders of the biliary tract and pancreas
14.24 Diseases of the gallbladder and biliary tree

PRAVAN SUNTHARASAMAI

Associate Professor, Department of Clinical Tropical Medicine, Mahidol University, Bangkok, Thailand
7.14.9 Gnathostomiasis

R. SUTTON

Consultant Cardiologist and Director of Pacing and Electrophysiology, Royal Brompton Hospital, London, UK
15.3.5 Syncope and palpitation
15.8.2 Pacemakers

J.D. SWALES

Professor of Medicine, University of Leicester, UK
15.27 Essential hypertension

R.H. SWANTON

Consultant Cardiologist, University College London, UK
15.4.6 Cardiac catheterization
15.10.3 Angina and unstable angina

D.M. SWIRSKY

Senior Lecturer in Haematology, Royal Postgraduate Medical School; Honorary Consultant, Hospital, London, UK
22.5.4 The spleen and its disorders

D.A. TABERNER

Clinical Director, Thrombosis Reference Centre, University Hospital of South Manchester, UK
22.6.7 Thrombotic disease

I.C. TALBOT

Consultant Pathologist, St Mark's Hospital, London, UK
14.16 Tumours of the gastrointestinal tract

C.R. TAYLOR

Charles P. Lyman Professor of Biology, Harvard University, Cambridge, Massachusetts, USA
17.2.1 Functional anatomy of the human lung

D. TAYLOR-ROBINSON

Professor of Genitourinary Microbiology and Medicine, St Mary's Hospital Medical School, Paddington, London, UK
7.11.41 Chlamydial infections
7.11.43 Mycoplasmas

G.M. TEASDALE

Professor of Neurosurgery, Institute of Neurological Sciences, University of Glasgow, UK
24.14 Head injuries

P.J. TEDDY

Consultant Neurosurgeon, The Radcliffe Infirmary, Oxford, UK
24.12 Intracranial tumours
24.15.4 Intracranial abscess

H.J. TESTA

Consultant in Nuclear Medicine, Royal Infirmary, Manchester, UK
15.4.4 The clinical assessment of cardiovascular function: nuclear techniques

A.C. THOMAS

Senior Specialist and Consultant in Tissue Pathology, Institute of Medical and Veterinary Science, Adelaide, South Australia
20.4.1 IgA nephropathy, Henoch-Schönlein purpura, and thin membrane nephropathy

P.K. THOMAS

Emeritus Professor of Neurology, Royal Free Hospital School of Medicine and Institute of Neurology, London, UK
24.3.6 Neurology: organization and features of dysfunction; other cranial nerves
24.8 Neurology: inherited disorders
24.17 Peripheral neuropathy

H.C. THOMAS

Professor of Medicine, St Mary's Hospital Medical School, Imperial College of Science, Technology and Medicine; Consultant Physician and Hepatologist, St Mary's Hospital, London, UK
14.26 Clinical features of viral hepatitis

J.E.P. THOMAS

Formerly Professor of Medicine, University of Zimbabwe, Harare, Zimbabwe
7.16.1 Schistosomiasis

D.G. THOMPSON

Senior Lecturer in Medicine and Consultant Physician, Hope Hospital, Salford, UK
14.2.5 Constipation
14.13 Functional bowel disease and irritable bowel syndrome

M.O. THORNER

Kenneth R. Crispell Professor of Medicine; Chief, Division of Endocrinology and Metabolism, University of Virginia School of Medicine, Charlottesville, USA
12.2 Anterior pituitary disorders

A.J. THRASHER
Honorary Lecturer and Wellcome Training Fellow, University College London Medical School, UK
22.5.1 Leucocytes in health and disease

P. THULLIEZ
Head, Laboratoire de la Toxoplasmose, Institut de Puériculture de Paris, France
7.13.4 Toxoplasmosis

P. TOOKEY
Research Fellow, Department of Epidemiology and Biostatistics, Institute of Child Health, London, UK
7.10.18 Rubella

P.P. TOSKES
Professor and Associate Chairman for Clinical Affairs; Director, Division of Gastroenterology, Hepatology and Nutrition, Department of Medicine, University of Florida College of Medicine, Gainsville, USA
14.23.2 Chronic pancreatitis

T.A. TRAILL
Associate Professor of Medicine, Johns Hopkins University School of Medicine, Baltimore, Maryland, USA
15.19 Cardiac myxoma

D.F. TREACHER
Consultant Physician, Department of Intensive Care, St Thomas's Hospital, London, UK
16 Intensive care

T. TREASURE
Consultant Cardiothoracic Surgeon, St George's Hospital, London, UK
15.10.6 Coronary artery bypass grafting

G.S. TREGENZA
Associate Specialist, Division of Addictive Behavior, St George's Hospital Medical School, University of London, UK
28.3.5 Drug misusers and addicts in accident and emergency

J.D. TREHARNE
Reader in Virology, Institute of Ophthalmology, University of London, UK
7.11.41 Chlamydial infections

SIR LESLIE TURNBERG
Section of Gastroenterology, Hope Hospital, Salford, Lancashire, UK
14.2.4 Diarrhoea

P.C.B. TURNBULL
Head, Anthrax Section, Centre for Applied Microbiology and Research, Porton Down, Salisbury, Wiltshire, UK
7.11.18 Anthrax

R.C. TURNER
Clinical Reader, Nuffield Department of Clinical Medicine, Diabetes Research Laboratories, Radcliffe Infirmary, Oxford, UK
11.12 Hypoglycaemia

F.E. UDWADIA
Emeritus Professor of Medicine, Grant Medical College and J.J. Group of Hospitals; Consultant Physician, Breach Candy Hospital and Parsee General Hospital, Bombay, India
7.11.20 Tetanus

S.R. UNDERWOOD
Senior Lecturer in Cardiac Imaging, National Heart and Lung Institute; Honorary Consultant, Royal Brompton Hospital NHS Trust, London, UK
15.4.5 Magnetic resonance and computed X-ray tomography

C.G. URAGODA
Physician, Chest Hospital, Welisera; Course Director of Clinical Studies, Postgraduate Institute of Medicine, University of Colombo, Sri Lanka
7.11.23 Particular problems of tuberculosis in developing countries

J.A. VALE
Director, National Poisons Information Service (Birmingham Centre), West Midlands Poisons Unit, City Road Hospital, Birmingham; Senior Clinical Lecturer, University of Birmingham, UK
8.1.1 Poisoning: introduction and epidemiology
8.1.2 Poisoning: clinical and metabolic features and general principles of management
8.2.1 Poisoning caused by analgesic drugs
8.2.2 Poisoning from antidepressants, hypnotics, antihistamines, anticonvulsants, and antiparkinsonian drugs
8.2.3 Poisoning from cardiovascular drugs
8.2.4 Poisoning caused by respiratory drugs
8.2.5 Poisoning caused by drugs acting on the gastrointestinal system
8.2.6 Poisoning by haematinics and vitamins
8.2.7 Poisoning by endocrine drugs
8.2.8 Poisoning from antimicrobials
8.2.10 Poisoning from drugs of abuse
8.2.11 Poisoning due to miscellaneous drugs
8.3.1 Poisoning from household products
8.3.2 Poisoning from alcohols and glycols
8.3.3 Poisoning from hydrocarbons and chlorofluorocarbons, and volatile substance abuse
8.3.4 Poisoning by inhalational agents
8.3.5 Poisoning due to corrosive substances
8.3.6 Poisoning from metals
8.3.8 Pesticides

P. VALLANCE
Senior Lecturer and Honorary Consultant in Clinical Pharmacology, St George's Hospital Medical School, London, UK
15.9.2 Vascular endothelium, its physiology and pathophysiology

SIRIVAN VANIJANONTA
Associate Professor, Head, Department of Clinical Tropical Medicine, Faculty of Tropical Medicine, Mahidol University, Bangkok, Thailand
7.16.3 Lung flukes (paragonimiasis)

D.J.T. VAUX
Lecturer in Experimental Pathology, Sir William Dunn School of Pathology, University of Oxford, UK
4.2.2 Cell biology of organelles and the endomembrane system

P.J.W. VENABLES

Reader in Rheumatology, Charing Cross and Westminster Medical School; Consultant Rheumatologist; Charing Cross Hospital, London, UK
18.11.5 Sjögren's syndrome

M.P. VESSEY

Professor of Public Health, Department of Public Health and Primary Care, University of Oxford, UK
3.2 Health and sickness in the community
13.1 Benefits and risks of oral contraceptives

P.D. WAGNER

Professor of Medicine, University of California San Diego, La Jolla, California, USA
17.4 Pathophysiology of lung disease

D.H. WALKER

Professor and Chairman, Department of Pathology, University of Texas Medical Branch at Galveston, USA
7.11.37 Rickettsial diseases including the ehrlichioses

J.A. WALKER-SMITH

Professor of Paediatric Gastroenterology, Medical College of St Bartholomew's Hospital and Queen Elizabeth Hospital for Children, London, UK
14.15 Congenital abnormalities of the gastrointestinal tract

J.R.F WALTERS

Senior Lecturer, Gastroenterology Unit, Royal Postgraduate Medical School, Hammersmith Hospital, London, UK
14.9.1 Mechanisms of intestinal absorption

LORD WALTON OF DETCHANT

President, World Federation of Neurology; Former Professor of Neurology, University of Newcastle on Tyne; Honorary Consultant Neurologist, Oxford, UK
18.11.6 Polymyositis and dermatomyositis
25.1 Disorders of voluntary muscle: introduction
25.2 The muscular dystrophies
25.3 The floppy infant syndrome
25.4 Myotonic disorders
25.5 Inflammatory myopathies
25.6 Miscellaneous disorders (of voluntary muscle)

R.J.A. WANDERS

Senior Biochemist and Associate Professor, University Hospital Amsterdam, Academic Medical Centre, Amsterdam, The Netherlands
11.9 Peroxisomal disorders

C.P. WARLOW

Professor of Medical Neurology, University of Edinburgh, UK
24.6 Cerebrovascular disease

D.A. WARRELL

Professor of Tropical Medicine and Infectious Diseases, University of Oxford
7.8 Travel and expedition medicine
7.10.15 Rhabdoviruses: rabies and rabies-related viruses
7.10.16 Colorado tick fever and other arthropod-borne reoviruses
7.11.29 Rat bite fevers
7.11.31 Other Borrelia infections
7.11.44 Bartonellosis
7.13.2 Malaria
7.13.5 Cryptosporidium and cryptosporidiosis
7.18 Pentastomiasis (porocephalosis)
8.4.1 Injuries, envenoming, poisoning, and allergic reactions caused by animals
24.15.1 Bacterial meningitis
24.15.2 Acute viral infections of the central nervous system
25.10 Tropical pyomyositis (tropical myositis)

M.J. WARRELL

Clinical Virologist, Centre for Tropical Medicine and Infectious Diseases, John Radcliffe Hospital, Oxford, UK
7.10.15 Rhabdoviruses: rabies and rabies-related viruses
7.10.16 Colorado tick fever and other arthropod-borne reoviruses

J.A.H. WASS

Professor of Clinical Endocrinology, St Bartholomew's Hospital Medical College, London, UK
12.11 Endocrine manifestations of non-endocrine disease

M.F.R. WATERS

Consultant Leprologist, Hospital for Tropical Diseases, London; sometime Member of the Medical Research Council External Scientific Staff, Middlesex Hospital, London, UK
7.11.25 Leprosy (Hansen's disease, hanseniasis)
7.11.26 Mycobacterium ulcerans infection

G. WATT

Chief, Department of Medicine, AFRIMS, Bangkok, Thailand
7.11.38 Scrub typhus

R.W.E. WATTS

Royal Postgraduate Medical School Visting Professor and Honorary Consultant Physician, Hammersmith Hospital, London, UK
11.1 The inborn errors of metabolism: general aspects
11.8 Lysosomal storage diseases
11.10 Disorders of oxalate metabolism
20.9.3 Hypercalcaemic nephropathy
20.12.2 Urinary stone disease (urolithiasis)

SIR DAVID WEATHERALL

Regius Professor of Medicine and Honorary Director of the Institute of Molecular Medicine, University of Oxford, UK
2.1.2 Scientific method and the art of healing
4.1 Molecular biology and medicine
4.2.1 Medical applications of cell biology: introduction
15.26 Pulmonary embolism
22.1 Disorders of the blood: introduction
22.3.8 Polycythaemia vera
22.3.9 Myelosclerosis
22.3.10 Primary thrombocythaemia
22.4.1 Erythropoiesis and the normal red cell
22.4.2 Anaemia: pathophysiology, classification, and clinical features
22.4.5 Normochromic, normocytic anaemia
22.4.7 Disorders of the synthesis or function of haemoglobin
22.4.8 Other anaemias resulting from defective red cell maturation
22.4.9 Haemolytic anaemia: the mechanisms and consequences of a shortened red cell
22.4.11 Haemolysis due to red-cell enzyme deficiencies
22.4.14 The relative and secondary polycythaemias
22.7 The blood in systemic disease

A.D.B. WEBSTER
MRC Immunodeficiency Research Group, Royal Free Hospital Medical School, London, UK
5.3 Immunodeficiency

E.R. WEIBEL
Professor of Anatomy Emeritus, University of Bern, Switzerland
17.2.1 Functional anatomy of the lung

R.A. WEISS
Professor of Viral Oncology, Institute of Cancer Research, London, UK
7.10.27 Viruses and cancer
7.10.28 Human immunodeficiency viruses

I.V.D. WELLER
Professor and Head of the Academic Department of Genitourinary Medicine, University College London Medical School, UK
7.10.29 HIV infection and AIDS

L. WESTRÖM
Associate Professor of Obstetrics and Gynaecology, University of Lund, Sweden
21.5 Pelvic inflammatory disease

N.J. WHITE
Director, Wellcome-Mahidol University, Oxford Tropical Medicine Research Programme, Faculty of Tropical Medicine, Mahidol University, Bangkok, Thailand
9 Principles of clinical pharmacology and drug therapy

H.C. WHITTLE
Deputy Director, Medical Research Council Laboratories, The Gambia, West Africa
7.10.12 Measles

D.E.L. WILCKEN
Consultant Physician, The Prince Henry and Prince of Wales Hospitals, Sydney, Australia
15.2 Clinical physiology of the normal heart

P.J. WILKINSON
Consultant Medical Microbiologist and Director, Public Health Laboratory, University Hospital, Nottingham, UK
7.11.35 Listeria and listeriosis

D.G. WILLAMS
Professor of Medicine, United Medical and Dental Schools of Guy's and St Thomas's Hospitals, University of London, UK
20.5.2 Infections and associated nephropathies
20.5.6 Rheumatological disorders and the kidney

R.C. WILLIAMS
Chief Medical Officer, GKN plc, Redditch, Worcestershire, UK
8.5.5(j) Environmental factors and disease: noise

A.C. de C. WILLIAMS
Consultant Clinical Psychologist, INPUT Pain Management Unit, St Thomas's Hospital, London, UK
28.3.7 Management of pain in the drug abuser

R. WILLIAMS
Director, Institute of Liver Studies and Consultant Physician, King's College Hospital, London, UK
14.31 Liver transplantation

C.B. WILLIAMS
Consultant Physician in Gastrointestinal Endoscopy, St Mark's Hospital, Northwick Park, London, UK
14.16 Tumours of the gastrointestinal tract

D.H. WILLIAMSON
Medical Research Council, External Scientific Staff, Nuffield Department of Clinical Medicine, Oxford University, UK
10.2 Biochemical background

BRIGADIER GENERAL KYAW WIN
Director and Consultant Physician, Directorate of Medical Services, Ministry of Defence, Union of Myanmar
7.11.38 Scrub typhus

C.G. WINEARLS
Consultant Nephrologist, Churchill Hospital, Oxford, UK
20.16 Acute renal failure
20.17.1 Chronic renal failure

D.L. WINGATE
Professor of Gastrointestinal Science, London Hospital Medical College, University of London, UK
14.12 Disorders of motility

P.A. WINSTANLEY
Senior Lecturer in Clinical Pharmacology, Department of Pharmacology and Therapeutics, University of Liverpool, UK
8.2.9 Poisoning from cinchona alkaloids and other antimalarials

F. WOJNAROWSKA
Consultant Dermatologist and Senior Clinical Lecturer, Churchill Hospital, Oxford, UK
13.14 The skin in pregnancy

A.J. WOODROFFE
Renal Physician, Royal Adelaide Hospital, Australia
20.4.1 IgA nephropathy, Henoch-Schönlein purpura, and thin membrane nephropathy

H.F. WOODS
Sir George Franklin Professor of Medicine, University of Sheffield, UK
11.14 Disturbances of acid-base homeostasis

B.P. WORDSWORTH
Clinical Reader in Rheumatology, Nuffield Department of Clinical Medicine, University of Oxford, UK
18.4 Rheumatoid arthritis

V.M. WRIGHT
Consultant Paediatric Surgeon, Queen Elizabeth Hospital for Children and University College London Hospitals, London, UK
14.15 Congenital abnormalities of the gastrointestinal tract

D.J.M. WRIGHT
Reader in Medical Microbiology, Charing Cross and Westminster Medical School, London, UK
7.11.34 Syphilis

F.C.W. WU
Senior Lecturer, Department of Medicine, University of Manchester, UK
12.8.2 Disorders of male reproduction

M.A.S. YASUDA

Associate Professor, Department of Infectious and Parasitic Diseases, São Paulo University School of Medicine (USP), Brazil
7.12.4 Paracoccidioidomycosis

A. YOUNG

Professor of Geriatric Medicine, Royal Free Hospital School of Medicine, London, UK
30 Sports medicine

V. ZAMAN

Professor of Microbiology, Aga Khan University, Karachi, Pakistan
7.13.7 Sarcocystosis
7.13.9 Blastocystis hominis
7.14.6 Other gut nematodes
7.14.7 Toxocariasis and visceral larval migrans

A.J. ZUCKERMAN

Dean and Professor of Medical Microbiology and Director of the World Health Organization Collaborating Centre for Reference and Research on Viral Diseases, Royal Free Hospital School of Medicine, London, UK
7.10.26 Viral hepatitis

J.N. ZUCKERMAN

Clinical Research Fellow, Royal Free Hospital School of Medicine, London, UK
7.10.26 Viral hepatitis

Plates for Section 7

Chapter 7.10.2

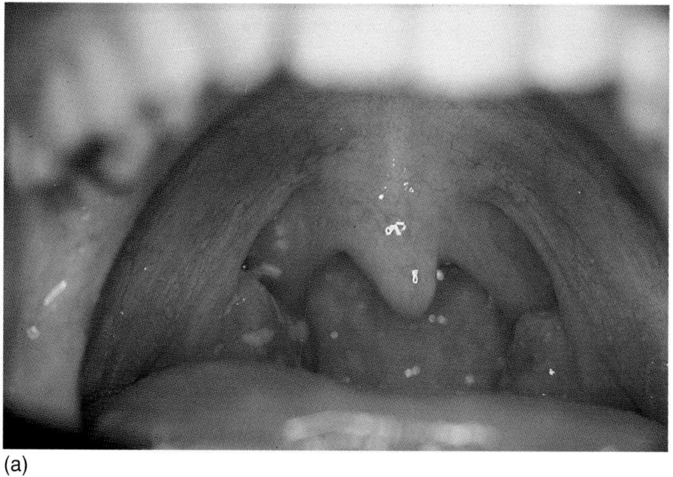

(a)

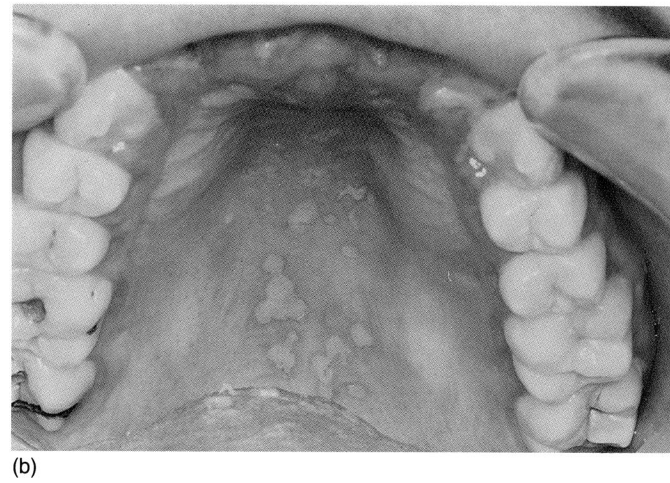

(b)

Plate 1 (a) Primary herpetic gingivostomatitis, part of generalized HSV-2 infection. The lesions on the soft palate are indistinguishable from the 'herpangina' in certain coxsackievirus infections. (b) Primary herpetic gingivostomatitis.

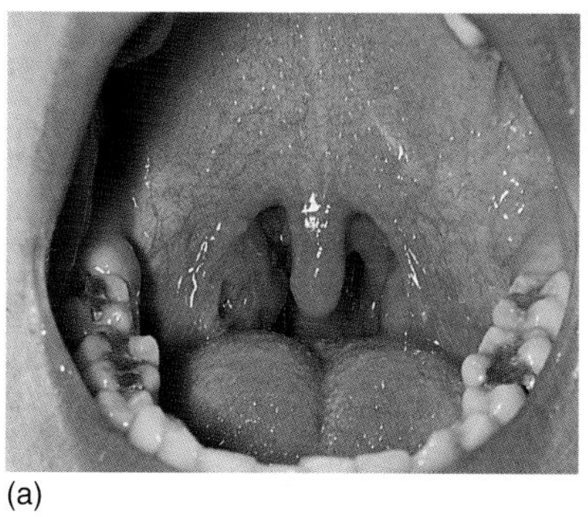

(a)

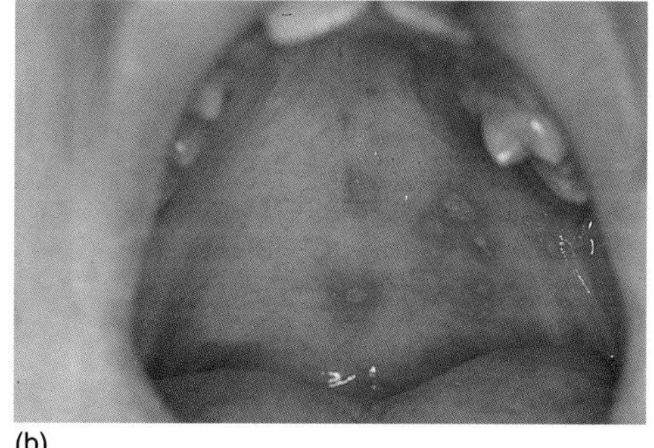

(b)

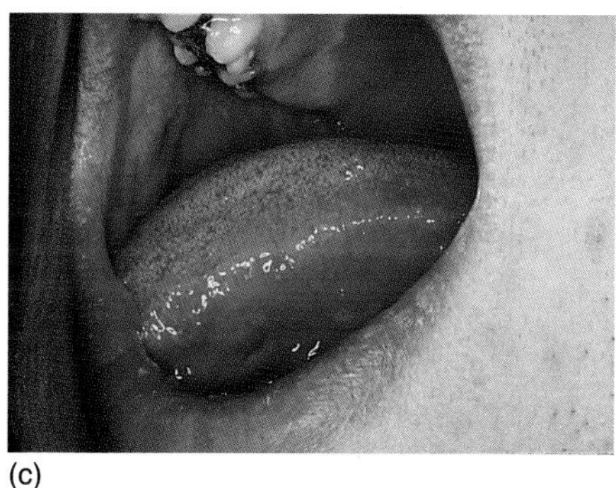

(c)

Plate 2 Differential diagnosis of herpes simplex lesions of the mouth (and see Fig. 3): (a) infectious mononucleosis; (b) herpes zoster; (c) hand, foot, and mouth disease (Coxsackie A16 infection)

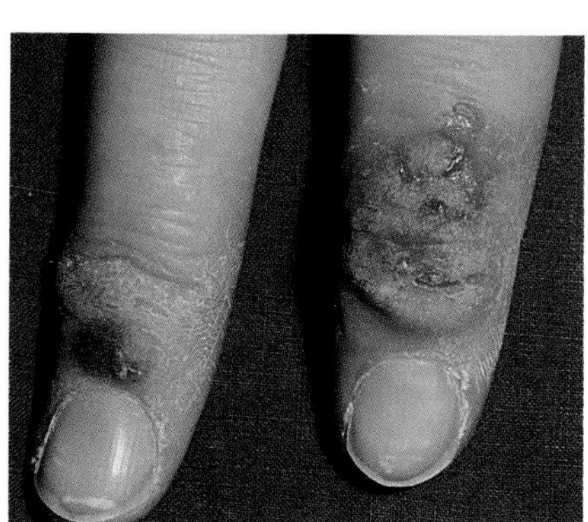

Plate 3 Herpetic whitlow with spread to an adjoining finger.

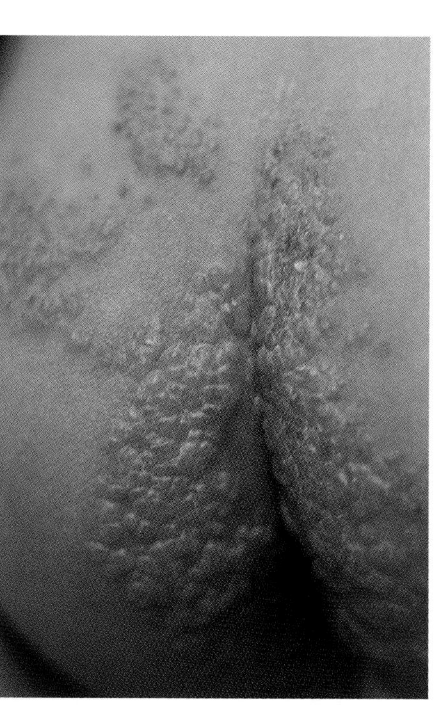

Plate 4 Primary HSV-2 of the buttocks (and see Fig. 6).

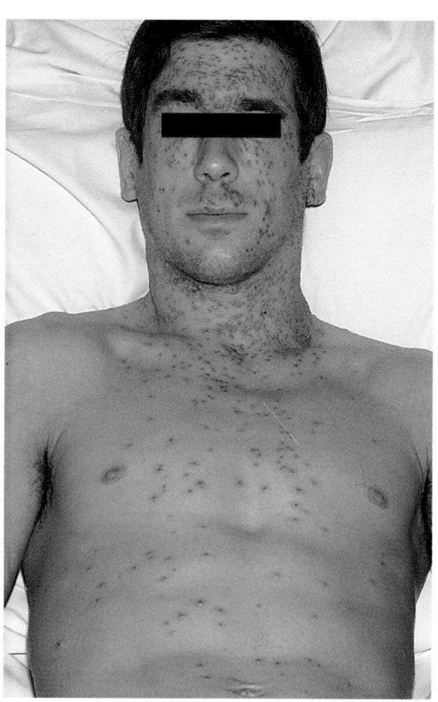

Plate 5 Eczema herpeticum in a man of 28 years.

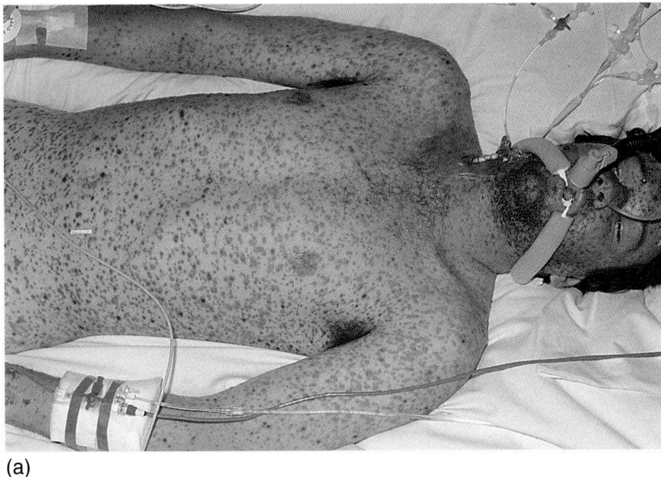
(a)

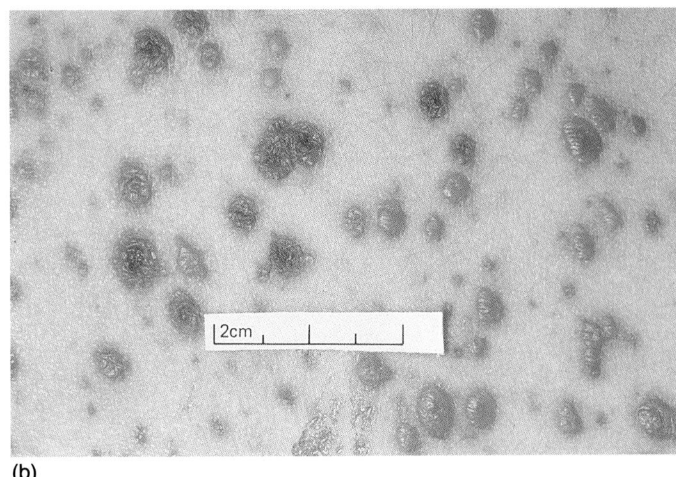

(b)

Plate 1 (a) Dense chickenpox eruption in a young man with severe infection also involving the lungs. (b) Detail of the rash.

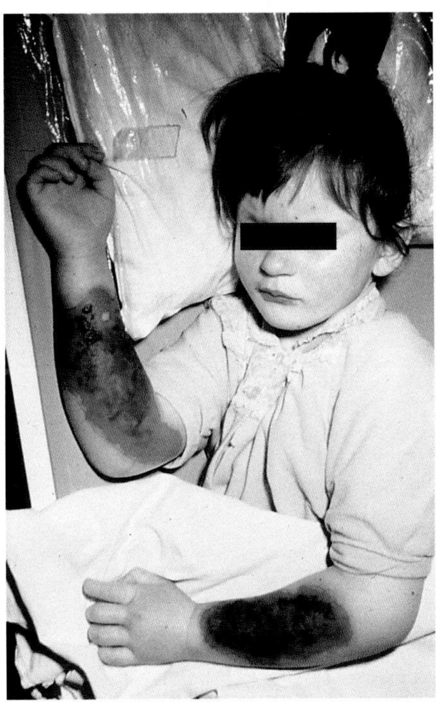

Plate 2 Purpura fulminans in a 9-year-old girl. (Reproduced by courtesy of the late Dr A. A. Sharp.)

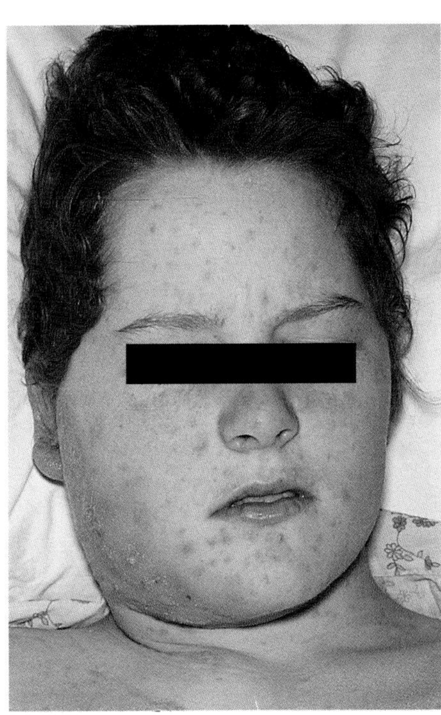

Plate 3 Zoster of the mandibular nerve with generalized spread in girl following marrow transplantation after whole body irradiation for acute myeloid leukaemia.

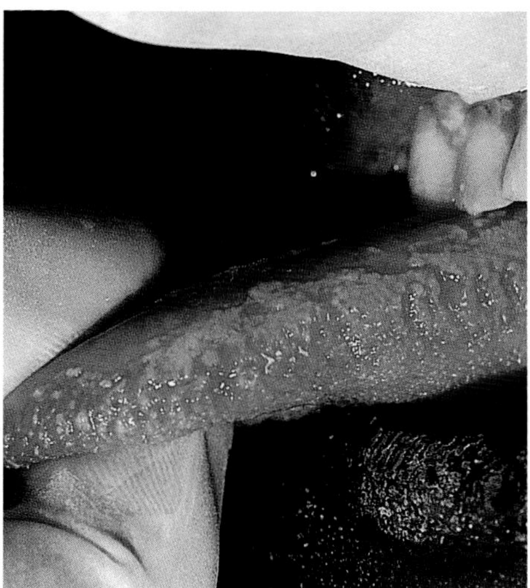

Plate 1 Typical hairy leukoplakia of the tongue (copyright C.F. Gilks).

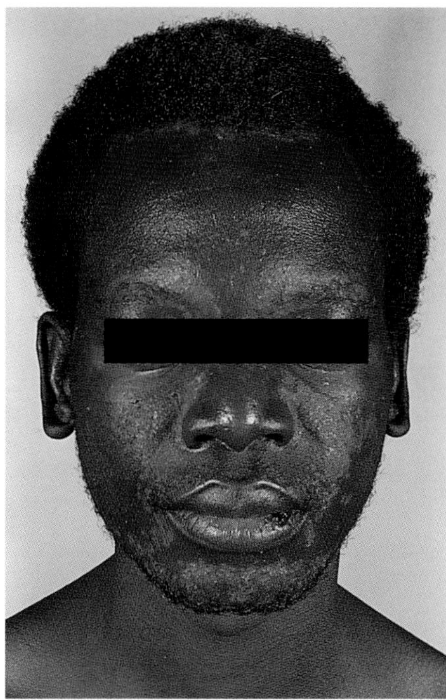

Plate 2 Seborrhoeic dermatitis (by courtesy of M.A. Ansary and C. Conlon, Lusaka).

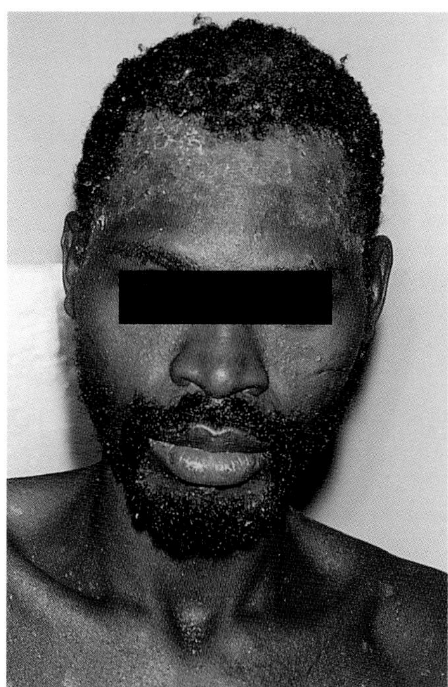

Plate 3 Exacerbation of psoriasis associated with AIDS (by courtesy of M.A. Ansary and C. Conlon, Lusaka).

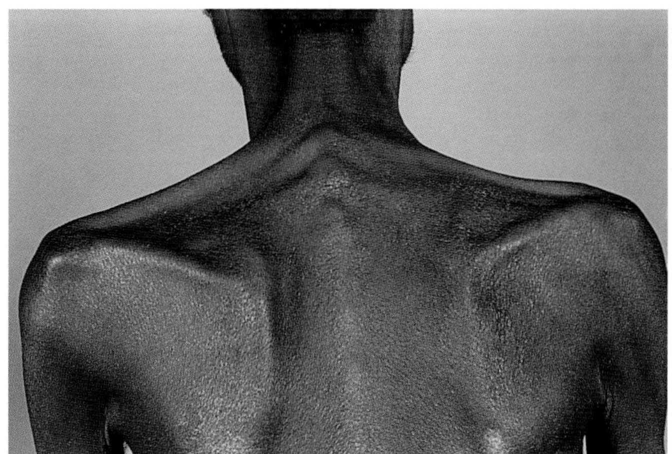

Plate 4 Severe wasting associated with HIV enteropathy ('slim disease') (by courtesy of M.A. Ansary and C. Conlon, Lusaka).

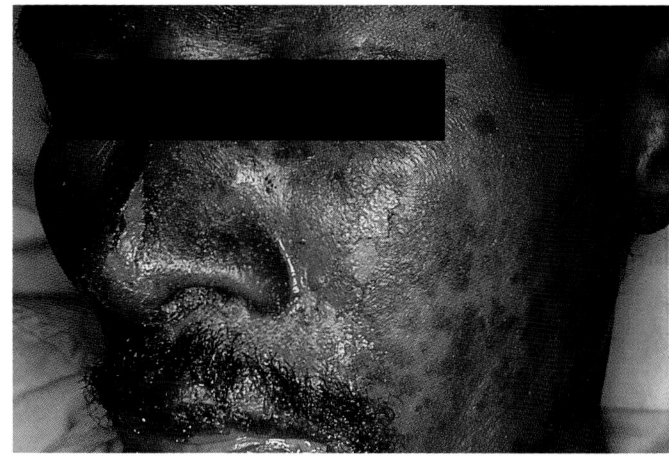

Plate 5 Severe Stevens–Johnson syndrome caused by thiacetazone treatment in an HIV-seropositive patient with tuberculosis in Kenya (by courtesy of Dr Paul Nunn, Geneva).

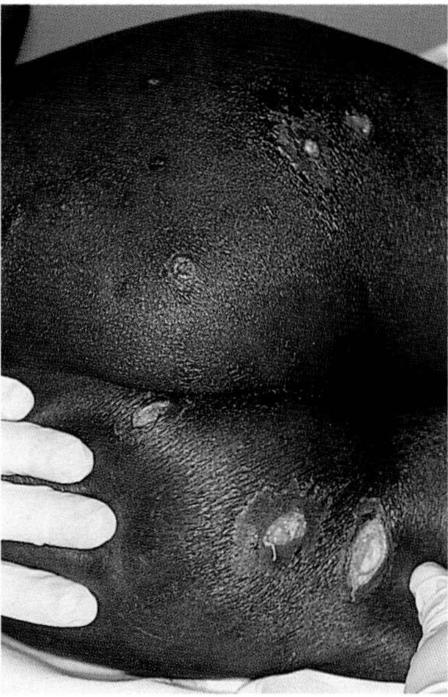

Plate 6 Multiple extending *Staphylococcus aureus* skin ulcers in an HIV-seropositive woman.

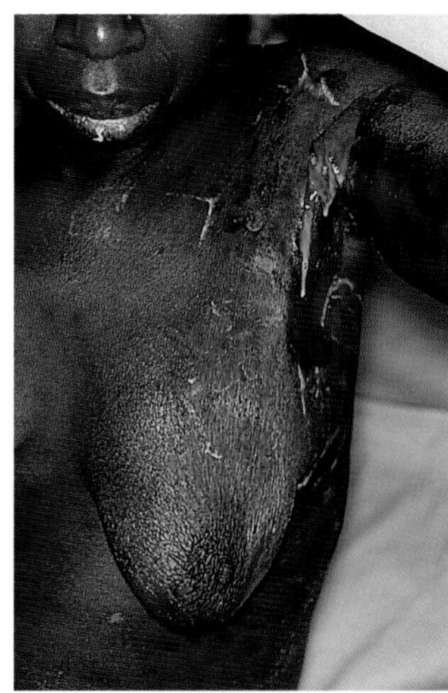

Plate 7 Extensive ulceration and subcutaneous abscess formation attributable to *Staphylococcus aureus* in an HIV-seropositive woman.

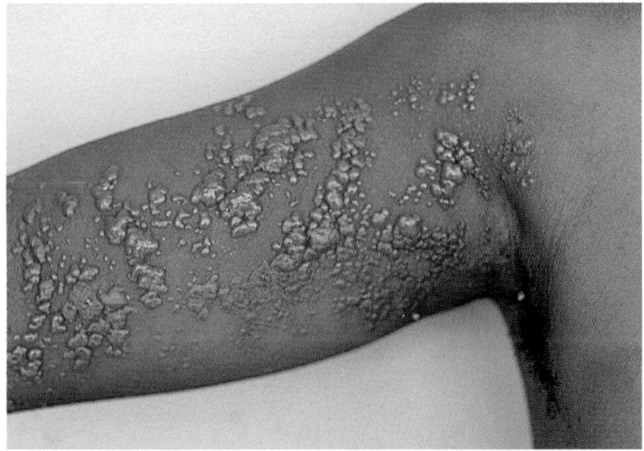

Plate 8 Acute herpes zoster in an HIV-seropositive patient (copyright C.F. Gilks).

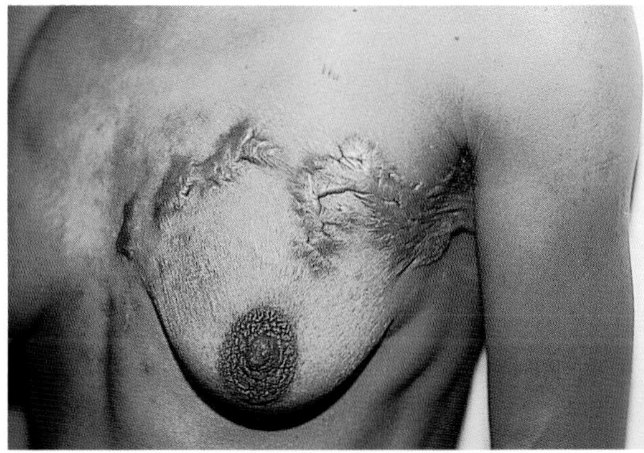

Plate 9 Keloid formation at the site of herpes zoster in an HIV-seropositive patient (copyright C.F. Gilks).

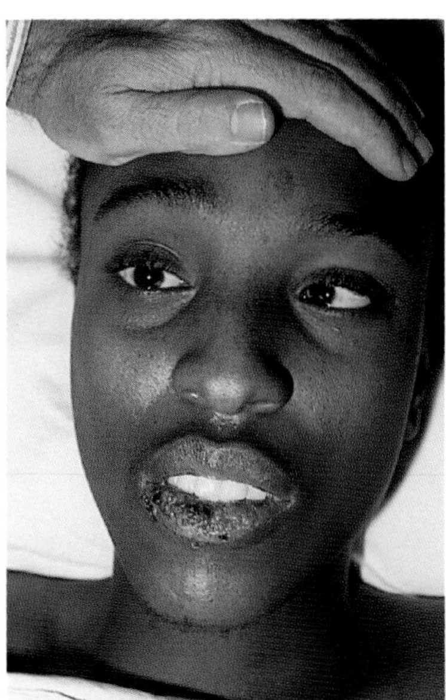

Plate 10 Cryptococcal meningitis in an HIV-seropositive patient with right VIth cranial nerve lesion (the patient is endeavouring to look to his right).

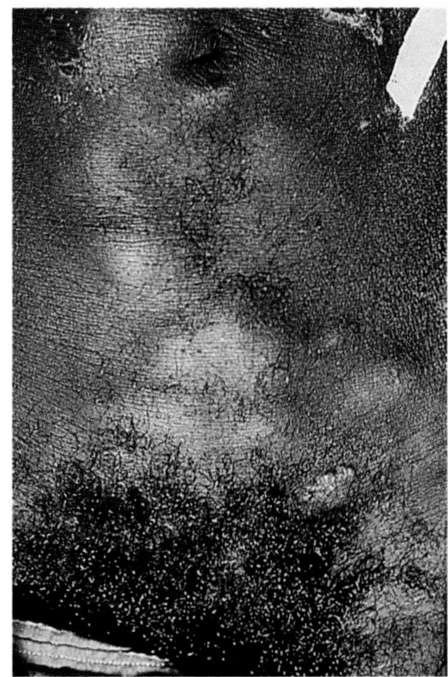

Plate 11 Subcutaneous masses of *Histoplasma duboisii* in the lower abdomen of a Nigerian patient (by courtesy of Mr Peter Cheese, Zaria).

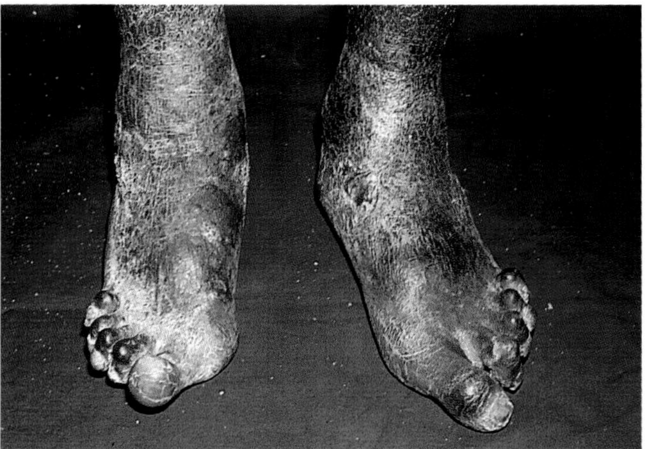

Plate 12 Endemic Kaposi's sarcoma (by courtesy of M.A. Ansary and C. Conlon, Lusaka).

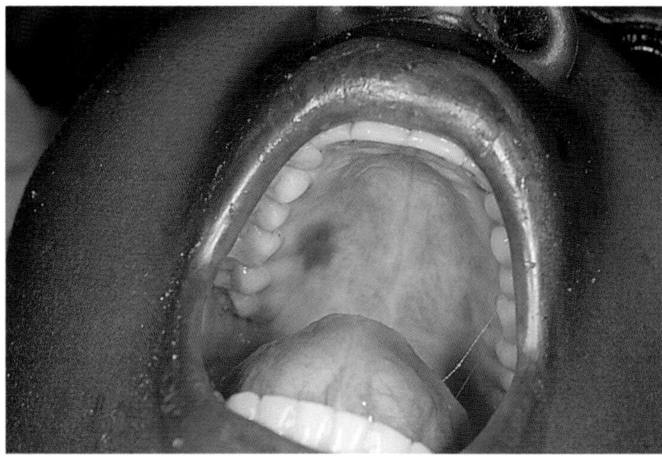

Plate 13 Kaposi's sarcoma of the palate in a seropositive patient.

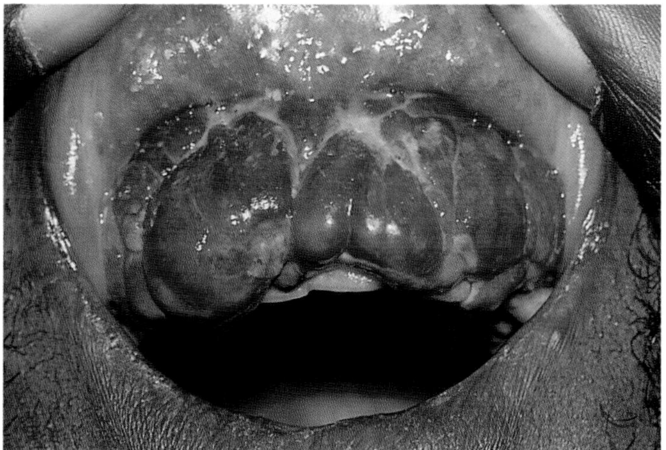

Plate 14 AIDS-associated Kaposi's sarcoma of the gum (copyright M.A. Ansary and C. Conlon, Lusaka).

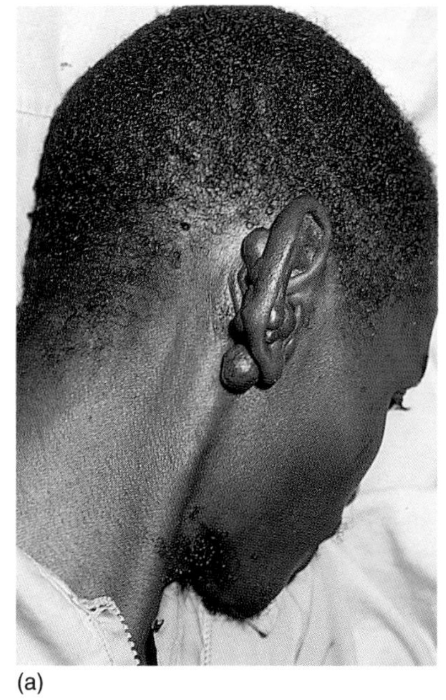

(a)

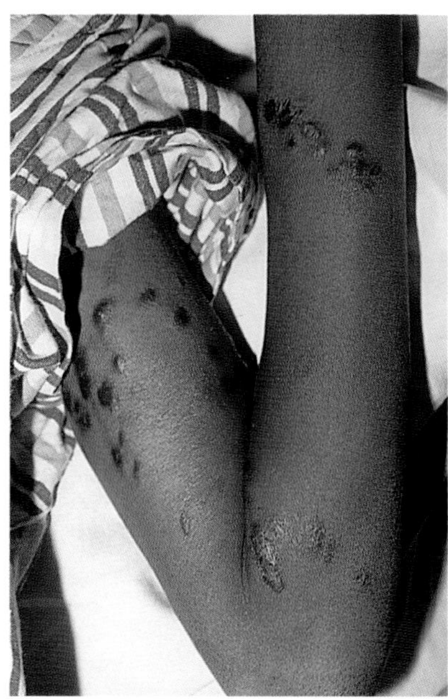

Plate 15 Multiple cutaneous Kaposi's sarcomas in an HIV-seropositive woman.

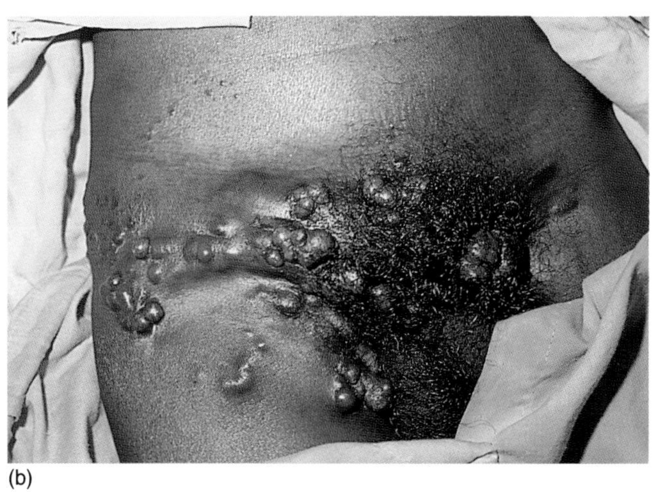

(b)

Plate 16 (a) and (b) Extensive invasive Kaposi's sarcomas in an HIV-seropositive man.

Chapter 7.11.1

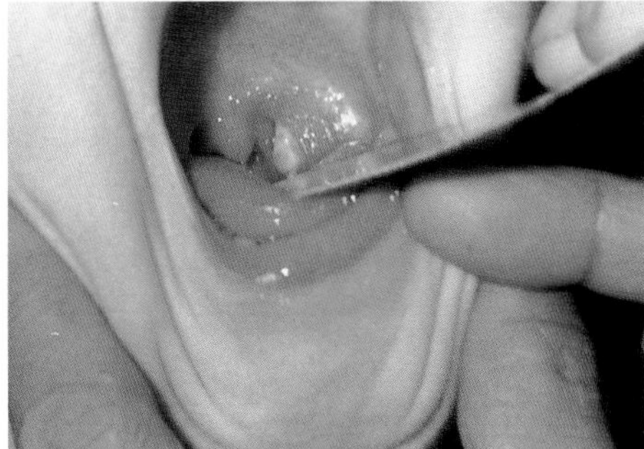

Plate 1 Early faucial diphtheria in a Vietnamese child.

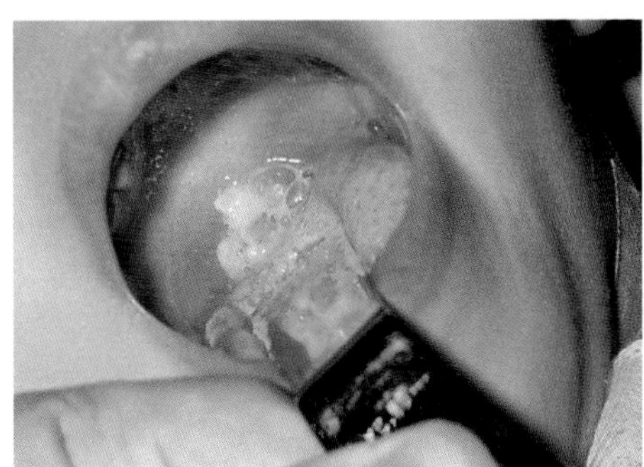

Plate 2 Spread of membrane to involve the hard palate.

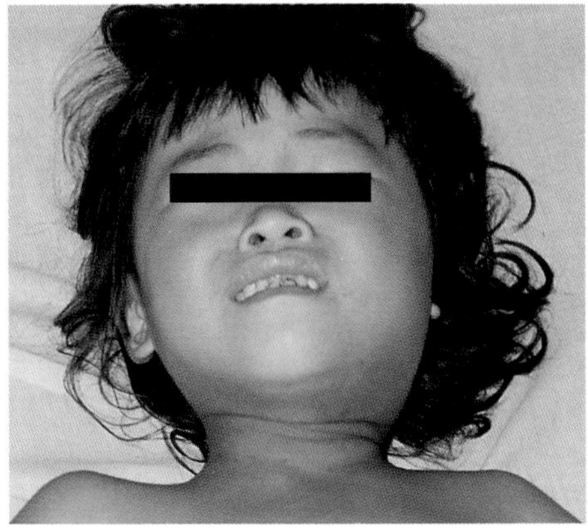

Plate 3 'Bull neck' of malignant diphtheria.

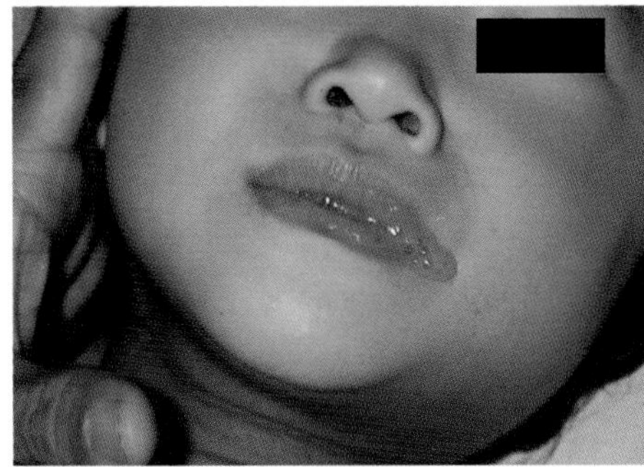

Plate 4 Bleeding from the mouth in malignant diphtheria.

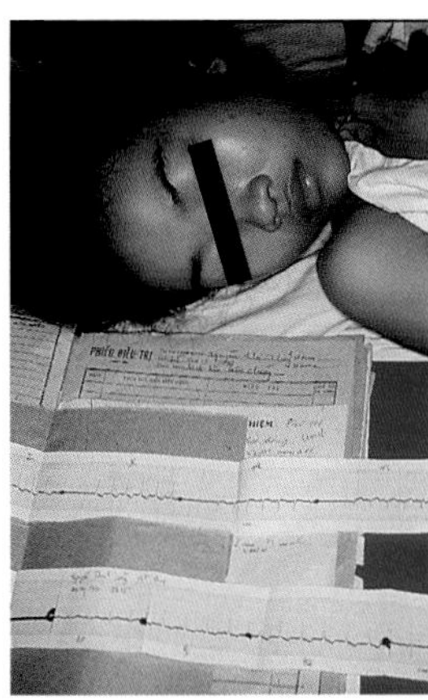

Plate 5 Fifteen-year-old Vietnamese girl with diphtheritic myocarditis (T-wave inversion, prolonged $Q–T_c$) and IXth, Xth, and VIIIth cranial-nerve lesions, 4 weeks after the acute illness. (Copyright D.A. Warrell.)

Chapter 7.11.6

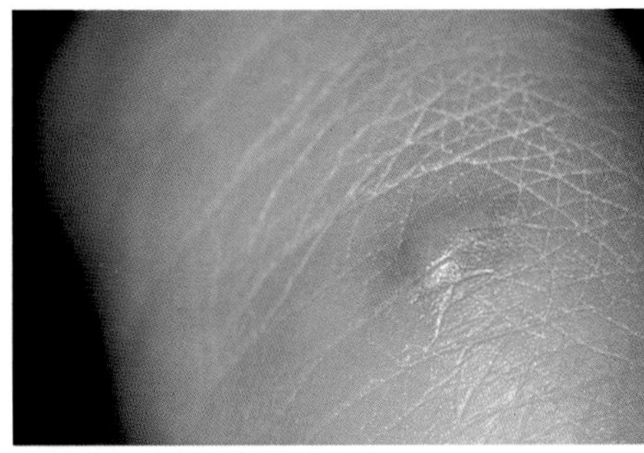

Plate 1 Disseminated gonococcal infection: haemorrhagic vesiculopustule.

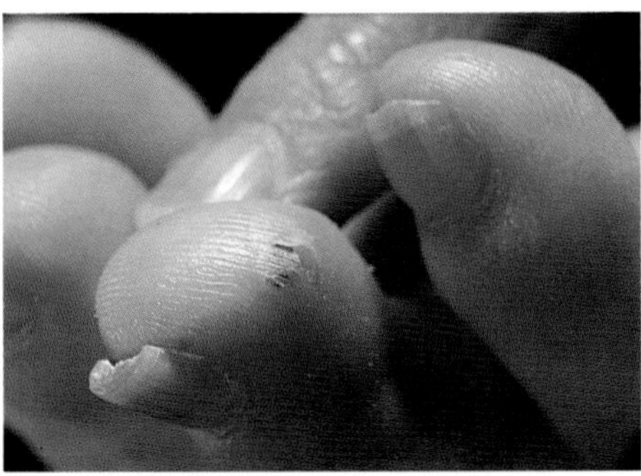

Plate 2 Disseminated gonococcal infection: healing lesion with desquamation and deposition of haemosiderin.

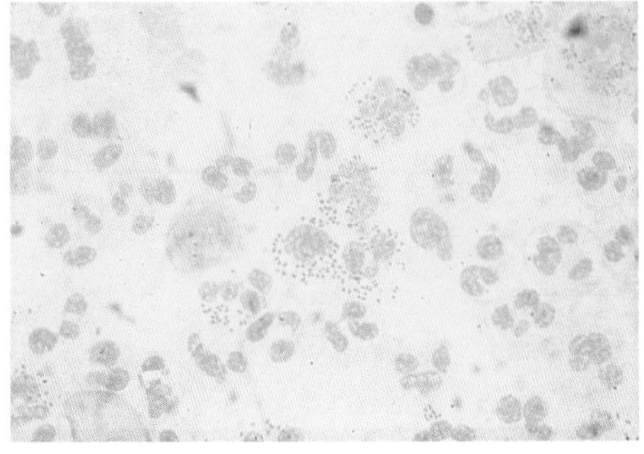

Plate 3 Gram-stained urethral discharge showing Gram-negative, intracellular diplococci.

CHAPTER 7.11.17(a)

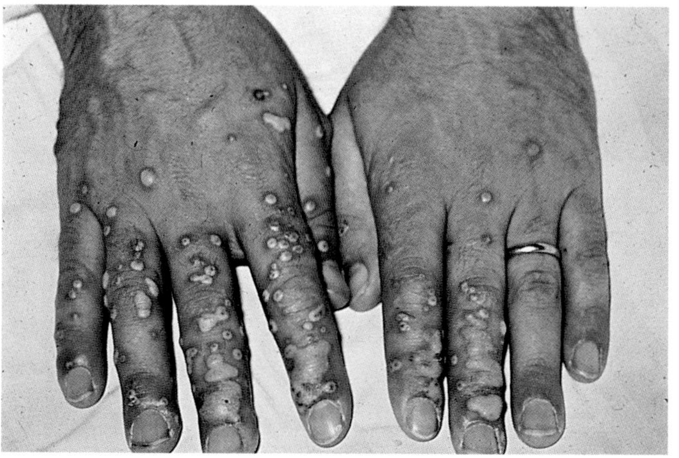

Plate 1 Hands in a case of ulcero-(cutano)-glandular tularaemia (by courtesy of A. Berglund, Falund, Sweden).

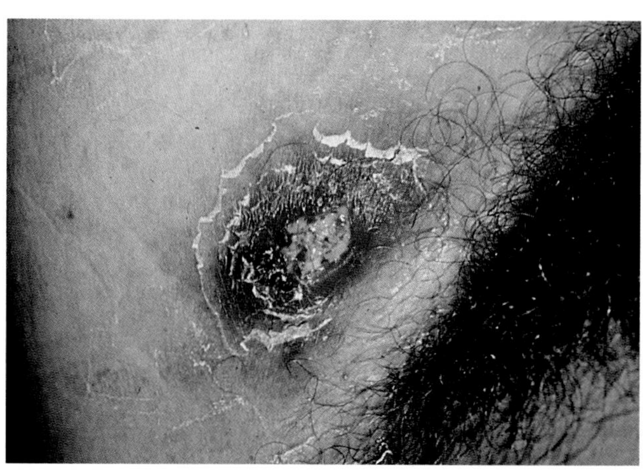

Plate 2 Inguinal lymphadenopathy in ulceroglandular tularaemia (by courtesy of A. Berglund, Falund, Sweden).

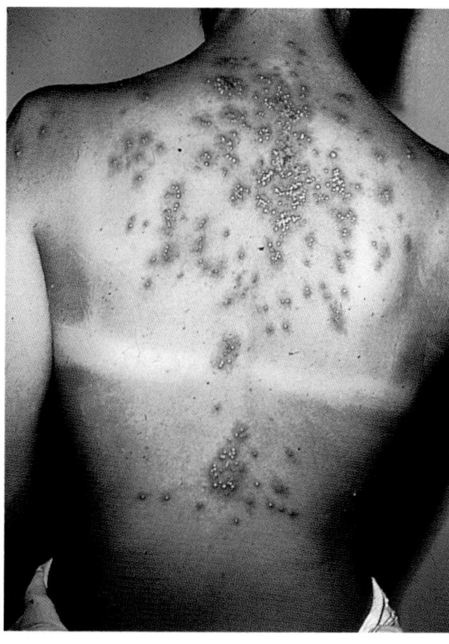

Plate 3 Hypersensitivity reaction in infection with *F. tularensis* subsp. *holarctica* (type B) in Scandinavia (by courtesy of A. Berglund, Falund, Sweden).

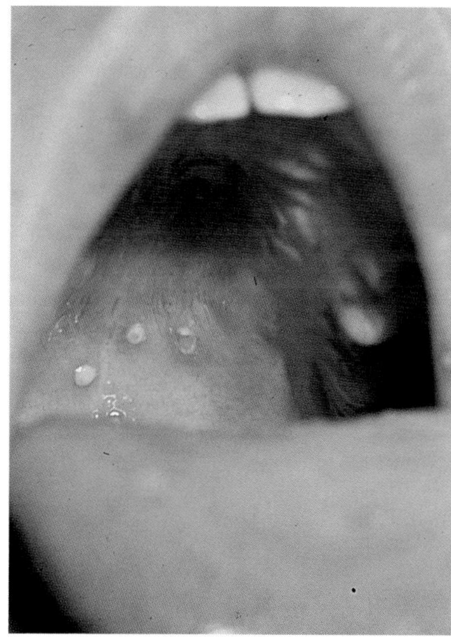

Plate 4 Oral tularaemia in a case from northern Sweden (by courtesy of A. Berglund, Falund, Sweden).

CHAPTER 7.11.41

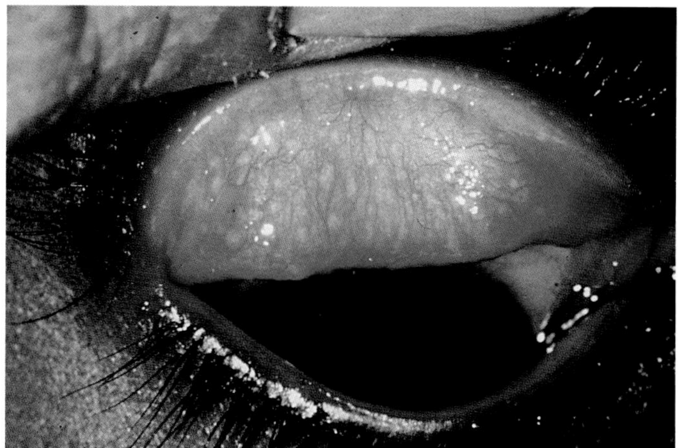

Plate 1 Everted upper eyelid showing follicular trachoma (TF).

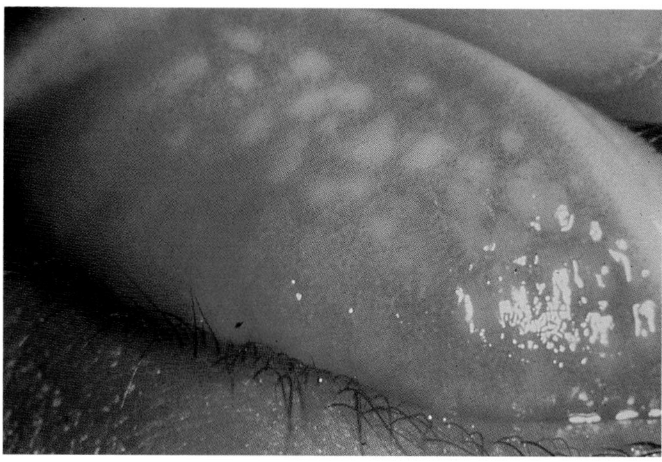

Plate 2 Everted upper eyelid showing intense inflammatory trachoma (TI).

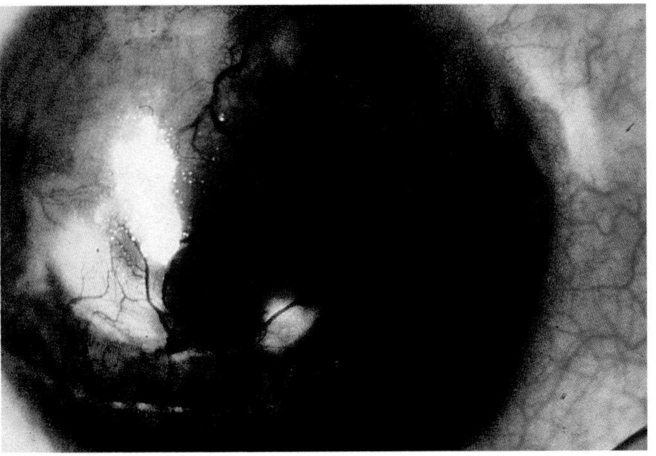

Plate 3 Extensive neovascularization of the cornea (pannus) due to trachoma.

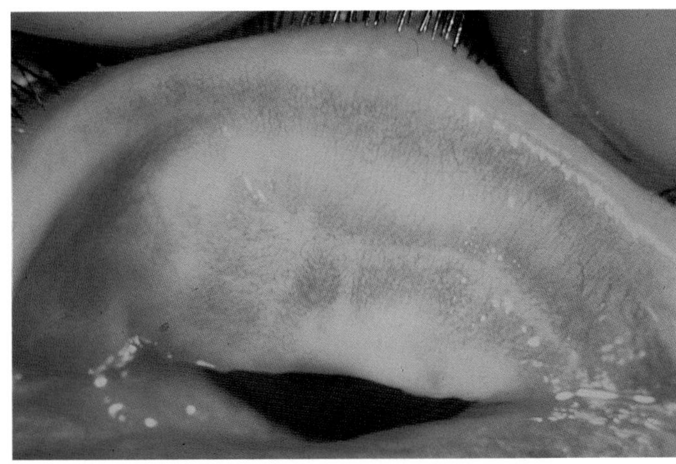

Plate 4 Everted upper eyelid showing trachomatous scarring (TS).

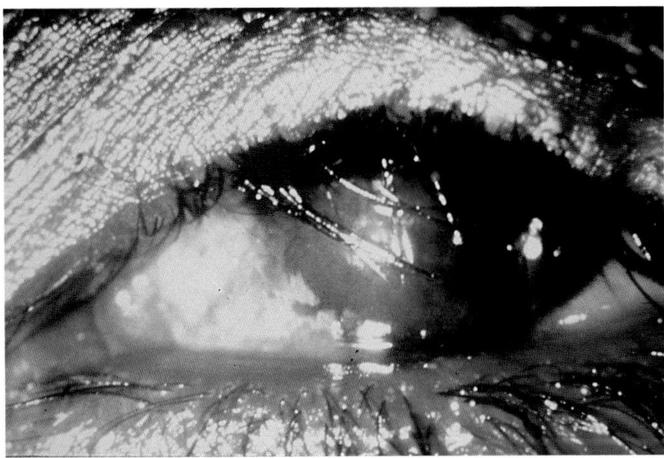

Plate 5 Trachomatous trichiasis (TT).

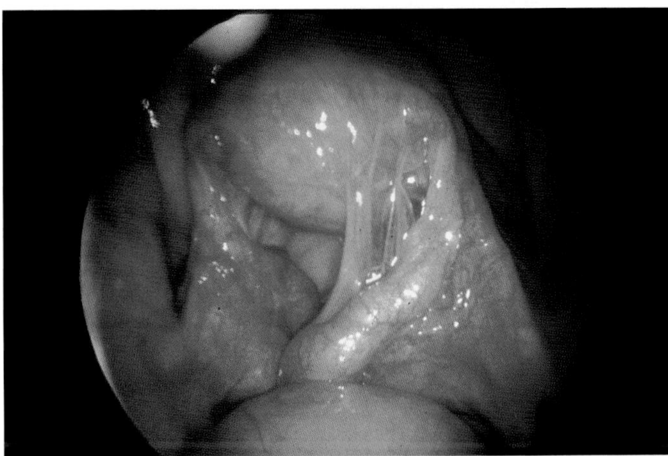

Plate 7 Laparoscopic view of inflamed fallopian tube due to *C. trachomatis*. (By courtesy of P. Greenhouse.)

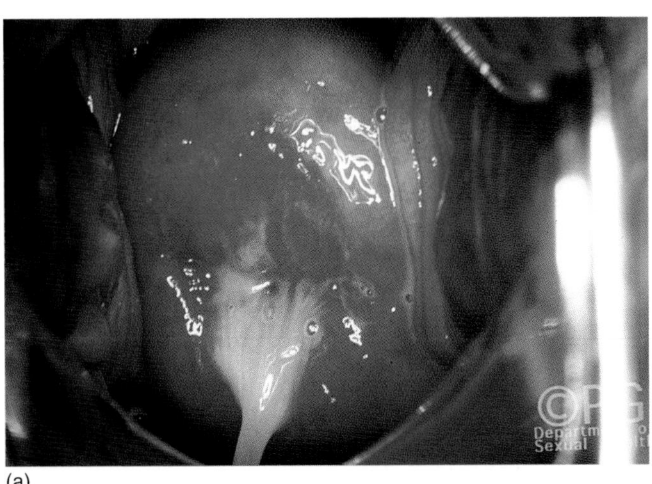

(a)

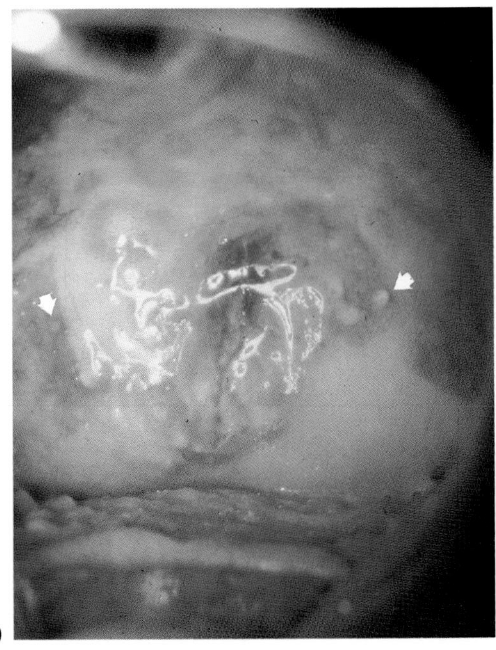

(b)

Plate 6 (a) Mucopurulent cervicitis; (b) follicular cervicitis.

Plate 8 Adhesions in perihepatitis (Curtis Fitz-Hugh syndrome) due to *C. trachomatis*. (By courtesy of P. Greenhouse.)

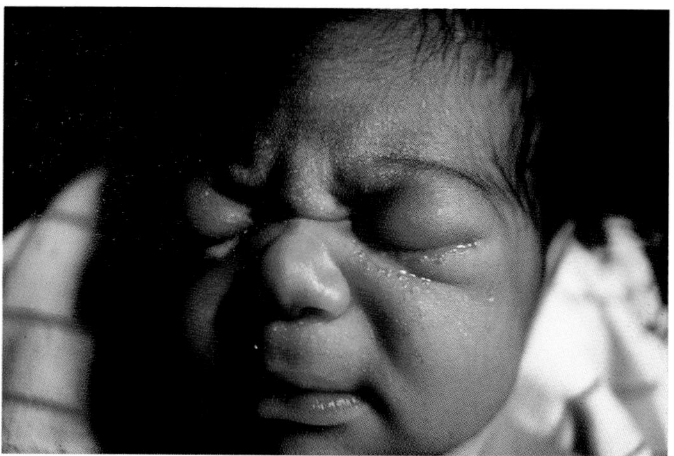

Plate 9 Mucopurulent neonatal conjunctival discharge due to *C. trachomatis*.

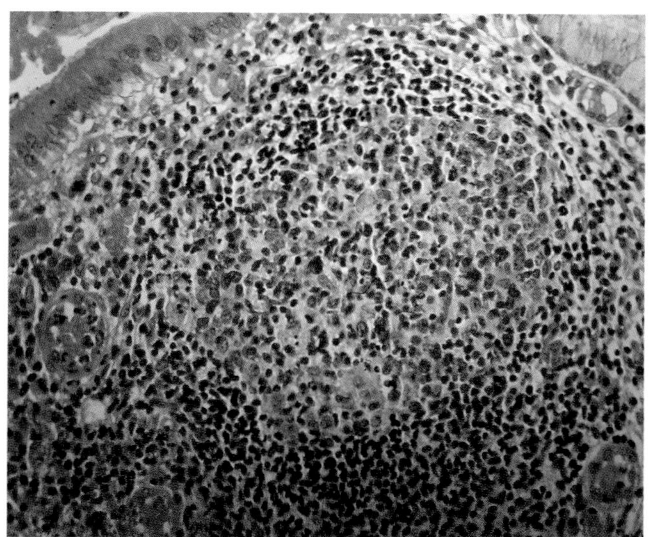

Plate 10 Germinal centre formation in lymphoid follicle of cervicitis due to *C. trachomatis*.

CHAPTER 7.11.44

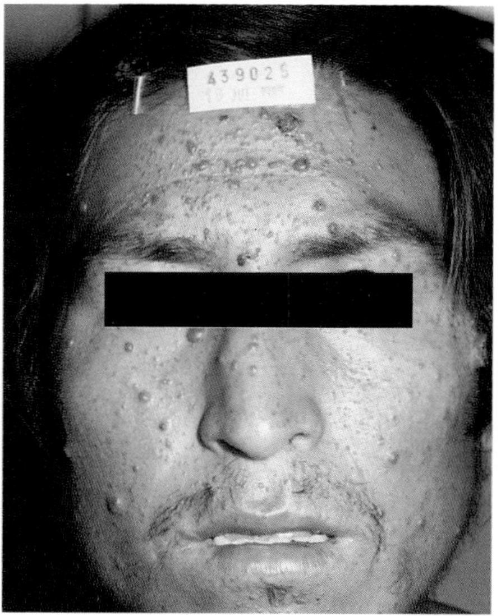

Plate 1 Miliary haemangioma-like lesions of 'verruga peruana'.

(a)

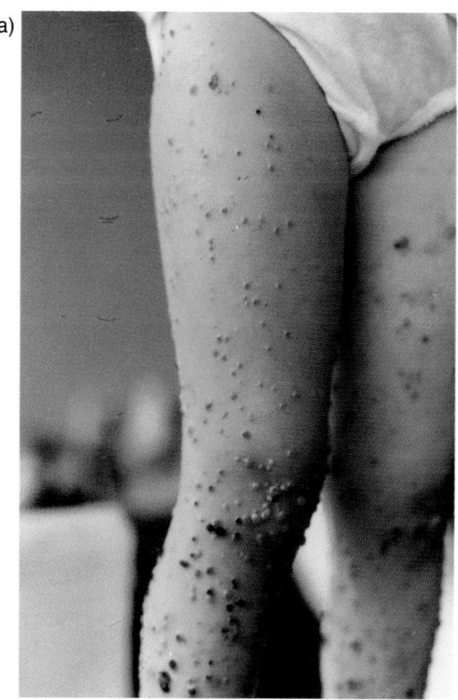

(b)

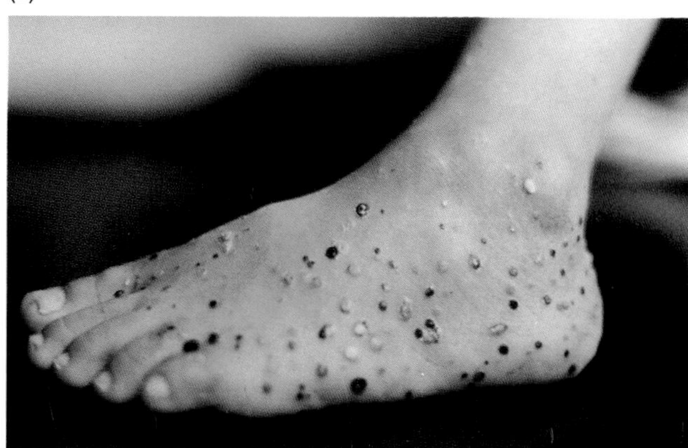

Plate 2 (a, b) Nodular lesions of 'verruga peruana'.

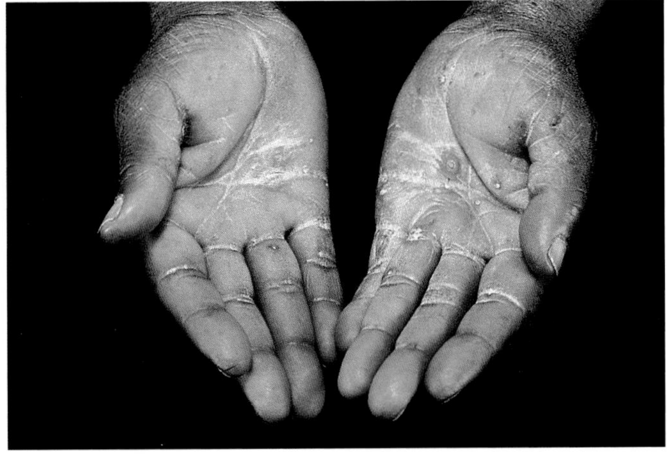

Plate 1 Palmar scaling due to *Trichophyton rubrum*.

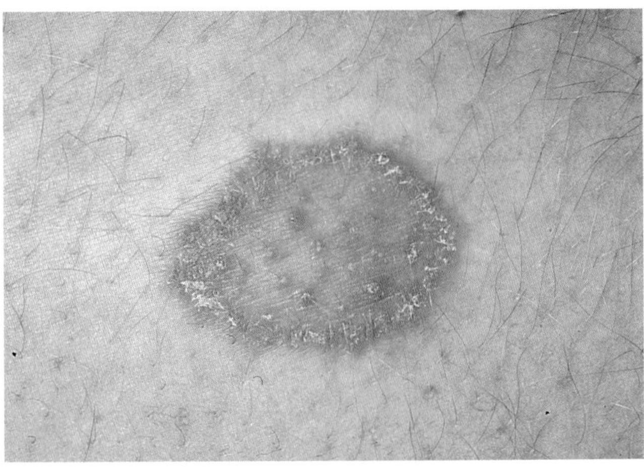

Plate 2 Tinea corporis due to *Microsporum gypseum*.

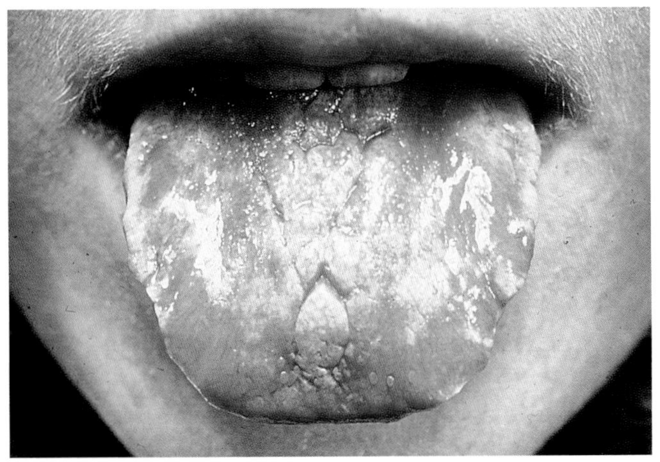

Plate 3 Oral candidosis in a patient with chronic mucocutaneous candidosis.

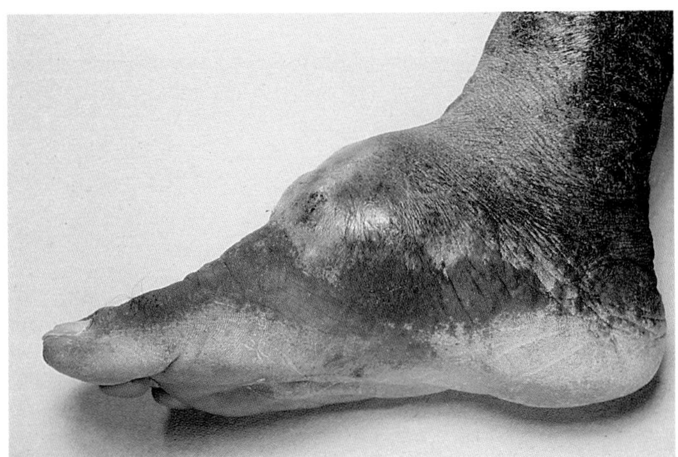

Plate 4 A mycetoma caused by *Madurella grisea*.

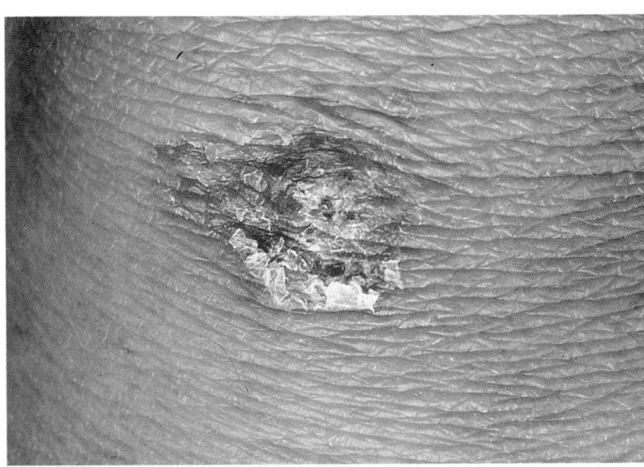

Plate 5 An early lesion of chromoblastomycosis.

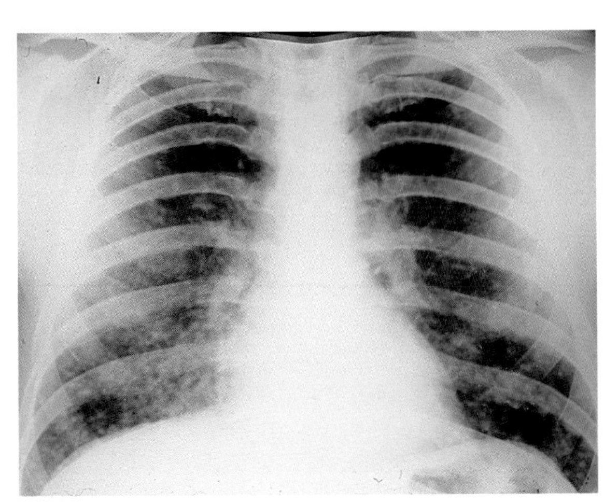

Plate 6 Acute pulmonary histoplasmosis.

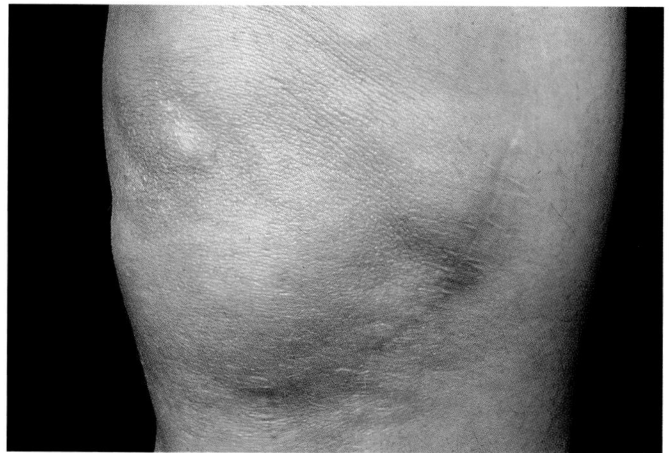

Plate 7 Arthritis due to disseminated coccidioidomycosis.

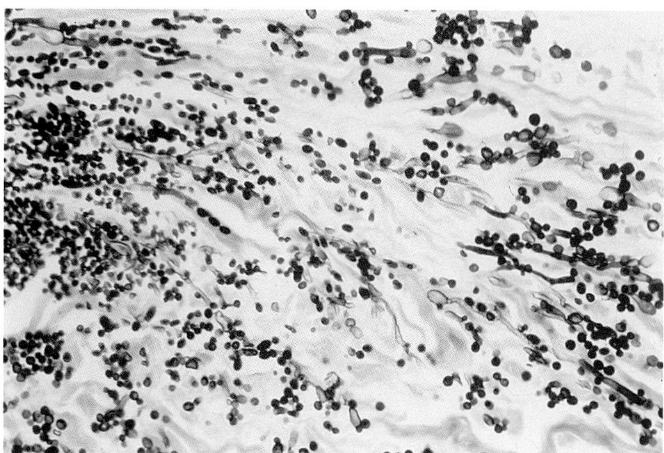

Plate 8 Candidosis disseminated to skin (methenamine silver × 516).

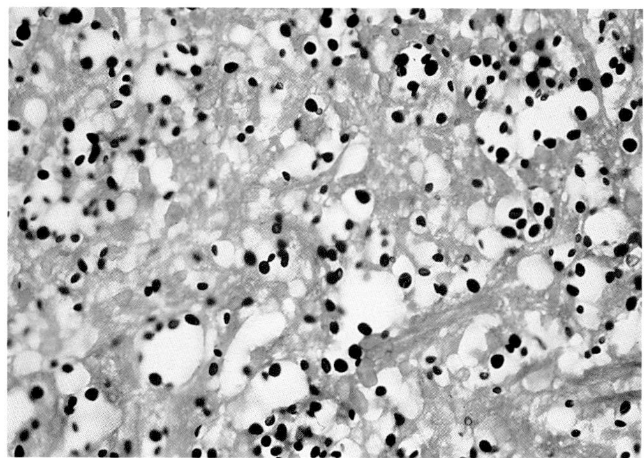

Plate 9 Disseminated cryptococcosis (methenamine silver × 52).

Chapter 7.13.2

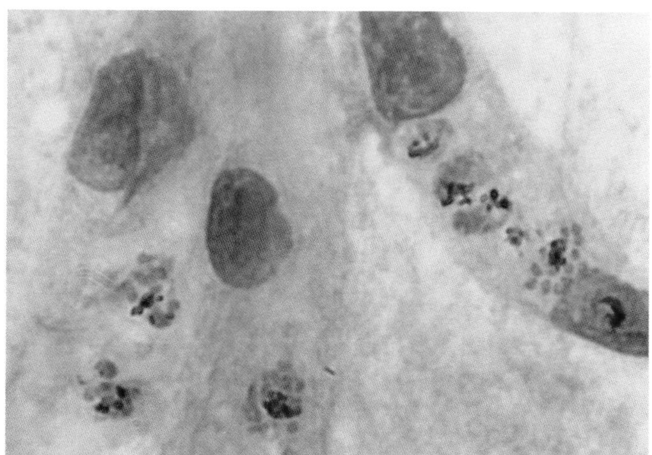

Plate 1 Impression smear made from a needle necropsy of the brain of a patient who died of cerebral malaria. Note capillary endothelial nuclei (N), parasitized red blood cells choking lumen (arrow), and malaria pigment (P). (By courtesy of Dr M.J. Warrell.)

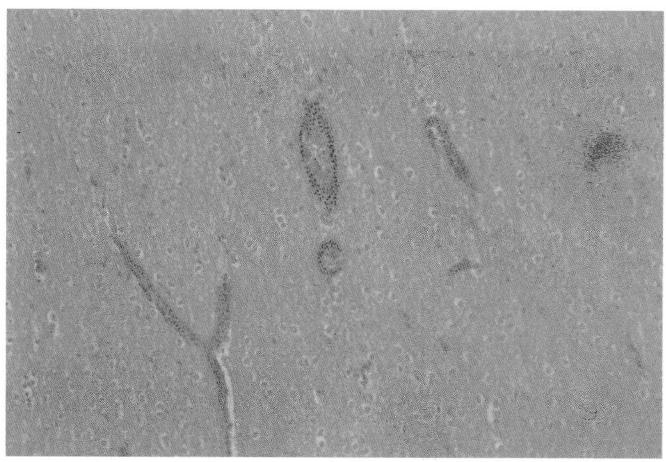

Plate 2 Section of frontal cortex from a Vietnamese patient who died of cerebral malaria, showing margination of parasitized red blood corpuscles along the endothelial lining of blood vessels and occlusion of a small vessel with parasitized red blood corpuscles (by courtesy of Dr Gareth Turner, Oxford).

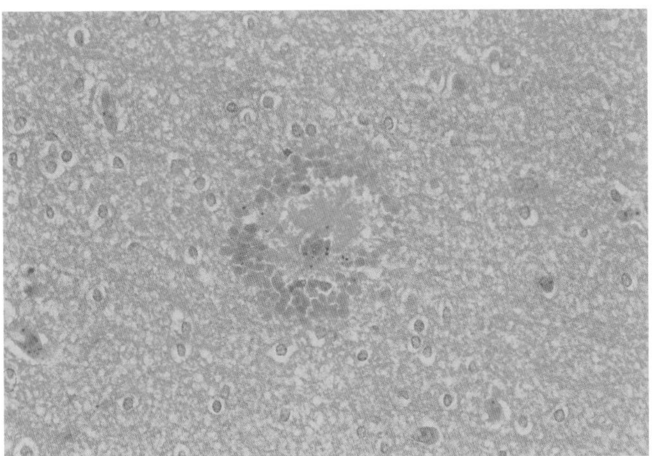

Plate 3 Section of the temporal lobe in a Vietnamese patient who died of cerebral malaria showing a resolving ring haemorrhage with parasitized red blood corpuscles in the occluded central vessel and predominantly unparasitized red blood corpuscles in the surrounding ring haemorrhage (by courtesy of Dr Gareth Turner, Oxford).

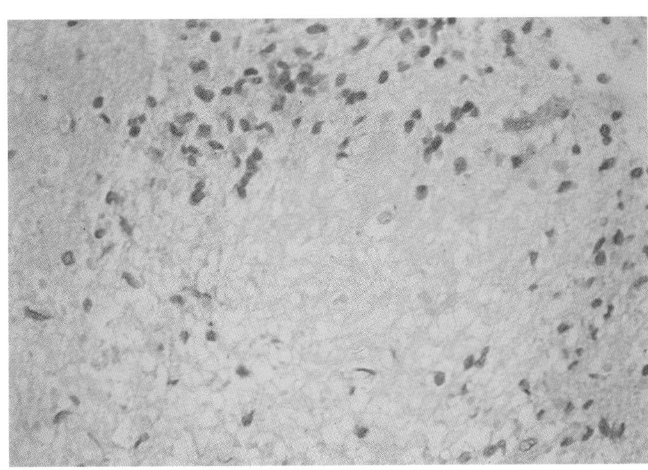

Plate 4 Dürck's granuloma: demyelinized central part with ring of microglial cell proliferation. The small central vessel lumen is visible and parasitized red blood corpuscles in marginal small vessels are also visible. (By courtesy of Dr N. Francis, London.)

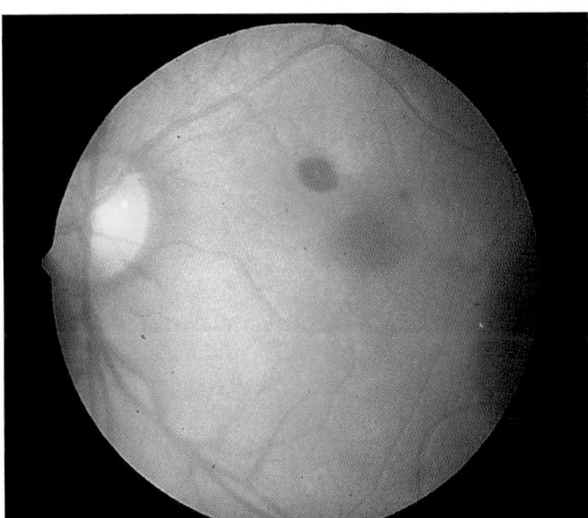

Plate 5 Retinal haemorrhages close to the macula in a Thai patient with cerebral malaria. (Copyright D.A. Warrell.)

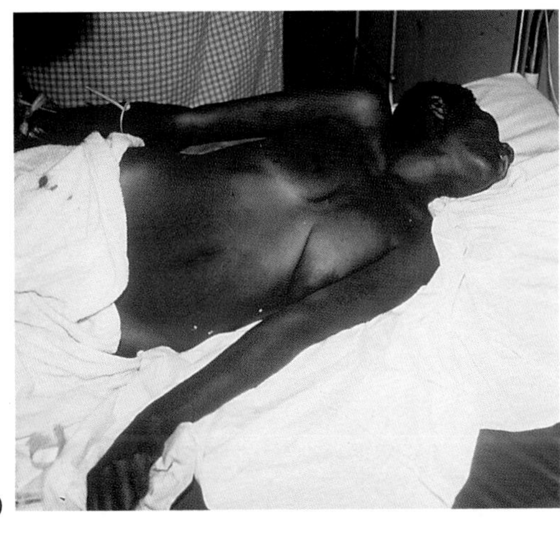

(a)

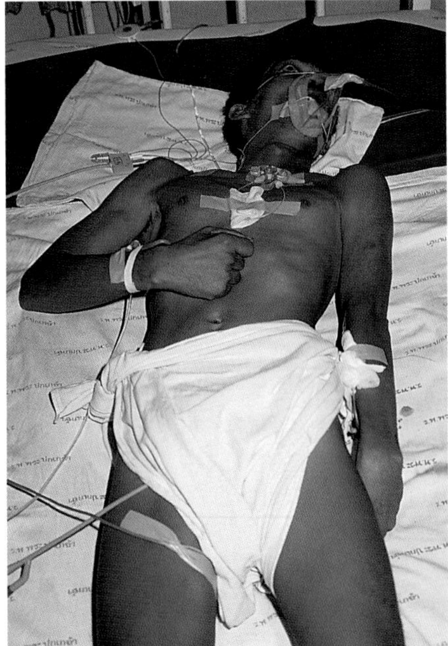

(b)

Plate 7 Extensor posturing. (a) Decerebrate rigidity in a Papuan New Guinean woman with cerebral malaria complicated by hypoglycaemia (by courtesy of Dr D. G. Lalloo, Oxford). (b) Decorticate rigidity in a Thai man with cerebral malaria. (Copyright D.A. Warrell.)

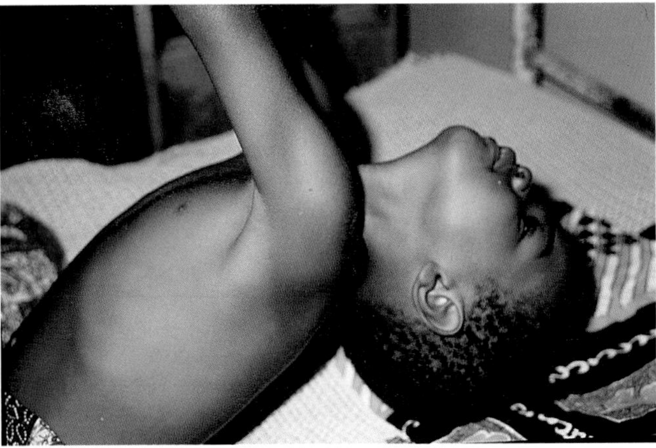

Plate 6 Generalized reduction in muscle tone ('broken neck sign') in a Kenyan child recovering from cerebral malaria. (Copyright D.A. Warrell.)

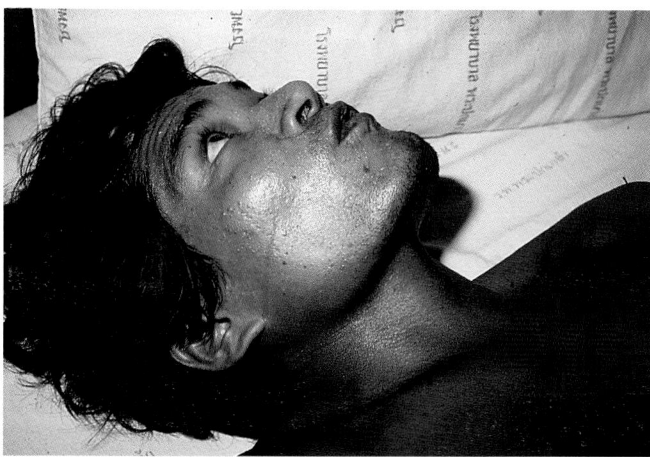

Plate 8 Pouting and sustained upward deviation of the eyes accompanied by stertorous respiration in a Thai man with cerebral malaria complicated by hypoglycaemia. (Copyright D.A. Warrell.)

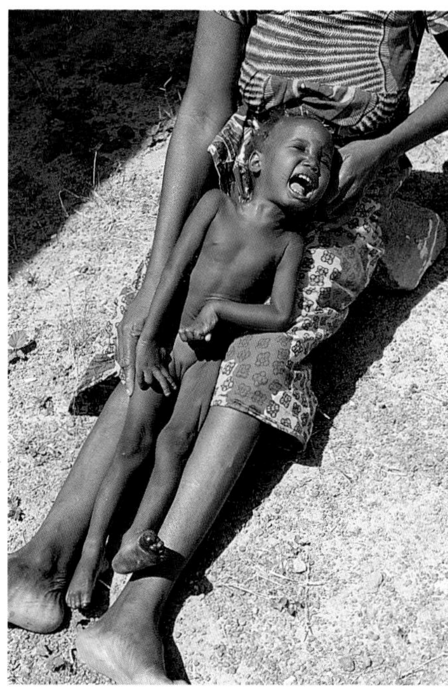

Plate 9 Hemiplegia and other severe residual neurological sequelae in a Nigerian child who survived an attack of cerebral malaria. (Copyright D.A. Warrell.)

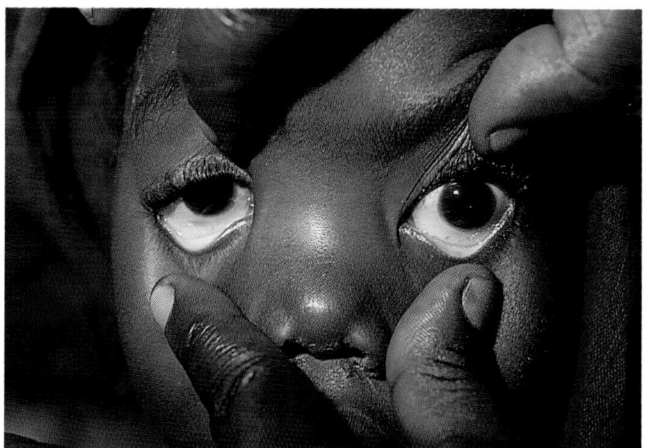

Plate 10 Profound anaemia (haemoglobin 1.2 g/dl) in a Kenyan child with *P. falciparum* parasitaemia. (Copyright D.A. Warrell.)

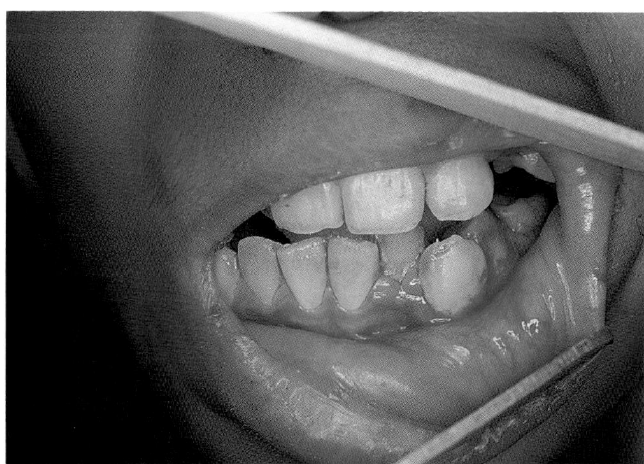

Plate 11 Cerebral malaria. Spontaneous systemic bleeding from the gingival sulci in a Thai patient with disseminated intravascular coagulation. (Copyright D.A. Warrell.)

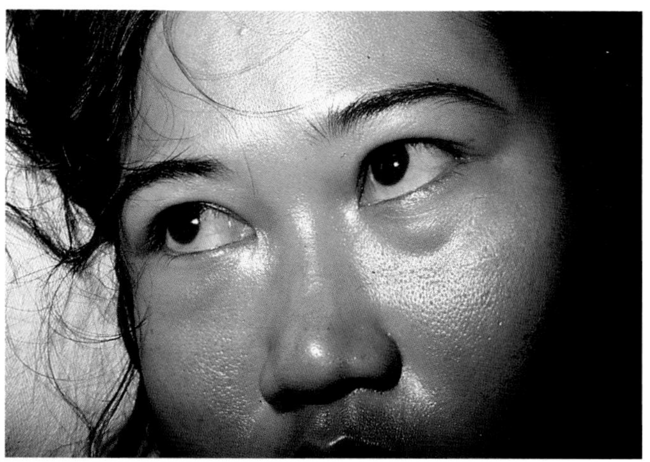

Plate 12 Deep jaundice in a Thai woman with severe falciparum malaria. (Copyright D.A. Warrell.)

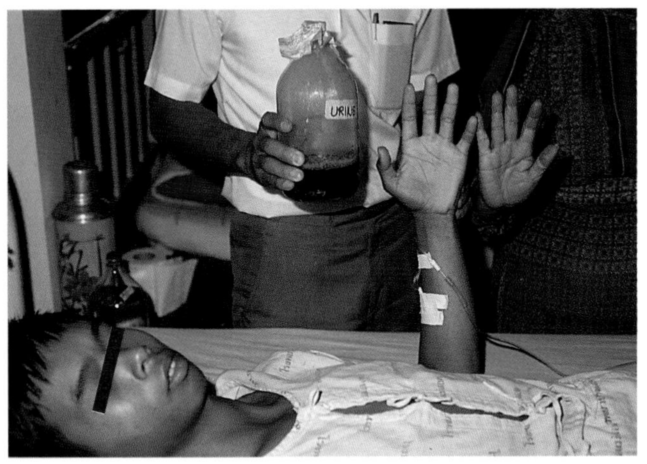

Plate 13 Intravascular haemolysis in a Karen patient with glucose 6-phosphate dehydrogenase deficiency resulting in haemoglobinuria and anaemia. (Copyright D.A. Warrell.)

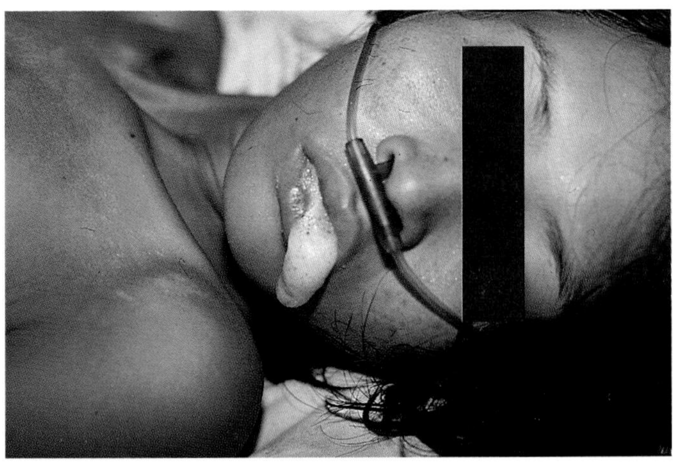

Plate 14 Fatal pulmonary oedema developing 3 h postpartum in a Thai woman with cerebral malaria; the fetus was stillborn (by courtesy of Professor Sornchai Looareesuwan, Bangkok).

Gametocytes		Schizonts		Trophozoites		
Female	Male	Mature	Immature	Old	Young	
						P. falciparum
						P. vivax
						P. malariae
						P. ovale

Plate 15 Malaria parasites developing in erythrocytes (by courtesy of the Wellcome Trust, London).

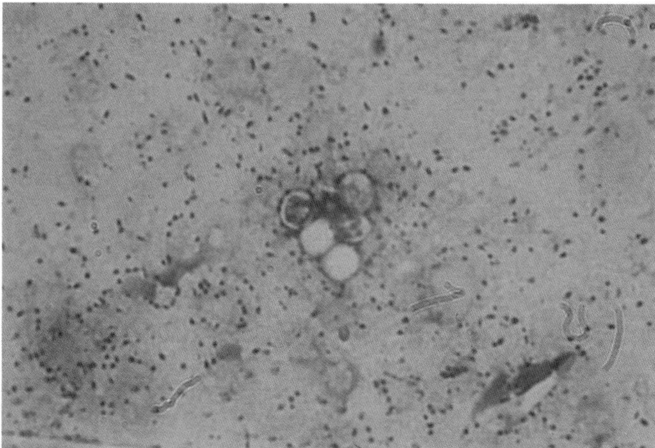

Plate 1 Modified Giemsa-stained faecal smear showing oocysts of *C. parvum*, examined with × 100 oil-immersion objective lens. The uniformity of size (4.5–5 μm) but variability of staining of oocysts can be seen. The eosinophilic nuclei and basophilic bodies of the sporozoites can be clearly seen within the oocysts that have taken up the stain. (Plates 1 to 10 of Chapter 7.3.5 provided from photographs by A. Curry and D.P. Casemore.)

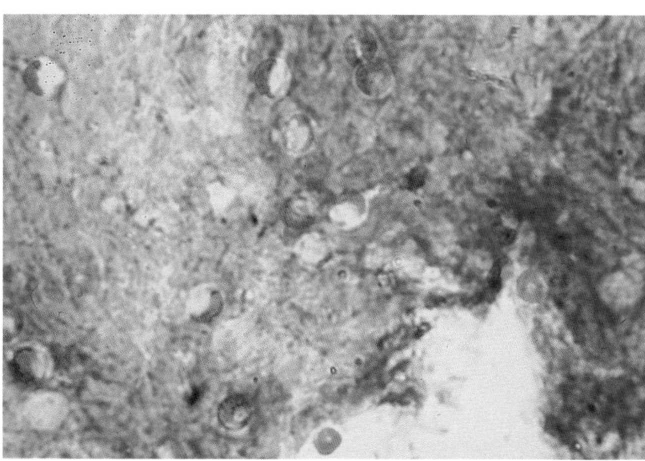

Plate 2 Modified Ziehl–Neelsen-stained faecal smear showing oocysts of *C. parvum* examined with × 100 oil-immersion objective lens. The uniformity of size (4.5–5 μm) but variability of staining of oocysts can be seen.

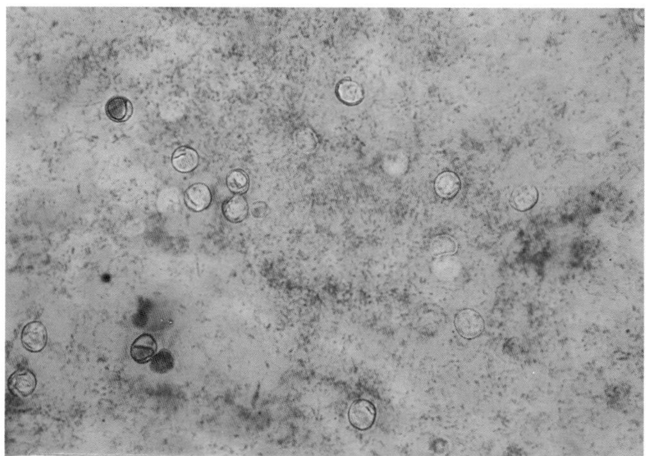

Plate 3 Modified Ziehl–Neelsen-stained faecal smear showing oocysts of *C. parvum*. The uniformity of size (4.5–5 μm) is apparent but the oocysts in this preparation show a definite increase in refractility and marked failure to take up the stain (identity confirmed by immunofluorescence and electron microscopy).

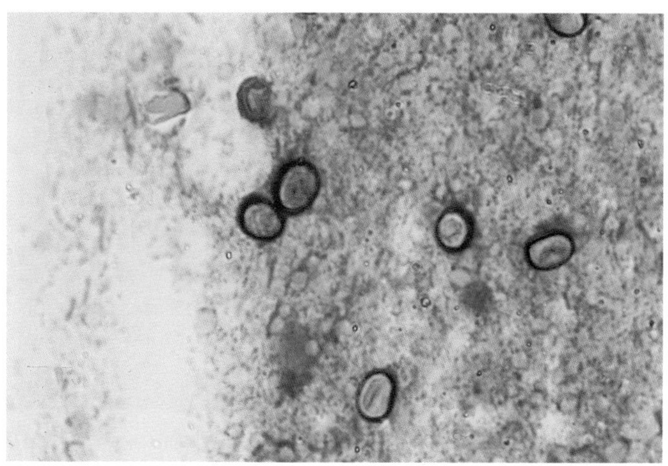

Plate 4 Modified Ziehl–Neelsen-stained faecal smear showing oocyst-like bodies (mushroom spores) examined with × 100 oil-immersion objective lens (from specimen submitted to Reference Unit for identification).

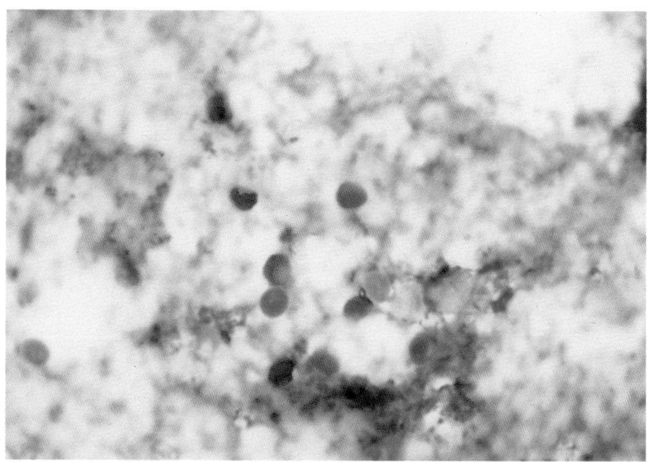

Plate 5 Modified Ziehl–Neelsen-stained faecal smear showing oocyst-like bodies (mould spores) examined with × 100 oil-immersion objective lens. The spores are uniform in size but a little smaller (4.0 μm) than oocysts of *C. parvum*. They are generally more uniform in their acid-fast staining (identity confirmed by mycological culture and electron microscopy).

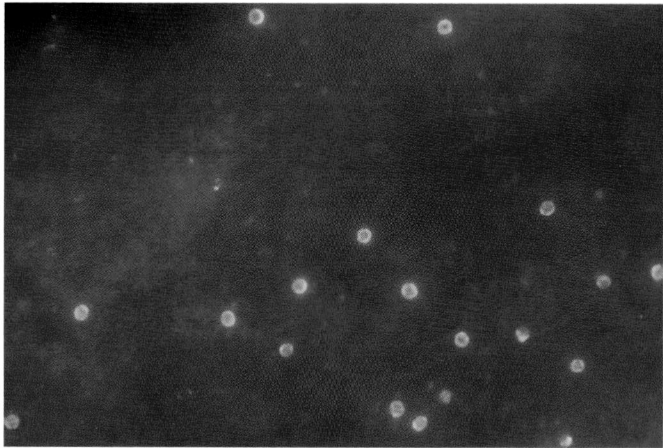

Plate 6 Phenol–auramine/carbol fuchsin-stained faecal smear showing oocysts of *C. parvum*, examined with × 20 dry objective lens (screening magnification) on a fluorescence microscope.

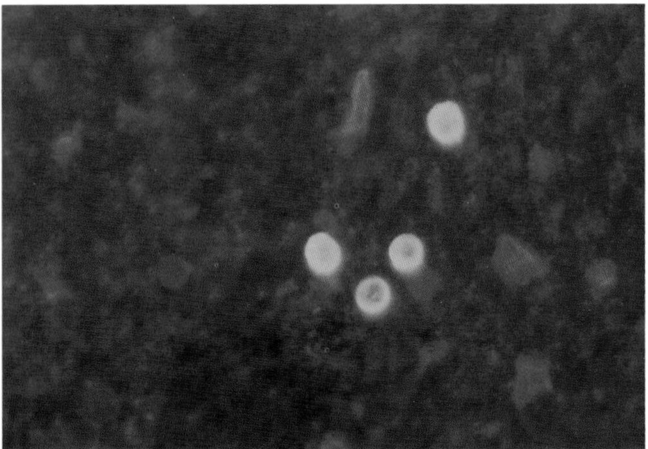

Plate 7 Phenol–auramine/carbol fuchsin-stained faecal smear showing oocysts of *C. parvum*, examined with × 100 oil-immersion objective lens on a fluorescence microscope.

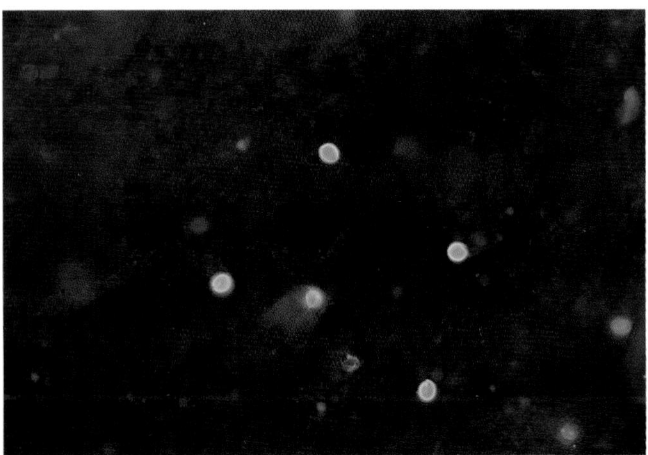

Plate 8 Fluorescent dye-tagged monoclonal antibody-stained faecal smear showing oocysts of *C. parvum*, examined with × 50 oil-immersion objective lens on a fluorescence microscope. The suture or associated surface cleft or fold, through which the sporozoites are released, can be seen.

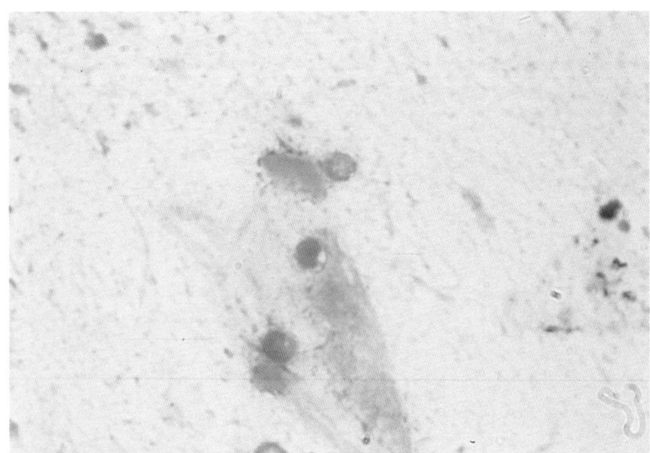

Plate 9 Modified Ziehl–Neelsen-stained sputum smear from an AIDS patient with respiratory involvement (examined with × 100 oil-immersion objective lens). The *C. parvum* bodies present may include endogenous (tissue) stages attached to exfoliated cells. For this reason, oocyst wall-specific indirect immunofluorescence may show a poor reaction. There may also be less uniformity of size and differences in the staining appearance of the internal structures.

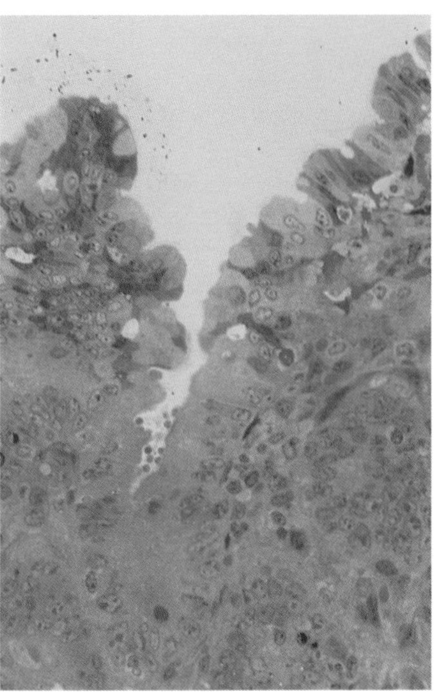

Plate 10 Toluidine blue-stained, semithin section of human rectal biopsy tissue of an AIDS patient with cryptosporidiosis. The apparently pseudo-external location of the parasite can be seen, the true location being intracellular but extracytoplasmic.

CHAPTER 17.13.6

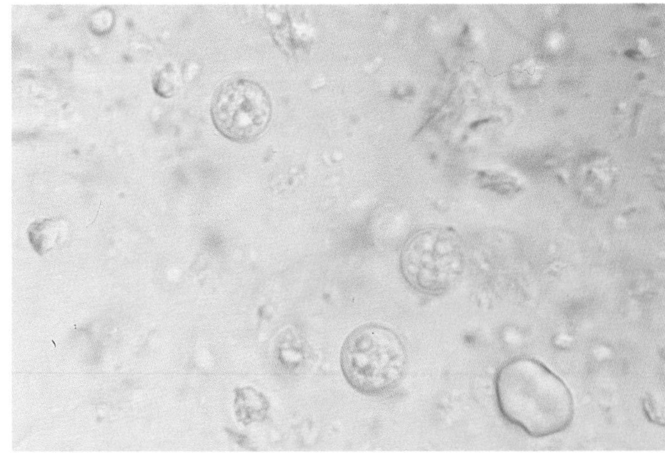

Plate 1 Unstained wet preparation of human faecal material showing oocysts of *Cyclospora* sp., examined with × 100 water-immersion objective lens by phase-contrast microscopy. The uniformity of size (8–10 μm) and the morular (mulberry) internal structure of the oocysts can be seen.

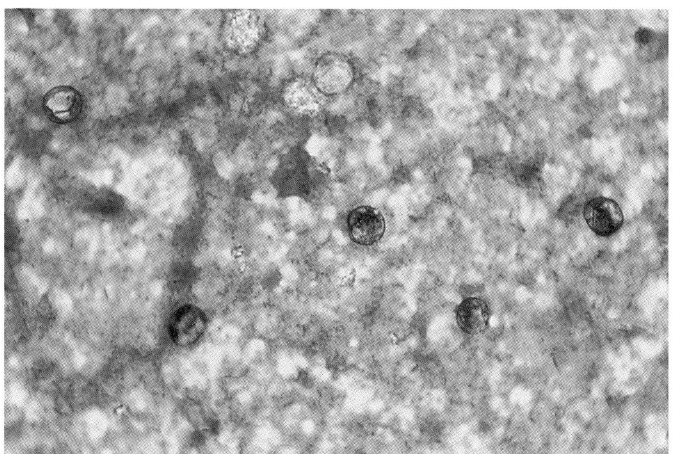

Plate 2 Modified Ziehl–Neelsen-stained faecal smear showing oocysts of *Cyclospora* sp. examined with × 50 oil-immersion objective lens. The uniformity of size (8–10μm) but variability of staining of the oocysts can be seen. Apart from the greater size, the oocysts can be distinguished from those of *Cryptosporidium parvum* by the different pattern of acid-fast staining. Unstained oocysts within the smear sometimes show the morular structure apparent in wet preparations.

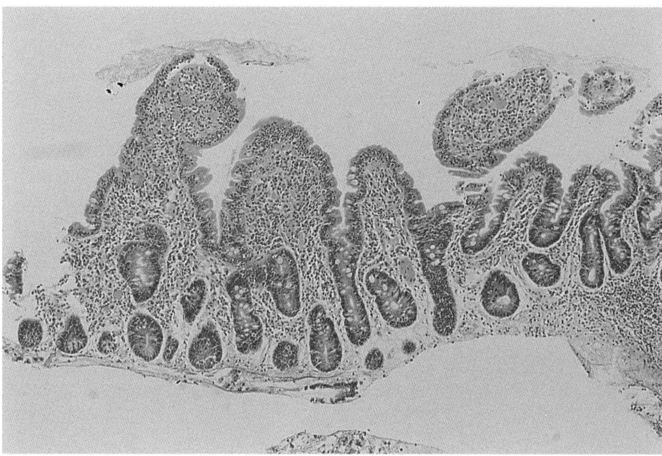

Plate 3 Jejunal biopsy from a patient with cyclosporiasis showing jejunitis with blunting of villi (low power H&E stain). (By courtesy of Dr. Sebastian Lucus, London.)

Plates for Section 8

Chapter 8.4.1

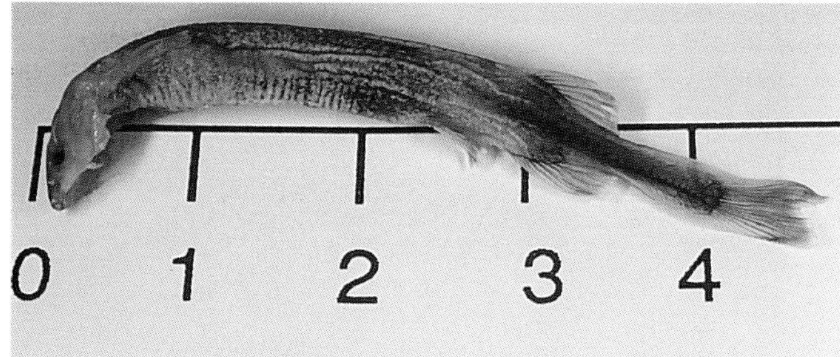

Plate 1 Parasitic catfish or candirú (*Vandelia species from the Amazon region of Brazil.*

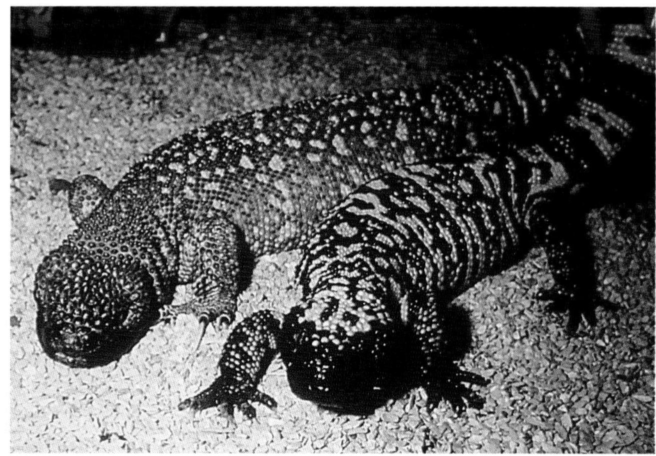

Plate 2 Two species of venomous lizards: left, Mexican beaded lizard (*Heloderma horridum*); right, Gila monster (*H. suspectum*). (By courtesy of the Zoological Society of London.)

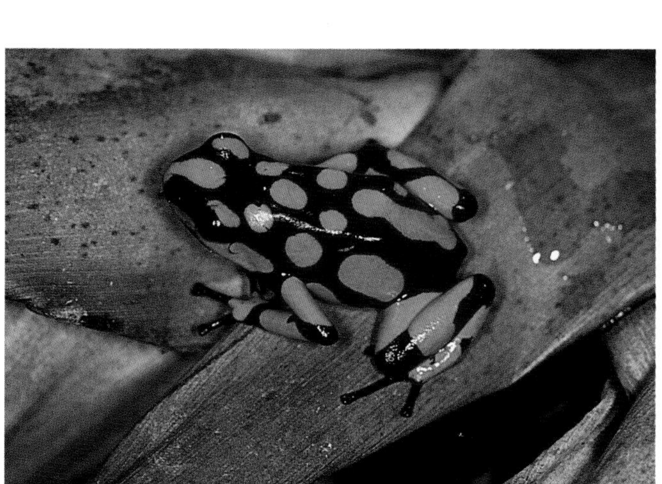

Plate 3 'Poison dart frog'—*Dendrobates histrionicus* family Dendrobatidae, from Bahia Solauo, Colombia. (Copyright D.A. Warrell.)

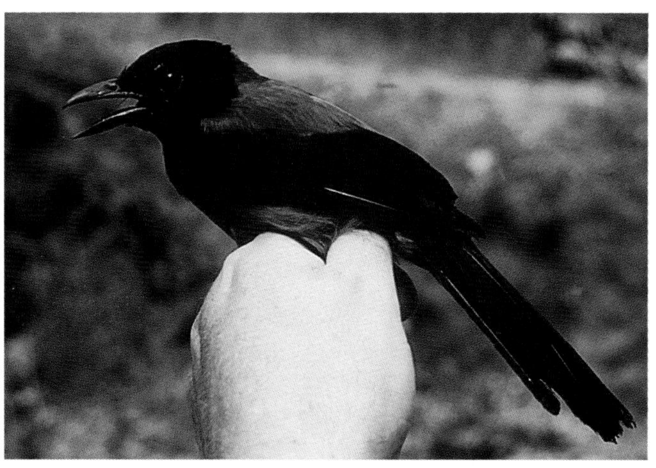

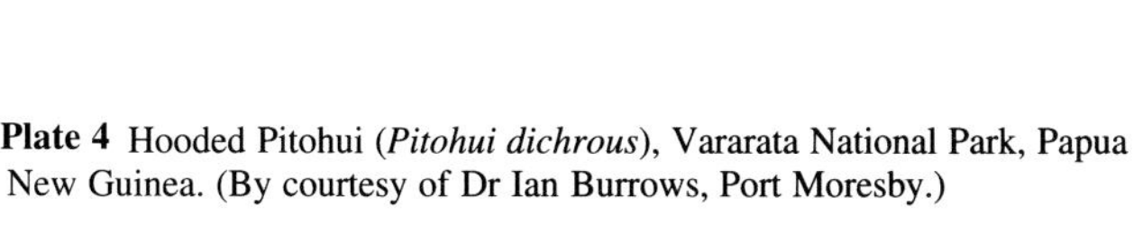

Plate 4 Hooded Pitohui (*Pitohui dichrous*), Vararata National Park, Papua New Guinea. (By courtesy of Dr Ian Burrows, Port Moresby.)

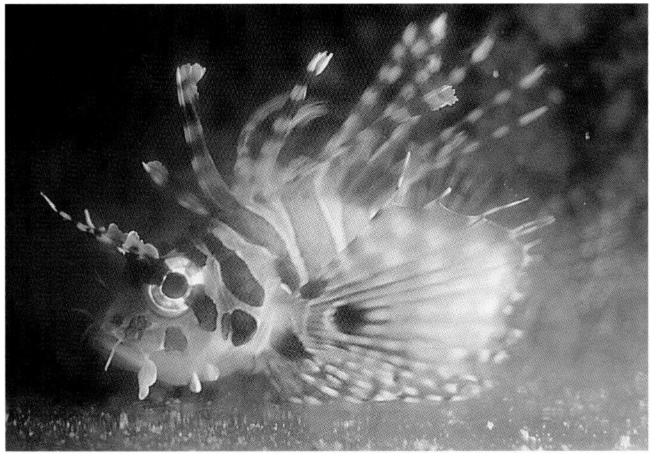

Plate 5 Venomous lion fish or butterfly cod (*Brachirus* or *Dendrochirus zebra*), from Madang, Papua New Guinea. (Copyright D.A. Warrell.)

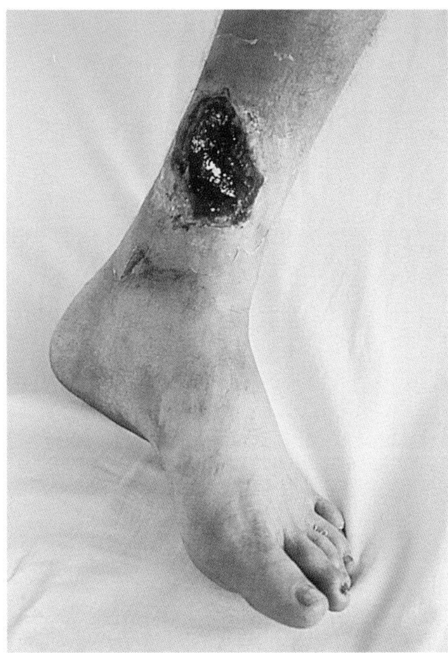

Plate 6 Necrotic and secondarily infected wound at the site of a sting by a freshwater ray (*Potamotrygon hystrix*) in a Brazilian patient. (By courtesy of Dr João Luiz Costa Cardoso, São Paulo, Brazil.)

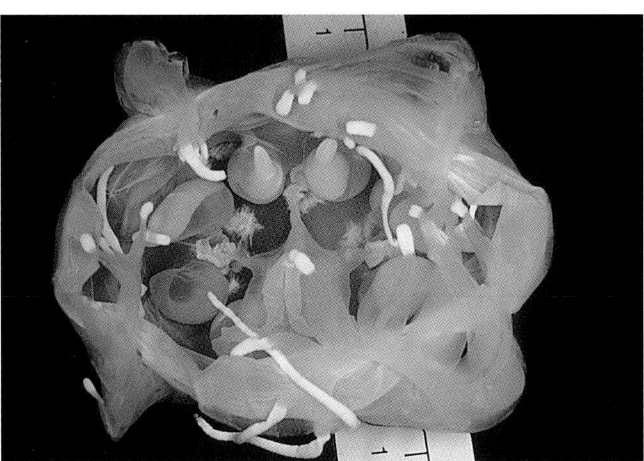

Plate 7 Under surface of chirodropid (box jellyfish) (*Chiropsalmus buitendijki*) collected from Dehiwala, Sri Lanka, by Dr Malik Fernando. (Copyright D.A. Warrell.)

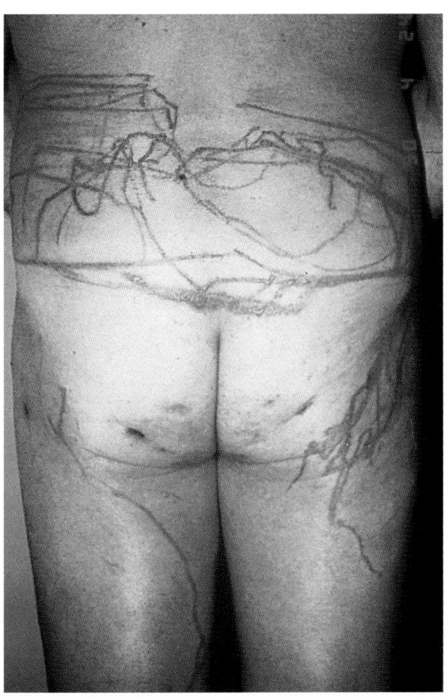

Plate 8 Extensive weals from contact with the stinging tentacles of the box jellyfish (*Chironex fleckeri*) in an Australian patient stung in Darwin. (By courtesy of Drs B. Currie and P. Nitschke, Darwin.)

(a)

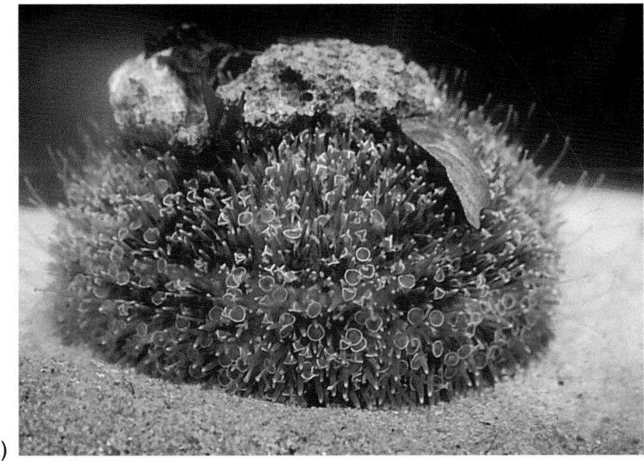

(b)

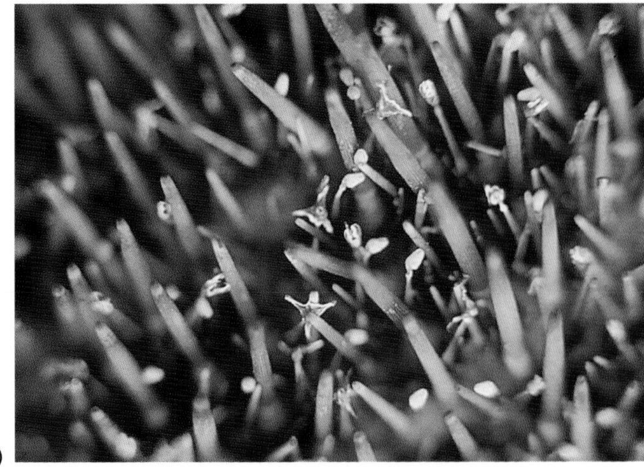

Plate 9 (a) Flower or felt cap sea urchin (*Toxopneustes pileolus*) from Unawatunne, Sri Lanka. (b) Stinging apparatus (pedicellariae) of *T. pileolus*. (By courtesy of Dr Malik Fernando, Colombo, Sri Lanka.)

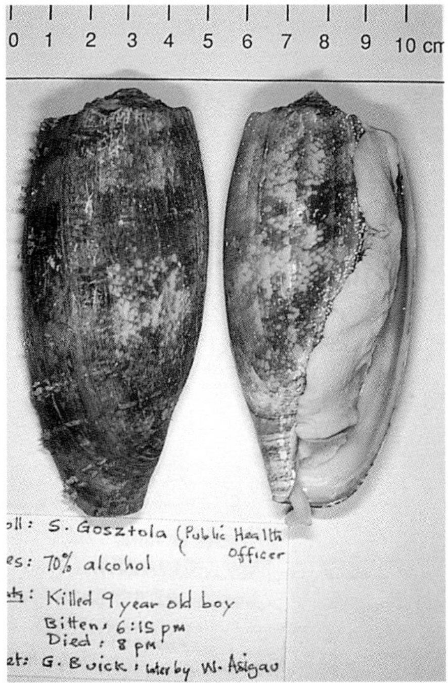

Plate 10 Geography cone shell (*Conus geographus*) 10 cm long, responsible for killing a 9-year-old boy at Samarai, Papua New Guinea. (Copyright D.A. Warrell.)

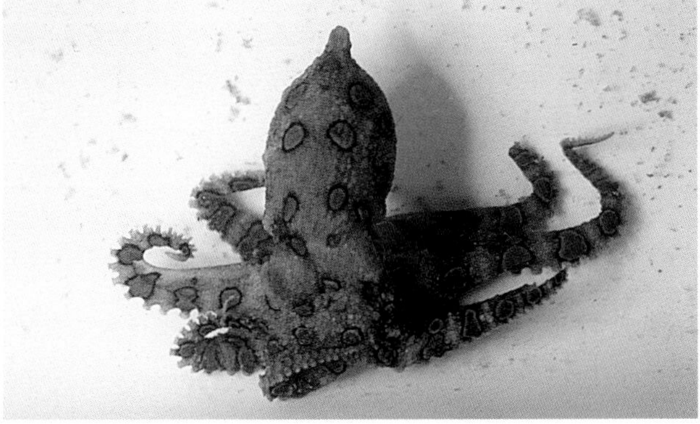

Plate 11 Spotted octopus (*Octopus lunulatus*) from Madang, Papua New Guinea. (Copyright D.A. Warrell.)

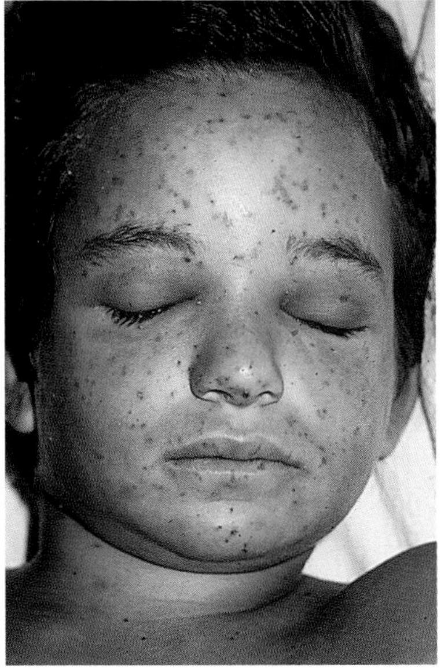

Plate 12 Fourteen-year-old Brazilian boy severely envenomed after more than 1000 stings by Africanized honey bees (*Apis mellifera scutellatus*).

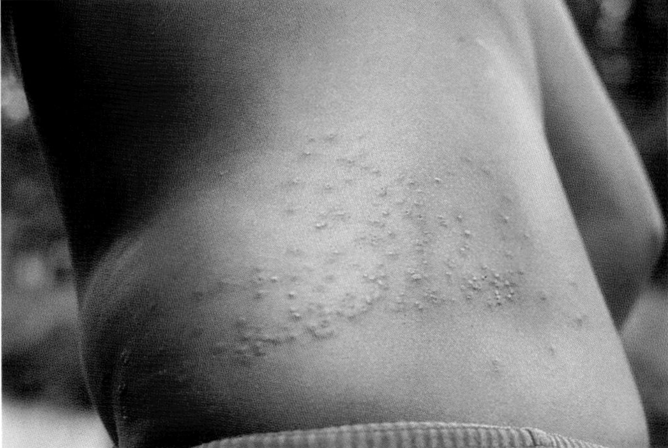

Plate 13 Multiple stings by fire ants (Solenopsis) in a Brazilian patient. (By courtesy of Dr João Luiz Costa Cardoso, São Paulo, Brazil.)

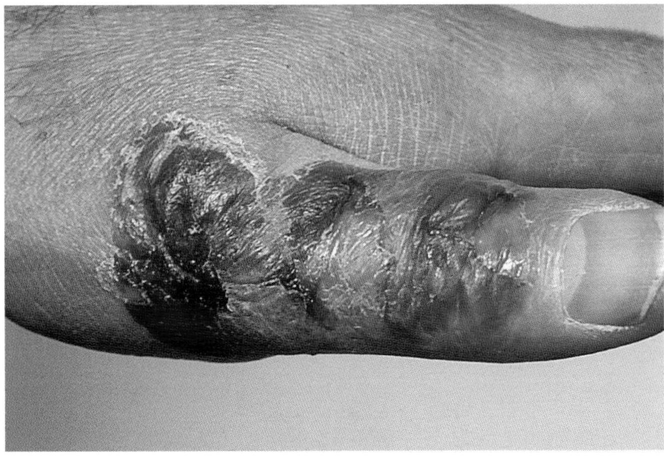

Plate 14 Secondarily infected wasp sting. Because they are carnivorous, wasps may contaminate their stings with bacteria acquired while feeding on rotting meat. (Copyright D.A. Warrell.)

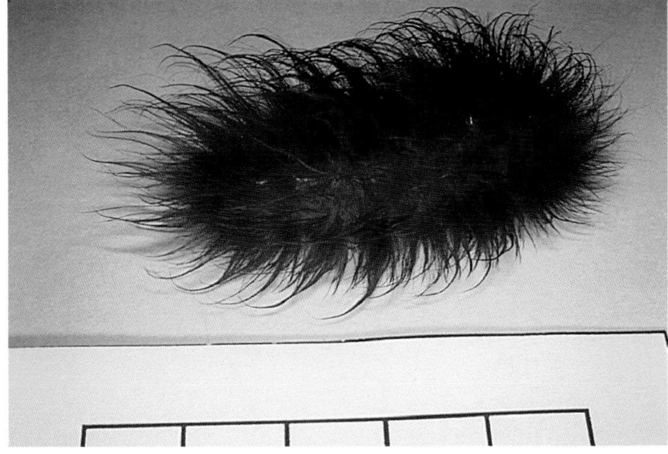

Plate 15 Caterpillar of South American 'pussmoth' (*Megalopyge lanata*). Its hairs can cause severe urticating lesions. (Copyright D.A. Warrell.)

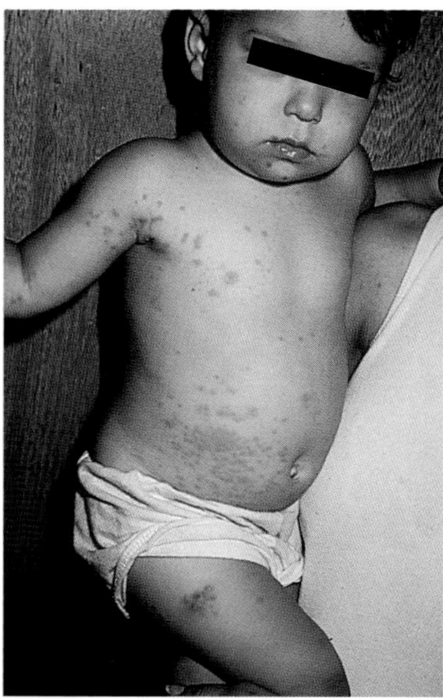

Plate 16 Lepidopterism. Child with lesions caused by urticating abdominal hairs of female moths (*Hylesia* sp.) during an epidemic on the coast near São Paulo. (Copyright D.A. Warrell.)

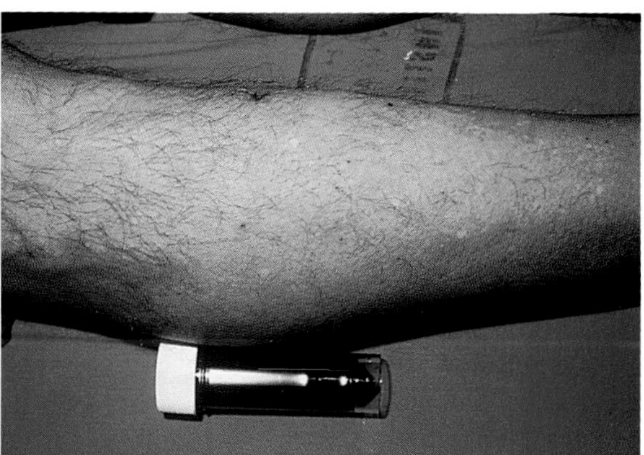

Plate 17 Erucism. Shin of Brazilian patient showing lesions made by caterpillars of Lonomia moths. He developed bleeding gums and haematuria (in the specimen tube). (Copyright D.A. Warrell.)

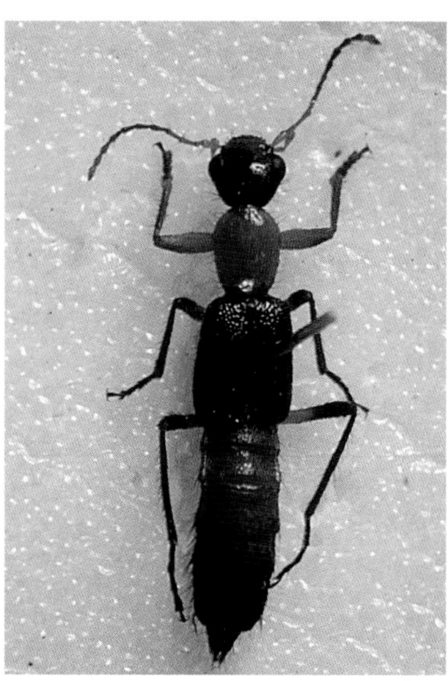

Plate 18 Beetle (Paederus, Staphylinidae) responsible for causing 'Nairobi eye'. (By courtesy of Dr John Paul, Oxford.)

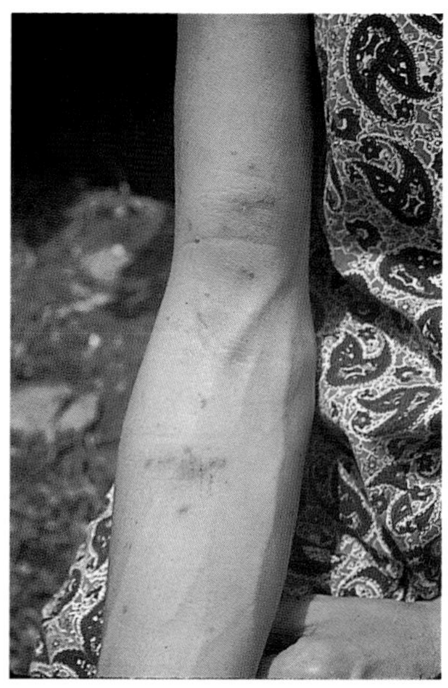

Plate 19 Dermatitis linearis caused by inadvertently trapping a blister beetle in the antecubital fossa in Nigeria. (Copyright D.A. Warrell.)

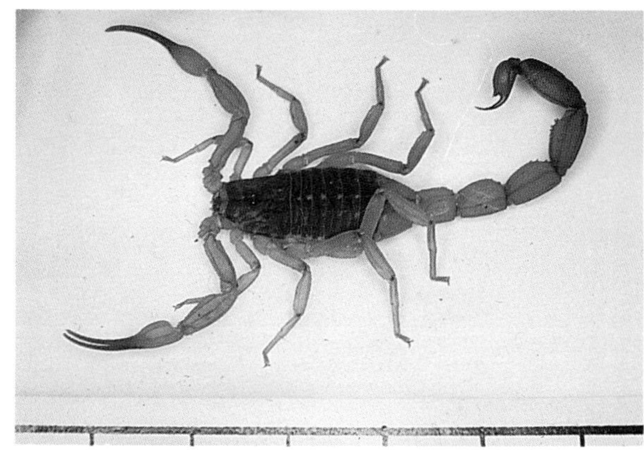

Plate 20 Scorpion (*Tityus serrulatus*) from Brazil. (Copyright D.A. Warrell.)

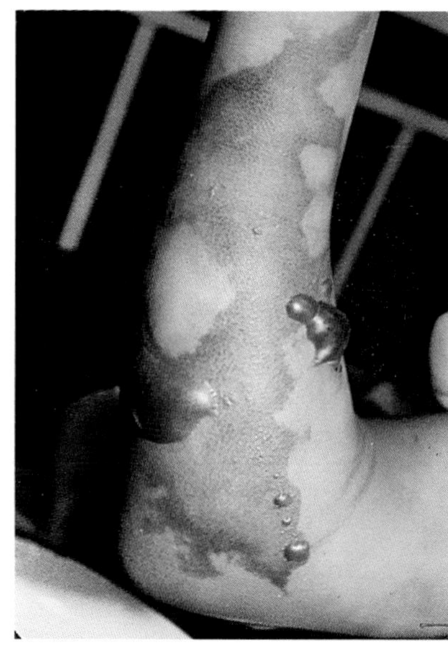

Plate 21 Local blistering and necrosis caused by the sting of the scorpion *Hemiscorpius lepturus* (Scorpionidae) found in Iran and Iraq. (By courtesy of Dr M. Radmanesh, Shiraz, Iran.)

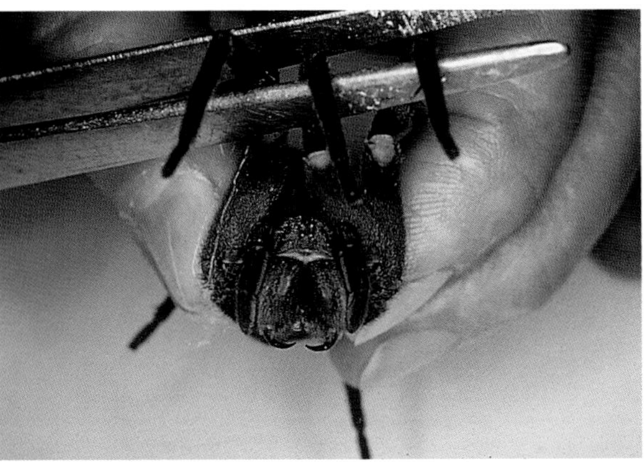

Plate 22 Banana spider (*Phoneutria nigriventer*) from Brazil showing fangs (chelicerae). (Copyright D.A. Warrell.)

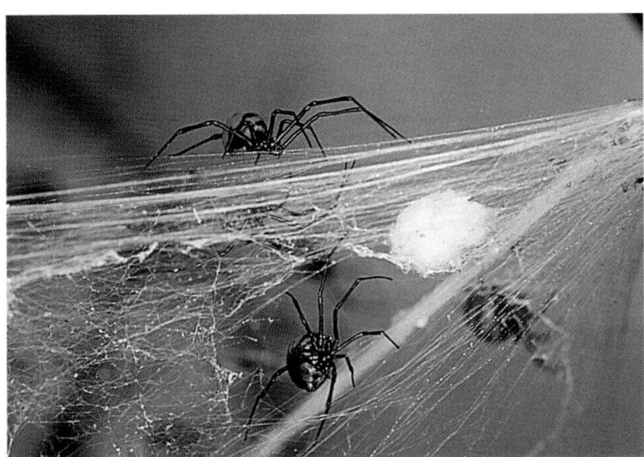

Plate 23 'Black widow' spider (*Latrodectus curacaviensis*) from Brazil. (Copyright D.A. Warrell.)

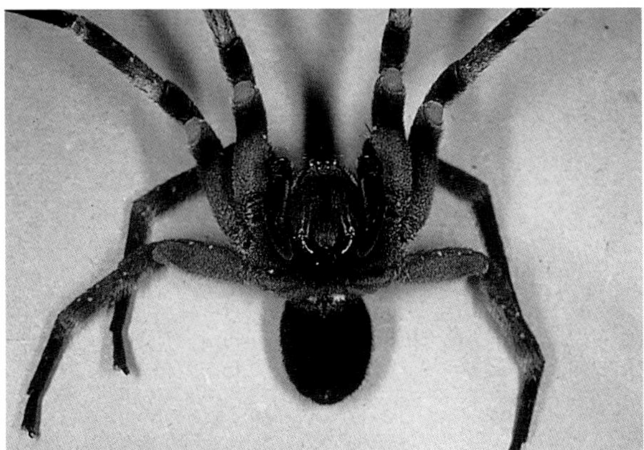

Plate 24 Threatening posture of a female Brazilian 'banana spider' (*Phoneutria nigriventer*). Note multiple eyes and large chelicerae. (Copyright D.A. Warrell.)

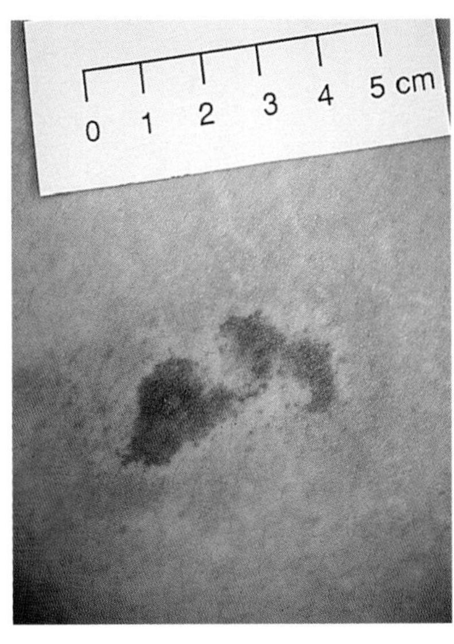

Plate 25 Necrotic araneism. Early ischaemic and prenecrotic lesion following a bite by *Loxosceles gaucho* in Brazil. (Copyright D.A. Warrell.)

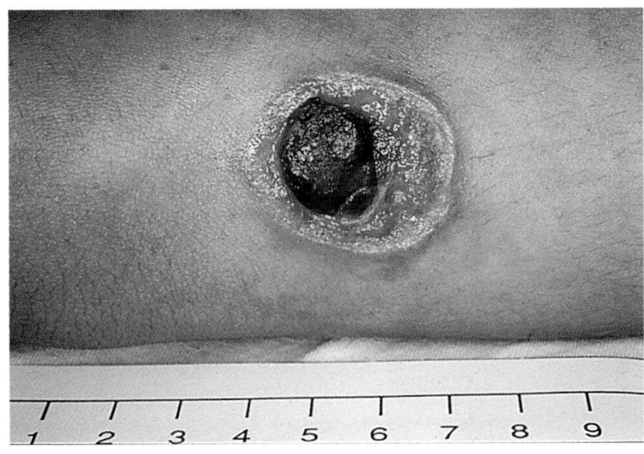

Plate 26 Necrotic slough 6 weeks after a bite by *Loxosceles gaucho* in Brazil. (Copyright D.A. Warrell.)

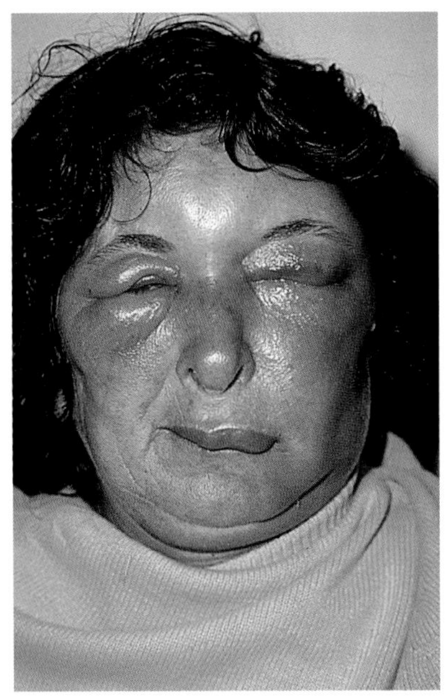

Plate 27 Extensive inflammation and oedema 24 h after a bite on the right upper eyelid by *Loxosceles gaucho* in Brazil. (Copyright D.A. Warrell.)

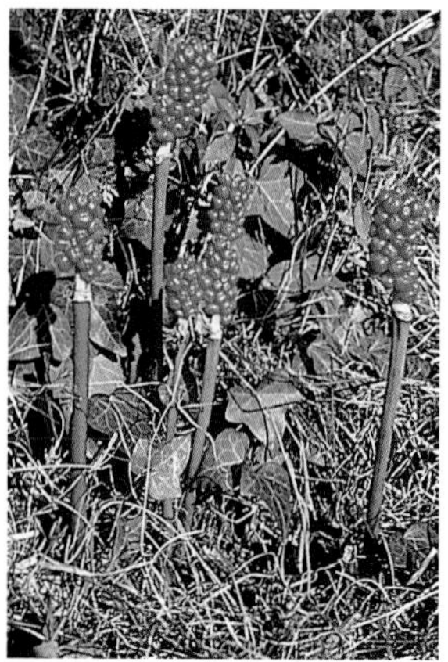

Plate 1 Wild arum, cuckoo pint, *Arum maculatum* (ARGM).

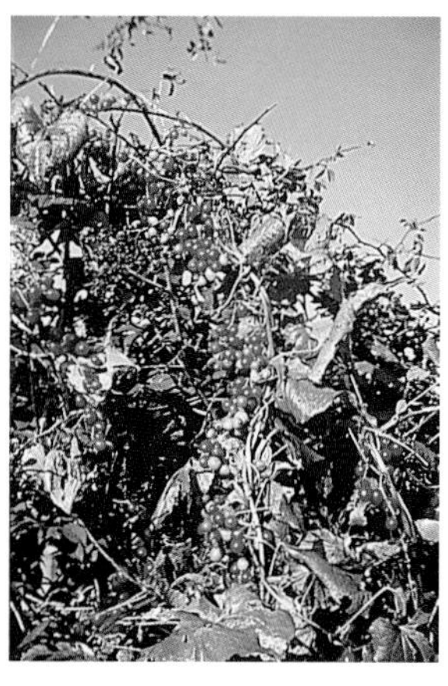

Plate 2 Black bryony, *Tamus communis* (ARGM).

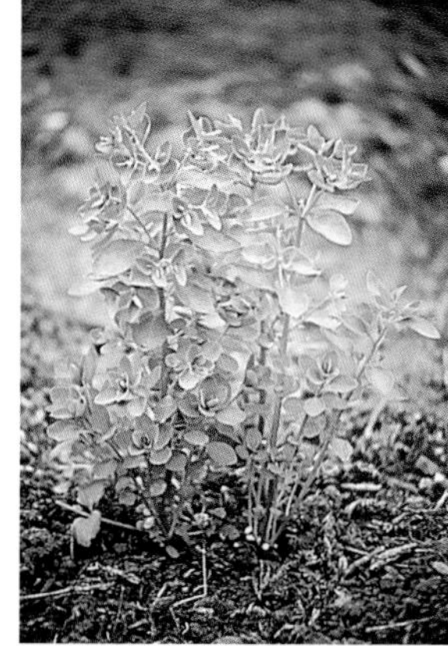

Plate 3 Petty spurge, *Euphorbia peplus* (GTC).

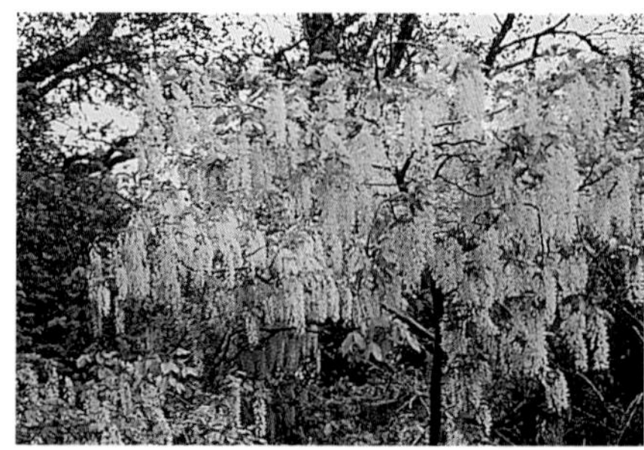

Plate 4 Laburnum, *Laburnum anagyroides* (GTC).

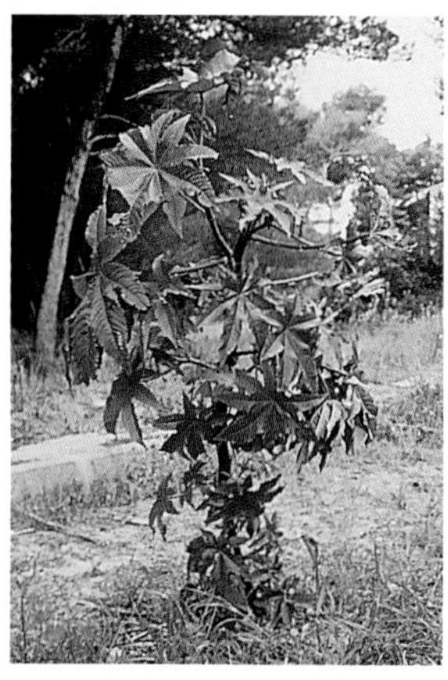

Plate 5 Castor oil plant, *Ricinus communis* (SB).

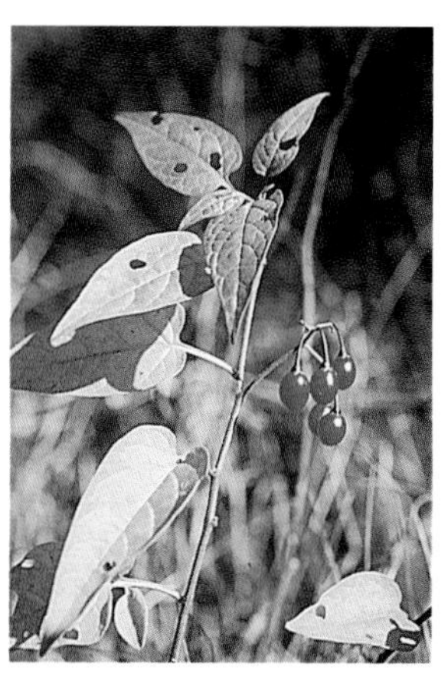

Plate 6 Woody nightshade, bittersweet, *Solanum dulcamara* (ARGM).

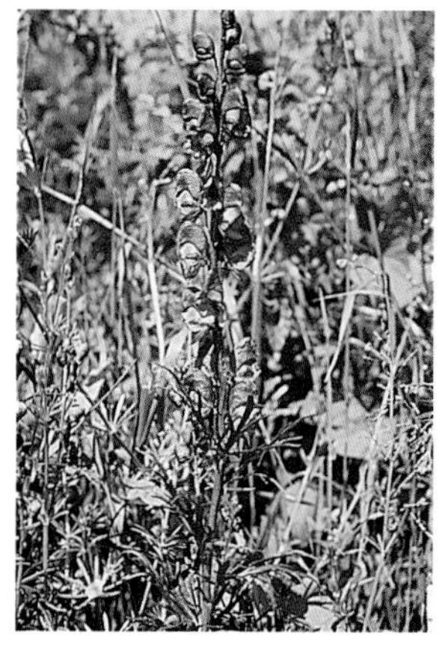

Plate 7 Monkshood, *Aconitum napellus* (ARGM).

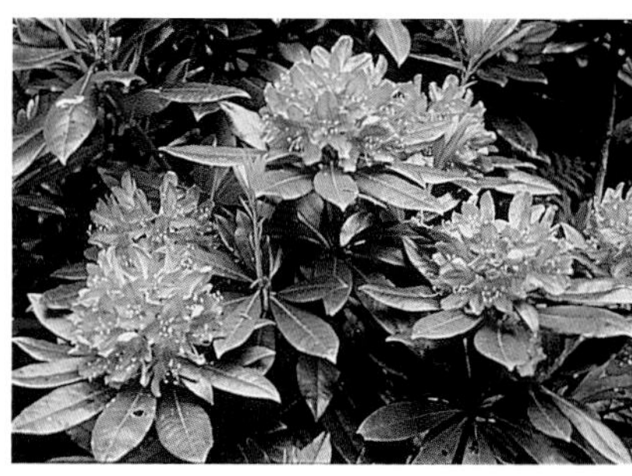

Plate 8 Rhododendron, *Rhododendron ponticum* (GTC).

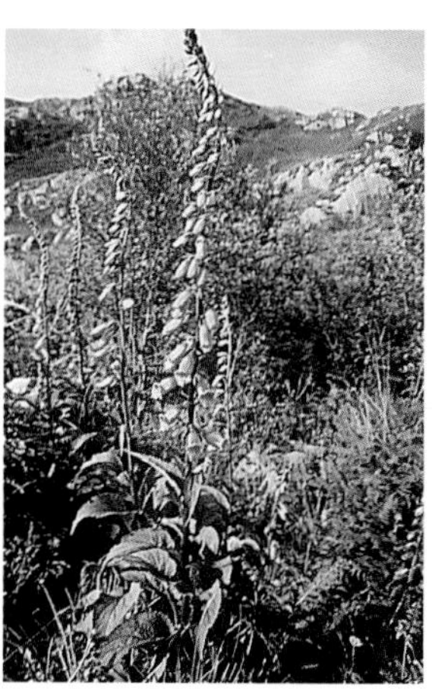

Plate 9 Foxglove, *Digitalis purpurea* (GTC).

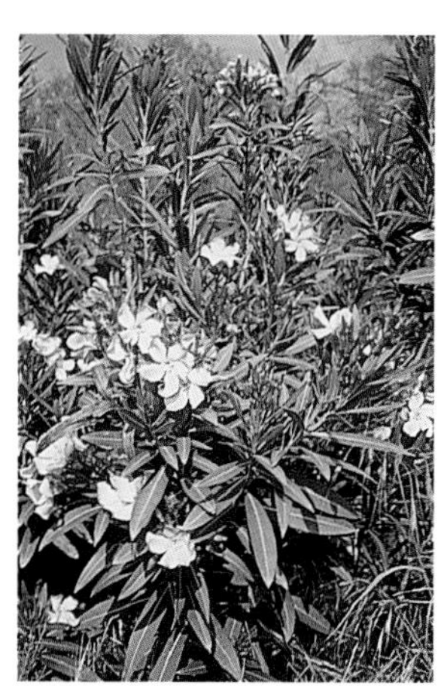

Plate 10 Oleander, *Nerium oleander* (ARGM).

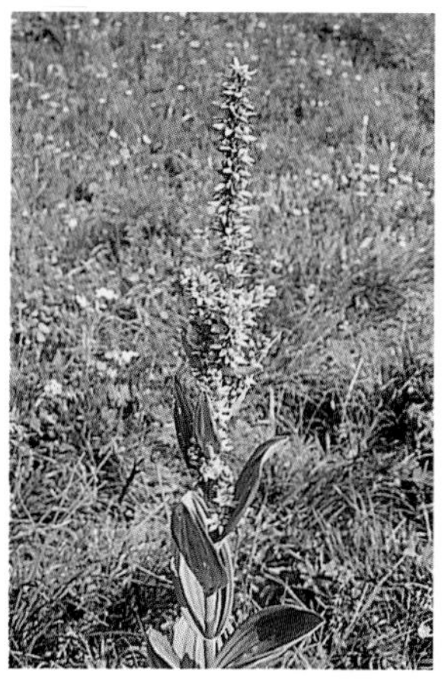

Plate 11 False hellebore, *Veratrum album* (ARGM).

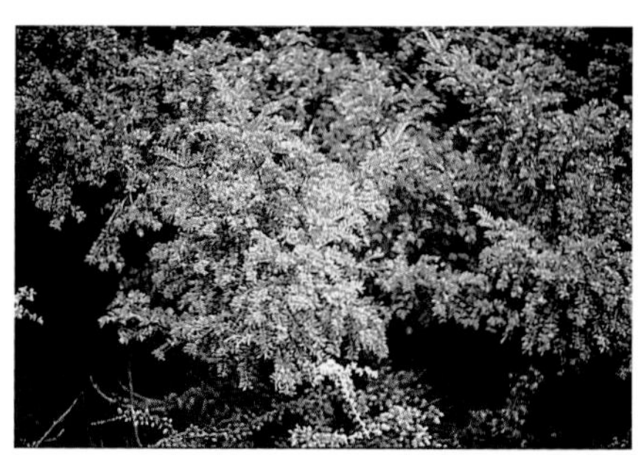

Plate 12 Yew, *Taxus baccata* (DPD).

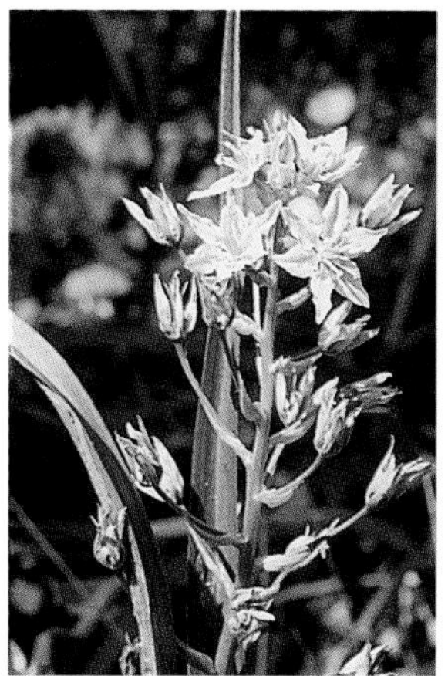

Plate 13 Death camas, *Zigadenus elegans* (ARGM).

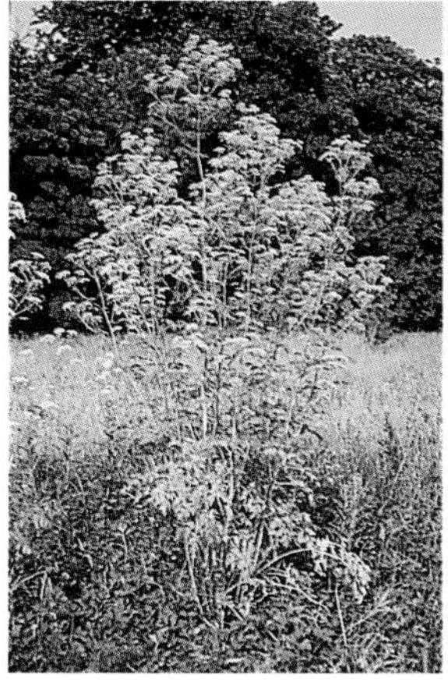

Plate 14 Hemlock, *Conium maculatum* (GTC).

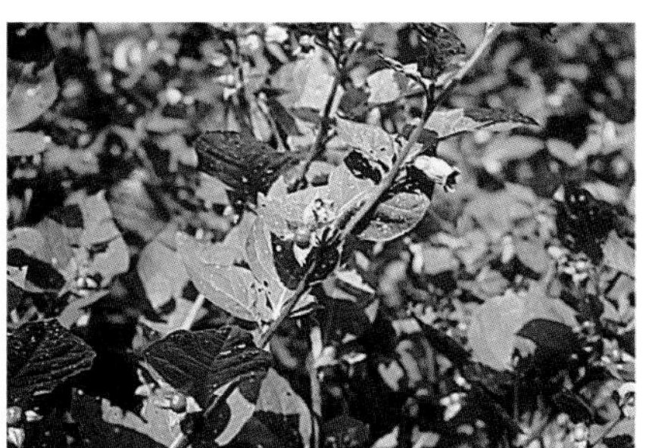

Plate 15 Deadly nightshade, *Atropa belladonna* (berries black when ripe) (GTC).

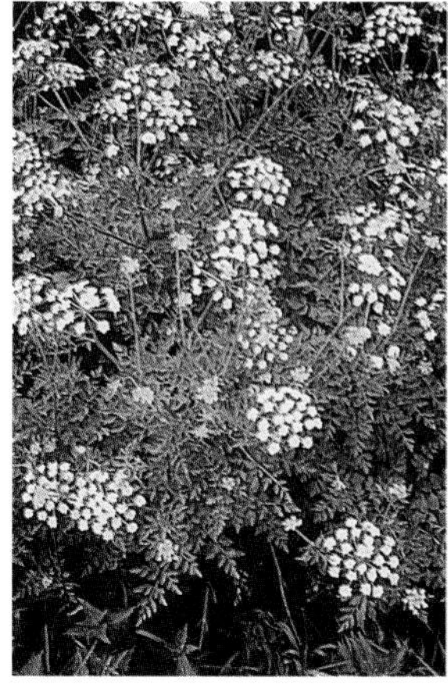

Plate 16 Hemlock water dropwort, *Oenanthe crocata* (SB).

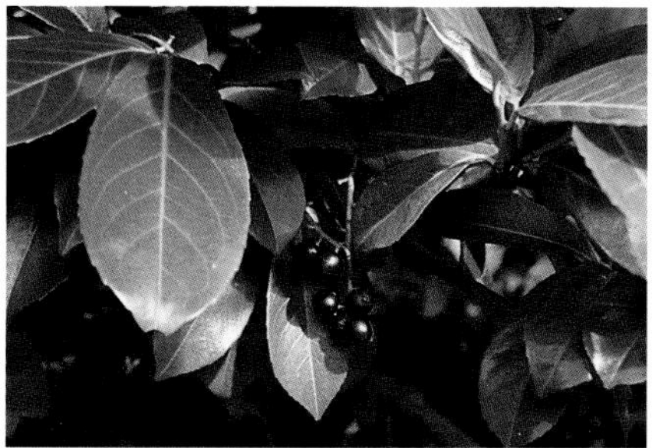

Plate 17 Cherry laurel, *Prunus laurocerasus* (GTC).

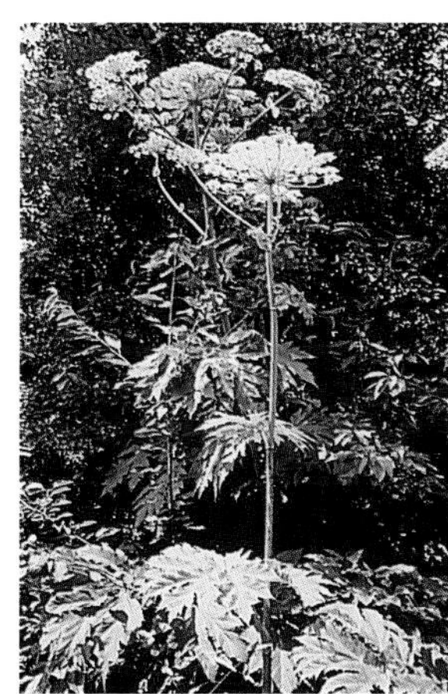

Plate 19 Giant hogweed, *Heracleum mantegazzianum* (Haslemere Educational Museum) (GTC).

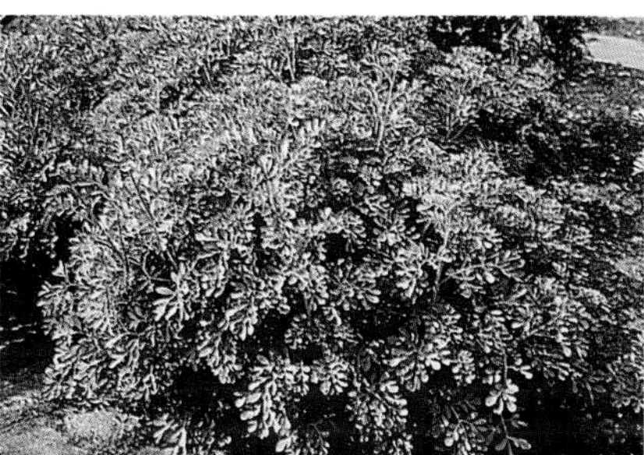

Plate 20 Rue, *Ruta graveolens* (SB).

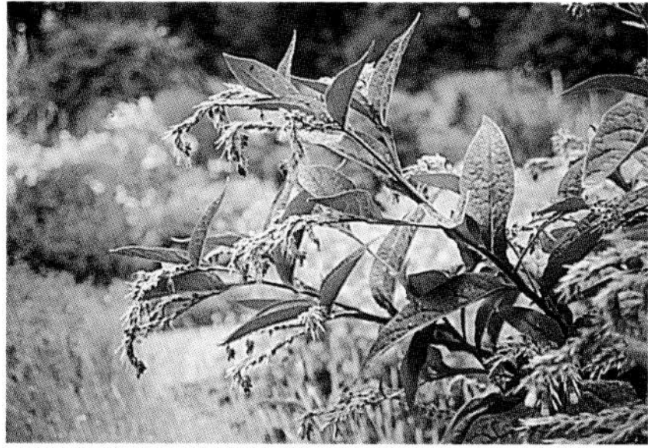

Plate 18 Comfrey, *Symphytum officinale* (GTC).

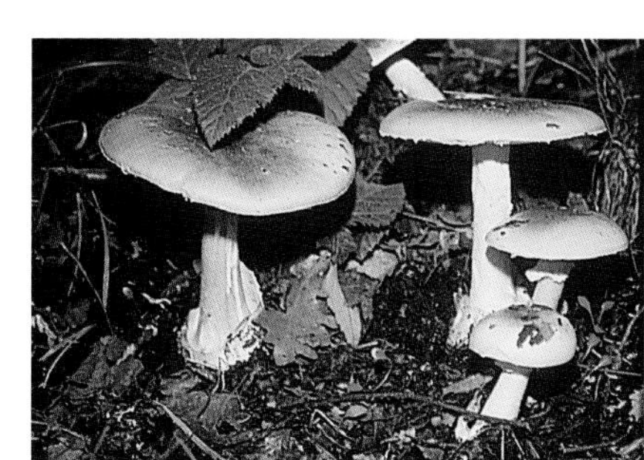

Plate 21 Deathcap, *Amanita phalloides* (ARGM).

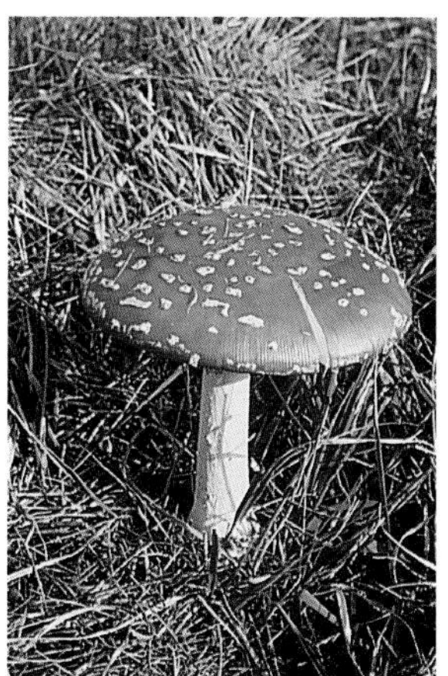

Plate 22 Fly agaric, *Amanita muscaria* (ARGM).

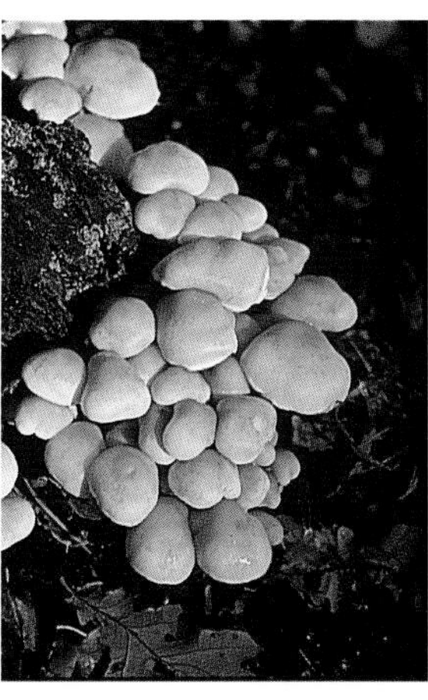

Plate 23 Sulphur tuft, *Hypholoma fasciculare* (ARGM).

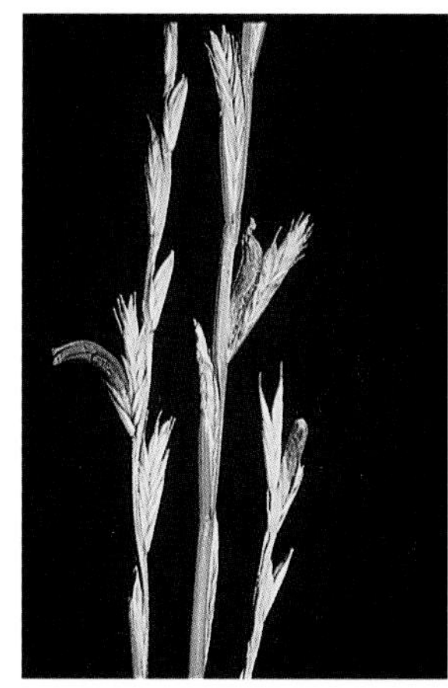

Plate 24 Ergot, *Claviceps purpurea* (on ryegrass) (ARGM).

Chapter 8.5.1

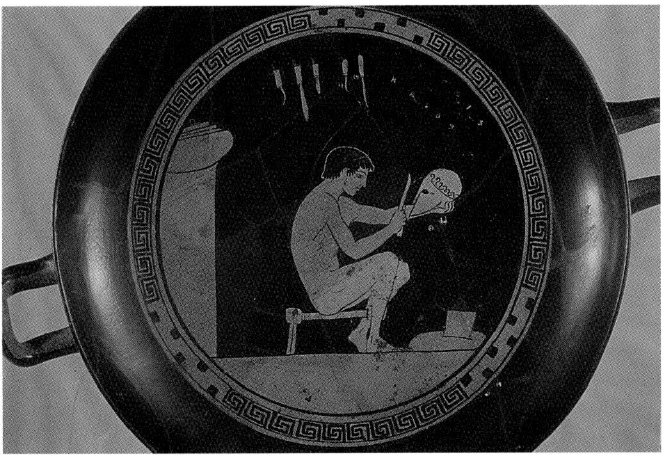

Plate 1 A 5th century BC Greek helmet maker finishing a bronze helmet. Lead exposure was likely from impurities in the silver used for decoration. (Reproduced with permission of the Ashmolean Museum, Oxford.)

Chapter 8.5.3(a)

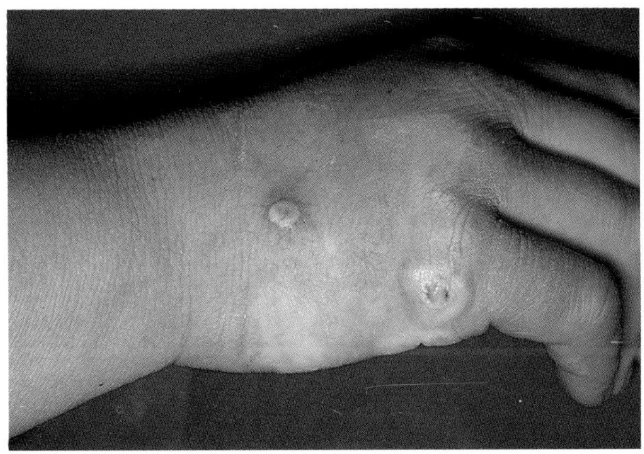

Plate 1 Orf, a sheep pox virus, is a common zoonosis in agriculture.

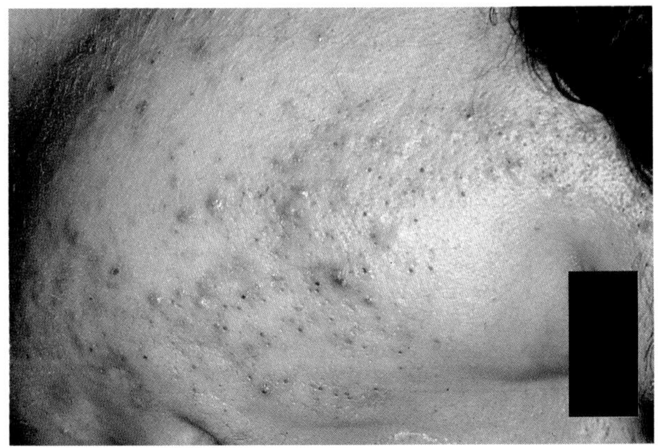

Plate 2 Chloracne may occur with prolonged exposure to halogenated aromatics.

Chapter 8.5.5(l)

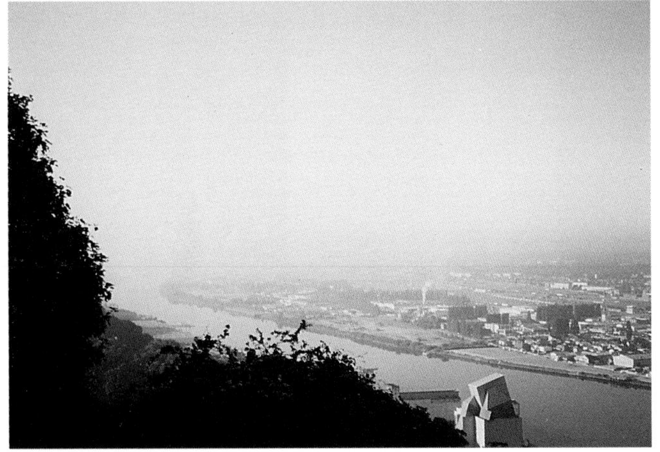

Plate 1 Photochemical pollution in Rouen, France, 1992.

Chapter 8.5.5(m)

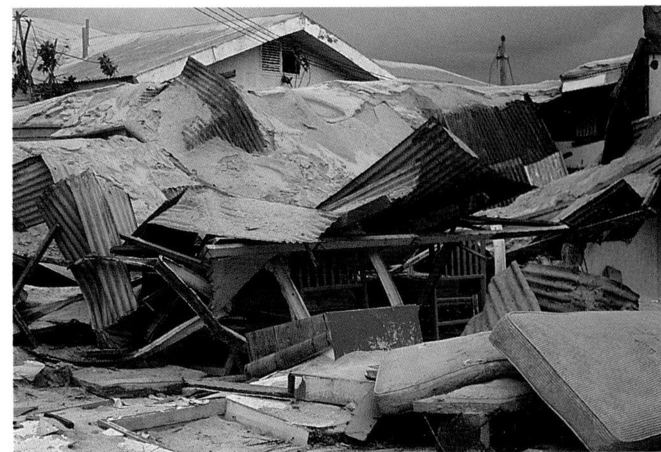

Plate 1 Mount Pinatubo eruption, Philippines 1991. Hospital roof collapsed under the weight of ash and eight people were killed.

Section 1 *On being a patient*

1 On being a patient

C. Clothier

'Patior' – 'I am suffering' – one recalls being taught at school. Every student knows that a patient is generally, but not always, one who is suffering, and perhaps not very patiently. Only by derivation has the word become associated with the bearing of pain or sorrow without complaint. Yet this secondary meaning is important in medicine because it reminds us that the great majority of patients do in fact suffer their illnesses with remarkable fortitude and endurance. Might this be another facet of the urge to survive and to minimize disability in the essentially competitive struggle of life? Is it this instinct, perhaps, which leads the average healthy person who stumbles and falls in the street to declare: 'It's nothing really' or 'I'll be all right in a minute', as they try to rise quickly from the fallen position of the vanquished? For falling to the ground in combat is usually fatal, and voluntary prostration of the body usually signifies submission and defeat.

So when otherwise healthy persons seek help from a doctor, or are admitted to hospital, it may be assumed that they are in some perturbation of mind as well as of body. It is this suffering in the mind that makes every patient different, even when their condition is familiar and well recognized, because the mental element in any illness varies enormously with circumstance and temperament.

Visiting the family doctor is usually less of an ordeal for the patient than admission to hospital. The patient often retains the dignity of an upright position *vis-à-vis* the doctor. But the element of personal distress may still be there and may mask or distort the objective signs and symptoms for which the doctor is trained to look. The 'dependent well' may only be seeking a listening post for the torments of family dissension, personal tragedy, or just old age. Other patients enjoy being examined, manipulated, or injected because of the personal contact and attention involved, which they otherwise lack. How much time to give to each of the greatly diverse patients of a practice or a hospital is a matter of delicate judgement: most will deserve a sympathetic response but some will seem to merit a rather positive rejection. And yet one must be careful; for there have been recorded instances of patients who complained of bizarre symptoms, signifying no identifiable illness, who were rejected as malingerers but subsequently were shown to have suffered greatly from insidious disease or poison. Those who are truly ill may be brave, or craven, or something in between, depending upon age, circumstance, or personal quality. But one thing is certain, each patient will think himself or herself to be reacting normally to the predicament of illness, real or imaginary, and will be expecting the same degree of medical attention. If they do not get it they will be offended and angry: whether that reaction should provoke sympathy or dismissal from the doctor may be as crucial a judgement as writing a prescription.

On the other hand, admission to hospital is a fundamentally different experience both for patients and those caring for them. Here the dominant factor is the concession of defeat and the abandonment of the safe haven of home. To lie down in the presence of others in a strange place, to get undressed in the middle of the day, to give specimens of urine or blood, all on the orders of those who remain upright, are acts of submission. The arrival in hospital is accompanied by feelings of anxious apprehension, fear, isolation, and general mental turmoil which caused Osbert Sitwell to speak of 'First depressions on arrival'. Mingled with these feelings may also be some sense of relief in having finally admitted defeat and agreed to surrender one's body into other hands. When one adds to these varied emotions anxiety about work, about the home, or about the patient's spouse or children, it is a wonder that the admitting doctor gets any sensible or accurate answer out of a patient for the first 24 hours after admission. When histories are taken, these widely variable responses to stress, for the most part concealed, should be in the doctor's mind. Even the lay patient is likely to be aware that blood pressure and heart rate are raised when first they are measured in hospital. Symptoms may be minimized, exaggerated consciously or unconsciously, invented, or simply forgotten. Dates and times of episodes or onsets may be so wide of the mark as to be of little use in diagnosis, if not positively dangerous.

The risk, then, is that the hospital patient becomes merely an interesting focus of medical attention rather than a person with all those confusions of mind that make him or her an individual. This is a very real danger in modern hospital practice, the more so as we are now equipped with the most sophisticated apparatus for diagnosis, facilities that may be seen by some as reducing the need for any contribution from the patient. The feeling of personal unimportance is a marked cause of unhappiness among hospital patients and a frequent source of complaint against doctors and nurses. Doctors can and sometimes do speak and look as if the patient was no more than an interesting clinical object and nurses can exacerbate the grievance by discussing their private affairs across the bed of the patient to whom they are attending.

In teaching hospitals, the patient's sense of worthlessness may be greatly increased by the ordeal of the professional ward round. It has to be stated that even now, close to the start of the twenty-first century, there are consultants who persistently treat patients as the fortunate recipients of their attentions, whose views and feelings are of little relevance in the pursuit of a learned profession. Besides being a technical breach of obligation under the terms of a consultant's National Health Service contract, such conduct is rude. A good doctor, who engages the patient's attention and participation in a discussion of their case, may learn a great deal, besides giving the patient immense satisfaction and inspiring confidence. 'Encourage the patient to talk', said a wise old practitioner, 'and he will eventually tell you what is the matter with him'. It is regrettable that those who practise an excessive clinical detachment are not only the old and authoritarian, but include those who have grown up in a world where medical omniscience is no longer taken for granted. Doctors who cannot naturally feel a surge of sympathy for the body prostrated before them should perhaps consider a career in research.

The patients of today are very different from those of half a century ago. Until the advent of the mass media, the relationship between patient and doctors resembled that between parishioner and pastor, schoolmaster and pupil, or lawyer and client. It was impious to question the wisdom or judgement of the learned professional adviser. The remarkable expression 'sapiential authority' sought to encapsulate this ascendancy of doctor over patient. Such a relationship was often quite a happy one for both parties, and perhaps more conducive to treatment and cure than a less trusting one. But the mass media, and supremely, television, have changed all that. Behind the camera we have all penetrated into the operating theatre and other private places and there seen what doctors and their assistants actually do in the attempt to cure illness or repair damage. And, however skilful and ingenious, it is obviously not miraculous, and some of it is rather pedestrian. The curtains have been parted and the magic revealed. The magicians themselves have often admitted their humanity and confessed to their failures. When mystery is dispersed, the questions come thick and fast.

It is of no use to resist the tide of doubt and curiosity that now threatens to overwhelm not just medicine but all the learned professions. Family doctors must now expect patients to ask quite penetrating questions about the treatment proposed for them and the drugs it is intended to use. These questions must be answered with some candour if mutual trust is to be maintained. Nothing more disturbs a patient, who may be very intelligent even though not learned in medicine, than hearing their doctor seeking to disguise his own ignorance or doubt by prevarication or deviousness, often easily detected. Besides all of which, it sometimes does professionals in any discipline a great deal of good to be closely questioned about beliefs and practices that they have long held to be unassailably correct; and they should listen to their own explanations and audit them for intelligibility and rationality.

For almost every patient, the general anaesthetic and surgical operation engender particular anxieties which must be recognized and accommodated. It is no small thing to surrender one's consciousness into the hands of others, with all the vulnerability which unconsciousness brings. The intrusion of hands and instruments into the previously intact body equally induces dark fears in many minds. Doctors may not fully appreciate these anxieties, familiar as they are with the procedures used and their general safety and success. Most patients of reasonably resolute temperament face up to these prospects with good enough courage: but having done so, find a postponement of the day especially demoralizing. It is important that surgeons try to arrange lists so that patients do not wait many hours in a state of some tension, only to be told that they must face it all again on another day.

Modern practice and health economics combine nowadays to reduce the patient's stay in hospital to a minimum. Perhaps doctors do not sufficiently realize how much dependence may develop between patients who have been really ill and those who have rescued them from suffering, or even from death, and subsequently cared for them. The cheerful words 'Well, you can go home tomorrow' are not invariably greeted with joy. It is not merely that for some, the attention they receive in hospital, is better than anything they get elsewhere: those who have been really ill are often haunted by the prospect of relapse or recurrence and feel a security in hospital, amplified by care and kindness, which they cannot feel at home. Some introductory words of sympathy for the patient's anxiety and reassurance for their ability to survive outside the hospital are often necessary.

An essay entitled 'On being a patient' ought to contain not merely adjurations for doctors but at least some directions for patients. And the foremost of these could be to remember the meaning of the newly acquired status and title. Many patients are irritable and demanding, even when those attributes are not produced or justified by some disease process. They are very unattractive qualities in those who have, after all, been obliged to submit themselves to the care and skill of their fellow beings, sometimes through their own fault or neglect. A little humility and gratitude seem called for and no less because the patient is paying for some part of the services rendered, or believes that he has already done so. It is perhaps one of the least likeable of human attitudes to believe that money buys everything and that plenty of it entitles one to special care and attention. Doctors and nurses do not for the most part do what they do in the expectation of great worldly reward. Patients likewise should recognize and appreciate human kindness when they see it and be grateful for it whether or not they are paying for their treatment.

Finally it is necessary to reflect that, as man is a social animal, the illness of any member of a family affects most of the others. Obviously enough, the spouse of a sick person is liable to be deeply affected by sorrow and by anxiety about the future. Such feelings spring not merely from love and affection but from fear of a future either robbed of economic support or burdened by care for an invalid or disabled person. So a good doctor has more than just the patient to consider and should try to speak to the relatives and to offer them proper and helpful explanations of present treatment and future prospects. It may seem unreasonable to suggest that the doctor should treat the relatives of their patients as well as the patients themselves, but human beings are highly interactive and the sick person is sensitive to the sorrows and anxieties of his or her family. If a patient's relatives are much cast down and obviously anxious, this is perceived by the patient and greatly affects morale and the peace of mind that is conducive to recovery.

It is only too easy to avoid the patient's relatives. Besides being upright and healthy, in contradistinction to the patient, their sorrows and anxieties may make them noisy and demanding. They are apt to ask questions which seem absurd to the doctor and impossible to answer in simple lay terms. But the effort must be made, not only for humanitarian reasons but because it may rightly be regarded as part of the treatment.

In sum, the patient views those who care for him or her as being in a relationship every bit as confidential and trusting as that which exists within the patient's family, probably more so. And the patient has no hesitation in imposing this burdensome connection on one who has hitherto been a total stranger. That is the enormous measure of a doctor's voluntarily assumed responsibilities to the human race.

Section 2 *On modern scientific medicine*

2.1 Scientific method and the art of healing

D. J. Weatherall

When Henry Dale, the distinguished British physiologist and pharmacologist, arrived at St Bartholomew's Hospital as a medical student in 1900 he was told by his first clinical teacher, Samuel Gee, that, as medicine was not a science but merely an empirical art, he must forget all the physiology that he had learnt at Cambridge. This advice reflects a deep-rooted tension between the art and science of clinical practice, which still permeates the medical profession.

Patient care, from its earliest beginnings to the present day, has always been a mixture of sympathy and kindness backed up with a well-meaning but often empirical effort to alter the natural course of events. In this sense it has been, and still is, an art, practiced against a background of incomplete scientific knowledge about the nature of disease processes. Human beings, like all living things, are immensely complex biological systems. Even today, with all our knowledge of their chemistry and physiology, we have a very limited understanding of the mechanisms that underlie most of the diseases that we encounter in day-to-day practice. Caring for sick people involves making considered judgements based on limited evidence and information. At best, we are slowly reaching the stage at which we are aware of how little we know.

In view of the remarkable progress in the biological sciences over the last few hundred years, today's doctors must try to establish the extent to which the balance of medical practice has shifted from 'craft' to 'science'. How far do the contents of a modern textbook of medicine reflect genuine scientific knowledge as compared with received wisdom and experience? And, of particular relevance to current medical practice and its future development, to what extent have advances in patient care in the twentieth century depended on progress in the basic sciences rather than improvements in our environment and lifestyles? In short, how much of our day-to-day clinical practice depends on a scientifically-based understanding of the diseases that we encounter? It is important that we address these questions at a time when there is growing public and governmental disillusion with high technology scientific medicine, and when many believe that the medical profession has lost its way and become more interested in diseases than in those who suffer from them. Before we tackle these difficult questions it may be helpful to define what we mean by 'scientific medicine' and to outline the way in which it has developed over the years.

Philosophers and historians of science and medicine always seem unhappy when it comes to deciding what is meant by 'scientific medicine'; this is dangerous country for the unwary! Here we shall take a pragmatic (if circular) approach, and use the term simply to describe the prevention and management of illness using methods that have been subjected to the same kinds of rigorous experimental, statistical and observational scrutiny that are applied in other branches of science.

The earliest documentary evidence to survive from the ancient civilizations of Babylonia, Egypt, China, and India, suggests, not surprisingly, that longevity, disease, and death are among our oldest preoccupations. From ancient times to the Renaissance, knowledge of the living world changed very little and the distinction between animate and inanimate objects was blurred. The Babylonians and Egyptions believed that water, air, and earth were the primary constituents of the world; a fourth, fire, was added later. This notion of the all-pervading influence of the four elements was extended to form a theory about how the human body is constituted. In short, it was thought to consist of four humours, blood, phlegm, yellow bile, and black bile. The notion that disease results from an imbalance of the humours permeated Graeco-Roman medicine and persisted until the seventeenth century. Health was viewed as a harmonious balance of the humours, while disease was thought to reflect an imbalance, or dyscrasia, leading to an abnormal mixture of the humours. This view of pathology, which provided an explanation for both mental and physical illness, formed the basis for what, at the time was a rational approach to treatment by bleeding, purging, and dietary modification.

The extraordinary developments in natural philosophy in the seventeenth century created an environment that led to the birth of scientific medicine as we now understand it. Modern physics was founded by Isaac Newton, and the work of Boyle and Hooke finally disposed of the Aristotlean elements of earth, fire, and water. The shape of medical and biological thinking was moulded by the French mathematician, philosopher, and biologist René Descartes, who held that material things, whether animals, plants, or inorganic objects, are ruled by the same mechanical laws. All living things, he held, can be looked on as machines. A sick man is like an ill-made clock; a healthy man a well-made clock. And it was during this time that William Harvey published an almost complete description of the circulation of the blood, work that involved many years of animal experimentation and the application of simple statistical methods to determine the output of blood from the heart, and which, in effect, formed the foundation for modern investigative physiology and, later, medicine.

During the eighteenth and nineteenth centuries, the sciences that underpin medicine were further developed. In particular, the concept of the cell became the centrepiece of biology. As perceived by the French Nobel laureate, Francois Jacob, 'with the cell biology discovered its atom'. In 1858 Rudolph Virchow published his celebrated *Di Cellular Pathologie*, in which cell theory was applied to the study of pathology. All diseases, he held, are diseases of cells. This was the dawning of modern cellular pathology and the study of disease at the microscopic, and later submicroscopic levels. The nineteenth century also saw the gradual decline of vague theories about life forces and a growing belief, helped by the emergence of organic chemistry, that living processes can be understood in terms of chemistry and physics working through complex interactions between the many different types of cells that constitute all living things, a movement that was to culminate in the extraordinary achievements in biochemistry and molecular biology in the twentieth century.

This was also the time when a start was made at assessing the value of therapeutic practices that had gone on largely unchanged for centuries. For despite these rapid advances in the biological sciences, very little could be done for the majority of the disorders that doctors faced in every day practice. Blood-letting and the administration of a variety of useless and potentially harmful treatments were still rife, and although a few drugs of genuine value had been found, foxglove extract and quinine for example, much of the doctors' armamentarium was of unproven value. In the mid-nineteenth century a French clinician, Pierre Charles Alexandre Louis, pioneered the application of statistical analysis to medical practice. One of his earliest ventures was to compile sufficient data to prove that blood-letting, which had been practised for centuries, was not only useless but positively harmful in the management of many diseases. During the latter half of the nineteenth century the focus of medical science moved from France to Germany. It was here that, during the late nineteenth and early twentieth centuries, laboratories were set up where men and women could devote their time to research in the blossoming basic sciences, anatomy, physiology, and, later, biochemistry. In this atmosphere a new generation of clinical scientists evolved who became interested in physiological medicine, that is in understanding the fundamental mechanisms of disease.

These developments led to the establishment of university medical schools in the United States and other parts of Europe, based on the German tradition. In 1910 the American educationalist Abraham Flexner, after visiting several German medical schools, wrote a withering critique of medical education and science in North America. This attack stimulated the development of specialist clinical departments in many American and European medical schools. Flexner's revolutionary study advocated that medical education should begin with a strong foundation in the basic sciences followed by the study of clinical medicine in an atmosphere of critical thinking and with adequate time and facilities for research. His philosophy was widely accepted, not only in North America but in many European medical schools.

The development of university clinical academic departments in the period between the two world wars, and particularly after the second, led to the emergence of 'clinical science', experimentation on patients or laboratory animals on problems that stemmed directly from observations made at the bedside. Ultimately, this led to a remarkable improvement in our understanding of disease mechanisms. Together with the expanding pharmaceutical industry, it set the scene for the development of modern, high technology medical practice. Not surprisingly, it also had a profound effect on medical education. Indeed, those who criticize modern methods of teaching doctors, in particular its Cartesian approach to the study of human biology and disease, believe that the organization of university clinical academic departments along Flexner's lines may have done much to concentrate the minds of doctors on diseases rather than those who suffer from them.

The twentieth century has seen a revolution in the basic sciences, which started in physics, spread to chemistry, and, ultimately, completely changed the face of biology. Remarkable developments in physics at the end of the nineteenth century paved the way to an understanding of the way in which atoms are joined together to form molecules and for the development of a new kind of chemistry, which would start to explain the structure of the molecules that make up living things. The amalgamation of physics and chemistry spawned a new discipline, molecular biology, which was to unravel the way in which genetic information is passed from generation to generation and how individual cells function, both as self-contained units and as part of the complex communication network which is the basis of life itself. In the last 20 years there has been a slow shift of emphasis in medical research from the study of disease at the level of patients or their diseased organs to their cells and molecules. Although major scientific achievements do not always have practical benefits for many years, it is already apparent that molecular and cell biology have enormous potential for the future of medical research and practice.

There is no doubt that a combination of improvements in the environment combined with the fruits of scientific medicine have greatly improved the health of Western industrialized societies. In England a century ago, four out of ten babies did not survive to adult life, the life expectancy at birth was only 44 years for boys and 47 for girls, and even as recently as the 1930s 2500 women died each year during pregnancy or childbirth. Today, life expectancy at birth is about 73 years for boys and 78 years for girls. The major triumph for scientific medicine and public health has undoubtedly been the control of many infectious diseases. Consequently, the proportion of deaths due to infection and respiratory diseases has declined dramatically and the major causes of mortality in the West are now vascular disease and cancer. Although relatively little progress has been made towards their prevention, their management has been transformed by the ingenuity of the pharmaceutical industry combined with development of high technology medical practice based on a better understanding of disease mechanisms.

Modern scientific medicine is not without its detractors however. Early this century George Bernard Shaw, in his brilliant Preface to *The Doctor's Dilemma*, derided medical research of his time. His cry 'stimulate the phagocytes' came straight from the laboratory of Almroth Wright at St Mary's Hospital Medical School. But this work was written with style and humour and was concerned mainly with debunking the pomposity of the medical profession. This was not the case in the book, *Medical Nemesis*, written by the philosopher and theologian Ivan Illich, which first appeared in 1975. Using a mass of statistics, Illich set out to show that modern medical practice in general, and scientific medicine in particular, has had no effect whatever on the health of society. His thesis holds that common infections such as tuberculosis and poliomyelitis were disappearing long before the advent of antibiotics and vaccines, and, even worse, that modern medicine is a threat to society as well as to individual patients. It is, he believes, more harmful than good because it generates demands for its services and encourages aspects of behaviour that lead to more ill health and reduce our ability to cope with illness and to face suffering and death. Illich concludes that the medical profession, at least in its present form, should be disbanded.

A series of much more thoughtful critiques of modern medicine were published in the late 1970s by Thomas McKeown and others. McKeown extended Illich's thesis that the advent of vaccination, immunization, and antibiotics has had little effect on the control of infectious disease. He argued that the dominance of the mechanistic approach to the problems of disease, which started in the seventeenth century, had caused doctors to overlook important messages that the patterns of disease origins in the past had left for them, and that it had led them to underestimate their potential value for the organization of health care in the future. McKeown believed that the vast majority of diseases are environmental in origin and that if we had been thinking of disease origins rather than mechanisms it would not have taken us so long to suspect the importance of environmental agents or lifestyles in the genesis of our current killers, smoking or lack of exercise as the cause of heart disease for example. In short, writers like Illich and McKeown believe that, because practically all disease stems from the environment, modern scientific medicine, with its accent on disease mechanisms rather than origins, has had little effect on the health of society. While flawed in many ways, particularly with respect to their lack of appreciation of the relative roles of nature and nurture in the genesis of disease, arguments of this kind have had an important influence on current perceptions of the role of science in medicine.

These criticisms of modern scientific medicine have been mirrored by increasing disenchantment with modern medical practice on the part of the public, media, politicians, and even some doctors themselves. Paradoxically, the origins of this mood of disillusionment can be traced to some of the extraordinary successes of scientific medicine earlier this century. In the period after the Second World War, which saw the emergence of vaccines and antibiotics and the control of many infectious diseases, it appeared that medical science was capable of almost anything. The virtual disappearance overnight of scourges like smallpox, diphtheria, and poliomyelitis led to the expectation that similar successes would soon follow. In effect, society came to expect a state of constant rude health as its right. But this did not happen. The diseases that replaced infection, heart attacks, strokes, cancer, rheumatism, and psychiatric disorders, turned out to be much more intractable. Granted there were some remarkable advances in their symptomatic control but these new killers could not be prevented or cured. As this became clear there was a move on the part of society to alternative medicine; if medical science could not cope with chronic backache or lung cancer why not turn for help to those who claimed they had the answers? Dietary manipulation, food allergy, herbal remedies, and a variety of other approaches to chronic illness were taken up with enthusiasm.

Yet coincident with this disillusionment with modern medicine and the search for better alternatives, it became apparent that the revolution in the biological sciences, stemming from applications of molecular and cell biology, promised to change completely the face of health care in the future. Today, hardly a week goes by without a new breakthrough being splashed all over our television screens and newspapers; another human gene has been isolated and the cause of a disease of which we have never heard is announced. New cures for heart disease or cancer appear to be just round the corner. Whenever these new remarkable discoveries are announced excited scientists or journalists tell us that they will have a major impact on health care 'within the near future'. Yet time goes by and this doesn't seem to happen. There is a growing feeling that much which goes on in modern science is motivated more by scientists' wish for self-glorification rather than by any practical goals. Furthermore, many believe that modern science, whether it involves the manipulation of human genes or enquires into the origins of the universe, is a debasing activity that is damaging our environment and moving into areas of knowledge that are best left alone. There is a growing fear about the increasing reductionist approach to medical research. This, combined with concerns about the dehumanizing effect of modern hospitals and the feeling that doctors must return to a more holistic approach to their patients, that is to treat them as individuals rather than diseases, is causing increasing concern to our medical educationalists.

Clearly, younger readers of this book are learning their trade at a time when the whole ethos of scientific medicine is being questioned, and when thoughts are turning more to preventive medicine by modification of our environment and lifestyles, with less emphasis on understanding the basic mechanisms of disease. What are they to make of this confusing scene?

In effect, the doctors of today find themselves in a similar position to their predecessors at the beginning of this century. It was already apparent that many of the infectious diseases that were killing their patients could be partly controlled by better housing, hygiene, and other improvements in the environment; a few could be prevented by vaccination. Yet it was far from clear how far measures of this kind would be successful in controlling these diseases. In the meantime there was little that they could do for their patients with tuberculosis, meningitis, poliomyelitis, or puerperal sepsis, except improve their general well-being and manage their symptoms. They knew that there were some exciting developments in the basic biological sciences, microbiology, and, in particular, immunology, which promised to provide the solution to their problems. Yet these fields had been on the move for over half a century and still appeared to be of limited practical value. Hopes for the development of a cure for tuberculosis, following Koch's discovery of the tubercle bacillus in the 1880s, had still come to nothing. In the event it was to be another 60 years before the discovery of streptomycin provided a definitive cure for tuberculosis.

The situation is more or less the same today. We know that we can reduce the frequency of heart disease and cancer by changes in our environment and lifestyles, stopping cigarette smoking for example. But we have no idea of the extent to which we can control our major killers. For this reason it is essential that we continue to support the basic sciences and to provide the doctors of the future with sufficient understanding of them so that, as practical applications come along, as they certainly will, they are in a position to take advantage of them. If the story of the development of scientific medicine from the seventeenth century onwards has anything to tell us it is simply this. The bulk of our major advances in health care have stemmed from advances in both public health *and* scientific research, the latter quite often stemming from fields that were driven by curiosity rather than any practical end in view. Harvey's discovery of the circulation of the blood had no practical value for patients with heart disease at the time; it was to be several hundred years before advances stemming from the disparate sciences of physiology, anatomy, pharmacology, and biochemistry, together with the discovery of anaesthesia and remarkable developments in surgical technology, laid the ground for modern cardiological practice. We must not neglect the role of the basic sciences in medical education and practice simply because they do not appear to have any immediate benefits.

As scientifically trained clinicians we try and analyse our patients' illnesses as far as we can with the tools of modern medical science, but frequently we find ourselves in a situation in which knowledge is incomplete and some form of therapy, even if it is of unproven value, has to be tried. The further scientific knowledge increases, the more difficult it is for caring clinicians to dissociate their scientific training from the practical necessity of doing something to relieve suffering, even though they are aware that they are rarely sure about what they are doing. Medicine has remained an art, but one that has become increasingly difficult to practice as knowledge of the scientific ignorance that underlies it has increased. The central problem for those who educate doctors of today is, on the one hand, how to encourage a lifelong attitude of critical, scientific thinking to the management of illness, yet, at the same time, recognize that moment when the scientific approach, because of ignorance, has reached its limits and must be replaced by sympathetic empiricism. Doctors have to learn to live with uncertainty. For many, this can be one of the most difficult and disturbing aspects of their work.

Textbook descriptions of disease are, of necessity, misleading. Even in the case of the most straightforward of illnesses, for which we know the cause down to the last building-block of DNA, the presentation, course, and management is never the same in any two patients. Not only are they modified by the protean physiological adaptations that occur in response to disease, but also by an individual's reaction to illness, depending on their personality, degree of family support, and many other factors that we do not understand. If, as is frequently done in our better teaching hospitals, we attempt to analyse all the features of a patient's illness and explain them in terms of current scientific knowledge, we always fail. And because we know so little about the mechanisms that underlie most of the illnesses that we encounter, a great deal of what we do must still remain empirical. It is the sheer complexity of the manifestations of illness that is responsible for the notion that medicine is still an art. And if this is the case for the relatively well-defined diseases that we see in hospital; the situation is even more complex in the community. The bulk of a family doctor's work involves non-specific complaints that seem totally foreign to anything that they learnt in the laboratory or lecture theatre as a student, often reflecting an individual patient's reactions to stresses of work, family, and environment rather than clearly defined organic disease.

Thus, apart from pastoral qualities, good doctoring requires an ability to cut through many of the unexplained manifestations of disease, to appreciate what is important and what can be disregarded, and hence to get to the core of the problem, knowing when scientific explanation has failed and empiricism must take over. This is the real art of clinical practice. It comes naturally to some doctors, but for others the difficult transition from theory to practice, from the relative certainty of the preclinical sciences to complexities of sick people, is never quite accomplished. This may be the reason for the notion that good medical practice depends more on the acquisition of experience based on long years of practice, rather than on methods of prevention, diagnosis, and treatment based on sound scientific principles. Unfortunately, this view, which may partly reflect doctors' defence mechanisms against continued ignorance, has been responsible for a great deal of poor practice, often based on fashion and anecdote rather than anything more substantive. An over-exaggerated perception of the importance of medicine as a craft may also have been responsible for the dogmatism, unhealthy respect for received wisdom of the past, and extreme pomposity that has characterized many aspects of medical practice over the years. Like most human endeavours, the art of medicine has both its good and bad aspects.

In 1941 Sir Arthur Hall wrote:

> Medicine–however much it develops–must always remain an 'applied science' and one differing from all the rest in its applications to man himself. Were there no sick persons there would be no need for Medicine, either the Science or the Art. So long as there are both, both will be necessary. The application of its Science, to be of value, must be made in such a way that it will produce the maximum relief to the sick man. This calls for certain qualities in the practising physician which differ entirely from anything required in the practice of the other applied sciences. Herein lies the Art of Medicine. The need for it is as great today as it ever was, or ever will be, so long as human sickness continues.

As we have seen, our greatest difficulty is to recognize that moment in caring for a sick patient when the scientific approach, because of ignorance, has reached its limits and has to be replaced by sympathetic empiricism. It is the ability to choose that moment, partly by instinct and partly by experience gained by caring for sick people, that is the main characteristic of a good doctor. Undoubtedly, modern medical science, with its increasingly reductionist approach to the study of disease, has tended to focus our attention more on disease mechanisms than on those who are suffering from the diseases that fascinate us so much. We must redress this balance, and return to a more holistic approach to medical care, without, at the same time, allowing ourselves to develop those uncritical attitudes and reliance on received wisdom which permeated the medical profession for so many centuries. For genuine advances in medicine have stemmed from science, as defined at the beginning of this chapter, regardless of whether it involved cells and molecules, or people and populations.

REFERENCES

Booth, C. (1993). History of science in medicine In *Science in medicine: how far has it advanced*? (ed. G. Teeling-Smith) pp. 11–22. Office of Health Economics, London.

Illich, I. (1977). *Limits to medicine. Medical nemesis: the expropriation of health*. Penguin Books, Middlesex.

McKeown, T. (1988). *The origins of human disease*. Blackwell, Oxford.

Weatherall, D.J. (1995). *Science and the quiet art. The role of research medicine*. Norton, New York.

2.2 Medical ethics

G. R. DUNSTAN

Introduction

Two initial obstacles now face a writer on medical ethics. First, the object of study lacks definition. A basic ethics of practice has been expanded first verbally into 'biomedical ethics' and then substantially into 'bioethics', a term that can be stretched to cover all life. So our consciences are engaged with everything from the primary manifestations of organic life to 'the global environment' and space beyond.

Secondly, observation is coloured with social theories, ideologies of various sorts, which bring their own values to the analysis and impose their own language on the discussion. Rights theories confuse expectations and the respective constraints of ethics and law. Together with the promotion of consumerism and of health care as a marketable product, they arouse feelings of conflict and the resort to litigation. The pressures of feminism and for 'openness' in society, even without their exaggerated manifestations, impose new patterns of constraint within which clinical decisions are taken: they can no longer be taken as though these pressures did not exist. Financial constraints on a health service funded from taxation and national insurance bring medicine into the national economic and political debates. Administrative changes are perceived as threats to career structures and professional self-regulation. The ethics of politics, economics, and management require study in their own right; they are different from the studies of the ethics of conduct within medical practice.

Attempts by philosophers and others to clarify vision have in some ways further obscured it. When, in the mid-1950s, philosophers and theologians in Britain began to sit with doctors to discuss ethical issues arising in new areas of practice, they brought with them the experience of their own disciplines, but they did not impose them, as theories or even in language, upon the discussions. Their purpose was pragmatic: to work out together a method of moral reasoning by which those responsible for clinical decisions could formulate an ethics of practice apt to the new choices opened by advances in medical science and technology. When legislation was in prospect, on suicide or abortion for instance, they sought an ethical basis to the law. Their method was specific: to open out the empirical features of the practice contemplated and the indications for it, to isolate the moral claims, and to ask how these claims could be met consistently with the values assumed to be held in common in the community, and with the ethics of the profession – both evolving, both destined for marked change in a newly fluid society. They created no new language, no new patterns of jargon, no schematic grid on to which every question had to be stretched before it could be answered. This method persists in Britain today. It proved itself as new issues called for elucidation: transplant surgery in the 1960s, *in vitro* fertilization (IVF), new embryology and new treatments for infertility in the 1970s and 1980s, gene therapy in the early 1990s. In each case the aim was to achieve a consensus by moral reasoning; to formulate this in appropriate guidance or codes for professional practice; then to open the subject to national debate in terms appropriate for legislation, when that was called for.

Elsewhere it was not so. Philosophers in the United States extended their discussions into medical questions and created a career structure of 'medical ethicists' or 'bioethicists' to do so. They set out to teach their principles in medical schools, they set up consultancies, and attached themselves to departments of medicine as experts in providing solutions, argued from principle, to ethical questions arising in practice. To observers from outside the extent of this infiltration was surprising, and internal observers are now alarmed to discern a shift in decision-making from the primary physician to the ethical consultant: the pretension, indeed the credibility, of 'ethicists' is now under challenge. British moralists and clinicians have steadily resisted that shift. They have insisted that the doctor alone is the responsible moral agent in clinical decision: consult as they will and must – with patients, medical, nursing, and laboratory colleagues – doctors in the end must decide what to advise or do, and answer for their decisions. Even the British Courts will not order medical practitioners to undertake treatment that, in their clinical judgement, is contraindicated as not in the patient's interest. This has been a consistent judgment in a series of decisions in the Court of Appeal and House of Lords from 1981 to 1993, authorizing, but never ordering, clinical decisions to treat or not to treat, whichever the interest of the patient required.

Doctors are entrusted, therefore, with an accountable freedom to practice their art according to the ethics of their profession. 'Clinical autonomy' is an inept term for this freedom. It is philologically inept and it invites collision with 'patient autonomy' and hence a conflict of 'rights'. 'Autonomy' means living by one's own laws; and this neither doctor nor patient may do. Patients have rights: not only, in the United Kingdom, a statutory right to medical consultation and to available and appropriate treatment, but also natural rights to bodily integrity and freedom to consent or not to what is advised. Doctors have a duty to serve patients' interest in health while fully respecting those rights.

A natural right is a claim to the recognition of a vital capacity grounded in human nature, for example, liberty to think, to speak, to move, to marry, recognized by competent authority as capable of being protected and enjoyed. (The competent authority may be a sovereign legislature or established system of common law; or it may be a moral consensus recognized internationally by convention or protocol.) Interests relevant to health care are grounded in these capacities, but their discernment is subjective. Is it worse to be born with grave handicap than not to be born at all? Is duration of life more important than comfort in it? Medical practice now is more considerate of patients' own perception of their interest in such cases and, where ethical options are available, patients have a liberty of choice. Tensions arise when mere wishes are invested arbitrarily with the language of rights and are advanced in conflict with professional duty and discretion. This is an issue still seeking resolution. It requires that the public refines its expectations of medicine and that the profession clarifies its own understanding of its role.

Ethical judgements are not arbitrary judgements. Doctors' consciences are their own; but the ethics by which doctors are governed are those of their profession, corporate though personally embodied. The corporate obligation has been restated powerfully in the last half of the twentieth century. Among its products are codes or guidelines for medical practice and, for medical research, peer review and supervision by Research Ethics Committees (in the United States, Institutional Review Boards). International Codes have been promulgated by the World Medical Association (WMA), following upon the Declaration of Geneva (1948), and by the Council for International Organizations of Medical Sciences (CIOMS). National initiatives have been taken, in the United Kingdom by the Royal Medical Colleges, especially the Royal College of Physicians, by specialist faculties and associations, and by the Medical Research Council. Similar initiatives were taken in Australia, Canada, and the United States. Medical practice, as distinct from research, has not been subjected to the scrutiny of ethics committees, except in two sensitive areas of innovative therapy. The first was *in vitro* fertilization and embryo transfer. These were established at first by consensual agreement between practitioners and the Voluntary (Interim) Licensing Authority, and were then made statutory by the Human Fertilization and Embryology Act (1990). Since 1993 innovative gene therapy has been similarly governed. Research Ethics Committees were also initially set up by professional initiative – that of the Royal College of Physicians. The Department of Health has now required their establishment in all National Health Service authorities and trusts, and has taken a formal, though non-statutory, role in their oversight and regulation. Innovative measures, first tentative experiments to improve on established methods of treatment, are still within medical discretion, with the concurrence of peers. Once there is reason to believe that they may succeed in wider practice, there is a moral obligation, now generally insisted upon, to evaluate them by proper research, and so to submit them, in formal protocol, to a Research Ethics Committee for review and approval.

Application

Ethics and belief

Ethical conduct is action consistent with belief or with principle grounded in belief. Belief in human worth or dignity will determine the quality of the relationship between doctors and their patients, and of the health care that the State provides for its people. Beliefs about the value or worth of each human life will determine the extreme limits of a doctor's duties in critical areas of practice, from reproductive medicine to terminal care. The belief that each human life has absolute value entails a strict or absolute duty to preserve it in all circumstances, regardless of other consideration. Belief, however, that there is a strong but rebuttable presumption in favour of each human life will entail a *prima facie* duty to preserve life, but leave the doctor with a discretion, and often a duty, to change the management, in the patient's interest, from active prolongation to palliative terminal care. There are those who hold the 'absolutist' view in relation to the beginning of life – in embryology, for instance, fetal medicine and neonatal care – and those who profess it for the prolongation of life at the end; but not all are consistent in applying it to both.

Neither the ethics nor the law governing accepted medical practice puts an absolute value on life nor imposes a strict duty to preserve it. Both rest on a presumption in favour of life from the cleaving embryo onwards, a presumption growing in strength with embryonic development and fetal growth until legal personality and rights are attributed at birth. The duty of care for the child in the womb advances *pari passu*, and antedates and stands independently of the attribution of rights. In recent decades tension between these beliefs has engendered ethical conflict, as new knowledge and technical skills have opened new possibilities for medical intervention and new options for patients.

Reproductive medicine

The ethics of assisted and donor insemination have been debated for nearly half a century. In the 1970s, advances in the understanding and control of ovulation brought *in vitro* fertilization and embryo replacement to the fore; the first IVF birth occurred in 1978. Variations of method, in the collection of oöcytes, the management of fertilization and the replacement of embryos or of gametes, continue, with the microinjection of single sperm into ova now at the leading edge. The Human Fertilization and Embryology Act (HFEA) (1990) established that the doctor had a duty of care for the resulting child as well as for the potential mother. The ethics of risk pertain to both.

For the mother there are not only the physical risks attending ovarian stimulation, hormonal preparation and oöcyte recovery; there is also the emotional risk that her intense wish for a child may be exploited, in the interest of research or technical advance, or for financial gain in the commercialized private sector, when her chances of a successful pregnancy are demonstrably low. The highest risk is of disappointment.

For the child the main risk is in high multiple pregnancy – the incidence of congenital defect being statistically normal. Doctors may replace more gametes or embryos than the best assessment of clinical need may indicate or the HFEA guidelines now permit. They may do so either from miscalculation, or in a calculated gamble, or by yielding, against clinical judgement, to insistent patients' demands. When multiple pregnancies are established, either by this means or by hyperstimulation for coital conception, both mother and babies, if born, are put at a more severe risk. Selective feticide is then seen as an option justified by expediency: it is better to kill some than to lose all, or suffer a multiple birth with the likelihood of morbidity and social deprivation. Selective termination to obviate iatrogenic error or complication invites attack as a further erosion of the value put upon life and encourages the hostility of opponents of 'interference' in procreation.

The conflict of views on the value of life dominated the national and Parliamentary debates on the Human Fertilization and Embryology Bill. 'Absolutist' opponents argued that, because in the IVF process embryos are necessarily discarded, or diverted into medical research, doctors fail in their strict duty to preserve life, which is 'sacred' 'from the moment of conception'. This indeed is the view dogmatically asserted by authority in the Roman Catholic Church. The rejection by Parliament of this doctrine as a principle for the nation and its laws was consistent with common law, the ancient canon law, and a continuing moral tradition grounded in Aristotelian embryology and philosophy; it was enshrined in the Greek version (LXX) of the Old Testament at Exodus 21:22; it was enunciated authoritatively by Catholic theologians, moralists, canonists, and Popes until repudiated, for the Roman Catholic Church, by Pope Pius IX in 1869. In juridical terms, homicide was not committed in the termination of 'unformed' and therefore 'unanimated' embryonic life, but only when the embryo was morphologically so developed as to be recognizably human. The Act of 1990 gave statutory protection to embryonic life at the end of 14 days, instead of the old canonical setting of upwards of 40. But by its provisions for the regulation of embryonic manipulation before 14 days it recognized the distinctive character of the genetically human organism from the appearance of the zygote onwards.

Debate continues on the ethics and social policy concerning various extramarital applications of assisted reproduction, as with lesbian couples or varieties of surrogate maternity. For the doctor, except where the law has imposed restriction (as for commercial involvement with surrogacy), practice is discretionary: no doctors are obliged to assist if they do not wish to. And as doctors are obliged to have regard for the welfare of any child to be born, the relationship in which the child would be reared cannot be a matter of indifference.

Antenatal care

Between conception and birth come new techniques for fetal observation, investigation, and intervention; non-invasive means of measuring not only fetal structure but also organ function, like the velocity of cardiac blood flow, advancing DNA technology based on expanding knowledge of the human genome and chromosomal distribution, and advances in fetal medicine and surgery. In all of this, the direct object of clinical attention is the embryo or fetus. But as the embryo is located, in total dependence, in the mother's womb, it is accessible only through her and with her consent. Not even a Court of Law can authorize any intervention upon a woman's body, in the interest of her unborn child, without her consent. (The exceptional declaration by the President of the Family Division in Re S (Adult: Refusal of Medical Treatment) (1992) 4 All ER 671, in which he authorized the performance of a caesarean section on a woman who refused consent, startled the legal and medical professions alike. It is unlikely to be followed as a precedent.) Any decision to act, therefore, must be a joint decision, between mother and doctor. (A decision not to act may be taken by the doctor alone.) Both mother and doctor must resolve the tensions of principle that have been seen to inform the ethics of reproductive medicine.

Morbidity may be disclosed or predicted by appropriate tests at any stage from the first polar body and early embryonic cleaving to the viable fetus. Cellular biopsy may confirm a genetic defect in an embryo, *in vitro*, of parents who may have reason to suspect the transmission of a heritable disorder. The parents are then free to decide whether to have the embryo replaced in the womb, or to discard it in the hope of having another, uncompromised, embryo. Later tests, from trophectoderm, chorionic villi, or amniotic fluid, giving positive indications of congenital disorder, invite the possibility of terminating the pregnancy. For parents holding the strict view of the inviolability of human life, these options – discarding the embryo or terminating the pregnancy – are closed. The Vatican Declaration of 1987, at I.2, stated that a woman who sought antenatal diagnosis with the deliberate intention of aborting a fetus found defective 'would be committing a gravely illicit act'; even to counsel such a diagnostic procedure 'would be acting contrary to the moral law'. Although these proscriptions have no standing in accepted professional ethics, doctors should respect this scruple in patients presenting with it. But first, they should assist their patients to exercise their undoubted civil liberty of choice by giving and interpreting the relevant information and assuring, so far as possible, their freedom of consent or refusal.

Antenatal testing does not, in fact, always end in a stark choice between continuance or termination. More commonly it may assure, when no evidence of genetic defect is found. It may give indications for fetal intervention, medical or surgical, or for dietary advice. It may enable the planning of neonatal management before birth.

Medical genetics

As genome analysis yields more knowledge it may enable predictions, which raise other ethical questions. Genes may be detected for a 50 per cent chance of a disease of late onset, like Huntingdon's chorea, unpreventable and incurable. Should parents be told of this possibility? Some clinical geneticists argue firmly against. There is no need to invent a new 'right not to know' in order to recall the duty to respect a settled wish not to know. The counsellor would consider with patients the clinical details; the prospects of palliation; the capacity to transcend anxiety and to live with the knowledge and uncertainty and to help the child to do the same; and any wish the parents might have to make prudent provision for future contingencies.

A negative answer is by no means decisive or universal; it may vary from case to case. A similar question will present itself with the disclosure of genes indicating a susceptibility to serious polygenic disorders, the expression of which may depend on later environmental or other influences. It would be foolish to excite groundless anxiety; on the other hand it might be opportune to offer prudential advice, dietary or occupational, which might be for a patient's good.

The practice of clinical genetics, though focused on individual patients, extends – in those patients' interest – into families as well; and ethical norms are capable of extension with them. Enquiries through the family of the index patient with a defective gene may identify members who carry that gene unawares, and who may transmit it. A good clinical relationship may gain ready consent to the disclosure necessary for the familial search to begin. If consent is withheld, the clinician's wish to prevent, if possible, avoidable suffering will be frustrated by the ethics of professional secrecy, as it is in France, and perhaps elsewhere, by the criminal law. Is it time to extend the obligation of confidence from the traditional one-to-one relationship into the family relationship in such cases? As a gene is, in fact, a corporate possession of the family, so might the knowledge of it be. If the risk is high and the potential for help is available, a duty to other members of the family may outweigh the duty of confidence to one patient. Compulsory screening is not in question. All that is suggested is that potential carriers are entitled to such knowledge as will enable them to make choices for themselves. It may be asked: can a claim to 'autonomy' by one person infringe the 'autonomy' of others by denial of knowledge of themselves?

A point of practical importance is entailed. When family contact is sought, or when, perhaps for research purposes, a child on a genetic register is recalled, the contact should be made through the doctor known to the patient and who knows the patient's circumstances: the general practitioner or the original consultant. Clumsiness can harm, not only the child and family relations, but also the public acceptance of the medical or research endeavour.

GENE THERAPY

The new genetics offers more than enhanced diagnostic skills; it opens the possibility of gene therapy. Among other studies of the ethics of this stands the Report of the United Kingdom Department of Health, published in 1992. It is commonly held that, for the immediate future, the genetic manipulation of somatic cells should be regarded ethically as research leading to a potentially innovative therapeutic procedure, and should be supervised and regulated as such. As genes or genetic segments are recognized as coding for serious clinical disorders for which remedies either do not exist or are gravely burdensome and far from effective, and as *in vitro* and animal studies give grounds for confidence in the possibility of success, with low risk of escape from control or other ill-consequence, so licensed practice with patients has begun in a few specialist centres. The range of intervention would be extended, step by step, under supervision, as experience warrants. If ill-consequence did follow, the harm would be limited to one generation, that is, to the patient subjected to the procedure. Ill-consequence from intervention in the germ cells, by contrast, would not be so limited; it could be transmitted to further generations. Desirable as it might be to eliminate a defective gene from a family's future, as well as counteracting it in one generation, intervention in the human germ line – and this would include intervention in the cleaving embryo – should not be licensed until control, knowledge of possible consequences, and safety have all been assured. The embryonic cells are already protected under the Human Fertilization and Embryology Act (1990). For patients offered somatic gene therapy, the ethical protections normal to research and innovative procedures apply. Despite popular misgivings, it is nowhere established that old ethical principles are violated or that new ones are involved.

Neonatal care

Advances in neonatal paediatrics prompt attempts to prolong the life of babies of very low birth weight, prematurely born, and of babies born severely malformed or handicapped. (Earlier practice, with home delivery attended at most by an understanding midwife, would have been not to resuscitate when the omens forbade; and this would have been accounted merciful. Modern practice and sentiment alike make that resort now improbable.) Those who equate life itself with good, reckon prolongation of life, however achieved, a benefit. And perceptions of what is tolerable in handicap and suffering vary beyond belief. There are parents whose spirit, determination, and capacity to cherish enable them to accept prospects from which others would turn away. Clinicians must recognize this possibility and welcome it, and assess it as highly pertinent to the interest of the child.

But there are studies that conclusively relate higher morbidity with lower birth weight; and these must be borne in mind by paediatricians as, with instruments and tests, they monitor the infant in intensive care. Must that life be sustained at all costs, regardless of outcome?

Given the presumption in favour of life, paediatricians would try (they would say) to do what they could. They would know, from studies and experience, that their *attempts* were *tentative*, truly *experimental* for this particular child (three words derived from Latin words for *to try*). It would follow that if these tentative measures were proving not to be for the child's benefit, paediatricians are not bound to pursue them; indeed, they ought not to pursue them, even for the sake of research or advancement of skill, if they were proving adverse to the baby's interest. The paediatrician is at liberty, and sometimes under duty, to desist. Consultation with parents, and consideration for them, are axiomatic requirements. But the decision to desist, if it has to be taken, must remain a professional one, the doctor's alone. And if the decision, given the clinical indications, was in accord with the professional opinion of the doctor's peers, that action would be defensible in law.

The ethics of practice, as distinct from the principles of ethics, are inextricably related to knowledge and available skill, and so must change with them. Research brings about such changes. Although contentious, the criteria for the management of babies with meningomyelocele and high lumbar paraplegia at birth, established after 10 years of research by Lorber, Zachary, and colleagues in the Sheffield Children's Hospital, were widely accepted, and left their mark on the statistics of infant mortality. Further research in Newcastle upon Tyne afforded ground to modify those criteria. The modifications gave doctors more time to decide whether to operate or not; they established that involvement of parents in early care, with or without surgery, extended life expectancy, and this without necessarily diminished intellectual capacity. Good science and observation thus pointed to more positive and conservative management – conservative in that the presumption in favour of life was strengthened. Nevertheless, the ethics of discretion persisted: if, taking all positive factors into account, surgical intervention would carry the prognosis of a life of foreseeable minimum grave handicap and suffering, intensified with adolescent awareness and requiring increasingly invasive palliative surgery, with no expectation of long-term alleviation or cure, the initial surgical intervention might, ethically, be withheld: the child's interest could be better served by good nursing and palliative terminal care. There is neither a strict obligation to prolong life by all available means, nor a licence to kill. The ethics of the decision whether to persist in or to desist from active intervention have also been formulated in the technical but unfortunate language of 'ordinary and extraordinary means'. These are discussed in the next section.

Palliative medicine and terminal care

In this field also, research and its medical application have softened the starkness of ethical decision. Pharmaceutical advances have given doctors the means to alleviate pain and most of the distresses of chronic and acute illness without obliterating consciousness and distorting personality. Experience and training in the required skills needed a hospitable context, provided initially by the Hospice movement and developed in Continuing Care Units and the Macmillan home nursing service. It needed also a radical change of perception in the objectives of medicine as perceived in a high-technology hospital mentality. A determined will to cure, to preserve life, and to seek new means to this praiseworthy end has so possessed some of the most vigourous minds as to close them to the unexpressed interests and wishes of patients; indeed, patients were neither expected nor enabled to articulate them. Intervention – invasive, painful, disfiguring, and distressing – could be imposed, for the prolongation of life, long after it became in the patient's interest to be comforted and allowed to die. As long ago as 1957 even the Roman Catholic Church, committed as it is to an absolute view of the sacredness of human life, could distinguish through Pope Pius XII between 'ordinary' and 'extraordinary' means of prolonging life. The distinction was not between what is and what is not medically prescribable for given indications, but between what is and what is not apt for particular patients. Ordinary procedures, those which offer *this* patient reasonable hope of benefit without excessive expense, pain, or other serious inconvenience, the physician would be bound ethically to offer and the patient to accept. 'Extraordinary' procedures, which would impose undue suffering or expense, distortion of personality, a barrier to relationships, or a lessening of human capacity, need not be offered or accepted.

In terminal care, therefore, as in neonatal intensive care, the criterion determining appropriate management is the interest of the patient; the presumption in favour of life is rebutted if the patient's interest is in being allowed to die comfortably. In the tradition of Rabbinic Judaism, the recognition of the patient's interest is delayed until the death process has begun, although pain should be alleviated meanwhile. A well-titrated balance of analgaesic and other distress-relieving drugs need not lead now to respiratory failure. However, should such necessary treatment lead to a shortening of life by a brief period, the treatment is not deemed a culpable contribution to the death. It is not the moral equivalent of 'euthanasia', the intentional killing of a patient. The death is reckoned to be an unintended secondary consequence or effect of a necessary action directed to a proper end and effective to that end, the comfort of a patient moribund.

Looking forward

Emphasis on the primacy of the patient's interest over the full deployment of all possible medical and surgical techniques in no way diminishes the obligation to pursue research and innovation designed to give doctors better means of preventing, curing or alleviating disease. Conventions and institutions for the ethical control of such research have been noted; the process will continue. As science and skills advance, the ethics of decision require more than the simple application of old formulae. New practical possibilities require a reshaping of the ethical kaleidoscope to find new patterns with a moral fit. Ahead lie a series of AIDS vaccine trials, ethical conditions for which have already been set out. Behind lies the history of organ transplantation, in which ethical response to new demands may be traced over the last 30 years.

The main focus has been on consent. Some countries presume the consent of the deceased to the removal of cadaveric organs unless there has been a stated wish to the contrary. This is called the principle of 'contracting (or opting) out'. In the United Kingdom the prior consent of the deceased, or that of the nearest available kin, is required: the principle of 'contracting in'. For the British system to succeed there must first be an ethical relationship between those administering intensive care and those seeking viable organs, of such a sort that cooperation is possible without threat to patients' interests; and, secondly, sensitivity in the approach to relatives when consent has to be sought. It requires also public confidence in the integrity of the procedures – an assurance that the interest of the dying patient is protected and that the donor is truly dead – and a willingness to donate, a morally higher act, surely, than a mere submission to the exaction assumed in the 'opting out' system.

For live donors – a regrettable necessity while cadaveric organs cannot meet demand – the freedom of consent is also paramount. It must be given without pressure, familial, social, financial, religious or emotional: a sense of fear, or guilt, or self-abasement can masquerade as altruism and be exploited. The United Kingdom Human Organ Transplant Act (1990) prohibited commercial dealings in human organs and established the unrelated Live Transplants Regulatory Authority to regulate transplants between genetically unrelated living persons. (Trade in organs, although repudiated by international convention, is still practised, and indeed defended, in some countries.)

These basic rules are long established. Additions were called for when a diagnosis of brain-stem death had excluded, with moral certainty, all possibility of recovery, while a heart beat mechanically maintained could keep organs in better condition for successful grafting. The ethics require sufficient certainty in the diagnosis so that (despite appearances) the brain-dead patient whose circulation is maintained artificially is indubitably dead before organ retrieval. To this end, the United Kingdom Conference of Royal Medical Colleges issued guidelines, later refined, conformity with which would give this assurance. The criteria do not permit the use of abortuses or anencephalic neonates as sources of organs because their brains are not developed enough to meet the tests. Neither may patients in a persistent vegetative state be so used: their brain stems are demonstrably functioning. To take organs from these three groups while heart beat continued spontaneously would be ethically impermissable and would discredit validated procedures for transplanting from genuinely dead patients. Research leading to the transplanting of fetal cells has already received authoritative ethical guidelines. Here the ethics of the clinical relationship are complicated by the ethics of abortion: fears, real or exaggerated, that women might be persuaded to conceive and abort for the sake of producing usable fetal material had to be met and guarded against.

Xenografting, the transplanting or organs from animals transgenically adapted towards histocompatibility with man, will soon be attempted clinically. Ethical discussion has already shown that, once again, the public debate will be complicated by a side-issue, this time the propriety of this use of animals. There is probably a gap between public perception of the practice, and medical opinion, which would regard it as a legitimate advance upon established lines.

Research acumen, and a high output of research publications, is not in itself a commendation for good clinical practice. Yet clinicians must be open to innovation and judge critically its suitability for patients in their care. The primary responsibility must rest upon practitioners themselves, aware that a necessary condition of change is public trust. A public slowly being educated must therefore be a party to the ethical debate.

REFERENCES

British Paediatric Association. (1991). *Diagnosis of brain stem death in infants and children.* British Paediatric Association, London.

British Paediatric Association. (1992). *Guidelines for the ethical conduct of research involving children.* British Paediatric Association, London.

Byrne, P., *et al.* (1991). Hospice care: Jewish reservations considered in a comparative ethical study. *Palliative Medicine*, **5,** 187–200.

Campbell, A.G.M. (1989). Some ethical issues in neonatal care. In *Doctors' decisions: Ethical conflicts in medical practice* (ed. G.R. Dunstan and E.A. Shinebourne), pp. 51–66. Oxford University Press.

Cartwright, W. (1991). The ethics of xenografting in man. In *Organ replacement therapy: Ethics, justice, commerce* (ed. W. Land and J.B. Dosster), pp. 519–27. Springer-Verlag, Berlin.

Congregation for the Doctrine of the Faith (1987). *Instruction on respect for human life in its origin and on the dignity of procreation.* The Vatican, 22 February 1987.

Court of Appeal: Re B 1981; 3 All ER 927. Re C 1989; 2 All ER 78. Re J 1990; 3 All ER 330. Re R 1991; 4 All ER 177. Re B 1991; *The Times* 27 May 1991. Re J 1992; *The Times* 12 June 1992. cf. House of Lords, Re KD, 18 Feb. 1988. House of Lords, Airedale NHS Trust *v.* Bland, 4 February 1993.

Department of Health. (1983). *Cadaveric organs for transplanting.* A Code of Practice including the diagnosis of brain death. Department of Health, London

Department of Health. (1992) *Report of the committee on the ethics of gene therapy.* Cm 1788. H.M.S.O. London.

Department of Health. (1992). *Local research ethics committees.* Department of Health, London.

Duncan, A.S., Dunstan, G.R., and Welbourn, R.B.(ed.) (1981). *Dictionary of medical ethics*, (2nd edn). Darton, Longman and Todd, London.

Dunstan, G.R. (1987). The authority of a moral claim: Ian Ramsey and the practice of medicine. *Journal of Medical Ethics*, **13,** 189–94.

Dunstan, G.R. (ed.) (1990). *The human embryo: Aristotle and the Arab and European traditions.* University of Exeter Press, Exeter.

Dunstan, G.R. and Seller, M.J. (ed.) (1988). *The Status of the human embryo: Perspectives from moral tradition.* King Edward's Hospital Fund for London, London.

Dunstan, G.R. and Shinebourne, E.A. (ed.) (1989). *Doctors' decisions: Ethical conflicts in medical practice*, pp. 1–9, 228–43. Oxford University Press.

Elliott, C. (1991). Good to be beside the bedside. *Times Higher Educational Supplement*, **16 August,** 17.

Elliott, C. (1992). Solving the doctor's dilemma? *New Scientist*, **17 January,** 42–4.

Fentiman, I. (1992). Testing times. *Science and Public Affairs*, **Summer 1992,** 25–7.

Fishel, S. and Symonds, E.M. (ed.) (1993). *Gamete and embryo micromanipulation in human reproduction.* Edward Arnold, London.

Ford, N.M. (1988). *When did I begin? Conception of the human individual in history, philosophy and science.* Cambridge University Press.

Harper, P.S. and Clarke, A. (1990). Should we test our children for 'adult' genetic diseases? *Lancet*, **335,** 1295–6, 1406.

Hoffenberg, R. (1987). *Clinical freedom.* The Rock Carling Lecture for 1986. Nuffield Provincial Hospitals Trust.

Jakobovits, I. (1983). The doctor's duty to heal and the patient's consent in the Jewish tradition. In *Consent in medicine: Convergence and divergence in tradition*, (ed. G.R. Dunstan and M.J. Seller), pp. 32–6. King Edward's Hospital Fund for London, London.

Kennedy, I. (1991). A woman and her unborn child. In *Treat Me Right: Essays in medical law and ethics*, 2nd edn. (ed. I. Kennedy), pp. 364–84. Clarendon Press, Oxford.

Lamb, D. (1990). *Organ transplants and ethics.* Routledge, London.

Lorber, J. (1971). Results of treatment of myelomeningocele. *Developmental Medicine and Child Neurology*, **15,** 279.

Menzies, P.C., Parkin, J.M., and Hey, E.N. (1985). Prognosis for babies with meningomyelocele and high lumbar paraplegia at birth. *Lancet*, **ii,** 993–5.

Medical Research Council. (1963). *Responsibility in investigations on human subjects*, Cmnd 2382. HMSO, London.

Medical Research Council. (1991). *The ethical conduct of research on children.* Medical Research Council, London.

Medical Research Council. (1991). *The ethical conduct of research on the mentally handicapped.* Medical Research Council, London.

Medical Research Council. (1991). *The ethical conduct of AIDS vaccine trials.* Medical Research Council, London.

Polkinghorne, J. (1989). *Review of the guidelines on the research use of fetuses and fetal material.* The Report of a Committee under the chairmanship of John Polkinghorne, Cm. 762. HMSO, London.

Royal College of Obstetricians and Gynaecologists (1994). *A consideration of the law and ethics in relation to Court-authorized intervention.* Royal College of Obstetricians and Gynaecologists, London.

Royal College of Physicians. (1986). *Research in Healthy Volunteers.* Royal College of Physicians, London.

Royal College of Physicians. (1990). *Research Involving Patients.* Royal College of Physicians, London.

Royal College of Physicians. (1995). *Guidelines on the Practice of Ethics Committees in Medical Research involving Human Subjects*, 3rd edn. Royal College of Physicians, London.

Saunders, C. and Sykes, N. (ed.) (1993). *The management of terminal malignant disease*, 2nd edn. Edward Arnold, Sevenoaks.

Silver, C.A. (1991) Ethicists in medicine. *Lancet*, **338,** 1325.

Wilkes, E. (1989). Ethics in terminal care. In *Doctors' Decisions: Ethical conflicts in medical practice*, (ed. G.R. Dunstan and E.A. Shinebourne), pp. 197–204. Oxford University Press.

Zachary, R.B. (1968). Ethical and social aspects of treatment of spina bifida. *Lancet*, **ii,** 274–6.

2.3 Evaluation of clinical method

D. L. SACKETT

Our first moments with a patient are packed with visual, auditory, tactile, and sometimes olfactory information that determines both the effectiveness and the costs of our subsequent care. Of all the diagnoses that ever will be made, most are made during the history, and most of the rest during the physical examination. Even when patients are referred to specialist centres after exhaustive examination elsewhere, attention is appropriately refocused on the key clinical enactment: the patient's 'story' and the physical examination.

Obtaining an accurate history and making a proper physical examination are venerated elements of the art of medicine. But there is a science to this art. One of its cornerstones is the recognition that the important tasks we carry out as clinicians require the particularization, to an individual patient, of our prior experiences (not just as individual clinicians, but as a profession) with groups of similar patients. Thus, the rational evaluation of a symptom, sign, or laboratory result in today's patient demands our critical appraisal of how this finding has behaved previously among groups of patients with the same differential diagnosis. Similarly, the rational selection of a treatment for today's patient requires appraisal of how similar patients have fared on various treatments in the past. No wonder, then, that the scientific strategies and tactics developed for dealing with large numbers of patients—derived from epidemiology and biostatistics—have been so valuable in the diagnosis and management of the individual patient.

The four strategies of diagnosis

Clinicians assign diagnoses in one of four ways.

1. Pattern recognition (Gestalt)

This happens when a patient's illness, and especially their physical appearance, conforms to a previously learned picture (or pattern) of disease. The face of a child with Down's syndrome, the parkinsonian gait of a psychotic patient on phenothiazines, and the voice of a woman with hypothyroidism can evoke an immediate diagnosis in a seasoned clinician. Laboratory tests are often unnecessary unless required to confirm the diagnosis or to guide therapy. This strategy, which comes into increasing use with clinical experience, relies on the very high specificity of the findings (that is, their rarity in all other conditions but this one). When the specificity of findings is lower, attempts to apply the strategy of pattern recognition will frequently result in misdiagnoses.

2. Arborization (algorithm)

Some illnesses lend themselves to a strategy in which diagnosis can proceed down but one of a large number of potential, preset paths by a method in which the response to each diagnostic inquiry automatically determines the next inquiry to be carried out and, ultimately, the correct diagnosis or course of action. The use of these carefully constructed algorithms is becoming widespread, especially when diagnostic responsibility is delegated from physicians to other health workers. The example shown in Fig. 1 also illustrates how this method sequentially employs clinical findings with the highest degrees of specificity. As with pattern recognition, the differential occurrence of each pertinent sign and symptom must be known for each of the competing diagnoses.

3. The complete 'history and physical' (exhaustion)

Early in their training, medical students are taught how to painstakingly search for all medical facts that could be extracted from performing a history and physical examination. By means of this exhaustive approach, students gain competence in both identifying and pursuing any and all diagnostic leads. However, this method of the novice, required for the mastery of 'subroutines', is prohibitively inefficient. Effective clinicians soon abandon it for the fourth and final strategy.

4. The hypothetico-deductive method

In this strategy, the one used by nearly all clinicians, nearly all the time, the clinician formulates, from the earliest clues about the patient, a 'short list' of potential diagnoses or courses of action, followed by the performance of those clinical (from the history and physical examination) and paraclinical (from the laboratory) manoeuvres that will best reduce the length of the list. The hypotheses come from our understanding of human biology and pathophysiology and, with greater experience, from prior encounters with similar illnesses (perhaps by pattern recognition of a 'short list' rather than a single diagnosis). The key to accurate, efficient diagnosis is the identification of clinical findings (which can be elicited by applying one of the 'subroutines' memorized in earlier training in the method of exhaustion) that render a diagnosis very unlikely, so it can be abandoned and the list further shortened. In this case, it is the absence of a finding that is virtually always present in the diagnosis of interest (i.e. a finding with high sensitivity) which permits its removal from the short list.

Once again, and as with pattern recognition and algorithms, a thorough knowledge of the differential occurrence of specific items in the history and physical examination in the competing diagnostic conditions distinguishes the superior clinician from her colleagues. To succeed in clinical diagnosis, one needs to understand the precision (reproducibility) and accuracy (e.g. sensitivity and specificity) of individual elements of the clinical examination.

The precision and accuracy of the clinical examination

In addition to developing rapport with, and understanding of, our patients, the clinical examination allows us to execute three other powerful acts. First, for many conditions it supplies us with everything we need to clinch a diagnosis. Secondly, it often permits us to rule out diagnostic hypotheses. Finally, the examination often allows us to identify patients at an early stage of their disorder, which, if left unattended, can lead to disability or untimely death. These acts require that the elements of the clinical examination be both precise (so that two competent clinicians who independently examine the same patient will agree on the presence or absence of an important sign or symptom) and accurate (so that the conclusion drawn from the examination would be verified by an autopsy, operation, or other 'gold standard' of diagnosis).

Precision

For an item of the clinical history or physical examination to be accurate, it first must be precise. That is, we need to have some confidence that two clinicians examining the same, unchanged patient would agree with one another on the presence or absence of the symptom or sign.

Suppose two clinicians recorded whether they found spider naevi when they independently examined the same 100 patients suspected of having liver disease, and generated the data shown in Fig. 2. The two clinicians agreed that 23 of the patients (cell *a*) had spider naevi, and that 66 patients (cell *d*) did not; thus, they agreed on $(23 + 66)/100 = 89$ per cent of the patients that they examined. However, 6 patients (cell *c*) judged to have spider naevi by the first clinician were judged not to have naevi by the second, and 5 patients (cell *b*) judged to have spider naevi by the second clinician were judged not to have naevi by the first. How should we interpret this precision? Is this degree of clinical agreement good, or should we expect better?

We might begin by recognizing that some clinical agreement always occurs by chance alone. For example, if the second clinician merely tossed a coin for each patient instead of carrying out an examination, reporting naevi if the coin came up 'heads' and no naevi if it came up 'tails', agreement would be 50 per cent. We should begin, then, by determining how much of the observed agreement of 89 per cent was due to chance, so that we can find out how much real clinical skill (agreement beyond chance) was displayed by these clinicians. Chance agreement can be calculated by the formal process of 'marginal cross-products' shown in Fig. 2, but it also can be thought of as a coin toss in which, for example, the first clinician's coin came up heads 29 per cent of the time (based on $(a + c)/(a + b + c + d)$). Thus, 29 per cent of the 28 patients judged to have spider naevi by the second clinician $(a + b)$ would also be judged to have them by the first clinician, and 29 per cent of 28 is 8 (the number of patients we would expect to find in

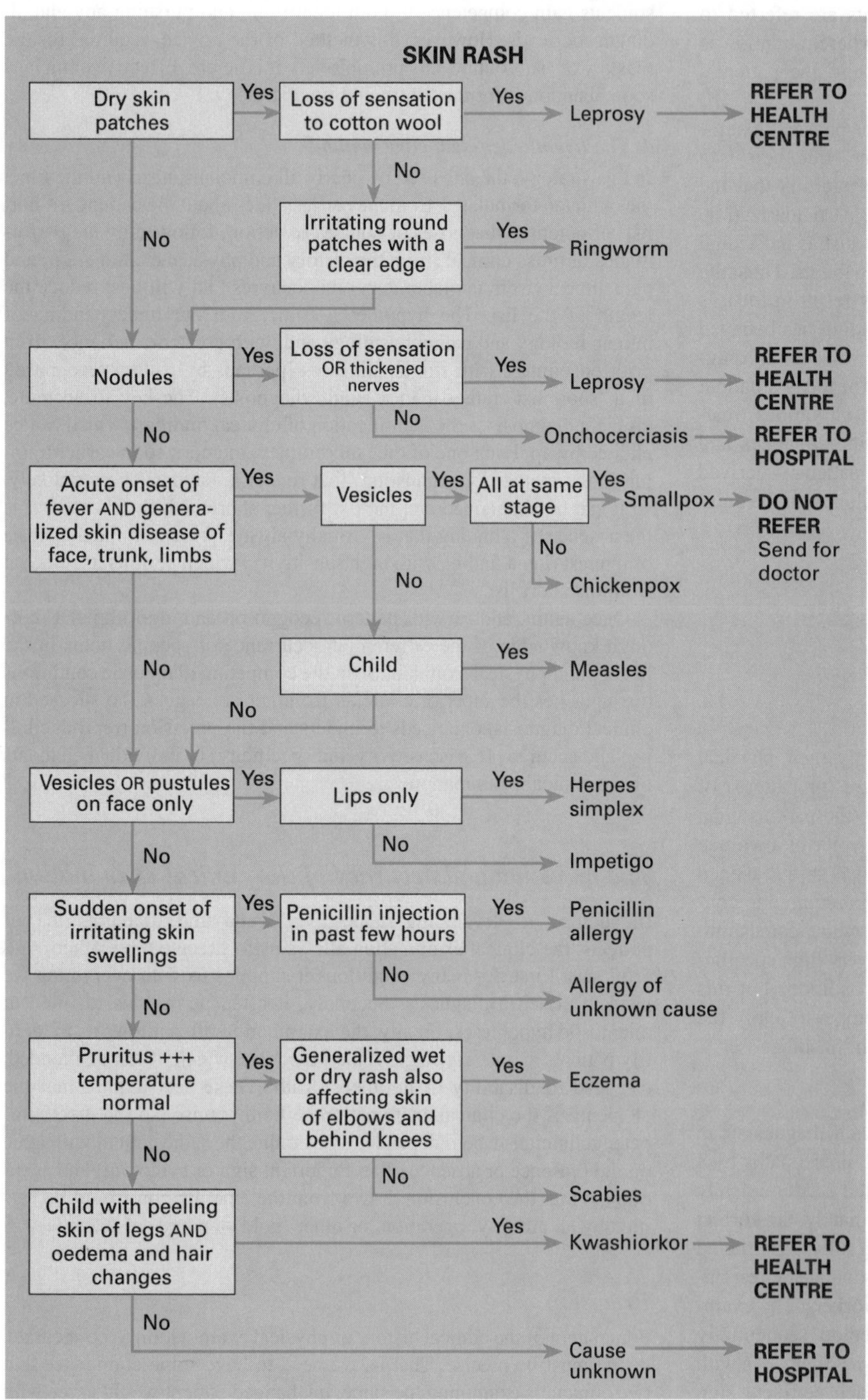

Fig. 1 The 'skin rash in Tanzania algorithm' from B. J. Essex. (1976) *Diagnostic pathways in clinical medicine*. p. 134. Churchill Livingstone, Edinburgh. (Reproduced with permission.) This algorithm will have been updated with the eradication of smallpox.

cell *a* by chance alone). Similarly, the first clinician's coin came up 'tails' 71 per cent of the time $[(b + d)/(a + b + c + d)]$, and 71 per cent of the 72 patients judged to be free of spider naevi by the second clinician $(c + d)$ is 51 (the expected value for cell *d*). As a result, we would expect the two clinicians to agree (8 + 51)/100 or 59 per cent of the time on the basis of chance alone, and the remaining potential agreement beyond chance is therefore 100 − 59 per cent or 41 per cent.

How much of this 41 per cent potential agreement beyond chance was achieved? This is determined by comparing it to the actual agreement beyond chance of 89 − 59 per cent or 30 per cent, and 30 per cent/41 per cent comes to 0.73, which means that about three-quarters of the potential agreement beyond chance was achieved by our two clinicians. This measure of agreement goes by the name kappa, and is rather like a correlation coefficient. It ranges from − 1.0 (where two clinicians would be in total disagreement), through 0.0 (where only chance agreement was accomplished), to + 1.0 (where two clinicians would be in perfect agreement). As you can see in the listing of 'conventional levels of kappa' that appears at the bottom of Fig. 2, the agreement between our two clinicians is considered 'substantial', and this is the case for many 'present/absent' aspects of the physical examination. As you might imagine, agreement is greater still when the two examinations are made by the same clinician.

Fig. 2 Precision of the clinical examination for spider naevi.

		First clinician's examination for spider naevi: Positive	Negative	
Second clinician's examination for spider naevi	Positive	23 (expect 8)	5	28
		a	b	a+b
		c	d	c+d
	Negative	6	66 (expect 51)	72
		a+c	b+d	a+b+c+d
		29	71	100

Observed agreement:
- $(a+d)/(a+b+c+d) = (23+66)/100 = 89$ per cent

Expected agreement:
- For cell a: $([a+b]\times[a+c])/(a+b+c+d) = (28\times29)/100 = 8$
- For cell *d*: $([c+d]\times[b+d])/(a+b+c+d) = (72\times71)/100 = 51$
- (expected a + expected d)$/(a+b+c+d) = (8+51)/100 = 59$ per cent

Agreement beyond chance = kappa:

$$\frac{\text{Observed agreement (\%)} - \text{expected agreement (\%)}}{100\% - \text{expected agreement (\%)}} = \frac{89-59}{100-59} = 0.73$$

Conventional levels of kappa:
- 0.0–0.2, 'slight agreement'
- 0.2–0.4, 'fair agreement'
- 0.4–0.6, 'moderate agreement'
- 0.6–0.8, 'substantial agreement'
- 0.8–1.0, 'almost perfect agreement'

Other aspects of the clinical examination do not fare as well. For example, in one study of examination of the chest, the kappas for cyanosis, tachypnoea, and whispering pectoriloquy were 0.36, 0.25, and 0.11, respectively.

The conclusion here is clear. Proficiency in clinical skills includes knowing which signs and symptoms are sufficiently precise to be clinically useful. However, precision is not enough; the symptoms and signs we seek must also accurately detect the patient's underlying anatomy, physiology, and disease state.

Accuracy

For example, questioning patients about their use of alcohol provides notoriously inaccurate accounts of their actual consumption of alcohol. For this reason, clinicians have sought more accurate methods of taking an alcohol history, and many now use a simple, four-question approach:

1. Have you ever felt you should *C*ut down on your drinking?
2. Have people *A*nnoyed you by criticizing your drinking?
3. Have you ever felt bad or *G*uilty about your drinking?
4. Have you ever had a drink first thing in the morning to steady your nerves or to get rid of a hangover (*E*ye-opener)?

This quick and easy approach, known by its acronym CAGE, has now been studied in several settings, and a typical result is shown in Fig. 3,

Fig. 3 The CAGE questions for alcohol abuse/dependency.

		Alcohol abuse or dependency: Yes	No	
Number of positive answers to the 4 CAGE questions	3 or 4	60 (true +)	1 (false +)	61
		a	b	a+b
		c	d	c+d
	2,1, or none	57 (false −)	400 (true −)	457
		a+c	b+d	a+b+c+d
		117	401	518

Characteristics:
- $a/(a+c) = 60/117 = 0.51$ or 51 per cent = sensitivity
- $d/(b+d) = 400/401 = 0.998$ or 99.8 per cent = specificity

Predictions:
- $a/(a+b) = 60/61 = 0.98$ or 98 per cent = positive predictive value or post-test probability of having the target disorder (alcohol abuse/dependency) for patients with three or four positive responses
- $d/(c+d) = 400/457 = 0.88$ or 88 per cent = negative predictive value or post-test probability of not having the target disorder for patients with two or fewer positive responses
- $c/(c+d) = 57/457 = 0.12$ or 12 per cent = post-test probability of having the target disorder for patients with two or fewer positive responses

Pre-test probability (prevalence):
- $(a+c)/(a+b+c+d) = 117/518 = 23$ per cent = prevalence or pre-test probability of having the target disorder

which shows the number of positive answers to the CAGE questions from two different groups of patients admitted to the orthopaedic or medical services of a community-based teaching hospital in Boston, Massachusetts. In the left-hand column are the responses from patients whose extensive examination (including, where indicated, detailed social histories, follow-ups, and liver biopsies) provided acceptable 'proof' that they were alcohol abusers or alcohol dependent. In the right-hand column are patients whose examination showed that they were not. These extensive confirmatory investigations often are referred to as 'gold standards' of diagnosis, and typically consist of definitive findings at angiography, operation, autopsy, and the like.

How to read an article about diagnosis

This study is useful to clinicians because the CAGE history and the extensive ('reference' or 'gold' standard) investigations were made independently among a wide range of well-described patients in whom it was clinically reasonable to inquire about alcohol abuse. It thus satisfies the first criterion of a valid, clinically useful article on diagnostic strategies that appears in Table 1 (was there an independent, 'blind' comparison with a 'gold standard' of diagnosis?). Note that the guides in Table 1 can be applied to any clinical articles that make claims about the usefulness of (especially new) diagnostic tests, whether done at the bedside on the whole patient or in the laboratory on body fluids or other samples from the patient. The study that generated Fig. 3 also satisfied the second, common-sense guide as well, for it was made on a sample of patients that included an appropriate range of mild and severe, treated and untreated alcoholics, plus individuals with different but commonly confused disorders. The questions were presented with their exact wording in the article, satisfying the fourth guide, permitting their exact application in the reader's own practice.

Having evaluated the validity of an article on diagnostic testing, and interpreted the results (more details to follow), the reader is left with the question: 'How will this article help me in caring for my patients?' Another set of questions addresses this issue (Table 1). The setting for the CAGE study (a large, urban general hospital) was described, satisfying the seventh guide and permitting us to determine the applicability of the results to our own setting. The eighth guide (will the results of this test change my management?) is satisfied to the extent that the CAGE questions recognized far more alcoholics and, especially, alcohol abusers than routine clinical diagnosis, and made them candidates for treatment and counselling. (We will return to the sixth guide of reproducibility later.)

In summary, the CAGE study observed most of the methodological standards required for a valid and clinically useful description of the usefulness of any diagnostic information, whether it comes from the history, the physical examination, or the diagnostic laboratory.

Table 1 *Readers' guides for an article about a diagnostic test*

I. *Are the results in the study valid?*
A. Primary guides
1. Was there an independent, blind comparison with a 'gold' or 'diagnostic' standard?
2. Did the patient sample include an appropriate range of the sort of patients to whom the diagnostic test will be applied in clinical practice?
B. Secondary guides
3. Was the decision to preform the reference standard independent of the results of the test being evaluated?
4. Were the details of the test described in sufficient detail to permit their exact replication?

II. *What are the results?*
5. Are likelihood ratios for a different level of test results presented, or data necessary for their calculation included?

III. *Will the results help me in caring for my patients?*
6. Will the test be interpreted reproducibly and consistently in my setting?
7. Are the results applicable to my patient?
8. Will the results change my management?
9. Will patients be better off as a result of the test?

SENSITIVITY, SPECIFICITY, AND PREDICTIVE VALUE

Returning our attention to Fig. 3, we can examine the accuracy characteristics of the CAGE questions. The 60 patients in cell a of Fig. 3 answered 'yes' to three or four of the CAGE questions, and constitute 51 per cent or 0.51 of all the 117 patients $(a + c)$ with a positive diagnosis of alcohol dependency/abuse. The shorthand term for this proportion of 0.51, or $a/(a + c)$ is 'sensitivity', and it is a useful measure of how well a diagnostic test (whether a symptom, sign, or laboratory test) detects a target disorder when it is present. The closer the sensitivity to 100 per cent, the more 'sensitive' the clinical or laboratory finding.

In the right-hand column of Fig. 3 are the responses from patients in whom the 'gold standard' ruled out the diagnosis of problem drinking. The 400 patients in cell d answered 'yes' to two, only one, or none of the CAGE questions, and constitute 99.8 per cent or 0.998 of all the 401 patients $(b + d)$ who did not have alcohol dependency/abuse. The shorthand term for this proportion of 0.998 or $d/(b + d)$ is 'specificity', and it is a useful measure of how often a symptom, sign or other diagnostic test is absent when the target disorder is not present. The closer the specificity to 100 per cent, the more 'specific' the clinical or laboratory finding.

You will note that the sensitivity of the CAGE questions is not very impressive. The number of 'true positives' in cell a are almost equalled by the number of 'false negatives' in cell c, and the sensitivity of only 51 per cent confirms that it 'misses' about half the problem drinkers. On the other hand, the specificity of the CAGE questions is outstanding. The number of 'true negatives' in cell d vastly outnumbers the number of 'false positives' in cell b, and the specificity of 99.8 per cent confirms that it almost never labels a patient as a problem drinker erroneously.

Now we can consider the 'predictions' we make about our patient based on the foregoing characteristics. Because of the very high specificity, virtually every patient in cell a who answered 'yes' to three or four of the CAGE questions $(a + b)$ has the target disorder, alcohol abuse/dependency. The shorthand term for this proportion $a/(a + b)$, which is 60/61 or 98 per cent, is the 'positive predictive value' or 'post-test probability of having the target disorder' (among patients with three or more positive answers). Moreover, despite the rather unimpressive sensitivity, most of the patients in cells c and d who answered 'yes' to none, just one, or two of the CAGE questions were in cell d and did not have the target disorder. The shorthand term for this proportion $d/(c + d)$, which is 400/457 or 88 per cent, is the 'negative predictive value' or 'post-test probability of not having the target disorder' among those patients with two or fewer positive answers. The complement of this negative predictive value, or $c/(c + d)$, describes the post-test probability of having the disorder among those patients with two or fewer positive answers, and this other way of saying the same thing is found useful by some clinicians.

The effect of prevalence on predictive value

The reason that the negative predictive value looks relatively high, despite the low sensitivity, lies in the fact that the proportion of all patients in this study who had alcohol dependency/abuse, $(a + c)/(a + b + c + d)$ or 117/518, was only 23 per cent to begin with. That is, 100 − 23 per cent (or 77 per cent) of the patients were not alcohol dependent before they were asked any questions. The shorthand term for the prior knowledge contained in this $(a + c)/(a + b + c + d)$ is 'prevalence' or, more usefully, the 'pre-test probability' of the target disorder. (Because this pre-test probability is the starting point for making clinical use of the test characteristics, we will place it above the 'predictions' entries in subsequent figures.)

In contrast to the pre-test probability of 23 per cent in the clinical article describing the CAGE questions, suppose that you judge that the pre-test probability of alcohol abuse/dependency in your patient is 50 per cent. How would the CAGE questions perform in patients like yours? If the patients in the study summarized in Fig. 3 were like your own patient, you should expect the result shown in Fig. 4. Sensitivity and specificity would remain constant, despite changes from the study's to our patient's pre-test probability of the target disorder. Thus, the sensitivity (51 per cent) and specificity (99.8 per cent) in Fig. 4 are the same as those in Fig. 3.

Notice, however, that the negative predictive value has fallen from 88 per cent to 67 per cent. This is because predictive values must change with changes in the prevalence of the target disorder. One useful way to think about this is to carry through this concept of prevalence. After all, the predictive value of a positive test result is simply the prevalence of the target disorder among those patients with positive test results. Similarly, the negative predictive value is the prevalence of not having the target disorder among patients with a negative test result. No wonder, then, that predictive values must change with a change in the overall prevalence of the target disorder.

LIKELIHOOD RATIOS

Many articles on the accuracy of diagnostic information describe not only the sensitivity and specificity of specific symptoms and sign, but also their 'likelihood ratios'. This method of describing the accuracy of diagnostic information, once mastered, is much faster and more powerful than the sensitivity and specificity approach. It is shown in Fig. 5 for the CAGE questions. In brief, a likelihood ratio (or **LR** for short) expresses the odds that a given finding on the history or physical examination would occur in a patient with, as opposed to a patient without, the target disorder. When the likelihood ratio of a finding is above 1.0, the probability of disease goes up (because the finding is more likely among patients with, than without, the disorder); when the likelihood ratio is below 1.0, the probability of disease goes down (because the finding is less likely among patients with, than without, the disorder); finally, when the likelihood ratio is close to 1.0, the probability of disease is unchanged (because the finding is equally likely in patients with, and without, the disorder).

Likelihood ratios are related to sensitivity and specificity, but possess some advantages for clinicians. In a 'two-by-two' table such as Fig. 3, the likelihood ratio for a positive CAGE questionnaire is equal to sensitivity/(1 − specificity) or 0.51/0.002 or 255, indicating that a positive history is over 250 times as likely to be obtained from a patient with, as opposed to a patient without, an alcohol problem. The likelihood ratio for a negative CAGE questionnaire is equal to (1 − sensitivity)/specificity or 0.49/0.998 or .49, indicating that a negative history is about half as likely to be obtained from a patient with, as opposed to a patient without, an alcohol problem.

The first advantage of likelihood ratios is that the likelihood ratio for a given finding, when applied to the pre-test odds of the target disorder, generates the post-test odds for that disorder. As the likelihood ratio is expressed as an odds, this may at first appear cumbersome, for it means that the pre-test probability must also be expressed as an odds. However, the necessity for converting probability to odds and back again can be obviated by using the nomogram shown in Fig. 6. Suppose that your patient, in whom you judged the pre-test probability of alcohol abuse to be 50 per cent, answers two of the four CAGE questions with a 'yes'. Anchoring a straight edge at 50 per cent along the left margin of the nomogram, and rotating it until it intersects the centre LR line at 8, the post-test probability can be found at the right margin, and it is almost 90 per cent (88.9 per cent), making the diagnosis highly likely.

The second advantage of likelihood ratios becomes apparent when we see that the nomogram permits us to determine the probability of alcohol abuse when the pre-test probability changes from patient to patient. We can simply re-anchor the straight edge at any pre-test prob-

Fig. 4 The CAGE questions for alcohol abuse/dependency when the pre-test probability is 50 per cent.

		Alcohol abuse or dependency: Yes	Alcohol abuse or dependency: No	
Number of positive answers to the 4 CAGE questions	3 or 4	510 (true +) *a*	2 (false +) *b*	512 *a+b*
	2,1, or none	490 (false −) *c*	998 (true −) *d*	1488 *c+d*
		1000 *a+c*	1000 *b+d*	2000 *a+b+c+d*

Characteristics:
- *a*/(*a*+*c*) = 510/1000 = 0.51 or 51 per cent = sensitivity
- *d*/(*b*+*d*) = 998/1000 = 0.998 or 99.8 per cent = specificity

Pre-test probability (prevalence):
- (*a*+*c*)/(*a*+*b*+*c*+*d*) = 1000/2000 = 50 per cent = prevalence or pre-test probability of having the target disorder

Predictions:
- *a*/(*a*+*b*) = 510/512 = 0.996 or 99.6 per cent = positive predictive value or post-test probability of having the target disorder for patients with three or four positive responses
- *d*/(*c*+*d*) = 998/1488 = 0.67 or 67 per cent = negative predictive value or post-test probability of not having the target disorder for patients with two or fewer positive responses
- *c*/(*c*+*d*) = 490/1488 = 0.33 or 33 per cent = post-test probability of having the target disorder for patients with two or fewer positive responses

Fig. 5 Multiple levels of responses to the CAGE questions for alcohol abuse/dependency.

		Alcohol abuse or dependency: Yes	Alcohol abuse or dependency: No	Likelihood ratios
Number of positive answers to the 4 CAGE questions	4	23 (0.20)	0 (0)	∞
	3	37 (0.32)	1 (0.002)	160
	2	28 (0.24)	14 (0.03)	8
	1	11 (0.09)	28 (0.07)	1.3
	0	18 (0.15)	358 (0.89)	0.17
		117 (1.00)	401 (1.00)	

ability and run it across the LR that corresponds to the diagnostic test result.

The third advantage of likelihood ratios is that, unlike sensitivity and specificity (which limit the number of test results to just two levels, 'positive' and 'negative'), likelihood ratios can be generated for multiple levels of the diagnostic test result. This is particularly useful for test results expressed as continuous rather than dichotomous variables. At each level, the proportion of patients with the target disorder at this level is divided by the proportion of patients who do not have the target disorder at this same level; the result is the likelihood ratio for this level. This was shown in Fig. 5, where likelihood ratios for four, three, two, one, and no positive responses to the CAGE questionnaire are shown (the awkward, infinitely high likelihood ratio for four positive answers can be avoided if three and four positive answers are combined, generating a likelihood ratio of 255 for the combination).

The fourth advantage of the likelihood ratio strategy is that the post-test probability of the target disorder (say, the nephrotic syndrome) obtained from the first item of diagnostic information (say, a history of ankle swelling) is the pre-test probability of that diagnosis for the next item of diagnostic information (say, the physical examination for ankle oedema). The post-test probability (after physical examination) of nephrotic syndrome then becomes the pre-test probability for the next test (say, a 24-h urine analysis). This example also identifies the problem we always face when we combine diagnostic information from the history, physical, laboratory, and radiological tests: the results of the history and physical examination are not independent of each other. Thus, a patient with a positive history of swollen ankles is far more likely to have pedal oedema than a patient with a negative history, and we must either employ a likelihood ratio that considers both the two items as a pair, or modify the likelihood ratio for the second, based on the results of the first.

Fig. 6 The likelihood ratio nomogram. (Reproduced from Sackett, D. L., Haynes, R. B., Guyatt, G. H., and Tugwell, P. (1991). *Clinical epidemiology: a basic science for clinical medicine*. 2nd edn. p. 124. Little, Brown, London.)

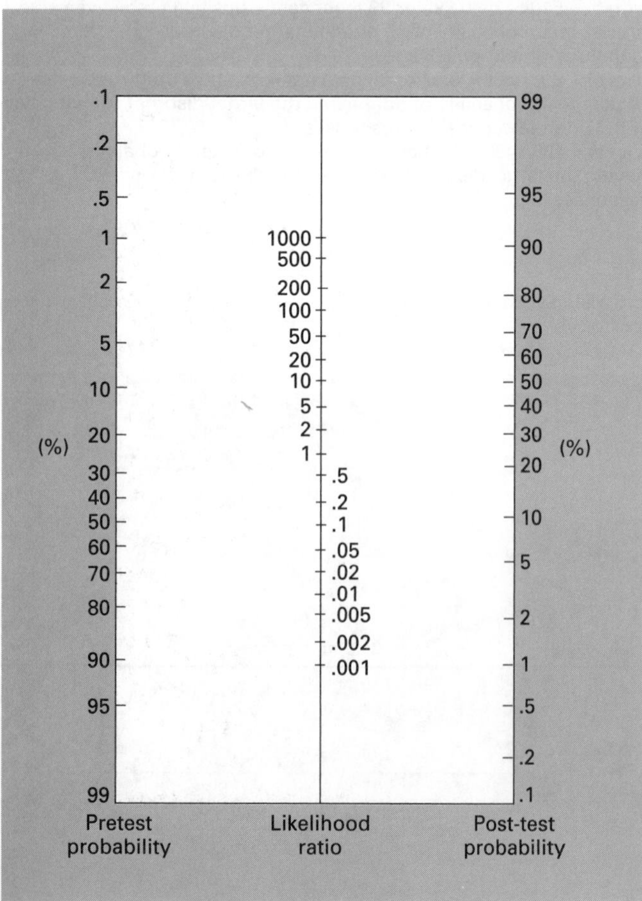

The use of likelihood ratios in interpreting diagnostic (laboratory and radiological) test results is very empowering for the clinician. Textbooks are now available that provide access to more and better information on pretest likelihoods and likelihood ratios for continuous and multilevel test results for a broad range of clinical problems.

Let us suppose that a 54-year-old man with congestive heart failure develops dyspnoea and hypoxaemia (Po_2 of 50 mmHg on room air) without any new significant changes on his electrocardiogram or chest radiograph. If the pre-test probability estimate for pulmonary embolism is high (80 per cent), a high-probability finding on a ventilation/perfusion scan (LR 15) would result in a post-test likelihood of 98 per cent. An indeterminate (LR 1) or low-probability (LR 0.3) ventilation/perfusion scan would result in a post-test probability of 85 and 60 per cent, respectively. If the pre-test probability of a pulmonary embolism were lower (50 per cent), and a high-probability, intermediate- or low-probability lung scan were found, the post-test likelihoods would be 95, 50 and 25 per cent, respectively. A completely normal lung scan would exclude the diagnosis.

Conclusion

Over the last decade, there have been important advances in clinical methods. We are moving from intuitive, informal judgement based on experience alone to a more formal process in which evidence from studies of groups of similar patients increasingly influences the practitioner's judgement. This formal process is gaining momentum through several routes, both in the training of physicians in 'evidence-based medicine' and in the publication of overviews of the most precise and accurate diagnostic tests and the most efficacious treatments. While the interplay of careful history-taking skills, expertise in conducting a physical examination, intuition, sensitivity, understanding of pathophysiology, and clinical experience will always create and mould the superior physician, the addition of some practical strategies and tactics of clinical epidemiology will prepare the contemporary physician for the year 2000.

REFERENCES

Barrows, H.S., Norman, G.R., Neufeld, V.R., and Feightner, J.W. (1982). The clinical reasoning of randomly selected physicians in general medical practice. *Clinical and Investigative Medicine*, **5**, 49–55. This article nicely summarizes the thought processes of clinicians who were captured on videotape as they examined a group of 'programmed' patients.

Bush, B., Shaw, S., Cleary, P., Delbanco, T.L., and Aronson, M.D. (1987). Screening for alcohol abuse using the CAGE questionnaire. *American Journal of Medicine*, **82**, 231–5. The raw data used in this chapter, and a good example of the modern approach to the evaluation of clinical method.

Chalmers, I., Enkin, M., and Keirse, M.J.N.C. (ed.) (1989). *Effective care in pregnancy and childbirth*. Oxford University Press. This landmark text provides authoritative overviews of thousands of randomized trials of interventions in pregnancy and childbirth, and is the harbinger of similar texts in other fields.

Evidence-based Medicine Working Group, McMaster University Faculty of Health Sciences. (1992). Evidence-based medicine: a new approach to teaching the practice of medicine. *Journal of the American Medical Association*, **268**, 2420–5. This article describes a paradigm shift in postgraduate medical education: the rise of evidence-based medicine, which complements clinical judgement and pathophysiological rationale with efficient literature searching and the application of formal rules of evidence in evaluating the clinical literature.

Kuhns, L.R., Thornbury, J.R., and Fryback, D.G. (1989). *Decision making in imaging*. Yearbook Medical, Chicago. This text summarizes the sensitivities, specificities, likelihood ratios, and rational use of xrays and other diagnostic imaging procedures.

Panzer, R.J., Black, E.R., and Griner, P.F. (1991). *Diagnostic strategies for common medical problems*, (2nd edn). American College of Physicians,

Washington DC. This text presents the sensitivities, specificities, and likelihood ratios for a wide array of diagnostic tests, as well as typical pretest probabilities for the target disorders which prompt their execution. It is an example of the modern era in medical texts.

Sackett, D.L. (1992). A primer on the precision and accuracy of the clinical examination. *Journal of the American Medical Association*, **267,** 2638–44. This article inaugurated a new series on 'The Rational Clinical Examination' in this journal.

Sackett, D.L., Haynes, R.B., Guyatt, G.H., and Tugwell, P. (1991). *Clinical epidemiology: a basic science for clinical medicine*, (2nd edn). Little, Brown, London. This book forms much of the chapter, and provides an expanded discussion and bibliography for those who wish to read further.

Williams, J.W. and Simel, D.L. (1992). Does this patient have ascites? How to define fluid in the abdomen. *Journal of the American Medical Association*, **267,** 2645–8. One of a series of overviews describing the precision and accuracy of individual components of the history and physical examination, appearing in this journal under the title 'The Rational Clinical Examination'.

2.4 Large-scale randomized evidence: trials and overviews

R. Collins, R. Peto, R. Gray, and S. Parish

INTRODUCTION AND SUMMARY

This chapter is intended principally for practising clinicians who need to use the results of clinical trials in their routine practice, and who want to know why some types of evidence are much more reliable than others. It is concerned with treatments that might improve survival (or some other major aspect of long-term disease outcome) and its chief point is that, as long as doctors start with a healthy scepticism about the many apparently striking claims that appear in the medical literature, trials do make sense. The main enemy of common-sense is over-optimism: there are a few striking exceptions, where treatments for serious disease really do turn out to work extremely well, but in general most of the claims of vast improvements from new therapies turn out to be evanescent. Hence, clinical trials need to be able to detect or to refute more moderate differences in long-term outcome. Once this common-sense idea is explicitly recognized, the rest follows naturally and it becomes obvious what types of evidence can and cannot be trusted. Although the chapter may also be of some interest or encouragement to doctors who are considering participating in (or even planning) large trials, its main intended readers are practising clinicians. For, even the most definite results from large-scale randomized evidence cannot save lives unless such practitioners accept and apply them. The chapter does not include large amounts of statistical detail: instead, it tries to communicate the spirit that underlies the increasing emphasis on large-scale randomized evidence that has developed over the last decade.

Unrealistic hopes about the chances of discovering large treatment effects can be a serious obstacle not only to appropriate patient care but also to good clinical research. For, such hopes may misleadingly suggest to some research workers or funding agencies that small or even non-randomized studies may suffice. In contrast, realistically moderate expectations of what treatment might achieve (or, if one treatment is to be compared with another, realistically moderate expectations of how large any difference between these treatments is likely to be) should tend to foster the design of studies that aim to discriminate reliably between (a) differences in outcome that are realistically moderate but still worthwhile, and (b) differences in outcome that are too small to be of any material importance. Studies with this particular aim must guarantee strict control of bias (which, in general, requires proper randomization and appropriate statistical analysis, with no unduly 'data-dependent' emphasis on specific parts of the overall evidence) and strict control of the play of chance (which, in general, requires large numbers rather than much detail). The conclusion is obvious: moderate biases and moderate random errors must both be avoided if moderate benefits are to be assessed or refuted reliably. This leads to the need for large numbers of properly randomized patients, which in turn leads to both large simple randomized trials (or 'mega-trials') and large systematic overviews (or 'meta-analyses') of related randomized trials.

Non-randomized evidence, unduly small randomized trials, or unduly small overviews of trials are all much inferior as sources of evidence about current patient management or as foundations for future research strategies. They cannot discriminate reliably between moderate (but worthwhile) differences and negligible differences in outcome, and the mistaken clinical conclusions that they engender could well result in the undertreatment, overtreatment, or other mismanagement of millions of future patients worldwide. In contrast, hundreds of thousands of premature deaths each year could be avoided by seeking appropriately large-scale randomized evidence about various widely practicable treatments for the common causes of death, and by disseminating such evidence appropriately. Likewise, appropriately large-scale randomized evidence could substantially improve the management of many important, but non-fatal, medical problems.

The value of large-scale randomized evidence is illustrated in this chapter by the trials of fibrinolytic therapy for acute myocardial infarction, antiplatelet therapy for a wide range of vascular conditions, hormonal therapy for early breast cancer, and drug therapy for lowering blood pressure. In these examples proof of benefit that could not have been achieved by either small-scale randomized evidence or non-randomized evidence has led to widespread changes in practice that are now preventing tens of thousands of premature deaths each year.

MODERATE (BUT WORTHWHILE) EFFECTS ON MAJOR OUTCOMES ARE GENERALLY MORE PLAUSIBLE THAN LARGE EFFECTS

Some treatments have large, and hence obvious, effects on survival: for example, it is clear without randomized trials that prompt treatment of diabetic coma or cardiac arrest saves lives (and, indeed, a plaque at the entrance to our own hospital records the first clinical use of penicillin). However, perhaps in part because of these striking successes, for the past few decades the hopes of large treatment effects on mortality and major morbidity in other serious diseases have been unrealistically high. Of course, treatments do quite commonly have large effects on various less fundamental measures: drugs readily reduce blood pressure, blood lipids, or blood glucose; many tumours or leukaemias can be controlled temporarily by radiotherapy or chemotherapy; in acute myocardial infarction, lidocaine can prevent many arrhythmias and streptokinase can dissolve most coronary thrombi; in early HIV infection, antiretroviral drugs substantially reduce viraemia. However, although all these effects are large, any effects on mortality are much more modest; indeed, there is still dispute as to whether any net improvement in survival is provided by the routine use of radiotherapy for common cancers, lidocaine for acute myocardial infarction, or antiretroviral agents for early HIV infection.

Table 1 *Requirements for reliable assessment of moderate effects: negligible biases and small random errors*

NEGLIGIBLE BIASES
(i.e. guaranteed avoidance of moderate biases)
- **Proper randomization**
(non-randomized methods might suffer moderate biases)
- **Analysis by allocated treatment**
(including all randomized patients: 'intention-to-treat' analysis)
- **Chief emphasis on overall results**
(no unduly data-dependent emphasis on particular subgroups)
- **Systematic overview of all relevant randomized trials**
(no unduly data-dependent emphasis on particular studies)

SMALL RANDOM ERRORS
(i.e. guaranteed avoidance of moderate random errors)
- **Large numbers in any new trials**
(to be really large, trials should be 'streamlined')
- **Systematic overviews of all relevant randomized trials**
(which yield the largest possible total numbers)

In general, if substantial uncertainty remains about the efficacy of a practicable treatment, its effects on major end-points are probably either negligibly small, or only moderate, rather than large. Indirect support for this rather pessimistic conclusion comes from many sources, including: the previous few decades of disappointingly slow progress in the curative treatment of the common chronic diseases of middle age; the heterogeneity of each single disease, as evidenced by the unpredictability of survival duration even when apparently similar patients are compared with each other; the variety of different mechanisms in certain diseases that can lead to death, only one of which may be appreciably influenced by any one particular therapy; the modest effects often suggested by systematic overviews (see later) of various therapies; and, in certain special cases, observational epidemiological studies of the strength of the relationship between some disease and the factor that the treatment will modify (for example, blood pressure, blood cholesterol, or blood glucose: see later).

Having accepted that only moderate reductions in mortality are likely with many currently available interventions, how worthwhile might such effects be if they could be detected reliably? To some clinicians, reducing the risk of early death in patients with myocardial infarction from 10 per 100 patients down to 9 or 8 per 100 patients treated may not seem particularly worthwhile, and if such a reduction was only transient, or involved an extremely expensive or toxic treatment, this might well be an appropriate view. Worldwide, however, several million patients a year suffer an acute myocardial infarction, and if just one million were to be given a simple, non-toxic, and widely practicable treatment that reduced the risk of early death from 10 per cent down to 9 or 8 per cent (i.e. a proportional reduction of 10 or 20 per cent), this would avoid 10 000–20 000 deaths. (For example, about half a million patients a year now receive fibrinolytic therapy for acute myocardial infarction, avoiding about 10 000 early deaths, and large trials have shown that this difference in early mortality persists for several years afterwards.) Such absolute gains are substantial, and might considerably exceed the numbers of lives that could be saved by a much more effective treatment of a much less common disease.

RELIABLE DETECTION OR REFUTATION OF MODERATE DIFFERENCES REQUIRES AVOIDANCE OF BOTH MODERATE BIASES AND MODERATE RANDOM ERRORS

If realistically moderate differences in outcome are to be reliably detected or reliably refuted, then errors in comparative assessments of the effects of treatment need to be much smaller than the difference between a moderate but worthwhile effect and an effect that is too small to be of any material importance. This in turn implies that moderate biases and moderate random errors cannot be tolerated. The only way to guarantee very small random errors is to study really large numbers, and this can be achieved in two main ways: make individual studies large, and combine information from as many relevant studies as possible in systematic overviews (Table 1). However, it is not much use to have very small random errors if there may well be moderate biases, so even the large sizes of some non-randomized analyses of computerized hospital records cannot guarantee medically reliable comparisons between the effects of different treatments.

AVOIDING MODERATE BIASES

Proper randomization avoids systematic differences between the types of patient in different treatment groups

The fundamental reason for randomization is to avoid moderate bias by ensuring that each type of patient can be expected to have been allocated in similar proportions to the different treatment strategies that are to be compared, so that only random differences should affect the final comparisons of outcome. Non-randomized methods, in contrast, cannot generally guarantee that the types of patient given the study treatment do not differ systematically in any important ways from the types of patient given any other treatment(s) with which the study treatment is to be compared. For example, moderate biases might arise if the study treatment was novel and doctors were afraid to use it for the most seriously ill patients or, conversely, if they were more ready to use it for those who were desperately ill. There may also be other ways in which the severity of the condition differentially affects the likelihood of being assigned to different treatments by the doctor's choice (or by any other non-random procedure).

It might appear at first sight that by collecting enough information about various prognostic features it would be possible to make some mathematical adjustments that would correct for any such differences between the types of patients who, in a non-randomized study, receive the different treatments that are to be compared. The hope is that such methods (which are sometimes called 'outcomes analyses') might achieve comparability between those entering the different treatment groups, but they cannot be guaranteed to do so. For, some important prognostic factors may be unrecorded, while others may be difficult to assess exactly and hence difficult to adjust for. There are two reasons for this difficulty. First, it is often not realized that even if there are no systematic differences between one treatment group and another in the accuracy with which prognostic factors are recorded, purely random errors in assessing prognostic factors can introduce systematic biases into the statistically adjusted comparison between treatments in a non-randomized study. Second, in a non-randomized comparison the care with which prognostic factors are recorded may differ between one treatment group and another. Doctors studying a novel treatment may investigate their patients particularly carefully, and, perhaps surprisingly, this extra accuracy can introduce a moderate bias. For example, an unusually careful search of the axilla among women with early breast cancer will sometimes result in the discovery of tiny deposits of cancer cells that would normally have been overlooked, and hence some women who would have been classified as stage I will be reclassified as stage II. The prognosis of these 'down-staged' women is worse than that of those who remain as stage I but better than that of those already classified as stage II by less intensive investigation. Paradoxically, therefore, such down-staging improves not only the average prognosis of stage I breast cancer but also the average prognosis of stage II breast cancer, biasing any non-randomized comparison with other average women with stage I or stage II disease for whom the staging was less careful.

The machinery of a properly randomised trial: no foreknowledge of treatment allocation, no bias in patient management, unbiased outcome assessment, and no post-randomization exclusions

No foreknowledge of what the next treatment will be

In a properly randomized trial, the decision to enter a patient is made irreversibly and in ignorance of which of the trial treatments he or she will be allocated. The treatment allocation is made after trial entry has been decided upon. (The purpose of this sequence is to ensure that foreknowledge of what the next treatment is going to be cannot affect the decision to enter the patient; if it did, those allocated one treatment might differ systematically from those allocated another.) Ideally, any major prognostic features should also be irreversibly recorded before the treatment is revealed, particularly if these are to be used in any treatment analyses. For, if the recorded value of some prognostic factor might be affected by knowledge of the trial treatment allocation, then treatment comparisons within subgroups that are defined by that factor might be moderately biased. In particular, treatment comparisons just among 'responders' or just among 'non-responders' can be extremely misleading unless the response is assessed before treatment allocation.

No bias in patient management or in outcome assessment

An additional difficulty, in both randomized and non-randomized comparisons of various treatments, is that there might be systematic differences in the use of other treatments (including general supportive care) or in the assessment of major outcomes. A non-randomized comparison may well suffer from moderate biases due to such systematic differences in ancillary care or assessment, particularly if it merely involves retrospective review of medical records. In the context of a randomized comparison, however, it is generally possible to devise ways to keep any such biases small. For example, placebo tablets may be given to control-allocated patients and certain subjective assessments may be 'blinded' (although this is less important in studies assessing mortality).

'Intention-to-treat' analyses with no post-randomization exclusions

Even in a properly randomized trial, unnecessary biases may be introduced by inappropriate statistical analysis. One of the most important sources of bias in the analysis is undue concentration on just one part of the evidence, i.e. on 'data-derived subgroup analyses' (see below). Another bias, which is easily avoided, is caused by post-randomization exclusion of patients, particularly if the type (and prognosis) of those excluded from one treatment group differs from that of those excluded from another. Therefore the fundamental statistical analysis of a trial should compare all those originally allocated one treatment (even though some of them may not have actually received it) with all those allocated the other treatment (i.e. it should be an 'intention-to-treat' analysis). Additional analyses can also be reported: for example, in describing the frequency of some very specific side-effect it may be preferable to record its incidence only among those who actually received the treatment. (This is because strictly randomized comparisons may not be needed to assess extreme relative risks.) However, in assessing the overall outcome, such 'on-treatment' analyses can be misleading, and 'intention-to-treat' analyses are generally a more trustworthy guide as to whether there is any real difference between the trial treatments in their effects on long-term outcome.

Problems produced by data-dependent emphasis on particular results

Treatment that is appropriate for one patient may be inappropriate for another. Ideally, therefore, what is wanted is not only an answer to the question 'Is this treatment helpful on average for a wide range of patients?', but also an answer to the question 'For which recognizable categories of patient is this treatment helpful?'. However, this ideal is difficult to attain directly because the direct use of clinical trial results in particular subgroups of patients is surprisingly unreliable. Even if the real sizes of the effects of treatment in specific subgroups are importantly different, standard subgroup analyses are so statistically insensitive that they may well fail to demonstrate these differences. Conversely, even if there is a highly significant 'interaction' (i.e. an apparent difference between the sizes of the therapeutic effects in different subgroups) and the results seem to suggest that the treatment works in some subgroups but not in others (thereby giving the appearance of a 'qualitative interaction'), this may still not be good evidence for subgroup-specific treatment preferences.

Table 2 *False-negative mortality effect in a subgroup defined only by the astrological birth sign: the ISIS-2 (1988) trial of aspirin among over 17 000 acute myocardial infarction patients*

Astrological birth sign	No. of 1 month deaths (aspirin vs. placebo)	Statistical significance
Libra or Gemini	150 vs. 147	NS
All other signs	654 vs. 869	$2P < 0.000001$
Any birth sign*	804 vs. 1016 (9.4%) (11.8%)	$2P < 0.000001$

*Appropriate overall analysis for assessing the true effect in all subgroups.

Questions about such interactions between patient characteristics and the effects of treatment are easy to ask, but are surprisingly difficult to answer reliably. Apparent interactions can often be produced by the play of chance and, in particular subgroups, can mimic or obscure some of the moderate treatment effects that might realistically be expected. To demonstrate this, a subgroup analysis was performed based on the astrological birth signs of patients randomized in the very large Second International Study of Infarct Survival (ISIS-2) trial of the treatment of acute myocardial infarction. Overall in this trial, the 1 month survival advantage produced by aspirin was particularly clearly demonstrated (804 vascular deaths among 8587 patients allocated aspirin versus 1016 among 8600 allocated control; 23 per cent reduction, two-sided P value < 0.000001). However, when these aspirin analyses were subdivided by the patients' astrological birth signs, to illustrate the unreliability of subgroup analyses, aspirin appeared totally ineffective for those born under Libra or Gemini (Table 2). It would obviously be unwise to conclude from such a result that patients born under the sign of Libra or Gemini should not be given this particular treatment. However, similar conclusions based on 'exploratory' data-derived subgroup analyses that, from a purely statistical viewpoint, are no more reliable than these are often reported and believed, with inappropriate effects on practice.

There are three main remedies for this unavoidable conflict between the reliable subgroup-specific conclusions that doctors want and the unreliable findings that direct subgroup analyses can usually offer. However, the extent to which these remedies are helpful in particular instances is one on which informed judgements differ.

First, where there are good *a priori* reasons for anticipating that the effects of treatment might be different in different circumstances then a limited number of subgroup analyses may be *pre*-specified in the study protocol, along with a prediction of the direction of such proposed interactions. (For example, it was expected that the benefits of fibrinolytic therapy for acute myocardial infarction would be greater the earlier patients were treated, and so some studies pre-specified analyses subdivided by time from onset of symptoms to treatment: see later.) These pre-specified subgroup-specific analyses are then to be taken much more seriously than other subgroup analyses.

The second approach is to emphasize chiefly the overall results of a trial (or, better still, of all such trials) for particular outcomes as a guide to—or at least a context for speculation about—the qualitative results in various specific subgroups of patients, and to give less weight to the actual results in each separate subgroup. This is clearly the right way to interpret the findings in Table 2, but it is also likely in many other circumstances to provide the best assessment of whether one treatment is better than another in particular subgroups. Of course, the extrapolation needs to be performed in a sensible way. For example, if one treatment has substantial side-effects, it may be inappropriate for low risk patients. (In this case, the side-effects in a particular subgroup and the proportional benefit in that subgroup should be estimated separately, but the estimation for both might be more reliable if based on an appropriate extrapolation from the overall results rather than on the results in that one subgroup alone.)

The third approach is to be influenced, in discussing the likely effects on mortality in specific subgroups, not only by the mortality analyses in these subgroups but also by the analyses of recurrence-free survival or some other major 'surrogate' outcome. For, if the overall results are similar but much more highly significant for recurrence-free survival than for mortality, subgroup analyses with respect to the former may be more stable and may provide a better guide as to whether there are any major differences between subgroups in the effects of treatment (particularly if such subgroup analyses were specified before results were available).

AVOIDING MODERATE RANDOM ERRORS

The need for large-scale randomization

To distinguish reliably between the two alternatives that there is no worthwhile difference in survival or that treatment confers a moderate, but worthwhile, benefit (for example, 10 or 20 per cent fewer deaths), not only must systematic errors be guaranteed to be small (see above) compared with such a moderate risk reduction, but so too must any of the purely random errors that are produced just by chance. Random errors can be reliably avoided only by studying large enough numbers of patients. However, it is not sufficiently widely appreciated just how large clinical trials need to be in order to detect moderate differences reliably. This can be illustrated by a hypothetical trial that is actually quite inadequate—even though by previous standards it is moderately large—in which a 20 per cent reduction in mortality (from 10 to 8 per cent) is supposed to be detected among 2000 heart attack patients (1000 treated and 1000 controls). In this case, one might predict about 100 deaths (10 per cent) in the control group and 80 deaths (8 per cent) in the treated group. However, even if this difference were observed, it would not be conventionally significant ($P = 0.1$), indicating that even if there is no real difference between the effects of the trial treatments, it would still be relatively easy for a result at least as extreme as this to arise by chance alone. Although the play of chance might well increase the difference enough to make it conventionally significant (for example, 110 deaths vs. 70 deaths, $2P < 0.001$), it might equally well dilute, obliterate (for example, 90 deaths vs. 90 deaths), or even reverse it. The situation in real life is often even worse, as the average trial size may be only a few hundred patients rather than the several thousand that would ideally be needed.

Mega-trials: how to randomize large numbers

One of the chief techniques for obtaining appropriately large-scale randomized evidence is to make trials extremely simple, and then to invite hundreds of hospitals to collaborate. The first of these large simple trials (or mega-trials) were the ISIS and GISSI studies of heart attack treatment, and a few other mega-trials have now been undertaken. However, in terms of medically significant findings, what has been achieved so far is only a fraction of what could quite readily be achieved by the assiduous pursuit of such research strategies. Any obstacle to simplicity is an obstacle to large size, and so it is worth making enormous efforts at the design stage to simplify and streamline the process of entering, treating, and assessing patients. Many trials would be of much greater scientific value if they collected 10 times less data, both at entry and during follow-up, on 10 times more patients. It is particularly important to simplify the entry of patients, for if this is not done then rapid recruitment may be difficult. The current fashions for unduly complicated eligibility criteria, overly detailed 'informed' consent, excessive 'quality-of-life' assessments, extensive auditing of data, and measurements of the economic costs of treatment are often inappropriate.

Inappropriate inclusion of cost and of 'quality-of-life' indices

Eventually, the cost-effectiveness of various treatments needs to be assessed, but this does not necessarily imply that costs should be assessed in the same studies in which effectiveness is to be assessed, particularly if attempts to assess costs seriously damage attempts to assess the effects on mortality and major morbidity reliably. Moreover, what really matters is the cost of a treatment in routine practice, not its cost when given in the particular circumstances of a randomized trial.

Likewise, of course, any important ways in which treatments affect the quality of life need to be understood, but again this does not necessarily imply that quality-of-life indices should be assessed in the same trials that assess the main effects of treatment. For, although 20 000 patients may be required for reliable assessment of the effects of treatment on mortality and major morbidity, only a few hundred are likely to be needed for sufficiently reliable assessment of the effects of treatment on various proposed quality-of-life measures (or on costs of treatment). It may be possible to incorporate such assessments within a large mortality study as small sub-studies. But, this may be difficult in practice, and there are many instances where what should be a large simple trial of clinical efficacy should not be jeopardized by the measurement of such factors. Moreover, the effects of a treatment on quality of life in a trial when both the doctors and the patients are uncertain about any clinical benefits of the treatment may differ substantially from its effects on quality of life after the treatment has been shown to improve survival. Hence, it may be better to assess these other outcome measures only after having determined whether the treatment has any worthwhile effects on mortality and major morbidity, and if (as is often the case) it does not then any costs and adverse effects on quality of life may be largely irrelevant.

Simplification of entry procedures for trials: the 'uncertainty principle'

For ethical reasons, patients cannot have their treatment chosen at random if either they or their doctor are already reasonably certain what treatment is preferred. Hence, randomization can be offered only if both doctor and patient feel substantially uncertain as to which of the trial treatments is best. The question then arises: 'Which categories of those about whose treatment there is such uncertainty should be offered randomization?' The obvious answer is all of them, welcoming the heterogeneity that this will produce. (For example, either the treatment of choice will turn out to be the same for men and women, in which case the trial might as well include both, or it will be different, in which case it is particularly important to study both sexes.) In large trials, homogeneity of patients is generally a defect, while heterogeneity is generally a strength. Consider, for example, the trials of fibrinolytic therapy for acute myocardial infarction. Some had restrictive entry criteria that allowed inclusion of only those patients who presented 0–6 h after onset of pain, and so those trials contributed almost nothing to the key question of how late such treatment can still be useful. In contrast, trials with wider and more heterogeneous entry criteria that included some patients with longer delays between pain onset and randomization assessed this question prospectively, and were able to show that fibrinolytic therapy can have definite protective effects when given not only 0–6 but also 7–12 h after onset of pain (see later).

This approach of randomizing a wide range of patients in whom there is substantial uncertainty as to which treatment option is best was used in the Medical Research Council's European Carotid Surgery Trial (ECST), which compared a policy of immediate carotid endarterectomy with a policy of 'watchful waiting' in patients with partial carotid artery stenosis and a recent minor stroke in that part of the brain supplied by the carotid artery. If a patient was prepared at least to consider surgery, then the neurologist and surgeon responsible for that individual's care considered in their own way whatever medical, personal, or other factors seemed to them to be relevant (Fig. 1), including, of course, the patient's own preferences and values.

1. If they were then reasonably certain, for any reason, that they *did wish* to recommend immediate surgery for that particular patient, the patient was ineligible and was not part of ECST.
2. Conversely, if they were reasonably certain, for any reason, that they *did not wish* to recommend immediate surgery, the patient was likewise ineligible.
3. If, but only if, they were *substantially uncertain* what to recommend, the patient was automatically eligible for randomization between immediate versus no immediate surgery (with all patients receiving whatever their doctors judged to be the best available medical care, which generally included advice to stop smoking, treatment of hypertension, and the use of aspirin as an antithrombotic drug).

Fig. 1 Example of the 'uncertainty principle' for trial entry: the chief eligibility criterion for the European Carotid Surgery Trial (ECST) was that the doctors and patient should be substantially uncertain whether to risk immediate or deferred surgery. (Partly because this criterion was appropriately flexible, ECST became the largest ever trial of vascular surgery.)

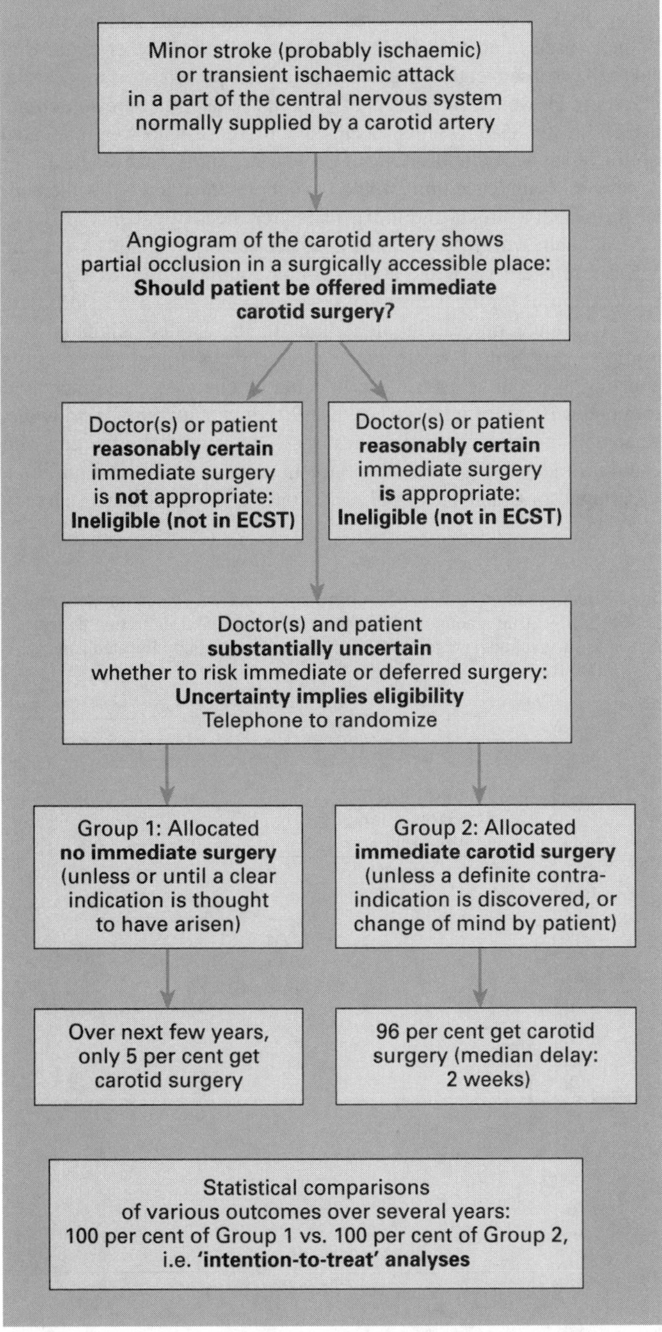

There were substantial differences between individual doctors in the types of patients about whom they were uncertain (in terms of the severity of carotid stenosis, as well as various other characteristics). This guaranteed that no category—mild, moderate, or severe stenosis—would be wholly excluded, and hence that the trial would yield at least some direct evidence in each case. As a result of the wide and simple entry criteria adopted by ECST, 3000 patients were randomized and therefore the study was able to provide some clear answers about who needed carotid endarterectomy. For patients with only mild carotid artery stenosis (0–29 per cent) on their pre-randomization angiogram there was little risk of ipsilateral ischaemic stroke, even in the absence of surgery, so that any benefits of surgery over the next few years were small and outweighed by its early risks. Conversely, for patients with severe stenosis (70–99 per cent), the risks of surgery were significantly outweighed by its later benefits over the next few years. The trial stopped early for both of these categories, but for the intermediate category of patients with moderate stenosis (30–69 per cent) the balance of surgical risk and eventual benefit remained uncertain, and so recruitment into the study continued with entry still governed by the 'uncertainty principle' as before.

The 'uncertainty principle' simultaneously meets the requirements of ethicality, heterogeneity, simplicity, and maximal trial size. It states that the fundamental eligibility criterion is that both patient and doctor should be substantially uncertain about the appropriateness of each of the trial treatments for the particular patient. With such uncertainty as the fundamental principle of eligibility, informed consent can also be simplified, for the degree of 'informed consent' that is appropriate in a randomized comparison of different treatments that is governed by the 'uncertainty principle' should probably not differ greatly from that which is applied in routine practice outside trials when treatment is being chosen haphazardly—or, to put it another way, 'double standards' between trial and non-trial situations are not appropriate. The haphazard nature of many non-randomized treatment choices is reflected in the wide variations in practice between and within countries. Even when practice is similar it may be similarly wrong: for example, before the ISIS-2 results became available (see later), almost no doctors were using fibrinolytic therapy for acute myocardial infarction. Provided that trials are governed by the 'uncertainty principle', there is an approximate parallel between good science and good ethics. Indeed, in such circumstances excessively detailed consent procedures (which can be distressing and inhumane, and so would not be considered appropriate in routine practice) would not be either scientifically or ethically appropriate.

This 'uncertainty principle' is just one of many ways of simplifying trials and thereby helping them to avoid becoming enmeshed in a mass of wholly unnecessary traditional complexity. If randomized trials can be substantially simplified, as has already been achieved in a few major diseases, and hence made very much larger, then they will play an appropriately central role in the development of rational criteria for the planning of health care throughout the world.

MINIMIZING BOTH BIAS AND RANDOM ERROR: SYSTEMATIC OVERVIEWS (META-ANALYSES) OF RANDOMIZED TRIALS

Cochrane was one of the first people to emphasize the need to bring together, by speciality, the results from all relevant randomized trials and the Cochrane Collaboration is now attempting to do this systematically. When several trials have all addressed much the same therapeutic question, the traditional procedure of choosing only a few of them as the basis for practice may be a source of serious bias, since chance fluctuations for or against treatment may affect which trials are chosen. To avoid this, it is appropriate to base inference chiefly on a systematic overview (or meta-analysis) of all the results from all the trials that have addressed a particular type of question (or on an unbiased subset of such trials) and not on some potentially biased subset of the trials. Such overviews will also minimize random errors in the assessment of treatment since, in general, far more patients are involved in an overview than in any individual trial that contributes to it.

The separate trials may well be heterogeneous in their entry criteria, their treatment schedules, their follow-up procedures, their methods of treating relapse, etc. In view of this heterogeneity, at one extreme each trial might be considered in virtual isolation from all others, while at the opposite extreme all might be considered together. Both these extreme views have some merit, and the pursuit of each by different people may prove more illuminating than too definite an insistence on any one particular approach. However, the heterogeneity of the different trials merely argues for careful interpretation of any overviews of different trial results, rather than arguing against any such overviews. For, whatever the difficulties of interpretation of overviews may be, without them moderate biases and random errors which may obscure any moderate treatment effects (or, conversely, may imply effects where none exists) cannot reliably be avoided.

Which overviews are trustworthy?

Over the past two decades, a large (and rapidly increasing) number of meta-analyses of the results of randomized trials have been reported, not all of which are trustworthy. The two fundamental questions are how carefully the overview has been performed and how large it is. The simplest approach is merely to have collected and tabulated the published data from whatever randomized trial reports are easily accessible in the literature, and sometimes this may suffice. At the opposite extreme, extensive efforts may have been made by those organizing the overview to locate every potentially relevant randomized trial, to collaborate closely with the trialists to seek individual data on each patient ever randomized into those trials, and then (after extensive checks and corrections of such data) to produce, in collaboration with those trialists, agreed analyses and publications. The results of some of the largest such collaborations will be described later: the Antiplatelet Trialists' (APT) Collaborative Group, the Fibrinolytic Trialists' (FTT) Collaborative Group, and the Early Breast Cancer Trialists' Collaborative Group (EBCTCG). Collaboration of the original trialists in the overview process, with collection of individual patient data, can help to avoid or minimize the biases that could be produced by missing trials (for example, owing to the greater likelihood of extremely good, or extremely bad, results being particularly widely known and published), by inappropriate post-randomization withdrawals, or by failure to allocate treatment properly at random. If randomization was performed properly in the first place, then post-randomization withdrawals can often be followed up and restored to the study for an appropriate 'intention-to-treat' analysis. Knowledge of the exact methods of treatment allocation (backed up by checks on whether the main prognostic factors recorded are non-randomly distributed between the treatment groups in a particular trial) may help to identify trials that were not properly randomized and hence should be excluded from an overview of randomized trials. Overviews based on individual patient data may also provide more information about treatment effects than the more usual overviews of grouped data, for they allow more detailed analyses—indeed, if they are really large then they may actually yield statistically reliable subgroup analyses of the effects of treatment in particular types of patient.

Conversely, even a perfectly conducted overview may not be large enough to be reliable. An overview that brings together complete data from all the trials of a certain treatment that have ever been performed but still (because the trials were all small) includes a total of only 100 deaths will have random errors that are no smaller than those for a single trial with 100 deaths among such patients. Small-scale evidence, whether from an overview or from one trial, is often unreliable and will often be found in retrospect to have yielded wrong answers. What is needed is large-scale randomized evidence; it does not matter much whether that evidence comes from a properly conducted overview or a properly conducted trial. The practical medical value of such evidence will now be illustrated by a few recent examples.

SOME EXAMPLES OF IMPORTANT RESULTS IN THE TREATMENT OF VASCULAR AND NEOPLASTIC DISEASE THAT COULD HAVE BEEN RELIABLY ESTABLISHED ONLY BY LARGE-SCALE RANDOMIZED EVIDENCE

Definite result from a single very large trial: *benefit from medium-dose aspirin for patients with suspected acute myocardial infarction (and benefits among other groups of patients indicated by overviews of trials)*

In the ISIS-2 trial, half of 17 000 patients with suspected acute myocardial infarction were allocated aspirin tablets (162 mg/day for 1 month, which virtually completely inhibits cyclo-oxygenase-dependent platelet inhibition) and half were allocated placebo (i.e. dummy) tablets. Before 1988, when the ISIS-2 results were published, aspirin was not routinely used in acute myocardial infarction, and no other major trial had (or has subsequently) assessed aspirin in suspected acute myocardial infarction. However, the effects of 1 month of aspirin were so definite in ISIS-2 (804/8587 vascular deaths among those who were allocated aspirin versus 1016/8600 among those who were not) that even the lower 99 per cent confidence limit would have represented a worthwhile benefit from such a simple and inexpensive treatment (Fig. 2).

As a result, worldwide treatment patterns changed sharply when the ISIS-2 results emerged, and aspirin is now routinely used in many different countries for the majority of emergency hospital admissions with suspected acute myocardial infarction. In the United Kingdom, for example, two British Heart Foundation surveys found cardiologists reporting that routine aspirin use in acute coronary care had increased from under 10 per cent in 1987 to over 90 per cent in 1989. Worldwide, the annual number of patients with suspected myocardial infarction who would nowadays be given such treatment must be well over a million a year, suggesting that in this clinical context alone aspirin is already

Fig. 2 Effect of administration of aspirin for 1 month on 35-day mortality in the 1988 ISIS-2 trial among over 17 000 acute myocardial infarction patients. (Absolute survival advantage: 24 SD5 lives saved per 1000 allocated aspirin, $2P < 0.00001$.)

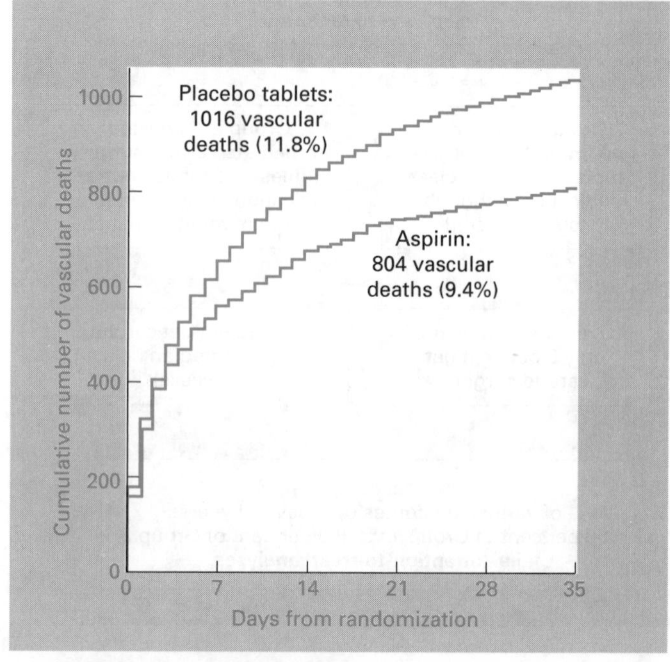

Table 3 *Summary of the overall results of trials of aspirin (or other antiplatelet drugs)* for the prevention of vascular events: the Antiplatelet Trialists' Collaboration (1994), involving a total of about 100 000 randomized patients in over 100 trials*

Type of patient	Average scheduled treatment duration (approximate no. of patients randomized)	Proportion who suffered a non-fatal stroke, non-fatal heart attack, or vascular death during the trials: Antiplatelet	Control	Events avoided in these trials
High risk:				
Suspected acute heart attack	**1 month** (20 000)	**10%**	**14%**	**40 per 1000** ($2P < 0.00001$)
Previous history of heart attack	**2 years** (20 000)	**13%**	**17%**	**40 per 1000** ($2P < 0.00001$)
Previous history of stroke or TIA	**3 years** (10 000)	**18%**	**22%**	**40 per 1000** ($2P < 0.00001$)
Other vascular disease**	**1 year** (20 000)	**7%**	**9%**	**20 per 1000** ($2P < 0.00001$)
Low risk:				
Primary prevention in low risk people	**5 years** (30 000)	**4.4%**	**4.8%**	**4 per 1000** ($2P > 0.05$)

*The most widely tested regimen was medium dose aspirin, involving an average daily dose of 75–325 mg, and no other antiplatelet regimen appeared to be significantly more or less effective than this in preventing such vascular events. (For comparison, in the United Kingdom or United States, a child's aspirin tablet contains about 75–80 mg of aspirin, while an adult tablet contains 300–325 mg.) Pharmacological evidence suggests that, after the first few days, all daily doses of aspirin in the range 75–325 mg are likely to be approximately equivalent in their effects on platelets and on the vascular endothelium. Hence, to limit any gastric discomfort with long-term use, a daily dose at the lower end of this range, such as 75, 80, or 100 mg (depending on what is conveniently available), might be slightly preferable. However, in acute emergencies such as suspected myocardial infarction or unstable angina, at least the initial dose should perhaps be at the upper end of the range, such as 250, 300 or 325 mg, so as to achieve a virtually complete antiplatelet effect within less than 1 hour (which could then be maintained by a lower daily dose).

**For example, angina, peripheral vascular disease, arterial surgery or angioplasty, etc.

preventing tens of thousands of premature deaths each year. However, if the ISIS-2 trial had been a factor of 10 smaller (i.e. 1700 instead of 17 000 patients), then exactly the same proportional reduction in mortality as shown in Fig. 2 would not have been conventionally significant and therefore would have been much less likely to influence medical practice—indeed, the result might by chance have appeared exactly flat, greatly damaging future research on aspirin in this context. Likewise, if the ISIS-2 trial had been non-randomized, then it might well have produced the wrong answer (since in a non-randomized study doctors might tend to give active treatment to patients who were particularly ill, or who were rather different from those not given active treatment in various other ways). In addition, even if a non-randomized study did happen to produce an unbiasedly correct answer, it would be impossible to be sure that it had actually done so, and hence again a non-randomized study might have had much less influence on medical practice than did ISIS-2.

In the ISIS-2 trial aspirin significantly reduced the 1 month mortality, but it also significantly reduced the number of non-fatal strokes and non-fatal reinfarctions that were recorded in hospital. Combining all these three outcomes into 'vascular events' (stroke, death, or reinfarction), 13 per cent of those who were allocated aspirin and 17 per cent of those who were not were known to have suffered a vascular event in the month after randomization (Table 3)—an absolute difference of 40 events per 1000 treated (or, perhaps more relevantly, of 40 000 per million). The randomized trials of aspirin, or of other antiplatelet regimens, in other types of high risk patients (for example, a few years of aspirin for those who have survived a myocardial infarction or stroke) have not been as large as ISIS-2, and so, taken separately, most have yielded false-negative results. However, when the results from many such trials are combined, statistically definite reductions in 'vascular events' are seen (Table 3). Since such treatments do not appear to increase non-vascular mortality, all-cause mortality is also significantly reduced.

In principle, these findings could, if appropriately widely exploited, prevent about 100 000 premature vascular deaths a year in developed countries alone, and there are probably at least as many vascular deaths in less developed as in developed countries. Hence, with realistically achievable levels of use of 'medium dose' aspirin (75–325 mg/day) for the secondary prevention of vascular disease, it might well be possible in practice to ensure that aspirin is used in enough high risk patients to prevent, or substantially delay, at least 100 000 vascular deaths per year worldwide, and such use of aspirin would, in addition, prevent a comparable number of non-fatal strokes or heart attacks. (Medium dose aspirin was the least expensive and most widely tested antiplatelet regimen: it is of proven efficacy, and on review of all the antiplatelet trials no other antiplatelet regimen has been shown to be of greater efficacy in preventing vascular events; see notes to Table 3.) This large-scale randomized evidence about medium dose aspirin is now changing worldwide clinical practice in ways that will, at low cost, prevent much death and disability in high risk patients. However, small trials, small overviews, or non-randomized studies (however large) could not possibly have provided appropriately reliable evidence about such moderate risk reductions.

Definite result from a very large overview of trials: *benefit from 'adjuvant' therapy with tamoxifen for patients with 'early' breast cancer (and possible benefit suggested with ovarian ablation in younger women)*

By definition, in 'early' breast cancer all detectable deposits of disease are limited to the breast and the locoregional lymph nodes, and can be removed surgically. However, experience shows that undetectably small deposits may remain elsewhere that eventually cause clinical recurrence at a distant site, perhaps after a delay of several years, which is then usually followed by death from the disease. These micrometastatic deposits may have been stimulated by the body's own hormones during the years before recurrence became detectable. Therefore, among women who have had the detectable deposits of breast cancer removed by surgery (or by surgery with radiotherapy), there have been many trials of 'adjuvant' treatments that either reduce the production of endogenous oestrogens (for example, various forms of ovarian ablation) or block the access of those oestrogens to the tumour cells (for example, tamoxifen, which blocks the oestrogen receptor protein in some breast cancer cells).

Taken separately, most of these adjuvant trials have been too small to provide reliable evidence about long-term survival. However, if the results of all of them are combined, some very definite differences in 10 year survival emerge (Fig. 3). Among women with stage II disease who are less than 50 years old (and therefore generally pre- or perimenopausal), ovarian ablation appears to produce about a 10 per cent absolute difference in 10 year survival (for example 50 per cent vs. 40 per cent). This finding is based on the analysis of only a few hundred deaths so it is still not as reliable as might ideally be wished and, because substantial uncertainty remains, much larger trials are now in progress. Among older stage II women ovarian ablation is unlikely to be of much relevance (since most of the endogenous oestrogen at older ages comes from sources other than the ovaries) but, in aggregate, the randomized trials among such women have shown very definitely that a few years of tamoxifen also produces about a 10 per cent absolute difference in 10 year survival. A smaller, but still highly significant, reduction in mortality by tamoxifen is also seen among the 10 000 randomized women with stage I disease. Taken separately, however, 37 of the 42 tamoxifen trials were too small to have yielded statistically reliable evidence on their own ($2P > 0.01$), and the five other trials were significant only because, by chance, they had results that were too good to be true.

These tamoxifen overview results have already changed clinical practice substantially, and have redirected research towards large randomized trials of the effects of different durations of tamoxifen: should tamoxifen in asymptomatic women continue for 2 years, for 5 years, or indefinitely? Large randomized studies of the primary prevention of breast cancer among high risk women by tamoxifen are only just beginning, but they have been encouraged by the results from the tamoxifen trials overview in 30 000 patients with established cancer (stage II or stage I) in one breast, among whom there has been a highly significant reduction of one-third in the likelihood of development of contralateral breast cancer (but a small absolute increase in endometrial cancer). Again, this degree of trustworthy detail would not have been attainable without large-scale randomized evidence.

Promising overview of small trials confirmed by a large trial: ***benefit from fibrinolytic therapy as emergency treatment for a wide range of patients with acute myocardial infarction***

Fibrinolytic drugs that dissolve a thrombus that may be blocking a coronary artery, thereby causing an acute myocardial infarction, were introduced into clinical research in the late 1950s. However, the trials of fibrinolytic drugs in the 1960s and 1970s were too small to be statistically reliable (none involved even 1000 patients). So, by the early 1980s the haemorrhagic side-effects were obvious, the benefits had not been convincingly demonstrated, and these agents were generally considered to be dangerous, ineffective, and hence not appropriate for routine coronary care. Overviews published in the mid-1980s of the previous small trials (involving a total of only about 6000 patients in two dozen trials) indicated a statistically definite benefit, but were not really believed by cardiologists and so such treatments were still not widely used. The situation has been saved by two large randomized trials, ISIS-2 and GISSI-1, both of which involved more than 10 000 patients (and by their aggregation with the seven other randomized trials that involved more than 1000 patients; see below). In ISIS-2, not only were patients randomly allocated to receive aspirin or placebo tablets as described earlier (Fig. 2), but they were also separately allocated to receive intravenous streptokinase (1.5 million units infused over about 60 min) or a placebo infusion. In this 'factorial' design (which allows the separate assessment of more than one treatment without any material loss in the statistical reliability of each comparison), a quarter of the patients were allocated aspirin alone, a quarter were allocated streptokinase alone, a quarter were allocated both streptokinase and aspirin, and a quarter were allocated neither (i.e. placebo tablets and placebo infusion). Streptokinase, like aspirin, produced a highly significant reduction in mortality, and the combination of streptokinase and aspirin was highly significantly better than either aspirin or streptokinase alone (Fig. 4).

The results shown in Fig. 4 might suggest that there was no need to collect any more randomized evidence about fibrinolytic therapy, but this ignores the potential hazards of such treatment and the heterogeneity of patients. Taken separately, even ISIS-2, the largest of these trials, was not large enough for statistically reliable subgroup analyses, but when the nine largest trials were all taken together they included a total of about 60 000 patients, half of whom were randomly allocated fibrinolytic therapy. Those entering a coronary care unit with a diagnosis of suspected or definite acute myocardial infarction range from patients who are already in cardiogenic shock with low blood pressure and a fast pulse (half of whom will die rapidly) to those who have merely had a history of chest pain and no very definite changes on their ECG (of whom 'only' a small percentage will die before discharge). Fibrinolytic

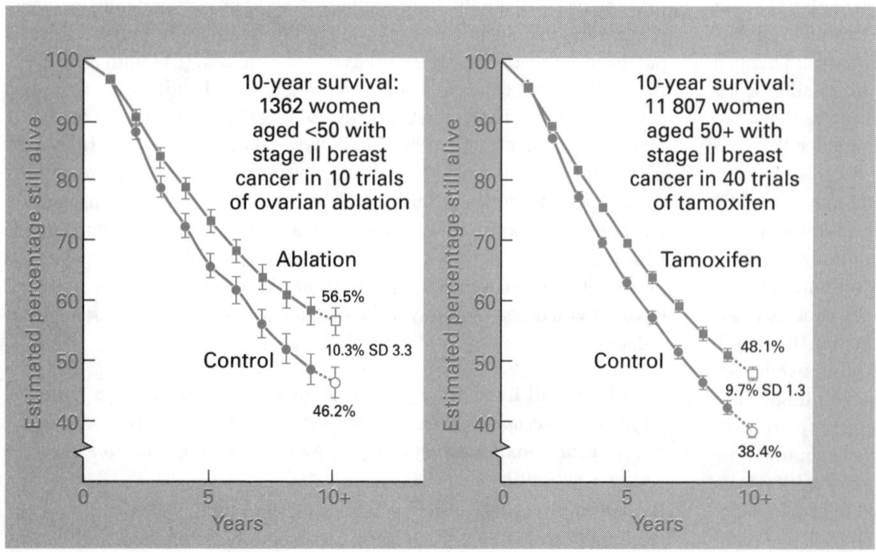

Fig. 3 Effects of hormonal adjuvant treatments for early breast cancer on 10 year survival in a worldwide overview of randomized trials. (Early Breast Cancer Trialists' Collaborative Group, 1992.)

therapy often causes a frightening blood pressure drop: should it be used in patients who are already dangerously hypotensive? It occasionally causes serious strokes: should it be used in patients who are elderly or hypertensive, and therefore already have an above-average risk of stroke (or who have only slight changes on their ECG, and therefore have only a low risk of cardiac death)? Finally, if the coronary artery has been occluded for long enough, the heart muscle that it supplies will have been irreversibly destroyed: how long after the heart attack starts is fibrinolytic treatment still worth risking—3 hours? 6 hours? 12 hours? 24 hours?

These questions needed to be answered reliably before appropriate and generally accepted indications for and against such an immediately hazardous but potentially effective therapy could be devised. To address them, all fibrinolytic therapy trialists have collaborated in a systematic overview of the randomized evidence. On review of the 60 000 patients randomized between fibrinolytic therapy and control in trials of more than 1000 patients, some of the therapeutic questions were relatively easy to answer satisfactorily. For example it appears that most of those whose ECG is still normal (or shows a pattern that indicates only a low risk of death) can be left untreated, leaving open the option of starting fibrinolytic treatment urgently if their ECG changes suddenly for the worse in the following few hours. Conversely, among those who already had 'high risk' ECG changes when they were randomized, the absolute benefit of immediate fibrinolytic therapy was, if anything, slightly greater than is indicated by Fig. 4, and age, sex, blood pressure, heart rate, diabetes, and previous history of myocardial infarction could not identify reliably any group that would not, on average, have their chances of survival appreciably increased by treatment.

The longer that fibrinolytic treatment for such patients was delayed, the less benefit it seemed to produce. Among those whose ECG showed definite ST-segment elevation or bundle branch block, the benefit was greatest (about 30 lives saved per 1000) among those randomized 0–6 h after the onset of pain (Fig. 5). However, the mortality reduction was still substantial and significant (about 20 per 1000, $2P < 0.003$) when such patients were randomized 7–12 h after onset of pain. Indeed, if they were randomized 13–18 h after onset of pain there still appeared to be some net reduction in mortality (about 10 per 1000, but not statistically definite). The regression line in Fig. 5 reinforces these separate subgroup analyses in a more reliable way. Yet, before these large trials, it was forcefully, but mistakenly, argued that such treatments could not possibly be of any worthwhile benefit if given more than a few hours after the onset of symptoms.

Such detailed inferences are difficult enough with large-scale properly randomized evidence, and would be impossible without it; because of their unknowable biases (see above), non-randomized database analyses are simply not a viable alternative to large-scale randomized evidence. Nor would randomization of 'only' several thousand patients have been sufficient. Indeed, in several important respects what is still needed is more, rather than less, randomized evidence about the effects of fibrinolytic therapy in various particular types of patient. First, it is still not clear whether patients who have definite ECG changes such as ST elevation or bundle branch block, but who present 12–18 h, or even 18–24 h, after the onset of pain should be treated; more randomized evidence is still needed (Fig. 5). Second, for one particular poor-prognosis ECG category (ST depression) the 1 month mortality results still appear unpromising even when all currently available trials are combined (15 per cent dead among those allocated fibrinolytic therapy versus 14 per cent dead among controls, but based on only 4000 patients). Analogy with the results in other high risk categories suggests that this result for patients with ST depression may well be a false-negative. Perhaps it has arisen from unduly data-dependent emphasis on what may in retrospect prove to have been a random irregularity in the results in this particular subgroup which included only a few thousand individuals. Again, more randomized evidence is needed. Nevertheless, substantial progress has been made by the past decade of mega-trials of fibrinolytic agents. Worldwide, in the mid-1990s, about half a million patients per year are being given fibrinolytic therapy, avoiding about 10 000 early deaths each year.

Fig. 4 Effects of a one-hour streptokinase infusion (and of 1 month of aspirin) on 35 day mortality in ISIS-2 (1988) among 17 187 acute myocardial infarction patients who would not normally have received streptokinase or aspirin, divided at random into four similar groups to receive aspirin only, streptokinase only, both, or neither. (Any doctor who believed that a particular patient should be given either treatment gave it, and did not include that patient in ISIS-2.)

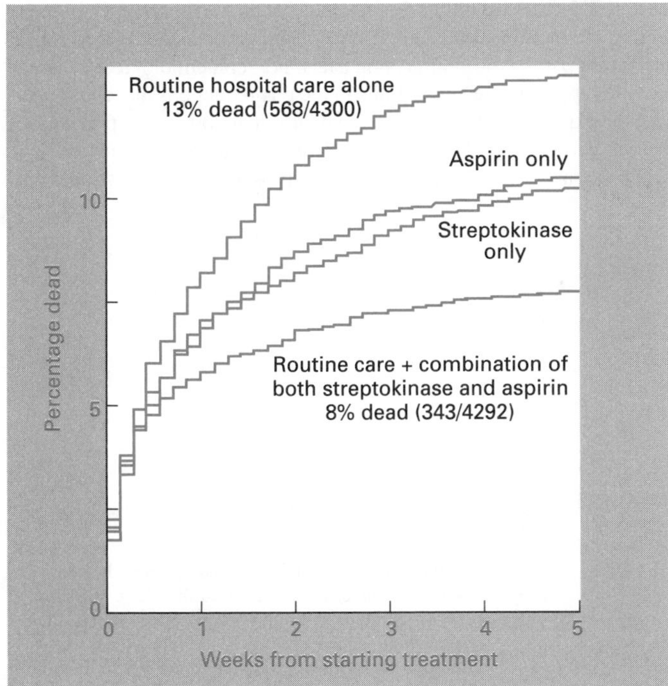

Small trials refuted by a mega-trial: *lack of significant benefit from magnesium infusion in suspected acute myocardial infarction*

It had been suggested that an infusion of a magnesium salt might reduce early mortality in patients with suspected acute myocardial infarction.

Fig. 5 Benefit versus delay (0–1, 2–3, 4–6, 7–12, or 13–24 hours) in the nine largest randomized trials of fibrinolytic therapy versus control in patients with acute myocardial infarction. One-month mortality results for 45 000 patients with ST elevation or bundle branch block when randomized, showing the definite net benefit even for the 9000 randomized 7–12 hours after the onset of pain. (Fibrinolytic Therapy Trialists' Collaboration, 1994.)

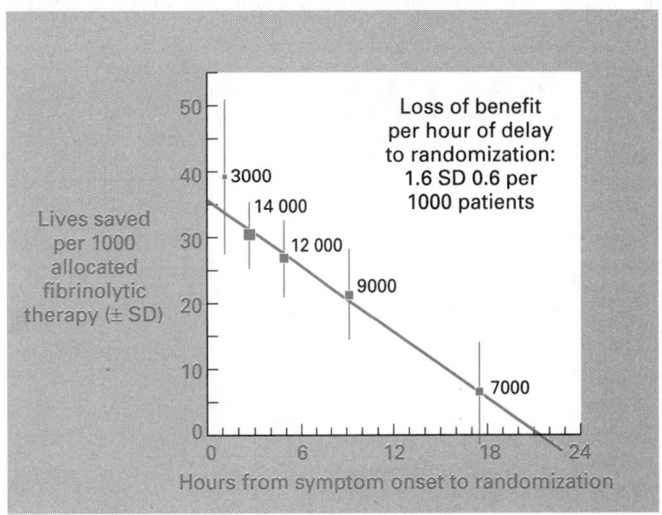

Table 4 *Magnesium in acute myocardial infarction: contrast between the results of the smaller and the larger randomized trials*

	No. of patients randomized	1 month mortality			
		Allocated magnesium		Allocated control	
9 small trials	1500	42/754	(5.6%)	86/740	(11.6%)
LIMIT-2 trial	2300	90/1159	(7.8%)	118/1157	(10.2%)
ISIS-4 trial	58 000	2216/29 011	(7.6%)	2103/29 039	(7.2%)
All trials	**62 000**	**2348/30 924**	**(7.59%)**	**2307/30 936**	**(7.46%)**

There is highly significant heterogeneity ($P < 0.001$) between the group of small trials whose 'hypothesis-generating' results led to the testing of magnesium in ISIS-4 and the pair of larger trials (ISIS-4 and LIMIT-2) whose results tested that hypothesis.

Several small trials, involving between them a total of only about 1500 patients, had addressed this question, and their aggregated results indicated a statistically significant, but implausibly large, benefit (42/754 deaths among those allocated magnesium versus 86/740 among the controls, $2P < 0.001$). Some argued that such results constituted proof beyond reasonable doubt that magnesium was of sufficient value to justify widespread usage without seeking further randomized evidence, but others remained sceptical, arguing that the apparent results were far too good to be true.

Therefore two trials, one (LIMIT-2) involving 2000 patients and one (ISIS-4) involving 58 000 patients, were set up to test the possible effects of magnesium more reliably. The former yielded a moderately promising result (Table 4), indicating avoidance of about a quarter of the early deaths, but because of its small size this result was statistically compatible with a true benefit that ranged from no effect to about a halving of early mortality. The much larger ISIS-4 trial yielded a completely unpromising result, and so the overall evidence, based on about 60 000 randomized patients, is now non-significantly adverse.

In view of the striking disparity between the apparent effects of magnesium before and after ISIS-4 had provided large-scale randomized evidence, it is of interest to recall some of the expert views that were expressed while ISIS-4 was in progress. Some felt so strongly that magnesium was already of proven benefit (and hence that further randomization was unethical) that the data-monitoring committee of ISIS-4 was lobbied to try to have the study stopped early and all future patients given magnesium. In contrast, the ISIS-4 steering committee was sufficiently sceptical to want large-scale randomized evidence. They believed that the available evidence was consistent with a negligible benefit, or even a small net hazard, although they all thought it more likely that at least some net benefit would be seen. Even after the LIMIT-2 result was available they continued to hold these opinions, and thought that if there was any real benefit then this was likely to be less than LIMIT-2 had suggested (and hence very much less than the other small trials had suggested).

Those who had trusted the implausibly extreme results from the previous small trials may well have been disappointed by the results of the ISIS-4 mega-trial, which now provide strong evidence that the routine use of magnesium has little or no effect on mortality in acute myocardial infarction. However, in a world where moderate benefits are much more plausible than large benefits, striking results in small-scale trials, in small-scale overviews, or in small subgroups will frequently prove evanescent. The medical assumption that both a moderate mortality difference and a zero mortality difference may be plausible, but that an extreme mortality difference is much less so, has surprisingly strong consequences for the interpretation of randomized evidence. In particular, it implies that even quite highly significant (e.g. $2P = 0.001$) mortality differences that are based on only relatively small numbers of deaths may provide untrustworthy evidence of the existence of any real difference.

Trials in their epidemiological context: *effects of lower, and of lowering, blood pressure on the risk of stroke and coronary heart disease*

The quantitative epidemiological evidence about the effects of long-term differences in risk factors such as blood pressure or blood cholesterol can help to interpret the results from trials of the effects of reducing these risk factors for only a few years. This may help not only in interpreting the previous trials but also in planning the size and duration of any future risk factor modification trials. For, epidemiological evidence provides approximate upper limits to the risk reductions that could plausibly be expected in the trials and may also help to identify populations that are particularly likely to benefit from risk factor modification.

For example, appropriate analyses of prospective observational epi-

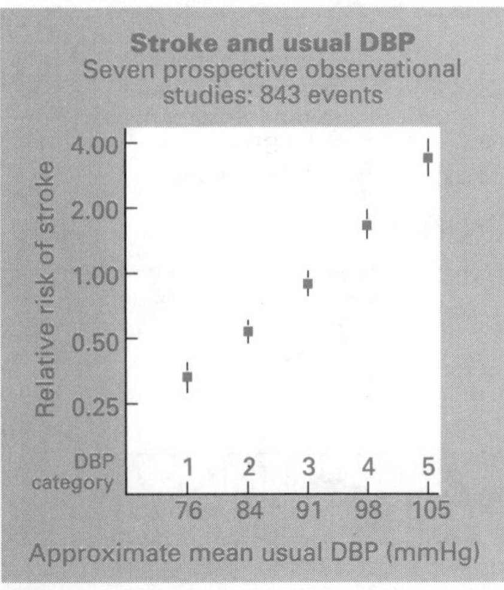

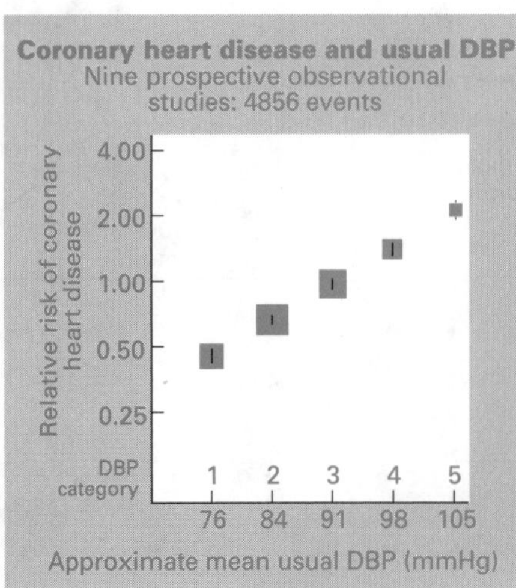

Fig. 6 Relative risks of stroke and coronary heart disease for five categories of diastolic blood pressure from the combined results of prospective observational studies. Solid squares represent the relative risks of disease in each category relative to the risk in the whole study population and 95 per cent confidence intervals are denoted by vertical lines. (MacMahon, 1994.)

demiological studies of diastolic blood pressure and disease indicate that, throughout the range of usual diastolic blood pressure in the populations studied (i.e. about 70–110 mmHg), a lower value was associated with a lower risk of suffering a first stroke or episode of coronary heart disease (i.e. there did not seem to be any 'threshold' or 'J-shape' Fig. 6). The steepness of this continuous relationship between blood pressure and vascular disease suggests that the eventual reductions in risk produced by practicable blood pressure reductions (for example with antihypertensive treatment) may well be worthwhile not only among certain 'hypertensive' individuals but also among certain individuals who, although considered 'normotensive', are at high risk for some reason (for example as a result of a previous stroke or myocardial infarction).

After making due allowance for the substantial and systematic extent to which the true relationship is diluted by purely random fluctuations in the baseline measurements of blood pressure (i.e. the 'regression dilution' bias), the prospective studies suggest that a *prolonged* difference of only 5 mmHg in usual diastolic blood pressure is associated with avoidance of at least one-third of the risk of stroke and at least one-fifth of the risk of coronary heart disease in late middle age. However, although non-randomized prospective observational studies may be more relevant to the eventual effects of prolonged differences in blood pressure, despite the possibility of confounding by other factors, randomized trials of blood pressure reductions that last for only a few years may be more relevant to assessing the speed with which the epidemiologically expected reductions in stroke or coronary heart disease risk are produced by reducing blood pressure. By comparing the results of a systematic overview of all randomized trials of antihypertensive therapy with the observational epidemiological evidence, it may be possible to estimate the extent to which the eventual effects of a lower blood pressure on disease incidence rates can be achieved within just a few years of treatment in middle or old age. (Ideally, these age ranges should be considered separately, as the fractional avoidance of risk may well be substantially different in middle and in old age.)

Over the past few decades, numerous trials of the treatment of hypertension have been conducted to determine whether blood pressure reduction in middle age reduces the risk of stroke and coronary heart disease. However, although it was fairly rapidly accepted that the treatment of severe hypertension could at least prevent stroke, until recently there has been controversy as to whether the treatment of even severe hypotension could also prevent coronary heart disease, and questions have also persisted about the effects on stroke of the treatment of mild to moderate hypertension. This continuing uncertainty about the benefits of lowering blood pressure may chiefly have reflected the inability of individual trials, even those with several hundred coronary heart disease events, to detect moderate coronary heart disease reductions reliably, rather than from any important heterogeneity of the real effects of treatment. The mean difference in diastolic blood pressure between treatment and control groups in the trials was only about 5–6 mmHg, and the epidemiological evidence suggests that a long-term difference of this magnitude is associated with only about 20–25 per cent less coronary heart disease (and about 35–40 per cent less stroke). Even if such trial treatments would eventually produce 20–25 per cent less coronary heart disease after many years, the effects seen within the 2 or 3 years that are available on average between randomization and death in a 5 year trial might well be somewhat smaller (for example, 15 per cent). Considered separately, however, none of the trials had recorded enough coronary heart disease events (or enough vascular deaths) for statistically reliable assessment of 15 per cent risk reductions.

For stroke, the overview of randomized trials provides direct and highly significant evidence that most or all of the stroke avoidance associated with a prolonged difference in usual diastolic blood pressure appears soon after the blood pressure is lowered (Fig. 7). In contrast, the significant reduction in coronary heart disease seen in the trials (16 per cent SD 4, 95 per cent confidence interval of 8–23 per cent, $2P$ = 0.0001) falls somewhat short of the difference of about 20–25 per cent suggested by the observational epidemiological evidence for a prolonged 5–6 mmHg difference in usual diastolic blood pressure. However, this coronary heart disease reduction is substantial and real ($2P$ = 0.0001). Therefore it is reasonable to hope that trials of antihypertensive regimens that can reduce blood pressure to a greater extent than the 5–6 mmHg diastolic blood pressure reduction seen in these trials will demonstrate even greater reductions in stroke and coronary heart disease.

The proportional reduction in vascular disease risk observed in the trials appeared to be similar in high and low risk individuals, so that the absolute size of the reduction that is produced by treatment may be largely dependent upon the absolute risk. Therefore, for high risk individuals, the absolute reduction in risk produced by antihypertensive treatment might be substantial even among those who are only moderately 'hypertensive'. Indeed, in view of the epidemiological evidence that, for stroke and coronary heart disease risk, there is no 'threshold' level of diastolic blood pressure within the normal range, large randomized trials might even show that blood pressure reduction is of substantial value among many 'normotensive' individuals at high risk of stroke (such as those with a history of cerebral vascular disease) or of coronary heart disease (such as patients with a history of myocardial infarction, angina, peripheral vascular disease, diabetes, or chronic renal failure).

RESULTS FROM LARGE ANONYMOUS TRIALS ARE RELEVANT TO REAL CLINICAL PRACTICE

A clinician is used to dealing with individual patients, and may feel that the results of large trials somehow deny their individuality. This is

Fig. 7 Reduction in the odds of stroke and coronary heart disease in all unconfounded randomized trials of antihypertensive drug treatment (mean diastolic blood pressure differences of 5–6 mmHg for 5 years). Solid squares represent the odds ratios (treatment:control) for the four larger trials and the properly stratified odds ratio for the combination of the 13 smaller trials. 95 per cent confidence intervals are denoted by horizontal lines (for individual large trials or the combined small trials) and by diamonds (for overviews of all trials). (Collins and Peto, 1994.)

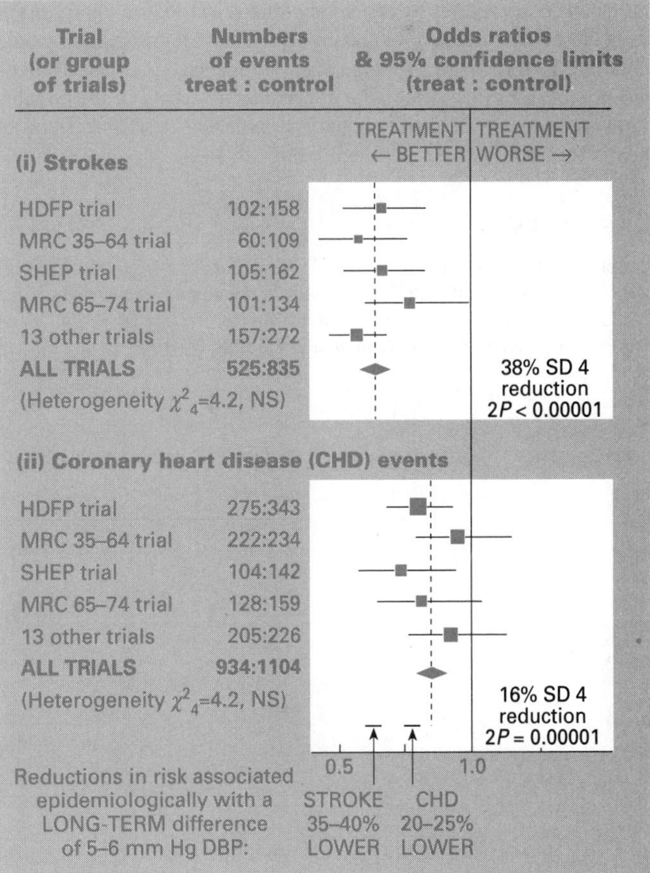

almost the opposite of the truth, for one of the main reasons why trials have to be large is just because patients are so different from one another. Two apparently similar patients may run entirely different clinical courses, one remaining stable and the other progressing rapidly to severe disability or early death. Consequently, it is only when really large groups of patients are compared that the proportion of patients with truly good and bad prognosis in each can be relied on to be reasonably similar. One commonly hears statements such as: 'If a treatment effect isn't obvious in a couple of hundred patients then it isn't worth knowing about'. As the previous examples demonstrate, such statements may reveal not clinical wisdom but statistical naïvety.

It is also said that what is really wanted is not a blanket recommendation for everybody, but rather some means of identifying those few individuals who really stand to benefit from therapy. If any criteria (for example, short-term response to a non-placebo-controlled course of some disease-modifying agent) can be proposed that are likely to discriminate between people who will and will not benefit, then these can be recorded prospectively at entry and the eventual trial results subdivided with respect to them. However, there is a danger in too detailed an analysis of the apparent response of small subgroups chosen for separate emphasis because of the apparently remarkable effects of treatment in these subgroups. Even if an agent brought no benefit, it would have to be acutely poisonous for it not to appear beneficial in one or two such subgroups! Conversely, if an intervention really avoids an approximately similar proportion of the risk in each category of patient, it will, by chance alone, appear not to do so in some category. The surprising extent to which this happens is evident from the example in Table 2. A large anonymous trial will at least still help to answer the practical question of whether, on average, a policy of widespread treatment (except where clearly contraindicated) is preferable to a general policy of no immediate use of the treatment (except where clearly indicated). Moreover, without a few really large trials it is difficult to see how else many such questions could be resolved over the next few years. For example, digitalis has already been in use for over two centuries, and there is still no reliable consensus as to its net long-term effects on mortality. Trials are at least a practical way of making some solid progress, and it would be unfortunate if desire for the perfect (i.e. knowledge of exactly who will benefit from treatment) were to become the enemy of the possible (i.e. knowledge of the direction and approximate size of the effects of the treatment of many large categories of patient).

REFERENCES

Antiplatelet Trialists' Collaboration (1994). Collaborative overview of randomised trials of antiplatelet therapy. I: Prevention of death, myocardial infarction, and stroke by prolonged antiplatelet therapy in various categories of patients. *British Medical Journal,* **308,** 81–106.

Armitage, P. and Berry, G. (1994). *Statistical methods in medical research.* (3rd edn) Blackwell Science, Oxford.

Chalmers, I. (1994). The Cochrane Collaboration: preparing, maintaining and disseminating systematic reviews of the effects of health care. *Annals of the New York Academy of Sciences,* **703,** 156–63.

Chalmers, T.C. and Lau, J. (1993). Meta-analytic stimulus for changes in clinical trials. *Statistical Methods in Medical Research,* **2,** 161–72.

Cochrane, A.L. (1979). 1931–1971: a critical review, with particular reference to the medical profession. In: *Medicines for the year 2000,* pp 1–11. Office of Health Economics, London.

Collins, R. and Peto, R. (1994). Antihypertensive drug therapy: effects on stroke and coronary heart disease. In: *Textbook of hypertension,* Ch. 69, p. 1156. Blackwell Science, Oxford.

Collins, R., Gray, R., Godwin, J. and Peto, R. (1987). Avoidance of large biases and large random errors in the assessment of moderate treatment effects: the need for systematic overviews. *Statistics in Medicine,* **6,** 245–50.

Collins, R., Doll, R., and Peto, R. (1992). Ethics of clinical trials. In: *Introducing new treatments for cancer: practical, ethical and legal problems,* Ch. 4, p. 49. Wiley, New York.

Early Breast Cancer Trialists' Collaborative Group (1992). Systemic treatment of early breast cancer by hormonal, cytotoxic, or immune therapy: 133 randomised trials involving 31,000 recurrences and 24,000 deaths among 75,000 women. *Lancet,* **339,** 1–15, 71–85.

European Carotid Surgery Trialists' Collaborative Group (1991). MRC European Carotid Surgery Trial: interim results for symptomatic patients with severe (70–99%) or with mild (0–29%) carotid stenosis. *Lancet,* **337,** 1235–43.

Fibrinolytic Therapy Trialists' Collaborative Group (1994). Indications for fibrinolytic therapy in suspected acute myocardial infarction: collaborative overview of early mortality and major morbidity results from all randomised trials of more than 1000 patients. *Lancet* **343,** 311–22.

ISIS-2 (Second International Study of Infarct Survival) Collaborative Group (1988). Randomised trial of intravenous streptokinase, oral aspirin, both, or neither among 17,187 cases of suspected acute myocardial infarction: ISIS-2. *Lancet,* **ii,** 349–60

ISIS-4 (Fourth International Study of Infarct Survival) Collaborative Group. (1995). ISIS-4: A randomised factorial trial assessing early oral captopril, oral mononitrate, and intravenous magnesium sulphate in 58050 patients with suspected acute myocardial infarction. *Lancet,* in press.

MacMahon, S. (1994). Blood pressure and the risks of cardiovascular disease. In: *Textbook of hypertension,* Ch. 3, p. 46. Blackwell Science, Oxford.

Peto, R., Pike, M.C., Armitage, P., Breslow, N.E., Cox, D.R., Howard, S.V., *et al.* (1976). Design and analysis of randomized clinical trials requiring prolonged observation of each patient. Part I: Introduction and design. *British Journal of Cancer,* **34,** 585–612.

Peto, R., Pike, M.C., Armitage, P., Breslow, N.E., Cox, D.R., Howard, S.V., *et al.* (1977). Design and analysis of randomized clinical trials requiring prolonged observation of each patient. Part II: Analysis and examples. *British Journal of Cancer,* **35,** 1–39.

Yusuf, S., Collins, R., and Peto, R. (1984). Why do we need some large, simple randomized trials? *Statistics in Medicine,* **3,** 409–20.

Section 3 *The spectrum of disease and clinical practice*

3.1 The diseases of gods: some newer threats to health

M. H. King and C. M. Elliott

Une difficulté est une lumière.
Une difficulté insurmontable est un soleil.
Paul Valéry

It has been said that not until about 1900 did the average patient benefit from consulting the average doctor. This book is a monument to what scientific medicine has achieved since then—for those lucky enough to receive such care. Some of its most senior readers will have been born before the invention of salvarsan (Ehrlich 1910), or perhaps even before man first flew (the Wright brothers 1903). We have all seen more scientific, technical, and social change in our lifetime than any previous generation. For 99 per cent of our existence as a species we have been upper palaeolithic hunter–gatherers, which physiologically is what we still are. Both the blessings and the curses of our present condition are increasingly bound up with the speed and the scale of the change that *Homo sapiens* is now undergoing. The science-based industrial economy that is driving this change has given most of the developed world a standard of material wealth that was only achieved by very few in previous ages. The world's élites now live like gods. We can land on the moon, and disentangle the chemistry of our own genes, and there have been undreamed of advances in the scientific basis of medicine; but a variety of discomforting social, economic, and geophysical factors continues to make for sickness in individuals and in society.

Our industrial economy has not only made many of our species richer, it has also made us healthier, albeit substituting one set of diseases, particularly the infections of childhood, for another, the degenerative and neoplastic diseases of old age. It may seem therefore both churlish, and unduly pessimistic, to question what the industrial economy, which is the engine for the generation of wealth, is now doing for health. Paradoxically, having in the past done so much to improve our well-being, it is now showing us some of its more subtle deleterious effects. Its more obvious ones, the industrial diseases and accidents, are now well understood, and in some countries well controlled. Some of the newer ones are barely even suspected, and when they are, there is often considerable reluctance to confront them.

The maladies of modernization

Mortality is still the most common yardstick of health, since there is no convenient index of morbidity, nor any practical way of measuring the 'well-being' that is such an important part of the World Health Organization's definition of health as a state of 'complete mental social and physical well-being, and not merely the absence of disease and infirmity'. As medicine deals better and better with disease and infirmity, new threats are becoming evident that in different ways reduce well-being and increase morbidity.

A modern, science-driven industrial economy affects health in complex ways, sometimes with the gravest ethical implications: (i) it is treating the global environment as an infinite source of resources, and as an infinite sink for pollutants; (ii) it is destroying the concept of family (especially the nuclear family) in a way that is unique in human history; (iii) it is also destroying traditional community values; (iv) it has replaced the environment in which we evolved and which determined our physiology with another one that has afflicted us with a variety of 'Western diseases' that were rare or absent among our forebears, and still are in preindustrial societies; (v) it has triggered unprecedented population growth, with the result that some communities are in danger of exceeding the carrying capacity of their ecosystems; (vi) having created wealth and employment in one community, labour-intensive manufacturing industry soon moves to other more competitive ones where wages are lower, leaving serious unemployment and misery in its wake, with all that this does to impair health and reduce the tax base from which to finance health care; (vii) technology has come to dominate medicine, and in doing so has made it a disproportionate consumer of wealth; (viii) in the industrial world, much health expenditure is now spent on prolonging the existence of those whose quality of life is so low that it has made euthanasia an important issue.

The difficulties in changing these trends are formidable. The critical factors and their interrelationships are hard to untangle and, even if identified, very difficult to alter. Our inability to make an adequate policy on cigarette smoking is a good illustration. The problems may be definable in 'scientific' terms but ultimately require political and sociological solutions.

Sickness in the system itself

Between 1950 and 1986, gross world product and fossil-fuel consumption quadrupled while population doubled. Growth benefits some people while imposing great (and perhaps greater) costs on others, and on the biosphere itself. Economics has emphasized the material aspects of human existence at the expense of even more fundamental ones. It is not surprising, therefore, that there is a growing feeling that, like medicine, economics has created new problems in the process of solving others.

The destruction of the community and the environment stems from the urge to maximize physical production in a finite ecosystem. Economic growth is still too readily assumed to be the universal objective, and the alternatives to it remain poorly defined. Unfortunately, conventional economics forgets that the industrial economy is only part of 'the great economy', which is the ecosystem on which all life depends. In trying to simplify the real world, reductionist economics has had to remove from its models as 'externalities' everything it considered inessential—including the effect of the industrial economy on the family and the environment, which it either considers unimportant or indestructible. Simplification has too often reduced the environment to land, social institutions to the market, and economic success to growth in production. Such simplifications are only now being seen to ignore some critically important aspects of economic reality. The remedy is not to sweep away all classical economics, but to temper it with a proper consideration of the values that it previously considered so marginal.

Economics is capable of alteration by changing what we do—which is determined in large part by what we think, wherein lies both the cause and the solution of the problem. Alas, for many, that thinking is now, *de facto,* increasingly controlled—by the media and the advertisers.

THE MEDIA AS DISEASE AGENT

The argument that the media merely entertain and educate without influencing values, ethics, and behaviour is no longer seriously defensible. The questions now are: in what way and how does this influence health, and if harm is being done, what can be done about it? That the media inform, and that planned health education programmes can have some useful effect, is not in doubt. What is questioned is the potentially untoward effects on health of the multiplicity of uncontrolled, commercially motivated channels to which an increasing proportion of humanity is progressively being exposed.

The ill effects of the media would appear to include: (i) *The relentless promotion of a high resource consuming, excessively polluting lifestyle,* that the planet is unable to support; (ii) *The erosion of traditional culture.* The expense of producing an hour of television, the increasing number of channels to be filled, the ease of satellite transmission, and the widespread use of English are causing North American culture, in particular, to erode those elsewhere, especially the diverse cultures of the developing world. The web of traditional family relationships is particularly at risk. (iii) *The encouragement of violence.* The average North American is said to have witnessed several thousand murders in his sitting room by the time he is 15—it seems unlikely that this will have had no effect. (iv) *The steady erosion of the norms of traditional sexual behaviour and with it the stability of the family,* as discussed below, not so much by purveying the patently pornographic, deleterious though this probably is, but by presenting such an impossible supposed ideal of marriage, particularly in matters physical, that the viewer feels let down if his (or her) partner does not meet it, and by continually portraying infidelity in a way that makes it seem inevitable, desirable, and normal.

Cooling a fevered earth

Industrialization is altering the climate of the earth through the 'greenhouse effect'. Six of the seven warmest years in the 140-year period since records began have occurred since 1980, with 1988 and 1990 the hottest years. Differences of scientific opinion now concern only the extent and timing of the warming. The 'best guess' of one scientific panel was that, if emissions grow at current rates, there will be a 1 °C rise in temperature above today's average by about 2025, and a rise of about 3 °C by 2100, with an upper estimate of 5 °C; rates of increase which are 10 to 100 times faster than any in the past. Carbon dioxide in the atmosphere, which has increased by 25 per cent since industrialization began, contributes about half the effect, with chlorofluorocarbons, methane, and nitrous oxide accounting for the rest. The picture is complicated by feedback mechanisms that could dampen or accelerate change, the most sinister one being the positive feedback loop that could arise out of the release of frozen methane from thawing permafrost.

Regional changes are difficult to predict. Most models suggest a rise in temperature and a fall in rainfall in middle latitudes, especially in the centre of continents, causing drought and reduced grain harvests. Hunger and famine could follow, especially in poor tropical communities where human survival is already marginal, and in the many communities fed from the North American grain belt. Rises in sea level of between 0.3 and 1.1 m are expected by 2100, with the permanent flooding of low-lying communities in Bangladesh, Egypt, Pakistan, Indonesia, and Thailand.

Rising average temperatures are expected to increase the incidence of communicable diseases, especially those that are vector borne, notably malaria. Above 32 °C, and especially above about 38 °C, mortality increases, especially among the aged or already chronically ill, from heart disease, stroke, heat stress, and heat stroke. The incidence of basal- and squamous-cell carcinoma, melanoma, and probably also cataracts is expected to increase as the ozone layer is destroyed and ultraviolet irradiation increases.

There is now almost unanimous scientific agreement that emissions must be reduced, but how much, how fast, and at what cost? The Intergovernmental Panel on Climatic Change (**IPCC**) concluded that emissions of carbon dioxide, the main greenhouse gas, need to be reduced by 60 to 80 per cent worldwide to stabilize the climate, and even this may not be enough. To reach the IPCC target the average household in the United Kingdom will have to cut its emissions of carbon dioxide from 27.3 to 2.2 tonnes.

The global destruction of the family—'physician heal thyself'

Anthropologically, there are many kinds of family, so that the traditional nuclear family with two stably married parents living at home is not the only one, and might not even be the best one for industrial and post-industrial societies. However, one of the most notable features of being human, particularly in an industrial society, is the need for continuing support by carers close to us, ideally our parents, until we are at least 20, and thereafter support by a spouse 'in sickness and in health . . . till death do us part'. Before this actually happens we need care in our 80s and 90s by our children. To be deprived of such support is to be in a large measure isolated, with all that this means for well-being, for development of children, and for our chances of being cared for at home in acute and chronic sickness, and in old age. Not only is the traditional family the tested arrangement for safeguarding the welfare of children, but it is much cheaper than any of its alternatives in providing care and housing. The loneliness and single parenthood that result from broken families may have substantial effects on health.

There are also signs that even 'normal' family life is deteriorating; a study in the United States found that fathers only spend 40 seconds a day interacting with their children. The headmaster of a British public school found it necessary to remind parents to eat with their children. In Britain the family only started to succumb seriously in the 1960s, but is now doing so increasingly fast. Every year now, 150 000 British children under 16 are added to the number who experience the divorce of their parents; on present trends a quarter of all children will be subject to its short- and long-term effects. Never-married mothers quadrupled to 360 000 over the period 1971–89. In 1980, 12 per cent of births took place outside marriage; in 1990, 28 per cent did so. Only 10 per cent of mothers with a prenuptial conception now marry, compared with 20 per cent a decade ago. One-parent families now comprise 19 per cent of all families, and 28 per cent of births now take place outside marriage.

In the United States the epidemic of teenage pregnancy—'children having children'—has become a public health crisis, and the divorce rate has doubled in 10 years and increased 700 per cent this century. Two-fifths of children will live in single-parent homes for at least part of their youth; and more than half the mothers of school-age children work outside the home, with all that this means for family life. One year after divorce the average man's standard of living has increased 42 per cent, while that of his spouse—and usually their children—has fallen 73 per cent, with the result that the 40 per cent of the population in poverty are children, often very young ones.

Divorce and the health of children

It is not that individual children from single-parent families cannot prosper, but that well into adult life they do worse *on average* than those from traditional families in every dimension in which they are measured—physically, emotionally, behaviourally, educationally, economically, and in terms of smoking and drinking—disadvantages that are not adequately explained by their often lower standard of living. They die earlier, do less well at school, are less well nourished, suffer more unemployment, and are more prone to deviance and crime. They are between two and five times more susceptible to psychiatric illness, and run a higher risk of physical and psychological ill health from the time of parental separation well into adult life. Even their bone age is delayed. If they are under 5 when their parents divorce, they are particularly vulnerable. It is hardly surprisingly therefore that the suicide rate in British children aged 10 to 14 has doubled, and in adolescents aged 15 to 19 has tripled in the last 20 years.

Given, then, that stable families are so strongly associated with health and well-being, why are they declining? Which factors in the modern industrial economy are the likely culprits? The complex web of factors includes contraceptive technology, especially 'the pill'; women working outside the home; women's careers; the financial stresses that follow from ever greater material expectations; families not eating together; the stress and difficulty of 'coping' in a complex modern society; excessive mobility and the alienation from genuine community; changes in interpersonal relations and in the ethics of sex and marriage, the decline of religion, and the advance of the media.

So what is to be done? Will more enlightened employment policies (flexitime and parental leave), education in personal relationships for teenagers, or early intervention and better counselling be enough? Or will the preservation of the family require something much more radical?

The destruction of community

The community is in one sense only the family writ large. Loss of community finds expression in crime, drugs, vandalism, and violence—in the course of a year 10 per cent of inner-city women in western Philadelphia sustained injuries that ended in death, or the accident and emergency department; for those aged between 15 and 34 years the figures were even higher, 16 per cent. There is now increasing evidence that a strong local community is essential to psychological well-being, personal growth, and social order. Modern industry is destroying the community in many ways, but especially by its demand for excessive mobility of employment, such that the average house in England and the United States changes hands about every 5 years, and in doing so breaks the family and neighbourhood ties that require many years to establish. The workers that it so easily declares redundant commonly suffer such severe collapse of their living standards, and self-image, that physical and emotional morbidity follow.

The extent of family and community breakdown, *anomie,* and deculturation in the most severely affected areas is better experienced than described. There is so much crime, vandalism, violence, teenage pregnancy, incest, substance abuse, and alcoholism (and smoking): and so little employment or stable relationship. There is a vanishing sense of either family or community.

This is one result of the industrial economy, and is found in the worst housing estates rather than in the inner cities, often with striking differences between adjacent streets, so that the condition of the worst areas is hidden in aggregate data. It is particularly common in the oldest industrial towns, where the industrial process has now proceeded over six generations. Those with ability have moved away, leaving those who remain highly dependent on the social services (they would starve if there were none), and also making heavy demands on the health services. Although mortality rates are disproportionately high from malignant, respiratory, and heart disease, psychological and emotional morbidity and 'unwell-being' are the greater problem. Some of the premature ageing that was recorded among the workers of the early industrial revolution seems to have reappeared. The increasing speed of the process is alarming—when in the depression of the 1930s 'rowdies broke the place up', they subsequently worked to pay for repairs—such social solidarity is unthinkable now. Much of the individual and community damage now appears irreparable, particularly in the absence of a viable political philosophy that can embrace such problems. Not surprisingly, the social workers in such communities are run off their feet and can barely begin to cope.

Demographic entrapment

The problems of the industrial world are at least partly recognized. The same cannot properly be said of many parts of the developing world. The numbers of the human species are expected to double and could triple, with medicine partly responsible for the increase. Will rapidly growing populations in the developing world outgrow the carrying capacity of their ecosystems, and what will happen if they do?

A local population is demographically trapped if it has exceeded, or is projected to exceed the combination of: (a) the carrying capacity of its own ecosystem, (b) its ability to obtain the products, and particularly the food, produced by other ecosystems except as food aid, and (c) its ability to migrate to other ecosystems in a manner which preserves (or improves) its standard of living (voluntary migration). Items (b) and (c) describe the links that a population has with other ecosystems, and are crucial, so they are most easily thought of as 'connectedness', and its opposite 'disconnectedness'. A severely trapped population has a choice of five possible entrapment options in varying combination. Depending on local cultural, political and ecological factors it can: (i) migrate in misery to a refugee camp or urban slum (involuntary migration); (ii) become progressively stunted, and/or starve; (iii) slaughter itself or its neighbours; (iv) die from disease; (v) be supported indefinitely by food aid (if food is available). Since endangered populations are growing rapidly, the critical part of the definition is '. . . is projected to . . .', and concerns the ultimate size of a population at the end of its demographic transition when its demographic momentum is exhausted, in relation to its carrying capacity and its connectedness. The major constraint is time, and particularly whether there is yet time to bring the birth rate down before carrying capacity and connectedness are exceeded.

Population pressure was already so high in Rwanda that it was well up in the list of trapped countries before its recent tragedy. The scale and nature of the slaughter, with neighbour killing neighbour, suggest that population pressure was a major factor in the initiation of the genocide and its manifestation at village level. What other countries are trapped in that they can be expected to follow Rwanda? We should have answered this question long ago, but have not done so because it confronts us with a formidable list of dilemmas that we would prefer to forget.

The concept of entrapment is 'politically incorrect', especially in North America. The result is a curious state of 'doublethink', in which private and official United Nations views of reality drift further apart. Entrapment brings 'the population problem' from being something 'out there' which we can more easily forget, to being something 'down here', which is much more threatening. It confronts us with the problem of 'who is going to starve (or slaughter his neighbour) and when is this going to happen? It forces us to think about 'population control'. It points out the failure of conventional family planning programmes down to a two-child norm. It threatens some 'human rights', especially those of a woman to have as many children as she wishes, regardless of the interests of her community. It threatens the pro-life position on abortion, and some aspects of the feminist movement. Unfortunately, the ecological constraints on population of territory, food, and water fail to recognize such rights. It is not that such rights do not exist, but that they have to be modified to take account of entrapment. Put bluntly, the choice may be between aborted fetuses and starving adults. If entrapment is severe there is a conflict between the interests of the child and his or her community, in that one more child mouth to feed means less to eat for someone else. This is only serious when child mortality is high (as presently in Rwanda). Entrapment also questions the high status of the child in contemporary western liberalism. It forces us to re-examine one of the fundamental assumptions of public health, which is that diseases which could be eradicated or controlled should be. The eradication of smallpox contributed to the entrapment of Rwanda. It threatens some research programmes, such as those for a malarial vaccine. Entrapment especially threatens 'the Northern lifstyle', and it reminds us that the richest eat at least four times as much as the poorest, in terms of grain equivalent. It requires that constraints on the migration of ecological refugees need to be eased for flows of at least tens of millions. It questions the priorities of many agencies, including those of the United Nations system. It presents us with some new ethical problems: (i) should a seriously trapped community be faced with the proposition 'if you don't limit your families to one child, you will starve'; (ii) 'if starvation is to occur, would suffering be minimized if it were slow or fast?'

THE CONTAINING MORAL CONTEXT AND THE RETREAT TO EGO

One of the superstitions of modern society is that if *ego* maximizes his or her choices we are all better off—the fallacy that individual freedom is a collective good. We forget that a society and its members require mutual civility for mere survival, that its moral capital is at least as important as capital of any other kind, and is transferred (or lost) between one generation and another. In many societies there are signs that this capital is being destroyed by increasingly uncontrolled self-interestedness. How closely retreat to *ego* in the family is connected with the industrial economy *per se* is arguable.

Western diseases—epidemiological 'proof' and public health policy

Before white settlers came to East Africa many diseases were either rare or absent: essential hypertension, obesity, non-insulin-dependent diabetes, cholesterol gallstones, cerebrovascular disease, coronary heart disease, peripheral vascular disease, and carcinoma of the colon, for example. They have all appeared since. Evolutionary pressure has been unable to eliminate the genes that predispose to these diseases. Hitherto, only élites have been affluent enough to suffer them. But which factors in this lifestyle are responsible for which disease, and when is epidemiological 'proof' a sufficient basis for public health policy?

The hypothesis here is that our physiology evolved during the millennia that we were hunter-gatherers and is ill adapted to some current lifestyles. For instance, exposure to high energy Western diets and associated lack of exercise must be of considerable importance in the generation of conditions such as coronary artery disease and diabetes mellitus in populations that are genetically poorly adapted to such environmental hazards.

Some of the most potentially remediable of Western diseases and deficiencies of well-being are often forgotten—those that follow from the replacement of mother's milk by formula, and of breast by bottle feeding. These range from impaired bonding and death from diarrhoea, to the absence of lactational amenorrhoea, and the effect this has in shortening birth intervals and increasing the birth rate. It has been said that breast feeding prevents more pregnancies than all the other family planning methods combined.

Intoxication by wealth, imiseration by absolute poverty

The number of people in absolute poverty struggling to remain alive on less than $370 a year has risen, and is presently about a fifth of the world, or about a billion—the world's bottom billion. At the same time the difference between the rich and poor has been increasing. The richest and ever richer fifth, including the European Union, North America, and Japan, enjoys more than 80 per cent of the global product, while those in the poorest fifth do their best to survive on 1 per cent of it. These are figures for entire countries, but if the maldistribution within countries is included, the disparity between richest and poorest fifth increases to a factor of 150. As money buys more in Ougadougu than it does Geneva, the actual difference in purchasing power is a mere 50-fold—and steadily increases; it was only 30-fold in 1960. It is the old problem—wealth begets wealth, just as poverty begets poverty. Wealth also extracts wealth—from the poor—such that in 1983–89 rich creditors received a staggering $214 billion in net transfers on long-term lending from the indebted developing world, with all that this means for the increase or the diseases of poverty.

THE MEDICINE OF WEALTH

Now that medicine can do so much, it is tragic that those who could benefit from it, by contributing regularly to an insurance scheme while they are healthy, often don't get the health care they need when they are sick. This is especially unfortunate because many interventions are, or could be, so cheap, and so much money is spent on health—often inefficiently. In the United States, spending per person in current prices has tripled over the past 12 years from about $1000 in 1980, or 9.1 per cent of gross national product **(GNP)**, to about $3000 in 1992, a total of $800 billion or well over 13 per cent of GNP. Forecasts for the year 2000 are $1.7 trillion and 18 per cent of GNP. Health care costs are rising at more than double the rate of inflation. As President Clinton said 'these costs are overwhelming society . . . they are seriously undermining industrial competitiveness of the USA and are the number one cause of bankruptcy (particularly of the middle classes), and of labour disputes . . . they also add $1000 to the cost of every car made in America'. Despite this massive expense, 12 per cent of the United States population is, at the time of writing, completely uninsured, and a quarter have no regular cover.

If health care is to be universal and efficient, and is not to impoverish society, the following appear essential. (1) Some form of health insurance has to be compulsory, so that steady contributions by all economically active wage earners during health are available to buy care in sickness. The number of insurers also has to be limited—the United States at present has 1500, all requiring different forms, and said to consume 15 per cent of health care expenditure in administrative costs. (2) Some mechanism has to be found for capping total expenditure in a global budget—in the United Kingdom 'cash limits' on the National Health Service are set at Cabinet level. (3) Health care has to be planned, particularly so that expensive health installations are not duplicated unnecessarily. (4) Procedures need to be delegated to the least expensive worker capable of doing them satisfactorily. Why should anaesthetics that can be given by nurses in Sweden and the United States need doctors in Britain? (5) Salaries should not be disproportionate. Sadly, in some of the more affluent societies the salaries earned by doctors are an unnecessary burden on society and an impediment to the care of the sick, especially the sick poor. From 1982 to 1990 the average take home pay of doctors in the United States rose from $98 000 to $164 000, while the average pay for all full-time workers rose from $18 500 to $25 900. Should a general practitioner earn more than a schoolmaster, and is any superspecialist really worth half a million dollars a year (see below)? It is not surprising, therefore, that the British system of merit awards is under threat—the take-home pay associated with a top award is about £90 000 a year, with an additional £38 000 for the two-thirds of consultants who do private work. In a country where average earnings are less than £15 000, the £300 000 that doctors in full-time private practice can earn causes much national envy. (6) All technologies, especially new ones, need to be evaluated, so that only the cost-effective ones are applied. (7) Drugs are second only to salaries in the cost of health care, so the rule must be to use the least expensive ones capable of achieving a given end. The medicines in the World Health Organization's list of essential drugs are also the cheapest, and should be the first choice where possible. (8) Resources must be directed towards health promotion and prevention, and the support of carers in the community.

The temptations of technological immortality

A huge and increasing fraction of all health expenditure is now spent at the very ends of life, often on *tours de force* of technical expertise—more than a quarter is spent on those in the last year of life. In England and Wales in 1984 23 per cent of non-psychiatric beds were occupied by patients who died before discharge. One of medicine's challenges is to find out who these patients are, to realize that not everything that might be done for them has to be done, and to do its best, ethically and wisely, to redirect the resources that are freed.

Another challenge concerns the care of those patients who don't want to live any more. An increasing number for whom life has become an intolerable burden are finding it difficult to die—when they want to; hence a growing movement in many countries to make euthanasia easier. The Netherlands' government is codifying what has hitherto been an informal concordat between the medical profession, the coroners, and the public prosecutors. Although euthanasia is legally criminal, prosecutions are rare, provided doctors abide by strict guidelines. A recent study found that medical decisions concerning the end of life (MDEL) were taken in 54 per cent of all non-acute deaths, and 38 per cent of all deaths. In 17.5 per cent of these, such high doses of opioids were used to alleviate pain and symptoms that the patient's life was probably shortened. In another 17.5 per cent, non-treatment decisions were made. In a further 1.8 per cent, lethal drugs were given at the patient's request (euthanasia), including 0.3 per cent in which he took them himself (assisted suicide). Altogether 54 per cent of doctors were found to have used euthanasia (96 per cent only on explicit and persistent request), and another 34 per cent said that they could conceive of situations where they might. The reasons for requesting it included loss of dignity, unworthy dying, dependency, tiredness of life, and pain. Each year, 25 000 patients in The Netherlands ask their doctors to make sure that they will be given assistance if suffering becomes unbearable. Altogether, there are nearly a thousand explicit requests for euthanasia each year, of which less than a third are agreed to.

Should euthanasia (strictly defined) be decriminalized altogether? Should it remain a criminal act in principle with clear rules about when and when not to prosecute? Or should the *status quo* continue? All societies, including Britain, where no informal concordat exists, are going to have to decide. Here, although the withdrawal of dialysis is allowed, illogically the withdrawal of tube feeding is not. National decisions will be easier when there has been as thorough a study, and as much public debate, as in Holland. Discussion needs to start from the premise that, in the best interests of the dying, MDEL are already being taken.

Epilogue—'health is an ecosustainable state'

There seems to be no panacea for sickness in the body economic, beyond a steely resolve to stare the facts in the face, and the certain need for sacrifice—the foregoing of present material gratification for much greater good. 'Deep ecologists' argue for no economic growth, for simpler lifestyles, for lowered material standards of living, and for a global economic consciousness. It seems that we shall need a 'carbon tax', or a 'carbon ration', or both. We shall also need 'the bicycle lifestyle', to recycle everything, and to live in much more locally self-sufficient communities. Population growth must slow, forests be replanted, and, most controversial of all, will we also need a media policy ('control of the media'), in the interests of the ecosustainability and the stability of the family? All these measures are in the end ideological. What is wanted, therefore, is a full onslaught on all the ethical presuppositions of late capitalism—which include *inter alia* that the West has the right to go on consuming the world's resources at a disproportionate rate, that migratory population flows from areas of ecological breakdown can and should be stopped; that a sophisticated form of aid-by-triage is morally acceptable; and that we can use a full but largely invisible battery of financial and economic devices to extract wealth and welfare from the poor countries in order to buttress our own standard of living. The ethic of global solidarity, which should now be mandatory, is devastatingly demanding of us in the West.

So it is a challenging era in which to be practising medicine—especially for those born since the discovery of the double helix. The psalmist wrote: 'Whither shall I go from my spirit, whither shall I flee from they presence? If I ascend into heaven thou art there, if I make my bed in hell, behold thou art there. If I take the wings of the morning and dwell in the uttermost parts of the sea, even there shall thy hand lead me, and my right hand shall hold me.' Let us never forget that many of our patients do, in fact, lie in beds in hell. Especially, let us never allow such beds to be made for them, either by society, or by the health care system, or by ourselves.

REFERENCES

Anderson, D.C. (ed.) *Loss of virtue, moral confusion and social disorder in Britain and America.* Social Affairs Unit, distributed from 2 Spey Close, Altringham, Cheshire.

Bloom, A. (1987). *The closing of the American mind.* Simon and Schuster, New York.

Daly, H.E. and Cobb, J.B. (1980). *For the common good* (1980 Greenprint). Merlin Press, London.

Dennis, N. and Erdos, G. (1992). *Families without fatherhood.* IEA Health and Welfare Unit, 2 Lord North Street, London SW1P 3LB.

Editorial (1993). Rise and fall of diseases. *Lancet,* **341,** 151–2.

Haines, A. (1991). Global warming and health. *British Medical Journal,* **302,** 669–70.

King, M.H. (1990). Health is a sustainable state. *Lancet,* **336,** 664–7.

King, M.H. and Elliott, C. (1993). Legitimate doublethink. *Lancet,* **341,** 669–72.

Ravetz, J.R. (1990). *The merger of knowledge with power; essays in critical science.* Mansell, London and New York.

Morgan, T. (1992). Sodium and blood pressure revisited. *Medical Journal of Australia,* **156,** 4–5.

Townsend, P., Phillimore, P., and Beattie, A. (1989). *Health and deprivation, inequality and the north.* Routledge, London.

Trowell, H.C. and Burkitt, D.P. (1981). Western diseases: their emergence and prevention. Edward Arnold, London.

Van der Maas, P. *et al.* (1992). Euthanasia and other medical decisions concerning the end of life. *Lancet,* **338,** 669–74.

3.2 Health and sickness in the community

M. J. Goldacre and M. P. Vessey

The World Health Organization has defined health as a state of 'complete physical, mental, and social well-being and not merely the absence of disease and infirmity'. This definition emphasizes that our attitude towards health should be a positive one but, for practical purposes, heavy reliance is placed on negative indices—mortality, morbidity, and disability—in measuring the health status of communities.

Mortality in the United Kingdom

Mortality statistics have been collected and analysed routinely in the United Kingdom since 1838. They occupy a special place in the measurement of disease because of their ready availability both for geographical and historical comparison. Tables 1 and 2 show annual death rates for England and Wales, expressed per 1000 individuals within each age group, at various times during the twentieth century. Mortality rates declined substantially at all ages, although the changes are more impressive in those under 45 years of age than in older people. Analysis of mortality rates by cause leaves no doubt that numerically the most important factor in the decline has been the fall in deaths from infectious diseases. The reasons for this are to some extent a matter of speculation, although it is clear that for many diseases the greater part of the reduction occurred before the introduction of specific medical interventions, such as immunization or antimicrobial chemotherapy, directed to the

Table 1 *Annual death rates per 1000 people within each age group for selected years, England and Wales: males*

Age (years)	1901–5	1931–5	1951–5	1961–5	1971–5	1981–5	1986–90
Less than 1[a]	151	70	30	23	19	11	10
1–4	20.1	6.9	1.2	0.9	0.7	0.5	0.4
5–9	3.7	2.3	0.6	0.5	0.4	0.3	0.2
10–14	2.1	1.4	0.5	0.4	0.3	0.3	0.2
15–19	3.2	2.5	0.9	1	0.9	0.8	0.7
20–24	4.4	3.2	1.2	1.1	1	0.8	0.9
25–34	5.9	3.3	1.4	1.1	1	0.9	0.9
35–44	9.7	5.4	2.7	2.5	2.2	1.7	1.7
45–54	17	11	7.9	7.4	7.2	5.7	4.9
55–64	32	24	23	22	20	17	16
65–74	65	57	55	54	51	45	41
75–84	138	135	127	121	115	104	96
85 and over	275	279	266	253	237	221	195
All ages	17.1	12.7	12.5	12.4	12.3	11.9	11.5
SMR[b]	234	127	98	95	89	78	72

[a]Deaths under 1 year of age per 1000 live births.

[b]Standardized mortality ratio (base years, 1950–2 = 100).

Source: Office of Population Censuses and Surveys (1992). *1841–1990 mortality statistics: serial tables*, Series DH 1 no. 25. HMSO, London.

Table 2 *Annual death rates per 1000 people within each age group for selected years, England and Wales: females*

Age (years)	1901–5	1931–5	1951–5	1961–5	1971–5	1981–5	1986–90
Less than 1[a]	124	54	23	18	15	9	8
1–4	19.2	6.2	1	0.8	0.6	0.4	0.4
5–9	3.8	2.1	0.4	0.3	0.3	0.2	0.2
10–14	2.2	1.4	0.3	0.3	0.2	0.2	0.2
15–19	3	2.2	0.5	0.4	0.4	0.3	0.3
20–24	3.7	2.8	0.7	0.5	0.4	0.3	0.3
25–34	5	3.1	1.1	0.7	0.6	0.5	0.5
35–44	8.1	4.3	2.1	1.8	1.6	1.2	1.1
45–54	13	8	4.9	4.4	4.4	3.6	3.1
55–64	25	17	12	11	10	9.6	8.9
65–74	55	43	33	30	26	24	23
75–84	120	109	92	84	75	64	60
85 and over	249	245	222	207	189	176	161
All ages	15	11.4	10.9	11.2	11.4	11.4	11.3
SMR[b]	264	141	95	87	80	73	69

[a]Deaths under 1 year of age per 1000 live births.

[b]Standardized mortality ratio (base years, 1950–2 = 100).

Source: see Table 1.

care of the individual patient (Fig.1). McKeown has suggested that the main reasons for the downward trend in mortality have been, in order of importance, rising standards of living (of which possibly the most significant factor was improvement in diet), developments in hygiene and the control of the physical environment, limitation of population growth, and the introduction of preventive and therapeutic medical measures.

The infant mortality rate (i.e. deaths under 1 year of age per 1000 live births) declined dramatically in the United Kingdom during the twentieth century (Tables 1 and 2). None the less, death rates are still higher in the first year of life than in any other single year below the age of 55 in males or 60 in females. The main causes of death in the neonatal period (the first 4 weeks of life) are now those associated with low birth weight, complications of pregnancy and childbirth, and congenital malformations. The main causes of death in the postneonatal period (from the end of the fourth week to the end of the first year of life) are respiratory and other infective diseases, congenital malformations, the sudden infant death syndrome, and accidents.

Death rates in children aged 1 to 14 years have shown about a 10-fold decline since the beginning of the twentieth century, mainly due to the reduction in deaths from infectious diseases, and now stand at very low levels. Accidents presently account for about one-third of all deaths in this age group and neoplasms for one-fifth. Other numerically important causes of death include congenital malformations and respiratory infections.

For adolescents and young adults, mortality has fallen more steeply in females than in males (see Tables 1 and 2). The importance of accidents as a cause of death in young adults, especially in males, is shown in Table 3.

In older age groups, neoplasms and circulatory diseases are now the dominant causes of death (Table 4). Mortality rates among men in middle- and late middle-age showed a marked improvement during the early part of the twentieth century (Fig.2) but began to level off in the 1920s and showed only modest changes from then until the 1970s. Mortality rates among women in these age groups declined much more strikingly than those in men. This period saw the emergence of two conditions in

Fig. 1 Standardized mortality ratios for tuberculosis: England and Wales.

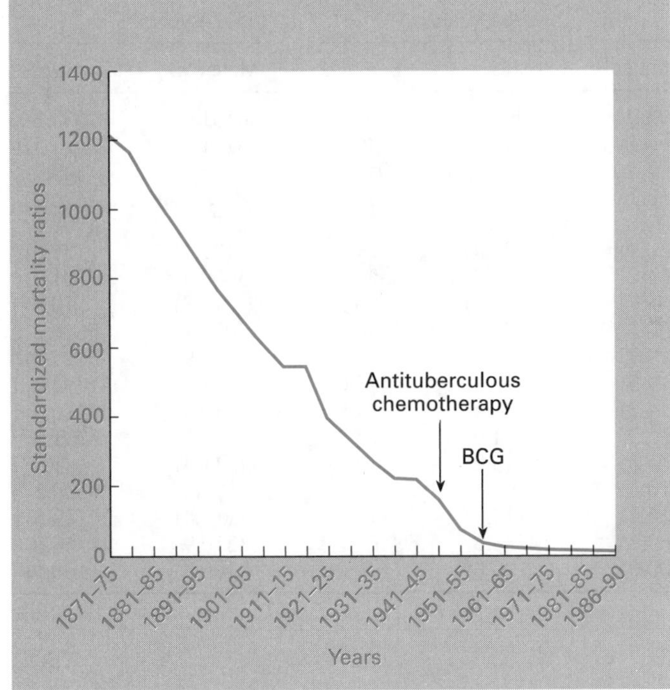

particular, ischaemic heart disease (notably acute myocardial infarction) and lung cancer, which have increased substantially as causes of death and which, at present, are both more common in men than women. During the 1980s, overall death rates in men in these age groups started to decline again (in particular, male death rates from lung cancer and myocardial infarction have started to fall) whilst those in women have started to level off.

Morbidity in the United Kingdom

THE HOSPITAL PERSPECTIVE

Most routinely available information on morbidity in the population comes from statistics about the contact of people with health services. Some of the most common causes of death are also among the most common reasons for hospital admission—for example, acute myocardial infarction, other manifestations of ischaemic heart disease, cerebrovascular disease, and cancers. But other conditions are also prominent: these include head injuries, adverse effects of medicinal agents (mainly self-poisoning), diabetes mellitus, bronchitis, asthma, and admissions for tonsillectomy, appendicectomy, herniorrhaphy, termination of pregnancy, uterine dilatation and curettage, prostatectomy and cholecystectomy.

Detailed information on the use made of outpatient services in the United Kingdom is not routinely collected but much specialist care is provided without admission to hospital; outpatient attendances exceed inpatient admissions in the acute specialties by an overall ratio of about 5 : 1.

THE GENERAL PRACTITIONER'S PERSPECTIVE

Hospital patients constitute a small proportion of all contacts between doctors and patients. An estimated 98 per cent of all episodes of illness that result in medical consultation are managed wholly within general practice. In addition, the majority of patients who are seen in hospital are referred from general practice. Some of the most common and some of the serious but less common reasons for consultation in general practice are shown in Table 5.

THE INDIVIDUAL'S PERSPECTIVE

Data on illnesses that do not result in contact with the health service are relatively sparse but some information on self-reported illness is available from the General Household Survey, in which samples of the population are interviewed about various matters including health. In the most recent survey, 14 per cent of the population said that they had had an acute sickness, causing a restriction of normal activity, in the 14 days prior to interview. Self-reported long-standing illness was recorded for 33 per cent of males and 35 per cent of females and, as might be expected, the percentage of respondents with self-reported illness rose with advancing age. Some common conditions that accounted for self-reported, long-standing illness are shown in Table 6.

Sources of information about disease in the community

Sample surveys are undertaken from time to time by research workers to determine the occurrence of particular diseases in the community.

Table 3 *Death rates in people aged 15–24 and 25–34 years per million people of each sex in each age group: England 1990*

	Males		Females	
Causes	15–24 years	25–34 years	15–24 years	25–34 years
Neoplasms	63.0 (7.6)	118.2 (12.7)	40.6 (14.0)	140.9 (32.5)
Circulatory diseases	29.8 (3.6)	82.8 (8.9)	21.3 (7.3)	43.7 (10.1)
Respiratory diseases	17.9 (2.2)	41.5 (4.5)	17.8 (6.1)	16.2 (3.7)
Accidents	576.2 (69.8)	507.8 (54.7)	128.7 (44.2)	130.2 (30.0)
All other causes	138.4 (16.8)	178.6 (19.2)	82.5 (28.4)	102.5 (23.6)
TOTAL	825.3 (100.0)	928.9 (100.0)	290.9 (100.0)	433.5 (100.0)

Percentage of all deaths within each age group in parentheses.

Source: Office of Population Censuses and Surveys (1992). *1990 morbidity statistics: general*, Series DH 1 no. 24. HMSO, London.

Table 4 *Death rates in people aged 35–74 years per million people in each age group for selected causes of death: England, 1990.*

	35–44 years		45–54 years		55–64 years		65–74 years	
Causes	Males	Females	Males	Females	Males	Females	Males	Females
Malignant neoplasm of lung	64.8 (3.8)	44.1 (4.0)	401.4 (8.8)	193.0 (6.7)	1797.7 (12.6)	763.4 (9.0)	4531.3 (11.8)	1634.8 (7.5)
Malignant neoplasm of female breast		211.6 (19.2)		577.8 (20.1)		1017.2 (12.0)		1343.7 (6.2)
All other neoplasms	308.0 (18.1)	331.9 (30.1)	1050.1 (23.1)	873.1 (30.4)	3332.2 (23.4)	2315.3 (27.3)	8072.4 (21.1)	4708.6 (21.6)
Cerebrovascular disease	60.0 (3.5)	60.5 (5.5)	209.1 (4.6)	164.2 (5.7)	772.3 (5.4)	535.5 (6.3)	3000.5 (7.8)	2301.2 (10.6)
Ischaemic heart disease	350.8 (20.6)	53.2 (4.8)	1513.2 (33.3)	306.3 (10.7)	5105.1 (35.9)	1670.7 (19.7)	13003.1 (33.9)	5646.2 (25.9)
Other circulatory diseases	73.6 (4.3)	31.7 (2.9)	209.2 (4.6)	119.5 (4.2)	774.0 (5.4)	412.6 (4.9)	2487.4 (6.5)	1492.1 (6.9)
Accidents	478.3 (28.1)	150.8 (13.7)	452.1 (9.9)	165.3 (5.8)	451.9 (3.2)	205.7 (2.4)	538.6 (1.4)	331.9 (1.5)
All other causes	366.2 (21.5)	217.7 (19.8)	709.3 (15.6)	470.4 (16.4)	2005.4 (14.1)	1546.7 (18.3)	6677.6 (17.4)	4309.5 (19.8)
All causes	1701.7 (100.0)	1101.5 (100.0)	4544.4 (100.0)	2869.6 (100.0)	14238.6 (100.0)	8467.1 (100.0)	38310.9 (100.0)	21768.0 (100.0)

Percentage of all deaths within each age/sex group in parentheses.
Source: see Table 3.

However, most systematic information comes from routinely collected statistics and these are usually worth consulting before embarking on special studies. In addition to the sources of information referred to so far, there are some diseases that are recorded in systems of notification and registration. Notification of certain infectious diseases was introduced gradually in England and Wales around the turn of the twentieth century as a means of controlling individual outbreaks and of monitoring the occurrence of infectious disease. Statistics are published regularly. Registration of cancers is undertaken in a number of countries, including the United Kingdom. International data from cancer registries are now pooled and the latest publication from the International Association of Cancer Registries provides data on cancers from over 100 populations in 36 countries. Many studies that make interpopulation comparisons in cancer epidemiology use this source of information. There are also registration or notification systems for congenital malformations, some industrial diseases, and certain forms of handicap.

Diseases in the community: the epidemiological approach

The physician engaged in clinical practice is concerned with the diagnosis, treatment, and care of patients as individuals. There are, however, circumstances where it is important to relate the illness of individuals to the populations from which they are drawn. Epidemiology is the study of disease and its distribution in defined populations. The hallmark of epidemiology is that it is concerned with both identifying the individuals who have the disease under study and with enumerating those who do not. In this way it is possible to calculate rates of occurrence of disease and to estimate whether the disease is more common in people with particular characteristics than in others, whether it is more common in one place than another, and whether its occurrence has changed over time. The term 'population' means more to the epidemiologist than simply a geographically defined group of people: it includes, for example,

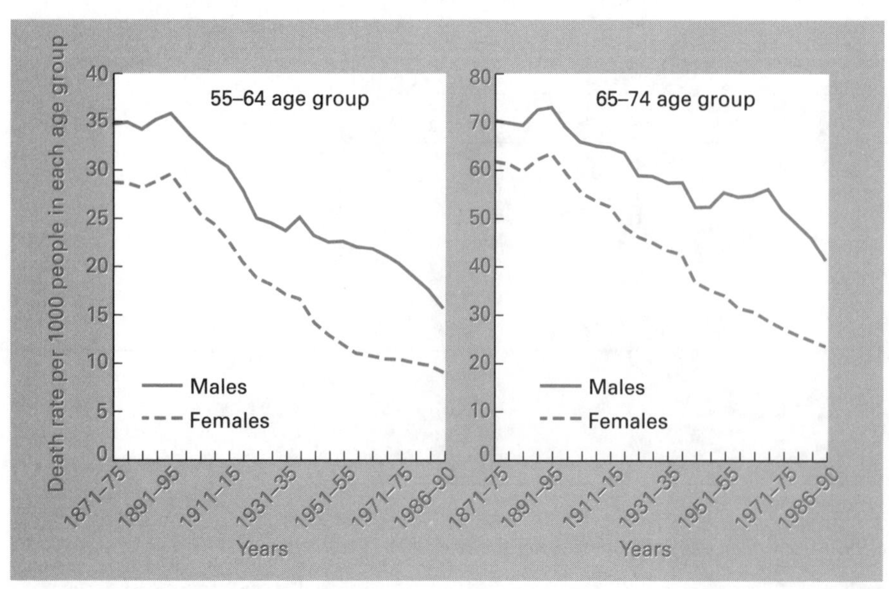

Fig. 2 Annual death rates in people aged 55–74 years: England and Wales.

Table 5 *Average number of people who consulted general practitioners per year per 1000 population, tabulated by reason for consultation*

Disease	No. of patients
Selected broad disease groupings	
Diseases of the respiratory system	407.8
Diseases of the nervous system and sense organs	182.6
Diseases of the musculoskeletal system	167.8
Diseases of the skin	140.5
Infections	138.1
Accidents	133.0
Neoplasms	14.2
Selected specific reasons for consultation	
Upper acute respiratory infection	156.1
Contraceptive advice	69.1
Bronchitis, bronchiolitis	67.6
Anxiety, depression	57.6
Tonsillitis	48.9
Hypertension	41.4
Intestinal infection	35.7
Abdominal pain	32.1
Back pain	31.1
Conjunctivitis	30.3
Diabetes mellitus	7.7
Stroke	4.3
Acute myocardial infarction	4.3
Appendicitis	1.5
Neoplasm of lung	0.9
Lymphoma, leukaemia	0.6

Source: Office of Population Censuses and Surveys (1986). *Morbidity statistics from general practice. Third national study, 1981–1982*, Series MB5 no. 1. HMSO, London.

Table 6 *Chronic sickness rates: number of people who reported long-standing illness per 1000 population for selected conditions*

	Age in years			
Conditions	16–44	45–64	65–74	75 and over
Musculoskeletal	77	177	241	331
Heart and circulatory	17	124	238	251
Respiratory	60	55	84	94
Digestive	21	47	60	88
Eye complaints	8	18	50	115
Ear complaints	10	23	45	60
Endocrine and metabolic	13	38	61	68

Source: Office of Population Censuses and Surveys (1989). *General household survey*, Series GHS no. 20. HMSO, London.

groups of people defined by their age, sex, or occupation, or who share particular social, behavioural, or environmental characteristics.

Measurement in epidemiology

Several general measures are commonly used in epidemiology. The incidence of a disease is the number of new cases occurring during a specified period of time. The incidence rate is this number per specified unit of population. A conventional expression of an incidence rate would be the number of new cases of the disease that occurred per year per thousand (or million) population. The prevalence of a disease is the total number of cases of the disease existing in the population at a specified time; and the prevalence rate is this number expressed per unit of population, say, per thousand individuals. There is an obvious numerical relation between the measures of incidence and prevalence: the prevalence of a disease varies according to the product of its incidence and duration. In circumstances where the incidence of a disease and its duration—the length of time from onset to recovery or death—remain constant over time, the prevalence of the disease equals the product of its incidence and duration.

The occurrence of most diseases and death varies considerably with age. It is usually more appropriate, therefore, to calculate age-specific mortality, incidence, or prevalence rates than 'all ages' rates. Indeed, a comparison of, say, mortality rates between populations of different age compositions that does not take account of age-specific rates can be very misleading. For example, whilst mortality rates have declined in every single age group over the past 50 years, the 'all ages' mortality rate has shown little change (Tables 1 and 2). The reason for this seeming paradox is that the percentage of elderly people in the population has increased over the years; and that, because the risk of dying is much higher in the elderly than in the young, the population has contained a greater percentage of people at 'high risk' of dying by virtue of their age in recent than in earlier years.

In practice, a comparison between populations across a whole range of age-specific rates is usually rather cumbersome. Statistical methods have therefore been developed to summarize the disease experience of populations in a single figure that is standardized for differences in the age structure of the populations. One statistic commonly used for this purpose is the standardized mortality ratio. This is the ratio of the number of deaths actually observed in a study population to the number of deaths that would have occurred in the population if it had experienced the age-specific death rates of a standard population. The standardized mortality ratios in Table 1 indicate that the age-standardized death rate for males in 1931–5 was 27 per cent higher, and that in 1986–90 was 28 per cent lower, than that in 1950–2. The methods of standardization can be applied to the study of morbidity as well as mortality rates, can be used to take account of differences between the sexes as well as differences in age, and can be used to compare populations defined by any number of characteristics.

Epidemiology in the study of causes and risks

The main application of epidemiology has been to study the determinants of the distribution and spread of disease in populations. The aim of this approach to disease, aetiological epidemiology, is to identify factors that are causally associated with the occurrence of disease and may be manipulated in order to prevent it.

A classic example is the demonstration by John Snow in mid-nineteenth century London that mortality from cholera was higher in areas that received their water supply from a particular company which obtained its water from a part of the river Thames heavily polluted with sewage. Snow recognized that factors other than differences in water supply might be correlated with the geographical differences in mortality from cholera. He took account of this possibility in the design of his studies, which, indeed, finally implicated contaminated water as an important means by which cholera had spread. More recent examples of aetiological epidemiology include (among many others) the studies of the association between smoking and lung cancer; between the use of oral contraceptives and the risk of cardiovascular disease; between X-irradiation and leukaemia; between maternal rubella and congenital malformations; between work in the dye and rubber industry and cancer; and between dietary factors, exercise, and ischaemic heart disease.

The concept of a causal association is one of profound importance in epidemiology. First, an observed association may be causal (factor A causes disease B) either directly or indirectly, such that a change in the factor will result in a change in the frequency of the disease. Secondly, the possibility must sometimes be considered that the disease has caused the factor associated with it, rather than vice versa, as when the occurrence of the disease itself leads to a change in (say) the dietary, behavioural, or physiological variable under study. Thirdly, an observed association may be non-causal. For example, if factor A influences both factor B and disease C, factor B and disease C will be associated statistically. The association between B and C will, however, be non-causal and there would be no hope of producing a change in disease C by manipulating factor B. Awareness of the possibility of obtaining spurious associations, through 'confounding' variables, is a central feature in the design, analysis, and interpretation of epidemiological studies.

Descriptive studies

Descriptive epidemiological studies are undertaken to determine whether a disease varies in frequency from place to place, has changed in frequency over time, and whether particular characteristics of populations with a high frequency of the disease distinguish them from populations in which the frequency of the disease is low. Examples of geographical variation in disease frequency are legion—see, for instance, Chapter 6.2 in relation to cancers and heart disease—and, indeed, all countries exhibit their own patterns of disease.

Studies of variation in disease frequency over time may be concerned with long-term trends (for example, changes in the occurrence of lung cancer or coronary heart disease over decades), with the cyclical changes characteristic of an infectious aetiology, or with short-term fluctuations in association with other environmental factors (e.g. atmospheric pollution).

Some data on the type of person affected by particular diseases are often available from routine health statistics and, in assembling epidemiological information about a disease, these usually receive early consideration both because of their ready availability and because of the clues they may give to aetiology. They include such factors as patients' age, sex, socioeconomic status, occupation, and marital status. For example, the facts that death rates from cancer of the lung and ischaemic heart disease are strikingly higher among men than women (see Table 4) indicate that aetiological factors exist that predispose males to, or protect females from, these diseases.

Descriptive studies are useful for generating or testing the plausibility of aetiological hypotheses and may occasionally go far towards implicating a particular exposure. However, the investigator will usually wish to proceed to analytical studies (Fig. 3) to test whether the observations made on populations as a whole can be confirmed in groups of people defined according to whether they, as individuals, manifest the disease and have experienced the aetiological factor under study.

Case-control, cohort, and prevalence studies

The starting point for a case-control study is the identification of a group of individuals who have the illness under study and of an appropriate 'control' group of individuals who do not (Fig. 3). Information about prior exposure to the suspected cause is then sought. The exposure of each group to the suspected cause is compared to determine whether it is any more common among the cases than the controls. In a case-control study the diagnostic criteria for the inclusion of cases must be carefully defined; and the control subjects should be chosen such that they are comparable with the cases in all relevant respects except that they do not manifest the disease under consideration. Information about exposure to the suspected cause should be obtained in the same way for both cases and controls. Case-control studies are commonly used to investigate a specific hypothesis—for example, that there is a relation between thromboembolic disease in young women and the use of oral contraceptives. Sometimes, however, if a specific hypothesis is not apparent, case-control studies may be used to explore a wide range of possible aetiological variables.

In a cohort study, groups of people are identified according to whether or not they have been exposed to a factor (or possess a characteristic) that is thought to be related to the subsequent development of a disease. People in the non-exposed cohort are chosen such that they are comparable with the exposed cohort in all relevant respects except that they have not been exposed to the factor under study. These groups of people are then observed over a period of time to determine and compare the frequency of disease among the exposed and non-exposed groups.

Case-control and cohort studies each have advantages and disadvantages. Case-control studies involve many fewer patients than cohort studies; they are usually fairly quick, cheap, relatively easy to undertake, and they are the only feasible way to study rare diseases. Cohort studies usually need observations on large numbers of individuals and may require a period of follow-up over many years. They are therefore usually slow, expensive, and relatively difficult to undertake, and are only practicable for fairly common diseases. The smaller numbers in a case-control study will often permit study of individual cases in depth, whilst the large numbers in a cohort study usually preclude collection of very detailed information on each subject. A case-control study is usually concerned with only a single disease but many possible aetiological factors may be sought. A cohort study is usually concerned with only one type of exposure but allows the study of many different diseases that may subsequently develop in association with the exposure.

Case-control studies are dependent on obtaining information about events that occurred in the past; they may be subject to deficiencies and biases in patients' recall of past events and/or deficiencies of recording in old medical records. They are also sometimes subject to problems of bias in the selection of cases and controls. The problems of recall and some of the problems of bias can be avoided in cohort studies. Case-control studies cannot be used to study variables (such as physiological measurements) that may be altered by the disease; such factors can be studied in cohort studies. Case-control studies usually provide an estimate of relative risk only; cohort studies provide information on both relative and absolute risk (see below).

In a prevalence study the investigator studies individuals within a defined population to discover those with a disease (or with various levels of a quantitative attribute, e.g. blood pressure, serum cholesterol) and, at the same time, also measures the presence or absence of factors suspected to be related to the existence of the disease (or level of the attribute). The investigator then assesses whether the disease and the suspected causative factor coexist more commonly than would be expected by chance. Prevalence studies can avoid some of the biases inherent in the selection of cases in a case-control study, or in the identification of exposed individuals in a cohort study, because the whole population is sampled. Uniform criteria can be used readily in both the measurement of disease and of factors associated with it because both are studied simultaneously. As with cohort studies, prevalence studies usually require large numbers of individuals and are only appropriate for common conditions with a chronic course; but, unlike cohort studies, information on the occurrence of disease in relation to the factors associated with it does not need to await the passage of years. A common problem with prevalence studies, however, is that of distinguishing whether the disease preceded the factor associated with it or vice versa. A prevalence study may be indispensable when no means exists through available records of identifying cases of the disease or of individuals with a particular exposure. In these circumstances a prevalence survey may be the essential first step in identifying cases for a case-control study or cohorts of individuals for further follow-up.

Interpretation of observational studies

The results of the methods of observational study described so far must be interpreted with due regard to the validity of the observations made and to the possibility of bias and confounding. For example, the investigator who uses routine sources of data such as death certificates must consider the likely accuracy of certification of the cause of death. Interpretation of studies based on patients' recall must include the possibility that diseased individuals may be more likely than others to recall past events that they believe could be associated with their current disease. Bias in the identification of cases must also be considered as when, for example, subjects exposed to a suspected cause of illness are under more intensive medical surveillance than controls because of their exposure. The possibility that an association between a disease and a factor has arisen through the influence of a confounding variable related to both must always be considered.

If an association does not seem to be attributable either to chance or to methodological problems in the design of the study, a causal interpretation can be considered. The likelihood that an observed association is causal is strengthened by (a) an appropriate temporal relation in which the exposure clearly preceded the onset of the disease; (b) a high relative risk; (c) a dose response and/or duration response such that the risk of disease is associated with the degree of exposure; (d) consistency with findings from other epidemiological studies, with the results of laboratory research, and with other known facts about the disease.

Intervention studies

An intervention study, if practicable and ethical, is the definitive experimental way of testing an aetiological hypothesis. The effect of the removal of a factor thought to be related to the development of a disease, or the addition of a factor thought to confer protection, is tested (preferably in a randomized, controlled trial) to see whether the expected changes in disease frequency occur.

Risk

The risk of acquiring a disease can be expressed in several ways (Table 7). The absolute risk of developing a disease per year is given by the annual rate at which the disease occurs. The absolute risk over a period of years can be estimated simply by accumulating the successive annual incidence rates for the period required. The relative risk of acquiring a disease in association with an exposure is given by the incidence rate of disease in the exposed group divided by the incidence rate in the non-exposed group. The attributable risk is given by subtracting the incidence rate in the non-exposed group from the incidence rate in the exposed group.

Uses of epidemiology to complete the clinical picture

The experience of disease gained in clinical practice, and notably in hospital practice, is often incomplete for a number of reasons. Patients with an illness who are seen in one hospital or locality may not necessarily be representative of all patients with the illness. Selective factors, such as a unit's special interests and reputation, may influence whether a patient is admitted to a particular hospital. Selective factors, such as the severity of the illness, whether its presentation is typical, and whether treatment can be given outside hospital, will influence whether a patient is admitted to hospital at all. Patients vary in the extent to which they seek medical services for symptoms: some with even quite marked symptoms do not seek medical help. Information about disease

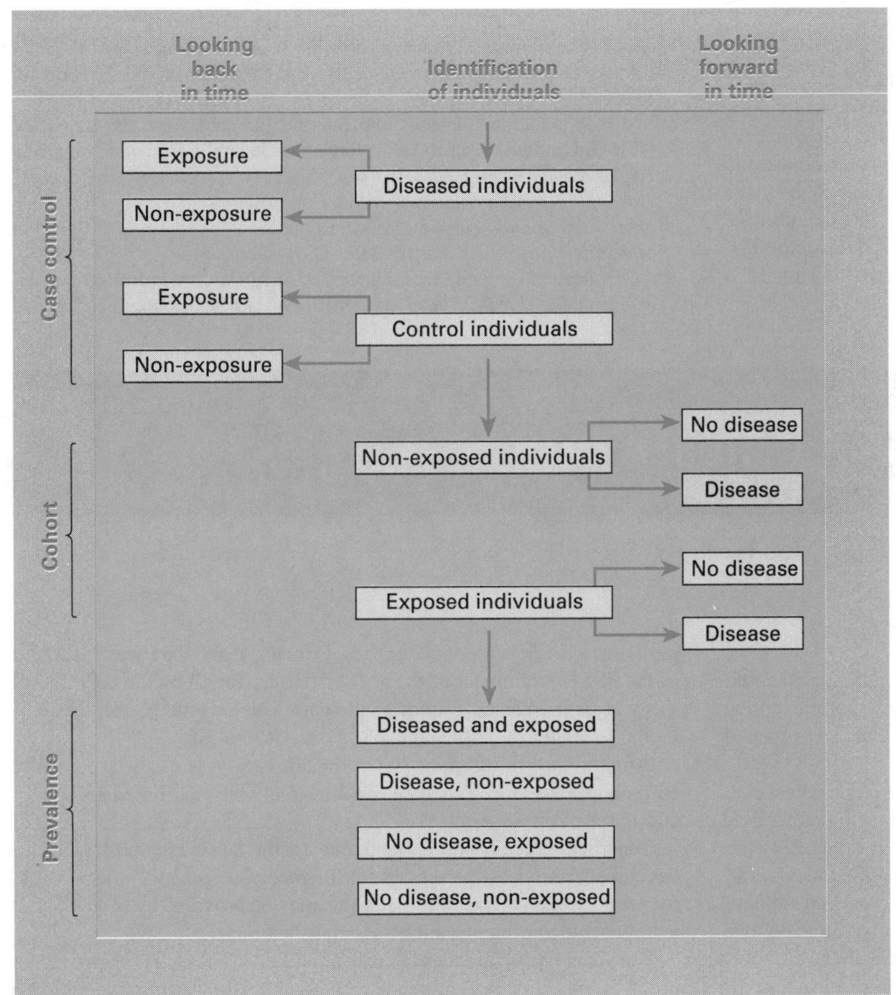

Fig. 3 Comparison of methods of case-control, cohort, and prevalence studies.

Table 7 *Annual death rates, relative and attributable risks: death from lung cancer and ischaemic heart disease in non-smokers and heavy smokers*

	Death rate among non-smokers per 100 000 men	Death rate among heavy smokers per 100 000 men	Relative risk	Attributable death rate per 100 000 men
Cancer of lung	10	251	25.1	241
Ischaemic heart disease	413	792	1.9	379

Based on figures reported by Doll and Peto (1976).

in the community as a whole, as well as from particular medical institutions, may greatly aid understanding of the natural history of disease as the following examples illustrate.

1. Community-based studies of fatal acute myocardial infarction show that the majority of deaths occur outside hospital and that many of these occur very soon after the onset of the acute attack. Thus the outcome of heart attacks is considerably worse than would be apparent from observations made only on patients admitted to hospital. Furthermore, it cannot be assumed that hospital patients, who constitute only a selected proportion of all patients with the disease, are necessarily typical of all patients in respect of, say, factors that precipitated their attack. The findings also have implications for the organization of coronary care services; and, since a proportion of patients with coronaries are always likely to die before the arrival of care, they underline the importance of seeking means to prevent the disease.
2. The search for methods of early detection of presymptomatic disease, in order to screen for and prevent the development of disease, by definition requires the study of individuals in the community rather than of patients with manifest illness.
3. With some attributes (e.g. blood pressure, serum cholesterol) the distinction between disease and normality cannot be made from the study of clinical populations alone. The definition of levels of low, intermediate, and high risk of developing disease depend on observations made on normal individuals as well as those made on patients with the disease.

Epidemiology in managing health services

The clinical management of a patient requires a clinical diagnosis. Management of medical resources to meet the medical needs of the community requires knowledge of the occurrence and distribution of disease in the community. The epidemiological approach can be used to monitor the health of the community, to show changing patterns of disease in the community, to identify groups of people who are at special risk, to assess local health problems, and to quantify needs for local health services. In these ways, epidemiological knowledge can be applied to the provision and management of health services.

REFERENCES

Doll, R. and Peto, R. (1976). Mortality in relation to smoking: 20 years' observations on male British doctors. *British Medical Journal*, **ii,** 1525–36.

McKeown, T. (1979). *The role of medicine*. Basil Blackwell Ltd, Oxford.

Muir, C., Waterhouse, J., Mack, T., Powell, J., and Whelan, S. (eds.) (1987). *Cancer incidence in five continents*, Vol. 5. International Agency for Research on Cancer, Lyon.

Office of Population Censuses and Surveys (annual). *Mortality statistics*. HMSO, London. (Prior to 1974: Registrar-General's *Statistical review of England and Wales, medical tables*.) Also:
Hospital in-patient enquiry. HMSO, London.
General household survey. HMSO, London.
Statistics of infectious disease. HMSO, London.

Royal College of General Practitioners (1986). *Morbidity statistics from general practice, 1981–2: third national study*. HMSO, London.

3.3 Primary care

G. H. Fowler

DEFINITION

Primary health care has been defined by the World Health Organization (**WHO**) as 'advice given to a person or group of persons for preventive or therapeutic purposes by one or more members of the health or related professions, acting alone or in a team'.

Primary health care is more comprehensive than primary medical care in that it includes health promotion and disease prevention as well as curing, caring for, and rehabilitating those who are ill. It is generally the first level of contact with the health care system for individuals, the family, and the community; after self-care, it constitutes the first element of the health care process. Following the Alma Ata International Conference on primary health care in 1978, a joint WHO/UNICEF report called for urgent and effective national and international action to develop and implement primary health care throughout the world and particularly in developing countries. Primary health care was identified as the key to attainment of the goal of 'Health for all by the year 2000'; this was defined as 'a level of health care which would permit the individual to lead a socially and economically useful life'.

Primary care is essential in any health care system. It is generally community-based, complementing the largely hospital-based secondary and tertiary care systems.

General practice or family medicine are the labels applied (at least in developed countries) to the branch of medicine generally responsible for primary care—though some of this may be provided by accident and emergency departments and by specialists directly.

The general practitioner or family practitioner/doctor has been defined as: 'A licensed medical graduate who gives personal, primary, and continuing care to individuals, families, and a practice population, irrespective of age, sex, and illness. It is the synthesis of these functions which is unique. He [sic] will attend in his consulting room and in their homes and sometimes in a clinic or hospital. His aim is to make early diagnosis. He will include and integrate physical, psychological, and social factors in his considerations about health and illness. This will be expressed in the care of his patients. He will make an initial decision about every medical problem which is presented to him as a doctor. He will undertake the continuing management of his patients with chronic, recurrent or terminal illness. Prolonged contact means that he can use repeated opportunities to gain information at a pace appropriate to each patient and build up a relationship of trust which he can use professionally. He will practise in cooperation with other colleagues, medical and non-medical. He will know how and when to intervene through treatment, prevention, and education to promote the health of his patients and their families. He will recognise that he also has a professional responsiblity to the community.' (Royal College of General Practitioners 1969)

Health care systems and primary care

Different systems of health care have evolved in different countries; history, geography, political, and cultural factors, and availability of resources have influenced developments.

In the United Kingdom, where health services are funded almost entirely from taxation, there is a centrally planned National Health Service with some delegation to regions and districts. Comprehensive community and hospital services, essentially free at the time of use, are available to everyone. General practitioners are 'independent contractors', paid largely by capitation fees; hospital doctors are salaried. Recent changes have increased autonomy at the periphery, especially for 'fund holding' general practitioners and hospital 'trusts'. Basically similar health services exist in Australia, Canada, New Zealand, and Scandinavia, but with less centralized planning and more direct charges to patients.

In North America, medical care is generally part of a 'free enterprise' system, though federal and state funds now contribute about half the cost. The system is essentially fee-for-service, with fees paid directly by patients or through prepaid insurance schemes; or through Medicare (for the elderly) or Medicaid (for the poor). Doctors' incomes are largely derived from fees. Primary care is often provided by specialists as well as family physicians, while in poor urban areas much primary care is provided by public hospitals through emergency rooms.

In the former Soviet Union and some other countries, community services are provided through polyclinics, staffed by primary care doctors and specialists. A non-medical personnel, especially in rural areas, provides some primary care services. In developing countries, the tendency has been for the limited financial and manpower resources available to be devoted to development of 'Western style' medical services, largely hospital-based, doctor intensive, and cure orientated. While providing sophisticated medical care for a minority affluent urban population, such systems ignore the needs of the majority—the poor and those living in rural areas. In such systems, there is a need for greater emphasis on primary care with a preventive orientation, which is more widely dispersed, and makes greater use of an auxiliary personnel.

Levels of health care and special features of primary care

Self-care of many medical problems is common; even in countries with sophisticated health care systems like that in the United Kingdom, at least three-quarters of medical problems are managed by individuals themselves, without reference to any medical agency.

The levels of medical care, categories of provision, and average size of populations served by each group, in the United Kingdom are illustrated in Fig. 1.

The acknowledgement that primary care has special characteristics which distinguish it from that of the hospital-based specialist is relatively recent. Not only does primary care have its own core of knowledge, but its methods of diagnosis, treatment, and management are somewhat different from those generally provided by hospitals. Some of the conditions seen in primary care for instance are not seen by specialists, while others are seen across a wider spectrum of severity.

Effective primary care has the following features:

- availability and direct accessibility to the population served;
- provision of first-contact, continuing, and long-term care;
- ability to deal with undifferentiated problems;
- comprehensive care concerned with both sexes, all ages, and conditions that may be minor or major, acute or chronic;
- personal care (prior knowledge of the patient allows provision of appropriately tailored management for each individual);
- coordination of the services provided by specialists and others;
- preventive care;
- community care for a small, defined population.

The content of primary care

In a developed country, the content of primary care is largely determined by the 'consumer'—by what the population considers are the problems for which medical advice should be sought. This in turn will be influenced by the attitudes of society towards medicine and by the availability of medical services. But although there are substantial differences between developed countries in the provision of medical care, the pattern of primary care in them is remarkably similar. About 90 per cent of health problems presented to doctors in such countries are dealt with entirely at a primary care level.

SEVERITY OF CONDITIONS

About two-thirds of the problems for which a patient consults a general practitioner may be classified as minor in that they are generally self-limiting and without risk to life, or pose no likelihood of permanent disability. Of the remaining third, the majority are chronic, causing some degree of permanent disability. Overall, only about 1 in 10 of the problems presenting to general practitioners is major/acute, some of which may be potentially life threatening.

CLINICAL CONTENT

The pattern of clinical disorders and specific conditions seen in the average group practice of five doctors and about 10 000 patients in the

Fig. 1 Levels of care (adapted from Fry (1978)).

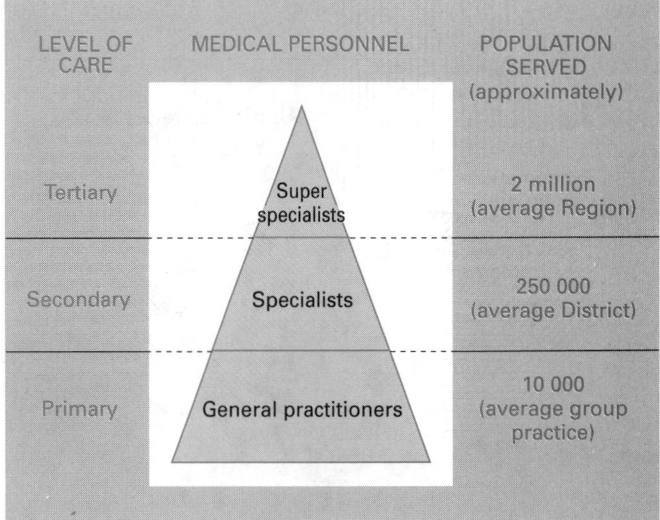

United Kingdom is illustrated in Fig. 2 and Tables 1 to 4. The most common conditions about which patients consult doctors in the United Kingdom are respiratory infections, skin disorders, emotional problems, trauma, gastrointestinal and musculoskeletal problems. Rather rarely seen are many more serious conditions that are commonplace in hospital practice. The number of new cancers seen annually in the average group practice is shown in Table 5. In recent years, general practice in Britain has seen a growth in preventive medicine providing advice for instance on life-style, cancer screening (in particular cervical cytology), and on factors increasing the risk of cardiovascular disorders.

CONSULTATION RATES

At least three-quarters of the population consult a general practitioner at least once a year and over 90 per cent do so at least once in 5 years. The annual consultation rate is about three or four per patient per year (with a range of 2 to 7). The young, the old, and people from lower social classes seek advice more frequently, and women consult about twice as often as men. Some of the variation is due to factors attributable to the doctor rather than the patient. The average general practitioner, looking after a nominal 2000 patients, does about 7000 consultations annually, averaging about 30 each day, of which not more than five will be home visits.

Relationship between primary and secondary (hospital) care

In any given year, about 1 in 6 of the population of the United Kingdom attends a hospital outpatient department and about 1 in 10 is admitted to hospital, compared to the two-thirds who consult their general practitioner at least once. In Britain, general practice has a 'gatekeeper' role in that most hospital attendances and admissions are through referral by the general practitioner. This system exercises a major influence over the use of hospital services. Rates of referral of patients to hospital by general practitioners vary, as illustrated in Fig. 3. Although such variations may be explained partly by differing demography and morbidity of populations, much depends on the characteristics of the general practitioner and practice concerned.

Fig. 2 Percentage distribution of common minor conditions.

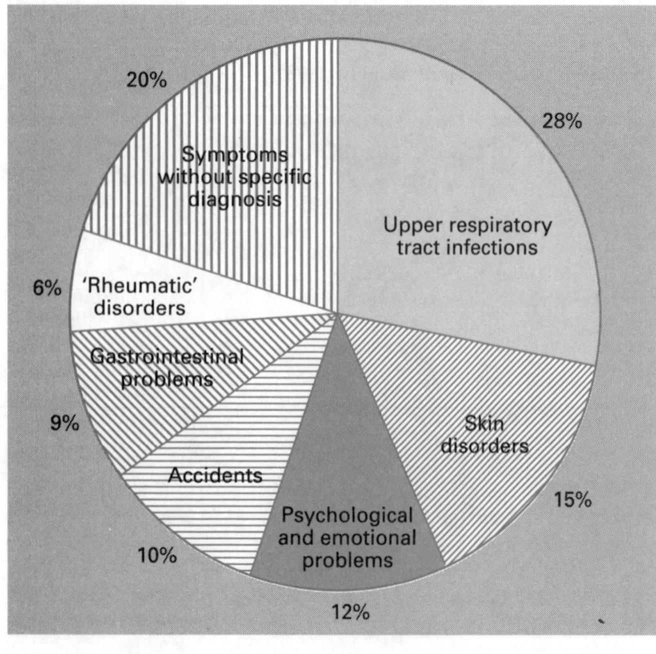

Table 1 *General minor conditions in general practice*

Conditions	Persons consulting annually per 10 000
Upper respiratory infections	2400
Skin disorders	1400
Psychoemotional problems	1000
Minor accidents	1000
Gastrointestinal conditions	800
Rheumatic 'aches and pains'	600
Vague symptoms	1500

Reproduced from Fry (1983), with permission.

Table 2 *Specific minor conditions in general practice*

Condition	Persons consulting annually per 10 000
Acute throat infections	400
Lacerations	400
Eczema/dermatitis	400
Acute otitis media	300
Ear wax	200
Urinary tract infections	200
Acute backache	200
Vaginal discharge	120
Migraine	100
Hayfever	100
Vertigo	80
Hernia	60
Piles	60

Reproduced from Fry (1983), with permission.

Table 3 *Chronic diseases in general practice*

Conditions	Persons consulting annually per 10 000
High blood pressure	1000
Chronic 'rheumatism'	400
Chronic psychiatric problems	400
Ischaemic heart disease	200
Obesity	200
Congestive cardiac failure	160
Anaemia	120
Cancers under care	120
Diabetes	120
Varicose veins	120
Strokes	80
Thyroid disorders	40
Epilepsy	40
Multiple sclerosis	12
Parkinsonism	12
Chronic renal failure	2

Reproduced from Fry (1983), with permission.

REFERRALS

The evolution of the referral system prevailing in Britain was an historical accident rather than a planned development and was the outcome of competition for patients between the physician or surgeon (consultants) and the apothecaries (general practitioners) in the nineteenth century. The general practitioner retained 'control' of the patient but was, in turn, excluded from hospitals. The introduction of National Insurance

Table 4 *Major diseases in general practice*

Condition	Persons consulting annually per 10 000
Acute bronchitis	400
Pneumonia	80
Severe depression	40
Acute myocardial infarction	40
Acute strokes	20
All new cancers	20
Acute appendicitis	15

Reproduced from Fry (1983), with permission.

Table 5 *New cancers in general practice*

Cancer	Persons consulting annually per 10 000
All	20
Lung	8
Breast	4
Large bowel	3
Stomach	2
Prostate	2
Bladder	1
Cervix	1
Ovary	<1
Oesophagus	1 in 2 years
Brain	1 in 3 years
Lymphoadenoma	1 in 4 years
Thyroid	1 in 5 years

Reproduced from Fry (1983), with permission.

in 1911 and of the National Health Service in 1948 firmly established the distinction between general practitioners and specialists and reinforced this referral system.

In other countries, particularly in North America where the general practitioner/specialist relationship does not have this historical basis, the differentiation is less clear and the referral system less well defined. Patients frequently 'shop around' themselves to select the specialist of their choice.

Reasons for referral from general practitioner to specialist include:

- for help with diagnosis, not only because of the greater expertise of the specialist, but also because of the availability of more sophisticated diagnostic techniques;
- for advice on management where diagnosis is already known, but management difficult;
- for hospital treatment of a known condition (e.g. surgery for a hernia) because treatment must necessarily be carried out by a specialist in hospital;
- for 'second opinion' reassurance in a situation where the patient's (or doctor's!) anxiety needs to be allayed.

One of the problems with the referral system is the tendency for the hospital team to continue management long after the objectives of the initial referral have been achieved. This may cause a number of problems. It may lead to duplication of effort and be wasteful of both the doctor's and patient's time. It may result in a situation where neither doctor accepts responsibility for the care of the patient, each assuming that the other adopts this role. There may be failure of communication, differing information and advice given to patients, and even different treatments, all leading to confusion—not least to the patient. It is sometimes, but seldom, wise for two doctors to be managing a patient at the same time.

Hospital follow-up clinics are increasingly scrutinized to ensure that unnecessary follow-up is eliminated, allowing more supervision in the community of patients with chronic diseases, such as diabetes and hypertension. The approximate number of new outpatient referrals and inpatient admissions for a group practice of about 10 000 patients, and the specialities to which they are referred, are illustrated in Tables 6 and 7.

The primary health care team

At the inception of the National Health Service in 1948 about half of all general practitioners were working single handed, often unsupported except by their wives. Now, fewer than 1 in 6 of general practitioners practises single handed and almost half are in partnerships of four or more.

The building of health centres was one factor in the growth of partnerships and about one-fifth of general practitioners now practise in health centres. Alongside of the growth in partnership size, there are other developments that have contributed to the evolution of primary health care teams. The first of these was the attachment of health authority-employed community (district) nurses, health visitors, and midwives to general practices. The other was the increased employment by practices of more staff—receptionists, secretaries, practice managers, practice nurses, and others—as a result of financial incentives introduced in the mid-1960s. The composition of a typical primary health care team for 10 000 'registered' patients is:

- 5 general practitioners ('principals')
- 1 trainee general practitioner

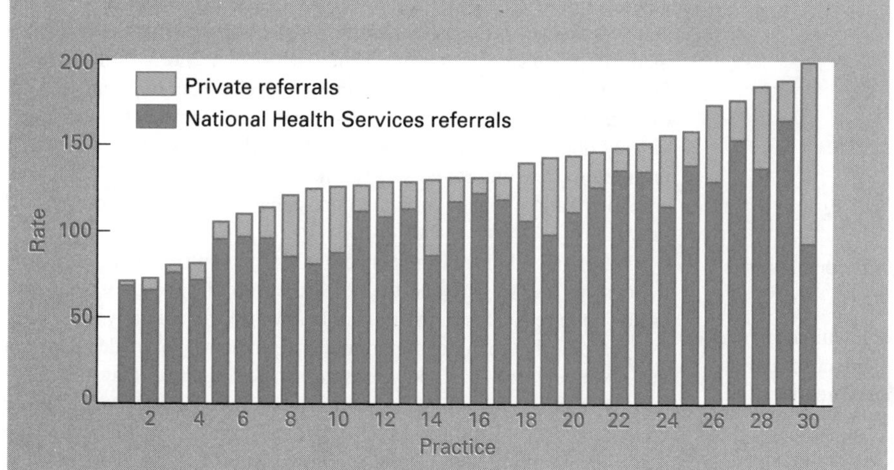

Fig. 3 Outpatient referral rates from 30 practices in the Oxford Region. Annual rates per 1000 registered patients. (Source: Coulter and Roland (1992).)

Table 6 *Annual new referrals to outpatient departments*

Speciality	Referrals per 10 000 patients
Surgical	
General surgical	200
Gynaecological	120
Trauma/orthopaedics	240
Ear, nose, and throat	120
Ophthalmology	120
Others	20
SUBTOTAL	1000
Medical	
General medical	100
Paediatrics	40
Psychiatry	48
Dermatology	100
Chest	60
Others	92
SUBTOTAL	440
Obstetrics	120
Others	100
TOTAL	1660

Table 7 *Annual hospital admissions*

Speciality	Admissions per 10 000 patients
Surgical	
General surgery	216
Gynaecology	104
Trauma/orthopaedics	100
Ear, nose, and throat	60
Others	80
SUBTOTAL	560
Medical	
General medical	160
Paediatrics	48
Psychiatry	44
Geriatrics	40
Others	28
SUBTOTAL	320
Obstetrics	120
Others	100
TOTAL	1100

- 1 practice manager
- 1 or 2 secretaries
- 3 or 4 receptionists
- 2 or 3 practice nurses
- 2 community nurses
- 1 or 2 health visitors
- 1 midwife
- Others (possibly): counsellor, psychologist, chiropodist, physiotherapist, dietitian, 'attached' social worker.

The concept of a team implies that different people, each with their own special knowledge and skills, contribute to the achievement of a common goal. The advantages of a primary health care team are that:

- Care given by a group is greater than the sum of care by individuals.
- Rare skills are used more appropriately.
- Informal teaching and peer influence within the group raises the standards of care.
- Team members have increased job satisfaction.
- Team working encourages coordinated activities.

However, evaluation of the effectiveness of primary health care teams is difficult. Some would argue that, while development of teams has had advantages to primary health care providers (particularly doctors) in enabling the sharing and delegation of tasks, there have been disadvantages to patients. These may include 'barriers' restricting access to the doctor, reductions in personal care, and interference with continuity of care.

Health promotion and prevention

The 1980s saw a growth in prevention and health promotion in primary care. The potential of each primary care contact for dealing with not only the presenting health problem and the supervision of any continuing problems but also for health education and preventive medicine became acknowledged. Increasing awareness of the contribution of unhealthy lifestyles and behaviour, especially smoking and unhealthy diets, to much present-day illness and premature death encouraged this shift in attitude. Moreover, evidence of some degree of efficacy of the advice of general practitioners in helping people to stop smoking, for example, encouraged the view that lifestyle advice in general practice could be effective. In 1990, it became a formal requirement of National Health Service general practitioners in Britain to incorporate health promotion and disease prevention into their work. Because of financial incentives, this requirement has often been fulfilled by practice nurses conducting 'health promotion clinics'; but evidence of the efficacy of such activities, compared with opportunistic prevention as part of patient-initiated consultations, is lacking. Doctors should therefore be cautious about abdicating their health educational role.

The future

For a decade or more after the introduction of the National Health Service in 1948, general practice appeared to be in decline. Isolation from hospitals (where rapid advances in medical treatment were taking place), recruitment to general practice of doctors who were deemed to have 'failed' in hospital medicine, low morale, poor conditions of work (including inadequate premises, equipment and staff) and, seemingly unlimited demand, were some of the factors that contributed to this. However, improvements in premises, equipment, and staffing arising from changes in the way National Health Service general practitioners were paid in the mid-1960s, and the development of primary health care teams, saw the beginning of a renaissance in British general practice. Vocational training for general practice became the norm and was made mandatory in 1980. The status of general practice steadily improved and this contributed to the recruitment of many able and highly motivated medical graduates. General practice became a more professionally rewarding occupation and the continuing development of primary health care teams, with practice-employed nurses doing some of the work previously done by doctors (particularly in field of prevention and health promotion), and improved record and information systems, including computerization, have continued to enhance the status of general practice.

Moreover, with increasing concern in many countries about escalating the costs of health care and the need to ensure the most cost-effective use of finite resources, primary care is now seen as crucially important. It is realized that many common medical problems can be dealt with in this relatively low-cost, low-technology setting, and that the more expensive, high-technology hospital services must be reserved for those patients and problems for which they are essential. In the future the management of chronic disease such as asthma, diabetes, hypertension and psychiatric disorders will become increasingly the responsiblity of primary care. For many reasons, therefore, primary care will have a vital role in medical education.

REFERENCES

Coulter, A. and Roland, M.O. (1992). *Hospital referrals*. Oxford University Press.

Fowler, G., Gray, M., and Anderson, P. (1992). *Prevention in general practice*. Oxford University Press.

Fry, J. (1978). *A new approach to medicine*. MTP Press, Lancaster.

Fry, J. (1983). *Present state and future needs in general practice*. Royal College of General Practitioners, London.

Horder, J. and Horder, E. (1954). Illness in general practice. *Practitioner 1973*, **173,** 177–87.

Office of Population Censuses and Surveys. (1994). Morbidity Statistics from General Practice 1991/92. *OPCS Monitor MB5 94/1, 17 February 1994*. HMSO, London.

Royal College of General Practitioners. (1969). The educational needs of the future general practitioner. *Journal of the Royal College of General Practitioners*, **18,** 358–60.

Royal College of General Practitioners (with OPCS and DoH) (1986). *Morbidity statistics from general practice*, Third National Morbidity Survey 1980–2. HMSO, London.

Stott, N.C.H. and Davis, R.H. (1979). The exceptional potential in each primary care consultation. *Journal of the Royal College of General Practitioners*, **29,** 201–5.

World Health Organization (1978). *Primary health care*, Report of a conference Alma Ata. WHO, Geneva.

3.4 Health care in developing countries

H. Annett and A. Cassels

Health and demographic status

Changing patterns of ill health

Slow but sustained progress in the improvement of health status is evident in many developing countries. At the same time, they are undergoing important demographic and epidemiological transitions. Overall, mortality and fertility rates are declining, and disease patterns are shifting. Childhood morbidity and mortality caused by communicable diseases, particularly the diarrhoea–malnutrition–pneumonia complex, are becoming less dominant, while chronic and degenerative diseases among adults and the elderly are becoming more prevalent.

These shifts in disease patterns are most marked in Latin America and Asia, much less so in Africa. Even in Latin America and Asia the transitions suggested by aggregate data obscure the vast differentials in health experience of the least healthy and the healthiest sections of the population. Thus health status in many of the poorest countries, and among the poorest members of the population in the more developed countries of the Third World, is not improving. The gap between developed and developing countries continues to widen. Infant mortality rates in the 25 United Nations-defined least developed countries are estimated to average 125/1000 live births, as compared to 15/1000 in developed countries. Disease in infancy and early childhood accounts for at least half of all deaths. Life expectancy at birth in least developed countries remains less than 50 years, compared to 74 years in the developed world. Children die of vaccine-preventable disease; half a million women in developing countries die every year in childbirth. In short, the absolute number of people living in poverty continues to grow and despite shifts in the patterns of mortality, the cycle of poverty, malnutrition, communicable disease, and lack of access to safe water continues to take its heavy toll.

Population growth

In mid-1992 the world population was estimated at 5.48 billion and over the next decade annual additions will average 97 million. The rate at which the population continues to grow and the final stable population of the world will have a profound impact on global ecology and the progress of national economies. Recent figures show that rates of demographic growth in less developed countries not only exceed rates of economic growth, but are higher than those of the group of developing countries as a whole.

In 1965, Sir Dugald Baird argued that 'freedom from the tyranny of excessive fertility' should be placed in the same category as the four other basic human freedoms (freedom of speech and worship, freedom from want and fear). Possibly the crucial element in making this 'fifth freedom' a reality is universal access to effective family planning. Potts and Rosenfield have remarked that 'population growth is no longer a problem looking for a solution; it is a solution looking for resources'. Identifying and utilizing those resources effectively is a major task for the 1990s. For the world population to stabilize at 8 billion, according to one recent estimate, there must be: universal access to contraception; universal access to voluntary surgical contraception, universal access to safe, cheap abortion, and quadruple the resources for family planning services by the year 2000.

Migration, war, and natural disasters

The breakdown of traditional society, particularly in the vast periurban slums that are multiplying throughout the developing world, is associated with social problems on a colossal scale. The numbers of homeless and exploited children and abandoned elderly people run into millions. In many countries this is compounded by the effects of war, civil unrest, and natural disaster. Today the world has about 20 million refugees. In addition, approximately 30 million people are displaced from their homes or under stress, but not afforded refugee status. The political situation in many poor countries, made worse by international tensions, makes it likely that this number will increase rather than decrease in the next decade. The displaced represent an 'underclass' of the world's poor, with the worst health experience; child mortality rates for recently arrived refugees can rise to over 100/1000.

The evolution of health policy in developing countries

From the early 1900s, colonial administrations and the national governments of developing countries began to establish organized systems of health care. Although government health facilities were usually supplemented by those run by missionaries, large segments of the population continued to rely upon traditional health practitioners, and had limited or no access to allopathic medicine. Extensive public-health legislation relating to environmental health and control of communicable diseases was introduced from the 1930s. The 1950s and 1960s saw strong international backing for communicable disease control programmes; justified by the eventual eradication of smallpox, but later called into question by the failure to eradicate malaria. The middle years of the century also saw an increasing emphasis on basic health services, as opposed to hospital-based care, with the enthusiastic promotion of the health-centre concept as a means of increasing health-care coverage in rural areas. By the 1970s, it had become clear that it was inefficient to run separate vertical disease-control programmes. The need to develop a more integrated, multipurpose health service, which included both preventive and curative activities, emerged as a critical policy issue.

The emergence of primary health care

The 1970s saw concern and debate about effectiveness of health care in industrialized and in developing countries. At the 1974 World Health Assembly in Geneva, the World Health Organization presented a critical report that highlighted the wide gaps in health status both between and within countries. Delegates were reminded that health services were failing to achieve a level of coverage adequate to meet needs; that escalating costs were not being accompanied by improved services; and that 'consumers' perceived that health systems were driven by the interests of health professionals rather than community needs. For the first time the World Health Organization acknowledged that poverty is a primary determinant of disease, and that the health of deprived populations can only be significantly improved when poverty is successfully tackled.

These concerns and debates culminated in a conference at Alma Ata in 1978, which promulgated primary health care, subsequently popularized under the slogan 'Health for All by the Year 2000'. Arguably one of the most important influences on public health in the second half of the twentieth century, at least in the developing world, primary health care is a complex and often confusing concept. Thus, while the Alma Ata Declaration was influential throughout the 1980s in securing apparent political commitment to primary care, its ambiguities bedevilled the development of health-care systems. For example, the emphasis placed on 'community participation' in the Alma Ata document was frequently equated with the creation of village health committees and the training of volunteer community health workers, with scant regard for how a particular community normally organized its activities or remunerated its healers.

A concern for equity

Fundamentally, primary health care is concerned with equity (allocation of resources on the basis of need) as the guiding principal for socioeconomic development in general, and health systems in particular. Understood as such it remains a central concern in the field of health development. Apart from the ethical concern for social justice, it is argued that health policies which promote a more equitable health system will yield greater health benefits for society as a whole. From an equity perspective, change that benefits the poor should be encouraged but where the benefits of change go instead to the better off and leave the poor at an even greater disadvantage than before, it should be resisted.

The term primary health care is commonly used to denote primary as compared to secondary or tertiary care, or promotive and preventive rather than curative health activities. The concern for equity does indicate that priority should be given to health activities close to and in a community, and that a proper balance should be achieved between promotive, preventive, and curative interventions. But this emphasis is often mistaken to mean that primary health care is a 'cheap option for the poor', an alternative to 'high-tech' hospital-based care. Rather, it needs to be understood as a concern to achieve more equitable health systems, and is a means of improving the health status of populations in cost-effective ways.

Contemporary health systems

The ultimate objective of any intervention in the health sector is to improve overall health. It is important not to forget the systems responsible for the delivery of health care. Much of the debate about health policy in the 1980s, particularly concerning the different approaches to primary health care, has overlooked the importance of institutional and organizational issues. It is now clear that medical training alone is no longer sufficient preparation for working in developing countries. An understanding of the importance of issues relating to systems of care in dealing with health status is critical for any health professional working in the development of health care.

The term health system is used here in its broadest sense to describe the framework of policies, organizations, institutions, programmes, and technologies that have as a common purpose the general improvement of health. To illustrate some of the major organizational problems, this section sketches the key characteristics of systems used in developing country. It is followed by an outline of current trends and unresolved issues.

The characteristics of health systems in developing countries

Systems that provide for health care in poor countries have several common features. The core is the ministry of health or its equivalent. The ministry is generally taken to mean not just a central government department but the complete organization, from political head to health facilities in the villages. It is often difficult to separate political, administrative, managerial, and technical roles; as a result, they are a frequent source of conflict. The main departure from a single, vertically integrated bureaucracy occurs in countries where local government takes responsibility for aspects of service delivery. Health policies in many countries are still based on an implicit assumption that government remains ultimately responsible for all aspects of the financing and provision of health care. As a result, voluntary and private-sector organizations, which may be responsible for between 30 to 40 per cent of all spending on health, operate independently without regulation, and according to their own agenda.

ABSOLUTE SCARCITY OF CASH

In many countries, even if the total funds available from public and private sources were spent as cost-effectively as possible, they would be insufficient to meet critical needs for health. Absolute scarcity makes it hard to deal with relative imbalances—between preventive and curative care or urban and rural health, for example. If a government can only afford between US$5–10 *per capita* (equivalent to about 5 per cent of health spending in most industrialized countries), it is difficult to specify spending priorities that are both managerially realistic and politically acceptable.

RIGID FINANCIAL SYSTEMS

Poverty, however, is not just a question of money. It is common to find that ministries of health are not able to spend all of the money available to them. Rigid and outmoded systems for disbursing and accounting for government funds limit the capacity of governments to absorb more resources, and to get them to where they are needed. Dysfunctional financial management systems, which make it hard to track how money is spent, have encouraged donors to set up their own parallel systems, adding to the administrative burden of overstretched managers.

FRAGMENTED MANAGEMENT STRUCTURES

Despite the widely acknowledged need for better management, authority is commonly fragmented between two sets of interrelated vertical systems: those organized around technical programmes and those organized around particular cadres of technical staff (doctors, nurses, public-health inspectors etc.). At best, management relies on 'trade-offs' between different groups, more often the lack of unitary authority and structural disarray leads to managerial paralysis.

INCREASING PRESSURE ON OPERATING COSTS

The public service continues to be a major source of secure employment and ministries of health are often among the largest employers. In many of the poorest countries, salaries account for up to 80 per cent of the recurrent budget, leaving inadequate funds for other costs of running services. If health workers do not have access to drugs or to fuel for vehicles, their capacity to function is seriously constrained. If there are no funds allocated for maintenance, buildings, vehicles and equipment will rapidly deteriorate.

DONOR-DRIVEN DEVELOPMENT

Donor concerns for accountability and quantifiable results have tended to favour discrete projects in selected districts or vertically managed disease-control programmes. The former often bypass the management systems they are designed to strengthen, and the latter reinforce the fragmented vertical management structures of the ministry of health. Many donors have also preferred to support only capital expenditure. However, unstaffed hospitals, unused equipment, and poorly maintained vehicles have shown the need for a balance between investment and recurrent-cost support. In recent years, many donors have come round to the view that it is important to support the development of more broadly based planning and management systems to improve the functioning of government services as a whole. Others, however, continue to link their funding to a specific set of health interventions such as immunization and family planning.

INAPPROPRIATE MODELS

Government primary health-care programmes worldwide have been influenced by the experience of non-government organizations or small-scale pilot projects run as research programmes. However, the culture and values of these organizations are very different from those of large, state-funded bureaucracies. People or programmes that thrive in one culture, such as voluntary community health workers—the mainstay of primary health care in many countries—may not take root in the other. Similarly, rational approaches to planning and budgeting fail to recognize how large organizations really work.

Trends and issues

DISTRICT HEALTH SYSTEMS

The district has been promoted, particularly by international agencies, as the most important focus for the development of health care. The district (or its administrative equivalent) is said to be the level at which managers can integrate the activities of vertical programmes and coordinate non-government providers. It is also the level at which community representatives can have an input into planning ('where top-down and bottom-up meet'), and at which collaboration between different government departments (such as education and agriculture) can take place. But there is a limit to what can be achieved by treating the district in isolation. In practice, health-service staff have limited room to manoeuvre and few discretionary powers. Real progress in making health services both more efficient and more responsive to peoples' needs will require that governments address the management problems facing the health system as a whole.

DECENTRALIZATION

For districts to function effectively, a greater say in how resources are allocated is necessary. Decentralization features prominently in documents of health policy, and is seen as a way of increasing local accountability. In practice, decentralization can take make many forms, but few countries have succeeded in fully translating policies into practice. It is rare to find that local managers have control over significant amounts of money or the numbers of staff that work in their area. Where power has been transferred to locally elected bodies, inequalities at local level can be reinforced. The involvement of local politicians may actually increase the demand for facility-based curative services rather than preventive or promotive care.

DISEASE ERADICATION

There is mounting pressure on governments and donor agencies to repeat the success of the campaign to eradicate smallpox. Current targets for eradication include dracunculiasis and polio. From an epidemiological perspective the case for eradication can be compelling, and well-run campaigns for control of disease can attract badly needed resources to the health sector in poor countries. However, there is a price to pay. Concentration on particular diseases, or pursuit of over-ambitious immunization programmes in health systems with limited capacity, can tie up scarce resources, thereby seriously disrupting other areas of work. There is likely to be a continuing tension between advocates of disease control working often to an internationally determined agenda and those concerned with developing the capacity to set local priorities and develop planning systems that address the wide range of health problems facing populations in developing countries.

CHANGES IN HEALTH-CARE FINANCING

It is widely accepted that in most developing countries, tax revenues alone will be insufficient to fund a credible health service. A number of important developments are taking place, as follows.

User fees The most widespread change in health-care financing in developing countries over the last decade has been the introduction of user fees for government services. In several African countries, the Bamako Initiative has linked user fees to the purchase of drugs and suggested that a proportion of income be used to give community groups some control over the management of facilities. It had been hoped that fees might cover between 10 to 20 per cent of operating costs. However, experience in several subSaharan countries has shown the average cost–recovery ratio from user fees to be approximately 4 per cent. Higher rates are possible in hospitals, but for fees to become a more significant source of income, requires that they be implemented in conjunction with a system of health insurance.

Even if user fees have limited potential in relation to the overall financing of health care, they are an extremely important source of funds locally. Experience shows that even very small sums can make a big difference to the performance of health centres, if fee income can be used to cover expenses (for soap, paper, kerosene etc.) for which funds would otherwise might not be available.

Social insurance Social insurance systems, in which contributions are related to income and benefits provided according to need, are well established in Europe and Latin America. They probably represent the most promising means of increasing substantially the resources available for health care in developing countries. If, however, there is no income tax system, it is very difficult to collect contributions from the self-employed and thus equity becomes a major issue. Nevertheless, the potential of compulsory insurance as means of alleviating the constraints on resources of the health systems of developing countries is likely to be major issue during the next decade.

ROLE OF HOSPITALS

Hospitals will continue to absorb a large proportion of government spending on health and demand for hospital services will continue to increase. There is a need therefore, on one hand, to safeguard public funding for primary care and, on the other, to enable hospitals to improve efficiency and the quality of services on offer. Referral hospitals are often the only part of the health system that can raise significant amounts of money from fees. Several countries have therefore decided to establish semi-autonomous boards to take over the management of large referral hospitals from the ministry of health. The constitution of these boards usually confers the right to determine staffing needs and fee levels, independent from the rest of the health service. The government contracts with the hospital to provide services on the basis of a global budget. Hospital managers are then required to run services within the limits imposed by this budget and the income they generate from fees. Experience suggests that the actual degree of autonomy granted to boards is less than intended and that conflicts between clinical and managerial interests persist.

HEALTH-SECTOR REFORM

Recent experience has shown the limitations of many previously accepted assumptions about strengthening the capacity of national health systems. First, there are limits to what can be achieved by interventions within the ministry of health itself. Several constraints to effective performance are common to all ministries and need to be dealt with in relation to the management of the public sector as a whole. Secondly, traditional bureaucratic structures do not necessarily provide sufficient incentives to guarantee either cost-effective or 'user-friendly' public services. Thirdly, it is recognized that there are several functions, previously assumed to be the responsibility of government, which can be better fulfilled by organizations in the private sector. Reform programmes in the health sector address these issues through reform of the civil service and public-sector management programmes; through changes in the financing of health care; and by introducing competition between providers as a means of increasing efficiency and responsiveness to service users.

REFERENCES

Able-Smith, B. (1992). Health insurance in developing countries: lessons from experience. *Health Policy and Planning*, **7,** 215–26.

Akin, J.S., Birdsall, N., and de Ferranti, D. (1987). *Financing health services in developing countries: an agenda for reform.* World Bank, Washington DC.

Bennett, S. (1992). Promoting the private sector: a review of developing countries. *Health Policy and Planning*, **7,** 97–110.

Cassels, A. and Janovsky, K. (1991). Management development for primary health care: a framework for analysis. *International Journal of Health Planning and Management*, **6,** 109–24.

Creese, A. (1991). User charges for health care: a review of recent experience. *Health Policy and Planning*, **6,** 309–19.

Janovsky, K. (1988). *The Challenge of implementation: district health systems for primary health care.* WHO, Geneva.

Nabarro, D. and Mosley, W.H. (1989). Aid for primary health care: a decade of experience. In *Strengthening Development Co-operation for Primary Health Care: a DAC concern*, pp. 13–43. OECD, Geneva.

Potts, M. and Rosenfield, A. (1990). The fifth freedom revisited: I. Background and existing programmes. *Lancet*, **ii,** 1227–31.

Potts, M. and Rosenfield, A. (1990). The fifth freedom revisited: II. The way forward. *Lancet*, **ii,** 1293–5.

World Bank. (1993). *World Development Report 1993: investing in health.* World Bank, Washington DC.

World Health Organization (1993). *Evaluation of recent changes in the financing of health services: Report of a WHO Study Group.* WHO Technical Report Series. WHO, Geneva.

Section 4 *Medical relevance of molecular and cell biology and genetics*

4.1 Molecular biology and medicine

D. J. WEATHERALL

Over the next few years, molecular and cell biology are likely to play an increasingly important part in clinical practice. Here I shall summarize briefly what we might expect to achieve and discuss briefly some of the wider implications of the new science of human molecular biology. It will only be possible to highlight a few aspects of this exciting field; for more extensive discussion the reader is referred to the monographs and reviews cited at the end of this section.

The structure and function of human genes

Proteins consist of one or more peptide chains folded into a three-dimensional structure, the exact shape of which is critical for their normal function, as enzymes or building blocks of tissues for example. Their conformation depends on the interactions of the different amino acids from which they are constructed. The genetic information that determines the order of amino acids in a peptide chain is encoded in the DNA which constitutes the gene for that chain. This information is transported from nuclei of cells to their cytoplasm by means of a form or ribonucleic acid (RNA) called messenger RNA (**mRNA**), which has a structure exactly complementary to that of the DNA from which it is copied, or transcribed. The process whereby a protein chain is synthesized on its mRNA template is called translation. Thus, the flow of genetic information in cells can be written:

$$\text{DNA} \xrightarrow[\text{transcription}]{} \text{RNA} \xrightarrow[\text{translation}]{} \text{protein}$$

The structure of DNA and genes

DNA consists of two chains of nucleotide bases wrapped around each other. There are four bases: adenine (A), guanine (G), cytosine (C), and thymine (T). The building blocks of each chain are deoxyribonucleotides, which consist of a base, deoxyribose, and a phosphate, covalently joined. The backbone of DNA, which is constant throughout the whole molecule, consists of deoxyribose molecules linked by phosphates. Thus the only variable part of a DNA chain is the sequence of bases, which can be in any order along the sugar–phosphate backbone. Because of their particular shapes, A always pairs with T, and C with G. Genetic information is encoded by the order of bases; it is a triplet, non-overlapping code in which three bases determine a particular amino acid.

DNA replication is an extremely complex process whereby the strands are separated and each one is copied to produce new daughter strands. Because one of each parent strand remains intact after replication the process is said to be semiconservative. Through the action of enzymes called DNA polymerases each new strand is synthesized in a $5'\rightarrow3'$ direction by the stepwise addition of the four deoxyribonucleotide triphosphates; these bases are added to complementary bases on the parental template strand so that the replication produces two identical copies of the original molecule.

A gene is defined as a length of DNA that carries the information to make a single peptide chain. This information must include not only instructions about the amino acid sequence of the chain but also to ensure that the protein product is made in appropriate amounts in the correct tissues at a particular time during development. Although some genes are transcribed in many tissues at all stages of development, and are therefore called 'housekeeping' genes, many are only expressed in specific tissues at particular times of development. Although the 'one gene–one peptide chain' rule is generally true, there are some exceptions. For example, some genes are able to produce more than one product as a result of complex post-transcriptional modification of their mRNAs or by post-translational processing of their protein products.

Almost all mammalian genes that have been analysed so far have their coding sequences interrupted by sequences of unknown function called intervening sequences or introns, at varying positions along their length (Fig. 1). Their number and size, often considerably longer than the coding sequences or exons, varies from gene to gene. At the $5'$ and $3'$ ends of genes there are specific triplets that determine the initiation (AGG) and termination (TAA, TAG, or TGA) of protein synthesis on mRNAs. There are also sequences of varying lengths at both ends that determine the structure of untranslated regions of mRNA. The highly conserved AATAAA sequence in the $3'$ non-coding region of all mammalian genes is essential for the normal processing of mRNA.

Most mammalian genes have blocks of sequences in their $5'$-flanking regions that are similar to those found in Drosophila and many other species. The first, ATA, is located 26 to 30 nucleotides upstream from the RNA initiation site. Another conserved box, CCAAT, is found about 72 to 77 nucleotides upstream. These regions and another with the general structure CACCC, which occurs twice 80 to 110 nucleotides upstream from the beginning of the gene, are involved in the regulation of transcription of mRNA. For this reason they are called promoters, or upstream promoter elements, regions of DNA to which RNA polymerases bind and initiate gene transcription.

There are other major regulatory elements that are involved in determining whether genes are transcribed in particular tissues. Some of these are *cis*-acting, that is they modify the activity of genes on the same chromosome. The most important regulatory elements of this type are called enhancers, sequences that are often at some distance from the structural genes but are brought into apposition with their promoters to form an activation complex. There is another important family of regulatory proteins, which may be encoded on other chromosomes, and which are *trans*-acting, that is they are involved in activation or suppression of genes on both pairs of homologous chromosomes. Many of these regulators are DNA-binding proteins. There appears to be hierarchy of such molecules, some of which are ubiquitous while others may be involved in tissue or developmental stage-specific gene activation.

Transcription and processing of mRNA

Messenger RNA is synthesized on its DNA template in a $5'\rightarrow3'$ direction by the action of enzymes called RNA polymerases. Chemically, RNA is similar to DNA except for two differences: the sugar of DNA is deoxyribose while in RNA it is ribose, and instead of thymine (T) RNA contains the closely related pyrimidine, uracil (U). The synthesis of RNA on its DNA template is similar in principle to the process of DNA replication and involves the formation of complementary base pairs, in this case G pairs with C, but A pairs with U instead of T. In this way, mRNA carries the faithful replica of the DNA strand from which it is transcribed.

The primary transcript is a large mRNA precursor that contains the entire gene complex, including exons and introns. This molecule undergoes a series of processing steps before it is ready for delivery to the cytoplasm (Fig. 1). The introns are cut out and the exons are spliced together in a two-stage progress. First, the mRNA precursor is cut at the

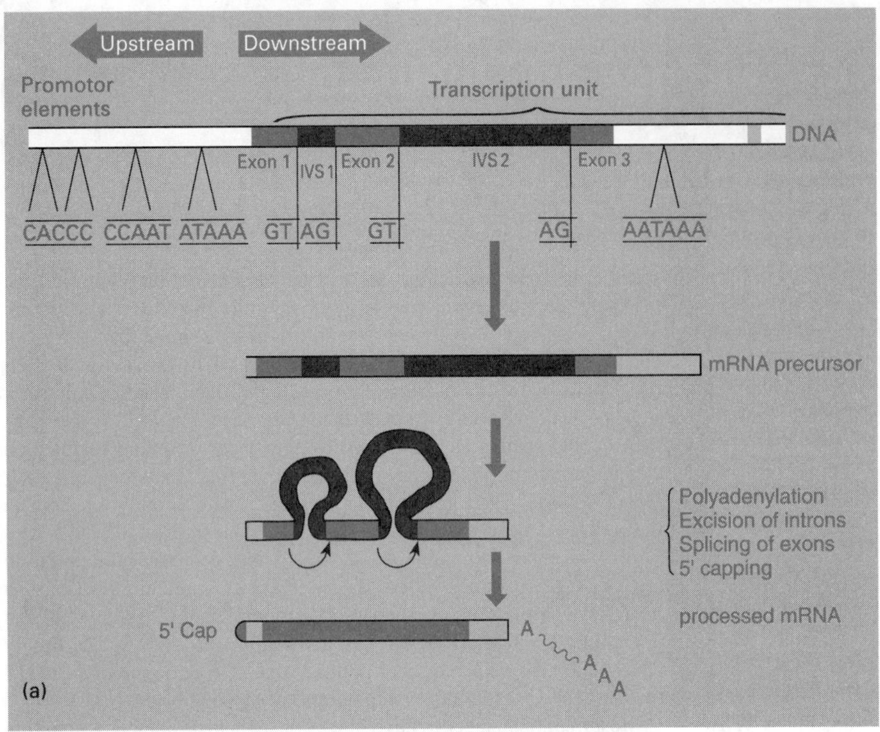

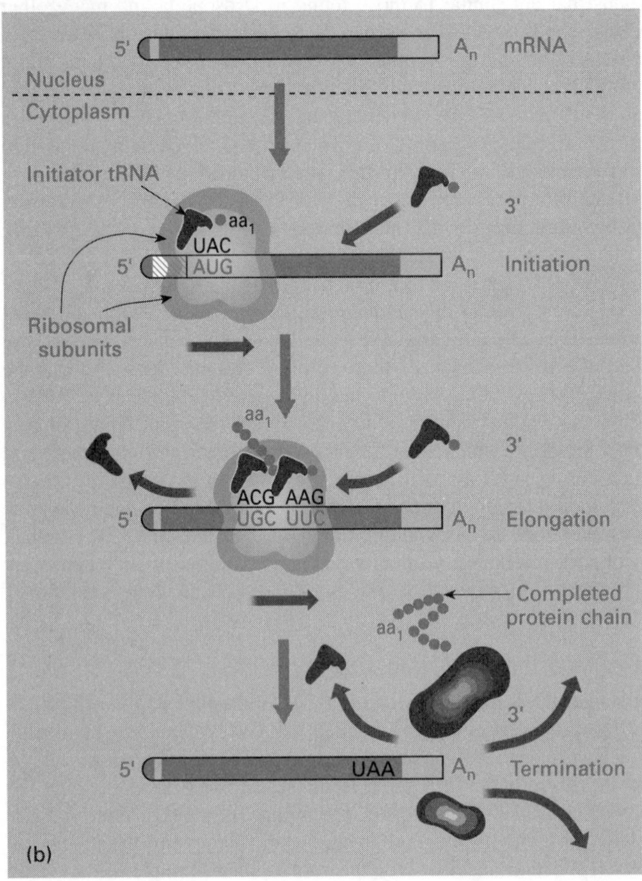

Fig. 1 Gene action. (a) The structure of a gene and the processing of its transcript. (b) The different steps in the translation of messenger RNA.

5′ prime site to generate two intermediates, a linear first exon and a branched, lariat-shaped molecule containing the intron and second exon. Second, the 3′ splice site is cleaved, the lariat intron released, and the two exons joined. This process involves the interaction of several enzymes and other nuclear proteins. While it is in the nucleus mRNA undergoes further processing, including a chemical modification of its 5′ end and the attachment of a string of adenylic acid residues (polyA) at its 3′ end, which may serve to stabilize it during its passage to the cytoplasm.

Once in the cytoplasm mRNA acts as a template for protein synthesis. Amino acids are brought to mRNA attached to another type of molecule called transfer RNA (**tRNA**). There is a family of different tRNAs, specific for a particular amino acid and for three bases (anticodons) that are complementary to the appropriate mRNA codons for their amino acids. Protein synthesis occurs on ribosomes, each of which consists of two different-sized subunits. The initiation of protein synthesis occurs when a ribosome is bound to the region of the initiation codon, AUG, and when an initiator tRNA base pairs with this codon. As each amino acid is brought to its appropriate place by its tRNA it forms a peptide bond with its fellow which is already in place, and hence a peptide chain is formed and gradually lengthens as the ribosomes move along the mRNA (Fig. 1). The ribosomes move over the mRNA in a 5′→3′ direction, from codon to codon, until the termination codon is reached. The completed chain is then released from the mRNA and ribosomes.

The relation between the DNA bases and their RNA equivalents that carry the information to make a peptide chain is called the genetic code. It is a triplet, non-overlapping code. Because there are more codewords than amino acids it follows that several amino acids can be encoded by more than one triplet. Thus the code is said to be degenerate.

Many proteins have to undergo a considerable amount of post-translational modification before they are functional. Insulin, for example, is first synthesized as a molecule called preproinsulin, which is 110 amino acids long. The first 24 amino acids constitute a signal peptide that facilitates entry of the molecule into the endoplasmic reticulum; many secreted proteins have signal or leader peptides of this type. The signal peptide is cleaved to produce a shorter molecule called proinsulin, which is then further modified to form the functional, two-chain insulin molecule.

Regulation

DNA exists in a highly compressed form in nuclei, complexed with histones and the other proteins, which constitute chromatin. For this reason its transcriptional activity in individual cells is quite limited. For example, in erythroid cells only a small percentage of the total DNA sequence is capable of being expressed, or active. This variability is reflected by extensive alterations in chromatin structure, which can be demonstrated experimentally as an increased sensitivity to digestion by various nucleases, notably DNAase 1. Another useful indicator of the state of activity of genes is their degree of methylation; actively transcribed genes are hypomethylated, and vice versa. Very little is known about the regulation of chromatin structure that leads to genes being in active or closed conformations. However, at the level of DNA there is some knowledge about the sequences involved in gene activation. We have already seen that there are promoter and enhancer elements. In recent years some evidence about how these regions interact with *trans*-acting regulatory proteins has been obtained.

Many DNA-binding proteins have been purified from nuclear extracts. There are several different classes identified by particular structural motifs. They bind to specific regulatory regions close to, or at a distance from, particular genes; in this way they regulate their activation or suppression. The emerging overall pattern of regulation is that there is a complex network of genes, which code for regulatory proteins and which can respond to external signals, so ensuring the synchronous interaction of the activity of many genes with similar functions in different tissues and at different stages of development.

The tools of recombinant DNA technology

Before considering the clinical applications of molecular and cell biology it is important to outline briefly some of the methods involved, particularly as they will play an increasingly important part in medical research and practice over the next few years.

Molecular hybridization and gene probes

The two strands of DNA can be dissociated and reassociated *in vitro* by heating and cooling. It is also possible to form double-stranded DNA/RNA molecules in this way. This reannealing process is highly specific, and under suitable conditions occurs only between DNA or RNA strands that have identical or almost identical base sequences. If we wish to look for a particular gene buried away in a large amount of DNA we can make a length of DNA with a complementary sequence that will anneal to the gene but not to the rest of the DNA. This is the principle that underlies the construction of gene probes.

There are various ways of making gene probes. An enzyme called reverse transcriptase can be used to synthesize a DNA copy (complementary DNA, or **cDNA**) from any mRNA that can be isolated from human cells. If radioactive bases are added to the reaction the cDNA can be labelled and hence used as a hybridization probe to 'look for' its partner sequences in genomic DNA or cellular RNA. If cDNA probes are made from cellular RNA they may represent several different mRNA species. However, it is possible to clone cDNA into bacterial plasmids. This is done by synthesizing a second DNA strand on newly synthesized cDNA using a bacterial DNA polymerase. In this way, small cDNA duplexes are made that can be incorporated into plasmids and then grown in bacterial cells (see below). It is also possible to generate genomic probes by cloning fragments of genomic DNA into plasmids or

Fig. 2 Some restriction enzymes which are commonly used for analysing human DNA.

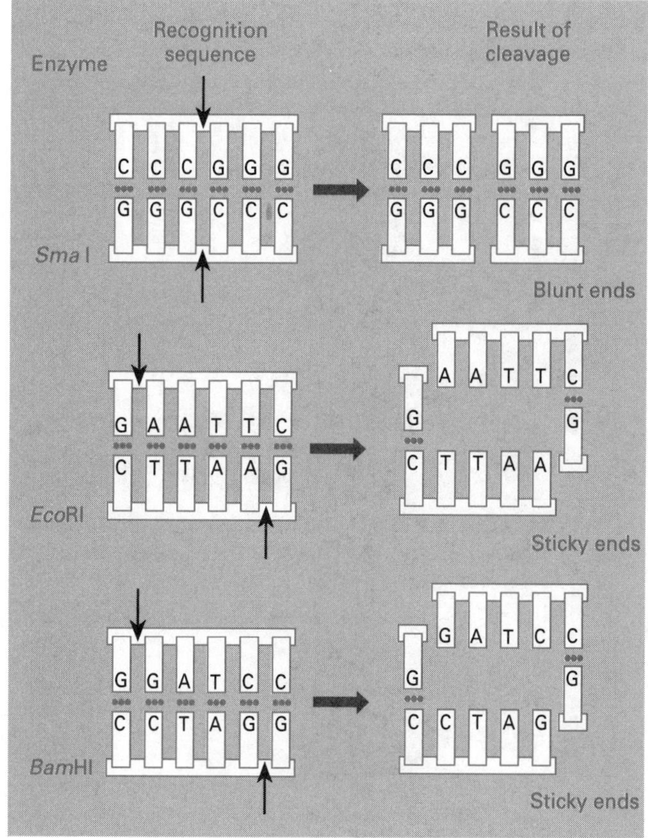

bacteriophage and amplifying individual genes in *Escherichia coli*. Thus, there are three main sources of gene probes: cDNA, cloned genomic DNA, or DNA fragments prepared from genomic DNA.

In order to label DNA to make a hybridization probe, a technique called nick translation is used. Appropriate nicks can be introduced into double-stranded DNA with various nucleases. So treated, DNA can act as a template for the enzyme DNA polymerase 1. Appropriate nicks are introduced with nucleases, and the DNA is labelled by incorporating a ^{32}P-labelled deoxyribonucleoside 5-triphosphate at the 3′-OH terminus of the nick by the action of the DNA polymerase. In this way it is possible to prepare highly radioactive probes.

DNA fractionation: restriction endonucleases

Restriction endonucleases are enzymes that occur naturally, mainly in bacteria, and that cleave DNA. They are called restriction endonucleases because they restrict their activity to foreign DNA. For example, if DNA from one strain of *E. coli* is introduced into another strain it is fragmented by the host restriction endonucleases; the bacterium's own DNA is not attacked because its vulnerable sites are protected by methylation. The restriction enzymes used most commonly in genetic engineering recognize signals consisting of six bases, often palindromes. Over 400 restriction enzymes with 100 different specificities have now been isolated, many of which are in regular use for recombinant DNA technology. They are named according to their organism of origin; *Eco*R1 is derived from *E.coli* for example (Fig. 2).

Gene mapping

Restriction-endonuclease mapping, or Southern blotting as it is usually called, after its inventor Edward Southern, has become an important tool for analysing genetic diseases (Fig. 3). DNA is obtained from any available tissue, usually from peripheral-blood white cells, and, after purification, is treated with a particular restriction enzyme. The mixture of fragments is then subjected to electrophoresis on an agarose gel. After separation of the fragments according to their size, the DNA in the gel is denatured by alkali treatment and the separated fragments are transferred to a nitrocellulose filter. The filter is then exposed to a radioactively labelled gene probe. The position of the fragments containing the gene of interest is then determined by autoradiography. By using a series of different enzymes that cleave DNA either within or outside the gene or genes we are studying, and by orientating some of the fragments in the appropriate direction, it is possible to build up restriction-enzyme maps of areas of the genome. The power of this technique for studying human diseases is quite remarkable. Out of the white cells from as little as 5 ml of blood it is possible to obtain sufficient DNA to analyse any normal or mutant gene for which we happen to have an appropriate probe.

Fig. 3 Restriction enzyme mapping (Southern blotting).

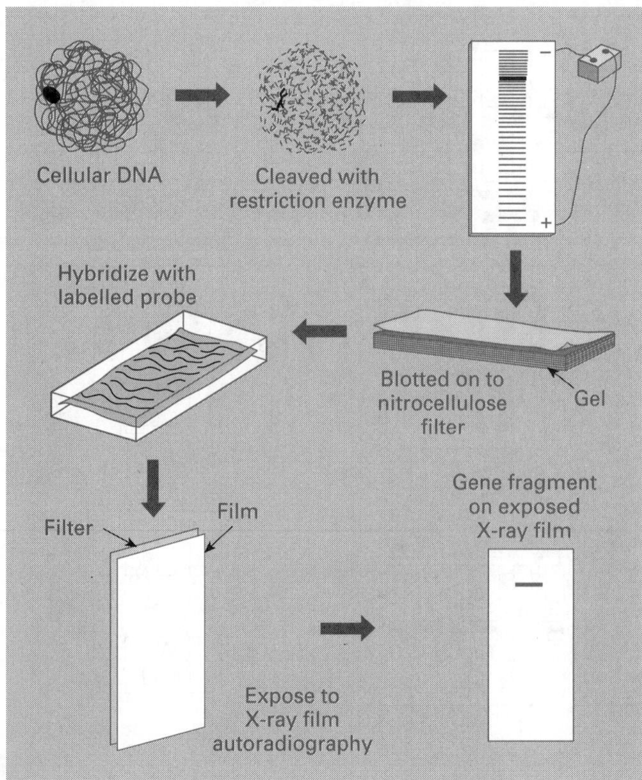

Gene cloning and the preparation of gene libraries

The insertion of foreign DNA into bacterial plasmids or bacteriophage is the keystone of recombinant DNA technology. Plasmids are closed, circular DNA molecules that replicate autonomously in bacteria. A plasmid commonly used for this type of work is illustrated in Fig. 4. It has an origin of replication, which means that it can be replicated in a bacterium by exploiting the latter's DNA-synthesizing machinery. It usually contains one or two genes for antibiotic resistance, and sites where restriction enzymes can cleave the DNA circle, so opening it up to produce a linear molecule. The DNA to be inserted into the plasmid is fragmented by the same restriction enzyme (Fig. 5). Plasmid and DNA fragments are then mixed and associate with each other by virtue of the sticky ends of the DNA. A permanent union is achieved by adding an enzyme called DNA ligase. Some plasmids rejoin and form the original circular DNA but others, recombinants, incorporate the foreign DNA. Suitable bacteria are then transformed by the plasmids, that is, plasmids and bacteria are mixed and a small number enter the bacteria. The frequency of transformation is such that each bacterium usually contains only one plasmid. The transformed bacteria are selected by a variety of microbiological tricks, usually by allowing the recombinant plasmids to confer antibiotic resistance on their bacterial hosts and growing the bacteria on selected media. Bacterial colonies can be screened by hybridization with appropriate gene probes for the presence of foreign DNA inserts, and when such a colony is identified it can be grown in large quantities to provide the particular DNA fragment required.

In this way it is possible to prepare gene libraries. To make a genomic library, DNA is prepared so that it consists of fragments of greater than 100 kb (a kilobase (kb) is 1000 nucleotide bases). These pieces are then digested with restriction enzymes so as to provide a random assortment of pieces of DNA. The fragments are inserted into an appropriate vector.

Fig. 4 A typical plasmid used in recombinant DNA technology.

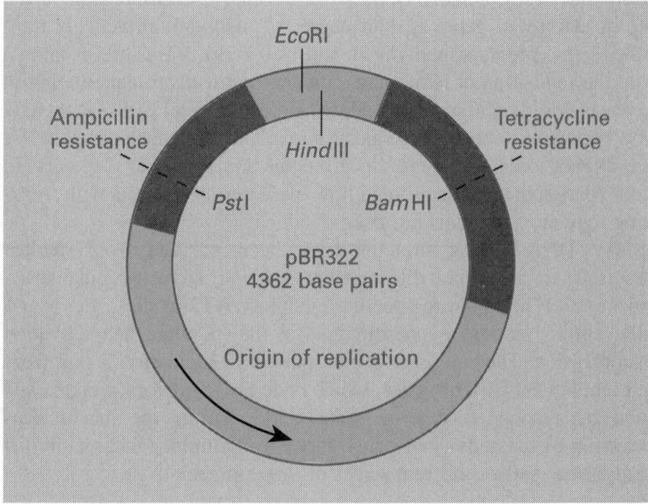

Three types of vectors are now commonly used: plasmids, bacteriophage, and cosmids. Plasmids have the disadvantage that they can only be used to clone a piece of DNA of fewer than 10 kb. On the other hand, bacteriophage (bacterial viruses) can accommodate fragments of 10 to 20 kb. As this field has progressed it has been necessary to handle even larger DNA fragments. A number of ingenious approaches have been developed. One particularly valuable system involves cloning in cosmids. A cosmid is an artificial vector, produced by genetic engineering, which consists of plasmid DNA packaged into a phage particle. Another valuable technique has been derived from yeast genetics and makes use of methods for taking apart and putting together entire chromosomes. It has been possible to exploit this technology in a novel and ingenious way to develop cloning vectors called yeast artificial chromosomes. It turns out that these vectors can accommodate human DNA fragments of hundreds of kilobases in length.

Gene libraries may contain hundreds of thousands of different recombinants, each representing roughly one gene attached to a plasmid or a bacteriophage DNA. In order to select a particular colony or plaque containing a particular gene from a bacterial plate, a technique called colony hybridization is used. A nitrocellulose filter is placed over the bacterial colonies or phage plaques. This absorbs a small amount of DNA. The filter is then incubated under hybridization conditions with a radioactive DNA probe complementary to the sequence of the gene being sought. After the excess probe has been washed away the filter is exposed to an X-ray plate; the position of the colony being sought is indicated by a mark on the plate. In constructing libraries, care is taken to ensure that the entire genome is accurately represented.

Various ingenious methods have been developed for constructing probes for screening libraries. I have already mentioned how it is possible to make cDNA probes, provided that purified mRNA is available from the gene we wish to find. However, this is often not the case and other approaches are required. For example, in many cases we will wish to identify a gene whose mRNA constitutes only a very tiny percentage of the total RNA of the cells in which it is expressed. One way round this problem is to try to determine at least part of the amino acid sequence of the particular gene product and then to synthesize short (oligonucleotide) probes with sequences deduced from the structure of the particular protein. But sometimes nothing is known about the amino acid sequence of the product of a particular gene. This problem can be overcome by immunological purification of the appropriate mRNAs. Newly formed proteins start to fold into their three-dimensional structures as they are being assembled on ribosomes. If a suspension of polyribosomes is incubated together with antibodies against the protein product of a gene we wish to find, antigen–antibody complexes form only with those polyribosomes that are producing the particular protein. By using affinity chromatography it is possible to harvest the polysomes that are bound to the antibody and then to isolate mRNA from them. Other extremely ingenious methods have been devised to isolate low-abundance mRNA. Finally, it is sometimes possible to isolate human genes by transferring genomic DNA into mouse fibroblasts; genes coding for proteins that are expressed on the cell surface, such as T cell-specific antigens, can be identified on the transformed mouse cell membranes by fluorescent-antibody screening of the cell population.

Cloned DNA can be used for many purposes. Individual genes can be isolated and sequenced, probes for gene mapping can be prepared, and a start has been made in devising transcription systems for analysing the function of abnormal genes in the test-tube. Finally, and with enormous potential for the future, cloned genes can sometimes be persuaded to transcribe their products in bacteria.

Fig. 5 The construction of a bacterial plasmid containing a foreign DNA insert for propagation in a bacterial cell.

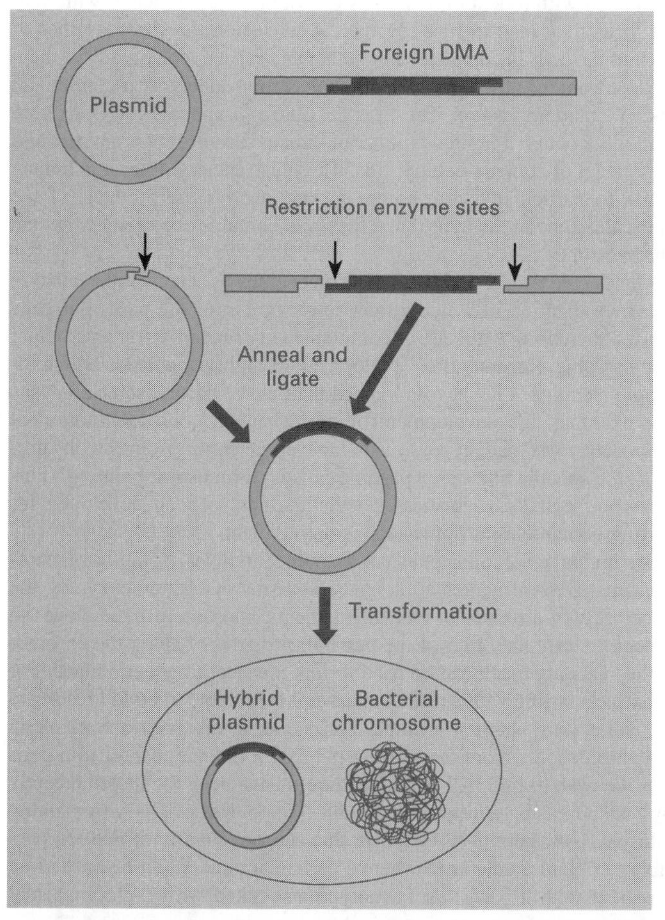

Gene sequencing

Now that genes can be isolated by cloning, the development of rapid methods for DNA sequencing has made it possible to determine the molecular basis for many single-gene disorders. There are two commonly used methods for DNA sequencing, developed independently by Maxam and Gilbert in the United States and Sanger in England. Both require the initial fractionation of DNA but from then on they are fundamentally different. Maxam and Gilbert use a degradative technique while Sanger uses a synthetic method based on stopping synthesis of a DNA chain at a particular point, rather than breaking it. Readers who wish to learn more about these methods are referred to the monographs cited at the end of this chapter.

Speeding up the analysis of human genes

Recently, various ingenious techniques have been developed for increasing the speed of analysis of human DNA. The most important is called the polymerase chain reaction (**PCR**), which is designed to amplify any short DNA sequence over a period of a few hours. Indeed, such is its power that it is possible to amplify sufficient DNA from one or two cells to obtain a genetic diagnosis within 24 h. The principle of PCR is illustrated in Fig. 6. This method has already had many important uses, including the development of extremely rapid methods for gene sequencing. It has also allowed short regions of DNA containing mutations to be amplified and analysed with oligonucleotide probes, thus greatly facilitating the diagnosis of genetic diseases.

Studying the function of genes

There are several ways to study the function of isolated genes, none entirely satisfactory. First, using what are called transient expression systems it is possible to insert genes into cells and to study both the quantity and structure of their mRNA transcripts. DNA can be inserted into a cell in the form of calcium microprecipitates, although this is very inefficient. More recently, several types of virus-derived vectors have been used to study the expression of human genes in mammalian cells.

A completely different approach is to introduce genes into established cultures of cells of appropriate lineage for the genes we wish to study. For example, human haemoglobin genes can be inserted into mouse erythroleukaemia cells. This can be done either by using purified genes or by transferring intact human chromosomes by techniques of cell fusion. The latter approach usually entails making use of a product of the particular human chromosome to ensure that it confers a selective property which will allow the hybrid cells to grow in culture. Finally, genes can be introduced into embryos by microinjection so that their patterns of integration and expression can be studied over several generations. Currently, the study of transgenic mice derived by this method is providing some extremely important information about the regulation of the expression of genes in different tissues.

Searching for genes

As early as 1927, J.B.S. Haldane reasoned that if it were possible to map 50 or more inherited characters they could be used as markers for predicting whether children would carry genes for conditions such as Huntington's disease. The idea is very simple. Supposing we want to follow the progress of a particular genetic trait through a family but have no way of identifying it. The thing to do is to find a gene that we can easily identify and that is linked to the gene we are looking for. If the two are so close together on the same chromosome that they always pass together through successive generations we now have a 'handle' on the gene that we can't identify; if the marker gene is inherited so must the gene that is closely linked to it. It follows, therefore, that if we know the chromosomal location of our marker gene we can use this approach to find any gene that happens to be linked to it. This is the idea behind the idea of generating a complete map of the human genome in which there are linkage markers spread at convenient distances that could lead us to any gene we wish to find. Such a map would be called a genetic map. The other type of map that we could prepare would be

Fig. 6 The polymerase chain rection. Specific DNA sequences are amplified in the following way. The double-stranded DNA is heated and the separated chains are allowed to bind the primers. The latter then initiate the sequences of two new chains complementary to the originals. This series of events is repeated 20 to 30 times, with each cycle giving a doubling of the DNA.

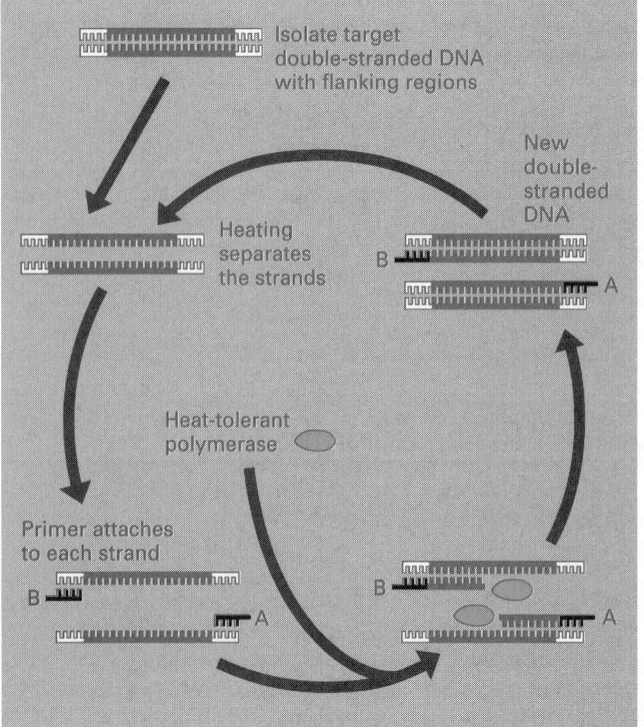

a physical map, that is one which shows us the structure of the genome. The ultimate physical map would, of course, entail sequencing the entire genome. These are the current goals of the Human Genome Project, which are expected to be achieved in the next 20 to 30 years.

Before setting out to produce a map of anything it is useful to have a rough idea what kind of distances are involved. In fact they are very large. Current estimates of the human genome put it between 3 and 3.5×10^9 bp. It has also been estimated that there may be somewhere between 50 000 and 100 000 important genes to be found and mapped. Furthermore, it is apparent that much of the human genome consists of non-coding DNA of no known function, so-called junk DNA. Given these rather daunting statistics, where might we start in our efforts to map the human genome?

Before the techniques of recombinant DNA became available the main difficulty for gene mappers was the lack of markers. There were a few protein variants, such as blood-group antigens, serum protein polymorphisms, and so on but they were never sufficient even to start making a map. However, as soon as restriction enzymes were discovered and human DNA was digested it became clear that all of us show remarkable variability in the structure of our DNA. Single-base changes that are in themselves harmless can be identified by altered cutting sites for restriction enzymes. Thus the size of the fragments of DNA generated by such enzymes will vary. This is the basis for what are called restriction fragment length polymorphisms (**RFLPs**). If we can identify their chromosomal location, they are excellent markers for hunting genes by linkage analysis. But it turns out that things are even better than this, because scattered about the genome there are regions of DNA that are highly polymorphic. Such regions often represent blocks of repeated segments of DNA that vary in length from person to person. Such mini- or microsatellite DNA has turned out to be a particularly valuable source of linkage markers.

Physical mapping has also moved forward quickly. This can be done at various levels. At low resolution one of the most useful approaches has been a technique called somatic-cell hybridization. If human cells are mixed with rodent tumour cells grown in culture together with Sendai virus they tend to fuse together. After fusion the chromosomes of each of the cells become mixed together and subsequently many of them are lost from the now hybrid cell; human chromosomes are preferentially lost in a random fashion. Thus it is possible to propogate cells in culture that only contain a limited number of human chromosomes and to build up a panel of somatic-cell hybrids. These can be used to assign human genes to particular chromosomes by looking for the products of the particular gene in the hybrid line that only contains one or a few human chromosomes.

Genes can also be assigned to chromosomes by a technique called *in situ* hybridization in which a radioactive probe for the particular gene is used to hybridize directly to complementary sequences on a particular chromosome. Recently, the development of highly sophisticated microscopic techniques has revolutionized the field of chromosome analysis. For example, the development of multichannel, confocal fluorescent microscopy has made it possible to lable entire chromosomes with chromosome-specific libraries, a pastime called 'chromosome painting'. Furthermore, equally sophisticated techniques have been developed for sorting human chromosomes and isolating them.

At higher resolution, physical mapping involves isolation of chromosomal DNA, fragmentation of the DNA by restriction enzymes, the generation of a library of cloned fragments, and ordering the clones to reflect the original order of the particular fragments along the chromosome. This approach can be used to link physical to genetic maps. For example, starting with an RFLP marker it is possible to build up a series of overlapping phage or cosmid clones and, in essence, to walk along the chromosome from the starting-point of a linkage marker to a gene that we wish to find. All these techniques have been facilitated recently by our increasing ability to deal with large pieces of DNA by cloning into yeast, as mentioned earlier in this chapter. Finally, it is often possible to obtain a clue as to where a particular gene might be by finding a patient with a particular phenotype associated with a chromosomal

Table 1 *Some applications of recombinant DNA technology*

Single-gene disorders
Molecular pathology
Diagnosis
Treatment
Genetic basis of common polygenic diseases
Identification of susceptibility
Pathogenesis
Treatment
Diagnostics
Gene probes
Monoclonal antibodies
Therapeutics
Drugs
Vaccines
Growth factors; repair and regeneration
Monoclonal antibodies
Anti-sense DNA
Targeted cancer therapy
Broader aspects of human biology
Development
Ageing
Evolution

abnormality such as a deletion. In such cases it is reasonable to assume that the patient's clinical picture may be related to loss of particular genes in the deleted region of DNA. Thus the deletion can act as a starting-point for finding a particular gene.

Mapping techniques of this type have led to some remarkable success stories in clinical genetics. In particular, it has been possible to discover the cause for some important genetic diseases. The first step is to define an RFLP linkage, which may put us within a few million bases of the gene that we are looking for. Next, by various chromosome walking or jumping techniques it is possible to move towards the gene and finally to define it. The next step is to sequence the gene and to make an educated guess as to the kind of protein product that would be directed by such a sequence. Next, the mutations in the gene are determined and, finally, the function of the particular product is worked out from its protein sequence and insights are gained into how this might be affected by the particular mutations. The discovery of the genetic defects in Duchenne muscular dystrophy, cystic fibrosis, and Huntington's disease are prime examples of the power of this approach (see also Chapter 4.3).

Clinical applications of recombinant DNA technology

It is beyond the scope of this chapter to outline all the possible clinical applications of recombinant DNA technology. The main areas in which this technology will be applied to medical research and practice are summarized in Table 1. In the following sections we will consider a few examples.

The molecular pathology of single-gene disorders

Broadly speaking there are two main classes of mutations. First, there are those that result in an altered protein product, most of which involve a single base substitution that causes a single amino-acid substitution, so-called mis-sense mutations. In many cases they have no ill effects, but if they change the function or stability of the protein they may cause a clinical disorder. The other group is made up of mutations that cause defective synthesis of proteins without changing their structure.

Work on the thalassaemias, and more recently on other single-gene disorders, has told us how a single base change in a gene can profoundly modify its output. For example, it may produce a premature stop codon, so that when mRNA is translated, shortened and therefore functionally useless, peptide chains are produced (Fig. 7). Such lesions are called nonsense mutations. Because amino acids are encoded by a triplet code, loss or insertion of one, two or four bases in a gene throws the 'reading frame' out of sequence; its mRNA cannot be translated beyond the frameshift (Fig. 8). As mentioned earlier, most genes have their coding regions (exons) divided up into several pieces by lengths of DNA of unknown function called introns. As primary mRNA transcripts contain both intron and exon sequences, the introns have to be cut out and the exons precisely spliced together before mRNAs move into the cytoplasm. Several types of thalassaemia and some other single-gene disorders result from mutations that interfere with the splicing mechanism. Single base changes at the junctions between introns and exons may prevent splicing; no normal mRNA is produced. More surprisingly, it turns out that base changes within introns or exons can produce alternative splice sites which result in the production of both normal and abnormally spliced mRNA; the latter cannot be used as a template for peptide-chain synthesis. Finally, and as mentioned earlier, all mammalian genes have sequences in common at their 5′-flanking regions that play a critical part in the regulation of transcription. Base changes in these regions may reduce their rate of transcription.

Studies of the appropriate genes of patients with Christmas disease, haemophilia, Duchenne muscular dystrophy, cystic fibrosis, growth-hormone deficiency, antithrombin III deficiency, and low-density lipoprotein-receptor deficiency have shown that the molecular pathology of these disorders is similar to that of the thalassaemias.

This work has started to help us to understand why single-gene disorders may show such remarkably diverse phenotypes. For example, nonsense or frameshift mutations entirely inactivate a gene, while mutations involving splicing or promoter regions may result in a moderate to severe reduction in the output of a particular gene product. Thus homozygosity for severe or mild mutations, or compound heterozygosity for a mild and severe mutation, may give rise to a wide range of different clinical phenotypes for diseases involving a particular locus. However, work over recent years has revealed that there may be other novel mechanisms which may modify the phenotypic expression of single-gene disorders.

It is now clear that several chronic neurological diseases, including Huntington's disease, the fragile X syndrome, and others, result from a variation in the size of long tracks of trinucleotide repeats which are found either close to or within the genes that are involved in these conditions. These regions of DNA seem to be unstable and may increase in length over several generations. When they reach a critical size they

Fig. 7 A nonsense mutation. A tyrosine codon UAU has a single base change, U→A which produces a premature stop codon.

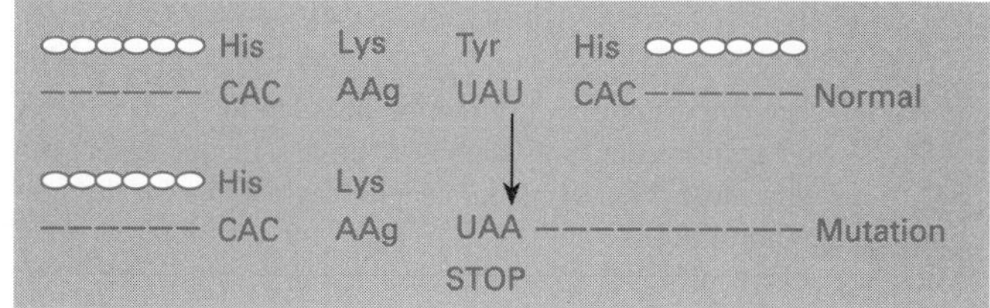

Fig. 8 A frameshift mutation. Two bases have been deleted from a threonine codon, ACU. This leaves a U which now links up with the next two bases of the next lysine codon to produce UAA, which is a stop codon.

Lys Ser Ile Thr Lys
AAG AGU AUC ACU AAG Normal
2 Base deletion
Lys Ser Ile
CAC AGU AUC U AAG Mutation
STOP

seem to interfere with normal gene expression and the clinical phenotype results. This phenomenon may explain changing phenotypes over different generations, or anticipation of, or even a reversion to, a normal phenotype. In the case of Huntington's disease it also seems to explain the particular time of onset of the clinical disorder. The phenotype of some monogenic diseases may also be modified according to which parent the disorder is inherited from. This strange phenomenon, called parental imprinting, may also be involved in the molecular pathology of a number of premalignant disorders.

Another mechanism for phenotypic diversity of genetic disease is exemplified by the mutations that involve mitochondrial DNA. Mitochondria have their own genetic material in the form of a 16.6 kb, double-stranded, circular DNA molecule. Although most mitochondrial proteins are encoded by nuclear DNA, a few are encoded only by mitochondrial DNA. These include 13 proteins that are involved in the respiratory chain required for oxidative phosphorylation. All our mitochondrial DNA is inherited from our mothers and hence mitochondrial DNA disorders are transmitted by females. But there is marked heterogeneity in the phenotypic expression of these conditions because of the phenomenon of heteroplasmy, that is the presence of a mixture of mutant and normal mitochondrial DNA in the same cell. Furthermore, tissues are affected differently on the basis of their energy requirements. This is the main basis for the remarkable heterogeneity of these conditions, which are described in detail in Section 25.

Common polygenic diseases

When we consider common disorders such as diabetes, degenerative arterial disease, autoimmune disease, and the major psychoses, the applications of recombinant DNA and cell biology are less obvious. Many of them have a complex polygenic basis and, in addition, environmental factors play an important part in their aetiology. Why do we want to try to determine the important genes involved in these disorders?

Studies that have analysed the occurrence of common diseases in identical twins have suggested that the genetic component varies considerably between disorders. For example, the common form of maturity-onset diabetes, type II diabetes, is a genetic disease; if one of a pair of identical twins is affected there is a very high likelihood that the other twin will become diabetic. Similar findings have been obtained in many common diseases, although often the genetic component is very much weaker. However, we know virtually nothing about the aetiology of these disorders except that in some cases environmental factors may play an important part, smoking and diet in vascular disease for example. It is likely, therefore, that if we were able to identify a few important genes that are involved in making us more or less susceptible to the action of these environmental agents, and we were able to understand the function of these genes and how it varies between susceptible or resistant individuals, we might gain considerable insights into the underlying causes of these diseases, and how such genetic variability interacts with the environment. Similarly, it might be possible for us to identify individuals who are particularly susceptible to environmental agents and hence to develop more focused public-health programmes for the prevention of these diseases.

There are several different approaches to attempt to define the major genes in these complex polygenic systems. One, and probably the least rewarding, is to find large families in which more than one member is affected. By using random, RFLP-linkage markers and making extensive family studies it might be possible to obtain a linkage to a susceptibility gene, which could then be identified by reverse genetics. This is extremely time-consuming and difficult, and so far has rarely been successful. A variation on this approach, and one that is particularly valuable for diseases in which it is difficult to find multiply affected generations of a particular disease, is the analyse the segregation of the disease with a particular marker in pairs of siblings. The finding of the association of the particular marker with a disease by such sib-pair analysis may offer a valuable clue due to a particular linkage.

Another approach is to try to make an educated guess about which genes might be involved. For example, in coronary arterial disease it would be reasonable to suppose that genes involved in cholesterol or vessel-wall metabolism might be important players. Thus, having isolated these so-called candidate genes and obtained appropriate RFLP markers, family studies can be used to see if any polymorphisms segregate with a particular disease. Another way to tackle this problem is through mouse genetics. A great deal is known about the location of genes in the mouse genome and there are many mouse models for common human diseases. Furthermore, although many genes in the mouse are on different chromosomes from those in man, there is already considerable information about the equivalent chromosomal locations of genes between mouse and man. It is relatively easy to do breeding experiments in mice and therefore quickly to define the loci involved in some of the diseases that resemble their human counterparts.

Using these different approaches, considerable progress has already been made in defining some of the genes that are likely to be involved in susceptibility or resistance to common diseases. For example, in type I diabetes it is clear that there are at least two major gene systems involved, one being the class II genes of the HLA-DR system and the other a locus close to the insulin gene, although probably not insulin itself. At least 10 loci have been found to be involved in producing the phenotype of non-obese diabetes in mice, a condition similar though not identical to human type I diabetes. All these mouse genes may have their human homologues. It is of particular interest that one of them seems to be involved in susceptibility or resistance to a variety of infections.

There has also been considerable progress towards defining some of the major genes involved in susceptibility to type II diabetes. By studying families with an unusually early onset of the condition, and in which the inheritance seems to be of a dominant variety, it has been possible to define a series of mutations of the glucokinase gene that seems to be responsible for some forms of this condition. Similarly, there is increasing evidence that in some families the glycogen synthase gene may be involved. Although these families have an unusual type of type II diabetes, these results are very encouraging and suggest that it should be possible to determine some of the genes involved in the more common forms of this condition that occur in later life.

Some of the major genes involved in susceptibility to coronary arterial disease have also been defined. This work was stimulated by the discovery of the molecular basis for monogenic hypercholesterolaemia, which turned out to be due to a variety of different mutations of the low-density lipoprotein-receptor gene. Other genes that involve cholesterol metabolism have been shown to be polymorphic. Some forms of coronary arterial disease appear to be due to mutations of the apolipoprotein b-100 locus. Information is being obtained about other polymorphisms that may modify the level of cholesterol in populations, variability at the apolipoprotein E locus for example, and genetic variability at the Apo(a) locus also appears to be responsible for some premature coronary arterial disease. The recent discovery that a particular polymorphism of the *ACE* gene, that is the locus which encodes for the angiotensin-converting enzyme, may be responsible for considerable numbers of cases of premature coronary arterial disease is of particular interest. It also appears that genetic variability at the fibrinogen locus may be involved with susceptibility to myocardial infarction.

Currently, we are going through a phase of development in which variability at many different individual loci is being studied with respect to susceptibility or resistance to coronary arterial disease. Sooner or later it will be important to try to derive genetic profiles that show how all these different variables interact with each other to produce particular risks for individual patients. This is slow and difficult work but progress will undoubtedly be easier once we have a detailed linkage map of the human genome.

Some of the most encouraging progress towards understanding the major genes in these complex polygenic systems has been made in the field of dementia, particularly Alzheimer's disease. The first break in

Table 2 *Examples of retrovirus oncogenes (v-onc) and the chromosomal location of their human cellular oncogene (c-onc) counterparts*

onc	v-*onc* origin	Virus disease	Product or activity	Human chromosome
abl	Mouse	pre B-cell leukaemia	PK (tyr)	9q34
*erb*B	Chicken	Erythroblastosis	Truncated EGF receptor	7p13-q11.2
fms	Cat	Sarcoma	M-CSF receptor	5q34
fos	Mouse	Osteosarcoma	DNA binding	14q21-31
Ha-*ras*1	Rat	Sarcoma	GTP binding	11p15
Ha-*ras*2	Rat	Sarcoma	GTP binding	X
Ki-*ras*1	Rat	Sarcoma	GTP binding	6p23-q12
Ki-*ras*2	Rat	Sarcoma	GTP binding	12p12
mos	Mouse	Sarcoma	PK (ser. thr)	8q22
myc	Chicken	Myelocytomatosis	DNA binding	8q24
sis	Monkey	Sarcoma	Truncated PDGF (β-chain)	22q12-q13
src	Chicken	Sarcoma	PK (tyr)	20q12-q13

EGF, epidermal growth factor; GTP, guanosine triphosphate; M–CSF, macrophage–colony-stimulating factor; PDGF, platelet-derived growth factor; PK, protein kinase.

this complex problem followed the discovery of mutations at the locus for the β-amyloid precursor protein on chromosome 21 in affected members of families with early-onset Alzheimer's disease. More recently, however, it has been found that a particular polymorphism of the apolipoprotein E-4 locus has a strong association with the likelihood of developing the later-onset form of the condition. Even more remarkably, it appears that the age of onset of dementia is closely related to whether an individual is homozygous or heterozygous for this particular polymorphism. Findings of this kind promise to provide extremely valuable information about the molecular pathology and causation of this distressing group of disorders.

Thus, although progress in this difficult field is slow, and particularly in the case of the important psychoses has often thrown up some false leads, we already know enough to suggest that over the next few years the study of the complex genetic basis for susceptibility or resistance to the environmental agents which undoubtedly cause many of these conditions may provide us with considerable insights into their pathogenesis and, hopefully, may provide better methods for their prevention or treatment.

Cancer (see also Chapter 6.3)

Another area of considerable potential for recombinant DNA technology is the study of the mechanisms of malignant transformation. Here we are moving into a different area of human genetics called somatic-cell genetics.

Undoubtedly the pathogenesis of cancer involves even more complex interactions between environment and genome. Familial cancers are rare and very little is known about inherited susceptibility to common cancers. However, it is becoming clear that malignant transformation involves fundamental changes in the genome of individual cells that are passed on to their progeny. The current excitement in the cancer field has arisen because the new tools of cell and molecular biology have made it possible to synthesize several long-standing observations about the epidemiology and cytogenetics of cancer into a working model of what may go wrong in a neoplastic cell.

One of the most important threads in the development of this story was the discovery of oncogenes. There is a variety of ways in which oncogenic viruses can produce neoplastic transformation. Although in some cases this is achieved by their insertion close to a critical host regulatory region (insertional mutagenesis), it is also clear that some of them carry specific genes that are involved in producing a neoplastic phenotype. The discovery which has transformed the cancer field was that these viral oncogenes have their equivalent in the cells of almost all species studied. It appears the viruses have picked up normal cellular genes during evolution, by recombination events, and that they have developed their oncogenic properties in their new home. The cellular homologues of viral oncogenes (v-*onc*), cellular oncogenes (c-*onc*), appear to be part of a cell's normal genetic machinery, responsible for the control of proliferation, differentiation, and development.

It is now clear that there are various ways whereby the action of cellular oncogenes may be modified such that a malignant phenotype may develop. First, they may be the site of point mutations or more extensive structural alterations such as amplification to many copy numbers. Presumably this is how the effect of many environmental carcinogens is mediated. In other cases, abnormal function of an oncogene may follow a change in their chromosomal location, as part of a translocation specific for a particular type of tumour for example. This type of mechanism undoubtedly causes abnormal oncogene expression in association with the Philadelphia chromosome that occurs in chronic myeloid leukaemia and as part of the particular chromosome changes characteristic of Burkitt's lymphoma. In recent years over 60 oncogenes have been identified. A few examples are summarized in Table 2. In many cases their sites and mechanisms of action have been identified. They include growth factors, growth-factor receptors, membrane and cytoplasmic transducers, and a number of DNA-binding proteins. Overall, abnormal function of these genes due to the mechanisms that we have just described leads to dominant stimulatory effects on cell growth and maturation.

It is apparent, however, that oncogenesis can be mediated by the loss of inhibitory function because of mutations which act in a recessive manner and involve another family of genes called tumour-suppressor genes. Evidence for the involvement of these genes in causing cancer has come from several different fields, cell hybrids, the inherited cancer syndromes, and the observation that there is loss of heterozygosity at different loci in tumours.

In the case of certain rare childhood cancers such as retinoblastoma or Wilms' tumour it appears that we may be born with a particular mutation. While we remain heterozygous for these lesions, these tumours do not develop; the presence of the normal allele, or tumour-suppressor gene, appears sufficient to maintain a normal phenotype. However, if there is a rearrangement or deletion of the normal allele, leading to its inactivation, the affected cells undergo neoplastic transformation. It turns out that this phenomenon is not restricted to rare childhood leukaemias and that loss of heterozygosity of this kind is a common feature in many different cancers. The functions of a number of tumour-suppressor genes, including those for retinoblastoma and one called are now known. They seem to be key players in the regulation of the cell cycle; products of both genes restrict cells at the G_1–S phase of the cycle, thus preventing the entry of the cells into the proliferative phase of the cycle.

Recent studies of the evolution and pathogenesis of colon cancer provide an excellent example of the way in which oncogenes and tumour-suppressor genes may be involved in the complex series of events leading to a neoplasm. Analysis of families with familial polyposis coli (**FAP**) has shown that this important premalignant condition is determined by a locus, *APP* or adenomatous polyposis coli, on the long arm of chromosome 5 (5q15.21). It seems likely that inherited mutations of this gene make it more likely that patients will develop ademonata of the colon. It is also clear from the study of sporadic colon cancers that a number of other gene loci are involved. One, called *MCC* (mutated in colon cancer), is close to APP on chromosome 5. Another locus that seems to be a major player in this disorder maps to the long arm of chromosome 17 and has been identified as the tumour suppressor, *p53*. Yet another locus that is also often involved in colon cancer maps to the long arm of chromosome 18 (18q21.22). This has been called the *DCC* gene, standing for *d*eleted *co*lon *ca*ncer locus. Its product appears to be similar to certain key adhesion molecules involved in the interactions between nerve cells. Finally, mutations of the *ras* oncogene occur very frequently in colon cancer. From analyses of different parts of particular cancers a picture is emerging which suggests that the development of colon cancer involves a minimum of six different mutations. Some of them, like that involving the *FAP* locus, may be inherited, while it is presumed that the majority reflect somatic mutations occurring during our lifetime, possibly as the result of environmental carcinogens. The precise order in which these mutations occur may not be important. It appears that what is essential for neoplastic transformation is a critical number of mutations.

It is clear, therefore, that even in the short time in which molecular technology has been applied to the study of cancer, some remarkable insights have been obtained about the general mechanisms of malignant transformation. Key genes involved in the regulation of growth and division of cells are involved. Sometimes we may inherit mutations that take us part of the way along the road to developing a cancer, a single mutation is rarely sufficient, and most cancers represent multiple different mutations and/or chromosomal rearrangements, which combine to reduce a cell's normal facility for orderly division and differentiation.

This remarkable story is continued in Section 6.

Development, differentiation, repair, and congenital malformation

The most interesting question in human biology is how a single, fertilized egg with its 10^9 bp of DNA turns into a human being. This field has enormous implications for all aspects of clinical practice. It is becoming clear that developmental work in such an apparently unpromising organism as the fruit fly, Drosophila, has important implications for understanding major developmental abnormalities in man. Like much modern biological research the ideas are not new but the availability of the tools of recombinant DNA technology is allowing them to be explored in a novel fashion. In 1894, Bateson suggested that the study of chance deviation in normal developmental patterns might provide clues about the rules that govern the regulation of development. This is turning out to be the case. For example it has been found that the homeotic genes of Drosophila, which regulate the development of body segments, have DNA sequences in common with many other species including man. Furthermore the products of these genes are expressed in different tissues during mammalian development. Homeotic mutations in insects result in major developmental abnormalities, including substitutions of one or more segments normally found elsewhere along the body axis. Thus the discovery of the human equivalent of the homeotic genes suggests a particularly promising new area of research in human development and its abnormalities.

Another large area of advance in developmental genetics is the isolation of genes for proteins involved in the regulation of growth and differentiation and, incidentally, of particular interest for surgery, of repair. As well as more general regulatory molecules such as the insulin-like growth factors, there are many proteins that are involved in the differentiation of specific tissues. For example, a whole battery of regulatory proteins plays a part in the complex programme in which haemopoietic stem cells divide and give rise to progeny that mature into red cells, white cells, and platelets. Similarly, many other important tissue-specific growth factors have been isolated and are available for the study of the regulation of growth and differentiation of particular cell populations. Further studies along these lines have important implications for such intractable problems as nerve repair and the control of regenerative and healing processes in general.

It has been known for many years that many congenital abnormalities result from chromosomal defects. Hitherto, it has only been possible to identify gross abnormalities of this type using light microscopy. Recently, however, it has become apparent that we may be able to identify much more subtle structural changes of chromosomes, submicroscopic deletions or insertions for example, using restriction-enzyme technology.

The diagnosis and prevention of disease

It seems likely that the applications of recombinant DNA technology and cell biology will have practical implications for all aspects of clinical practice. Indeed, the pharmaceutical industry has moved rapidly into this field and is putting a large effort into developing biotechnological facilities for producing diagnostic and therapeutic agents.

Diagnosis

Recombinant DNA and monoclonal antibody technology promise to revolutionize diagnostic medicine over the next few years. The earliest use of gene probes for diagnostic purposes was for the detection of carrier states for genetic diseases and for their prenatal detection using fetal DNA. This new technology promises to revolutionize preventative genetics and offers the possibility of controlling many inherited diseases.

Gene probes, together with the use of PCR, will have wide application in diagnostic pathology. Because of their extreme sensitivity and specificity they will be of particular value in microbiology and virology for the identification and taxonomy of micro-organisms. Various diagnostic kits have already been constructed for this purpose. And as more is learnt about the activation of oncogenes or the synthesis of abnormal gene products due to mutations of these genes as a cause of cancer, DNA probes will become increasingly valuable for screening and for monitoring treatment.

The other area of biotechnology with important implications for diagnosis is monoclonal antibody production. Diagnostic agents based on this have already been established for a wide range of applications including pregnancy testing, monitoring ovulation, ovarian function, and the identification of a variety of infections including AIDS, hepatitis and legionella. And as our understanding of the cell biology of cancer increases it should be possible to radiolabel specific probes or monoclonal antibodies for imaging and more precise localization of tumours.

Treatment

There is already enough information to suggest that therapeutics will be changed dramatically by the use of recombinant DNA and monoclonal antibody technology. The ability to clone and express genes for human proteins in micro-organisms provides a remarkably effective way of producing large quantities of absolutely pure products for therapeutic purposes. One of the first success stories in this field was the development of recombinant erythropoietin, which is now in routine use for treating the anaemia of chronic renal failure. A number of other valuable recombinant proteins are now being used in clinical practice, including interferon -α and -γ, tissue plasminogen activator, human growth hormone, human insulin, and human factor VIII for the treatment of haemophilia. In recent years a variety of growth factors, lymphokines and other biologically active mediators has been produced, and their value in therapeutics is being explored at the present time. They include haemopoietic growth factors, which promise to be extremely valuable in the management of patients with bone marrow depression following treatment for cancer or after transplantation.

Recombinant DNA technology also offers many possibilities for the development of new vaccines or for the replacement of vaccines in present use. Recent innovations include synthetic peptide vaccines or cloning the genes for particular peptide antigens in yeast; a vaccine against hepatitis B made in yeast was one of the first successes for this branch of biotechnology. Various monoclonal antibodies have been developed for therapeutic use, and by some ingenious genetic engineering it has been possible to 'humanize' rat monoclonal antibodies. These agents have a wide range of uses in treating infectious disease and cancer.

Recombinant DNA technology has provided the basis for the newly developing field of human gene therapy. It is possible to insert genes into foreign cells, either directly or by using vectors such as retroviruses. The discovery of the major regulatory regions for many human genes, together with the development of safer and more effective retrovirus vector systems, have raised the possibility that gene therapy may be with us in the near future. Indeed, it has already been possible to insert the defective gene into the lymphocytes of children with an immune-deficiency disorder and improve their function so that these children are protected against infection. It seems likely that many single-gene disorders will be amenable to gene therapy, particularly those that are expressed in haemopoietic stem cells.

There are numerous other potential products from the biotechnology industry. The dream of harmless alternatives for blood products is closer with the recent finding that it is possible to persuade yeast to synthesize human haemoglobin. Vascular implants can be made more compatible by treatment with cells, growth factors, and collagen. The problem of graft rejection is being tackled by removing T cells, using a specific antibody bound to magnetite to permit cell separation in a magnetic field. And, as described in Section 6, many different ways are being explored to reverse abnormal oncogene action as an approach to cancer therapy.

But perhaps the most promising potential of molecular therapeutics is the development of 'designer drugs'. Now that it is possible to isolate individual genes, and to study their products in detail, rapid progress is being made towards an understanding of the precise mechanisms by which various effectors bind to their cell surface receptors and how information is passed through the interior cell to its nucleus. Although there are still many difficult problems to be solved, particularly a better understanding of the rules of protein folding, it is clear that we are moving towards a time when drug design can be directed at modifying cellular function. Thus the pharmacology of the future will change from the rather hit-and-miss approach of medicinal chemistry to a more precise form of tailor-made drug design.

The overall impact of human molecular biology

The overall effect of molecular medicine on clinical practice in the developed countries is difficult to forecast; it is unlikely to change it overnight. Nor will it lessen the need for skill at the bedside or the holistic approach to patient care. The most immediate impact will be in preventative genetics, and the production of diagnostics, vaccines, blood products, and a wide variety of therapeutic agents. It is too early to predict whether a greater understanding of the molecular pathology of degenerative arterial disease, autoimmune disease, cancer, congenital malformation, or neuropsychiatric illnesses, which should follow the application of DNA technology to these problems, will have a large impact on their prevention or management. But as we have largely failed to control these diseases, except by high-technology patch-up procedures, this is surely the way that basic medical research must go in the future. Epidemiological studies have already taught us how we might reduce the prevalence of some of these diseases by changes of diet, stopping smoking, and other modifications of lifestyle; we now need to understand the molecular and cellular basis of individual susceptibility to these bad habits and, based on this information, to find out whether the diseases that they cause can be better controlled.

What will the new tools of biotechnology do for the problems of the developing countries? In a world in which millions of children die each year of starvation, the major medical application of recombinant DNA technology should be for improving food supplies and for developing vaccines and diagnostic agents for parasitic and infectious diseases, which, together with malnutrition, still look like being the main killers of the twenty-first century.

The advent of recombinant DNA technology has raised the expectation that, as we gradually gain control over our genome, we may be able to modify the human phenotype, more or less as we please. We have been regaled by television accounts of potential parents walking round 'gene supermarkets' stocking up their trolleys with genes that they would like to see expressed in their children, and fears of eugenics, and memories of Nazi Germany, have been raised again. Biological determinism is already having a large effect on sociobiology and the dubious science that underlies this philosophy is providing a convenient peg on which extremist political groups are hanging their views on how society should be regulated. But we do not have the faintest idea about the nature of the complex interactions of genome and environment that underlie human behaviour. Indeed, it is debatable whether we shall ever be able to explain much of human behaviour in terms of a DNA sequence. Perhaps in the long term our exploration of the human genome will provide some real insights into why we are what we are but it would be unwise to pin our hopes for the future on this expectation. For the moment we need to develop an open debate with the public about how far we wish to move in modification of our genomes for medical advances.

REFERENCES

Alberts, B., Bray, D., Lewis, J., Raff, M., Roberts, K., and Watson, J.D. (1994). *The molecular biology of the cell*, (3rd edn). Garland, New York and London.

Gelehrter, T.D. and Collins, F.S. (1990). *Principles of medical genetics*. Williams and Williams, Baltimore.

Lewin, B. (1994). *Genes V*. University Press, Oxford.

Singer, M. and Berg, P. (1991). *Genes and genomes*. University Science Books, California and Blackwell Scientific Publications, Oxford.

Trent, R. (1993). *Molecular medicine: an introductory text for students*. Churchill Livingstone, Edinburgh.

Weatherall, D.J. (1991). *The new genetics and clinical practice*, (3rd edn). University Press, Oxford.

4.2 Medical applications of cell biology

4.2.1. Introduction

D. J. WEATHERALL

Hand in hand with the exciting developments in molecular biology that were described in the previous section, over recent years there have been equally spectacular advances in cell biology, many of which are having increasing applications in the clinic. This rapidly expanding field is likely to change the way we think about pathology and therapeutics over the next few years.

The scope of modern cell biology is enormous. In the previous chapter we discussed how proteins are produced under the control of their respective genes. Cell biology explains how they are transported to the particular cellular compartments where they function, enzymes of the Krebs' cycle to the mitochondria and degradative enzymes to liposomes for example. All this is achieved by an extensive membrane-bound system in the cytoplasm, particularly the endoplasmic reticulum and the Golgi apparatus. Much has been learnt about the so-called signal sequences of proteins that are involved in these key transport processes, and a start is being made in understanding the fate of abnormal proteins that cannot be handled by these sophisticated transport systems, and about the transport of proteins that are secreted from cells.

Another major area in cell biology of increasing clinical relevance is an understanding of the cytoskeleton of cells, their scaffolding, and how a cell can alter its shape appropriately and, in some cases, adapt its mobility to its physiological function. Much is now known about the microanatomy of the cytoskeleton, including its actin filaments, microtubules, and intermediate filaments, and how it is related to the plasma membrane. Similarly, the properties of the extracellular matrix, which is secreted by cells and also has a vital role in determining their behaviour, can now be explored.

As well as all this new information about the function and microanatomy of cells a great deal has been learnt about the molecular and biochemical basis for differentiation and the regulation of cell division and maturation. This has extremely important consequences for the cancer field. Furthermore, the discovery of cytokines, a class of regulatory molecules, is providing valuable information about the ways in which cell populations are controlled and about how they mediate their many different physiological functions.

Clearly it would be impossible to cover this enormous field as part of an introduction to a textbook of medicine. The three chapters that follow will, however, serve to introduce clinicians to some of the important areas in modern cell biology that will be of particular relevance to medical practice over the next few years.

4.2.2 Cell biology of organelles and the endomembrane system

D.J.T. VAUX

The endomembrane system: a unique feature of eukaryotic cells

A cardinal feature of the evolutionary advance from prokaryotic bacterial cells to eukaryotic animal cells is the acquisition of internal membranes that serve to subdivide the interior of the cell. This leads to efficient compartmentalization of cellular processes into organelles within which the environment is independently controlled and optimized for the specialized functions carried out there. George Palade suggested in the 1970s that these membrane-bound intracellular structures are not static islands, but exist in dynamic equilibrium with a continuous flux of membrane and content moving between them in the form of shuttling vesicles. This insight has turned out to be very powerful, and colours many subsequent efforts to understand the way in which the internal-membrane economy of a cell can be regulated.

The internal membranes of mammalian cells may be divided into two types. One class of membrane includes the organelles that form the 'conveyor belt' system running out of the cell from the endoplasmic reticulum (the secretory or exocytic pathway) and the organelles that form the 'conveyor belt' system running into the cell from the plasma membrane to the lysosome (the endocytic pathway). These two pathways interact at multiple points, and are characterized by a series of local recycling circuits and branch-points at which sorting of membrane and soluble content occurs. The morphology of these pathways varies widely between cells: neurones are a clear example of cells exquisitely specialized for regulated exocytosis and have a far more complex set of exocytic membranes than a muscle cell, for example; conversely, the macrophage is specialized for endocytic uptake and has an especially well-developed endosomal and lysosomal system.

The second class of membrane-bound organelles is of discrete structures that exist as end-destinations for families of characteristic resident components. Examples of this class include the mitochondrion and the microbodies, such as peroxisomes. The nucleus falls uneasily between these groups, as it is a single-copy organelle whose bounding membrane is part of the endoplasmic reticulum, which forms the first station of the exocytic pathway.

The exocytic pathway: producing and distributing

The exocytic pathway can be regarded as a production line in which components are first introduced into the system by cotranslational translocation into the endoplasmic reticulum. There then follows a series of discrete stages involving the product passing through a number of organelles; at each stage characteristic post-translational modifications occur until the mature form of the protein is released by exocytosis at the plasm membrane. Nascent proteins are inserted into the membrane of the endoplasmic reticulum in the correct topology, and the topology of proteins that span the membrane more than once is also determined at this step. All of the subsequent vesicular transport events are topologically conservative and preserve the integrity of both donor and acceptor membranes. For this reason, vesicular budding requires a true membrane-fission event, and the delivery of the contents of a transport vesicle requires not only appropriate recognition of and docking to the correct acceptor membrane, but also a true membrane fusion event.

The exocytic pathway begins when a nascent polypeptide chain emerges from a free cytosolic ribosome translating the mRNA of a secretory protein. The aminoterminal region of proteins destined to enter the exocytic pathway bears a signal called a 'signal sequence' or 'leader sequence'. Comparison of many signal sequences reveals little obvious conservation, although variability is limited and a short (10 ± 3 residues) hydrophobic core is the critical feature; exact sequence is less important and about 20 per cent of random sequences will function as a signal sequence in yeast.

Translocation of a hydrophilic polypeptide chain across a hydrophobic lipid bilayer is energetically expensive so it is not surprising that the translocation pore should be small. This requires that the nascent protein be translocated as an unfolded, extended chain. Recent evidence from a yeast system suggests that a mechanism is required to prevent premature folding of the nascent polypeptide chain even as it lies within the ribosome groove. In the cytoplasm, heat-shock proteins (e.g. hsp70) can act as molecular chaperones to ensure appropriate folding of nascent cytoplasmic polypeptides. It seems that similar heat-shock protein homologues may be required to prevent premature folding of proteins destined for translocation; yeast contain hsp70 homologues called Ssb1/2p that are associated with actively translating ribosomes and appear to be important in nascent chain-binding.

The appearance of the signal sequence from the ribosome groove triggers rapid binding of a multi-subunit signal recognition particle, or **SRP**, which halts chain elongation and ensures targeting of the complex to the rough endoplasmic reticulum by specific interaction with the SRP receptor or docking protein.

Docking protein is a GTP/GDP-binding heterodimer of α- and β-subunits; binding of an SRP complex triggers GDP/GTP exchange, and the signal sequence and the ribosome are released from the SRP. GTP hydrolysis occurs to complete a unidirectional cycle that ends with the release of SRP from docking protein. This is an important example of the way in which GTP hydrolysis promoted by an activating protein operating on GTPases with low spontaneous enzyme activity can be used to control rate and vectoriality of intracellular interactions.

Cross-linking studies using short (70-residue) nascent polypeptide chains reveal that the signal sequence is now in close proximity to the α- and β-chains of a heterodimeric complex in the membrane of the rough endoplasmic reticulum (**SSR**, or signal sequence receptor) and an abundant, similarly sized (36 kDa) multiple membrane-spanning protein (TRAM). Reconstitution of microsome membrane proteins depleted of TRAM resulted in vesicles incompetent for translocation of β-lactamase and prepro-α-factor. However, translocation of preprolactin continued, suggesting that this pathway may be even more complex than expected.

Early conclusions from the observation of cotranslational translocation suggested that the emergence of the nascent polypeptide chain provided the driving force for translocation, but this view lost favour when experimental systems uncoupling translation from translocation were found. These observations are complicated by the possibility that there exists an SRP/docking protein/SSR independent pathway for translocation across the membrane of the endoplasmic reticulum, which is also ATP and cytosol requiring, and shares common internal endoplasmic reticulum proteins with the conventional pathway.

Very recently it has been possible to demonstrate bidirectional movement of nascent polypeptide across microsomal membranes. This result suggests that chain elongation (translation) drives inward movement, but does not explain why it should be vectorial. Early post-translational folding or modification events in the lumen of the endoplasmic reticulum have been suggested to prevent retrograde movement of the chain in the so-called Brownian ratchet model.

FUNCTION OF THE PROTEIN TRANSLOCATION PORE

Although the composition of the protein translocation pore remains controversial, recent elecrophysiological studies have greatly improved our understanding of its function. By fusing isolated microsomal membranes into an artificial lipid bilayer, Blobel and colleagues have been able to measure the conductance of single protein pores (about 220 pS) and demonstrate that they can remain open after release of nascent peptide provided that the ribosomes remain associated with the membrane. Using a bacterial translocation system the same group have recently shown that a putative protein translocation pore can be opened by signal peptides, confirming the multiple roles of this signalling sequence.

A brief mention should also be made of a peptide-transporting system in the membranes of early exocytic organelles that is involved in the translocation of peptides from the cytoplasm to the lumen of the secretory pathway for loading major histocompatibility complex (**MHC**) class I molecules (see also Section 5). Genetic evidence suggests that a translocation machinery composed of a hetero-oligomer of two membrane proteins encoded by genes lying within the MHC cluster (*RING4* and *RING11*, also known as *TAP-1* and *TAP-2*) may be required for presentation of intracellular antigens via MHC class I. Recent evidence suggests that this transporter system may not be located in the membrane of the endoplasmic reticulum itself, but rather in a later compartment prior to the Golgi apparatus.

ALTERNATIVE TRANSLOCATION MECHANISMS

There is at least one completely separate eukaryotic secretory pathway that does not involve the endoplasmic reticulum or Golgi apparatus at all. For example, the yeast *a*-type mating factor undergoes a series of proteolytic and fatty acylation events in the cytoplasm and is then directly translocated across the plasma membrane via a pore encoded by the gene *STE6*. *STE6* has homology with a family of multiple membrane-spanning, ATP-driven, transport ATPases found in mammalian cells, including the p-glycoprotein associated with mammalian multidrug resistance and the cystic fibrosis gene product. A possible role for these types of channels/transporters in secretion in mammalian cells is eagerly sought. Candidates for such transport include interleukin 1 and both basic and acidic forms of fibroblast growth factor; these proteins lack a signal sequence, are not glycosylated, are secreted when the normal exocytic pathway is blocked by drugs such as brefeldin A, and are secreted at different rates (excluding cell lysis as the mechanism of release).

TOPOGENESIS OF MEMBRANE PROTEINS

Secretory proteins translocate completely across the bounding membrane of the endoplasmic reticulum and are released into the lumen as soluble proteins. Membrane-protein biogenesis requires that translocation be arrested to leave transmembrane domains traversing the membrane; subsequent vesicular shuttling steps preserve the topology of membrane proteins established at this early step through all the subsequent compartments of the exocytic pathway.

The orientation of the first transmembrane domain to interact with the membrane of the endoplasmic reticulum determines the topology of all the rest; the disposition of charged residues immediately adjacent to the hydrophobic transmembrane region is critical in determining orientation.

EARLY EVENTS IN THE LUMEN OF THE ENDOPLASMIC RETICULUM

A complex series of modifications to the newly made polypeptide occurs during the exocytic pathway, many of them in the lumen of the endoplasmic reticulum. This includes the cotranslational removal of the N-terminal signal sequence by a multicomponent endopeptidase of the endoplasmic reticulum membrane called signal peptidase. Not all proteins that enter the endoplasmic reticulum with a signal sequence have this sequence removed; ovalbumin is a good example of a major secretory protein with an internal, uncleaved signal sequence.

Disulphide-bond formation is also an early event in the endoplasmic reticulum, along with folding of the newly translocated polypeptide chain into the mature conformation. Many proteins contain multiple cysteine residues and so have many potential disulphide linkages, only one set of which is compatible with stable folding into the mature conformation. The various possibilities are sampled randomly, but arrival at the lowest-energy conformation is facilitated by a soluble luminal enzyme of the endoplasmic reticulum, protein disulphide isomerase (**PDI**), which catalyses the breakage and reformation of disulphide bonds.

An important consequence of this enzymatic activity of PDI is that the lumen of the endoplasmic reticulum is not a suitable environment for the assembly of large disulphide-linked structures from many separate polypeptide chains. Assembly of such structures—the surface antigen particle of hepatitis B virus, for example—has recently been localized to a downstream 'intermediate compartment' from which the PDI is excluded.

Oligosaccharide side-chains may be added to polypeptides via O-glycosidic bonds to serine or threonine (O-linked) or by N-glycosidic bonds to asparagine residues within the consensus sequence Asn-X-Ser or Asn-X-Thr (N-linked). O-linked glycosylation does not begin until the protein has reached the *cis* side of the Golgi complex. N-linked glycosylation, on the other hand, begins in the endoplasmic reticulum with the transfer of a preformed, 14-sugar complex to asparagine residues in the protein from a lipid-anchored precursor, dolichol phosphate. Three glucose residues and one mannose residue of this precursor are rapidly trimmed by enzymes within the endoplasmic reticulum, and the protein is ready for onward transport.

QUALITY CONTROL AND THE EXOCYTIC PATHWAY

There is a finite failure rate for any biological process and the synthesis and folding of a polypeptide chain is no exception. This implies that some of the proteins translocated into the endoplasmic reticulum will be defective. The level of malfolding is kept low by a series of protein–protein interactions between the nascent chain as it emerges into the lumen of the endoplasmic reticulum and a 'reception committee' of enzymes (such as signal peptidase, oligosaccharyl transferase, and PDI) and 'chaperone' proteins (such as the heavy chain-binding protein, **BiP**). Together these help to ensure that the early post-translational events go to completion and folding takes place in the correct order.

Many proteins function as oligomeric complexes; the endoplasmic reticulum is the site for the assembly of these complexes. The assembly of heterodimers such as heavy and light chain of immunoglobulin is controlled by interaction of the heavy chain with BiP, another soluble resident protein of endoplasmic reticulum, until released by ATP hydrolysis upon the arrival of a light chain. For membrane proteins, the rate of oligomer formation depends on the lateral mobility of the monomer subunits and their density in the membrane; it can be a much slower process than translation or translocation. In the case of multi-subunit hetero-oligomers, the completion of a mature complex depends on the expression level of the least abundant subunit. This means that there will be many complexes complete but for the last subunit in the endoplasmic reticulum at any given moment.

Thus the endoplasmic reticulum will contain an appreciable level of incompletely translated, improperly folded, or incompletely or incorrectly oligomerized proteins at any given moment. Some of these will go on to achieve the mature form with the passage of time, but some will always remain defective. This gives rise to two problems. Firstly, it would be wasteful and in some cases potentially dangerous to deliver the damaged and non-functional proteins to their normal destinations. Secondly, the cell now has the problem of selectively disposing of the permanently defective products that would otherwise accumulate in the endoplasmic reticulum. Therefore, the exocytic pathway requires a quality-control test for all nascent products, and a scavenger system to remove and destroy all that consistently fails this test.

A quality-control mechanism forms a gate at the exit from the endoplasmic reticulum; only correctly folded, complete, appropriately glycosylated and disulphide-bonded proteins that have completed oligomer formation may pass from the endoplasmic reticulum to the later stages of the exocytic pathway. One mechanism for this quality control involves persistent binding of proteins involved in polypeptide folding and resolution of disulphide bonds to nascent chains that are not yet fully folded or disulphide bonded. These normally resident proteins prevent unready nascent chains from passing on down the exocytic pathway, probably by the operation of the same machinery that would promptly retrieve the resident proteins alone from a proximal downstream compartment. For example, single chains of multichain complexes like the T-cell receptor may be expressed in fibroblasts, but the translated protein, although translocated into endoplasmic reticulum and post-translationally modified, never arrives in the Golgi apparatus. Instead, it is singled out for degradation at a rate that is characteristic for each polypeptide chain and at a site that may be a subset of the rough endoplasmic reticulum, or a separate compartment to which these malfolded or improperly oligomerized proteins are delivered for degradation.

Very recently a second type of quality-control system has been hinted at by the observation that the budding of transport vesicles from the endoplasmic reticulum appears to depend on a heterotrimeric G protein. This is of interest because the usual function of a G protein is to amplify the transduction of a signal across a membrane, classically the plasma membrane. This has given rise to the suggestion that there may be transmembrane proteins capable of recognizing transport-competent proteins and transmitting this recognition to the cytoplasmic budding machinery via a G protein.

The scavenger system that permits the removal of components which repeatedly fail the quality-control test is not well understood. Evidence from experiments in which a single chain of a multichain complex is expressed in cells not making the other chains suggests that the rate of removal of these 'orphan' chains depends on the polypeptide itself. The removal of some aberrant polypeptides exhibits a lag phase and a dependence on metabolic energy, functional vesicular transport and intact pH gradients, implying transport to a separate acid organelle, presumably a lysosomal compartment, for degradation. When none of these requirements is found, degradation of the polypeptide presumably does not require vesicular transport and may be the result of local aggregation within the endoplasmic reticulum, followed by autophagic engulfment of these subdomains. Isolated fragments of endoplasmic reticulum can certainly be found in low-pH, autophagic vacuoles containing acid hydrolases. These routes leave unexplained the pathway of degradation for polypeptides that continue to be degraded in cells with no low-pH compartments. A search for endogenous proteases in the lumen of the endoplasmic reticulum is under way, but this plausible solution raises the question as to how such a degradation machinery could be made specific for malfolded proteins. The questions are central to an understanding of the effects of genetically abnormal proteins on the cells in which they are produced (see Section 22).

SELECTIVE TRANSPORT OR SELECTIVE RETENTION

We must now consider a fundamental problem of the exocytic pathway. A huge flux of secretory proteins and newly synthesized membrane proteins passes from the endoplasmic reticulum through the Golgi complex to their destinations, and yet these organelles retain their characteristic morphology and composition. Simply put, how does a resident protein of any of these compartments not get swept out to the cell surface?

Two possible solutions may be envisaged—either all proteins remain in any given organelle unless they contain a signal enabling them to leave (selective transport) or all proteins are transported from the organelle unless they bear specific retention signals (selective retention). A model of selective transport was initially suggested by the widely varying rates of transport of individual protein through the exocytic pathway.

Arguments against this model include the observation that often heterologous proteins (even prokaryotic proteins) can pass through the exocytic pathway, and that comparisons of sequences of secretory proteins fail to reveal any obvious signals for transport. Strong experimental evidence for a signal-independent bulk flow through the exocytic pathway came from an experiment using a synthetic substrate. A radiolabelled tripeptide consisting of an N-linked acceptor consensus was modified with hydrophobic groups and allowed to diffuse into cells. Esterases within the cells removed the side-groups trapping the charged peptide within the cytoplasm and the intraluminal space of the organelle. Peptide in the lumen of the endoplasmic reticulum was a substrate for glycosylation, and the glycosylated peptide could be easily detected in cell lysates or medium. As the peptide is too small to carry a specific transport signal, its secretion suggests that there is a bulk flow. This in turn implies that there should instead be specific retention signals on resident proteins of the endoplasmic reticulum and Golgi apparatus.

TRANSPORT THROUGH THE GOLGI STACK

Correctly folded, oligomerized proteins that carry no retention signals are transported by vesicular shuttling mechanisms to the Golgi stack. Here the high-mannose form of the N-linked oligosaccharide side-chains is further trimmed and then built up to form the mature, complex, N-linked structure.

The exact distribution of the enzymes responsible for this sequential processing within the cisternae of the Golgi apparatus varies from cell type to cell type and probably with the state of the cell as well. None the less, the sequential nature of the modifications of the N-linked sugars provides a very important tool in the analysis of transport through the Golgi apparatus. Recently, it has been suggested that sequential processing of N-linked oligosaccharides may be a consequence of the fine specificities of the enzymes involved rather than their compartmentalization into a series of separate cisternae; this model accepts the possibility of long-term luminal continuities between the visible stacked elements of the Golgi apparatus. Such connections have been observed in Golgi stacks from a number of species.

TARGETING FROM THE *TRANS* FACE OF THE GOLGI APPARATUS

Evidence to date suggests that all secretory and membrane proteins, regardless of their destination, follow the same route (albeit at different rates) through the endoplasmic reticulum and the Golgi stack. However, it is necessary at some stage to separate membrane proteins destined for intracellular organelles from membrane proteins destined for the cell surface, and soluble proteins required in intracellular organelles from those to be secreted. This is the task of the *trans*Golgi network.

Fig. 1 The organization of the exocytic pathway. Where multiple arrows leave a compartment a branch-point is required and the compartment must contain a sorting mechanism (see text). The bulk-flow pathway in red is the default route through the cell; deviations from this route require positive sorting signals.

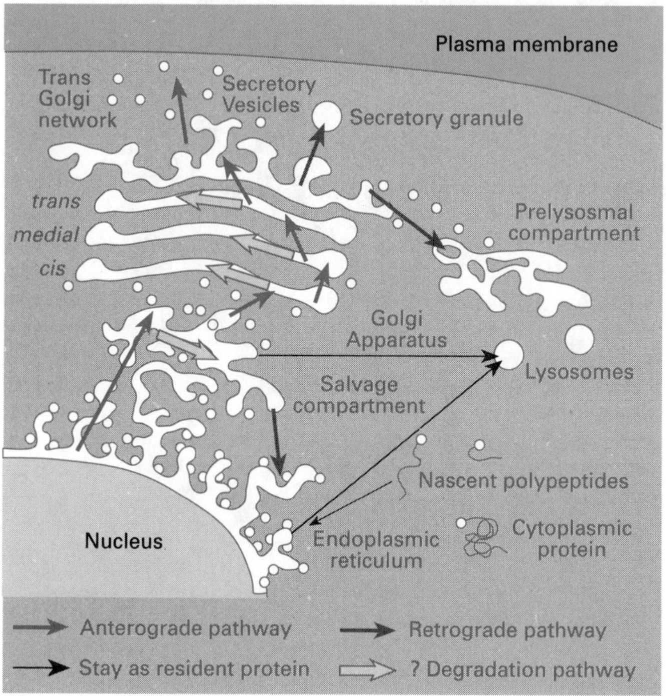

The delivery of material to the plasma membrane is the default pathway in the majority of cell types. The situation is a little more complex in differentiated epithelial cells that have developed two separate plasma-membrane domains, the apical and the basolateral. In such cells the basolateral surface may be the default and the apical a new destination that requires additional sorting machinery to service. However this machinery works, it is clear that the task of separating apical and basolateral proteins is carried out in the *trans*Golgi network. This contention is supported most strongly by studies on polarized cells such as hepatocytes, which appear to lack any direct apical delivery route to the bile canalicular membrane, instead relying on basolateral delivery and sorting by endocytosis/transcytosis to provide secondary apical targeting. These observations confirm that the exocytic pathway is not a single, unidirectional flow and imply the need for branch-points on the pathway. At each branch-point, sorting machinery separates components into the required vesicles for onward transport to the appropriate branch of the pathway. Figure 1 demonstrates the complexity of the exocytic pathway and identifies several branch-points. The current consensus is that the sorting signals reside in the proteins, glycoproteins or glycolipids themselves and are recognized by receptors for these signals which then interact specifically with one class of budding vesicle rather than another.

Polarized sorting in epithelia in which cells have distinct apical and basolateral domains has been recently reviewed. A specific role has been suggested for proteins that are anchored in the membrane not by a transmembrane domain but by a covalently attached glycosylphosphatidylinositol (**GPI**) moiety acquired as a post-translational modification. The selective delivery of such GPI-anchored proteins to the apical domain of polarized epithelial cells has suggested possible sorting mechanisms. Simons *et al.* hypothesized that GPI-anchored proteins might be gathered into glycolipid-rich subdomains of membrane at the *trans*Golgi network, and that this might account for apical targeting. The recent isolation of a GPI-anchored protein associated with a detergent-insoluble sheet of glycolipids containing other GPI-anchored proteins but no basolateral proteins from polarized epithelial cells provides strong indirect support for this model.

The presence of microdomains of specific phospholipid composition in apically targeted vesicles results in differences in detergent solubility; these differences have been exploited to isolate a protein of the apical vesicles budding from the *trans*Golgi network. VIP21 is a 21-kDa, integral membrane protein present at high levels in the *trans*Golgi network and in apically directed transport vesicles—it has recently been shown to be identical to caveolin, a membrane protein localized to specialized regions of the plasma membrane called caveolae. Caveolae are implicated in a number of uptake processes mediated by GPI-anchored, plasma-membrane proteins in a process that has been called potocytosis; these structures may be to GPI-anchored proteins what coated pits are to transmembrane receptor proteins involved in receptor-mediated endocytosis. Caveolae are clinically significant not only because they are the site of uptake of folate, but also because they are the route of entry for cholera and tetanus toxins. The physical properties of some membrane lipids, such as the sphingolipids, promote local microdomain formation and this may explain the observed associations between sphingolipid trafficking and protein sorting.

RETENTION OF RESIDENT PROTEINS IN ORGANELLES OF THE EXOCYTIC PATHWAY

Conceptually, the retention of a protein in a particular compartment is simply another example of a branch-point on the exocytic pathway. Retention of resident proteins can be shown often to consist of efficient retrieval from a proximal downstream compartment, as illustrated in Fig. 2; in this case the side-branch consists of a vesicle travelling retrogradely 'up' the pathway to return escaped resident proteins to their correct organelle. Although the exact mechanisms are not fully resolved for any retention step, receptors have been identified for several 'retention signals', and in the case of the receptor for the retrieval signal on soluble resident proteins of the endoplasmic reticulum the intracellular itinerary for the candidate receptor molecule is a local recycling circuit, which fits the model very well.

CONSTITUTIVE VERSUS REGULATED SECRETION

Some secretory proteins follow the exocytic pathway and are released immediately from the cell. This is the constitutive pathway. Other secretory proteins are stored late in the exocytic pathway in secretory granules and are only released at the plasma membrane by exocytosis in response to specific stimuli—this is the regulated secretory pathway.

Sorting between the constitutive and regulated secretory pathways occurs in the *trans*Golgi network and involves collection of proteins destined for regulated secretion by aggregation with specialized families of proteins known as secretogranins. The aggregation event depends on the intraluminal environment of the *trans*Golgi network; a lowered pH and an increased free calcium-ion concentration have both been implicated. The aggregation of regulated secretory proteins and the subsequent budding of immature secretory granules from the *trans*Golgi network has recently been reconstituted in a cell-free system.

THE EXOCYTIC FUSION EVENT

The exocytic pathway ends with the fusion of the transport vesicle to the appropriate domain of the plasma membrane, releasing the luminal contents into the external medium and delivering vesicle-membrane proteins into the plasma membrane. Despite its importance this process is still very poorly understood. Recently, major advances have been made by using electrophysiological techniques such as patch clamping to study rapid electrical changes during exocytic fusion events. For example, the addition of membrane area to the cell surface by fusion of a secretory vesicle with the plasma membrane results in a detectable change in the capacitance of the cell. A 10-fF capacitance step corresponds to the addition of about 1 μm^2 to the surface area of the cell, which is the approximate equivalent of one 0.5 μm-diameter secretory vesicle. A combination of electrophysiological and fast-freeze electron microscopy is now rapidly expanding our knowledge of this critical step.

The endocytic pathway: collecting and sorting

The endocytic pathway is illustrated in outline in Fig. 3. A primitive endocytic pathway may have begun as a compensatory system for retrieving the excess area added to the plasma membrane by fusion of exocytic vesicles during secretion. Endocytosis now has many more functions than simply the homeostatic control of cell surface area. The simplest role for endocytosis is seen even in free-living unicellular organisms—internalization of complex nutrients permits the local release of hydrolytic enzymes into a closed compartment for digestion. This process is more efficient than the prokaryotic approach of secreting enzymes and using plasma-membrane permeases to take up any released hydrolytic fragments.

The endocytic pathway is similar to the exocytic pathway in a number of ways. In particular, it consists of a series of interconnected, local recycling circuits and a series of branch-points such that a flux of material may pass through it while resident components of the organelles themselves remain concentrated in distinct places. The schematic diagram illustrates the pathway, together with some branch-points and examples of species following particular paths through the endocytic compartment (Fig. 4).

Fig. 2 Resident proteins in a compartment may be retained by recycling. Recent results suggest that most resident proteins, whether soluble or attached to the membrane, leave their compartment in bulk-transport vesicles and arrive in the next compartment. From here they are recognized and retrieved back to their resident compartment by a specific retrieval mechanism. Thus, at steady state, components resident in compartment A may have modifications characteristic of passage through compartment B.

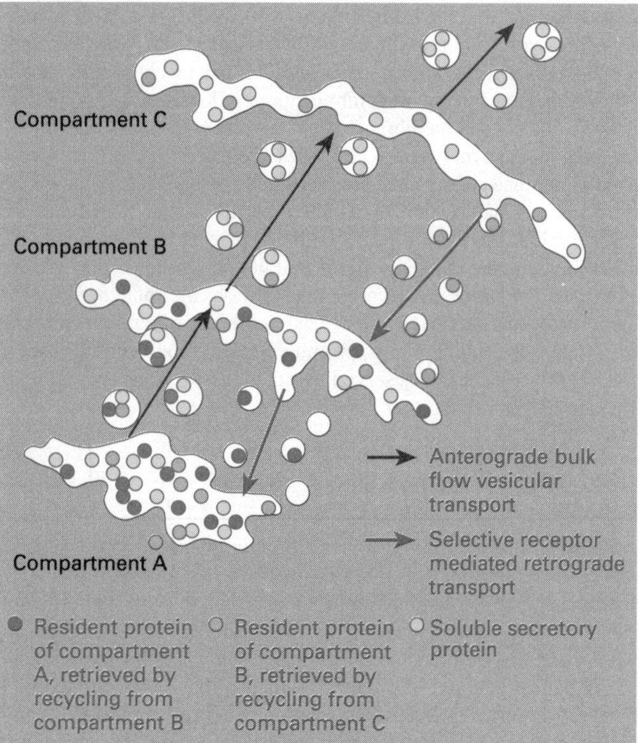

Fig. 3 Schematic outline of the endocytic pathway. Like the exocytic pathway, the endocytic pathway has multiple branch-points at which internalized ligand may be separated from its receptor and receptors destined for degradation may be singled out from those bound for the cell surface.

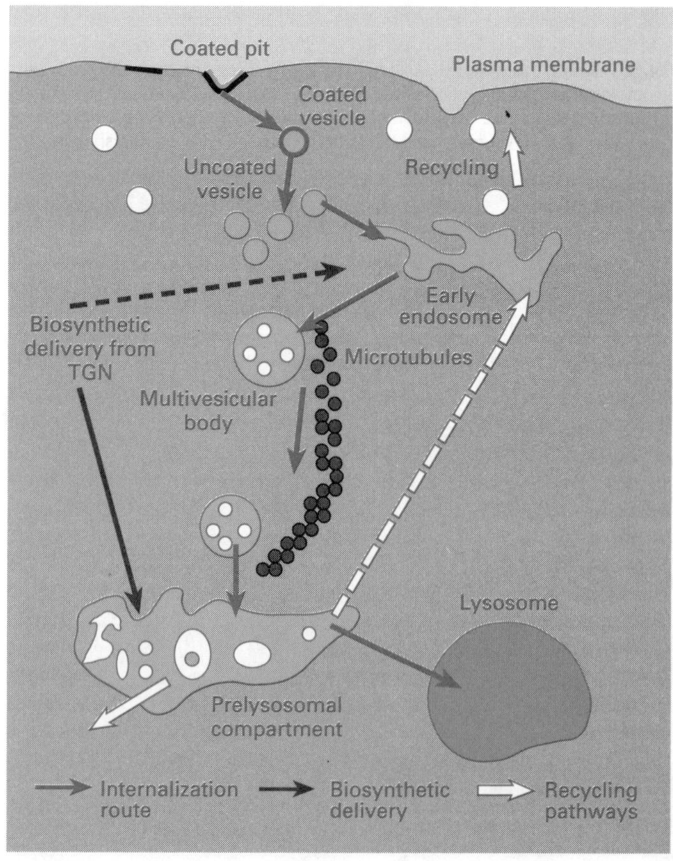

RECEPTOR-MEDIATED ENDOCYTOSIS

The most efficient uptake mechanism requires a receptor in the plasma membrane to sweep out a large volume of the extracellular space and concentrate a ligand on the cell surface before endocytosis. This process can be made even more efficient if the receptors then cluster into small areas of the plasma membrane that are subsequently selectively internalized. This occurs in the process of receptor-mediated endocytosis. The specialized regions of plasma membrane involved are morphologically distinct because of a concave curvature and an electron-dense coat on the cytoplasmic face, resulting in a structure called a coated pit. A wide range of ligands are internalized bound to receptors that enter the cell via coated pits, and the surface density of many hormone receptors (eg. receptors for insulin and epidermal growth factor) is maintained as a balance between biosynthetic delivery and loss by internalization in coated pits. The steps involved in endocytosis via a coated pit and the redeployment of recycling receptors are shown in (Fig. 5).

A number of the steps in receptor-mediated endocytosis are now understood at the molecular level and progress is rapid. The electron-dense coat consists of a pair of polypeptides, the clathrin heavy and light

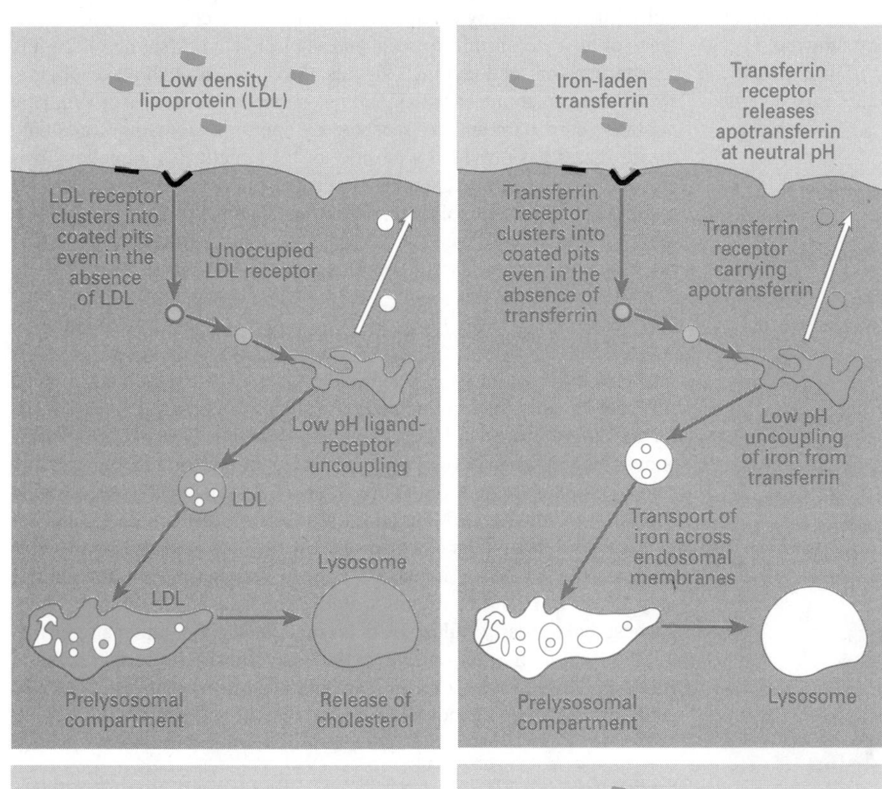

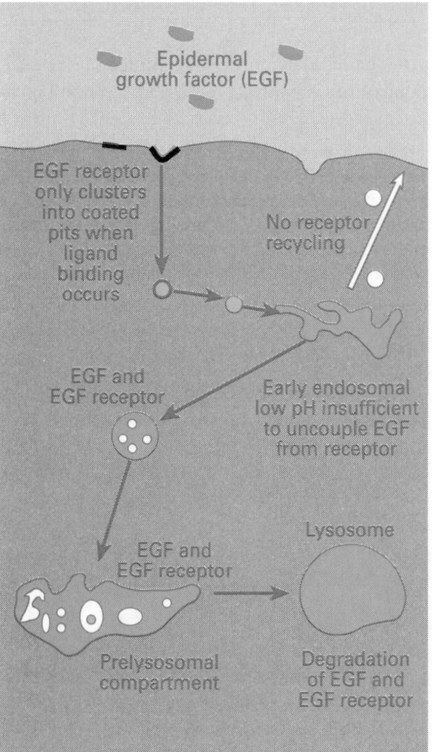

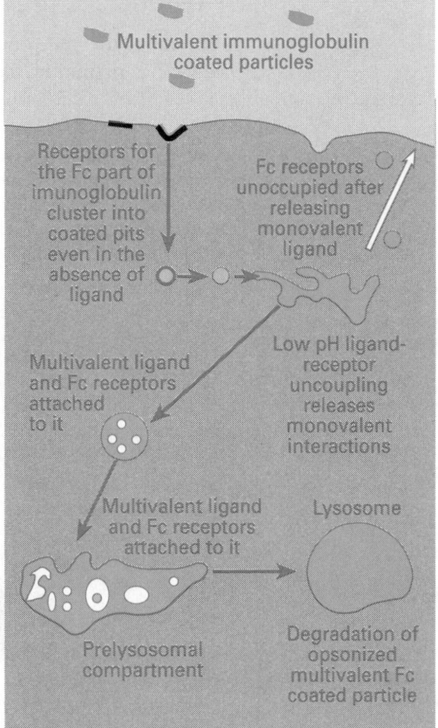

Fig. 4 Different routes through the endocytic pathway. The uptake of low-density lipoprotein (LDL) (top left) involves a receptor that recycles independently of ligand. Internalized LDL receptor is unloaded of any ligand in the endosome before recycling and the ligand follows the pathway to the lysosome for degradation. The transferrin receptor (top right) binds iron-laden transferrin at the cell surface and delivers it to the early endosome where the reduced pH releases the iron. The transferrin itself remains attached to the receptor and is recycled with it back to the plasma membrane. Here, the neutral pH causes release of the apotransferrin and the cycle begins again. Growth-factor receptors such as the epidermal growth factor (EGF) receptor (bottom left) are down-regulated by ligand after a single use; they are not recruited to the coated pit until ligand is bound, and they do not recycle, but are degraded along with the ligand after transduction of the hormonal signal. Immune cells internalize opsonized ligands via receptors for the Fc part of immunoglobulin (bottom right); monovalent ligands are released by low endosomal pH and the Fc receptors are redeployed to the plasma membrane like LDL receptors. However, if the ligand is multivalent the complex is not disassembled in the early endosome but passes through the pathway to the lysosome for degradation.

chains, which form a polyhedral lattice connected to the plasma membrane via a heterotetrameric adaptor complex. Although clathrin-coated structures are found at the plasma membrane and in the membrane of the *trans*Golgi network, these sites are differentiated by containing distinct adaptor complexes. The interaction of an adaptor complex with the cytoplasmic domain of a transmembrane receptor glycoprotein is thought to mediate the clustering of receptors into coated pits.

The cell-surface receptor for low-density lipoprotein particles (the **LDL$_R$**) is the best understood example of this pathway. The LDL$_R$ was the first receptor shown to cluster into coated regions of the plasma membrane before internalization, and the first endocytic receptor shown to cause serious disease when defective (see Section 11). The normal pathway for the receptor-mediated endocytosis of LDL is shown in Fig. 4. The dimeric receptor follows this pathway whether LDL is present or not, makes one round trip about every 10 min and does this several hundred times in a lifetime of about 20 h. Clinically significant hypercholesterolaemia results if this receptor is defective; the cloning of the gene for the LDL$_R$ and the classification of loss-of-function mutations were major milestones in molecular cell biology. A particularly informative mutation results in the replacement of the tyrosine from the cytoplasmic domain of the LDL$_R$ with a non-aromatic residue; this produces a receptor that is present on the cell surface in a normal copy number and with a normal affinity for LDL, and yet uptake is markedly decreased. Electron microscopy of fibroblasts from patients homozygous for this mutation reveal that the bound LDL is dispersed over all the cell surface, and not clustered into the coated pits as in control cells. Subsequent studies by a number of groups have confirmed the importance of the cytoplasmic domain, and suggested the existence of specific 'clustering' or 'endocytosis' signals. Most recently, high-resolution, two-dimensional nuclear magnetic resonance spectroscopy of synthetic peptides corresponding to receptor cytoplasmic domains containing these signals has provided a glimpse of the structure of an endocytosis signal. The cognate receptor in the coated pit is probably the adaptor complex but the exact polypeptide responsible remains elusive, although there is indirect evidence for the asialoglycoprotein receptor that it is the β-subunit of the adaptor complex that plays this part.

Fig. 5 The steps involved in internalization via coated pits.

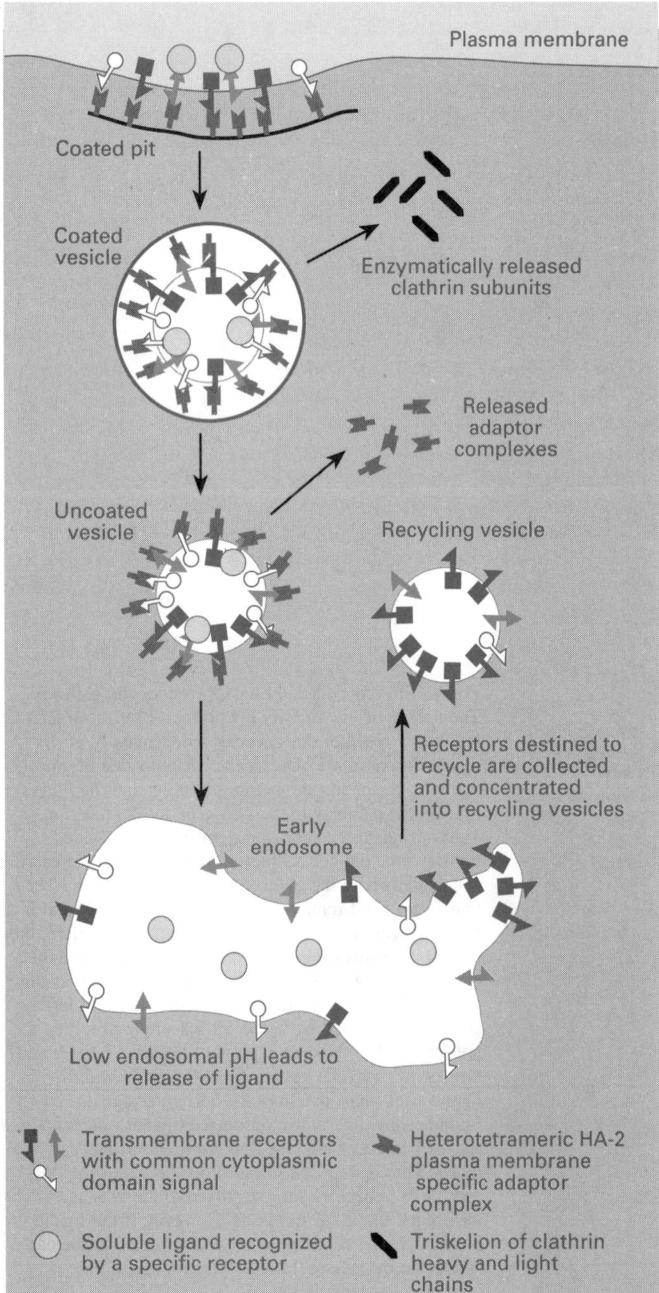

ACIDIFICATION OF THE ENDOCYTIC PATHWAY

The endocytic pathway is progressively acidified by the action of an ATP-dependent proton pump and this falling pH is crucial to the normal functioning of many endogenous receptor systems. The pH in the early endosome has fallen only as far as about 6.5, but this is still significantly acidic compared to the external medium and is sufficient to release many ligands from their receptors, permitting sorting of ligand and receptor to separate intracellular destinations. In the later prelysosomal compartment the pH falls to about 5.0–5.5, whereas in the lysosome the pH may be as low as 4.6. Inhibitor studies on isolated early endosomes suggest that the early endosome pH is prevented from falling any further by the action of internalized, plasma-membrane, sodium–potassium ATPase, which creates a membrane potential against which the electrogenic proton pump cannot pump effectively.

PATHOGENS AND THE ENDOCYTIC PATHWAY

The endocytic pathway provides an efficient uptake route for the cell, as well as permitting the control of cell surface area and the number of

Fig. 6 Internalized virus may modify the organelles of the endocytic pathway. Some enveloped viruses gain access to cells via the endocytic pathway. After internalization the low endosomal pH results in a conformational change to the viral glycoproteins resulting in membrane fusion. The micrograph shows the result of this process in cells infected with Semliki Forest virus (an alphavirus); the resulting structure is known as a type I cytopathic vacuole.

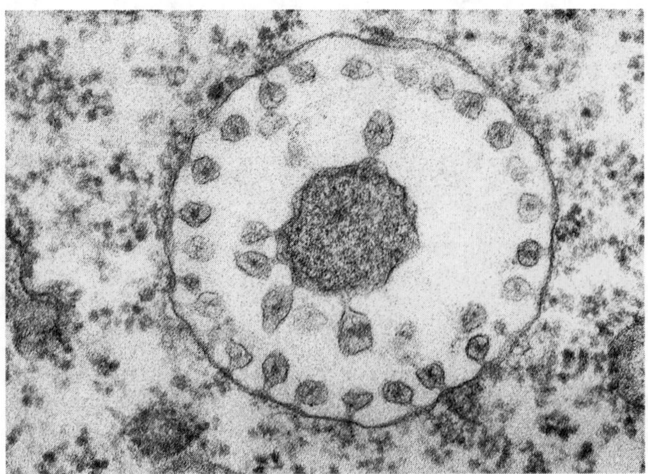

hormone and growth-factor receptors at the surface. However, the very efficiency of uptake that it allows makes this a serious chink in the cell's armour against attack by pathogens. The specialized role of the macrophage puts this cell type especially at risk from pathogens that are able to exploit the endocytic pathway to enter cells (See Macrophage section for a discussion of this problem with bacterial and protozoal pathogens.)

The acid pH of endocytic compartments is essential for unidirectional uptake of ligand by recycling receptors, and is therefore beneficial to the cell. However, the acidic environment of the endocytic pathway has been exploited by a wide range of viruses that infect mammalian cells. Productive infection with these viruses is prevented when drugs are used to abolish the endosomal pH gradient, and in some cases infection via the cell surface can only occur when the external pH is lowered. Virus binding at the cell surface involves surface proteins of the virus recognizing specific extracellular domains on the target cell. Once binding has occurred, endocytosis follows and the virus is enclosed within an endosome that is progressively acidified by the action of ATP-dependent proton pumps as usual. The falling pH causes a conformational change in the viral surface glycoproteins, exposing hydrophobic fusion peptides that promote fusion of the viral envelope with the bounding endosomal membrane. The viral genome may then be released to the cytoplasm without being exposed to low pH, extracellular medium or hydrolytic enzymes. Because this process only occurs in live cells with sufficient metabolic energy to internalize and acidify the virion, the virus can ensure that it does not attempt to infect a cell that will be unable to sustain virion production.

In some cases the genome is not released free into the cytoplasm but remains close to the site of penetration and a virally modified endosomal structure results. This is the origin of the cytopathic vacuole type I that can be found in the cytoplasm of cells infected with alphaviruses, for example (such as Semliki Forest virus, see Fig. 6) (see also Section 7).

Intracellular transport: molecular machinery for communication within the endomembrane system

The individual elements of the endomembrane system are in continuous connection via shuttling transport vesicles, and yet fluxes of membrane and content are controlled and unidirectional rather than random. This implies that there are many different types of transport vesicle, one for each possible connection between two organelles, and yet they are all specifically delivered to the appropriate destination. A major focus of contemporary cell biology is to understand the budding, targeting and docking/fusion mechanisms of these transport vesicles at the molecular level. Reconstitution of single transport steps in cell-free systems and the use of selection strategies and genetic analysis in yeast have been two of the most powerful tools in this work.

RECONSTITUTION STUDIES

Many intracellular transport events have now been reconstituted *in vitro*, either using isolated organelle components or 'semi-intact' cell systems. The first of these involved intercisternal transport within the Golgi apparatus. The system relies on scoring the transfer of a viral glycoprotein marker from a donor Golgi stack obtained from a mutant cell line lacking the enzyme *N*-acetyl glucosamine transferase I to an acceptor Golgi stack derived from uninfected wild-type cells. Transport is scored by the acquisition of *N*-acetyl glucosamine on the viral glycoprotein. A critical control included the demonstration that the marker protein remained sequestered in closed, membrane-bound organelles by protease protection and electron-microscopic immunocytochemistry.

Using this experimental system it was possible to dissect the events of a single round of vesicle formation from a donor compartment, followed by its delivery to, and subsequent fusion with, an acceptor compartment. The assay system was also used as a tool for the purification of the cytosolic factors involved, including the cytosolic protein that confers sensitivity to the sulphydryl-modifying reagent *N*-ethyl maleimide (NEM-sensitive factor, **NSF**). In addition a late-acting cytosolic factor required for the maturation of bound vesicles on the acceptor membrane before fusion has also been identified and purified.

NSF is a homotetramer of a 76-kDa polypeptide; its function appears to be highly conserved during evolution, because yeast cytosol supports the mammalian *in vitro* assay in an ATP-dependent and NEM-sensitive manner.

The cDNA sequence reveals the reason for this—mammalian NSF is highly homologous to a yeast protein that had already been identified by a genetic approach to be involved in vesicular transport in yeast (Sec18p, see below). In fact, yeast Sec18p alone replaces the requirement for NSF in the *in-vitro* assay, showing them to be functionally equivalent.

This result was unexpected because NSF was originally identified in an assay that reconstituted Golgi–Golgi transport, and analysis of the yeast Sec18 mutant revealed a defect in endoplasmic reticulum to Golgi transport. Recently, it has become clear that NSF has no role in determining the targeting of vesicles to the acceptor membrane, but rather has a general role in vesicular transport. NSF has also now been shown to be essential for endoplasmic reticulum–Golgi transport in a semi-intact cell assay system. An even bigger surprise was the demonstration that vesicle fusion after receptor-mediated endocytosis also required NSF. Thus, NSF appears to be involved in a late step of vesicular transport in both the endocytic and exocytic pathways.

Further clues to NSF function came from the cDNA sequence, which revealed a consensus ATP-binding site, and from biochemical studies which showed that NSF was partitioned between the cytosol and the outer face of the Golgi membrane in an ATP-dependent manner. *In vitro* binding studies revealed that NSF binds specifically and saturably to Golgi membranes, but requires additional cytosolic components to do so. This led to an assay which identified three soluble NSF attachment factors (**SNAPs**) that bind to NSF after themselves binding to an unidentified 'SNAP receptor' in the Golgi membrane. The relevance and importance of SNAPs for transport processes has been recently underlined by the demonstration that the yeast Sec17p (see below) has α-SNAP activity.

These results have led to a model in which vesicle fusion with the target acceptor membrane requires the assembly of a 'fusion machine' consisting of NSF, SNAPs, and the SNAP receptor at the site of a pre-targeted vesicle. The 'fusion machine' ensures that membrane fusion only occurs when a vesicle has been specifically targeted to the appropriate destination; prompt disassembly after fusion, probably involving hydrolysis of ATP, ensures that no illegitimate fusion events occur.

This is clearly an oversimplification and other components are probably required as well, as palmitoylation via fatty acylCoA is also essential at this step, and there is no evidence that the polypeptides implicated so far are modified in this way. Why the fusion mechanism for intracellular transport vesicles should be so much more complex than the single-component system used by viruses remains unexplained.

The inhibitory effect of non-hydrolysable analogues of GTP on uncoating of docked vesicles implicates low molecular-weight GTP-binding proteins with inducible GTPase activity in the transport process (see below) and provides a route for the purification of the coated transport vesicle. The coat proteins of these vesicles share similar molecular weights to the major coat proteins of classical coated vesicles derived from coated pits at the plasma membrane, but clathrin itself is not present. None the less, the 110 kDa protein associated with Golgi-derived transport vesicles has homology to the 100 kDa β-adaptin of clathrin-coated vesicles. In addition, the four major proteins of the coat of Golgi-derived transport vesicles can be isolated from the cytosol as a stable 'coatomer complex' in much the same way as the adaptor complex of clathrin-coated vesicles, suggesting a broadly similar organization.

In the same way that the role of adaptor complexes in nucleation of coated pits has been discussed in the context of endocytosis, the role of the coatomer complex in the budding of intracellular transport vesicles has aroused great interest. Two models have been proposed (see Fig. 7). In coat-mediated budding the assembly of a coatomer coat on an organelle membrane provides the essential driving force for budding, whereas, in the membrane-mediated budding model, the production of buds is an intrinsic property of the organelle membrane. In this second model the coatomer serves to convert the tips of spontaneously forming tubules into vesicles. In a recent study involving serial-section electron microscopy on an *in vitro* Golgi budding system that could be immunodepleted of coatomer, the loss of coats resulted in reduced vesicle formation and no tubule production. This supports the coat-mediated budding hypothesis, and calls into question the physiological significance of long tubules that have been seen to emerge from the Golgi apparatus.

Analysing the membrane proteins involved in vesicular transport is much more difficult, as they cannot be freely removed from, or added back to, a reconstituted transport assay. In order to study the membrane proteins involved in these vesicular transport events a different approach was required. The first isolation of such a membrane receptor was achieved recently using affinity isolation.

The 20 *s* fusion particle was assembled *in vitro* from NSF and α and γ-SNAP using the SNAP receptor from a crude detergent extract of bovine brain. The particle was then isolated using an anti-NSF column and disassembled by permitting NSF to hydrolyse ATP. Four major proteins were released and identified; all are proteins associated with synapse function that have been implicated in exocytosis [syntaxin A, syntaxin B, synaptobrevin-2 and SNAP-25 (the name is a pure coincidence—it was isolated as a 25 kDa protein associated with the synaptosome)]. These are very exciting results that fit beautifully with previously puzzling observations in yeast that several proteins implicated in intracellular transport steps had already been found to have unexpected homologies with syntaxin (e.g. SED5 and SEC22). If specific SNAP receptors, or **SNARE**s, are restricted to individual donor and acceptor compartments, then a budded vesicle will carry a donor SNARE; this has been called the v-SNARE. The target membrane may carry a second SNARE, the target- or t-SNARE. To ensure specificity of transport, one specific v-SNARE/t-SNARE pair is required for each step. Thus, these recent results are the first evidence that the machinery unravelled by this biochemical approach may be capable of coding for specificity in intracellular transport.

Fig. 7 Models for role of coat proteins in vesicle formation. In the first model, vesicle production follows recruitment of coat proteins to the cytoplasmic face of the donor membranes, followed by selection of ligand for transport (shown in red in the diagram). The coat proteins may be instrumental in determining the rate of budding and the size, shape and content of the vesicles. In the second model the formation of vesicles is an intrinsic property of the membranes, and may only be consequent on formation of a patch of ligands for transport. In this model, coat proteins are not involved in the formation of the vesicles or the selection of their content, but are recruited at a late stage.

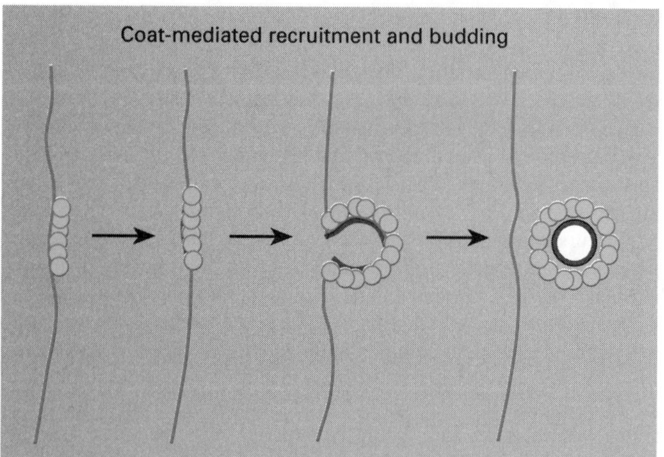

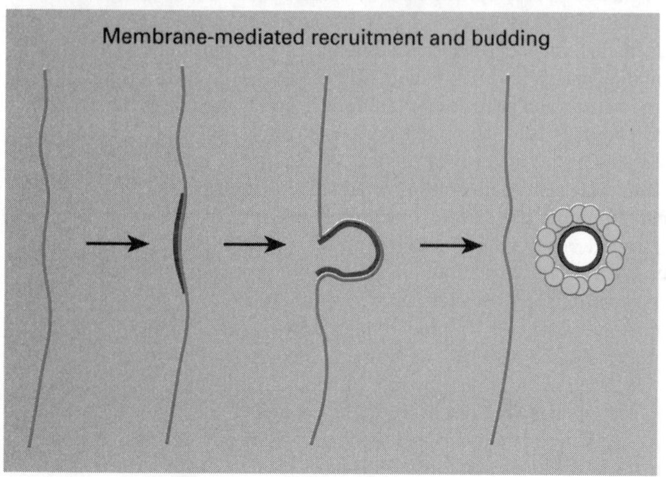

STUDIES OF VESICULAR TRANSPORT IN YEAST

In 1980 a spectacularly fruitful experiment in yeast genetics showed that *S. cerevisiae ts*-mutants defective for secretion and plasma-membrane expansion become dense at the non-permissive temperature, permitting the simple isolation of large numbers of mutants by mutagenesis and density-gradient fractionation. The 188 mutant clones identified fell into 23 complementation groups, which were named Sec1 to Sec23. Electron-microscopic analysis showed that most of these mutants accumulated novel membrane-bound structures at the non-permissive temperature, often vesicles of about 50 nm diameter. Most of the mutants were freely thermoreversible and return to the permissive temperature resulted in a rapid loss of these vesicles and the reappearance of secreted proteins. Later studies involving both biochemical measurement (e.g. glycosylation state of transported proteins) and quantitative electron-microscopic morphology in single and double mutants implicated seven different Sec gene products in early exocytic events in yeast. The studies also separated these mutations into two groups based on the properties of the double mutants (see Fig. 8).

This grouping makes sense when we recall that Sec18 is the yeast NSF and Sec17 is the yeast α-SNAP, and that the mammalian homologues of these proteins are required for a late step in vesicular transport, when a docked transport vesicle fuses with the acceptor membrane. The recent recognition that SEC22 is related to mammalian synaptic-vesicle proteins implicated as membrane receptors for the NSF–SNAP complex completes the story.

Similarly, the reconstitution of endoplasmic reticulum to Golgi transport in yeast using techniques developed for mammalian cells permitted the demonstration that the Sec23 defect is located on the acceptor membranes. A mammalian homologue for Sec23 has not yet been found.

Fig. 8 Functional location of yeast *sec* mutant phenotypes. A combination of biochemical and morphological assays permits the grouping of early sec mutants in yeast. The Sec 12, 13, 16, 23 group blocks endoplasmic reticulum to Golgi transport but the cells do not contain transport vesicles (i.e. vesicle formation is blocked), whereas the Sec17, 18, 22 group blocks the same transport step but result in accumulation of large numbers of transport vesicle (i.e. vesicle consumption is blocked).

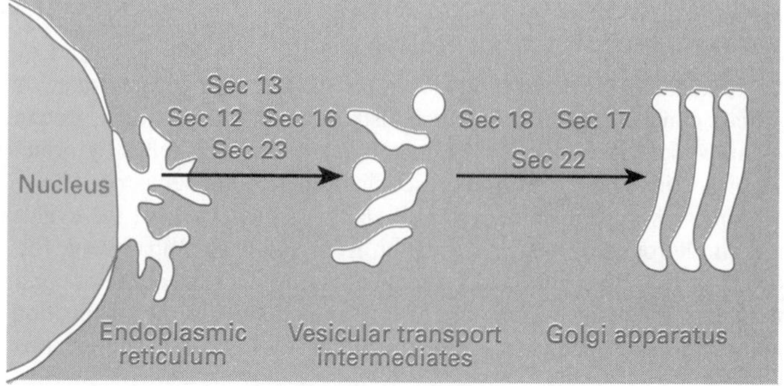

Apart from the Sec mutants that cause early transport defects, other Sec mutants cause changes in Golgi morphology (e.g. Sec 7 and 14) or blocks in late (i.e. post Golgi) steps in the secretory pathway (e.g. Sec4, see below).

Another important yeast transport mutant was identified by chance as an open reading frame adjacent to the yeast actin gene (*YPT1*). The open reading frame was of interest because of a homology to the GTP-binding *ras* oncogene product. *YPT1* mutants have a partial defect in secretion, and the protein has been shown to be required at the time of maximal bud growth (i.e. when transport of new membrane proteins to the cell surface is greatest). Subsequently, it was shown that the *YPT1* protein is a GTP-binding protein required in an early transport step between endoplasmic reticulum and Golgi in yeast, and that the protein is membrane bound in wild-type Golgi membranes. The ability of wild-type cytosol to reconstitute transport in a system where the acceptor membranes were from *YPT1* mutant strains suggested the presence of an additional soluble pool. Immunofluorescence studies suggested a Golgi localization for the *YPT1* protein in yeast and hinted that a mammalian homologue might exist, also localized to the Golgi region. This has been subsequently confirmed, and the mouse homologue (*Rab1*) shown to functionally replace the yeast *YPT1* gene product.

A powerful feature of the yeast genetic approach is the ability to study interactions between proteins by means of isolation of extragenic suppressors, or by studying the phenotype of double mutants. For example, a series of extragenic suppressors of *YPT1* deletion have been identified, and shown in some cases to restore endoplasmic reticulum–Golgi transport. Amongst these are membrane proteins similar to synaptic-vesicle membrane proteins called synaptobrevins (Sly2p and Sly12p) and a protein that seems to be related to the chloroplast phosphate translocator (Sly41p) and may function to control the ionic environment of exocytic compartments.

A second *ras*-like GTP-binding protein was implicated in a late step in the yeast exocytic pathway when the Sec4 gene was sequenced and the Sec4 protein studied in detail. Strong genetic interactions were detected between Sec4 and Sec2, Sec8 and Sec15. The Sec15 protein is a 105-kDa hydrophilic protein that shows a pH-dependent ionic interaction with microsomal membranes, and is found in a small patch within yeast cells, similar to the patch seen with antibodies to the Sec4 protein. It has been suggested that these low molecular-weight GTP-binding proteins function in targeting transport vesicles to the correct acceptor membrane, where the fusion machinery can then be assembled. Up to this point, we have not considered how such a targeting system both ensures unidirectional transport for vesicle content, but also retrieval of the machinery necessary for further rounds of transport.

Table 1 *Intracellular location of Rab proteins*

Protein*	Organelle distribution
Rab 1 (YPT1 in yeast)	Endoplasmic reticulum and Golgi complex
Rab 2	Intermediate or salvage compartment
Rab 3A	Regulated secretory vesicles
Rab 4	Early endosomes
Rab 5	Plasma membrane and early endosomes
Rab 6	Golgi complex (medial and *trans* and the *trans*Golgi network
Rab 7 (YPT7 in yeast)	Late endosomes
Rab 8	*Trans*Golgi network and basolateral transport vesicles
Rab 9	*Trans*Golgi network and late endosomes
Rab 12	Golgi complex (from *cis* stack to *trans*Golgi network
Rab 17	Transport vesicles in polarized epithelia
Rab 22	Early and late endosomes, plasma membrane
Rab 24	Endoplasmic reticulum, intermediate compartment and late endosomes
SEC4	Post-Golgi secretory vesicles
AFT$	Golgi complex, significant cytoplasmic pool
SAR1	Endoplasmic reticulum

*Sequential numbering of Rab proteins is based on sequence identification; rab proteins omitted from the table have not yet been localized at the protein level.

$ADP ribosylation factor, ARF, is now recognized as a member of a new gene family in its own right. Specific localization of individual members is not yet clear.

THE ROLE OF LOW MOLECULAR-WEIGHT GTP-BINDING PROTEINS

Some proteins that are important for vesicular transport have sequence homology to the *ras* oncogene product; this homology is especially striking in the four regions most important for GTP binding. Reconstituted systems for a variety of intracellular transport steps share several common features—a requirement for cytosolic factors, a temperature dependence, a requirement for metabolic energy in the form of ATP, and a common sensitivity to non-hydrolysable analogues of GTP, such as GTPγS. The importance of small GTP-binding proteins similar to those identified in yeast in mammalian transport events is a major growth area in cell biology and has been recently reviewed.

A plausible function for these small GTP-binding proteins was suggested in a brief review by Henry Bourne, who suggested that the GTP-binding proteins might provide target information and ensure vectorial transport. He used an analogy with the mammalian elongation factor EF-Tu, which uses the switch between the GTP-and GDP-bound states to ensure unidirectional transport of the amino acid residue in an amino-acyl-tRNA complex to the nascent polypeptide chain at the ribosome.

The analogous model for vectorial vesicular transport makes several predictions, including the existence of membrane-specific recognition proteins that recruit the GTP-binding protein to the site of bud formation on the donor membrane, the existence of docking sites on the acceptor membrane that specifically bind the GTP-binding protein–vesicle complex, and a mechanism for promoting GTP hydrolysis or GTP–GDP exchange. Only one candidate rab docking protein has been identified so far; rabphilin 3 is a rab 3-binding protein related to the synaptic-vesicle membrane protein synaptotagmin. Specific proteins promoting GTP hydrolysis (*G*TPase-*a*ctivating *p*roteins, or GAP proteins) as well as proteins regulating GTP/GDP exchange have now also been found.

A further consequence of this model is that a single GTP-binding protein could ensure the directionality of all vesicular shuttling events in the cell, provided that the targeting of a vesicle from a given donor membrane to its correct acceptor membrane was mediated by other recognition molecules.

In this case, the GTP-binding protein would act in a similar way to the components of the putative 'fusion machinery'. However, we have already seen that in yeast there are at least two, low molecular-weight, *ras*-like, GTP-binding proteins with different cellular locations (YPT1 on intracellular structures, especially the Golgi, and Sec4p on the inner face of the plasma membrane and the outer surface of late secretory vesicles). This introduces the possibility that there are many small GTP-binding proteins, and that they have a role in targeting as well as ensuring unidirectional vesicular transport.

Recent, polymerase chain reaction-based, cloning experiments have identified multiple low molecular-weight GTP-binding protein in mammalian cells, and some of these have been localized to distinct intracellular locations (Table 1). The hypervariable C-terminal region of the rab proteins has been shown to be responsible for targeting to specific intracellular locations. This suggests that the donor membrane-docking site recognizes signals found in the short, hypervariable C-termini, and suggests an experimental approach for identifying these predicted docking sites.

Recently, a clear role for one of these low molecular-weight GTP-binding proteins, rab5, in an intracellular transport event has been directly demonstrated. These experiments also showed that rab5-depleted cytosol could be restored by addition of recombinant wild-type rab5, but not by a mutant rab5 carrying a mutation that locks it into one conformation, preventing the GTP–GDP conformational switch. These results strongly suggest that it is the GTP–GDP switch that is essential for the low molecular-weight GTP-binding proteins to mediate vectorial transport. The existence of multiple rab proteins with distinct intracellular locations suggests that these proteins may also have a role in controlling targeting of transport vesicles to acceptor membranes.

Additional components are presumably required to act as effector proteins responding to rab protein signals on acceptor membranes. Recent studies have made use of an analogy with the solved crystal structure of *ras*. The crystal structure is available for both the GTP- and GDP-bound forms; superimposition of these structures identifies two major regions that alter in conformation as a result of hydrolysis of GTP. These regions have been called switch I and switch II. Synthetic peptides corresponding to these switch domains inhibit vesicular transport in semi-intact transport assays, although a confusing aspect of the result is that a rab3 peptide is needed to inhibit the rab1/rab2-dependent endoplasmic reticulum to Golgi transport step.

There has been a recent interesting twist to the story of GTP-binding proteins in intracellular transport. Initially, intracellular transport was thought not to involve the heterotrimeric membrane-associated G proteins that are important in signal transduction across membranes. It was widely believed that the effects of GTPγS could be explained completely in terms of *ras*-like, low-molecular weight GTP-binding proteins. However, this belief was challenged by the demonstration that aluminium fluoride, which activates heterotrimeric G proteins but has no effect on members of the *ras* family, inhibits vesicular transport.

The transport of proteins from the endoplasmic reticulum to the Golgi is strongly inhibited by a wasp-venom peptide called mastoparan, which is known to activate and uncouple heterotrimeric G proteins from their cognate receptors. This inhibition occurs at the step of exit from the endoplasmic reticulum and has led to the suggestion that heterotrimeric G proteins may gate exit from the endoplasmic reticulum and thus form an important part of the quality-control system during secretion.

THE CONTROL OF VESICULAR TRANSPORT DURING MITOSIS

When cells divide, the chromosomes segregate and all the other cellular components are partitioned between the daughter cells. For single-copy organelles in mammalian cells, such as the endoplasmic reticulum and the Golgi apparatus, there is an obvious problem to be overcome to ensure that both daughter cells receive part of each organelle. Long-standing morphological observations suggest that mitosis is associated with a fragmentation of these organelles, together with dispersal throughout the cytoplasm. In this way both daughter cells are ensured of receiving at least part of each of the membrane-bound organelles that they require and cannot synthesize *de novo*.

Considerable interest has been shown in the effects of mitosis on intracellular vesicular traffic because it has been regarded as a possible approach to study the overall control of these pathways. A variety of experiments on mitotic cells has demonstrated that processes involving intracellular vesicular transport are inhibited at this stage of the cell cycle. These include endocytosis, receptor recycling to the plasma membrane, secretion, and the transport of newly synthesized plasma-membrane proteins to the cell surface. The block to secretion and transport of membrane proteins is before the first vesicular transport step out of the endoplasmic reticulum.

The requirement for organelle fragmentation and the inhibition of vesicular transport events during mitosis led to the suggestion that fragmentation might be the result of vesicle budding continuing after vesicle fusion had been inhibited. Thus, an organelle would bud itself out of existence and the vesicles produced would not be able to fuse because of a mitotic block to this process.

Direct evidence for this model is now available. When cell-free, endosome–endosome fusion assays are reconstituted using mitotic cytosol, fusion activity is less than that seen when interphase cytosol is added.

Interphase cytosol could be made to mimic mitotic cytosol by the addition of the cell-cycle control protein kinase cdc2. This is the first evidence coupling a cell-cycle regulator with a membrane-fusion event. If this result turns out to be general it may explain how vesicle consumption by fusion is inhibited in the mitotic cell.

The nucleus: an unusual, self-replicating, single-copy organelle

The nucleus is the repository of the genetic information of the cell and contains the genome organized into chromosomes. The major functions of the nucleus centre around the preservation and inheritance of the genetic information, together with its utilization to provide information for synthesis of the proteins necessary for cell function. The process of replication of the genome occurs during the S-phase of the cell cycle—unscheduled replication outside this 'window' is the result of DNA repair mechanisms correcting accumulated defects in the double-stranded DNA genome. During G_1 and G_2, active genes are transcribed to give a primary RNA transcript, which then undergoes a series of post-transcriptional modifications including capping, polyadenylation, and splicing. There is increasing evidence to suggest that these processes are consecutive and occur at specific sites within the nucleoplasm; an analogy with the postsynthetic processing of nascent polypeptides is not too far fetched, although the RNA does not have to pass between membrane-bound compartments by vesicular shuttling. Indeed, this is an important difference; nascent RNA moves from its point of primary transcription in the nucleoplasm to its place of utilization in the cytoplasm without crossing a lipid bilayer because it passes through the nuclear pore (see below). The machinery necessary to get a secretory or membrane process from its initial site of synthesis in the cytoplasm to its final destination across a lipid bilayer is not needed for nucleic acids.

ENTRY OF PROTEINS INTO THE NUCLEUS

The nuclear envelope consists of a closely spaced pair of lipid bilayer membranes; the luminal space between the membranes is in continuity with the lumen of the endoplasmic reticulum. This organization provides a permeability barrier between nucleoplasm and cytoplasm, and enables them to maintain distinct compositions. None the less, a large flow of RNA from nucleus to cytoplasm and an equally large bidirectional movement of proteins are required. Specializations in the nuclear envelope called nuclear pores are responsible for mediating this transport. Although the nuclear pores may be freely permeable to some ions and small molecules they have an exclusion limit at about 9 nm, which translates to roughly 60 kDa for a globular protein. The nuclear transport of most proteins, including all those larger than the diffusion limit, is selective and mediated by signal recognition and an active transport mechanism.

The first evidence for a nuclear localization signal (**NLS**) came from studies on a highly abundant, pentameric nuclear protein of about 165 kDa called nucleoplasmin. Microinjection of this protein into the cytoplasm is followed by rapid transport into the nucleus. Proteolysis, which removes the ends of each of the pentameric chains, results in a defective complex that remains in the cytoplasm after microinjection. Interestingly, the released tail fragments were transported into the nucleus, suggesting the existence of a specific, localized signal. This experiment could not differentiate between selective transport and selective nuclear retention after random active transport. However, a subsequent experiment showed that nuclear injection of the proteolysed fragment resulted in nuclear retention.

Detailed studies on a large number of nuclear proteins revealed motifs that were subsequently shown to act as NLSs. A seven-residue linear sequence from the SV40 large-T antigen is often regarded as the prototypical NLS—the sequence is PKKKRKV (Pro-Lys-Lys-Lys-Arg-Lys-Val). Transfer of this sequence on to a cytosolic protein results in it being relocalized to the nucleus. Even single mutations within this sequence gives rise to a T antigen that no longer accumulates in the nucleus.

There is now evidence that not all NLSs are like the T-antigen one, although most are rich in basic amino acids. There is also some evidence that the SV40 T-antigen NLS is only efficient if another basic cluster 15 residues N-terminal to the heptapeptide is also present. This has been fitted to a model of local protein unfolding by a 70-kDa heat-shock protein (**hsp**) that binds to these two basic regions and presents the NLS to an NLS-binding protein at the nuclear pore.

NLS sequences also operate outside the context of the parent protein; colloidal gold particles can be imported into the nucleus if they carry a synthetic peptide corresponding to an NLS.

IDENTIFICATION OF A RECEPTOR FOR NLS SIGNALS

The above experimental approach, involving a cell-free nuclear import assay, has been used to study the requirements for uptake. Import is found to be a two-stage process—binding to the nucleus requires only an intact NLS, but import requires physiological temperatures, cytosol, and a supply of ATP.

Together with the demonstration that the nuclear uptake rate is saturable, these results suggested that there might be a specific NLS receptor. (A model for the operation of such a NLS receptor is shown in Fig. 9). The model shown involves the entry of the NLS receptor into the nucleus and its subsequent return to the cytoplasm; an alternative model involves the NLS receptor passing the nuclear protein on to the import machinery at the nuclear-pore complex, but not itself entering the nucleus.

Various experimental approaches have been used to identify NLS receptors, including affinity methods using synthetic NLS peptides, cross-linking, searches with antibodies raised against short, very acidic sequences, and genetic approaches in yeast. A number of plausible candidates identified by these approaches are found to be cellular proteins not expected to be involved in nuclear transport (PDI, ERp72, and tubulin). The only common feature that they share is a highly acidic domain, and this may be the reason for their interaction with the basic NLS. Thus, the ability to bind to NLSs is necessary but not sufficient for a functional NLS receptor. Cytosolic erythrocyte proteins of 54 and 56 kDa are strong candidates for NLS receptors. These proteins bind an SV40 T-antigen NLS peptide but not a peptide consisting of the same residues in reverse order (i.e. not just a basic stretch) and stimulate cytosol-dependent nuclear import in digitonin-permeabilized cells.

Another important NLS-binding protein is found localized to the nucleolus. This is a heavily phosphorylated 140-kDa protein, Nopp140, which has a very unusual motif structure repeated 10 times. This protein has recently been demonstrated to shuttle between the cytoplasm and the nucleolus. When labelled antibodies to Nopp140 are injected into the cytoplasm they are carried into the nucleus and concentrate in the nucleolus, whereas antibodies against other nuclear proteins do not show this behaviour.

Electron-microscopic immunocytochemistry suggests that the Nopp 140 in transit is aligned along curved tracks within the nucleus emanating from the dense core of the nucleolus. Interestingly, there is evidence that transport of some newly synthesized mRNA also involves distinct tracks within the nucleus. Whether these two apparent track systems are the same remains to be determined. A number of early studies on the nuclear-pore complex commented on the presence of fibres extending from the pore both into the nucleus and into the cytoplasm. When high concentrations of colloidal gold particles are used in nucleus import assays they accumulate in lines perpendicular to the nuclear pore, suggesting that the first binding step may occur on filamentous extensions remote from the pore itself.

In permeabilized mammalian cells there is a requirement for cytosol for nuclear import and the factors involved are sensitive to *N*-ethyl maleimide (cf. NSF and the fusion particle in vesicular transport; see Mechanisms of vesicular transport above). However, yeast apparently do not require such NEM-sensitive factors for nuclear import. Recent evidence suggests that the NEM-sensitive factors, which have been called NIF-1 and NIF-2, are involved in binding of NLSs to the nuclear pore and may form part of a fibrillar network.

Fig. 9 Schematic for the operation of a nuclear location sequence receptor. Newly synthesized proteins bearing a nuclear location sequence (NLS) are transported into the nucleus by a two-step process requiring ATP, physiological temperatures, and cytosol. One or more NLS receptors are probably involved in this process, and recent evidence suggests that some may shuttle between the cytoplasm and the nucleus to escort nuclear proteins through the nuclear-pore complex.

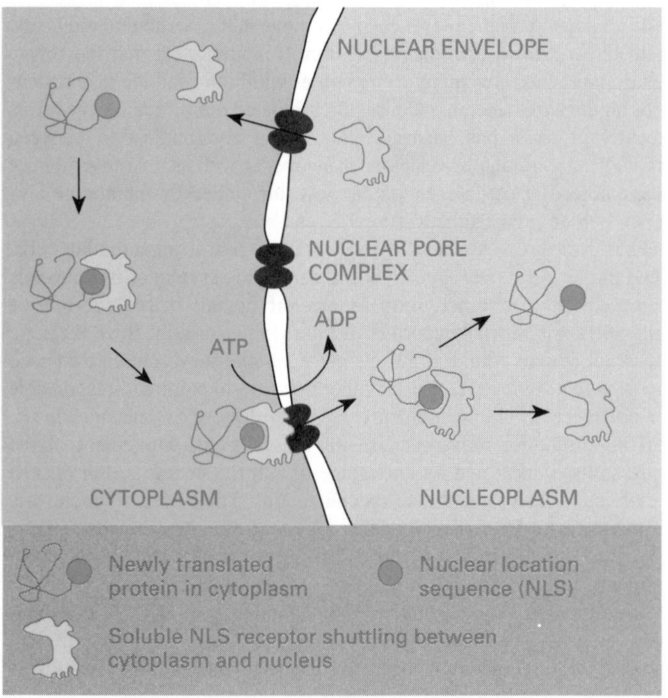

REGULATION OF NUCLEAR TRANSPORT

Some proteins are required in the nucleus only at certain stages of the cell cycle or in response to stimuli such as hormonal binding. Little is known about the regulation of the transport of these proteins into the nucleus, but what evidence there is suggests that there is an additional cytosolic factor that binds to the nuclear protein, obscures the NLS, and prevents nuclear import. This appears to be the case for the glucocorticoid receptor, where the role of the additional cytosolic factor is mediated by hsp90 in the cytoplasm.

Some viruses also have the problem of organizing bidirectional movement of ribonucleoprotein particles (**RNP**s) across the nuclear boundary. In the case of influenza virus, replication occurs in the nucleus and budding at the plasma membrane. This means that early during infection, incoming RNPs must get into the nucleus, but later in infection newly synthesized RNPs must leave the nucleus before budding at the plasma membrane. Recent evidence suggests that this switch is mediated by a viral protein called M1. Newly synthesized RNPs become associated with M1 and are exported from the nucleus, whereas incoming RNPs lose the M1 protein during virus uncoating and are then competent for nuclear import.

This result provides an explanation for the anti viral effect of amantadine, a drug that blocks the proton-channel activity of another influenza protein, M2. RNP–M1 dissociation occurs rapidly at low pH, so when virus enters the endosome and M2 is functioning the pH also falls inside the virus, allowing RNP–M1 dissociation and delivery of the RNPs to the nucleus. In the presence of amantadine the virus enters the endosome but in the absence of the M2 pore the pH does not fall inside the virion itself and so RNP–M1 dissociation does not occur, the RNPs cannot be imported, and no infection results.

THE NUCLEAR-PORE COMPLEX

The nuclear envelope is studded with specialized structures about 0.13 μm in diameter, 0.07 μm thick, with eightfold rotational symmetry and a molecular weight of approximately 125×10^6 Da. These are the nuclear pores; they span the double nuclear membrane and can be isolated as complex structures after detergent treatment to disrupt the nuclear membranes.

The rotational symmetry of nuclear pores has made them attractive objects for study by computational methods in conjunction with electron microscopy. This approach has been used with images of negatively stained, isolated nuclear-pore complexes and images of membrane-associated and detergent-solubilized complexes examined in a frozen, hydrated state. Figure 10 shows a reconstruction based on rendered, symmetrized density maps obtained from electron-microscope images of isolated nuclear pores.

The structure shown is symmetrical about the membrane and missing the central plug or transporter that is involved in active nuclear transport. It forms a framework upon which is then built the asymmetrical elements that control vectorial transport. All of the wheatgerm agglutinin-binding, O-linked glycoproteins are absent from the nuclear pores as isolated, so they are also absent from this model. None the less, it does show how the nuclear-pore complex locks the inner and outer nuclear membranes in position, and suggests that active transport passes through the central channel (colloidal gold always passes close to the central axis, not at the periphery) while passive diffusion of small molecules could occur via the peripheral openings.

The structural asymmetry of the nuclear-pore complex reflects the asymmetrical transport processes it mediates—a predominant export of RNA and a predominant import of protein (although as we have seen some components recycle). A major role of the nuclear pore is to control the nucleocytoplasmic trafficking of snRNPs and ribosomes, both catalytic RNPs that are assembled in a different compartment from that in which they eventually function.

Fig. 10 The nuclear-pore complex (NPC). This rendered image of an isolated nuclear-pore complex is the result of computational reconstruction from images of frozen, hydrated NPCs. The eight-fold symmetry and the presence of a central pore and central plug are clearly visible. (Reproduced from Akey and Radermacher (1993), with permission.)

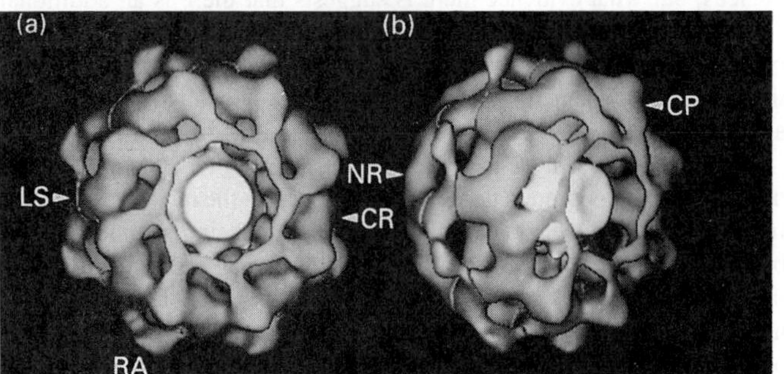

ASSEMBLY OF THE NUCLEAR ENVELOPE

At the onset of mitosis in most eukaryotic cells the nuclear envelope vesiculates and detaches from the chromatin, probably as a result of phosphorylation of lamin B. The numerous small vesicles that result undergo partition between the daughter cells and at the end of mitosis reform a nuclear envelope by binding to chromatin (probably via lamin A and B) via vesicle-bound lamin B. Several *in vitro* systems have been developed to study the reassembly of the nuclear envelope, using chromatin or naked DNA as the nucleating material and isolated mitotic-vesicle fractions (or Xenopus oocyte postnuclear supernatant) to provide the membrane.

In a Xenopus system, a specific fraction of 70-nm vesicles binds to chromatin in an NEM-insensitive, ATP-independent manner via a protein–protein interaction, but no fusion occurs unless cytosol is present. Electron-microscopic quantitation suggests that one vesicle is bound per 100 kb DNA.

Further experiments showed that both GTP and ATP were required for fusion of chromatin-bound vesicles, and that the membranes contained an NEM-sensitive factor required for fusion. It is not yet known whether this is the same NSF that is involved in fusion events in the endocytic and exocytic pathways.

Not all vesicles positive for endoplasmic reticulum markers such as BiP and PDI are capable of binding chromatin in these *in vitro* systems—in fact, only about 20 per cent of such vesicles will. However, the non-chromatin-binding vesicles can contribute to the reassembling nuclear envelope by interaction with a vesicle that is already bound, and this process also requires both ATP and GTP. These results suggest that at the onset of mitosis a subset of vesicles in endoplasmic reticulum are formed that carry specific chromatin-attachment signals. The form in which the nuclear-pore complexes pass through mitosis remains very unclear.

The cytoskeleton: girders, nets, cables, and motors

The cytoplasm is not a simple homogeneous space in which organelles are free floating. Rather, the cytoplasm is itself highly organized and shows marked local variations in both composition and physical properties. The shape of the entire cell, its ability to move and to respond to external signals from soluble molecules, extracellular matrix or other cells all depend on the presence of a complex net of structural elements, collectively known as the cytoskeleton. It is now clear that the shape, positioning, and movement of organelles within the cell are also dependent on the cytoskeleton and a highly regulated motor machinery. Most recently of all it has been recognized that communication between organelles by tubular or vesicular structures as well as the movement of macromolecular complexes that are not surrounded by membrane also depend on an intact, functional cytoskeleton.

There are three classes of cytoskeletal element in mammalian cells. The familiar actin- and myosin-based contractile system of muscle cells is present in a modified form in most if not all cells. Non-muscle cells still contain filaments of actin, but do not usually form the long myosin filaments found in muscle cells. Instead they contain truncated myosins (e.g. myosin I) that lack the long, rod-like domain responsible for polymerization into filaments. None the less, actin and myosin are still important for movement of non-muscle cells. Movement of the entire cells is mediated by anchorage of actin filaments to the plasma membrane at local membrane specializations. Thus, actin filaments are important in control of cell shape. The attachment of small myosins (myosin I) to organelles permits intracellular movements along actin filaments.

Microtubules are made up from tubulin and form continuously remodelled, polarized filaments that may change length only by recruitment and loss of subunits from the ends. The filaments are not themselves contractile but motor proteins may use metabolic energy to move up and down the outside of the tubules. If the motor protein is attached to an organelle, then the organelle may be rapidly drawn through the cytoplasm along a microtubule highway; anterograde and retrograde movement are both possible because there are two motor proteins, cytoplasmic dynein and kinesin. Modulation of binding sites on the organelle surface permits selection of anterograde or retrograde movement; interphase cells usually have a Golgi apparatus that lies close to the microtubule organizing centre (**MTOC**) and this is because the cisternae of the Golgi apparatus interact with cytoplasmic dynein, the negative end-directed motor. When the motor protein complex attaches to two adjacent microtubules, then relative movement may occur; this is manifest as bending, and provides the motion generation for flagella and cilia. The microtubules of the interphase cell are rearranged by the MTOC during cell division to provide a platform for the alignment and subsequent separation of the daughter chromosomes. In this case the force of movement is probably provided by treadmilling of microtubules through the stationary kinetochore.

The third class of cytoskeleton is the intermediate-filament network. Intermediate filament are composed of subunits in the same way as actin microfilaments and microtubules, but they differ in that they can assemble and disassemble by recruitment along their length and not only at their ends. The subunit proteins of microfilaments and microtubules are members of multigene families α-, β-, and γ-actins are known, and there are at least α-, β-, and γ-tubulins (we do not know if this is a complete list). Strikingly, intermediate filament subunit proteins are derived from a very large gene family and the usage of particular subunit genes is a hallmark of the differentiated state of a cell. For this reason, analysis of the phenotype of intermediate filament expression provides valuable information about the differentiation state of a cell. The analysis of keratin subtypes has great importance in immunodiagnostic analysis of tumours of epithelial origin, for example.

The selection of particular subunits of intermediate filaments by different cell types implies that there is a functional significance to this choice, but this observation has been of limited use in understanding the functions of intermediate filament in cells. Some correlations are clear; epithelial cells that suffer repeated mechanical stresses express high levels of keratin intermediate filament. These intermediate filaments are anchored in membranes at sites of specialized cell–cell contact and permit the formation of a supracellular network without the loss of membrane integrity or cellular autonomy.

INTERMEDIATE FILAMENTS

Intermediate filaments are ubiquitous, 8 to 10 nm diameter filaments that are especially prominent in cells subjected to mechanical stress, such as epithelial cells. They characteristically form a basket-like network around the nucleus and extend to the cell periphery where they make cell–cell contacts with the intermediate filament network of the adjacent cell via desmosomes. A given cell type may contain more than one intermediate filament subunit protein and they may form independent networks in the cytoplasm. The subunit proteins of intermediate filament are encoded by a large multigene family and show tissue and cell type specific distributions.

A characteristic feature of intermediate filament subunits is a central α-helical region that can form a coiled coil rod structure. A dimer of these elongated subunits assembles by lateral interactions into an antiparallel tetramer and then into protofilaments. Unlike microtubules and microfilaments (see below), intracellular intermediate filaments seem to have a steady-state equilibrium with the cytosolic pool of subunits throughout their length, rather than just at the ends.

Intermediate filaments undergo profound structural changes during mitosis. These changes differ from subunit to subunit and even from cell type to cell type but in each case the evidence suggests that phosphorylation of their subunits is an important step. The breakdown of the nuclear lamina at the onset of mitosis is the result of phosphorylation of the N-terminal domain of lamin B by cdc2 kinase, the cell-cycle control kinase. Vimentin filament networks are also disrupted by cdc2 kinase-mediated phosphorylation.

The functions of intermediate filaments remain uncertain. Their anchorage at sites of cell–cell contact and their prominence in cells subject to mechanical stress suggest a structural role in maintaining the mechanical integrity and organization of epithelia, but they are also found in cells that are not obviously subject to mechanical stress. Increased phosphorylation of intermediate-filament subunits in response to external stimuli such as chemotactic peptides has led to the suggestion that intermediate filaments might be involved in signal-transduction mechanisms.

There is little evidence to link intermediate filaments with vesicular transport, although their subunits often copurify with intracellular organelles.

MICROFILAMENTS

Muscle-cell contraction depends on the interaction of highly ordered arrays of actin and myosin filaments. Non-muscle cells also contain both actin and myosin and use these proteins for force generation, but lack the highly ordered structures characteristic of muscle cells. Actin is a globular protein of 42 to 44 kDa, which is expressed from a multigene family in tissue-restricted patterns. Monomeric actin polymerizes to form a microfilament of 8 nm diameter; these filaments form a network throughout the cytosol of non-muscle cells, concentrating in a zone just beneath the plasma membrane (the cortex) and as thick filament bundles near the basal membrane of adherent cells. The cores of microvilli are composed of bundled, non-contractile microfilaments whose organization is maintained by fimbrin, a 68-kDa actin-binding protein.

The characteristic behaviour of microfilaments is modulated by a wide array of actin-binding proteins in the same way as the behaviour of microtubules depends on a range of microtubule-associated proteins. A characteristic feature of many actin-binding proteins is that their effects are calcium dependent, thus helping to ensure that actin and myosin activity in non-muscle cells is modulated by local calcium concentration (as it is in muscle cells). In non-muscle cells, actin and myosin II form a contractile actomyosin gel that is important for control of cytoplasmic viscosity and for the organization of cell movement on a substrate, as well as the specialized variant of this movement required for phagocytosis. Actin and myosin II are also important for the process of cytokinesis by which two daughter cells separate after mitosis. The calcium-dependent gel–sol transitions in the cytoplasmic actomyosin network are coupled to plasma-membrane movement by focal, actin-microfilament anchorage sites. These sites have a characteristic complement of polypeptides that serve to link the intracellular actin-microfilament network both to the plasma membrane and to the extracellular matrix via receptors for extracellular matrix components such as fibronectin.

In 1986, Pollard showed that isolated Acanthamoeba organelles could be propelled along actin microfilaments derived from the alga Nitella in an ATP-dependent manner. The rate of movement was only 0.24 μm/s, which was much less than the 40 μm/s recorded for endogenous organelles. However, they were able to clear up a long-standing problem. Non-muscle cells were known to contain a myosin very similar to that found in muscle cells (myosin II), but they also contained a smaller myosin (myosin I), which lacks the long α-helical tail domain and does not dimerize. The function of this myosin I or minimyosin was unclear. Using monoclonal antibodies specific for myosin I or myosin II, Pollard showed that the movement of organelles along microfilaments was dependent on myosin I. In sucrose gradients a significant fraction (around 20 per cent) of the myosin I coisolated with the fraction that contains organelles motile in the *in vitro* assay. Pollard demonstrated that the Acanthamoeba organelles which moved included endocytic structures by preinternalizing a fluorescent tracer, but was unable to identify other organelles. Subsequent experiments confirmed that the endoplasmic reticulum could also move along actin microfilaments in a cell-free system. Many smaller organelles were seen to be entrapped in the network of endoplasmic reticulum, this offers a plausible explanation for the puzzling observation that the organelle streaming movement appeared coordinated. The streaming was known to be sensitive to the drug cytochalasin, which interferes with microfilament function, but this was the first study that showed by electron-microscopic freeze fracture the association of cisternae of endoplasmic reticulum with bundles of actin microfilaments.

Very recently, a completely different mechanism for the movement of organelles in the cytoplasm has been described. The Gram-positive bacterium *Listeria monocytogenes* is a facultative intracellular pathogen that shows rapid movement in host cell cytoplasm (up to 0.4 μm/s). An actin-rich, phase-dense tail is seen behind the moving bacterium. Using a sophisticated experimental approach involving microinjection of actin labelled with a caged fluorochrome into infected cells, Mitchison and colleagues have demonstrated that this movement is the result of recruitment of actin monomer at the back of the bacterium followed by local polymerization into filaments. The speed of bacterial movement is related to the length of the microfilament tail and the slope of this line estimates the persistence time for the new filaments at 42 s (which agrees well with bulk filament-turnover measurements).

Within the last few years a developing theme in cell biology has been the importance of small (20–25 kDa) GTP-binding proteins with similarities to the protein product of the *ras* oncogene (see Section 6 Molecular mechanisms). Control of the actin cytoskeleton has recently been recognized as yet another cellular activity controlled, at least in part, by small, *ras*-like, GTP-binding proteins. For example, the ability of serum-starved mouse fibroblasts to produce focal adhesions and new actin-microfilament bundles ('stress fibres') depends on the normal function of the *rho* protein, whereas the membrane ruffling response appears to depend on the related but distinct GTP-binding protein, *rac*.

Yeasts were the first organisms to be shown to have an additional actin-like protein with only 40 to 50 per cent identity to the consensus actin sequence, but this is very highly conserved. The yeast protein, the product of the *ACT2* gene, is essential for growth, and mutant strains are arrested during bud formation. In addition, the yeast *S. cerevisiae* contains a myosin-like protein encoded by the gene *MYO2* and a tropomyosin homologue encoded by the *TPM1* gene. Disruption of either of these gene results in defects in polarized secretion, strongly suggesting a role for an actomyosin system in yeast vesicular transport. Surprisingly, a search for multicopy suppressors of mutations in the yeast myosin gene produced a gene, *SMY1*, which encodes a protein related to kinesin, a microtubule motor protein (see below). This result was the first hint that there may be an unexpected connection between the microfilament-and microtubule-based motility systems.

This hint has now been startlingly confirmed in mammals. Two groups using different approaches have identified a mammalian actin homologue that associates with the dynactin complex, a 20 *s* particle required for stimulation of cytoplasmic, dynein-dependent movement of organelles along microtubules, and which is concentrated at the MTOC.

MICROTUBULES

The third major class of cytoskeletal elements in the cytoplasm of eukaryotic cells is the microtubule, a complex, labile, tubular structure with a diameter of about 25 nm. The subunit of the microtubule is a heterodimer of a 50-kDa polypeptide called tubulin.

In the interphase cell, microtubules are usually found to radiate from a single centre, the centrosome or MTOC, which contains the paired centrioles that will define the poles of the metaphase plate during mitosis. Microtubules have a characteristic polarity; although they are dynamically unstable through continuous polymerization and depolymerization at both ends, the 'plus' end of the microtubule grows and shrinks fastest. The negative end of the microtubule is stabilized by anchorage in the MTOC while the plus end grows and shrinks rapidly unless it is stabilized by capping or capture by a peripheral structure. (Several characteristic patterns for microtubule organization within cells are shown in Fig. 11).

There are a number of drugs that disrupt microtubules by inhibiting monomer addition and thus promoting net depolymerization (these include nocodazole and colchicine). The effects of these drugs include the loss of normal positioning and morphology of organelles, including the Golgi apparatus and mitochondria. This suggested that these organelles required an intact microtubule network for normal organization. A comparison of the distribution of microtubules and cisternae of endoplasmic reticulum in cells which the microtubule pattern has been simplified by cold depolymerization strongly suggests that the endoplasmic reticulum is also a microtubule-dependent organelle.

The assembly of morphologically convincing networks of endoplasmic reticulum can be carried out *in vitro* by adding microsomes and ATP to taxol-stabilized microtubules on a glass substrate. Based on the*in vitro* reconstitution experiments, Sheetz and colleagues suggested that microtubule-dependent tethering and extension, together with fusion of extensions, could give rise to the characteristic network of the endoplasmic reticulum. Very similar movements of tubule extension, sliding, branching, and fusion are seen *in vivo* when the endoplasmic reticulum is stained with the vital lipid label $DiOC_6$.

The intracellular positioning of the Golgi apparatus also involves the

Fig. 11 Characteristic patterns of microtubule distribution in animal cells. (a) In cells with flagella a column of orientated microtubules emanates from the basal body and terminates with the plus end at the tip of the flagellum. (b) During mitosis the separation of the duplicate chromosome sets is mediated by a symmetrical array of microtubules organized by the centrosomes. (c) In interphase the microtubule network originates from the centrioles or microtubule organizing centre (MTOC). Organelles positioned by negative end-directed motors such as the Golgi apparatus and the prelysosomal compartment tend to cluster in the vicinity of the MTOC. (d) In neurones the long distances involved in axonal transport are traversed by microtubules with their plus ends at the tip of the axon. Rapid plus end-directed movement is required for delivery to the presynaptic region. Notice that the shorter dendrites may contain microtubules in either orientation.

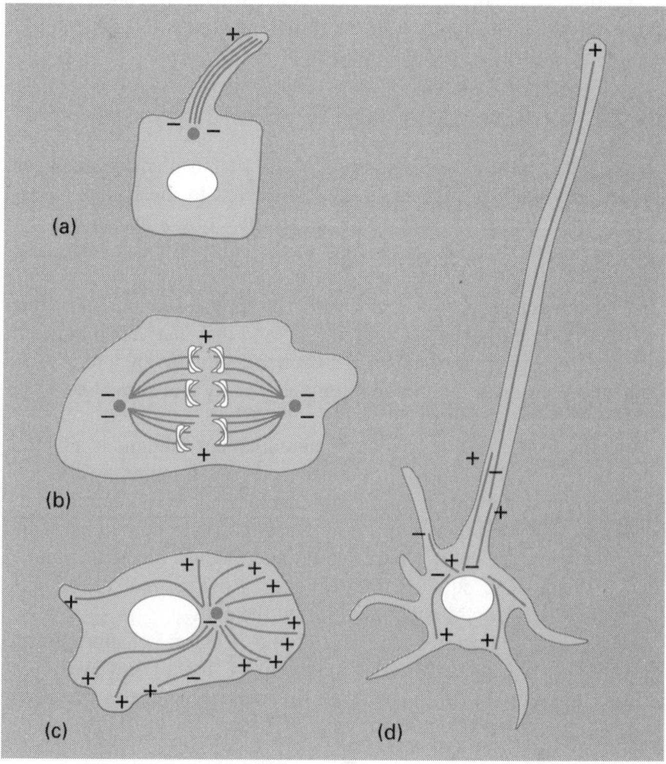

microtubule network. In interphase cells the Golgi apparatus is found in the vicinity of the MTOC, raising the possibility that it is held there by the constitutive activity of a minus end-directed, microtubule-associated motor protein. An ingenious experiment based upon the capture of isolated, biotinylated Golgi membranes by semi-intact cells confirmed that exogenous Golgi membranes could be captured by the microtubule network and concentrated near the MTOC. This activity required ATP, physiological temperatures, cytosol, and the minus end-directed motor protein, cytoplasmic dynein.

MOTOR PROTEINS

When microtubules are attached to a glass substrate and salt-washed organelles from squid axoplasm are added, the organelles bind to the microtubules but no movement is seen. If cytosol and ATP are added, then organelle movement occurs. This provided the assay by which the microtubule-associated protein (**MAP**) kinesin was shown to be a motor protein. The cytosol-induced movement was lost if the cytosol was first immunodepleted of kinesin with an antibody.

Kinesin is a heterotetramer consisting of two 124-kDa heavy chains and two 64-kDa light chains; it exhibits microtubule-stimulated ATPase activity. Interestingly, pure kinesin alone was not sufficient to restore the activity of the immunodepleted cytosol, suggesting that additional soluble factors are needed. Similar assays in which the microtubules were polymerized from centrosomes so that their orientation was known revealed that kinesin generates force towards the plus end of microtubules. That is to say, kinesin-powered movement takes organelles away from the MTOC towards the cell periphery.

A similar assay system using chick embryo fibroblasts as the source of organelles and cytosol resulted in predominantly minus end-directed movement, and this was subsequently shown to be mediated by the MAP, cytoplasmic dynein. Dynein is also known as MAP1c. It consists of several polypeptides with an overall molecular mass of about 1000 kDa. The largest subunit is about 400 kDa.

As in the case of the kinesin assay, organelle movement was not seen with purified dynein alone, but required a high-speed cytosol fraction. This was subsequently shown to include a 20 *s* particle called the dynactin complex (see above).

A third class of protein important in the association of organelles with microtubules is not a motor protein itself, but is required for the binding of organelles to microtubules. An example of such a protein is CLIP170, which is a 170-kDa, nucleotide-dependent MAP that is the prototype of a class called the cytoplasmic linker proteins (hence **CLIP**). It was identified using monoclonal anti-MAP antibodies and shown to be required for endosome binding to microtubules in an *in vitro* assay similar to that for the motor proteins. The functional form of CLIP170 is a homodimer with globular N-and C-terminal domains separated by a very long coiled coil domain containing intermediate filament-like heptad repeats.

A plausible, static, organelle–microtubule attachment protein must exhibit modulatable binding within the cell or no motor-protein movement would be possible, nor could organelle release from microtubules occur. CLIP170 offers a possible mechanism for this, as it no longer binds to microtubules when phosphorylated, and it is found to be heterogenously phosphorylated *in vivo*.

Because motor proteins exist as soluble complexes, there must be a means of attaching them not only to microtubules but also to specific organelles for directed transport. A long search for such molecules has recently been successful, and a 160-kDa, integral-membrane protein that binds kinesin has recently been identified and named kinectin. The successful approach involved immobilizing kinesin with a monoclonal antibody against the motor domain, leaving the tail exposed for interaction with kinesin membrane receptors. Kinectin is located on the cytoplasmic face of intracellular organelle membranes, especially the endoplasmic reticulum. This result supports the view that the morphology of the endoplasmic reticulum is maintained by kinesin-mediated centrifugal forces acting on its tubules. A membrane receptor for cytoplasmic dynein is not yet known, but a similar experimental approach using isolated Golgi membranes and immobilized dynein might provide candidates.

The peroxisome: an independent multicopy organelle?

In 1954, a graduate student named Rhodin described a novel organelle in mouse kidney cells. The organelle consisted of a single, membrane-bound structure of about 500 nm diameter containing an electron-dense granular matrix, which was often crystalline. The organelle remained mysterious until the demonstration in 1966 that it contained the enzyme catalase and two oxidases, both of which produce hydrogen peroxide. As a result the organelle became known as the peroxisome, although it is now clear that the enzymes responsible for the β-oxidation of fatty acids are also localized to this organelle.

For many years peroxisomes were thought to arise from the endoplasmic reticulum by budding, based on the result of electron-microscopic studies. However, as more peroxisome luminal proteins were studied it became clear that they do not carry signal sequences and do not acquire N-linked oligosaccharide modifications, making a route through the endoplasmic reticulum less likely.

Furthermore, the characteristic proteins of the peroxisome membrane could be shown to be translated on free ribosomes, and therefore must be post-translationally inserted into the organelle membrane in a process very unlike that for endoplasmic reticulum-mediated incorporation. Finally, it was shown that the lipid composition of the peroxisome membrane is unlike that of the endoplasmic reticulum membrane.

These results led to the idea that peroxisomes resemble mitochondria and chloroplasts and originate by direct division and subsequent incorporation of new membrane and content proteins by specific transport and recognition processes.

SIGNALS FOR PEROXISOMAL IMPORT

The search for a specific peroxisomal import signal was accelerated by the observation that firefly luciferase accumulates in peroxisomes when expressed in mammalian cells (it is a peroxisomal protein in fireflies as well). Gene deletion, gene fusion, and linker-insertion experiments were then used to locate the import signal in the luciferase protein.

The C-terminal tripeptide was found to be necessary and sufficient for peroxisomal targeting, and mutagenesis studies suggested a consensus sequence—(S or C or A)–(K or H or R)–LCOOH. Although this signal is widespread it is not found in all peroxisomal proteins, and this is especially true for non-mammalian peroxisomal proteins.

There is additional evidence for possible internal import signals, although the original SKL motif is non-functional if it is extended by even two residues. As a final complication it is now known that at least one peroxisomal protein, thiolase, is processed during import and contains a cleaved, N-terminal import signal that is not related to the C-terminal signal described above.

CYTOSOLIC FACTORS IN PEROXISOMAL IMPORT

The presence of an import signal at the C-terminus of a protein implies that it will have been translated to completion before the targeting signal can be acted upon. This in turn implies that the protein is either imported in a folded state or that it is unfolded by interaction with a cytosolic factor until import can take place. The unfolded state is the most likely for translocation processes, and there is good evidence in the case of the mitochondrion that proteins are imported post-translationally after unfolding by cytosolic hsp homologues.

Interestingly, a protein of 72 kDa has been identified that binds to clofibrate, a drug which induces proliferation of peroxisomes in liver cells, and is a member of the hsp70 family.

Table 2 *Proteins involved in peroxisomal import*

Name	Species	Protein	Function
PAF1	Human/rat	34 kDa	Complements mutant CHO cells
Pas3	Yeast	48 kDa	Required for peroxisome biogenesis
Pas1	Yeast	117 kDa	Required for peroxisome biogenesis
pmp70	Rat/human	70 kDa	ATP-binding peroxisome membrane protein

MEMBRANE PROTEINS IN PEROXISOMAL IMPORT

The membrane-associated import machinery of the peroxisome remains poorly understood. Four genes have been identified on the basis of rescuing peroxisome import-defective cells (Table 2). Both pas1 and pmp70 have consensus ATP-binding sequences, although ATP-binding has been shown only for pmp70. Clofibrate and thyroxine, both drugs that induce β-oxidation and cause peroxisome proliferation, cause a marked induction of the pmp70 protein.

Two mutant cell lines expressing normal levels of peroxisomal proteins such as thiolase and catalase but lacking detectable peroxisomes have been isolated after mutagenesis. The gene for the defect in one of these cell lines (Z65) has been identified using cDNA expression-library rescue of peroxisome function. This resulted in isolation of the *PAF1* gene, which produces a 35 -kDa protein that restores peroxisome biogenesis to the Z65 CHO cell line. Immunolocalization showed that peroxisomal proteins now accumulated in morphologically normal peroxisomes, which also contain the 35 kDa PAF1 protein in the form of an integral membrane component.

CLINICAL SYNDROMES ASSOCIATED WITH PEROXISOME DEFECTS (SEE ALSO SECTION 11)

There are a number of clinical syndromes associated with generalized abnormalities of peroxisomes. These include Zellweger syndrome, infantile Refsum's disease and an X-linked condition manifest in childhood as adrenoleukodystrophy and in adults as adrenomyeloneuropathy.

Zellweger syndrome is a fatal, autosomal recessive disease with clinical evidence of severe neurological disorders including profound hypotonia and psychomotor retardation, dysmorphic facial features, hepatomegaly, and multiple renal cysts. It is not compatible with survival beyond early childhood. Biochemically the syndrome is characterized by the absence of catalase-positive organelles in the cytoplasm, and a range of abnormalities that follows from the destruction of the fatty acid β-oxidation pathway. No peroxisomes can be seen morphologically. The condition is not genetically homogenous, but one of the complementation groups of human Zellweger syndrome is now known to correspond to a defect in the *PAF1* gene.

The principal biochemical defect in adrenoleukodystrophy and adrenomyeloneuropathy results from accumulation of very long-chain fatty acids due to loss of peroxisomal β-oxidation capacity. Biochemical analysis of fibroblasts from patients with adrenoleukodystrophy suggested that the defective gene might encode very long-chain fatty acid CoA synthase, but the result of a successful positional cloning approach was quite unexpected. This approach mapped one of the genes that can be responsible for adrenoleukodystrophy to Xq28 and identified a gene disrupted in eight patients with the condition. Rather than encoding the CoA synthase, the gene encodes a protein that closely resembles the human 70 -kDa PMP, a protein already identified as involved in peroxisomal import and known to be a member of the ATP-binding, cassette family of transporter proteins.

REFERENCES

Akey, C.W., and Radermacher, M. (1993). Architecture of the *Xenopus* nuclear pore complex revealed by three dimensional cryo-electron microscopy. *Journal of Cell Biology*, **122,** 1–19.

Balch, W.E. (1990). Small GTP-binding proteins in vesicular transport. *Trends in Biological Science*, **15,** 473–7.

Balch, W.E., *et al.* (1994). Vesicular stomatitis virus glycoprotein is sorted and concentrated during export from the endoplasmic reticulum. *Cell,* **76,** 841–52.

Barr, F.A. *et al.* (1992). Trimeric G proteins and vesicle formation. *Trends in Cell Biology*, **2,** 91–4.

Bourne, H.R. (1988). Do GTPases direct membrane traffic in secretion? *Cell*,**53,** 669–71.

Dingwall, C. and Laskey, R. (1992). The nuclear membrane. *Science*, **258,** 942–7.

Gerace, L. (1988). Functional organisation of the nuclear envelope. *Annual Review of Cell Biology*, **4,** 335–74.

Hinshaw, J.E. *et al.* (1992). Architecture and design of the nuclear pore complex. *Cell*, **69,** 1133–41.

Mellman, I., and Simons, K. (1992). The Golgi complex: in vitro veritas? *Cell*, **68,** 829–40.

Monck, J.R., and Fernandez, J.M. (1992). The exocytic fusion pore. *Journal of Cell Biology*, **119,** 1395–404.

Mosser, J. *et al.* (1993). Putative X-linked adrenoleucodystrophy gene shares unexpected homology with ABC transporters. *Nature*, **361,** 726–30.

Orci, L. *et al.* (1993). *Nature*, **362,** 648–52.

Schroer, T. *et al.* (1988). *Journal of Cell Biology*, **107,** 1785–92.

Skalli, O. *et al.* (1992). Intermediate filaments: not so tough after all. *Trends in Cell Biology*, **2,** 308–12.

Söllner, T., *et al.* (1993). SNAP receptors implicated in vesicle targeting and fusion. *Nature,* **362,** 318–24.

van Meer, G., and Burger, K.N.J. (1992). Sphingolipid trafficking—sorted out? *Trends in Cell Biology*, **2,** 332–7.

Warren, G. (1993). Bridging the gap. *Nature*, **362,** 297–8.

4.2.3 The mononuclear phagocyte system and tissue homeostasis

S. GORDON

INTRODUCTION

Macrophages, together with their precursors in haemopoietic organs and blood, form a heterogeneous family of specialized cells that help to control the physiological integrity of the host, but also contribute to its disruption by many disease processes. The definition of the mononuclear phagocyte system is based on common cell lineage and differentiation,

Work in the author's laboratory is supported by grants from the Medical Research Council, UK and the Arthritis and Rheumatism Research Council (ARC). This chapter is dedicated to the memory of Zanvil A. Cohn.

phagocytic efficiency, and widespread distribution of macrophage-related cells throughout tissues. By virtue of their extensive repertoire of receptors and versatile secretory responses, macrophages interact with other cells of the body as well as with a range of micro-organisms and foreign antigens. The mononuclear phagocyte system is a dispersed, biosynthetically active, adaptive organ that is implicated in the host response to most forms of endogenous or environmental injury. Table 1 lists some conditions in which macrophage dysfunction contributes to the overall disease process. In dealing with the role of macrophages in the pathogenesis of many different types of disease it is possible to discern common, stereotypical effects on the host, irrespective of aetiological agent or tissue localization, as well as organ-specific variations in macrophage activity. Our knowledge of macrophage functions and abnormalities comes mainly from studies in cell culture and in experimental animals, many of which can be readily extended to man, although our knowledge of macrophage function in the human clinical setting is still rudimentary. In this chapter I shall review some of the cellular and biochemical properties that illustrate the central role of macrophages in human disease and bring out general principles concerning the response of the mononuclear phagocyte system to changes within the host microenvironment.

Origin, distribution, and tissue heterogeneity of macrophages

RESIDENT AND RECRUITED MACROPHAGES

Mature macrophages in adult tissues are derived from bone-marrow progenitor cells (Fig. 1) that proliferate and differentiate into cells committed to the myeloid lineage, eventually giving rise to non-dividing, terminally differentiated mononuclear phagocytes (see also Section 22). Relatively mature macrophages retain a limited ability to replicate in peripheral tissues or in response to selected stimuli, depending on the presence of specific growth factors such as macrophage colony-stimulating factor (**M-CSF**) and granulocyte/macrophage (**GM**)-CSF. Other cytokines, including interleukin(**IL**)-3, -4, and -13 also promote multiplication of immature and mature macrophages to a variable extent (see also Section 22). Monocytes circulate for 1 to 2 days before constitutive distribution to tissues of the normal adult host as 'resident' mature macrophage populations. Resident macrophages are present in substantial numbers in the liver (sinus-lining Kupffer cells), lung (alveolar macrophages), bone marrow, spleen and other lymphoid organs, lamina propria of the gut, connective tissue, dermis and the nervous system (microglia). Interstitial macrophages are readily detectable in normal kidney, testis, ovary, and pancreas, and in smaller numbers in most organs of the body. These locations bring macrophages into intimate contact with all major cell types—endothelium, epithelium, connective tissue, neurones/macroglia, muscle, bone—as well as with other haemopoietic cells, including granulocytes, mast cells, T and B lymphocytes. Local cellular interactions are markedly altered by the recruitment of blood monocytes to sites of injury, inflammation, immune or metabolic stimulation. It is useful to distinguish 'elicited' macrophages, recruited by non-immune inflammatory stimuli, from those that have been 'activated' by immunologically stimulated T lymphocytes and their products, consequently expressing enhanced antimicrobial and cytotoxic activities. Recent studies in the mouse have shown that Th1 and Th2 CD4+ lymphocyte subsets exert distinct actions on macrophages via lymphokines such as interferon-γ (Th1), IL-4, IL-13 and IL-10 (Th2), as considered further below, and it is likely that analogous heterogeneity of macrophage phenotype will be present in man.

The microenvironment in each tissue contains different cell types and products that influence the properties of resident macrophages and of recently recruited monocytes. For example, microglia, the resident macrophages found within the parenchyma of the nervous system, are markedly down-regulated with regard to many characteristic macrophage properties and can therefore be distinguished from more typical macrophages present in the choroid plexus and meninges; monocytes newly recruited in response to death of neurones during development or following excitotoxin treatment adopt a similar morphology to that of microglia within 3 to 5 days of entering the neuropil. The distinction between initially resident macrophages and more recently recruited monocytes becomes progressively more difficult because local injury and inflammation up-regulate many properties of resident cells, which therefore come to resemble monocytes in the same microenvironment. Whilst perhaps seen in its most extreme form in the nervous system, similar difficulties in interpreting the origin of macrophage heterogeneity arise at most sites of local injury outside the nervous system.

The lifespan of tissue macrophages can vary from months (resting microglia turn over most slowly)to less than a day, for example at sites of delayed-type hypersensitivity. Factors that regulate macrophage death are ill-defined—CSFs in low concentration enhance survival, even in the absence of growth, and macrophages are susceptible to their own cytotoxic products as well as those generated by other myeloid and lymphoid cells. Unlike polymorphonuclear leucocytes, in which senescence and resultant apoptosis are readily evident, macrophages can remain viable and biosynthetically active for long periods. Naturally occurring and inflammation-induced death of macrophages presumably results in phagocytosis by other macrophages in the vicinity, with resultant transfer of their undegraded inclusions in a continuous chain.

HAEMOPOIETIC AND LYMPHOID ORGANS

Mature macrophages in haemopoietic organs regulate the development of other haemopoietic lineages as well as their own. In the adult, macrophages in bone marrow constitute part of the haemopoietic stroma and form clusters with developing erythroblasts and myeloid cells that can be isolated as intact aggregates by collagenase digestion and gentle physical methods. Clusters of stromal macrophages and haemopoietic/lymphoid cells are also present in spleen and lymphoid organs. Two haemagglutinins are known to be involved in haemopoietic cell-cluster formation by stromal macrophages: sialoadhesin, a lectin-like molecule with specificity for sialylated glycoconjugates that is concentrated at sites of contact with developing myeloid cells; and **EbR**, a divalent cation-dependent receptor for erythroblasts, myeloid, and lymphoid subpopulations that is independently expressed by selected tissue macrophages in haemopoietic and lymphoid organs. The functions of these receptors are not clear—they do not mediate cell engulfment, but promote trophic interactions between stromal macrophages and adherent cells, perhaps signalling via specific ligands or cytokines that regulate haemopoietic cell growth and differentiation. In spleen and lymph nodes, sialoadhesin is prominent in the marginal metallophil zone and subcapsular sinus, entry sites for circulating cells and other potential ligands from blood and afferent lymph, and may thus be implicated in cell trafficking and clearance. The EbR is the major adhesion receptor for haemopoietic cells in fetal liver. During development, macrophages appear during mid-gestation and play an important part in tissue remodelling and organogenesis, in the nervous system, for example, as well as in erythropoiesis. The earliest macrophages in yolk sac do not asso-

Table 1 *Physiological and pathological processes involving macrophages*

Process	Examples of disease or syndrome
Phagocytosis	Antibody-mediated haemolytic anaemia, thrombocytopenia
Monocyte recruitment/complement opsonization (CR3)	Leucocyte adhesion-deficiency syndrome
Respiratory burst	Chronic granulomatous disease (oxidase deficiency)
Antigen processing and presentation	Induction of immunity, adjuvants, secondary immune response
Cell-mediated immunity and delayed-type hypersensitivity	Listeriosis, tuberculosis, leprosy, AIDS, berylliosis
Autoimmune injury	Multiple sclerosis, diabetes
Intracellular pathogen entry and persistence	Infection by mycobacteria, legionellae, leishmanias
Chronic inflammation	Crohn's disease, ulcerative colitis, rheumatoid arthritis
Tissue remodelling, repair, and injury	Emphysema, pneumoconiosis
Acute or persistent secretory activity (endogenous pyrogen, neutral proteinases, cytokines, arachidonate metabolites)	Fever, septic shock, dengue haemorrhagic shock, wasting, amyloidosis
Recruitment to lipid accumulation/ cell degeneration	Atherosclerosis, ageing, e.g. central nervous system
Lysosomal digestion	Storage diseases, mucopolysaccharidoses, e.g. Gaucher's disease
Growth and differentiation	Leukaemia, histiocytosis, e.g. Langerhans-cell histiocytosis
Promotion of malignant cell growth	Asbestosis, mesothelioma

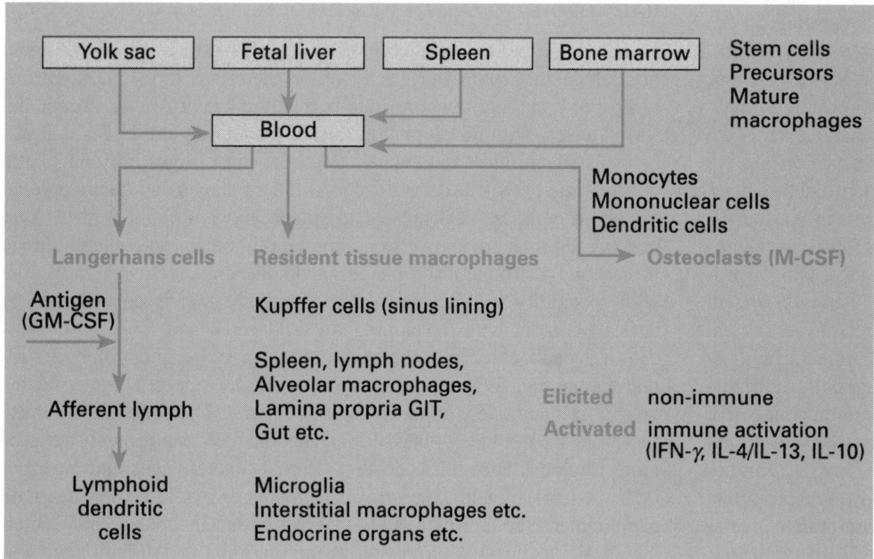

Fig. 1 Differentiation and tissue distribution of macrophages and related cells. GIT, gastrointestinal tract; IFN, interferon; other abbreviations in text.

ciate with primitive nucleated erythroblasts also present at that site. Stromal macrophages associating with erythroblasts appear first in fetal liver, in parallel with the production of more mature, enucleated erythroblasts. Subsequently, stromal macrophages in bone marrow bind viable erythroid cells before their release into the circulation, whilst engulfing discarded erythrocyte nuclei by poorly understood mechanisms.

The development of lymphoid organs is accompanied by the expansion and turnover of macrophage populations. Naturally dying thymocytes are phagocytosed by macrophages; in secondary lymphoid organs such as spleen, the postnatal increase in T and B lymphocytes is associated with the appearance of distinctive macrophage populations in the red pulp, marginal zone, and white pulp. Maturation of the spleen is accompanied by a complex balance between entry of blood monocytes, local proliferation, redistribution within the organ, local death, and possibly emigration of macrophages. The functions of these regionally differentiated subpopulations of macrophages are obscure, but include the phagocytic clearance of senescent erythrocytes, neutrophils and lymphoid cells, trapping of particulate and other antigenic substances including micro-organisms, and interactions with immunologically stimulated T and B lymphocytes. Macrophages in lymph nodes, bronchial and gut-associated lymphoid tissue (tonsil, Peyer's patches) share many properties; these cells come from haematogenous and local sources as well as from lymphoid drainage.

DIFFERENTIATION OF LYMPHOID DENDRITIC CELLS AND OSTEOCLASTS

The general outline above suggests a relatively simple life history and migration pathway for macrophages compared with that of lymphocytes: mainly haematogenous distribution, irreversible differentiation of specialized cells with increased refractoriness to growth factor-induced proliferation, and limited migration in afferent lymph from tissues to lymph nodes. Evidence for these events comes mainly from immunocytochemical studies using a range of plasma-membrane differentiation markers, such as F4/80 antigen in the mouse. The identification in several species of a group of macrophage-related cells (Langerhans, veiled, interdigitating, lymphoid, and blood dendritic cells) as specialized antigen-presenting cells has complicated our relatively simple description of the mononuclear phagocyte system. For example, dendritic cells isolated from spleen lack the F4/80 antigen, are poorly adherent and minimally phagocytic, and therefore can no longer be regarded as classical macrophages. These cells constitutively express high levels of major histocompatibility complex (**MHC**) class II antigens and are uniquely potent in stimulating primary immune responses in naive T lymphocytes, for example during the mixed leucocyte reaction. More typical macrophages can be induced to express class II antigens, by interferon-γ for example, but, like B lymphocytes, which express class II antigens constitutively, are only able to function as antigen-presenting cells for previously sensitized T lymphocytes in secondary responses. Further evidence for a specialized role in antigen presentation comes from studies showing that isolated lymphoid dendritic cells readily form clusters with T lymphocytes and express high levels of leucocytic adhesion receptors and known co-stimulatory molecules, such as B7 antigen(s), which have been implicated in T-cell activation.

However, there is good reason to believe that the lymphoid dendritic cell is a derivative of the mononuclear phagocyte system. Langerhans cells, which are found within epidermis and other complex epithelia, are specialized macrophages with a reduced phagocytic as well as low antigen-functioning capacity. They originate from circulating mononuclear cells, express the F4/80 macrophage differentiation antigen, and are able to transport antigenic peptides to draining lymph nodes, where they become highly efficient antigen-presenting cells. Langerhans cells isolated from tissues also differentiate into F4/80 negative, potent mixed leucocyte reaction-stimulatory, dendritic cells when cultivated in the presence of GM-CSF. Lymphoid dendritic cells, which are highly motile, may therefore be uniquely migratory derivatives of mature macrophages. Functionally mature dendritic cells present in blood may be migrating from, as well as to, lymphoid and other organs, especially spleen.

Recently, it has become possible to generate cells with a dendritic cell phenotype from bone marrow and blood precursors in GM-CSF-supplemented cell-culture systems. *In vitro*-derived dendritic cells coexist with typical macrophages and express many macrophage markers at low levels, whilst strongly positive for MHC class II antigens and antigen-presenting functions. Taken together, these studies suggest that in the host, lymphoid dendritic cells comprise a further differentiation pathway derived from common as yet undefined precursors of the mononuclear phagocyte system via Langerhans cells. The dendritic-cell phenotype *in vitro* is critically dependent on GM-CSF and is unaffected by M-CSF; tumour necrosis factor (**TNF**)-α may also contribute to dendritic-cell migration and differentiation.

The osteoclast, a specialized bone-resorbing multinucleate cell, is an analogous F4/80-ve, but M-CSF-dependent, sublineage of the mononuclear phagocyte system. Mutations in the M-CSF gene result in osteopetrosis, in which animals lack mature osteoclast function as well as selected, but not all, macrophage populations, and the bone and some of the other deficiencies can be corrected by exogenous M-CSF. Multinucleated macrophage giant cells can be distinguished from osteoclasts (tartrate sensitivity of acid phosphatase, lack of calcitonin response) and some progress has been made in deriving osteoclasts from poorly defined precursors in cell-culture systems using stromal cell lines, M-CSF, and vitamin D metabolites.

CONSTITUTIVE AND INDUCED MIGRATION OF MONOCYTES

Monocytes enter developing and normal adult tissues selectively and their anatomical location (sinus lining, interstitial, intraepithelial) implies specific control of adhesion and migration within each organ. Many questions about the constitutive delivery of circulating cells to particular sites are unsolved: the nature of the recruitment stimulus, predetermination or random recruitment from the circulating pool of monocytes, the adhesion molecules and endothelial ligands involved, and so forth. Naturally occurring cell death may initiate monocyte-specific recruitment to the developing nervous system, but cannot account for extensive continuous replacement of Kupffer cells in normal adult liver from blood monocytes. Recruitment by local tissue injury, infection, and other stimuli is more amenable to study; progress has been made in identifying candidate cytokines that evoke monocyte entry (chemokines), adhesion receptors involved in this process (selectins, integrins) and the mechanism of transendothelial diapedesis (Fig. 2). Resident macrophages appear to play a key part in initiating an acute inflammatory response after phagocytosis of invading micro-organisms. A family of small chemokine proteins produced by macrophages and other local cells in injured tissue may account for migration of monocytes, with or without lymphocytes or other myeloid cells. Monocyte chemotactic protein-1 and RANTES are chemokines that show considerable selectivity for monocytes and T lymphocytes, whereas IL-8, macrophage inflammatory protein-1α and other chemoattractants such as leukotrienes, formylated small peptides, and the complement-cleavage polypeptides C5a and C3a favour recruitment of neutrophils, presumably because of the relatively selective expression of plasma membrane receptors for different chemotaxins by different leucocytes.

Adhesion receptors known to interact with inflamed endothelium include L-selectin, present on several types of leucocytes, and the β_2-integrins, especially complement receptor type 3 (**CR3**), which is expressed by neutrophils and natural killer cells as well as monocytes. Human inborn deficiency of a family of three β_2-integrins (leucocyte adhesion-deficiency syndrome) results in failure of circulating myelomonocytic cells to adhere to cytokine-activated endothelium and to enter sites of inflammation. Experimentally, monoclonal antibodies directed against epitopes of CR3 involved in cell adhesion, such as the 5C6 rat anti-mouse monoclonal antibody, are able to inhibit recruitment of myelomonocytic cells to immunologically non-specific stimuli, such as injection of thioglycollate broth into the murine peritoneal cavity. Induced recruitment of leucocytes has been shown to depend on CR3-mediated adhesion to endothelium in several species and in a wide range of inflammatory conditions, for example reperfusion injury after surgically induced myocardial infarction. The effects on monocyte recruitment tend to be overshadowed by the inhibition of neutrophils, but have been found after treatment with 5C6 in murine models of T-cell-dependent inflammation such as listeriosis (highly detrimental) and autoimmune diabetes (beneficial). T-lymphocyte-induced recruitment of monocytes recovers in the presence of 5C6 after a lag period, indicating the subsequent utilization of CR3-independent pathways. Constitutive migration of monocytes during development and in the normal adult is resistant to blockade by the 5C6 antibody and is therefore thought to depend on unidentified adhesion molecules. Receptors involved in monocytic recruitment to sites of degeneration or metabolic injury have also not been identified in experimental model systems or man.

Adhesion involves sequential activation of receptors (weak binding via leucocyte (L) and endothelial (E) selectins as leucocytes roll over endothelium, stronger binding via integrins as cells adhere and flatten before diapedesis). Known ligands on leucocytes and endothelium include specific carbohydrate Lewis blood group-related antigens for selectins and intercellular adhesion molecule-1 for leucocyte β_2-integrins. CR3 is known to bind many proteins relatively promiscuously, including iC3b and fibrinogen, and several plasma-derived and endothelial ligands might therefore contribute to myelomonocytic migration. Other plasma-membrane receptors that play a part in monocytic recruitment include the vitronectin receptor (β_1, α_4-integrin), CD31 (PECAM-1, an immunoglobulin superfamily glycoprotein responsible for migration through endothelial-cell junctions), and CD44, a widely distributed adhesion molecule for components of extracellular matrix.

MACROPHAGE HETEROGENEITY IN RELATION TO NATURAL AND ACQUIRED CELLULAR IMMUNITY

Resident macrophages at portals of entry such as skin, lung and gut, or in direct contact with blood and lymph, constitute an important early line of defence against invading micro-organisms, but can contribute to further spread by transporting pathogens. These resident macrophages, particularly the Kupffer cells in normal liver, are not well equipped to deal with rapidly growing virulent organisms such as Listeria; host survival then depends critically on rapid mobilization of monocytes able to express more potent antimicrobial activities than Kupffer cells, which are thought to be deactivated by chronic exposure to lipopolysaccharide from the gut. Enhancement of monocytic effector mechanisms by interferon-γ plays a critical part in resistance to a range of intracellular pathogens including mycobacteria. The concentration of newly recruited and activated monocytes and T lymphocytes within granulomas localizes invading organisms in the immunocompetent host, but cannot form such lesions or limit mycobacterial growth in interferon-γ-deficient mice.

'Epithelioid' macrophages in granulomas are thought, on morphological grounds, to be poorly phagocytic but active secretory cells. *In situ* hybridization studies confirm that these cells uniformly express high levels of mRNA for lysozyme; only a subpopulation of macrophages and activated T cells contains mRNA for more tightly regulated proinflammatory cytokines such as TNFα, which also plays a part in granuloma formation and host resistance, and whose production by macrophages is boosted by interferon-γ. These and other properties (see below), such as induction of MHC class II antigens, serve to distinguish recruited, granuloma macrophages from resident macrophages. Multinucleated Langhans giant cells, a feature of tuberculous and other granulomas, result mainly from macrophage fusion, although DNA synthesis and aberrant cytokinesis may contribute to polykaryon formation. Interferon-γ is produced by the Th1 subset of CD4+ lymphocytes and by natural killer cells upon stimulation by IL-12, a product of phagocytosing macrophages (Fig. 3). Activated Th2 CD4+ lymphocytes produce other lymphokines, such as IL-4 and -13, which are implicated in the shift from cellular to humoral immunity. These cytokines modulate cellular immunity and delayed-type hypersensitivity responses induced by Th1 lymphocytes, contribute to macrophage growth and giant-cell formation, and may initiate concurrent repair of the granulomatous lesion by stimulating fibroblast activities. IL-10, a Th2 cytokine also produced by stimulated macrophages, inhibits proinflammatory cytokine production and the antigen-presenting functions of macrophages, thus deactivating delayed-type responses.

Kupffer cells in liver are not the only resident macrophage population with a limited ability to contain invading micro-organisms. Resident macrophages in many tissues including bone marrow and the central

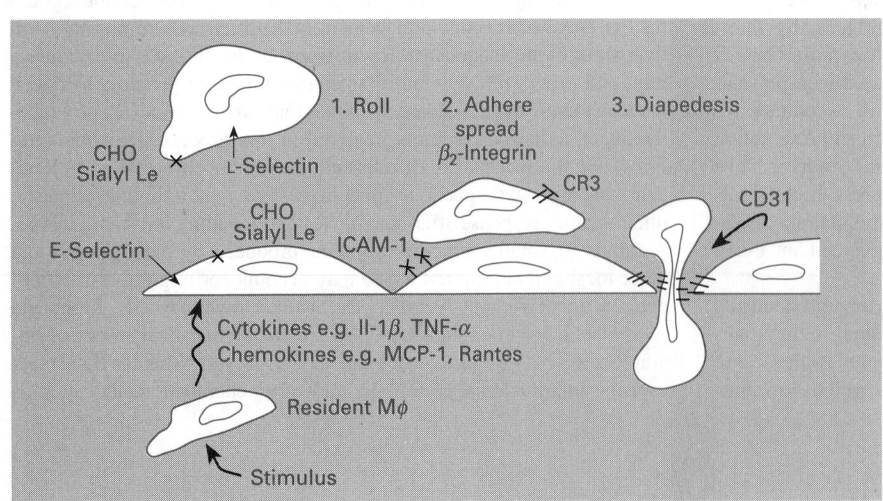

Fig. 2 Monocyte–endothelium interactions involved in induced migration.

nervous system are down-regulated and susceptible to infection; one possible exception is lung, where alveolar macrophages are continually stimulated via airway particulates and 'spontaneously' express proinflammatory cytokines, such as TNF-α, and antimicrobial enzymes such as lysozyme. Down-regulation of surface-receptor expression, endocytosis and secretory activities of microglia, Langerhans cells, and other resident macrophages results from local interactions in each microenvironment. Transforming growth factor-(**TGF**)β and interferons-α/β are cytokines present in many tissues that are able to deactivate macrophages, as do glucocorticoids. However, poorly defined, tissue-specific, plasma-membrane and matrix constituents can also influence the phenotype of macrophages; the microenvironment of the central nervous system, for example, exerts a highly localized, reversible anti-inflammatory effect on recruited and immunologically stimulated macrophages, which may involve as yet unidentified components of neurones and/or macroglia.

Cellular basis for macrophage interactions with other cells and pathogens

PLASMA-MEMBRANE RECEPTORS

Table 2 provides a list of some of the receptors known to be present on the surface of macrophages, although not necessarily expressed by all cells *in situ*. These receptors account for macrophage interactions with other cells and their products, and control a wide range of macrophage activities including growth, differentiation and activation, recruitment, adhesion and migration, phagocytosis, pinocytosis, and recognition of various target cells. Surface receptors play a part in the destruction and clearance of potential pathogens and other ligands, and in interactions with extracellular matrix, plasma-derived proteins and peptides of the coagulation, complement, and kinin cascades. Other receptors mediate regulation of macrophage activities by a multiplicity of cytokines, inflammatory mediators, hormones, and drugs. Conversely, receptors provide potential routes for cellular entry by a wide range of pathogens. Engagement of receptors that induce phagocytic ingestion and macrophage cytotoxicity determines the viability and fate of modified host cells and micro-organisms. Only a few aspects of plasma membrane-receptor function will be selected to illustrate the diversity of interactions and functions mediated by these macrophage molecules.

Fig. 3 Modulation of macrophage activation.

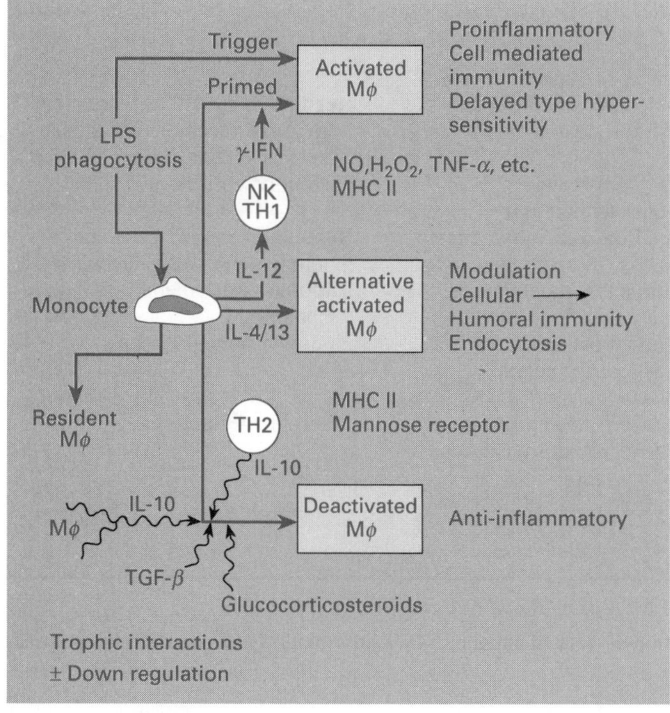

Discrimination of self and non-self

Specific antibodies (most classes except IgM, and many isotypes) provide a powerful array of opsonins for recognition of many diverse antigens by a limited number of Fc receptors. Molecular studies have defined structural determinants of Fc receptors on macrophages and other cells, and have begun to characterize their ability to initiate intracellular and secretory responses. Utilization of Fc receptors for different immunoglobulin isotypes can be regulated by Th2 and Th1 lymphokines, which control humoral responses and/or macrophage-receptor expression. Cleaved C3, deposited on a target via the classical or alternative pathway of complement activation, provides a ligand for several adhesion and phagocytic receptors (CR3, p150/95, CR1). Recognition by the macrophage therefore depends on the initiation and control of complement activation, for example by repeating carbohydrate structures, and on the availability of C3 and other alternative-pathway components, most of which can be produced locally by macrophages themselves. Expression of the CR3 molecule and control of its ability to mediate ingestion depend on the functional state of the macrophage and is regulated by matrix and adhesion proteins such as fibronectin acting via other macrophage integrins. In the absence of opsonins, foreign or aberrantly expressed sugars can be recognized directly by lectin-like receptors, of which the macrophage mannosyl receptors are best characterized. These contain multiple carbohydrate-recognition domains and promote clearance of cellular and macromolecular ligands; their expression on macrophages can be modulated by interferon-γ (decrease) or IL-4 and IL-13 (increase). Other receptors that may be implicated in phagocytic recognition include receptors for C1q and various collectins (soluble lectins with collagenous domains, e.g. mannose-binding protein, surfactant proteins), and the macrophage scavenger receptor, which mediates adhesion to and uptake of denatured, low-density lipoproteins and a range of polyanionic ligands, including polynucleotides and polysaccharides.

Control of growth and other functions by M-CSF

The proto-oncogene c-*fms* (see Chapter 6.3) is the macrophage receptor for M-CSF and controls normal growth and differentiation; the viral oncogene v-*fms* encodes a mutated receptor that is constitutively active even in the absence of exogenous M-CSF and results in uncontrolled growth. M-CSF is predominantly produced as a proteoglycan form on the surface of fibroblasts; direct contact with M-CSF-bearing mesenchymal cells is therefore able to influence the properties of macrophages in haemopoietic organs and at sites of chronic inflammation. The role of M-CSF in osteoclast differentiation and in osteopetrosis was noted above; other effects of M-CSF on macrophages include increased cell survival and spreading, and enhanced adhesion and endocytosis via up-regulation of scavenger-receptor expression. The latter may contribute to macrophage retention in atherosclerotic lesions.

Sialoadhesin

This macrophage-specific, non-phagocytic lectin is found on stromal macrophages in haemopoietic and lymphoid organs as noted above. It is a 185 kDa, single-chain glycoprotein that mediates rosetting of unopsonized sheep erythrocytes in experimental systems, as well as binding immature and inflammatory neutrophils and other sialylated ligand-bearing cells via a carbohydrate-recognition domain. The molecule has multiple immunoglobulin-type domains and is homologous to CD22, a B-lymphocyte lectin for sialylated structures. Although murine peritoneal macrophages express only low levels of sialoadhesin and of rosetting activity, cultivation in the presence of murine plasma or serum induces high levels of both, through an autocrine mechanism involving interferon-β. Both interferon-γ and IL-4 strongly down-regulate rosetting. Thus, stromal macrophages, through the expression and function

Table 2 *Macrophage plasma-membrane receptors and ligands*

Receptor(R)	Ligand(s)	Functions	Comment
FcR (several)	IgG, IgE	Opsonic phagocytosis cytotoxicity, release inflammatory mediators	Ig superfamily (IgSF)
CR3	iC_3b, ICAM-1, promiscuous	Opsonic phagocytosis Non-opsonic pathogen entry Migration Cell activation	β_2-integrin (also LFA-1, p150,95)
C1qR	C1q, collectins (mannose-binding protein, surfactant protein A)	?Opsonic	Ligands, lectins with collagenous sequences
Macrophage scavenger R (MSR)	Modified lipoproteins Selected polyanionic macromolecules	Adhesion and endocytosis	Expressed by selected tissue macrophages
AGE R	Advanced glycosylation end-products	Endocytosis, cytokine release	Interacts with non-enzymatically glucosylated proteins, e.g. diabetes
VLA 1,2,4,5,6	Matrix/coagulation components, laminin, fibrinogen	Adhesion/migration	Several β_1- and possibly β_3-integrins
VnR (CD51)	Vitronectin		α_v β_3
CD31	Endothelial cells, platelets	Diapedesis	Homophilic—IgSF
CD44	Hyaluronic acid	Adhesion/migration	Haemopoietic variant
CD36	Thrombospondin	Adhesion	
L-selectin	Lectin: sialyl-Lewis *x* antigen	Rolling on inflamed endothelium	Monocytes also express ligand for E,P selectins
Sialoadhesin	Lectin: Neu Acα2→3 Galβ1→3 Gal NAc on sialoproteins and gangliosides	Interactions with haemopoietic cells	Stromal macrophages in bone marrow and lymphoid organs Carbohydrate recognition and multiple IgGSF domains
Macrophage mannose receptor (MMR)	Lectin: mannosyl glycoconjugates	Endocytosis, phagocytosis, and secretion	Multiple C-type carbohydrate recognition domains
Cytokine receptors	M-CSF	Growth, differentiation of macrophages and osteoclasts, endocytosis	IgSF, macrophage-restricted c-*fms*
	GM-CSF	Growth, differentiation of macrophages and dendritic cells	Haemopoietin receptor superfamily (low- and high-affinity polypeptides)
	IFNγ	Activation of macrophages MHC class II antigen ↑, induction of i-NOS respiratory burst	Regulation by Th1 cells; two polypeptides
	IL-4	Alternate differentiation and activation, fusion	Regulation by Th2 cells related to IL-13 receptor, which has similar effects
	TNFα	Granuloma formation, antimicrobial activity	Two polypeptides (p75, p55)
	IL-10	Deactivation, anti-inflammatory	Regulation by Th2 cells and stimulated macrophages
	MCP-1, RANTES	Recruitment of monocytes	Multiple—transmembrane spanning
α_2-Macroglobulin		Clearance proteinases	Non-macrophage-specific
Urokinase		Localization fibrinolysis	
Transferrin		Endocytosis	
CD14		Receptor for plasma LPS-binding protein transduces LPS activation	Macrophage-specific
Peptides (many)		Modulation of inflammatory functions	
Drugs (many)			

Modified from Fraser, I. and Gordon, S. (1993). An overview of receptors of MPS cells. *Blood Cell Biochemistry*, **5**, 1–27.

IgSF, immunoglobulin superfamily; IFN, interferon; LFA, lymphocyte function-associated antigen; NOS, nitric oxide synthase; LPS, lipopolysaccharide; all other abbreviations in text.

of sialoadhesin, provide a potential link between products of activated T lymphocytes and haemopoietic-cell interactions.

PHAGOCYTOSIS, RECEPTOR-MEDIATED ENDOCYTOSIS, AND PATHOGEN ENTRY

Figure 4 illustrates some of the events involved in endocytic uptake of particles by phagocytosis, a highly specialized property of macrophages; pinocytosis resembles the process seen in other cell types, although it can be extremely active in mature macrophages. Attachment of a particle via specific receptors to a local segment of the macrophage plasma membrane results in engulfment if sequential interactions with surface ligands proceed all the way round the circumference of the particle, the so-called zipper mechanism. Ingestion is temperature dependent and sensitive to cytochalasin, which disrupts the actin filament network beneath the site of attachment. A source of glucose can be a critical requirement for uptake of selected particles. The membrane of the phagosome is coated with clathrin and differs only subtly in composition from bulk plasma membrane. Macrosialin (CD68), a heavily glycosylated glycoprotein, is selectively concentrated in phagosomes and endosomes, and may provide a protective function in acidic compartments. After ingestion of a particle, the pH of the phagosome falls progressively as it fuses with lysosomes to form phagolysosomes. Acidic hydrolases delivered to this compartment degrade macromolecular substrates, leaving only residual, non-degradable material. Membrane is recycled to the surface, and newly added to the phagosome/phagolysosome by fusion of endocytic vesicles. Receptor-mediated pinocytosis resembles phagocytosis except that large-scale local membrane and cytoskeletal reorganization is not required. Both endocytic activities involve extensive membrane flow, fusion and fission, activation of pumps to maintain fluid and membrane balance, and interactions with the trans-Golgi network, as a source of newly synthesized membrane and vesicular contents.

Fig. 4 Phagocytic pathway and pathogen invasion of macrophages.

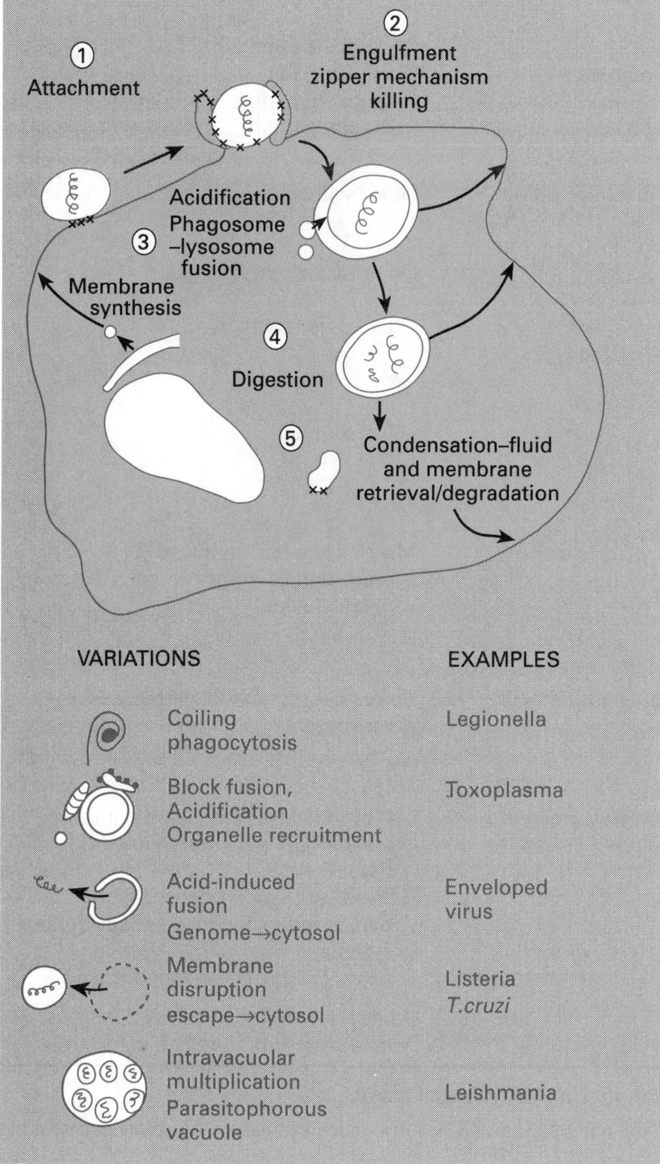

The phagocytic pathway plays a central part in intracellular parasitism of macrophages, induction of natural and acquired immunity, and induction of secretory and cytotoxic activities. A wide range of micro-organisms is taken up by macrophages through different surface receptors via the zipper mechanism; in contrast, organisms such as legionellae induce a bizarre, alternative coiling process of ingestion. Pathogens employ various strategies to evade killing by the macrophage and to replicate in the appropriate intracellular compartment. Examples include inhibition of acidification and phagosome–lysosome fusion (mycobacteria, Toxoplasma, legionellae), replication within parasitophorous vacuoles (Leishmania) and lysis of the phagosomal membrane (Listeria). Viral agents infect macrophages by utilizing receptors common to many cell types, influenza for example, or by receptors relatively restricted to macrophages; for example, Fc receptor-dependent binding can enhance infection by flaviviruses in the presence of selected antiviral antibody. (The actual entry receptors have not been identified.) CD4 is an important entry receptor for human immunodeficiency virus (**HIV**)-1 in macrophages, as in CD4+ T lymphocytes, although other membrane molecules may contribute to its binding, fusion or uncoating. Cytokines such as TNF-α are able to slow HIV-1 entry into macrophages, in parallel with down-regulation of CD4 expression, whilst up-regulating subsequent viral replication. Endocytosed viruses, enveloped and otherwise, can escape into the cytosol by translocating their genomes across the endosomal membrane, a process catalysed by acidification. Mitochondria and portions of the endoplasmic reticulum surround unfused vacuoles containing legionellae, *Toxoplasma gondii*, and other pathogens, although the mechanism or significance of organelle recruitment is unknown. *Listeria monocytogenes*, once free within cytoplasm, initiates a striking assembly of an actin tail, which propels the escaping organism into adjacent macrophages as well as other cells.

The outcome of macrophage–pathogen interactions is crucial to the survival and spread of the organism within the host and depends on many factors. Resistance to a range of intracellular organisms (mycobacteria, salmonellae, Leishmania) is controlled by a single gene, N-*ramp*, which has recently been cloned in mouse (chromosome 1) and man (chromosome 2). The cDNA has limited homology to a nitrite transporter (see role of NO in macrophage cytotoxicity below), but the presumed transmembrane, macrophage-specific gene product has not yet been localized to a particular cell compartment. Other host factors that modulate host resistance and the activation state of the macrophage include lymphokines, particularly interferon-γ, IL-4/IL-13, and IL-10, and the presence of opsonins, such as specific antibody, which can direct the invading organism into a degradative pathway. Virulence factors of the organism can subvert macrophage responses, for example by inactivation of signal-transduction pathways that involve G-proteins (e.g. pertussis) or by phosphorylation/dephosphorylation of plasma membrane and intracellular intermediates (e.g. salmonellae, yersinia). The host response to lipopolysaccharide depends on several macrophage gene products including the CD14 antigen, the receptor for a circulating, lipopolysaccharide-binding protein, as well as cytoplasmic proteins involved in intracellular signalling and cytoskeletal function.

The nature of resultant macrophage responses depends on the particular plasma-membrane receptors utilized for entry/capture. Most Fc receptors mediate ingestion and initiate cytotoxic responses, whereas

Table 3 *Macrophage-derived secretory products*

Product	Function	Comments
Enzymes		
Lysozyme	Antimicrobial	Constitutive *in vitro*, inducible *in vivo*; myelomonocytic and Paneth cells
Urokinase	Plasminogen activation and fibrinolysis, neutral proteinase activation	Inducible by macrophage activation, and phagocytosis, cytokines.
Collagenase	Connective tissue	Inducible
Elastase	catabolism	
Angiotensin-converting enzyme	Pressor	Steroid inducible
Acid hydrolases (many)	Lysosomal digestion	Mainly intracellular
Cytokines		
IL-1β	Multiple local and systemic host defence functions e.g. endothelium,	Endogenous pyrogen, tissue injury, weight loss
TNF-α	leucocytes, connective tissue	Superinducible
IFN-α/β	Antiviral, immune modulation	
IL-6	Acute-phase response	
IL-10	Inhibitor pro-inflammatory cytokines and APC function	Also product of Th2 cells
IL-12	Stimulates IFN-γ production by NK, Th cells	
FGF	Fibroblast growth	
TGF-β	Inhibitor of macrophage activation, other targets	
GM-CSF	Granulocyte, macrophage, and dendritic-cell growth and differentiation	
IL-8	Granulocyte chemoattractant	Chemokine family
MIP-1α,β	Chemoattractant, haemopoietic regulator	Chemokine family
MCP-1	Monocyte recruitment	Chemokine family
RANTES	Recruitment of monocytes and Th cells	Chemokine family
Complement proteins		
Most components of classical and alternative pathways	Local opsonization and complement activation	Other sources, e.g. liver
Coagulation factors:		
Several, including tissue factor	Local initiation and regulation clotting	Other major sources
Adhesion, matrix molecules:		
Fibronectin, thrombospondin, proteoglycan	Localization, migration Modulation of cellular interactions and phagocytosis	Other major sources
Transport proteins:		
Transferrin, B_{12}-binding protein, apolipoprotein E, α_2-macroglobulin	Transport of Fe, vitamin, lipid Proteinase inhibitor	Other sources
Bioactive lipids		
Cyclo-oxygenase, lipoxygenase products of arachidonate	Mediators of inflammation, e.g. effects on leucocytes, small vessels	Macrophage has high level of arachidonate in membranes, therefore potent source
PAF	Platelet activation	
Reactive oxygen intermediates		
Superoxide anion, hydrogen peroxide, singlet oxygen, hydroxyl radicals	Killing and stasis of micro-organisms and cells by activated macrophages	Tissue injury, modulated by radical scavengers
Reactive nitrogen intermediates		
Nitric oxide, nitrites, nitrates	Killing microbial, parasitic and cellular targets by IFN-γ-activated macrophages	i-NOS inducible, compared with low levels NOS constitutive in other tissues. **NB:** NO not readily detectable in human monocyte/macrophage culture systems
Defensins		
(Polypeptides)	Antibacterial	Produced only by some macrophages, as well as PMN, Paneth cells

Adapted from Gordon S. (1992) *Oxford textbook of pathology*, Vol. **1**, pp. 336–45. University Press, Oxford.

APC, antigen-presenting cell; FGF, fibroblast growth factor; IFN, interferon; NK, natural killer; NOS, nitric oxide synthase; PAF, platelet activating factor; other abbreviations in text.

CR3 ligation can effect engulfment of a target without triggering a respiratory burst or the release of arachidonate products by the macrophage. Organisms such as Toxoplasma exploit an entry pathway that does not induce a respiratory burst, but the receptors by which these and many other organisms invade macrophages alone, or with other cell types, remain obscure. Entry into macrophages via selected receptors induces extensively altered glycosylation of the endosomal antigen macrosialin (CD68), thus prolonging its half-life. Association of exogenous immunogenic peptides with MHC class II antigen is thought to occur in the endosome after partial proteolysis of phagocytosed particulates. This may account for induction of secondary immune responses by antigen-presenting macrophages; however, as discussed above, the phagocytically active macrophages are poor antigen presenters for naive T lymphocytes compared with dendritic cells, which express only limited phagocytic activity. The rudimentary vacuolar apparatus of dendritic cells, which are constitutively MHC class II+, may be an important differentiation step to avoid extensive degradation of foreign antigens by macrophages, which express the more labile MHC class II antigen. It is also possible that macrophages transfer peptides of phagocytic origin to dendritic cells for presentation to T cells.

SECRETORY RESPONSES

Table 3 lists some of the products that macrophages are able to generate *in vitro*, often in response to a surface-acting stimulus such as lipopolysaccharide acting directly or via a circulating lipopolysaccharide-binding protein and the CD14 receptor for the lipopolysaccharide–protein complex. Macrophages can potentially release a very large variety of products, including cytokines (monokines), pro-enzymes, and antagonists for these (soluble receptors or antiproteinases), as well as low molecular-weight metabolites derived from oxygen, nitrogen or arachidonate. These play a part as mediators of inflammation, local intercellular communication and repair (e.g. IL-1β and TNFα, acting on endothelial and haemopoietic cells), systemic responses (e.g. IL-6, hepatocytes, hypothalamic neurones), growth promoters (e.g. IL-1β, fibroblasts, T lymphocytes) and growth inhibitors (interferon-β, TGFβ), antimicrobial agents (lysozyme, H_2O_2, NO), and connective tissue catabolism (e.g. urokinase). Other cell types, hepatocytes for example, produce larger amounts of complement and coagulation-cascade proteins, but the widely distributed macrophages are major local sources of monokines in chronic granulomatous inflammation and degenerative diseases. Although most products are generated in small amounts (lysozyme, the most abundant, comprises about 10 per cent of extracellular product/day in culture) and products are not usually stored preformed in secretory granules, the cells are relatively long-lived and responsive to environmental signals, such as phagocytosis of poorly degradable particulate substances, and hence constitute a major inducible secretory organ. Macrophages that have been immunologically activated, by mycobacterial infection for example, become primed by interferon-γ to respond more explosively to triggers such as lipopolysaccharide and can then release lethal amounts of vasoactive substances such as TNF-α and IL-1β. IL-10 and, to a lesser extent, other Th2 lymphokines (IL-4, IL-13) inhibit production of such proinflammatory cytokines by macrophages. *In situ* hybridization studies show that many resident tissue macrophages *in vivo* do not express high levels of message for lysozyme, a 'constitutive' product in cell culture, but that all newly recruited monocytes in granulomas, for example, are induced to do so. By contrast, fewer cells express high levels of proinflammatory cytokines (e.g. IL-1β, TNF-α, IL-6), even after an additional lipopolysaccharide stimulus. These cytokines are also regulated translationally but it is often difficult to detect the protein products by immunochemical methods (they can be released/taken up by other cells) or by functional assays (often undetectable in the circulation, or masked by inhibitors).

The mechanisms by which macrophage products act on targets are complex. For example, urokinase can bind to macrophage receptors and/or extracellular substrate-bound inhibitors. Circulatory plasminogen becomes bound to fibrinogen/fibronectin and greatly amplifies potential proteolysis by formation of local plasmin, again limited by antiplasmin and α_2-macroglobulin. Thus proteolysis, able to activate the zymogens of plasma cascades as well as latent enzymes such as procollagenase, initiates inflammation and repair, but also contributes to catabolism of connective tissues when produced in excess, or in combination with cytotoxic products of macrophages and other cells. Proteolysis by chronically stimulated macrophages can generate insoluble polypeptides from immunoglobulins and other host proteins that accumulate extracellularly in various types of secondary amyloidosis. Excessive production by macrophages of growth factors for connective tissue cells, small blood vessels and smooth-muscle cells, in atherosclerotic arteries for example,

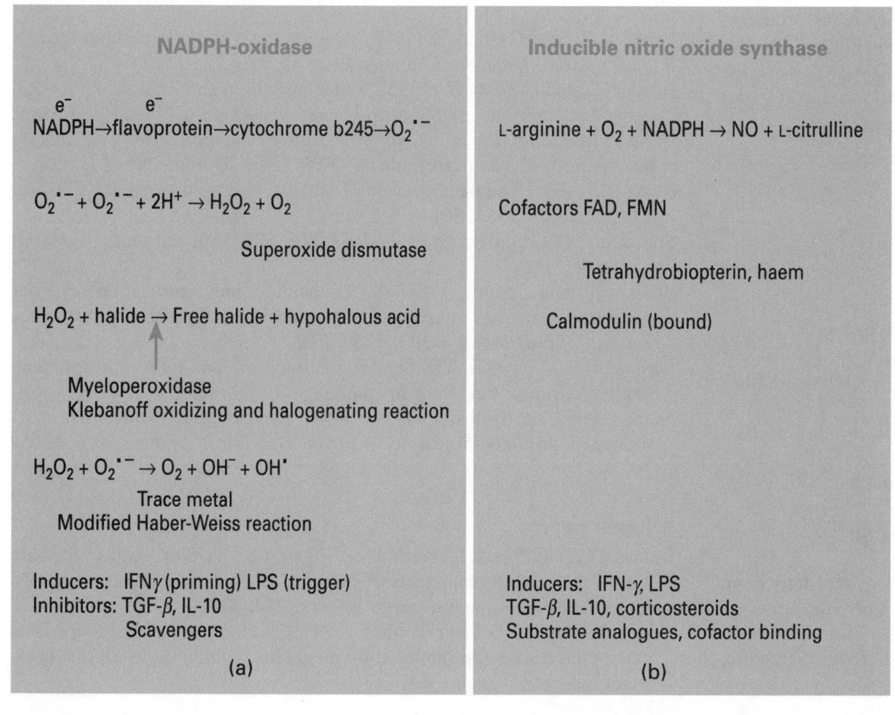

Fig. 5 Oxygen-dependent killing systems.

contribute to the fibrotic and vascular complications of prolonged inflammatory/metabolic injury.

KILLING MECHANISMS

Oxygen- and nitrogen-based antimicrobial and cytotoxic activities generated by activated macrophages are outlined in Fig. 5. Oxygen- and nitrogen-dependent antimicrobial killing systems are complemented by oxygen-independent killing by enzymes (e.g. lysozyme) and other polypeptides (e.g. defensins), although there is considerable heterogeneity in the ability of different macrophages to produce these agents. TNF-α, acting on broadly distributed cellular receptors, may contribute to cellular cytotoxicity and to septic shock by endothelial-cell injury. The assembly of an active oxidase in the plasma membrane of leucocytes involves several cytoplasmic and membrane molecules; autosomal and X-linked inborn errors in these proteins give rise to deficient oxidase activity, and susceptibility to persistent microbial infections in patients with chronic granulomatous disease. The inducible nitric oxide synthase of myelomonocytic cells has only been discovered recently, and its control and contribution to antimicrobial resistance are less well understood. A distinct nitric oxide synthase is constitutively present in many cell types, including endothelium and neurones, and NO generated by this enzyme is thought to be important in vasodilation and neurotransmission.

Conclusion

There are few diseases in man in which the macrophage is exclusively involved, and few diagnostic tests that are specific indicators of excessive, inappropriate, or deficient macrophage functions. Nevertheless, the properties of the cells, and their widespread tissue localization, indicate that they are major contributors to pathogenesis of many common, chronic conditions in which they are known to accumulate in various locations (Table 1). These include inflammatory and autoimmune diseases in lung, joints, gut and the nervous system, acute and persistent infection by agents such as tuberculosis, HIV, legionellae and leishmania, and disorders of lipid metabolism, such as atherosclerosis, where macrophages are selectively recruited to arterial-wall lesions. Apart from their local activities, macrophages have the capacity to act on distal organs that regulate systemic responses of the host to numerous diseases. The mechanisms by which macrophages contribute to fever, malaise, weight loss, and other metabolic disorders so common in clinical disease are not entirely clear. However, as outlined in this chapter, the macrophages of the body play a general role in a wide range of environmental responses of the host, contribute to homeostasis of all tissues, and provide a suitable target to treat many clinical condition of major importance.

REFERENCES

Books

Austyn, J.M., and Wood, K.J. (1993). *Principles of cellular and molecular immunology*. Oxford University Press.

Gordon, S. (ed.) (1988). *Macrophage plasma membrane receptors: structure and function*, *Journal of Cell Science*, Suppl. 9.

Horton, M.A. (ed.) (1993). *Macrophages and related cells*, *Blood Cell Biochemistry 5*. Plenum, New York.

Lewis, C., and McGee, J.O'D. (ed.) (1992). *The macrophage*. IRL Press, Oxford.

Metcalf, D. (1984). *The hemopoietic colony stimulating factors*. Elsevier, Amsterdam.

Russell, S. and Gordon, S. (ed.) (1992). Macrophage biology and activation. In *Current topics in microbiology and immunology*, Vol. 181. Springer Verlag, Berlin.

van Furth, R. (ed.) (1970). *Mononuclear phagocytes*. Blackwell Scientific, Oxford.

van Furth, R. (ed.) (1975). *Mononuclear phagocytes in immunity, infection and pathology*. Blackwell Scientific, Oxford.

van Furth, R. (ed.) (1980). *Mononuclear phagocytes, functional aspects I* and *II* Martinus Nijhoff, Amsterdam.

van Furth, R. (ed.) (1992). *Mononuclear phagocytes. Biology of monocytes and macrophages*. Kluwer, Boston.

Zembala, M. and Asherson, G.L. (ed.) (1989). *Human monocytes*. Academic Press, London.

Zucker-Franklin, D., Greaves, M.P., Grosin, C.E., and Marmont, A.M. (ed.) (1988). *Atlas of blood cells: function and pathology*, (2nd edn). Fischer, Stuttgart.

Review articles

Clark, R.A. (1990). The human neutrophil respiratory burst oxidase. *Journal of Infectious Diseases*, **161,** 1140–7.

Cohn, Z.A. (1978). The activation of mononuclear phagocytes: fact, fancy, and future. *Journal of Immunology*, **121,** 813–16.

Crocker, P.R., Morris, L., and Gordon, S. (1988). Novel cell surface adhesion receptors involved in interactions between stromal macrophages and haematopoietic cells. *Journal of Cell Science*, Suppl. **9,** 185–207.

Gordon, S. (1992). The mononuclear phagocyte system and host defence. In *Oxford textbook of pathology*, (ed. J.O'D. McGee, N.A. Wright, and P.G. Isaacson), Vol. 1, pp. 336–45. Oxford University Press.

Gordon, S. (1992). Monocytes/phagocytes. In *Oxford textbook of pathology*, (ed. J. O'D. McGee, N.A. Wright, and P.G. Isaacson) Vol. 1, pp. 236–58. Oxford University Press.

Gordon, S., Fraser, I., Nath, D., Hughes, D., and Clarke, S. (1992). Macrophages in tissues and *in vitro*. *Current Opinions in Immunology*, **4,** 25–32.

Gordon, S., Lawson, L., Rabinowitz, S., Crocker, P.R., Morris, L., and Perry, V.H. (1992). Antigen markers of macrophage differentiation in murine tissues. In *Macrophage biology and activation*, (ed. S. Russell and S. Gordon), *Current topics in microbiology and immunology*, Vol. 181. pp. 1–37. Springer-Verlag, Berlin.

Gordon, S., Perry, V.H., Rabinowitz, S., Chung, L-P., and Rosen, H. (1988). Plasma membrane receptors of the mononuclear phagocyte system. *Journal of Cell Science*, **Suppl. 9,** 1–26.

Kaplan, G. (1993). Recent advances in cytokine therapy in leprosy. *Journal of Infectious Diseases*, **167, Suppl. 1,** 18–22.

Nathan, C. (1987). Secretory products of macrophages. *Journal of Clinical Investigation*, **79,** 319–26.

North, R.J. (1978). Opinions. The concept of the activated macrophage. *Journal of Immunology*, **121,** 806–9.

Perry, V.H., Andersson, P-B., and Gordon, S. (1993). Macrophages and inflammation in the central nervous system. *Trends in Neurosciences*, **16,** 268–73.

Perry, V.H., and Gordon, S. (1988). Macrophages and microglia in the nervous system. *Trends in Neurosciences*, **11,** 273–7.

Rosen, H., and Gordon, S. (1992). The contribution and limitations of CR3-dependent recruitment of macrophages to inflammatory and lymphoid sites. In *Mononuclear phagocytes. Biology of monocytes and macrophages*, (ed. R. van Furth), pp. 21–30. Kluwer, Dordrecht and Boston.

Ross, R. (1993). The pathogenesis of atherosclerosis: a perspective for the 1990's. *Nature*, **362,** 801–9.

Schall, T.J. (1991). Biology of the RANTES/SIS cytokine family. *Cytokine*, **3,** 165–83.

Sherry, B., and Cerami, A. (1988). Cachectin/tumor necrosis factor exerts endocrine, paracrine, and autocrine control of inflammatory responses. *Journal of Cell Biology*, **107,** 1269–77.

Steinman, R.M. (1991). The dendritic cell system and its role in immunogenicity. *Annual Review of Immunology*, **9,** 271–96.

Nathan, C.F., and Hibbs, J. (1991). Role of nitric oxide synthesis in macrophage antimicrobial activity. *Current Opinion in Immunology*, **3,** 65–70.

Selected papers

Dalton, D., Pitts-Meek, S., Keshav, S., Figari, I.S., Bradley, A., and Stewart, T.A. (1993). Multiple defects of immune cell function in mice with disrupted interferon gamma genes. *Science*, **254,** 1739–42.

Fraser, I., Hughes, D., and Gordon, S. (1993). Divalent cation-independent macrophage adhesion inhibited by monoclonal antibody to murine scavenger receptor. *Nature*, **364,** 343–6.

Kindler, V., Sappino, A.P., Grau, G.E., Piguet, P.F., and Vassalli, P. (1989). The inducing role of tumor necrosis factor in the development of bacterial granuloma during BCG infection. *Cell*, **56,** 731–40.
Salgame, P. *et al.* (1991). Differing lymphokine profiles of functional subsets of human CD4 and CD8 T cell clones. *Science*, **254,** 279–82.
Vidal, S.M., Malo, D., Vogan, K., Skamene, E., and Gros, P. (1993). Natural resistance to infection with intracellular parasites: isolation of the candidate for *BCG. Cell*, **73,** 469–85.

4.2.4 Cytokines

S. KESHAV

Introduction

Cytokines is the term given to the relatively recently characterized group of peptides that permit contact-independent communication between cells involved in immunity, inflammation, growth, and healing. They are similar biochemically and in mode of action to endocrine peptides such as human growth hormone. However, they are distinguished by originating primarily from cells of the lymphohaemopoietic system rather than specialized cells in an endocrine organ. Furthermore, while endocrine hormones normally circulate in the bloodstream before reaching their target organs, cytokines act mainly in a paracrine fashion, that is to say, by diffusion, on other cells within the same tissue microenvironment. Indeed some cytokines act back on the producing cell (autocrine action), while others have, in addition to the secreted form, a membrane-bound form that probably acts only when direct cell-to-cell contact is achieved (Fig. 1).

No comprehensive definition or listing is entirely satisfactory, although certain common features of cytokines are apparent. They are all small to medium-sized proteins (generally less than 200 amino acids), secreted by immune and other cells in response to specific stimuli, which act by binding to specific cell-surface receptors. All cytokines are involved in immunological or inflammatory reactions. Redundancy is widespread, with most cytokines having multiple biological targets and activities, and most specific biological activities being shared by more than one cytokine. The physiologically relevant actions or roles of many cytokines are still undecided. Table 1 shows an abbreviated list of some of the most important cytokines, with their predominant actions, and molecular characteristics.

Fig. 1 Paracrine action of cytokines. Cytokines released from the cells that produce them may diffuse across capillary walls and enter the bloodstream to be carried to distant sites of action (such as the brain and liver), producing systemic effects (endocrine action). Most cytokine actions, however, are probably local, with the cytokine binding to receptors on the same cell that produced the cytokine (autocrine action), or binding to receptors on nearby cells (paracrine action). In addition, there is some evidence that some cytokines remain bound to the producing cell, and are only active when two cells make close physical contact.

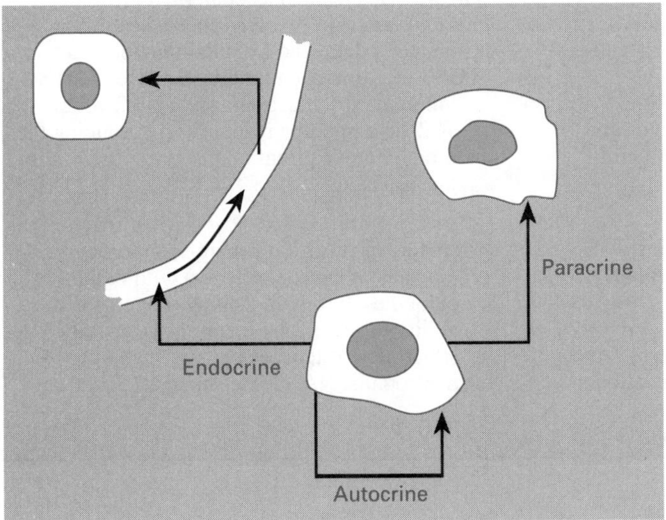

Classification

INTERLEUKINS

This is the prototypical group of cytokines. The term interleukin was given in 1979 to the growing number of proteins with immunological and inflammatory actions that were being biochemically characterized and were soon to be molecularly cloned. For many of these, biochemical characterization had enabled researchers to ascribe a number of diverse biological actions to a single protein. Interleukin (**IL**) 1 was thus shown to be the same as leucocyte endogenous pyrogen, lymphocyte-activating factor, and leucocyte endogenous mediator. The term interleukin conveys the idea of chemical communication between leuc(k)ocytes, but interleukins are produced and secreted from many cell types, and act on equally diverse target cells.

Interleukins comprise most of the important growth- and differentiation- promoting factors for T and B lymphocytes (IL-1,-2,-4,-5,-7,-9,-10,-11,-12,-13), a growth factor for platelets and other haemopoietic cells (IL-3), a growth factor for eosinophils (IL-5), inflammation-provoking factors (IL-1,-2,-6,-8,-12), and inflammation-reducing factors (IL-4,-10,-13).

There are now at least 15 named interleukins, and the list grows at the rate of about one a year. In addition, there are a number of cytokines that merit interleukin numbers, but which for historical reasons are better known by another name. The situation may be rationalized by adopting a new nomenclature.

TUMOUR NECROSIS FACTOR (TNF)

TNF was named for its ability to induce haemorrhagic necrosis of certain experimental tumours. TNFα is produced mainly by macrophages, and induces fever, hypotension, hypercoagulability, and cardiovascular collapse when released into the circulation. At the cellular level, TNFα stimulates leucocyte microbicidal activity, induces adhesion receptors on endothelial cells, and appears to regulate cell growth and apoptosis. TNFβ has similar actions but is produced mainly by T lymphocytes. The uncontrolled release of TNF (and probably other proinflammatory cytokines) from macrophages may be largely responsible for the shock syndrome following Gram-negative septicaemia or intravascular release of bacterial endotoxins. While excessive release of TNF is associated with morbidity and mortality, the production of TNF has also been shown in experimental animals to be necessary for resistance to infection. The effective *in vivo* level of TNF must be related to TNF-binding proteins, which are produced under inflammatory conditions. TNF also binds to two distinct TNF receptors, which may result in different effects on target cells. The clinical value of inhibitors of TNF is being actively investigated.

INTERFERONS

The interferons are a group of proteins with the property of interfering with the spread of viral infection from one cell to another, by enhancing cellular resistance. The main members of this group are interferons-α and -β (known as type I interferons). Their synthesis and release is triggered by viral infection of cells, and their protective effect is exerted on neighbouring, uninfected cells, in which antiviral biochemical adaptations are induced. Thus the spread of a viral infection from cell to cell within a tissue may be inhibited.

Interferon-γ, a type II interferon, has weak antiviral action, and plays

Table 1 *The important cytokines*

Cytokine	Biochemistry	Major actions
Interleukins (IL)		
IL-1	Two forms—α and β. Closely related receptor antagonist (IL-1ra) Two forms of receptor that α,β, and IL-1ra bind	Released from activated macrophages and other cells Pyrogen, proinflammatory
IL-2	Single form	Released from stimulated T lymphocytes; major T-cell growth factor
IL-4, IL-10, IL-13	IL-4 and IL-13 are related 'Th2' cytokines and may bind the same receptor protein.	Promote IgE production and inhibit cell-mediated immunity and production of proinflammatory cytokines by macrophages
Tumour necrosis factor	Closely related α and β forms Genes closely linked, in MHC class III region Two forms of receptor, which may transduce different intracellular signals Soluble receptor may increase plasma half-life of trimeric active form	Major proinflammatory cytokine, together with IL-1, and IL-6, responsible for many features of inflammation, fever, and septic shock syndromes High levels are correlated with increased morbidity and mortality, but moderate levels appear necessary for resistance to infection Cytotoxic effects important in cytotoxic T-lymphocyte-mediated killing, apoptosis, and programmed cell death
Interferons (IFN)		
Type I interferons (IFNα and β)	α and β families of related proteins	Produced by many cells, responsible for enhancing natural cellular resistance to viral infection
IFNγ	Single molecular form; binds single, multicomponent receptor	Major activator of macrophage microbicidal and cytotoxic activity Vital for effective cell-mediated immunity, and inhibition of inappropriate B-lymphocyte proliferation and antibody production
Colony-stimulating factors	Macrophage, granulocyte, and macrophage/granulocyte CSFs have been characterized: all are unique proteins that bind cognate receptors on their target cells IL-3 may be regarded as a 'multilineage' CSF, while IL-5 has growth-promoting effects on eosinophils	Promote growth and differentiation of the relevant haemopoietic cell lineage, and also have activating and chemoattractant properties in some cases (e.g. IL-5) Role in normal, steady-state haemopoiesis is not clear
Growth factors	Large number of diverse proteins with growth promoting effects (e.g. platelet-derived growth factor, fibroblast growth factor, keratinocyte growth factor) A number of common oncogenes are related to growth factors and their receptors Transforming growth factor-β (TGFβ) is a family of homo- and heterodimers with its own family of receptors.	Fibroblast and endothelial cell proliferation is an integral part of the inflammatory response, under the influence of growth factors Growth factors such as epidermal growth factor are also involved in the healing of epithelia damaged by inflammation TGFβ has a profound inhibitory effect on inflammatory reactions, and also favours Th2-type immune responses by reducing the production of proinflammatory cytokines by macrophages
Chemokines		
(IL-8, monocyte chemotactic peptide, macrophage inflammatory protein 1, RANTES, and others)	Two families of small proteins with conserved, cysteine-containing amino acid sequences characterize this group A large family of receptors has been discovered, but the relation of individual chemokines to receptors is still ill understood	Members of this group share some properties (such as induction of fever) with other cytokines, but their striking property is the ability to recruit, by chemotaxis, specific subgroups of leucocytes: e.g. IL-8—neutrophils, RANTES—memory T cells

a pivotal part in promoting cell-mediated immune responses. It is released by natural killer cells and T lymphocytes. It promotes macrophage activation to an enhanced antimicrobial and tumouricidal state, while inhibiting the proliferation and differentiation of B lymphocytes. Interferon-γ is the major 'Th1' cytokine, whose effects are opposed by and opposed to 'Th2' cytokines such as IL-4,-10, and -13 (see below).

CHEMOKINES

This term refers to two related families of relatively small, cysteine-rich proteins with strong sequence homology between family members. Most of the members of this group, which includes IL-8, monocyte chemotactic peptide (**MCP**) and macrophage inflammatory proteins 1α and β, are potent and specific chemoattractants for different groups of leucocytes. For instance, IL-8 is a specific chemoattractant for neutrophils, while MCP attracts predominantly monocytes. Another member of this group, known as RANTES, has the interesting property of attracting monocytes and memory T cells.

HAEMOPOIETIC GROWTH FACTORS (SEE ALSO SECTION 22)

The discovery of soluble factors that encouraged the growth and differentiation of specific cell types from undifferentiated precursors in the bone marrow led to the cloning and characterization of colony-stimulating factors (**CSF**): M-CSF for monocyte CSF, G-CSF for granulocyte CSF and GM-CSF for granulocyte–monocyte CSF, which encourages the growth of mixed colonies of cells. In addition, IL-3, which stimulates the growth of multiple lineages including megakaryocytes, is known as multiCSF. IL-5, which enhances the production of eosinophils, may also be included in this category.

In addition to their effects on growth and differentiation, the CSFs have other proinflammatory actions, and while increased levels of G-CSF and GM-CSF may be detected during illness, it is not clear what the role of the CSFs is in normal haemopoiesis. G-CSF, GM-CSF, and IL-3 are all being evaluated for use clinically, to overcome the effects of bone marrow suppression from whatever cause.

Erythropoietin arguably is a member of this group, but appears distinct in having a discrete source in the kidney, and the apparently single biological activity of stimulating erythropoiesis.

GROWTH FACTORS

Classical growth factors such as platelet-derived growth factor (**PDGF**) are included in the cytokine scheme because they are derived from similar cell sources, in response to similar stimuli, and act on similar targets in the same microenvironment as the other cytokines. The growth factors have multiple biological actions in addition to the promotion of cell multiplication. Transforming growth factor-β (**TGFβ**) appears particularly important in reducing the intensity of acute inflammatory reactions, promoting humoural rather than cell-mediated immune reactions, and favouring fibrosis as the end-result of inflammation. The release of PDGF, as well as other cytokines, from platelets, may play a key part in the generation of atheromatous plaques.

Mode of action

Like peptide hormones, cytokines act by binding to cell-surface receptors, which then transduce intracellular signals that result in modifications of the target cell—ultimately by changes in the pattern of gene transcription. The intracellular second-messenger systems used vary depending on the particular cytokine and its receptor or receptors. An emerging theme is that dimerization of receptors upon binding of the cytokine agonist is an important step in signal transduction.

The general idea of one cytokine–one receptor is complicated in many cases by the existence of a family of closely related cytokines, which may all bind the same receptor, or a family of related receptors. The complexity is further increased by the existence of binding proteins and soluble forms of the receptor(s), which may bind cytokines, and receptor-blocking proteins, which resemble the cytokine and bind to its receptor without transducing a signal.

The potential molecular interactions involved when a cytokine is released are shown in Fig. 2. In this scheme, the net effect of a given concentration of the cytokine is a complex function of the relative concentration of α- and β-forms, the presence of different forms of receptor, the concentration of soluble antagonists and/or binding proteins, and the binding-affinity constants of all these molecular species for each other. The corollary of this daunting complexity is that therapeutic strategies using recombinant proteins may involve recombinant cytokines, antagonists, soluble receptors, or even mutant forms of the cytokine that bind one or other receptor preferentially. Similarly, antibodies and pharmacological agents may be targeted at any part of the network.

Physiological role

To understand the physiological role of cytokines, it is necessary to describe briefly the process by which a cytokine characterized. The first step in studying a new cytokine involves the production of a soluble factor from cells, such as leucocytes, which have been suitably stimulated, for example by adding bacterial endotoxin.

The factor is then shown to have a potent biological action, for example causing fever. Such a factor might be provisionally named 'leucocyte pyrogen'. Further biochemical purification and characterization lead to molecular cloning of the gene for 'leucocyte pyrogen', which might show it to be a unique protein not previously described, and it would then be assigned an official name (preferably an interleukin number). The 'gold standard' for assigning particular biological activities to newly described cytokines would be reproduce the activities of the original 'factor' using pure recombinant protein, and to block the activities of the protein using specific antibodies. In certain cases it is also possible to produce transgenic animals that have an excess of, or entirely lack, the cytokine in question.

Fig. 2 Cytokine–receptor interactions. Cytokines act by binding to cell-surface receptors, which then transduce intracellular signals using a variety of second-messenger systems. The simple case of a single cytokine interacting with its cognate receptor on the responding cell is often complicated in reality by the existence of multiple biochemical subtypes of a single cytokine (shown here as cytokine a and cytokine b, and a cell membrane-bound form of cytokine a); multiple species of receptors (shown here as receptor I and receptor II); and physiological antagonists, either in the form of homologues of the cytokine, which bind to the receptors without transducing a signal (receptor antagonists), or in the form of soluble receptors, which bind to and inactivate or modify the cytokine. The relative abundance of each of these interacting molecular species and their respective binding affinities determine the final effect on the target cell. While this complicated network makes the study of cytokine effects difficult, it also provides multiple opportunities for pharmacological intervention.

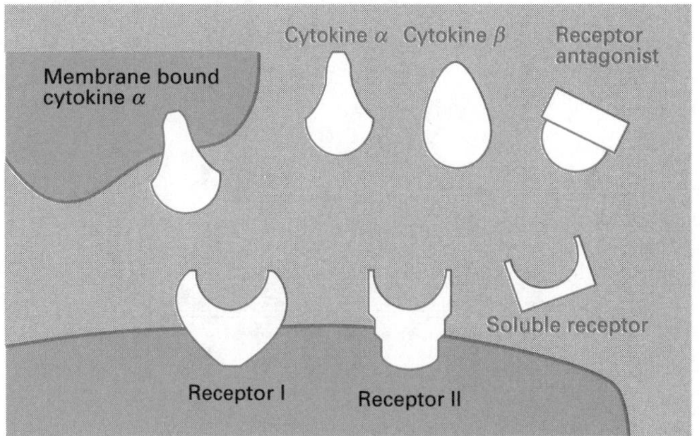

INFLAMMATORY REACTIONS

It is impossible to describe the well-known cellular phenomena of acute inflammation—leucocyte migration, phagocytosis of micro-organisms, removal of debris from injured tissue, formation of new blood vessels, and healing—without reference to cytokines (Fig. 3).

IL-1 and TNFα are responsible for inducing the expression of receptors on endothelial cells that permit adhesion of leucocytes to the vessel wall. Endothelial cells may in turn produce increased amounts of CSFs, signalling the need for increased haemopoiesis in the bone marrow, while IL-1 and -6, together with TNFα, released into the bloodstream by macrophages, act on the central nervous system and liver to induce pyrexia and the hepatic acute-phase reaction, respectively. Other consequences of inflammation, such as arthralgia, myalgia, muscle wasting, and increased slow-wave sleep, are also caused by systemic release of proinflammatory cytokines.

The recruitment of leucocytes to sites of injury and infection may be partly achieved by microbial chemoattractants and tissue breakdown products, but the recruitment of specific groups of leucocytes (neutrophils, eosinophils, monocytes) is probably due to the selective release of specific chemotactic cytokines such as the chemokines. The microbial factors that determine which predominant subgroup of leucocytes is recruited are not known. Chemoattractant cytokines may be produced by local inflammatory cells as well by parenchymal cells of the affected tissue, and by fibroblasts in the connective tissue. Parenchymal cells may also respond to inflammatory cytokines by enhancing cellular defence mechanisms, the production of heat-shock proteins for example.

In the resolution phase of inflammation, growth factors produced by macrophages, fibroblasts, and parenchymal cells play a part in inducing angiogenesis, fibroblast proliferation, collagen production, and epithelial healing. Inadequate inflammatory responses, as much as over-exuberant responses, prevent proper repair and healing.

IMMUNOLOGICAL REACTIONS (SEE ALSO SECTION 5)

The production of adequate cell-mediated or humoral immunity requires a complex interaction between antigen-presenting cells, helper T lymphocytes, B lymphocytes, and effector cells such as cytotoxic T lymphocytes and macrophages. This interaction involves cell–cell contact via cell-surface proteins as well contact-independent signalling via soluble cytokines (Fig. 4).

The initial interaction of antigen-presenting cells with T cells involves the secretion of IL-1, which is a costimulatory factor for T-cell proliferation. The major cytokine stimulus for T-cell proliferation following recognition of an antigen is IL-2, which is produced by proliferating T cells, and acts in an autocrine manner to increase both IL-2 receptor levels and IL-2 secretion.

T-helper cells proliferating in response to antigen produce a large number of cytokines, and the regulation of T-cell cytokine production is the subject of intensive research. Helper T cells can produce cytokines such as IL-5, which has eosinophil chemotactic and growth-promoting activities, GM-CSF, which promotes the production of monocytes and neutrophils, IL-4,-7, and -10, which promote the differentiation and proliferation of B lymphocytes, T-lymphocyte growth factors such as IL-9 and -12, and IFNγ which activate macrophages and greatly enhance their ability to ingest and kill.

Helper T cells produce two main groups of cytokines: those promoting cell-mediated immunity (i.e. enhanced proliferation of T cells, activation of macrophages) and those promoting humoural immunity (i.e. enhanced proliferation of B cells and maturation of the antibody response, recruitment of eosinophils). The first type of response is known as Th1, while the second type is known as a Th2. While the stimuli favouring one or other response are not completely understood, it is known that certain antigens tend to provoke humoral responses (e.g. common allergens) while others provoke cell-mediated immunity (e.g. mycobacteria). Understanding and manipulating this aspect of the immune response, in diseases as wide ranging as asthma, HIV infection, and leprosy, may be of great clinical benefit in the near future.

OTHER ROLES

Cytokines such as PDGF have been implicated in the pathogenesis of atheromatous plaques. The role of other cytokines that may specifically recruit monocytes and modify their lipid uptake and metabolism is under

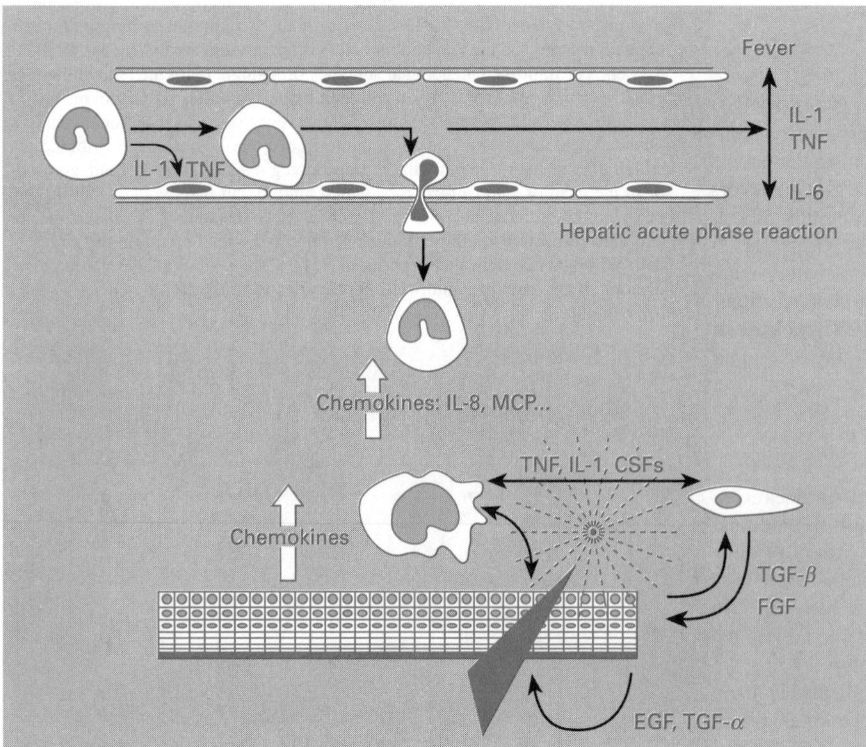

Fig. 3 Role of cytokines in acute inflammation. Classical proinflammatory cytokines IL(interleukin)-1, tumour necrosis factor (TNF), and IL-6 play a major part in acute inflammation, as shown here following a thorn prick to the skin. Resident inflammatory cells, including mast cells, natural killer cells and macrophages, all release preformed inflammatory mediators, such as histamine and cytokines, which attract new leucocytes to the area (chemokines). Injured blood vessels contribute to this initial burst of cytokine release through the release of platelet granule contents. Locally released cytokines act on endothelial cells in the vicinity to increase their adhesiveness for circulating leucocytes. This is achieved by increasing the surface expression of adhesion molecules. Leucocytes adhering to altered endothelial cells migrate out of the blood vessels and enter the inflamed tissue, moving towards released chemokines. Release of cytokines such as IL-1 and IL-6 from these leucocytes into the bloodstream is responsible for the systemic signs of inflammation (e.g. fever and production of acute-phase serum proteins). Fibroblasts and tissue cells such as epithelial cells contribute to the resolution of inflammation by producing growth factors, including transforming growth factor-β, which profoundly limits the inflammatory reaction. This is very important for healing and prevention of damage by excessive inflammation.

investigation. Cytokines undoubtedly play a part in the development of lymphohaemopoietic cells in the bone marrow, thymus, spleen, and peripherally. However, the precise cytokines involved, their cellular sources, and mode of action are not well understood.

Therapeutic uses

Despite the availability of pure recombinant material, cytokine-based therapies have not yet found their place in everyday practice, but remain an area of active research. One of the major obstacles to using cytokines clinically is the extreme multiplicity of their actions, resulting in excessive side-effects. There are also no clearly defined deficiency or excess states in which one single cytokine may be implicated—this is due at least in part to the overlap in function between many cytokines. In addition, the appropriate dosages, routes, and modes of delivery for therapeutic trial are difficult to predict, as cytokines are normally produced at high levels only at local sites of inflammation for short periods of time.

Fig. 4 Cytokines in immune reactions. Cytokines are involved at all stages of the generation of an immune response to an antigen. The presentation of antigen to T cells by dedicated antigen-presenting cells (APC) is accompanied by the production of IL(interleukin)-1, which acts as a costimulatory molecule for lymphocyte proliferation. The main stimulus for lymphocyte proliferation is IL-2, which is produced by proliferating lymphocytes themselves. The initial 'cytokine environment' in which antigen presentation occurs is determined by the production of cytokines such as IFN(interferon)-γ, IL-12, IL-4, and transforming growth factor-β (TGFβ) by APC, natural killer cells (NK cells), and parenchymal tissue cells. It is thought that immune reactions are biased towards Th1 or Th2 type reactions by this initial interaction. T-helper cells produce cytokines that influence the further development and proliferation of the T cells themselves, and effector cells such as B cells and macrophages. Th1 cells produce cytokines that inhibit the production of cytokines by Th2 cells and vice versa. In the effector phase of immunity, cytotoxic T cells (CTL) produce TNFβ, which induces DNA fragmentation and death in susceptible target cells. Macrophages stimulated by Th1 cytokines produce proinflammatory cytokines and cytotoxic products that help to combat infections and kill tumour cells.

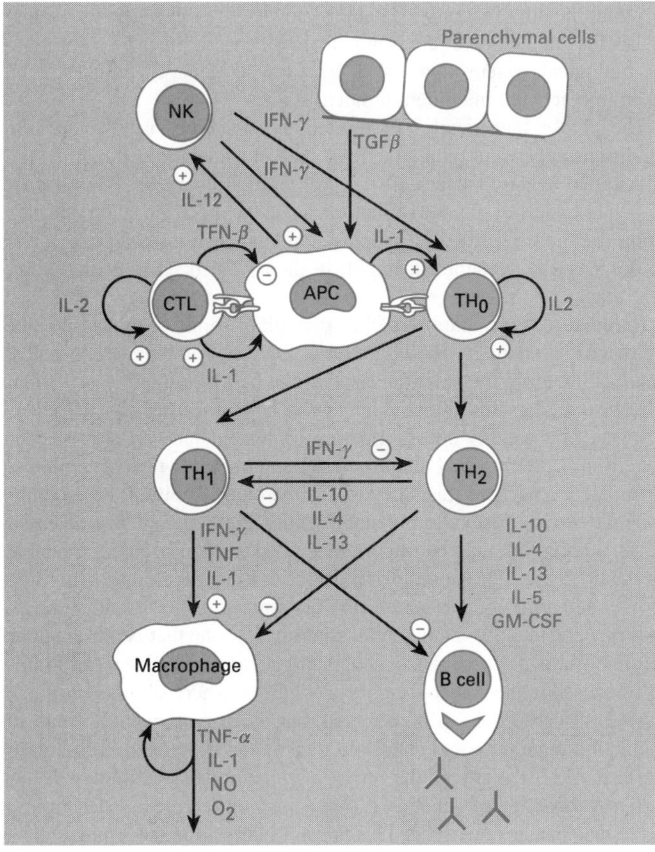

Recombinant human G-CSF and GM-CSF have been used with some success in increasing neutrophil counts following high-dose, marrow-ablative chemotherapy. However, no clear benefit in overall outcome has been demonstrated. Recombinant proteins with active moieties from both IL-3 and GM-CSF are now being studied in relation to boosting neutrophil and platelet counts following marrow ablation.

Some success has been achieved in the use of recombinant human IFNγ for the treatment of patients with chronic granulomatous disease, a variably inherited deficiency in the superoxide-generating pathway of neutrophils. The mechanism of action of IFNγ in this setting is not clear. A novel approach aimed at avoiding the side-effects of systemically administered cytokines involves the removal of lymphocytes from patients with tumours, *in vitro* treatment with IL-2, which activates the lymphocytes, and reinfusion of the cells. Reinfused, cytokine-treated cells home in on the tumour, where their enhanced cytotoxicity may result in tumour regression.

Cytokine-blocking therapies have been advocated for a number of illnesses in which excessive inflammation is the major problem. A variety of approaches are being pursued, including the use of antibodies against cytokines and their receptors, and recombinant natural inhibitors such as soluble TNF receptor and IL-1 receptor antagonist (**IL-1ra**). Both soluble TNF receptor and recombinant IL-1ra have proved beneficial in small initial trials in the treatment of endotoxic shock. The use of inhibitors (such as antibodies) of Th2 cytokines to switch dysfunctional allergic responses towards protective cell-mediated immunity is another potential therapeutic option. Another promising avenue is the use of non-protein, low molecular-weight compounds such as the bicyclic imidazoles, which interfere with the production of proinflammatory cytokines.

REFERENCES

Arai, K. *et al.* (1990). Cytokines: coordinators of immune and inflammatory responses. *Annual Review of Biochemistry*, **59,** 783.

Balkwill, F.R., and Burke, F. (1989). The cytokine network. *Immunology Today*, **10,** 299.

Clemens, M.J. (1991). *Cytokines.* BIOS Scientific Publications, Oxford.

Dalton, D.K. *et al.* (1993). Multiple defects of immune cell function in mice with disrupted interferon-γ genes. *Science*, **259,** 1739–42.

De Maeyer, E., and De Maeyer-Guignard, J. (1988). *Interferons and other regulatory cytokines.* Wiley, New York.

diGiovane, F.S., and Duff, G.W. (1990). Interleukin 1: the first interleukin. *Immunology Today*, **11,** 13.

Nicola, N. (1989). Hemopoietic cell growth factors and their receptors. *Annual Review of Biochemistry*, **58,** 45.

Meager, A. (1990). *Cytokines.* Open University Press, Milton Keynes.

Wardle, E.N. (1993). Cytokines: an overview. *European Journal of Medicine*, **3,** 417–23.

4.3 Genetic factors in disease

M. E. Pembrey

Genetics and medicine

INTRODUCTION

The relative decline in the prevalence of infectious and nutritional deficiency diseases in many populations over the years has highlighted the contribution that inherited disease makes to the suffering of humans.

At least 1 per cent of all live babies have a disorder inherited in a simple mendelian fashion that is manifest at birth, or will develop later. If one includes multifactorial conditions where there are substantial genetic influences, the proportion rises to 2 to 5 per cent. It has been estimated that genetic causes account for 75 per cent of all severe handicapping disorders in childhood, and increasingly these children are surviving into adult life. Genetic factors can also greatly influence the susceptibility, or resistance, to many of the chronic mental and physical illnesses of later life. Not only are patients with inherited diseases encountered in virtually all clinical disciplines, but an understanding of gene activity at the cellular level is essential for a full understanding of the pathogenesis of many diseases. In short, genetics is an integral part of modern medicine.

Over the last few years, the many technical developments have allowed rapid progress towards mapping and characterizing the 75 000 or so genes in the human genome, an international effort that is known collectively as the Human Genome Project. Much of this advance in human molecular genetics has come from biomedical research focused on particular diseases, an activity that demands the closest of collaboration between clinicians and molecular biologists. In return, this liaison allows the very rapid translation of research discoveries into service for patients and their families. This chapter includes some of these improvements in diagnostic precision, prognostication, clinical management, and genetic prediction as part of genetic counselling. Figure 1 summarizes the lively interface between the domains of clinical and laboratory science when the focus is on the cloning (i.e. isolating the length of DNA corresponding to at least the coding region) of a gene that is defective in a particular disease. The thick arrows emphasize the elements that are critically dependent on the input of practising clinicians.

The molecular aspects of gene structure and function are outlined in Chapter 4.1

Is it genetically determined?

This is a common question that often cannot be answered in a simple yet meaningful way. Clearly, the growth, development, and maintenance of health in any individual is dependent on the constant interaction of the genes that were inherited and an environment that varies within certain limits. However, in medicine as in human biology generally, what usually concern us practically are the differences between individuals. Given the same general environmental circumstances, why was this child born deaf and the brother not, or why did this woman develop diabetes mellitus, whilst many people never do? It is helpful to think of several categories of disorder. At one extreme there is complete hereditary determination. The abnormality, or failing health in early life, is determined at conception; the course of events is altered little by environmental factors. The condition arises in people of a certain genetic constitution, always occurring in those people and in those people only. This is the case with most chromosomal abnormalities and the so-called monogenic conditions inherited in a simple mendelian fashion. The second category of disorder occurs only in people with a certain genetic constitution, but not in everyone with that constitution. The third category of disorder occurs with varying frequency that is dependent on the person's genetic constitution. Finally, there is complete environmental determination, for practical purposes uninfluenced by the person's genetic constitution.

Some people fear that the Human Genome Project and advances in molecular genetics generally are leading to undue focus on the genetic component of diseases of complex aetiology, when useful interventions are likely to come from an understanding of the non-genetic factors. Two points should be made in reply. First, as an adverse environmental change becomes more marked and challenging, so there will be a phase when any genetic differences in people's ability to deal with it will tend to be revealed, although eventually, of course, an extreme environmental stress will overwhelm all genotypes. Thus, paradoxically, demonstration of genetic differences between those who develop a common mutifactorial disease and those who do not does not necessarily diminish the likely importance of environmental influences in that disease, rather it may actually indicate rising environmental pressure of great importance to public health. Secondly, detailed knowledge of the genetic factors assists the elucidation of environmental influences, either by pointing to the biological system involved or by allowing genetic variables to be taken into account in epidemiological studies.

The phrase 'genetically determined' is sometimes used to include conditions dependent on a genetic change in a somatic cell that is then transmitted to descendant cells as proliferation proceeds. Such a phenomenon underlies tumour formation, a genetic mutation being one step along the multistep road to neoplasia. Whilst such a phenomenon can be described as 'genetic', it is not, in the accepted sense of the word, hereditary.

Hereditary determination implies that all, or some, of the germ cells, the ova or sperm, carry the mutation or relevant combination of genes. There is therefore the potential for these to be transmitted to offspring. In some disorders this potential may never be realized because the severity of the abnormality does not permit prolonged survival or reproduction. Many chromosomal abnormalities, and probably many rarer lethal birth defects, fall into this category. In the clinical setting these conditions are usually just called 'genetic', although the hereditary potential exists, a point that may be important if the condition becomes treatable for the first time. The sporadic occurrence of a disorder tells you nothing about whether or not it is genetically determined. Likewise, it is important to appreciate that a congenital abnormality, one that is present at or before birth, is not necessarily genetically determined. The term 'familial' was used in the past to describe a condition where siblings (brothers or sisters) were likely to be affected, but the parents were normal, in distinction to an inherited condition transmitted from one generation to the next. Whilst many of the terms just mentioned are still used, our current knowledge of genetics allows a much more precise description of the mechanisms involved. This is particularly so in the simple inherited disorders and chromosome defects.

A useful distinction when considering genetic factors is the actual combination of particular genes inherited, the genotype, and the observable effect the activity of these genes produce in the individual, the corresponding phenotype. In molecular terms, genotype refers to DNA and phenotype to proteins as they naturally appear in the tissues. The terms genotype and phenotype are usefully limited to the discussion of one particular gene (or a few) and its effect.

Fig. 1 A flow diagram illustrating the various contributions to cloning a disease gene and the various clinical benefits that can follow. The clinicians' involvement is indicated by the thick arrows.

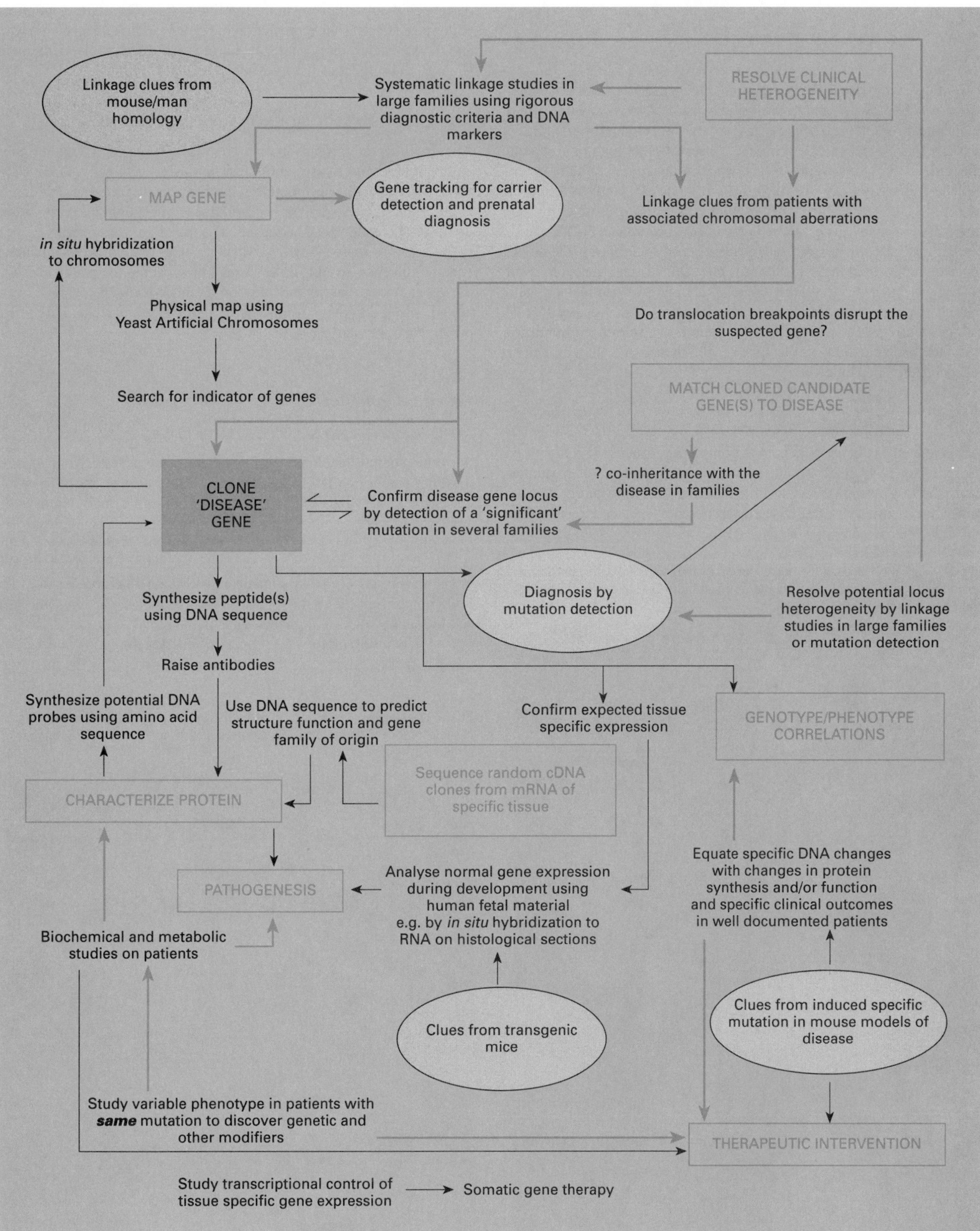

There are three basic approaches to elucidating genetic factors in disease: twin studies, family studies, and direct analysis of chromosomes or genes.

TWIN STUDIES

The simplest of these is the comparison of concordance in monozygotic (identical, **MZ**) twins, and in dizygotic twins. MZ twins have inherited an identical complement of genes and will be concordant for a condition that is wholly genetically determined. Observation of high or complete concordance in monozygotic twins, whilst indicating hereditary determination, does not provide information about the number of genes involved. The key features of the human face are determined by the interaction of many genes; there is complete concordance in MZ twins but because of the number of independent genes contributing, the recurrence of an identical face in siblings is rare. On the other hand, albinism is the consequence of the inheritance of a single pair of mutant genes; there is complete concordance in MZ twins and a high (usually 1 in 4) risk of recurrence in siblings. It is the pattern of recurrence in families that yields information on the type of inheritance and the number of independent genes involved.

FAMILY STUDIES

Pedigree analysis is the cornerstone of medical genetics. The advent of recombinant DNA technology, with the ability to look at particular genes directly, has in no way lessened the importance of family studies; rather it has emphasized it. Disease associations, such as the discovery that a particular HLA type is more common in a specific patient population than expected, tell us little about the genetic influences on the disease without complementary family studies. The starting point for pedigree analysis is an appreciation of the way individual chromosomes and the genes they carry segregate during the formation of ova or sperm (Fig. 2), the subject of the next main section.

Fig. 2 Diagram illustrating the behaviour of a single chromosome pair during the reduction division, or meiosis, and fertilization. (Reproduced from Roberts and Pembrey (1985) with permission.)

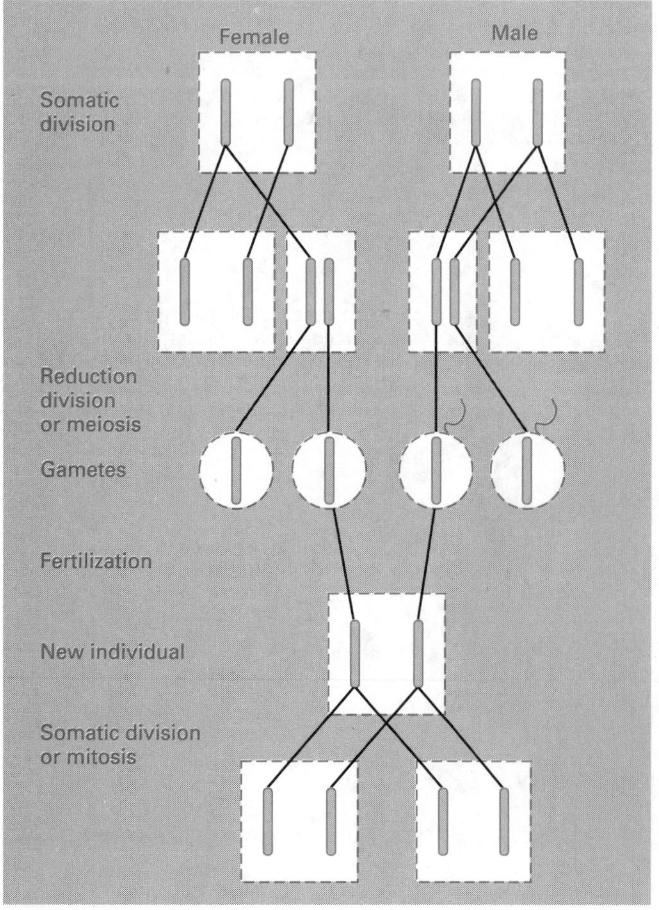

DIRECT ANALYSIS OF CHROMOSOMES OR GENES

Abnormalities in chromosome number, and increasingly smaller alterations in chromosome structure, can be observed directly. Analysis of the DNA with gene-specific DNA probes can indicate the deletion of all, or parts of, genes and may also detect certain significant alterations in DNA nucleotide-base sequence. The consistent co-inheritance of a specific DNA segment with a disease within families establishes a genetic influence, even if little else is known about the pathogenesis.

Any attempt to answer the question 'Is this disorder genetically determined, and if so how is it inherited?' requires an understanding of the principles of human genetics.

Essential genetics

ASSORTMENT AND SEGREGATION OF GENES

A working definition of the word 'gene' will emerge later, but in essence it is that part of the DNA double helix within the chromosome which codes for a particular RNA molecule that, in turn, usually dictates the synthesis of a polypeptide chain at ribosomes in the cell cytoplasm. The transmission of genes from parent to offspring is dependent on the behaviour of the chromosomes during the formation of gametes, the ova or sperm (Fig. 2). Ordinary somatic cells contain 46 chromosomes (diploid complement), 22 pairs of autosomes, and a sex chromosome pair, XX in females and XY in males. Thus in the female there are 23 homologous pairs and therefore two copies of every gene, one maternal and one paternal in origin. It is the same in males except for the difference

Fig. 3 The stages of mitosis illustrating the movement of two non-homologous chromosomes (as opposed to 46). (Reproduced from Roberts and Pembrey (1985) with permission.)

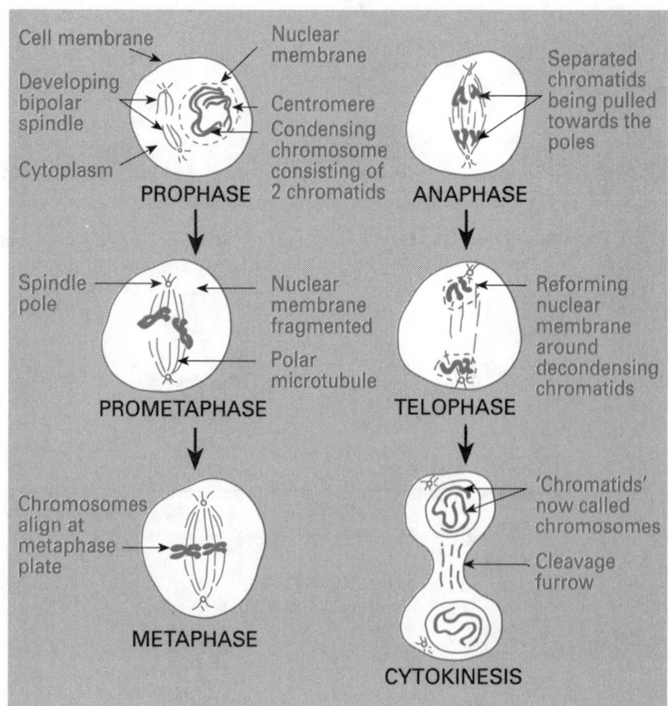

in the sex chromosome pair, which in essence means the genes carried on the X are present as a single copy. During somatic division, mitosis (Fig. 3), each chromosome and with it every gene along its length replicates faithfully, so that broadly speaking all nucleated cells of the body, except gametes, have 46 chromosomes and the same genetic make-up. Gamete formation, however, involves a special reduction division, meiosis (Fig. 4), which results in cells with a single set of 23 chromosomes (haploid complement). Which chromosome of a pair ends up in a particular gamete is essentially a matter of chance and is uninfluenced by whether it was maternal or paternal in origin, or the movement of the members of other pairs of chromosomes. In other words chromosome pairs assort independently giving 2^{23} possible combinations in the gametes. Further mixing of maternally and paternally derived genes results from the exchange, or crossing over, that occurs between chromosomes of the same (homologous) pair when they align alongside each other during the early stages of meiosis, as illustrated in Fig. 4. With all this assortment of genes it is important not to lose sight of the fact that genes, like chromosomes, are paired; only one of a pair, not both, will end up in any particular gamete. This last point is of no practical consequence if the genes of the pair are exactly same, but of great importance if they differ in some way. The word allele is used to describe an alternative form of one of the gene pair, and this concept together with the term gene locus is best explained by an example.

β-Globin contributes to the formation of adult haemoglobin (α_2 β_2; see Section 22). There is one β-globin gene on each of the pair of chromosomes 11. The two β-globin genes together constitute the β-globin gene locus. So alleles are alternative forms of a gene at a single locus. One of the nucleotides in one of the two β-globin genes is altered

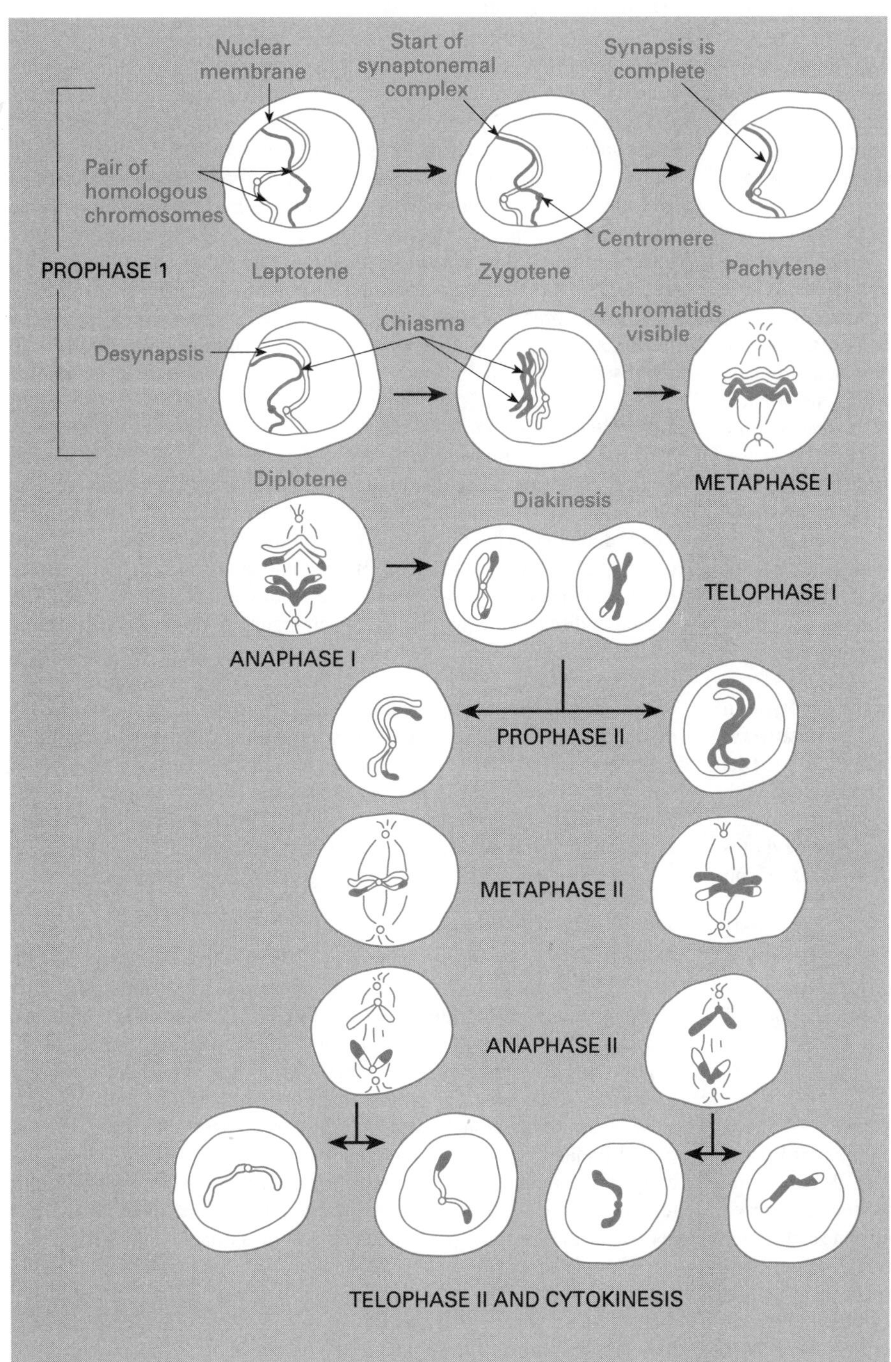

Fig. 4 The stages of meiosis illustrating one pair of homologous chromosomes (as opposed to 23 pairs). Paternally derived chromosome, black; maternally derived chromosome, white. Note how the four haploid cells at the end each contain a chromosome derived from one of the four chromatids visible at diakinesis of prophase I. The consequences of two crossovers involving the same two chromatids are illustrated. (Reproduced from Roberts and Pembrey (1985) with permission.)

in people with the sickle-cell trait, and therefore the sickle, or β^s, gene and the normal β-gene are alleles (see Section 22). Such a person cannot pass on the normal β- and the β^s-gene to a particular child because the gamete involved carries either one or the other, but not both; in other words, the two alleles segregate. Obviously, with only two DNA sites any one individual can only have two alleles at any one locus. However, in the population there may be numerous alleles and indeed over a hundred variants of β-globin chain have been described. In summary, genes at different loci assort whilst alleles segregate.

LOCI AND ALLELES

A meaningful classification of disease is essential for good clinical practice. As more and more genes are mapped and sequenced (or at least their exons and exon/intron junctions are sequenced), the closer we can get to a definitive classification of the simply inherited, or Mendelian, disorders. The first requirement is to know which gene locus (or loci—see Locus heterogeneity below) is involved in a particular disease phenotype. To date, nearly all the normal genetic variation in human populations seems to be confined to small changes in DNA sequences rather than in the actual position of a particular gene on the chromosome; a fact that allows universal human gene maps to be constructed. As indicated above, this relatively constant chromosomal position of a gene is known as the gene locus.

Where the alleles at an autosomal locus are the same, the term homozygous is used. Where one is the normal, common or 'wild type' allele and the other a mutant, the individual is said to be heterozygous. Where an individual has two different mutant alleles, they are called compound heterozygotes. This terminology works well in clinical genetics where one is dealing with harmful mutations and simple mendelian inheritance. Now that it is becoming possible to characterize the mutations in autosomal recessive disorders at the level of DNA sequence, it turns out that many affected individuals are not homozygotes in the strictest sense, that is homoallelic, but compound heterozygotes. Nevertheless, because both alleles are clinically significant mutants, the person has no normally functioning allele and is clinically affected. In Britain, about 60 per cent of patients with cystic fibrosis are true homozygotes with a deletion of codon 508 of the *CFTR* gene on each chromosome 7, whilst the remainder are nearly all compound heterozygotes (e.g. Δ-508 on one chromosome 7 and a point mutation at codon 551 on the other chromosome 7, or other combinations).

In clinical genetics one needs to be able to describe the genotype in a meaningful way when it comes to DNA analysis, and so it is useful to use the term compound heterozygote for distinguishing these patients from healthy carriers or heterozygotes. However, when dealing with highly polymorphic loci, with numerous normally functioning alleles (e.g. the *HLA* genes), the distinction between the terms heterozygotes and compound heterozygotes becomes meaningless and serves no purpose.

The term hemizygous refers to the situation when there is just a single chromosome involved. A male that carries a mutant gene on his only X chromosome is often called hemizygous as is a person who has had a whole gene locus deleted from one of an autosomal pair of chromosomes.

Allele-specific disease phenotypes

The protein product (or products, produced by differential RNA splicing) of the same gene may serve a different role during embryological development than in the maintenance and functioning of the fully differentiated tissue. Distinct domains of the protein product can serve separate purposes and so different mutations of the same gene can sometimes produce different clinical outcomes; indeed, so different that, from the clinical point of view, there would be little to suspect that the two diseases were due to mutations at the same gene locus. Some types of mutations in the *RET* oncogene at 10q11.2 can produce Hirschsprung's disease, where there is inadequate neuronal migration down the colon during development, whilst other mutations in the same gene are responsible for the dominantly inherited cancer syndrome, multiple endocrine neoplasia type 2A. Sometimes the allele-specific disease phenotype arises because the point mutation enhances an existing tendency, the sickle mutation enhancing the tendency of deoxygenated adult haemoglobin molecules to aggregate for example. Sickle-cell disease, with its painful, vasculo-occlusive crises, presents a very different clinical picture from the transfusion dependence of β-thalassaemia, yet both are due to mutations in the β-globin gene at 11p15. Sickle-cell disease is unusual in that it always involves exactly the same mutation at codon 6 of the β-globin gene, usually on both the chromosomes of the pair, although sickle/thalassaemia compound heterozygotes may present a very similar clinical picture. However β-thalassaemia is much more typical of genetic disorders and can be caused by over 60 different mutations in the β-globin gene; in other words, it shows allelic heterogeneity.

Allelic heterogeneity

Allelic heterogeneity is where the same clinical condition can be produced by different mutations but at the gene locus. It is the rule rather than the exception with genetic diseases. Haemophilia B provides a striking example. A study in Britain of 216 unrelated individuals with haemophilia B found four gross deletions and 135 different, small, causal mutations in the factor IX gene. The different classes of mutations and their effects on function are listed later, but it is easy to imagine that any mutation that effectively knocks out gene expression will produce the same result, whilst two mutations that modify the protein product in very different ways could result in quite distinct phenotypes.

From the practical point of view, allelic heterogeneity poses problems for mutation detection. Defining the specific mutation in one family with the disease does little to predict what will be found in the next family.

Locus heterogeneity

This form of genetic heterogeneity refers to the apparent same or similar clinical condition being due to mutations at entirely different gene loci. One fairly obvious way this can arise is if the mature functional protein that is defective in the disease is a heterodimer where the two component polypeptide chains are products of different genes. A mutation in either gene could lead to a non-functional heterodimeric protein and therefore the same disease phenotype. Locus heterogeneity obviously causes difficulties when it comes to genetic counselling and predictive tests based on DNA analysis, whether mutation detection or gene tracking, as discussed later. There are many diseases that are difficult, if impossible, to distinguish clinically and yet are due to mutations at one of two or more gene loci. Table 1 lists a few important examples. These loci may be on one or more autosomes, and sometimes the X chromosome as well. Retinitis pigmentosa is an example of a disorder that can be inherited in either an X-linked or autosomal fashion.

The nature of the human genome

Figure 5 shows the human genome as it has been viewed for the last few decades. Each chromosome is an enormous DNA double helix of complementary nucleotide sequences. The DNA molecule is bound into chromatin by coiling around a protein complex, called a nucleosome, about every 200 nucleotide base pairs (bp) and then packing further in a supercoiled fashion. The only striking, normal variation in the appearance of the chromosomes is the sexual dimorphism—XY in males and XX in females. The most important Y-linked gene, *SRY,* which diverts early development along the male route by turning fetal gonads into testes, has already been cloned. However, apart from some genes concerned with spermatogenesis, there are presumably no other really important genes carried exclusively on the Y chromosome for the simple reason that half the human race manages very well without it! It follows that Y-linked genetic diseases do not feature large in medicine. It also indicates that most of the Y chromosome does not consist of expressed genes but some other form of DNA.

Table 1 *Some examples of locus heterogeneity, where indistinguishable diseases can be due to different mutant genes*

Disorder	Gene	Chromosomal location
Osteogenesis imperfecta type 1	Collagen 1 A1	17q21.31–q22.05
	Collagen 1 A2	7q21.3–q22.1
Tuberous sclerosis:		
TSC1	?	9q33–q22.1
TSC2	Tuberin	16p13
Epidermolysis bullosa simplex	Keratin 5	12q11–13
	Keratin 14	17q12–21
Retinitis pigmentosa:		
RP1	?	8p11–q21
RP2	?	Xp11–3
RP3	?	Xp21.1
RP4	Rhodopsin	3q21–q24
(RP5)		
RP6	?	Xp21.3–p21.2
RP7	Peripherin/RDS protein	6p21.1–ter
RP8	?	7q31–35
RP9	?	7q15.1–p13

MOST DNA IS REPETITIVE SEQUENCE

It is estimated that only a few per cent of the DNA comprising the whole human genome consists of genes encoding proteins. Much of the remainder is made up of repetitive DNA sequences, either dispersed throughout the genome like the minisatellite DNA of 'DNA fingerprinting' fame or contained in huge blocks, such as the heterochromatin that flanks the centromere of each chromosome. Some types of dispersed repeat sequence (e.g. di- or tetranucleotide repeat 'microsatellites') are particularly valuable as DNA markers in genetic linkage studies. This is because they not only define a particular position on a chromosome, but also the number of repeats varies considerably between individual copies of that chromosome in the general population. This in turn means that in most people the two chromosomes of the pair can be distinguished and their inheritance traced (see below).

Why the repeat sequences are there and what part they play in human disease is uncertain. What is certain is that this so-called junk DNA cannot be dismissed as being of no medical importance. The dispersed, 300-bp long, Alu sequence, which is repeated 500 000 to 1 million times throughout the human genome, can predispose to misalignment and unequal crossing over between chromosomes of the pair during egg or sperm formation, causing gene deletions or duplications. Furthermore, the haphazard 'jumping' of an Alu sequence (via a transcribed RNA product) into the middle of the *NF1* gene has been shown to be the causative mutation in at least one case of neurofibromatosis. Thus there is medical interest beyond just those nucleotide sequences that are transcribed and processed into mRNA molecules for translation into proteins, the regular expressed genes.

AN EVOLUTIONARY PERSPECTIVE ON GENE SEQUENCES

Unique identifier sequences of human genes (expressed sequence tags) are now being generated at the rate of many thousands per year. The way this is done, using the retroviral enzyme, reverse transcriptase, to

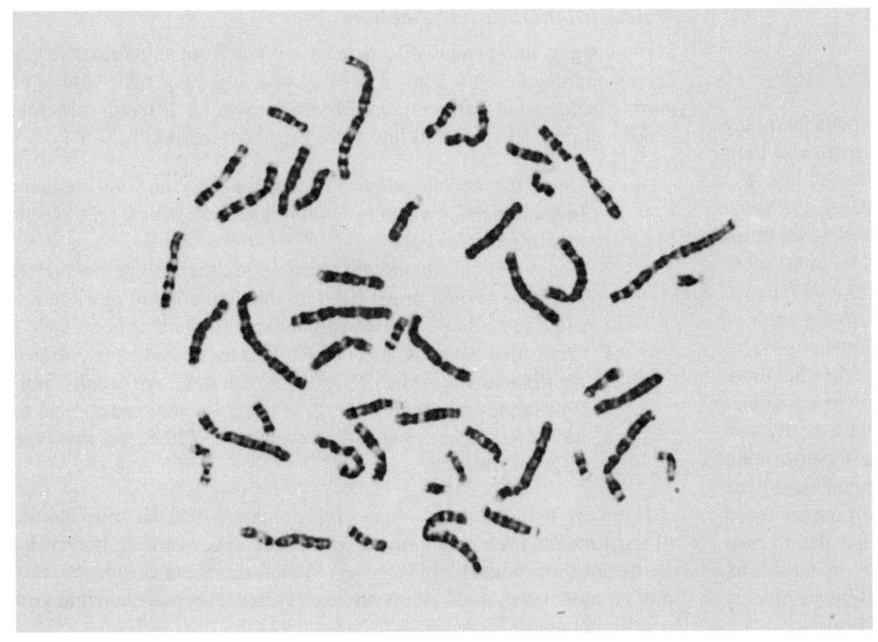

Fig. 5 The human genome in the form of 46 metaphase chromosomes. (Reproduced from Roberts and Pembrey (1985) with permission.)

generate DNA copies (cDNA) from mRNA molecules harvested from the tissue of choice, is described elsewhere. What is instructive for an understanding of the human genome is how the thousands of short (approx. 400 bp), partial gene sequences that are generated are being sorted out in a meaningful way. That any sense at all can be made of these random DNA sequences is a consequence of the evolutionary process. As one might expect, human evolution was not so much a matter of design but one of modification, reshuffling, and rejigging of pre-existing DNA sequences, the direction and speed of change being largely driven by natural selection. This has resulted in many entirely different genes sharing bits of DNA sequence in common.

Over evolutionary time these shared DNA sequences of different genes tend to accumulate different neutral or adaptive changes, but still retain sufficient DNA sequence homology for computer searches to detect some similarity. This means that analysis of the nucleotide-base sequence of a randomly cloned cDNA may well predict the gene's function and allow its tentative classification to a gene family. DNA sequence homology also allows the identification of equivalent genes across species. We share most of our genes with the mouse, which allows mouse models of human genetic diseases to be engineered (or discovered) to facilitate the elucidation of molecular pathology or develop new treatments.

Another evolutionary process that ran in parallel with exon shuffling was whole-gene duplication. Once duplicated, the two genes could gradually change, taking on slightly different, but still similar, functions. As further duplications occurred so a large gene family could emerge, such as the Ig superfamily embracing the immunoglobulin, *HLA,* and T-cell receptor genes amongst others. Gene families may remain clustered at one or two chromosomal locations, or become more dispersed. Some members of a gene family may accumulate disabling mutations, stop functioning, and become a pseudogene—a troublesome relic of the past that can predispose to deletions and duplications by unequal crossing over. Processed pseudogene is the name given to a pseudogene whose sequence resembles mRNA in that it has no introns and has a run of adenines at the 3′ end. These have clearly been incorporated into the genome by the reverse transcription of a mRNA intermediate. Thus, on an evolutionary timescale, and indeed for some genes even over a few generations (as occurs in the trinucleotide repeat expansions, described later), the human genome is far from fixed. Its structure reflects a dynamic process in which conservation of important sequences is set against a natural tendency for DNA replication and normal exchange between DNA molecules to go awry, with genetic disease as the consequence.

GENETIC LINKAGE AND GENE MAPPING

The transmission of genes from parents to offspring is dependent on the behaviour of the chromosomes that carry them, and in particular their behavior during gamete formation or meiosis, as illustrated in Fig. 4.

The term synteny is used to describe genes that are on the same chromosome. If there was no crossing over between homologous chromosomes during meiosis, then all syntenic genes would be transmitted *en bloc;* and all that would have been necessary to track the inheritance of any mutant gene would have been one or two markers for each of the 23 chromosomes. In fact, some 30 or so recombinations occur throughout the chromosome pairs in male meiosis (it is somewhat more in females), and so only genes or DNA markers that are close together on the chromosome would be expected to co-inherit consistently and not become separated by recombination. This means that demonstration of co-inheritance (i.e. demonstration of linkage) between a mutant gene and markers of known chromosomal location in a set of families maps the disease gene to that chromosomal region. It also means that to map all the disease genes of interest, a large number of markers ordered along each chromosome would be needed. Producing such a reference linkage map was one of the prime aims of the Human Genome Project.

Modern linkage maps represent an array of highly informative, easy-to-use, DNA markers along all the chromosomes, such that the transmission of any small chromosome region (and the genes within it) can be reliably tracked through the family pedigree. By 'highly informative' it is meant that in any one individual the DNA marker probe is very likely to reveal a naturally occurring DNA sequence variation (e.g. tandem-repeat polymorphism) that can be used to distinguish the two chromosomes of the pair. Use of such a high-resolution genome map of DNA markers will permit the mapping of the 'disease gene' (the genetic locus containing the mutation) by linkage analysis in any suitably large family affected by a simply inherited disease with a distinct phenotype. The limiting factors in mapping unmapped diseases are fast becoming access to large families, obtaining the family blood samples, and completing the clinical work-up to determine who is affected and who is not.

Consanguineous families can be particularly useful for mapping rare autosomal recessive mutation by what has become known as homozygosity, or more precisely, autozygosity mapping. When a child of first-cousin parents has a rare autosomal recessive disease, it is reasonable to assume that just one great-grandparent was a carrier and the mutant gene was transmitted down both sides of the family to come together as a 'double dose' in the affected child. Any DNA markers close to the mutation on the original great-grandparental chromosome will tend to co-inherit with the mutation and be present in the child, but in a double dose. Furthermore, because it is a double dose of a single ancestral chromosome, the DNA sequence of these closely linked markers will be exactly the same on both chromosomes of the pair (i.e. homo- or autozygous). Any DNA marker sequence that is heterozygous in the affected child must have become separated from the region containing the mutation by recombination during one of the six meioses in its journey down both sides of the family from great-grandparent to child. The ability to exclude all heterozygous markers in the affected child from close linkage to the disease mutation makes this a very efficient mapping method. It has already been used to map alkaptonuria to 3q2, and one non-syndromic autosomal recessive deafness locus to 13q1.

The statistical evaluation of whether or not the co-inheritance of disease and DNA marker is due to chance alone or reflects true genetic linkage, and some other aspects of linkage studies, are described elsewhere.

As indicated in the summary Fig. 1, the rare occurrence of a visible, chromosomal deletion or translocation in an affected subject can provide an initial linkage clue in autosomal dominant and X-linked diseases.

A developmental perspective

Many insights into genetic disorders have come from an increase in our understanding of embryological development and the genetic control of morphogenesis and differentiation. There are several different roles that genes can play and they fall into three broad categories.

1. Genes that encode proteins needed for tissue and cell structure (e.g. collagen, myosin or myelin) and metabolism (e.g. receptors or enzymes).
2. Genes that encode protein transcription factors that bind DNA and have as their prime function the regulation of other genes, often in response to extracellular signals such as hormones.
3. Genes that have untranslated RNA as their product (e.g. transfer RNA or ribosomal RNA), of which there are usually multiple copies in the genome. A few single-copy genes seem to have no protein product, for example *XIST,* the gene involved in X-inactivation.

There are many metabolic and other functions that all cells require all the time, and the genes involved in these processes are known by the quaint term housekeeping genes. Whilst their rate of transcription may be modulated, these genes are not permanently inactivated as part of differentiation.

A group of developmental genes, usually encoding transcription factors, is of particular interest. So fundamental is the laying down of the body plan during early embryological development that the organization and sequence of key genes controlling morphogenesis are highly conserved between mouse and man, a fact that facilitated the genetic study of Waardenburg syndrome type 1, for example. This condition is characterized by deafness and pigmentary disturbances, typically a white forelock, and genetic linkage studies in affected families mapped the mutation to the q35 region of chromosome 2. A naturally occurring mutation in the mouse, called Spotch because of its depigmented patches, was shown to be due to a mutation in the developmental gene, *Pax3*. *Pax3* maps to that part of mouse chromosome 1 which is known to be homologous to human chromosome region 2q35. Thus the human *PAX3* gene (capital letters are used for the human gene) became a prime 'candidate gene' for Waardenburg syndrome type 1. Mutations were duly found in some patients. Interestingly the *PAX3* gene has also been found to be rearranged in the consistent translocation between chromosome 2 and 13—t(2;13)(q35;14) that arises in conjunction with the childhood solid tumour, alveolar rhabdomyosarcoma. This example emphasizes the links that can exist between genes involved in development and mutations implicated in cancer. After all, in the final analysis, cancer is the loss of regulation of cell growth. There are other examples. We noted earlier that Hirschsprung's disease and multiple endocrine neoplasia type 2A can both be due to constitutional mutations in the *RET* proto-oncogene.

There is still an enormous amount to learn about how combinations of transcription factors interact to modulate gene expression during development, and the subsequent maintenance and function of differentiated tissues. It is now clear that DNA methylation, methylation of the carbon atom of the pyrimidine ring of cytosine, represents one mechanism for the regulation (usually repression) of gene expression mammals.

DNA methylation

The long-term silencing of genes that underpins differentiation and the inactivation of one or other of the two X chromosomes in female cells (X-inactivation, see later) is probably consolidated by shifts in DNA packing that serve to limit the access of RNA polymerase, the enzyme responsible for gene transcription. How are such changes regulated in the first place? A key challenge for any such mechanism for sustaining differentiation is how to cope with successive cell divisions, as DNA replication is likely to disrupt protein–DNA binding. DNA methylation is a system that meets this challenge, the methylation pattern being maintained during DNA replication by a maintenance methylase. DNA methylation goes through dynamic changes during embryogenesis and, at least in the mouse, the entire genome is known to be highly undermethylated at the preimplantation stage. A wave of *de novo* methylation before gastrolation establishes two different patterns depending on the type of genes involved, with the housekeeping genes remaining unmethylated.

In general there is preferential methylation of the cytosine of CpG dinucleotides and these have an interesting distribution within the genome. They tend to cluster, in what are called CpG islands, in the promoter region (usually upstream) of housekeeping genes. It is these that seem to escape the *de novo* wave of methylation and this unmethylated state is associated with the housekeeping genes remaining active. Tissue-specific genes, on the other hand, are initially methylated in all cell types in the embryo, becoming selectively demethylated in association with being expressed as part of tissue-specific differentiation. The above is just a crude overview and there are local variations on the theme presented. Exactly how methylation/demethylation plays a part in appropriate gene expression, via methyl-CpG-binding proteins for example, has still to be elucidated.

One aspect of gene expression that is assuming increasing importance in medical genetics is genomic imprinting. The general expectation is that both genes (one inherited from each parent) are expressed, but it is clear that this 'joint operation' does not apply to all genes. With some normal genes there is different expression depending on the sex of the parent who transmits it. When this is observed, it implies that the gene must have carried a parent-of-origin 'tag' or imprint that was placed during spermatogenesis or oogenesis, and this results in modulation (usually silencing) of gene expression in the developing embryo. DNA methylation is involved in at least some aspects of this selective modulation of gene expression and possibly in the 'imprint' itself. The medical aspects of this normal phenomenon arise when imprinted genes are involved in mutation or aberrant chromosomal segregation, and these are discussed in detail later.

Types of mutational mechanisms

MUTATIONS MAY BE CONFINED TO A SUBSET OF CELLS

It is worth remembering that the patient we see represents the end-result of an almost countless number of cell divisions, during which errors in DNA replication or chromosomal segregation can occur at any time. If a lethal mutation occurs in a cell in relatively differentiated tissue, it is of no significance. The cell dies and that's that. However, a mutation that perturbs the regulation of cell growth can predispose to cancer. When mutations at gene, or chromosomal, level occur early in development they can predispose to congenital disorders, with the end-result being a reflection of (a) how early the error occurred; (b) the extent to which the proliferative advantage of the normal cells over the mutant ones can offset the damage; and (c) the degree to which the placental function is involved and therefore the chance of miscarriage.

Somatic mosaicism is the term used when an organism (derived from a single zygote) develops with two or more major cell lines of different genotypes. Somatic mosaicism may result in all or some of the germ cells carrying a mutation. When the mosaicism is confined to the gonads so that just some of the germ cells are affected, the term gonadal mosaicism is used. Another possibility, of course, is that just a single sperm or egg mutates and it happens to be the one involved in a conception. Given the number of germ cells, particularly sperm, it has been claimed, rather fancifully, that men, especially older men, are walking around with the potential for the whole of McKusick's catalogue of mendelian disorders in their scrotum! True or not, there are certainly some types of mutation that occur relatively frequently and these are discussed below. It should be remembered, however, that the mutations (and the diseases they cause) that do see the light of day are the end-result of a balance between DNA damage/misreplication and DNA repair, and DNA repair systems are themselves dependent on genes that can mutate.

DNA REPAIR

DNA repair systems have been extensively studied in lower organisms, and their importance in man is highlighted by several inherited disorders characterized by the inability to correct specific types of DNA damage. Perhaps the best known is the heterogeneous, autosomal recessive group of conditions called xeroderma pigmentosa in which there is hypersensitivity to ultraviolet (**UV**) light and a high incidence of UV-induced skin cancers. Most have a defect of excision repair of the UV-induced pyrimidine dimers, where adjacent thymidine or cytosine bases link up with each other rather than to bases on the other DNA strand.

A striking recent addition to the list of human DNA repair defects is hereditary non-polyposis colon cancer, where there is an inherited defect in mismatch repair. The gene h*MSH2* was mapped to chromosome 2p by linkage studies, and the gene was then cloned by the candidate-gene approach using DNA homology to a similar gene in yeast. Mutagenesis experiments on the yeast gene induced remarkable instability in DNA repeat sequences in the yeast genome, and similar instability of microsatellite DNA markers had been found in tumour tissue from patients with hereditary non-polyposis colon cancer.

SOME DNA SEQUENCES ARE PRONE TO MUTATION

CpG as a mutational 'hot spot'.

The nature of some DNA sequences makes them liable to mutate. As indicated earlier, the cytosine of the dinucleotide CpG is often methylated, and 5-methyl-C naturally tends to deaminate to thymine. This results in a C to T (or G to A) substitution and is a potent cause of point mutations. One estimate is that it accounts for a third of all single base-pair substitutions causing human diseases; in the British study of 217 unrelated patients with haemophilia B referred to earlier, 74 of 191 single base-pair substitutions were at a CpG. Not only does this mutational 'hot spot' cause a substantial proportion of known disease mutations, but is also accounts for the fact that the dinucleotide CpG is under-represented in the genome.

Unstable trinucleotide repeats

The recent discoveries of the mutational events underlying the fragile X syndrome, Huntington's disease, and myotonic dystrophy have illustrated just how unstable some stretches of trinucleotide repeats (CGG, CAG, and CTG, respectively) can be. The genetics of each disorder is described later (pp. 00 and 00), but they share a progressive lengthening of the trinucleotide repeat sequence from one generation to the next and at some critical length the associated gene malfunctions. In the fragile X (FRAX A) syndrome and myotonic dystrophy, the DNA repeat becomes highly unstable in somatic cells expanding to enormous size. Whilst the number of repeats can get smaller, in general it does seem that there is some mechanism that makes increases more likely.

Unequal crossing over

A third class of mutation-prone DNA sequence is on a larger scale and has already been mentioned. When homologous chromosomes (the paternally and maternally derived copy of a chromosome) pair up during the first division of meiosis, they must align precisely because recombination between chromatids of the pair will occur. If this crossing over takes place when two chromatids are misaligned, a chromatid with a deletion and one with a corresponding duplication will be generated, plus two normal chromatids. A prerequisite for unequal crossing over is the existence of local repeated homologous or very similar DNA sequences, for it is in these situations that misalignment due to 'mistaken identity' can occur (much like partnership errors in square dancing with many sets of identical twins!). The repeated sequences can be duplicated active genes (e.g. α-globin genes on chromosome 16), neighbouring inactive pseudogenes (e.g. 21-hydroxylase/C4 loci on chromosome 6) or dispersed non-coding repeat sequences such as the 300-bp Alu repeat that are known to cause some deletions in the low-density lipoprotein receptor gene for example.

LARGER-SCALE REARRANGEMENTS

The past, apparent separation of genetic defects into chromosomal aberrations and mendelian disorders with small mutations at the DNA level was, in part, just a reflection of the limitations of our methods for analysis. There were chromosomal abnormalities visible by light microscopy and DNA sequence changes easily detected with gene-specific probes, but little else in between. Clearly, segregation abnormalities of whole chromosomes are in a class of their own, but structural rearrangements of chromosomes come in all shapes and sizes. In reality, mutations range in size from single-nucleotide substitutions to deletions, duplications or other rearrangements involving one, a few, or many genes. For the most part, these probably arise as errors of the natural process of recombination, enhanced no doubt by misalignment of similar DNA sequences.

About 5 per cent of mutations causing Duchenne muscular dystrophy are due to duplications of some 1 to 500 kb within the huge dystrophin gene, whilst the mutation causing autosomal dominant Charcot–Marie–Tooth disease (hereditary motor and sensory neuropathy, type 1) is always due to a 2-mb duplication at 17p11.2. Occasionally, a stretch of DNA is inverted, or back-to-front. The first example was encountered in a patient with thalassaemia (see Section 22). More recently it has been found that an inversion causes about 50 per cent of cases of severe haemophilia A. A gene residing in a large intron(22) in the factor VIII gene is similar to one close to the tip of Xq. Some form of mispairing and recombination between these two genes results in a large inversion within Xq28 and consequent disruption of the factor VIII gene. This inversion occurs *de novo* quite frequently; about 10^{-5} per gamete per generation, or 1 in 40 000 males born.

Table 2 *Some examples of microdeletions that are often at or beyond the limit of cytogenetic visualization and require molecular (cyto)genetic analysis*

Disorder	Chromosomal region
Alagille syndrome	20p11.23–12.1
Angelman syndrome	15q11–13
Cri-du-chat syndrome	5p15
Di George syndrome (Velocardialfacial)	22q11.2
Langer–Giedion syndrome	8q24.1
Miller–Dieker syndrome (isolated lissencephaly)	17p13.3
Prader–Willi syndrome	15q11–13
Rubinstein–Taybi syndrome	16p13.3
WAGR syndrome[1]	11p13
Williams syndrome	7q11.2
Wolf syndrome	4p15.32

[1]WAGR is an acronym for the contiguous deletion syndrome comprising Wilms' tumour, aniridia, genital abnormalities, and growth/developmental retardation.

MICRODELETIONS

More and more genetic disorders are being revealed as microdeletions (Table 2). They represent some of the most frequent mutations. It is now known that the 22q11.2 deletion found in the Di George or velocardio-facial syndrome is also a cause of just congenital heart defect on its own and probably occurs *de novo* at a rate exceeding 1 in 10 000 pregnancies. A syndrome due to a deletion that extends to remove more than one gene is called a contiguous gene disorder or contiguous deletion syndrome, with the combination of features being a reflection of the number and function of genes knocked out.

POINT MUTATIONS

The ways single nucleotide-base substitutions and other changes involving one or very few bases affect gene function are discussed elsewhere.

TRANSPOSABLE ELEMENTS

We have already noted an example of a copy of the repeat sequence, Alu, disrupting the *NF1* gene and causing neurofibromatosis 1. Although not a proper gene as such, most, if not all, Alu sequences are transcribed into RNA. The presence of a poly(A) tail at the 3′ end of the genomic Alu repeats suggests that they have integrated at new genomic positions through an RNA intermediate, and the *NF1* mutation is just such a spontaneous genomic integration. An Alu repeat had 'jumped' into the intron between exons 5 and 6. This caused skipping of exon 6 in the mRNA and the splicing of exon 5 to 7, which resulted in a frameshift, and which in turn generated a premature stop codon such that the *NF1* protein (normally 2818 amino acids long) would be missing 771 amino acids from the C-terminus. Disruption of genes by transposable elements may not be so very rare.

Genotype/phenotype correlations

CLASSIFICATION OF MENDELIAN DISORDERS BY LOCUS

Advances in molecular genetics are having an enormous impact on our understanding of the pathogenesis of the simply inherited disorders and are also beginning to illuminate the common diseases of complex inheritance. The Human Genome Project, by eventually listing all the 75 000 or so expressed genes, will greatly aid the classification of mendelian diseases, although it should be remembered that there is not a 'one to one' relationship between human genes and genetic diseases as seen in clinical practice. With 5000 mendelian disorders now delineated, it does not mean we still have 70 000 to discover! Some genes can be deleted with no significant clinical effect, whilst mutations in others are likely to be incompatible with even the earliest development. Admittedly, some of the latter may underlie disorders that manifest only as somatic mosaics (see later).

Genetics has been full of surprises, and it is still too early to predict when and how knowledge of the genotype will inform prognosis and clinical management, but some general points can be made.

With the prospect of defining all single-gene disorders at the DNA sequence level, there has to be a gradual convergence of the existing clinical classifications with the standardized listing of all monogenic disorders in McKusick's catalogue *Mendelian Inheritance in Man.* This catalogue has been adopted as the main clinical listing for the Human Genome Project and is increasingly arranged on a gene-locus basis, so it does seem logical for the primary classification of monogenic disorders to also be by gene locus. The role of the clinician will be to compare similar diseases known to arise as a result of mutations at two different loci to detect subtle differences in the clinical phenotype. These features will then serve as clinical guides to which gene locus is mutant in the patient and where DNA analysis should be focused. It is likely that biochemical data or histological features will be an even better guide to which molecule is primarily involved in the pathogenesis of the disease and therefore which gene locus is mutant. For example, haemophilia A (factor VIII deficiency) had been distinguishable from haemophilia B (factor IX deficiency) by coagulation studies long before the two X-linked loci were mapped to Xq27 and Xq28, respectively.

Whilst classification at the locus level will have to be incorporated into disease definitions, it will often be insufficient by itself for clinical purposes. As indicated earlier, two mutations in the same gene can sometimes give quite different diseases. It should also be noted that different mutations of the same gene locus can not only lead to different clinical manifestations but also different patterns of autosomal inheritance. One mutation may only produce disease in the homozygous state (autosomal recessive inheritance) whilst another does so in the heterozygous state (autosomal dominant inheritance). It follows that just because two diseases are inherited in a different mendelian fashion, it should not necessarily be assumed that different gene loci are involved.

One consequence of being able to define the mutation at the DNA level in individual patients is that genotype/phenotype correlations can be studied. These will reveal as much about the function of the normal gene product as the pathogenesis of the genetic disease; one illuminates the other.

POINT MUTATIONS MAY ENHANCE EXISTING TENDENCIES

To understand the way a single amino-acid substitution can produce a dramatic clinical effect may require detailed knowledge of the normal structure and functions of the protein. In sickle-cell anaemia the GAG $\rightarrow$ GTG base change at the sixth codon position of the β-globin gene results in the normal glutamic acid being replaced by valine. This single amino-acid substitution on the surface of the haemoglobin molecule enhances the tendency for molecular aggregation that already exists with deoxygenated adult haemoglobin. The phenomenon of an amino acid substitution enhancing a tendency that already exists in the normal protein can sometimes be understood in an evolutionary context.

The elucidation of the point mutation underlying the bleeding disorder associated with the abnormal α_1-antitrypsin Pittsburgh provides a fascinating insight into the link between α_1-antitrypsin and antithrombin III. These plasma proteins share a similar structure, whose genes arose by divergent evolution from an ancestral gene some 500 million years ago. α_1-Antitrypsin protects the body against released elastase and its synthesis is increased in response to trauma, whilst antithrombin III controls coagulation by inhibition of thrombin and remains at a constant concentration in the plasma and requires activation by heparin. α_1-antitrypsin Pittsburgh arises as a result of an ATG $\rightarrow$ AGG base change at codon position 358. This change from the normal methionine to arginine occurs at the reactive centre and in effect changes the α_1-antitrypsin into an antithrombin III, that is independent of heparin activation. However, this mutant α_1-antitrypsin still retains the short-term genetic regulation appropriate to normal α_1-antitrypsin, and so the unfortunate patient responded to trauma by producing what was, in effect, antithrombin III, with disastrous and ultimately fatal consequences.

DOMINANT–NEGATIVE EFFECTS

In considering genotype/phenotype correlations, it is worth noting the most common way in which a mutation in a single dose can cause the full clinical effect, that is, why the condition is inherited in a dominant fashion. This phenomenon goes by several different names, such as protein suicide, included/excluded mutants or dominant–negative effect, but in essence it is a case of a faulty gene product being more trouble than its worth when it comes to assembling multimeric proteins. It is better to do without, or use an unconventional but correctly formed protein as a partner. Osteogenesis imperfecta is due to defects in type 1 collagen, a trimer of two α_1-chains and one α_2-chain. It provides an illustration of why heterozygotes for a mutation causing an abnormal α_1-chain of type 1 collagen end up worse off than those heterozygous for an α_1-gene deletion. In the former situation, not half but three-quarters of the collagen trimers 'include' one or two defective α_1-chains. It is better to build a thinner wall than lay half-baked bricks in three courses out of four. The general principle is well illustrated by 'mutant' wheels on bicycles (Fig. 6) or tricycles for that matter.

Disabling a multimeric protein is not the only way to produce a dominant effect. Specific mutations in a receptor can result in it being 'locked' on, in the presence of little or no agonist. Familial male precocious puberty is a gonadotrophin-independent disorder that is inherited in an autosomal dominant, male-limited fashion. It can be caused by a point mutation (Asp 578 to Gly in the sixth transmembrane helix) in the luteinizing-hormone receptor.

GENETIC SUSCEPTIBILITY

Genotype/phenotype correlations are much more problematical when it comes to common disorders of complex aetiology, and yet great practical benefit is likely to be derived from defining genetic variations (particular alleles) that either predispose to a common disease or protect against it. In the past, for want of a more specific way into the pathogenesis, there was considerable reliance on disease association studies; namely, taking a major polymorphic system (e.g. the HLA system) in which patient and health populations can be apportioned according to the alleles they carry, and seeing if there are any disease associations. An alternative approach stemmed from knowledge of the pathogenesis of the disorder. Various subclinical indicators of the disease, such as hypercholesterolaemia in ischaemic heart disease, were sought in all relatives to see if they segregated in a mendelian fashion. If so, genes known to be involved in the relevant metabolic or physiological function became 'candidates' for the gene locus at which susceptibility alleles might exist. From time to time a subgroup of cases was shown to be due to the action of a single mutant gene. This was useful information for the affected families, and the removal of such specific subgroups from the general pool of patients also helped reduce the heterogeneity that so often confounds research into common diseases.

The recent advances in human molecular biology, both technical and conceptual, have led to a coming together of the two approaches outlined above. Disease association studies in populations are increasingly testing candidate genes suggested by more direct molecular investigations of patients and affected families. Nevertheless, if one is to make sense of the large amount of disease-association data that is generated, certain basic principles need to be born in mind, in particular the relation between genetic linkage, susceptibility genes, and association.

The difference between linkage and association

Close linkage between a disease-specific gene locus, such as factor VIII, and a gene showing considerable protein polymorphism, such as glucose-6-phosphate dehydrogenase **(G6PD)** does not in any way mean that people with haemophilia are more likely to have one particular G6PD type. In other words, genetic linkage does not necessarily mean association between two particular alleles at the respective gene loci.

A mild dominant disorder, the 'nail–patella syndrome', shows genetic linkage with the blood-group *ABO* locus, both the *ABO* and the disease gene locus being situated on chromosome 9. If the nail–patella syndrome mutation happens to be on a chromosome 9 that carries the allele for group A, then the disease and the blood group A will tend to be inherited together. However, because of eventual crossing over, or independent mutations leading to different affected families, the nail–patella syndrome may be linked with blood group O in another family or group B in a third family. Thus there is genetic linkage, but no association with a particular blood group. Genetic linkage is a phenomenon demonstrable within families. By contrast, association is a phenomenon demonstrated by comparing a population of affected individuals with a control population.

People with blood group A are more likely to get cancer of the stomach than are people with blood group O. This is an association between the group A allele and the cancer, but this does not necessarily mean that a cancer susceptibility gene is situated on chromosome 9 close to the *ABO* gene locus.

LINKAGE DISEQUILIBRIUM AS AN EXPLANATION OF AN ASSOCIATION

Having emphasized the risk of confusing linkage with association, it is necessary to describe certain special situations where the two phenomena may indeed be interrelated; and the genetics of the HLA histocompatibility antigens provide the example.

The region on chromosome 6 that carries the major histocompatibility complex is designated *HLA*. The different gene loci are designated by the letters *A*, *B*, *C*, *D*, and the specificities or alleles at each locus are identified by the numbers *1*, *2*, *3*, etc. This is not the place to discuss the number of actual loci that may be involved; for the sake of simplicity discussion will be confined to the *HLA-A* and *HLA-B* specificities.

The particular combination of alleles (and the specific antigens they determine) on a single chromosome is called a haplotype, and because the *HLA-A* and *HLA-B* loci are closely linked, the parental haplotypes are generally passed on unchanged. However, during meiosis, about once in a 100 times, cross-over between the two number 6 chromosomes occurs at a site between loci *A* and *B*, and the ovum or sperm will then carry a recombinant haplotype. A particular haplotype is not 'fixed' for evermore, even if it is transmitted unchanged for many generations. Given enough time and random mating, every combination of alleles at loci *A* and *B* should arise; and in theory the frequency of the combinations, or haplotypes, should be a reflection (actually the product) of the

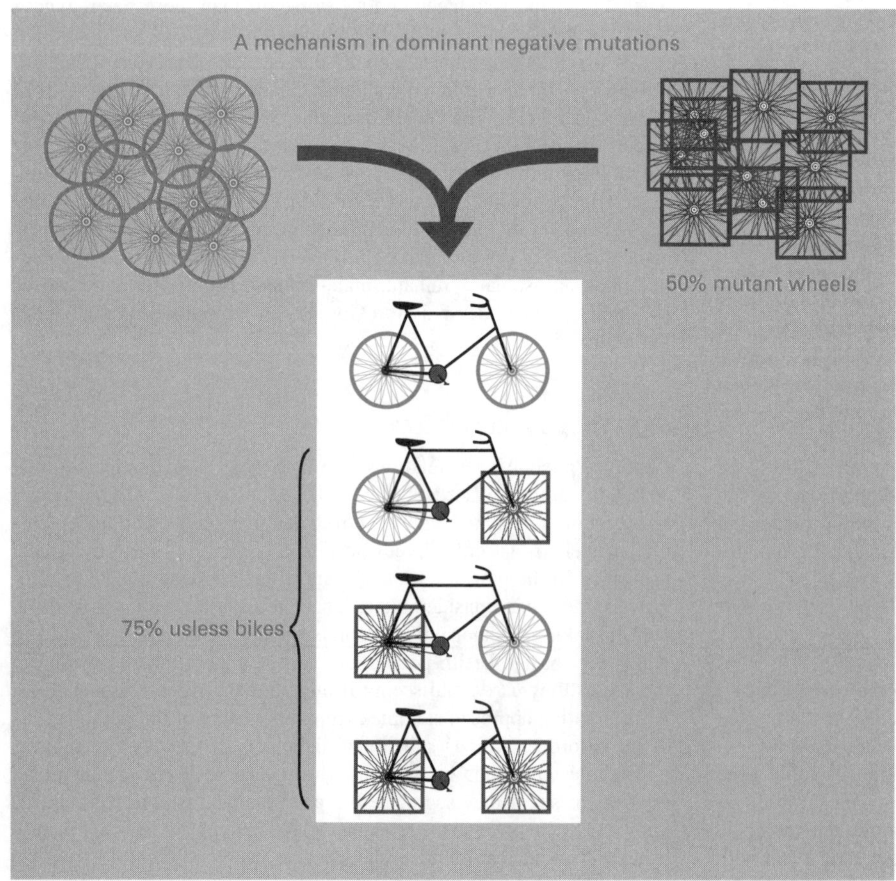

Fig. 6 Polypeptide gene products often associate in dimers or multimers to form the functional protein. When half the polypeptides are mutant, 75 per cent (or more with multimers) of the protein molecules are non-functional and the phenotype is likely to be inherited as a dominant.

frequencies of the individual alleles. Where this is the case the alleles are said to be in linkage equilibrium.

When two alleles occur together more frequently or less frequently than expected from the individual frequencies, they are said to be in linkage disequilibrium. Linkage disequilibrium can arise in a variety of ways. One allele may have arisen by mutation relatively recently (on the evolutionary time-scale) and not yet achieved equilibrium, still reflecting the original combination. A particular combination may have a selective advantage or disadvantage and achieve disequilibrium by natural selection. The same principles of equilibrium and disequilibrium can apply to alleles of any two linked gene loci. The haplotype *A1–B8* occurs more frequently than the individual frequencies would predict, and therefore these two alleles show linkage disequilibrium.

Confusion between genetic linkage and disease associations can arise because in cases of an association between a particular HLA antigen and a disease, one of the explanations for the association is genetic linkage between the *HLA* locus and a disease susceptibility gene plus linkage disequilibrium involving the particular allele at the *HLA* locus. Linkage disequilibrium is an essential part of this explanation because genetic linkage *per se* cannot account for the association.

In interpreting an association between a disease and a particular 'allele' of a polymorphic DNA marker system, the nature of the DNA polymorphism must be borne in mind. If the DNA marker used is actually a polymorphically expressed gene, where the different protein variants might have different functions, then the marker itself could be the susceptibility gene. This could well be the situation in the recently described association between Alzheimer's disease and the *4* allele of apolipoprotein E.

If the marker is an untranscribed, dinucleotide repeat sequence for example, then clearly this is very unlikely to be the actual gene for which there is the disease-susceptibility allele. The probable explanation is that there is a closely linked gene locus containing the susceptibility allele and this allele is in linkage equilibrium with a particular 'allele' at the DNA marker. The way forward, as always with mere associations, is to move on to family linkage studies to try and map the susceptibility locus. In conditions where the inheritance does not approximate to a simple mendelian pattern, such linkage studies are likely to take the form of 'affected sib pair' analysis. In essence this method asks the question 'Which bit of DNA have affected siblings inherited in common, more often than can be explained by chance?'

Linkage disequilibrium and gene mapping

Although quite removed from defining susceptibility genes for common diseases, this is as good a place as any to mention the important part linkage disequilibrium has played in mapping mendelian, particularly autosomal recessive, disorders. Linkage analysis in families suffers from the law of diminishing returns. Because the 'genetic distance' represented by 1 per cent recombination between disease locus and marker is a physical distance of about 1 million bases, family linkage studies are not good at getting very close. Given limited family material, all fairly close markers tend to show no recombination. However, if (and only if) the affected people in a population carry the same mutation derived from the distant ancestor in which the mutation originally occurred, then the alleles at DNA markers that are very close to the disease locus are likely to show linkage disequilibrium. These markers are so close that there has been insufficient time for recombination to establish equilibrium between the marker alleles and the disease mutation. For the gene mappers this meant that the stronger the linkage disequilibrium with successive markers, the closer they were getting to the disease locus.

Relative risk

Although research into the aetiology of common diseases is best set in prospective, longitudinal studies of the whole population, disease associations are always demonstrated by comparing a population of patients who have suffered the disease with a control population who have not.

Sometimes the associations are weak, the gene having an almost incidental influence on the disease risk, and knowledge of the association is of little practical value. The association of blood group O with duodenal ulceration is in this category. It has certain academic interest, for it confirms the existence of genes that have a small additive effect, in the way predicted for polygenes. Other associations, like that between ankylosing spondylitis and *HLA-B27,* are not only of value in elucidating the pathogenesis, but also in predicting an individual's risk. In practice the absence of the *B27* allele is as much use, or perhaps even more use, in advising individuals as is its presence. Indeed, more might be usefully made of negative associations, or quite independent protective factors, in exploring the pathogenesis of multifactorial diseases.

What should be emphasized is that finding a disease association with a genetic marker like an *HLA* allele can only be regarded as a starting point for a genetic study, not an end in itself. Some of the strongest associations to date are with the *HLA* alleles, where that between narcolepsy and *HLA* heads the list.

These disease associations can be expressed as a relative risk, which is really another term for relative incidence. If P is the number of patients with the marker, and p is the number of patients without; and C is the number of presumably healthy controls with the marker, and c those without, then the relative incidence is:

$$\frac{P/p}{C/c} = \frac{Pc}{pC}.$$

Taking ankylosing spondylitis and *HLA-B27,* for example, one study showed that 90 per cent of patients had *HLA-B27* whilst only 8 per cent of health controls had *HLA-B27.* Thus $P/p = 90/10$ and $C/c = 8/92$:

$$\frac{P/p}{C/c} = \frac{Pc}{pC} = 103.5.$$

The association of ankylosing spondylitis with *HLA-B27* shows a relative risk of about 100.

Practical intervention

Medicine is concerned directly, or indirectly, with practical intervention. The provision of information may be no less of an intervention than administering a powerful drug, and liable to the same misuse by the ill informed. The diagnosis of a serious disease is a matter not only for the patient but for those with whom they share their everyday lives. If the disease is also inherited it may be a matter for the whole extended family. The birth of a severely handicapped child damages the family by distorting or disrupting relationships between family members, and between the family and the community of which it is part. There is a process of healing for the family during which adjustments to relationships are made that take account of what can and cannot be done to correct or overcome the child's disabilities; in other words there is restoration of family life. Genetic prediction often plays a vital part in this healing, whether it involves a general discussion of recurrence risks, carrier exclusion or detection, or prenatal diagnosis and selective abortion.

Whilst the most lasting impact of an understanding of monogenic disorders will be the opportunity for people to modify their reproductive behaviour, there is an immediate need to emphasize specific treatments because there is a tendency to think that because the disorder is genetic it is unlikely to be treatable or only treatable by gene therapy (discussed in the next section). Table 3 summarizes the main types of treatment, listing selected examples. However, the greatest benefits in the future are likely to be derived from our increased understanding of genetic influences in the common multifactorial disorders such as neural-tube defects, congenital heart disease, diabetes mellitus, coronary arterial disease, rheumatoid arthritis, psychotic illnesses, and the dementias.

Table 3 *Approach to treatment of genetic disorders*

Approach	Example
Avoidance of risk factors	Avoidance of fava beans in glucose-6-phosphate dehydrogenase deficiency
Symptomatic treatment	Anticonvulsant therapy in tuberous sclerosis
Surgical correction before irreversible damage:	
Postnatal	Ramstedt's operation in infantile pyloric stenosis
Prenatal	Vesicoamniotic shunt in urethral obstruction
Dietary restriction of a substrate that cannot be metabolized	Phenylalanine restriction in phenylketonuria
Replacement of a missing or inactive product	Factor VIII replacement in haemophilia A
Removal of a toxic metabolite	Penicillamine treatment in Wilson's disease (hepatolenticular degeneration)
Pharmacological doses of a cofactor	Pyridoxine treatment in homocystinuria
Pharmacological doses to overcome a specific malabsorption	Zinc treatment in acrodermatitis enteropathologica
Tissue transplants:	
To replace defective tissue	Bone marrow transplant in severe combined immunodeficiency
For enzyme augmentation	Renal transplant in Fabry's disease
Gene therapy	Severe combined immunodeficiency (ADA deficiency) treated by 'corrected' T-cells

Because genetic and non-genetic influences operate together to cause these diseases there is the possibility of elucidating those environmental components that can be modified in such a way as to prevent the disorder developing, or at least delay its onset and reduce its severity. However, this obvious strategy is bedevilled by the fact that the relative contribution of genetic and environmental factors varies from one case to another. The interpretation of intervention studies will be greatly enhanced if those individuals with the greatest and least genetic predisposition can be identified. In time it will be possible to identify those individuals with a high, average, or minimal risk of developing a particular common disease. Those at low risk can be reassured and those at high risk can be offered active, preventative measures once such measures are discovered. This knowledge will also allow dietary advice, health education, and possibly certain vaccination programmes to be 'targeted' more precisely. The development of tests to give individuals a genetic susceptibility profile can only encourage them to take more responsibility for their own health and also, through periconceptional care, reduce the risks to their unborn children.

Gene therapy

The strategy for this new approach to treatment depends on a detailed knowledge of the pathogenesis of the disease. If it is an absence or deficiency of gene product, any system that delivers that product to the right part of the appropriate cells in sufficient quantity is likely to work. The mutant gene does not have to be replaced, just supplemented; and this supplementation, or augmentation, could come from one or more normal genes inserted anywhere in the genome, provided that they were transcribed properly and the insertion itself did not cause new genetic problems for the patient. The new gene(s) need not be inserted into the hosts chromosomes at all, provided they were packaged in a relatively stable vector that allowed them genes to be transcribed. Such a strategy might be particularly appropriate if the cells to be treated were long-lived, terminally differentiated cells, so the question of ensuring that the new gene replicates along with ordinary cell division is not a major issue.

If the genetic problem stems from a troublesome, mutant gene product, adding extra normal genes is unlikely to work and true gene replacement is required. However, replacing a mutant gene with a normal one is technically much more difficult than just adding new genes. It has been achieved by homologous recombination at a low rate in cultured cells, but there is a world of difference between laboratory (usually animal) experiments and getting something to work clinically in a patient.

It is probably the everyday success of the specific manipulation of animal genes that led to exaggerated expectations for gene therapy in the clinical setting. It is worth remembering that generating transgenic animals (i.e. with new genes added or a specific one replaced) involves introduction of the new DNA into very early embryos or embryonic stem cells, followed by a major selection process in which the few successes are distinguished from the large number of failures. Introduction of new genes into human embryos is rightly outlawed (in most instances, the same clinical goal could be achieved by preimplantation diagnosis and selective embryo transfer) and anyway a very high rate of abortive attempts would be clinically unacceptable.

Many discussions of gene therapy refer to the distinction between somatic and so-called germline gene therapy, but these phrases are rather misleading and deserve brief comment. The concern has never been about a specific targeting of the germline cells or gonads, rather than some strategies to ensure that the new DNA gets into the tissue of clinical interest will incidentally also allow it to get into the germline. The most obvious example is incorporation into very early embryos, along the lines of making transgenic mice, but it would also be true of direct injection of some forms of 'infectious' vector into the bloodstream. In distinction, the term 'somatic' emphasizes that the germline has been specifically avoided. The main reason for the current outlawing of gene therapies that could incidentally alter the germline is that we know far too little about the risks to offspring (rather than because of some vague objection to changing the genetic make-up for generations to come). Insertion of new DNA into the genome has some risk of disrupting the function of an existing gene, as animal studies have shown. This insertional mutagenesis in the germline could lead, of course, to genetic abnormalities in the offspring. In somatic cells the new insertional mutation is likely to just kill that cell or be inconsequential, although there must be some risk, as yet unquantifiable, of inducing malignant change.

INTRODUCING NEW GENES INTO CELLS

There are two types of methods for introducing cloned genes into cells, physical and viral. Physical methods of gene insertion include co-precipitation of DNA with calcium phosphate, the use of polycations or lipids to complex the DNA, cell fusion techniques utilizing liposomes, erythrocyte ghosts or protoplasts, and microinjection and electroporation techniques. Recent experiments have exploited receptors on the cell that specifically bind and internalize particular proteins. The new DNA is complexed with the particular protein (e.g. transferrin) and is taken up by the appropriate receptor along with the protein. The main disadvantage of the physical methods is that the integration rate is still low and when integration does occur, multiple copies of the DNA are often incorporated.

Viruses have often been used to introduce DNA into cells in culture, the first so-called expression vectors utilizing the tumour viruses SV40 and polyoma. More recently, work in this area has focused on the murine retroviruses Moloney leukaemia virus and myeloproliferative sarcoma virus, and also on adenoviruses. Retroviruses have a number of features that make them suitable for use as vectors for gene therapy. It is possible to establish permanent, viral- producing cell lines suitable for efficient infection of target cells. The retroviral-expression vector is constructed so that the new human DNA replaces the viral genes necessary to make infectious capsules, thereby making the expression vector unable to infect further cells once in the target cell. The initial infection of the target cell is achieved by using a cell line containing a mutant retrovirus that can only produce empty viral capsules; when the expression vector is added to this cell, just a single round of infectious particles is produced (Fig. 7). This approach can infect up to 100 per cent of target cells and the DNA is usually integrated as a single copy. Once integrated into the host genome the new transgene acts as a cellular gene in that it is faithfully passed on to progeny cells.

Whilst most is known about the use of retroviral vectors and these vectors were used for the first clinical trials, there are some problems. First, only about 7 kb of DNA can be incorporated into the retroviral vector and it still work. Many genes, plus their necessary regulatory sequences, are much longer than 7 kb. Secondly, retroviruses appear not to infect non-dividing cells, posing constraints on what target tissues can be used. In particular, bone-marrow stem cells do not readily divide in culture and yet these would be the preferred target cells for many types of gene therapy. Thirdly, there is a theoretical potential for producing replication-competent (helper) virus during the production of the retroviral vector based on some form of recombination between the vector and the packaging-deficient mutant or some endogenous virus in the packaging cell. There are ways of minimizing this potential and infective virus has not arisen so far in practice. If it did, it should be efficiently neutralized by complement present in the patient's own serum. Additional potential problems relate to the 'random' insertion of retroviral vectors into the genome. The insertion site may reduce expression of the gene in the vector for some reason or, as mentioned above, the retroviral vector might activate an endogenous gene concerned with cell replication and cause a malignancy.

Fig. 7 A packaging cell containing a packaging-defective retrovirus allows one round of infection of the target cells by the vector carrying the new DNA. Thereafter the vector cannot infect further cells because it does not carry genes for the viral protein coat.

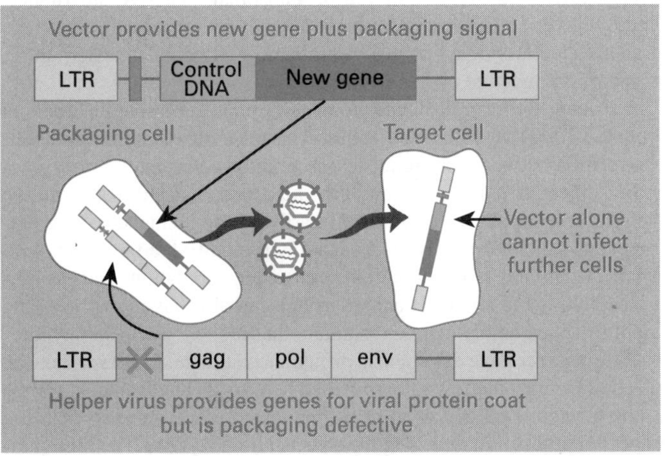

Recent work suggests that adenovirus vectors may be useful in gene therapy. Important advantages are their potential to carry large segments of DNA (possibly up to 36 kb) and their ability to infect non-replicating cells, including lung tissue, *in situ.* Whilst natural adenoviruses, in contrast to retroviruses, are believed to integrate at one particular region of chromosome 19 rather than at random, the current adenovirus-based vectors do not integrate into chromosomal DNA at all. This avoids the potential problem of insertional mutagenesis but may result in instability of gene expression as cell division proceeds.

TARGET TISSUES

Getting genes into cells and to function properly is just the first step in gene therapy. If a long-term treatment or a cure is the aim, then the gene has to be introduced into sufficient numbers of self-renewing stem cells or very long-lived cells of the right tissue.

Whilst considerable attention has been paid to targeting muscle tissue and a clinical trial has been approved for low-density lipoprotein **(LDL)** receptor gene transfer into hepatocytes of patients suffering from LDL-receptor deficiency, bone marrow is currently the main target for gene therapy. Haemopoietic stem cells occur at low frequency in bone marrow. Enrichment can be achieved using a system of stem-cell 'capture' that exploits the cell-surface marker CD34. As indicated earlier, efficient integration of retroviral vector into stem cells is proving difficult, and the first clinical trial has used reinfusion of the patients T lymphocytes into which a retroviral vector expressing adenosine deaminase had been introduced.

THE FUTURE

The results of the first attempts at gene therapy have been encouraging, but many problems remain to be resolved. Ultimately this new form of treatment should have applications in many areas of clinical practice.

Clinical genetics

Mendelian inheritance

Autosomal dominant disorders

In medical genetics the term autosomal dominant refers to the situation where a monogenic disorder manifests clinically in the heterozygous state, that is there is usually inheritance from one parent only. A family pedigree can be so characteristic as to establish the mode of inheritance, without reference to any other information (Fig. 8). Affected individuals have a 1 in 2 chance of passing it on to a child. This is regardless of sex, so there can be male-to-male transmission, which rules out X-linked inheritance. Unaffected individuals do not pass the condition on to their children or further descendants; but some qualification of this statement is given later. In Britain the overall incidence of autosomal dominant disorders is about 7/1000 live births. The more common ones are listed in Table 4.

In the rare instance of the marriage of two affected individuals, there is the opportunity for a child to receive the mutant gene from each parent, but it would be wrong to assume on the basis of the classical definition of dominant that the child will be no more severely affected than either parent. Achondroplasia, one of the most common non-lethal

Table 4 *Estimates of birth frequencies of some more common dominant conditions (symptomatic and asymptomatic) in Britain per 1000 live births*

System	Disorder	Frequency
Nervous system	Huntington's disease	0.5
	Neurofibromatosis	0.3
	Myotonic dystrophy	0.2
	Hereditary motor and sensory neuropathy (Charcot-Marie-Tooth disease)	0.2
Intestines	Multiple polyposis coli	0.1
Kidney	Polycystic disease of the kidneys	0.8
Skeleton	Diaphysical aclasis	0.5
Sight	Dominant forms of blindness	0.1
Hearing	Dominant forms of early childhood onset deafness	0.1
	Dominant otosclerosis (adult onset, severe)	1.0
Circulation	Monogenic hypercholesterolaemia	2.0
Teeth	Dentinogenesis imperfecta	0.1
Blood	Congenital spherocytosis	0.2

forms of short-limbed dwarfism, is just one of an increasing list of autosomal dominant disorders where the homozygote is more severely affected than the heterozygote. On average 1 in 4 of the offspring of an achondroplastic couple has an extreme form of limb shortening that is lethal. By contrast, in Huntington's disease, homozygotes are no more severely affected than heterozygotes. The above discussion apart, autosomal dominant inheritance is, in theory, extremely simple and straightforward as you can actually track the inheritance of the mutant gene by just looking at the pedigree.

Unfortunately, in clinical practice the matter is complicated by two things, variation in the expression of the gene and new mutation. Both points are illustrated by neurofibromatosis, which has an incidence of about 1 in 3000. The manifestations in someone carrying the gene vary from just a few characteristic pigmented patches on the skin, so-called *café au lait* spots, to gross disfigurement with a mass of cutaneous and subcutaneous tumours, and mental handicap. In neurofibromatosis, as in many autosomal dominant disorders, a mildly affected person has to be warned that any child inheriting the gene may not be so lucky as they have been. It can also be seen that a person with minimal manifestations may be regarded as normal, and give rise to the view that the condition has 'skipped a generation'. Some progress has been made in understanding the variable expression in conditions like myotonic dystrophy and this is discussed later. In some situations there will be no manifestations of the gene carried by some family members; that is, the gene has less than 100 per cent penetrance. Reduced penetrance as a concept distinct from variable gene expression is not very helpful in practice. The important message is that you cannot advise someone until you have made a careful physical examination, a general rule in clinical medicine. If they

Fig. 8 Pedigree illustrating the characteristic nature of autosomal dominant transmission. (Reproduced from Roberts and Pembrey (1985) with permission.)

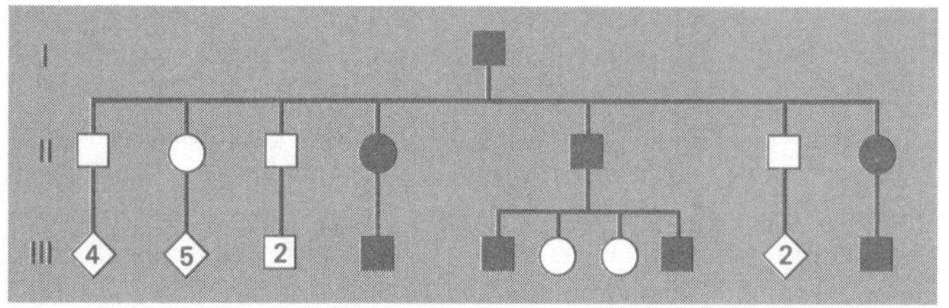

are clear, one may be reassuring about risks to children, but you may not be able to give an absolute guarantee.

All dominant disorders have to start at some time as new mutations in the ovum or sperm; obviously, the more severe the type of disease the less likely the patient is to reproduce, and the greater proportion of affected individuals will be the result of a new mutation. In the mild dominant disorders, or those of late onset, the vast majority of patients have inherited the condition from an affected parent. New mutations and variable gene expression can combine to create difficult clinical decisions. If a single child in the family has overt neurofibromatosis, the apparently healthy parents will want to know the risk to further children. If it is decided the child is the result of a new mutation, then the risk of recurrence is very low. However, if an examination reveals convincing minimal signs of neurofibromatosis in one parent, then the couple face a 1 in 2 risk with each pregnancy. This demonstrates the importance of knowing what the minimal signs of the disorder are, and the difficulties that could arise in doubtful cases.

It is estimated that about half the cases of neurofibromatosis are due to new mutations and this represents an estimated mutation rate of about 10^{-4}; that is, 1 in 10 000 germ cells mutate per generation, or 1 in 5000 babies have neurofibromatosis as a result of a new mutation. This is one of the highest mutation rates in humans, and estimated mutation rates for dominant conditions usually lie between 10^{-5} and 10^{-6}.

Autosomal recessive disorders

In autosomal recessive inheritance the disorder is only manifest clinically when the patient has a double dose of the abnormal gene, that is in the homozygous (or compound heterozygous) state. The patient has no normal allele at the particular locus involved, having inherited one abnormal gene from each parent. Usually both parents are heterozygous for the gene in question, and are clinically normal, the action of their normal allele at the locus being sufficient to compensate. Rarely, one or even both parents are themselves affected homozygotes. Even rarer still is the situation where only one parent is a carrier and the child represents a case of uniparental disomy (see later). In the usual situation, where both parents are heterozygous, a child has a 1 in 4 chance of being an affected homozygote, there is a 2 in 4 chance of being a heterozygote like the parents, and a 1 in 4 chance of being normal. For practical purposes, particularly with the modern tendency to have small families, there is no characteristic pedigree of autosomal recessive inheritance in the way that there is for autosomal dominant and X-linked disorders. Even the instance of an affected boy and girl born to first-cousin parents is not absolute proof of autosomal recessive inheritance, although suggestive. In many parts of the world a third or more of couples are first cousins and affected siblings could, for example, be due to an unbalanced chromosome translocation carried in balanced form by one parent. The pedigree in autosomal recessive disorders is not used to establish the mode of inheritance, but rather to predict the probability of a relative being a carrier on the assumption of autosomal recessive inheritance. Figure 9 gives some illustrative probabilities; note that healthy siblings of an affected individual have a ⅔ probability of being a carrier, not ½ as one might imagine on casual inspection.

In Britain, the overall incidence of autosomal recessive disorders is about 2.5/1000 live births, and Table 5 lists the more common examples. The relation between the frequency of heterozygotes and homozygotes is the subject of a later section. The incidence at birth of a recessive disorder in a population depends primarily on the incidence of the heterozygous state. Obviously, early death will modify the frequency with which the disease is encountered in an older population, and, as discussed below, the rate of cousin marriage can also have an effect. The extent to which new mutations maintain the frequency of heterozygotes for different recessive disorders is difficult to estimate. However, natural selection for the heterozygote, so-called heterozygote advantage, can be a most powerful influence on gene frequency, much more so than the reduced reproductive fitness in the affected homozygote. The high incidence of sickle-cell anaemia in people of African origin is related to the fact that heterozygotes, those with the sickle-cell trait, are less likely to die of malignant tertian malaria *(Plasmodium falciparum)* than are normal homozygotes. Indeed, when a recessive disorder is common in a population it is generally assumed that some heterozygote advantage is, or has been, operating; although there can be other explanations.

The heterozygous state can be detected by DNA analysis or biochemical tests in some autosomal recessive disorders and this can play an important part in genetic counselling. This fact also raises the question of whether a condition is fully recessive if the gene produces a detectable effect in the heterozygous state. In practice the heterozygote is generally healthy and there is such a vast difference between the clinical manifestation in the heterozygous and the abnormal homozygous state that the use of additional categories such as intermediate or co-dominant disorders is unhelpful. Sickle-cell anaemia and β-thalassaemia major (Cooley's anaemia) can be regarded as autosomal recessive disorders even though the heterozygote or sickle-cell trait may have some *in vivo* sickling of their red cells with extreme anoxia, and people with β-thalassaemia trait may be slightly anaemic.

Table 5 *Estimates of birth frequencies of some more common recessive conditions in Britain per 1000 live births*

System	Disorder	Frequency
Metabolism	Cystic fibrosis	0.5
	Phenylketonuria classical	0.1
Nervous system	Neurogenic muscle atrophies	0.1
Red blood cells	Sickle-cell anaemia	0.1
Endocrine glands	Adrenal hyperplasias	0.1
Hearing	Severe congenital deafness	0.2
Sight	Recessive forms of blindness	0.1
Mental retardation severe	Non-specific recessive forms	0.5

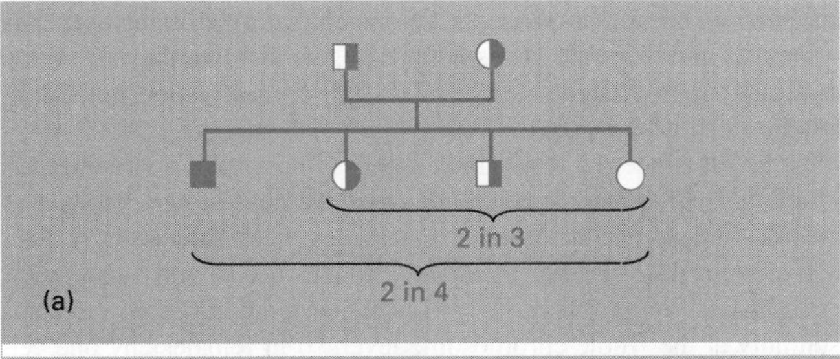

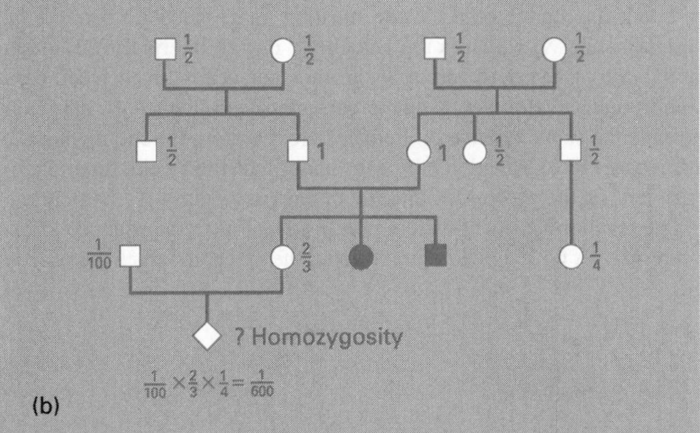

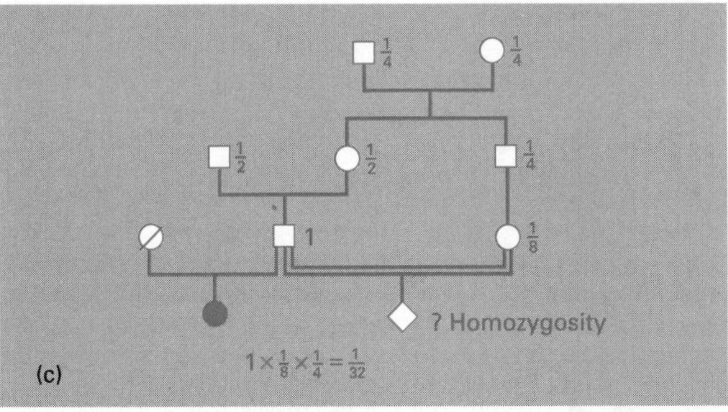

Fig. 9 Pedigrees of autosomal recessive inheritance illustrating the chance that particular relatives of an affected homozygote are carriers. (a) A schematic pedigree showing the proportion of heterozygous offspring (◐ ◨) from a marriage between two heterozygotes for an autosomal recessive trait. Healthy siblings of a homozygote (■) have a ⅔ chance of being heterozygous. (b) The figures represent the probability of being heterozygous for a rare autosomal recessive mutation (carrier frequency 1 in 100) and the chance of the healthy sibling of two affected individuals having an affected child herself, given marriage to an unrelated male. (c) The figures represent the probability of being heterozygous for a rare autosomal recessive mutation, and the chance of a first-cousin marriage involving one known carrier producing an affected child.

From Fig. 9 it can be seen that first cousins share ⅛ of their genes in common. If a person is heterozygous for a recessive condition their first cousin will have a 1 in 8 chance of possessing the same mutation by virtue of their common grandparents. This fact is essentially independent of the frequency of the particular recessive gene in the population. As a consequence, the rarer the gene the more likely it is that when a marriage between two heterozygotes does occur, it will be a marriage between blood relatives. However, in general, the frequencies of harmful recessive mutations in a population are sufficiently low to make the absolute prospective risk to the children of first cousin parents acceptably small (about 3 per cent) when compared to other causes of handicap. It must also be appreciated that with respect to the risks to a child, it is only the relationship of the parents that is important. The fact that grandparents or other ancestors married relatives has virtually no influence on the risks if the parents themselves are not related.

X-linked disorders

X-linked recessive inheritance produces a characteristic family pedigree, where males are affected and the gene is passed on by unaffected females (Fig. 10). It is easy to satisfy oneself that an abnormal gene carried on one of the X chromosomes in a female will be passed on to half of her daughters, who would be heterozygous like herself, and to half of her sons, who would manifest the disease because they have no compensating X chromosome. An affected male would produce only heterozygous daughters, but cannot pass the gene on to his sons, who only receive his Y chromosome. In a population where the X-linked red-cell enzyme defect G6PD deficiency is common, an affected man may have an affected son, but only because his wife is also a heterozygote. Such a mating results in half the girls being affected homozygotes.

In some X-linked disorders a proportion of female heterozygotes are mildly affected, and this is the case with G6PD deficiency. Cytochemical staining of the red cells shows that about half are G6PD deficient and half are normal. The explanation lies in the fact that only one of the X-chromosome pair is active in any one cell. The random inactivation of one or other X chromosome in each cell early in embryonic development is discussed below. By chance, some women heterozygous for G6PD deficiency have the normal X chromosome inactivated in 80 to 90 per cent of their cells, and can therefore develop haemolysis, like the affected hemizygous males, when exposed to certain drugs such as sulphonamides and antimalarials.

In Britain the incidence of X-linked disorders is about 1.4 per 1000 total male live births (Table 6). Two important examples are Duchenne muscular dystrophy (1 in 4000 males) and the fragile X syndrome (1 in 1500). Duchenne muscular dystrophy is due to mutations in the dystrophin gene that result in no protein product in the muscle (when there is a reduced amount or truncated dystrophin present, the patient suffers the milder Becker muscular dystrophy). The dystrophin gene has the distinction of being the largest gene yet described in man. It has 79 exons distributed over about 2400 kb within the p21 region of the X chromosome. About 60 per cent of boys with Duchenne muscular dystrophy have intragenic deletions, which are readily detected by DNA analysis, although the presence of the normal X makes detection of deletions in female carriers more difficult. Even so, new molecular genetic methods, such as fluorescent *in situ* hybridization (outlined later), look very promising. New methods to detect truncated dystrophin molecules (after *in vitro* translation of cDNA made from patient lymphocyte mRNA!) also looks promising as a means of detecting some of the point mutations. As a group, carriers have a higher level of plasma creatine kinase. Measurement of this enzyme, pedigree analysis taking into account the presence of healthy males, and mutation detection and gene tracking by DNA analysis are used in various combination to determine the carrier status of female relatives seeking help.

The pedigree may indicate that a woman must be a carrier but this may not be quite as often as one might first think. The first affected male in a family may represent a new mutation in the ovum that leads to his conception, and neither his mother or other female relatives are carriers. For an X-linked lethal disorder like Duchenne muscular dystrophy, such a boy represents the beginning and end of the disorder in the family. From considerations of population genetics we can infer that about ⅓ of isolated affected boys represent new mutations, whilst in the remaining ⅔ the mothers are carriers. Heterozygous women have a ½ chance of being a new mutation and a half chance of having inherited it from their mother. These figures are appropriate for X-linked lethal disorders assuming equal mutation rate in sperm and ova. This seems to approximate to the truth in Duchenne muscular dystrophy, although in haemophilia A, for example, more than ⅔ of mothers of isolated boys appear to be carriers. The probability of a woman being a carrier can be modified by taking into account the normal boys in the family, and the sister of a boy with Duchenne muscular dystrophy can occasionally be reassured because of her normal brothers and sons.

One unexpected aspect revealed by the use of DNA analysis in counselling families with Duchenne muscular dystrophy is the relatively high frequency of (gonadal) mosaicism in mothers of isolated affected boys. As indicated above, the two obvious possibilities are that the mother is a carrier (but just happens to have only one affected son) and has a 50 per cent risk with a future son, or the boy represents a new mutation—the result of a 'one off' mutation in an egg—with very little chance of recurrence in the family. Now it is clear that a third possibility has to be entertained; that a substantial proportion of the mother's eggs carry the mutation, but not some of her other tissues, including the white cells that are used for DNA analysis. This mosaicism came to light as families were found where the two or more affected boys had a dystrophin gene deletion, but mother did not, based on the fact that both copies were intact on blood analysis. Mosaicism is a feature of many cases of unexpected inheritance and is discussed later.

Table 6 *Estimate of birth frequency in males of the more common X-linked conditions in Britain per 1000 live births*

System	Disorder	Frequency
Locomotor system	Duchenne muscular dystrophy	0.25
Blood clotting	Haemophilia A	0.1
Skin	Ichthyosis	0.1
Mental retardation	Fragile X syndrome	0.75

The term X-linked dominant has been used for the very few rare conditions where the heterozygous female is regularly affected. However, the hemizygous male is always more severely affected and in some instances, affected males rarely survive gestation to be born, so only female patients are encountered in clinical practice.

X-INACTIVATION

The Y chromosome carries very few genes compared to the X. However, these chromosomes do pair during meiosis, with synapsis between homologous DNA sequences on the tip of the short arm of the X and the short arm of the Y. This pairing region is called the pseudo-autosomal region, because there is at least one obligatory crossing over during meiosis and therefore genes here segregate just like they do on the autosomes. Appropriately, these genes escape X-inactivation; both sexes have the same gene dosage.

For the remainder of the X-linked genes, most have no counterpart on the Y and so females would have twice the dose of gene product as males do, unless one or other of the alleles were 'silenced'. In fact, inactivation of one or other of the alleles does occur with most genes, just as Mary Lyon proposed in 1961. The inactivation process operates essentially at the whole chromosome level, so in females any one cell has either one or the other X chromosome inactivated (to become the late replicating X, which is the Barr body during interphase). Random inactivation of one or the other X chromosome occurs in each cell early in embryonic development, and thereafter the descendants of a particular cell have the same inactive X. Females are therefore functional mosaics with respect to X-linked genes, with about half their cells functionally dependent on the paternal X and the others operating with the maternal X. This random X-inactivation process is of no consequence if the woman carries no X-linked mutation, but the extent to which the process

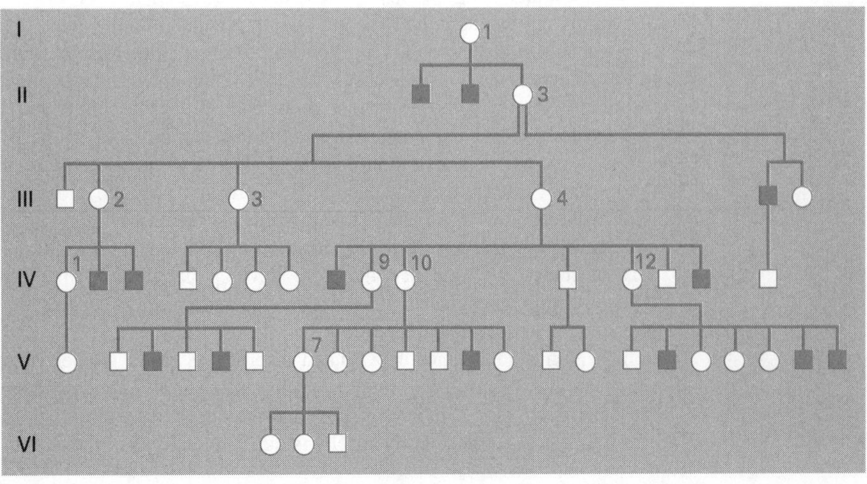

Fig. 10 Pedigree illustrating the transmission of a recessive X-linked trait. (Reproduced from Roberts and Pembrey (1985) with permission.)

Table 7 *Selected examples of a two allele genetic system showing the relationship between the gene (allele) frequency and the frequency in the population of heterozygotes and homozygotes given random mating*

Usual type of genetic trait involved	Gene frequency (rare allele)	Frequency of heterozygotes	Frequency of homozygotes
Common genetic	50%	50%	25%
polymorphisms	30%	42%	9%
OR	25%	37.5%	6.25%
Restriction fragment length	20%	32%	4%
polymorphisms	10%	18%	1%
Autosomal	1 in 30	1 in 15	1 in 900
recessive	1 in 50	1 in 25	1 in 2500
traits	1 in 100	1 in 50	1 in 10 000
	1 in 300	1 in 150	1 in 90 000
	1 in 500	1 in 250	1 in 250 000
Autosomal	1 in 5000	1 in 2500	1 in 25 000 000
dominant	1 in 20 000	1 in 10 000	1 in 400 000 000
traits	1 in 50 000	1 in 25 000	1 in 250 000 000

deviates from 50:50 can be critical if she does. Unfavourable X-inactivation is the most likely cause of a female heterozygote suffering more marked clinical manifestations of an X-disease than usual, and vice versa.

How X-inactivation happens is not really known. It spreads from an inactivation centre located at Xq12 and a candidate for the key gene located there has been cloned. This gene, *XIST*, is only transcribed when on the inactive X and appears to have no protein product, functioning at the RNA level. What is known is that some alleles on the active and inactive X can be distinguished by their pattern of DNA methylation.

There is an interesting clinical result in those rare instances when a balanced X/autosome reciprocal chromosomal translocation disrupts a critical gene on the X. In this situation the normal X is inactivated and the cells are therefore reliant on the translocated X, which lacks expression of the disrupted gene. The woman is functionally the same as an affected male and suffers to the same extent. It is likely that this distortion of random X-inactivation stems from the selective loss of those cells in which the translocated X is the inactive one. The inactivation process may spread to the attached bit of autosome to fatally silence gene expression there. Alternatively, that bit of the translocated X without the inactivation centre cannot inactivate as it should and the cell's function is compromised. One always has to remember that in the patient we see only the end-result of the long cell-proliferation (and selection) process of embryological development. These X/autosome translocations provide valuable clues to the location of X-linked disease loci and have provided the initial mapping information for many genes.

Gene frequencies

The concept of gene frequency is useful when thinking of the genetic make-up of whole populations, and for relating the frequency of people who are heterozygous at a particular locus to the frequency of homozygotes. The latter is described by the Hardy–Weinberg equilibrium, which, in essence, states that given a large population and random mating, in the absence of mutation and selection, the genetic constitution of the population remains the same from one generation to the next.

It is important, of course, to remember that with the exception of X-linked genes in the male, chromosomes and the genes they carry come in pairs. When considering gene frequencies we think of a 'pool' or population of chromosomes (chromosomes 11 for example) rather than individuals. Taking a single chromosome-11 locus with two alleles we let the proportion of normal alleles (e.g. normal β-globin, A) be p, and the proportion of mutant alleles (e.g. sickle β-globin, S) be q, so that $p + q = 1$. If one imagined taking pairs of chromosome 11 from the pool at random, the probability of getting two S genes would be $q \times q$, two A genes would be $p \times p$, and either one A gene plus an S gene or one S gene plus an A gene would be $pq + qp$. The proportion of normal homozygotes, heterozygotes, and abnormal homozygotes can therefore be written as follows:

$$\underset{AA}{p^2} + \underset{AS}{2pq} + \underset{SS}{q^2} = 1$$

If the sickle gene, S, frequency was 10 per cent, q would equal 0.1, and SS homozygotes, those with sickle-cell anaemia, would be $0.1 \times 0.1 = 0.01$. Because $p + q = 1$, $p = 0.9$ and therefore normal AA homozygotes would be $0.9 \times 0.9 = 0.81$. The proportion with sickle-cell trait AS, would be $2 \times 0.9 \times 0.1 = 0.18$. Note that the S gene frequency is not the same as the frequency of heterozygous individuals, it is nearly half the value, and would approximate closer to half as the gene frequency falls. This is easy to visualize; if the disease is at all rare, as most monogenic disorders are, virtually all the mutant alleles in the population will reside in heterozygous individuals. The gene frequency determines the chance of any one chromosome carrying that allele, but as individuals have two of the relevant chromosomes there is twice the chance of having the allele on either one or other chromosome. Thus, for practical purposes the heterozygote frequency is twice the gene frequency. In autosomal recessive disorders the gene frequency is the square root of the abnormal homozygote frequency. For example, galactosaemia occurs with a frequency of about 1 in 40 000; $\sqrt{(1/40\,000)} = 1/200 =$ the gene frequency, and therefore $1/200 \times 2$, or 1 in 100 individuals in the population will be heterozygous. Table 7 shows the relation of homozygote to heterozygote frequencies at different gene frequencies. It will be seen that in a recessive disease with a 1 in 10 000 frequency, such as phenylketonuria, the chance of a homozygote marrying a carrier is 1 in 50, giving a small but not negligible risk of 1 in 100 of an affected child.

The frequencies of particular matings in a population may be of clinical interest, for example, in predicting the proportion of all matings that could produce rhesus or ABO incompatibility. The frequency of a mating is the product of the frequencies of the genotypes involved. Taking the sickle-cell example where the gene frequency, $p = 0.1$, the frequency of AS × AS matings would be $2pq \times 2pq$ or $0.18 \times 0.18 = 0.0324$.

The Hardy–Weinberg equilibrium can describe a three allele system, such as blood group alleles *A*, *B*, and *O* with gene frequencies p, q, and r, by the equation:

$$\text{Genotype} \quad \underset{OO}{r^2} + \underbrace{p^2 + 2pr}_{AA\ AO} + \underbrace{q^2 + 2qr}_{BB\ BO} + \underset{AB}{2pq} = 1.$$

$$\text{Blood group} \quad \text{O} \qquad \text{A} \qquad \text{B} \qquad \text{AB}$$

Consideration of gene frequencies is important in planning population screening programmes, and these are discussed later.

Chromosomal abnormalities

Chromosomal disorders fall into two broad groups: those due to the abnormal segregation of whole chromosomes during meiosis (or mitosis), and those caused by abnormalities/rearrangements of chromosome structure. Each of these broad groups covers several categories.

The most clinically prominent of the segregation abnormalities are those errors of meiosis resulting in an extra chromosome, the trisomies, but there may be a missing chromosome as in Turner's syndrome, or even a disorder due to uniparental disomy such as in some patients with the Prader–Willi syndrome where the chromosome number is normal. Segregation errors after conception lead to mosaicism, which can underlie disorders ranging from intrauterine growth retardation to congenital malformations and predisposition to malignancies.

In discussing mutational mechanisms in an earlier section, it was pointed out that, now analytic methods can cover all levels from whole chromosomes down to DNA sequence, many structural chromosomal abnormalities, such as deletions, duplications and inversions, merge with classical mendelian disorders showing autosomal dominant or X-linked inheritance. However, structural chromosomal abnormalities also include translocations of material between different chromosomes, which again may be there at conception, affecting all cells, or may occur later on during mitosis, when it may be associated with cancer.

In their widest sense, chromosomal abnormalities represent a huge field of great clinical relevance. Here, we can only cover the general principles with a few illustrative examples, starting with the methods of analysis.

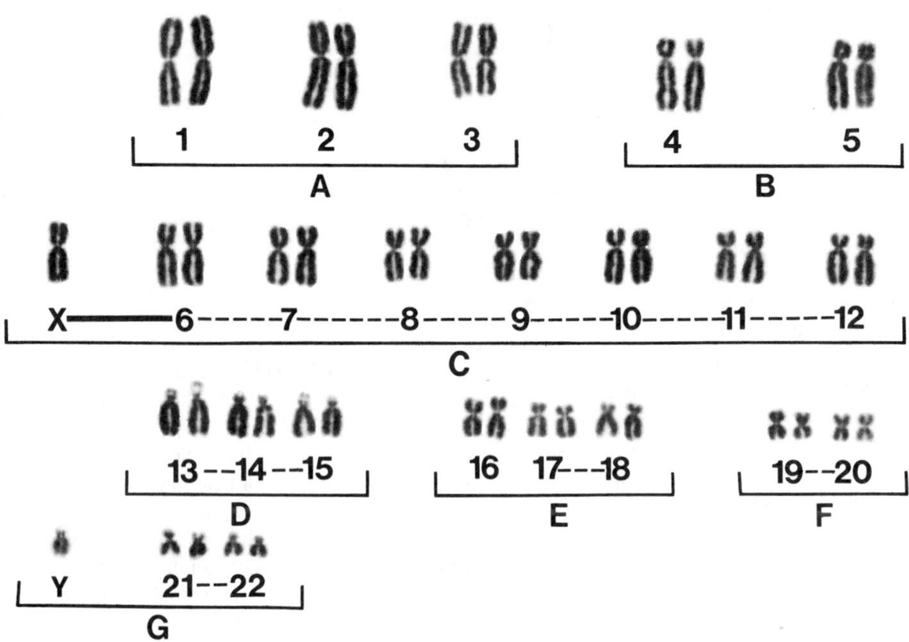

Fig. 11 A normal male karyotype, 46,XY. Orcein-stained metaphase chromosomes with the Denver classification superimposed. The dotted lines indicate uncertainty, and the solid line between X and 6 great uncertainty, of individual chromosome identification by this technique. The centromere joining the two chromatids of each chromosome is readily seen. (Reproduced from Roberts and Pembrey (1985), with permission.)

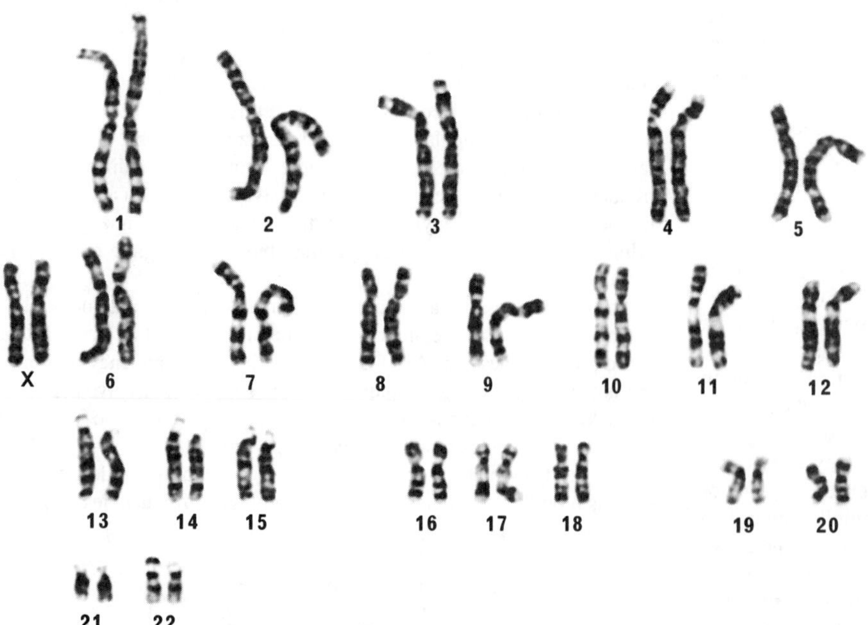

Fig. 12 A karyotype of a normal female, stained with one of the Giemsa banding techniques that permit individual chromosome identification. Large satellites, a normal chromosome variant, are present on one homologue of chromosome 22. (Reproduced from Roberts and Pembrey (1985), with permission.)

CHROMOSOME ANALYSIS

Chromosomes are only visible by light microscopy when contracted during mitotic cell division (see Fig. 3). Blood lymphocytes stimulated to divide by phytohaemagglutinin are the usual source of material for chromosome analysis, but direct analysis of bone marrow or chorionic villus, or the study of cultured skin or amniotic cells, are also possible. Because division is usually arrested by the use of colchicine at metaphase, each chromosome is often clearly seen as two chromatids held together at the centromere (Fig. 11).

The first technique, orcein staining, as used in Fig. 11, could not distinguish the individual chromosomes within the groups A–G, and the facility to do this had to await the so-called banding methods that stain only selected regions of the chromosomes, probably depending on the concentration of adenine/thymine base pairs in the DNA.

The standard banding techniques used on metaphase chromosomes reveal about 300 to 400 bands, but so-called high-resolution banding on the much less contracted prometaphase chromosomes can show 1200 bands, although such analyses are not usually routinely available. Figure 12 shows a good-quality, G-banded karyotype of a normal female. Figure 11 shows that chromosomes 13, 14, 15, 21, and 22 are acrocentric, with the centromere close to one end. The short arm consists only of some ribosomal genes that can be lost without ill-effect. Incidentally, Fig. 12 shows that one of the 22 chromosome pair has an additional band on the short arm. These are called satellites (not to be confused with repetitive or 'satellite' DNA) and are a normal, familial variation of no clinical significance. It is essential that the clinician is appropriately advised about these normal variations, which include variation in heterochromatin at the centromeres of chromosomes 1, 9, and 16.

Whilst much can be done by banding techniques and simple light microscopy, the advent of molecular cytogenetics, in which the classical analysis of metaphase spreads (or even interphase nuclei) are combined with the use of DNA probes, is providing greatly enhanced resolution and revolutionizing both research and clinical investigation. It is now possible to hybridize fluorescently labelled DNA probes directly to the kind of metaphase spreads shown in Fig. 12 and see where they 'light up'. This technique goes by the acronym FISH, fluorescent *in situ* (suppression) hybridization and can be used two ways. By using a mixture of many probes specific for a particular chromosome, the whole of both chromosomes of the pair can be 'painted' with a specific fluorochrome. Other chromosomes can be painted with fluorochromes giving different colours. Chromosome painting is very helpful for revealing the chromosomal origin of fragments attached to other chromosomes or lying free. It also helps to resolve the nature of complex translocations, important in both general clinical genetics as well as cancer cytogenetics. An alternative approach is use of a gene- or marker-specific probe to determine its rough location on the chromosome and its relation to other sequences. Not only is this a very powerful way to map newly cloned DNA sequences, it can also be used in clinical practice to look for the deletion or relocation of known genes, or parts of large genes.

Shorthand description of karyotypes

The normal male and female karyotypes are written: 46,XY and 46,XX. Where there is an extra whole chromosome, for example, Down's syndrome, the karyotype is written 47,XX+21, or 47,XY+21 if male. It will be seen that the total chromosome count (based on the number of centromeres) is given first, followed by the sex chromosomes, and, if necessary, this is followed by some further detail. Klinefelter's syndrome is written 47,XXY and Turner's syndrome 45,X. With structural anomalies it is necessary to specify whether it is the long arm or the short arm that is affected, and so p (think of *petit*) represents the short arm and q the long arm. 46,XY,4p− describes a male with the short arm of chromosome 4 shorter in length than normal. The notation p+ or q+ indicates that the chromosome arm is longer than normal but does not indicate where the extra material has come from (this will have to be determined by chromosome painting). If the change occurs in a heterochromatic region and therefore likely to be of little clinical significance, the symbol h is used before the + sign; for example, 16qh+, When a particular rearrangement is to be described, the symbol for this is placed after the sex chromosome notation and before the chromosome(s) involved, which are placed in parentheses. A reciprocal translocation between chromosomes 1 and 3 could be as follows: 46,XX,t(1;3)(q32;p24), where the breakpoints on the long arm of 1 and the short arm of 3 are given in the last set of parentheses. The description of the breakpoints uses the numbering for the chromosome region and band that has been internationally agreed; an example of a chromosome idiogram indicating the numbered bands is seen in Fig. 16 below.

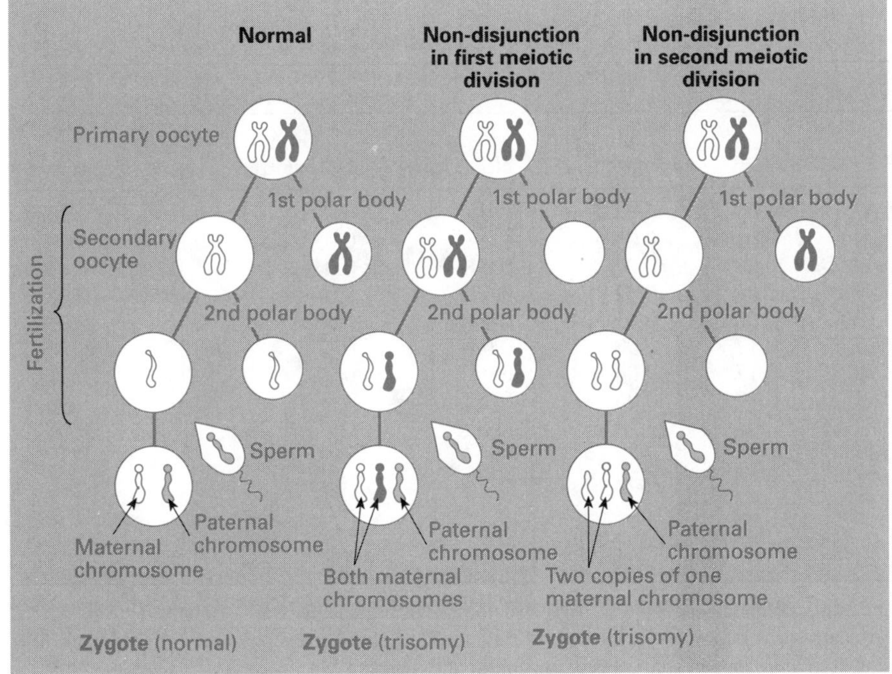

Fig. 13 A diagram to illustrate the consequences of: normal disjunction during oogenesis; non-disjunction at the first meiotic division; and non-dysjunction at the second meiotic division. Only the pair of homologous chromosomes involved in the non-disjunction is shown. (Reproduced from Roberts and Pembrey (1985) with permission.)

Table 8 *The usual chromosomal complements and key clinical features of the common sex chromosome anomalies*

Syndrome	Chromosomal abnormality karyotype		Frequency (%)	Clinical features
Turner's syndrome	Monosomy X	45,X	55	Female; lymphoedema of hands and feet (infant). webbed neck; low hair line; broad shield-shaped thorax with wide-spaced nipples; cardiovascular malformations usually coarctation of aorta; renal malformation; short stature; ovarian dysgenesis; hearing loss; slight reduction in expected IQ range, but great majority in the normal range
	Mosaicism	46,XX/45,X 47,XXX/45,X etc.	10	
	Isochromosome X	46,X,i(Xq) 46X,i,(Xq)/45,X etc.	20	
	Other karyotypes X deletions etc.		15	
Triple-X syndrome		47,XXX		Female; in most patients phenotype, puberty, and fertility normal; head circumference, reduced, 8% microcephalic; delayed language development in 50%; IQ below 70 in 15% (Rare 48, XXXX females have mental retardation in 80%)
Klinefelter's syndrome		47,XXY	80	Male; often no distinctive features in childhood, but increased incidence (15–20%) of various congenital malformations; eunuchoid habitus; testicular atrophy; infertility; gynaecomastia in 25–30%; delayed language development in 50%; IQ below 90 in 30%, but very few below IQ 80
	Mosaicism etc.	47,XXY/46,XY 47,XXY/46,XX 48,XXXY etc.	20	
Double-Y-syndrome		47,XYY		Male with no distinctive phenotype; usually tall (> 180 cm) and fertile; delayed language development in 30%; IQ below 90 in about a third, few below IQ 80; some with mental retardation have antisocial behaviour leading to an over-representation in institutions for dangerous mentally ill subjects (The rare 48, XXYY males have a Klinefelter's syndrome with mental retardation and antisocial behaviour being common)

Table 9 *Crude maternal age specific rates (%) for chromosome abnormalities in pregnancies monitored because of a maternal age ≥ 35 years*

Maternal age (years)	Number of pregnancies	Autosomal aberrations +21	+18	+13	Extra marker	Mosaics etc.	Un-bal.	Bal.	t13:14
35	5409	0.35	0.07	0.05	0.04	0.04	0.02	0.26	0.07
36	6103	0.57	0.08	0.03	0.03	—	0.05	0.21	0.08
37	6956	0.68	0.09	0.03	0.07	0.07	0.04	0.18	0.03
38	7926	0.81	0.15	0.04	0.02	0.02	0.04	0.19	0.08
39	7682	1.09	0.19	0.06	0.05	0.03	0.05	0.16	0.03
40	7174	1.23	0.25	0.12	0.08	0.03	0.07	0.17	0.06
41	4763	1.47	0.36	0.17	0.06	0.04	0.02	0.17	0.02
42	3156	2.19	0.63	0.19	0.06	0.13	—	0.19	0.06
43	1912	3.24	0.78	0.05	0.10	0.10	0.05	—	0.05
44	1015	2.95	0.49	—	—	—	—	—	0.10
45	508	4.53	0.39	0.20	0.39	0.20	—	—	—
46	232	8.19	0.43	—	—	—	—	—	—
>46	129	2.33	0.77	—	—	—	—	—	—
≥35	52 965	1.16	0.23	0.07	0.06	0.04	0.04	0.18	0.05

+21, +18, +13—Autosomal trisomies. Un-bal.—Duplication deficiencies resulting from structural rearrangements. Bal.—Balanced structural rearrangements (translocations, inversions, excluding pericentric inversions of 9). *De novo*—Balanced structural rearrangements arising from new mutation. Abn—All unbalanced aberrations. From Collaborative European study. Ferguson-Smith and Yates (1984).

FREQUENCY OF CHROMOSOMAL ABNORMALITIES

The overall incidence in live births is about 5–6/1000 and it is estimated that about 50 per cent of early spontaneous abortions are chromosomally abnormal; of 1000 recognized pregnancies there are about 75 fetal or neonatal deaths due to chromosome abnormalities, the great majority arising as new mutations in the ovum, sperm, or early zygote. If preimplantation embryos are included, perhaps up to 20 per cent of conceptuses are chromosomally abnormal. These high rates, particularly of trisomy and monosomy, are relevant to the surprising prevalence of uniparental disomy considered later. It will be appreciated that the frequency of certain anomalies at birth is largely determined by their relative chances of survival to term. The most common trisomy in man appears to be trisomy 16, but all abort.

DISORDERS OF CHROMOSOME NUMBER

During meiosis, the reduction division that leads to the ovum and sperm having a single, haploid set of chromosomes, homologous chromosomes pair up before moving apart to the opposite poles of that dividing cell (see Fig. 4). Failure of the pair to associate in the first place, or failure to dissociate, can lead to an ovum or sperm with an extra chromosome, or one missing. The term non-disjunction, which assumes the latter mechanism, is often used for this error of chromosome segregation. The causes of non-disjunction are largely unknown, but the chance of it having occurred in the ovum increases with maternal age. The resulting fetus will either have three copies of a particular chromosome (trisomy) or only one (monosomy). In practice the trisomies are the most important, monosomies in general being non-viable. Figure 13 is a generalized diagram of the consequences of non-disjunction during oogenesis. Non-disjunction can occur at the first or second meiotic division and the timing can sometimes be deduced from using chromosome or DNA markers, provided these are close to the centromere. Figure 13 does not show recombination between chromatids, for simplicity's sake, but for regions away from the centromere recombination obscures the origin of the non-disjunction. Knowledge of when the non-disjunction occurred will be important in attempts to elucidate the cause of Down's syndrome, for example. In females the first meiotic division of oogenesis begins when the woman herself was a fetus, whilst the second meiotic division occurs at fertilization.

Anomalies of sex-chromosome number (see Table 8)

Trisomies involving the X or Y chromosome are relatively common (see table 9) and lead to surprisingly minor physical abnormalities considering the size of the X chromosome and the many genes it carries. The explanation resides in the phenomenon of X-chromosome inactivation described earlier. Only one X chromosome remains active in any one cell beyond an early stage of development and the inactive X chromosome becomes the X-chromatin body (formerly known as the Barr body), which is visible close to the nuclear membrane in a proportion of cell nuclei in females. XXX females have two X-chromatin bodies in their cell nuclei, and the much rarer XXXX females have three X-chromatin bodies.

Down's syndrome due to primary trisomy 21

Down's syndrome, always due to an extra chromosome 21, is the most common, viable autosomal trisomy, presumably because of the small size of the chromosome involved. Overall about 96 per cent are due to a primary non-disjunction, and about 95 per cent of these involve errors in the formation of the ovum rather than the sperm. In the other 4 per cent the extra chromosome 21 is attached to another chromosome and will be discussed in the next section. The incidence of Down's syndrome increases from about 1 in 1200 in mothers under 30 years to about 1 in 100 at the age of 39 years (Table 9), and at present accounts for about a third of all cases of severe mental handicap in children of school age.

It is likely that some people are predisposed to non-disjunction, although they cannot be identified, and overall a couple who have had one Down's child have a 1 in 100 chance of the next child having a trisomy, usually Down's.

Other trisomies

Trisomy 18, Edwards' syndrome, is the next most common after Down's, followed by trisomy 13, Patau syndrome. Death is usual in infancy but survival for many years can occur rarely, particularly if there is no severe heart defect. There is always severe mental retardation. The incidence for all trisomies appear related to maternal age and Table 9 gives the collaborative European data on age-related risks based on amniocentesis results. Despite some earlier claims to the contrary, it now seems clear that there is no independent paternal-age effect.

Although the absolute risk to a couple does not reach a high level if they delay having children, the overall effect on the population incidence

Sex chromosome aberrations							Totals			
XXX	XXY	XYY	XO	Mosaics etc.	Un-bal.	Bal.	Abn.	Bal.	*De novo*	All aberrations
0.07	0.09	0.05	0.05	—	0.05	0.05	0.91	0.39	0.02	1.29
0.08	0.08	0.02	0.10	0.05	—	0.02	1.09	0.31	0.03	1.41
0.07	0.04	0.03	0.06	0.06	—	0.03	1.24	0.26	0.04	1.50
0.08	0.08	0.02	0.08	0.04	0.02	—	1.39	0.26	0.04	1.65
0.12	0.16	0.04	0.03	0.04	0.01	0.04	1.87	0.22	0.05	2.10
0.06	0.15	0.03	0.04	0.04	0.03	—	2.13	0.22	0.01	2.36
0.15	0.29	0.04	—	0.04	—	2.64	0.19	0.02	2.83	
0.28	0.35	0.03	0.03	0.03	—	—	3.77	0.24	0.03	4.01
0.31	0.31	—	—	—	0.05	—	5.02	0.05	—	5.07
0.49	0.39	—	—	—	—	—	4.33	0.10	—	4.43
0.39	0.98	0.20	—	—	—	7.28	—	0.20	7.28	
0.43	1.29	—	—	—	—	—	10.34	—	—	10.34
1.55	1.55	0.77	—	—	—	—	6.98	—	—	6.98
0.12	0.16	0.03	0.04	0.04	0.02	0.02	2.01	0.25	0.03	2.26

of Down's syndrome, for example, is greatly influenced by the age at which women choose to start a family.

CHROMOSOMAL TRANSLOCATIONS

There are broadly two types of translocation, a robertsonian translocation and a reciprocal translocation.

Robertsonian translocation

This occurs when two acrocentric chromosomes join at their centromeres and the clinically unimportant short-arm material is lost from the cell, in other words there is a centric fusion. Such people, who now have 45 chromosomes, are healthy, and because there is no significant loss or gain of genetic material they are said to carry a balanced translocation. There is, however, a risk of an unbalanced arrangement in their offspring, the risk, for some unknown reason, depending on the acrocentric chromosomes involved. Although carriers of a $^{13}/_{14}$ translocation are the most common (approximately 1 in 2000), unbalanced offspring such as trisomy 13 are rare. A clinically more important situation arises with robertsonian translocations involving chromosome 21, of which the most common is $^{14}/_{21}$. Figure 14 shows the karyotype of a woman carrying a $^{14}/_{21}$ translocation and that of her daughter with Down's syndrome. In essence the woman has passed on her normal 21, and the composite 14^{21} chromosome in place of her normal 14. Because of the complicated 'pairing' of the 14, 14^{21} and the 21 chromosomes during meiosis and the resultant difficulties in segregation, a number of different types of gamete can be formed, although only four are commonly observed. A gamete may contain chromosomes 14 and 21 and on fertilization produce a normal child. The gamete may contain just the composite 14^{21} chromosome and produce a carrier like the parent. A gamete containing just chromosome 14 and no 21 will produce a non-viable 21 monosomy. Finally, a gamete with the 14^{21} and 21 chromosome will produce a Down's child. Selection at various stages means that the theoretical risks are not realized in real life. A woman with a $^{14}/_{21}$ translocation has approximately a 1 in 8 risk of a Down's baby, whilst a male translocation carrier has perhaps only a 1 in 50 risk. Both have a high

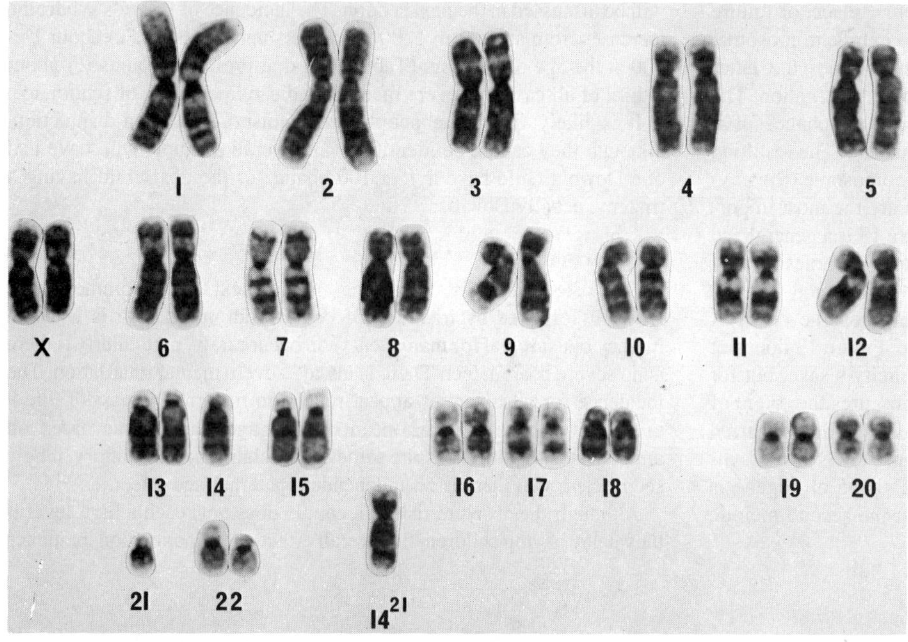

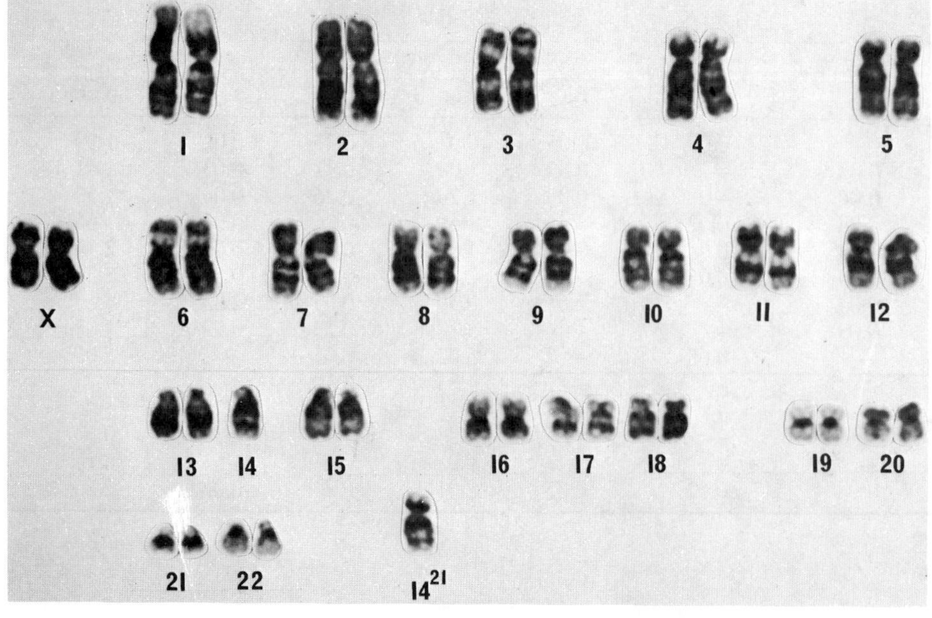

Fig. 14 Karyotype of a healthy woman (above) and that of her Down's syndrome child (below). The mother has a chromosome count of 45 because of a robertsonian translocation between chromosomes 14 and 21, written 45,XX,t(14q21q). Her child has inherited both the composite $^{14}/_{21}$ chromosome and the normal 21 from her, and therefore effectively has three 21 chromosomes. The karyotype is written 46,XX,t(14q21q). (Reproduced from Roberts and Pembrey (1985), with permission.)

risk, approaching 50 per cent, of producing a carrier like themselves, and herein lies the importance of family studies to alert relatives, especially females, to their risk of a Down's baby and the need to check their chromosomes.

Clinically, a translocation of Down's is no different from the primary trisomy 21 case. About two-thirds represent *de novo* translocations, both parents having normal karyotypes. In the remainder one or other parent, usually the mother, will be a carrier. Although Down's syndrome due to a translocation, being independent of maternal age, is over-represented in younger mothers (8–10 per cent of cases when the mother is under 30 years), it is still good practice to examine the chromosomes of all cases of Down's syndrome, regardless of maternal age. For many years to come there will be relatives seeking reassurance about their own risk and a karyotype on the affected family member is most helpful.

Not all translocation Down's cases are $^{14}/_{21}$ and other robertsonian translocations, such as $^{15}/_{21}$, $^{21}/_{21}$ and $^{21}/_{22}$, can be responsible for familial Down's syndrome. For a parent with a $^{21}/_{21}$ translocation the only viable offspring will have Down's syndrome. This is one of the rare situations in clinical genetics where there is no chance of normal offspring, the mating of two individuals with the same recessive condition being another.

Reciprocal translocation

The choice of the centric fusion between chromosome 14 and 21 as the example of a robertsonian translocation was an easy one, for this is by far the most common one of clinical importance. There is no such obvious candidate as an example of a reciprocal translocation; they may involve any two chromosomes, and no one translocation stands out as more important than another. Figure 15 gives the pedigree of a family in which there was a reciprocal translocation between the short arm of chromosome 5 and the long arm of 1 (see Fig. 16). The clinical story began with the youngest son, II-7, of the couple, I-1 and I-2. He was found to have an absence of much of the short arm of one chromosome 5, or 5p−. At that time (1964) it was only possible to say there was an absence of part of the short arm of a B-group chromosome; but the clinical picture was typical of the *cri-du-chat* syndrome. The patient had typical facies, was severely mentally and physically retarded, and died in infancy. At that time his mother, I-2, and his three healthy brothers II-3, 4, and 6, were found to have a similar abnormality of one B chromosome; and because of their normal development it was assumed that the missing bit was translocated to another chromosome, although which one could not be identified for certain at that time.

Despite a recommendation that these boys should be referred for genetic advice when they grew up, communication across the generation gap failed, and II-6 produced a daughter, III-4, who also suffered from the *cri-du-chat* syndrome. Prenatal diagnosis was offered to the wife of II-3 and her first fetus had the alternative, unbalanced arrangement; not a loss of 5p material but an additional copy (partial trisomy) of 5p material. The parents opted for termination of the pregnancy and autopsy confirmed the presence of multiple malformations. Fortunately the daughter, III-3, of the translocation carrier, II-4, was shown to have an entirely normal karyotype. Thus all four common combinations involving chromosome pairs 1 and 5 have been realized in this family.

It can be appreciated from Fig. 16 that a person with a balanced reciprocal translocation has one normal chromosome 1, one normal chromosome 5, a chromosome 1 with a bit of 1q missing but a bit of 5p attached, and a chromosome 5 with a bit of 5p missing but a bit of 1q attached. This complement results in no loss or gain of genetic material and therefore the person is healthy. However, when that person forms gametes there are four possible combinations that result in a normal chromosome count and these are illustrated in Fig. 16. Rarer combinations producing 45 or 47 chromosomes could occur. The actual risks vary according to the reciprocal translocation and the viability of fetuses with unbalanced chromosome complements. Overall the risk of a translocation carrier of either sex producing an unbalanced fetus at midtrimester diagnosis is about 1 in 9 (the risk is about 1 in 5 if the carrier was ascertained through a previous unbalanced, malformed child; and 1 in 26 if ascertained through previous early miscarriages). There is, of course, a high chance, 1 in 3 to 1 in 2, of producing a healthy child with a balanced translocation, and this raises the important point of offering to screen healthy family members to exclude the balanced translocation state before reproduction.

Translocation arising in somatic cells can be associated with a variety of malignancies and these are described in conjunction with the individual diseases.

Fig. 15 Pedigree of the transmission of a balanced reciprocal translocation between the end of the long arm of chromosome 1 and the short arm of chromosome 5, from a woman to three of her sons. All four combinations involving the chromosome pairs 1 and 5 are realized in this family; both unbalanced arrangements, the balanced arrangement, and the normal karyotype. (Reproduced from Roberts and Pembrey (1985), with permission.)

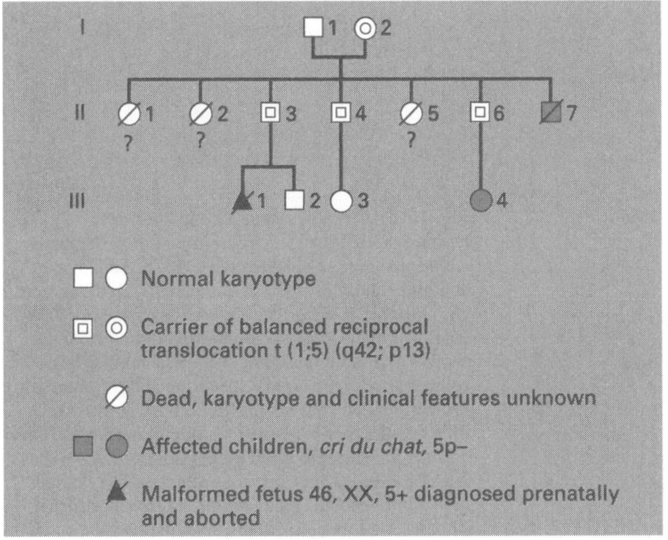

OTHER ABNORMALITIES OF CHROMOSOMAL STRUCTURE

Invertions do not usually cause any problem *per se* but can lead to difficulties with 'pairing' at meiosis. If the inversion spans the centromere (pericentric inversion), a cross-over at meiosis can lead to gametes with either a deletion or duplication. Sometimes inversions disrupt genes, as with a common mutation causing haemophilia A discussed earlier.

Some specific deletions cause distinct, recognizable malformation syndromes, including an increasing number of clinical entities not previously thought to be chromosomal defects, summarized in Table 2.

Mosaics

Although the type of mutation in a somatic cell that initiates the mosaicism may vary from a whole-chromosome segregational error to a point mutation in some gene critical for cellular growth and function, some general aspects are common to all mosaics. The effects are often visible in the skin. Many of the trivial circumscribed lesions on the skin, depigmented patches for example, are probably due to somatic mutations either at the DNA level or involving whole chromosomes. It is also likely that genes may become 'silenced' by the sort of factors involved in imprinting (epigenetic factors) in some somatic cells during life.

When the mosaicism arises early in development the abnormal cell line may be widely distributed throughout the tissues, causing malfunction in several organs. An important example here is the group of disorders subsumed under the term hypomelanosis of Ito **(HI)**, in which pigmented and depigmented whorls on the skin, often along Blaschko's lines, are associated with body asymmetry and sometimes serious eye and brain malformations. In the minority of cases of HI, chromosomal mosaicism can be demonstrated by a combination of blood and skin fibroblast karyotyping. If one were able to take multiple biopsies, no doubt the proportion of HI patients showing chromosomal or genetic mosaicism (demonstrable by DNA fingerprinting) would be much greater. In keeping with the chromosomal mosaic pathogenesis is the wide variety of associated malformations and the sporadic nature of the disorder. With regard to sporadicity, the assumption must be that it is the normal cell line that rescues the embryo from lethality (or an established trisomic phenotype) and therefore any offspring inheriting the abnormal genotype from a mosaic parent would not be viable. In theory, such affected offspring could themselves become mosaic by losing the additional chromosome, but such 'transmission' of mosaicism from one generation to the next must be rare. Happle has proposed that sporadic disorders where cutaneous lesions tend to follow the lines of Blaschko, such as the McCune–Albright, Schimmelpenning–Feurerstein–Mims (linear sebaceous naevus) and Proteus syndromes, might be due to lethal mutations that can only exist in a mosaic state, which in turn explains the patchy distribution of lesions along Blaschko's lines.

The nature of Blaschko's lines is itself unclear. They are thought to reflect the dorsoventral outgrowth of two functionally different populations of cells during early embryogenesis. It is proposed that the two different populations of cells can be generated by either random X-inactivation in a female carrying an X-linked mutation (e.g. as incontinentia pigmenti) or mosaicism. How the presence of two different cell lines leads to the pigmentary disturbances is not known but presumably stems from altered developmental signals concerned with melanocyte migration.

Another area where chromosomal mosaicism has a clinical impact is when it is discovered on placental biopsy, in conjunction with prenatal diagnosis for example. It is estimated that about 2 per cent of all pregnancies are associated with confined placental chromosomal mosaicism (i.e. without obviously extending to the fetus). The extent to which this underlies some intrauterine growth retardation due to a malfunctioning placenta is under investigation. Placental mosaicism may raise the suspicion of uniparental disomy in the baby, if it has a normal karyotype, but some growth or developmental problem. Uniparental disomy is described later in conjunction with genomic imprinting.

Non-classical inheritance

Unstable trinucleotide repeats, premutations, and anticipation

Just when we thought it was safe to say that we had probably seen the full repertoire of mutations causing human diseases, expanding tri-

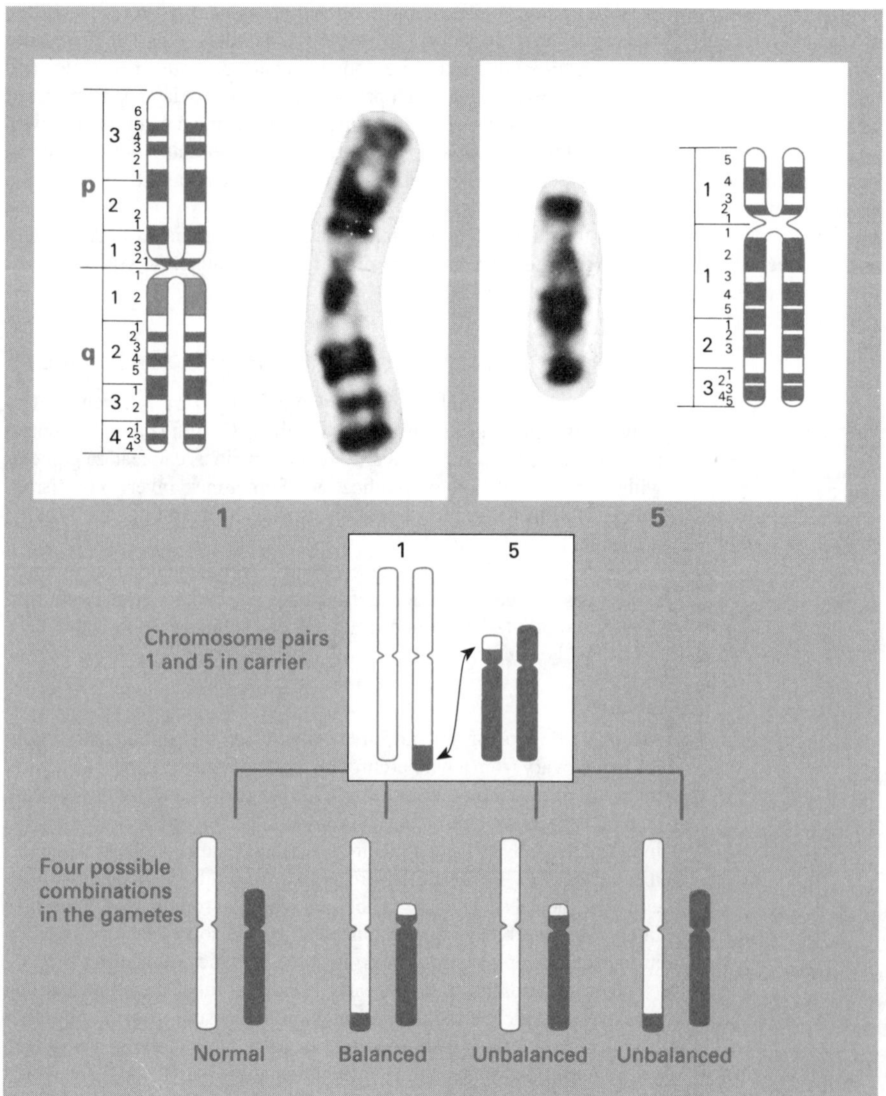

Fig. 16 The reciprocal translocation between chromosomes 1 and 5 that was found in the family whose pedigree is illustrated in Fig. 15. Top: The abnormal chromosome 1 is compared with the normal chromosome 1 ideogram: it clearly has an extra dark band near the end of the long arm (derived from the short arm of a chromosome 5). The abnormal 5 is compared with the normal ideogram and the short arm is clearly reduced in length. Bottom: A diagram to illustrate the four combinations of chromosomes 1 and 5 in the gametes produced by a carrier of the translocation. Rare errors of segregation can produce other chromosome combinations. (Reproduced from Roberts and Pembrey (1985), with permission.)

Table 10 *The first seven examples of diseases due to dynamic mutations where there is expansion of a trinucleotide repeat*

	Fragile X syndrome	Spinobulbar muscular atrophy	Myotonic dystrophy	Huntington's disease	Spinocerebellar ataxia type 1	FRAX E (? mild mental retardation)	Dentatorubral pallidoluysian atrophy (DRPLA)
Inheritance	X-linked with normal transmitting males (anticipation)	X-linked recessive Variable severity	Autosomal dominant Anticipation	Autosomal dominant Anticipation	Autosomal dominant Anticipation	X-linked	Autosomal dominant Anticipation
Sex bias for transmission of early onset/ severe form	Maternal (full mutation)	Maternal (due to X-linked inheritance)	Maternal (congenital DM)	Paternal (early onset)	Paternal ?	?	Paternal ?
Protein/ expression	Putative RNA-binding protein mRNA widely expressed	Androgen receptor	Putative protein kinase	Unknown function, mRNA widely expressed	mRNA widely expressed	?	?
Disease-causing mechanism	Transcription shut down; abnormal DNA methylation	Abnormal protein gain of function?	Altered level of mRNA/protein	Abnormal protein gain of function?	Abnormal protein gain of function?	?	?
Repeat/location	CGG 5′UTR	CAG Protein coding (Gln)	CTG 3′UTR	CAG Protein coding (Gln)?	CAG Protein coding (Gln)?	GCC ?UTR	CAG Protein coding (Gln)?
Number of repeats (normal)	10–50	11–31	5–35	9–34	25–36	6–25	8–25
Linkage disequilibrium	Yes	Not known	Yes	Yes	?	?	?
Disease alleles	52–200 (premutation) 200–2000 (full mutation)	40–62	50–80 (protomutation) 80–2000 affected	30–100	43–81	?>25>200 premutation ?>200 full mutation	54–68

nucleotide repeat sequences were discovered. What's more, these discoveries go a long way towards explaining the unusual inheritance in important diseases such as fragile X syndrome, myotonic dystrophy, and Huntington's disease. Table 10 summarizes some key features of seven diseases where this class of 'dynamic' mutation occurs.

FRAGILE X SYNDROME

The fragile X syndrome, the most common inherited form of mental retardation, gets its name from the unstainable gap or 'fragile site' seen at Xq27.3 in 5 to 50 per cent of cells, when lymphocytes are cultured in folic acid-deficient or other special media (Fig. 17). It is still not clear how the mutational events cause the fragile site. However, discovery of the role of expansion of the polymorphic CGG repeat at the 5′ end of the *FMR1* gene in causing the mental retardation has explained both the unusual inheritance of this condition and revolutionized genetic services for affected families. A striking feature of many pedigrees is that affected cousins have inherited the condition from the maternal grandfather who is fragile site-negative and clinically normal. It is now known that these 'normal transmitting males' carry a premutation which corresponds to a small expansion of the CGG repeat from the normal range of 5–?50 to ?55–200 repeats. The daughters of normal transmitting males are also phenotypically normal because in this condition, as opposed to myotonic dystrophy, the premutation only progresses to the full mutation when transmitted by a female.

Fig. 17 A metaphase spread showing the appearance of the fragile site (arrowed) near the tip of the long arm of the X chromosome [fra(X)(q28)]. The presence of the fragile site is dependent on the composition of the tissue culture medium; low folic acid levels inducing fragile sites. (Reproduced from Roberts and Pembrey (1985), with permission.)

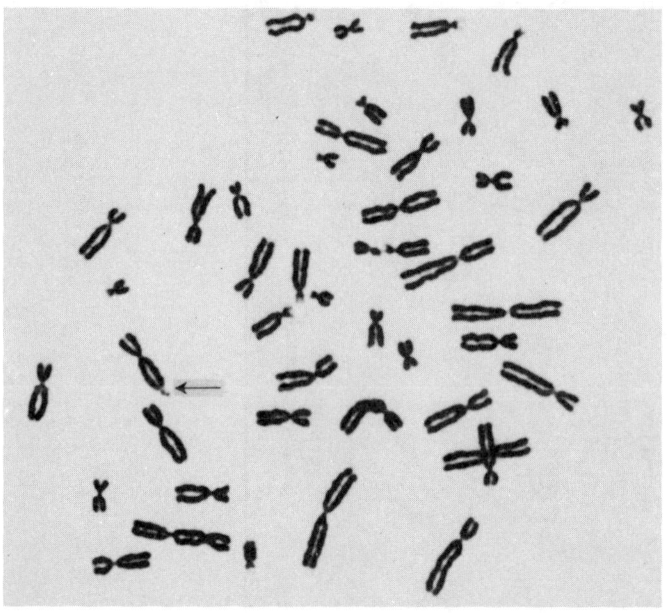

As illustrated in Fig. 18, the full mutation that correlates with mental retardation is characterized by a massive expansion of the CGG repeat sequence. It seems that when a critical repeat size is reached, two important things happen. Firstly, the DNA becomes somatically unstable, so that different cells have different sized CGG repeat expansions and give a smear rather than discrete band on DNA analysis. Secondly, the CGG repeat and other cytosines become methylated and transcription of the *FMR1* gene ceases. As one might expect, with this methylation 'threshold', the level of *FMR1* protein and clinical severity do not relate closely to the number of CGG repeats; the gene works (premutation) or not (full mutation). However, a subset of patients, who as a group are less severely affected, do have a substantial line of cells with just the premutation and an unmethylated, active gene. These 'mosaic' situations raised the question of when during maternal transmission does the premutation progress to the full mutation. There is now evidence that this occurs soon after fertilization, and therefore is a postzygotic, somatic event. Sperm from affected males (with methylated full mutations on blood analysis) show only CGG repeats in the premutation range.

About 30 to 50 per cent of sisters of affected males are clinically affected (showing the full mutation on one X), although on average the intellectual deficit is less than in males. DNA analysis now allows simple carrier testing for female relatives of affected individuals and much more reliable prenatal diagnosis for those who want it. To date, testing earlier generations in affected families has not revealed the progression from normal to premutation. Where a female relative has a premutation of more than 90 repeats, then progression to the full mutation on transmission of that X chromosome seems inevitable. Preliminary studies on the general population indicate about 1 in 500 women have repeat numbers in the premutation range that one might expect to be unstable on transmission (although prospective studies will be needed). The existence of linkage disequilibrium (see above) between specific 'alleles' at neighbouring DNA markers and the full mutation suggests that all modern-day affected families derive from only a few ancestral X chromosomes. This is quite remarkable and it is conceivable that there is some other explanation of the allelic association.

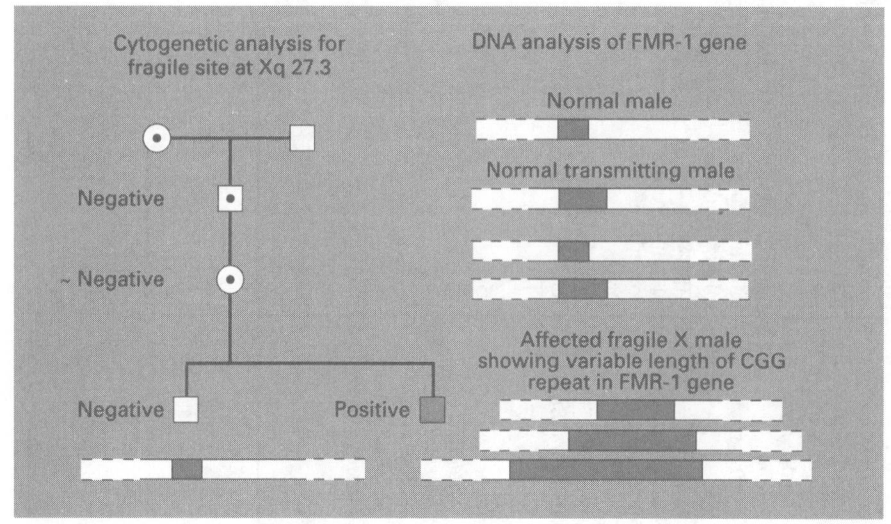

Fig. 18 A diagramatic representation of the progressive change in the CGG repeat in the *FMR-1* gene as the X chromosome is transmitted from a normal transmitting male to his grandson.

MYOTONIC DYSTROPHY AND ANTICIPATION

Myotonic dystrophy is a disease that has long fascinated clinicians. It is inherited as an autosomal dominant, but also shows the phenomenon of anticipation, in which there is increased severity/earlier age of onset with successive generations. The grandparent may just have cataracts and not be diagnosed until the offspring present with classical myotonia in early adult life (indeed it is sometimes difficult to decide which grandparent is the affected one!). The grandchild, on the other hand, may be congenitally affected, particularly if the transmitting parent is the mother. Recognized by physicians since 1911 and formally demonstrated by Julia Bell in 1947, who compared sib and parent/child age-of-onset correlations, anticipation has in recent years been largely dismissed as being due to ascertainment bias. Discovery of the expanding CTG repeat as the mutational basis of myotonic dystrophy also provided a molecular genetic explanation for the anticipation. There is a fair correlation between the age of onset and the length of the CTG repeat in the untranslated 3′ end of the myotonin protein kinase gene *(DM),* which even holds true on the rare occasion in which there is a reversal of the usual progression on transmission to give a reduction rather than an expansion in the repeat. It should be stressed, however, that unlike fragile X, expansion of the repeat can occur in both male and female transmissions, and so CTG expansion alone cannot explain the fact that congenitally affected babies nearly always inherit the DM mutation from an affected mother not father. The other striking feature of myotonic dystrophy is that DNA marker evidence indicates that all families share a particular ancestral chromosome 19 (or rather the *DM* gene region of it), raising the question of what it is that triggers expansion to very high levels (over 1000 repeats) after many generations of slight expansion (40–60 repeats) above the normal (5–30 repeats).

HUNTINGTON'S DISEASE

All typical patients with this autosomal dominant neurological disorder have a CAG repeat expansion mutation within the coding region of the *IT15* gene for the 'huntington' protein. As indicated in Table 10, the expansion is much less extreme than in fragile X or myotonic dystrophy, with the repeat number rarely exceeding 100. There does not appear to be much somatic instability and analysis of sperm (which show a wider spread of repeat sizes than in somatic cells) indicates that, unlike fragile X, the progression of the mutation is prezygotic. It has been known for some time that patients with a juvenile onset of Huntington's disease nearly always inherit the mutation from their fathers. Furthermore, anticipation, in which the age of onset gets earlier with succeeding generations, has been demonstrated, particularly down the male line. Both these aspects of the inheritance of Huntington's disease have been shown to tie in with mutation size. Despite the rather restrictive range of the CAG expansion, there is a clear inverse correlation between the CAG repeat size and the age of onset of Huntington's disease, which persists even when juvenile cases are removed from the analysis.

Mutation detection has greatly simplified the laboratory aspects of presymptomatic diagnosis, but of course the major counselling issues remain. They are discussed briefly later.

Parent-of-origin effects and genomic imprinting

We have already noted that the increase in the size of the trinucleotide expansion in Huntington's disease, myotonic dystrophy, and the fragile X syndrome can explain the clinical variability within pedigrees and anticipation, but what of the parent-of-origin effects? In fragile X (FRAX A) the premutation expands to the full mutation after fertilization, but only on the maternally derived X, which must therefore be different in some way from a paternally derived premutation carrying X. In Huntington's disease the repeat seems especially unstable in sperm, whilst in myotonic dystrophy there seems to be a constraint on fathers transmitting very large expansions. The basis for these parent-of-origin effects is unknown but such effects, particularly genomic imprinting, are turning out to be an important component of the variation in gene expression seen in a number of diseases.

The term genomic imprinting refers to different expression of a normal or mutant gene, depending on the sex of the parent who transmits it. When this is observed, it implies that the gene carries a 'tag', or imprint, that was placed during spermatogenesis or oogenesis and can modulate gene expression in the developing embryo. The imprint often acts to silence the allele from one parent, so that normal development is dependent solely on the function of the allele from the other parent. That this silencing is not a DNA mutation is shown by the fact that the same gene transmitted in a later generation by someone of the opposite sex is no longer silenced; the imprint has been erased at some time between generations.

There are to date few characterized genes that are normally subject to imprinting, but clearly more exist. Only the paternal copy of the insulin-like growth factor 2 *(IGF2)* gene is active during fetal development. Very close to the *IGF2* gene on human chromosome 11p15.5 lies another gene, *H19*, that is also imprinted, but the other way round, being only expressed from the maternal copy. An intriguing feature of *H19* is that it does not seem to encode any protein, but its RNA product has tumour-suppressor activity. A gene *(SNRPN)* encoding a peptide involved in RNA splicing, the small nuclear ribonucleoprotein polypeptide N, is currently a candidate gene for the Prader–Willi syndrome (see below). It maps to 15q12 and is only active on the paternal chromosome.

As with many normal phenomenon, imprinting is most clearly revealed when the system goes wrong. Not only will it modify the inheritance pattern, it also allows new disease mechanisms to be entertained, including relaxing of imprints on the alleles that should be silent or silencing alleles that should be active. Even where the disease gene is unknown and direct study not possible, there are three informative situations: large pedigrees, microdeletions, and uniparental disomy.

Dominant transmission of a mutation involving an imprinted gene through several generations and by people of different sex will reveal a parent-of-origin effect. In this situation, the mutation will be inconsequential when transmitted by the parent that is silencing the gene anyway; the child is unaffected. However, when the same mutant gene is transmitted by a person of the other sex and becomes the 'active' allele, the child will be affected, because the allele from the other parent is normally silenced. Genomic imprinting does not mean that the affected patients are of one sex, only that the transmitting parent is. Neither does it matter whether the transmitting parent is affected or not.

Syndromes due to *de novo* microdeletions can also be informative, because the parental origin of the deleted chromosome can be determined by polymorphic DNA markers. If an imprinted locus is deleted, the deletion will be inconsequential (with respect to that locus) if it occurs on one parental chromosome but cause the disorder if it involves the other parental chromosome. As a consequence, in clinical practice the syndrome will always be associated with microdeletions of one parental origin.

The third situation involves a recently recognized chromosomal aberration, uniparental disomy. If indeed a gene is silenced when transmitted by one parent, then if both chromosomes come from the parent of that sex, there will be no active alleles and the child should be affected. Uniparental disomy, namely both intact chromosomes of a pair coming from the same parent (e.g. arising from the loss of one chromosome from a trisomic conceptus) is discussed later.

The Angelman and Prader–Willi syndromes are good examples. Angelman syndrome is a disorder associated with mental retardation, absent speech, jerky ataxic movements, fits, a low laughter threshold, and subtle but characteristic facial features. To date, it is the one condition that shows all the above types of evidence for genomic imprinting. Large pedigrees exist, where a mutation in the *AS* locus has been transmitted by males to their daughters with no ill effect, but when these daughters have children, 50 per cent suffer Angelman syndrome. Microdeletions within the q11–13 region of chromosome 15 are found in about 75 per cent of sporadic cases of Angelman syndrome and, without exception, all have arisen in the maternal 15. Finally, about 3 per cent of cases have shown uniparental paternal disomy (with no chromosome 15 from mother but two from father), confirming that the *AS* locus is silenced by an imprint during spermatogenesis. The remaining 20 to 25 per cent of cases of this syndrome presumably have a point mutation or very tiny deletions; it is within this group that the familial cases arise.

It happens that genomic imprinting also occurs at the Prader–Willi locus (very close to, but distinct from *AS* at 15q12) where in contrast to Angelman syndrome, it is the maternally transmitted allele that is silenced. Again about 75 per cent of patients have a microdeletion, but now it is the paternal 15 that is deleted. All the remainder have uniparental maternal disomy. The Beckwith–Weidemann locus mapping to 11p15.5 provides another example and is discussed below.

Parent-of-origin effects have been detected in relation to a number of tumours, including a bias for the paternal chromosome 9 and maternal 22 to be involved in the 'Philadelphia chromosome' translocation of chronic myeloid leukaemia. Wilms' tumour is particularly informative because the imprinted gene *IGF2* seems to be implicated and its activity can be studied directly. Normally the maternal *IGF2* allele is imprinted and therefore silent, but in more than half of the cases studied the maternal allele was also active in the Wilms' tumour tissue. Intriguingly, a constitutional relaxation of the maternal *IGF2* imprint, demonstrable in blood leucocytes, has been found in a child with a Wilms' tumour and excessive growth.

Uniparental disomy

In uniparental disomy, diploid offspring inherit both homologues of a pair from one parent—a fact that seems to fly in the face of Mendel. There are several possible mechanisms by which this might arise. Firstly, non-disjunction during meiosis can produce gametes that, on fertilization, could give rise to a diploid zygote with uniparental disomy by three mechanisms, as follows.

1. *'Gamete complementation'* Conception with one gamete missing a particular chromosome (nullisomic) and the other gamete with two copies of that chromosome (disomic).
2. *'Monosomy duplication'* Conception with one normal gamete and one nullisomic gamete. This zygote would be non-viable unless the single chromosome duplicated itself, resulting in isodisomy for that chromosome.
3. *'Trisomy rescue'* Conception with one normal gamete and one disomic gamete producing a regular trisomic zygote. If there was early, random loss of one of the three chromosomes (which might well provide that cell with a selective advantage), in one-third of cases uniparental disomy would result.

There have been several reported examples of trisomic rescue leading to a child with the Prader–Willi syndrome. Typically, a chorionic villus sample, taken for other reasons, reveals mosaic trisomy 15 and then a later amniocentesis or fetal blood sample shows the fetus to have a normal-looking diploid karyotype. However, it eventually transpires that the baby has Prader–Willi syndrome with uniparental disomy revealed by DNA analysis using chromosome 15 markers (the disomy in this syndrome involves the whole chromosome 15). Given that 1 to 2 per cent of pregnancies show confined placental mosaicism, often with a trisomic cell line, trisomic rescue causing uniparental disomy is something that has to be considered in clinical management of such pregnancies. However, much still had to be done to discover what developmental abnormalities, if any, arise from maternal and paternal, uniparental disomy for each of the chromosomes. Trisomy 16 accounts for about 30 per cent of trisomic spontaneous abortions and confined placental trisomy/mosaicism has been associated with maternal, uniparental disomy 16 in the fetus. They all suffered intrauterine growth retardation, although it is not easy to distinguish the effect of the disomy from poor placental function. Maternal, uniparental disomy 7 is associated with short stature.

Postzygotic mitotic non-disjunction may also result in uniparental isodisomy if one homologue of the pair is lost and the other duplicates, ensuring survival of the cell lineage. However, it may be an even more complicated somatic event as indicated by the findings in Beckwith–Wiedemann syndrome. In familial forms of this syndrome the full clinical picture occurs only when transmitted by the mother. This can be interpreted in two ways and the current evidence is inconclusive. Either the maternal allele is normally silenced by the imprint and the syndrome is due to a gene overdose (familial Beckwith–Wiedemann syndrome—mutation causing relaxation of the imprint), or the paternal allele is normally silenced and the syndrome is due to gene malfunction (familial Beckwith–Wiedemann syndrome—regular mutation). In any event, some 20 per cent of sporadic cases of the syndrome show evidence of paternal isodisomy from markers on 11p. However, there is often evidence of mosaicism, indicating that the uniparental disomy arose as a postzygotic event and fitting with the hemihypertrophy so often found in patients with Beckwith–Wiedermann syndrome. What is all the more remarkable is that there is evidence for the paternal isodisomy being sometimes confined to just the distal part of the short arm of chromosome 11, indicating a somatic exchange between the two chromosomes 11. Presumably this unusual event results in an embryonic cell with proliferative advantage.

Finally, it should be mentioned that if the chromosome involved in uniparental isodisomy happens to carry a harmful recessive allele, then a child can be affected with a recessive disease, even when only one parent is a carrier. This has been seen with cystic fibrosis.

Mitochondrial gene defects (see also Section 24)

Mitochondria contain their own genetic material; between two and ten copies of a double-stranded, circular DNA molecule that is 16 569 bp in length. The mitochondrial chromosome encodes 13 subunits of the mitochondrial respiratory-chain and oxidative phosphorylation system, as well as the mitochondria's own translational machinery, there being two ribosomal RNA and 22 transfer RNA (tRNA) genes. An increasing number of diseases (typically variable, multiorgan energy failure over time) are being recognized as due to mitochondrial mutations.

A mature ovum has about 2000 mitochondria, but during the passage from one generation to the next the number of mitochondria in the germ-cell lineage is thought to go through a 'bottleneck' of less than 10 mitochondria. Whilst both eggs and sperm have mitochondria, none from the sperm survives fertilization, so mitochondrial inheritance is exclusively maternal. What is true of normal mitochondria is true of mutant mitochondria, and exclusive maternal transmission characterizes those diseases due to mutation in the mitochondrial chromosome. The mitochondria accumulate mutations at a relatively fast rate and, owing to the 'bottleneck' effect, some offspring of a woman carrying one or a few mutant mitochondria can end up with the majority, even all, of their mitochondria of the mutant variety. A mutation or polymorphism that is present in all copies of the mitochondrial chromosome is said to be homoplasmic, whilst the term heteroplasmy refers to a mixture of mutant and normal mitochondrial chromosomes. The proportion of mutant mitochondria in any particular tissue can account for much but not all of the variable expression seen within and between families.

Perhaps the best known mitochondrially inherited disorder is Leber's hereditary optic neuropathy **(LHON),** which gives rise to acute or subacute blindness affecting males more commonly than females. Although the majority of LHON families have a point mutation at base-pair position 11 778, which changes a conserved arginine to histidine in subunit 4 in respiratory complex 1, this does not explain the male excess. There is some evidence that interaction with a regular X-linked polymorphic gene is necessary. Like nuclear-encoded genetic disease, mitochondrially inherited disorders also show genetic heterogeneity. There are now a total of several high-risk, intermediate and low-risk 'LHON' mutations affecting respiratory complexes I, II, and IV. Some patients have combinations of 'LHON' mutations.

Multifactor causation

The correlation between the height of parents and their children's eventual height is clear for all to see. The inheritance of quantitative characters such as height has been the subject of careful study for over a century, and it can be shown that the correlation between various relatives can be explained on the basis of many genes, each of small effect, segregating in a normal mendelian fashion.

Indeed, alleles at several independent gene loci that have a small, additive effect will segregate to produce a phenotype distribution within the population that approximates to the well-known gaussian or normal curve. Two loci each with two alleles of simple, additive effect produce the distribution of phenotypes 1:4:6:4:1. If one is dealing with a quantitative character showing continuous variation that is solely genetically determined, then the term polygenic inheritance would be appropriate. However, in medicine, even if the genetic component is determined by the combination of several genes of small effect, one or more environmental factors are also likely to be affecting the outcome and so the use of the term polygenic inheritance may be misleading and the term multifactorial inheritance preferred. Some people even object to this, on the grounds that within a single clinical entity the relative contribution of genetic and environmental factors may vary so widely from case to case that some are essentially non-genetic and the word inheritance is therefore inappropriate.

The title multifactor causation is chosen to emphasize these points, although the term multifactorial inheritance is the one most widely used. Diseases appear more or less as 'all or none' pheonomena and this is particularly true of the more common congenital malformations.

It has been long thought that polygenic inheritance might produce an underlying 'distribution of susceptibility' with those individuals beyond a particular threshold being affected by a common malformation or later-onset disorder. Whilst this may indeed be the basis for some disorders, it is equally possible that the inherited tendency observed can be accounted for by just one or a few susceptibility genes of major effect, with other genetic modifiers being only minor influences. It is likely that the genetic contribution in common disorders will range from true polygenic inheritance right through to subsets due to dominant genes of barely reduced penetrance. Those cases or families where the latter is so are likely to have their genetic susceptibility elucidated first, and this is beginning to happen. It has been known for some time that within coronary arterial disease in general, familial hypercholesterolaemia due to mutations in the low-density lipoprotein **(LDL)** receptor represents a susceptibility gene of major effect.

It should be emphasized that such genes of major effect may lead to quite a range of phenotypes from a clinical viewpoint. For example, a proportion of patients with just congenital heart defects are now known to have submicroscopic deletions at 22q11.2, the region that is deleted in those with the Di George and velocardiofacial syndromes. This is particularly so if there is a family history of congenital heart disease, and interestingly the type of disease can range from a right aortic arch to Fallot's tetralogy or a relative may just have a cleft palate. Variation in the type of cancer associated with some inherited predispositions is well established. Constitutional mutations in the p53 gene (Li Fraumeni syndrome) can predispose to a range of different cancers, perhaps because of the likely role of the p53 protein in preventing malignant proliferation in cells stressed by genetic or other damage. On a similar theme of loss of protective mechanisms, mutations in the h*MSH2* gene on chromosome 2, normally responsible for DNA mismatch repair, can be associated not only with hereditary non-polyposis colon cancer (the conditions usual name) but also urinary-tract and female genital-tract cancers.

It can be seen that two complementary processes of discovery are at work, one teasing out genetic heterogeneity within a clinical entity, the other defining a wider range of phenotypic expression of mutations of a known gene. Each genetic subset due to known mutations at a gene of major effect that is removed from the pool of clinical cases leaves the remainder somewhat less heterogeneous, allowing, amongst other things, a more refined empirical recurrence risk or prognosis to be calculated for clinical use. Furthermore, each rarer mendelian disorder or major genetic susceptibility that is characterized at the molecular genetic level almost always suggests other functionally interacting candidate genes to be explored in the common form of the condition.

Whilst progress in elucidating the genetics of common disorders is steady, empirical data on recurrence within families will provide the basis of genetic advice for some years to come, particularly in the common congenital malformations.

Congenital malformations as examples of multifactorial inheritance

There is a significant genetic contribution to the cause of some common congenital malformations like spina bifida, cleft lip and/or palate, or congenital heart disease. First-degree relatives (brothers and sisters, or children) of an affected person have a considerable risk of being affected, but this increased risk diminishes rapidly when one moves to second-degree relatives (nephews, nieces, and grandchildren) and is almost back to the general population incidence for third-degree relatives (cousins). This general point about multifactorial inheritance is illustrated by cleft lip and/or palate, which has an incidence of about 1/1000 live births in Britain. In first-degree relatives of an affected case the incidence is about 40/1000, but falls to 7/1000 for second-degree relatives and 2–3/1000 for third-degree relatives. When a couple has had two affected children, the risk to a further child is higher, about 14 per cent. In reality, of course, the risk has been the same for each pregnancy; what has increased is our information about how susceptible the children of this couple are to the malformation. It must be emphasized that largely unknown environmental factors also play an important part in the cause of these common malformations, and 'preventative measures' around the time of conception and in early pregnancy might be possible in the future. There is evidence that maternal folic-acid supplementation is associated with a reduction in the recurrence risk for spina bifida and anencephaly.

Additional observations fit with predictions made for multifactorial inheritance. The sibling recurrence risk of any form of cleft lip and/or palate is 5 to 6 per cent if the index case has a bilateral cleft lip and palate, and 2 to 3 per cent if the index case has a unilateral cleft lip only.

In conditions where one sex is particularly susceptible, one may observe another phenomenon suggestive of multifactorial inheritance. For every girl with infantile pyloric stenosis there are five affected boys. There is a similar overall increased risk to siblings or offspring, but when regard is paid to sex it is found that the brothers and sons of affected men show a frequency of 10 times the population average; sisters and daughters of affected men, 25 times; brothers and sons of affected women, 30 times; and sisters and daughters of affected women, 100 times. Women who are affected are so in spite of the protection conferred by their sex; they are more extreme deviants in terms of the presumed underlying continuous distribution of susceptibility, and this is faithfully reflected in the greater incidence found in their relatives. Incidentally, no fewer than about 16 per cent of sons and brothers of affected women are affected. This is an order of magnitude hardly approached with any other relatively common congenital malformation.

To summarize briefly, multifactorial inheritance is likely if: (i) the condition is relatively common; (ii) the incidence in relatives is low; (iii) the incidence falls off rapidly as one passes to more distant relatives; (iv) the risk to first-degree relatives is about the square root of the population incidence; (v) the risk to sibs is similar to the risks to offspring; (vi) the incidence in relatives rises as the manifestations become more severe in the index case; (vii) the incidence in relatives is higher when the index case is the least commonly affected sex; and (viii) the risk is greater after the birth of two affected children.

Biochemical genetics, pharmacogenetics, and teratogens

Characteristic biochemical disturbances have now been described in so many disorders in which genetic factors play a major part that some aspect of biochemical genetics will often be included in the general description of a disorder. There is a whole branch of medicine concerned with disorders of metabolism (Section 11). Indeed, there are good reasons to try and understand all diseases at a biochemical level whether the disturbance is confined to a particular cell, clone or one tissue, or has a general effect on metabolic homeostasis, even if it means cloning the relevant genes first. It is appropriate in this chapter to just extract a few general principles.

Inborn errors of metabolism (see also Section 11)

Elucidation of an inherited defect in an enzyme that is part of a well-understood metabolic pathway often allows a clear description of how the genetic defect produces its manifold clinical effects. At its simplest, the clinical manifestations of an enzyme defect can be seen as a combination of deficiency of substances beyond the block in the metabolism pathway and accumulation of substances before the block. Sometimes, alternative metabolic pathways will allow the block to be bypassed, but with this compensatory mechanism failing under conditions of stress.

One enzyme defect may cause problems soon after the newborn has lost the protection afforded by the transplacental removal of toxic metabolites, whilst another may interfere with the degradation of macromolecules, like mucopolysaccharides, and produce a slowly progressive 'storage' disorder. The natural course of most untreated inborn errors of metabolism is early death. Whilst several respond dramatically to dietary control, the long-term outlook for 'successfully' treated individuals has still to be assessed. It is now clear that some cases of galactosaemia, apparently successfully treated by dietary restriction of galactose and lactose, are developing neurological deterioration in their third and fourth decade. There is now concern that some difficult to control sufferers of phenylketonuria are developing demyelination in later life despite remaining on a diet.

The mischief caused by high levels of intermediate metabolites may be critically dependent on the individual's stage of development. The brain in particular may be more susceptible to damage when immature, and this has important implications for maternal–fetal interactions. A fetus deficient in phenylalanine hydroxylase activity has classical phenylketonuria. It will be protected by transplacental removal of phenylalanine by its mother until the time of birth. During childhood, strict dietary control of phenylalanine intake is necessary to prevent brain damage, but later in life many individuals with phenylketonuria can tolerate a relaxation of the diet with no significant neurological sequelae. However, this is not true for any fetus such a woman may be carrying. Untreated maternal phenylketonuria is likely to have disastrous consequences for her fetus, regardless of its genotype, with the great majority suffering from microcephaly and mental retardation with increased risk of congenital heart disease and other malformations. There is evidence that even mild, asymptomatic hyperphenylalanaemia in a woman, which would not have been diagnosed before the days of neonatal screening, may put her fetus at risk, although the degree of risk is unclear.

What is clear is that those caring for girls with phenylketonuria have a responsibility to ensure that they appreciate the need to go on strict dietary control before they become pregnant. Other examples of maternal metabolic disorders that are known to put the fetus at risk of brain or other malformations are the carrier state for ornithine carbamoyl transferase deficiency, where maternal hyperammonia may be damaging, and maternal diabetes mellitus where the known increased risk of fetal abnormality can only be eliminated by meticulous diabetic control from conception onwards.

Metabolic causes of fetal malformation may not always be maternal in origin. Some rare inborn errors of metabolism inherited by a fetus may result in a toxic metabolite accumulating so early during gestation that it disturbs its own morphogenesis or disturb morphogenesis in some other way. Recently, it has been shown that the Smith–Lemli–Opitz syndrome is due to a block in the synthesis of cholesterol from 7-dehydrocholesterol.

Pharmacogenetic polymorphisms

Pharmacogenetic polymorphism can be of considerable practical importance, but space permits only a few key points to made here. Two examples concern genetic variation in acetylation by *N*-acetyltransferase, and variation in metabolic oxidation by the cytochrome P450 enzyme CYP2D6.

Acetylation is a controlling factor in the rate of metabolism of several drugs, the acetylated drug being more easily excreted by the kidney than the free drug. In Western populations about half the population are rapid acetylators and half slow acetylators, the latter being homozygous for a 'slow' allele and having low *N*-acetyltransferase activity in the liver. As one might expect with a common polymorphism, there are two sides to the acetylator coin. Slow acetylators are more likely to develop the cumulative toxicity, peripheral neuritis, with the antituberculous drug, isoniazid, whilst rapid acetylators are more likely to develop hepatitis as a reaction to this drug.

CYP2D6 is one of a large family of cytochrome P450 enzymes involved in the elimination of noxious foreign compounds, including drugs. Originally described as a debrisoquine oxidation polymorphism, genetic variation in the CYP2D6 results in about 5 per cent of the Western population being 'poor metabolizers'—the phenotypic state for those homozygous for the deficiency allele(s). Amongst other drug effects, 'poor metabolizers' do not get pain relief from codeine. It is becoming clear that this enzyme has endogenous substrates, suggesting a role beyond detoxification of noxious substances, and it has been shown that mutations in the the *CYP2D6* gene are unduly common in Parkinson's disease. 'Extensive metabolizers' are more likely to get hepatocellular carcinoma in Nigeria and interstitial endemic nephropathy in Bulgaria.

The most important genetic polymorphism of drug response concerns G6PD deficiency. This X-linked character has an incidence of 25 per cent in males in some areas and predisposes these subjects to haemolysis in response to a large variety of drugs. They are also prone to haemolysis on eating the bean *Vicia faba,* giving the syndrome of favism, and to neonatal jaundice (see Section 8).

What have been described briefly are variations in the metabolism of drugs that show simple mendelian inheritance. It would be wrong to imagine that pharmacogenetic influences are necessarily monogenic. With much of the variation in response to drugs the genetic influences will be complex and extremely difficult to elucidate. This difficulty is made worse when it is the influence of maternal drugs on the development of the fetus. Not only are there two distinct genotypes (maternal and fetal) to consider for any particular polymorphism, but also variation in susceptibility of the fetus at different stages of gestation.

Teratogens

It would be very surprising if genetic factors did not influence the effect of maternal ingestion of drugs or other chemicals on the development of the human fetus, for this has been clearly demonstrated in experimental animals. Until more is understood the clinician has to follow some general guidelines, steering a course between sensible anticipation of danger and giving in to unsubstantiated claims that drugs used for many years are now to be regarded as teratogenic. The need for good data becomes critically important when a choice of drug has to be made because stopping treatment during pregnancy is regarded as too dangerous.

Once descriptions of the teratogenic effects of phenytoin had been published there was a tendency for epileptic women to be switched during pregnancy to a new drug such as sodium valproate, until eventually this drug too was shown to have teratogenic effects. Table 11 lists those drugs currently regarded as established teratogens, although only a proportion of fetuses exposed will be affected. Whilst these drugs should not normally be prescribed during pregnancy, inadvertent treatment during early pregnancy is not necessarily cause for great alarm or, for example, an indication for termination of pregnancy. It would be important to seek specialized advice in this situation.

Table 11 *Teratogenic drugs*

Thalidomide
Antineoplastic drugs*
Aminopterin
Methotrexate
Azauridine
Cyclophosphamide
Busulphan and probably others
Vitamin A analogue
Etretinate
Cis-retinoic acid
Anticoagulants
Warfarin and other coumarins
Anticonvulsants
Phenytoin
Primidone
Sodium valproate
Phenobarbitone
Trimethadione
Steroid hormones
Methyl testosterone
Ethiterone
Norethisterone
Diethylstilboestrol
Lithium
Antibiotics
Streptomycin
Tetracycline
Alcohol
Methyl mercury
Radioactive iodine
L-penicillamine

*Azathioprine appears to have only a very small, if any, teratogenic potential

Genetic counselling, testing, and services

Genetic counselling is now regarded as part of the health services in many countries. A genetic centre often serves a population of 3 million, and clinicians have a responsibility to either give counselling in consultation with the centre or make the appropriate referrals.

The object of genetic counselling is to provide information on the risk to offspring, at a time appropriate to the options available for modifying the outcome, and to put the risk into perspective. It will be noted that the object of genetic counselling is not a reduction in the incidence of genetic disorders. This may be, indeed often is, a consequence of genetic counselling, but what action is taken in the light of the information provided is up to the person or couple concerned. It should be remembered that the concept of 'risk' combines two components, chance or probability and extent of damage or burden. Genetic counselling is concerned with both. It is usually the professional who is best placed to determine the actual probability of some outcome or genetic status and they have a responsibility to be as precise as possible, although when it comes to carrier or presymptomatic testing it is essential that this is only done after adequate counselling and when requested by the person being tested. Assessment of the burden comes as a result of a dialogue with the person or couple concerned and is very much dependent on their own experiences, beliefs, and the support they can rely upon.

The non-directive nature of genetic counselling is not merely a particular stance adopted during discussions, but reassurance that you will actively support any decision (within the law) the couple may make and mobilize the necessary services to help them. It is this element of commitment or 'availability' to the family that makes genetic counselling a major undertaking.

Like most branches of clinical practice, genetic counselling calls for considerable sensitivity and psychological insight, whether it concerns the timing of an interview after a stillbirth, or how to protect a young couple from undue family pressures to follow a particular course of action. Realization of the inherited nature of a child's handicap can add guilt and blame to an already stressful situation for the family. A couple may have feelings of hopelessness, believing they can never have a normal child, and if the condition is sporadic the mother may be blaming some trivial action of hers during pregnancy.

It would be wrong, however, to underestimate the importance of correct factual information, and the first responsibility of the clinical geneticist is to ensure that the diagnosis in the propositus is correct. A propositus is the name given to the affected family member who is the immediate reason for the family being referred for genetic advice. The term consultand is often used for the person actually seeking advice.

DIAGNOSIS

Verification of the diagnosis in the propositus may just mean obtaining copies of appropriate hospital reports. It may be that further specialist consultation should be arranged, or some histological preparations reviewed with a particular feature in mind that will serve to distinguish an inherited form of the disorder from others.

In the case of multiple congenital malformations the clinical geneticist is often expected to make the diagnosis. There are over 2500 different multiple malformation or dysmorphic syndromes, many very rare and often, but not always, inherited in a mendelian fashion. In addition to specialist books and access to the genetic journals, the modern dysmorphologist is increasingly using the assistance of a computerized database, such as a London dysmorphology database.

PEDIGREE

The clinical geneticist will record a family history, and the most efficient way to do this is to draw up a pedigree (usually three generations) using standard symbols (Fig. 19). All affected and unaffected individuals are recorded. As emphasized earlier, in certain autosomal dominant disorders careful examination of the parents or other relatives of the propositus is necessary to detect minimal signs of the condition, before accepting that they are, indeed, not carrying the mutant gene.

THE RECURRENCE RISK

The risk to offspring is given as odds or a percentage, a 1 in 4 risk or 25 per cent chance of the next child having cystic fibrosis for example. It is often helpful to present the figure in more than one way. Note that 1 to 4 or 1:4 is not the same as 1 in 4, but 1 in 5. The couple may need reminding that chance has no memory, that it is a 1 in 4 risk with each pregnancy regardless of previous outcomes, and the ambiguous phrase 'one out of four children will be affected' does not mean that of their four children one will be affected.

Deriving the recurrence risk may be more than just recalling the mendelian ratios. It may require a calculation of the frequency of heterozygotes in the population as illustrated in Fig. 9, and if the probability of a new mutation comes into the equation, as in X-linked disorders, then the calculation may be complicated. In autosomal dominant disorders of late clinical onset, such as Huntington's chorea or adult polycystic disease of the kidney, someone who began life with half a chance of inheriting the gene obviously has a falling residual risk of carrying the gene the older they become without manifesting the disease. Such calculations of the residual risk combine age of onset data with the prior genetic risk to give a final risk figure.

Genetic advice on the disorders of multifactorial cause depend on empirical recurrence risks for siblings or children based on careful unbiased family studies. These figures can differ between populations and examples given in Table 12 should not be used without confirmation with the local genetic service.

Sometimes the clinical geneticist deliberately gives a composite risk, where an inherited form of the disease cannot be distinguished from sporadic cases. In a particular form of mental retardation with microcephaly, half the cases are autosomal recessive and half sporadic, so a 1 in 8 recurrence risk is given. It is of no help to the couple to say the recurrent risk is either 1 in 4 or less than 1 per cent, but we don't know which. Finally, the risks should be put in some perspective. A useful yardstick is the overall incidence of some error of development manifest at birth, or soon afterwards (i.e. mental retardation), which is about 1 in 30, or to put it the positive way round, 97 per cent of babies are perfectly normal.

CARRIER DETECTION

Heterozygote, or carrier, testing is offered in two rather different situations: as part of counselling a family into which an affected person has been born, or as part of a defined population-screening programme for carriers of a common disorder. The former may involve either an autosomal recessive or an X-linked disease, and where the offer is extended, in successive steps, to more and more distant relatives as they are revealed to have a high chance of being a carrier, the term 'cascade' counselling is sometimes used. The approach is an extension of the standard genetic services offered to a family at risk and is valid no matter how rare the disease is, provided of course there is a useful carrier test. Even in a condition like cystic fibrosis, where usually only some 85 per cent of the mutations can be detected, relatives and their partners can be substantially reassured, or forewarned should both be carriers.

Fig. 19 Symbols commonly used in the drawing of human pedigrees.

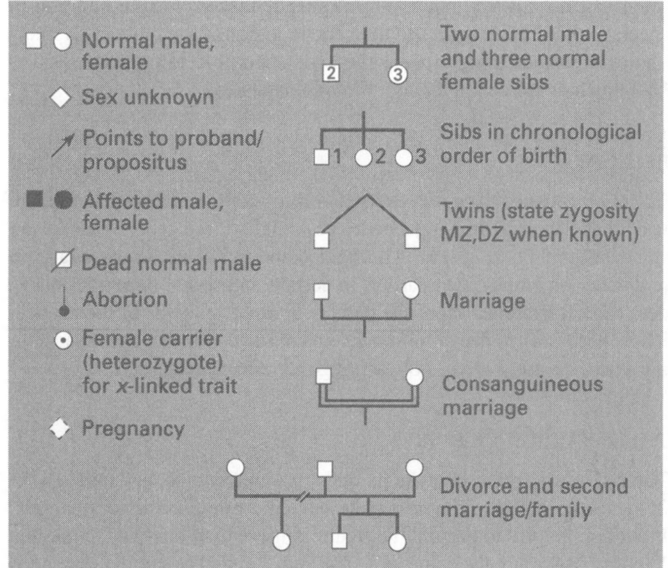

The word screening (which tends to be used rather indiscriminately for all types of genetic testing) is best reserved for a programme where carrier testing is offered to a defined population with a specific disorder in mind. In screening it is usually the health professional who approaches the individual or couple rather than the other way round, and this in itself is a challenge. There is a need to explain what is available, whilst avoiding undue pressure to have the test. An 'opt in' is more likely to achieve the latter than a programme where the person has to 'opt out'. Above all, the whole process must be supported by adequate education and counselling. The aim is to maximize informed choice and minimize unwarranted anxiety. Various screening programmes for the detection of cystic fibrosis carriers are under evaluation. Table 13 summarizes the established population screening programmes for common autosomal recessive disorders. Tay–Sachs screening is still done by biochemical testing, although it is known that some 'pseudo-deficiency' false positives can occur due to an allele that does not cause disease but reduced activity with artificial substrate. Positive results are best checked by DNA analysis. In the strictly Ashkenazi Jewish population about 98 per cent of carriers have one of three mutations, making screening by DNA analysis a possibility. However, in other situations the pros and cons of a functional assay versus mutation detection by DNA analysis have to be carefully assessed. The former may pick up more, particularly when a substantial minority of carriers have one of several rare mutations for which screening is impractical.

The screening of all children with learning difficulties for fragile X through special schools or even 'well baby' developmental assessment clinics falls somewhere between regular genetic counselling and screening. Although the parents may be aware of the child's educational needs, the move to investigate the genetic aspects is being initiated by the health professional.

GENETIC REGISTERS

The extended family counselling, maintained from one generation to the next, that characterizes the support needed for families with X-linked or autosomal dominant disorders is often best achieved with the aid of a register for that condition. The register would normally be kept by the regional genetics centre, which would liaise with those providing clinical management, such as annual colonoscopy in individuals who have inherited a mutation for familial polyposis coli. The register allows the children at risk of being affected themselves in later life (e.g. Huntington's disease), or of having affected children, to be offered counselling when they reach a suitable age. In general, genetic testing is not appropriate until the individual involved is old enough to request it, unless it has some immediate relevance to his or her own health care. This policy does not preclude parents from initiating discussion of the family disorder and its inheritance with their children.

Genetic prediction by DNA analysis

DNA ANALYSIS AND TRADITIONAL TESTS CAN COMPLEMENT EACH OTHER

Carrier exclusion and carrier detection might, at first, appear to be two sides of the same coin, but in practice this is not so. Results of biochemical tests, such as a high creatine phosphokinase level in a woman at risk of Duchenne muscular dystrophy or a low factor VIII activity to protein ratio in a woman at risk of haemophilia A, may confirm the carrier state, but a 'normal' result cannot reliably exclude it. On the other hand, gene tracking can exclude the carrier state in more instances than it can confirm it and two examples are given in Fig. 20. Thus the

Table 12 *Empirical risks for some common disorders (in percentages)*

Disorder	Incidence	Sex ratio M:F	Normal parents having a second affected child	Affected parent having an affected child	Affected parent having a second child
Anencephaly	0.20	1:2	5*	—	—
Cleft palate only	0.04	2:3	2	7	15
Cleft lip ± cleft palate	0.10	3:2	4	4	10
Club foot	0.10	2:1	3	3	10
Congenital heart disease (all types)	0.50	—	1–4	1–4	—
Diabetes mellitus (early onset)	0.20	1:1	8	8	10
Dislocation of hip	0.07	1:6	4	4	10
Epilepsy ('idiopathic')	0.50	1:1	5	5	10
Hirschsprung's disease	0.02	4:1			
Male index			2	—	—
Female index			8	—	—
Hypospadias (in males)	0.20	—	10	—	—
Manic-depressive psychoses	0.40	2:3	—	10–15	—
Mental retardation ('idiopathic')	0.30	1:1	3–5	—	—
Profound childhood deafness	0.10	1:1	10	8	—
Pyloris stenosis	0.30	5:—			
Male index			2	4	13
Female index			10	17	38
Renal agenesis (bilateral)	0.01	3:1			
Male index			3	—	—
Female index			7	—	—
Schizophrenia	1–2	1:1	—	16	—
Scoliosis (idiopathic, adolescent)	0.22	1:6	7	5	—
Spina bifida	0.30	2:3	5*	3*	—

*Anencephaly or spina bifida.

From Emery (1979). *Elements of medical genetics.* 5th edn. Churchill Livingstone, Edinburgh, by courtesy of the author.

Table 13 *Population screening for heterozygotes in selected populations*

Condition	Populations	Carrier frequency	Preliminary test	Comments on further testing
β-Thalassaemia[1]	Many populations in the Mediterranean, Middle East, India, and south-east Asia	Up to 20%	Reduced red cell indices (MCH, MCV) Elevated HbA_2	If HbA_2 normal or borderline, α-thalassaemia, coexistent iron deficiency, etc. need to be excluded
Sickle-cell anemia[1]	Populations of African origin, some populations in the Middle East	Up to 30%	Solubility sickling test confirmed by Hb electrophoresis	
Tay–Sachs disease	Ashkenazi Jewish origin	About 3%	Reduced ratio of hexosaminidase A to total hexosaminidase activity in serum Overlap between carriers and non-carriers results in about 10% with indeterminate result	Indeterminate serum values plus subjects who are pregnant, on the contraceptive pill, or have diabetes require assay of hexosaminidase A activity in leucocytes Confirmation of mutation by DNA analysis useful

[1]In many populations a screening strategy is needed to detect a variety of common haemoglobinopathies either singly or in combination.

traditional biochemical tests and the new gene tracking approaches often complement each other.

TWO TYPES OF DNA ANALYSIS IN GENETIC PREDICTION

There are two distinct approaches to using DNA analysis to predict the genotype of a family member, or fetus during prenatal diagnosis: mutation detection and gene tracking. Table 14 compares the advantages and disadvantages of each approach.

Mutation detection

This is the ideal. In a simple mendelian disorder, defining the mutation at the DNA level provides the definitive diagnosis. There would only be a need to refine the genotype analysis if there is considerable phenotypic variation in expression due to modifying genes. One such example is the variation in severity of homozygous (compound heterozygous) β-thalassaemia due to co-inheritance of α-thalassaemia, or the coexistence of a DNA sequence variation that enhances γ-globin chain synthesis.

The various approaches to a mutation search or detection of a specific known mutation have been described earlier. The final step in a mutation search is generally DNA sequencing, but this is often preceded by a screening step designed to reveal if any differences exist between the subject's DNA and normal; usually indicated by the presence of an aberrant band on electrophoresis. Single-stranded conformational polymorphism analysis, denaturing gradient-gel electrophoresis or chemical-mismatch cleavage methods are the common preliminary mutation screens currently employed.

The main drawbacks to mutation detection in clinical practice are allelic heterogeneity and the unreliability of existing techniques and knowledge in discovering the mutation. A clinical service should be able to know in advance that a clear-cut result will be obtained in the great majority of cases. This ideal may be achieved where the mutation is essentially the same in all patients, trinucleotide expansions in myotonic dystrophy or Huntington's disease for example, or where a handful of known mutations accounts for nearly all the mutant chromosomes in the local population, as in cystic fibrosis. However, even in the latter case, it is necessary to have suitable markers for gene tracking as a back-up. Analysis of the parents of a child with cystic fibrosis may reveal a common mutation in only one of them, and they need prenatal diagnosis or a relative on the 'unresolved' side of the family needs a carrier test because their partner has turned out to be a carrier for a known mutation. Searching for a rare mutation in these circumstances would be a very open-ended business, with no reassurance if the 'test was negative'. We noted earlier that for many years the causative mutation in about half the patients with severe haemophilia A could not be found, despite the factor VIII gene having been cloned in 1984. However, once the inversion involving sequences in the large intron between exons 22 and 23 and elsewhere was discovered, mutation detection in this important group of patients became easy. It can be seen that progress in mutation detection is a combination of both new, disease-specific information and technological advance.

It is instructive that the above discovery in haemophilia A arose out of reverse-transcriptase, polymerase chain-reaction analysis of factor VIII mRNA transcripts in the patient's lymphocytes; some tissue-specific genes do show a little 'illegitimate' transcription in lymphocytes. The RNA was truncated and therefore so was the protein product. In general, truncated proteins more commonly arise from point and other mutations that stop translation. With genes that show 'illegitimate' transcription in lymphocytes, it is now possible to make a lot of cDNA from this little amount of mRNA and then use an *in vitro* transcription/translation system to make the protein. In this way a truncated protein may be seen, establishing the existence of a mutation that, because it is roughly localized with respect to exons, can more easily be confirmed on DNA analysis. Such a diagnostic approach looks promising in Duchenne muscular dystrophy.

Fig. 20 Pedigrees from families in which female relatives may have been at risk of carrying the haemophilia A mutation and how RFLP analysis with the factor VIII DNA probe can exclude the carrier state. Errors due to recombination would be negligible. (a) The mother is heterozygous for the Bc1 I RFLP, and both her affected and normal son have inherited the same X chromosome carrying the 0.9 kb band. This means that the affected boy represents a new mutation and neither his mother nor his sister are at risk. (b) The woman seeking advice (homozygous for the 1.1 kb band) and her affected uncle (hemizygous for the 0.9 kb band) share no RFLP alleles, and therefore no X chromosome, in common. In this instance carrier exclusion is possible even though intermediate relatives are dead.

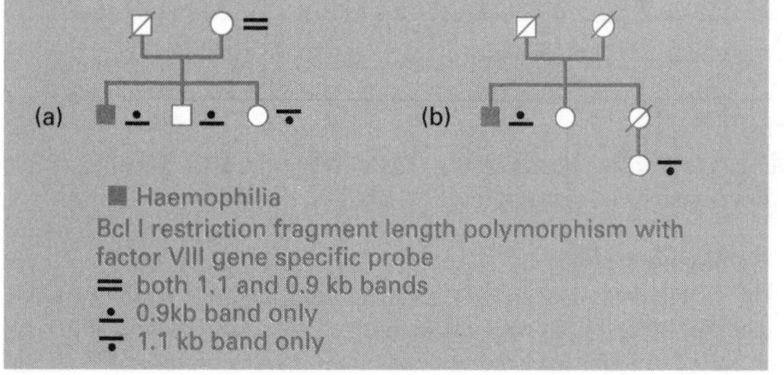

Table 14 *Two approaches to genetic prediction by DNA analysis*

	Mutation detection	Gene tracking
Advantages	Definitive DNA diagnosis	Mutation independent
	Population screening (AR, XL) possible	Can be used as soon as disease locus is mapped
	Presymptomatic screening (AD) possible	Exclusion of risk often achieved
	Few, if any, family studies	
Disadvantages	Allelic heterogeneity	Affected families only
	Exclusion of risk may be difficulty	Family studies needed
	Causative mutation or not?	Uninformative markers
		Recombination errors
		Paternity?

AD, autosomal dominant; AR, autosomal-recessive; XL, X-linked.

Gene tracking

Gene tracking asks the question 'Has the family member or fetus inherited the same relevant chromosome region(s) as a previous affected member?' There are variations to this question, but all depend on formulating a simple linkage study with the family members available. Rather than try to detect the causal mutation, the path of transmission of the mutant chromosome(s) through the family is tracked using polymorphic DNA markers that are closely linked to the disease gene locus. One of the drawbacks of gene tracking is the small chance of a wrong prediction due to recombination between the DNA marker used and the actual mutation. Given that such a recombination is possible, clearly it is desirable to know when it has happened during any clinical analysis, and the best safeguard is to use two markers that flank the disease gene locus being tracked. Such a strategy will detect a single recombination between the flanking markers and it will be clear that genetic prediction is not possible on that occasion without further analysis. Only with very large genes, such as dystrophin, and in certain other situations where double recombinations between these flanking markers could occur with an appreciable frequency, will gene tracking approaches fail to detect recombinations that invalidate the result.

One of the difficulties in using flanking markers in the past was the limited availability of highly polymorphic markers sufficiently close to the disease gene locus under study. This is becoming less of a problem as more 'microsatellite' or VNTR type markers are defined. In gene tracking it is essential that certain key family members are not only available to give a sample but are heterozygous for the DNA markers used, so the two chromosomes of the pair can be distinguished. When this is not so, the particular marker(s) in that particular situation is said to be 'uninformative'. It is important that the stated father is the real biological father. This is particularly so in autosomal dominant and X-linked transmission, where one is likely to deduce linkage phase from the result in 'father', and where the person seeking genetic prediction would usually be ignorant of any questionable paternity. Where critical to the genetic prediction, most laboratories check the paternity with suitable markers. Clearly this matter can raise challenging counselling issues if suspected or discovered on DNA analysis, and may be one situation where testing without automatically disclosing the result is justified. The commonly used phrase 'non-paternity' is quite ridiculous (with its implication of virgin births!) and one should use the term wrong or unexpected paternity.

The final point to bear in mind when using gene tracking is new mutations, and the associated matter of gonadal mosaicism. This has already been mentioned in discussing genetic prediction in Duchenne muscular dystrophy. Figure 20 illustrates a situation (which could equally apply to Duchenne muscular dystrophy) in which the mother does not appear to be a carrier (so all her mother's other descendants can be reassured), although the possibility remains that she is a gonadal mosaic and offspring inheriting the same X chromosome as the affected son have a significant chance of inheriting the mutation. Those inheriting the other X chromosome can be reassured, illustrating how gene tracking can be used for risk exclusion, even when the carrier or gonadal status of the mother is uncertain.

The reader can be forgiven for thinking that gene tracking has so many potential pitfalls that nothing should be offered other than mutation detection, but this would be to underestimate the current difficulties (in clinical as opposed to research practice) of defining the mutation in many disorders even where the relevant gene is known. Gene tracking still has an important part to play as an adjunct to genetic counselling and in prenatal diagnosis.

Prenatal diagnosis of genetic disorders and congenital malformations

As with the different approaches to carrier detection, a distinction has to be made between prenatal screening offered to all women of a particular population, and prenatal diagnosis in selected, at-risk families.

PRENATAL SCREENING

The most widespread specific screening procedure is the offer of fetal karyotyping to an older mother with the express purpose of detecting Down's syndrome. The actual 'screening' procedure is really the selection of the mothers by age with respect to a predetermined cut-off point; usually 35 to 40 years depending on the services available. Increasingly, the levels of some serum biochemical markers in the mother are taken into account (see below). This is followed by a definitive diagnostic test in the 'at-risk' mothers who wish to have the option of selective termination of pregnancy should the fetus be affected.

One of the drawbacks of using just the mother's age as the screening measure is that despite the increasing individual risk of a baby with Down's syndrome as the mother gets older (Table 9), only a small proportion of all babies are born to women over 35 years. In many populations, age-alone screening using 35 to 38 years as the cut-off would, at best, detect only a third of pregnancies where the fetus has Down's syndrome. This fact highlighted the importance of the chance observation that the maternal serum alpha-fetoprotein (being used as a screening test for fetal, open neural-tube defects, where the level is high) was low when the fetus had trisomy 18. It was quickly shown that a low maternal serum alpha-fetoprotein was a risk factor for the more common trisomy, Down's syndrome, and other maternal serum markers, high human chorionic gonadotrophin and low unconjugated oestriol, also had predictive value. A judicious combination of these maternal biochemical markers at 16 weeks' gestation can detect some two-thirds of Down's pregnancies with cut-offs set to maintain an overall amniocentesis rate of about 5 per cent.

Although screening for maternal serum alpha-fetoprotein was initially developed to help detect fetal spina bifida and anencephaly (and continues due to its added role in Down's screening), these neural-tube defects are increasingly being picked up by a routine ultrasonographic examination of the fetus at 16 to 18 weeks of gestation. A fetus with spina bifida generally has a narrowed frontal cranium (lemon sign) and a distorted fourth ventricle (banana sign). Indeed, sonographic (ultrasound) markers, such as nuchal-fold thickening, may come to be combined with maternal serum biochemical markers as part of Down's syndrome screening.

In many ways, routine ultrasound examination of the fetus is becoming a form of screening for congenital abnormalities. Some important points are, however, emerging. Any deviation from normal has to be assessed against the prior risk. In a woman known to have a 1 in 4 risk of a fetus with a syndrome that includes short limbs, limb lengths on the third percentile are very significant. However, in a woman with no increased prior risk such an observation by itself is no cause for great alarm.

Certain abnormalities, such as exomphalos where the gut remains in a sac outside the abdominal cavity, are an absolute indication to check the fetal chromosomes. A high proportion of such cases will have chromosome defects and this knowledge will obviously be needed before the parents can make a choice between abortion and planned neonatal surgery.

There are risks associated with widespread ultrasonographic screening, the greatest of which is the clinician, on discovering a structural abnormality, giving an unwarranted poor prognosis for the baby's future development, which in turn leads to the parents choosing to terminate the pregnancy. This is not just a matter of inexperience on the clinician's part, but a lack of information on the natural outcome of certain 'abnormalities' that appear alarming. About 1 in 1500 midtrimester fetuses have a choroid-plexus cyst 'in the brain', which naturally caused concern until the proper follow-up studies were done. Virtually all the cysts disappear as the pregnancy progresses. When associated with other risk factors (maternal age above 35 years or minor structural abnormalities such as dilation of the renal pelvis) about 15 per cent turn out to have a chromosomal defect. As an isolated finding, only 1 in 300 have an associated chromosomal defect. In the absence of a chromosomal abnormality, there is no indication of clinically significant intellectual deficit in the child, but follow-up studies are needed. Natural history studies are needed on fetal renal-pelvic dilation, brain ventriculomegaly, and so on, if parents are to be truly informed and the appropriate management offered.

PRENATAL DIAGNOSIS

Prenatal diagnosis is possible in a great many different genetic diseases or malformations when it is already known that the woman is at risk for a particular disorder. The conditions are too numerous to list and any list will be immediately out of date. As a general guide, prenatal diagnosis is likely in any condition in which (a) there is a chromosome abnormality, or (b) there is a gross physical abnormality internal or external, or (c) a biochemical diagnosis can be made on fibroblasts/serum, or (d) there is a disease-specific DNA probe.

However, certain practical points have to be noted. A precise diagnosis in the affected family member is obligatory. Material from the affected individual may be necessary and every effort should be made to prepare for a prenatal test in collaboration with the obstetricians and laboratories concerned before the pregnancy. Gene tracking in particular may not be possible in all females at risk.

A variety of procedures are used by obstetricians to examine the structure of the fetus or obtain fetal-tissue analysis. Ultrasound examination, or sonography, plays a central part in prenatal diagnosis. It is a necessary component of all the other procedures and the resolution of the images obtained by the latest machines is remarkable. The experience of the operator is equally; if not more, important in getting a reliable prediction. Prenatal diagnosis is based on several interrelated approaches: detection of structural abnormalities, detection of abnormal growth by serial examinations during early pregnancy, and sometimes detection of a physiological function such as emptying of the fetal bladder.

The next most commonly used procedure is amniocentesis at about 16 weeks' gestation. The cells in the amniotic fluid are fetal in origin and can be used for cytogenetic, DNA, and some types of biochemical analysis. The risk of causing a miscarriage that would otherwise not have happened is of the order of 1 in 100 to 1 in 200.

Chorionic villus sampling can be done at about 10 weeks' gestation. One technique involves aspiration via a cannula inserted through the cervix under ultrasound guidance. A transabdominal route can also be used and is preferable if the developing placenta is accessible. The chorionic villi are inspected under a dissecting microscope and contaminating maternal decidua removed if present. The villi can be used for chromosome analysis, for certain biochemical investigations, and for fetal DNA analysis.

The great advantage of chorionic villus sampling is the prospect of the couple getting an early diagnostic result on the fetus, often before they are obliged to disclose the pregnancy to others and in time for a termination of pregnancy by vacuum extraction if it comes to an abortion. There are, however, some disadvantages compared to amniocentesis, the principal one being the 1 to 2 per cent chance of confined placental mosaicism, where serious chromosomal abnormalities are detected but turn out to not involve the baby. There is an anxious wait until the situation can be clarified by amniocentesis or fetal blood sampling. Chorionic villus sampling at 10 to 12 weeks' gestation has a 1 to 2 per cent chance of causing a miscarriage that would not have otherwise occurred. More serious has been preliminary evidence that very early villous sampling, at about 8 weeks' gestation, which is no longer done, was associated with limb-reduction defects, possibly as a result of inducing fetal hypotension and underperfusion of the limb extremities.

Ultrasound-guided fetal blood sampling, usually from the placental insertion site of the umbilical cord, has an important back-up role in prenatal diagnosis, particularly in assessing the likely impact of placental or amniocyte mosaicism on the baby, or dealing with a pregnancy where the risk is only realized late. Analysis of fetal blood can often be the quickest route to the most reliable result.

Prenatal diagnosis is not always made with selective abortion in mind. Advance warning of structural abnormalities, such as heart defects, can ensure that delivery occurs at an appropriate treatment centre. Some fetal therapies are under trial. There is evidence that maternal dexamethasone administration from 6 weeks' gestation can reduce virilization of the genitalia in females with the autosomal recessive disorder 21-hydroxylase deficiency. However, such maternal corticosteroid treatment should not be continued unnecessarily, and early prenatal diagnosis by villus sampling and DNA analysis is essential.

Fig. 21 Biopsy of preimplantation embryos for genetic analysis and selective uterine transfer.

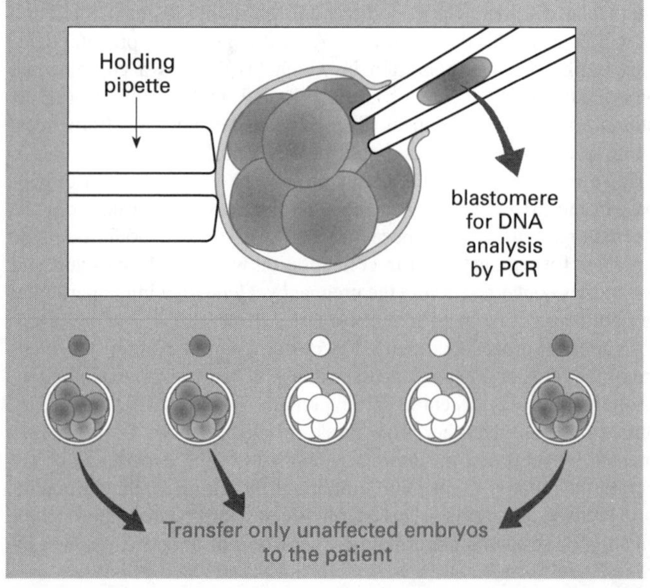

Couples seeking to achieve a healthy family in the face of a known genetic risk carry a great 'burden of choice'. They have to weigh the pain of termination of a planned pregnancy against the natural desire to have children of their own and their belief that it would be wrong to deliberately risk bringing a child into the world to suffer. Many say they would dearly love to start a pregnancy knowing that their chance of a healthy baby is the 'same as everyone else'; a pregnancy they can welcome with confidence. It was these sentiments that led to the development of preimplantation diagnosis.

PREIMPLANTATION DIAGNOSIS

Preimplantation diagnosis combines *in vitro* fertilization (**'IVF'**) with genetic analysis of the early (usually 3 days' postfertilization) embryos, before selective transfer of unaffected embryos to the woman's uterus. Given that 50 per cent or more offspring of nearly all couples facing a genetic risk are unaffected, preimplantation diagnosis and selective transfer provides them with the prospect of starting a pregnancy with their specific genetic risk excluded. It also obviates, in most people's opinion, the need to contemplate genetic manipulation of the human preimplantation embryo as a means of coping with genetic disease. Difficult though it is, preimplantation diagnosis is a much simpler and safer alternative to any future, embryo gene therapy with its added concern of affecting the germline. The promising developments in preimplantation diagnosis did much to reassure people that the general ban on embryo gene therapy is not 'closing the door' on research aimed at helping families with genetic disease.

Preimplantation diagnosis is made possible by the exquisite sensitivity of the polymerase chain reaction, such that the starting material can be just one or two DNA molecules from a single cell. This same sensitivity means that extreme care is needed to avoid errors due to contaminating cells/DNA. There are various biopsy approaches under trial, but the one used for most of the 16 babies born in clinical trials at the time of writing followed the strategy outlined in Figure 21. After the ordinary IVF procedure, during which there is hyperstimulation of the woman's ovaries to generate up to 12 or so mature eggs, those successfully fertilized are cultured until about the 8-cell stage. With the embryo on a holding pipette, a hole is 'drilled' in the zona pellucida with acid tyrose and one or two cells (blastomeres) are sucked into a pipette. After the biopsy of all the embryos, they remain in culture for an additional day compared to regular IVF, whilst the genetic analysis is made.

The type of genetic analysis depends on the disease. The simplest is embryo sexing, using Y- and X-specific DNA probes, which can allow only female embryos to be transferred to the uterus of a woman who is carrying an X-linked disease. A child has been born after embryo screening for the common Δ-508 mutation in a couple at risk of another child with cystic fibrosis. There are many technical challenges to be overcome before preimplantation begins to feature as a significant option for 'at-risk' couples, but, like somatic gene therapy, it is something that is likely to really benefit the next generation.

Genetic services and the use of genetic information

JUDGING THE SUCCESS OF GENETIC SERVICES

The broad objective of medical genetics is to help people with genetic diseases and their families to live and reproduce as normally as possible. More specifically, clinical genetic services aim to maintain or restore family life and reproductive confidence in the face of a perceived or known recurrent heritable risk. We have seen already that, to make a reduction in the birth incidence of genetic disease, the object or 'mission' of genetic services is to undermine the guiding principle in the use of genetic information, namely informed choice of the person or couple concerned, provided it is within the law. This provision of informed choice is achieved by a precise diagnosis, clinical referral if necessary, genetic counselling, carrier testing, and the offer of prenatal diagnosis and selective abortion as a means of having healthy children whilst avoiding the birth of a child destined to suffer a severe genetic disease. It is only achievable in an equitable, nationwide health service accessible to all.

Public-health statements sometimes talk of prevention of genetic disease, without making clear what is meant by prevention. True prevention, such as reducing the recurrence risk of neural-tube defect by maternal, periconceptional, folic-acid supplements, is welcomed by all. Provision of genetic counselling to forewarn those at high risk, but without effective treatment or the option of prenatal diagnosis and selective abortion, may be viewed very differently. There is evidence with respect to β-thalassaemia, Huntington's disease, and cystic fibrosis that genetic counselling alone led to many couples foregoing having (further) children, so fearful were they of risking a pregnancy. This impact of genetic counselling reduces the birth incidence of the disorder and in doing so may achieve a public-health aim. It may well be welcome news for couples who already have some healthy children and are happy to avoid further pregnancies, but for childless couples or those with just an affected child it may represent a tragic impasse, and certainly no 'success' for genetic services. In many people's eyes, the introduction of prenatal diagnosis provided the first chance to plan a healthy family. For them it is the healthy children born in the face of genetic risks that are the 'successes' of genetic services. For others who wish to continue the pregnancy even though the baby is affected, the benefits of the genetic services are more in terms of time to prepare for the birth, and support in the care and treatment of their beloved child. A cost–benefit analysis that accords with the hopes and fears of the families (the only analysis of any worth) would always count an abortion as a cost—not a beneficial saving on health resources—and the birth of a wanted baby, whatever its genetic status, as a benefit. Not only is counting the number of terminations of pregnancies after prenatal diagnosis an inappropriate measure of 'prevention', it is also a fallacious measure of money saved on health care, because many mothers would not have dared to get pregnant in the first place if they had not already decided to seek prenatal diagnosis and selective abortion.

The combined, overall impact of the introduction and development of modern genetic services results in both more healthy children born and less affected children born to families at risk, and consequently a redistribution of resources rather than an absolute increase. It is one of the few areas where meeting the rising demand for services can be met without imposing a significant burden on public funds.

QUALITY MEASURES IN GENETICS SERVICES

Measures of the quality of genetic services are concerned with the following questions:

1. Where it is possible, and proper, to identify those who are at risk, are they informed of the risk in good time, and enabled to cope with it?
2. Are those at risk enabled to benefit from the advice that is given, and from the interventions available?
3. Are reproductive confidence and family life restored towards normal?
4. Is life restored towards normal for those who are at risk of developing a specific genetic disorder?
5. Is the uncertainty that accompanies statistical estimates of risk reduced as far as possible?

Ethical dilemmas

Whilst, for the most part, clinical genetics does not raise entirely new types of ethical dilemma, new challenges in this area are arising thick and fast. It is important to distinguish between a true ethical dilemma and just bad clinical practice. To do genetic tests without any counselling is just bad practice and everyone more or less agrees that this is so. Whether or not to disclose the incidental discovery, during DNA analysis, of an unexpected paternity is a dilemma; there are conflicting views. On the one hand, one usually discloses the results of DNA analysis, but on the other what right has one to disclose information that another family member has chosen to keep secret. Table 15 summarizes, under broad headings, some of the opposing views that generate the tensions typical of the ethical dilemmas commonly encountered in clinical genetics.

Table 15 *Summary of where ethical dilemmas arise in the use of genetic information*

COPING		
	Prenatal diagnosis	
1. Selection abortion		Care/treatment
	Placement	
2. Exclusion from mainstream		Integration
PRIVACY		
	Family ties	
3. Keeping your genotype secret		Obligation to share family information
	Disclosure	
4. Protecting individual interest		Protecting the legitimate interests of others
TOLERANCE		
	Social regulation	
5. Legislation		Family responsibility
	Genetic variation	
6. High-risk genotype		Valued sensitivity
JUSTICE		
	Research	
7. Protection of research subjects		Medical advance
	Health care	
8. Equitable services		'Market forces'

The ethical dilemmas are characterized by tension between conflicting claims represented here by the two catchphrases.

Only three will be highlighted here. First, integration or not: this is a familiar one in all areas involving people with disabilities. How best to provide for their special needs? There are some couples with profound hearing impairment who wish to see a separate 'deaf community' develop. What if they seek to have many children all of whom will be deaf, or even avoid the birth of children with 'normal hearing'?

Secondly, family ties and confidentiality: this is perhaps the one area that typically raises genetic ethical problems. The ethical principle of autonomy emphasizes individual choice. We are used to this being a starting point in discussing ethical issues, but where genetic matters are concerned the information in some way belongs to the family as well as the individual. What right does one family member have to genetic results of another family member?

Finally, what responsibility does the medical genetic community have to counter the tendency (which stems from the case-control types of studies amongst other things) to define genetic variation—polymorphisms—by disease risk. Are there dangers in labelling common alleles in this way; in the 'medicalization' of genetic variation? Will injustice be done by only designing studies to detect medical risk factors rather than benefits? Will there be loading of medical and life insurance, not to mention the commercial promotion of specific lifestyles, for years before counterbalancing benefits are discovered? But will the study of non-medical outcomes itself be problematical for those wishing to avoid any accusation of a drift towards positive eugenics? We do not refer to people with fair hair as 'at risk of sunburn/skin cancer'. Indeed, their sensitivity to the sun may have played a valuable role in convincing people at large to accept the danger of losing the ozone layer. Some people even dream about blondes! Can we maintain such wholesome attitudes to our genetic variation as the genetic revolution unfolds.

In 1992, the 'deletion' allele of the angiotensin-converting enzyme was hailed as a 'potent risk factor' for myocardial infarct. In 1994 the same allele was found to be over-represented in French centenarians! It is a long journey from the discovery of genetic variations to a full and balanced description of their impact on an individual's development and health. Considerable care will be needed in the use of the information that is generated along the way.

REFERENCES

Ash, P., Vennart, J., and Carter, C.O. (1977). The incidence of hereditary disease in man. *Lancet*, **i**, 849–51.

Bodmer, W., Bishop, T., and Karran, P. (1994). Genetic steps in colorectal cancer. *Nature (Genetics)*, **6**, 217–19.

Brock, D., Rodeck, C., and Ferguson-Smith, P. (1992). *Prenatal diagnosis and screening.* Churchill Livingstone, Edinburgh.

Carter, C.O. (1977). Monogenic disorders. *Journal of Medical Genetics*, **14**, 316–20.

Emery, A.E.H. and Rimoin, D.L. (ed.) (1990). *Principles and practice of medical genetics.* Churchill Livingstone, Edinburgh.

Hall, L.G. (1990). Genetic imprinting: review and relevance to human diseases. *American Journal of Human Genetics*, **46**, 857–73.

Harper, P.S. (1993). *Practical genetic counselling*, (4th edn). Butterworth-Heinemann, Oxford.

McKusick, V.A. (1994). *Mendelian inheritance in man*, (11th edn). The Johns Hopkins University Press, Baltimore.

Roberts, J.A.F. and Pembrey, M.E. (1985). *An introduction to medical genetics.* 8th edn. University Press, Oxford.

Royal College of Physicians (1989). *Prenatal diagnosis and genetic screening. Community services implications.* RCP, London.

Saunders, A.M. *et al.* (1993). Association of apolipoprotein E allele *e4* with late-onset familial and sporadic Alzheimer's disease. *Neurology*, **43**, 1462–72.

Schächter, F. *et al.* (1994). Genetic associations with human longevity at the *APOE* and *ACE* loci. *Nature (Genetics)*, **6**, 29–32.

Sutherland, G.R. and Richards, R.I. (1993). Dynamic mutations on the move. *Journal of Medical Genetics*, **30**, 978–81.

Wald, N.J., Kennard, A., Densem, J., Cuckle, H.S., Chard, T., and Butler, L. (1992). Antenatal maternal serum screening for Down's syndrome: results of a demonstration project. *British Medical Journal*, **305**, 391–4.

Weatherall, D.J. (1991). *The new clinical genetics.* Oxford University Press.

Wilkie, A.O.M. (1994). The molecular basis of genetic dominance. *Journal of Medical Genetics*, **31**, 89–98.

Wilson, D.I., Goodship, J.A., Burn, J., Cross, I.E., and Scambler, P.J. (1992). Deletions within chromosome 22q11 in familial congenetical heart disease. *Lancet*, **340**, 573–5.

Section 5 *Immune mechanisms in health and disease*

5.1 Principles of immunology

A. J. McMichael

INTRODUCTION

Two features distinguish immune responses from the non-specific defence mechanisms such as inflammation. The first is the specificity of the reaction, which is easiest to appreciate in terms of antibody responses but is also true of the cellular immune responses; an essential part of this specificity is the remarkable ability to distinguish between self and non-self. The second is memory, by which a second challenge with a stimulus provokes a more rapid and more vigorous immune response. In the last 25 years the cellular and molecular basis of these two characteristics has become clear.

Immune reactions have important roles in most disease processes. Much of what is observed at the bedside involves immune responses, although the visible, palpable, or audible end-result can be quite distant from the primary event. End-immune reactions can be divided into those dependent on antibody secreted by B lymphocytes and their plasma-cell progeny (humoral responses) and those dependent on T lymphocytes (cell-mediated immune responses). Antibody reactions themselves are normally quite 'silent' *in vivo* (e.g. neutralizing virus infectivity), but sometimes antibodies may trigger various secondary events that become literally visible (e.g. anaphylaxis) or revealed on investigation (e.g. haemolysis). Cell-mediated immune responses may also be silent (e.g. clearing of some virus infections by T cells lysing infected cells or releasing interferon), visible (e.g. delayed hypersensitivity reactions in the skin), or revealed by investigation (e.g. kidney graft rejection).

These two different types of immune response are indicative of the basic division of lymphocytes into two types, B and T cells. They interact with each other and with a third important cell, the antigen-presenting cell. The following sections explain how these cells work, as far as possible at a molecular level.

Antigens

Both B and T lymphocytes make the fundamental distinction between self and non-self. This is quite remarkable; consider, for example, the immune response to cytochrome *c*. If immunized, each species will make antibody to cytochrome *c* of other species but not self, even though they are closely related proteins differing in very few amino acids. Similarly, T cells respond to all HLA (transplantation) antigens of other members of the species but not self. The mechanisms that underlie this self tolerance are complex and will be explained later. First, the nature of antigens recognized by B and T cells needs to be examined, because there are important differences.

Antigens recognized by B cells

B lymphocytes recognize antigen through their surface antibody receptors. In chemical terms the recognition is identical to that by secreted antibody. The antibody reacts with antigenic macromolecules (proteins, polysaccharides, or nucleic acids) in their native conformation. The availability of large amounts of purified antibodies, particularly those secreted by hybridomas (see below), has facilitated detailed analysis of how protein or carbohydrate macromolecules are recognized. By using small sugars to inhibit antibody reactivity to polysaccharides, it was shown that an antibody binds to a small part (epitope) of a macromolecule, about the size of seven sugars. For protein antigens, knowledge of structure has helped to define their antigen epitopes. A good example is the haemagglutinin of influenza A virus. The amino acid sequence and the three-dimensional structure of this molecule are known. In addition, the amino acid sequences of variant haemagglutinin molecules that react with different antibodies have been determined. It is possible thereby to locate the parts of the molecule that bind to antibody. Four have been identified in this way, situated on the outside of the globular head of the molecule, each involving fewer than 10 amino acids; because the antibodies bind to a folded molecule these amino acids are not in continuous sequence. Thus, for both protein and polysaccharide, the epitopes that react with antibodies and B cells are discrete and small.

A protein antigen must be greater than about eight amino acids in size to stimulate an immune response. It is possible, however, to make antibodies to smaller molecules if these are coupled to larger carrier proteins. In this way, antibodies can be made to virtually all drugs and other small chemical (hapten) groups. This implies a further very special feature of the humoral immune response: it can recognize molecules that do not occur in nature or that have not been previously synthesized. This is because the spatial configuration of many small molecules may be similar in the sense that they fit antigen-binding sites of antibodies. Such molecular mimicry has been invoked to explain some autoimmune reactions, for instance the cross-reaction between streptococcal and cardiac antigens in rheumatic carditis.

B cells can react with antigen in its natural form, and special processing is not required. However, the signal delivered to B cells by antigen is on its own insufficient to activate them to proliferate and secrete antibody. Other signals, which are now known to be growth and differentiation factors, must be provided, normally by 'helper' T lymphocytes. As discussed below, T lymphocytes respond to processed antigen. Certain carbohydrate antigens, however, which have multiple repeating units that can function as epitopes, can stimulate B cells directly to divide and secrete IgM antibody. Some polysaccharide carbohydrates achieve this by non-specifically activating cells to which they bind, lipopolysaccharide from Gram-negative bacteria for example.

Antigens recognized by T cells

In principle, T cells can recognize as antigen the same range of molecules as are seen by antibodies. However, they are more fastidious about the nature of antigen and its presentation: they do not respond to soluble or free antigen, but to antigen at cell surfaces. The antigen is always protein derived. On the presenting cells the antigen has to be associated with histocompatibility (HLA) molecules. As foreign antigens are invariably presented *in vivo* with self HLA antigen, the T cells show specificity for self HLA plus foreign antigen. T cells so activated will not recognize the same foreign antigens if presented with foreign HLA *in vitro*. However, foreign HLA molecules can themselves provoke very strong immune reactions. There is therefore something very special about T-cell recognition of HLA antigens.

Foreign protein antigens are presented to **Th** cells (helper T cells that will stimulate B cells to make antibody) by specialized antigen-presenting cells. When the parts of the protein molecule that T cells respond to are analysed, it is clear that these are often different from those seen by antibody. Using the same example as above, the Th cells can often recognize parts of the influenza A virus haemagglutin that are buried in the molecule. They respond well to short (15–20 amino acid residues) synthetic peptides that represent fragments of the known amino-acid sequence. Experiments have indicated that if antigen-presenting cells (macrophages) are lightly fixed with paraformaldehyde they will successfully present peptide fragments but not whole protein antigens to T cells of the Th type. All this implies that helper T cells see digested fragments of protein antigens, rather than native proteins, in association with self HLA molecules. The role of the antigen-presenting macrophage or monocyte is to capture protein, or other antigen, ingest it, and present it in processed from on its surface in association with HLA class II (Fig. 1).

The other chief subset of T cells, the cytotoxic T lymphocytes, see foreign antigen at the surface of non-specialized presenting cells, particularly virus antigen on infected cells. Cytotoxic T cells recognize peptide fragments of virus antigens at the surface of target cells bound to HLA class I molecules. In this form, antigen would not be recognized by antibody specific for the intact protein. This suggests a reason for this apparently complicated process of T-cell recognition. If T cells could react with native antigen free from cell surfaces, they would be inactivated because the receptor would be engaged but the secondary signals needed for T-cell activation, provided by the antigen presenting cell, would be lacking.

Histocompatibility antigens

These antigens, HLA in man, play a central part in T-lymphocyte function because, as described above, they associate with foreign antigen to stimulate T cells. HLA antigens are encoded by the major histocompatibility complex (**MHC**), which is a cluster of genes on the short arm of chromosome 6 (Fig. 2). There are two types of MHC antigen, class I and II.

Class I antigens are dimers with a 45 000-Da heavy chain, encoded in the MHC, and an invariant light chain, β_2-microglobulin, that is coded on chromosome 15. In 1987 the three-dimensional structure of HLA-A2 was determined, a finding that has had a profound impact on our understanding of T-cell recognition. The heavy chain is divisible into extracellular three domains of about 90 amino acids, of which the membrane-proximal α3 domain resembles one of the domains that make up the immunoglobulin structure. The heavy chain associates with β_2-microglobulin, which is also immunoglobulin-like. Together these form a stalk on which sits a structure made up by the α-1 and -2 domains. This part of the molecule is folded to form a groove, bordered on its sides by two α-helices and on its floor by an eight-stranded β-sheet; nearly all of the amino acids that differ between class I molecules of different HLA type contribute to the fine structure of this groove. The ends of the groove are closed and contain tyrosines and threonines that are conserved in nearly all class I molecules. The crystal structure showed that the groove contains bound peptides, now known to be derived from degraded cytoplasmic proteins. Because different class I molecules (types) have differently shaped grooves, they bind different peptides. The peptides are usually nine amino acids in length and are bound as extended chains with the amino and carboxy termini fitting into the conserved ends of the groove. Between two and four of the side chains of the amino acids that make up the peptides are involved in binding to the HLA molecule, fitting into pockets in the groove. These anchoring residues are different in different class I molecules: for instance, all nonamer peptides that bind to HLA-B27 have arginine at position two, whereas those binding to HLA-A2 have leucine or isoleucine at this position and those binding to HLA-B35 have proline. The class I molecules on a given cell probably bind several hundred peptides, almost all of which share these common anchor residues; these give the cell a 'signature' that is monitored by T cells, which are tolerant to normal self peptides. If a foreign peptide, derived from an intracellular parasite or mutated self protein, enters the system, T cells can react and destroy the cell. The class I molecules thus serve the function of displaying abnormalities within the cell at its surface.

Most nucleated cells express class I HLA, although trophoblast is negative and very low amounts are expressed on hepatocytes, muscle cells, and nerve cells. Some tumours are negative, which may be one way in which they evade T-cell immunity. However, expression on many cell types is increased by the action of interferon-γ released by activated T cells.

Class I heavy chains are encoded in the MHC. Products of two loci, HLA-A and -B, are expressed on cell surfaces in large amounts (10 000–100 000 molecules per cell), a third series, HLA-C, is expressed at much lower levels. Products of some other class I loci, HLA-E, -F, and -G, do not reach the surface or are restricted in their expression to a few cell types (for instance, HLA-G is expressed on extravillous trophoblast); their role is not understood. The HLA-A, -B, and -C antigens are highly polymorphic with multiple alleles at each locus (Table 1). As described

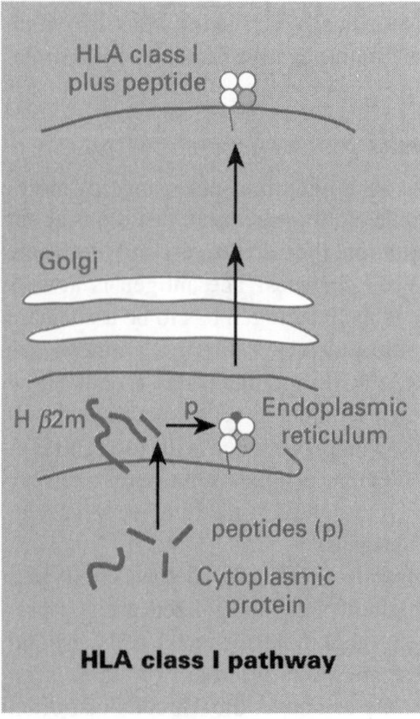

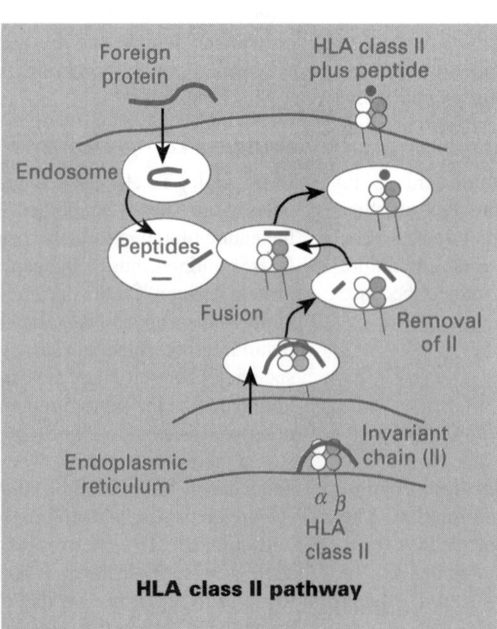

Fig. 1 Antigen processing: the two pathways are shown, through HLA class I on the left and through HLA class II on the right. For the class I route, cytoplasmic (e.g. virus) proteins are degraded to peptides in the cytosol. The peptides are transported to the lumen of the endoplasmic reticulum. Here, nonamer peptides bind to the newly synthesized class I molecules, stabilizing folding with β_2-microglobulin. The stable complex is translocated to the cell surface where foreign peptides as well as self peptide are displayed. For the class II route, foreign protein antigen is ingested by the cell and degraded to peptides in the endosome. The newly synthesized class II molecules fold in the endoplasmic reticulum and the groove is protected by binding to a polypeptide, 'invariant chain'. As the complex formed is transported towards the cell surface the invariant chain is digested away by proteases exposing the groove. HLA class II-containing endosomes fuse with peptide-containing vesicles and peptide binds to the class II HLA groove, stabilizing the structure. The HLA class II molecules reach the cell surface and display foreign peptides. (For further details see Townsend, A. and Trowsdale, J. (1993). The transporters associated with antigen presentation. *Seminars in Cell Biology*, **4**, 53–61.)

above, class I antigens present peptide fragments of foreign antigens, usually derived from viruses, on the surface of normal cells to cytotoxic T lymphocytes. It is likely that the extreme degree of HLA polymorphism results from selection of HLA alleles, because individually they vary in their efficiency in presenting particular intracellular parasite antigens to cytotoxic T lymphocytes.

HLA class II molecules have many similarities with Class I molecules. Class II antigens have two chains, α and β. Each is of around 30 000 Da and is composed of two extracellular domains (Fig. 2). At least four different members of the family are expressed on cells and most are polymorphic. The best-studied series are the DR antigens, which have a highly polmorphic β-chain (from the *DRB1* locus) giving rise to over 20 DR types (Table 1). There is a second, less polymorphic DR β-chain giving the specificities DR51,52, and 53 encoded by the *DRB3, DRB4,* and *DRB5* loci, respectively. The DQ molecules are polymorphic in both α- and β-chains, which means that hybrid molecules can occur in heterozygotes. The DP molecules are polymorphic in the β-chain and are expressed in smaller amounts. The HLA class II molecules are expressed on a limited set of cells, normally B lymphocytes, monocytes, activated T lymphocytes and some epithelial cells, but can be induced on many other cell types, thyroid and gut epithelia for example, by interferon-γ.

The three-dimensional structure of HLA-DR1 has recently been determined (Plate 1). It is remarkably similar to that of HLA class I. The main difference is that the groove is open ended, allowing the bound peptides to hang out; thus they are longer, 12 to 16 amino acids (Plate 1). Like class I bound peptides, there are anchor residues, determined by the fine structure of the groove. There is a particularly prominent pocket in the floor at the left-hand end of the groove, which binds large aromatic side chains in some instances. These binding motifs in amino acid sequence differ for different class II molecules and are currently being worked out in detail.

The function of the class II antigens is to present foreign processed antigen to helper T cells. As discussed above, this process is mediated by specialized antigen-presenting cells, although wider expression of class II antigens induced by interferon suggests that other cells may be able to process and present under certain circumstances. The DQ and DP molecules are not expressed on as many cell types as are DR molecules. Differential expression of DP or DQ macrophages, for instance, may influence the type of T-cell response.

Fig. 2 The HLA gene complex. The horizontal line represents the short arm of chromosome 6 with the centromere on the left. Vertical bars represent genes for the different HLA chains. The diagram is drawn roughly to scale in terms of distance between genes (centimorgans), with breaks to indicate long gaps between genes. Terminology of the genes is explained in the text. In the lower part of the figure a more detailed map of the class II region is shown, together with the genes contribution to the class II proteins. Also shown are the protease components LMP2 and MP7, which are thought to be involved in the generation of peptides in the cytosol, and the transporter genes *TAP1* and *TAP2,* which code for the transporter that takes peptides from the cytoplasm into the lumen of the endoplasmic reticulum. There is some polymorphism in the *TAP* genes.

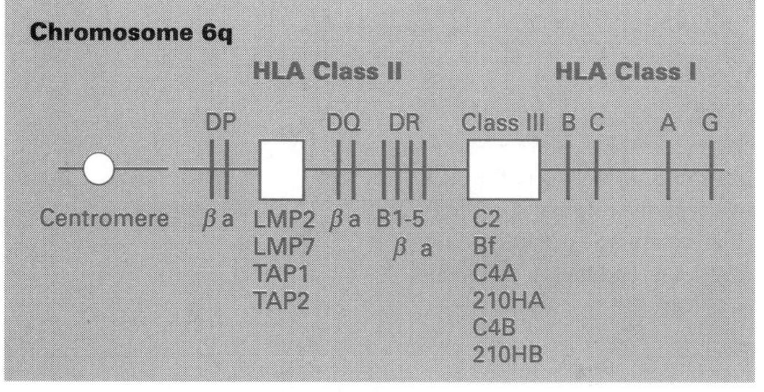

Humans differ in the epitopes of an antigen that they recognize according to their HLA class II type. The effects of this could be manifest, for instance, in the degree of cross-reactivity between related viruses that stimulate antibody responses. Similarly, HLA class II type could determine whether antigens that differ from self in only a few amino acids are recognized. Self antigens that are slightly altered could fall into this category and it is striking that several organ-specific autoimmune diseases are associated with HLA-DR3. However, the exact reasons for this and other HLA and disease associations (Table 2) remain unresolved. It should be noted that the disease associations demonstrated imply either a direct role for the HLA molecule or that there is a nearby disease-susceptibility gene in linkage disequilibrium with the HLA marker. In the case of *HLA-DR3* there is strong linkage disequilibrium with *HLA-B8* and everything in between, including a complement C4 null allele and at least 50 genes, most of which are non-polymorphic and are of unknown function.

The action of HLA class II antigens in presenting antigens to helper T cells gives them a key role in initiating immune responses. In contrast, class I antigens are involved at a later and more specialized stage. This is important in transplantation, where matching class II antigens is more important than matching class I, although the final damaging activity of cytotoxic T cells and antibody is largely directed at class I antigens.

Antigen processing

There are two pathways of antigen processing, generating the peptides that bind to HLA class I and II molecules, recognized by cytotoxic T cells (which carry the CD8 surface marker) and Th (CD4+), respectively.

As indicated above, class I HLA molecules present short peptides derived from cytoplasmic proteins. The most likely pathway by which this happens is shown in Fig. 1. Proteins in the cell are naturally turning over, broken down by cytoplasmic proteases. The multicatalytic proteasesome complex is a major contributor to this process. It degrades proteins that have been coupled to ubiquitin and digests them to small fragments. It is made up of some 28 components; two of these are encoded in the MHC in the class II region, and may affect the protease specificity. The peptides generated are transported into the endoplasmic reticulum by an ATP-dependent transporter made up of two chains, TAP-1 and TAP-2, both encoded in the class II region of the MHC. In the lumen of the endoplasmic reticulum, peptides are degraded further unless they bind to newly synthesized class I HLA molecules and are then taken to the cell surface bound in the groove (Plate 1). Expression of class I molecules at the cell surface is dependent on the integrity of this pathway.

Processing of antigens to be presented by class II HLA takes place in specialized antigen-presenting cells. Protein antigens are taken into the cell from outside. Monocytes may take up antigen passively by endocytosis or by receptor-mediated uptake, acquiring proteins bound through complement or Fc receptors. The former complex with antibody bound to antigen, bringing the antigen to the presenting cells. The latter bind to the constant regions of antibodies and so also mediate uptake of proteins bound to cells as immune complexes; antigen may bind to small amounts of 'natural antibody' or the early specific antibody (giving an early positive feedback). Also, B lymphocytes with specific antibody receptors can bind foreign proteins directly, endocytose, and process antigen to present peptides bound to class II molecules. Digestion of proteins takes place in an endosomal compartment, which later fuses with class II HLA-carrying vesicles. The newly synthesized class II molecules do not bind peptides in the endoplasmic reticulum; instead they bind to a protein known as the 'invariant chain'. This protects the groove from peptide binding and the complex is exported through the Golgi complex where glycosylation and addition of sialic acid residues to both the class II molecules and the invariant chain take place. In a

Table 1 *HLA antigens*

A	B	C	DR (B1)	DR (Bx)	DQ	DP
A1	B5	Cw1	DR1	DR51	DQ1	DPw1
A2	B7	Cw2	DR103	DR52	DQ2	DPw2
A203	B703	Cw3	DR2	DR53	DQ3	DPw3
A210	B8	Cw4	DR3		DQ4	DPw4
A3	B12	Cw5	DR4		DQ5(1)	DPw5
A9	B13	Cw6	DR5		DQ6(1)	DPw6
A10	B14	Cw7	DR6		DQ7(3)	
A11	B15	Cw8	DR7		DQ8(3)	
A23(9)	B16	Cw9(w3)	DR8		DQ9(3)	
A24(9)	B17	Cw10(w3)	DR9			
A2403	B18		DR10			
A25(10)	B21		DR11(5)			
A26(10)	B22		DR12(5)			
A28	B27		DR13(6)			
A29(19)	B35		DR14(6)			
A30(19)	B37		DR1403			
A31(19)	B38(16)		DR1404			
A32(19)	B39(16)		DR15(2)			
A33(19)	B3901		DR16(2)			
A34(10)	B3902		DR17(3)			
A36	B40		DR18(3)			
A43	B4005					
A66(10)	B41					
A68(28)	B42					
A69(28)	B44(12)					
A74(19)	B45(12)					
	B46					
	B47					
	B48					
	B49(21)					
	B50(21)					
	B51(5)					
	B5102					
	B5203					
	B52(5)					
	B53					
	B54(22)					
	B55(22)					
	B56(22)					
	B57(17)					
	B58(17)					
	B59					
	B60(40)					
	B61(40)					
	B62(15)					
	B63(15)					
	B64(14)					
	B65(14)					
	B67					
	B70					
	B71(70)					
	B72(70)					
	B73					
	B75(15)					
	B76(15)					
	B77(15)					

This table shows the full listing of HLA serological specificities, grouped according to the locus for each allelic series. Some of the original types have been split into related types, shown with the original specificity in parentheses. (This is necessary because some of the older names persist in the literature (e.g. DR2, which is now DR15 or DR16)). The DR antigens are shown for specificities at the *BRB1* locus and the second locus *DRBx* (x = 3, 4, or 5 according to the haplotype).

Data from Sasazuki, T. *et al.* (ed.) (1993). *HLA typing.* Oxford University Press.

Table 2 *HLA and disease associations: relative risks*

Locus	Antigen	Disease	Percentage antigen frequency		Relative risk[a]
			Normal	Patients	
A	A3	Id haemochromatosis	28	76	8
B	B5	Behçet's syndrome	10	41	6
	B27	Ankylosing spondylitis	9	90	87
		Reiter's syndrome	9	79	37
	B35	Subacute thyroiditis	15	70	14
C	Cw6	Psoriasis	33	87	13
D	DR2	Narcolepsy	26	100	>50
		Goodpasture's syndrome	26	88	16
		Multiple sclerosis	26	59	4
	DR3	Dermatitis herpetiformis	26	85	15
		Coeliac disease	26	79	11
		Sjögren's (sicca syndrome)	26	78	10
		Id Addison's disease	26	69	6
		Graves' disease	26	56	4
		Myasthenia gravis	26	50	2
		SLE	26	70	6
		Id membranous nephropathy	26	75	12
		IDDM	26	56	3
	DR3 and/or 4	IDDM	57	99	8
	DR4	IDDM	20	75	6
		Rheumatoid arthritis	20	50	4
	DR5	Pernicious anaemia	6	25	5

Abbreviations: Id, idiopathic; IDDM, insulin-dependent diabetes mellitus; SLE, systemic lupus erythematosus; RR, relative risk.

[a]Relative risk is the factor of increased risk of developing the disease by individuals with the HLA antigen. Data compiled from Svejgaard, A., Platz, P. and Ryder, L.P. (1983). *Immunology Review,* **70,** 192.

late endosomal compartment, at low pH, the invariant chain is degraded and removed from the class II molecules. At this pH, binding of peptides is optimal and these endosomes are thought to fuse with those in which the peptides have been generated. Binding of peptide stabilizes the class II structure and the class II molecule containing the peptide reaches the surface. As for class I HLA, several peptides derived from normal proteins are displayed and elicit no T-cell response because of tolerance. Foreign peptides that stimulate T cells with appropriate receptors initiate Th responses.

Priming the immune response

It is becoming clear that antigen presentation by class I or class II MHC on its own is insufficient to initiate a T-cell immune response. Specialized cells have a role, particularly B lymphocytes, dendritic cells, and others of the monocyte series. In addition to presenting peptides on their MHC molecules they display other accessory molecules on their surface, important for cell-to-cell interactions. As well as the adhesion molecules that are also necessary for T-cell recognition of target cells, such as LFA-1 and CD2, a molecule called B7 (not to be confused with HLA-B7) is especially important. This binds to the T-cell glycoprotein CD28 and delivers a signal to naïve T cells initiating their response. Once activated in this way these T cells can interact with antigen-presenting cells, such as virus-infected epithelial cells, and react; this effector stage no longer requires CD28:B7, but does need LFA-1 and CD2. The importance of this pathway is that there could be cells in the body that display potentially antigenic peptides and do not suffer immune attack unless some other event primes the responding T cells; thus a virus infection could initiate an autoimmune response to a cross-reacting self peptide epitope.

Antibodies

Structure

The basic structure of an antibody molecule is illustrated in Fig. 3. An IgG molecule consists of four chains, two identical heavy chains (50 000 Da) and two identical light chains (25 000 Da). The immunoglobulin molecule can be broken into segments by enzymes, giving the peptides illustrated in Fig. 3. Sequence analysis of light and heavy chains and crystallographic studies have revealed that they are composed of domains of about 100 amino acids, held by a disulphide loop between two cysteines (a domain structure that has been found to be present in many other cell-surface molecules). There are two for each light chain (**L**) and four for an IgG γ heavy chain (**H**). The N-terminal domains of both L and H chains are highly variable when different antibody molecules are compared: they contain the antigen-binding site. The constant domains of the heavy chain define the isotype of the antibody, IgG, A, D, M or E, each of which has particular functions. The main differences between the various heavy-chain constant regions are described in Table 3. The isotypes determine essential properties of the antibodies, particularly binding of C1q of the complement system, binding of the Fc receptor that enables antibody to cross the placenta, and binding of Fc receptors on mast cells and basophils. IgA binds to a specific Fc receptor, known as a secretory component, which is on the epithelial membranes. The antibody can then be endocytosed and transported across these cells and released on the outside, that is the gut lumen, biliary tract, respiratory tract or milk duct. Light-chain constant regions are one of two classes, κ or λ. There are no known differences in function between the two.

The N-terminal domains of L and H chains are variable regions. They vary between different antibodies to a remarkable degree. Sequence comparison of several variable regions has shown that there are three short hypervariable patches between amino acids 28–34, 45–56, and 91–97 in both light and heavy chains. The crystalline structure of antibody indicates that these hypervariable regions form a surface to which antigen binds. In agreement with the studies on antigen epitopes, this is the right size to make contact with about six amino acids on the surface of the antigen. Sequence analysis has also revealed that there must be multiple (hundreds of) genes for variable regions because of the enormous variability. Estimates, by various methods, agree that an individual must be capable of generating over 1 million different antibody molecules, probably 10^8 or even higher. As the variability is contributed by both the L and the H chains, which appear to associate independently, this means that there must be between 10^3 and 10^4 VL and VH sequences. How these are generated is discussed below.

Polyclonal or monoclonal antibodies

A normal antibody response includes multiple antibody molecules that bind to each epitope on a given antigen. B-cell activation requires binding of antigen, so that any B cell that binds antigen with an affinity above a certain threshold can be stimulated (with appropriate signals from helper T cells) and ultimately secrete antibody. A single antigen epitope can evoke a response comprising several hundred antibody molecules. This means that each antibody must be capable of binding more than one antigen, which is not surprising considering that antibodies recognize surfaces rather than sequences. An antiserum made up of hundreds or thousands of different molecular species of antibody maintains its specificity because the immunogen is the common denominator. As each antibody molecule is the product of a single clone of B lymphocytes, and many are involved, this type of response is known as polyclonal (Fig. 4).

Under certain circumstances a monoclonal antibody response is generated. This may happen when the stimulating antigen is limited in its variation from self or when it is present in extremely low amounts, thus selecting out only cells with the receptor with the highest binding avidity. Oligoclonal responses are also found in the cerebrospinal fluid in multiple sclerosis, possibly as a consequence of limiting the immune response to the few clones of cells that manage to cross the blood–brain barrier. More commonly, a monoclonal immunoglobulin *in vivo* is the product of abnormal proliferation of a single clone of B cells or plasma cells.

Kohler and Milstein in 1975 devised a way of fusing normal (mouse) B lymphocytes to cultured plasmacytoma cells to generate immortal hybrid cell lines (hybridomas) that secrete the antibody of the B-cell parent. Because the donor of the spleen cells can be immunized at will, these monoclonal antibodies can be generated to any antigen. They have been used to explore the structure of human cells, particularly their surfaces, because unlike polyclonal antibodies made in another species, each monoclonal antibody reacts with a single component of the immunogen. They also have a multitude of practical applications in the study of growth factors, cell-surface receptors, micro-organisms, and many other antigens. They have become routine tools for many diagnostic assays and increasingly their therapeutic applications are being explored.

Fig. 3 Basic structure of an immunoglobulin, IgG, molecule. Two identical light (L) and two identical heavy (H) chains are shown. At the amino terminal (N) there is a variable (V) domain of 110 amino acids. In the light chain (L) this is connected to one constant domain of 100 amino acids which is one of the two types: λ or κ. The heavy-chain variable domain links to three constant-region domains, Cl1, Cl2, and Cl3. Between Cl1 and Cl2 is the hinge region, which gives the binding site (VL + VH) flexibility and contains interchain disulphide (—S—S—) bridges (see Table 3). The site of cleavage by the proteolytic enzymes papain and pepsin are shown, which give the antigen-binding fragments Fab and $F(ab)_2$ and the constant fragment Fc.

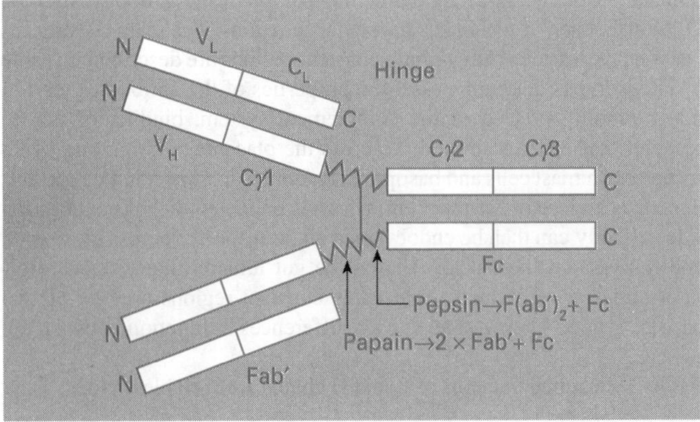

Genetics of antibody production

(The principles of gene structure are described in Section 4).

The development of methods for DNA cloning and rapid sequencing have had a big impact on our understanding of immunoglobulin genes. The genes are arranged, as shown in Fig. 5, on three chromosomes: 14 for heavy chain, 22 for κ, and 2 for λ. The antibody genes are arranged in exons, each coding for a single immunoglobulin domain, with further exons for the hinge and transmembrane regions. The constant-region exons are grouped according to antibody class. There are additional exons for the leader sequence, which takes the newly synthesized antibody chain across the membrane (and is then cleaved off), and a transmembrane exon, which is only expressed on antibody that is attached to cell surfaces.

The variable *V* genes are on the 5′ side of the constant genes (i.e. upstream, as DNA is read from 5′ to 3′). There are many of these and it appears that any variable gene can combine with a constant gene on the same region of the chromosome. The antibody genes are therefore unusual and complex in their arrangement. Besides the multitude of variable genes there are also *D* (diversity) (for heavy chains but not light chains) and *J* (joining) genes, which are short coding sequences (exons) found between *V* and *C*. The arrangement of the genes in B lymphocytes and plasma cells is different from that in all other cells. Early in B-cell development, a single heavy-chain variable gene joins to a *D* and *J* gene to make a *VDJ* rearrangement. Similarly, in one light-chain gene region a *VJ* rearrangement is made. Coupling of *VDJ* or *VJ* to the *C* gene occurs after transcription to nuclear RNA, which is then processed to make mRNA, where, for both heavy- and light-chain transcripts, J is connected to C, and this is translated. The *D* segment, which is 1 to 3 amino acids long, is in the third hypervariable and the very many combinations of VD and J that are possible contribute substantially to antibody diversity. In addition to this it has been shown that breaks in this region may occur in early B cells and be repaired in a random fashion by an enzyme called terminal deoxynucleotide transferase, which again adds further diversity.

Even further variation in both heavy- and light-chain variable regions occurs by somatic mutation as B lymphocytes proliferate in large numbers in the germinal centres of lymphoid organs. This involves selection by antigen and a special (and as yet poorly understood) mechanism that localizes the mutations to particular sites in the antigen-binding regions. As the concentration of antigen declines, only high-avidity B-cell clones will be stimulated to divide and this exerts selective pressure on mutations in the hypervariable regions. It is now known that developing B lymphocytes divide rapidly in the germinal centres and that a large proportion die by apoptosis (programmed cell death), a process not unlike that occurring in the thymus as T cells develop.

The above process of gene rearrangement occurs on only one of the chromosomes encoding the heavy chain, and a similar process occurs on just one of the four chromosomes encoding a light chain (allelic exclusion). A B cell is therefore committed to making one antibody, one heavy-chain VDJC and one light chain VJC, by the time it is immu-

Table 3 *Human immunoglobulins*

Isotype	Chain structure[a]	Number of H domains	M_r (kDa)	Serum concentration (mg/ml)	$t_{1/2}$[b]	Clq[c]	Placenta[d]	Mast cells[e]
IgG1		4	146	9	21	+	+	±
IgG2		4	146	3	20	+	+	–
IgG3		4	165	1	7	+	+	±
IgG4		4	146	0.5	21	–	+	±
IgM	$(\;)_5$ +J	5	970	1.2	5	+	–	–
IgA1		4	160	2	6	–	–	–
IgA2		4	160	0.5	–	–	–	–
sIgA	$(\;)_{2+S}$ +J	4	405	0.5	–	–	–	–
IgD		4	170	0.06	3	–	–	–
IgE		5	190	0.0002	3	–	–	+

[a]To show light and heavy chains with disulphide bridges. (Derived from Nisonoff, A. *Introduction to Molecular Immunology*. Sinauer, Massachusetts.)

[b]Half-life in days.

[c]Binding of complement component Clq.

[d]Ability to cross the placenta.

[e]Ability to bind to and activate mast cells.

nocompetent. It is not clear why this only happens on one chromosome for each chain; there may be some suppressive signal generated once a successful VDJ arrangement has occurred. This property provides a useful way of determining whether proliferating or infiltrating lymphocytes (e.g. in a tissue section) are polyclonal or monoclonal. The latter will all express either a κ or λ chain; the former will include both light-chain types in roughly equal numbers.

The heavy-chain *VDJ* sequence is attached to the *C* genes in an orderly progression during B-cell development. The gene order is $C\mu$, $C\delta$, $C\gamma3$, $C\alpha1$, $C\gamma1$, $C\gamma2$, $C\gamma4$, $C\epsilon$, and $C\alpha2$. All the B cells appear to go through a $C\mu$ stage, most go through $C\delta$, and $C\gamma$ but may end up at one of the γ subtypes, or α or ϵ, probably jumping segments in the process. This progression involves deletion of DNA coding the no longer used *C* genes as the B-cell develops. It is therefore a one-way process. Switching of B cells from production of IgM to IgG is a striking and normal feature of a simple antibody response. The process is regulated by external factors, particularly T helper cells, interacting with the CD40 molecule on B cells, and by the cytokines interleukin (**IL**)-4 and IL-5. IL-4 drives the switch towards IgE, and IL-4-secreting T cells (Th2 cells) probably have a key role in the development of allergic responses. It is also of practical importance that fetal and cord B lymphocytes do not switch from IgM to IgG production.

Fig. 4 Polyclonal antibodies. An antigen such as a protein has many antigenic sites (epitopes) on the surface of the molecule. To each can bind a set of antibodies with a range of affinity depending on the amino acid sequence of their variable regions. These are indicated diagrammatically by the shape of the binding site that binds to epitope. Each species of antibody is the product of one clone of B lymphocytes that can only make antibody with that shape, i.e. V-region sequence.

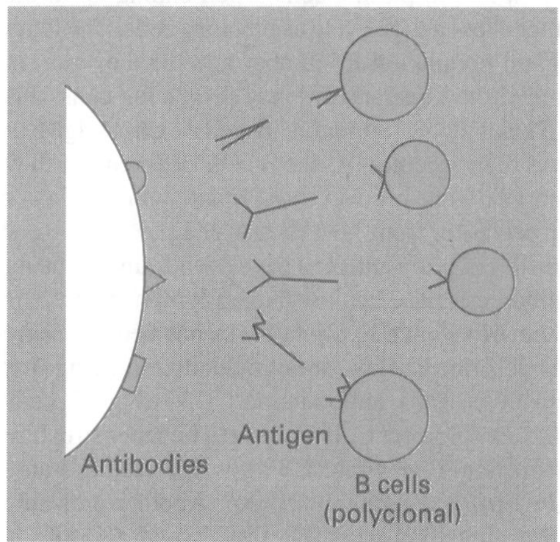

Fig. 5 Arrangement of the immunoglobulin genes. These are arranged on three chromosomes, chromosome 2 for *L* κ, 22 for *L* λ, and 14 for the heavy chain. The basic arrangement of the human genes are shown. *L*κ is arranged with a large number (*n*) of *V* genes, each preceded for a gene for the leader sequence L. Downstream are five *J* genes and further on the one *C* gene. *L*λ is arranged in an unknown number (*n*) of sets, with a group of *x* (?*x* > 20) *L–V* pairs followed by one *J* and *C*. There may be six to nine such sets. *H* is arranged with a large number (>100) of *L–V* pairs followed by a set of *D* minigenes and a set of *J* genes. Downstream are the constant-region *C* genes, each split into separate exons for each domain, and an optional membrane segment, which are placed in the order shown.

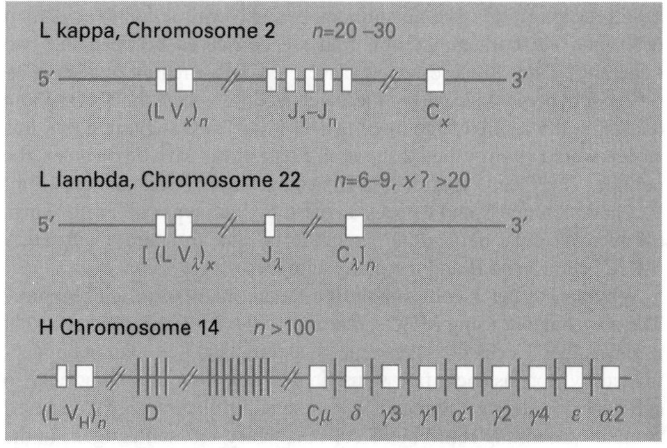

Table 4 *Differentiation antigens on B cells*

Antigen	Synonym	M_r (kDa)	Distribution	Function
Surface Ig		150	All B cells	Antigen receptor
CD9	BA2	24	Pre-B → Virgin B	
CD10	CALLA	100	Pre-B	
CD19	B4	95	Pre-B → P-blasts	Signalling
CD20	B1	35	Pre-B → P-blasts	Signalling
CD21		140	B subset	C3d and EBV receptor
CD22		135	All B cells	Adhesion, ligand CD45RO,CD75
CD23	B2	45	B subset	IgE receptor, signalling
CD24		45–55–65	All B cells	Signalling
CD37		40–52	Mature B cells	
CD40		50	Mature B cells	Ig-class switching
CD72		40	B cells	Activation, ligand CD5
CD80	B7,BB1	60	B subset, act-B	Priming T cells Ligand CD28

Abbreviations: act-B, activated B cells; EBV, Epstein–Barr virus; P-blasts, plasmablasts. Further concise details of leucocyte differentiation antigens can be found in Barclay *et al.* (1993).

The T-cell receptor

Although the T-cell receptor was elusive for many years, recent developments have led to its characterization in all aspects except its three-dimensional structure. Early studies with monoclonal antibodies revealed a two-chain glycoprotein. When its DNA was cloned it was found to rearrange in ways similar to that described above for B-cell immunoglobulin receptors. Unexpectedly, two families of T-cell receptors were found, the αβ-receptor present on all conventional T cells and the γδ-receptor present on a subset of T cells whose function is still not clearly defined.

Both chains of αβ T-cell receptors have been sequenced from several T-cell clones of known antigen specificity. Both chains are similar to immunoglobulin light chains, with two external domains, each of about 100 amino acids. The N-terminal domains of both α- and β-chains are variable. They include V and J segments, with a D segment for the β-chain. Several families of Vβ, Jβ, Vα, and Jα have been identified. The genes for these rearrange as T cells develop whilst the cells are in the thymus. There are two constant-region classes for the β-chain, *C*β1 and *C*β2, which are very similar in structure. The number of possible T-cell receptors has been estimated to be a staggering 10^{14}, generated by the multiple combinations of the gene segments on the two chains. A substantial part of this diversity comes from the activity of the enzyme terminal deoxy nucleotide transferase creating much variability at the V–(D)–J junction.

There are three hypervariable regions (complementarity-determining regions, **CDR**) that would form an antigen-binding site if the molecule were folded like an antibody; a persuasive case has been made that the T-cell receptor folds like an antibody because critical amino acids that determine the immunoglobulin fold are conserved between the two structures. This structure would place the CDR-3 region, made up by the most hypervariable part of the T-cell receptor where the V-(D)-J join occurs, at the centre of the binding site. It has been suggested that this region would sit over the most variable part of the MHC molecules, the peptide. The T-cell receptors on Th and cytotoxic T cells are very similar, and the same *V* and *J* genes are used by both types of T cell. Thus, the receptor must be flexible enough to be able to interact with HLA (MHC) class I and II and the many allotypes.

Why do not the T cells simply use the antibodies as their receptor? The advantage of using MHC molecules as the antigen presenter is that it means that T cells do not see native antigen and thus cannot be inactivated by, for instance, free virus. In addition, by responding only to cell-surface antigens the response can be controlled by signals derived from the presenting cell. Thus T cells that react with self antigens in the thymus may be eliminated while those that react with foreign antigens in the periphery are stimulated.

The function of the T cells that carry the γ∂-receptor remains enigmatic. In mice, but not man, they are abundant in the intestinal mucosa. In humans they have been found at sites of chronic inflammation. It has been suggested that they are involved in antibacterial immunity, but further evidence is needed.

Lymphocytes

Lymphocytes mediate immune reactions and can be divided into two main subtypes, B and T cells.

B lymphocytes

B lymphocytes are the precursors of antibody-secreting plasma cells. They express immunoglobulin on their surface, which acts as antigen receptor. The B cell expresses only one pair of immunoglobulin VH and VL gene products and thus one receptor. The progeny, or clone, of this cell retains the same commitment and the antibody secreted uses the same variable genes. Thus, antigen on first immune challenge selects B cells that already express appropriate receptors. These divide and mature to antibody-producing cells and memory cells. This process occurs in lymphoid organs through a pathway that involves migration to germinal centres, proliferation of immature B cells, somatic mutation of the receptors, selection of those with high affinity for antigen, and apoptosis of the rest. Some B cells progress to plasma cells, often ending up in the bone marrow; others enter a less active cycle as memory cells. The latter greatly exceed the original population in number and, as they can, in turn, be activated by antigen to generate antibody-producing cells, this explains the memory phenomenon. Immature B cells express IgM or IgM plus IgD antibody as their receptor. As the B cells differentiate they switch their heavy-chain *VDJ* gene product to associate with a γ-, α- or ϵ chain and thus switch secretion from IgM to IgA or IgE.

A number of B-cell differentiation antigens have been found by using murine monoclonal antibodies raised against human lymphocytes. The best characterized of them are shown in Table 4. As has been the case with the T-cell antigens described below, it is gradually emerging that these have important functions. Thus, antibodies to CD20 trigger B cells to divide and CD21 is the complement C3b receptor. The latter structure is also the receptor for Epstein–Barr virus (**EBV**), which readily transforms B lymphocytes *in vitro* and probably *in vivo*. Another molecule that is crucial in B-cell signalling is CD40; its ligand CD40L is expressed on T lymphocytes. In the hyper-IgM syndrome, where there is a failure of B cells to switch to IgG production, CD40L is mutated, implying a role for CD40 in signalling immunoglobulin-gene switching.

Activation of B lymphocytes requires antigen and a signal from Th lymphocytes, which are themselves responding to the same antigen. Cells of the Th2 subset (see below) release cytokines (including IL-4 and IL-5) as well as initiating signals through the CD40–CD40L interaction; these activate B lymphocytes in the presence of antigen to divide and differentiate. Note that two kinds of signal are needed, an antigen-specific trigger through the antigen receptor and a second type mediated in a non-antigen-specific fashion. Inappropriate signalling, such as an antigen signal in the absence of the second type, can lead to inactivation of the B cells.

Besides secreting antibody, B cells have a role in antigen presentation that is increasingly recognized as important. B cells can bind foreign antigen directly through their immunoglobulin receptor or as an immune complex through the Fc or complement receptors (immune complexes bind complement; see Chapter 5.4). Such antigen can be internalized and digested in endosomes to generate peptides that bind to class II MHC.

The ontogeny of B lymphocytes is of some clinical relevance because various leukaemias and lymphomas express surface antigens characteristic of B cells at various stages of development. Figure 6 gives the scheme for B-cell differentiation indicating the corresponding leukaemias and lymphomas. Studies on the immunoglobulin light chains expressed indicate that these malignancies are monoclonal diseases.

Burkitt's lymphoma is a B-cell malignancy caused by EBV. In addition to the presence of EBV DNA in the malignant cells, there are chromosomal rearrangements. The c-*myc* oncogene on chromosome 8 is translocated to chromosome 2, 14, or 22. There it comes into close proximity with one of the three sets of immunoglobulin genes. There is a tissue-specific enhancer present between the *J* and *C* exons, which probably activates the displaced oncogene.

T lymphocytes

T lymphocytes require the thymus for their development and show a set of characteristic surface glycoproteins and their own form of receptor, as described above. They can be divided into types: cytotoxic T lymphocytes that carry the CD8 glycoprotein and helper T cells that carry CD4 in mice. The latter can be divided according to the cytokines they release on antigen contact into Th1 (IL-2 and interferon-γ) and Th2 (IL-4, -5, and -10).

T cells may also be divided into those in an inactive state (virgin T cells) and preactive state (memory T cells) by the CD45 glycoprotein isotype on the cell surface. Thus, there is a very high proportion of CD45RA positive (virgin) in cord blood, and CD45RO (memory) T cells appear during early life. *In vitro,* T-cell proliferation to recall antigens (e.g. tetanus toxoid) involves CD45RO T cells, whereas T-cell proliferation to alloantigens involves both CD45RA and -RO populations.

T-CELL DIFFERENTIATION ANTIGENS

Hybridoma-generated monoclonal antibodies have been used to explore the surface of T lymphocytes and have revealed a series of molecules that have essential accessory roles in antigen recognition by T cells (Table 5). Monoclonal antibodies to these structures are now often used to define T-cell subpopulations or leukaemias and are being used therapeutically so that some knowledge of their role is important. Their expression on T cells as they develop is described in Fig. 7.

CD3

The CD3 antigen is present on T-cell surfaces in association with the T-cell receptor. Antibodies to one will precipitate the other from detergent-solubilized cell membranes. The antigen, which is made up of three chains of 19 000, 20 000, and 29 000 Da, is important in T-cell activation. *In vitro,* antibodies to CD3 stimulate T cells to divide by causing

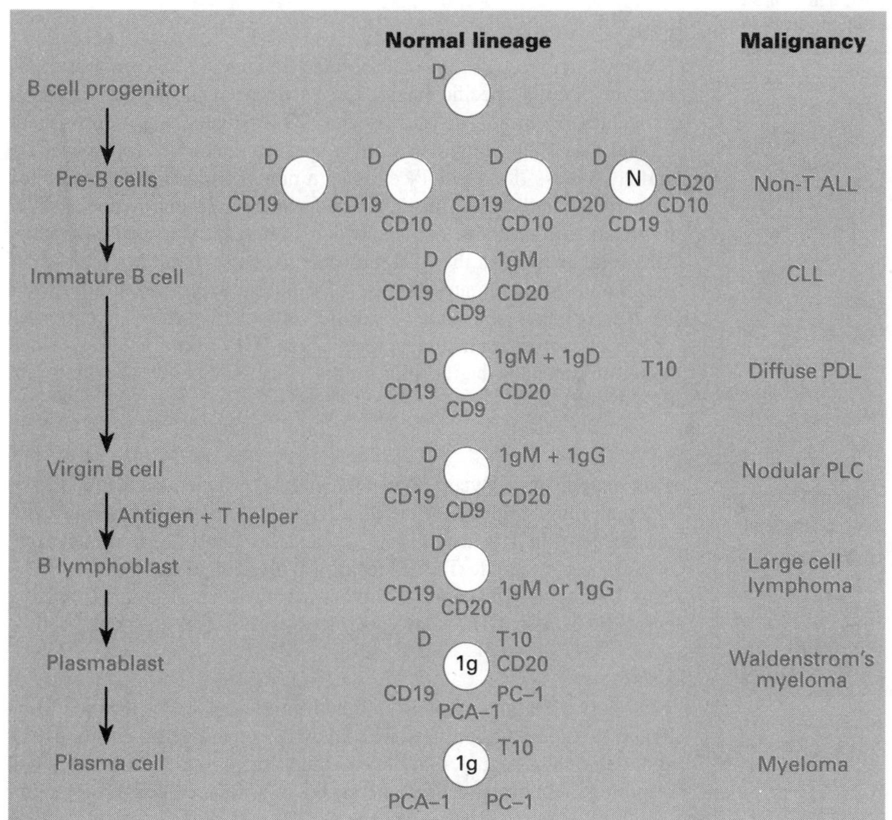

Fig. 6 Expression of B-lymphocyte differentiation antigens on the surface of differentiating B cells. The circles represent developing B cells. The CD antigens are listed in Table 4. In addition, D is HLA class II, μ is an intracellular immunoglobulin μ-chain. IgM, IgD, and IgG are surface immunoglobulins. Plasmablasts and plasma cells are shown with intracellular immunoglobulin (Ig). On the right are the B-cell malignancies that are thought to arise at the levels shown. They express the surface antigens indicated for their level. The B cell lymphomas and their abbreviations are described in Chapter 22.5.3.

Table 5 *T-lymphocyte differentiation antigens*

Antigen	Synonym	M_r (kDa)	Distribution	Function
CD1	T6	47+12	Cortical thymocytes Langerhans cells	?Antigen presentation
CD2	T11, E-rec	50	T cells	Activation, adhesion Ligand LFA-3(CD58)
CD3/Ti	T3/TCR	26,21 19,30	T cells	Antigen receptor plus signalling (CD3)
CD4	T4	55	Th cells	Binds HLA class II HIV receptor
CD5	T1,Leu-1	60	T cells, B subset	Activation, ligand CD72
CD6	T12	120	T cells	Signalling
CD7		40	Pre-T and T cells	
CD8	T8, Lyt-2	33	CTL	Binds HLA class I
CD11a/18	LFA-1	180–95	All leucocytes	Adhesion, essential for T cell and leucocyte functions Ligands: ICAM-1, -2, -3.
CD25	IL-2R	35	Activated T cells	α-chain of IL-2 receptor
CD26		110	Activated T cells	Dipeptidyl peptidase IV
CD27		50	T cells	?activation,(nerve-growth factor receptor family)
CD28		44	T cells	Priming T cells; ligand B7
CD29		110	T_{mem}, activated leucocytes	Adhesion
CD45	LCA	180–240	All leucocytes	Activation, phosphatase
CD45RA			Virgin T cells	
CD45RO			Memory T cells	Binds CD22
CD40L			T cells	Binds CD40 on B cells

Abbreviations: CTL, cytotoxic T lymphocytes; ICAM, intercellular adhesion molecules; IL, interleukin; LFA, lymphocyte function-associated antigen; TCR, T-cell receptor; T_{mem}, memory T cells. Further concise details of leucocyte differentiation antigens can be found in Barclay *et al.* (1993).

Fig. 7 Expression of T-lymphocyte differentiation antigens on differentiating T cells. The arrows indicate the probable pathway of T-cell development in the thymus and periphery. The CD antigens are described in Table 4 and in the text. Ti is the T-cell receptor. D is HLA class II. Negative selection (deletion of self-reactive T cells) occurs at the double positive (CD4+CD8+) stage and is followed by positive selection as either CD4 or CD8 is selected.

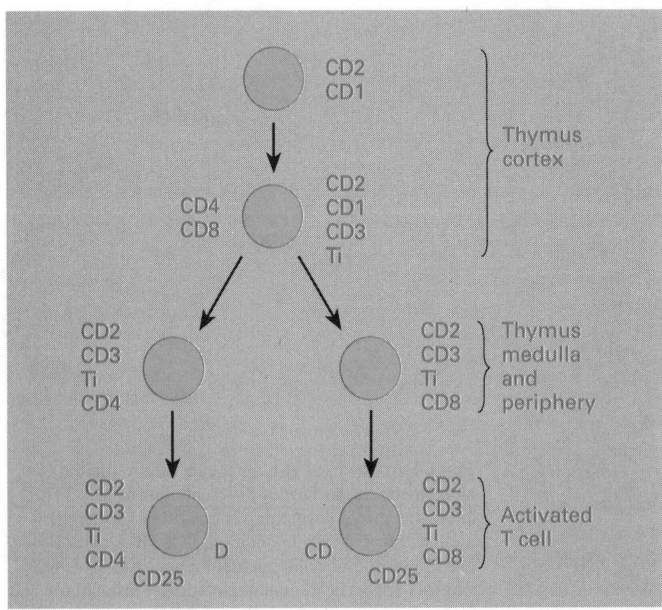

release of the lymphokine IL-2, which binds to the IL-2 receptor on T cells. It is the IL-2 that actively stimulates division.

CD4

Helper T-cell recognition of processed antigen on antigen-presenting cells involves a specific interaction between CD4 and HLA class II molecules. Helper T cells carry the CD4 antigen, a glycoprotein of 55 000 Da. There is evidence for a specific interaction between CD4 and HLA class II. Helper T-cell recognition of antigen can be inhibited by antiCD4 antibodies. Inside the cell, the cytoplasmic region of CD4 is linked to the kinase p56lck, which is important in cell activation. Structural analysis of the CD4 molecule indicates that it is a member of the immunoglobulin superfamily. CD4 is also expressed at low levels on macrophages and some dendritic cells. The surface glycoprotein gp120 of human immunodeficiency virus (**HIV**) bind to CD4, which therefore serves as the receptor for the virus; HIV shows specificity for CD4+ cells.

CD8

This antigen is a glycoprotein of 33 000 Da. This also has a single, external, immunoglobulin-like domain and a transmembrane and cytoplasmic portion. It is heavily glycosylated. It seems to be the counterpart of CD4 for cytotoxic T cells, being involved in recognition of HLA class I antigens. Thus anti-CD8 blocks recognition of target T cells by cytotoxic T cells. CD8 is also associated with p56lck inside the cell.

CD28

This 43 000-Da glycoprotein is found on most T cells. It binds to its ligand B7 (not to be confused with HLA-B7) on antigen-presenting cells and delivers a signal that is essential for the initiation of T-cell responses. Abnormal cells that lack B7 (e.g. tumour cells) may therefore fail to initiate T-cell responses, although they can still be targets for attack by cytotoxic T cells as the CD28–B7 interaction is not required for recognition of targets by mature, effector, cytotoxic T lymphocytes.

CD11a/18

This antigen, also known as leucocyte function-associated antigen 1 (**LFA-1**), is strictly speaking not a T-cell differentiation antigen, being expressed on other leucocytes. However, it is involved non-specifically but vitally in T-cell adherence to antigen-presenting cells without forming part of the receptor complex. The glycoprotein has two chains, one of 180 000 and one 95 000 Da. It is also implicated in the functions of monocytes and granulocytes. Two other glycoproteins, which are receptors for fragments of complement C3 and expressed on monocytes and granulocytes, share the same light chains. There is evidence that two of these molecules are receptors for fragments of the complement component C3. A number of patients who lack these glycoproteins on the surface of their cells have been described. They are immunodeficient and also suffer severely from chronic bacterial infections due to impaired granulocyte function.

CD2

This antigen was known before the advent of monoclonal antibodies because it binds fortuitously to sheep red cells and forms the basis of the E-rosetting method of counting and purifying human T lymphocytes. The antigen has a single chain of 55 000 Da. Functionally, antibody to CD2 has very similar properties to the anti-CD18 reagents, blocking most T-lymphocyte functions; the ligand for CD2 is a molecule called LFA-3 (CD58). CD2 is involved in both adhesion of T cells to targets and activation of T cells.

CD25

This is one of the chains of the IL-2 receptor. IL-2 is a peptide of 25 000 Da that is made by helper T cells and, on binding to the IL-2 receptor CD25, stimulates T-cell division. T-cell proliferation is normally mediated by IL-2. In the rare form of T-cell leukaemia caused by the human T-cell leukaemia/lymphoma virus type 1 there is a high level of CD25 expression and it has been suggested that this contributes to the proliferation.

CD45

This glycoprotein is widely distributed on leucocytes. It has several isoforms generated by differential splicing of small exons within the gene. T lymphocytes can be divided into two populations according to whether they carry the CD45RA or -RO forms. The former are considered to be naïve T cells and the latter memory T cells. The cytoplasmic tail of CD45 is large and is thought to be a phosphatase that is involved in activating p56lck.

CD44

This glycoprotein is also complex, with many isoforms. Its function appears to be as homing receptor for recirculating T cells.

T-CELL SUBPOPULATIONS

Functionally, as outlined above, T lymphocytes can be divided into helper (Th) cells, which carry the CD4 glycoprotein and recognize antigens presented by class II HLA, and cytotoxic (**CTL**) cells which carry CD8 and respond to peptides presented by HLA class I. Th cells may be divisible into two subtypes with different functions, Th1 and Th2, which stimulate T-cell and antibody responses. At one time a third population of suppressor T cells was thought to exist; although this notion still has its advocates, most of the suppressive phenomena can now be explained in terms of cytokine actions or effects on antigen-presenting cells. Suppressor T cells have not been well characterized.

Helper T cells (Th)

Helper T cells are essential for normal activation of B cells and of CTL. They express a clonally restricted receptor (see above), the CD4 antigen, and recognize foreign antigen in association with HLA class II antigens on presenting cells. In response to antigen, Th cells divide and release lymphokines. In mice there are two subpopulations of Th cells, which have different profiles of cytokine release: Th1 cells that secrete IL-2 and interferon-γ and Th2 cells that secrete IL-4, -5, and -10. The former mediate cellular immunity, that is they stimulate CTL and initiate inflammation (delayed-type hypersensitivity). The latter are more involved in activating B cells, giving the second signals that cause them to divide, differentiate, and switch immunoglobulin isotype. These distinctions are not quite so clear in man but it is apparent that T-cell clones grown *in vitro* may secrete differing patterns of cytokines that correspond to these types. What may be important in setting the pattern could be the nature of the antigen studied and the environment in which it is delivered. The balance between the Th1 and Th2 types may be important in many diseases. As IL-4, a Th2 cytokine, drives the immunoglobulin switch towards IgE, it has been argued that atopy represents overactive Th2 cells. Similarly, lepromatous leprosy results from an antibody-mediated and hence Th2 immune response, whereas tuberculoid leprosy is Th1-mediated resulting in stimulation of CTL and activation of macrophages. In HIV infection, it has been argued that a switch from Th1 to Th2 response heralds the onset of AIDS.

One special response of Th cells is the mixed lymphocyte reaction. A relatively high proportion (approximately 1 per cent) of Th cells can respond strongly to a foreign HLA class II antigen without prior sensitization. The latter must be presented by live cells and the mechanism of response is probably similar to the Th response to foreign protein plus self HLA class II. The strength of the T-cell response probably reflects the large variety of peptide antigens that stimulate the response. *In vivo* the reaction probably contributes substantially to graft-versus-host disease.

CYTOTOXIC T LYMPHOCYTES

The effector T cells that mediate cellular immune responses are the CTL and Th cells that secrete cytokines such as interferon-γ and tumor necrosis factor (**TNF**) (Th1 cells). CTL recognize antigen plus class I HLA antigen on presenting cells. In life, these include virus-infected cells and cells infected with intracellular bacteria and parasites (e.g. liver cells infected with the malaria parasite). The majority of CTL are CD8+ and recognize peptides presented by class I MHC, as described above. The CTL response has also been studied in great detail in several virus infections. For instance, in HIV infection CTL appear just before seroconversion and then are present at high levels throughout the asymptomatic phase. Levels decline dramatically when AIDS develops. These observations, experimental findings in the simian model of AIDS, and direct evidence *in vitro* suggest that CTL play a part in controlling HIV infection, although ultimately unsuccessfully. Most CTL are CD8+ and class I MHC restricted, a minor population are CD4+ and class II restricted.

On contact with virus-infected cells, CTL memory or precursor clones with appropriate receptors are activated to divide and differentiate. It takes about 3 days for the cytotoxic property to develop fully. Division is dependent on IL-2, which CTL do not make; this is provided by Th1 cells, which are therefore essential for initiating CTL responses.

On binding antigen at the cell surface, CTL lyse the target cell. The mechanism involves specific molecules released by T cells, such as perforin, which punches holes in the membrane of target cells. CTL can also release lymphokines, particularly interferon and TNF. They are thus potent in their ability to terminate virus infections, killing infected cells before they release infectious particles and, through the effects of γ interferon-γ, inhibiting virus replication, increasing HLA expression on target cells (and hence enhancing T-cell recognition), and activating natural killer cells (see below).

Table 6 *Cytokines important for T-cell function*

Cytokine	M_r (kDa)	Made by:	Receptor on:	Function
IL-1(αβ)	15.5	Monocytes	Type I: T,thy,fib,cho,syn, hep,end,ker Type II: B,mac,mono	T activation, acute-phase reaction, inflammation
IL-2	15–20	Th1	Act-T, (B,mono)	T activation/proliferation
IL-3	14–30	T	BM stem—all lineages	Growth, differentiation
IL-4	15–19	Th2	B,T,BM,fib,epi,end	Switch to IgG1, IgE Macro activation
IL-5	2 × 21.5	Th2	eo,baso	Growth and differentiation
IL-6	21–28	Th2	act-B,PC (epi,fib,hep,neur)	Growth factor, acute-phase IgA selection
IL-7	25	T	Pre-B,thy,T,mono	Activation,proliferation
IL-8			N,baso,T subset, mono,ker	Chemotaxis, activation, adhesion
IL-9	32–39		T	Proliferation
IL-10	19	Th2	T,B,mono	Ig switch, T and B activation
IL-11	23		BM	Haemopoiesis
IL-12	35,40		T,B	IgE selection, T proliferation
IFN-γ	20–24	Th1,CTL	mac,mono,B,fib,epi,endo	Activation, proliferation → HLA I and II Ig2a (mice)
TNF	3 × 17	T	Most cells	Activation, apoptosis

The genes for all of the cytokines listed have been cloned, as have those for their receptors in most cases. The functions are summarized and in most cases are still under intense investigation. Abbreviations: act, activated; B, B cells; BM, bone marrow cells; baso, basophils; cho, chondrocytes; end, endothelial cells; epi, epithelial cells; eo, eosinophils; fib, fibroblast; hep, hepatocyte; ker, keratinocytes; mac, macrophages; mono, monocytes; neur, neuronal cells; PC, plasma cells; T, T cells; thy, thymocytes; TNF, tumour necrosis factor. For further details see Burke *et al.* (1992).

Evidence that CTL clear virus infections has been gained by studies on influenza virus in mice. Congenitally athymic mice are more likely to be killed by influenza virus, and survivors excrete virus chronically; passive, specific antibody does not cure them but injection of specific CTL does. More directly, intravenous injection of virus-specific CTL clones has substantially reduced the amount of virus. There is experimental evidence that this type of immunity is also important in influenza virus, EBV, and cytomegalovirus infections in man. It is also clear that T-cell immunity, and by inference CTL immunity, is vital in many other acute virus infections in man including measles, herpesvirus infections, and smallpox. However, it is also possible that CTL could cause damage under certain circumstances. In lymphocytic choriomeningitis virus infections in mice, encephalitis correlates with the presence of CTL activity in the brain. Similar observations have been made in the rare mumps encephalitis where active CTL have been found in the cerebrospinal fluid of patients. In HIV infection, CTL may contribute to associated neurological diseases.

Graft rejection is the classical cellular immune response. The evidence indicates that both CTL and Th cells are involved, and that activation by HLA class II is essential to induce T-helper cells and thus to activate T cells. This reaction is discussed in detail in Chapter 5.5.

THE ROLE OF THYMUS IN T-CELL FUNCTION

T lymphocytes by definition are thymus derived. Thymectomized or congenitally athymic animals lack mature T cells and T-cell-mediated functions. Athymic (nude) mice and human infants with thymic hypoplasia (Di George syndrome) show no cellular immune responses and impaired antibody responses; B cells, however, can respond by secreting IgM to some polysaccharide antigens in the absence of T cells. Normal thymocytes carry the T-cell differentiation antigens described above and also CD1, which has some similarities to an HLA class I antigen, but is not MHC encoded, and has an unknown function. The T-cell-receptor genes rearrange in early, cortical, thymocytes, with the β-gene reorganizing first.

Immature thymic T cells lack CD4 and CD8 when they start to rearrange their receptor genes. Then, both CD4 and CD8 glycoproteins are expressed together with T-cell receptor. At this stage, negative selection, that is deletion by apoptosis of self-reactive T-cell clones, occurs. Self peptides presented by MHC class I and II molecules on dendritic cells, which may enter the thymus from the periphery, seem responsible for this apoptotic signal. At this stage more than 90 per cent of thymocytes die. This process is followed by a step of positive selection and expression of either CD4 or CD8. Expression of CD4 implies selection by class II MHC and CD8 by class I MHC. If either is lacking, as in CD4- or CD8-gene-inactivated (knock-out) mice, positive selection of class II- or class I-restricted T cells, respectively, is grossly impaired. Thymic epithelial cells are thought to be important in this selective process; it is likely that these cells express MHC molecules containing self peptides that react with low affinity with the T-cell receptors; obviously the interactions at this stage must be different in some way from those that stimulate apoptosis. It is at this last stage that the restriction of the T-cell response to self MHC (plus peptide) is imprinted.

Some T cells may escape to the periphery but are still self reactive. Some of these may be deleted but there is a second mechanism termed anergy. T cells that carry self-reactive receptors are inactivated. It is possible that under some circumstances they could be reactivated and trigger autoimmune reactions.

A third way of preventing autoreactivity is for the self cell to be immunologically inert. This may occur at certain sites that are inaccessible to the immune system, e.g. in the eye. It may also happen on cells that fail to express the costimulatory molecules, such as B7, that are necessary to initiate T-cell responses.

Cytokines (see Chapter 4.2.4)

A number of cytokines have already been referred to, particularly in the context of understanding the fuanction of Th cells and immunoglobulin-class switching. They are small polypeptides, released by immunocytes and other cells, with normally short-range functions on target cells that carry the appropriate receptor. Specificity is therefore conferred by the nature and state of activation of the cell that makes the cytokine and by the cell that bears the receptor. The actual effects of cytokines tend to be pleiomorphic—activating cells, triggering general differentiation, and activation of specific genes (e.g. of the HLA complex genes by interferon-γ). Of particular interest is the control of immunoglobulin isotype switching by cytokines (see Table 6) as well as by the CD40–CD40L interaction. Cytokine activity in terms of T-cell function can be described by the Th1–Th2 division. Although this seems clear in mice, it is more complex in human cells, possibly because the original activation of the T cells *in vivo* is usually not under experimental control and also because the source of cells, peripheral blood lymphocytes in man and spleen cells in mice, is different. Nevertheless, it is probably a useful distinction, implying that the response of Th cells may be set at the time of activation, and with implications for understanding of disease processes. The cytokines relevant to the immune response are listed in Table 6. Because all have been cloned, they are being tried for therapy (e.g. interferon and IL-2), with mixed results. Also, antibodies to cytokines or their receptors are being used (e.g. antiTNF), with some preliminary encouraging results. This area of therapeutic activity is likely to become more active in the near future.

Accessory cells in the immune response

Antigen-presenting cells

Besides T and B lymphocytes, certain accessory cells have crucial roles in immune responses. Antigen-presenting cells are clearly important. B cells and CTL can react with antigen directly or on some specialized cells, respectively, but both require signals from Th cells, which are dependent on specialized presenting cells. The specialized cells are related to monocytes and macrophages but must carry HLA class II antigens and molecules such as B7 that are essential for the initiation of the immune response by binding to CD28 on T cells. A set of cells known as dendritic cells plays a key part. They express large amounts of HLA class II antigens on their surface and are potent activators of Th cells, delivering the necessary other signals. They are found not only in the T-cell areas of lymph nodes (see below) but are also widely distributed in many organs. Here they may be important in activating local immune responses, for example to localized virus infection.

In the B-cell area of lymph nodes, the secondary follicles, there is a network of follicular dendritic cells (see also Section 23). Unlike the dendritic cells referred to above, they are HLA class II negative but display receptors for C3b (of complement) and immunoglobulin Fc. They can therefore capture immune complexes, which are particularly good at initiating primary antibody responses. They are probably able to capture small amounts of antigen percolating through the sinuses of lymphoid organs. They can hold antigen at their surface for long periods, possibly many months or even years.

Adjuvants are chemicals given with antigen that are able to localize antigens at the site of injection, giving a local inflammatory response, activating macrophages and antigen-presenting cells, and thus initiating immune responses more effectively. An example that is clinically important is the potassium alum added to diphtheria and tetanus toxoids. By triggering non-specific inflammatory reaction at the site of injection, adjuvants may direct the type of immune response (e.g. Th1 or -2) as well as enhancing the level.

Mast cells (see Section 23)

In addition to antigen-presenting cells there are other accessory cells at the other end of the immune response, which might be termed enhancers. The best characterized of these is the mast cell which has a receptor for the Fc portion of the ϵ-chain of IgE. When this antibody binds antigen, cross-linking the Fc receptor causes the mast cell to degranulate. This results in the release of histamine, kinins, and leukotrienes, which give the anaphylactic type of allergic reaction. Mast cells also have receptors for some of the peptides released during complement activation.

Natural killer cells

Interferon is a potent activator of natural killer cells. These are large, granular lymphocytes, not classical T or B cells, which lyse cultured tumour cells and virus-infected cells very efficiently *in vitro*. Their role *in vivo* is uncertain but they have been implicated in rejection of histocompatible bone-marrow grafts, tumour immunity, and antivirus immunity. They may thus form a general surveillance system, eliminating tumour cells and virus-infected cells as they arise. Although these effects are non-specific, antigen-specific T cells, by releasing interferon-γ, could activate them to give a vital enhancement of T-cell killing. A large puzzle still remains as to the nature of the receptor on the surface of natural killer cells. They do show some specificity, for instance, lysing MHC class I-negative cells and not class I-positive cells.

Macrophages

Macrophages are derived from monocytes and are long-lived, potently phagocytic cells. Differentiation to macrophages and their activation are a response to local events such as contact with foreign material, lectins, and complement fragment C5a, but are also under the control of immune cells, with immune complexes and interferon-γ (which is released by antigen-specific T cells) being potent activators. Macrophages are larger

Fig. 8 Schematic representation of the structure of a lymph node. The drawing is not to scale but shows the main components. The cell types found in each region are indicated: Bδ, B cells expressing surface IgD; Bμ/γ, B cells expressing surface IgM or surface IgG; FDC, follicular dendritic cells; T, T cells (a few T cells are also found in the germinal centres where B cells may present antigen).

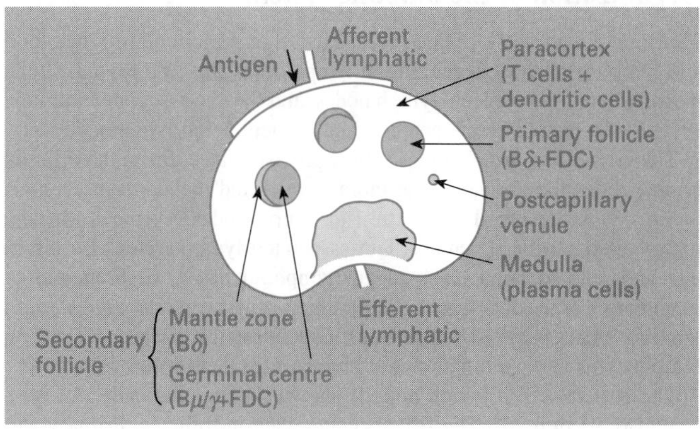

Fig. 9 Lymphocyte recirculation. Antigen enters the lymph node by the afferent lymphatics. Lymphocytes enter the tymph node through the walls of the postcapillary (high endothelial) venules. They leave by the efferent lymphatics, whence they go to the thoracic duct and the superior vena cava.

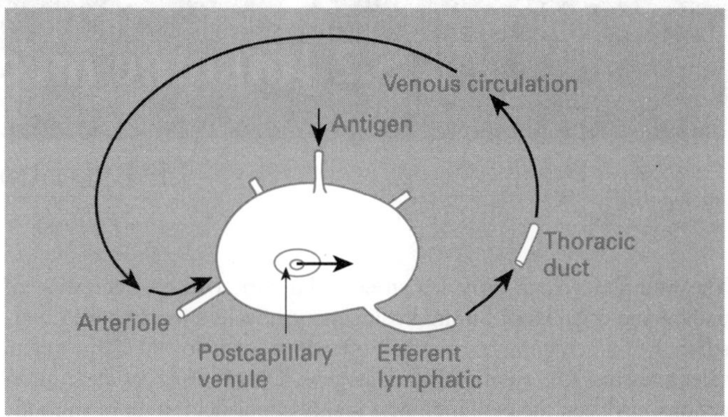

than monocytes and differ in their surface glycoproteins with less HLA class II antigen and increased amounts of receptors for immunoglobulin Fc fragments and complement. Within the cells, lysosomes are increased in number.

The chief function of macrophages, and also granulocytes, is phagocytosis. This is greatly enhanced (several thousandfold) if the foreign material is coated with antibody and/or the complement fragment C3b. Ingested particles are taken into the cell in a phagosome, which fuses to a lysosome. A similar process in granulocytes is associated with a respiratory burst, with sudden uptake of oxygen and generation of superoxide, hydrogen peroxide, hydroxyl radicals and nitric oxide, which are toxic to micro-organisms. This also occurs, but less prominently, in macrophages. Activated macrophages also produce a variety of enzymes that are important in inflammatory processes, including proteases, elastase, collagenase, plasminogen activator, and procoagulants. The last may account for the deposition of fibrin that is responsible for the characteristic induration of delayed-type hypersensitivity reactions.

Macrophages also release monokines and synthesize complement components. The former include IL-1 and TNF (Table 6). The latter may help to amplify the local inflammatory responses. Other bioactive molecules, including prostaglandins and leukotrienes, are also made.

Macrophages are thus highly active cells that are crucially important in converting immune responses into inflammatory reactions. They feature prominently in granuloma formation, in which antigen persists or forms immune complexes. Mycobacteria are thought to inhibit fusion between phagosomes and lysosomes and thus evade the toxic mechanisms. Under these circumstances the macrophages form epithelioid and giant cells in forming the granuloma.

Organization of the immune system

The immunocytes are divided into those that are circulating in blood and lymph, and those localizing in lymphoid organs: the thymus, bone marrow, fetal liver, spleen, lymph nodes, and the gut-associated immune system of tonsils, Peyer's patches, and intraepithelial lymphocytes.

The circulating lymphocytes follow precise routes. From the efferent lymph nodes they travel to the thoracic duct and thence to the venous blood. From the blood they return to lymph nodes or spleen through high-walled capillary venules. Gut-associated lymphocytes also circulate and tend to home back to gut lymphoid tissue, or bronchial or mammary tissue, thus distributing antigen-sensitive cells widely to all possible sites of entry of organisms. Glycoproteins, such as CD44, on lymphocytes and endothelium are important in these routings.

The structure of a lymph node is shown diagrammatically in Fig. 8 (see also Section 23). The B cells congregate in follicles. Primary follicles contain mostly early B cells with IgD on their surface. Activation of B cells by an immune response in a germinal center results in their division and accumulation to generate secondary follicles, which contain mostly IgG-bearing B cells. Scattered through the follicle are helper T cells and follicular dendritic cells. From the follicles, stimulated B cells mature to plasma cells in cords in the medulla where they secrete immunoglobulin.

The majority of T cells in the lymph nodes are in the paracortex surrounding the follicles. The T helper cells and CTL are found there. They are clearly associated with the HLA class II-positive dendritic cells. Antigen enters by the afferent lymphatics and percolates through the lymph nodes, activating immune cells via the antigen-presenting cells.

The spleen is similarly organized in the white pulp that surrounds the end arterioles, whence the cells and antigen enter. Circulating lymphocytes leave by venous sinuses (Fig. 9).

Conclusions

Immune responses are continuously occurring in healthy individuals. The immune system should be thought of as an essential part of the homeostatic mechanism, continually keeping out and destroying invaders and abnormal cells as they appear. At the same time it is regulating its own cells as they develop and circulate. Although the immune system has been described in terms of its individual components, they do not react in isolation. Thus, an infecting virus for instance will evoke an antibody response, activate complement through the classical and alternative pathways, stimulate T-cell immunity involving both regulatory and effector T cells, stimulate lymphokine release, and activate natural killer cells. In the following chapters the consequences of abnormal immune responses are described, both where there is a deficiency in immune reactivity and where for various reasons the immune reaction itself is harmful.

REFERENCES

Alberts, B. *et al.* (1994). *Molecular biology of the cell,* (3rd edn). Garland, New York.

Barclay, A.N. *et al.* (1993). *The leucocyte antigen facts book.* Academic Press, London.

Bjorkman, P.J., Saper, M.A., Samraoui, B., Bennett, W.S., Strominger, J.L., and Wiley, D.C. (1987). Structure of the human class I histocompatability antigen, HLA-A2. *Nature,* **329,** 506–12.

Burke, F., Naylor, S., Davies, B., and Balkwill, F. (1993). The cytokine wall chart. *Immunology Today,* **14,** 147–65–70.

Davis, M.M. and Bjorkman, P.J. (1988.). T-cell receptor genes and T-cell recognition. *Nature,* **334,** 395–402.

Elliott, T., Smith, M., Driscoll, P., and McMichael, A.J. (1993). Peptide selection by class I molecules of the major histocompatibility complex. *Current Biology,* **3,** 854–66.

5.2 Immune mechanisms of disease

J.I. BELL AND R.E. O'HEHIR

The immune system provides an essential barrier to a large range of pathogenic organisms. Strong evolutionary selective forces have diversified the human immune response, often in reaction to equally powerful selective pressures on microbial pathogens. The net effect of these interactions has been the evolution of a highly sophisticated set of immune effector pathways. The development of a complex immunological network has the coincident liability that the defence system may become directed at self rather than foreign antigens. Such immunologically mediated damage accounts for much human pathology, although often the precise mechanism remains obscure.

Although 'autoimmunity' is the term used to describe this process, the evidence that this represents an 'aberrant' immune response has been substantiated in only a few circumstances. The clinical similarity between normal immune responses to a foreign antigen and an autoimmune disease indicates that the lack of a recognizable pathogen is insufficient evidence that these disorders result simply from a loss of tolerance to self antigens. For example, the inflammatory arthritis seen after infection with *Borrelia burgdorferi* (Lyme disease) has considerable similarity to rheumatoid arthritis, commonly considered to be autoimmune in origin. Similarly, there is still some evidence that an immune response to chlamydia may result in reactive arthritis and Reiter's syndrome. The immune-complex diseases of the kidney accompanying subacute bacterial endocarditis have much in common with other forms of less well-understood immune-complex diseases in which the antigens have been poorly defined and which are usually assumed to be autoimmune in origin. It remains possible, therefore, that at least some of the currently recognized autoimmune disorders may eventually emerge as diseases in which infection with an undefined pathogen has led to a normal immune response and its accompanying tissue damage. This possibility has led to a search for a range of fastidious organisms in autoimmune disorders (e.g. *Mycobacteria paratuberculosis* in Crohn's disease, retroviruses in Sjögren's syndrome and multiple sclerosis, or mycoplasma in rheumatoid arthritis).

Immune tolerance

Regardless of the initiating event, the progress of most autoimmune disease relies on inappropriate reactivity of components of the immune response with self antigens, leading to tissue damage. This suggests that the breakdown of discrimination between self and non-self is essential for the progress of all such diseases.

Tolerance is maintained to self antigens in both the T- and B-cell components of the immune system (Table 1). There is now substantial evidence for the central deletion of T cells recognizing self antigens during their 'education' in the thymus. This is likely to be true for T cells recognizing ubiquitous cellular antigens and for antigens present in high concentrations in serum, which also have access to the thymic environment. Other mechanisms of tolerance must also exist, however, to account for the normal lack of responsiveness to a large range of antigens present exclusively in peripheral organs. The explanation for this lack of responsiveness may lie simply in the fact that many peripheral antigens are seldom exposed to the immune system (e.g. antigens on the cornea and sperm), and are present in insufficiently high concentrations to provoke an immune response. Inaccessibility may also be relevant to the tolerance that is present with tissue-specific antigens that can be immune targets in the course of organ-specific autoimmune diseases such as type I diabetes and thyroid disease.

Other mechanisms of T-cell peripheral tolerance have been suggested by experimental work. These include anergy (the presence of reactive T cells that have lost their ability to expand and respond to antigen), peripheral deletion, and suppression. Evidence for anergy has been supported by the observation that if T cells are stimulated through the T-cell receptor without a second signal provided by surface molecules such as CD28 or CTLA-4, these cells will be unable to respond normally to antigen. Convincing evidence for mechanisms of T-cell peripheral deletion and suppression has been more difficult to generate and there is no evidence that any one mechanism predominates *in vivo*.

B-cell tolerance may result from a combination of anergy and deletion. It is now clear that B cells which carry antibodies specific for soluble self antigens may exist *in vivo* but are anergic and are unable to differentiate beyond IgD-positive cells, and hence are not capable of producing self-reacting antibodies. Deletional mechanisms may also account for B-cell tolerance in some circumstances. In some species it appears that extensive deletion of the B-cell repertoire occurs in the gut-associated lymphoid tissue. This form of deletion does not appear to be important in mouse or man; however, there is firm evidence for other peripheral deletional mechanisms that eliminate B cells carrying immunoglobulin specific for cell-surface antigens.

Table 1 *Mechanisms by which immune tolerance is maintained to self antigens*

Hidden antigens
Clonal deletion:
T cells
B cells
Clonal anergy:
T cells
B cells
Active suppression

Table 2 *Sequences shared between human proteins and bacterial or viral pathogens*

Protein	Sequence
Human cytomegalovirus IE2	PDPLGRPDED
HLA-DR molecule	VTELGRPDAE
Papillomavirus E2	SLHLESLKDS
Insulin receptor	VYGLESLKDL
Rabiesvirus glycoprotein	TKESLVIIS
Insulin receptor	NKESLVISE
Klebsiella pneumoniae nitrogenase	SRQTDREDE
HLA-B27 molecule	KAQTDREDL
Adenovirus 12 E1B	LRRGMFRPSQCN
α-Gliadin	LGQGSFRPSQQN
Human immunodeficiency virus P24	GVETTTPS
Human IgG constant region	GVETTTPS

After Oldstone (1987). *Cell,* **50,** 819.

Breaking tolerance in autoimmunity

Clearer understanding of T- and B-cell tolerance has provided insights into methods by which tolerance might be overcome to produce autoimmune disease. The explanations most commonly suggested include (a) cross-reacting epitopes, (b) loss of active suppression, (c) release of 'hidden' antigens, (d) generation of modified antigen, (e) T-cell 'bypass', and (f) superantigen stimulation of T-cell populations.

Cross-reacting epitopes

The observation that T cells are activated by the recognition of short peptides in the context of HLA molecules has led to the suggestion that human proteins having sequence homology with proteins of infectious pathogens might be the targets of an autoimmune response after an episode of infection. Heat-shock proteins form one such family of proteins that is highly conserved between prokaryotes and higher eukaryotes. Immune responses to heat-shock proteins have been implicated in experimental diabetes and arthritis. A range of other bacterial and viral proteins with weak homologies to human proteins has been identified (Table 2). For example, sequences in *Klebsiella pneumoniae* are shared with HLA-B27, and a cytomegalovirus-IE2 protein sequence has homology to HLA-DQw3. An adenovirus-12 peptide is homologous to a sequence in α-gliadin and might have a role in coeliac disease. These sequence similarities are usually not extensive and none has been shown to be the restricted peptide recognized by T cells. Serological cross-reactivity has been demonstrated but its significance is uncertain. The importance of some pathogens in activating some autoimmune states does suggest that cross-reactivity may be involved, however. For example, the association of hepatitis B infection with polyarteritis nodosa or of chlamydia, shigella, and salmonella infections with reactive arthritis or ankylosing spondylitis suggest a role for cross-reacting epitopes in the pathogenesis of these autoimmune disorders.

Loss of active suppression

Active suppression has long been thought to have a controlling influence on the immune response, and defects in this regulatory process could be important in diseases such as type I diabetes. However, clear identification of the cell population responsible or definition of the biochemical nature of the 'factors' involved have proved impossible.

Release of hidden antigens

Tissue damage may result in the exposure of the immune system to a range of antigens normally not visible to T cells. Given an appropriate genetic background, this can lead to an immunological response to tissue-specific antigens. The initial damage may be secondary to infection or may be induced by other mechanisms of cell death. Dressler's syndrome, which develops after episodes of myocardial ischaemia, may represent such a phenomenon. It is accompanied by an elevated erythrocyte sedimentation rate, fever, and evidence of an immune response to cardiac and pericardial tissues. Similarly, the wide range of antibody responses to B-cell-specific antigens during the course of type I diabetes may represent an immune response to otherwise hidden antigens.

Generation of modified antigens

Peptide epitopes may be modified so that novel structures are recognized by T cells that have not been previously rendered tolerant. Such modification might include novel patterns of glycosylation, or might result from somatic mutations in coding regions. In theory, somatic mutation in immunoglobin loci is likely to produce a large range of antigens to which the immune system is intolerant. Similarly, frameshift somatic mutations at other loci may produce new T-cell epitopes, leading to autoreactivity. Although hypothetically possible, there is no direct evidence that this process leads to an autoimmune response.

T-cell bypass

Although self-reactive B cells require both immunoglobulin molecules specific for self antigen and help from T cells, there are several mechanisms through which B cells can be activated by a foreign antigen associated with a self antigen. The ability of a low-affinity immunoglobulin molecule to acquire a higher affinity through somatic mutation makes it possible for even low-affinity B cells eventually to result in an autoimmune response. An example of this might be the association between viral proteins to DNA and DNA-binding proteins, which would permit B cells capable of recognizing self proteins (i.e. histones or other nuclear proteins) to receive help from T cells activated against the associated viral protein.

This mechanism could account for the observation that many of the known autoreactive humoral responses are to proteins associated with DNA in the nucleus (e.g. anti-DNA antibodies, antiribonuclear antibodies, anticentromere antibodies), or with cell-surface receptors (acetylcholine receptor, thyroid-stimulating hormone receptor) that may associate with viral particles to allow them to enter cells. Such associations may provide an important mechanism for bypassing normal tolerance mechanisms.

Superantigen-induced autoreactivity

Superantigens have the capacity to expand individual T-cell subsets defined by Vβ sequences that are bound via superantigens to major histocompatibility complex (**MHC**) class II proteins. This process is mediated by a range of proteins, usually bacterial exotoxins, and it might provide an explanation for the variations in expression of particular Vβ elements that may be seen in autoimmune diseases such as rheumatoid arthritis. Streptococcal exotoxins are superantigens, giving rise to speculation about their role in the pathogenesis of rheumatic fever; staphylococcal exotoxins have been implicated in Kawasaki disease.

Effector mechanisms in autoimmunity

The conventional description of effector mechanisms in immune-mediated disease was based on four types of hypersensitivity (Table 3). Type I hypersensitivity referred to IgE-mediated disease, type II to antibody-mediated disease, type III to immune complex-mediated disease, and type IV was associated with delayed-type hypersensitivity. Although helpful, this classification has been superseded by a clearer understanding of the cellular and biochemical components of the immune response. The different forms of effector mechanisms can, therefore, be discussed in the context of specific immune-mediated diseases or syndromes.

Table 3 *Hypersensitivity reactions*

Reaction type	Mediation	Typical reactions
Type I Immediate	IgE mediated	Anaphylaxis Asthma Atopy
Type II Cytotoxic	IgG mediated	Autoimmune Autoimmune haemolytic anaemia Goodpasture's syndrome Pemphigus vulgaris Transfusion reactions
Type III	Immune complex mediated	Extrinsic allergic alveolitis Serum sickness Glomerulonephritis
Type IV Delayed type	Cell mediated	Contact sensitivity

IgE-mediated immunological diseases

Introduction

In 20 to 30 per cent of the population, exposure to common environmental allergens may result in potentially pathogenic inflammatory responses, which are characterized by the production of specific IgE antibodies and the activation of most cells and polymorphonuclear leucocytes. The term 'allergy' is used to describe these exaggerated responses to external substances, which are regulated by the interaction between heterogeneous cell populations and their soluble products. It is important that specific IgE production has a protective role in response to helminthic infestation and occurs in individuals with a healthy cellular immune system.

Allergens are antigens that trigger IgE-mediated allergic responses, either when in their native form or as haptens. The ability to synthesize specific IgE to common environmental allergens such as house-dust mite, grass, tree or weed pollen, animal proteins, or fungi defines the atopic state. However, not all atopic individuals suffer from allergic disease and only approximately 25 to 50 per cent develop one or more of the principal allergic diseases, with symptoms ranging from allergic rhinitis and extrinsic asthma to atopic dermatitis. In general, the immune mechanisms of allergic diseases are IgE mediated or anaphylactic, but in a minority of cases these may be anaphylactoid or non-IgE mediated.

A primary event in the induction of all allergic inflammatory immune responses is the activation of CD4+ T lymphocytes, which follows the recognition by T-cell antigen receptors (**TCR**) of complexes formed between specific peptide fragments of allergens and HLA class II molecules. Both the production of allergen-specific IgE by B cells and the differentiation and expansion of the non-specific polymorphonuclear granulocytes, including mast cells, eosinophils and basophils, requires CD4+ T-cell-derived cytokines. This emphasizes the central part played by CD4+ T lymphocytes in the pathogenesis of allergic diseases (Fig. 1).

Antigen-specific mechanisms of allergic inflammation

CD4+ T LYMPHOCYTES

CD4+ T cells initiate and regulate the specific and the non-specific effector mechanisms of allergic immune responses. Following their activation by antigen-presenting cells bearing antigenic complexes of allergen-derived peptides and MHC class II molecules, selected antigen-specific clones of T cells expand and synthesize cytokines, some of which promote isotype switching to IgE production by B cells. Allergen-specific IgE is the principal effector molecule of allergic diseases. Other cytokines promote non-specific effector mechanisms, including chemotactic activity, that contribute to the overall allergic inflammatory response.

Knowledge of physicochemical properties and molecular sequences in a variety of allergens has made it possible to define regions (T-cell epitopes) within allergens that are critical for T-cell activation. The route of allergen contact may affect the outcome of allergen exposure, for different antigen-presenting cells are important in different sites. The T-cell 'help' induced by allergens in atopic subjects is an 'IL-4 dominant' response analogous to the biological activity exhibited by murine T-helper type 2 (**Th2**) cells. Interleukin 4 (**IL-4**) promotes IgE production. However, why T cells from non-atopic individuals fail to secrete IL-4, and subsequently to support IgE synthesis after stimulation by allergens, remains unclear. Differences at the level of antigen presentation, TCR gene-product usage, and a genetic predisposition to allergy may all contribute.

Murine CD4+ T-cell populations are clearly distinguishable by their cytokine profile. T helper 1 (**Th1**) cells produce IL-2 and interferon (IFN)-γ, but no IL-4 or IL-5, while, in contrast, Th2 cells produce IL-4 and IL-5 but no IFN-γ or IL-2 after activation. Both populations secrete IL-3, tumour necrosis factor (**TNF**)-α, and granulocyte–macrophage-colony-stimulating factor (**GM-CSF**). Delayed-type hypersensitivity is primarily mediated by Th1 cells; Th2 cells provide better help for antibody production by B cells. A third T-helper subset, designated Th0, produces an array of cytokines including the classical Th1 and Th2 forms. Th1 and Th2 populations have cross-regulatory effects, with IFN-γ produced by Th1 cells down-regulating the proliferation and function of Th2 cells. In contrast, murine IL-10, which is produced by Th2 cells, inhibits proliferation and cytokine production by Th1 cells. In man, however, IL-10 is produced by Th0, Th1-like, and Th2-like cells, and the different populations of T-helper cells are less clearly demarcated.

Fig. 1 Type 1 allergic reactions are initiated by antigen being presented to CD4 T cells by antigen-presenting cells. These T cells produce cytokines, including IL4, that stimulate B cells to produce IgE. IgE is then bound and cross-linked to high-affinity Fc receptors on the surface of mast cells, which degranulate and release a variety of mediators leading to vascular smooth-muscle reactivity, bronchoconstriction, endothelial leakage, and recruitment of other inflammatory cells.

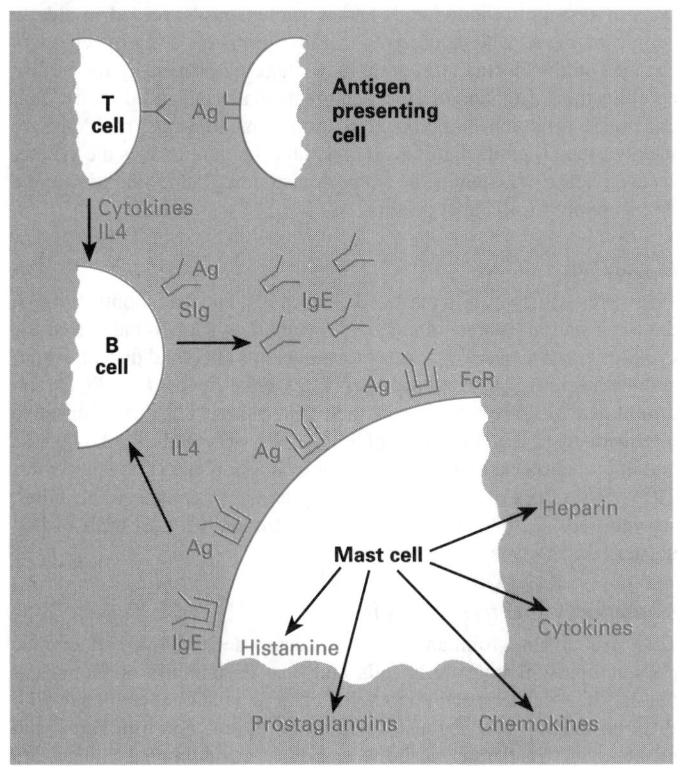

B CELLS AND IMMUNOGLOBULINS IN ALLERGY

As well as differentiating into plasma cells that secrete specific IgE, B lymphocytes may also function as antigen-presenting cells. Interactions between B and T cells, the production of IL-4 in allergic individuals, and the B-cell surface molecules CD23 (the low-affinity IgE receptor) and CD40 are important for allergen-specific IgE production. In non-atopic individuals, IgE is the least abundant of the immunoglobulins, with serum levels of 0.1 to 0.4 mg/l, but its synthesis may be markedly increased in sensitized allergic individuals or in those with helminthic infections. Particularly high levels of IgE are found in the serum of patients with atopic dermatitis. The presence of high levels of allergen-specific IgE, together with the clinical history, contribute to the diagnosis of allergic diseases, which may be demonstrated by skin-prick testing in the clinic or by measurement of specific IgE antibody in serum in the laboratory.

CYTOKINES REGULATING IgE SYNTHESIS AND ALLERGIC INFLAMMATION

Cytokines influence all phases of allergic inflammatory responses including specific IgE production, early mediator release, and late-phase responses. IL-4 is required for IgE synthesis by antigen-primed B cells. Ongoing IgE synthesis may also be enhanced by IL-5, which increases the IL-4-dependent production of IgE, and by IL-6, which indirectly up-regulates the production of immunoglobulin in an isotype-non-specific manner. Other cytokines, such as IFN-γ, down-regulate IgE synthesis.

T-cell-derived cytokines influence the immediate allergic response by their action on non-specific effector cells. GM-CSF and IL-3, -4, and -9 promote the differentiation and expansion of mast cells, whereas IFN-γ inhibits their growth. Another functional group of cytokines, the histamine-releasing factors, was first identified in monocytes. They prime mast cells and basophils for the release of histamine. It now appears that mast cells and eosinophils themselves may synthesize cytokines, including IL-3, -4, -5, -6, and GM-CSF.

The role of T-cell-derived cytokines in the delayed phase of the allergic response is less clear, however. The recently identified T-cell-derived proinflammatory cytokine RANTES, which is a member of the family of SIS cytokines, is chemotactic for eosinophils and appears to be more potent than either IL-5 or TNF-α. Therefore, T-cell cytokines are clearly capable of recruiting inflammatory cells to sites of allergic responses. Other T-cell-derived cytokines, including IL-8, have direct neutrophil chemotactic effects.

CD8+ CYTOTOXIC T LYMPHOCYTES

The role of CD8+ T lymphocytes in atopy and allergic diseases remains controversial. It has been suggested that the failure of non-atopic individuals to synthesize IgE after exposure to allergens is due to specific suppressor T-cell activity. The molecular characterization of this functional subset of T cells has been slow and evidence to support this hypothesis is still lacking. There is increasing interest in CD8+ T cells that appear to have a regulatory role through the profile of cytokines they secrete, including IFN-γ and transforming growth factor-β.

ALLERGENS

Over the last few years, DNA technology and refined biochemical techniques have allowed considerable advances in the isolation and characterization of important allergens. Sequence data have enabled the mapping of B- and T-cell epitopes. Interestingly, an increasing number of major and minor allergens, as defined by specific IgE levels in patients' serum, have been found to have enzyme activity, which may contribute to their ability to penetrate mucosal surfaces and so become accessible to elicit an immune response. For example, of the major house-dust mite allergens, the group I antigens are cysteine proteases, the group II antigens are lysozymes, the group III antigens are serine proteases, and group IV antigens are amylases.

Allergen preparations are used for diagnosis and have also been used as immunotherapy, in which increasing doses are given to the patient subcutaneously in order to induce specific unresponsiveness. The lack of purity and standardization of the extracts has resulted in variable efficacy and unacceptable complications of anaphylactic reactions or even death. This has caused a marked decline in the use of this therapeutic approach in Britain. Now, emphasis is being placed on the quality control of extracts, and the mapping of T-cell epitopes has promoted interest in the potential of peptide vaccines for immunotherapy. The advantage of such a strategy is that using immunodominant peptides or bioengineered proteins, which do not contain B-cell epitopes, should minimize the possibility of allergic reaction. Alternative routes and vectors for allergen administration are also being investigated.

GENETIC BASIS OF ATOPIC DISEASE

The quantity, quality, and route of exposure may determine allergenicity and a genetic predisposition to allergy has been identified in some cases. For example, responsiveness to allergens of *Lolium perenne* (rye grass) is associated with the HLA-DR3 haplotype of the MHC located on the short arm of chromosome 6, while certain ragweed allergens, *Amb a* V and *Amb a* VI, are recognized in association with HLA-DR2,Dw2 and HLA-DR11 haplotypes, respectively. It is now appreciated that allergen-reactive T cells are detectable in primary *in vitro* stimulation in both atopic and non-atopic subjects, but the functional activity of these cells is qualitatively different, those from atopic individuals in general being of 'IL-4 dominant' phenotype.

Population analysis of the inheritance of allergic diseases argues against sole regulation by gene products encoded by the HLA gene complex. It has been known for sometime that allergic diseases tend to have a familial disposition. Perhaps the antigenic complexity of the common environmental allergens has been responsible for the difficulty in identifying a clear mendelian pattern of inheritance. Recently, however, lineage studies of large families have suggested autosomal dominant inheritance. Rather than focusing only on atopic individuals, initial studies looked for associations with one or more criteria: high total serum IgE, positive skin-prick tests to allergens, or clinical allergic diseases. Linkage data suggested the presence of an atopy gene on the long arm of chromosome 11 (11q), and this has recently been shown to result from mutations in the high-affinity receptor for IgE that codes to this region. This suggests that non-MHC-linked genes may determine the overall predisposition to allergic diseases whilst MHC gene products control the specificity of the allergic response. Current work seeks to identify putative atopy genes, but the promise of specific gene therapy against allergic diseases remains a goal for the future.

Antigen non-specific, immediate-hypersensitivity mechanisms

MAST CELLS AND BASOPHILS

The tissue mast cell and the circulating basophil are the important effector cells causing immediate-hypersensitivity responses. Although their biological function is not fully identified, both cell types originate from bone marrow precursors and share the features of abundant cytoplasmic granules and high-affinity IgE surface receptors. Human tissue mast cells are mostly found in the lungs, skin, and gastrointestinal mucosa, which are the main foci of immediate-hypersensitivity reactions. IL-3, which is derived from T cells, is required for the growth, differentiation, and survival of mast cells and basophils. In contrast, T-cell-derived GM-CSF is antagonistic and inhibits mast-cell differentiation. Fibroblast-derived factors are also required for mast-cell maturation.

Two phenotypically distinct subsets of mast cell have been identified: the connective tissue mast cell, containing tryptase, chymase, carboxypeptidase and heparin, is particularly abundant in the intestinal submucosa and the skin; the mucosal mast cell, which particularly secretes tryptase and chondroitin sulphate, is more common in the lung and intestinal lamina propria. Basophils, which are mainly found as circulating leucocytes, contain mainly chondroitin sulphate proteoglycans.

Cross-linking of cell-bound IgE by allergen triggers the cells. Intracellular signals mediated by increased levels of intracellular calcium with activation of protein kinase C lead to phosphorylation of a granule-membrane protein. Preformed mediators, including histamine, are released from cells by degranulation. Activation also induces the synthesis of membrane phospholipid mediators, including the eicosanoids or arachidonic acid metabolites (particularly prostaglandin D_2, leukotriene C_4, and platelet-activating factor. Mast cells may themselves synthesize small amounts of cytokines (including IL-3, -4, -5, -6, and TNF-α), suggesting the possibility of autocrine regulation.

MEDIATORS OF ALLERGIC DISEASE (TABLE 4)

Histamine

This is the main mediator of immediate hypersensitivity synthesized by mast cells and basophils. Three specific histamine receptors are now recognized. H_1 mediates hypersecretion of mucus, pruritus, contraction of non-vascular smooth muscle (uterus, bronchi, and small intestine), and relaxation of vascular smooth muscle. The new non-sedating H_1-antihistamine drugs, terfenadine, astemizole, loratidine, and cetirizine for example, are important for controlling manifestations of allergic disease. High-dose terfenadine infrequently induces ventricular arrhythmias in susceptible individuals and is perhaps best avoided in elderly people or those with underlying cardiac problems. Non-specific QT changes on the electrocardiogram may suggest a propensity for cardiac complications. Ligation of H_2-receptors mediates enhanced gastric acid and mucus secretion, and bronchodilation. Cimetidine and ranitidine are widely used H_2-antihistamines. H_3-receptor ligation induces the synthesis and release of histamine and neurotransmitters, but H_3-antihistaminic drugs are not available at present.

Eicosanoids

These are synthesized by mast cells, basophils, and eosinophils through the oxygenation of arachidonic acid metabolites via two pathways; the cyclo-oxygenase pathway forms prostaglandins (**PG**) and thromboxanes and the 5-lipoxygenase pathway generates leukotrienes (**LT**). PGD_2 and thromboxane A_2 are bronchoconstrictors in asthma. LTA_4 is an unstable intermediate in the formation of LTB_4, -C_4, -D_4, and -E_4. LTB_4 is a potent bronchoconstrictor and is chemotactic for phagocytic leucocytes. The leukotrienes induce increased systemic vascular permeability, smooth-muscle contraction, and mucus secretion. Clinical trials of leukotriene antagonists are under way.

Platelet-activating factor (PAF)

This is a potent proinflammatory molecule derived from membrane phospholipids in lung mast cells and also eosinophils, mononuclear phagocytes, platelets, and endothelial cells. Inhalational challenge with PAF promotes bronchoconstriction even in the non-asthmatic, and increases in vascular permeability and release of pulmonary mucus are

Table 4 *Mediators of allergic reactions*

Mediator	Cell source	Target tissue
Histamine	Mast cells, basophils	Vascular smooth muscle (relaxation) Non-vascular smooth muscle (contraction)
Eicosanoids		
Prostaglandins	Platelets	Vascular smooth muscle Bronchial smooth muscle
Leukotrienes	Basophils, eosinophils Macrophages	Vascular smooth muscle, mucous glands
Thromboxanes	Neutrophils, mast cells Basophils, eosinophils	Vascular and non-vascular smooth muscle
Platelet-Activating Factor	Basophils, eosinophils Platelets, endothelium Macrophages	Bronchi Vascular smooth muscle
Heparin	Mast cells	Platelets
Chemokines	Macrophages, lymphocytes Mast cells	Chemoattraction
Kallikrein	Basophil	Vascular smooth muscle
Hagemann factor	Basophil	Vascular smooth muscle

also induced. PAF is a strong chemoattractant for eosinophils and neutrophils, thereby supplementing the inflammatory cell infiltration following IgE-triggered mast-cell degranulation. Receptor antagonists are currently under development.

EOSINOPHILS

Blood and tissue eosinophilia are features of allergic inflammation and helminthic infestation. Morphologically, the bone marrow-derived eosinophils have prominent cytoplasmic granules that stain red with eosin and a characteristic electron-dense crystalline core on electron microscopy. IL-3, IL-5, and GM-CSF, which are predominantly derived from T cells, are critical for eosinophil differentiation, growth, and maturation. Eosinophils usually comprise less than 3 per cent of the circulating granulocyte population and have a brief circulatory phase, being a hundredfold more abundant in the tissues. The site of tissue retention is determined by chemotactic factors including histamine, leukotrienes (especially LTB_4), PAF, and the complement component C5a. The activation of eosinophils by engagement of their low-affinity IgE receptors induces the generation of lipid mediators (LTC_4) and PAF, together with granule exocytosis of the highly cationic proteins: major basic protein, eosinophil cationic protein, eosinophil-derived neurotoxin, and the enzyme eosinophil peroxidase. The eosinophil cationic proteins have been causally implicated in the denudation of the bronchial epithelium in asthma and in injury to pneumocytes, cardiac cells, and neural cells. Pathognomonic Charcot–Leyden crystals, the crystallized membrane-associated eosinophil enzyme lysophospholipase, may be found in asthmatic sputum or in the stool of patients with parasitic infestation. IL-5 is important for the enhancement of eosinophil degranulation, antibody-dependent cytotoxicity, adherence, and superoxide generation.

NEUTROPHILS

Neutrophils seem to have a minor role in the pathogenesis of allergic disease. They are non-specifically recruited to the site of inflammation by ligation of specific neutrophil receptors. Certain bacterial products, C5a, products of arachidonate metabolism, particularly LTB_4 and IL-8, which are secreted by T cells and monocytes, are all neutrophil chemotaxins. Activated neutrophils then produce superoxide radicals and eicosanoids, including LTB_4, which is itself a potent bronchoconstrictor. Neutrophil-derived LTB_4 is a possible trigger for the amplification of exercise-induced asthma.

MONOCYTES AND MACROPHAGES

Mononuclear phagocytes may also contribute to the non-specific inflammation of allergic diseases. They may be activated by allergen binding to low-affinity IgE surface receptors expressed on up to 20 per cent of peripheral blood mononuclear cells and lung macrophages in atopic asthmatic subjects. Stimulated monocytes and macrophages then produce a variety of proinflammatory mediators and cytokines including lysosomal enzymes, superoxide anions, lipid mediators (LTB_4, LTC_4, PAF, and thromboxane A_2) and the cytokines GM-CSF, TNF-α, IL-1, -6, and -8, which may be important for cellular priming and perpetuating the chronic inflammatory response.

Allergic diseases

ANAPHYLAXIS

Anaphylaxis, which results from the rapid degranulation of mast cells and basophils, constitutes a medical emergency that can result in cardiovascular collapse and death. IgE-triggered reactions (anaphylactic) may result from exposure to certain antibiotics (commonly penicillin or other β-lactam drugs), insect stings (especially bees, wasps, fire ants, hornets), food allergens (shellfish, nuts), and drugs (including immunoglobulins, blood products, and anaesthetic agents). IgE-mediated reactions (anaphylactoid) may be triggered by acute complement activation, resulting in the induction of the anaphylatoxins C3a and C5a, and also C4a to a lesser extent, after the ingestion of aspirin or non-steroidal anti-inflammatory drugs, or the injection of radiocontrast media, metabisulphites, or opiates. When no trigger factors can be identified a diagnosis of idiopathic anaphylaxis may be made.

Clinical manifestations range through flushing, urticaria, angioedema, laryngeal oedema, sneezing, rhinorrhoea, bronchoconstriction, abdominal pains, nausea, vomiting, diarrhoea, pruritus, metallic taste, burning and itching of the perineum, tachycardia, arrhythmias, hypotension, myocardial or cerebral infarction to cardiac or respiratory arrest. Rapid diagnosis should be followed by removal of the inciting agent where possible and prompt therapy with subcutaneous or intramuscular adren-

Table 5 *Management of anaphylaxis*

Age (years)	Volume of adrenaline 1 in 1000 (1 mg/ml)
Under 1	0.05 ml
1	0.1 ml
2	0.2 ml[a]
3–4	0.3 ml[a]
5	0.4 ml[a]
6–12	0.5 ml[a]
Adult	0.5–1 ml

[a]Suitable for robust children in these age groups: for underweight children use half these doses (British National Formulary, 1994).

1. Administer **adrenaline** by intramuscular injection
   Repeat every 15 min until blood pressure stable
2. **Antihistamines**—(e.g. chlorpheniramine maleate 10–20 mg by slow intravenous injection over 1 min)
   Maintain antihistamine cover for 24–48 h.
3. **Corticosteroids** are helpful in preventing late deterioration in severely affected individuals
4. Persistent symptoms may require intravenous fluids, aminophylline, salbutamol

aline (1:1000; 0.5 ml) for prompt vasoconstriction and bronchodilatation. If complete cardiovascular shock has occurred, intravenous adrenaline may be given (1:10 000 dilution at a SLOW rate of 1 ml/min). Repeated doses at 15-min intervals may be required for intractable or rebound anaphylaxis. H_1-antihistamines and corticosteroids should then be given, with airway and cardiovascular support as required (oxygen, intravenous fluid, and even vasopressor agents as necessary). Patients should be observed for a minimum of 24 h. The management of anaphylaxis is outlined in Table 5. Important differential diagnoses include vasovagal reaction, diabetic hypoglycaemic episode, seizures, cerebrovascular accidents, arrhythmias, and pulmonary embolus. Prompt diagnosis and intervention are essential.

Radiocontrast reactions occur in up to 1:40 000 injections and prophylaxis may be instituted in those patients with a history of adverse reaction. Premedication should be given with corticosteroids and H_1-antihistamines (prednisolone, 60 mg, 6-hourly for three doses before the procedure with an H_1-antihistamine at the time of the last prednisolone tablet 30 min before the radiocontrast injection). Wherever possible the trigger should be identified to facilitate avoidance of subsequent episodes. This prophylactic regimen may also be useful in avoiding recurrent adverse allergic reactions to some blood products such as immunoglobulin. Laboratory diagnosis may be helpful in identifying specific IgE against drugs, certain foods or insect venoms. Patients who are prone to anaphylactic reactions should avoid aspirin, non-steroidal anti-inflammatory drugs or β-blocking medications, which may precipitate mast cell or basophil degranulation. Prepacked adrenaline syringes and metered-dose adrenaline inhalers should be carried by patients at high risk of life-threatening recurrences, but it is essential that thorough instruction be given in the use of these first-aid preparations. Risks associated with insect venom allergy may be decreased by allergen desensitization injections.

ALLERGIC RHINITIS

Allergic rhinitis affects approximately 10 per cent of the population and may be seasonal or perennial. The condition is usually accompanied by conjunctivitis and is characterized by sneezing, nasal congestion interspersed with profuse watery rhinorrhoea, pharyngeal and conjunctival pruritus, and lacrimation. Inspection of the nasal passages usually reveals a pale mucosa with swollen turbinates and the conjunctiva is often reddened and oedematous. Clinical manifestations, which are due to IgE-mediated degranulation of mast cells and basophils, often present before the fourth decade and decrease gradually with ageing. Grass, tree, and weed pollens are usually responsible for seasonal rhinitis and may be predicted by pollination calendars, although published pollen counts usually follow the event. In Britain, tree pollens peak from March to May, grass pollens follow in June and July, and weed pollens peak in late July and early August. House-dust mite antigens and animal salivary protein allergens are associated with perennial symptoms. Allergenic particles of 10 to 100 μm in diameter are particularly prone to nasal trapping. Not uncommonly, atopic individuals may suffer from perennial symptoms with seasonal exacerbations due to multiple allergies. In severe cases, swelling may be sufficient to obstruct the sinus ostia and eustachian tubes, resulting in secondary bacterial infection with associated purulent nasal discharges. Nasal polyps may accompany the mucosal oedema of, in particular, perennial rhinitis and so increase the nasal blockage. They are semitransparent mucosal sacs of grape-like appearance that contain oedema fluid, mast cells, and eosinophils. Nasal polyps challenged with specific allergen are able to release histamine, leucotrienes, and peptides chemotactic for eosinophils. Vasomotor or non-allergic rhinitis has many of the clinical symptoms of perennial allergic rhinitis but occurs in non-atopic individuals. Nasal polyposis and eosinophilia may also accompany this non-allergic condition.

A diagnosis of allergic rhinitis requires a convincing clinical history and examination, evidence of specific IgE by skin-prick testing or the presence of specific serum IgE in laboratory assays, and is usually accompanied by a positive family history of allergic diseases.

Skin-prick testing

Skin-prick testing was described in the 1860s when Charles Blackley, while investigating summer catarrh, scarified skin on his forearm and applied moist pollen to elicit an immediate weal and a late cutaneous reaction. Sites for allergen testing on the volar aspect of the forearm are marked with points and labelled. A saline (negative control) is placed at the antecubital region and histamine hydrochloride (as a positive control) is placed at the wrist. A drop of allergen extract is placed on the skin at each marked point and then, using a blood lancet, the drop is penetrated at a 45 ° angle and the skin lifted to create a small break in the epidermis. Excess allergen extract is blotted with absorbent paper. Results are read at 15 to 20 min by measurement of the diameter of the weal (mm), which is the positive response. Antihistamines will induce false-negative results and increasing age is also associated with decreased positive responses. Large numbers of skin tests are unhelpful and the clinical history should suggest the relevant allergens for testing. Intradermal (intracutaneous) testing may be more useful for drug or insect-venom allergy testing but is more painful, technically more difficult, and carries a real risk of anaphylactic reaction. The identification of food-specific IgE is less reliable by skin testing and is best done in the laboratory by measurement of specific serum IgE.

In vitro tests for specific IgE antibodies: radioallergosorbent testing (RAST)

Small amounts of allergen-specific IgE may be measured in serum samples by this method. Allergen extracts are immobilized on to an insoluble particle, frequently cellulose or paper, and then allowed to react with the patient's serum. Binding occurs between the specific IgE, if present, and the immobilized allergen; complexes may then be detected by a further incubation with a radiolabelled antihuman IgE antiserum. The radioactivity, usually of ^{125}I bound to the particles, reflects the amount of allergen-specific IgE. Non-radioactive methods, for example enzyme-linked immunosorbent assays, are also available.

Treatment

The most effective treatment is allergen avoidance but this is often not practical. Medical treatment with the combination of a long-acting, non-sedating H_1-antihistamine (terfenadine, loratidine, cetirizine) and a topical corticosteroid nose spray (flunisolide or beclomethasone) is effective in most individuals. Topical vasoconstrictors are not recommended for other than very short periods, owing to rebound chemical rhinitis. For pharmacologically unresponsive, seasonal allergic rhinitis, immunotherapy involving weekly injections of gradually increased doses of specific allergen was efficacious in some patients. However, this practice is now unpopular in the United Kingdom because of the risk of anaphylaxis with the currently licensed preparations. Atopic individuals frequently have many clinically relevant allergens, which renders specific immunotherapy less feasible. The underlying immunological mechanisms of successful allergen immunotherapy have not been determined, although a good clinical outcome is associated with an eventual decrease in specific IgE and an increase in specific IgG subclasses. The induction of peripheral T-cell anergy to the allergen has been suggested and the outcome of research into new approaches for immunotherapy is encouraging. Treatment with antihistamines and topical corticosteroids is often also effective for symptoms of vasomotor rhinitis.

ALLERGIC CONJUNCTIVITIS

Allergic conjunctivitis usually accompanies allergic rhinitis but may occur in isolation. The five main allergic eye diseases are seasonal allergic conjunctivitis, perennial allergic conjunctivitis, vernal keratoconjunctivitis, atopic keratoconjunctivitis, and giant papillary conjunctivitis. The first form, 'hayfever', is the most common and is usually due to grass pollens, tree pollen, or weeds. Symptoms are mainly pruritus and excessive lacrimation, and there may be minimal hyperaemia or no clinical signs. Good responses are usually obtained with systemic H_1-antihistamines combined with topical applications of sodium cromoglycate 2 per cent eyedrops thrice or four times daily as required. Topical corticosteroids are contraindicated because of possible sight-threatening complications. Perennial allergic conjunctivitis may be due to house-dust mite allergens or cat salivary-protein allergy. Symptoms, signs, and treatment are as for seasonal conjunctivitis. Cases of vernal keratoconjunctivitis, atopic keratoconjunctivitis, and giant papillary conjunctivitis should be suspected when symptoms are more severe and signs are present. These patients should be referred to an ophthalmologist for management as the conditions are potentially sight threatening.

EXTRINSIC ASTHMA (SEE SECTION 17)

Asthma is a heterogeneous disease that affects 10 per cent of children and 3 to 5 per cent of adults, ranging from wheezy bronchitis to a severe, life-threatening, obstructive ventilatory disease. By definition, asthma is manifested by widespread narrowing of the airways, which is reversible either spontaneously or as a result of treatment. However, chronic asthma may ultimately result in a degree of fixed airway obstruction. Allergic or extrinsic asthma is often associated with a personal or family history of allergic diseases and there may be a clear history of offending allergens precipitating an attack. Like allergic rhinitis and conjunctivitis, perennial symptoms are frequently due to allergens of house-dust mites or cats, with seasonal symptoms induced by tree pollens, grass pollens, and weeds. Specific IgE to these allergens is detectable by skin-prick or blood testing, but positive results should only be considered relevant in association with the full clinical picture.

Environmental pollution has been suggested as a possible cause for the recently increasing mortality from asthma. However, other important factors are incorrect diagnosis, underperception of asthma severity, failure to implement systemic corticosteroid therapy, and non-compliance with treatment.

Allergen bronchial-provocation tests have demonstrated that extrinsic asthma has two phases, with an immediate response within 30 min due to mast-cell degranulation of preformed mediators. Asthmatic individuals have heightened non-specific irritability of the tracheobronchial tree and show bronchoconstriction in response to preformed mediators, including histamine. Infiltration of mononuclear and polymorphonuclear cells and the release of secondary mediators then induce a delayed secondary response in 6 to 8 h, with an intense inflammatory response resulting in bronchoconstriction, vascular congestion, and oedema. The major basic and cationic proteins of the eosinophil are particularly important for cilial damage and epithelial desquamation. Exfoliated cells may block the airways as Creola bodies.

The diagnosis and management of asthma are discussed in Section 17.

INSECT-VENOM ALLERGY (SEE ALSO SECTION 8)

Insect-venom hypersensitivity is an important cause of IgE-mediated anaphylaxis and results in approximately 4 deaths in the United Kingdom and 40 in the United States per year. Adverse reactions have been associated with the order Hymenoptera, including honeybees (family Apidae), hornets, yellow jackets and wasps (Vespidae), and fire ants (Formicidae), and may occur in atopic or non-atopic individuals. Typically, there is a history of a prior systemic reaction to an insect sting, although patients may not recall previous episodes. Usually those patients who have only experienced large local reactions continue with similar responses on subsequent stings and as such are not candidates for desensitization.

Diagnosis depends on the history supported by evidence of specific IgE as determined in the laboratory or by careful skin-prick testing with dilute preparations of specific venoms. Adrenaline should be available if skin testing is used as there is a small risk of anaphylaxis with this procedure.

Treatment should be instituted promptly, as outlined for anaphylaxis in Table 5, and patients often subsequently carry emergency kits. Simple avoidance measures, such as wearing shoes and long-sleeved clothing, are recommended. Fatalities associated with further stings tend to occur in adults and a history of a life-threatening episode with confirmatory specific venom IgE is sufficient to recommend venom immunotherapy, which is highly efficacious. Particularly stringent observation, with adrenaline and resuscitation equipment to hand, is essential as therapy may precipitate adverse reactions. Maintenance therapy is usually continued monthly for 5 years and then reassessed.

ALLERGIC SKIN DISEASES (SEE ALSO SECTION 23 FOR MAIN COVERAGE)

Atopic dermatitis

Atopic dermatitis, which is synonymous with the term eczema, describes an inflammatory skin reaction that frequently affects flexural regions, the neck, and the hands. It is absent at birth but may develop within 2 to 4 months and be associated with profound pruritus; severe cases may manifest as erythema, oedema, papules, vesicles, and exudation. Chronic disease results in lichenification or thickening of the epidermis, and painful fissures may develop over joints. Responses to profound pruritus may cause excoriation and secondary bacterial infections. Other complications may include viral warts, molluscum contagiosum, and herpes simplex infection.

There are many forms of eczema but in some cases an external allergen may trigger the disease. Often, affected individuals also have rhinitis or asthma and serum IgE levels are usually markedly elevated; in others there is no associated allergic disease. Skin biopsies in allergic dermatitis have revealed cellular infiltrates of T cells, eosinophils, mast cells, and Langerhans cells and macrophages bearing surface IgE. The Langerhans cells are capable of antigen presentation to T cells. T cells isolated from sites of atopic dermatitis appear to have the 'IL-4 dominant' phenotype characteristic of allergic immune responsiveness. The ability to isolate and culture T cells from skin biopsies of affected tissues allows detailed investigation of allergen recognition by T cells, T-cell function, and novel therapeutic approaches. The possibility of a bacterial enterotoxin being important in eczema has been recently suggested by the demonstration of antibodies against specific staphylococcal enterotoxins in the serum of affected patients that are not found in the serum of patients with other dermatological disorders.

Allergic contact dermatitis (see also Section 23)

Substances such as nickel (nail polish, costume jewellery), colophony (some adhesive plasters), chromates (cement, leather goods), rubber additives, shoe and hair dyes, topical medicaments including suntan lotions, antibiotics, and lanolin may result in contact hypersensitivity. Some plants are particularly prone to sensitize, including poison ivy, primulae, and rhus trees. Agents tend to have a low molecular weight and easily form haptens with serum and skin proteins. Presentation of these antigenic complexes to skin T cells by HLA class II-positive Langerhans cells, expressing HLA class II molecules, may then evoke an immune response. Diagnosis depends on a careful history and confirmation by patch skin testing. Avoidance of the offending agent is the mainstay of treatment but corticosteroid creams may be helpful for acute lesions.

Urticaria/angioedema (see also Section 23)

The urticarias form a spectrum of heterogeneous conditions. The weals of urticaria, commonly known as hives, are well-defined areas of transient dermal oedema, demarcated by a red, serpiginous border, which usually resolve spontaneously within a few hours. If the oedema spreads through the underlying epidermis then the term angio-oedema is used. Common sites for subcutaneous spread include the periorbital region, the lips, the tongue, and oropharynx. In these instances, dangerous pharyngeal obstruction may rapidly develop. Mast-cell degranulation, whether immunologically or non-immunologically mediated, causes vasodilation and leaky vessels. Histamine may also cause secondary bronchoconstriction. Biopsies of urticarial lesions demonstrate oedema, neutrophil and eosinophil infiltration, and perivascular mononuclear cells.

Particularly common causes of urticaria are plants, for example 'stinging nettles', animal fur, certain foods (strawberries, egg white, shellfish, nuts, chocolate) and drugs, including antibiotics, aspirin-containing compounds, and non-steroidal anti-inflammatory agents. Underlying atopy is not a prerequisite for urticarial eruptions and mast cells may be degranulated directly to release their mediators.

Acute urticaria usually resolves within hours or days. If crops of lesions persist for more than 6 weeks the term chronic urticaria is used. While aetiological agents can often be identified for acute urticaria, they are seldom identified in the chronic form. However, antihypertensive drugs, antirheumatoid arthritis drugs, and hormone-based medications (oral contraceptives and hormone replacement therapy) are increasingly recognized as triggering agents.

Other forms of urticaria may have physical triggers. Weals following skin scratches are benign lesions described as dermographism. Cholinergic urticaria is associated with the tendency to excessive perspiration, and urticaria may also be evoked by cold, heat, pressure, solar light, or water. Urticarial vasculitis is rare; the lesions resolve to leave a bluish scar that gradually fades. A biopsy diagnosis confirms a leucocytoclastic vasculitis with immunoglobulin and complement deposition. The rare condition of hereditary angio-oedema is an autosomal dominant disorder in which severe episodic attacks of intractable angio-oedema occur. A quantitative or qualitative deficiency of the protein C1 inhibitor is associated with uncontrolled activation of complement components C4 and C2. A detailed family history provides an essential clue to the diagnosis. Urticaria as such does not occur in this condition, which does not respond to antihistamines or corticosteroids. As it is potentially fatal it is very important to make the diagnosis and institute appropriate prophylaxis and treatment.

If attacks of urticaria are recurrent with no obvious precipitating factors, patients should be advised to keep a diary and document food, beverages, drugs, contacts, and activity at half-hourly intervals for 24-h periods, which will at times precede the onset of attacks. In this way, common triggers may be identified. Identifiable agents should obviously be avoided but the possibility of underlying systemic disease should be entertained, for example lymphoma, systemic lupus erythematosus. Aspirin, non-steroidals, and β-blocking medications should all be avoided, and susceptible individuals usually benefit from the avoidance of perfumed products and the use of non-biological washing detergents. The new non-sedating H_1-antihistamine preparations have proved useful (cetirizine, loratidine, terfenadine or astemizole). Occasionally, if these are ineffective, benefit may be achieved with the use of one of the older, sedating, H_1-antihistamine preparations such as cyproheptadine. Acute attacks usually settle within a few days but chronic attacks should be controlled with continuous therapy for 3 to 4 months before gradually withdrawing the drugs. If severe urticaria/angioedema occurs with airway obstruction, management should be instituted with adrenaline as described under 'Anaphylaxis'. Systemic corticosteroids are usually not necessary in the urticarias but may be required in severe cases. Vasculitic urticaria can usually be controlled by a combination of H_1-antihistamines and dapsone.

Other conditions in which urticaria or related manifestations occur are considered elsewhere: hereditary angio-oedema (Chapter 5.4); systemic mastocytosis (Section 22); and the hypereosinophilic syndromes (Sections 15 and 22).

IgE-mediated allergic drug reactions

Adverse drug reactions may result from excessive dosage, recognized side-effects, idiosyncratic reactions, and interactions with other medications. True immunological drug reactions are rare but IgE-mediated reactions are the most common of these, with antibiotics, local anaesthetic agents, insulin, and allogeneic antisera being well-recognized causes. Penicillin has major and minor determinants that may all induce allergic responses. Erythromycin usually offers a suitable, safe alternative but, if a specific need for penicillin arises, skin-prick testing with dilute preparations of the determinants may be done, increasing gradually to intradermal testing. Progression to oral doses and then gradually increasing intravenous doses at 15- to 20-min intervals may induce short-term tolerance and successful treatment. Adrenaline and resuscitation facilities should always be available to combat possible severe adverse reactions. Cephalosporins, which have a similar nuclear structure to penicillin, have also been associated with drug allergy, with cross-reactivity between them and penicillins varying from 10 to 50 per cent. Cephalosporins should only be given with caution to penicillin-sensitive patients.

Food allergy/intolerance (see also Section 14)

True IgE-mediated food allergy is rare and often tends to be associated with nut allergy and the ingestion of shellfish. In sensitized subjects this may result in anaphylaxis or even death. Treatment of acute anaphylactic episodes is with adrenaline and the sufferer should be educated in the self-administration of adrenaline and carry an emergency kit. Food intolerance, which is usually milder and non-IgE mediated, occurs more commonly and may manifest as respiratory (asthma), neurological (migraine), gastrointestinal (diarrhoea/vomiting) or skin (urticaria/angioedema) disturbances. True food intolerance is rather uncommon and non-specific symptoms are usually not due to food allergy. Where a clear trigger is identified, it is logical to eliminate those foods from the diet but radical elimination diets are seldom indicated and should be discouraged. Skin-prick testing is usually unhelpful in the diagnosis of food allergy but specific serum IgE may be detected in the laboratory.

IMMUNOTHERAPY (DESENSITIZATION)

Allergen immunotherapy, which is commonly known as desensitization or hyposensitization, has been used as therapy for some IgE-mediated disorders since its empirical introduction by Noon in 1909. Despite the widespread popularity of the practice of subcutaneously injecting increasing doses of soluble allergen extract up to a maximally tolerated maintenance dose in order to induce specific tolerance, the mechanisms involved were unknown. Controlled studies have shown varying efficacy and a significant placebo effect. The venom preparations for wasp- and bee-venom hypersensitivity have been the most standardized extracts and have unequivocally been efficacious. In contrast, many of the pollen and house-dust mite allergen extracts have been poorly standardized, with varying clinical response and often troublesome local side-effects, occasionally anaphylaxis, and even some deaths. This practice is, therefore, not currently recommended in Britain other than for insect hypersensitivity and for severe summer hayfever, with a minimal observation period of 2 h postinjection and full resuscitation facilities available. In particular, allergen immunotherapy is not suitable for asthmatic patients, in whom severe attacks may be precipitated and clear benefit has not been demonstrated.

Although the efficacy of desensitization has been controversial, in controlled studies, immunotherapy with standardized extracts has been shown to be effective under optimal conditions, but this may not preclude a need for additional pharmacological intervention. Despite reports of increased membrane stability of mediator-releasing cells, activation of anti-idiotypic networks, altered lymphocyte reactivity, generation of suppressor T cells, tolerance induction, and reduced IgE synthesis accompanied by protective antibodies of other immunoglobulin isotypes to account for the clinical effectiveness of immunotherapy, the underlying mechanisms determining hyporesponsiveness remain ill-defined. Variation in allergen preparation, patient selection, and experimental protocols could account for the different mechanisms proposed. Furthermore, the ability of hyposensitization to modulate cytokine release, as now seems to be the case, could account for the wide range of immunological changes attributed to protective immunity induced by immunotherapy.

Current research into novel immunotherapeutics has targeted the potential use of peptides and recombinant allergen proteins as a means for redirecting or desensitizing the functional T-cell repertoire of allergic individuals.

Autoantibodies and disease

Although autoantibodies have been defined in a wide range of diseases, establishing a specific role in disease pathogenesis has been considerably more difficult. Antibodies may mediate the pathology of disease or they may simply be markers of an active inflammatory process. Differentiating these two possibilities has often proved problematical.

To be definitively linked to the pathogenesis of a disease, it must be possible to produce an experimental model of the disease either by passive transfer of antibody or by immunization with antigen. In addition, the presence of the antibody must coincide with the disease and reduction in antibody level must correlate with improvement in the disease. These criteria have been met in very few diseases and in a large range of disorders the pathogenic role for antibodies is highly suggestive but unproved.

ANTIBODIES TO CELL-SURFACE RECEPTORS

The presence of antibodies to acetylcholine receptors (**AChR**) provides an example *par excellence* of antibody-mediated autoimmune disease. Myasthenia gravis is the disease that results from the presence of such antibodies, which may disrupt ion-channel function or may lead to a reduction in receptor number. Experimental models can be produced in animals either by immunizing with AChR or by transfer of antiAChR antibody. Other antireceptor antibodies are also associated with well-documented clinical syndromes. Graves' disease results from antibodies to the thyroid-stimulating hormone receptor on thyroid epithelial cells. These antibodies may stimulate the gland through the receptor, although it has been reported that such antibodies occasionally produce hypothyroidism by blocking the receptor. The exact role in pathogenesis of these long-acting thyroid stimulators has never been precisely defined but they clearly have a role in disease pathogenesis. Other hormone receptors are occasionally also the target of autoantibodies. Anti-insulin receptor antibodies may produce diabetes or hypoglycaemia. Antibodies to a range of red-cell surface glycoproteins may lead to autoimmune haemolytic anaemia, secondary to the premature destruction of antibody-coated red cells by the spleen. Similarly, idiopathic thrombocytopenic purpura is associated with rapid destruction and sequestration of platelets coated with antiplatelet antibodies, often seen in patients with systemic lupus.

ANTIBODIES TO ADHESION MOLECULES AND EXTRACELLULAR MATRIX

Pemphigus vulgaris provides an example of a disease mediated by antibodies to a member of the family of cellular adhesion molecules. Antibodies in this disease can be used to transfer the disease passively to mice and the disease may also be transferred to the children of an affected mother by transplacental antibody. The pathogenic antibodies are specific for a desmoglein, which is a member of the cadherin family of calcium-dependent cell-adhesion molecules. Antibodies to type IV collagen are important in mediating the destruction of renal and pulmonary basement membranes in Goodpasture's syndrome; models of arthritis have also been described using type II collagen as an immunogen, but its precise role in the pathogenesis of human arthritis is uncertain.

ANTIBODIES TO CIRCULATING SERUM PROTEINS

The best example of a pathogenetic antibody specific for a circulating protein is the antiphospholipid syndrome. Often associated with systemic lupus, but frequently occurring in the absence of another underlying disease, this disease is associated with arterial and venous thrombosis. These antibodies are common in young individuals suffering from stroke and may also play a part in recurrent abortions. Although these antibodies were at one time thought to bind phospholipids, it may be that these effects are in part mediated by the binding of β_2-glycoprotein I a molecule implicated in platelet function and coagulation.

ANTIBODIES TO CYTOPLASMIC ANTIGENS

Antibodies to mitochondrial antigens are invariably found in individuals with primary biliary cirrhosis, and are not seen in other examples of bile-duct damage or destruction. These antibodies are components of dihydrolipoylacetyl transferase on the mitochondrial membrane. Antibodies to aminoacyl-tRNA synthetases have been associated with myositis but have not yet been shown to have a role in pathogenesis. Autoantibodies to myosin are seen after heart-muscle damage but again have no clear role in disease pathogenesis. Antibodies to cellular components of β-cells in the pancreas are recognized as important markers of the β-cell damage in type I diabetes. For example, antibodies to glutamic acid decarboxylase have been found very early in the course of type I diabetes, but again there is no clear evidence for a role in the pathogenesis. Other antibodies seen during the course of type I diabetes include anti-insulin antibodies and antibodies specific for granule proteins.

One group of autoantibodies that has received much attention as a marker for inflammatory disease is the antineutrophil cytoplasmic autoantibodies (c-ANCA). Specific for the proteinase 3 found in primary lyosomes, these antibodies are markers for Wegener's granulomatosis, crescentic nephritis, and vasculitis.

ANTIBODIES TO NUCLEAR ANTIGENS

A wide range of autoantibodies to nuclear proteins is recognized. Antibodies are seen to centromere antigens, mRNA-splicing components, ribonucleoproteins (Ro and La), DNA, and histones. There is no direct evidence of a pathogenic role for these antibodies in disease, and it has even been suggested that cross-reaction of anti-DNA antibodies with glycosaminoglycans may account for their pathogenicity.

Mechanism of antibody-mediated tissue damage

Antibody may produce pathological effects through a variety of mechanisms. The ability to fix complement, leading to the formation of a membrane-attack complex, is the most important mechanism of antibody-mediated pathology. Another mechanism is through antibody-dependent cell-mediated cytotoxicity. This most probably relies on non-T-, non-B-cell populations acting in concert with antibody to produce cellular damage.

In some cases, the pathological effort of the antibody may rely on its binding altering the biological function of the molecule. Pathogenic antibodies in pemphigus vulgaris bind to the N-terminal adherent domain of a cadherin, perhaps disrupting its function. Antibodies to the thyroid-stimulating hormone receptor in Graves' disease have a range of effects, from stimulation to blocking of the receptor. This may in part reflect the specific antibody epitopes. In myasthenia gravis, antibodies to the AChR lead to its defective function. Although damage to the motor end-plate is one explanation for these effects, it is clear that receptor modulation by antibodies also has an important role. Finally, antibodies may also directly alter the channel activity of the receptor.

The mechanism by which antibodies to intracellular proteins, particularly nuclear antigens, might influence disease processes remains unclear. Although these antibodies may represent epiphenomena rather than pathogenic agents, some animal models suggest that they may contribute to tissue damage. Interestingly, infants born to mothers with systemic lupus and anti-Ro antibodies are prone to develop heart block, suggesting that the development of cardiac conduction pathways may be altered by passive transfer of antibody from mother to fetus.

Immune complex-mediated diseases

In addition to diseases in which antibodies play a primary or secondary part in pathogenesis, antibodies can produce a disease process secondary to the effect of antibody–antigen immune complexes (Fig. 2). This mechanism was established when it was observed that serum sickness produced vasculitis and nephritis in rats. These experiments led to a clear recognition that many forms of glomerulonephritis were mediated through the accumulation of complexes in the glomerulus. In bacterial endocarditis, nephritis is thought to result from accumulation of antigen–antibody complexes; the antigens are thought to be derived from the infectious pathogen. Extrinsic allergic alveolitis results from the accumulation of immune complexes in the lung. In some cases these complexes contain the relevant external antigen (e.g. *Micropolyspora faeni* in farmer's lung). In most circumstances, however, the antigen responsible for these immune complexes is poorly defined. Some diseases associated with multiple autoantibodies, such as systemic lupus erythematosus, are complicated by vasculitis and nephritis as a result of immune-complex deposition. The factors responsible for such deposition, and its tissue localization, remain obscure. Complement components might have an important part to play in solubilizing immune complexes. Hence individuals in whom complement consumption is prominent (systemic lupus), and in whom hereditary defects in complement synthesis are present, have a marked predisposition to both vasculitis and nephritis. Defects of complement components, such as C4a deficiency, are found in up to 50 per cent of patients with systemic lupus.

Drugs are well known to induce immune-complex disease in some individuals; the mechanism is not clear, but it is now recognized that these effects may result from the drug altering the ability to clear immune complexes. Some drugs, such as penicillamine, inhibit the covalent binding of C4 to complement-activating surfaces and in some cases the drugs bind to C4 itself. This leads to a failure to solubilize immune complexes, as seen in the hereditary deficiencies of C4.

Fig. 2 Immune complex-mediated disease (type 3 hypersensitivity reactions) begin with antibody complexes, which are deposited in a variety of sites. These complexes are able to bind and activate complement, leading to the attraction and binding of macrophages and neutrophils. The binding of these cell populations leads to their degranulation, releasing a range of enzymes and mediators. These in turn lead to increased vascular permeability, swelling, and tissue damage. Platelets are similarly activated, leading to the additional release of vascular mediators.

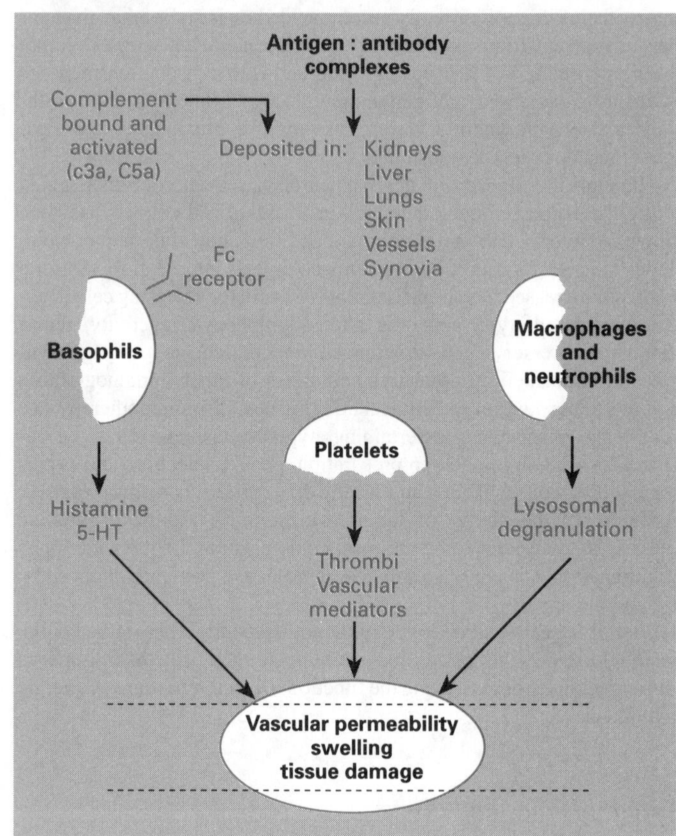

Fig. 3 Delayed (type 4) hypersensitivity involves the activation of T cells by 'professional' antigen-presenting cells in the skin. These Langerhan's cells activate T-cell populations which in turn release cytokines and chemokines. This in turn leads to the recruitment of monocytes and macrophages, and produces swelling, reddening, and necrosis at the site.

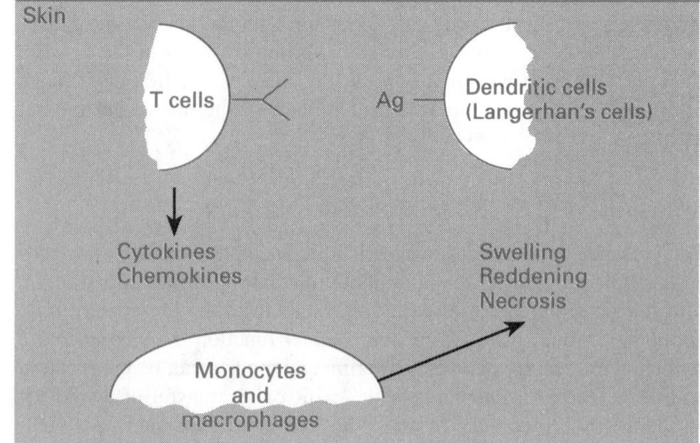

Table 6 *Delayed-type hypersensitivity reactions*

	Organ affected
Tuberculin	Skin
Contact	Skin
Chrome, nickel, cosmetics	
Urushiol:	
poison ivy *Rhus toxicodendron*	
poison oak *Toxicodendron radicans*	
Granuloma	Multiple organs
Mycobacterial infection	
Schistosomiasis	
Fungal infections	
Silica	

The sites of immune-complex deposition effect major foci of injury in disorders associated with immune activation. Immune complexes collect in the kidney adjacent to the glomerular basement membrane and account for the nephritis seen in a wide range of immune disorders, including some infectious diseases where the antigen load is large. Other sites of deposition of immune complexes include the joints and the anterior chamber of the eye. These sites are commonly found to be inflamed in autoimmune disorders.

Cellular mechanisms of immune-mediated disease

All aspects of immune-mediated disease rely to some extent on cellular components, particularly T cells. Antibody-mediated disease, immune-complex disease, and IgE-mediated disease all rely on help provided by CD4 T lymphocytes. These cells are central to the humoral immune responses and also contribute to disease pathogenesis through the action of cytokines. Other cell populations that may contribute to autoimmunity include CD8 cytotoxic populations of T cells, macrophages, which release a host of inflammatory cytokines, and natural killer cells, which are involved in non-MHC-restricted lymphotoxicity.

Classically, cell-mediated mechanisms of hypersensitivity involve T cells and monocytes and are referred to as delayed-type hypersensitivity reactions (Fig. 3). The T cells are predominently CD4 cells and recognize antigen in the context of MHC molecules on the surface of Langerhan's cells in the skin. These T cells produce cytokines, including IFN-γ, and these increase the capacity of monocytes and macrophages to invade the site. This delayed-type hypersensitivity is classically seen in the tuberculin reaction and may reflect the immune response occurring at the site of the tubercle infection itself. Contact sensitivity is another example of a cellular delayed-type response, as are the granulomatous hypersensitivity responses seen with *Mycobacterium tuberculosis, M. leprae,* and schistosomiasis (Table 6).

In many autoimmune diseases, T-cell populations predominate in the cellular infiltrate of the organ. These cells are occasionally of one predominant phenotype, such as the CD8 intraepithelial lymphocytes that accumulate in coeliac disease. In other diseases, such as type I diabetes, both CD4 and CD8 lymphocytes appear to have an important role. The HLA class II associations seen in the majority of autoimmune disorders have provided strong evidence for a role for CD4 class II-restricted cells in disease. It is now clear, however, that help can be generated by non-CD4 populations of T cells and cytotoxicity may result from cells with a CD4, rather than CD8, phenotype.

T-cell populations are obviously important in a range of diseases that are antibody mediated. This population need not be present at the site of tissue damage, as antibodies produced by these cells at distant sites provide an effective mechanism. Most inflammatory infiltrates associated with autoimmunity also contain macrophages. Elimination of these populations with specific antibodies can prevent the development of diabetes in animal models. It is likely, therefore, that these cells have an important role in disease pathogenesis. These are a common cell population in inflammatory infiltrates in joints during the course of reactive or rheumatoid arthritis. They do not express antigen-specific receptors but play an important part in presenting antigen, particularly to MHC class II-restricted T-cell populations.

T cells have received much attention as cellular mediators of autoimmune disease. Studies in most autoimmune conditions have sought to establish whether T cells at the site of lesions express CD4 or CD8. Most diseases show a combination of CD8+ and CD4+ cells. The TCR sequences present on cells at the site of inflammation have also received attention. The rationale for these studies has been the suggestion that T cells responding to a specific antigen–MHC combination may show restricted usage of TCR components or that a superantigen, if involved in the disease process, might lead to a specific expansion of T cells expressing a particular Vβ sequence. With the exception of superantigen-mediated T-cell expansions, there is little reason to believe that a response to a particular peptide–MHC combination will lead to the expansion of a single TCR V-region. Indeed, much evidence suggests that such expansions are heterogeneous. Findings in the mouse model of demyelinating disease, extrinsic allergic encephalomyelitis, suggest that clonal populations of T cells which can initiate the disease are scarce at the site of inflammation in the central nervous system, and that most of the inflammatory infiltrate represents a second level of immune responsiveness to antigens other than the initiating antigen, or may even represent cells recruited to the site that have antigen specificities irrelevant to the disease. This makes it unlikely that single populations of T cells bearing similar TCRs are likely to be present in the cellular populations in autoimmune infiltrates.

In addition to conventional T-cell populations, two populations sharing the morphology of large granular lymphocytes are also often seen in autoimmunity. These may possess the natural killer phenotype and be involved in non-MHC-restricted cytotoxicity, or alternatively may express CD3, CD8 and CD57, making them an αβ TCR-positive T-cell population with a large granular lymphocyte (**LGL**) morphology. The role of these cells in the normal immune response remains uncertain, but interestingly they appear to show oligoclonal patterns of expansion in a wide range of individuals. These expansions may account for 20 to 30 per cent of peripheral CD8+ cells. Some of these populations expand after viral infections such as cytomegalovirus, while others appear to be present in response to B-cell proliferations such as myeloma and benign paraproteinaemia. Individuals with very large expansions of these cells, previously referred to as LGL leukaemias, often have a phenotype of severe rheumatoid arthritis, similar to Felty's syndrome. Expansions of these populations in rheumatoid arthritis may therefore be important in the pathogenesis of the disease.

Although all the cellular populations can be found at the site of autoimmune damage, the importance of any single population remains to be determined. It is likely, however, that many populations act in concert to damage tissue and that it would prove difficult to identify single populations that are predominately responsible for disease.

REFERENCES

Allergy and immunology (1991). *Medical knowledge self-assessment programme IX.* American College of Physicians, Washington DC.

Clinical allergy (1992). Royal College of Physicians position paper.

Holgate, S.T. and Church, M.K. (1993). *Allergy.* Gower, London

Klein, J. (1990). *Immunology.* Blackwell Scientific, Boston.

Naporstek, Y. and Plotz, P.H. (1993). The role of autoantibodies in autoimmune disease. *Annual Review of Immunology,* **11,** 79–104.

O'Hehir, R.E., Garman, R.D., Greenstein, J.L., and Lamb, J.R. (1991). The specificity and regulation of T-cell responsiveness to allergens. *Annual Review of Immunology,* **9,** 67–95.

Rose, N.R. and Bona, C. (1993). Defining criteria for autoimmune disease. *Immunology Today,* **14,** 426–30.

5.3 Immunodeficiency

A.D.B WEBSTER

Introduction

The study of primary immunodeficiencies has provided valuable insight into the mechanisms for protection against infection. Delays in the diagnosis of immunodeficiency are common, probably because of the false sense of security provided by modern antibiotics. This section describes defects in lymphocytes, and aims to stimulate clinicians to consider the diagnosis of immunodeficiency in all patients with recurrent infections. Defects in complement and phagocytes, which are an integral part of the immune system, are described in Chapter 5.4 and in Section 22.

CLASSIFICATION

It is useful to classify immunodeficiency as primary or secondary despite confusion as to how some disorders should be categorized. Most of the primary immunodeficiencies are inherited single-gene disorders presenting in infancy or early childhood, many of which are now understood at a molecular level. However, common variable (varied) immunodeficiency sits uneasily within this classification because of its clinical heterogeneity and frequent presentation after childhood. Secondary immunodeficiency is associated with a wide range of disorders, with the immune defect in many cases only playing a minor part in the overall prognosis. The World Health Organization (**WHO**) sponsors a Committee to meet every 5 years to update these classifications.

HISTORY AND EXAMINATION

The family history is important, as it may suggest X-linked or autosomal inheritance. There are few characteristic physical features, but the total absence of tonsils in infants and children is a feature of X-linked agammaglobulinaemia and severe combined immunodeficiency, the latter also being associated with failure to thrive and an absent thymic shadow on chest radiographs. Signs of chronic otitis media, sinusitis, conjunctivitis, and bronchitis are typical, and splenomegaly is common in some types.

Primary immunodeficiency

Antibody-deficiency syndromes

Prevalence

The life-time prevalence of the severe antibody deficiency syndromes is about 16 per million of the population in the West but there is no reliable information on the Third World; there are currently about 1000 diagnosed patients in the United Kingdom. However, partial antibody deficiency is common in the West, and occurs in about 1 in 700 of Caucasians, the majority of whom are healthy.

Aetiology

Various blocks in the maturation and differentiation of B lymphocytes have been identified in many of the syndromes, and the relevant genes cloned (Fig. 1).

Nomenclature (Table 1)

Most of the known inherited single-gene disorders are clearly defined but there is difficulty with the most common primary immunodeficiency, now called 'common varied immunodeficiency' by the WHO. This term covers a range of immunopathological disorders of varying severity, for which there is no consensus on whether they represent a spectrum of a single disease or separate, inherited, autosomal recessive disorders.

X-LINKED (BRUTON'S) AGAMMAGLOBULINAEMIA (XLA)

Patients with classical disease develop recurrent infection in the first 2 years of life, usually at about 3 months when maternal IgG is exhausted. In fact, none of the patients is truly agammaglobulinaemic, and all have some plasma IgG (usually less than 50 mg/100 ml). Affected children have normal numbers of circulating T cells and normal cellular immunity, but very few circulating B cells. The *XLA* gene has been cloned, and probes are available to confirm the diagnosis in the fetus or young child, and to identify female carriers. The *XLA* gene codes for a B-cell-specific tyrosine kinase that appears to be crucial for the proliferation of pre-B cells in the bone marrow. There are clinically mild *XLA* variants where the block at the pre-B-lymphocyte stage is incomplete. There are a few children with classical XLA and growth hormone deficiency, but the cause of the latter is still not known.

X-linked immunodeficiency with hyper-IgM

This rare condition is characterized by very low levels of serum IgG, IgA, and IgE, but markedly raised levels of IgM and sometimes IgD. The relevant gene codes for the ligand (on some T cells) for the B-cell CD40 surface antigen, through which signals are delivered to switch B cells from IgM to IgG production. The defect is not confined to B cells, however, as affected boys often have T-cell lymphopenia and neutropenia, and suffer from opportunistic fungal and viral infections.

X-linked lymphoproliferative syndrome

Affected boys have a defect in the control of Epstein–Barr virus replication and are prone to severe and fatal acute infectious mononucleosis, Burkitt's-like B-cell lymphomas, and moderate hypogammaglobulinaemia. The mechanism is unknown, and there is currently no treatment or prophylaxis available except immunoglobulin replacement therapy for those who develop hypogammaglobulinaemia.

Transient hypogammaglobulinaemia in infancy and childhood

Maternal IgG crosses the placenta in the last trimester of pregnancy and helps protect the infant against infection for the first few months of life. Between 4 and 6 months of age the normal infant will develop an increasing repertoire of IgG antibodies, mainly of the IgG1 subclass. The capacity to make IgG2 and IgA antibodies is not fully developed until adolescence. This sequence may be retarded in some infants, who present in early childhood with infections and hypogammaglobulinaemia. The mechanism is unknown, and full recovery later in childhood differentiates the condition from common varied immunodeficiency (see below). Mild variants of the condition are probably common.

Common varied immunodeficiency (CVID) (synonym: common variable hypogammaglobulinaemia)

Patients present at any age, with a peak incidence in early childhood and in late adolescence. Serum immunoglobulin levels are variable, but usually serum IgA is virtually absent, the IgG is below 2 g/l, and the IgM below 0.2 g/l. However, some patients have normal or even raised

IgM levels. There is an increase in the incidence of selective IgA deficiency and/or autoimmune disease in first-degree relatives, and occasionally a parent and offspring may both develop CVID. The condition is associated with the major histocompatibility complex **(MHC)** haplotype, C4A*QO, DR3 in about 50 per cent of patients; the same haplotype is associated with systemic lupus erythematosus, coeliac disease, and a poor prognosis in human immunodeficiency virus **(HIV)** infection. A third of patients are severely lymphopenic, with circulating CD4+ T-cell counts below 0.4×10^9/l, low numbers of circulating B cells, and a relative increase in CD8 T cells; similar phenotypic changes are seen in AIDS.

Lymphopenic patients tend to have splenomegaly and sometimes hypersplenism, and a few have recurrent lymphadenopathy. Despite the depletion of CD4+ T cells and other evidence of functional defects in cellular immunity, the prognosis is relatively good and only about 10 per cent die from opportunistic fungal and viral infections within 30 years from onset of symptoms.

Despite the heterogeneity of CVID, there are subgroups of patients with similar clinical and laboratory features, suggesting a single aetiological mechanism. One subgroup (type 1) comprises patients with CD4 T- and B-cell lymphopenia, evidence of chronic T-cell activation, splenomegaly, and failure of the remaining circulating B cells to produce immunoglobulins *in vitro* when stimulated with interleukin 2 **(IL-2)**. In another major subgroup (type 2) there are normal T-cell numbers and function, and the circulating B cells produce both IgG and IgM *in vitro* with IL-2; in general the prognosis is better in these patients. The sequence of events in some patients with type 1 CVID suggests a viral aetiology or trigger. A mononucleosis-like illness with lymphadenopathy may occur in adolescence, sometimes associated with autoimmune thrombocytopenia or haemolytic anaemia, followed by infections and hypogammaglobulinaemia. Some patients with CVID may have rare, unknown, inherited metabolic disorders of T and B lymphocytes that only become clinically apparent when the immune system is persistently activated by chronic infection (e.g. Epstein–Barr virus). A recent report of two adults with recurrent infections and autosomal-recessive adenosine deaminase deficiency supports this view.

Thymoma and hypogammaglobulinaemia

This has some distinctive features but many clinical and laboratory similarities with CVID. The thymoma, usually benign and well encapsulated, occurs in patients over 40 years of age, with hypogammaglobulinaemia at the time or some years later. There may be autoimmune phenomena such as neutropenia, haemolytic anaemia, and red-cell aplasia. The patients have a poorer prognosis than with CVID and usually die within 15 years from opportunistic viral or fungal infections due to associated defects in cellular immunity. Surgical removal of the thymoma has no effect on the immunodeficiency or the prognosis.

Infections associated with hypogammaglobulinaemia

Patients with X-linked agammaglobulinaemia and CVID are prone to mycoplasmas and certain bacterial, protozoal, and viral infections (Fig. 2). However, they recover uneventfully from most common childhood viral infections (e.g. measles, varicella, and mumps) and are not prone to fungal disease.

BACTERIA

Non-capsulated *Haemophilus influenzae* is the most important cause of infection in these patients. This is a semicommensal organism that colonizes the upper respiratory tract of many normal individuals, overgrowth being commonly associated with bronchitis following viral infections. Patients with antibody deficiency suffer from chronic infec-

Fig. 1 Various blocks in the maturation and differentiation of B lymphocytes in some of the primary immunodeficiency syndromes. Hatched bars identify blocks in lymphocyte differentiation/proliferation: (A) reticular dysgenesis; (B) X-linked severe combined immunodeficiency; (C) adenosine deaminase, purine nucleotide phosphorylase, *RAG NF-AT,* and *ZAP-70* gene defects, and lymphocyte class II deficiency; (D) common varied immunodeficiency (CVID) type I; (E) X-linked agammaglobulinaemia and *RAG* gene defects; (F) immunodeficiency with hyper-IgM; (G) CVID type I and II, block confined to IgA or IgG subclasses in selective deficiencies. Note that differentiation and maturation of pre-T and immature T cells takes place within the thymus.

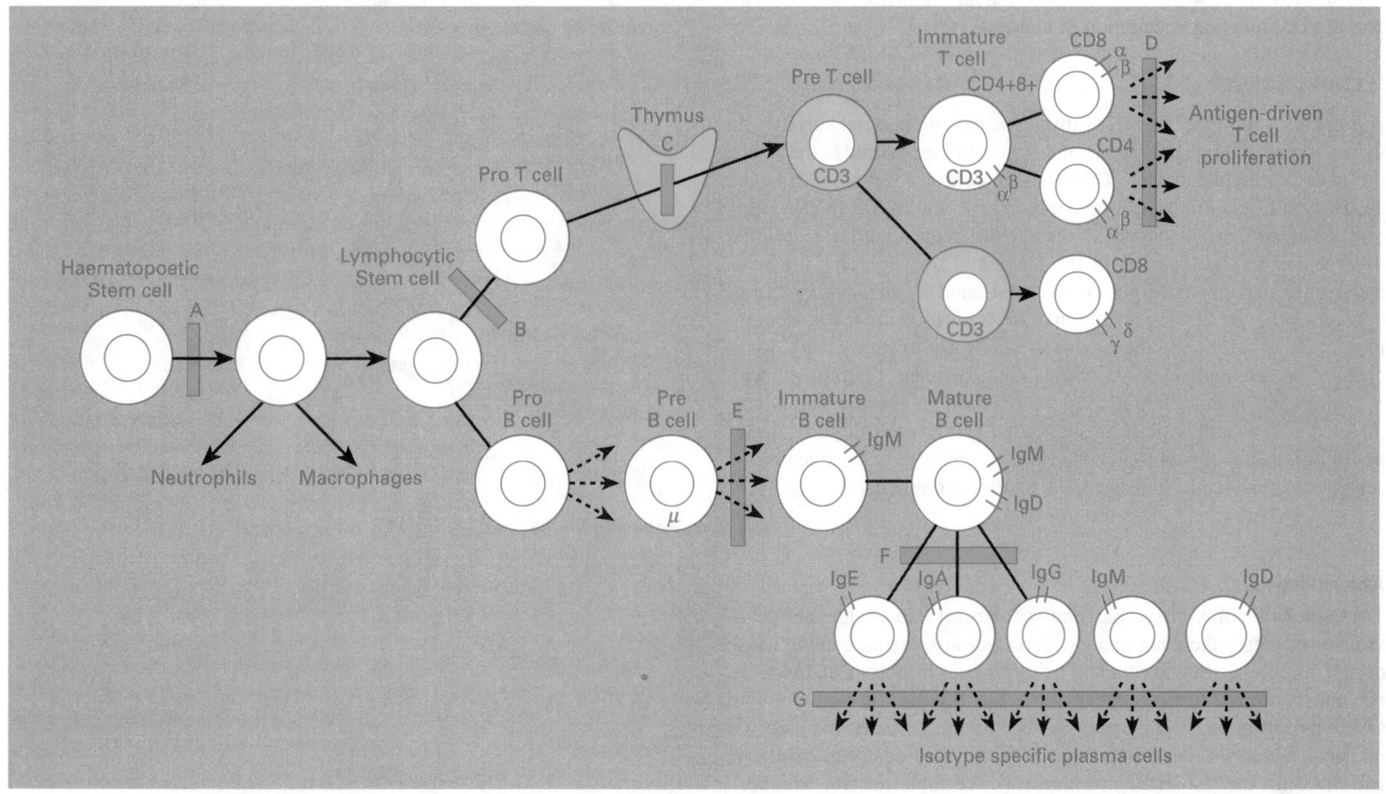

Table 1 *Classification of primary immunodeficiency*

Antibody deficiency
X-linked agammaglobulinaemia
Common varied immunodeficiency
Thymoma with hypogammaglobulinaemia
Selective IgA deficiency
Selective IgG subclass deficiencies
Transient hypogammaglobulinaemia of infancy
Selective T-cell deficiency
Thymic aplasia
Purine nucleoside phosphorylase deficiency
T-cell-receptor defects
Mixed T- and B-cell defects
Severe:
Severe combined immunodeficiency:
• X-linked
• adenosine deaminase deficiency
• lymphocyte class II deficiency
• *RAG* gene defects
• defects in *RAG* genes
ZAP-70
NP-AT
Reticular dysgenesis
Moderate:
Immunodeficiency with hyper-IgM
Ataxia telangiectasia (Nijmegen breakage syndrome)
Wiskott–Aldrich disease
TAP (class 1) transporter defect
X-linked lymphoproliferative syndrome
Short-limbed dwarfism and immunodeficiency
Bloom's syndrome
Ligase-1 deficiency

tion in the ears, sinuses and bronchi, often leading to bronchiectasis and deafness. Patients may also present with pneumococcal, *H. influenzae* (capsulated) or meningococcal septicaemia and arthritis, and staphylococcal skin infection is common in children.

MYCOPLASMAS

Antibodies inhibit the growth of mycoplasmas on mucosal surfaces. In their absence, overgrowth occurs and organisms are carried to the joints, probably within phagocytes. This leads to a chronic septic arthritis and destruction of the joints. The mycoplasma species known to cause disease are *M. salivarium,* which is a commensal in the mouth, *Ureaplasma urealyticum* and *M. hominis* in the urogenital tract (chronic urethritis and cystitis may precede joint involvement), and *M. pneumoniae,* a recognized pathogen causing pneumonia. Mycoplasmas are the most common cause of arthritis in these patients, and early treatment with doxycycline is recommended to avoid joint damage. Treatment with hyperimmune animal serum may be required in those rare patients infected with an antibiotic-resistant strain. Most laboratories do not routinely culture for mycoplasmas and few are able to test for antibiotic sensitivities; advice from a specialist unit is recommended.

VIRUSES

Enteroviruses

These include polio, coxsackie, and echoviruses. Coxsackie and echoviruses, of which there are many different strains, are a common cause of self-limiting mild enteritis and/or meningitis in normal individuals, but cause chronic meningoencephalitis and myositis in patients with severe hypogammaglobulinaemia. Echoviruses are usually involved, the classical features being convulsions, VIIIth nerve deafness, headache and myositis, the last leading to fibrosis of the limb muscles with contractures. The disease slowly progresses, sometimes for up to 8 years, finally causing death from damage to a vital centre in the brainstem. The diagnosis is made by culturing the virus from cerebrospinal fluid or muscle. Cultures are often negative in patients on immunoglobulin replacement therapy, possibly due to partial neutralization of the virus by passively administered antibody. The diagnosis may then depend on demonstrating enteroviral RNA (by polymerase chain reaction) in cerebrospinal fluid. Most patients eventually die from the disease and there is no specific therapy available. It is likely that intravenous immunoglobulin therapy every 2 weeks will reduce the risk of infection.

There is a raised incidence of paralytic poliomyelitis and patients must not be immunized with live polio vaccine. Fortunately, regular immunoglobulin therapy appears to prevent poliovirus infection from recently immunized family members, probably because enough neutralizing IgG leaks into the saliva.

Other viruses

Patients with CVID are prone to recurrent varicella-zoster skin infection (shingles) but this rarely recurs after they are treated with immunoglobulin. A few with CVID and associated T-cell defects are prone to recurrent reactivation of herpes simplex with skin and nerve involvement, but not to Epstein–Barr virus or cytomegalovirus.

GASTROINTESTINAL INFECTIONS

Giardia lamblia

This is the only protozoal parasite that commonly infects these patients. Mild to severe malabsorption may follow, with some patients complaining of abdominal distension, colicky pain, and flatulence. A secondary lactose intolerance is common. Patients often relapse after a standard course of metronidazole (2 g daily for 3 days) and may need treatment for 10 days. In addition, patients should be given high-dose immuno-

Fig. 2 Pattern of infections associated with immunodeficiency. Prior to bone marrow transplantation, most infants with SCID require prophylactic cotrimoxazole for pneumocystis, and sometimes acyclovir for herpes viruses, and fluconazole for candida.

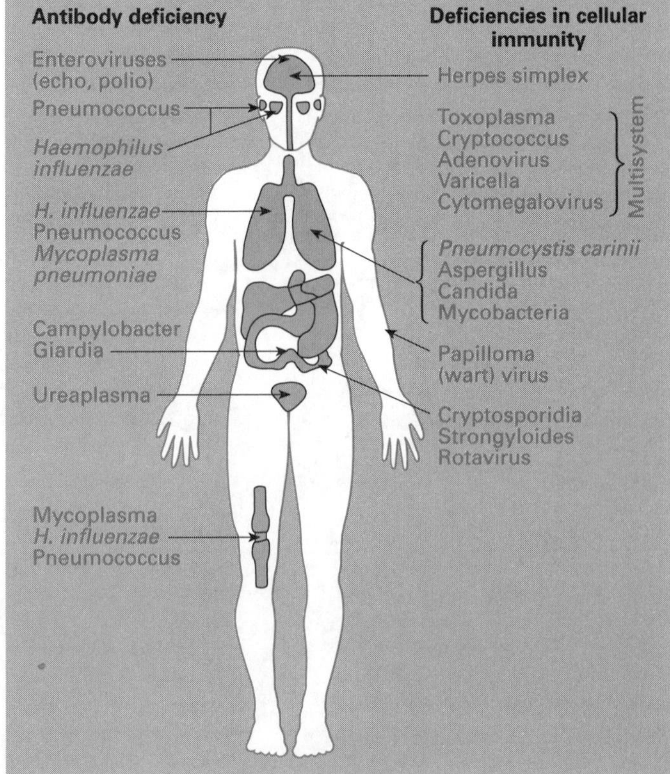

globulin therapy, preferably intravenously at a dose of 200 mg/kg body weight every 2 weeks. Giardiasis is rare in antibody-deficient patients on intravenous immunoglobulin, which suggests that enough specific IgG reaches the intestine to prevent infection.

Campylobacter

Campylobacter infection, usually *C. jejuni,* is the most frequent cause of bacterial-associated diarrhoea. Chronic or recurrent infection occurs but is easily treatable with erythromycin (in adults, 500 mg, four times a day for 10 days). Infection is rare in patients on immunoglobulin therapy. Chronic diarrhoea due to shigellae or salmonellae is unusual in X-linked agammaglobulinaemia but can occur in CVID when there are additional defects in cellular immunity.

Liver disease

Chronic hepatitis is common but is usually due to hepatitis C virus **(HCV)** infection. Most patients with HCV were infected in the 1970s and early 1980s from contaminated immunoglobulin or plasma therapy, but sexually transmitted infection is also possible. The incidence of HCV hepatitis has declined since the introduction of safer therapy in the late 1980s. There is also a raised incidence of chronic hepatitis B infection. Mild chronic hepatitis, often associated with hepatic granulomas, is common in CVID, and there are rare patients with sclerosing cholangitis of unknown aetiology who may have a distinct syndrome.

Special features associated with CVID

A large subset of patients with CVID (about 70 per cent) have special features not usually seen in X-linked agammaglobulinaemia which contribute to morbidity and mortality. In general, these are related to chronic inflammation in various organs with evidence of persistent T-lymphocyte activation and CD4 T-cell lymphopenia.

Chronic inflammatory bowel disease

Chronic or recurrent diarrhoea, not related to known pathogens, occurs in at least 20 per cent of patients with CVID. Most have a mild to moderate colitis with an excess of T lymphocytes infiltrating the mucosa. Ileitis is less common but usually causes the most severe symptoms, with abdominal pain and malabsorption. Surgery may be required for obstruction due to fibrosis. These features are similar to classical Crohn's disease but florid granulomatous changes are rare. Inflammation may also occur in the jejunum, with histological features of partial to severe mucosal atrophy. In rare cases this is due to gluten sensitivity, with complete recovery on a gluten-free diet. For the rest, antimobility drugs such as codeine phosphate or loperamide hydrochloride may be adequate, but an elemental diet and/or low-dose corticosteroids may be required in severe cases. Nodular lymphoid hyperplasia involving the submucosa of the small intestine, and sometimes the stomach and large bowel, is common in CVID but is usually of no clinical significance and does not predispose to gut lymphoma. This is probably yet another manifestation of chronic immune activation. Chronic gastritis, affecting all regions of the stomach, is common and may rarely cause anaemia due to deficiency of vitamin B_{12}. Gastric and duodenal ulceration is rare, and *Helicobacter pylori* appears to play no part in the gastritis.

Lymphoid system

Splenomegaly is common; in some patients the spleen gradually increases in size to cause hypersplenism with thrombocytopenia and neutropenia. Splenectomy may be necessary. Lymphadenopathy, both peripheral and involving mediastinal or mesenteric nodes, may occur, with histological signs of chronic immune stimulation with scattered granulomas.

Autoimmune disease

About 10 per cent of patients develop autoimmune disease, particularly haemolytic anaemia, thrombocytopenia, neutropenia, vitiligo, and alopecia. Immunosuppressive therapy may be required. The tendency to autoimmune disease is probably due to the associated T-cell abnormalities, as autoimmunity is also a feature of other selective T-cell deficiencies (see below).

Malignancy

There is about a 50-fold increase in the incidence of gastric cancer and lymphoma in CVID, probably due to the combination of chronic inflammation in the stomach and lymphoid system, and failure of adequate T-cell immune surveillance.

Prognosis

Recent surveys show that about 70 per cent of patients with CVID survive for up to 30 years. However, those with thymoma usually die from opportunistic infections within 15 years. The prognosis for X-linked agammaglobulinaemia is much better, with over 90 per cent survival for 30 years, which will probably improve with earlier diagnosis and treatment. Pneumonia and bronchiectasis remain the most common causes of death, although liver failure due to chronic HCV infection and malignancy (gastric carcinoma, lymphoma) are important causes in CVID.

Diagnosis

The value of the lymphocyte count in the differential diagnosis of low serum immunoglobulins is outlined in Fig. 3. The diagnosis is straightforward when there is severe panhypogammaglobulinaemia, but lymphoma is often suspected when serum immunoglobulin levels are only moderately depressed in patients with lymphadenopathy and/or splenomegaly. In these cases a lymph node biopsy is useful, and sometimes a diagnostic splenectomy is required. Secondary immunoglobulin deficiency due to protein-losing enteropathy can sometimes be difficult to distinguish from CVID, but the presence of normal numbers of IgG, IgM, and IgA plasma cells in the intestinal mucosa is good evidence against a primary immunodeficiency. *In vitro* tests of B-lymphocyte function can be helpful, and secondary immunodeficiency is likely if the patient's circulating B cells produce normal amounts of IgG, IgM, and IgA when stimulated with IL-2 *in vitro.* The interpretation of low immunoglobulin levels in children under 1 year of age is difficult and confirming a diagnosis of CVID may not be possible until the child is older.

Treatment

IMMUNOGLOBULIN REPLACEMENT THERAPY

Immunoglobulins for therapeutic use are manufactured from large pools of donor blood (about 20 000 donations). Those used for intramuscular **(IMIG)** or subcutaneous injection are 16 per cent solutions that do not contain stabilizing sugars to prevent IgG aggregation. Preparations for intravenous use **(IVIG)** are less concentrated (6–10 per cent solutions) and some manufacturers have incorporated procedures for viral inactivation (heat inactivation or solvent detergent treatment) into the process to improve safety. The basic steps in the manufacture involve alcohol precipitation of plasma to produce an IgG concentrate with very little IgA or IgM remaining. Fortunately, HIV is very sensitive to alcohol, and there is no convincing evidence that HIV has ever been transmitted in IMIG or IVIG treatment, contrasting with the major epidemic of AIDS in haemophiliacs given factor VIII. However, there have been outbreaks of HCV infection associated with contaminated batches of IVIG, although most of the currently licensed preparations have good safety records.

Immunoglobulin prophylaxis prevents pneumococcal and *H. influenzae* septicaemia, staphylococcal skin infection, giardia and campylobacter enteritis, but only partially protects against mycoplasma and enteroviral infection. It reduces the frequency of bronchitis, probably by preventing common respiratory viral infections. There is poor penetration into the respiratory mucosa with little effect on the growth of *H. influenzae* in the respiratory tract.

Indications

The serum IgG level is not a good guide to the frequency or dose of immunoglobulin required. In general, patients with evidence of bronchiectasis, chronic sinusitis, recurrent otitis media, recurrent giardiasis, mycoplasma urethritis, cystitis and/or arthritis should be treated with regular IVIG at a dose of at least 200 mg/kg body weight every 2 weeks; doses of 400 mg/kg body weight every 4 weeks are commonly used in the United States but there are no comparative trials to show which is the best regimen. Infants and young children with difficult veins can be successfully managed in the first few years of life with antibiotics and weekly intramuscular immunoglobulin injections (25 mg/kg body weight), but the risk of chronic enteroviral infection can probably only be reduced by higher-dose immunoglobulin therapy. For this reason, some paediatricians surgically implant a permanent infusion reservoir, although the long-term complications of this in immunodeficient children have not been properly assessed. Regular subcutaneous infusions, which are gaining popularity in both children and adults, may be a safer alternative. IMIG injections are suitable for some patients with less frequent infections but can be painful. Furthermore, about 10 per cent of patients on IMIG experience severe anaphylactoid reactions from time to time, probably due to the inadvertent injection of aggregated immunoglobulin into a vein.

IVIG therapy is currently the most popular procedure. Patients with hypogammaglobulinaemia are prone to mild anaphylactoid reactions during the first few IVIG infusions, probably due to the sudden interaction of antibodies with antigens. This can usually be prevented by giving hydrocortisone intravenously before the first three infusions, and by slowing the infusion rate to about 1 ml/min. There are no absolute contraindications to immunoglobulin therapy, but care should be taken in those patients with high levels of polyclonal anti-IgA antibodies in their serum. Those particularly at risk have selective IgA deficiency (see below), although there is a poor correlation between the presence of such antibodies and reactions. There is no requirement to screen for anti-IgA antibodies in patients with panhypogammaglobulinaemia, but facilities for resuscitation and trained personnel should always be available during the first few infusions.

GENERAL MANAGEMENT

Patients should be encouraged to take antibiotics early for bronchitis, and those with structural lung damage may require long-term prophylaxis. The quinolones (e.g. ciprofloxacin) are particularly effective because they are concentrated in the mucous layer lining the respiratory tract and have a very low minimal inhibitory concentration for non-typable *H. influenzae*. Amoxycillin, alone or in combination with clavulanic acid, or cotrimoxazole, is a useful alternative. Postural drainage and regular exercise are useful in promoting removal of secretions from the lungs. Patients should be educated in the appropriate treatment for various complications, and many countries now have patient support groups which provide assistance.

Fig. 3 A scheme for the differential diagnosis of patients with immunoglobulin deficiency, with useful diagnostic tests and features for the more common disorders. Secondary immunodeficiency can usually be excluded by standard laboratory tests. The circulating lymphocyte count can be a useful guide to the type of primary immunodeficiency.[a] Usually in infants and young children; ADA, adenosine deaminase; EBV, Epstein–Barr virus; FH, family history.

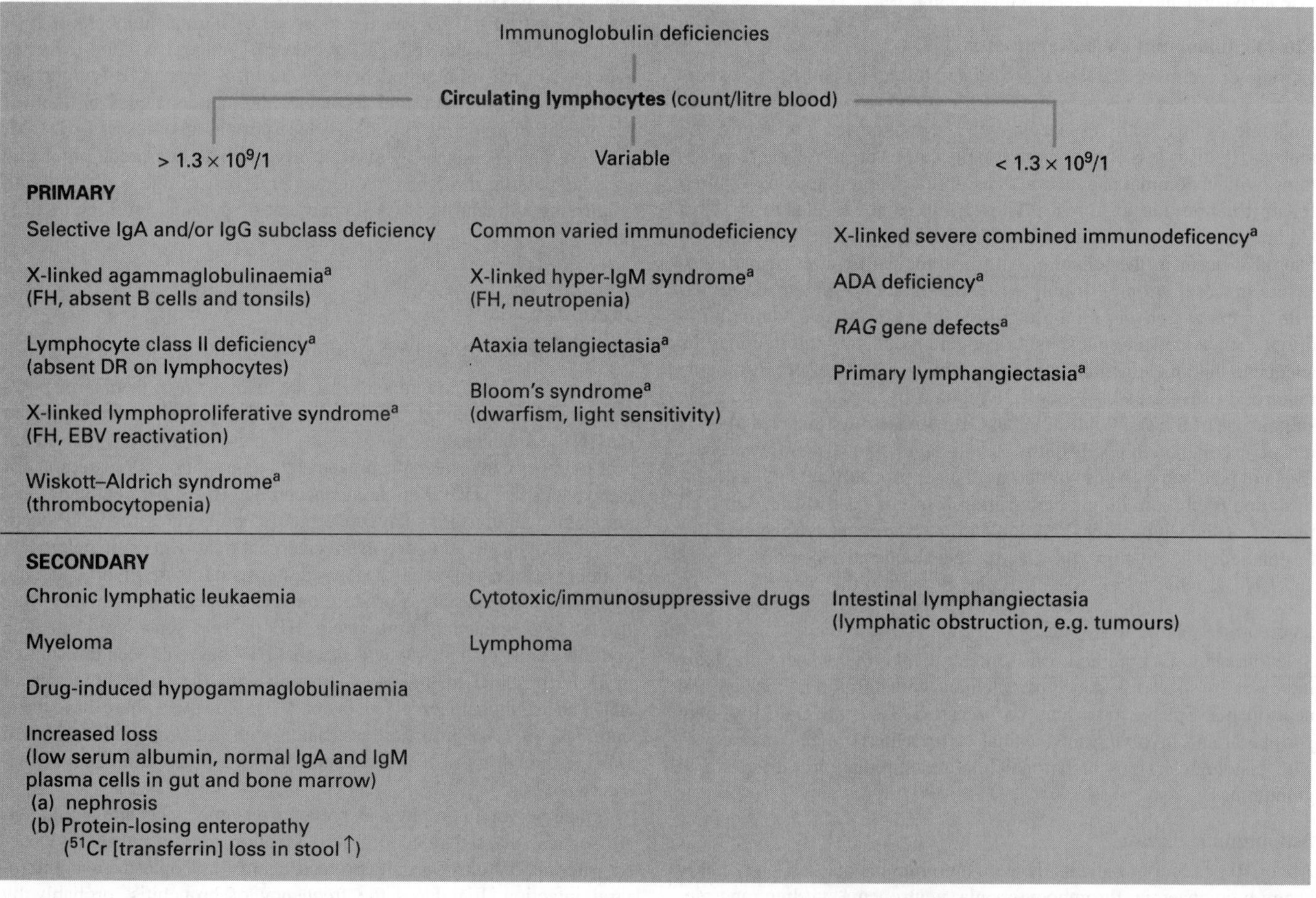

Selective and functional immunoglobulin deficiency

SELECTIVE IGA DEFICIENCY

Complete absence of IgA (<0.01 g/l) occurs in about 1 in 700 Caucasians but only in 1 in 18 500 Japanese. Most remain healthy and are not prone to infection, but probably about 5 per cent suffer from respiratory infections; some of these have additional functional deficiencies in IgG antibody production despite normal total serum IgG levels (see below). The mechanism of selective IgA deficiency is not understood, but in the majority it is due to a failure of terminal differentiation of B cells into IgA-producing plasma cells, with no abnormality in the α-chain gene itself. In most cases the condition is probably part of the spectrum of CVID; there is a raised incidence of selective IgA deficiency in family members of CVID patients, and both conditions are associated with the MHC haplotype HLA-A1, B8, C4A*QO, DR3.

Disease associations

There is a small increase in IgA deficiency in coeliac and Still's disease and in rheumatoid arthritis, but sometimes this may be due to drugs such as sulphasalazine, gold or pencillamine, all of which are known causes of IgA deficiency or panhypogammaglobulinaemia. There is also a raised incidence of IgA deficiency in epileptics, but this is partly due to phenytoin therapy.

IgG SUBCLASS DEFICIENCIES

The clinical significance of IgG subclass deficiency is controversial. IgG2 deficiency has received most attention because it is probably as common as selective IgA deficiency, and the two deficiencies may occur together. Moreover, IgG2 deficiency is compatible with normal health and many healthy children have unrecordable levels of this subclass in the first year of life. Selective deficiencies in the other subclasses (IgG1, IgG3, and IgG4) have been reported and may be associated with recurrent respiratory infection. Selective IgG4 deficiency is probably clinically irrelevant.

In general, IgG1 and IgG3 antibodies are stimulated by protein antigens, with the IgG3 response to viral proteins being relatively high. IgG2 antibodies are mainly directed against polysaccharides. However, selective deficiencies in either IgG1, IgG2 or IgG3 are usually compensated for by the others. In early life, IgG1 antibodies to polysaccharides normally compensate for the relative lack of IgG2, although this does partly explain the weak response to polysaccharide vaccines in infants. Most IgG subclass deficiencies probably represent the milder end of the spectrum of CVID, but there are rare patients who are homozygous for deletions in the heavy-chain coding genes for IgG1, IgG2, or IgG4. Measuring serum IgG subclasses in patients with recurrent respiratory infections may help identify a clinically relevant defect, but in practice it rarely helps in the management. The important issue is whether patients can make functional IgG antibodies to protein and polysaccharide antigens (see below).

OTHER SELECTIVE DEFICIENCIES

Complete selective IgM deficiency is very rare and is due to mutations in the μ-chain coding gene. Most cases of incomplete IgM deficiency are secondary to lymphoma or associated with rare syndromes such as Bloom's or Wiskott–Aldrich syndrome. Selective IgE deficiency has been described but is not clinically important.

FUNCTIONAL IMMUNOGLOBULIN DEFICIENCIES

Functional deficiency is defined as complete or partial failure to produce antibodies to specific proteins/peptides or polysaccharides, in the presence of normal total serum immunoglobulin levels. The mechanism is not known. In practice, only functional IgG immunoglobulin deficiency is currently recognized as clinically important. The diagnosis should be considered in patients with recurrent respiratory infections who are not neutropenic, lymphopenic or complement deficient. The standard practice is to test immunize with tetanus toxoid, (0.5 ml adsorbed vaccine by deep subcutaneous injection), and pneumococcal polysaccharide vaccine (e.g. Pneumovax) and measure the response after 3 weeks. Published reports of deficiencies are anecdotal, but evidence is accumulating that there are significant numbers of children and adults with recurrent infections, many of whom have selective IgA deficiency, who fail to respond to immunization and subsequently benefit from immunoglobulin therapy. Some patients respond to protein antigens but not to polysaccharides; the clinical significance of this is not yet clear.

TREATMENT OF SELECTIVE AND FUNCTIONAL DEFICIENCIES

Some patients may benefit from immunoglobulin replacement therapy (IMIG or IVIG), while in others the early use of antibiotics for respiratory symptoms is adequate. There are no clear guidelines as to the best approach, but those with evidence of chronic bronchitis, sinusitis or otitis probably require immunoglobulin therapy.

Selective T-cell deficiency

The selective T-cell deficiencies are very rare but have provided valuable information on the role of T cells for human survival. In general, children with grossly depleted levels of T cells can remain relatively healthy in the Western world. Only when the defect is associated with macrophage dysfunction and antibody deficiency is the condition potentially fatal.

Thymic aplasia (Di George syndrome)

This is caused by fetal malformation of the third and fourth branchial arch at about 4 to 6 weeks of gestation, usually associated with other developmental defects such as micrognathia, dysmorphic facies, cardiac malformations, and absence of the parathyroid glands causing hypocalcaemic convulsions and tetany in infancy. Until recently it was considered to be an acquired defect but many cases are associated with structural defects of chromosome 22. Severely affected infants often die early from the associated cardiac abnormalities. Those that survive usually have a few circulating T lymphocytes (less than 10 per cent), suggesting the presence of some thymic tissue. Such infants may remain healthy, with their circulating T-cell numbers gradually increasing throughout childhood. Serum immunoglobulin levels and specific antibody production are usually adequate. Severely affected infants are prone to recurrent bacterial, fungal, and viral infections, and have a tendency to develop life-threatening chronic cytomegalovirus and varicella infections; in the past some children died from chronic vaccinia infection following immunization. Patients with both the severe and mild clinical phenotype are prone to autoimmune disease, particularly haemolytic anaemia or thrombocytopenia.

TREATMENT

A fetal thymus graft, surgically inserted into the rectus sheath, has been successful in severe cases. The graft releases factors that promote the differentiation of prethymic T cells into mature T lymphocytes. The use of synthetic thymic factors as an alternative is controversial. Patients with mild clinical disease should be tested carefully over the first 2 years of life and a thymic graft considered if there is evidence of clinical deterioration. Affected patients should not be immunized with live vaccines.

Purine nucleoside phosphorylase (PNP) deficiency

This autosomal recessive disease is characterized by T-cell deficiency, susceptibility to severe cytomegalovirus and varicella infection, autoimmune blood dyscrasias, lymphoma, and neurological disease with spasticity and muscle weakness. Most affected patients present in infancy, although there are milder variants with residual enzyme activity presenting later in childhood. The defect causes the accumulation of the substrates for PNP (guanosine and deoxyguanosine) in the plasma, which prevents the normal development of T cells, leaving the B cells relatively unaffected. Attempts have been made to lower the plasma deoxyguanosine level by infusing red cells containing PNP from normal donors. This may partially reverse the immunological defect, but has no effect on the neurological disease. Bone marrow transplantation from an HLA haploidentical family member is the best treatment. The *PNP* gene has been cloned on chromosome 14, and gene therapy may be feasible in the future.

Severe combined immunodeficiency disease (SCID)

Most SCID is due to rare inherited or spontaneous mutations of genes that influence the maturation of lymphocytes, particularly T cells (Fig. 1). Infections are much more severe than those seen in selective T-cell deficiency or primary hypogammaglobulinaemia, probably because macrophage function is also depressed. Although HIV infection in infancy may lead to combined immunodeficiency, there is no evidence yet of other viruses causing this syndrome.

CLINICAL FEATURES

Symptoms usually start in infancy with failure to thrive, diarrhoea due to parasitic or viral infection, *Pneumocystis carinii* pneumonia, and mucocutaneous or systemic candidiasis. Immunization with live vaccines (e.g. polio, BCG) may cause a fatal infection. Most patients die within 2 years without a successful bone marrow graft.

IMMUNOLOGY

With one exception (see below), there is a severe depression of circulating T-lymphocyte numbers, with a failure of T cells to proliferate with mitogens *in vitro.* T-lymphocyte and natural killer cytotoxicity is often severely depressed. B-lymphocyte function is variable, and some patients have normal levels of serum immunoglobulins, sometimes with functional antibodies. The differential diagnosis of lymphopenia with normal serum immunoglobulins is summarized in Table 2.

Table 2 *Differential diagnosis, in order of probability worldwide, in patients with lymphopenia ($<1.3 \times 10^9$/l), normal serum immunoglobulin levels and opportunistic viral, fungal and protozoal infections*

Transient (viral infections e.g. herpes simplex, varicella, measles)
Severe nutritional deficiency
AIDS
Cytotoxic/immunosuppressive drugs
Severe combined immunodeficiency (some types)[a]
Thymic aplasia[a]
Purine nucleoside phosphorylase deficiency (very rare)[a]

[a]Nearly always in infants.

TREATMENT

Regular transfusions of normal red cells, containing ADA, have been useful in some patients with residual ADA activity, although in the long term this may lead to iron overload. The red cells metabolize the excess deoxyadenosine in the plasma to inosine. Weekly injections of purified ADA from calf thymus linked to polyethylene glycol (ADA-PEG) have been more successful. Gene therapy is a radical approach, and trials are in progress using viral vectors to transfect the human *ADA* gene into lymphocyte precursors in patients' bone marrow. Bone marrow transplantation is an alternative.

Adenosine deaminase (ADA) deficiency

Although rare, this autosomal recessive disease has achieved notoriety because affected patients have been the first to receive gene therapy. A variety of mutations in the *ADA* gene on chromosome 20 cause the disease. Heterozygotes have half-normal levels of red-cell ADA activity but are healthy. The enzyme is present in both red and white cells and there are healthy individuals who lack red-cell ADA but retain residual activity in their lymphocytes. Most patients present in infancy with classical symptoms of SCID, but a few present later in childhood, and rarely in adolescence or as young adults. Lack of ADA causes deoxyadenosine to accumulate in the plasma, and this inhibits the proliferation of T lymphocytes. Macrophage, and probably antigen-presenting cell, function is also impaired. The effect on B cells is variable, and although some patients may have normal or even raised levels of serum immunoglobulins, there is usually evidence of a functional antibody defect. The diagnosis is made by measuring ADA activity in red cells. Heterozygote detection and prenatal diagnosis are best done using molecular probes for the *ADA* gene.

X-linked SCID

This is a severe form of SCID presenting in infancy with lymphopenia, hypogammaglobulinaemia, and early death. There is evidence of a clinically milder disease presenting later in childhood. The relevant gene codes for the gamma chain of the receptors for interleukin 2, 4, and 7. Molecular probes are available for prenatal diagnosis and to identify carriers.

Lymphocyte MHC class II deficiency

The underlying defect is a mutation in a gene coding for one of the factors involved in the regulation of class II *(DR)* gene transcription. The inheritance is autosomal recessive and many affected families are of North African descent. The immunological abnormalities are not typical of SCID, with a normal circulating lymphocyte count and normal *in vitro* lymphocyte proliferation with mitogens; however, there is no proliferation with antigens. The diagnosis can be confirmed by demonstrating lack of lymphocyte class II expression. Affected infants have a clinically severe type of SCID, underlining the importance of class II in generating protective immunity against infection.

A defect in the expression of MHC class I (originally called the bare lymphocyte syndrome) has been associated with either severe or mild immunodeficiency, and has even been reported in healthy individuals. Defects in the TAP2 peptide transporter genes have been found in some patients.

Reticular dysgenesis

This very severe form of SCID is due to failure of an early stem cell in the bone marrow to differentiate into the white-cell series. Affected infants are neutropenic, lymphopenic, and have no circulating monocytes or macrophages.

Multiple interleukin deficiency

This rare autosomal recessive condition is probably due to mutations in one of the transcriptional regulating proteins for a variety of interleukins, particularly IL-2, which is of central importance for lymphocyte proliferation. One family has been described where there appears to be a defect in the NF-AT transcriptional protein. Patients have a severe immunodeficiency that may respond to regular injections of IL-2 linked to polyethylene glycol (IL2-PEG).

Other syndromes

There are likely to be other rare autosomal recessive conditions involving the function of T cells and macrophages. Omenn's syndrome (SCID with hypereosinophilia), and T-cell deficiencies associated with short-limbed dwarfism or ectodermal dysplasia are examples that are still not well defined. There are also more general metabolic disorders that have a profound effect on the immune system, but these are described under 'Secondary immunodeficiency'.

RAG 1 *and* 2 *gene defects*

The *RAG* genes control the rearrangement of immunoglobulin and TCR genes. Mutations in these genes have been found in about 20 percent of SCID patients, leading to a severe B-cell and variable T-cell deficiency.

Treatment and prognosis

All SCID patients, with the exception of those with IL-2 or ADA deficiency, require early bone-marrow transplantation for survival. The outcome continues to improve, with a 97 per cent survival for those receiving HLA-identical sibling marrow and about 55 per cent long-term survival for those receiving T-cell-depleted parental marrow. Patients with immunodeficiency are ideal candidates for gene therapy and we look forward to technical advances for improving the efficiency of transfecting the relevant genes into bone marrow stem cells.

Syndromes associated with moderate immunodeficiency

Wiskott–Aldrich disease

Wiskott–Aldrich disease is an X-linked disease characterized by thrombocytopenia, lymphopenia with depressed cellular immunity, and lymphoid malignancy: there is usually a mild antibody deficiency, with a low serum IgM and depression of IgM antibody production to polysaccharides. Allergic eczema is common and many patients have a very high serum IgE. Some are prone to infections, mainly bacterial and viral. There are variants with thrombocytopenia and minimal immunodeficiency. Splenectomy is recommended for those with severe thrombocytopenia and haemorrhagic tendency. The diagnosis is confirmed by demonstrating that the platelets are small in size, and that the lymphocytes have a deficiency of sialophorin (CD43) on their surface, an adhesion molecule that belongs to the integrin superfamily. However, the *CD43* gene is not on the X chromosome, so the underlying defect involves the regulation and expression of CD43 on cell surfaces. The relevant gene on the short arm of the X chromosome has recently been cloned.

Defects in DNA repair

Rapid and efficient repair of DNA damage is fundamental to cell survival. The cascade involved in the excision of damaged nucleotides, insertion of new nucleotides, and rejoining (ligation) of the DNA strands is not well understood. However, inherited defects involving excision and rejoining are associated with immunodeficiency.

Ataxia telangiectasia

An autosomal recessive disease characterized by progressive cerebellar ataxia and telangiectasia on exposed areas of skin, particularly on the conjunctivae: the immunodeficiency is variable, but IgA and IgG2 deficiency occurs in about a third, with a few patients having severe panhypogammaglobulinaemia. Lymphopenia is common, with depressed cellular immunity and T-lymphocyte cytotoxicity. The patients are particularly prone to lymphomas, associated with translocations between chromosome 7 and 14, and other malignancies at an early age. Most die from progressive neurological disease, infection, or tumours before the third decade. It is estimated that at least 1 in 200 of the general population is heterozygous for ataxia telangiectasia, and there is evidence that they are also at increased risk of malignancy.

The gene for ataxia telangiectasia has been localized to chromosome 11 but is not yet cloned. The defect involves a failure to excise nucleotide bases damaged by γ-irradiation, and diagnostic and therapeutic irradiation should be kept to a minimum. The Nijmegen breakage syndrome, identified in Dutch patients, appears to be a similar disorder with additional microcephaly and growth retardation

DNA ligation defects

Bloom's syndrome, which is associated with hypersensitivity to ultraviolet light, T-cell defects, poor IgM antibody production, and lymphomas and other tumours at an early age is caused by a defect in regulating the transcription or expression of the ligase-1 gene. One patient with growth retardation and severe immunodeficiency has been described with inherited mutations in a non-functional ligase-1 gene.

T-cell-receptor (TCR) defects

The TCR complex consists of α- and β-chains complexed with the CD3 γ-, δ-, ϵ-, and ζ-chains. Mutations in any one of these genes could theoretically compromise function of the whole complex. Two brothers with IgG2 deficiency and inherited mutations in the *CD3-*γ gene have been described;, one died at 3 years with severe autoimmune haemolytic anaemia following a viral pneumonia, and the other is alive and healthy at 10 years. One child with mutations in the *CD3-*ϵ genes has a clinically mild immunodeficiency. There appears to be redundancy in the TCR complex, and defects in the δ- and ζ-chains are unlikely to be clinically important. Inherited functional defects in the ZAP-70 cytoplasmic protein tyrosine kinase, which is involved in signalling from the CD3 complex, is a rare cause of SCID.

Secondary immunodeficiencies

Lymphoid malignancies, immunosuppressive agents, and AIDS are common causes of severe immunodeficiency, while nutritional deficiencies, metabolic disturbances (e.g. uraemia), and trauma have a less severe affect on the immune system (Table 3). In many of these conditions the primary disease usually overshadows the immunodeficiency, although attention to the latter can improve the quality of life, the best example being the use of immunoglobulin replacement therapy in chronic lymphatic leukaemia.

Recurrent pneumonia and bronchitis suggest antibody deficiency, whereas varicella-zoster and herpes simplex reactivation, oral candida, and rapid growth of skin warts are often early indications of a defect in cellular immunity. The presence of lymphopenia, often overlooked, indicates that the immune system is compromised but is a poor guide to the clinical significance of the defect (Table 4). In practice, circulating CD4+ T-cell counts and serum immunoglobulin levels may influence management, with functional antibody tests (i.e. responses to test immunization) likely to become more widely used.

Lymphoid malignancy

Various types of lymphoreticular malignancy can be associated with both humoral and cellular immunodeficiency, exacerbated by the use of cytotoxic drugs. However, chronic lymphatic leukaemia is the most

Table 3 *Classification of secondary immunodeficiency*

Lymphoreticular malignancy
Chronic lymphatic leukaemia[a]
Myeloma[a]
Therapeutic agents
Corticosteroids[b]
Cyclophosphamide[b]
Azathioprine[b]
Cyclosporin[b]
Anti-T-cell antibodies[b]
Gold[a]
Phenytoin[a]
Penicillamine[a]
Sulphasalazine[a]
Methotrexate[b]
Bleomycin[b]
Vincristine[ab]
cis-platinum[b]
Viruses
HIV[b]
Rubella[a]
Metabolic and vitamin deficiencies
Vitamin A[a]
Zinc (acrodermatitis enteropathica)[b]
Selenium[b]
Transcobalamin II deficiency[a]
Orotic aciduria[ab]
Biotin-dependent carboxylase deficiency[ab]
Renal and liver failure[ab]
Trauma[ab]
Hypercatabolism or increased loss of immunoglobulin
Nephrotic syndrome
Protein-losing enteropathy:
Lymphangiectasia
Inflammatory bowel disease
Dystrophia myotonica

Predominant effect on antibody production[a] or cellular immunity[b].

Table 4 *Differential diagnosis in patients with lymphopenia ($<1.3 \times 10^9/l$) and opportunistic viral, fungal and protozoal infections*

Primary immunodeficiency
Severe combined immunodeficiency
PNP deficiency
Thymic aplasia
CVID type I
X-linked hyper-IgM
DNA repair defects:
Ataxia telangiectasia
Bloom's syndrome
Exclude secondary immunodeficiency
AIDS
Drugs
Lymphoma
Severe nutritional deficiency
Intestinal lymphangiectasia

CVID, common varied immunodeficiency; PNP, purine nucleoside phosphorylase.

important, with most patients developing hypogammaglobulinaemia during the course of their disease. Many suffer from recurrent infections, particularly of the upper and lower respiratory tract, and benefit from regular immunogloblin replacement therapy. The cause of the antibody deficiency is not understood, but is unlikely to be solely due to a 'crowding out' of the normal lymphoid apparatus by malignant cells.

Myeloma

This may also be associated with profound antibody deficiency, which explains the predisposition to pneumococcal pneumonia and septicaemia. Modern cytotoxic therapy can now induce prolonged remissions, so it is worth treating these patient with immunoglobulin during the induction period. The cause of the antibody deficiency is not known but the malignant plasma cells appear to produce factors that inhibit antibody production from normal cells.

Drugs

The extensive literature on the immunological effects of cytotoxic agents and steroids will not be reviewed here. Many of these drugs have a profound effect on cellular immunity, as shown by the severity of varicella in patients on corticosteroids, and the risk of cytomegalovirus infection with cytotoxic agents. Some of these drugs, particularly cyclophosphamide and azathioprine, will compromise antibody production and may lower the serum immunoglobulins after prolonged use. Gold commonly lowers the serum IgM and IgG and occasionally causes IgA deficiency or severe hypogammaglobulinaemia with infections. Penicillamine, sulphasalazine, and phenytoin may also cause severe hypogammaglobulinaemia, but more commonly selective IgA deficiency. The effects of these drugs are reversible, but it may take up to 2 years for antibody production to recover. It is not clear whether this is an idiosyncratic reaction or whether the drugs trigger CVID in susceptible individuals.

Viruses

HIV is the most important immunosuppressive virus, and is described in Section 7. Many other viruses may cause moderate immunosuppression during active infection, the best known being measles and cytomegalovirus, which depress cellular immunity. Fetal infection with rubella virus may rarely lead to permanent depression of IgG and IgA antibody production, sometimes with high total and specific non-neutralizing IgM antibodies.

Nutritional immunodeficiency

This is probably the most common cause of immunodeficiency worldwide and contributes to the high infant death rate in the Third World. Protein-calorie malnutrition and deficiency of vitamins and trace elements, particularly vitamin A, zinc, and probably selenium, can lead to significant depression of T-lymphocyte function as well as poor antibody production. Vitamin A supplementation has been shown to reduce childhood mortality from infection in New Guinea. Rare autosomal recessive conditions compromising the absorption of crucial vitamins and elements have highlighted their importance; a deficiency of transcobalamin II causes severe vitamin B_{12} deficiency in infancy, with neutropenia, megaloblastic anaemia, and hypogammaglobulinaemia; a primary failure to absorb zinc causes acrodermatitis enteropathica, with a characteristic skin rash, malabsorption, and infections. There is some evidence that vitamin deficiencies, particularly B_{12} in vegans, may contribute to a predisposition to tuberculosis in Indian Asians.

Severe trauma and thermal injury

Both humoral and cellular immune depression is common in these conditions, but the antibody deficiency is of little importance in modern intensive-care units where broad-spectrum antibiotics are used routinely. The longer the patient remains critically ill, the more likely the effects of cellular immunodeficiency will become clinically important, such patients often dying from cytomegalovirus or fungal infections. Immunosuppression may be more pronounced in young children, particularly after burns when antibody production may be severely depressed.

Increased catabolism/loss of immunoglobulin

Loss of immunoglobulin from the kidney or bowel is an important cause of mild hypogammaglobulinaemia, but is rarely of clinical significance. Serum IgM, being a larger molecule, is usually normal, with low IgA and IgG. The nephrotic syndrome and protein-losing enteropathy are common causes, the latter being difficult to diagnose when the serum albumin is normal. Leakage of protein and lymphocytes occurs in primary or secondary intestinal lymphangiectasia, the combination of hypogammaglobulinaemia, low serum albumin, and lymphopenia being a useful clue to this diagnosis. An increase in the catabolism of many proteins occurs in chronic infection/inflammation, but this is never severe enough to cause hypogammaglobulinaemia unless there is a primary defect in immunoglobulin synthesis. Increased catabolism of IgG occurs in dystrophia myotonica but the mechanism is unknown.

REFERENCES

Cooper, M.D. and Butler, J.L. (1989). Primary immunodeficiency diseases. In *Fundamental immunology,* (2nd edn), (ed. W.E. Paul). Raven Press, New York.

Primary immunodeficiency diseases—report of a WHO Scientific Group. (1995). *Clinical Experimental Immunology,* **99**, Suppl. 1.

5.4 Complement and disease

H.M. Chapel

Basic physiology

Introduction

The existence of complement pathways that increase the effects of the immune system has been known for almost 100 years. The alternative pathway was discovered first but the importance of the system was not appreciated at first. The details of the classical pathway were described originally in the 1940s and then more precisely in the 1950s and 1960s. The demonstration in the 1960s that animals who were deficient in classical-pathway components still showed complement activation led to the rediscovery of the alternate pathway; hence the name. It is phylogenetically older and supplements the non-antigen-specific immune system, that is it is independent of immunoglobulins and immune complexes (Fig. 1) and enhances the action of phagocytic cells (macrophages and neutrophils), mast cells, eosinophils, and basophils. It has been suggested that this evolved before the development of the antigen-specific lymphoid system. The alternate pathway is not only older but also less efficient, although the positive feedback loop provides amplification.

The terminology of the complement systems is confusing. Components are numbered in the order in which they were discovered and not in the order in which they take an active role in any given pathway. Components of the classical and final lytic pathways are numbered, where those of the alternate pathway have letters. Many components are pre-enzymes (Fig. 2), which become activated by the preceding component; activated enzymes are distinguished from their precursors by a bar drawn above the component, for example $\overline{C1}$. The activated enzyme will then act on the next component in the sequence of the pathway. An individual component is usually fragmented into two parts: the new active enzyme is the larger fragment, suffixed with a 'b'; the smaller component has biological activity and is suffixed with an 'a'. (The Complement Committee of the World Health Organization has yet to bring C2 into line; for consistency we will use the suggested logical terminology of C2a for the small fragment and C2b for the larger fragment.)

The complement pathways, like the clotting pathways, are cascades, in which a great deal of functional amplification can occur as a result of the activation of a few molecules. Regulation is therefore crucial and is provided in two ways. If an activated enzyme does not find its substrate rapidly, there is spontaneous decay, the active site of the component is non-functional, and the sequence is terminated. There are also specific inhibitors for each component, which regulate ongoing activation.

The two complement pathways are initiated by different stimuli, but both result in activation of C3, which, in turn, provokes the activation of the final lytic pathway (Fig. 1). The classical pathway is activated by immune complexes, composed of IgG or IgM and the relevant antigen. The sequential activation of C1, C4, C2 results in the production of C3 convertase, an enzyme that then activates C3. In contrast, the alternate pathway is activated by bacterial products and other non-immune substances. Small amounts of C3 are continuously activated by hydrolysis; the presence of alternate-pathway activators stabilizes the active C3b fragment, which results in more C3 being broken down via the positive feedback loop (see Fig. 1).

There are at least three main functions of the complement system (Fig. 3): opsonization, lysis of pathogenic organisms, and the production of inflammatory mediators. The attachment of C3 to such as immune complexes, bacteria or bacterial products is a process known as opsonization. The resulting macromolecules containing C3 fragments are recognized by complement receptors, particularly those on phagocytic cells. The binding of these substances to complement receptors activates the phagocytes and the macromolecules are ingested by the cell and usually destroyed. Opsonization is probably the most important function of the complement system. This is underlined by the fact that individuals with deficiencies of C3 suffer recurrent pyogenic infections as well as immune-complex diseases. Activation of the final lytic pathway, also known as the membrane-attack pathway, is demonstrated traditionally by lysis of red cells, though this may not be an important physiological function *in vivo*. It is only known to be involved in cold autoimmune haemolytic anaemia. On the other hand, failure to lyse bacteria, owing to a deficiency of a component of the final lytic pathway, results in recurrent pyogenic infections, thus demonstrating the importance of such lysis in preventing infections, particularly neisserial infections.

Inflammation is vital for host defence and repair of tissue damage. It is too important to be dependent on a single pathway and inflammation can be initiated by several different systems, of which the complement system is one. Many steps in that system are associated with the production of small fragments that have an influence on inflammation.

The chief site of synthesis of complement components is the liver. This has been formally shown for C3, C6, C8, and factor B by demonstrating a change of allotypes of these components in the plasma of recipients of liver transplants; other components have also been shown to be synthesized by hepatocytes and monocytes in culture. The liver is the primary site of the acute-phase reaction and complement components C3, C4, C5, C6, and factor B act as acute-phase proteins. This means that the rate of synthesis of these components is increased during inflammation, as a result of increased production of interleukin (**IL**)-1 and -6. The practical consequences of acute-phase synthesis is a raised concentration of these components in the serum during inflammation. This may mask complement consumption, which results in a decrease of an individual component involved (Fig. 4).

Pathways

As shown in Fig. 1, there are two activation pathways in the complement system, as well as the final lytic pathway, which is triggered by either of the activation pathways.

Fig. 1 The three complement pathways (reproduced from Chapel and Haeney (1993), with permission).

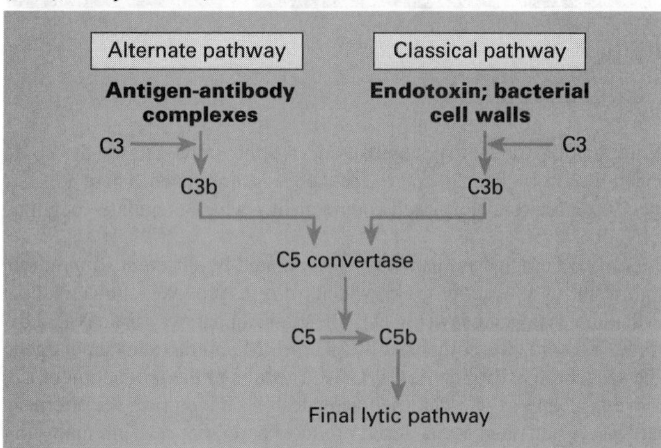

Fig. 2 Cleavage of complement components (reproduced from Chapel and Haeney (1993), with permission).

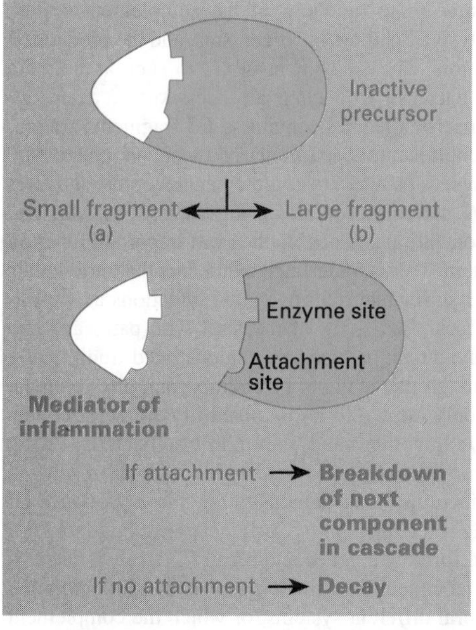

CLASSICAL PATHWAY

The classical pathway provides an efficient mechanism for the removal of specific antigen–antibody complexes. It is activated by the change in shape of antibodies once they are complexed with their specific antigen; this allows the binding of the multiple globular domains of C1q. Thus the pentameric head of IgM in an immune complex is most efficient at binding C1q whereas IgG molecules only bind C1q if they are in close proximity to each other and provide an appropriate binding site for C1q (Fig. 5). Non-complement-fixing IgG antibodies (e.g. anti-Rhesus antibodies) bind to epitopes that are too distant from each other to allow C1q to bridge the gap. Activated C1q binds with C1r and C1s to form

Fig. 3 Functions of complement pathways (reproduced from Chapel and Haeney (1993), with permission).

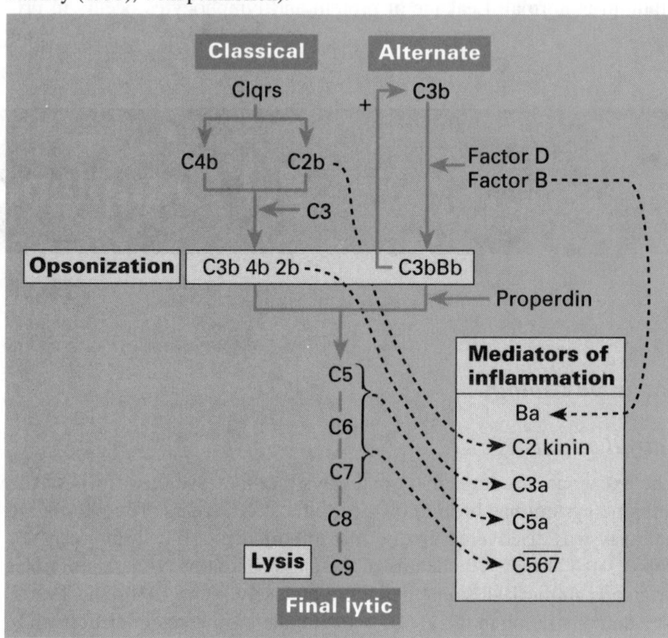

Fig. 4 Acute-phase complement components.

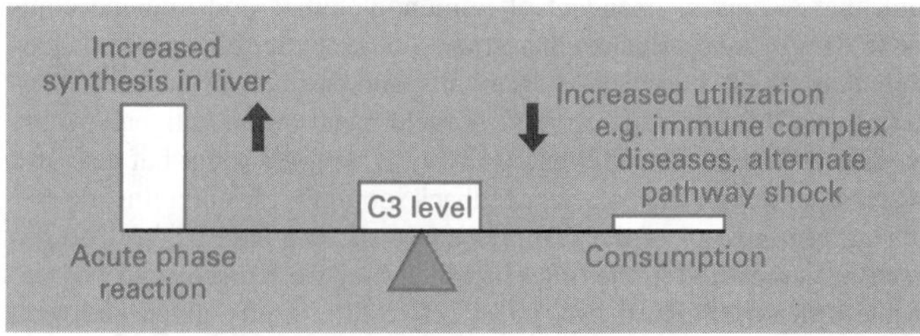

Fig. 5 Classical pathway generation of C5 convertase.

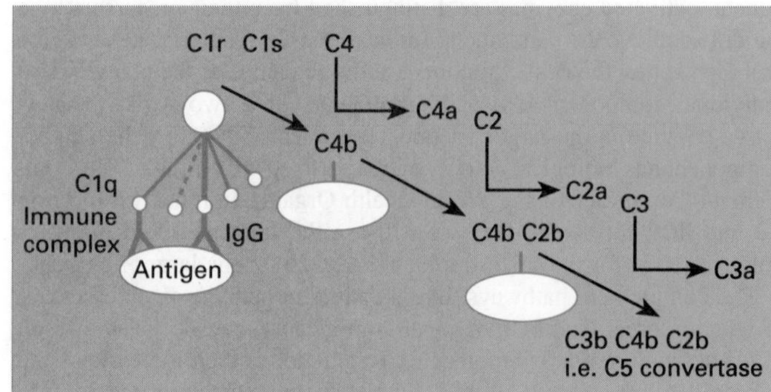

C4 convertase, an enzyme that will break down C4. C4 molecules are fragmented to C4a, an inflammatory mediator, and C4b, which becomes convalently bound to the surface of the antigen–antibody complex where it acts as both a binding site for C2 and a C2 convertase. The resulting C4b2b complex is the classical-pathway C3 convertase, the enzyme that goes on to break down C3.

C1q is closely homologous to mannan-binding protein. This protein can bind to micro-organisms, such as mycoplasma, and then bind with C1r and C1s to initiate the classical pathway. The plasma concentration of mannan-binding protein in adults is much lower than that of C1q and therefore this protein is probably not of clinical significance in adults; however, in young infants, where the level of C1q is low in association with low serum IgG levels, mannan-binding protein may be an important protective mechanism.

ALTERNATE-PATHWAY ACTIVATION

Although some of the components of the alternate pathway are individually analogous to those of the classical pathway, the mechanism of activation is quite different. Small amounts of C3 are activated continually by proteolysis *in vivo.* In the absence of an activating substance, the resultant C3b is rapidly catabolized and no further activation takes place. In the presence of an activating surface, such as a bacterial product, bacterial cell wall or, in particular a yeast cell wall, C3b is concentrated and this enables factor B to be broken down (Fig. 6). Factor B is cleaved into two fragments by factor D: factor Ba, an inflammatory protein, and factor Bb, which binds with C3b to form C3bBb, the alternate-pathway C3 convertase (Fig. 6). C3bBb is a naturally unstable enzyme and spontaneously dissociates into its individual components. However, the complex can be stabilized by properdin, which slows the dissociation, allowing the positive feedback loop to cycle (Fig. 6). Factors B and D are normally present in low concentrations in the tissues and alternate-pathway activation usually takes place only in plasma.

Other substances stabilize C3bBb and thus permit amplification of the pathway. One is an autoantibody to this complex, known as C3 nephritic factor. This is present in some patients with membranoproliferative glomerular nephritis (type II) (see Section 20); these patients have low or undetectable serum levels of C3 and normal levels of C4. The role of this autoantibody in the actual pathogenesis of the renal lesion (C3 deposits in the mesangium and glomerular basement membrane) is unclear, as is the clinical association between the presence of C3 nephritic factor and partial lipodystrophy (see Section 20).

FINAL LYTIC PATHWAY (OR MEMBRANE-ATTACK COMPLEX)

In contrast to the initiation pathways, the final lytic pathway depends on the complexing of different complement components rather than enzymatic activity. Once C5 has been cleaved by C5 convertase into C5a and C5b (Fig. 3), the larger fragment, C5b, complexes with C6 and C7 and the complex $\overline{C567}$ is then inserted into lipid bilayers. C8 and C9 bind alongside the complex to form a tubular membrane plug, which can be seen by electron microscopy. This results in loss of membrane integrity and the death of the cell or organism.

Fig. 6 Alternate pathway generation of C5 convertase.

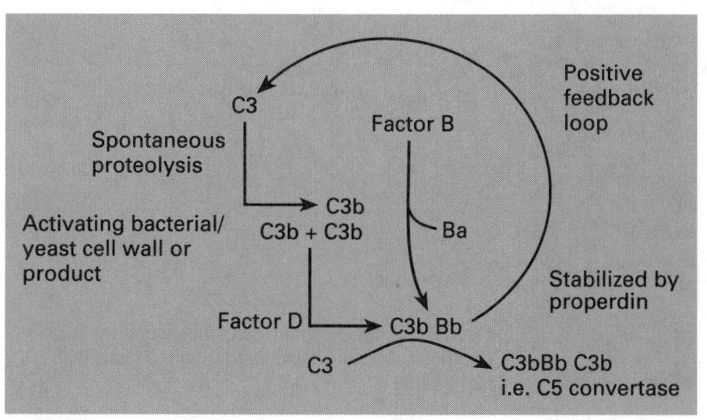

Regulation

Control of activation of the classical pathway is largely due to a specific inhibitor for C1 esterase that inactivates the whole C1 complex. Deficiency of this inhibitor, whether congenital or acquired, results in recurrent attacks of angio-oedema. The inherent instability of C2b prevents excessive activation; in the absence of C4 the enzyme rapidly decays. Decay of C4b is promoted by specific C4b-binding protein, which acts as a soluble cofactor for the enzyme factor I (I for inhibitor). In addition, a membrane analogue of the C4-binding protein, namely CR1 (see below), accelerates the C4b2b decay, as do the membrane proteins DAF (decay accelerating factor) and membrane cofactor protein (CD46).

The alternate pathway feedback loop is controlled by the catabolism of C3b to the inactive fragment, iC3b, which can no longer bind factor B. This is achieved by binding factor H, which competes with factor B for the active binding site, and then acts as a cofactor for the enzyme, factor I. Factor I breaks C3b into iC3b and then iC3b rapidly into C3c and C3dg. Continued activation of the feedback loop therefore depends on C3b binding factor B in preference to factor H; conversely, inhibition depends on the binding of factor H preferentially.

As in the classical pathway, CR1, a close analogue of both C4-binding protein and factor H, can inhibit the formation of C3bBb.

Regulation of the final lytic pathway involves the inherent instability of the complexes as well as specific inhibitors of the individual components. The insertion of C5bC6C7 complexes into cell membranes can be inhibited by a variety of plasma proteins not yet well classified. Cell membranes themselves contain regulatory proteins for C8 and C9 binding. The absence of these in patients with paroxysmal nocturnal haemoglobinuria results in acute sensitivity of the red cells of these patients to complement-mediated lysis (see Section 22).

Receptors

Receptors for activated complement components are important for opsonization and phagocytosis (Fig. 7) as well as inflammation. Those so far described recognize various fragments of C3 or soluble inflammatory mediators C5a, C3a, and C4a (Table 1). Membrane complement receptors for C3 are of two types: regulatory proteins, namely complement receptors (**CR**)1 and CR2, and those that belong the β_2-integrin supergene family, adherence proteins CR3 and CR4 (Table 1). Complement receptors may be either anchored to, or inserted in, cell membranes. They may have other functions depending on the cell on which they are expressed and, in addition, they may react with other substances (ligands) in order to be effective. Thus the function of CR1 (CD35) on erythrocytes is not only to inactivate C3b and C4b in order to prevent further inflammation; it also transports inactivated immune complexes on the erythrocytes to the liver for disposal. When CR1 on phagocytic cells react with C3b, endocytosis or even phagocytosis are initiated. In addition, CR1 are present on the renal podocytes, where they are thought to play a part both in inactivation and endocytosis, thus preventing renal damage by immune complexes and providing another means of clearance. The role of CR2 on B lymphocytes is less clear, as B-cell proliferation and antibody production may be both stimulated or inhibited through this receptor.

CR3 and CR4 (Table 1) are present on myeloid and monocytic cells, combine not only with C3 fragments but also with other ligands such as lipopolysaccharide or *Escherichia coli,* and provoke binding and ingestion of these substances.

Receptors for other components of complement include those for the C1q inhibitor (whose function remains unclear) and for C5a and C3a, which are present on a variety of cells but known to be involved in the degranulation of mast cells and basophils; in addition the C5a receptor on neutrophils is known to be involved in mobilization from the bone marrow, chemotaxis, and aggregation.

Biological functions of complement

Figure 1 shows that there are three major functions of complement: opsonization, lysis, and inflammation. As mentioned in the Introduction, the most important function is probably opsonization. This is important physiologically not only for the removal of the soluble immune complexes formed as a result of antibody–antigen interaction but also for the removal of bacteria and bacterial products. Furthermore, the rapid clearance of antigen from the site of entry following formation of immune complexes and complement activation, and the concentration of the complexed antigen by cells such as dendritic cells in lymph nodes, enable antigens to be localized in germinal centres, which is ideal for provoking antibody production.

C3 is central to opsonization and individuals with low or undetectable C3 are prone to all types of bacterial infection, but in particular to infections with encapsulated bacteria. Similarly, deficiencies of classical (C4 or C2) or alternate components (properdin) result in reduced opsonization and increased risk of bacterial infection. In addition, failure of the classical pathway results in immune-complex diseases (Fig. 8). The physiological importance of bacterial lysis by the complement system is demonstrated by the susceptibility of patients with deficiencies of final lytic-pathway components to infection with pyogenic bacteria, even though their C3 levels are normal.

The complement system is one of several involved in the production of inflammation. It interrelates with other enzyme cascades, particularly those for coagulation and fibrinolysis as well as the kinin system. Some of the small complement fragments have been identified as biologically active in inflammation (see Fig. 3). Circulating C3a and C5a fragments can be detected in overwhelming complement activation such as occurs in sepsis, meningitis, severe trauma, shock lung, Gram-negative septicaemia, or shock following renal dialysis or pulmonary bypass operations.

Failure of 'inflammatory' signs in infection, such as the absence of pus, is indicative of a major defect in neutrophil numbers or function. Neutropenia is the most common cause but lack of complement receptors on inflammatory cells, such as neutrophils, which then fail to migrate to the inflammatory site, should be considered if circulating neutrophil numbers are normal.

Genetics

Although many of the complement proteins show inherited structural polymorphisms, these allotypes are rarely related directly to disease, other than when the components are missing (see below). The polymorphisms have been detected by differences in molecular weight or antigenicity, and most of the components function normally. Complement components are the products of single genes. There are two loci for C4, *C4A* and *C4B;* their products differ slightly in structure and function. Thus each individual has four genes that are responsible for the production of serum C4, which explains the wide variability of C4 levels in normal individuals. The most common malfunctioning gene is *C4AQO,* which is often associated with the particular HLA-A1, B8, DR3 haplotype that is associated with several autoimmune diseases. Whether or not the absence of functioning *C4A* genes is involved in the pathogenesis of these diseases is unknown.

Genes for C2 and factor B are closely linked with *C4A* and *C4B* within the major histocompatibility complex **(MHC)** on chromosome 6. Both C2 and factor B show polymorphisms, though that of C2 is less variable. In practice, other than frank deficiencies, these polymorphisms of complement are not thought to have clinical significance, though this may yet turn out to be an unfounded assumption.

Several of the complement components are members of a supergene family (Fig. 9). Members of such families share one or more homologous domains, sequences of similar DNA structure that may have similar functions, though not always. Because members of the supergene family are often susceptible to the same inhibitors, it may be that the homologous domains offer a common inhibitory mechanism. An example is C1 esterase inhibitor, which blocks not only C1s and C1r but also plasmin, clotting factor XIIa, clotting factor X1a, and kallikrein.

Members of a given supergene family may have arisen by gene duplication, particularly those that are present in the same area of a given chromosome. Genes for C4 and C2 (of the classical pathway) and factor B (of the alternate pathway) are clustered together as class 3 antigens of the MHC on human chromosome 6. They have similar functions: C4 and C2 are principal components in activation of the classical pathway and factor B is a principal component of activation of the alternate pathway. These genes have almost certainly arisen by duplication.

Another example is the clustering of the regulators of complement activation, a group of proteins whose production is coded on chromosome 1 (Fig. 9). These proteins include transmembrane proteins, which are fixed to cell surfaces in order to protect them from excessive complement activation. Examples are CR1 and membrane cofactor protein, both of which help the enzyme factor I in the breakdown of C3b to iC3b; CR1 ensures that iC3b is rapidly broken down to harmless C3dg.

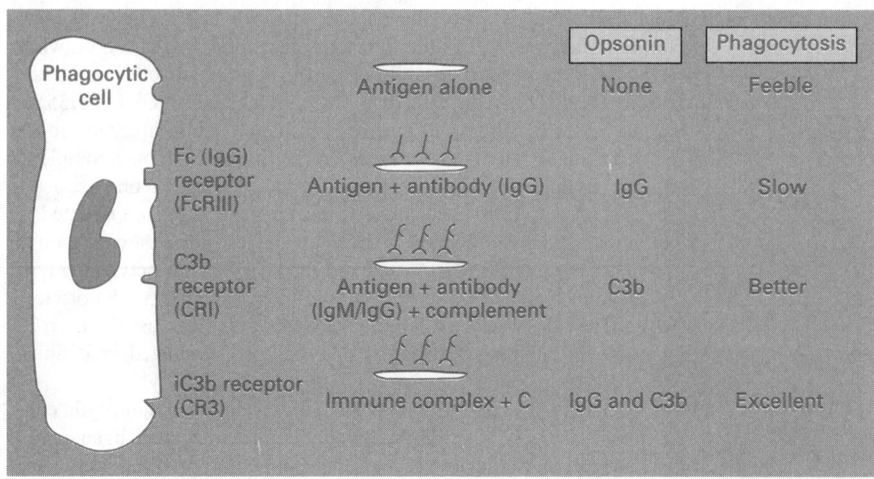

Fig. 7 Phagocytic-membrane complement receptors (reproduced from Chapel and Haeney (1993), with permission).

Table 1 *Three families of receptors for activated complement fragments*

Complement receptors	C3 fragment that is ligand	Main cellular distribution	Function	Leucocyte antigen workship number
1. Regulatory proteins				
CR1	C3b	Erythrocytes	Cofactor for C3b cleavage—C3dg + C3c Transport of immune complexes	CD35
		Monocytes	Adherence of immune complexes and (with other surface ligand–receptor interactions) phagocytosis	
CR2	C3d	B cells Renal podocytes	Protection against immune complexes	CD21
		B cells, dendritic cells	Involved in B-lymphocyte differentiation	
2. *β_2-integrins* (adherence proteins)				
CR3	iC3b	Neutrophils, monocytes	Probably several types of receptors (freely mobile, linked to cytoskeleton etc.) for phagocytosis	CD716/ CD18
CR4	iC3b	Tissue macrophages	Also needed for crossing endothelium at sites of inflammation	CD11c/ CD18
3. Receptors for soluble inflammatory mediators				
C5aR	C5a	Mast cells, neutrohils	Trigger mast cells to release mediators	
C3/4aR	C3a/4a	Mast cells, eosinophils	Trigger to release mediators	
C1qR	C1q	B cells, neutrophils monocytes, fibroblasts	?	

Fig. 8 Inherited complement deficiencies (reproduced from Chapel and Haeney (1993), with permission).

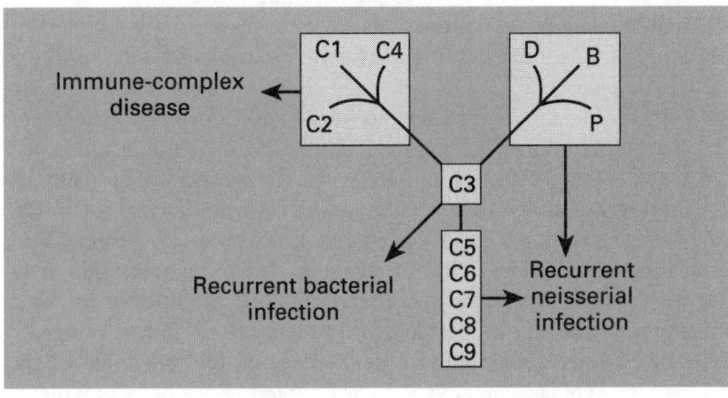

Fig. 9 Regulators of complement activation coded on chromosome 1 (reproduced from Lachmann *et al.* (1993) with permission).

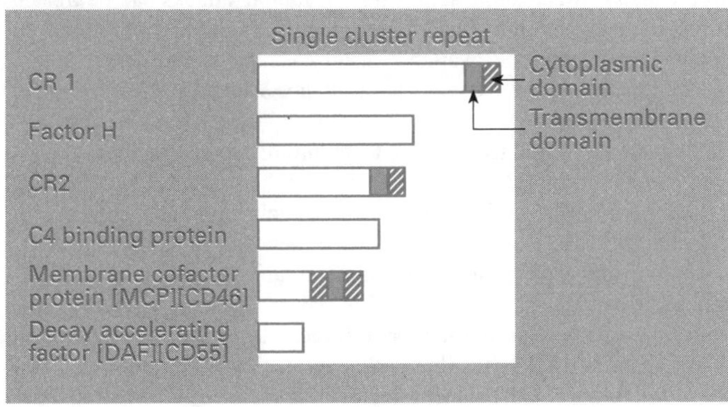

Decay accelerating factor is anchored to the cell surface and is a regulatory component of the complement system in that it accelerates the decay of both C4bC2b and C3bBb. The cofactor of factor I for the breakdown of C4 is a soluble protein, C4-binding protein; it, too, is coded in the same region of chromosome 1.

Diseases of the complement systems

Role of complement in immunopathogenic mechanisms

Complement-mediated disease may result either from a deficiency in the system or from excessive, prolonged, or persistent activation.

As with other components of the immune system, a deficiency of an individual complement component can lead to a variety of diseases. Deficiency may be inherited, as in congenital deficiencies of individual components, or acquired if a process has led to the total consumption of an individual or several components. Deficiencies may lead to persistent infection, owing to failure of opsonization or bacterial lysis, or continued inflammation following physiological activation, perhaps as the result of failure to complete the process of opsonization to remove soluble complexes. Inflammatory mediators are liberated from the activation pathways as far as the missing component; the accompanying failure to remove the immune complexes results in persistent activation of the classical pathway. Thus a deficiency of one component may allow the continuous activation of others, resulting in inflammation.

In a similar way an intact complement system may cause disease if activated persistently or by excessive stimuli. Failure to clear immune complexes fast enough in the presence of continually renewed antigen (such as in malaria) results in inflammation and immune-complex disease. Excessive activation, for example by large number of Gram-negative bacteria, can cause shock; the carbohydrate moieties on the surface of the organisms provide binding for the alternate-pathway components with subsequently massive activation and release of vascular mediators. Shock lung is associated with rapid and excessive production of C5a anaphylotoxin, resulting in aggregation and trapping of neutrophils in the pulmonary vasculature accompanied by a peripheral-blood neutropenia. A similar type of activation was seen with the earlier forms of renal dialysis membranes and cardiopulmonary bypass through first-generation oxygenators.

Deficiency of components

Unlike the specific immune system, where a defect in antibody production leads to recurrent bacterial infections and a deficiency of T cells to recurrent infections with fungi and viruses, deficiencies of complement components were originally described in otherwise healthy individuals. This underlines the fact that there are several mechanisms resulting in inflammation, opsonization, and phagocytosis so that failure of one does not jeopardize these important functions. The complement system is particularly important in the prevention of infection soon after invasion of the pathogen, when there is little IgG antibody, as complement is well activated by IgM, the first isotype of antibody produced to a pathogenic organism. Later, high levels of IgG antibody provoke additional phagocytosis though IgG Fc receptors on neutrophils and tissue macrophages (Fig. 7). Treatment of patients who have deficiencies of complement components is difficult. Replacement of components is impractical because most have a very short half-life (less than 24 h). Furthermore, there is a balance to be maintained, as discussed above, between helpful inflammation to remove immune complexes and the pathogenic activation resulting in disease.

The earliest descriptions of complement-component deficiencies, usually reporting only one such deficiency in any one individual, were made in the 1960s. These deficiencies can be roughly divided into three groups (Fig. 8). Failure of the classical pathway, owing to an individual component deficiency of C2, C4, or any of the components of C1, results in immune-complex disease, the systemic lupus erythematosus (**SLE**)-like syndromes (Fig. 8). These may be accompanied by recurrent, severe infections. Failure of C3, whether congenital or acquired, is associated with pyogenic infection. Congenital deficiency of C3 production is very rare; most C3 deficiencies are secondary to an autoantibody, such as C3 nephritic factor, or a deficiency of factor 1, resulting in rapid consumption of C3. Defects in the alternate-pathway components and those of the final lytic pathway are associated with recurrent neisserial infections (Fig. 8).

C1q deficiency may be due to total absence of C1q or due to normal synthesis of an abnormal, dysfunctional protein. The effect of the dysfunctional protein is a high incidence of immune-complex disease and of severe skin infections. C1r and C1s deficiencies have been described but are very rare.

C2 deficiency is the most common isolated deficiency of a complement component amongst Caucasians, being found in approx. 1:10 000 of the population; it is not been found in Japanese. It is probable that one-third of patients with C2 deficiency are healthy, that a further third have SLE, and a third have another immune-complex disease, with or without infection.

C4 deficiency is associated with the HLA-A1, B8, DR3 haplotype; this haplotype carries not only the susceptibility genes for SLE but also those for coeliac disease and autoimmune endocrine diseases. However, C4-deficient individuals have an increased risk for SLE but not the latter two diseases. Furthermore, C4 deficiency is also associated with SLE in those ethnic groups who do not have the A1, B8, DR3 haplotype, suggesting that it is the C4 deficiency, rather than the MHC associations, that are immunopathogenic in SLE.

Known deficiencies of the alternate pathway components are restricted to properdin deficiency, which was originally described as associated with severe, often fatal neisserial infections. More recently, families have been found in Israel in whom these neisserial infections have been less severe. There is currently only one family with factor D deficiency; as yet no individuals with factor B deficiency have been described.

Deficiencies of the final lytic-pathway components, although rare among Caucasians, are associated with recurrent neisserial infections. C6 deficiency is common in the black population of South Africa. The marked prevalence of homozygous C6 deficiency may be associated with protection against the high infant mortality that follows gastroenteritis and shock, as C6 deficiency protects against endotoxic shock. C7 and C8 deficiencies are well described in the Middle East, particularly Israel; they are associated with recurrent, non-fatal, meningococcal meningitis. C9 deficiency is common among Japanese, with a prevalence of 1:1000, although the association with susceptibility to meningococcal disease in that population is only slight.

Deficiency of complement regulators

As with deficiency of complement components, deficiency of complement regulators may be congenital or acquired and partial or total. A good example is the deficiency of C1 esterase inhibitor, which is associated with angio-oedema. The hereditary form of angio-oedema was described first but, more recently, acquired deficiencies have been found in two types of patients, elderly individuals with a covert B-cell lymphoma where an abnormal monoclonal autoantibody may have anti-idiotypic activity, and young women with polyclonal autoimmune antibodies that cleave C1 esterase inhibitor *in vivo*.

Hereditary angio-oedema is due to a deficiency of C1 esterase inhibitor. Inheritance follows a dominant autosomal pattern. Lack of sufficient quantities of functional protein results in episodic attacks of oedema, which characteristically last between 12 and 24 h, are not itchy, and are not associated with urticaria. These episodes usually affect the subcutaneous tissues but may involve the bowel, resulting in abdominal pain, or rarely produce a potentially fatal laryngeal oedema. Though some attacks are triggered by a known factor, such as dental extraction or trauma, many have no obvious predisposing cause.

Uninhibited activation of the classical pathway generates a high concentration of C2 kinins, C2 fragments with kinin-like activity, resulting in increased vascular permeability and tissue oedema. C2 kinins are produced by plasmin, which degrades C2a and C2b in the absence of C1 esterase inhibitor. Once the circulating C2 has been consumed, the attack aborts spontaneously and there is a rest period whilst synthesis of C2 allows a sufficient concentration of C2 to build up again. The diagnosis of hereditary angio-oedema depends on a low serum C4 in association with low levels of C1 esterase inhibitor demonstrated by a functional assay. Antigenic measurements alone are insufficient, as a small proportion (10–15 per cent) of patients have normal antigenic levels of C1 esterase inhibitor in the presence of low functional levels, owing to the synthesis of a dysfunctional protein. Both types of patients respond to treatment with modified androgens such as danazol or stanozolol. The side-effects of these drugs, such as delayed puberty in children, the prevention of pregnancy, or abnormal liver enzymes, may require alternative treatment with plasmin inhibitors such as ϵ-aminocaproic acid or tranexamic acid. Life-threatening attacks can be treated by replacing the inhibitor intravenously and C1 esterase inhibitor concentrate should now be available in all casualty departments. A less effective alternative if the concentrate is not at hand is an infusion of fresh-frozen plasma.

Deficiency of C3 is usually due to failure of factor I or the presence of an autoantibody, C3 nephritic factor; in either case, C3 is consumed by lack of inhibition of the positive feedback loop. The presence of nephritic factor is associated with dense deposits of C3 in the renal mesangium and glomerular basement membranes of patients with membranoproliferative glomerulonephritis (type II), but whether the nephritic factor has an immunopathogenic role is doubtful, as not all patients with low C3 levels due to this autoantibody develop renal disease. Furthermore, C3 nephritic factor is associated with partial lipodystrophy, which tends to come on after virus infections in children; all children with lipodystrophy who have a positive C3 nephritic factor should be followed for the development of nephritis (see Sections 20 and 23).

Deficiencies of receptors

There are only two complement receptors whose absence is at present known to be associated with disease, CR1 and the β_2-integrin family. Low numbers of CR1 are found on red cells in patients with SLE. Although there is genetic variation in numbers as well as polymorphisms of the proteins, whether either of these have a role in disease susceptibility in lupus remains controversial because low CR1 erythrocyte numbers and raised C3dg levels are found in a variety of diseases associated with complement activation, particularly in active phases of disease. Immune complexes are normally transported to the liver by CR1, which also assist in the breakdown of C3b to C3dg. This enables circulating complexes to be removed in the liver without involvement of the lymphoid system and possible enhancement of antibody formation. Failure of CR1 in patients with lupus results in inappropriate deposition of immune complexes in a variety of tissues (Fig. 10) (see Section 18), leading to excessive complement activation and inflammation; subsequent release of autoantigens thus perpetuates immune complexes.

Another disease in which complement receptors are missing is paroxysmal nocturnal haemoglobinuria (Section 22). This is a rare disease in which a clone of haemopoietic cells is abnormally sensitive to complement, owing to a failure of development of membrane-associated complement regulators, CD59 and C8-binding protein. Intravascular haemolysis, haemoglobinuria, and occasional episodes of venous thrombocytosis precede marrow aplasia or leukaemia.

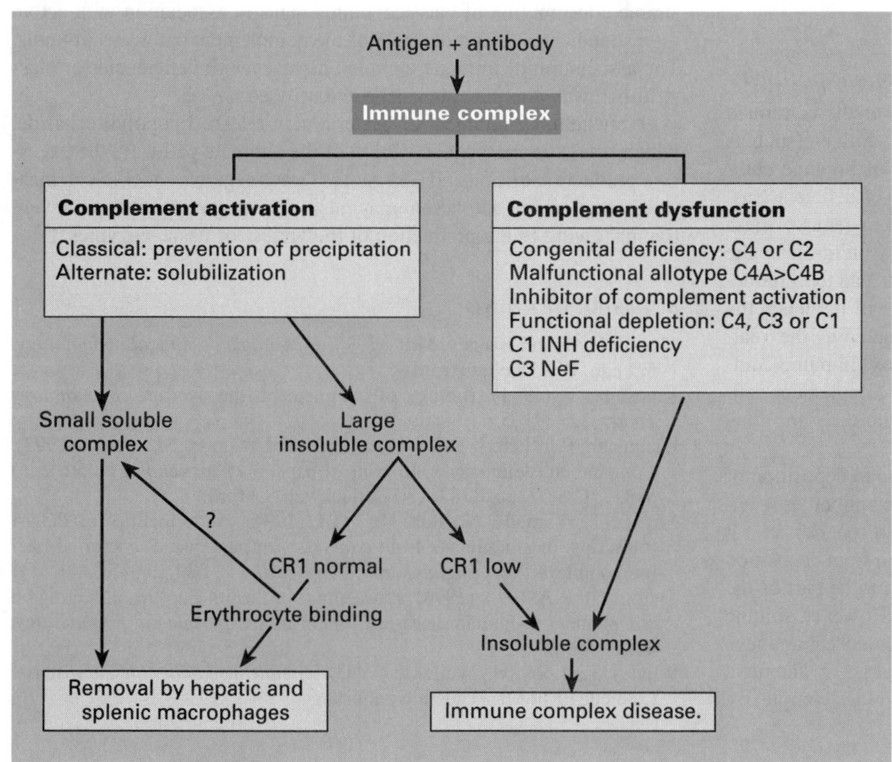

Fig. 10 Role of complement in prevention of immune-complex disease.

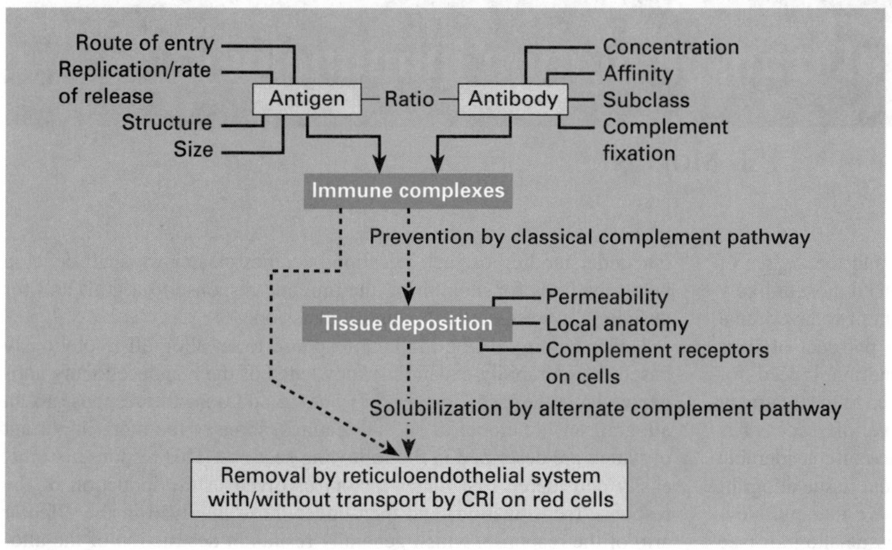

Fig. 11 Factors influencing the development of immune-complex disease (reproduced from Chapel and Haeney (1993), with permission).

Table 2 *Diseases in which complement activation is pathogenic**

Reaction of complement with membrane-fixed specific antigens
Myaesthenia
Goodpasture's syndrome
Cold autoimmune haemolytic anaemia
Reaction of complement with deposited, previously circulating, antigen or immune complexes
Infection of ventriculoatrial shunts
Subacute bacterial endocarditis
Post-streptococcal glomerulonephritis
Systemic lupus erythematosus

*This list is of examples only and is not intended to be exhaustive.

Persistent or excessive activation of complement pathway

Persistent antigen may be due either to the presence or the continued production of an autoantigen or a replicating extrinsic antigen (such as in infection). Either can provide a continuing source of immune complexes in immunocompetent patients. In the presence of deficient classical-pathway components or defective CR1, failure to remove these immune complexes with sufficient speed results in a build-up in the circulation and their deposition in the tissues. This can lead to immune-complex disease, as discussed. A number of factors will influence the development of immune-complex disease (Fig. 11), including the quality and nature of the antibody involved in the complex. Immune complexes containing low-affinity antibody or with poor complement-activating properties are not rapidly cleared by phagocytic cells and may lead to inappropriate deposition.

It is important to try to distinguish inflammation due to deposition of preformed immune complexes from that due to specific antibodies reacting with antigens already fixed in tissues (Table 2). In renal disease it is particularly difficult to distinguish trapping of antigen from deposition of preformed complexes. Where the antigen is known to be part of the membrane, as in Goodpasture's syndrome, it is clear. However, soluble products such as malaria antigen or nephrotoxic streptococcal antigens may bind to basement membrane for reasons of charge or chemical nature, and subsequently bind antibody to form immune complexes. That complement activation is involved in the pathogenesis of many of these diseases is not in doubt, as classical components are found *in situ* in renal biopsy material. Furthermore, it is likely that infiltration by inflammatory cells, such as in Goodpasture's syndrome, is mediated by complement activation following *in situ* formation of immune complexes.

The role of complement in systemic immune-complex diseases is exemplified by SLE. Deposition of preformed complexes was thought to account for renal, cerebral, joint, and skin manifestations, as well as circulating cytopenias, when deposition of IgG, C3, C4, and sometimes DNA were demonstrated in biopsy material. However, specific autoantibodies to endothelial cells, platelets, and erythrocytes also contribute to these manifestations. In addition, DNA has an affinity for glomerular basement membrane and collagen; trapped DNA may act as a fixed antigen for immune-complex formation. However, as before, the demonstrable consumption of classical components in association with active disease indicates the pivotal role of the complement pathways in lupus. The association of immune-complex diseases with deficiencies of classical-pathway components has been discussed above.

Overwhelming numbers of bacteria may release lipopolysaccharide, which results in massive activation of the alternate pathway; the excessive production of C3a and C5a causes Gram-negative shock. Such massive complement activation may also follow pancreatitis or severe trauma, owing to the production of the variety of tissue enzymes.

FURTHER READING

Chapel, H.M. and Haeney, M.R. (1993). *Essentials of clinical immunology.* 3rd edn. Blackwell, Oxford.

Kinoshita, T. (1991). Biology of complement: the overture. *Immunology Today,* **12,** 291–5.

Lachmann, P.J., Peters, D.K., Rosen, F.S., and Walport, M.J. (eds). (1993). Complement deficiencies. In *clinical aspects of immunology.* (5th edn) Vol. 1, Ch. 67, pp. 1287–1304. Blackwell, Oxford.

Miyata, T., Yamada, N., Iida, Y., *et al.* (1994). Abnormalities of PGI-A transcripts in granulocyte from patients with paroxysmal nocturnal haemoglobinuria. *New England Journal of Medicine,* **330,** 249–55.

Thompson, R.A. (ed.). (1994). Proceedings of the 5th European Meeting on complement in human disease. *Clinical and Experimental Immunology,* **47,** Suppl. 2.

Whaley, K., Loos, M., Weiler, J. (1993). *Complement in health and disease.* (2nd edn) Kluwer Academic publishers.

5.5 Principles of transplantation immunology

P.J. Morris

Transplantation of organs is now common practice, and the degree of success that has been achieved today would have seemed most unlikely even as little as 10 years ago. For example, 80 per cent of cadaver renal allografts, 80 per cent of cardiac allografts, and 70 per cent of liver allografts will be functioning at 1 year after transplantation. Indeed, for many years now, renal transplantation has been accepted as the treatment of choice for end-stage renal failure. The present level of success has been reached slowly over the past 30 years, in the face of considerable ignorance about the nature of the immune response to a tissue allograft that may result in rejection despite immunosuppressive therapy. Nevertheless, knowledge of the mechanism by which a tissue allograft (see Table 1 for terminology) is rejected continues to grow rapidly, and as our understanding of such rejection becomes clearer we shall develop better methods for monitoring the immune response to a graft and for designing more specific immunosuppression.

Understanding of the immune response to an allograft is obviously based on the rapidly expanding knowledge of the response to any antigenic challenge (see Chapter 5.1) but, in addition, the response to an allograft has a number of special features, some of the more important of which are described in the following sections. This response is most easily considered first under factors involved in the induction of the response (sensitization) and then under those involved in the effector arm of the response, which generally results in destruction of the allograft in an unmodified host (Table 2).

Table 1 *Terminology*

Autograft (autologous)
Transplantation of an individual's own tissue to another site, e.g. the covering of third-degree burns with skin from unburnt areas or a saphenous vein femoropopliteal graft

Isograft (isogeneic or syngeneic)
Transplantation of tissues between genetically identical members of the same species, e.g. kidney transplant between monozygotic identical twins or skin grafts between mice of the same inbred strain

Allograft (allogeneic)
Transplantation of tissues between genetically non-identical members of the same species, e.g. a cadaveric renal transplant or skin graft between mice of different inbred strains

Xenograft (xenogeneic)
Transplantation of tissues between members of different species, e.g. a baboon kidney transplanted into a human

Table 2 *Factors that determine the immune response to an allograft*

Afferent limb
(a) Major histocompatibility antigens:
Immunogenicity
- class I
- class II

(b) Minor histocompatibility antigens
(c) Antigen processing and presentation:
- dendritic cells
- macrophages

(d) Site of sensitization—peripheral or central
(e) Privileged sites and tissues
(f) Genetic control

Effector limb
(a) Specificity
(b) Specific humoral:
- complement fixation
- antibody-dependent cellular cytotoxicity

(c) Specific cellular—T_c
(d) Non-specific:
- delayed-type hypersensitivity
- natural killer cells

Induction phase of the immune response to an allograft

Major histocompatibility antigens (see also Chapter 5.1)

DEFINITION

It is the histocompatibility antigens, glycoproteins present on the cell membrane, that determine the outcome of tissue allografts between members of the same species. As described in earlier sections, the influence of such antigens on the fate of a tissue allograft is only a by-product of their basic biological role in immunological cellular interactions. In all vertebrate species, histocompatibility antigens can be divided into major and minor, the major being under the genetic control of one system known as the major histocompatibility complex **(MHC),** and the minor under the control of numerous systems, at least 40, and probably several hundred in the mouse for example. The definition of a histocompatibility antigen as major or minor is based on the behaviour of a tissue allograft transplanted across an incompatibility for that antigen. It is incompatibility for the MHC between a donor and recipient that, in general, leads to the immune response to an allograft and its destruction. Minor histocompatibility antigens probably do not play a part in the presence of incompatibility for the MHC, but where there is no incompatibility for the MHC, multiple minor differences or the presence of prior sensitization against minor histocompatibility antigens can be responsible for a very vigorous rejection reaction in rodents. In man the MHC is known as HLA. We know relatively little about minor histocompatibility systems in man, other than they must exist, as evidenced by the occasional rejection of renal transplants between HLA-identical siblings and the occurrence of graft-versus-host **(GVH)** reactions after bone marrow transplantation between HLA-identical siblings.

GENETIC CONTROL OF THE MHC

There is a remarkable homology between the MHC in different species both from the immunogenetic and biochemical aspects. The MHC in man, HLA, is described in Chapter 5.1. The antigens of the MHC in each species are divided into class I and class II, the former being relatively ubiquitous in their tissue distribution, while the latter show a limited distribution, being expressed primarily on B lymphocytes, macrophages, activated T cells, dendritic cells, and endothelium. Class I antigens are represented in man by the products of the *HLA-A, -B* and *-C* loci; class II antigens are the products of the D-region loci, *DP, DQ,* and *DR.* However, class I antigens may be expressed more densely and class II antigens may be induced on cells not previously expressing those antigens in the presence of an immune reaction, such as graft rejection. This induction of MHC antigen expression is triggered primarily by interferon-γ produced by T cells responding to the graft.

IMMUNOGENICITY

Many factors, including the type of tissue, the method of graft vascularization, and the site of transplantation, influence the immunogenicity of histocompatibility antigens, and therefore the ultimate fate of a tissue allograft. But the *sine qua non* for rejection to occur is, in the first instance, incompatibility for antigens of the MHC. Incompatibility for either class I or class II antigens can give rise to an immune response resulting in graft rejection, as has been shown clearly in congenic strains of mice differing only for class I or II antigens. However, in general, class II antigen incompatibility causes a more marked response to an allograft than class I incompatibility, for reasons discussed later.

What does seem apparent is that MHC antigens of themselves are not immunogenic unless presented to the recipient on the surface of a viable cell, and perhaps only a lymphoid cell. Presentation of antigen in the form of a soluble membrane extract or in liposomes does not produce an immune response. Furthermore, presentation of antigen on cells that do not express class II antigens (i.e. red cells or platelets) does not produce a primary immune response, suggesting that class II antigens must be present on cells of the immunizing tissue for the immune response to be generated. Indeed, not only does such presentation of class I antigen fail to evoke a primary immune response but it also seems, in many instances, to result actively in donor-specific unresponsiveness. This donor-specific unresponsiveness induced by pretreatment with cells expressing class I antigen may also be induced by cells expressing class II antigen, although not so readily. The phenomenon is dependent on the intravenous route of antigen presentation as well as the dose and timing of pretreatment in relation to the subsequent graft, and this is usually a vascularized organ graft rather than a free skin allograft. The unresponsiveness is characterized in most experimental models by a state of specific clonal anergy in the responding T cells, perhaps maintained by an imbalance of cytokines. For example, in one such model in our own laboratories, anergy has been shown to be due to the lack of production of interleukin 2 **(IL-2)** as well as lack of expression of high-affinity IL-2 receptors. Furthermore, this unresponsiveness can be transferred by T cells to a syngeneic host, the so-called suppressor-cell phenomenon, the nature of which still remains unclear. However, as mentioned earlier, congenic strains of mice will reject skin allografts where differences exist only for class I or class II antigens of the MHC, which means that although class II antigens are necessary for the induction of the allograft response, they do not have to be incompatible with the host. For the class II antigens of the host may participate in the induction of the response where donor and host are compatible for MHC class II, as explained below.

MATCHING FOR HLA

From what has been said, it would thus seem necessary to try to match donors and recipients of organ allografts for HLA, the MHC in man. In renal transplantation, matching for HLA has been sought for the past 20 years. This has become increasingly difficult in cadaver transplantation as the complexity of the HLA system has continued to unfold. Within families the inheritance of HLA can be determined very precisely and the outcome of transplantation between family members is determined to a considerable extent by the genetic disparity between donor and recipient. For example, renal transplants between HLA-identical siblings have very few rejections (which must be due to minor histocompatibility antigens) and at least 85 per cent of such grafts will be functioning 5 years after transplantation.

In the time before cyclosporin the outcome of renal allografts between siblings who shared neither of the parental HLA haplotypes and who therefore were completely mismatched for HLA was little better than that achieved in cadaveric transplantation, with parent-to-child (sharing one HLA haplotype) showing a graft survival intermediate between the two. However, in the cyclosporin era, graft survival of a living related transplant mismatched for one or even two HLA haplotypes has improved dramatically and now approaches that achieved with HLA-identical sibling transplants.

In cadaveric renal transplantation the value of matching for HLA has a controversial history. Suffice it to say that in the azathioprine era there was an undoubted benefit in terms of graft survival achieved by transplantation of kidneys well matched for HLA-A, -B, and -DR. As first shown in Oxford, this better outcome was largely due to matching for the class II antigens, HLA-DR. However, in the cyclosporin era the benefits of matching have become much less apparent, although registry data from large cohorts of transplants are still able to show a better graft survival for very well-matched donors and recipients. In our own centre the beneficial matching effect of HLA-DR is no longer apparent in terms of survival for first cadaveric grafts, but is for the survival of cadaveric regrafts. However, in first cadaveric grafts there are still highly significant differences in the outcome of grafts that are matched for HLA-DR as assessed by other features, namely fewer episodes of acute rejection, less treatment for rejection either with high-dose corticosteroids or anti-T-cell reagents, and less time in hospital. Thus attempts to match donor and recipient, at least for HLA-DR, are still worthwhile. The two other loci of the class II region of HLA, *HLA-DQ* and *-DP,* have not been shown to influence graft outcome in the presence of compatibility for *HLA-DR.* Now that the molecular structure and amino acid sequence of MHC antigens have been largely defined, studies of matching for HLA in transplantation are now directed at examining the influence of sequence differences between HLA molecules that might be seen by antibody or T cells, as these would seem to be logical candidates for refining the influence of HLA matching on graft outcome.

THE PRESENTATION OF MHC ANTIGENS TO THE RECIPIENT

This is obviously a key factor in the induction of the immune response to an allograft. In contrast to the host response to other exogenous antigens that are processed by host antigen-presenting cells, such as dendritic cells and macrophages, and are presented to the T-helper (**T_H**) cell in association with host class II antigen (MHC restriction), a tissue allograft may induce a response in a different manner. For in the tissue allograft there are leucocytes of donor origin, which for years have been defined functionally as passenger leucocytes, but more recently characterized as a specialized cell, the interstitial dendritic cell, which is not of the macrophage lineage. These cells are widely distributed throughout the body, and in particular express large amounts of class II MHC antigen. In the skin they are known as Langerhans cells. They probably play an important part in the recognition of the allograft by the recipient.

The role of the passenger leucocyte in the induction of an allograft response has been known for some years and has been demonstrated by two types of experiments. In one, passenger leucocytes were removed from an allograft before transplantation by pretreatment of the donor with either irradiation or cyclosphosphamide. This was followed by prolonged survival of the subsequent allograft. In the other, radiation or drug chimeras were made such that the parenchymal and stromal tissue of the allograft chimeras were of different MHC specificity to that of the passenger leucocytes. This allowed allografts to be implanted in recipients differing in specificity either for the parenchymal tissue or the passenger leucocytes. Furthermore, retransplantation of long-surviving renal allografts in the rat (where the passenger leucocytes of the donor organ would have been replaced by cells syngeneic with the host) into a fresh recipient, syngeneic with the original recipient, leads to prolonged survival of the retransplanted kidney. That this is not due to replacement of donor endothelium by host endothelium has been clearly demonstrated in our laboratories, again supporting the role of these cells in the induction of the response leading to rejection. However, this phenomenon is very dependent on the strain combination used and the homozygosity or heterozygosity of the donor tissue in relation to the recipient.

Undoubtedly, in the *in vitro* mixed lymphocyte reaction in the mouse and the rat, the dendritic cells are potent inducers of the proliferative response against the stimulator cell population. This response can be produced by very small numbers of dendritic cells, and in their absence it does not occur. Furthermore, in the rat, when a long-surviving kidney allograft is retransplanted into a fresh allogeneic host in which it is normally not rejected, it can be made to reject by the injection of a small number of dendritic cells syngeneic with the retransplanted kidney. In these experiments, injection of T- and B-lymphocyte populations either has no effect or large numbers are required to produce any evidence of rejection. In addition, Lafferty and his colleagues, in a series of elegant experiments, produced prolonged survival of thyroid and pancreatic islet allografts in mice after a period of tissue culture in a high-oxygen environment. This was attributed to the loss of dendritic cells from the allogeneic endocrine tissue during the culture period, thus preventing the second signal necessary for T-cell activation, the first signal being provided by the T-cell receptor interaction with alloantigen. Thus, in the mouse and the rat, there is a good deal of evidence, both *in vitro* and *in vivo,* to suggest an important role for the dendritic cell in the induction of the immune response. More recently, a molecule known as B7 on the dendritic cell (the so-called professional antigen-presenting cell) has been shown to react with a molecule on the T_H cell, CD28. B7 has a restricted tissue distribution, being largely confined to dendritic and B cells. This B7–CD28 interaction may be the source of the hypothetical second signal needed for activation of the T_H cell, and explain the requirement for dendritic cells in the induction of an alloresponse.

These observations suggest then that incompatibility for class II MHC antigens expressed on donor dendritic cells in the allograft can be recognized directly by the CD4+ T_H cells of the recipient. This direct presentation of alloantigen is a feature of the alloresponse, in contrast to the classical presentation of exogenous antigen by host dendritic cells to host T_H cells, and is felt to be the major pathway for recognition of foreigness in the alloresponse. It is probable that T cells can recognize different class II MHC antigens bearing a variety of self peptides, thus providing an explanation for the large number of T cells in any given individual that are capable of reacting to a given alloantigen. However, indirect presentation of MHC alloantigen (as for any exogenous antigen) undoubtedly does also occur in the absence of donor dendritic cells in the allograft or in the presence of compatibility for class II MHC antigen between donor and recipient, but this does not appear to be the principal pathway of sensitization in normal circumstances.

However, the relevance to man of these observations in the rodent must be questioned, for in the rodent class II antigens are not expressed on endothelium whereas they are in man. There is now some evidence that endothelium can present antigen in the same way as an accessory cell, be it a dendritic cell or a macrophage, in endothelial–lymphocyte reactions *in vitro*. If this were so it would mean that attempts to rid the donor tissue of dendritic cells would be of no value as the endothelium of the allograft would still be able to act as a presenting cell to host T_H lymphocytes. Of considerable interest in this respect are the observations that in the presence of an inflammatory reaction, class II antigen may be expressed on cells that do not normally do so. For example, we have shown expression of class II antigen on renal tubular cells and an increased density of class II antigen on endothelium during a rejection episode in human kidneys. Perhaps this class II antigen may be capable of enhancing the recognition of alloantigen.

Thus, at present, there is a considerable body of evidence which suggests that the interstitial dendritic cell plays a prominent part in the induction of the immune response to an allograft in the rodent, but it is clear that an immune response can still occur in the absence of this cell. However, in man the presence of class II antigens on endothelium and the possibility that endothelium may present alloantigen must raise some doubt about the significance of the role of dendritic cells in graft rejection in a clinical setting.

SITE OF SENSITIZATION

The induction of the immune response may take place both peripherally in the allograft itself or centrally in the lymphoid system. The classical dogma of transplantation immunology has suggested that, in the case of a vascularized graft such as a kidney, the induction of the response occurs primarily in the graft itself, while in the case of a secondarily vascularized free graft such as a skin allograft, sensitization occurs in central lymphoid organs, such as draining lymph nodes. However, recent evidence now challenges this dogma.

Certainly, in the case of a free graft such as skin, revascularization of the graft takes several days, and it seems probable that sensitization takes place centrally either by the passage of donor dendritic cells or by the transport of incompatible antigen in host macrophages via host lymphatics to central lymphoid organs. Indeed, if one places a skin allograft in a site where there is no lymphatic connection with the host, as, for example, in the hamster cheek pouch or on an artificially contrived pedicle flap, the survival of the allograft is markedly prolonged. However, it now seems that even in the case of a vascularized graft, sensitization also may occur centrally, for in a cardiac transplant model in the mouse we have shown that donor dendritic cells in the transplanted heart have migrated from the heart within 24 h of transplantation, and may then be demonstrated in the recipient spleen in association with host T cells. Thus it would appear that, although there is a physiological difference in the traffic of donor dendritic cells to central lymphoid organs, namely via lymphatics to draining lymph nodes in the case of a skin allograft and via the blood stream to the spleen in the case of a vascularized graft, in both instances sensitization is essentially a central phenomenon.

MINOR HISTOCOMPATIBILITY ANTIGENS

Minor histocompatibility antigens may have a prominent role in graft rejection either in a recipient who is given an MHC-compatible graft and where pre-existing sensitization to minor histocompatibility antigens exists, or where there are multiple minor differences. This can be demonstrated clearly in the rodent and probably explains the not infrequent rejections that are seen in renal transplants between HLA-identical siblings, as well as GVH reactions that occur after bone marrow transplantation between HLA-identical siblings. Indeed, in this latter situation, several minor histocompatibility antigens recognized by T cells have been defined that appear to influence the development of GVH reactions. Allogeneic tissue-specific antigens may well be common and such systems have been demonstrated for mouse skin and rat kidney. However, in the rat, incompatibility for the kidney system alone was not capable of causing rejection of a renal allograft, even where the recipient had been presensitized to the system. Similarly an endothelial–monocyte system has been demonstrated in man, and here there is evidence that prior sensitization can cause graft damage. In man a number of the minor blood groups have been considered to be minor histocompatibility antigens, Lewis, Rh, P for example, but the evidence for this, not surprisingly, is not strong. The structure and function of minor histocompatibility antigens have been difficult to elucidate, for they are only recognized by T cells. It appears that these minor histocompatibility antigens represent MHC antigens carrying self peptides in their groove and that these peptides are derived from self proteins that vary between different members (e.g. mitochondrial protein) or sexes (e.g. H-Y) of the same species.

PRIVILEGED SITES AND PRIVILEGED TISSUE

Tissue allografts placed in certain sites may not evoke an immune response and the allografts may survive for prolonged periods or even indefinitely. The anterior chamber of the eye is one such site, and numerous reports indicate that it is a privileged site not only for allografts but also xenografts of a variety of tissues and tumours (nevertheless, there are reports that no prolongation of survival of allografts was obtained in this site). Certainly, sensitization of the recipient by a prior tissue allograft, such as skin, leads to rapid destruction of an allograft from the same donor on implantation into the anterior chamber. In man the cornea represents another privileged site, as seen by the success of corneal grafting in clinical practice. Vascularization of the cornea or prior sensitization of the recipient will lead to early failure of such grafts. The brain represents another privileged site, as does the testis to some extent. Probably the best known experimental site is the cheek pouch of the Syrian hamster in which a skin allograft will survive indefinitely, provided that the host has not been specifically sensitized against donor histocompatibility antigens.

What these sites have in common, to a greater or lesser extent, is a lack of or an abnormal lymphatic drainage, which seems to play such an important part in sensitization of the host against a free graft, such as skin, as discussed already in the case of an artificial privileged site. Although there are undoubtedly well-documented privileged sites in many species, it appears that no site is uniformly privileged for all tissues, even in the same species.

Not only are certain sites more favourable to graft acceptance but also certain tissues seem less susceptible to rejection. Cartilage appears to survive for a long time, probably because the chondrocytes are protected by the ground substance or matrix surrounding them. As a result they are not only feebly immunogenic but also resistant to destruction even in the sensitized animal. The hamster cheek pouch skin itself is not only privileged *in situ* but is also a privileged tissue when transplanted to the chest wall, where it survives for twice as long as a skin allograft. This is also thought to be due to the protective effect of the connective tissue moiety of the pouch allograft, which remains alymphatic.

Fetal or neonatal skin allografts in certain strain combinations may also show prolonged survival, while certain endocrine tissues such as the ovary, pituitary, and parathyroid glands may survive and function for a long time. There has been considerable investigation of transplantation of isolated pancreatic islets in the rodent, but there is no evidence of lack of immunogenicity of either adult or fetal islet allografts when implanted in diabetic recipients.

Finally, the liver is a vascularized graft that often behaves as a privileged tissue. Calne first showed that certain outbred pigs failed to reject orthotopic liver allografts; moreover, kidney allografts transplanted at the same time, and which are normally rejected, also showed prolonged survival. Furthermore, in certain strain combinations in the rat in which an orthotopic liver allograft is not rejected, the liver allograft has been shown to abrogate an existing state of sensitization of the host against donor histocompatibility antigen, a truly remarkable finding. In this case the liver appears to induce an active state of suppression that is associated with the secretion of large amounts of donor soluble MHC class I antigen by the transplanted liver as well as the migration of large numbers of donor dendritic cells from the donor liver into the host. Whether this association is the cause of this reduced immunogenicity of liver allografts in experimental animal models remains to be confirmed.

In man, liver allografts behave as if they may be less immunogenic than the kidney, for example, but this difference is not as striking as once thought, and acute rejection is a common occurrence after liver transplantation.

GENETIC CONTROL

There is good evidence in the rat that the immune response to an allograft is genetically controlled. This control appears to be due to Ir (immune response) genes linked to the MHC and influences the induction phase of the response rather than the effector phase. There is also some evidence showing that the effector arm of the response to minor histocompatibility antigen may be restricted by class I antigens of the MHC of the recipient. In the mouse we have shown that rejection of vascularized cardiac allografts is genetically controlled by both MHC and non-MHC genes. There is even some evidence suggesting that there may be some HLA-linked genetic influence in rejection of human kidney allografts, but none of these observations suggesting HLA associations (e.g. HLA-DR6, HLA-A1) has been irrefutably confirmed.

The effector arm of the immune response to an allograft

The effector limb of the response to a tissue allograft is complex, comprising both specific and non-specific components. The specific response can be divided into an antibody-mediated or humoral response and a cellular response. Although antibody to the target allograft is produced by B lymphocytes, this humoral response to an allograft is T_H cell dependent. The cellular response is a T-cell response, but considerable controversy exists as to the nature of the T-cell involvement, which might be either the T-cytotoxic (**T_C**) cell or the T_H cell as part of a delayed-type hypersensitivity reaction to the graft. T_H and T_C cells are recognized phenotypically by the expression of the CD4 and CD8 molecules, respectively).

The non-specific response includes macrophages, natural killer cells, and possibly killer cells, which *in vitro* lyse targets specifically sensitized by antibody (antibody-dependent cellular cytotoxicity). This non-specific response may in part be the inflammatory response consequent on the release of cytokines by cells participating in the initial specific reaction to the graft and thus can be considered as a delayed-type hypersensitivity reaction.

SPECIFIC CELLULAR RESPONSE

That the T cell has a major role in the effector limb of the immune response resulting in graft rejection is beyond question; the athymic nude mouse will not reject a skin allograft, and B rats and mice (rats and mice that have been thymectomized, lethally irradiated, and reconstituted with syngeneic B lymphocytes) will not reject skin or renal allografts. But there has been considerable controversy over the years concerning the nature of the effector T cell in the cellular immune response. Is graft rejection due to the lysis of the target cells of the donor tissue by the T_C cell? Or is rejection a delayed hypersensitivity reaction in which the specificity of the reaction is due to the activation and proliferation of the T_H cell and tissue destruction is produced by the non-specific cellular response to this initial reaction?

There is evidence that the T_C cell is able to mediate allograft rejection, and that this reaction is exquisitely specific. For example, a very early, but little cited, experiment by Mintz and Silvers showed that individual allogeneic cells were destroyed by a process that left neighbouring cells unharmed. In their experiments, skin grafts from allophenic mice produced by the fusion of blastomeres of two different H-2 strains (H-2 being the MHC of the mouse) were transferred to recipients from one of the parental strains. Melanoblasts and hair follicles that expressed the same H-2 antigens as the host survived, while those expressing the foreign H-2 antigens were destroyed. In a different type of experiment in our own laboratories, intimate mixtures of allogeneic and syngeneic pancreatic islets were implanted beneath the kidney capsule of rats, and, although the allogeneic islets were rapidly destroyed, there was no evidence of damage to the syngeneic islets in the mixed implant.

In the absence of any 'bystander' cytotoxicity it is difficult to implicate a delayed-type hypersensitivity reaction as being responsible for rejection of the allogeneic cells, although obviously the T_C cell cannot be directly implicated. However, cytotoxic T-cell clones have been shown to eliminate susceptible tumour-cell grafts in mice and to produce local tissue necrosis when injected intradermally into mice expressing the minor, skin-specific tissue antigen to which the T_C cell alone was directed. Furthermore, rejection of heart allografts in sublethally irradiated rats, where host and donor were incompatible only for class I MHC antigens, was produced only by T cells of the T_C phenotype. Further evidence in support of an important role for the T_C is provided by a comparison between the ability of infiltrating mononuclear cells harvested from rejecting renal allografts and from healthy allografts in cyclosporin-treated animals to lyse ^{51}Cr-labelled target cells. In these experiments from our laboratories, cells were extracted from renal allografts of rats 5 days after transplantation both from untreated animals and animals treated with cyclosporin. Large numbers of mononuclear cells were extracted in each case (5–7 $\times$ 10^7 cells in both treated and untreated animals). In untreated animals these cells exhibited both specific killing by T_C as well as non-specific killing, due to macrophages and natural killer cells, of appropriate targets. However, cells extracted from the kidney allograft of an animal treated with cyclosporin (at a dose that completely prevents rejection) showed no specific killing, but non-specific killing was unchanged. Despite the demonstration *in vitro* of considerable non-specific killing by these mononuclear cells from the cyclosporin-treated rats, there was no evidence of graft rejection.

On the other hand a number of experiments suggest that T_C cells are not essential for graft rejection, at least in the rodent. For example, B mice are tolerant of skin allografts. Injection of syngeneic T lymphocytes of the T_C phenotype does not result in rejection of tolerated skin allografts whereas the injection of T_H cells does. Similarly, in the B rat, skin allografts are rejected after reconstruction with T_H but not T_C lymphocytes. More recently, experiments in our own and other laboratories have shown that deletion of the T_H cells in naïve recipients with monoclonal antibodies against CD4 leads to prolonged survival of allografts; this is in contrast to animals in which T_C cells have been depleted with an anti-CD8 antibody, where only a modest prolongation of survival was achieved. However, the most effective prolongation of allograft survival is achieved by depletion of both populations. It is also of interest that in a sensitized recipient, depletion of T_C cells leads to prolonged survival where depletion of T_H cells has no effect whatsoever.

However, considerable caution must be exercised in interpreting much of these data, for it is not clear, for example, that in the reconstituted host, cytotoxic T-cell precursors are absent from these B animals. Furthermore, it has now been demonstrated that within the T_H-phenotype population of lymphocytes there are cytotoxic precursors that can mature into cytotoxic cells with specificity for class II antigens on the target cell. Although these experiments clearly show that the T_H cell is essential for rejection to occur, either because this subpopulation is needed for the generation of the T_C or because it triggers a delayed-type hypersensitivity, they do not exclude the role of the T_C in graft rejection, especially as the T_C may have the helper phenotype.

Of particular interest in view of the possibility that there are cytotoxic T cells of the T_H phenotype, are the relatively recent observations that class II MHC antigens may be expressed on cells that do not normally do so in the presence of inflammatory reactions such as a GVH or rejection. The induction of class II antigen expression is mediated by interferon-γ and has been observed both on skin allografts in the rodent as well as on the tubular cells of the human kidney during an acute rejection reaction. It is possible that the class II expression precedes the reaction and enhances the induction of the immune response to the allograft, but the more likely explanation is that it appears as a result of the initial response and provides an increased target for T_C (probably of the T_H phenotype) directed at MHC class II antigens.

The cells infiltrating a rejecting graft are a heterogeneous population. Both in rat and human kidney allografts the mononuclear cell infiltrate seen in a rejecting graft has been shown to comprise macrophages, natural killer cells, B lymphocytes, plasma cells, and T lymphocytes of both the T_H and T_C phenotype. These populations have been identified both by functional assays and by monoclonal antibodies, although one must be cautious in attributing function to the phenotype, especially in respect of T cells, in view of the above observations.

SPECIFIC HUMORAL RESPONSE

The role of antibodies in graft rejection is difficult to establish. Undoubtedly, in most species, a graft performed in the presence of antibody against donor-specific class I, and perhaps class II, antigens will immediately be destroyed, as illustrated by the white skin allograft or the hyperacutely rejected renal allograft in a specifically sensitized recipient. However, in the non-sensitized recipient the role of antibody in graft rejection is uncertain. It is possible to cause rejection of an established allograft by passive transfer of donor-specific antibody, but it is difficult, and usually rather artificial experimental models have been used. However, lymphocytotoxins with donor MHC specificity can be demonstrated in the serum of patients who are rejecting or have rejected renal allografts, and antibodies can be shown to be deposited in rejecting kidneys and can be eluted from rejected kidneys.

Many of the histological changes associated with severe rejection in the human renal allograft, namely interstitial haemorrhage, fibrinoid necrosis, and arteriolar thrombosis, could be considered as the expected outcome of damage by antibody rather than by cells. This is also true of the extensive intimal fibrosis of arteries seen in kidneys or hearts undergoing chronic rejection. Antibody would be expected to bind to endothelium and fix complement, thus producing endothelial damage with subsequent platelet and fibrin deposition, and eventually thrombosis, all of which are compatible with the histological findings. Antibody could also produce damage to an allograft by the mechanism of antibody-dependent cellular cytotoxicity, where target cells coated with specific antibody are killed by so-called killer (K) cells. Although this latter phenomenon is well-established *in vitro,* it is difficult to be sure that it has a role in rejection *in vivo.*

NON-SPECIFIC RESPONSE

The role of the non-specific cellular response in graft rejection has already been discussed and although there is no doubt that both macrophages and natural killer cells are found in considerable numbers in a rejecting allograft in experimental models, these cells probably play little part in the initial damage to an allograft but represent the inflammatory response to tissue damage produced by the specific cellular response. They are thus an indication of the severity of a rejection reaction but do not contribute to it except in its final stages.

The role of complement can be considered here also and may be important in determining the effect of antibody on an allograft. For example, in the rat, complement appears to be inefficient *in vivo,* in that damage to an allograft by passively transferred alloantibody needs the administration of heterologous guinea-pig complement. This may explain the failure of most, but not all, rat strain combinations to reject hyperacutely a renal allograft in the presence of high-titre, donor-specific, cytotoxic antibody.

CYTOKINES AND THE ALLORESPONSE

Cytokines are soluble proteins secreted by a wide variety of cells apart from those involved in the immune response. They include the interleukins, interferons, tumour-necrosis factors **(TNF),** and transforming growth factors. A considerable body of data is beginning to accumulate concerning the role of various cytokines and their receptors in the alloresponse, but it is going to be some time before what must be an extraordinarily complex interaction of cells and cytokines is unravelled. Nevertheless, some more recent observations are accessible to interpretation. This, to a great extent, has been made possible by application of the polymerase chain reaction, which can now be semiquantitated, to detect mRNA for a variety of cytokines and their receptors in the allograft itself. For example, in our own laboratory, in a cardiac transplant model in the mouse, we have been able to show that the appearance of message for IL-2, IL-4, and TNF precedes overt evidence of rejection by several days. Messages for other cytokines can also be detected (e.g. IL-1, -3, -6, and -8) but these are also seen in syngeneic transplants, no doubt induced in response to non-specific damage to the graft as a result of ischaemia. Early studies of cytokines in human renal allografts using fine-needle aspirates, again in our own department, suggest also that message for IL-2 can be detected several days before there is biochemical evidence of rejection, while in contrast no IL-2 is seen in grafts that show no evidence of rejection. The role of cytokines in tolerance induction has also been referred to briefly, but evidence from our own laboratories in a tolerance model induced by prior blood transfusion shows a decreased production of IL-2 by cells that are essentially anergic, whereas a similar observation has been made by others for interferon-γ. Administration of IL-2 or interferon-γ in these models certainly abrogates the induction of tolerance. In other tolerance models, induced by cyclosporin or anti-CD4 monoclonal antibodies, for example, we and others have shown an imbalance between certain cytokines, such as IL-2 and interferon-γ, which are down-regulated, and IL-4 and -10, which are up-regulated. This is of considerable relevance for there are two populations of T_H cells in the rodent with different cytokine profiles, namely T_{H1} cells, which produce IL-2 and interferon-γ, and T_{H2} cells, which produce IL-4 and -10. Moreover, these two populations regulate the activity of each other. Thus it is possible that in the rodent model tolerance is mediated by the down-regulation of T_{H1} cells by the expansion of the T_{H2} population. However, for the time being this attractive concept must be regarded as speculative.

THE TARGET OF THE IMMUNE RESPONSE

The principal target of the immune response, be it cellular or humoral, against a vascularized graft such as a kidney must be the endothelium of the allograft, at least in the first instance, bearing in mind that endothelium in man expresses both class I and class II antigens. This explains the predominantly vascular changes that are seen in rejection of a vascularized organ allograft.

The more recent recognition of a variety of adhesion molecules and their ligands on leucocytes and endothelium (selectins and integrins) changes our earlier concept of the endothelium in a vascularized organ allograft as being merely a passive target for the immune response to one in which the endothelium in the presence of activation through both non-specific or specific damage actively participates in and enhances the response to the allograft.

Summary

The immune response to a tissue allograft is a very complex phenomenon, both in the manner in which allogeneic histocompatibility antigen is recognized and in the response to this recognition, which generally results in graft damage. In the recognition of antigen the dendritic cell (passenger leucocyte) plays a prominent but not all-important part, while the effector arm is mediated both by cells and antibody.

The immune response is exquisitely specific and is mediated both by T cells and antibody. The T_H cell is the pivotal cell in the alloresponse in a naïve recipient, while T_C cells have a role but are probably not essential, in contrast to the sensitized recipient where T_C cells are the key effectors. Other cells such as macrophages have a secondary role in the alloresponse. Antibody also plays a part in both acute and chronic rejection, but it is difficult to dissect the role of antibody from that of cells. Intermingled with both the cellular and humoral responses are a host of cytokines, the messages between the cells, and many of these cytokines, such as IL-2 and interferon-γ, play a prominent part in the alloresponse.

In certain situations the immune response may be aborted, leading to a state of unresponsiveness rather than alloagression. Again, in most experimental models this unresponsiveness is maintained as an active phenomenon and is not due to deletion of an alloreactive clone of cells. This phenomenon of unresponsiveness represents a form of clonal anergy, mediated by an altered immunoregulation by different populations of T cells and their cytokine profiles.

Because of the complex interaction of so many factors involved in the immune response to a tissue allograft it is impossible to define a mechanism of rejection clearly, or indeed to determine the mechanism by which a graft is not rejected. Nevertheless, the picture is gradually becoming less blurred, and it is possible to describe the phenomenon of rejection even if the precise relations of the many factors involved remain to be defined.

REFERENCES

Baldwin, W.M.I., Pruitt, S.K., and Sanfilippo, F. (1991). Alloantibodies: basic and clinical concepts. *Transplantation Reviews,* **5,** 100–9.

Barker, C.F. and Billingham R.E. (1968). The role of afferent lymphatics in the rejection of skin homografts. *Journal of Experimental Medicine,* **128,** 197–221.

Dallman, M.J. *et al.* (1991). Peripheral tolerance to alloantigen results from altered regulation of the interleukin 2 pathway. *Journal of Experimental Medicine,* **173,** 79–87.

Dallman, M.J. *et al.* (1992). Sequential analysis of IL-2 gene transcription in renal transplants. *Transplantation,* **53,** 683–5.

Fuggle, S. *et al.* (1986). Sequential analysis of HLA-Class II antigen expression in human renal allografts. *Transplantation,* **42,** 144–50.

Goulmy, E. (1985). Class I restricted human cytotoxic T lymphocytes directed against minor transplantation antigens and their role in organ transplantation. *Progress in Allergy,* **36,** 44–72.

Gracie, J.A. *et al.* (1990). T Cell requirements for the rejection of renal allografts bearing an isolated class I disparity. *Journal of Experimental Medicine,* **172,** 1547–57.

Kamada, N., Davies, H., and Roser, B.R. (1981). Reversal of transplantation of immunity by liver grafting. *Nature,* **292,** 840–2.

Lafferty, K.J. *et al.* (1976). Effect of organ culture on the survival of thyroid allografts in mice. *Transplantation,* **22,** 138–49.

Larsen, C.P., Morris, P.J., and Austyn, J.M. (1990). Migration of dendritic leucocytes from cardiac allografts into host spleens: a novel pathway for iniation of rejection. *Journal of Experimental Medicine,* **171,** 307–14.

Lechler, R.I. and Batchelor, J.R. (1982). Restoration of immunogenicity to passenger cell-depleted kidney allografts by the addition of donor strain dendritic cells. *Journal of Experimental Medicine,* **155,** 31–41.

Loveland, B.E. and McKenzie, I.F.C. (1982) Cells mediating graft rejection in the mouse. *Immunology,* **46,** 313–20.

Mason, D.W. and Morris, P.J. (1986). Effector mechanisms in allograft rejection. *Annual Reviews of Immunology,* **4,** 119–45.

Mason, D.W., Dallman, M.J., Arthur, R.P., and Morris, P.J. (1984) Mechanisms of allograft rejection: the roles of cytotoxic T-cells and delayed type hypersensitivity. *Immunology Reviews,* **77,** 167–84.

Mintz, B. and Silvers, W.K. (1970). Histocompatibility antigens on melanoblasts and hair follicle cells. Cell-localized homograft rejection in allophenic skin grafts. *Transplantation,* **9,** 497–505.

Morris, P.J. (1994). *Kidney transplantation: principles and practice,* (4th edn), Saunders, Philadelphia.

Morris, P.J. and Ting, A. (1982). Studies of HLA-DR with relevance to renal transplantation. *Immunology Reviews,* **66,** 103–31.

Morris, P.J. *et al.* (1969). Serotyping for homotransplantation XXII specificity of cytotoxic antibodies developing after renal transplantation. *British Medical Journal,* **1,** 758–9.

Mosmann, T.R. and Coffman, R.L. (1989). TH1 and TH2 cells: different patterns of lymphokine secretion lead to different functional properties. *Annual Reviews of Immunology,* **7,** 145–73.

Peugh, W.N. *et al.* (1986). The role of H-2 and non-H-2 antigens and genes in the rejection of murine cardiac allografts. *Immunogenetics,* **23,** 30–7.

Pober, J.S. and Cotran, R.S. (1991). Immunologic interactions of T lymphocytes with vascular endothelium. *Advances in Immunology,* **50,** 261–302.

Strober, S. and Gowans, J.C. (1965). The role of lymphocytes in the sensitisation of rats to renal homografts. *Journal of Experimental Medicine,* **122,** 347–60.

Welsh, K.I., Burgos, H., and Batchelor, J.R. (1977). The immune response to allogeneic rat platelets; Ag-B antigens in matrix form lacking Ia. *European Journal of Immunology,* **7**, 267–72.

Wood, K.J., Evins, J., and Morris, P.J. (1985). Suppression of renal allograft rejection in the rat by class I antigens on purified erythrocytes. *Transplantation,* **45,** 759–67.

Section 6 *Clinical oncology*

6.1 General characteristics of neoplasia

H. Harris

The control of cell multiplication

A tumour is produced by the growth of cells that have become in some measure insensitive to normal growth control mechanisms. Some consideration of these mechanisms is thus a prerequisite of any informed discussion of the cancer problem. The fundamental principles were first elucidated by the analysis of regeneration in epidermis and especially, for an interesting biological reason, the epidermis of insects. In insects, once the cuticle has been laid down, the epidermis is composed of a single layer of contiguous epithelial cells which do not undergo further multiplication during the life of the adult insect unless the epidermis is wounded. This tissue thus provides an initially static two-dimensional system that lends itself to more precise analysis than is normally possible in the heterogeneous three-dimensional arrays of which most animal tissues are composed. In a classic study, Wigglesworth showed that, when insect epidermis is wounded, a wave of mitoses is induced in the cells near the wound and that this mitotic activity is controlled in a quite specific way. The initial response is a migration of epithelial cells to the edge of the wound. This redistribution of the cell population occurs well before any multiplication of cells begins, with the result that the cell density immediately adjacent to the wound is increased, whereas, further away, a zone is produced in which the cell density is reduced. When, later, the cells begin to multiply, the mitoses are observed not in the region of high cell density adjacent to the wound, but in the region of reduced cell density further away. The cells continue to multiply until the cell density is restored to normal, then multiplication ceases. Throughout the whole process of repair, the epidermal cells remain in contact with one another through cytoplasmic bridges. The multiplication of the cells is therefore initiated not by diffusible factors generated at the edge of the wound, nor by the disruption of cell contact, but by some mechanism associated with a reduction in the normal cell density. Similar experiments on young insects in which the volume of the body is reduced by starvation provide strong support for this interpretation. The reduction in body volume produces a greatly increased density of cells in the epidermis. In this crowded epidermis, the migration of cells to the edge of a wound does not generate an outer zone in which cell density is reduced below normal; and the healing of the wound is achieved without the intervention of a wave of cell multiplication.

These simple experiments delineate a cardinal property of metazoan cells: their ability to register and respond to cell density. It will be obvious that the acquisition of this property during evolution must have been essential for the development of metazoan life. If cells within a tissue were not able to sense changes in cell density and respond to them by increasing or decreasing the rate of cell multiplication, it is difficult to see how organized metazoan forms could ever have evolved. We are therefore dealing here with a very primitive cell response. The process of differentiation, of course, imposes on the basic density-sensing mechanism specializations and refinements appropriate to the tissue architecture in which particular cells find themselves; but the long evolutionary history of this mechanism makes it reasonable to suppose that certain elements in it might well be common to all metazoan cells. Cells in which the density-sensing mechanism is intact maintain a density appropriate to the tissue in which they function; they do this by limiting their rate of multiplication to what is necessary to replace, and no more than replace, the cells that are lost. Thus, in tissues such as the intestine or bone marrow, where the rate of cell loss under physiological conditions is high, the basal rate of cell multiplication is also high; where the physiological rate of cell loss is low, as, for example, in the adult liver, the basal rate of cell multiplication is also low. Non-physiological destruction of cells in any tissue, provided that the cells in that tissue remain capable of mitosis, initiates a wave of cell multiplication, and this ceases when normal cell density is restored. The whole process is a paradigm of balanced feedback control.

IMPAIRMENT OF THE DENSITY-SENSING MECHANISM

Disease processes may impair the density-sensing mechanism in various ways. Cells may fail to respond, or may respond inadequately, to a reduction in cell density or a disruption of tissue architecture. In this case, a wound may fail to heal or may heal imperfectly. Cells may respond in the appropriate way, but they may fail to stop multiplying when normal cell density has been restored. Exuberant masses of superfluous tissue may then be produced. Or cells may be induced to multiply even though cell density and tissue architecture remain normal. Some viruses, for example, may initiate a wave of mitotic activity in certain cells without first perturbing their topological interrelationships. In some way the virus renders the cell insensitive to the normal restraints on its multiplication. The gratuitous cell multiplication induced by viruses is usually limited: the cells either recover their sensitivity to growth controls or they die. Under certain conditions, however, cells may undergo a more stable change. Not only do they become insensitive to normal growth controls, but this insensitivity becomes heritable. Cells so affected beget daughter cells that are also insensitive and hence continue to multiply without responding to changes in cell density, and without respect for the integrity of tissue architecture. This kind of rogue growth is called a tumour. The cardinal biological characteristic of a tumour cell is thus the presence of a heritable lesion that determines insensitivity to the normal restraints governing cell multiplication.

The nature of the heritable lesion

These days, when one talks about heritable lesions, one thinks naturally of alterations in the nucleotide sequences of DNA or RNA; and the simplest explanation of the heritable cellular aberration that produces a tumour is that it is caused by a mutational event or series of events in the genetic material of the cell. This idea, which is sometimes called the 'somatic mutation' theory of cancer, is so consonant with our present understanding of cell biology, and with our knowledge of the behaviour of tumours, that it is perhaps difficult to see why other kinds of explanation should be entertained. There are two essential reasons: first, the argument, based on histological appearances, that tumours do not arise from a single cell, as would be expected for a mutational event, but by the large scale transformation of a 'field' of cells; and second, the observation that the tumour cell phenotype can, under certain conditions, apparently be restored to normal. These considerations have led some authors to propose that the heritable lesions that determine the tumour cell phenotype are not genetic in the classic sense, but epigenetic, that is, akin to the cellular changes that determine stable forms of differentiation. A tumour is then envisaged as an aberration of the normal process of differentiation.

With respect to the 'field' theory of carcinogenesis, it seems surprising that it is still necessary to say that histological methods cannot, in principle, resolve questions of this kind. A single cell, provided it retains the ability to undergo appropriate forms of differentiation, may generate a population of cells that can organize itself into an easily recognizable tract of differentiated tissue. This has been formally demonstrated *in vitro*, where clonal populations of cells have been grown for long periods of time without losing the ability to form, under appropriate conditions, specialized tissues such as muscle, cartilage, or lens. There is no way of telling, simply by looking at the histology of the tumour, whether it arose from a single cell or by the wholesale transformation of a 'field' of normal tissue. But it is clearly of cardinal importance to determine whether tumours do indeed arise from single cells or from large numbers of contiguous cells, for, if the latter were the case, a somatic mutation model for carcinogenesis would be difficult to sustain. Mutations are rare and, to a first approximation, random events which could not reasonably be held to explain a co-ordinate change occurring more or less simultaneously in a large group of cells. The best available evidence indicates, however, that in the great majority of cases, tumours, whether they form recognizable tissues or not, are clones that arise from the proliferation of a single cell.

Evidence for the clonal origin of human tumours

Three main lines of evidence support the conclusion that tumours are usually clonal growths.

THE PRESENCE OF MARKER CHROMOSOMES

It often happens that all, or almost all, of the cells in a tumour carry the same specific marker chromosome. Morphologically recognizable marker chromosomes are generated by chromosomal rearrangements, such as breaks and translocations, which are comparatively rare events. It is hardly conceivable that within a tumour the same rearrangement could occur independently but simultaneously in a high proportion of the cells. When one finds such a situation, the only plausible explanation is that all the cells bearing the specific marker are the progeny of a single cell in which that particular chromosomal rearrangement occurred initially. Cells carrying a diagnostic chromosome marker may, of course, generate subpopulations that have lost it, so that the presence in the tumour of cells not carrying the marker is no argument against a clonal origin. Nor is the fact that there are tumours that do not show consistent chromosomal abnormalities; for one would not expect that every cell capable of giving rise to a tumour would necessarily show a chromosomal abnormality that could be recognized in cytological preparations. It is, however, notable that as the resolution of cytogenetic techniques improves, marker chromosomes are discovered in tumours with increased frequency. In the case of some leukaemias, lymphomas and other malignancies of the haemopoietic system, the presence of certain specific chromosome translocations is so regularly found that they may serve as reliable diagnostic criteria. The cytogenetic evidence does not exclude the possibility that initially more than one cell might have escaped growth control, but it does indicate that during the growth of the tumour the progeny of one such cell has an overwhelming selective advantage.

TUMOURS THAT FORM SINGLE ANTIBODIES

It is now well established that once a cell is committed to antibody production, it can produce only one kind of antibody; and its descendants form a clone in which all the cells produce the same antibody. The heterogeneity of antibody molecules seen in the natural immune response of an animal to an antigen is due to contributions from a number of different antibody-forming clones. Myelomas, which are tumours derived from antibody-forming cells, often synthesize and secrete antibodies. It has, however, been shown that each myeloma produces an antibody that is chemically homogeneous and distinct from the antibody produced by any other myeloma. The homogeneity of the antibody has been formally established by the analysis of amino-acid sequence. This provides compelling evidence for the conclusion that myelomas are clones derived from single antibody-forming cells.

TUMOURS ARISING IN MOSAIC TISSUES

In placental mammals, such as man, the cells of the female normally contain two X chromosomes, but one of these is rendered inactive at an early stage of embryological development. Inactivation affects the paternal and the maternal X chromosome in a random fashion, so that the tissues of the adult female are an intimately mixed mosaic of two populations of cells, one containing an inactive maternal X, the other an inactive paternal X. This mosaicism may be revealed where X-linked enzymes show polymorphisms that permit the paternal form of the enzyme to be distinguished, usually by its electrophoretic mobility, from the maternal form. The tissues of the adult female, and even the smallest fragments of them that can be analysed, will then show both the paternal and the maternal forms of the enzyme. If a tumour arose by conversion of a substantial number of cells in such a tissue, then one would expect that the tumour would also show the mosaicism of the tissue of origin. But if the tumour arose from a single cell (or from a very few, depending on how intimately mixed the two cell populations were in the tissue), then one would expect the cells of the tumour to contain only one form of the enzyme, either the paternal or the maternal. The X-linked enzyme most extensively used for this sort of analysis is glucose 6-phosphate dehydrogenase, which shows an easily demonstrable polymorphism in man. A very wide range of human tumours of different kinds taken from individuals whose tissues contain a mixture of two electrophoretic variants of glucose 6-phosphate dehydrogenase have now been examined. The majority of these tumours have been found to contain only one form of the enzyme. This again argues strongly for the view that most tumours arise from single cells, or, at the very least, from the selective overgrowth of a very small number of cells.

The cumulative weight of all this evidence effectively eliminates the idea that tumours are produced by the wholesale conversion of large 'fields' of cells. An animal may be exposed to ionizing radiation at a dose sufficient to ensure that every cell in it is subjected to multiple ionizing events; a chemical carcinogen may be administered at a concentration that ensures that every cell in the target tissue receives many thousands of molecules; a tumorigenic virus may be injected in an inoculum large enough to ensure that every accessible cell is infected with many viral particles. But, in each case, only an occasional cell among the huge numbers of like cells at risk gives rise to a tumour. The heritable change that renders a cell insensitive to normal growth control is thus a rare and, at least superficially, a random event. In this respect it clearly resembles a mutation rather than a form of differentiation. For differentiation is not a clonal event. It is, on the contrary, the process *par excellence* in which an induced change affects a 'field' of cells, not a single cell; and there is nothing random about the character of the transformation.

Evidence from hereditary abnormalities of DNA metabolism

There is a group of hereditary diseases that are produced by defects in the enzymes involved in the replication or repair of DNA. These diseases are associated with an extremely high incidence of malignant tumours, and, in some cases, these tumours arise inevitably if the patient lives long enough. The best studied condition of this kind is xeroderma pigmentosum, in which the inherited defect involves one of the enzymes responsible for the repair of damage produced in DNA by ultraviolet light. Those parts of the body that are exposed to ultraviolet light become progressively disfigured by chronic inflammatory processes, and eventually generate multiple carcinomas. Malignant tumours are not notably more common than usual in those parts of the body that are not exposed to ultraviolet light. In the case of ataxia telangiectasia and Bloom's syndrome, the enzymatic basis of the defect in DNA metabolism has not been delineated as precisely as in xeroderma pigmentosum, but here again aberrant DNA synthesis or repair leads to a very high incidence of malignant disease, especially leukaemia. These observations make it very difficult to escape the conclusion that the generation of a tumour must involve some alteration in the structure of the DNA.

The correlation between carcinogenicity and mutagenicity

Earlier studies, which, on the whole, had failed to establish a good correlation between carcinogenicity and mutagenicity have been undermined by the discovery that many carcinogens require metabolic activation before they are effective. If metabolic activation systems that convert inert carcinogens to more reactive intermediates are incorporated in the test procedure, then an astonishingly good correlation between carcinogenicity and mutagenicity emerges. The most extensively used test is that devised by Ames, which measures reversion in auxotrophic histidine mutants of *Salmonella typhimurium.* A liver homogenate is added to the bacterial culture to achieve metabolic activation of the compound being tested. Several hundred carcinogens have now been screened by this procedure, and some 90 per cent of them have been found to be highly mutagenic. Animal cells growing *in vitro* can also be used as screens for mutagens. Although the data so far obtained with animal cells are not very extensive, the correlation between carcinogenicity and mutagenicity holds. The importance of the small proportion of cases in which the correlation breaks down should not be overestimated. It is always possible that the metabolic activation system incorporated in the test is not the appropriate one for any particular carcinogen, or that other special conditions operating in the whole animal are not mimicked in the *in vitro* tests. What is impressive is that the results of simple *in vitro* tests for mutagenicity should correlate so well with a phenomenon as complex as the generation of a tumour *in vivo*. This striking correlation further strengthens the argument that tumours are produced by cellular events that involve structural alterations in DNA.

The problem of reversibility

The main support for the idea that tumorigenicity might be determined by epigenetic events comes from experiments in which the insensitivity to growth control is suppressed or reversed by the process of differentiation: cells known to be tumorigenic cease to be so when they undergo certain specialized changes. In a sense, this is a very old piece of information. The whole of tumour histopathology is based on the fact that tumour cells may undergo recognizable forms of differentiation, and, in many tumours, differentiation generates cells that are no longer capable of continued multiplication. In extreme cases, for example keratinization of skin tumours or the generation of enucleated erythrocytes by erythroid tumour cells, differentiation actually results in cell death. There is, therefore, no problem about accepting the fact that differentiation can override whatever it is that produces the unphysiological growth of tumour cells; but this fact does not in itself constitute evidence for the view that tumorigenicity is determined by epigenetic mechanisms.

In both plants and animals it has been demonstrated that the progeny of certain kinds of tumour cells can contribute to many, if not all, of the specialized tissues of the developing organism. The experiments that have been done with plant cells are more dramatic than those with animal cells. Single cells isolated from crown gall tumours of *Nicotiana tabacum* are capable of generating apparently normal, and fertile, tobacco plants. This striking observation clearly demonstrates that the malignant phenotype can be suppressed in every one of the cells that go to form the mature plant. But again, this fact is not a decisive argument for the view that tumorigenicity is determined by epigenetic mechanisms. Further investigation of the cells that form the regenerated plants shows that they are not normal cells: when they are reexplanted *in vitro*, these cells are found to have retained the biochemical and cultural abnormalities characteristic of crown gall tumour cells. In fact the whole problem has been transformed by experiments of another kind. It has been shown that the production of a crown gall tumour involves the incorporation into the plant cell of a plasmid normally carried by the tumorigenic bacterium *Agrobacterium tumefaciens*; and there is strong genetic and biochemical evidence that specific DNA sequences in the plasmid are responsible for certain critical steps in the generation of the neoplastic state. Moreover, the plasmid DNA is still present in the somatic cells of the phenotypically normal plants generated from the crown gall tumour cells. We must therefore conclude either that the process of differentiation can over-ride the expression of the plasmid DNA sequences that contribute to the production of the malignant phenotype, or that the process of plant growth selects for cells in which the plasmid DNA sequences are not expressed. In any case, it is now difficult to avoid the conclusion that the formation of the crown gall tumour does involve genetic changes in the classical sense, that is, changes in DNA nucleotide sequence.

We cannot yet generate a phenotypically normal adult individual from a single somatic animal cell, but the experiments that have been done on the reversibility of the malignant phenotype during animal development, and the interpretations that have been given to them, are very reminiscent of the work with crown gall tumour cells. It has been shown that embryonal teratocarcinoma cells injected into mouse blastocysts may generate progeny that contribute to the apparently normal development of many different tissues. As in the case of the crown gall tumour, this observation has been used as an argument for the view that tumorigenicity is determined by epigenetic mechanisms, but, once again, these experiments merely show that the insensitivity to growth control can be suppressed by the process of differentiation. It is altogether possible that if the cells derived from the injected embryonal carcinoma cells were reisolated from the chimaeric tissues and grown again *in vitro*, they might, as in the comparable case of the crown gall tumour, retain or regain elements of the tumour cell phenotype. In this connection, it is of interest that, under certain conditions, many of the animals derived from blastocysts that have received embryonal carcinoma cells eventually develop embryonal carcinomas and other tumours at various sites.

Compared with the massive circumstantial evidence supporting genetic mechanisms for the generation of tumours (the fact that tumours arise as rare and essentially random events, the correlation between the carcinogenicity of chemical agents and their mutagenicity, the inordinately high incidence of tumours in patients with inherited defects of DNA metabolism), the case for epigenetic mechanisms is very weak.

Genetic analysis of the cellular lesions determining tumour growth

It was the introduction of cell fusion techniques that first made it possible to apply genetic methods to the analysis of somatic cells. This approach involves the construction of hybrid cells in which the genomes of two different parent cells are initially combined, and in which different genes are subsequently segregated by chromosome loss and rearrangement. Consistent cosegregation of a particular marker with a particular chromosome usually permits the assignation of the gene specifying the marker to that chromosome. A very large number of human genes have now been mapped in this way. Regional mapping within a chromosome, which establishes the order of genes and the distance between them, can be achieved by techniques that combine cell fusion with radiation-induced chromosome rearrangement. These new genetic techniques have been applied to the problem of tumour growth, and some interesting findings have emerged.

When various highly malignant transplantable mouse tumour cells was fused with normal diploid cells, it was found that the resulting hybrids, so long as they retained something close to the sum of the two parental chromosome sets, were unable to grow progressively in immunosuppressed genetically compatible hosts. On continued cultivation *in vitro*, however, these hybrid cells, like all others, underwent chromosome losses and rearrangements; and, with a variable frequency, they generated subsets of cells which regained the ability to grow progressively *in vivo*. Interpreted in simple Mendelian terms, these findings suggested that, if they are mutational events, the lesions determining escape from growth control behave as if they were recessives. This conclusion is in line with a good deal of circumstantial evidence derived from the incidence of tumours in human populations. As dominant mutations occurring in one of two homologous genes would be expressed in diploid cells, it is difficult to see how any of us could ever reach adult life without developing a tumour if tumours were determined by dominant mutations occurring at a frequency within the normal range. If only one or two dominant mutations were required, we would rarely, if ever, survive fetal life. The literature does contain some experiments in which tumorigenicity appears not to have been suppressed when tumour cells were fused with diploid cells; but these experiments have not been analysed in enough detail to provide convincing evidence for the view that, in these cases, the genetic determinants of tumorigenicity are transmitted in a dominant fashion. The reappearance of tumorigenicity in hybrids in which it was initially suppressed is sometimes associated with the loss of identifiable chromosomes derived from the diploid parent cell. This chromosome loss forms the basis of attempts to map the genetic determinants of the tumour phenotype. This has proved to be a more difficult task than might have been anticipated, but it has none the less been shown that certain specific genetic loci are indeed commonly involved even in different kinds of tumour. This conclusion is supported by two additional pieces of evidence derived from hybrid cells. The first of these is based on complementation tests in which different tumour cells are fused with each other. These tests also suggest that many different kinds of tumour may have lesions at the same genetic locus. The second is based on the analysis of hybrids in which parent cells of different morphological types are fused together. If, for example, a lymphoma is fused with a normal fibroblast, the subsets of tumorigenic cells that arise in the hybrid cell population may produce either lymphomas or sarcomas when injected into the animal. This indicates that the same genetic lesions may determine tumorigenicity in both lymphoid cells and cells of fibroblastic type. Similar observations have been made with other parental combinations in hybrid cells.

Cell fusion experiments have also thrown some light on the mode of action of oncogenic viruses. Tumorigenicity may also be suppressed in hybrids produced by the fusion of virus-induced tumour cells with normal diploid cells. Such hybrid cells may be unable to grow progressively *in vivo* even though they can be shown to carry the oncogenic virus, and even though the normal parent cell is known to be susceptible to the virus. This finding indicates that at least some oncogenic viruses must act indirectly by inhibiting or modifying certain cellular genes whose defective function is made good in the hybrid by the activity of homologous genes contributed by the normal parent cell.

TUMOUR SUPPRESSOR GENES

Shortly after the demonstration by cell fusion that the genetic lesions determining malignancy were recessive to the wildtype, the proposal was made that in the case of retinoblastoma, a malignancy for which a predisposition is inherited as an autosomal dominant, the genetic events responsible for the formation of the tumour were not dominant mutations, but homozygous recessives. It was suggested that one of the relevant alleles was mutated in the germ line and that the second allele was inactivated by some event that took place in the cells of the retina. Sporadic cases of retinoblastoma would then be expected to occur very infrequently because two inactivating events at the same allele would be required to generate the tumour, whereas in the inherited form of the disease the tumour would arise with much greater frequency because only a single inactivating event would be required, one of the alleles being already inactivated in all tissues. This model was soon extended to Wilms' tumour and eventually to other tumours whose incidence was governed by a strong hereditary component. At about the same time, it was discovered that, in Drosophila, some mutations at the lethal-2-giant larvae locus produced malignant tumours of the nervous system. These mutations were found to be recessive, and, again, the tumour was produced only when the recessive mutations were present in the homozygous condition.

None the less, in the analysis of tumorigenesis, two decades elapsed before the importance of recessive mutations, and especially homozygous recessives incurring functional losses in cells, finally percolated into the general consciousness. The impulse came from cytogenetic studies that provided a chromosomal localization for the principal gene involved in the genesis of retinoblastoma. It was shown in a patient with the hereditary form of the disease that one of the alleles at this locus was indeed deleted in the germ line and that, in the tumour itself, the second allele was also inactivated. These findings unleashed a major effort to identify and characterize the gene responsible, and, with the help of not a little luck, the effort was crowned with success. This gene (Rb1) was the first of its kind to be isolated and sequenced. About ten such genes have since been identified and characterized fully, including, in man, the gene responsible for one form of Wilms' tumour, the neurofibromatosis gene, and the gene determining familial adenomatous polyposis coli. Genes that contribute to tumorigenesis when they are inactivated or eliminated are now termed tumour suppressor genes. Although most of those that have been characterized fully are involved in the formation of tumours with a strong hereditary component, it is becoming increasingly clear that recessive mutations, especially in the homozygous form, are implicated in an important way in the genesis of the great majority of human tumours. With the possible exception of some malignant tumours of the haemopoietic system, there is widespread agreement that several genetic events must occur before the fully malignant phenotype emerges. It now seems probable that most of these events entail losses of cell function that act cumulatively. We do not yet know in molecular terms what the normal function of any of these tumour suppressor genes is, but there is increasing evidence that at least some of them are implicated in executing critical steps in the process of differentiation. If this proves to be generally true, then there is a case for regarding malignancy as a genetically determined aberration of differentiation.

Oncogenes

The term 'oncogene' was originally used to denote a hypothetical class of cellular genes which, it was proposed, were dormant in normal cells but became activated in tumour cells. The idea was that the progressive multiplication of tumour cells was driven by the abnormal activity of these postulated genes. More recently, the term has been transferred to a class of real cellular genes that have in common the property that they share at least some measure of homology with the genes of oncogenic retroviruses (RNA viruses whose replication requires the synthesis of a strand of DNA complementary to the viral RNA). A large number of such genes have now been identified. Their nomenclature is based on abbreviations of the names given to the retroviruses with which they show homology. Thus, v-*myb* is the gene found in avian myeloblastosis virus and c-*myb* the cellular homologue; v-*myc* the gene found in avian myelocytomatosis virus, c-*myc* the cellular homologue; v-*abl* the gene found in Abelson murine leukaemia virus, c-*abl* the cellular homologue; and so on. It is generally thought that the evolutionary history of the retroviruses involved the capture and subsequent modification of genetic sequences of host origin.

Cellular genes homologous with the retroviral genes have been detected by two general procedures. The first involves screening the cellular DNA with polynucleotide probes derived from, and complementary to, the viral genes. The second is based on a functional test done with a highly unusual cell line bearing the name NIH3T3. NIH3T3 is an established fibroblastic mouse cell line which, despite an aneuploid subtetraploid chromosome constitution, has retained some of the properties of a normal diploid fibroblast, in particular, a regular pattern of growth as a monolayer *in vitro*, density-dependent inhibition of cell multiplication, and an inability to grow in semi-solid media. When genes from certain tumours or tumorigenic cell lines are introduced (transfected) into NIH3T3 cells, either directly as preparations of cellular DNA or as fragments isolated in plasmid vectors, the treated cell populations may generate foci composed of cells that grow irregularly, do not show density-dependent inhibition of cell multiplication and multiply in semi-solid media. Such cells are said to be 'transformed', and some of them may be, or become, tumorigenic. The first genes to be isolated by means of the NIH 3T3 cell transformation assay were found to be homologous with genes of the Harvey or the Kirsten strains of murine sarcoma virus, and were hence given the names H-*ras* or K-*ras*. *Ras* oncogenes isolated from tumours often show point mutations within certain restricted domains, but no *ras* oncogene, mutated or otherwise, can alone confer the transformed, to say nothing of the malignant, phenotype when transfected into normal diploid cells. The co-operation of other mutated genes is necessary to achieve transformation, and the intervention of an unknown number of additional events is required before a fully malignant phenotype emerges.

The polypeptides specified by oncogenes show enormous structural and functional heterogeneity. They range in molecular mass from about 20 000 to more than 150 000. Some of them are found in solution in the cell cytoplasm, others are apparently membrane-bound; some bind to the cellular DNA. Some have phosphokinase activity, others do not. Some have structural homology with polypeptide growth factors of one kind or another or with the cell membrane receptors for growth factors, although it is a feature of some malignant tumours that they lose functional receptors for polypeptide growth factors. In a small number of cases, it has been shown that there is a measure of homology between the oncogenes detected in mammalian somatic cells and genes present in the cells of Drosophila and even in yeast cells, an observation that has prompted the suggestion that at least some c-oncogenes have important biological roles requiring substantive conservation of the structure of the gene product throughout evolution. If all these different gene products do indeed have a role in determining malignancy, their immense heterogeneity of structure and function raises a profound problem, for it is very difficult to see how such a heterogeneous collection of molecules could act to produce the same systematic change in phenotype unless they acted indirectly, by different routes, to modify the activity of some common set of cellular genes. But if the action of oncogenes is indirect, it is important to establish just how indirect it is. Ionizing radiation, for example, can be oncogenic, but it acts non-specifically by producing a large number of random changes that destabilize the genome and thus greatly increase the probability that the specific changes responsible for malignancy will eventually arise in the irradiated cell population. In the case of some of the oncogenic viruses, the quantitative information available makes it unlikely that the virus acts as indirectly as this. A crucial unresolved problem is whether continued activity of the transfected oncogene is required for the maintenance of the malignant phenotype once it has been established. On this point present evidence is meagre, but at least in some systems it is clear that continued activity of a mutated oncogene is not necessary for the maintenance of the malignant state. It appears that in generating a tumour, some oncogenes operate by a 'hit-and-run' mechanism.

Because some oncogenes isolated from malignant cells can, at a variable frequency, induce transformation *in vitro* in NIH3T3 cells, which are presumed to have homologous c-oncogenes that are functioning normally, it has been argued that the oncogenes derived from the malignant cells act in a genetically dominant fashion. There are two reasons for supposing that this may be a rather naive interpretation of the data. First, it has been shown that cells transformed by oncogenes have often lost, or otherwise inactivated, their homologous normal c-oncogenes, a situation reminiscent of what has been found in retinoblastoma; and second, fusion of such transformed cells with non-transformed, or normal diploid, cells, usually yields hybrids in which the transformed phenotype is lost. It is clear that the mode of action of transfected oncogenes in producing transformation *in vitro*, and, *a fortiori*, tumorigenicity, is complex; and a great deal of careful somatic cell genetics will be required to elucidate the dominance relationships of oncogenes introduced into cells in this way. Evidence continues to accumulate that, in many cases, mutations in c-oncogenes, like mutations in tumour suppressor genes, induce losses of cell function, and some of these functional losses also involve differentiation processes. If this is found to be generally the case, then the distinction between oncogenes and tumour suppressor genes will become increasingly difficult to define and might eventually be reduced to differences in the methodologies that led to their detection.

The natural history of a tumour

Once a cell has undergone the heritable change that confers insensitivity to growth control, it generates within the tissues of the affected animal a subpopulation of cells whose subsequent evolution is governed by principles that are very familiar to population geneticists. A population of this kind is subjected to extreme selection pressure which continually favours the emergence of cells with increased growth potential. Thus, any cellular change, mutational or other, which results in an increased rate of multiplication confers a selective advantage: the progeny of a cell that has undergone such a change will progressively increase its representation in the growing tumour. A cell may undergo a change affecting substrate utilization; this may endow it with the ability to survive under conditions that inhibit the growth of other cells. A cell may lose the ability to maintain normal coadaptation with its neighbours. It might then move away from the primary tumour mass, where conditions are crowded, and thus gain for itself an increased nutrient supply. A detached cell, or group of cells, may be translocated by lymph or the blood stream to other sites in the body. If these new sites provide a favourable milieu for cell multiplication, a secondary growth or metastasis is produced. Thus, the tumour cell population, like any other growing population, continually generates variants, and the tissues of the body select those variants that are best fitted for growth at the particular site where they find themselves. It is this Darwinian process that determines the histopathology of a tumour and ultimately its clinical course.

Tumour histopathology rests on the fact that, in general, tumour cells retain enough of the morphological characteristics of differentiation to permit their tissue of origin to be recognized. Thus, for example, tumours arising from muscle cells or cartilage cells are usually composed of tissue that unmistakably resembles muscle or cartilage. The histological appearances of very early tumours suggest that the event that determines initial escape from growth control does not, in general, produce a gross alteration in the morphology of the cell affected. Some tumours never lose the specific morphological characteristics of their tissue of origin; but others, at some stage of their development, do. This loss is often called 'dedifferentiation', which is a rather misleading term as it implies the reversal of the process of differentiation, that is, a wholesale conversion of a population of cells from one phenotype to another. There is, in fact, every reason to believe that 'dedifferentiation' is simply the selective overgrowth within the tumour of cells that have lost a particular morphological marker or group of markers that permits the differentiated state of the tissue of origin to be recognized. If the loss of any particular marker of differentiation results in an increased rate of cell multiplication, then cells lacking the marker will eventually come to dominate the tumour. As expression of most differentiated states involves the synthesis of molecules that are not essential to cell survival, it will be obvious that changes that determine the loss of differentiated markers will very commonly confer a growth advantage. It is for this reason that a broad correlation is found between the degree of 'dedifferentiation' of a tumour and its rate of growth.

From the clinical point of view, the most important property of a tumour cell population is whether it has the ability to generate secondary deposits elsewhere in the body. Cancer would be a trivial disease if tumour cells did not sometimes have this ability. There is very little information about either the biochemical or the genetic basis of metastasis. Cell fusion experiments have demonstrated that the heritable determinants of metastasis are different from those that determine progressive growth: hybrids between the cells of tumours that metastasize and normal diploid cells generate subsets of tumorigenic cells that do metastasize and others that do not. Attempts are being made to use genetic methods to delineate the biochemical basis of metastasis, but these are at a very preliminary stage, more preliminary, indeed, than the comparable analysis of progressive growth.

REFERENCES

Ames, B.N., Durston, W.E., Yamasaki, E., and Lee, F.D. (1973). Carcinogens are mutagens: a simple test system combining liver homogenates for activation and bacteria for detection. *Proceedings of the National Academy of Sciences, U.S.A.* **70,** 2281–2285.

Bishop, J.M. (1983). Cellular oncogenes and retroviruses. *Annual Review of Biochemistry,* **52,** 301–54.

Braun, A.C. and Wood, H.N. (1976). Suppression of the neoplastic state with the acquisition of specialized functions in cells, tissues, and organs of crown gall teratomas of tobacco. *Proceedings of the National Academy of Sciences, U.S.A.* **73,** 496–500.

Cavenee, W.K. *et al.* (1983). Expression of recessive alleles by chromosomal mechanisms in retinoblastoma. *Nature, London,* **305,** 779–784.

Cleaver, J.E. (1968). Defective repair replication of DNA in *Xeroderma pigmentosum. Nature, London,* **218,** 652–656.

Dyson, P.J., Quade, K. and Wyke, J.A. (1982). Expression of the ASV *src* gene in hybrids between normal and virally transformed cells. *Cell,* **30,** 491–498.

Fiaklow, P.J. (1976). Clonal origin of human tumours. *Biochimica et Biophysica Acta. Reviews on Cancer,* **3,** 283–321.

Gateff, E. (1982). Cancer, genes and development – The *Drosophila* case. *Advances in Cancer Research,* **37,** 33–74.

Godbout, R. *et al.* (1983). Somatic inactivation of genes on chromosome 13 is a common event in retinoblastoma. *Nature, London,* **304,** 451–453.

Harris, H. (1971). Cell fusion and the analysis of malignancy. The Croonian Lecture. *Proceedings of the Royal Society,* **B179,**1–20.

Harris, H. (1990). The role of differentiation in the suppression of malignancy. *Journal of Cell Science,* **97,** 5–10.

Huberman, E. and Sachs, L. (1976) Mutability of different genetic loci in mammalian cells by metabolically activated carcinogenic hydrocarbons. *Proceedings of the National Academy of Sciences U.S.A.* **73,** 188–192.

Illmensee, K. and Mintz, B. (1976) Totipotency and normal differentiation of single teratocarcinoma cells cloned by injection into blastocysts. *Proceedings of the National Academy of Sciences, U.S.A.* **73,** 549–553.

Jonasson, J., Povey, S., and Harris, H. (1977) The analysis of malignancy by cell fusion. VII. Cytogenetic analysis of hybrids between malignant and diploid cells and of tumours derived from them. *Journal of Cell Science,* **24,** 217–254.

Klein, G. (ed.) (1990). *Tumor Suppressor Genes.* Marcel Dekker Inc., New York.

Knudson, A.G., Strong, L.C., and Anderson, D.E. (1973) Heredity and cancer in man. *Progress in Medical Genetics,* **9,** 113–158.

Lund, H., Parada, L.F., and Weinberg, R.A. (1983). Cellular oncogenes and multistep carcinogenesis. *Science,* New York, **222,** 771–778.

McCann, J., Choi, E., Yamasaki, E., and Ames, B.N. (1975). Detection of carcinogens as mutagens in the *Salmonella*/microsome test: assay of 300 chemicals. *Proceedings of the National Academy of Sciences, U.S.A.* **72,** 5135–5139.

Marshall, C.J. (1980) Suppression of the transformed phenotype with retention of the viral 'src' gene in cell hybrids between Rous sarcoma virus transformed rat cells and untransformed mouse cells. *Experimental Cell Research,* **127,** 373–384.

Miller, D.A. and Miller, O.J. (1983). Chromosomes and cancer in the mouse: studies in tumours, established cell lines and cell hybrids. *Advances in Cancer Research,* **39,** 153–182.

Mintz, B. (1978). Gene expression in neoplasia and differentiation. *Harvey Lecture,* **71,** 193–246.

Nowell, P.C. (1976) The clonal evolution of tumour cell populations. *Science,* New York, **194,** 23–28.

Papaioannou, V.E., Gardner, R.L., McBurney, M.W., Babinet, C., and Evans, M.J. (1978) Participation of cultured teratocarcinoma cells in mouse embryogenesis. *Journal of Embryology and Experimental Morphology,* **44,** 93–104.

Papaioannou, V.E., McBurney, M.W., Gardner, R.L., and Evans, M.J. (1975) Fate of teratocarcinoma cells injected into early mouse embryos. *Nature, London,* **258,** 70–73.

Sager, R. (1985) Genetic suppression of tumour formation. *Advances in Cancer Research,* **44,** 43–68.

Santos, E. *et al.* (1984). Malignant activation of a K-ras oncogene in lung carcinoma but not in normal tissue of the same patient. *Science,* New York, **223,** 661–664.

Schell, J., Van Montagu, M., de Beuckeleer, M., de Block, M., Depicker, A., de Wilde, M., Engler, G., Genetello, C., Hernalsteens, J.P., Holsters, M., Seurinck, J., Silva, B., van Vliet, F., and Villarroel, R. (1979). Interactions and DNA transfer between *Agrobacterium tumefaciens,* the Ti-plasmid and the plant host. *Proceedings of the Royal Society,* **B204,** 251–266.

Slamon, D.J. *et al.* (1984). Expression of cellular oncogenes in human malignancies. *Science,* New York, **224,** 256–262.

Stanbridge, E.J. *et al.* (1981). Specific chromosome loss associated with the expression of tumourigenicity in human cell hybrids. *Somatic Cell Genetics,* **7,** 699–712.

Stanbridge, E.J. *et al.* (1982). Human cell hybrids: analysis of transformation and tumourigenicity. *Science,* New York, **215,** 252–259.

Stoker, M.G.P. (1972) Tumour viruses and the sociology of fibroblasts. *Proceedings of the Royal Society,* **B181,** 1–17.

Turgeon, R., Wood, H.N., and Braun, A.C. (1976). Studies on the recovery of crown gall tumour cells. *Proceedings of the National Academy of Sciences, U.S.A.* **73,** 3562–3564.

Wiener, F., Cochran, A., Klein, G., and Harris, H. (1972) Genetic determinants of morphological differentiation in hybrid tumours. *Journal of the National Cancer Institute,* **48,** 465–186.

Wiener, F., Klein, G., and Harris, H. (1971). The analysis of malignancy by cell fusion. III. Hybrids between diploid fibroblasts and other tumour cells. *Journal of Cell Science,* **8,** 681.

Wiener, F., Klein, G., and Harris, H. (1974a). The analysis of malignancy by cell fusion. V. Further evidence of the ability of normal diploid cells to suppress malignancy. *Journal of Cell Science,* **15,** 177–183.

Wiener, F., Klein, G., and Harris, H. (1974b). The analysis of malignancy by cell fusion. VI. Hybrids between different tumour cells. *Journal of Cell Science,* **16,** 189–198.

Wigglesworth, V.B. (1937). Wound healing in an insect (*Rhodnius prolixus* Hemiptera). *Journal of Experimental Biology,* **14,** 364.

6.2 Epidemiology of cancer

R. DOLL and R. PETO

Note: readers of this chapter may, on first examination, wish to pass over the central part, which lists separately the epidemiological features of each separate type of cancer, as the preceding and subsequent parts may be read without much reference to it.

Introduction

The epidemiology of cancer, by which is meant the study of the incidence of the disease in man under different conditions of life, has a history dating back nearly 300 years to Ramazzini's observation that cancer of the breast occurred more often in nuns than in other women and to Pott's observation, 200 years ago, that scrotal cancer in young men occurred characteristically in chimney sweeps. Both observations have been confirmed many times since, but whereas the reason for the first is still incompletely understood (except insofar as it is attributable to the avoidance of pregnancy), the second led to the realization that the combustion products of coal could cause cancer on any part of the skin with which they came into repeated contact, and became the foundation stone on which our knowledge of chemical carcinogenesis was built. One hundred years ago, lung cancer was found in the miners of Schneeberg and Jachymov (who, it has subsequently been realized, were heavily exposed to radon), and then skin cancer was found in radiologists and radiographers exposed to X-rays and in farmers and seamen exposed to ultraviolet light, bladder cancer in aniline dye workers, and buccal cancer in betel chewers. Until the interwar years, however, such observations depended for the most part on the acumen of individual physicians, surgeons, and pathologists who were struck by seeing a cluster of cases of a particular type of cancer in patients with a similar occupational or cultural background, and they provided almost all that was known about the causes of cancer. Gradually, however, the epidemiological methods that are described in Section 2 began to be applied to the study of cancer and other non-infectious disease. Many other causes were identified with sufficient certainty to justify preventive action and data were obtained to suggest hypotheses that would be tested in the laboratory.

Biological factors

Certain biological characteristics of cancer have constrained speculations about its causes and the mechanisms that lead to its occurrence. These include the relationships between incidence and age and sex, and the length of the 'latent period' between the first exposure of an individual to a carcinogenic agent and the appearance of clinical disease. These characteristics vary from one type of cancer to another and sometimes also, for a given type, between communities and at different times.

AGE

Some risk of cancer occurs at every age, but the risk of developing any particular type varies with age in many different ways. The most common relationship is a progressive increase in incidence from near zero in childhood to a high figure in old age. This type of relationship is shown by carcinomas of the skin, lung, and gastrointestinal and urinary tracts, and by myelomatosis and chronic lymphatic leukaemia. The rate of increase is rapid, being typically proportional to the fourth, fifth, or sixth power of age, so that cancers that affect only 1 or 2 persons per 1 000 000 each year at around 20 years of age may affect 1 or 2 per 1000 each year at age 80. With most of these cancers, the recorded rate of increase diminishes after about 75 years of age and the recorded incidence may stabilize, or even decrease, in the oldest age groups; but this is partly or wholly an artefact due to incomplete investigation of the terminal illnesses of old people. With the continuing development of medical services, the increasingly intensive investigation of the old, and the collection of progressively more complete data, the cancer incidence rates that are recorded in old age may be expected to increase still more, even if there is no real change in the risk of developing the disease at a given age. This pattern of a rapidly increasing incidence with age is observed for skin carcinoma due to exposure to ultraviolet light and for bronchial carcinoma both in non-smokers and in men who regularly smoke a constant number of cigarettes a day, and can, under certain circumstances, be observed in the laboratory in skin-painting experiments on mice. It is probable that it reflects the cumulative effect of processes that operate steadily throughout life, starting at around the time of birth (or, for lung cancer among habitual smokers, adolescence).

Two much less common patterns are a peak incidence early in life followed by a decline virtually to zero, or a slow rise to a second peak in old age. Retinoblastomas and nephroblastomas occur only in childhood, with peak incidences (respectively) in the first and second years of life. Teratomas and seminomas of the testis have peak incidence rates at about 20 and 30 years of age, respectively, and later almost cease to occur, while osteogenic sarcoma has a peak incidence in adolescence and then shows a slow increase with age from a lower rate in young adult life.

The remaining cancers show a bewildering variety of patterns. Carcinomas of the breast and cervix uteri of women, for example, begin to appear in adolescence and become rapidly more common up to the menopause. After the menopause the incidence of carcinoma of the breast may remain approximately constant, or may even become slightly less common for a few years, before increasing in incidence again with age, though at a slower rate. Carcinoma of the cervix continues to increase fairly steeply for a few years after the menopause, before showing a stable or declining rate. Hodgkin's disease, on the other hand, appears in childhood and then continues to occur more or less evenly throughout life with only minor peaks in young adult life and in old age, while connective tissue sarcomas become progressively more common from childhood on, but with a much slower rate of increase than is shown by the common carcinomas.

Some of these patterns, like that for retinoblastoma, are invariant, being the same everywhere and, as far as is known, at all times. Others vary from community to community, or from time to time. Cancer of the breast, for example, becomes progressively less common with increasing age after the menopause in parts of Asia, while carcinoma of the lung used to show a peak incidence at about 60 years of age in the United Kingdom, which gradually moved to older ages, and it still does show a pattern with a peak in late middle or early old age in many developing countries.

All these various patterns provide information, either about the period of activity of the stem cells from which the cancers derive, or about the times when exposure to the causative agents occurs and the duration of the exposure. Some of this variation has already helped to explain the causes of cancer, as has been the case with the shift in the peak incidence of bronchial carcinoma; but much of it still awaits elucidation.

Sex

Cancer used to be more common in women than in men in nearly all countries due to the great frequency, 70 years ago, of carcinoma of the cervix uteri and the rarity of bronchial carcinoma, and this is still the case in populations for which these conditions hold, as in parts of Latin America. Elsewhere, cancer is now more common in men. This overall male preponderance hides, however, a wide range of sex ratios for cancer of different organs. If the sites of cancer that are peculiar (or almost peculiar) to one sex are ignored, the ratio of the rates varies in Britain from a male excess of about 6 to 1 for pleural mesothelioma and carcinoma of the larynx, through many types of cancer with a small male preponderance, to carcinomas of the right side of the colon, thyroid, and gallbladder, which may be up to twice as common in women.

For many types of cancer the sex ratio is much the same in different countries and at different times. For some, however, and particularly for cancers of the mouth, oesophagus, larynx, and bronchus, the sex ratio may be extremely variable—not only between countries and at different times, but sometimes also between different ages at the same time and in the same country. The most marked variation is shown by cancer of the oesophagus, which may affect both sexes equally or be 20 times more common in men than in women. As with the various patterns of incidence with age, these different sex ratios and the variation between countries and times can provide useful clues to the causation of the particular type of cancer, not all of which have yet been successfully followed up.

Latent period

One reason why it has been difficult to recognize causes of cancer in humans is the long delay that characteristically occurs between the start of exposure to a carcinogen and the appearance of the clinical disease. This 'latent period', as it is commonly, but rather misleadingly, called is often a few decades, although it may be as short as 1 year or as long as 60. The exact relation between the date of exposure and the date of the appearance of different cancers is still uncertain, partly because the interval is subject to random factors, partly because few cancers are induced by a single, brief exposure, and partly because there are still very few sets of quantitative data with detailed information about the dates when exposure began and ended.

When cancer is induced by short but intensive exposure to ionizing radiation, as in Hiroshima and Nagasaki following the explosions of the atomic bombs or in patients treated by radiotherapy, the excess incidence of solid tumours rises for 15 to 20 years and then may continue to rise, level off, or decline. In the case of acute leukaemia, however, a peak incidence occurs earlier (about 5 years after exposure) and few cases appear after more than 30 years.

Short, intensive exposure to a carcinogen is, however, exceptional. The more usual situation is for exposure to a carcinogen to be prolonged for years—perhaps a decade or two in the case of occupational exposure, several decades in the case of tobacco smoking, and a lifetime in the case of ultraviolet sunlight. In this situation the incidence of cancer increases progressively with the length of exposure. In the last two cases cited, the incidence appears to vary approximately in proportion to the fourth power of the duration of exposure so that the effect after (say) 40 years is about 10 to 20 times as great as that after 20 years, and two or three hundred times as great as that after 10 years. Whether the same holds for occupational exposure is not known; but it has been shown to hold in some skin-painting experiments on mice and it may prove to be a general biological rule for many types of tumour and many carcinogens.

There is still less quantitative information about what usually happens when exposure ceases; but in the case of cigarette smoking the annual risk stabilizes and remains at approximately the same level for one or two decades before increasing again slowly. The ex-smoker, therefore, avoids the enormous progressive increase in risk suffered by the continuing smoker. Such quick benefits will, however, be conferred only by stopping exposure to agents that affect at least one of the later stages of the process that culminates in clinical cancer and cannot always be anticipated, particularly if the carcinogen persists in the body (as may happen following exposure to asbestos). For initiating agents that affect only an early stage in the process, it may be safer to assume that the risk continues to increase for some time after exposure stops, though at a slower rate.

These findings accord with the idea that the appearance of clinical cancer is the end-result of a multistage process in which different effects are exerted by initiating and promoting agents. From the point of view of the clinician the important conclusions are that cancer is more likely to occur after prolonged exposure to a carcinogen than after short exposure, that it is seldom likely to appear within 5 years after first exposure (except in the case of leukaemia and the specific cancers of childhood), that it commonly occurs several decades after first exposure, and that it may continue to occur for many years after exposure has ceased. The exact relation may differ for different carcinogens and different types of tumour. Bladder tumours, for example, began to appear within 5 years of intensive exposure to 2-naphthylamine in the dye industry, while mesotheliomas of the pleura have seldom, if ever, appeared within 10 years of exposure to asbestos, but they continue to increase in incidence for up to 50 years after first exposure, even if the exposure was relatively brief.

Preventability of cancer

Perhaps the most important result of epidemiological observation has been the realization that the common cancers occur, in large part, as a result of the way people behave and the circumstances in which they live and are, therefore, at least in principle, preventable. This does not mean that we can envisage a society in which any of the common cancers are completely eliminated (although this may prove to be possible when we understand more clearly the mechanisms by which the disease is produced). What it does mean is that we can envisage a society in which the risk of developing cancer at any particular age is greatly diminished.

The evidence that much human cancer is preventable can be summarized under four heads: differences in the incidence of a particular type of cancer between different settled communities (especially if these are obviously correlated with some quantitative characteristics of the ways those communities live); differences between migrants from a community and those who remain behind; variation with time within particular communities; and the actual identification of a large number of specific and controllable causes.

Differences in incidence between communities

Evidence of variation between communities has not been easy to establish because of differences in the provision and utilization of medical resources and changes in terminology and methods of diagnosis. Detailed clinical and pathological comparisons backed up by surveys of limited populations have, however, shown that the sort of differences now reported by good cancer registries throughout the world are for the most part real, particularly if comparisons are restricted to the limited range of ages between 35 and 64 years. This excludes the youngest ages, at which cancer is rare, and the oldest ages, at which the records of the diagnosis are least reliable.

Table 1 shows for selected types of cancer the range of variation recorded by cancer registries that have produced data sufficiently reliable for the purpose of international comparison (International Union Against Cancer, 1970; International Agency for Research on Cancer,

Table 1 *Range of incidence rates of common cancers (men, unless specified otherwise)*

Site of origin of cancer	High-incidence area	Cumulative incidence (%) in high incidence area[1]	Low-incidence area	Ratio of rates in high- and low-incidence areas[2]
Skin	Australia (Queensland)	> 20	India (Bombay)	> 200
Oesophagus	Iran, N.E.	20	Nigeria	300
Lung	England	11	Nigeria	35
Stomach	Japan	11	Uganda	25
Cervix uteri[3]	Columbia	10	Israel	15
Prostate	USA (blacks)	9	Japan	40
Liver	Mozambique	8	England	100
Breast[3]	Canada (British Columbia)	7	Israel (non-Jewish)	7
Colon	USA (Connecticut)	3	Nigeria	10
Corpus uteri[3]	USA (California)	3	Japan	30
Buccal cavity	India (Bombay)	2	Denmark	25
Rectum	Denmark	2	Nigeria	20
Bladder	USA (Connecticut)	2	Japan	6
Ovary[3]	Denmark	2	Japan	6
Nasopharynx	Singapore (Chinese)	2	England	40
Pancreas	New Zealand (Maori)	2	India (Bombay)	8
Larynx	Brazil (São Paulo)	2	Japan	10
Pharynx	India (Bombay)	2	Denmark	20
Penis	Parts of Uganda	1	Israel (Jewish)	300

[1]By age 75 years, in the absence of other causes of death.

[2]At ages 35–64 years, standardized for age.

[3]Women.

1976). Types of cancer have been included if they are common enough somewhere to have a cumulative incidence among men or women of at least 1 per cent by 75 years of age. The ranges of variation shown are for incidence rates between 35 and 64 years (see above). The range of variation is never less than sixfold and is sometimes more than a hundredfold. Despite the selection of reliable registries, some of this tabulated variation may still be an artefact, due to different standards of medical service, case registration, and population enumeration; but in many cases the true ranges will be greater. First, there are still large gaps in the cancer map of the world so that some extreme figures may have been omitted, because no accurate surveys have been practicable in the least developed areas and it is just these areas that are likely to provide the biggest contrasts (both high and low) with Western society as Chen *et al.* have shown in China. Secondly, the figures cited refer to cancers of whole organs and do not distinguish between different histological types or different locations within the organ. This does not matter for cancer of the oesophagus because this is nearly always squamous and the various causes thus far discovered all produce cancer in the same part of the organ (the lower two-thirds), but it does matter for many other types of cancer. It is, for example, not satisfactory to compare the aggregates of non-melanomatous skin cancers with each other, for these include such unrelated diseases as basal-cell carcinomas of the face, which affect more than half the fair-skinned population of Queensland by 75 years of age, scar epitheliomas of the leg, which develop on the site of old ulcers in Africa and account for 10 to 20 per cent of all cancers seen in some hospitals in Malawi and Rwanda Burundi, '*dhoti*' cancers of the groin in India, and occupational cancers on the forearm due to exposure to tar and oil in industrialized countries.

The variation in incidence that is shown in Table 1 is not limited to the common cancers, but is also shown by many others. Burkitt's lymphoma, for example, never affects more than 1 in 1000 of the population, but it is at least 100 times as common among children in parts of Uganda as it is in Europe and North America; while Kaposi's sarcoma, which was extremely rare in most of the world until the advent of the acquired immunodeficiency syndrome (**AIDS**), is so common in children and young adults in parts of Central Africa that it accounted for 16 per cent of all tumours seen in one of the African hospitals surveyed by Cook and Burkitt. Some few cancers occur with approximately the same frequency in all communities; but, if any do, they are never common. Acute myeloid leukaemia at 15 to 25 years of age is one such type of cancer and nephroblastoma is another, except that it is only half as common in Japan as elsewhere.

The figures that have been cited so far all refer to the incidence of cancer in different communities defined by the area in which they live. Communities, can, however, be defined in other ways and no matter what method is used, including categorization by ethnic origin, religion, or socioeconomic status, substantial differences may be found. Jewesses, for example, have a low incidence of cervical cancer irrespective of the country in which they live, and the Mormons of Utah and the Seventh Day Adventists of California suffer fewer cancers of the respiratory, gastrointestinal, and genital systems than members of other religious groups living in the same American States.

It does not seem likely that the large differences observed between communities can be explained by genetic factors, apart from some of the differences observed in the incidence of cancer of the skin, the risk of which is much greater for whites than blacks, and possibly also some of the differences in the incidence of chronic lymphocytic leukaemia, which rarely affects people of Chinese or Japanese descent. Genetic factors, moreover, cannot explain the differences observed on migration or with the passage of time, which are discussed below, nor can they explain the correlations that are often observed between the national rates for particular types of cancer and some measures of the lifestyle of the different countries.

Changes in incidence in migrant groups

That changes in the incidence of cancer occur on migration is certain. Many groups have been studied, including Indians who went to Fiji and South Africa, Britons who went to Fiji and Australia, and Central Europeans who went to North America. Among the most reliable data are those for the black Africans whose ancestors were taken to America and the Japanese who went to Hawaii. The former experience incidence rates

Table 2 *Comparisons of cancer incidence rates in migrants and residents in homelands and adopted countries (men, unless otherwise specified)*

	Annual incidence per million persons[1]					
		Hawaii			USA	
Primary site of cancer	Japan[2]	Japanese	Caucasians	Nigeria (Ibadan)	Blacks[2]	Whites[2]
Oesophagus	131	46	75			
Stomach	1311	397	217			
Colon	83	371	368	34	351	315
Rectum	93	297	204	34	204	225
Liver				272	77	36
Pancreas				55	225	124
Larynx				37	193	141
Lung	268	379	962	27	1532	981
Prostate	14	154	343	134	651	275
Breast[3]	315	1221	1869	337	1187	1650
Cervix uteri[3]	364	149	243	559	569	276
Corpus uteri[3]	26	407	714	42	222	568
Ovary[3]	53	160	274			
Non-Hodgkin's lymphoma				133	8	4

[1]Rates are standardized for age among men aged 35–64 years unless otherwise specified. Data are provided only for those types of cancer where there are marked differences in incidence between residents of countries of origin and of destination.

[2]Average of rates in two regions.

[3]Women.

for internal cancers that are generally much more like those of white Americans than those of the black populations in West Africa from which most came, while the latter have experienced rates that are much more like those of the Caucasian residents in Hawaii than those of the Japanese in Japan (Table 2). The ancestors of black Americans and Hawaiian Japanese will have come from many different parts of West Africa and Japan, some of which are likely to have cancer rates somewhat different from those that have been cited in Table 2. Nevertheless, the contrasts are so great that there can be no doubt that new factors were introduced with migration.

Changes in incidence over time

Changes in incidence with time can provide conclusive evidence of the existence of preventable factors. Such changes may, however, be difficult to be sure about, chiefly because it is difficult to compare the efficiency of case finding at different periods and partly because few incidence data have been collected for long enough, so that we have to compare mortality rates and these may be influenced by changes in treatment as well as by changes in incidence.

There are no simple rules for deciding which of the many changes in recorded cancer incidence and mortality rates are reliable indicators of real changes in incidence. Each set of data has to be assessed individually. It is relatively easy to be sure about changes in the incidence of cancer of the oesophagus as the disease can be diagnosed without complex investigations and its occurrence is nearly always recorded, at least in middle age, because it is nearly always fatal. It is much more difficult to be sure about changes in the incidence of many other types. The common basal-cell carcinomas of the skin, for example, are also easy to diagnose, but they seldom cause death and can be treated effectively outside hospital, so that they often escape registration. What appears to be a change in incidence may, therefore, be a change only in the completeness of registration. Cancers of the pancreas, liver, and brain, and myelomatosis, in contrast, are usually fatal, but may be overlooked or misdiagnosed as cancer of another type, so that an increased incidence or mortality rate may be wholly or partly due to improvements in diagnosis, in the availability of the medical services, or in the readiness of physicians to inform cancer registries of the cancers they find. Such changes are particularly likely to affect the rates recorded for people over 65 years of age, as many old people who are terminally ill used not to be intensively investigated.

Despite these difficulties, however, some changes have been so gross that there can be doubt about their reality. These include the increase in oesophageal cancer in the black population of South Africa, the increase in lung cancer throughout most of the world, the increase in mesothelioma of the pleura in males in industrialized countries, the decrease in cancer of the tongue in Britain, and the decrease in cancers of the cervix uteri and stomach throughout western Europe, North America, and Australasia. For a fuller account see *Trends in the Incidence of Cancer* (Doll *et al.*, 1994).

Identification of causes

Finally, it has been possible to obtain evidence of the preventability of cancer by defining agents or circumstances that are a cause of the disease and are capable of control. The most straightforward evidence would be the demonstration by scientific experiment that an alteration led to an alteration in the incidence of the disease. Such evidence is, however, difficult to obtain and we often have to be content with the type of strong circumstantial evidence that would be sufficient to secure a conviction in a court of law. Action, based on such evidence, has in practice often been followed by the desired result—for example, a reduction in the incidence of bladder cancer in the chemical industry on stopping the manufacture and use of 2-naphthylamine and the reduction in the incidence of lung cancer that has occurred in men in England and Wales following the change in smoking habits. Cancer research workers have, therefore, accepted that the type of human evidence that has been obtained (often, but not invariably, combined with laboratory evidence that the suspected agents are carcinogenic in animals) is strong enough to conclude that a cause of human cancer has been identified and that, as a corollary, the disease can be prevented by controlling the conditions under which it is produced. Such causes, which amount altogether to about 50, are described under the specific types of cancer they are known to produce and in later sections on medicinal drugs and occupation.

Epidemiology of cancer by site of origin

In the preceding discussion, cancers arising in different anatomical sites have been treated as if they were diseases as different from each other as the different infectious diseases. They have certain obvious pathological and clinical characteristics in common, but they are in many ways aetiologically distinct, as the avoidable causes are different and there is no evidence that the prevention of any one type of cancer augments the age-specific risk of any other. It is, therefore, impossible to review the epidemiology of cancer as a whole. One must rather examine separately the epidemiology of each type. There are a few exceptions, when one agent does or may cause cancer at all or many sites (e.g. ionizing radiations, overnutrition, and deficiency of some micronutrients) but, in general, the agents responsible for the production of human cancer vary with the organ in which the tumour arises and with the tissue within it.

Not surprisingly, the large majority of all human cancers arise from the epithelial cells that line those parts of the human body that communicate, directly or indirectly, with the external environment and are subject to wear and tear. Endothelial or mesodermal cells, in contrast, although they account for most of the human body, are the source of only a small proportion of human cancers. In the account that follows, cancer always implies a carcinoma arising from epithelial tissue unless specified otherwise.

The description of each type is preceded by notes showing its importance in England and Wales. One figure gives the proportion of all cancers that arise in the site, as indicated by the national cancer register for England and Wales for 1987 (Office of Population Censuses and Surveys, 1993*a*) and another gives the proportion of all cancer deaths allocated to the site in the national mortality statistics for 1991 (Office of Population Censuses and Surveys, 1993*b*). A third gives the ratio of the age-standardized incidence rates for each sex. The way in which the incidence of the disease varies with age in each sex is shown in a series of graphs, using the data for England and Wales over the 5-year period 1983–87. The rates at ages under 25 years frequently vary irregularly due to chance variation of small numbers. (The occurrence of one case in a 5-year age group of young people over this 5-year calendar period corresponds to an annual rate of approximately 0.01/100 000.)

Major differences between Britain and other countries are commented on in the text and are described more fully in the report on *Cancer Risks by Site* by the International Union Against Cancer (1980) and by the International Agency for Research on Cancer (1990).

Lip

0.1 per cent of all cancers and 0.02 per cent of cancer deaths.
Sex ratio of rates 4.5 to 1. Age distribution like skin (non-melanoma)

Carcinoma of the lip was one of the first types of cancer to be related to an extrinsic cause when, more than 200 years ago, it was noted to occur characteristically in pipe smokers. Many years later it was realized that the disease could also be produced by smoking in other ways, so that it must be produced by the chemicals in smoke rather than by the non-specific effect of local heat. It is also much more common in outdoor than in indoor workers and is evidently induced by ultraviolet light in the same way as other cancers of the exposed skin. Ultraviolet light and tobacco account, between them, for the great majority of all cases in Britain, probably multiplying each other's effects. The disease is much less common than it used to be, because of the decrease in pipe smoking and outdoor work.

Oral cavity and pharynx (excluding salivary glands and nasopharynx)

1.0 per cent of all cancers and 1.1 per cent of cancer deaths.
Sex ratio of rates 2.1 to 1. Age distribution, see Fig. 1.

Cancers of the tongue, mouth, and pharynx (other than nasopharynx) are all related to smoking (of pipes, cigars, and cigarettes) and to the consumption of alcohol. The two factors act synergistically and cancers in these sites are extremely rare in non-smokers who do not drink alcohol.

Cancer of the tongue is much less common in Britain than it was early this century, but the reason for the sharp decline in incidence is unknown. One explanation could be the decrease in syphilis, which was commonly believed to be a predisposing factor because of the clinical association with syphilitic leucoplakia, but this hypothesis is still unproven.

Cancers that occur low in the hypopharynx are distinguished by a tendency to affect women who have suffered from iron-deficiency anaemia and dysphagia.

Cancers of the buccal cavity and pharynx (excluding nasopharynx) are particularly common in South-East and Central Asia where tobacco smoking is largely replaced by chewing tobacco, betel nut or leaf, and lime (calcium hydroxide). A close association with such chewing habits has been established by studies which have shown that the cancers tend to originate in the part of the mouth in which the quid is usually held—a characteristic that varies both between individuals and between areas. The materials chewed differ in different places and, although the disease is commonly described as 'betel chewer's cancer', betel is not invariably a component of the quid and the most characteristic constituent seems to be a small amount of lime and, in most cases, some form of tobacco. In parts of Asia the disease is so common that it accounts for 20 per cent of all cancers and in those populations the abandonment of chewing would be the single most effective means of reducing the total incidence of cancer—so long as the habit was not replaced by an increase in tobacco smoking. (Moreover, among habitual quid chewers, the risks are particularly elevated in those who both chew and smoke—indeed, in parts of India the majority of deaths from 'betel chewer's cancer' could have been avoided even if the chewing habits remained unchanged, if those affected had not also been smokers.) The incidence might also be reduced by improved nutrition, as the disease in Southern Asia tends to be associated with vitamin A deficiency.

In parts of India where women tend to smoke local cigars and cigarettes with the burning end inside the mouth to prevent them going out, the habit is associated with cancer of the palate.

Salivary glands

0.1 per cent of all cancers and 0.1 per cent of cancer deaths.
Sex ratio of rates 1.6 to 1. Age distribution like non-Hodgkin's lymphoma.

Fig. 1 Annual incidence of cancers of the oral cavity and pharynx by age and sex (excluding cancers of the salivary glands and nasopharynx).

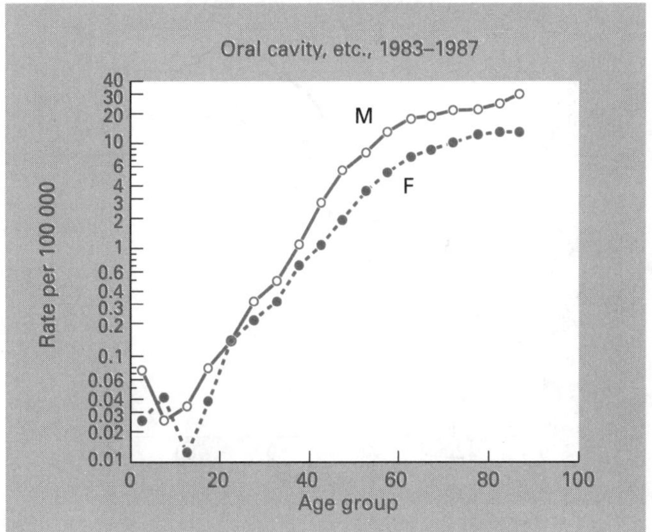

The salivary glands are not common sites for cancer anywhere. They are, however, relatively more common in the Asiatic populations of Hawaii and in Canadian Indians than elsewhere. A small proportion of cases occurs specifically in families that also have a high incidence of breast cancer. No causative factors are known and no notable changes in incidence over time have been reported.

Nasopharynx

0.1 per cent of all cancers and 0.09 per cent of cancer deaths.
Sex ratio of rates 1.3 to 1. Age distribution, see Fig. 2.

Cancers of the nasopharynx, unlike those in other parts of the pharynx, are not strongly related to alcohol or to tobacco. They are rare in most populations but are common in those that originated from parts of Guangdong, in southern China, where the disease is the most common type of cancer. Moderately high rates have been observed in Alaskan Eskimos and American Indians, and intermediate rates in Malaysia, Kenya, and North Africa. A weakly significant relationship with HLA type has been reported from Singapore, but the existence of a specific genetic predisposition remains to be proved. Incidence rates appear to have been decreasing among Chinese Americans.

DNA characteristic of the Epstein–Barr virus (**EBV**) has been detected in the nuclei of nasopharyngeal cancer cells and patients with the disease tend to have unusually high antibodies against EBV-related antigens. Among adults, sudden increases in certain EBV antigens in the blood often precede by a few years the appearance of a pathological cancer. Infection with the EBV is, however, almost universal and can be only one of several agents that act in combination to produce the disease. One such agent in Southern China occurs in the 'salted fish' on which children are commonly weaned. This strongly flavoured delicacy bears little relation to the salted fish eaten elsewhere, and might better be described as decomposing fish: it contains various mutagens, and it has been suggested that exposure of children to it at the same time as their first EBV infection alters the usual lifelong balance between host and virus in some hazardous way.

Oesophagus

2.2 per cent of all cancers and 3.6 per cent of cancer deaths.
Sex ratio of rates 2.0 to 1. Age distribution like gastric cancer.

Cancer of the oesophagus, like other cancers of the upper respiratory and digestive tracts, is closely related to prolonged smoking and consumption of alcohol. All types of smoking have comparable effects and, so it appears, do all alcoholic drinks, although spirits may be slightly more effective per gram of ethyl alcohol than other alcoholic drinks. Alcohol and tobacco act synergistically and, in the absence of either, the incidence of the disease in Britain would be greatly reduced. In France, where the consumption of alcohol is greater than in Britain, it would be reduced even more. A few cases originate from the scars produced by poisoning with corrosive substances and a very few in conjunction with a particular hereditary form of tylosis (presenting with keratoses of the palms and soles). The relatively small excess in men probably reflects the existence of other unknown causes in women, possibly nutritional in origin and similar to those responsible for cancers of the hypopharynx. Mortality (which, because of the high fatality rate, approaches incidence) fell progressively in the first half of the twentieth century *pari passu* with the fall in the consumption of alcohol, and rose again after 1950 when the trend in the consumption of alcohol reversed. Since pipe smoking affects oesophageal cancer risks at least as strongly as cigarette smoking, no large effects on male oesophageal cancer trends could be predicted from the male switch from pipes to cigarettes, although the switch by females from non-smoking to cigarettes should, other things being equal, produce a large upward trend. It appears, however, that other things are not equal and some other, possibly nutritional, cause of oesophageal cancer seems to have decreased, for any upward trends in oesophageal cancer are moderate.

In Africa and Asia the epidemiological features are quite different and present some of the most striking unsolved problems in the field of cancer epidemiology. In parts of China (particularly in North Henan but also elsewhere) and on the east coast of the Caspian Sea in Turkmenistan and Iran, oesophageal cancer is the most common type of cancer, with incidence rates in both sexes that are equal to the highest rates observed for lung cancer in men in European cities. Within China, the disease varies more than 10-fold from one county to another; alcohol and tobacco cannot account for these geographic differences, but when people within one particular Chinese county or city are compared with each other the disease is more common among those who smoke. In parts of Africa, particularly in the Transkei region of South Africa and on the east coast of Lake Victoria in Kenya, extremely high rates are also observed, sometimes equally in both sexes and sometimes only in men. In these and several other areas, as in Asia, the high incidence zones are strictly localized and the incidence falls off rapidly over distances of two or three hundred miles.

When tobacco and alcohol are used, they increase the hazard, but they are not the principal agents in these high-incidence areas. Many causes have been proposed, including molybdenum deficiency in the soil (resulting in a deficiency of the plant enzyme nitrate reductase and a build-up of nitrosamines), contamination of food and pickled vegetables by fungi (particularly by species of *Fusaria*) with the production of carcinogenic metabolites, an agent associated with the production of beer from maize, and the residues left behind in pipes from smoking opium (which are commonly swallowed). None, however, is supported by any impressive epidemiological data. The high incidence area in Iran, which has been intensively investigated, is characterized by extreme poverty and a restricted diet consisting chiefly of home-made bread and tea, with some sheep's milk and milk products, and very little meat, vegetables, or fruit. In this area the disease has been common for centuries. In Southern Africa, however, it seems to have become common only since the First World War. In China, where cancer of the oesophagus was the second most important neoplastic cause of death in the 1970s, large decreases in the disease are beginning to be reported.

Fig. 2 Annual incidence of cancer of the nasopharynx by age and sex.

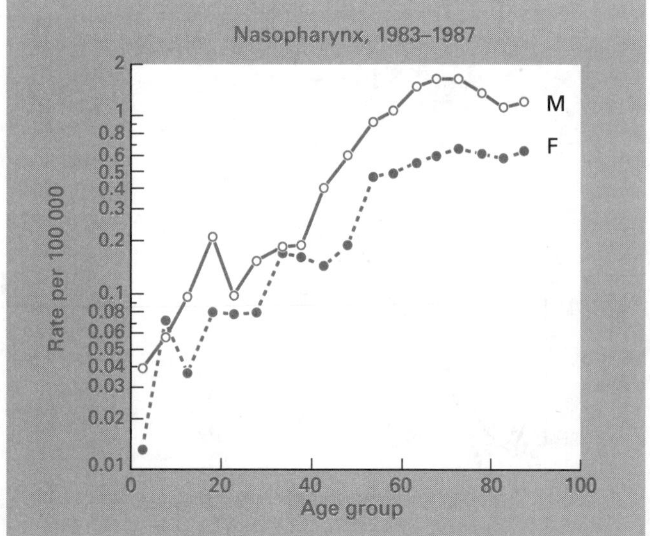

Stomach

5.0 per cent of all cancers and 5.8 per cent of cancer deaths.
Sex ratio of rates 2.4 to 1. Age distribution, see Fig. 3.

Until about 1980, gastric cancer was responsible for more deaths from malignant disease worldwide than any other type. Over the last 50 years, however, the incidence has declined in Western Europe, North America, and Australasia and recently it has begun to do so in South America and Japan. High rates are now confined to China, Japan, Russia and other countries of the old Soviet Union, and Central and South America, while the lowest rates are, perhaps surprisingly, found equally in North America, Australasia, and some of the least developed parts of Africa. Irrespective of whether the incidence is high or low, the sex ratio is between 1.5 and 3 to 1.

Within Britain, cancer of the stomach is most common in North Wales and becomes progressively less common from north to south and from west to east. Over the last 70 years it has consistently been some five times more common in unskilled labourers than in members of the major professions, a gradient with socioeconomic status that has been one of the most marked for any disease. Relatively high rates have been observed in coal miners and in some chemical workers; but no specific occupational hazards have been identified and the excess in coal miners was paralleled by a similar excess in their wives. A hazard has been suspected from exposure to asbestos, but the apparent excess may be due to misdiagnosis of lung cancer and mesothelioma.

Four factors are known to predispose to the disease: blood group A constitution, gastritis associated with infection by *Helicobacter pylori* (sometimes leading to atrophic gastritis), a diet deficient in fruit and green and yellow vegetables, and a poor diet with large amounts of salt and salt-preserved food. Chronic infection with *H. pylori* is a major cause of peptic ulcer, a finding that is of considerable practical value in patients with ulcers, because the infection can generally be eliminated from the stomach by a short course of appropriate antibiotic therapy, providing long-term protection against recurrence. It is not yet known, however, whether such treatments would have any material effect on the incidence of stomach cancer. Whether smoked foods also increase the risk is less clear; if they do, they are certainly less important than the other dietary factors referred to. How these various factors influence the production of the disease is unclear. One possibility is that they encourage or discourage the formation of carcinogens *in vivo*, particularly perhaps the production of nitrosamines; but if they do, the intake of nitrates (which can be converted into nitrites by bacterial enzymes) is not a rate-limiting factor. Changes in all the three environmental factors could have contributed to the decline in the incidence of the disease, but it is difficult to see how they could have brought about such a large and widespread reduction in risk, and it seems probable that the better preservation of food, resulting from the extensive use of refrigeration, has played a major part.

No risk has been detected from the consumption of mutagens produced by the different methods of cooking meat and fish, nor from food additives or pesticide residues. Some food additives may, on the contrary, have served to reduce risk (by avoiding food spoilage and hence improving nutrition, by avoiding contamination by carcinogen-producing micro-organisms, or by some antioxidant or other protective effect on the gastric epithelium).

Large bowel

11.6 per cent of all cancers and 11.3 per cent of cancer deaths.
Sex ratio of rates 1.4 to 1. Age distribution, see Fig. 4.

Cancers of the colon and rectum ought to be considered separately, as their causes are not identical. Cancer of the colon, for example, tends to occur more often in women than in men, particularly when it occurs on the right side, while cancer of the rectum is nearly twice as common in men. The geographical distribution also differs slightly, colonic cancer varying in incidence more than rectal cancer. Separate consideration may, however, sometimes be misleading as cancers occur commonly at the rectosigmoid junction and the site of origin of these cases is not recorded consistently. Moreover, there is a growing tendency to describe both diseases merely as 'cancers of the large bowel', which, according to the internationally agreed rules, are classed with cancers of the colon. The two diseases will, therefore, be considered together.

Over the past few decades in the United Kingdom and United States the male rates have been approximately constant, while the female rates have decreased slightly. More recently, decreases in early middle age have begun to be seen in both sexes. In contrast, the incidence in Japan, which used to be very low, has begun to increase and the disease in Japanese migrants in Hawaii has become as common as in Caucasians. In most other parts of Asia, and in Africa and Eastern Europe, large-bowel cancer continues to be relatively uncommon (except in areas where chronic schistosomal infestation of the large intestine is common; for example, high rectal cancer rates are found in those Chinese counties where *S. japonicum* was, until recently, a major cause of death). Incidence rates in different countries correlate closely with the per caput consumption of fat and meat and crudely with the consumption of processed foods from which the natural fibre has been removed. Ways in which these and several other dietary constituents might influence the development of the disease are discussed later.

Within Britain there is no clear relation to socioeconomic status and no occupational hazard has been established. The association that has been reported with exposure to asbestos may be due to misdiagnosis as in the case of cancer of the stomach. Cases in childhood or early adult

Fig. 3 Annual incidence of cancer of the stomach by age and sex.

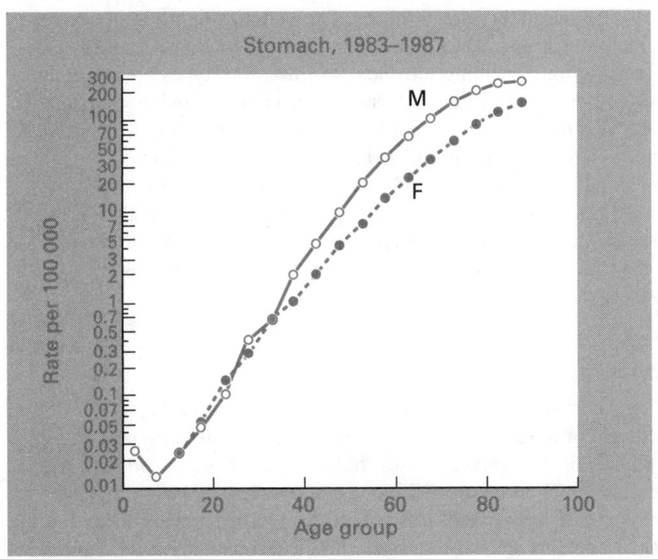

Fig. 4 Annual incidence of cancer of the large bowel by age and sex.

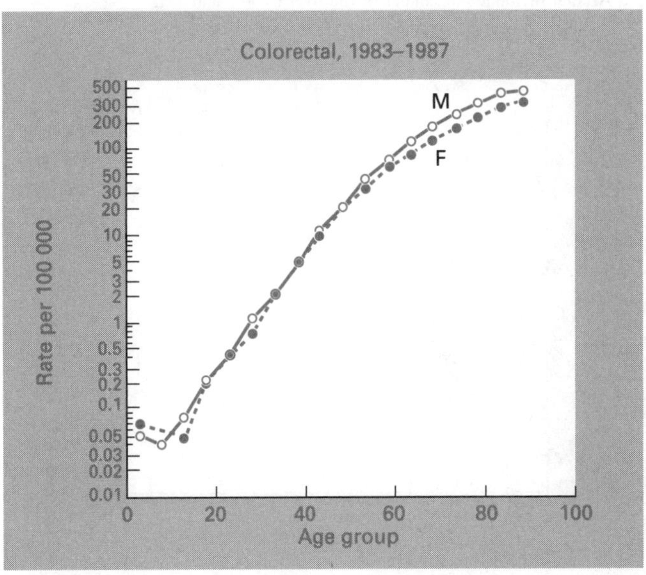

life occur as a complication of polyposis coli or (more rarely) Gardner's syndrome. These conditions are determined by dominant genes, which so increase the susceptibility to the disease that it almost invariably develops before middle age. Many other cases develop from adenomatous polyps and a few occur as a complication of long-standing ulcerative colitis.

Anal intercourse causing infection with type 16, type 18 or some other specific types of the human papillomavirus is a probable cause of some anal carcinomas, but patients who merely have sexually transmitted anal warts that are due to other types of human papillomavirus are not thereby placed at risk of cancer.

Liver

0.5 per cent of all cancers and 1.1 per cent of cancer deaths.
Sex ratio of rates 2.1 to 1. Age distribution, see Fig. 5.

Incidence rates tend to be overestimated in developed countries because the primary condition is often confused with metastases to the liver from cancer in various other organs, particularly over 65 years of age when carcinomas of the gastrointestinal and respiratory tracts are common. Changing standards of medical services make reliable assessment of trends difficult, so although the death rates attributed to liver cancer are, if anything, still decreasing in the United States, this gives no reason to suppose that there are at present any appreciable changes in liver cancer rates either in the United States or in Britain, where current rates are among the lowest anywhere. Compared with Britain and America, however, liver cancer is much more common in South-East Asia, including parts of China, and in large parts of tropical Africa it is the most common type of cancer in men.

Most cases derive from the main cells of the organ (hepatocellular carcinomas) and are attributable primarily to chronic active infection, established early in life, with the hepatitis B virus, exacerbated by some specific metabolite (e.g. aflatoxin) of particular types of fungal contamination of stored foods. Neonatal vaccination against the virus has been begun in Japan and parts of China and tropical Africa, and produces a marked decrease in the proportion of children who, at 5 years of age, are chronically infected, but it will be some years before its efficacy in the prevention of hepatocarcinoma can be seen.

In developed countries such as Britain it is uncertain whether the minute amounts of aflatoxin that are consumed could account for any of the few cases of liver cancer. A more important cause of hepatocellular carcinoma is cirrhosis, irrespective of whether it is due to hepatitis, chronic alcoholism, or haemochromatosis. Occasionally, liver cancer is

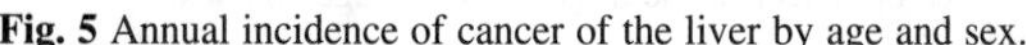

Fig. 5 Annual incidence of cancer of the liver by age and sex.

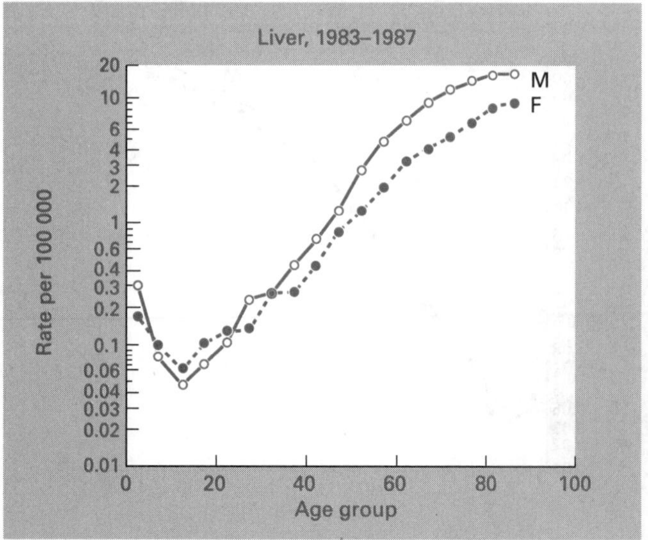

produced by drugs. A few cases have occurred in young men who have taken androgenic–anabolic steroids to increase their muscular strength and a few from the use of steroid contraceptives, either by causing them to arise *de novo* or by complicating the development of the benign adenomas of the liver, which are themselves rare complications of the use of steroid contraceptives.

A second histological type (cholangiosarcoma) arises from the intrahepatic bile ducts, tends to occur at a somewhat later age than hepatocellular carcinoma, and, although generally less common than hepatocellular carcinoma, nevertheless accounts for an appreciable proportion of cases. In China, Thailand, and other parts of Asia it can be produced by chronic infection with liver flukes (*Clonorchis sinensis* or *Opisthorchis viverrini*).

A third histological type that is extremely uncommon everywhere has been variously described as reticuloendothelioma or angiosarcoma. It was first recognized as a complication of the use of 'Thorotrast' as a contrast agent in neuroradiology, a long-abandoned practice that led to chronic retention of insoluble thorium radionuclides in the marrow, spleen, and liver. In 1973 it was found to be an occupational hazard for men exposed to vinyl chloride. A few hundred cases have occurred throughout the world in men who were heavily exposed in the manufacture of vinyl chloride polymer, and it seems improbable that the minute amounts that have leached out of the plastic consumer products can have caused more than a dozen cases altogether in the general public, if indeed they have produced any. A third, and even rarer, cause is prolonged exposure to inorganic arsenic, such as used to result from the medical prescription of Fowler's solution. Despite these multiple causes only three or four cases of hepatic angiosarcoma occur each year in Britain, which is why the recognition of new causes has been so easy.

Cancer of the liver is almost uniformly fatal and it is fortunate that it should be so rare in developed countries. The fact of its rarity is intriguing, since most of the carcinogens thus far discovered in experimental animals induce, perhaps *inter alia*, tumours of the liver, so the lack of any high or increasing liver cancer rate in Britain and America suggests that, on average, the populations have not been substantially exposed to the sort of chemical carcinogen that is currently recognized by such studies.

Gallbladder and extrahepatic bile ducts

0.5 per cent of all cancers and 0.6 per cent of cancer deaths.
Sex ratio of rates 0.9 to 1. Age distribution like colorectal cancer.

Cancers of the gallbladder and extrahepatic bile ducts are nearly always classed together, which is unfortunate as the causes are certainly different. The former is more than twice as common in women as in men, is strongly associated with obesity, and is usually preceded by (and probably caused by) cholelithiasis. The latter is slightly more common in men and is increased in incidence by clonorchiasis and (to a less extent) by long-standing ulcerative colitis. Both types are uncommon, and their aggregate varies only slightly from one population to another. Relatively high rates are recorded among Jewesses in Israel, especially among those born in Europe and America.

The incidence of cancer of the gallbladder has fallen sharply in the United States in the last 20 years, which may be due to the decreased consumption of animal fat or, perhaps more importantly, to an increase in the rate of cholecystectomy in people who, having gallstones, are at greatest risk of cancer of the gallbladder.

Pancreas

2.7 per cent of all cancers and 4.2 per cent of cancer deaths.
Sex ratio of rates 1.5 to 1. Age distribution like stomach cancer.

Cancer of the pancreas is two to three times more common in regular cigarette smokers than in lifelong non-smokers. The mechanisms by which cigarette smoke causes pancreatic cancer are not known, but the smoke contains several thousand chemicals including minute amounts of volatile nitrosamines and some pancreatic carcinogen could well be absorbed from the alveoli and carried to the pancreas in the bloodstream. The disease is twice as common in diabetics as in the population as a whole. It should not, therefore, be surprising that the highest rate recorded is among New Zealand Maoris, who smoke heavily and are prone to obesity, hypertension, myocardial infarction, and diabetes.

Cancer of the pancreas is generally regarded as a disease of the developed world, but the diagnosis is difficult in the absence of a well-developed medical service and some of the relatively small geographical and temporal variations may be due to variation in diagnostic standards. Mortality rates in Britain and the United States have begun to decrease under 65 years of age, and this is more likely to reflect a real reduction in incidence (due perhaps to changes in diet and smoking habits) than to improvement in treatment, as the 5-year survival rate remains well under 10 per cent.

Nose and nasal sinuses

0.2 per cent of all cancers and 0.1 per cent of cancer deaths.
Sex ratio of rates 1.6 to 1. Age distribution like non-Hodgkin's lymphoma.

Surprisingly, in view of the widespread exposure of the human nose to tobacco smoke and other airborne toxins, cancers of the nasal cavity itself are extremely rare and most of the cancers in this group arise from the paranasal sinuses. Several occupational hazards have been recognized, including the refining of nickel, the manufacture of isopropyl alcohol and hardwood furniture, and some aspect of the manufacture of leather goods. It would be wrong, however, to conclude that all contact with nickel, hardwood dust, etc. creates a hazard. The hazards have been observed in special occupational situations in which exposure has been intensive and prolonged, and probably also in which specific physical and chemical conditions have occurred. The nickel-refining hazard was first observed in South Wales where the nickel carbonyl process was used, but similar hazards were subsequently observed with other processes in Canada, Norway, and the then USSR. In the Welsh refinery the workplace exposures were much heavier before the Second World War, and (despite the continued use of the nickel carbonyl process in Wales) no hazard of nasal sinus cancer has yet been observed among men first employed there since 1950. The hazard in furniture workers was first observed in High Wycombe and appears to have followed the introduction of high-speed wood-working machinery early in the twentieth century. It certainly affects some other groups but should not be assumed to affect furniture workers in general.

Most occupational and other cancers in this group are squamous carcinomas, but the hazard from hardwood dust characteristically produced adenocarcinomas. In some of the exposed groups as many as 5 per cent of the men developed the disease. This meant that the risk of adenocarcinoma was increased 1500 times (as this histological type of the disease is normally very rare) and the hazard was, in consequence, easy to confirm once suspicion had been aroused.

Chromate workers are sometimes said to experience a hazard of nasal cancer, but this is perhaps an error due to confusion with the characteristic 'chrome ulcer' of the nasal septum. These ulcers have not been shown to become malignant.

Larynx

0.8 per cent of all cancers and 0.6 per cent of cancer deaths.
Sex ratio of rates 5.9 to 1. Age distribution, see Fig. 6.

Cancers of the larynx, like cancers of the oesophagus and buccal cavity, are closely associated with tobacco smoking and with the consumption of alcohol. The two agents act synergistically and in the absence of either the disease is rare. Cancers of the glottis (like cancers of the lung) are associated particularly closely with cigarette smoking, while all types of tobacco smoking may equally cause cancers of the extrinsic larynx.

In Scandinavia the incidence has increased *pari passu* with the increase in cancer of the lung. A similar increase has not, however, been seen in Britain and it seems probable that some other aetiological factor, perhaps nutritional in character, has become less prevalent. That there are other causal factors is evident from the relatively high incidence rates in parts of India, Turkey, North Africa and Brazil, which cannot be accounted for by tobacco and alcohol.

The disease has also occurred as an occupational risk in the manufacture of mustard gas and possibly also from exposure to asbestos.

Lung

16.8 per cent of all cancers and 23.7 per cent of cancer deaths.
Sex ratio of rates 3.5 to 1. Age distribution, see Fig. 7.

Nearly all lung cancers are bronchial carcinomas and should properly be so described. The term 'lung cancer' is, however, in such common use that it will be used here as synonymous with bronchial carcinoma, although it actually includes a very small proportion of alveolar-cell carcinomas and other rare types of cancer with different characteristics.

Until the 1920s, lung cancer was uniformly rare (except in the Hartz mountains, see below). In the next two decades, German and then British

Fig. 6 Annual incidence of cancer of the larynx by age and sex.

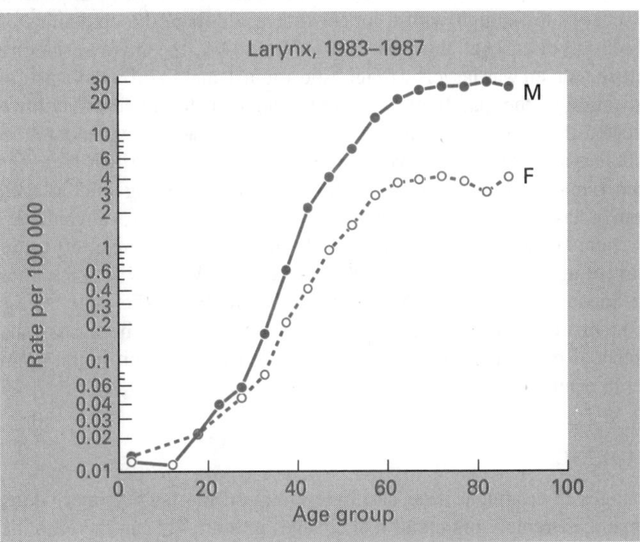

Fig. 7 Annual incidence of cancer of the lung by age and sex.

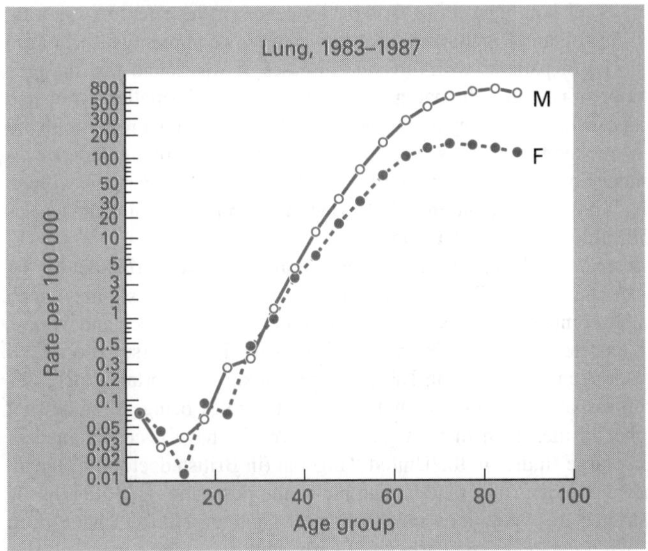

Table 3 *Mortality from lung cancer in the United States by cigarette smoking and sex (study of the American Cancer Society)*

Sex	Death rate per 100 000 persons per year[1]				
			Continuing regular cigarette smokers number of cigarettes smoked per day		
	Lifelong non-smokers	Ex-cigarette smokers	1–14	15–24	25 or more
Male	5	38	74	115	160
Female	5	16	28	59	93

[1]Standardized for age on age distribution of man-years at risk of male doctors.

pathologists began to comment on an apparent increase, but this tended to be dismissed as an artefact of the greatly improving methods of diagnosis and the establishment of special centres for thoracic disease, and at that time much of the increase in the incidence of the disease was indeed artefactual. Gradually, however, the increase became so pronounced, and the change in the sex ratio so marked, that it could no longer be dismissed as being wholly artefactual in males, and by the late 1940s, when the age-standardized mortality rate in men in the United Kingdom had increased 20 times, it was clear that the developed world had begun to see an epidemic of lung cancer that was comparable in severity to, though with a longer time scale than, the epidemics of infectious disease of the past. Up to the 1940s, the increase among British women was largely a diagnostic artefact, and so provides a useful indication of the quantitative extent to which such artefacts may have affected the male rates. Since 1950, however, diagnostic standards in middle age have changed very little, the increase in British men has been replaced by a decrease, while the increase among middle-aged women has continued for longer, before also reversing. As a result, the sex ratio (male rate divided by female rate) at, for example, 50 to 54 years of age, which rose from 1.8 after the First World War to 8.9 after the Second World War, was reduced to 2.2 in 1991. The male excess in the first quarter of the century may have existed partly because of the effects of pipe smoking (an almost exclusively male habit in the nineteenth century).

SMOKING

Changes in treatment have had little effect on the fatality rate, which remains extremely high, and real changes in mortality can therefore be regarded as reflecting real changes in incidence. These can be almost entirely explained by the effects of smoking tobacco, particularly in the form of cigarettes, which in the early 1990s caused more than 90 per cent of all lung cancers in Britain. Evidence of the effect of smoking was first obtained in the middle of the century by comparing the smoking histories of patients with different diseases. It was found that the proportion of patients who had never smoked was much smaller if they had lung cancer than if they had some other disease, and the proportion who had smoked heavily was correspondingly greater. Further evidence was obtained by asking large numbers of apparently healthy men and women what they smoked, and then following them up to determine the causes of death of those that had died.

Interim results of a study of over 1 million people carried out by the American Cancer Society and the National Cancer Institute, which enable comparisons to be made of the mortality of both men and women are reported by Clark Heath Jr. and Michael Thun (personal communication) and are shown in Table 3. In both sexes, the mortality increases progressively with the amount smoked, the rates being all somewhat higher in men than in women. Similar results have been obtained in other large studies in the United Kingdom (in British doctors) in Japan, and in Sweden (in a random sample of the population). If attention is restricted to populations in which most cigarette smokers have been smoking cigarettes regularly since early adult life, lung cancer eventually becomes about 20 times more common in regular cigarette smokers than in lifelong non-smokers and up to 40 times more common in very heavy smokers. At present the differences appear to be less marked in women than in men, but this difference may be only a temporary phenomenon, arising mainly because most female smokers who are now old enough to have a high risk of cancer either did not begin smoking cigarettes so early in adult life or smoked them less intensively when they began.

No other exposures have been identified that can account for the extreme difference in lung cancer risk between regular cigarette smokers and lifelong non-smokers, and so most or all of the excess must be taken as having been caused by smoking. Further quantitative studies have found that the relative risk of lung cancer increased with decreasing age of starting to smoke and decreased with the number of years that smoking had been stopped; that the national increase in incidence appeared at an appropriate time after the increase in cigarette sales (after due allowance was made for a spurious increase due to improved diagnosis) and with an appropriate lag in time in both men (who started to smoke cigarettes early in the twentieth century) and women (who started a few decades later); and that there is a general parallelism between the incidence of the disease in different countries and social and religious groups and the prolonged consumption of cigarettes. Furthermore, it was found that when extracts of cigarette smoke were applied repeatedly to the skins of laboratory mice many tumours developed. Finally, and most encouragingly, the trend in mortality at young ages reversed following reduction in smoking and the change to a type of cigarette that delivers substantially less tar. By 1991, the mortality from lung cancer among men in their 30s in Britain, many of whom had smoked low-tar cigarettes for a greater part of their smoking lives, was only about a quarter of that of men in their 30s some 40 years earlier, the smokers among whom had always smoked high-tar cigarettes. At older ages the decreases are less striking, but they are now seen at all ages in British men, and up to 60 in British women.

OCCUPATION

Several other causes of lung cancer have been discovered as a result of observations in industry. Many thousands of men and women have experienced significant hazards from exposure to asbestos or to polycyclic hydrocarbons (from the combustion of fossil fuel). The former has given rise to hazards in asbestos mines, asbestos textile works, and in a wide variety of insulation work in the shipbuilding and construction industries. The latter gave rise to specific hazards in the manufacture of coal gas in coking ovens, in steel works, in aluminium foundries, and wherever else substantial amounts of incompletely combusted fumes were released into the working environment. Much smaller numbers of men have experienced substantial hazards from radon in the air of mines (not only when mining radioactive materials but also when mining haematite and fluorspar under conditions in which radon seeped into the mine air from streams and the surrounding rock), from the manufacture of chromates and chrome pigments, from the refining of nickel, from arsenic (in the manufacture of arsenical pesticides and in the refining of copper, which is always contaminated with arsenic), and from the manufacture of mustard gas. In one extreme situation, the absolute risk of contracting lung cancer due to the occupational hazard of radon exposure was so large that more than half the workers contracted the disease (in the cobalt mines of the Hartz mountains in Central Europe, which were subsequently mined for radium and uranium). In several other situations with heavy exposure to asbestos or the early stages of nickel refining the occupational hazard has affected as many as 20 to 30 per cent of the exposed men.

ATMOSPHERIC POLLUTION

Some of the materials responsible for these occupational hazards—particularly the combustion products of fossil fuels—are or have been widely distributed in the air of towns and it is still uncertain how far they, in this way, contributed to the production of the disease in the general population. That lung cancer was more common in big towns than in smaller towns and rural areas is certain, but this held as strongly for Oslo and Helsinki, two relatively unpolluted cities, as for London, Birmingham, Manchester, Chicago, Los Angeles, and Pittsburgh. Differences between the largest towns and the least populated areas have seldom been more than threefold and it is difficult to estimate how far these differences can be accounted for by past differences in cigarette smoking, a habit which has tended to spread outwards from the major cities. Attempts to 'allow for' cigarette smoking are probably inadequate, as it is impossible to take full account of such factors as the age of starting to smoke cigarettes, the amount smoked daily at different periods, and the method of smoking (number of puffs, depth of inhaling, etc.). The results of a large study carried out by Hammond and Garfinkel (1980) for the American Cancer Society showed some small differences between residents of the different areas after standardizing for current cigarette smoking to the best of the authors' ability, but they concluded that the data offered 'little or no support to the hypothesis that urban air pollution has an important effect on lung cancer'. One thing is certain, that in the absence of cigarette smoking any effect of urban pollution is relatively so small that it has been impossible to measure it reliably. Some synergism between smoking and urban air pollution, however, is possible, and estimates based on extrapolation from the effects observed in heavily polluted factories suggest that previous levels of atmospheric pollution may, by aggravating the hazards of tobacco, have contributed to as much as 10 per cent of all lung cancers in certain big cities. (Among non-smokers, however, any excess risk from urban air pollution is, in absolute terms, small.) In Britain the present levels of air pollution by benzo[a]pyrene and various other components of smoke are much lower than the levels of half a century ago, and their effects on future lung cancer rates are, therefore, likely to be even smaller.

GEOGRAPHIC DIFFERENCES

The development of the male lung cancer epidemic and the early signs of its departure have been most prominent in Britain and Finland, since the switch of young men to cigarettes was largely complete in these countries by the 1920s. In the United States, where cigarette consumption doubled during the Second World War, the benefits of recent reductions in tobacco exposure are superimposed on the increasing lung cancer rates due to the delayed effects of past increases in smoking in early adult life by those who are now reaching middle and old age. Hence, it is thus far only among younger men in the United States that the benefits of reduced smoking and a switch to low-tar cigarettes are causing net decreases in lung cancer mortality. In some other developed countries the development of the epidemic is still further behind and it is only just beginning to appear in many developing countries. Chinese males, for example, who now consume about 30 per cent of the world's cigarettes, experienced a threefold increase in cigarette consumption during the 1980s that may well eventually cause almost a million cancer deaths a year when the young men of today reach middle age. In women, the development of the epidemic has been later. Only in the Maori population of New Zealand did it occur at the same time as in men. In the United Kingdom, United States, and a few other developed countries, the female lung cancer rates are already substantial, but in others, such as France and Spain, the epidemic in women has scarcely begun. A relatively high risk has long been noted in Chinese women who are non-smokers, irrespective of their country of residence, which is probably due to their exposure to mutagens in the fumes from oils used in cooking with a wok, and from the coal smoke with which many Chinese homes are heavily polluted.

Pleura and peritoneum

0.3 per cent of all cancers and 0.4 per cent of cancer deaths.
Sex ratio of rates 6.0 to 1. Age distribution like laryngeal cancer.

The existence of a specific type of tumour arising from the pleura or peritoneum was debated by pathologists until 1960 when Wagner and his colleagues reported that six African patients with a similar type of 'peripheral lung cancer' had all lived in villages that were heavily polluted with dust produced by the mining of blue asbestos (i.e. crocidolite). Since then, many cases have been reported throughout the world, the great majority of which have been specifically associated with exposure to asbestos at work. A few cases arise from neighbourhood pollution with asbestos or secondary contamination (e.g. from household contact with asbestos workers) and some in Turkish villages are due to the weathering into the general atmosphere of mineral fibres in local rock that are physically similar to, but chemically different from, asbestos. A few cases have been caused by radiotherapy and natural ionizing radiations may be responsible for most of those that are not associated with asbestos. Most mesotheliomas arise from the pleura, but some originate from the peritoneum. They are much less likely to occur after exposure to white asbestos (chrysotile) than after exposure to brown asbestos (amosite) or blue, which persist for longer in the lungs.

Mesothelioma seldom occurs less than 15 years after first exposure to asbestos, commonly occurs 25 to 30 years afterwards, and may be delayed for 50 years or more. Almost all cases are fatal, so that the mortality would reflect incidence, if all cases were correctly diagnosed. Due to the rarity of the disease and the possibility of confusion with lung or other types of cancer, it is still uncertain how many cases occur each year. The recorded rate is still rising and, although the disease may now be somewhat overdiagnosed, the pattern of increase is alarming, as it still continues even in young adults, suggesting that it will be several decades before the maximum effects are seen.

Pleural mesothelioma is not related to cigarette smoking and the occupational hazard affects cigarette smokers and non-smokers alike.

Bone

0.2 per cent of all cancers and of cancer deaths.
Sex ratio of rates 1.1 to 1. Age distribution, see Fig. 8.

Sarcomas can affect any bone, but characteristically affect the long bones in adolescence. After 45 years of age they occur most commonly in bones affected by Paget's disease (osteitis deformans), which predisposes to sarcoma so strongly that as many as 1 per cent of all affected people eventually develop one.

Many different histological varieties occur, some of which appear to have different causes. Osteogenic sarcomas and chondrosarcomas are the most common, the former accounting for nearly all the adolescent peak. One rare type (Ewing's tumour) occurs only in childhood and adolescence and is almost unknown in black people, irrespective of the society in which they live.

Ionizing radiations are the only known extrinsic cause. Cases have been produced after intensive radiotherapy or the medicinal use of thorium (a bone-seeking radionuclide). In industry they have occurred in 'luminizers' who, in previous decades, used delicate paint brushes to apply radium compounds, and ingested radium, possibly as a result of 'pointing' the paint brushes in their mouths.

National statistics record a reduction in mortality over the last 50 years, but are unreliable indicators of incidence as many deaths attributed to tumours of bone are in reality due to cancers that have metastasized from other sites. The recorded decrease in mortality is, therefore, largely an artefact due to improved diagnosis (though it has been contributed to in recent years by higher survival rates in childhood) and the true incidence may have remained roughly constant.

Connective tissues

0.4 per cent of all cancers and of cancer deaths.
Sex ratio of rates 1.2 to 1. Age distribution, see Fig. 9.

Sarcomas of the soft tissues include a variety of different diseases, all of which are rare everywhere. Some are caused by ionizing radiations, others may be caused by intensive immunosuppression, and a few may result from exposure to chlorophenols, but the evidence for this is inconclusive.

Fig. 8 Annual incidence of cancer of bones by age and sex.

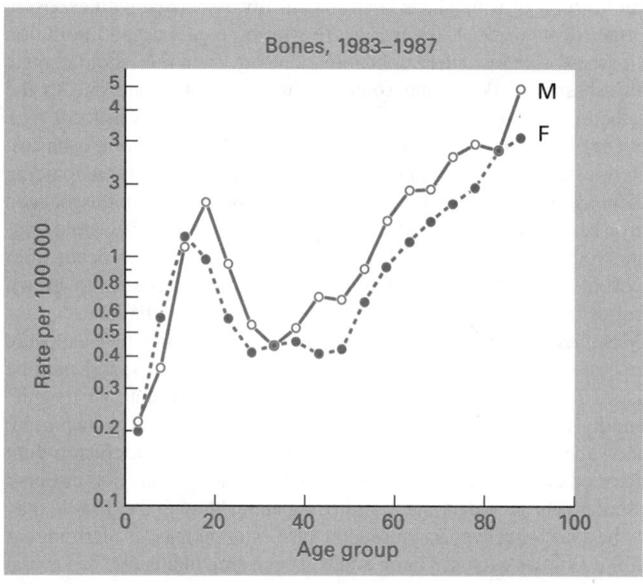

Fig. 9 Annual incidence of connective tissue sarcoma by age and sex.

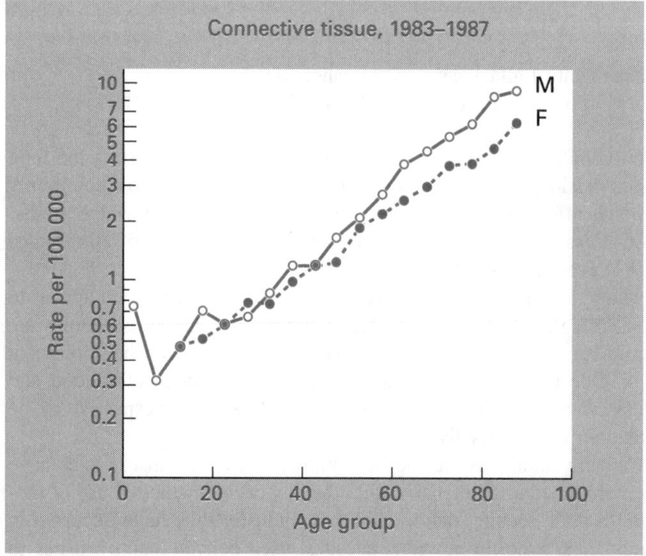

Skin (melanoma)

1.5 per cent of all cancers and 0.8 per cent of cancer deaths.
Sex ratio of rates 0.6 to 1. Age distribution, see Fig. 10.

The incidence of the disease varies inversely with the amount of skin pigmentation. In white people the tumour occurs most commonly on the legs (in women) and the trunk, head, and neck (in men). It is extremely rare in blacks in the United States, but is more common in Africa, where it occurs at the junction of the pigmented and unpigmented skin on the sole of the foot. Like basal-cell and squamous carcinoma of the skin, it is particularly common in sufferers from xeroderma pigmentosum.

Incidence rates in white people vary roughly in proportion to the flux of ultraviolet light in the countries in which they live. It is not, however, more common in outdoor than indoor workers (rather the reverse, in fact, perhaps due to the protective effects of a semipermanent suntan) and it seems to be associated with periodic bouts of sunbathing and sunburn. Incidence and mortality rates have increased in Britain, the United States, and in many other countries with mainly white populations. The increase began in cohorts born early this century, who exposed their skin more readily to the sun than their predecessors had, and still continues. The totality of the evidence suggests that ultraviolet light is the principal cause, but the relationship is not simple and other factors may also be important.

Skin (non-melanoma)

12.2 per cent of all cancers and 0.3 per cent of cancer deaths.
Sex ratio of rates 1.7 to 1. Age distribution, see Fig. 11.

Non-melanomatous skin cancers are of two main types, basal-cell and squamous carcinomas. The former, also known as rodent ulcers, are produced by ultraviolet light. They occur mainly on parts of the body that are regularly exposed to the sun and, in particular, on the face, head, and neck. They are more common in outdoor workers, such as seamen and farmers, than in indoor workers, more common in fair-skinned than in dark-skinned people, and are almost unknown in blacks (except those who suffer from albinism). Some few cases have been produced by exposure to X-rays, but the risk is very small unless the dose is very large and they seldom occur after normal courses of radiotherapy. People who suffer from xeroderma pigmentosum, a hereditary condition in which there is a defect in the enzyme responsible for the repair of the damage done to DNA by ultraviolet radiation, develop large numbers of skin tumours at an early age in response to even quite mild exposure to diffuse sunlight (see Section 23).

Fig. 10 Annual incidence of melanoma of the skin by age and sex.

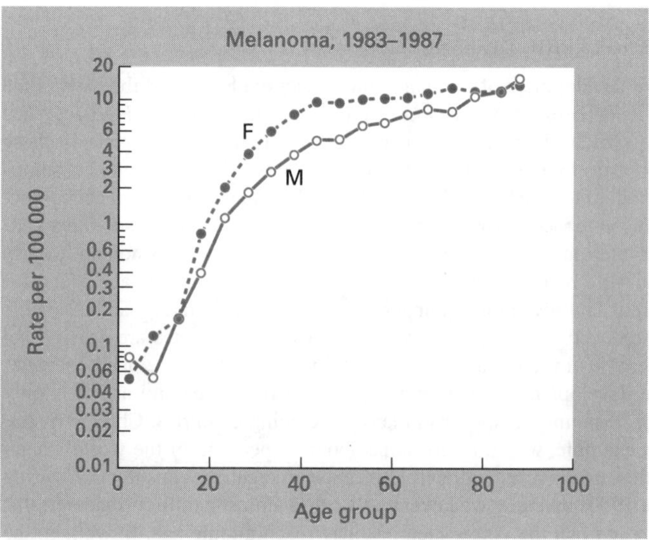

Squamous carcinoma is also produced by ultraviolet light, but less easily, so that it accounts for only about 20 per cent of cancers on the exposed skin. It is, however, the principal type of skin cancer produced by various carcinogenic chemicals, and particularly by polycyclic hydrocarbons in the combustion products of coal. These chemicals have been responsible for the scrotal cancers of chimney sweeps, who accumulated soot in the folds of the scrotal skin, of mule spinners, whose clothes were saturated with carcinogenic oils, and of various other groups of workers whose clothes were contaminated with tar. They have caused (and still do cause) cancers of the forearm in industrial workers whose arms are regularly splashed with tar or carcinogenic oils, cancers of the groin in India, localized by the continued friction of the *dhoti* cloth, and cancers of the abdomen in Kashmir that are associated with the habit of carrying a *kangri*, or small stove, inside the clothes in winter to keep warm.

Squamous carcinoma has also been due to prolonged exposure to arsenic, which is excreted by the skin and in the hair, when it may be accompanied by arsenical pigmentation and keratoses. All these conditions have been produced by prolonged medical treatment with inorganic arsenic, which used to be prescribed for a variety of chronic conditions, by the consumption of well water from arsenic-rich soils, and by occupational exposure, sometimes to as much as 1000 μg of arsenic/m^3 of air, in the smelting of copper and cobalt (the ores of which often contain arsenic), and in the manufacture of arsenical pesticides.

How large a part human papillomavirus plays in the development of squamous carcinoma of the skin is unclear. The type 5 virus is responsible for the warty lesions of epidermodysplasia verruciformis, some of which progress to cancer, and a role for other types of the viruses may account for the increased risk that follows the intensive immunosuppression given to permit the survival of organ transplants.

Kaposi's sarcoma, now classed as a skin cancer, may also result from infection by an unrecognized virus. The association with AIDS is common only when AIDS results from homosexual intercourse and probably only when this is accompanied by orofaecal contact. Frequent at first, particularly in the United States, the association has become progressively less common. Before the advent of AIDS, Kaposi's sarcoma was common in some parts of Central Africa, where it occasionally affected children, progressed rapidly, and could account for as many as 10 per cent of all hospital patients with cancer. Elsewhere it was rare, but indolent cases occurred occasionally in developed countries, principally on the legs of middle-aged and elderly men.

Breast

11.1 per cent of all cancers and 9.6 per cent of cancer deaths.
Sex ratio of rates 0.01 to 1. Age distribution, see Fig. 12.

Cancer of the breast was the most common fatal cancer in women throughout most of the developed world, but is now being displaced by lung cancer in some areas. It is less common in Eastern Europe and much less common in Asia and in black African populations south of the Sahara. Incidence rates have tended to rise slowly in many countries but the changes are relatively small and decreases have recently been recorded in young age groups. The geographical differences are unlikely to be chiefly due to genetic factors as black women in the United States and Japanese women in Hawaii have rates that are similar to those in their white American compatriots and much greater than those in their countries of origin.

Hormonal factors are important in the production of the disease, but it has not been possible to define them precisely. The duration of ovarian activity appears to be relevant as the disease is particularly common in women who have an early menarche and a late menopause (the former being more important than the latter). Pregnancy produces a short-term increase in risk, followed after a few years by a lifelong decrease, particularly with teenage or early adult pregnancies. The incidence in later life increases progressively with a woman's age at the time of her first full-term pregnancy, being about three times greater when the first birth occurs after 35 years of age than when it occurs before 18 years. Full-term pregnancies after the first have an additional protective effect. Pregnancies that end in abortion have little or no effect, however, suggesting that the effects of pregnancy depend on the induction of lactation. The duration of lactation, however, has only a minor additional productive effect.

Parity and menstrual differences are insufficient to account for the large variations in the incidence of the disease in different countries, which seem to be correlated with a 'high' standard of living: that is, with life in a developed country. Diet may play an important part, but the evidence is complex and is discussed later. Obesity is associated with a reduced risk before the menopause, as it tends to be associated with ovarian dysfunction. After the menopause obesity increases slightly both the incidence and probably the fatality of the disease. Oestrogens prescribed medically, as hormone replacement therapy after the menopause, increase the risk slightly; combined with progestogens, as in the contraceptive pill, they increase it by about 50 per cent during, and for a few years after, use, but do not appear to affect the risk later in life. Tamoxifen, an anti-oestrogen prescribed for breast cancer patients, reduces the subsequent incidence of cancer in the unaffected breast.

Fig. 11 Annual incidence of non-melanomatous skin cancer by age and sex.

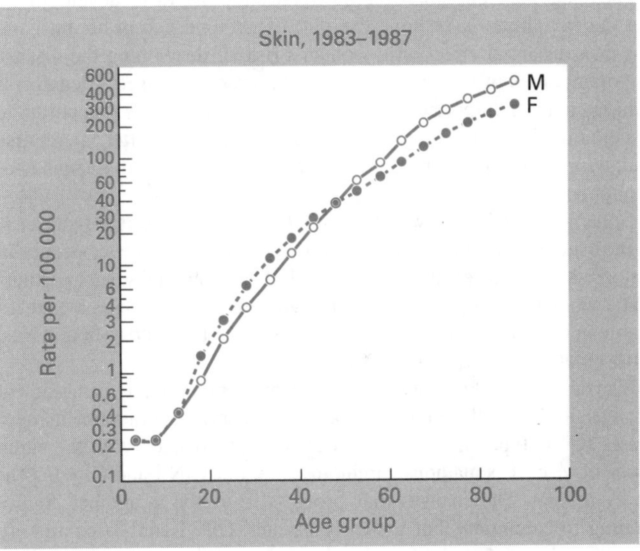

Fig. 12 Annual incidence of breast cancer in women by age.

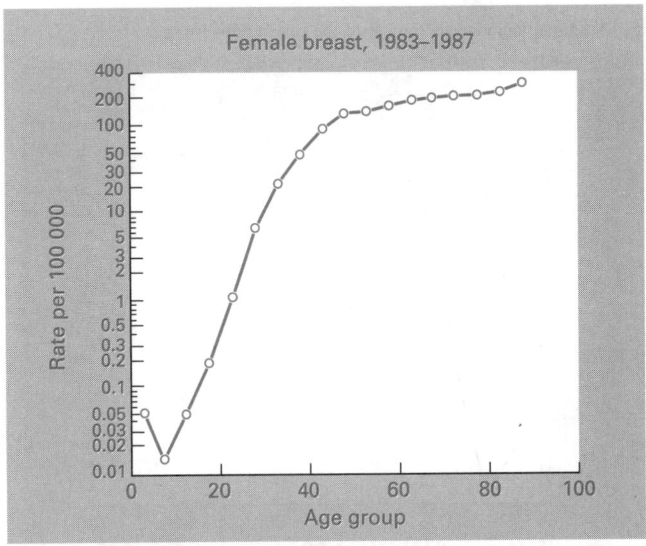

Cervix uteri

1.8 per cent of all cancers and 1.2 per cent of cancer deaths.
Occurs only in women. Age distribution, see Fig. 13.

Carcinoma of the cervix is the most common type of cancer throughout much of Africa, Asia, and Latin America, and used also to be common in Europe and North America. It has always been rare in Jewesses and has tended to be less common in Muslim women than in women of other faiths living in the same country (as, for example, in Hindu women in India).

Changes in incidence have been difficult to assess, partly because mortality data have not always distinguished between deaths due to cancer of the cervix and those due to cancer of the corpus uteri (or endometrium), partly because the introduction of screening programmes has made it possible to diagnose and treat premalignant lesions (see below), and partly because hysterectomy before the onset of the disease has become progressively more common, with a corresponding reduction in the number of uteri in which the disease could occur. Despite these complications there can be no doubt that the disease has become substantially less common in Europe and North America than it used to be before the Second World War.

The rarity of the disease in Jewesses and its relative rarity in Muslims suggest that male circumcision may reduce the risk of its development, but this is unlikely to be so as the state of circumcision of her husband has no substantial effect on a woman's risk of developing the disease in communities in which only some men are circumcised. Cleanliness is likely to be an important factor, as the disease is relatively uncommon in communities that practise ritual ablution before and after intercourse and, within each community, it becomes less common with rising socioeconomic status.

Squamous carcinoma, which constitutes the vast majority of all cases, is intimately connected with sexual activity. It almost never occurs in virgins, and increases in frequency with the number of sexual partners that a woman or her partner have. The great majority of cases are attributable in part to infection with some types of the human papillomavirus, most notably with types 16 and 18.

The development of squamous carcinoma is preceded by pathological changes limited to the epithelium, known as cervical intraepithelial neoplasia (**CIN**) types I, II, and III. CIN III is associated with the same types of virus as squamous carcinomas are, but CIN I and CIN II generally are not. The changes may progress from one to another, finally leading to carcinoma, but the early lesions (CIN I and II) commonly regress and even CIN III (previously known as carcinoma *in situ*) may do so occasionally. The lesions can be recognized in cervical smears and destroyed by lasers or extensive biopsy, and the occurrence of clinical disease can be greatly reduced by the examination of all sexually active women every 2 or 3 years and the treatment of advanced CIN lesions.

Fig. 13 Annual incidence of cancer of the cervix uteri by age.

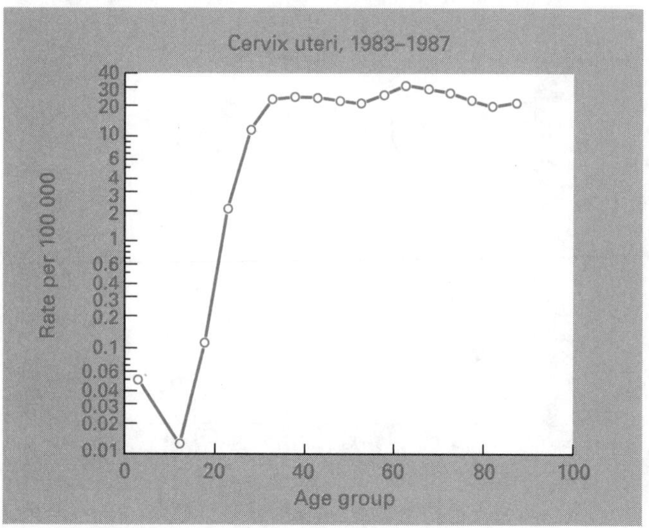

Other factors associated with the production of the disease are the use of oral contraceptives and cigarette smoking. Both tend to be associated with behaviour conducive to venereal infection, but it is difficult to explain the observed associations completely in this way.

Adenocarcinoma of the cervix uteri is generally rare, but it may have become somewhat more common recently. Its causes are unknown.

Endometrium (corpus uteri)

1.5 per cent of all cancers and 0.7 per cent of cancer deaths.
Occurs only in women. Age distribution like cancer of ovary.

The epidemiological features of endometrial cancer are in many respects the opposite of those of cervical cancer. Histologically, it is nearly always an adenocarcinoma. It is common in developed countries, rare in poor, and is, if anything, becoming more common with the passage of time. It is inversely related to parity, but not otherwise related to coitus, and is unaffected by the number of sexual partners. Like cancer of the breast, it is positively associated with early menarche and late menopause.

The one factor known to produce the disease is regular exposure to oestrogens, unopposed by progestogens. This leads to endometrial hyperplasia and eventually, in some cases, to cancer. Known causes include oestrogen-secreting tumours of the ovary, the use of oral contraceptives in which oestrogens and progestogens are prescribed sequentially (which have now been abandoned), the use of 'natural' conjugated oestrogens to relieve menopausal and postmenopausal symptoms, and adiposity. The last causes the disease because oestrogens are produced in the body after the menopause in adipose tissue from the adrenal hormone, androstenedione. Tamoxifen, an analogue of the natural oestrogens, which, in the breast, blocks the hormone receptor and hence generally acts as an antioestrogen, can, due to differences between the hormone receptors in different tissues, have a pro-oestrogenic effect in the endometrium, and may therefore increase the incidence of endometrial cancer.

It is improbable, however, that oestrogens are initiating agents. They are not mutagens *in vitro* and the changes that took place in the incidence of the disease in the United States following the increase and the subsequent reduction in the use of premarin (a conjugated oestrogen) for the treatment of menopausal symptoms occurred so quickly that they make sense only if oestrogens act on some late stage(s) of the carcinogenic process.

Ovary

2.3 per cent of all cancers and 2.7 per cent of cancer deaths.
Occurs only in women. Age distribution, see Fig. 14.

Cancer of the ovary is not one disease but many, each of which is defined by its histological appearance. Most types are too rare to have been considered separately in epidemiological studies and the few characteristics that have been recognized may refer only to adenocarcinoma, which is the most common type. These characteristics resemble those of endometrial cancer, in that the risk of developing the disease is greatest in countries with a high standard of living, increases with the length of time from menarche to menopause, and decreases progressively with increasing number of children. The incidence of the disease is substantially reduced by the use of oral contraceptives and seems to depend on the number of ovulations.

Prostate

5.0 per cent of all cancers and 6.2 per cent of cancer deaths.
Occurs only in men. Age distribution, see Fig. 15.

Cancer of the prostrate is more characteristically a disease of old age than any other cancer, so that it comes to play a much larger part in clinical experience as the proportion of old people in the population increases. It is also unusual in that foci of cells resembling cancer can be found in a high proportion of clinically normal prostates, so that the recorded incidence is increased dramatically by increasing the number of prostatic biopsies. Some increase in mortality has been recorded recently in Britain and North America, but the weight of evidence suggests that the disease is due to factors that have affected society for many years. What these factors are remains obscure. Associations have been reported with both increased and decreased sexual activity. On general grounds it seems likely that the disease is dependent on hormonal imbalance (particularly as castration slows the progression of clinical disease), but the nature of the imbalance is unknown. Vasectomy may cause an increase in incidence two decades later, but the limited evidence is inconclusive.

Two epidemiological observations stand out: the high incidence in black populations throughout the world, and the low incidence in Japanese. Both may be partly due to genetic factors, but they are not wholly so, as both Japanese and blacks have higher rates in the United States than in Japan and Africa.

Testis

0.5 per cent of all cancers and 0.1 per cent of cancer deaths.
Occurs only in men. Age distribution, see Fig. 16.

Fig. 14 Annual incidence of cancer of the ovary by age.

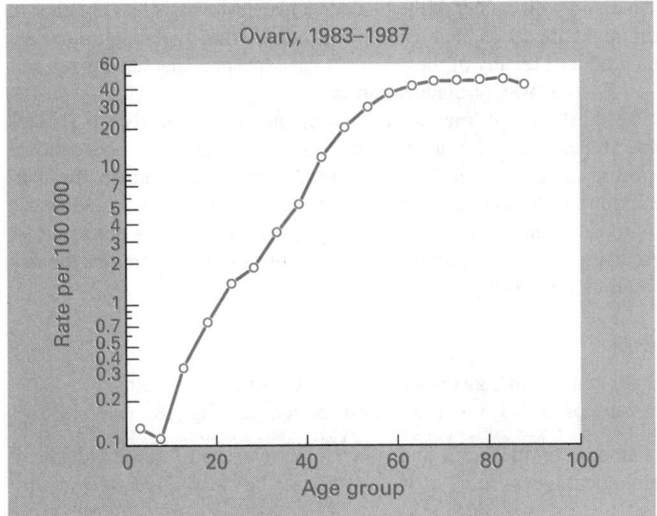

Fig. 15 Annual incidence of cancer of the prostate by age.

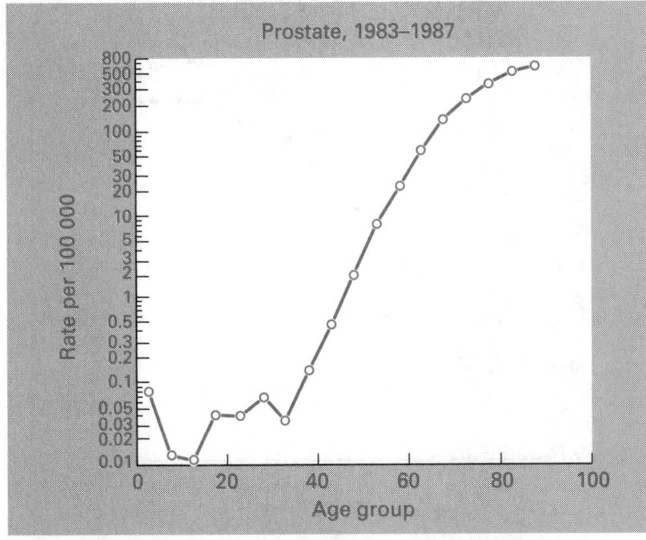

Testicular cancers are of two main types. Seminomas, which are the more common, have a peak incidence at about 30 years and teratomas, which are more often called embryomal carcinomas in the United States, have a peak incidence about 10 years earlier. Tumours after 50 years of age are mostly lymphomas. Both genetic and environmental factors are important. On the one hand, the disease is uniformly rare in black populations, whether in Africa or in the United States. On the other, it has increased in incidence in many countries, notably in Denmark and Britain. In Britain, the increase began in the 1920s and affected first the higher socioeconomic groups. The increase trebled the mortality at 15 to 34 years of age, producing a sharp peak in young adult life that had not previously been present. The increase started later and has been less marked in the United States. The disease is much more likely to occur in an undescended than in a normal testis, but otherwise its causes are unknown.

Penis

0.1 per cent of all cancers and of cancer deaths.
Occurs only in men. Age distribution like skin (non-melanoma)

Cancer of the penis is at all common only in some parts of tropical Africa and Brazil, in which it may account for 10 per cent of all cancers in men. It is avoided almost entirely by circumcision at birth and is very rare if circumcision is carried out in boyhood. In developed countries it is rare even in the absence of circumcision if the glans, coronary sulcus, and foreskin are kept clean.

The oncogenic types of the human papillomavirus (principally types 16 and 18) can usually be identified in the malignant cells and are probably an important cause of the disease.

Bladder

4.6 per cent of all cancers and 3.4 per cent of cancer deaths.
Sex ratio of rates 3.8 to 1. Age distribution like gastric cancer.

Cancer of the bladder can be produced by cigarette smoking, occupational exposure to a group of chemicals classed together as aromatic amines, infestation of the bladder with *Schistosoma haematobium*, and the medical prescription of chlornaphthazine (*N,N′*-bis(2-chloroethyl)-2-naphthylamine) and cyclophosphamide. It is not surprising that the bladder should be affected by many chemicals, as any noxious small molecules in the blood will tend to be found at greatly increased concentration in the urinary tract. For example, cigarette smoke contains various mutagenic chemicals that enter the bloodstream and thence the bladder, so that, when tested *in vitro* on bacterial DNA, the urine of

Fig. 16 Annual incidence of cancer of the testis by age.

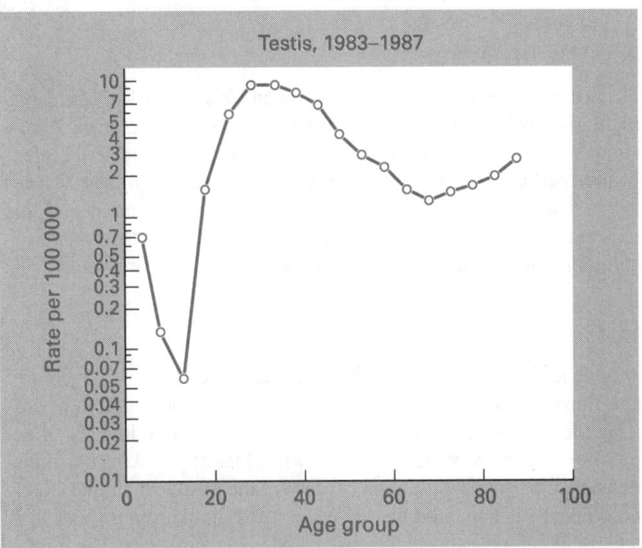

cigarette smokers is found to be mutagenic, while that of non-smokers is barely active.

SMOKING

Of all these causes, the most important numerically is cigarette smoking, which probably accounts for about half the total number of cases in Britain and North America. 2-Naphthylamine and 4-aminobiphenyl are present in cigarette smoke but whether the amounts are sufficient to account for the carcinogenic effect is uncertain.

OCCUPATION

An occupational cause was first suspected in 1898 in Germany, when Rehn commented on a cluster of cases in men using aniline for the manufacture of dyes. Aniline, however, is not carcinogenic in experimental animals, more recent studies have failed to incriminate it epidemiologically, and it seems likely that other carcinogenic chemicals were present as impurities. Four aromatic amines that are carcinogenic in experimental animals have been shown to cause bladder cancer in man: 2-naphthylamine, benzidine, 3,3′-dichlorobenzidine, and 4-aminobiphenyl. The first is one of the most powerful human carcinogens so far discovered and was responsible for the development of bladder cancer in all the 19 men who were employed in distilling it in a British factory. Its manufacture was stopped in Britain in 1949, but small amounts continued to be imported until the 1960s. Other aromatic amines that may cause bladder cancer include auramine, magenta, and, perhaps, 1-naphthylamine. The last is dubiously carcinogenic in experimental animals and it seems probable that the cases associated with its use have been due to a few per cent of 2-naphthylamine present as an impurity in the commercial material. These chemicals were used in the manufacture of dyes, in the rubber industry as antioxidants (1-naphthylamine and 4-aminobiphenyl) and hardeners (benzidine), and in laboratories as a reagent (benzidine). 2-Naphthylamine is also found in the combustion products of coal and may have been responsible for the hazard of bladder cancer in men who made coal gas. As many as 10 per cent of cases have been attributable to occupational causes in Britain and North America; but the proportion should now be less.

MEDICINES

The two medicinal causes have, by contrast, been responsible for only a handful of cases. Chlornaphthazine was used briefly for the treatment of myelomatosis, until it was found to be metabolized into 2-naphthylamine. Cyclophosphamide is used primarily for the treatment of malignant disease but also as an immunosuppressant. In large doses it may cause sloughing and, occasionally, cancer of the bladder mucosa.

PARASITIC INFECTION

The association between schistosomiasis and cancer of the bladder is particularly marked in Egypt and Tanzania. The schistosomes start a chain of events that may lead to cancer through chronic bacterial infection and, perhaps, the formation of nitrites and nitrosamines. Cancer associated with schistosomiasis is characteristically squamous and this type is predominant in countries where *S. haematobium* schistosomiasis is common. Others are predominantly transitional-cell carcinomas.

DIET

The evidence linking bladder cancer to diet is weak. Several case-control studies have suggested a positive relation with the consumption of coffee, but the results are inconsistent and it is difficult to exclude the effect of confounding by the stronger relation with cigarette smoking. Artificial sweeteners came under suspicion because of the results of animal experiments in which first mixtures of cyclamates and saccharin and then saccharin alone were shows to cause bladder cancer in rats. The human use of cyclamates was banned before saccharin came under suspicion, but it now appears that the 'positive' results of animal experiments with cyclamates alone were due to impurities. Saccharin has been shown to cause cancer of the bladder in rats in straightforward feeding experiments, especially when given over two generations and when given after a single instillation into the bladder of a powerful carcinogen. In both instances the quantities that had to be given were large, constituting a few per cent of the feed. The human evidence is extensive and, in sum, could hardly be more negative (although it is still possible that lifelong use of saccharin will produce a measurable risk).

Kidney

1.6 per cent of all cancers and 1.8 per cent of cancer deaths.
Sex ratio of rates 2.2 to 1. Age distribution, see Fig. 17.

Cancers of the kidney are of three main types: nephroblastomas (or Wilms' tumours), adenocarcinomas (or hypernephromas), and transitional- and squamous-cell carcinomas of the renal pelvis. The first are limited to childhood, occur with almost equal frequency everywhere, and apart from a few of genetic origin, are of unknown aetiology. The second constitute by far the majority of all cases, are more common in Western Europe and North America than in Africa and Asia, and have been slowly increasing in incidence. Cigarette smoking may account for a quarter of the cases but the association is weak and the conclusion that it is causal would not be regarded as probable were it not for the mutagenicity of the urine of cigarette smokers and the strong association of smoking with cancer of the bladder. This, however, is less conclusive than might appear as there is no firm evidence that hypernephromas are also produced by any of the occupational exposures that have given rise to substantial risks of bladder cancer.

The third type of renal cancer (carcinoma of the pelvis) constitutes some 10 per cent of all cases. Three established causes are occupational exposure to the chemicals that cause cancer of the bladder, the consumption of large enough amounts of phenacetin to produce analgesic nephropathy, and smoking. In all three cases the hazards are small. A third cause, Balkan nephropathy (see Chapter 20.9.4), increases the risk several hundredfold.

Brain

1.3 per cent of all cancers and 1.8 per cent of cancer deaths.
Sex ratio of rates 1.5 to 1. Age distribution, see Fig. 18.

Tumours of the brain and nervous system are of several different histological types, some of which may not be clearly benign or malig-

Fig. 17 Annual incidence of cancer of the kidney by age and sex.

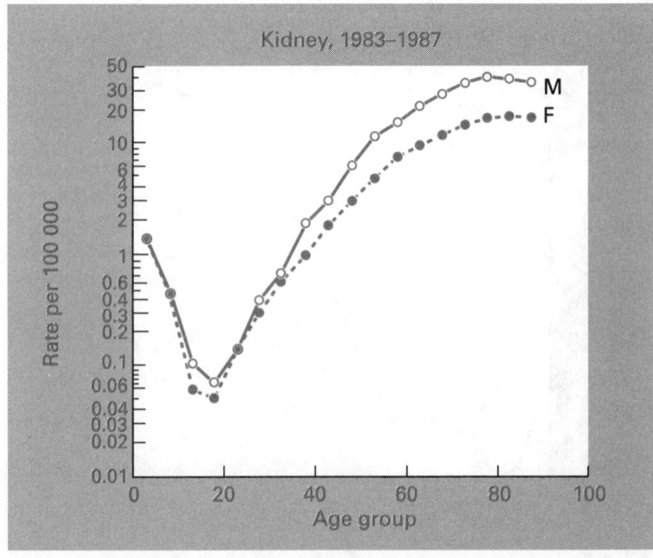

nant. One type occurs characteristically in childhood (medulloblastoma), another in adult life (glioblastoma), and a third (astrocytoma) at all ages. Despite the overall male excess, one type (meningioma) is more common in women.

A moderately large increase in incidence in old age has been recorded in many countries, which can be attributed to improved diagnosis with computerized tomographic scans and nuclear magnetic imaging. Little or no increase in mortality in or before middle age has been reported, however, and it is possible that the apparent increases in incidence are largely or wholly artefactual. No new environmental cause has been established, but many have been suspected, including electromagnetic fields associated with the use of electricity (50–60 Hz).

Thyroid

0.4 per cent of all cancers and 0.2 per cent of cancer deaths.
Sex ratio of rates 0.5 to 1. Age distribution, see Fig. 19.

The thyroid is particularly sensitive to ionizing radiation in childhood. Substantial numbers of cases have occurred among the survivors of the atomic explosions in Hiroshima and Nagasaki, children who were exposed to large amounts of radioactive iodine following the Chernobyl accident, and young people whose necks were irradiated in infancy for the treatment of an enlarged thymus (a condition now considered to be perfectly normal, but at one time thought to be a cause of sudden death). Fortunately, the thyroid tumours produced by ionizing radiations are nearly all of the papillary and follicular types, which respond well to treatment. No causes are known of the medullary and anaplastic types, which have a high fatality and occur only in adult life.

The disease is several times more common in Iceland, northern Norway, Hawaii, Fiji, and Israel than elsewhere.

Hodgkin's disease (Hodgkin's lymphoma)

0.5 per cent of all cancers and 0.3 per cent of cancer deaths.
Sex ratio of rates 1.4 to 1. Age distribution, see Fig. 20.

Hodgkin's disease is, perhaps, best thought of as at least two diseases, one affecting primarily youths and young adults, the other primarily the middle aged and elderly. This division is suggested partly by the existence of two peaks in the age-specific incidence rates, partly by the histological appearances (younger patients tending to have the nodular sclerotic form of the disease and older patients the mixed cellular form), and partly by the clinical distinction that young patients show mediastinal involvement in more than 50 per cent of cases and infradiaphragmatic involvement in less than 5 per cent, while the reverse tends to be true in the elderly.

No specific causes are known, but there are several reasons for thinking that the type characteristic of young people may be at least partly infective in origin. In developing countries, Hodgkin's disease occurs in childhood, but as the standard of living rises, the childhood cases disappear and are replaced by a larger number in young adults. This changing pattern is reminiscent of what happened to poliomyelitis in the first half of the century and suggests that the disease may be due to a ubiquitous infective agent that becomes less widespread as hygiene improves. The Epstein-Barr virus (EBV) that causes infectious mononucleosis may cause some cases, as the disease has been followed by a slightly increased incidence of Hodgkin's disease between 5 and 20 years later, and the virus has been detected in some of the malignant cells.

Non-Hodgkin's lymphoma

2.4 per cent of all cancers and 2.6 per cent of cancer deaths.
Sex ratio of rates 1.5 to 1. Age distribution, see Fig. 21.

Fig. 18 Annual incidence of cancer of the brain by age and sex.

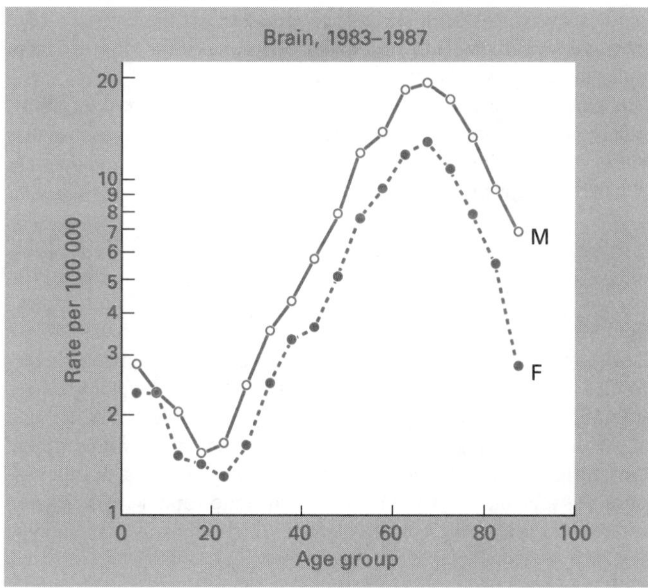

Fig. 19 Annual incidence of cancer of the thyroid by age and sex.

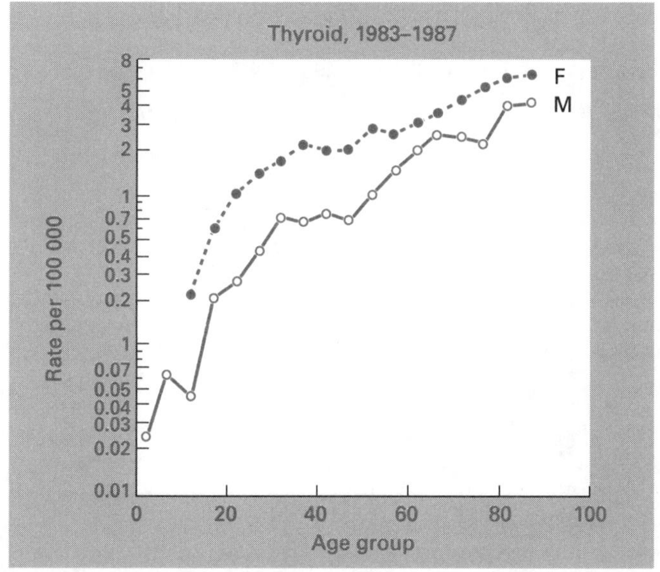

Fig. 20 Annual incidence of Hodgkin's lymphoma by age and sex.

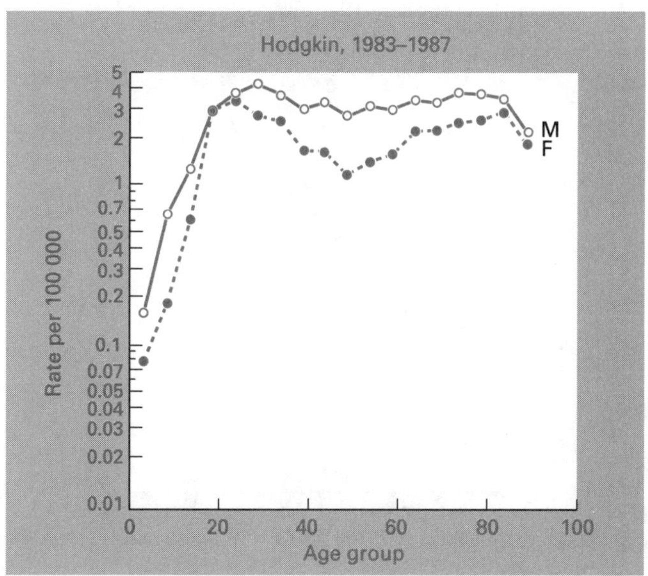

Non-Hodgkin's lymphoma is a non-specific term that embraces several diseases with different histological appearances. The histological classification has, however, varied from place to place and from time to time, and it has been difficult to collect epidemiological information about the individual types.

One type that has been clearly distinguished is Burkitt's lymphoma, derived from B lymphocytes. This affects children everywhere, but is common only in a few areas in which malarial infection is both heavy and widespread. In parts of Uganda, Tanzania, and Nigeria the disease is 100 times more common than in Europe and North America. In these high incidence areas, EBV can nearly always be recovered from the lymphomatous cells and part of its genome is identifiable in the cells' DNA. Infection with the virus is, however, not necessary for the development of the disease, as some cases occur in its absence; nor is it sufficient, as infection is almost universal and occurs at a very young age in high incidence areas. It seems, therefore, that EBV is a potential cause and that its carcinogenic effect is precipitated by the intense stimulation of the reticuloendothelial system that is characteristic of heavy and chronic malarial infection.

Another type occurs as part of the adult T-cell leukaemia–lymphoma syndrome that follows infection with the human T-cell leukaemia–lymphoma virus (**HTLV-1**). The disease is common in South Japan and the Caribbean, but may occur occasionally anywhere.

A third type, primary upper small-intestinal lymphoma (PUSIL), affects young people in many populations with a low standard of living, not only in North Africa and the Middle East (where its frequency gave it its earlier name of Mediterranean lymphoma) but also in South Africa and Central and South America. Malnutrition is not, however, a sufficient cause as it is uncommon in Bangladesh and several other malnourished populations.

The remaining lymphomas, which constitute the majority in developed countries, should probably be divided further. (Some in childhood, for example, might be better classed with acute lymphatic leukaemia from which they are distinguished arbitrarily only by the number of lymphocytes in the blood.) At present, however, they have to be considered as a group. As such they constitute one of the few types of cancer that have been increasing in incidence at all ages.

Two factors that have contributed to the increase, but which cannot account for it all, are the use of immunosuppressive drugs and the spread of AIDS. Intense immunosuppression is followed within 1 or 2 years by an increase of the order of 50- to 100-fold in the incidence of non-Hodgkin's lymphoma, and smaller increases follow the less intensive use of immunosuppressive drugs for the medical treatment of patients with arthritis, Crohn's disease, and other similar conditions. Many, but not all, of the lymphomas that occur in these circumstances are associated with EBV and some of them may, unusually, arise in the brain. Greatly increased incidence rates are also seen in a variety of rare hereditary disorders characterised by major immunological impairment, such as the Wiskott–Aldrich syndrome.

The rare hairy-cell leukaemia is now classed as another type of lymphoma rather than as leukaemia.

Myelomatosis

1.1 per cent of all cancers and 1.5 per cent of cancer deaths.
Sex ratio of rates 1.5 to 1. Age distribution like large bowel cancer.

Myelomatosis has been much easier to diagnose since marrow puncture and then serum electrophoresis became standard diagnostic tools and since the management of renal failure, which is often the presenting symptom, has improved. As a result it is difficult to be sure whether the increase that has been recorded in both incidence and mortality rates, and which has now stopped in all but the oldest age groups, is due solely to improved diagnosis, or whether it also reflects the introduction of major new causes into Europe and North America between the two World Wars. In southern Sweden, where there has been a long-standing interest in, and search for, cases of myeloma over the past few decades, no large increase has been seen; a few decades ago the rates recorded there were higher than in other developed populations, but in recent decades the other populations have caught up.

The disease is uncommon in undeveloped areas, where it is almost certainly underdiagnosed. Genetic factors could be important, as it is twice as common in blacks in the United States as in whites and is rare in Japanese irrespective of where they live.

Leukaemia

2.1 per cent of all cancers and of cancer deaths.
Sex ratio of rates 1.7 to 1. Age distribution, see Fig. 22.

Leukaemia may be divided primarily into chronic lymphatic leukaemia (**CLL**), chronic myeloid leukaemia (**CML**), acute myeloid leukaemia (**AML**), and acute lymphatic leukaemia (**ALL**). CML, AML, and ALL are, in turn, amalgams of two or more different types, with different causes, different age distributions, and different prognoses, but the distinction between them is still undergoing evolution and, with the exception referred to later, the epidemiological descriptions of each subtype are unclear.

CLL increases progressively with age in the same way as myelomatosis and most of the common epithelial cancers. It is extremely rare in

Fig. 21 Annual incidence of non-Hodgkin's lymphoma by age and sex.

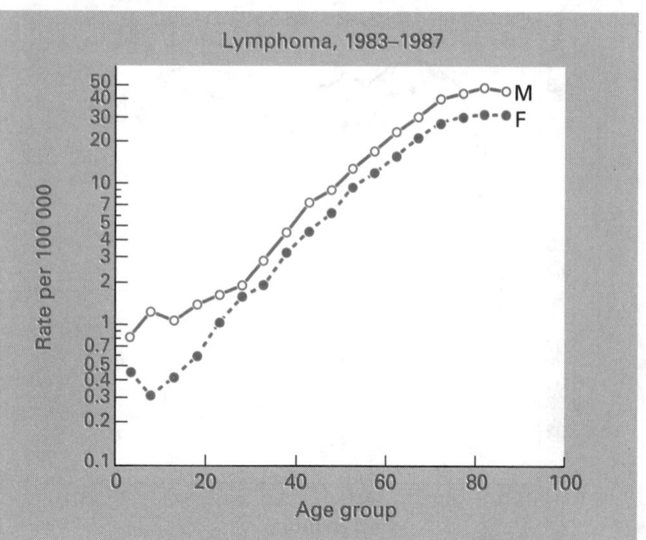

Fig. 22 Annual incidence of leukaemia by age and sex.

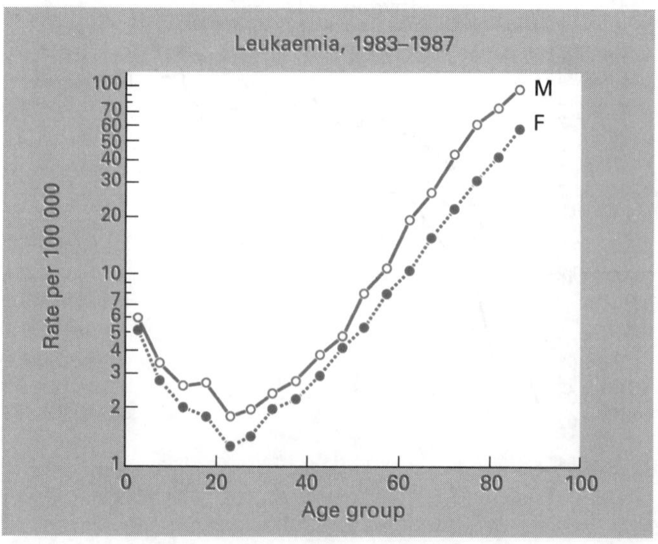

Chinese, Japanese, and Indians, which is presumably due to genetic differences in susceptibility as it continues to be rare in these racial groups even when they migrate to other countries. Unlike nearly every other type of cancer, CLL does not appear to be induced by ionizing radiations. This may be because the relevant stem cells are so radiosensitive that they are killed by small doses that would otherwise be carcinogenic.

In contrast with CLL, the other three main types are induced by ionizing radiation more easily than most other types of cancer and they constitute about 10 per cent of the risk of fatal cancer from whole-body irradiation.

AML occurs at all ages. It becomes slowly but progressively more common from childhood on and is the most common type in young adult life. In this age group, its incidence is probably less variable throughout the world than that of any other reasonably common type of cancer. CML, by contrast, is very rare in youth, but becomes more common than AML in later middle age. The few cases that occur in childhood should perhaps be regarded as constituting a separate disease, as they lack the Philadelphia chromosome that normally characterizes CML in adult life.

ALL is the most common type of childhood cancer. Three main types can be distinguished. Common (c) ALL arises from B-lymphocyte precursors and is responsible for a peak incidence of the disease at 2 to 3 years of age. Null ALL also arises from B-cell precursors, but lacks the common antigen and accounts for most cases in the first year of life. T-cell ALL occurs more or less equally at all ages in childhood. ALL in adult life can be either B cell or T cell. One type (adult T-cell leukaemia/lymphoma) which occurs commonly in the south island of Japan (Kyushu) and in the West Indies and rarely elsewhere, is caused by the human HTLV-1 (see Section 22).

Other causes of leukaemia include several chemicals and genetically determined diseases. The most important is benzene, which is used widely in industry. Prolonged occupational exposure to large amounts has caused a substantial risk of AML (particularly one of its subtypes, erythroleukaemia) and, less commonly, acute lymphatic leukaemia. Many cases are preceded by periods of aplastic anaemia and there is still some doubt whether leukaemia can be caused by small doses.

Two other chemicals, melphalan and busulphan, are used in the treatment of cancer and the small risk of AML that follows their use in unimportant in relation to the benefit obtained if they are used appropriately. Melphalan is an alkylating agent and so presumably mutagenic. Busulphan, however, has been observed to produce a substantial risk of leukaemia only after being given in such high doses that it produces aplastic anaemia.

Of the hereditary causes of leukaemia, Down's syndrome is the most common and, for this reason, is probably responsible for the greatest number of cases, although the relative risk in some of the other syndromes may be greater than the 20-fold increase in childhood leukaemia that occurs with Down's disease. Ataxia telangiectasia and Bloom's syndrome predispose to ALL, while Fanconi's anaemia predisposes to AML.

General factors

In this review of cancers of different organs it has not been possible to examine in detail the evidence relating to pervasive causes that affect many different types of cancer. Some of these are, therefore, examined separately in the following sections before an estimate is made of the proportion of cancers attributable to each category of cause.

Ionizing radiations

Ionizing radiations, of whatever sort, share the characteristic of being able to penetrate animal tissues and damage DNA. It is not surprising, therefore, that they have been found to increase the incidence of cancer in practically every organ. It has not been possible to detect by direct observation the effect of the small amounts of radiation that adults receive as a result of exposure to (for example) radiological examination, atmospheric pollution, and natural background; but it has been possible to make an estimate of their effect by extrapolating from the observed effects of the much larger doses received by the survivors of the atomic explosions at Hiroshima and Nagasaki, patients given radiotherapy or repeatedly screened radiologically, and people exposed occupationally to radium or to high concentrations of radon in mines. Theoretical considerations and the dose–response relation observed with these relatively large doses both indicate that there is unlikely to be any threshold below which no effect is produced. This conclusion is reinforced by the discovery that children who received doses of 10 to 20 mGy *in utero* (because their mothers were irradiated for diagnostic purposes whilst they were pregnant) were subject to an added risk of developing cancer in childhood of approximately 1 in 2000. At low doses (less than about 20 mGy) it seems probable that the carcinogenic effect is linearly proportional to the dose; at higher doses the same is true for most cancers other than leukaemia, for which the risk is approximately proportional to the square of the dose. It is unlikely, however, that we should be far out in our estimate if we accepted the conclusions of the International Committee on Radiological Protection (1991) and assumed that the lifetime risk of developing a fatal cancer is approximately 10 per cent per Gray (or per Sievert) to the whole body if the radiation is given acutely and about half that if the dose is low and spread out over time (for example 5 per 100 000 per mGy (or mSv)), with corresponding reductions if only part of the body is exposed.

People are exposed to different amounts of radiation in different countries, depending principally on the build up of radon in the air in domestic houses and the medical use of radiation for diagnosis and therapy. In the United Kingdom, the average annual dose is about 2.6 mSv, which in a population of about 55 million is estimated to cause about 7000 deaths from cancer, about 5 per cent of the total. In the United States, the average annual dose is about 50 per cent greater. These estimated hazards depend critically on the effects of chronic exposure to radon, and these have not yet been reliably assessed. The biggest contribution comes from radon in houses, which, on average, contributes about half the total dose of all forms of radiation exposure. In some parts of the country, however, most notably Devon and Cornwall, the average radon dose is three or four times greater and in a few houses it may be 10 times greater or even more. Nearly all the rest comes from natural radiation from other sources (35 per cent) and medical uses (14 per cent). The last, however, causes less cancer than would be deduced from the dose since much is received by old or ill people who will not survive for long enough for a radiation-induced cancer to appear or because the doses given radiotherapeutically are so large that most of the cells that might have been made cancerous are destroyed. Less than 0.5 per cent of all radiation can be attributed to occupational exposure, fall-out from past bomb tests, and man-made products or radioactive waste.

Medical drugs

Apart from ionizing radiations, some 20 agents have been used therapeutically that are known to cause cancer in humans. These are listed in Table 4. That so many carcinogenic agents should have been prescribed medically is not surprising when it is borne in mind that treatment often requires modification of cellular metabolism and is sometimes intended to interfere with DNA. The hazard of cancer, however, need not necessarily be a bar to the use of a drug if the risk of life due to iatrogenic cancer is materially less than the chance of saving life that is brought about by its use—as is commonly the case with antineoplastic agents, immunosuppressive drugs, and radiotherapy.

Some of the agents listed in Table 4 were soon abandoned, while others have continued to be used for the treatment of uncommon conditions, and the sum of the cancers that they all now produce cannot amount to more than a hundred or so a year. Two, however, are used extensively: oestrogens and steroid contraceptives. The former were used almost routinely for the treatment of postmenopausal symptoms

Table 4 *Carcinogenic agents used in medical practice (other than ionizing radiations)*

Agent	Type of cancer
Antineoplastic agents:	
Busulphan	Leukaemia[1]
Chlorambucil	Leukaemia[1]
Chlornaphazine	Bladder
Cyclophosphamide	Bladder, leukaemia[1]
Melphalan	Leukaemia[1]
MOPP[2]	Leukaemia[1]
Thiotepa	
Treosulphan	Leukaemia[1]
Arsenic	Skin, liver (angiosarcoma), lung
Immunosuppressive drugs:	
Azathioprine	Non-Hodgkin's lymphoma,
Cyclosporin	
Methoxypsoralen (plus UV light)	Skin
Phenacetin	Renal pelvis
Polycyclic hydrocarbons (coal-tar ointment)	Skin
Oestrogens:	
Unopposed	Endometrium, breast
Transplacental	Vagina (adenocarcinoma)
Steroids:	
Oxymetholone	Liver (hepatoma)
Oral contraceptives (combined)[3]	Liver (hepatoma), breast

[1]Acute non-lymphocytic.

[2]Combination of nitrogen mustard, vincristine, procarbazine, and prednisone.

[3]See text for value in preventing cancer.

and the prevention of osteoporosis in some parts of the United States. This led to an 'epidemic' of endometrial cancer, which, at one time, may have doubled the normal incidence. Their prolonged use may also cause a small increase in the risk of cancer of the breast, just as a late menopause would do, although this might be outweighed by a decrease in myocardial infarction. Oestrogens also caused some cancers of the endometrium when given unopposed by a progestogen as a component of the sequential type of contraceptive pill.

The current contraceptive pills, which combine both types of drug, not only do not cause endometrial cancer, but actually diminish the risk of the disease and of ovarian cancer as well. This does not, however, conclude the tale. Firstly, they very rarely cause cancer of the liver either *ab initio* or as a complication of a benign adenomas. Secondly, they may well increase the risk of cancer of the cervix. Thirdly, prolonged use increases, perhaps by about one-third, the risk of cancer of the breast in young women who are current pill users. The increased risk does not, however, persist after the menopause and the total increase in the risk of fatal cancers of the liver, cervix, and breast is less than the reduction in risk from cancers of the ovary and endometrium.

Taken altogether it seems unlikely that medically prescribed drugs can be responsible for more than 1 per cent of all today's fatal cancers.

Occupation

In the years that followed Pott's observation that chimney sweeps tended to develop cancer of the scrotum, many other groups of workers have been found to suffer from specific hazards of cancer and more substances that are known to be carcinogenic to humans have been unearthed by the search for occupational hazards than by any other means. These hazards, many of which were described in relation to individual types of cancer, are listed in Table 5. Many of the hazards that have been recognized caused large, or at least relatively large, risks and it may well be that other occupational hazards exist that have not yet been detected, either because the added risk is small in comparison with that due to other causes, or because only a few men have been exposed, or simply because they have not been suspected and so not looked for. It must also be borne in mind that cancer in humans seldom develops until one or more decades after exposure to the carcinogen first occurs and it is, therefore, too soon to be sure whether agents that have been introduced into industry only during the last 20 years are carcinogenic or not.

Many groups of workers other than those listed in Table 5 have been suspected of having a special risk, but it has not yet been possible to decide whether the risk is real and attributable to their work. Such groups include lead workers and coal miners (gastric cancer), and professional chemists and agricultural workers (lymphoma). Some of the excess mortality rates that have been described may be due to chance. Many types of cancer have been examined in each occupational group and, in these circumstances, some differences that are conventionally 'statistically significant' (that is to say, likely to turn up by chance less than once in 20 times) are bound to be observed by chance alone. Such differences should be regarded as pointing to the presence of a hazard only if highly significant ($p< 0.001$), or if excess rates are confirmed in other studies, or if a risk of the specific type of cancer was predicted from the nature of the agent to which they were exposed.

Other excess rates may be due to confounding; that is, they may be produced by social factors that are associated with the occupation in question rather than by the occupation itself. The potential importance of such confounding was illustrated by Fox and Adelstein's analysis of the occupational mortality statistics for England and Wales over the period 1970–72. They aggregated the occupations of men aged 15 to 64 years into 25 major categories and found that the lung cancer rates in these categories differed up to twofold, a spread that was far too wide to be attributed to chance alone. However, data obtained from random samples of the general population showed that the proportions of men who smoked in each of these 25 large occupational categories varied from about 65 per cent of the national average to about 130 per cent, and that these proportions correlated closely with the mortality rates from lung cancer and could account for nearly all the variation among them.

Given sufficient details and the ability to repeat the observations, it is usually possible to obtain a fairly clear idea of whether or not a marked excess incidence in an occupational group does or does not reflect an occupational hazard by (for example) seeing whether the effect is related to the length of employment, the time after first exposure, and to any specific type of work within the industry. Unfortunately these details are not always available and the reasons for many of the moderate excesses of cancer that have been reported in certain industries are still uncertain.

Although occupational hazards may not account for a large proportion of the total number of cancers in the nation as a whole, such hazards may be of great importance to the groups of individuals concerned. Even in the absence of conclusive proof, it is often advisable to err on the side of safety by restricting exposure if any strong suspicion of a hazard has been aroused, particularly if the occupation involved substantial in exposure to an agent that can be shown by animal or other laboratory tests to be potentially carcinogenic. The closure of an industry may, however, have serious social implications, which also have to be taken into account, and it is no help to government, the employers, or the employees at risk if judgements about the existence of a hazard are made on anything other than strict objective criteria.

At present it seems unlikely that occupational hazards account for more than 2 or 3 per cent of all fatal cancers in developed countries. The three principal causes are probably previous exposure to asbestos dust (lung and pleural cancer), the combustion products of fossil fuels (skin and lung cancer), and ionizing radiations (any cancer). The quantitative evidence is, however, uncertain and this estimate could be out by a factor of two.

Table 5 *Occupational causes of cancer*

Agent	Site of cancer	Occupation[1]
Aromatic amines:	Bladder	Dye manufacturers
4-Amino-diphenyl		Rubber workers
Benzidine		Coal-gas manufacturers
2-Naphthylamine		Some chemical workers
Arsenic	Skin, lung	Copper and cobalt smelters
		Pesticide manufacturers
		Some gold miners
Asbestos	Lung, pleura, peritoneum, larynx	Asbestos miners
		Asbestos textile manufacturers
		Insulation workers
		Shipyard workers
Benzene	Marrow	Workers with glues and varnishes
Beryllium[2]	Lung	Beryllium refiners and machiners
Bis-chloromethyl ether	Lung	Makers of ion-exchange resins
Cadmium[2]	Lung	Cadmium refiners
Chromium[2]	Lung	Manufacturers of chromates from chrome ore; pigment manufacturers
Ionizing radiations	Lung	Uranium and some other miners
	Bone	Luminizers
	Marrow, all sites	Radiologists, radiographers
Mustard gas	Larynx, lung	Poison-gas manufacturers
Nickel[2]	Nasal sinuses, lung	Nickel refiners
Polycyclic hydrocarbons in soot, tar, oil	Skin, scrotum, lung, and sometimes bladder	Coal-gas manufacturers, roofers, asphalters, aluminium refiners, and many groups exposed to tars and selected oils
Sulphuric acid mists (strong acid)	Nasal sinuses, larynx	Many industries, isopropanol manufacture, 'steel pickling'
Ultraviolet light	Skin	Farmers, seamen
Vinyl chloride	Liver (angiosarcoma)	PVC manufacturers
?	Nasal sinuses	Hardwood furniture manufacturers
?	Nasal sinuses	Leather workers

[1]Typical occupations with proven hazards.

[2]Certain compounds or oxidation states.

Pollution

The idea that pollution might be an important cause of cancer has been in the forefront of the minds of cancer research workers since it was realized that the incidence of lung cancer tended to be higher in towns than in the countryside and that the combustion products of coal, which used to produce a pall of smoke over all large cities in Britain, contained carcinogenic hydrocarbons. More recently, with the rapid expansion of the chemical industry and the discovery that some of its products are mutagenic *in vitro* and carcinogenic in laboratory animals, anxiety has increased about the possible effects of distributing such products ubiquitously in the air we breathe, the water we drink, and the food we eat.

The effects of pollution of this sort are, however, peculiarly difficult to assess directly by epidemiological methods, as pollutants are likely to be present in each area, the absolute risk from each is likely to be small, and there may be little difference in the extent to which individuals are exposed over a wide area. Reliance is, therefore, often placed on two indirect methods: extrapolation from the effects of chronic exposure to much larger amounts in an occupational setting, and prediction of the effects on humans from laboratory tests. Both have their difficulties and it is essential, whenever the situation permits, to check the results obtained against the actual experience of people living in the polluted areas.

So far as atmospheric pollution is concerned, the epidemiological picture is complicated by the personal pollution produced by tobacco smoke and the social distribution of smoking habits; but, despite this complication, the various methods that have been discussed under lung cancer all lead to the conclusion that the pollution of the past may have contributed to the production of a few per cent of all lung cancers; but that the levels over the last three decades (principally from the combustion of fossil fuels, but also from asbestos, dioxins, and various other materials) are unlikely to be responsible for more than a fraction of 1 per cent of future cancers—although there may be exceptions awaiting discovery in the neighbourhood of particular factories.

The effect of polluted drinking water and food is even more obscure. Until recently no serious consideration had been given to the possibility that either might be important, except for the possible effect of the contamination of food with smoke from urban air. Now, however, analytical techniques permit the detection of chemicals at concentrations of less than 1 p.p.b. (billion) in both food and water and, in consequence, many have been detected that might arguably be carcinogenic, including pesticide residues and a variety of halogenated organic materials produced by the chlorination of water supplies. Relationships have been reported between the concentrations of some of these compounds in water and the mortality from cancers of the bladder and, possibly, the large intestine, in different localities; but it is extremely difficult to know what these relationships mean as there are so many potentially confounding factors.

Mortality rates from cancers of the liver and gastrointestinal and urinary tracts are, for the most part, stable or decreasing in early middle age, when the effects of new agents might be expected to show themselves first, and, in the absence of more specific evidence, it seems unlikely that chemical pollution of water and food could have a greater effect than the small effect already estimated for pollution of the air. It is important, however, to monitor the situation and, in particular, to seek an explanation for any definite increase in incidence (as has occurred

Table 6 *Some indirect ways in which diet may influence the incidence of cancer indirectly*

Possible ways	Example
Affecting the formation of carcinogens in the body	Providing substrates for the formation of carcinogens (e.g. nitrites, secondary amines)
	Inhibiting formation of carcinogens (e.g. vitamin C in the stomach)
	Altering intake or excretion of cholesterol and bile acids and hence the production of carcinogenic metabolites in the bowel
	Altering the bacterial flora and hence the capacity to produce carcinogenic metabolites
Affecting contact of carcinogens with stem cells	Altering transport of carcinogens (e.g. alcohol, fibre)
	Altering concentration of carcinogens (e.g. effect of fibre on faecal mass)
Affecting activation or deactivation of carcinogens	Induction or inhibition of enzymes that affect metabolism of carcinogens (e.g. indoles in Brassica)
	Deactivation or prevention of formation of short-lived intracellular species (e.g. by selenium and vitamin E, by otherwise trapping free radicals, by quenching singlet oxygen with β-carotene, or by antioxidants used as preservatives)
Affecting 'promotion' of cells that are already initiated	Possible effect of β-carotene, or of determinants of lipid 'profiles'
Affecting secretion of hormones	Increasing amount of adipose tissue

with non-Hodgkin's lymphoma not attributable to AIDS) and any definite irregularities in the geographical distribution of any type of cancer that may be observed.

Diet

For many years there has been suggestive evidence that most of the cancers that are currently common could be made less so by modification of the diet; but, with few exceptions, there is still little reliable evidence as to the modifications that would be of major importance. If we define diet to include all materials that occur in natural foods, are produced during the processes of storage, cooking, and digestion, or are added as preservatives or to give food colour, flavour, and consistency, the ways in which diet could influence the development of cancer are legion.

INGESTION OF PREFORMED CARCINOGENS

The most obvious is the ingestion of small amounts of powerful carcinogens or precarcinogens. Several have been identified in foodstuffs but only two have been related at all clearly to the production of cancer in humans: that is aflatoxin, a metabolic product of *Aspergillus flavus*, which contaminates stored or oily foods in many countries, and is a major cause of liver cancer in the tropics, and the salted fish eaten extensively in South China, which acts synergistically with EBV to cause nasopharyngeal cancer. A third possible source is bracken fern, an extract of which is carcinogenic in animals. It is eaten extensively in Japan and has been linked with the development of oesophageal cancer. The polycyclic hydrocarbons and other mutagens that are produced in food by grilling or smoking have often been suspected of playing a role, but intensive investigation has failed to detect it. It seems, therefore, that if diet does affect the incidence of cancer in the Western world in any material way, it is likely to do so by some more indirect means.

INDIRECT MECHANISMS

Some of the indirect ways in which diet could influence the incidence of cancer are summarized in Table 6. Only the effect of overnutrition has been established with certainty; but the evidence to suggest that others are important is mounting.

Overnutrition

That overnutrition could affect the incidence of cancer was first suggested by Tannenbaum's experiments on mice during the Second World War. These showed that the incidence of spontaneous tumours of the lung and breast, and of a variety of tumours produced experimentally, could be halved by restricting the intake of food without modifying the proportions of the individual constituents. This protective effect has been demonstrated repeatedly since, but it has attracted little attention (perhaps because reports of such results emphasized the benefits of restriction rather than the harm of overeating). It is now clear, however, that what is considered normal nutrition in developed countries increases the risk of breast cancer (by bringing forward menarche and increasing body size) and possibly also that of testis cancer. With greater consumption leading to obesity, the risks of breast and endometrial cancer after the menopause are increased by the formation of oestrogen from androstenedione in adipose tissue (when it becomes significant in the absence of ovarian oestrogen) and the risk of gallbladder cancer is increased by the increased excretion of bile salts.

Meat and fat

Figures for food consumption and cancer incidence and mortality rates in different countries show a close correlation between the consumption of fat and, to a less extent, the consumption of meat and the rates for several different types of cancer. The correlations are closest for breast cancer followed by those for cancers of the large bowel, and, less closely, cancers of the endometrium, pancreas, and prostate. When, however, attempts are made to associate the consumption of either type of food with cancer in individuals within a country the evidence is conflicting. This could be because the correlations are misleading, indicating only that the risks are correlated with something that is correlated with fat and meat consumption (for example, a high gross national product), but it could be partly because of the inaccuracy of dietary histories and partly because people in developed countries, and particularly in North America, eat such similar diets. Overviews of the published data, however, strongly suggest that a high consumption of fat is associated with a high risk of colorectal cancer and that a high consumption of saturated fat is associated with a high risk of breast cancer after the menopause, but not before it.

Whether meat increases the risk of any type of cancer, apart from the contribution it makes through its content of saturated fat, is more uncertain. The low incidence of several types of cancer that is commonly observed in vegetarian communities is not necessarily due to the absence of meat from the diet, as it can generally be explained by the increased consumption of protective foods (vegetables and fruits) and commonly by associated behavioural characteristics (below average use of tobacco and alcohol). Some studies that make allowance for these confounding factors suggest that meat specifically increases the risk of large-bowel cancer, but the evidence is weak and the increase in risk, if any, is small.

Fibre

That fibre may play a part was suggested by Burkitt's observation that several intestinal diseases, including cancer of the colon, were common in countries in which cereals were processed to remove the fibre and rare in rural Africa and Asia where they were not. The term is better replaced by the broader term 'non-starch polysaccharides', as there are many such polysaccharides that share some of the characteristics which Burkitt attributed to fibre. All pass through the small bowel unchanged and some also pass through the large bowel; some are partially degraded (15 per cent) by the flora of the large bowel and others are almost wholly degraded (85 per cent). For physiological purposes some starch, known as 'resistant starch', should be classed with the non-starch polysaccharides, as it also passes through the small bowel unchanged.

Non-starch polysaccharides are found in whole-grain cereals, vegetables, and fruit, and resistant starch most notably in green bananas and cold potatoes. In the large bowel these materials serve as pabulum for the gut flora and protect against the development of cancer mechanically by increasing faecal bulk (by increasing the number of bacteria) and increasing the speed of transit through the bowel, hence both diluting any carcinogens present and diminishing the length of time they are in contact with the mucosa. Their metabolic products, most notably butyrate, also help the normal growth and differentiation of colonic mucosal cells, perhaps by inducing apoptosis.

Retinoids and carotenoids

Experiments on animals and on cell cultures *in vitro* have suggested that vitamin A (retinol) and its esters and analogues (retinoids) may, in appropriate circumstances, reduce the risk of cancer by reducing the probability that partially transformed cells become fully transformed and proliferate into clinically detectable tumours, although in other circumstances they appear to have opposite effects. Human studies, however, fail to support the idea that serum levels of retinol are related to the risk of any type of cancer, at least in countries in which clinical symptoms of vitamin A deficiency seldom or never occur. Such studies suggest that the risks are inversely related to the serum level of β-carotene, which acts as an antioxidant and is broken down to produce retinol. The finding that patients with many different types of cancer commonly report intakes of vitamin A (usually taken to include β-carotene) which are lower than those reported by other patients or healthy control subjects is probably explained by confounding between vitamin A and other protective factors in vegetables including, but not necessarily limited to, β-carotenes.

Other components

Many other components of the diet, including the indoles in cabbages and sprouts, vitamins C and E, and calcium and selenium have also been proposed as protective agents; while nitrates, nitrites, secondary amines, and the preservation of food by salting, have been thought to increase the risk of cancer. For a few of these chemicals the evidence is strong: notably for vitamin C, which reduces the risk of gastric cancer, and for salt-preserved foods, which increase it. For calcium it is less strong, but it may well help to reduce the risk of cancer of the large bowel. For the rest, the evidence is too weak to justify any firm conclusion, except that nitrates and nitrites cannot be of more than marginal significance.

Conclusion

Some of the uncertainties about the effect of diet can probably be resolved only by means of controlled diets in which volunteers are allocated at random micronutrient supplements (like vitamins C and E, β-carotene and other carotenoids, calcium and selenium) or a dietary schedule that requires a substantial reduction in the consumption of fat. Several such studies are under way and if such factors affect the later stages of cancer induction, then clear answers may well be obtained to some of the outstanding questions within a few years. Meanwhile, it seems likely that practicable modifications of the diet should provide the means for reducing cancer deaths in developed countries by a third; but the range of uncertainty about this figure is large. The uncertainty about the specific factors that cause or prevent the disease means that there is substantial uncertainty as to what dietary changes to recommend, other than a general increase in the use of fresh fruit and vegetables.

Interaction of agents

Attribution of the risk of cancer to different causes is complicated by the fact that some agents interact with others to produce effects that are much greater than the sum of the separate effects of each on its own. An example is provided by smoking and asbestos, which multiply each other's effects so that, compared with non-smokers in general, the incidence of cancer of the lung was increased sixfold among a group of insulation workers in the United States who did not smoke, 10- to 20-fold among cigarette smokers in general who did not work with asbestos, and nearly 90-fold among asbestos insulation workers who also smoked cigarettes regularly (Hammond *et al.*, 1979). Other examples are provided by smoking and radon (which interact similarly to produce cancer of the lung), by smoking and alcohol (which interact to produce cancer of the oesophagus), and by infection with the hepatitis B virus and aflatoxin (which interact to produce cancer of the liver).

Such interactions may come about through some analogue of the dual mechanism of initiation and promotion that was suggested some 50 years ago by the experiments of Rous and Kidd and Berenblum and Shubik, and has since been extended to include the concept of 'antipromotion'. They could, however, also be produced in many other ways, some of which have been discussed in the section on diet (see above). From a statistical point of view, they complicate the attribution of risk, as we may find ourselves appearing to claim that more cancer can be prevented than actually occurs by attributing, say, 80 per cent of lung cancers in men heavily exposed to asbestos to their occupational exposure and 90 per cent of the same cancers to cigarette smoking. Interactions, however, greatly facilitate the task of the specialist in preventive medicine, as they provide a choice between two methods of prevention, one of which may be simpler or more acceptable than the other or, perhaps, quicker acting if, as seems likely, some act as promoting or antipromoting agents in the late stage of the development of the disease.

Role of genetic susceptibility (see also Chapter 6.3)

The factors that determine whether a person of a given age will develop cancer in the course of the year are of three types: 'nature', 'nurture', and 'luck' or the play of chance. The first describes people's genetic make-up at conception and affects their liability to react to a given environment by developing a specific type of cancer. The second is the sum of the effects of everything that people do or have done to them in the womb, in childhood, and in adult life, and has been the main topic of this chapter. The third is commonly ignored. Luck, however, is the reason why two animals of identical genetic constitution that have been treated in the same way do not, in general, develop cancer in the same place at precisely the same age. It reflects the element of chance that determines whether a particular series of events all occur in an appropriate relation to each other in the same cell and may be as important in determining who next develops cancer as it is in determining who is next involved in a traffic accident. For any one individual the role of good or bad luck in determining the occurrence of cancer may be large; but in a population of a million it has only a trivial effect on the incidence of cancer and only nature and nurture are important.

The existence of genetic differences in susceptibility may, in principle, be recognized in two ways: by laboratory demonstration of a close connection between chromosome abnormalities, gene mutations, and enzyme variants or other biochemical characteristics of cells, and the occurrence of specific types of cancer, or by epidemiological observation that specific types of cancer tend to cluster in families or are associated with genetically determined factors like blood groups. A mass of laboratory evidence has accumulated over recent years, which is discussed elsewhere. The epidemiological evidence, for its part, has consisted mainly of two sorts: (i) the recognition of clusters that are so marked that no statistical analysis is needed to show the reality of their existence, and (ii) the demonstration that if one member of a family develops a specific type of cancer, other members are somewhat more likely to develop that particular type than would be expected from the experience of a control series.

The first has shown that several rare genes have such a great effect on susceptibility that bearers of one such gene (if it is dominant) or two (if they are recessive) almost invariably develop a particular type of cancer. Examples include the dominant genes for retinoblastoma and for polyposis coli and Gardner's syndrome, leading to cancer of the large bowel, and the recessive genes for xeroderma pigmentosum leading to squamous carcinoma and melanoma of the skin. Similar evidence has also shown that other genetic syndromes frequently, but not invariably, lead to cancer, such as von Recklinghausen's neurofibromatosis leading to fibrosarcoma, the Peutz–Jeghers syndrome leading to carcinoma of the small bowel, the Wiskott–Aldrich syndrome leading to non-Hodgkin's lymphoma, and ataxia telangiectasia, Bloom's syndrome, and Fanconi's anaemia leading to leukaemia. The recognition of these syndromes is important to the individual, as it may provide an opportunity for prophylactic surgery, or enable the diagnosis of malignancy to be made at an early stage when treatment is more likely to be effective, or (rarely) enable precautions to be taken to prevent exposure to the relevant carcinogens, as in the case of sufferers from xeroderma pigmentosum and albinism, who can be protected against sunlight. The proportion of all cancers that occur in people who are highly susceptible to cancer in this way is, however, very small.

The second sort of epidemiological evidence has shown that there is no material tendency for cancer as such to cluster in families and that there are no genes that increase the risk of developing cancer in all organs (although mutations in the p53 gene may increase the risk in many). It has also shown, however, that all the common types of cancer do tend to cluster in families to a small extent, in that a sibling of an affected patient commonly has about twice the normal risk of developing a cancer in the same site. Differences of this sort do not necessarily imply that the familial clusters are genetic in origin: they could be due to familial similarities of behaviour in regard to smoking, drinking, eating, infection or other exposures. Nor, however, do they necessarily imply that any genetic difference in susceptibility is particularly small. Calculations show that they are compatible with 50- to a 100-fold differences in genetic susceptibility if the genes for high susceptibility have an appropriate prevalence in the population. That important genetic variants exist is demonstrated by the greatly increased risk of developing basal-cell and squamous carcinomas of the exposed skin in fair-skinned populations compared with dark-skinned, and there may be other genes associated with localized populations, which, for example, diminish the risk of chronic lymphatic leukaemia and myelomatosis in Chinese, Japanese, and Indians. Other genes may have only a minor effect, such as the gene for blood group A, the possession of which increases the risk of gastric cancer by about 20 per cent over that of people belonging to blood groups O or B.

Discovery of genetic factors that affect particular types of cancer is unlikely to explain much of the differences in the social and geographical distribution of cancer that have been described previously, but it may help to elucidate mechanisms, and focus health education and costly methods of early diagnosis on the sections of the populations that are most at risk.

Conclusion

Estimates of the proportions of fatal cancers that can be attributed to environmental (including behavioural) causes of cancer are given in Table 7. For this purpose, individual causes (such as the various carcinogenic drugs and occupational hazards) have been grouped into 13 main categories. The evidence on which these estimates are based is summarized in previous sections of this chapter and in greater detail by Doll and Peto (1981) and the International Agency for Research on Cancer (1990).

The sum of the best estimates in Table 7, it will be noted, amounts to less than 100 per cent, despite the fact that some of the listed agents interact with one another to augment each other's effect and that some fatal cancers are consequently counted twice. The total would be somewhat more than 100 per cent, however, if the true proportions attributable to some of the categories turn out to be nearer the upper end of the acceptable estimates and it would be a great deal more than 100 per cent if it had been possible to characterize the factors that have been classified as 'other and unknown'.

These estimates do not distinguish between factors that are sufficiently understood to enable specific action to be taken with a guarantee of success and those that are not. They should not, therefore, be taken as guides to the proportion of cancer deaths that can now be prevented by practicable means.

Relative roles of laboratory investigation and epidemiology

Until some years ago all the known causes of human cancer, or the circumstances that gave rise to them, had been discovered by clinicians, or pathological or epidemiological observation, and the specific agents responsible had been identified (if they had been identified) by subsequent laboratory investigation. More recently, a variety of laboratory and statistical methods has been developed that claim to be able to predict which chemicals would be likely to cause cancer in man, and how great the risks might be, if men and women were exposed to them acutely in a few high doses or chronically in repeated low doses.

Laboratory tests

Many methods of testing have been proposed and the most favoured ones are reviewed by the International Agency for Research on Cancer (1980). These include not only 'long-term' tests involving repeated application of the test chemical to living animals, but also a variety of 'short-term' tests that are both quicker and cheaper to perform. In a long-term test, a few dozen, small, laboratory animals are fed or otherwise repeatedly exposed to the test chemical, usually in very high doses throughout a substantial part of their lives, to see if they develop an excess of tumours of any particular type. In most short-term tests, the chemicals are applied to isolated cultures of bacterial or mammalian cells to see whether the cellular DNA can be made to suffer a permanent change that can be detected by allowing selective proliferation of the changed cells, by causing certain cellular side-effects, or by 'transforming' some of the cells so that they appear cancerous and have a selective advantage over their unaltered neighbours. Alternatively, the test chem-

Table 7 *Proportion of cancer deaths attributable to different environmental and behavioural factors in countries such as the United States or United Kingdom*

Factor or class of factors	Best estimate of proportion (%)	Range of acceptable estimates (%)
Ionizing radiation:		
Background	3.5	2 to 6
Medical procedures	0.5	
Industry	< 0.1	
Ultraviolet light	1	0.5 to 1
Occupation	3	2 to 4
Industrial products	< 1	< 1 to 2
Pollution:		
Atmospheric	< 1	< 1 to 2
Water	< 1	
Medical drugs	< 1	< 1 to 2
Diet	30	20 to 60
Food additives	< 1	− 2 to 1
Tobacco	33	25 to 40
Alcohol	3	2 to 4
Hormones	7	5 to 10
Infection	9	5 to 15
Other and unknown	?	?

icals may be given to animals that are killed a few hours later, to see if the DNA extracted from any particular organ shows signs of recent damage.

The use of these tests has led to the discovery of a few agents that have subsequently been shown to be carcinogenic to man, together with hundreds of other substances that are carcinogenic to one or more animal species. Many of these chemicals have, as a result, not been manufactured for general use. Others, however, are already in deliberate use or are found as unintended pollutants of air, water, food, or industrial products, and the question arises how far efforts should be made to remove them from the environment.

Unfortunately, it is not always possible to answer this question clearly, as quantitative knowledge of the mechanisms of carcinogenesis is too incomplete. Alteration of a normal cell into the seed of a growing clone of cancerous cells seems to require at least two qualitatively different types of change and the chief causes of one may not be important causes of the other, and vice versa. Agents that increase the risk of cancer may, therefore, do so in a variety of ways: by, for example, facilitating early changes, by conferring a selective advantage on partially altered cells relative to their normal neighbours, by facilitating later changes, or by interfering with any hypothetical host defence factors that may exist to restrain fully cancerous cells from proliferating. There are, moreover, important differences between man and the small, short-lived animals that laboratory workers must necessarily study, not only in the ways in which particular chemicals are metabolized and detoxified (which differ somewhat haphazardly in different species) but also in the ways that humans have evolved to allow most people to remain free of cancer despite having a far larger body size and a far longer lifespan than that of laboratory animals.

Direct evidence that the short- and long-term tests are of some predictive value is provided by the qualitative observation that most chemicals that have been found to be carcinogenic in both rats and mice also damage DNA in one or more short-term tests for mutagenicity, whereas most chemicals that have been found not to cause any excess of cancer in either species are inactive in the short-term tests. It has not yet been possible, however, to demonstrate reliably any quantitative relation between the results of short- or long-term laboratory tests and the risk of human cancer over the whole range of conditions that are known to cause human cancer. Nor, according to the International Agency for Research on Cancer (1980), are we yet even at the point where useful quantitative estimates of animal risk in long-term feeding studies can be derived from the findings in the various short-term tests.

Epidemiological observation

Epidemiological observation, for its part, may be displaced almost entirely by laboratory investigation in the course of time, if the mechanisms by which cancer is produced ever come to be completely understood. Meanwhile, epidemiological observation has many advantages.

Firstly, observations of the vagaries of human behaviour may suggest ideas that might never occur to a laboratory investigator. Historically, they provided the starting point for a large part of all cancer research by pinpointing many specific risks, and they are continuing to provide new ideas by, for example, pointing to the role of non-starch polysaccharides and vegetables in the diet and to the role of pregnancy, menarche, and the menopause.

Secondly, study of national trends in age-specific mortality from particular diseases draws attention to types of cancer likely to be due to newly introduced factors (as happened in the 1940s with cancer of the lung and in the 1960s with melanoma of the skin). Similarly, study of the recent trends in incidence among occupational or other groups in which an excess of cancer had previously been shown to be present for reasons that were incompletely understood provides a monitoring system to check whether the measures that have been instituted have effectively reduced exposure to the actual cause of the disease.

Thirdly, positive epidemiological observations provide quantitative data relating directly to the species whose cancers we are trying to prevent, and to some of the doses to which humans are actually exposed (for example, from ionizing radiations). By so doing they avoid or reduce the pitfalls in extrapolating from one species to another and from one dose level to an extremely different one, and so may provide estimates of human risk that are reliable enough for a rational comparison of risks and benefits. Moreover, such large numbers of people can be studied that direct evidence of quite small risks can sometimes be obtained. Humans feed and house themselves and arrange their own medical care at no cost to the epidemiologist, so that observations can be made on hundreds of thousands of individuals, while comparable-sized studies on experimental animals would be prohibitively expensive.

Fourthly, apparently negative epidemiological observations (that is, ones that are consistent with the absence of risk) may provide a useful upper limit to the effect that certain agents which have been shown to be carcinogenic in the laboratory can be expected to have in a human population. Epidemiology cannot prove that an effect could never occur; but it may be able to provide data for so many people who have been heavily exposed for such a long time that it is possible to conclude that the effect is small enough to be neglected (as with limited use of isoniazid, phenobarbitone, and saccharin).

Trustworthy epidemiological evidence nearly always requires the demonstration that a relation holds for individuals (or at least for small groups) within a population, as well as between large population groups as a whole. Correlations between the incidence of cancer in whole towns or whole countries and, say, air or water pollution or the consumption in those areas of certain items of food are unlikely to provide reliable evidence, although they may provide hypotheses for testing by other means. In such 'ecological' studies, attempts to separate the role of causative and confounding factors by statistical analysis are often made, but the information obtained in this way is, at best, of only marginal value.

In practice the danger of reaching wrong conclusions is slight when observations are made on individuals rather than on whole populations and when the risk of the disease is increased many times by exposure to the agent under suspicion. In these circumstances, risks have been detected that are quite small in absolute terms (affecting perhaps 1 in 1000 exposed people) and some have been detected after only a handful of cases of a rare type of cancer have occurred. The situation is very different, however, when the induced disease is as common as cancer of the lung or cancer of the breast. In these circumstances, risks that will ultimately kill as many as 1 per cent or more of the exposed population may be overlooked or attributed to chance, unless the population studied is very large. In these circumstances, too, when cancer rates are only a moderate multiple of those among the unexposed (that is, when the relative risk lies between 1 and 2, as it does for kidney cancer in smokers), problems of interpretation become acute and it may be extremely difficult to disentangle the various contributions of biased information, confounding with other factors, and cause and effect. There is, moreover, a special difficulty in the study of cancer, because the disease is seldom induced within 5 years of starting exposure and may not be induced to any great extent until exposure has continued for a few decades. In short, unless epidemiologists have studied reasonably large, well-defined groups of people who have been heavily exposed to a particular substance for a long time, they can offer no guarantee that continued exposure to moderate or low levels will be without material risk.

Conclusion

Epidemiology and laboratory investigation complement each other and both are needed to understand the important causes of cancer and learn how to prevent the disease. The latter is essential if risks of cancer are to be predicted before they occur and so avoided; it must, therefore, be expected that laboratory investigation will gradually replace epidemiology as we come to learn more about the mechanism by which cancer is produced. The former, meanwhile, has the advantage that it starts not with the 10 000 trace chemicals that may be found in one or other organ of the body or in the environment of a particular city, but with the 10 000 deaths that occur in that city each year. Epidemiology is more likely to overlook many small effects of a variety of chemicals than is laboratory investigation: but it is much less likely to overlook the main determinants of cancer rates and trends, especially if these are not simple industrial products or environmental pollutants. Further information about the epidemiology of cancer is given in reviews by the International Union Against Cancer (1980); Doll and Peto (1981) and the International Agency for Research on Cancer (1990).

REFERENCES

Chen, J., Campbell, T.C., Li, J., and Peto, R. (1990). *Diet, life-style, and mortality in China: a study of the characteristics of 65 Chinese counties*. Oxford University Press.

Doll, R., and Peto, R. (1981). The causes of cancer: quantitative estimates of avoidable risks of cancer in the United States today. *Journal of the National Cancer Institute*, **66,** 1191–308. (Also reprinted as an Oxford University Press paperback, published in 1981.)

Doll, R., Fraumeni, J., and Muir, C. (1994) *Trends in cancer incidence and mortality. Cancer Surveys*, Vol. 19 and 20, (ed. R. Doll, J. Fraumeni, and C. Muir). Cold Spring Harbor Laboratory Press, New York.

Fox, A.J., and Adelstein, A.M. (1978). Occupational mortality: work or way of life? *Journal of Epidemiology and Community Health*, **32,** 73–8.

Hammond, E.C., and Garfinkel, L. (1980). General air pollution and cancer in the United States. *Preventive Medicine* **9,** 206–11.

Hammond, E.C., Selikoff, I.J., and Seidman, H. (1979). Asbestos exposure, cigarette smoking, and death rates. *Annals of the New York Academy of Sciences*, **330,** 473–90.

International Agency for Research on Cancer (1976). *Cancer incidence in five continents*, Vol. 3 (ed. J. Waterhouse, C. Muir, P. Correa, and J. Powell). IARC, Lyon.

International Agency for Research on Cancer (1980). *Molecular and cellular aspects of carcinogen screening tests.* IARC Scientific Publications No. 27. IARC, Lyon.

International Agency for Research on Cancer (1990). *Cancer causes, occurrence and control.* IARC Scientific Publications No. 100, (ed. L. Tomatis). IARC, Lyon.

International Commission on Radiological Protection. (1991) Recommendations of the International Commission on Radiological Protection. Publication 60. *Annals of the ICRP*, **21,** Nos. 1–3.

International Union Against Cancer (1970). *Cancer incidence in five continents*, Vol. 2, (ed. R. Doll, C.S. Muir, and J.A.H. Waterhouse). IARC, Geneva.

International Union Against Cancer (1980). *Cancer risk by site*, (ed. T. Hirayama, J.A.H. Waterhouse, and J.F. Fraumeni, Jr). International Union Against Cancer, Geneva.

Office of Population Censuses and Surveys (1993a). *Registrations of cancer diagnosed in 1987, England and Wales.* HMSO, London.

Office of Population Censuses and Surveys (1993b). *Review of the Registrar General on deaths by cause, sex and age, in England and Wales, 1991.* HMSO, London.

6.3 Growth factors and oncogenes

W. J. GULLICK

INTRODUCTION

Cancer is an accumulation of tumour cells in the body as a result of alterations in the balance between their rates of growth, differentiation, and death. Cancer research has for many years attempted to explain the mechanisms underlying this altered behaviour. With the development of techniques in molecular biology, this goal is now within sight. Such knowledge should help in diagnosis, prognosis, and in obtaining the maximum benefit from therapies. Most excitingly, it will allow the rational design and evaluation of new, systemic chemotherapeutic drugs.

The expression and function of many molecules alter during cell transformation. The central issue of molecular cancer research is to identify and distinguish those changes that are causing transformation (the conversion of a normal to a malignant cell) from those that represent associated or adaptive change (such as the need for a greater nutrient supply). The convergence of two areas of research in the early 1980s resulted in a great step forward on the way to this objective. These were the studies of oncogenic retroviruses and of polypeptide growth factors.

The simple genomes of type C retroviruses facilitated research into their mechanisms of transformation. It was found that oncogenic variants contained additional nucleic acid sequences very similar to expressed genes in mammalian cells. It rapidly became clear that these were acquired by recombination from host DNA and that their presence in the virus and their expression following infection were critical for transformation. Viral transformation was thus identifying individual genes, now called oncogenes, present normally in human DNA and with the potential to transform cells.

At the same time, largely independent work had begun to elucidate the structure and function of polypeptide growth factors and their receptors, whose normal function is to regulate cell division. The discovery that genes acquired by retroviruses encoded activated growth-regulatory molecules bridged these fields and provided a model for cell transformation. Thus, expression of a growth-promoting protein from the genome of the retrovirus superseded the cell's own regulatory systems, leading to sustained cell replication. These discoveries rapidly led to evaluation of these systems in human cancers, which generally develop without retroviral infection. The same types of growth-regulatory molecules were also found to be altered by overexpression or mutation exclusively in tumour cells and in particular tumour types. Proof of their central importance in oncogenesis has come from experiments in which overexpression or activation of these molecules, in normal cells and in transgenic animals, leads to the predictable development of cancer in affected tissues.

Growth factors and their receptors represent the upper two tiers of the growth-signalling pathway from the cell surface to the nucleus. It is now clear that molecules which convey signals downstream from receptors through the cytoplasm, called second-messenger systems, and transcription factors, which receive these messages in the nucleus, may also be activated aberrantly in cancer, achieving the same end result. Other systems that regulate apoptosis (the programmed death of cells) may also be altered. Finally, molecules such as cell-adhesion proteins may also be mutated, which might contribute to metastasis.

Several genes are altered during the progress of a normal to a fully malignant cell. Some of these are effectors of transformation, such as the signal-pathway molecules described above. These genes have generally been termed oncogenes. Others may be considered as facilitators of transformation, in that changes to their function allow either the more frequent occurrence or the increased incorporation of mutations in other genes. These genes are often called tumour-suppressor genes (Table 1). The most well studied of these molecules is the p53 gene, whose normal function appears to be to halt the cell in its cycle before DNA replication if the chromosomal DNA has been damaged. This pause allows time for DNA repair, preventing the mutation becoming incorporated permanently. Other as yet poorly characterized genes, such as cause the inherited predisposition to cancer called ataxia telangiectasia, may also be involved in the repair of damaged DNA. Very recently, another clue to possibly similar genes has been obtained from studies on the inherited predisposition to non-polyposis colorectal cancer. Here genes that control the fidelity of DNA replication are mutated leading to DNA instability perceived by replication errors to microsatellite repeat sequences, clearly offering the opportunity for an increased rate of mutation in expressed genes.

Table 1 *Some examples of oncogenes and tumour-suppressor genes*

Growth factors
TGF-α
Amphiregulin
PDGFs
FGFs
IGF-1
Growth-factor receptors
EGF-R
c-*erb*B-2/*HER2*
c-*erb*B-3/*HER3*
Met
PDGF-R
IGF-1-R
FGF-Rs
Ret
Cytoplasmic proteins
ras
abl
Nuclear proteins
myc
fos
jun
ski
rel
myb
Tumour suppressors
RB
p53

EGF, epidermal growth factor; FGF, fibroblast growth factor; IGF, insulin-like growth factor; PDGF, platelet-derived growth factor; R, receptor; TGF, transforming growth factor.

Oncogenes and tumour-suppressor genes in human cancer

GROWTH FACTORS

Two observations from animal viruses indicate the importance of growth factors in cell transformation. First, the oncogenic Simian sarcoma virus was found to contain a gene, v-*sis*, which was nearly identical to the β-chain of platelet-derived growth factor (**PDGF**). After viral infection cells produce PDGF, which can bind to cell-surface receptors, promoting growth by a process known as autocrine stimulation. Secondly, mouse mammary tumour virus, which causes cancer by insertion of a promoter sequence next to an oncogene, was found adjacent to the *int-2* [*FGF* (fibroblast growth factor)-*3*] or *hst* (*FGF-4*) genes, which encode related growth factors. Again, this led to overexpression of the growth factor and transformation. Laboratory studies of human cancers have provided a complementary line of evidence in that cancer cells tend to grow more autonomously in tissue culture than normal cells, and produce and secrete growth-stimulatory molecules. Treatment of some cells with antisense oligonucleotides that suppress growth-factor expression can revert them to a more normal phenotype.

So far, no reliable example of a single instance of genetic change to a growth-factor gene leading to overexpression (such as amplification) or expression of an altered molecule (by mutation) has been reported in human cancer. The expression in human tumours and tumour-derived cell lines of a range of growth factors has, however, been examined by radioimmunoassay, immunocytochemistry, and functional assays and in many instances elevated levels have been observed, presumably due to increased gene transcription. The interpretation of these sorts of analyses is rather complex, as an individual growth factor may bind to more than one receptor (for instance, FGF-1 binds to all four known FGF receptors). Equally a single growth-factor receptor may possess several distinct ligands (such as the epidermal growth-factor (**EGF**) receptor, which binds EGF, transforming growth factor-α (**TGF-α**), amphiregulin, heparin-binding EGF, and betacellulin). In addition, the location of a growth factor detected by immunohistochemical staining at the protein level may not necessarily be the same as its site of synthesis. Finally, some growth factors are fully stimulatory at picomolar concentrations, at which they are very difficult to detect. Thus, the analyses of growth-factor expression in normal tissues and tumours provide an incomplete picture of these complex systems. The most impressive evidence for the importance of deregulation of growth-factor expression as one of the underlying causes of cancer has come from transgenic animal experiments. Expression of TGF-α in mice, under the control of tissue-specific promoters, results in a much higher incidence of cancers in the affected organs than in control animals. The notion of the multistep model of cancer is supported by the much more rapid and certain development of tumours when these animals are crossed with other transgenic strains bearing the *myc* gene or SV40T antigen. Thus, both direct and indirect evidence confirms the important role of growth factors in the development of human tumours.

GROWTH-FACTOR RECEPTORS

The role of growth-factor receptors in transformation of cells is more manifest. Several receptor genes, such as EGF receptor, c-*erb*B-2/*HER2*, and the platelet-derived growth factor (**PDGF**) receptor are amplified in human cancer cells, leading to greatly elevated levels of mRNA and protein expression. Increased mRNA transcription of growth-factor receptor genes has now been convincingly demonstrated in cancer cells, both with and without gene amplification. In certain tumour types, particularly brain tumours, growth-factor receptor genes are not only amplified but rearranged, leading to the expression of altered receptor proteins. The EGF receptor gene is amplified in about 40 per cent of glioblastoma multiforme, but much less frequently in grade II and III glioma. In about half of these cases the amplified copy contains a deletion of exons that normally encode part of the extracellular ligand-binding domain. In a smaller fraction of cases the gene is also deleted in its 3′ region, resulting in a protein lacking part of its cytoplasmic domain. It is likely that these altered receptor proteins are at least partially activated in the absence of ligand.

The EGF receptor gene is also amplified in a proportion of squamous lung cancers, bladder cancers, gastric and head and neck tumours, and rarely, in breast cancers. In these tumours the level of EGF receptor mRNA and protein is higher than in normal tissue. In other cases, gene amplification is not found but high levels of receptor mRNA and protein are present, probably due to increased gene transcription. The c-*erb*B-2 gene is amplified in about 20 per cent of breast, stomach, ovary, and bladder cancers, resulting in elevated levels of protein expression. The gene is rarely amplified in pancreatic cancer, although increased levels of receptor mRNA and protein are observed in about 20 per cent of cases. The PDGF receptor gene was found amplified and apparently rearranged in a small proportion of brain tumours, but so far not in other tumour types. The Met receptor, which binds hepatocyte growth factor/scatter factor, is amplified in a small number of stomach and colorectal cancers, but may be overexpressed by increased gene transcription in a higher proportion of cases. Some members of the FGF receptor gene family may also be amplified in human cancers, notably FGFR-1 and -2 in breast cancer. It is not yet clear if these are the important genes in the amplicon.

Several lines of evidence support the importance of alterations to growth-factor receptors in causing malignant transformation. Experimentally induced expression of high levels of growth-factor receptors or of mutationally activated receptors can at least partially transform cells, and induce cancer in transgenic animals. Reduction of their expression in human cancer cells using antibodies or antisense oligonucleotides causes partial reversion of these cells to an untransformed phenotype, supporting their importance as cancer-causing genes.

The association of overexpression, which generally occurs in only a fraction of any tumour type, with disease outcome and thus their value in prognosis has been explored. Elevated levels of EGF receptor proteins are generally measured by radioreceptor assays using radioactive EGF of known specific activity and tissue homogenates. Until recently, immunohistochemical evaluation was limited to analysis of frozen tissue sections, owing to the lack of antibodies capable of recognizing the receptor in formalin-fixed, paraffin-embedded tissue. Antibodies have now been developed that do react under these conditions, which may lead to the more frequent use of this technique. Antibodies that detect the c-*erb*B-2 protein in formalin-fixed material have been available for some years, and many thousands of cases have been evaluated in this way. Some studies have examined gene amplification by Southern blotting; however, it is now clear that overexpression may occur without amplification and analysis of DNA copy number will tend to underestimate the frequency of positivity. As research progresses, antibodies are becoming available for newly identified receptors such as c-*erb*B-3 and the FGF receptors, allowing more comprehensive studies of their pattern of expression in normal and malignant tissues.

Overexpression of the EGF receptor or the c-*erb*B-2 protein was reported as being an indicator of short relapse-free interval and overall survival in several types of cancer, in particular in breast cancer. In such studies it is critical to evaluate the additional information provided by a new marker, using a multivariate analysis that includes the conventionally used clinical factors such lymph node status, tumour grade, size, age at diagnosis, and any molecular analyses such as oestrogen-receptor status. In addition, many published studies have had too few patients with too short a follow-up to determine the value of the measurement. In the case of c-*erb*B-2 overexpression, some studies of breast cancer have now examined in excess of 1500 cases, providing a reliable estimate of the association of growth-factor receptor expression and disease outcome. These have demonstrated that overexpression is indicative of short relapse-free interval and overall survival in node-positive disease. Unfortunately, it is still controversial whether this effect also applies to node-negative patients, in whom such information would be of the greatest value. In other cancers, where studied, EGF receptor or c-*erb*B-2 overexpression tends to be associated with poor prognosis. In general, these associations have been demonstrated less reliably, owing to the smaller number of cases studied or to the lower prevalence of overexpression. Other examples of growth-factor receptor overexpression, such as the PDGF receptor in brain tumours or the Met gene in gastric cancers, occur too rarely to be evaluated and indeed, for the same reason, would be of relatively little clinical significance. The value of new markers such as c-*erb*B-3 has yet to be determined. Whatever emerges as the final consensus on the prognostic power of growth-factor receptor expression, they are very promising targets for the development of new therapeutic agents and should these prove of value the determination of an 'oncogene profile' of an individual patient will become a commonplace.

CYTOPLASMIC ONCOGENES

Growth factors send signals to the cell nucleus via a chain of interacting proteins. Very recently, members of a direct and uninterpreted sequence of signal transduction have been identified. Within this cascade are found several proteins that are the product of cytoplasmic oncogenes (Fig. 1). The specific proteins that are activated by individual growth-factor receptors are currently a subject of intense research, but some general principles may already be discerned. Most growth-factor receptors with tyrosine kinase activity dimerize in response to ligand binding. Their catalytic activity is increased, causing transphosphorylation of a receptor pair. These phosphorylated tyrosine residues create binding sites for proteins containing a sequence called an **SH2** domain (standing for *src*-homology region-2—a sequence first found in the *src* oncogene). SH2 domains recognize, in addition to phosphorylated tyrosine, a short surrounding linear sequence, often of about four amino acids, providing

Fig. 1 A signal-transduction pathway from the cell surface to the nucleus.

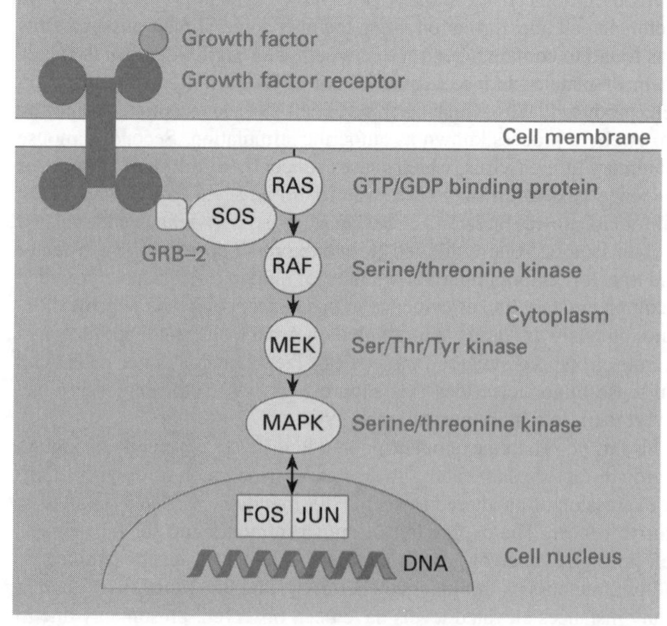

their specificity of interaction. SH2 domain-containing proteins may themselves have an enzyme activity (such as in phospholipase Cγ) or act as 'adaptor' proteins forming a bridge with another enzyme (such as the p85 subunit, which is associated with the p110 catalytic element of phosphatidyl inositol-3 kinase). On binding to the receptor, the enzyme may become phosphorylated on tyrosine or, in some cases, interaction itself seems to be activating, perhaps by inducing a conformational change. The signal is then passed on to downstream molecules. In the main pathway so far identified, a receptor such as for EGF binds to the *GRB-2* SH2 domain-adaptor protein (Fig. 1). This then interacts with the SOS protein, which functions to regulate the *ras* proteins; *ras* binds guanine nucleotides and can interact with either GDP or GTP, the latter being the 'active' form. SOS appears to regulate the rate of GDP/GTP exchange on *ras*.

Mutations have been found in *ras* genes in many human tumour types, often with a high prevalence. These mutant *ras* proteins are found predominantly in the GTP-bound, activated state; *ras* binds to *raf*, a serine/threonine kinase, which has also been found as a retroviral oncogene; *raf* binds to MEK, an unusual protein with both threonine and tyrosine kinase activity; this phosphorylates MAP kinase, which in turn phosphorylates a number of proteins including transcription factors. Thus, at various levels in the signal-transduction pathway, individual proteins have been found to be altered by mutation in human cancers. It is apparent, therefore, that aberrant activation of this information-transfer cascade at many levels can result in the same end-point of excessive growth stimulation.

Some studies have examined the incidence of mutant cytoplasmic oncogenes in particular tumour types and their association with disease outcome. Mutations in the three members of the *ras* gene family (H-*ras*, K-*ras*, and N-*ras*) have been found quite commonly. Mutations in K-*ras* are particularly prevalent in pancreatic cancer (75 per cent of adenocarcinomas) and colonic cancers (35 per cent), whereas all three *ras* proteins have been found mutated in thyroid cancers (50 per cent of cases). In other tumour types such as breast cancer, *ras* mutations are extremely rare. Mutations in the K-*ras* gene occur in about 30 per cent of lung adenocarcinomas and are reportedly associated with short relapse-free interval and survival.

Another cytoplasmic oncogene called *abl* is altered in 90 per cent of chronic myelogenous leukaemias. In this instance, the gene is apparently activated by chromosomal rearrangement with another gene called *bcr*, resulting in the expression of a hybrid *bcr*/*abl* protein. The most commonly observed rearrangement is a reciprocal translocation of a small portion of the long arm of chromosome 9 and the long arm of chromosome 22. The altered chromosome 9 was first detected at the cytogenetic level and has been called the Philadelphia chromosome after the city in which it was discovered. Other more complex but rarer translocations have also been reported. Although *abl* possesses tyrosine kinase activity that is apparently activated in the *bcr*/*abl* fusion protein, it is not yet clear how this fits in to a normal growth-regulatory signal pathway.

Many other second-messenger proteins and signal-transduction pathways are now being identified, which will allow a greater understanding of this vital biological system. The mechanisms used by non-tyrosine kinase receptors are, for instance, just beginning to be determined. It is likely, also, that new oncogenes may be identified and roles defined for others (such as *mos*, *cot*) whose functions are currently obscure.

NUCLEAR ONCOGENES

Several oncogenes have been identified whose products are expressed in the cell nucleus. Some, such as *fos*, *jun*, and *erbA*, are known to function as transcription factors. These bind to DNA elements in the promoters of specific genes, enhancing (or occasionally inhibiting) gene expression. Each of these has been found as an oncogene in transforming retroviruses, but there is little evidence for alterations in their structure or function in human tumours. The control of gene transcription into mRNA is often very complex and the exact nature of the groups of proteins that can interact, both with themselves and with nuclear DNA, is currently the subject of much basic research. It is generally agreed to be one of the great achievements of modern molecular biology that signals in the form of growth factors acting at the cell surface can now be traced to the activation of expression of individual genes.

One nuclear oncogene remains tantalizingly enigmatic. The *myc* gene family consists of c-*myc*, N-*myc*, and L-*myc*, and is activated by more mechanisms than any other in cancer. Overexpression occurs as a result of chromosomal translocation or gene amplification, or in model systems by promoter insertion (by avian leucosis virus). The functions of the *myc* proteins are poorly understood, but recently it has been proposed that c-*myc* plays a part in regulating apoptosis, the programmed death of cells. Another oncogene, *bcl-2*, has also been implicated in this process. Apoptosis involves a characteristic condensation and fragmentation of nuclear DNA, changes in cell shape and gene expression, and the ultimate death of the cell. Alterations in genes such as *bcl-2* and *myc* may affect the balance between cell division and death, which in concert with aberrant growth stimuli may result in the growth of malignant cell populations.

Oncogenes and tumour-suppressor genes as targets for new anticancer drugs

GROWTH FACTORS

The clinical exploitation of aberrant expression of growth factors is now being explored. Associations between growth-factor expression and measures including relapse-free interval and survival of cancer patients have been sought but usually not found. Hybrid growth factors fused to cytotoxic agents with the potential for killing tumour cells are being evaluated, but several problems remain to be overcome, particularly their influence on normal tissues. Alternatively, the completely different usage of exogenous growth factors is already common in cancer treatment. Loss of haemopoietic-cell production due to marrow toxicity following treatment with some common chemotherapeutic agents has limited their use. Growth factors such as stem-cell factor and granulocyte–macrophage colony-stimulating factor, often in combination with other cytokines, are now being optimized for stimulating haemopoietic-cell regeneration after chemotherapy.

GROWTH-FACTOR RECEPTORS

The use of monoclonal antibodies directed to the extracellular domain of the c-*erb*B-2 protein is currently the most advanced use of growth factor receptors for diagnosis. Antibodies have been used to image primary breast cancer and lymph node metastases using technetium-99, iodine-125, or indium-111, and with iodine-124 for positron-emission tomography. Various approaches are being explored to exploit growth-factor receptors as therapeutic targets. One strategy involves the passive use of overexpression to accumulate selectively, on cancer cells, antibodies or growth factors generally linked to toxic molecules such as plant-derived enzymes, radionucleotides or conventional chemotherapeutic molecules. A second approach is to decrease the expression level or enzyme activity of the receptor by using monoclonal antibodies, antisense oligonucleotides, or tyrosine kinase and dimerization inhibitors. Another suggestion is to exploit the increased transcription of the receptor in cancer cells. In this case, introduction of a hybrid gene bearing the receptor's promoter sequence but specifying some form of toxic activity could selectively kill cancer cells.

Monoclonal antibodies are the reagents that have been most frequently studied for their antitumour properties both in experimental animals and in patients. In some cases, bispecific antibodies have been created with one combining site directed to c-*erb*B-2 and the other to molecules such as CD3, a T-cell-specific surface antigen, with the intention of activating cytotoxic lymphocytes adjacent to the tumour cells.

In perhaps the most sophisticated application of this approach so far, a monoclonal antibody, 4D5, has been 'humanized' by grafting its specificity-determining sequences on to a human antibody framework with the intention of avoiding the human antimouse immune response that normally occurs when using mouse monoclonal antibodies and prevents repeated treatment. Clinical trials of monoclonal antibodies to the c-*erb*B-2/*HER2* protein are already underway, but it may be several years before it can be determined if any of these approaches produce clinically useful drugs.

CYTOPLASMIC ONCOGENES

Several strategies are being explored to develop specific inhibitors of the *ras* proteins. Normally, H-*ras* and K-*ras* are modified by the post-translational addition of a farnesyl group to their C-terminal region, which acts as an anchor to fix them to the cell membrane. Mutation of critical residues that prevent this modification inactivates both wild-type and mutant *ras*, emphasizing the importance of their localization to the inner surface of the plasma-cell membrane. Compounds that inhibit the farnesyl transferase enzyme have been developed and are being explored for their effect on mutant *ras*-transformed cells. Other approaches include the use of antisense oligonucleotides and ribozymes to suppress *ras* expression and the development of antibody and cellular immune responses to the mutant proteins.

NUCLEAR ONCOGENES

The development of inhibitors of transcription factors is a growth area. Two fundamental strategies are proposed, targeted either at the protein factor or at the DNA sequence forming its binding site. Most transcription factors can be activated either by post-transcriptional modifications (such as phosphorylation) or by binding activating ligands (such as steroid hormones). An excellent example of the latter as a target for therapy is the development of the drug tamoxifen, which binds to and (in the presence of oestrogen) inhibits the function of the oestrogen receptor. The main strategy currently proposed for influencing the DNA-binding site is the use of triple-helix-forming oligonucleotides that sterically hinder transcription-factor binding.

Summary

Genes have now been identified that are involved in signal transduction, DNA replication and repair, and apoptosis whose functions are increased or diminished in particular types of human cancers. Experimental evidence supports their direct role in cell transformation. Analysis of the genetic changes present in an individual patient's tumour may allow more accurate prediction of the likely course of the disease and optimization of therapy. Most excitingly, these changes are being explored as targets for new forms of cancer therapies.

REFERENCES

Aaltonen, L.A. *et al.* (1993). Clues to pathogenesis of familial colorectal cancer. *Science*, **260,** 812–16.

Bishop, J.M. (1991). Molecular themes in oncogenesis. *Cell*, **64,** 235–48.

Bos, J.L. (1989). *ras* oncogenes in human cancer: a review. *Cancer Research*, **49,** 4682–9.

Brunton, V.G., and Workman, P. (1993). Cell-signalling targets for antitumour drug development. *Cancer Chemotherapy and Pharmacology*, **32,** 1–19.

Cantley, L.C. *et al.* (1991). Oncogenes and signal transduction. *Cell*, **64,** 281–302.

Cross, M., and Dexter, T.M. (1991). Growth factors in development, transformation and tumorigenesis. *Cell*, **64,** 271–80.

Fantl, W.J., Johnson, D.E., and Williams, L.T. (1993). Signalling by receptor tyrosine kinases. *Annual Review of Biochemistry*, **62,** 453–81.

Fearon, E.R. and Vogelstein, B. (1990). A genetic model for colorectal tumorigenesis. *Cell*, **61,** 759–67.

Gullick, W.J. (1991). Prevalence of aberrant expression of the epidermal growth factor receptor in human cancers. *British Medical Bulletin*, **47,** 87–98.

Hunter, T. (1991). Cooperation between oncogenes. *Cell*, **64,** 249–70.

Hunter, T. and Karin, M. (1992). The regulation of transcription by phosphorylation. *Cell*, **70,** 375–87.

Lofts, F.J. and Gullick, W.J. (1991). c-*erb*B2 amplification and overexpression in human tumors. In *Genes, oncogenes, and hormones: Advances in cellular and molecular biology of breast cancer*, (ed. R.B. Dickson and M.E. Lippman), pp. 161–79. Kluwer, Boston.

Marshall, C.J. (1991). Tumor suppressor genes. *Cell*, **64,** 313–26.

Sandgren, E.P., Luetteke, N.C., Qiu, T.H., Palmiter, R.D., Brinster, R.L., and Lee, D.C. (1993). Transforming growth factor alpha dramatically enhances oncogene-induced carcinogenesis in transgenic mouse pancreas and liver. *Molecular Cell Biology*, **13,** 320–30.

Varmus, H. (1988). Retroviruses. *Science*, **240,** 1427–35.

Weinberg, R.A. (1991). Tumor suppressor genes. *Science*, **254,** 1138–46.

6.4 Tumour immunology

P. C. L. BEVERLEY

Historical perspective

Underlying all immunological approaches to cancer is the idea that tumour cells must differ from normal cells, and that these differences must be detectable by the immune system. Tumour immunologists have tried to exploit this in two main ways. The first is to use antibodies produced in another species to distinguish between tumour and normal cells; this difference can then be exploited for diagnostic, prognostic, or therapeutic purposes. The second is to stimulate the host's own immune system by specific or non-specific immunization to react more vigorously to autologous tumour. These avenues have been pursued for nearly one hundred years, so that it is pertinent to ask why it is that immunology has had such a minor impact in oncology.

The early years of the twentieth century saw many experiments in tumour transplantation, and the description of tumour rejection. Non-specific stimulation with bacterial products (Coley's toxin) was tried as therapy. Later it was realized that the tumour rejection experiments were documenting allograft rejection, and more rigorous examination of the effect of immunostimulation showed that the success rate was extremely low. In the postwar period the development of inbred animals allowed properly controlled experiments on tumour-specific immune responses to be performed and the development of the theory of immune surveillance provided a stimulus and a theoretical basis for a new wave of experiments in tumour immunology. Nevertheless, although tumour-specific immune responses were soon detected, it remained difficult to define their target antigens until the development of monoclonal antibodies and methods for gene cloning. One other advance was also essential for understanding of antitumour immune responses—the realization that thymus-derived (T) lymphocytes can recognize only those antigens processed inside cells and displayed at the cell surface in association with major histocompatibility complex (MHC) antigens.

IMMUNE SURVEILLANCE

The theory of immune surveillance postulated that tumours arise frequently but that the majority are eliminated by the immune system before becoming clinically apparent. A variety of evidence was adduced in support of the theory (Table 1) and many experiments performed to test it. The majority were studies of the effects of either genetic or induced immunosuppression, as the strongest prediction of the theory was that tumours should arise with overwhelming frequency in the absence of an immune response. Initially, the results were confusing. Very few tumours were seen in a large study of congenitally athymic nude mice. In contrast, a higher frequency of tumours was observed in mice deliberately immunosuppressed with antilymphocyte globulin than in controls, but these were all characteristic of tumours caused by polyoma virus (later found to have been inadvertently introduced into the mice in the antilymphocyte globulin). Similarly, in man, both deliberately immunosuppressed individuals and AIDS sufferers have a greatly increased risk of tumours (Table 2), but not of the common types. The data are clearly not in accord with a straightforward immune surveillance hypothesis; if they were, all tumours should be increased. It is also striking that viruses are implicated in the aetiology of several of the tumours types arising in immunocompromised individuals (Table 3). These observations have led to a modified view of immune surveillance, which may be stated as follows; tumours arise infrequently and the immune response is a late event. Effects attributed to surveillance against tumour cells are most likely due to immune responses against potentially oncogenic viruses.

As immunological intervention has usually been most effective when employed prophylactically, the best approach to virus-induced tumours may be by immunization against the oncogenic virus, preventing infection and therefore transformation. Immunization against hepatitis B virus should greatly decrease the worldwide incidence of liver cancer, and the development of vaccines against Epstein–Barr virus (EBV) and papillomaviruses is the subject of active research (see Section 14). Nevertheless, in the case of many of the most common tumours there is no evidence for a viral aetiology, so that for these tumours the question of the existence and importance of immune responses to tumour-associated antigen remains.

Table 1 *Evidence for immune surveillance*

Tumours arise frequently in the young and old, periods of relative immunoincompetence
Tumours arise frequently in genetically immunodeficient individuals
Tumours arise frequently in immunosuppressed individuals
Tumours usually show infiltrating lymphocytes
Immune responses to tumours can be demonstrated *in vivo* and *in vitro*
Spontaneous regression of tumours occasionally occurs and is often associated with lymphoid infiltration

Table 2 *Tumours and immunosuppression*

Tumour type	Approximate relative risk
Kaposi's sarcoma	50–100
Non-Hodgkin's lymphoma	25–45
Carcinoma of the liver	20–35
Carcinoma of the skin	20–50
Carcinoma of the cervix	2.5–10
Melanoma	2.5–10

Figures for relative risks vary considerably in different studies. This may be due to differences in length of follow-up as well as variation in cofactors (e.g. sunlight) in different parts of the world.

Table 3 *Viruses and human tumours*

Tumour	Virus
Burkitt's lymphoma	Epstein–Barr virus
Nasopharyngeal carcinoma	Epstein–Barr virus
Transplant lymphomas	Epstein–Barr virus
Liver carcinoma	Hepatitis B virus
Cervical carcinoma	Human papillomaviruses
Adult T-cell leukaemia	Human T cell leukaemia virus 1

In the tumours in the table, all or a part of the viral genome is present in tumour cells. In other tumours, such as Kaposi's sarcoma or skin carcinoma, viruses may be involved but the evidence is less direct.

Tumour-specific immunity

The first convincing evidence that there were tumour-specific antigens came from experiments in inbred mice using chemically-induced tumours. Figure 1 illustrates such an experiment. Mice were immunized by grafting a tumour fragment and then excising the growing tumour. Mice challenged with the same tumour showed resistance, while those challenged with a different tumour of the same type did not. Immunity was later shown to be T-cell-mediated. Many experiments of this type confirmed the original findings but, interestingly, spontaneously arising tumours were usually found to be much less immunogenic, raising the possibility of tumour escape mechanisms.

In man, early data showed that lymphocytes of many patients could kill tumour cells and it was also suggested that 'blocking factors' present in serum might be responsible for the progressive growth of tumours in the face of a cellular tumour-inhibitory response. Later results raised doubts as to the specificity of the early data and it became clear that the lymphocytes of both normal and cancer patients could often inhibit the growth of tumour targets. This led to the definition of natural killer cells. Although the main function of this cell population remains obscure, there is little to suggest that it plays a major role in protection against tumours.

More persuasive evidence of specific T cell responses to tumours was obtained after it was realized that T cells can only recognize antigen in the context of self-major histocompatibility complex (see Section 5), and that specific immune responses can often be revealed only after an *in vitro* boost. A number of authors have since shown that both major histocompatibility complex class II restricted tumour-specific T helper, and class I restricted T cytotoxic responses can be generated by coculture of lymphocytes and autologous tumour cells (Fig. 2). Although it is clear that these responses occur in many tumour-bearing patients, the fact that they have been difficult to detect reproducibly indicates that there is probably a low frequency of responding T cells. Nevertheless, the possibility that even weak responses might be boosted by immunization led to efforts to define the molecular nature of tumour antigens.

WHAT ARE TUMOUR ANTIGENS?

The nature of the tumour-specific antigens of non-viral experimental tumours and of most human tumours remained inaccessible until the development of gene cloning methods made possible a series of important experiments by Boon and his colleagues. They first set out to identify tumour antigens of a mouse tumour, P815. The tumour was initially non-immunogenic in syngeneic DBA/2 mice, so that it grew readily even in preimmunized mice. A set of tumour variants were produced by treating the tumour with a mutagen. Some of these were highly immunogenic and unable to grow in preimmunized mice (tum$^-$ variants). From mice immunized with tum-variant cells it was possible to isolate cytotoxic T cell (CTL) clones, which could kill only the immunizing tumour variant and not parental P815 or other tum$^-$ variants. The cytotoxic T cell clones were used to screen parental P815 cells that had been transfected with a cosmid library constructed from tum$^-$ variant cells (Fig. 3). Eventually tum$^-$ antigen-positive transfectants were identified, the cosmid recovered, and, after subcloning, transfecting the subclones, and rescreening, the gene coding for the cytotoxic T cell target antigen could be identified.

Several different tum$^-$ antigens have now been cloned in this way and it has become clear that they fall into two categories (Table 4). The first is due to a genetic alteration in the coding sequence of a gene and the second to altered expression of a normal gene product. That there can be a response to the second type of antigen implies that there are self antigens to which tolerance is at least incomplete.

Boon and his colleagues have gone on to investigate human tumour antigens in a similar fashion. Melanoma stimulates a relatively strong host T cell response and cytotoxic T cell clones specific for a melanoma antigen designated MZ2E were therefore produced and used to screen a melanoma cDNA library. The properties of the melanoma antigen gene (Mage-1) eventually cloned are listed in Table 5. Mage-1 belongs to the category of unaltered tumour antigens abnormally expressed. More remarkably, the gene belongs to a large previously undiscovered family, which is widely expressed in tumours and seldom in normal tissues.

The results of the studies detailed above lead to the conclusion, hardly surprising in retrospect, that most tumour antigens are similar to other antigens recognized by T cells. They are short peptides presented by major histocompatibility complex molecules. Just as in the case of other T cell-recognized antigens, two main factors will determine whether a tumour antigen stimulates an immune response in the host. First, processed peptides from the molecule must reach the cell surface in association with major histocompatibility complex molecules. Whether a particular peptide does so will in turn depend on the amount produced by processing enzymes, its ability to reach intracellular compartments where it may bind to major histocompatibility complex molecules and its affinity for the major histocompatibility complex alleles expressed by the cell. Second, there must be T cells capable of responding. It is likely that there are many peptides transported to the cell surface to which the host is unable to respond because potentially responsive T cells have been deleted during thymic education. It is therefore quite possible that many alterations in the sequence or amount of proteins expressed in tumours cells will not induce a T cell immune response.

Fig. 1 Fibrosarcomas are readily induced in inbred mice by subcutaneous injection of the carcinogen methylcholanthrene. These tumours do not readily metastasize, so mice with growing tumours can be cured by local excision. Following tumour excision mice may be challenged with the same or a different tumour induced by the same carcinogen in the same inbred strain. The immunized mice are immune to challenge with the same tumour but not others.

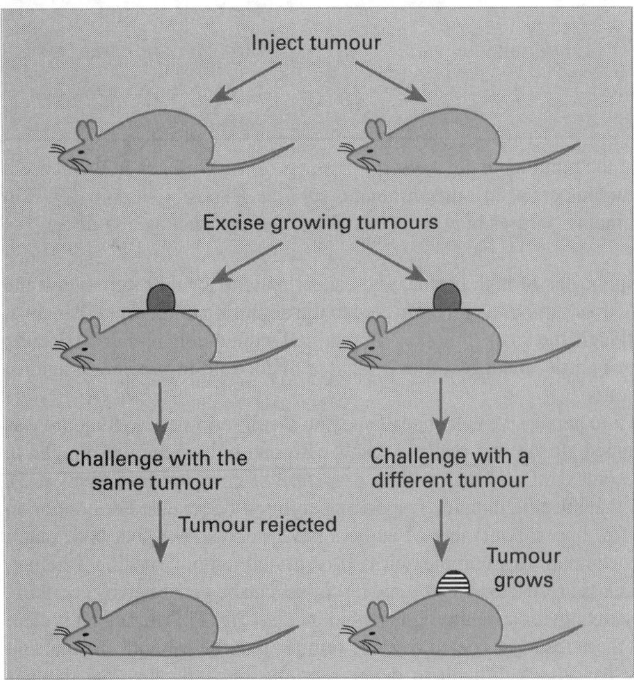

Fig. 2 Tumour cell lines can sometimes be established from enzyme-disaggregated surgical specimens. Alternatively, viable tumour cells can be stored in liquid nitrogen for use in *in vitro* assays. Lymphocytes may be obtained from blood, lymph nodes, or disaggregated tumour (tumour infiltrating lymphocytes; TILs). After initial mixed lymphocyte–tumour culture (MLTC), *in vitro* boosted lymphocytes may be assayed or alternatively cloned and expanded by growth in interleukin-2.

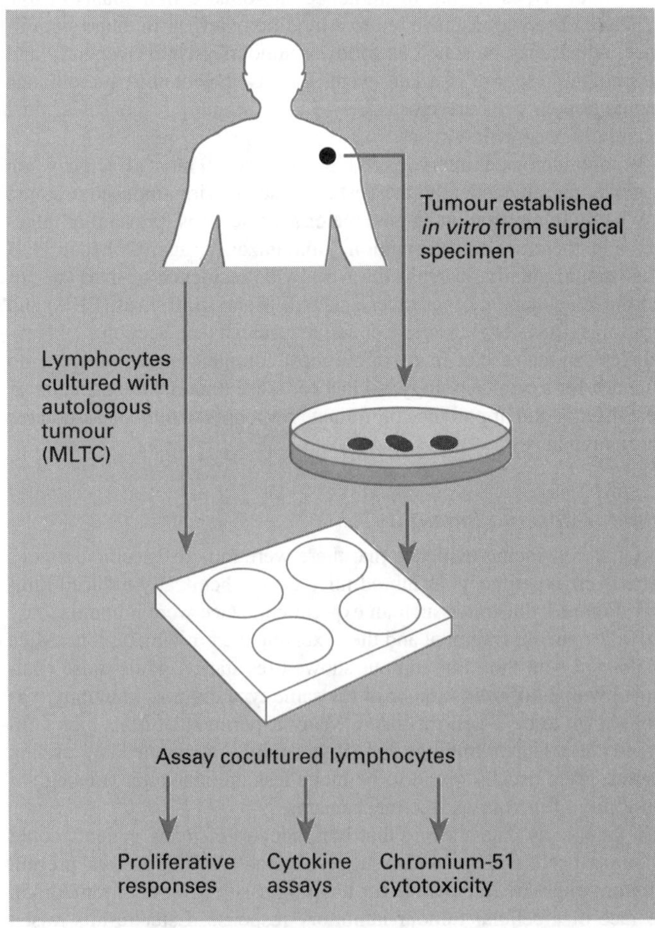

Furthermore the frequency of T cells able to respond to a single epitope, as in the case of a point mutation, or a small number of epitopes when a protein is produced in excessive amounts, is likely to be low. This may explain the generally weak immune response to spontaneous tumours.

However, the elucidation of the nature of tumour antigens does provide a means of identifying potential target antigens in tumour cells and this has been exploited in experimental models and in man. Mutations and genetic rearrangements creating new sequences are common in tumours (Table 6) and may be immunogenic. Thus it has been shown that humans and mice can respond to peptides of mutant *ras* oncogene and an ovarian cancer patient was shown to be able to generate cytotoxic T cell to the *neu* (neuroblastoma) oncogene product. Similarly, mice could respond to peptides derived from the joining region of the bcr–abl chimeric oncogene product found in human chronic myeloid leukaemia.

One other form of T cell antitumour response is of interest. Polymorphic epethelial mucin (PEM) is a heavily glycosylated molecule that is expressed at the surface of many epithelial cells and corresponding tumours. Cytotoxic T cells generated from breast cancer patients lyse tumour cells expressing the mucin but in an unrestricted fashion. The cytotoxic T cell may be CD4 or CD8 and have an αβ T cell receptor but, unusually, killing can be blocked by a monoclonal antibody (mAb) to the tandem repeat structure of the protein core. Exactly how these unusual cytotoxic T cells recognize their antigen remains to be determined.

This evidence suggests that many tumours may have potential T cell target antigens. In most cases it is unclear whether immune responses to these antigens play an important role in modifying tumour growth, although the common occurrence of total or allele specific loss of major histocompatibility complex molecules in as many as 50 per cent of human tumours can be taken as evidence for immunoselection. That there appear to be potential targets for T cell responses encourages the view that rational use of therapeutic vaccines may eventually become possible.

Fig. 3 Cloned cytotoxic T cells respond to tum$^-$ antigen transfected into parental P815 cells by proliferation or cytokine production, which are readily assayed. Stimulatory transfectants can be recovered and the cosmid DNA extracted. This can be subcloned into plasmids, retransfected and the transfectants rescreened for transmission of tum$^-$ antigen. Eventually after several rounds of subcloning, screening and transfection the gene for the tum$^-$antigen can be isolated and sequenced. Usually at least 10 000 cosmid clones had to be screened.

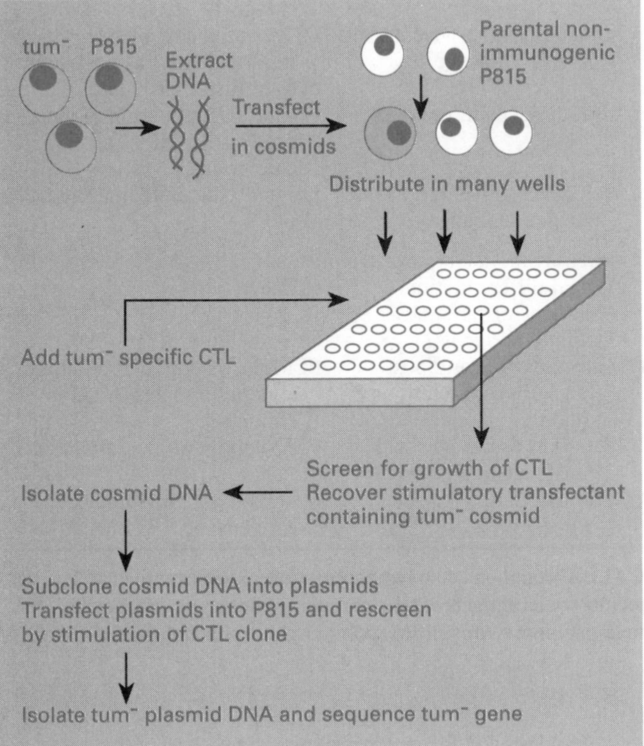

Table 4 *The properties of two types of mouse tumour antigens*

Altered antigen	Overexpressed antigen
Tumour sequence has a point mutation	Sequence identical to the germ line gene
Not necessarily expressed at a high level	Expressed at high level in tumours
Normal gene expressed in mouse tissue(s)	Expressed at very low level in normal tissues
Antigen is a nonapeptide recognized in association with class I molecules	Antigen is a nonapeptide recognized in association with class I molecules

Table 5 *Properties of a human melanoma antigen*

Mage-1 tumour sequence is identical to genomic Mage-1
Mage-1 has no homology to known genes
The antigen is an internal cellular protein
Mage-1 is part of a large gene family
One or another family member are expressed in most melanomas and some other tumours
The antigen is only expressed in testis among normal tissues surveyed
The peptide epitope detected by MZ2E-specific CTL is HLA-A1 restricted

CTL, cytotoxic T cell; HLA, human leucocyte antigen.

ANTIBODIES TO TUMOUR CELLS

The exquisite specificity of antibodies has long persuaded investigators that it should be possible to use them to distinguish between tumour and normal cells. However until the development of monoclonal antibodies there had been few successful examples. Since that time it has become clear that, in contrast to T cells, the vast majority of monoclonal antibodies raised against tumour cells recognize not tumour antigens, but normal differentiation antigens (Table 7). There are a few exceptions. Thus antibodies to the idiotype of T and B cell tumours are tumour specific and antibodies to mutant forms of the p53 tumour suppressor gene product identify this as a tumour associated molecule. In spite of this apparent failure, monoclonal antibodies have proved extremely useful in studying the biology of tumours and lack of absolute specificity for tumour cells does not preclude their use as diagnostic or therapeutic agents.

Carcinoembryonic antigen: the history of a tumour-associated antigen

Carcinoembryonic antigen (CEA) provides an instructive example of the evolution of information and ideas about a molecule initially considered to be tumour associated. Carcinoembryonic antigen, discovered by Gold and Freedman in the early 1960s, was first defined by polyclonal antisera raised against perchloric acid extracts of colon carcinoma. The molecule was found not only in carcinoma extracts but also in the serum

Table 6 *Some genetic alterations in human tumours*

Oncogene alteration	Function of protein	Tumour type
Point mutations		
FMS	CSF-1 receptor	AML, myelodysplasia
ras	GTP-binding protein	Carcinomas and others
p53	Tumour suppressor, cell cycle control	Many including lung, colon, and breast
RB1	DNA binding protein	Bladder
Chromosomal translocations		
BCR-ABL	Tyrosine kinase	CGL, ALL
E2A-PRL	Transcription factor	Pre-B cell ALL
H4-RET	Growth factor receptor, tyrosine kinase	Thyroid carcinoma
MYL-RAR α	Retinoic acid receptor	APL
TPR-MET	Growth factor receptor tyrosine kinase	Gastric carcinoma
L MYC-RLF	Transcription factor	SCLC
Deletion mutations		
ERB-B	Growth factor receptor	Gliomas
Amplification		
ERB-B2	Growth factor receptor	Breast
ERB-B	Growth factor receptor	Brain
C-MYC	Cell cycle control	Breast

ALL, acute lymphoblastic leukaemia; AML, acute myeloid leukaemia; CSF, colony stimulating factor; GTP, guanosine triphosphate; SCLC, small cell lung cancer; APL, acute promyelocytic leukaemia; CGL chronic granulocytic leukaemia.

of patients with colon carcinoma. At first it was not thought to be present in normal adult tissue or other tumours, although it was found in fetal gut and gut-associated tissues. However, as more sensitive assays using mAbs to carcinoembryonic antigen were introduced, raised serum carcinoembryonic antigen levels were found in a wide range of patients with carcinoma and in several non-neoplastic conditions, including heavy smoking. This limits the value of carcinoembryonic antigen as a diagnostic test, although it may be useful for monitoring treatment.

While carcinoembryonic antigen was being studied empirically by clinicians as a tumour marker, others were attempting to understand the biology of the molecule. Initial immunochemical studies showed that carcinoembryonic antigen was a member of a family of heavily glycosylated and heterogeneous molecules, which included several antigenically related entities such as non-specific cross-reacting antigen (NCA). Gene cloning clarified this confusion and showed that carcinoembryonic antigen is a member of a family of molecules, which in turn belong to the immunoglobulin gene superfamily (Fig. 4).

Many immunoglobulin superfamily members are cellular adhesion molecules (CAMs), and carcinoembryonic antigen is no exception. Studies using transfected cells show that it can function as a homotypic adhesion molecule and may also interact with other family members. In the normal colon, carcinoembryonic antigen is found on the luminal surface of epithelial cells, while in both (multilayered) fetal epithelium and in tumours it is more evenly distributed. While this change in distribution is likely to alter the behaviour of the tumour cells, it is not clear whether it is a primary or secondary abnormality. Nevertheless, changes in other surface adhesion molecules are a common feature of tumour cells, presumably providing survival advantages (see below).

Changes in tumour cells detected by antibodies

Just as for carcinoembryonic antigen, so the focus on other tumour antigens has shifted from regarding them simply as markers of malignant transformation to attempting to understand their role in the behaviour

Table 7 *Types of tumour antigen*

Types of alteration	Example
Detected by host response	
Normal gene products expressed abnormally	P1 antigen of P815 mouse mastocytoma Human melanoma antigen (Mage-1)
Mutated or otherwise altered protein sequence	P91A antigen of mouse mastocytoma, ras oncogene bcr-abl fusion protein of CGL
Viral antigens in tumours	E6 and E7 transforming gene products of HPV in cervical carcinoma
Molecules showing post-translational alterations	Polymorphic epithelial mucin
Detected by monoclonal antibodies	
Normal differentiation antigens of rare cells	CALLA.
Oncofetal antigens	CEA, α-fetoprotein
Molecules showing post-translational alterations in tumours	PEM has altered carbohydrate epitopes and new peptide epitopes
Mutations associated with transformation	P53 suppressor gene mutations
Viral antigens	Epstein–Barr virus nuclear antigens

CALLA, common acute lymphoblastic leukaemia antigen; CEA, carcinoembryonic antigen; CGL, chronic granulocytic leukaemia; HPV, human papilloma virus; PEM, polymorphic epithelial mucin.

of tumour cells. Because metastasis is so important, much effort has been devoted to attempting to understand molecules involved in cell adhesion and migration. Cellular adhesion molecules belong to several families of surface molecules. Prominent among these are the immunoglobulin superfamily, the integrins, cadherins, and the cartilage link protein family. While it is possible to alter expression of such molecules in experimental tumours by gene transfection, it is more difficult in man to obtain direct evidence for their role in the behaviour of tumours. Nevertheless, strong correlations can be obtained by studying the expression of particular molecules in tumours at different stages, known to be predictive of prognosis.

Melanoma provides a favourable model because the depth of cutaneous melanomas is highly predictive of the likelihood of metastasis. In one study there was a strong association between the depth of lesions and the expression of intercellular adhesion molecule-1 (ICAM-1, a member of the immunoglobulin superfamily), implying that this may play some role in escape of tumour cells from the primary site. At present the mechanisms remain open to speculation. Intercellular adhesion molecule-1 expression is correlated with the presence of leucocytes in lesions, and not only do these produce cytokines (interferons), which can upregulate intercellular adhesion molecule-1, but they also express its counter-receptor, the leucocyte function antigen (LFA-1), one of the integrins. It has been suggested that interaction between intercellular adhesion molecule-1 on melanoma cells and leucocyte function antigen on leucocytes may allow the tumour cells to 'hitch a ride' out of the epithelium and into lymphatics. Intercellular adhesion molecule-1 also shows sequence homology with known complement binding proteins so that increased expression may also provide protection against immune attack by antibody.

Another widely distributed and heavily glycosylated adhesion molecule, CD44, belonging to the cartilage link protein family, may play an important role in the metastatic process. CD44 is a receptor for hyaluronate, a major component of extracellular matrix, but almost certainly interacts also with other ligands, some of which may be cell bound. Comparison of CD44 expression on metastatic and non-metastatic variants of a rat model tumour, showed that there was a difference in CD44 molecular weight, although the amount of CD44 at the cell surface was the same. Molecular analysis showed that CD44 undergoes alternative splicing and in the metastatic tumour a short extra sequence is inserted into the molecule. How this affects tumour behaviour is not yet clear, but it seems likely that adhesion of the tumour cells must be altered. Molecular analysis of mouse and human CD44 shows that similar alternative splicing occurs, but as yet there is little information on the distribution of different isoforms in spontaneous tumours. Interestingly, other adhesion molecules exhibit alternative splicing, the neural and vascular cell adhesion molecules (NCAM and VCAM), for example, so that this appears to a common mechanism for subtle regulation of the adhesive and migratory properties of cells. Gene mutations that affect the expression of adhesion molecules in tumours are likely to have a profound affect on tumour progression and metastasis.

In contrast to these molecules, which are normal in structure although they may be expressed aberrantly, others may show structural alterations due to well understood genetic events, the *bcr–abl* fusion protein of chronic granulocytic leukaemia, for example. Other changes are less well understood but nevertheless well documented. One example is the change in glycosylation that occurs in many tumour cells, giving rise to sugars that are shorter than normal and often lacking terminal sialic acid (Fig. 5). These changes are quantitative not qualitative, but nevertheless truncated carbohydrate antigens may provide targets for therapy. Another consequence of altered glycosylation is that new protein epitopes may be revealed. This is well recognized in the breast tumour associated polymorphic epithelial mucin. Much of the extracellular domain consists of a 20-amino-acid repeat sequence containing several O-glycosylation sites. In the tumour-associated form of the molecule, an epitope identified by a monoclonal antibody is revealed in the repeat structure, which is hardly detectable in the molecule in normal breast

Fig. 4 Members of three of the major adhesion molecule families are shown. ○, N-linked carbohydrate; ⬭ O-linked carbohydrate; —, glycose amino glycan; s s, the presence of disulphide bonds; CEA, phosphoinositol linkage while the integrins and CD44 are transmembrane glycoproteins.

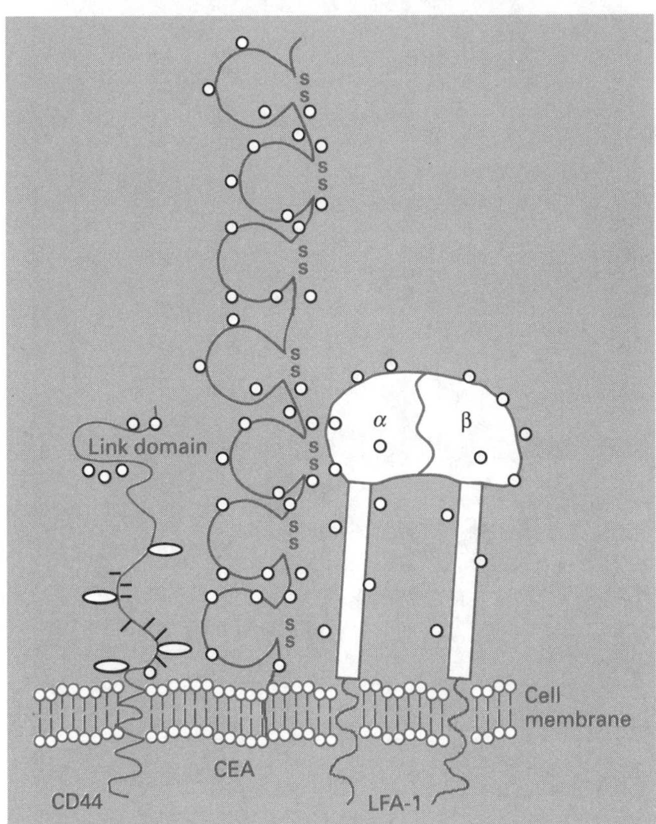

Fig. 5 The figure shows typical branched chain O-linked carbohydrate of normal, and the shorter and less branched chains, of tumour-associated mucin. As well as new carbohydrate epitopes, the alteration in carbohydrates reveals new peptide epitopes of the mucin core protein.

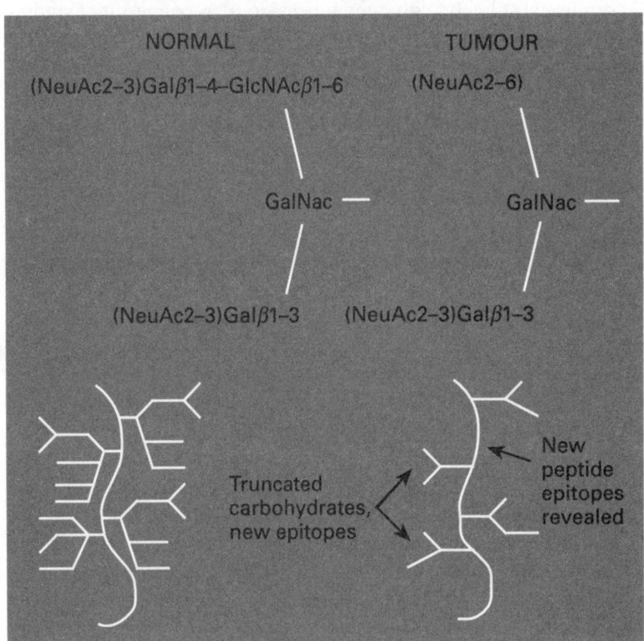

Table 8 *Antibodies for tumour typing*

Antibody specificity	Tissue recognized	Tumour example
Vimentin	Connective tissue	Sarcoma
Cytokeratins	Epithelia	Carcinoma
Epithelial membrane antigen	Epithelia	Carcinoma
Neurofilaments	Nervous tissue	Neuroblastoma
Desmin	Muscle	Myosarcoma
Glial fibrillary acidic protein	Glia	Glioma
Leucocyte common antigen (CD45)	Leucocytes	Lymphoma
S100	Nervous tissue	Melanoma
Placental alkaline phosphatase	Germ cells	Teratoma, choriocarcinoma

epithelial cells. Again the neoepitope is a potential target for immunotherapy.

The potential for immunodiagnosis and immunotherapy

ANTIBODIES *IN VITRO*

Monoclonal antibodies have already found a place in the diagnosis of malignant disease (summarized in Table 8) although they seldom play much role in determining whether a cell is malignant. So far, perhaps the most exploited use is that of cell identification. Monoclonal antibodies readily allow identification of single gene products in sections or smears, and this is often a simple way of assigning a cytologically undifferentiated cell to a cell lineage. Thus a relatively small panel of monoclonal antibody (Table 8) allows the identification of most tumours, which might otherwise cause diagnostic confusion. An extension of this is the detection of rare malignant cells. Thus monoclonal antibodies to epithelial cells (anticytokeratins or mucins) have been used to identify micrometastases in lymph nodes or bone marrow that are below the limit of detection by conventional histology or cytology, indicating that the presence of micrometastases at the time of diagnosis is much more common for many carcinomas than had been appreciated before.

Monoclonal antibodies may also be used to provide prognostic information. Estimation of the proportion of cells expressing molecules associated with progression through cell cycle such as the transferrin receptor or nuclear cyclins does correlate to some degree with the malignancy of tumours. However, it is unlikely that expression of any single marker will correlate absolutely with tumour behaviour, as one result of studies with monoclonal antibodies is to reinforce the view that tumours are very heterogeneous. Nevertheless, it is possible that, as understanding of the function of gene products expressed in tumour cells improves, studies of tumours with carefully designed panels of monoclonal antibodies will provide increasingly useful prognostic information.

ANTIBODIES *IN VIVO*

Few antibodies identify molecules that are truly tumour specific, but this is not essential for *in vivo* use. What is needed for diagnostic and therapeutic use is to obtain a useful 'signal-to-noise' ratio. The first requirement is to achieve penetration of the monoclonal antibody into tumour, which depends on the size of the molecule, its half-life in the serum, the vascularity of the tumour, and the abundance and availability of the antigen. The second problem is that heterologous antibody is immunogenic, as are most of the larger molecules, which are commonly attached to it, such as plant toxins. Both of these problems have been addressed by immunochemical or molecular engineering methods. Thus it is possible to produce a variety of sizes of antibody fragments and to replace most of a rodent immunoglobulin by human sequences (Fig. 6). This will reduce greatly the immunogenicity of the antibody (although the idiotypic epitopes associated with the antibody binding site may remain immunogenic) but will not affect the ability of attached toxins to generate an antibody response. Strategies designed to circumvent this problem include further engineering of toxin moieties to render them less immunogenic, induction of tolerance to immunogenic molecules, and the use of a succession of different antibody–toxin or drug conjugates. None of these strategies has been explored fully. It should also be noted that the anti-idiotype response to an antitumour monoclonal antibody can generate a further anti-idiotypic response (Ab3), which may react with the original tumour antigen. The presence of Ab3 has been associated with a favourable outcome in some studies.

Present experience in man with antibodies for diagnosis suggests that their sensitivity is of the same order as that of computer assisted tomography. However, optimization of antibody and radioisotope selection

Fig. 6 The figure illustrates several of the possibilities for engineering mouse and human antibodies. Fab, antibody binding fragment; Fv, variable fragment; scFv, single chain variable fragment; dAb, domain antibody; mru, minimal residual unit.

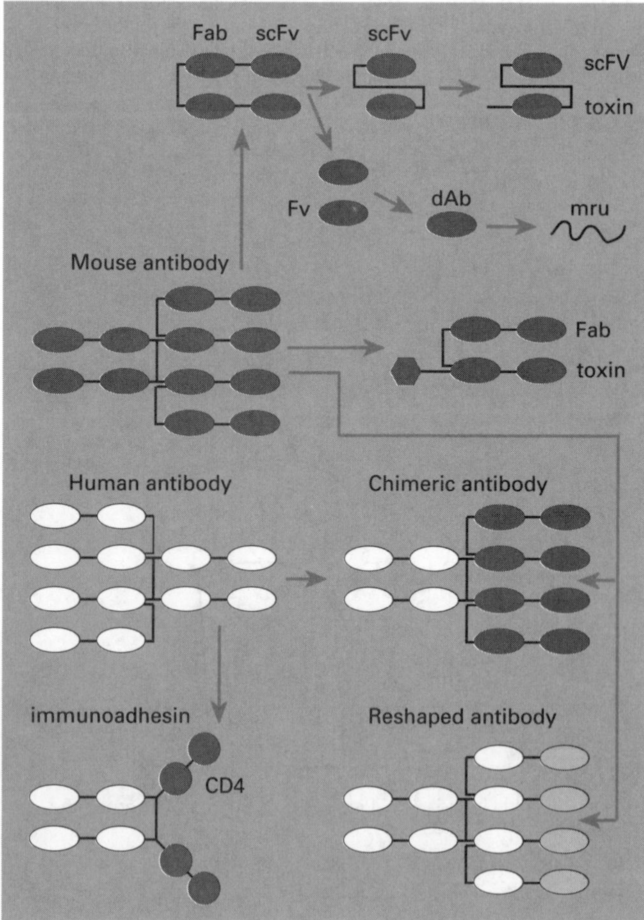

and coupling procedures will undoubtedly yield improvements. For therapy, the problem of penetration into large tumour masses may dictate that antibodies are most useful in an adjuvant setting. Results of a randomized trial of antibody given at the time of surgery to colon cancer patients are encouraging. Here the target is micrometastases, which would be expected to be relatively easily reached by serum antibody, and indeed it could readily be demonstrated that antibody had bound *in vivo* to tumour cells in the bone marrow.

One possible avenue of progress with the problem of antibody penetration is to target, not the tumour itself, but tumour vasculature. Endothelial cells respond to their microenvironment by changes in surface phenotype and the vessels of tumours may therefore express molecules, which could be targeted. Initial animal experiments are encouraging. So also is the successful treatment of melanoma by limb perfusion with very high dose tumour necrosis factor (TNFα), to which the tumour vasculature appears to be susceptible while normal endothelium remains unscathed.

T CELL IMMUNOTHERAPY

For those tumours in which a virus is implicated (see Table 3), prophylactic vaccination would be the most obvious long-term solution. For other common cancers where there is no obvious viral target, T-cell-based therapy, if it has a role, will have to be directed at established tumours.

As discussed earlier, there is now good evidence for a specific T-cell response to at least some human tumours. In principle, an altered or even a normal but overexpressed gene product may be recognized as a tumour antigen. It seems likely that most tumours will accumulate several possible tumour antigens during their evolution, although not all will be immunogenic in a particular individual because of the necessity for peptides of the tumour antigen to bind to self-human leucocyte antigen (HLA) molecules (genetic restriction). Although cataloguing the target epitopes present in tumours is a major task it is certainly now possible, and methodology will continue to improve. Given this information how can it be exploited?

One possibility will be to attempt active immunization against the antigens identified. This is not a trivial task, as cytotoxic T-cell epitopes need to be introduced into the endogenous pathway of antigen processing. This can be done with recombinant viruses, peptides with lipid tails, or cells of appropriate human leucocyte antigen type expressing the antigen. Initial experiments are under way using the MZ2E antigen of melanoma but, if this strategy is to be effective, several distinct epitopes must be targeted to minimize the possibility of tumour escape. New adjuvant procedures, including the insertion of cytokine or accessory molecule genes into immunizing cells, may greatly increase the effectiveness of active immunization.

An alternative may be to develop passive immunization. T-cell lines can be grown to very large numbers *in vitro* and at least in animal models tumour specific cells can be effective, especially when given with recombinant interleukin-2 (IL-2). Definition of tumour antigens will make it easier to isolate tumour specific clones and grow the large numbers of cells required for this strategy. One potential advantage is that the cells grown *in vitro* can be used to carry damaging molecules to the tumour. Initial experiments using marker genes have shown some localization of *in vitro* expanded tumour infiltrating lymphocytes (TILs). A disadvantage is that this method will always be labour intensive and will have to be carried out individually for each patient.

CYTOKINE THERAPY

Once cytokines became available, after their genes had been cloned and expressed, many clinical studies were carried out. So far the results have not been dramatic, although high dose interleukin-2, with or without lymphokine activated killer (LAK) cells, appears to cause some remissions of renal carcinoma, but not without considerable toxicity. In retrospect, it is not surprising that the effects of high dose cytokine therapy have been less than dramatic. Few cytokines are directly cytotoxic to tumour cells, although they may be cytostatic, and their effects are often transient because of receptor downregulation. In addition, the indirect *in vivo* effects of high doses of cytokines are little understood. Much more work on the biology of cytokines is needed to be able to use them for tumour therapy in a rational fashion although preliminary studies suggest that low dose locoregional therapy may have some effect.

Of course, cytokines have found other applications in cancer therapy, as colony stimulating factors can shorten significantly the period of aplasia following bone marrow transplantation. Another possibility is to use cytokines as vehicles for targeting. A recombinant interleukin 2–diphtheria toxin molecule has been engineered and shows some promise as an immunosuppressive agent. In principle, such a recombinant molecule can be used to target interleukin-2 receptor-bearing tumours, such as those caused by human T-cell lymphoma 1 (HTLV-1).

CONCLUSIONS

In non-malignant disease, immunological manoeuvres have been most effective when applied prophylactically. It is not to be expected, therefore, that immunotherapy of established tumours will be easy. Antibody-based therapy shows some promise and genetic engineering is capable of ameliorating the problem of immunogenicity, but in the near future antibodies are most likely to be useful in an adjuvant setting. The future of T-cell-based therapy is less clear. Although active immunization against tumour antigens will soon become possible, its effectiveness will depend on the frequency of responding T cells and how quickly tumour escape mutants develop. More sophisticated forms of gene therapy for tumours all ultimately depend on targeting tumour cells. As yet it is clear that there remains a great deal to learn before this will become a matter of routine.

REFERENCES

Adair, J.R. (1992). Engineering antibodies for therapy. *Immunological Reviews*, **130**, 5–39.

Browning, M.J. and Bodmer, W.F. (1992). MHC antigens and cancer: implications for T-cell surveillance. *Current Opinion in Immunology*, **4**, 613–18.

Kinlen, L. (1982). Immunosuppressive therapy and cancer. *Cancer Surveys*, **1**, 565–83.

Kinlen, L. (1992). Immunosuppressive therapy and acquired immunological disorders. *Cancer Research* (supplement), **52**, 5474s–6s.

Riethmuller, G. and Johnson, J.P. (1992). Monoclonal antibodies in the detection and therapy of micrometastatic epithelial cancers. *Current Opinion in Immunology*, **4**, 647–55.

Urban, J.L. and Schreiber, H. (1992). Tumour antigens. *Annual Reviews of Immunology*, **10**, 617–44.

van der Bruggen, P. and van den Eynde, B. (1992). Molecular definition of tumour antigens recognised by T lymphocytes. *Current Opinion in Immunology*, **4**, 608–12.

6.5 Medical imaging in oncology

S. J. GOLDING

INTRODUCTION

Radiology and other forms of medical imaging are fundamental to the diagnosis of tumours, being in most cases the primary method of disease detection and localization. The final element of diagnosis, characterization, is less well achieved by imaging, being more the province of the histologist and biochemist (Fig. 1).

The diagnostic role of imaging will be found throughout this book. It is not considered here because the oncologist's work begins after diagnosis has been made. Instead, the oncologist is concerned with establishing the extent of disease in order to define treatment (i.e. staging), and with monitoring response to treatment and detecting recurrence. A further diagnostic role for radiology does, however, exist when intercurrent conditions complicate treatment.

The golden rule of investigational medicine is that patients are examined only when the results will influence clinical management. This is particularly true in oncology, where clinical and psychological pressures are significant and where the temptation to overinvestigate is understandable but unjustified.

This is one of the fastest growing areas of medicine; new treatments are continually becoming available and the technology of imaging changes progressively to meet new clinical needs.

Disease staging—the basis of treatment

The prospect of effective tumour control depends heavily on the extent at presentation, which therefore defines the appropriate treatment. The following rules apply:

- Staging intervenes between diagnosis and treatment and therefore should be as quick as possible. Tumours grow exponentially; there is no case for wasting time.

Fig. 1 CT scan of the upper abdomen demonstrating disease localization but poor characterization. The patient presented with upper abdominal pain; CT showed a mass (M) expanding the pancreas, and low-attenuation lesions in the liver (arrows), consistent with pancreatic carcinoma metastasizing to liver. However, percutaneous biopsy of the liver revealed disseminated malignant melanoma.

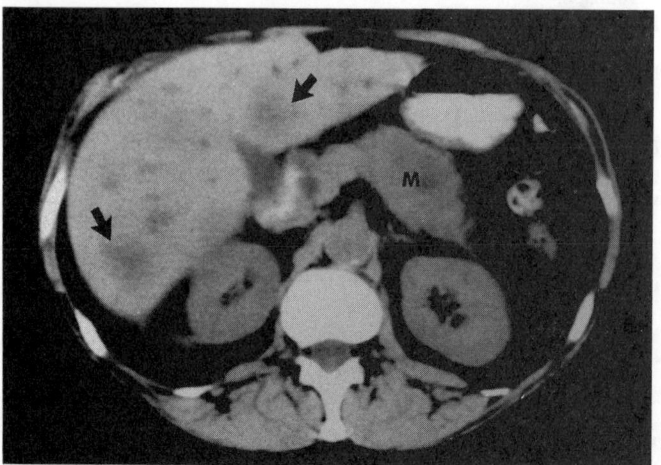

Fig. 2 Chest radiograph showing right upper-zone consolidation due to carcinoma of the bronchus. There is erosion of the ribs posteriorly (arrow), indicating that disease is unresectable.

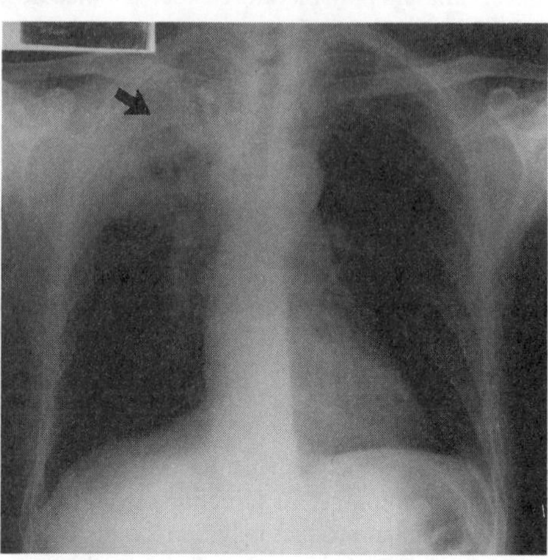

Fig. 3 The use of ultrasound to detect and stage carcinoma of the kidney. (a) A longitudinal section of the right kidney shows expansion of the lower pole by a mass (M) of altered echogenicity. (b) A transverse section through the upper abdomen shows that the inferior vena cava (arrow) is expanded by tumour thrombus. (Reproduced by courtesy of Dr D.R. Lindsell.)

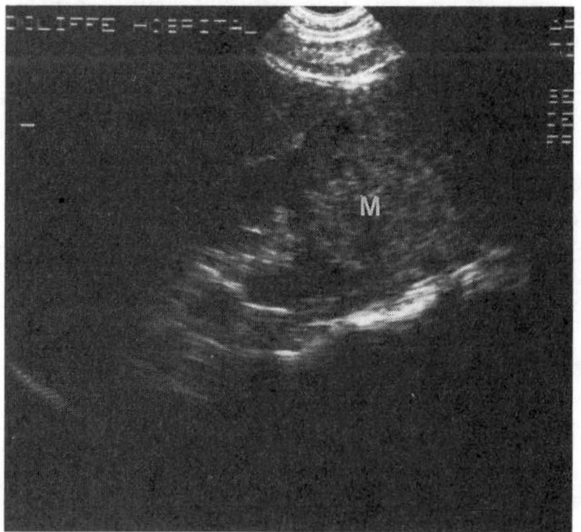

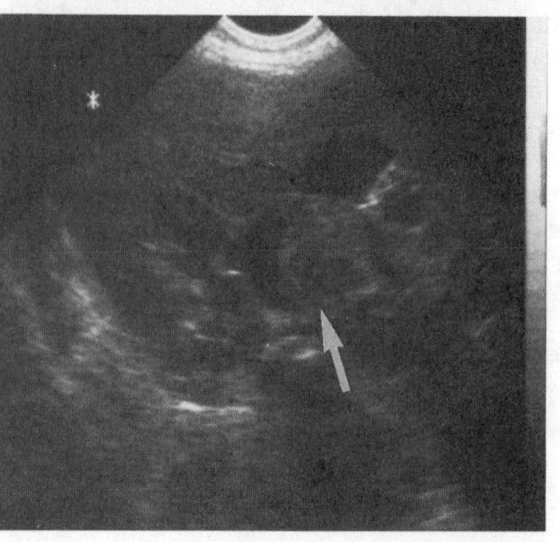

- Staging investigations are pointless if no treatment is appropriate; especially important in the patient presenting with disseminated disease (see below).
- The philosophy of staging differs from that of diagnosis in that the conventional diagnostic 'work-up', from simple, non-invasive, inexpensive tests does not apply. Instead, an imaging protocol is defined that excludes disease spread to the probable sites as far as is possible with current technology.
- Staging protocols are therefore tumour-specific. There is no point in starting a series of staging investigations until a histological diagnosis has been made.

STAGING SCHEMES

Many clinical staging schemes have been devised for individual tumours but the most accepted and applicable to imaging is the TNM system, where:

- T represents the extent of the primary tumour;
- N represents the extent of lymph node involvement;
- M represents the degree of distant metastasis.

Schemes are specific to each neoplasm and full details are given in the UICC *TNM Atlas* (Spiessel *et al.*, see References).

The aim of staging is to exclude spread of disease so that radical treatment can be given. The clinician therefore asks, 'How can I assess all the likely sites of spread accurately and as quickly as possible?' It is impractical to screen all sites for each patient, so staging schemes are based on current knowledge of tumour behaviour.

Fig. 4 Skeletal scintigram showing multiple, asymmetrical areas of increased radionuclide uptake in keeping with skeletal metastases. (Reproduced by courtesy of Dr F.V. Gleeson.)

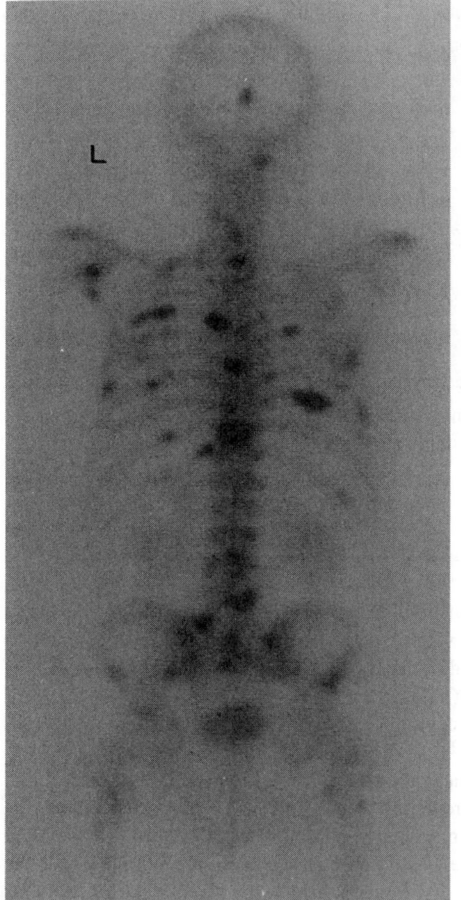

Although clinical examination is important and biochemical tests have a place, imaging is the mainstay of tumour staging and the full range of techniques is used, including conventional radiographs (Fig. 2), ultrasound (Fig. 3) and nuclear medicine, or scintigraphy (Fig. 4). However, the two techniques that have made the most impact are computerized tomography (**CT**) and magnetic resonance imaging (**MRI**). CT (Fig. 5) offers clear, cross-sectional images that are excellent maps of tissues and therefore valuable in assessing the extent of primary tumours. CT is not impeded by bone or by gas in lungs or bowel, which gives it an advantage over ultrasound. MRI, like CT, is a sectional imaging technique but has the additional advantage of multiplanar display and a contrast discrimination between soft tissues that is unrivalled by any other imaging technique (Fig. 6).

As no single imaging technique can be expected to be the most accurate investigation for each site of possible tumour spread, imaging protocols have been defined to evaluate these in the smallest number of steps (Table 1). For convenience the rest of this chapter describes the use of imaging in the order of TNM stages but in practice many staging protocols begin by excluding distant metastasis by simple tests, there

Fig. 5 CT scan in a patient with carcinoma of the bronchus, for disease staging. Contrast-medium enhancement has been used to distinguish the blood vessels from a mass (M) at the right hilum, which extends into the subcarinal area (arrow).

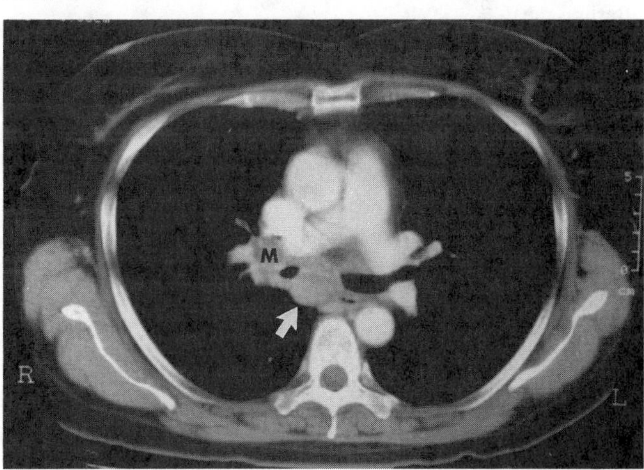

Fig. 6 MRI section of the pelvis in a patient with carcinoma of the cervix. A mass within the cervix is identified as an area of high signal intensity. The normal, dark fibrous stroma of the cervix (arrow) is eroded posteriorly but the outline of the cervix is intact (FIGO stage Ib). This is the most accurate form of disease staging currently available.

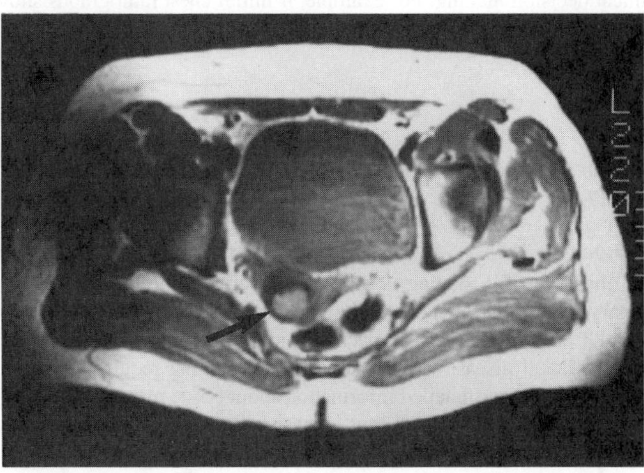

Table 1 *Recommended staging schemes for some common neoplasms*

Carcinoma of the larynx and pharynx
Chest radiograph
MRI (primary and regional nodes)
(or CT if MRI unavailable)

Carcinoma of the thyroid
Chest radiograph
Skeletal scintigram
Thyroid scintigram (if tumour accumulates nuclide)
If T staging required, ultrasound
(or CT if very extensive clinically)

Carcinoma of the bronchus
Chest radiograph
Skeletal scintigram
CT (primary, mediastinal nodes, adrenal glands)
MRI only if CT equivocal, or resection of central tumour considered

Carcinoma of the oesophagus
Chest radiograph
Barium swallow
CT (primary, liver, coeliac nodes)
(MRI may replace CT if available)

Carcinoma of the stomach
Chest radiograph
Barium meal
CT (primary, liver and coeliac nodes)
(MRI of liver for greatest accuracy, e.g. when considering radical gastrectomy)

Carcinoma of the pancreas
Chest radiograph
CT (primary, liver and coeliac nodes)

Carcinoma of the kidney
Chest radiograph
Ultrasound (primary, nodes and draining veins)
(or MRI if ultrasound findings indefinite)
Skeletal scintigram
(Some clinicians also require CT of the chest)

Carcinoma of the bladder
Chest radiograph
Excretory urogram
Skeletal scintigram
CT (primary, pelvic and abdominal nodes)
(lymphography is sometimes used for additional nodal investigation)

Carcinoma of the rectum
Chest radiograph
Barium enema
CT (primary, pelvic and abdominal nodes, and liver)
(MRI may be used for more accurate liver evaluation)

Carcinoma of the ovary
This neoplasm is usually staged by laparotomy. A chest radiograph should be obtained before surgery
Further imaging is required to provide a baseline for adjuvant treatment; CT (pelvis, abdominopelvic nodes, and liver) is most commonly used

Carcinoma of the cervix and uterine corpus
Chest radiograph
MRI (primary, pelvic nodes)
(CT may replace MRI if primary is advanced clinically or extensive abdominal lymphadenopathy suspected)
(Lymphography sometimes performed for further nodal evaluation)

Carcinoma of the prostate
Chest radiograph
Skeletal scintigram
EITHER: transrectal ultrasound (primary)
plus CT (pelvic nodes)
OR: MRI (primary and nodes)
(CT or MRI should include the abdomen if pelvic nodes abnormal)

Testicular tumours
BEFORE RESECTION: chest radiograph
ultrasound (primary)
AFTER RESECTION: CT (lungs, thoracoabdominal nodes)

Lymphomas
Chest radiograph
CT (region of primary, mediastinal and abdominopelvic nodes)
Investigation of specific organs by appropriate technique required if visceral involvement

Sarcoma of bone
Chest radiograph
Skeletal scintigram
MRI (primary)
CT (lungs)

Sarcoma of soft tissues
Chest radiograph
MRI (primary)
(include regional nodes if synovial, neural, or myogenic cell type)
CT (lungs)

Note that not all investigations should be obtained in each case; each scheme should proceed until sufficient information has been obtained for clinical decision making. For example, if initial chest radiographs show pulmonary metastases, T staging will not be required in most patients.

Non-imaging procedures such as biochemical assay are not included in this Table.

being no point in undertaking detailed T staging if disease is disseminated (Table 1).

T staging

The objective of T staging is to define accurately the margins of the primary tumour. No imaging technique can detect microscopic disease and all T staging is based on macroscopic findings only.

Unless local disease is very advanced, T staging requires imaging techniques that give detailed information about tissue planes. For example, in carcinoma of the bronchus a chest radiograph may be all that is needed if tumour has eroded the ribs (Fig. 2), but only CT or MRI can reveal lesser degrees of involvement of the chest wall or mediastinum (Fig. 5). In practice, T staging depends largely on CT or MRI, and to a lesser extent ultrasound in the abdomen and pelvis (Fig. 3). The ease of distinguishing between soft tissues on MRI means that where it is available it becomes the T-staging technique of choice in most tumour types (Figs 6 and 7).

In many tumours, radical surgery is the treatment of choice and T staging is a basis for predicting resectability. This requires accurate display of all the tumour margins, in particular the relation to surrounding structures. An accurate prediction can be made in most cases but the radiologist must not discourage surgery on equivocal or dubious grounds. In practice, therefore, the radiologist reports either that there are no signs to preclude an attempt at resection, or that definite findings indicate that surgical intervention would be pointless.

The demonstration of obviously inoperable disease, while usually of grave prognostic significance to the patient, spares them a pointless invasive procedure, and spares the hospital a waste of resources; this is the most significant economic benefit of modern tumour staging.

Where radiotherapy is the treatment of choice, T staging is less stringent, needing to document only the margins of the tumour so that treatment portals can be defined. CT also provides a basis for computerized treatment planning (RT plan); this is more accurate than the traditional method based on clinical examination and radiographs alone.

N staging

Large lymph-node masses may be detectable clinically or on simple investigations such as chest radiographs but only lymphography (Fig. 8(a)), ultrasound, CT, and MRI can detect smaller degrees of regional lymph-node involvement. Ultrasound is used the least because, although it can certainly detect lymphadenopathy in the abdomen and pelvis, accurate staging depends on the confident exclusion of lymphadenopathy; in many patients interference from bowel gas makes it difficult to examine all abdominopelvic nodal sites with ultrasound.

There are important differences between lymphography and the sectional techniques. CT and MRI display all node sites whereas lymphography is limited to iliac and abdominal para-aortic groups (Fig 8(a)). On CT and MRI (Figs 8(b) and 9) nodal enlargement is the only criterion of abnormality; metastases cannot be excluded in nodes of normal size. Lymphography opacifies the nodal parenchyma and may detect intranodal metastases but unlike CT and MRI is invasive. It is usual, therefore, to examine first with CT or MRI, reserving lymphography for abdominopelvic disease where no nodal enlargement has been shown.

Because of their ease of detecting lymph node enlargement, CT and MRI have become the techniques of choice in assessing the extent of primary nodal neoplasia such as lymphoma (Fig. 10).

Reactive hyperplasia of nodes can produce false-positive findings with all three sectional techniques, especially when inflammation accompanies the primary tumour.

M staging

In practice, M staging often precedes T staging (Table 1), as finding distant metastasis obviates evaluation of the primary tumour. It is also conventional practice to start M staging with simple tests; if a chest radiograph shows multiple pulmonary or osseous metastases, further investigation is pointless.

All patients with known or suspected neoplasia must undergo chest radiography, even if metastasis from the site in question is known to be unlikely. If this simple test shows disseminated disease, the patient falls into a different management category (see below). Moreover, metastases from carcinoma of the bronchus may mimic many other primary neoplasms.

The technique of choice for detecting pulmonary metastases in patients with normal chest radiographs is CT. This is capable of showing pulmonary metastases greater than 2 mm in diameter (Fig. 11).

Skeletal radiographs are very insensitive to the presence of metastases and should not be used to screen patients. Skeletal scintigraphy is the method of choice (Fig. 4). Although increased uptake of radionuclide is a non-specific sign, multifocal, asymmetrical abnormalities in a patient

Fig. 7 MRI section of the pelvis in a patient with Ewing's sarcoma of the left ilium. The ilium is expanded by tumour and there is considerable extraosseous infiltration. The sequence used to create this image readily distinguishes the tumour from the surrounding muscles.

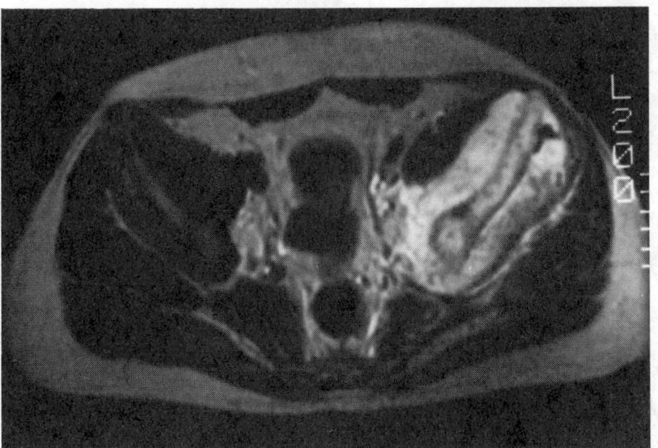

Fig. 8 (a) Bipedal lymphogram in a patient with carcinoma of the cervix. Both common iliac and para-aortic node groups have been opacified. There is an enlarged node in the left common iliac group, showing a central filling defect due to a metastasis (arrow). (b) MRI section in the same patient shows the mildly enlarged node (arrow) lying between the femoral artery and vein. Compare with the contralateral vessels.

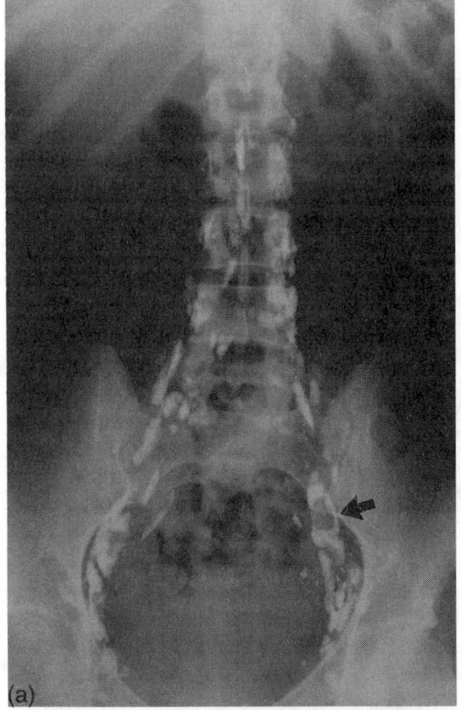

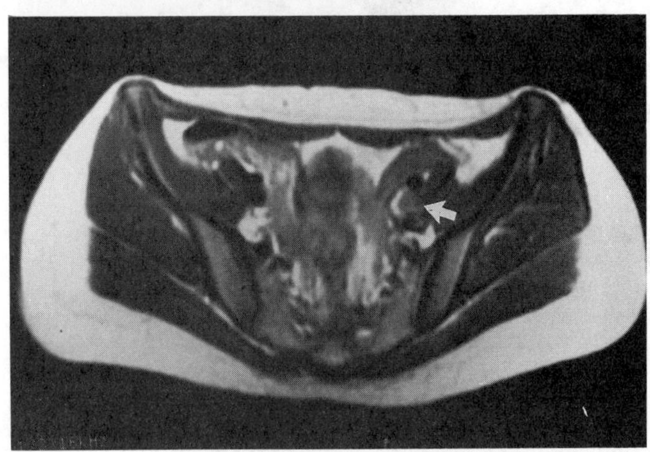

Fig. 9 CT scan of the chest in a patient with carcinoma of the bronchus (note the mass in the right upper lobe). The section shows lymphadenopathy in the pretracheal group of nodes (arrow). This was not shown on the chest radiograph as it is contained within the mediastinal silhouette.

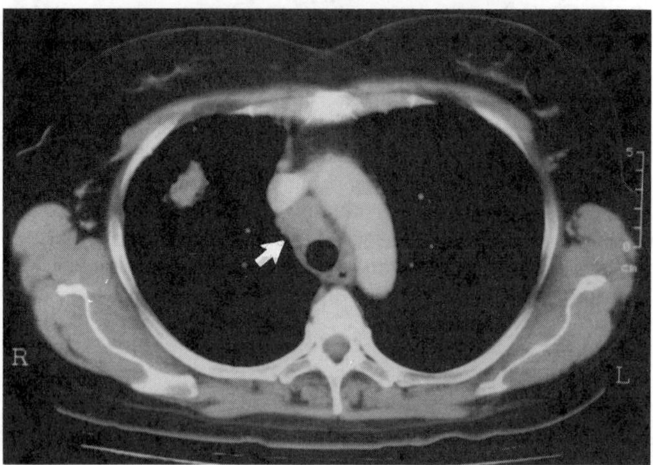

Fig. 10 CT scan of the abdomen in a patient with non-Hodgkin's lymphoma. The image shows numerous enlarged lymph nodes (arrows) surrounding the abdominal aorta. There is also enlargement of the spleen (S).

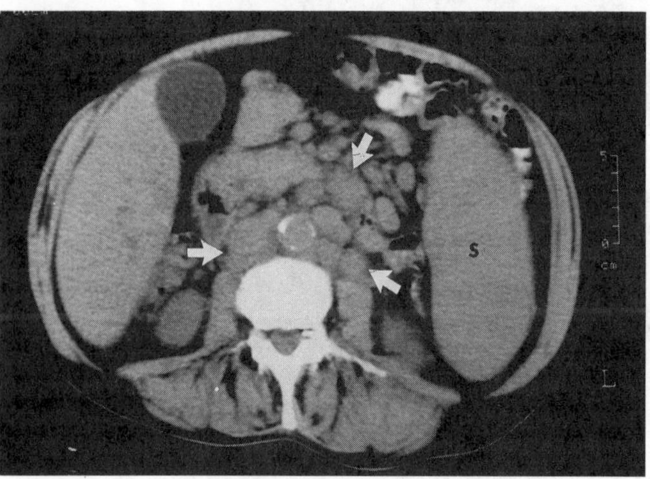

Fig. 11 CT scan showing pulmonary metastases. This enlarged view of the left lung field shows multiple nodules (arrows) lying between the pulmonary vessels. The smallest of these is approximately 2 mm in diameter.

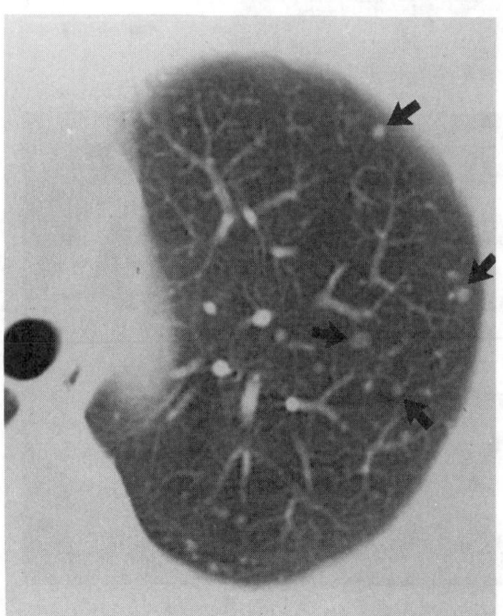

with known neoplasia are virtually pathognomonic of metastases. Solitary areas of increased activity may be due to benign or malignant disease and CT or MRI are used to distinguish these, and also to elucidate equivocal scintigraphic findings (Fig. 12). MRI has proved particularly valuable as a confirmatory test, as it is the only technique that reliably displays abnormal tissues in bone marrow (Fig. 13). This facility, and the multiplanar display and non-invasive nature of MRI, have made this technique the investigation of choice in suspected spinal-cord compression due to spinal metastases (Fig. 14).

Techniques of choice for other sites of distant spread are shown in Table 2. These recommendations are included in the protocols suggested in Table 1.

Fig. 12 The value of MRI in confirming skeletal metastases in a patient with carcinoma of the breast. (a) Skeletal scintigram showing poorly defined areas of increased activity in the thoracic spine. The lumbar region shows some increase in uptake but is not definitely abnormal. (b) MRI section of the thoracolumbar spine showing definite multifocal infiltration of the vertebral bone marrow. This provides unequivocal confirmation of metastatic spread and also a baseline for monitoring treatment.

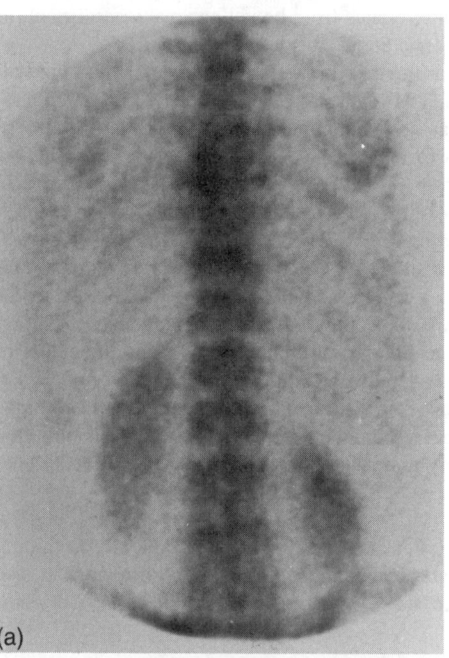

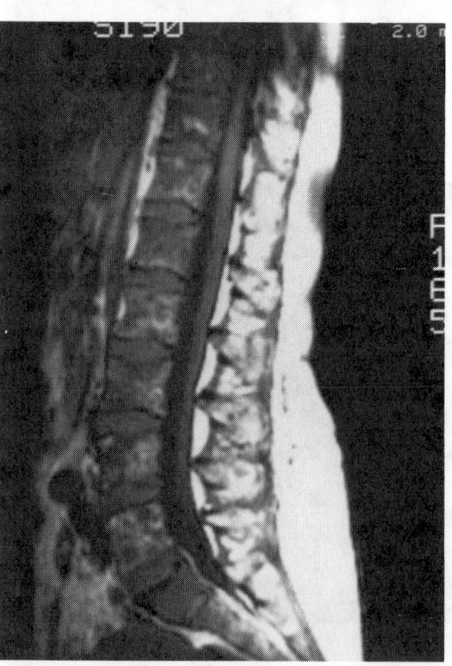

The patient presenting with disseminated disease

This is a different clinical situation. When disseminated malignancy presents as a diagnostic problem, for example as abdominal pain or jaundice due to hepatic metastases, or pathological fracture, there is no case for attempting to identify the primary site; any mass found elsewhere is just as likely to be another metastasis (Fig. 1). The likelihood of effective treatment being available to such patients depends almost entirely on the cell type. If no easily accessible site for percutaneous biopsy has been identified, it may be worth imaging further to see if a suitably sited lesion can be identified, before resorting to open biopsy. Otherwise, further imaging is a waste of time and resources.

Fig. 13 The value of MRI in detecting disease of bone marrow: an MRI section of the lumbar spine in this young man with low back pain shows abnormal signal from the L4 vertebral body (arrow), due to Hodgkin's lymphoma. Radiographs and CT scan of L4 were normal.

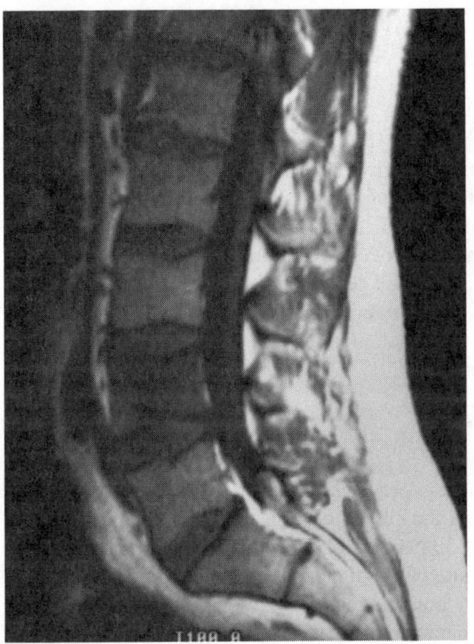

Fig. 14 MRI scan in a patient with carcinoma of the prostate, showing spinal-cord compression. The patient's symptoms and signs suggested lower thoracic-cord compression. MRI shows abnormal signal intensity in several vertebrae, with two definite points of compression (arrows). The sequence used to obtain this image readily distinguishes the spinal cord from cerebrospinal fluid.

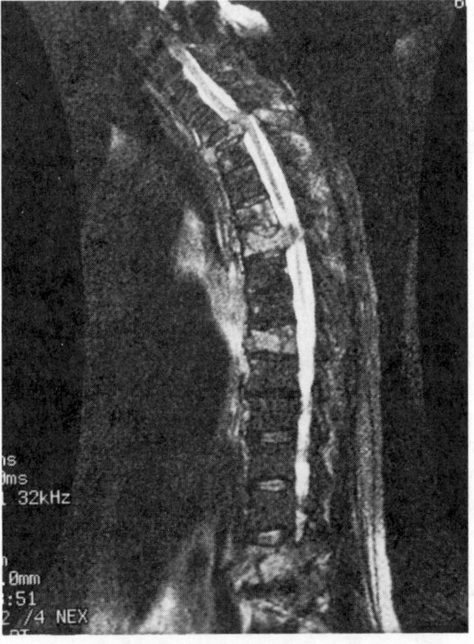

Table 2 *Recommended techniques for demonstrating distant metastases*

	Technique of choice	Alternative
Lung	CT (if chest radiograph normal)	None
Skeleton	Skeletal scintigraphy	MRI if local symptoms or signs
Liver	MRI	CT (technique-dependent; CT arterioportography the most accurate)
Brain	MRI	CT

Note that, although MRI is recommended for examination of some areas individually, when these form part of staging schemes covering a large area it may be more convenient, if using CT to stage the primary tumour, to extend the CT study to include the organ of distant metastasis also.

Monitoring response to treatment and detecting recurrence

In many patients, symptomatic response is the most important arbiter of successful treatment. Imaging is only required when a management change, for example use of a different therapeutic agent in the case of failed response, would follow investigation. In general, the most appropriate technique for monitoring is that used for initial staging.

Neoplasms in which effective therapy is available for recurrent disease may justify post-treatment screening. This is only practicable where the time of possible recurrence can be predicted from the natural history of the disease. The best current example is testicular teratoma, where frequent screening by CT for 2 years after initial treatment may identify recurrence at an early stage and with good prospect of cure. Patients with this disease who remain well at 2 years are very unlikely to relapse after this time.

MRI has proven value in distinguishing residual masses due to fibrosis from those due to active neoplasm, provided that the inflammatory response to necrosis during treatment has resolved. In practice this means that an accurate prediction can only be made several months after treatment; before that time, guided biopsy should be used in cases of doubt.

Diagnostic problems complicating treatment

Patients undergoing radiotherapy or chemotherapy are subject to a range of intercurrent diseases. These may be local, in the case of unavoidable damage to surrounding tissues from radiotherapy, or systemic, resulting from immunosuppression. Imaging plays an important part in the diagnosis of these conditions and often requires a radiologist with special expertise in this area. The field is too extensive to be described in detail here but an account will be found in the references.

REFERENCES

Baert, A., Felix, R., Musemeci, R., Semmler, W., and Sze, G. (1990). *Magnetic resonance in oncology.* Springer-Verlag, Berlin. An informative overview of the impact of MRI on oncology.

Glazer, G.M. (1986). *Staging of neoplasms.* Churchill Livingstone, New York. A useful monograph, largely concerned with CT.

Johnson, R., Eddleston, B., and Hunter, R.D. (1990). *Radiology in the management of cancer.* Churchill Livingstone, Edinburgh. The standard British textbook on oncological imaging, relating this well to clinical management.

Sobin, L.H., and Ros, P. (1990). Radiology and the new TNM classification of tumors: the future. *Radiology*, **176,** 1–4. The case for a standardized approach to staging.

Spiessel, B., Scheibe, O., and Wagner, G. (1990). *TNM atlas; illustrated guide to the classification of malignant tumours*. Springer-Verlag, Berlin. The oncological radiologist's vade-mecum.

Vanel, D. and Stark, D. (1993). *Imaging strategies in oncology*. Dunitz, London. A comprehensive and informative book with an international cast of authors.

Williams, C. (1983). *All about cancer: a practical guide to cancer care*. Wiley, Chichester. A useful paperback giving an overview of cancer medicine; includes some imaging advice but excludes modern techniques.

6.6 Cancer: clinical features and management

R. L. SOUHAMI

Introduction: cancer in general medical practice

Cancer is a common disease – the second largest cause of death after vascular disorders. Approximately 20 per cent of the population of the United Kingdom will die of cancer. It is a source of concern and perplexity to oncologists that so many of their patients are referred to them late in the disease. Often symptoms have been present for a long period of time, during which their significance has been overlooked, or when multiple (and sometimes futile) investigations have been performed with a failure to appreciate the need for speed in diagnosis and management. To this can be added a frequent lack of understanding on the part of the possibilities of treatment both by general practitioners and by specialists in hospital medicine, and a failure to inform patients either of the nature of the diagnosis or of its implications and possibilities for therapy.

The problem is that almost every specialist sees patients with cancer affecting their particular field; unfortunately, these specialists may not have been taught the principles of cancer medicine as part of their speciality training. Oncologists therefore frequently see patients with advanced disease, who have not had a proper explanation of their illness, and who have little idea of what treatment might involve. The size of the problem may be illustrated by the fact that 60 per cent of all patients dying with lung cancer in the United Kingdom have never seen a specialist in cancer medicine at any stage in their illness. While it is possible that some of them had disease so far advanced that nothing but palliative treatment was needed, it is also possible that some may have been denied the opportunity for treatment and some prolongation of life. The principles of cancer management are therefore of great importance for every physician.

Management of patients would be improved greatly if the following simple rules were adhered to:

1. Cancer should be suspected with any unexplained illness, especially in the elderly.
2. Imaging with isotopic and computer tomography (CT) and magnetic resonance (MR) scanning (see Chapter 6.5), will often speed the process of diagnosis. However a tissue diagnosis cannot be made by these means and every attempt should be made to make a histological or cytological diagnosis as quickly as possible.
3. Once the diagnosis is obtained, for many tumours patients should start a planned programme of treatment within days and not weeks. Patients should not spend long periods waiting for results of investigations and for clinic appointments. The need for speed in diagnosis and treatment is tacitly recognized in specialist centres for breast cancer where patients can, in well-regulated clinics, reasonably expect to have a diagnosis made within a few days of first consultation and to begin definitive treatment within 2 weeks. This admirable efficiency should be the norm for all cancers.

Common symptoms and signs of cancer

Many of the symptoms and signs of cancer are due to the local effects of the tumour infiltrating surrounding tissues and causing pressure and distortion of neighbouring structures. In addition to these local site-specific symptoms, tumours produce symptoms that are, to some extent, common to all cancers. These are general symptoms due to the metabolic disturbances caused by the tumours and to specific symptoms related to hormonal effects and immunological effects of the tumour: so-called paraneoplastic syndromes.

PAIN

Most patients with cancer experience pain at some stage in their illness, either as a direct result of the tumour or of its treatment. Pain is a feature at presentation in about 30 per cent of cancer patients, but the incidence varies greatly with the site of the tumour. For example, over 90 per cent of patients with primary bone tumours or with metastases to bone have pain, and this has the characteristic feature of being worse at night time. In contrast, only 5 per cent of patients with leukaemia develop pain. Pain also varies according to the rate of progression of the disease and is more likely to occur with rapidly growing tumours. No symptom of cancer causes greater demoralization than unremitting pain. Any patient with unexplained, persistent pain should be suspected of having malignant disease and appropriate investigations performed. In pain clinics, 80 per cent of patients seen with cancer have pain due to direct tumour infiltration. If the pain is due to neurological infiltration it may be felt at the distribution of the nerve root. Certain pain syndromes are sufficiently common and misleading to warrant separate consideration.

Direct tumour infiltration of bone

The origin of the pain that occurs with tumour infiltration of bone is not fully understood. The periosteum is a pain-sensitive structure and may be the source in many patients. It is probable that osteolytic processes involving prostaglandins are also involved. Pain is a common feature of metastasis at the base of the skull. If the tumour is situated around the jugular foramen, pain is often referred to the vertex of the head and the ipsilateral shoulder and arm. Movement of the head may exacerbate the pain and, later, cranial nerve involvement may cause hoarseness, dysarthria, and dysphasia. Involvement of the 9th to the 12th cranial nerves, and the development of ptosis and Horner's syndrome indicates involvement of the sympathetic nervous system extracranially adjacent to the jugular foramen. When metastases occur in the sphenoid sinus, severe headache, usually felt in both temples or retro-orbitally, is a common feature. There may be a full sensation in the head, nasal stuffiness, and a 6th nerve palsy.

When metastases occur in vertebral bodies the pain frequently precedes neurological signs and symptoms. Persistent thoracic vertebral pain and a positive bone scan is an indication for urgent investigation and treatment. In small cell lung cancer, for example, a patient with thoracic vertebral pain and a positive bone scan has a 30 per cent chance of developing a paraplegia. Ninety per cent of patients who have epidural spinal cord compression have vertebral body metastasis as the source of the epidural tumour (the management of spinal compression is described later). With metastasis to the odontoid process, patients complain of severe neck pain and stiffness radiating over the skull, up to the vertex. This is then followed by progressive neurological signs, often associated with autonomic dysfunction. In the lower cervical vertebrae pain is felt as an aching sensation, often radiating over both shoulders. If nerve root compression occurs at this site, there will be pain in the root distribution felt in the back of the arm, the elbow and the ulnar aspect of the hand. The association with Horner's syndrome suggests involvement of the paravertebral sympathetic system. Lumbar metastases are associated with local pain, worse on lying or sitting and relieved by standing. In lesions in L1 the pain is often felt over the superior iliac crests. In the sacrum, pain may be accompanied by neurological signs with symptoms of bowel and bladder dysfunction and perianal sensory loss and impotence.

When tumours infiltrate peripheral nerves they are often accompanied by an alteration in sensation, with hyperaesthesia, dysaesthesia, and sensory loss. This is a particularly common presentation when tumours invade the paravertebral or retroperitoneal region. Here the pain is often in a root distribution and is unilateral. Another common site is when a metastasis in a rib entraps the intercostal nerves. When tumour infiltrates the brachial plexus the pain is felt in the C7 or T1 distribution. Pain in this site is particularly common with the Pancoast syndrome, where an apical lung cancer infiltrates the lower brachial plexus roots. Pain in the C5 distribution occurs with upper root infiltration.

Visceral pain is a frequent symptom of cancer; it can cause diagnostic confusion and be difficult to control when it is part of a previously diagnosed tumour. Poorly localized abdominal pain is a frequent feature of ovarian and pancreatic cancer and of peritoneal carcinomatosis. Retroperitoneal pain may be particularly difficult to diagnose. It may vary greatly in position (being relieved on leaning forwards) and be felt variably in the back. Left upper quadrant pain may be a presenting feature of carcinoma of the tail of the pancreas involving the mesentery of the splenic flexure of the colon.

WEIGHT LOSS

Weight loss is an invariable accompaniment of advanced cancer and a frequent presenting symptom. Often it results from the physical presence of the tumour interfering with gastrointestinal function, such as with carcinoma of the stomach, pancreas, or colon, or with peritoneal carcinomatosis. Mechanical obstruction of the bowel and loss of appetite are common accompaniments of these tumours. Loss of appetite is a frequent symptom of any cancer that has metastasized to the liver and usually appears at a point when metastasis is replacing much of the normal liver tissue. The mechanism is not known. Pancreatic cancers and cancers metastatic to the porta hepatis cause weight loss from a malabsorption syndrome due to obstructive jaundice or blockage of the pancreatic ducts.

Nevertheless, many tumours cause weight loss without direct involvement of digestive organs. It is well recognized that a weight loss of more than 5 per cent is a very adverse prognostic feature in almost all cancers. Usually it indicates that the disease is more widespread than is apparent on clinical investigation but the mechanisms of this symptom, which is often accompanied by alteration of taste, anorexia, and a general feeling of ill health, are obscure. Sometimes quite profound weight loss can accompany non-metastatic tumours, which are relatively small in size. As with advanced cancer, the cachexia syndrome is then accompanied by anorexia and change in taste. These tumours may produce circulating factors responsible for the weight loss and loss of appetite. Tumour necrosis factor (TNFα) and interleukin-1β have both been shown to produce cachexic syndromes experimentally. Tumour necrosis factor is identical to cachectin, previously described as a substance inducing weight loss in animals transplanted with human tumours.

Tumours may also themselves contribute to weight loss by alteration in protein and energy metabolism. Negative nitrogen balance has been frequently documented in patients with cancer, particularly when advanced. An increase in whole body glucose recycling via pyruvate and lactate has also been reported in cancer patients.

The loss of body weight is therefore due to an accumulation of events involving direct interference with digestive function, production of factors leading to weight loss and anorexia by the tumour, and possible alteration in protein and energy metabolism. Later in the course of the illness, antineoplastic treatment with chemotherapy, radiation, and surgery may exacerbate these problems.

TUMOUR MASS

It is astonishing how often patients report the appearance of a swelling only to have the significance of the finding overlooked by their doctors. The appearance of any mass should lead to prompt investigation. Although imaging techniques can sometimes distinguish benign from malignant swellings, a biopsy will usually be necessary and should be undertaken at once. Nowadays it is often unnecessary to undertake surgical excision biopsy. Indeed, doing so may sometimes make subsequent management almost impossible. Where there is doubt about the nature of a swelling the correct procedure will usually be to undertake needle biopsy. Biopsy is in general preferable to aspiration cytological diagnosis because the precise diagnosis of many cancers depends on architecture as well as on cytology. The great advantage of early biopsy diagnosis is that a planned approach to treatment can then be undertaken by oncologists, radiotherapists, and surgeons together. Injudicious, and often marginal, surgical excision may lead to a greatly increased risk of local recurrence of the tumour – a particularly frequent occurrence in sarcomas. Furthermore, for some tumours chemotherapy may be the first line of treatment and will allow assessment of response to drug treatment before surgery is undertaken and major response may modify the surgery.

FEVER

In cancer, fever is usually caused by infection. However, about 30 per cent of patients with cancer develop fever at some stage in their illness and it may be the presenting feature of some tumours, particularly lymphomas, renal carcinoma, and any cancer metastatic to the liver. The fever may be accompanied by sweating, particularly at night. The characteristic feature of the sweats that accompany malignant lymphomas and other cancers is that the patient falls asleep and wakes in the middle of the night to find themselves drenched with sweat. Rigors are very uncommon with febrile episodes in cancer, and should always lead to a suspicion that an infective complication is present. Characteristic patterns of fever are seldom observed; usually it is of a low grade remittent type. The Pel–Ebstein fever of Hodgkin's disease, in which febrile periods are interspersed with several days of normal temperature, is very uncommon.

The cause of the fever of malignant disease is unknown. Endogenous pyrogens are possibly liberated from cells of the mononuclear phagocyte series in the liver or bone marrow. Tumour cells have also been shown to produce 'pyrogens'. The nature of the cytokines responsible is not clear. Exogenously administered tumour necrosis factor and interleukin-2 both produce fever and may be produced in cancer patients.

The fever of malignant disease may respond to simple antipyretics such as aspirin or paracetamol. In malignant lymphoma it will disappear with successful treatment of the tumour. In advanced cancer most steroidal anti-inflammatory agents may also help, but corticosteroids are more effective, at least for a period of time.

ANAEMIA

The anaemia of malignant disease is multifactorial (see Section 22). Chronic blood loss may occur in cancer of the gastrointestinal tract, as a result of vaginal bleeding, or because of malabsorption of iron. Usually the anaemia is normochromic, or slightly hypochromic in nature, and the plasma transferrin and serum iron are low. The iron stores are not reduced as judged by stainable iron in the bone marrow. The mechanism is discussed in Section 22.

HYPERCALCAEMIA

Malignant disease is responsible for most of the very severe cases of hypercalcaemia seen in clinical practice. The patient will usually have widespread skeletal metastases but occasionally the syndrome is paraneoplastic (see below). Hypercalcaemic symptoms include anorexia, weight loss, and mental confusion, all of which may simulate metastatic disease. The symptoms and signs of hypercalcaemia and its management are discussed in Sections 12 and 22.

Paraneoplastic syndromes

Many patients with cancer have complications that are not due to direct invasion of adjacent tissues by the cancer or its metastases. The tumour produces hormones or cytokines, which are responsible for symptoms at a remote site. Alternatively, the tumour provokes an immune response to altered cellular constituents and the paraneoplastic syndrome arises from the resulting immunological reaction. Taken together, paraneoplastic syndromes are not rare. However, each syndrome only occurs in a minority of cancer patients. Furthermore although some syndromes, such as the production of parathyroid hormone-related peptide, are found in a wide variety of cancers, others, such as Cushing's syndrome, are found in a very restricted range of tumours and these are of neuroendocrine type.

It is important to be aware of paraneoplastic syndromes in cancer medicine because their appearance may be the first sign that malignant disease is present. Furthermore, they may lead the physician into believing that the patient has metastases and thus alter management inappropriately. The syndromes themselves may cause considerable disability, which is amenable to treatment. The wide variety of paraneoplastic syndromes means that only a brief description of these can be given in this chapter. A summary, in which some of these syndromes are divided according to their major clinical manifestation is shown in Table 1.

The range of paraneoplastic syndromes is very wide indeed. A simple generalization is that cancer can cause almost any clinical syndrome, however bizarre, and should, therefore, enter the list of differential diagnosis in any unusual clinical disorder. There are, however, dangers in the diagnosis of paraneoplastic syndromes. For example, most neurological problems in cancer are not due to paraneoplastic manifestations but to the direct physical presence of the tumour. This means that spinal cord signs in a patient with cancer are much more likely to be due to direct compression of the cord than due to transverse myelitis as a paraneoplastic syndrome. Prompt treatment of the space-occupying lesion is essential and a mistaken diagnosis of paraneoplasia is potentially disastrous. Similarly, endocrine syndromes from cancer are often caused by endocrine cancers themselves. These may be resectable. Anaemia or thrombosis may be paraneoplastic in origin but more frequently a deep venous thrombosis is due to a direct compressive affect of cancer in the pelvis and iron deficiency anaemia should always raise the possibility that occult bleeding is occurring. Unless obviously paraneoplastic in nature, symptoms from cancer should, in the first instance, be regarded as likely to be produced by a direct effect of the tumour since this distinction has important therapeutic consequences. Some of these syndromes are described in detail in later sections; endocrine in Section 12, renal in Section 20, and neurological in Section 24.

Genetic cancer syndromes

A wide variety of cancers are inherited in a typical Mendelian fashion, both autosomal (dominant and recessive) and sex-linked (Table 2). Their importance is that, taken together, they are not rare. They form parts of syndromes that require vigilance in the early detection of the associated cancer. They have important implications for patients with respect to genetic counselling, and they will ultimately give great insight into genes that are important in the regulation of normal tissue growth and that, when missing or aberrant, predispose towards cancer development. At present, most of the syndromes are themselves rare, but it is likely that this will change with the growth of modern molecular genetics. Germ line mutations have already been shown to be present in the Li-Fraumeni syndrome (a cancer family syndrome in which sarcomas in children are accompanied by a variety of cancers in close relatives). Although at first considered rare, it is now apparent that some children with sarcoma in childhood carry the germ line p53 mutation even in the absence of the familial syndrome. There is clearly a strong genetic component in both breast and ovarian cancer in which typical Mendelian patterns of inheritance are not manifest, perhaps due to partial penetrance of the gene or a multifactorial causation of the tumour. Recently, the locus for one familial type of breast cancer has been defined and since this may occur with the frequency of 1 in 200, there will be major ethical, financial, and clinical implications when the gene is identified.

The cancer-inducing effects of treatment, such as the delayed onset of bone cancer after irradiation, and of leukaemia after cytotoxic chemotherapy, might also occur more frequently in genetically predisposed individuals. This will clearly be an important issue as 1200 patients are cured of cancer in childhood and adolescence each year in the United Kingdom alone. If they have a normal life expectation this means that there will soon be 50 000 adults with a history of being cured of cancer in the early years of life. Genetic predisposition to tumours and to the late effects of treatment will therefore become an exceedingly important issue in the follow-up of these patients and in advising them about having families of their own. Table 2 presents a summary of some major genetic syndromes in cancer. Some cancers are directly inherited and others develop as part of an hereditary preneoplastic syndrome in which cancers develop in most, but not all, patients.

Investigation and staging

HISTOPATHOLOGICAL DIAGNOSIS

The first and most important investigation of a cancer is to verify that the diagnosis is correct. Oncologists are completely dependent on the quality of the histopathological examination. Errors are not common but may be very serious, as they may lead to inappropriate investigation or the denial of curative treatment. The latter is so important that it is worth considering the two circumstances in which this might occur.

Misdiagnosis of a lymphoma

Lymphomas may present with histological appearances very similar to anaplastic or undifferentiated carcinoma. The diagnosis should therefore always be considered when this is the pathology report. Nowadays diagnosis of lymphoma has been made much easier as a result of immunohistochemical techniques. An example is shown in Figure 1. The use of leucocyte common antigen is an invaluable diagnostic tool. If negative, it makes lymphoma unlikely, but does not rule out the possibility. If positive, the diagnosis of lymphoma is virtually certain. Nevertheless, histologists may have difficulty either because the immunohistochemical technique is not sufficiently standardized in the laboratory, or because they mistake infiltrating lymphocytes for the tumour cells. Some undifferentiated pleomorphic lymphomas may be leucocyte common-antigen negative. These present formidable diagnostic difficulties,

Table 1 *Paraneoplastic syndromes*

Syndrome	Clinical features	Tumour	Comments
*Endocrine syndromes**			
Cushing's syndrome	Metabolic features (BP ↑ K^+ ↓ glucose ↑) are severe. Obesity, etc. occur in slower growing SCLC tumours	SCLC, carcinoid, other neuroendocrine tumours	Pro-opiocortin produced by tumour Occurs in 0.5% of cases Immunoreactive ACTH ↑ in many more. In SCLC, chemotherapy may help the syndrome. In other tumours resection is curative
Antidiuretic hormone excess	Low plasma sodium (less than 130 mmol/l with continued urine sodium excretion. Below 120 mmol/l altered mental state, confusion, fits, coma, death	SCLC	Tumour produces ADH. Slightly low plasma Na is common feature of all advanced cancer (due to pituitary ADH release). Treatment is by water restriction and demeclocycline. Hypertonic saline in emergency
Hypercalcaemia	Symptoms of hypercalcaemia often very severe	Squamous cancers T-cell leukaemia Some lymphomas	Immunoreactive PTH-related peptide. Possibly release of cytokines (IL-1β, osteoclast activating factors) in some cases. Treatment described in Chapter 12.6
Gonadotrophin excess	Gynaecomastia in men, oligomenorrhoea, thyroid overactivity	Gestational trophoblastic tumours Germ cell tumours Adenocarcinoma of the lung Hepatoblastoma Other adenocarcinomas	β-HCG produced in excess. Clinical syndromes are uncommon. Mechanism of clinical syndrome is incompletely understood
Hypoglycaemia	Clinical features are of hypoglycaemia Tumours are usually large	Sarcoma Mesothelioma Hepatoma Adrenal carcinoma	Major mechanism is non-suppressible insulin-like activity (NSILA, somatomedins) and insulin-like growth factors. Mesothelioma is usually abdominal
Osteomalacia	Vitamin-D-resistant rickets with bone pain, phosphaturia	Benign mesenchyme tumours, fibromas, haemangiomas in soft tissue and bone	Low 1.25-OH vitamin D, low PTH. Treatment requires large doses of vitamin D and removal of tumour
Neurological syndromes			
Dementia	Variable onset dementia	Lung cancer (SCLC)	May be due to vascular endothelial disorder induced by the tumour
Cerebellar degeneration	Subacute and progressive associated with dementia	SCLC, prostate, colorectal cancer	CSF[1] protein raised and lymphocytosis
Limbic 'encephalitis'	Dementia	SCLC Hodgkin's disease	Pathologically there is hippocampal degeneration
Optic neuritis	Visual failure, papilloedema often bilateral	SCLC	Produced by antibodies (? to altered tumour-related proteins) which bind to retinal ganglion cell
Myelopathy	Rapid onset cord degeneration often mid-thoracic. Usually quickly fatal	SCLC	CSF[1] protein elevated
Amyotrophic lateral sclerosis	Lower motor neurone weakness combined with spasticity fasciculation. Mostly in men. Slow course	Various	Cancer found in 5–10% of cases of ALS
Peripheral neuropathy	Either pure sensory neuropathy or a severe sensorimotor neuropathy	SCLC. Other intrathoracic tumours (thymoma, oesophageal cancer, lymphoma)	CSF[1] protein may be elevated. May antedate tumour. Often does not improve if tumour removed. Sensory neuropathy is due to dorsal root ganglion degeneration and specific antibodies have been found
Guillain–Barré syndrome	Typical clinical features	Lymphomas	Association frequently noted but ? genuine

Table 1 *Paraneoplastic syndromes (continued)*

Syndrome	Clinical features	Tumour	Comments
Dermatological syndromes			
Acanthosis nigricans	Hyperkeratosis and pigmentation in axillae neck and flexures	Gastric, other intra-abdominal	There is a congenital form which must be distinguished
Seborrhoeic keratoses	Sudden onset of keratoses (Leser–Tralat syndrome)	Gut, non-Hodgkin's lymphoma	Keratoses appear quickly in large numbers
Exfoliative dermatitis	Severe erythema and scaling	Lymphomas, especially T-cell type	Common cause of exfoliative dermatitis Responds to steroids and treatment of lymphoma
Migratory erythema	Blistering, necrotic erythema	Glucagonoma	
Panniculitis	Crops of tender, subcutaneous lesions which look like erythema nodosum	Pancreas	Probably due to fat inflammation caused by liberation of pancreatic lipases
Porphyria cutanea tarda	Nodular or erythematous skin lesions. Photosensitive	Hepatocellular carcinoma	Very uncommon
Ichthyosis	Dry scaly skin with hyperkeratosis of palms and soles	Lymphomas	Different from congenital form, which may be accompanied by carcinoma of oesophagus
Musculoskeletal			
Finger clubbing and hypertrophic pulmonary osteoarthropathy	Clubbing of finger nails. Tenderness over distal ends of radius and ulna, and tibia and fibula. Periosteal reaction on radiography	Bronchial carcinoma (not SCLC), benign mesothelioma, diaphragmatic neurilemmoma	One of the great unsolved mysteries of medicine. Cause unknown
Dermatomyositis	Erythema of face – cheeks, eyelids – and over backs of hands	Wide variety of cancers, especially adenocarcinoma	May precede cancer by 6–24 months. In middle age approx 30% of cases have underlying malignancy
Lambert–Eaton syndrome	A myasthenic syndrome with muscle weakness, especially in thighs and pelvis. Ptosis, dysarthria, double vision occur. EMG shows increase in action potential with repeated stimulation	SCLC	Syndrome often antedates cancer. Muscle strength does not deteriorate with exercise. An IgG autoantibody to voltage-gated calcium channels reduces acetylcholine release. Responds to treatment of tumour and to guanidine
Haematological syndromes			
Autoimmune haemolytic anaemia	Anaemia may be the presenting symptom. Splenomegaly may occur. Response to steroids is poor. May be associated with ITP	Non-Hodgkin's lymphoma (B-cell type), wide variety of epithelial cancers	Antibodies to red cell antigens. ? cross-react with altered tumour surface antigens. Remits with successful treatment
Microangiopathic haemolytic anaemia	Mild forms are common, clinically apparent cases rare	Mucin-producing adenocarcinomas	May respond to anticancer treatment. Procoagulant appears to be produced by the tumour
Thrombocytosis	Usually asymptomatic. Mild elevation of platelet count is common. Thrombosis of haemorrhage is rare	Carcinoma, Hodgkin's disease	The tumour associated cytokine has not yet been identified
Granulocytosis	Usually asymptomatic. Modest elevations frequently found with liver metastases	Adenocarcinomas, melanoma	Blood film does not show immature forms. CSFs[2] are assumed responsible, but IL-1 and IL-3 have been implicated in some tumours
Erythrocytosis	Elevated Hb with normal $Pa\text{O}_2$ and Hb electrophoresis	Renal carcinoma, Wilms' tumour, adrenal tumours, hepatomas	Erythrocytosis resolves with removal of primary. Erythropoietin is made by the tumour or its release is stimulated

These are some of the most common paraneoplastic syndromes.

*The endocrine syndromes are those where the hormonal syndrome is produced by a non-endocrine cancer.

ACTH, adrenocorticotrophic hormone; ADH, antidiuretic hormone; ALS, amyotrophic lateral sclerosis; BP, blood pressure; CSF[1], cerebrospinal fluid; CSF[2], colony-stimulating factor; Hb, haemoglobin; hCG, human chorionic gonadotrophin; IL interleukin; ITP, idiopathic thrombocytopenia purpura; $Pa\text{O}_2$, arterial partial pressure of oxygen; PHT, parathyroid hormone; SCLC, small cell lung cancer.

Table 2 *Some inherited cancer syndromes*

Clinical abnormality	Cancer
Immune deficiency	
Ataxia-telangiectasia (AR)	Non-Hodgkin's lymphoma, gastric cancer
Agammaglobulinaemia (XLR)	Non-Hodgkin's lymphoma
Lymphoproliferative syndrome (XLR)	Non-Hodgkin's lymphoma
Wiskott–Aldrich syndrome (XLR)	Non-Hodgkin's lymphoma, acute leukaemia
Cutaneous disorders	
Neurofibromatosis (AD)	Sarcomatous change
Dysplastic naevus syndrome (AD)	Melanoma
Tylosis palmaris (AD) (hyperkeratosis of palms and soles)	Oesophageal cancer
Bloom's syndrome (AR) (photosensitivity)	Squamous carcinoma of skin
Chediak–Higashi syndrome (AD) (defective skin and hair pigmentation)	Lymphoma and leukaemia
Naevoid basal cell carcinoma (AD)	Basal cell carcinoma, medulloblastoma, ovarian fibroma
Intestinal disorders	
Polyposis coli (AD)	Carcinoma of colon
Gardner's syndrome (AD) (epidermal cysts and dermoids)	Carcinoma of colon
Peutz–Jeghers syndrome (AD) (mucocutaneous pigmentation)	Gut cancers and ovarian cancers
Neurological syndromes	
Retinoblastoma (AD)	Retinoblastoma, osteosarcoma
Tuberous sclerosis (AD)	Glioma
Retinal–cerebellar angiomatosis (AD)	Phaeochromocytoma, renal cell carcinoma, ependymoma

AD, autosomal dominant; AR, autosomal recessive; XLR, X-linked recessive.

Fig. 1 (a) H & E section of excision specimen of a retroperitoneal mass. The tumour is poorly differentiated, with fibrosis and infiltration of retroperitoneal fat. (b) Immunostaining with an antibody of CD20 (a B lymphocyte marker) shows intense staining of tumour cells confirming that this is a B-cell non-Hodgkin's lymphoma.

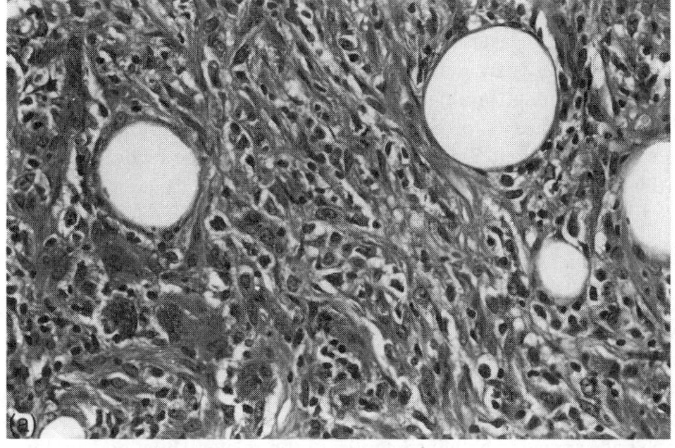

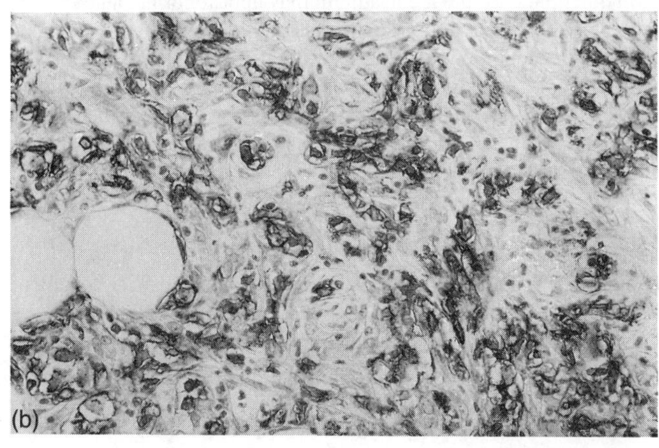

which may be resolved by examination of the tissue by molecular genetic techniques looking for rearrangement of the T-cell receptor genes or for immunoglobulin gene rearrangement. Other situations in which lymphoma may be overlooked or mistaken diagnosis made are in the pulmonary lesions (or metastases) from small cell carcinoma, which may be mistaken for lymphoma, or in biopsies from gastric ulcers where malignant lymphoma cells may be regarded as chronic inflammatory cellular infiltrate. As non-Hodgkin's lymphomas can present in many different sites, where the diagnosis is not clear, a prudent physician will always ask the pathologist whether the diagnosis of lymphoma has been firmly excluded.

Mediastinal or metastatic germ cell tumours

These tumours may be mistaken for anaplastic carcinoma. This is an exceedingly important diagnosis, as many of them are curable. Mediastinal germ cell tumours typically present in young adults and may present with cervical node metastases. Special stains for α-fetoprotein (AFP) or β-HCG (human chorionic gonadotrophin) may be very helpful but, if negative, do not exclude the diagnosis. Several recent reports have indicated that the use of intensive combination chemotherapy, as for germ cell tumours, may result in lasting remissions of mediastinal poorly differentiated tumours in young adults, even when there were no other features of the germ cell nature of the neoplasm. In contrast, poorly differentiated adenocarcinoma in the mediastinum of young adults is seldom ascribable to germ cell tumour, although occasional cases may respond dramatically to chemotherapy.

INVESTIGATING THE LOCAL EXTENT OF THE TUMOUR

Clinical staging is the most important first procedure. Clinical examination will often establish the likely extent of the tumour. This may require specialized techniques such as ear, nose, and throat (ENT) examination and bronchoscopy. The extent of infiltration and fixation to surrounding structures is assessed. Computer tomography and magnetic resonance scanning have greatly improved the preoperative determination of tumour extent. They have largely replaced more invasive techniques such as angiography and lymphangiography. Magnetic resonance scanning is particularly valuable in the staging of sarcomas and central nervous system tumours. Both techniques show the extent of the tumour and infiltration of surrounding structures (Fig. 2(a) and (b)). Computer tomography is particularly valuable for needle biopsy diagnosis of deep-seated tumours.

STAGING OF LYMPH NODE SPREAD

Spread to adjacent lymph nodes may be noted clinically or on straightforward investigations, such as chest radiography. Lymphangiography was used to examine pelvic and lower para-aortic nodes but has largely been supplanted by computer tomography scanning. In fact the two techniques give slightly different information, as a computer tomography scan will show enlarged lymph nodes (the assumption being that these are replaced by tumour when the lymph nodes become more than 2 cm in size), while lymphangiography may show abnormal appearances even when the nodes are not enlarged but contain foci of tumour cells within them.

Fig. 2 (a) Longitudinal MR scan of lower thigh. A large, soft tissue mass is seen displacing the muscle groups posteriorly. It lies behind the femur and the femoral artery is in close proximity to the mass, which at one point surrounds it. (b) CT scan of abdomen. A carcinoma of the body of the pancreas is shown (arrowed). The liver contains numerous small metastases.

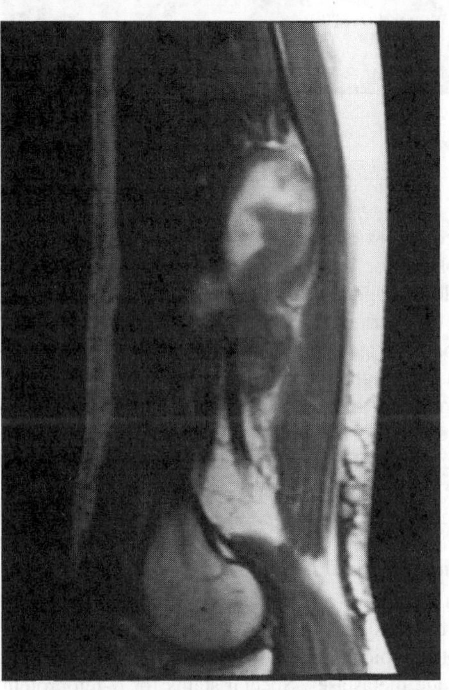

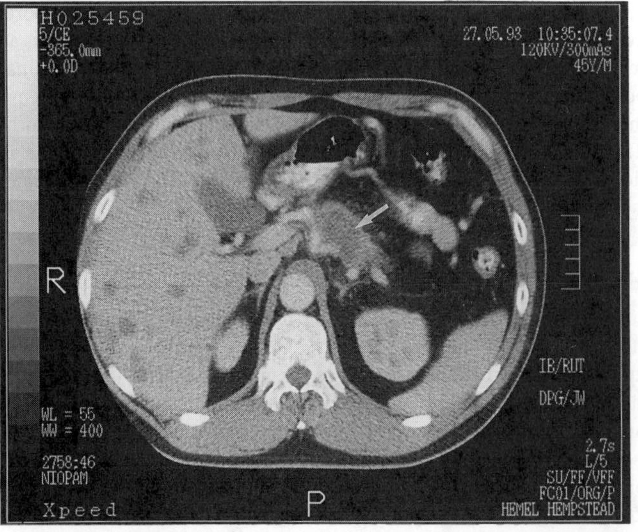

STAGING FOR DISTANT METASTASES

Bone metastases are usually demonstrated by ^{99}Tc polyphosphate isotopic scanning. The sensitivity of the examination is high and abnormalities frequently precede detectable changes on plain radiography. However, the specificity is rather lower because any traumatic or inflammatory disorder in bone can give areas of increased uptake. When areas of increased uptake are seen on technetium scanning it is important to follow up with plain skeletal radiography, particularly in the long bones of the limbs. This is because isotope scanning gives no indication of the structural integrity of the bone and the risk of pathological fracture in a limb cannot be assessed on an isotope scan.

Liver metastases are detected by an increase in circulating enzyme levels, particularly alkaline phosphatase and serum glutamate-oxaloacetic transaminase (SGOT). Lactic dehydrogenase (LDH) is also elevated in a somewhat greater frequency. Nevertheless, liver metastases can be present without alteration in serum enzyme levels and ultrasound scanning is an invaluable non-invasive method of detecting liver metastases. Computed tomography and modern ultrascanning are approximately equal in sensitivity. Metastases down to 1 cm in size can be detected reliably.

Pulmonary metastases may be detected on chest radiograph but may be present even when the chest radiograph is normal if they are below 1.5 cm in size. Metastases larger than this may also be overlooked if they are situated behind the heart or behind the diaphragm. Computer tomography scanning is the best method for demonstrating pulmonary metastases and lesions as small as 0.4 cm in diameter may be seen. Computer tomography scanning is therefore an essential investigation in patients who are to undergo extensive or mutilating surgery, such as for sarcomas where metastases to the lungs is particularly frequent and the presence of metastases may influence the surgical decision.

Brain metastases are detected by computer tomography or magnetic resonance scanning. In a patient who is neurologically normal there is only a low chance of detecting asymptomatic cerebral metastasis by these methods (about 5 per cent). For this reason the technique is not worthwhile as a routine in the investigation of most cancers.

SURGICAL STAGING OF CANCER

Surgery specifically for staging rather than treatment is reserved to a few specific tumour sites. In lung cancer, investigation of the mediastinum is extremely important in deciding whether a tumour is operable. Computer tomography scanning may demonstrate inoperability either because the tumour is infiltrating the mediastinum or because there is lymph node spread to both ipsilateral and contralateral hilar nodes. However, in other patients, the mediastinum may appear normal and a mediastinoscopy may reveal tumour in mediastinal nodes implying the inoperability of the condition. Staging laparotomy used to be performed in localized Hodgkin's disease, but is now reserved for specific indications. In ovarian cancer thorough surgical staging is performed at the time of the initial resection but surgical staging is here (as in many other tumour resections) part of the treatment.

THE USE OF A STAGING NOTATION

This has been valuable in the reporting of results of cancer treatment and is also helpful, in an individual patient, in focusing attention on the extent of the disease and the subsequent planning of treatment. A widely used system is the T (tumour) N (nodes) M (metastasis) system. This is particularly valuable for tumours that follow an orderly progression of spread from the primary site to adjacent lymph nodes and then to met-

Table 3 *Staging of non-small cell lung cancer*

T_1	< 3 cm diameter		
T_2	> 3 cm diameter but > 2 cm distal to carina may be visceral pleural invasion		
T_3	Involves chest wall or mediastinum		
T_4	Invades heart, great vessels, trachea or oesophagus, malignant pleural effusion		
N_0	No involved nodes		
N_1	Isilateral peribronchial or hilar nodes		
N_2	Ipsilateral mediastinal or subcarinal		
N_3	Contralateral nodes or supraclavicular nodes		
M_0	No distant metastases		
M_1	Distant metastases		
Stage grouping			
Stage 1	$T_{1,2}$	N_0	M_0
Stage 2	$T_{1,2}$	N_1	M_0
Stage 3a	$T_{1,2}$	N_2	M_0
	T_3	N_{0-2}	M_0
Stage 3b	Any T	N_3	M_0
	T_4	Any N	M_0
Stage 4	Any T	Any N	M_1

Table 4 *The management of tumours*

Chemotherapy (including endocrine therapy)	Radiotherapy
May be curative in	*May be curative in*
Hodgkin's disease	localized Hodgkin's disease
non-Hodgkin's lymphoma	non-Hodgkin's lymphoma
germ cell tumours	stage II seminoma
Wilm's tumour	head and neck cancer
Ewing's sarcoma	
osteosarcoma	
rhabdomyosarcoma	
leukaemia	
Adds to cure rate in	*Adds to cure rate in*
stage II breast cancer	Ewing's sarcoma
? colorectal cancer	localized breast cancer
ovarian cancer	small cell lung cancer
small cell lung cancer	anal cancer
	cervical cancer
	skin cancer
	rectal cancer
Produces remission and/or prolongs survival in	*Produces remission and/or prolongs survival in*
small cell lung cancer	non-small cell lung cancer
advanced breast cancer	glioma
prostate cancer	prostate cancer
ovarian cancer	biliary tract cancer
myeloma	
Palliates	*Palliates*
non-Hodgkin's lymphoma (when incurable)	bone metastases
small cell lung cancer (extensive)	non-small lung cancer
	brain metastases
	rectal cancer
	oesophageal cancer

astatic sites. Thus, tumours of the head and neck, breast, non-small-cell lung cancer, renal carcinoma, bladder carcinoma, and rectal carcinoma are all well-defined by these means. In addition to the TNM system, many classifications contain a stage grouping, by which tumours with varying TNM assignments are grouped together because of equivalence of prognosis or similar approaches to management. An example of the TNM staging system and stage grouping for lung cancer is given in Table 3.

Not all tumours can be summarized by the TNM system. For example, small cell lung cancer is usually widely metastatic at the time of presentation and a simpler classification into limited (confined to one side of the thorax with ipsilateral supraclavicular node) or extensive (disease that is bilateral within the chest or metastatic). This simple classification serves to separate patients in whom radiation treatment may be worthwhile and those in whom it is unlikely to have any benefit. In leukaemia and myeloma, other staging criteria, which are based on prognostic factors and are not related to anatomical stage, have been developed. In Hodgkin's disease and non-Hodgkin's lymphoma, the presence (B) or absence (A) of constitutional symptoms is added to the anatomical staging system, which is used to define the degree of lymph node spread. These additions were made because the presence of constitutional symptoms confers an adverse prognostic significance in addition to the prognosis related to the anatomical stage (see also Section 22).

Principles of cancer management

The principles and details of cancer chemotherapy are discussed elsewhere. This section summarizes an integrated approach towards cancer management.

Nowadays the management of cancer will nearly always involve more than one specialist and more than one type of treatment. Increasingly, cancer patients are being seen in joint clinics where surgeons, medical oncologists, and radiotherapists plan treatment. Often there will be several possible approaches towards treatment, and these require discussion and assessment by the appropriate experts. It is of inestimable value if a patient is referred for expert opinion before any definitive procedure is undertaken. For example, more information about gynaecological malignancy can often be obtained if a patient with abdominal swelling and ascites and an ultrasound demonstrable mass in the pelvis is assessed preoperatively by a gynaecological oncologist. The subsequent laparotomy is likely to reveal much more information than if it is carried out as an emergency by an inexperienced surgeon. Similarly, a mass on a limb should be investigated thoroughly, including a biopsy diagnosis, before surgery is undertaken, because the nature of the histological diagnosis may profoundly alter management in the case of a sarcoma. Table 4 lists tumours in which radiotherapy and chemotherapy have an important part to play in management and where these modalities of treatment may sometimes be curative.

SURGERY

Surgeons see over 80 per cent of patients presenting with cancer for the first time. Following diagnosis and staging to exclude metastases, curative surgery may be undertaken, for example in breast or colorectal cancer. The aim of the operation is complete excision of the tumour with a margin of normal, uninvolved tissue around the main tumour mass. The risk of local recurrence is very high with a marginal excision in which a tumour has been 'shelled out' because the pseudocapsule around the tumour is likely to be infiltrated with tumour cells. Removal or sampling of the draining lymph nodes will often be undertaken, for example in breast cancer and other tumours where involvement of draining lymph nodes is likely. In some cancers, such as breast cancer, it has become clear that very extensive primary tumours are usually accompanied by distant metastasis. The role of surgery is therefore to prevent local recurrence rather than to be curative. With other tumours, of the head and neck, for example, extensive surgery may be the only means of gaining effective control and in these cases a high degree of surgical expertise is necessary. In some situations the tumour may be approached either by surgery or by radical radiotherapy and there may be little to choose between the results. Examples are in stage III, non-small lung cancer, where long-term results of radical radiation and surgery are probably equivalent (although randomized comparison has not been performed), and in operable oesophageal cancer, particularly of squamous histology, where long-term results of radiation appear to be equivalent to those of surgery.

Nowadays local treatment frequently involves both surgery and radiation in order to maximize the chances of local control. Wide local excision is increasingly practiced in carcinoma of the breast and radiation to the breast and to axillary nodes is used as an adjunct. Radiation reduces the risk of local relapse, both in the breast and in the axilla. 'Lumpectomy' and radical radiotherapy have now replaced mastectomy for many patients with small primary breast cancers. Preoperative radiation of soft tissue sarcoma may increase the chance of successful compartmental excision of the tumour, and postoperative radiation decreases the risk of local recurrence in patients in whom the excision has been marginal. These are two examples of the way in which the definitive local management of the primary tumour is a matter of discussion between surgical and radiation oncologists.

Optimum local management has become further complicated by the successful use of chemotherapy in many tumours. An example is the treatment of Ewing's tumour. In this highly malignant round cell tumour of childhood, initial chemotherapy usually produces a prompt regression of the main tumour mass, both in the bone and in the surrounding soft tissues. However, the tumour permeates widely through the bone, and local irradiation, given after initial chemotherapy, is a standard means of maintaining local control. There is an increasing tendency to continue both chemotherapy and radiation synchronously. However, in large tumours, even with full dose radiation, the risk of local relapse is still present. For this reason surgery is being used increasingly, provided that the cosmetic and functional results are reasonable. Surgical excision alone may be successful after chemotherapy but, frequently, because of the permeating nature of the tumour, viable tumour is present right up to the resection margins of the bone. In this situation radiation will be needed in addition to the chemotherapy and surgery. In these tumours, very detailed planning of the approach to treatment by experienced specialists is essential for optimum results.

PRINCIPLES OF CHEMOTHERAPY

The cure of many cancers by combination chemotherapy has been a considerable achievement. The tumours that have been cured are those that were shown to be very sensitive to anticancer drugs when these were first introduced in 1950–60. These tumours, such as lymphomas and leukaemias, showed marked sensitivity even to single agents. The use of single agents did not, however, lead to cures of these diseases, and it was not until combination chemotherapy was introduced that a substantial proportion of cures was achieved.

It can be seen from Table 4 that some tumours are sensitive to cytotoxic drugs and others are not. The remarkable thing about the sensitivity of tumours to cytotoxic agents is that sensitivity or resistance is a property of tumour types, and not of the chemical nature of the cytotoxic agent being used. Lymphomas, for example, are sensitive to a wide variety of agents, whether they are alkylating agents, anthracyclines, or antimetabolites. Pancreatic cancer and melanoma, on the other hand, are resistant to all these agents. Of course, there are individual examples of tumours that show unexpected sensitivity or resistance, but it is a remarkable fact of chemotherapy, and radiation therapy, that different tumours are vulnerable or resistant to a wide variety of seemingly unrelated types of chemical attack. The reasons for sensitivity are not well understood. Many biochemical mechanisms of drug resistance mechanisms have been described. These include induction of enzymes blocked by cytotoxic agents, overexpression of drug efflux proteins (such as the multiple drug resistance protein), and expression of enzymes such as O6 alkyltransferase, which repairs DNA damage due to nitrosoureas. It is probable that, in an individual tumour, a variety of mechanisms of resistance are present. Nevertheless, there is no generally satisfactory explanation for why tumours differ in drug sensitivity in the way that is outlined in Table 4. A possible explanation is that, in some tumours, there is deficient repair of drug-damaged DNA. In recent years techniques that will allow further study of this problem have become available but at the moment it is not clear why we are fortunate enough to be able to cure some tumours with cytotoxic agents.

Table 5 *Commonly used cytotoxic agents*

Alkylating agents
oxazophosphorines – cyclophosphamide, ifosfamide
melphalan
busulphan
nitrosoureas – CCNU, BCNU
platinum compounds – cisplatin, carboplatin
Anthracyclines
doxorubicin
daunorubicin
Antimetabolites
purine analogues – 6-mercaptopurine, azathioprine
pyrimidine analogues – 5-fluorouracil, cytosine arabinoside
antifolates – methotrexate, edatrexate
Vinca alkaloids
vincristine
vinblastine
vindesine
Topoisomerase inhibitors
etoposide
teniposide
Antitumour antibiotics
bleomycin dactinomycin
distamycin
mithramycin

Table 5 lists some of the commonly used chemotherapeutic agents according to the class of chemical. It is important to realize that alkylating agents, whose main cytotoxic effect appears to be the result of a drug binding to DNA, do not attack DNA in a random fashion. Extreme chemical sensitivity is shown in the formation of the drug–DNA adduct. Furthermore, the resulting biological consequences to normal tissues differ widely from one alkylating agent to another. For example, cyclophosphamide causes an acute, readily reversible, depression of the white count, with relatively less effect on platelets. Nitrosoureas, on the other hand, typically produce delayed, slow onset, neutropenia and, particularly, thrombocytopenia, which may take many weeks to recover. Cisplatin is associated with severe nausea, vomiting, renal toxicity, and deafness. Its analogue, carboplatin, binds to DNA with similar nucleotide specificities, but at a slower rate. Its pattern of toxicity is different from cisplatin in that it produces prolonged myelosuppression, but much less renal toxicity and nerve damage. It is not possible to predict, from the chemical structure of the analogues, that this widely different pattern of toxicity would occur.

One side-effect that many cytotoxic drugs have in common is that they produce nausea and vomiting. Again, the way in which such widely differing chemicals are able to produce a common symptom is not understood. It is not clear if the effect is primarily central, or peripheral on the gastrointestinal tract. Similarly, hair loss, which is a troublesome and universal feature of treatment with some drugs (such as etoposide, doxorubicin, and cyclophosphamide), does not occur with drugs such as cisplatin, carboplatin, and methotrexate.

The toxicities of chemotherapy can be divided into both short-term and long-term effects, and these are summarized in Table 6. These toxicities are a further reason why chemotherapy should always be given by those expert in its use.

Table 6 *Toxicity of chemotherapeutic agents*

Short term
- nausea and vomiting (many agents, especially cisplatin)
- alopecia (alkylators, anthracyclines, etoposide)
- bone marrow suppression (alkylators, anthracyclines, etoposide)
- cardiac toxicity (anthracyclines)
- renal impairment (especially cisplatin)
- peripheral neuropathy (cisplatin, vinca alkaloids)
- pulmonary fibrosis (bleomycin)

Long term
- peripheral neuropathy (cisplatin, vinca alkaloids)
- cardiac toxicity (doxorubicin)
- male infertility (alkylators)
- reduction of female fertility (especially in older women)
- oncogenesis (e.g. leukaemia induced by nitrosoureas and etoposide)
- deafness (cisplatin)

The intention behind combination chemotherapy is to circumvent drug resistance by using drugs that interfere with the reproductive integrity of cells via a variety of biochemically different pathways. The larger the tumour, the more likely it is that somatic mutation will have given rise to cells with widely differing sensitivities. The intention behind combination chemotherapy is to subvert this resistance. The principles of combining drugs are:

1. To use drugs that are known to be effective when used as single agents in advanced or relapsed disease.
2. To use these effective agents in the optimum dose and schedule.
3. To combine agents that are known to work through different biochemical mechanisms (for example agents that cross-link DNA combined with drugs that are antimetabolites).
4. To combine agents with differing, or non-additive, toxicity.
5. To combine agents where the mechanisms of resistance, if known, are different (for example the combination of drugs where resistance is mediated through the multiple drug resistance (mdr) mechanism, with other agents where DNA damage is repaired by excision of drug–nucleotide adducts).

Although combination chemotherapy is based on the above principles, in practice a considerable degree of empiricism lies behind the development of successful regimens. In general these combination regimens have had dose limitations set by toxicity (usually on the bone marrow and gut). For these reasons the drugs are given in cycles of treatment, allowing time for marrow and gut recovery.

The successful use of combination chemotherapy depends on considerable expertise and experience. There is no place for the use of combination chemotherapy by those whose major speciality lies elsewhere (for example, in general surgery or gynaecology). Cytotoxic chemotherapy is part of the specialist services that a hospital has to offer in the same way as a coronary care unit or an endoscopy unit. Lack of familiarity with chemotherapy either leads to excessive toxicity or to the avoidance of toxicity by using drugs in inadequate dosage, thus comprising the chances of cure.

Specific management problems

SPINAL CORD AND CAUDA EQUINA COMPRESSION

Cord and cauda equina compression are common and devastating complications of metastatic cancer. For successful diagnosis and management it is essential to remember one rule – every hour counts. Even if early treatment is not always successful, delay ensures that the patient will end his or her days bed- or chair-bound, paralysed, and incontinent.

The metastasis often develops in a vertebral body, from which it spreads backwards or via the intervertebral foramina to compress the cord (or cauda equina below L1) from the extradural space (Fig. 3(a)). Alternatively, the malignant mass may originate in a mass of retroperitoneal nodes, or the primary tumour (for example a bronchial carcinoma) may be in the posterior mediastinum or retroperitoneum (Fig. 3(b)). Damage to the cord is by direct compression and by interruption of the arterial supply leading to infarction. It is uncommon for the tumour to be metastatic to the cord itself, although meningeal spread occurs and may cause compression (see carcinomatous meningitis, below). Cord compression may be the first manifestation of cancer but more commonly arises with metastases from a known primary.

Pain often precedes the onset of neurological symptoms. In the case of cord compression it is felt in the thoracic and cervical vertebrae. It is worse on coughing. An exceedingly sinister symptom is vertebral pain with a root distribution. A patient with this symptom needs urgent investigation, as cord compression may be imminent. The next symptom is usually weakness of the legs combined with sensory loss, of which loss of proprioception is especially characteristic. Loss of bladder and bowel sensation is late and once weakness and bladder disturbance begins progression to irreversible paraplegia occurs in hours or a few days.

The patient often has a sensory level, motor weakness, brisk leg reflexes, and extensor plantar responses. The bladder may be palpable. Radiography of the spine often shows vertebral destruction – loss of a pedicle or compression of the body being typical. Myelography will demonstrate the block but magnetic resonance scanning (and, less reliably, computer tomography scanning) is very valuable and can replace or supplement myelography. Treatment usually consists of surgical decompression, although for radiation-sensitive tumours such as lymphoma or Ewing's sarcoma, high dose corticosteroids and radiation will produce quick relief of compression. If there are multiple sites of block, radiation and steroids may be the only feasible option. The surgical approach to decompression varies according to the nature of the lesion – whether anterior or posterior, cervical or thoracic. Anterior decompression may involve removal of part of the vertebral body but the risk of destabilization of the spine means that immediate stabilization may be necessary. It is not clear whether radiation is inferior to surgical decompression in patients with tumours that show sensitivity to radiation. Radiation is, in any event, usually given after laminectomy.

Outcome is crucially dependent on the functional state of the patient before treatment. Less than 10 per cent of those who are paraplegic

Fig. 3 MR scan of thoracic vertebrae showing destruction of the body of T10 by a mass of Hodgkin's disease. The tumour extends posteriorly and compresses the spinal cord. The tumour mass has passed to the side of the vertebra (not shown), and is also compressing the cord posteriorly after infiltrating into the intervertebral foramen.

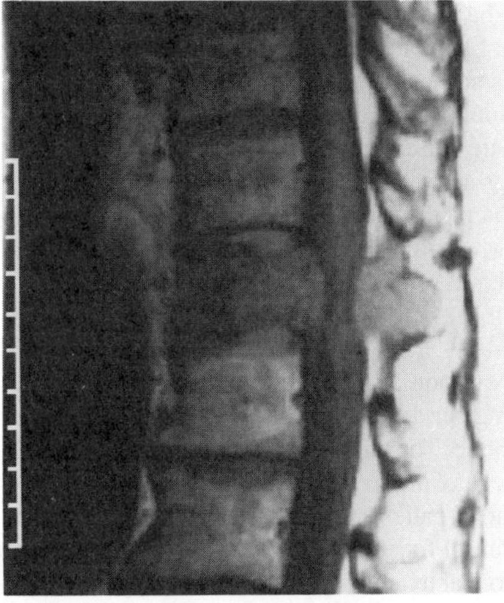

before treatment will be able to walk later, 25 per cent will do so if they have some motor function preserved, while almost all patients who can still walk will continue to be able to do so.

CEREBRAL METASTASIS

Cerebral metastasis is an exceptionally serious complication of cancer occurring in about 30 per cent of all patients. Metastases are over 10 times as common as primary brain tumours. About 15 per cent of cancer patients will develop symptomatic brain metastases during life. Thus, there will be approximately 15 000 deaths each year in the United Kingdom of patients with symptomatic cerebral metastasis. Metastasis at this site is life-threatening and disabling, causing severe deterioration in quality of life and great difficulty for the patient and his or her carers.

The majority of cerebral metastases are intradural, usually in the substance of the brain extending to the meningeal surface. About 80 per cent of these are situated in the cerebrum and the rest in the cerebellum and other regions. Lung cancer and breast cancer are the most common primary sites, and certain tumours are particularly associated with single metastases (cancer of the breast, ovary, and kidney). Usually cerebral metastases occur following diagnosis and treatment of a primary tumour.

In the brain substance, the metastases are vascularized from the cerebral circulation, but there is no evidence that a vascularized metastasis maintains a 'blood–brain' barrier. Indeed, capillary leakiness appears to be a feature of cerebral metastasis and is responsible for the substantial amount of oedema of the brain, which typically accompanies cerebral metastasis. The blood–brain barrier may be an important impediment to cytotoxic treatment when the metastasis is being established before it is vascularized and will be a significant factor in leptomeningeal spread of cancer.

Symptoms and signs

The typical signs are headache, disturbance of cognitive function and affect, focal fits or grand mal convulsions, and limb paresis. Headache usually reflects a rise in intracranial pressure. It is typically present in the morning and increases in duration and frequency until other signs of raised intracranial pressure become apparent. Focal weakness is present in about half of all patients, and disturbance in higher cerebral function in about 60 per cent.

Investigation

Computer tomography or magnetic resonance scanning is the essential diagnostic investigation. On a computer tomography scan most metastases appear hypodense but enhance with contrast material. Typically there will be oedema around the metastases. Occasionally computer tomography scans may be normal even in patients whose symptoms strongly suggest cerebral metastasis and where cerebral metastasis is sometimes proven by further scanning some weeks later or at autopsy. In these patients there may be multiple small metastases without oedema or leptomeningeal spread. Magnetic resonance scanning has a greater degree of sensitivity and is particularly valuable in detecting leptomeningeal spread of tumour. Both magnetic resonance and computer tomography have largely supplanted arteriography as a diagnostic method. In the presence of a known primary it is not necessary to subject patients to histological confirmation of the tumour. However, after a very long disease-free interval, or where the primary is unknown, histological diagnosis will be essential.

Treatment

Dexamethasone is started as soon as the diagnosis is made. The usual dose is approximately 16 mg per day, although higher doses can be used if the patients does not respond. The clinical effects are rapid and usually noticeable within 24 h. The maximum effect is achieved in about 4 days. Approximately 80 per cent of patients will respond. Phenytoin or carbamazepine are used to control focal fits.

The most useful non-surgical treatment is radiation therapy. The therapeutic doses depend on the likely primary site, but usually consist of 30 Gy in 10 fractions in 2 weeks, or 40 Gy in 15 fractions in 3 weeks. The former is the most widely used schedule in the United Kingdom and no schedule has been proven to be superior over another. Solitary cerebral metastases may be removed if they are in an accessible site. The criteria for operation are usually that a solitary metastasis is present, that the diagnosis is uncertain, or that the response to radiation is unpredictable because of doubt about the nature of the primary tumour. The patient must be clinically fit in other respects to undergo surgery, and without metastatic disease elsewhere.

In recent years there has been some interest in the use of chemotherapy in the treatment of cerebral metastasis, as it is now clear, in tumours such as small cell lung cancer, that the response to chemotherapy in cerebral metastases is equal to that in metastases at other sites. Responses to chemotherapy in tumours such as small cell lung cancer may be rapid and dramatic, but brain radiation will usually be necessary as an adjunct to chemotherapy.

Prognosis

The prognosis depends on the clinical setting. If there is a solitary metastasis with no disease elsewhere then a long disease-free interval may result, particularly if the metastasis has occurred after a considerable interval following the primary treatment. In other tumours, where multiple metastases occur either synchronously with the primary tumour or after a short disease-free interval, and where the tumour is a particularly difficult type to treat (such as melanoma and non-small-cell lung cancer), the prognosis is very poor indeed. Overall, only 30 per cent of patients will be alive at 1 year and the median survival is about 7 months. A recent randomized trial has confirmed that surgical resection of a solitary metastasis adds to survival when compared with radiation and steroids alone.

CARCINOMATOUS 'MENINGITIS'

Leptomeningeal spread of cancer seems to be increasing in frequency. In autopsy series about 4 per cent of patients dying of advanced cancer have leptomeningeal spread. The frequency is higher in breast cancer (5–10 per cent). This complication is increasing in lymphoma, small cell lung cancer, ovarian cancer, and some sarcomas. Curiously, adenocarcinomas seem to have a greater propensity for this form of metastasis than other epithelial tumours. There may or not be intracerebral metastasis at the same time. Malignant cells may enter the cerebrospinal fluid from intracerebral tumour via the arachnoid, or from vertebral deposits growing along nerve roots into the subarachnoid space. However, the most likely source of seeding appears to be directly from the bloodstream. Tumour is present as a thin covering of malignant cells, but in some cases the tumour cells penetrate deeper into the substance of the brain along blood vessels. The tumour may also penetrate cranial and spinal cord nerves as they pass through the subarachnoid space.

Clinical features

The onset is usually over a few weeks and may be subtle at first. Headache is often severe and is due to raised intracranial pressure. Cranial nerve dysfunction is frequent, with diplopia, hearing loss, and facial numbness. There is often back pain and sometimes bladder and bowel dysfunction. A change in mental state may occur. Focal fits are uncommon. On examination there may be an abnormal mental state, signs of raised intracranial pressure, and extensive plantar responses. Focal neurological signs in the limbs are uncommon. Cranial nerve weaknesses are frequent, the commonest being ocular muscle palsy, facial weakness and hearing loss.

Diagnosis and treatment

The diagnosis is made by examining the cerebrospinal fluid. Typically, the opening pressure is high, the white count is raised, the cerebrospinal fluid sugar low, and the protein increased. Cytological confirmation on the first lumbar puncture is obtained in about 60 per cent of patients, but a negative examination does not exclude the diagnosis. Myelography may show typical appearance of multiple small tumour seeds in the subarachnoid space, but MR scanning is proving invaluable and is the preferred initial investigation if cerebrospinal fluid cytology is negative and the diagnosis strongly suspected.

Treatment is difficult and often unsuccessful. Temporary improvement can be obtained by the insertion of an intraventricular reservoir to deliver chemotherapy. Chemotherapy administered by lumbar puncture is uncomfortable and may not be effective if there is meningeal involvement supratentorially, since the drugs do not penetrate in high concentration beyond the foramen magnum. In breast cancer and lymphoma, intrathecal methotrexate is effective and may be administered in combination with thiotepa or, in the case of lymphoma, cytosine arabinoside. In addition, whole brain irradiation is often given if the patient is improving and the clinical situation indicates that this treatment would produce further benefit. In general, however, the prognosis is poor when the meningeal infiltration is from an epithelial tumour, with a median survival of only 4 months.

PLEURAL EFFUSION

Malignant pleural effusions occur either as a sign of metastasis or due to direct invasion of the pleural space from an underlying primary bronchial carcinoma, or pulmonary metastasis. The effusions are typically exudates with a protein content of more than 3 g/dl. There is increased capillary permeability through inflammation and abnormal capillary endothelium in the tumour lining the pleural space. Typical primary sites are breast and ovarian cancer, as common epithelial tumours metastasize into the pleural space; lung cancer, as a cause of pleural effusion with underlying lung disease; and sarcomas, as a cause of pleural effusion due to invasion of the pleura by pulmonary metastasis.

Clinical features

The typical features are dyspnoea, which is directly related to the size of the effusion, dry cough, and chest wall discomfort. Even a small effusion may cause dyspnoea in a patient who has underlying lung disease such as chronic bronchitis and emphysema. Many patients have asymptomatic pleural effusions detectable on chest radiograph. The sequence of radiological appearances includes blunting of the costaphrenic angle, (with volumes of 2–3 ml) increasing effusion, and, finally, mediastinal shift, which usually occurs when amounts in excess of 2 litres have accumulated. Ultrasound examination is of help in localizing the effusion and any loculi, which may be important in planning aspiration.

Diagnosis

The diagnosis, if the primary tumour is not known, is made by demonstrating malignant cells in the pleural fluid. The rate of positivity, in patients known to have an underlying cancer, is about 60 per cent with a low false positive rate. If pleural cytology is negative on the first aspiration this should be repeated. Occasionally, pleural biopsy will be necessary to make a diagnosis, and the combination of the two increase the diagnostic yield to about 90 per cent. If both techniques fail thoracoscopy is more successful, but is, of course, more invasive.

Treatment and prognosis

The primary tumour should be treated if possible. When a pleural effusion persists after treatment of the primary tumour, or if such treatment has been unsuccessful, treatment may need to be directed to the effusion itself. Frequently the effusion will need to be aspirated in order to make the patient comfortable, and pleural sclerotherapy considered. For best results of sclerotherapy it is important to drain the pleural cavity as completely as possible. A small flexible chest drain is ideal and is left in place for some time (12 to 24 h if possible) to allow the fluid to drain as far as possible. If there has been loculated effusion, the insertion of the drain is best done under ultrasound control. Sclerosis of the two pleural surfaces can be achieved by a variety of means; all give approximately equivalent results. The most favoured techniques are the instillation of tetracycline, bleomycin, or *Corynebacterium parvum.* They all cause an inflammatory reaction in the pleural space and have an approximately 60 per cent success rate in preventing immediate recurrence of the effusion. When pleural effusion complicates an underlying bronchial carcinoma it is more difficult to control than when it is a metastasis manifestation of a distant neoplasm, such as ovarian cancer. If the effusion is recurrent and is the major cause of morbidity, pleuroperitoneal shunting can be carried out, whereby the pleural fluid drains into the peritoneal cavity.

PERICARDIAL EFFUSION

The most common malignancies to cause pericardial effusion are breast, lung, and gastrointestinal cancers and non-Hodgkin's lymphomas. Pathologically, the pericardium may be infiltrated with tumour or diffusely nodular. The accumulation of fluid is due to obstruction of lymphatic and venous drainage of the pericardium.

Symptoms and signs

The symptoms are usually vague in onset, including orthopnoea, dyspnoea, and cough. Fatigue and dizziness also develop. If cardiac tamponade occurs it is associated with severe dyspnoea, vague central chest pain, and anxiety. The physical signs are usually minimal, although when tamponade occurs there will be jugular venous distension, pulses paradoxus, hypotension and tachycardia.

Investigation

Investigations include a chest radiograph, which shows enlargement of the cardiac silhouette, and echocardiography, which is a rapid non-invasive technique for demonstrating pericardial effusion.

Diagnosis and management

The diagnosis is made by finding malignant cells in the pericardial fluid. False negative results occur and the test may need to be repeated. Once the diagnosis has been established, the pericardial fluid may need drainage using a small rubber catheter. Installation of sclerosants can be carried out as for pleural effusions, but troublesome pericardial effusions can be controlled by the formation of a pericardial window through a small left anterior thoracotomy. Some patients, particularly those who have lymphoma, will respond to external beam radiation with a dose of approximately 30 Gy given in 15 fractions over a 2- to 3-week period. Radiation is also considered for control of chronic pericardial effusion in breast cancer. The management of cardiac tamponade is discussed in Section 15.

CANCER FROM AN UNKNOWN PRIMARY SITE

Approximately 3 per cent of patients present with a metastasis from a cancer where the primary site is not known after full history, physical examination, blood count, and chest radiograph. This clinical situation requires considerable clinical expertise, as the diagnosis creates especial anxiety for the patient. The clinician has to decide on the most effective therapy and to sustain the patient without indulging in futile, invasive, and expensive investigations which will not alter management. The problem with extensive investigations is that they seldom alter management and the overall prognosis in this position is poor (4 to 6 months median survival). As one investigation after another fails to reveal the primary site, the patient and the doctor may come to consider this a failure and confidence can be badly shaken. Nevertheless, some tumours are potentially curable, and for these investigation is justified. The common primary sites, when one is discovered, are cancers of the lung, pancreas, liver, gut, and stomach. The tumours for which therapy is

Table 7 *Metastasis from an unknown primary site. Possibilities for treatment*

Potentially curable tumours
germ cell tumours
lymphomas
trophoblastic tumours
Effective palliative chemotherapy
breast cancer
small cell lung cancer
ovarian cancer
Palliative hormonal therapy
prostate cancer
breast cancer
endometrial cancer
Effective (potentially curative) local therapy
head and neck cancer

possible, and which therefore must not be overlooked, are listed in Table 7.

Presentation

If the presentation is exclusively in cervical nodes, a full ear, nose, and throat examination is mandatory as local treatment with surgery and/or radiation may produce prolonged survival or even cure. The higher the cervical node, the more likely it is that and ear, nose, and throat tumour is the primary source. Supraclavicular lymph nodes carry a worse prognosis because the likely primary site on the right-hand side is the lung or breast, and on the left-hand side intra-abdominal malignancy via the thoracic duct. Patients presenting with lymph node enlargement in the axilla are likely to have breast cancer as the primary site and this may not be excluded even with normal mammograms. Malignant melanoma is another possibility at this site and a careful examination for skin lesions should be made. Inguinal lymph nodes usually point to a primary site in the pelvis, vulva or rectum, or prostate. Malignant melanoma may present with an inguinal mass. Cutaneous metastasis typically occurs from carcinomas of the lung, breast, and melanomas. A pulmonary metastasis may arise from a variety of different sites, including breast, kidney, gut, melanoma, and sarcoma. In the liver, the likely source for the primary will be the gastrointestinal tract, although breast and lung primaries are other possibilities. A metastasis presenting in bone is particularly likely to occur from a cancer of the lung, breast or prostate, the last being particularly likely if there is a mixed lytic and osteoblastic appearance.

Investigation

The most important single investigation is a review of the histology. The clinician should discuss the situation with the pathologist so that appropriate tests can be carried out. It is absolutely essential to distinguish between an epithelial tumour, a sarcoma, and a lymphoma. Immunohistochemistry may be invaluable in this respect. If there is any question of a germ cell tumour the section should be stained for α-fetoprotein, β-human chorionic gonadotrophin (β-hCG), and placental alkaline phosphatase. If the histology is that of adenocarcinoma, the diagnosis will be more difficult and special stains may not serve to elucidate the diagnosis further. Where possible the tissue should be examined for the presence of oestrogen or progesterone receptor, as this would make carcinoma of the breast or ovary more likely. The protein S100 is typically present in melanoma and may be invaluable in distinguishing this diagnosis from anaplastic carcinoma.

Further investigation and management

Investigation must be selective. As there is specific treatment available for breast and prostate cancer, these diagnoses must always be considered when the histology is adenocarcinoma. Mammography is therefore justifiable, and measurement of serum acid phosphatase and prostatic specific antigen are simple and non-invasive. A pelvic ultrasound may show an ovarian mass, which may influence management as platinum-based combination chemotherapy might then be used, whereas it would not be contemplated in many patients with metastasis from an unknown primary site in view of its toxicity. The possibility of a germ cell tumour must always be considered in a young person, and in these circumstances full investigation is necessary if this diagnosis is possible.

Treatment follows pragmatic lines. Locally troublesome or painful metastases are treated with irradiation. If breast cancer seems a possible diagnosis a trial of hormone therapy is fully justified and, similarly, hormone treatment of prostatic cancer should be introduced if this seems a likely diagnosis. As mentioned above, radiation is frequently given to patients with enlarged cervical nodes when the diagnosis is poorly-differentiated carcinoma, even if a head and neck primary has not been found.

The use of combination chemotherapy when the primary site is not known is much more controversial. In general, responses are infrequent and are not long lasting. This drug treatment should be reserved for patients with more than one lesion and particularly when symptoms occur. It is important not to be dogmatic about this issue because many patients find it quite unacceptable to be told that no treatment of any kind is available to them, and are willing to accept the possible toxicities of chemotherapy in exchange for the chance of response. Most chemotherapy programmes will include an alkylating agent and some include doxorubicin, although this last drug has the disadvantage of hair loss.

Supportive care of the cancer patient (see also Section 32)

PSYCHOLOGICAL SUPPORT

All clinicians should be aware that patients do have a life outside the consulting room! They will all have had friends or relatives who have had cancer and who may have died of it, and they will have read articles and seen television programmes about cancer and its management. Many patients will have been worried about the possibility of cancer before they ever consult their general practitioner, or are subjected to a series of diagnostic tests, the effect of which may be to increase their anxiety. At each stage in the diagnostic process physicians should be aware of patients' feelings and be prepared to talk openly to them about why investigations are being performed. When the diagnosis is established it is essential for the physician to sit quietly with the patient, explaining the nature of the diagnosis and the broad principles that treatment will follow. Sometimes patients will like to have a member of the family with them during this conversation, in case they forget aspects of what is said. The conversation should take place quietly, not on a ward round, with both the patient and the physician seated and the physician calm and unhurried in their approach. Avoidance of the word 'cancer', body language that indicates discomfiture or embarrassment, evasion, and vagueness, are very likely to be interpreted by the patient as signs of a serious or hopeless outlook.

Many patients will be unable to take in all that is said in the first conversation, and the physician needs to make it quite plain that he or she will be very pleased to talk again the next day, to go over points that need further clarification. There is much useful literature for the patient to take home, there are professional and expert support groups that the patient can contact and, in many hospitals, skilled counsellors who can provide follow-up support after the physician has outlined the basis of treatment. It is essential that all members of the medical team understand what was said and what words were used. The members of the family also need to understand exactly what information has been imparted. It may be necessary to hold back on a precise prognosis, first, because one may not be known until treatment starts, and second, because patients tend to become fixated on the numerical prognosis, which is likely to be extremely inaccurate. If referral to an oncologist is to be made it is important to indicate exactly what has been said to the patient. Oncologists are put in an extremely difficult position when patients arrive with a diagnosis of cancer, without any indication at all of whether they know the diagnosis, or what words have been used.

When treatment is to be palliative, after relapse, or with widespread metastatic disease, it should none the less be made clear to the patient that it is 'treatment'. Patients dislike feeling that they are being abandoned. Indeed, many oncologists see their patients more frequently when they are having palliative treatment than they do during routine treatments or follow up. This is because palliative treatment requires extreme attention to detail, both with respect to control of pain and other symptoms, and also to provide psychological support for the patient and the family. One of the most common reasons for patients seeking second opinions is that they have been given no feeling that there are possibilities for treatment in their case. Continuity in management is one of the most rewarding aspects of cancer medicine both for the physician and for the patient. There is no place for impersonal clinics where patients see different doctors each time they attend, and where the emotional component of their illness cannot be properly explored.

MANAGEMENT OF CANCER PAIN

Pain is a common and distressing feature of cancer. It is usually due to local infiltration of soft tissues or bone, often involving entrapment of a nerve. A careful history is essential to determine the exact site and nature of the pain and to establish a close and trusting relationship with a patient who feels that the symptom is being taken seriously. Exacerbating factors should be noted and an anatomical diagnosis made as far as possible. If the pain is arising in a bone it may be quickly and effectively helped by radiation treatment. The primary tumour or metastasis may be responsive to treatment with irradiation or chemotherapy. If specific antitumour treatments of this kind are not appropriate then the only approach is to control the pain with analgesics.

Non-narcotic analgesics are used for mild or moderate pain. Useful agents include aspirin, paracetamol, and non-steroidal anti-inflammatory drugs such as ketoprofen or naproxen. A combination may be useful. Combination drugs such as co-proxamol or co-dydramol are also helpful. Although prescribing each drug separately allows greater control over the constituents, in practice this may not be helpful, particularly for elderly patients who often find it difficult to take multiple medication. The aim of treatment should be to prevent pain as far as possible by taking regular analgesics, and to have additional analgesics on hand for an acute exacerbation. Side-effects of non-opiate analgesics include gastric irritation (and they should therefore be used cautiously if steroids are being used as the same time), nausea, and constipation, particularly with codeine, oxycodone, or propoxyphene.

If these analgesics do not control the pain, opiate analgesics are essential. Two preparations have made an enormous contribution to pain relief. The first is long-acting morphine sulphate, which can be given twice daily, and the second is short-acting morphine sulphate (sevredol). The former has a duration of action of 8 to 12 h and the latter of about 4 h. One curious feature of the use of morphine-like drugs is that the dose required to control pain varies greatly from person to person. It must therefore be found by trial and error and the patient must be prepared to increase the dose under medical supervision. The aim is to produce background pain relief for most of the day and night. Sevredol is particularly useful for dealing with acute exacerbations of pain.

If oral opiates are unable to control pain fully, continuous subcutaneous infusion is a useful alternative. This approach is particularly valuable in patients who cannot tolerate oral analgesics because of gastrointestinal symptoms, or where the tumour causes nausea or intestinal obstruction. Many pumps are now available, which are designed for continuous infusion through a small gauge butterfly needle implanted subcutaneously. Patients can manage at home with these infusion pumps, with a nurse calling daily to change the infusion mixture.

Specialized forms of analgesia

A detailed discussion is beyond the scope of this chapter. Amongst the specialized techniques available are continuous epidural and intrathecal opiode infusion, nerve block procedures (including coeliac plexus block, peripheral nerve block and epidural blocks), neurosurgical procedures, such as ablation of the peripheral nerve by neurectomy or, more radically, interruption of pain pathways by cordotomy. Each of these procedures has its value and limitations and the advice of specialists in the field of pain relief will be necessary.

REFERENCES

deVita, V.T., Hellman, S., and Rosenberg, S.A. (1993). *Cancer: Principles and practice of oncology*, 4th edn. Lippincott, Philadelphia.

Souhami, R.L. and Tobias, J.S. (1994). *Cancer and its management*, 2nd edn. Blackwell, Oxford.

Tobias, J.S. and Williams, C.J. (1991). *Cancer: A colour atlas*. Gower, London.

6.7 Role of radiotherapy in the treatment of cancer

A. Horwich

INTRODUCTION

Radiotherapy has been used to treat cancer since the early years of the twentieth century. It may be toxic to normal as well as malignant tissue, but therapeutic benefit can be achieved by fractionation of the dose and by accurate spatial localization. Clinical radiotherapy is based on three supporting subjects – imaging, medical physics, and radiobiology. Computer tomographic scanning and, more recently, magnetic resonance imaging have greatly improved the accurate staging of tumour extent and also the localization of tumours within the body contour. These advances over the last two decades have been accompanied by a corresponding increase in the sophistication of radiotherapy treatment machines, which are able to deliver a high dose accurately to a localized, irregular target volume of tissue.

Radiation biology has a long history dating from observations at the beginning of this century, when the anatomist Regaud first showed selectivity of radiotherapy for a particular cell type. During experiments on irradiated rams' testes he was able to demonstrate a greater cytotoxicity in spermatogonia than in spermatozoa, which was attributed to an increased sensitivity of cycling cells. This led to a proposal that radiation of cancers be protracted, and in the 1920s Coutard transformed this concept into fractionated radiotherapy and reported successful treatment of tumours of the head and neck. Detailed studies correlating dose of radiation, number of fractions of treatment and overall treatment time allowed the derivation of formulae to make adjustments for differences in overall treatment times. More recently it has been appreciated that these formulae need to be adjusted for individual tissues and tumours, if accurate prediction either of normal tissue tolerance or of tumour control is to be achieved for a particular radiotherapy prescription. Although at present the dose prescription for a particular tumour tends to be based on institutional practice, radiotherapy is entering the era of predictive testing, when treatment will be based on assessment of radiobiological parameters in the individual patient and tumour.

Biological principles underlying radiotherapy

Radiotherapy is conventionally administered in 15 to 35 fractions, delivering one fraction per day and three to five fractions per week. The overall treatment course lasts between 3 and 7 weeks. The biological bases of fractionated radiotherapy are five principles known as the 'Rs' of radiobiology:

1. *Radiosensitivity.* This refers to the intrinsic radiosensitivity of cells, thought to be based on the extent of damage caused by a particular dose of radiotherapy. The major target for this damage is nuclear DNA and it is thought that the critical lesion for cytotoxicity is a double-strand-break.
2. *Repair of sublethal damage.* It can be shown both by biochemical assay and by studies of cell survival that considerable recovery can occur within the first 6 h after a single dose of radiation. Thus if a second fraction of radiotherapy is given in less than this time there will be an increased risk of tissue damage; this may be a particular problem for spinal cord where repair times are longer.
3. *Repopulation.* Replenishment by stem cells is a source of treatment resistance in tumours and is a protective mechanism in normal tissue, especially epithelial tissues. The longer the overall course of radiotherapy the more replenishment can occur and the ideal overall treatment time would be based on knowledge of the proliferative capacity of the tumour and the treated normal tissues.
4. *Reoxygenation.* It can be shown in laboratory experiments that hypoxic cells are approximately three times more resistant to a dose of radiation than are well-oxygenated cells. This is particularly relevant to tumours because their blood supplies are usually poorly organized, with large areas of inadequate vascularity. In contrast, the majority of normal tissue have a tissue architecture designed to ensure high oxygenation. Thus hypoxia may be a cause of tumour radiation resistance. It is envisaged that an initial fraction of radiotherapy would lead to cytotoxicity in the well-oxygenated part of a tumour, leaving the remainder in a relatively radioresistent stage. It is therefore the timing of reoxygenation of this remaining tumour that may determine the sensitivity to fractionated radiotherapy.
5. *Reassortment.* Cellular sensitivity to irradiation varies in different phases of the cell cycle. Thus the cells in phases G2 or M are radiosensitive, whereas those in S phase are considerably more resistant. Protraction of radiation may allow cells to move from a more resistant to a more radiosensitive phase of the cell cycle.

Differences between the magnitude and kinetics of these radiobiological processes in tumours and in normal tissues contribute to the therapeutic ratio achieved by radiotherapy. Repair of radiation damage between fractions and repopulation both reduce the cytotoxicity of radiotherapy, whereas processes of reoxygenation and of cell cycle reassortment increase cytotoxicity. Knowledge of these principles has led to a variety of areas of research in radiotherapy, such as the use of hyperbaric oxygen or of hypoxic cell radiosenitizing drugs to mitigate the effects of tumour hypoxia. Radiotherapy using neutron beams rather than X-rays or gamma-rays has been investigated because this form of radiotherapy is less sensitive to the oxygenation status of the irradiated cells and also allows less repair. Clinical experience of these approaches has not thus far been encouraging.

Current trials involve two forms of altered fractionation regimens. Accelerated fractionation is based on the shortening of the overall treatment time in order to reduce the possibility of tumour stem cell repopulation. The overall time reduction is achieved by giving two or three fractions per day instead of only one fraction per day. Hyperfractionation is a different form of altered fractionation in which a very small fraction size is employed, because this has a sparing effect on the possibility of long-term radiation damage, and thus allows a modest degree of total dose escalation. As a smaller fraction size is employed, many more fractions are required to give the same total dose of treatment and, in order to avoid making the treatment time very long, these small fractions are also given more than once per day. Both of these altered fractionation approaches have shown some encouraging results in trials, but their place in oncology has not been firmly established. It seems likely that the correct choice of fractionation should be based on measurement of individual tumour characteristics, such as the capacity for rapid proliferation, which would suggest the use of an accelerated fractionation regimen.

Physical principles and treatment planning

The purpose of radiation treatment planning is to deliver radiation selectively to a defined tissue volume. Within this volume the radiation dose should be homogeneous, or otherwise 'peak' doses will increase the risk of normal tissue damage and 'trough' doses may allow survival of cancer cells. The tissue that the radiotherapist designates to be treated is termed the target volume and is defined by the following factors:

1. *Tumour stage and type.* Some tumours, such as carcinoma of the prostate, tend to extend along nerves, whereas others such as head and neck cancers or Hodgkin's disease tend to spread to adjacent lymph node areas. It is important to consider whether the target volume should include these areas. However, increasing the target volume also will reduce the dose of radiation that normal tissue can tolerate.
2. *Tumour localization.* Superficial tumours can often be located accurately by visual inspection or palpation; more deep-seated tumours need to be pinpointed within the body in relationship to a superficial mark, such as bony landmark or, preferably, a medical pinprick tattoo. The most accurate form of localization of the tumour within an axial body outline is based on computer tomographic scanning and radiation planning computers can now be linked directly to computer tomography images (Fig. 1).

Fig. 1 Three-field radiation isodose plan for treatment of a patient with bladder cancer, displayed directly on axial computer tomograph through the centre of the target volume.

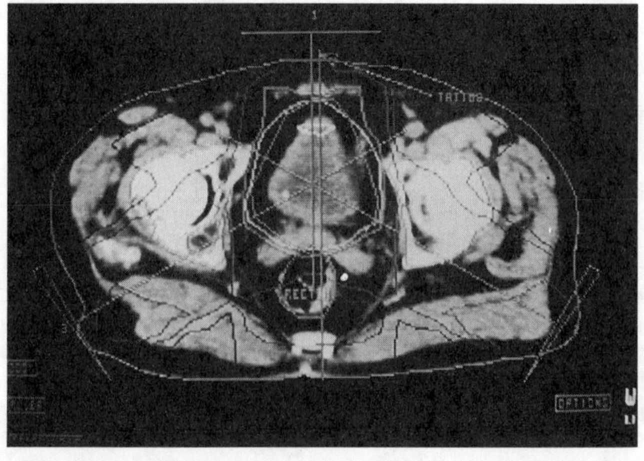

3. *Adjacent normal structures.* The dose of radiotherapy that can be tolerated is determined by normal tissues within the irradiated volume. Normal tissue damage can be severe and chronic and, as some tissues are more sensitive than others, it is necessary to be aware of the dose received by each tissue within the radiation fields. For example, the spinal cord may be close to the target volume in the treatment of head and neck tumours, or of intrathoracic tumours. It may be desired to treat the tumour to a dose of 60 Gy in 30 fractions over 6 weeks, but it is known that doses to the spinal cord of more than 45 Gy may be associated with a risk of radiation myelitis and consequent paraplegia. The arrangement of radiation fields and the dose delivered from each field must be designed to allow the required tumour dose while avoiding overdose to the spinal cord.

Therefore, the process of radiotherapy planning must identify accurately and reproducibly an exact target volume within the patient for each fraction of radiotherapy with which the patient is treated. The following considerations are important for accuracy:

1. *Patient positioning and immobilization.* Stable positioning can often be achieved by the use of cushions, but for more critical sites, such as treatment of brain, or head and neck tumours, a perspex shell is made individually for each patient. The cast of the appropriate area is taken using a fast-setting dental alginate, which is then filled with plaster. The plaster reproduction is then used to make a perspex shell that can be fitted around the appropriate part of the patient and then clipped to the radiotherapy treatment couch.
2. *Beam alignment and localization.* The position of the patient in relation to the treatment machine is achieved by fixed laser lights in the treatment room. To facilitate accurate initial positioning of the radiation beam the skin is usually tattooed vertically above the center of the target volume. In an 'isocentric set-up' the axis of rotation of the radiotherapy machine is centred in the middle of the target volume, such that any rotation of the radiation machine head will align the beam through the centre of the target volume. Alternatively, the alignment of the radiation beam can be checked by front and back pointers along the axis of the beam, which can be aligned with entry and exit marks.

For deep-seated tumours the target volume is defined radiologically. In the past this involved the use of orthogonal radiographs with radio-opaque rulers placed within the field to allow calculation of magnification factors. The modern alternative is to plan directly on a computer tomographic scan, which gives the overall outline of the patient, together with the organs and tumour volumes. The radiotherapist can identify the target volume directly on an axial slice image using a light-pen on the computer monitor and at the same time can identify critical normal structures. A computer-assisted calculation of the radiation distribution then allows a variety of combinations of field direction and number size to be tested to find the optimal arrangement. A range of technical modifications to the radiation beam might improve the distribution, such as, for example, of the insertion of a 'wedge' to change the distribution of radiation from a single beam.

RADIATION PLANNING

This is usually carried out on a specially constructed diagnostic X-ray machine termed a treatment simulator, which is designed to mimic the geometry of a radiotherapy treatment machine. The patient is positioned on the simulator couch and the simulator is set-up in a fashion identical to that proposed for treatment. The ability of the simulator to take good quality diagnostic X-rays allows the treatment plan to be checked in advance without using valuable time on the treatment machine (Fig. 2).

TREATMENT

The patient is placed in exactly the same position on the treatment couch as defined during the planning procedure on the treatment simulator. A light-beam from the treatment machine aids positioning and is usually centred on the pin-prick skin tattoo used to mark the field centre during treatment simulation. Usually, having set up the initial position of the radiotherapy machine in relationship to the patient, a series of treatment fields can then be treated and with a modern linear accelerator actual treatment times are usually less than 5 min per fraction.

Radiation practice

TYPES OF MEDICAL RADIATIONS

X-rays

The usual radiation used for therapy is provided by X-rays from a linear accelerator, although tissues close to the skin surface can be treated with X-rays from a much similar lower energy apparatus.

Gamma-rays

These are generated from some isotopes such as cobalt-60. A telecobalt apparatus is used in a manner somewhat similar to a linear accelerator.

Electron beams

This form of particle radiotherapy is available either from specialized radiotherapy machine or from high energy linear accelerators. Electrons are particularly useful in some circumstances because there is a relatively sharp reduction of dose beyond a certain depth in the tissue, the depth being defined by the electron energy.

Neutron irradiation

This form of particle radiotherapy is little used nowadays because it is extremely expensive and there is little evidence of any improvement compared with conventional X-rays.

Brachytherapy

This is the delivery of radiotherapy by placing radioactive sources close to the tumour. As the dose distribution close to a source is determined

Fig. 2 Simulator radiograph used in planning parallel opposed anterior and posterior fields to para-aortic and ipsilateral pelvic lymph nodes following right orchidectomy for stage I seminoma. The hatched areas represent lead blocks, and the circles are aligned on pinprick skin tattoos.

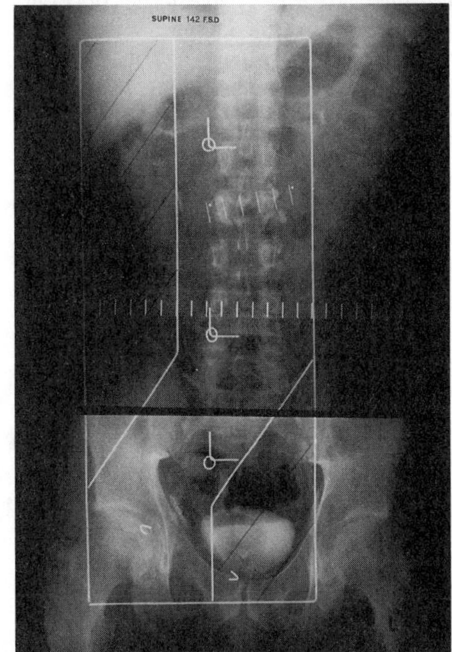

by the inverse square law, very little radiation affects tissues at any distance from the radioactive source. Therefore, when it is possible to use brachytherapy, a very confined radiation distribution is achieved. Iridium-192 wires, iodine-125 seeds, and caesium-137 have replaced radium for staff safety reasons, and occasionally cobalt-60 is employed for rapid brachytherapy treatments. The most common example of brachytherapy is in the insertion of sources next to the cervix and into the uterine cavity for cancer of these sites. To avoid accidental exposure of staff, techniques have been designed to allow the emplacement of small catheters adjacent to the tumours. These can be inserted into the correct position, adjusted, and checked without the need for radiation protection, as the actual radioactive source is transmitted along the tubes subsequently, a technique termed 'afterloading'.

Systemic radioisotopes

Some unsealed isotopes can be used for systemic therapy. An example is iodine-131, which is concentrated in thyroid tissue and can be used in the treatment of differentiated thyroid cancers. Similarly strontium-89 is taken up in areas of bone formation and is used in the treatment of widespread bone metastases, especially those from carcinoma of the prostate, which are known to be associated frequently with an osteoblastic reaction. Both metabolic and antibody targeting of radiation isotopes are being investigated as methods to achieve selective radiation.

RADIATION DOSE

The dose of radiation is defined in terms of energy deposited per unit mass (1 Gy = 1 J per kg). In the past the standard unit of radiotherapy was 1 rad, and 1 Gy = 100 rads. A conventional curative dose of external beam radiotherapy would be to administer 55 to 65 Gy in fractions of 1.6 to 2.5 Gy, five times per week over a time period of 4 to 6 weeks. Some radiosensitive tumours, such as Hodgkin's disease or seminoma, require lower doses over a shorter period of time. For palliative radiotherapy where relief of symptoms requires only a moderate degree of tumour cell kill, a single dose of 6 to 8 Gy often suffices, or in some cases slightly higher doses given in five to ten fractions over 1 to 2 weeks.

There is no international consensus on the ideal radiotherapy prescription for a particular tumour type. A number of prescriptions are in current use based either on the principle of administering a high dose which requires multiple fractions over relatively long time period (for example 64 Gy in 32 fractions over 6½ weeks) or, alternatively, on the principles of short treatment time and relatively large fraction (for example 52 Gy in 15 fractions over 3 weeks). In some settings these approaches are clearly equivalent in terms of tumour cure rates and risk of normal tissue complication, but in other sites there is considerable controversy and it is likely in the future that an appropriate prescription will be based on assessments of the individual tumour rather than institutional practice.

RADIATION TOXICITY

The side-effects of radiotherapy are usually divided into acute side-effects, occurring during or soon after the course of radiotherapy, and late side-effects, occurring 6 months or more after radiotherapy has been completed. Acute side-effects are usually transient and thus late side-effects, representing permanent loss of function, are usually clinically more serious and are thus dose-limiting. Although some patients describe rather general side-effects such as tiredness, the majority of normal tissue effects relate entirely to the tissues within the treated area. Tables 1 and 2 list a number of radiation side-effects and it can be seen that there is a range in the sensitivity of normal tissue to radiation. It should be emphasized that the risk of normal tissue damage, especially late side-effects, is dependent upon the fraction size at any particular dose of radiotherapy. The figures in Tables 1 and 2 indicating dose thresholds for side-effects are presented for simplicity, assuming that radiation is given at 2 Gy per fraction, and present the dosage at which less than 5 per cent of patients would be predicted to have a side-effect.

Table 1 *Acute toxicity of radiotherapy*

Organ	Toxicity	Timing*
Stomach	Nausea	1 h
Pharynx and bowel	Mucositis and ulceration	2 weeks
Skin	Erythema and desquamation	2–3 weeks
Bladder	Cystitis	3–4 weeks
Central nervous system	Somnolence	1–2 months
Lung	Pneumonitis	2–4 months

*From start of radiotherapy.

Table 2 *Late side-effects of radiotherapy*

Organ	Effects	Threshold dose (Gy)*
Lens	Cataract	5
Kidney	Nephritis/atrophy	15
Lung	Fibrosis	20
Spinal cord	Paraplegia	45
Bowel	Stricture	50–60
Bladder	Contracture	60
Skin	Atrophy/telangiectasia	50+
Limb	Oedema	50+*

*Assumes 2 Gy daily fractions.

It can be seen from Table 1 that acute side-effects are usually caused by transient loss of integrity of an epithelial lining. These can be mitigated by anti-inflammatory drugs such as steroids; however, it is also important to prevent secondary infection. A brief period of inpatient supportive care may be required in severe cases.

Late side-effects represent partial or total organ failure, depending upon the proportion of the critical normal organ within the high dose irradiation volume. These are usually not reversible. When radiation doses are taken close to the levels of normal tissue tolerance it is important to exclude as much normal tissue as possible from the high dose volume.

Clinical roles of radiotherapy

RADICAL THERAPY

Radiotherapy may be used as the sole curative modality of treatment of some cancers (radical radiotherapy) and, as shown in Table 3, this role is especially important in early cancers of the head and neck, cervix, vagina, anal canal, bladder, and prostate. Lower doses of radiation are sufficient to cure early Hodgkin's disease and testicular seminoma. Although radiotherapy is used in the attempted cure of some more common cancers, such as lung cancer, in practice it is rare for inoperable cases to be sufficiently small to be cured by radiotherapy. It should be appreciated that although the results in Table 3 are of local control, survival may be much lower due to metastatic recurrence. For example, in T3 cancers of the prostate, 5-year local control can be achieved in 75 per cent of patients, but within the same time period 50 per cent will have suffered metastatic relapse in lymph nodes on the skeleton. In cancer of the oesophagus, approximately 10 per cent of patients are cured; the results of radiotherapy are somewhat similar to those of surgery.

Table 3 *Examples of radical radiotherapy results*

Local tumour control at 5 years (%)	Cancer sites				
	Head and neck	Gynaecology	Urology	Lymphoma and skin	Lung
100			Seminoma (II)		
	Larynx (T1/2)	Cervic (I)		Basal cell carcinoma Hodgkin's disease Non-Hodgkin's lymphoma Squamous carcinoma	
			Prostate (T1/2)		
80	Oral cavity and tongue (T1/2)	Vagina (I)			
			Prostate (T3) Bladder (T2)		
	Nasopharynx	Cervix (II)			
60					
		Vagina (II)			
	Larynx (T3/4)		Bladder (T3)		
40					
		Cervix (III)			
	Tongue (T3/4)				Squamous or adenocarcinoma (T1–T3)
20					
0					

Stage in parentheses.

ADJUVANT THERAPY

As surgical failure often occurs at the margin of excised tumour, radiotherapy can improve both local control rates and also can allow a more limited surgical procedure thus reducing the morbidity of cure. Results are illustrated in Table 4; as discussed previously, success may be compromised by metastatic recurrence and, in breast cancer, for example, it is unclear that radiotherapy influences survival at all. Radiotherapy is often used preoperatively, when it may reduce the size and extent of an otherwise inoperable tumour; however, it is more commonly employed postoperatively, when the full pathological extent and grading of tumour is available. Adjuvant radiotherapy reduces local recurrence rates following conservative treatment of breast cancer, and following resection of rectal cancers, soft tissue sarcomas, and some brain tumours, such as medulloblastoma.

In some settings radiotherapy is used as an adjuvant to chemotherapy. For example, in acute lymphoblastic leukaemia the blood–brain barrier limits access of chemotherapy to the central nervous system, and prophylactic cranial irradiation (PCI) of patients in remission greatly reduces the risk of meningeal relapse and has been shown to improve survival. Also in the treatment of myeloid leukaemia, whole body irradiation is employed prior to bone marrow transplantation.

PALLIATIVE RADIOTHERAPY

It has been estimated that approximately 25 per cent of radiotherapy resources are used in the palliation of incurable malignant disease. The most common indication is the relief of pain from bone metastases, where radiotherapy is effective in all histological types of tumour. As the prognosis of patients with widespread malignancy is so poor, palliative radiotherapy should be administered as quickly and simply as possible and, in practice, it is rare to employ more than ten fractions and for most patients with bone pain a single fraction of treatment is sufficient. As with all radiotherapy treatments, accurate localization of the metastases causing a particular symptom is important to ensure that treatment is appropriate and effective.

Palliative radiotherapy is required urgently in a number of other settings such as a superior vena caval obstruction from non-small-cell lung cancer or other solid tumours. For some tumours such as lymphomas, small cell lung cancer, or mediastinal germ cell tumour, urgent chemotherapy is an alternative approach.

Spinal cord compression

This is one of the most distressing complications of malignant disease and, as recovery of mobility is related to duration of symptoms, the clinical suspicion of cord compression should lead to urgent assessment and treatment. Radiotherapy is usually the treatment of choice, especially in the presence of widespread metastatic disease. However, for patients with localized cord compression from a previously undiagnosed tumour, or in patients who have had previous radiotherapy to the site of compression or who have tumours that respond poorly to radiation, such as adenocarcincomas of the lung or bowel or renal cell cancers, surgical decompression is an alternative approach.

Table 4 *Radiotherapy combined with surgery: results*

Local control at 5 years (%)	Cancer sites			
	Head and neck	Breast cancer	Gastrointestinal tract	Sarcoma
100				
		Breast cancer (T1/2)	Rectum (B/C)	
				Limb sarcoma
80	Node metastases			
		Breast cancer (T3)		
				Limb girdle sarcoma
60				
	T3 tumours			
				Trunk sarcoma
		Oesophagus		
40				
20				
0				

Early radiotherapy for cord compression allows about 60 per cent of patients to retain mobility and self-dependence; however, it is rare for patients who have complete paralysis to achieve sufficient recovery to be mobile.

Multidisciplinary care

As with all aspects of cancer management, radiotherapy should be considered in conjunction with medical, surgical, and psychosocial supportive measures with consideration for the needs of the patients and their families. Appropriate initial therapy cures approximately half of all cancers, although the proportion is smaller if skin cancer and *in situ* cancers are excluded. Clinical judgement relating to the balance of treatment with surgery, drugs, or radiation is critical to mitigate long-term toxicity in patients who are cured and to ensure the best quality of life where cure is impossible.

REFERENCES

Horwich, A. (ed) (1992). *Combined radiotherapy and chemotherapy in clinical oncology*. Edward Arnold, London.

Sikora, K. and Halnan, K.E. (1990). *Treatment of cancer*, 2nd edn. Chapman and Hall, London.

Steel, G.G., Adams, G.E. and Horwich, A. (1989). *The biological basis of radiotherapy*, 2nd edn. Elsevier Science, Amsterdam.

6.8 New approaches to cancer therapy

A. L. Harris and J. Carmichael

Introduction

Current treatment of the majority of the common solid tumours remains unsatisfactory. Most tumours present with locally advanced or metastatic disease, making local approaches such as surgery or radiotherapy unlikely to result in cure or long-term remission. Major advances have been achieved in the systemic treatment of germ cell tumours, lymphomas, and leukaemias, but there has been less success with the common solid tumours, such as lung cancer, breast cancer, and colorectal cancer.

As a result of advances, particularly in molecular biology, there has been an enormous increase in our understanding of malignant growth and metastasis. As the mechanisms relating to transformation; local invasion and metastasis; escape from immunological surveillance; and resistance to drug, hormone, or radiation therapy have become defined, a wide range of new approaches to treatment has been produced, including the identification of many new rational therapeutic targets. It has also become apparent that there are multiple mechanisms at each step of the process involved in tumour progression. We have attempted below to highlight areas where there are clinical trials planned or in progress against these new targets. This should provide a basis for understanding future drug development and how these therapies may be added to, or substitute for existing therapies.

Prognostic factors and tumour markers

There is wide variability in outcome for patients with the same tumour type. Some of this can be related to expression of different oncogenes or growth factor receptors that may confer a more aggressive phenotype.

Measuring these in the initial tumour biopsy may help select patients for more intensive therapy, which is likely to be of particular benefit in the adjuvant setting. Examples include the epidermal growth factor receptor in bladder and breast cancer and the nuclear oncoprotein p53 in breast cancer. The ability to identify patients at highest risk of relapse and, potentially, patients with the greatest chance of response, would result in more selective use of existing treatments, reducing unnecessary toxicity of these drugs.

Some of the products of oncogenes are released into the circulation. These may be of value in screening and also help in monitoring disease response and the effects of adjuvant therapy when a tumour is not detectable by conventional means. p53 and the external domains of growth factor receptors and cell adhesion molecules are currently being assessed. The polymerase chain reaction has been used recently to detect circulating melanoma cells. This method may be used to detect patients with occult metastasis in the future, although the clinical relevance of such occult metastases would need to be closely monitored.

Agents in current use are more effective when tumour bulk is low, and most of the new therapies are likely to be more effective in this setting.

Advances in cytotoxic drug treatment

Several new anticancer drugs are under development, most aimed at new targets, although still basically interfering with DNA metabolism.

TOPOISOMERASE INHIBITORS

The topoisomerases represent a class of nuclear enzymes that are actively involved in multiple cellular processes, including DNA replication and separation of daughter chromosomes. The topoisomerases can be divided into type I and type II proteins. The type II proteins consist of products of two distinct genes, topo IIα and topo 2β.

Type II topoisomerases

A number of the currently used cytotoxic drugs have inhibition of topoisomerase II as their major mechanism of action, although many have additional mechanisms. These drugs include epipodophyllotoxins, such as etoposide; anthracyclines, such as doxorubicin; amsacrine derivatives; and the anthrapyrazole group of compounds, including the new agent, CI-941.

These drugs are effective in the treatment of solid tumours; etoposide is one of the most active drugs in lung cancer treatment and doxorubicin is the most active single agent in breast cancer. Unfortunately, resistance to these agents occurs via many biochemical mechanisms, including development of the classic multidrug resistance phenotype, decreased expression of topoisomerase II protein by mutation of its gene and altered phosphorylation status.

Laboratory studies have focused on the mechanisms underlying the development of drug resistance and regulation of gene expression. These investigations, in different tumours and tissues, may help to explain the specificity of the currently available inhibitors for tumours and normal tissues, and will help with the rational design of new inhibitors.

Type I topoisomerases

Inhibitors of topoisomerase I are less widely available, the lead compound being camptothecin, which underwent clinical evaluation many years ago. Although an antitumour effect was seen, clinical studies were not pursued, as unacceptable gastrointestinal toxicity was observed. Recently, new topoisomerase I inhibitors have been developed, and these are under clinical evaluation. Of particular interest, an analogue of camptothecin, 9-aminocamptothecin, has been shown to have significant activity in colon cancer xenografts, an area where inhibitors of topoisomerase II have had minimal impact.

NEW ANTIMETABOLITES

Antimetabolites, as a class of anticancer drugs, have been in use for more than 40 years. Initial work focused on the antifolates, of which methotrexate has been the most widely used. Later, a number of new targets were explored. For instance, agents have been developed to target inhibition of thymidylate synthase. Recently, a deoxycytidine analogue, difluoro-deoxycytidine (gemcitabine), has been developed. This drug is converted to metabolites that inhibit DNA polymerase. Gemcitabine, as a single agent is active in non-small-cell lung cancer and breast cancer.

Modulation of drug resistance

There are many ways by which cancer cells may become resistant to cytotoxic drugs. Early studies focused on the importance of the multidrug resistance phenotype in drug resistance. The *mdr*1 gene has been shown to encode a 170-kDa membrane glycoprotein, which functions as an energy dependent efflux pump for a number of cytotoxic drugs. A number of drugs have been shown to modify the activity of this glycoprotein, the first of which were the calcium-channel blockers, such as verapamil, although toxicity prevented the attainment of clinically relevant levels known to modify resistance *in vitro*. Subsequently, other modifiers have been identified, including calmodulin antagonists, progestagens, anti-oestrogens, and immunosuppressant drugs such as cyclosporin A. It is possible to achieve clinically relevant levels of these drugs, particularly anti-oestrogens.

The major problem with modifiers of multidrug resistance relates to normal tissue expression of *p*-glycoprotein. This protein is expressed highly in renal tubules and biliary canaliculi in particular, which is important because inhibition of this protein could lead to alteration in pharmacokinetics of many cytotoxic drugs.

New drug targets

INHIBITORS OF SIGNAL TRANSDUCTION AND SECOND MESSENGER SYSTEMS

Overexpression of growth factor receptors, and mutations in *ras* and in G proteins regulating adenylate cyclase, all lead to increased intracellular signalling by second messenger systems. These include protein kinase C and cyclic-AMP-dependent protein kinase, which make potentially selective targets for therapy. There is extensive *in vitro* and *in vivo* experimental work demonstrating that cyclic AMP analogues can selectively inhibit tumour growth with little normal tissue toxicity. They appear to increase the activity in a particularly regulatory subunit, RIIb, which may have an intranuclear regulatory role in cell growth. Phase I clinical studies are now starting with the compound 8-chlorocyclic AMP.

Phase I trials using a novel compound, bryostatin, which can antagonize activation of protein kinase C, are ongoing. Several agents of this kind are being developed.

Tyrosine kinases are another major target because many, when inappropriately activated, have a transforming role. The epidermal growth factor receptor, IGF1 receptor, and erbB-2 are kinases for which there have been attempts to obtain selective inhibitors. Most so far have been tyrosine analogues and it may be possible to distinguish between the kinases.

ANGIOGENESIS

Angiogenesis has become a major target for therapy following the pioneering work of Judah Folkman. It is an essential step in tumour growth, as tumours cannot grow above approximately 2 mm^3 without developing a new blood supply. This also opens up the route for metastasis, and several studies have shown a poor prognosis and high metastasis rate in tumours with focal areas of high vascularization. Normal endothelial cells have an extremely low rate of turnover, approximately once in 10 years. Thus, targeting rapidly proliferating endothelium in tumours should provide differential toxicity to tumours. A range of approaches are being studied, including antibodies to proliferating endothelium, suramin analogues and two new classes of agents, angioinhibins and collagenase inhibitors.

This type of approach may be used in combination with hypoxically activated drugs. The latter are a group of drugs that are activated under reducing conditions to generate toxic metabolites that can bind to DNA and generate strand breaks.

RECEPTOR TARGETING

Inhibition of second messenger systems has been discussed, but the external domain of the receptors provides another target. Recombinant DNA methodology allows large scale preparation of the ligand alone, or as a fusion protein with another molecule. This provides high specificity and affinity for targeting the active anticancer agent. Examples of high receptor expression providing targets include the interleukin-6 receptor in myeloma, interleukin-2 receptor in lymphomas and c-erbB-2 or the epidermal growth factor receptor in breast cancer. The toxins providing the anticancer component of the fusion proteins include diphtheria and pseudomonas exotoxin. Animal models have shown a differential effect against tumours compared to normal tissues and phase I studies have started in bladder cancer.

NEW DEVELOPMENTS IN MONOCLONAL ANTIBODIES

As the problems of using monoclonal antibodies have emerged, new strategies have been developed. One is to use much smaller molecules, single chain proteins comprising variable heavy and light chains, to enhance access to tumours with a poor vasculature. Another is to use two-step strategies allowing the first antibody to localize for several days. A second binding protein, which recognizes the first and which has the therapeutic agent attached, is then administered. An example of this approach is to have biotin on the first antibody and streptavidin as the second protein. Allowing time for the first antibody to bind and for non-specific binding to clear greatly enhances the tumour/normal tissue ratio when the second protein is used. Humanizing antibodies may present antibody responses against existing monoclonals that are murine.

Although there is much interest in using toxins such as ricin or gelonin attached to antibodies, other approaches are under development. One of these is antibody dependent enzyme prodrug therapy (ADEPT). In this case, the toxin is generated by an enzyme attached to the antibody from a non-toxic precursor. A non-human enzyme is used. This has the advantage of producing a cytotoxic drug locally that will be active against tumour cells that have not bound the antibody well, and can allow repeated daily doses of the prodrug.

IMMUNOTHERAPY AGAINST TUMOUR ANTIGENS OR MUTANT ONCOGENES

Non-specific immunotherapy with BCG has been ineffective in systemic cancer therapy. However, specifically activated cytotoxic T cells can be very effective in eliminating experimental tumours. There is circumstantial evidence of escape from immunological surveillance in many common cancers. Endogenous antigens are presented by human leucocyte antigen (HLA) class I molecules. In all types of epithelial tumours studied, there is evidence of selective loss of class I human leucocyte antigen alleles. The more comprehensive the studies, the greater the frequency reported. This appears to be a tumour-specific phenomenon and is not due to deletion of the genes. One interpretation is that there are tumour antigens that would allow destruction of tumours at an early stage, but by down regulation of human leucocyte antigen class I molecules they can escape.

Potential antigens include mutant oncogenes that are specific to tumours. Examples include mutant *p53*, mutant H-*ras*, and mutant K-*ras*. If the immunodominant epitopes can be defined, recent advances in vaccine technology may allow immunization against tumours, providing human leucocyte antigen class I molecules could be upregulated. The latter can be carried out *in vivo* in patients with interferons, hence allowing combined therapy.

MOLECULAR TARGETS

Improvements in molecular biological techniques allow for the development of a wide range of new anticancer treatments. These range from the use of antisense oligonucleotides that downregulate mRNA expression, to gene transfer usually via retroviral vectors.

Oligonucleotides

The predominant aim of oligonucleotide therapy is to downregulate expression of important genes that may be overexpressed in cancer cells, such as certain oncogenes. This can be achieved by either using an antisense approach, targeting specific mRNAs, or by an antigene approach aimed at blocking transcription at its genetic location. Oligodeoxynucleotides are used in preference to ribonucleotides as they are more resistant to degradation by ribonucleases. Normally, oligonucleotides of 15 to 20 bases in length are used to combine greatest selectivity with ease of access. For the antisense approach, inhibition of translation is achieved either by degradation of the mRNA by RNase H or by inhibition of binding of ribosomal subunits if the oligonucleotide is targeted to the 5′ untranslated region of the selected mRNA. The antigene approach requires oligonucleotides of around 17 bases to form a triple helix, and various modifications can be included to enhance the stability of the complex. This approach has been used to block *c-myc* transcription.

There are a number of important challenges to overcome before this technology is likely to have significant impact in cancer therapy. The most important include identification of 'tumour-specific targets' and cellular penetration of the oligonucleotides in order to achieve effective intracellular concentrations of the molecules.

Human solid tumours contain multiple genetic defects, including amplification of proto-oncogenes (*c-myc*) point mutations K-*ras* and deletions of growth suppressor genes such as *p53*. Many of these abnormalities can be present in the same tumour, best described in colorectal carcinoma. Although multiple defects may be present in solid tumours, growth inhibition appears feasible targeting only one defect.

Gene therapy (see also Section 4)

There are a number of ways by which foreign DNA material can be transferred into human cells. These include calcium phosphate precipitation, microinjection, and electroporation techniques, although recently attention has focused on the use of viral vectors. There are many potential pitfalls to the latter approach, although it represents the most realistic approach for the stable integration of these sequences into the host genome. The majority of approaches using gene therapy have concentrated on the introduction of material into cells outside of the host, but the potential exists to develop more selective approaches whereby genetic material could be introduced directly into the host. Different routes of administration have been used for in vivo gene transfer.

Gene therapy in cancer patients to date has concentrated on immunomodulating approaches using tumour infiltrating lymphocytes focusing predominantly on malignant melanoma.

Targeting of cytokine genes is potentially achieved by the selective uptake of tumour infiltrating lymphocytes cells back into the tumour. Other targeting approaches utilize the fact that certain genes are transcribed in fetal and malignant tissues that are not transcribed in normal adult tissues. These include α-fetoprotein in hepatomas and germ cell tumours, and carcinoembryonic antigen in a range of adenocarcinomas, particularly colonic tumours. Vectors can thus be constructed using promoters to these particular proteins. It is, however, possible that, by introducing a drug activating enzyme into only a subpopulation of cells, nearby cells can also be killed by transfer of active drug metabolites.

The multiple genetic abnormalities frequently observed in cancer patients does not, at first impression, suggest that gene replacement therapy would be a viable approach. There are many potential pitfalls to overcome before these approaches are likely to be a realistic possibility for cancer patients.

Conclusions

This is not a comprehensive survey of new treatments, but highlights the wide range of new approaches already tested experimentally, either in phase I or planned. These treatments will not replace surgery but proper handling of tumour specimens—collection of fresh tumours and their analysis—will become much more important for optimum therapy. As with existing cancer treatments, combined approaches are most likely to be successful, especially when applied as adjuvants. This will require much larger numbers of patients to be entered in clinical trials. This is a choice that should be available to patients.

REFERENCES

Bicknell, R. and Harris, A.L. (1992). Anticancer strategies involving the vasculature: vascular targeting and the inhibition of angiogenesis. *Seminars in Cancer Biology*, **3**, 399–408.

Cell (1991). Special issue on Oncogenes. *Cell*, **64**, 235–326.

Fearon, E.R. and Vogelstein, B. (1990). A genetic model for colorectal tumorigenesis. *Cell*, **61**, 759–67.

Rosenberg, S.A. (1992). The immunotherapy and gene therapy of cancer. *Journal of Clinical Oncology*, **10**, 180–99.

Section 7 *Infection*

7.1 Clinical approach to the patient with suspected infection

H. P. Lambert

The ecological context

Infectious diseases are among the most prevalent and important causes of ill health throughout the world and at all ages, but viewed in a larger context they are unusual events in the close and generally uneventful relationship between man and the microbial world, a relationship that begins at birth when the normally sterile infant is rapidly colonized by a huge number and variety of micro-organisms

The nature of the encounter between pathogenic organisms and their human host varies greatly from case to case. At one extreme the life of an organism such as *Clostridium tetani* has no connection with man unless the bacterium is implanted at a potentially anaerobic site, when tetanus may develop. By contrast, obligate human pathogens such as measles virus, herpes simplex hominis, *Bacillus pertussis, Vibrio cholerae, Neisseria gonorrhoeae*, and many others have co-evolved with their human hosts, developing highly adapted mechanisms that enable them to attach to their target mucosal surfaces, to survive and multiply at specific sites in the host, to evade host defence systems, and to be transmitted from host to host. Some parasites have evolved two separate life-cycles, in man and in arthropod, with consequent advantages for parasite transmission. Another important group are the zoonoses such as the salmonelloses, brucellosis, and rabies, with their main ecological niche in other animals but with the capacity to cause disease in man. It is often said that the most highly adapted microbial parasites are the least pathogenic, as their advantage lies with a well rather than an ill or dead host. Certainly, a very wide range of organisms, including viruses, bacteria, fungi, and protozoa, are capable of establishing subclinical infection and many organisms can achieve a state of long-term latency in the human host. For some organisms, however, the human illness confers advantage to the parasite by facilitating multiplication and transmission. In the respiratory tract, measles, and in the alimentary tract, cholera, may be cited as examples of this amplification mechanism.

Host and parasite variables both contribute to determine the consequences of infection. Many organisms widespread in the environment, some of them normal human commensals, are able to cause disease only in the presence of some impairment of host defences. Thus, *Staphylococcus epidermidis* rarely causes disease in normal people, but is important as a cause of endocarditis in patients with prosthetic valves, and of infection in cerebrospinal fluid shunts. Many other examples of specific or general immune defects leading to infection could be cited such as *Pneumocystis carinii* in human immunodeficiency virus (**HIV**) infection, disseminated candidiasis and Gram-negative bacillary pneumonia in profound neutropenia, and *Pseudomonas aeruginosa* in burns. Perhaps of more common concern are the 'grey areas' of immune impairment, the infections of infancy and old age, those that complicate many chronic, non-infectious diseases, and host factors in hospital infection. In an evolutionary context, more important still are genetic polymorphisms related to resistance to infection. The advantage conferred by the sickle-cell trait in resistance to *Plasmodium falciparum* is familiar, but other relationships, notably between HLA haplotypes and susceptibility to infection, are now being revealed.

The adaptations undergone by parasites in the course of evolution are also being elucidated, especially among bacteria, which, by virtue of mobile extrachromosomal elements (plasmids and transposons), are able to exhibit great genetic flexibility. One example of this is plain to see in day-to-day clinical practice, the progressive loss of valuable antimicrobial agents by the emergence and spread of resistant strains. The adaptive capacities of bacteria are shown most vividly in the changes they undergo in response to different environmental conditions. Different phenotypic characters may be of optimal survival advantage under the varying environments that bacteria must inhabit in order to survive and to spread. For example the metabolic requirements most suited to the survival of *V. cholerae* in brackish water are unlikely to be the same as those optimal for survival and multiplication in the human gut. Most pathogens possess a number of virulence factors mediating such properties as mucosal attachment and toxin production. The genes controlling these functions are often part of a global regulatory network by which an array of regulatory genes is switched on or off in response to changes in environmental conditions such as temperature or the concentration of various ions. The functional significance of such mechanisms has been clearly shown in infections such as cholera, bacillary dysentery, and pertussis.

The long human generation time makes it difficult to demonstrate directly the mutually adaptive character of host–parasite relationships in the way so clearly achieved for myxomatosis in rabbits, in which the virus has become less virulent and the host more resistant. Nevertheless, much historical evidence, and increasing evidence from studies of the molecular genetics of micro-organisms, indicates that similar processes of co-evolution also take place in man and his pathogens.

The clinical approach

HISTORY

The approach to the patient with a suspected infection generally follows the pattern of any medical consultation, but some points stand out as especially important in the task of amplifying and translating the patient's account to yield fruitful diagnostic hypotheses. One problem, often encountered in history taking, is to reach agreement on the meaning ascribed to various words and phrases in common use. Thus 'fever', 'a virus', 'gastroenteritis', even 'diarrhoea', have surprisingly different connotations for different people. 'I have a fever' may denote a feeling of warmth, a feeling of chilliness, sweating, or perhaps that the body temperature has actually been measured and found to be raised. 'Flu', another word in common use, usually denotes aching muscles and sometimes chills and shivering, but some people use the word for specific respiratory symptoms such as a runny nose or scratchy throat, or for fever. Some words may unwittingly lead to false assumptions on the part of the doctor. Thus, 'gastroenteritis', used to equate with diarrhoea, may lead the unwary to assume an infective illness, whereas diarrhoea and vomiting can, of course, have a host of non-infectious causes.

The history in suspected infection must include a careful 'systems inquiry'. Although the value of this traditional component of the medical history has been questioned, minor system-related clues in a patient with obscure febrile illness may sometimes provide the only localizing evidence. Thus, a half-forgotten episode of abdominal pain may be the first lead to the diagnosis of an intra-abdominal abscess, or a recent dry cough the clue leading to pulmonary tuberculosis or an atypical pneumonia. And, as in all histories, an accurate sense of the timing and duration of symptoms is enormously valuable in pondering the diagnostic possibilities. Perhaps the best example of this is the frequent attribution to, and search for, viral infection in patients with prolonged fever. Certainly many viruses cause prolonged or recurrent illnesses, either directly or by provoking immunopathological processes, but acute fevers of viral origin unaccompanied by other gross features rarely last longer than a few weeks at most, indeed most run their course in less than a week or two. Prolonged fever of uncertain origin is certainly often microbial in origin, but its cause is rarely viral. Although the search for localizing symptoms has been stressed, they may also deceive. Muscle and joint pains are often hard to interpret in a febrile patient, dark urine may denote dehydration of fever rather than liver involvement, and some people suffer headache when they are febrile, so that a neurological cause of their fever may be wrongly supposed. At this stage, many system clues must be assigned a provisional status only.

Travel and occupation are other elements of the medical history of great potential importance when infection is suspected. The enormous scale and frequent infective risks of world travel make this a common issue, but the recurrent reports of death from *P. falciparum* malaria diagnosed as influenza or 'a virus' until too late reveal a frequent omission in history taking. Timing is important because the dates of travel and possible exposure are often well known and can be related to known incubation periods. Thus, a febrile illness beginning 1 month after return from, say, India or Indonesia, is unlikely to be typhoid but might well still be hepatitis A. A careful travel history has an importance beyond that of helping the immediate diagnosis; it may also assist provisional antibiotic choice when the patient's condition demands treatment before the diagnosis can be confirmed. Thus *Salmonella typhi* from many parts of Asia is now resistant to formerly effective agents such as amoxycillin, co-trimoxazole, and chloramphenicol so that the fluorinated quinolones have become agents of first choice for typhoid originating in these areas. Likewise the distribution of the different patterns of drug resistance in malaria must always be taken into account, especially as, unlike bacterial infections, direct evidence about resistance of the infecting strain will not be available during the patient's acute illness. Travel histories tend to direct attention towards exotic disease, but travellers also acquire infections which are not specifically tropical, notably sexually transmitted and respiratory infections. Here, too, knowledge of drug resistance can be important, for example, penicillin resistance would be assumed in a patient developing pneumococcal pneumonia soon after visiting certain countries such as Spain and Hungary.

The travel history may carry implications of importance for public health as well as for the individual patient, as it frequently did before smallpox was eradicated. For example, a febrile illness starting within 3 weeks of a visit to certain mainly rural areas of West Africa, especially if the visit included hospitals or clinics, will demand that Lassa fever be considered in the differential diagnosis.

Occupation provides occasional but sometimes important leads towards the diagnosis of infectious disease. Some dramatic and specific ones are easily borne in mind, such as anthrax in hide workers, psittacosis in bird handlers, or *Streptococcus suis* infections in abattoir workers, but the less obvious, including tuberculosis and hepatitis A, may be forgotten and health care personnel must be firmly included in the occupations at special risk of infection. Some infections regarded as occupational in some places, for example leptospirosis in Britain, may in other areas, such as many parts of the Far East, be common causes of infection in any rural area.

The history of previous medication is important and sometimes relevant to difficulty in establishing diagnosis, but is especially significant in patients developing new or recurrent fever during the course of treatment

PHYSICAL EXAMINATION

As with history taking so, too, physical examination in patients with suspected infection follows the standard routine but, again, certain aspects take on special importance. Of these, fever takes pride of place because, although not all fever is caused by infection and not all infections produce fever, fever is one of the most common manifestations of infection, and infection is the most frequent cause of fever. The pathophysiology of this important sign is discussed in Chapter 7.3. Caveats about 'fever' as a word used in the history have already been given. As a physical sign the fact of fever and its pattern is easily established in patients admitted to hospital but even here there are pitfalls. In severely ill patients with the tachypnoea of pneumonia or impending bacterial shock syndrome the mouth is dry and cool, and in shock peripheral vasoconstriction makes measurement of oral or skin temperature unreliable; in these circumstances a measurement of core temperature must always be used. At the other end of the spectrum of severity, in patients complaining of minor fevers of long standing, pathological fever has to be differentiated from the normal, cyclical variations of body temperature.

Patterns of fever, beloved of classical diagnostic texts, are in practice seldom helpful chiefly because classical fever charts are of low sensitivity for the relevant diagnosis. While an undulant pattern may be suggestive of brucellosis or of Hodgkin's disease, most patients with lymphoma and many with brucellosis do not show this pattern. Another reason for their limited value is that 'classical' temperature patterns are easily altered by treatment. Antibiotics, often given before admission or during the diagnostic process, may have such an effect. So, too, can antipyretics given for symptomatic relief. In this way the step-ladder 'classical' chart of enteric fever can be converted into something resembling a silhouette of the Alps.

Some more specific points about febrile patterns are worth noting. Perhaps the most dangerous misconception is associated with malaria. The regular tertian (meaning every other day) or quartan (fever every third day) cycles are not found in the early days of the illness and often not at all in the most dangerous, *P. falciparum* infections; the temperature pattern is often quite erratic and malaria must be considered in all febrile (and some non-febrile) patients in or from a malarial area. Hectic fever, with large variations in the body temperature accompanied by chills and even rigors, is certainly a feature of pyogenic infections such as acute pyelonephritis or pyogenic abscesses, but can be seen in many other conditions, for example, with lymphoma, and sometimes in tuberculosis, and even in drug fever.

Examination of the skin can be enormously helpful in the diagnosis of infectious diseases. Sometimes the skin lesion is pathognomonic, for example erythema chronicum migrans of Lyme disease. Other rashes are pathognomonic in context; thus a morbilliform rash in an unimmunized child who has been febrile, snuffly, and coughing for 2 or 3 days and has Koplik's spots adds up to measles, whereas the same rash in a young adult who was given ampicillin a week ago and who turned out to have infectious mononucleosis denotes a drug reaction. Table 1 shows some of the ways in which skin lesions can make, or contribute to, the diagnosis of infection. Remember, though, that infections associated with specific rashes can also cause less specific ones. The early rash of meningococcal septicaemia may be macular or maculopapular rather than petechial, and Lyme disease is associated with non-specific rashes as well as with erythema chronicum migrans.

The mouth, too, can provide useful diagnostic information such as the enanthems of some of the classical infectious diseases, the raw red tongue of scarlet fever, toxic-shock syndrome and Kawasaki disease, the vesicles of some enteroviral infections and the many important oral signs of HIV disease (see Chapter 7.10.29).

Some other signs are worth special notice. Suspected endocarditis clearly demands careful examination of the heart and a search, including that of the fundi, for evidence of embolism or autoimmune phenomena. Enlarged lymph nodes can be an important clue; here the main snags are to distinguish between abnormal nodes and enlargements, so common in the neck and inguinal areas, that are residual from past infections. Another error is omitting to search carefully in the relevant drainage areas, for example, the area of skin drained by the abnormal node or the nasopharynx in relation to cervical nodes, and thus missing an important primary source. By contrast, splenic enlargement is often unhelpful, chiefly because it may be found in so many diverse causes of possible infection, and in so many non-infectious febrile illnesses. Patients who turn out to have meningitis, encephalitis, or brain abscess usually have

Table 1 *Rashes associated with infectious diseases*

Causal agent	Rash or syndrome	Comment
Measles	Measles	
Rubella	Rubella	
Varicella-zoster	Chickenpox Shingles	
Herpes simplex	Disseminated herpes Eczema herpeticum	
Herpesvirus 6	Roseola infantum	
Parvovirus B19	Erythema infectiosum	
Enteroviruses	Various	Usually macular or maculopapular but may be petechial or vesicular
HIV	Various	In early disease especially follicular and seborrhoeic rashes, herpes zoster, and Kaposi's sarcoma
Viral haemorrhagic fevers	Petechial/purpuric rashes	
N. meningitidis	Petechial/purpuric rashes	Also non-haemorrhagic rashes
N. gonorrhoeae (disseminated)	Petechial/purpuric rashes	Also papulovesicular
Staph. aureus	Petechial/purpuric rashes	In staphylococcal endocarditis
Haemophilus aegyptius	Petechial/purpuric rashes	Brazilian haemorrhagic fever
Rickettsia spp.	Petechial/purpuric rashes	Some also show primary eschar (*tache noire*)
Leptospira icterohaemorrhagica	Petechial/purpuric rashes	Weil's disease
Salmonella typhi	Rose spots	
Ps. aeruginosa	Ecthyma gangrenosum	Also in Aeromonas and other Gram-negative bacillary infections
Borrelia burgdorferi	Erythema chronicum migrans	Lyme disease, also non-specific rashes
Strep. pyogenes	Toxic erythema	
Staph. aureus	Toxic erythema	
Kawasaki	Toxic erythema	
Treponema pallidum	Various	

initial clinical features, such as neck stiffness or changes in cerebration, that at least steer the doctor in the direction of the central nervous system, but this is not invariable. To the widely recognized problem of diagnosing meningitis in neonates, infants, and occasionally the elderly must now be added the often extremely insidious onset of cryptococcal meningitis, sometimes a first manifestation of AIDS. A common general omission, in the examination of adults, and obviously relevant especially if brain abscess is suspected, is that of the ears, a normal routine in the examination of children not everywhere extended to adults.

Whatever local signs are or are not found, however, a most important principle in suspected infection, and especially in prolonged undiagnosed fever, is to make repeated and detailed examinations. This is more than a general exhortation to thoroughness; in such patients it is easy to plan further investigations, and to become discouraged by the often elusive diagnosis in spite of them, so that re-examination is forgotten, when a changing heart murmur, a new skin lesion, or the finding of an abdominal mass may immediately redefine and narrow the diagnostic possibilities.

LABORATORY INVESTIGATIONS

Laboratory investigation plays a crucial part in investigating infection, for it must be conceded that, if we except classical infectious diseases such as measles, varicella, pertussis, and the like, enormous numbers of infectious illnesses have no specific features definable by clinical examination, however carefully done, and that their elucidation relies entirely on laboratory study. As the vast majority of microbial disease worldwide afflicts patients with minimal or no access to laboratory tests, it follows that diagnosis of infectious disease is often a rough inference from the available evidence rather than a precise diagnosis. However, the addition of even a very modest number of laboratory or bedside investigations, some of them of low cost and not requiring long training in their use, greatly enlarges the possibilities of aetiological diagnosis. Microscopy of blood films, and of urine, pus, and some skin specimens (such as slit skin smears for leprosy) and of the stool by suitably trained people, is of enormous value, including, as it does, the diagnosis of malaria. Other specific diagnoses that can sometimes be achieved by direct microscopy of the blood include trypanosomiasis, some forms of filariasis, leptospirosis, relapsing fever, and bartonellosis. Apart from specific diagnoses such as these, examination of blood films has other and more common benefits. The differential leucocyte count is an important staging post in the diagnosis of febrile patients. Neutrophilia is found in pyogenic bacterial infections, in amoebiasis, leptospirosis, thromboembolism, various forms of connective tissue disease, rheumatic fever, Still's disease, in exacerbations of chronic hepatitis, and in mechanical tissue damage. Neutropenia, by contrast, is often seen in malaria, visceral leishmaniasis, typhoid, brucellosis, rickettsial disease, and in many viral infections including HIV. Eosinophilia, especially if substantial, can be an invaluable lead, so, too, can other specific appearances such as a high proportion of atypical mononuclear cells or the presence of primitive precursors. Microscopy of a fresh urine specimen reveals pus cells and bacteria, important because the urinary tract is an important site of infection and one from which focal symptoms may be entirely absent.

At a somewhat more elaborate level, diagnostic possibilities are further increased by the ability to culture urine, blood, pus, stools, and occasionally other specimens, while the addition of a chest radiograph makes another big inroad into the diagnosis. These investigations are singled out because they are often the most readily available tests, but also because they are all of high diagnostic yield in suspected infection.

Where more sophisticated laboratory and imaging facilities are available, investigation of suspected infection is, of course, much more extensive, and often includes initial serology and antigen detection tests for suspected pathogens, and relevant imaging methods. In particular, ultrasonographic scanning, computerized tomographic and magnetic resonance imaging, and radionucleide techniques (especially endogenous-labelled leucocyte scanning using indium or technetium isotopes) have greatly aided diagnosis of the more elusive and prolonged illnesses.

Above all, however, the value of biopsy and culture of a suspect tissue or organ must be stressed, and here too ultrasound-guided biopsy of the suspect site has much facilitated the diagnosis of difficult problems. Decisions about the extent and timing of further investigation, and the frequency with which investigations are repeated, call for fine judgement of costs and benefits. On one side are the discomforts, occasional dangers, and the financial costs of further tests that may or may not in the event contribute to the diagnosis; on the other are the possible risks in delayed treatment of a treatable condition and the certain added anxiety of prolonged uncertainty for patients and families. Whatever decisions are made about the pace and scope of further investigations, every effort should be made to avoid unnecessary multiplication of blood tests and other investigations, which are all-too-often repeated because of poor organization rather than medical necessity.

ISOLATION PROCEDURES

Management of infectious disease involves a decision additional to those common to other branches of medicine—whether or not the patient needs to be isolated and, if so, how to do it. Very many microbial diseases are not dangerous to other people; they may have arisen because of particular susceptibility of the host, or most of the surrounding population may already be immune by reason of past exposure and subclinical infection. But some infections are easily transmitted and hospitals present particular dangers, as in them patients ill with infection are congregated with patients at special risk in an environment conducive to the selection of virulent and antibiotic-resistant pathogens. Attention is often focused on highly susceptible hosts, for example people with profound neutropenia during treatment for leukaemia, but the problem of cross-infection is universal in hospitals, with neonates, the elderly, and surgical patients among the most vulnerable groups.

Formal isolation facilities are not available in many parts of the world, but some precautions against cross-infection are possible wherever any kind of health facility exists. The three fundamental steps are physical separation of the patient—if possible in a separate room—careful attention to hand washing by all staff including doctors, and routines for the safe disposal of infected materials including blood and secretions. This type of standard isolation, properly executed, is highly effective for gut and skin-borne pathogens, but face masks are also sometimes necessary when respiratory pathogens are involved. The more elaborate and expensive forms of isolation, either in the containment mode for the protection of contacts or the protective mode for the benefit of at-risk patients, are necessary only for an extreme minority of hospital patients. The essential requirement of all isolation systems, simple or complex, is to establish agreed and preferably simple methods, to train staff in their use, and to monitor their performance. In institutions with full facilities the roles of the control-of-infection nurse and the microbiology laboratory are crucial in implementing efficient infection control procedures.

REFERENCES

Brock, T.D. (ed.) (1990). Microorganisms—from smallpox to Lyme disease. *In Readings from* Scientific American *magazine*. Freeman, New York.

Christie, A.B. (1987). *Infectious diseases. Epidemiology and clinical practice*, 4th edn. Churchill Livingstone, Edinburgh.

Farrar, W.E., Wood, M.J., and Innes, J.A., (1992). *Infectious diseases—text and color atlas*, (2nd edn). Gower Medical, London.

Mandell, G.L., Douglas, R.G., and Bennett, J.E. (1995). *Principles and practice of infectious diseases*, (4th edn). Churchill Livingstone, Edinburgh.

Mims, C.A., Playfair, J.H.L., Roitt, I.M., Wakelin, D., and Williams, R. (1993). *Medical Microbiology*. Mosby-Year Book Europe Ltd.

7.2 Biology of pathogenic micro-organisms

7.2.1 Introduction to the diversity of bacterial pathogens

P. J. SANSONETTI

Introduction

Among the enormous number of bacterial species that can be associated with the human body (i.e. 10^{13} bacteria constitute our intestinal flora), only a few of those encountered are pathogenic, in other words, able to cause infection in a non-immunocompromised host. The first contact between pathogenic bacteria and their human host varies depending upon the route of inoculation. Pathogenic species such as *Francisella tularensis* are able to penetrate transcutaneously, whereas *Staphylococcus aureus* requires a breach in the skin layer. Other pathogens such as *Yersinia pestis* (the plague bacillus), Borrelia, and Rickettsia (the causative agents of various forms of typhus) are transmitted by the bites of haematophagous arthropods.

In a large majority of infections, however, the initial event is at mucosal surfaces. Bacteria such as *Mycobacterium tuberculosis*, *Legionella pneumophila*, and *Bordetella pertussis* are ingested by inhalation and cause respiratory infections; others, such as Salmonella, Shigella, and *Vibrio cholerae* are ingested orally and cause enteric infections. The urogenital tract can also be infected by sexually transmitted pathogens such as *Neisseria gonorrhoeae*, *Chlamydia trachomatis*, and mycoplasmas, or by ascending spread of uropathogenic *Escherichia coli* or *Proteus mirabilis*, which are naturally part of the faecal flora. All these pathogenic species express attachment or invasion factors that allow specific colonization and/or invasion of their respective mucosal surfaces. Initiation of the infection process depends also on the size of the inoculum. Some agents, such as *M. tuberculosis* and *Shigella dysenteriae*, are extremely infectious, their 50 per cent infectious doses (ID_{50}) being equal to or less than 100 bacteria in man; *Salmonella typhi* or *V. cholerae* on the other hand, are less infectious, their ID_{50} being equal to or greater than 10^7 micro-organisms.

However, pathogenicity ultimately remains a relative concept that depends on the balance between the local or general immune status of the host and the degree of pathogenicity of the bacterial species.

Determinants of bacterial pathogenicity

In Table 1, pathogenic bacteria have been classified according to classical bacteriological criteria. In Table 2, classification is based on their major pathogenic properties.

COLONIZATION OF HOST SURFACES

Association, adhesion, and invasion are the major ways by which bacteria can interact with host surfaces.

Table 1 *Principal human bacterial pathogens*

Micro-organisms	Diseases	Other characteristics
Gram-positive cocci		
Staphylococcus aureus	Skin infections, septicaemia, food poisoning, toxic-shock syndrome, nosocomial infections	Common skin commensal
Streptococcus pyogenes Group A	Skin infections, tonsilitis, scarlet fever, septicaemia, toxic shock	Immunopathological complications: rheumatic fever, acute glomerulonephritis
	Group C and G also cause upper respiratory, skin and septicaemic infections	
Streptococcus agalactiae Group B	Neonatal infections: septicaemia, meningitis, nosocomial infections	Commensal in intestine and female genital tract
Enterococci Group D and non-typable streptococci	Infective endocarditis, nosocomial infections	Oral commensals (non-typable streptococci), intestinal and urogenital commensals (enterococci)
Streptococcus mutans	Dental caries	Oral commensal
Streptococcus pneumoniae	Pneumonia, septicaemia, meningitis, otitis	Commensal of the human upper respiratory tract
Gram-positive bacilli		
Listeria monocytogenes	Neonatal infections: granulomatosis infantiseptica, flu-like syndrome in pregnant women, meningitis (~50% in immunocompromised patients)	Ubiquitous in soil, animals, foods
Corynebacterium diphtheriae	Diphtheria: pseudo-membranous tonsilitis, systemic manifestations of diphtheria toxin diffusion (myocarditis)	Interhuman transmission; healthy carriage is possible
Bacillus anthracis	Anthrax	Pathogenic in cattle after ingestion of spores
Clostridium spp.		
C. perfringens	Gas-gangrene, food poisoning	Ubiquitous in soil, intestinal flora
C. tetani	Tetanus	
C. botulinum	Botulism	
C. difficile	Diarrhoea, pseudomembranous colitis	
Gram-negative cocci		
Neisseria gonorrhoeae	Gonorrhoea, rarely septicaemia	Obligate human pathogen
Neisseria meningitidis	Meningitis, purpura fulminans, upper respiratory tract infections	Obligate human pathogen; nasopharyngeal carriage
Gram-negative bacilli		
Enterobacteriaceae		
Escherichia coli	Urinary tract infections, gastrointestinal infections, nosocomial infections, neonatal infections (K1 capsular type)	Commensal of human intestine except for ETEC, EPEC, EHEC and EIEC*
Salmonella spp.	Enteric fever (*S. typhi*), food poisoning	*S. typhi*: man is exclusive host, other salmonellae are animal pathogens or commensals
Shigella spp.	Bacillary dysentery	Obligate pathogen for man and some monkeys
Yersinia spp.		
Y. pseudotuberculosis	Gastrointestinal infections, mesenteric lymphadenitis	Largely present in soil, water and animals
Y. enterocolitica		
Y. pestis	Plague	Flea-borne pathogen of rodents; transmitted to man
Opportunistic Enterobacteriaceae (Klebsiella, Enterobacter, Serratia)	Respiratory infections, urinary tract infections, septicaemia	Commensals of human intestinal flora Largely present in environment
Proteus spp.	Urinary tract infections	Commensals of human intestinal flora
Other Gram-negative bacilli		
Vibrio cholerae	Cholera	Man is the only natural host but contaminated water is the major source of infection
Other vibrios		
V. parahaemolyticus	Diarrhoea Septicaemia Skin infections	As above

Table 1 (*cont.*)

Micro-organisms	Diseases	Other characteristics
Aeromonas	Diarrhoea	As above
Campylobacter jejuni	Diarrhoea, dysenteric syndromes	Ubiquitous in animals
Helicobacter pylori	Type B gastritis, gastroduodenal ulcer?	Unknown reservoir
Pseudomonas aeruginosa	Urinary tract infections, wound infections, septicaemic infections in immunocompromised patients	Commensal of human intestinal flora
Haemophilus influenzae	Otitis, pneumonia, meningitis	Commensal of human upper respiratory tract
Bordetella pertussis	Whooping cough	Obligate pathogen of human respiratory tract
Brucella spp.	Septicaemia, undulant fever Localized infections: arthritis, meningitis	Animal products
Pasteurella multocida	Subcutaneous infections after animal bite	Commensal of vertebrate respiratory and intestinal tract
Francisella tularensis	Tularaemia: acute lymphadenitis	Ubiquitous in animals, especially rodents
Legionella pneumophila	Legionnaires' disease	Often acquired from air-conditioning units
Acinetobacter	Agent of nosocomial infections	Ubiquitous in environment
Gram-negative anaerobes		
(Bacteroides, Capnocytophaga, Fusobacterium)	Agents of infection after surgery of intestinal, genital or urinary tract	Commensal of the intestinal and genital flora
Acid-fast bacilli		
Mycobacterium tuberculosis	Tuberculosis	Obligate pathogen of human respiratory tract
Mycobacterium leprae	Leprosy	Obligate pathogen of man
Mycobacterium avium-intracellulare	Respiratory and intestinal infections in immunocompromised patients (AIDS)	Ubiquitous in environment
Miscellaneous		
Spirochaetes		
Treponema pallidum	Syphilis	Obligate human pathogen
Leptospira spp.	Leptospirosis	Mostly pathogenic in animals: rodents, dogs, etc.
Borrelia spp.	Relapsing fever (tick and louse-borne)	Rodent reservoir (tick-borne relapsing fever)
Borrelia burgdorferi	Lyme disease (tick-borne disease)	Animal reservoir
Actinomyces		
Actinomyces israelii	Actinomycosis	Commensal of human mouth
Nocardia asteroides	Pneumonia, brain abscesses in immunocompromised patients	Ubiquitous
Rickettsiales		
Rickettsia spp.	Typhus and related diseases (arthropod-borne disease)	Rodent reservoir
Coxiella burnetti	Q fever (air-borne disease)	Large animal reservoir
Rochalimea henselae	Cat-scratch disease; bacillary angiomatosis (AIDS)	Cat
Bartonella bacilliformis	Oroya fever	Human reservoir, transmitted by sandflies
Chlamydiaceae		
Chlamydia trachomatis	Urethritis, conjunctivitis, chronic salpingitis	Obligate human pathogen
Mycoplasmas		
Mycoplasma pneumoniae	Pneumonia	Commensal of the human respiratory tract
Ureaplasma urealyticum	Genital infections	Commensal or pathogen of the human urogenital tract
Mycoplasma hominis		

*ETEC, enterotoxigenic *E. coli*; EPEC, enteropathogenic *E. coli*; EHEC, enterohaemorrhagic *E. coli*; EIEC, enteroinvasive *E. coli*.

Association

This is a process by which bacteria can interact with proteins of the cellular matrix such as fibronectin, laminin, or collagen. Such proteins are recognized as secretion products or as structures exposed after tissue destruction. Many pathogenic bacteria, particularly those that are Gram-positive, such as staphylococci and streptococci, produce surface proteins allowing such associations.

Adhesion

This is the consequence of a specific interaction between pathogenic bacteria and host cells. The process requires the bacterial ligand called adhesin to bind to a cell-surface receptor. The host cell receptor usually corresponds to the sugar moiety of a glycoprotein or a glycolipid; therefore, bacterial adhesins are usually lectins. It is among the various enteropathogenic and uropathogenic subtypes of *E. coli* that adhesion

Table 2 *Human bacterial pathogens classified according to their chief pathogenic properties*

Colonization of surfaces		
Association		
Binding to extracellular matrix proteins (collagen, fibronectin, etc.)	Tissue destruction by local production of toxins and enzymes	*Staphylococcus aureus* *Streptococcus pyogenes*
Adhesion		
DAMAGE DUE TO LOCAL SECRETION OF BACTERIAL PRODUCTS		
Binding of bacterial adhesin to cell-surface receptor (glycolipid, glycoprotein)	Activation or blockage of ion channels by local production of cytotonins (CT, LT, ST)	*Vibrio cholerae* ETEC
	Tissue production by local production of cytotoxins (SLT etc.)	EHEC *Clostridium difficile* *Clostridium perfringens*
	Tissue destruction by local production of toxins (LPS, Hly) and enzymes (urease)	Uropathogenic *Escherichia coli* *Proteus mirabilis* *Helicobacter pylori*
DAMAGE DUE TO SYSTEMIC DIFFUSION OF BACTERIAL PRODUCTS		
Binding to mucosal or skin surfaces followed by systemic intoxination	Production of neurotoxins (DT, TT, BT)	*Clostridium tetani* *Clostridium botulinum* *Corynebacterium diphtheriae*
	Production of cytotoxins (SLT1–2)	EHEC (HUS)*
	Production of superantigens, TSST1, erythrogenic toxins, enterotoxins	*Staphylococcus aureus* *Streptococcus pyogenes*
	Production of adenylate cyclase and other toxins	*Bacillus anthracis* *Bordetella pertussis*
Invasion of surfaces		
Mechanical		
Invasive devices (catheters etc.); nosocomial infections		*Staphylococcus aureus*, *Serratia marcescens*, *Pseudomonas aeruginosa*, *Acinetobacter*, etc.
Translocation		
Normal uptake through mucosal surfaces without further control in immunocompromised patients	Passage through M cells, virus- or chemotherapy-induced ulcerations	Opportunistic bacteria
Invasion		
Capacity to invade cells of epithelial surfaces	Production of invasion proteins	*Yersinia* spp. *Salmonella* spp. *Shigella* spp. *Listeria monocytogenes* *Neisseria gonorrhoeae*
Life inside cells		
Survival and multiplication within macrophages and related cells	Blockage or survival to phagolysosomal fusion	*Legionella pneumophila* *Mycobacterium tuberculosis* *Mycobacterium leprae*
Survival, differentiation and growth within epithelial cells		*Chlamydia trachomatis*
Systemic dissemination		
Several attributes allow systemic dissemination	Resistance to serum killing (wall of Gram +ve, LPS of Gram −ve)	*Klebsiella pneumoniae* *Staphylococcus aureus*
	Resistance to phagocytosis (expression of LPS and capsule)	
Ultimate localization: bacterial meningitis	Factors leading to CNS tropism unknown	*Escherichia coli* *Streptococcus agalactiae* *Haemophilus influenzae* b *Neisseria meningitidis* *Streptococcus pneumoniae* *Listeria monocytogenes*

*HUS; haemolytic uraemic syndrome.

mechanisms have been best studied. These strains often produce surface appendages (fimbriae or pili) that support the adhesion. Many other Gram-negative pathogenic species, such as vibrios, pseudomonads, moraxellae, and bacteroides, also produce fimbriae.

Certain pathogens, such as *Bordetella pertussis*, have evolved extremely sophisticated adhesion systems, which are probably adapted to the various environments encountered in the human host. This pathogen that causes whooping cough produces seven independent adhesion systems, including four fimbriae, the fibrillar haemagglutinin, pertussis toxins, and pertactin. Fibrillar haemagglutin contains a selectin-type domain that adheres to surface polysaccharides of respiratory cells and an Arg-Gly-Asp (RGD) sequence allowing adhesion to the receptor for C3 on macrophages.

Invasion

For certain pathogenic micro-organisms, adhesion to mucosal surfaces is simply a precursor to internalization into epithelial cells. Intracellular life allows these invasive micro-organisms to survive and multiply. After internalization has occurred, often through a process closely related to phagocytosis, bacteria such as salmonellae and yersinia must be able to survive the hostile environment of the endocytic vacuole whereas some pathogenic species, such as shigellae and *Listeria monocytogenes*, lyse their membrane-bound phagocytic vacuole and escape to the cytoplasm. It is likely that the clinical differences observed between the pathogenic processes caused by these various micro-organisms depend very much on their intracellular behaviour.

INTERACTION WITH PHAGOCYTIC CELLS

The way pathogenic bacteria interact with phagocytic cells is critical for the development of the infectious process. There are several different possible behaviours. Some species are obligate intracellular parasites. This is the case for *Chlamydia trachomatis* and mycobacteria, particularly *M. leprae* and *M. tuberculosis*. These mycobacteria multiply almost exclusively within macrophages and related cells by both inhibiting phagolysosomal fusion and resisting the lethal activity of lysosomal products.

Other species, such as salmonellae, *Legionella pneumophila*, and *L. monocytogenes*, are facultative intracellular parasites that usually escape being killed by phagocytic cells by expressing on their surface proteins that confer resistance to lysosomal products. This is particularly true for *S. typhimurium*, in which mutants have been obtained that no longer resist lysosomal compounds, such as defensins.

Many pathogenic species are true extracellular bacteria. Encapsulated micro-organisms, such as *Klebsiella pneumoniae*, *Neisseria meningitidis*, *Haemophilus influenzae*, *S. typhi*, *Streptococcus pneumoniae*, and septicaemic *E. coli* expressing K*1* capsular serotypes, are naturally resistant to phagocytosis by polymorphonuclear cells and macrophages. Only the presence of specific anticapsular antibodies allows opsonization and subsequent efficient phagocytosis. Other micro-organisms can prevent phagocytosis by using sophisticated strategies such as the inactivation of the complement cascade by M protein in group A streptococci.

PRODUCTION OF TOXINS

Bacterial toxins can be classified into different groups, according to their localization in the growing micro-organisms.

Endocellular toxins are associated with the bacterial body and are released only with the death of the micro-organism. This is the case for the bacterial endotoxin that corresponds to the lipid moiety (lipid A) of the bacterial lipopolysaccharide of Gram-negative bacteria. Components of the cell wall (peptidoglycan) of Gram-positive bacteria also have toxic properties for the host. Both lipid A and fragments of the bacterial wall may activate overproduction of inflammatory cytokines such as interleukins 1 and 6 and tumour necrosis factor-α, which are particularly deleterious for the host and may cause septic shock.

Extracellular toxins are proteinaceous toxins secreted by bacteria during their growth phase. These toxins are enormously diverse in their size, structure, number of component subunits, and pharmacological mode of action. Some bacterial exotoxins may cause cell death by blocking host-cell protein biosynthesis, as it is the case for Shiga toxin produced in large amounts by *S. dysenteriae* 1 and diphtheria toxin produced by *Corynebacterium diphtheriae*.

Other toxins cause ADP-ribosylation of regulatory proteins such as G proteins, thus causing severe dysfunction of important membrane enzymes such as adenylate cyclase. This is the case for cholera toxin and pertussis toxin. On the other hand, haemolysins, which are produced by Gram-positive and Gram-negative pathogens, are pore-forming proteins that are able to lyse membrane-bound phagocytic vacuoles as well as cytoplasmic membranes.

REFERENCES

Alouf, J.E. and Freer, J.H. (1991). *Sourcebook of bacterial protein toxins*, (ed. J.E. Alouf and J.H. Freer). Academic Press, New York.

Beachey, E.H., Giampapa, C.S., and Abraham, S.N. (1988). Bacterial adherence: adhesin receptor-mediated attachment of pathogenic bacteria to mucosal surfaces. *American Review of Respiratory Diseases*, **138**, S45–8.

Bone, R.C. (1991). The pathogenesis of sepsis. *Annals of Internal Medicine*, **115**, 457–69.

Cooper, N.R. (1991). Complement evasion strategies of microorganisms. *Immunology Today*, **12**, 327–31.

Falkow, S. (1991). Bacterial entry into eukaryotic cells. *Cell*, **65**, 1099–102.

Finlay, B.B. (1990). Cell adhesion and invasion mechanisms in microbial pathogenesis. *Current Opinion in Cell Biology*, **2**, 815–20.

Ganz, T., Selsted, M.E., Babior, B.M., and Curnette, J.T. (1988). Neutrophils and host defense. *Annals of Internal Medicine*, **109**, 127–42.

Hoepelman, A.I.M. and Tuomanen, E.I. (1992). Consequences of microbial attachment: directing host cell functions with adhesins. *Infection and Immunity*, **60**, 1729–33.

Isberg, R.R. (1991). Discrimination between intracellular uptake and surface adhesion of bacterial pathogens. *Science*, **252**, 934–8.

Finlay, B.B. and Falkow, S. (1989). Common themes in microbial pathogenicity. *Microbiological Review*, **53**, 210–30.

Mims, C.A. (1987). *The pathogenesis of infectious diseases*, (3rd edn). Academic Press, London.

Moulder, J.W. (1985). Comparative biology of intracellular parasitism. *Microbiological Review*, **49**, 298–337.

7.2.2 Molecular taxonomy of bacterial pathogens

P. J. SANSONETTI

Introduction

Definition of a species is a difficult task in the case of prokaryotic micro-organisms because taxonomists cannot rely on the phylogenetic studies that are used in the eukaryotic world. These are:

(1) demonstration of phenotypical similarities between natural groups;
(2) demonstration of a genetic relationship between these groups, which is usually by the occurrence of fertile crossings between individuals among a given species;
(3) definition, based on phylogenetic models, of morphological and physiological similarities that link the lineages of individuals through evolution;

(4) confirmation of these models by tracing the evolution of relevant fossils.

Except for phenotypical comparisons, no such analysis can be made with bacteria for which classical phylogenetic studies are impossible, due to incomplete sexual recombination and lack of informative fossils.

Consequently, a specific taxonomic analysis had to be developed for prokaryotic micro-organisms. It is based on phenetic relations, in other words, classificational systems based on the overall similarity of many characters regardless of the evolutionary history of the micro-organisms, and on cladogenetic relations (*klados*, branch) in which taxonomists try to reconstitute evolutionary pathways in order to design tree-like branching of taxa based on comparison of molecular sequences (DNA, RNA, proteins).

Definition of a bacterial species (from molecular taxonomy to bacterial identification)

Modern methods of molecular taxonomy, based on the comparison of genomic sequences, have allowed unambiguous definition of a bacterial species.

A bacterial species can be phylogenetically defined as 'a group of strains that share DNA–DNA homology such that their hybridization values are equal or superior to 70 per cent with a ΔTm value equal or inferior to 5°C'. ΔTm (i.e. difference in thermal stability) is the difference between denaturation temperatures of homologous and heterologous DNA heteroduplexes. This is an extremely technical definition. It basically says that micro-organisms that share more than an overall 70 per cent identity of their genome belong to the same species. DNA–DNA hybridization methods are based on natural properties of DNA strands, which can renature *in vitro* if their nucleotidic sequences are complementary, thus allowing formation of double-stranded DNA molecules. If two heterogeneous bacterial genomes are compared, the extent of renaturation that occurs between their denatured DNA defines a degree of homology corresponding to the percentage of complementary sequences, as compared to the total sequences. Reciprocal DNA–DNA hybridization must be done as a control of relatedness as well as of genome size, as reciprocal relatedness values are considered only when compared bacteria have genomes of similar size.

However, if genomic characters reflect the hereditary message more faithfully than expression of phenotypic characters, two genomes are likely to hybridize only if the micro-organisms share sufficient identity and therefore express a high degree of phenotypic similarity. In consequence, two bacterial species that are identified only on the basis of DNA–DNA hybridization and not on the basis of phenotypic characters cannot be named until discriminative phenotypic properties are identified. Joint study of phenotypic and genotypic traits is the only way to establish a balanced classification.

On the other hand, an easy approach to the every-day practice of clinical microbiology relies on grouping related bacteria on the basis of their expressed phenotypes. However, for the clinician involved with infectious diseases and the clinical microbiologist, there is another level of complexity because 'classical species' that have been established on expressed phenotypic characters, such as *Escherichia coli* and Shigella, actually belong to the same genomic species. The same is true for Salmonella and Arizona as well as for *Yersinia pestis* and *Yersinia pseudotuberculosis*. In other words, two taxa form a single species and these two taxa are still considered independently as they clearly cause distinct pathological entities. It is understandably hard for a clinician to contemplate that the micro-organism responsible for the Black Plague belongs to the same species as that responsible for a usually mild pseudoappendicular syndrome.

One must consequently separate the concept of bacterial classification, which is now essentially based on modern methods of molecular taxonomy, and bacterial identification, which can ignore these methods and remain based on the recognition of a set of phenotypic characters expressed by all the members of this group—Gram staining, motility, morphology, metabolic markers, common immunological properties (serotypes).

In addition, if one considers the clinical aspects as a major factor in bacterial classification, even inside a single genomic species such as *E. coli*, groups exist that correspond to pathovars. For instance, *E. coli* encompasses at least three different pathovars for human beings: enteric strains; septicaemic strains or strains that cause meningitis; uropathogenic strains. Even among enteric strains, there are at least five subgroups: enterotoxigenic (ETEC), enteropathogenic (EPEC), enterohaemorrhagic (EHEC), enteroaggregative (EAgEC), enteroinvasive (EIEC). These pathovars have occurred by acquisition of genes encoding adherence factors, toxins or capsules that may be located on plasmids, bacteriophages or integrated within the chromosome. Other bacterial pathogens such as *Staphylococcus aureus* also encompass several pathovars. DNA probes have become very convenient tools to detect the virulence sequences that characterize a given pathovar, as genes encoding virulence factors are often cloned. DNA may be labelled by radioactive or non-radioactive elements and subsequently hybridized to the bacterial genome. Such techniques may, under certain circumstances, be used for the diagnostic of such pathogens within a culture or an infected fluid or tissue. They are also often used to perform epidemiological studies on a pathovar in a given clinical state.

16s ribosomal RNA (rRNA) and rRNA gene sequencing: from the phylogeny of eubacteria to the molecular diagnosis of uncultivable or even unknown micro-organisms

Diversity is written into the bacterial genome, thus making the study of nucleic acid sequences more convenient than phenotypic cataloguing. If DNA–DNA hybridization has allowed better definition of a bacterial species, more specific areas of the genome can be selected and their variation considered as 'molecular clocks'. DNA sequences encoding 16*s* or 23*s* rRNA are currently considered as the most suitable region to study. Polymerase chain reaction (**PCR**) can even be used in order to amplify and sequence limited fragments among variable portions of these regions, the sequence of the primers being based upon the highly conserved portions flanking these variable regions. Unlike DNA–DNA hybridization techniques and complementary to approaches studying restriction profiles of the genes encoding rRNA, PCR amplification of 16*s* RNA gene sequences does not require primary isolation and cultivation of the bacteria.

It is now possible, by comparing catalogues of sequences, to establish a phylogenetic tree of the bacterial world. A bacterium can currently be located in the phylogenetic tree even before classical identification has been made. Pushed to its limits, sequencing of a PCR-amplified fragment of 16*s* rRNA from a non-cultivated micro-organism may replace bacterial isolation and identification. 16*s* rRNA genes are suitable for these approaches for several reasons.

1. They are present in all bacteria.
2. Their sequences contain zones that are identical in all bacteria but different in eukaryotic DNA and mitochondrial DNA.
3. These sequences contain zones that are identical in bacteria belonging to a given phylum.
4. These sequences also contain variable zones that are specific to a given species.

About 2000 16s rRNA sequences are now available in gene banks, thus allowing accurate phylogenetic positioning of newly discovered micro-organisms.

Based on these rRNA approaches, 10 phylogenetic groups can be identified among Eubacteria. The five of them that are relevant to human infections are summarized in Table 1. The close relatedness that appears between micro-organisms responsible for totally different diseases (i.e.

Table 1 *Five major phylogenetic groups of Eubacteria defined by analysis of 16s rRNA sequences*

1. Gram-positive bacteria
   Clostridies and related:
   Bacillus, Staphylococcus, Streptococcus, Lactobacillus, Erysipelothrix, Clostridium, Peptostreptococcus, Mycoplasma.
   Actinomycetes and related:
   Bifidobacterium, Propionibacterium, Actinomyces, Streptomyces, Arthrobacter, Cellulomonas, Corynebacterium, Brevibacterium, Nocardia, Mycobacterium
2. Photosynthetic bacteria, purple bacteria, and related
   α branch:
   Aquaspirillum, Agrobacterium, Nitrobacter, Rickettsiae, Rochalimea, Bartonella, Brucella, Afipia felis, Ehrlichia
   β branch:
   Pseudomonas acidovorans, Alcaligenes, Neisseria
   γ branch:
   Enterobacteriaceae, *Vibrios, Aeromonas hydrophila, Pasteurella multocida, Pseudomonas fluorescens,* Legionella
   δ branch:
   Desulfovibrios, Bdellovibrios, Myxobacteria
3. Bacteroides, flavobacteria, and related
   Bacteroides group, Fusobacterium
   Flavobacterium group, Cytophaga
4. Spirochetales and related
   Spirochetales:
   Spirochaeta, Treponema, Borrelia
   Leptospirales:
   Leptospira
5. Chlamydiaceae
   Chlamydia psittaci, Chlamydia trachomatis

From Stackebrandt and Woese (1981); Woese *et al.* (1985)—examples of genera are not exhaustive.

Staphylococcus and Mycoplasma) and the close vicinity between bacteria that are highly pathogenic and others that are totally avirulent (i.e. Mycobacteria and Bifidobacteria) is certainly surprising.

The combination of PCR and molecular phylogenetics, based on 16s rRNA sequencing, has recently offered new openings in microbiological diagnosis. This approach may engage some of the major problems that remain in this area such as:

- absence or extremely fastidious growth of some bacterial pathogens *in vitro* (e.g. *Treponema pallidum*, Mycobacteria);
- suspicion that a bacterial micro-organism is responsible for a syndrome or a disease, due to suggestive histopathological lesions such as microabscesses, presence of bacterial inclusions in phagocytes (e.g. Whipple's disease, cat-scratch disease);
- lack of proper or accessible phenotypical characters allowing identification of a cultivable micro-organism (e.g. many anaerobic bacteria);
- lack of description of the corresponding species.

This technique has allowed successful identification of the likely aetiological agents of cat-scratch disease, although some arguments remain about *Afipia felis* or *Rochalimea henselae* being the actual causative agent. The situation appears clear, on the other hand, for bacillary angiomatosis and hepatic pelliosis, particularly in patients with acquired immune deficiency syndrome, where 16*s* rRNA gene sequencing reveals the presence of *Rochalimea henselae* or *Rochalimea quintana*. Similarly, a non-cultivable pathogen now known as *Tropheryma whippelii* is proposed as the aetiological agent for Whipple's disease.

Conclusion

Molecular taxonomy has become an essential component of modern clinical microbiology. It is an obligatory tool for ascertaining the classification of bacteria, particularly the pathogenic species. It is also now used to develop new techniques of diagnosis that not only may allow us to identify new pathogenic species, but also in the near future, to identify pathogens from clinical products on which classical bacteriological techniques have failed.

REFERENCES

Brenner, D.J., Fanning, G.R., Miklos, G.V., and Steigerwalt, A.G. (1973). Polynucleotide sequence relatedness among *Shigella* species. *International Journal of Systematic Bacteriology*, **23,** 1–7.

Brenner, D.J. (1978). Characterization and clinical identification of Enterobacteriaceae by DNA hybridization. *Progress in Clinical Pathology*, **7,** 71–117.

Johnson, J.L. (1973). Use of nucleic-acid homologies in the taxonomy of anaerobic bacteria. *International Journal of Systematic Bacteriology*, **23,** 308–15.

Relman, D.A., Loutit, J.S., Schmidt, T.M., Falkow, S., and Tomkins, L.S. (1990). The agent of bacillary angiomatosis. An approach to identification of uncultured pathogen. *New England Journal of Medicine*, **323,** 1573–80.

Relman, D.A., Schmidt, T.M., Mac Dermott, R.P., and Falkow, S. (1992). Identification of the uncultured bacillus of Whipple's disease. *New England Journal of Medicine*, **327,** 293–301.

Sneath, P.H.A. (1974). Phylogeny of microorganisms. *Symposiums of the Society for General Microbiology*, **24,** 1–39.

Sneath, P.H.A. (1984). Numerical taxonomy. In *Bergey's manual of systematic bacteriology* (ed. N.R. Krieg and J.G. Hold), pp. 5–7. Williams & Wilkins, Baltimore.

Stackebrandt, E. and Woese, C.R. (1981). The evolution of prokaryotes. In *Molecular and cellular aspects of microbial evolution* (ed. M.J. Carlile, J.F. Collins, and B.E.B. Moseley), pp. 1–31. Cambridge University Press.

Wayne, J.G. *et al.* (1987). Report of the *ad hoc* committee on reconciliation of approaches to bacterial systematics. *International Journal of Systematic Bacteriology*, **37,** 463–4.

Woese, C.R. (1987). Bacterial evolution. *Microbiology Reviews*, **51,** 221–71.

Woese, C.R., Stackebrandt, E., Macke, T.J., and Fox, G.E. (1985). A phylogenic definition of the major eubacterial taxa. *Systematic Applied Microbiology*, **6,** 143–51.

7.3 The host's response to infection

B. M. GREENWOOD

Introduction

Man is exposed constantly to potentially pathogenic micro-organisms, yet clinical infections are rare events and fatal infections even rarer. Why does one individual exposed to an organism such as the meningococcus experience an asymptomatic infection whilst another exposed to the same bacterium develops an illness that kills within a few hours of the first appearance of symptoms? 'Why me not him' is a question that the unfortunate victim could reasonably have asked. Occasionally there is an obvious answer, for example the patient with fulminating meningococcal disease might have had a complement deficiency, but in many cases there is not. The problem of the variable response of man to an infection has been resolved in many traditional societies by invoking the power of supernatural forces. Thus, whilst the concept of an infectious cause of an illness such as AIDS may be accepted, the reason why one person develops the disease but another who is equally at risk does not is attributed to the fact that the former has offended the spirits in some way or been rendered susceptible to the disease by someone who wishes him ill. In societies where this kind of explanation is no longer accepted there is a tendency to fall back on the concept of 'chance' or 'bad luck'. Whilst random selection of victims must occur, the invocation of chance is usually an expression of our ignorance about the many complex variables that influence the course of an infection in a particular individual. While a great deal is now known about the organisms responsible for common infections and the way in which they are transmitted, there is still much to be learnt about the factors that influence the host's response to infection. The nature of some of these factors and the ways in which they can be modified are the subject of this chapter.

The host–parasite interaction

The outcome of exposure of a susceptible host to a potentially pathogenic organism is determined by both the characteristics of the pathogen and by those of the host (Fig. 1).

The two most important microbial determinants that need to be considered are (i) the virulence of the individual strain of microbe and (ii) the dose of infection. It is not proposed to discuss determinants of microbial virulence in any detail. In the case of some microbes there are clearly defined virulence factors that differentiate one strain from another, for example toxin production, but it is likely that there are still many more subtle variables that remain to be identified.

Fig. 1 Factors influencing the host/parasite balance.

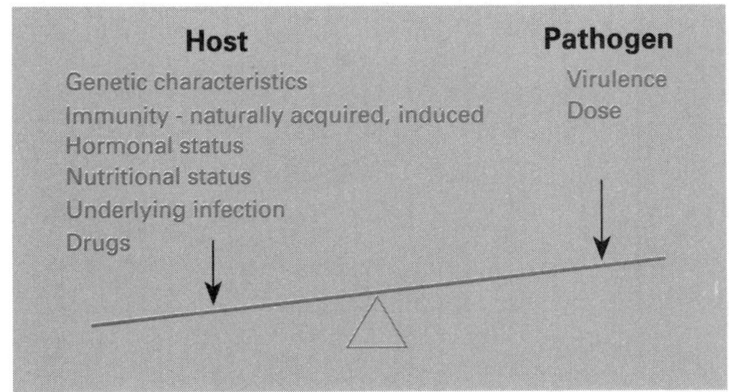

The importance of infecting dose as a determinant of the outcome of infection has probably been underestimated, perhaps because in naturally acquired infections it is rarely known. However, studies in animals and in human volunteers have shown clearly the importance of dose in determining the severity of gastrointestinal infections. Cleaning one's teeth in contaminated water may be relatively safe whilst to drink it would be disastrous. Infective dose is probably also an important factor in determining the outcome of infections spread by respiratory droplets. The high mortality of measles seen in secondary cases infected by an older sibling is probably a reflection of the large dose of virus to which these children have been exposed.

To cause disease a pathogen must be able to overcome the surface defence mechanisms and, if it is to cause systemic disease, it must be able to survive the powerful non-specific and specific protective immune responses that the host will direct against it (Fig. 2). The nature of these protective mechanisms are the subject of the following sections.

The immune response to infection

Surface barriers and protection against infection

Skin and mucosa provide an important mechanical barrier to invasion by many pathogenic organisms. Secretion of bactericidal substances, such as free fatty acids and lysozyme, on to the surface of the skin increases its protective properties. Damage to the skin, for example by burns, may make an individual susceptible to systemic infection by an organism that would not usually be pathogenic.

The mechanical barrier to infection provided by the gastric epithelium is aided by the acid pH of the contents of the stomach. People with achlorhydria, a common consequence of malnutrition and of smoking

Fig. 2 Three lines of defence against infection.

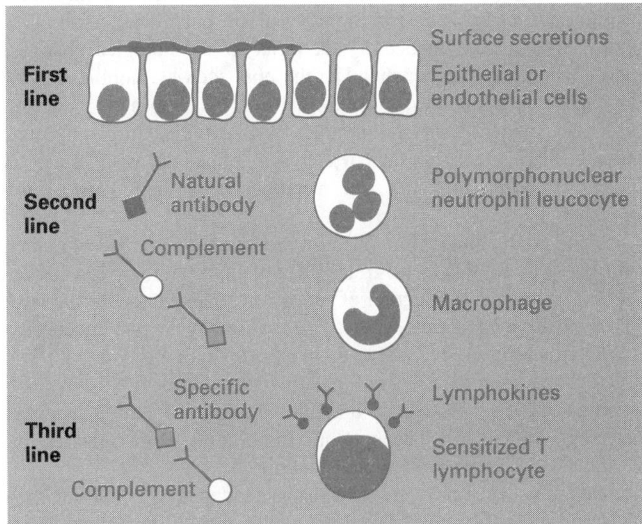

marijuanha, have an increased susceptibility to infection with organisms such as *Vibrio cholerae* and *Giardia lamblia*.

Organisms that invade through the respiratory tract must be able to overcome a number of mechanical defence mechanisms. Inhaled organisms are frequently trapped by respiratory mucus, carried upwards by the cilia of respiratory mucosal cells, and either expectorated or swallowed. Factors that impair the function of the clearance pathway, such as cold, smoking, excessive intake of alcohol, and anaesthetics, predispose to infection of the lower respiratory tract. If organisms succeed in reaching pulmonary alveoli they may be ingested and destroyed by alveolar macrophages. Respiratory secretions contain small amounts of antibody, mainly of the IgA class, and of complement, which may aid the phagocytosis of organisms by alveolar macrophages. However, large amounts of specific antibody are required for phagocytosis of virulent organisms such as capsulated pneumococci.

Damage to the defence mechanisms of the respiratory tract by adverse climatic factors is one of the features responsible for the seasonal variations in incidence shown by many infections that are spread by respiratory droplets. In countries with a temperate climate, serious respiratory infections occur most frequently during the winter, whilst in tropical countries infections spread by the respiratory route are seen most often at the hottest and driest time of the year. Atmospheric absolute humidity is low under both these sets of climatic conditions. A low absolute humidity may predispose to respiratory infection by impairing the secretion of respiratory mucus and antibody, and by impairing the function of ciliated respiratory-tract epithelial cells.

Non-specific protective mechanisms

The acute-phase reaction

Many infections lead to a series of physiological changes, of which fever is one of the most prominent. These changes include anorexia, general malaise, polyarthralgia, an increase in basal metabolic rate, and an increase in cardiac output. Biochemical changes include a fall in serum iron and zinc, and an increase in certain plasma proteins such as C-reactive protein, α_1-glycoprotein, and orosomucoid. During the past few years, considerable progress has been made in elucidating the mechanisms of the acute-phase response. It is now clear that the majority of these changes are brought about by the action of cytokines secreted by cells of the macrophage/monocyte lineage. Interaction between the various cytokines involved in the acute-phase response is complex but tumour necrosis factor appears to have a central role. In both experimental and human Gram-negative infections, levels of tumour necrosis factor rise before those of interleukin (**IL**) 1 and IL-6 and, in experimental animals, septic shock can be prevented by prior administration of antitumour necrosis factor monoclonal or polyclonal antibodies. Tumour necrosis factor induces a wide variety of physiological changes, some of which may be beneficial to the host such as mobilization of endogenous energy sources, and some detrimental such as the induction of vascular damage. Excessive production of cytokines probably contributes to the severe illness seen in a minority of patients with infections caused by *Escherichia coli*, the meningococcus, and *Plasmodium falciparum*.

Cytokine production is stimulated by structural components of micro-organisms or by soluble factors released by them. Endotoxin is a powerful stimulator of the production of tumour necrosis factor. In the case of Gram-positive infections, such as those caused by the pneumococcus, cell-wall structures are the main stimulus for cytokine production. The characteristic intermittent fever of malaria is associated with the cyclical production of cytokines, in particular tumour necrosis factor, that occurs at schizogony (Fig. 3). The cytokine-stimulating factor released by malaria parasites is probably a phospholipid.

Whilst many of the physiological changes induced by cytokines such as IL-1 and tumour necrosis factor are unpleasant for the patient, there is evidence that sometimes they have a protective effect. The therapeutic effect of fever on neurosyphilitic infections was so pronounced that malaria-induced fever was introduced as a therapy for this condition and some recent evidence suggests that the fever of malaria plays a part in controlling unrestrained multiplication of this parasite. Fever has also been shown to have a protective effect in experimental infections with leishmaniasis and leprosy.

The rapid fall in serum iron that accompanies many acute infections may have a protective role by depriving iron-dependent bacteria of this essential nutrient. Acute-phase proteins inhibit the growth of malaria parasites and may have a harmful effect on other microbes. Small doses of tumour necrosis factor are directly harmful to malaria parasites and to some bacteria.

Thus, from the point of view of the host, the acute-phase response to infection comprises a mixture of harmful, protective, and indifferent responses.

Polymorphonuclear neutrophil leucocytes and macrophages

Polymorphonuclear neutrophil leucocytes (**PMN**) are usually the first cells to be brought into action against an invading micro-organism. They are attracted to sites of invasion by chemotactic factors produced either directly by the organism or as a result of complement activation. The way in which PMNs ingest and destroy micro-organisms is described in Section 5. PMNs can phagocytose some organisms unaided but many virulent bacteria can be phagocytosed only if they have been trapped against a mechanical barrier, such as a pulmonary alveolar membrane, or if they have been coated with antibody or complement. Patients with neutropenia or with PMNs that are functionally defective show an increased susceptibility to infection with many bacteria, including species that are not usually pathogenic. Defective PMN function may result from a hereditary defect, such as chronic granulomatous disease, or from environmental factors such as an overwhelming infection or diabetes.

Organisms that are not destroyed by PMNs may be taken up by fixed, tissue macrophages or by phagocytic cells derived from blood monocytes. Such cells are attracted to sites of infection by organisms, such as *Mycobacterium tuberculosis*, that produce monocyte chemotactic factors. Phagocytosis and killing of micro-organisms by macrophages follows similar lines to those described for PMNs except that the myeloperoxidase enzyme system is not as well developed in macrophages as it is in PMNs. Some micro-organisms, for example *M. leprae* and *Toxoplasma gondii*, can survive unharmed in macrophage phagosomes, thus escaping the harmful effects of antibody, unless the macrophages have

Fig. 3 The relationship between fever (closed circles) and plasma levels of tumour necrosis factor (open triangles) in a patient with *P. vivax* malaria (reproduced from Karunaweera *et al.* (1992). *Proceedings of the National Academy of Sciences* (USA), **89,** 3200, with permission).

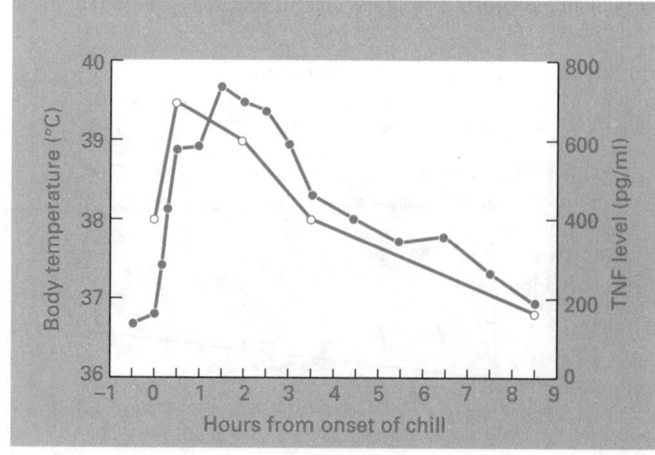

Table 1 *Methods by which specific antibody can protect against infection*

Mechanism	Examples
Neutralization of a toxin	Diphtheria, tetanus
Prevention of attachment of an organism to the surface membrane of a cell	Many viral and bacterial infections of the gastrointestinal and respiratory tracts
Prevention of spread of a micro-organism from cell to cell	Many viral infections, malaria
Immune lysis with complement	*E. coli* infections, neisserial infections, African trypanosomiasis
Enhancement of phagocytosis by PMNs or macrophages	Most coccal infections
Antibody-dependent cellular cytotoxicity in conjunction with:	
K cells	Some viral infections, malaria
Eosinophils	Schistosomiasis, trichinellosis

been activated by cytokines produced as a consequence of a specific cell-mediated immune reaction.

The macrophages of the spleen play an important part in protection against pneumococcal infection, malaria, and babesiosis. Patients without a spleen or with a non-functioning spleen, as may occur in sickle-cell disease, have an increased susceptibility to these infections. It is likely that the unusual vascular anatomy of the spleen provides an environment in which circulating micro-organisms can be brought into close proximity to tissue macrophages, which can then ingest and destroy them.

Natural antibodies

Some individuals possess antibodies that act against organisms to which they have not been exposed previously. These 'natural' antibodies, which belong mainly to the IgM class, are probably formed as a result of exposure to a cross-reacting antigen present in another organism. Thus, infection with the harmless bacterium *Neisseria lactamica* can induce the formation of antibodies that are bactericidal to the meningococcus. However, in most instances protective antibodies are formed only as a result of direct exposure to the organism in question.

Complement

The complement pathway is described in detail in Chapter 5.4. Complement activation commonly accompanies systemic infections as a result of activation of the classical complement pathway by immune complexes, as a result of activation of the alternative complement pathway by microbial products such as pneumococcal polysaccharides or endotoxin, or as a consequence of direct digestion of complement components by bacterial proteases. Activation of complement by any of these pathways can aid in protection against infection in three main ways: (i) attracting white cells to the site of the infective agents, (ii) facilitating their phagocytosis or (iii), by destroying them directly by punching holes through their cell walls.

Patients with C3 deficiency suffer from recurrent pyogenic infections. Patients with deficiency of late complement components (C5, 6, 7, and 8) show an increased susceptibility to infections with Neisseria.

Specific protective immune responses

Antibodies

Production of specific protective antibodies takes 7 to 10 days from the time of first exposure to antigen, unless the immune system of the host has been primed by previous infection or by vaccination. During this interval, death or irreparable tissue damage may occur. Antibody can aid recovery from infection, or prevent reinfection, by a number of mechanisms summarized in Table 1. Prevention of reinfection may be dependent upon a different mechanism from that used to achieve recovery.

Patients with a primary or an acquired defect in antibody production show an increased susceptibility to infection with many species of bacteria, including some which are not usually pathogenic.

Antibody-dependent cellular cytotoxicity

The synergistic action of antibody and PMNs in the destruction of bacteria has long been recognized. More recently it has been shown that other types of cell can cooperate with antibody in killing micro-organisms. Killing of protozoa, bacteria, and virally infected cells by a subpopulation of lymphocytes acting in conjunction with antibody has been demonstrated *in vitro*, but it is still uncertain how important this mechanism is in life. Eosinophils can kill schistosomula of *Schistosoma mansoni* and larvae of *Trichinella spiralis* with the aid of antibody. Eosinophils obtained from patients with schistosomiasis are more effective killers than eosinophils obtained from controls.

Cellular immune responses

Parasites within a cell are safe from the harmful effects of antibody. Recovery from infection with many intracellular organisms is thus dependent upon specific cell-mediated immune mechanisms mediated by thymus-dependent (T) lymphocytes. Sensitized T lymphocytes, usually of the CD8 subtype, can destroy an infected host cell by direct cytolytic action. Direct contact between the T lymphocyte and the target cell is required and the effector cell must be metabolically active. Neither antibody nor complement are required. Killing is only achieved when the effector cell and the target cell share the same class I histocompatibility antigens (HLA), the effector cell recognizing a peptide HLA complex on the surface of the target cell.

Sensitized lymphocytes can also protect against infection through their influence on macrophages. Macrophages activated by lymphokines produced as a result of contact between sensitized lymphocytes and the appropriate antigen are able to destroy organisms against which they were previously impotent. Such activated macrophages show enhanced activity against organisms other than the one which induced the cell-mediated immune reaction that led to their formation.

Patients with deficient cell-mediated immunity have an increased susceptibility to infection with many viruses, some intracellular bacteria, and protozoa, and they are susceptible to infection with fungi and yeasts.

Protective mechanisms acting at mucosal surfaces

As many pathogenic organisms invade through either the alimentary or respiratory tracts, protective mechanisms acting at these sites play an especially important part in determining susceptibility to infection.

Organisms that survive the acid pH of the stomach and thus reach the small bowel are susceptible to attack by IgA antibodies produced by plasma cells in the lamina propria of the gut. These cells produce secretory IgA antibodies (two IgA molecules linked by a polypeptide secretory piece) that are resistant to digestion by small-bowel enzymes. Some helminths induce an IgE-mediated immune response in the gut, which

Table 2 *Some examples of type 1 allergic reactions complicating infections and their different clinical manifestations*

Peripheral circulatory collapse	Pulmonary infiltration or asthma	Rashes
Onchocerciasis (treatment reaction)	Aspergillosis	Animal hookworm larvae (cutaneous larva migrans)
Ruptured hydatid cyst	Migrating roundworm larvae	Animal schistosome cercariae
	Migrating schistosomulae	Hookworm larvae (ground itch)
	Tropical eosinophilia	Onchocerciasis (treatment reaction)
		Trypanosomiasis

may contribute to their expulsion. The epithelium of the gut is capable of mounting a specific cell-mediated immune reaction but the role of cell-mediated immunity in protection against gastrointestinal infections has been little studied.

Breast milk protects an infant from gastrointestinal infection in several ways. It provides a relatively sterile source of food and it contains IgA antibodies, lysozyme, and other less clearly defined substances that have an adverse effect on the growth of many bacteria and viruses. Cell-mediated immune responsiveness may also be transferred from mother to baby through breast milk. Bottle-fed babies experience gastrointestinal infections more frequently than breast-fed babies, especially in developing countries, where preparation of uncontaminated bottle feeds is difficult.

Harmful immune response to infection

Introduction

The value of the immune response in achieving recovery from infection and in preventing reinfection is illustrated clearly by the serious consequences that ensue when the integrity of the immune system is impaired. However, there is often a price to be paid for elimination of micro-organisms by the immune system. Destruction of an intracellular parasite can often be achieved only at the cost of destruction of the host cell within which the parasite resides. At sites such as the liver, where cell regeneration is rapid, damaged cells are easily replaced. However, immunologically mediated recovery from infections of the nervous system can often be achieved only at the expense of irreversible tissue damage.

It is convenient to describe immunopathological responses to infection under one of four classical headings of immune response (see Section 5) but such responses are not mutually exclusive and tissue damage may be the result of several immune responses occurring concurrently. Furthermore, in the case of some infections it is apparent that immunopathological processes are involved in the pathogenesis of the disease but it is not clear by what mechanism these are brought about. Infection with the human immunodeficiency virus (**HIV**) provides a topical example. It is generally accepted that most of the clinical features of AIDS are brought about as a result of loss of CD4-bearing cells brought about by HIV infection but there is controversy about how this is achieved. The HIV virus can be detected in only a small proportion of the CD4 cells of infected individuals and it has been argued that this level of infection is insufficient to cause a fall in the blood CD4 count. Thus, it has been suggested that the HIV virus induces some kind of an autoimmune reaction directed against uninfected CD4 cells or induces apoptosis.

The factors that determine why immunopathological complications are associated with some infections but not with others are poorly understood. Thus, immune complex-mediated arthritis and vasculitis are well-recognized complications of meningococcal infection but they are rarely seen as a complication of pneumococcal infection. Further uncertainties surround the question of why only a small proportion of patients with a particular infection develop immunopathological complications. Acute nephritis complicates only a small proportion of group A α-haemolytic streptococcal infections and progressive glomerulonephritis is an ever rarer complication of *P. malariae* malaria.

Immediate hypersensitivity reactions

Immediate hypersensitivity reactions result from the release of histamine and other vasoactive amines from basophils and mast cells that have been sensitized with IgE antibody and then exposed to the relevant antigen. Such reactions often complicate helminthic infections, which are associated with enhanced synthesis of IgE antibody.

Some examples of type 1 reactions complicating an infection are shown in Table 2. The clinical features of type 1 allergic reactions, which are largely those of histamine poisoning, vary in severity from a mild skin lesion to peripheral circulatory collapse and death.

Eosinophilia is a frequent accompaniment of infections that are complicated by immediate hypersensitivity reactions. Eosinophils can inactivate histamine and other vasoactive compounds, such as slow-reacting substance, released by mast cells. Thus, in patients with a helminthic infection, eosinophils may have a protective function by modulating some of the harmful effects of an immunopathological response to the infection.

Antibody-mediated tissue damage

Sensitization of host cells by microbial antigens may render such cells susceptible to immune attack. Such a process probably plays a part in the pathogenesis of the haemolytic anaemia associated with *Mycoplasma pneumoniae* and with some other viral infections. The anaemia of malaria has a complex aetiology, since non-parasitized cells as well as parasitized cells are destroyed more rapidly than normal during this infection. It is possible that binding of malaria antigen to the surface of non-infected red cells renders them susceptible to immune attack by antibody and complement and to their subsequent elimination by phagocytic cells.

Tissue damage by antibody may occur during the course of other infections. Antibodies that react with myocardial cells and with Schwann cells are often found in sera obtained from patients with South American trypanosomiasis but it is uncertain whether these antibodies play any part in bringing about the cardiac and neurological damage characteristic of this infection.

Immune complex-mediated tissue damage

Tissue damage as a result of immune-complex deposition is one of the most frequently encountered immunopathological complications of infection. Immune complex-mediated tissue damage can be produced in two ways. Immune complexes formed within the circulation during the course of an infection may be trapped in the kidneys, skin, or synovium where, as a result of complement activation, they induce an acute inflammatory reaction. Deposition in the kidneys is favoured by their high blood flow and by the presence of C3b receptors on the basement membrane of renal capillaries. During the course of other infections, for example, lepromatous leprosy, large amounts of antigen accumulate in the peripheral tissues; such aggregates may be the site of local immune-complex formation (an Arthus reaction). Such a mechanism is respon-

Table 3 *Some examples of immune complex-mediated tissue damage arising as a complication of an infection*

Shock syndrome	Acute glomerulonephritis	Chronic glomerulonephritis	Rashes and/or arthritis
Dengue	Bacterial endocarditis Dengue Hepatitis B infection Leprosy *P. falciparum* infection Pneumococcal infection Schistosomiasis mansoni Streptococcal infection Syphilis Typhoid	*P. malariae* infection Streptococcal infection	Hepatitis B infection Meningococcal infection* Leprosy* Syphilis

*Due to local formation of immune complexes.

sible for erythema nodosum leprosum and for the arthritis associated with meningococcal disease. Immune complexes can cause a variety of clinical syndromes, dependent upon the site at which they are formed, ranging in severity from a mild rash to peripheral circulatory collapse and associated disseminated intravascular coagulation. Table 3 lists some of the most frequently encountered clinical manifestations of immune-complex disease and the infections with which they are associated.

Delayed hypersensitivity reactions

Damage to host cells is inevitable whenever a cell-mediated immune attack is directed against an intracellular parasite. For some infections, tissue damage produced in this way is more important than that produced by the causative micro-organism itself (Table 4). Thus, in experimental animals, the outcome of some viral meningoencephalitides is less serious in immunodeficient animals than in animals with an intact immune system, even though the virus is not eliminated by the animals with defective immunity.

Cell-mediated immune damage plays an important part in the pathogenesis of the clinical features of tuberculoid leprosy. Patients with this form of leprosy are able to contain, and eventually to eradicate *M. leprae* but this may be achieved only at the expense of severe and irreversible damage to peripheral nerves. A sudden deterioration in the clinical features of patients with borderline leprosy may follow an increase in the patient's ability to mount a cellular immune response after the start of treatment or as a consequence of other less clearly defined factors.

Factors influencing the host's response to infection

Introduction

A large number of factors, some genetic and some acquired, can influence the host's response to infection (see Fig. 1). Thus, it is not surprising that a host–parasite encounter can result in a wide range of outcomes, depending on interactions between these many variables. Whilst the role of individual risk factors in influencing susceptibility to many infections has been clearly established by epidemiological investigations, such as case-control studies, it is often not clear how these effects are achieved. It is probable that many act by modulation of specific immune responses. Recent immunological studies indicate the kind of ways in which this could be achieved. It has been shown that CD4 helper T lymphocytes can be subdivided into two types, Th1 and Th2 cells, that are associated with the production of different cytokines (interferon-γ and IL-1 for Th1 cells and IL-5, IL-6, and IL-10 for Th2 cells). Each of these cytokines induces its own characteristic effector response. Thus, it is easy to imagine how a genetic or environmental factor that could

Table 4 *Some examples of cell-mediated tissue damage arising as a complication of an infection*

Viral	Bacterial	Protozoal	Helminth
Encephalitides	Tuberculosis Leprosy Brucellosis Salmonellosis	Leishmaniasis Toxoplasmosis	Schistosomiasis

influence the magnitude or timing of Th1 and Th2 responses could have an important influence on the clinical features of an infection. This is likely to be just one of the ways in which the immune response and clinical pattern of an infection can be modulated.

Genetic factors and susceptibility to infection

Introduction

Studies with inbred strains of experimental animals have indicated clearly that genetic factors influence susceptibility to infectious diseases and their clinical outcome; in some instances, the mechanism of this genetic influence has been defined. Demonstrating the importance of genetic factors in determining susceptibility to infections in man has proved to be more difficult. Racial differences in the pattern of individual infectious diseases, for example the tendency of Indian patients with tuberculosis to show bone involvement and the severity of yellow fever in Europeans, suggest that genetic factors have an influence on the clinical course of an infection but, in these situations, it is difficult to differentiate between the influence of genetic and environmental factors such as diet. Studies of identical twins have provided stronger evidence. Such studies have shown that the twin of a patient with tuberculosis or leprosy has a higher risk of contracting the infection than a control, even when the twin is brought up in a different environment from his or her sibling.

HLA and infection

Studies made during the past few years have shown that susceptibility to a variety of diseases, most of which involve some kind of immunological abnormality, is associated with the possession of specific HLA antigens. The association between the HLA system and susceptibility to infection has been investigated in several ways. At a population level it has been shown that the distribution of certain HLA antigens is related to the geographical distribution of widespread infections such as malaria. At the individual level it has been demonstrated that patients with some infections, for example tuberculosis and leprosy, possess certain HLA haplotypes significantly more frequently than carefully matched controls, but caution is needed in the interpretation of such findings because the large number of alleles involved means that some apparently statistically significant associations will be found by chance. Appropriate corrections are needed to take this into account. Further evidence comes from the fact that in families with more than one case of the infection, affected siblings carry the same haplotype as the index cases significantly more frequently than do non-affected siblings, although the haplotype involved may vary from family to family.

Histocompatibility-related factors may influence the clinical outcome of an infection as well as its incidence. HLA-determined factors may determine whether a patient infected with *M. leprae* develops the lepromatous or tuberculoid form of the disease. The likelihood that hepatitis B infection will progress to chronic liver disease is HLA related, as is the development of hepatic fibrosis in patients with schistosomiasis. Some, but not all studies, have shown that progression of HIV infection to AIDS is accelerated in those carrying the HLA-DR3 antigen and possession of the antigen B27 increases the likelihood that arthritis will develop after gastrointestinal infection with yersiniae, salmonellae, or shigellae.

Other genetic markers and susceptibility to infection

Immune responsiveness is related to the possession of certain genetically determined allotypes of immunoglobulin molecules. In man, immune responsiveness to meningococcal and *H. influenzae* polysaccharides is related to the presence of a specific κ_m allotype of IgG and responsiveness to flagellin is influenced by γ_m allotype, perhaps because the genes controlling these alleles are in linkage disequilibrium with an immune-response gene. Some studies, although not all, have shown a decreased incidence of bacterial meningitis in κ_mI-positive subjects.

Possession of specific blood-group antigens also influences susceptibility to some infections. Severe infection by *Schistosoma mansoni* and Giardia are encountered more frequently in blood-group A individuals than in subjects with other ABO blood groups; the association may be due to the fact that hypochlorhydria is found more frequently in group A subjects than in individuals with other ABO blood groups. Non-secretors of blood-group antigens have an increased risk of becoming meningococcal nasopharyngeal carriers. The association between Duffy blood-group antigens and *Plasmodium vivax* is discussed below.

Mechanisms by which genetic factors increase susceptibility to infection

Genetic factors can influence susceptibility to infection in at least three ways.

1. INFLUENCE ON SURFACE RECEPTORS

Invasion of a host cell by an intracellular parasite initially involves attachment of the micro-organism to the surface of its new target. This attachment is often achieved by binding to a specific surface-membrane receptor. The presence or absence of a suitable membrane receptor may be under genetic control. This situation has been demonstrated most clearly in man in connection with *P. vivax* infection. Red cells can be infected with this malaria parasite only if they possess a surface receptor closely related to the Duffy red-cell antigen. Most West Africans lack Duffy antigens, thus offering the probable explanation for the infrequent occurrence of *P. vivax* malaria in West Africa. It is likely that genetic factors influence susceptibility to other infections by a similar mechanism.

2. INFLUENCE ON HOST CELL CONSTITUENTS

An intracellular parasite is dependent for its nutrition upon the constituents of the host cell that it has invaded. The nature of these constituents may be under the influence of genetic factors. Malaria offers an example of this phenomenon also. Epidemiological studies indicate that subjects who possess the haemoglobin genotype AS are partially protected against *P. falciparum* malaria but it is still not certain exactly how this protection is brought about (see Chapter 7.13.2.)

3. INFLUENCE ON THE SPECIFIC IMMUNE RESPONSE

A number of clearly defined, genetically determined, primary immunodeficiency syndromes that are associated with an increased susceptibility to infection have been described. Lymphocytes, immunoglobulins, complement, and PMNs may all be involved. These well-characterized primary immune deficiencies are responsible for only a small fraction of all severe infections. It is possible that more subtle genetically determined defects of the immune system, which have not yet been defined, contribute to the pathogenesis of a much larger proportion of cases of infectious disease.

Recent studies have provided evidence of how HLA genes might exert their disease-modifying effect through an influence on specific immune responses. It has been shown that stimulation of T lymphocytes is brought about by interaction between a lymphocyte carrying the appropriate receptor and a peptide of about 15 amino acids held in the cleft of the HLA class II antigen on the surface of an antigen-presenting cell (see Section 5). Most peptides will bind to only one specific HLA antigen. Thus, if the peptide in question is an important one in inducing a protective response to the organism from which it was derived, then carriers of that HLA antigen will be protected against that infection.

In a similar way, HLA class 1 antigens on infected cells can present smaller peptides, derived from cytoplasmic breakdown of proteins to cytotoxic T lymphocytes. These cells, predominantly of the CD8 type, can kill cells carrying on their surface the appropriate peptide, provided that these cells also carry the same HLA class 1 antigens as the effector T cells. Thus, subjects carrying a particular HLA type may be particularly effective at mounting a cytotoxic reaction against infected cells. This may result in either diminished or enhanced disease severity depending upon the balance between destruction of the micro-organism and destruction of host cells.

The specificity of peptide binding to HLA has recently been used to try to determine which antigens may be important in producing protection against malaria. Epidemiological studies have shown that Gambian children who possess the HLA class I antigen Bw53 have a reduced risk of developing severe malaria. Therefore, a series of peptides derived from pre-erythocytic malaria antigens was screened to see which bound most avidly to this HLA antigen. One peptide corresponding to a region of the liver-stage antigen LSA1 gave particularly strong binding. Cells expressing this peptide are attacked by cytotoxic T cells from malaria immune individuals so that this peptide may be an important inducer of this kind of immunity.

Constitutional factors and susceptibility to infection

Introduction

Environmental, as well as genetic, factors play an important part in determining susceptibility to infection and in determining its severity. Some of the most important of these constitutional factors are considered below.

Age

Many infectious diseases show a characteristic age distribution. Age exerts an influence on susceptibility to infection in various ways. Infants are usually protected against infection with ubiquitous organisms by antibody transmitted across the placenta, so that the peak incidence of many infections such as measles, mumps, and whooping cough is in

Table 5 *Some common infections seen more frequently, -or with increased severity, in the malnourished*

Protozoa	Bacteria	Viruses	Yeasts
Amoebiasis	Cholera	Herpes simplex	Candidiasis
Giardiasis	Gram-negative sepsis	Infectious hepatitis	
Pneumocystis	Infectious diarrhoea	Measles	
	Tuberculosis		

Table 6 *The harmful effects of protein-energy malnutrition on defences against infection*

Surface defences	Damage to the skin and other epithelial surfaces; achlorhydria
Non-specific immunity	Impaired microbial killing by PMNs; depression of serum complement levels
Specific cellular immunity	Diminished cutaneous delayed hypersensitivity; depletion of T lymphocytes; diminished proliferative response of lymphocytes *in vitro*; diminished cytokine production; inhibitory serum factors
Humoral	Impaired antibody production to some antigens

early childhood. Susceptibility to infection increases in the old in association with a decline in immune responsiveness.

The age distribution of many infectious diseases is determined by age-dependent occupational or social activities. Venereal infections are an obvious example. Other examples of age dependence are determined by more subtle changes in social behaviour. Thus, in endemic areas, the clinical features of schistosomiasis are seen more frequently in young boys than in adults. Gradual acquisition of protective immunity is one explanation for this phenomenon but the fact that children, unlike adults, bathe frequently in infected water is also important.

Age influences not only susceptibility to infection but also its clinical severity. Thus, in endemic areas, malaria is a milder infection in adults than in children because adults have acquired some protective immunity as a result of numerous previous infections. The converse applies to many viral infections. Measles is usually mild in young infants, perhaps because of the protective effects of maternally transmitted antibody. Poliomyelitis, yellow fever, hepatitis A infection, Epstein–Barr virus infection, and mumps are all milder infections in children than in adults. Why this should be the case has never been explained satisfactorily. It is possible that immunopathological reactions are more marked in adults than in children, because of maturation of the immune system or because of previous exposure to cross-reacting antigens, but this is unlikely to be the only explanation for this phenomenon.

Sex and hormonal factors

Variation in the sex distribution of infectious diseases may be brought about by both social and hormonal factors. Some infections are more common in men than in women because men come into close contact with the source of the infection more frequently than women as a result of their occupation. However, for reasons that are not obvious, young women are more susceptible to tuberculosis than young men. Certain infections, for example hepatitis, pneumococcal infection, amoebiasis, and malaria, are more severe when they occur during pregnancy than when they occur at other times. An enhanced susceptibility to infection during pregnancy may be a reflection of the generalized impairment of immunity that occurs at this time.

An excess of glucocorticosteroids, resulting from adrenal hyperplasia, an adrenal tumour, or steroid therapy, increases susceptibility to many infections and increases their severity. Herpes simplex and herpes zoster can cause severe, and sometimes fatal, infections in patients who are receiving large doses of corticosteroids. Tuberculosis, amoebiasis, and strongyloidiasis can all be activated by these drugs and strongyloidiasis may be fatal when it occurs in such circumstances. Corticosteroids probably exert their effect by their action on the immune response. In large doses they cause depletion of T lymphocytes, impairment of cell-mediated immunity, and impairment of some functions of PMNs.

Patients with diabetes, especially when the condition is poorly controlled, show an increased susceptibility to several infections. Boils, abscesses, and urinary tract infections are common. Tuberculosis may be activated, and pulmonary infections with yeasts or fungi may occur. Cell-mediated immune reactions and chemotaxis by PMNs are impaired in patients with diabetes and these defects may contribute to the increased susceptibility to infection shown by those with this condition.

Trauma

Trauma predisposes to infection in several ways. Damage to the surface defences, for example by a severe burn, opens the way to systemic invasion by organisms normally confined to the surface of the body. Severe burns have a depressive effect on the immune system also. Tissue destruction as a result of mechanical trauma or vascular damage can create an environment in which anaerobic organisms, such as *Clostridium tetani* and *C. perfringens*, can thrive. Thus, pulmonary and bone infarcts may become infected by organisms that have difficulty in establishing themselves in normal tissue. This is likely to be one of the reasons for the high incidence of salmonella osteomyelitis observed in patients with sickle-cell disease. Tonsillectomy and intramuscular injections predispose to paralytic poliomyelitis but the mechanism of this association is uncertain.

Malnutrition

Numerous studies in experimental animals have shown that dietary deficiency of protein, of individual vitamins, and of trace elements increases susceptibility to infection by a wide variety of organisms. Similarly, in man, clinical studies have shown that certain infections are more frequent or more severe in malnourished subjects than in healthy controls (Table 5). Children with kwashiokor are much more susceptible to infection than those with marasmus. The pathogenesis of the enhanced susceptibility to infection shown by subjects with protein-energy malnutrition is complex, for this form of malnutrition affects adversely nearly all host defence mechanisms (Table 6).

In man, severe isolated deficiencies of metals and vitamins are rarely encountered, but it has been shown that iron deficiency increases susceptibility to certain bacterial infections. Deficiency of vitamin A predisposes to infection at epithelial surfaces and increases the severity of measles.

Studies in severely malnourished refugees have shown that refeeding may be associated with an increased prevalence of tuberculosis, brucellosis, amoebiasis, malaria, and herpes. Furthermore, some studies have shown that treatment of iron-deficient subjects with iron increases their susceptibility to malaria. Thus, dietary deprivation may under some circumstances protect against infection.

Table 7 *Examples of conditions in which one infection predisposes to another*

Primary infection	Secondary infection	Likely mechanism of susceptibility
Bartonellosis	Salmonella septicaemia	Haemolysis
HIV	Pneumocystis, tuberculosis and many other infections	↓ Cell-mediated and other immune functions
Influenza	Bacterial pneumonia	Damage to epithelium
Malaria	Salmonella septicaemia	↓ PMN function ↓ Humoral immunity Haemolysis
Measles	Bacterial pneumonia, gastroenteritis herpes simplex, tuberculosis	Severe impairment of cellular and humoral immunity
Meningococcal disease	Herpes simplex	↓ Cell-mediated immunity
Pneumococcal disease	Herpes simplex	↓ Cell-mediated immunity
Schistosomiasis	Salmonella septicaemia	Adult worm acts as a focus
Septic abortion	Tetanus, gas gangrene	Tissue damage
Tuberculosis	Aspergillosis	Tissue damage
Trypanosomiasis	Pneumococcal pneumonia	↓ Humoral immunity

Infection

The fact that one infection frequently follows hard upon the heels of another is well known and illustrated dramatically by HIV infection. Some other examples of this are shown in Table 7. The mechanisms underlying these associations vary from infection to infection and they are, in some instances, very complex. A large parasite can act as a nidus for infection by a smaller one. Thus, salmonellae can colonize the cuticle of adult schistosomes and, from this protected site in the portal vein, cause recurrent episodes of septicaemia. Tissues damaged by one organism may provide a favourable environment for invasion by another. Thus, *C. tetani* can colonize infected wounds that are the site of a pyogenic infection, and tetanus may follow a guinea-worm infection. Old tuberculous cavities may be colonized by moulds such as Aspergillus. Damage to the epithelium of the respiratory tract by viruses may predispose to subsequent pulmonary infection with bacteria. However, the most important mechanism by which one infection predisposes to another is by depressing the immune response of the host.

Some degree of immunosuppression accompanies most infections; it is the rule rather than the exception. In some cases immunodepression produced in this way is of interest to the immunologist but is of little importance to the patient. However, in a few instances, suppression of the immune response of the host regularly leads to a secondary infection that has a large influence on the outcome of the patient's illness. Measles is an important example of this phenomenon. Children with this infection frequently develop secondary bacterial infections, such as pneumonia and severe gastroenteritis. Tuberculosis may be activated and activation of herpes simplex may result in severe ulceration of the mucosa of the mouth and of the cornea or, occasionally, an overwhelming viraemia. Children probably remain at increased risk of death for many months after they have apparently recovered from measles.

The pathogenesis of the immunosuppression that accompanies infection is complex and varies considerably from infection to infection. In some instances, the immune defect is very specific; for example, patients with lepromatous leprosy have a specific cellular immune defect to products of *M. leprae* but they are able to respond normally to other antigens. In contrast, many components of the immune response are impaired in patients with HIV infection or with measles. In general, cellular immune reactions are depressed more frequently by infections than are humoral immune mechanisms but both these components of the immune response, as well as PMNs and macrophages, may be adversely affected. Activation of one component of the immune response by a previous infection may result in the immune response to a second being driven in an ineffective or harmful direction rather than in a beneficial one. The complex interactions that may arise between infection, nutrition, and immunity are well illustrated by measles (Fig. 4).

Drugs

The problem of infection in patients receiving cytotoxic or immunosuppressive drugs is considered in Chapter 7.19.3. Alcohol in excess increases susceptibility to many infections, especially when cirrhosis of the liver has supervened. Septicaemia is a common terminal event in intravenous drug addicts who neglect simple hygienic precautions. Smoking, by damaging the epithelium of the respiratory tract, predisposes to respiratory infections.

Malignant disease

Immune responsiveness is impaired in patients with widespread malignant disease, and such patients have an increased risk of infection, sometimes with organisms of low virulence. The risk of infection may be increased further by extensive radiotherapy or by treatment with cytotoxic drugs.

Conclusion

In this section some of the numerous environmental factors that can influence susceptibility to infection have been considered. This list must be borne in mind whenever a patient with a serious infection is seen. In such a situation the first task of the physician is to identify correctly the causative organism and to start an appropriate form of treatment. However, s/he must also try to establish how and why the patient became infected. Failure to recognize an underlying systemic illness may lead to failure of an apparently appropriate course of chemotherapy.

Fig. 4 The complex interaction between infection, nutrition, and impaired immunity seen in measles.

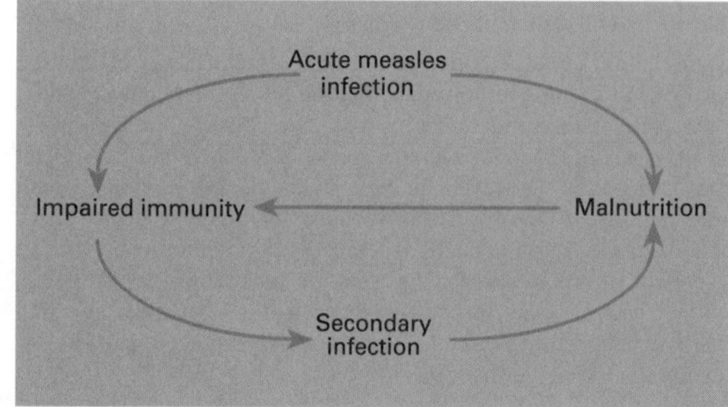

Modulation of the host response to infection

Suppression of the immune response

When an immunopathological response dominates the clinical features of an infection, it may be necessary to depress the immune response of the host, even if this carries the risk of allowing enhanced growth of the causative organism. Such severe reactions are prone to occur at the time at which chemotherapy is started, for this may result in the release of large amounts of antigen from dead or dying micro-organisms. The drugs used most frequently to prevent or control immunopathological complications of infection are the corticosteroids. Some examples of this use of corticosteroids are given in Table 8.

Enhancement of the host's response

There are a number of ways in which the resistance to an infection of an individual, or of a community, can be enhanced, as follows.

Correction of predisposing factors

Improvement in general living standards is sometimes as important a factor in controlling an infectious disease as specific immunoprophylaxis. This point is clearly illustrated by study of the incidence of major infectious diseases in industrialized countries throughout the twentieth century (see Chapter 7.4). In many cases, for example, whooping cough, the incidence of the infection and the mortality that it caused fell considerably before the discovery of antibiotics and before the introduction of vaccination (Fig. 5). This decline probably resulted from improvements in housing, nutrition, and sanitation. Conversely, increasing poverty, as well as HIV infection, have probably contributed to the recent resurgence of tuberculosis in several industrialized countries. The importance of correcting underlying nutritional deficiencies has recently been demonstrated by trials of vitamin A supplementation. In several, although not all studies, vitamin A supplementation of children led to a reduction in overall mortality and in morbidity from gastrointestinal and respiratory diseases.

Chemoprophylaxis

Chemoprophylaxis has a valuable role to play in increasing host resistance to infection in specific circumstance (see Section 9). A decision as to whether to embark upon chemoprophylaxis in a particular situation requires careful balancing of potential benefits and risks. Nearly all drugs used for chemoprophylaxis have the potential to cause serious side-effects and there have been several fatalities following the use of malaria chemoprophylactics. Further widespread use of antimicrobials for chemoprophylaxis encourages the emergence of resistant organisms. Chemoprophylaxis is most effective when used in a subject at high risk of infection for a short period.

Passive immunoprophylaxis

POLYVALENT GAMMAGLOBULIN

Polyvalent gammaglobulin, given by regular intramuscular or by less painful intravenous injections, is of proven value in protecting patients with agammaglobulinaemia or severe hypogammaglobulinaemia from a variety of infections. Its value in the management of patients with an increased susceptibility to infection associated with less clearly defined immune defects has not been established clearly.

SPECIFIC ANTISERA

Antisera with a high titre of antibody against defined microbial products have been used for the treatment of infections since the beginning of the century and, until the discovery of powerful antimicrobial chemotherapeutic agents, immune sera were the only effective form of treatment for conditions such as meningococcal and pneumococcal meningitis. The discovery of antibiotics led to an almost complete loss of interest in serum therapy but the realization that death from many common infections is frequent in spite of prompt treatment with an effective antibiotic has led to a resurgence of interest in this approach, especially in the treatment of septic shock. Recent treatment trials of both polyvalent and monoclonal anti-endotoxin antisera have given promising results, although interpretation of the results of some of these trials is controversial.

Although largely abandoned for therapy, antisera are still used widely to provide protection against a limited number of infections. Antisera with a high titre of antibodies to tetanus toxin effectively prevent tetanus, although not infection with *C. tetani*. Antitetanus serum is used less widely than in the past now that a large proportion of the population of areas where tetanus is prevalent has been actively immunized against tetanus in infancy. However, if there is doubt as to whether a patient

Table 8 *Some examples of the use of corticosteroids to diminish the immunopathological response to an infection*

Condition	Comments
Acute rheumatic carditis	Short-term beneficial effect; no protection against valve damage
African trypanosomiasis	Protect against melarsoprol treatment reactions
Chronic hepatitis B infection (chronic active hepatitis)	Corticosteroids given with azathioprine increase survival
Mumps orchitis	Symptomatic relief; no protection against sterility
P. malariae nephritis	Ineffective in most patients
Acute schistosomiasis (Katayama fever)	Reported to be effective
Tuberculous meningitis	Probably reduces late sequelae

Fig. 5 Whooping-cough deaths per million population in England and Wales in relation to the introduction of antibiotics and whooping-cough immunization (modified from Dick (1978). In *New trends and developments in vaccines* (ed. A. Voller and H. Friedman). MTP Press, Lancaster).

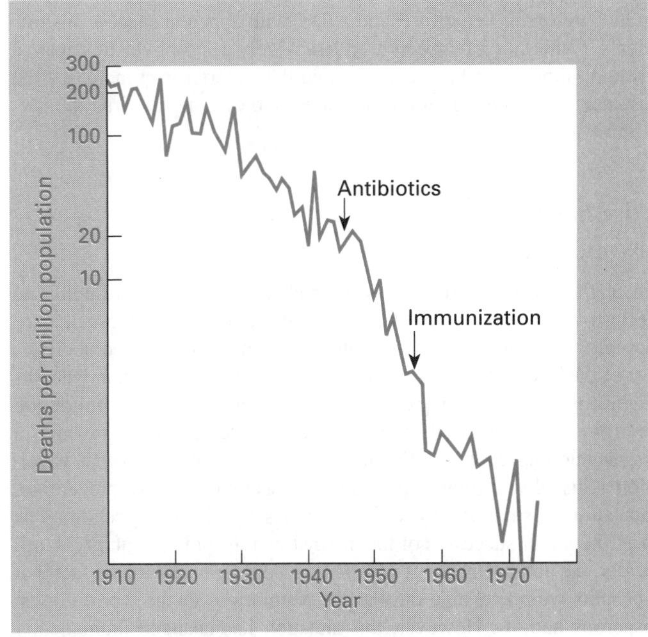

with a dirty wound has been actively immunized, then antitetanus serum should be given together with tetanus toxoid. High-titre rabies antiserum is recommended for patients with a high risk of infection because they have been bitten on the face or neck or bitten by a wild animal. Administration of rabies antiserum together with rabies vaccine does not interfere significantly with the response to active immunization. Gammaglobulin has been used extensively in the past to provide short-term protection against hepatitis A infection but it is likely to be used less frequently for this purpose in the future now that a hepatitis A vaccine is commercially available.

Antisera with high titres of antibody against specific micro-organisms have been used to provide short-term protection for immunocompromised children exposed to a potentially dangerous infection such as herpes zoster. Recently, an antiserum with high titres of antibodies against the meningococcus, pneumococcus and *H. influenzae* type b (BPIG) was tried in Navajo infants, who are at high risk from these infections during the first few months of life.

Antisera for prophylactic use are produced either by selection and pooling of donor serum samples with a high titre of the appropriate antibody produced as a result of natural exposure or by immunizing volunteers with the relevant antigen and obtaining serum by plasmapheresis. Antisera prepared from animals may cause severe anaphylaxis and this risk is reduced by using human antisera. There is natural concern that use of pooled antisera could result in transmission of infections such as hepatitis C or HIV. However, through a combination of screening tests and inactivation procedures during production, the risks of the transmission of any infection through commercially prepared antisera are now extremely small. In future, it may be possible to produce humanized antibodies for use in treatment or prophylaxis by genetic engineering of micro-organisms, thus completely eliminating this risk.

POLYMORPHONUCLEAR NEUTROPHIL LEUCOCYTES

Transfusions of granulocytes can help to provide short-term protection against infection in patient with severe leucopenia resulting from cytotoxic drug therapy, malignant disease, or infection. However, a cell separator is required to produce the large number of leucocytes required and this is a very expensive and not very effective form of prophylaxis.

CYTOKINES

Cytokines, including transfer factor and interferon, have been used to treat a variety of infections including leprosy, cutaneous leishmaniasis, systemic mycoses, hepatitis B and AIDS, with apparent success in some patients. Cytokines have been used less widely as prophylactics against infection, although it has been reported that interferon-γ increases the resistance of immunocompromised patients to cytomegalovirus and herpes infections.

Active immunization

INTRODUCTION

One of the most effective ways of modifying the host's response to infection is by vaccination. Vaccines have played an important part, although not the only one, in abolishing from industrialized societies most of the infectious diseases that were responsible for so many deaths and serious illnesses among children in Victorian times, when childhood mortality was substantially higher than the level that now prevails in most developing countries. Numerous studies have shown that vaccination is usually a highly cost-effective means of disease prevention. Eradication of smallpox by vaccination has rightly been acclaimed as one of the major successes of the international health community. Until recently, the achievements of vaccination were tarnished by the fact that its benefits were available only to the populations of the world's most prosperous nations. However, this situation has changed dramatically during the past decade as a result of sustained efforts by international organizations such as WHO and UNICEF and, in 1993, it was estimated that approximately 80 per cent of all the world's children now receive the basic childhood vaccines. A system is now in place through which the many new vaccines that are being developed could be delivered effectively to communities where they are needed most at low cost.

VACCINATION

The principles of vaccination are described in detail in Chapter 7.7, together with some exciting new advances in this rapidly developing field. Two new vaccines, hepatitis B and *H. influenzae* type b vaccines, have recently been introduced into the (**EPI**) programmes of several countries and other new vaccines are making good progress. Development of new methods of vaccine delivery, such as the incorporation of vaccines into biodegradable microspheres and the development of attenuated poxvirus able to express up to 10 different foreign antigens, indicate that further new breakthroughs are on their way.

However, it would be naive to assume that the next decade of vaccinology will be a continuing success story without any setbacks. It has yet to be shown that the present success of the global EPI programme, which is heavily aid dependent, can be sustained at a time when there are many other demands on donor agencies. Furthermore, interruption of the normal balance between host and parasite by vaccination is a chancy business and the ultimate outcome of mass vaccination campaigns cannot be predicted with certainty. Mathematical modelling can help in providing information as to what is likely to happen when different levels of vaccine coverage are achieved in different epidemiological conditions and modelling can help in pointing out potential danger areas. Dangerous conditions are particularly likely to arise in infections whose clinical manifestations are heavily age dependent, for example yellow fever or hepatitis A. For such infections it is relatively easy to model conditions in which a partially effective vaccination programme could, by shifting the age distribution of cases, make things worse. There is some evidence to suggest that this occurred during some early polio vaccination programmes.

Finally, it must be assumed that micro-organisms subject to a massive immune assault are going to fight back. Two main options are open to an organism faced with this situation if it is to survive—to change its antigens or to change its host. The latter is difficult, although not impossible, but many micro-organisms are adept at changing their antigens in the face of immune pressure, although they may not be able to accomplish this sufficiently well to evade a broad-based immune attack. The recent description of mutant hepatitis B viruses in vaccinated subjects may be the first sign that this virus is adopting this strategy.

Conclusion

Experience in many industrialized countries has shown that the best way of improving resistance to infection is through a combination of measures such as improvement of housing and nutrition as well as by vaccination. Unfortunately, the chances of improving living conditions for much of the world's expanding population in the near future are small unless there is a major change in world attitudes. In these circumstances, vaccination offers the best and most cost-effective means of preventing many infectious diseases.

REFERENCES

Bloom, B.R. (1989). Vaccines for the third world. *Nature*, **342,** 115–20.

Fong, Y. and Lowry, S.F. (1990). Tumour necrosis factor in the pathophysiology of infection and sepsis. *Clinical Immunology and Immunopathology*, **55,** 157–70.

Frank, M.M. (1987). Complement in the pathophysiology of human disease. *New England Journal of Medicine*, **316,** 1525–30.

Hill, A.V.S. (1992). HLA and infection. *Journal of the Royal College of Physicians of London*, **26,** 11–16.

Rodbard, D. (1981). The role of regional body temperature in the pathogenesis of disease. *New England Journal of Medicine*, **305,** 808–14.

Wenzel, R.P. (1992). Anti-endotoxin monoclonal antibodies—a second look. *New England Journal of Medicine*, **326,** 1151–53.

7.4 Epidemiology and public health

R. T. MAYON-WHITE

Introduction

The epidemiology of infectious diseases may be said to have started with Dr John Snow's studies on the transmission of cholera, published in 1854. Snow made an orderly collection of facts about disease in a population of people, and used these facts to devise and test theories. The value of this scientific approach was shown by the consequent actions, when stopping the polluted water supply ended an epidemic. In the 60 years that followed Snow's work on cholera, public health, and infectious disease epidemiology developed rapidly in many countries. The development was due to a combination of political and scientific advances. The growth of local democratic government gave people the means to organize safe sewerage and water supplies, and better housing and services to manage infectious disease problems. In Britain, local Medical Officers of Health were appointed to lead this organization of local public-health services. At the same time, Pasteur, Koch, and their successors were establishing the microbiological knowledge that complemented the epidemiological findings. By the end of this 60-year period, the prospects of improving health by the control of infection seemed limitless, if vaccines, antitoxins, antimicrobial chemotherapy, good hygiene, safe sanitation, adequate housing, and better nutrition could be developed as public-health tools.

These hopes were partly realized in Europe and North America in the first half of the twentieth century. The discovery of antibiotics seemed to give to human beings all the powers needed to control microbial disease. This and the major public-health work in the developing countries (for example to eradicate malaria) suggested to many doctors that communicable disease epidemiology would have little importance in the second half of the century. By 1975, this common view was changing. Although smallpox was close to being eradicated, malaria was far from being controlled. Antibiotic resistance was an established problem in hospital-acquired infections and some of the treatable diseases, like gonorrhoea, were on the increase. Unfamiliar infections were recognized, either as imported disease, like Lassa fever, or as opportunistic infections in immunocompromised hosts. Some diseases that have probably been present for a long time were identified as infections, for example campylobacter diarrhoea and legionella pneumonia. The lack of a sustained public-health interest in infection control resulted in poor management of outbreaks in Britain. Publicity about these incidents and the excitement of the 'new' diseases have stimulated a renaissance of this type of epidemiology, leading to the systems described in this chapter. The British organizations are used as one example of public-health services. Other countries have similar arrangements.

The relation between host, agent, and environment

Why do some people become infected and others do not? This question is often asked by patients seeking an explanation for their illness. For a person to become infected, they must be susceptible to the micro-organism in question, the micro-organism must be in an infective dose delivered in a way that can set up a pathogenic state, and host and micro-organism must be brought together by environmental factors. The chances of this happening are not high, and infection is relatively uncommon considering the ubiquity of many pathogenic micro-organisms. Food poisoning by *Clostridium perfringens* will serve as an example of this. *C. perfringens* is a normal resident of the large intestines of human beings and food animals. Meat used in catering will commonly be contaminated by Clostridia. Normal cooking will kill the vegetative bacteria but strains vary in their resistance to heat and spores will survive. Meat dishes left at warm temperatures for several hours after cooking provide good conditions for the spores to germinate and for rapid bacterial multiplication, to reach infective doses of enterotoxic Clostridia. If such a meat dish with its clostridial contamination is eaten, resulting in an outbreak of food poisoning, it is probable that the attack rate will be between 30 and 70 per cent. This less than complete infection rate is despite a fairly uniform exposure. Prior exposure to the infecting strain, variation in gastric acidity, the possible effect of other foods eaten at the same time, the individual's disposition to feel gastrointestinal symptoms, and chance all play their parts in determining who presents as ill. Poor food hygiene, like leaving meat dishes too long in warm conditions, is not uncommon but outbreaks are rare in relation to the frequency of meals. So chance plays a significant part in bringing together susceptible hosts and pathogenic organisms in the right circumstances.

From an evolutionary perspective, the advantages to a micro-organism in not causing a high attack rate of disease in its hosts are clear. For most parasites, the death of the host means the death of the parasite and its means of reproduction. More subtle relationships are common: for example, the time that a person with measles is most infectious is in the prodromal stage, when symptoms are mild and the type of illness undeclared, so that the infected person will still be mixing with others and transmitting the causative virus. This results in measles having a high rate of spread, so that susceptible family and school contacts can be expected to become infected. Such adaption is important to maintain the measles virus species, which has no reservoir apart from infected individuals.

The spread of infection

Knowledge of the means by which micro-organisms get from one host to another is fundamental to the control of disease. The route most commonly used by human pathogens is by respiratory droplets. The respiratory-tract infections, common childhood infections like measles and chickenpox, and the main causes of meningitis are transmitted by this route. The micro-organisms are attached to small drops of the liquids and cellular debris covering the respiratory mucosa, which are expelled by coughing, sneezing, and speech. The droplets travel for a distance of 1 to 2 m before falling to the ground. Most of these pathogens will die as the droplets dry, so the risk of infection is chiefly to people in close contact by inhaling infective droplets.

Direct contact with an infected skin or mucosal lesion is an obvious source of infection. Impetigo, scabies, herpes simplex, and cutaneous fungal infections provide examples. The micro-organisms vary between two extremes, from the staphylococci that can survive on dust particles and so spread indirectly from wound to wound, through scabies that normally requires close and warm skin contact to move from host to host, to gonorrhoea that is only transmitted by intimate contact.

Spread by the faecal–oral route is another common method, used by enteric viruses, giardia, and shigellae. Organisms excreted in faeces, especially during episodes of diarrhoea, contaminate hands and surfaces. The organisms on unwashed hands may reach food ingested by susceptible people, who then become part of the chain of infection to others. This method of spread is readily observed in children of nursery and toddler ages.

The faecal–oral route is not the only means of spread for these micro-organisms, which share with others the ability to contaminate food and water. As a general rule, the organisms that spread directly from person to person have lower infective doses than the common causes of food poisoning, when food offers the bacteria an opportunity to multiply. Similarly the infective dose for water-borne infections is often lower than for food-borne disease. The epidemic patterns observed with these three different means of spread of gastrointestinal infection is often a clue to the cause of an outbreak. A food-poisoning outbreak is typically short and sharp with infection occurring at one time (i.e. one meal). A water-borne outbreak has a lower but more persistent incidence, because the smaller chances of consuming an infected dose in a single drink of water, but the exposure is frequent. Person-to-person faecal–oral spread will produce the classical epidemic curve, with the numbers of cases being small at first, then rising exponentially as the infection spreads from case to case, and finally falling sharply when most of the susceptibles have been infected and recovered.

Some infections are spread by animal bites. The most common is malaria, but there is a wide variety of arbovirus infections similarly spread by mosquitoes and other insects, in addition to louse- and tick-borne rickettsial disease. Rabies is the infection that will come to most people's mind as caused by an animal bite, and it is justly feared as a zoonosis, the term for an infection transmissible from vertebrate animals to human beings. Other zoonoses are spread by the various routes discussed here; they include enteric infections such as salmonellosis, fevers such as brucellosis, and skin infections such as orf.

Some organisms pathogenic to man are free-living in the environment, or survive as spores in soil. Infection is relatively uncommon, unless the skin of a host is injured or the organism can gain access to a more easily penetrated mucous membrane. Examples of wound infections are tetanus and anthrax. Free-living environmental organisms include legionella and leptospira in water. Hospitals create special environments with risks of infection by the insertion of urinary catheters and intravascular lines and by surgical operations.

Variation in the occurrence of disease

Another facet of infectious disease that attracts public interest is the occurrence of epidemics or outbreaks, when the incidence of disease is abnormally high. The term outbreak is used for small and relatively confined epidemics. An outbreak can be one case of a rare disease, for example poliomyelitis in developed countries, or two or more associated cases of any disease. When it is not known whether the observed cases are associated, reference must be made to the expected incidence in order to decide whether there is an outbreak. The most predictable variation in incidence is seasonal. Respiratory infections occur more often in winters of both the Northern and Southern hemispheres. Of the respiratory infections, influenza has the most distinct epidemiological pattern, in which there are periods of one or two winter months when deaths from pneumonia, sickness, absence from work, admissions to hospital, consultations for influenza-like symptoms to general practitioners, and the isolation of influenza viruses rise to a peak together. The exact timing varies from year to year, but an indication of a forthcoming influenza epidemic can be gained from the types of influenza virus isolated in the other hemisphere during its winter season, and from the early isolations of influenza in the current winter. The events in the opposite hemisphere are soon enough to help decide on influenza vaccine composition, but it is too late for vaccination to influence the course of an epidemic if action is left until the first signs of influenza activity in the winter. The exact mechanism for the seasonality of respiratory infections is not known, although cold, damp conditions may favour the survival and thus the transmissibility of infecting organisms in respiratory droplets.

Interactions between different organisms play a part in seasonal and geographical variation. Staying with the example of influenza, there is some evidence that the increased incidence of meningococcal infection in winter time is partly due to the effects of influenza virus. Viral damage to the pharyngeal mucosa may facilitate the invasion of meningococci, resulting in bacteraemia and meningitis instead of a non-pathogenic colonization. In the 'meningitis belt' of subSaharan Africa, meningococcal disease has a marked seasonal incidence, with epidemics coming at the end of the dry season, possibly because dust acts as the preliminary irritant to the nasal mucosa. Malaria with its dependence on the Anopheles mosquito is a more obvious example of an infection with a marked geographical and seasonal variation. Within tropical areas, high altitude reduces the number of mosquito vectors. In the subtropics, malaria is much less common in winter months when insect activity is reduced. In temperate regions, the summer conditions are too short to sustain the necessary pool of infected mosquitoes and people to make malaria an endemic disease.

In addition to the fairly predictable variations caused by climate, there are unexpected fluctuations in the incidence of infection. Persistent investigations show those to be the result of two events: either the arrival of a new infection in a susceptible population or a fault in the normal control mechanisms. If a child in the prodromal stage of measles goes into a school where few of the other children have had measles or measles vaccine, an outbreak will probably occur. If proper methods of food handling are not followed in a kitchen, the chances are that an outbreak of food poisoning will occur sooner or later. In the former example, the likelihood of transmission is so high that an outbreak is to be expected; the variation comes from the chances of one of the children acquiring measles in the first place and the possibilities that some or most of the other children are immune. In the latter example, the variation comes from the probabilities of several factors occurring in the right sequence: the introduction of a food-borne organism into the kitchen, a failure of cooking to eliminate the pathogen, the right conditions to allow the pathogen to reach infective doses, and the consumption of the contaminated food by people who are susceptible. In a way that is parallel to the individual susceptibility discussed above, populations vary in their susceptibility, through past exposure, vaccination, education, and the environments that they inhabit and modify.

Surveillance

Public interest in the occurrence of outbreaks depends on, and itself determines, the surveillance of infection. Surveillance is the systematic collection and analysis of information about disease. Most of the surveillance methods are based on medical events, such as a consultation with a doctor, the discharge from hospital or death with a diagnosis of an infectious disease, the laboratory recognition of a pathogen or diagnostic serological response to infection. To be used in surveillance, these medical events must be recorded routinely, and reported to a local or central office for analysis. The information loop must be completed by reporting the results of the surveillance back to the recorders and to the public. Occasionally, special surveys are made to get directly to the population from which information is required. As an example, a cross-section of the population of children at school and women at antenatal clinics may be sampled and blood specimens taken for rubella virus antibodies to see how well the combined effects of natural infection and vaccination are protecting girls against rubella in pregnancy.

The longest-established method of surveillance is the statutory notification of infectious disease. By public-health legislation, a doctor who is treating a patient for one of the notifiable diseases should report the fact to the local public-health office. In the past in Britain, the office was that of the Medical Officer of Health employed by the local government. This has now become the responsibility of consultants in communicable disease control (**CCDCs**), employed by local health authorities. The official notification form gives the name, age, sex, and address of the patient, the date of onset of illness, the diagnosis, and the name of the reporting doctor. These details may be seen as a breach of medical confidentiality, but the legal position is that public health has to be considered as well as interests of the individual patient. In practice, the details on the notification form are kept confidential by CCDCs, who are keen to encourage more reporting. There is scope for improvement in notification systems, which are usually incomplete: only a third of the cases of measles and whooping cough and a half of the cases of meningococcal meningitis are reported despite an active interest in all three infections. In England and Wales, summaries of the local collections of notifications are sent weekly to the Office of Population, Census and Surveys, to form a national picture of the incidence of infectious disease. Although the reporting is incomplete, the level of incompleteness can be sufficiently consistent for trends in notification rates to have epidemiological significance. Such findings should be interpreted with caution and not accepted unless supported by independent evidence. Examples of worthwhile observations from notifications are the dramatic decline in diphtheria and poliomyelitis in Britain after the introduction of specific vaccination programmes. This was confirmed by a parallel reduction in cases admitted to hospital.

The list of notifiable infectious diseases can be divided into those that are reported for immediate investigation and those that are being monitored in the long term. In the first group are acute poliomyelitis, anthrax, cholera, diphtheria, dysentery, food poisoning, leprosy, leptospirosis, meningitis, meningococcal septicaemia, paratyphoid fever, plague, rabies, relapsing fever, smallpox, tuberculosis, typhoid fever, typhus, viral haemorrhagic fever, viral hepatitis, yellow fever. In the second group are acute encephalitis, AIDS (included in the list so that legal controls can be applied if necessary, but not notified as individual named cases), malaria, measles, mumps, ophthalmia neonatorum, rubella, scarlet fever, tetanus, whooping cough. The list is difficult to remember and has surprising omissions, like brucellosis, Q fever, chickenpox, and legionellosis, all with public health importance equal to or greater than some of those on the list.

The incompleteness of routine notifications, which is not confined to Britain, has led to the development of alternatives. Sentinel or 'spotter' practices are general practitioners who have agreed to record all new cases of selected infections observed by them. In Britain, sentinel practice records have been a sensitive and rapid way of detecting influenza epidemics. The advantage of this method of surveillance is that the denominator is well defined by the population registered with the general practitioner, reporting is near complete and timely, and confidentiality is preserved because patients' names are not required. A further advantage is that the system can be adapted to run research projects, either by collecting additional information on a disease or by using a diagnostic register to follow-up on cases. By not being a statutory system, the list of recorded diseases can be changed easily to match new interests. Sentinel practice schemes are limited by the number of participating practices, which may be too small for studies on rare but important infections. The chosen practices may not be representative of the whole population, especially in areas where a significant part of the population are not registered with general practitioners.

Surveillance based on clinical diagnoses, as in the notifiable diseases and the sentinel practices, can be strengthened by using case definitions. In Britain, there has been less interest in case definitions than elsewhere, perhaps because of the vigorous alternative surveillance system of laboratory reports to a central epidemiological agency. In this system, most medical microbiological laboratories report weekly to the Communicable Disease Surveillance Centre for England, Wales, and Northern Ireland, or to the Communicable Diseases (Scotland) Unit in Scotland. The reports include summary statistics on the laboratory-confirmed infections of epidemiological interest. The reports include all virological diagnoses, food- and water-borne diseases, meningitis, and outbreaks of infection. The system allows for additional information to be collected on selected conditions. One of the reasons for its success has been the high quality of feedback in weekly reports. It has been extended to collect information about the incidence of AIDS by asking clinicians to report new AIDS cases and deaths in strict confidence using a code for patients' names.

Mortality statistics are now less useful in the study of communicable diseases, because of the low case-fatality rates. Information derived from hospital records is not easy to gain access to, if the intention is to survey a wide area. The arrangements differ from place to place, which often makes it necessary to make individual approaches to every hospital. Moreover, the hospital medical records usually omit the epidemiological information that is wanted. This last weakness can be improved by planning surveys in which the information requirements are agreed in advance by the clinicians who are involved. This is achieved by the British Paediatric Surveillance Unit.

For some diseases, no single system of surveillance is sufficient. Tetanus is notifiable, but is not always reported by that system. A microbiological laboratory may isolate the *C. tetani*, but sometimes the causative wound is closed. Most cases should survive with modern therapy. The disease is so rare in Britain that surveillance would have to cover every hospital admission to be effective. Only by using a combination of systems can the incidence of tetanus be properly monitored.

INVESTIGATION OF OUTBREAKS

One of the key functions of surveillance is to detect outbreaks in time to investigate their causes and to apply preventive measures. In Britain, the responsibility to lead the investigation of a suspected outbreak rests with the local CCDC. The local authority's environmental health department will be involved if food, water, or other environmental factors are suspected. An outbreak that extends over a large area or involves the whole country will need the services of a national agency, like the Communicable Disease Surveillance Centre, to coordinate the investigation. So a preliminary requirement is to have a system of communications that promptly alerts the CCDC and quickly brings in the other agencies if required. The telephone has proved invaluable in doing this and has not been supplanted by facsimile machines and electronic mail.

Legionnaires' disease will serve as an example for an outbreak investigation. Once an outbreak is suspected, the first step is to check the diagnosis on the index (first reported) case. It may be that the diagnosis is based on a clinical and radiological picture of pneumonia for which legionellosis is one of several possible microbiological causes. Exposure to an air-conditioning plant or the occurrence of other cases of pneumonic illness in the same building may have triggered the suspicion of legionnaires' disease. If there are only one or two possible cases, more definite evidence of legionellosis will be needed before a full investigation is justified. On another occasion, the local laboratory may have diagnosed three or four cases of legionella infection in a recent short period. In these circumstances, the question is whether the cases are an outbreak or a coincidence of sporadic cases. If the answer is not obvious from preliminary enquiries (perhaps the few cases came with their infections from three or four different places), the investigation should go on. Knowledge of the incubation period (the time between the moment of infection and the onset of disease) will indicate the time when infection could have occurred. Interviews with the index and other early cases will often reveal several leads to the possible causes, and show where there may be further cases to study. At this point, it is worth writing down the case definition that will be used in the investigation, and to decide what and how information will be collected, stored, and analysed. In the example, anyone with serological evidence of a recent infection by the same type of legionella as the index case might be counted as a definite case, and anyone with pneumonia who did not have serum collected at the appropriate time as a possible case, and all other cases would be excluded. The information could be collected by interview, to include age, sex, home and work address, occupation, recent travel away from home, route to work and shops, recreation, and activities known to be shared with other cases. The data could be recorded on a questionnaire form, and handled by one of several database and statistical programmes for computers. The clues found in the first round of enquiries might indicate an air-conditioned building used by some of the cases and passed by some of the others on their way to work or shopping. A more precise investigation would be mounted to test the hypothesis that the air-conditioning plant was the source of infection. This would entail microbiological tests on the water in the air-conditioning plant, a search for further cases amongst the people who had been exposed in and around the building, and a case-control study to examine the strength of the association between legionellosis and the presumed source. If some or all of these supported the hypothesis, the investigation could be concluded with a report that explained the outbreak and recommended how similar problems could be prevented. It may be that some of the cases remain unexplained and appear to be sporadic, or that some parts of the investigation cannot be completed (for example, the epidemiological information may be very limited for a person who dies from the disease under investigation). So conclusions may be tentative, but helpful when similar outbreaks occur in future. In an outbreak like this example, the press will take a very active interest, so that public relations form an important part of the outbreak management. In any outbreak, the people who are the subjects of the investigation should be told about the enquiries and the results.

Methods of infectious disease control

Determining the cause of an outbreak of infection is only one part of the practice of communicable disease epidemiology. The primary objective is to learn how endemic and epidemic infection can be controlled. The two traditional methods of prevention are hygiene rules and various forms of quarantine. It is unclear how these practices were started, but their force in religious and political affairs should not be underestimated. The worldwide epidemic, or pandemic, of AIDS has stimulated some senior officials to state publicly the concept that adverse natural events represent the wrath of God, and others to try to stop infected people from entering their country.

HYGIENE

At their simplest, hygiene rules are conventional modes of behaviour, like hand-washing after defecation or avoiding coughing directly into somebody's face. These simple rules are taught in childhood and their purpose is commonly understood. Most of the rules make epidemiological sense, that is they fit in with what is known about methods of spread of infection. However, inadequate facilities, such as a shortage of soap or water, and poor discipline can make the rules difficult to observe.

At a more elaborate level, good hygiene is determined by codes of practice. The earliest codes were folklore or religious practices, like the avoidance of pork in the Jewish and Moslem faiths (presumably to prevent tapeworm infections). In modern times, codes of practice have been established to prevent hospital infection, food poisoning, and occupational diseases. Typically, these codes are written and adopted after much discussion. Often they are good sense but contain one or two items for which there is little scientific justification, for example the wearing of face-masks in minor invasive procedures in hospital or wearing a hat in kitchens. The codes gain force by becoming references of good practice should a complaint be made against the hospital, caterer, or employer. They incur costs, not just to provide the materials required, but also in consuming time and restricting activities. Codes of practice are helpful when they are prepared by expert groups for widespread use, but their limitations should be recognized.

Sterilization and disinfection are elements of good hygiene. The complete removal or killing of all micro-organisms that might contaminate a substance is sterilization. It can be achieved by heat, usually combined with pressure and moisture in order to kill organisms more rapidly at lower temperatures, by radiation, and by chemicals like ethylene oxide. It is used for medical equipment. Disinfection, by chemicals, lesser degrees of heat, filtration of fluids or simply by soap and water, removes pathogens to well below an infective dose.

Good hygiene is also the principle behind harm minimization, which has its clearest expression in the prevention of the spread of the human immunodeficiency virus (**HIV**). Injecting drug users have an increased incidence of blood-borne infections due to HIV and hepatitis B virus. In controlling these infections, it is accepted that education against illicit drug use has a limited effect. The public-health action is to persuade drug users that if they are going to inject themselves, at least they should do it with clean needles and syringes, that they should not share equipment, and that the 'sharps' should be safely disposed. Less controversially, but with the same principle, travellers to tropical countries are advised on how to reduce the harm that may come from exposure to malaria and other 'tropical' infections.

Critical-point control

The catering trade has developed hygiene practice to a higher level with hazard analysis and critical control points. In this system, the process of preparing food on a large scale in examined carefully in the light of microbiological and epidemiological knowledge of where and how things can go wrong. Control measures are focused on the critical points thus identified. The process is monitored to ensure that the control measures are working. Risk management of hospital infection is developing along the same lines.

Attention to the critical points in the chain of infection is not new. In the control of cholera associated with contaminated water from the Broad Street pump in London in 1854, Dr John Snow's action was to have the pump handle removed. In the eradication of smallpox in the 1970s, vaccination, the restrictions on travel, and follow-up were applied to the contacts of the index case and the ring of close contacts of the primary contacts. Mass immunization, which had been useful when smallpox was more common, had become a dangerous distraction when full control was possible.

VACCINATION

A vaccination programme is different in some respects from control by good hygiene. Vaccination, a term now used synonymously with active immunization, is a compact series of medical interventions offering long-term protection, unlike hygiene, which has to be constantly applied by non-medical people. Vaccination is specific for each type of infection, whereas hygiene protects against many infections. Vaccination is less effective for people with impaired immunity for whom good hygiene is important. However, there are similarities in the need for public education about the value of both vaccination and hygiene.

Vaccination starts in infancy, at a time when mothers are likely to attend clinics for advice and welfare benefits. The first doses of vaccine can be given at the age of 2 months, or sooner in some cases (see below). The aim should be to get children fully immunized as soon as possible within the capability of the immune system. In Britain, the present schedule is a combined diphtheria, tetanus, and pertussis vaccine given at the same time as live oral poliovirus vaccine and a conjugated *Haemophilus influenzae* type b vaccine, at the age of 2, 3, and 4 months. Variations on this schedule are used in other countries, with a slightly later timing of 2, 4, and 6 months or a killed injected polio vaccine. The purpose of the earlier British schedule is to give infants some protection against whooping cough in the most vulnerable first year of life. A live attenuated measles, rubella, and mumps virus vaccine is given at the age of 13 to 15 months, after maternal antibodies have left the infant's blood. In developing countries where measles in infancy is a serious hazard, a first dose of measles vaccine may be given at the age of 6 weeks and then repeated a year later. The tetanus and diphtheria immunity is boosted either by a single dose at the age of 18 months in some countries or at the time of entry to primary school, as in Britain. Some countries require by law that all children starting school should have been vaccinated.

In Britain, schools are also used as a setting to give rubella vaccine to girls aged 10 to 13 years and a booster of tetanus and polio vaccines at about the age of 15 years. The point that emerges from these different policies is that vaccination programmes are designed to take advantage of social organizations as well as adapting to differing incidence of disease. An important objective is to raise vaccination uptake to the levels at which a sufficient proportion of the population is immune, so stopping the circulation of the pathogenic organism—what is known as herd immunity. Herd immunity protects those who cannot be effectively vaccinated, because of adverse reactions to vaccine or impaired immunity.

In places where tuberculosis is common, BCG vaccine may be given at or soon after birth. The role of routine BCG vaccination is less well established than that of the other childhood vaccines. Trials in Indian children did not show good protection. In some British cities, BCG was given to all infants, but now the national policy is one of selective use in neonates (babies born into families with an increased risk of tuberculosis) plus a programme of vaccination of tuberculin-negative schoolchildren around the age of 11 to 13 years.

CHEMOTHERAPY

The United States of America has not used BCG vaccine in its regular programme. Instead there has been a greater reliance on control by chemotherapy, not only for patients with active disease but also as prophylaxis for close contacts who may have become tuberculin-positive as a result of this exposure to infection. Antimicrobial chemotherapy has a small but significant role in public health. In addition to the control of tuberculosis, the treatment of typhoid fever and diphtheria reduces the risk of further cases. It is uncertain whether the wide use of antibiotics for pharyngitis has played a part in the reduction of the sequelae of streptococcal infection (rheumatic fever and acute glomerular nephritis), but a marked decline in puerperal sepsis followed the introduction of sulphonamides into obstetric practice. Regular penicillin prophylaxis for patients who have rheumatic fever, antimalarial drugs for travellers to warmer climates, and rifampicin for the close contacts of patients with meningococcal meningitis are three preventive uses of chemotherapy that are generally recommended.

ISOLATION

When there are no other methods of infection control, isolation of the infected individual has a part to play, if used selectively and sensitively. The most acceptable form of isolation is the single-bedded hospital room for acutely ill infected patients. This common practice can become irksome to isolated patients when they are recovering and wanting to see more than the four walls of one room. Old or mentally ill patients may be made more confused by the lack of normal contact with other people. The intentions of the isolation may be bypassed by hospital staff and relatives if they do not follow the correct procedures. A more extreme form of isolation is a plastic tent with controlled ventilation, used in high-security infectious disease units for patients with viral haemorrhagic fevers. It has been questioned whether this is necessary, after patients with Lassa fever were nursed in ordinary single rooms without infection spreading to staff or other patients. British law provides for the compulsory admission to hospital of patients with notifiable infectious diseases to prevent the spread of infection, but this power of enforced isolation is very rarely used and can be applied only for short periods. Therefore, it is not possible to control the risk of infection from someone who is persistently infectious (e.g. HIV infection or untreated tuberculosis) by enforced admission. Attempts to control infection by reverse isolation, that is the exclusion of infected people, are also prone to failure. Quarantine at seaports failed to exclude plague or cholera from European countries, and health screening at immigration desks in airports fails to exclude tuberculosis or HIV today. Infected schoolchildren may provoke demands that they be excluded from school, despite the higher risk of transmission from the unexcluded children who have not had their infections recognized. Food handlers who have become convalescent carriers of non-typhoid salmonellae face exclusion from work from overstrict interpretation of codes of practice. The threat of isolation and exclusion tends to make people frightened and hide their infections.

REFERENCES

On the legal aspects of infectious disease and the organisation of public health in Britain:

Committee of Inquiry into the Future of the Public Health Function (1988). *Public health in England.* HMSO, London.

Department of Health (1989). *Review of law on infectious disease control* [Consultation document, DoH, London.]

On the management of outbreaks:

Beneson, A.S. (1990). *The control of communicable diseases in man*, (15th edn). American Public Health Association, Washington DC.

Bres, P. (1986) *Public Health action in emergencies caused by epidemics.* World Health Organization, Geneva.

On practical public health methods:

Bassett, W.H. (ed.) (1992). *Clay's handbook of environmental health.* Chapman & Hall, London.

Vaughan, J.F. and Morrow, R.H. (1989). *Manual of epidemiology for district health management.* World Health Organisation, Geneva.

7.5 Physiological changes in infected patients

P. A. Murphy

The physiological responses that are observed in infected patients are generally divided into the local inflammatory response and systemic features such as fever, neutrophil leucocytosis, and shock. However, it is becoming clear that this distinction is invalid; bacterial shock simply represents a large-scale version of local inflammation, and the same cells and enzymatic cascades participate in both. Both systemic and local inflammation are fundamentally due to mediators of host origin whose initial effects are on vascular endothelium and on phagocytic cells. Rubor, calor, and tumor are caused by dilated and leaky small vessels whose surfaces have become sticky and promote adhesion by platelets and neutrophils. Dolor is caused by interactions between bradykinin, prostaglandins, and substance P. When infection is systemic, the same mediators and cells promote the hypotension and progressive tissue oedema of sepsis.

That both local inflammation and sepsis are caused by the reactions of host proteins and cells to invading micro-organisms has several important consequences. First, although bacteria certainly have components that can initiate inflammatory reactions, the reactions may also be triggered by non-infectious stimuli. Clinical sepsis is most commonly caused by bacterial infection, but may also result from non-bacterial infections, or from major trauma without evidence of infection. Second, because inflammation progresses through multiple cascades of host-mediated reactions, removal of the bacteria after inflammation has been initiated may not affect the outcome. This is why patients still die of pneumococcal pneumonia even though the pneumococcus is exquisitely sensitive to penicillin. Third, if we understood how inflammation progressed, we might be able to interfere with some crucial mediator, and save patients who are too far gone to respond to antibiotics alone.

Triggers for inflammation

BACTERIA AND FUNGI

All bacteria are recognized as foreign and cause inflammation immediately on entry into tissue. The mechanisms are multiple and primitive, and do not require previous experience of the organism. They include recognition of bacterial carbohydrates by the alternative pathway of complement fixation; this depends on the fact that most mammalian carbohydrates terminate in sialic acid residues whereas bacterial ones do not. Bacterial proteins are recognized as foreign because the initial amino acid is *N*-formyl methionine. Bacterial cell-wall polymers, endotoxin or peptidoglycan, depending on Gram-stain reaction, cause inflammation because they are recognized by receptors on macrophages. Fungi are recognized as foreign because of the carbohydrates in the cell wall, but are less phlogistic than bacteria because they do not contain endotoxin or peptidoglycan.

IMMUNOLOGICAL FACTORS

Immunological responses, mediated either by antigen–antibody complexes, or by sensitized T cells, contribute in varying degrees to the inflammation caused by bacteria, viruses, fungi, parasites, and tumours. There are infectious conditions in which the mere presence of the parasite in tissue is inconsequential but tissue destruction results from the immune response to parasite antigens. Immune responses are particularly important in chronic infections with the tubercle bacillus, *Histoplasma capsulatum* and similar fungi, and tissue helminths such as schistosomes. These are all characterized by little local reaction at first, followed by chronic, fibrosing, destructive lesions. Especially in tuberculosis, patients may die when the local lesions have not compromised respiration or some other vital function. This 'toxicity' is generally unexplained, but may be a response to widespread, T-cell-mediated, macrophage activation.

TISSUE DAMAGE

Tissue damage and cell death are also important inflammatory stimuli. Burns, fractures, and myocardial infarcts are examples of conditions that cause local and systemic inflammation in the absence of infection. Most viruses do not contain components that are directly inflammatory, and signs of disease only arise after extensive cell death has occurred, or as a consequence of immunological reactions. Obviously, severe inflammation of any type may be enhanced by cell death. A small minority of cases do not fit into any of these three categories; thus, fever in Hodgkin's disease is attributable to the production of pyrogens by the tumour cells.

Changes caused by particular organisms

There are a few infections where the symptoms and signs are mostly attributable to specific properties of the causative organism. The production of toxin by the diphtheria bacillus or the binding of poliovirus to receptors on spinal motoneurones determine the course of those diseases. Infectious diseases such as these, and others such as measles, tetanus, leptospirosis, and whooping cough have unique and characteristic symptoms and signs, and can be diagnosed simply on the basis of the history, the physical examination, and a thorough knowledge of epidemiology. However, even when there are distinctive features, some aspects of the illness are shared in common with other infections. Almost always there is fever; generally, inflamed areas hurt.

Infection without specific features

Most of the infections met with in ordinary clinical practice do not have symptoms and signs that enable one to make an organism-specific diagnosis. Rather, the features suggest acute or chronic inflammation in a particular organ or organs. One diagnoses pneumonia, meningitis, urinary-tract infection, or endocarditis. The species of organism responsible may be guessed at, but the only safe method of diagnosis is through the laboratory. Competent clinicians cannot diagnose streptococcal sore throat, and experienced radiologists shown only a radiograph have great difficulty in deciding whether a pneumonia is due to a bacterium, a virus or a mycoplasma. The fact is that the lung or the pharynx can react to infection in a rather limited number of ways, and that the symptoms, signs, and pathological appearances are very similar whatever the causative organism.

Importance of bacterial numbers

Both locally and systemically, the crucial variable in determining outcome is the number of micro-organisms present. This has been established for bacterial infections, but the available evidence, as well as common sense, suggest that it must also be true for viral and other infections. Numbers are important because the reactions of bacterial and viral components with host enzymes and cells follow log dose–response laws. A minimum weight of endotoxin or peptidoglycan is required to elicit an inflammatory response: the quantity is of the order of 1 to 10 μg. A minimum weight of antigen is required to elicit any immunological response: this varies from a few milligrams for an Arthus reaction to a few nanograms for an IgE-mediated, mast-cell degranulation. In all cases, the required weight greatly exceeds that of one organism (about one picogram for a bacterium). Weights that exceed the minimum produce graded responses: in the case of serum components, more molecules are activated; in the case of cells, the response of each cell is proportional to log concentration, and in addition more cells may become activated.

All bacteria produce very similar inflammatory responses because all bacteria have very similar cell-wall constituents. The chief irritant of Gram-negative organisms is endotoxin; Gram-positive organisms have peptidoglycan and teichoic acid. The inflammatory actions of these polymers can be measured in various ways; endotoxin proves to be more toxic than peptidoglycan by one to three orders of magnitude depending on the test used. Experimental studies in human skin showed that dead Gram-negative bacteria caused a standardized inflammatory response when injected in a dose of 10^6 organisms. The species of bacteria was not important, and pathogens produced no more inflammation than non-pathogens. Gram-positive organisms were less effective; they had to be injected in a dose of 10^7 organisms to produce the same histological response. *Lactobacillus casei* was as effective as the pneumococcus. This kind of evidence strongly suggests that the main difference between 'pathogens' and 'non-pathogens' is that pathogens have devices such as capsules and leucocidins which frequently enable them to multiply to a titre that will cause clinically obvious infections. It also accounts for the fact that almost any organism can cause pneumonia, endocarditis, or meningitis on occasion, and that people with grossly compromised defences frequently develop serious or fatal infections with 'non-pathogens'.

A great deal of clinical evidence supports the view that most of the features of bacterial infection are responses to large numbers of organisms, and that species is of little consequence, provided a critical population is attained. The best systemic example is the accidental intravenous infusion of infected fluids. Fluids infected with Gram-negative organisms frequently cause severe shock and sometimes death; fluids infected with Gram-positive organisms cause high fever, but deaths are rare. This observation corresponds to the measured difference in toxicity between endotoxin and peptidoglycan. Many of the bacteria causing these accidents are of unusual, or even unnamed, species, which are incapable of causing any kind of spontaneous disease. Furthermore, antibiotics do not lessen the symptoms, and if the patient dies there is generally no evidence of bacterial multiplication in the tissues at autopsy. The only important variable is the number of bacteria given to the patient before the situation is recognized and the infusion stopped. If that number is high enough, death will result. A local example of the same phenomenon is respirator-associated pneumonia. If organisms are allowed to multiply in the nebulizer reservoir and large numbers are subsequently blown straight down the trachea, pneumonia will develop, even though the organism may be ordinarily non-pathogenic.

Of course, the idea that one bacterium is much the same as another provided an adequate population is attained is something of an exaggeration. There are clinically valid differences between the thick, localized pus of *Staphylococcus aureus*, and the rapidly spreading, thin pus of *Streptococcus pyogenes*. *Bacteroides fragilis* does have a penchant for invading veins. In each case, the organism secretes a specific enzyme that may explain the observed behaviour. But on the whole the similarities between organisms of the same Gram class are much more impressive than the differences.

Inflammatory reactions of endotoxin

Endotoxin fixes complement by the alternative pathway, causes activation of factor XII of the plasma clotting system, and binds to a specific receptor on the cell membrane of macrophages. However, there is now general agreement that activation of clotting, fibrinolysis, the kinin system, and the complement system are of relatively minor importance. The key cell in inflammatory responses, both local and systemic, is the macrophage. The key mediators that initiate the inflammatory cascade are interleukin (**IL**) 1, IL-6, and tumour necrosis factor (**TNF**)-α, which are proteins secreted by macrophages (monokines).

The evidence that macrophage-mediated reactions to endotoxin are more important than activation of plasma-protein cascades comes primarily from studies of the concentrations of endotoxin required to elicit various reactions. Macrophages react to 10^{-15} g/ml of endotoxin, and are fully activated by concentrations of about 10^{-9} g/ml. Other reactions mediated by endotoxin require concentrations measured in μg/ml.

IL-1 and TNF separately produce effects on vascular endothelium, but relatively large quantities are required. However, minute amounts of these monokines work together to induce large effects. Activated endothelium displays adhesion molecules for phagocytic cells. They include E selectin, which is synthesized; and P selectin, which is mobilized from Weibel–Palade bodies.

IL-1 and TNF also induce soluble inflammatory mediators. Both cause activation of phospholipase A_2 in many tissues and cells. This enzyme liberates arachidonic acid from cell-membrane lipids. Arachidonic acid supply is rate-limiting for prostaglandin, thromboxane, and leukotriene synthesis. Another important soluble mediator is platelet-activating factor (**PAF**). Both enzymes on the PAF synthetic pathway are indirectly activated by IL-1 and TNF, probably through phosphorylation. Finally, both IL-1 and TNF induce synthesis of the highly chemotactic protein, IL-8.

The ligands for selectins are integrins, membrane proteins expressed on the membranes of phagocytic cells. Phagocytic cells, especially neutrophils, adhere to each other and to activated endothelium. In mild inflammation, most of the adherent cells migrate through the endothelium without inducing large increases in permeability. In severe inflammation, the endothelial cells are damaged or destroyed by activated polymorphonuclear neutrophils. The final destructive agents are proteases, and various free radicals and activated forms of oxygen that are ultimately derived from superoxide. The most important may be the hydroxyl radical, .OH, which peroxidates cell-membrane lipids. Hydroxyl radical can be generated either from superoxide and hydrogen peroxide, or through an interaction between superoxide and nitric oxide. It is of some interest that endothelium contains nitric oxide synthetase, and that the activity of that enzyme is up-regulated by IL-1 and TNF.

All of the multitudinous actions of endotoxin, including the sepsis syndrome, can be understood as the consequence of activation of this series of host-mediated reactions. At the local level, these reactions are protective. They allow antibodies, complement, and phagocytic cells to gain access to infected tissue and set about eliminating the invading organism. If the organism escapes local control, and invades the bloodstream, small vessels all over the body become inflamed, and the peripheral circulatory failure is likely to induce a downward spiral to death. As Lewis Thomas said, 'Sepsis is the response to a situation which was not supposed to happen.'

Inflammatory reactions provoked by Gram-positive bacteria components

The principal irritative components of Gram-positive bacteria are peptidoglycan and teichoic acid. Peptidoglycan is rather efficient at causing abscesses: 10 μg in the skin of a man is an adequate dose. There is some doubt as to whether it fixes complement by the alternative pathway at all; certainly if it does it is grossly inefficient. However, all normal sera contain antibodies against peptidoglycan, so it does fix complement by the classical pathway. There is no evidence as to whether it activates the Hageman factor. Peptidoglycan is a powerful activating stimulus for macrophages, but concentrations of 10 to 100 ng/ml are required (compare endotoxin). The active group appears to be *N*-acetyl muramyl-1-ala-D isoglutamine (**MDP**). This compound activates macrophages in solutions of 10 to 100 μg/ml, and is at least 100 times more active when coupled to an inert carrier. Macrophages activated by MDP secrete the same substances as do macrophages stimulated with endotoxin.

Teichoic acids are efficient activators of complement via the alternative pathway. In addition, antibodies to teichoic acids are present in all normal sera after infancy, sometimes in large quantities. Teichoic acids have many negatively charged groups and therefore ought to activate the Hageman factor. Something about Gram-positive organisms probably promotes clotting, as they are frequently observed adhering to the surface of platelets, and disseminated intravascular coagulation occasionally complicates Gram-positive sepsis.

Inflammation in non-bacterial infections

It is common clinical experience that the local inflammation of viral infections, and the consequences of viraemia, are much less dramatic than those of bacterial infections. The reason appears to be that most of the damage is due to cell death: few viruses contain components that promote inflammation directly. Large particles such as myxoviruses can activate macrophages, but the concentrations required are huge, and the degree of activation achieved is modest. Later in disease, virus components may be demonstrable in antigen–antibody complexes. However, very large quantities of complexes are required to produce clinically evident inflammatory changes, and as soon as large quantities of antibody are synthesized, viral infections tend to be suppressed, cutting off the supply of antigen. Dengue haemorrhagic fever is thought to be produced by the effects of antigen–antibody–complement complexes on neutrophils. Focal glomerulonephritis appears to be an immune-complex disease in which the antigen is often viral. Some cases of periarteritis nodosa are caused by complexes containing hepatitis B antigens. None of these conditions is common compared to the total incidence of infection with those viruses.

The most serious acute viral infections, such as measles and smallpox, are those in which there is widespread activation of cell-mediated immunity. It is probably no accident that sensitized T cells exposed to antigen secrete a lymphokine that is a powerful activating stimulus for macrophages.

Shock

Shock is a condition in which vital tissues are inadequately perfused with blood. Tissue ischaemia leads to further changes that cause progressive deterioration of the circulation, with steadily falling blood pressure. Unless something happens to break this vicious circle, death is inevitable. Death is most usually due to a cardiac arrhythmia, but it is only apparently sudden, and attempts at resuscitating septic patients who have sustained cardiac arrest almost invariably fail.

Shock may be caused by pump failure, as in myocardial infarction; or by severe loss of intravascular volume, as in haemorrhage or dehydration. These conditions are characterized by low cardiac output and high systemic vascular resistance. Apart from anaphylaxis, which is rare, the sepsis syndrome is the only important cause of peripheral circulatory failure, with high cardiac output and low systemic vascular resistance. This is so reliable that sepsis is often diagnosed from the haemodynamic measures, in the absence of any other evidence of infection (Table 1).

As previously discussed, bacteria can cause hypotension in several ways, initially by activating the complement and kinin cascades. Histamine release caused by bacterial stimulation of platelets is important in dogs and rabbits but apparently not in man. Other soluble mediators of hypotension that have been demonstrated in septic patients, and may be important, include products derived from arachidonic acid such as prostaglandins, thromboxane A_2 and leukotrienes, endogenous opioids, and nitric oxide.

Table 1 *Typical haemodynamic variables in shock states*

	Left atrial pressure (mmHg)	Cardiac output (l/min)	Systemic vascular resistance, (dyn/s/cm^5)
Normal	10	5	1200
Left ventricular failure	25	2	3000
Bleeding	0	3	3000
Sepsis	2	12	400

Note: Left atrial pressure is only available if the patient has been fitted with an indwelling pulmonary arterial catheter.

Table 2 *A simplified pathogenesis of sepsis*

Bacteria
Macrophages and endothelial cells
TNF-α, IL-1, IL-6
Arachidonate metabolites and platelet-activating factor
Leaky, sticky, small-vessel walls lined with activated polymorphonuclear leucocytes
Endothelium destroyed by leucocyte proteases and reactive oxygen derivatives
Vessel-wall destruction causes adult respiratory distress syndrome and multiple organ failure

In shocked animals, it has been possible to raise blood pressure by using antagonists of most of the mediators above. Sometimes it has been possible to change outcome, especially if the shock stimulus was endotoxin rather than a live, replicating bacterium. In people, there are no promising studies of soluble-mediator antagonists, and some completely negative ones. For example, a controlled trial of naloxone during clinical sepsis produced transient increases in blood pressure in some patients but no change in mortality.

There has been much better luck in changing outcome in animals by interfering with the sepsis chain that goes through macrophages (Table 2).

Before going into specifics, some general comments about animal experiments can be made. Experimental animals are healthy individuals challenged with organisms or bacterial products. Sepsis virtually never occurs in a completely healthy human, and the most important determinant of the outcome of human sepsis is the severity of the underlying disease that was present before the patient got septic. Also, because the moment of challenge is known, animals can be treated with antagonists of inflammation very soon after, or before the bacteria are given. Patients often present in far-advanced circulatory failure after having been septic for many hours. Because of these caveats, the fact that a given antagonist changes mortality in animals does not mean that it will necessarily change mortality in people. However, experiments in animals have conclusively validated the pathogenesis of sepsis given in Table 2.

Antibody to endotoxin, given before bacterial challenge, prevented neutropenic rabbits from dying from infection with Gram-negative rods that had been placed in the drinking water. Steroids, given before or with bacterial challenge, prevented death from sepsis in a large number of experimental models. Antibody against TNF-α, with no other treatment of any kind, prevented death from sepsis in baboons infused with live *Escherichia coli*. Similarly, the IL-1 receptor-antagonist protein, which binds to the IL-1 receptor but has no agonist activity, reduced by

90 per cent deaths from sepsis in rabbits. Monoclonal anti-IL-6 reduced mortality from peritonitis caused by live *E. coli* in mice. In a variety of animals, TNF-α and IL-1, separately or together, can induce all the features of the septic syndrome, including shock and death. IL-6 alone is seldom lethal, but induces the changes in hepatic protein synthesis that are collectively referred to as the acute-phase response.

In septic people, circulating levels of TNF-α, IL-1, and IL-6 are generally elevated, although correlation is not precise. Furthermore, patients with extremely high serum levels of these mediators do not survive. Although experiments in man cannot be carried to the lengths they are in animals, intravenous infusions of small doses of IL-1, Il-6, and TNF have made it clear that all three of these mediators can induce features of sepsis in man.

The best evidence that arachidonic acid products have something to do with mortality in sepsis is the arachidonic acid-deficient rat, which is relatively resistant to endotoxin poisoning but becomes sensitive again if given purified arachidonic acid. In people, the most important cyclo-oxygenase product seems to be thromboxane A_2 (TXA_2), which is usually measured as its stable metabolite thromboxane B_2. Non-survivors of sepsis had plasma levels of the metabolite 10 times higher than those who did survive. The levels were particularly high in patients with adult respiratory-distress syndrome and multiple organ failure. Also there was a suggestion in a small human trial that indomethacin could reverse the hypotension of advanced sepsis. As regards leukotrienes, they are certainly liberated in septic animals and man, and there is evidence in animals that inhibitors of 5-lipoxygenase, or leukotriene-receptor antagonists, attenuate some of the hypotensive and pulmonary features of sepsis. So far, the effects on mortality have been unimpressive.

PAF is not an arachidonic acid derivative, but it is liberated from cell membranes by the action of two enzymes that are both up- regulated by IL-1 and TNF-α. The first enzyme is phospholipase A_2; the second is a specific PAF synthetase. PAF is an important mediator of the adhesion of polymorphs to vessel walls, and of their subsequent activation to secrete proteolytic enzymes and activated forms of oxygen. PAF antagonists have reduced the pathological manifestations in several models of local and systemic infection in animals. In addition, PAF antagonists have attenuated vascular damage in several non-infectious conditions such as reperfusion injury.

The evidence reviewed above, and a large body of information not discussed here, leaves little doubt that the main outlines of the pathogenesis of sepsis given in Table 2 are correct. How far this information has been translated into useful clinical treatment will be discussed in the chapter on septiaemia (Chapter 7.19.2).

The endstages of sepsis

The earliest event in septic shock is generalized peripheral vasodilation. But most of the increased flow seems to occur in arteriovenous anastomoses, with stagnation in the true capillaries. If shock is long continued, blood is readmitted to the capillaries but flow remains stagnant. The capillary walls leak fluid and protein, and there is a progressive loss of intravascular volume. Shocked patients usually, though not always, have evidence of disseminated intravascular coagulation, and small vessels all over the body may be obstructed by fibrin thrombi as well as by masses of agglutinated platelets and polymorphonuclear leucocytes.

In the lungs, alveoli steadily fill with fluid exuding from leaky capillaries. Hypoxaemia and tachypnoea are early symptoms of sepsis; advanced stages of the same process cause the adult respiratory distress syndrome.

Myocardial failure supervenes quite early, probably because the heart normally extracts almost all oxygen from the blood supplied to it. There is some evidence that left-ventricular failure in sepsis is due to a circulating myocardial toxin rather than directly caused by ischaemia. In any event, myocardial function is depressed from the outset of sepsis. The high initial cardiac output is supported mostly by tachycardia rather than by increased stroke volume. With continuing sepsis, left-ventricular stroke output declines, and cardiac output falls into the normal range, or below.

Important organs such as the brain, kidneys, intestine, and liver are subjected to progressive anoxia because of small-vessel obstructions, and because of oedema related to their leaky capillaries. Added to this is low oxygen delivery related to worsening pulmonary and cardiac function. Clinically, one sees various degrees of clouding of consciousness, ranging from lethargy to stupor, and from slight disorientation to frank delirium. Urine flow first diminishes and then ceases. Jaundice may occur if the patient survives long enough. Chemically, there is evidence of progressive liver and renal failure. Lactic acid accumulates in the blood because of glycolysis in the anoxic tissues. The serum pH is lowered, and the heart is even further compromised. Lysosomes are destabilized and their enzymes released in many tissues. This vicious circle soon leads to death. It is thought that the final event may be massive endotoxin influx from the ischaemic bowel.

The endstage is referred to as multiple organ failure, and is seen in the terminal stages of all forms of shock, although sepsis is the most common cause. It is generally lethal, with mortalities of about 50 per cent for sepsis plus adult respiratory-distress syndrome, and over 80 per cent for sepsis with failure of three or more organs. It is apparent that patients in this state are unlikely to be helped by antagonists of early mediators of sepsis.

Fever

The cause of fever in infectious illnesses can now be regarded as settled. Fever is due to a resetting of the anterior hypothalamic thermostat so that the body temperature is regulated with the same exquisite sensitivity as in the normal person, but the regulation is at a higher level. Fever in infectious illness is a purposeful reaction, which evolved because it potentiated the immune and inflammatory responses to infection. If the nervous system is intact, fever in infectious illness never exceeds about 41°C, and is usually lower.

The resetting of the thermostat is due to synthesis of prostaglandin(s), probably PGE_2, in the brain, There are no presynthesized stores of prostaglandins, in the brain or elsewhere. The is site of synthesis is probably the organum vasculosum laminae terminalis. This area has permeable blood vessels, which would allow stimuli to enter from the bloodstream; it is exquisitely sensitive to PGE_2, and it projects to the anterior hypothalamus.

It would be expected that if PGE_2, or another arachidonic acid derivative, were an essential part of the development of fever, then cyclo-oxygenase inhibitors would antagonize fever. And indeed aspirin and similar drugs have been well-known antipyretics for more than a century, long before we knew how they worked.

The stimuli for prostaglandin synthesis are the three monokines IL-1, TNF-α, and IL-6, which have been discussed above. Each of these mediators alone is pyrogenic, and each has been shown to stimulate prostaglandin synthesis in the anterior hypothalamus. TNF-α is doubly pyrogenic because it also induces synthesis and secretion of IL-1 and -6. These three proteins are secreted by macrophages stimulated by bacteria and by a variety of other substances.

The list of substances that cause macrophages to secrete IL-1, TNF-α, and IL-6 is very long. It includes whole bacteria, both Gram-positive and Gram-negative, as well as bacterial cell-wall components such as endotoxin and peptidoglycan. Certain bacterial toxins, such as the toxic-shock toxin of *Staph. aureus*, can activate macrophages at very low concentration. In the toxic-shock syndrome, the patient shows all the features of sepsis, but blood cultures are negative. Macrophages are activated to secrete proteins by intact fungi, fungal cell walls, and by certain large viruses. Macrophages are also activated by T cells that have responded to antigen displayed on the macrophage surface, and by antigen–antibody complexes and complement components.

Fever, like sepsis, is therefore another manifestation of the leakage of inflammatory mediators into the bloodstream from a local site of infection. If the organism is in the bloodstream, mediators are released directly into blood by circulating monocytes and by tissue macrophages, such as Kupffer cells, which line blood sinusoids. Virtually all clinical fevers can be so explained. The exceptions are fever seen in neurological diseases that in one way or another damage the temperature-regulating centres or pathways; heat stroke, which is caused by inability to cool the body fast enough to compensate for the existing heat load; and certain fevers accompanying leukaemias or lymphomas, in which IL-1 and other pyrogens are synthesized by the tumour cells.

Other systemic changes associated with fever

Changes in plasma proteins

Infected people usually show a stereotypical array of changes in their plasmas proteins. The erythrocyte sedimentation rate is raised because of increased synthesis of fibrinogen by the liver. Several other proteins present in normal plasma or serum are also synthesized in increased quantity during infection; they include the haptoglobins and caeruloplasmin. In addition, some proteins that are not present at all in normal serum are synthesized in very large quantities by the liver. Twenty-four hours after the onset of an infection, the concentration of C-reactive protein in serum may reach 3 mg/ml. This represents the synthesis of about 15 g of protein in a 70-kg man. Another protein synthesized *de novo* in even larger quantities is the serum amyloid-associated protein. Proteins whose concentration increases during infection are known as the 'acute-phase reactants'; most have α_2-globulin mobility, and they are responsible for the increased density of this area in serum electrophoretic strips from infected people.

C-reactive protein binds to phosphoryl choline residues; these are commonly present in bacterial cell walls. Both teichoic acids and endotoxins may contain such residues. Bound C-reactive protein fixes complement and facilitates phagocytosis of organisms. It is thus a kind of primitive antibody, non-specific, and inefficient, but available in large quantity shortly after the onset of infection. Serum amyloid-associated protein is an apolipoprotein, and its relative insolubility may lead to its deposition in tissue as amyloid fibrils in chronic suppurative states such as bronchiectasis and osteomyelitis. It presumably has an adaptive function also, but what that might be is unknown. Nor is it clear why increases in fibrinogen and haptoglobins might be useful.

The obverse of increased synthesis of some proteins by the liver is a lessened synthesis of other proteins normally made by the liver, especially albumin. In severely infected animals, synthesis of albumin mRNA in hepatocytes essentially stops within a few hours. As the half-life of serum albumin is about 5 days, there is no immediate fall in serum albumin level. However, as sepsis continues, albumin is lost into the tissues and is not replaced. The consequence is severe hypoalbuminaemia.

The main cause for the shift in liver protein synthesis is IL-6. IL-1 serves a synergic function, but is relatively ineffective by itself, and may in fact work by stimulating IL-6 synthesis by hepatocytes.

Changes in serum iron

Sick people also show a marked fall in serum iron and serum zinc. The fall in serum iron is clearly adaptive, because all organisms need iron to grow, and the virulence of several pathogenic bacteria can be enhanced by many orders of magnitude if enough ferric iron to saturate serum transferrin is given intravenously. As regards zinc, no evidence is available. Finally, sick people generally show a neutrophil leucocytosis, which again is obviously adaptive. These changes appear to be primarily mediated by IL-1.

Changes during prolonged infection

A prolonged infection always results in major nutritional problems. Sick people have an elevated energy requirement: fever raises the metabolic rate approximately 15 per cent for each 1°C of temperature elevation. In addition, there is an increased metabolic rate, out of proportion to fever, in serious infections such as peritonitis. Sick people seldom have good appetites, and they tend to eat mostly fluid and carbohydrate. Rarely is the caloric intake sufficient to balance the increased metabolic load, and the protein intake is almost always subnormal.

However, the nutritional changes of prolonged infection are not just due to starvation. There is an apparently obligatory breakdown of protein in muscle and bone, mainly mediated by adrenal corticosteroids. The amino acids are deaminated and the skeletons are used for gluconeogenesis in the liver. The ammonia is converted to urea and excreted in the urine. Normal urea nitrogen is 6 to 15 g/day, but may rise to 30 g/day during severe systemic infection, in the absence of any protein intake. Muscular wasting and loss of bone matrix are always seen in prolonged infections. Loss of calcium from bone may cause semispontaneous fractures or renal calculi.

Fat is also broken down at an increased rate. The glycerol is used for liver gluconeogenesis and the fatty acid portions are mostly burned in muscle. The respiratory quotient during prolonged sepsis is 0.7 to 0.8, indicating a significant use of fat as fuel. Fat synthesis essentially stops because TNF-α down-regulates transcription of the gene for lipoprotein lipase.

The nutritional response to prolonged infection is identical to the response to major trauma, major surgery, or burns. The response is so stereotypical that it must have adaptive value. However, during prolonged infections some clearly maladaptive changes occur. The changes can be partially overcome by aggressive feeding, and unless one can clearly see that the infection will be controlled within a week or so, that should be considered. It is especially important if the patient was malnourished before the infection developed. Exactly what should be repleted is still being determined. Most people would agree with providing calories and protein, and correcting severe anaemia or hypoalbuminaemia. However, there may be specific nutritional defects worth correcting. There is evidence from animal experiments that glutamine deficiency causes increased intestinal permeability, and that enteral glutamine repletion may reduce the frequency and severity of the multiple organ-failure syndrome.

Summary

It is easy to forget that mediators of inflammation have the primary function of protecting the host. What we see as clinical disease always represents a failure of local control of infection. The most important functions of TNF-α, IL-1, and IL-6 are to initiate the local inflammatory reaction, and attract phagocytes to the area to dispose of the invading organisms. IL-1 is also fundamentally important in mediating the activation of T cells and indirectly of B cells, which underlie the specific immune responses to infection. These processes go on in everyone every day and are normally so efficient that they never rise to the level of clinical notice.

What happens in a clinical infection is a function of how far the invading organism succeeds in multiplying. Single organisms are disposed of by phagocytosis without any other response, and even a few thousand bacteria cause only microscopic inflammation. A few million organisms incite the generation of substances that cause enough vasodilation, increased capillary permeability, and chemotaxis to be clinically visible as inflammation. Many millions of organisms are required to cause local abscesses; the tissue destruction is actually caused by proteolytic enzymes liberated from dead and dying polymorphs. In chronic bacterial infections such as tuberculosis, local tissue destruction is a result of gross overstimulation of macrophages.

If the local lesion is extensive, then IL-1, TNF-α, IL-6, and other mediators leak into the bloodstream. This induces systemic changes such as fever, the acute-phase serum protein changes, and neutrophil leucocytosis. Septicaemia occurs when large numbers of organisms enter the bloodstream, and there is systemic activation of the plasma enzyme cascades and macrophages. The clinical hallmark of sepsis is peripheral circulatory failure, with raised cardiac output, low systemic vascular resistance, and generalized capillary leakage. The damage to vessel walls is initially pharmacologically mediated by substances such as kinins, histamine, and anaphylatoxins derived from complement. However, the lethal endothelial damage that leads to adult respiratory-distress syndrome and multiple organ failure is initiated by the action of bacterial products on macrophages. Principal macrophage-derived mediators of endothelial damage are TNF-α, IL-1, and IL-6. Although these proteins have multiple effects, the most important appears to result in adhesion of polymorphonuclear leucocytes to vessel walls. One important intermediate step is IL-1/TNF-directed synthesis of PAF by endothelial cells. Vessel walls are finally destroyed by polymorph enzymes and activated forms of oxygen.

Knowledge of these reaction sequences can be expected in the near future to lead to better management of infected patients.

REFERENCES

General reading

Gallin, J.I., Goldstein, I.M., and Snyderman, R. (1992). *Inflammation: basic principles and clinical correlates*, (2nd edn). Raven Press, New York.

Mackowiak, P.A. (1991). *Fever: basic mechanisms and management*. Raven Press, New York.

Neugebauer, E.A. and Holaday, J.W. (1993). *Handbook of mediators in septic shock*. CRC Press, Boca Raton, FA.

Detailed topics

Baum, T.D. *et al.* (1990). Endotoxin induced myocardial depression in rats: effect of ibuprofen and SD2 64–688, a platelet activating factor antagonist. *Journal of Surgical Research*, **48,** 629–34.

Beasley, D., Schwartz, J.H., and Brenner, B.M. (1991). Interleukin 1 induces prolonged L arginine dependent cGMP and nitrite production in rat vascular smooth muscle. *Journal of Clinical Investigation*, **87,** 602–8.

Bevilacqua, M.P. *et al.* (1985). Interleukin 1 acts on cultured human vascular endothelium to increase the adhesion of PMN, monocytes and related cell lines. *Journal of Clinical Investigation*, **76,** 2003–11.

Braude, A.E. (1958). Transfusion reactions from contaminated blood. Their recognition and treatment. *New England Journal of Medicine*, **258,** 1289–93.

Breese, B.B. and Disney, F.A. (1954). The accuracy of diagnosis of beta streptococcal infections on clinical grounds. *Journal of Pediatrics*, **44,** 670–3.

Bussolino, F., Camussi, G., and Baglioni, C. (1988). Synthesis and release of platelet activating factor by human vascular endothelial cells treated with TNF or IL-1. *Journal of Biological Chemistry*, **263,** 11856–61.

Bussolino, F. *et al.* (1987). Intravascular release of platelet activating factor in children with sepsis. *Thrombosis Research*, **48,** 619–20.

Cannon, J.G. *et al.* (1990). Circulating IL-1 and TNF in septic shock and experimental endotoxin fever. *Journal of Infectious Diseases*, **161,** 79–84.

Faist, E. *et al.* (1988). Immune protective effects of cyclo-oxygenase inhibition in patients with major surgical trauma. *Journal of Trauma*, **30,** 8–18.

Greisman, S.E. and Hornick, R.B. (1972). Cellular inflammatory responses of man to bacterial endotoxin. A comparison with PPD and other bacterial antigens. *Journal of Immunology*, **109,** 1210–22.

Leeman, M. *et al.* (1985). Administration of dazoxiben, a selective thromboxane synthetase inhibitor in the adult respiratory distress syndrome. *Chest*, **87,** 726–30.

Luedke, C.E. and Cerami, A. (1990). Interferon gamma overcomes glucocorticoid suppression of TNF alpha biosynthesis by murine macrophages. *American Society of Clinical Investigation*, **86,** 1234–40.

Matsushima, K. *et al.* (1988). Molecular cloning of a human monocyte derived neutrophil chemotactic factor (IL-8) and the induction of IL-8 mRNA by IL-1 and TNF alpha. *Journal of Experimental Medicine*, **167,** 1883–93.

Ohllsson, K. *et al.* (1990). Interleukin 1 receptor antagonist reduces mortality from endotoxin shock. *Nature*, **348,** 550–2.

Okusawa, S. *et al.* (1988). IL-1 induces a shock-like state in rabbits: synergism with TNF alpha and the effect of cyclo-oxygenase inhibition. *Journal of Clinical Investigation*, **87,** 1162–72.

Paul, W.E. (1989). Pleiotropy and redundancy: T cell derived lymphokines in the immune response. *Cell*, **57,** 521–4.

Reines, H.D. *et al.* (1982). Plasma thromboxane concentrations are raised in patients dying with septic shock. *Lancet*, **21,** 174–5.

Tew, J., Calanoff, C., and Berlin, B.S. (1971). Bacterial or non-bacterial pneumonia: accuracy of radiological diagnosis. *Radiology*, **124,** 607–12.

Tracey, K. *et al.* (1987). Anti-cachectin/TNF monoclonal antibodies prevent septic shock during lethal bacteraemia. *Nature*, **330,** 662–4.

Wakabayashi, G. *et al.* (1991). *Staphylococcus epidermidis* induces complement activation, TNF and IL-1, a shock-like state, and tissue injury in rabbits without endotoxemia. *Journal of Clinical Investigation*, **87,** 1925–35.

Wallace, J.L. *et al.* (1987). Evidence for platelet activating factor as a mediator of endotoxin induced gastrointestinal damage in the rat. *Gastroenterology*, **93,** 765–73.

Ziegler, E.J. *et al.* (1973). Treatment of *E. coli* and klebsiella bacteremia in agranulocytic animals with antiserum to a UDP-GAL epimerase deficient mutant. *Journal of Immunology*, **111,** 433–8.

7.6 Antimicrobial chemotherapy

P. G. Davey

Introduction

All doctors regularly prescribe antimicrobials and there has been an understandable desire to establish some simple general principles that will help doctors to decide whom to treat, what drug to select, and the appropriate dose, route of administration and duration of therapy. With time these general principles achieve the status of rigid laws that bury the complexity of the problem beneath the attractive simplicity of a single right answer. This in turn leads to complacency, which is communicated from doctors to public. A media interviewer in the United States recently asked: 'How is it that we have conquered most infectious diseases but are unable to find a cure for AIDS?' In fact, infectious diseases kill more people than either cardiovascular diseases or cancer. Moreover, amongst infectious diseases, the single organism responsible for most deaths is *Mycobacterium tuberculosis*. Globally, there are 8 million new cases and 2.9 million deaths from tuberculosis per year, almost twice as many deaths as caused by AIDS (1.5 million/year).

Antimicrobials are unique among drugs in that overuse may lead to development of drug resistance. The failure of antimicrobial chemotherapy to control infectious diseases is due in part to the emergence of drug-resistant microbes. However, it is also due to inadequacies of prevention through public health systems and of failure of individual prescribers to use drugs in the most effective manner. There are not, and never have been, any grounds for complacency about antimicrobial chemotherapy.

Prescribers should maintain a proper respect for the complexity of chemotherapy. Prescribing should be based on a knowledge of the scientific principles underlying chemotherapy, together with a constant review of existing practice and a willingness to change. Written policies for antimicrobial chemotherapy can help the prescriber. Ideally these policies should be drawn up and continuously revised by multidisciplinary groups that are willing to encourage a scientific and critical evaluation of the wide range of choices available for antimicrobial chemotherapy.

The majority of antimicrobial prescribing is for the treatment of bacterial infection, although there is an increasing range of drugs available for the treatment of infections caused by protozoa, fungi, and, in particular, viruses. It would be impossible to provide a comprehensive review of all these drugs in a single chapter. This is a review of general principles and the illustration of these principles is based on selected examples only.

Pharmacology of antimicrobial drugs

Mechanisms of action

All antimicrobial drugs rely on the principal of selective toxicity. Antimicrobial drugs are so commonly prescribed that it is easy for the prescriber to take selective toxicity for granted. However, in the decades leading up to the development of sulphonamides, 'magic bullets' was used as a somewhat disparaging metaphor for the whole idea of chemotherapy. In fact there already existed a range of natural products which were capable of killing bacteria, fungi, and protozoa within humans without major adverse effects. The term antibiotic was introduced by Waksman in 1942 to describe substances which are produced by micro-organisms and which are antagonistic to the growth of others in high dilution. The last clause is necessary to exclude substances like gastric juices, hydrogen peroxide, and alcohol, which are naturally occuring antiseptics. The evolutionary role of antibiotics is not entirely clear. In some cases antibiotics may have protected one organism against another, but the role of many antibiotics was probably to regulate the metabolism and reproduction of the organism which produced them. More recently improved molecular techniques have led to the synthesis of drugs which have been specifically designed to attack identified targets in micro-organisms. Strictly speaking, synthetic antimicrobial drugs are not antibiotics.

ANTIBACTERIAL DRUGS

Bacteria have a cell wall as well as a cell membrane. This fundamental difference from mammalian cells is the principal target for β-lactam antibiotics (penicillins and cephalosporins) and for other, less commonly prescribed drugs as well (Table 1). The other principal targets for antibacterial drugs are intracellular (Table 1). The precise sequence of events leading to the death of bacteria is still the subject of research, even for drugs such as the aminoglycosides, which have been in clinical use for over 40 years. Aminoglycosides interfere with protein biosynthesis, but their ability to kill bacteria also relies on a complex sequence of events including two energy-dependent phases of uptake of aminoglycosides across the cell membrane and into the bacteria.

The mechanism of action of some older drugs has been little investigated. For example, the molecular mechanism of isoniazid has recently been described but the precise mechanism of other antituberculosis drugs remains unknown. Research on new drugs is inextricably linked with the commercial priorities of the developed world and there is little appreciation of the threat that tuberculosis poses to the public health of developed nations. Perhaps the increase in tuberculosis and the alarming increase in drug-resistant strains will stimulate a re-evaluation of the priorities for development of new antibacterials.

The fluoroquinolones are exceptional among the antibacterials in that their development has owed more to chemical analysis and drug design than to screening of naturally occurring products. The synthesis of nalidixic acid, a 4-quinolone, was reported in 1962. Together with other similar drugs it had a place in chemotherapy in the 1960s and 1970s that was limited by a combination of poor activity against Gram-positive bacteria, development of resistance amongst Gram-negative bacteria and adverse effects including stimulation of the human central nervous system and photosensitive skin reactions. Continued research on these molecules showed that fluorination of position 6 of the 4-quinolone nucleus had beneficial effects and led to the development of numerous fluoroquinolones (ciprofloxacin, enoxacin, norfloxacin, and ofloxacin are already licensed in the United Kingdom). Continued research with molecular techniques has shown that manipulations of the molecule at positions 1, 5, 7, and 8 can be used further to refine antibacterial spectrum, pharmacokinetic behaviour, and adverse effects.

The fluoroquinolones that are now undergoing clinical trial are therefore examples of drugs which have been designed from an understanding of some of the important relationships between structure and activity. However, new drugs bring new problems. Temafloxacin, licensed in the United Kingdom, United States, Spain, and Sweden early in 1992, was withdrawn because of serious adverse effects within 6 months. Although carefully designed to take advantage of existing knowledge linking structure with adverse effects, its clinical use was associated with rare (fewer than 1 : 1000 prescriptions) reports of a severe clinical syndrome, including haemolysis and renal failure, that has not been associated with other fluoroquinolones. This occurrence serves as a reminder that knowledge about the structure and activity of a new drug is limited to what is already known about existing drugs of the same class. While this knowledge may help in the design of drugs with improved antimicrobial activity, there is always the risk that the new drug will have completely new adverse effects that are impossible to predict with existing experimental techniques.

ANTIFUNGAL AND ANTIPROTOZOAL DRUGS

Fungi and protozoa are nucleated, eukaryotic cells and, like mammalian cells, they do not have a cell membrane. None the less there are a number of drugs that do have selective toxicity for these organisms, including folate antagonists and other antibacterial drugs that act by modification of energy metabolism (Table 1).

Almost all the clinically useful antifungals act by binding to ergosterol or by blocking its synthesis, making the cell membrane leaky. Ergosterol is the predominant sterol within the membrane of fungal cells but is relatively unimportant in mammalian cells, but the extent of selectivity is quite variable and the most effective antifungal (amphotericin) has dose-related adverse effects on mammalian cells. Other mechanisms of antifungal action include interference with protein synthesis (flucytosine) or mitosis (griseofulvin).

Many of the drugs used to treat protozoal infections are antibacterial antibiotics (Table 1) or have similar mechanisms of action to these drugs. Some of the most useful antiprotozoal agents are derived from ancient herbal remedies and their mechanism of action remains unclear. These include emetine, derived from ipecacuanha and used for treatment of amoebiasis or giardiasis, as well as the antimalarials quinine and artemisinine. The mechanism of action of the antimalarial chloroquine is also unclear. Inhibition of microbial glucose catabolism is the mechanism of action of pentamidine (used for treatment of *Pneumocystis carinii* infections), as well as the arsenical or antimonial compounds

Table 1 *Mechanism of action of antibacterial, antifungal and antiprotozoal drugs*

Mechanism of action	Antibacterial drugs	Antifungal drugs	Antiprotozoal drugs
Inhibition of synthesis or damage to cell wall	Amoxicillin (penicillin)* Cefuroxime (cephalosporin) Aztreonam Imipenem Bacitracin Vancomycin (glycopeptide) Cycloserine Fosfomycin	Fungi do not have a cell wall	Protozoa do not have a cell wall
Inhibition of synthesis or damage to cytoplasmic membrane	Polymyxin	Amphotericin Nystatin (polyenes) Ketoconazole (imidazole) Fluconazole (azole) Terbinafine (allylamine) Amorolfine	Amphotericin Ketoconazole Fluconazole
Inhibition of synthesis or metabolism or function of nucleic acids	Ciprofloxacin (quinolone) Rifampicin Nitrofurantoin Metronidazole	Griseofulvin	Metronidazole
Protein biosynthesis	Gentamicin (aminoglycoside) Tetracycline Chloramphenicol Clindamycin Erythromycin (macrolide) Fusidic acid	Flucytosine	Tetracycline Clindamycin Azithromycin Clarithromycin (macrolides)
Modification of energy metabolism	Sulfonamides Trimethoprim Isoniazid	No example	Dapsone Sulfonamides Pentamidine Pyrimethamine Antimonials Arsenicals Eflornathine

*Where there are several other related drugs, the class of drug is given in addition to the name of a commonly used representative agent.

used to treat leishmaniasis and trypanosomiasis. Although they are relatively selective for microbial glucose catabolism, they do have dose-related adverse effects in man. Eflornithine is a relatively recently introduced drug for African trypanosomiasis, which also acts by selective inhibition of energy metabolism.

In addition to the antimicrobials listed in Table 1 there are a number of other drugs that have been developed for other purposes but appear to have useful antiprotozoal activity. These include the xanthine-oxidase inhibitor allopurinol and the calcium antagonist verapamil.

ANTIVIRAL DRUGS

Development of drugs with selective toxicity against host cells that have been infected by viruses is analogous to the problems of development of cytotoxic drugs for cancer chemotherapy. It is remarkable that, within 11 years of the clinical description of the acquired immunodeficiency syndrome, drugs have been developed to attack the human immunodeficiency virus (**HIV**) at a number of different sites (Fig. 1). Most of the currently available antiviral drugs act by interfering with nucleic acid metabolism.

Although the life-cycle of the HIV virus has important differences from that of other viruses, it can be used as a model for understanding the problems associated with design of antiviral drugs. Prevention of viral infection by inhibition of binding or uptake to the host cell are mechanisms of drug action that could prevent infection of cells (Fig. 1, site 1). Unfortunately, the drugs produced so far have been disappointing. The drugs in routine clinical use act by inhibition of reverse transcriptase (Fig. 1, site 2). However, drugs that act at sites 3 to 5 (Fig. 1) are currently in clinical trial.

Selective toxicity has been the major limitation to development of chemotherapy for the common cold and other infections due to RNA viruses. Currently there are no available drugs with acceptable efficacy and toxicity for the treatment of these common infections. The DNA viruses, which include the herpesviruses and the hepatitis B virus, present an additional problem. Like the HIV virus, DNA viruses are integrated within the genome of the infected cell. Infected cells can survive for months or years in a latent phase during which no viral replication takes place and the cell functions normally. The targets for available antivirals are only expressed in cells in which viral replication is taking place. Acyclovir, which is the most commonly prescribed antiviral, is selectively toxic for cells infected with herpesviruses provided that these cells are producing the enzyme thymidine kinase, which phosphorylates and activates acyclovir. Cells that have latent infection with herpesviruses do not express thymidine kinase and therefore acylovir does not prevent recurrent infection unless it is given continuously.

Mechanisms of resistance

Mechanisms of resistance to antibacterial drugs are generally well characterised. The three most common mechanisms are production of drug-inactivating enzymes, alteration of the target site, and mechanisms that prevent access of the drug to the target site.

The drug-inactivating enzymes, which are such a common mechanism of bacterial resistance probably, have a natural function because there is evidence to show that some bacteria were producing β-lactamases in the pre-antibiotic era. However, the clinical use of antibiotics has dramatically increased the prevalence of strains that produce drug-inactivating enzymes. Moreover, the ability to produce these enzymes has been transferred from one bacterial species to another by transfer of genetic information encoded in plasmids. Production of drug-inactivating enzymes is a common mechanism of resistance to aminoglycosides, β-lactams, macrolides, and chloramphenicol.

Alteration in target site is becoming an increasingly common mechanism of drug resistance. An alteration of a single amino acid in a bacterial enzyme can render it resistant to inhibition by antibacterial drugs. This is the principal mechanism of resistance to newer synthetic antibacterial drugs such as quinolones.

Amongst bacteria, change in permeability is a resistance mechanism largely confined to Gram-negative bacteria, which have a much more complex outer membrane than Gram-positive bacteria. The outer membrane of Gram-negative bacteria contains lipoproteins, which present a natural barrier to hydrophilic antibacterial drugs. Benzylpenicillin is relatively inactive against Gram-negative bacteria in comparison with ampicillin because it crosses this outer membrane less readily. Certain species, notably *Pseudomonas*, have become progressively more resistant to aminoglycosides, β-lactams, and quinolones because of reduced permeability of their outer membranes. Some bacteria are resistant to tetracycline because they have an active transport pump that removes tetracycline from within the bacteria.

Fig. 1 Schematic representation of the lifecycle of the HIV virus and potential targets for antiviral chemotherapy.

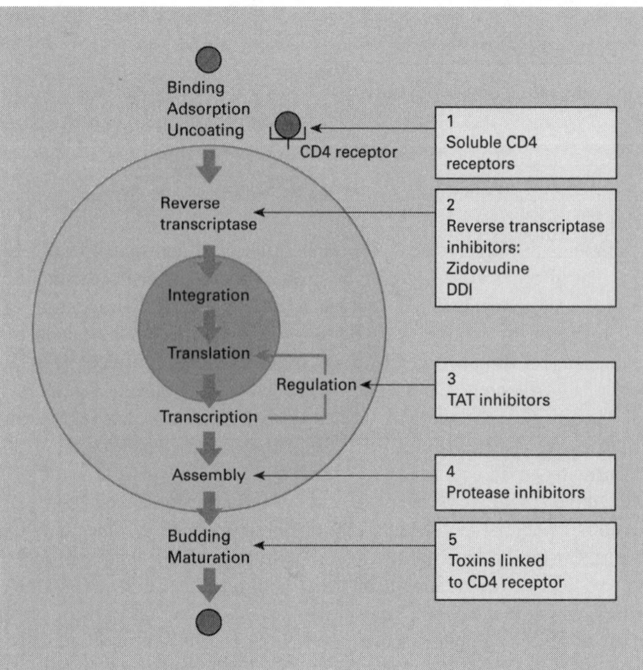

It is important to distinguish between intrinsic and acquired resistance. Intrinsic resistance means that a bacterial species is inherently resistant to the effects of the antibacterial drug. An example is that streptococci and anaerobic bacteria both lack the respiratory quinones required for energy-dependent uptake of aminoglycosides. Acquired resistance means that a bacterial species has acquired a mechanism of resistance since the introduction of antibacterial drugs into clinical medicine. An example is the growing proportion of gonococci that produce penicillinase. Before the introduction of penicillin there were no β-lactamase-producing gonococci. Acquisition of resistance can occur either by mutation or by transfer of genetic information between bacteria on plasmids. Plasmids can transfer complex mechanisms of resistance, including the active efflux pump that renders some bacteria resistant to tetracyclines.

Prescribers should be aware of which bacteria are intrinsically resistant to the antibacterial drugs they use regularly. However, knowledge of acquired resistance requires careful collaboration between laboratories and clinicians. By definition the situation is constantly changing and may show quite marked geographical differences, even within one hospital. The information presented in Fig. 2 is only a guide. The most important point to note is that, with the single exception of β-haemolytic streptococci, all bacterial species have acquired resistance to a wide variety of drugs. Of all the drugs listed in Fig. 2, only metronidazole has been little affected by development of resistance since its introduction.

Acquired resistance to antiviral drugs occurs by alteration in the target site. Acquired resistance to antifungal and antiparasitic drugs is relatively poorly understood but increasingly common. Resistance of fungi to amphotericin or azoles occurs because of reduction in the ergosterol component of the cell membrane, or impaired binding of drugs to ergosterol. Mechanisms of resistance to other antifungals have not been fully characterized. Some malaria parasites have become resistant to chloroquine by development of an efflux mechanism, whereas resistance to folate antagonists occurs because of alteration in the target site. Testing drug susceptibility of fungi or protozoa presents formidable technical problems. Moreover, the mechanisms of action of most of the antiparasitic drugs are relatively poorly understood. It follows that the mechanism of drug resistance is also poorly understood.

Tests for resistance

Laboratory testing of susceptibility to antibacterial drugs is based on measurement of inhibition of bacterial growth. There is a variety of techniques in use in different laboratories and efforts are being made nationally and internationally to standardize these tests. It may seem unnecessary for the prescriber to understand technical aspects of these tests. However, some understanding is essential to an informed discussion about resistance.

Measurement of the effects on bacterial growth of increasing concentration of a drug establishes the minimal inhibitory concentration (**MIC**). This is the minimum concentration that completely inhibits bacterial growth.

The problems inherent in susceptibility testing can best be illustrated by considering a specific example. Some strains of *Haemophilus influenzae* are resistant to ampicillin because they produce β-lactamase (Fig. 3). This results in a bimodal distribution of MICs with β-lactamase producers having higher MICs than non-producers. However, it can be seen that the two populations overlap (Fig. 3). It is necessary to decide on a breakpoint to separate strains that are assumed to be sensitive from those that may be resistant. In the United Kingdom, the breakpoint for ampicillin is 2 mg/l. However, it can be seen that 16 (7 per cent) of the 228 β-lactamase producers have MICs of below 2 mg/l (Fig. 3). The reason is probably that they produce relatively small quantities of β-lactamase under the growth conditions used for the test. Moreover, 26 (1 per cent) of the β-lactamase non-producers have MICs in excess of 2 mg/l. These strains are either intrinsically resistant to ampicillin or have acquired other mechanisms of resistance such as reduced permeability or altered target site. This example illustrates two important principles. One is that a known mechanism of resistance (i.e. β-lactamase production) is not always fully expressed during *in vitro* susceptibility testing, although it may well be expressed *in vivo* and lead to treatment failure. The second is that there are several mechanisms of resistance, so that testing for β-lactamase production cannot completely replace susceptibility testing. The prevalence of ampicillin resistant strains of *H. influenzae* is highly variable in the United Kingdom. A recent survey of 2212 strains from 22 laboratories found 8.6 per cent to be β-lactamase producers and 5.8 per cent to be amipicillin resistant by other mechanisms. However, the range for individual laboratories was 0 to 23.0 per cent for β-lactamase producers and 0.4 to 12.7 per cent for ampicillin-resistant non-producers.

The situation is becoming rapidly more complex with the introduction of new drugs and with the spread of a wide variety of mechanisms of resistance into different bacteria. Interpretation of results is further complicated by the fact that the best method for establishing whether or not an organism is resistant to one drug may be to test it against a different drug. Methicillin-resistant *Staphylococcus aureus* are an excellent example of this apparent paradox. These bacteria have altered penicillin-binding proteins that make them resistant to all penicillins, cephalosporins, and other β-lactams. The best way to detect this alteration in penicillin-binding proteins is to test the susceptibility of the bacteria to methicillin or oxacillin, drugs that are never used clinically in the United Kingdom. Testing susceptibility to cloxacillin or cephalosporins may well give misleading results. Unfortunately, to quote Courvalin, 'not all Medical Microbiologists are Experts in Antibiotics'. The result is that some laboratories may report what are, in effect, impossible antibiotic resistance phenotypes. An example would be *S. aureus* reported to be resistant to oxacillin but sensitive to co-amoxiclav or cefuroxime. The correct sequence of reasoning required can be described as observation of a phenotype, inference of a mechanism, and prediction of overall phenotype. In this case the phenotype observed was oxacillin resistance, the inferred mechanism is the posession of altered penicillin-binding proteins by this strain of *S. aureus*, and the predicted phenotype is that it will be equally resistant to all β-lactam drugs.

Advances in understanding of the molecular mechanisms of drug resistance will help to ensure that *in vitro* susceptibility testing identifies

Fig. 2 Development of resistance to antimicrobials.

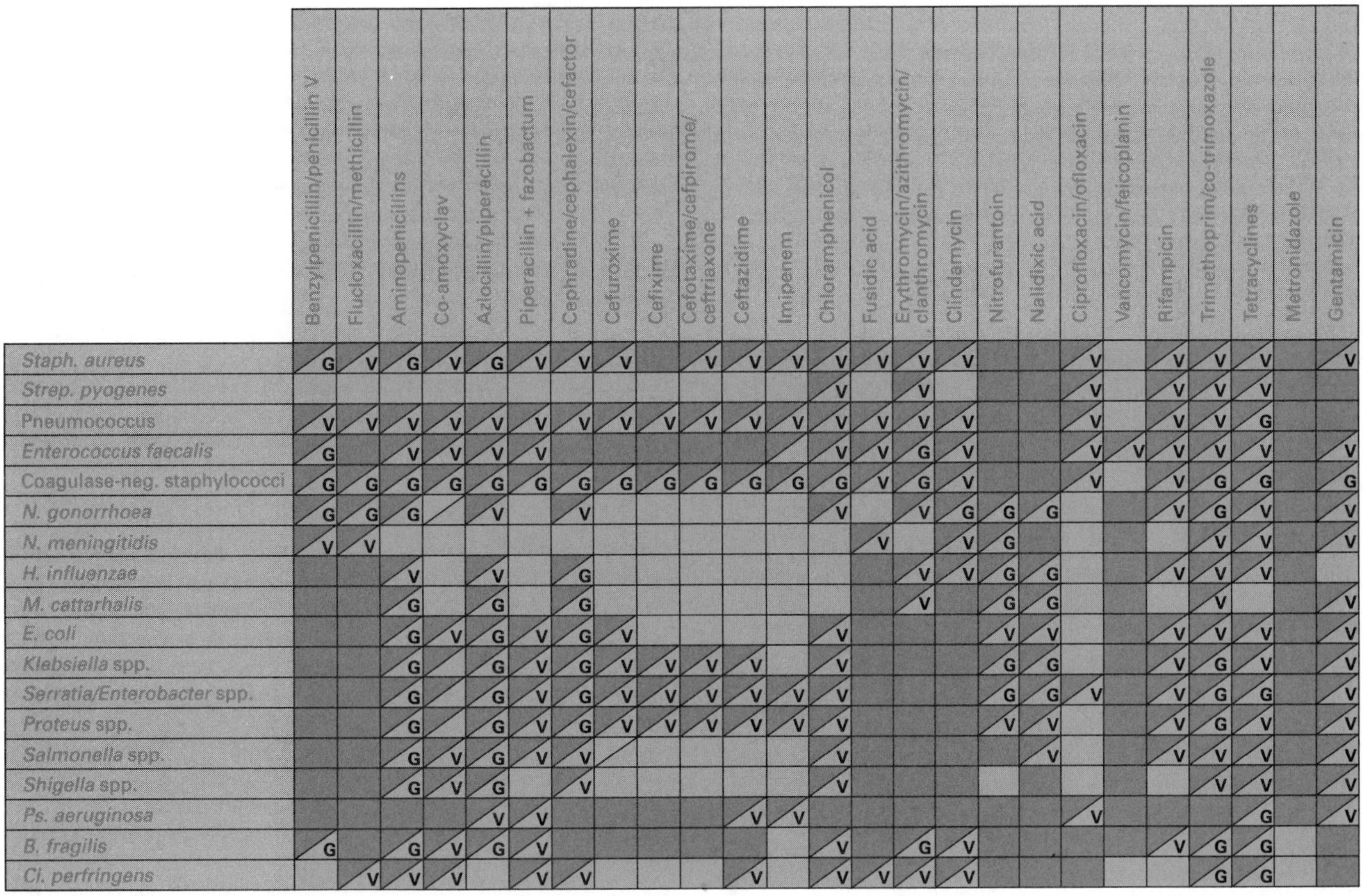

	Benzylpenicillin/penicillin V	Flucloxacillin/methicillin	Aminopenicillins	Co-amoxyclav	Azlocillin/piperacillin	Piperacillin + tazobactum	Cephradine/cephalexin/cefactor	Cefuroxime	Cefixime	Cefotaxime/cefpirome/ceftriaxone	Ceftazidime	Imipenem	Chloramphenicol	Fusidic acid	Erythromycin/azithromycin/clanthromycin	Clindamycin	Nitrofurantoin	Nalidixic acid	Ciprofloxacin/ofloxacin	Vancomycin/teicoplanin	Rifampicin	Trimethoprim/co-trimoxazole	Tetracyclines	Metronidazole	Gentamicin
Staph. aureus	G	V	G	V	G	V	V	V		V	V	V	V	V	V	V			V		V	V	V		V
Strep. pyogenes													V		V				V		V	V	V		
Pneumococcus	V	V	V	V	V	V	V	V	V	V	V	V	V	V	V	V			V		V	V	G		
Enterococcus faecalis	G		V	V	V	V							V	V	G	V			V	V	V	V	V		V
Coagulase-neg. staphylococci	G	G	G	G	G	G	G	G	G	G	G	G	G	V	G	V			V		V	G	G		G
N. gonorrhoea	G	G	G		V		V						V		V	G	G	G			V	G	V		V
N. meningitidis	V	V												V		V	G					V	V		V
H. influenzae			V		V		G								V	V	G	G			V	V	V		
M. cattarhalis			G		G		G								V		G	G				V			V
E. coli			G	V	G	V	G	V					V				V	V			V	V	V		V
Klebsiella spp.			G		G	V	G	V	V	V	V		V				G	G			V	G	V		V
Serratia/Enterobacter spp.			G		G	V	G	V	V	V	V	V	V				G	G	V		V	G	G		V
Proteus spp.			G		G	V	G	V	V	V	V	V	V				V	V			V	G	V		V
Salmonella spp.			G	V	G	V	V						V					V			V	V	V		V
Shigella spp.			G	V	G		V						V									V	V		V
Ps. aeruginosa					V	V					V	V							V				G		V
B. fragilis	G		G	V	G	V							V		G	V					V	G	G		
Cl. perfringens		V	V	V		V	V				V		V	V	V	V						G	G		

Intrinsically resistant.

G Global acquired resistance: >10% of strains in any country have acquired resistance or drug unsuitable for treatment of infections with this organism.

V Variable resistance: prevalence of resistance is highly variable; >10% in some countries.

Negligible acquired resistance: acquired resistance is rare in any country.

drug-resistant strains. However, even if practical methods for analysis of genotype become available, they are unlikely completely to replace susceptibility testing as new mechanisms of resistance evolve continuously. Moreover, drug resistance may be conferred by more than one mechanism. For example, a combination of loss of an outer-membrane porin protein plus production of a broad-spectrum β-lactamase may make a Gram-negative bacillus resistant to relatively β-lactamase stable drugs such as cefotaxime. It is likely that the interpretation of laboratory testing of antimicrobial susceptibility will become increasingly complex. It is important that prescribers of antibacterial drugs and people responsible for antibiotic policies are aware of the difficulties involved in susceptibility testing. It is no longer a simple process of testing one organism against the drug the patient is receiving; indeed, that approach may give dangerously misleading results. There is an urgent need to standardize techniques and interpretation nationally. The technical aspects are being addressed by a number of national working parties. Failure to invest in good quality testing could be a very short-sighted economy if it leads to increased treatment failure through failure to identify drug-resistant strains correctly.

Routine susceptibility testing is not yet available for antifungal, antiprotozoal, and antiviral drugs. Compared with testing of antibacterial drugs, the technical problems involved in testing other antimicrobials are formidable. Furthermore, mechanisms of resistance are relatively poorly understood so that it is difficult to validate the results of tests based on expression of phenotype.

Pharmacokinetics

Dosing of antimicrobials is based in part on a knowledge of their absorption, distribution, and elimination from the body. In this respect, antimicrobials do not differ from other drugs and the general principles of pharmacokinetics will not be discussed further here. However, in comparison with other drugs, information about intestinal elimination and distribution into tissues has special relevance to antimicrobials.

INTESTINAL ELIMINATION

The human body contains a large number of bacteria that have important functions, particularly in the gut. Consequently, knowledge about the amount of an antimicrobial that is excreted through the gut is relevant to its potential adverse effects, in addition to explaining its elimination from the body. The adverse effects of antibiotics on the normal flora include emergence of resistant strains from among that flora, and its replacement by more harmful organisms. Examples of the latter include colonization of the colon by pathogenic fungi or *Clostridium difficile*, a cause of antibiotic-associated colitis.

Antimicrobials reach the gut by three principal mechanisms. After oral administration a proportion of the dose is not absorbed and passes directly through the gut. The term bioavailability is used to describe the amount of drug absorbed and varies quite widely amongst commonly prescribed antibacterials (Table 2). Acyclovir and other antiviral nucleosides (e.g. zidovudine and dideoxyinosine) have dose-dependent bioavailability. The higher the dose administered, the lower the proportion of the dose absorbed.

In general, drugs with low bioavailability have a more profound effect on the normal flora of the colon. However, after absorption of an antimicrobial from the gut it may be eliminated from the body by secretion into bile or by secretion by enterocytes. Thus, even intravenously admin-

Fig. 3 Distribution of MICs of 2529 strains of *Haemophilus influenzae* isolated from 78 laboratories in nine European countries. The number of strains is shown at the end of each bar. The strains are divided according to the breakpoint for resistance to ampicillin in the UK (≥ 2 mg/l). The strains are divided into β-lactamase producers (Beta-lac + ve) and non-producers (Beta-lac − ve). (Redrawn from data in Kayser, *et al.* (1990). *European Journal of Clinical Microbiology and Infectious Disease*. **9**, 810–17, with permission.)

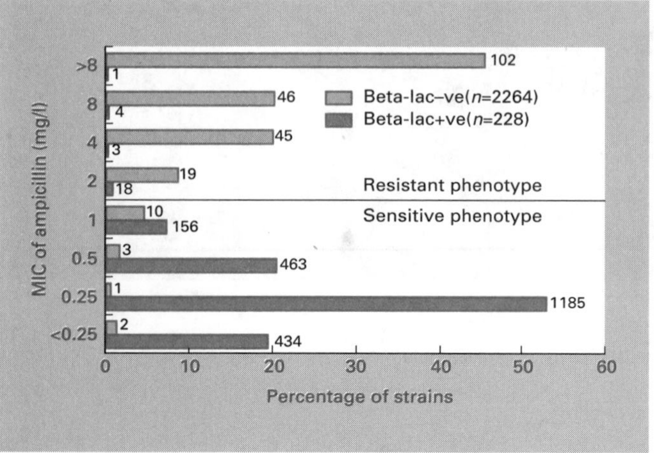

Table 2 *Bioavailability and intestinal elimination of some commonly prescribed antibacterial drugs after oral administration*

Drug	Bioavailability (%)	Intestinal elimination
Penicillins		
Amoxicillin	80–90	Concentrated up to 10-fold in bile
Ampicillin	50	Concentrated up to 10-fold in bile
Flucloxacillin	80–90	Negligible
Cephalosporins		
Cephalexin	80–100	Concentrated up to 3-fold in bile
Cefuroxime axetil	30–40	Bile concentrations of up to 80% of serum
Cefixime	40–50	Concentrated up to 50-fold in bile
Quinolones		
Nalidixic acid	90–100	Biliary concentrations similar to serum
Ciprofloxacin	70–85	Concentrated up to 10-fold in bile; additional enteral secretion
Other antibacterials		
Erythromycin	18–45	Concentrated up to 300-fold in bile
Chloramphenicol	75–90	Concentrated up to 3-fold in bile
Metronidazole	80–95	Concentrations in bile similar to serum
Rifampicin	90–100	Concentrated up to 1000-fold in bile
Sulfamethoxazole	70–90	Concentrations in bile 40–70% of serum
Tetracycline	75	Concentrated up to 10-fold in bile
Trimethoprim	80–90	Concentrated up to 2-fold in bile

*Note that drugs which are well absorbed may still achieve high concentrations in the faeces because of secretion into bile or other enteral secretions.

istered antimicrobials reach the gut in sufficient quantities to cause harmful effects on the normal flora. Quinolones such as ofloxacin are almost completely absorbed after oral administration but still have a profound effect on the normal flora of the gut because quinolones are secreted from the blood in the lower small intestine and caecum.

TISSUE DISTRIBUTION

Infections occur in every tissue in the body, therefore information is required about distribution of antimicrobials throughout the body. Most bacteria are located in the extracellular fluid. However, bacteria including *M. tuberculosis* and *Legionella pneumophila* survive within cells and drugs which are used to treat these infections must be capable of entering into and functioning within mammalian cells. Viruses and the malaria parasites are essentially intracellular organisms.

Distribution in extracellular fluid of non-specialized tissues

Most tissues are supplied by fenestrated capillaries, which allow the free diffusion of antimicrobial drugs from plasma to the extracellular fluid.

Fig. 4 Distribution of drug from serum into rapidly equilibrating interstitial fluid (a), a collection or reservoir of tissue fluid (b), and a specialized site with non-fenestrated capillaries and/or a transport efflux pump (c). (Reproduced from Barza, M. (1993), with permission.)

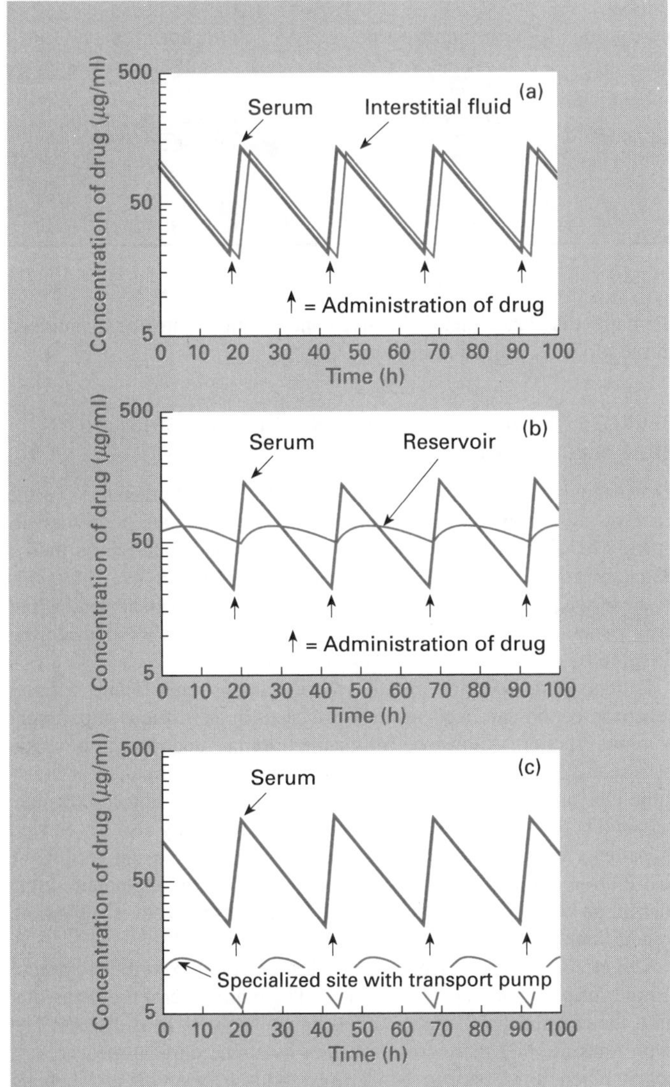

In this case the average drug concentration in plasma is the same as in the extracellular fluid. However, the profile of drug concentrations may be different in plasma and extracellular fluid (Fig. 4). The profile of drug concentrations in extracellular fluid is a function of the physical dimensions of the space containing the fluid. Specifically, the higher the ratio of surface area to volume, the more rapid the equilibration of concentrations between plasma and extracellular fluid (Fig. 4(a)). Peritoneal fluid is a good example of a rapidly equilibrating fluid. Peritoneal fluid is secreted over the whole surface of the peritoneum but does not form large accumulations of fluid under normal circumstances. In contrast, a sphere, such as a fluid-filled cyst or any large collection of fluid, has a relatively low ratio of surface area to volume and drugs diffuse slowly into and out of extracellular fluid occupying a spherical space (Fig. 4(b)).

Although the average drug concentration in extracellular fluid is unaffected by the speed of diffusion of drug into the extracellular space, the peak drug concentration is affected (Fig. 4(a),(b)). This may be relevant if the effects of drugs are directly linked to peak concentration (see Pharmacodynamics).

Distribution of drugs into extracellular fluid of specialized tissues

In contrast to the situation in other tissues, the capillaries supplying the central nervous system, the posterior chamber of the eye, and the prostate are non-fenestrated. The tight junctions between the endothelial cells of these capillaries can only be crossed by lipid-soluble drugs, which are capable of passage through the cells. In addition to this barrier to diffusion into these sites, the choroid plexus and the posterior chamber of the eye also have active efflux pumps that remove β-lactam drugs from the site. Concentrations of antimicrobials within these specialized sites cannot be predicted from a knowledge of plasma concentrations (Fig. 4(c)). In addition to these naturally occurring specialized sites, infection may occur in avascular sites. These may be avascular because of trauma or because of collection of fibrin, as in the cardiac vegetations that result from bacterial endocarditis. There is evidence that drug diffusion into these vegetations is both incomplete and uneven.

Another feature of the barrier to free diffusion of molecules across capillaries in specialized tissues is the potential for pH partition. This has been documented in the prostate, in that prostatic fluid has a lower pH than plasma. Consequently, weak basic drugs, such as macrolides and quinolones, may accumulate in prostatic fluid because they will be ionized at acidic pH and this will impede back diffusion across the cells of the prostatic capillaries.

Intracellular fluid

Penetration of drugs into intracellular fluid depends on the lipid solubility of the drug. Beta-lactams and aminoglycosides have poor lipid solubility and do not achieve high concentrations in cells. In contrast, lipid-soluble drugs like macrolides, quinolones, and rifampicin may achieve higher concentrations within cells than in the plasma or extracellular fluid. Distribution of these drugs within the cells is uneven. This may be due in part to pH partition within the cell, in that macrolides and quinolones are weak bases and accumulate within the acid environment of the phagolysosome. The pH of intracellular fluid also has implications for the activity of the drug (see Pharmacodynamics).

Monitoring of drug concentrations in tissue fluid

In the majority of bacterial infections the organisms are contained in the extracellular fluid (Table 3). For these infections it can be assumed that the average concentration in the plasma is a reasonable indication of the average drug concentration at the site of infection and a knowledge of plasma kinetics is all that is required.

For intracellular pathogens information about intracellular drug concentration is clearly relevant. If the pathogen is contained within cells of the blood (malaria parasites within red cells, for example), this information is relatively easy to obtain. The concentration of drugs in tissue biopsies gives some indication of intracellular drug concentrations but

Table 3 *Kinetic requirements for treatment of bacterial infections at different anatomical sites*

Anatomical site of infection	Relevance of blood levels?	Natural barrier from blood to interstitial fluid?	Intracellular penetration desirable?	Extracellular pathogens	Penetration into luminal secretions required?
Meningitis	Yes	Yes, all infections	*Listeria monocytogenes*	*H. influenzae* *N. meningitidis* *Strep. pneumoniae*	Effective CSF concentrations crucial
Biliary infection	Yes	No	None proven, causative organisms do not survive in cells	*E. coli* Other coliforms (anaerobic bacteria rarely involved)	High biliary concentrations probably not necessary
Respiratory infections	Bacteraemia common for pneumonia only	No	*Chlamydia psittaci* *Chlamydia pneumoniae* *Coxiella burnettii* *Legionella pneumophila* *Mycoplasma pneumoniae*	*Strep. pneumoniae* *Strep. pyogenes* *H. influenzae* *M. catarrhalis*	High concentrations in bronchial secretions may be desirable when part of the aim of treatment is reduction of bacterial load in sputum (e.g. cystic fibrosis)
Bone	Yes	No	None proven	Staphylococci *Strep. pyogenes* Gram-negative bacteria in chronic infections	Relevance of bone concentrations unproven; bacteria probably located in interstitial fluid
Urinary tract	Bacteraemia common with pyelonephritis	Only for prostatitis	*Chlamydia trachomatis* (prostatitis/epididymo-orchitis)	*E. coli* Other coliforms *Staph. saprophyticus* *Enterococcus faecalis*	Effective urinary concentrations essential; drugs that achieve low concentrations in interstitial fluid (nitrofurantoin) are relatively ineffective in pyelonephritis

only 60 to 80 per cent of the weight of a tissue biopsy is contributed by cells, the remainder being extracellular fluid. Thus if the drug concentrations in extracellular and intracellular fluids are 10 mg/l and 1 mg/l, the concentration in a homogenized tissue biopsy will be 2.8 mg/kg, assuming that 20 per cent of the biopsy is extracellular fluid and cells make up the remaining 80 per cent. In contrast, if the drug is concentrated within cells the extracellular and intracellular fluid concentrations might be 1 mg/l and 10 mg/l, in which case the concentration in tissue homogenate would be 8.2 mg/kg. In general, if the average concentration in tissue homogenate is 20 to 40 per cent of average concentration in plasma, the drug is probably only equilibrating in extracellular fluid.

Most intracellular bacterial infections occur in the lung, where distribution of antibacterials has been relatively well characterized. This information is of direct relevance to the management of infections caused by obligate intracellular pathogens, such as *Legionella pneumophila*, *Chlamydia pneumoniae*, or *M. tuberculosis*. Ability to penetrate eukaryotic cells is a prerequisite for drugs aimed at infections by these organisms. However, high lung-tissue concentrations are of less certain relevance in the majority of lung infections, which are caused by extracellular pathogens. It could be argued that drug contained within cells is irrelevant because it is excluded from contact with the bacteria. However, it is possible that intracellular drug provides a reservoir that slowly diffuses back into the extracellular fluid as plasma concentrations decline, so prolonging the period of contact between the drug and bacteria. This possibility requires further investigation. However, the concept of an intracellular drug reservoir is appropriate only if effective drug concentrations are maintained in extracellular fluid at all times. If the patient is bacteraemic, effective concentrations must be maintained in the blood as well as in the lung.

EFFECTS OF INDIVIDUAL PATIENT CHARACTERISTICS ON PHARMACOKINETICS

Pharmacokinetics are profoundly affected by age and pregnancy. In the very young, systems for drug binding or metabolism are poorly developed, whereas in the very old they may no longer function normally. Separate kinetic studies will be required for drugs used to treat infections in these age groups. Information about kinetics in pregnancy and about drug penetration into breast milk should be sought when considering drugs to be used during pregnancy or lactation.

Patients with infection may have pre-existing renal failure but any severe infection can itself result in transient or permanent impairment of renal function. Allowance for changing renal function can be made with relatively simple general rules, the key being estimation of creatinine clearance from serum creatinine concentrations adjusted for age, sex, and body weight. Clearance of antimicrobials may also be reduced in patients with severe infection because of changes in the volume of distribution of the drug (Fig. 5). Clearly, it is important to obtain information on kinetics of antimicrobials from patients with severe infection, in addition to normal volunteers.

The effects of liver disease on kinetics are complex and there are no simple rules to guide dose adjustment. There are several problems that limit the usefulness of kinetic studies in patients with liver disease. The main ones are that there are no readily available clinical measures of portal blood flow, hepatic blood flow, biliary excretion and hepatic metabolism, and that different liver pathologies do not affect these variables uniformly.

Pharmacodynamics

PHARMACODYNAMICS OF ANTIMICROBIAL ACTION

Inhibition of microbial growth

In general, increasing concentrations of antimicrobials have a progressive effect on microbial growth. These have been well characterized for antibacterial drugs, starting from a measurable reduction in the rate of growth, through complete inhibition of growth (bacteristatic effects) to reduction in numbers of bacteria (bactericidal effects). Dose-related antimicrobial effects have also been documented for antivirals (Fig. 6) and antiparasitic drugs (Fig. 7).

The distinction between bacteristatic and bactericidal drugs is relative, and is of doubtful relevance to the management of most bacterial infections. The definition of a bactericidal effect is a 99.9 per cent reduction in bacterial numbers. However, if there are a million bacteria to start with then there will still be 1000 left after 99.9 per cent are killed. Increasing concentrations of β-lactams have little additional effect on the extent or rate of bacterial killing. Drugs such as chloramphenicol, which are regarded as being primarily bacteristatic, may reduce bacterial numbers by 90 or 99 per cent, without reaching the somewhat arbitrary cut-off of 99.9 per cent reduction.

There are few clinical situations in which drugs that are primarily bactericidal have been shown to be more effective than bacteristatic drugs. Possible exceptions include infections in patients with significantly impaired host defences (neutropenia) or infections at sites that are inaccessible to phagocytic cells (endocarditis). However, even these situations are not clear-cut. For example, vancomycin is frequently used to treat patients who are neutropenic and those with endocarditis yet its bactericidal action is slow and variable under different culture conditions. In most infections, there is no evidence that drugs which are only weakly bactericidal (e.g. chloramphenicol, clindamycin, erythromycin or other macrolides, tetracyclines, and vancomycin or other glycopeptides) are inferior to those which have more rapid or complete bactericidal effects (aminoglycosides, β-lactams, and quinolones).

Fig. 5 Average plasma quinine concentrations following administration of a loading dose of 20 mg (salt)/kg to patients with severe and uncomplicated malaria, compared with those predicted to occur in normal subjects. (Reproduced from White (1992), with permission.)

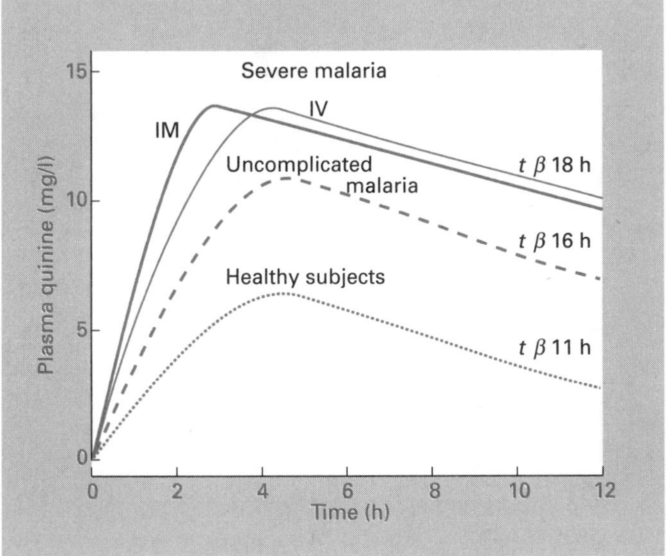

Antimicrobial effects other than inhibition of growth

Concentrations of antibacterial drugs below those required measurably to inhibit growth do have demonstrable effects on bacterial metabolism and morphology (Fig. 8). Both Gram-positive cocci and Gram-negative bacilli increase enormously in size after exposure to subMIC concentrations of β-lactam drugs. The concentration is not sufficient to prevent cell-wall synthesis but is sufficient to prevent septation and division of the bacteria after mitosis. These grossly enlarged organisms are essentially multiple genomes within a single cell wall. Because of their size they are readily phagocytosed by host cells and may well be deficient in other ways that diminish virulence. The interaction of microbe and host is complex and concentrations of antimicrobials below the *in vitro* MIC may have significant effects on these interactions *in vivo*.

Fig. 6 Relation between the suppression of p24 antigen and the steady-state area under the plasma concentration–time curve of dideoxyinosine (ddI). The relation between ddI exposure and suppression of p24 from the baseline value was analysed using a sigmoid E_{max} model ($r^2 = 0.94$; $p < 0.001$). (Reproduced from Drusano, G.L. *et al.* (1992). *Annals of Internal Medicine*, **116,** 562–6, with permission.)

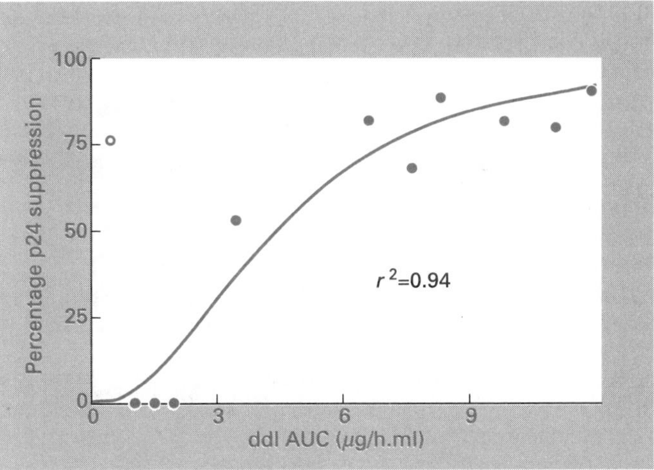

Fig. 7 Slope of the log-linear portion of parasite clearance curves (hs− 1) vs. area under the blood concentration–time curves (mg/l per 1 h) for quinine in children ($n = 42$) with severe falciparum malaria ($r = 0.3807$, $p < 0.02$, 40 d.f.). (Reproduced from Winstanley and Watkins (1992), with permission.)

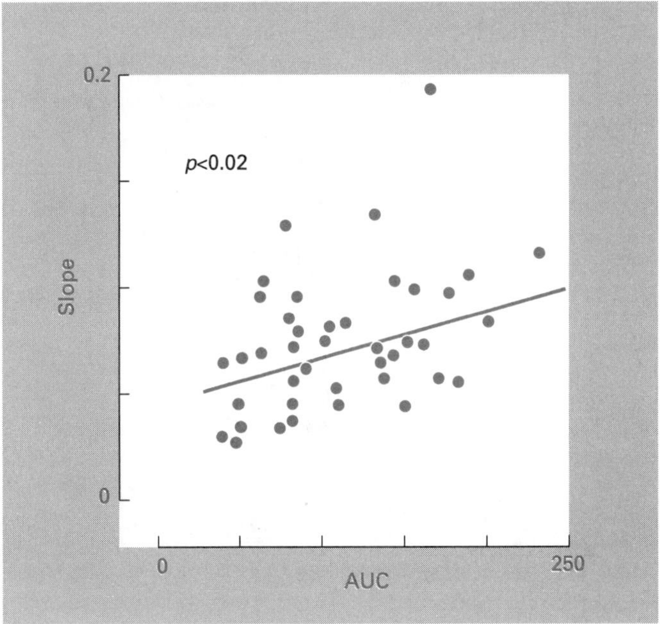

Post-antibiotic effects

It is possible to observe the effects *in vitro* of exposure to antimicrobial drugs on organisms that have survived. A population of bacteria is exposed to the drug for a short time and the culture is then diluted 1000-fold to allow resumption of growth, which is monitored either by counting viable organisms or by measurement of metabolism such as synthesis of ATP. The most pronounced post-antibiotic effects have been demonstrated with aminoglycosides such as gentamicin (Fig. 9). The post-antibiotic effect of gentamicin is dose related over the range of concentrations likely to be achieved in clinical practice (Fig. 9). Re-exposure to gentamicin while the organism is recovering from a previous exposure results in relatively little measurable bactericidal effect from the second dose. The reason is probably that the energy-dependent uptake systems required for gentamicin to enter bacteria will not be functioning during the period of recovery after exposure to a previous dose of gentamicin. These observations have been partly responsible for the move towards single daily dosing of aminoglycosides (see Design of dosing regimens).

In comparison with aminoglycosides, the post-antibiotic effect for β-lactams is both relatively short and unpredictable. The effect lasts for 1 to 2 h for Gram-positive cocci and there is no consistent effect for Gram-negative bacilli. Quinolones do have a measurable, dose-related, post-antibiotic effect on most bacteria. However, the clinical relevance of the post-antibiotic effect of quinolones has yet to be established.

Fig. 8 Morphological features of *Bacteroides fragilis* grown in the absence of antibiotic (A and B) in 1/2 MIC of cefoxitin (C and D), in 1/2 MIC of clindamycin (E and F), and in 1/2 MIC of penicillin (G and H). Staining with methylene blue shows cell structure (A, C, E, and G); negative staining with nigrosin shows the capsule (B, D, F and H). (Reproduced from Gemmell, C.G. *et al.* (1983). *European Journal of Clinical Microbiology*, **2**, 1–4, with permission.)

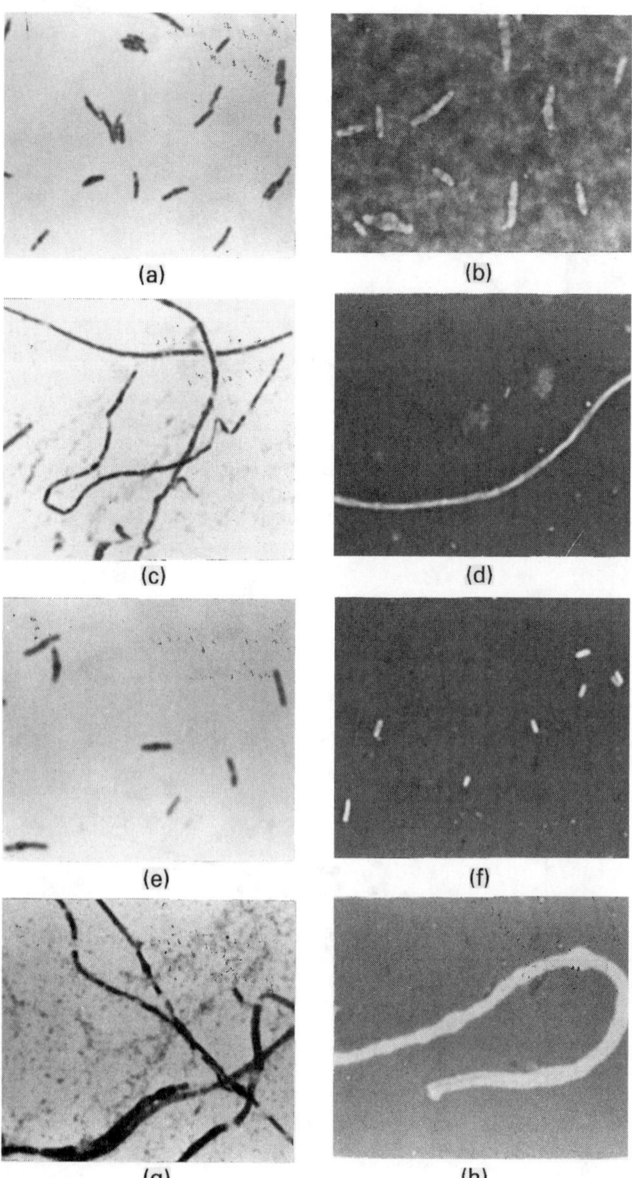

Importance of microbial growth phase

Bacterial numbers in a culture increase exponentially until there are about 10^9 bacteria/ml. This exponential growth phase lasts 6 to 12 h, depending on the growth conditions. The exponential growth phase is followed by a stationary growth phase during which bacterial numbers remain constant but there may be some limited growth to replace bacteria that die. The same is observed *in vivo* when bacteria are growing in a confined space (Fig. 10).

Both *in vitro* and *in vivo*, all antibacterials have relatively little bactericidal effect on bacteria in the stationary phase of growth (Fig. 10). It is technically difficult to perform similar studies with fungi or parasites but limited evidence suggests that the dynamics of antimalarial drugs are different *in vitro* and *in vivo*.

Other factors that influence the pharmacodynamics of antimicrobial action

Almost any change in the milieu in which microbes grow will influence their growth rate and this in turn may influence the action of antimicrobials. Important influences on microbial growth include temperature, pH, po_2, and the type and concentration of nutrients.

In addition to their effects on microbial growth, pH and po_2 can influence antimicrobials directly. For example, the antimicrobial effects of macrolides are highly pH dependent, being markedly reduced once the local pH falls below 7, as is likely in an abscess. The same is true of quinolones once the pH falls below 5. This is unlikely to occur in the extracellular environment but does occur in lysosomes within phagocytes, where quinolones and macrolides are known to concentrate.

The pharmacodynamics of intracellular drugs are potentially very complex. The effect of any given intracellular drug concentration depends on the precise location of the bacteria and the drug within the cell and also on the local pH. Mycobacteria localize in the lysosome but infection causes a rise in lysosomal pH. Consequently, macrolides and

Fig. 9 Post-antibiotic effect of gentamicin on *Escherichia coli*. After 1 h of exposure to the drug the culture was diluted 1000-fold and resumption of bacterial synthesis was monitored. (Redrawn from Isaksson, B. (1988). *Journal of Antimicrobial Chemotherapy*, **22**, 23–33, with permission.)

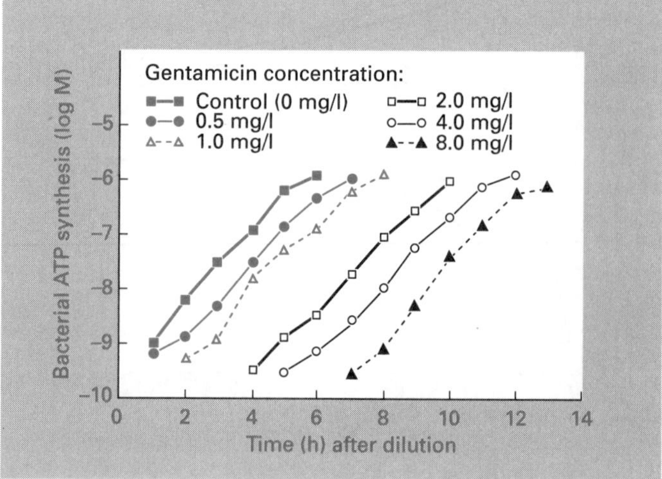

quinolones remain active against mycobacteria within the phagolysosome. In contrast, the phagolysosome remains acidic when infected with *Brucella* spp. and quinolones have been relatively disappointing in clinical trials of brucellosis, despite promising *in vitro* activity.

Oxygen is critical to the bactericidal effect of aminoglycosides because they enter bacteria via an oxygen-dependent transport system. Many aerobic bacteria are facultative anaerobes, that is they can grow in an anaerobic environment. *Escherichia coli* and *S. aureus*, which are normally sensitive to gentamicin, will be resistant when growing anaerobically.

In vivo, microbes tend to attach to surfaces and to form biofilms. These are complex microenvironments in which one or more different organisms are protected by a film composed of mucopolysaccharides. The biofilm probably acts as a physical barrier to antimicrobials and, in addition, the organisms within the biofilm are in the stationary phase of growth and are therefore less susceptible to the actions of antimicrobials.

Binding of antimicrobials to other molecules may neutralize their antimicrobial effect. Albumin and α_1-acid glycoprotein bind antimicrobials in the blood. Moreover, the concentration of these proteins may be influenced by the infection itself or by other disease. For example, concentrations of α_1-acid glycoprotein are increased in patients with severe malaria, leading to a reduction in the proportion of total quinine concentration that is free and active. The action of many antimicrobials is reduced in pus. This may be due to binding to proteins or nucleic acid fragments in pus, in addition to the effects on antimicrobial action of acid pH and slow microbial growth rate.

Fig. 10 Comparative efficacy of early and late treatment of rat granuloma pouches infected with *Pseudomonas aeruginosa*. The granuloma pouch is a fluid-filled, superficial cyst. The drugs were injected directly into the cyst to achieve local concentrations equivalent to 10 times the *in vitro* minimal bactericidal concentration. The drugs were ciprofloxacin (a), gentamicin (b), and imipenem (c). Administration of all three drugs 24 h after infection produced a statistically significant reduction in bacterial numbers whereas the effect of all of the drugs was markedly reduced when administered 48 h after infection. Each point is the mean pm SE of data from six animals. (Reproduced from Davey, P.G. *et al.* (1988). *Journal of Antimicrobial Chemotherapy*, **21**, 395–404, with permission.)

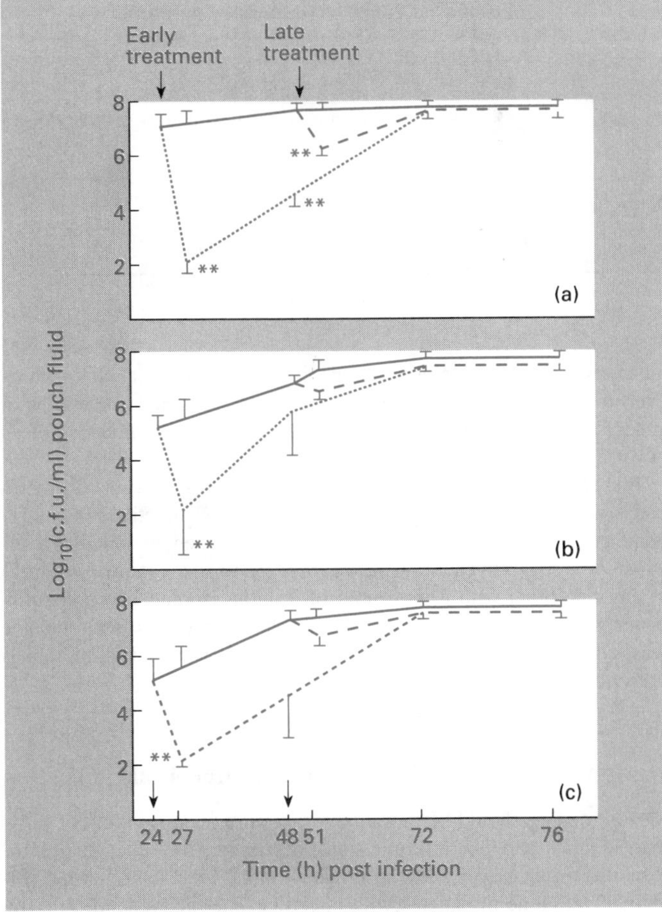

Relevance of pharmacodynamics to* in vitro *susceptibility testing

Many factors affect the relationship between drug concentration and antimicrobial effect *in vivo*. It is therefore not surprising that it is difficult to predict the sensitivity of microbes to treatment from the results of *in vitro* tests alone. In contrast, *in vitro* definition of microbial genotype and the presence of specific mechanisms of resistance provide laboratory information of direct relevance to the selection of drugs for treatment.

PHARMACODYNAMICS OF ADVERSE EFFECTS ON THE PATIENT

Selection of resistance and the risk of superinfection following suppression of normal flora are both dose related and will be considered in more detail later.

All antimicrobials have some dose-related adverse pharmacological effects (Table 4). Fortunately, with a few exceptions, such effects are rare at clinical doses. Exceptions include aminoglycosides, amphotericin, quinine, and zidovudine. For other antimicrobials, such as β-lactams, the most common adverse events are idiosyncratic. By definition these are unpredictable from a knowledge of the basic pharmacology of the drug and do not show any simple dose–response relations. The mechanism may be immunological (penicillin allergy) but may also be due to accumulation of a toxic metabolite because of altered metabolism (insoniazid induced hepatotoxicity, chloramphenicol myelotoxicity) or photodegradation (photosensitive reactions associated with quinolones).

Patients should always be asked about previous exposure to antimicrobials and about any adverse effects that they experienced. If a patient reports allergy to penicillin or another antimicrobial, it is important to obtain as much information as possible from the patient or from their medical records. Rashes are common in patients with infection and are not necessarily attributed to drug allergy. For example, of 198 children with a history of rashes associated with penicillin therapy, 110 received subsequent treatment with a penicillin but only 7 (6 per cent) had any obvious rash after re-exposure. In contrast, a history of anaphylactic reaction suggests genuine immediate hypersensitivity. The term anaphylactic reactions includes urticarial rash, asthma, angio-oedema, and full anaphylactic shock. If a patient has a history suggesting an anaphylactic reaction to penicillin they should avoid all β-lactam drugs if at all possible (i.e. penicillins, cephalosporins, carbapenems, and monobactams). If prescription of a β-lactam is considered essential, then it should only be done with full resuscitation facilities at the ready. Fortunately, there is a wide range of alternative drugs. Less common hypersensitivity reactions include serum sickness and reactions such as interstitial nephritis. As with immediate hypersensitivity, there is likely to be cross-reaction between drugs with similar chemical structures. Unfortunately, there is no reliable method for skin testing for allergy to antimicrobials.

DRUG INTERACTIONS

In 1952, Jawetz and Gunison suggested that the result of an interaction between two or more antimicrobial drugs might be synergistic, additive, indifferent or antagonistic. This terminology is often misused to say that a particular drug combination is synergistic or antagonistic. The distinction may seem subtle but it is important.

Synergy means that the combined effect of the drugs is greater than the sum of their individual effects, additive that it is equal to the sum of the individual effects, indifferent that it is equal to the effect of one drug alone, and antagonistic that it is less than one of the drugs acting alone. These terms are meaningless without precise description of the experimental conditions. For example, exposure of bacteria to chloramphenicol stops protein synthesis and subsequent exposure to an ami-

Table 4 *Dose-related adverse effects of selected antimicrobials*

Drug	Adverse effect	Comment
Antibacterial drugs	Superinfection by yeasts or *Clostridium difficile*; selection of drug-resistant bacteria from the normal flora	These are universal adverse effects of antibacterial drugs and are related to the duration of exposure
β-lactams	Myelosuppression	Neutropenia may occur after 1–2 weeks high-dose i.v. therapy
	Drug fever	Occurs during prolonged (> 1 week), high-dose i.v. therapy (e.g. endocarditis)
	Central nervous stimulation/convulsions	Intrathecal injection dangerous and probably unnecessary; can occur with overdose in renal failure
Aminoglycosides	Nephrotoxicity; ototoxicity	Monitoring of serum concentrations minimizes but does not avoid toxicity
		Risk of toxicity is related to the duration of treatment
Glycopeptides (e.g. vancomycin, teicoplanin)	Nephrotoxicity; ototoxicity	May potentiate aminoglycoside nephrotoxicity; evidence for direct glycopeptide nephrotoxicity or ototoxicity is weak
	Histamine release ('red man syndrome')	Related to the rate of infusion of vancomycin; does not occur with teicoplanin
Macrolides (e.g. erythromycin)	Gastrointestinal stimulation	This is a pharmacological effect that occurs with i.v. or oral administration of erythromycin but does not occur with all macrolides
	Ototoxicity; cardiac arrhythmias	Only with high-dose i.v. therapy
	Drug interactions	Increased serum concentrations of theophylline and cyclosporin
Quinolones (e.g. ciprofloxacin)	Central nervous stimulation	Quinolones are weak GABA antagonists; this effect is potentiated by co-administration with NSAIDs, especially fenbufen
	Drug interactions	May inhibit metabolism of theophylline
Antifungal/antiprotozoal/antiviral drugs		
Amphotericin	Nephrotoxicity	Decreased creatinine clearance and renal potassium wasting are universal at clinically effective doses
	Rigors/hyperthermia/hypotension	Related to the rate of infusion
Ketoconazole	Inhibition of steroid synthesis	Occurs with prolonged (> 1 week) high-dose therapy
Acyclovir	Central nervous adverse effects; crystalluria	Rare except with high-dose i.v. therapy
Zidovudine	Gastrointestinal; myelosuppression; myopathy	All related to unit dose and to duration of treatment
Quinine	Hypoglycaemia	

GABA, γ-aminobutyric acid; NSAID, non-steroidal anti-inflammatory drug.

noglycoside may have relatively little effect. Under these conditions, chloramphenicol has antagonized the bactericidal action of the aminoglycoside but the aminoglycoside has an indifferent effect on the antibacterial action of chloramphenicol. If the bacteria are exposed to the aminoglycoside first, the effect of chloramphenicol may be additive. It is clearly wrong to state categorically that chloramphenicol plus gentamicin is an antagonistic combination.

The most reproducible example of synergy is the combined action of penicillins and aminoglycosides on streptococci and enterococci. These bacteria are resistant to aminoglycosides because they do not possess the respiratory quinones needed for active uptake of these drugs. Exposure to a penicillin disrupts the cell wall and allows the aminoglycoside to enter the bacteria and kill them. This interaction is reproducible under a variety of *in vitro* and *in vivo* conditions and may occur in enterococci that are not killed by exposure to the penicillins alone.

For all drugs, the relation between the risk of an adverse drug event and the number of drugs prescribed is non-linear. That is, the risk of an adverse event after exposure to two drugs is more than twice the risk after exposure to one, and the risk after exposure to four drugs is more than twice the risk after exposure to two. For antimicrobials, the possible adverse events include mutual antagonism of antimicrobial effect. However, even when two antimicrobials are being combined in the hope of synergism, the very fact of their combination increases the risk of an adverse event.

A specific example of the potential adverse interactions of antimicrobials was provided by an audit of management of infections in neutropenic patients. Each course of anti-infective treatment included an average of 4.9 drugs and each patient was exposed to an average of 3.4 drugs at any one time, with a maximum of 7 antimicrobials given simultaneously. The risk of hepatic or renal adverse events and fatal outcome was all significantly correlated with the number of antimicrobials prescribed.

Design of dosing regimens for antimicrobials

Ideally, dosing should be based on a thorough understanding of pharmacokinetics and pharmacodynamics. However, for older antimicrobials there may be very little information about kinetics in normal volunteers, let alone in patients with infection. The recommended dosing regimens for some of these drugs are difficult to justify. For example, recent kinetic evaluation of a new oral formulation of sodium fusidate showed that this drug has an elimination half-life of 10 h after intravenous administration and 16 h after oral administration. The currently recommended dosing regimen of 500 mg every 8 h will inevitably lead to accumulation, which is even greater than predicted because clearance of sodium fusidate decreases with multiple dosing (Fig. 11). Metronidazole is another example of a drug with a prolonged elimination half-life (4.95–42.4 h) for which the recommended dose interval of 8 h may lead to accumulation. Fortunately, deficiencies in understanding of the pharmacology of older antimicrobials are being addressed and used to produce more effective dosing strategies. In particular, the application of clinical pharmacology to antiprotozoal therapy has led to clinically significant improvements in dosing strategies.

In vitro, experimental and clinical information shows marked differences in the dose response of infections to treatment with aminoglycosides in comparison with β-lactams (Table 5). The experience with aminoglycosides in particular illustrates the importance of considering both pharmacodynamics and pharmacokinetics in the design of dosing regimens (Fig. 12). There are three measures relating plasma drug concentrations to the *in vitro* MIC: ratio of peak plasma concentration to MIC; time during which plasma concentrations exceed MIC, and the area under the curve (**AUC**) of plasma concentrations above MIC. Single daily dosing maximizes ratio of peak to MIC, whereas more frequent dosing maximizes time above MIC. For AUC above MIC, the total AUC above baseline is identical if the same dose is given as a single injection or as multiple injections. However, the AUC above MIC after single daily dose will be greater than the AUC above MIC for divided daily doses (Fig. 12). The dose response to aminoglycosides is primarily determined by the ratio of peak concentration to MIC, hence they are best given as single daily injections, despite having a relatively short serum half-life (2 h). In contrast, for β-lactams the time above MIC appears to be critical. Consequently, a drug with a serum half-life of 1.5 h should probably be given at least three times daily (Fig. 12).

THE IMPORTANCE OF OUTCOME MEASURES IN DESIGNING DOSING REGIMENS

Infections for which dose–response relations are clear

Information about dose responses of antimicrobials *in vitro* and in experimental infections forms a sound basis for design of dosing regimens for clinical practice. However, dosing regimens should ultimately be based on measures of outcome of treatment (Table 6). For some infections there are clear biological measures of outcome. These infections are fatal if untreated and there is a clear relation between the biological outcome measure and mortality. Examples include clearance of malaria parasites from the blood (Fig. 7) and reduction in P24 antigen in patients with HIV infection (Fig. 6).

The shape of most dose–response curves can be described by a sigmoid E_{max} model (Fig. 6). As the dose is increased from zero there is initially little or no response to increasing dose. After this initial plateau there is a steep, linear section to the curve where response is sensitive to small alterations in dose. The linear portion of the curve continues until the maximum effective concentration is reached (E_{max}). Further increases in dose above E_{max} do not alter response; this will also apply to dose-related adverse effects.

It follows that it should be relatively easy to establish dosing regimens for infections for which unsuccessful treatment carries a high risk of serious consequences, particularly when treatment also has serious, dose-related side-effects. Examples include use of aminoglycosides for treatment of endocarditis, quinine for treatment of falciparum malaria, and zidovudine for treatment of HIV infection. The components that need to be determined are the daily dose and the duration of treatment. Increase in either of these may increase the probability of successful outcome but will also, inevitably, increase the probability of adverse effects. Finally, it is essential to recognize the need to consider multiple outcome measures in assessing overall response to treatment (Table 6).

Infections for which dose–response relations are unclear

Many infections that are commonly treated with antimicrobials would resolve spontaneously if they were not treated. Moreover, many commonly prescribed antimicrobials do not have dose-related side-effects within the dose range prescribed. Otitis media provides an excellent example of the issues involved. Even today, the consequences of inadequately treated otitis media can be severe (Fig. 13). However, the probability of this type of outcome was low even in the pre-antibiotic era, and mastoiditis is now estimated to occur in only 0.04 per cent of cases. Treatment with antimicrobials produces measurable benefits (Fig. 14). However, in this example of secretory otitis media, 50 per cent of the treated children still had middle-ear effusions after treatment and after a few months there was no difference in outcome between the children who did or did not receive antibiotic. There is no international consensus about any aspect of the treatment of otitis media (Table 7). There is even an example of a placebo-controlled trial that resulted in totally opposite conclusions being reached by two of the investigators. The saga of the original clinical trial, the legal trials that followed it, and the eventual publication of the dissenting view after an interval of 4 years is a graphic illustration of the difficulties involved in assessing outcome of treatment of otitis media. All the investigators agreed that there were some short-term benefits from antibiotic treatment, although they disagreed about the magnitude of these benefits. However, the major source of disagreement was that the original trial report failed to mention that patients who were treated with amoxicillin were two to six times more likely to have a recurrence within 4 weeks after completion of all treatment than patients who had received placebo.

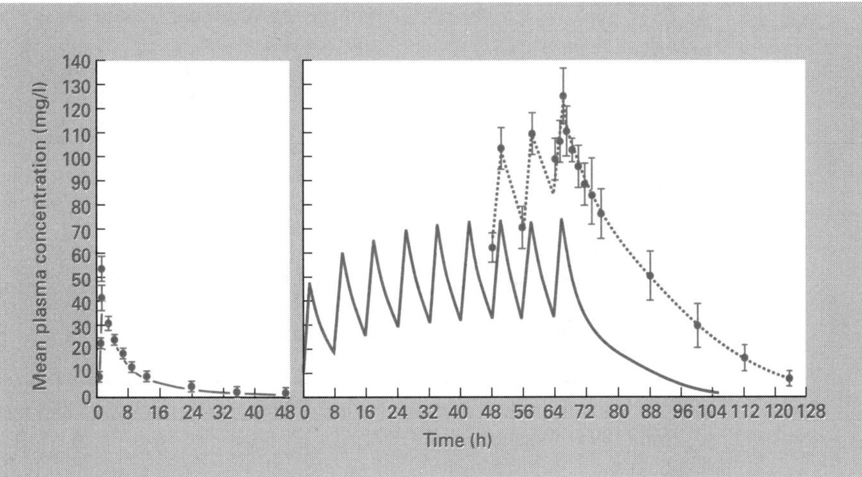

Fig. 11 Mean plasma concentrations of sodium fusidate after a single i.v. infusion (left-hand figure) and measured following repeated administration of 500 mg every 8 h for 3 days (----). The solid lines in the right-hand figure show the predicted serum concentration based on the information obtained after administration of a single dose. Clearly the currently recommended dosing interval of 8 h for sodium fusidate leads to marked accumulation of the drug, which is aggravated by reduced clearance after multiple dosing. (Redrawn from Taburet, A.M., *et al. Journal of Antimicrobial Chemotherapy*, **25,** (Suppl. B), 23–31, with permission.)

Table 5 *Summary of major pharmacodynamic differences between aminoglycosides and β-lactams*

Pharmacodynamic measurement	Aminoglycosides	β-lactam
Rate of killing of bacteria	Rapid and dose related	Slower with little or no increase in rate at higher doses
Number of bacteria killed per dose administered	Concentration-dependent over a wide concentration range	Little increase in extent or rate of killing of bacteria at concentrations above the minimum bactericidal concentration (MBC)
Post-antibiotic effect	Consistent for Gram-positive and Gram-negative bacteria; concentration-dependent over a wide concentration range (Fig. 9)	Unpredictable in Gram-negative bacteria; always short (< 3 h) with little or no increase related to concentration
Most effective method of administration of a daily dose in experimental models of Gram-negative infection	Large, infrequent doses more effective than smaller, more frequent doses. Allowing for kinetic differences between small animals and man, support once daily dosing	Frequent (hourly) injection or constant infusion most effective
Clinical trials	Ratio between peak serum concentration and *in vitro* minimal inhibitory concentration (MIC) is strongly related to outcome of treatment of Gram-negative bacteraemia or pneumonia Clinical trials with amikacin, gentamicin, and netilmicin have shown single daily dosing to be effective	Limited clinical data in patients with neutropenia or nosocomial pneumonia support dosing regimens that keep serum concentrations above the MIC throughout the dosing interval

Fig. 12 Simulation of serum concentrations for an antimicrobial after single daily dosing or administration of the same daily dose in three injections at 8-hourly intervals. The daily dose is 1 g, the serum half-life 1.5 h, and the volume of distribution 21 l. The simulation has calculated three pharmacodynamic measures for a microbe with an *in vitro* MIC of 2 mg/l: ratio of peak serum concentration (C_{max}) to MIC, time above MIC, and area of serum concentrations (AUC) above MIC. (Simulation performed by Dr Terry Moreland, Drug Development Scotland, Dundee.)

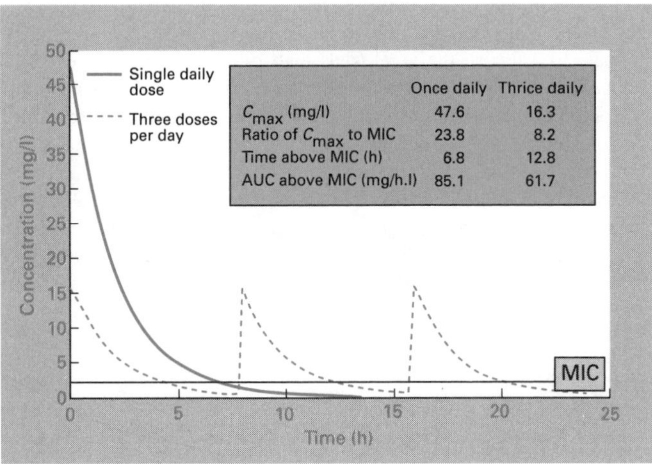

Table 6 *Outcome measures for assessment of chemoprophylaxis or chemotherapy*

Type of outcome measure	Examples
Risk marker	Primarily biological measures of presence of infection (culture of micro-organisms, measurement of antigen levels) or of host responses that are assumed to be protective (serum antibody titres)
Occurrence	Primarily clinical measures describing or quantifying symptoms or signs (number of wound infections as defined by a wound-scoring system)
Severity	May be biological or clinical *Biological*: resolution of local inflammation (e.g. chest radiograph in pneumonia) or general acute-phase response (e.g. C-reactive protein) *Clinical*: symptom scores; duration of hospital stay; other measures of consumption of health-care resources; days off work.
Death	*Discontinuous*: deaths prevented *Partially continuous*: number of life years saved
Combined measures of disability and distress	SF26 Health Profile Medical Outcomes Study Instrument
Combined measures of death and severity	Quality-adjusted life years saved

For further examples and discussion see Davey *et al.* (1993), Garratt *et al.* (1993), Wachtel *et al.* (1992).

Differences in interpretation of data about the effectiveness of antimicrobial treatment should be explicitly acknowledged and resolved through scientific appraisal of published trials, audit of existing clinical practice and, if necessary, new prospective clinical trials.

Table 7 *International variation in prescribing practices for acute otitis media*

	UK	USA	Holland	Australia
Proportion (%) of patients prescribed any antibiotic	97	98	31	98
Use of aminopenicillins (% of total prescriptions)	76	74	92	64
Duration of treatment (% patients):				
5 days	55	1	30	25
6–7 days	38	6	68	46
8–10 days	7	93	2	29

Source: Froom *et al.* (1990).

Note that in Denmark the Danish Medical Association recommends penicillin V rather than aminopenicillins for this condition and 68 per cent of doctors comply with this recommendation (see Friis *et al.* 1989).

Clinical aspects of antimicrobial use

Control of resistance to antimicrobials

Epidemiology of antimicrobial resistance

Every common bacterial pathogen has developed resistance to at least one commonly prescribed antibacterial drug (see Fig. 2) and resistance to antiviral, antiprotozoal, and antifungal drugs is also increasing. There is no doubt that development of resistance is linked to use of antimicrobials. There are quite marked international differences in the prevalence of resistance (Table 8) and these can be explained in part by the relative consumption of drugs in these countries. Development of resistance is particularly common in Third World countries in which antibiotics are freely available without prescription. For example, resistance to trimethoprim among the Gram-negative bacteria that cause urinary-tract infections is as high as 34 per cent in Chile and 63 per cent in Nigeria. In developed countries, emergence of resistance amongst pneumococci is strongly related to geographic variation in penicillin consumption. For example, in Spain both penicillin consumption and the prevalence of penicillin-resistant pneumococci have been rising steadily since 1983, at which time penicillin consumption was already 27 million units per year, compared to 5 million units in the United Kingdom. At the same time there was a decline in consumption of, and pneumococcal resistance to, chloramphenicol and tetracycline in Spain.

What factors determine the emergence of resistance? Clearly, characteristics of the bacteria themselves are important. *Pseudomonas* spp. have always been relatively resistant to antibacterial drugs and have been successful in acquiring mechanisms of resistance to all of the antipseudomonal drugs which have been developed (see Fig. 2). In contrast, strains of *Streptococcus pyogenes* have acquired resistance to erythromycin and other macrolides but remain sensitive to the other drugs that have been used to treat streptococcal infections. In particular, *S. pyogenes* has not acquired β-lactamases. The likely sequence of events is that a minority of strains of a bacterial species either possess a resistance mechanism or acquire it by plasmid transfer from another species. The prevalence of the resistance mechanism within the species is then determined by the selective pressure exerted by antimicrobial use.

Fig. 13 Computerized tomographic scan showing a large cerebral abscess in a 24-year-old man who had a 6-week history of discharge from the right ear. Note that the mastoid process was opaque on the left side (copyright P.G. Davey).

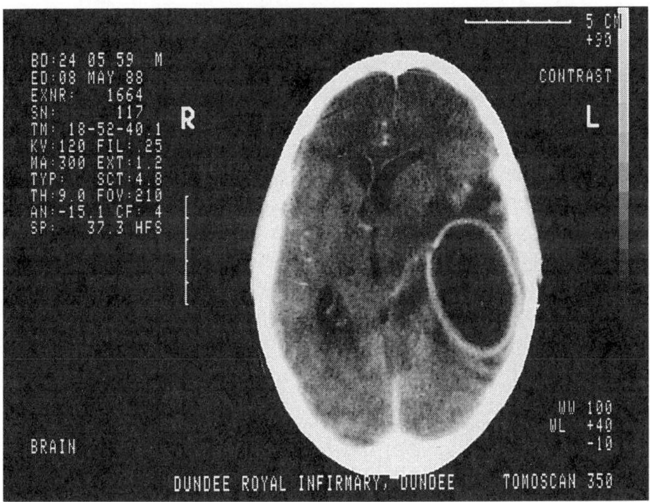

Fig. 14 Incidence of secretory otitis media in 131 children treated for 1 month with co-amoxyclav (——) versus 133 children who received placebo (----). There is a statistically significant difference between the groups at 1, 3, and 5 months after initiation of treatment. (Redrawn from Thomsen, J. *et al.* (1989). *Archives of Otolaryngology and Head and Neck Surgery*, **115**, 447–51, with permission.)

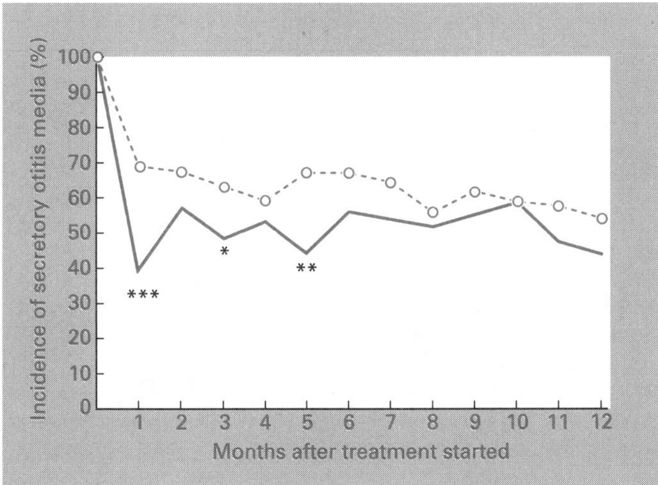

RESERVOIRS OF RESISTANCE, ANIMATE OR INANIMATE

Examples of animate reservoirs of resistance include countries, hospitals, individual clinical units, individual patients, and animals. Intercontinental spread of penicillin-resistant pneumococci has been documented, and there are many published examples of resistant bacteria emerging under selective pressure in one clinical unit and spreading to other units in the same hospital or to other hospitals. There are also well-documented cases linking outbreaks of infection with drug-resistant strains to a single individual, or to emergence of resistance in animals through veterinary use of antimicrobials. Examples of inanimate reservoirs include surfaces, clothing, and even the apparatus used to dispense antiseptics.

What factors predispose to emergence of resistance? The best method

Table 8 *Variation in resistance of* Staph. aureus *and* Pseudomonas *spp. to selected antibacterials in Europe*

Organism	Antibiotic	Mean (range) % resistance		
		Northern Europe	Central Europe	Southern Europe
Staph. aureus	Cefazolin and other β-lactams	2 (0–4)	3 (0–18)	16 (1–24)
	Ciprofloxacin	1 (0–13)	2 (0–5)	8 (0–18)
	Gentamicin	2 (0–4)	3 (3–23)	14 (4–58)
Pseudomonas spp.	Ceftazidime	6 (0–15)	13 (8–29)	14 (0–29)
	Ciprofloxacin	4 (0–10)	7 (4–8)	16 (0–25)
	Ceftazidime	6 (0–15)	14 (8–29)	14 (0–29)
	Imipenem	10 (0–15)	13 (0–15)	10 (3–14)
	Piperacillin	18 (0–30)	29 (13–43)	34 (19–56)

Susceptibility tests were made on consecutive blood culture isolates by 37 laboratories in Northern, Central, and Southern Europe. Northern Europe: Sweden, Finland, Denmark and United Kingdom; Central Europe: Belgium, The Netherlands, West Germany, Austria; Southern Europe: France, Spain, Portugal, Italy, Greece.

After Dornbusch (1990) and Dornbusch *et al.* (1990).

for selecting drug-resistant strains in the laboratory is to expose a dense culture of bacteria (10^9/ml) continuously to subinhibitory concentrations of antibiotic. The same is probably true in clinical practice. Sufficiently dense populations are found in the normal gut and in abscesses. It may not be the organism being treated that becomes resistant. A published example concerns a child prescribed long-term prophylactic co-trimoxazole for recurrent *E. coli* urinary infections who acted as the source of an outbreak of co-trimoxazole-resistant shigellosis. In addition, selection of resistance with one drug may have implications for other drugs. An example includes the veterinary use of apramycin, which has been shown to select for gentamicin resistance in strains of salmonellae that have subsequently infected man. Thus, although apramycin is not used in man, its use in animals has implications for the treatment of human infections.

Principles of antimicrobial chemotherapy

Emergence of drug resistance is related to the number of patients exposed to antimicrobials and to the duration of treatment of individual patients. It follows that spread of resistance may be reduced by treating as few patients as possible with as few drugs as possible for as short a time as possible. This can only be achieved if there is informed debate about the need for antimicrobial treatment. An economic model for assessment of needs is required. According to this model the primary determinant for using antimicrobials should be the patients' capacity to benefit, rather than the severity of their disease. Capacity to benefit should be defined by a range of outcome measures (see Table 6) rather than a single biological end-point such as elimination of a potential pathogen. Demonstration that micro-organisms are present in parts of the body in which they do not normally reside is neither a necessary nor sufficient reason for chemotherapy. Patients who have clinical signs of septicaemia but sterile blood cultures may well benefit from prompt chemotherapy. However, transient bacteraemia occurs in completely asymptomatic people with no measurable harmful consequences so that the presence of bacteria in a blood culture does not mean that the patient will benefit from chemotherapy.

CHEMOPROPHYLAXIS

Chemoprophylaxis should be considered if there is a well-defined high risk of infection (e.g. wound infection after colonic surgery) or if the risk is low but the consequences are dire (e.g. infection of a prosthetic joint). Definition of the precise costs and benefits of prophylaxis requires the same rigorous measure of outcome as chemotherapy (see Table 6). Unfortunately, much existing practice is based on little, poor-quality information about the occurrence and severity of infection and about the efficacy of prophylaxis. In particular, there is very little information about actual, as opposed to potential, benefits of prevention of infection. For example, wound infection is associated with prolonged hospital admission. It does not follow that prevention of wound infection shortens hospital stay. Risk of wound infection is related to many factors, including the patient's underlying condition, which may independently influence length of hospital admission. Ultimately, the benefits of prevention of infection can only be properly quantified by controlled clinical trials.

Recognized indications for prophylaxis are constantly changing. For example, the effectiveness of chemoprophylaxis for endocarditis has been challenged, while recent evidence suggests that prophylaxis against

Fig. 15 Wound infection rate corresponding to the timing of administration of prophylaxis in relation to the time of incision. Data from 2487 patients undergoing elective clean or clean–contaminated surgical procedures. (Redrawn from Classen, *et al.* (1992). *New England Journal of Medicine*, **326**, 281–6, with permission.)

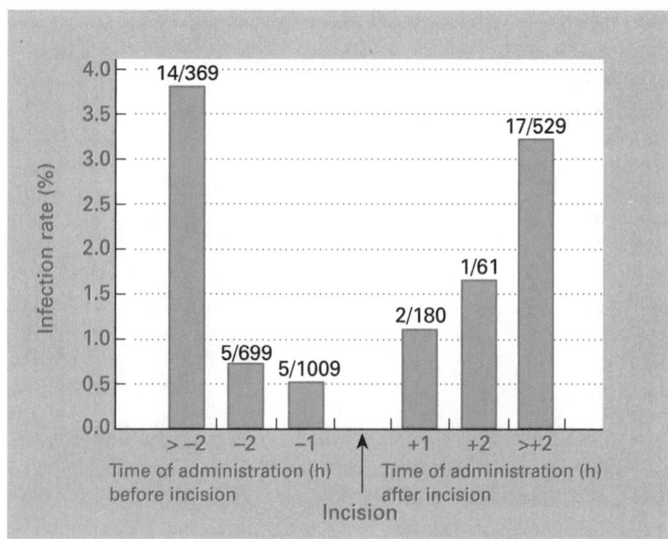

Table 9 *International variation in prescribing antibacterial drugs in hospitals based on records completed by doctors for between 1000 and 1900 patients per country*

	France	Germany	Italy	Spain	UK
Route of administration (all infections)*:					
Oral	50	45	12	30	60
i.m. injection	5	1	48	10	2
i.v. injection	45	54	40	60	38
Mean duration of therapy (days, all infections):					
Therapeutic	9.8	10.7	11.4	10.7	7.1
Surgical prevention	4.8	5.8	6.5	6.3	4.4
Use of individual drugs for lower respiratory-tract infection*:					
Aminopenicillins	50	25	26	20	55
Cephalosporins	10	25	40	22	10
Macrolides	22	5	2	12	25
Quinolones	2	8	4	2	2
Tetracyclines	2	15	1	1	0
Other drugs	14	22	27	43	8

*Data are percentages.

(Data from Mr. G. Halls, Medical Market Studies Ltd., UK, with permission).

wound infection after hernia repair may be cost-effective. It is not possible to review all the indications for chemoprophylaxis in this chapter. However, two important general principles will be discussed.

Timing of chemoprophylaxis

It should be self-evident that prophylaxis is likely to be most effective if it is administered when the risk of infection is maximal. However, audit of surgical prophylaxis shows that many patients receive drugs at inappropriate times (Fig. 15). The aim of surgical prophylaxis should be to ensure that effective drug concentrations are present at the time of surgery. For most drugs this means that intravenous administration should occur within 2 h of the incision being made (Fig. 15). Earlier administration means that most of the dose is in the urine at the time of surgery, whereas delay in administration clearly diminishes effectiveness (Fig. 15). The efficacy of chemoprophylaxis is dependent on the drug preventing the microbe from reaching the potential site of infection.

Duration of chemoprophylaxis

Continuation of prophylaxis beyond the period of likely exposure is, with few exceptions, unnecessary. An obvious exception is the chemoprophylaxis of malaria, which should be continued for 4 weeks after leaving the area where malaria is prevalent. However, for surgical prophylaxis there is very little evidence that continuing prophylaxis beyond the end of the operation is beneficial. Despite this, audit of antibiotic use consistently reveals so-called prophylaxis being continued for days after surgery. It is really alarming that a recent European survey showed that the average duration of 'surgical prevention' was from 4.4 to 6.5 days (Table 9). As well as being wasteful, this unnecessary prolongation of surgical prophylaxis must be increasing the risk of drug resistance.

CHEMOTHERAPY

The principles of pharmacokinetics, pharmodynamics, and measurement of outcome can be drawn together into a series of questions that the prescriber should answer before starting chemotherapy. There is certainly little current consensus in Europe about the most appropriate route of administration, duration of therapy or choice of drug (Table 9).

Does the clinical presentation warrant consideration of a treatable infection? Acute respiratory symptoms are the most common reason for acute consultations in community practice but the majority are not caused by organisms for which there is effective treatment. Systematic recording of symptoms and signs has been used to help doctors to assess the probability that the patient will benefit from antimicrobial treatment. This approach has been successful in developed and developing countries. More general use of simple, standard methods for recording symptoms and signs of infection is essential for audit of antimicrobial prescribing.

Should cultures be taken or should treatment be given empirically? The answer to this question depends on the quality of sampling, the facilities for storage and transport to the laboratory, the quality of laboratory services, and the evidence that the information obtained affects clinical decision making. With respect to decision making, it is important to recognize that the information obtained may have epidemiological importance, in addition to its relevance to the person from whom the sample was obtained. Finally, it is important to recognize that the answer may depend on who is asking the question. These points can best be addressed with some specific examples.

Example 1: microbiology services in developing countries

Antibiotic resistance is particularly prevalent in developing countries in which drugs are available freely in the community without prescription. Doctors treating serious infections in hospital may have few facilities for diagnostic culture and sensitivity testing, and therefore tend to use relatively expensive drugs in order that empirical treatment will be effective against drug-resistant bacteria. Apart from being relatively expensive, widespread use of broad-spectrum drugs is likely to exacerbate the problem of resistance. It may be more cost-effective in the long run to improve diagnostic facilities if this allows increased use of cheaper, narrow-spectrum drugs.

Example 2: surgical peritonitis

An audit of the management of surgical peritonitis showed a clear relation between outcome and the appropriateness of initial antimicrobial therapy (Table 10). The decision about the appropriateness of treatment was based on whether or not the bacteria isolated from peritoneal pus were sensitive to the drugs prescribed empirically. Correction of antimicrobial treatment according to culture results did not significantly improve outcome (Table 10). However, the results obtained do provide important information that should influence clinical decision making. In this case the main utility of the intraoperative cultures is to provide

Table 10 *Outcome of surgical peritonitis according to appropriateness of empirical antimicrobial chemotherapy in relation to culture of bacteria from operative samples*

Outcome measure	Group 1: Empirical therapy appropriate for bacteria isolated from operative specimens (n = 180)	Group 2: inappropriate empirical therapy (n = 49)	Group 2a (n = 13), appropriate change in empirical treatment in response to culture results	Group 2b (n = 36), no change or inappropriate change in treatment in response to culture results
Length of stay (days)	9.6	18.5	17.7	18.8
Wound infection*	26 (14.4)	13 (26.5)	2 (15)	11 (31)
Abscess*	19 (10.5)	17 (34.7)	3 (23)	12 (33)
Reoperation*	25 (13.9)	18 (36.7)	3 (23)	15 (42)
Total complications*	34 (18.9)	25 (51.0)	4 (31)	16 (44)
Deaths*	10 (5.6)	6 (12.2)	3 (23)	3 (8)

*Data in parentheses are percentages.

Source: Mosdell *et al.* (1991).

information on which to base the selection of effective empirical therapy and, if necessary, convince errant prescribers that their current practice is inappropriate.

Example 3: urinary tract infection

Several studies from the United States on the management of urinary infection have concluded that the most cost-effective approach is to give empirical treatment and ask the patient to return if the symptoms do not improve. However, while this approach may be appealing to insurance companies and other third-party payers in the United States, it is effectively transferring costs from these third-party payers to the patient. Moreover, if this possibility were adopted widely it would lead to potentially misleading information about the sensitivity of bacteria causing urinary infection, because these would usually have been isolated from patients whose empirical treatment had failed. This may encourage more widespread use of broad-spectrum drugs and ultimately increase drug resistance.

Example 4: diagnostic sampling of abscesses

Several studies have shown that bacteria from swabs of pus draining from deep collections bear little or no relation to the bacteria isolated from pus obtained directly from the collection itself. The reasons include contamination of the pus by the normal flora of the skin and the difficulties in isolating anaerobic bacteria from swabs. In this case, culture of a swab may yield results that are actively misleading to the correct management of the patient and to the rational choice of empirical therapy for other patients. Instead, if the clinical condition permits, antimicrobial therapy should be withheld until adequate specimens of pus or tissue have been obtained for culture. Drainage of pus is also essential for successful treatment of most abscesses (Fig. 10, Table 11).

These are just a few selected examples to illustrate the complexities of this particular question. It is essential that the procedures for taking and transporting clinical samples are reviewed regularly by microbiologists and clinicians. As clinical budgeting becomes more widespread, provision needs to be made for resourcing and encouraging pretreatment sampling that will provide the epidemiological information necessary for studying antibiotic-resistance patterns and so ensure the rational management of subsequent patients.

Should empirical treatment cover all likely infecting strains or is it reasonable to prescribe a drug to which some strains are resistant? The answer to this question clearly depends on the consequences of failure of empirical treatment. The data on surgical peritonitis (see Table 10) show that, for this infection, it is important to get it right first time. Even if the patient survives a period of inappropriate treatment, appropriate treatment may not be effective if it is delayed until abscesses have formed (Fig. 10). Other examples for which prompt appropriate treatment is essential include meningitis, septicaemia, infections in the neutropenic patient, herpes encephalitis, and falciparum malaria. Chemotherapy is only part of the management of these infections and success is equally dependent on general resuscitation, particularly the proper assessment of fluid requirements.

Table 11 *Questions to be answered before prescribing antimicrobial chemotherapy*

Does the clinical presentation warrant consideration of treatable infections?
Should cultures be taken or should treatment be given empirically?
Should empirical treatment cover all likely infecting strains or is it reasonable to prescribe a drug to which some strains are resistant?
Is parenteral treatment necessary?
Should serum concentrations be monitored?
How long should treatment be continued?
What should be done if the clinical response is not satisfactory?

Information about the prevalence of resistance must be related to the benefit that the patient is likely to derive from treatment. Penicillin resistance is increasing amongst pneumococci but, fortunately, penicillin-resistant strains respond to treatment with cefotaxime. If the resistance rate reaches 10 per cent, should cefotaxime become the treatment of choice for suspected pneumococcal infection? The answer will clearly be different if the patient has meningitis compared with an acute exacerbation of chronic bronchitis. It depends on both the probability of good and bad outcomes, and on their relative utility.

Formal decision analysis has been used to address the question of empirical treatment of gonorrhoea in the face of rising prevalence of penicillin-resistant strains. In this case the consequences of ineffective treatment include spread of infection to other people, as well as the outcome of the original patient. It has been concluded that empirical use of ciprofloxacin would be cost-effective if the prevalence of penicillin-resistant isolates exceeded 3 per cent of all isolates of *Neisseria gonorrhoeae*. The technique of decision analysis merits wider application in assessment of need for antimicrobial chemotherapy.

Is parenteral treatment necessary? Parenteral administration certainly improves the bioavailability of a drug, but it is more expensive than oral therapy because parenteral formulations are always more expensive, sometimes by as much as 10-fold, and there are a number of additional, significant expenses including costs of preparation and administration.

Parenteral therapy also increases the risk of adverse effects. Parenteral therapy should be reserved for initial therapy of patients who are severely ill and in whom there is reason to doubt the adequacy of oral absorption. With very few exceptions, oral therapy should be substituted as soon as clinical signs have stabilized (temperature, pulse rate, blood pressure) and the patient is taking normal diet and/or other oral medication. Possible exceptions include infections at specialized sites at which average concentrations in extracellular fluid are below average serum concentrations (endophthalmitis, endocarditis, meningitis), although even these infections can be treated with oral agents that have good bioavailability (see Table 2).

Should serum concentrations be monitored? The answer is only if there is a clear relation between serum concentrations and either outcome or adverse effects. In practice it may be preferable to obtain good-quality kinetic data from a relatively small number of patients, which can then be used to design dosing regimens based on body weight and renal function, especially when facilities for drug monitoring are not generally available. Monitoring of aminoglycoside therapy is essential because audits of clinical practice show that the majority of patients do not achieve effective serum concentrations at the doses that are prescribed initially. Use of single daily dosing of aminoglycosides will improve this situation. Otherwise, monitoring of serum concentrations is essentially a research procedure that should be actively encouraged in a few selected centres in order to supplement information about the kinetics and dynamics of antimicrobial therapy.

How long should treatment be continued? This is one of the most difficult questions. In general, the longer treatment continues, the more likely it is that the original infection will be eradicated. However, for every infection there must be a maximum effective length of treatment (see Fig. 8) and prolonging treatment also increases the risk of selecting resistant strains, of encouraging superinfection by other microbes and of dose-related, pharmacological adverse effects. The duration of treatment should be planned at the outset, either as a fixed duration or dependent on response (e.g. for 2 days after the temperature is normal). Overall, the duration of treatment of many common infections is probably unnecessarily long.

What should be done if the clinical response is not satisfactory? The answer is emphatically not an empirical change in chemotherapy, or even worse the prescription of one or more additional drugs. Instead, the prescriber should work systematically through a checklist of possible reasons for poor response.

1. Is the clinical diagnosis wrong? The patient may be receiving an antibacterial drug for a viral infection, or may not have an infection at all (two-thirds of cases of pyrexia of unknown origin are caused by malignancy or connective tissue disease rather than infection).
2. Does the patient have an abscess that requires surgical or percutaneous drainage?
3. Is the prescribed drug likely to reach the anatomical site of infection?
4. Are the dose and route of administration appropriate?
5. If the answer to all of the above is yes, is it possible that the patient's infection is caused by a drug-resistant organism?

If the possibility of drug resistance remains, then it would be advisable to discuss the patient with a microbiologist or infectious diseases physician to consider the need for further samples for culture as well as the most appropriate alternative treatment.

Proposals for improvement of current practice

Prescribers should address a few simple questions whenever they plan to initiate chemotherapy (Table 11). Unfortunately, the extreme variations in current practice both in the community (Table 7) and in hospitals (Table 9) suggest that there is little consensus about the answers to them. However, it is vital that doctors, pharmacists, and administrators resist the temptation to resolve these differences through hasty imposition of consensus documents that are, in reality, spurious endorsements of essentially arbitrary current practice. Instead, the questions posed in Table 11 should be addressed through audit of current practice and decision analysis of the relative cost-effectiveness of the many alternatives that exist. There is an extensive literature about methods for influencing prescribing of antimicrobials. Peer review of prescribing and feedback of information to prescribers are highly effective. Limited data from hospitals suggest that continued review of prescribing reduces overall use of antimicrobials and the prevalence of drug-resistant bacteria. A more systematic review of community prescribing might have equally beneficial effects.

REFERENCES

Mechanism of action

Lambert, H.P., and O'Grady, F.W. (1992). *Antibiotic and chemotherapy.* Churchill Livingstone, Edinburgh.

Mechanisms and tests for resistance

Baquero, F. (1990). European standards for antibiotic susceptibility testing: toward a theoretical consensus. *European Journal of Clinical Microbiology and Infectious Diseases*, **9**, 492–5.

Courvalin, P. (1992). Interpretive reading of antimicrobial susceptibility tests. Molecular analysis and therapeutic interpretation of *in vitro* tests to improve antibiotic therapy. *ASM News*, **58**, 368–75.

Finch, R.G. (1991). A guide to sensitivity testing. *Journal of Antimicrobial Chemotherapy*, **27** (suppl.D), 1–50.

Lambert, H.P., and O'Grady, F.W. (1992). *Antibiotic and chemotherapy.* Churchill Livingstone, Edinburgh.

Pharmacokinetics

Baldwin, D.R., Honeybourne, D., and Wise, R. (1992). Pulmonary disposition of antimicrobial agents: in vivo observations and clinical relevance. *Antimicrobial Agents and Chemotherapy*, **36**, 1176–80.

Barza, M. (1993). Pharmacokinetics of antibiotics in shallow and deep compartments. *Journal of Antimicrobial Chemotherapy*, **31**, (suppl. D), 17–27.

Davey, P.G. (1988). Pharmacokinetics in liver disease. *Journal of Antimicrobial Chemotherapy*, **21**, 1–5.

Maderazo, E.G., Sun, H., and Jay, G.T. (1992). Simplification of antibiotic dose adjustments in renal insufficiency: the DREM system. *Lancet*, **340**, 767–70.

Plaisance, K.I., Quintiliani, R., and Nightingale, C.H. (1988). The pharmacokinetics of metronidazole and its metabolites in critically ill patients. *Journal of Antimicrobial Chemotherapy*, **21**, 195–200.

White, N.J. (1992). Antimalarial pharmacokinetics and treatment regimens. *British Journal of Clinical Pharmacology*, **34**, 1–10.

Pharmacodynamics of antimicrobial effect

Cremieux, A-C. and Carbon, D. (1992). Pharmacokinetic and pharmacodynamic requirements for antibiotic therapy of experimental endocarditis. *Antimicrobial Agents and Chemotherapy*, **36**, 2069–74.

Drusano, G.L. (1991). Human pharmacodynamics of β-lactams, aminoglycosides and their combination. *Scandinavian Journal of Infectious Diseases*, **74** (suppl.), 235–48.

Drusano, G.L. *et al.* (1992). Impact of bioavailability on determination of the maximal tolerated dose of 2′,3′-dideoxyinosine in phase I trials. *Antimicrobial Agents and Chemotherapy*, **36**, 1280–3.

Dudley, M.N. (1991). Pharmacodynamics and pharmacokinetics of antibiotics with special reference to quinolones. *American Journal of Medicine*, **91** (suppl. A), 45–50S.

Gilbert, P., Collier, P.J., and Brown, M.R.W. (1990). Influence of growth rate on susceptibility ot antimicrobial agents: biofilms, cell cycle, dormancy, and stringent response. *Antimicrobial Agents and Chemotherapy*, **34**, 1865–8.

Merluzzi, V.J. *et al.* (1990). Inhibition of HIV-1 replication by nonnucleoside reverse transcriptase inhibitor. *Science*, **250**, 1411–13.

Young, L. (1993). The Garrod Lecture. Mycobacterial diseases in the 1990s. *Journal of Antimicrobial Chemotherapy*, **32**, 179–94.

Adverse events

Davey, P.G. and McDonald, T. (1993). Postmarketing surveillance of quinolones, 1990 to 1992. *Drugs*, **45** (suppl.3), 46–53.

Graff-Lonnevig, V., Hedlin, G., and Lindfors, A. (1988). Penicillin allergy—a rare paediatric condition? *Archives of Disease in Childhood*, **63,** 1342–6.

Park, B.K., Pirmohamed, M., and Kitteringham, N.R. (1992). Idiosyncratic drug reactions: a mechanistic evaluation of risk factors. *British Journal of Clinical Pharmacology*, **34,** 377–95.

Drug interactions

Rahal, J.J. (1978). Antibiotic combinations: the clinical relevance of synergy and antagonism. *Medicine*, **57,** 179–95.

Design of dosing regimens

Winstanley, P.A. and Watkins, W.M. (1992). Pharmacology and parasitology: integrating experimental methods and approaches to falciparum malaria. *British Journal of Clinical Pharmacology*, **33,** 575–81.

Controversies in assessment of response to antimicrobials/ international variation in medical practice

Cantekin, E.I., McGuire, T.W., and Griffith, T.L. (1991). Antimicrobial therapy for otitis media with effusion ('secretory' otitis media). *Journal of the American Medical Association*, **266,** 3309–17.

Froom, J. *et al.* (1990). Diagnosis and antibiotic treatment of acute otitis media: report from International Primary Care Network. *British Medical Journal*, **300,** 582–6.

Mandel, E.M., Rockette, H.E., Bluestone, C.D., Paradise, J.L., and Nozza, R.J. (1987). Efficacy of amoxicillin with and without decongestant-antihistamine for otitis media with effusion in children: results of a double-blind, randomized trial. *New England Journal of Medicine*, **316,** 432–7.

Rennie, D. (1991). The Cantekin affair. *Journal of the American Medical Association*, **266,** 3333–7.

Epidemiology and control of resistance to antimicrobials

Dornbusch, K. for the European Study Group on Antibiotic Resistance. (1990). Resistance to β-lactam antibiotics and ciprofloxacin in Gram-negative bacilli and staphylococci isolated from blood: a European collaborative study. *Journal of Antimicrobial Chemotherapy*, **26,** 269–78.

Dornbusch, K., Miller, G.H., Hare, R.S., Shaw, K.J. for the ESGAR Study Group. (1990). Resistance to aminoglycoside antibiotics in Gram-negative bacilli and staphylococci isolated from blood. Report from a European collaborative study. *Journal of Antimicrobial Chemotherapy*, **26,** 131–44.

Lamikanra, A. and Ndep, R.B. (1989). Trimethoprim resistance in urinary tract pathogens in two Nigerian hospitals. *Journal of Antimicrobial Chemotherapy*, **23,** 151–4.

Montefiore, D., Rotimi, V.O., and Adeyemi-Doro, F.A.B. (1989). The problem of bacterial resistance to antibiotics among strains isolated from hospital patients in Lagos and Ibadan, Nigeria. *Journal of Antimicrobial Chemotherapy*, **23,** 641–51.

Powell, M., Fah, Y.S., Seymour, A., Yuan, M., and Williams, J.D. (1992). Antimicrobial resistance in Haemophilus influenzae from England and Scotland in 1991. *Journal of Antimicrobial Chemotherapy*, **29,** 547–54.

Urbina, R., Prado, V., and Canelo, E. (1989). Trimethoprim resistance in enterobacteria in Chile. *Journal of Antimicrobial Chemotherapy*, **23,** 143–9.

Consequence of resistance

Bloom, B.R., and Murray, C.J.L. (1992). Tuberculosis: commentary on a reemergent killer. *Science*, **257,** 1055–64.

Cohen, M.L. (1992). Epidemiology of drug resistance: implications for a post-antimicrobial era. *Science*, **257,** 1050–5.

Viladrich, P.F. *et al.* (1991). Evaluation of vancomycin for therapy of adult pneumococcal meningitis. *Antimicrobial Agents and Chemotherapy*, **35,** 2467–72.

Principles of chemoprophylaxis

Davey, P.G., Parker, S.E. and Malek, M.M. (1993). Pharmacoeconomics of antimicrobial prophylaxis. *Journal of Antimicrobial Chemotherapy* **31** (suppl. B), 107–18.

Editorial (1992). Chemoprophylaxis for infective endocarditis: faith, hope, and charity challenged. *Lancet*, **339,** 525–6.

Finch, R.G. (1993). Prophylaxis at the margins. *Journal of Antimicrobial Chemotherapy*, **31,** (suppl. B).

Principles of chemotherapy

Deciding who to treat

Cebul, R.D., and Poses, R.M. (1986). The comparative cost-effectiveness of statistical decision rules and experienced physicians in pharyngitis management. *Journal of the American Medical Association*, **256,** 3353–7.

Isenberg, H.D. (1988). Pathogenicity and virulence: another view. *Clinical Microbiology Reviews*, **1,** 40–53.

Pandey, R.M., Daulaire, N.M., Starbuck, E.S., Houston, R.M., and McPherson, K. (1991). Reduction in total under-five mortality in western Nepal through community-based antimicrobial treatment of pneumonia. *Lancet*, **338,** 993–7.

Decision analysis applied to drug selection

Davey, P.G., Parker, S.E., and Malek, M.M. (1992). Pharmacoeconomics of antibacterial treatment. *PharmacoEconomics*, **1,** 409–37.

Davey, P.G., Parker, S.E. and Malek, M.M. (1993). Pharmacoeconomics of antimicrobial prophylaxis. *Journal of Antimicrobial Chemotherapy* **31** (suppl. B), 107–18.

Nettleman, M.D., Smith, V., and Moyer, N.P. (1990). Penicillin resistant *Neisseria gonorrhoeae* in low prevalence areas: implications for cost-effective management. *Sexually Transmitted Diseases*, **17,** 175–180.

Intravenous versus oral

Davey, P.G., Parker, S.E., and Malek, M.M. (1992). Pharmacoeconomics of antibacterial treatment. *PharmacoEconomics*, **1,** 409–37.

Measuring outcome

Garratt, A.M., Ruta, D.A., Abdalla, M.I., Buckingham, J.K., and Russell, I.T. (1993). The SF36 health survey questionnaire: an outcome measure suitable for routine use within the NHS? *British Medical Journal*, **306,** 1440–4.

Mosdell, D.M. *et al.* (1991) Antibiotic treatment for surgical peritonitis. *Annals of Surgery*, **214,** 543–9.

Wachtel, T., Piette, J., Mor, V., Stein, M., Fleishman, J., and Carpenter, C. (1992). Quality of life in persons with human immunodeficiency virus infection: measurement by the medical outcomes study instrument. *Annals of Internal Medicine*, **116,** 129–37.

Auditing antibiotic prescribing

Moss, F., McNicol, M.W., McSwiggan, D.A., and Miller, D.L. (1981). Survey of antibiotic prescribing in a district general hospital 1. Pattern of use. *Lancet*, **ii,** 349–52.

Moss, F., McNicol, M.W., McSwiggan, D.A., and Miller, D.L. (1981). Survey of antibiotic prescribing in a district general hospital II. Lower respiratory tract infection. *Lancet*, **ii,** 407–9.

Moss, F., McNicol, M.W., McSwiggan, D.A., and Miller, D.L. (1981). Survey of antibiotic prescribing in a district general hospital III. Urinary tract infection. *Lancet*, **ii,** 461–2.

O'Hanley, P., Easaw, J., Rugo, H., and Easaw, S. (1989). Infectious disease management of adult leukemic patients undergoing chemotherapy: 1982 to 1986 experience at Stanford University Hospital. *American Journal of Medicine*, **87,** 605–13.

7.7 Immunization

D. Isaacs and E. R. Moxon

Introduction

The germ theory of disease is now so entrenched in the thinking of contemporary society that it is as well to remember that it was highly controversial as little as 100 years ago. Achievements in the late nineteenth and early twentieth centuries—the golden era of microbiology—built on the discovery of the causal role of microbes in disease and resulted in the development of several vaccines (active immunization) and strategies for immunoprophylaxis using antisera (passive immunization). Although it must be emphasized that improved socioeconomic circumstances, especially clean water and sanitation, resulted in drastic reductions in mortality from many infectious diseases, vaccination has been decisive in the control of at least nine major microbial diseases—smallpox, diphtheria, tetanus, yellow fever, pertussis, polio, measles, mumps, and rubella. Programmes of immunization have undoubtedly provided one of the most compelling examples of the profound impact of public health measures on mortality and morbidity. These successes must be tempered by an appreciation of the enormous unfulfilled potential for preventing microbial diseases. To mention but a few examples; at the time of writing, the World Health Organization has recognized the increase in tuberculosis as a global health emergency—a disease which, in many parts of the world, has never been controlled; there is a pandemic of disease caused by human immunodeficiency viruses (**HIV**) that poses a radical threat to the infrastructure of many of the most populous nations; millions of children die each year as the result of diarrhoeal disease or lower respiratory infections; there is no successful immunoprophylactic strategy against any human parasite despite the infection of about two-thirds of the world's population with various macroparasites that are collectively responsible for enormous morbidity.

There is a dual challenge. First, the development of safe, effective, and inexpensive vaccines; secondly, their successful implementation. There can be many impediments to overcome in developing a successful vaccine (Fig. 1). The rapid generation (doubling times) of many microbes, together with their capacity to generate genetic and epigenetic variation, facilitates their ability to avoid host defences. Despite the relatively small size of the genome of many of the most virulent microbes, for example viruses, their capacity to vary surface structures has made the task of developing effective vaccines extremely difficult, a problem that has been long appreciated for influenza virus and has been more recently emphasized by HIV. Bacteria can vary surface structures through intragenomic rearrangements of genes (molecular switches) or intergenomic exchange of DNA (e.g. plasmids). Parasites also have extraordinary prowess in this regard. For example, trypanosomes have a gene pool running into the thousands, each encoding an antigenically distinct surface glycoprotein—a target for protective antibodies. Parasites have also evolved numerous mechanisms for subverting host defences; these include the elaboration of molecular signals that down-regulate the activity of host defences, disguising themselves by mimicking self antigens on the parasite cell surface, or adorning themselves with host structures. Some microbes present special difficulties because of their intrinsic biological characteristics. Herpesviruses exhibit latency, so that once a host is infected the presence of the virus in perpetuity makes it imperative that there be some reasonable assessment of the potential for reactivation or, in some cases, of oncogenic potential. Some pathogenic microbes present particular technical limitations, for example, our inability to grow them *in vitro* (hepatitis B, *Pneumocystis carinii*). Finally, the interplay between host and microbial factors can be subtle, as in areas of holoendemic *Plasmodium falciparum* malaria where individuals can be immune to illness but remain susceptible to parasitaemia. Taken together, the pathogenic personality and other characteristics of microbes pose troublesome—in some instances, seemingly insurmountable—problems.

Immunity from disease may result from the eclectic effect of many quite different mechanisms, which can be categorized as adaptive and non-adaptive. Until recently, the manipulation of adaptive mechanisms has been the major focus of strategies of immunoprophylaxis. Adaptive mechanisms involve two classes of lymphocytes, B cells and T cells. B cells produce antibodies, proteins that are capable of preventing infection. Antibodies can be produced naturally, actively induced, passively acquired by injection, or transferred from mother to fetus/infant via the placenta or breast milk. Antibodies can neutralize, facilitate removal of, or kill, microbes when they are outside host cells. Alternatively, antibodies can eliminate infected cells (antibody-mediated cellular cytotoxicity) directly or in conjunction with lysis by complement. This radical function of antibodies is achieved through the specific recognition of conformational structures (i.e. the three-dimensional shape) on the sur-

Fig. 1 Developing a successful vaccine (Reproduced with kind permission of P.H. Lambert, World Health Organization.)

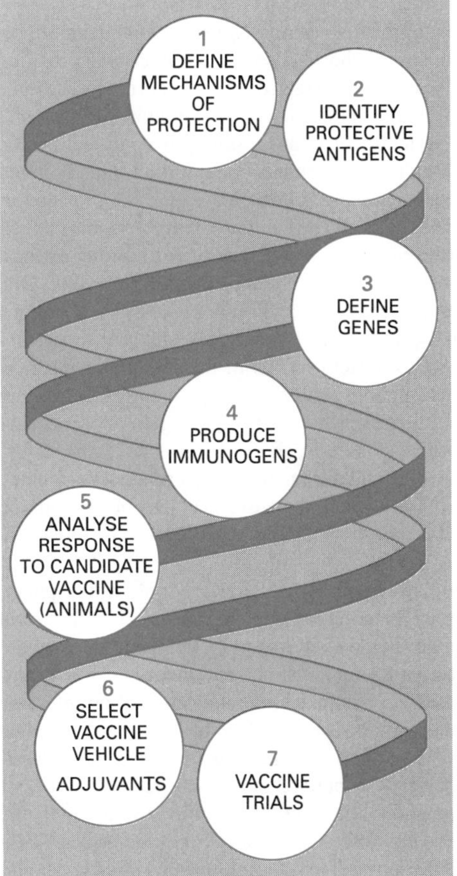

face of microbes. A good example is the neutralization of influenza virus haemagglutinin. The limitations of this strategy are as follows. Because only a limited number of domains (epitopes) are candidates for recognition by antibodies, this strategy tends to fail when there is antigenic shift or drift; this can be countered by frequently changing the vaccine. For some antigens, the genetically determined repertoire of germ-line genes of a particular individual's lymphocytes may be unfavourable and limit the potential for an optimal response. In contrast to B cells, neither T cells nor their products, acting alone, can prevent infection. Their role is most prominent in facilitating the quality and quantity of antibody production through regulating the ability to make antibodies ('helper' and 'suppressor' functions) and through effector functions that include delayed-type hypersensitivity, cytotoxicity, and augmentation of non-adaptive immune responses (interferons and cytokines). In contrast to B cells, T cells can recognize a wide variety of microbial structures irrespective of their location (e.g. surface, internal), thereby overcoming to an extent the constraints imposed by the genetic variations of microbes. Although the T-cell repertoire and function are genetically restricted for each individual, allelic variation (polymorphisms) helps to ensure that at least some individuals within the population are favourably endowed to resist lethal infection with any particular microbe. Crucial to the adaptive function of B and T cells in immune function is the concept of biological memory. Lymphocytes acquire and 'fine tune' their affinity for particular microbial determinants through an evolutionary process that involves genetic rearrangements, somatic mutation, and subpopulation selection. Biological memory resides in the prior selection (priming) of lymphocyte clones with specific receptors so that persistence of the relevant microbial antigen or re-exposure to it maintains, mobilizes, and expands the availability of the relevant immune-effector functions. Strategies that augment non-adaptive immune mechanisms, such as those associated with natural killer cells, polymorphonuclear phagocytes, or proteins such as the interferons and cytokines, are receiving more attention but these activities can only supplement, not pre-empt, the cardinal role of adaptive mechanisms in disease prevention.

Most pathogens show tropism for particular tissues so that an important consideration is the specific host cells in which microbial infection is initiated, or to which disease is targeted; one which may determine the degree of difficulty and the optimal strategy in attaining a successful vaccine. In contrast to systemic infections resulting from dissemination of microbes or circulating toxins, pathogens that initiate infection and cause disease at mucosal surfaces—as in the case of cholera or gonorrhoea—have proved to be especially difficult problems in vaccine development. This is in part because our knowledge of the biology of local immunity has lagged behind that of systemic immune functions. Oral immunization, for example, may occur through processing of antigen by specialized epithelial (M) cells that are located adjacent to submucosal lymphoid tissue. This system results in the production of local antibodies (e.g. IgA) in secretions such as saliva or breast milk. We are still profoundly ignorant of the developmental and regulatory aspects of the modulation of these responses, such as the effects of the nature and timing of exposure to antigenic, nutritional, and genetic factors. Local immune responses are often short-lived, a sensible adaptation of this host function, but one not obviously favourable to long-term protection.

The availability of an effective vaccine is clearly only a first phase, just one of many steps, in the complex implementation of a successful immunization programme (Fig. 1). An important appreciation is of the non-linear relation between host populations and microbes. For example, as a population doubles its numbers, the incidence of an infection may increase more than twofold. It is therefore of the utmost practical importance to consider major variables such as the geography, distribution (urban or rural), age distribution, and sexual habits (number of partners) of target populations. For any infection to sustain itself, the average number of secondary infections arising from one primary case must exceed unity, and the most effective immunization strategy should be based upon sound epidemiological principles. It is well known that not everyone in a population needs to be immunized to eliminate disease—often referred to as herd immunity (see below). This is because successful immunization reduces the number of susceptibles in the population and this effectively reduces the efficiency with which the microbe is transmitted from one person to another. This has the same effect on the incidence of infection as a reduction in the number of individuals in a population; the microbe cannot sustain itself and disease disappears at some level of vaccine coverage that is less than 100 per cent. On the other hand, coverage below that needed to prevent disease may have little impact on the total number of susceptibles—as has been predicted using mathematical models and verified, in the case of rubella, by observation. The implementation of immunization programmes needs to be accompanied by case surveillance, in conjunction with analysis of appropriate serological samples both before and after the introduction of the vaccine. If such data are not carefully scrutinized, the consequences may be dire. For example, an immunization programme may reduce the number of cases but at the same time may increase the average age at which infection occurs. If the severity of disease increases with age at acquisition, as in rubella (the risk of an infected fetus in an infected woman) and polio (the risk of paralytic disease), an immunization programme may actually be less useful than none at all.

Passive immunization

Passive immunization is the administration of preformed antibodies in an immune serum, human or animal, and is used to prevent or modify disease following exposure to an organism or toxin. Passive immunization is used where there is exposure of an immunocompromised individual to an organism that is normally relatively benign, varicella-zoster immune globulin to prevent or modify chickenpox, for example, or following exposure of a normal host to a particularly virulent organism such as rabies. Passive can be combined with active immunization, particularly if the incubation period is long; for example, hepatitis B immunoglobulin and vaccine are both given to neonates or after accidental exposure to virus.

In the above examples, passive immunization is used prophylactically to prevent infection or modify the severity of infection. It may also be used therapeutically to neutralize toxins, such as those of diphtheria and tetanus. Specific diphtheria and tetanus antitoxins have been produced in horses and are available for treatment of cases. The use of intravenous immunoglobulin to treat Kawasaki disease may be a form of passive immunization, in that the globulin may be acting by toxin neutralization, although this is unproven.

There are three main types of sera used for passive immunization. First, normal human immunoglobulin, which is purified, pooled serum from normal individuals; this can be given intramuscularly or intravenously. It is used prophylactically in immune-deficient patients, but also following some exposures to infection (see Table 1). Second, hyperimmune serum, which is serum pooled from humans known to have a high titre of antibodies to a given organism, varicella-zoster immune globulin for example. Third, animal sera, which are generally used as antitoxins to neutralize potent toxins. Examples of the use of these three types of sera are given in Table 1.

NORMAL HUMAN IMMUNOGLOBULIN

Normal human immunoglobulin is prepared by Cohn alcohol fractionation of pooled human serum, which is known to kill HIV-1 and -2, and hepatitis B viruses. The use of early intravenous preparations to treat immune-deficient patients was associated with an illness that was described, before hepatitis C virus had been identified, as non-A, non-B hepatitis.

Intravenous immunoglobulin has been treated to eliminate high molecular-weight immune complexes. Both intramuscular and intrave-

Table 1 *Products used for passive immunization*

Product	Origin[1]	Indication for use
Normal human immunoglobulin		
Intravenous immunoglobulin	H	Prophylaxis of neonatal infections
Intramuscular immunoglobulin	H	Prophylaxis of infections following exposure, particularly measles and hepatitis A
Hyperimmune serum globulin		
Hepatitis B (HBIG)	H	Prophylaxis following exposure
Varicella-zoster (ZIG or VZIG)	H	Prophylaxis of immunocompromised
Rabies (RIG)	H	Prophylaxis following dog bite
Cytomegalovirus (CMV-IVIG)	H	Prevention and treatment of infection in immunocompromised
Tetanus (TIG)	H	Prophylaxis of major wounds if not adequately immunized Treatment of tetanus
Animal sera		
Rabies antiserum (EARS)	E	When RIG unavailable
Tetanus antitoxin (TAT)	E	When TIG unavailable
Diphtheria antitoxin (DAT)	E	Prevention of diphtheria if not adequately immunized Treatment of diphtheria
Botulism antitoxin	E	Treatment of botulism
Snake, fish, scorpion, tick, jelly-fish, and spider antivenoms	E/O	Various antivenoms, mono- or polyspecific, for treatment of bites/stings

[1]H, human; E, equine; O, ovine.

nous immunoglobulins are over 95 per cent γG, with traces of γA, γM, and other serum proteins. They are very safe, but may cause reactions resembling serum sickness, and very rarely can cause anaphylactic reactions. The mechanism of these reactions is complement activation by IgG polymers or type I hypersensitivity. The half-life of immunoglobulin is 3 to 4 weeks.

HYPERIMMUNE GLOBULIN

The efficacy of different types of hyperimmune globulin, administered as soon as possible after exposure, has been known for nearly a century. In 1907, Cenci prevented measles in children by the prophylactic administration of convalescent serum. Since then, early administration of normal human immunoglobulin has been shown to prevent measles and, if given late, to reduce its severity. Therefore, normal human immunoglobulin rather than a hyperimmune preparation is used for measles.

The use of hyperimmune preparations will prevent or modify varicella-zoster infections and prevent cytomegalovirus infections. Treatment of established infections such as cytomegalovirus or respiratory syncytial virus with hyperimmune globin is less well established and more controversial.

ANIMAL SERA

Animal sera are much more likely to cause anaphylaxis, and human sera are preferable, if available. It has been estimated that equine tetanus antitoxin causes fatal anaphylaxis at a rate of 1 in 100 000 doses. Intradermal skin testing will only detect type I hypersensitivity and is unreliable in predicting the more common reactions resulting from complement activation by Fc and IgG aggregates. Adrenaline (1 : 1000) should always be available for immediate administration in case of anaphylaxis.

Active immunization

Edward Jenner is often credited with being the father of modern immunization having developed systematic immunization against smallpox. However, variolation, the technique of inoculating pustular smallpox material on the arm, was practised in China at least as long ago as the sixth century AD. It is important that, as diseases become rare through effective immunization programmes, the side-effects of immunizations do not become overemphasized and the severity of the diseases forgotten. Evidence of the efficacy of immunizations and their continued need, despite improvements in living standards, which it has been argued by some have made the diseases less severe, comes from two main sources. One is the recurrence of whooping cough in the late 1970s in the United Kingdom and Japan when the numbers of individuals immunized against pertussis had fallen: the resultant severe epidemics resulted in hundreds of infant deaths and many more children left handicapped as a result of whooping cough with encephalopathy. The second source of evidence is from communities or sects that do not immunize themselves for religious or other reasons, such as the Amish, who are at high risk for outbreaks of measles, pertussis, and poliomyelitis.

Primary vaccination schedules

The vaccines commonly used in the primary immunization schedule in many developed and developing countries are shown in Table 2. In 1974, as the global smallpox eradication programme neared successful completion, the Expanded Programme on Immunization (**EPI**) was launched by the World Health Organization (**WHO**). The goal of EPI was global immunization of children against tuberculosis, diphtheria, tetanus, pertussis, polio, and measles. Within 20 years, 80 per cent of the world's children had been immunized against these six diseases, through the efforts of the WHO, the United Nations, and local governments. It is estimated that 3.2 million children's lives are saved each year by this increased level of immunization. In the United States the incidence of all these vaccine-preventable diseases has been reduced by over 95 per cent since immunization was introduced.

TOXOIDS

Diphtheria and tetanus are toxin-mediated diseases, caused by exotoxins released by *Corynebacterium diphtheriae* and *Clostridium tetani*. The toxoid vaccines against these diseases are prepared by treating a cell-

Table 2 *Vaccines in common use in primary immunization schedules*

Vaccine	Nature	Route[1]	Age[2]	Indications
Bacille Calmette–Guérin (BCG)	Live bacteria	i.d., s.c.	Birth or 12–13 years	Neonatal period in developing countries
Diphtheria-tetanus-pertussis (DTP)	Toxoids of diphtheria and tetanus; inactivated pertussis	i.m.	2,3,4 months or 2,4,6, months Boosters at 18 months, 5 years DT every 10 years	Triple vaccine Three doses and boosters
Hepatitis B	Surface antigen (yeast or plasma derived)	i.m.	0,1,6 months or starting later Booster every 5 years	Three doses and boosters
Haemophilus influenzae type b (Hib) conjugate vaccines	Hib polysaccharide conjugated to protein	i.m.	2,3,4 months or 2,4,6 months Booster at 18 months	Immunogenic in infancy
Measles-mumps-rubella (MMR)	All live, attenuated viruses	s.c.	12 months	One or two doses
Poliovirus	Live, attenuated (OPV) Inactivated (IPV)	Oral s.c.	2,3,4 months or 2,4,6 months Booster at 5 years	Three doses and booster(s)

[1]i.d., intradermal; i.m., intramuscular; s.c., subcutaneous.

[2]The ages at which these vaccines are given and the exact schedules vary from country to country.

free preparation of the respective toxin with formaldehyde. Immunization with toxoid protects against the disease, but does not prevent colonization. A primary course of three doses of diphtheria and tetanus toxoids, with two boosters, provides long-lasting protection. Boosters of tetanus and diphtheria toxoids are recommended every 10 years for adults.

PERTUSSIS VACCINES

The most commonly used pertussis vaccines are whole-cell suspensions of killed *Bordetella pertussis* organisms. These cause a relatively high incidence of local side-effects, fever, and rarely even neurological events. Whether pertussis vaccine causes encephalopathy (or possibly merely uncovers underlying brain damage) is controversial, although it is clear that the risk of brain damage from the disease is many hundreds or thousands of times greater than from the vaccine.

Acellular pertussis vaccines, which contain various combinations of one or more *B. pertussis* enzymes, have been used in Japan since 1981 and are being tested by clinical trials in many other countries. They are either made by purifying antigens or by genetic engineering. They are less reactogenic than whole-cell vaccines. However, it is not known which antigens are most important in immunity to pertussis, so the ideal formulation is not yet known. It is likely that acellular pertussis vaccines will replace whole-cell vaccines in the near future.

POLIO VACCINES

There are two types of vaccine against poliomyelitis, live attenuated oral polio vaccine, first developed by Albert Sabin, and inactivated polio vaccine, as first developed by Jonas Salk. These vaccines contain the three serotypes of poliovirus that can cause paralytic poliomyelitis. An enhanced-potency inactivated polio vaccine is now available.

Oral polio vaccine induces a secretory immune (IgA) response to polio not seen with inactivated vaccine. It spreads readily within families, boosting levels of immunity. It is also considerably cheaper than inactivated vaccine, a factor of major importance in developing countries. On the other hand, the oral vaccine causes vaccine-induced paralytic poliomyelitis at a rate of approximately 1 in 1 000 000 doses, although estimates of the frequency vary. Inactivated vaccine does not cause vaccine-induced polio. Some countries use oral vaccine, some use inactivated, and there is a growing interest in the option, already used in France, to commence immunization with inactivated polio vaccine and then change to oral.

HEPATITIS B VACCINES

Hepatitis B vaccines consist of the surface antigen of the virus (HBs) purified from plasma or derived by genetic engineering. In the United States it is now recommended that immunization of all children should start at birth. Vaccine-induced immunity wanes after 3 to 5 years, so booster doses will be needed. Most other Western countries screen pregnant women for hepatitis B and immunize the babies of hepatitis B antigen-positive mothers and babies from ethnic groups with a high prevalence of hepatitis B infection. Universal hepatitis B immunization will have most impact when it is introduced in countries such as those in South-East Asia and Africa where the prevalence is extremely high.

HAEMOPHILUS INFLUENZAE TYPE B CONJUGATE VACCINES

Protection against *Haemophilus influenzae* type b (**Hib**) infection is mediated primarily by antibody to the polysaccharide capsule of the organism, the type b antigen. However, this polysaccharide is poorly immunogenic in children under 2 years of age, and the maximum age for infection is the first year of life. The Hib conjugate vaccines are the first effective example of vaccines using the hapten principle, whereby a poorly immunogenic molecule is bound to an immunogenic protein, thus converting the poor immunogen to a good one. The different Hib conjugate proteins used include diphtheria toxoids, tetanus toxoid, or outer-membrane proteins of *Neisseria meningitidis*. This is an important advance in vaccine development and conjugate vaccines are being developed for other weak immunogens such as pneumococcal and meningococcal polysaccharides.

MEASLES–MUMPS–RUBELLA VACCINE

Measles-mumps-rubella (**MMR**) vaccine is now the most common formulation used for childhood measles immunization, although previously each of these viral vaccines was used on its own. All are live, attenuated

Table 3 *Vaccines available for special indications*

Vaccine	Nature	Indication
Adenovirus	Live attenuated virus (oral)	US Armed Forces
Cholera	Inactivated *V. cholerae*	Travel to epidemic area (but protection poor)
Epidemic typhus	Inactivated *Rickettsia prowazekii*	Workers in epidemic areas
Hepatitis A	Inactivated virus	Travel to endemic area
Influenza	Inactivated virus	High risk, e.g. chronic disease, elderly, immunocompromised
Japanese encephalitis virus	Inactivated virus	Travel to area during epidemic or residence in endemic area
Meningococcal	Polysaccharide	Protection during outbreaks, travel to endemic area
Plague	Inactivated *Yersinia pestis*	Laboratory and field workers in enzootic areas
Pneumococcal	Polysaccharide	Protection against pneumonia, e.g. elderly, asplenic, sickle-cell disease
Q fever	Inactivated *Coxiella burnetii*	Laboratory, veterinary, and abattoir workers in endemic areas
Rabies	Inactivated virus	Laboratory and veterinary workers in endemic areas, *not* routine for travellers to endemic areas
Typhoid	Inactivated bacteria. Live, attenuated, oral (Ty 21a)	Travel to endemic area
Yellow fever	Live, attenuated virus	Travel to endemic area

viruses. A single dose given at 12 months gives long-term protection, although some countries such as Sweden, the United States, and Australia recommend a second dose, which is given either at 5 years or 12 to 13 years of age.

Vaccines with special indications

A list of vaccines with special indications is given in Table 3. Many of these are used for travel to endemic areas or to protect laboratory workers working with the live organism.

HEPATITIS A

Inactivated hepatitis A virus vaccines have been developed, and are immunogenic in children and adults. However, their protective efficacy has not yet been proven and indications for their use have yet to be determined.

INFLUENZA VACCINES

Influenza vaccines are inactivated virus vaccines containing A and B strains, Because of antigenic drift and occasionally shift of wild influenza virus, the vaccines are revised each year in the light of prevailing epidemic strains. They provide about 70 per cent protection for a year and are recommended for high-risk individuals. Examples are adults over 65 years old; adults and children with chronic debilitating disease, especially cardiac, pulmonary, renal, and metabolic disorders; residents of nursing homes; and immunocompromised patients.

MENINGOCOCCAL VACCINES

Meningococcal polysaccharide vaccines contain polysaccharides from serogroups A and C, and sometimes groups W and Y, but not serogroup B, which is non-immunogenic. The vaccines are poorly immunogenic in children under 2 years of age. They are indicated for travellers to endemic areas where the prevalent strain is included in the vaccine (usually serogroup A). They can be useful to prevent transmission of meningococcal infection in outbreaks due to serogroups A or C in closed communities. They are also indicated for patients with immune deficiency with an increased risk of meningococcal sepsis, such as those with defects in one of the terminal components of the complement pathway and patients with congenital or acquired asplenia. The response to unconjugated polysaccharide vaccines is T-cell independent so there is no T-cell memory and the response does not boost with repeated doses.

PNEUMOCOCCAL VACCINES

Pneumococcal polysaccharide vaccines contain polysaccharides from the most common of the many pneumococcal serotypes known to cause disease. Response is poor in children under 2 years of age. Pneumococcal vaccine can be given safely to asplenic children under 2 years of age, but does not provide protection; it should therefore be given at or after 2 years. The main indication for pneumococcal vaccine is for children with congenital asplenia, those with functional asplenia as in sickle-cell disease, and for children and adults who have had a splenectomy. Where splenectomy is elective, pneumococcal vaccine should be given before surgery, but the immune response is only marginally better than if given after. Other indications for pneumococcal vaccine are elderly people in chronic care; chronic diseases, particularly cardiac, renal or pulmonary disease; diabetes; alcoholism; patients with cerebrospinal—fluid leaks (at risk of pneumococcal meningitis); and immunocompromised patients such as those with nephrotic syndrome, lymphoma, Hodgkin's disease, multiple myeloma, HIV infection, and immunosuppressed post-organ transplant. The vaccine is not completely protective and penicillin prophylaxis may also be indicated.

Vaccines being developed

There are some infections for which new or improved vaccines have already been developed and are undergoing clinical trials of safety, immunogenicity, and efficacy. Varicella vaccine is one such new vaccine, while acellular pertussis vaccines are examples of improved vaccines.

For other infections, vaccines are desperately needed, but development has so far been unsuccessful. Perhaps the outstanding infections to fall into this category are malaria, HIV, respiratory syncytial virus, and rotavirus infections.

There is a third group of infections for which vaccines are available, but where problems with safety or efficacy of the existing vaccine mean

Table 4 *Diseases or pathogens for which vaccines are being improved or developed, or for which development should be considered*

Chlamydias
Cholera (improved)
Coronaviruses
Cytomegalovirus
Dengue
Escherichia coli
Filariasis
Giardia lamblia
Group A streptococcus
Group B streptococcus
Haemophilus ducreyi
Hepatitis C
Herpes simplex 2
HIV-1
HIV-2
Influenza A and B (improved)
Japanese encephalitis (improved)
Leishmaniasis
Malaria
Meningococcus A/C (improved)
Meningococcus B
Mycobacterium leprae
Mycobacterium tuberculosis (improved)
Mycoplasma pneumoniae
Neisseria gonorrhoeae
Norwalk agent
Parainfluenza
Pertussis (improved)
Poliovirus (improved)
Rabiesvirus (improved)
Respiratory syncytial virus
Rotavirus
Salmonella typhi (improved)
Schistosomiasis
Shigella
Streptococcus pneumoniae (improved)
Treponema
Trypanosomiasis
Varicella-zoster
Yellow fever virus (improved)

Unpublished report by G. L. Ada (printed with permission).

that new vaccines urgently need to be developed. Examples are cholera and tuberculosis.

A comprehensive list of infections for which vaccines are being or need to be developed is given in Table 4. However, effective vaccines are unlikely to be developed for many of these diseases in the next few years, although varicella vaccine is an exception.

VARICELLA VACCINE

The OKA strain of live attenuated varicella vaccine was first used in clinical trials in Japan in 1973. It is immunogenic in normal children and in children with leukaemia. The reason varicella vaccine is not in routine use is that certain lots were associated with vaccine-induced chickenpox, which was sometimes severe.

Combination vaccines

Vaccines already in regular use which are combinations of two or more vaccines include diphtheria/pertussis/tetanus (**DPT**) and MMR vaccines. Quadrivalent vaccines with DPT and a Hib conjugate vaccine are being introduced and similarly DPT is being combined with hepatitis B vaccine.

Dr Stanley Plotkin has been so bold as to predict a vaccine schedule for 2025, which makes liberal use of combined vaccines yet to be developed (Table 5).

Immunization in developed countries

Most developed countries employ a primary immunization schedule similar to that shown in Table 2, with the exception that neonatal BCG is given only to babies whose ethnic background or family history puts them at high risk of tuberculosis, and universal hepatitis B vaccination from birth is only used in a small number of developed countries. The exact extent of immunization coverage required to achieve 'herd immunity', that is the inability of an organism to cause epidemic spread to susceptibles because of the high number of immunes, varies for different diseases. For example, outbreaks of measles in highly immunized populations (over 95 per cent immunized) in the United States suggest that almost 100 per cent immunization may be needed to prevent spread of measles if it continues to be introduced to the population. In contrast, because immunization with Hib conjugate vaccines decreases colonization with Hib, much lower levels of immunization produce substantial herd immunity.

In most developed countries, immunization is provided by the government as part of a comprehensive health-care system, although in North America and Australia a substantial proportion of children are immunized at private cost. Measures that appear to increase immunization rates are computerized notification of appointments for immunizations, easy access to and ready availability of immunization clinics, and an encouraging approach to immunization by health-care professionals. Parent-held child health records have been successfully used in some regions. Rapid knowledge of local immunization rates and the delineation of community health staff responsible for immunization in areas of a manageable size have been highly successful in raising immunization levels in the United Kingdom.

Legislation, either requiring immunization before entry to child-care facilities or school, as in parts of the United States, or requiring evidence of immunization status at child care or school entry with exclusion of susceptibles during outbreaks, as in parts of Australia, is controversial. Education of parents and health-care professionals about the continued importance of immunizing against vaccine-preventable diseases is vital. Many children have gaps or delays in immunization because of false contraindications, perpetuated by family, friends, or health professionals.

Opportunistic immunization is one way in which immunization levels can be improved. This requires all health-care personnel to ask about immunization status at any health-care visit, and either to immunize or arrange appointments for children whose immunizations are not up to date. In the United States, up to 30 per cent of unimmunized children who developed measles had been seen previously by a health-care professional and could have been immunized, while 57 per cent of women who delivered a baby with congenital rubella syndrome had one or more missed opportunities for rubella vaccination.

Immunization in developing countries

The impact of the EPI on mortality in developing countries has been discussed above. There are certain priorities in developing countries that differ from those in developed countries (Table 6). Tuberculosis is a major problem and kills over 3 million people annually in the world. Neonatal BCG provides 75 to 80 per cent protection against disease and 85 to 100 per cent protection against severe manifestations such as tuber-

Table 5 *Predicted vaccine schedule of the year 2025*

Age	Vaccines
0–2 months	Respiratory syncytial virus (RSV): hepatitis B; tuberculosis
2–6 months	Diphtheria/tetanus/acellular pertussis (DPT)/ *Haemophilus influenzae* type b (Hib)/inactivated polio vaccine (IPV)/pneumococcus/meningococcus/hepatitis A,B,C (combination); RSV/parainfluenza virus types 1–3 (combination); rotavirus; adenovirus types 1,2,5–7 (combination)
Added in developing world	Measles; malaria; dengue fever; hepatitis E; oral enterotoxigenic *Escherichia coli*/cholera/Shigella/Campylobacter (combination)
1–2 years	Measles/mumps/rubella/varicella; DTP/IPV/Hib/hepatitis B (combination); Lyme disease
Added in developing world	Schistosomiasis; rabies; typhoid
4–6 years	Boosters for some of the above; live influenza virus
11–12 years	Cytomegalovirus/Epstein–Barr virus/parvovirus (combination); human immunodeficiency virus/ human papillomavirus/herpes simplex virus type 2 (combination)
Adults	Killed influenza virus; pneumococcus; varicella (to prevent zoster)

Reproduced from Plotkin, S.A. (1993). Vaccination in the 21st century. *Journal of Infectious Diseases*, **168,** 29–37, with permission.

Table 6 *The immunization schedule for developing countries recommended in the Expanded Programme of Immunization of the World Health Organization*

Age	Vaccines
Birth	BCG and OPV
6 weeks	DPT and OPV
10 weeks	DPT and OPV
14 weeks	DPT and OPV
9 months	Measles
Women of childbearing age	Tetanus toxoid

BCG, bacille Calmette–Guérin; DPT, diphtheria-pertussis-tetanus; OPV, oral polio vaccine.

culous meningitis. Exposure to poliovirus may occur early, and polio immunization is commenced at birth. Neonatal tetanus kills about 800 000 babies annually in developing countries, but does not occur if the mother is immune to tetanus. Therefore, immunization of women of child-bearing age against tetanus is incorporated in the EPI. Measles occurs at younger age than in developed countries, and maternal antibody interferes less with immunization. Children in cities in developing countries are at particular risk of early measles. Measles immunization is recommended at 9 months of age. A more potent measles vaccine, Edmonston–Zagreb vaccine, was given to some children at 4 to 8 months of age, but has been withdrawn because of worries about increased mortality from causes other than measles in recipients.

There are problems with delivering immunization in developing countries. Even so, the proportion of children immunized in The Gambia compares favourably with that in many Western countries. The first problem is the obvious one of cost, not just of the vaccines themselves, but of delivering them to children in remote areas. The organizational structure needs to be there for vaccine delivery. A further problem is maintenance of the 'cold chain', so that vaccines are not damaged by excessive heat. It has been shown, using special thermometers, that the chain generally can be maintained, and modern vaccines have been made more heat stable. War is extremely disruptive of health services, and immunization levels are lowest, often disastrously low, in countries ravaged by long wars.

REFERENCES

American Academy of Pediatrics Committee on Infectious Diseases (1991). The relationship between pertussis vaccine and brain damage: reassessment. *Pediatrics*, **88,** 397–400.

Beale, A.J. (1990). Polio vaccines: time for a change in immunisation policy? In *Modern vaccines*, (ed. E.R. Moxon), pp. 59–66. Arnold, London.

Cenci, F. (1907). Alcune esperienze di siero-immunizzazione e sieroterapia nel morbillo. *Rivista di Clinica Pediatrica*, **5,** 1017–25.

Clarke, A., and Rudd, P. (1992). Neonatal BCG immunisation. *Archives of Diseases in Childhood*, **67,** 473–4.

Edwards, K.M. (1993). Acellular pertussis vaccines—a solution to the pertussis problem? *Journal of Infectious Diseases*, **168,** 15–20.

Isaacs, D., and Menser, M. (1990). Measles, mumps, rubella and varicella. In *Modern vaccines* (ed. E.R. Moxon), pp. 50–8. Arnold, London.

Lever, A.M. *et al.* (1984). Non-A, non-B hepatitis occurring in agammaglobulinaemic patients after intravenous immunoglobulin. *Lancet*, **ii,** 1062–4.

Margolis, H.S. (1993). Prevention of acute and chronic liver disease through immunization: hepatitis B and beyond. *Journal of Infectious Diseases*, **168,** 9–14.

Miller, D., Wadsworth, J., Diamond, J., and Ross, E. (1985). Pertussis vaccine and whooping cough as risk factors for neurological illness and death in young children. *Developments in Biological Standardization*, **61,** 389–94.

Peckham, C.S. and Bedford, M.E. (1990). Factors influencing uptake of preschool immunisation. In *Control of virus diseases*, (ed. N.J. Dimmock, P.D. Griffiths, and C.R. Madeley), pp. 155–65. Cambridge University Press.

Peter, G. (1992). Childhood immunizations. *New England Journal of Medicine*, **327,** 1794–800.

Gardner, P., and Schaffner, W. (1993). Immunization of adults. *New England Journal of Medicine*, **328,** 1252–8.

Robbins, A., Freeman, P., and Powell, K.R. (1993). International childhood vaccine initiative. *Pediatric Infectious Diseases Journal*, **12,** 523–7.

Sixbey, J.W. (1987). Routine immunizations and the immunosuppressed child. *Advances in Pediatric Infectious Diseases*, **2,** 79–114.

UNICEF (1992). *State of the world's children 1992*, p. 14, Oxford University Press.

7.8 Travel and expedition medicine

C. P. Conlon and D. A. Warrell

INTRODUCTION

Over the past couple of decades the advent of relatively cheap air travel has meant that many millions of people travel every year for work or pleasure. Increasingly, many people from developed countries go to live and work for prolonged periods in less well-developed areas of the world. This increased movement around the globe has important health implications. Not only are individuals risking the acquisition of new diseases in endemic areas but physicians everywhere must be aware of the possibility of imported diseases with which they may be unfamiliar.

Advice for international travellers can be categorized into pretravel advice, including immunizations and assessments of individual risks, advice about dealing with particular problems when abroad, and an approach to managing the problems of the traveller who returns home and becomes ill or who returns home because of illness.

Pretravel advice

GENERAL PRINCIPLES

One of the most important aspects of pretravel advice is finding sources of information. Travel medicine is not yet a well-developed speciality and there are few clinics specializing in providing travel advice and help. Nevertheless, travellers should seek advice from physicians with an interest and knowledge in the subject and, if appropriate, ask their primary physicians to refer them. Some embassies of the countries to be visited will be able to provide information about health requirements but will not usually be able to provide a critical appraisal of the health risks to travellers to their country. Independent advice should be sought.

Many countries do have immunization requirements and demand that travellers should have a certificate to prove that they have had the statutory vaccinations. International Certificates of Vaccination are yellow booklets, which should be carried together with the passport. These certificates record yellow fever vaccinations and can be used to document other immunizations, known allergies, blood group etc. Patients with chronic illnesses on regular medication should have a note about the drugs they require and, ideally, should carry the name and contact address of their physician at home in case of emergency.

Most travellers will want to have adequate insurance to cover accidents and medical emergencies in addition to cancellation or baggage-loss insurance. Sometimes this will be part of a pre-existing policy but often the insurance will need to purchased specially. Considerations such as the geographical area to be visited, the age and health of the applicant, and any special risks of the journey (e.g. mountain climbing) need to be taken into account. In remote areas or those with inadequate health facilities, some form of medical evacuation policy may be desirable.

GENERAL ADVICE ABOUT HEALTH

Many people will want advice about what to take as a first-aid kit. In addition to antiseptic solution, bandages and plasters, proprietary drugs to treat pain, diarrhoea, dyspepsia, and allergy should be taken. More specific drugs might be included, depending on the individual traveller and their itinerary. Sunscreen preparations are often needed, as are water purification tablets and insect repellents; the last should contain permethrin (for application to clothes or nets) or **DEET** (*N,N*-diethyl-*m*-toluamide) (for skin application) as active ingredients.

Motion sickness may be a problem for some people, especially if the journey is by sea. A variety of antiemetic drugs, such as cyclizine, is available but most are mildly sedative and often cause anticholinergic symptoms like dry mouth. More recently, long-acting transdermal skin patches containing scopolamine have become available. Long-haul air flights are increasingly popular but lead to jet lag. This may cause sleep disturbance, fatigue, and poor concentration. Some travellers may find it useful to use a short-acting benzodiazepine, such as temazepam, for the first couple of nights after flying in order to re-establish a regular sleeping pattern. In addition, diabetics may need advice on how to alter their insulin regimen or diet to adjust to the changes in time zones.

Extremes of climate may be experienced. Travellers should be warned particularly about the dangers of ultraviolet light and sunburn. Snow blindness and severe sunburn can occur even at very low ambient temperatures under clear skies at high altitude. The problems of heat, dehydration, and salt depletion should be discussed. People intending to go to areas of high altitude should be advised to acclimatize themselves slowly and to build up their level of physical activity gradually. They should be aware of the symptoms and signs of altitude sickness. Acetazolamide may be useful prophylaxis for mountain sickness but there is no substitute for rapid descent if symptoms arise. Special advice will be needed, depending on the destination and type of activity (for example how to avoid frostnip and frostbite in polar regions, and special precautions for scuba divers or cave explorers).

It is standard advice to take care when eating and drinking in countries with relatively poor sanitation. However, the old adage of 'boil it, peel it, or forget it' is rarely followed. Water purification tablets are now readily available, as are many types of portable water filters. Beverages made with boiled water are generally safe, whereas bottled water and, particularly, ice cubes may not always be reliable. Treated water should be used even for tooth brushing.

The potential dangers to travellers of used needles and blood transfusions, should they need emergency hospital treatment, have been much publicized since the advent of AIDS. In many tropical developing countries, blood-borne pathogens, such as hepatitis B and C viruses, human immunodeficiency viruses (**HIV**) types 1 and 2, human T-leukaemia/lymphoma virus type 1, and in some areas malaria parasites, trypanosomes and other organisms are prevalent. Screening of donated blood may not be rigorous and needles are commonly reused, sometimes without adequate sterilization. As a result, travellers have been advised to take 'AIDS kits' of varying size and complexity, usually containing needles, cannulas, intravenous giving sets, syringes, and artificial plasma expanders. These are usually too bulky and expensive for most travellers, but it is worth taking a few 21-gauge needles and 10-ml syringes in case blood must be taken for a laboratory test. A covering letter from a doctor may allay the suspicion of customs officials that they are to be used for drug abuse.

Particularly when on holiday, travellers may become less inhibited and engage in sexual activity with new partners. This may be more likely if alcohol or other drugs are involved. Travellers should be warned that the risks of sexually transmitted diseases, including HIV, are increased in these circumstances. At the very least, good-quality condoms, often not available when travelling, should be carried and used.

Patients with chronic illnesses, such as diabetes or asthma, should take with them a generous supply of their current medications and should not rely on being able to buy these abroad.

Table 1 *Immunizations*

Vaccine	Type	Route	Primary course	Booster
Routine				
Polio (Sabin)	Live virus (attenuated)	p.o.	3 doses at monthly intervals	10 years
Polio (Salk)	Killed virus	i.m.	As above	10 years
Tetanus	Adsorbed toxoid	i.m.	3 doses at monthly intervals	10 years (max. 5 doses)
Diphtheria	Adsorbed toxoid	i.m.	3 doses at monthly intervals	Single low dose if > 10 years
Haemophilus influenza b	Conjugated polysaccharide	i.m.	2–3 doses 2-monthly	Single dose
Pneumococcal	23-valent polysaccharide	i.m.	Single dose	Repeat in those at high risk
Influenza	Killed virus	i.m.	Single dose	Yearly
Travel				
Yellow fever	Live virus (attenuated)	i.m.	Single dose	10 yearly
Typhoid	Killed bacteria	i.m.	2 doses a month apart	3 yearly
Typhoid	Live Ty21a strain (attenuated)	p.o.	4 doses on alternate days	5 yearly
Typhoid	Capsular Vi polysaccharide	i.m.	Single dose	3 yearly
Meningococcal	Polysaccharide types A,C,(Y,W)	i.m. or s.c.	Single dose	3 yearly
Rabies[1,2]	Killed virus	i.m. or i.d.	3 doses on days 0, 7 and 28	2–3 yearly
Japanese (B) encephalitis	Killed virus	i.m.	3 doses on days 0, 7 and 28	1 year, then 4 yearly
Hepatitis A	Killed virus	i.m.	2 doses 2–4 weeks apart	6–12 months, then ? 5-yearly
Hepatitis B[1]	Adsorbed	i.m.	0, 1 and 6 months	3–5 yearly
BCG	Attenuated	i.d.	Single dose	None
Gammaglobulin	Pooled immunoglobulins (mainly IgG)	i.m.	Single dose	6-monthly (while at risk)

[1]Should not be given into buttock; deltoid or anterior thigh preferred.
[2]Efficacy reduced if given with chloroquine antimalarial prophylaxis.

Immunizations

When someone comes for travel advice, their record of routine immunizations should be reviewed. Many adults will require booster doses for tetanus and polio, and, because of the increase in reports of diphtheria in some countries, including those in Eastern Europe, diphtheria immunization may need updating. Influenza vaccine, pneumococcal vaccine, and the new conjugate *Haemophilus influenzae* vaccines are also worthwhile for those at increased risk of the complications of chest infections, such as the elderly or those with chronic heart or lung disease.

Yellow fever is the only vaccine for which there is still an international requirement before entry to some countries. Yellow fever is endemic only in tropical Africa and South America, not in Asia. Cholera vaccine used to be required but this is no longer recommended by the World Health Organization as its efficacy is poor and the risks of adverse effects probably outweigh its usefulness.

Other immunizations may be recommended to travellers, depending on the risk of exposure to certain pathogens. Some of the more commonly administered ones are shown in Table 1. Typhoid vaccines are among the most commonly given; most travellers still receive the killed whole-bacteria vaccine. In many instances the risk of typhoid is exaggerated and the vaccine is probably not necessary. A critical assessment of the risks may reduce the number of vaccinations and hence lead to fewer adverse effects and financial savings.

Hepatitis A is a common risk for travellers to less-developed areas. Traditionally, prophylaxis has taken the form of injections of gammaglobulin before travel. Gammaglobulin is from pooled blood donations from individuals with past exposure to hepatitis A and is effective and safe. However, the need for repeated injections every 6 months makes it inconvenient for the frequent traveller or long-term resident abroad. Now active immunization is available against hepatitis A ('Havrix'), which has been shown to be safe, effective, and durable. It is likely that this will replace gammaglobulin in the near future if its cost can be decreased.

In some parts of the world, such as subSaharan Africa and Central and South Asia, meningococcal meningitis outbreaks are common so travellers are advised to be immunized. The standard vaccine is effective against types A and C but not against type B meningococcus, the most common cause of meningitis in developed countries.

Rabies vaccine is being used increasingly to protect travellers to regions where the disease is endemic. Although the risk of transmission is fairly low, the lack of effective treatment for rabies encephalitis makes consideration of immunization important. The biggest risk is from dog bites as canine vaccination programmes are often inadequate. Pre-expo-

Table 2 *Antimalarial chemoprophylaxis*

Generic drug	Trade names	Usual tablet dose	Prophylactic dose
Prophylaxis in areas with chloroquine resistance			
Mefloquine[1]	Lariam	250 mg	1 tablet weekly
OR			
Proguanil **plus** choloroquine	Paludrine	100 mg	2 tablets daily
	Nivaquine	150 mg (base)	2 tablets weekly
	Avloclor		
OR (in some areas)			
Dapsone/pyrimethamine[2]	Maloprim	100 mg + 12.5 mg	1 tablet weekly
plus chloroquine	Nivaquine	150 mg (base)	2 tablets weekly
	Avloclor		
Prophylaxis in areas without drug resistance			
Proguanil	Paludrine	100 mg	2 tablets daily
OR			
Chloroquine	Nivaquine	150 mg (base)	2 tablets weekly

[1]Contraindicated in first trimester of pregnancy; avoid during pregnancy and lactation if possible; do not use if history of epilepsy or psychiatric disorder.

[2]Give folic acid supplements if used during pregnancy.

sure vaccination by the intradermal route has been shown to be effective and cheaper than the intramuscular route. However, intradermal injections may lead to an inadequate immune response in those who are concurrently taking chloroquine for antimalarial prophylaxis. It is best, therefore, to ensure that all the immunizing doses are given before antimalarial drugs are started.

Less commonly required vaccines include those against hepatitis B, Japanese B encephalitis, and plague. These are expensive and are only necessary in special circumstances. Plague vaccine is effective but may give rise to serious side-effects. An alternative in endemic areas is prophylactic or post-exposure doxycycline treatment. Japanese (B) encephalitis vaccine is safe but the risk of infection is low unless travellers spend a long time (more than 3 months) in certain rural parts of Asia in the rainy season. Hepatitis B is a risk primarily for those, like clinical and laboratory staff, whose work involves contact with human blood.

The physician should critically assess the balance of risk–benefit for individual travellers depending on their destination, intended activities, and background medical problems. Increasingly, the cost of immunization must be taken into account.

Prevention of malaria

Perhaps the most important way to reduce the risk of malaria is to educate both the traveller and the non-specialist physician. Cases of imported malaria in Britain, and elsewhere, continue to rise, with an increasing proportion due to *Plasmodium falciparum*. Every year there are about 10 deaths in England and Wales due to malaria in people returning from endemic areas. Many cases and most deaths result from travellers' ignorance of preventive measures and from doctors' failing to think of malaria as a cause of symptoms in non-endemic countries. Prevention encompasses three main areas; antimosquito measures, chemoprophylaxis, and awareness of symptoms and signs of infection.

Antimosquito measures

The anopheline mosquitoes that transmit malaria bite at dusk and at night. Bed nets have been shown to be an effective means of reducing transmission of malaria, especially if the nets are impregnated in the insecticide permethrin. Insect repellents containing DEET may also be applied to exposed skin to reduce the chances of mosquito bites. Additionally, vaporized permethrin from mosquito coils used in bedrooms may help.

Travellers should be advised to dress appropriately during the evenings. Long-sleeved shirts with button-up necks, long trousers, and socks all limit the area of skin exposed to the biting mosquito.

Chemoprophylaxis

There is a variety of chemoprophylactic drugs available but none is 100 per cent effective (Table 2). In some geographical areas, malaria parasites are highly resistant to chloroquine and to other, newer agents. Risk–benefit analysis favours the combination of chloroquine weekly and daily proguanil for many endemic areas. However, in coastal East Africa, West Africa, and parts of South-East Asia the risk of transmission of chloroquine-resistant malaria is high. Weekly mefloquine is preferred in Africa and either mefloquine or daily doxycycline for South-East Asia. Travellers and their physicians should seek expert advice before travelling to areas endemic for malaria. Some form of chemoprophylaxis is generally better than none.

Recognition of symptoms and signs

People travelling in endemic areas, particularly those intending to spend long periods in remote regions, should be told of the possible symptoms of acute malaria so that they may take early action. Fever is a common symptom, often associated with chills and rigors, headache, and joint and muscle pains. Diarrhoea and vomiting are also common. If symptoms persist for more than 24 h, travellers should seek medical help. It may be appropriate for the traveller to have some antimalarial drugs in reserve for presumptive treatment of acute malaria if medical help is not readily available. Mefloquine, halofantrine or pyrimethamine-sulfadoxine (Fansidar) may be the best drugs for this purpose.

Travellers' diarrhoea

Surveys of international travellers indicate that diarrhoea is their most common health problem. Although the symptoms are usually mild and last only about 3 to 5 days, holiday and business plans may be disrupted as a result. The most common cause of travellers' diarrhoea is infection with enterotoxigenic *Escherichia coli* (ETEC). Other bacteria can also cause problems; especially *Salmonella* spp., *Campylobacter* spp., *Shigella* spp., and other pathogenic *E. coli*. Protozoan pathogens, such as *Giardia lamblia, Entamoeba histolytica*, and *Cryptosporidium parvum* are less common aetiological agents, as are viruses.

Most infective agents are food and water borne so obsessive adherence to food and water precautions should minimize the risks of gastroenteritis. However, experience shows that the vast majority of travellers fail to follow advice about dietary precautions. Heating water to 100°C will kill most pathogens, as will chemical treatment using either chlorine or iodine. Water filters are useful additions. Chemoprophylaxis for travellers' diarrhoea has been proposed as an alternative strategy. Evidence from clinical trials shows that some antimicrobials such as co-trimoxazole, doxycycline, and the 4-fluoroquinolones have a protective effect. However, these drugs are generally not cheap, may cause side-effects, cannot be taken for prolonged periods, and may lead to the emergence of antimicrobial resistance in some pathogens. Colloidal bismuth salts may be cheaper, safer, and reasonably effective but large volumes are needed so they are inconvenient and they may interfere with other medication. There are no effective vaccines available.

Although not easily preventable, travellers' diarrhoea is usually treatable. The maintenance of an adequate fluid intake should be emphasized to the traveller. It is helpful to carry sachets of rehydration salts that can be made up with boiled water. Antidiarrhoeal agents, such as loperamide, often relieve symptoms sufficiently for normal activities to be continued. Short courses of empirical antimicrobials, for example ciprofloxacin, can be useful, particularly for patients with underlying medical conditions. If there is localized abdominal pain or bloody diarrhoea, patients should be advised to seek local medical help.

Immunocompromised travellers

Advances in medical therapy have given many people with chronic diseases an opportunity to travel. Some patients will be immunosuppressed, either because of their underlying disease or because of the drugs they are prescribed. In practice, the groups to consider are people on long-term steroids, those having (or who have recently had) cancer chemotherapy, organ transplant recipients, those with anatomical or functional asplenia, and, increasingly, those infected with HIV.

In general, the above patients (except the asplenic group) should not be given live vaccines such yellow fever, oral polio, and oral typhoid. Killed vaccines and peptide or polysaccharide vaccines are safe. However, the main concern is whether on not the individual will be able to mount an immune response to the antigen administered. Those patients with little to moderate immune suppression, including those with early HIV infection, will probably make a reasonable response to immunization; those with more severe immunosuppression may still make a useful, though less durable response. In addition to routine immunizations, many of these patients will benefit from influenza vaccine, pneumococcal vaccine, and the *Haemophilus influenzae* b (Hib) conjugate vaccine, as the risk of respiratory infection and bacteraemia is increased. Gammaglobulin is the preferred prophylaxis against hepatitis A in these patients, as the response to the new hepatitis A vaccine is unknown and likely to be suboptimal. Asplenic individuals should be on prophylactic antibiotics, such as amoxycillin, particularly if travelling. Overwhelming infections with malaria may occur in the asplenic patient so they should be dissuaded from travelling to areas with high rates of malaria transmission.

Immunocompromised patients should carry antimicrobials with them for treating respiratory or gastrointestinal infections. They should have a low threshold for seeking medical help when abroad and should carry a letter from their physician outlining their condition and medication.

Pregnancy and travel

Most pregnant women remain well throughout their pregnancy and many now travel on business or on holiday. Commercial airlines will not normally convey a woman who is 36 weeks or more pregnant without a covering letter from her physician. Although the risks of modern air travel are minimal, the 36-week limit should be borne in mind when booking return flights. Clearly, insurance to cover the costs of delivery abroad should be considered.

The risk–benefit assessment of immunizations and chemoprophylaxis is of particular importance for the pregnant woman and the fetus. Generally, live vaccines should be avoided, but, if there is a genuine risk of yellow fever, the vaccine should be given as there is no recognized associated teratogenicity. Inactivated polio vaccine may be given parenterally and tetanus immunization is safe. Because of anxieties about febrile reactions to heat-killed typhoid vaccine stimulating premature labour, this is probably best avoided. Pneumococcal and meningococcal vaccines are probably safe in pregnancy and should be given to women who would normally require them. Gammaglobulin is safe in pregnancy, as is hepatitis B vaccine.

Pregnant women are at much more than average risk of complications if they acquire malaria and there is an increased risk of fetal loss. The only drugs for malaria chemoprophylaxis that are known to be safe in pregnancy are chloroquine and proguanil. In areas with intense transmission of chloroquine-resistant falciparum malaria, it is best to advise pregnant women not to travel. If such travel cannot be avoided, strict antimosquito measures should be used in conjunction with chloroquine and proguanil. Stand-by antimalarial treatment with quinine may be needed; in normal therapeutic doses it is safe in pregnancy. Pregnant women should take special care with food and drink when abroad, as dehydration may threaten the fetus. There are concerns about congenital goitre when pregnant women use iodine to purify water. The maximum recommended daily intake is 175 μg. Loperamide as an antidiarrhoeal agent is safe but antimicrobials such as tetracyclines and quinolones should be avoided.

Extremes of age

It is important to be sure that young children have had their routine immunizations before travelling. Children are at particular risk from malaria so chemoprophylaxis is recommended for all ages with appropriate dose reduction for a given age or weight. Yellow fever vaccine should probably only be given to those older than 9 months as a few cases of vaccine-associated encephalitis have occurred in younger children. Most other vaccines, including rabies, are safe. Because hepatitis A is rarely symptomatic in children under 5 years old, gammaglobulin is not usually offered before this age. Families that are planning to spend prolonged periods living in less well-developed countries should be offered BCG vaccination for their children to reduce the risk of tuberculous meningitis.

The elderly should have the same immunizations as younger adults and should take antimalarial drugs. They are more prone to respiratory infection and should, therefore, be given influenza and pneumococcal vaccines. Jet lag may present more problems for old people and time-zone changes may provoke confusion. Older people are more likely to have an underlying medical condition that requires medication. It is important that sufficient supplies of medicines are taken abroad and that the patient has a detailed list of these medicines and their dosages in case the tablets are lost or stolen.

Explorers and expeditions

By their very nature, expeditions are likely to involve exposure to greater environmental extremes and hazards than other types of travel. As expeditions are usually to areas remote from hospitals or even rural health centres and dispensaries, greater responsibility for dealing with medical problems will fall on the members of the expedition. The explorer's greatest fear may be a dramatic tropical disease or an attack by a wild animal, but most mortality in recent years has been from road traffic accidents, mountaineering disasters, drowning, and attacks by humans. Prevention and treatment of medical problems must be considered well in advance. Advice and information can be obtained from a number of useful reference books (see below), organisations such as the Expedition Advisory Centre of the Royal Geographical Society in London (Tel: 0171-581-2057; Fax 0171-584-4447) and from clubs specializing in mountaineering, cave exploring, diving, and other activities. All expeditions should have a designated medical officer and as many members

Table 3 *Causes of fever in returning travellers*

Tropical (short incubation; < 3 weeks)
African trypanosomiasis
Brucellosis
Dengue
Haemorrhagic fevers (Lassa)
Hepatitis A
Leptospirosis
Malaria
Relapsing fevers
Tick/scrub typhus
Typhoid
Tropical (long incubation; > 3 weeks)
Amoebic abscess
Brucellosis
Filariasis
Hepatitis A, B, or C
HIV
Leishmaniasis
Malaria
Tuberculosis
Typhoid
Other infections
Endocarditis
Pneumonia
Prostatitis
Sexually transmitted disease
Sinusitis
UTI[1]
Non-infective causes of fever
Connective tissue disease
Drug reaction
Factitious
Inflammatory bowel disease
Malignancy

[1]UTI, urinary-tract infection.

Table 4 *Causes of rash in returning travellers*

Infective
Cutaneous larva migrans, myiasis
Cutaneous leishmaniasis
Dengue
Dermatophytes
Lyme disease
Meningococcus
Mycobacterial
Scabies/lice
STDs[1]
Tick/scrub typhus
Tinea versicolor
Typhoid
(Enterovirus, mycoplasma, streptococcal infection etc.)
Non-infective
Drug reaction
Erythema multiforme
Insect bites
Sunburn

[1]STD, sexually transmitted disease.

Table 5 *Infective causes of eosinophilia in travellers*

Ascariasis
Echinococcus
Filaria
Hookworm
Schistosomiasis
Strongyloides
Trichinosis
Trichuris
Visceral larva migrans
(Angiostrongylus, Gnathostoma, and other nematodes)

as possible should attend first-aid training, which, ideally, should be aimed at particular needs of the expedition. At the very least, this training should deal with clearing the airway, controlling blood loss, treating shock, relieving pain, and the safe movement of the injured. Expedition medical kits have to be much more comprehensive than those carried by ordinary tourist travellers. Lightweight emergency insulation must be taken if there is any risk of exposure in severe weather conditions, and an adequate water supply must be assured or taken if the expedition is into desert areas. A lightweight collapsible stretcher should be included for mountaineering and caving expeditions. Lists of essential drugs are given in *Expedition Medicine* (1994). Scissors, and a generous supply of large triangular and crepe bandages and adhesive plasters, are important. A covering letter on official notepaper, signed by a doctor, may be helpful in getting drugs through customs (for example into the Russian Federation). The hospitals or medical stations nearest to the site of the expedition must be identified and contacted in advance. An emergency plan must be drawn up for evacuation of severely ill or injured expedition members. In some areas, such as East Africa, organizations such as 'Flying Doctor' services (AMREF) may agree to be responsible for evacuation of casualties. Insurance cover must include a generous allowance for medical care and repatriation of the injured. Before leaving their home country, expedition members should have a thorough dental check and treatment for any unresolved medical or surgical problems. In selecting members for an expedition, experience, possession of the necessary skills (for example diving and mountaineering), physical fitness, and a reputation for psychological stability under stress are among the most important criteria. It is always advisable to appoint a reliable local agent in the country where the expedition will take place.

Problems of the returning traveller

Most travellers survive their time abroad without illness, but some will experience symptoms related to their travels at some stage after returning home. It is essential that physicians take a detailed travel history in order not to be caught out by unusual diseases in non-endemic countries. Histories should include countries visited, activities while travelling, immunization record, and antimalarials taken. It is also a good idea to enquire about the route of returning home, as diseases such as malaria may be acquired even during the briefest of stop-overs, or waiting on the runway in an endemic area.

The most common problems are fever, rash, diarrhoea, and eosinophilia. All the possible causes of fever and rash cannot be discussed in detail here, but Tables 3 and 4 outline the more common causes.

Patients returning with diarrhoea may have either an acute problem or they may have chronic diarrhoea persisting for more than 10 days. Those with acute diarrhoea should be worked up in the usual way, with a dietary history, an assessment of hydration state, and stool microscopy and culture. Abdominal films and sigmoidoscopy may sometimes be needed. Patients with chronic diarrhoea may have a persistent infection with such parasites as Giardia, Cryptosporidium or *Entamoeba histolytica*. Sometimes bacterial causes, such as shigellae or salmonellae, may cause persistent symptoms. Investigations should include a search for *Clostridium difficile* and its toxin, especially if the patient had antimicrobials while abroad. A minority of patients may develop a postinfective enteropathy, with the most common problem being a secondary lactose intolerance. Rarely, bacterial overgrowth or tropical sprue develop.

Eosinophilia can arise from a large number of causes; allergic reactions are probably the most common causes. However, in the returning traveller it is possible that eosinophilia is due to a parasitic infection. In general, only metazoan parasites (i.e. helminths) give rise to eosinophilia, and these are not usually acquired unless the patient has spent a few months or more in endemic areas. The common infective causes of eosinophilia are shown in Table 5. The majority can be diagnosed by careful stool examination or by appropriate serological tests.

REFERENCES

Auerbach, P.S., and Geehr, E.C. (ed.) (1983). *Management of wilderness and environmental emergencies.* Colin Macmillan, Oxford.

Behrens, R.H., and McAdam, K.P.W.J. (ed.) (1993). Travel medicine. *British Medical Bulletin*, **49,** 257–478.

Bradley, D. (1993). Prophylaxis against malaria for travellers from the United Kingdom. *British Medical Journal*, **306,** 1247–52.

Dawood, R. (ed.) (1992). *Travellers' Health: how to stay healthy abroad*, (3rd edn). Oxford University Press.

Edholm, O.G., and Gunderson, E.K. (1973). *Polar human biology.* Heinemann, London.

First Aid Manual (1993). The Authorised Manual of St John Ambulance, St Andrew's Ambulance Association and the British Red Cross Society.

Gilles, H.M. and Warrell, D.A. (ed.) (1993). *Bruce Chwatt's essential malariology*, (3rd edn). Arnold, London.

Gormly, P. (1992). *ANARE first aid manual.* Publications Office, Australian Antarctic Division, Kingston 7050, Australia.

Hackett, P.H. (1980). *Mountain sickness: prevention, recognition and treatment*, (2nd edn). American Alpine Club, New York. Available from Cordee Mountain Books, Leicester.

Hatt, J. (1993). *The tropical traveller*, (3rd edn). Penguin, London.

HMSO (1967). *The ship captain's medical guide*, (20th edn). HMSO, London.

Ilingworth, R.N. (1984). *Expedition medicine: a planning guide*, (3rd edn). Blackwell Scientific, Oxford.

Juel-Jensen, B., and Warrell, D. (1994). *Expedition medicine*, (5th edn). Expedition Advisory Centre, Royal Geographical Society, London. Available from EAC/RGS, 1 Kensington Gore, London SW7 2AR.

Kirby, N.G. (1981). *Field surgery pocket book.* HMSO, London.

Melville, K.E.M. (1984). *Stay alive in the desert*, (2nd edn). Lascelles, London.

Miles, S., and Mackay, D. (1976). *Underwater medicine*, (4th edn). Granada, London.

Mitchell, R. (1978). *Mountaineering first aid*, (4th edn). The Mountaineers, Seattle. Available from Cordee Mountain Books, Leicester.

Potter, S.A. (ed). (1992). *Anare Antarctic Field Manual.* 4th edn. Australian Antarctic Division, Kingston, Tasmania.

Renouf, J., and Hulse, S. (1978). *First aid for hillwalkers and climbers.* Penguin, Harmonsworth.

Steele, P. (1976). *Medical care for mountain climbers.* Heinemann Medical, London.

US Department of Health, Education and Welfare (1978). *The ship's medicine chest and medical aid at sea*, Publications No. HSA-78-2024. United States Government Printing Office, Washington DC.

Vallotton, J., and Dubas, F. (ed.) (1991). *A colour atlas of mountain medicine.* Wolfe, London.

Ward, M.P. (1975). *Mountain medicine: a clinical study of cold and high altitude.* Crosby Lockwood Staples, London.

Ward, M.P., Milledge, J.S., and West, J.B. (1989). *High altitude medicine and physiology.* Chapman and Hall Medical, London.

Watt, D.G. (1975). *Emergency dentistry (intended for those who must treat the occasional dental patient).* Clausen Publications, Weybridge.

Wilson, M.E. (1991). *A world guide to infections. Disease, distribution, diagnosis.* Oxford University Press, New York.

World Health Organization (1989). *The treatment and prevention of acute diarrhoea.* (ISBN 924 154243 8). From WHO Publications, CH-1211, Geneva 27, Switzerland.

PERIODICALS

Journal of Wilderness Medicine (1990–). Paul Auerbach, MD and Oswald Oelz, MD (ed.). Published for the Wilderness Medical Society by Chapman and Hall Medical, 11 New Fetter Lane, London. EC4P 4EE.

Travel Medicine International (1983–). H.L'Etang (ed.). Mark Allen Publishing Ltd, 288 Croxted Road, London. SE24 9DA

EXPEDITION ADVISORY CENTRE PUBLICATIONS

Expedition planners' handbook & directory 1993–94 (1992). S. Winser and N. McWilliam (ed.).

Caving expeditions (1993). D. Willis (ed.)
Desert expeditions (1988). T. Sheppard
Insurance for expeditions (1993). J. Berridge
Polar expeditions (1990). D. Rootes (ed.)
Tropical forest expeditions (1993). A.C. Jermy
Underwater expeditions (1990). R. Palmer (ed.)

7.9 Nosocomial infections

D. W. M. Crook and I. C. J. Bowler

DEFINITION

Hospital-acquired or nosocomial (Gk. νοσοκομειον, hospital) infections are distinct from community-acquired infections. They may affect patients and hospital staff. Most are readily recognized because they develop while a patient is in hospital, but others are not so clearly seen as hospital acquired; for example, hepatitis B infection may be acquired in hospital but, because of the prolonged incubation period, may not become clinically apparent until months after the patient has been discharged. A number of terms are used to describe aspects of nosocomial infection. Iatrogenic infections are those acquired as the direct consequence of a therapeutic intervention (e.g. insertion of a urinary catheter). Opportunistic infections are those caused by organisms that do not ordinarily harm healthy people; they occur in people with impaired defences. Endogenous (autogenous) infections are produced by the patient's normal flora, while exogenous infections result from transmission of organisms to the patient from elsewhere. In practice, it may not always be possible to distinguish endogenous from exogenous infections. However, it is important to attempt differentiation between these two sources of infection as it has significant implications for deciding how to control them.

HISTORY

Before the Middle Ages there was little institutionalized health care. During the Middle Ages, infirmaries attached to monasteries first appeared and by the late Middle Ages, institutions comparable to hospitals, run by religious orders but organized by local authorities, appeared in Europe. The transition from these institutions to modern hospitals typical of the developed world has seen profound changes in the practices aimed at reducing infection among patients in hospital. The realization that hospital-acquired diseases were important and could be controlled began to emerge in the mid-nineteenth century. The magnitude of the problem is exemplified by early hospitals, such as the Hôtel de Dieu in Paris, founded in the seventh century, where virtually all wounds became infected and mortality after amputations was about 60 per cent. Death from puerperal sepsis was commonplace.

During the nineteenth century a number of factors that raised the risk of death from admission to hospital were recognized and various measures to control these infectious diseases were devised. During the period 1840–1870, work by Ignaz Semmelweiss, Florence Nightingale, William Farr, and James Simpson had a profound effect on improving the understanding of diseases acquired in hospital. This work clearly indicated that sepsis was passed from person to person and that mortality rates could be decreased by interrupting spread using simple measures such as improved hygiene, hand washing, and separation of patients by space. The benefit of these interventions was shown by remarkable studies that measured the frequency of clinical problems and the effects of treatment before and after an intervention. Such analyses of recorded data were the beginning of the statistical methods used today in clinical studies of the epidemiology and control of infection.

In the 1860s, Pasteur's discovery of 'living germs' provided the explanation for the transmissibility of sepsis and gave a rational basis for the concept of infection. Soon, measures such as treating wounds with the antiseptic carbolic, introduced by John Lister, became widely used. They were aimed at killing living micro-organisms locally in the wound and successfully reduced infection and mortality. Other measures to prevent the transfer of organisms to patients, such as wearing gloves, gowns and masks, hospital hygiene, control of ventilation, and sterilization of surgical instruments, medical devices and infusion fluids, were introduced later and are now adhered to rigidly. Nosocomial infection had been reduced dramatically by the early twentieth century and fear of admission to hospital diminished. With the introduction of antibiotics it seemed inevitable that hospital infection would be abolished. This optimism was short-lived, as there were serious epidemics of hospital-acquired, penicillin-resistant *Staphylococcus aureus* infections, with fatalities, in the 1950s. These severe epidemics provided the impetus for the establishment of hospital infection control as a speciality.

SCALE AND COST OF NOSOCOMIAL INFECTIONS

The World Health Organization (**WHO**) has recognized the serious global problem of nosocomial infections. Epidemic nosocomial infections frequently receive greater attention because of the alarm caused by the obvious spread of an infectious disease. A common point source or person-to-person spread are usually involved. Immediate application of control measures to prevent transmission often curtails such outbreaks. However, it is estimated that only 3 per cent of all nosocomial infections are accounted for by epidemic infection. Endemic nosocomial infections are 'usually' acquired in hospital and account for 97 per cent. Susceptibility of the host, the infectious risk of medical procedures, and the type of hospital environment (e.g. intensive-care unit) are responsible. Methods for reducing endemic nosocomial infections focus on reducing identifiable risk factors for infection (e.g. use of prophylactic antibiotics for contaminated surgical procedures).

Table 1 *Rates and sites of nosocomial infection reported from three countries*

	Canada (1976)	UK (1981)	USA (1986)
Rates (cases/100 admissions)			
	8.2[1]	9.2[1]	5.7[2]
Sites (% of all infections)			
UTI	39	30	42
SWI	24	19	24
LRI	26	16	11
Other	11	35	23

[1]Cases/100 admissions (prevalence).

[2]Cases/100 admissions/year (incidence).

UTI, urinary-tract infection; SWI, surgical wound infection; LRI, lower respiratory-tract infection.

Table 2 *Estimated cost to countries of nosocomial infections*

Continent*	Average no. of patients	5% of patients with nosocomial infections	Cost estimate for 5 days ($US)
Africa	4 900 000	245 000	55 125 000
America	46 500 000	2 325 000	523 125 000
Asia	17 500 000	875 000	196 875 000
Europe	56 000 000	2 800 000	630 000 000
Oceania	490 000	24 500	5 512 500
TOTAL	125 390 000	6 269 500	1 410 637 500

*Statistical data are not available from 16 countries in Africa—Egypt, Equatorial Guinea, Ethiopia, Kenya, Mali, Mauritania, Mozambique, Namibia, Niger, Nigeria, Réunion, Seychelles, Sierra Leone, Somalia, United Republic of Cameroon and Zaire; 15 countries in the Americas—Anguilla, Argentina, Belize, Bolivia, Brazil, Dominica, Guadelupe, Haiti, Mexico, Antilles, Paraguay, Peru, Suriname, US Virgin Islands, Venezuela; 14 countries in Asia—Afghanistan, Bangladesh, China, Democratic Kampuchea, East Timor, India, Korea, Lebanon, Nepal, Oman, Pakistan, the Philippines, Quatar, Yemen; 8 countries in Europe—Albania, Belgium, Bulgaria, German Democratic Republic, Isle of Man, Malta, Rumania, the USSR; 5 countries in Oceania—Australia, New Hebrides, Tuvalu, Papua New Guinea and Solomon Islands.

(Reproduced from Kereselidze, T. and Mangay Maglacas, A. (1984). *Journal of Hospital Infection* **5** (Supplement A), 7–11, with permission)

On a national scale, the number, severity, and cost of nosocomial infections have been difficult to measure. Rates of between 5.7 and 8.2 infections per 100 admissions have been reported. The urinary tract, surgical wounds, and the lower respiratory tract are the first, second, and third most common sites for these nosocomial infections. (see Table 1). Mortality associated with nosocomial infection has been difficult to determine, but in the United States it is estimated that, of 200 000 deaths in patients with nosocomial infections, 20 000 were attributable directly to the infection. In a further 60 000, it contributes to death. The cost of nosocomial infections was approximately £120 million per year in England and Wales in 1987, based on an average additional stay of 4 days for each hospital-acquired infection. This is likely to be an underestimate of the true cost. The WHO published comparative worldwide costs in 1984 based on an extra 5 days of hospitalization per infection and a minimum cost of a hospital stay, per day, of $45.00 (Table 2). For a developed country, this is an artificially low cost for a hospital stay per day.

HOST

The principal factor contributing to the risk of nosocomial infection is the severity of the underlying disease (e.g. neutropenia, organ system failure). To a lesser extent, extremes of age, male sex, previous community-acquired infection, and length of preoperative hospital admission are associated with an increased risk of infection.

MICRO-ORGANISMS

The main aetiological agents are bacteria. Viruses, fungi, and protozoa play a minor part. The five leading bacterial groups or species associated with nosocomial infections, in decreasing order of frequency are *Escherichia coli, Staphylococcus aureus, Enterococcus* spp., *Pseudomonas* spp., and coagulase-negative staphylococci.

Whether endogenously or exogenously acquired, the organisms that cause nosocomial infection are usually part of a patient's colonizing flora. Therefore, it may be difficult to distinguish by bacteriological tests alone, organisms causing infection from those merely colonizing a surface. These bacteria are frequently resistant to many antimicrobials. A shift towards a more resistant colonizing flora occurs in hospitals, particularly in burns and intensive-care units. Empirical antibiotic therapy must therefore accommodate the likely antibiotic-resistance patterns of the infecting flora. For example, *Pseudomonas aeruginosa*, methicillin-resistant *Staph. aureus* (**MRSA**), and enterococci are organisms that exhibit multiresistance to antimicrobials and are difficult to treat.

Principles of hospital infection control

The main goal of hospital infection control is to prevent nosocomial infection. The first step is to identify hospital-acquired infections and determine if they are endemic or epidemic by clinical recognition and careful epidemiological investigation of the relation between cases. The identification and typing of isolates causing nosocomial infection provides an additional powerful tool for recognizing organisms that are epidemiologically linked. Invasive multiresistant organisms, for example MRSA, are organisms that often require application of infection control measures to prevent their spread.

Epidemic outbreaks are usually amenable to measures that interrupt the spread of infection. These may include the use of gowns and gloves by those attending patients and careful hand washing after patient contact. Transfer of colonized or infected patients to a single room or an isolation ward is a physical means of preventing spread. Patients infected with the same organism can be grouped together and attended to by a cadre of nurses who do not care for uninfected patients. Identification of additional carriers and elimination of colonization may be necessary for some epidemic outbreaks. Controlled trials demonstrating the efficacy of such measures have not been made, but many observational studies support their use.

Control and reduction of endemic nosocomial infections is a less tractable, but not insurmountable, problem. Control measures include the use of prophylactic antimicrobials and meticulous sterile technique for high-risk invasive procedures (e.g. prosthetic joint-replacement surgery).

Nosocomial infections by site

Nosocomial urinary-tract infection

Identification is by urine culture. A bacterial count of 10^5 organisms or more per ml is usually interpreted as indicating infection. However, counts as low as 10^2 organisms/ml have been regarded as indicative by some investigators. Urinary-tract infection accounts for between 30 and 40 per cent of all nosocomial infections. Most patients remain asymptomatic, but 20 to 30 per cent develop the symptoms of urinary-tract infection, of which a small proportion, about 1 in 100, develops bacteraemia. The types of organisms that cause nosocomial urinary-tract infections are listed in Table 3.

Table 3 *Micro-organisms causing nosocomial urinary-tract infections (%)*

	UK	USA
Escherichia coli	43	32
Proteus spp.	13	7
Kebsiella spp.	8	9
Enterococci	7	14
Pseudomonas aeruginosa	5	11
Coagulase-negative staphylococci	3	3
Enterobacter spp.	1	4
Other	14	22

Indwelling urinary catheters account for 80 per cent of nosocomial urinary-tract infections, which is scarcely surprising, as 50 per cent of patients catheterized for longer than 7 to 10 days develop bacteriuria. Most of the other urinary-tract infections are accounted for by instrumentation of the urinary tract. The main source of organisms is the periurethral flora. Bacteria gain access to the bladder, usually by spreading up the outside of the lumen of the catheter. Occasionally, the infecting organisms are acquired from an exogenous source, as part of an epidemic nosocomial infection. Most symptomatic or bacteraemic urinary-tract infections occur within 24 h of the organisms gaining access to the bladder. Early recognition, by daily urine culture, of a urinary-tract infection before it becomes symptomatic is not helpful.

Clinically, symptomatic cases present with dysuria, frequency, lower abdominal discomfort, loin pain, fever, and sometimes features of septic shock. Treatment of a symptomatic patient requires broad-spectrum antimicrobials administered empirically after obtaining appropriate cultures. Treatment should later be adjusted according to the results of bacteriological studies. There is no need to treat asymptomatic patients.

Prevention of nosocomial urinary-tract infections has received much attention. Prophylactic antimicrobial treatment does not have a significant role, but it is important to avoid urinary catheterization or reduce the period of catheterization. Catheters should be inserted aseptically, and closed sterile drainage systems, uninterrupted gravity drainage, or intermittent or suprapubic catheterization should be used.

Surgical wound infection

As there is no objective test for the diagnosis of a surgical wound infection, no precise definition is available. One acceptable definition requires the presence of a purulent discharge in, or exuding from, a wound. The two leading causes of this infection are *Staph. aureus* (15–33 per cent of all wound infections) and *E. coli* (12–19 per cent). A wide range of other aerobic and anaerobic bacterial species can also be implicated.

There are a number of risk factors for surgical wound infection. The main risk is the degree of wound contamination at operation. Operations can be classified as 'clean' (e.g. herniorrhaphy), 'clean contaminated' (e.g. appendicectomy which requires incision of bowel) and 'contaminated' (e.g. gross spillage from the gastrointestinal tract during surgery). The risk of wound infection obviously increases from 'clean' to 'contaminated'. Other risk factors include the length of the operation, obesity, a remote infection, and underlying disease. Most wound infections follow the direct inoculation of organisms into the wound at the time of surgery or spread of bacteria to open wounds such as burns.

Clinically, wound infections present with local symptoms and signs at the site of the wound and produce general features of infection such as fever. Management consists first of taking appropriate cultures, including blood cultures, draining pus if it is present, and empirically giving broad-spectrum antimicrobials effective against the likely flora. Treatment can subsequently be changed according to the bacteriological results. Prevention of wound infection depends largely on meticulous aseptic technique, good surgical technique, and the use of 24 h of prophylactic antimicrobials.

Nosocomial pneumonia

Pneumonia is defined clinically. Features include the production of purulent sputum, chest signs, a fall in arterial Po_2 and the appearance of infiltrates on the chest radiograph not ascribable to pulmonary emboli, collapse, or pulmonary oedema. Between 0.55 and 1.5 per cent of patients admitted to hospital are estimated to develop lower respiratory-tract infections. The mortality attributable to pneumonia has not been reliably determined because many of the patients with pneumonia have serious underlying illnesses that are independently associated with death. Crude case fatalities of between 20 and 30 per cent are quoted. Intubated and ventilated patients have the highest risk of acquiring pneumonia. The source of the organisms is the bacteria colonizing the gastrointestinal and upper respiratory tracts. They probably gain access to the lung by aspiration. This infecting flora is frequently acquired by the patient after admission to hospital. The types of organisms cultured from bronchoscopic samples are listed in Table 4.

Clinically, these patients will present with general signs and symptoms of infection and new physical signs typical of pneumonia or bronchopneumonia. Chest radiography should reveal a new infiltrate and blood gases show evidence of an increasing arterial alveolar oxygen gradient (a–A gradient). Culture of expectorated sputum or tracheal aspirate is poorly predictive of the bacterial cause of nosocomial pneumonia, which is best determined by quantitative culture of specimens obtained by sampling the terminal airways (e.g. by bronchoalveolar lavage). Initially, broad-spectrum antimicrobials appropriate for the likely infecting flora should be given empirically. Once the susceptibility of the causative pathogen has been determined, specific antimicrobial treatment can be applied. Prevention of endemic nosocomial infections has attracted considerable attention. However, despite reducing the occurrence of these infections using measures such as selective decontamination of the digestive tract, no reduction in the mortality of ventilated patients has been seen. Epidemic nosocomial infections that usually result from bacterial contamination of respiratory equipment such as nebulizers, ventilators or bronchoscopes can be prevented by meticulous control measures.

Intravascular device-associated infections

The most important clinical outcome of intravascular device-associated infection is bacteraemia, which varies in its incidence from a low of about 0.04 per cent for subcutaneous central venous ports to about 0.2 per cent for peripheral intravenous cannulae to a high of approximately 10 per cent for central venous haemodialysis catheters.

Bacteria usually gain access to the blood by direct spread from the skin surface along the subcutaneous catheter tunnel to its tip in the blood vessel. Bacteraemia from intraluminal bacteria results from contamination of connecting devices. This is particularly important in catheters with subcutaneous cuffs, such as Hickman catheters, where the periluminal route of infection is less likely. The leading organisms causing intravenous device-related sepsis are *Staph. aureus*, *Pseudomonas* spp., and *Candida* spp. In patients with haematological malignancies, coagulase-negative staphylococci and enterococci are, in addition, frequently implicated.

Line-related sepsis can present with local inflammation around the catheter or occasionally with signs of thrombophlebitis. Usually, it presents with features of bacteraemia. Management involves obtaining blood cultures, removing and culturing the affected catheter, and giving empirical antimicrobials. In some circumstances, long-term intravenous catheters, such as Hickman lines, can be 'sterilized' by giving parenteral antibiotics down the line. Intravascular catheter sepsis is prevented by using aseptic technique when inserting catheters, maintaining a high standard of line care, and removing catheters as soon as possible. The insertion site should be disinfected with a reliable disinfectant such as an iodine-containing agent, 70 per cent alcohol or 2 to 4 per cent chlorhexidine. At the time of insertion the operators should wash their hands, and for long-line insertion, wear gloves. Peripheral intravenous cannulae should not be left in for more than 3 days. Central venous catheters should be removed before 7 days. Central lines dedicated to a single purpose, such as giving total parenteral nutrition, can be left in for longer. Lines can be left in place for prolonged periods by using subcutaneous tunnelling, insertion of a subcutaneous cuff (Hickman line), or by burying them subcutaneously (e.g. portacaths). These manoeuvres reduce the infection rate significantly. Replacing the entire intravenous delivery set every 72 h is sufficient to reduce sepsis secondary to the intraluminal contamination of 'giving' sets.

Table 4 *Causative organisms identified in samples drained at bronchoscopy by protected specimen brush (percentage of all pneumonias)*

	France	Spain
Pseudomonas aeruginosa	31	35
Acinetobacter spp.	15	30
Proteus spp.	15	
Moraxella catarrhalis	10	
Haemophilus spp.	10	
Staphylococcus aureus	33	25
Streptococci	15	20
Other species	37	60
Polymicrobial	21	50

Prosthetic device-related infection

A wide range of prosthetic devices such as heart valves, vascular grafts, cerebrospinal-fluid shunts, artificial lenses, and joints is used in medical practice. Infections of these devices are usually caused by the normal skin flora, for example coagulase-negative staphylococci. Most prosthetic devices become coated with a layer of host-derived macromolecules such as fibronectin. Fibronectin, and possibly other molecules, (e.g. fibrin) have receptors specific for adhesion to organisms, particularly staphylococci. Once attached, these organisms multiply on the surface of the coated prosthesis forming a film ('biofilm'). Bacteria in this state appear to be physiologically different from rapidly dividing, 'free' micro-organisms. In particular, they are inherently more resistant to antimicrobials, which may explain the frequent failure of antimicrobial treatment of these infections. Bacteria gain access to prosthetic devices by direct inoculation, which usually occurs at the time of surgery and therefore often presents early, and by settling on a prosthesis after bacteraemic spread. This is probably the mode by which many late prosthetic-device infections occur. Except for organisms that are exquisitely susceptible to antimicrobials, these infections are seldom cured with antimicrobial agents; therefore, surgical removal of the device is frequently necessary. The exception, fortunately, seems to be infection of artificial lenses in the eye, where antimicrobial treatment is frequently curative.

Prosthetic device-related infections can be reduced by avoiding contamination of the wound at the time of surgery, by using strict aseptic measures, and by good surgical technique. In some circumstances, such as when inserting prosthetic joints, a small benefit can be achieved by using operating theatres provided with ultra-clean air. Prophylactic antimicrobials have been shown to reduce the risk of some prosthetic devices becoming infected during insertion.

Nosocomial bacteraemia

Bacteraemia may occur secondarily to the infections mentioned above. The incidence is approximately 3/1000 hospital discharges. The case fatality is about 40 per cent, but varies depending on the severity of the underlying disease and is as low as about 2 per cent in obstetric patients. The management is directed towards identifying the focus, removing it surgically if possible, and by giving appropriate antimicrobials after obtaining blood and other relevant cultures.

Other nosocomial infections

There are numerous other nosocomial infections including viral infections (e.g. varicella-zoster, human immunodeficiency virus, hepatitis B, Norwalk and rotaviruses). Bacterial infections such as tuberculosis and legionellosis, and fungal infections such as aspergillosis are also encountered. Specific control measures are used to prevent their occurrence or spread; they depend on identifying the source and interrupting the transmission of these infectious agents.

REFERENCES

Ayliffe, G.A.J., Lowbury, E.J.L., Geddes, A.M., and Williams, J.D. (ed.) (1992). *Control of hospital infection*: a practical handbook, (3rd edn). Chapman & Hall, London.

Bennett, J.V. and Brachman, P.S. (ed.) (1992). *Hospital infections*, (3rd edn). Little, Brown, New York.

Meers, P., Jacobsen, W., and McPherson, M. (1992). *Hospital infection control for nurses*. Chapman & Hall, London.

Wenzel, R.P. (ed.) (1993). *Prevention and control of nosocomial infections*, (2nd edn). Williams & Wilkins, Baltimore.

7.10 Viruses

7.10.1 Respiratory tract viruses

D. Isaacs

Introduction

Acute respiratory infections are estimated to result in 2 to 3 million childhood deaths in the world each year and, in an unknown but significant proportion of these infections, viruses cause the infection or predispose to bacterial superinfection. In developed countries, respiratory virus infections are responsible for significant childhood morbidity and absence from work.

DEFINITION

The term respiratory virus is vague. A number of viruses may be transmitted via the respiratory route and cause prominent respiratory signs and symptoms as part of a systemic illness, for example measles, chickenpox, enteroviruses, mumps. The term respiratory viruses conventionally refers to those viruses whose main manifestations are respiratory.

EPIDEMIOLOGY

Respiratory viruses are ubiquitous, and can be grown in tissue culture from respiratory secretions from subjects with infections throughout the world. Most preschool children in developed countries will experience about six to eight respiratory viral infections per year, predominantly with rhinoviruses. The major determinant of the number of infections is exposure (see Table 1): preschool children in day care or attending kindergarten contract significantly more infections than those at home with an older sibling at school, who in turn have more infections than preschool children at home and with no school-aged siblings. Urban children have more infections than rural ones. Passive smoking has been shown to increase the incidence and severity of respiratory virus infections and clinical syndromes such as otitis media and pneumonia in infancy. Breast-feeding protects against respiratory virus infections. The popular belief that getting cold or wet causes colds has not been borne out by experimental studies, which have shown that significant lowering of the body temperature of volunteers by immersion in cold water does not increase their susceptibility to infection. There is, however, a clear seasonality for many respiratory viruses, which generally but not always cause more infections in the colder months of the year. Psychological stress increases susceptibility to respiratory viral infections more than it increases the perceived severity of the infections. Susceptibility to infection by several different, unrelated respiratory viruses increases linearly with increasing stress.

MODES OF TRANSMISSION (TABLE 2)

Traditionally, respiratory viruses are believed to be transmitted by respiratory droplet spread. During the Second World War a British poster proclaimed 'Coughs and sneezes spread diseases. Stop the germs by using your handkerchief.' Most of the evidence, obtained from inventive and often bizarre experiments carried out by the Common Cold Research Unit in Salisbury and more recently at the University of Madison, favours droplet spread (see Table 1).

Table 1 *Factors associated with increased incidence of respiratory infections*

Age: maximum 6 months to 4 years
Day-care or kindergarten attendance
Siblings: school-age > preschool; number of siblings
Urban > rural
Maternal smoking
Bottle > breast-feeding
Psychological stress

There is evidence that infections may also be spread by passage of infected secretions on hands, either by direct contact with a child's nose, in the case of staff caring for children with respiratory syncytial virus (**RSV**) infection, or by contact with intermediate objects or fomite spread. Viruses can then be inoculated by fingering the nasal mucosa or conjunctiva. For RSV infection such spread appears to be more important than droplet spread, and hand-washing is an important and effective means of preventing spread of RSV infection within hospitals. For other viruses, droplet spread is the most important but not the only means of transmission (Table 2). It has proved surprisingly difficult to spread colds experimentally, but spread increases with increasing duration of exposure.

PATHOGENESIS

Respiratory viruses infect cells by taking advantage of natural host-cell receptors. For example, almost all rhinoviruses bind to the intercellular adhesion molecule receptor, **ICAM-1**, to gain entry to fibroblasts and other cells. Most respiratory viruses replicate locally in the respiratory tract and cause relatively little viraemia. In contrast, influenza A virus infection can cause viraemia, which results in interferon-α appearing in the serum, and probably causing many of the symptoms of 'flu', since interferon alone can cause fever, headaches, myalgia, and malaise.

The local symptoms of respiratory viral infections are caused largely by inflammatory mediators, particularly bradykinins. Rhinoviruses cause very little destruction of the nasal mucosal epithelium, but RSV is more destructive and can cause necrosis of respiratory epithelium.

IMMUNITY

Immunity against reinfection with a respiratory virus usually correlates better with the presence of specific secretory IgA antibody than with serum IgG antibody, presumably because these are mainly local infections. Cellular immunity may also be important in preventing reinfection. Immunity against one serotype of a virus (e.g. rhinovirus) does not confer cross-protection against other serotypes. The vast number of serotypes (over 100 rhinovirus serotypes alone) explains the seemingly endless number of infections suffered by children. Immunity appears to wane with time: paediatricians starting to work on the wards initially seem to catch every respiratory virus but gradually become immune. If they do research for a year or two, and then return to the wards they are again highly susceptible.

Recovery from acute infection is different from immunity against reinfection. Antibody is usually produced too slowly to be effective, although local specific IgA antibody may contribute to recovery. In general, cellular immunity is the most important mechanism for recovery,

Table 2 *Studies on the transmission of respiratory viruses*

Study	Source of cold	Recipients	Result	Conclusion
Lovelock *et al.* (1952)	(i) Children with natural colds	Volunteers played table games with children; or across room from them with blanket screen and fan blowing air	Volunteers got colds	Droplet spread
	(ii) Cards contaminated with nasal secretions from above children	Volunteers played with cards but not with children	No colds	No fomite spread
Bynoe *et al.* (1961)	Direct inoculation of rhinovirus	Volunteers	Inoculation on to nasal epithelium or conjunctiva, but not external nares or pharynx, caused colds	Suggested spread by respiratory droplet or by rubbing secretions into eyes
Buckland *et al.* (1965)	Artificial 'sneeze' of coxsackievirus into wardrobe	Volunteers poked their heads into wardrobe	Got colds	Droplet spread
D'Alessio *et al.* (1984)	Donor with rhinovirus cold	Kissed donor for 1 to $1\frac{1}{2}$ min	Only 1 of 13 got a cold	Kissing to be encouraged (or at least not discouraged)
Hall and Douglas (1981)	(i) Babies with RSV infection	Adults changed nappies and fed babies: the 'cuddlers'	Most adults (5 of 7) infected	Spread of secretions on hands and from fomites more important than droplet spread
	(ii) Room emptied of baby with RSV infection	Adults touched cot-sides and surfaces and rubbed their eyes and nose: the 'touchers'	4 of 10 adults infected	
	(iii) Babies with RSV infection	Adults sat 1.8 m away: the 'sitters'	None of 14 adults infected	
Dick *et al.* (1986)	Donor with rhinovirus cold playing cards	Played cards with donor but wiped cards with virucidal wipes	Prevented colds if used wipe (otherwise colds)	Transmission by secretions on hands
Dick *et al.* (1987)	Donor with rhinovirus cold playing cards	(i) Played cards but wore splints to prevent touching eyes or nose	Got as many colds as if no splints	Both airborne and fomite spread important, but airborne more so
		(ii) Played cards but frequent changes of cards	No colds	

and children with isolated antibody deficiency recover normally from respiratory viral infections whereas children with pure T-cell deficiency are at increased risk of life-threatening infections with RSV, parainfluenza and and influenza viruses. Interferon-α is produced locally, appearing in nasal secretions as viral titres fall, and is probably another important factor in recovery from most acute respiratory viral infections. In contrast, specific serum and secretory antibody is the most important factor in preventing reinfection with respiratory viruses.

DIAGNOSIS

Inoculation of respiratory secretions on to tissue culture has long been the mainstay of the diagnosis of respiratory virus infections. This was because the large number of serotypes of rhinoviruses and the wide range of other respiratory viruses made antigen detection less attractive.

Where a single virus is largely responsible for a clinical syndrome, rapid diagnosis is now possible by detection of viral antigen in respiratory secretions, either by immunofluorescence using a fluorescein-labelled specific antibody, or by enzyme immunoassay, and may virtually replace tissue culture. RSV bronchiolitis is the prime example, but others are influenza virus (immunofluorescence used in outbreaks), parainfluenza viruses (immunofluorescence or enzyme immunoassay for summer croup or summer bronchiolitis), and rhinoviruses (enzyme immunoassay for common antigens).

Secretions aspirated by gentle suction from the back of the nose (nasopharyngeal aspirates) are the preferred specimens for respiratory viral detection. Nose and throat swabs give a lower yield. If throat swabs are taken, the fauces should be rubbed vigorously with the swab, which can be done, without making the patient gag, by swabbing the lateral pharynx. It is always important that cells are obtained, as these are the site of viral replication.

Serology is useful for diagnosing many infections, but generally much less so in babies and infants. IgG antibodies are usually sought, using complement fixation tests. Acute and convalescent sera taken at least 10 to 14 days apart are needed for detection of at least a fourfold rise in IgG antibody titre.

Specific viruses

Rhinoviruses

Rhinoviruses, together with the enteroviruses (coxsackie, echo, and polio), comprise the picornaviruses (pico (= small) RNA viruses). The RNA is infectious and can act as mRNA, so that replication is entirely cytoplasmic. Rhinoviruses, unlike enteroviruses, are destroyed by acid. Thus they do not cause enteritis, and their acid liability is used in tissue culture to distinguish them from enteroviruses.

EPIDEMIOLOGY

Rhinoviruses exhibit great antigenic diversity. There are over 100 serotypes distinguishable serologically. Infection with one strain does not generally confer cross-protection against other strains. Several serotypes usually circulate simultaneously in a community, and infections occur throughout the year, but particularly from late autumn to spring. The infection rate is highest in preschool children, declining from school age throughout the rest of life.

Rhinoviruses are difficult to grow in conventional tissue culture, although the Ohio strain of HeLa cells supports their growth well. Some fastidious rhinoviruses will grow only on organ cultures. This probably explains the variation in incidence of rhinovirus infections reported in different studies. Stringent efforts at isolation indicate that they may be the most important cause of colds, or wheezing illnesses complicating coryza, and of viral pneumonia.

TRANSMISSION

Transmission depends on prolonged close contact, and is probably by droplet spread, although it is surprisingly difficult to reproduce experimentally. Spread via contaminated nasal secretions hand-to-hand or fomite-to-hand and thence to nasal mucosa or conjunctiva is also an important mechanism of transmission (see Table 2). It has been estimated that a susceptible adult has a 50 per cent chance of being infected by 100 h of close exposure to someone with a moderately severe cold.

IMMUNITY

Rhinoviruses stimulate nasal production of interferon-α and specific nasal IgA, both of which appear within about 24 h of infection, and probably contribute to recovery. Serum IgG may appear after 1 to 2 weeks, but rhinoviruses are often poor at stimulating a humoral immune response. Cellular immunity to rhinoviruses can also be detected but its role in recovery is unknown.

Protection against reinfection correlates best with the presence of specific nasal IgA antibody against the infecting serotype, and to a lesser extent with serum IgG antibody.

PATHOGENESIS

Rhinoviruses replicate mainly in the upper respiratory tract. Most serotypes attach to the ICAM-1 receptor on fibroblasts and other cells to gain entry, and replicate mainly in ciliated epithelial cells. They generally elicit little local mucosal damage, and cause rhinorrhoea with mucus production through the action of local inflammatory mediators such as bradykinins, which are potent endogenous vasoactive peptides. Histamine is not involved.

Rhinoviruses are an important cause of wheezing in asthma. High titres of virus can be isolated from the sputum of school-age asthmatic children who wheeze during rhinovirus infections. This suggests that lower respiratory-tract replication may be important. Rhinoviruses can also be isolated from the nasopharynx in many children with viral pneumonia, providing further circumstantial evidence of replication in the lower respiratory tract.

CLINICAL MANIFESTATIONS

The most common manifestation of rhinovirus infection is the common cold, but rhinoviruses have also been detected in the middle-ear fluid of children with acute otitis media, and in sinuses during acute sinusitis. They are an occasional cause of infantile bronchiolitis, producing a clinical syndrome indistinguishable from RSV bronchiolitis. They can precipitate wheezing in asthmatic children, sometimes called wheezy bronchitis, although this term has fallen into disrepute as it is now recognized that most children who wheeze with respiratory infections have asthma. Rhinoviruses are a common cause of wheezing in school-age children, and intensive studies have shown that they are also an important cause of recurrent wheezing in preschool-aged asthmatics. Rhinoviruses can cause pneumonia in children, occasionally severe, and very rarely fatal, and in studies of childhood pneumonia they are usually the second most important virus implicated after RSV. They have also been implicated in exacerbations of cystic fibrosis.

TREATMENT

There is no effective specific therapy for rhinoviruses, and so treatment is symptomatic. William Osler is credited with saying that the only way to treat a cold is with contempt. Controlled trials of vitamin C have shown no clear-cut benefit, while aspirin actually enhances viral shedding. Nasal interferon-α sprays are effective when given to asymptomatic family members of a rhinovirus-infected subject as 'contact prophylaxis', but are ineffective as treatment. As the side-effects of nasal interferon sprays include nasal irritation and epistaxis, they are unlikely to be clinically useful, except perhaps for prophylaxis of high-risk subjects, such as children with cystic fibrosis.

Coronaviruses

Coronaviruses, so-called because of the sun-like crown appearance seen under the electron microscope (Fig. 1), are even more fastidious in their growth than rhinoviruses. The first coronavirus was isolated by Tyrrell and Bynoe in 1965, working in Salisbury, using organ cultures of human embryonic trachea and nasal epithelial mucosal cells. This strain was subsequently termed 229E. A second coronavirus strain was later grown in organ culture and called OC43. Antigens from these two prototype strains have been used to develop serological assays, and serosurveys have contributed greatly to understanding coronavirus epidemiology. Detailed analysis of coronaviruses has shown quite marked antigenic variation, which is largely mediated through a high frequency of recombination of their RNA.

Fig. 1 Electron micrograph of human coronavirus (× 200 000).

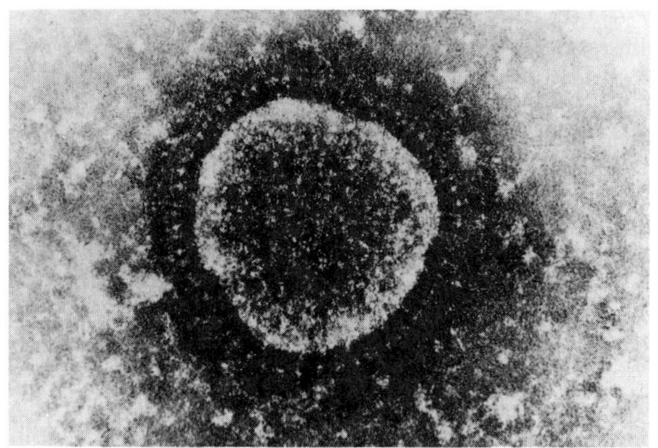

DIAGNOSIS

Human coronavirus infections have usually been diagnosed serologically, but human coronavirus antigens can be detected in nasopharyngeal secretions by enzyme immunoassay, a technique that is particularly useful in children.

EPIDEMIOLOGY

Human coronaviruses cause mid-winter outbreaks of respiratory infection. The same coronavirus strain does not circulate each year. Sporadic cases occur throughout the rest of the year. Reinfections with human coronavirus, demonstrated by a rise in antibody titre in adults with prior antibody, are common. Human coronaviruses have been found throughout the world.

TRANSMISSION

Human coronaviruses are infectious by the respiratory route, and volunteers can be infected by intranasal inoculation. Both aerosol and large-droplet spread are thought to be important routes of transmission.

IMMUNITY

Coronavirus infection stimulates nasal production of secretory IgA and interferon-α, both of which are probably important in recovery from acute infection. Immunity appears to be transient, as seropositive individuals can be reinfected with the same strain, although immunity against reinfection has been shown to last at least 1 year.

PATHOGENESIS

Human coronavirus infections cause quite marked destruction of the ciliated epithelium of the nasal mucosa and trachea. Coronaviruses, like rhinoviruses, can cause wheezing.

CLINICAL MANIFESTATIONS

The most frequent manifestation of human coronavirus infection is the common cold: coryza, nasal soreness and congestion, and sneezing. In adults, OC43 can cause sore throat and cough. Pharyngitis is frequent in children, and cervical adenitis, coryza, and low-grade fever are also common.

Human coronaviruses are a frequent cause of wheezing in asthmatic children. They are a less common cause of childhood pneumonia. They can cause exacerbations of chronic obstructive bronchitis in adults.

TREATMENT

There is no specific therapy.

Adenoviruses

Adenoviruses are non-enveloped DNA viruses, with a virion in the form of an icosahedron (Fig. 2). Most adenoviruses can cause respiratory infections, and can be cultured readily in tissue culture. Enteric adenoviruses are not cultivable but are seen on electron microscopy of faeces. Over 40 different adenoviral serotypes have been described: they share a generic antigen that can be identified by complement fixation or enzyme immunoassay, and can be divided into strains by identifying distinct surface antigens by neutralization by specific antibody. Diagnosis is by culture, antigen detection, or serology.

EPIDEMIOLOGY

Adenovirus infections can occur at any age but are most common in infants and preschool children. Epidemics can occur, primarily in institutions such as day-care centres and orphanages, but also among adults in close proximity, and in association with swimming pools, schools, and military barracks. Lower socioeconomic groups have a higher incidence, probably because of overcrowding.

Infections with adenoviruses occur worldwide. Epidemics are most frequent from winter through to early summer, but sporadic cases can occur throughout the year.

TRANSMISSION

Transmission is by aerosolized spread, mainly through small droplets, which infect the nose, throat, or conjunctiva, from where the virus can be isolated. In swimming-pool epidemics of pharyngoconjunctival fever, the virus survives in the water and can infect conjunctivae. Adenoviruses may be carried asymptomatically in the nasopharynx of children for several months following acute infection, and may act as a source of spread.

IMMUNITY

Local secretory IgA is produced in the nasopharynx from about 3 days after adenovirus infection, followed by specific nasal IgG at 7 days and then serum neutralizing antibody. The role of cellular immunity in recovery is unclear. Infants may sometimes develop severe adenovirus pneumonia (Fig. 3), which may progress to disseminated disease with

Fig. 2 Electron micrograph of adenovirus (× 150 000).

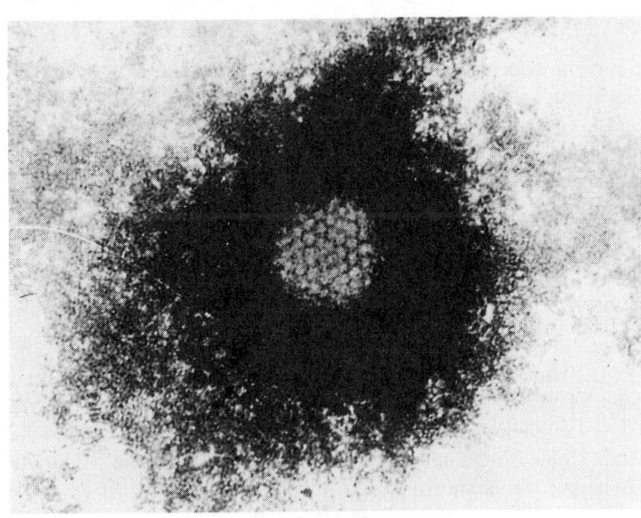

Fig. 3 Necrotizing bronchiolitis due to adenovirus (× 200).

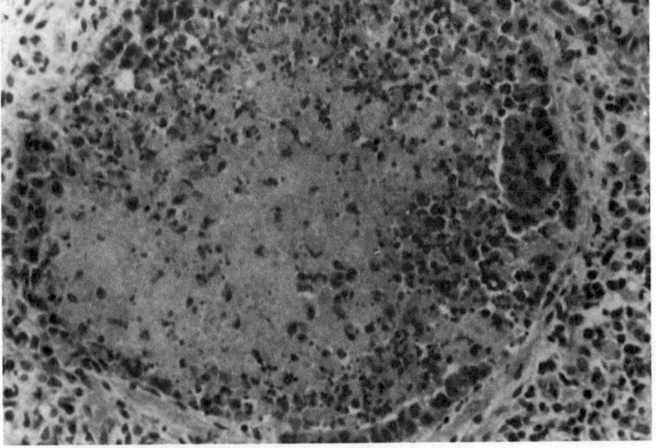

Table 3 *Respiratory infections caused by adenoviruses*

Illness	Comments	Most common types
Tonsillitis or pharyngitis	Common; epidemics	1, 2, 3, 5, 7
Pharyngoconjunctival fever	Common; epidemics	2, 3, 4, 5, 7, 14
Common cold	Rare; sporadic	1, 2, 3, 5, 7
Pneumonia	Common; epidemics	3, 7, 21
Acute respiratory disease	Epidemics in military recruits	4, 7
Laryngotracheitis (croup)	Rare; sporadic	1, 2, 3, 5, 6, 7
Bronchiolitis	Rare; sporadic	3, 7, 21
Bronchiectasis	Rare complication	3, 7, 21
Bronchiolitis obliterans	Very rare; late complication	7, 21

hepatitis and meningoencephalitis. Certain serotypes, notably 7 and 21, are more likely to disseminate. Severe disease has been described following measles, suggesting that T-cell immunity, which is depressed after measles, may be important in preventing dissemination. Adenovirus pneumonia may also occur in malnourished children, but many cases of severe adenovirus infection occur in infants who appear immunologically normal.

Adenovirus early protein can bind major histocompatibility complex class I molecules, and thus evade immune surveillance by T cells.

PATHOGENESIS

Respiratory adenoviruses invade the ciliated epithelium of the respiratory tract causing a degree of damage depending on the virulence of the infecting strain. Spread to the bloodstream may occur early, resulting in rashes and viraemic dissemination to other organs. Lung and pleural involvement could be due to local or viraemic spread. In severe pneumonia there is necrotizing bronchiolitis (Fig. 3) with necrosis and hyaline membrane formation.

CLINICAL MANIFESTATIONS

The respiratory manifestations of adenovirus infection are shown in Table 3. Adenovirus type 7 is the strain most commonly reported to cause disseminated disease and has been found to cause rashes, which may be morbilliform or petechial (rarely of Stevens–Johnson type), hepatitis, meningoencephalitis, myocarditis, nephritis, and rarely arthritis.

Tonsillitis is frequently follicular or exudative, with high fever, and may mimic group A streptococcal infection. Conjunctivitis, either alone or in conjunction with pharyngitis, and occurring in epidemics is frequently due to adenoviruses. Pneumonia is less frequently due to adenovirus than to RSV, rhinoviruses or parainfluenza viruses, but severe and often fatal cases in children under 18 months have been attributed to types 3, 7, and 21. Severe infantile adenovirus pneumonia may result in bronchiectasis, bronchiolitis obliterans or unilateral hypertranslucent lung (McLeod's syndrome). Acute respiratory disease was described in the Second World War, occurring in epidemics in military recruits. It is characterized by fever, dry cough, which may become paroxysmal, pharyngitis, laryngotracheitis, and often wheezing. The disease may progress to pneumonia.

TREATMENT

There is no proven specific treatment for systemic adenovirus infections. Topical interferon-β was effective in adenovirus keratoconjunctivitis in a comparative trial. There are anecdotal reports of the successful use of nebulized ribavirin to treat adenovirus pneumonia in children and of immune globulin for an immunodeficient child with pneumonia. It has been suggested that ganciclovir might be effective but this has not yet been evaluated.

Parainfluenza viruses

The parainfluenza viruses are paramyxoviruses, RNA viruses that, despite their name, are not closely related to influenza viruses. They do not produce a marked cytopathic effect in tissue culture, and are identified there by their ability to agglutinate red blood cells (haemagglutination). There are three main serotypes, parainfluenza viruses 1, 2, and 3, which show little antigenic variation. Type 4 is subdivided into 4A and 4B.

EPIDEMIOLOGY

Parainfluenza virus infections occur worldwide. Type 3 infections occur early, so that 60 per cent of infants are seropositive by 12 months of age. Type 1 and 2 infections occur later in childhood. Almost all adults have antibodies to types 1 and 3, and most to type 2.

Parainfluenza 1 virus tends to cause autumn outbreaks of laryngotracheitis (croup) in alternate years in the Northern hemisphere, or sporadic cases for a few years. In the Southern hemisphere the biennial epidemic nature is not always so clear-cut. Parainfluenza 2 virus causes less well-defined autumn or winter epidemics of croup every 1 to 2 years. Parainfluenza 3 virus is endemic or causes annual summer epidemics of croup and bronchiolitis.

TRANSMISSION

Person-to-person contact is the main route of transmission, with spread by large droplets or infected secretions. Parainfluenza viruses can survive for prolonged periods in the environment.

IMMUNITY

Immunity is at best partial, and reinfections occur. Children with impaired cellular immunity suffer prolonged, symptomatic infections, suggesting that T cells are important in recovery from acute infection. Local nasal interferon-α is produced in acute infection and may contribute to recovery. Maternal antibody is partially protective, but after recovery from acute infection, secretory antibody appears to be more important than serum antibody in protecting against reinfection. Specific IgE antibody is found in the nasal secretions of children with more severe parainfluenza virus infections with wheezing or croup, and may be important in the pathogenesis of wheeze.

PATHOGENESIS

Parainfluenza viruses infect the respiratory epithelium by attaching to specific receptors, penetrating the cell by fusion, and being phagocytosed. Local respiratory-tract spread is mainly by cell-to-cell transfer but viraemic spread may also occur. In severe infections there is extensive epithelial necrosis and inflammation throughout the respiratory tract, even involving the alveoli.

CLINICAL MANIFESTATIONS

Laryngotracheitis or croup is the most commonly recognized clinical manifestation of parainfluenza virus infection, mainly due to types 1 and 2. Infection may also involve the large airways, causing wheezing and producing laryngotracheobronchitis. Febrile, upper respiratory-tract infections, often with rhinitis and sore throat, are actually more common than croup. Other important manifestations are infantile bronchiolitis and pneumonia, usually due to type 3 and occurring throughout the year but often in summer (unlike RSV). Type 4 can cause colds or infections of the upper respiratory tract. Reinfections with parainfluenzaviruses are common and are usually successively milder. These viruses can precipitate wheezing in asthmatics, exacerbate cystic fibrosis and chronic bronchitis, and are a rare cause of pneumonia in military recruits. They have been known to cause acute parotitis. Patients with T-cell deficiency may develop severe giant-cell pneumonitis, which is sometimes fatal.

TREATMENT

Nebulized ribavirin can suppress chronic parainfluenza virus infection in children with severe combined immunodeficiency. Although infection recurs when treatment is stopped, infections have been suppressed long enough in such children to allow curative bone-marrow transplantation, following which the children were able to clear the virus themselves.

Influenza viruses

Influenza was once attributed to divine influence, hence its name, which is said to have come from Florence in the fifteenth century. Influenza A viruses are renowned for causing pandemics with a very high mortality: the pandemic of 1918–19 killed an estimated 20 million, more people than both World Wars combined.

The influenza viruses are RNA orthomyxoviruses, with three main types, A, B, and C, and multiple subtypes. Influenza surface proteins include haemagglutinin (**H**) and neuraminidase (**N**). Viruses are described by the type, origin, strain, year, and H and N subtypes: hence, influenza virus A/Shanghai/6/90 (H_3N_2).

EPIDEMIOLOGY

Influenza viruses are renowned for their ability to escape host immune surveillance by antigenic changes. These are either minor changes in H or N, called antigenic drift, which occur with influenza A and B, or major changes in the H and/or N proteins to a new subtype, antigenic shift, which is the sole property of influenza A strains.

Sporadic cases of influenza are rare, and influenza viruses cause epidemics of varying degree. These may be small local outbreaks, nationwide epidemics or global pandemics. Pandemics have probably occurred for over 2000 years, and a possible epidemic was described by Hippocrates and Livy in 412 BC. Recently there have been pandemics every 10 to 20 years, the largest being in 1918–19. Continuous worldwide surveillance of influenza virus strains is maintained by the World Health Organization.

The highest attack rate for influenza is in young children, but the highest mortality is in the elderly. Mortality is higher in the immunocompromised and those with heart disease, chronic lung disease, diabetes, and chronic renal disease.

Influenza virus infections occur almost exclusively in the winter in temperate climates, and may spread around the world with the change of season, affecting Australasia, for example, 6 months after Western Europe.

TRANSMISSION

Large-droplet spread from coughs and sneezes is probably the main mode of spread. Experimentally, a fine aerosol reaching the alveoli is more infectious than nasal deposition. Virus may also spread in nasal secretions on hands.

Influenza A virus can be found in nasal secretions up to 6 days before symptoms, influenza B for only 1 day. High titres of virus, 10^6/ml or more, are present in respiratory secretions at the start of symptoms, but the infectious dose is far lower. Infected individuals continue to shed virus for 1 to 2 weeks. The incubation period is short, usually only 2 to 3 days. All these factors contribute to rapid epidemic spread. Closed communities such as schools, military barracks, residential homes, and even hospitals are likely to suffer dramatic outbreaks.

IMMUNITY

A number of different immunological mechanisms are important in influenza infections. In recovery from acute infection, cellular immunity (specific cytotoxic T cells), nasal interferon-α production, and nasal IgA all appear to play important roles. Studies have shown that protection against reinfection is correlated, partially but not absolutely, with pre-existing specific ('memory') cytotoxic T cells, specific serum IgG antibody, and specific nasal IgA antibody.

The doctrine of 'original antigenic sin', whereby infection with one strain of influenza stimulates an anamnestic antibody response specific for the strain causing that person's first ever influenza infection, is true for fairly closely related strains. Where there has been antigenic shift of H and N antigens, no anamnestic response occurs.

Interferon-α appears in nasal secretions and also in the bloodstream during acute influenza; the systemic clinical manifestations of influenza may well be due to interferon because parenterally administered interferon-α causes influenza-like symptoms.

Natural immunity following acute infection lasts for about 4 to 6 years, but is variable in duration, and depends in part on the degree of antigenic variation. Vaccine-induced immunity, using an inactivated influenza vaccine, lasts for only one influenza season, but the vaccines contain the strains that the World Health Organization predicts are likely to circulate in the coming winter.

PATHOGENESIS

The principal site of influenza virus infection is the ciliated columnar epithelial cell. Necrosis of nasal and tracheal ciliated cells occurs early, often within the first day, and impairment of the mucociliary escalator predisposes to bacterial superinfection. Influenza virus infection also impairs chemotaxis and phagocytosis by macrophages and neutrophils. Secondary bacterial pneumonia is an important contributor to illness and death. Primary influenza pneumonia, particularly in immunocompromised or other high-risk patients, without bacterial superinfection, may also be fatal. It is characterized by bronchiolar epithelial necrosis with haemorrhagic alveolar exudate and lymphocytic infiltration of the alveoli, peribronchial areas, and interstitium.

CLINICAL MANIFESTATIONS

Influenza A virus is unusual in causing a similar febrile illness in children and adults. Characteristically there is sudden fever, with chills, headache, myalgia, and dry cough. Sore throat and rhinitis or nasal stuffiness are common. Influenza B and C cause an almost identical illness, but B may be milder and is more likely to cause ocular symptoms: conjunctivitis, eye pain, or photophobia. In children, abdominal pain and vomiting are common. The illness usually lasts 2 to 3 days, rarely up to 1 week.

In neonates, influenza causes apnoea, lethargy, pulmonary infiltrates, and tachypnoea with increased oxygen requirements. This clinical picture is indistinguishable from neonatal RSV or rhinovirus infection.

In children, influenza A virus is the second most common cause of viral croup, producing a more severe illness than parainfluenza viruses, with a greater likelihood of requiring respiratory support. Influenza viruses can cause febrile convulsions in preschool children. They do not appear to be an important cause of exacerbations of asthma.

Influenza viruses can cause primary pneumonia, particularly in immunocompromised patients or those with pre-existing heart disease, and this may be progressive. Bacterial superinfection can occur, usually with pneumococci or *Staphylococcus aureus*. The latter is particularly fulminant, with haemoptysis and dyspnoea, pneumatoceles and empyema, and often a rapid demise.

Cardiac complications of influenza virus may be asymptomatic. Myocarditis and pericarditis are well described. Sudden deaths from influenza have occurred, either spontaneously during exercise, or merely on getting out of bed. Some of these are due to subclinical myocarditis.

Myalgia is normal in influenza, but if severe may indicate true myositis. The serum levels of muscle enzymes are usually grossly elevated in myositis. Rhabdomyolysis with myoglobinuria occurs rarely. Influenza B is a more common cause of myositis than influenza A.

Rare complications of influenza virus infection include Reye's syndrome (fatty liver, hypoglycaemia, and encephalopathy) and neurological conditions, such as Guillain–Barré syndrome and transverse myelitis. Glomerulonephritis and parotitis have been described.

PREVENTION AND TREATMENT

Current influenza vaccines are formalin inactivated, usually contain two influenza A strains and one B strain, and are chemically treated to reduce pyrogens ('split' vaccines) or untreated ('whole' vaccines). Vaccination is recommended for those at high risk of severe disease, particularly the elderly and immunocompromised, and for staff caring for high-risk persons. Immunization of normal healthy children is not recommended, as immunity due to infection with wild virus lasts longer. Immunization is probably not indicated for asthma, but should be considered for children with cystic fibrosis and those with severe heart disease, especially if they have pulmonary hypertension.

Chemoprophylaxis using the antiviral drug amantidine (or the related drug rimantidine) reduces the incidence of influenza A infection, but is ineffective against B. Amantidine has been used in boarding schools and geriatric and other homes for routine winter prophylaxis or to limit spread during outbreaks. It has been used for winter prophylaxis of children with cystic fibrosis. Amantidine can cause central nervous side-effects, such as difficulty in concentrating, while both amantidine and rimantidine can result in gastrointestinal effects, nausea, and anorexia.

Specific treatment of severe influenza A infections is possible using oral amantidine or rimantidine, both of which have been shown to be effective. The adult dose of amantidine is 200 mg once, followed by 100 mg once daily for 5 to 7 days. The child dose is scaled down proportionately.

Nebulized ribavirin has been shown to be effective against both influenza A and B virus infections in adults.

Respiratory syncytial virus (RSV)

RSV was isolated in 1955 from a chimpanzee with a cold, and was rapidly recognized as one of the most important pathogens in the world. The name derives from the tendency to cause syncytia, or multinucleate giant cells, in tissue culture. RSV is an enveloped RNA virus of the paramyxovirus group. There are two major groups of RSV, A and B or 1 and 2. There is some antigenic variation within these groups so that subgroups can be defined.

RSV was one of the earliest viruses that could be diagnosed rapidly. Fluorescein-labelled antisera were used to detect RSV antigen in nasopharyngeal secretions. The antisera are specific for RSV (direct immunofluorescence) or directed against an antibody to RSV (indirect). Enzyme immunoassay is also commonly used for detecting RSV antigen.

EPIDEMIOLOGY

RSV infection occurs worldwide. In temperate climates there are epidemics every winter, lasting about 4 months, while in equatorial climates RSV epidemics occur in the rainy season. The epidemics occur when the days are shortest and the weather coldest, although the timing is not a function of absolute temperature because the temperature of an English summer and an Australian winter are comparable. Sporadic cases of RSV occur outside the winter peak, but are rare, and it is a mystery where the virus goes between each epidemic. Group A or B may predominate in different years, or a group A and a group B strain may circulate concurrently.

RSV infection is unique in that the peak incidence is at 2 to 6 months of age, when it might be expected that passively acquired maternal IgG would be protective. In fact, serum IgG is at best only partially protective, and reinfections with RSV are extremely common. Infections under 2 months of age are less common, perhaps because babies of this age tend to be protected against exposure. Adults can readily be reinfected, and can act as a source of infection for spread to children at home and in hospitals.

The incidence of RSV infection increases with exposure to other children (urban environment, overcrowding, day care) and with passive exposure to tobacco smoke, particularly maternal smoking. The incidence is lower in breast-fed than in bottle-fed babies.

There is an association between RSV infection and recurrent wheezing, but it is not known whether RSV bronchiolitis causes asthma, or whether the virus merely causes bronchiolitis in atopic children who were destined to be asthmatic.

TRANSMISSION

Close contact is necessary for efficient spread of RSV, which is carried in large droplets and secretions, and survives for some hours on metal or plastic surfaces. RSV infection can occur by inoculation of the nasal mucosa or conjunctiva. An experimental study by Hall and Douglas (see Table 2) indicated that hand-washing might be an important way to prevent hospital-acquired infection.

The incubation period is 2 to 8 days (median 5 days). Infants with RSV infection usually shed virus for up to 10 days although sometimes for 3 to 4 weeks, or even longer, particularly if immunocompromised.

PATHOGENESIS

RSV infects the respiratory epithelium primarily, but can also infect alveolar macrophages and blood mononuclear cells. Viraemia is unusual. Severe RSV infection causes necrosis of the bronchiolar epithelium, and RSV antigen can be demonstrated in epithelial cells throughout the respiratory tract. The alveoli are spared, unless there is RSV pneumonia. Obstruction of small airways by cell debris results in hyperinflation.

It has long been felt that the host immune response may contribute to pathogenesis of RSV infection. In the 1960s a number of infants in the United States were given a formalin-inactivated RSV vaccine. Although the vaccine resulted in IgG antibody formation it was not protective against natural RSV infection, and immunized babies who were subsequently infected naturally with wild-type RSV experienced more severe disease than unimmunized babies, frequently requiring admission to hospital. Some died. One possible explanation for this surprising phenomenon is that the vaccine enhanced cellular immunity, although another possibility is that the vaccine resulted in a partial immune paresis rendering the vaccinees unable to recognize wild-type RSV when subsequently exposed.

Nasopharyngeal cells from some infected infants have RSV-specific IgE bound to their surface, and this correlates with subsequent wheezing. Alveolar macrophages produce tumour necrosis factor and mononuclear cells produce platelet-activating factor when stimulated with RSV, both of which may contribute to disease.

IMMUNITY

Children with impaired T-cell immunity are susceptible to more severe RSV infection and, as with parainfluenza viruses, infection can be prolonged and symptomatic with wheezing, and may be fatal. Examples are children with severe combined immune deficiency, those with isolated T-cell defects, and those with human immunodeficiency virus infection. Cytotoxic T cells appear in the peripheral blood early in infection, even in babies, and their numbers correlate with milder disease and with recovery. In a mouse model of RSV, moderate numbers of cytotoxic T cells will clear RSV infection whereas large numbers potentiate disease, suggesting that there may be a critical level of T-cell response.

Secretory IgA appears in the nasopharynx early and may contribute to recovery, and to resistance to further infections. RSV is a poor stimulator of local interferon-α. Serum IgG is only partially protective. Children with high levels of maternal IgG tend to have milder infections than those with low levels, but some of the most severe infections occur in those with very high levels. Most RSV-infected children produce circulating RSV-specific IgE antibody.

Reinfections are common and most adults can be infected readily. About half of a group of volunteers could be reinfected with RSV within 2 months and two-thirds within 8 months of natural RSV infection, and most could be reinfected with the same strain on two or more occasions.

CLINICAL MANIFESTATIONS

Almost all children (90–95 per cent) have been infected with RSV by the age of 2 years. Initial infections are nearly always symptomatic, and about 40 per cent cause clinical bronchiolitis, with wheeze, cough, rhinorrhoea, and fever. RSV is by far the most important cause of bronchiolitis. Most babies with bronchiolitis have patchy pulmonary consolidation, although some authorities make a distinction between RSV bronchiolitis, in which wheeze predominates, and RSV pneumonia. The diagnosis of RSV infection in infancy is made by rapid antigen detection in nasopharyngeal secretions, using indirect or direct immunofluorescence or enzyme immunoassay, or by viral culture. Serology can be useful in older children and adults.

RSV bronchiolitis is particularly severe in immunocompromised children, those with underlying cardiopulmonary disease including congenital heart disease, bronchopulmonary dysplasia and cystic fibrosis, and babies born prematurely. Preterm babies may present with apnoea as a major feature.

RSV is an important precipitant of asthma attacks in older children. Infections with RSV otherwise tend to become progressively milder. Children under 5 years old may develop otitis media, or, rarely, pneumonia. School-age children and adults are likely to have a febrile upper respiratory infection with pharyngitis and cough. The elderly may develop pneumonia.

PREVENTION

There is no effective vaccine against RSV. It is an important cause of nosocomial (hospital acquired) infection in children's hospitals, neonatal units, and homes for the elderly. The spread of RSV may be reduced by use of gloves and gowns, cohorting (isolating) RSV-positive patients, and improved hand-washing (Fig. 4).

TREATMENT

Nebulized ribavirin results in modest improvements in the clinical severity and oxygen saturation, and sometimes in viral shedding. The morbidity is slightly reduced in children with congenital heart disease or bronchopulmonary dysplasia, but mortality has not been affected. Ribavirin can precipitate in ventilator tubing and cause fluctuations in pressure. It is extremely expensive. There is no good evidence that ribavirin

Stop Bronchiolitis:-

* Your baby is in hospital with a condition called bronchiolitis.

* This is caused by a virus called respiratory syncytial virus (RSV).

* The disease is very infectious and is passed on by infected nasal secretions carried on hands or toys but not usually by coughing. The secretions are rubbed into the nose or eyes to cause infections.

* The best way of preventing spread of RSV infection is, therefore, by washing your hands after handling your baby. If you have a cold yourself try to wash your hands before handling other children.

* Many children on the ward have conditions such as heart disease which can be made much worse by RSV infection. To prevent these children being infected please wash your hands. If you have an older child with a cold do not let them play in the play areas on the ward until they are better.
Thank you

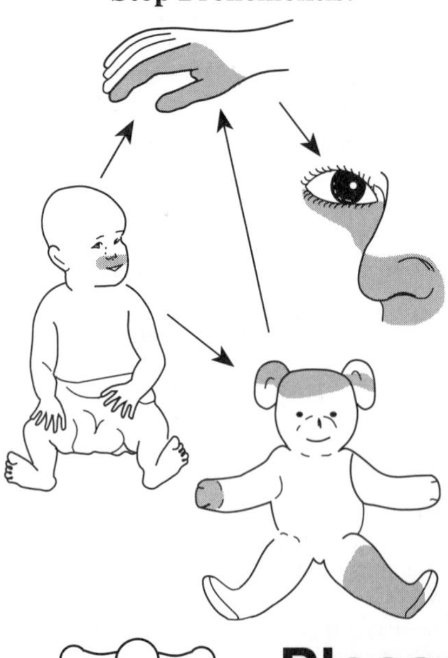

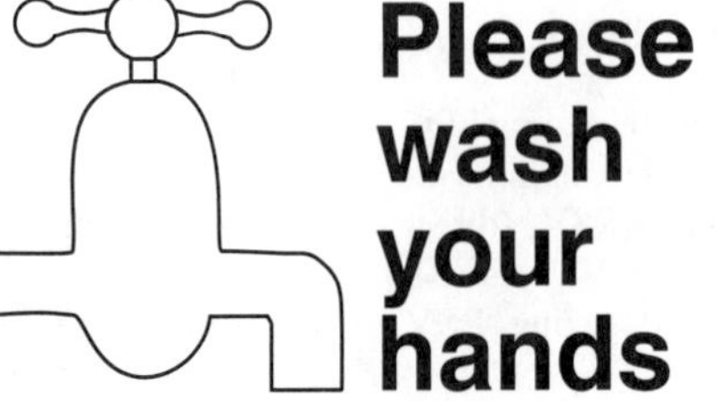

Information leaflet given to parents.

Fig. 4 Leaflet handed to parents of child admitted to hospital with respiratory syncytial virus infection (reprinted from Isaacs, D. *et al.* (1991). *Archives of Diseases of Childhood*, **66**, 227–31, with permission).

Table 4 *Features of respiratory virus infections*

Viruses	DNA or RNA	Incubation period (days)	Modes of transmission	Main diseases	Comments
Rhinoviruses	RNA	1–3	Secretions on hands Large droplets Infect nasal mucosa or conjunctiva	Colds, URTIs, sinusitis, otitis media, wheeze, pneumonia	More than 100 serotypes
Coronaviruses	RNA	2–4	Large droplets Aerosols (small droplets)	Colds, URTIs, wheeze, pneumonia	Two main serotypes Reinfections common
Adenoviruses	DNA	3–7	Small droplets Large droplets Nose, pharynx, or conjunctiva	See Table 3	Over 40 serotypes Asymptomatic shedding can persist for months
Parainfluenza	RNA	1–4	Large droplets Secretions on hands	Type 1 croup, pneumonia Type 2 croup Type 3 croup, bronchiolitis, pneumonia Type 4 cold, URTI	Autumn epidemics every 2nd year Autumn every 1–2 years Summer epidemic Sporadic Reinfections common
Influenza viruses	RNA	1–6	Large droplets Small droplets Secretions on hands	Influenza, croup, pneumonia	Types A, B, C Type A can cause pandemics Amantidine only effective against type A
Respiratory syncytial virus	RNA	2–8	Secretions on hands Fomites	Bronchiolitis, pneumonia, otitis media, wheeze	Two major groups, A and B Reinfections common

URTI, upper respiratory-tract infection.

should be used for previously healthy babies with RSV infection, but it should be considered for children with underlying immune deficiency or cardiopulmonary disease.

Treatment of RSV infection is otherwise supportive. The need for supplemental oxygen is best assessed by pulse oximetry.

Summary

A comparison of features of respiratory virus infections is shown in Table 4.

REFERENCES

Buckland, F.E., Bynoe, M.L., and Tyrrell, D.A.J. (1965). Experiments on the spread of colds. II. Studies in volunteers with coxsackievirus A21. *Journal of Hygiene (Cambridge)*, **62,** 365–77.

Bynoe, M.L., Hobson, D., Horner, J., Kipps A., Schild, G.C., and Tyrrell, D.A.J. (1961). Inoculation of human volunteers with a strain of virus isolated from a common cold. *Lancet*, **i,** 1194–6.

Cohen, S., Tyrrell, D.A.J., and Smith, A.O. (1991). Psychological stress and susceptibility to the common cold. *New England Journal of Medicine*, **325,** 606–12.

D'Alessio, D.J., Meschievitz, C.K., and Peterson, J.A. (1984). Short-duration exposure and the transmission of rhinoviral colds. *Journal of Infectious Diseases*, **150,** 189–94.

Dick, E.C., Hossain, S.U., and Mink, K.A. (1986). Interruption of transmission of rhinovirus colds among human volunteers using virucidal paper handkerchiefs. *Journal of Infectious Diseases*, **153,** 352–6.

Dick, E.C., Jennings, L.C., Mink, K.A., Wartgow, C.D., and Inhorn, S.L. (1987). Aerosol transmission of rhinovirus colds. *Journal of Infectious Diseases*, **156,** 442–8.

Editorial (1988). Splints don't stop colds—surprising! *Lancet*, **i,** 277–8.

Feigin, R.D. and Cherry, J.D. (1992). *Textbook of pediatric infectious diseases*, (3rd edn.). Saunders, Philadelphia.

Hall, C.B. and Douglas, R.G., Jr. (1981). Modes of transmission of respiratory syncytial virus. *Journal of Pediatrics*, **99,** 100–3.

Lovelock, J.E., Porterfield, J.S., Roden A.T., Sommerville T., and Andrewes, C.H. (1952). Further studies on the natural transmission of the common cold. *Lancet*, **ii,** 657–60.

Ruuskanen, O., Meurman, O., and Sarkkinen, J. (1985). Adenoviral diseases in children: a study of 105 hospital cases. *Pediatrics*, **76,** 79–83.

Herpes viruses

7.10.2 Herpes simplex virus infections

T.E.A. PETO and B.E. JUEL-JENSEN

Since antiquity, medical writers have used the term herpes to describe cutaneous manifestations of infection with herpes simplex virus and varicella-zoster virus. The skin lesions of herpes simplex virus and zoster are sometimes similar, the pathological changes at cellular level produce the same type of intranuclear inclusions, and both viruses have affinities for nervous tissue. The term herpes zoster, referring to the reactivation of varicella-zoster virus, is therefore confusing. Infection with the two strains of herpes simplex viruses (**HSV-1** and **HSV-2**) causes a primary infection in the non-immune; subsequently the patient is at risk from reactivation, causing cold sores.

Epidemiology

There are no animal vectors for herpes simplex virus and humans are the only natural reservoir. It has a worldwide distribution. The capacity of these viruses to establish lifelong latent infections with intermittent reactivation and shedding ensures their survival in small, isolated pop-

Table 1 *Incidence of antibodies to herpes simplex virus (HSV) (complement-fixing), and, for later years, for comparison, to cytomegalovirus (CMV) (complement-fixing), Epstein-Barr virus (EBV) (fluorescent antibody), and varicella-zoster (V/Z) virus in Oxford clinical students. Figures in parentheses show numbers tested*

	1964–68	1976	1977	1978	1979	1980	1981	1982	1983	1984
HSV	32.8% (131)	26.7% (60)	16.9% (65)	16.4% (67)	20.3% (69)	23.5% (85)	20.5% (88)	29.3% (99)	26.7% (101)	26.7% (105)
CMV		57.4% (61)	38.3% (65)	29.2% (65)	26.9% (67)	16.4% (85)	19.3% (88)	13.4% (99)	24.8% (101)	24.8% (105)
EBV				60.0% (65)	62.3% (69)	68.2% (85)	80.7% (88)	65.7% (99)	67.3% (101)	80.0% (105)
V/Z							86.4% (88)	96.0% (99)	88.1% (101)	91.4% (105)

ulations which are otherwise too small to support the continuous circulation of viruses that cause epidemic diseases. Transmission is through direct contact with infected secretions via mucocutaneous sites or traumatized or diseased skin. Herpes simplex virus is labile and there is no evidence that transmission can occur from inanimate objects or by aerosols. Spread of HSV-1 is predominantly by contact with oral secretions and HSV-2 by genital secretions. Spread from oral secretions to other areas of skin is an occupational hazard of dentists, medical health workers, and in certain contact sports (wrestlers, exponents of judo and rugby football players). The virus can be transmitted from the genital tract sexually, during birth to the neonate, and by autoinoculation to hands, thighs, and buttocks.

Transmission can occur both from people with active herpetic lesions and from asymptomatic excretors but the actively infected person is the more infectious. Surveys have shown that between 0.65 and 15 per cent of adults are excreting herpes simplex virus at any one time. The majority of new herpes simplex virus infections (1 and 2) are transmitted from asymptomatic carriers. Because more than 80 per cent of primary infections are asymptomatic the prevalence of the disease is best assessed by serological surveys, although standard complement-fixing antibody tests cannot distinguish HSV-1 from HSV-2. The prevalence of infection is changing. Until the 1950s, seroepidemiological studies showed a seroprevalence of about 90 per cent by the fourth decade of life. Since then, rates in the higher socioeconomic groups have shown a slow decline. For instance, in 1953 in the United Kingdom, 85 per cent of a sample of children aged between 3 and 15 years had antibodies compared to only 41 per cent when the survey was repeated in 1965. In the period 1964–8, 33 per cent of 181 British-born Oxford clinical students had antibodies, contrasting with 62 per cent of 42 students born in Third World countries. Only a third gave a history of recurrent cold sores or other herpetic manifestations. Table 1 shows that the trend has continued. It will be noted that the incidence of cytomegalovirus has dropped over the 10-year period 1976–85, possibly because an increasing proportion of students have been to day schools where the incidence of this infection is lower than in boarding schools. These studies indicated that in the past most primary infections of HSV-1 occurred in early childhood. In recent years, however, a second peak of transmission has appeared in early adult life. For example, in a study of college students in the United States, only 30 per cent were seropositive for HSV-1 infection on admission and primary infection subsequently occurred in about 10 per cent a year of the susceptible students.

In contrast to HSV-1, HSV-2 is the predominant cause of genital herpes. The highest rate of infection occurs between the ages of 15 and 25 years. The prevalence of HSV-2 antibodies is dependent on sexual activity, ranging from 0 per cent in celibate adults to over 80 per cent in prostitutes.

Pathogenesis

Herpes simplex viruses (herpes hominis) (HSV-1 and -2) are members of the herpesvirus family, which in man includes varicella-zoster virus, Epstein–Barr virus, human cytomegalovirus, and herpesvirus type 6. The virus has an internal core containing a double-stranded DNA of about 150 kbp encoding about 33 virion proteins; a further 30 proteins are expressed during cellular infection. HSV-1 and -2 share about half their nucleotide sequence and express functionally equivalent proteins. The two strains differ antigenically and biologically.

On entry into skin sites, herpes simplex virus replicates locally in parabasal and intermediate epithelial cells, causing cell lysis resulting in a local inflammatory response. The early papules are associated with multinucleated giant cells formed by the fusion of infected and uninfected neighbouring cells. The typical vesicles are caused by cell degeneration and oedema fluid, which elevates the stratum corneum. The vesicle fluid contains degenerating cells, multinucleated giant cells, and cell-free virus. Evolution of vesicles into pustules is associated with invasion by inflammatory cells.

After the primary infection, herpes simplex virus may invade sensory nerves and become latent within their ganglia. The exact mechanism of latency remains unclear. Work on animal models and neuronal cell-culture systems suggests that latent virions are present not only in neuronal but also in non-neuronal cells of the sensory ganglion. Metabolically, the virus in the latent phase does not transcribe genes responsible for its reproduction but it does transcribe a family of RNAs (latency-associated transcripts). The function of these sequences is unclear. One theory suggests that they are the antisense sequence of a protein critical for the activation of the virus; another suggestion is that they encode for a protein which may be responsible for the maintenance of latency. Reactivation of the virus can be triggered by fever, trauma, stress, sunlight, and menstruation but the precise mechanism for this is not yet understood, although increased blood flow in the nerve cells may be a common factor.

Clinical manifestations

The clinical manifestations of HSV-1 and -2 overlap. Both types cause genital and orofacial infections, and these infections are clinically indistinguishable. However, the frequency of future reactivations is influenced by the anatomical site and the type of virus. Recurrence of genital HSV-2 infection is more common than genital HSV-1 infection, whereas orofacial HSV-1 infection recurs more frequently than orofacial HSV-2 infection.

The primary infection is frequently asymptomatic but, especially in adults, may be serious and occasionally fatal. Any skin site may be involved, although perioral and genital areas are most commonly affected.

OROFACIAL INFECTION

Primary infection

The incubation period ranges from 2 to 12 days and in symptomatic cases is followed by high fever, sore throat, and pharyngeal oedema. The disease can be trivial, especially in children (Fig. 1), but more severe, painful vesicles may appear a few days later on the pharyngeal and oral mucosa, spreading to an extensive gingivostomatitis (Fig. 2 and Plate 1). Hypersalivation and drooling often occur. Lesions may extend to the lips and cheeks. In adults the disease is sometimes confined to the pharynx and tonsils. The high fever, toxicity, and severe mouth pain can persist for several days. The fever is accompanied by generalized muscle pains and sometimes rigors. There is cervical lymphadenopathy and sometimes splenomegaly. In some cases, patients cannot eat or drink. Without treatment the illness subsides after about 10 to 14 days and the vesicles heal slowly. Occasionally, autoinoculation occurs to other sites, especially on the fingers.

The diagnosis is usually made clinically from the widespread oral lesions together with a severe systemic disease. The diagnosis is often missed simply because it is not considered. The main differential diagnosis is severe Stevens–Johnson syndrome or severe, non-specific, aphthous ulceration. A good many cases of so-called 'Vincent's angina' are probably examples of herpetic gingivostomatitis. The other three herpesvirus infections must be excluded. Zoster of the second branch of the trigeminal nerve confined to the mouth has caught the unwary (Fig. 3). It is, of course, unilateral. Infectious mononucleosis may give an identical picture (Plate 2(a)), as may cytomegalovirus infection. Coxsackie and echoviruses must also be excluded (Plate 2(b),(c)), and bacterial infections, particularly β-haemolytic streptococcal infection and diphtheria, should be considered.

Fig. 1 Primary herpetic stomatitis. A single lesion on the tongue of a 6-year-old boy.

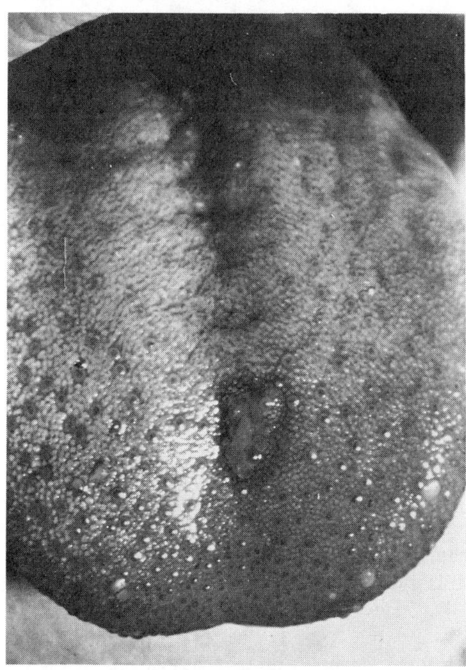

Fig. 2 Primary herpetic gingivostomatitis in a man of 25. Lesions on the tongue and gums.

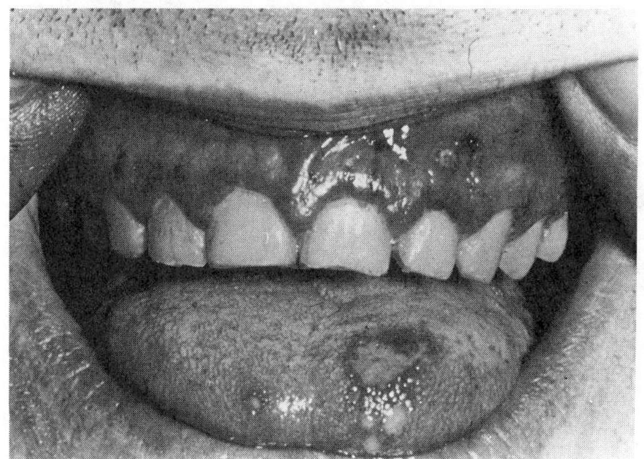

Recurrent infections (cold sore; herpes labialis, fever blisters)

Recurrent lesions usually occur on the skin innervated by the cutaneous branches of the maxillary and mandibular branches of the trigeminal nerve. They usually recur in the same site for each patient. Recurrent herpes labialis usually starts with localized prodromal symptoms (pain, burning, tingling or itching) lasting from 6 to 48 h. Vesicles most commonly occur on the lips or skin around the mouth, and in the nostrils, and are often painful. There are usually no systemic symptoms associated with recurrences. After several days the lesions crust; complete healing takes about 10 days. Sometimes the lesions are secondarily infected.

Recurrent cold sores due to HSV-1 occur in about 30 per cent of the seropositive population but are less frequent in those with HSV-2. The frequency of recurrences varies greatly and has not been well documented. Fewer than 10 per cent have more than one attack per month, while about half the seropositive population have fewer than two attacks per year. There appears to be a decrease in the frequency of recurrences with time. Trigger factors for reactivation include sunlight, menstruation, fever, stress, and local trauma.

Diagnosis is usually easy. The main differential diagnosis includes zoster, which rarely recurs in the same site. In hand, foot, and mouth disease (Plate 2(c)), caused by a coxsackievirus, there are usually vesicular lesions on the hands and feet as well. Impetigo can be confused with infected herpetic lesions, just as herpetic lesions may be secondarily infected with staphylococcal abscesses.

HERPETIC WHITLOW

The herpetic whitlow is an occupational disease of medical personnel, dentists, nurses, and physiotherapists. Patients with a high fever or those with a tracheostomy are particularly likely to excrete virus in their secretions. In children, whitlows can result from autoinoculation. The skin of the hand is rarely intact, allowing the virus to invade. Usually only one finger is infected, although infection may spread to an adjoining finger (Plate 3).

The incubation period of the primary infection is about 2 to 7 days. The whitlow is extremely painful. The digit swells, becomes red, and, like all primary infections, is accompanied by painful lymphadenopathy, high fever, and systemic disease. A day or two later the typical vesicle develops, with clear fluid evolving into a cloudy fluid and then into a yellow, crusty lesion. Without treatment, recovery from the systemic illness takes about 2 weeks, while the skin may take up to 4 weeks to heal and virus may be recovered from the finger for about 3 weeks. Very occasionally a toe may be affected (Fig. 4).

A good history should lead to the correct diagnosis. The main differential diagnosis is a bacterial infection and, unfortunately, because of the intense pain and systemic toxicity, incision for drainage is often

Fig. 3 Lesions in mouth of a patient with zoster (and see Plate 2).

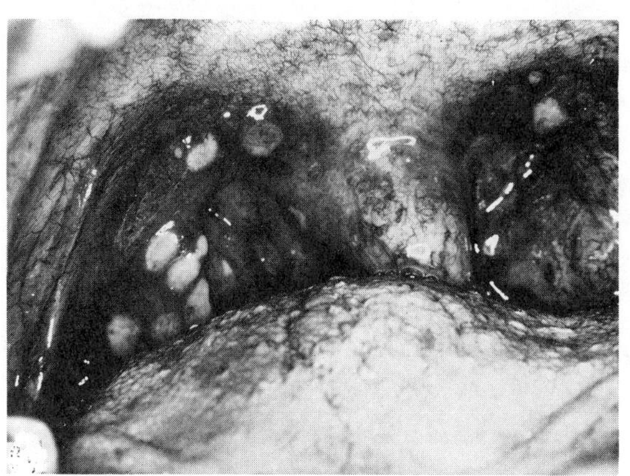

attempted, which will only spread the infection. On rare occasions, it can be confused with orf and vaccinia.

Recurrent whitlows are less common than recurrent cold sores. They are often heralded and accompanied by severe neuralgic pain in the hand and arm, and the vesicles are associated with oedema of the hand, lymphangitis, and regional lymphadenopathy.

TRAUMATIC HERPES; HERPES GLADIATORUM; SCRUM POX

Primary herpes can occur in any part of the skin if it is traumatized. The clinical course is similar to that of the herpetic whitlow. Herpes gladiatorum occurs in contact sports such as wrestling, judo or rugby football in players whose faces come into close contact with other parts of the body (Fig. 5). If the cheek is affected the differential diagnosis includes cellulitis, impetigo, and trigeminal zoster. There may be recurrence at the site of the primary infection.

GENITAL HERPES (SEE ALSO CHAPTER 21.3)

Primary genital herpes occurs after sexual contact. The illness is similar to other primary infections. In women there is often a vaginal discharge with severe genital pain, dysuria and urinary retention. Herpetic lesions involve the vulva, perineum, buttocks (Plate 4), cervix, and vagina. Extragenital lesions are common. Whereas women often have severe systemic illness, men usually have a milder primary attack. An accompanying sacroradiculomyelitis can cause urinary retention, neuralgia, and constipation. In men the vesicles occur on the shaft of the penis (Fig. 6) or the glans, together with an associated urethritis. Herpes simplex proctitis occurs after anorectal intercourse: symptoms include anorectal pain and discharge, tenesmus, constipation, sacral paraesthesiae, impotence, and urinary retention. Sigmoidoscopy reveals ulcerative lesions up to 10 cm.

About 70 per cent of cases will have recurrent infections within the first year of primary infection. The rate of recurrence is about 0.33 attacks per month for HSV-2 and less than 0.1 attacks per month for HSV-1. Recurrence rates tend to decrease with time. Recurrent attacks are less severe than the primary attack and more severe in women than in men.

Fig. 4 Herpetic whitlow of the big toe of a man aged 24.

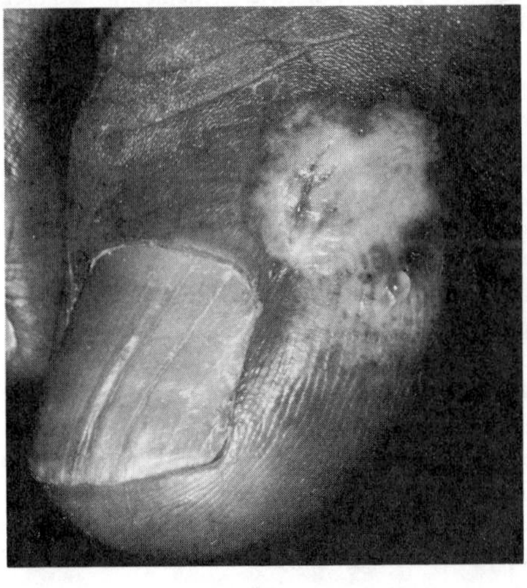

Fig. 5 Herpes gladiatorum in a sixth-form public school rugby football player.

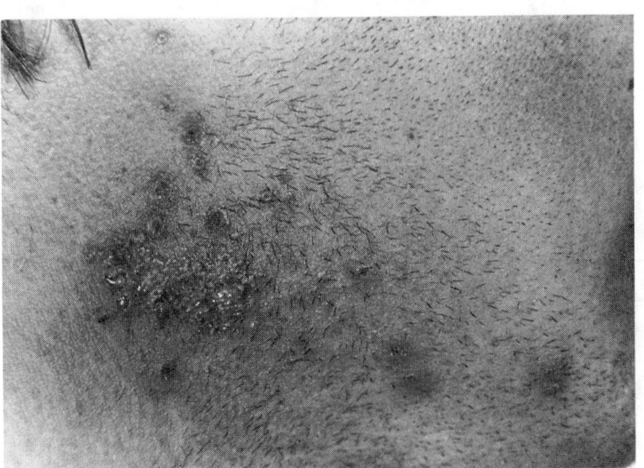

OCULAR HERPES

Primary infections present with fever and constitutional symptoms, together with a unilateral follicular conjunctivitis, or a blepharitis with vesicles on the lids, and preauricular lymphadenopathy. There is associated photophobia, chemosis, excessive lacrimation, and oedema of the eyelids. In uncomplicated cases, the symptoms spontaneously resolve completely within 2 to 3 weeks. However, in some cases there is involvement of the cornea, producing acute herpetic keratoconjunctivitis to form the characteristic branching ('dendritic') lesions. There is pain and a foreign-body sensation. Occasionally the underlying stroma is affected, which can lead to corneal ulceration or corneal scarring. The use of topical cortico steroids may exacerbate the symptoms and make permanent corneal damage more likely.

Recurrences happen in about 25 per cent of cases and are a serious ophthalmological problem. Recurrent infections usually present as a keratitis with dendritic ulceration, seen with fluorescein stains, or stromal involvement. Repeated attacks can lead to corneal scarring and neovascularization, with eventual loss of vision.

Ophthalmic herpes should be managed and treated by specialist ophthalmologists.

INFECTIONS OF THE CENTRAL NERVOUS SYSTEM (SEE ALSO CHAPTER 24.15.2)

Herpes simplex encephalitis

This is an acute necrotizing viral encephalitis with a mortality, untreated, of over 70 per cent, and a high incidence of neurological sequelae in survivors. Except in newborns, the infection is usually caused by HSV-1. Serological data suggest that about 50 per cent of cases are due to primary infection. It is a rare disease with an estimated frequency in

Fig. 6 Primary genital herpes due to type 2 virus (and see Plate 4).

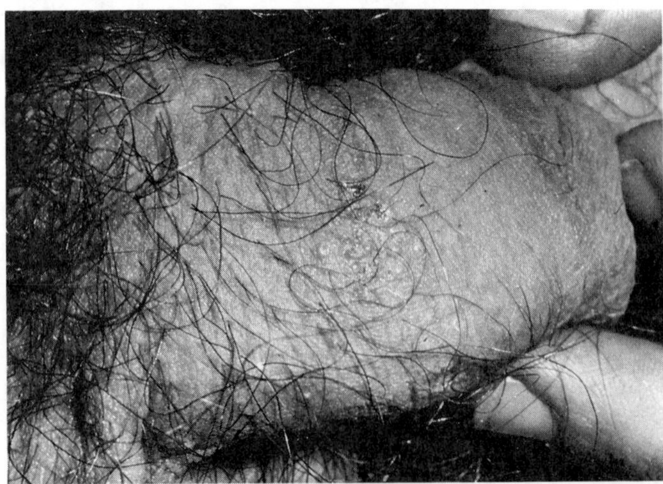

the United States of about 1 in 400 000 persons per year. It can occur at any age and does not appear to be more frequent in the immunosuppressed host.

Presentation is with high fever, headache, nausea, and vomiting, followed by reduced consciousness and seizures. Sometimes there are signs of meningeal irritation. Focal neurological signs typically involve the temporal, orbitofrontal cortex, and limbic systems. Patients have dysphasia, hallucinations, peculiar behaviour, and memory loss. In some cases there is rapid progression to coma and death. There are usually no skin manifestations of herpes simplex infection. In other cases, progression is slower, with several days of lethargy and bizarre behaviour, which can be confused with acute psychosis or delirium tremens. The differential diagnosis includes other cases of encephalitis including simian herpes virus encephalitis (see Chapter 7.10.5), cerebral abscess, and meningitis. Computerized tomographic scanning or magnetic resonance imaging of the brain will show typical features of changes in the temporal lobes. Lumbar puncture should only be attempted if the clinician is certain there is not significant cerebral oedema. Examination of the cerebrospinal fluid shows a moderate pleocytosis, mildly elevated protein concentration, and normal glucose concentration. Virus is only rarely isolated from the fluid but may be detected by polymerase chain reaction. Definitive diagnosis can be made by demonstrating virus in a brain biopsy but this is rarely indicated clinically. Characteristically the serum (and cerebrospinal fluid) complement-fixing antibody rises from zero to titres of greater than 1/1000.

Herpes simplex meningitis

In contrast to herpes simplex encephalitis, herpes simplex causes a relatively benign lymphocytic meningitis in normal adults, often in association with HSV-2 genital herpes. The virus can occasionally be isolated from the cerebrospinal fluid. Symptoms usually resolve in about a week. About 20 per cent of cases recur, usually in association with genital herpes.

Idiopathic neurological syndromes

Herpes simplex has been implicated in the aetiology of Bell's palsy, trigeminal neuralgia, atypical pain syndromes, ascending myelitis, Mollaret's recurrent meningitis, and temporal-lobe epilepsy. However, these associations depend mainly on serological evidence and the precise role of herpes simplex virus in the aetiology of these syndromes has not been definitely established, but there is increasing evidence, from the use of polymerase chain reaction, that Mollaret's meningitis may be caused/associated with HSV-1 or -2 infection.

VISCERAL AND DISSEMINATED INFECTIONS

Infection of visceral organs occurs only rarely. Oropharyngeal herpes can extend into the oesophagus, especially in the presence of nasogastric tubes, causing dysphagia, substernal pain, and weight loss. Ulcers are seen on endoscopy. Similarly extension can occur, following endotracheal intubation, to the bronchial tree and lungs, causing pneumonia. Very rarely, herpes simplex virus is a cause of hepatitis and, in a few cases, especially in pregnant women in the third trimester or transplant recipients, can be part of a fulminating, disseminated infection. There is associated leucopenia, thrombocytopenia, and disseminated intravascular coagulation.

NEONATAL INFECTIONS

Infection in the newborn ranges from a mild disease to a fatal disseminated infection. In the United States the incidence is about 1 in 2500 to 1 in 10 000, while in the United Kingdom the disease is less common. Most infections are caused by spread of herpes simplex virus from the maternal genital tract or sometimes postnatally from nurses with oral herpes or herpetic whitlows. It is unclear to what extent infection occurs either before the onset of labour or during passage of the fetus through the birth canal. The use of fetal scalp monitoring may increase the risk of transmission. Infection can also occur with asymptomatic infections. The risk of neonatal infection is about 40 per cent with active primary infection but less than 8 per cent with recurrent infections at the time of delivery.

Neonatal infection appears several days or even weeks after birth. It presents as a neonatal sepsis syndrome, often with vesicles or conjunctivitis. If untreated, it rapidly progresses to seizures, cranial-nerve palsies, lethargy, and later visceral dissemination. Overall the mortality is 65 per cent, with only 10 per cent escaping neurological sequelae.

Congenital infection, a consequence of primary infection early in pregnancy, can cause severe abnormalities, which, in the absence of vesicles, are difficult to distinguish from similar syndromes caused by rubella, toxoplasmosis or cytomegalovirus.

HERPES SIMPLEX VIRUS IN THE IMMUNOCOMPROMISED HOST

Patients with impaired cellular immunity are at risk from severe disease. They include organ transplant recipients on immunosuppressive chemotherapy, patients with lymphoreticular malignancies, haematological malignancies and AIDS, and children with congenital immunodeficiencies or malnutrition.

Immunosuppressed patients are at risk from disseminated disease following primary infection. Recurrences are also more frequent in these patients. Although recurrent herpes often resolves spontaneously, the vesicles sometimes enlarge slowly, ulcerate, and become necrotic, extending to deeper tissues (Fig. 7). The lesions spread slowly both on the skin and into the oesophagus and trachea. In spite of this spread, dissemination following recurrent infections is rare.

HERPES SIMPLEX IN SKIN DISORDERS

Eczema herpeticum; Juliusberg's pustolosis acuta varioliformis; Kaposi's varicelliform eruption

Herpes simplex infections are much more severe and extensive in patients with underlying skin disorders. Patients with eczema, burns, pemphigus, Darier's disease, and Sezary's syndrome are unable to contain the infection, which causes widespread cutaneous dissemination (Plate 5). As these patients are often on corticosteroid treatment, the spread of the lytic herpes simplex is further facilitated. There are usually systemic symptoms: fever, rigors, general adenopathy, and enlargement of the liver and spleen. Untreated the condition is likely to recur, although the systemic symptoms may be less severe.

Fig. 7 Severe herpetic stomatitis in a woman of 64 on immunosuppressive doses of steroid.

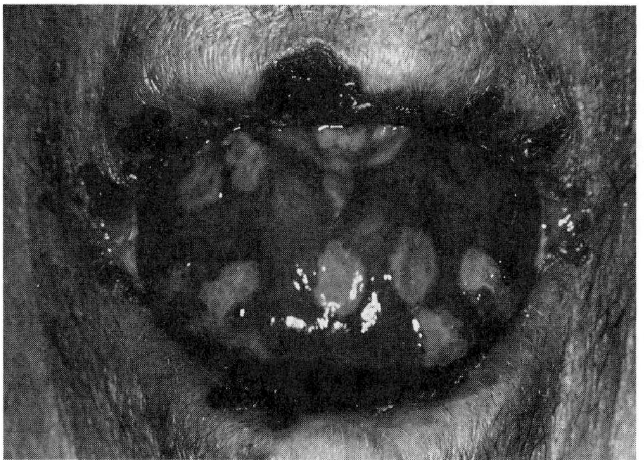

The term 'Kaposi's varicelliform eruption' is misplaced, not least because Moricz Kaposi* was not the first to notice the condition, which he thought was a complication of infantile eczema, possibly caused by fungi. It had been described earlier by Fritz Juliusberg, who thought it was caused by staphylococci. The use of an eponym has led to further confusion, for the term 'Kaposi's varicelliform eruption' has, without justification, been used to describe eczema vaccinatum.

Herpes simplex and erythema multiforme

Recurrent herpes simplex infections may be associated with erythema multiforme. About 15 per cent of all cases of erythema multiforme are preceded by a symptomatic attack of recurrent herpes simplex. In susceptible individuals, the skin rash can be induced by the intradermal inoculation of inactivated herpes simplex virus antigen. The rash starts several days after the onset of the herpetic vesicles. In severe cases the rash can involve the mucous membranes (Stevens–Johnson syndrome). The frequency of these attacks can be reduced by acyclovir prophylaxis.

Diagnosis

Most cases of herpes simplex infection can be made on clinical grounds alone. Confirmation is best made by the isolation of the virus from vesicles. Direct examination of the fluid by electron microscopy may demonstrate herpesvirus particles. Virus in vesicle fluid or other infected bodily secretions can be grown in tissue culture, and typical cytopathic effects are seen sometimes within a few hours with high inocula but may rarely take up to 2 weeks for low-titre specimens. A variety of methods is available for more rapid and specific identification techniques, including monoclonal antibodies specific to HSV-1 and -2 antigens and DNA-typing methods. Serological tests using complement-fixation or the more sensitive neutralization tests depend on the demonstration of rising titres of antibody to herpes simplex virus in paired sera. This test can only be used for the retrospective diagnosis of primary infection and for epidemiological surveys. Only about 5 per cent of patients with recurrent attacks show a greater than fourfold rise in antibody titre.

Treatment

The treatment of herpes simplex has been revolutionized by the development of antiviral drugs. Acyclovir is the most commonly used antiviral in herpes simplex virus infection, and because it is usually effective at non-toxic concentrations it has replaced vidarabine and other earlier antiviral drugs. It is safe—neurotoxicity has been described rarely. The drawback is unpredictable absorption from the gut, so that relatively high doses need to be given. If the drug is given intravenously too quickly, reversible renal dysfunction can occur. Intravenous acyclovir (10–15 mg/kg, 8-hourly for 10 days) reduces the mortality and morbidity of herpes simplex encephalitis and neonatal herpes simplex infections. In contrast, oral acyclovir (200 mg, five times day for 7 days) is sufficient for the treatment of uncomplicated primary infections. If swallowing is difficult, intravenous acyclovir (5 mg/kg, 8-hourly) may need to be given. Acyclovir reduces the severity of infection, the duration of symptoms, and the duration of viral shedding. The expense of the drug is the main disadvantage for its widespread use in herpes infections. Unfortunately, there is only the slightest evidence that treatment of primary infections reduces the incidence of recurrent infections.

Treatment of recurrent infections in the immunocompetent host is often unnecessary as the symptoms are usually very mild. However, acyclovir can shorten the duration of symptoms if it is given very early in the course of the recurrence. Oral acyclovir is effective and anecdotal reports suggest that topical acyclovir is effective symptomatically. In view of the cost, treatment should be considered if the recurrences are particularly distressing or if they are complicated by erythema multiforme.

Long-term acyclovir is undoubtedly successful in preventing most recurrent infection. In many cases a low dose (200mg/day) is sufficient to prevent recurrences; the minimum dose varies between individuals. Because of the cost and an obvious reluctance to prescribe drugs for long-term prophylaxis, this is not routinely recommended. However, patients who are in great distress from frequent recurrent attacks should be considered for treatment as there is no evidence that there is any toxicity from long-term use.

Immunocompromised patients often have more severe recurrent disease and therefore benefit more from acyclovir treatment. In some cases, patients with AIDS develop chronic mucocutanous herpes simplex disease. In this setting, where the virus is continuously replicating, suppressive treatment with acyclovir can lead to resistant strains, with the development of thymidine kinase-deficient mutant strains. These are usually still sensitive to vidarabine or foscarnet.

Prevention

Avoidance of exposure to herpes simplex is difficult because many carriers are asymptomatic shedders of virus, and their mild primary infection has gone unnoticed. However, medical, paramedical, and dental staff should be advised to wear gloves every time they are in contact with bodily secretions. Newborn infants are at particular risk from infection, and medical personnel who have herpetic whitlows should not handle these babies.

The prevention of neonatal herpes infection is controversial. Mothers with primary genital infections shortly before birth are at high risk of infecting their babies. Although caesarian section is commonly done, its efficacy in preventing neonatal infection has not been proven. Regardless of the mode of delivery it is probably prudent to treat the mother, antenatally, for primary infection. The management of healthy newborn babies of mothers with active genital lesions (primary or secondary) is unclear. Some clinicians prefer to treat all such children with acyclovir emperically while others prefer to only treat once symptoms in the infant develop.

REFERENCES

Corey, M.D. and Spear, P.G. (1986) Infections with herpes simplex viruses. *New England Journal of Medicine,* **314,** 686–91; 749–57.

Juel-Jensen, B.E. and MacCallum, F.O. (1972) *Herpes simplex, varicella and zoster.* Heinemann, London.

Puchhammer-Stockl, E. *et al.* (1993). Evaluation of the polymerase chain reaction for diagnosis of herpes simplex encephalitis. *Journal of Clinical Microbiology,* **31,** 146–8.

Rooney, J.F. *et al.* (1993). Oral acyclovir to suppress frequently recurrent herpes labialis. A double-blind placebo controlled trial. *Annals of Internal Medicine,* **118,** 268–72.

Symposium (1993). Herpes: a global challenge. *Journal of Medical Virology,* Supplement 1.

Wagstaff, A.J., Faulds, D., and Goa, K.L. (1994). Acyclovir. A reappraisal of its antiviral activity, pharmacokinetic properties and therapeutic efficacy. *Drugs,* **47,** 153–205.

7.10.3 Varicella-zoster virus infections: chickenpox and zoster

T.E.A. Peto and B.E. Juel-Jensen

Varicella-zoster virus causes two distinct clinical entities, chickenpox (varicella) and zoster (shingles). The primary infection in the non-immune host is chickenpox. After the acute, often trivial, primary infec-

* Kaposi is pronounced 'Kawposhi' with the accent on the first syllable as in all Hungarian words (Rothman, S. (1963). Some remarks on Moricz Kaposi and on the history of Kaposi's sarcoma. In *Symposium on Kaposi's sarcoma,* (ed. L.V. Ackerman and J.F. Murray), pp. 9–12. Karger, Basel.)

tion, the virus becomes latent in nerve cells. In the 'immune' host, reactivation of the virus results in zoster, a predominantly dermatomal infection.

Epidemiology

Humans are the only known reservoir of infection. Varicella-zoster virus is the most infectious of the human herpesviruses. Transmission is by droplets from nasopharyngeal secretions (chickenpox) or from vesicular fluid (chickenpox or zoster). Patients are infectious for 2 days before the onset of the rash until the skin lesions are crusted. The incubation period is about 15 days (range 10–21 days). The attack rate within household non-immune contacts is about 90 per cent after chickenpox but only 15 per cent after zoster. In temperate countries about 90 per cent of the population are seropositive by early adulthood, but in tropical countries only 50 per cent of young adults are seropositive. The reasons for this difference are unknown. Outbreaks of chickenpox can occur in clusters, although transmission occurs throughout the year. Contact histories with index cases are commonly found.

Following the primary infection there is a relatively increased risk of zoster in the first year of life and in elderly people. Outbreaks of zoster are sporadic and do not occur in clusters, although some seasonal variation is found. Trauma, of whatever kind, which leads to increased blood flow to ganglia may be responsible for reactivation. The chance of young, seropositive adults acquiring zoster is about 0.7/1000 per year, rising to 10/1000 per year in people over 80 years old. Overall, at least 20 per cent of all adults suffer from zoster at some time and about 1 per cent suffer two attacks. The risk of zoster is greatly enhanced by immunosuppression or in patients infected with the human immunodeficiency virus (**HIV**).

Pathology

Varicella-zoster virus is a member of the herpesviridiae. The virus has icosahedral symmetry containing 125 000 bp of double-stranded DNA with a surrounding envelope. The DNA encodes about 71 proteins. Only enveloped virions are infectious and the envelope is sensitive to air drying, detergents, and ether. The virus can infect a variety of cell cultures, particularly those derived from human embryos or foreskin. The virus does not readily infect other animals, consequently much of the pathophysiology has been determined from autopsy examination or inferred from animal infections with other herpesviruses.

After primary infection the virus enters the host, spreads locally in the upper respiratory tract, and there is thought to be a primary viraemia in the first week spreading to the reticuloendothelial system. Shortly before the clinical illness, a secondary viraemic phase has been described, resulting in spread to the skin and the mucosal surfaces. Virus spreads to endothelial cells of the skin and then infects the basal and deep spinous layers of the epidermis. Local extracellular oedema results in vesicles. In addition, multinucleation occurs, with condensation of viral proteins within the nuclei resulting in intranuclear inclusions. The infection is contained by the appearance of both humoral and cell-mediated immune responses.

Following the primary infection, the virus becomes latent in the sensory ganglia and in motor neurones. Recent *in situ* hybridization studies with varicella-zoster virus-specific RNA probes suggest that the virus lies dormant predominantly in perineuronal rather than neuronal cells. The molecular basis for latency and the trigger for the reactivation of the virus are unknown. Histopathological studies have shown that the ganglion is the site of intense inflammation, with haemorrhagic necrosis of nerve cells and destruction of portions of the ganglion. There is degeneration of axons and myelin, and virus particles occur in the cytoplasm and nuclei of epidermal cells, in the cytoplasm of perineural cells, and in both cytoplasm and nuclei of Schwann cells. Both cytoplasm and nuclei of ganglion cells are full of virus particles. The development of live, attenuated vaccines has led to speculation that repeated exposures to natural or vaccine strains of virus in immune individuals can enhance the immune status of the host and delay reactivation and hence the development of zoster.

Chickenpox

In children, there are usually no or minimal prodromal symptoms and the characteristic centripetal rash is the first manifestation of the illness. It may be so slight—like a few drops of water on the skin—that it is missed. In older children the rash itches and the child recovers without complications.

In adults, the prodromal symptoms are more common and occasionally severe. Severe headaches, general aches and pains, severe backaches, fever, and extreme malaise are typical. There may be a transient pink rash before the vesicles erupt. The vesicles tend to be irregular (Plate 1(a),(b)). Within 12 h the vesicles become papular and then progress to pustules and subsequently to scabs. Normally the scabs fall at the end of 10 days. No scar is left unless the scabs have been scratched. Characteristically, different crops of vesicles appear over 3 to 4 days, starting with the head and progressing to the trunk and limbs. All stages of the exanthem are seen in the same region of the skin. The infection is not only limited to the skin and therefore can lead to more serious complications.

COMPLICATIONS IN THE IMMUNOCOMPETENT HOST

Overall, the mortality of chickenpox in immunocompetent individuals is low. Mortality is age dependent. Neonates are at highest risk, while the mortality in children aged 1 to 14 years is only about 1 in 70 000 cases. In adults the mortality rises to 1 in 3000 and is probably much higher in older patients, although this has not been studied systematically. Pregnant women are at increased risk from serious infections and a mortality as high as 1 per cent has been reported in some series.

Pneumonitis

Pneumonitis is uncommon in children but reaches an incidence of about 0.3 per cent in immunocompetent adults. Smokers are particularly susceptible. Patients present with breathlessness, cough, hypoxia, and bilateral chest infiltrates on the chest radiograph a few days after the onset of the chickenpox (Fig 1). In severe cases the disease can rapidly progress, with increasing shortness of breath, pulmonary oedema, cyanosis, and chest pain. The pneumonitis can be fatal, even with mechanical ventilation and intensive care. The clinical picture can be mistaken for carcinomatosis or miliary tuberculosis. If patients survive, their long-term pulmonary prognosis is excellent. Minor chest radiographic changes occur asymptomatically in about 16 per cent of young adults and, if not associated with hypoxia, have an excellent prognosis: the chest radiographic changes occasionally progress to those of benign nodular calcification.

Encephalitis

Mild encephalitis is not uncommon and can occur within 10 days before and several days after the onset of the rash. Patients commonly present with cerebellar signs or encephalopathy, and the condition is associated with a pleocytosis and elevated protein in the cerebrospinal fluid. Severe encephalitis is uncommon; cerebellar ataxia has an excellent prognosis and, in contrast to herpes simplex encephalitis, varicella-zoster viral encephalitis is less serious, with a mortality of about 5 per cent.

Thrombocytopenia and bleeding disorders: purpura fulminans

Both disseminated intravascular coagulation and idiopathic thrombocytopenia are rare but potentially life-threatening disorders in chickenpox. At least 20 cases have been described. Following typical chickenpox, ecchymoses appear symmetrically in the lower extremitites, and occasionally on the arms (Plate 2) from 5 to 18 days after the rash began.

Large areas of skin slough, and there is extensive tissue necrosis. Four out of a group of 18 patients died in renal failure, shock or sepsis, and 11 lost some part of their limbs. There is a low prothrombin and reduced factors V, VII, VIII, and X. Intravascular coagulation takes place in the peripheral vessels and the picture is one of thrombotic purpura. The best treatment is unclear but fresh-frozen plasma combined with heparin have been used.

Recurrent chickenpox

Recurrent chickenpox in otherwise healthy individuals is extremely rare. In Oxford, one family has been seen where four brothers had many attacks. The index case, a boy of 15, had a second, very severe attack of chicken pox (Fig. 2). A brother of 19 had two, one of 18 and one of 16 three attacks, all of increasing severity. The parents and two sisters had had only one attack of mild chickenpox. In other respects the boys were normal.

Secondary bacterial infection

Secondary infection with bacteria, particularly staphylococci and streptococci, is not uncommon, particularly if the lesions are scratched. Although secondary bacterial infections of the respiratory tract can occur, the incidence is much lower than after other viral infections such as influenza or measles.

CHICKENPOX IN THE IMMUNOCOMPROMISED HOST

Patients on corticosteroids, receiving immunosuppression for organ transplants or vasculitis, receiving intensive chemotherapy for lymphoproliferative disorders or with late HIV disease are at greater risk from severe chickenpox. The skin lesions can continue cropping for much longer and the patients are at risk from a generalized systemic illness. The mortality in children on treatment for leukaemias has reached 18 per cent in some series, even when treated with antiviral drugs.

MATERNAL, CONGENITAL, AND PERINATAL INFECTION (SEE ALSO CHAPTER 13.12.1.)

Pregnancy increases the risk of chickenpox and a mortality of 1 per cent with an incidence of pneumonitis of 10 per cent have been reported in some series. There is also a risk to the fetus and newborn child. Chickenpox in the first and second trimester is associated with a rare varicella syndrome of skin scarring, hypoplastic extremities, eye abnormalities, and evidence of central nervous impairment. The precise risk of congenital abnormalities is unknown but is likely to be about 1 per cent. Chickenpox in the newborn following maternal infection in the third trimester is serious; about 10 per cent have severe disease. The overall mortality has not been fully assessed but may not be as large as early reports suggested. If possible, delivery should be delayed to allow time for antibodies to appear in the maternal plasma, thereby protecting the newborn.

Fig. 1 Chest radiograph of the young man shown in Plates 1(a) and (b), who had severe chickenpox infection also involving the lungs. There are scattered infiltrates, which, in the course of the next few days, coalesced, giving a clinical picture of adult respiratory distress syndrome. The patient survived.

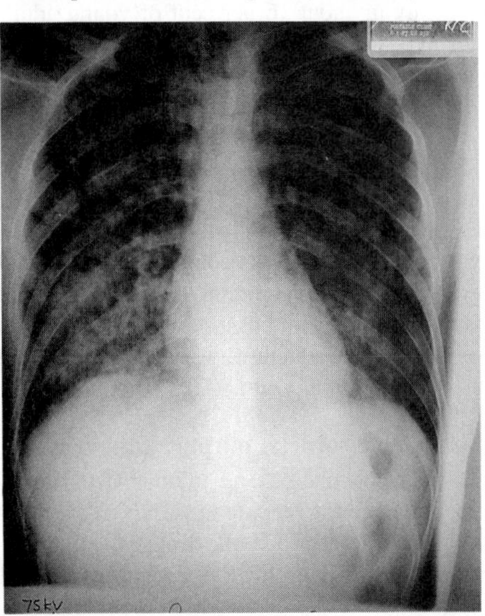

Zoster

Shingles and zoster both mean 'a belt'; the Norwegians call it 'belt of roses from hell'; the Danes call it 'hellfire', a very apt description. It is usually preceded by paraesthesia over the affected dermatome, in most, perhaps two-thirds of all patients, by shooting pains, which precede the eruption by 2 to 3 days but sometimes as much as 3 weeks. A few patients get pain at no stage of the illness. Erythematous, maculopapular lesions appear that rapidly evolve into a vesicular rash. In the normal host, these lesions continue to form over a period of 3 to 5 days (Fig. 3). The rash is often accompanied by a mild systemic illness with a low-grade fever but no haematological or biochemical changes. The vesicles normally scab after 3 to 7 days, and all dry scabs have separated at the end of a fortnight. Untreated, the lesions often become infected with *Staphylococcus aureus.*

The eruption varies greatly. In the young it is often trivial, with a single or a few groups of vesicles and, in particular on the face, it may be mistaken for herpes simplex. In severe cases a whole or several dermatomes may be involved, with an oedematous base and a dense rash covering the entire segment. The rash is characteristically unilateral and bilateral zoster is very rare. Zoster can occur on any dermatome. Often there are some outlying lesions—varying from a few to a dense eruption. These eruptions occur in the early days of the disease before antibodies

Fig. 2 Severe recurrent chickenpox.

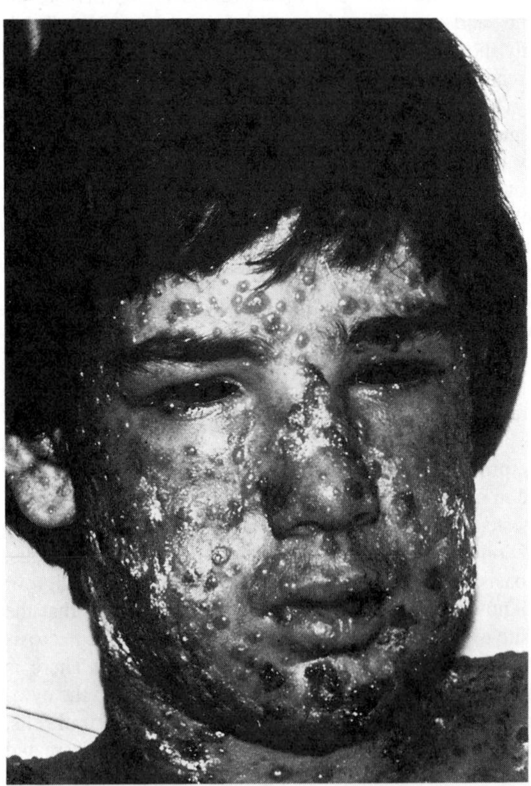

have reappeared. Except in the immune deficient, dissemination is not necessarily serious. Rarely, reactivation occurs without a rash—zoster sine herpete. Patients can present with pain that has a dermatomal distribution. There are case reports implicating zoster as the cause of polyneuropathy, myelitis, aseptic meningitis, and severe hepatic necrosis.

COMPLICATIONS

Ophthalmic zoster

When zoster affects the first division of the trigeminal nerve, and especially the nasociliary branch, the eye may be involved. Conjunctivitis is common and keratitis can occur. Fortunately, sight-threatening complications such as glaucoma secondary to uveitis or cataract are relatively rare. Ophthalmic zoster is often accompanied by widespread periorbital oedema, sometimes spreading bilaterally. This is not a sign of dissemination or infection but arises because the fluid in the skin of the forehead, which is tightly bound, emigrates to the lower tissues round the eye.

Motor zoster

Zoster is not confined to the sensory nerves and often associated motor nerves are affected. Clearly, transient palsies of the thoracic motor nerves are not clinically obvious. With careful clinical examination, motor palsies associated with other dermatomes are sometimes found. Zoster of C5 and C6 may lead to diaphragmatic palsy, and motor zoster of the upper limb (usually of the deltoid) and lower limbs is occasionally a complication of sensory zoster at that level. Zoster of the cranial nerves III, IV, and VI is not uncommon. We found it in 3 of 56 patients with ophthalmic zoster.

In contrast, a facial-nerve paralysis is more dramatic, although the accompanying pain and vesicles in the external auditory meatus and loss of taste in the anterior two-thirds of the tongue can easily be missed (Fig. 4). It is associated with zoster of the auriculotemporal branch of the trigeminal nerve or the tympanic branch of the glosspharyngeal, or the auricular branch of the vagus, and of the great auricular and lesser occipital branches of the cervical plexus. The suggestion that zoster of the geniculate ganglion (Ramsay Hunt syndrome) affected vestigial motor fibres of the VIIth cranial nerve was wrong.

Apart from facial nerve palsy, where the outcome is variable, the prognosis of motor zoster is good.

Autonomic zoster

Zoster of the S2 and below can be particularly distressing, with acute retention of urine due to paralysis of the bladder. A haemorrhagic cystitis can occur, owing to zoster vesicles on the wall of the bladder that can be demonstrated on cystoscopy. Lumbar zoster can be associated with bowel atony. If this occurs at the stage of segmental pain but before the rash appears, the condition can be confused with an acute abdomen.

Zoster encephalomyelitis

A mild encephalitis is not uncommon and is similar to that found in chickenpox. It can occur both before or up to 6 weeks after the onset of the illness and is probably due to an immune-mediated mechanism. There is little information on the cerebrospinal fluid in uncomplicated zoster. It is possible that many cases have an abnormal fluid. The prognosis is good. Very rarely, the encephalomyelitis can be severe and life threatening. In these cases, cerebellar involvement is not uncommon.

Purpura fulminans

This very rare condition can lead to alarming tissue loss. It follows a similar course to the condition in chickenpox. In the patient in Fig. 5 the purpura appeared at the end of a week.

Immunocompromised host and disseminated zoster

Dissemination can follow a segmental lesion. In the normal host the disease is usually mild, with a single crop of extradermatomal vesicles presumably arising from an early viraemic phase that is rapidly arrested by the redevelopment of immunity. In the immunocompromised host, zoster is more likely to occur and to disseminate (Plate 3). Usually the disease is self-limiting, but on rare occasions, when the degree of immu-

Fig. 3 Frontal and maxillary zoster.

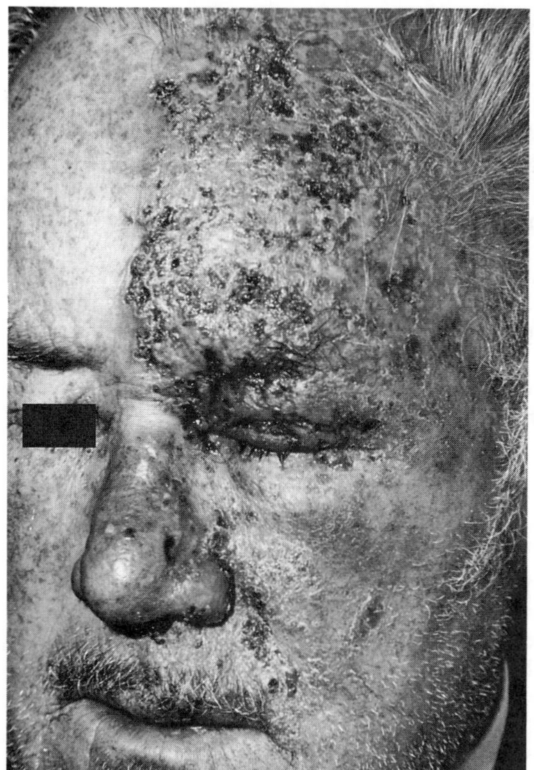

Fig. 4 Motor zoster of the left facial nerve.

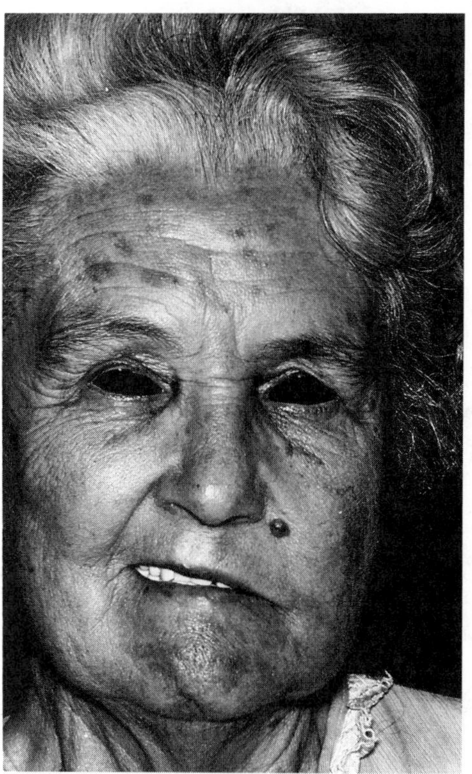

nodeficiency is very great, dissemination can be fulminating and a life-threatening disease occurs.

Acute retinal necrosis

Patients present with blurring of the vision and pain in the affected eye. There is a progressive necrotizing retinitis, which can lead to permanent visual impairment and retinal detachment. Immunocompetent patients can present with no other manifestation of zoster reactivation. In contrast, acute retinal necrosis in HIV-infected patients commonly occurs following cutaneous zoster infection. In one study, in 17 per cent of HIV-seropositive patients with ophthalmic zoster there was retinal necrosis. Specific antiviral treatment can prevent the progression of the disease; retinal complications may require surgery.

Postherpetic neuralgia

Postherpetic neuralgia is the most dreaded of the complications of shingles. As the pain tends to fade with time, any definition is arbitrary. One month after the acute attack, pain is still present in some 10 per cent of all untreated patients. The prevalence of pain rises with the age of the patient. About 50 per cent of patients over 60 years of age experience pain, while about 75 per cent do at 70. In one study of patients over 65, 22 per cent had had pain for over 1 year. Two types of pain have been described: a steady burning, aching pain and a paroxysmal, jabbing pain sometimes with an associated area of hypoaesthesia. The pain can occur spontaneously or may be triggered. The incidence of pain is lowest in lumbar zoster and highest in ophthalmic zoster.

Diagnosis

The diagnosis of both chickenpox and shingles is usually made by history and physical examination. Patients with chickenpox often have a history of exposure 2 weeks previously. A unilateral segmental distribution suggests shingles. The differential diagnosis includes poxviruses (exposure to smallpox virtually impossible, to monkeypox and camelpox unlikely but always ask: 'Where have you been?'). Bacterial impetigo due to streptococci can occasionally cause vesicles. Eczema herpeticum caused by herpes simplex can be mistaken for chickenpox but the vesicles tend to be all at the same stage of development. Rarely, disseminated coxsackievirus infections produce widespread vesicular lesions ('hand, foot, and mouth disease'); the lesions are most common on the palms of the hands and soles of the feet, while chickenpox usually has a centripetal distribution of lesions.

If necessary, the diagnosis of chickenpox can be confirmed serologically, by a greater than fourfold rise in paired sera. A serological boost follows shingles, but the sensitivity and specificity of this response have not been fully assessed in immunosuppressed individuals, where the diagnosis is particularly important. If facilities are available, diagnosis can be established more directly by the isolation of virus from vesicular fluid. Herpesvirus particles can be demonstrated immediately by electron microscopy and varicella-zoster virus positively identified after 3 to 5 days in tissue culture. Other diagnostic methods available in research laboratories include immunostaining of cells obtained from the base of skin lesions.

As both uncomplicated chickenpox and shingles are systemic infections, the diagnosis of a complicating pneumonitis or encephalitis cannot be confirmed by viral isolation techniques. Such complications are essentially diagnosed clinically.

Fig. 5 Purpura fulminans in zoster of the maxillary nerve.

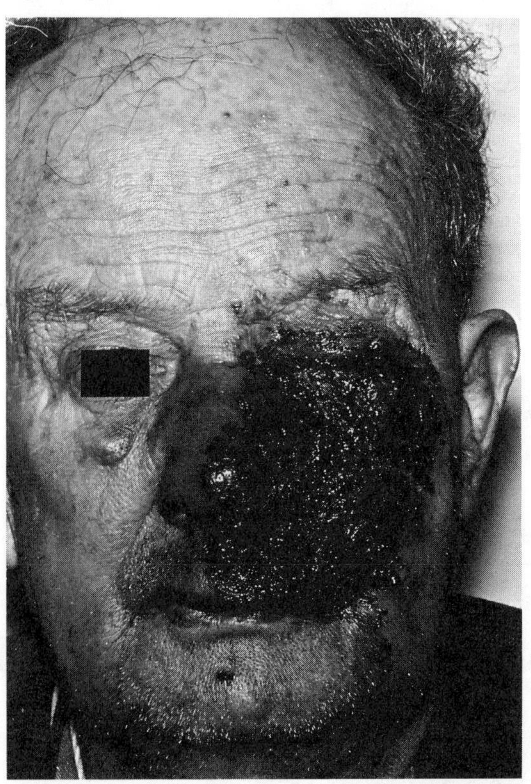

Management and treatment

Symptomatic treatment

In the majority of cases, the illness is mild and no specific treatment is required. Patients with chickenpox should be given calamine lotion to ease the itch and warned not to scratch in order to avoid secondary infection and scarring. Pruritus can also be eased by warm baths containing baking soda or by antihistamines. Skin care is important to avoid secondary bacterial complications. Patients with zoster require more careful skin care to avoid infection and often require pain relief during the acute attack.

Antiviral therapy

The aim of antiviral treatment is to alleviate and shorten the symptoms of infection, to prevent the development of severe, life-threatening complications of the virus, and finally, with shingles, to prevent the establishment of postherpetic neuralgia. Vidarabine and acyclovir have been shown to be clinically effective in placebo-controlled trials of varicella-zoster infections. Vidarabine is too toxic and famciclovir, recently introduced, is too new to be recommended for routine use. Acyclovir has been extensively used and is relatively non-toxic. High doses are required to obtain virucidal blood levels. (The oral dose is 800 mg, five times a day, and the intravenous dose is 10 mg/kg 8-hourly). Treatment should be continued until 48 h after the last skin eruption (usually about 5 days). Because of the variability of the absorption of oral acyclovir intravenous therapy should be considered for serious infections. Unfortunately, the best use of antiviral drugs has yet to be described. The policy in our unit is described in Table 1 and is somewhat arbitrary.

The indications for oral treatment represent a compromise between the inconvenience and expense of intravenous treatment and no treatment. The use of acyclovir in uncomplicated shingles as prophylaxis against postherpetic neuralgia is most controversial. There is only limited evidence of efficacy but the low toxicity of the drug and the great morbidity suffered by some patients makes treatment tempting. The main reason why it is not commonly prescribed is the expense of the drug. If more effective and better absorbed antizoster agents become generally available, it is likely that all patients with chickenpox and zoster will be routinely treated.

Table 1 *Use of acyclovir in varicella-zoster infections*

Indications for intravenous acyclovir (10 mg/kg, 8-hourly)
Chickenpox:
Immunocompromised patients
Neonatal chickenpox
Chickenpox with systemic complications
Severe chickenpox in adults and in pregnancy
Shingles:
Severe shingles in immunocompromised patients
Multidermatomal shingles
Shingles complicated by ocular, motor, autonomic, or systemic involvement
Infections not requiring active antiviral treatment
Patients presenting more than 48 h after the appearance of the last lesion or when all the lesions have crusted
Postherpetic neuralgia
Uncomplicated, mild chickenpox in children
Uncomplicated shingles in patients under 45 years
***Indications for oral acyclovir* (800 mg, 5 per day)**
Uncomplicated chickenpox
Shingles
Uncomplicated shingles in patients over 45 years
Uncomplicated shingles in immunosuppressed patients
Shingles presenting with severe pain

TREATMENT OF COMPLICATIONS

There is no specific treatment of the complications of varicella-zoster infection. The use of varicella specific antibodies is not indicated. Complications should be therefore treated on their merits. Patients with severe pneumonitis or encephalitis may benefit from intensive care and ventilation.

Ophthalmic zoster

All patients with zoster of the first division of the trigeminal nerve should be examined ophthalmologically with the aid of a slit lamp and the complications treated appropriately with topical steroids, antimicrobials, and mydriatics. Steroids given in the active phase of the infection must be accompanied by antiviral therapy.

PREVENTION AND TREATMENT OF POST-HERPETIC NEURALGIA

Information on the prevention of postherpetic neuralgia is difficult to obtain. Controlled trials require long-term follow up and depend on the subjective assessment of pain. A number of different agents including steroids, amantadine, interferon-α, as well as acyclovir, have been studied in the early phase of the illness in an effort to prevent the onset of postherpetic neuralgia. Unfortunately, the relative merits of these drugs are still unclear.

The treatment of postherpetic neuralgia, once established, is notoriously difficult. In many cases conventional analgesia, though unsatisfactory, is relied on. A large number of alternative remedies, including tricylic antidepressants, anticonvulsants (carbamazepam, phenytoin, or valproate), phenothiazines and even thalidomide (which may destroy or damage nerve fibres), have been used but with only limited success. Similarly, various physical treatments, including ethyl chloride spray, vibration, transcutaneous electrical nerve stimulation and stellate ganglion blockade, occasionally produce some relief but none is predictably successful. A most important aspect of management is to provide patients with continual support and sympathy. They should be reassured that most people will improve with time. Some patients are grateful for the hope provided by the use of apparently 'active' treatment.

Prevention

PREVENTION OF SPREAD OF VARICELLA-ZOSTER IN HOSPITAL

Patients with varicella infections are highly infectious and it is essential that non-immune, immunocompromised patients be protected. Infectious patients should be isolated and nursed by immune staff. Non-immune staff who are accidentally exposed should, in turn, avoid contact with non-immune, immunocompromised patients.

VARICELLA HYPERIMMUNE GLOBULIN

There is some evidence that varicella-zoster immune globulin, if given early after exposure to non-immune individuals, can attenuate the infection. Because it is in short supply, therapy is usually restricted to neonates born to mothers with chickenpox 5 days before and up to 48 h postpartum, to immunodeficient children under 15 years of age, or to bone marrow-transplant recipients. It has also been offered to non-immune pregnant women.

VACCINATION

A live, attenuated varicella vaccine (Oka strain) has been available since 1974 and was first licensed in Japan. It is not yet licensed in Europe and North America. Protection from clinical disease is found in about 90 per cent of healthy children, 85 per cent of leukaemic children, and 70 per cent of healthy adults. The frequency of mild chickenpox associated with the Oka strain is about 5 per cent of healthy children, 50 per cent of leukaemic children, and 10 per cent of adults. The incidence of zoster in vaccinated, immunocompromised children is lower than in unvaccinated children who have had natural infection. Vaccination of healthy older patients with a past history of chickenpox boosts the response to varicella skin tests, indicating an increase in cell-mediated immunity. Whether this response will translated into protection against zoster must await the results of clinical trials.

REFERENCES

Christie, A.B. (1988). Chickenpox (varicella). In *Infectious diseases,* (4th edn). Churchill Livingstone, Edinburgh.

Enders, G., Miller, E., Cradock-Watson, J., Bolley, I., and Ridehalgh, M. (1994). Consequences of varicella and herpes zoster in pregnancy: prospective study of 1739 cases. *Lancet,* **343,** 1547–50.

Gershon, A.A. (1992). First International Conference on the Varicella-Zoster Virus. *Journal of Infectious Diseases,* **166,** Supplement 1.

Gilden, D.H. (1994). Herpes zoster with postherpetic neuralgia—persisting pain and frustration. *New England Journal of Medicine,* **330,** 930–4.

Harding, S.P. (1993). Management of ophalmic zoster. *Journal of Medical Virology,* (suppl. 1), 97–101.

Hellinger, W.C., Bolling, J.P., Smith, T.F., and Campbell, R.J. (1993). Varicella-zoster virus retinitis in a patient with AIDS-related complex: case report and brief review of the acute retinal necrosis syndrome. *Clinics in Infectious Diseases,* **16,** 208–12.

Huff, J.C. *et al.* (1993). Effect of oral acyclovir on pain resolution in herpes zoster: a reanalysis. *Journal of Medical Virology,* (suppl. 1), 93–6.

Juel-Jensen, B.E. and MacCallum, F.O. (1972). *Herpes simplex, varicella and zoster.* Heinemann, London

Pastuszak, A.L. *et al.* (1994). Outcome after varicella infection in the first 20 weeks of pregnancy. *New England Journal of Medicine,* **330,** 901–5.

Wagstaff, A.J., Faulds, D., and Goa, K.L. (1994). Acyclovir. A reappraisal of its antiviral activity, pharmacokinetic properties and therapeutic efficacy. *Drugs,* **47,** 153–205.

Wallace, M.R., Bowler, W.A., Murray, N.B., Brodine, S.K., and Oldfield, E.C. (1992). Treatment of adult varicella with oral acyclovir—a randomized placebo-controlled trial. *Annals of Internal Medicine,* **117,** 358–83.

Wood, M.J., Johnson, R.W., McKendrick, M.W., Taylor, J., Mandal, B.K., and Crooks, J. (1994). A randomized trail of acyclovir for 7 days or 21 days with and without prednisolone for treatment of acute herpes zoster. *New England Journal of Medicine,* **330,** 901–5.

7.10.4 The Epstein–Barr virus

M. A. Epstein and D. H. Crawford

Background

The virus

Epstein–Barr virus (**EBV**) was discovered in 1964 during a search for potentially causative agents in an unusual, newly described tumour of children in Africa, Burkitt lymphoma. EBV is one of the seven herpesviruses of man, and like all herpesviruses, has a relatively complex structure consisting of an outer, cell-derived envelope surrounding an icosahedral protein capsid of about 86 nm in diameter, which encloses a 172 kb, double-stranded linear DNA genome. The entire nucleotide sequence of the genome has been determined.

Two viral types, A and B (or 1 and 2), have been differentiated but neither shows any particular disease association.

Viral infectious cycle

Natural infection with EBV is strictly limited to man and the cellular host range is determined by the expression on the surface of susceptible cells of the CR2 molecule (the C3d complement component receptor), to which the virus attaches. Target cells are therefore B lymphocytes and squamous epithelial cells of the oral cavity, pharynx, and genital tract. Infection of epithelial cells leads to a lytic infection with production of viral progeny and cell death. In contrast, the virus causes a latent infection of B cells *in vivo* and has the ability to transform normal B lymphocytes *in vitro* into continuously growing, latently infected, immortalized lymphoblastoid lines. These two types of infection (lytic and latent) are characterized by the expression of specific sets of viral genes, and in lymphoblastoid cell lines the latent infection can be induced into the lytic cycle by certain stimuli, phorbol esters for example, which cause B-cell differentiation.

Immortalization of lymphocytes by EBV is used to generate a steady supply of such cells in culture both for general study and, from individual patients, for many types of research.

Treatment with acyclovir holds lytic infection in check during the time the drug is being given but does not affect latent infections.

Virus-coded proteins

Although the EBV genome is large enough to code for about 100 proteins, only a small number have been identified to date. These can be categorized according to the time of their appearance during the infectious cycle as latent, early, or late antigens.

LATENT ANTIGENS

These are expressed in EBV-immortalized B lymphocytes in culture. Such cells are said to be latently infected because the infectious process has been arrested at an early stage which is compatible with continued cell proliferation and which does not proceed to the production of virus particles. Six EB viral nuclear antigens (**EBNA**s) and three membrane proteins (latent membrane protein (**LMP**) and terminal proteins (**TP**) 1 and 2) have been defined, and in addition, two small EBV-coded RNAs (EBERS 1 and 2) are transcribed but not translated. Although the latent gene products are all clearly involved in the immortalization process, their functions are mostly unknown. EBNA 1 is required for maintenance of the viral genome within the infected cell, while EBNA 2 and LMP act as viral oncogenes *in vitro*. All the latent antigens are recognized by the immune system since antibodies to each can be found in the serum under certain conditions and all except EBNA 1 have been shown to elicit cytotoxic T-cell responses. Antigen expression in latently infected B cells *in vivo* has not yet been clarified.

EARLY ANTIGENS (EA)

These are expressed early in the lytic cycle before viral DNA replication and their presence is not compatible with continued viability of the cell. These antigens are non-structural and are generally assumed to be enzymes involved in viral DNA replication. Immunocytochemical techniques using human sera have shown staining patterns which are described as diffuse (**D**), involving the whole cell, and restricted (**R**), which is confined to the cytoplasm. The EA complex is currently being investigated and so far DNA polymerase, ribonucleotide reductase, protein kinase, alkaline exonuclease, and thymidine kinase have been identified as components. Serum antibodies to EA-D and EA-R can be detected in certain disease states and may be used for diagnostic and/or prognostic purposes (see below).

LATE ANTIGENS

These are expressed in the infected cell after DNA replication has been initiated, and they form the structural components of the viral capsid and envelope. The viral capsid antigen (**VCA**) complex elicits an antibody response early in primary infection which is maintained for life and can readily be detected; these antibodies are therefore used in epidemiological studies undertaken to determine seropositivity rates (see below). The virus-coded envelope glycoproteins (**gp**) are synthesized late in the virus cycle and are inserted into the cell membrane through which the viral capsid buds out to acquire its envelope. These glycoprotein antigens are designated by their molecular weights (gp340, gp270, and gp85) and are involved in virus binding and entry into susceptible cells, gp340 binding in particular to the CR2 molecule on the cell surface being a prerequisite for virus infection. Each of these envelope glycoproteins elicits an antibody response and in the case of gp340 the antibodies neutralize viral infectivity by preventing binding to CR2.

General epidemiology

The virus is widespread in all human populations. Natural primary infection usually occurs in early childhood, is not accompanied by obvious clinical manifestations, and leads only to the generation of antibodies to the viral and virus-determined antigens, and to the development of specific cytotoxic T lymphocytes. A lifelong carrier state ensues, in which both humoral and cellular immune responses are maintained continuously. The virus persists as a latent infection in a few circulating B lymphocytes and as a productive, lytic infection in epithelial cells of the mouth, pharynx, urogenital tract, and perhaps the salivary glands. EBV is shed into the buccal fluid in considerable amounts in about 20 per cent of those who have been infected and in small amounts in almost all the remainder; the virus has also been detected in genital secretions. However, it appears that virus in the buccal fluid provides the main source for transmission of the infection in the population, by droplets and casually contaminated objects in children, and by salivary transfer during kissing amongst the sexually active. In developing countries, 99.9 per cent of all children are infected by the second to the fourth year of life, depending on geographical location, but in industrialized countries with high standards of hygiene a considerable number of individuals do not meet the virus as young children. The percentage of each age cohort remaining free of infection as teenagers or young adults in Western societies depends on socioeconomic group—the higher the standard of living, the greater the percentage; amongst the very affluent as many as 50 per cent of young adults may never have been infected.

Tests to determine EBV status

It is usual for infected carriers to remain perfectly healthy and such people can only be distinguished from those who have never been infected by laboratory investigations. The quickest and easiest tests are those to determine serological status, since all healthy people who have been previously infected by EBV have serum IgG antibodies to VCA. Antibodies to EBNA 1 and often to the other EBNA components can also be detected, but are not generally used for routine screening. Other indicators of EBV infection such as the presence of virus in throat washings and in circulating B lymphocytes, and the presence of EBV-specific cytotoxic T cells, are time consuming to demonstrate and are therefore only used in experimental investigations.

Disease associations

The virus causes acute infectious mononucleosis (see below) and is also associated with a variety of lymphomas and with diseases of squamous epithelial cells, including the following (also discussed below): Burkitt lymphoma, lymphoma in the immunocompromised, a subset of Hodgkin lymphomas, some T-cell lymphomas, undifferentiated nasopharyngeal carcinoma, and oral hairy leukoplakia. In addition, the virus will induce multiple, rapidly growing, malignant lymphomas if a sufficient dose is injected experimentally into the cottontop tamarin, a New World non-human primate.

Infectious mononucleosis

It is well established that EBV is the aetiological agent of classical infectious mononucleosis. Those who miss the clinically silent infection by the virus in childhood are likely sooner or later to undergo delayed primary infection, and although 50 per cent of such delayed infections are symptom free as in childhood, the other 50 per cent are accompanied by the manifestations of classical infectious mononucleosis. The fact that it is the teenagers and young adults in the more affluent classes of Western countries who escape infection as children explains why infectious mononucleosis is predominantly a disease of upper socioeconomic groups and why it is exceptionally rare in developing countries. Although most cases of infectious mononucleosis occur in adolescents and young adults, children and the middle aged may sometimes develop the disease, and rarely also the elderly. Infectious mononucleosis has long been known to be associated with kissing and the usual pattern of acquisition depends on a healthy carrier, who will be shedding virus in his/her saliva, passing this during close buccal contact directly into the oropharynx of a partner who has not been primarily infected in the usual way as a child. This method of spread explains why case-to-case infection and epidemics are not seen in infectious mononucleosis and why the incubation period, perhaps 30 to 50 days, is difficult to calculate. Primary EBV infection giving infectious mononucleosis-like symptoms may also be transmitted by blood transfusion or organ grafting from a seropositive (i.e. infected) donor.

SYMPTOMS

Classical infectious mononucleosis may be preceded by some days of vague indisposition or may have a fairly abrupt onset. Sore throat, fever with sweating, anorexia, headache, and fatigue are the principal presenting symptoms, together with malaise quite out of proportion to the other complaints. Actual dysphagia may be noticed and orbital oedema may be present for a brief time. An erythematous rash occurs in a small number of patients but affects the majority of those who have been taking ampicillin. Rarely, tonsillar and pharyngeal oedema can be so severe as to cause pharyngeal obstruction.

SIGNS

The fever may rise to 40 °C during the day but high levels and marked swings are not usually seen. There is redness and oedema of the pharynx, fauces, soft palate, and uvula, and about half the patients develop a greyish exudate. In addition, generalized lymphadenopathy is almost always present, most marked in the cervical region; the glands are symmetrical, discrete, and slightly tender, and accompanied by splenomegaly in about 60 per cent of cases and an enlarged liver in 10 per cent. There is usually a moderate bradycardia. Besides the rash, a characteristic palatal enanthem consisting of crops of reddish petechiae is found in about one-third of patients, and some jaundice can be detected in about 8 per cent.

CLINICAL COURSE

Mild cases of infectious mononucleosis may resolve in days, but the disease usually lasts for about 1 to 2 weeks and is often followed by a period of lethargy before complete recovery. The duration of this convalescence may be influenced by psychological factors, particularly the speed with which patients are encouraged to resume full activity. About 1 case in 2000 may continue in a truly chronic or recurrent form for several months or even years, and where some of these patients have been exhaustively investigated immunological defects have been found. However, a currently growing number of cases of so-called chronic infectious mononucleosis are in all probability manifestations of 'chronic fatigue syndrome' (sometimes designated 'chronic active EBV infection', 'myalgic encephalomyelopathy', 'yuppie disease') but it is highly controversial as to whether these are indeed true entities rather than belief disorders; credible connections with EBV have not been established. In contrast, there is an extremely rare, genetically determined, X-linked, lymphoproliferative condition (**XLP** disease, or Duncan syndrome after the first family to be recognized) in which the affected young males of certain kindred die from infectious mononucleosis owing to a specific inability to respond normally to EBV during primary infection; the disease progresses inexorably, with necrotic destruction of vital organs and multisystem failure. Although the exact cause of the massive necrosis of vital organs is not known, there is evidence to suggest that an aberrant immune response to EBV in XLP results in unregulated natural killer-cell and cytotoxic T-cell activity being directed against the normal cells of organs instead of concentrating solely on EBV-infected cells displaying EBV antigens.

COMPLICATIONS

Minor non-specific complications may result from the symptoms. Rarely, true infectious mononucleosis-related complications may be serious in nature, namely secondary bacterial throat infections, traumatic rupture of the enlarged spleen, asphyxia from pharyngeal oedema, massive hepatic necrosis, Guillain–Barré syndrome, and autoimmune manifestations such as thrombocytopenia and haemolytic anaemia.

DIFFERENTIAL DIAGNOSIS

Classical infectious mononucleosis, especially in adolescents and young adults, presents few diagnostic difficulties and even the somewhat atypical cases in younger and older age groups will not be missed if the clinical picture of fever, sore throat, generalized lymphadenopathy, and splenomegaly is considered in conjunction with serological and haematological laboratory investigations (see below). However, an infectious mononucleosis-like disease can occur in primary cytomegalovirus infection and in toxoplasmosis, but in both conditions the sore throat is much less severe and with cytomegalovirus the lymphadenopathy may be minimal or absent.

LABORATORY DIAGNOSIS

During acute infectious mononucleosis, serum IgM and IgG antibodies to VCA and IgG antiEA antibodies appear very early; antiEBNA 1 antibodies usually only become detectable during the convalescent period.

On recovery, IgM antiVCA and IgG antiEA disappear, whereas IgG antibodies to VCA and EBNA 1 are maintained for life at detectable levels. Because it is not usually possible to document a seroconversion or even a significant rise in IgG antiVCA antibody titres in infectious mononucleosis, the presence of IgM antibodies to VCA is regarded as the most reliable diagnostic test. This may be corroborated by the finding of anti-EA antibodies (usually of D type) and/or the absence of antibodies to EBNA 1. However, these tests, which are best done by immunofluorescence staining of B-cell lines expressing viral antigens, are time consuming and therefore usually only available in larger laboratories. For this reason a rapid screening test (Monospot test) has been introduced, which detects the presence of heterophil antibodies in the patient's serum. This test has been adapted from the previously used Paul–Bunnell test for IgM antibodies which agglutinate red blood cells from species other than man. Although these heterophil antibodies are not directed against viral-coded proteins they are present in up to 85 per cent of infectious mononucleosis sera. Cases of Monospot-negative infectious mononucleosis tend to be those outside the classical 15 to 25 year age range, and false-positive tests may occur in pregnancy and autoimmune disease. An additional classical feature of infectious mononucleosis is the presence of lymphocytosis of up to 15×10^9/l, with the majority of cells having an 'atypical' morphology. Thus, infectious mononucleosis can generally be diagnosed by a combination of the clinical and haematological findings, and a positive Monospot test. If the latter is negative and infectious mononucleosis is still suspected, then confirmation should be sought by testing for IgM antiVCA antibodies. A retrospective diagnosis may sometimes be made if samples are available that allow seroconversion to be detected or a rising titre of IgG antibodies to EBNA 1.

TREATMENT

Bedrest and aspirin for headache and pharyngeal discomfort are the only treatments required in uncomplicated cases. As soon as the fever resolves the patient should be encouraged to get up and resume some activities as fast as is practicable, although violent exercise should be avoided for 3 weeks after an enlarged spleen ceases to be palpable. Only complications need active therapy: splenic rupture requires surgery, bacterial infections call for appropriate antibiotics, airway obstruction must be relieved by tracheostomy, and corticosteroids should be given for life-threatening pharyngeal oedema and neurological and haematological complications.

PATHOGENESIS

Exactly why children do not react with symptoms to primary EBV infection whereas adolescents and young adults frequently become ill with infectious mononucleosis when they meet the virus for the first time is not fully understood, but there are likely explanations. The immunological reactions of young adults on first encountering EBV are clearly more exuberant than those of children and it has been suggested that this reflects a physiological difference in responsiveness. The mode of infection and consequent size of infecting dose also play an important part; children coming into contact with saliva from a shedder in droplets or casually contaminating some sucked object will receive a much smaller quantity of virus than a young person taking in large amounts of virus-containing saliva from a carrier during kissing. An exaggerated immunological response to a large infecting dose of EBV fits well with the changes seen in infectious mononucleosis and it appears that large numbers of reactive T cells stimulated by the infected B cells in the circulation, in lymph nodes, in tonsils, in lymphoid tissue of the mouth and pharynx, in spleen, and in other organs such as liver are responsible for causing the sore throat, fever, malaise, lymphadenopathy, and hepatosplenomegaly by immunopathological mechanisms.

Endemic (or 'African') Burkitt lymphoma

The classic form of this B-cell tumour is found in certain parts of Africa and Papua New Guinea where the temperature does not fall below 62 °F or the rainfall below 55 cm; it is perhaps also present in tropical South America where these conditions are fulfilled, but the data from these regions are incomplete. The original description of the tumour was given by Burkitt in the late 1950s and has not required revision; endemic Burkitt lymphoma is distinct from the so-called Burkitt-like tumours that occur sporadically everywhere in the world (sometimes called 'American' Burkitt lymphoma) and that have a different age incidence, anatomical distribution, and response to therapy, and arise from B cells with different phenotypic characteristics. The term 'Burkitt type' is also sometimes applied to certain leukaemias, but this is merely on the basis of the morphology of the malignant cells.

The association between EBV and endemic Burkitt lymphoma is so close that it is generally accepted that the virus is a necessary but not sufficient element in the aetiology of the disease, an essential link along with cofactors in a complicated chain of events which leads to the malignancy. Hyperendemic malaria has been identified as an important cofactor, and its spread by anopheline mosquitoes requiring warmth and moisture explains the climate dependence of Burkitt lymphoma.

Burkitt lymphoma is overwhelmingly a disease of childhood, is extremely rare over the age of 14 years, and in the endemic areas it is more common than all other childhood tumours added together. There is no evidence in the tumour belt for any particular tribal susceptibility and cases occur in all races in the ratio to be expected from the population proportions.

SYMPTOMS

The tumour is usually multifocal and can present in a variety of different sites, or in several sites, and the symptoms depend entirely on anatomical location. Jaw tumours, in maxilla or mandible, are present in 70 per cent of patients, are the presenting feature in most of these, may be multiple in two, three, or even all four quadrants, and are almost always accompanied by tumours elsewhere; a rapidly growing mass, loosening of teeth, and exophthalmos from orbital spread are the main consequences. Abdominal tumours are also common, involving retroperitoneal nodes, liver, ovaries, intestine, and kidneys. Burkitt lymphoma may sometimes present in the thyroid, the adolescent female breast, the testicles, and the salivary glands; extradural tumours in the spine cause paraplegia of rapid onset, and skeletal lesions are also seen. A most unusual and characteristic feature of this lymphoma is its failure to involve the spleen and peripheral lymph nodes.

SIGNS

The tumours are firm, very rapidly growing, remarkably painless, and even when large cause minimal constitutional disturbance. The tumour sites determine the clinical signs.

CLINICAL COURSE

The lymphoma grows relentlessly and death ensues within a few months of onset in the absence of treatment.

DIFFERENTIAL DIAGNOSIS

In endemic zones, Burkitt lymphoma can usually be diagnosed on the basis of its clinical picture. Unlike Burkitt lymphoma, retinoblastoma is intraocular in origin, rhabdomyosarcoma is extraorbital and does not involve teeth, nephroblastoma rarely involves both kidneys and is not multifocal, and neuroblastoma and ovarian tumours can be distinguished histologically. As regards paraplegia, that of tuberculous origin causes vertebral collapse, whilst acute transverse myelitis is preceded by pain and fever. Other lymphomas can be distinguished by their dissimilar anatomical distribution.

LABORATORY DIAGNOSIS

Although the diagnosis of Burkitt lymphoma in an endemic area can often be made on clinical grounds, this should be confirmed by the histological examination of a biopsy specimen. The tumour shows a characteristic histological picture of a poorly differentiated, non-cleaved lymphocytic lymphoma of B-cell origin, which is infiltrated with histiocytes giving the classical 'starry sky' appearance.

Serological studies of antibodies to EBV antigens show a unique pattern in Burkitt lymphoma, which may be useful diagnostically. Antibody titres vary as the disease progresses and with tumour regression in response to treatment; they may therefore be used to assess disease outcome. IgG antibodies to VCA are found at 8 to 10 times higher geometric mean titres than in healthy controls matched for age and sex. In addition, IgG antibodies to EA-R and membrane antigens (**MA**) are also detectable and likewise vary with disease progression; successful treatment causes a rise in anti-MA and a fall in anti-EA-R, whereas the reversal of this pattern may herald a recurrence of the tumour.

TREATMENT

Surgery and radiotherapy are not effective and are contraindicated because excellent results are obtainable with moderate courses of chemotherapy. Cyclophosphamide is the drug of choice because Burkitt lymphoma is extremely sensitive to it, and rapid and sustained resolution is not uncommon where tumours are small and circumscribed.

PATHOGENESIS

The molecular mechanisms underlying the capacity of EBV to immortalize human B lymphocytes *in vitro* into continuously growing cell lines have recently become accessible to investigation, and a likely scenario for the sequence of viral gene expression responsible for the immortalization can be outlined. There are also now credible explanations as to how the viral genes, in combination with cofactors, cause Burkitt lymphoma. According to one view, EBV infection in the presence of the impaired immunological control brought about by hyperendemic malaria leads to a high level of EBV-driven B-cell proliferation. This in turn increases the chances of one or another of three Burkitt lymphoma-specific chromosomal translocations (t8:14; t8:22; t2:8) occurring, each of which can activate the c-*myc* oncogene whose deregulation causes malignant change in the affected cell and the emergence of a rapidly growing tumour clone. An alternative hypothesis suggests that the first step is the generation, through the chronic immunological stimulation of hyperendemic malaria, of a high turnover of B cells; then, one or more of these dividing lymphocytes acquires one of the three chromosomal translocations involving c-*myc* activation, which renders the affected cell responsive to growth-promoting signals. Infection of such a cell by EBV finally provides viral functions conferring malignancy and a tumour clone grows out unchecked.

Lymphomas in immunosuppressed states

The lifelong EBV infection present in all normal seropositive individuals is controlled by cell-mediated immune mechanisms. In primary and secondary suppression of cellular immunity there is a loss of this control of persisting EBV infection, which leads to increased virus replication in the oral cavity, increased numbers of circulating, virus-carrying B lymphocytes, and increased levels of serum antibodies to lytic-cycle EBV antigens (VCA, EA). When this occurs it is sometimes described as a 'reactivated infection' although the condition is clinically silent. However, on occasions the loss of control leads to the development of EBV-associated lymphomas.

1. In organ graft recipients

It has been known for many years that organ graft recipients who receive lifelong immunosuppressive drugs to prevent graft rejection have an increased risk of developing lymphoproliferative disease and lymphoma (28 to 100 times that of normal controls) and that most of these conditions are of B-cell origin, and contain the EBV genome and express viral antigens in their cells. Lymphoproliferative disease has two forms of clinical presentation: in about 50 per cent of cases it occurs within the first year after transplantation in a young age group, has infectious mononucleosis-like symptoms, and is associated with primary EBV infection in patients who were seronegative at the time of grafting; the second type of presentation occurs in older patients late after transplantation and takes the form of a localized mass, commonly in the gut, central nervous system, or transplanted organ. Biopsy of the lesion shows large-cell lymphoma, which is usually monoclonal in origin, although progression from a polyclonal B-cell proliferation probably occurs early in the disease. The fact that all the EBV latent viral genes are expressed in lymphoproliferative disease, just as with lymphoblastoid cell lines immortalized by the virus *in vitro*, suggests that EBV is of prime importance in the aetiology of these lesions, although other events, perhaps cytogenetic abnormalities, may be necessary to cause the monoclonal growth.

Reduction of immunosuppressive therapy, with or without acyclovir therapy, has been shown to cause complete and often sustained regression of the tumours in many cases. This has therefore become the first line of treatment, with cytotoxic drugs and/or radiotherapy being used only where there is no response or after recurrence.

2. In acquired immunodeficiency syndrome (AIDS)

Two types of lymphoma are being seen with increasing frequency in AIDS patients; large-cell lymphoma and Burkitt lymphoma, and both of these may be associated with EBV.

Large-cell lymphomas similar to those seen in organ graft recipients (see above) occur in severely immunocompromised AIDS patients; their distribution is extranodal and involves many unusual sites, the most common being the central nervous system. These lymphomas show a strong association with EBV, which reaches 100 per cent in cerebral tumours. The clinical presentation depends on the site involved; the progress is rapid, with a mean survival time from diagnosis of 3 to 4 months. The treatment of choice is radiotherapy, but the results are disappointing mainly because patients in the terminal stages of the underlying AIDS are in such poor condition.

Burkitt lymphoma usually occurs earlier on in the course of human immunodeficiency virus (**HIV**) disease while the immune system is still relatively intact and is therefore more amenable to treatment. About 50 per cent of these lymphomas contain EBV DNA.

Hodgkin disease and T-cell lymphomas

There has long been a suspicion that EBV may play some part in the induction of Hodgkin disease because of the similar socioeconomic epidemiology of Hodgkin disease and infectious mononucleosis, and because of the well established fact that within 5 years of infectious mononucleosis there is a four- to sixfold increase in the likelihood of developing Hodgkin disease. In recent years, evidence has been obtained that in a proportion of patients with Hodgkin disease, EBV DNA is carried and expressed in both Reed–Sternberg and the tumour reticulum cells. Although such findings are intriguing, they are as yet insufficient to implicate EBV in the aetiology of Hodgkin disease, but point to the need for further investigation of a possible relationship.

A similar situation exists with some T-cell lymphomas where a few, particularly oral T-cell lymphoma in AIDS patients and nasal T-cell lymphomas, have been shown to carry the virus genome and express viral latent genes in the malignant cells.

Nasopharyngeal carcinoma

This is a tumour strictly restricted to the postnasal space and arising from the squamous epithelial cells lining this small, well-defined cavity. About 60 per cent of nasopharyngeal carcinoma is undifferentiated in type, often even anaplastic, whilst the remainder show squamous differentiation with foci of keratinization. The tumour is seen in small numbers throughout the world but has a remarkably high incidence in southern Chinese wherever they reside and in the Inuit and related races of North America and Greenland; whether the circum-Arctic inhabitants of the Russian Federation are similarly prone is not known. In these high incidence areas, nasopharyngeal carcinoma is the most common cancer of men and the second most common of women. In addition, there is a rather high incidence of nasopharyngeal carcinoma amongst Malays, Dyaks, Indonesians, Filipinos, and Vietnamese, and a medium-high incidence belt stretching across North Africa, down through the Sudan, and into the Kenya highlands. In most parts the tumour is a disease of middle or old age, but in the African medium-high incidence areas it has bimodal age peaks, the first involving children and young people up to 20 years of age and a second much later in life. Irrespective of geographical region, undifferentiated nasopharyngeal carcinoma always carries the EBV genome in the tumour cells; patients with this carcinoma, and even healthy individuals destined to develop the tumour, always show a specific pattern of antibody responses to EBV antigens.

SYMPTOMS

The principal local symptoms of nasopharyngeal carcinoma are nasal obstruction, discharge, or bleeding; deafness, tinnitus, or earache; headache; ocular paresis from tumour spread to involve cranial nerves. About one-third of patients presents with a single symptom caused locally by the tumour, about one-third presents with several such symptoms, and about one-third complains only of cervical lymph-node enlargement due to metastatic spread from a primary tumour which is frequently occult.

SIGNS

Direct spread from the primary tumour may involve neighbouring soft tissues, bone, parotid gland, buccal cavity, and oropharynx, where distortion of architecture or firm, fixed swellings will result. Anteriorly, the neoplasm may extend into the nasal fossae, the paranasal sinuses, or the orbit, again giving distortion and swelling. Lateral spread can invade the eustachian canal, which may become blocked, or the parapharyngeal space, where cranial nerves IX, X, XI, and XII can be involved; superior extension leads to invasion of the skull or cranial foramina with damage to cranial nerves II, IV, V and VI; cranial nerve palsies, often causing dysfunction of eye movements or ophthalmoplegia, will be detected.

Lymphatic spread causes enlarged cervical lymph nodes, mobile at first but hard and fixed later, and subsequently extends to the supraclavicular glands as well. If blood-borne metastases occur they are most frequent in bones, liver and lungs, but may be in any organ; the signs will depend on the site.

CLINICAL COURSE

If nasopharyngeal carcinoma is left untreated it progresses inexorably to death.

DIFFERENTIAL DIAGNOSIS

Nasopharyngeal carcinoma must be distinguished from other tumours of the nasal cavities, namely adenocarcinomas, sarcomas, malignant lymphomas, and rare malignancies such as chordoma, teratoma, and melanoma. In high-incidence areas, nasopharyngeal carcinoma is about 100 times more common than all the other tumours added together; the classical presenting symptoms taken in conjunction with laboratory tests (see below) form the basis for diagnosis.

LABORATORY DIAGNOSIS

The diagnosis of nasopharyngeal carcinoma is made histologically on a biopsy sample either from the primary tumour or from an enlarged cervical lymph node. In addition, serum antibody titres to EBV antigens can be used to confirm the diagnosis because, regardless of geographical location, they show a characteristic reaction pattern—IgG and IgA antibodies to VCA and EA-D are raised, with the titre correlating with the tumour burden. Uniquely, IgA antibodies to VCA and EA are also found in the saliva from patients with nasopharyngeal carcinoma. In the high-incidence areas of southern China, success in detecting very early cases of nasopharyngeal carcinoma has been achieved by mass screening of susceptible populations for serum IgA antibodies to VCA and following up those with persistently positive results; this has proved important because such early lesions are usually amenable to treatment.

TREATMENT

Nasopharyngeal carcinoma responds well to radiotherapy and this therefore is the treatment of choice. Several systems have been described for classifying nasopharyngeal carcinoma on the basis of the clinical stage of the disease in order to guide planning of the radiotherapy and to give some indication of prognosis. Each of these systems takes account of the extent of the primary tumour and its local spread, the extent of regional lymph-node involvement, and the clinical evidence for the presence or absence of distant metastases.

In the earliest stages of the disease, radiotherapy gives 5-year survival rates of 50 per cent or more, and of those surviving 70 per cent remain permanently free of relapse. More advanced stages of nasopharyngeal carcinoma have correspondingly worse prognoses.

PATHOGENESIS

The association of EBV with nasopharyngeal carcinoma is so consistent that it is widely accepted that the virus plays a part in causation, as with Burkitt lymphoma, as a necessary agent that is not sufficient on its own. Besides the racial predisposition of southern Chinese and the Inuit, amongst the former a modest but definite genetic factor has been demonstrated; thus, those with an A_2BW_{36} haplotype are four to six times more likely to have nasopharyngeal carcinoma than others in the population.

There is also an environmental cofactor associated with the Chinese way of life that has been revealed by epidemiological studies on migrants, and two likely candidates have been identified:

(1) traditional herbal medicines taken as snuff and made from dried plants of the Euphorbiaceae and Thymeliaceae families that contain tumour-promoting substances of phorbol ester type;

(2) traditional salt fish, which has been shown to contain carcinogenic nitrosamines.

As EBV replicates in nasopharyngeal squamous epithelial cells of all carriers, and southern Chinese invariably undergo primary infection as very young children, the taking into the nose of phorbol ester-containing herbal snuffs is significant because phorbol esters in addition to their tumour-promoting effects are also powerful activators of EBV replication when virus genome-containing lymphoid cells are treated *in vitro*. If virus production is likewise greatly increased in the nasopharynx in those with a genetic predisposition to nasopharyngeal carcinoma there will be a greatly increased pool of EBV-infected cells exposed to the chance of undergoing other essential events in the progression to malignancy.

Hairy leukoplakia in AIDS

This rather recently described lesion occurs in HIV-positive homosexual men, usually before the features of AIDS develop but sometimes heralding or accompanying the onset of clinical AIDS. Hairy leukoplakia presents as painless white patches on the tongue and sometimes also on the lateral buccal mucosa. The lesions are slightly raised, poorly demarcated, and have a 'hairy' or corrugated surface; the patches are usually multiple and measure from 1 or 2 mm up to 3 cm in diameter.

The squamous epithelial cells of this condition contain large amounts of actively replicating EBV. Treatment with acyclovir arrests the EBV replication and the lesions regress, but only for as long as the drug is continued. Hairy leukoplakia is not of great significance clinically, but it has given important insights into the role of oral and pharyngeal squamous epithelial cells in supporting EBV production.

Smooth muscle tumours in immunosuppressed patients

Recently EBV has been implicated in leiomyomas and leiomyosarcomas in children immunosuppressed by AIDS or after organ transplantation.

FURTHER READING

Burkitt, D. (1958). A sarcoma involving the jaw in African children. *British Journal of Surgery*, **46,** 218–23.

Burkitt, D. (1963). A lymphoma syndrome in tropical Africa. In *International review of experimental pathology* (ed. G.W. Richter and M.A. Epstein), Vol. 2, pp. 67–138. Academic Press, New York.

Carter, R.L. and Penman, H.G. (ed.) (1969). *Infectious mononucleosis*, pp. 1–258. Blackwell Scientific, Oxford.

de Thé, G., Ito, Y., and Davis, W. (ed.) (1978). *Nasopharyngeal carcinoma: etiology and control*, pp. 1–606. International Agency for Research on Cancer, Lyon.

de Thé, G. *et al.* (1978). Epidemiological evidence for causal relationship between Epstein–Barr virus and Burkitt's lymphoma: results of the prospective Ugandan study. *Nature*, **274,** 756–61.

Epstein, M.A. and Achong, B.G. (ed.) (1979). *The Epstein–Barr virus*, pp. 1–459. Springer Verlag, Berlin.

Epstein, M.A., Achong, B.G., and Barr, Y.M. (1964). Virus particles in cultured lymphoblasts from Burkitt's lymphoma. *Lancet*, **i,** 702–3.

Farrell, P. (1989). Epstein–Barr virus genome. In *Advances in viral oncology* (ed. G. Klein), Vol. 8, pp. 103–32. Raven Press, New York.

Greenspan, J.S. *et al.* (1985). Replication of Epstein–Barr virus within the epithelial cells of oral hairy leukoplakia, an AIDS-associated lesion. *New England Journal of Medicine*, **313,** 1564–71.

Henle, G., Henle, W., and Diehl, V. (1968). Relation of Burkitt's lymphoma tumor-associated herpesvirus to infectious mononucleosis. *Proceedings of the National Academy of Sciences (USA)*, **59,** 94–101.

Kieff, E. and Liebowitz, D. (1990). Epstein–Barr virus and its replication. In *Virology* (ed. B.N. Fields and D.M. Krupe), pp. 1889–920. Raven Press, New York.

Lenoir, G.M., O'Conor, G.T., and Olweny, C.L.M. (ed.) (1985). *Burkitt's lymphoma:a human cancer model*, pp. 1–484. International Agency for Research on Cancer, Lyon.

Liebowitz, D. (1995) Epstein-Barr Virus—an old dog with new tricks. *New England Journal of Medicine,* **332,** 55–7.

Luxton, J.C., Thomas, J.A., and Crawford, D.H. (1991). Aetiology and pathogenesis of non-Hodgkin lymphoma in AIDS. *Cancer Surveys*, **10,** 103–19.

Miller, G. (1990). Epstein–Barr virus. In *Virology* (ed. B.N. Fields and D.M. Krupe), pp. 1921–58. Raven Press, New York.

Rickinson, A.B., Murray, R.J., Brooks, J., Griffin, H., Moss, D.J., and Masucci, M.G. (1992). T-cell recognition of Epstein–Barr virus associated lymphomas. *Cancer Surveys*, **13,** 53–80.

Shanmugaratnam, K. (1971). Studies on the aetiology of nasopharyngeal carcinoma. In *International review of experimental pathology* (ed. G.W. Richter and M.A. Epstein), Vol. 10, pp. 361–413. Academic Press, New York.

Stein, H., Herbst, H., Anagnostopoulos, I., Niedobitek, G., Dallenbach, F., and Kratzsch, H-C. (1991). The nature of Hodgkin and Reed–Sternberg cells, their association with EBV, and their relationship to anaplastic large-cell lymphoma. *Annals of Oncology*, **2,** (suppl. 2), 33–8.

Thomas, J.A., Allday, M.J., and Crawford, D.H. (1991). Epstein–Barr virus-associated lymphoproliferative disorders in immunocompromised individuals. *Advances in Cancer Research*, **57,** 329–80.

7.10.5 Human infections caused by simian herpesviruses

L. E. CHAPMAN and C. J. PETERS

Most of the more than 30 herpesviruses isolated from non-human primates have no known medical significance for humans. Only Cercopithecine herpesvirus 1 is clearly recognized to have significant human pathogenicity. This is an alpha herpesvirus of macaque monkeys first isolated by Sabin and Wright in 1932 from the brain and spinal cord of a researcher who died of rapidly progressive meningoencephalitis after a bite from a macaque monkey. Cercopithecine herpesvirus 2 (simian agent 8, or SA8), a closely related alpha herpesvirus of baboons and African green monkeys, has been possibly but not unequivocally implicated in one fatal human case of encephalitis.

Cercopithecine herpesvirus 1 (formerly Herpesvirus simiae, commonly known as B virus) is closely related to herpes simplex virus (**HSV**), and in many ways is an analogous virus in its natural host, monkeys of the genus Macaca.

Epidemiology

B virus is enzootic among Old World *Macaca* monkeys, in which it causes minimal morbidity. Natural infections have been most frequently reported in rhesus (*M. mulatta*) and cynomolgus (*M. fascicularis*) macaques, but B virus has also been isolated from bonnet (*M. radiata*), Japanese (*M. fuscata*), Taiwan (*M. cyclopis*), and stump-tail (*M. artoides*) macaques. No other Old World or New World monkeys have been reported as harbouring B virus naturally. Fatal disease associated with B-virus infections has been reported among several non-macaque species of primates in addition to humans.

Like human HSV infection, the prevalence of B-virus infection among macaques is low in populations of immature animals, increases rapidly as animals reach sexual maturity, and approaches 80 per cent or higher in adult populations. Vesicular oral lesions have been seen in some cases thought to represent acute infections. Chronically infected monkeys shed virus only intermittently. In one study of a group of macaques with 100 per cent seroprevalence of B-virus infection, only 2 to 3 per cent were shedding virus at any given time. Monkeys are more likely to shed B virus when they are ill, under stress, or during the breeding season. Virus can be cultured with equal frequency from the conjunctiva, buccal mucosa, and genital areas of shedding monkeys, although there are generally no lesions present. Macaca monkeys, native to Asia and northern Africa, are housed in research facilities, zoos, and private homes throughout the world. Humans who have contact with these animals or their products may be exposed to B virus through bites, scratches, and other routes.

Most reported human infections are from the United States, with the remainder from Great Britain and Canada. Human B-virus infections usually occur as single cases, but two clusters have been described: one in Florida in 1987 and a second in Michigan in 1989. The only reported human-to-human transmission of B-virus infection, documented in 1987, occurred through direct, repeated inoculation of drainage from active primary B-virus herpetiform lesions on to skin disrupted by contact dermatitis. Transmission was possibly facilitated by use of corticosteroid cream. Humans have most frequently been infected through injuries sustained while working in the biomedical research industry. Increases in reports of human cases occurred in the late 1950s at the time when rhesus monkeys were being used increasingly for polio vaccine testing in biomedical research laboratories, and again in the 1980s with their use in retrovirus research. B-virus infection in humans remains an uncommon result of bites, scratches, and other exposures to monkeys.

Clinical manifestations

Fewer than 30 human B-virus infections have been discussed in detail in the literature. In well-documented human cases, clinical evidence of B-virus infection has developed between 3 and 30 days after exposure.

The most common presentation is with rapidly ascending encephalomyelitis following a prodrome characterized by non-specific febrile malaise, variably accompanied by herpetic blisters and/or peripheral neuraesthesia near the site of injury and infection. Herpetic blisters, when present, may occur within days of injury. One patient presented with an ophthalmic zoster-like rash, interpreted as recrudescent human herpes. More commonly, a non-specific systemic febrile illness, which may include respiratory symptoms or mild abdominal colic, follows infection by a couple of weeks and may proceed or occur with the start of neurological symptoms. Neurological features may include paraesthesia of the limbs, followed by weakness or loss of reflexes. Neck stiffness, facial paralysis, dysphagia, or diplopia are ominous signs, rapidly followed by respiratory arrest and coma. Some patients have developed involvement of the central nervous system without preceding peripheral symptoms.

Without treatment with a herpes-specific antiviral drug, the infection has a fatality rate of approximately 70 per cent, comparable to that of herpes simplex encephalitis. However, the clinical symptoms and signs of at least five laboratory-confirmed human B-virus infections have resolved following high-dose intravenous therapy with acyclovir or ganciclovir, suggesting a response to treatment.

The virus replicates at the site of inoculation, with local inflammation followed by lymphangitis and lymphadenitis. Viraemia has not been detected in humans. The virus appears to spread primarily by neuronal routes, although spread via lymphatics, particularly to abdominal viscera, is possible, and evidence of visceral congestion and focal haemorrhagic necrosis (particularly of liver and lung) may be found at autopsy. However, the virus is strongly neurotropic for the central nervous system, and unlike HSV, does not tend to localize regionally. Myelitis, encephalitis, encephalomyelitis, or combinations of the above may also occur.

Diagnosis

Diagnostic techniques for human B virus, which include viral culture and serology, are complicated by both the extensive cross-reactivity between antibodies to HSV and B virus, and biosafety requirements for propagation of B virus.

Serological tests for B virus were originally developed for simians. In human populations, in which the prevalence of B-virus infection is low and that of HSV-1 and HSV-2 high, the predictive value of serological testing is lower, and the likelihood of a false-positive result is higher than that obtained when testing macaques. The reproducibility of positive serological test results in blind studies using human sera has been uneven. Any apparent human seroconversion should be confirmed by using a third serum specimen.

Prevention

Most injuries inflicted by monkeys are preventable. All macaques should be presumed to be shedding B virus and handled accordingly, as described in guidelines published by the United States Centers for Disease Control and Prevention.

The adequacy and timeliness of wound decontamination are important factors in minimizing risk of infection once exposed. The eyes, mouth, nose, or other exposed mucosal surfaces should be irrigated for at least 15 min with sterile saline solution or rapidly flowing water only. For injuries in other locations, any concentrated solution of soap or detergent, povidone-iodine, or chlorhexidine may be used.

Evaluation and treatment

Detailed guidelines for the evaluation of human exposures to or treatment of human infections with B virus have been developed by the Centers for Disease Control and Prevention.

Injuries associated with monkeys other than macaques should not raise concerns about B-virus infection. With injuries associated with macaques, prompt debridement and prophylaxis against tetanus, rabies, and bacterial infection should be considered. Postcleansing culture specimens should be obtained, and a full-thickness skin biopsy specimen for culture may be appropriate, depending upon the site and nature of the injury. Evaluation of acute- and convalescent-phase sera is useful for detecting seroconversion.

All potentially exposed people should be educated about the early symptoms and signs suggestive of B-virus disease. It is prudent to instruct patients to take precautions with their blood and other body fluids until absence of seroconversion has been documented.

The clinical and virological status of a macaque associated with a human injury has prognostic implications. If the animal is ill or has herpetiform lesions, the injury should be considered high risk. However, B-virus shedding can occur in clinically healthy animals. Exposure-directed cultures should be collected from the monkey's buccal mucosa (for saliva exposures), conjunctiva or, if urine contamination is a concern, the urogenital areas.

Some experts recommend presumptive acyclovir therapy immediately after macaque-related injuries in the hope of preventing actual B-virus infection. Presumptive therapy is of unclear efficacy, may complicate diagnostic issues by suppressing seroconversion, and is unnecessary after most such injuries. Clear evidence of viral shedding by the monkey may merit consideration of presumptive therapy for persons who received inadequately cleansed, high-risk injuries.

The treatment of choice is acyclovir. The 50 per cent inhibitory dose of acyclovir for B virus in tissue culture (ID_{50}) is about 10-fold higher than that for HSV-1. The recommended dosage for presumptive therapy is in the range of 800 mg by mouth five times a day for at least 14 days.

The development of suggestive neurological symptoms or signs in persons exposed to B virus warrants immediate admission to hospital and strict barrier precautions to avoid contact with blood, any body fluids, or wound drainage. The history should carefully note exposure, onset, and progression of symptoms. The physical examination should include evaluation of skin lesions as well as a baseline assessment of sensory and motor function (with particular attention to the originally injured limb), and cerebellar and cortical function. In view of the potential toxicity of high-dose antiviral therapy, the minimal laboratory evaluation should include a complete blood count, differential cell count, and a serum creatinine measurement.

Bites from non-human primates bred in captivity and housed without access to feral animals pose virtually no risk of rabies infection. However, paralytic rabies must be considered in the differential diagnosis of anyone who presents with neurological disease following bites from free-living primates, newly imported captive primates, or primates housed in outdoor facilities allowing potential contact with raccoons and other rabies carriers.

Bilateral conjunctival swabs, posterior oropharyngeal swabs, and swabs (or, if clinically appropriate, full-thickness biopsy specimens) from the bases of any vesicular or ulcerative lesions may yield B virus in culture.

Magnetic resonance imaging or, if unavailable, computerized tomography are useful in the evaluation of central nervous lesions. Median somatosensory-evoked potentials may help identify early evidence of brainstem and cervical spinal-cord involvement. Electroencephalography or radionuclide brain scans may be helpful in differentiating B-virus encephalitis from HSV encephalitis; the latter frequently localizes in the temporal lobe areas. Rising B-virus antibody titres have been identified in cerebrospinal-fluid specimens collected serially from two patients.

Acyclovir in doses of at least 10 mg/kg given intravenously every 8 h is recommended for patients with only peripheral neurological symptoms and signs or herpetiform lesions limited to the trunk or extremities. If central nervous symptoms or signs or herpetiform lesions of the head or neck are present, maximal intravenous acyclovir dosages of 15 mg/kg given every 8 h (45 mg/kg per day) should be used, and the use of ganciclovir (5 mg/kg every 12 h) should be considered. The *in vitro* ID_{50} of ganciclovir for B virus is somewhat lower than that of acyclovir; however, the increased toxicity of ganciclovir makes it less suitable for initial use.

When the patient is clinically improved and serial cultures are consistently negative, therapy may be switched to acyclovir 800 mg by mouth five times per day (4 gm/day). The patient should be closely monitored for clinical deterioration and continued suppression of viral shedding should be confirmed.

The required duration of acyclovir therapy in patients with documented, previously symptomatic, B-virus infection is controversial. The propensity of herpesviruses to establish chronic infections and to reactivate, the late onset of disease in a rabbit model with premature discontinuation of acyclovir, and the existence of human cases with features suggestive of reactivation of chronic latent infections has led some experts to argue that lifelong therapy is imperative. Conversely, the persistently asymptomatic state of at least one long-term survivor, in the absence of acyclovir therapy, and the absence of disease in a rabbit model when acyclovir was discontinued after a 14- to 21-day course has led others to argue that lifelong acyclovir therapy and the attendant risk of drug-associated side-effects may be unnecessary.

The discontinuation of acyclovir therapy for any reason should be done with the informed consent of the patient and with continuous monitoring for evidence of resumed viral shedding or symptoms.

B-virus-infected people who have no evidence of viral shedding by culture should be advised that transmission to their intimate contacts is unlikely but possible. One instance of human-to-human transmission was identified in Florida in 1987. There have been no other instances reported of secondary spread to others from at least five surviving persons infected with B virus between 1987 and 1989.

REFERENCES

Artenstein, A.W., Hicks, C.B., Goodwin, B.S., and Hilliard, J.K. (1991). Human infection with B virus following a needlestick injury. *Reviews of Infectious Diseases*, **13,** 288–91.

Boulter, E.A., Thornton, B., Bauer, D.J., and Bye, A. (1980). Successful treatment of experimental B virus (*Herpesvirus simiae*) infection with acyclovir. *British Medical Journal*, **280,** 681–3.

Breen, G.E., Lamb, S.G., and Otaki, A.T. (1958). Monkey bite encephalomyelitis: Report of a case with recovery. *British Medical Journal*, **2,** 22–3.

Davenport, D.S., Johnson, D.R., Holmes, G.P., Jewitt, D., Ross, S.C., and Hilliard, J.K. (1994). Diagnosis and management of human B virus (*Herpesvirus simiae*) infections in Michigan. *Clinical Infectious Diseases*, **19,** 33–41 .

Davidson, W.L., and Hummeler, K. (1960). B virus infection in man. *Annals of the New York Academy of Sciences*, **85,** 970–9.

Fierer, J., Bazeley, P., and Braude, A.I. (1973). Herpes B virus encephalomyelitis presenting as ophthalmic zoster: a possible latent infection reactivated. *Annals of Internal Medicine*, **79,** 225–8.

Holmes, G.P. *et al.* (1990). B virus (*Herpesvirus simiae*) infection in humans: epidemiologic investigation of a cluster. *Annals of Internal Medicine* **112,** 833–9.

Holmes, G.P. *et al.* and the B Virus Working Group. (1995). Guidelines for preventing and treating B virus infections in exposed persons. *Clinical Infectious Diseases*, **20,** (in press).

Palmer, A.E. (1987). B-virus, *Herpesvirus simiae*: historical perspective. *Journal of Medical Primatology*, **16,** 99–130.

Sabin, A.B. and Wright, A.M. (1934). Acute ascending myelitis following a monkey bite, with the isolation of a virus capable of reproducing the disease. *Journal of Experimental Medicine*, **59,** 115–36.

Weigler, B.J. (1992). Biology of B virus in macaques and human hosts: a review. *Clinical Infectious Diseases*, **14,** 555–67.

Zwartouw, H.T., Humphreys, C.R., and Collins, P. (1989). Oral chemotherapy of fatal B virus (*Herpesvirus simiae*) infection. *Antiviral Research*, **11,** 275–84.

7.10.6 Cytomegalovirus

S. STAGNO

Cytomegalovirus is a group of agents within the herpesvirus family known for their wide distribution among man and other mammals. *In vivo* and *in vitro* infections with these viruses are highly species-specific and produce a typical cytopathology of greatly enlarged (cytomegalic) cells containing intranuclear and cytoplasmic inclusions. Cytomegalovirus causes diverse clinical manifestations in both children and adults. Most infections are subclinical. Occasionally it causes a syndrome of cytomegalic inclusion disease in newborns and a mononucleosis-like syndrome in normally immunocompetent adults. In contrast, among immunosuppressed individuals, recipients of organ transplants, premature infants, and patients with AIDS, it causes significant disease. The infection that occurs in a seronegative, virgin host is referred to as primary infection while recurrent infection represents reactivation of latent infection or reinfection in a seropositive, immune host. Disease may result from primary or recurrent infection but the former usually causes more severe disease. Following a primary infection, viral excretion from one or multiple sites persists for weeks, months, or even years before it becomes latent. As with other herpesvirus infections, episodes of recurrent infection with renewed viral shedding are common even years after the primary infection.

Epidemiology—transmission

Seroepidemiological surveys have found evidence of cytomegalovirus infection in every human population examined. (Fig. 1). The prevalence of antibody to cytomegalovirus increases with age but the increment is quite different among various populations. Prevalence of infection is higher in developing countries and among lower socioeconomic strata of the more developed nations. Transmission occurs by direct person-to-person contact. Sources of cytomegalovirus include saliva, milk, cervical and vaginal secretions, urine, semen, tears, stools, and blood. Indirect transmission is possible with contaminated fomites, such as children's toys. Climate does not affect infection rates. As cytomegalovirus is very labile, spread requires very close or intimate contact.

The incidence of congenital infection ranges from 0.2 to 2.2 per cent. Transmission can occur *in utero* as a consequence of viraemia during primary or recurrent infections. Recurrence is common in lightly immune populations and is presumed to result from reactivation of cytomegalovirus.

Transmission of cytomegalovirus during the perinatal period is quite common, with rates of infection reaching 10 to 60 per cent by 6 months of age. The two most important sources of virus during this period are exposure to infected genital-tract secretions at delivery and breast milk. The risk of infection for infants exposed to these two sources is 57 and 63 per cent, respectively. Typically, children with congenital and perinatal infections excrete virus for years in the oropharynx and in urine. After the first year of life the rate of infection is highly dependent upon child-rearing practices. Day-care centres, where infection rates of 50 to

80 per cent are common, and similar facilities contribute to the rapid spread of cytomegalovirus.

For children who are not exposed to other toddlers the rate of infection increases very slowly throughout the first decade of life. During adolescence a second spurt may be noticed, particularly among population groups with more seronegative subjects. This is partly the result of sexual transmission. Cytomegalovirus is frequently isolated from semen and cervical or vaginal secretions. In populations with high rates of cytomegalovirus infection in childhood, sexual transmission plays a minor part as a source of primary infection, but its importance in reinfection is unclear.

Seronegative parents of young children shedding cytomegalovirus and seronegative day-care workers exposed to infected children have a 20 to 40 per cent annual risk of acquiring cytomegalovirus, compared with a 1 to 3 per cent annual risk for the general population. Despite the belief that health-care workers are also at increased risk, the data show that this is not the case even for nurses working with patients with AIDS, recipients of organ transplants, or with children and infants with documented congenital cytomegalovirus infection.

Nosocomial cytomegalovirus infection is a significant hazard of transfusion of blood and blood products. The risk is highest in populations with a high prevalence of cytomegalovirus infection. In a population with 40 to 50 per cent seroprevalence the risk of transmission has been estimated at 2.7 per cent per unit of whole blood, but it is substantially higher with leucocyte transfusions. Infection is usually asymptomatic but even in children and adults who are well there is a definite risk of disease if they are seronegative and receive multiple transfusions. In immunosuppressed patients and seronegative premature infants the hazard of significant disease is much higher (10–30 per cent). The risk of infection can be eliminated or significantly decreased by selecting seronegative donors, or using leucocyte-depleted, filtered or cryopreserved blood.

After organ transplantation many patients excrete cytomegalovirus. The most important sources for a primary cytomegalovirus infection are transplanted tissues or organs and to a lesser degree, blood or blood products such as leucocytes and platelets. Recurrent cytomegalovirus infections are more likely to result from reactivation of latent infection, although the above sources may also contribute.

Clinical manifestations

The clinical manifestations of cytomegalovirus infection vary with age, route of transmission, and the immune competence of the subject. In the great majority of cases, including those with congenital infection, cytomegalovirus infection is subclinical.

CONGENITAL INFECTION

Only 5 per cent of all congenitally infected infants have typical cytomegalic inclusion disease, another 5 per cent have atypical involvement, and 90 per cent are born with subclinical but chronic infection. The most common and characteristic signs and symptoms are given in Table 1. With cytomegalic inclusion disease, mortality may reach 20 per cent and the outlook for normal development is poor. More that 90 per cent of all symptomatic patients develope central nervous and sensory defects in later years (Table 2). In infants with subclinical infection the outlook is much better, but 5 to 15 per cent will develop some sequelae such as sensorineural hearing loss, developmental abnormalities, microcephaly, chorioretinitis, and neurological defects that are generally less severe than in infants with symptomatic infection at birth (Table 2). Most symptomatic congenital infections and those resulting in sequelae are the result of primary infection acquired during gestation (10–25 per cent) rather than recurrent (0.5–2 per cent) infections in pregnant women. The risk of *in utero* transmission following a primary infection appears to be constant throughout gestation.

PERINATAL INFECTIONS

Infections resulting from exposure to cytomegalovirus in the maternal genital tract at delivery or to breast milk occur in the presence of mater-

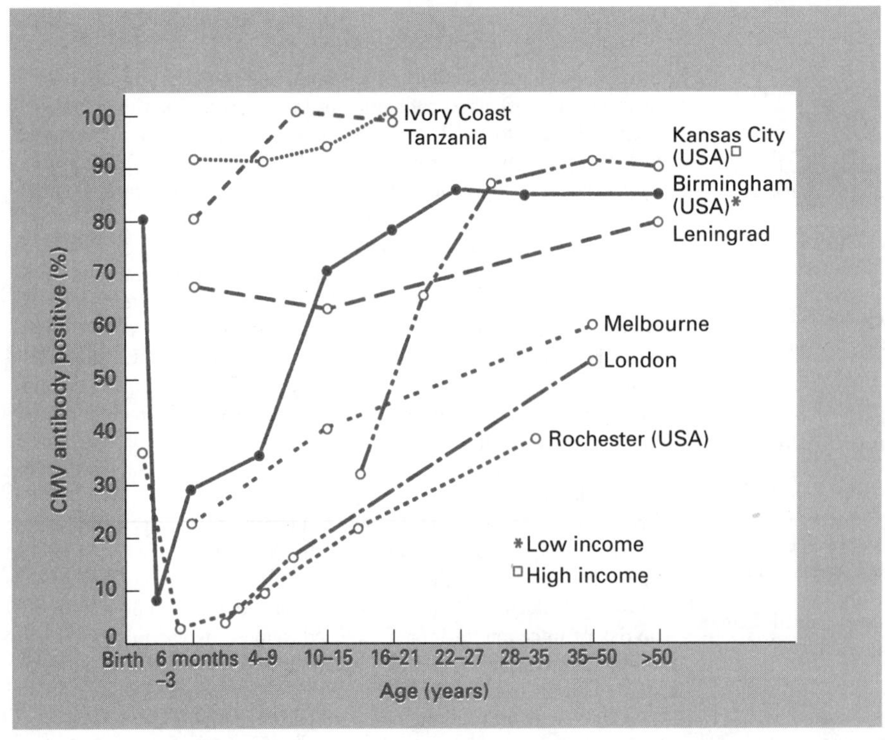

Fig. 1 Seroepidemiology of cytomegalovirus (CMV) infection.

Table 1 *Clinical and laboratory findings in 106 infants with symptomatic congenital cytomegalovirus infection in the neonatal period*

Abnormality	Positive/total examined (%)
Prematurity (< 38 weeks)	36/106 (34)
Small for gestational age	53/106 (50)
Petechiae	80/106 (76)
Jaundice	69/103 (67)
Hepatosplenomegaly	63/105 (60)
Purpura	14/105 (13)
Neurological findings	
One or more of the following:	72/106 (68)
Microcephaly	54/102 (53)
Lethargy/hypotonia	28/104 (27)
Poor suck	20/103 (19)
Seizures	7/105 (7)
Elevated ALT (> 80 u/l)	46/58 (83)
Thrombocytopenia:	
$< 100 \times 10^3$ /mm^3	62/81 (77)
$< 50 \times 10^3$ /mm^3	43/81 (53)
Conjugated hyperbilirubinemia: direct serum bilirubin, 4 mg/dl	47/68 (69)
Haemolysis	37/72 (51)
Increased CSF protein (120 mg/dl)*	24/52 (46)

*Determinations in the first week of life.

ALT, alanine aminotransferase; CSF, cerebrospinal fluid.

Table 2 *Sequelae in children after congenital cytomegalovirus infection*

Sequelae	Symptomatic % (*N*)	Asymptomatic % (*N*)
Sensorineural hearing loss	58.0 (58/100)	7.4 (22/299)
Bilateral hearing loss	37.0 (37/100)	2.7 (8/299)
Speech threshold moderate to profound (60 to > 90 db) for better ear	27.0 (27/100)	1.7 (5/299)
Chorioretinitis	20.4 (19/93)	2.5 (7/281)
IQ less than 70	55.0 (33/60)	3.7 (6/159)
Microcephaly, seizures, or paresis/paralysis	51.9 (54/104)	2.7 (9/330)
Microcephaly	37.5 (39/104)	1.8 (6/330)
Seizures	23.1 (24/104)	0.9 (3/330)
Paresis/paralysis	12.5 (13/104)	0.0 (0/330)
Death (after neonatal period)	5.8 (6/104)	0.3 (1/330)

nally derived, passively acquired antibody. The majority of infants infected in these ways remain asymptomatic and do not suffer long-term complications. Occasionally, perinatally acquired cytomegalovirus infection is associated with a protracted pneumonitis syndrome that is clinically and radiographically indistinguishable from other causes of afebrile pneumonia in young infants. In premature and sick full-term infants, naturally acquired cytomegalovirus infection may have neurological sequelae and psychomotor retardation. However, the risk of hearing loss, chorioretinitis, and microcephaly does not appear to be increased.

Transfusion-acquired, perinatal cytomegalovirus infection can cause significant illness and death, particularly in premature infants (birth weight less than 1500 g) born to mothers seronegative for the virus. Seronegative infants given blood from seropositive donors have a nearly 20 per cent risk of acquiring cytomegalovirus, and if they become infected, nearly 40 per cent develop a syndrome of hepatosplenomegaly, deterioration of respiratory function, grey pallor, thrombocytopenia, atypical lymphocytosis, and or haemolytic anaemia. The syndrome, which is self-limiting, lasts 2 to 3 weeks; but the mortality is 20 per cent.

YOUNG CHILDREN

Most cytomegalovirus infections acquired in childhood are asymptomatic. Occasionally they cause hepatosplenomegaly with abnormal 'liver function tests' or respiratory illnesses.

ADOLESCENTS AND ADULTS

Serologically-proven cytomegalovirus infection becomes increasingly frequent with advancing age, with a burst in adolescence. While cytomegalovirus has been implicated in disease of virtually every organ system, well-established clinical syndromes are few. A heterophile antibody-negative mononucleosis syndrome occurs spontaneously in adults and can develop following infection acquired by blood transfusion at any age (Fig. 2). In contrast to the Epstein–Barr virus-induced syndrome, tonsillopharyngitis, lymphadenopathy, and splenomegaly are less common. There is malaise, myalgia, fever, abnormal liver function, and lymphocytosis with a significant increase in the proportion of atypical lymphocytes. The course of cytomegalovirus mononucleosis is generally mild, but occasionally patients may present with high persistent fever, or with clinically apparent hepatitis, generalized lymphadenopathies, and/or morbilliform rashes. Rare complications of acute primary cytomegalovirus infection include pneumonitis, myocarditis, pericarditis, neuritis, and myelitis (Guillain–Barré syndrome), encephalitis, aseptic meningitis, thrombocytopenic purpura, haemolytic anemia, and retinitis. In normal hosts, recurrent infections are asymptomatic. In immunocompromised individuals the risk of illness and death is increased, especially in primary but also in recurrent infections. Clinically, pneumonitis is most common, but hepatitis, chorioretinitis, gastrointestinal disease, and fever with leucopenia occur individually or in combination, leading to combination generalized disease often associated with a fatal outcome.

The greatest risk is in patients undergoing transplantation and those with AIDS. As with other populations, primary infections are clearly more virulent. In patients with AIDS, common problems include pneumonitis, involvement of the gastrointestinal and central nervous systems, and chorioretinitis, which may be devastating.

In transplant recipients, cancer patients, and other immunosuppressed groups the clinical manifestations are quite variable and depend largely on the degree of immunosuppression. Common findings include a mononucleosis-like illness with fever, myalgia, hepatosplenomegaly, liver enzyme elevations, and, unlike in cytomegalovirus mononucleosis in normal hosts, leucopenia, thrombocytopenia, and anaemia. Pneumonitis is a hallmark of cytomegalovirus disease in this group, particularly in bone-marrow transplant patients. Hepatic dysfunction is common but frank hepatitis is rare. In liver transplant recipients, hepatitis must de distinguished from rejection episodes. Gastrointestinal complications are difficult to evaluate yet may cause significant problems in the immunosuppressed. Submucosal ulcerations can occur anywhere in the gastrointestinal tract from oesophagus to rectum. Haemorrhage and perforation are known complications, so are pancreatitis and cholecystitis. Cytomegalovirus retinitis is a serious complication that may occur at any time after transplantation or during immunosuppression.

Laboratory diagnosis

In neonates, children and adults, whether healthy or immunocompromised, the diagnosis of cytomegalovirus infection requires laboratory confirmation. The best means of demonstrating an active infection is by virus isolation from urine, saliva, milk, cervical secretions, buffy coat, or other tissues obtained by biopsies or at autopsy. Rapid (24 h) viral diagnosis is now possible with monoclonal antibodies to specific early antigens. Virus isolation alone cannot distinguish between primary and recurrent (reactivation/reinfection) infections.

A primary infection is confirmed by seroconversion (*de novo*) appearance of IgG antibodies), or the simultaneous detection of IgG and IgM antibodies, provided that the measurement is done with a specific and sensitive assay. Rising IgG antibody titres may follow primary or recurrent infections and so must be interpreted with caution. Several sensitive and specific serological tests for measurement of IgG antibodies are readily available. However, clinicians must remember that to define rises in antibody titres, complement fixation, neutralization, anticomplement immunofluorescence, and indirect immunofluorescence assays are preferable because they are quantitative and have well-defined end-points. In contrast, radioimmunoassay and enzyme immunoassay are less reliable at demonstrating significant changes in titres, as most laboratories establish binding ratio (radioimmunoassay) and absorbance units (enzyme immunoassay) at a fixed serum dilution to compare the quantities of antibodies present in two sera. A simple rise in antibody titres in initially seropositive subjects must be interpreted with caution as these are occasionally seen years after primary infection. IgG antibodies persist for life. IgM antibodies can be demonstrated transiently (4–16 weeks) during the acute phase of symptomatic or asymptomatic primary infection in adults. Radioimmunoassay, enzyme immunoassay, and an IgM-capture radioimmunoassay have acceptable specificity and sensitivity to detect primary infections. With these assays IgM antibodies are not found, or are only transiently detected in patients with recurrent infection.

A recurrent infection is defined by the reappearance of viral excretion in a patient known to have been seropositive in the past. The distinction between reactivation of endogenous virus and reinfection with a different strain of cytomegalovirus is difficult and requires restriction enzyme analysis of viral DNA to demonstrate homology between viral isolates.

In immunocompromised patients, excretion of cytomegalovirus rises in IgG titres and even the presence of IgM antibodies is common, making the distinction between primary and recurrent infections more difficult. Determining the serological status of patients before transplantation and immunosuppressive treatment helps future management. Viraemia (cultured from buffy coat) implies active disease and a worse prognosis whether the type of infection is primary, recurrent or unknown.

The decisive way of distinguishing congenital from perinatal cytomegalovirus infection is by isolating virus during the first 2 weeks of life. Urine and saliva are the best specimens to submit to the laboratory. An IgG antibody test is of little diagnostic value. A negative result excludes the diagnosis but a positive result generally reflects maternal immunity. Demonstration of stable or rising titres during the first year of life does not help because perinatal infections are common. In general, IgM tests lack sensitivity and specificity, and are technically demanding. No reliable test is commercially available.

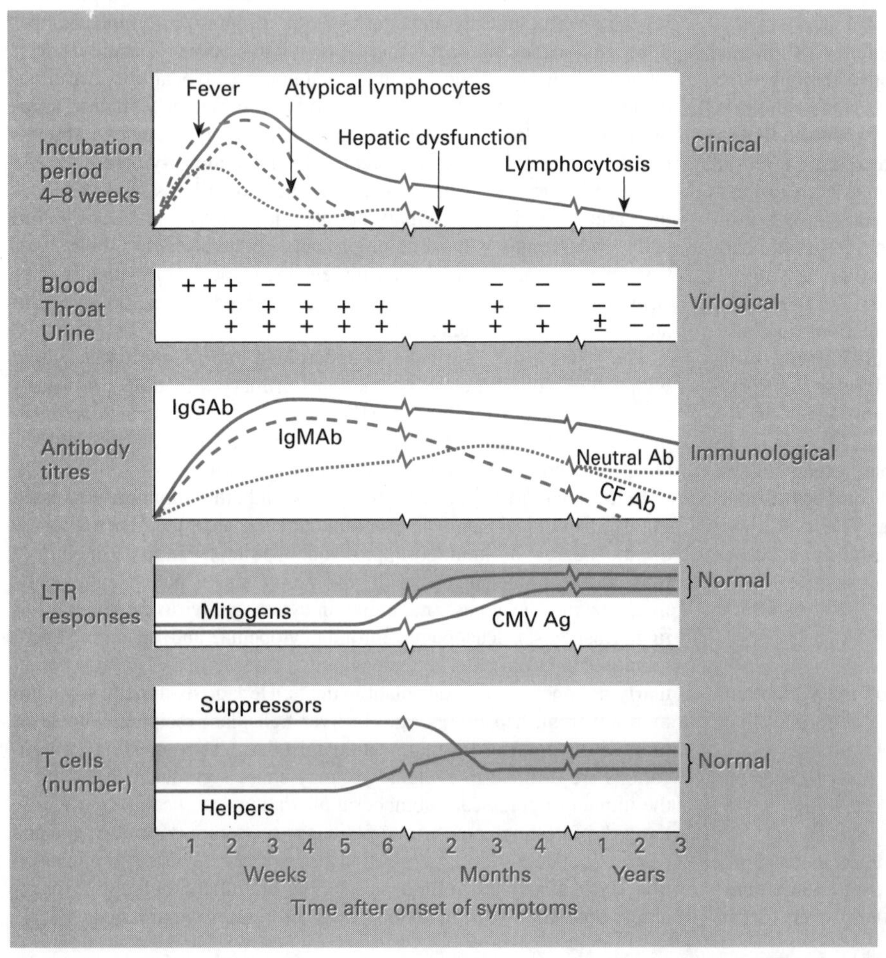

Fig. 2 Findings with symptomatic primary cytomegalovirus (CMV) infection (mononucleosis syndrome) in normal hosts. (Reproduced from Alford, C.A. and Britt, W.J. (1990). Cytomegalovirus. In *Virology* (ed. D.M. Knipe, *et al.*) 2nd edn. pp. 1981. Raven Press, New York, with permission.)

Treatment

Cytomegalovirus is unusually recalcitrant; adeninarabinoside, acyclovir, and interferon have failed but ganciclovir, the most recent antiviral to undergo clinical trials, has produced some encouraging results. It has been used to treat life-threatening cytomegalovirus infections in immunocompromised hosts (such as those with bone marrow, cardiac, and kidney transplants, and with AIDS). A regimen of 10 mg/kg per day, with individual doses given at 12-h intervals for 2 or 3 weeks, followed by a once-a-day maintenance of 5 mg/kg given until regression of clinical manifestations, has proved to have some efficacy. Cytomegalovirus retinitis and gastrointestinal disease appear to be clinically responsive to therapy, but like viral excretion, recur upon cessation of therapy. The results are even less encouraging with cytomegalovirus pneumonitis.

Drug toxicity with ganciclovir is extensive and includes neutropenia, thrombocytopenia, liver dysfunction, reduction in spermatogenesis, and gastrointestinal and renal abnormalities. No results of controlled studies of treatment for congenital cytomegalovirus infection are yet available. One phase I/II study has shown encouraging results at a dose of 12 mg/kg/day for a total of 6 weeks. A randomized study of symptomatic congenital infection is under way.

Prevention

Passive immunoprophylaxis

The use of prophylactic hyperimmune plasma or globulin in recipients of transplants has resulted in a significant reduction of symptomatic disease but not in prevention of infection. The efficacy of immunoglobulin is more striking in situations in which the risk of primary cytomegalovirus infection carry a high risk of morbidity such as in bone marrow transplantation. One recommended regimen is 1.0 g/kg of immunoglobulin given as a single intravenous dose beginning within 72 h of transplantation and once weekly there after until day 120 after transplantation.

ACTIVE IMMUNIZATION

The beneficial role of acquired immunity to cytomegalovirus is substantial as illustrated by the fact that the most severe disease generally follows primary infection in seronegative patients. This is particularly true in congenital infection, transfusion-acquired infection, and infection in transplant recipients. The most important targets for a vaccination are seronegative women of childbearing age and seronegative transplant recipients. Vaccine trials however, have been disappointing. Live attenuated vaccines are immunogenic but immunity wanes quickly. The Towne attenuated vaccine produces self-limiting asymptomatic infection resulting in humoral and cell-mediated immune responses in almost all healthy volunteers. Vaccine virus does not seem to be transmissible. Vaccinees are protected when challenged with low but not with high dosage of virus. In renal transplant recipients the vaccine does not protect against cytomegalovirus infection but appears to reduce the virulence of primary infection. In a recent study of vaccine efficacy in normal adult women the Towne vaccine did not provide protection against naturally acquired infection.

In summary, live attenuated cytomegalovirus vaccines have at best a marginal effect in preventing primary cytomegalovirus disease and their use remains controversial. Subunit and recombinant vaccines remain to be developed.

OTHER PREVENTIVE MEASURES

The use of cytomegalovirus-free blood and blood products, and when possible the use of organs from cytomegalovirus-free donors, represent important measures to prevent cytomegalovirus infection and disease in non-immune patients.

The screening of pregnant women to identify those at risk of primary infection remains controversial because the risk is relatively low and there are no proven means of identifying the infected fetuses that will go on to develop significant disease.

REFERENCES

Adler, S.P. (1986). Molecular epidemiology of cytomegalovirus: evidence for viral transmission to parents from children enrolled in a day care center. *Pediatric Infectious Diseases*, **5,** 315–18.

Adler, S.P. (1989). Cytomegalovirus and child day care: evidence for an increased infection rate among day care workers. *New England Journal of Medicine*, **321,** 1290–300.

Adler, S.P., Chandrika, T., Lawrence, L., and Baggett, J. (1983). Cytomegalovirus infections in neonates due to blood transfusions. *Pediatric Infectious Diseases*, **2,** 114–18.

Alford, C.A. and Britt, W.J. (1990). Cytomegalovirus. In *Virology*, (2nd edn), (ed. B.N. Fields *et al.*), pp. 1981–2010. Raven Press, New York.

Balfour, H.H., Jr., Welo, P.K., and Sach, C.W. (1985). Cytomegalovirus vaccine trial in 400 renal transplant candidates. *Transplant Procedures*, **17,** 81–3.

Gold, E. and Nankervis, G.A. (1976). Viral infections of humans: epidemiology and control. In *Cytomegalovirus*, (ed. A.S. Evans), pp. 143–61. Plenum, New York.

Griffiths, P.D. *et al.* (1984). Rapid diagnosis of cytomegalovirus infection in immunocompromised patients by detection of early antigen fluorescent foci. *Lancet*, **ii,** 1242–5.

Handsfield, H.H. *et al.* (1985). Cytomegalovirus infection in sex partners evidence for sexual transmission. *Journal of Infectious Diseases*, **151,** 344–8.

Ho, M. (1990). Cytomegalovirus. In *Principles and practice of infectious diseases* (3rd edn.) (ed. G.L. Mandell, *et al.*) pp 1159–72. Churchill-Livingstone, Edinburgh.

Kangro, H.O., Booth, J.C., Bakir, T.M.F., Tryhorn, Y., and Sutherland, S. (1984). Detection of IgM antibodies against cytomegalovirus: comparison to two radioimmunoassays, enzyme-linked immunosorbent assay and immunofluorescent antibody test. *Journal of Medical Virology*, **14,** 73–80.

Pass, R.F. and Stagno, S. (1988). Hospital acquired infection in the pediatric patient. In *Cytomegalovirus*, (ed. L.G. Donowitz), pp. 174–87. Williams & Wilkins, Baltimore.

Pass, R.F., August, A.M., Dworsky, M.E., and Reynolds, D.W. (1982). Cytomegalovirus infection in a day-care center. *New England Journal of Medicine*, **307,** 477–9.

Pass, R.F., Hutto, C., Ricks, R., and Cloud, G. (1986). Increased rate of cytomegalovirus infection among parents of children attending day care centers. *New England Journal of Medicine*, **314,** 1414–16.

Plotkin, S.A. *et al.* (1984). Towne-vaccine-induced prevention of cytomegalovirus disease after renal transplants. *Lancet*, **i,** 528–30.

Stagno, S., Reynolds, D.W., Pass, R.F., and Alford, C.A. (1980). Breast milk and the risk of cytomegalovirus infection. *New England Journal of Medicine*, **302,** 1073–6.

Stagno, S., Pass, R.F., Dworsky, M.E., and Alford, C.A. (1984). Maternal cytomegalovirus and perinatal transmission. In *Clinical obstetrics and gynecology*, (ed. G.E. Knox), pp. 563–76. Lippincott, Philadelphia.

Stagno, S., Britt, M.D., and Pass, R.F. (1989). *Cytomegalovirus*, 12, *Diagnostic procedures for viral, rickettsial and chlamydial infections*, (ed. N.J. Schmidt and R.W. Emmons), pp. 321–78. American Public Health Association, Washington DC.

Stern, H. (1984). Live cytomegalovirus vaccination of healthy volunteers: eight-year follow-up studies. In *Cytomegalovirus: Pathogenesis and prevention of human infection*, (ed. S.A. Plotkin, S. Michelson, J.S. Pagano, and F. Rapp). *Birth defects*, Original article series, Vol. 20, no. 1, pp. 263–9. Liss, New York.

Strangert, K., Carlstrom, G., Jeansson, S., and Nord, C.E. (1976). Infections in pre-school children in group day care. *Acta Paediatrica Scandinavica*, **65,** 455–63.

Weller, T.H. (1971). The cytomegaloviruses: ubiquitous agents with protein clinical manifestations. *New England Journal of Medicine*, **285,** 203–14; 267–74.

Yeager, A.S., Grumet, F.C., Hafleigh, E.B., Arvin, A.M., Bradley, J.E., and Prober, C.G. (1981). Prevention of transfusion-acquired cytomegalovirus infections in newborn infants. *Journal of Pediatrics*, **988,** 281–7.

7.10.7 Human herpesvirus 6

P. E. Pellett and J. A. Stewart

Human herpesvirus 6 (**HHV-6**) is common throughout the world. It is predominantly tropic for T cells both *in vitro* and *in vivo*, although it can grow in other cell types, including macrophages, cells of neural origin, fibroblasts, and epithelial cells. Two groups of HHV-6 isolates have been identified by physical and biological properties: variants A and B (HHV-6A and HHV-6B). HHV-6A has not been specifically associated with human disease, while HHV-6B is aetiologically associated with roseola (exanthem subitum or sixth disease) and is a leading cause of febrile illness in children. HHV-6 infections are easily misdiagnosed, for example as antibiotic sensitivity or post-transplant graft-versus-host disease, so it is important to understand the range of clinical features associated with the virus.

Epidemiology

Primary infection with HHV-6 usually occurs 6 months to 2 years after birth. It persists latent in the host, like other herpesviruses. Current serological assays cannot distinguish antibodies to HHV-6A from those to HHV-6B; in most populations, over 90 per cent of people over 2 years old are seropositive for at least one HHV-6 variant.

The rapid acquisition of the virus after loss of maternal antibody implies that HHV-6 is common in the household environment; the virus has been detected in salivary glands, saliva, and urine. Breast-feeding has not been ruled out as a possible route of transmission, but breast-fed and non-breast-fed children acquire primary infection at the same age and viral DNA was detected in none of 120 breast milk specimens by polymerase chain reaction.

Several diseases are associated with HHV-6 activity. Acute primary infection with HHV-6 can cause roseola and other febrile illnesses in children, and reactivated infections or reinfection may lead to post-transplant complications. Its association with chronic diseases, such as lymphoid malignancies and chronic fatigue syndrome is unproven. Elevated antibody titres, increased frequency of virus isolation, and even the presence of the virus in the affected tissue do not establish aetiology.

Clinical features

PRIMARY INFECTION

The most common clinical manifestation of primary HHV-6 infection is childhood roseola. This is characterized by 3 or 4 days of fever, followed by rapid defervescence and then the appearance of a rash that persists for 1 to 3 days. High fever (frequently over 40°C) in an otherwise healthy child is characteristic. The rash may be either patchy, rubella-like, and maculopapular or a more severe measles-like eruption. A transient viraemia present during the febrile period seldom persists through the rash phase. Diarrhoea, bulging fontanelle, and bronchopneumonia are frequently observed. Convulsions, hepatocellular dysfunction, and intussusception are less frequent. The illness generally resolves untreated without complication. Approximately 30 per cent of all children are estimated to experience roseola.

Primary HHV-6 infection can lead to a variety of other conditions, including subclinical infections and a rash without fever, or fever following or without rash. Primary HHV-6 infection is a leading cause of febrile illness in children. In one study of children less than 2 years old, 34 (14 per cent) of 243 febrile admissions to a paediatric emergency department had HHV-6 viraemia. Only one child was still viraemic after 30 days. In most cases, HHV-6 IgG titres rose significantly within 30 days. Viraemia was associated with higher average temperatures (39.7°C vs. 39.1°C), lower white-cell counts (8900 vs. 13 200/mm^3), and significantly more frequent malaise and irritability. The HHV-6-positive children were less likely to have inflamed tympanic membranes, nasal congestion, or vomiting. Only three of the children had clinical courses similar to classical roseola; approximately one-third were reported to have had a rash at the time of, or within a week of, the initial visit.

A rash following antimicrobial treatment for fever of unknown origin can be mistaken for hypersensitivity to the antimicrobial when the actual cause is primary HHV-6 infection. A diagnosis of drug allergy should not be made without good evidence in view of its long-term consequences.

Rare associations with probable primary HHV-6 infection include liver dysfunction, fatal fulminant hepatitis, fatal haemophagocytic syndrome, hepatosplenomegaly, heterophile antibody-negative mononucleosis, induction of spontaneous abortion, meningoencephalitis, encephalitis, and fatal disseminated infection. Viral activity in these conditions has been suggested by a serological response to HHV-6 but not to other potential pathogens, virus isolation during the acute phase of disease, and detection of virus in biopsy materials.

HHV-6 AND ORGAN TRANSPLANTATION

HHV-6 activity has been detected during the immune suppression that follows bone-marrow, cardiac, hepatic, and renal transplantation. In one study, viral antigen was detected in 30 per cent of rejected kidneys. In another, 12 of 25 bone-marrow transplant recipients showed evidence serologically or by virus isolation of HHV-6 reactivation. Symptoms associated with reactivation or reinfection included fever, severe interstitial pneumonitis, and rashes. HHV-6 episodes have been mistaken for acute graft-versus-host disease; correct differential diagnosis is important as the immunosuppressive therapy for graft-versus-host disease may prolong or increase HHV-6-associated symptoms. The emergence of each herpesvirus following transplantation occurs after a characteristic period of time. Most HHV-6 activity occurs 2 or 3 weeks after bone marrow transplantation.

HHV-6 AND AIDS

Several of the initial isolates of HHV-6 were obtained from lymphocytes of patients with AIDS. Both HHV-6 and human immunodeficiency virus type 1 (**HIV-1**) replicate in and can dually infect CD4+ T lymphocytes. HHV-6 and HIV-1 can exert synergistic effects on cytopathology *in vitro*. Although its role in the progression of HIV-1 infection or the course of AIDS is uncertain, dissemination of HHV-6 has been observed to lung, lymph nodes, liver, spleen, retinas, and the brain in necropsy tissues from AIDS patients. In addition, the virus has been associated with pneumonitis in some patients.

HHV-6 AND HAEMATOLOGICAL MALIGNANCY

The role of HHV-6 in the development and progression of haematological malignancies is not clear. The virus has been isolated from patients with lymphoproliferative disorders, including B-cell lymphoma, T-cell lymphoma, angioimmunoblastic lymphadenopathy, and acute lymphocytic leukaemia. HHV-6 nucleotide sequences have been detected in fewer than 5 per cent of biopsy specimens from patients with leukaemia and lymphoma, and in some positive specimens the level of viral DNA varied independently from the tumour content. *In vitro* cell transformation does not result from infection with HHV-6, although it has been observed following transfection of the viral genome and several cloned genomic subfragments, even in the absence of detectable viral DNA in the resulting transformed cells. If a 'hit and run' mechanism operates *in vivo*, as suggested by the *in vitro* results, retrospective analysis of tumours may not illuminate the role of the virus in their development. Although HHV-6 nucleic acids are infrequently found in tissues from lymphoproliferative diseases, they were present in tissues from seven of nine patients with sinus histiocytosis with massive lymphadenopathy

(Rosai–Dorfman disease). It is not known whether the virus is a passenger or agent of this disease.

HHV-6 AND CHRONIC FATIGUE SYNDROME

There is no clear evidence of an aetiological association between HHV-6 and chronic fatigue syndrome. Higher HHV-6 antibody titres (as well as higher antibody titres to other viruses) were found in patients with this syndrome than in controls in some studies but not in others. Virus was isolated more frequently from patients in one study. The discrepancies between the studies may be the result of differences in study design, including case definitions and identification of control populations, as well as differences in laboratory procedures. There is no clinical value in determining HHV-6 antibody status in patients with chronic fatigue syndrome, as most people are seropositive and there is no diagnostically useful antibody titre.

Laboratory diagnosis

Diagnostic tests for HHV-6 infections are not widely available. Rapid and simplified methods need to be developed. HHV-6 can be detected by culture of patient's lymphocytes either alone or by cocultivation with activated human cord-blood lymphocytes. The virus may induce a cytopathic effect characterized by the appearance of large refractile cells during the first week of culture, but this effect cannot be distinguished from that induced by HHV-7 and enlarged lymphocytes can appear spontaneously. The virus is identified using commercially available HHV-6-specific monoclonal antibodies, or by *in situ* hybridization with an HHV-6-specific probe sequence. Several primer sequences suitable for use in the polymerase chain reaction have been described, including some that discriminate between HHV-6A and -6B. Rapid detection by DNA amplification may be particularly valuable in monitoring sequential specimens from transplant recipients. It is the change in status that is important because viral DNA is frequently detected in healthy people.

Serological assays are useful epidemiologically and in prospective studies of the role of HHV-6 in specific diseases. They are less useful in the diagnosis of an individual patient because paired sera collected at least 10 days apart are needed to show a significant rise in antibody level. The most widely used assays for HHV-6 antibodies are the indirect immunofluorescence assay and the anticomplement immunofluorescence assay. Both can be accurate and sensitive, but skilled interpretation is essential. Several microplate-based enzyme immunoassays that use infected cell extracts as antigen have been described. These provide objective and quantitative readings and are more easily standardized from batch to batch.

Often HHV-6-specific IgG can be detected within 2 weeks of primary infection, and titres can rise significantly in response to reactivation or reinfection. Neutralizing IgM antibodies appear 5 to 7 days after onset of exanthem subitum, reach maximum levels after 2 to 3 weeks, and then become undetectable by 2 months. These IgM antibodies are detectable in the second and third month after organ transplantation and persist for 2 to 3 months. About 5 per cent of adults also have IgM neutralizing antibody, possibly indicating either intermittent reactivation or reinfection.

Temporally coincident antibody responses have been described for HHV-6 and human cytomegalovirus, as well as for HHV-6 and measles virus. Adsorption tests have shown that these responses are not due to cross-reactive antibodies. The nature of these viral interactions is not known.

Treatment

Several antiviral drugs have been tested. The most effective *in vitro* growth inhibitors are gancyclovir, phosphonacetic acid, and phosphonoformate. Their effectiveness *in vivo* has not been tested, but they may be useful in immunosuppressed patients in the future.

REFERENCES

Ablashi, D.V., Krueger, G.R.F., and Salahuddin, S.Z. (ed.) (1992). *Human herpesvirus-6: epidemiology, molecular biology and clinical pathology.* Elsevier, London.

Aubin, J. *et al.* (1991). Several groups among human herpesvirus 6 strains can be distinguished by Southern blotting and polymerase chain reaction. *Journal of Clinical Microbiology*, **29,** 367–72.

Bernstein, D.I. (1991). Human herpesvirus-6 and exanthem subitum. In *Advances in pediatric infectious diseases*, Vol. 6, (ed. S.C. Aronoff, W.T. Hughes, S. Kohl, W.T. Speck, and E.R. Wald), pp. 179–92. Mosby Year Book, St. Louis.

Knox, K.K. and Carrigan, D.R. (1994). Disseminated active HHV-6 infections in patients with AIDS. *Lancet*, **343,** 577–8.

Levine, P.H., Jahan, N., Murari, P., Manak, M., and Jaffe, E.S. (1992). Detection of human herpesvirus 6 in tissues involved by sinus histiocytosis with massive lymphadenopathy (Rosai–Dorfman disease). *Journal of Infections Diseases*, **166,** 291–5.

Okuno, T. *et al.* (1990). Human herpesvirus 6 infection in renal transplantation. *Transplantation*, **49,** 519–22.

Pellett, P.E., Black, J.B., and Yamamoto, M. (1992). Human herpesvirus 6: the virus and the search for its role as a human pathogen. *Advances in Virus Research*, **41,** 1–52.

Pruksananonda, P. *et al.* (1992). Initial human herpes virus-6 infection in American children. *New England Journal of Medicine*, **326,** 1445–50.

Schirmer, E.C., Wyatt, L.S., Yamanishi, K., Rodriguez, W.J., and Frenkel, N. (1991). Differentiation between two distinct classes of viruses now classified as human herpesvirus 6. *Proceedings of the National Academy of Sciences (USA)*, **88,** 5922–6.

Yamanishi, K. *et al.* (1988). Identification of human herpesvirus-6 as a causal agent for exanthem subitum. *Lancet*, **i,** 1065–7.

Yoshikawa, T., Kojima, S., and Asano, Y. (1992). Human herpesvirus-6 infection and bone marrow transplantation. *Leukemia and Lymphoma* **8,** 65–73.

Poxviruses

7.10.8 Poxviruses

G. L. SMITH

Poxviruses are a group of large DNA viruses that replicate in the cytoplasm of infected cells. The most infamous member of this group was variola virus, the aetiological agent of smallpox. Smallpox was a greatly feared disease that caused devastating epidemics, with up to 40 per cent mortality, which have significantly affected history. The disease was eradicated in 1977 by extensive immunoprophylaxis with vaccinia virus, a related orthopoxvirus. Subsequently, human diseases caused by poxviruses have been restricted to molluscum contagiosum and rare zoonoses such as monkeypox, cowpox, orf, pseudocowpox, yaba tumour virus, and tanapox. Despite this, poxvirus research remains intense, because vaccinia virus, and now other poxviruses, are being developed as molecular cloning and expression vectors. These recombinant poxviruses are widely used laboratory research tools and also have the potential to be used as live vaccines against diseases other than smallpox.

Classification

Poxviruses are divided into the entomopox and chordopoxvirus subfamilies. Discussion here is limited to the chordopoxviruses, which are subdivided into eight genera of which the orthopoxviruses have been the most important for man (Table 1). Genera are antigenically distinct, while members within a genus share cross-reactive antigens and are broadly cross-protective. Different species of orthopoxvirus have traditionally been distinguished by their biological properties, such as pock type and ceiling temperature on the chorioallantoic membrane, or by the

Table 1 *Poxvirus classification*

Subfamily	Genus	Species
Entomopox		
Chordopox	Orthopox	Variola virus*
		Vaccinia virus*
		Monkeypox virus*
		Cowpox virus*
		Ectromelia virus
		Rabbitpox virus
	Capripox	Sheeppox virus
		Goatpox virus
		Lumpy skin disease virus
	Parapox	Orf virus*
		Pseudocowpox virus*
	Avipox	Fowlpox virus
		Canarypox virus
	Suipox	Swinepox virus
	Leporipox	Myxoma virus
		Shope fibroma virus
		Malignant rabbit virus
	Molluscipox	Molluscum contagiosum virus*
	Yatapox	Yaba tumour virus*
		Tanapox virus*

*Viruses that infect man.

restriction pattern of genomic DNA, but with the availability of increasing amounts of nucleotide-sequence data, species-specific probes may soon be available. Four of the nine poxviruses that infect man are orthopoxviruses. These are cowpox, variola, monkeypox, and vaccinia. Vaccinia has no known natural animal reservoir and its origin remains a mystery. It caused human disease only as a rare complication of its former use as the smallpox vaccine. Cowpox and monkeypox viruses were named according to the species in which they were first isolated but in each case the natural reservoir of the virus may be rodents. Infections in cows or monkeys, like the occasional transmission to man, are rare. Cowpox, monkeypox, and vaccinia virus have a broad host range, while variola virus naturally infected only man. This lack of an animal reservoir contributed greatly to the success of the smallpox eradication campaign.

Poxvirus biology

Most DNA viruses replicate in the host nucleus and can use the host transcriptional and replicative machinery. However, poxviruses have evolved to replicate in the cytoplasm and consequently encode their own enzymes necessary for these processes. Other distinguishing features of poxviruses are the large and complex virus particle (Fig. 1) and the large double-stranded DNA genome of more than 150 kbp, with inverted terminal repeats and terminal hairpins. Much of our knowledge of poxvirus molecular biology has derived from the study of vaccinia virus and what follows pertains to vaccinia unless otherwise stated. The genome of vaccinia virus strain Copenhagen is 192 kbp and encodes approximately 200 genes. These are of three classes (early, intermediate, and late), which are expressed in a strictly regulated manner with transcription of each class being dependent upon the prior expression of the previous class. Early genes are transcribed immediately after infection by the virus-associated, DNA-dependent RNA polymerase. Intermediate genes require prior early-gene expression and their transcription commences with the onset of virus DNA replication. Late genes encode the majority of the virus structural proteins and their expression requires transcription factors encoded by intermediate genes.

Virus morphogenesis is a complex process that occurs in cytoplasmic factories (Fig. 2a) and produces two forms of infectious virus: (i) intracellular mature virus **(IMV),** which remains within the cell cytoplasm and represents the majority of infectious progeny; (ii) extracellular enveloped virus **(EEV),** which is released from the cell and forms only a few percent of infectivity (Fig. 2(b)). EEV possesses an additional lipid envelope that is absent from IMV, with which several virus-encoded proteins are associated. These confer on EEV distinct immunological and biological properties. Thus, although EEV is less abundant than IMV, it is the form of the virus that mediates the long-range spread of virus *in vitro* and *in vivo* and most protective immune responses are directed against antigens unique to EEV. The major vaccinia glycoproteins of the EEV outer envelope have recently been genetically mapped. Genes encoding very highly conserved homologues have been discovered in variola major virus, providing an explanation for the effectiveness of vaccinia virus as a vaccine against smallpox.

Pathogenesis

Poxvirus infections cause either a local skin lesion or a generalized pustular rash, as seen in smallpox (Fig. 3). Detailed experimental analysis of human smallpox was impossible, but generalized poxvirus infections have been studied in experimental models, namely monkeypox in monkeys, rabbitpox (a neurovirulent vaccinia virus that became endemic in rabbits) in rabbits, and ectromelia virus in mice. The spread of human smallpox through the body is believed to have been similar to that of ectromelia virus in mice, as studied by Fenner and colleagues, and is characterized by sequential phases of virus infection, replication, and release accompanied by cell necrosis.

Virus entry was either through minute skin abrasions (ectromelia in mice or cowpox in man and cows) or through the inhalation of airborne virus and establishment of respiratory infection (ectromelia in mice, rabbitpox in rabbits, and smallpox in man). In smallpox the respiratory route was the most important, as airborne virus was sometimes the only possible route of transmission from index cases to contacts, and patients became infectious only after enanthem developed. Rabbitpox virus is similarly transmitted to other rabbits via nasal and pharyngeal secre-

Fig 1. Electron micrograph of material from smallpox lesion, viewed by negative contrast, showing a clump of poxvirus particles (by courtesy of the late Henry Bedson).

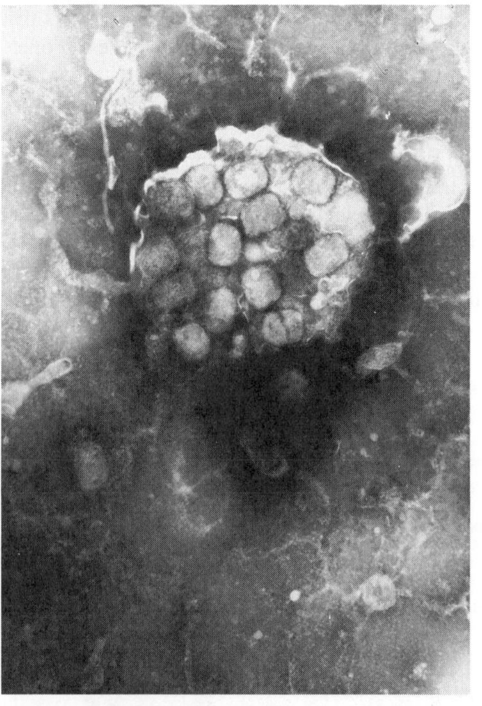

tions. A respiratory infection was established by the virus replicating first in the epithelial cells of the alveoli and small bronchioles. Here, alveolar macrophages became infected and transmitted the virus via lymphatics to local lymph nodes where further replication occurred. Virus released into the blood (primary viraemia) was mostly cell associated and enabled the spread to other organs of the reticuloendothelial system, notably the liver, spleen, and lymph nodes. Extensive replication in these tissues was followed by release of larger amounts of virus into the blood (secondary viraemia), which allowed the virus to infect other internal organs such as the kidneys, lungs and intestines, and to reach the skin and produce the skin lesions with the characteristic centrifugal distribution. These lesions started with a papule that became pustular and then crusted; after 2 to 3 weeks the scab was shed leaving a scar. For smallpox the incubation period before the onset of symptoms was approximately 12 days, during which time considerable virus replication occurred. Symptoms included headache, fever, malaise, vomiting and, in severe cases, prostration, toxaemia, and hypotension. A delayed onset of the skin eruptions generally correlated with a grave prognosis. Haemorrhagic or flat, confluent-type smallpox had very high mortality rates.

Fig 2. Electron micrographs showing (a) a cytoplasmic vaccinia virus factory containing maturing virus particles; numbers 1 to 4 indicate the stages of virus morphogenesis from lipoprotein crescents (1) to intracellular mature virus (IMV) (4). (b) Fully enveloped virus particles, one of which is leaving the cell: 1, fully enveloped mature virus within cytoplasm; 2, EEV leaving the cells.

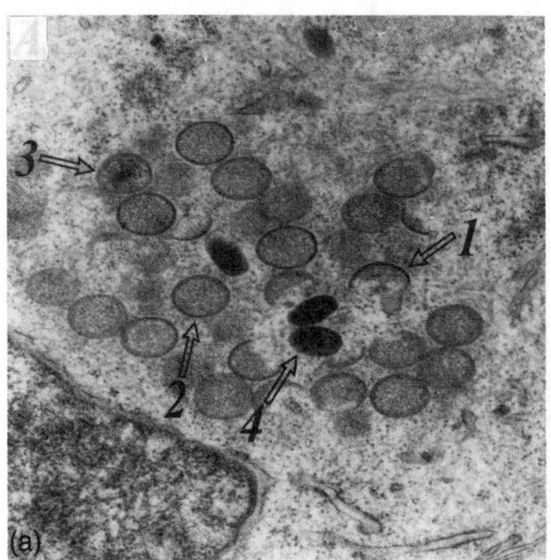

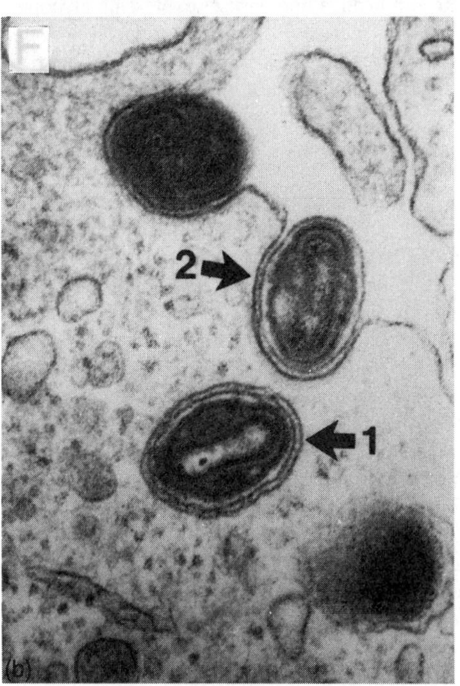

The outcome of infection depended upon a number of factors, notably the age and physiological and immunological status of the patient and the strain of virus. During the late nineteenth century in the United States and South America and the early twentieth century in United Kingdom it was recognized that some smallpox epidemics produced higher mortality rates than others. These were caused by distinct viruses. Variola major was more virulent and produced fatality rates in unvaccinated patients of between 5 and 40 per cent, while the milder variola minor, called alastrim in the Americas, caused only 0.1 to 2 per cent mortality. The viruses were morphologically indistinguishable from each other and other orthopoxviruses, and vaccination with vaccinia was equally effective in preventing infection by either virus, but they could be distinguished by biological tests such as their thermostability and ceiling temperature on the chorioallantoic membrane. Alastrim virus was consistently more thermolabile and had a lower ceiling temperature of 37.5 °C compared to 38.5 °C for variola major, 39 °C for monkeypox, 40 °C for cowpox, and 41 °C for vaccinia.

The very young and elderly patients were most susceptible to infection and those aged 5 to 20 years most resistant. Pregnancy was also a factor that predisposed to more severe infections and pregnant women were more likely than any other group to develop haemorrhagic-type smallpox, which was usually fatal. This greater susceptibility was possibly due to the increased levels of the anti-inflammatory and immunosuppressive steroid hormones (e.g. 17-dihydroxycorticosteroids), as cortisone administration in experimental poxvirus infections or corticosteroid treatment of humans receiving smallpox vaccination greatly increased the severity of infection.

The consequence of infection was also determined by the integrity of the immune response. A deficiency of cell-mediated immunity in particular was associated with severe disease. The greater importance of cell-mediated immunity than antibody in recovery from poxvirus infec-

Fig 3. Smallpox in a nine month-old boy in Pakistan, photographed on the eight day of the rash (by courtesy of the WHO).

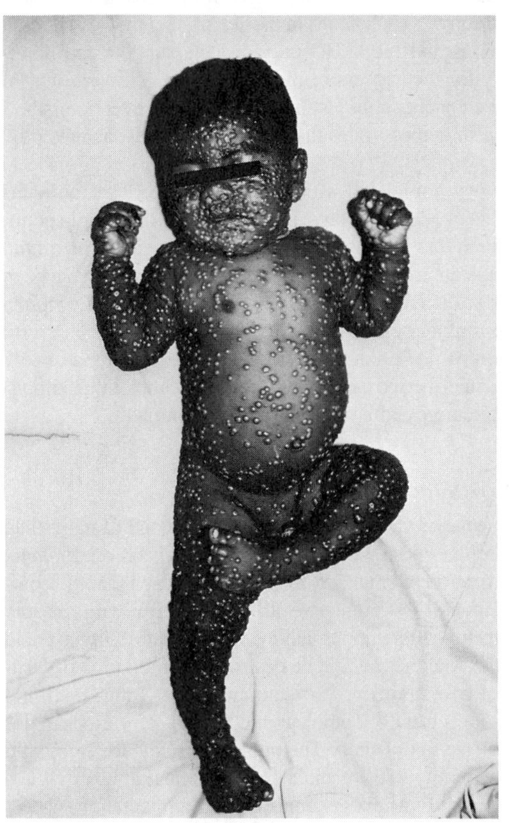

tions was illustrated in children with severe defects in cell-mediated immunity. Vaccination with vaccinia resulted in a progressive and uncontrolled virus replication from the vaccination site, which was usually fatal. In contrast, defects in antibody production were usually tolerated if the cell-mediated immune response was vigorous.

The eradication of smallpox

For centuries smallpox was a universally dreaded, incurable disease that afflicted all mankind. Early attempts at control relied upon the practice of 'variolation' or 'inoculation' practised by the ancient Chinese and Indians. To prevent natural infection with smallpox, those daring enough would infect themselves by sniffing or scratching material isolated from a patient who had suffered a mild smallpox infection. This was a dangerous practice but with a fatality rate at less than 1 per cent was acceptable in view of the possible 40 per cent mortality from natural infection. Variolation remained the only protection available against smallpox and was widely used in the United Kingdom until Edward Jenner introduced vaccination in 1798. Jenner noticed that the milkmaids often acquired poxvirus infections on their hands from the teats of cows and were subsequently protected from smallpox epidemics. He performed the famous experiment of infecting a boy (James Phipps) with poxvirus material (probably cowpox), derived indirectly from a cow via a milkmaid (Sarah Nelmes), and subsequently challenging him with smallpox. Protection was achieved, and due to the efficacy and greater safety of this procedure it rapidly replaced variolation. At some time between 1798 and the twentieth century, vaccinia virus replaced cowpox virus as the vaccine used for smallpox vaccination. In 1959 the World Health Organization (**WHO**) adopted a recommendation to achieve the global eradication of smallpox. With fresh funding in 1968 and a plentiful supply of potent, freeze-dried vaccine, this goal was finally achieved in 1977. Two years later the WHO certified that eradication was complete. Several features contributed to the success of this eradication campaign: the vaccine was cheap and potent as a single dose, stable without refrigeration, easily administered by medically unskilled personnel, and stimulated long-lasting antibody- and cell-mediated immunity; the disease was acute, easily recognized and distinguised from chickenpox by the centrifugal distribution of skin lesions; in particular, there was no animal reservoir for the virus and the WHO provided the support and determination necessary for the success of the programme. This triumph of preventive medicine conclusively justifies the saying 'prevention is better than cure' but also demonstrates that prevention is best achieved by eradication.

The eradication was completed without a knowledge of the antigens of vaccinia virus that evoked protective immunity or of the variola counterparts against which this immunity was directed. Recently, the amino acid sequences of the outer-envelope proteins of these viruses have been determined and are sufficiently similar to explain the efficacy of vaccinia virus for smallpox immunoprophylaxis. For vaccinologists it is worth recording that smallpox was eradicated without an understanding of why vaccinia virus was an effective vaccine and paradoxical that this knowledge is being acquired only after eradication was complete.

Sequencing of orthopoxvirus genomes

The complete sequence of vaccinia virus Copenhagen and of more than 95 per cent of vaccinia virus Western Reserve have been determined. Following the eradication of smallpox the WHO proposed that the complete sequence of several representative strains of variola virus should be determined and thereafter the remaining virus (held at Atlanta and Moscow) and all DNA clones should be destroyed. At the time of writing the sequence of two strains of variola major virus (India 1967 and Bangladesh 1975) are virtually complete and 22 kbp of variola major strain Harvey have been published. The published sequence shows 96 per cent nucleotide identity with vaccinia virus. A remarkable difference between the vaccinia and variola genomes is the fragmentation of several open reading frames in variola that are intact in vaccinia. It is possible that the functional disruption of such genes of an ancestral poxvirus, which hitherto may have moderated its virulence, may have contributed to the evolution of variola major as a highly pathogenic virus for man.

Poxvirus expression vectors

In the early 1980s, techniques were developed for the insertion of foreign genes into vaccinia virus by marker rescue. Placement of these protein-coding regions downstream of a vaccinia virus promoter ensured expression of the foreign protein during vaccinia virus replication. The relatively high levels of expression obtained and the broad host range of the virus have made vaccinia vectors a widely used laboratory expression system. Vaccinia recombinants have also been proposed as live vaccines for human or veterinary diseases. Inoculation of a recombinant virus allows expression and simultaneous delivery of the antigen to the host's immune system without the need for antigen purification. The large capacity of vaccinia virus allows the expression of multiple foreign genes from a single recombinant, so creating polyvalent vaccines.

A disadvantage of the proposed application of vaccinia virus recombinants as new live vaccines is the rare postvaccinial complications that were recognized during the smallpox eradication campaign. These were eczema vaccinatum, generalized vaccinia, progressive vaccinia in patients with deficiencies in cell-mediated immunity, or neurological complications of encephalopathy (below 2 years of age) or encephalitis (over 2 years). While the low frequency of these complications was tolerated in the face of life-threatening smallpox, it is no longer acceptable in a modern vaccine that might be directed against diseases with morbidity or mortality less than those of smallpox. Consequently, there is a clear need to achieve virus attenuation and several laboratories have identified vaccinia genes that contribute to virulence. In most cases, deletion of these genes has considerably attenuated the virus and the prospects of producing suitably attenuated vaccine strains is very promising.

An alternative strategy to achieve safety is to utilize other poxviruses that establish only abortive infections in human cells as the antigen delivery system. The avipoxviruses, such as fowlpox virus and canarypox, have been proposed. These infect the host cell, synthesize the foreign antigen, and deliver it to the host's immune system in the context of a live infection, but the infection cannot spread to other cells and thereby cause disease. Recombinant avipoxviruses expressing glycoproteins derived from rabies or measles virus have induced immune responses in man. Strains of vaccinia virus that establish only abortive infections in human cells due to the deletion of host range genes represent a similar approach.

Human monkeypox (Fig. 4)

Monkeypox was discovered in 1958 in captive non-human primates in Copenhagen and during the next 10 years caused similar outbreaks in other primate colonies. Similar viruses were isolated in 1970 from humans with generalized poxvirus rashes visibly very similar to smallpox in tropical rain forests of West and Central Africa. If this was reintroduction of smallpox from an animal reservoir into man it constituted a real threat to the success of the smallpox eradication campaign. Fortunately, the virus was shown to be distinct from smallpox by its pock morphology, ceiling temperature, and its ability to produce large, indurated lesions with haemorrhagic centres in rabbit skin and to be passed indefinitely in mouse brain. Variola virus is negative by the last two tests. The genome also had a restriction endonuclease pattern distinct from that of variola and vaccinia virus. Although monkeypox produced a disease very similar to smallpox in man, person-to-person transmission was too rare to enable the establishment of epidemics. Thus human monkeypox infections are single or multiple sporadic cases restricted to dense tropical rain forest in Central and West Africa.

Clinically, human monkeypox closely resembles ordinary, discrete-type smallpox except that there is a pronounced lymph-node enlargement. Mortality rates in unvaccinated patients between 1970 and 1986 were 11.2 per cent but these were all in children under 8 years old and the highest rate, 18.7 per cent, was in infants of less than 2 years. The virus is probably acquired from infected monkeys or rodents such as squirrels.

Cowpox and pseudocowpox

Cowpox virus has a broad host range and although it was first recognized in cows, hence the name, is not enzootic in cattle but merely an incidental infection. It has been isolated from several other large mammals including man, captive felines, and even elephants, but its natural host is probably one or more species of rodent. Cowpox is famous as the virus that Jenner used to prevent smallpox. It has often been confused with vaccinia virus and other viruses that produce lesions on cow's teats such as pseudocowpox virus and bovine alphaherpesvirus 2. Vaccinia may have been transmitted to cows from man; it is clearly distinguishable from cowpox by the pock type, ceiling temperature, and rate of replication in tissue culture. The cowpox virus genome is considerably larger than that of vaccinia and has a different restriction pattern. Cowpox virus produces cytoplasmic A-type inclusion bodies while vaccinia does not.

Pseudocowpox is enzootic in cattle, unlike cowpox. It was important historically because it was often mistakenly used for smallpox vaccination. Being a parapoxvirus, and hence ineffective in preventing orthopoxvirus infections, its misuse compromised Jenner's correct conclusion that true cowpox was effective in preventing smallpox.

In man and cow the lesions produced by cowpox are more severe than those of pseudocowpox. In man, cowpox causes an acutely inflamed local lesion, similar to a primary smallpox vaccination. There is usually fever, enlargement of the local lymph nodes, and pain. Unlike vaccinia, which occasionally produced a generalized infection, cowpox lesions are always local. Human lesions caused by pseudocowpox virus (milker's nodules) are extremely rare and are less painful than those caused by cowpox.

Fig 4. Moderately severe monkeypox in a girl of seven years from Equateur Province, Zaire (by courtesy of the WHO).

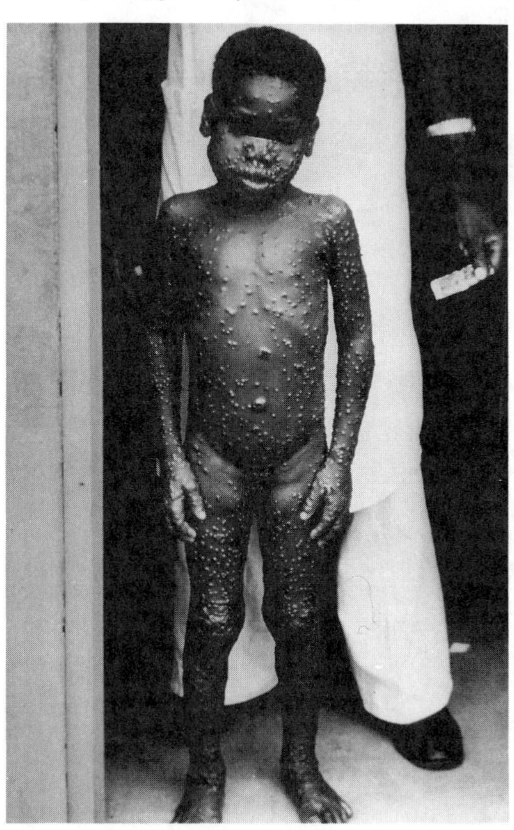

Tanapox and yaba tumour virus

Tanapox virus was first isolated from the Tana valley in Kenya from humans with localized skin lesions typical of poxviruses. A similar virus was subsequently found in humans in Zaire during surveillance for monkeypox and in a non-human primate colony in the United States after animal handlers became infected. It is a rare zoonosis of monkeys, and in Kenya, may have been transmitted by mosquitoes. It is serologically related to yaba tumour virus but not monkeypox. In man it usually produces a solitary lesion that follows a few days of mild fever. The lesion takes 5 to 6 weeks to clear and is distinguished from other poxvirus lesions by the failure to become pustular. This virus cannot be cultured on the chorioallantoic membrane.

Yaba tumour virus is a monkey virus that can cause histiocytomas if injected subcutaneously or intradermally into man. The lesions are not neoplastic and are cleared by the immune response.

REFERENCES

Aguado, B., Selmes, I.P., and Smith, G.L. (1992). Nucleotide sequence of 21.8 kbp of variola major virus strain Harvey and comparison with vaccinia virus. *Journal of General Virology,* **73,** 2887–902.

Binns, M.M. and Smith, G.L. (1992). *Recombinant poxviruses.* CRC Press, Boca Raton, FA.

Cadoz, M. *et al.* (1992). Immunisation with canarypox virus expressing rabies glycoprotein. *Lancet,* **339,** 1229–432.

Fenner, F. (1990). Poxviruses. In *Virology,* (ed. B.N. Fields and D.M. Knipe), pp. 2113–33. Raven Press, New York.

Fenner, F., Anderson, D.A., Arita, I., Jezek, Z., and Ladnyi, I.D. (1988). *Smallpox and its eradication.* World Health Organization, Geneva.

Fenner, F., Wittek, R., and Dumbell, K.R. (1989). *The orthopoxviruses.* Academic Press, London.

Lane, J.M., Ruben, F.L., Neff, J.M., and Millar, J.D. (1969). Complications of smallpox vaccination, 1968. National surveillance in the United States. *New England Journal of Medicine,* **281,** 1201–8.

Moss, B. (1990). Poxviridae and their replication. In *Virology, op. cit.,* pp. 2079–111.

7.10.9 Orf

T.E.A. Peto and B.E. Juel-Jensen

Contagious pustular dermatitis, or orf, is a poxvirus disease. It usually affects lambs but also cattle and goats. In lambs, the mucosa of the lips is usually involved but any part of the skin can be infected (Fig. 1). The virus is fairly resistant and may survive in the environment in dust and wool, on hooks, and the wood of sheep pens. The mortality among lambs and kids is less than 1 per cent. Similar infections with related parapoxviruses occur in the teats of cows (milker's nodule) and in reindeer and musk ox.

The virus is a brick-shaped poxvirus that on electron microscopy has a characteristic 'ball of wool' appearance (Fig. 2). It may sometimes be grown with difficulty in tissue culture, and serological tests (neutralization and complement-fixing antibody) are not always reliable. An attenuated vaccine for use in animals has been developed.

Human orf

Orf is an occupational hazard of farmers, shepherds, sheep handlers, abattoir workers, veterinary surgeons, and physiologists experimenting on sheep. Person-to-person transmission is unusual.

CLINICAL FEATURES

After an incubation period of 3 to 4 days a macular rash develops, which then turns papular. A vesicle forms, the skin breaks down, and the vesicle evolves into a hyperplastic, nodular mass. The whole lesion disappears after about 5 weeks. During the initial maculopapular stage the lesion may have a red centre surrounded by a white ring, in turn surrounded by a red halo (the target stage) (Figs 3 and 4). Usually the lesions are painless until they break down. There may be just one lesion, but usually there are several on one or both hands and arms. Infections can occur on the nostrils, the eye at the canthus, or the external auditory meatus (Fig. 4) if the infection is caught by facial contact with a pet lamb.

In most cases the patients remain well. If many lesions are present, the patient may have some fever. Generalized disease is very rare, although a severe infection ('giant orf') has been reported in a patient with lymphoma. Erythema multiforme complicates orf in some patients (Fig. 5). Humoral immunity seems to be irrelevant to recovery or prevention of recurrent infections, which may be common in those who continue to be exposed to sheep. Orf acquired from animal (usually sheep) bites may be complicated by other infections such as erysipeloid.

DIFFERENTIAL DIAGNOSIS

The diagnosis is usually made from the history of contact with an obviously infected animal. In many cases, sheep handlers are more familiar

Fig. 1 Contagious pustular dermatitis ('orf') in a lamb.

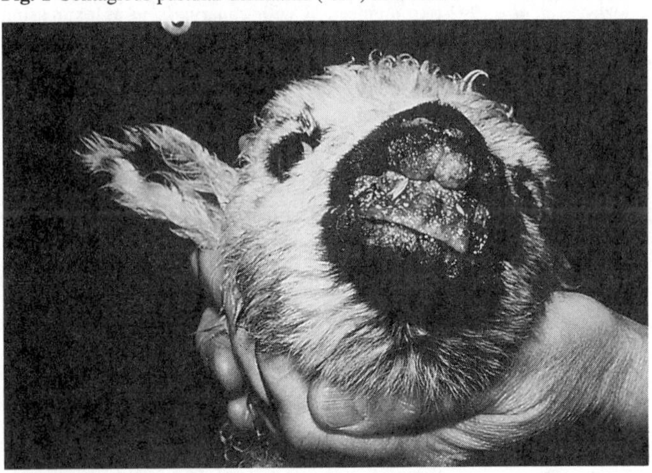

Fig. 2 Electron micrograph of two orf virions showing 'ball of wool' appearance.

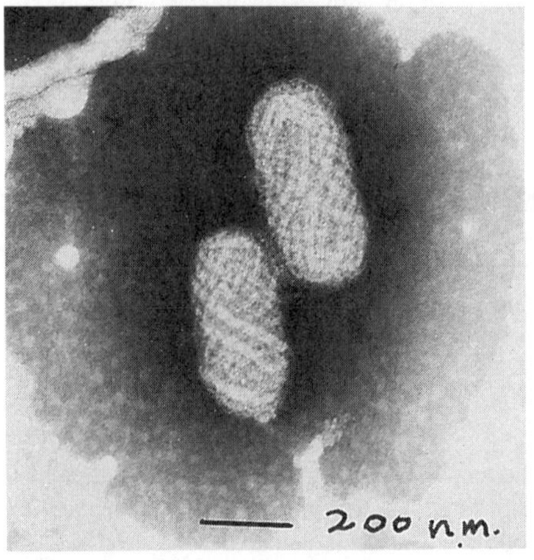

Fig. 3 Human orf of hand.

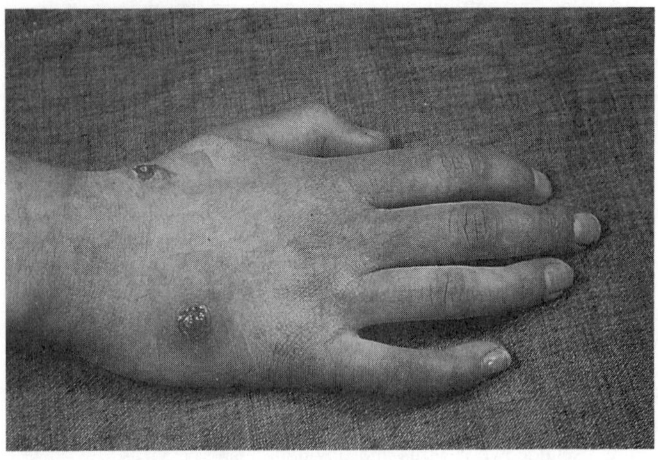

Fig. 4 Human orf of ear.

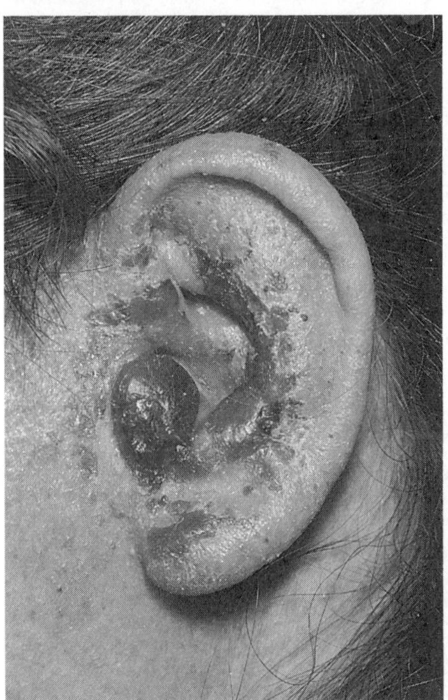

Fig. 5 Erythema multiforme complicating orf of the left middle finger in a veterinary student.

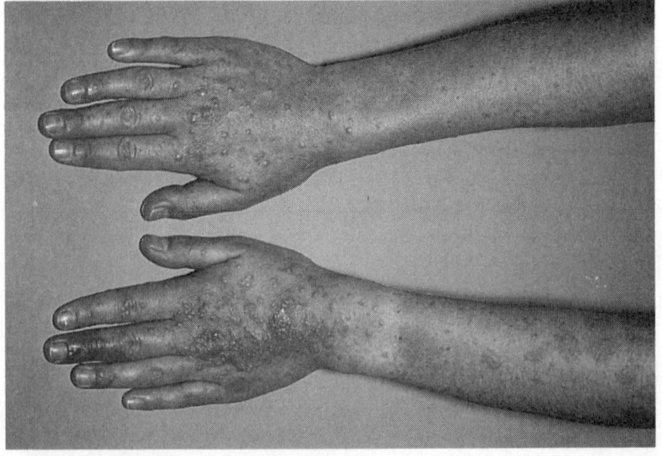

with orf than the doctor because most cases are not sufficiently severe to warrant medical attention. The lesions can be mistaken for herpetic whitlow, vaccinia whitlow, milker's node virus (pseudo-cowpox), anthrax and impetigo. Diagnosis can be confirmed by electron microscopy.

TREATMENT

Most cases do not require treatment. Analgesia and antimicrobials to prevent secondary infection may be required. Patients need to be reassured that the infection is self-limiting and that they will probably acquire sufficient immunity to avoid a second attack. Topical idoxuridine in dimethylsulphoxide has been used in some cases.

REFERENCES

Falk, E.S. (1978). Parapoxvirus infections of reindeer and musk ox associated with unusual human infections. *British Journal of Dermatology,* **98,** 647–54.

Freeman, G., Bron, A.J., and Juel-Jensen, B. (1984). Ocular Infection with orf virus. *American Journal of Ophthalmology,* **97,** 601–4.

Leavell, U.W. *et al.* (1968). Orf: report of 19 cases with clinical and pathological observations. *Journal of the American Medical Association,* **204,** 657–64.

Robinson, A.J. and Balassu, T.C. (1981). Contagious pustular dermatitis (orf). *Veterinary Bulletin,* **51,** 772–82.

Savage, J. and Black, M.M. (1972). 'Giant' orf of finger in patient with a lymphoma. *Proceedings of the Royal Society of Medicine,* **64,** 766–8.

7.10.10 Molluscum contagiosum

T.E.A. PETO and B.E. JUEL-JENSEN

Molluscum contagiosum is a common infection of the skin caused by a member of the poxvirus group. On electron microscopy, the virus is brick shaped and measures 200 × 300 μm (Fig. 1). The virus has not been cultured *in vitro,* and attempts at demonstrating antibodies in the serum have been disappointing.

Fig. 1 Virus particles in molluscum contagiosum (× 155 550).

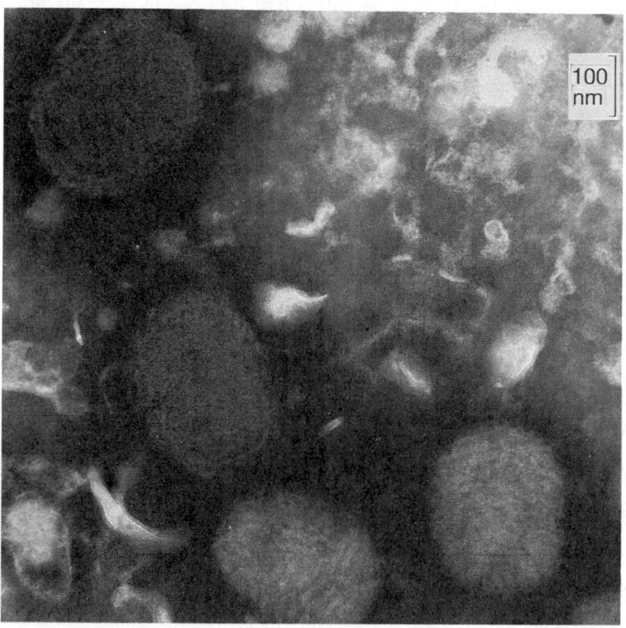

EPIDEMIOLOGY

The virus is transmitted from person to person. There is no evidence of an animal reservoir. The infection is common in children and in individuals seropositive for the human immunodeficiency virus. It is transmitted by close bodily contact, and can be transmitted venereally.

CLINICAL PRESENTATION

After an incubation period of 2 to 7 weeks, characteristic lesions develop (Figs 2 and 3). The abdomen, the buttocks, the genitals, the face, and arms are common sites. There are rarely lesions inside the mouth, or on the soles of the feet or the palms. The lesions vary in size from 1 to 5 mm in diameter.

Small, pearly-white, umbilicated bodies are scattered over the affected parts. The lesions may recover spontaneously after several months, but in the meantime further seedlings have often developed elsewhere. The superficial cells of the lesion are filled with large, hyaline, granular masses known as the molluscum body, which displaces the nucleus.

More extensive lesions occur in patients with AIDS and on immunosuppressive therapy. Although these patients do not develop systemic symptoms, these lesions often do not resolve spontaneously and can sometimes recur, even after treatment.

TREATMENT

Specific treatment is normally unnecessary, as the lesions mostly resolve spontaneously, occasionally leaving small depigmented areas. If necessary, individual lesions can be treated with cryotherapy. Curettage and

Fig. 2 Molluscum contagiosum on skin.

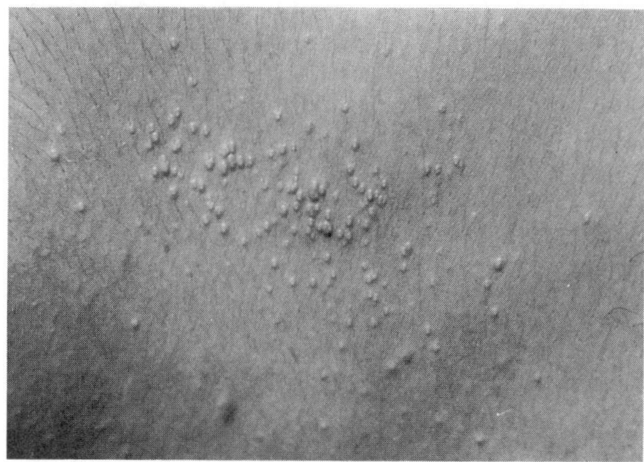

Fig. 3 Single lesion on eyelid.

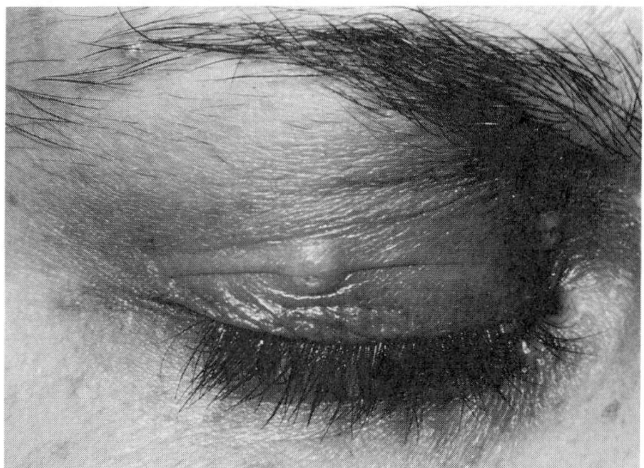

diathermy are appropriate for large lesions, especially if histological confirmation of diagnosis is wanted. Physical disruption, or enucleation with a Volkman's spoon, and touching the base with silver nitrate, phenol or a strong iodine solution may also be effective.

REFERENCES

Katzman, M. *et al.* (1987). Moluscum contagiosum and the acquired immunodeficiency syndrome: clinical and immunological details of two cases. *British Journal of Dermatology,* **20,** 76–82.

MacCallum, F.O. (1967). Molluscum contagiosum and warts. In *Virus and rickettsial disease of man,* (45th edn), (ed. S. Bedson, A.W. Downie, F.O. MacCallum, and C.H. Start-Harris), pp. 143–4. Edward Arnold, London.

Paramyxoviruses

7.10.11 Mumps: epidemic parotitis

B. K. RIMA and A. B. CHRISTIE

Mumps is an acute, generalized, communicable virus infection of children and young adults. The virus can infect almost any organ: the salivary glands, the pancreas, the testes or ovary, the brain, the breast, the liver, the joints, and the heart. The swelling of the face is only one of the symptoms of the disease, albeit the most common one.

Epidemiology

The incubation period lies between 14 and 18 days; much shorter or longer periods are quoted. In any outbreak, as many as 30 to 40 per cent of those exposed excrete virus and show a rise of antibody but have no clinical illness. In any assessment of the infectivity of mumps, these inapparent excreters must be included, and mumps can then be seen to be a highly infectious condition, though less so than measles or chickenpox. Spread may seem much slower than in measles but its incubation period is longer. Environment is important; in a classroom or troop-ship the virus spreads rapidly. When introduced into an island population with no recent exposure to mumps, the virus rapidly spreads and causes severe disease. All epidemiological evidence shows that transmission depends on close personal contact with a patient who is excreting virus in the saliva. In the pre-vaccine era, the peak incidence was in the late winter or early spring months, in 3- to 7-year cycles.

Virology

CULTURE

Mumps virus can be grown in tissue culture of chick embryo, monkey kidney, human amnion, or Hela cells, and cytopathic changes may be seen as early as the third day. With immunofluorescence techniques, virus replication can be detected in hours rather than days. The virus can also be cultured in the yolk sac or embryonic cavity of chick embryos.

RESISTANCE OF VIRUS

Mumps virus can remain infective for weeks or months if stored below 10°C, or for years at lower temperatures. Infectivity is lost in 3 or 4 days at room temperature. Heating the virus at 55°C for 20 min abolishes infectivity, as does 0.2 per cent formalin at 4°C for 2 h or dilute ether for 30 min; intense ultraviolet radiation destroys it at once. None of these processes destroys the antigens responsible for complement fixation, haemagglutination, or reactivity in the skin test.

Dr. A.B. Christie died in 1987. Much of his second edition chapter has been retained in this edition.

SOURCE OF VIRUS

Mumps virus can be grown during the acute illness from saliva, throat washings or a swab of the Stensen's duct orifice, from urine in every case, and from cerebrospinal fluid when there is meningitis. It has been cultured from breast milk, and at autopsy from brain tissue. It is likely that virus could be isolated from any infected organ.

A patient excretes virus in the saliva for between 2 and 6 days before the parotitis and for up to 4 days after it. Virus can be detected in the urine for up to 14 days around the onset of the illness: it can be cultured almost as easily as from saliva, especially from ultracentrifugates, but there is no evidence of spread of the disease by urine. In the blood it can be detected and isolated only for a day or two at the onset of the disease. Virus can be isolated from the cerebrospinal fluid for the first 3 or 4 days of the meningeal illness.

ANTIBODY RESPONSE TO VIRUS

Mumps virus contains several different antigenic components, which provoke distinct antibodies in infected patients. It is an enveloped RNA virus with a genome of 15 384 nucleotides. Its inner core contains the RNA genome of negative polarity encapsidated by the major nucleocapsid (**N**) protein. The nucleocapsid has the herring-bone structure characteristic of paramyxoviruses (Fig. 1(a)). Attached to this ribonucleoprotein structure are two proteins involved in transcription and replication of the virus: the phosphoprotein (**P**) and the large replicase protein (**L**). The nucleocapsids are surrounded by a lipid bilayer membrane derived from the host cell (Fig. 1(a, b)). On the inner surface there is a membrane or matrix protein (**M**), which plays a part in virus budding. On the outer surface two viral glycoproteins, one carrying the haemagglutinin–neuraminidase activity (**HN**) and the other responsible for the fusion activity (**F**). The gene order (Fig. 1(c)) leads to an expression gradient in which the abundance of mRNA decreases with increasing distance from the 3′ end of the genome so that the mRNA encoding the N protein is most abundant, the one encoding the L protein least abundant.

The HN protein was previously called the V antigen and the N protein the S antigen. Both antigens can fix complement in the presence of corresponding specific antibody. S antibody rises in the first 2 weeks of infection but then declines rapidly. V antibody appears at the end of the first week, usually in high titre: it may persist for years and is an index of past infection. Titration of acute and convalescent sera for V and S antibody is a reliable method of diagnosis, especially in patients who do not have parotitis. There is usually a four-fold rise in haemagglutination-inhibiting antibody during the illness. Neutralizing antibodies also develop. Complement fixation, haemagglutination-inhibiting antibodies, and neutralization measure different combinations of viral antibodies and these may give different results, depending on the immune responses of individual patients.

For early diagnosis, mumps-specific IgG and IgA may be measured by indirect immunofluorescence tests. IgA can be detected in saliva or mouth washings on about the fourth day after infection, and in the serum early in the disease; the method is as sensitive as virus culture.

SKIN TEST

Viral antigen produces a tuberculin-like reaction when injected into the skin of people who have been infected with mumps virus before, with or without clinical symptoms. The test will not diagnose a clinical attack but is of value in assessing immunity or the need for vaccination.

VIRUS SPREAD IN THE BODY

Mumps virus causes a systemic infection in which viraemia leads to infection of many organs, most often the salivary glands. This is preceded by an infection of the upper respiratory tract. If mumps virus is injected experimentally into the orifice of the parotid duct, the patient often gets parotitis within 8 days, whereas after natural exposure this takes nearer 18 days.

Pathology

CHANGES IN SALIVARY GLANDS

Because mumps is not often lethal, there is little information about the changes caused in organs by the virus. In the salivary glands there is some lymphocytic infiltration of periductal tissue, and oedematous changes or vacuolar degeneration in the cells lining the ducts. These cells become detached and, with leucocytes and other debris, they block the duct and cause dilatation above the block. Sometimes the whole gland is affected but more often the changes are in some lobules only. The lymphatics in the tissues surrounding and lying over the glands become obstructed, producing a gel-like oedema that may spread down over the chest wall, especially when the swelling of the salivary glands is severe. The parotitis may be caused by a reaction between virus and antibody, and not by simple inflammation, because antibody is often already present when parotitis develops. In non-parotitic cases, where the virus first declares its presence in the testis or the meninges, there may be a delay in antibody formation, for virus is often present in the saliva some days before the orchitis or meningitis, yet there is no parotitis. The same delay in antibody formation may explain the many cases of inapparent mumps.

CHANGES IN THE GENITALIA

In mild orchitis there is only oedema and serofibrinous exudate in the interstitial tissues, but when the infection is severe there is intense lymphocytic infiltration and destruction of the cells lining the seminiferous tubules, which leads to blocking. Partial atrophy of the testes may follow and the epididymis, spermatic cord, and prostate may all be affected by the inflammatory reaction. All this is bound to affect function, but complete sterility is not a common sequel of mumps (see below). Women sometimes complain of ovarian pain during an attack of mumps, but it is rarely as severe as in men with orchitis. There is no evidence that it affects fertility. Mastitis is more common, both in females and males, but it is usually mild and fleeting.

CHANGES IN THE NERVOUS SYSTEM

Mumps virus frequently invades the nervous system: changes can be detected by electroencephalography or by examination of the cerebrospinal fluid in at least half the patients with mumps. In most cases with electroencephalographic or cerebrospinal-fluid changes, there are no nervous symptoms or signs. Mumps virus is one of the most common known causes of lymphocytic meningitis. It is a self-limiting disease and so there are no autopsy reports, but neuronal damage probably does occur and explains the occurrence of quadriplegia or single-nerve paralysis in some patients. Apart from transient weakness of the facial nerve, which may be due to pressure of a swollen gland or damage by mumps virus, these complications are all very rare.

Mumps encephalitis is a different entity; cerebrospinal fluid is normal and contains no virus. At autopsy there is perivascular demyelination exactly the same as in other forms of postinfectious encephalitis (see Chapter 7.19.4).

CHANGES IN THE PANCREAS AND OTHER ORGANS

Mild upper abdominal pain is common in mumps and may be related to viral changes in the pancreas. One author writes of subclinical pancreopathy, but there is little firm evidence of pathological changes in the pancreas in mumps. The amount of amylase in duodenal fluid may be less than normal in patients with mumps who have abdominal pain, and this might be caused by blocking of the ducts in the pancreas, just as in the salivary glands or the testes.

There are some anecdotal reports of diabetes occurring after an attack of mumps, but in these cases the virus may simply have precipitated clinical signs of a pancreatic defect which would have led to diabetes eventually. There is no virological or immunological evidence for a direct link with mumps virus.

Mumps virus has been isolated on biopsy from a patient with subacute

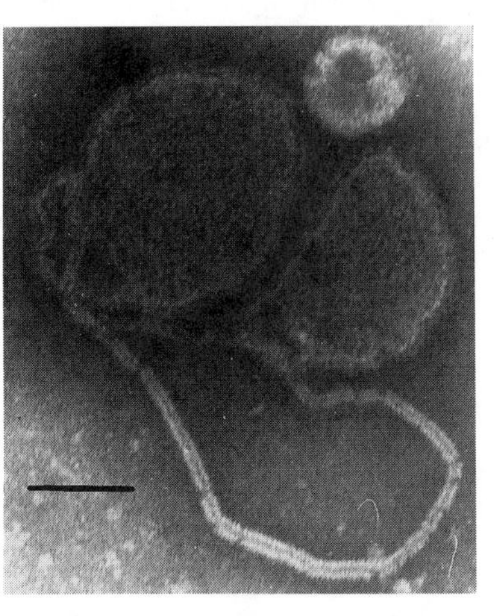

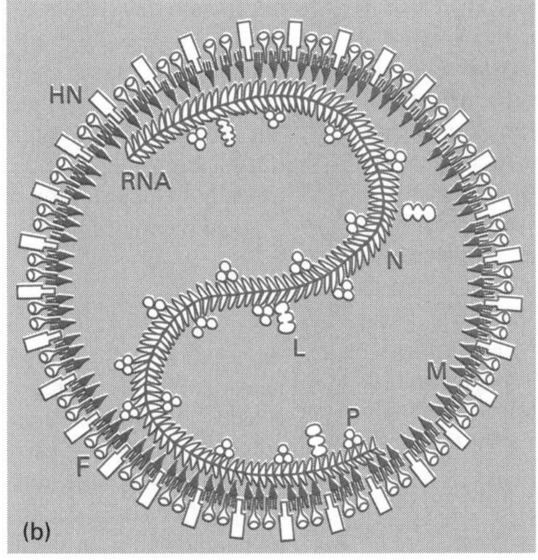

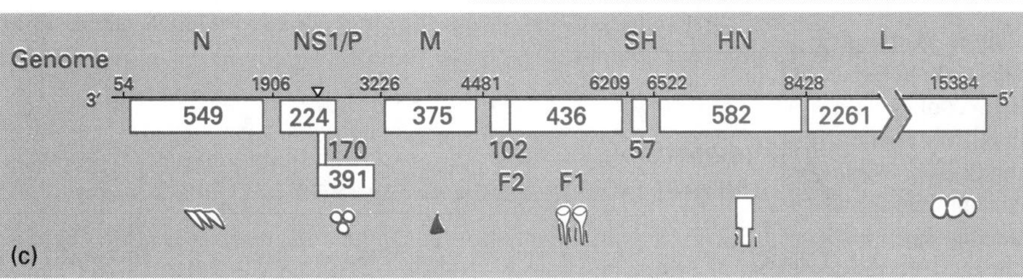

Fig. 1 Structure and genome organization of mumps virus. (a) A disrupted, negatively stained mumps virion. The viral nucleocapsid protrudes from the particle and the fringe of viral spikes is visible (bar = 100 nm). (b) Diagram of the localization of the nucleocapsid (N), phospho- (P), large (L), matrix (M) and haemagglutinin–neuraminidase (HN), and fusion (F) proteins in the mumps virion. (c) Structure of the genome of mumps virus indicating the localization of the genes, the nucleotide number of their starting and stopping position, and (in boxes) the numbers of amino acid residues in each of the viral proteins.

thyroiditis, and there is a report of several cases in Israel. Myocarditis has been seen in one fatal case, but otherwise the evidence for any heart damage comes from electrocardiographic changes and these are usually fleeting. Mild hepatic changes have been seen on biopsy of patients with jaundice, a very rare manifestation of mumps. Arthritis is also rare: the complement fixation test may be positive in aspirated joint fluid but nothing is known of any changes in the joint. Mumps virus can probably invade any other organ, but it usually only causes fleeting damage.

MUMPS IN THE FETUS AND INFANT

Mumps vaccine virus has been isolated from placental tissue, but in the one recorded case in which mumps virus was isolated from a 10-week fetus there was no pathological evidence that the virus had caused the death of the fetus. Abortion may occur in women with mumps in the first 3 months of pregnancy, but this is not common; there is no evidence that it is caused by virus damage to the fetus. The connection between primary endocardial fibroelastosis and mumps is rather vague. Mumps virus has not been isolated from heart tissue at autopsy and these infants have no mumps antibody in their blood. They may show a delayed hypersensitivity response to the skin test. It has been suggested that in these cases the mother's attack of mumps is a secondary one to which she already has some antibody, and that antibody and virus both pass to the fetus, where their collision in infant tissue causes a hypersensitivity reaction. Or there may be some immune defect in the fetus, an absence of B-lymphocyte humoral response perhaps, and this causes myocarditis and the laying down of the thick layer of collagen and elastic tissue under the endocardium.

In the normal infant, maternal IgG passes to the fetus and seems to protect the infant against mumps during the first year of life. The typical disease of mumps in infants is a rare clinical finding, and even in populations with no previous experience of the disease and thus presumably no maternal antibody, mumps in the first year is very uncommon. The reason for this is unknown. Orchitis has been reported in infants, and mumps virus may be isolated in vague respiratory infections in infants.

Clinical manifestations

PAROTITIS

A patient with mumps parotitis is ill and uncomfortable. The temperature may be as high as 40 to 40.5°C, although 37.2 to 38.3°C is usual. The patient feels chilled but does not have rigors, and has pain near the angle of the jaw. Next day the gland begins to swell, and within another day the face and neck are distorted with swelling. The skin over the gland is hot and flushed but there is no rash as in the swelling of erysipelas. Usually both glands swell, sometimes with a day or two between the sides, but sometimes only one is affected. The swelling begins at the zygomatic bone on the face and goes down and back beneath the auricle and into the neck, covering the bony angle of the jaw on the way. The neck swelling is ill defined and the angle of the jaw is impalpable, in contrast to cervical lymph nodes that are swollen from some other cause. If the swelling is severe, the mouth cannot be opened for pain and tightness, and is dry because the flow of saliva is blocked. This discomfort lasts for 3 or 4 days. Sometimes as one side clears, the parotid on the other side swells and this prolongs the illness.

SUBMAXILLARY MUMPS

The symptoms are similar to those in parotitic mumps, but it is difficult or impossible to distinguish the swelling from other forms of submaxillary swellings. Some of the lymph nodes in the neck lie in contact with the salivary gland, some within its substance. In submaxillary mumps there is sometimes a great deal of oedema of the overlying tissues, which may spread down over the sternum, but this is not a constant finding. If the parotid gland is also swollen, diagnosis is easy. Otherwise one must try to examine the fauces for signs of tonsilitis that might cause cervical adenitis, and laboratory tests are needed for definite diagnosis.

SUBLINGUAL MUMPS

The sublingual salivary glands lie below the floor of the mouth on either side of the frenulum of the tongue near the symphysis of the mandible. When they swell, they push up into the mouth below the tongue, forcing it up against the hard palate, and also down under the chin as a very tender swelling. It is acutely uncomfortable, often accompanied by severe general symptoms. It usually subsides after a few days, and is fortunately uncommon.

ORCHITIS

Orchitis may occur 4 or 5 days after the onset of parotitis, just when that swelling is beginning to subside and the patient thinks his trouble is over. But quite often it occurs without preceding parotitis. It is an acute condition, with chills, sweats, headache, and backache, and a swinging temperature as well as severe local testicular pain and tenderness. The scrotum is swollen and oedematous, and the testicles are impalpable. Most often only one testicle is affected but sometimes both: the second testicle may become affected just as the swelling of the first is subsiding. The illness lasts 3 or 4 days before the swelling begins to subside.

Orchitis is unusual before the age of puberty, though it has occurred in young boys and even in infants. In adolescent and young males it develops in 1:5 cases. Some degree of atrophy of the testicle occurs in at least one-third of patients with orchitis. It may be detected by a shrinking and softening of the affected testicle. In one series of 39 patients with atrophy, only one had azoospermia: the others had sperm counts very little different from normal. Azoospermia after mumps may be only temporary, and the fear of sterility after mumps orchitis has been exaggerated, so the doctor can reassure the patient.

MENINGITIS AND ENCEPHALITIS

Mumps is a relatively common cause of lymphocytic or viral meningitis. It may develop a few days after the start of parotitis, but almost as often it occurs in the absence of parotitis. In the cerebrospinal fluid, protein and lymphocytes are both increased and mumps virus can be isolated in the first few days. The meningitis is usually mild and self-limiting. Occasionally the patient develops paralysis of limbs but, unlike poliomyelitis, this usually disappears in time.

Polyneuritis, neuritis of the trigeminal or facial nerve, and retrobulbar optic neuritis have been described in mumps but all are rare.

In encephalitis the outlook is different. The patient is mentally disturbed and may lapse into coma and remain comatose for days, weeks, or months. This is a form of postinfectious encephalitis like that which occurs in measles; but it is much rarer after mumps than after measles.

OTHER COMPLICATIONS

Deafness is sometimes reported after mumps: in one outbreak 13 of 298 Finnish soldiers with mumps became deaf but only one of them permanently. Virus was once cultured at operation from inner-ear perilymph, proving that it can invade the inner structure of the ear. Labyrinthitis has also been reported with tinnitus, vertigo, and nystagmus during outbreaks of mumps. If this is due to mumps virus, it is a very rare complication. In the army outbreak, there may have been special features connected with dosage or virulence of virus that increased the rate of ear complications in the soldiers.

Diagnosis

DIPHTHERIA AND OTHER SWELLINGS

When there is bilateral parotitis, clinical diagnosis is usually obvious. One condition that must be excluded is bull-neck diphtheria (see Chapter 7.11.1), which can, at a careless glance, look very like mumps. Inflammation of various groups of lymph nodes may cause some difficulty. Those that drain the pinna of the ear and side of the scalp, the preauricular group, lie superficial to the parotid, but those draining the front of the scalp and the eyelids lie within its substance; the swelling is less uniform and does not go into the neck. Other groups that drain parts of the pharynx lie deep to the parotid and may swell bilaterally; one must examine the pharynx carefully. Enlargement of the cervical lymph nodes is confined to the neck; one can feel round the swelling and the angle of the jaw is above it. In infectious mononucleosis the glands stand out distinctly and the parotid is not affected. The lymph nodes in contact with the submaxillary and sublingual salivary glands drain the corner of the eye, the side of the nose, the cheeks, the lips, and the floor of the mouth. One must look for lesions there, for otherwise diagnosis from submaxillary or sublingual mumps is difficult.

In septic parotitis there is more parotid tenderness; there may be fluctuation, and pus exudes from the orifice of Stensen's duct. Calculus causes spasmodic pain and swelling and may be detected radiographically. Recurrent parotitis and Mikulicz's syndrome are unlikely to be confused with mumps except in the earliest stages, nor are uveoparotid fever and tumours of the gland, for they are chronic conditions. In erysipelas the condition clearly affects the skin and subcutaneous tissue, not the deeper parotid gland.

Orchitis when it occurs without parotitis is difficult to diagnose from gonococcal epididymo-orchitis unless there has been contact with mumps. The rare case of orchitis in infancy may resemble torsion of the testis and perhaps it is safer to operate than risk a serious misdiagnosis.

LABORATORY DIAGNOSIS

Virus isolation and serological tests have already been discussed. In cases without parotitis, especially meningitis, and in the absence of contact history, they are the only means of reaching a firm diagnosis. The skin test and serum amylase levels are not helpful.

Treatment

There is no specific treatment. Symptomatic treatment includes simple analgesics, but for the severe pain of orchitis, morphia (15–30 mg) may be required for a day or two. Corticosteroids are worth trying in severe cases of parotitis, more especially in orchitis. A dose of 300 mg cortisone or its equivalent daily for 2 or 3 days sometimes gives dramatic relief from pain though it may not reduce the swelling. There is no need to taper off the dose. The inflamed scrotum should be supported on wads of cotton wool, not wrapped in bandages, for the patient sweats a lot and the bandages becomes sodden. Immune globulin treatment is not costeffective and is no longer commercially available.

Prevention

The mainstay of prevention is vaccination of susceptible individuals. Isolation is not effective, except in closed communities, as the patient has been infectious for days before parotitis occurs and inapparent cases are not detected at all.

Killed vaccine gave only short-term protection, and killed vaccines of other paramyxoviruses have given rise to enhanced or atypical clinical symptoms and are no longer used. Attenuated live vaccine, licensed since 1967, gives 95 per cent seroconversion, and protection lasts for at least 15 years. In developed countries, live attenuated mumps vaccine is currently given between 14 and 16 months of age as one component of a trivalent mumps/measles/rubella (**MMR**) vaccine with live attenuated strains of measles and rubella virus. This has succeeded in suppressing the incidence of mumps by 98 per cent in the United States. Introduction of the MMR vaccine in the United Kingdom has had similar effects. The live attenuated Urabe strain of mumps has been shown to be associated with unacceptable levels of meningitis in vaccines and this virus has now been replaced by other live attenuated strains in MMR vaccine used in the United Kingdom. Mumps infection is confined to man, so that widespread vaccination might lead to eradication of the disease. Mumps vaccination is contraindicated in patients with immunodeficiency due to immunosuppressive therapy or disease, but human immunodeficiency virus-positive children should be vaccinated with the MMR vaccine.

REFERENCES

Annotation (1966). Mumps embryopathy. *Lancet, ii*, 692–3.

Christie, A.B. (1980). *Infectious diseases: epidemiology and clinical practice*, (3rd edn). Churchill Livingstone, Edinburgh.

Feldman, H.A. (1989). Mumps. In *Viral infections of humans*, (3rd edn), (ed. A.J. Evans), pp. 471–91. Plenum Medical, New York.

Gordon, J.E. and Kilham, L. (1949). Ten years in the epidemiology of mumps. *American Journal of Medicine, 218,* 338–59.

Hanshaw, J.B. and Dudgeon, J.A. (1978). In *Viral diseases of the fetus and the newborn*. Saunders, Philadelphia.

Kurtz, J.B., Tomlinson, A.H., and Pearson, J. (1982). Mumps virus isolated from a fetus. *British Medical Journal, 284,* 471.

Rima, B.K. (1994). Mumps virus. In *Encyclopedia of Virology* (ed. R.G. Webster and A. Granoff) pp.876–83. Academic Press, London.

Weibel, R.E. (1988). 'Mumps vaccine'. In *Vaccines* (ed. S.A. Plotkin and E.A. Mortimer), pp. 223–34. Saunders, Philadelphia.

Wolinsky, J.S. and Waxham, M.N. (1990). Mumps virus. In *Virology*, (2nd edn), (ed. B.N. Fields *et al.*), pp. 989–1011. Raven Press, New York.

7.10.12 Measles

H. C. WHITTLE and P. AABY

Measles is an acute, highly transmissible viral infection of man causing much death and suffering, especially among children of the so-called Third World. Its severity varies according to host and socioeconomic factors, not to antigenic variation or alteration in virulence of the virus. There is no reservoir of infection other than in man and no evidence of a carrier state. The virus causes a generalized infection coupled with severe immunosuppression. The chief clinical features result from infection of the skin, mucous membranes, and respiratory tract. Attack rates in home contacts are very high (of the order of 90 per cent), subclinical infection is infrequent, and children are the main victims. Long-life immunity follows the disease. In 1987 measles was estimated to kill 2 million children annually. Global coverage by measles immunization has now increased to 80 per cent, with a corresponding drop in deaths to 900 000 annually.

Epidemiology

The epidemiology of this global infection varies markedly between developed and developing countries.

In the West most children are infected between 3 and 6 years of age, when in nursery and primary schools. Mortality is low (under 0.05 per cent) and morbidity, although considerable when compared to many other common viral infections, is limited. Most cases occur in the winter and spring, with a biannual epidemic pattern. Recently the epidemicity has been influenced by widespread immunization (Fig. 1), which has dramatically reduced both the number of cases and complications. However, even in the United States of America, which has the longest experience of systematic immunization, there is now evidence of resurgence of measles with a higher case fatality (0.3 per cent) in non-immunized subgroups of the population such as religious minorities who do not believe in vaccines, refugees, illegal immigrants, and the poor in the inner cities.

In the Third World, measles is severe and different: it kills between 3 and 15 per cent of children in the community and some 10 to 20 per cent of those admitted to hospital. Mortality from measles is considerably higher in Africa (5.0–15.0 per cent) than in Asia or South America (1.0–3.0 per cent); within Africa, West Africa has the highest case fatality rates. Contrary to the early European experience, when the highest mortality was among the overcrowded urban poor, studies from the developing world indicate a higher mortality in rural rather than urban populations. In communities where females tend to stay at home and are more constrained in their social contacts, mortality is higher in girls than boys. There is a high fatality rate in children with chronic disease, including kwashiorkor, tuberculosis and human immunodeficiency virus (**HIV**) infection.

There are many reasons for this increase in severity: children are infected at a young age (median age, 12–24 months); severe malnutrition leads to prolonged, severe measles that kills up to 40 per cent of those infected. Overcrowding is another strong determinant of outcome, for secondary and tertiary cases in large families are at great risk of death. Exposure to a large dose of the virus when in close contact with the index case may be an important factor. Furthermore, the severity of measles and the chances of the secondary case dying are dependent on the severity of disease in the index case. Transmission of measles from one sex to the other has been found to increase mortality two- to threefold compared to transmission from the same sex. The high mortality found in West Africa is likely to be due to the very large, polygamous and extended families, which increase the risk of intense exposure.

The epidemiology of measles in the developing world varies according to the degree of urbanization. Remote villages suffer outbreaks every 3 to 5 years in which a wide range of age groups from young children to adults are infected and mortality, which can be high, occurs at a later age. In such outbreaks there are many susceptible children in each family and hence a high risk of exposure. These outbreaks resemble the severe epidemics that in the past have devastated the remote island populations of the Faeroes, Greenland, and Tristan da Cunha. In urban areas, migration, overcrowding, and poverty have led to a hyperendemic pattern of infection. The median age of infection may be less than 2 years, 5 to 10 per cent of children under 9 months old contract the disease, and mortality is greatest in those between 6 and 18 months of age. Hospital wards and clinics in the developing world are important centres of infection; in a hospital in the north of Nigeria, 35 per cent of children with measles had acquired the infection by attending the outpatient clinic 2 to 3 weeks before. Acute measles is often less severe among children under 6 months of age, among previously immunized children, and among those who have received immunoglobulin when exposed. The course of infection, which is modified by antibody, is characterized by a prolonged incubation period, a short prodrome, mild symptoms, and a favourable outcome.

Long-term morbidity and mortality may be considerable, especially in young children, for several studies from West Africa have suggested that the relative risk of dying in the year after measles, compared to vaccinated controls, is in the order of 10. The causes of death are not well documented but are likely to be due to a combination of malnutrition and secondary infections occurring as a result of prolonged immunosuppression after measles.

Popular beliefs

In most cultures, measles has a specific local name and is a much feared disease. Popular understanding is centred around the rash, which if it stays within the body will lead to severe disease. This belief has some basis in truth for the prodrome is prolonged in severe cases and in very severe epidemics a proportion of deaths reportedly occur before the appearance of the rash. Therapeutic practices, such as rubbing the skin with palm oil or kerosene, are aimed at eliciting the rash quickly. In West Africa it is believed that cooling keeps the rash within the body, so the child may be bedded in warm sand or covered with blankets, and is not washed or given cold water to drink. Such habits may aggravate dehydration. In West Africa, as a result of popular awareness of measles, good correspondence exists between parental diagnosis and that based on clinical and immunological assessments. The mother's diagnosis, which can be used for epidemiological surveillance, is nearly always correct.

The virus and its antigens

Measles, a paramyxovirus that contains a single strand of RNA, is highly pleomorphic, ranging from 100 to 300 nm in diameter. The virus propagates by budding from the cell membrane, from which it acquires an envelope. The membrane of infected cells and the virion envelope contain two surface glycoproteins, the haemagglutinin (**H**) and fusion (**F**)

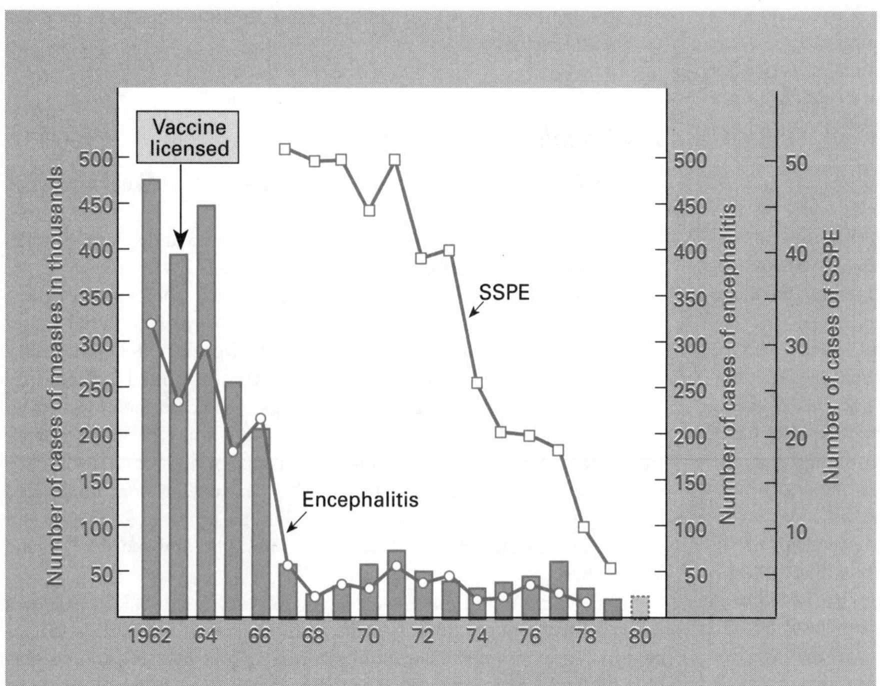

Fig. 1 Incidence of measles, measles encephalitis, and subacute sclerosing, panencephalitis (SSPE) since the introduction of live attenuated measles vaccine. (Reproduced by courtesy of S. Krujim, from Marshall (1983). Measles, in *Oxford Textbook of Medicine*, Oxford University Press.)

proteins, and a non-glycosylated matrix (**M**) protein, which forms the inner layer. The H protein, which allows attachment of the virus to cells, is the main target for neutralizating antibodies; the F protein is responsible for fusion and syncytium formation of infected cells. The internal components or nucleocapsid consist of RNA, the nucleoprotein (**N**), which is the major protein, the phosphoprotein (P) and the large protein (L). The F protein is remarkably stable, the H protein shows minor antigenic variation but the N protein, which contains a variable region in the C terminus, is highly divergent among different strains of virus. There is also variation in the M protein, which some claim is related to persistent infection. The replication and assembly of measles virus is shown in Fig. 2.

Pathogenesis and the immune response

The course of infection and the immune response to this invasion are shown in Fig. 3. The measles virus, which is thermolabile and survives best at low humidities, is spread to susceptible contacts in droplets during sneezing and coughing. First it infects and multiplies in the epithelium of the upper respiratory tract or the conjunctivae. Some 4 to 6 days later the virus is found in the reticuloendothelial tissue of the liver and the spleen after passage through lymph nodes and spread via the blood. Here it multiplies, causing fusion of cells to form giant cells with many nuclei. Viral antigens, which can be found by immunofluorescent techniques in and on the surface of both these cells and lymphocytes, now induce the immune response. First, natural killer cells and cytotoxic T cells mount a cell-mediated reaction that contains the virus and limits its spread within cells. Later, B cells are primed to produce antibody. Defects in the cellular immune system, as in severe malnutrition, cancer or primary immunodeficiencies, allow widespread multiplication of the virus to cause fatal giant-cell pneumonia.

Around day 8 the measles virus is carried by the blood, either free or in mononuclear cells, to the target tissue which are the epithelia of the eye, lung, and gut. Again, the agent multiplies to cause a bright redness of the mucosa and Koplik's spots (see below), which are foci of viral multiplication. At this stage, measles virus may be cultured from nasopharyngeal secretions and antigen can be detected by immunofluorescent techniques in the characteristic giant cells of the buccal mucosa, in epithelial cells, and in both B and T lymphocytes in the blood.

The rash, appearing around days 14 to 16, is in fact the sign of a strong and complicated allergic reaction to the virus in the epithelia. The extent and severity of the rash, which is largely responsible for the clinical severity of the disease, is determined by the number of target cells infected. Histological examination shows virus in the disrupted epidermis, in the corium, and in capillary endothelium. These tissues are infiltrated by mononuclear cells together with antibody, immune complexes, and complement. An intact cell-mediated immune response is essential to generate the rash and clear the virus, for if impaired, as in the case of children with leukaemia, or occasionally in severe kwashiorkor, the virus multiplies unchecked and no rash appears. Two or three days after the start of the rash, around day 17 or 18, the virus can no longer be cultured in the epithelia, for infected cells have been disrupted and the free virus neutralized by antibody. The first antibody to appear is to the nucleoprotein antigens. The second, which is largely responsible for neutralization of the virus, is to the haemagglutinin.

Fig. 3 Pathogenesis of measles. + Denotes amount of virus, ab = antibody. (Reproduced from Parry (1984). *Principles of medicine in Africa*, 2nd edn, University Press, Oxford.)

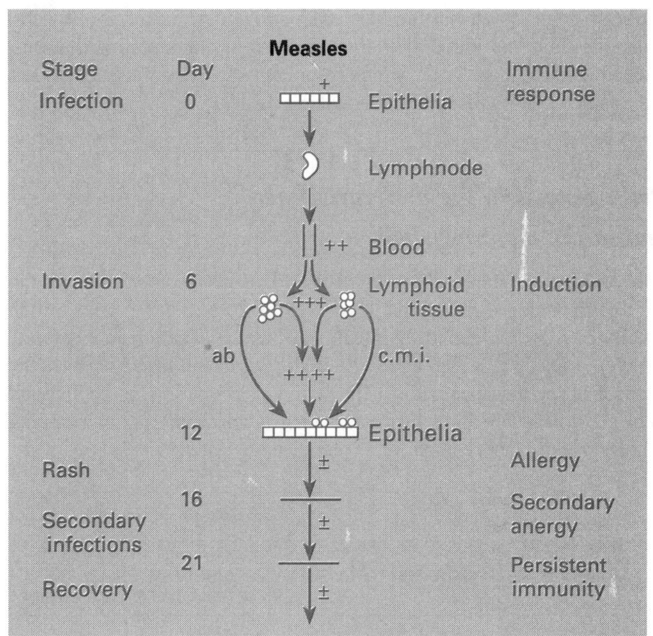

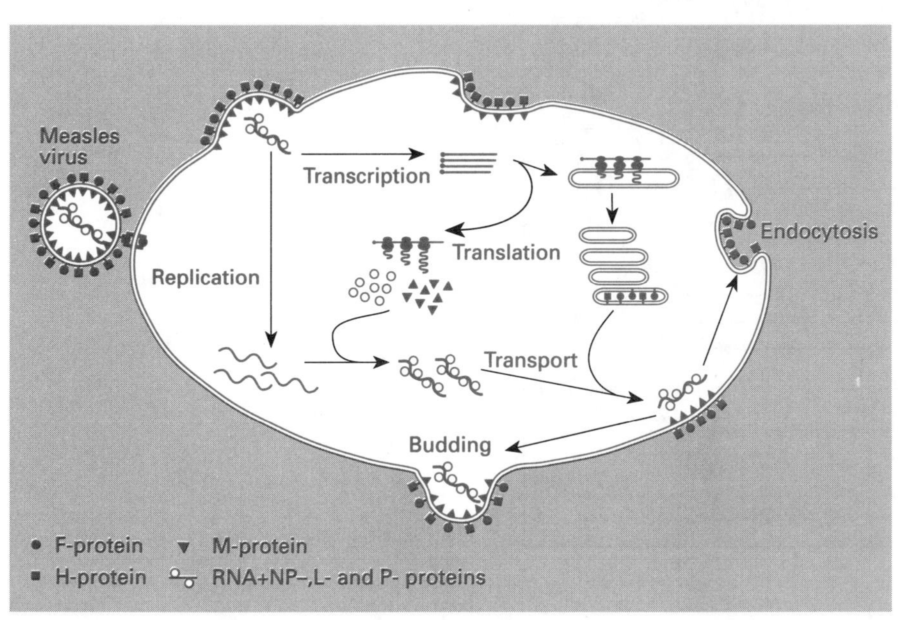

Fig. 2 Replication and assembly of measles virus (reproduced by courtesy of van Binnedijk (1992). T-cell function in measles. PhD thesis. University of Utrecht, Holland).

Finally the antibody to the fusion glycoprotein appears in a low titre. This antibody stops cell-to-cell spread of the virus. At this stage the child is markedly immunosuppressed and thus susceptible to secondary infections of eye, mouth, gut, and lung. The mechanism of immunosuppression is complex: T lymphocytes, especially the T-helper subset, are infected with the virus and depleted, antigen processing is defective, as is the production of lymphokines, and a suppressor factor, possibly an immune complex, circulates in the serum. Latent viruses such as herpes simplex or cytomegalovirus may be reactivated and in turn cause further immunosuppression. The delayed hypersensitivity reaction as measured by skin tests to old tuberculin or candida antigen is absent or severely impaired.

By the third week, day 21, as the patient recovers, antibody is in full production. Levels remain elevated for the rest of the patient's life, either because of repeated subclinical infections or because the virus persists in latent form in the spleen and other organs, so stimulating antibody. Occasionally the virus persists in the brain in a damaging form to cause subacute sclerosing panencephalitis (see below). In this rare condition, virus can be isolated from the brain up to 8 years after measles, and antibody levels to all but the M protein antigen are raised in the cerebrospinal fluid and blood. The immune system, for unknown reasons, has failed to clear the virus, which is probably aberrant, for such strains are unable to produce normal amounts of protein.

Pathogenesis in the underprivileged and in the malnourished

Measles in the children of the Third World, as was formerly the case in the underprivileged in Europe, is severe, prolonged, and carries a high fatality rate due to secondary infections. Two explanations are offered. Crowding leads to a high dose of measles virus and also increases the chances of secondary infection. The period of incubation has been found to be short in severe and fatal cases, which is consistent with the emphasis on dose as a mechanism of severe disease. Alternatively, or in tandem, malnutrition diminishes the immune response to the virus allowing great proliferation of virus and subsequent damage to the host. There is experimental evidence, although only in severely malnourished children with marasmus or kwashiorkor, that lymphocytes of these patients may be more readily infected during the induction phase. A normal immune response follows, which generates a severe and widespread rash followed by prolonged immunosuppression. Secondary bacterial infections such as with *Streptococcus pneumoniae* or latent infections like herpes simplex or with *Mycobacterium tuberculosis* follow in the wake of this intense immunosuppression, often killing or maiming the child. Virus persists in lymphocytes and epithelial cells for up to 30 days after the start of the rash. Antibody production occasionally fails and secretory IgA is deficient, which may explain why the virus persists for so long in the gut. Anorexia, increased catabolism, protein loss from the gut, and further malnutrition compound the problem, which is worst in the weanling child (Fig. 4).

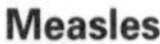

Fig. 4 Interaction of malnutrition and measles. (Reproduced from Greenwood and Whittle (1981). *Immunology of medicine in the tropics*, Edward Arnold, London, with permission.)

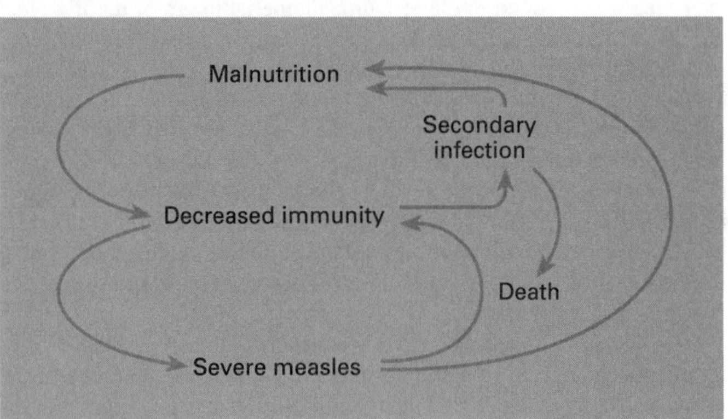

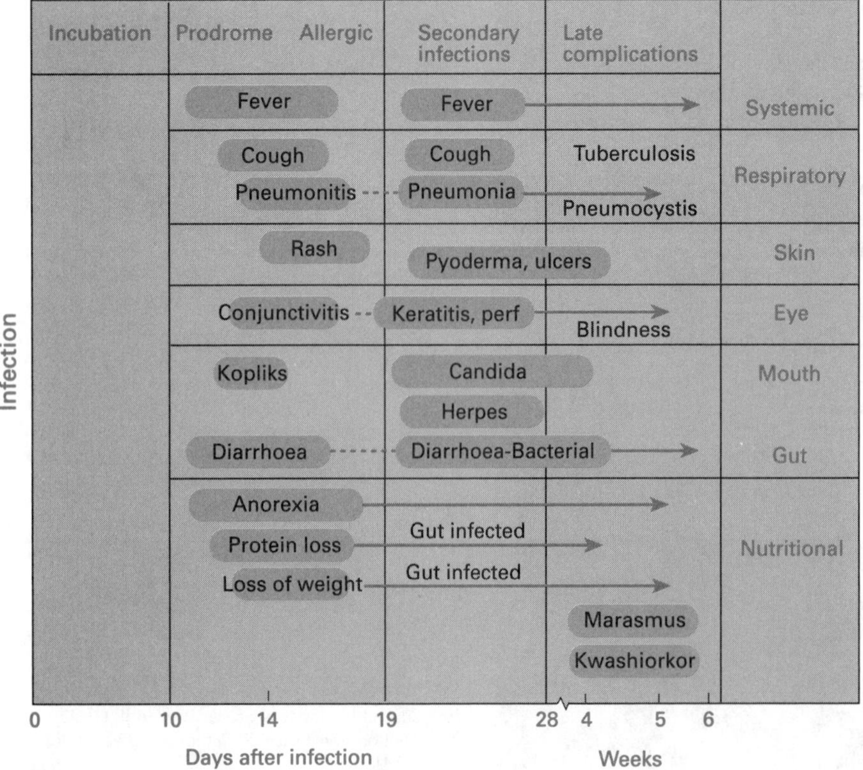

Fig. 5 Clinical features of measles and some of its complications. (Reproduced from Parry (1984). *Principles of medicine in Africa*. 2nd edn, University Press, Oxford.)

Clinical features and complications

There is a spectrum of severity that ranges from mild in the privileged and well nourished to severe in the blatantly malnourished or immunosuppressed. However, the rule is not inviolate and other factors such as the age and dose of infection are probably as important in determining the severity of disease. Measles, often severe, occasionally infects unvaccinated young adults or individuals who have lived in isolated communities. The clinical features of measles and some complications are shown in Fig. 5.

Prodrome (days 10–14)

Diagnosis is often missed at this stage, when fever coupled with runny nose and sometimes complicated by convulsions is the main feature. Other signs are mild conjunctivitis, red mucosa, Koplik's spots, and diarrhoea. Koplik's spots are found in the buccal mucosa. They are 'small irregular spots of bright red colour; in the centre of each spot is seen a minute bluish-white speck'. A useful diagnostic test is to scrape the buccal mucosa with a spatula, place the scraping on a microscope slide, stain with Leishman's stain, and examine for giant cells with a microscope. The prodrome is prolonged in severe cases and reduced in individuals with modified measles due to maternal antibodies or prophylactic use of immunoglobulin.

Rash (days 14–18)

The morbilliform rash first appears on the forehead and neck and then spreads, over a period of 3 to 4 days, to involve the trunk and finally the limbs.

In Africa and other parts of the developing world the rash is often red, confluent, raised, very extensive, and sometimes accompanied by bleeding into the skin and gut. Later the rash blackens, then the skin peels causing extensive desquamation. Other epithelial surfaces are inflamed, the severity matching that of the rash. Cough, a cardinal sign, may be hoarse and coupled with difficulty of inspiration if the larynx and trachea are inflamed. Signs of pneumonitis are apparent, which in severe cases may cause cyanosis or be complicated by mediastinal and subcutaneous emphysema. Conjunctivitis, especially in those who are vitamin A deficient, can be severe; enteritis may cause profuse diarrhoea with resulting loss of protein, and malabsorption of food and water. The mouth is painful and red, which adds to the misery of the child, who becomes anorexic and may even refuse to suck the breast. In the uncomplicated case, as is usual in the West, the convalescent period is short, usually lasting less than a week. If fever persists while the rash is fading or desquamating, complications should be suspected.

Early complications (days 18–30)

As a result of the widespread, severe allergic reaction to the measles virus signified by the rash, the patient is left severely immunosuppressed and is susceptible to infection.

PNEUMONIA

This causes most deaths (Table 1) and is heralded by a rise in fever, leucocytosis, and respiratory difficulties. Lobar pneumonia is usually cause by *Strep. pneumoniae* but bronchopneumonia, which is more common, results from other bacteria, such as *Staphylococcus aureus*, or secondary viral infections such as with herpes simplex or adenovirus. A variety of other organisms such as Gram-negative bacteria, cytomegalovirus, fungi, *M. tuberculosis*, and *Pneumocystis carinii* should be considered as potential pathogens of the lung in the malnourished or immunocompromised child.

Table 1 *Complications and mortality in patients with measles in hospital, northern Nigeria, July–December 1978*

	Number	Died	Percentage dead
Pneumonia	169	32	18.9
Gastroenteritis	65	9	13.8
Marasmic kwashiorkor	25	6	24.0
Laryngotracheobronchitis	21	4	19.0
Encephalitis	10	4	40.0

Reproduced from Parry (1984). *Principles of medicine in Africa.* 2nd edn. University Press, Oxford, with permission.

STOMATITIS AND ENTERITIS

Chronic diarrhoea and a sore mouth caused by candidal infection are common complications of measles in children in the Third World. The gut is often superinfected with bacteroides, *Escherichia coli*, Pseudomonas, and *Staph. aureus*, which results in malabsorption and protein loss. Deep ulcers caused by herpes simplex virus erode the corners of the mouth, gums, and inner surface of the lips causing much misery, illness, and pain (Fig. 6).

EYE INFECTIONS

Corneal ulceration leading to impaired vision or blindness is common after measles, especially in malnourished and vitamin A-deficient children. Several studies from Africa have shown that more than half of childhood blindness is related to measles. The mechanisms are still under discussion. In northern Nigeria, herpes simplex was found in 47 per cent of active corneal ulcers after measles and measles virus in 12 per cent: the children often had evidence of oral herpes. In a study in

Fig. 6 Herpes simplex ulceration of lips and gingiva following measles.

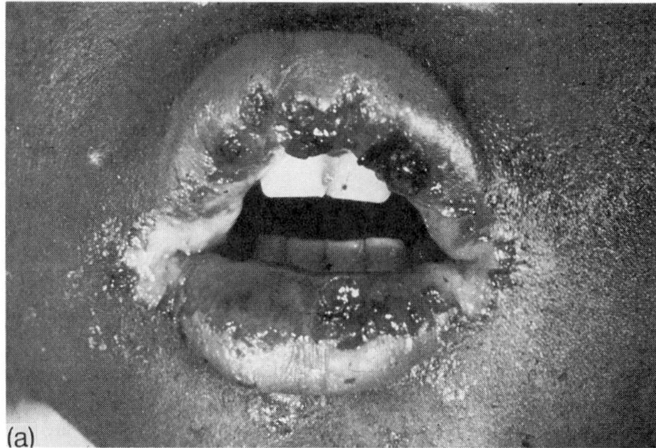
(a)

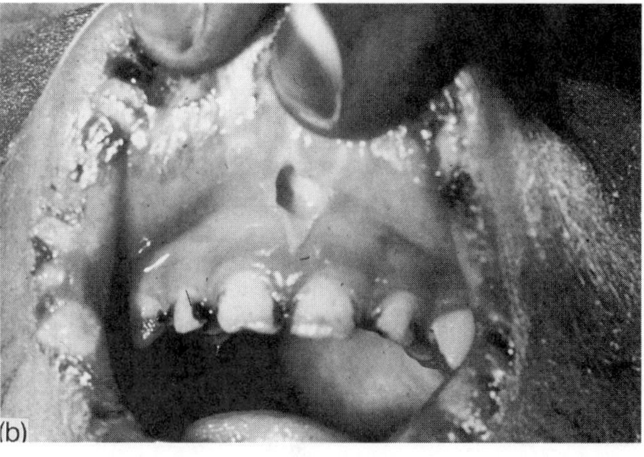
(b)

Tanzania, blindness precipitated by measles was associated with vitamin A deficiency (50 per cent), herpes simplex infection (21 per cent), and the use of traditional eye medicine (17 per cent).

SKIN AND OTHER INFECTIONS

Pyoderma is common after measles. In the malnourished, deep eroding ulcers may bore through the skin even into bone. Otitis media is also common.

Encephalitis

This is a rare but much feared complication found in approximately 1 to 2 per 1000 cases. The onset is usually between 4 and 7 days after the start of the rash but rarely it may occur within 48 h or up to 2 weeks from the onset. In addition to seizures there is often fever, irritability, headache, and a disturbance in consciousness that may progress to profound coma. The disorder is probably attributable to a neuroallergic process: lymphocytes from the cerebrospinal fluid have been shown to respond to myelin basic protein, as in experimental allergic encephalomyelitis. The virus cannot be isolated from cerebrospinal fluid, which contains lymphocytes and raised levels of IgG but normal levels of measles antibody. Mortality and morbidity is high: 10 to 15 per cent of victims die and 25 per cent of children are left with permanent brain damage. Treatment is supportive; dexamethasone has no convincing beneficial effect.

Late complications

MALNUTRITION

This is the most frequent complication, for children of the developing world often lose much weight during measles and may take many weeks to regain it. Those originally underweight, who have had severe measles, are at greatest risk, for in these children anorexia is prolonged, much protein is lost from the gut, and secondary infections, which lead to marasmus or marasmic kwashiorkor, are frequent. Measles has been shown to persist in the epithelia and lymphocytes of the severely malnourished for 30 or more days after the rash.

Persistent infection

PNEUMONITIS

A giant-cell pneumonia is found in patients with defects in cell-mediated immunity; children with leukaemia or kwashiorkor are particularly vulnerable. The lung disease may develop weeks after measles, and in most cases the rash of measles has been absent and thus the diagnosis may not be suspected. The diagnosis is made by virological and/or histological examination of lung tissue. Most of these children die.

SUBACUTE SCLEROSING PANENCEPHALITIS (SSPE)

Persistent measles virus infection is responsible for this rare, progressive disease of the brain, which is found in 0.1 to 1.4 per million children after measles. The virus is detected in the brain by electron microscopy and by immunofluorescent methods, and has been isolated only by cocultivation techniques. The child with SSPE has usually experienced normal measles, albeit at a young age, 5 to 10 years earlier. The first indication is a disturbance in intellect and personality; behaviour disorders and deterioration in school work are frequently mentioned. There then follows, over a period of weeks and months, seizures akin to myoclonus, signs of extrapyramidal and pyramidal disease, and finally a state of decerebrate rigidity followed by death. The electroencephalogram shows a characteristic regular series of high-amplitude, spike-like waves. Very high titres of measles complement-fixing and haemagglutinin inhibitory antibody are present both in serum and cerebrospinal fluid; the haemagglutin inhibitory antibody is probably produced within the nervous system. Treatments for SSPE have included transfer factor, plasmapheresis, and antiviral drugs, but to no avail.

MULTIPLE SCLEROSIS

There is no convincing evidence that measles virus or immune responses to it have a causative role in this disease.

Treatment of measles and its complications

No effective antimeasles drug exists, yet some children do benefit from treatment in hospital. The following criteria indicate severe measles and a need for admission: a widespread, confluent rash darkening to deep red or purple, signs of laryngeal obstruction of subcutaneous emphysema, marked dehydration, blood in the stool or more than five stools a day, convulsion or loss of consciousness, severe secondary pneumonia, corneal ulceration, or severe ulceration of the mouth and skin. These signs should be taken particularly seriously when the child is underweight or frankly malnourished.

Hydrate the child orally or intravenously. Treat lobar pneumonia with benzylpenicillin, and bronchopneumonia with combined antibiotics such as gentamicin and cloxacillin, or with co-trimoxazole. Antibiotic eye ointments relieve discomfort and possibly prevent secondary infections of measles conjunctivitis. Antibiotics, topical and systemic, and vitamin A should be given routinely for eye ulcers. If herpes simplex virus is the cause, use acyclovir topically or, when severe, systemically. Candidal infections of the mouth or gut often respond dramatically to nystatin. Feeding, by tube if necessary, needs careful planning and presentation, for the anorexic infected child will be in severe negative energy balance due to a greatly increased catabolic rate. Case fatality rates are 30 to 50 per cent lower in children in hospital treated with vitamin A. This should be given orally at the time of diagnosis in dose of 100 000 i.u. for children below 12 months of age and in a dose of 200 000 i.u. for older children. If eye signs of vitamin A deficiency are present the initial dose should be repeated the next day and again 1 to 4 weeks later. No specific effective treatment for encephalitis or SSPE exists.

Prevention

Passive immunization with human immunoglobulin is highly effective if given within 2 or 3 days of exposure, in a dose for children of 0.2 ml/kg. Immunoglobulin should be given to those for whom vaccination is contraindicated: children immunosuppressed by kwashiorkor, by malignancies such as leukaemia or lymphoma, or by steroids or cytotoxic drugs. Passive immunization is also used to protect the pregnant and those with active tuberculosis.

The currently used vaccines are live strains, attenuated by culture in chick fibroblasts. The complications of vaccination are few and generally mild. Fever of moderate severity is infrequent, and a mild rash with some signs of upper respiratory tract infection occurs rarely. Encephalitis or SSPE is exceedingly rare after vaccination, which drastically reduces these fearsome complications of natural measles (Fig. 1). Underweight children respond normally to the vaccine as do ill children in the outpatient department and on the ward. As clinics and hospitals are major sites of transmission of the virus in the developing world, all susceptible children in these places, unless seriously immunocompromised as in leukaemia or kwashiorkor, should be vaccinated. Failures of vaccination are usually due to heat rendering the vaccine impotent or to maternal antibody, which neutralizes the vaccine.

The first measles vaccines introduced in the United States and Europe in the 1960s were inactivated with formalin. Although they produced high levels of H antibody they failed to raise antibody to the F protein.

This gave poor protection, and on exposure a severe local reaction at the site of injection or a bizarre form of measles resulted. The rash was unusual, having urticarial and vesicular features, fever was high, oedema of the limbs frequent, and severe pneumonia present. This syndrome is still occasionally seen in adults who were vaccinated with killed vaccine during childhood.

The optimal age for vaccination in the developed world is 14 to 16 months, when maternal antibody, which neutralizes the virus to cause vaccine failure, has disappeared. This counsel does not apply to children in the Third World, because there measles infects at an early age. The World Health Organization (**WHO**) recommends vaccination at 9 months of age but, by then, 5 to 15 per cent of children may have had measles. Edmonston–Zagreb, a different strain of vaccine, passaged in human diploid cells, and given in high dose (in excess of 10^5 infectious particles) subcutaneously, has proved to be immunogenic at the age of 4 to 6 months. Subsequently the WHO recommended its use at 6 months of age in areas of the world with a high incidence of measles below 9 months of age. However, long-term follow-up demonstrated lower survival rates among female recipients of high-titre vaccine than among female recipients of standard-dose measles vaccine. Although the biological explanation for this unexpected finding is unknown, the use of high-titre vaccines is now no longer recommended.

Some scientists have argued that measles vaccines will have a limited impact on childhood survival, for disadvantaged children, saved from measles by vaccination, will only die at a later date from other infections or malnutrition. However, a variety of epidemiological studies has documented remarkable reductions in mortality after standard measles vaccine. In Bangladesh, measles vaccination was associated with a 36 per cent reduction in all-cause mortality from the age of 9 months despite the fact that acute measles only accounted for 4 per cent of deaths in the community. The reason for this unexpected benefit is unknown.

New vaccines, which can be given in early infancy, or two-dose strategies using the standard vaccine at 6 and 9 months of age will be necessary to contain measles in the developing world. Eradication, which has nearly been achieved in the United States by insistence that children be immunized before going to school, will be difficult on a global scale for measles is highly infectious. Coverage of at least 95 per cent of all susceptible children, including those between 6 and 9 months of age, with a vaccine that is at least 95 per cent effective will be necessary if the virus is to be eradicated. Current vaccines do not meet these standards. New vaccines now in the developmental stage, much as the combination of F and H proteins with immune-stimulating complexes (ISCOMs) or the canarypox recombinant virus expressing these proteins may possibly fulfil such exacting requirements.

REFERENCES

Aaby, P. (1991). Determinants of measles mortality: host or transmission factors? In *Medical virology 10* (ed.) L.M. de la Maza and E.M. Peterson, pp. 83–116. Plenum Press, New York.

Aaby, P. (1992). Influence of cross-sex transmission on measles mortality in rural Senegal. *Lancet*, **340,** 388–91.

Aaby, P., Butch, J., Lisse I.M., and Smits, A.J. (1983). Measles mortality, state of nutrition, and family structure. A community study from Guinea-Bissau. *Journal of Infectious Disease*, **147,** 6593–701.

Aaby, P. *et al.* (1993). Long-term survival after Edmonston–Zagreb measles vaccination: increased female mortality. *Journal of Pediatrics* **122,** 904–8.

Bech, V. (1962). Measles epidemics in Greenland. *American Journal of Disease in Children*, **103,**, 252–3.

Dossetor, J., Whittle, H.C., and Greenwood B.M. (1977). Persistent measles infection in malnourished children. *British Medical Journal*, **1,** 1633–5.

Enders, J.F., McCarthy, K., Mitus A., and Cheatham, W.J. (1959). Isolation of measles viruses at autopsy in cases of giant-cell pneumonia without rash. *New England Journal of Medicine*, **261,** 875–81.

Fenner, F. (1948). The pathogenesis of the acute exanthems. An interpretation based on experimental investigations with mouse-pox (infectious ectromelia of mice). *Lancet*, **ii,** 915–20.

Fraser, K.B. and Martin, S.J. (1978). *Measles virus and its biology*. Academic Press, London.

Fulginiti, V.A., Eller, J.J., Dowine, A.W., and Kemp, C.H. (1967). Altered reactivity to measles virus, atypical measles in children previously immunized with inactivated measles virus vaccines. *Journal of the American Medical Association*, **202,** 1075–80.

Johnson, R.T. *et al.* (1984). Measles encephalomyelitis—clinical and immunologic studies. *New England Journal of Medicine*, **310,** 137–41.

Hussey, G.D. and Klein, M. (1990). A randomized, controlled trial of vitamin A in children with severe measles. *New England Journal of Medicine*, **323,** 160–4.

Horta-Barbosa, L., Fucillo, D.A., Sever, J.L., and Zeman, W. (1969). Subacute sclerosing panencephalitis: isolation of measles virus from a brain biopsy. *Nature*, **221,** 974.

Kaschula, R.O.C., Druker, J., and Kipps, A. (1983). Late morphologic consequences of measles: a lethal and debilitating lung disease among the poor. *Review of Infectious Disease*, **5,** 395–404.

McChesney, M.B. and Oldstone, M.B.A. (1989). Virus-induced immunosuppression with measles virus and human immunodeficiency virus. *Advances in Immunology*, **45,** 335–80.

Morley, D. (1969). Severe measles in the tropics. *British Medical Journal*, **1,** 297–300; 363–5.

Merz, D.C., Scheid, A., and Choppin, P.W. (1980). Importance of antibodies to the fusion glycoprotein of paramyxoviruses in the prevention of spread of infection. *Journal of Experimental Medicine*, **151,** 275–88.

Smythe, P.M. *et al.* (1971). Thymolymphatic deficiency and depression of cell-mediated immunity in protein calorie malnutrition. *Lancet*, **ii,** 939–43.

Scheifele, D.W. and Forbes, C.E. (1972). Prolonged giant cell excretion in African measles. *Pediatrics*, **50,** 867–73.

Ward, B.J., Johnson, R.T., Vaisberg, A., Jauregui, E., and Griffin, D.E. (1991). Cytokine production *in vitro* and the lymphoproliferative defect of natural measles virus infection. *Clinical Immunology and Immunopathology*, **61,** 236–48.

Whittle, H.C., Dossetor, J., Oduluju, A., Bryceson, A.D.M., and Greenwood, B.M. (1978). Cell-mediated immunity during natural measles infection. *Journal of Clinical Investigation*, **62,** 678–84.

Whittle, H.C., Sandford Smith, J., Kogbe, O.I., Dossetor, J., and Duggan, M. (1979). Severe ulcerative herpes of mouth and eye following measles. *Transactions of the Royal Society for Tropical Medicine and Hygiene*, **73,** 66–9.

7.10.13 Enteroviruses

N. R. Grist and E. J. Bell*

Enteroviruses are common infectious agents spread characteristically by the faecal–oral route and capable of causing a variety of clinical syndromes. Typical picornaviruses, they have a non-enveloped virion of icosahedral symmetry, 25 to 30 nm in diameter, containing a genome of single-stranded RNA of 'positive' (mRNA) sense. The molecular weight of the nucleic acid is 2.5×10^6. The viral capsid is composed of 60 protamers, each made up of one molecule each of four viral proteins designated VP1 to VP4. The epitopes that elicit neutralizing (protective) antibody are located on three of these structural proteins (VP1,2,3).

As befits their gastrointestinal habitat, enteroviruses are relatively stable, resisting treatment with deoxycholate, ether, and other fat solvents, and acid (pH 3 for 1 h). They survive for long periods in water at low temperature but are inactivated by drying or exposure to heat (50 °C for 1 h unless stabilized by magnesium chloride) or free residual chlorine (0.3–0.5 parts 10^6). There are numerous types, some infecting mammalian species other than man. The enteroviruses of man were classified as polioviruses (causing paralytic disease in primates); coxsackieviruses (causing paralytic disease if inoculated into newborn mice, in which

*Dr Eleanor Bell died suddenly in November 1993.

Table 1 *The enteroviruses*

Group	Major disease
Poliovirus types 1–3	Paralytic poliomyelitis
	Viral ('aseptic') meningitis
Coxsackievirus types A1–A24[1]	Viral ('aseptic') meningitis
	Herpangina
	Hand, foot, and mouth disease
	Conjunctivitis (type A24)
Coxsackievirus types B1–B6	Viral ('aseptic') meningitis
	Pleurodynia (Bornholm disease)
	Myopericarditis
	Fatal neonatal disease
Echovirus types 1–34[1]	Viral ('aseptic') meningitis
	Skin rashes
	Febrile illness
Enterovirus types 68–72[1]	Conjunctivitis (type 70)
	Poliomyelitis-like disease (type 71)
	Hepatitis (type 72)

[1]Coxsackie A23 = echovirus 9; coxsackie A24 = echovirus 34; echovirus 10 = reovirus 1; echovirus 28 = rhinovirus 1A; enterovirus 72 = hepatitis A.

Table 2 *Main pattern of infection by a typical enterovirus*

Portals of entry
Oral
Respiratory
Primary site of multiplication
Pharynx
Alimentary tract
Viraemia—in some cases
Secondary sites of viral multiplication and damage
CNS (meningitis, poliomyelitis, encephalitis)
Heart (myocarditis, pericarditis)
Muscles (Bornholm disease)
Skin and mucosae (exanthem; enanthem)
Respiratory tract (upper, lower)
Liver (hepatitis A)
Liver, pancreas and other viscera in generalized infections—mainly in infants
Portals of exit
Faeces
Pharyngeal and respiratory secretions

group A types cause severe generalized myositis whereas group B types cause patchy myositis but severe brain damage); and echoviruses, which can be isolated in cell cultures but are not usually pathogenic for newborn mice. Antigenic types are distinguished by neutralization tests with specific antisera. Some anomalous enteroviruses share properties of more than one of these classical groups. Those most recently discovered have been designated 'higher enterovirus types' instead of being fitted into the original groups. Hepatitis A virus, now designated enterovirus type 72, is not considered further here (see Chapter 7.10.26). Table 1 summarizes the currently recognized enteroviruses and their main disease associations.

Pattern of infection

Typically, enteroviruses infect by the oral route, resist stomach acid, infect cells in the throat and lower alimentary tract, and are excreted in faeces (Table 2). Sometimes they penetrate systemically, with brief viraemia and fever. They may then reach and infect cells in other organs such as the nervous system, heart, and muscles. Some infect mainly the respiratory tract and can be transmitted by respiratory droplet infection; others infect the eye and spread mainly by contagion. Recovery is accompanied by development of humoral immunity protective against symptomatic reinfection by the same virus type—both serum antibodies and also secretory IgA 'coproantibodies' inhibitory to reinfection of the gut. The role of cellular immunity is less well understood. At cellular level, infection is cytolytic; virus multiplies within cells, which burst liberating progeny virus, as seen in infected cell cultures. No clinically effective antiviral agents are available for enterovirus infections, although interferon suppresses enteroviruses *in vitro*.

Epidemiology

Enterovirus infections are most prevalent in young children and under conditions of overcrowding and poor hygiene, especially in warm seasons and hot climates. In such circumstances, spread occurs mainly by faecal pollution of people and the environment, water, and food as the virus is stable for long periods in moist organic matter, sewage, and contaminated water. In many such warm-climate communities, unless controlled by vaccination, paralytic poliomyelitis is prevalent at all seasons and every year, affecting mainly young children. In smaller populations and with improved hygiene, spread of infection is slowed down; poliovirus and some other enteroviruses then show epidemic activity at intervals of 3 or commonly 4 years, which allow the emergence of non-immune children to support fresh outbreaks. In large conurbations in temperate climates, 20 or more different enteroviruses may be active in a single year with one or two dominating the summer–autumn epidemic season. In sparse and isolated communities where standards of hygiene are high, infection tends to die out. This allows a non-immune population to build up, which then, if infection is reintroduced, may support an epidemic with broad age distribution. Older and adult non-immune people often suffer more severe disease than children, although most enterovirus infections are silent or trivial in effect. Infants, however, if unprotected by maternal passive immunity, may develop severe and life-threatening disease. Where hygienic standards are high enough to prevent significant faecal–oral transmission, limited spread may still occur by the respiratory route because acute infections entail brief infectivity of nasopharyngeal secretions, but this route is less effective as enteroviruses do not withstand desiccation.

Antibody responses to first infections in life are type specific, but cross-reactions are common in older children and adults because some antigens are shared by different enteroviruses. Infection induces immunity to the same serotype of enterovirus. Transient reinfections of the gut by poliovirus of a type to which the individual already has antibody are not uncommon, showing that 'gut immunity' is neither absolute nor permanent.

For poliomyelitis the situation is altered by the influence of vaccination. Circulation of 'wild' polioviruses in crowded populations of the tropics and subtropics remains common, with unvaccinated individuals or groups at high risk of exposure to infection. Even in countries with high uptake of vaccine, the remaining cases of poliomyelitis involve unvaccinated or incompletely vaccinated persons, as in The Netherlands in 1992. Improved living standards postpone the average age of first infection and probably explain the emergence of epidemic poliomyelitis first in the developed countries of northern Europe and North America. Improved hygiene exerts selection pressure in favour of the more vigorously multiplying strains of poliovirus, which are also more virulent. Urbanization of populations from relatively isolated rural areas of many developing countries provides opportunities for epidemic spread among persons not previously exposed to the particular poliovirus (or other enterovirus). Thus the epidemiological situation throughout the world is complex and changing, requiring constant surveillance and efficient use of available poliomyelitis vaccines.

Virological diagnosis

Diagnosis of acute enterovirus infections is best achieved by isolating virus from faecal extracts by inoculation of cell cultures, or, when infection with a group A coxsackievirus is suspected, of newborn mice. Virus excretion in faeces begins a few days after infection and continues for 1 or 2 weeks in adults or longer in young children. As enteroviruses are relatively stable in faeces, samples can yield virus after mailing or vehicular delivery to the laboratory. In respiratory illness, isolation of virus from throat swabs (placed immediately into virus transport medium) is possible up to a week after the first symptom. Isolation of virus from cerebrospinal fluid in neurological illness carries greater diagnostic significance than from faeces alone and, where possible, should be attempted. Despite their affinity for central nervous tissue, polioviruses are rarely isolated from cerebrospinal fluid, whereas in some epidemics of enterovirus infection (e.g. echovirus 6 or 9) up to 80 per cent of specimens of cerebrospinal fluid may yield virus.

Neutralization tests with type-specific antisera are the best means of identifying the virus isolated. Primary serological diagnosis is usually impracticable because of the profusion of enteroviral serotypes. However, paired sera from acute and convalescent stages of illness should be collected, especially from suspected poliomyelitis cases, as tests with particular suspected viruses are possible. Cardiac cases of suspected coxsackieviral origin may show unusually high or rising antibody titres to one or more of these viruses.

Because of the large number of enteroviral serotypes, rapid diagnosis of these infections has lagged far behind the advances made in other viral infections such as hepatitis B, rubella, or rotaviruses. This problem is now being overcome by application of enzyme immunoassay techniques to detect viral antigen or specific antibody such as IgM. These assays are sensitive, can be automated, and give objective results. Most work in this field has concentrated on coxsackieviruses.

Other methods under development involve probing clinical specimens for the presence of viral nucleic acid by dot-blot hybridization or *in situ* hybridization. Polymerase chain reaction is the latest development and can detect a single viral genome in a cell suspension or tissue section. These new methods are unlikely to provide first-line tests but are powerful investigative tools and should become more readily available as commercial kits are developed.

Diseases caused by enteroviruses

Non-specific, febrile, and respiratory illnesses

Most enteroviruses cause silent, minor, or transient symptoms, mainly upper respiratory, for example sore throat, with or without rhinitis, often with fever. In the United Kingdom, enteroviruses make only a small contribution to the total of respiratory illnesses. In hospital these affect mainly preschool children; in the community, children of school age. They also cause pharyngitis, tonsillitis, and 'influenzal' fevers in adults. Early studies in the United States showed that enteroviruses, particularly coxsackieviruses, were often incriminated in 'summer grippe' and similar febrile catarrhs in their summer–autumn season of peak incidence. Even polioviruses can sometimes cause purely respiratory symptoms.

The most clear-cut association of enteroviruses with acute respiratory illness is found in young children. The youngest are most vulnerable to the more serious, lower respiratory tract diseases. In closed communities and where nutrition and housing conditions are poor, outbreaks of serious disease may occur. Coxsackie B viruses have caused outbreaks of upper respiratory tract disease in young children in nurseries, camps, and residential homes. Echoviruses have also caused outbreaks, particularly among neonates and infants in hospitals and institutions. Echovirus 11 was isolated from children with croup during outbreaks in Sweden and has caused upper and lower respiratory tract infections in many parts of the world.

Table 3 *The main enteroviruses associated with exanthems and enanthems*

Syndrome	Coxsackievirus types A	Coxsackievirus types B	Echovirus types	Enterovirus type
Herpangina	1–10	1–5	6,9,16,17	
Lymphonodular pharyngitis	10			
Hand, foot, and mouth disease	5,10,16	2,5		71
Erythematous rashes	2,4,5,9, 16	1,3,4,5	1–7,9,11, 14,16,etc.	

Outbreaks of infection causing characteristic illness such as paralysis (poliovirus), meningitis (echovirus 30, coxsackievirus A9), or exanthem (echovirus 9) are accompanied by many cases of non-specific minor febrile and respiratory illness in the community, especially in close and family contacts of patients with more serious and typical disease.

Mucocutaneous syndromes

Enterovirus infections are sometimes accompanied by rashes and/or vesicular oropharyngeal lesions from which the virus can often be isolated as well as from faeces. Each syndrome can be due to any of several enteroviruses, each of which can cause a variety of mucocutaneous manifestations as well as other types of disease (Table 3). During an outbreak, most cases are due to the same enterovirus.

Enanthems

These may be considered as more florid and localized forms of the non-specific respiratory diseases considered above, but the high titres of mainly IgG antibodies found in the acute-phase sera of some patients suggest the possibility of an underlying Arthus-type reaction due to previous infection with a different but antigenically related enterovirus.

HERPANGINA

This acute, febrile illness with vesicular enanthem mainly affects young children. There is rapid onset of fever, headache, and painful sore throat. The fauces and soft palate show inflammation, with small, initially vesicular lesions that macerate into punched-out aphthae surrounded by reddened areas. These persist for about 2 days before healing. Lesions may also involve the uvula and palate. Illness usually lasts for 2 or 3 days only. Abdominal pain, nausea, and transient neck stiffness are sometimes present. Coxsackieviruses mainly of group A are the usual causes of herpangina. Echoviruses have been isolated from sporadic cases.

LYMPHONODULAR PHARYNGITIS

This is a similar but uncommon condition from which coxsackievirus A10 has been isolated. The yellowish or white oral lesions are nodular instead of vesicular and do not ulcerate.

HAND, FOOT, AND MOUTH DISEASE

This acute illness has been reported in outbreaks or epidemics from many parts of the world. Coxsackievirus A16 or enterovirus 71 are the most common causes. Children are mainly affected, typically by rapid onset of fever and sore throat. Small, superficial ulcers develop rapidly from vesicles on the gums, tongue, buccal mucosa, and palate. One or two days later, punctate and usually fleeting maculopapular skin lesions appear, as greyish, oval vesicles on the palms of hands, soles of feet, often on nail folds, sometimes on the dorsa of fingers and toes, and occasionally on the buttocks, axillae or other areas. Skin lesions may be very few. Fever and rash subside rapidly but mouth lesions may last more than a week, during which time adults often continue to be unwell.

Exanthems

Various transient and erythematous (rubelliform, maculopapular, rarely morbilliform or vesicular) skin rashes may accompany infections by many types of echovirus and occasionally coxsackieviruses, particularly in young children, among whom outbreaks of fever and rash can occur. Rashes are most common in infancy and may be petechial or purpuric in severe infections of the newborn.

Echovirus 9 can cause epidemics of rubella-like disease in children during community outbreaks in which others affected, particularly adults, have febrile illnesses and many have aseptic meningitis. After an incubation period of about 5 days the onset is sudden, with headache, fever, and often vomiting, most severe in older patients but often trivial in young children, in whom the rash may be the first or only notable feature. The rash typically presents as pink or red maculopapules, sometimes confined to the face, and also as minute pink or pale papules, usually on the trunk or limbs. Cervical, axillary, and inguinal lymph nodes may be enlarged. Illness usually subsides in 4 or 5 days. Differentiation from rubella may require laboratory investigation by attempted virus isolation from throat or faeces plus serological tests. Unlike rubella, echovirus 9 does not damage the fetus.

BOSTON EXANTHEM

Echovirus type 16 causes this, the first enteroviral eruptive fever recognized in children. The maculopapular rash on face, trunk, and extremities tends to appear after defervescence of the fever.

OTHER RASHES

Petechial, purpuric, urticarial, and telangiectatic rashes have been described in children infected usually with echoviruses but sometimes with coxsackieviruses.

Neurological diseases (see also Chapter 24.15.2)

Paralytic poliomyelitis was the first enteroviral disease to be recognized. Originally isolated in monkeys, polioviruses were the first members of the group to be identified. Further studies of paralytic and non-paralytic meningeal illnesses led to isolation of the 'Coxsackie' viruses in newborn mice. Subsequently cell culture techniques revealed '*E*nteric *C*ytopathic *H*uman *O*rphan' (ECHO) viruses.

In a country that originally had low but now has rising standards of living and hygiene there is typically evolution from a hyperendemic or endemic condition, with poliomyelitis essentially confined to suscepti-

Fig. 1 Poliomyelitis notifications illustrate transition from the stage of endemic 'infantile paralysis' to epidemic paralytic poliomyelitis in 1947, brought under control by vaccination with inactivated vaccine (IPV) from 1958 and oral vaccine (OPV) from 1962 up to the present. Virological tests became available in time to identify Type 1 poliovirus as the cause of the last three epidemics. (Statistical data from the Information Services Division of the Common Services Agency, Scottish Home, and Health Department; virological data from publications of the Virus Laboratory, Ruchill Hospital, Glasgow. Illustration prepared by Department of Audio Visual Services, Stobhill General Hospital, Glasgow.)

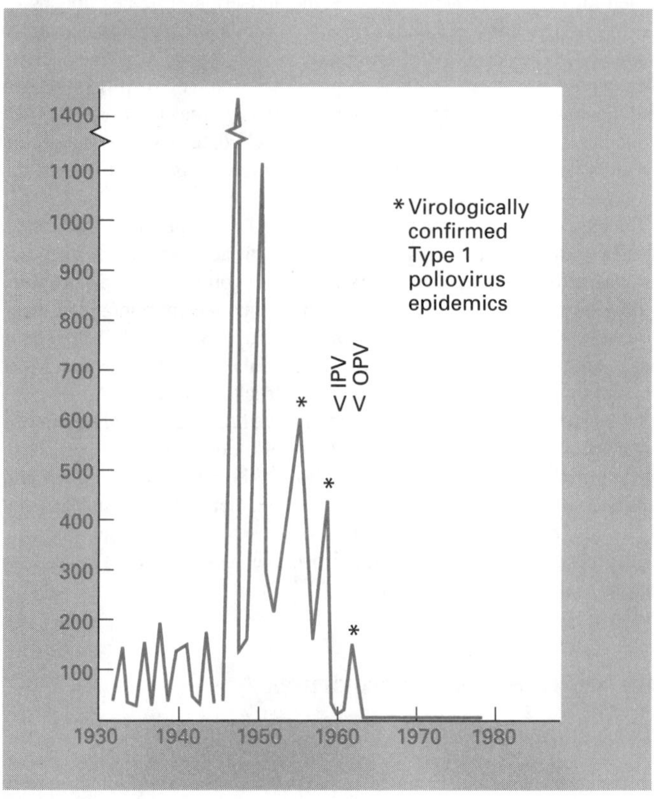

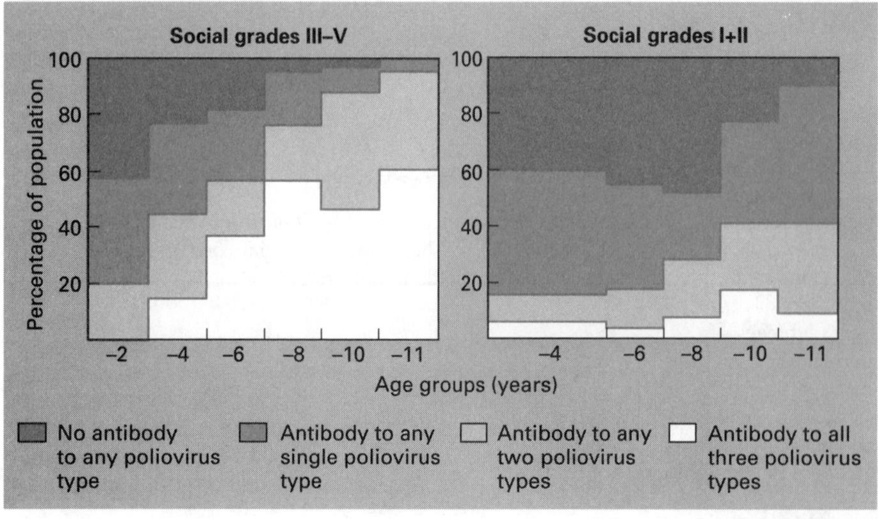

Fig. 2 Poliovirus antibody surveys before the introduction of vaccination: they showed marked differences between the lower and higher social grades of the same population. Children in grades III–V show progressive acquisition of immunity during preschool and school years, most of them acquiring antibodies to at least two or all three types by natural exposure to infection. Those in grades I and II acquired antibodies slowly and incompletely, most of them remaining susceptible to two or three of the polioviruses types. (Data from MacLeod *et al.* (1958). *Scottish Medical Journal* **3**, 76–81. Illustration prepared by Department of Audio Visual Services, Stobhill General Hospital, Glasgow.)

Table 4 *Main associations of enteroviruses with acute neurological diseases*

Syndrome	Poliovirus	Coxsackie virus	Echovirus	Enterovirus
Paralytic disease	+++ (especially types 1 and 3)	+ (especially type A7)	+/−	+ (type 71)
Meningitis	+ (types 1,2,3)	++ (especially types A9,B5,etc.)	++ (especially types 9,30, etc.)	+ (type 71)
Encephalitis	+	++	+/−	+ (type 71)

ble children under 5 years old and a relatively inconspicuous penalty of disease ('infantile paralysis'), although surveys in tropical Africa showed serious residual rates of paralysis of 2 to 11/1000 children. As improving conditions postpone the average age of primary infections, recurrent epidemics of paralytic poliomyelitis develop as a serious public health problem. These affect a wide age range and inflict a heavy burden of lifelong disability until controlled by vaccination (Fig. 1). Different socioeconomic groups of the same population may simultaneously be at different stages of this evolution (Fig. 2).

The main patterns of neurological disease caused by enteroviruses comprise acute paralytic poliomyelitis, non-bacterial 'aseptic meningitis' (the most common syndrome), and encephalitis (Table 4). Intermediate syndromes (meningoencephalitis; polioencephalitis) also occur.

Paralytic poliomyelitis

Typically, a minor prodromal illness lasts several days, with fever, sore throat, anorexia, and occasionally nausea, vomiting, and diarrhoea. If the later stages of the disease do not develop, this minor illness is known as 'abortive poliomyelitis', which cannot be diagnosed by clinical criteria alone. With or without a few days of well-being there follows abrupt onset of major neurological illness. The patient is anxious, irritable, often sweating, with fever (38–39 °C), headache, stiffness, and pains in the neck, trunk, and limbs. Nuchal rigidity and a positive Kernig sign are present. In about a third of patients that reach this stage the condition resolves in about a week and is then known as 'non-paralytic poliomyelitis', that is, aseptic meningitis due to poliovirus. The remainder progress rapidly to paralysis, which may be preceded by pain and fasciculations in the muscles to be affected. Paralysis usually appears during the fever, rarely afterwards, and may be the first sign of poliomyelitis in infants or very young children. It may evolve rapidly or progress gradually over a week or so. The pattern of paralysis is variable, typically asymmetrical, and usually affects the lower limbs more seriously than other muscles. Bulbar and encephalitic signs may appear. The paralysis is of lower motor-neurone type, flaccid with absent tendon reflexes. It tends to be more severe, extensive, and possibly progressive if there was strenuous physical exercise in the incubation period. Paralysis may be more severe or localized in a traumatized area, for example following irritating vaccine injection ('provocation poliomyelitis') or recent tonsillectomy, which may provoke severe bulbar paralysis. Paralysis classically presents as follows.

Spinal form

Muscles innervated by spinal nerves are affected by paralysis, often preceded by diminution or loss of deep reflexes a few hours before weakness is detectable. Paralysis is more widespread in early stages because many temporarily injured anterior horn cells may recover function. Some muscle groups usually escape serious damage and slow functional recovery can progress over many weeks or months. Most commonly affected, in order of frequency, are:

in the lower limb
- quadriceps
- tibialis anterior
- peroneal muscle

in the upper limb
- deltoid
- biceps
- triceps

in the trunk
- abdominal muscles
- back
- intercostals
- diaphragm.

Respiratory paralysis can cause life-threatening impairment of ventilation, commonly associated with involvement of shoulder muscles.

Bulbar form

This most severe and dangerous form of poliomyelitis results from damage in the brain-stem, particularly the medulla. Any case of poliomyelitis with unusually rapid and stormy onset and development, drowsiness or marked apprehension should be watched for signs of medullary involvement, which may progress rapidly to death despite therapy. The main patterns are as follows.

1. Cranial nerve nuclei involved:
   (a) IIIrd to VIIth nerve nuclei, with good prognosis and recovery usual;
   (b) IXth to XIIth nerve nuclei, with difficulties in swallowing and clearing the pharynx, where pooled saliva and mucus can obstruct airways or be inhaled. Airway clearance and maintenance of ventilation are essential to preserve life.
2. Respiratory centre impaired: irregularities of rate and rhythm of breathing may lead to respiratory failure and sudden collapse.
3. Circulatory centre impaired: hypertension or peripheral circulatory failure can occur, sometimes with hyperpyrexia.

Multiple neurological signs may coincide with hypoxia and hypercapnia from ventilatory dysfunction, and death with acute myocarditis. Encephalitic forms of poliomyelitis are often combined with bulbar or bulbospinal features.

In preparalytic and paralytic stages the cerebrospinal fluid is usually clear, rarely hazy, with increased cells (10–500/mm^3), predominantly lymphocytic. The cell count is maximal in the preparalytic stage, when polymorphs transiently predominate. A raised protein level persists for some time after the cell count has reverted to normal, an example of 'albumino-cytological dissociation' to be distinguished from the Guillain–Barré syndrome.

AETIOLOGY

The most common cause of the paralytic poliomyelitis syndrome is a poliovirus:

- type 1 causes the major epidemics and outbreaks before vaccination has been instituted;
- type 3 tends to predominate among any cases occurring after general vaccination;
- Type 2, the least neurovirulent both as 'wild' and attenuated vaccine virus, tends to establish itself in the gut more efficiently than types 1 and 3.

A few sporadic cases of similar paralytic disease are caused by other enteroviruses, mainly of the coxsackie groups, with paralysis usually milder and recovery more rapid, with encephalitic features sometimes more prominent. Coxsackie A7 virus caused outbreaks of meningitis, paralysis, and some deaths mainly in children in Kazakhstan and Scotland but has not established itself as a serious threat. Enterovirus 71 also caused large outbreaks in children in Eastern Europe, with paralytic, bulbar, and fatal cases. In order to monitor such occurrences and distinguish possible failures of poliovaccination control programmes, in addition to notification at least a sample of cases should be investigated virologically using all available techniques and recording epidemiological details including vaccination history and contact with recently vaccinated persons. Where poliomyelitis is usually absent and vaccine coverage is good, every paralytic case should be thus investigated.

Aseptic meningitis (benign lymphocytic meningitis; viral meningitis)

Enteroviruses are the most common cause of this benign infective form of meningitis, which outnumbers bacterial meningitis except during epidemics of meningococcal disease. Outside the epidemic season for enteroviruses, arboviruses are important where they are endemic. The general pattern of cases in different enteroviral epidemics varies according to the virus concerned.

This, either in meningitis cases or in associated non-meningeal cases, may cause rash (especially echovirus 9) and myalgia (especially coxsackievirus B). Most infections involve children but the age distribution differs from outbreak to outbreak, with higher proportions in older and adult groups for those viruses (e.g. echovirus types 4, 30) that recur in epidemics at longer intervals.

The onset is usually sudden but may be preceded by brief prodromal illness. Fever, headache, stiff neck, and often nausea, vomiting, sore throat, myalgia or photophobia develop, subsiding usually with a few days to a week, with complete recovery the rule. Transient, mild encephalitic features or paresis may rarely be noted, and there may be extraneural manifestations such as maculopapular eruptions, especially in infants.

The main clinical feature is nuchal stiffness with fever and often faucial redness. The cerebrospinal fluid is clear or cloudy with lymphocytic pleocytosis up to 500/mm^3, though higher counts with polymorph preponderance may be found in the earliest stages, especially in echovirus 9 infections. Protein levels are moderately increased but sugar levels are normal.

Differental diagnosis is important to distinguish other and treatable causes of meningeal irritation including tuberculosis and other types of bacterial meningitis. Virus isolation should be attempted with cerebrospinal fluid and faeces. Paired sera should be checked for an antibody response to identify mumps, leptospirosis, and other infections. Bacteriological tests, including culture, should be made.

Encephalitis

Encephalitis or ataxia, with or without sequelae, is a rare complication seen mainly in generalized neonatal coxsackieviral disease. It is usually associated with other features (e.g. meningoencephalitis; polioencephalitis). Coxsackieviruses are mainly involved, and encephalitis was a marked feature of the enterovirus 71 epidemics. Cases are also seen during epidemics of paralytic poliomyelitis. The clinical pattern is not specific and laboratory investigation is required to identify the enteroviral aetiology by isolating virus from faeces, cerebrospinal fluid or brain, and testing paired sera for antibody responses.

Myalgic encephalitis ('ME'); postviral fatigue syndrome (see also Chapter 7.19.4)

Outbreaks of this debilitating illness have been reported from many parts of the world during the past 50 years. In most outbreaks, women were more often affected than men, with curious susceptibility in nursing staff. The wide variety of symptoms always includes severe muscle fatigue after even slight exertion, muscle pain, and psychological upset. The lack of objective physical signs makes it easy to dismiss the illness as hysterical. Recovery may take months or years and relapses are common during periods of physical or mental stress. No specific treatment is available, only rest and symptomatic relief.

Viral aetiology has been postulated but not proven. Recent studies of well-characterized cases suggest association with Coxsackie B infection in some patients. By the more sensitive techniques now available, virus-specific IgM has been found in some of them; long-term (over a year) faecal excretion of the same virus serotype has been shown and enterovirus-specific RNA sequences in muscle biopsies reported. Active research continues.

The heart and muscles

Coxsackieviruses show myotropic properties both in experimentally infected newborn mice and in man, affecting both skeletal and cardiac muscles. A few echoviruses can rarely do the same, and myocarditis has been reported in fatal poliovirus infections. In addition to sporadic cases, incidence rises during epidemics of, for example, coxsackievirus B5 infection, when many patients may manifest Bornholm disease (epidemic myalgia) and/or acute myopericarditis.

Acute myocarditis and pericarditis

The term 'myopericarditis' is sometimes used because probably neither myocarditis nor pericarditis of enteroviral origin occur in pure form. However, usually the illness is mainly myocarditic (especially in young children) or pericarditic (especially in older children and adults). Severe pancarditis can complicate generalized infections of the newborn (see below) with tachycardia, heart enlargement, and progressive congestive failure with liver swelling, sometimes arrhythmias, or heart block. Mortality in these infants is high but recovery appears complete in those who survive the first weeks of stormy illness. Cardiac effects of enteroviruses are shown in Table 5.

CARDITIS IN EARLY CHILDHOOD

Prodromal fever and throat congestion may precede the major illness. Weakness, dyspnoea, precordial pain, tachycardia with or without irregularities, feeble pulse, and sometimes heart block are typical. Radiographic examination may show cardiomegaly. Electrocardiographic examination shows signs of myocarditis, usually without pericarditis unless in later childhood. Death from heart failure may occur in the acute stage or after months of persisting failure, but most children recover fully after a few weeks of serious illness.

Pericarditis can predominate in later childhood, typically with fever and precordial pain similar to Bornholm disease, with which it may be associated. Dyspnoea and heart failure may become severe from cardiac tamponade by pericardial effusion. Constrictive pericarditis can be a late complication.

CARDITIS IN OLDER CHILDREN AND ADULTS

Acute pericarditis is the most common presentation. There may be prodromal fever and upper respiratory symptoms. Often onset is rapid, with precordial pain, palpitations, dyspnoea, and feelings of weakness and oppression. Bornholm disease may coexist. The pericarditis is detectable by electrocardiographic examination and sometimes by clinical signs of friction. Pericardial effusion is often demonstrable radiographically. Recovery is usually good after a few weeks of illness, but a few patients suffer recurrent pericarditis with renewed effusions at intervals of a few months for several years. Constrictive pericarditis is a rare late sequel.

Table 5 *Effects of enteroviruses on the heart*

1. Nil
2. Transient ECG changes only
3. Myopericarditis
(a) Acute (< 1% fatal)
(b) Acute with recovery, complete or with residual ECG changes
(c) Relapsing, with recovery or with chronic sequelae: dilated cardiomyopathy, constrictive pericarditis, endocarditis
(d) Persisting myopericarditis

Acute myocarditis may also be heralded by fever and perhaps myalgia. Illness can be severe, with dyspnoea, congestive failure, tachycardia, arrhythmias, and sometimes heart block, often with associated pericarditis. Electrocardiographic changes and sometimes enzyme abnormalities reflect the myocarditis, which may be difficult to distinguish from myocardial infarcation. Stormy, febrile illness may last several weeks or months. Recovery may be complicated by relapses or persisting illness. Mortality is less than 1 per cent but death may occur either in the acute stage or later.

VIROLOGICAL DIAGNOSIS

Virological tests are useful, especially for differential diagnosis of acute cases in young adults with no previous cardiac illness or signs of vascular disease. Faeces should be collected for virus isolation as early as possible in the illness; a throat swab in viral transport medium may also yield virus if taken during the first few days of febrile illness. Pericardial fluid may also be a source of virus. Because virus excretion has often ceased by the time the patient comes to attention, paired acute and convalescent sera should be taken for tests for antibodies to group B coxsackieviruses (serological tests for the numerous other enteroviruses are impracticable unless the type has already been identified by virus isolation).

Using nucleic acid hybridization techniques, replicating enteroviral RNA has been found in myocardial biopsies from patients with myocarditis but not in controls. In another study, all those with active or healing myocarditis who showed significant levels of coxsackievirus B IgM antibody also had detectable enteroviral RNA in biopsy tissue. The importance of group A coxsackieviruses is probably underestimated because of present difficulties in isolating them in, or preparing specific antigens from, newborn mice; also, echoviruses are implicated in some cases, especially in young children.

Chronic cardiac disease

Recurrent and constrictive pericarditis have been referred to above. Congestive cardiomyopathy of adults is often associated with unusually high titres of antibody to group B coxsackieviruses, inflammatory cells in the myocardium, and defective cellular immunity. This suggests that a minority of patients with this immune defect may be predisposed to develop congestive cardiomyopathy from infection that has no such effect in most persons. There are conflicting reports of a possible relation of these infections to non-streptococcal 'rheumatic' heart disease. Immunofluorescence tests were reported to show coxsackieviral antigens in diseased endocardium and heart valves, and there are suggestions of viral damage to the aorta and coronary vessels, though a relation to myocardial infarction has not been satisfactorily confirmed.

Nucleic acid hybridization techniques revealed enterovirus-infected cells in 7 of 39 patients with chronic dilated cardiomyopathy, including 4 of 19 with heart transplants; 30 with myocardial disease inconsistent with viral aetiology were negative. Autoimmunity also contributes to enteroviral heart disease.

Myositis: Bornholm disease

Bornholm disease (epidemic myalgia; epidemic pleurodynia; 'devil's grip') is named after a classical description of an early epidemic on the Danish island of Bornholm. Sporadic cases can also occur as well as those during epidemics, usually of coxsackievirus B but sometimes of group A, or rarely echovirus (especially type 6) infection. Mostly children but often young adults are affected, and infection may involve any age. Illness usually begins suddenly with severe abdominal or thoracic chest pain, usually fever and headache, and sometimes sore throat. In children, pain is commonly abdominal, often periumbilical or right sided suggesting appendicitis, with superficial muscle tenderness but not usually nausea or vomiting. In adults and older children, pain is more often thoracic, substernal, or localized on either side, often with local intercostal tenderness and sometimes transient pleuritic friction. This often suggests pneumonia, acute pneumothorax or cardiac infarction. Definite pericarditis or myopericarditis may complicate the disease; orchitis or aseptic meningitis are less frequent complications. Association of myalgia with myocarditis is close and a high proportion of patients with myalgia during acute viral infections have been reported to show electrocardiographic changes. There is usually improvement to full recovery in a week or so but relapses sometimes occur.

For virological diagnosis, faeces should be taken for virus isolation, also paired sera for tests for the corresponding antibody.

Gastrointestinal tract and associated organs

Diarrhoea

One might expect that viruses which infect the gut would cause diarrhoea, but there is no clear evidence that enteroviruses do so. Occasional reports of the isolation of an enterovirus from stools of infants or children involved in an outbreak of diarrhoea may merely reflect high prevalence of enteric viral infections in children with illness due to another cause, or undetected agent in circulation, the diarrhoea then helping to disseminate any infectious agents present in the faeces. The extent of damage by enteroviruses to the rapidly replaced cells of the gastrointestinal mucosa is probably not sufficient to disturb normal alimentary function.

Hepatitis

Apart from hepatitis A (type 72), other enteroviruses may be isolated during outbreaks of hepatitis, but as in diarrhoea they probably represent mere 'epidemiological passengers', not causal agents. In generalized infections of the newborn, usually with coxsackieviruses, severe and necrotic hepatitis is common (see below).

Pancreatitis

Acute pancreatitis is a rare manifestation of infection with coxsackieviruses, mainly of type B4. Coxsackie B3 and B4 antibodies have been reported as more prevalent in cases of recent acute pancreatitis than in controls, and raised serum and/or urine amylase levels suggesting pancreatic damage were reported in about a quarter of cases in coxsackievirus B5 and A9 outbreaks. Although rarely recognized as a complication of enteroviral infections in man, pancreatitis is a characteristic effect of group B coxsackieviruses in experimentally infected mice.

DIABETES MELLITUS

Reports of an excess prevalence of coxsackieviral antibodies suggest that insulin-dependent diabetes mellitus can be a late consequence of infection, particularly with type B4 coxsackievirus. Persons with certain HLA serotypes (DR3 in males; DR4 in females) are particularly predisposed to develop insulin-dependent diabetes, and damage to B cells by coxsackievirus B infection may precipitate onset of frank diabetes in such persons. The causal role of coxsackie B viruses may be clarified by application of immunological and viral probe techniques to histopathological studies of the pancreas of recent-onset cases of insulin-dependent diabetes mellitus.

Acute conjunctivitis

The ability of some enteroviruses to cause eye infections was hardly realized until the sudden pandemic of acute haemorrhagic conjunctivitis in several countries of Africa and south-east Asia in 1969. Infection spread to many other countries in the next few years but failed at that time to establish itself in northern Europe, Australia, New Zealand, or the Americas. From 1970, epidemics of a similar disease due to a different enterovirus were reported from Singapore and Hong Kong. 'Picornavirus epidemic conjunctivitis' has been proposed as a term for both these diseases, distinguishing them from epidemic keratoconjunctivitis due to adenoviruses.

Acute haemorrhagic conjunctivitis

This term was applied to the pandemic disease from which a previously unknown enterovirus, type 70, was isolated and shown to be the cause. There were explosive outbreaks in densely populated areas. Spread of the highly contagious infection within families was common, transmitted mainly by contaminated fingers and fomites, and it spread within eye clinics. Onset is sudden after an incubation period of about 24 h. A gritty, painful, lachrymating eye becomes red and inflamed, with acute subconjunctival haemorrhage complicating the severe, blinding conjunctivitis. Both eyes are usually affected. Despite severe, incapacitating acute illness, complete recovery is usual within a week or two. Neurological complications, mainly lumbar radiculomyelopathy, were reported. Enterovirus 70 can be isolated with difficulty from conjunctival swabs or scrapings, or rising antibody titres in paired acute and convalescent phase sera may provide the diagnosis.

Epidemic conjunctivitis due to coxsackievirus A24

This has been mainly reported from the Far East, sometimes concurrently with enterovirus 70 epidemics. The acute conjunctivitis tends to be less severe than enterovirus 70 disease, subconjunctival haemorrhage is unusual, and the prognosis is good. Neurological complications have not been reported. The virus spreads like enterovirus 70 by eye–hand–fomite routes, and can be isolated from the eye or throat.

Infections of the unborn and newborn child

Viraemic enterovirus infections in pregnancy may reach the fetus, but significant developmental defects rarely ensue. Serological studies in the United States showed somewhat more evidence of coxsackievirus B infections in infants with congenital heart disease than in comparison groups, and in mothers of infants with cardiovascular abnormalities.

Perinatal and neonatal disease

The effects of intrauterine infection range from a silent process without obvious disease to severe, generalized infection usually due to a group B coxsackievirus and affecting particularly the liver, nervous system and heart, often fatally. Maternity and neonatal units are vulnerable to outbreaks after introduction of infection by a patient, visitor, or member of staff whose symptoms have often been minor or inapparent. Several such outbreaks with deaths were caused by echovirus 11 in Britain. Features of severe enterovirus infection can be difficult to differentiate clinically from bacterial sepsis, but viral aetiology is suggested when birth was not associated with trauma or other factors known to predispose to bacterial infection, when bacteriological tests are negative, when birth took place during a community or hospital outbreak of enterovirus infection, or when the mother has a history of febrile illness within a week before the birth.

Usual presenting features are fever and gastrointestinal disturbances (feeding difficulty, abdominal distension, vomiting, diarrhoea), often with lethargy or irritability and occasionally convulsions. Hepatomegaly may be accompanied by jaundice. A maculopapular skin rash often appears after a few days; petechial rash with thrombocytopenia carries a poor prognosis. Disseminated intravascular coagulation and haemorrhages may occur. The throat is often red, and tachycardia and tachypnoea may suggest cardiac involvement. Other effects include meningitis or meningoencephalitis, mild or severe respiratory infection including interstitial pneumonitis, carditis, hepatitis, pancreatitis, focal adrenal cortical necrosis, and renal medullary haemorrhage, which has been reported particularly in type 11 echovirus infections.

Leucocytosis with polymorph preponderance is common, resembling bacterial infection. The cerebrospinal fluid often shows pleocytosis and virus may be isolated from it, even though clinical signs of meningitis are often absent. Thrombocytopenia and elevations of liver enzymes may be found.

Prematurity, low birth weight, and onset of illness within the first week of life are factors that increase the risk of the most severe forms of disease. Later in infancy, meningitis and acute carditis are the major presentations of enterovirus infections, which more often produce only minor febrile or respiratory illness or may be inapparent.

Other diseases due to enteroviruses

Orchitis

Bornholm disease is occasionally complicated by acute orchitis, from which testicular biopsy has yielded coxsackievirus B5.

Renal disease

The occasional reports of infection with several types of enterovirus in cases of acute renal failure, mainly in children, probably represent rare effects of enteroviruses.

Parotitis

Reported in coxsackievirus B3 infections, this also is probably a rare complication.

Control of enterovirus infections

Personal prophylaxis

Specific vaccines are available for poliovirus and hepatitis A infections but are impracticable for the numerous other enteroviruses. The only general measure to minimize risk of infection is adoption of high standards of personal hygiene, avoidance of consumption of faecally polluted food or drink unless adequately cooked, boiled or chlorinated, and avoiding contagion from likely excretors such as young and sick children.

Poliomyelitis vaccination

Poliomyelitis is preventable, but despite the availability of effective vaccines since the early 1960s it is estimated that at least 116 000 cases of

Table 6 *Characteristics of current poliomyelitis vaccines*

Characteristics	Live, attenuated vaccine (OPV)	Enhanced, inactivated vaccine (eIPV)
Seed virus source	Attenuated (Sabin strains)	Virulent strains
Cell substrate	Human diploid cells	Monkey kidney or human diploid cells
Administration route	Oral	Injection
Primary course	Three doses at monthly intervals starting age 2 months (plus preliminary dose at birth in endemic areas)	Two doses at 2-month intervals
Immunity produced		
(a) systemic	IgA,IgM,IgG	IgM,IgG,(IgA)
(b) local	IgA	Minimal
Booster doses required	At school entry and between ages 15 to 19 years; also in adult life if exposed to risk when last dose 10 years or more ago	Yes
Reliability of effect	Good in temperate climates; variable in tropics	Good if antigenicity satisfactory
Spread to contacts	Yes	No
Vaccine-associated paralysis	1.5–2/million first doses	No (unless faulty inactivation process)
Cost (in 1992)	0.07$	0.7$
Personnel	Need not be highly trained	Trained and skilled
Combination with other vaccines	No	Possible
Use in immune deficiency	Contraindicated	Acceptable

poliomyelitis occurred worldwide during 1991 (the World Health Organization estimates that under 15 per cent of cases are reported). Global eradication of poliomyelitis and elimination of indigenous transmission of wild polioviruses by the year 2000 is now an objective of the World Health Organization through its Expanded Programme on Immunization (**EPI**).

Two effective vaccines are in current use: live, attenuated, oral poliovaccine (**OPV**) developed by Sabin, and enhanced-potency, inactivated poliovaccine (**eIPV**) developed and refined by Salk. Their characteristics, advantages, and disadvantages are listed in Table 6. Both vaccines contain all three viral serotypes. Although eIPV has achieved successful control in several European countries, OPV is the generally recommended vaccine especially for poorly immunized communities.

LIVE, ATTENTUATED, ORAL VACCINE

The preference for OPV is based on cost, ease of administration, superior production of intestinal immunity, and ability to infect contacts and so extend vaccine coverage. Because progeny virus excreted by vaccinees tends to revert slightly towards higher virulence, it can very rarely cause paralytic disease in non-immune contacts; it is therefore advisable to give vaccine at the same time to the parents of a child being vaccinated if their immune status is doubtful. The very rare cases of paralysis in recipients of vaccine are not necessarily due to the vaccine, and all such cases should be reported and fully investigated. In countries where poliomyelitis is endemic, OPV should be given at birth and at 6, 10, and 14 weeks of age; supplemental measures such as use of national or local immunization days, outbreak control, and identification of groups at high risk or underserved may be required. Although rates of seroconversion by three or more doses of OPV have been good in developed countries, results in developing countries have been suboptimal. Recent epidemics in several such countries despite high vaccine coverage have heightened concern about vaccine immunogenicity and efficacy. Possible factors related to failure of vaccine to protect include imbalance of serotypes in the vaccine formulation, failure to maintain the 'cold chain' in transit from supplier to point of use, intercurrent enteric pathogens, diarrhoea, breast feeding, and seasonality. Current EPI studies aim to determine improved formulations of OPV and to investigate the number of doses and optimal intervals between these. In developed countries, additional doses of oral vaccine are advisable at school entry and later (Table 6) to ensure immunity to all three serotypes.

ENHANCED-POTENCY, INACTIVATED VACCINE

This is more immunogenic than the original 'Salk vaccine' and can provide protection after only two injections, though boosters in later life are advisable. Despite cost, eIPV has the advantage of carrying no risk of causing paralysis (important in countries where poliomyelitis has been eliminated) and can be combined with other inactive vaccines (e.g. diphtheria, pertussis, and tetanus). Its role in eradicating poliomyelitis merits further investigation, especially in countries where transmission of 'wild' poliovirus has been interrupted. However, its current cost prohibits its use in developing countries, and it may not eliminate spread of 'wild' polioviruses as it does not stimulate intestinal immunity as effectively as oral vaccine.

Combined (sequential) administration of OPV and eIPV may have a future role, mucosal immunity induced by OPV being complemented by the strong antibody response to eIPV. As global eradication comes closer, eIPV alone could provide immune defence while residual poliovirus in the environment is sought.

Community preventive measures

GENERAL MEASURES

Appropriate hygiene and sanitation reduce faecal pollution and the spread of enteric infections and provide water supplies unpolluted or adequately purified. Enteroviruses survive many of the sewage treatments devised to reduce or eliminate pathogenic bacteria. Increase of human populations with limited water supplies necessitates recycling and reuse of water contaminated by faecal effluents upstream. Waterborne transmission may then allow enteroviruses to cause outbreaks or sporadic infections.

IMMUNIZATION POLICY

Apart from hepatitis A, this concerns only poliomyelitis. The immediate target is to achieve at least 80 per cent coverage of children in all countries by poliovaccine. Choice of vaccine depends on local circumstances and national policies. Combinations of OPV and eIPV, used successfully in some countries (e.g. Denmark), are being considered in the United States, but such complex schedules pose logistic problems in most developing countries. In tropical countries with limited resources, OPV can be given by 'pulse vaccination', on the same day to as many children as possible in the community. This strategy has succeeded dramatically in the Americas, reducing poliomyelitis from 1 case/100 000 in 1975 to less than 0.05/100 000 by the end of 1992, with simultaneous decline in detection of 'wild' poliovirus.

Special efforts may be needed to identify and offer vaccine to highly susceptible groups such as those that have not accepted vaccination through ignorance or prejudice. Antibody surveys help to identify such groups and to direct the control programme generally.

If a traveller's immune status is unknown or in doubt, OPV should be given at least 2 weeks before departure to an area where poliomyelitis is endemic. Similarly, those travelling to areas with poor hygiene and sanitation with high risk of hepatitis A can be protected either passively for up to 6 months by injecting hepatitis A immune globulin or by two injections of hepatitis A vaccine; a third dose of vaccine protects for up to 10 years.

Outbreak control

Because silent infections outnumber those with meningitis or paralysis, poliovirus spreads more widely than the distribution of clinical cases suggests. Live oral vaccine (trivalent or monotypic of the same type as the epidemic strain) can be given to known and secondary contacts, and even to whole communities, with priority to young children, in order to inhibit the epidemic virus by interference as well as by immunization. Faecal samples for virus isolation should be taken from representative cases and also from others in the community before they receive vaccine; if possible, blood samples should also be collected to study the prevaccination immune status of the population.

Surveillance

Poliomyelitis is one of the diseases under surveillance by the World Health Organization. National administrations should report outbreaks. Within countries, cases of paralytic poliomyelitis should be notified on clinical criteria. Where possible these cases should be investigated virologically using both stool culture and serology. In some developing countries where poliomyelitis is significantly under-reported, lameness surveys of crippling sequelae may provide an alternative measure of the impact of poliomyelitis.

It is important to investigate virologically any case of paralysis in a recent recipient or contact of poliomyelitis vaccine so as to distinguish those whose illness has a cause other than vaccine and to give early warning of defective vaccine (which rigorous testing before release makes highly improbable).

As mentioned above, antibodies can guide the most effective and economic use of vaccine. Ongoing serological surveillance gives a check on the continued effectiveness of the vaccination programme once control of the disease has rendered surveillance by notifying clinically recognizable cases ineffective. In a developed country it should not be necessary to wait for the appearance of cases to signal inadequate herd immunity!

REFERENCES

Behan, P.O. and Behan, W.M.H. (1988). The postviral fatigue syndrome. *CRC Critical Reviews in Neurology*, **4,** 157–78.

Fegan, K.G., Behan, P.O., and Bell, E.J. (1983). Myalgic encephalomyelitis—report of an epidemic. *Journal of Royal College of General Practitioners*, **33,** 335–7.

Grist, N.R., Bell, E.J., and Assaad, F. (1978). Enteroviruses in human disease. In *Progress in medical virology*, Vol. 24 (ed. J.L. Melnick), pp. 114–57. Karger, Basel.

Lemon, S.M. and Robertson, S.E. (1991). Global eradication of poliomyelitis: recent progress, future prospects, and new research priorities. In *Progress in medical virology*, Vol. 38 (ed. J.L. Melnick), pp. 42–55. Karger, Basel.

Minor, P.D. and Bell, E.J. (1990). Picornaviridae (excluding Rhinovirus). In *Topley and Wilson's principles of bacteriology, virology and immunity*, (9th edn) (ed. M.T. Parker and L.H. Collier) *4: Virology*, pp. 323–57. Arnold, London.

7.10.14 Viruses in diarrhoea and vomiting

C. R. MADELEY

Introduction

Viruses are now well established as causes of diarrhoea and probably account for nearly half the episodes in infants and young children, particularly in the poorer, overcrowded parts of the world. However, it is only since the early 1970s that individual viruses have been identified as probable causes. Before then, several studies, based on attempts to culture from stools, failed to identify any viruses with sufficient frequency to incriminate them. A variety were isolated, including serotypes of enteroviruses, reoviruses, and adenoviruses. From time to time echoviruses or adenoviruses were recovered from outbreaks of diarrhoea and/or vomiting and the presence of a single serotype pointed to a common source. Unfortunately the serotypes concerned (for example echovirus type 11 and adenovirus type 7) were not uncommon and were more commonly not associated with gastrointestinal upsets.

Nevertheless, the patterns of spread suggested that viruses were involved but a new technique for identifying them would be needed.

Fig. 1 Some of the viruses associated with diarrhoea as seen by electron microscopy directly on stool extracts: (a) rotavirus, (b) astrovirus, (c) calicivirus, (d) small round structured virus (SRSV). The SRSVs are very similar in appearance (and may be identical) to the Norwalk group of viruses. The adenoviruses of type 40 and 41 are identical with other serotypes whose appearance is well known. The viruses are shown by negative contrast with uranyl acetate (a) or potassium phosphotungstate (b–d) and at a magnification of 200 000 ×.

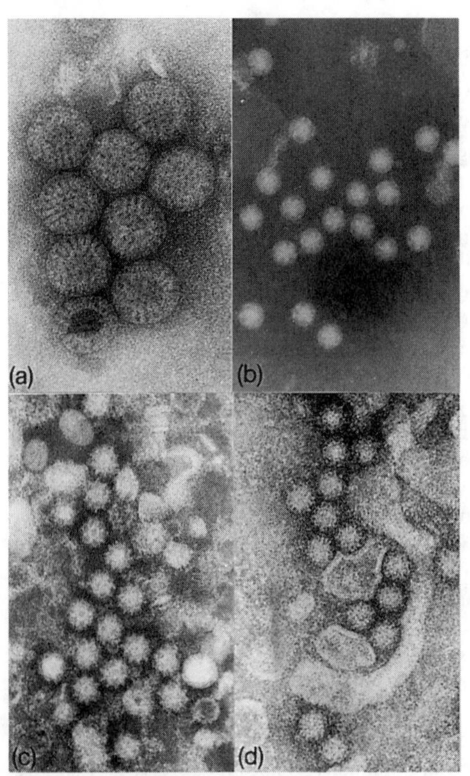

Table 1 *Summary of stool viruses*

Virus	Number of human serotypes	Found in stool of normal babies	Animal species with similar viruses	Approximate size (nm)	Infection of adult volunteers	Antibody prevalence in general population (%)
Norwalk and SRSVs	Probably multiple	NR[a]	NR	35	Diarrhoea	0–60
Rotavirus	9	Yes	Many species Diarrhoea caused	60–75	Minimal infection: little or no diarrhoea	80–100
Adenovirus	2 (40, 41)	Yes	Many species[b]	75	NR	Variable—up to 100
Astrovirus	5	Yes	Several species; diarrhoea caused	28	Minimal infection; little or no diarrhoea	60–80
Calicivirus	5	Yes	Few species; diarrhoea may be caused	33–35	NR	60–80
SRVs[c]	?	Yes	?	22–30	NR	NR
Coronavirus	?	Yes (adults)	Few species; diarrhoea caused	Pleomorphic, > 100	NR	NR
Reovirus	3	Yes	Many species; no diarrhoea caused	70–75	NR	NR

[a]NR, not reported; [b] reported widely but association with diarrhoea uncommon; [c]a heterogeneous group of, probably, several viruses.

This was provided by electron microscopy applied directly to stool extracts. Almost immediately two novel viruses were discovered—Norwalk virus by immune electron microscopy (using convalescent-phase sera to react with stool extracts obtained from a school outbreak) in the United States in 1970, and rotavirus in thin sections cut from duodenal biopsies taken from infants in Australia in 1973. It was soon found that rotavirus could be observed directly in extracts of faeces using the simple negative-contrast technique, and a search for these and other viruses began whenever virologists could find an adequate electron microscope (EM) (Fig. 1).

The list of different new viruses has gradually lengthened and the search has been helped by the finding of similar viruses in the faeces of domestic animals with diarrhoea, as in the case of rotaviruses.

The list of hitherto unknown viruses discovered by electron microscopy since 1977 now includes, as well as Norwalk and rotavirus: adenovirus; astrovirus, calicivirus, coronavirus, and a variety of small, spherical particles that may be seen under the microscope as featureless spheres (small round viruses) or as having an ill-defined, 'hairy' surface (small round structured viruses). Further attempts to grow these viruses have confirmed their reluctance to replicate in the routine cell cultures used for enteroviruses, reoviruses, and adenoviruses. Surprisingly, the adenoviruses seen by electron microscopy frequently do not grow in cell culture, though adenoviruses may be cultured from electron-microscopically negative stools. This paradox is discussed further below. The list of the viruses identified by electron microscopy may still be incomplete but no new candidates have been reported for several years.

Finally, typical lollipop-shaped bacteriophages are frequently observed in human faeces, sometimes in very large numbers, and some of the small round viruses may also be bacteriophages. Neither the host bacteria nor the significance of finding them are known.

Disease associated with stool viruses

Viruses have been found in babies' and young children's stools of any consistency between 'normal' stools and severe watery diarrhoea with vomiting. With considerable variations in the severity of the disease associated with each of the viruses, it is not possible to define exactly the syndrome caused by each. There is also evidence that some types of rotavirus are less or more virulent than others—the so-called avirulent nursery strains and those causing adult outbreaks.

Where disease is associated, it takes the form of a loose or watery diarrhoea of abrupt onset, frequently but not invariably preceded or accompanied by vomiting. It is normally self-limiting, with a peak incidence between 12 and 18 months of age and with both sexes equally affected. Occasionally, in temperate climates, and more frequently in tropical ones, babies may become more severely ill, with increasing dehydration leading to circulatory collapse and death. There may be a rise in body temperature but this is not invariable and may reflect the amount of tissue damage in the gut, although there is no direct evidence for this. Early descriptions of rotavirus infections included reports of a mild respiratory involvement but babies frequently have respiratory secretions and rotaviruses have never so far been recovered from the nasopharynx. The detection methods available are, however, not very sensitive and it seems unlikely that faecal–oral spread can account for all the epidemiological evidence. Other gut-infecting viruses such as enteroviruses may be recovered from throat swabs and a respiratory infection with or without overt signs may therefore occur.

Viruses involved

Rotavirus

This is a comparatively large virus (see Table 1) with a characteristic structure that can be recognized readily by electron microscopy. It has been found to be endemic in every country in which it has been sought and is one of the most common viruses in man. Moreover, strains have been found to infect virtually every animal species in which they have been sought, both domestic and wild. In faeces, the number of rotavirus particles is often very large and the ease with which rotavirus can be recognized has focused considerable attention on it, possibly with some neglect of viruses that are smaller and more difficult to recognize.

Rotavirus has been found much more frequently in the stools of children with diarrhoea than in non-diarrhoeal stools and was originally observed in the epithelial cells of duodenal biopsies taken from children recovering from diarrhoea. The human virus, like animal strains, causes diarrhoea in gnotobiotic newborn animals, a very artificial system. Rotaviruses very commonly cause infections in animal species, most of them producing significant disease only in the very young. Adult human volunteers may be infected and excrete virus but few show evidence of disease. Most, however, already possess serum antibody and this may prevent overt disease, although the mechanism is not clear.

There is thus good evidence for pathogenicity but three additional observations suggest that the story is not quite so simple. Firstly, there are several reports of excretion of rotavirus by normal neonates, particularly at an age when gnotobiotic newborn animals are very susceptible; excretion has been reported in both breast- and bottle-fed babies, although the bottle-fed were more likely to have diarrhoea. Secondly, a small-scale community follow-up study showed that excretion by normal neonates may also be found at home. This finding has also been indirectly confirmed by the third observation. Several serological surveys have found that between 80 and 100 per cent of the population over the age of 3 years have antibody to rotavirus. The techniques used in these surveys included complement fixation, which normally detects only short-term antibodies detectable for up to a year after the stimulus. This suggests that infection with the virus is widespread and repeated contact with rotaviruses (perhaps by subclinical infection) may be common.

Rotavirus of man and animals can be classified into six groups (A–F) with two subgroups of group A (I and II), which are further subdivided into 9 serotypes. Only rotaviruses of groups A to C have been found in man and only serotypes 1 to 4, 8, and 9 of group A. It is not yet clear whether there are any barriers to spread between man and animals. As with strains of influenza A virus, it does not appear to happen readily.

So far the vast majority of identified human strains have been of group A, with group B mostly found in mainland China. The epidemiological patterns of rotavirus are still being explored and understanding them will be essential to developing a successful vaccine (see below).

Astrovirus

Astroviruses are spherical particles about 28 nm in diameter with a five- or six-pointed surface star visible on about 10 per cent. The virus is smaller and less easily recognized than rotavirus by electron microscopy. It has consequently not been recorded either so frequently or so widely. Whether this reflects a genuinely lower frequency or difficulty in recognizing it among faecal debris is still unclear. In routine diagnosis over several years, astroviruses were observed with about a quarter the frequency of rotaviruses.

The evidence linking it with childhood diarrhoea is both as strong and as weak as that for rotavirus: it is found more commonly in the stools of diarrhoeal patients than in normal people; it can be present in very large numbers; adult volunteers can be infected but do not develop marked symptoms; a serological survey has shown similar high proportions of antibody positives in different age groups throughout life; and morphologically similar viruses have been found in the stools of neonatal animals (lamb, pig, calf) with diarrhoea. It is not uncommon to find both astroviruses and rotaviruses in the same stool but there is no evidence that a baby with a dual infection is made more ill as a result, nor that the two viruses are related.

Calicivirus

Unlike the two preceding viruses, the calicivirus was not a 'new' virus when discovered by electron microscopy. Its morphology was familiar because strains had been recognized in cats, pigs, and sea-lions for some years previously, although no strains had been found infecting man. A human virus was first described in 1976 in preparations of faeces from a group of babies, most of whom had diarrhoea. Subsequently, caliciviruses have been found in association with common-source outbreaks of vomiting and diarrhoea in adults and children; more rarely in the stools of normal babies. There is some evidence that particular serotypes are more likely to be associated with outbreaks but this has to be confirmed. One small serological survey in Japan has shown that the majority of older children and adults possess antibody to this virus.

Other small spherical viruses

When examined by electron microscopy, stools contain a large amount of debris about the size and shape of virus particles. Most can be dismissed as non-viral but a proportion of stools contain spherical objects that look convincingly virus-like, often being present as small or large clusters. They can be divided into two groups morphologically, depending on whether their outer surface is smooth or rough (the SRSVs).

NORWALK AND RELATED SMALL ROUND STRUCTURED VIRUSES (SRSVs)

The Norwalk viruses were originally thought to be parvoviruses coated with antibody. As such they would be DNA-containing viruses about 22 nm in size. They are now known to contain RNA, to be larger (35 nm), and to be SRSVs in appearance, with the surface fuzziness being part of the structure of the virus and not antibody attached to it.

Norwalk was the first SRSV to be described, but similar viruses have now been found in outbreaks in many areas, notably in Hawaii and Montgomery County, Maryland. The Norwalk and Montgomery County viruses have been shown to be related antigenically but Hawaii is probably unrelated. Though morphologically indistinguishable from Norwalk, further antigenic typing has been prevented by difficulty in obtaining sufficient purified virus and by SRSVs' failure to grow in cell cultures. No animal strains have been described.

Serological studies in the United States have shown a different pattern of acquisition of antibody with age compared to rotaviruses, astroviruses, adenoviruses, and caliciviruses. Unlike these, antibody is apparently acquired later, as the majority of the population studied does not have antibody until after the age of 50. This suggests that this is a virus which affects all ages and that a considerable number of infections are silent. Although most observed cases are from outbreaks, SRSVs are sometimes found in the faeces of endemic diarrhoea. They are likely to be under-reported because the virus particles lack a clearly identifiable structure and are present in faeces in comparatively small numbers even at the acute stage. Their appearance in the electron microscope is similar to that of caliciviruses but no unequivocal calicivirus particles have been observed among the Norwalk virus particles.

SMALL ROUND VIRUSES (SRVs)

The smooth particles (SRVs) may vary in size between one stool and another but are consistent within each stool. Some of them may be spherical bacteriophages, others appear similar to enteroviruses, and some have been associated with outbreaks. They are a heterogeneous group whose role in disease is still unclear but have a claim to be considered part of the pattern. Their endemic presence provides the background to outbreaks involving similar particles that have been called W agent, Cockle virus, Ditchling agent, etc. (see Food poisoning below). It should also be noted that astroviruses on which no characteristic surface stars were seen would be called SRVs.

Coronavirus

Until recently, coronaviruses in man have been known only as causes of a proportion of the common cold syndrome, although similar viruses caused diarrhoeal diseases in animals, particularly in pigs and cows. Coronavirus-like particles in stool are similar in general structure to respiratory strains but differ in detailed morphology. They have been observed more often in the stools of adults than children in the United Kingdom, India, and Australia. Prolonged excretion, lasting up to several months, can be detected and this has raised doubts as to whether they are genuine causes of diarrhoea. Virus-like particles with morphological and antigenic similarities to the Breda virus of calves have been described in diarrhoeal faeces. Their identity and significance have yet to be established.

Reovirus

First discovered over 20 years ago, reoviruses are viruses in search of a disease. They belong to the same family (Reoviridae) as rotaviruses, which they resemble closely in appearance. They can be distinguished by careful inspection and there is no doubt that the two viruses are different. There are three human reovirus serotypes and similar viruses have been isolated from animals and plants. They may occasionally be detected in small numbers in stool extracts by electron microscopy but the virus is usually grown without difficulty. There is no good evidence that they cause diarrhoea.

Adenovirus

These have been left to last because they illustrate well the paradoxes in this topic. Adenoviruses have been regularly isolated from stool specimens since the advent of cell cultures, but cultivable strains are rarely implicated in diarrhoea. Such adenoviruses have rarely been isolated from common-source outbreaks, but in these cases it is not clear whether the virus initiated the outbreak or was spread as a consequence of the diarrhoea. Isolates from faeces have been common serotypes (numbers 1, 2, 5, 6, and 7), and it came as a surprise, with the use of electron microscopy on stool extracts, to find that there was a substantial number of apparently typical adenoviruses that did not grow in cell culture. These were often present in very large numbers (up to 10^{11} particles/g of faeces) and were sometimes the only potentially pathogenic microorganism common to a number of cases of diarrhoea. Further investigations confirmed that they did not grow in routine cell cultures but a considerable proportion of these fastidious strains have now been grown in less frequently used cell types, such as Graham 293 cells, which are continuous human embryo kidney cells transformed by the presence of part of an adenovirus type 5 genome. It is now accepted that two hitherto unknown serotypes, 40 and 41, can cause a gastrointestinal upset. Further serotypes (42–47) have now been recovered from the faeces of AIDS patients, several of whom had chronic diarrhoea, but there is no evidence that these higher numbered serotypes are of significance in either endemic or epidemic diarrhoea.

It is paradoxical that the more adenovirus there is in the stool, the less likely it is to grow in cell culture. The reason for this is unknown and it is unlikely to be due to antibody on the virus surface, inhibitors in the stool, or an incomplete form of adenovirus.

The role of adenoviruses in the pathogenesis of gastrointestinal disease is uncertain because prolonged excretion occurs from the gut of children (as well as the nasopharynx). In Sweden, adenoviruses are regarded as gut pathogens second in importance only to rotaviruses because they are found in acute-phase diarrhoeal stools, but the possibility that the child was already excreting adenoviruses should be borne in mind.

Diagnosis

The only method capable of detecting all known types of virus in a stool is electron microscopy and this is essential in the investigation of any outbreak of vomiting or diarrhoea. This technique suffers from the disadvantages of being both insensitive and unsuitable for screening large numbers. Other methods using antibodies have therefore been developed for individual viruses including detection of partial growth in cell culture by immunofluorescence, enzyme immunoassay, and latex agglutination. Commercial kits based on the last two are now available for rotaviruses and, to a lesser extent, adenoviruses. Antibody-based tests for some of the other viruses (Norwalk, astrovirus) have been developed but are not yet available commercially. Whether laboratories could afford to repeat tests for each possible virus is doubtful and many have concentrated on rotaviruses alone. A stool specimen is always necessary for the detection of virus and attempts have been made to find virus in other body fluids and secretions. With the exception of Norwalk agent in vomitus, these attempts have not been successful.

Tests for antibody, including those for the different classes (IgG, IgM and IgA), are available in some laboratories and seroconversion has been demonstrated. Whether this adds to the recognition of virus in the stool is debatable.

It is difficult to interpret the results from one stool or one patient, so it is important to contact the laboratory before deciding to send specimens.

Epidemiology

Viruses found in large numbers in the faeces are likely to be spread by the faecal–oral route, but the acquisition of virus by neonates, including those only a few days old, makes it likely that other routes may also be involved. It is probable that adults, in particular, may spread rotavirus in respiratory droplets, and a large outbreak affecting all ages in a town in Sweden may have been water-borne, although this was not confirmed. The methods available for detecting these viruses are insensitive, and we know too little of the natural ecology of these viruses to draw conclusions about mechanisms of spread.

Preventing spread

As with other transmissible agents, this is a combination of good hygiene and common sense. These faecal viruses may spread even in children's wards divided into cubicles and using barrier precautions; circumstantial evidence suggests that the mechanism may be asymptomatic adult carriers, although this has not been demonstrated. Hand-washing is important and has been shown to limit spread of rotavirus, but the use of alcohol rubs afterwards does not add further protection.

There have been several assessments of the activity of antiviral disinfectants, particularly on rotaviruses. These inevitably use very artificial systems and, because the results were not completely predictable, cannot be reliably extrapolated to other viruses or day-to-day practice. Further, with those that cannot be grown in cell culture (the majority), direct assessment of inactivation is impossible.

It is very unlikely that any virus will withstand strong bleach (hypochlorite) or glutaraldehyde for long but reliance on alcohols and detergents as disinfectants cannot be recommended. Nevertheless, thorough washing of hands and surfaces will both dilute any virus and physically remove most of it.

Food poisoning

A considerable number of outbreaks have been associated with small spherical viruses, both SRVs and SRSVs. Some have been water-borne (for example, at summer camps in the United States) but others have been food-borne. Many have involved raw or partly cooked shellfish. These are filter feeders and accumulate virus from the surrounding water, although they are probably not infected themselves. Contamination by human sewage occurs because the shellfish are grown too close to outfalls or because abnormal weather conditions spread sewage to new areas. Oysters and other shellfish should be checked regularly for risk factors according to government food regulations.

Investigation of outbreaks must be early, because virus excretion is usually very transient, and must involve the use of electron microscopy if the cause is not to be missed.

General conclusions

Gastrointestinal upsets can occur both endemically and epidemically, although this distinction is blurred at the interface. Endemic viral diarrhoea is mostly in children under five, is rarely life-threatening in the temperate, more wealthy regions of the world (Europe, North America, Australasia) but more serious in the tropical, poorer regions. It is mostly due to rotavirus, adenovirus, and astrovirus.

Epidemic viral diarrhoea can affect all ages, is short-lived, and uncomfortable. The common source may be an index case, though good evidence for this is scanty. Much more often the virus is food- or water-borne. Such outbreaks are usually due to SRSVs (including Norwalk-like viruses) or SRVs.

This distinction is a rough guide only; for example, rotaviruses have been recovered from outbreaks and SRSVs from endemic cases.

The position of epidemic winter or summer vomiting is now more uncertain. The recognition of specific gut-associated viruses has meant that fewer epidemics have been noted, perhaps because it is no longer acceptable to assume a viral cause without attempting to prove it. Some common-source outbreaks are likely to be due to Norwalk and related viruses or to caliciviruses. Otherwise no clear associations have emerged so far.

Treatment

There is no specific treatment for virus infections of the gut. Management of resulting diarrhoea depends on restoration of hydration and electrolyte balance, in some cases by the use of oral fluids (solutions of glucose or sucrose plus electrolytes) and intravenous fluids if necessary, as outlined elsewhere (see Chapter 14.2.4).

Prevention

Substantial efforts have been made to develop a vaccine against rotaviruses. These began with a bovine strain used in Finland providing some protection in an area of relatively low challenge. This and other vaccines based on human or monkey strains, or genetically engineered variants and/or combinations of them, have been used experimentally in various parts of the world. All have shown some promise and also deficiencies in practice. The main problems are that: a single 'protective' antigen has not been identified; it seems to be necessary to incorporate locally significant serotypes; and the very young age of infection in highly endemic, overcrowded, and poor regions. Whether components of groups B and C should be included is also undecided. It is still too early to say whether these problems can be overcome but veterinarians faced with significant economic consequences of rotavirus infections in calves have also failed to solve the technical problems so far. Vaccines against the other viruses (including adenoviruses and Norwalk) have not been attempted.

Following experimental work in lambs where protection was obtained, a trial of pooled human gammaglobulin given orally showed that neonates could be protected from disease associated with rotavirus in endemically affected nurseries, although it did not prevent the babies from becoming infected.

REFERENCES

Carter, M.J., Milton, I.D., and Madeley, C.R. (1991). Caliciviruses. *Reviews in Medical Virology*, **1,** 177–86.

Champsaur, H. *et al.* (1984). Rotavirus carriage, asymptomatic infection and disease in the first two years of life. I. Virus shedding. *Journal of Infectious Diseases*, **149,** 667–74.

Cubitt, W.D. *et al.* (1987). Antigenic relationships between human calicivirus and Norwalk virus. *Journal of Infectious Diseases*, **156,** 806–13.

Desselberger, U. (1989). Molecular epidemiology of rotaviruses. In *Viruses and the gut*, (ed. M.J.G. Farthing), pp. 55–64. Smith Kline and French, Welwyn Garden City.

Estes, M.K. and Cohen, J. (1989). Rotavirus gene structure and function. *Microbiological Reviews*, **53,** 410–49.

Flores, J. *et al.* (1986) Conservation of the fourth gene among rotaviruses recovered from asymptomatic newborn infants and its possible role in attenuation. *Journal of Virology*, **60,** 972–9.

Greenberg, H.B. and Kapikian, A.Z. (1978). Detection of Norwalk agent antibody and antigen by solid phase radio-immunoassay and immune adherence haemagglutination assay. *Journal of the American Veterinary Medical Association*, **173,** 620–3.

Hall, G.A. (1987). Comparative pathology of infection by novel diarrhoea viruses. In *Novel diarrhoea viruses*, (ed. G. Bock and J. Whelan), pp. 192–207. Wiley, Chichester.

Hardy, D.B. (1987). Epidemiology of rotaviral infection in adults. *Reviews in Infectious Diseases*, **9,** 461–9.

Madeley, C.R. (1983). Viruses and diarrhoea: problems of proving causation. In *Medical virology 2*, (ed. L.M. de la Maza and E.M. Peterson), pp. 81–104. Elsevier Biomedical, New York.

Madeley, C.R. (1994). Viruses associated with acute diarrhoeal disease. In *principles and practice of clinical virology*, (3rd edn), (ed. A.J. Zuckerman, J.E. Banatvala, and J.R. Pattison), in press. Wiley, Chichester.

Nakagomi, O. and Nakagomi, T. (1991). Genetic diversity and similarity among mammation rotaviruses in relation to interspecies transmission of rotavirus. *Archives of Virology*, **120,** 43–55.

Parrino, J.A. *et al.* (1977). Clinical immunity in acute gastroenteritis caused by Norwalk agent. *New England Journal of Medicine*, **297,** 86–9.

Rannig, R.F. (ed.) (1994). The Rotaviruses. In *Current Topics in Microbiology and Immunology*, vol. 185, pp. 380. Springer-Verlag, Berlin.

Ward, R.L. *et al.* (1990). Evidence for natural reassortants of human rotaviruses belonging to different genogroups. *Journal of Virology*, **64,** 3219–25.

Willcocks, M.M., Carter, M.J., and Madeley, C.R. (1992). Astroviruses. *Reviews in Medical Virology*, **2,** 97–106.

7.10.15 Rhabdoviruses: rabies and rabies-related viruses

M. J. WARRELL and D. A. WARRELL

Virology

The Rhabdoviridae are a family of more than 100 rod- or bullet-shaped RNA viruses found in vertebrates, insects, and plants (Fig. 1). Two genera infect animals: Vesiculovirus and Lyssavirus. The type species of the genus Vesiculovirus is vesicular stomatitis virus of cattle and horses, which occasionally causes an influenza-like illness in farmers or laboratory workers. The genus Lyssavirus comprises more than 30 viruses, some of which are grouped into six genotypes (Table 1). The type species, rabies viruses, form genotype 1, and the remaining genotypes are antigenically related and morphologically similar rabies-related viruses. Genotype 2, Lagos bat virus, is not known to infect man, unlike genotype 3 (Mokola virus), genotype 4 (Duvenhage virus), and genotypes 5 and 6 (European bat lyssaviruses).

The rabies virion is approximately 180 × 75 nm. Its core is a single negative strand of non-segmented RNA, associated with a nucleoprotein (N), a phosphoprotein (NS), and an RNA polymerase (L) to form a helical ribonucleoprotein complex (RNP). The enveloping membrane consists of inner matrix (M) protein covered by a coat of glycoprotein (G) and host cell-derived lipid. This G molecule bears numerous spikes or knobs, 10 nm long, and its composition determines viral virulence.

The virus is readily inactivated by sunlight, ultraviolet or X-radiation, drying, heating, (especially at pH values outside the range 4 to 10), by most organic lipid solvents including 45 per cent ethanol, soap solution, detergents, proteolytic enzymes (e.g. 0.1 per cent tryspin), and hypochlorite and glutaraldehyde solutions.

Virus isolated from naturally infected animals is known as 'street' virus. Repeated intracerebral passage in rabbits produces 'fixed' virus, with a shortened incubation period, and reduced pathogenicity for other species. This is used for vaccine production. The use of monoclonal antibodies or genetic sequencing techniques allows the identification of strains of rabies and rabies-related viruses (see below). These methods confirm the geographical and vector-related diversity of strains of rabies virus.

RABIES-RELATED VIRUSES KNOWN TO INFECT MAN

Mokola virus, Duvenhage virus and European bat lyssavirus are the three rabies-related viruses that have been proven to infect man (Table 1). Mokola virus (genotype 3), which has been isolated from shrews (*Crocidura* spp.) in Nigeria and Cameroon, and cats, dogs and rodents in Zimbabwe, caused a febrile illness with respiratory-tract symptoms in a child who recovered, and a fatal encephalitis in another. Duvenhage virus (genotype 4) caused a fatal illness, with clinical features identical to furious rabies, in a South African of that name who was bitten by a bat and had then received a full course of rabies vaccine. The rabies fluorescent antibody test was negative in the Duvenhage case and weakly positive in the Mokola cases. The G protein of Mokola virus shows less antigenic homology than Duvenhage with genotype 1 rabies virus. Tissue-culture rabies vaccines have not protected animals against challenge with Mokola virus and their effect against Duvenhage virus is uncertain (see Post-exposure vaccine).

Fig. 1 Rhabdoviruses. Virions of (a) vesicular stomatitis virus; (b) Lagos bat virus; (c) Nigerian horse virus; and (d) rabies virus. (Electron micrographs by courtesy of Mr C. J. Smale and Dr Joan Crick.)

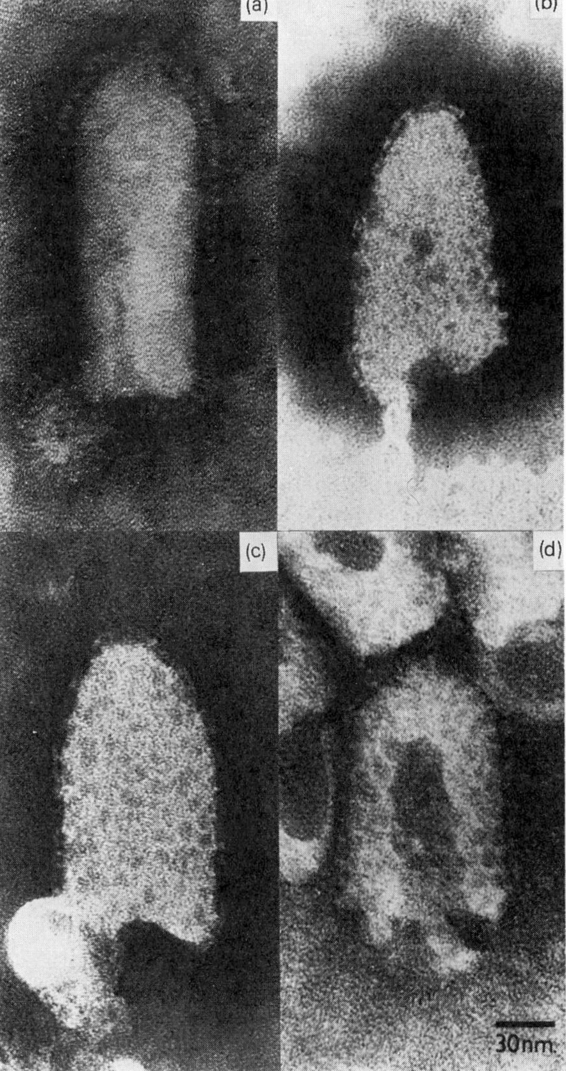

European bat lyssaviruses (genotype 5) have been recognized in the last decade. Rabid bats had been found occasionally in Europe since 1954. In 1985, a woman was bitten by a rabid, *Eptesicus serotinus* insectivorous bat in Denmark, and an extensive search revealed many rabid bats there and in Germany and The Netherlands, a few in Russia, and one or two in Poland, Spain, and France. These viruses are similar to, but antigenically distinct from, Duvenhage virus (genotype 4) and form the European bat lyssavirus (**EBL**) group. Two Russian girls died of rabies following bat bites, and one was definitely an EBL strain. A zoologist in Finland, bitten by a bat from an unknown source, died of furious rabies-like encephalitis. The virus isolated from him could be distinguished from other EBL viruses but was similar to two isolates from Dutch Myotis bats and these form a second biotype of EBL strains (genotype 6).

Epidemiology

Rabies is a zoonosis that remains endemic in most parts of the world (Fig. 2). Currently, the following countries are rabies free: the British Isles, Iceland, mainland Norway, Sweden, Finland, Spain (except Ceuta in North Africa), Portugal, Cyprus and other Mediterranean islands, Australia, New Guinea, Bali, New Zealand, Antarctica, Oceania, peninsular Malaysia, Singapore, Japan, South Korea, Taiwan, Hong Kong islands (but not the New Territories), and Caribbean islands with the notable exceptions of Cuba, the Dominican Republic, Grenada, Haiti, Trinidad and Tobago. Some other countries have no indigenous rabies but infected animals cross land borders.

Primarily an infection of wild mammals, rabies is spread by bites and to a much lesser extent by inhalation of aerosols in bat caves and by ingestion of infected prey. The ecology of rabies virus can be divided into urban and sylvatic phases, which overlap to a varying extent in different countries. The sylvatic phase has different wild-mammal reservoir species in different geographical areas: in the United States, striped skunks (*Mephitis mephitis*) and to a lesser extent spotted skunks (*Spilogale putorius*) in the central States and California; the gray fox (*Urocyon cineroargenteus*) in central areas and red fox (*Vulpes vulpes*) in the east; raccoons in mid-Atlantic and south-east states; and insectivorous bats, especially the Mexican free-tailed bat (*Tadarida brasiliensis mexicana*) in the south-west, the red bat (*Lasiurus borealis*) in the south-east, and the big brown bat (*Eptesicus fuscus*) in the north-east; in the Arctic, the fox *Alopex lagopus*; in Grenada and Puerto Rico mongooses (*Herpestes auropunctatus*); in Trinidad, Mexico, and Central and South America, vampire bats, especially *Desmodus rotundus*; in most of Africa and Asia, wolves, jackals and small carnivores of the families *Mustelidae* and *Viverridae* (e.g. the yellow mongoose *Cynictis penicillata* in South Africa and the palm civet *Paradoxurus hermaphroditus* in Indonesia); and in Europe foxes, wolves, raccoon dogs (*Nyctereutes procyonoides*) and insectivorous bats (e.g. *Eptesicus serotinus*). There are reports of rabies virus being isolated from wild rodents in many countries including the Russian Federation, Germany, Egypt, Nigeria, Thailand and the United States, but the significance of this finding is uncertain.

In a particular area, transmission in the sylvatic phase tends to occur predominantly within a single species. For example, in the United States, rabies in foxes, skunks, and bats exists in separate ecological compartments. Each vector, such as the raccoon, may have a separate virus strain and a distinctive method of transmission. In many parts of Africa and Asia, and in urban areas elsewhere (including Britain and Japan before the disease was eradicated), domestic dogs are the principal reservoir of rabies. The prevalence of rabies among stray dogs in Bangkok is thought to be as high as 3 per cent.

Humans are occasionally infected by wild mammals, but domestic dogs and cats, the principal vectors in the urban phase of rabies, are responsible for more than 90 per cent of human cases worldwide. In

Table 1 *Lyssaviruses that have infected man*

Genotype	Virus	Source	Known geographical area	Human disease
1	Rabies	Mammals, predominantly dog, cat, fox, raccoon, skunk, bat and man	Widespread (see Fig. 2)	Encephalitis with either furious symptoms and hydrophobia or paralytic signs (especially from bat bite)
3	Mokola	Shrews (*Crocidura* spp.)	Nigeria, Cameroon	
		Harsh furred mouse (*Lophuromys sikapusi*)	Central African Republic	
		Cat	South Africa	
		Cat, dog, rodents	Zimbabwe	
		Man	Nigeria	Pharyngitis + recovery; fatal encephalitis (no hydrophobia)
4	Duvenhage	Insectivorous bat	South Africa	
		Human	South Africa	Furious rabies-like encephalitis
		Insectivorous bat (*Nycteris thebaica*)	Zimbabwe	
5	European bat lyssavirus (biotype 1)	Insectivorous bat (predominantly *Eptesicus serotinus* in Western Europe)	Germany, Denmark, Netherlands, Russia, Poland, Spain, France	Two Russian cases resembled furious rabies
6	European bat lyssavirus (biotype 2)	*Myotis dasycneme*	Netherlands	None known
	Finland virus	Human from bat	Unknown	Fatal encephalitis with paralytic and furious signs

Genotype 2, Lagos bat virus, has not been detected in man.

Western Europe, 86 per cent of all isolates of rabies are from foxes, yet about 75 per cent of cases of human exposure result from dog bites, a reflection of the intimate relation between dogs and man. Rabies control programmes can reduce the risk of rabies in domestic animals to such an extent that wild animals, for example, skunks in the United States, become the principal vectors.

The three species of true vampire bats, *Desmodus rotundus*, *Diaemus youngi*, and *Diphylla ecaudata* (*Desmodontinae*), occur from sea level to over 3500 m but usually below 1500 m, only in Mexico, Central and South America, and some Caribbean Islands (Fig. 3). Carnivorous bats of the family Megadermatidae, such as the Indian 'vampire' (*Megaderma lyra*), are usually responsible for the myth that vampires occur outside this area. In Latin America, between 500 000 and 1 000 000 head of cattle are lost each year from vampire bat-transmitted paralytic rabies (derriengue). This entails a financial loss of more than $US 100 million each year. One hundred and seventy-seven humans are known to have died from vampire bat-transmitted rabies since 1980. Non-haematophagous bats have been responsible for a few cases of human rabies in North America, India, a recent case in Finland, and the case of Duvenhage virus infection in South Africa.

Cyclical epizootics of rabies, such as the current fox epizootic in Europe, result from an uncontrolled increase in the population of the key reservoir species. This epizootic started in Poland at the end of the Second World War. Initially it advanced at a rate of about 40 km a year, but recently has slowed considerably. Although the fox is one of the most susceptible species to rabies, about 3 per cent of animals survive the infection and become immune. In the Caribbean island of Grenada, almost half of the mongooses have serum neutralizing antibody against rabies. Seropositive raccoons, bats, and very occasionally dogs have also been found.

INCIDENCE OF HUMAN RABIES

The true incidence of human rabies throughout the world is not reflected in official figures, such as those reported by the World Health Organization, which have always been less than 2000 cases each year. In 1992, in India alone, the estimated mortality was 30 000, and in Bangladesh, it was 2000 (1.8/100 000 population). In the same year in Nepal, 200 deaths (1.1/100 000) and in Sri Lanka, 112 (0.64/100 000) deaths were reported. The true mortalities were probably considerably higher. Unof-

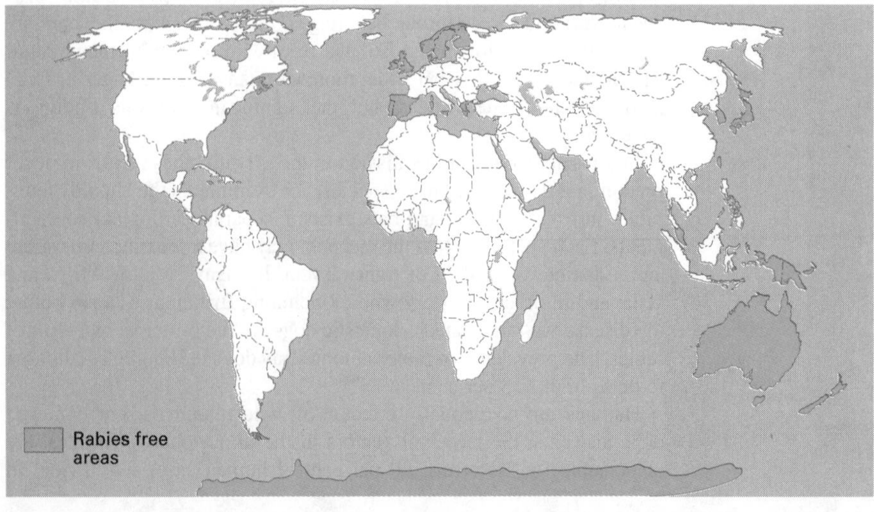

Fig. 2 Global distribution of rabies.

ficial estimates include 6500 in Pakistan and 2000 in North Vietnam. In Cali, Columbia almost 2 per cent of a large series of autopsies showed evidence of rabies. In the United States there were more than 25 human deaths each year in the 1940s, but since 1960 this has decreased to less than 6 per year. Rabies was eradicated from Britain by 1903. The last two patients to develop rabies, after being infected in this country, died in 1902, but there had been 173 deaths in England and Wales in the preceding 15 years. In the last 20 years, 11 people have died of rabies in England. Ten were infected in the Indian subcontinent, and one in Africa. In continental Europe only a few cases are now reported each year.

Transmission

Virus can penetrate broken skin and intact mucosae. Humans are usually infected when virus-laden saliva is inoculated through the skin by the bite of a rabid dog or other mammal (Figs 4 and 5). Dog bites are common in most parts of the world (Chapter 8.4.1). Saliva from a rabid animal can infect if the skin is already broken, by the animal's claws for example. Animals can be infected through the gastrointestinal tract, but there is no evidence that this happens in man, despite a 4 per cent prevalence of rabies in apparently healthy cattle slaughtered in Mexico City.

Inhalation of rabies virus may be an important method of transmission among cave-dwelling bats. In Texas, two men died of rabies after visiting caves inhabited by millions of Mexican free-tailed bats, many of which were rabid. They probably inhaled an aerosol created by the bats' infected nasal secretions. Two laboratory workers in the United States developed rabies after inhaling fixed strains of rabies virus during the preparation of vaccines. The accidental use of vaccine in which the virus was not inactivated has led to fixed virus rabies (*rage de laboratoire*): for example, in Fortaleza, Brazil in 1960, 18 people developed paralytic rabies 4 to 13 days after their first injection of vaccine.

Transmission of rabies from one person to another has been proved only in six patients who received infected corneal grafts. Considering that the saliva, respiratory secretions, tears, and urine of rabies patients contain virus it is surprising that the disease has not been spread to people in close contact with these patients. The cases involving infected

Fig. 3 (a) Distribution of the three species of true vampire bats (*Desmodontinae*). (b) Vampire bat (*Desmodus rotundus*) (By courtesy of the Zoological Society of London.)

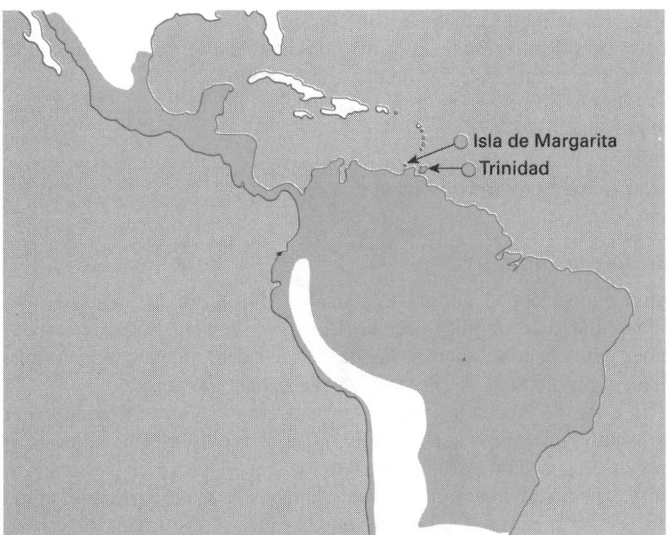

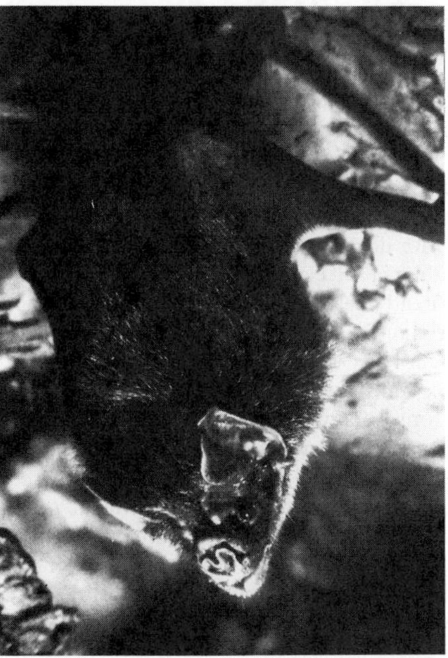

Fig. 4 and 5 Children bitten on the face by rabid dogs. These wounds carry a high risk of rabies with a short incubation period. (Copyright D.A. Warrell.)

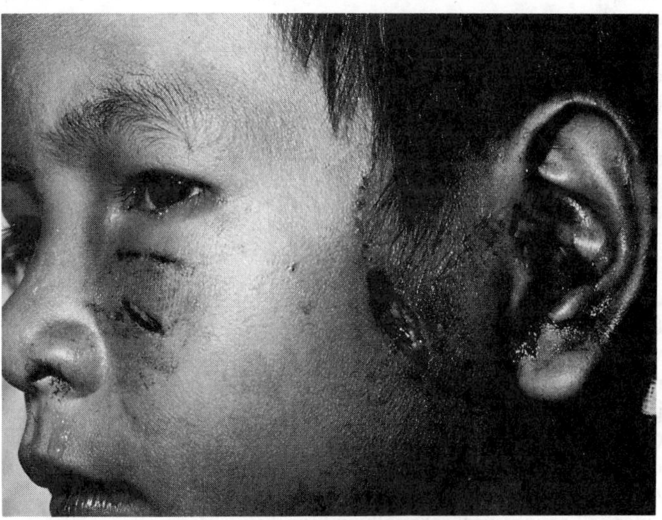

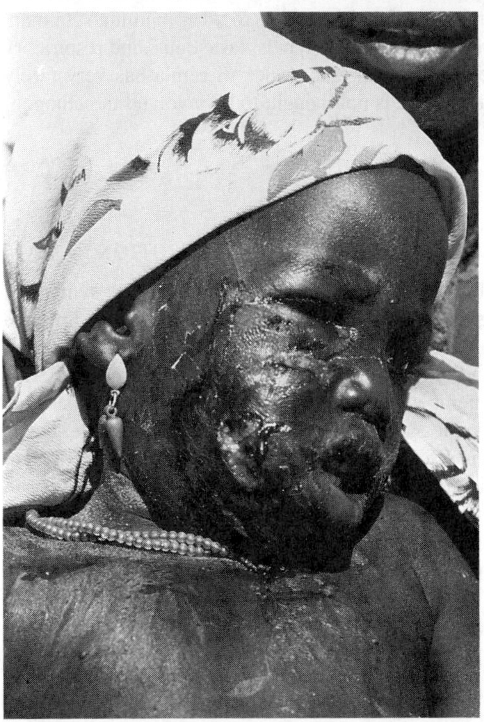

corneal grafts occurred in France, the United States, Iran and Thailand. The three donors had died of undiagnosed neurological diseases, such as Guillain–Barré syndrome and flaccid quadriplegia. Twenty-two to 39 days after transplantation, the recipients noticed retro-orbital headache on the side of the graft and died of rabies. In a seventh recipient, in Morocco, rabies was prevented by vigorous postexposure prophylaxis. Other infections spread by corneal grafts are Creutzfeldt–Jacob disease and cryptococcosis. Clearly, tissues from patients who die of undiagnosed neurological illnesses should not be transplanted.

Transplacental infection has been observed in animals but until recently had not been reported in man. A number of women with rabies encephalitis have been delivered of healthy babies. The transmission of rabies from mother to suckling infant via the breast milk has been suspected in at least one human case and is well known in animals.

Pathogenesis

The mechanism by which the highly neurotropic rabies virus enters the nervous system, travels into the brain and out again to many organs is intriguing. Rabies virus may replicate locally in muscle cells or attach directly to the motor or sensory nerve endings. Its preferential attachment to postsynaptic acetylcholine receptors at motor end-plates is blocked by α-bungarotoxin, whose structure has homologous sequences with rabies glycoprotein. Having gained access to peripheral nerves it travels centripetally within the axoplasm. This progression can be blocked experimentally by local anaesthetics, metabolic inhibitors, and nerve section. No complete virus can be seen in the axons by electron microscopy. A current hypothesis is that the virus travels in an incomplete form, perhaps as naked ribonucleoprotein complexes, at this stage. Rabies virus is experimentally inaccessible to humoral antibodies while inside the peripheral nerve.

On reaching the central nervous system, there is massive viral replication on membranes within neurones and direct transmission of virus from cell to cell occurs across synaptic junctions. Centrifugal spread of virus from the central nervous system in the axoplasm of many efferent nerves, including those of the autonomic nervous system, deposits virus in virtually every tissue. These include skeletal and cardiac muscle, adrenal medulla, where infection may be clinically significant, kidney, retina, cornea, pancreas, and nerve twiglets in the hair follicles (see below). At this stage, productive viral replication occurs, with budding from outer cell membranes, especially in the salivary glands, and is essential for the further transmission of rabies by bites to other mammals. In man, virus is also delivered to the lacrimal glands, taste buds, and respiratory tract. Virus may be shed in milk and urine. Viraemia has very rarely been detected in animals and is not thought to be involved in pathogenesis or spread.

Immunology

IMMUNOLOGICAL RESPONSE TO RABIES INFECTION IN MAN

There is no detectable immune response until encephalitic symptoms develop, suggesting that rabies virus avoids or suppresses the immune system. Neutralizing and other antibodies become detectable in serum after about 7 days and in cerebrospinal fluid a little later. They may rise to high levels in patients whose lives are prolonged by intensive care. A small amount of rabies-specific IgM is sometimes detectable, but is not useful as a means of diagnosis.

There is little evidence of a lymphocyte-mediated immune response to rabies encephalitis. A pleocytosis appears in only 60 per cent of patients, with a mean leucocyte count of 75×10^3/mm. Peripheral-blood lymphocyte transformation has been shown in some patients with furious rabies, but not in those with paralytic disease. Experimentally, in fatal rabies there is suppression of the cytotoxic T-lymphocyte response to unrelated viral antigens and a T-cell response is associated with survival in mice.

Interferon is induced by rabies infection, but appears to be at a very low level in human patients. In animals, latent infections can be reactivated by corticosteroids and stress. This provides a possible explanation for occasional reports of long incubation periods (see below).

IMMUNOLOGICAL RESPONSE TO RABIES VACCINATION

Sensitive assay techniques may detect neutralizing antibody as early as seven days after the start of primary immunization. The surface glycoprotein of the virus is the only molecule capable of inducing neutralizing antibody, which protects against subsequent challenge with rabies virus in animals. The titre of these antibodies shows a better correlation with protection than any other measure of immune response.

Rabies nucleoprotein antigens also stimulate protective immunity in animals, through non-neutralizing antibody, helper T lymphocytes and interferon-γ induction. This protection is effective against a variety of rabies and rabies-related strains, unlike the glycoprotein-mediated immunity.

In human vaccinees, peripheral-blood lymphocyte transformation occurs in response to a variety of rabies and rabies-related virus antigens. The role of helper and cytotoxic T lymphocytes in protection against disease is unclear.

Neutralizing antibody is undoubtedly protective in the early stages after inoculation of virus, but in experimental animals a very low level of rabies antibody accelerates the terminal phase of the encephalitis. This 'early death' phenomenon might be caused by enhancement of viral replication by antibody, as demonstrated *in vitro*.

A low level of interferon may be induced briefly after the first dose of rabies vaccine. In animals, interferon induced by viruses or synthetic inducers, or the administration of exogenous interferon, was effective postexposure prophylaxis against rabies.

Rabies in animals

Any warm-blooded animal (mammal or bird) can be infected with rabies, but susceptibility decreases in the following order: foxes and other wild Canidae, skunks, Felidae, Viverridae, rodents, lagomorphs, man, domestic dogs, herbivores, chickens, and opossums.

In dogs the incubation period ranges from 5 days to 14 months, but is usually between 3 and 12 weeks. The compulsory quarantine of 6 months imposed on dogs imported to the United Kingdom is a compromise. The first symptom, as in many humans, is intense irritation at the site of the infection. Despite the popular idea of the 'mad' rabid dog, only 25 per cent develop furious rabies. There is an early and marked change in behaviour. Clinical features include dysphagia, ptosis, altered bark, paralysis of the jaw, neck and hind limbs (Fig. 6), hypersalivation, congested conjunctivae, pruritus, shivering, trembling, snapping at imaginary objects, pica, and extreme restlessness, causing the animal to wander miles from home. Dogs with furious rabies attack inanimate objects, often seriously injuring their mouths in the process. Virus may be excreted in the saliva 3 days before symptoms appear, and the animal usually dies within the next 7 days. This is the basis for the traditional 10-day observation period for dogs that have bitten humans. There are rare reports, from India, Ethiopia and elsewhere, of chronic excretion of virus in the saliva of apparently healthy dogs. *Oulou fato* is a clinical variant of canine rabies seen in West Africa 50 years ago. It was probably caused by a strain with reduced virulence for man. After a short incubation dogs with *oulou fato* showed progressive paralysis and diarrhoea and some survived for several weeks.

Rabid foxes lose their fear of man and the majority develop the paralytic form of the disease. An extreme degree of furious rabies is seen in 75 per cent of infected cats. Cattle usually develop paralytic symptoms, with dysphagia, hypersalivation, groaning, trembling, colic, diarrhoea, tenesmus, and rectal prolapse. Most other domestic ungulates develop paralytic symptoms. Horses often show furious features with sexual excitement. Most wild animals, like foxes, lose their fear of man and may appear tame. Rabid skunks, raccoons, badgers, martens, and mongooses may become very aggressive. Dysphagia and inability to drink is common in rabid animals, but they do not exhibit hydrophobia.

Clinical features in man

The incubation period ranges from 4 days to many years, but it is between 20 and 90 days in three-quarters of cases. It tends to be shorter after bites on the face (average 35 days) than after those on the limbs (average 52 days). The incubation period is short when infection is transmitted by corneal transplantation (22–39 days), inhalation (approx. 21 days) or by accidental inoculation of live virus (4–13 days).

PRODROMAL SYMPTOMS

In many patients, the first symptom is itching, pain, or paraesthesia at the site of the healed bite wound (Fig. 7). Non-specific prodromal symptoms include fever, chills, malaise, weakness, tiredness, headache, photophobia, myalgia, anxiety, depression, irritability, and symptoms of upper respiratory-tract and gastrointestinal infections. Subsequently, symptoms of either furious or paralytic rabies will develop, depending on whether the spinal cord or brain are predominantly infected.

FURIOUS RABIES

Furious rabies is the more common presentation. Most patients have the diagnostic symptom of hydrophobia: a combination of inspiratory muscle spasm, with or without painful laryngopharyngeal spasm, associated with terror (Fig. 8). Initially provoked by attempts to drink water, this reflex can be excited by a variety of stimuli including a draught of air ('aerophobia'), water splashed on the skin, irritation of the respiratory tract or, ultimately, the sight, sound, or even mention of water. The inspiratory spasm is violent and jerky. The neck and back are extended, the arms thrown up, and the episode may end in generalized convulsions with cardiac or respiratory arrest.

Patients experience hyperaesthesia and at times generalized arousal, during which they become wild, hallucinated, fugitive, and sometimes aggressive, alternating with lucid intervals. Despite these dramatic symptoms, attributable to brain-stem encephalitis, neurological examination may prove surprisingly normal. Reported abnormalities include meningism, cranial-nerve lesions (Fig. 9) (especially III, VI, VII, IX, X, XI, and XII), upper motor-neurone lesions, fasciculation, and involuntary movements. Disturbances of the hypothalamus or autonomic nervous system are reflected by hypersalivation (Fig. 10), lacrimation, sweating, hypertension or hypotension, hyperthermia or hypothermia, inappropriate secretion of antidiuretic hormone, or diabetes insipidus and, rarely, priapism with spontaneous orgasms.

Fig. 6 Dog with paralytic rabies showing paralysis of the hind limbs and hypersalivation. (Copyright D.A. Warrell.)

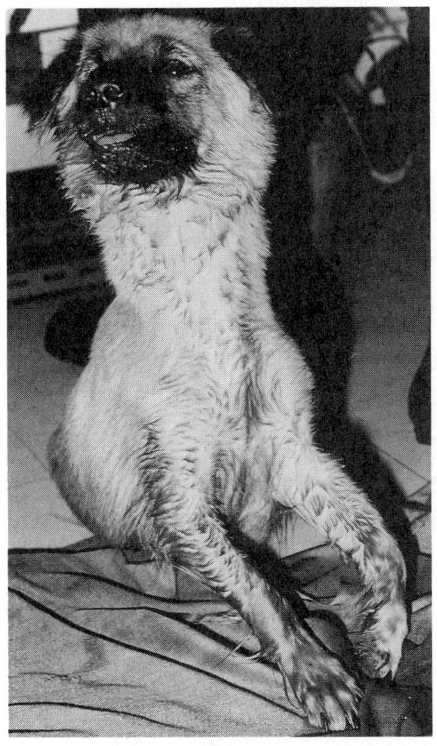

Fig. 7 Excoriation caused by frenzied scratching in a patient who developed intense itching of the left leg 2 months after being bitten on the calf by a mad dog (note pigmented healed bite wounds). She became hydrophobic and died a few days later. (Copyright D.A. Warrell.)

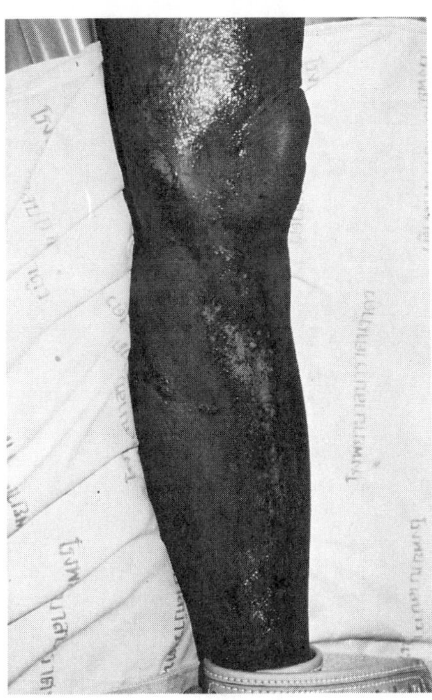

Fig. 8 Hydrophobic spasm in a 14-year-old Nigerian boy with furious rabies. Note the violent contraction of inspiratory muscles: sternomastoids and diaphragm (depressing xiphisternum). (Copyright D.A. Warrell.)

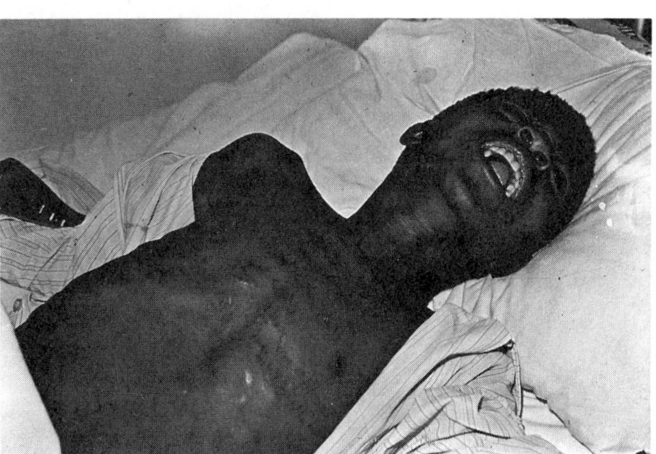

Without supportive treatment, about one-third of the patients will die during a hydrophobic spasm in the first few days. The rest lapse into coma and generalized flaccid paralysis, and rarely survive for more than a week without intensive care.

PARALYTIC OR DUMB RABIES

This is the clinical pattern in less than a fifth of human cases except in the case of vampire bat-transmitted rabies (Fig. 11), which is invariably paralytic. The largest reported outbreak was in Trinidad between 1925 and 1935, when there were 89 human cases; others have been described from Mexico, Guyana, Brazil, Peru, Bolivia and Argentina. The paralytic form of rabies was also seen in patients with postvaccinal rabies, in the two patients who inhaled fixed virus, and in two of the four patients infected by corneal grafts, and is said to be more likely to develop in patients who have received antirabies vaccine. After the usual prodromal symptoms, especially fever, headache and local paraesthesiae, flaccid paralysis develops, usually in the bitten limb, and ascends symmetrically or asymmetrically with pain and fasciculation in the affected muscles and mild sensory disturbances. Paraplegia and sphincter involvement then develop, and finally fatal paralysis of deglutitive and respiratory muscles. Hydrophobia is unusual, but may be represented by a few pharyngeal spasms in the terminal phase of the illness. Even without intensive care, patients with paralytic rabies have survived for up to 30 days. In future, the use of monoclonal antibodies may allow identification of the strains of rabies virus (e.g. fixed virus and isolates from insectivorous and vampire bats) responsible for the paralytic form of rabies.

Fig. 9 Left IIIrd cranial nerve palsy in a Thai patient with rabies encephalitis. (Copyright D.A. Warrell.)

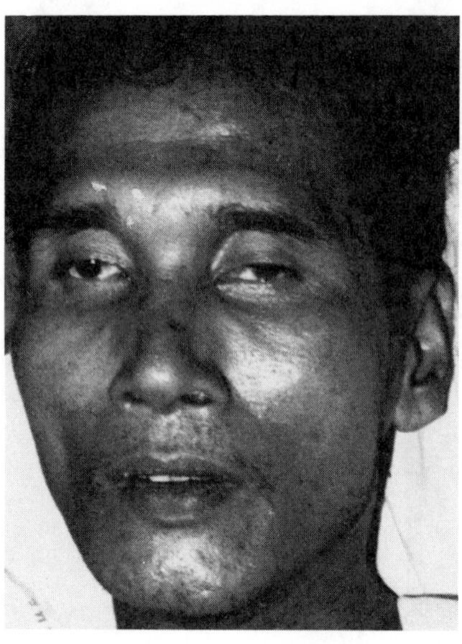

Fig. 10 Hypersalivation, sweating, and haematemesis in a 5-year- old Thai boy with furious rabies. (Copyright D.A. Warrell.)

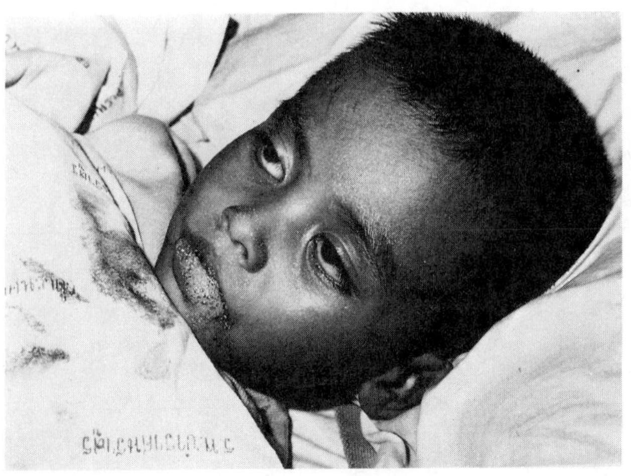

OTHER MANIFESTATIONS AND COMPLICATIONS

Renewed interest in the treatment of rabies encephalitis has led to better understanding of the systemic manifestations and complications of the disease.

Respiratory system

Asphyxiation and respiratory arrest may complicate the hydrophobic spasms or generalized convulsions of furious rabies and the bulbar and respiratory paralysis of dumb rabies. Bronchopneumonia is an expected complication and a primary rabies pneumonitis may occur. Various abnormal patterns of respiration have been described, including cluster and apneustic breathing. There are some similarities to respiratory myoclonus. Pneumothorax may complicate inspiratory spasms.

Cardiovascular system

A variety of dangerous cardiac arrhythmias has been reported, including supraventricular tachycardias, sinus bradycardia, atrioventricular block, and sinus arrest. Hypotension, pulmonary oedema, and congestive cardiac failure are attributable to myocarditis (Fig. 12).

Nervous system

Raised intracranial pressure resulting from cerebral oedema or internal hydrocephalus has been reported in a few cases, but spinal-fluid opening pressure is usually normal and papilloedema rarely found. Evidence of diffuse axonal neuropathy is consistent with histological appearances of degeneration of peripheral nerve ganglia and axons.

Gastrointestinal system

'Stress' ulcers and Mallory–Weiss syndrome are possible explanations for the haematemesis often reported in rabies (Fig. 10).

Fig. 11 Vampire bat bite inflicted on the ear of a sleeping child in Brazil (by courtesy of Dr João Luiz Costa Cardoso, São Paulo).

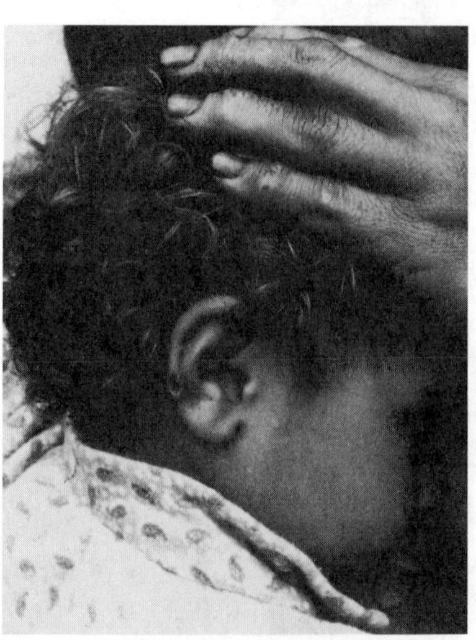

DIFFERENTIAL DIAGNOSIS

Rabies should be suspected whenever a patient develops severe neurological symptoms after being bitten by a mammal in a rabies endemic area. Some patients fail to remember that they have been bitten. Hydrophobia is pathognomonic of rabies and is unlikely to be mimicked accurately by the hysteric. Inspiratory spasms with associated emotional response are produced by asking the patient to swallow accumulated saliva or by directing a draught of air on to their face. Patients are sometimes misreferred to otolaryngologists or psychiatrists.

Tetanus, which can also follow an animal bite, is similar to rabies in some respects, especially the pharyngeal form of cephalic tetanus ('hydrophobic tetanus'). It is distinguished by its shorter incubation period (usually less than 15 days), the presence of trismus, the persistence of muscle rigidity between spasms, the absence of meningoencephalitis (cerebrospinal fluid is universally normal), and a better prognosis. Hydrophobia does not occur in other encephalitides; the combination of intense brain-stem encephalitis and furious behaviour in a conscious patient would be most unlikely except in rabies. Delirium tremens and some plant toxins (e.g. *Datura fastuosa*) and drugs (phenothiazines and amphetamines) may enter the differential diagnosis.

Paralytic rabies can be confused with other causes of ascending (Landry-type) paralysis. Postvaccinal encephalomyelitis (see below) usually develops within 2 weeks of the first dose of the older types of rabies vaccines. In poliomyelitis, objective sensory disturbances are absent and fever rarely persists after paralysis has developed. Examination of cerebrospinal fluid may help to distinguish acute inflammatory polyneuropathy (Guillain–Barré syndrome). *Herpes simiae* (B virus) encephalomyelitis is transmitted by monkey bites, but the incubation period (3–4 days) is usually shorter than in rabies. Vesicles may be found in the monkey's mouth and at the site of the bite. The diagnosis can be confirmed virologically and the patient treated with acyclovir.

Pathology

The brain, spinal cord, and peripheral nerves show ganglion-cell degeneration, perineural and perivascular mononuclear cell infiltration, neuronophagia, and glial nodules. Inflammatory changes are most marked in the midbrain and medulla (Fig. 13) in furious rabies and in the spinal cord in paralytic rabies. The diagnostic Negri bodies (Fig. 14) are eosinophilic, intracytoplasmic inclusions predominantly consisting of masses of viral ribonucleoprotein, with a basophilic inner body, containing fragments of cellular organelles including ribosomes and occasional virions. They can be demonstrated by haematoxylin and eosin or Schleiften's stains in histological sections of grey matter in up to 75 per cent of human cases, especially in hippocampal pyramidal cells and cerebellar Purkinje cells.

In view of the appalling prognosis of rabies encephalitis, neuronolysis is often surprisingly mild and patchy, and death can occur without any inflammatory response. Vascular lesions such as thrombosis and haemorrhage have also been described. The brain-stem, limbic system, and hypothalamus appear to be most severely affected. Outside the nervous system, there is focal degeneration of salivary and lacrimal glands, pancreas, adrenal medulla, and lymph nodes. An interstitial myocarditis, with round-cell infiltration, is found in about 25 per cent of cases (Fig. 12).

Fig. 12 Interstitial myocarditis in a patient with rabies who presented with supraventricular tachycardia. Myocytes show nuclear swelling and focal degeneration of nuclei and fibres with interstitial mixed inflammatory cell infiltration. Haematoxylin and eosin stain (× 400). (Copyright D.A. Warrell.)

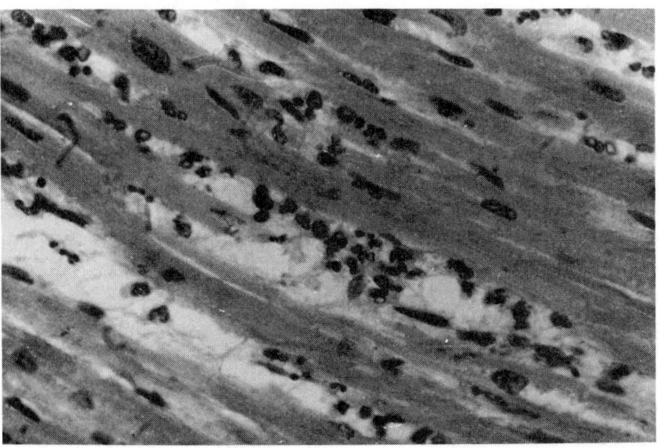

Laboratory diagnosis

A suspect rabid animal that might have infected a patient should be killed and the brain examined without delay. Rabies antigen can be detected within a few hours by a direct immunofluorescent antibody test on acetone-fixed, brain impression smears or using a rapid enzyme immunodiagnosis kit if a fluorescent microscope is not available. Virus

Fig. 13 Inflammatory cells around neurones in the central medulla (paraambigualis region) of a patient who died of rabies encephalitis (× 400). (Reproduced by courtesy of Dr P. Lewis, London.)

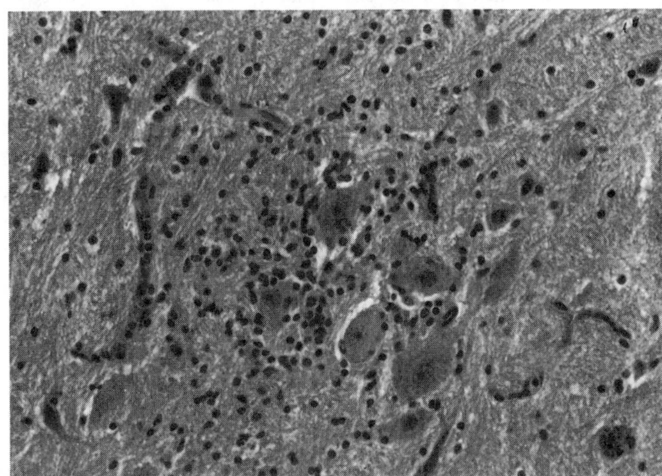

Fig. 14 Street virus in human brain as seen with the light microscope. Many Negri bodies can be seen (one is arrowed). The section is from Ammon's horn of the hippocampus, stained with haematoxylin and eosin (× 1000). (Reproduced by courtesy of Professor P. Atanasiu, Institut Pasteur, Paris.)

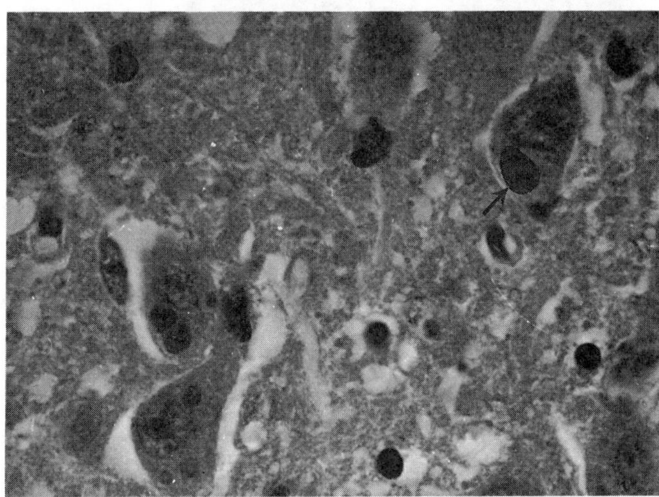

isolation takes up to 3 weeks by intracerebral inoculation of mice, or about 4 days in murine neuroblastoma cell culture.

In man, rabies can be confirmed early in the illness by demonstration of viral antigen by immunofluorescence in nerve twiglets in skin biopsies (Fig. 15). This rapid method is positive in 60 to 100 per cent of cases, and no false-positive results have been reported. Viral antigen can also be detected in brain biopsies or, occasionally, in corneal impression smears, but this last test is usually falsely negative. The use of newer techniques to identify rabies antigen, for example the polymerase chain reaction, are being evaluated.

During the first week of illness virus may be isolated from saliva, brain, cerebrospinal fluid, and rarely urine. Rabies antibodies are not usually detectable in serum or cerebrospinal fluid before the eighth day of illness in unvaccinated patients. Rabies neutralizing antibody may leak into the cerebrospinal fluid in patients with postvaccinal encephalomyelitis, but a very high titre suggests a diagnosis of rabies. A specific IgM test has not proved useful diagnostically.

The cerebrospinal fluid is normal in 40 per cent of patients in the first week of illness; a mild lymphocytic pleocytosis is usual. A peripheral neutrophil leucocytosis is common in the early stages of the disease.

Treatment

Patients with rabies must be sedated heavily and given adequate analgesia to relieve their pain and terror. Rabies was formerly regarded as a universally fatal disease, but there have now been four well-documented cases of recovery. The most recent was a Mexican boy with severe dog bites given post-exposure vaccination. These successes were achieved by intensive care, which is the only known method for prolonging or saving life once rabies encephalomyelitis has developed.

The aim is to prevent complications such as cardiac arrhythmias, cardiac and respiratory failure, raised intracranial pressure, convulsions, fluid and electrolyte disturbances including diabetes insipidus and inappropriate secretion of antidiuretic hormone, and hyperpyrexia. Antiserum, antiviral agents, interferon-α, corticosteroid, and other immunosuppressants have proved useless.

Fig. 15 Diagnosis of human rabies during life. Vertical section through a hair follicle and shaft showing brilliant fluorescence of nerve cells around the follicle indicating the presence of rabies antigen (× 250). (Copyright M.J. Warrell.)

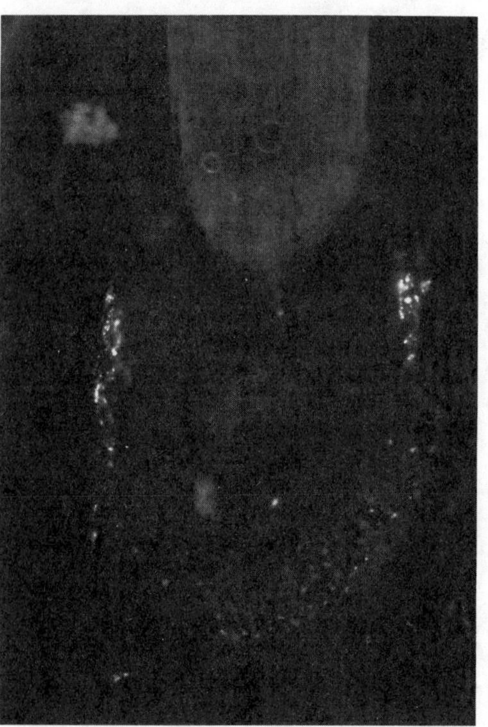

Prognosis

Despite the limited success of intensive care, the prognosis of rabies encephalomyelitis is still virtually hopeless. At the time of the bite, however, before virus has invaded the nervous system, correct cleaning of the wound (see below) and the use of optimum postexposure immunization reduce the risk of rabies developing from about 35 to 67 per cent in untreated cases to near zero. The risk varies with the biting species and the site and severity of the bites. It is highest following head bites by proved rabid wolves, when the mortality in unvaccinated people may exceed 80 per cent.

Prevention and control

IN COUNTRIES WHERE RABIES IS ENDEMIC

Control strategy is based on gathering information about the prevalence and host range of rabies in wild and domestic animals. This requires laboratory facilities for confirming the diagnosis. Domestic animals can be protected by yearly vaccination. Dogs are muzzled and kept off the streets; strays are eliminated. People should be discouraged from keeping wild carnivores, such as skunks, raccoons, coatimundis, and mongooses, as pets. Unnecessary contact with mammals should be avoided (e.g. stroking stray dogs, exploring bat-infested caves). Reduction of wild-animal reservoir populations may be attempted, but this is difficult to achieve and likely to cause ecological chaos. An alternative approach is to attempt the vaccination of key reservoir species by using live oral vaccines distributed in bait. Rabies is most likely to be controlled or eradicated where the principal reservoir is the domestic dog, as in nineteenth century Britain, Malaysia, and Japan.

Humans who are particularly at risk, such as veterinarians and dog catchers, can be given pre-exposure vaccination and those bitten by animals must be given postexposure prophylaxis (see below). Clinics and dispensaries must be adequately supplied with vaccine and antiserum to deal with this problem, but in the developing countries where rabies is most prevalent this may be difficult because of expense, supply, and preservation.

Education and publicity about rabies is always needed. For example, in Bangkok 88 per cent of a series of 328 patients admitted with rabies had not received vaccine, so were possibly ignorant of the risk of dog bite.

IN COUNTRIES WHERE RABIES IS NOT ENDEMIC

Importation of potential vectors, especially domestic dogs and cats and wild bats and carnivores, should be strictly controlled and, where feasible, imported mammals should be vaccinated against rabies and kept in quarantine for an adequate period.

Pre-exposure vaccination is needed only by those who handle imported animals before and during quarantine in kennels, stables, farms, zoos, and laboratories; those who work with rabies virus in laboratories; and those who intend to travel to rabies-endemic areas and will be particularly at risk (e.g. veterinarians, cave explorers, naturalists, and animal collectors).

Postexposure prophylaxis may be required for people who were exposed to the risk of rabies while abroad. Travellers should be educated to seek local medical help if they are bitten, scratched or licked by animals. Action may then be taken to confirm rabies in the animal and postbite prophylaxis can be started promptly, depending on what is known about the local prevalence of rabies.

Many travellers wait until they return to their homeland, sometimes weeks or months after the bite, before asking for medical advice. It is important to determine the precise geographical location of the exposure; when it occurred; its severity—whether it was a bite or lick on broken skin; the nature, appearance, behaviour, and fate of the biting animal, and, if possible, whether it had been vaccined against rabies within the last year. This information may allow proper assessment of risk; but if there is any doubt the patient should be given full postexposure prophylaxis, even if the bite is several months old.

PRE-EXPOSURE IMMUNIZATION REGIMENS

A course of three doses of tissue-culture rabies vaccine is given on days 0, 3, and 28 (or 21) intramuscularly into the deltoid or the anterolateral thigh in children. An economical alternative for human diploid-cell vaccine (**HDCV**) (Pasteur–Mérieux), which was introduced in 1973, and more recent products, purified chick embryo-cell vaccine (**PCEC**) (Behring) and purified vero cell vaccine (Pasteur–Mérieux) is intradermal injections of 0.1 ml of vaccine at the same intervals. To avoid nosocomial viral infection, a sterile needle and syringe must be used for each patient sharing an ampoule. The neutralizing antibody response is so predictable that it need not normally be checked. However, a failure of pre-exposure vaccination following intradermal immunization in Kenya was partly attributed to immunosuppression by chloroquine that was being taken for malaria prophylaxis. In this or other cases of suspected immunosupression, the intramuscular route must be used. Booster doses may be given intramuscularly or intradermally, or the antibody level checked (minimum 0.5 i.u./ml), at intervals depending on the risk of infection. Rabies laboratory staff at continuous risk should be tested every 6 months and those at frequent risk after 2 years. A late booster dose, 6 to 24 months after the primary course, is likely to prolong the duration of antibody to 5 years or more. Unnecessary vaccine treatment should be avoided because of possible hypersensitivity (see below).

POSTEXPOSURE PROPHYLAXIS

The aim is to neutralize inoculated virus before it can enter the nervous system. Wound cleaning and active and passive immunization must be implemented as soon as possible.

Wound cleaning

This is effective in killing virus in superficial wounds and is therefore of great importance, but is often neglected. First aid consists of scrubbing the wound with soap or detergents and water under a running tap for at least 5 min. Foreign material should be removed and the wound rinsed with plain water. A viricidal agent such as 40 to 70 per cent alcohol, povidone iodine, or 0.01 per cent aqueous iodine should be applied liberally. Quarternary ammonium compounds, such as 1 per cent benzalkonium chloride, are inactivated by soap and may become contaminated with pathogens such as *Pseudomonas cepacia* and are no longer recommended. Hospital treatment of wounds involves thorough exploration, debridement, and irrigation of deep wounds with saline, if necessary under local or general anaesthetic (see Chapter 8.4.1). Suturing should be avoided or delayed and the wound should be left without occlusive dressings. Attention should be given to tetanus prophylaxis and the range of bacterial and other pathogens, particularly associated with mammal bites (Table 2). Most of the bacteria are sensitive to amoxicillin/clavulanic acid, cephoxitin, or tetracycline.

Specific prophylaxis

This consists of active and passive immunization. The indications are given in Table 3.

Active immunization

Tissue–culture vaccines

Products such as HDCV, PVRV, and PCEC are now the vaccines of choice for postexposure immunization. The recommended postexposure course of these vaccines is 5×1 ml intramuscular doses on days 0, 3, 7, 14, 30, although for PVRV each dose is only 0.5 ml. An economical regimen of HDCV, which proved effective in a large group of Thai patients bitten by proved rabid dogs, requires eight intradermal injections of 0.1 ml (deltoids, suprascapular, lower-quadrant abdominal wall, and thighs) on day 0, four intradermal injections of 0.1 ml (deltoids and thighs) on day 7, and a single intradermal dose of 0.1 ml on days 28 and 91. This regimen uses only 40 per cent of the volume of vaccine demanded by the conventional course, and has the added advantages of fewer hospital attendances and a very rapid induction of neutralizing antibody.

Side-effects of tissue culture vaccines are mild and transient: local itching, redness or pain at the site of injection, influenza-like symptoms, and occasionally a rash. More serious allergic reactions include rare, type I immediate hypersensitivity during primary courses, and type III immune-complex hypersensitivity. This was reported in 6 per cent of those receiving booster doses of HDCV in the United States and consisted of urticaria, rash, angio-oedema and arthralgia 3 to 13 days after injection, but none has been fatal. A few cases of polyneuritis, Guillain–Barré syndrome or local limb weakness have been reported in patients receiving tissue-culture vaccines. These events are very rare and recovery usually rapid.

Nervous-tissue vaccines

Initially introduced by Pasteur 100 years ago and developed by Semple and Hempt, these are still the most widely used in Africa and Asia. In India, an estimated 3 million people receive postexposure courses of Semple vaccine each year. Doses of 2 or 5 ml of 5 per cent brain suspension are given on 14 or 21 consecutive days, followed by booster doses, the abdomen often being used as a suitable target for these numerous subcutaneous injections. Semple-type vaccines produce neurological reactions, including postvaccinal encephalomyelitis (see below). In Central and South America, suckling mouse brain (Fuenzalida) vaccine is the most widely used, but, despite the relative absence of myelin protein in the immature brains of the young mice used in its production, neuroparalytic reactions still occur.

In Western countries, duck embryo vaccine (**DEV**) replaced nervous-tissue vaccines for about 20 years until the introduction of tissue-culture vaccines. Recently, a new, highly purified DEV has been produced in Switzerland. It is of similar potency and as safe as tissue culture vaccines. It is given by the same regimens.

Neurological reactions to nervous tissue vaccines occur in up to 1 in 220 courses of Semple type, with a 3 per cent mortality, and are an allergic response to myelin and related neural proteins in the vaccine. In Latin America, neuroparalytic reactions complicated 1 : 7865 to 1 : 27 000 courses of suckling mouse brain vaccine with a 22 per cent mortality. Most reactions to Semple vaccine affect the central nervous system, whereas at least 70 per cent of those following suckling mouse brain vaccine involved the peripheral nervous system.

The incubation period ranges from 3 to 35 days after the first injection of vaccine, but in most cases it is between 7 and 14 days. Clinical forms include a rapidly reversible mononeuritis multiplex involving particularly the facial nerve but also the oculomotor, vagus, radial, brachial and sciatic nerves; a dorsolumbar transverse myelitis with fever, paralysis and sensory loss in the lower limbs, with sphincter involvement, loss of tendon reflexes, extensor plantar responses and severe girdle and thoracic pain; an ascending paralysis (Landry type), which ends in fatal bulbar paralysis in a third of cases; and meningoencephalitic and meningoencephalomyelitic reactions. The overall mortality of these reactions is 15 to 20 per cent. Most survivors make a complete recovery in 2 to 3 weeks, but a few are left with permanent neurological sequelae.

A moderate lymphocyte pleocytosis and elevated cerebrospinal-fluid protein is usual. Pathological changes consist of swelling and chromatolysis of neurones with extensive perivascular demyelination and lymphocytic infiltration in the spinal cord. These features resemble experimental allergic encephalitis, postvaccinal encephalomyelitis of

Table 2 *Some infections associated with bites by humans, dogs, and other mammals*

Organism	Particular mammalian species	Cross-reference (chapter)
Viruses		
Rhabdoviruses		
Herpes simiae (B virus) etc.	Monkey	7.10.5
Lymphocytic choriomeningitis and other Arenaviruses	Rodent	7.10.22
Orf	Sheep	7.10.9
Cowpox	Cat	7.10.8
Bacteria		
Aeromonas hydrophila	(Leech)	8.4.1
Acinetobacter spp.		
Actinomyces spp.		7.11.27
Actinobacillus lignieresii	Horse	7.11.46
A. equuli, A. suis,		7.11.46
A. actinomycetemcomitans		7.11.46
Arachnia propionica	Human	7.11.46
Bacillus spp.		7.11.10
Bacteroides spp. (and other anaerobes)		7.11.19
Brucella canis	Dog	7.11.46
Capnocytophaga canimorsus (DF-2)	Dog	7.11.46
C. cynodegmi (DF-2 like)	Dog	7.11.46
Cat-scratch disease bacillus	Cat	7.11.40
Chromobacterium spp.		
Clostridium tetani		7.11.20
Corynebacterium spp.		7.11.1
EF-4	Dog	7.11.46
Eikenella corrodens (HB-1)	Human	7.11.46
Erysipelothrix indiosa		7.11.46
E. rhusiopathiae		7.11.46
Enterobacter cloacae		7.11.46
Escherichia coli		7.11.7
Eubacterium plantii	Dog	
Francisella tularensis	Rodent, cat	7.11.17(a)
Fusobacterium spp.		7.11.10
Haemophilus aphrophilus (HB-2)	Dog, human	7.11.46
Klebsiella spp.		7.11.7
Leptospira spp.	Rodent, dog, cattle	7.11.32
Leptotrichia buccalis		7.11.46
M-5	Dog	7.11.46
Micrococcus spp.		7.11.46
Moraxella spp.	Human	7.11.46
Mycobacterium leprae	? vampire bat	7.11.25
M. marinum	Dolphin	7.11.24
Neisseria canis	Cat	7.11.46
Pasteurella multocida (septica)	Dog, cat, lion, tiger, rodent, Tasmanian devil	7.11.17(b)
P. pneumotropica	Dog, cat	7.11.17(b)
P. stomatis		7.11.17(b)
Peptostreptococcus		7.11.7
Propionibacterium		7.11.7
Proteus mirabilis		7.11.7
Pseudomonas fluorescens		7.11.7
Simonsiella	Dog	7.11.7
Spirillum minor	Rodent	7.11.29
Staphylococcus aureus		7.11.4
S. epidermidis		7.11.4
S. intermedius		7.11.4
Streptobacillus moniliformis	Rodent	7.11.29
Streptococcus α, β, γ		7.11.2
Veillonella parvula		7.11.46
Weeksella zoohelcum	Dog	7.11.46
Yersinia enterocolitica	Pig, dog	7.11.17(c)
IIj, IIr	Dog	7.11.46
Fungi		
Blastomyces dermatitidis	Dog	7.12.1
Sporotrichosis	Rodent	7.12.1

Table 3 *Specific postexposure prophylaxis for use in a rabies endemic area*[1] *following contact with a domestic or wild rabies vector species, whether or not the animal is available for observation or diagnostic tests*

	Treatment
Minor exposure (including licks of broken skin, scratches, or abrasions without bleeding)	• Start vaccine immediately • Stop treatment if animal remains healthy for 10 days • Stop treatment if animal's brain proves negative for rabies by appropriate laboratory tests
Major exposure (including licks of mucosa, minor bites on arms, trunk or legs, or major bites—multiple or on face, head, fingers, or neck)	• Immediate rabies immune globulin and vaccine • Stop treatment if domestic cat or dog remains healthy for 10 days • Stop treatment if animal's brain proves negative for rabies by appropriate laboratory tests

[1]This scheme is a simplification of the recommendations of the WHO Expert Committee on Rabies (1992).

smallpox, postinfectious encephalomyelitis, and acute multiple sclerosis. Corticosteroids, for example, prednisolone 40 to 60 mg/day, are thought to be helpful, and the use of cyclophosphamide has been suggested. Vaccination should be stopped as soon as symptoms appear and the course continued with a tissue-culture vaccine.

Passive immunization

Rabies immune globulin (**RIG**) has proved valuable in protection, presumably by neutralizing rabies virus during the first week after initial vaccination, before neutralizing antibody has appeared, and it enhances the T-lymphocyte response to vaccine experimentally. Its use is recommended at the start of all primary postexposure courses of rabies vaccine, but it is vital following severe bites (on the head, neck, hands, and multiple or deep bites).

The dose of the original equine RIG is 40 i.u./kg body weight. Hypersensitivity reactions occur in 1 to 6 per cent of those treated, but these are not reliably predicted by a previous intradermal test. Human rabies immune globulin (**HRIG**) may also be available. The dose is 20 i.u./kg body weight. Serum sickness has not been reported after HRIG treatment.

The RIG is infiltrated into the tissues around the bite wound, and any remaining is injected intramuscularly into the thigh, not the buttock. If RIG is given hours or days before the first dose of vaccine, the immune response will be impaired. RIG is prohibitively expensive and is not available or affordable to 99 per cent of Africans and 95 per cent of Thai patients receiving postexposure treatment.

Postexposure prophylaxis in people who have received previous vaccination

If a complete pre- or postexposure course of a modern potent tissue-culture vaccine has been given, or if the neutralizing antibody level has been over 0.5 i.u./ml, only two doses of tissue-culture vaccine should be given on days 0 and 3, with a third dose on day 7 for severe bites. Passive immunization is not required. Otherwise, full postexposure treatment must be given.

Failures of postexposure prophylaxis

Deaths from rabies have occured despite vaccine treatment. These may be attributable to the use of low-potency nervous-tissue vaccines, delay in starting vaccination, an incomplete vaccine course, omission of passive immunization, failure to infiltrate RIG around the wound, injection of vaccine into the buttock, or decreased immune responsiveness of the vaccinee. So far, in the few cases in which the virus strain could be typed with monoclonal antibodies, tissue-culture vaccine failures could not be attributed to failure of neutralization of the particular infecting strain of virus by antibody induced by the vaccine. However, it is probable that vaccine-induced immunity would not neutralize the rabies-related Mokola virus and that it would be less efficent against European bat lyssaviruses than against genotype 1 street rabies viruses.

A reduced or delayed immune response to vaccine can sometimes be predicted. If treatment is started late (e.g. more than 2 days after exposure), no RIG is available for severe bites, the patient is immunocompromised, or a rabies-related virus infection is suspected, the immune stimulus can be enhanced either by doubling the initial dose of vaccine, or by dividing the first dose of tissue culture vaccine between eight sites intradermally, as for the economical HDCV regimen (see above).

REFERENCES

Advisory Committee on Immunization Practices (1991). Rabies prevention—United States. 1991. *Morbidity and Mortality Weekly Report*, **40,** RR-3, 1–19.

Baer, G.M. (ed.) (1991). *The natural history of rabies*, (2nd edn). CRC Press, Boca Raton, FA.

Baer, G.M., Bridbord, K., Hui, F.-W., Shope, R.E., and Wunner, W.H. (1988). Research towards rabies prevention. *Reviews of Infectious Diseases*, **10** (suppl. 4), S1–815.

Bourhy, H., Kissi, B. and Tordo, N. (1993). Molecular diversity of the *Lyssavirus* genus. *Virology,* **194,** 70–81.

Campbell, J.B., and Charlton, K.M. (ed.) (1988). *Rabies*. Kluwer Academic, Boston.

Kaplan, C., Turner, G.S., and Warrell D.A. (1986). *Rabies, the facts*, (2nd edn). Oxford University Press.

King, A.A., and Turner G.S. (1993) Rabies: a review. *Journal of Comparative Pathology*, **108,** 1–39.

Kuwert, E. *et al.* (ed.) (1985). *Rabies in the tropics*. Springer Verlag, Berlin.

Helmick, C.G., Tauxe, R.V., and Vernon, A.A. (1987). Is there a risk to contacts of patients with rabies? *Reviews of Infectious Diseases*, **9,** 511–18.

Rupprecht, C.E., Dietzschold, B. and Koprowski, H. (eds) (1994). *Lyssaviruses,* Springer-Verlag, Berlin.

Thomson, G., and King A. (eds) (1993). Rabies in southern and eastern Africa. *Onderstepoort Journal of Veterinary Research,* **60** (4), 263–512.

Tsiang, H. (1993). Pathophysiology of rabies virus infection of the nervous system. *Advances in Virus Research*, **42,** 375–412.

Warrell, D.A. *et al.* (1976). Pathophysiologic studies in human rabies. *American Journal of Medicine*, **60,** 180–90.

Warrell, M.J. and Warrell D.A. (1995). Rhabdovirus infections of man. In *Handbook of infectious diseases*, Vol. 3 Exotic viral infections. (eds. J.S. Porterfield & D.A.J. Tyrrell). 1995. Chapman & Hall, London, (in press).

Warrell, M.J. *et al* (1985). Economical multiple-site intradermal immunisation with human diploid-cell-strain vaccine is effective for post-exposure rabies prophylaxis. *Lancet*, **i,** 1059–62.

World Health Organization (1992). *WHO expert committee on rabies eighth report*, Technical Report Series No. 824. WHO, Geneva. (The revised recommendations for postexposure immunization will be published by WHO in 1996.)

7.10.16 Colorado tick fever and other arthropod-borne reoviruses

M. J. WARRELL and D. A. WARRELL

The large family of Reoviridae includes the vertebrate-specific viruses: reoviruses types 1 to 3 and rotaviruses. Five arthropod-borne reoviruses are known to infect man:

• Colorado tick fever	genus *Coltivirus* (previously *Orbivirus)*
• Kemerovo	genus *Orbivirus*
• Changuinola	genus *Orbivirus*
• Orungo	unclassified
• Lebombo	unclassified.

Colorado tick fever

The reovirus responsible for Colorado tick fever or 'mountain fever' is an 80-nm, double-shelled particle, covered with capsomeres. The icosahedral core contains 12 segments of double-stranded, negative-sense RNA. Colorado tick fever virus produces a cytopathic effect on several cell lines, but culture in suckling mice is more sensitive for diagnostic isolation. The virus has the unique ability to infect human erythrocytes.

Colorado tick fever is a zoonosis involving hard (ixodid) ticks (principally *Dermacentor andersoni*, but also *D. occidentalis*, *D. variabilis*, *D. parumapertus*, *D. albipictus*, etc.) and wild mammals including porcupines, coyotes, squirrels, chipmunks, deer, mice and other rodents. Ticks pass Colorado tick fever virus trans-stadially, but not transovarially.

EPIDEMIOLOGY

Colorado tick fever is acquired from tick bites in western and northwestern parts of the United States (including California), British Columbia, and Alberta. Very rarely, it has been caused by an infected blood transfusion. Several hundred cases are reported each year in the United States, but the true incidence is thought to be at least 10 times higher than that. Hikers, campers, and other people invading the wild rodent and tick-infested terrain are at special risk; for example, among shepherds, the prevalence of antibody to Colorado tick fever was 32 per cent. The highest incidence is from May to July when ticks are most active. Infection usually confers lasting immunity.

CLINICAL FEATURES

In adults, the infection is nearly always mild, but in children it is occasionally severe or even fatal. Three to six days after the tick bite (extreme range, 1–19 days) there is a sudden fever associated with rigors, generalized aches, myalgia, headache, and backache. In half the bitten patients there is a remission of fever, followed by recrudescence ('saddleback' fever). A maculopapular or petechial rash appears in about 10 per cent of cases and gastrointestinal symptoms in 20 per cent. The illness usually resolves in about 10 to 14 days, but convalescence may be prolonged. Severe manifestations result from infection of the central nervous system, haemostatic abnormalities, and direct or immunological effects on other organs and tissues. Meningism and drowsiness, sometimes associated with gastrointestinal symptoms, are seen in patients who develop aseptic meningitis or encephalitis. Spontaneous bleeding, thrombocytopenia, and disseminated intravascular coagulation have been described in severe or fatal cases. Late, possibly immunological effects, include myocarditis, pericarditis, pleurisy, arthritis, and epididymitis. In pregnant women, Colorado tick fever may precipitate abortion but the transplacental infection and teratogenic effects reported in mice have not been observed in man.

LABORATORY FINDINGS

These include leucopenia with relative lymphocytosis, occasional thrombocytopenia, and mild lymphocyte pleocytosis.

DIAGNOSIS

Viral antigen may be detected in erythrocytes by immunofluorescence 1 to 120 days after the start of symptoms. Erythrocytes are infected in the marrow; their survival is apparently not affected. The virus is cultured in suckling mice by intracerebral injection of ground blood clot, or preferably washed erythrocytes. An indirect fluorescent antibody test can provide early serodiagnosis. Neutralizing antibody and specific IgM enzyme immunoassays become positive after 14 to 21 days and the IgM disappears after 45 days.

DIFFERENTIAL DIAGNOSIS

Many other tick-borne acute febrile illnesses, some with rashes and nervous-system involvement, can be acquired in the endemic area for Colorado tick fever. These include Rocky Mountain spotted fever, tularaemia, Lyme disease, and relapsing fever. Rocky Mountain spotted fever is now much less common than Colorado tick fever in Colorado. The rashes are different in the two diseases and the remission/recrudescence is not seen in Rocky Mountain fever. Tick paralysis caused by *D. andersoni* and other ixodid ticks presents as a poliomyelitis-like, ascending, flaccid paralysis that is unlikely to be mistaken for the meningitic or encephalitic syndromes of Colorado tick fever.

TREATMENT

The symptomatic treatment of fever and pain should exclude salicylates in case of thrombocytopenia. Tribavirin (ribavirin) inhibits the replication of Colorado tick fever virus experimentally but its use in man has not been reported.

Other arthropod-borne reoviruses

Kemerovo

The orbivirus serogroup Kemerovo contains three viruses that have been isolated from Ixodes and Hyalomma ticks in Russia and Central Europe. They may cause benign febrile illnesses and, occasionally, meningitis or encephalitis in spring and early summer, when ticks are active. Rodents and birds are involved in the zoonotic cycle.

Changuinola

There is a single report of human febrile illness with the orbivirus Changuinola in Panama. The virus has been isolated from phlebotomine flies and mammals in that area.

Orungo

The untyped reovirus Orungo is found mainly in West Africa but also in Uganda and the Central African Republic. Up to 75 per cent of some populations are seropositive. The clinical effects are unknown but fever and diarrhoea occur in some people, perhaps with encephalitis, as in experimental mice. There is no rash or jaundice. Orungo virus is transmitted by Anopheles, Aedes, and other mosquitoes. Monkeys, sheep, and cattle may be infected but not rodents.

Lebombo

This reovirus was isolated from one febrile child in Nigeria. Lebombo is also found in mosquitoes and rodents.

REFERENCES

Brown G.S. (1988). Colorado tick fever, In *The arboviruses: epidemiology and ecology*, Vol II (ed. T.P. Monath), p. 159–76. CRC Press, Boca Raton, FA.

Burgdorfer, W. (1977). Tick-borne diseases in the United States: Rocky Mountain spotted fever and Colorado tick fever. A review. *Acta Tropica*, **34**, 103–26.

Emmons, R.W. (1981). Colorado tick fever. In *Handbook series in zoonoses*, Section B, *Viral zoonoses*, (ed. J.H. Steele), p. 113. CRC Press, West Palm Beach, FA.

Knudson, D.L. and Monath, T.P. (1990). Orbiviruses. In *Virology*, Vol. 2, (ed. B.N. Fields *et al.*), pp. 1405–33. Raven Press, New York.

Libikova, H., Heinz, F., Ujhazyova, D., and Stunzner, D. (1978). Orbiviruses of the Kemerovo complex and neurological diseases. *Medical Microbiology and Immunology*, **166**, 255–63.

Togaviruses

7.10.17 Alphaviruses

D. I. H. Simpson

There are currently 28 members of the genus Alphavirus (formerly group A arboviruses), which all replicate in and are transmitted by mosquitoes. Although 12 alphaviruses have been known to infect man, only eight produce significant disease (Table 1).

The virion has a diameter of 60 to 70 nm and contains a single strand of positive-sense RNA enclosed in an icosahedral nucleocapsid, surrounded by a lipid membrane.

The type of illness produced by alphaviruses varies from a mild febrile illness, which may or may not be accompanied by a rash, myalgia and arthralgia, to frank encephalitis. The mild fever, which is often unrecognized, occurs during the initial viraemic stage. This may be followed by a much more serious form of illness at which stage viraemia may have ceased and immunological responses, including the formation of antibodies, taken place. Generally, only a small proportion of people infected with potentially encephalitogenic arboviruses during epidemics develop encephalitis in the second phase. The great majority develop only the first phase or the infection may be asymptomatic.

Chikungunya

Chikungunya virus was first isolated from patients and mosquitoes during an epidemic in the Newala district of Tanzania in 1952–53. The native name is derived from the main symptom, being 'doubled-up' as a result of excruciating joint pains. Since then, chikungunya virus has been frequently isolated from humans and mosquitoes during epidemics in India and South-East Asia as well as in eastern, western, central, and southern Africa. The largest epidemics in recent years have been in cities of the Indian subcontinent and it has been estimated that there were 300 000 cases of illness in a population of nearly 2 million in Madras.

Chikungunya virus is transmitted in Africa by *Aedes africanus* and *Ae. aegypti*, while the latter transmits the disease in the urban centres of India and South-East Asia. No vertebrate host other than man has been confirmed, although evidence has been found that monkeys might be a maintenance host in Africa.

CLINICAL FEATURES

Following an infective mosquito bite, there is an incubation period of 2 to 12 days followed by the sudden onset of fever and crippling joint pains, which may incapacitate the patient within a few minutes to a few hours of onset. The pain in the limbs and spine is so severe as to cause patients to be doubled up and immobile. Headache is usually mild, there is no retro-orbital or eye pain, and patients have anorexia and constipation. The disease has a biphasic course; following 1 to 6 days of fever, the temperature returns to normal for 1 to 3 days and then there is a second period of fever for a few days. In the second phase of illness, 80 per cent of patients develop a maculopapular pruritic rash on the trunk and extensor surfaces of the limbs. After 6 to 10 days patients recover completely, although, rarely, arthralgia can persist for months. A leucopenia is the only unusual laboratory finding.

In India and South-East Asia, chikungunya virus has been implicated in outbreaks of haemorrhagic fever, often in association with dengue viruses. It was isolated repeatedly, along with all four dengue serotypes, from patients during outbreaks in Thailand and Singapore, but haemorrhagic disease due to chikungunya virus is rare. Accumulated evidence indicates that it is not severe enough to cause shock. No haemorrhagic complications in chikungunya infections have ever been reported in Africa.

Diagnosis by isolation of virus from the blood, in suckling mice or tissue culture, is possible in the first 4 or 5 days of illness. Thereafter haemagglutination inhibiting and neutralizing antibodies can be detected, but serological cross-reactions occur with other alphaviruses. A virus-specific IgM enzyme immunoassay has proved useful. No vaccine is produced commercially.

Mayaro virus

This virus has been isolated from humans and various mosquito species in Trinidad, Brazil, Bolivia, and Surinam. The virus causes a benign, 2- to 6-day illness with fever, headache, conjunctivitis, prostration, joint and muscle pains, and a rash. The arthralgia can last for 2 months. A high-titre viraemia favours viral isolation from the blood.

O'nyong nyong virus

This virus caused a major epidemic that began in Uganda during 1959 and quickly spread to Kenya, Tanzania and Malawi, involving an estimated 2 million people. The virus was isolated again in 1979 and may still be active in western Kenya. O'nyong nyong is closely related to chikungunya and the disease it produces also resembles this infection. This virus is transmitted to man by *Anopheles gambiae* and *A. funestus*, which are also malaria vectors.

CLINICAL FEATURES

After an incubation period of up to 8 days, illness begins abruptly with fever, rigors and sometimes epistaxis, followed by backache, severe joint pains, headache, pain in the eyes, generalized lymphadenopathy, and an irritating rash beginning on the face and spreading to the trunk and limbs. High fever is uncommon. The rash generally lasts for 4 to 7 days but the joint pains and malaise are protracted. There are no sequelae and no deaths have been directly attributable to the infection.

Ross River virus

This virus has caused 'epidemic polyarthritis' in Australia, south-western Pacific Islands, and more recently Fiji. Ross River virus was isolated from *Ae. vigilax* in Australia and New Guinea and from *Ae. aegypti* in Fiji. Epidemics in the Murray Valley, Australia have involved several thousand people.

The patients present with arthralgia of the small joints of the hands and feet, sore throat, rash, and paraesthesiae of the palms and soles of the feet. The rash, which sometimes covers the whole body, may begin as discrete macules and progress to papules and occasionally to small vesicles. Petechiae and an enanthem have also been seen. Fever is not marked and may be absent. Arthritis lasts for 2 to 28 days, but may persist for months. There is no evidence that the arthropathy is immunopathological.

Table 1 *Alphaviruses known to cause human disease*

Virus	Geographical distribution of viruses	Effect on man
Chikungunya	Tropical Africa, S and SE Asia	Epidemics of painful arthritis E Africa, India, SE Asia
Mayaro	Trinidad, Brazil, Bolivia, Surinam	Transient febrile illness
O'nyong nyong	E and W Africa, Zimbabwe	Epidemics of febrile illness E Africa and Zimbabwe only
Ross River	Australasia, Fiji	Epidemics of polyarthritis
Sindbis	Africa, E Mediterranean, S and E Asia, Australia	Disease only recognized in Africa
Okelbo	Sweden, restricted areas N Europe	Outbreaks of polyarthritis
Eastern equine encephalitis	N and Central America, Trinidad, Guyana, Brazil, Argentina	Sporadic with severe encephalitis in N America
Western equine encephalitis	N America, Mexico, Guyana, Brazil, Argentina	Encephalitis, epidemics only in N America
Venezuelan equine encephalitis	Northern countries S America, Central America, and southern USA	Epidemics of febrile illness, encephalitis, mainly in children

Sindbis virus

Although this virus is widely distributed in Africa, India, tropical Asia, and Australia, it has only occasionally been associated with overt human disease. Sindbis is the prototype species of the genus Alphavirus, and a member of the western equine encephalitis virus complex. It has been isolated from several *Culex* mosquito species—*C. tritaeniorhynchus*, *C. pseudovishnui* and *C. inivittatus*—and from wild and domestic birds.

The variety of associated clinical features includes fever, rash, arthralgia, myalgia, malaise, and headache. The maculopapular rash progresses from trunk to extremities and vesicles can occur on the palms and soles. Virus has been isolated from vesicle fluid.

Viruses closely related to Sindbis also occur in northern Europe: Okelbo virus is responsible for outbreaks of rash, arthritis and sometimes fever, across central Sweden in the late summer. It has been isolated from *Culiseta* mosquitoes. Pogosta disease is a similar illness seen in Finland and likewise Karelian fever in Karelia.

Eastern equine encephalitis virus

Eastern equine encephalitis carries a high mortality and occurs widely along the eastern seaboard states of the United States and South America. Small outbreaks have occurred in the United States, the Dominican Republic, Cuba, and Jamaica. In the United States, equine cases occur each summer in coastal regions bordering the Atlantic and the Gulf of Mexico and in other eastern states. Cases in eastern Canada were first recorded in 1972. Outbreaks in man are generally sporadic with a low infection rate and only a small number of severe cases, but in horses and pheasants there is considerable morbidity and mortality. The virus is probably maintained by wild birds and mosquitoes, but the maintenance species in tropical areas have not been elucidated. *Culiseta melanura* seem to be the main mosquito infecting birds in North America; outbreaks are often associated with *Ae. sollicitans* and *Ae. vexans*. In the tropics, *Ae. taenioryrnchus*, *C. taeniopus*, and *C. nigripalpus* appear to be involved.

CLINICAL FEATURES

In the United States, encephalitis occurs mainly in young children. Inapparent cases are rare. Onset is abrupt with high fever (39–41°C), headache, and vomiting followed by drowsiness, coma, and severe convulsions. On examination there is neck stiffness, spasticity, and, in infants, bulging fontanelles. Oedema of the legs and face and cyanosis have been described. The cerebrospinal fluid is under pressure and contains increased protein and up to 1000 cells/mm. The mortality rate reaches 70 per cent and death can occur within 3 to 5 days of onset. Sequelae are common in non-fatal cases and include convulsions, paralyses, and mental retardation. Older patients usually recover more completely. Systemic illness without central nervous signs is also possible. Eastern equine encephalitis is usually diagnosed by finding either a rise in haemagglutination inhibiting or neutralizing antibody level, or virus-specific IgM by enzyme immunoassay.

Vaccines have been used successfully in horses and an inactivated vaccine is available for laboratory staff.

Western equine encephalitis virus

The virus has been isolated in the United States, Canada, Mexico, Guyana, Brazil, and Argentina, but human disease is rare outside North America and Brazil. Summer epidemics of western equine encephalitis have occurred in the United States where there was a large outbreak in 1975 in North Dakota, Minnesota, and adjacent Manitoba. This epidemic was precipitated by extensive flooding in early summer, which encouraged the breeding of *Culex tarsalis*, the principal vector in western parts of the United States. Further outbreaks appeared in this region in 1977, 1981 and 1987. The western equine encephalitis virus isolated in the eastern United States is the antigenically distinct Highland J (HJ) strain. This virus is less pathogenic in animals and the usual vector is *Culiseta melanura*.

The virus has been isolated from a variety of wild birds, which appear to be the maintenance hosts at least in North America. Equine epizootics generally precede the appearance of human cases but horses play no part in the transmission cycle. Little is known about the maintenance cycle of the virus in tropical regions.

CLINICAL FEATURES

The disease varies with age but fever and drowsiness are common at all ages. Children are highly susceptible and all infant infections seem to cause illness, whereas less than 1 per cent of adult infections are symptomatic. There is typically headache, vomiting, stiff neck, and backache. Restlessness and irritability are often seen in children. Convulsions occur in 90 per cent of affected infants and in 40 per cent of children between 1 and 4 years old, but are rare in adults. Drowsiness, severe occipital headache, mental confusion, and coma are seen in up to 40 per cent of adults. In milder cases recovery takes place in 3 to 5 days and in severe cases within 5 to 10 days. Convalescence may be protracted. In adults, sequelae are rare but become more common with decreasing age. In infants, almost half are left with convulsions. Mortality varies from outbreak to outbreak from 2 to 15 per cent.

The virus can be isolated from brain tissue and rarely from cerebrospinal fluid or serum, but serology is the usual means of diagnosis in life. Inactivated vaccine is available for laboratory staff and horses.

Venezuelan equine encephalitis virus

This virus causes large epizootics of encephalitis in horses, mules, and donkeys in northern countries of South America and Central America, sometimes reaching the southern United States. In humans, encephalitis occurs in a small proportion of cases but the majority have only a non-fatal, 'influenza-like', febrile illness.

Six subtypes within the Venezuelan equine encephalitis virus complex are separable by serological and physicochemical means. Five antigenic variants can be distinguished within subtype I, designated IAB, IC, ID, IE and IF. Venezuelan equine encephalitis viruses IAB and IC have been found in equine **epizootics** and are more pathogenic for man and horses than the **enzootic** strains ID–F, subtypes II (Everglades), III (Mucambo), IV, V, and VI. These enzootic strains may occasionally produce sporadic disease but asymptomatic infection is common in man.

Epizootic strains of the virus appeared in Guatemala and spread in huge epizootic waves, reaching north to southern Texas in 1971 and south to Costa Rica. Over 200 000 horses died in this outbreak and there were several thousand human infections.

A wide variety of mosquitoes including *Aedes*, *Mansonia* and *Psorophora* spp. can transmit the virus. Enzootic strains are continually active in subtropical and tropical areas of the Americas, having small rodent and marsupial hosts, and are transmitted by *Culex* (*melanoconion*) mosquitoes. Birds may also act as hosts.

CLINICAL FEATURES

After an incubation period of 1 to 6 days, there is a brief febrile, occasionally 'influenza-like' illness of sudden onset, characterized by malaise, nausea or vomiting, headache, which may be severe, and myalgia. Fever lasts up to 4 days and convalescence may take 3 weeks with generalized asthenia. About 4 to 14 per cent of human cases caused by epizootic viruses develop neurological symptoms, which occur particularly in children below the age of 15 years, and the fatality rate of encephalitis can be 20 per cent. A similar spectrum of disease from inapparent infection with fever to fatal encephalitis is seen in equines.

The virus can be isolated from serum early in infection, otherwise the diagnosis is made serologically. Finding viraemia in nearby horses may accelerate specific identification. Transmission between humans has not been documented, although there have been several laboratory-acquired infections.

Live attenuated and inactivated vaccines have been used in laboratory workers. Equine immunization has been effective in controlling epizootic disease.

REFERENCES

Bartelloni, P.J., McKinney, R.W., Duffy, T.P., and Cole, F.E. (1970). An inactivated eastern equine encephalomyelitis vaccine propagated in chick embryo cell culture. II Clinical and serologic responses in man. *American Journal of Tropical Medicine and Hygiene*, **19**, 123–6.

Carey, D.E., Myers, R.M., De Ranitz, C.M., Jadhav, M., and Reuben, R. (1969). The 1964 Chikungunya epidemic at Vellore, South India, including observations on concurrent dengue. *Transactions of the Royal Society of Tropical Medicine and Hygiene*, **63**, 434–45.

Doherty, R.L., Barrett, E.J., Gorman, B.M., and Whitehead, R.H. (1971). Epidemic polyarthritis in eastern Australia, 1959–70. *Medical Journal of Australia*, **1**, 5–8.

Monath, T.P. (ed.) (1988,1989). *The arboviruses: epidemiology and ecology*, Vols I–III (1988) IV–V (1989). CRC Press, Boca Raton, FA.

Niklasson, B. *et al.* (1984). Association of a Sindbis-like virus with Okelbo disease in Sweden. *American Journal of Tropical Medicine and Hygiene*, **33**, 1212–17.

Pan American Health Organization (1972). *Venezuelan encephalitis*, Scientific Publication No. 243. PAHO, Washington, DC.

Peters, C.J. and Dalrymple, J.M. (1990). Alphaviruses. In *Fields virology*, (2nd edn), (ed. B.N. Fields, *et al.*), Vol.1, pp. 731–61. Raven Press, New York.

Sarkar, J.K., Chatterjee, S.N., Chakravarti, S.K., and Mijram, A.C. (1965). Chikungunya virus infection with haemorrhagic manifestations. *Indian Journal of Medical Research*, **53**, 921–5.

7.10.18 Rubella

S. LOGAN and P. TOOKEY

Introduction

Rubella infection usually causes a mild exanthematous disease of little clinical significance. Infection in the early months of pregnancy may result in multiple congenital abnormalities in the fetus, but, as a result of the widespread use of rubella vaccine, congenital rubella syndrome has become uncommon in most countries with developed health services.

The enveloped RNA virus of rubella is classified in a separate genus, Rubivirus, within the family Togaviridae. There are a number of strains of rubella; these show differences in virulence and other biological characteristics but are serologically indistinguishable.

Epidemiology

Humans are the only known host for rubella virus. In temperate zones the infection is seen predominately in spring and early summer, although sporadic cases occur throughout the year. Before the introduction of a vaccine, rubella was endemic in virtually all countries. Epidemics were superimposed on the endemic infection every 6 to 9 years in the United States and every 4 to 5 years in Europe, with major epidemics at intervals ranging from 10 to 30 years. In some parts of the world, for example Japan, Panama, rural Peru, and Hawaii, relatively large proportions of the adult population remain susceptible to rubella. This may be due to low population density or to genetic factors, including a lower propensity to spread the virus. In most populations, unless there is a mass immunization programme, around 10 per cent of women reach child-bearing age still susceptible to rubella infection.

Infection is rare below the age of 1 year. The incidence rises slowly during the first 4 years and then rapidly with a peak between 5 and 9 years of age. Outbreaks of infection are described among groups of young adults, typically students, prisoners, and service personnel.

Postnatally acquired infection

The most prominent feature of rubella infection is the rash, which usually begins on the face and spreads to the trunk and later to the extremities. The rash is pink and maculopapular; initially the lesions are discrete but they later tend to coalesce. The suboccipital and posterior cervical lymph nodes are characteristically enlarged. Mild fever, sore throat, coryza, cough, and conjunctivitis may be present; symptoms are usually mild and last only 3 to 7 days. There may be a prodrome with malaise and fever, especially in adults. There is no specific treatment.

Arthralgia affecting the ankles, knees, hips, fingers, and intervertebral joints is a common complication in older patients. Frank arthritis is unusual but the incidence increases with age. Both arthralgia and arthritis are normally transient but recurrent or persistent symptoms have been reported, mainly in older women. Less common complications include purpura, thrombocytopenia, post-infectious encephalitis, transverse myelitis, and the Guillain–Barré syndrome.

None of the signs or symptoms of rubella is sufficiently characteristic for it to be distinguishable clinically from picornavirus, myxovirus, adenovirus, and streptococcal infections. A history of clinically diagnosed rubella infection is not therefore an adequate reason for withholding rubella vaccine. At least half of all infections may be clinically inapparent or produce only mild, non-specific signs.

The incubation period is 14 to 21 days with a mean of 17 days. The exact mode of transmission is not known but the virus can be found in oropharyngeal secretions. Spread by airborne infection through the respiratory route is likely and close contact is usually necessary for transmission. Patients are infectious from 5 to 7 days before to 3 to 5 days after the start of symptoms but infectivity is highest immediately before, and on the first day of, symptoms. Congenitally infected infants shed large amounts of virus from the oropharynx and may continue to be a source of infection for many months after birth.

Infection usually produces lifelong immunity but reinfection has occasionally been reported. This is usually asymptomatic and viraemia is uncommon.

Congenital infection

Although rubella had been recognized clinically in Germany in the eighteenth century and in other countries by the 1880s, it was not until 1941 that its role as a congenital infection was first suggested. Sir Norman Gregg, an Australian ophthalmologist, noticed a sudden increase in referral of children with congenital cataract, often associated with cardiac lesions, in the months following a widespread rubella epidemic in Australia. Many of the mothers gave a history of rubella infection in the first trimester of pregnancy. His suggestion that a mild illness during pregnancy might be the cause of the lesions in the fetus evoked general scepticism, as it did not fit in with the accepted views of the origin of congenital abnormalities. His hypothesis was later confirmed by similar reports from other countries.

The classical triad of abnormalities associated with congenital rubella is cataracts, cardiac anomalies, and deafness. However, the teratogenic effects may result in a wide range of defects (Table 1). Sensorineural deafness alone or in combination with other abnormalities is the most common problem; congenital cataracts, cardiovascular anomalies, microcephaly, mental retardation, or growth retardation may also occur. The picture in an individual child is largely determined by the stage of pregnancy at which infection occurred; the earlier the infection the more likely the child will have severe, multiple problems (Table 2). The risk of damage to a child infected in the first 10 weeks of pregnancy is around 90 per cent. This drops rapidly thereafter; following infection at 13 to 16 weeks only about one-third of infants are damaged and most have only sensorineural hearing loss. After 16 weeks' gestation the only associated abnormalities are sensorineural hearing loss and growth retardation, and even these are rare; no abnormalities have been demonstrated in children of mothers with serologically confirmed infection after 18 weeks' gestation. Congenitally infected infants who are growth retarded at birth but have no other abnormalities usually grow and develop normally during childhood. It has been suggested that rubella infection acquired just before conception might result in congenital infection but none of these reports has been confirmed.

It is important to recognize that some of the defects associated with congenital rubella syndrome may not develop or reveal themselves until later infancy or childhood (Table 3). Deafness, in particular, may develop in a child with previously normal hearing. This emphasizes the importance of careful long-term follow-up of all children with congenital rubella infection. Hearing loss and other central nervous problems may worsen as the child gets older. A progressive rubella panencephalitis, like that after measles, has occasionally been reported but is rare.

It is possible that a number of other conditions caused by congenital rubella infection may arise in late childhood or early adult life (Table 3). Reports from the United States suggest that diabetes mellitus may affect up to 20 per cent of congenitally infected individuals by the time they are adults, although this has not yet been confirmed in a British cohort. Thyroid dysfunction has been reported in 5 per cent of patients. Autism and other behavioural and psychiatric disorders have also been reported to be more common in these children.

Not all maternal rubella infection results in transmission to the fetus. Transmission is most likely during the first trimester, the rate then diminishes until the last few weeks of pregnancy when it rises again. It is not known what determines whether or not an infection will be transmitted.

Table 1 *Defects associated with congenital rubella*

Classic triad
Sensorineural deafness
Abnormalities of the cardiovascular system:
- Persistent ductus arteriosus
- Pulmonary stenosis
- Aortic and renal artery stenosis
- Tetralogy of Fallot
- Ventricular septal defect
- Myocarditis

Abnormalities of the eye
- Retinopathy
- Cataracts
- Microphthalmos
- Glaucoma

Other defects
Growth retardation
Microcephaly
Mental retardation

Other signs in infancy and the neonatal period
Hepatosplenomegaly
Jaundice
Rash
Purpura
Thrombocytopenia
Osteopathy
Hypogammaglobulinaemia
Pneumonitis

Table 2 *Risk of rubella-associated defects after infection at different stages of pregnancy*

Gestation (weeks)	Risk of defects (%)
< 10	90
11–12	34
13–16	17
17–18	3
> 18	0

Adapted from Miller (1990*b*).

Many cases of congenital rubella syndrome occur after inapparent maternal infection. Most prospective studies of the risk to the fetus have been carried out on women with symptoms but the risk after inapparent infection is thought to be similar.

A few cases of congenital rubella syndrome have been reported in infants born to women previously shown to be immune. The risk of fetal infection following maternal reinfection is not known but is likely to be extremely low as prospective studies of asymptomatic reinfection have not demonstrated any cases of intrauterine infection. Maternal reinfection associated with a rash is rare, but in these circumstances viraemia is more likely and the risk to the fetus is likely to be significant.

The diagnosis of congenital rubella infection is relatively easy if suspected early but more difficult to confirm in older infants and young children. In most congenitally infected infants, virus can be isolated from multiple sites including the oropharynx, urine, and conjunctival fluid during the first months of life. Although viral shedding may occasionally persist for years, only about 10 per cent of infants are still shedding virus at 12 months. The isolation of virus in a young child not

Table 3 *Late-appearing conditions associated with congenital rubella infection*

Sensorineural hearing loss
Cerebral palsy
Diabetes mellitus
Thyroid dysfunction
Panencephalitis (rare)

obviously acutely ill with rubella is diagnostic of congenital infection. The presence of IgG antibody alone is not diagnostic, as this may be due to either passively transferred maternal antibody or to postnatally acquired rubella infection, but the persistence of high levels of IgG is highly suspicious. The presence of rubella IgM antibody in early infancy is virtually diagnostic of congenital infection because acquired infection is rare at this age. Unfortunately, as the abnormalities associated with congenital rubella may present late, a presumptive diagnosis may have to be made on the basis of a clinical picture compatible with congenital rubella syndrome and the presence or persistence of rubella IgG antibodies. The introduction of **MMR** (the triple measles, mumps and rubella vaccine) in the United Kingdom in 1988 for children in the second year of life means that confirmation of congenital rubella is now even more difficult. The diagnosis is important for an accurate prognosis to be given to the child and to provide appropriate genetic counselling to the parents of a child with disabilities.

Management of possible rubella during pregnancy

A woman presenting with suspected rubella infection during the first 4 months of pregnancy must be offered investigation. Any asymptomatic woman who has been exposed to rubella during this period also requires investigation; because of the possibility of laboratory error and of reinfection, most virologists now recommend that even women previously reported to be immune should be investigated. A blood sample should be tested for the presence of IgG and IgM antibodies, with a repeat sample being tested after 2 weeks if the results are equivocal. A rise in IgG or the presence of IgM antibody is diagnostic of recent infection.

There are a number of reports of cases where the diagnosis of congenital infection has been missed as a result of poor communication between clinicians and laboratory leading to the wrong tests being performed or misinterpretation of results. Investigations must be done in consultation with a virologist, who should be made aware of the date and type of contact and the stage of pregnancy.

The use of immunoglobulin in women who have been exposed to rubella in early pregnancy is of no proven value. Although large doses of immunoglobulin may attenuate the course of the infection, there is no evidence that this reduces the likelihood of transmission to the fetus. Treatment should therefore be restricted to seronegative women in recent contact with rubella who definitely intend to continue with the pregnancy. As viraemia is present up to a week before the onset of symptoms, immunoglobulin should be given as soon as possible after contact, once susceptibility is confirmed.

Vaccination

Three strains of live, attenuated rubella vaccine were developed and were licensed in 1969. The RA27/3 strain is now the one in common use. The vaccine is given subcutaneously and results in an immune reaction similar to that following wild virus infection. Protective levels of antibody are produced in around 95 per cent of recipients; protection is expected to be lifelong in most individuals, and has been shown to persist for up to 18 years in long-term studies. Nevertheless, reinfection can occur both naturally and after vaccine challenge, and there are occasional well-documented reports of loss of immunity. A small number of cases of congenital rubella syndrome have been reported in the offspring of women in whom rubella antibody had been demonstrated after vaccination.

Different approaches to vaccine strategy have been pursued. In some countries, including the United States, there was mass immunization of children of both sexes at between 12 and 15 months of age in an attempt to eliminate rubella from the community. This strategy has the advantage not only of protecting those who are vaccinated but also reducing the risk of infection in susceptible pregnant women. In the United States the programme was supplemented by the immunization of all children under 12 years to begin with, and combined with the immunization of susceptible women identified by screening during pregnancy or at work. The danger with this strategy is that if the uptake of vaccine in childhood is low the spread of wild virus in the community is slowed down but not eliminated: the effect is to push the peak age of incidence of infection into an older age group, which could, paradoxically, lead to an increase in the number of cases of congenital rubella syndrome.

In other countries, including the United Kingdom, concern about the dangers of low uptake and about the duration of vaccine-induced immunity led to the adoption of a selective strategy of immunizing schoolgirls after the age of peak incidence, and susceptible women. This approach depends on the continued circulation of wild virus ensuring that most women are protected by natural immunity acquired during childhood, with most of those who remain susceptible being covered by the schoolgirl and adult immunization programmes. A third method was implemented in Sweden in 1982, when MMR vaccine was introduced for all children in the second year of life. A second dose was given to 12-year-

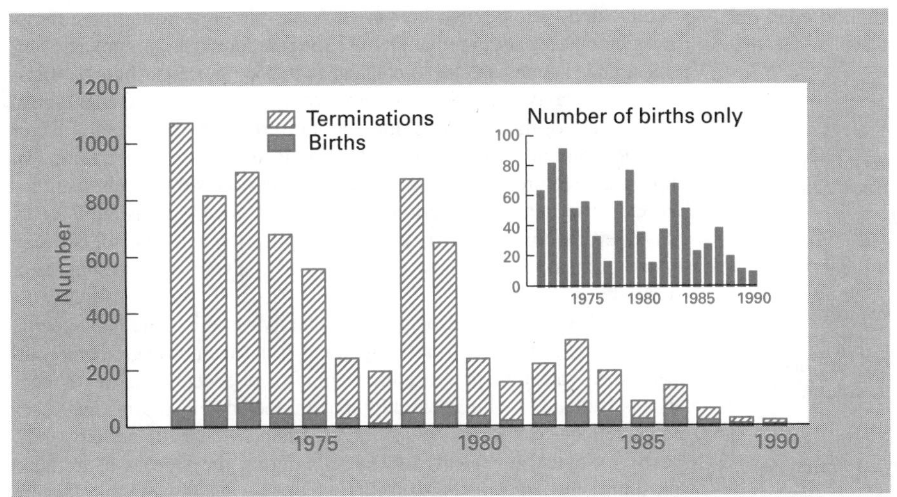

Fig. 1 Congenital rubella in England and Wales 1971–1990: terminations (disease/contact) and births.

olds, irrespective of a history of disease or vaccination, in order to reach those who did not receive vaccine as young children or failed to respond, and to boost antibody status in the rest.

In 1988, in the United Kingdom, reassuring data on the persistence of immunity after vaccination and the generally increasing levels of vaccine uptake led to the introduction of mass immunization of young children with MMR. Schoolgirl immunization and the identification and immunization of susceptible adult women will be maintained for some time, but a booster dose for all young people is not envisaged at present. The strategy to be adopted in any country seeking to control congenital rubella by vaccination must depend on the projected uptake of vaccination and the long-term prospects for continuing the programme. An important part of any strategy is the screening and immunization of susceptible health personnel, particularly those who may come into contact with pregnant women.

Vaccination has led to dramatic declines in the number of pregnant women susceptible to rubella infection, in rubella-associated terminations, and in the number of children born with congenital rubella. In the United Kingdom only 12 congenitally infected infants born in 1990 have so far been identified, compared with an average of 58.5 in the 1970s (when diagnostic methods and case ascertainment were less efficient) while in the United States comparable figures are 11 and 44.2. However, 47 cases of congenital rubella were registered in 1991 in the United States; the explanation for this rise has not so far been identified. Terminations of pregnancy for rubella disease or contact averaged 612 a year in England and Wales during the 1970s, but in 1991 this had plummeted to 10 (Fig. 1).

In children, rubella vaccine causes few side-effects. Low-grade fever and rash are occasionally reported, and transient arthralgia has been seen in about 3 per cent of vaccinees; there have also been rare reports of myositis and vasculitis. Joint symptoms are common in adult women, affecting up to 40 per cent of vaccinees, though they are less frequent and less severe than following naturally acquired rubella infection. These symptoms are generally mild and transient but a handful of cases of apparently recurrent or persistent arthritis after rubella immunization have been described.

There have been persistent concerns that the vaccine virus might be teratogenic if given during pregnancy. The virus can be isolated from the nasopharynx 1 to 3 weeks after administration and from the blood 7 to 10 days after inoculation. Although vaccinees cannot infect other susceptible individuals, it has been shown that the virus can cross the placenta. Data pooled from studies of children born to several hundred women inadvertently vaccinated up to 3 months before conception or during pregnancy show less than 3 per cent with serological evidence of congenital infection, and no infant born to any of these vaccinated women was reported to have abnormalities attributable to congenital rubella. Over 80 of these infants were born to women vaccinated in the month of conception, probably the period of greatest vulnerability. Although the risk of damage due to vaccine virus cannot be ruled out, these data suggest that the likely maximum theoretical risk is less than 5 per cent.

REFERENCES

Anonymous (1991). Increase in rubella and congenital rubella syndrome—United States, 1988–1990. *Morbidity and Mortality Weekly Report* **40,** 93–9.

Banatvala, J.E. and Best, J. (1990). Rubella. In *Topley and Wilson's principles of bacteriology, virology and immunity*, (8th edn), (ed. L. Collier and M. Timbury), pp. 501–31. Arnold, London.

Department of Health (1992). *Immunisation against infectious disease*, pp. 57–75. HMSO, London.

Enders, G., Miller, E., Nickerl-Pacher, U., and Cradock-Watson, J.E. (1988). Outcome of confirmed periconceptional maternal rubella. *Lancet*, **i,** 1445–7.

Gregg, N.M. (1941). Congenital cataract following German measles in the mother. *Transactions of the Ophthalmological Society Australia*, **3,** 35–46.

International Symposium on Prevention of Congenital Rubella Infection (1985). *Reviews of Infectious Diseases*, **7**(suppl. 1).

Lindegren, M.L., Fehrs, L.J., Hadler, S.C., and Hinman, A.R. (1991). Update: rubella and congenital rubella syndrome, 1980–1990. *Epidemiologic Reviews*, **13,** 341–8.

Miller, E. (1990*a*). Rubella reinfection. *Archives of Disease in Childhood*, **65,** 820–1.

Miller, E. (1990*b*). Rubella infection in pregnancy. In *Modern antenatal care of the fetus*, (ed. G. Chamberlain), pp. 247–70. Blackwell Scientific, Oxford.

Miller, E., Cradock-Watson, J.E., and Pollock, T.M. (1982). Consequences of confirmed maternal rubella at successive stages of pregnancy. *Lancet*, **ii,** 781–4.

Miller, E. *et al.* (1991). Rubella surveillance to December 1990: a joint report from the PHLS and National Congenital Rubella Surveillance Programme. *Communicable Disease Report*, **1,** R33–7.

Munro, N.D., Smithells, R.W., Sheppard, S., Holzel, H.G., and Jones, G. (1987). Temporal relations between maternal rubella and congenital defects. *Lancet*, **ii,** 201–4.

O'Shea, S., Best, J.M., Banatvala, J.E., Marshall, W.C., and Dudgeon, J.A. (1984). Persistence of rubella antibody 8–18 years after vaccination. *British Medical Journal*, **288,** 1043.

Preblud, S.R. and Alford, C.A. (1990) Rubella. In *Infectious diseases of the fetus and newborn infant*, (3rd edn), (ed. J.S. Remington and J.O. Klein), pp. 196–240. W.B. Saunders Company, Philadelphia.

Special Feature (1991). The epidemiology and control of rubella virus infection. *Epidemiology and Infection*, **107,** 1–68.

Tingle, J.T., Allen, M., Petty, R.E., Kettyls, G.D., and Chantler J.K. (1986). Rubella-associated arthritis. I. Comparative study of joint manifestations associated with natural rubella infection and RA 27/3 rubella immunisation. *Annals of the Rheumatic Diseases*, **45,** 110–14.

Tookey, P.A., Jones, G., Miller, B.H.R., and Peckham C.S. (1991). Rubella vaccination in pregnancy. *Communicable Disease Report*, **1,** R86–8.

7.10.19 Flaviviruses

T.P. MONATH

INTRODUCTION

The family Flàviviridae comprises at least 68 viruses, of which 29 cause human illness. The prototype virus, yellow fever (L. *flavus,* yellow) was isolated in 1927. New flaviviruses continue to be isolated from arthropod vectors and wild animals, and this group of agents is certainly among the 'emerging viruses'. Flaviviruses are transmitted by mosquitoes or ticks, and some are zoonotic infections spread between rodents or bats without involving arthropod vectors. All important human infections are caused by flaviviruses transmitted by mosquitoes or ticks. In two cases, dengue and yellow fever, humans serve as viraemic hosts in the transmission cycle, but the remainder use intermediate wild or domestic animals, and humans are 'dead-end' hosts that do not contribute to transmission. Flavivirus infections are not communicable. Geographical distribution of the disease is often circumscribed by the range of vector and host and provides a clue to the diagnosis of human infections. An important feature of arthropod virus transmission is the requirement for an extrinsic incubation period in the vector, generally lasting 7 to 14 days, representing the interval of virus replication in the vector between feeding on a viraemic host and ability to transmit by refeeding on a second host.

Disease syndromes associated with flaviviruses include non-specific febrile illness, fever with arthralgia and rash, haemorrhagic fever, and central nervous infection (aseptic meningitis or encephalitis). Pathogenesis is mediated by direct viral injury to infected cells or, in some cases (e.g. dengue haemorrhagic fever; see Chapter 7.10.20) perhaps indirectly by cytokines released from cells during the process of immune clearance. Because the clinical illness is rarely pathognomonic (except in an epidemic), the physician must use epidemiological information and specific laboratory tests to arrive at an accurate diagnosis. Vaccines are available or in advanced development for prevention of a number of flavivirus infections, but no effective antiviral drugs have been discovered and treatment is supportive and symptomatic.

Flaviviruses are small (37–50 nm) spherical particles consisting of a lipid–protein bilayer envelope surrounding a nucleoprotein core containing the single-stranded, positive-polarity RNA genome. Viruses attach to as yet undefined cell receptors by means of the envelope (**E**) protein spike protruding from the virion surface. After virus entry and uncoating, replication occurs in the cytoplasm. Virions mature and accumulate in the endoplasmic reticulum and are released by exocytosis or cell lysis. The genome organization has been fully elucidated and consists of approximately 11 000 nucleotides that encode 10 viral proteins, three of which make up the virus particle and seven of which are non-structural proteins remaining in the infected cell. From the medical standpoint, the most important gene products are the E protein, which subserves virus attachment and contains antigens stimulating humoral immunity, and two non-structural (**NS**) proteins, NS1 and NS3, that serve as targets for immune clearance.

Dengue (see also Chapter 7.10.20)

The clinical disease was described as early as 1780. Mosquito transmission was demonstrated in 1905, and a viral aetiology established by passage of filtered serum to man in 1906. The virus was not isolated, however, until 1944. It is now known that four antigenically distinct viruses (types 1–4) cause dengue fever.

EPIDEMIOLOGY

Dengue fever is the most prevalent flavivirus infection of man. In areas such as south-east Asia, where all four dengue types are hyperendemic, seroprevalence approaches 100 per cent by young adulthood. Although homotypic immunity is complete and lifelong, cross-protection between virus types is minimal and, hence, it is possible to sustain multiple, sequential infections. Worldwide morbidity is unknown, but probably exceeds 10 million cases annually. Epidemics in the Americas, where immunologically susceptible populations have been affected after introduction of the virus, have involved over 1 million cases with attack rates exceeding 50 per cent. Dengue viruses are transmitted principally by the bite of *Aedes aegypti* mosquitoes, a species that is abundant in and around human habitations. Viraemic humans serve as the source of virus for mosquito infection. The vector, and hence the disease, has a worldwide distribution in the tropics and warm areas of the temperate zone. The disease is most prevalent in south-east Asia, India, the American tropics, and the Horn of Africa, but recent epidemics have affected northern Australia and even the southern United States. Southern Europe, particularly the Adriatic region, is at risk of introduction. Movement of viraemic humans provides the principal means of spread, and rapid air travel is a factor in recent epidemic emergences. Air passengers often travel during the incubation period (2–7 days) of the disease. One hundred or more imported cases of dengue are reported annually in the United States and Europe.

CLINICAL FEATURES

The clinical manifestations include sudden onset of fever, accompanied by headache, retro-orbital pain and lumbosacral pain, and followed by severe malaise, myalgia, and joint or bone pain. The pulse rate is slow in relation to the fever, which may reach 41 °C. A transient macular rash or mottling of the skin is often seen during the first 1 to 2 days of illness. Between the second and sixth day, patients experience anorexia, nausea, vomiting, and, often respiratory symptoms (sore throat, rhinitis, cough), cutaneous hypersensitivity, and altered taste sensation. Defervescence occurs between days 3 to 6 and is followed by the appearance of a secondary, maculopapular or morbilliform, non-pruritic rash on the trunk, spreading to limbs and face, sparing palms and soles, lasting 1 to 5 days, and often resolving with desquamation. The fever may rise again after appearance of the rash, producing a 'saddle-back' fever curve. Other physical findings include generalized lymphadenopathy. Haemorrhagic phenomena (e.g. petechiae, purpura, epistaxis) occur in a few patients. Laboratory abnormalities include leucopenia (neutropenia) and thrombocytopenia. There are no fatalities; the disease resolves in the second week, but patients often experience prolonged convalescence with generalized asthenia and depression lasting several weeks. Persistent or recurrent musculoskeletal complaints or arthritis are not complications of dengue.

DIAGNOSIS AND DIFFERENTIAL DIAGNOSIS

The differential diagnosis includes influenza, measles, rubella, and other arboviral infections with rash, such as chikungunya, o'nyong nyong, West Nile fever, Sindbis fever, and Ross River fever (epidemic polyarthritis). Specific diagnosis is made by virus isolation or detection of viral genome in blood by polymerase chain reaction (during the first few days of illness), or by serological tests, including IgM enzyme immunoassay on paired acute and convalescent serum samples. Advice on the availability of these tests and on handling and transport of specimens should be sought from local or national health authorities.

TREATMENT

Treatment is symptomatic. Salicylates should be avoided because of the potential bleeding diathesis and because dengue has been associated with Reye's syndrome in a few cases.

PREVENTION

In areas infested with *Ae. aegypti,* patients should be safeguarded from mosquito bite. An intensive effort is under way to develop vaccines. Live, attenuated vaccines against all four serotypes have been tested clinically, but none is licensed yet.

Japanese encephalitis (B-encephalitis)

This encephalitic disease was described clinically in 1871. The virus was isolated from brain tissue in 1935, and mosquito transmission was proven in 1938. The virus exists as a single serotype, but strains circulating in distinct geographical regions are distinguishable by RNA sequencing. The lower disease incidence in Indonesia, for example, may be due to reduced virulence of local virus strains. Among the flaviviruses, Japanese encephalitis is closely linked antigenically to St Louis encephalitis, Murray Valley encephalitis, and West Nile viruses.

EPIDEMIOLOGY

Japanese encephalitis virus causes disease in man, horses, and pigs. The virus is widely distributed in Asia, from Japan and eastern Siberia to Indonesia and westward to India. The annual morbidity exceeds 50 000 cases, with highest incidence in temperate and subtropical regions of China, northern Thailand, and India, where epidemics occur in the summer months coincident with abundance of the principal vector, *Culex tritaeniorhynchus.* Recent outbreaks have occurred in Saipan and Okinawa, the first in over 40 years. Between 1978 and 1992, a total of 24 cases has occurred in United States expatriates visiting or living in endemic areas. The vector breeds in irrigated rice fields, and the distribution of human cases is linked to exposure in this ecological setting. Culex vectors bite preferentially at sunset and sunrise. Pigs and certain bird species are the amplifying, viraemic hosts in the transmission cycle, and man and equids are incidental, 'dead-end' hosts. Children suffer the highest attack rates in endemic areas, presumably because of cumulative immunity with age in the population. Elderly non-immune people are at higher risk of severe disease than young adults. Infection in pigs results in abortion and stillbirth, whereas horses develop encephalitis.

CLINICAL FEATURES

Most human infections are asymptomatic or so mild as to escape medical attention. Although estimates vary, only approximately 1 in 300 infections results in typical encephalitis. In such cases, after an incubation period of 6 to 16 days, illness begins with a non-specific prodrome lasting 2 to 3 days, followed by abrupt onset of high fever, chills, severe headache, meningism, photophobia, nausea, vomiting, abdominal pains, dizziness, restlessness, hyperexcitability, or drowsiness and obtundation. Generalized seizures occur in a high proportion of childhood cases. As the disease progresses, objective neurological signs appear, including cranial-nerve palsies, tremors, ataxia, rigidity and parkinsonian manifestations, abnormal reflexes, and upper motor-neurone paralysis, most commonly of the upper extremities. Neurological signs fluctuate and are highly variable, particularly alterations of consciousness, which include delirium, confusion, and ultimately coma. Lumbar puncture reveals elevated cell counts, generally under 1000/ mm^3 (polymorphonuclear initially, followed by lymphocytic), and mildly elevated protein and normal glucose levels. Respiratory dysregulation, coma, abnormal plantar reflexes, prolonged convulsions, and advanced age are associated with poor prognosis. Computerized tomography has revealed areas of low density and magnetic resonance scans have shown abnormal signals in deep areas of the brain (thalamus and basal ganglia). Japanese encephalitis is a much feared disease, with a lethality in excess of 25 per cent. Neuropsychiatric sequelae including parkinsonism, paralysis, and retardation occur in 30 to 70 per cent of survivors. In pregnant women infected during the first or second trimester, spontaneous abortion, and fetal death have been documented and the virus isolated from the conceptus. Data are insufficient to determine the quantitative risk of congenital infection or the risk of infection in the third trimester. There are several reports of recurrent encephalitic disease in children, with intervals of up 6 to 12 months between these occurrences. These episodes require further investigation, especially as latent infections have been documented experimentally in mice.

TREATMENT

No specific treatment is available. Uncontrolled trials of intrathecal interferon-α are inconclusive. Treatment is supportive, and includes attention to fluid management, respiratory support if required, avoidance of infection and bed sores, and use of anticonvulsants. Cerebral oedema may represent an important complication and requires prompt diagnostic evaluation and intervention (see Chapter 24.15.2).

DIAGNOSIS AND DIFFERENTIAL DIAGNOSIS

The differential diagnosis includes other viral encephalitides (especially herpes encephalitis for which antiviral therapy is available), as well as cerebral malaria and treatable bacterial, mycobacterial, and fungal infections of the central nervous system. Epidemiological features (place of travel or residence, season of the year, and occurrence of other cases in the community) provide important clues to the diagnosis. Specific diagnosis is by serological tests, particularly IgM enzyme immunoassay, which should be done on acute and convalescent sera and cerebrospinal fluid. From fatal cases, virus may be isolated from brain tissue or demonstrated by immunofluorescence. Virus is very rarely recoverable from blood during the acute phase.

PREVENTION

A formalin-inactivated purified vaccine derived from mouse brain has been in routine use for childhood immunization in Japan and some other Asian countries since the 1960s. Vaccine prepared by one producer (Biken, Osaka, Japan) is licensed and distributed in the United States (JE-VAX™, Connaught Laboratories Inc., Swiftwater, PA) and in Britain (Cambridge Selfcare Diagnostics Ltd), and is widely used in other developed countries to protect travellers. Although postvaccinal encephalitis is so rarely reported as to be a negligible risk, the vaccine has recently been associated with a variety of allergic complications (generalized urticaria, angio-oedema) at a rate of 0.1 to 1 per cent. Use of the vaccine to protect travellers should be restricted to those at highest risk of exposure (travel to an epidemic area, residence in an endemic area for more than 30 days, or extensive outdoor exposure in rural areas of Asia.) In endemic areas, it is estimated that the risk of acquiring encephalitis may approach 1 in 5000 per month of exposure. Tissue culture-based vaccines (inactivated and live, attenuated vaccines) are used in China, and second-generation genetically engineered vaccines are under development.

Kyasanur Forest disease

EPIDEMIOLOGY

In 1957, this virus was isolated during an outbreak in Karnataka (then Mysore) State, India of a new disease clinically characterized as haemorrhagic fever, affecting monkeys and man. The virus is antigenically linked to members of the tick-borne encephalitis complex (see below). Since the initial epidemic in 1957, annual outbreaks have occurred, involving 400 to 500 cases/year, with a case-fatality rate of 10 to 15 per cent. In 1983 a record 1555 cases and 150 deaths occurred. The disease has a limited geographical distribution, principally affecting villagers engaged in occupations requiring forest exposure in Karnataka State. Antibodies, but no disease, have been found in people living further north (in the Kutch area of India). The peak seasonal incidence of human cases is between February and May. The virus is amplified by transmission between immature ixodid ticks *(Haemaphysalis spinigera)* and small mammals (rodents, porcupines), passes to the adult tick stage during moulting, and is spread to man and wild monkeys by the bite of adult ticks.

CLINICAL FEATURES

The clinical illness appears after an incubation period of 2 to 7 days, with abrupt onset of fever, chills, severe headache and myalgia, abdominal pain, nausea, vomiting, and diarrhoea. Patients often present markedly dehydrated. Haemorrhage (purpura, epistaxis, menorrhagia, gastrointestinal bleeding) occurs in a minority of patients after about 72 h. Hypotension is frequently noted towards the end of the acute stage. Fatal cases develop signs of circulatory failure, pulmonary oedema, and acute respiratory distress. During the acute phase of illness, physical examination reveals relative bradycardia, cervical lymphadenopathy, conjunctival injection, and papulovesicular lesions on the soft palate. A biphasic illness is not uncommon, with resolution of the first phase in about 5 to 12 days, and return of fever and signs of meningoencephalitis after an interval of 1 to 3 weeks. This presentation resembles that of Central European encephalitis (see under Tick-borne encephalitis below); localizing neurological signs are infrequent, and residual deficits rare. Convalescence is prolonged.

Laboratory abnormalities include leucopenia, thrombocytopenia, and elevated serum transaminases during the acute phase of illness. Pathological findings in fatal cases have not provided clear explanations of pathogenesis. Diagnosis is made by virus isolation from blood collected during the first week after onset or by serological tests on paired sera.

The best source of information about the disease is the Virus Research Institute, Pune, India. Outside India, only a few laboratories with biocontainment level 4 facilities (Public Health Laboratories, Porton Down, Salisbury; Centers for Disease Control, Atlanta) are able to provide diagnostic assistance, because of the high risk of laboratory infections with this agent.

TREATMENT

No specific treatment is available; general supportive care, oxygen fluid replacement, and management of hypotension are appropriate.

PREVENTION

A formalized tissue culture vaccine developed in India has undergone successful field trials.

Louping ill

EPIDEMIOLOGY

This is a disease of veterinary importance, causing encephalitic illness in sheep and to a much lesser extent in cows, horses, farmed deer, sheepdogs, and pigs. Red grouse experience outbreaks of fatal disease. The virus was first isolated in 1931, is a member of the tick-borne encephalitis complex, and is transmitted by *Ixodes ricinus* (the same vector transmits Central European encephalitis (see under Tick-borne encephalitis below). Louping ill occurs principally in the hill country along the western coast of Scotland and northern England, and in Ireland. Cases in sheep have also been documented in Norway.

CLINICAL FEATURES

Natural infections resulting in human disease have been rare, although numerous laboratory infections are recorded. Ten naturally occurring cases are documented, including a veterinarian, abattoir workers, and farmers. Some of these cases undoubtedly were acquired by contact with sheep blood. The clinical disease in man is characterized by aseptic meningitis or encephalitis; no fatal infections have occurred.

PREVENTION

Vaccines for sheep have been developed. An experimental louping ill vaccine was used in man many years ago; it is probable (but unproven) that the licensed tick-borne encephalitis vaccine would be cross-protective against this infection.

Omsk haemorrhagic fever

This disease was first recognized in 1945, and the virus isolated from blood of a patient with haemorrhagic fever in 1947 during an epidemic in western Siberia. Cases were frequent between 1945 and 1949, with morbidity rates of 500 to 1400/100 000, but subsequently have been rare and sporadic. The virus is a member of the tick-borne encephalitis complex. Human infections are acquired by tick bite or contact with infected muskrats. Muskrat trapping is an occupational risk factor for infection. Muskrats (an introduced species) sicken and die of encephalitis. The human disease is characterized by abrupt onset of fever, headache, myalgia, facial flushing and oedema, conjunctival suffusion, minor haemorrhagic manifestations, and leucopenia. Recovery occurs in the second week, and the case-fatality rate is low (0.5–3 per cent). The differential diagnosis includes tularaemia, rickettsial infection, and leptospirosis. Specific diagnosis is made by virus isolation from blood during the acute phase, or by serological tests. Only a few laboratories outside Russia with biocontainment level 4 facilities are capable of providing laboratory assistance (Public Health Laboratories, Porton Down, Salisbury; Centers for Disease Control, Atlanta). Evidence suggests that the tick-borne encephalitis vaccines cross-protect against Omsk haemorrhagic fever.

Murray Valley encephalitis

This disease, originally labelled 'Australia X disease' was first recognized during an epidemic of severe encephalitis in New South Wales, Queensland, and the Murray Valley of Victoria in 1917–1918. The virus was isolated from human brains in a subsequent outbreak in the Murray Valley in 1951 and found to be antigenically linked to members of the Japanese encephalitis virus complex. Another outbreak occurred in 1974, and sporadic cases have been recorded in other years. Such cases have occurred also in the Kimberley region of Western Australia. The total recorded number of cases is only approximately 300, but with a case-fatality rate of 40 per cent. Children and elderly people appear to be at highest risk, and male cases exceed female. The virus is transmitted by *Culex annulirostris* mosquitoes, with wild birds, particularly water birds, implicated as principal amplifier hosts. Humans are tangential (dead-end) hosts. Asymptomatic infection is the rule, with serosurvey data suggesting one clinical case per 800 to 1000 infections. Those who become ill, however, experience severe disease similar to Japanese encephalitis. Diagnosis is by serological tests; the diagnostic assays must distinguish Murray Valley virus infection from that due to a closely related sympatric virus (Kunjin), which also causes encephalitis illness. Virus isolation from brain affords a postmortem diagnosis. Treatment is supportive. No vaccine is available.

Powassan encephalitis

The virus was first isolated from the brain of a fatal case in Powassan, Ontario in 1958. Since then, 20 human cases have been recognized in eastern Canada and the eastern United States, primarily in children, with a case-fatality rate of 10 per cent and a high incidence of residual neurological dysfunction. Incidence of the disease is extremely low, and it accounts for only 0.1 to 0.3 per cent of cases of encephalitis in the eastern United States and Canada subjected to diagnostic evaluation. Serological surveys of human populations indicate antibody prevalence of 1 to 3 per cent. The distribution of the virus in North America is considerably wider than indicated by human cases, however, and the diagnosis should be suspected in any case of summer or autumn encephalitis. Asymptomatic infection occurs in the former Soviet Union, and one human fatality has been reported. Transmission is by the bite of infected Ixodes ticks, with rodents serving as viraemic hosts in the transmission cycle. Milk-borne infection (from unpasteurized goat's milk) is a potential source of infection (see also under Tick-borne encephalitis below). The clinical features are those of viral encephalitis. Localizing neurological signs and convulsions are frequent. Diagnosis is by serological tests, which should include analysis of local (IgM) responses in cerebrospinal fluid. There is no specific treatment or vaccine.

Rocio encephalitis

The virus was first isolated in 1975 during an explosive epidemic of human encephalitis affecting the Ribeira Valley south-east of São Paulo, Brazil. The virus is more closely related to members of the Japanese encephalitis–West Nile complex than to other flaviviruses. Epidemics occurred between 1975 and 1977, resulting in 871 cases (an incidence of 3.8 per cent of the population), with the highest attack rate in young adult males engaged in outdoor agricultural work and fishing. Since 1978, only rare sporadic infections have occurred. Transmission was by mosquito bite, with wild birds as amplifying viremic hosts. The presumed principal vector is *Aedes scapularis.* The clinical disease is characteristic of viral encephalitis; 4 per cent of the cases died and 20 per cent were left with significant neuropsychiatric effects. Diagnosis is by serological tests (e.g. IgM enzyme immunoassay) on serum and cerebrospinal fluid. Virus is not recoverable from blood, but postmortem diagnosis is made by virus isolation from brain tissue. Treatment is supportive. There is no vaccine.

St Louis encephalitis

EPIDEMIOLOGY

The disease was discovered, and the virus was isolated from human brain during a large epidemic of encephalitis in Illinois and Missouri in 1932–33. The agent is a member of the Japanese encephalitis antigenic complex. Since 1955, over 5000 cases have been reported, representing 31 per cent of all cases of viral encephalitis diagnosed in the United States and 69 per cent of all cases of arboviral encephalitis. Cases occur annually as isolated events or in summer–autumn epidemics, the largest one in 1975 in the Mississippi–Ohio River basins (1815 cases). The case-fatality rate is 8 per cent overall, but 20 per cent in persons over 60 years, reflecting the increased severity of this infection in the elderly. Most infections are asymptomatic; the ratio of infection to clinical illness is high (ranging from 800:1 in children under 10 years to 85:1 in persons over 60 years). The disease occurs throughout the United States. Outbreaks have also occurred in southern Canada and northern Mexico. The virus has a much wider distribution in the Caribbean and Central and South America, where, however, only a few cases have been recorded. In North America, the virus is transmitted by several species of Culex mosquitoes, with wild birds serving as the amplifying viraemic host.

CLINICAL FEATURES

The clinical illness is recognized in three distinct forms of increasing severity; fever with headache, aseptic meningitis, and encephalitis. Because they are clinically less specific, the first two forms are generally recognized only in the setting of an epidemic. After an incubation period of 4 to 21 days, the typical case of encephalitis presents with an illness characterized at first by fever, headache, chilliness, anorexia, and nausea. Urinary-tract symptoms (frequency, urgency, dysuria) are frequent. Within 1 to 4 days, signs of central nervous infection intervene, with increasing headache, neck stiffness, drowsiness, and other signs of impaired consciousness and confusion. Tremor, abnormal reflexes, ataxia, and cranial-nerve palsies are often noted, but localizing motor or sensory signs are unusual. Convulsions are more frequent in children than adults. The cerebrospinal fluid shows fewer than 500 cells/mm^3, principally lymphocytes. The peripheral leucocyte count may be moderately elevated. Serum transaminase, aldolase, and creatine phosphokinase levels may be raised. The syndrome of inappropriate antidiuresis has been noted in up to one-third of patients. Deaths occur within 2 weeks of onset. Complications include bronchopneumonia, sepsis, stress ulcer, and pulmonary embolism. Underlying diseases (hypertension, diabetes, alcoholism) adversely affect outcome. Pathological study of fatal cases reveals inflammation and neuronal degeneration principally in the thalamus, midbrain, and brain-stem. Up to 50 per cent of patients who recover may have a prolonged convalescent syndrome (irritability, memory deficits, asthenia, ataxia) lasting several months, and some of these patients seem never to recover fully.

DIAGNOSIS AND DIFFERENTIAL DIAGNOSIS

The differential diagnosis includes other viral encephalitides (especially herpes encephalitis for which antiviral therapy is available), as well as treatable bacterial, mycobacterial, and fungal infections of the central nervous system. Some elderly patients have initially been diagnosed as having had a stroke. Epidemiological features (residence, season of the year, and occurrence of other cases in the community) provide important clues to the diagnosis. Specific diagnosis is by serological tests, particularly IgM enzyme immunoassay, which should be done on acute and convalescent sera and cerebrospinal fluid. From fatal cases, virus may be isolated from brain tissue or demonstrated by immunofluorescence. Virus is very rarely recoverable from blood during the acute phase.

TREATMENT

Treatment is supportive. Inappropriate antidiuresis is managed by water restriction. If signs of cerebral oedema are present, this condition should be treated. No antiviral agents are available.

TREATMENT

There is no vaccine. Prevention is aimed at surveillance and vector mosquito abatement.

Tick-borne encephalitis

EPIDEMIOLOGY

The disease was described in 1932 in the Far East of the former Soviet Union, and a virus (now called Russian spring–summer encephalitis, **RSSE**) isolated from blood of patients and from ixodid ticks in 1934. RSSE virus belongs to a medically important antigenic complex of the Flaviviridae, that includes the closely related Central European encephalitis **(CEE)** virus, as well as louping ill, Powassan, Kyasanur forest disease, and Omsk haemorrhagic fever viruses. In addition to being transmitted by ticks, viruses in this complex have certain other biological peculiarities: many are transmissible via the milk of infected domestic livestock, and they are notorious for producing laboratory infections via the aerosol route.

The distribution of RSSE and CEE viruses is determined by that of their vectors, *Ixodes persulcatus* and *I. ricinus,* respectively. RSSE causes human disease principally in the Far East, the Ural region, and western Siberia, whereas CEE occurs at highest incidence in Eastern and Central Europe, Moldavia, the Ukraine, and Byelorus, with smaller numbers of cases from Western Europe, the Balkan region, and Scandanavia. These infections are highly seasonal, occurring only during the period of tick activity, and incidence varies from year to year. Hundreds to thousands of cases occur annually, with morbidity rates approaching 20/100 000 in some areas. Occupational and vocational pursuits favouring tick exposure are risk factors. The transmission cycle involves immature ticks, insectivores and rodents; the virus is passed to the adult ticks through the moulting process, and then by tick bite to man and domestic animals, which do not contribute to virus transmission. Human infection may also be acquired by consumption of raw milk or cheese from goats, or more rarely, sheep or cows. Domestic livestock do not have observable symptoms; however, dogs may occasionally acquire clinical infections.

CLINICAL FEATURES

The incubation period is 7 to 14 days. The disease caused by RSSE virus is more severe than CEE. Onset is generally acute, with fever, headache, photophobia, chilliness, nausea and vomiting, followed by meningismus, and evolution of the encephalitic syndrome over several days. Asymmetrical lower motor-neurone paralyses, especially of the upper extremities, shoulder girdle, face and neck, are typical. Convulsions, tremors, ataxia, hyperaesthesia and sensory loss, and variable changes in sensorium accompany the syndrome. The case-fatality rate is approximately 20 per cent, and up to 60 per cent of survivors are left with neurological sequelae, including flaccid paralysis. CEE is a milder disease, which typically has a biphasic course. The first phase is a non-specific influenza-like illness with fever, headache, nausea, and vomiting lasting about a week. After a period of remission lasting a few days, fever returns, with aseptic meningitis or encephalomyelitis. The case-fatality rate is 1 to 5 per cent; about 20 per cent of survivors have neurological effects. Residual motor deficits are rare.

DIAGNOSIS AND DIFFERENTIAL DIAGNOSIS

The differential diagnosis of is similar to that described previously (see under Japanese encephalitis above); the pattern of flaccid paralysis may be confused with poliomyelitis. Epidemiological features of the case and history of tick exposure provide important clues; as in Lyme disease, however, a history of bite by small ixodid ticks is elicited in fewer than half the cases. Specific diagnosis is made by virus isolation from blood or cerebrospinal fluid during the first week of illness, or by serological tests, including IgM enzyme immunoassay, done on serum and cerebrospinal fluid.

TREATMENT

Treatment is supportive.

PREVENTION

Effective inactivated vaccines prepared in tissue culture are produced in Russia, Austria, and Germany. The vaccine produced against the CEE virus by Immuno AG, Vienna has been used to immunize the entire Austrian population, with a dramatic decline in disease incidence. A similar vaccine produced in Germany is in the late stages of regulatory approval. Cross-protection is probable (but not clinically established) between the CEE and RSSE vaccines. Use of a licensed vaccine (in Britain, obtainable from Immuno Ltd 0732 458101) should be seriously considered for tourists planning camping or extensive outdoor activities during the tick transmission season in endemic areas, particularly as Russia and Central Europe open up to tourism. In addition to the vaccine, commercial hyperimmune globulin preparations are available (in Britain, also from Immuno Ltd) for use after tick exposure or to provide short-term pre-exposure prophylaxis.

West Nile fever

Epidemiology

This virus was recovered from the blood of a fever patient in Uganda in 1937. The virus is antigenically related to Japanese encephalitis and other members of the Japanese encephalitis complex. Despite its prevalence and wide distribution, which includes Africa, the Middle East, Southern Europe, and Asia, human disease is relatively infrequent. Epidemics have occurred in Israel in the 1950s and 1960s, and in South Africa in the 1970s. Sporadic cases and small clusters of cases have been reported from India, Egypt, and subSaharan Africa. Encephalitis in horses has been described in southern France and Egypt. The transmission cycle involves mosquitoes (*Culex* spp.) and wild birds. Humans are incidental hosts.

CLINICAL FEATURES

Human infections are usually asymptomatic or so mild as to escape attention. The incubation period is 1 to 6 days. Disease may present as a dengue-like febrile illness, with or without rash. Headache, myalgia, anorexia and nausea, sore throat, epigastric pains, diarrhoea, lymphadenopathy, and leucopenia may accompany the fever, which lasts up to a week, and often exhibits a biphasic pattern. The rash is maculopapular or roseolar and non-pruritic; unlike dengue, desquamation does not occur. In its more severe form, West Nile virus infection may cause aseptic meningitis or encephalitis. The latter appears to be more frequent and severe in elderly people (like St Louis and Japanese encephalitis), but severe and fatal cases are also described in children. Unusual clinical presentations attributed to West Nile virus and described in single cases include myocarditis and pancreatitis. Four patients in the Central African Republic developed hepatitis. Virus strains from these patients were similar by molecular analysis to strains recovered from typical West Nile fever cases.

In the 1950s, infection with West Nile virus was tried as an experimental approach to cancer therapy. All patients developed fever and 10 per cent had mild, self-limiting encephalitic signs.

DIAGNOSIS AND DIFFERENTIAL DIAGNOSIS

The differential diagnosis includes influenza, sandfly fever, dengue, chikungunya, Sindbis, and other viral infections. Cases with meningitis or encephalitis must be distinguished from enteroviral infections, herpes, Japanese and tick-borne encephalitis, and other viral infections. Specific diagnosis may be made by virus isolation from blood in a high proportion of patients during the first few days of fever. Serologic diagnosis may be complicated by cross-reactivity with other flaviviruses, particularly in Africa and Asia.

TREATMENT AND PREVENTION

There is no specific treatment or vaccine. In an experimental non-human primate model, Japanese encephalitis virus induced cross-protection against West Nile (reciprocal protection was not found); the results suggest the possibility that Japanese encephalitis vaccine could be used to provide protection against West Nile. Epidemiological evidence also suggests that cross-protection occurs between these closely related agents.

Yellow fever

HISTORY AND EPIDEMIOLOGY

The disease was described in the seventeenth century and was one of the great plagues of mankind for over 200 years. In 1900, mosquito transmission and viral aetiology were proven, but the virus was not isolated until 1927. Control of the urban mosquito vector, *Aedes aegypti,* and vaccination have diminished the importance of yellow fever in this century. Epidemics still do occur, with devastating impact on human populations, especially in West Africa. For example, between 1986 and 1991, a series of outbreaks in Nigeria caused well in excess of 100 000 cases (although only about 5000 were officially reported), with attack rates in affected areas of 30/1000 and case-fatality rates exceeding 20 per cent. The most recent outbreak of yellow fever occurred in 1992–93 in western Kenya. Cases among unvaccinated travellers are reported, but, fortunately, rare.

The virus is present in tropical America and Africa, but does not occur in Asia. In South America, the disease affects 100 to 300 persons/year, principally young adult males engaged in agricultural or forest work and hence exposed to tree-hole breeding Haemagogus mosquito vectors (so-called jungle yellow fever). The virus transmission cycle involves these mosquitoes and monkeys. In the past 10 to 15 years, the domestic mosquito and historical yellow-fever vector, Ae. aegypti, has reinvaded South America, creating the potential for re-emergence of urban yellow fever, in which man serves as viraemic host in the transmission cycle. In Africa, a variety of tree-hole breeding (sylvatic) *Aedes* spp. play a part in virus transmission. The basic maintenance cycle involves these mosquitoes and monkeys, but, because of the abundance and biting habits of these vectors, transmission to man is much more frequent than in the Americas. Epidemics occur in moist savanna regions of Africa, involving sylvatic Aedes vectors and man as viraemic hosts. In dry areas and urban centres, where water-storage practices breed domestic *Ae. aegypti,* this mosquito has an important role in virus transmission.

CLINICAL FEATURES

Subclinical or abortive infections are frequent, and only about 1 in 10 to 20 infections results in clinical disease with jaundice. In its classical form, disease onset occurs abruptly after an incubation period of 3 to 6 days. The initial phase of illness ('period of infection'), during which time virus is present in the blood, is characterized by fever, chilliness, severe headache, lumbosacral pain, generalized myalgia, nausea, and severe malaise or prostration. On examination, the patient is febrile, with a relative bradycardia, conjunctival injection, and a coated tongue reddened along the edges. Within several days, the patient may recover transiently ('period of remission'), only to relapse ('period of intoxication') with increasing systemic symptoms, jaundice, albuminuria, oliguria, haemorrhagic manifestations (especially 'black vomit' haematemesis), delirium and stupor, metabolic acidosis, and shock. The prognosis in those who exhibit this full-blown syndrome is poor, and over 50 per cent succumb between the seventh and tenth day after onset. Clinical laboratory tests reveal leucopenia, and chemical signs of hepatic dysfunction and renal failure. The bleeding diathesis is believed due principally to decreased synthesis of clotting factors by the liver, but disseminated intravascular coagulation has been described in a few cases and may have a role. As yet unidentified vasoactive mediators are probably responsible for terminal events and shock. Pathological findings in the liver are characteristic, showing midzonal necrosis and eosinophilic degeneration of hepatocytes (Councilman bodies). The kidney shows acute tubular necrosis. Focal myocarditis, and brain swelling and petechial haemorrhages are found and may contribute to the pathogenesis of the disease. Some patients recover from the acute hepatic infection, only to die of complications of acute tubular necrosis and renal failure. Those who recover, do so without permanent effects or post-necrotic cirrhosis. Late deaths during convalescence have been attributed to cardiac arrhythmias, but this complication requires confirmation.

DIAGNOSIS AND DIFFERENTIAL DIAGNOSIS

The differential diagnosis is relatively simple in the setting of an epidemic, but is more difficult when presented with an isolated case. Exposure and travel history provide important clues to aetiology. Other causes of hepatitis, including hepatitis E, leptospirosis, dengue haemorrhagic fever, Rift Valley fever, Crimean–Congo haemorrhagic fever, and West Nile virus must be considered. Specific diagnosis may be accomplished during the period of infection by examination of serum for isolation of virus, demonstration of viral genome by polymerase chain reaction, or by antigen detection by monoclonal antibody–enzyme immunoassay. Serological methods (especially IgM enzyme immunoassay) are useful, but cross-reactions with other flaviviruses present problems for diagnosis, particularly in Africa where multiple heterologous flaviviruses abound. Postmortem diagnosis may be accomplished by histopathological examination of the liver, with or without immunocytochemical analysis to detect yellow-fever viral antigen. Liver biopsy should never be performed on living patients, as it may precipitate lethal haemorrhage.

TREATMENT

Treatment is symptomatic. Intensive care and countermeasures to acid-dosis, shock, and other pathophysiological disturbances would probably save lives but have not been available where most cases occur. Patients with renal failure may require dialysis. No specific antiviral drug is available.

PREVENTION

Yellow fever is a preventable disease. The live, attenuated 17D vaccine is produced in a number of countries from chicken embryos. The vaccine is delivered as a single 0.5 ml subcutaneous dose and induced long-lasting immunity in over 95 per cent of those immunized. Immunity is probably lifelong; for travel certification, revaccination is recommended every 10 years. Reactogenicity is minimal. Persons with documented egg allergy should not be immunized or should be skin tested with the vaccine (see package insert). The vaccine must not be given to children under 6 months of age, in whom there is a risk of postvaccinal encephalitis, and it is best to delay vaccination until 12 months of age if possible. On theoretical grounds, persons with immunosuppression (including those with clinical AIDS) should not be immunized but no case of harmful consequences of inadvertent immunization of these patients has been reported. The risk in pregnancy is uncertain; in one study, congenital infection (without adverse effect to the fetus) was found in 1 of 41 women immunized (inadvertently) during the first trimester. Immunization during pregnancy is contraindicated, but, if inadvertently performed, mothers should be reassured and followed.

Other flaviviral infections

Sporadic cases of illness caused by other flaviviruses have been reported. These associations are listed below.

Viruses causing febrile illness with myalgia/arthralgia, with or without rash: **Banzi** (Africa, mosquito-borne); **Bussuquara** (South America, mosquito-borne); **Dakar bat** (Africa, a bat virus, no arthropod vector); **Koutango** (Africa, mosquito-borne); **Sepik** (New Guinea, mosquito-borne); **Spondweni** (Africa, mosquito-borne); **Usutu** (Africa, mosquito-borne); **Wesselsbron** (Africa, Asia, mosquito-borne); **Zika** (Africa, Asia, mosquito-borne).

Viruses causing febrile illness, aseptic meningitis or encephalitis: **Ilheus** (South America, mosquito-borne); **Kunjin** (Australia, mosquito-borne); **Negishi** (China, Japan, tick-borne); **Rio Bravo** (United States, a bat virus, no arthropod vector).

REFERENCES

Centers for Disease Control (1993). Inactivated Japanese encephalitis virus vaccine. Recommendations of the Advisory Committee on Immunization Practices (ACIP). *Morbidity and Mortality Weekly Reports* **42,** 1–15.

Centers for Disease Control (1993). Recommendations of the Advisory Committee on Immunization Practices (ACIP): use of vaccines and immunoglobulins in persons with altered immunocompetence. *Morbidity and Mortality Weekly Reports* **42,** No RR–4.

Chambers, T.J., Hahn, C.S., Galler, R., and Rice, C.M. (1990). Flavivirus genome organization, expression, and replication. *Annual Reviews of Microbiology,* **44,** 649–81.

Halstead, S.B. (1989). Antibody, macrophages, dengue virus infection, shock, and hemorrhage: a pathologic cascade. *Reviews of Infectious Diseases,* **11,** S830–9.

Kurane, I. *et al.* (1991). Activation of T lymphocytes in dengue virus infections. High levels of soluble interleukin 2 receptor, soluble CD4, soluble CD8, interleukin 2, and interferon-γ in sera of children with dengue. *Journal of Clinical Investigation,* **88,** 1473–80.

Monath, T.P. (ed.) (1989). *The arboviruses: epidemiology and ecology,* Vols I–V. CRC Press, Boca Raton, FA.

Monath, T.P. (ed.) (1980). *St. Louis encephalitis.* American Public Health Association, Washington, DC.

Monath, T.P. (1987). Yellow fever: a medically neglected disease. *Reviews of Infectious Diseases,* **9,** 165–75.

7.10.20 Dengue haemorrhagic fever

SUCHITRA NIMMANNITYA and M. J. CARDOSA

DEFINITION

Dengue haemorrhagic fever is a severe form of dengue infection in which there is haemorrhage and a tendency to develop fatal shock (dengue shock syndrome).

THE VIRUSES

The dengue viruses are mosquito-borne viruses belonging to the family Flaviviridae, which gets its name from the prototype yellow fever virus. Four distinct serotypes of dengue virus have been defined; these are named dengue types 1 to 4 and abbreviated DEN1, DEN2, DEN3, and DEN4. The viral genome is a single-stranded, positive-sense RNA encapsidated by a single (12–14 kDa) core protein (C) with an envelope consisting of the major structural (55–60 kDa) envelope protein (E) and the 8-kDa membrane protein (M), which is cleaved late in maturation from the 19–23-kDa preM. The virions of the four serotypes of dengue virus share group-reactive epitopes and have flavivirus cross-reactive epitopes in addition to the epitopes that define each serotype. Most epitopic studies have concentrated on E, which bears the haemagglutinin as well as the epitopes involved in neutralization of virus infectivity. The virus genome also encodes a number of non-structural proteins including the three major non-structural proteins NS1 (44–49 kDa), NS3 (67–76 kDa), and NS5 (91–98 kDa), and a number of less well-defined, smaller proteins. All viral proteins are coded in a single, long open reading frame about 10.5 kb in length.

The sequences of all the dengue virus serotypes are now known, and an infectious clone of DEN4 has been generated. The question of whether differential virulence is associated with the different diseases that can be caused by dengue virus can now be addressed directly by manipulating the infectious clone. Neither the earlier studies of geographical and strain variations nor more recent studies of sequence variation have revealed associations of particular motifs or fingerprints with dengue fever, dengue haemorrhagic fever, or dengue shock syndrome.

THE VECTOR

Aedes aegypti is the main mosquito vector responsible for transmission of dengue (and yellow fever) virus infection. It has a domestic habitat and the female mosquito bites during the day. After the female *Ae. aegypti* has had a blood meal from a viraemic person, the virus multiplies in its salivary gland and can be transmitted after an incubation period of 8 to 10 days. It is also possible for the mosquito to transmit the virus immediately if its blood meal is interrupted and it bites someone else. Other known vectors are *Ae. albopictus*, *Ae. polynesiensis*, and several species of the *Ae. scutellaris* complex. Man is the principal mammalian host, but there is evidence of a sylvatic cycle that does not appear to be of great importance. Changes in economic activity of non-urban communities have led to the appearance of dengue virus transmission in unexpected situations, such as Sarawak after the introduction of cocoa as a cash crop. The cocoa pods proved to be a perfect breeding ground for *Ae. albopictus* and control measures have had to include advice to farmers about the handling of pods after the harvest.

HISTORY AND EPIDEMIOLOGY

Dengue haemorrhagic fever has been recognized as a separate disease entity from classical dengue fever since the second half of the twentieth century, with the first outbreak, called 'Philippine haemorrhagic fever', in 1953. This was followed by an outbreak in Thailand in 1958, which was referred to as 'Thai haemorrhagic fever'. The cause of these early outbreaks was at first unknown and there was considerable confusion and consternation until dengue viruses types 2, 3, and 4 were isolated from patients in the Philippines in 1956 and dengue type 1 in Thailand. Since then, dengue haemorrhagic fever has occurred in Malaysia, Singapore, India, Sri Lanka, Vietnam, Indonesia (1968), Burma/Myanmar (1970), Laos, Cambodia, several Pacific islands, Cuba and other islands in the Caribbean, Venezuela, and Brazil.

During the 25 years between 1956 and 1980 the mean number of cases of dengue haemorrhagic fever reported worldwide was about 30 000 per year, primarily in South-East Asia. This pattern, however, has been steadily changing. In the 5 years from 1981 to 1985 the mean number of cases of dengue haemorrhagic fever reported per year worldwide was 137 000 and this figure has doubled in the following 5 years. This dramatic increase reflects not only increased incidence in the countries of South-East Asia, but the emergence of the disease in countries of the Western Pacific, China and Taiwan, the Caribbean, and even in South America despite a large campaign to eradicate *Ae. aegypti* in many parts of that continent in the 1950s and 1960s. The first extensive epidemic of dengue haemorrhagic fever in the Americas was reported in Cuba in 1981, followed by another in Venezuela in 1989–1990, and today there is an increase in the incidence of sporadic cases of dengue haemorrhagic fever throughout the region. It is estimated that, since 1956, there have been 3 million hospital admissions and 45 000 deaths from dengue infection in the world.

Although dengue virus infections have been recognized for more than a century in many parts of the world, and dengue haemorrhagic fever has been of great importance in some countries of South-East Asia, it is now emerging as a principal endemoepidemic disease entity in the tropical and subtropical world. Just as the spread of dengue was influenced by movements of troops in the middle of the twentieth century, the world epidemiological picture is now being influenced by the explosion of international travel and trade, and by the forces of economic activity and cultural change.

Outbreaks are most frequent in areas where dengue infection occurs in early childhood and so classical dengue fever is rarely recognizable among the indigenous people. Annual outbreaks are observed in Burma, Indonesia, Thailand, and Vietnam. The vast majority of cases and deaths have been in children. Where environmental conditions are optimal for dengue transmission and multiple serotypes of dengue virus are simultaneously endemic or sequentially epidemic, infection with heterologous types is frequent. In endemic areas, dengue haemorrhagic fever occurs most frequently in children aged between 2 and 12 years, as older and many of the younger inhabitants are immune. However, cases in infants as young as 2 months and young adults in their twenties have been reported. This severe form of dengue is not confined to orientals, as shown by the recent outbreaks of dengue haemorrhagic fever in Cuba, other Caribbean islands, Venezuela, and Brazil. In these areas, where multiple serotypes of dengue virus have been reintroduced almost 30 years after their disappearance, dengue haemorrhagic fever occurred in adults in a relatively higher proportion than in Asian countries.

Dengue haemorrhagic fever is usually associated with secondary dengue infection but can appear during a primary dengue infection, especially in infants under the age of 1 year, all of whom possess maternal IgG dengue antibody. In Thailand, studies over the past 30 years have demonstrated transmission of all four dengue serotypes. Each serotype is capable of causing severe illness, but secondary infection with DEN2 was most common. In Cuba, the first outbreak of dengue haemorrhagic fever in 1981 occurred when DEN2 virus infected a large population immune to DEN1 following an outbreak of mild febrile illness in 1977. Based on epidemiological observations in many areas it has been suggested that the sequences of infecting dengue serotypes and probably the interval between the two infections may be important factors in determining the occurrence and severity of dengue haemorrhagic fever. A recent epidemiological study in Thailand revealed that a second infection with type 2 following type 1 infection is the highest risk factor.

THE HOST IMMUNE RESPONSE AND PATHOGENESIS

A person may be infected by dengue virus more than once. It is generally accepted that infection by one dengue virus serotype leads to an immune response that confers protection against reinfection by the same serotype. However, a second infection by a different serotype is possible, and is implicated in most patients who present with dengue haemorrhagic fever where the immune response is clearly secondary rather than primary. There are, of course, exceptions to this rule, but the epidemiological picture in South-East Asia supports the 'second infection hypothesis', which states that patients are more at risk of dengue haemorrhagic fever when they already have circulating antibodies against dengue virus. Subneutralizing levels of antidengue antibodies are thought to enhance the infectivity of the virus by increasing the efficiency of binding and uptake of virus–antibody complexes through Fc receptors present on cells of the monocyte–macrophage lineage, known to be the chief host cell in an infected person. The existence of this antibody-dependent enhancement has been well established *in vitro* but evidence of its relevance in patients relies on the observation that most cases of dengue haemorrhagic fever/dengue shock syndrome have, in the acute phase, antibodies capable of causing antibody-dependent enhancement *in vitro*. Further, it is argued that patients with dengue haemorrhagic fever below the age of 1 year, who clearly must have a primary immune response, have passively acquired maternal antibodies capable of causing antibody-dependent enhancement.

The role of antibody-dependent enhancement in pathogenesis is disputed by some but the shift in pattern of dengue fever to dengue haemorrhagic fever with increased circulation of different dengue virus serotypes in South America and the Caribbean mirrors the history of the rise of dengue haemorrhagic fever in South-East Asia. Increased population exposure to one viral serotype predisposes that population to dengue haemorrhagic fever when other serotypes are introduced.

A fascinating sequence homology has been observed between a 20-residue region of the E protein of DEN4 and plasminogen and other proteins of the blood coagulation pathway. Sera from patients with dengue haemorrhagic fever but not those from patients with Japanese encephalitis were found to contain antibodies that cross-reacted with plasminogen. This observation offers a fresh insight into the possible connection between dengue infection and perturbation of the coagulation pathway and associated homeostatic mechanisms.

Some attention has also been given to the study of cell-mediated immune responses and the role of cytokines in the pathogenesis of dengue haemorrhagic fever. It has been demonstrated that T lymphocytes are activated and produce interferon-γ and interleukin-2 *in vivo* during dengue haemorrhagic fever and dengue fever. While CD4+ T lymphocytes are activated at a higher level in dengue haemorrhagic fever than in dengue fever, CD8+ cells are significantly activated only in dengue haemorrhagic fever. These findings suggest that the rapid release of cytokines and chemical mediators caused by T-cell activation and by cytotoxic T-lymphocyte mediated lysis of dengue virus infected monocytes, and complement activation products trigger plasma leakage and coagulation derangement.

CLINICAL FEATURES

Typically the disease begins suddenly with high fever, facial flushing, and headache. Anorexia, vomiting, and abdominal pain are common. During the first few days, the illness resembles classical dengue fever in many respects but the maculopapular rash is infrequent. A haemorrhagic diathesis is frequently observed in the skin as scattered fine petechiae on extremities, axillae, trunk, and face. A positive tourniquet test and a tendency to bruise at venepuncture sites are invariably present. Bleeding from the nose, gums, and gastrointestinal tract is less common. Gross haematuria is extremely rare. The liver is often enlarged, soft, and tender.

The critical stage is reached after 2 to 7 days when the fever subsides. During or shortly after a rapid fall in the temperature there are circulatory disturbances of varying severity. The child may be sweating and restless, with cool extremities. In less severe cases, the changes in vital signs are minimal and transient, and the patient recovers spontaneously or after a brief period of fluid therapy. In more severe cases, shock ensues. The skin is cold, clammy, and sometimes cyanosed and the pulse pressure is often narrow (≤ 20 mmHg). The course of shock is short and stormy, and the patient may die within 24 to 48 h. Prolonged shock is often complicated by metabolic acidosis and severe bleeding, which indicate a poor prognosis. However, if the patient is properly treated before irreversible shock has developed, rapid, often dramatic, recovery is the rule. Infrequently, encephalitic signs associated with metabolic and electrolyte disturbances, intracranial haemorrhage, and hepatic failure (Reye's syndrome) occur and give rise to a more complicated course with a grave prognosis. Convalescence is generally short and uneventful. Sinus bradycardia is common and occasionally a confluent petechial rash is observed, mostly on the lower extremities. The illness lasts from 7 to 10 days in most cases.

A normal white blood-cell count or leucopenia are common initially and neutrophils may predominate. A relative lymphocytosis with more than 15 per cent of atypical lymphocytes is usually observed towards the end of the febrile period. Thrombocytopenia and haemoconcentration are constant findings. The platelet count drops shortly before, or at the same time as, the haematocrit rises; both changes occur before fever has subsided and before onset of shock. Clotting abnormalities are found, especially in patients with shock. Other changes include hypoalbuminaemia, hyponatraemia, and mild elevation of serum alanine aminotransferase.

Identification of these characteristic manifestations allows an accurate clinical diagnosis of dengue haemorrhagic fever, before the critical shock stage has developed. The World Health Organization (**WHO**) has established criteria for clinical diagnosis: high continuous fever for 2 to 7 days, a haemorrhagic diathesis, hepatomegaly, thrombocytopenia (≤ 100 000/mm^2) with haemoconcentration (haematocrit increased by 20 per cent or more), and shock. Four grades of severity are recognized: grade I uncomplicated, grade II with spontaneous haemorrhage, grade III shock, and grade IV profound shock with imperceptible pulse or blood pressure. Two laboratory changes, thrombocytopenia with concurrent haemoconcentration, are essential for the diagnosis of dengue haemorrhagic fever and its differential diagnosis from simple dengue fever and other infectious diseases.

PATHOPHYSIOLOGY (FIG. 1)

The hallmarks of the disease are leakage of plasma and abnormal haemostasis. Shock is caused by a critical loss of plasma volume, presumably resulting from increased vascular permeability. Evidence of plasma leakage includes the rapid rise in haematocrit, the development of pleural effusion, ascites and hypoproteinaemia, and the reduction in plasma volume. The acute onset of shock and the rapid and often dramatic clinical recovery when the patient is treated properly, together with the absence of inflammatory vascular lesions, suggest a transient change in vascular permeability. Immune complexes have been demonstrated and are thought to play a part in complement activation, which results in profound depression of C3 and C5 concentrations. Anaphylotoxins C3a and C5a, products of complement activation, are elevated at the same time as plasma leakage and their levels correlate with disease severity. The rapid inactivation and elimination of these anaphylotoxins from the circulation is consistent with the short duration of shock. Another factor is the enhancement by pre-existing heterotypic antibodies (antibody-dependent enhancement, see above) of virus multiplication in monocytes. This may trigger the monocytes, to produce chemical mediators of vascular permeability, and the activation of complement and tissue thromboplastin, which may initiate intravascular blood coagulation. Bradykinin has not been implicated in vascular permeability change.

The haemostatic disorder involves vascular change, thrombocytopenia, and coagulopathy. Increased fibrinogen consumption and decreased factor VIII concentration imply disseminated intravascular coagulation, which is probably responsible for the severe bleeding. The bone marrow shows maturation arrest of megakaryocytes during the early phase of the illness. At autopsy there are serous effusions and widespread petechial haemorrhages in many organs. Vascular changes include vasodilatation, congestion, oedema, and haemorrhage. Proliferation of reticuloendothelial cells and accelerated phagocytic activity of lymphocytes are frequently observed. Necrosis of hepatocytes and Küpffer cells may be seen. Cerebral oedema and intracranial haemorrhage are infrequently observed. There is no histological evidence of encephalitis.

AETIOLOGICAL DIAGNOSIS

Patients with dengue infection may have a primary or a secondary immune response, which is often referred to as primary or secondary dengue, although this is not strictly correct. The diagnosis of dengue fever, dengue haemorrhagic fever, or dengue shock syndrome is purely clinical, based on the criteria described, and it is important to remember that the role of the virology laboratory is to confirm the aetiological diagnosis. Assays are needed to confirm the diagnosis of dengue in patients with secondary as well as primary immune responses.

Detection of virus

Dengue virus may be propagated in mosquitoes as well as in cell lines. Adult mosquitoes can be used to detect the presence of dengue virus in patients' sera. The growth of virus in these mosquitoes is usually confirmed by detection of viral antigen in head squashes, using immunofluorescence techniques. Mosquito cell lines derived from *Ae. albopictus*, *Ae. pseudoscutellaris*, and *Toxorhynchitis* may also be used to isolate virus from patients' specimens. Virus is normally detected by using monoclonal antibodies and the immunofluorescence technique. Monoclonals specific for the four different serotypes may be used for serotyping and a flavivirus-reactive or group-reactive monoclonal antibody may be used for first-line screening to determine the presence of the virus. The real problem with this technique is that most clinical specimens do not yield detectable virus. Intrathoracic inoculation of adult mosquitoes yields positive results in up to 60 per cent only of serologically proven dengue cases, while inoculation of mosquito cell lines offers a 15 to 20 per cent positivity. These techniques are extremely demanding. They may be improved by the use of molecular biology. Radiolabelled RNA probes can detect, by molecular hybridization, the RNA of dengue virus in mosquito pools, and nucleic acid hybridization can detect dengue RNA in purified virus and in infected cell lines.

Detection of antibody

1. Haemagglutination inhibition test

This test requires the collection of paired sera 10 to 14 days apart. End-point titres against the four dengue serotypes must be determined to establish a fourfold seroconversion. This 'method of choice', described by the WHO Technical Advisory Group on dengue haemorrhagic fever/dengue shock syndrome, remains the reference test for confirmation of dengue virus infections. However, it is time-consuming and needs to be optimized with each batch of haemagglutinins and erythrocytes used because of the exquisite pH sensitivity of the dengue haemagglutinin-binding reaction to the goose erythrocytes now commonly used in this assay. Fresh reagents are required, making this a difficult test to use in a decentralized system of confirmation and control.

In primary dengue the acute-phase serum collected before the fourth day after onset of illness should have a titre not higher than 1:20, seroconverting after 2 to 3 weeks to a titre not higher than 1:1280. In secondary dengue, acute-phase sera often have titres greater than 1:20 and convalescent serum titres are expected to be higher than 1:1280. The acute-phase titres are often as high as 1:1280 and so no convincing seroconversion may be observed. Such cases are not presumptively considered to be recent dengue infections unless the presence of dengue-specific IgM can be established.

2. The IgM capture assay

The detection of antidengue IgM in serum has been successfully applied to confirm dengue infection, but as it is not always possible to detect IgM in the early or admission sera of patients with primary or secondary dengue, a second serum is often required. An IgM seroconversion is usually seen by the third or fourth day after defervescence. Experience in Thailand shows that 20 to 30 per cent of patients do not have detectable IgM in sera collected on admission. It is therefore advisable rou-

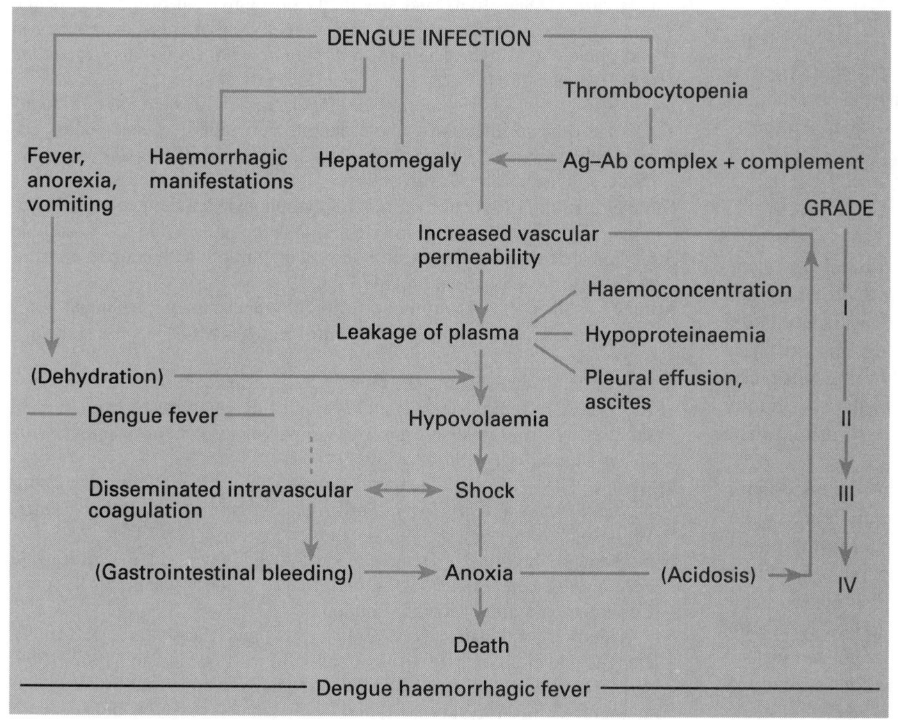

Fig. 1 Pathophysiology and disease severity.

tinely to collect serum specimens on admission and before discharge to confirm the initial laboratory diagnosis.

3. Dot enzyme immunoassay

Paired patient sera collected 3 to 5 days apart are tested at a single dilution, usually 1:500 or 1:1000. Either a strong IgG response (greater than 1:1280 haemagglutination inhibition equivalent) or seroconversion is observed, without the need to do doubling dilutions for testing against multiple serotypes as in the haemagglutination inhibition test.

Detection of the presence of the viral genome

As the dengue virus is a positive-strand RNA virus, cDNA must first be generated using reverse transcriptase and suitable downstream primers before polymerase chain reaction is possible. After amplification by that reaction, it is still necessary to confirm the presence of the correct sequences using nested primers, restriction analysis or probing with radiolabelled or non-radioactively labelled oligonucleotides that have sequences selected to confirm specificity.

These molecular techniques may be used to detect the presence of viral genomes and also to type the viruses detected for epidemiological purposes.

TREATMENT

The management of dengue haemorrhagic fever is entirely symptomatic and is aimed at correcting hypovalaemia during the period of leakage, that is for 24 to 48 h. Prognosis depends on early clinical recognition and frequent monitoring of patients for a drop in platelet count and rise in haematocrit. When the haematocrit rises sharply as plasma leaks out, early volume replacement can prevent shock. When shock has developed, satisfactory results have been obtained with the following regimen: replace plasma volume losses immediately and rapidly with isotonic saline and plasma or plasma expander in cases of profound shock, then continue to replace further plasma losses to maintain effective circulation for a period of 24 to 48 h; correct metabolic and electrolyte disturbances (acidosis and hyponatraemia); give fresh blood transfusions and occasionally platelet-rich plasma in cases of significant bleeding. It is important to stop replacement when the haematocrit returns to normal, the vital signs become stable, and diuresis ensues. Excessive fluid replacement at this stage can cause heart failure and pulmonary oedema when extravasated plasma is reabsorbed.

With this regimen the case-fatality rate of patients in shock at the Children's Hospital in Bangkok has fallen to below 1 per cent. There is no evidence that corticosteroid is of benefit in reducing the case-fatality rate. The efficacy of heparin in the treatment of cases with disseminated intravascular clotting has not been proved.

CONTROL

Of paramount importance is the control of the main vector, *Ae. aegypti*, by eliminating the breeding places in and around houses such as stagnant water in flower pots, old jars, tin cans, and old tyres. Larvicides should be used periodically for water stored in larger containers for household consumption and insecticide spraying should be used during outbreaks. Efforts should be focused on educating all members of the community to provide active participation and cooperation to reduce or eliminate the vector's breeding sites.

A live, attenuated, tetravalent dengue vaccine has been developed in Thailand and is currently undergoing phase II trials in children.

The possible role of antibody-dependent enhancement in the pathogenesis of dengue haemorrhagic fever must be taken into account in vaccine design. Antibodies able to bind to the virion may also be able to cause the enhancement. This has led to two main approaches to the design of a vaccine against dengue. In the first, where attenuated viruses are used as the candidate vaccine, a tetravalent vaccine consisting of all four serotypes is considered necessary. In the second, where the techniques of molecular biology are to be used, the candidate vaccines may be expected to exclude 'enhancing epitopes' in the E components, or else to use proteins other than E such as NS1. When it was shown in the mid-1980s that passively administered antibodies against NS1 could confer protection against flavivirus infection, there was a spurt in research activity into NS1, which is now known to be an important immunogen in the natural infection. More recently it has been demonstrated that dengue preM can also confer protective immunity.

REFERENCES

Bhamarapravati, N., Boonyapaknavik, V., and Nimsomburana, P. (1966). Pathology of Thai haemorrhagic fever. An autopsy study. *Bulletin of the World Health Organization*, **35,** 48–9.

Bundo, K., Chanyasanha, C., La Linn, M., Torres, C.A., and Igarashi, A. (1986). IgM capture ELISA for serodiagnosis on Japanese encephalitis virus and its differentiation from dengue virus infection. *Japanese Encephalitis and Haemorrhagic Fever Research Society Bulletin*, **1,** 27–35.

Burke, D.S. and Nisalak, A. (1982). Detection of Japanese encephalitis virus immunoglobulin M antibodies in serum by antibody capture radioimmunoassay. *Journal of Clinical Microbiology*, **15,** 353–61.

Cardosa, M.J. and Tio, P.H. (1991). Dot enzyme immunoassay: an alternative diagnostic aid for dengue fever and dengue haemorrhagic fever. *Bulletin of the World Health Organization*, **69,** 741–5.

Clarke, D.H. and Casals, J. (1958). Techniques for haemagglutination and haemagglutination inhibition with arthropod borne viruses. *American Journal of Tropical Medicine and Hygiene*, **7,** 561–73.

Edelman, R., Nimmannitya, S., Colman, R.W., Talamo, R.C., and Top, F.H. (1975). Evaluation of the plasma kinin system in dengue hemorrhagic fever. *Journal of Laboratory and Clinical Medicine*, **86,** 410–12.

Funahara, Y. *et al.* (1980). An acute type of disseminated intravascular coagulation characterized by decrease of α_2-plasmin inhibitor in dengue haemorrhagic fever. In *Proceedings of the first ICMR seminar 'Dengue haemorrhagic fever'*, pp. 217–19. International Center for Medical Research, Kobe, Japan.

Guzman, M.G., Kouri, G., Morier, L., Soler, M., and Fernandez A. (1984). A study of fatal hemorrhagic dengue cases in Cuba, 1981. *Pan-American Health Organization Bulletin*, **18,** 213–20.

Halstead, S.B. (1988). Pathogenesis of dengue: challenges to molecular biology. *Science*, **139,** 476–81.

Henchal, E.A., Polo, S.L., Vorndam, V., Yaemsiri, C., Innis, B.L., and Hoke, C.H. (1991). Sensitivity and specificity of a universal primer set for the rapid diagnosis of dengue virus infections by polymerase chain reaction and nucleic acid hybridization. *American Journal of Tropical Medicine and Hygiene*, **45,** 418–28.

Innis, B.L. *et al.* (1989). An enzyme-linked immunosorbent assay to characterize dengue infections where dengue and Japanese encephalitis cocirculate. *American Journal of Tropical Medicine and Hygiene*, **40,** 418–27.

Kurane, I. *et al.* (1991). Activation of T lymphocytes in dengue virus infections. High levels soluble interleukin-2 receptor, soluble CD4, soluble CD8, interleukin 2 and interferon in sera of children with dengue. *Journal of Clinical Investigation*, **88,** 1473–80.

Kurane, I., *et al.* (1994). Immunopathologic mechanisms of dengue hemorrhagic fever and dengue shock syndrome. *Archives of Virology (suppl.)*, **9,** 59–64.

Lanciotti, R.S., Calisher, C.H., Gubler, D.J., Chang, G.J., and Vorndam, A.V. (1992). Rapid detection and typing of dengue viruses from clinical samples by using reverse transcriptase–polymerase chain reaction. *Journal of Clinical Microbiology*, **30,** 545–51.

Malasit, P. (1987). Complement and dengue haemorrhagic fever/shock syndrome. *Southeast Asian Journal of Tropical Medicine and Public Health*, **18,** 316–20.

Nimmannitya, S. (1981). Dengue haemorrhagic fever. In *Paediatrics in developing countries*, (ed. G.J. Ebrahim), pp. 155–61. Macmillan Tropical Community Health Manuals, London.

Nimmannitya, S., Halstead, S.B., Cohen, S.N., and Margiotta, M.R. (1969). Dengue and chikungunya virus infection in man in Thailand 1962–1964. *American Journal of Tropical Medicine and Hygiene*, **18,** 954–71.

Nimmannitya, S., Tisayakorn, U., and Hemsrichart V. (1988). Dengue hem-

orrhagic fever with unusual manifestations. *Southeast Asian Journal of Tropical Medicine and Public Health*, **19,** 585–90.
Rice, C.M., Strauss, E.G., and Strauss, J.H. (1986). Structure of the flavivirus genome. In *The togaviridae and flaviviridae*, (ed. S. Schlesinger and M.J. Schlesinger), pp. 279–326. Plenum, New York.
Sangkawawhibha, N. *et al.* (1984). Risk factors in dengue shock syndrome: a prospective epidemiologic study in Rayong, Thailand. *American Journal of Epidemiology* **120,** 653–69.
Shope, R.E. (1990). Antigen and antibody detection and update on the diagnosis of dengue. *Southeast Asian Journal of Tropical Medicine and Public Health,* **21,** 642–5.
Srichaikul, T. *et al.* (1977). Fibrinogen metabolism and DIC in dengue hemorrhagic fever. *American Journal of Tropical Medicine and Hygiene*, **26,** 525–32.
Sumarmo, Talogo, W., and Asrin, A. (1982). Failure of hydrocortisone to effect outcome in dengue shock syndrome. *Pediatrics*, **69,** 45–9.
World Health Organization (1986). *Dengue haemorrhagic fever: diagnosis, treatment and control.* WHO, Geneva.

7.10.21 Bunyaviridae

J. S. Porterfield and J. W. LeDuc

The family Bunyaviridae currently contains around 300 viruses, and is divided into five genera (see Table 1). The family name, and that of the genus Bunyavirus, is derived from the type species, Bunyamwera virus, which was isolated in Uganda from Aedes mosquitoes. The other genera are also named after viruses, the genus Hantavirus after Hantaan virus, the causative agent of Korean haemorrhagic fever, the genus Nairovirus after Nairobi sheep disease virus, the genus Phlebovirus after Phlebotomus or sandfly fever virus and the genus Tospovirus after tomato spotted-wilt virus. All members of the family share certain structural, biochemical and genetic properties, such as a spherical, enveloped virion 80 to 120 nm in diameter (see Fig. 1), and a genome of single-stranded, negative sense RNA divided into three segments. Members of different genera vary substantially in their biological and biochemical properties and in the details of their mechanisms of replication. Bunyaviruses, nairoviruses and phleboviruses, which together make up the greater part of the family, are all *ar*thropod-*bo*rne animal viruses, or arboviruses; these circulate in nature in a wide variety of different vertebrate hosts and are biologically transmitted between vertebrates and to man by the bites of blood-sucking arthropods, principally mosquitoes for bunyaviruses, sandflies for phleboviruses, and ticks for nairoviruses. By contrast, hantaviruses are not arboviruses, but are zoonotic agents infecting rodents and other small mammals, which may spread to man if he is in close contact with their infected excreta, and tospoviruses are arthropod-transmitted plant viruses, of no known medical importance.

Viruses within the larger genera are further subdivided into serogroups of more closely related members, there being at least 18 serogroups within the bunyaviruses, and seven within the nairoviruses (see Table 1). Of over 60 Bunyaviridae that are known to infect man, the type species and those that cause major human diseases are shown in bold type in Table 1 and are described in more detail in the following sections. Table 2 lists the continental distribution of the remaining viruses that cause only minor human infections and also indicates the principal arthropod vector of each virus. The habitats in which the different viruses and their vectors occur range from arctic to tropical, with every intermediate form. The enzootic cycles by which arboviruses are maintained in nature are very imperfectly understood; most viruses undergo alternate cycles of replication in vertebrate and invertebrate hosts, but transovarial and trans-stadial transmission within some mosquitoes, ticks and phlebotomine flies, and venereal transmission from vertically infected male mosquitoes to uninfected females are also known to occur. Most arboviruses have a narrow host range, occur within a limited area, and are transmitted by specific vectors to a limited number of vertebrate hosts, but some viruses infect a wider host range, are transmitted by more than one type of vector, and may occur in more than a single continent. It is of interest that, for different members of the family, tick transmission predominates in Asia, but is unknown in South or Central America, and although some Bunyaviridae have been isolated in Australia, none is known to infect man in that continent. Further epidemiological details can be found in more specialized publications.

Following viral entry, whether through the skin after the bite of an infected arthropod or by another route, virus replicates in draining lymph nodes, which are frequently enlarged, and a viraemia follows. Symptoms develop when virus lodges in other sites and undergoes further replication cycles. Appropriate virucidal agents and methods include bleach, phenolic disinfectants and detergents, autoclaving or boiling, and the use of γ-irradiation. Various enzymes such as nucleases will also inactivate these viruses. For human pathogens with the ability to spread by the aerosol route, biosafety level 3 (hantaviruses, Oropouche virus, others) or 4 (Crimean–Congo haemorrhagic fever virus only) is recommended. Added precautions are necessary when handling hantavirus-infected animals.

REFERENCES

Centers for Disease Control and Prevention. (1994). Laboratory management of agents associated with hantavirus pulmonary syndrome: interim biosafety guidelines. *Morbidity and Mortality Weekly Report*, **43,** (No. RR-7), 1–7.
Francki, R.I.B., Fauquet, C.M., Knudson, D.L., and Brown, F. (ed.) (1991). Classification and Nomenclature of Viruses: Fifth Report of the International Committee on Taxonomy of Viruses. *Archives of Virology* (suppl. 2), 1–450.
Monath, T.P. (ed.) (1989). *The arboviruses: epidemiology and ecology*. CRC Press, Boca Raton, FA.
Smithburn, K.C., Haddow, A.J., and Mahaffy, A.F. (1946). Neurotropic virus isolated from *Aedes* mosquitoes caught in Semliki Forest. *American Journal of Tropical Medicine*, **26,** 189–208.

Genus Bunyavirus

Much of our knowledge about the family as a whole derives from intensive studies on the type species, Bunyamwera virus, and a few other members of this large genus. The three-segmented genome permits reassortment when two closely related viruses infect the same cell, either in nature or under controlled laboratory conditions. Such studies have been used to establish the genomic control of viral proteins, and to analyse the basis of virulence for both vertebrate and invertebrate hosts. Two bunyaviruses, Akabane and Aino viruses in the Simbu serogroup, are notable for their ability to produce congenital deformities in sheep, goats, and cattle in Japan, Australia, Africa, and in the Middle East. However, there is as yet no evidence that any member of the genus or family produces teratogenic effects in man, although there is evidence that Oropouche virus, an important Simbu serogroup pathogen of northern South America, may be a threat to pregnant women.

Bunyamwera virus

Symptoms

A mild, febrile illness, usually with headache, joint and back pains, sometimes associated with a rash, and occasionally with mild involvement of the central nervous system. Serological surveys indicated that infection of man is widespread in subSaharan Africa but most infections are unrecognized. Laboratory infections have been recorded.

Treatment and prognosis

No treatment is necessary and the prognosis is excellent.

Table 1 *The family Bunyaviridae: its genera, serogroups, vectors and viruses infecting man*

Genus	Serogroup	Vector	Viruses infecting man
Bunyavirus (over 150)	Anopheles A (12)	Mosquito	Tacaiuma
	Anopheles B (2)	Mosquito	
	Bakau (5)	Mosquito	
	Bunyamwera (32)	Mosquito	**Bunyamwera**[1], Calovo, Germiston, Ilesha, Maguari, Shokwe, Tensaw, Wyeomyia
	Bwamba (2)	Mosquito	**Bwamba**, Pongola
	C group (14)	Mosquito	Apeu, Caraparu, Itaqui, Madrid, Marituba, Murutucu, Nepuyo, Oriboca, Ossa, Restan
	California (14)	Mosquito	**California encephalitis**, Guaroa, **La Crosse**, **Inkoo**, **Jamestown Canyon**, **snowshoe hare**, **Tahyna**, trivittatus
	Capim (10)	Mosquito	
	Gamboa (8)	Mosquito	
	Guama (12)	Mosquito	Catu, Guama
	Koongol (2)	Mosquito	
	Minatitlan (2)	Mosquito	
	Nyando (2)	Mosquito	Nyando
	Olifanstsvlei (5)	Mosquito	
	Patois (7)	Mosquito	
	Simbu (24)	Mosquito	**Oropouche**, Shuni
	Tete (5)	Mosquito	
	Turlock (5)	Mosquito	
	Unassigned (3)	Mosquito	
Hantavirus (8)	Hantaan (8)	None	**Muerto Canyon**, **Hantaan**, Prospect Hill, **Puumala**, **Seoul**
Nairovirus (32)	Crimean–Congo (3)	Tick	**Crimean–Congo haemorrhagic fever**, Hazara
	Dera Ghazi Khan (6)	Tick	
	Hughes (10)	Tick	Soldado
	Nairobi S.D. (3)	Tick	Dugbe, Ganjam, Nairobi Sheep Disease
	Qalyub (3)	Tick	
	Sakhalin (7)	Tick	Avalon
	Thiafora (2)	Tick	
Phlebovirus (57)	Phlebotomus (44)	Sandfly[2]	Alenquer, Candiru, **Chagres**, Corfu, **Punta Toro**, **Rift Valley fever**[2], **Naples**, **Sandfly Fever**, and **Sicilian**,**Toscana**
	Uukuniemi (13)	Tick	Uukuniemi, Zalev-Terpeniya
Unassigned (53)		Mosquito	Bangui, Kasokero, Tataguine
		Tick	Bhanja, Keterah, Tamdy, Wanowrie
Tospovirus (1)		Thrip	

Numbers in parentheses indicate the approximate number of viruses in the genus or serogroup.

[1]Bold type indicates the type species and viruses causing major disease in man.

[2]Mosquito vector for Rift Valley fever virus.

California encephalitis virus, Inkoo, Jamestown Canyon, La Crosse, Tahyna, and snowshoe hare viruses

The viruses named above, and perhaps others currently unrecognized, are responsible for the clinical condition known as California encephalitis. The viruses are widely distributed in nature throughout many parts of North America, Europe, and Eurasia. Most recognized human infections in the United States are reported from Wisconsin, Iowa, Indiana, Minnesota or Ohio, but at least 20 states have reported one or more cases. The great majority of these occur in children, more often males than females, although Jamestown Canyon virus is unusual in that more adults are involved. There is nearly always a history of outdoor exposure in areas where woodland mosquitoes are prevalent. The incubation period is 5 to 10 days, and is followed by a gradual onset of symptoms, with fever, mild at first, and becoming more severe and frontal, leading to mental confusion and convulsions. Neck rigidity is common, as is nausea and vomiting. General lethargy may progress to coma, and although there may be meningeal signs, paralysis or permanent damage to the central nervous system is rare and the mortality is less than 1 per cent.

Fig. 1 Electron micrograph of Crimean–Congo haemorrhagic fever virus (× 400 000) (courtesy of Dr. D.S. Ellis).

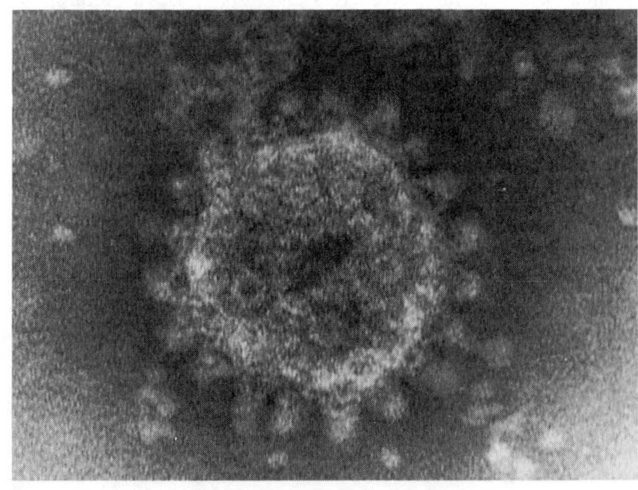

Table 2 *Bunyaviridae causing only mild or trivial infections in man, arranged on a geographical basis*

Africa	North America	Central America	South America	Europe	Asia
Bangui M[1]	Avalon T[2]	Madrid M	Alenquer P[3]	Bhanja T	Batai M
Bhanja T	Fort Sherman	Ossa M	Apeu M	Calovo M	Bhanja T
Bwamba M	Tensaw M	Restan M	Candiru P	Corfou P	Issyk-Kul T
Dugbe T	trivittatus M	trivittatus M	Caraparu M	Inkoo M	Ganjam T
Germiston M			Catu M	Tahyna M	Hazara T
Ilesha M			Guama M, P	Tamdy T	Keterah T
Kasokero M			Guaroa M	Uukuniemi T	Wanowrie T
Nyando M			Maguari M		Zaliv Terpeniya M, T
Pongola M			Marituba M		
Shokwe M			Murutucu M		
Shuni M			Restan M		
Tataguine M			Tacaiuma M		
Thiafora			Wyeomyia M		
Wanowrie T					

[1]M indicates that the virus is transmitted by mosquitoes.

[2]T indicates that the virus is transmitted by ticks.

[3]P indicates that the virus is transmitted by phlebotomine flies.

In Europe, Tahyna virus is widely distributed in Austria, the former Czechoslovakia, France, Germany, Italy, Norway, Romania, the former Yugoslavia, and the former USSR. Antibody rates can exceed 95 per cent in certain parts of Czechoslovakia, and are around 50 per cent in the Rhone valley in France and the Danube basin near Vienna; however, overt disease is seldom recognized. Inkoo virus is prevalent in Finland and in neighbouring regions of Russia, with the great majority of adult Lapps having antibodies; emerging information suggests that small children may have signs of central nervous involvement during acute infection. Antibodies reactive with California serogroup viruses have also been found in human sera collected in Sri Lanka, China, and in the far northern latitudes of Eurasia where a number of California serogroup viruses have been isolated from mosquitoes, some related to Inkoo and Tahyna viruses, but others to snowshoe hare virus. In another Russian study of some 50 persons, mainly 14 to 30 years of age, with infections caused by California serogroup viruses, about two-thirds had an influenza-like illness without central nervous involvement, while the remaining third had aseptic meningitis.

Control, treatment, and prognosis

Measures to limit mosquito breeding, particularly of *Aedes triseriatus*, are useful in endemic regions. No vaccines are available, and there is no specific treatment, although the fluid and electrolyte balance must be maintained, and anticonvulsive drugs may be required to control seizures. Between 5 and 15 per cent of patients may have recurrent seizures, but with a low case fatality rate the general prognosis is good.

REFERENCES

Butenko, A.M., Galkina, I.V., Kuznetsov, A.A., Kolobukhina, L.V., Lvov, S.D., and Nedyalkova, M.S. (1990). Serological evidence of the distribution of California serogroup viruses in the U.S.S.R. *Archives of Virology* (supp. 1), 235–41.

Kolobukhina, L.V., Lvov, D.K., Butenko, A.M., Nedyalkova, M.S., Kuznetsov, A.A., and Galkina, I.V. (1990). Signs and symptoms of infections caused by California serogroup viruses in humans in the U.S.S.R. *Archives of Virology* (suppl. 1), 243–9.

LeDuc, J.W. (1987). Epidemiology and ecology of California serogroup viruses. *American Journal of Tropical Medicine and Hygiene*, **37**, 60–8S.

Oropouche virus

Symptoms

Prior to 1961, Oropouche virus was known to have caused only a mild fever in a single forest worker in Trinidad, but that year it was responsible for a substantial epidemic in the Belem area of northern Brazil, with some 7000 individuals affected. Over the ensuing 30 years, massive epidemics of febrile illness have been recorded throughout the Amazon Basin, with perhaps as many as 200 000 persons infected. Symptoms include headache, generalized body pains, back pains, prostration, and moderately high fever (40 °C). Rash occasionally accompanies infection, as does meningitis or meningismus. Illness lasts from 2 to 5 days, occasionally with protracted convalescence. No fatalities have been reported.

Control, treatment, and prognosis

No vaccine is available. Transmission is probably by the biting midge, *Culicoides paraensis*, and outbreaks appear to be a long-term consequence of agricultural development of the Amazon Basin. Accumulated organic waste from cacao and banana production provide ideal breeding sites for Culicoides, leading to massive populations and subsequent epidemic Oropouche disease. Thus, measures to reduce Culicoides breeding may be of benefit. Treatment is supportive, and the prognosis is good, although convalescence may be protracted.

REFERENCE

Pinheiro, F.P. *et al.* (1981). Oropouche virus. I. A review of clinical, epidemiological, and ecological findings. *American Journal of Tropical Medicine and Hygiene*, **30**, 149–60.

Genus Hantavirus

The genus Hantavirus takes its name from Hantaan virus, the cause of Korean haemorrhagic fever in Korea. The name Hantaan in turn is from the Hantaan River near the demilitarized zone between North and South Korea, where the virus was first recovered from its rodent host, *Apodemus agrarius*. Hantaan virus was only isolated in 1976, although the clinical diseases it and related hantaviruses cause have been known much longer under many different synonyms; epidemic haemorrhagic fever, Korean haemorrhagic fever, nephropathia epidemica, haemorrhagic fever with renal syndrome, and others. The World Health Organization has adopted the term haemorrhagic fever with renal syndrome to serve as a common name for hantaviral disease. Three distinct viruses are responsible for most recognized haemorrhagic fever with renal syndrome: Hantaan virus, found primarily in Asia, with an enclave of disease in the Balkan region of Europe; Puumala virus, found in Scandinavia, western Russia, and recently in much of Europe; and Seoul virus, probably globally distributed wherever *Rattus norvegicus* populations exist uncontrolled. Hantaan virus causes a severe, life-threatening disease with mortality of about 5 per cent, reaching as high as 30 per cent in select populations. Puumala virus infections are less severe, although patients still require admission to hospital, with death in less than 1 per cent of admitted cases. Seoul virus is thought to be the least severe of the pathogenic strains of hantaviruses, although it too has been associated with human deaths.

Each hantavirus is specifically associated with a particular rodent host in nature: Hantaan virus with the striped field mouse, *Apodemus agrarius*; Puumala virus with the bank vole, *Clethrionomys glareolus*; and Seoul virus with the Norway rat, *Rattus norvegicus*. Human infection is from aerosols of infectious rodent excreta, and is occupationally associated. Most disease is seen among adult men in rural environments. Occupations at greatest risk include farmers, woodcutters, shepherds, and especially the military in the field. Most hantavirus disease is markedly seasonal, with peak incidence seen in the late fall and early winter, although the Balkan form is found most commonly during summer months in Greece and adjacent countries.

Symptoms

Incubation period for hantaviruses is rather variable, and may approach 2 months in some cases, but is generally 12 to 16 days. Severe disease, as typically associated with Hantaan virus infection in Asia or the Balkans, is characterized by five phases:

(1) febrile, of 3 to 7 days' duration;
(2) hypotensive, lasting from a few hours to 3 days;
(3) oliguric, 3 to 7 days;
(4) diuretic, from a few days to weeks;
(5) a prolonged convalescence.

Characteristic signs and symptoms of the febrile phase include fever, malaise, headache, myalgia, back pain, abdominal pain, nausea and vomiting, facial flushing, petechiae, and conjunctival haemorrhage (Fig. 2). The hypotensive phase is characterized by nausea, vomiting, tachycardia, hypotension, blurred vision, haemorrhagic signs and shock, with approximately one-third of the deaths occurring during this phase. In the oliguric phase, nausea and vomiting may persist, and blood pressure may rise, kidney failure presents, which may include frank anuria, and about one-third of the cases may experience severe haemorrhage as epistaxis, gastrointestinal, cutaneous or bleeding at other sites. Nearly one-half of deaths occur during the oliguric phase. In the diuretic phase urine output increases to several litres per day. Convalescence is protracted and may require months before full strength and function is regained.

Fig. 2 Patient with acute Korean haemorrhagic fever, showing extensive conjunctival haemorrhages (by courtesy of Professor H.W. Lee).

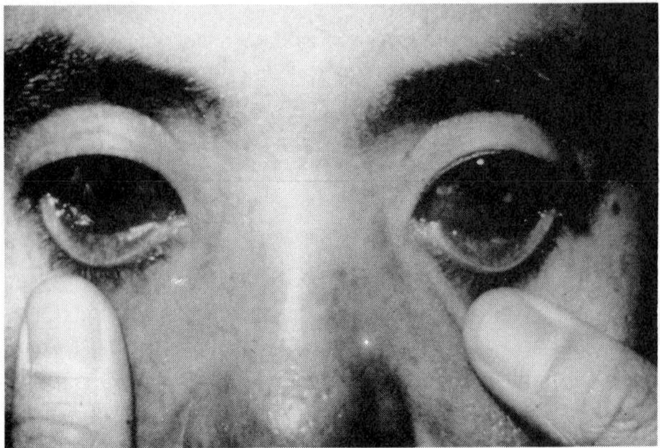

Less severe forms of the disease may skip phases, or spend less time in each phase. The milder forms of haemorrhagic fever with renal syndrome, such as nephropathia epidemica due to Puumala virus, follow a similar, but less severe course, with abrupt onset of fever of 38 to 40 °C, headache, malaise, backache, and generalized abdominal pain. Back or loin pain is especially common. Signs of renal failure are usually not as pronounced, and the need for renal dialysis varies. Transient blurred vision occurs in about 10 per cent of cases. Infection due to Seoul virus follows a similar course, but may present with more evidence of liver involvement. There is no evidence of person-to-person transmission.

Recently, hantavirus disease was reported from the United States affecting at least 68 people, mainly adults, from 17 states. More than half the identified cases have died. Most cases were reported from New Mexico, Arizona, Colorado, and Utah, and the newly recognized hantavirus thought to cause this disease has been named Muerto Canyon virus. This virus appears to be associated with deer mice (*Peromyscus maniculatus*) and is unusual in that symptoms are primarily those of acute unexplained adult respiratory distress syndrome, rather than renal disease. On admission, physical examination of confirmed cases reveals fever (> 38 °C), tachycardia (> 100/min), tachypnoea (> 20/min), and often hypotension (systolic < 100 mmHg), and rales. Laboratory findings include hypoxia, leucocytosis, haemoconcentration, thrombocytopenia, atypical lymphocytosis, elevated serum LDH and SGPT, and prolonged PTT (> 14 s).

Treatment, prognosis, and control

Admission to hospital, avoidance of trauma and unnecessary movement, close observation, and careful supportive care are essential to patient survival. Treatment is phase specific, with special attention to fluid balance and volume, and control of hypotension and shock. Dialysis may be required in cases of acute renal failure. Specific antiviral therapy using ribavirin has been shown to be efficacious if started early in disease. Recovery is protracted, but heretofore considered complete and without permanent complications. Recent evidence, however, suggests that persons previously infected with Seoul virus may be at increased risk of chronic renal disease, hypertension, or stroke.

Prevention involves avoidance of infected rodents, either through efficient rodent control programmes in urban settings for Seoul virus, or maintenance of clean campsites so that waste food is not allowed to accumulate and attract rodents. Vaccine development is under way, but at present none is available for routine use.

REFERENCES

Centers for Disease Control and Prevention. (1993). Update: Hantavirus Infection—United States, 1993. *Morbidity and Mortality Weekly Reports*, **42,** 517–19.

Glass, G.E., Watson, A.J., LeDuc, J.W., Kelen, G.D., Quinn, T.C. and Childs, J.E. (1993). Infection with a ratborne hantavirus in U.S. residents is consistently associated with hypertensive and renal disease. *Journal of Infectious Diseases*, **167,** 614–20.

Huggins, J.W. *et al.* (1991). Prospective double-blind, concurrent, placebo-controlled clinical trial of intravenous ribavirin in the therapy of hemorrhagic fever with renal syndrome. *Journal of Infectious Diseases*, **164,** 1119–27.

Nichol, S.T., Spiropoulou, C.F., Morzunov, S. *et al.* (1993). Genetic identification of a hantavirus associated with an outbreak of acute respiratory illness. *Science*, **262,** 914–7.

Genus Nairovirus

The genus Nairovirus is named after Nairobi sheep disease, an acute, haemorrhagic gastroenteritis affecting sheep and goats in East Africa, which was first described by Montgomery (1917), who correctly attributed the condition to a virus, and pointed out that transmission was due to the sheep tick, *Rhipicephalus appendiculatus*. In addition to the type species, which has caused laboratory infections, the genus also includes several other viruses known to infect man, of which the most important is Crimean–Congo haemorrhagic fever virus. Other nairoviruses causing less important human infections are Ganjam virus, almost indistinguishable from Nairobi sheep disease virus but first isolated in India from *Haemaphysalis intermedia* ticks collected from healthy goats; Hazara virus, recovered from *Ixodes redkorzevi* ticks collected from the vole *Alticola roylei*, in a subarctic habitat at an altitude of 12 000 feet (3660 m) in the Khaghan valley of Hazara district, Pakistan; Dugbe virus, isolated in Nigeria from *Amblyomma variegatum* ticks collected from healthy cattle; and Soldado virus, repeatedly isolated from a variety of bird ticks but recently linked to a mild illness in man.

REFERENCES

Begum, F., Wisseman, C.L., Jr., and Casals, J. (1970). Tick-borne viruses of West Pakistan. II. Hazara virus, a new agent isolated from *Ixodes redikorzevi* ticks from Kaghan valley, West Pakistan *and* IV. Viruses similar to, or identical with, Crimean haemorrhagic fever (Congo–Semunya), Wad Medani, and Pak Argas 461 isolated from ticks of the Chaga Manga forest, Lahore district, and of Hunza, Filgit Agency, West Pakistan). *American Journal of Epidemiology*, **92,** 197–202.

Chastel, C.G. *et al.* (1983). Are the arboviruses from seabird colonies in Brittany able to infect man? *Revue d'Epidemiologie Santé Publique*, **31,** 445–57.

Montgomery, R.E. (1917). On a tick-borne gastro-enteritis of sheep and goats occurring in British East Africa. *Journal of Comparative Pathology and Therapeutics*, **30,** 28–57.

Crimean–Congo haemorrhagic fever virus

Crimean haemorrhagic fever was described by Chumakov (1946) as an acute, febrile, haemorrhagic disease affecting man in the Crimean region of the former USSR, transmitted by ticks and carrying a mortality of 15 to 30 per cent. In Africa, Congo virus was first isolated in the then Belgian Congo (now Zaire) from the blood of a 13-year-old African boy, and it caused a moderately severe laboratory infection in a European; related viruses were isolated in Uganda, where more laboratory infections occurred, one of which ended fatally after a severe haematemesis. In Asia, a virus indistinguishable from Congo virus was isolated from pools of ticks collected from a variety of wild and domestic animals in Western Pakistan. Casals (1969) demonstrated that Crimean haemorrhagic fever virus was serologically indistinguishable from Congo virus, hence the use of the term Crimean–Congo haemorrhagic fever (**CCHF**) virus. Different strains of CCHF virus have been associated with outbreaks of severe and sometimes fatal disease in the Crimea, Rostov and Astrakhan regions of the former USSR, in Albania, Bulgaria and Yugoslavia, in East, West and South Africa, in Iran, Iraq and in Western Pakistan, and in China. Most infections are acquired by tick bites, but airborne infections have occurred in both hospital and laboratory environments. In South Africa an association with wild birds has been reported.

The incubation period is about 1 week. The onset of fever is usually sudden, and fever is usually continuous, although occasionally remittent or biphasic. Signs and symptoms include fever, headache, nausea, vomiting, joint pains, backache, photophobia, together with circulatory disorders, thrombocytopenia, and leucopenia. Haemorrhagic manifestations are common, with bleeding from nasal, gastric, intestinal, uterine and renal membranes (Fig. 3). Cases may present with acute abdominal pain, mimicking an acute surgical emergency, and operating-theatre staff have become infected and have died through contact with infected blood or secretions exposed at operation. The mortality is about 15 to 30 per cent, but may be as high as 40 to 80 per cent in hospital or nosocomial outbreaks. Transient hair loss has been reported.

Fig. 3 Patient with Crimean–Congo haemorrhagic fever showing extensive ecchymoses on the arms and thorax (by courtesy of Professor D.I.H. Simpson).

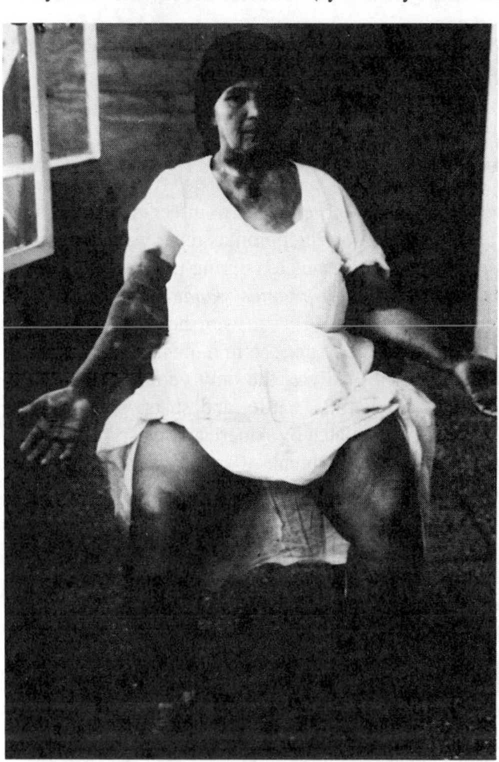

Control, treatment, and prognosis

No vaccine is available. Avoidance of tick bites may reduce the risk of infection. In hospital outbreaks, meticulous attention to the containment of infected secretions is essential and barrier nursing should be used. There may be neurological involvement, which usually indicates a poor prognosis. Those patients who recover may be left with a polyneuritis that persists for months, but eventual recovery is to be expected.

REFERENCES

Burney, M.I., Ghafoor, A., Saleen, M., Webb, P.A., and Casals, J. (1980). Nosocomial outbreak of viral haemorrhagic fever caused by Crimean haemorrhagic fever-Congo virus in Pakistan. *American Journal of Tropical Medicine and Hygiene*, **29,** 941–7.

Casals, J. (1969). Antigenic similarity between the virus causing Crimean haemorrhagic fever and Congo virus. *Proceedings of the Society for Experimental Biology and Medicine*, **131,** 233–6.

Chumakov, M.P. (1946) Crimean haemorrhagic fever. (In Russian.) *Izvestia Akademii Nauk SSSR*, **2,** 19–26.

Shepherd, A.J., Swanepoel, R., Shepherd, S.P., Leman, P.A., Blackburn, N.K., and Hallett, A.F. (1985). A nosocomial outbreak of Crimean–Congo haemorrhagic fever at Tygerberg Hospital. Part V. Virological and serological observations. *South Africa Medical Journal*, **68,** 733–6.

Shepherd, A.J., Swanepoel, R., Leman, P.A., and Shepherd, S.P. (1987). Field and laboratory investigations of Crimean–Congo haemorrhagic fever virus (*Nairovirus*, family Bunyaviridae) infection in birds. *Transactions of the Royal Society of Tropical Medicine and Hygiene*, **81**, 1004–7.

Simpson, D.I.H. *et al.* (1967). Congo virus: a hitherto undescribed virus occurring in Africa. *East Africa Medical Journal*, **44**, 87–92.

Genus Phlebovirus

At least nine different phleboviruses are known to infect man (see Table 1). Pappataci fever, sandfly fever, or Phlebotomus fever was recognized as a clinical entity in the Mediterranean area during the nineteenth century, and the association with *Phlebotomus papatasi* sandflies was clearly demonstrated by Doerr *et al.* (1909), who showed that filtrates of human blood would reproduce the disease in human volunteers. For many years it was thought that man was the only vertebrate host, but antibody studies indicate that gerbils, cattle, and sheep may also be infected. The Naples virus was isolated by American investigators from human serum collected during an outbreak of sandfly fever in Naples, and the Sicilian virus was isolated by the same workers from American troops with a similar fever in Palermo, Sicily. The two viruses have many common properties, but they are serologically quite distinct. Sandfly fever is widespread throughout the Mediterranean area, and also occurs in Egypt, Greece, Iran, Turkey, the former Yugoslavia, Bangladesh, India, Pakistan and the southern states of the former USSR. Toscana virus, serologically related to the Naples virus, has been isolated in Italy, Portugal, and in Cyprus; it is notable for its ability to infect the central nervous system. The viruses that cause classical sandfly fever do not occur in the New World, but in South and Central America a similar clinical condition follows infection with Alenquer, Candiru, Chagres and Punta Toro viruses.

Rift Valley fever has long been known as a disease of domestic animals, mainly sheep, in East Africa, which occasionally spreads to farm workers and others handling infected animals. The infection is endemic, but seldom recognized, in many wild game animals in Africa. Molecular studies have established that Rift Valley fever virus is very similar to sandfly fever viruses and Punta Toro virus in having an ambisense replication mechanism; this property distinguishes the genus Phlebovirus from other genera within the family. In its biological properties, Rift Valley fever virus differs from the sandfly fever viruses, Punta Toro viruses, and most other members of the genus, in being normally transmitted by mosquitoes rather than sandflies. When it was recognized that the tick-transmitted Uukuniemi and Zaliv-Terpeniya viruses also shared an ambisense replication strategy, these viruses were removed from their earlier classification in the genus Uukuvirus and were redesignated to the genus Phlebovirus. The only evidence that Uukuniemi virus can infect man is the finding of specific antibodies in some human sera collected in Estonia and in Czechoslovakia. Zaliv-Terpeniya virus was isolated from bird ticks collected on an island in the Sea of Okhotsk, Sakhalin region, and there is some evidence that it may be pathogenic to man.

REFERENCES

Doerr, R., Franz, K., and Taussig, S. (1909). *Das Pappatacifieber*. Deuticke, Leipzig.

Sabin, A.B., Philip, C.B., and Paul, J.R. (1944). Phlebotomus (Pappataci or sandfly) fever: a disease of military importance: summary of existing knowledge and preliminary report of original investigations. *Journal of the American Medical Association*, **125**, 603–8; 693–9.

Sandfly fever, Naples, and Sicilian viruses

Symptoms

After an incubation period of 2 to 6 days, there is an abrupt onset of fever, chills, nausea and vomiting, epigastric pain and often severe, generalized headache leading to incapacitating prostration. Fever of 38 to 40 °C usually resolves after 2 to 3 days, but may be biphasic and persist for a week. There is no rash, but small haemorrhages into the skin and mucous membranes may be seen. Photophobia and eye pain are not uncommon, lymphadenopathy is often seen, and the liver may be tender, although jaundice is rare. The disease is self-limiting, with complete recovery. No deaths have been attributed to either sandfly fever, Naples, or Sicilian viruses.

REFERENCE

Bartelloni, P.J. and Tesh, R.B. (1976). Clinical and serologic responses of volunteers infected with Phlebotomus fever virus (Sicilian type). *American Journal of Tropical Medicine and Hygiene*, **25**, 456–62.

Rift Valley fever virus

Following its initial isolation in 1930 as the agent of enzootic hepatitis of domestic animals in Kenya, Rift Valley fever virus was recognized as the cause of sporadic human infections in East, Central, and West Africa, with a particular capacity to infect those handling the virus in the laboratory. In East and Central Africa the virus has been isolated from a variety of mosquito species (Aedes, Culex, Eratmopodites, and Culicoides) and recent studies have shown that the virus is capable of persisting in mosquito eggs during the dry season, emerging when larvae hatch in the rainy season. From 1951 to 1956 there were severe epizootics in lambs in southern Africa, and many human cases occurred. Further human cases with several deaths were seen in South Africa in 1975.

In the Central African Republic in 1969 a virus isolated from *Mansonia africana* mosquitoes and named Zinga virus was associated with several cases of haemorrhagic fever; Zinga virus was later shown to be a strain of Rift Valley fever virus. In West Africa, Rift Valley fever virus was isolated from mosquitoes in Nigeria and from bats in Guinea, but despite the presence of antibodies in human sera collected in Nigeria and Senegal, human disease was unrecognized until 1987 when a substantial epidemic occurred in Mauritania, with further epidemics in following years. In 1977 the virus spread, apparently for the first time, into Egypt, producing a major epizootic in domestic animals, principally sheep and goats, but also cattle, and causing some 600 human deaths within a period of 3 months. In Egypt, the principal vector seems to have been *Culex pipiens*. It is of interest that both the Egyptian and the Mauritanian epidemics appear to be linked to major ecological changes following the construction of the Aswan Dam on the Nile and dams on the Senegal River.

Symptoms

After an incubation period of 3 to 6 days there is an abrupt onset of fever, shivering, nausea, and vomiting, epigastric pain, and often severe, generalized headache. The fever may be biphasic, with temperatures between 38 and 40 °C, and may remain elevated for at least a week. There is no rash, but small haemorrhages into the skin and mucous membranes may be seen. Photophobia and eye pains are not uncommon; there may be conjunctival inflammation, and a central serous retinitis, leading to central scotoma and sometimes to retinal detachment. The fundus may show macular exudates that are slow to disappear. There is often a lymphadenopathy, and although the liver is frequently involved and may be tender, jaundice is rare, but appears to have been more common during the recent outbreaks in Mauritania. Convalescence may be protracted, but is usually uncomplicated; however, a small percentage of patients may suffer severe complications such as haemorrhagic fever, encephalitis, or eye lesions. Haemorrhagic disease presents as above, but progresses with petechial, mucous membrane and gastrointestinal haemorrhage, severe liver involvement, and patients may die in shock.

Encephalitic patients typically recover from acute febrile disease only to present within a few days to 2 weeks later with headache, meningismus, confusion and fever, often leading to residua or ending in death. Ocular complications are characterized by rapid onset of decreased visual acuity due to retinal haemorrhage, exudates, and macular oedema. These are also seen after apparent recovery from the initial disease. About half of these patients suffer some degree of permanent vision loss. Deaths from Rift Valley fever were rare before the 1977 outbreak in Egypt and the later Mauritanian epidemics in which at least 25 persons died with jaundice and haemorrhagic manifestations.

Control, treatment, and prognosis

Veterinary vaccines have been used for a number of years, and formalin-inactivated vaccines have also had limited use for the prevention of disease in laboratory workers and others exposed to high risk of infection. Improved vaccines based on molecular techniques are under development. Although there are no reports of nosocomial transmission, barrier nursing would be a sensible precaution.

REFERENCES

Daubney, R., Hudson, J.R., and Garnham, P.C. (1931). Enzootic hepatitis or Rift Valley fever. An undescribed virus disease of sheep, cattle and man from East Africa. *Journal of Pathology and Bacteriology*, **34**, 545–79.

Digoutte, J.P. and Peters, C.J. (1989). General aspects of the 1987 Rift Valley fever epidemic in Mauritania. *Research in Virology*, **140**, 27–30.

Gear, J. (1977). Haemorrhagic fevers in South Africa. An account of two recent outbreaks. *Journal of the South African Veterinary Association*, **48**, 5–8.

Gear, J. *et al.* (1951). Rift Valley fever in South Africa. The occurrence of human cases in the Orange Free State, the north western Cape Province, the western and southern Transvaal. *South Africa Medical Journal*, **25**, 908–12.

Linthicum, K.J. *et al.* (1985). Rift Valley Fever virus (family Bunyaviridae, genus *Phlebovirus*). Isolations from Diptera collected during an inter-epizootic period in Kenya. *Journal of Hygiene (Cambridge)*, **95**, 197–209.

Meadors, G.F., Gibbs, P.H., and Peters, C.J. (1986). Evaluation of new Rift Valley fever vaccine: safety and immunogenicity trials. *Vaccine*, **4**, 179–84.

Meegan, J.M. (1979). The Rift Valley fever epizootic in Egypt 1977–1978. I. Description of the epizootic and virological studies. *Transactions of the Royal Society of Tropical Medicine and Hygiene*, **73**, 618–723.

Philippe, B. *et al.* (1989). Rift Valley fever in Southern Mauritania. *Bulletin de la Société du Pathologie Exotique*, **82**, 611–19.

Walsh, J. (1988). Rift Valley fever rears its head. *Science*, **240**, 1397–9.

World Health Organization (1983). The use of veterinary vaccines for prevention and control of Rift Valley fever: memorandum from a WHO/FAO meeting. *Bulletin of the World Health Organization*, **61**, 261–268.

Unassigned viruses and viruses causing only minor disease in man

The great majority of the viruses listed in Table 2 cause only a mild, febrile illness, but the following show certain additional features.

Bhanja virus (unassigned)

This virus was first isolated from *Haemaphysalis intermedia* ticks collected from healthy goats in India, but has since been isolated in Sri Lanka, in Africa, and in Europe. Infection of goats is widespread in Italy and in the former Yugoslavia, where there have been several reported human cases, including some with severe neurological disease, and at least two deaths. Laboratory infections have also occurred.

Bwamba virus (Bunyavirus)

This was first isolated in Uganda in 1941 and is very widespread in throughout subSaharan Africa. More than 75 per cent of adult human sera collected in Nigeria and over 95 per cent of human sera collected in Uganda and Tanzania have antibodies against Bwamba virus. The original cases showed fever, headache, generalized body pains, and conjunctivitis, but no rash, although a rash has been described in the Central African Republic. No fatalities have been reported.

Nyando virus (Bunyavirus)

This virus was first isolated from mosquitoes in Kenya; it has since been isolated from man in the Central African Republic, where it caused fever, myalgia and encephalitis.

Tataguine virus (unassigned)

This causes fever, rash, and joint pains in at least five African countries (Cameroon, Central African Republic, Ethiopia, Nigeria and Senegal).

Wanowrie virus (unassigned)

This virus was first isolated in India from *Hyalomma marginatum* ticks collected from sheep. It has also been isolated in Egypt and Iran, and in Sri Lanka, where it was recovered from the brain of a 17-year-old girl who died following a 2-day fever with abdominal pain and vomiting.

REFERENCES

Calisher, C.H. and Goodpasture, H.C. (1975). Human infection with Bhanja virus. *American Journal of Tropical Medicine and Hygiene*, **24**, 1040–2.

Vesenjak-Hirjan, J., Calisher, C.H., Beus, I., and Marton, E. (1980). First natural clinical human Bhanja virus infection. In *Arboviruses in the Mediterranean countries*, (ed. J. Vesenjak-Hirjan, E. Arslanagic, and J.S. Porterfield). *Zentralblatt für Bakteriologie, Parasitenkunde, Infektionsrankheiten und Hygiene* (suppl. 9), 297–301.

7.10.22 Arenaviruses

S. Fisher-Hoch and J. B. McCormick

General considerations

Ecology and epidemiology

Arenaviruses infect rodents in both the New and the Old World. There are at least 15 arenaviruses but only five produce significant human disease (Fig. 1); Lassa. Junin, Machupo, Guanarito, and lymphocytic choriomeningitis virus (**LCMV**), though a new virus from Brazil may shortly join this list, and others may be still to be found, as they tend to occupy circumscribed, sometimes remote, ecological niches. Rodents normally experience silent but persistent and lifelong infection, the viruses being passed in this highly successful ecological system by horizontal or vertical transmission at or near birth. Lifelong viraemia results in persistent viruria, the primary source of contamination of the environment.

The extent of intrusion into the rodents' ecologic niche usually determines the likelihood of human infection. Because this occurs mostly in rural areas with limited facilities for medical care, details of the clinical and pathogenic features of the diseases are scarce. The virus infects primarily through cuts and scratches, and possibly the mucosae, contaminated with rodent urine. Disease may be severe and haemorrhagic. Person-to-person spread is reported for Lassa fever in community and in hospital settings, but is apparently rare with the other pathogenic arenaviruses.

Virology

Arenavirus is taken from the Latin for sand (*arena*), as host-cell ribosomes included in the virion resemble grains of sand by electron microscopy (Fig. 2). The viruses are enveloped, pleomorphic, membrane viruses ranging in diameter from 50 to 300 nm, with a mean diameter of 110 to 130 nm, and virion density in sucrose of 1.17 g/cm^3. They contain two segments of single-stranded RNA, tightly associated with a nucleocapsid protein of 65 000 to 72 000 molecular weight. The large strand of ambisense RNA, of molecular weight $2.0 - 3.2 \times 10^6$, codes for the viral polymerase and a zinc-finger protein. The small ambisense single-strand RNA, molecular weight about 1.1 to 1.6×10^6, encodes the glycoprotein precursor and the nucleoprotein. The genome is enclosed in a membrane bearing two glycosylated proteins of about 34 000 to 44 000 (G1) and 54 000 to 72 000 (G2) molecular weight, derived from the glycoprotein precursor by post-translational cleavage. Antigenic cross-reactivity is conserved at least at one epitopic site across all known arenaviruses, but more cross-reactivity occurs between more geographically related viruses.

Lassa, Junin, and Machupo viruses are categorized as biosafety level 4 (**BSL**4) laboratory agents, and require high containment facilities for cultivation or animal studies. LCMV is a BSL3 agent.

Old world arenaviruses

Lassa fever

Epidemiology

DISTRIBUTION AND ECOLOGY

Lassa fever was first described in West Africa in the 1950s, although the virus was not isolated until 1969. It occupies a wide geographical area from Northern Nigeria to Guinea, encompassing perhaps 100 million population. The only known reservoir of Lassa virus is *Mastomys natalensis*, one of the most commonly occurring rodents in Africa. In southern Africa, a related Mastomys carries Mopeia virus. This is closely related to Lassa virus and can infect man, but is apparently unable to cause significant clinical disease. Mastomys are highly commensal with man. In some areas, 50 per cent of domestic rodents may be Mastomys, averaging 2.4 animals in each house, but they have limited movement within a village. Prevalence of Lassa virus infection is highly variable in Mastomys and tends to cluster in houses. Thus Lassa virus infection, although endemic, tends to be focal.

EPIDEMIOLOGY

It has been estimated that more than 100 000 infections with Lassa virus may occur each year in West Africa, with several thousand deaths. Lassa fever occurs in all age groups and sexes, and antibody prevalence increases with age, so it can be assumed that most virus transmission to man takes place in and around the home. Estimates of antibody prevalence range from 4 to 6 per cent in Guinea to 15 to 20 per cent in Nigeria, though in some villages in Sierra Leone as many as 60 per cent of the population have evidence of past infection. In prospective studies, seroconversion to Lassa virus ranged from 5 to 22 per cent/year of susceptible (seronegative) Sierra Leone villagers. Disease to infection ratios range from 9 to 26 per cent in Sierra Leone, and the proportion of febrile illness associated with seroconversion to Lassa virus from 5 to 14 per cent. Five to 8 per cent of infected people may be admitted to hospital, of whom 17 per cent may die if untreated. However, the fatality for all infections (admitted and not admitted to hospital) may be as low as 2 per cent. In endemic areas, Lassa fever may account for 10 to 16 per cent of all adult medical admissions and about 30 per cent of adult deaths in medical admissions.

TRANSMISSION

Direct contact between virus-contaminated articles and surfaces and cuts and scratches on bare hands and feet may be the most important and consistent mode of transmission in endemic areas. The sporadic pattern of human infection in the household community does not suggest aero-

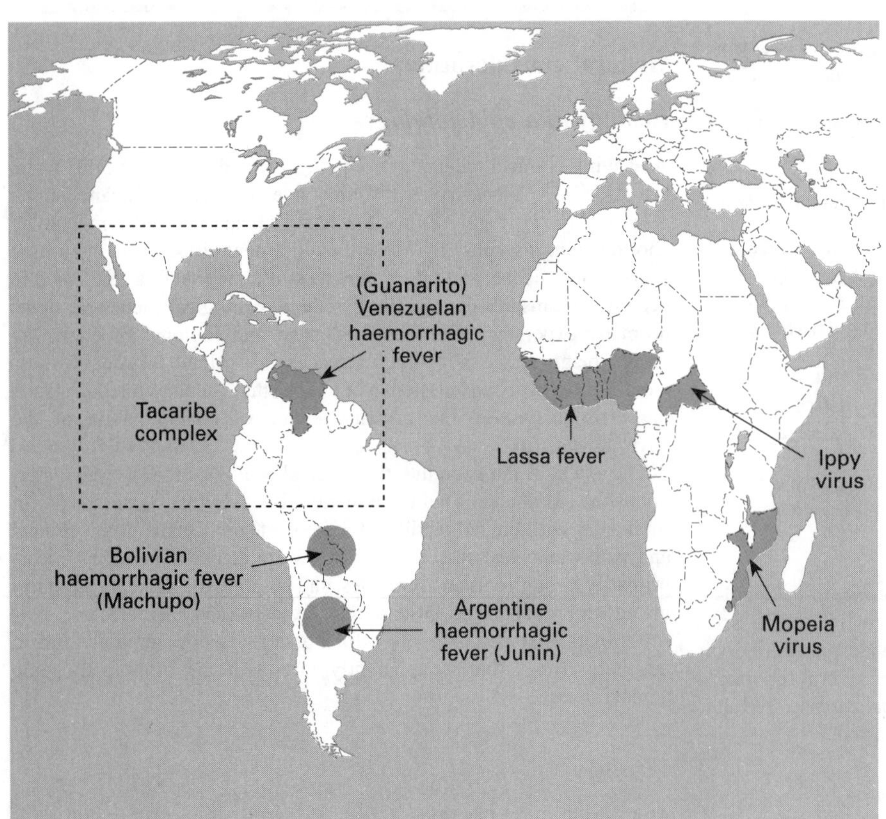

Fig. 1 World map showing the approximate distribution of arenaviruses.

sol transmission. Nosocomial spread in hospitals was, and continues to be, associated with inadequate disinfection and direct contact with infected blood and contaminated needles. Recently, increasing and indiscriminate use of routine intravenous therapy in West African hospitals, along with inadequate needle and syringe care, led to large-scale epidemics. Nevertheless, a prospective study in an endemic area in a hospital where simple but rigorous barrier nursing techniques were applied showed that Lassa virus infection occurred less frequently in hospital personnel handling Lassa fever patients, but aware of the risks, than in the less-educated populations of neighbouring villages. In another study in London, none of 159 unprotected hospital contacts of a severely ill Lassa fever patient was infected.

RISK FACTORS

Rodent to human infection is highly associated with indiscriminate food storage, and practices such as catching, cooking, and eating rodents. Person-to-person spread of Lassa virus in households is common. In villages, risk of infection is associated with direct contact, nursing care or sexual contact with someone during the incubation, acute, or convalescent phases of illness.

Fig. 2 Electronmicrographs of arenaviruses. (a) Machupo virus in tissue culture. Arrow shows virus budding through cell membrane. × 125 000. (By courtesy of F.A. Murphy and S.G.W. Whitfield.) (b) Lassa virus budding from cell membrane. × 74 000 (By courtesy of C. Goldsmith.)

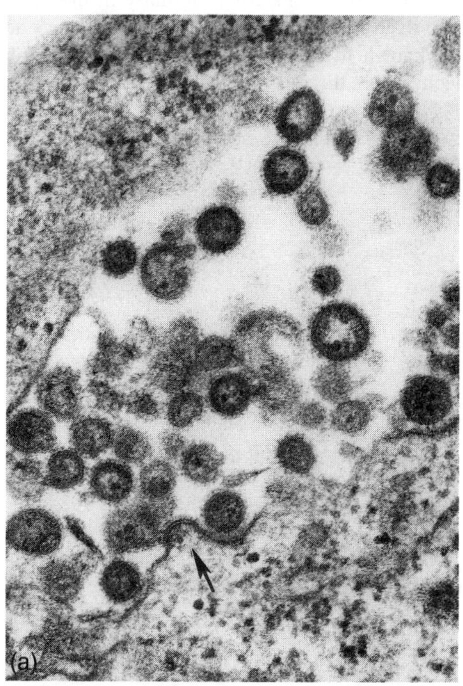

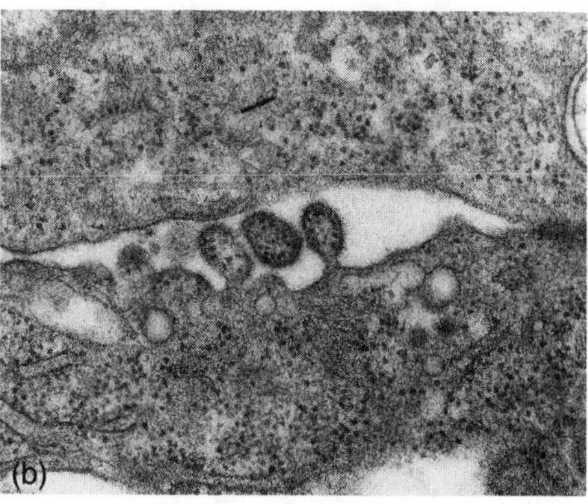

Clinical features

INCUBATION PERIOD AND PRODROME

After an incubation period of 7 to 18 days, Lassa fever begins insidiously, with fever, weakness, malaise, severe headache—usually frontal—and a very painful sore throat. Frequency of signs and symptoms is illustrated in Fig. 3. More than 50 per cent of patients then develop joint and lumbar pain and 60 per cent or more develop a non-productive cough. Many also develop a severe retrosternal chest pain, and about half will have nausea with vomiting or diarrhoea and abdominal pain.

On physical examination, respiratory rate, temperature, and pulse rate are elevated and blood pressure may be low. There is no characteristic skin rash in Lassa fever and petechiae and ecchymoses are not seen. About one-third of patients will have conjunctivitis. More than two-thirds have pharyngitis, half with exudates, diffusely inflamed and swollen posterior pharynx and tonsils, but few if any ulcers or petechiae. The abdomen is tender in 50 per cent of patients. Neurological signs in the early stages are limited to a fine tremor, most marked in the lips and tongue.

SEVERE DISEASE

Up to one-third of Lassa fever patients admitted to hospital progress to a prostrating illness 6 to 8 days after onset of fever, usually with persistent vomiting and diarrhoea. Patients are often dehydrated and the haematocrit is elevated. Proteinuria occurs in two-thirds of patients, and the blood urea may be moderately elevated. About half of Lassa fever patients will have diffuse abdominal tenderness but no localizing signs or loss of bowel sounds. The severe retrosternal or epigastric pain seen in many patients may be due to pleural or pericardial involvement. Bleeding is seen in only 15 to 20 per cent of patients, limited primarily to the mucosal surfaces or, occasionally, conjunctival haemorrhage or gastrointestinal or vaginal bleeding. Severe pulmonary oedema or adult respiratory distress syndrome is common in fatal cases with gross head and neck oedema, pharyngeal stridor, and hypovolaemic shock (Fig. 4).

Over 70 per cent of patients may have abnormal electrocardiograms (non-specific ST-segment and T-wave abnormalities, ST-segment elevation, generalized low-voltage complexes, and changes reflecting electrolyte disturbance), but none of these correlates with clinical or other measures of disease severity or outcome, or is associated with clinical manifestations of myocarditis. Neurological signs are infrequent, but carry a poor prognosis. There is progression from confusion to severe encephalopathy with or without general seizures, but without focal signs. Cerebrospinal fluid is usually normal, but with a few lymphocytes, and low titres of virus relative to serum. Pneumonitis, and pleural and pericardial rubs develop in early convalescence in about 20 per cent of patients admitted to hospital, occasionally in association with congestive cardiac failure.

LABORATORY MEASUREMENTS

Though the mean white blood-cell count in Lassa fever on admission to hospital is normal (6×10^9/l), there may be early lymphopenia and later relative or absolute neutrophilia, as high as 30×10^9/l. Though thrombocytopenia is moderate, even in severely ill patients, platelet function is markedly depressed or even absent. This abnormality is usually maximal on admission to hospital and is present even when circulating platelet numbers remain about 100×10^9/l. A circulating inhibitor of platelet function has been described, specifically inhibiting platelet dense-granule and ATP release but relatively sparing the thromboxane pathways. It also interferes with the generation of the superoxide induced by *N*-formyl-met-leu-phe in neutrophils.

A serum aspartate aminotransferase (**AST**) level in excess of 150 u/l is associated with a case fatality of 50 per cent, and there is a correlation between an increasing level and a higher risk of fatal outcome (Fig. 5). Alanine aminotransferase (**ALT**) is only marginally raised, and the ratio of AST:ALT in natural infections and in experimentally infected non-human primates is as high as 11:1. Prothrombin times, and glucose and bilirubin levels are near normal, excluding biochemical hepatic failure, and suggesting that some of the AST may be non-hepatic in origin.

Viraemia in excess of 3 $\log_{10}$ tissue-culture ID_{50}/ml is associated with increasing case fatality (Fig. 5). In addition to the liver, high virus titres occur in ovary, pancreas, uterus, and placenta, but no histological lesions compatible with organ failure are observed. Elevated viraemia and AST together carry a risk of death of nearly 80 per cent.

MORTALITY

The death rate for all Lassa virus infections may be as low as 2 per cent in some areas. Case fatality in hospitalized patients is about 16 per cent. However, in recent outbreaks in Nigeria, much higher death rates have been observed in patients admitted to hospital, possibly due to variation in virulence or to high-dose, parenteral transmission. The case fatality may be over 30 per cent in the third trimester of pregnancy, and 50 per cent in patients with haemorrhage.

COMPLICATIONS AND SEQUELAE

Nearly 30 per cent of patients with Lassa fever infection suffer an acute loss of hearing in one or both ears. The onset is invariably during the convalescent phase of illness, and its development and severity are unrelated to severity of the acute disease. It is unclear whether the damage is due to neurotropic virus strains, thrombosis, vasculitis, focal hemorrhage, or some other viral- or immune response-related phenomenon. The mean auditory threshold of these patients is 55 dB (normal $\leqslant$ 25dB), and the mean disability is over 20 per cent. About half of the patients show a near or complete recovery by 3 to 4 months after onset, but the other half continue with significant sensorineural deafness, which after about a year will be permanent. Many patients also exhibit cerebellar signs during convalescence from severe disease, particularly tremors and ataxia, but these usually resolve with time.

Infrequent complications are uveitis, pericarditis, orchitis, pleural effusion, ascites, and acute adrenal insufficiency. Renal and hepatic failure are not seen. A single case report describes an interesting complex of haemorrhagic pericarditis and cardiac tamponade with pleural effusions and ascites 6 months after acute Lassa fever. Repeated cultures failed to isolate virus from effusion fluids but these specimens contained high titres of Lassa-specific IgG and numerous lymphocytes.

LASSA FEVER IN PREGNANCY

Lassa fever may be a common cause of maternal death in many areas of West Africa, with a case fatality of about 20 per cent. However, there is a nearly twofold increase in the number of third-trimester Lassa virus infections requiring admission to hospital, compared to that in the first two trimesters, and a corresponding two-to threefold risk of maternal death from infection in the third trimester. Very high levels of virus replication have been found in placental tissue in third-trimester patients. A fourfold reduction was noted in case fatality among women with spontaneous or therapeutic abortions compared to those who were not aborted (odds ratio for fatality with pregnancy intact is 5.5 compared to uterine evacuation). Fetal loss is as much as 87 per cent, and does not seem to vary by trimester. The excess maternal mortality in the third trimester may be related to relative immunosuppression of pregnancy at that time. Lassa virus is known to be present in the breast milk of infected mothers, and neonates are therefore at risk of congenital, intra-

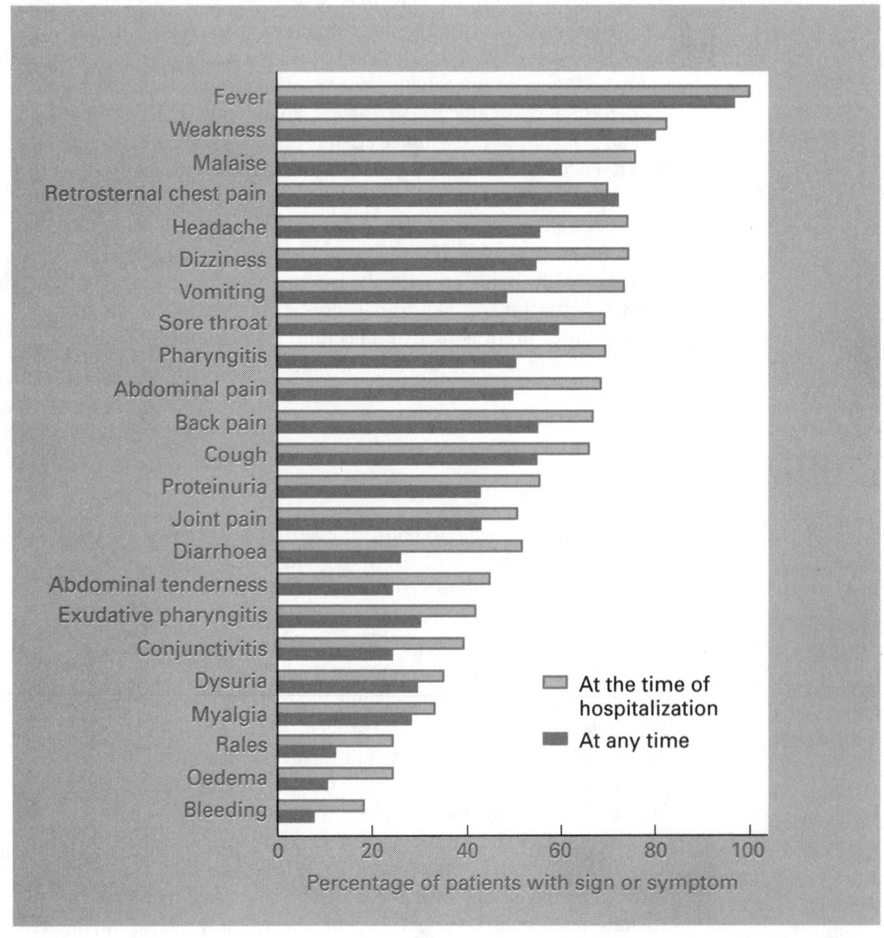

Fig. 3 Frequency of signs and symptoms of Lassa fever.

partum, and puerperal infection with Lassa virus. Relatives of patients with Lassa fever should be advised to seek help immediately if they develop a fever.

LASSA FEVER IN CHILDREN

Lassa fever is common in children, but may be difficult to diagnose because manifestations are so general. In very young babies, marked oedema has been reported. In older children the disease may manifest as diarrhoea or as pneumonia or simply as an unexplained prolonged fever. In one hospital study in Sierra Leone, 21 per cent of child admissions had Lassa fever, with 12 per cent fatality. A study of child outpatients in the same hospital found 24/435 (6 per cent) with evidence of previous Lassa infection and a further 68 who seroconverted (16 per cent).

DIFFERENTIAL DIAGNOSIS

The physician should be alerted to the diagnosis of Lassa fever by a history of potential exposure either to rodents or patients in or from West Africa. Failure to do so may have devastating consequences both for the patient and high-risk contacts. This said, common life-threatening infections such as cerebral malaria, or septicaemia must be considered, though double infections can occur, particularly Lassa fever and malaria. The clinical diagnosis of Lassa fever on presentation may be difficult, particularly early in the disease. In West Africa, extensive clinical studies of admitting signs and symptoms in febrile patients in hospital showed that fever with pharyngitis, proteinuria, and retrosternal chest pain had a predictive value for Lassa fever of 81 per cent and a specificity of 89 per cent. Similarly, a triad of pharyngitis, retrosternal chest pain, and proteinuria (in a febrile patient) correctly predicted Lassa fever 80 per cent of the time (in an endemic area). However, these triads of symptoms had sensitivities of only 50 per cent. Bleeding and sore throat had a specificity for fatal outcome of 90 per cent, but sensitivity of only 36 per cent. On the other hand, vomiting and sore throat had a specificity of only 47 per cent for fatal disease but a sensitivity of 89 per cent.

Fig. 4 Acute Lassa fever in a patient showing facial oedema, decerebrate posturing, and respiratory distress. This patient survived.

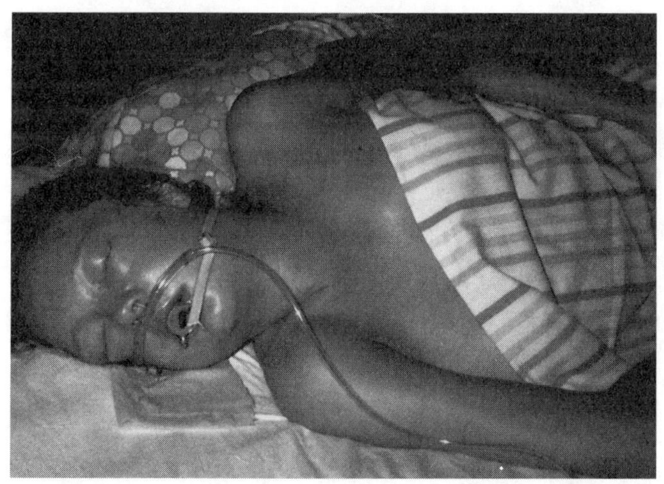

Pathogenic processes

PATHOGENESIS

The most common sites of initiation of human infection by the arenaviruses are not yet known, although they seem likely to be cuts and abrasions in the skin and thence to lymph nodes. Following the initiation of infection, all arenaviruses progress to generalized multiorgan infection, affecting especially the reticuloendothelial system. In Lassa fever, important clinical events in severe disease are intractable hypovolaemic shock, and/or severe central-nervous involvement, bleeding, and oedema of the face. The physiological correlates of this clinical picture are endothelial dysfunction and platelet dysfunction, (despite adequate numbers of circulating platelets). A marked decrease in prostacyclin production by endothelium has been found in non-human primates infected by Lassa virus. The inhibitor of platelet function identified in the serum of non-human primates and patients with severe Lassa fever appears to be a protein of undetermined molecular weight that is heat stable, and highly bioactive. Its origin is presumably the host because it cannot be reproduced with viral material nor can it be blocked by antibodies to Lassa virus. Its effect on platelets seems to be through interference with the second-messenger mechanisms, and it may well have a significant effect in the same way on other cells besides platelets and endothelial cells. Platelet and fibrinogen turnover are normal, and there is no increase in fibrinogen breakdown products nor evidence of platelet consumption, so that disseminated intravascular coagulation is not a significant component.

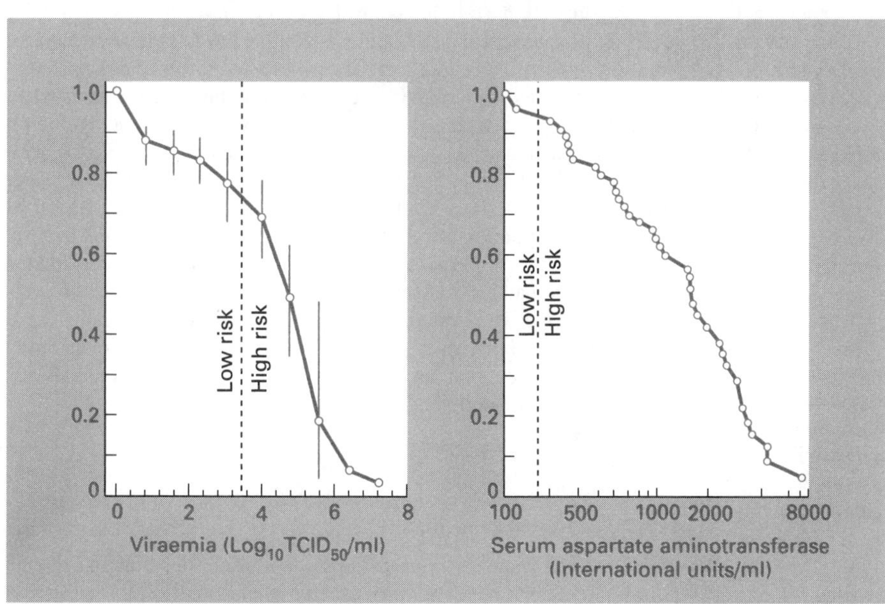

Fig. 5 Cumulative survival in Lassa fever related to serum viraemia and aspartate aminotransferase (AST) levels.

PATHOLOGY

The most frequently and consistently observed microscopic lesions in fatal human Lassa fever are focal necrosis of the liver, adrenal glands, and spleen. The degree of hepatocytic necrosis is variable, with concomitant necrosis and regeneration, but insufficient hepatic damage to implicate hepatic failure as a cause of death. A substantial macrophage response occurs in association with the liver necrosis, with little if any lymphocytic inflammatory response. Similarly, moderate splenic necrosis is a consistent finding, primarily involving the marginal zone of the periarteriolar lymphocytic sheath. Diffuse focal adrenocortical cellular necrosis has been observed less frequently. No significant light-microscopic lesions have been found in other organs, such as brain, ovary, pancreas, uterus, and placenta. Though there are few histological clues to the pathogenesis of Lassa fever, it is clear that its outcome is associated with the degree of viral replication, presumably by subtle biological effect on vascular endothelium, and perhaps other key cell systems.

IMMUNOLOGY

The immunological response to arenavirus infection is complex. In general, Lassa virus and LCMV appear to depend primarily on cytotoxic T-cell responses for clearance; neutralizing antibodies develop and are associated with clearance of viraemia due to the South American arenaviruses. There appears to be a brisk B-cell response with a classical primary IgG and IgM antibody response to Lassa virus early in the illness. By the sixth day of illness, IgG antibodies are found in 46 per cent of patients and IgM antibody in 59 per cent. By the 16th day of illness, both are found in 100 per cent of patients. These events do not, however, coincide with viral clearance, and high viraemia and high IgG and IgM titres often coexist in both man and non-human primates. Indeed, virus may persist in the serum and urine of man for several months after infection, and possibly in occult sites, such as renal tissue, for years.

Neutralizing antibodies to Lassa virus are absent in the serum of patients at the beginning of convalescence, and in most people they are never detectable. In a minority of patients some low-titre serum neutralizing activity may be observed several months after resolution of the disease. Passive protection from Lassa virus has been demonstrated in animals given selected antiserum at the time or soon after inoculation with virus. However, controlled clinical trials with human convalescent plasma containing high-titre antibodies have shown no protective effect. Thus the clearance of Lassa virus appears to be independent of antibody formation, and presumably depends on the cell-mediated immune response. This is supported by recent experience with experimental Lassa vaccines in non-human primates, where killed vaccine, and vaccinia-vectored vaccines expressing the nucleoprotein elicited high-level antibodies to Lassa virus, but no protection, while vaccinia-vectored glycoprotein vaccine elicited little antibody, but nevertheless provided protection. Reinfection following natural Lassa infection may occur in man, but clinical disease does not ensue.

Laboratory procedures

DIAGNOSIS

The laboratory diagnosis of arenavirus infections is by isolation of virus from serum, demonstration of a four-fold rise in antibody titre, or high-titre IgG antibody with virus-specific IgM antibody in association with compatible clinical disease. The most reliable and safe routine method for the laboratory at present is detection of virus specific antibody by immunofluorescent assay or enzyme-linked immunosorbent assay (**ELISA**). For immunofluorescence, slides of inactivated Lassa virus-infected tissue-culture cells may be stored at −20 °C for 6 months or at −70 °C for several years. An IgG titre of at least 16, and IgM titre of 4, both by immunofluorescent assay, are considered specific for Lassa infection. Routine virus isolation may be accomplished easily from serum or tissues in cell cultures, but should be done in BSL4 laboratory facilities. Specimens should preferably be drawn into a vacuum tube system to minimize risk of infection. Virus has also been isolated from breast milk, spinal fluid, pleural, and pericardial transudate, and from autopsy material. Virus may be recovered for 1 to 2 months in urine, but its presence in urine during acute disease is intermittent.

Viral protein may be detected by monoclonal antibodies in tissue imprints (usually liver) on a microscope slide. Efforts to detect antigen in conjunctival scrapings, buffy-coat preparations, cells from pharyngeal aspirates, and urinary sediment have not been successful. Recently, a polymerase chain-reaction assay on serum has been evaluated and shown to be both sensitive and specific in retrospective and prospective studies.

CONTAINMENT AND DISINFECTION

Lassa virus is robust, and withstands drying. Blood from severely ill patients may contain as many as 10^9 infectious units/ml, and rodent urine may contain up to 10^4 infectious units/ml. However, it can be inactivated by heat, detergents, chlorine, formalin, and ultraviolet radiation (including sunshine). Antigenic properties are best conserved by inactivation with γ-irradiation. Disinfection can be accomplished by washing with 0.5 per cent phenol in detergent (for example, Lysol), 0.5 per cent hypochlorite solution, formaldehyde, or paracetic acid.

Patient management

SUPPORTIVE CARE

Fluid, electrolyte, respiratory, and osmotic imbalances should be corrected, and full intensive-care support, including mechanical ventilation, offered if required. Every effort is justified because the crisis does not last longer than a few hours or days, and complete recovery can be expected in survivors. However, even vigorous support of this kind may be insufficient to prevent fatal progression of advanced disease. Pregnant women are a major challenge. They often present with absent fetal movements, and their survival may depend on aggressive obstetric intervention.

ANTIVIRAL THERAPY

Ribavirin (tribavirin), a guanosine analogue, is effective in treating acute Lassa fever, but must be given early in disease. It is given intravenously as a 2 g loading dose followed by 1 g every 6 h for 4 days, then 0.5 g every 8 h for 6 more days. Toxicity is confined to mild reversible anaemia. A 5- to 10-fold decrease in the case-fatality ratio was demonstrated in patients treated with ribavirin compared with untreated patients when therapy was given within the first 6 days of illness. Patients with high AST and viraemia, risk factors for unfavourable outcome (Fig. 5), who were treated within the first 6 days of illness experienced a 5 to 9 per cent case fatality. Those with the same risk factors receiving treatment more than 6 days after the onset of illness had a 26 to 47 per cent fatality, compared with 52 to 78 per cent untreated. Furthermore, patients treated with ribavirin had a significant reduction in viraemia regardless of outcome compared with untreated patients. Ribavirin is contraindicated in early pregnancy because of potential teratogenicity, but the fetus rarely survives the infection. It has been used in late pregnancy but its efficacy has not yet been determined.

Prevention

HOSPITAL CONTAINMENT

The key to prevention of person-to-person transmission both in endemic and non-endemic areas has consistently been good hospital and laboratory practice, with simple isolation of febrile patients and rigorous use of gloves and disinfection. Lassa fever is by far the most prevalent of the haemorrhagic fever viruses associated with person-to-person and nosocomial transmission, and the incubation period allows ample time for displacement of infected persons by modern transportation before onset. The importance of awareness by medical teams of the possibility of Lassa fever in patients in or from endemic areas presenting with classical clinical manifestations of Lassa fever as well as less obviously related conditions, such as fever with abdominal pain or septic abortion, cannot be overemphasized. Most important, complete support, including intensive care, or surgery, should not be denied because of the suspected diagnosis. Careful intensive care or surgery by informed and trained personnel using maximum precautions (double gloves, education of staff, limiting theatre personnel), does not carry large risks. Patient isolators should not be used as they induce loss of manual dexterity and fatigue, inhibit intensive-care procedures and communication, do not protect against injury by sharp instruments and have no provision for resuscitation. The 1988 Centers for Disease Control 'Guidelines for the Management of Patients with VHFs' recommends routine isolation in a single room, preferably but not necessarily with negative air-pressure gradient from the hallway, through an anteroom to the room. Staff education, use of gloves, gowns, masks, and rigorous disinfection with fresh liquids are mandatory. The recommendations issued for patient management and handling of clinical specimens from AIDS patients are adequate for containment of Lassa fever.

CONTACTS

High risk is only associated with direct percutaneous or mucosal contact with blood or body fluids. Medium-risk contacts (includes most unprotected contact with blood or body fluids) may safely be observed for development of persistent high fever for 3 weeks from the last date of contact by daily temperature measurement and telephone reporting. The practice of following up airline passengers and other low-risk contacts with Lassa fever has been discontinued.

PROPHYLAXIS

Though data on efficacy are lacking, it seems reasonable on present evidence to recommend the use of oral ribavirin as post-exposure prophylaxis as soon as possible after exposure, provided there is a good history of potential parenteral or mucosal contamination with blood or other material containing live Lassa virus (high-risk contacts). Ribavirin, 600 mg orally four times a day for 10 days, may be offered.

VACCINE

A candidate Lassa fever vaccine made by cloning and expressing the Lassa virus glycoprotein gene into vaccinia virus, has proved highly successful in preventing severe disease and death in monkeys lethally challenged with Lassa virus. At present, this is the most realistic and practical approach to control of this devastating public health problem, and a vaccine would be widely applicable in many West African populations, and in medical care personnel likely to encounter cases. However, the resources for vaccine development are currently not readily identifiable because of the limited economic impact of the disease internationally.

CONTROL

Elimination of contact with rodents has been shown to be very effective in trap-out studies in villages in Sierra Leone. However, the control of rodents as a broad approach to preventing Lassa fever in West Africa is not realistic. Improvement of housing and food storage might reduce the domestic rodent population, but such changes are not easily made without massive improvement in local economy.

Lymphocytic choriomeningitis virus (LCMV)

Epidemiology

DISTRIBUTION AND ECOLOGY

LCMV was isolated in 1933 from the cerebrospinal fluid of a patient suspected of having St. Louis encephalitis. Its natural host is *Mus musculis*, and its distribution is extensive. Transmission of virus from feral rodents to man rarely results in clusters of disease, as the frequency of contact between man and rodent excreta is low. The virus has acquired scientific importance in laboratory studies of immunological tolerance and virus-induced immunopathological disease.

EPIDEMIOLOGY

There are few studies of the prevalence of antibody to LCMV in the general population, but the available data suggest that it is probably between 1 and 5 per cent. Sporadic disease resulting from contact with feral rodents in rural areas appears to occur mostly during the colder months when rodents are driven indoors. The situation in urban areas plagued by large rodent populations may be different. A recent study in Baltimore reported that 54/1149 (4.7 per cent) attendees of a sexually transmitted disease clinic had antibodies to LCMV.

RISK FACTORS AND TRANSMISSION

Sporadic cases of human infection often occur after infection with feral mice; however, the most common sources of human infection are pet or laboratory rodents, particularly hamsters, white mice, or nude mice. Laboratory outbreaks of human disease have occurred in individuals in close contact with infected animals or handling the virus, and there is some suggestion that aerosol spread may have occurred in close proximity to highly infectious material, such as animal bedding.

Clinical features

INCUBATION PERIOD AND DISEASE

The incubation period is about 1 to 3 weeks, and the infection ranges from asymptomatic or mild to moderately severe with central nervous manifestations and admission to hospital. In the largest studies of human infections reported, 33 of 94 (35 per cent) infections were asymptomatic, 47 (50 per cent) were mild to moderate febrile illnesses without significant neurological manifestations, and 14 (15 per cent) had typical LCMV disease (disease to infection ratio 1:3). Typical lymphocytic choriomeningitis, from which the virus derives its name, begins with fever, malaise, weakness, myalgia, and headache that is often severe, retro-orbital, and associated with photophobia. Anorexia, nausea, and dizziness are common. Myalgia is marked in the lumbar region. As many as one-half of patients may have any combination of sore throat, vomiting, and arthralgias, with chest pain and pneumonitis. Although only two deaths are reported in the literature, disease can be severe, with a prolonged convalescence. Physical examination shows pharyngeal inflammation, usually without exudate, and in more severely ill patients, meningeal signs including nuchal rigidity.

LABORATORY FINDINGS

The initial white blood-cell count is often 3^9/l or less with a mild thrombocytopenia. Cerebrospinal fluid from patients with meningeal signs contains several hundred white cells, predominantly lymphocytes (over 80 per cent), with mildly increased protein and occasionally low sugar levels. Virus is often found in spinal fluids taken during acute disease.

COMPLICATIONS AND SEQUELAE

About one-third of patients with central nervous manifestations will develop encephalopathy while the rest exhibit primarily aseptic meningitis. An interstitial pneumonia has also been described in two atypical fatal human cases and in autopsy studies of non-human primates. Alopecia, orchitis, and transient arthritis of the hands have also been reported. Convalescence is prolonged, with persistent fatigue, somnolence, and dizziness; deafness similar to that observed in Lassa fever has been reported. Neurological sequelae to LCMV infection are unusual but include some unsubstantiated experimental and indirect epidemiological evidence of hydrocephalus in newborns following maternal LCMV infection.

DIFFERENTIAL DIAGNOSIS

LCMV disease should be considered in patients presenting with fever of unknown origin with persistent meningeal signs, particularly if a history of rodent contact is obtained (often only a history of observing rodents in the house may be given). Physicians should be particularly alert to the possibility of laboratory-acquired infection.

Pathogenic processes

PATHOLOGY

There are no published descriptions of the pathology of LCMV infection in man; presumably LCMV invades the meninges, followed by lymphocytic infiltration causing swelling and inflammation. In one report of a fatal case with primarily neurological manifestations, there was evidence of perivascular infiltration of macrophages in many areas of the brain. Antigen was observed in the meninges and cortical cells by immunofluorescent assay, consistent with viral replication in the central nervous system.

IMMUNOLOGY

In man, antibody to LCMV appears as early as the first week of illness, with titres peaking at 40 to 60 days. In animal studies, the leptomeninges show dense infiltration with lymphocytic cells, with little involvement of the brain parenchyma. In the natural host, the mouse, the immunology of natural and experimental infection has been extensively studied, but extrapolation to human disease should be made with caution.

The model of persistent and acute LCMV infection in the mouse has played a central role in the understanding of immunology, because of its unique ability to assess the interaction of specific viral gene products with mouse major histocompatibility complex (**MHC**) gene products. Three critical mechanisms are exploited by the virus in the mouse: tolerance, immunosuppression, and MHC restriction of the immune response. Persistent infection in mice is established *in utero* or at birth by a mechanism of immune tolerance. Viral antigen may appear in the fetal or neonatal thymus in early T-cell precursors. The maintenance of tolerance depends on the continued presence of antigen in the thymus of the adult mouse where it is found in immature T cells (CD4−, CD8−). Elimination of the antigen through adoptive transfer of immune virus-specific cytotoxic T-lymphocytes abrogates the tolerance, and the mouse is then able to mount a normal T-cell response to new infection. In the adult mouse, however, the regulation of susceptibility to lethal disease is dependent, in part, on MHC class I gene expression. Thus, some mouse MHC alleles confer dominant susceptibility, whereas others confer resistance.

In the adult, immunocompetent mouse, intracerebral inoculation of LCMV results in lethal destruction of choroid and meningeal cells, involving virus and host genetic components. Differences of a single amino acid at position 260 of the viral glycoprotein may be necessary (but not sufficient) to determine the tropism of the virus for the central nervous system, where it produces acute lymphocytic choriomeningitis on the one hand or persistent systemic infection on the other. Part of this determination has to do with the ability of the virus to augment the class I MHC response in the infected cells of the central nervous system. Expression of class I MHC antigens is required for an effective cytotoxic T-lymphocyte response, whereas failure to induce class I expression results in persistent infection and no disease. The disease of the central nervous system is, in fact, an immunopathological process mediated primarily by CD8+ cytotoxic T cells through interaction with MHC class I molecules on the surface of cells. In contrast, mice infected as newborns will establish persistent infection, with a low level of MHC class I expression in the brain, and little immunopathology.

Whether LCMV infection in mice results in persistence, mild disease with clearance, or fatal disease depends primarily on the balance between virus replication and the virus-clearing, cytotoxic T-cell (CD8+) response. The role of the B-cell response in clearing virus would appear to be minor. The extent of viral control over this is governed by genes determining the type of cell infected and the outcome of this infection. Viruses that infect parenchymal cells will induce a normal, brisk, cytotoxic T-cell response and be eliminated (producing disease in some instances). Other viruses, with as little as a single amino-acid difference in the glycoprotein, may infect lymphoid cells and result in immunosuppression by means of killing of infected CD4+ cells and perhaps macrophages by cytotoxic T-lymphocytes directed at viral antigens on these cells. The immunosuppression is broad, and includes other infections, and may, in part, be the result of impairment of antigen presentation to effector cells.

The level of LCMV replication in adult immunocompetent mice is also related to the production of interferon-α during the early stages of infection. Protection from lethal LCMV infection in adult immunocompetent mice can also be achieved through immunizing the mice with a peptide vaccine of 8 to 15 amino acids in length. The response to the vaccine is MHC class I dependent in the mouse, and it is effected through generation of CD8+ cytotoxic T-lymphocytes specific for killing *in vivo* as well as for restimulation *in vitro*. It should be pointed out that persistent infection by the non-lytic LCMV in mice may also cause a variety of diseases resulting from interference with differentiated cellular functions such as loss of production of growth hormone by infected pituitary or loss of insulin production by infected islet cells of the pancreas.

Laboratory diagnosis

Virus may readily be cultured from cerebrospinal fluid during the acute phase of disease. IgG and IgM antibody may be detected in serum by immunofluorescent assay.

Patient management

There is no standard treatment for LCMV infection; however, ribavirin is known to be effective *in vitro*, and might reasonably be used as it is for Lassa fever. The penetration of ribavirin into the cerebrospinal fluid is, however, poor.

Prevention

There has never been a reported case of person-to-person transmission. However, laboratory outbreaks continue to occur, particularly where persistently infected mice are handled by persons unfamiliar with infectious diseases. Of some concern are reports of a fatal disease produced by the WE strain of LCMV in rhesus and cynomolgus monkeys, similar to that caused by Lassa virus. The virus should be considered a major laboratory hazard, and care taken to avoid accidental infection. Although the viral peptides known to elicit a protective immune response are identified, there is no identifiable market for a vaccine.

New world arenaviruses

The New World arenaviruses causing human disease are Junin, (Argentinian haemorrhagic fever), Machupo (Bolivian haemorrhagic fever), and Guanarito (Venezuelan haemorrhagic fever). All are endemic in geographically limited areas, but new, related viruses may emerge in other yet unaffected areas. The major rodent hosts are *Calomys* spp., and the viruses are related to the Tacaribe virus isolated from Trinidad fruit bats, and numerous other non-pathogenic arenaviruses from South American rodents ('Tacaribe complex', Fig. 1).

Argentinian haemorrhagic fever

Epidemiology

DISTRIBUTION AND ECOLOGY

Argentinian haemorrhagic fever was first recognized in the 1950s in the fertile farmland of north-western Buenos Aires Province in Argentina, and Junin virus was first isolated in 1958. The major rodent hosts are *Calomys musculinus* and *C. laucha* which, unlike Mastomys or Mus, are affected by the virus, with up to 50 per cent fatality in infected suckling animals, and stunted growth in many others. These rodents occupy grain fields. Both of the South American viruses can cause illness and death in newborn mice, or induce persistence.

EPIDEMIOLOGY

About 21 000 cases have been reported over 30 years. The disease is seasonal, with peaks each May. Though the average number of cases each year is about 360, wide annual fluctuations result in totals from year to year ranging from 100 to 400, with peaks during the late summer and early autumn. The disease has spread over 30 years, but incidence in the earlier affected areas appears to diminish after 5 to 10 years, perhaps because of the effect of the virus on rodent populations. A serosurvey in the endemic area showed an overall human antibody prevalence of 12 per cent, with predominance in male agriculture workers, though data are not available from this study on the size of the population actually at risk of infection based on their occupation. One-third of the seropositive individuals had no history of typical illness, (disease to infection ratio 2:3).

TRANSMISSION

The main routes of virus transmission to man are probably through virus-infected dust and grain products, particularly from mechanical harvesters. There is no recorded person-to-person spread.

Clinical features

INCUBATION PERIOD AND PRODROME

After an incubation period of about 12 days there is insidious onset of malaise, high fever, severe myalgia, anorexia, lumbar pain, epigastric pain and abdominal tenderness, conjunctivitis and retro-orbital pain, often with photophobia and constipation. Nausea and vomiting frequently occur after 2 or 3 days of illness. There is no lymphadenopathy or splenomegaly, sore throat or cough, but there is marked erythema of the face, neck, and thorax, and conjunctivitis. Temperature is high, reaching 40 °C or above with little fluctuation. Unlike LCMV and Lassa fever, Argentinian haemorrhagic fever does not usually lead to respiratory symptoms and sore throat. On physical examination, patients appear toxic. Petechiae may be observed in the axillae by the fourth or fifth days of the illness. There may be a pharyngeal enanthem, but pharyngitis is uncommon. Relative bradycardia is often observed.

SEVERE DISEASE

The disease may begin to subside after 6 days of illness; if not, the second stage of illness supervenes, most commonly with epistaxis and/or haematemesis or acute neurological disease. In contrast to the relative infrequency of bleeding in Lassa fever and its absence in LCMV, the South American diseases are associated with haemorrhagic manifestations in nearly half of the patients; gingival haemorrhages, epistaxis, metrorrhagia, petechiae, ecchymoses, purpura, melaena, and haematuria. Severe cases progress with nausea, vomiting, intense proteinuria, microscopical haematuria, oliguria, and uraemia. Fatal cases develop hypotensive shock, hypothermia, and pulmonary oedema. Renal failure has been reported but glomerular filtration rates, renal plasma flow, and creatinine clearance are usually normal. There is some electrocardiographic evidence of myocarditis. Fifty per cent of patients with Argentinian and Bolivian haemorrhagic fevers also have neurological symptoms during the second stage of illness, such as tremors of the hands and tongue, progressing in some patients to delirium, oculogyrus, and strabismus. Meningeal signs and abnormalities of the cerebrospinal fluid are rare.

LABORATORY FINDINGS

A low white blood-cell count, under 10^9/l, and a platelet count under 100^9/l are invariable. Bleeding and clot retraction times are concomitantly prolonged. Though reductions of levels of fibrinogen and factors II, V, VII, VIII, and X are observed, in the main alterations in clotting functions are minor. Disseminated intravascular coagulation is apparently not a significant feature, despite some reports of the presence of fibrinogen degradation products and absence of fibrinolysis. Proteinuria is common and microscopical haematuria also occurs. Liver and renal function tests are only mildly abnormal. Virus titres in serum are not as high as in Lassa fever, but the infection is also apparently pantropic. Outcome may again be related to virus titre in blood or tissues, though definitive studies demonstrating this have not been published.

MORTALITY

Mortality is about 16 per cent in patients admitted to hospital with laboratory-confirmed, untreated Argentinian haemorrhagic fever. There are no estimates of overall mortality from population-based surveys.

COMPLICATIONS AND SEQUELAE

A late neurological syndrome has been described, consisting mainly of cerebellar signs, and associated with the high-titre antiserum used in treatment in about 10 per cent of cases. It begins between 4 and 6 weeks after onset of acute illness and lasts less than a week. It is characterized by fever, headache, ataxia and intention tremors, and a mild pleocytosis with anti-Junin virus antibody in the cerebrospinal fluid. However, death from this syndrome is rare, and most patients recover within 3 months. Mild permanent damage to acoustic centres has been detected in a small group of patients. Argentinian haemorrhagic fever is also reportedly severe in pregnancy, but no formal studies are available, and women are less frequently affected overall.

Pathogenic processes

PATHOGENESIS

Despite the different degrees of bleeding, there are sufficient similarities between the course of disease in Argentinian and Bolivian haemorrhagic fevers and Lassa fever to speculate that there exists a similar pathophysiological pathway underlying all of the diseases. Organ function, other than the endothelial system, appears to remain intact, and the critical period of shock is brief, lasting only 24 to 48 h. Hepatitis is mild and renal function is also well maintained. Bleeding is more pronounced with the South American than Lassa fevers, but it is not the cause of shock and death. Capillary leakage is significant, with loss of protein and intravascular volume being much more pronounced than loss of red cells. Proteinuria is significant, and dehydration with haemoconcentration appears to be an important process. The shock is not associated with evidence of disseminated intravascular coagulation, and even though there are petechiae suggesting some direct endothelial damage, no clear evidence of virus replication in, and damage to, endothelium has been demonstrated. Thus, clinical observations suggest that vascular endothelial dysfunction and subsequent circulatory failure may also occur in Argentinian and Bolivian haemorrhagic fevers. Persistent hypovolaemic shock in the face of intravascular volume expanders may be due to the loss of endothelial function and leakage of fluid into extravascular spaces. This notion is supported by the frequently observed tissue oedema, and more directly by the pulmonary oedema that may result from vigorous fluid therapy.

Two other observations have been made in Argentinian haemorrhagic fever: high levels of interferon in severely ill patients, and a decrease in complement. These are general phenomena observed in other severe infectious processes and are consistent with the events described above. Neither would dictate a substantially different pathophysiological explanation of these diseases.

PATHOLOGY

There are large areas of intraalveolar or bronchial haemorrhage, petechiae on the organ surfaces, and ulcerations of the digestive tract, though bleeding is not massive. Microscopical examination shows a general alteration in endothelial cells, mild oedema of the vascular walls, with capillary swelling and perivascular haemorrhage. Large areas of intra-alveolar or bronchial haemorrhage are often seen, with no evidence of an inflammatory process. Pneumonia with necrotizing bronchitis or pulmonary emboli is observed in half of the cases. Haemorrhage and a lymphocytic infiltrate have been observed in the pericardium, occasionally with interstitial myocarditis. The lymph nodes are enlarged and congested, with reticular-cell hyperplasia. Splenic haemorrhage is common, and medullary congestion with pericapsular and pelvic haemorrhages are frequently seen. Adrenal necrosis has not been reported. Renal damage occurs in about one-half of the fatal cases, and consists of severe structural damage in the distal tubular cells and collecting ducts with relative sparing of the glomeruli and proximal tubules. As in Lassa fever, the pathology of central nervous involvement is obscure, with no evidence of direct viral infection. Microscopically there is mild oedema of the vascular walls, with capillary swelling and perivascular haemorrhage. Viral antigen but no immunoglobulins or complement components are associated with the damage. Electron microscopy shows intracytoplasmic and intranuclear inclusions, and marked non-specific cellular damage in all organs examined.

IMMUNOLOGY

In marked contrast to Lassa fever, the antibody response to Junin virus is effective in clearing virus during acute disease, and may also be sufficient to protect against infection. Neutralizing antibody may be detectable at the time the patient begins to recover from the acute illness, and the therapeutic efficacy of immune plasma in patients with Junin infection is directly associated with the titre of neutralizing antibody in the plasma given. Nevertheless, like Lassa, Junin virus may persist.

DIFFERENTIAL DIAGNOSIS

Argentinian haemorrhagic fever should be considered in any individuals in the endemic area, particularly male agricultural workers, who present with fever of unknown origin and a bleeding diathesis. No cases have been reported outside Argentina.

Laboratory diagnosis

The immunofluorescent antibody test is the most commonly performed, and may be positive by the end of the second week of illness. Neutralizing and complement-fixing antibodies to Junin are usually detectable 3 to 4 weeks after onset. IgM is more difficult to read by immunofluorescence, and an ELISA system may be preferred. Virus may also be cultured from serum.

Patient management

SPECIFIC TREATMENT

In contrast to Lassa fever the use of convalescent-phase plasma is highly successful in Argentinian haemorrhagic fever, reducing the mortality from 16 to 1 per cent in patients treated in the first 8 days of illness. In treated patients, viraemia is reduced within 24 h and clinical symptoms and haematological alterations are less severe than in control cases receiving non-immune plasma. Efficacy is directly related to the concentration of neutralizing antibodies. Though immune plasma therapy is highly successful in patients treated early in disease, as with Lassa fever late initiation of therapy is less successful. Availability of appropriately screened plasma may be a problem. Ribavirin is effective in experimentally infected non-human primates, and therapeutic use of ribavirin late in disease is currently being explored. The late neurological syndrome of Argentinian haemorrhagic fever may be associated with therapy, particularly very high-titre immune plasma.

Prevention

The man–rodent encounter resulting in Argentinian haemorrhagic fever occurs during the crop harvests, and it is difficult to imagine how control of non-commensal feral rodents could be accomplished. A live attenuated vaccine against the virus is showing promise in field trials in Argentina. The target population for the vaccine is, however, limited.

Bolivian haemorrhagic fever

Epidemiology

Bolivian haemorrhagic fever is caused by Machupo virus isolated in 1965, limited to a portion of the department of Beni in Bolivia. The only known reservoir is *C. callosus*, found in the highest density at the borders of tropical grassland and forest, in the eastern Bolivian plains, northern Paraguay and adjacent areas of western Brazil. Infected rodents develop haemolytic anaemia and splenomegaly, with up to 50 per cent fatality among infected suckling animals, and stunted growth in many others. The virus renders *C. callosus* essentially sterile, with the young dying *in utero*. Transmission from rodent to rodent is horizontal, not vertical, and is believed to occur through contaminated saliva and urine.

By 1962 more than 1000 human cases had been identified in a confined area of two provinces. The largest known epidemic, involving several hundred cases, followed a marked and unusual increase in the Calomys population in homes in the town of San Joaquin in 1963 and 1964. This seems to have been a unique event, and there have been virtually no cases, and no increase in the geographical areas affected by Bolivian haemorrhagic fever in the last decade. Calomys is capable of living both in and around towns and human contact may occur in both places. As all ages and both sexes were affected, it can be assumed that most patients were infected in their homes. Person-to-person spread is rarely reported. Though human disease has apparently diminished, the virus is still found in rodents.

Clinical features

The incubation period, clinical disease, and pathology closely resemble those of Argentinian haemorrhagic fever, but no recent information on the Bolivian disease is available. Case fatality in the 1960s was reported as 22 per cent. Neurological sequelae are observed in experimentally infected non-human primates. Diagnosis can be made in the same way as for the Argentinian type. Machupo virus also induces a humoral immune response, which may include neutralizing antibody, in the face of persistent infection. Ribavirin would be a reasonable candidate for treatment.

The key to prevention and control is either to interrupt the contact between infectious source and susceptible persons or to avoid disease in the event of infection. The ideal method of prevention for these rodent-borne diseases is to prevent contact between rodent and man. The effectiveness of this was admirably shown in the outbreaks of Bolivian haemorrhagic fever in the 1960s, when rodent control programmes in the villages were highly successful in eliminating the epidemic.

Venezuelan haemorrhagic fever

Epidemiology

In contrast is the recent appearance of a new South American haemorrhagic fever virus, Guanarito virus, isolated from patients in central Venezuela in 1991. The epidemiological pattern of this disease has not yet been characterized, but the virus was isolated from the cotton rat (*Sigmodon hispidus*), and antibodies were detected in the rice rat (*Oryzomys* spp.). The occurrence of person-to-person transmission has not yet been demonstrated, but the low frequency of infection in family contacts and lack of disease in hospital workers caring for patients suggest that it is uncommon. The pattern of infection includes all ages and sexes, suggesting that transmission occurs in and around houses, similar to that of Lassa fever and Bolivian haemorrhagic fever, and unlike Argentinian haemorrhagic fever. Guanarito virus infection is endemic, and its epidemiology may resemble that of Lassa virus in Africa, which occurs throughout the year; however, there are insufficient data at present to confirm this impression. Though the ecology of the new virus has been studied, data on prevalence of infection in man or risk factors for infection are not available.

Clinical features

Little information is available on the spectrum of disease caused by Guanarito virus infection, but it seems to share similarities with both Argentinian haemorrhagic fever and Lassa fever. Patients admitted to hospital with severe disease are febrile, with prostration, headache, arthralgia, cough, sore throat, nausea/vomiting, and diarrhoea. Haemorrhage is manifest as epistaxis, bleeding gums, menorrhagia, and melaena. On physical examination, they are toxic, and usually dehydrated, with pharyngitis, conjunctivitis, cervical lymphadenopathy, facial oedema, or petechiae. Thrombocytopenia and neutropenia are common. Case fatality of the single group of 15 admitted patients was over 60 per cent; however, serum surveys suggest that the overall mortality to infection ratio is much lower. Observations at a limited number of autopsy dissections include pulmonary oedema with diffuse haemorrhages in the parenchyma and subpleura; focal hepatic haemorrhages with congestion and yellow discoloration; cardiomegaly with epicardial haemorrhages, splenic and renal swelling; and bleeding into numerous cavities including stomach, intestines, bladder, and uterus. Few data are available on antibody response, but, like Argentinian and Bolivian haemorrhagic fevers, antibodies to Guanarito virus seem to appear later in illness. Similarly, though no data are available, the disease might be expected to respond to ribavarin.

REFERENCES

Cummins, D. *et al.* (1989). A plasma inhibitor of platelet aggregation in patients with Lassa fever. *British Journal of Haematology*, **72,** 543–8.

Cummins, D. *et al.* (1990). Acute sensorineural deafness in Lassa fever. *Journal of the American Medical Association*, **264,** 2093–6.

Dykewicz, C.A. *et al.* (1992). Lymphocytic Choriomeningitis outbreak associated with nude mice in a research institute. *Journal of the American Medical Association*, **267,** 1349–53.

Enria, D., Franco, S.G., Ambrosio, A., Vallejos, D., Levis, S., and Maiztegui, J. (1986). Current status of the treatment of Argentine Hemorrhagic Fever. *Medical Microbiology & Immunology*, **175,** 173–6.

Fisher-Hoch, S.P., Mitchell, S.W., Sasso, D.R., Lange, J.V., Ramsey, R., and McCormick, J.B. (1987). Physiological and immunologic disturbances associated with shock in a primate model of Lassa fever. *Journal of Infectious Diseases*, **155,** 465–74.

Fisher-Hoch, S.P. *et al.* (1989). Protection of rhesus monkeys from fatal Lassa fever by vaccination with a recombinant vaccinia virus containing the Lassa virus glycoprotein gene. *Proceedings of the National Academy of Sciences (USA)*, **86,** 317–21.

Helmick, C.G., Webb, P.A., Scribner, C.L., Krebs, J.W., and McCormick, J.B. (1986). No evidence for increased risk of Lassa fever infection in hospital staff. *Lancet*, **ii,** 1202–5.

Holmes, G.P. *et al.* (1990). Lassa fever in the United States. Investigation of a case and new guidelines for management. *New England Journal of Medicine*, **323,** 1120–3.

Jahrling, P.B., Hesse, R.A., Eddy, G.A., Johnson, K.M., Callis, R.T., and Stephen, E.L. (1980). Lassa virus infection of rhesus monkeys: pathogenesis and treatment with ribavirin. *Journal of Infectious Diseases*, **141,** 580–9.

Johnson, K.M., McCormick, J.B., Webb, P.A., Smith, E.S., Elliott, L.H., and King, I.J. (1987). Clinical virology of Lassa fever in hospitalized patients. *Journal of Infectious Diseases*, **155,** 456–64.

McCormick, J.B. *et al.* (1986). Lassa fever. Effective therapy with ribavirin. *New England Journal of Medicine*, **314,** 20–6.

McCormick, J.B. *et al.* (1987). A case-control study of the clinical diagnosis and course of Lassa fever. *Journal of Infectious Diseases*, **155,** 445–55.

McCormick, J.B., Webb, P.A., Krebs, J.W., Johnson, K.M., and Smith, E.S. (1987). A prospective study of the epidemiology and ecology of Lassa fever. *Journal of Infectious Diseases*, **155,** 437–44.

Maiztegui, J.I. (1975). Clinical and epidemiological patterns of Argentine haemorrhagic fever. *Bulletin of the World Health Organization*, **52,** 567–75.

Mercado, R. (1975). Rodent control programmes in areas affected by Bolivian haemorrhagic fever. *Bulletin of the World Health Organization*, **52,** 691–6.

Monath, T.P., Newhouse, V.F., Kemp, G.E., Setzer, H.W., and Cacciapuoti, A. (1974). Lassa virus isolation from *Mastomys natalensis* rodents during an epidemic in Sierra Leone. *Science*, **185,** 263–5.

Price, M.E., Fisher-Hoch, S.P., Craven, R.B., and McCormick, J.B. (1988). A prospective study of maternal and fetal outcome in acute Lassa fever infection during pregnancy. *British Medical Journal*, **297,** 584–7.

Salas, R. *et al.* (1991). Venezuelan haemorrhagic fever. *Lancet*, **338,** 1033–6.

Speir, R.W., Wood, O., Liebhaber, H., and Buckley, S.M. (1970). Lassa fever, a new virus disease of man from West Africa. *American Journal of Tropical Medicine and Hygiene*, **19,** 692–4.

Walker, D.H. *et al.* (1982). Pathologic and virologic study of fatal Lassa fever in man. *American Journal of Pathology*, **107,** 349–56.

7.10.23 Filoviruses: Marburg and Ebola fevers

D. I. H. SIMPSON

History

MARBURG VIRUS

Marburg virus disease, sometimes referred to as 'vervet monkey' or 'green monkey' disease, is a severe, distinctive, haemorrhagic febrile illness of man. It was first recognized in August 1967 when it caused three simultaneous outbreaks in Europe, at Marburg, Frankfurt, and Belgrade. There were 31 cases, of which 25 were primary infections; seven of the primary cases died, but there were no deaths among the six secondary cases. All the primary cases were laboratory personnel who had come into direct contact with blood, organs or tissue cultures from one particular consignment of vervet monkeys (Cercopithecus aethiops) imported from Uganda. Four of the secondary infections were in hospital personnel who had come into close contact with patients' blood. The wife of a Yugoslav veterinary surgeon was infected through blood contact with her husband while the sixth case was the wife of a patient who transmitted the disease during sexual intercourse 83 days after the onset of illness. Marburg virus was detected in his seminal fluid. There were no tertiary cases and no spread of the disease to the community at large.

The disease next appeared in South Africa in 1975 in a young Australian man who had been hitch-hiking through Central and Southern Africa. He died shortly after his admission to a Johannesburg hospital. His female travelling companion and a nurse who looked after him also contracted the disease; both survived. Virological investigations confirmed that the virus isolated from these three cases was morphologically and antigenically identical to Marburg virus.

On 15 January 1980, Marburg reappeared, this time in Kenya. A 58-year-old man was admitted to the Nairobi Hospital with an 8-day history of progressive fever, myalgia, and backache. On admission he was in a state of peripheral vascular failure and bleeding profusely from the gastro-intestinal tract. He died within 6 h of admission. Marburg virus particles were seen by electron microscopy in liver and kidney tissues removed at autopsy. On 24 January, a male doctor who had attended this patient and had attempted resuscitation became ill with a similar disease syndrome. He survived after a stormy illness and Marburg infection was confirmed serologically.

EBOLA VIRUS

Between June and November 1976, outbreaks of severe and frequently fatal viral haemorrhagic fever occurred in the equatorial provinces of the Sudan and Zaire. In the Sudan there were 284 known cases with 151 deaths, a case fatality rate of 53 per cent, whilst in the Zaire outbreak there were 318 known cases with 280 deaths, a case fatality rate of 88 per cent. The virus strains isolated from patients in both these outbreaks were found to be morphologically identical to Marburg virus but antigenically distinct. The new strain was named Ebola, after a river in Zaire.

A second outbreak of Ebola haemorrhagic fever occurred in the southern Sudan during August and September 1979, in the same area as the original 1976 outbreak. There were 34 reported cases of which 22 were fatal. The clinical diagnosis was confirmed by both virus isolation and serology. Sporadic cases were also reported in Zaire in 1978 and Kenya in 1980.

EBOLA-RELATED, RESTON VIRUS

In late 1989, infections caused by a filovirus closely related to Ebola virus were detected in cynomolgus *(Macaca fascicularis)* monkeys imported in several different shipments from the Philippines and held in primate quarantine facilities at Reston, Virginia and other places in the United States. Many monkeys died. Several monkey handlers dealing with batches of Philippine monkeys encountered Ebola; virus was isolated from one but none had any clinical illness. A further instance of importation of filovirus-infected monkeys from the Philippines occurred in Siena, Italy in 1992.

The filovirus causing the outbreaks is clearly related to Ebola and was called Reston virus. This strain has also been identified in monkeys in the Philippines, confirming the occurrence of a filovirus in Asia.

Aetiological agent

Electron-microscopic studies have shown that both Marburg and Ebola viruses are structurally indistinguishable from one another (Figs 1, 2). The virus particles in both instances are pleomorphic, appearing in contrast preparations as long filamentous forms, U-shaped, or circular forms resembling a doughnut or torus. The length of these filamentous forms can vary from 130 nm to more than 2600 nm, and in some preparations virions of almost 14 000 nm in length have been observed. The diameter appears to be fairly uniform at 80 to 100 nm.

Studies on chemical composition have indicated that both Marburg and Ebola virions contain four to six proteins including one glycoprotein. The viral genome appears to be a single-strand, negative-sense RNA of approximately 4.0×10^6 Da.

Information on the stability of these viruses is based on the more extensive knowledge of Marburg virus. The virus is stable when stored at temperatures of −70 °C, and there appears to be very little reduction in infectivity when stored at room temperature for periods of up to 5 weeks. The virus is completely inactivated by heating at 60 °C for 1 hour but not at 56 °C over the same period. Rapid inactivation occurs under ultraviolet irradiation. Formalin, acetone, Chloros, diethyl ether, and Tego MGH completely inactivate the virus after 1 h exposure.

Marburg and Ebola viruses grow in a variety of primary and established cell-culture systems. In early passage neither produce specific cytopathic effects, but a more obvious cytopathic effect may appear after several passages. Most workers, however, have preferred to base their evidence of cell infection on the appearance of characteristic intracytoplasmic inclusion bodies demonstrated by immunofluorescent staining techniques.

Monkeys and guinea-pigs are susceptible to experimental infection with both viruses and Marburg was successfully adapted to baby hamsters after a course of several intracerebral or intraperitoneal passages.

Marburg and Ebola produce an illness in monkeys that in many ways closely resembles that found in man, with high fever, anorexia, haemorrhages, severe weight loss, and a distinctive skin rash, most pro-

Fig 1. Marburg virus (by courtesy of Dr F. A. Murphy).

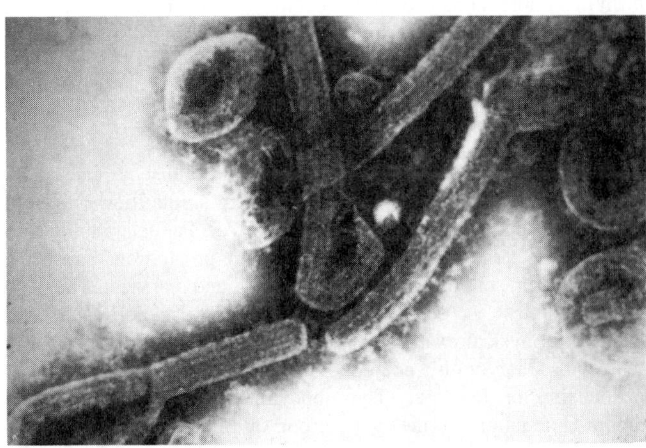

Fig 2. Ebola virus (by courtesy of Dr F. A. Murphy).

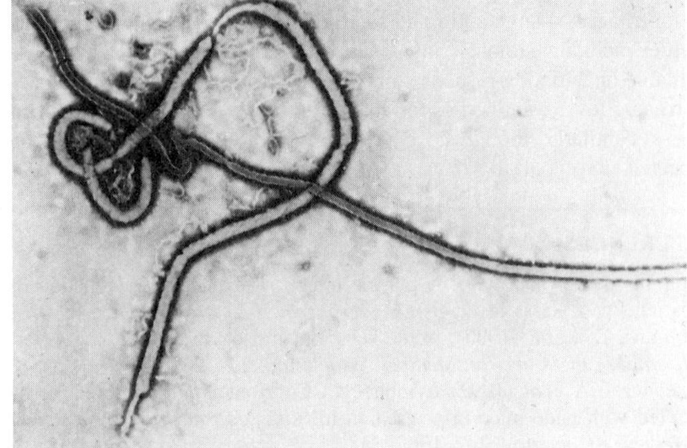

nounced on the forehead and face (where it is often confluent), on the chest, and on the medial aspect of the fore and hind limbs. Both viruses predominantly affect the liver, spleen, and lymph nodes, and, in addition, Ebola virus has some affinity for the lungs, intestines, and testes. Of particular interest is that the only monkey pancreas examined had high concentrations of virus. This accords well with the clinical observation of pancreatitis in man following Marburg infection during the South African outbreak.

Guinea-pigs inoculated with acute-phase blood become febrile (40.5–41 °C) after an incubation period ranging from 4 to 7 days. The febrile illness lasts for about 3 to 4 days, during which time the guinea-pigs fail to thrive and generally look ill. High concentrations of virus are found in the blood during the febrile period. The liver, spleen, and lymph nodes are the organs most consistently affected. Passage of the virus in guinea-pigs produces a uniformly fatal illness.

Clinical features

The illness caused in man by Marburg and Ebola viruses are virtually indistinguishable. The incubation period is about 4 to 10 days. Both infections have an abrupt onset with severe frontal and temporal headache, followed by high fever and generalized pains, particularly in the back. A relative bradycardia was often one of the early symptoms. The patient rapidly becomes prostrated and some develop severe watery diarrhoea leading to rapid weight loss and dehydration. Diarrhoea, abdominal pain with cramping, nausea, and vomiting often persist for a week. In the Sudanese Ebola outbreak, knife-like chest and pleuritic pain was an early symptom, and many patients complained of a very dry (rather than sore) throat, accompanied by cough. On white skin a characteristic, non-itching, maculopapular rash appears between days 5 and 7, lasts 3 or 4 days, and is followed by a fine desquamation (Figs 3,4). On black skin the rash, often described as being 'like measles', is not so obvious and can often only be recognized later with the appearance of skin desquamation. Conjunctivitis was a regular feature in all the outbreaks. An exanthema of the palate was reported in the Marburg outbreak in Germany, but was not seen in the three South African cases. In the Sudanese Ebola outbreak, pharyngitis was commonly noted and the throat was found to be dry accompanied by fissuring with open sores on the tongue and lips. Genital involvement with irritation and inflammation of the scrotum or labia majora was frequent and orchitis occurred in a few patients. Pancreatitis occurred in several instances.

Fig 3. Ebola fever—maculopapular rash (by courtesy of Dr R. T. D. Emond).

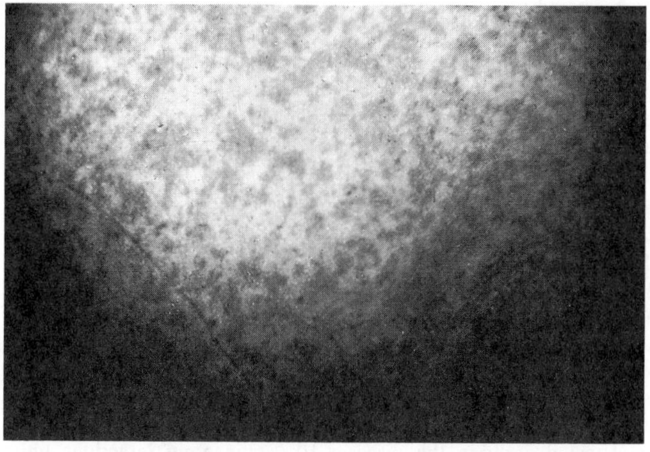

Fig 4. Marburg fever—maculopapular rash seen on patient in South Africa (by courtesy of Professor J. H. S. Gear).

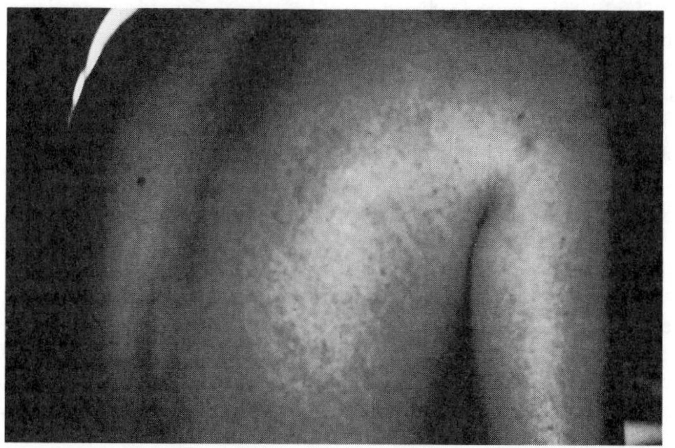

In both Ebola outbreaks, patients were generally admitted to hospital on the fifth day of illness and their appearance was described as 'ghost-like', with drawn, anxious features, expressionless faces, deep-set eyes, a greyish pallor, and extreme lethargy. Central nervous involvement may be apparent in a number of cases, with paraesthesia, lethargy, confusion, irritability, aggression, and signs of meningeal irritation.

A large number of patients in both the Marburg and Ebola outbreaks developed severe bleeding between days 5 and 7. The gastrointestinal tract and lungs were most frequently involved, with haematemesis, melaena, and sometimes the passage of fresh blood in the stools. There was also bleeding from the nose, gums, and vagina, and subconjunctival haemorrhages were common. Petechiae and bleeding from needle puncture sites are also very common. In some cases, laboratory investigation suggested profound haemostatic dysfunction with subsequent renal failure. In surviving patients recovery is slow, with considerable debility persisting for many weeks. Death generally occurred between days 7 and 16, usually preceded by severe blood loss and shock.

Laboratory features

Clinical laboratory studies have necessarily been limited to investigations on patients from the first two Marburg outbreaks. A leucopenia early in the course of illness has been a constant feature; this was followed by a leucocytosis and a low erythrocyte sedimentation rate. The acquired Pelger-Huet anomaly of the neutrophils together with atypical mononuclear cells was a feature in a number of patients. A considerable thrombocytopenia was recorded in most patients from about day 3 onwards, and platelet aggregation is abnormal.

Biochemical investigations showed that all patients had severe liver damage with both aspartate transaminase and alanine transaminase levels considerably, raised. In most of the fatal cases studied the levels of aspartate transaminase exceeded 2500 u/l. Bilirubin values were only slightly elevated, if at all. Serum alkaline phosphatase and creatinine phosphokinase remained normal. Creatine and urea increased only in cases of anuria. Electrocardiographic changes were compatible with a myocarditis or other damage to the myocardium.

Pathology

Marburg and Ebola viruses are pantropic and produce lesions in almost every organ, with the liver and spleen the most conspicuously affected. Severe degeneration of lymphoid tissue, spleen, and liver results in large accumulations of cellular and nuclear debris.

The pattern of disease is that of stimulation of the reticuloendothelial system, inhibition of the lymphatic system, and vascular changes leading to vascular occlusions and the formation of thrombi and haemorrhages. Macroscopic findings are similar in all cases. The stomach and parts of the intestines are usually filled with blood. Petechiae are seen in the mucosa of the stomach and the small intestines. In a number of cases the liver and spleen are enlarged and dark in colour. On section the spleen has no follicles and the pulp is soft and mushy. The liver is extremely friable and blood pours out freely on section, leaving the organ a light yellow colour. Histologically severe congestion and stasis are obvious in the spleen. There is proliferation of reticuloendothelial elements in the red pulp with the formation of large numbers of macrophages. Necrosis of the red pulp is accompanied by destruction of lymphoid elements. In the Malpighian bodies, lymphocytes are markedly depleted. There is widespread degeneration and necrosis of the liver cells, and hyaline changes are frequently seen. Hyaline-necrotic-eosinophil bodies similar to the Councilman bodies of yellow fever are often seen. The Kupffer cells are swollen and bulging, and full of cellular debris and red blood cells. Sinusoids are also full of debris, while mononuclear accumulation is seen in the periportal spaces. Even at the height of the necrotic process in the liver there is evidence of liver-cell regeneration.

Mononuclear transformation of lymphoid tissue as well as necrotic lesions are found not only in the liver and spleen but also in the pancreas, gonads, adrenals, hypophysis, thyroid, kidneys, and skin.

The lungs show few lesions except for circumscribed haemorrhages and evidence of endoarteritis, especially in the small arterioles. Neuropathological changes are confined mainly to glial elements scattered throughout the brain. No lymphocyte reactions have been observed but multiple haemorrhages into the brain have been seen. Glial lesions are either proliferative in the form of glial knots, nodules, and rosettes or degenerative in the form of nuclear pyknosis or karyorrhexis. All glial elements are affected, including astrocytes, microglia, and oligodendroglia. Cerebral oedema was found in all the human brain material examined.

Laboratory diagnosis

Specific diagnosis requires isolation and identification of the virus or evidence of antibody development between paired serum samples. The isolation of the virus is best achieved by the inoculation of acute-phase blood intraperitoneally into young guinea-pigs and into various tissue-culture cell lines. Identification is made by indirect immunofluorescent staining techniques. Attempts to isolate the virus must be carried out in high-containment laboratories.

Rapid detection of viral antigen is possible by immunoelectron microscopy or polymerase chain reaction on serum, enzyme immunoassay on tissue sections, and also by direct immunofluorescence on impressions of postmortem liver.

Antibody detection by an indirect immunofluorescence test has been used widely but there have been false-positive results at low concentrations. Other useful techniques include radioimmunoassay and enzyme immunoassay, but neutralizing antibody is not induced by filovivirus infections. Western blot analysis has been used to identify viral strains precisely.

Epidemiology

There is a strong suspicion that the disease is a zoonosis. Monkeys were originally implicated in the three Marburg outbreaks in 1967, but there was no real evidence to suggest that non-human primates were involved in the natural reservoir cycle of the virus. Following the South African outbreak in 1975, an extensive search for a reservoir was carried out without success. In 1977, large numbers of small mammals were caught in the epidemic areas of the Sudan and Zaire, and blood and tissues removed for virological investigation in an attempt to throw some light on the natural reservoir for these viruses, again without success.

The disease occurs in all age groups with a predominance in adults. The incubation period was from 3 to 9 days in both the German and South African outbreaks of Marburg disease, but in the two Ebola epidemics a wider range of 4 to 16 days was recorded.

Virological studies in both these virus infections have shown no evidence of significant virus shedding by any other route other than that of haemorrhage. There appears to be very little virus in the throat or urine but the persistence of virus in some body fluids for periods up to 83 days does pose a risk of late transmission. One of the South African Marburg patients developed a painful right eye. Uveitis was diagnosed and Marburg virus was cultured from fluid aspirated from the anterior chamber 2 months later.

The mechanism of transmission of infection in these outbreaks was mainly by direct contact with infected blood, by very close and prolonged contact with an infected patient, or by inoculation by accident or through the use of a contaminated syringe and needle. There was no evidence to suggest that there was any respiratory spread of infection in the community. Both in the Sudan and in Zaire there was serological evidence of small numbers of minor or even subclinical infections.

It may be assumed that sporadic cases of Marburg/Ebola virus-like disease occur from time to time and die off spontaneously without secondary spread. Exceptionally, as in the outbreaks in the Sudan and Zaire, unusual nosocomial transmission creates an amplifying cycle and causes epidemics. This happened in the former Federal Republic of Germany in 1967, whereas the South African cases in 1975 were more illustrative of the sporadic type of infection.

In the two Ebola epidemics the attack rate in infected communities varied from 3.5 per 1000 to 15.3 per 1000 in the Sudan and from 8 per 1000 in the infected community of Yandongi in Zaire to less than 1 per 1000 in neighbouring communities. This has indicated that the virus was not as highly transmissible as previously thought.

The secondary attack rate was about 15 per cent in Zaire. In the Sudan, active cases documented showed a secondary spread of 13 per cent, a tertiary spread of 14 per cent, and a quaternary spread of 9 per cent. Transmission stopped spontaneously after four generations, but in exceptional circumstances at least eight generations could be documented. The epidemics were readily brought under control by isolating the patients and instituting strict barrier nursing with gowns, gloves, masks, and the effective treatment of patients' excreta with disinfectants such as formaldehyde and hypochlorite.

Therapy

Therapy for these diseases has mainly been limited to nursing care and supportive measures. No vaccine is yet available, and ribavirin does not inhibit filovirus replication. In only a small percentage of cases has the use of specific therapy in the form of convalescent plasma been successful. The opportunity was taken to study the viraemic response in man following accidental laboratory infection with Ebola virus. Virus was detected early in the disease, $10^{4.5}$ guinea-pig infectious units **(GPIU)**/ml being detected on the first day of illness. No detectable change in the levels of circulating virus was evident on the day following initiation of interferon therapy. However within 12 h of administering 450 ml of Ebola immune plasma the viraemia had fallen to $10^{0.5}$ GPIU/ml. This much reduced level of circulating virus persisted throughout the acute stage of illness and virus became undetectable on the ninth day of illness. As both interferon and immunotherapy were administered together their respective merits cannot be assessed. There is no doubt that viraemia was dramatically reduced after the administration of immune plasma, but the patient's clinical condition did deteriorate despite the low virus levels in the blood.

During the South African outbreak, attempts were made to prevent the severe haemorrhage experienced in the first patient by giving the other two patients heparin early in the course of the disease and prevent disseminated intravascular coagulation. The results reported suggest that the prophylactic use of heparin in severe viral illnesses associated with haemorrhage may be warranted but only if continuous laboratory monitoring can be provided. However, the use of heparin in viral haemorrhagic fevers remains controversial.

REFERENCES

Edmond, R.T.D., Evans, B., Bowen, E.T.W., and Lloyd, G. (1977). A case of Ebola virus infection. *British Medical Journal*, **ii**, S41–4.

Feldman, H., Klenk, H-D., and Sanchez, A. (1993). Molecular biology and evolution of filoviruses. *Archives of Virology*, **7** (suppl.), 81–100.

Gear, J.S.S. *et al.* (1975). Outbreak of Marburg virus disease in Johannesburg. *British Medical Journal*, **iv**, 489–93.

Hayes, C.G. *et al.* (1992). Outbreak of fatal illness among captive macaques in the Philippines caused by an ebola-related filovirus. *American Journal of Tropical Medicine and Hygiene*, **46**, 664–71.

Murphy, F.A., Kiley, M.P., and Fisher-Hoch, S. (1990). Filoviridae. In *Fields virology*, Vol. 1, (2nd edn), (ed. B.N. Fields *et al.*), pp. 933–42. Raven, New York.

Simpson, D.I.H. (1977). *Marburg and Ebola virus infection: a guide to their diagnosis, management and control*, Offset Publication No. 36. WHO, Geneva.

World Health Organization (1978). Ebola haemorrhagic fever in Sudan, 1976. Report of a WHO/international study team. *Bulletin of the World Health Organization*, **56**, 247–70.

World Health Organization (1978). Ebola haemorrhagic fever in Zaire, 1976. Report of an international commission. *Bulletin of the World Health Organization*, **56**, 271–93.

7.10.24 Papovaviruses

K. V. SHAH

General description

Papovaviruses are small, spherical, non-enveloped, doubled-stranded DNA viruses that multiply in the nucleus. Viruses of the papovavirus family fall naturally into two subfamilies, papillomaviruses (wart viruses), and polyomaviruses. Viruses of each subfamily infect a wide variety of species including man and are largely host-specific. Papillomaviruses and polyomaviruses differ in many significant ways. The genetic information of papillomaviruses is carried on only one DNA strand but that of polyomaviruses is distributed over both strands. Papillomaviruses infect surface epithelia and produce disease at these sites. Polyomaviruses affect internal organs such as the kidney and the brain, where they are carried by viraemia after initial multiplication at the site of entry. Viruses of both subfamilies produce experimental tumors in laboratory animals but only papillomaviruses are related to naturally occurring cancers. Within each subfamily the viruses are immunologically related and share nucleotide sequences but there is no such relatedness between the two subfamilies.

So far, more than 60 human papillomaviruses have been recognized. About 35 types infect the skin and about 25 types infect mucous membranes (the genital tract, the respiratory tract, and the oral cavity). Human papillomaviruses are the aetiological agents of skin warts, genital warts, respiratory papillomatosis, and papillomas at other mucosal sites (e.g. mouth, eye). In addition, infection with some of the genital-tract human papillomaviruses is causally linked with cervical cancer, one of the most common female malignancies in the world. Human papillomaviruses may also contribute to cancers at other genital and non-genital sites.

Two polyomaviruses, BK virus and JC virus, infect man. JC virus is the aetiological agent of progressive multifocal leucoencephalopathy, a fatal demyelinating disease that occurs in people who are immunodeficient. Until recently, this encephalopathy was a rare disease that occurred at older ages, but because it is a complication of AIDS, it is now seen much more often and at younger ages. BK virus is associated with haemorrhagic cystitis in recipients of bone marrow transplants.

Human papillomaviruses

The remarkable plurality of human papillomaviruses was recognized in the 1970s, when techniques for molecular cloning of viral DNA became available. Human papillomaviruses still cannot be propagated in tissue culture and require nucleic-acid hybridization assays for their identification. Their double-stranded, circular genome contains about 8000 bp and is divided into an early region, which is necessary for transformation, a late region, which codes for capsid proteins, and a regulatory region, which contains control elements (Fig. 1). All of the open reading frames of the viral genome are located on one strand; E1 to E8 in the early region and L1 and L2 in the late region. The functions assigned to the different open reading frames are listed in Table 1.

Human papillomaviruses infect only man. They show a marked degree of cellular tropism. Mucosal human papillomaviruses do not readily infect cutaneous epithelia and cutaneous human papillomaviruses are rarely present on mucous membranes. Infection is initiated when, after minor trauma (e.g. during sexual intercourse or after minor skin abrasions), the basal cells of the epithelium come in contact with infectious virus particles. The virus stimulates the proliferation of basal cells. The early-region open reading frames are expressed in all layers of the infected epithelium, but expression of the late-region open reading frames and synthesis of viral particles occur only in the upper differentiating and keratinizing layers.

The most important disease associations and characteristics of mucosal human papillomaviruses are listed in Table 2; the genital tract is the reservoir for all but a few and genital human papillomavirus infections constitute the most common, viral, sexually transmitted disease. Genital human papillomaviruses may sometimes infect non-genital mucosal sites, for example, the respiratory tract, the mouth, and the conjunctiva. Transmission of genital-tract human papillomavirus (**HPV**) types 6 and 11 from an infected mother to the baby at birth results in juvenile-onset recurrent respiratory papillomatosis. Infection with two types, HPV-13 and -32, appears to be confined to the mouth.

Table 3 lists the disease association of cutaneous human papillomaviruses. They are transmitted from one person to another by direct contact with an infected tissue or by contact with a contaminated object.

Fig. 1 Genomic map of HPV-16. On the inner circle, P97 represents the transcriptional promoter and A_E and A_L designate early and late polyadenylation sites. The location of the early-region open reading frames (ORFs) (E1–E7), the late-region ORFs (L1–L2) and of the LCR (long control or regulatory region) are shown. (Reproduced from Shah and Howley (1990), with permission.)

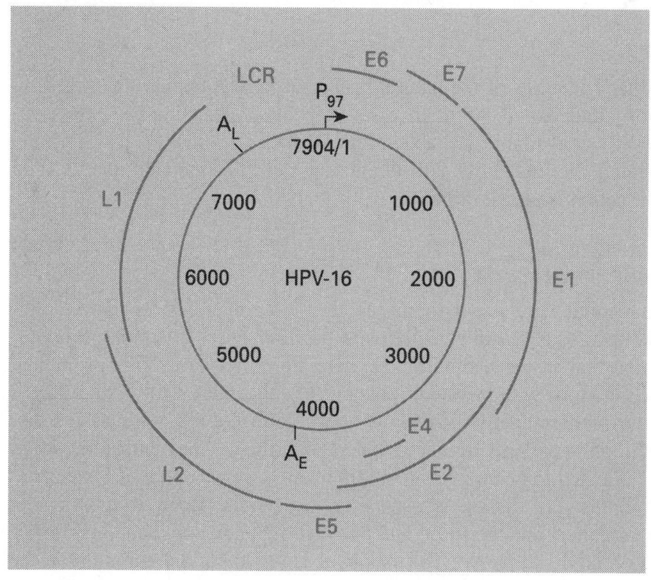

Table 1 *Functions of human papillomavirus open reading frames (ORF)*

Function	ORF
Replication of viral DNA	E1, E2
Regulation of transcription	E2
Coding for late cytoplasmic protein	E4
Cellular proliferation	E5*
Transformation	E6, E7
Not known	E3, E8

*In bovine papillomavirus, the major transforming activity is in E5.

Modified from Shah and Howley (1990).

Table 2 *Mucosal human papillomaviruses: chief clinical associations*

Clinical association	Viral type(s)
Exophytic condyloma; respiratory papillomas; oral and conjunctival papillomas.	HPV-6,-11
Cervical cancer	
'High-risk' infections	HPV-16,-18,-45,-56
'Intermediate-risk' infections	HPV-31,-33,-35,-39,-51,-52,-58
'Low-risk' infections	HPV-6,-11,-42,-43,-44
Focal epithelial hyperplasia of the oral cavity	HPV-13,-32

Table 3 *Cutaneous human papillomaviruses: chief clinical associations*

Clinical association	Viral type
Deep plantar wart	HPV-1
Common wart	HPV-2,-4
Mosaic wart (superficial spreading wart)	HPV-2
Flat warts	HPV-3,-10,-28,-41
Macular plaques of epidermodysplasia verruciformis	HPV-5,-8,-9,-12,-14,-15,-17,-19,-20, -21,-22,-23,-24,-25,-36,-47,-50

Modified from Shah and Howley (1990).

Many features of the natural history of human papillomaviruses are poorly understood. Antibody assays capable of detecting past infections are not yet available. Reliable information on questions such as duration of infection, infectivity at different stages of infection, and immunity to reinfection is also lacking.

Anogenital warts

Anogenital warts (condylomas) are the most commonly recognized clinical manifestations of genital human papillomavirus infections. It is estimated that in the United States there are more than a million annual consultations with private physicians for anogenital warts. Condylomas occur predominantly in sexually active young adults, with an age distribution of patients similar to that of gonorrhoea. The incubation period is estimated to be an average of 2.8 months with a range of 3 weeks to 8 months. The disease is transmitted to sexual partners in most cases. Condylomas may be florid and exophytic (condyloma acuminatum) or flat (condyloma plana). The exophytic condylomas are common on the external genitalia but rare on the cervix. They may increase in size and number during pregnancy and regress after delivery. Immunosuppressed individuals have a high prevalence of exophytic condylomas. Flat condylomas on the cervix are the precursor lesions of cancer and are indistinguishable from what is now classified as cervical intraepithelial neoplasia, grade 1, or low-grade squamous intraepithelial lesion of the cervix. HPV-6 and -11 are recovered from most exophytic condylomas; these two types are not associated with genital cancers. Flat condylomas (low-grade squamous intraepithelial lesion) are aetiologically more heterogeneous than exophytic condylomas and may contain any of the human papillomaviruses found in the genital tract.

Traditional therapies for anogenital warts have included application of caustic agents (e.g. podophyllin), cryotherapy, application of a DNA inhibitor (fluorouracil), surgical removal, and laser ablation. Intralesional and parenteral interferon therapy has often been successful in the treatment of refractory genital warts.

Cervical cancer

It is estimated that there are about 500 000 new cases of cervical cancers annually, worldwide. Cervical cancer is the most common female malignancy in the developing world. The lifetime risk of dying from cervical cancer varies as much as 10-fold between different countries. Cervical cancer has been recognized for over a century as having the characteristics of a sexually transmitted disease. It is almost never seen in virgins and is most frequent in women with multiple sexual partners. In the past, different sexually transmitted infections (e.g. herpes simplex virus) have been associated with cervical cancer but these associations have not proved to be aetiological. In the past decade, epidemiological and clinical studies of genital-tract specimens as well as laboratory investigations of human papillomaviruses for oncogenic potential have provided compelling evidence that infections with certain types of human papillomavirus are responsible for a large majority of cervical cancers in all parts of the world.

Human papillomavirus DNAs are recovered from 70 to 90 per cent of cases of invasive cervical cancer as well as from an equally high proportion of squamous intraepithelial lesions of the cervix, which precede invasive cancer. The viral genome is present in the tumour cells of primary as well as metastatic cervical cancer. The progression from low-grade squamous intraepithelial lesions to invasive cancer may take over 10 years; human papillomaviruses are found throughout this disease process. The viruses are recovered much less frequently from cytologically normal women of comparable age. In prospective studies of women with normal cervical cytology, the presence of human papillomaviruses is a strong risk factor for the subsequent development of squamous intraepithelial lesion.

Certain human papillomavirus types are preferentially associated with invasive cancers. From their distribution in normal individuals and in preinvasive and invasive cervical disease, genital-tract human papillomaviruses have been categorized as 'high-risk', 'intermediate-risk', and 'low-risk' types (Fig. 2; Table 2). HPV-16 and -18 are the predominant viruses in invasive cancers and account for 40 to 60 per cent and 5 to 20 per cent, respectively, of human papillomavirus-positive cancers in different studies. About a dozen additional types of human papillomavirus are found in small proportions of invasive cancers. Five to 10 per cent of the cancers contain as yet unidentified human papillomaviruses. The five 'low-risk' human papillomaviruses are almost never detected in invasive cervical cancers.

Comparisons of different human papillomavirus types for their ability to transform human keratinocytes *in vitro* show that HPV-16 and -18, those most clearly associated with naturally occurring cervical cancers, also have the greatest oncogenic potential in laboratory studies. The transforming functions of human papillomaviruses are localized to open reading frames E6 and E7; these are the frames consistently expressed in naturally occurring, human papillomavirus-positive cancers. The viral genome is integrated into the cellular DNA in most cervical cancers. The break in the circular viral genome that is required for integration occurs most frequently in the E1/E2 region and results in an enhanced expression of the transforming E6 and E7 open reading frames. The transforming human papillomavirus proteins E6 and E7 interact with cellular tumour-suppressor proteins p53 and Rb, respectively. It is likely that the oncogenic effect of human papillomaviruses is mediated partly by their ability to inactivate the tumour-suppressor proteins, which normally regulate the cell cycle.

Human papillomavirus infections of the genital tract are extremely common in sexually active populations. In young sexually active women, prevalence of human papillomavirus infection as measured by the detection of human papillomavirus DNA in genital-tract specimens by the sensitive polymerase chain reaction may be greater than 40 per cent. The prevalence decreases with increasing age. Most of these infections are found in women with normal cervical cytology and undoubtedly resolve without leaving a trace. Only a small proportion of infections progress to squamous intraepithelial lesions and then to invasive cancer. The cofactors that might be required for this progression are not conclusively identified, but smoking, use of oral contraceptives, parity, presence of other sexually transmitted diseases, and diet are incriminated to some degree, in some studies. Human immunodeficiency virus-infected women have a higher prevalence of human papillomavirus and of squamous intraepithelial lesions than women seronegative for human immunodeficiency virus.

Screening for cervical cytological abnormalities by Pap smear and treatment of preinvasive and invasive cancers identified by screening have been credited with the decrease in cervical cancer incidence and mortality that has been observed in many developed countries over the last 40 to 50 years. The possibility that diagnosis of human papillomavirus may be a useful adjunct to Pap smears in screening for cervical cancer has been raised. It has been suggested that if human papillomavirus testing and Pap smears were combined in a cervical cancer screening programme, positive tests for oncogenic human papillomaviruses would identify women with increased risk of cancer who were not identified by cytological screening, either because they had normal cytology or because they had a 'false-negative' Pap smear. On the other hand, screening the general population for human papillomaviruses would reveal a vast number of women who have transient infection of the genital tract and for whom, in the absence of an effective antiviral treatment, little can or need be done. The utility of human papillomavirus diagnosis in the management of patients with squamous intraepithelial lesions is under investigation. It has been proposed that low-grade squamous intraepithelial lesions of the cervix associated with 'low-risk' human papillomaviruses may require less follow-up and treatment than those associated with 'intermediate-risk' or 'high-risk' human papillomaviruses. The recognition of viral causation of cervical cancer has also opened future prospects of antigen-specific immunotherapy of established cervical cancer and of developing an effective vaccine against the virus to prevent cervical cancer.

Fig. 2 Distribution of human papillomavirus (HPV) types in normal women and in preinvasive (low-grade and high-grade squamous intraepithelial lesions (SILs)) and invasive cancer. In each diagnostic category, specimens are grouped as containing high-risk, intermediate-risk and low-risk HPV types (see Table 2), or as containing unclassified HPVs (Unc), or as negative (Neg). (Modified and reproduced from Lörincz *et al.*, (1992), with permission.)

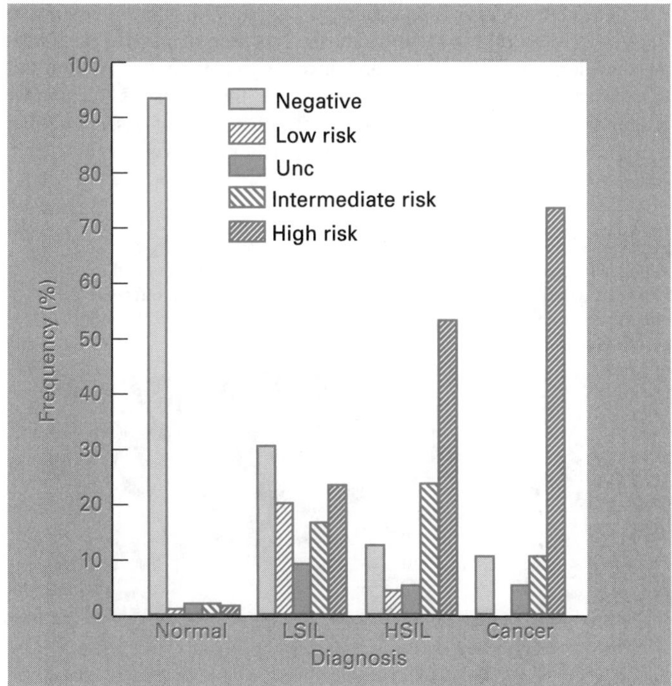

Cancers at other lower anogenital-tract sites

Human papillomavirus infections are very common on the vulva, the vagina, the penis, the perineum, and the anus. Synchronous neoplasia at multiple sites in the female lower genital tract is almost always associated with human papillomaviruses, especially HPV-16. Carcinoma of the vulva is aetiologically heterogeneous. Vulvar cancers occurring in younger women are associated with human papillomaviruses but the typical squamous-cell carcinoma of the vulva in older women is not. Neoplasia of the anal canal, seen frequently in homosexual men seropositive for human immunodeficiency virus, is strongly associated with human papillomaviruses.

Respiratory papillomatosis

This is a rare disease that may occur at any age but is most common in children under the age of 5 years. It may become life threatening if it obstructs the airways. The most common site of papillomatosis is the vocal cords and the most common presenting symptoms are hoarseness or voice change. Respiratory papillomas tend to recur after surgical removal.

HPV-6 and-11, genital-tract human papillomaviruses that are responsible for most of the exophytic genital warts, also cause respiratory papillomatosis. For juvenile-onset patients, transmission is thought to occur from mother to offspring during passage through an infected birth canal. In adult-onset cases, the transmission may occur by sexual contact. Respiratory papillomas very rarely progress to invasive cancer. Prior history of X-irradiation to reduce the size of the papilloma (a practice now discontinued) increases the risk of malignant progression.

Caesarean delivery for mothers who are found to have genital warts or are infected with HPV-6 or -11 would reduce the risk of juvenile-onset respiratory papillomatosis, but it is not generally recommended because the risk of developing respiratory papillomas for infants born to infected mothers is estimated to be quite small. Interferon therapy is not very effective in the treatment of respiratory papillomas.

Human papillomaviruses in the mouth and at other mucosal sites

The genital-tract human papillomaviruses may infect the oral cavity (Table 2). Genital human papillomaviruses, especially HPV-6 and -11, are readily recovered from oral lesions diagnosed histologically as condylomas or warty lesions. In addition, focal epithelial hyperplasia of the mouth, which is worldwide in distribution but highly prevalent in indigenous populations of Central and South America and of Alaska and Greenland, is aetiologically associated with HPV-13 and -32. These two types are found exclusively in the oral cavity. The role of human papillomaviruses in oral cancers and the frequency of asymptomatic human papillomavirus infections in the mouth are subjects of current investigations.

HPV-6 and -11 are associated with conjunctival papillomas and HPV-16 and -18 with conjunctival carcinomas. HPV-59 is associated with nasal papillomas.

Skin warts (see Section 23)

Skin warts and verrucas may occur at any location on the skin and have diverse morphological features. They are most common in older children and young adults. Except in the rare condition known as epidermodysplasia verruciformis (see below), they almost never become malignant. Most warts regress within 2 years. Specific human papillomavirus types are strongly associated with specific types of warts; for example, HPV-1 with deep plantar warts, HPV-2 and -4 with common warts, and HPV-3 and -10 with flat skin warts (Table 3).

EPIDERMODYSPLASIA VERRUCIFORMIS

This is a rare, life long disease in which a patient has extensive warty involvement of the skin that cannot be resolved. The disease generally begins in infancy or childhood with multiple, disseminated, polymorphic wart-like lesions on the face, trunk and extremities that tend to become confluent. The warts are of two different shapes: flat warts and reddish-brown macular plaques that resemble pityriasis versicolor. In about a third of the cases, foci of malignant transformation occur in the macular plaques located in areas of the skin exposed to sunlight. The tumours are slow growing and they rarely metastasize.

Epidermodysplasia verruciformis is often familial and patients sometimes have a history of parental consanguinity. The pattern of inheritance is suggestive of an X-linked recessive disease. It is thought that the genetic defect results in an immunological inability to resolve the warty infection. The flat warts yield the same human papillomavirus types as those of normal individuals but a very large number of human papillomaviruses that are seldom encountered in normal individuals are recovered from the macular plaques (Table 3). It is unclear how patients with epidermodysplasia verruciformis become infected with these specific human papillomaviruses. Carcinomas in such patients are associated with infection by specific human papillomavirus genotypes, for example, HPV-5 and -8. Thus, the factors that contribute to the occurrence of carcinoma in these patients include a genetic defect, infection with specific human papillomaviruses, and exposure of the affected area to sunlight.

Human polyomaviruses

BK virus and JC virus, the two polyomaviruses that infect man, were both recognized in 1971; BK virus was isolated from the urine of a renal transplant recipient and JC virus was recovered from the brain of a patient with progressive multifocal leucoencephalopathy. The viruses have a double-stranded DNA genome of about 5000 bp, which is divided into an early region that codes for viral T proteins, a late region that codes for viral capsid proteins, and a non-coding regulatory region. The early and late regions are transcribed from different strands of the viral DNA. BK and JC viruses have 75 per cent nucleotide-sequence homology, but the two infections are readily distinguishable from one another by conventional tests.

Infections with both viruses occur in childhood and are largely subclinical. Most of the children affected have antibodies to BK virus by the age of 10; infection with JC virus occurs at a somewhat later age. Acquisition of antibodies at an early age suggests that infection occurs by the respiratory route. Both viruses establish latent, often lifelong infection in the kidney and are occasionally excreted in the urine of normal individuals. Reactivation of the viruses in immunodeficient individuals is responsible for most of the associated illnesses. The viruses are reactivated in pregnancy but without any apparent harm to the mother or the newborn.

BK virus-associated illnesses

Reactivation of BK virus in renal transplant recipients is associated with some cases of ureteral obstruction, which is a late and uncommon complication of transplantation. Reactivation does not increase the risk of death or of loss of renal function. In bone-marrow transplant recipients receiving allogeneic marrow, late-onset haemorrhagic cystitis and BK viruria are strongly correlated. Primary infection with BK virus may be responsible for an occasional case of cystitis in normal children. A case of fatal tubulointerstitial nephritis in an immunodeficient child was ascribed to primary BK virus infection. The virus is reportedly present in pancreatic islet-cell tumours and in brain tumours but these observations have not been confirmed.

Progressive multifocal leucoencephalopathy

JC virus is the aetiological agent of progressive multifocal leucoencephalopathy, a subacute demyelinating disease of the central nervous system that occurs as a complication of illnesses known to impair cell-mediated immunity. Until recently, it was a rare disease found mainly in patients in the fifth or sixth decades of life who were suffering from lymphoproliferative disorders or chronic diseases. In the past decade, this encephalopathy has been seen much more frequently and in younger patients, because it occurs as a complication in 1 to 2 per cent of AIDS cases; Currently, progressive multifocal leucoencephalopathy in AIDS constitutes a majority of all cases of this encephalopathy, which has also been recognized in children who have inherited immunodeficiency diseases or AIDS.

The key pathogenetic event in the leucoencephalopathy is the cytocidal JC virus infection of oligodendrocytes, which are responsible for the production and maintenance of myelin. Destruction of the oligodendrocytes by JC virus leads to foci of demyelination that tend to coalesce over time and involve large areas of the brain. Infected oligodendrocytes, containing large inclusion-bearing nuclei filled with abundant numbers of virus particles, surround the foci of demyelination (Fig. 3). Enlarged astrocytes, which often show bizarre nuclear changes but are mostly virus negative, are found within the foci of demyelination. JC virus is disseminated haematogenously to the central nervous system, probably through virus-infected B lymphocytes. The brain may be seeded with JC virus either at the time of primary infection or when the virus is reactivated in times of immunological impairment.

Progressive multifocal leucoencephalopathy has an insidious onset. Early signs and symptoms indicate the presence of multifocal, asymmetrical lesions in the brain and involve impairment of vision and speech, and mental deterioration. As a rule, the disease is relentlessly progressive and results in death within 3 to 6 months of onset, although it can rarely become stabilized and the patient may survive many years.

Fig. 3 A lesion of progressive multifocal leucoencephalopathy showing oligodendrocytes with enlarged, deeply staining nuclei (arrow) and giant astrocytes (left). Crystalloid array of JC virus particles in an infected oligodendrocyte nucleus (right). (Reproduced from Shah (1992), with permission.)

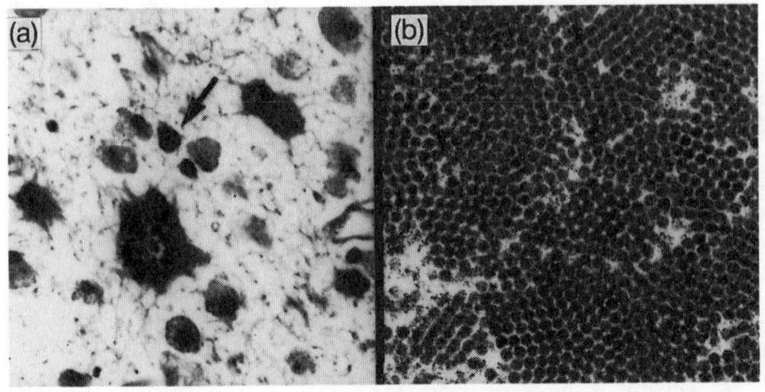

Non-invasive techniques such as computerized tomography and magnetic resonance imaging have been successful in its diagnosis, which until recently could be established only with a brain biopsy. Treatment with cytosine arabinoside and the presence of an inflammatory response in the brain have been associated with the few relatively successful outcomes.

REFERENCES

Bunney, M. (1982). *Viral warts: their biology and treatment.* Oxford University Press.

Hogan, T.F., Padgett, B.L., and Walker, D.L. (1991). Human polyomaviruses. In *Textbook of human virology*, (ed. R.B. Belshe), pp. 970–1000. Mosby Year Book, St. Louis.

Jenson, A.B. and Lancaster, W.D. (1991). Human papillomaviruses. In *Textbook of Human virology*, (ed. R.B. Belshe), pp. 947–69. Mosby Year Book, St. Louis.

Koutsky, L.A., Galloway, D.A., and Holmes, K.K. (1988). Epidemiology of genital human papillomavirus infection. *Epidemiological Review*, **10,** 122–62.

Ley, C. *et al.* (1991). Determinants of genital HPV infection in young women. *Journal of the National Cancer Institute*, **83,** 997–1003.

Lörincz, A.T., Reid, R., Jenson, A.B., Greenberg, M.D., Lancaster, W., and Kurman, R.J. (1992). Human papillomavirus infection of the cervix: relative risk associations of 15 common anogenital types. *Obstetrics and Gynecology*, **79,** 328–7.

Major, E.O., Amemiya, K., Tornatore, C.S., Houff, S.A., and Berger, J.R. (1992). Pathogenesis and molecular biology of progressive multifocal encephalopathy, the JC virus-induced demyelinating disease of the human brain. *Clinical Microbiology Reviews*, **1,** 49–73.

Muñoz, N., Bosch, F.X., Shah, K.V., and Meheus, A. (ed.) (1992). *The Epidemiology of human papillomavirus and cervical cancer*, Scientific Publication No. 119. International Agency for Research on Cancer, Lyon.

Shah, K.V. (1992). Polyomavirus, infection and immunity. In *Encyclopedia of immunology*, (ed. I.M. Roitt), pp. 1256–8. Academic Press, New York.

Shah, K.V. and Howley, P.M. (1990). Papillomaviruses. In *Virology* (ed. B.N. Fields *et al.*), pp. 1651–76. Raven Press, New York.

Zur Hausen, H. (1991). Human papillomaviruses in the pathogenesis of anogenital cancer. *Virology*, **184,** 9–13.

7.10.25 Parvoviruses

J. R. PATTISON

Members of the family Parvoviridae are small (18–25 nm), non-enveloped viruses with icosahedral symmetry, containing a single-stranded DNA molecule 5.5 kb in length. There are three genera, the parvoviruses (viruses of vertebrates capable of autonomous replication), the dependoviruses (again viruses of vertebrates but requiring coinfection with a helper virus, for example adenovirus, for replication) and the densoviruses (autonomous viruses of insects). The dependoviruses have not been linked with disease in man or animals but the parvoviruses have been shown to be the cause of a number of diseases in different species. Parvoviruses replicate most extensively in tissues undergoing relatively rapid division and disease is often related to gut epithelium (enteritis in cats, dogs, and mink) or bone marrow (panleucopenia in cats). In addition to acute diseases, a parvovirus causes Aleutian disease of mink, a persistent infection leading to hypergammaglobulinaemia and death in renal failure due to glomerulonephritis. In man, a parvovirus (Fig. 1) initially found by chance in the serum of asymptomatic blood donors has been shown to be associated with specific diseases (see below). It is also possible that some of the small, round viruses found in faeces are also human parvoviruses.

Pathogenesis of human parvovirus infection

Studies in normal volunteers have elucidated the sequence of events in human parvovirus infection (Fig. 2). Virus found originally in the serum of an asymptomatic blood donor leads to infection when given by the intranasal route. Approximately 1 week later there is a substantial (10^{11} particles/ml) viraemia and virus can be detected in upper respiratory-tract secretions, suggesting that the natural mode of spread is via the respiratory route. The disappearance of the viraemia is associated with a specific IgM antibody response (which persists for 2 to 3 months) and shortly afterwards by the appearance of specific IgG, which persists for life and correlates well with immunity to infection.

At the time of the viraemia there is a brief pyrexia and associated minor symptoms (itching, malaise, headache). During the second week after inoculation there is a transient reticulocytopenia and an associated small fall in haemoglobin concentration (of about 1 g/dl), neutropenia, lymphopenia, and a fall in platelet numbers. Normal values of these are restored during the third and fourth week after infection. Approximately 17 to 18 days after inoculation a second-phase illness occurs and this is characterized by a brief rash illness often associated with joint symptoms. Specific antibody but no viraemia is present at this time so the rash and joint symptoms are probably immune mediated.

Clinical features

Sixty to 70 per cent of adults have parvovirus antibody, the most frequent age at infection being 4 to 10 years. As with many common childhood virus infections there is a wide range of clinical consequences of these infections. In children about half the infections are asymptomatic and the next most common consequence is a non-specific respiratory-tract illness. These are generally mild but may be severe enough to suggest influenza and they coincide with the viraemic phase of the illness.

RASH ILLNESS

The most common specific clinical manifestation is an erythematous rash illness. In young children this tends to be recognized clinically when it occurs in outbreaks of erythema infectiosum (fifth disease). Classically, this begins with erythema of the cheeks (slapped-cheek appearance) and subsequently involves the trunk and limbs, with the rash having a lacy or reticular appearance and tending to fade and recrudesce for a week or so after its initial appearance. All outbreaks of erythema infectiosum so far investigated have been due to human parvo-

Fig. 1 Immune electron micrograph of parvovirus particles in serum from a case of aplastic crisis. Complete particles are 20–23 nm in diameter.

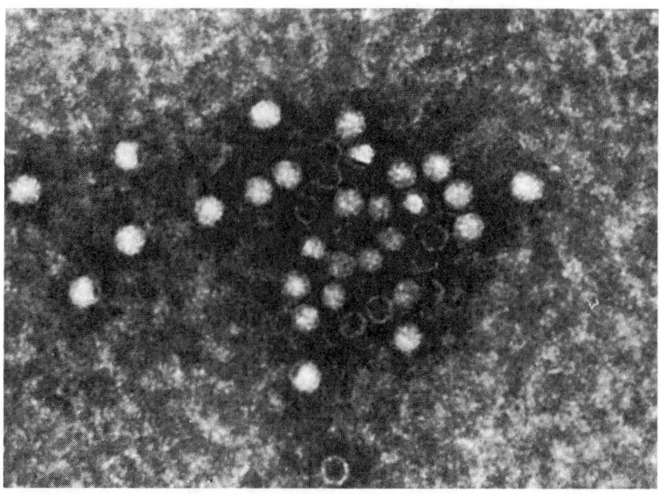

virus infection but other forms of rash illness may be produced. Sporadic cases occur in both adults and children; in many of these cases the rash is rubelliform and diagnosed clinically as rubella, allergy, or streptococcal infection. B19 infection occasionally presents as a purpuric rash, which may or may not be accompanied by transient thrombocytopenia.

JOINT DISEASE

Joint involvement is seen in less than 10 per cent of cases of infection in children but occurs in as much as 80 per cent of cases of infection in adult females. The joint involvement is similar to that seen in rubella and is generally a symmetrical arthralgia or arthritis involving most frequently the joints of the hands, with the wrists, ankles, and knees sometimes affected. In the majority of cases the symptoms and signs resolve within 2 weeks but occasionally persists for months and even years. Occasional cases resemble early rheumatoid arthritis but the patients will be rheumatoid factor negative and there is no relation between B19 virus infection and rheumatoid arthritis.

B19 infection in pregnancy

Clinical and laboratory studies have failed to detect any evidence that B19 causes birth defects, although the sample sizes of most studies have been too small to detect defects occurring at the rate of 1 per cent or less. However, there is an association between B19 infection in pregnancy and second-trimester fetal loss. Studies indicate that about 10 per cent of pregnancies complicated by B19 infection end in spontaneous abortion during the second trimester and this is approximately 10 times the incidence of abortion in unaffected pregnancies. The pregnancy is usually lost 4 to 6 weeks after the onset of the rash illness in the mother. Occasionally, infection during the second or third trimester of pregnancy results in hydrops fetalis in the infant. B19 is a likely cause if fetal hydrops is associated with a low haemoglobin in the absence of haemolytic disease. It would appear that approximately 10 per cent of cases of non-immunological hydrops fetalis are associated with B19 infection, although this will vary in relation to the epidemic pattern of B19 infection.

Aplastic crisis

The interruption of erythropoiesis for 5 to 7 days that occurs in volunteers is insufficient to produce clinically manifest anaemia in a normal individual with red blood cells whose lifespan is about 120 days. In patients with chronic haemolytic anaemia such an interruption leads rapidly to a more profound anaemia with clinical consequences. This event is termed an aplastic crisis (see Section 22) and in 1981 aplastic crises occurring in patients with sickle-cell anaemia were shown to be associated with human parvoviral infection. Since then, parvovirus-induced aplastic crises have been found in patients with sickle-cell anaemia in Europe, North America, and the West Indies, and in patients with hereditary spherocytosis, pyruvate-kinase deficiency, and β-thalassaemia intermedia. It is clear that the human parvovirus is the principal cause of the aplastic crisis of chronic haemolytic anaemia.

B19 infection in the immunosuppressed

Patients with underlying immunodeficiency states (Nezelof's syndrome, acute lymphatic leukaemia, and human immunodeficiency virus-infected individuals) fail to produce neutralizing antibody to B19 virus and infection becomes chronic. The clinical consequence of this is anaemia, which may be persistent or remitting and relapsing. The bone marrow picture is similar to that seen in aplastic crisis complicating haemolytic anaemia and there is usually an easily detectable viraemia during periods of anaemia. Intravenous administration of human immunoglobulin in these cases has proved effective in reducing viraemia and allowing haemoglobin concentrations to return to near normal.

Laboratory diagnosis

Human parvovirus infection can be confirmed by demonstrating the viraemia using either immunological or molecular biological techniques. Alternatively, recent infection can be diagnosed by demonstrating seroconversion or specific IgM antibody. Virus detection is suitable for the diagnosis of cases of aplastic crisis, of persistent infection in immunosuppressed patients, and persistent fetal infection. Otherwise the cornerstone of the diagnosis of rash illness and arthropathy is the detection of specific IgM antibody in serum, as in most individuals the viraemia has been cleared when the rash or joint symptoms develop (Fig. 2).

7.10.26 Viral hepatitis

A. J. ZUCKERMAN and J. N. ZUCKERMAN

Introduction

The last two decades have witnessed an explosion in knowledge of viral hepatitis, a major public health problem throughout the world affecting several hundreds of millions of people. Viral hepatitis is a cause of

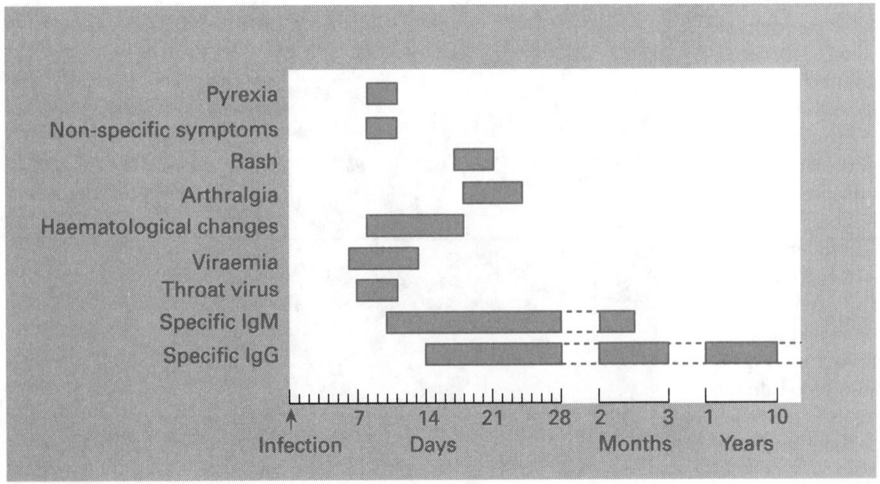

Fig. 2 Sequence of events following intranasal inoculation of volunteers with human parvovirus.

considerable illness and death in the human population both from acute infection and chronic sequelae, which include (with hepatitis B and hepatitis C infection) chronic active hepatitis, cirrhosis, and primary liver cancer.

The hepatitis viruses include a range of unrelated and often unusual human pathogens:

- Hepatitis A virus (**HAV**), a small, unenveloped, symmetrical RNA virus that shares many of the characteristics of the picornavirus family. This virus has been classified as enterovirus type 72, and is the cause of infectious or epidemic hepatitis transmitted by the faecal–oral route.
- Hepatitis B virus (**HBV**), a member of the hepadnavirus group of double-stranded DNA viruses that replicate by reverse transcription. HBV is endemic in the human population and hyperendemic in many parts of the world.
- Hepatitis C virus (**HCV**), an enveloped, single-stranded RNA virus that appears to be distantly related (possibly in its evolution) to flaviviruses, although hepatitis C is not transmitted by arthropod vectors. Infection with this virus is common in many countries, and it is associated with chronic liver disease and also with primary liver cancer at least in some countries.
- Hepatitis D virus (**HDV**) is an unusual, single-stranded, circular RNA virus with a number of similarities to certain plant viral satellites and viroids. This virus requires hepadnavirus helper functions for propagation in hepatocytes, and is an important cause of acute and severe chronic liver damage in some regions of the world.
- Hepatitis E virus (**HEV**) is an enterically transmitted, non-enveloped, single-stranded RNA virus that shares many biophysical and biochemical features with caliciviruses. HEV is an important cause of large epidemics of acute hepatitis in the subcontinent of India, central and south-east Asia, the Middle East, parts of Africa and elsewhere; and this virus is responsible for high mortality during pregnancy.

Many intriguing questions remain: is there a hepatitis F virus as the cause of sporadic fulminant hepatitis; what are the implications of the hepatitis B variants; and is non-B, non-C hepatitis awaiting discovery?

Hepatitis A

Outbreaks of jaundice have been described frequently for many centuries and the term infectious hepatitis was coined in 1912 to describe the epidemic form of the disease. HAV is spread by the faecal–oral route and continues to be endemic throughout the world and hyperendemic in areas with poor standards of sanitation and hygiene. The seroprevalence of antibodies to HAV has declined since the Second World War in many industrialized countries.

Fig. 1 Electron micrograph showing the large number of hepatitis A virus particles in faeces during the incubation period of the infection. × 200 000. (From a series by Anthea Thornton and A.J. Zuckerman.)

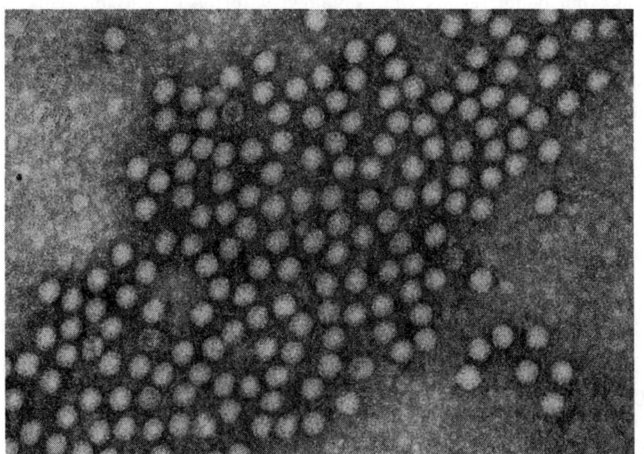

The incubation period of hepatitis A is about 4 weeks. The virus replicates in the liver. Very large quantities of virus are shed in the faeces during the incubation period before the onset of clinical symptoms (Fig.1). A brief period of viraemia occurs. The severity of illness ranges from the asymptomatic to anicteric or icteric hepatitis and rarely fulminant hepatitis. The virus is non-cytopathic when grown in cell culture. Its pathogenicity *in vivo*, which involves necrosis of parenchymal cells and histiocytic periportal inflammation, may be mediated via the cellular immune response. By the time of onset of symptoms, excretion of virus in the faeces has declined and may have ceased and anti-HAV IgM, which is diagnostic of acute infection, increases in titre. Anti-HAV IgG may be detected 1 to 2 weeks later and persists for years.

Classification

Examination by electron microscopy of concentrates of filtered faecal extracts from patients in the early stages of infection reveals 27-nm particles typical of the Picornaviridae. HAV was classified in 1983 in the genus *Enterovirus* (as enterovirus 72) of the family Picornaviridae, on the basis of its biophysical and biochemical characteristics, including stability at low pH. However, this classification pre-empted the isolation and analysis of complementary DNA (**cDNA**) clones leading to the determination of the entire nucleotide sequence of the viral genome. Comparison with other picornavirus sequences revealed limited homology to the enteroviruses or, indeed, the rhinoviruses; although the structure and genome organization is typical of the Picornaviridae. It is likely that HAV will be considered as a separate genus within the Picornaviridae as are the cardioviruses (of mice) and apthoviruses (foot-and-mouth disease viruses), and has recently been designated Hepatovirus.

Organization of the HAV genome

The HAV genome comprises around 7500 nucleotides of positive-sense RNA that is polyadenylated at the 3′ end and has a polypeptide (VPg) attached to the 5′ end. A single, large, open reading frame occupies most of the genome and encodes a polyprotein with a theoretical M_r252 000. An untranslated region of around 735 nucleotides precedes the open reading frame. Secondary structure within this region of the genome may be important for efficient translation of the RNA. There is also a short, untranslated region at the 3′ end of the HAV genome.

The viral polyprotein is processed to yield the structural (located at the aminoterminal end) and non-structural viral polypeptides. Many of the features of replication of the picornaviruses have been deduced from studies of prototype enteroviruses and rhinoviruses, in particular poliovirus type one.

The three-dimensional structures of a number of picornaviruses have been solved by high-resolution crystallography: polypeptides VP1 (1D), VP2 (1B), and VP3 (1C) are exposed on the surface of the virion, whilst VP4 (1A) is located internally. Following release of the structural domain from the polyprotein, the 3C protease cleaves the 1B/1C and 1C/1D junctions to yield VP0 (VP4 plus VP2), VP3, and VP1. The three polypeptides remain associated as a protomer and five protomers assemble to form a pentamer, so that the five copies of VP1 form the apex. Finally, 12 pentamers assemble around a molecule of viral RNA to form the icosahedral capsid. As the structure locks into place, most copies of VP0 cleave (presumably autocatalytically) to yield VP2 and VP4. However, in the case of HAV, it has not been possible to demonstrate VP4, which is predicted to comprise only 23 amino acids.

The functions of some of the other cleavage products of the polyprotein, such as 2B, 2C, and 3A, are less well understood. Product 3B corresponds to the genome-linked polypeptide VPg, which in other picornaviruses is the primer for the synthesis of both genome-sense

Table 1 *Passive immunization with normal immunoglobulin for travellers to highly endemic areas*

Person's body weight (kg)	Period of stay < 3 months	Period of stay > 3 months
< 25	50 i.u. anti-HAV (0.5 ml)	100 i.u. anti-HAV (1.0 ml)
25–30	100 i.u. anti-HAV (1.0 ml)	250 i.u. anti-HAV (2.5 ml)
< 50	200 i.u. anti-HAV (2.0 ml)	500 i.u. anti-HAV (5.0 ml)

RNA and the negative-sense RNA found in replicative intermediates. Polypeptide 3AB may be the precursor of VPg. Finally, the 3D product seems to be the viral replicase and contains the gly-asp-asp motif common to viral RNA-dependent RNA polymerases.

Prevention and control of hepatitis A

PASSIVE IMMUNIZATION

Control of hepatitis A infection is difficult. Because faecal shedding of the virus is at its highest during the late incubation period and the prodromal phase of the illness, strict isolation of cases is not a useful control measure. Spread of hepatitis A is reduced by simple hygienic measures and the sanitary disposal of excreta.

Normal human immunoglobulin, containing at least 100 i.u./ml of anti-hepatitis A antibody, given intramuscularly before exposure to the virus or early during the incubation period, will prevent or attenuate a clinical illness. The dosage should be at least 2 i.u. of anti-hepatitis A antibody/kg body weight, but in special cases such as pregnancy, or in patients with liver disease, that dosage may be doubled (Table 1). Immunoglobulin does not always prevent infection and excretion of HAV, and inapparent or subclinical hepatitis may develop. The efficacy of passive immunization is based on the presence of hepatitis A antibody in the immunoglobulin, but the minimum titre of antibody required for protection has not yet been established. Immunoglobulin is used most commonly for close personal contacts of patients with hepatitis A and for those exposed to contaminated food. Immunoglobulin has also been used effectively for controlling outbreaks in institutions such as homes for the mentally handicapped and in nursery schools. Prophylaxis with immunoglobulin is recommended for persons without hepatitis A antibody visiting highly endemic areas. After a period of 6 months the administration of immunoglobulin for travellers should be repeated, unless it has been demonstrated that the recipient has developed his or her own hepatitis A antibodies.

HEPATITIS A VACCINES

In areas of high prevalence, most children have antibodies to HAV by the age of 3 years and such infections are generally asymptomatic. Infections acquired later in life are of increasing clinical severity. Less than 10 per cent of cases of acute hepatitis A in children up to the age of 6 years are icteric but this increases to 40 to 50 per cent in the 6 to 14 age group and to 70 to 80 per cent in adults. Of 115 551 cases of hepatitis A in the United States between 1983 and 1987, only 9 per cent of the cases, but more than 70 per cent of the fatalities, were in those aged over 49 years. It is important, therefore, to protect those at risk because of personal contact with infected individuals or because of travel to highly endemic areas. Other groups to be immunized against hepatitis A infection include staff and residents of institutions for the mentally handicapped, day-care centres for children, sexually active male homosexuals, intravenous narcotic drug abusers, food handlers, sewage workers, health care workers, military personnel, and certain low socioeconomic groups in defined community settings. In some developing countries, the incidence of clinical hepatitis A is increasing as improvements in socioeconomic conditions result in infection later in life, and strategies for immunization are yet to be agreed.

Killed vaccines

The foundations for a hepatitis A vaccine were laid in 1975 by the demonstration that formalin-inactivated virus extracted from the liver of infected marmosets induced protective antibodies in susceptible marmosets on challenge with live virus. Subsequently, HAV was cultivated, after serial passage in marmosets, in a cloned line of fetal rhesus monkey kidney cells (FRhK6), thereby opening the way to the production of hepatitis A vaccines. Later, it was demonstrated that prior adaptation in marmosets was not a prerequisite for growth of the virus in cell cultures; various strains of virus have been isolated directly from clinical material using several cell lines, including human diploid fibroblasts, and various techniques have been employed to increase the yield of virus in cell culture. Safety and immunogenicity studies of formalin-inactivated hepatitis A vaccines with an adjuvant have been completed and the vaccine had been licensed in several countries by the end of 1992. Other preparations are under clinical trial.

Live, attenuated vaccines

The main advantages of live, attenuated vaccines (viz. the Sabin type of oral poliomyelitis vaccines) include the ease of administration on a large scale by the oral route, relatively low cost, and, as the virus vaccine strain replicates in the gut, the production of both local immunity in the gut and humoral immunity (thereby mimicking natural infection), and also longer-term protection. Disadvantages include the potential of reversion towards virulence, interference with the vaccine strain by other viruses in the gut, relative instability of the vaccine, and shedding of the virus strain in the faeces for prolonged periods.

The most extensively studied live attenuated hepatitis A vaccines are based on the CR326 and HM175 strains of the virus attenuated by prolonged passage in cell culture. Two variants of the CR326 strain have been investigated after passage in marmoset liver in FRhK6, MRC5, and WI-38 cells. Inoculation of susceptible marmosets demonstrated seroconversion, and protection on challenge. Biochemical evidence of liver damage did not occur in susceptible chimpanzees, although a number had histological evidence of mild hepatitis with the F variant and the vaccine virus was shed in the faeces for about 12 weeks before seroconversion. There was no evidence of reversion towards virulence. Studies in human volunteers indicated incomplete attenuation of the F variant, but better results were obtained with the F^1 variant, without elevation of liver enzymes. Studies with the HM175 strain, which was isolated and passaged in kidney cells of the African green monkey, showed that this strain was not fully attenuated for marmosets, although it did not induce liver damage on challenge. Further passages and adaptation of HM175 revealed some evidence of virus replication in the liver of chimpanzees and minimal shedding of the virus into faeces. Other studies are in progress in non-human primates.

As with vaccine strains of polioviruses, attenuation may be associated with mutations in the 5′ non-coding region of the genome that affect secondary structure. There is also evidence that mutations in the region of the genome encoding the non-structural polypeptides may be important for adaptation to cell culture and attenuation. However, markers of attenuation of HAV have not been identified and reversion to virulence may also be a problem. On the other hand, there is also concern that 'over-attenuated' viruses may not be sufficiently immunogenic.

Current candidate live, attenuated hepatitis A vaccines require injection; preparations that may be suitable for oral administration are not yet available.

Hepatitis E

Retrospective testing of serum samples from patients involved in various epidemics of hepatitis associated with contamination of water supplies with human faeces led to the conclusion that an agent other than HAV (or hepatitis B) was involved. Epidemics of enterically transmitted non-A, non-B hepatitis in the Indian subcontinent were the first reported in 1980, but outbreaks involving tens of thousands of cases were also documented in the then USSR, south-east Asia, northern Africa, and Mexico. The average incubation period is longer than that for hepatitis A, with a mean of 6 weeks. The highest attack rates are found in young adults and high mortality rates (up to 20 per cent) have been reported in women in the third trimester of pregnancy.

Virus-like particles have been detected in faecal extracts of infected individuals by immune electron microscopy using convalescent serum. However, such studies have often proved inconclusive because a large proportion of the excreted virus may be degraded during passage through the gut. The particles measure 32 to 34 nm in diameter. Cross-reaction studies between sera and virus in faeces associated with a variety of epidemics in several different countries suggest that a single serotype of virus is involved.

Studies on HEV have progressed following experimental transmission to susceptible non-human primates. HEV was first transmitted to cynomolgous macaques, a number of other species of monkeys and apes, including chimpanzees, also have been infected. Reports of transmission to pigs and rodents await confirmation. Attempts to amplify the virus by replication in cell culture have thus far proved unsuccessful.

The problem of degradation of HEV in the gut was circumvented when the bile of infected monkeys was found to be a rich source of virus. This material enabled the molecular cloning of DNA complementary to the HEV RNA genome and the entire 7.5-kb sequence was determined. The organization of the genome is distinct from the Picornaviridae, and the non-structural and structural polypeptides are encoded respectively at the 5′ and 3′ ends. HEV resembles the caliciviruses in the size and organization of its genome as well as the size and morphology of the virion.

Organization of the HEV genome

The HEVgenome is a polyadenylated, positive-sense RNA of around 7500 nucleotides. The genome of another calicivirus, vesicular exanthema of swine virus, has a polypeptide VpG attached to the 5′ end, which (unlike the Picornaviridae) is required for infectivity. Whether this holds true for HEV is not known. Hybridization of HEV cDNA probes to RNA isolated from infected liver reveals species of 7.5, 3.7, and 2.0 kb; it is likely that the smaller transcripts are subgenomic mRNAs for the capsid and other viral polypeptides.

Analysis of the sequence of the HEV genome reveals three open reading frames. The first, of approximately 5 kb, begins 28 nucleotides from the 5′ end of the genome and encodes motifs associated with nucleoside triphosphatase binding, helicase and RNA-dependent RNA polymerase activity. A second frame of around 2 kb begins 37 nucleotides downstream of the first, terminates 68 nucleotides from the polyA tail and is believed to encode the structural polypeptides. The third frame is very short (369 nucleotides) and overlaps the other two. The subgenomic RNAs are required presumably for translation of the second and third open reading frames and the products may be subject to proteolytic processing.

Sequencing of the HEV genome has resulted in the development of a number of specific diagnostic tests. For example, HEV RNA was detected, using the polymerase chain reaction (**PCR**), in faecal samples. An enzyme-linked immunosorbent assay (**ELISA**), which detects both IgG and IgM antiHEV, has been developed using a recombinant HEV–glutathione-*S*-transferase fusion protein and used to detect antibodies in sporadic cases of infection in children and adults.

Hepatitis B

HBV was originally recognized as the agent responsible for 'serum hepatitis', the most common form of parenterally transmitted viral hepatitis, and an important cause of acute and chronic infection of the liver. The incubation period of hepatitis B is variable, with a range of 1 to 6 months. The clinical features of acute infection resemble those of the other viral hepatitides. Frequently, acute hepatitis B is anicteric and asymptomatic, although a severe illness with jaundice can occur and acute liver failure may develop. The virus persists in about 10 per cent of infected immunocompetent adults, and in as many as 90 per cent of infants infected perinatally, depending on the ethnic group of the mother. About 350 million people worldwide are persistent carriers of hepatitis B. Liver damage is mediated by the responses of the cellular immune response of the host to the infected hepatocytes. Approximately 25 per cent of all patients with chronic hepatitis will progress to cirrhosis and about 20 per cent of those with cirrhosis will develop hepatocellular carcinoma. Hepatocellular carcinoma is one of the most common cancers worldwide.

During the first phase of chronicity, virus replication continues in the liver and replicative intermediates of the viral genome may be detected in DNA extracted from liver biopsies. Markers of virus replication in serum include HBV DNA, the preS1 proteins (see below) and a soluble antigen, hepatitis B *e* antigen (**HBeAg**), which is secreted by productively infected hepatocytes. In those infected at a very young age this phase may persist for life but, more usually, virus levels decline over time. Eventually, in most individuals, there is immune clearance of infected hepatocytes associated with seroconversion from HBeAg to anti-HBe. During the period of replication, the viral genome may integrate into the chromosomal DNA of some hepatocytes and these cells may persist and expand clonally. Rarely, seroconversion to anti-HBs follows clearance of virus replication but, more frequently, HBsAg persists during a second phase of chronicity as a result of the expression of integrated viral DNA.

Structure of the virus

The hepatitis B virion is a 42-nm particle comprising an electron-dense nucleocapsid or core, 27 nm in diameter, surrounded by an outer envelope of the surface protein (HBsAg) embedded in membraneous lipoprotein derived from the host cell (Fig. 2). The surface antigen is produced in excess by the infected hepatocytes and is secreted in the form of 22-nm particles (initially referred to as Australia antigen) and tubular structures with the same diameter.

The 22-nm particles are composed of the major surface protein in both non-glycosylated (p24) and glycosylated (gp27) form in approximately equimolar amounts, together with a minority component of the so-called middle proteins (gp33 and gp36), which contain the pre-S2 domain—a glycosylated, 55-amino acid, N-terminal extension. The surface of the virion has a similar composition but also contains the large surface proteins (p39 and gp42), which include both the pre-S1 and pre-S2 regions. These large surface proteins are not found in the 22-nm spherical particles (but may be present in the tubular forms in highly viraemic individuals) and their detection in serum correlates with viraemia. The domain that binds to the specific HBV receptor on the hepatocyte resides within the pre-S1 region.

The nucleocapsid of the virion consists of the viral genome surrounded by the core antigen (**HBcAg**). The carboxyl terminus of the core protein is arginine rich and this highly basic domain is believed to interact with the genome. The genome, which is approximately 3.2 kb in length, has an unusual structure and is composed of two linear strands of DNA held in a circular configuration by base pairing at the 5′ ends (cohesive end-region) (Fig. 3). One of the strands is incomplete and the 3′ end is associated with a DNA polymerase molecule that is able to complete that strand when supplied with deoxynucleoside triphosphates. In the past, this endogenous DNA polymerase reaction was used as a serological assay for the hepatitis B virion but this has now been superseded by DNA–DNA hybridization and the polymerase chain reaction. The 5′ ends of both strands of the genome are modified. The 5′ end of the complete strand is covalently linked to a protein and the 5′ end of the incomplete strand is an oligoribonucleotide. In both cases, these

Fig. 2 Hepatitis B virus. × 250 000. (From a series by A.J. Zuckerman *et al.*)

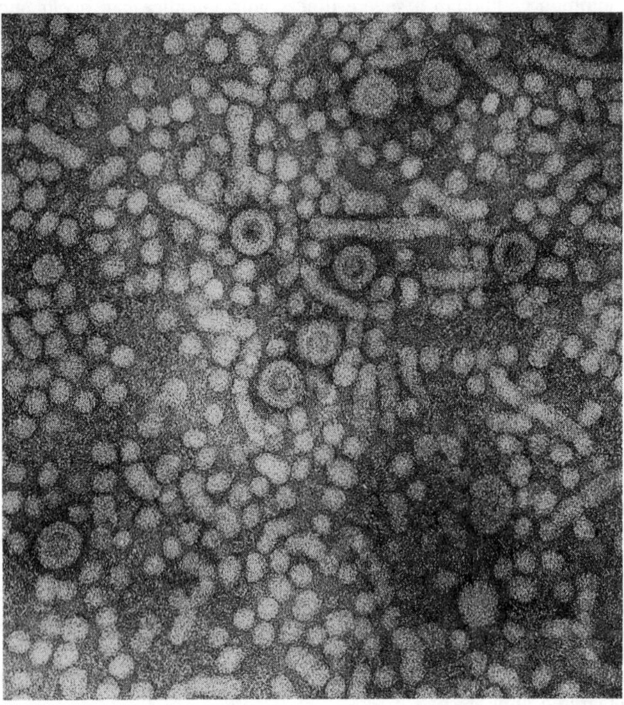

Fig. 3 Organization of the genome of hepatitis B virus.

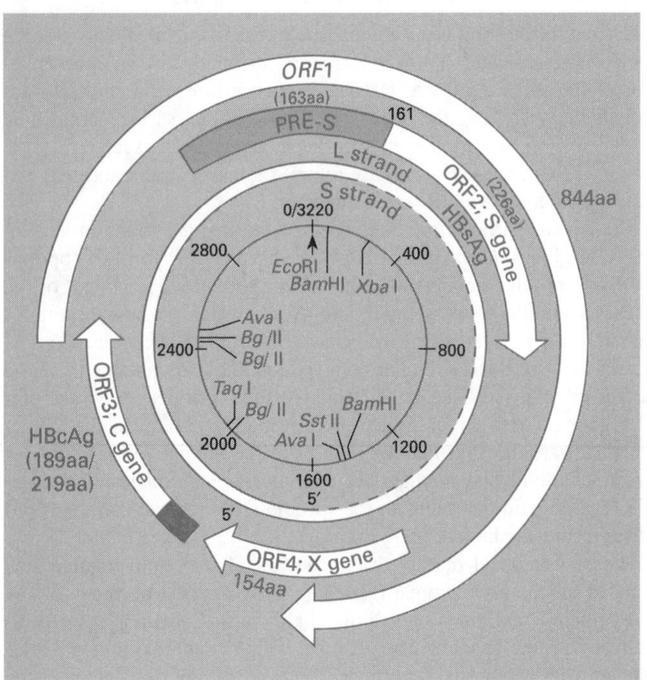

moieties seem to be primers for the synthesis of the respective strands during the genome replication. A motif of 12 bp is directly repeated in the genome near to the 5′ ends of the two strands (DR1 and DR2, respectively) and these sequences play an important part in replication.

Organization of the HBV genome

To date, the genomes of more than a dozen isolates of HBV have been cloned and the complete nucleotide sequences determined. Analysis of the coding potential of the genome reveals four open reading frames, which are conserved between all of these isolates. These have the same polarity as the incomplete strand of genomic DNA, which therefore has been designated the plus strand.

The first open reading frame encodes the various forms of the surface protein and contains three in-frame methionine codons that are used for initiation of translation. Both the middle (gp33 and gp36) and major (p24 and gp27) proteins are translated from a family of 2.1-kb mRNAs transcribed from a promoter located in the pre-S1 region and polyadenylated in response to a signal sequence located just downstream from the start of the core open reading frame.

A second promoter is located upstream of the pre-S1 initiation codon. This directs the synthesis of a 2.4-kb mRNA, which is coterminal with the other surface messages and is translated to yield the large (pre-S1) surface proteins. This promoter seems to be weak (or may be downregulated) so that the message is of low abundance and relatively little of the large surface proteins is synthesized. Unlike the middle and major surface proteins, the large surface protein is not secreted from the cell. In fact, its synthesis inhibits the secretion of the smaller proteins and may be a signal for virus assembly.

The core open reading frame also has two in-phase initiation codons. The 'precore' region is highly conserved, has the properties of a signal sequence, and is responsible for the secretion of HBeAg.

The third open reading frame, which is the largest and overlaps the other three, encodes the viral polymerase. This protein seems to be another translation product of the 3.5-kb RNA, and is synthesized apparently following internal initiation of the ribosome. The aminoterminal domain is believed to be the protein primer for minus-strand synthesis. There is then a spacer region followed by the (RNA- and DNA-dependent) DNA polymerase. The carboxyterminal domain has an RNase H-like activity. The fourth open reading frame was designated 'x', recently identified as a transcriptional transactivator and may be an 'early' gene product that functions to upregulate the viral promoters.

Replication of the HBV genome

Following infection of an hepatocyte, the single-stranded region of the virion DNA is repaired by the endogenous polymerase and the genome appears in a covalently closed, circular form in the nucleus. This DNA is the template for the transcription of all of the viral RNAs. Synthesis of minus-strand DNA is primed by a protein, now believed to be the amino-terminal domain of the polymerase, and proceeds with the concomitant degradation of the RNA template by the RNase H activity. Whether one or two copies of the polymerase molecule are involved and whether the primer domain is cleaved from the remainder of the polymerase remain unclear. There is no semiconservative replication of the covalently closed, circular DNA in the nucleus and a pool of up to 30 copies of template DNA is built up initially by transfer of some of the progeny DNA from the cytoplasm to the nucleus. The mode of replication of the viral genome resembles those of the phylogenetically related retroviruses and, more closely, a family of plant viruses (the caulimoviruses).

Prevention and control of hepatitis B

The discovery of variation in the epitopes presented on the surface of the virions and subviral particles identified subtypes of HBV that differ in their geographical distribution. All isolates of the virus share a common epitope, *a*, which is a domain of the major surface protein and seems to protrude as a double loop from the surface of the particle. Two other pairs of mutually exclusive antigenic determinants, *d* or *y* and *w* or *r*, are also present on the major surface protein. These variations have been correlated with single nucleotide changes in the surface open reading frame that lead to variation in single amino acids in the protein. Four principal subtypes of HBV are recognised: *adw*, *adr*, *ayw*, and *ayr*. Subtype *adw* predominates in northern Europe, the Americas and Australasia, and also is found in Africa and Asia. Subtype *ayw* is found in the Mediterranean region, eastern Europe, northern and western Africa, the Near East, and the Indian subcontinent. In the Far East, *adr* predominates but the rarer *ayr* occasionally may be found in Japan and Papua New Guinea.

The principal response to immunization with the current of hepatitis B vaccines is to the common *a* epitope, with consequent protection against all subtypes of the virus.

PASSIVE IMMUNIZATION

Hepatitis B immunoglobulin is prepared from pooled plasma with high titre of hepatitis B surface antibody and may confer temporary passive immunity under certain defined conditions. The principal indication for the administration of hepatitis B immunoglobulin is a single, acute exposure to HBV, such as occurs when blood containing surface antigen is inoculated, ingested, or splashed on to mucous membranes and the conjunctiva. The optimal dose has not been established but doses in the range of 250 to 500 i.u. have been used effectively. It should be given as early as possible after exposure and preferably within 48 h, usually 3 ml (containing 200 i.u. of antiHBs/ml) in adults. It should not be given 7 days or later after exposure. It is generally recommended that two doses of hepatitis B immunoglobulin should be given 30 days apart.

Results with the use of hepatitis B immunoglobulin for prophylaxis in babies at risk of infection with HBV are encouraging if the immunoglobulin is given as soon as possible after birth or within 12 h of birth; the chance of the baby developing the persistent carrier state is reduced by about 70 per cent. More recent studies using combined passive and active immunization indicate an efficacy approaching 90 per cent. The dose of hepatitis B immunoglobulin recommended in the newborn is 1 to 2 ml (200 i.u. of antiHBs/ml).

ACTIVE IMMUNIZATION

Immunization against hepatitis B is required for groups that are at an increased risk of acquiring this infection. These groups include individuals requiring repeated transfusions of blood or blood products, prolonged inpatient treatment, patients who require frequent tissue penetration or need repeated access to the circulation, those with natural or acquired immune deficiency, and those with malignant diseases. Viral hepatitis is an occupational hazard among health care personnel and the staff of institutions for the mentally handicapped and in some semi-closed institutions. High rates of infection with hepatitis B occur in narcotic drug addicts and drug abusers, male homosexuals who change partners frequently, and prostitutes. Individuals working in high endemic areas are also at an increased risk of infections. Women in areas of the world where the carrier state in that group is high are another segment of the population requiring immunization in view of the increased risk of transmission of the infections to their offspring. Young infants, children, and susceptible persons living in certain tropical and subtropical areas where present socioeconomic conditions are poor and the prevalence of hepatitis B is high should also be immunized.

The failure to grow HBV in tissue culture has directed attention to the use of other preparations for active immunization. Because immunization with HBsAg leads to the production of protective surface antibody, purified (22-mm spherical) surface antigen particles have been developed as vaccines. These vaccines have been prepared from the plasma of symptomless carriers. Trials on protective efficacy in high-risk groups have demonstrated the value of the vaccines and their safety. There is no risk of transmission of the acquired immune deficiency syndrome (**AIDS**) or any other infection by vaccines derived from plasma that meet the World Health Organization requirements of 1981, 1983, and 1987. Local reactions reported after immunization have been minor, occurring in less than 20 per cent of immunized individuals, and consisted of slight swelling and reddening at the site of inoculation. Temperature elevations of up to 38 °C were observed in only a few individuals.

Site of injection for vaccination

Hepatitis B vaccination should be given in the upper arm or the anterolateral aspect of the thigh and not in the buttock. There are over 100 reports of unexpectedly low antibody seroconversion rates after hepatitis B vaccination using injection into the buttock. In one centre in the United States a low antibody response was noted in 54 per cent of healthy, adult, health-care-personnel. Many studies have since shown that the antibody response rate was significantly higher in centres using deltoid injection than centres using the buttock. On the basis of antibody tests after vaccination, the Advisory Committee on Immunization Practices of the Centers of Disease Control, USA, recommended that the arm be used as the site for hepatitis B vaccination in adults, as have the Departments of Health in the United Kingdom.

A comprehensive study in the United States in 1989 by Shaw *et al.* showed that participants who received the vaccine in the deltoid had antibody titres that were up to 17 times higher than those of subjects who received the injections into the buttock. Furthermore, those who were injected in the buttock were two to four times more likely to fail to reach a minimum antibody level of 10 m.i.u./ml after vaccination. Recent reports have also implicated buttock injection as a possible factor in a failure of post-exposure prophylaxis for rabies using a human diploid-cell rabies vaccine.

The injection of vaccine into deep fat in the buttocks is likely with needles shorter than 5 cm, and there is a lack of phagocytic or antigen-presenting cells in layers of fat. Another factor may involve the rapidity of which antigen becomes available to the circulation from deposition in fat, leading to delay in processing by macrophages and eventually presentation to T and B cells. An additional factor may be denaturation by enzymes of antigen that has remained in fat for hours or days. The importance of these factors is supported by the finding by Cockcroft *et al.* at the Royal Free Hospital, London and elsewhere that thicker skinfold was associated with a lowered antibody response.

These observations have important public health implications, well illustrated by the estimate that about 20 per cent of subjects immunized against hepatitis B via the buttock in the United States by March 1985 (about 60 000 people) failed to attain a minimum level of antibody of 10 miu/ml and were therefore not protected.

Hepatitis B surface antibody titres should be measured in all individuals who have been immunized against hepatitis B by injection into the buttocks, and when this is not possible a complete course of three injections of vaccine should be given into the deltoid muscle or the anterolateral aspect of the thigh, the only acceptable sites for hepatitis B immunization.

INDICATIONS FOR IMMUNIZATION AGAINST HEPATITIS B

The current indications for the use of hepatitis B vaccines in low-prevalence areas are summarized below, although these recommendations are under revision. The recommendations for immunization against this infection in intermediate- and high-prevalence regions also include universal immunization of infants. Many countries, including the United States and Italy, introduced universal immunization for infants in 1992 and it is expected that most countries will implement this policy by 1996.

Current policy

1. All health care personnel in frequent contact with blood or needles and groups at the highest risk in this category including:
   (a) personnel, including teaching and training staff, directly involved over a period of time in patient care in residential institutions for the mentally handicapped where there is a known high risk of hepatitis;
   (b) personnel directly involved in patient care over a period of time, working in units giving treatment to known high risk of hepatitis B infection;
   (c) personnel directly involved in patient care working in haemodialysis, haemophilia, and other centres regularly performing maintenance treatment of patients with blood or blood products;
   (d) laboratory workers regularly exposed to increased risk from infected material;
   (e) health care personnel on secondment to work in areas of the world where there is a high prevalence of hepatitis B infection, if they are to be directly involved in patient care;
   (f) dentists and ancillary dental personnel with direct patient contact.
2. Patients:
   (a) patients on first entry into those residential institutions for the mentally handicapped where there is a known high incidence of hepatitis B;
   (b) patients treated by maintenance haemodialysis;
   (c) patients before major surgery who are likely to require a large number of blood transfusions and/or treatment with blood products.
3. Contacts of patients with hepatitis B:
   (a) the spouses and other sexual contacts of patients with acute hepatitis B or carriers of hepatitis B virus, and other family members in close contact.
4. Other indications for immunization:
   (a) infants born to mothers who are persistent carriers of HBsAg or are HBsAg positive as a result of recent infection, particularly if hepatitis B *e* antigen is detectable or HBV-positive mothers without antibody to *e* antigen (antiHBe)—the optimum timing for immunoglobulin to be given at a contralateral site is immediately at birth or within 12 h;
   (b) health care workers who are accidentally pricked with needles used for patients with hepatitis B; the vaccine may be used alone or in combination with hepatitis B immunoglobulin as an alternative to passive immunization with hepatitis B immunoglobulin only; studies on the efficacy of these different schedules of immunization are nearing completion.
5. Immediate protection:
   (a) Infants born to carrier mothers—whenever immediate protection is required, as, for example, for infants born to HBsAg-positive mothers (see 4(a)) or following transfer of an individual into a 'high risk' setting or after accidental inoculation, active immunization with the vaccine should be combined with simultaneous administration of hepatitis B immunoglobulin at a different site. It has been shown that passive immunization with up to 3 ml (200 i.u. of antiHBs/ml) of hepatitis B immunoglobulin does not interfere with an active immune response. A single dose of hepatitis B immunoglobulin (usually 3 ml for adults; 1–2 ml for the newborn) is sufficient for healthy individuals. If infection has already occurred at the time of the first immunization, virus multiplication is unlikely to be inhibited completely, but severe illness and, most importantly, the development of the carrier state of HBV may be prevented in many individuals, particularly in infants born to carrier mothers.
6. The immune response to the current hepatitis B vaccines is poorer in immunocompromised and in elderly people. For example, only about 60 per cent of patients undergoing treatment by maintenance haemodialysis develop anti-HBs. It is suggested therefore that patients with chronic renal damage be immunized as soon as it appears likely that they will ultimately require treatment by maintenance haemodialysis or receive renal transplant. Consideration should be given to the use of blood from healthy immunized donors with high titres of antiHBs for the routine haemodialysis of such patients who respond poorly to immunization against hepatitis B.
7. Other groups at risk of hepatitis B include the following:
   (a) individuals who frequently change sexual partners, particularly promiscuous male homosexuals and prostitutes;
   (b) intravenous drug abusers;
   (c) staff at reception centres for refugees and immigrants from areas of the world where hepatitis B is very common, such as south-east Asia;
   (d) although they are at 'lower risk', consideration should also be given to long-term prisoners and staff of custodial institutions, ambulance and rescue services, and selected police personnel;
   (e) military personnel are included in some countries.

DEVELOPING NEW HEPATITIS B IMMUNIZATION STRATEGIES

There is now strong support for the introduction of universal antenatal screening to identify hepatitis B carrier mothers and the vaccination of their babies. It is important that any other strategies do not interfere with the delivery of vaccine to this group. Immunization of this group will have the greatest impact in reducing the number of new hepatitis B carriers. For children outside this group it is difficult to estimate the lifetime risk of acquiring a hepatitis infection.

There are four main approaches:

(1) to continue vaccination of the 'high risk' babies as defined above;
(2) universal infant immunization;
(3) universal adolescent immunization;
(4) vaccinate everybody.

Vaccination of adolescents

This approach delivers vaccination at a time close to the time when 'risk behaviour' would expose adolescents to infection. Vaccination could be delivered as part of a wider package on health education in general, to include sex education, risk of AIDS, dangers of drug abuse, smoking, and benefits of a healthy diet and lifestyle.

The problems with this approach are as follows:

- persuading parents to accept vaccination of the children against a sexually transmitted disease, a problem they may not wish to address at that time;
- ensuring a full course of three doses is given;
- difficulty evaluating and monitoring vaccine cover—the systems for monitoring uptake of vaccine in this age group may not operate efficiently.

Vaccination of infants

The advantages of this approach are:

- It is known that vaccination can be delivered to babies.

- Parents would accept vaccination against hepatitis B along with other childhood vaccinations without reference to sexual behaviour.

The disadvantages of this approach are:

- Whether immunity would last until exposure occurred in later life—this was thought to become less of a problem as more people were vaccinated, as the chance of exposure to infection was reduced.
- That the introduction of further childhood vaccination would reduce the uptake of other childhood vaccinations—this problem would be avoided if hepatitis B vaccine could be delivered in a combined vaccine containing diphtheria/pertussis/tetanus and this proposal may have to await the production and evaluation of a suitable vaccine.

Vaccination of infants is preferable to vaccination of adolescents as there are sufficient mechanisms to ensure, monitor, and evaluate cover. A booster dose could be given in early adolescence combined with a health education package. A rolling programme could be introduced, giving priority to urban areas.

POLYPEPTIDE VACCINES

Hepatitis B polypeptide vaccines containing specific hepatitis B antigenic determinants of the major non-glycosylated peptide I of the surface antigen with a molecular weight of 22–24 000 and its glycosylated form, a polypeptide with a molecular weight in the range of 22–24 000 have been prepared in micellar form. The individual polypeptides of the surface antigen are immunogenic, and the purified 24 000 (designated as p24) and 27 000 (gp27) molecular-weight polypeptides are effective antigens. Clinical trials of the polypeptide micelle vaccine have been made.

PRODUCTION OF HEPATITIS B VACCINES BY RECOMBINANT DNA TECHNIQUES

Recombinant DNA techniques have been used for expressing HBsAg and core antigen in prokaryotic cells (*Escherichia coli* and *Bacillus subtilis*) and in eukaryotic cells, such as mutant mouse LM cells, HeLa cells, COS cells, CHO cells, and yeast cells (*Saccharomyces cerevisiae*).

Recombinant yeast hepatitis B vaccines have undergone extensive evaluation by clinical trials. The results indicated that this vaccine is safe, antigenic, and free from side-effects (apart from minor local reactions in a proportion of recipients). The immunogenicity is similar, in general terms, to that of the plasma-derived vaccine. Recombinant yeast hepatitis B vaccines are now been used in many countries. A vaccine based on HBsAg expressed in mammalian (CHO) cells is in use in the People's Republic of China.

HEPATITIS B VACCINES CONTAINING PRE-S EPITOPES

A disadvantage of plasma-derived and recombinant hepatitis B vaccines containing only the major protein of HBsAg (without pre-S sequences) is the lack of immune responsiveness of a minority of vaccinees. The identification of, and immunodominant domain, in the pre-S2 region of HBsAg and the observation that mice immunologically non-responsive to the major protein of HBsAg made antibodies to a synthetic peptide corresponding to this epitope stimulated interest in incorporation of pre-S sequences in hepatitis B vaccines. In 1986, Itoh *et al.* demonstrated that a synthetic peptide encompassing 19 amino acids from the pre-S2 regions, when coupled to keyhole limpet haemocyanin, elicited a protective antibody response when given to chimpanzees. The middle (pre-S2+S) and large (pre-S1+pre-S2–S) forms of HBsAg have been expressed in yeast using constitutive and inducible promoters, respectively. The former preparation has been evaluated for safety and immunogenicity. A vaccine containing all three (large, middle, and major) forms of HBsAg, synthesized in Chinese hamster ovary cells, has been tested in Singapore by Yap and colleagues; the preparation proved safe and immunogenic with a rapid antibody response in 96 per cent of the recipients.

HYBRID VIRUS VACCINES

Potential live vaccines using recombinant vaccinia viruses have been constructed for hepatitis B, and also for herpes simplex, rabies, and other viruses. Foreign viral DNA is introduced into the vaccinia virus genome by construction of chimeric genes and homologous recombination in cells, as the large size of the genome of vaccinia virus (185 000 bp) precludes gene insertion *in vitro*. A chimeric gene consisting of promoter sequences from vaccinia virus ligated to the coding sequence for the desired foreign protein is flanked by vaccinia virus DNA in a plasmid vector.

The recloned vaccinia virus containing HBsAg sequences has been used successfully for 'priming' experimental animals. At present, however, there is no accepted laboratory marker of attenuation or virulence of vaccinia virus for man, either in the host directly inoculated with the virus or after several passages in the same species. Alterations in the genome of vaccinia virus that are concomitant with the selection of recombinants may alter the virulence of the virus. Changes in host range or tissue tropism of vaccinia viruses may result from their genetic modification, and these could be caused by changes in the virus envelope as a result of the incorporation of gene products of the foreign viral genes inserted into the vaccinia virus.

The advantages of a vaccinia virus recombinant as a vaccine include low cost, ease of administration by multiple pressure or by the scratch technique, vaccine stability, long shelf-life, and the possible use of polyvalent antigens. The known adverse reactions with vaccinia virus vaccines are well documented and their incidence and severity must be carefully weighed against the adverse reactions associated with existing vaccines that a new recombinant vaccine might replace. There are also reports of spread of current strains of vaccinia virus to contacts and this may present difficulties. Other recombinant viruses as vectors are being explored, and in particular the oral adenovirus vaccines, which have been in use for some 20 years (reviewed by Zuckerman (1990)).

NOVEL HEPATITIS B VACCINES USING HYBRID PARTICLES

Other developments include the use of the envelope proteins of HBV (HBsAg) in a particulate form by expressing the proteins in mammalian cells. In-phase insertions of variable length and sequence of another virus (poliomyelitis virus type I) were made in different regions of the S gene of hepatitis B virus. The envelope proteins carrying the surface antigen and the insert are assembled with cellular lipids in the cultured mammalian cells after transfection. The inserted polio neutralization peptide was found to be exposed on the surface of the hybrid envelope particles and induced neutralizing antibodies against poliovirus in mice immunized experimentally. This approach may also be useful for studying the biological activity of other peptides incorporated into the surface of an organized, multimolecular complex. The expression and secretion of hybrid envelope particles by established cell lines may thus provide an efficient system for the production of potential new vaccines.

Another potentially excellent carrier vehicle for human and veterinary vaccines, in addition to hepatitis B, is the use of the core particles of HBV. The advantage of the core structure as a particle includes its ability to induce antibody with approximately 100-fold greater efficiency than the surface antigen particle, and an ability to augment T-helper cell function. The feasibility of this approach was recently demonstrated with synthetic and biosynthetic peptides of foot-and-mouth disease virus after fusion to hepatitis B core.

CHEMICALLY SYNTHESIZED HEPATITIS B VACCINES

The development of chemically synthesized polypeptide vaccines offers many advantages in attaining the ultimate goal of producing chemically uniform, safe, and cheap viral immunogens to replace many current vaccines, which often contain large quantities of irrelevant microbial antigenic determinants, proteins, and other material additional to the essential immunogen required for the induction of a protective antibody. The preparation of antibodies against viral proteins using fragments of chemically synthesized peptides mimicking viral amino-acid sequences is now a possible and attractive alternative approach to immunoprophylaxis.

Successful mimicking of determinants of HBsAg using chemically synthesized peptides in linear and cyclical forms has been reported by several groups of investigators. Peptides have been synthesized that retain biological function and appropriate secondary structure, even though they have a limited sequence homology with the natural peptide or are much smaller.

Various other studies also confirm that selected overlapping peptides corresponding to relevant epitopes of HBsAg may be useful as a synthetic vaccines when combined with adjuvants; antisera to these peptides cross-react with the native surface-antigen particles, and protective immunity has been demonstrated in limited experimental studies.

Enhancement of the immunogenicity of the preS region of HBsAg has been demonstrated in mice, using chemically synthesized amino-acid residues. The immune response to the pre-S2 region was shown to be regulated by H-2 linked genes, which are distinct from those that regulate the response to the S region. It was also demonstrated that immunization of a 'non-responder' murine strain with particles that contain both S and pre-S2 can circumvent non-responsiveness. More recently, a protein sequence that mediates the attachment of HBV to human hepatoma cells was identified. A synthetic peptide analogue, which is recognized by both cell receptors and viral antibodies, elicited antibodies reacting with the virus. Such a preparation may elicit protective antibodies by blocking the attachment of virus to the cells.

However, designing proteins with the correct tertiary structure and with functional activities is exceedingly difficult, as it is not possible to predict the tertiary structure of a protein from its amino acid sequence alone. X-ray crystallography and interactive computer graphics are essential and available tools. The first step is to obtain a highly purified protein that can be crystallized to diffraction quality. The electron density of the crystal can then be calculated and, as crystallography provides information on the non-hydrogen atoms in proteins, it is possible to build a scaffold model for fitting the known amino-acid sequence into this structure. The model can then be refined by using sets to test co-ordinates to improve the density map. More recent techniques using synchrotron X-ray sources may allow the collection of structural information from protein in solution.

Two-dimensional proton nuclear magnetic resonance techniques, which assign peaks to specific protons in the protein, are available now and the results can be converted to a set of co-ordinates for the molecule. An alternative approach is to develop comprehensive algorithms to simulate the mechanisms that determine protein structures, coupled with establishing libraries of protein database. Another approach is to design synthetic proteins based on the natural folding patterns of the α-helix configuration and the β-pleated sheet. However, there are no proven principles yet for *de novo* protein design, although it is equally clear that significant advances are being made in the construction of secondary patterns of proteins.

Nevertheless, several reports show that the modification of peptides based on secondary structure predictions and model building is now feasible. Peptides have been synthesized that remain biological function and appropriate secondary structure, even though they have a limited sequence homology with the natural peptide or are much smaller. For example, studies with hormones have shown that it is possible to stabilize a turn by cyclization of the molecule either by introducing a disulphide bond, or by designing a cyclic peptide.

Synthetic peptides may therefore be employed in due course as vaccines, although mixtures of more than one of the peptides may be required. Of the many questions that remain to be answered, the critical issues are whether antibodies induced by synthetic immunogens will be protective and whether protective immunity will persist. Some of the carrier proteins and some of the adjuvants that had been linked to the synthetic molecules cannot be used in man, and it is therefore essential to find acceptable and safe material for covalent linkage, or, alternatively, to synthesize sequences that do not require linkage. But the prospect of multivalent, chemically synthetic vaccines against a variety of microbial agents is within reach.

Hepatitis B antibody escape mutants

The emergence of mutants of HBV resistant to vaccine-induced antibody has been reported in Italy and in Singapore, and more recently elsewhere. In most cases in Italy and all in Singapore, the neonate of an infectious carrier mother became chronically infected despite circulating anti-surface antibody (anti-HBs) following combined immunoprophylaxis with hepatitis B immunoglobulin and vaccine. Nucleotide sequence analysis of the region of the HBV genome encoding the major antigenic domain of the surface protein revealed a point mutation (guanine to adenine) that specifies a coding change from glycine to arginine in the surface antigen. The amino acid residue involved is located in the second loop of the *a* determinant. Although it has not been possible to detect the variant in the mothers' sera, it is likely that their infecting dose of virus may have included the variant. It is possible then that the anti-HBs antibody present in the hepatitis B immunoglobulin neutralized wild-type virus, leaving the variant to become established in the neonate despite vaccination. This hypothesis is supported by a report from the United States by McMahon *et al.* of the identical mutation in an HBV variant isolated from an adult following transplantation for HBV-related liver disease. The human monoclonal antiHBs that was given in an unsuccessful attempt to prevent reinfection of the graft seems to have selected the mutant. Identical mutants have been reported from Japan, and preliminary studies suggest a similar mutant in Brazil.

HBV precore mutants

When DNA–DNA hybridization replaced the less sensitive assay of the endogenous DNA polymerase activity as a method for detecting hepatitis B virions in serum, it became clear that some patients with antiHBe were seropositive for virus. The early reports suggested that this finding was more common in Greece and other Mediterranean regions than elsewhere, raising the possibility of the involvement of a variant form(s) of HBV.

Vaudin *et al.* (1988) reported the nucleotide sequence of the genome of a strain of HBV cloned from the serum of a naturally infected chimpanzee. A surprising feature was a point mutation in the penultimate codon of the precore region that changed the tryptophan codon (TGG) to an amber termination codon (TAG). The nucleotide sequence of the HBV precore region from a number of anti-HBe-positive Greek patients was investigated by direct sequencing PCR-amplified HBV DNA from serum. An identical mutation of the penultimate codon of the precore region to a termination codon was found in seven of eight anti-HBe-positive patients who were positive for HBV DNA in serum by hybridization. In most cases there was an additional mutation in the proceeding codon. Similar variants were found in an Italian study by amplification of HBV DNA from serum from a further seven anti-HBe-positive patients, one of whom seemed to be coinfected with wild-type virus. These variants are not confined to the Mediterranean region; the same nonsense mutation (without a second mutation in the adjacent codon) has been observed in patients from Japan and elsewhere, along with rarer examples of defective precore regions caused by frameshifts or loss of the initiation codon for the precore regions.

Patients without HBeAg with high levels of HBV replication from various geographical areas may be infected frequently by viruses with variant precore regions. Presumably, these can replicate without secretion of HBeAg. The majority of patients who are infected with these variants are anti-HBe-positive, implying past infection with non-defective HBV. It is not clear whether these patients were infected originally with a mixture of wild-type and mutant viruses or whether the variants arose throughout the course of natural infection. The process of seroconversion from HBeAg to antiHBe seems to select the variant viruses and this may be related to the expression of HBeAg on the surface of hepatocytes infected by the wild-type virus.

In many cases, precore variants have been described in patients with severe chronic liver disease and who may have failed to respond to therapy with interferon. This observation raises the question of whether the variants are more pathogenic than the wild-type virus. For example, a nosocomial outbreak of fatal fulminant hepatitis B in Israel was associated with transmission of mutant HBV from a common source to five individuals; and in a study of British patients with fulminant hepatitis B, precore mutants were found in eight of nine HBeAg-negative patients but in none of six who were HBeAg positive on presentation.

HBV and hepatocellular carcinoma

Regions of the world where chronic carriage of HBV is common were found to coincide with a high prevalence of primary liver cancer. Furthermore, in these areas, patients with tumour almost invariably are seropositive for HBsAg. In a prospective study in Taiwan, 184 cases of hepatocellular carcinoma occurred in 3454 carriers of HBsAg at the start of the study, but only 10 such tumours occurred in the 19 253 control males who were HBsAg negative.

Southern hybridization of tumour DNA yields evidence of chromosomal integration of viral sequences in at least 80 per cent of hepatocellular carcinomas from HBsAg carriers. There is no similarity in the pattern of integration between different tumours, and variation is seen both in the integration site(s) and in the number of copies or partial copies of the viral genome. Sequence analysis of the integrants reveals that the direct repeats in the viral genome often lie close to the virus/cell junctions, suggesting that sequences around the ends of the viral genome may be involved in recombination with host DNA. Integration seems to involve microdeletion of host sequences and rearrangements, and deletions of part of the viral genome also may occur. When an intact surface gene is present, the tumour cells may produce and secrete HBsAg in the form of 22-nm particles.

Production of HBcAg by tumours is rare, however, and the core open reading frame is often incomplete and modifications such as methylation may also modulate its expression. Cytotoxic T cells targeted against core gene products on the hepatocyte surface seem to be the main mechanism of clearance of infected cells from the liver, and cells with integrated viral DNA, which are capable of expressing these proteins, may also be lysed. Thus, there may be immune selection of cells with integrated viral DNA that are incapable of expressing HBcAg.

The mechanism of oncogenesis by HBV remains obscure. HBV may act non-specifically by stimulating active regeneration and cirrhosis, which may be associated with long-term chronicity. However, HBV-associated tumours occur occasionally in the absence of cirrhosis and it is difficult to explain the frequent finding of integrated viral DNA in tumours. In rare instances, the viral genome has been found to be integrated into cellular genes such as cyclin A and a retinoic acid receptor. Translocations and other chromosomal rearrangements also have been observed. Although insertional mutagenesis of HBV remains an attractive explanation for oncogenicity, supportive evidence is lacking. In contrast with these findings for human hepatocellular carincoma, liver cancer in woodchucks associated with persistent infection with the woodchuck hepatitis virus frequently involves integration of the viral genome in or near to cellular *myc* genes.

An alternative possibility is that tumour formation is associated with a viral gene product. The product of the x gene is known to be a transactivator of transcription and so may cause inappropriate upregulation of cellular genes. Truncated forms of HBsAg, which may be produced from incomplete, surface open reading frames integrated in tumour cells, also can have transactivating activity, perhaps through interaction with receptors in the cell membrane. As with many other cancers, the development of hepatocellular carcinoma is likely to be a multifactorial process. The clonal expansion of cells with integrated viral DNA seems to be an early stage in this process and such clones may accumulate in the liver throughout the period of active virus replication. In areas where the prevalence of primary liver cancer is high, virus infection usually occurs at an early age and virus replication may be prolonged, although the peak incidence of tumour is many years after the initial infection.

Hepatitis D

Delta hepatitis was first recognized following detection of a novel protein, delta antigen (**HDAg**), by immunofluorescent staining in the nuclei of hepatocytes from patients with hepatitis B. HDV requires a helper function of HBV for its replication. HDV is coated with HBsAg, which is needed for release from the host hepatocyte and for entry in the next round of infection.

Two forms of delta hepatitis infection are known. In the first, a susceptible individual is coinfected with HBV and HDV, often leading to a more severe form of acute hepatitis caused by HBV. Vaccination against HBV also prevents coinfection. In the second, an individual chronically infected with HBV becomes superinfected with HDV. This may accelerate the course of the chronic liver disease and cause overt disease in asymptomatic HBsAg carriers. HDV itself appears to be cytopathic and HDAg may be directly cytotoxic.

Delta hepatitis is common in some areas of the world with a high prevalence of hepatitis B infection, particularly the Mediterranean region, parts of eastern Europe, the Middle East, Africa, and South America. It has been estimated that 5 per cent of HBsAg carriers worldwide (approximately 15 million people) are infected with HDV. In areas of low prevalence of hepatitis B, those at risk of HBV infection, particularly intravenous drug abusers, are also at risk of HDV infection.

Structure and replication of HDV

The HDV particle is approximately 36 nm in diameter and is composed of an RNA genome associated with HDAg, surrounded by an envelope of HBsAg. The virus reaches higher concentrations in the circulation than HBV, up to 10^{12} particles/ml have been recorded. The HDV genome is a closed, circular RNA molecule of 1679 nucleotides with extensive sequence complementarity that permits pairing of approximately 70 per cent of the bases to form an unbranched, rod structure. The genome thus resembles those of the satellite viroids and virusoids of plants, and similarly seems to be replicated by the host RNA polymerase II, with autocatalytic cleavage and circularization of the progeny genomes via *trans*-esterification reactions (ribozyme activity). Consensus sequences of viroids that are believed to be involved in these processes are also conserved in the delta virus.

Unlike the plant viroids, HDV codes for a protein HDAg. This is encoded in an open reading frame in the antigenomic RNA but four other open reading frames that are also present in the genome do not appear to be utilized. About 600 copies of a polyadenylated mRNA, approximately 800 nucleotides in length, may be detected in the cytoplasm of infected hepatocytes. The antigen, which contains a nuclear localization signal, was originally detected in the nuclei of infected hepatocytes and may be detected in serum only after removing the outer envelope of the virus with detergent.

Hepatitis C

Before the identification of HCV, transmission studies in chimpanzees established that the main agent of parenterally acquired non-A, non-B hepatitis was likely to be an enveloped virus some 30 to 60 nm in diameter. These studies provided a pool of plasma that contained a relatively high titre of the agent. In order to clone the genome, the virus was pelleted from the plasma. Because it was not known whether the genome was DNA or RNA, a denaturation step was included before the synthesis of cDNA so that either DNA or RNA could serve as a template. The resultant cDNA was then inserted into the bacteriophage expression vector λgt11 and the libraries screened using serum from a patient with chronic non-A, non-B hepatitis. This approach led to the detection of a clone (designated 5-1-1) that was found to bind to antibodies present in the sera of several patients with non-A, non-B hepatitis. This clone was used as a probe to detect a larger, overlapping clone in the same library. It was possible to demonstrate that these sequences hybridized to a positive-sense RNA molecule of around 10 000 nucleotides, which was present in the livers of infected chimpanzees but not in uninfected controls. By employing a 'walking' technique, it was possible to use newly detected overlapping clones as hybridization probes in turn to detect further virus-specific clones in the library. Thus, clones covering the entire viral genome were assembled and the complete nucleotide sequence determined. The organization of the genome closely resembles those of the enveloped RNA viruses, the pestiviruses, and flaviviruses, as discussed below.

Detection of HCV infection

Because the 5-1-1 antigen was originally detected by antibodies in the serum of an infected patient it was an obvious antigen for the basis of an ELISA to detect anti-HCVantibodies. A larger clone, C100, was assembled from a number of overlapping clones and expressed in yeast as a fusion protein using human superoxide dismutase sequences to facilitate expression. This fusion protein formed the basis of first generation tests for HCV infection. The 5-1-1 antigen comprises amino acid sequences from the non-structural, NS4, region of the genome and C100 contains both NS3 and NS4 sequences. It is now known that antibodies to C100 are detected relatively late after an acute infection. Furthermore, the first generation ELISAs were associated with a high rate of false positivity when applied to low-incidence populations and there were further problems with some retrospective studies on stored sera. Data based on this test alone should, therefore, be interpreted with caution.

Second-generation tests include antigens from the nucleocapsid and further non-structural regions of the genome. The former (C22) is particularly useful and antibodies to the HCV core protein seem to appear relatively early in infection. These second-generation tests confirmed that HCV is the major cause of parenterally transmitted non-A, non-B hepatitis. Routine testing of blood donations is now in place in many countries and prevalence rates vary from 0.2 to 0.5 per cent in northern Europe to 1.2 to 1.5 per cent in southern Europe and Japan. Most of those with antibody have a history of parenteral risk such as a history of transfusion, or administration of blood products, or of intravenous drug abuse. There is little evidence for sexual or perinatal transmission of HCV and the natural routes of transmission are yet to be identified.

The availability of the nucleotide sequence of HCV made possible the use of the PCR as a direct test for the genome of the virus itself. The first step is the synthesis of a cDNA copy of the target region of the RNA genome using reverse transcriptase (primed by the antigenomic PCR primer or, better, by random hexamers); the product of this reaction is then a suitable target for amplification. The concentration of virus in serum samples is often very low so that the mass of product from the PCR reaction is insufficient for visualization on a stained gel. Thus, either a second round of amplification (with nested primers) or detection of the primary product by Southern hybridization is required. There is considerable variation in nucleotide sequences among different isolates of HCV and the 5′ non-coding region, which seems to be highly conserved, is the preferred target for the PCR.

Current data suggest that about 50 per cent of infections with HCV progress to chronicity. Histological examination of liver biopsies from asymptomatic HCV carriers reveals that none has normal histological appearances and that up to 70 per cent have chronic active hepatitis and/or cirrhosis. Whether the virus is cytopathic or whether there is an immunopathological element remains unclear. HCV infection is also associated with progression to hepatocellular carcinoma. For example, in Japan, where the incidence of hepatocellular carcinoma has been increasing despite a decrease in the prevalence of HBsAg, HCV is now the principal risk factor. There is no DNA intermediate in the replication of the HCV genome or integration of viral nucleic acid and viral pathology may contribute to oncogenesis as a result of cirrhosis and regeneration of liver cells.

The organization of the HCV genome

The genome of HCV resembles those of the pestiviruses and flaviviruses in that it comprises around 10 000 nucleotides of positive sense RNA, lacks a 3′ poly A tract, and has a similar gene organization (Fig. 4). It has been proposed that HCV should be the prototype of a third genus in the family Flaviviridae. All of these genomes contain a single, large open reading frame that is translated to yield a polyprotein (of about 3000 amino acids in the case of HCV) from which the viral proteins are derived by post-translational cleavage and other modifications.

There is a short, untranslated region at the 5′ end of the genomic RNA and a further untranslated region at the 3′ end, the large open reading frame accounting for over 95 per cent of the sequence. The structural proteins are located towards the 5′ end and the non-structural proteins towards the 3′ end. The first product of the polyprotein is the non-glycosylated capsid protein, C, which complexes with the genomic RNA to form the nucleocapsid. As with the flaviviruses, a hydrophobic domain may anchor the growing polypeptide in the endoplasmic reticulum and facilitate cleavage by a cellular signalase releasing a nucleocapsid precursor (anchored C). The amino acid sequence of the nucleocapsid protein seems to be highly conserved among different isolates of HCV.

The next domain in the polyprotein also has a signal sequence at its carboxyl terminus and may be processed in a similar fashion. The product is a glycoprotein that is probably found in the viral envelope and is referred to as E1/S or gp35. The third domain may be cleaved by a protease within the viral polyprotein to yield what is probably a second surface glycoprotein, E2/NS1 or gp70. Other post-translational modifications, including further proteolytic cleavages, are possible. These proteins are the focus of considerable interest because of their potential use in tests for the direct detection of viral proteins and for HCV vaccines. Nucleotide sequencing studies reveal that both domains contain hypervariable regions. It is possible that this divergence has been driven by antibody pressure and that these regions specify important immunogenic epitopes.

Fig. 4 Hepatitis C viral genome. HV hypervariable region.

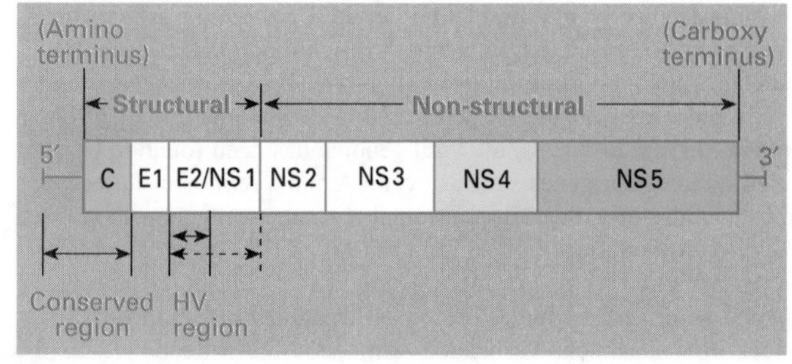

The non-structural region of the HCV genome is divided into regions NS2 to NS5. In the flaviviruses, NS3 has two functional domains, a protease that is involved in cleavage of the non-structural region of the polyprotein and a helicase that is presumably involved in RNA replication. Motifs within this region of the HCV genome have homology to the appropriate consensus sequences, suggesting similar functions. NS5 seems to be the replicase and contains the gly-asp-asp motif common to viral RNA-dependent RNA polymerases.

Other hepatitis viruses

It is likely that there are other human hepatitis viruses. Whilst HCV is clearly the major cause of parenterally transmitted non-A, non-B hepatitis, data from some of the original transmission experiments suggest that at least one other agent might be involved. A number of candidates are already emerging. Togavirus-like particles have been observed in the livers of patients with fulminant (candidate HFV?), sporadic (community-acquired), non-A, non-B hepatitis. A number of these patients proceeded to transplantation, with apparent reinfection of the graft with haemorrhagic manifestations. A severe form of sporadic hepatitis, characterized histologically by giant syncytial (candidate HGV?) hepatocytes and perhaps caused by a paramyxovirus, has also been described.

Treatment of viral hepatitis

Treatment of acute hepatitis

There is no specific treatment. General measures include bedrest and a generally nutritious diet. Patients should be encouraged to exercise regularly if they feel well. Consumption of alcohol should be avoided during the acute phase and should avoided during the acute phase and should be modest after convalescence.

Corticosteroids and non-steroidal anti-inflammatory drugs are not indicated and should not be used.

Treatment of chronic hepatitis B

Specific treatment is now available, following the demonstration that interferon-α inhibits replication of HBV and that prolonged treatment can lead to remission of the disease.

Antiviral therapy is aimed at patients with active disease and viral replication, preferably at a stage before signs and symptoms of cirrhosis or significant injury have occurred. Eradication of the disease is possible in only minority of patients. Permanent loss of HBV DNA and HBeAg results in an improvement in necroinflammatory change, and reduced infectivity. It is possible that the accompanying histological improvement reduces the risk of cirrhosis and hepatocellular carcinoma.

Unfortunately, treatment of chronic hepatitis with interferon is effective in less than half of the patients. It is relatively expensive, requires injection, and is not free from side-effects. None the less, recombinant interferon-α has been licensed for treatment of chronic hepatitis B in the United Kingdom, and several European countries.

The interferons act by interaction with specific membrane receptors, thereby inducing a number of enzymes and proteins, the best characterized of which are the 2′,5′-oligoadenylate synthetases (2′,5′ A synthetases) and protein kinases. The expression of the class 1 major histocompatibility antigen (**MHC**) genes is activated by all interferons, and those of the class II by interferon-γ, to increase the expression of MHC at the cell surface and thereby amplify viral antigen recognition and display. Interferons also modify the cellular and humoral immune response.

Three preparations of interferon-α are currently available, two of which are recombinant preparations and one of which is prepared from a lymphoblastoid cell line. Approximately 40 per cent of patients respond. Highest response rates are usually seen in carriers with higher baseline serum aminotransferase levels, lower levels of HBV DNA, and without AIDS. Although these factors provide some predictive information, none of these criteria is absolute, and individual carriers, for example, ethnic Chinese, with active disease, or those patients with anti-human immunodeficiency virus antibodies but normal CD4 lymphocyte counts may respond, making the prediction of treatment outcome somewhat difficult. The appropriate dose of interferon is not yet established, but 5 to 10 million units three times weekly for 3 to 4 months is currently prescribed.

The subclinical exacerbation of the hepatitis frequently seen in responders suggests that interferon acts by augmenting the immune response to HBV, perhaps triggered by the inhibition of viral replication as well as the effects of interferon on cytotoxic T cells. Although residual HBV DNA can be detected by PCR, the disease appears to be ameliorated. Approximately 20 per cent of patients who respond to treatment with clearance of HBeAg will also clear HBsAg within a year of treatment, and up to 65 per cent may later clear HBsAg after 6 years of follow-up.

Patients who do not respond to interferon-α represent a difficult management problem. Lower doses given for a longer period are currently being studied.

Pulsed corticosteroid treatment and interferon may also be of benefit in patients without elevated serum aminotransferases. This treatment regimen should be used with caution in those patients with decompensated hepatitis B because of the risk of inducing severe hepatic necrosis.

The main early side-effects of interferon include an influenza-like illness. Later side-effects include malaise, muscle aches, headaches, poor appetite, weight loss, increased need for sleep, irritability, anxiety and depression, hair loss, thrombocytopenia, and leucopenia. Unusual or severe side-effects include seizures, acute psychosis, bacterial infections, autoimmune reactions, thyroid disease, proteinuria, myocardiopathy, skin rashes, and interferon antibodies.

Other antiviral drugs

A number of other agents have been used for the treatment of hepatitis B. These include interferon-γ, acyclovir (acycloguanosine), 6-deoxyacyclovir, ganciclovir, forscarnet (tri-sodium phosphonoformate), azido-3′-deoxythymidine triphosphate, 2′,3′-dideoxycytidine and 2′,3′-dideoxyinosine, adenine arabinoside 5′-monophosphate (**ara-AMP**), *Phyllanthrus amarus*, interleukin-2, isoprinosine, thymosin, tumour necrosis factor, transfer factor, adenine arabinoside 5′-monophosphate conjugated with lactosaminated albumin, interferon-α and -γ, interferon-γ and -β, acyclovir and interferon, levamizole. Few of these drugs are useful clinically, but ganciclovir, ara-AMP, and foscarnet may suppress HBV in some patients.

Several newer nucleoside analogues suppress hepatitis B *in vitro*, and these drugs are undergoing clinical trial at present in man.

Treatment of chronic hepatitis C

Interferon-α treatment is indicated for patients with well-documented chronic hepatitis C in whom other causes of chronic hepatitis have been excluded, and who have at least a twofold elevation of serum ALT. Interferon-α reduces disease activity in hepatitis C after short courses (6 months) of treatment in approximately 50 per cent of patients. Liver biopsy provides useful information on the extent of liver damage. Treatment should be started at a dose of 3×10^6 units, three times per week, subcutaneously for 6 months. Treatment can be discontinued after 3 months if no response has occurred. However, approximately 50 per cent of responders relapse when treatment is stopped. Almost all of these relapses tend to respond again to retreatment.

Ribavirin, a nucleoside analogue that is taken orally, has also been shown to inhibit HCV. This drug may be a better choice for patients with cirrhosis, who respond poorly to interferon. The chief side-effect of ribavirin is haemolysis, and the drug is still under study.

REFERENCES

Anon. (1994). Prevention and control of hepatitis A. (1994). *Drug and Therapeutics Bulletin*, **32,** 9–11.

Beasley, R.P. and Hwang, L-Y. (1991). Overview on the epidemiology of hepatocellular carcinoma. In: *Viral hepatitis and Liver disease*, (ed. F.B. Hollinger, S.M. Lemon, and H.S. Margolis, pp. 532–5. Williams and Wilkins, Baltimore.

Bradley, D.W., McCaustland, K.A., Cook, E.H., Schable, C.A., Ebert, J.W., and Maynard, J.E. (1985). Posttransfusion non-A, non-B hepatitis in chimpanzees. Physicochemical evidence that the tubule-forming agent is a small, enveloped virus. *Gastroenterology*, **88,** 773–9.

Carman, W.F. *et al.* (1990). Vaccine-induced escape mutant of hepatitis B virus. *Lancet*, **336,** 325–9.

Cockcroft, A., Soper, P., Insail, C., Kennard, Y., Chapman, S., Gooch, C., and Griffiths, P. (1990). Antibody response after hepatitis B immunisation in health care workers. *British Journal of Industrial Medicine*, **47,** 199–202.

Choo, Q.L., Kuo, G., Weiner, A.J., Overby, L.R., Bradley, D.W., and Houghton, M. (1989). Isolation of a cDNA clone derived from a blood-borne non-A, non-B viral hepatitis genome. *Science*, **244,** 359–62.

Deinhardt, F.D. and Zuckerman, A.J. (1985). Immunization against hepatitis B: report on a WHO meeting on viral hepatitis in Europe. *Journal of Medical Virology*, **17,** 209–17.

Dusheiko, G.M. and Zuckerman, A.J. (1991). Therapy for hepatitis B. *Current Opinion in Infectious Diseases*, **4,** 785–94.

Fagan, E.A. *et al.* (1992). Toga virus-like particles in acute liver failure attributed to sporadic non-A, non-B hepatitis and recurrence after liver transplantation. *Journal of Medical Virology*, **38,** 71–7.

Hadziyannis, S.J., Lieberman, H.M., Karvountzis, G.G., and Shafritz, D.A. (1983). Analysis of liver disease, nuclear HBcAg, viral replication, and hepatitis B virus DNA in liver and serum of HBeAg vs. anti-HBe positive carriers of hepatitis B virus. *Hepatology*, **3,** 656–62.

Harrison, T.J., Hopes, E.A., Oon, C.J., Zanetti, A.R., and Zuckerman, A.J. (1991). Independent emergence of a vaccine-induced escape mutant of hepatitis B virus. *Journal of Hepatology*, **13,** (suppl. 4), S105–7.

He, L.F., Alling, D., Popkin, T., Shapiro, M., Alter, H.J., and Purcell, R.H. (1987). Determining the size of non-A, non-B hepatitis virus by filtration. *Journal of Infectious Diseases*, **156,** 636–40.

Hollinger, F.B., Trois, C., Heiberg, D., Sanchez, V., Dreesman, G.R., and Melnick, J.L. (1986). Response to hepatitis B polypeptide vaccine in micelle form in a young adult population. *Journal of Medical Virology*, **19,** 229–40.

Itoh, Y. *et al.* (1986). A synthetic peptide vaccines involving the product of the pre-S(2) region of hepatitis B virus DNA: protective efficacy in chimpanzees. *Proceedings of the National Academy of Science (USA)*, **83,** 9174–8.

Lieberman, H.M., LaBrecque, D.R., Kew, M.C., Hadziyannis, S.J., and Shafritz, D.A. (1983). Detection of hepatitis B virus DNA directly in human serum by a simplified molecular hybridization test: comparison to HBE-Ag/anti-HBe status in HBsAg carriers. *Hepatology*, **3,** 285–91.

McMahon, G., Ehrlich, P.H., and Moustafa, Z.A. (1992). Genetic alterations in the gene encoding the major HBs-DNA and immunological analysis of recurrent HBsAg derived from monoclonal antibody-treated liver transplant patients. *Hepatology*, **15,** 757–66.

Phillips, M.J. *et al.* (1991). Syncytial giant-cell hepatitis. Sporadic hepatitis with distinctive pathological features, a severe clinical course, and paramyxoviral features. *New England Journal of Medicine*, **324,** 455–60.

Shaw, F.E., Jr. *et al.* (1989). Effect of anatomic site, age and smoking on the immune response to hepatitis B vaccination. *Vaccine*, **7,** 425–30.

Skelly, J., Howard, C.R., and Zuckerman, A.J. (1981). Hepatitis B polypeptide vaccine in micelle form. *Nature*, **290,** 51–4.

Vaudin, M., Wolstenholme, A.J., Tsiquaye, K.N., Zuckerman, A.J., and Harrison, T.J. (1988). The complete nucleotide sequence of the genome of a hepatitis B virus isolated from a naturally infected chimpanzee. *Journal of General Virology*, **69,** 1383–9.

Yap, L., Guan, R., and Chan, S.H. (1992). Recombinant DNA hepatitis B vaccine containing pre-S components of the HBV coat protein—a preliminary study on immunogenicity. *Vaccine*, **10,** 439–42.

Zuckerman, A.J. (1973). Synthetic hepatitis B vaccine. *Nature*, **241,** 499.

Zuckerman, A.J. (1984). Who should be immunised against hepatitis B? *British Medical Journal*, **289,** 1243–4.

Zuckerman, A.J. (1990). Immunization against hepatitis B. *British Medical Bulletin*, **46,** 383–98.

Zuckerman, A.J. and Thomas, H.C. (eds.). (1993). *Viral hepatitis: scientific basis and clinical management.* pp. 1–590. Churchill Livingstone, Edinburgh.

Zuckerman, J.N., Cockcroft, A., and Zuckerman, A.J. (1992). Site of injection for vaccination. *British Medical Journal*, **305,** 1158.

Zuckerman, A.J., Harrison T.J., and Oon C-J. (1994). Mutations in S region of hepatitis B virus. *Lancet*, **343,** 737–8.

7.10.27 Viruses and cancer

R. A. Weiss

INTRODUCTION

Viruses are important in human cancer for two main reasons. First, it is estimated that 17 to 20 per cent of the worldwide incidence of cancer is attributable to a viral aetiology, including such common malignancies as carcinoma of the uterine cervix and hepatocellular cancer. As a transmissible agent is responsible for these cancers there is the prospect of eradication through screening and vaccination. Second, experimental studies of viral carcinogenesis in animals have led to the discovery of oncogenes and tumour-suppressor genes. Oncogenic viruses have therefore provided much insight into molecular mechanisms of carcinogenesis in the majority of cancers that do not have an infectious aetiology.

Viruses as aetiological agents of cancer

Table 1 lists the viruses implicated in human cancer. These viruses can establish persistence in the infected person. In most but not all cases the viral genome is present in the malignant cells; the exceptions appear to be those that promote cancer indirectly, such as human immunodeficiency virus (**HIV**) and possibly hepatitis C virus. The oncogenic viruses belong to many different virus families, and contain either DNA or RNA genomes. Their modes of transmission and mechanisms of cell transformation vary. For many of the viruses, malignancy is a rare effect and depends on other cofactors. For example, Epstein–Barr virus (**EBV**) is a ubiquitous infection yet children's Burkitt's lymphoma occurs only in areas of holoendemic malarial infection in Africa and Papua New Guinea, and undifferentiated nasopharyngeal carcinoma occurs mainly in Southern Chinese populations and in North Africa.

The epidemiological evidence linking particular viruses with particular cancers has accrued from different types of investigation. It has been recognized for more than 150 years that cervical cancer has a sexually transmissible component, as it is common in prostitutes and rare in nuns. During the 1960s and 1970s, herpes simplex virus type II was the chief suspect, but this association was not upheld to be causative. Human papillomaviruses (**HPV**) types 16 and 18 were not identified until 1983. As these papillomaviruses could not be propagated in culture, their discovery awaited DNA molecular hybridization and cloning. EBV was discovered in 1964 through electron microscopy of cultured cells from Burkitt's lymphoma. The link between EBV and nasopharyngeal carcinoma, on the other hand, was found serendipitously when cells from that tumour were used among others as controls for immunostaining of cells from Burkitt's lymphoma for EBV nuclear antigens (**EBNA**); nasopharyngeal carcinoma was EBNA positive. The possible link between EBV and some cases of Hodgkin's lymphoma is a recent observation and requires further investigation.

The correlation between a high incidence of primary hepatocellular carcinoma and hepatitis B virus (**HBV**) was noted over many decades, but the definitive evidence came from a longitudinal study of a large cohort of Taiwanese men. More than 98 per cent of those who subse-

Table 1 *Viruses implicated in human cancer*

Virus	Malignancy	Non-malignant disease
HPVs	Cervical cancer	Warts
	Skin cancer	
HBV	Primary liver cancer	Hepatitis
EBV	Nasopharyngeal carcinoma	Infectious mononucleosis
	Burkitt's lymphoma	
	Immunoblastic lymphoma	
HTLV-I	Adult T-cell leukaemia	Tropical spastic paraparesis
	Other T-cell lymphomas	
HIV-1	Non-Hodgkin's lymphoma	AIDS
	Kaposi's sarcoma	
HCV	Primary liver cancer	Hepatitis

Abbreviations of virus names are explained in the text.

quently developed liver cancer were HBV positive. The link between hepatitis C virus (**HCV**) and liver cancer is not yet as firm. Serological and polymerase chain-reaction assays for HCV have only recently been developed, yet it is becoming apparent that HBV-negative, HCV-positive persons have a significantly higher relative risk of liver cancer than uninfected persons.

The diseases associated with oncogenic viruses are not always malignancies. HBV and HCV cause chronic viral hepatitis. EBV causes infectious mononucleosis if infection is delayed beyond infancy. The human T-cell leukaemia virus (**HTLV**) type I is associated with tropical spastic paraparesis, known in Japan as HTLV-associated myopathy. HIV causes AIDS, and its associated malignancies are probably a secondary consequence of immune suppression, as discussed later.

Epidemiology and transmission

Oncogenic viruses establish persistent, lifelong infections, so that the event of infection may be far removed from the event of malignancy. That, and the difficulty of detecting latent or non-productive viral infection before the advent of molecular diagnostic assays, made it difficult to pin down their aetiological role. Moreover, cancer is often a rare outcome of virus infection, and many cofactors play a part in viral carcinogenesis.

As seen in Table 1, oncogenic viruses belong to many virus families. These have different routes of transmission. Some like HBV are frequently acquired perinatally or through subsequent exposure to blood. HTLV-I is similar except that the main vertical route of transmission is through infected cells in breast milk. HIV was present in cell-free blood fractions such as plasma and pooled clotting factors, whereas HTLV-I is almost exclusively cell associated. EBV is transmitted by saliva, whereas HIV has not been reported to pass from person to person in this way. Sexual transmission is common to HIV, HTLV-I (with a male to female bias), HBV, and HPV. Oncogenic viruses do not appear to be transmitted by the respiratory route, except adenoviruses, or via arthropod vectors, except some veterinary cases, bovine leucosis virus for example.

Whereas EBV occurs worldwide, viruses such as HBV and HTLV-I have a relatively high prevalence in particular population groups, and these are the ones in which the associated cancers occur. However, the individual risk of cancer differs according to the virus, and to other environmental and genetic cofactors. With persistent HBV infection, up to 50 per cent of infected persons may develop liver cancer if they live long enough. Other agents that damage the liver may exacerbate liver carcinogenesis, alcohol or dietary aflatoxins for example. The aflatoxins are carcinogenic in their own right, but recent evidence suggests that HBV plus aflatoxin, as is common in parts of Africa, may be synergistic in causing liver cancer.

With HTLV-I, less than 5 per cent of those with lifelong infection develop adult T-cell leukaemia, but the predisposing cofactors, if any, are not known. Tropical spastic paraparesis is also an unusual disease in HTLV-I-positive people but may occur more commonly after infection via contaminated blood transfusions. HTLV-I is prevalent in Japan, and among blacks in Africa and the Americas, but occurs sporadically elsewhere. HTLV-II is endemic in native American Indians, and in certain African groups; it has not been definitely linked to disease, but may be associated with a rare T-cell malignancy resembling hairy-cell leukaemia in blood smears.

An example of an essentially harmless virus causing cancer in a rare, predisposing condition is the recessive hereditary condition, epidermodysplasia verruciformis. The squamous cancers of patients with this condition only develop in sun-exposed areas of skin and harbour strains of papillomavirus (e.g. HPV-5) that are not commonly found in warts or skin cancers of normal people. Patients with epidermodysplasia verruciformis have a defect in cellular immunity that permits the virally infected cells to develop as benign warts and after ultraviolet exposure as malignant growths. Thus skin carcinogenesis in this condition is multifactorial; a host genetic defect, a papillomavirus and ultraviolet irradiation act in concert to cause these cancers. Because epidermodysplasia verruciformis is extremely rare, affecting less than 1 in 1 million people, it is inconceivable that HPV-5 is transmitted only between sufferers. HPV-5 is likely to be a relatively common yet inapparent skin infection. Indeed, recent evidence suggests that squamous skin cancers in other immunodeficient conditions such as AIDS are also attributable to the types of papillomavirus previously identified only in patients with epidermodysplasia verruciformis.

Kaposi's sarcoma is another tumour that occurs much more frequently in immunodeficient patients. The relative risk in recipients of organ transplants is about 400, and in persons with AIDS about 9000. However, there is a marked discrepancy in risk among different categories of AIDS patients. Those who acquired their HIV sexually are much more likely to develop the sarcoma than those who were infected by HIV parenterally. HIV probably contributes to Kaposi's sarcoma indirectly through immune suppression, although the tat protein of HIV may also play some part in the sarcoma-cell proliferation. Early studies implicated cytomegalovirus, but the evidence for the involvement of this agent and the more recently suggested HPV-18 has not been upheld. It seems more likely that an as yet unidentified micro-organism is the proximate cause of Kaposi's sarcoma, and that many immunocompetent persons may harbour the agent without ill effect. Presumably this agent would be more prevalent in those geographic areas where the sarcoma occurs among apparently immunocompetent people. The unknown agent is likely to be a virus, but it could be some other kind of micro-organism. The link between schistosomiasis and bladder cancer and the possible association of *Helicobacter pylori* with stomach cancer serves to remind us that viruses are not the only transmissible organisms with oncogenic potential.

Finally, in discussing epidemiological evidence for viruses causing cancer, mention should be made of common human viruses that are highly oncogenic in experimental animals but are not linked to human cancer, namely the polyomaviruses BK and JC, and the adenoviruses. Human adenovirus types 2 and 12 readily cause sarcomas and carcinomas in hamsters and other rodents. If the type 12 virus DNA were to be considered as a chemical rather than a biological agent, it would be classified as more carcinogenic on a molar basis than benzpyrene. The adenovirus genome persists in the animal tumours and the early genes, *E1A* and *E1B*, are implicated in carcinogenesis by sequestering the cellular p53 and Rb gene products. It is surprising, then, that there is no epidemiological evidence linking adenovirus infection with human cancer, and not for want of searching. One explanation is that human cells (in contrast to rodent cells) are fully permissive for viral replication, resulting in cell death. But during viral replication *in vivo*, millions of defective virions are produced. Some of these will express only the early, oncogenic genes, and spare the cells from cytopathic effects. The lack of association of these potent viral carcinogens with human cancer remains an enigma.

Mechanisms of viral carcinogenesis

Physical and chemical carcinogens are usually mutagens. They cause DNA mutations that contribute to the eventual malignant phenotype of the cancer. The tumour cells are derived as a clonal population from the mutated cells. The genes affected in cancer are broadly classified into two categories. If the mutations knock out the function of the protein encoded by the gene, so that the protein can no longer maintain the cell in a normal, growth-regulated state, that gene is called a tumour-suppressor gene. If the mutation activates a gene or causes its ectopic expression, so that the protein product actively contributes to the malignant phenotype by driving unregulated growth, then that gene is called an oncogene.

Oncogenes were first discovered in animal retroviruses, such as the Rous sarcoma virus of chickens. Later it was found that these oncogenes were not essential for the replication of the retrovirus, and had originated from cellular genes. The rare retroviruses that bear oncogenes cause tumours after a short latent period because they have transduced cellular oncogenes, which are then expressed from powerful viral promoter sequences. More commonly, retroviruses cause cancer not because they carry oncogenes but because the DNA provirus integrates into chromosomal DNA and promotes the activation of adjacent cellular oncogenes. In fact, retroviral genomes integrate randomly into cellular DNA, but if millions of cells become infected, one or two of them may have an integration site near an oncogene and that cell gives rise to the tumour. The activation of oncogenes by retroviruses is comparable to activation by chromosomal translocation. Many of the known oncogenes were first identified through the analysis of retroviral cancers in animals and were only later found in non-viral human cancers.

The mechanism of cell transformation by HTLV-I and -II is different from that of the majority of animal retroviruses, although the related bovine leucosis virus probably acts in a similar way. These viruses encode a viral gene, *tax*, which is essential to promote full viral gene transcription. The *tax* gene product is a protein that acts as a transcriptional activator, by associating with host-cell nuclear proteins to bind to promoter DNA sequences in the long terminal repeat of the viral genome. This results in a positive feedback, up-regulation of the viral genome. However, the viral *tax* gene also up-regulates certain cellular genes. One of these is the gene encoding the interleukin-2 (**IL-2**) receptor. If the infected T cells are already producing small amounts of IL-2, then the overexpression of the receptor results in autocrine T-cell proliferation. This one effect, however, cannot explain the whole pathogenesis of adult T-cell leukaemia following HTLV-I infection. Typically, the leukaemia does not become manifest until 40 or more years after HTLV-I infection, and in few of the infected people. However, HTLV-I and -II will 'immortalize' CD4+ T lymphocytes in culture through *tax* expression, rather as EBV immortalizes B lymphocytes, but this is only one step in the pathway to malignancy.

The cellular transformation by DNA viruses is best understood for polyomaviruses and adenoviruses, those viruses that, as already mentioned, appear not to cause human cancer. The transforming genes of these viruses are expressed early in the infection cycle. They activate cell proliferation, which aids viral replication. The genes encode viral proteins that bind to and sequester cellular proteins that normally control cell proliferation, thus triggering the cells into cycle. These cellular proteins are the tumour-suppressor proteins, such as Rb, which is missing in retinoblastoma, and p53, which is mutated in many human cancers, including a germ-line mutation in Li–Fraumeni syndrome. Instead of mutating the cellular tumour-suppressor genes, the DNA tumour viruses block the function of their proteins, which similarly results in unregulated cell proliferation.

To cause tumours, DNA tumour viruses and retroviruses (which form a DNA provirus) must persist in the tumour cells, often by integrating into chromosomal DNA, so that they are passed on through successive mitotic cycles as if they were cellular genes. Oncogenic herpesviruses, such as EBV, do not necessarily integrate into cellular DNA. They are maintained episomally. EBNA-1 is required for episomal replication, while other EBNA proteins and the latent membrane protein are responsible for the transformed cell phenotype. With HBV, integrated copies are found in many liver carcinoma lines, but a requirement for integration has not been unequivocally shown. HBV expresses transactivating functions, from the *X* gene and also possibly the envelope gene, so its transformation may resemble that of HTLV-I.

In all the mechanisms discussed so far the persistence and expression of the viral genome or part of it is assumed to be essential for maintaining the malignant phenotype of the tumour cell. However, it is conceivable that viruses could exert an oncogenic effect without persisting in (or in some cases even infecting) the cells destined to become the malignant clone. Viruses that have a mutagenic effect on host DNA could act in a 'hit-and-run' manner, like other mutagens. It was thought that herpes simplex virus and cytomegalovirus might act in this manner, but the evidence for their involvement in cancer is no longer considered strong.

Indirect carcinogenic effects are those in which damage to tissues by viruses may allow clones of premalignant cells to proliferate that would not otherwise do so. HCV and possibly HBV might do this by destroying normal liver cells, resulting in a much greater rate of liver-cell regeneration. Thus any stem cells initiated into a premalignant state by other carcinogens (e.g. aflatoxin) will have a greater chance of developing into malignant tumours. A severely immunosuppressive virus like HIV could be regarded as a special case of indirect viral carcinogenesis. Without being directly oncogenic, HIV may promote tumours by destroying helper T-cell immunity. The types of cancer seen in other immunodeficient conditions are also particularly common in AIDS, non-Hodgkin's lymphoma and Kaposi's sarcoma for example. The majority of tumours that occur in immunosuppressed individuals probably have a viral aetiology. The expression of viral proteins as foreign antigens may normally help to keep potential tumours under immunological control. It is noteworthy that it is this viral subset of cancers, rather than the most common malignancies, that becomes more prevalent under immunosuppression.

The foregoing discussions on epidemiology and on molecular mechanisms serve to emphasize that viral oncogenesis is multifactorial as is cancer in general. Many sequential events are needed before a patient presents with a fully malignant tumour. Yet if the virus plays a crucial part as an essential factor in oncogenesis, its elimination should prevent that type of cancer. Indeed, the final proof of the role of some viruses in cancer may come from the elimination of the malignancy through viral immunization programmes.

Treatment and prevention

Currently, there is no special approach to the treatment of cancers that have a viral aetiology. Among the lymphoid malignancies, for example, some often respond well to radiotherapy or chemotherapy, such as Hodgkin's disease, whereas others seldom show remission, such as adult T-cell leukaemia. One might expect those cancers that express viral antigens to be more responsive to immunotherapy. If immunosuppression promotes their presentation, then they should be susceptible to immune attack. Furthermore, for tumours in which viral proteins are required for the maintenance of the malignant state, molecular therapeutic strategies for those proteins or their genes should be potentially good targets, as any drugs that block them might be selected not to affect normal cellular functions. Molecular targets such as the *X* gene of HBV, *EBNA-1* of EBV, and *tax* of HTLV-I would be suitable as they are needed to maintain the transformed state of the cell or the persistence of the viral genome.

Prevention is preferable to cure, however, and it is in the field of prevention that viral tumours offer the greatest promise of reducing cancer mortality. Prevention could be accomplished by three strategies: (i) early screening for tumours, (ii) screening for the virus with prevention of transmission, and (iii) immunization.

Early screening is exemplified by cervical smears. The dyskaryotic cells recognized by the cytologist are in fact HPV-infected cells, showing virus inclusion bodies. Mostly, they detect cells infected with HPV-6 and -11, which are more closely associated with condylomata acuminata and other florid genital warts than with malignant cervical cancer. Colposcopy for flat, HPV-16- and -18-associated cervical carcinoma *in situ* comes closer to screening for malignant precursors. With rapid polymerase chain-reaction and enzyme immunoassay techniques for typing the HPV strains in smears and biopsies, more accurate prognosis of the lesion can be obtained. Another promising approach to early screening is for nasopharyngeal carcinoma in China. Early growth of the tumour in the nasopharynx is associated with elevated serum IgA levels to EBV antigens. Hence mass screening for EBV IgA identifies those persons with incipient tumours at a stage when surgery or radiotherapy is curative.

The prevention of viral transmission in the first place is possible even without vaccination where the virus is not ubiquitous. Screening against iatrogenic transmission via blood and blood products is routinely employed in many developed countries for potentially oncogenic viruses such as HBV, HCV, HIV, and HTLV-I. In Japan, particularly in Kyushu where infection is endemic, HTLV-I is being steadily eradicated through a policy of screening to prevent transmission. The major natural route of HTLV-I infection is from mother to child via breast milk. By testing pregnant mothers for HTLV-I antibodies, as well as the screening of all blood donations, the next generation of Japanese will be largely free of infection, so that the incidence of adult T-cell lymphoma/leukaemia, which today is the most common adult lymphoid malignancy, is likely to drop to almost negligible numbers. Unfortunately, in the other major endemic areas for HTLV-I, Africa and the Caribbean basin, feeding infants on formula milk in place of breast milk is likely to cause more deaths from enteric infections than the potential lives saved from the lymphoma.

Prevention of cancer by vaccination against oncogenic viruses is likely to have a major impact on world cancer mortality in the twenty-first century. At the time of writing, the only proven, mass-produced vaccine against a human oncogenic virus is the HBV vaccine based on surface antigen. Indeed, it is the first efficacious recombinant subunit vaccine against any virus. In the Far East, where HBV infection happens perinatally, and in Africa, where it occurs postnatally, transmission can be prevented by the administration of passive immune globulin at birth, shortly followed by subunit vaccine. Hepatocellular carcinoma is the world's sixth most common cancer and it is now largely preventable by vaccination, provided that the appropriate public-health and vaccination programmes can be implemented in developing countries.

Other vaccines currently under development that are likely to be successful within the next decade are for EBV, HCV, and HTLV-I. Intensive research is, of course, being undertaken on vaccines for HIV and HPV-16 and -18. However, there are likely to be some obstacles on the route to vaccination. For example, HIV is extraordinarily variable, and even the relatively constant HBV is showing evidence of immune-escape mutants in the face of vaccination programmes. Nevertheless, as our knowledge increases of the molecular biology of protective immune responses to viruses, these obstacles are likely to be surmountable. Vaccination against oncogenic viruses is likely to be the most effective cancer prevention strategy for many years to come.

Viruses as therapeutic agents

Another positive thought is that viruses may be put to iatrogenic use in the fight against cancer. First, some cytopathic viruses preferentially replicate in proliferating cells, parvoviruses for example. Some parvovirus strains are being investigated as specific oncolytic viruses that might reduce tumour load in conjunction with conventional treatments. Second, viruses as foreign antigens may aid the recognition of cancer cells by the host's immune system. Although the mechanism is ill understood, 'xenogenization' of tumour cells by virus infection can, in some cases, enhance immune control of non-infected cells of the same tumour. Third, viruses are favoured vectors of genes for gene therapy. Cancer is becoming a leading target for gene therapy, either by inducing enhanced immune responses through the expression of cytokine genes, or through the delivery of enzymes that locally convert prodrugs to active, chemotherapeutic agents. Ironically, the potentially oncogenic viruses, such as retroviruses, adenoviruses, and herpesviruses, are the leading candidate gene vectors, but other cancer treatments such as radiotherapy and much chemotherapy are also carcinogenic.

REFERENCES

Beral, V., Jaffe, H.W., and Weiss, R.A. (ed.) (1991). *Cancer, HIV and AIDS, Cancer Surveys 10.* Cold Spring Harbor Laboratory Press, N.Y.

Dalgleish, A.G., and Weiss, R.A. (ed.) (1990). *AIDS and the new viruses.* Academic Press, London.

Fields, B. (1990). *Virology.* Raven Press, New York.

Franks, L.M., and Teich, N.M. (ed.) (1995). *Introduction to the cellular and molecular biology of cancer,* University Press, Oxford.

Rickinson, A.L. (ed.) (1992). Viruses and human cancer. *Seminars in Cancer Biology,* **3,** 1–328.

Zur Hausen, H. (1991) Viruses in human cancers. *Science,* **254,** 1167–173.

Retroviruses

7.10.28 Human immunodeficiency viruses

R. A. Weiss

The human immunodeficiency viruses (HIV-1 and HIV-2) belong to the lentivirus subfamily of retroviruses. The two main types are distinct in origin: HIV-1 is closely related to an immunodeficiency virus isolated from chimpanzees, whereas HIV-2 is related to a simian immunodeficiency virus (SIV) naturally occurring in the sooty mangabey, an African monkey. The simian viruses exhibit little pathogenesis in their natural hosts, although they can cause AIDS in Asian macaque species. It is not known whether HIV-1 and HIV-2 represent recent zoonoses from simian hosts or whether small human populations have harboured HIV for thousands of years. What is clearly quite new is their epidemic spread, as AIDS is a new disease of mankind. HIV-1 is responsible for the worldwide pandemic. HIV-2 is mainly confined to West Africa and to people with contacts there, although it has recently started to spread rapidly in India.

Both HIV-1 and HIV-2 cause AIDS, but the incubation period and transmissibility of HIV-2 appear to be more attenuated. Some HIV-2 seropositive West African people in Liberia and Guinea Bissau harbour viral genomes that have more similarities to SIV than to HIV-2 isolated from AIDS patients; this SIV-like virus is present at low viral load in older as well as younger adults and may represent a non-pathogenic persistent virus. Understanding why certain SIV and HIV viruses are not pathogenic in their hosts may eventually help us to maintain HIV-positive individuals in good health.

As in all retroviruses, the genome in HIV particles is diploid, comprising two single-stranded RNA molecules (Fig. 1). Upon infection, the viral enzyme reverse transcriptase directs the synthesis of a haploid double-stranded DNA provirus, which is inserted into chromosomal DNA of the hose cell. This integrated provirus may remain latent in an expressed form. However, RNA transcripts and proteins are produced in activated cells, leading to the synthesis and release of progeny virus. The replication of HIV depends on an intimate interplay of viral and cellular factors, such as the host transcriptional regulator NF*k*B, and viral proteins, such as tat and rev.

HIV-1 and HIV-2 are transmitted parenterally and sexually. Hence it is necessary to test blood donors for evidence of infection, and hence these virus infections are particularly prevalent among intravenous drug users and persons with numerous sexual partners. HIV is also transmitted from mother to child. This route of infection mainly occurs perinatally, but transplacental transmission and milk transmission also occur.

HIV genes and proteins

The organization of the HIV-1 and HIV-2 proviral genomes is shown in Fig. 2. The genes and proteins are listed in Table 1. The long terminal repeats (LTRs) at each end of the genome are required for integration and contain the promoter and enhancer sequences necessary for gene expression. The *gag* (group-specific antigen) gene encodes the core proteins of the virion: p9 (nucleic acid binding protein (NC)), p24 (major capsid protein (CA)), p17 (matrix protein (MA)), and p6. The numbers represent the approximate size of the proteins, for example p24 has a molecular weight of 24 000. The gag proteins are responsible for the assembly of the virus particle, as shown in Fig. 3(a). The *pol* gene encodes three enzymes: viral protease, reverse transcriptase (RT), more properly called RNA-directed DNA polymerase (hence *pol*), and integrase. The *env* (envelope) gene encodes the membrane glycoproteins of the virion: gp41 (transmembrane protein (TM)) and gp120 (surface glycoprotein (SU)) (Figs 3(a) and 3(b)). Host membrane proteins such as major histocompatibility antigens are also present in the virion envelope.

The gag proteins are translated as a p55 precursor which becomes cleaved by the viral protease fairly late in virion maturation into p17, p24, and p9. The viral enzymes are similarly cleaved from a gag–pol precursor. The RT protein is a dimer of two cleavage products, p66 and p51. The *env* gene is transcribed from a singly spliced mRNA and is again translated as a precursor, gp160, cleaved by cellular enzymes into gp41 and gp120. The virion-associated proteins, vpr and vpu, and the regulatory proteins are translated from doubly spliced mRNA encoded by small genes.

Some retroviruses, such as the avian and murine leukaemia viruses, possess only *gag, pol,* and *env* genes, and the six accessory and regulatory genes of HIV and most other lentiviruses point to more subtle controls of the expression and assembly of these complex retroviruses. This is exemplified by the tat and the protein which acts to upregulate HIV gene expression by binding to the 'tar' sequence of viral RNA, permitting further transcripts to be initiated and transcribed by cellular RNA polymerase. It is a positive-feedback process whereby, if a small amount of tat is made, it acts on tar in the LTR to make more of itself as well as other viral proteins. However, the whole process will not proceed without the co-operation of other cellular transcriptional regulators, among them NF*k*B, which are only present in activated cells such as proliferating T lymphocytes and immunologically activated macrophages. Thus a silent HIV provirus can be switched to making many progeny virions by the physiological activation of the host cells.

The uniqueness of the viral replication cycle (Fig. 1) and the viral proteins (Table 1) provide opportunities for blocking virus production therapeutically, few of which have translated into clinical successes so far. Soluble receptor mimics can compete with the cell-bound CD4 receptor to block the initial step of the virus particle binding to its target cells. Other, currently unidentified, cell membrane proteins are required for viral penetration following binding, and sulphated sugars may block this step in virus entry. Once the HIV has entered the host cell, drugs that block reverse transcription, such as azidothymidine and dideoxyinosine, will prevent provirus synthesis, and others may be devised that block integration.

Inhibitors of later stages in the replication cycle may also eventually find use as antiviral drugs. Much research is devoted to inhibiting the action of tat in order to keep viral replication switched off. Rev inhibitors would prevent envelope glycoprotein synthesis. Inhibitors of the viral protease prevent progeny virions from becoming infectious by blocking gag precursor cleavage, and one of these is under clinical trial. Ultimately it is likely that the clinical control of viral replication will only be achieved through combination therapy of a number of antiviral drugs.

HIV variation

HIV and other lentiviruses show extraordinary genome variation during infection, both within a single infected individual and as the virus spreads through host populations. RNA viruses generally lack the proofreading mechanisms that DNA viruses have for checking mutations, but HIV is far more variable than, for example, human T-cell leukaemia virus, another retrovirus. This genetic variation has several implications for HIV control. It allows rapid antigenic diversification with escape from recognition by the humoral and cellular arms of the immune system, and will make vaccination more difficult to achieve. It also allows the relatively rapid evolution of resistance to antiviral drugs, as seen with zidovudine resistance. The variation is also reflected in spread of tropism for infection of different cell types that occurs following seroconversion.

Notwithstanding the foregoing discussion, many essential functions have to be conserved for HIV to remain viable and to replicate efficiently. Therefore there are restraints on variation for several functional epitopes of viral proteins, for example the CD4-binding regions of the

Fig. 1 Simplified replication cycle of HIV.

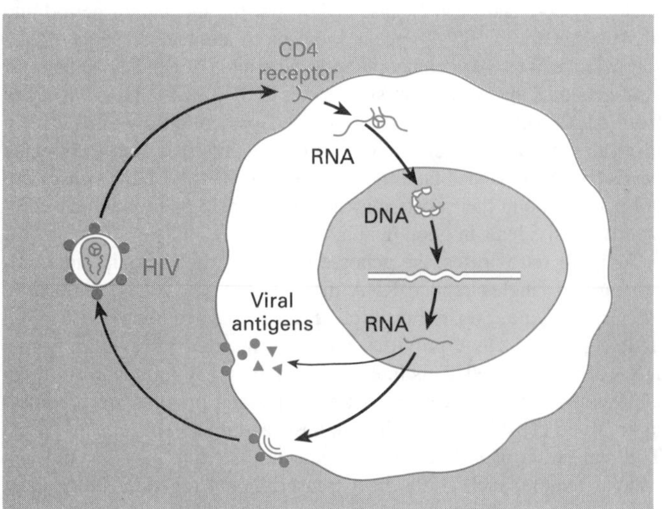

Fig. 2 Proviral genomes of HIV-1 and HIV-2.

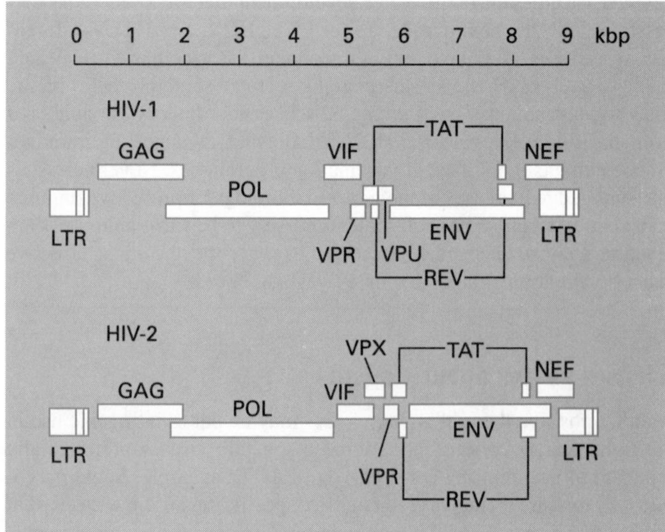

Table 1 *HIV genes and proteins*

Gene	Protein	Function
Virion proteins		
Gag	p17	Matrix protein: myristylated protein targeting gag precursor to plasma membrane; important for virion stability and maturation; role in uncoating and transport of the preintegration complex to the nucleus
	p24	Capsid protein: encapsidates viral RNA and replication enzymes; important for particle formation
	p9	Nucleocapsid protein: binds single-stranded RNA; important for RNA packaging
	p6	Proline-rich protien: important for virion assembly and release
Pol	p10	Protease: mediates gag and gag/pol precursor cleavage
	p66/p51	Reverse transcriptase; has DNA polymerase and RNase H activity; copies viral RNA into DNA
	p32	Integrase: essential for proviral integration
Env	gp41	Transmembrane envelope glycoprotein: anchors glycoprotein complex to the cell/virus membrane; mediates virus/cell fusion
	gp120	External envelope glycoprotein: important determinant of cell tropism, viral infectivity, and cytopathicity; mediates binding to CD4 receptor
VPr	P15	Component of the virus particle: functions early in the replication cycle; contains nuclear localization signals; important for efficient viral replication *in vivo*
Vpx	p16	Component of the virus particle: unique to HIV-2/SIV; functions early in the replication cycle; contains nuclear localization signals; important for efficient replication *in vivo*
Regulatory proteins		
Tat	p14	Transcriptional and post-transcriptional regulator of viral gene expression: mediates high level expression of all viral genes
Rev	p19	Post-transcriptional regulator of viral gene expression: facilitates nuclear export, stability, and translation of viral mRNA molecules which contain the rev response element (RRE)
Nef	p27	Myristylated cytoplasmic protein: reduces cell surface expression of the CD4 receptor; required for *in vivo* replication and pathogenesis
Vif	p23	Virus infectivity factor: facilitates efficient transmission of HIV; cell-type dependent and essential for replication in macrophages and primary T cells
Vpu	p15	Integral membrane protein: unique to HIV-1; facilitates viral maturation and release; destabilizes intracellular gp160–CD4 complexes

envelope glycoprotein gp120 are less variable than the principle epitopes V1, V2, and V3 that elicit neutralizing antibodies.

Vaccines

The prospects for developing safe efficacious prophylactic vaccines protecting against HIV infection is not helped by the high degree of viral variation and immune escape. Nevertheless, group-specific neutralizing antibodies and cross-reacting cytotoxic T-cell clones have been described. There is also evidence from human prostitutes repeatedly exposed to HIV and from monkeys exposed to low dose SIV that certain individuals can develop specific cytotoxic T-cell responses without evidence of persistent viral infection. These individuals may be protected from infection when exposed to live virus.

Non-infectious killed whole virus or recombinant subunit vaccines have not been successful to date in protecting chimpanzees from HIV infection or macaques from SIV infection and disease. However, certain live attenuated strains of SIV, with deletion mutations in *nef* and other regulatory genes, have established low grade persistent infections in monkeys that appear to protect adult animals from challenge with virulent SIV strains. There will be immense problems in attempting to introduce live attenuated HIV into humans (although it would represent an inexpensive vaccine), not least how long it takes to deem a vaccine strain attenuated when the mean incubation period from primary infection to AIDS for pathogenic HIV is 8 to 10 years. However, when the mechanism of protection by the attenuated strains is elucidated, it may offer a means of developing a similarly protective vaccine which is non-infectious and thought to be safe.

There is also considerable discussion about the possibility of developing postinfection ''therapeutic'' vaccines, although how such immunization would clear or allay infection is not clear.

HIV tropism

HIV infects T-helper lymphocytes and macrophages, gaining entry via the CD4 cellular receptor which specifically binds gp120. These are the cells mainly infected *in vivo* and also those susceptible to infection in culture. There is some confusion in the terminology over what are called T-lymphotropic and macrophage-tropic strains of HIV. In fact, all cultivable strains will propagate well in proliferating peripheral blood CD4+ T lymphocytes. Primary strains of HIV not adapted for serial propagation *in vitro* will not generally enter and replicate in immortalized CD4+ T-cell leukaemia cell lines. However, many primary isolates do infect monocytes and macrophages in addition to primary T cells, and hence are termed macrophage tropic.

In contrast, those HIV isolates which have been adapted to grow in immortalized T-cell lines have usually lost the capacity to replicate efficiently in macrophages. The major block appears to be in virus entry after binding to CD4. It involves the V1–V2 and V3 regions to gp120, which bear important determinants of viral tropism for different cell types. Since these epitopes also elicit neutralizing antibodies, which act after virus adsorption but before virus entry, the mechanism of neutralization may be to block the interaction of viral gp120 with secondary cellular receptor molecules.

HIV can also be subdivided into syncytium-inducing (SI) and non-syncytium inducing (NSI) strains. Generally speaking, SI strains tend to appear *in vivo* late in the progression to AIDS. These strains quickly adapt to growth in T-cell lines and are not generally macrophage tropic. Most primary HIV strains have the NSI phenotype, although transmission of SI virus from one individual to another has been observed. Because SI strains often appear shortly before stage IV disease develops, it has been suggested that the emergence of SI strains drives the final progression to AIDS. However, about 50 per cent of AIDS patients never develop SI viruses and a high virus load may develop *in vivo* without conversion to the SI phenotype. While SI strains may exacerbate disease, they are not essential for AIDS.

There is still controversy as to whether cells other than CD4+ T lymphocytes and macrophages become infected with HIV *in vivo,* although several CD4 positive and negative cell lines can be experimentally infected by SI strains *in vitro.* Follicular dendritic cells in the lymph nodes accumulate many HIV particles on the veiled cell surface and may present them to lymphocytes, but molecular studies suggest that they are passive absorbers of virions rather than active centres of replication. In contrast, blood dendritic cells and the related Langerhans cells of the skin and mucous membranes appear to be infectible with HIV *in vitro,* and budding replicating forms have been observed by electron microscopy from biopsies taken *in vivo.*

An alternative receptor to CD4 for binding HIV is the glycolipid galactosylceramide (galcer), which is present on astraglial cells in the brain and on some gut epithelial cells. While galcer avidly binds gp120 it is a weak receptor for HIV entry. Nevertheless, its interaction with gp120 may play a role in AIDS dementia; expression of gp120 in astraglia of transgenic mice leads to degenerative changes in the brain.

HIV pathogenesis

Figure 4 shows the typical course of HIV infection and the immune responses to it. Following infection, a primary viraemia develops before clearance by cytotoxic T cells and later antibodies to *gag, env,* and other viral antigens. During the long and variable asymptomatic period, viraemia is usually relatively low and sporadic with maintenance of good immune responses to the virus. However, low or falling titres of p24 antibodies are prognostic of early predisposition to AIDS. Later, virus load increases as AIDS develops, but whether at this late stage HIV is driving AIDS or represents an opportunistic activation of virus as a result of the onset of immunosuppression remains a moot point.

At the time of seroconversion and relatively high virus load in the plasma, the viral genome diversity remains low, perhaps owing to the rapid outgrowth and selection of one kind of variant. However, the genome diversity appears less conserved in gag proteins (e.g. p17) than in what later become highly variable epitopes, such as V3 of gp120. It would appear that there is positive selection for certain V3 motifs in primary infection of peripheral blood T lymphocytes, and that it diversifies more as new cell types become infected and as neutralizing antibodies to this epitope are mounted.

Specific CD8-positive cytotoxic T-lymphocyte cells are probably largely responsible for maintaining relatively low viral loads during the asymptomatic period, but plasma virus load, measured as culturable virus or by the polymerase chain reaction of RNA packaged in virions, varies over a 10 000-fold range in various asymptomatic patients. Recent studies have shown that there is enormous turnover of HIV, some 10^8 or more virus particles and infected lymphocytes daily, so it is not surprising that HIV eventually defeats the immune system, and gives rise to variants that become resistant to antibodies and antiviral drugs. Autopsies after deaths occurring in asymptomatic HIV-positive persons indicate very little HIV load in non-lymphoid organs, in contrast with autopsies of AIDS patients where considerable HIV colonization of the brain, liver, lungs, and gut are evident. Virus is present and actively replicates in several of the lymph nodes throughout the course of infection, as is evident from the persistent generalized lymphadenopathy seen in many HIV-positive individuals.

It is not at all clear why the infected individual eventually fails to keep HIV infection in check. A steady decline in CD4 T cells is generally seen, and opportunistic infections tend to set in when the total CD4 T-cell count falls below 400/μl. There is controversy as to whether HIV infection itself is sufficient to induce the immunosuppressive changes that lead to AIDS. Some investigators have postulated that other infections are necessary as cofactors in progression to AIDS. However, no specific second pathogen, be it mycoplasma, cytomegalovirus, or another virus, has been identified as a ubiquitous cofactor, although the overall number of infectious episodes is likely to hasten progression. Genetic cofactors are also likely to affect the pace of development of AIDS, and individuals with certain major histocompatibility antigens

Fig. 3 (a) Schematic structure of the HIV virion; (b) electronmicrograph of HIV-1 (reproduced by courtesy of H. Gelderblom).

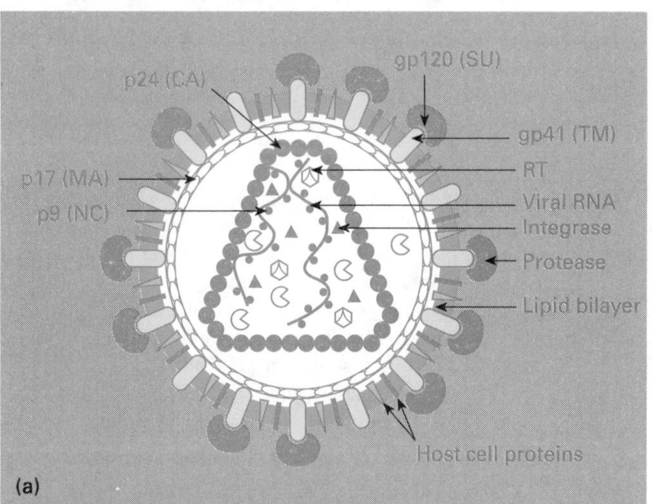

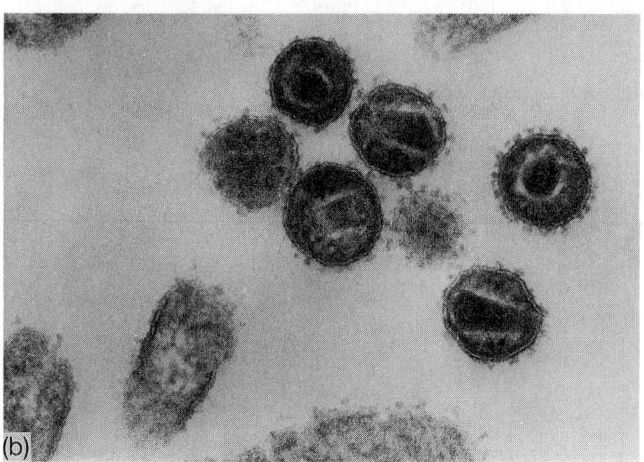

Fig. 4 Schematic course of HIV infection.

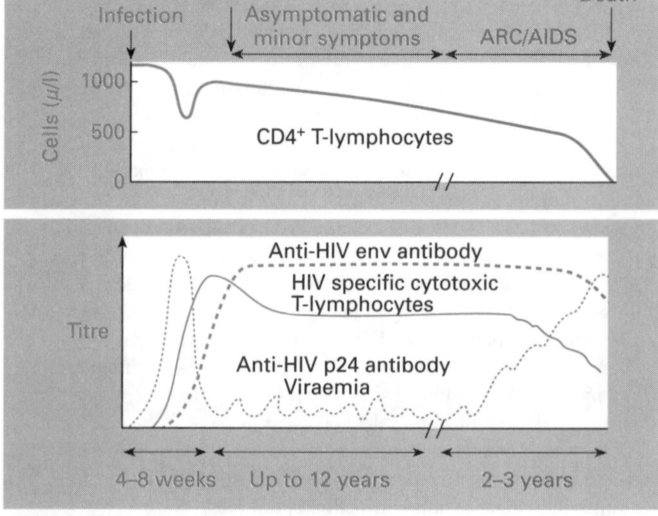

appear to be relatively protected or at relative high risk from early progression to AIDS. There is a widespread belief that a separate group of 'long-term survivors' exists among HIV-infected persons, but data are not yet sufficient to distinguish these from a Poisson distribution of chance survival. However, there exist a small proportion of HIV-positive ''non-progressors'' who have shown no decline in CD4 cells and remain in good health.

The proximate cause of CD4 T-helper cell depletion is also hotly debated. It would appear that direct killing by HIV (which kills activated lymphocytes when viral replication reaches high levels) may not be sufficient to account for the overall drop in CD4 cell numbers. Other HIV-infected CD4 cells will be killed by CD8+ cytotoxic T-lymphocytes specific for HIV peptide antigens. HIV-infected individuals also show enhanced levels of apoptosis (programmed cell death) when T lymphocytes are placed in culture and stimulated by phytohaemagglutin. Both CD4 and CD8 T cells from infected individuals proceed to apoptosis. However, the CD4 cell apoptosis is not evident in non-pathogenic immunodeficiency virus infections, such as HIV-1 in chimpanzees and SIV in African green monkeys. Thus programmed cell death of CD4 cells measured at an early time point *ex vivo* may be a useful marker of incipient pathogenic infection. Apoptosis could be a reflection of the generalized immune activation that precedes the immune collapse seen in late stage disease.

The role of macrophage and dendritic cell infection in AIDS is also a matter of debate. These cells are less susceptible to direct cytopathic effects of HIV and are able to sustain persistent infection and virus release, yet their cytokine release and signalling may be subtly or profoundly affected by HIV infection. One currently popular hypothesis is that HIV infection of antigen-presenting cells alters the balance of behaviour of CD4 T lymphocytes in favour of a greater proportion of T-helper-2-like phenotype and cytokine release (IL-4, IL-6, IL-10, and IL-13) at the expense of T-helper-1-like phenotype (IL-2, IFN-Y, TNF.ga). This would result in the B-cell hyperplasia seen in HIV infection and weaker T-helper activity for cell-mediated immune responses.

It should be borne in mind that the various tropisms of HIV may contribute differentially to the different attributes of the syndrome that comprises AIDS. Thus the central nervous system disease and wasting syndrome resemble the symptoms of diseased sheep infected with the visna-maedi virus, which infects macrophages but not T lymphocytes. In that case, tropism of HIV for the CD4+ T cells must contribute in a direct way to the depletion of these cells *in vivo*. It might also be recalled that in almost all other acute and persistent viral infections there are variations in virulence among individual virus strains. This is certainly true of SIV in macaques and is likely to be so for HIV. The emergence of SI variants possibly provides an example in which differentially pathogenic variants may emerge from the high viral genome diversity evident within a single infected individual.

A better understanding of the processes leading to AIDS following HIV infection may help to formulate therapies aimed at preventing progression to severe disease. Treatment aimed at restoring immune functions and the appropriate balance between different arms of the immune system may help to prevent the depletion of CD4 helper T lymphocytes. Such immune restoration will have to be combined with antiviral therapy, as HIV excels in replicating in immune-activated lymphocytes and macrophages.

REFERENCES

Broder, S., Merigan, T.C., and Bolognesi, D. (eds.) (1993). *A textbook of AIDS medicine.* Williams & Wilkins, Baltimore, MA.

Cao, Y., Qin, L., Zhang, L., Safrit, J., and Ho, D. (1995). Virologic and immunologic characterization of long term survivors of human immunodeficiency virus type 1 infection. *New England Journal of Medicine,* **332,** 201–8.

Donaldson, Y.K., Bell, J.E., Ironside, J.W., Brettle, R.P., Robertson, J.R., Busuttil, A., and Simmonds, P. (1994). Redistribution of HIV outside the lymphoid system with onset of AIDS. *Lancet,* **343,** 382–5.

Estaquier, J., Idziorek, T., De Bels, F., Barré-Sinoussi, F., Hurtrel, B., Aubertin, A.-M., *et al.* (1994). Programmed cell death and AIDS: the significance of T-cell apoptosis in pathogenic and non pathogenic primate models of lentiviral infection. *Proceedings of the National Academy of Sciences of the United States of America,* **91,** 9431–35.

Fauci, A.S. (1993). Multifactorial nature of human immunodeficiency virus disease: implications for therapy. *Science,* **262,** 1011–18.

Gao, F., Yue, L., White, A.T., Pappas, P.G., Barchue, J., Hanson, A.P., *et al.* (1992). Human infection by genetically diverse SIV_{SM}-related HIV-2 in West Africa. *Nature, London,* **358,** 495–9.

Haynes, B.F. (1993). Scientific and social issues of HIV vaccine development. *Science,* **260,** 1279–86.

Rowland-Jones, S., Sutton, J., Ariyoshi, K., *et al.* (1995). HIV-specific cytotoxic T-cells in HIV-exposed but uninfected Gambian women. *Nature Medicine,* **1,** 59–64.

Wei, X., Ghosh, S.K., Taylor, M.E., *et al.* (1995). Viral dynamics in human immunodeficiency virus type 1 infection. *Nature,* **373,** 117–22.

Weiss, R.A. (1993). How does HIV cause AIDS? *Science,* **260,** 1273–9.

7.10.29 HIV infection and AIDS

I.V.D. WELLER, C.P. CONLON, AND T.E.A. PETO

Introduction

The first recognition of the acquired immunodeficiency syndrome (AIDS) was in 1981 in the United States of America. Physicians in New York, Los Angeles, and San Francisco noted an increasing number of diseases in homosexual men which signified some form of cellular immunodeficiency. The most common manifestations were oral candidiasis, recurrent herpes simplex infections, *Pneumocystis carinii* pneumonia, and Kaposi's sarcoma, but a variety of other unusual infections and clinical presentations were observed. Epidemiological studies revealed that, although homosexual men formed the largest affected group, the new syndrome was also seen in injecting drug users, haemophiliacs, and recipients of blood transfusions. Various aetiologic agents were considered, including recreational drugs such as amyl nitrate and infections such as cytomegalovirus. Data from early epidemiological investigations strongly suggested a blood-borne infectious agent that was sexually transmissible. Late in 1983 the causative retrovirus was isolated from a patient in France. Initially referred to as lymphadenopathy associated virus (LAV) or human T-lymphotropic virus III (HTLV-III), it was renamed human immunodeficiency virus (HIV) in 1986 by the International Committee for Taxonomy of Viruses.

Although not initially appreciated, HIV was already present in at least four other continents at the time of the original descriptions of AIDS. The recognition of sexual intercourse as the most common means of HIV transmission followed the identification of the heterosexual epidemic in the developing countries of Africa and the Caribbean. It was also recognized that infected mothers could pass the virus on to their fetus or neonate, establishing vertical transmission as another important route of HIV infection.

In 1985 a second retrovirus causing AIDS was identified in West Africa and subsequently called HIV-2. This remains largely confined to West Africa, while HIV-1, the original 1983 isolate, is the cause of the world pandemic of AIDS. Over the past 15 years a vast amount has been learned about HIV and its clinical, psychological, and social consequences. Nevertheless, the HIV pandemic has led to increasing numbers of infected people, particularly in the rapidly growing populations of developing countries.

Figures 2 to 9 in this chapter are reproduced from Williams, I., Mindel, A., and Weller, I.V.D. (1989). *AIDS—an essential slide collection.* Mosby-Wolfe, London, with permission.

Definitions of AIDS and epidemiology

DEFINITIONS

Various case definitions of AIDS and classification systems for HIV infection have been used since 1982 and have been altered in the light of increased understanding of pathogenesis and natural history. In 1987 the Centers for Disease Control (CDC) defined AIDS as an illness characterized by one or more indicator diseases. In the absence of another cause of immune deficiency and without laboratory evidence of HIV infection (if the patient has not been tested or the results are inconclusive), certain diseases, when definitely diagnosed, are indicative of AIDS (Table 1). Regardless of the presence of other causes of immune deficiency, if there is laboratory evidence of HIV infection, other indicator diseases which require a definitive, or in some cases only a presumptive, diagnosis also constitute a diagnosis of AIDS (Table 2).

In 1993 an expanded definition of AIDS was used in the United States. This included individuals with proven HIV infection with a CD4 lymphocyte count of less than 200/μl, irrespective of clinical manifestation. Three new AIDS-indicator diseases (pulmonary tuberculosis, recurrent bacterial pneumonia in adults, and invasive cervical cancer) were added to the existing list. Adoption of this modified definition for national surveillance purposes has not been universal.

The World Health Organization (WHO) uses the CDC (1987) definition for surveillance in developed countries, but this is not ideal for developing countries where resources are insufficient to make definitive diagnoses or carry out widespread HIV testing. Other definitions based on clinical manifestations with or without laboratory confirmation of HIV infection have been proposed by the WHO for use in sub-Saharan Africa (Bangui definition) and by the Pan American Health Organisation and the WHO Global Programme for South America (Caracas definition).

GLOBAL EPIDEMIOLOGY

HIV has been isolated from lymphocytes in peripheral blood, cell-free plasma, semen, cervical secretions, cerebrospinal fluid, tears, saliva, urine, and breast milk. The major modes of transmission are perinatal, sexual through anal and vaginal intercourse, and the sharing of contaminated needles, transfusion of infected blood and blood products, and particularly infusion of infected factor VIII.

Accurate figures for the prevalence of HIV infection do not exist and all figures are estimates. The WHO has estimated that, by the year 2000, 40 million people worldwide will be infected. More than 90 per cent of them will live in developing countries in sub-Saharan Africa, South and Southeast Asia, Latin America, and the Caribbean. In addition, through the 1990s, mothers or both parents of more than 10 million children will have died prematurely from HIV-1 infection and AIDS.

The WHO has identified three distinctive epidemiological patterns of HIV infection globally.

Pattern 1 countries include North America, Western Europe, Australia, and New Zealand. In these countries the epidemic began in the late 1970s and early 1980s among homosexual men and injecting drug users. However, heterosexual transmission does occur and is increasing. Increasing numbers of AIDS cases amongst intravenous drug users have been reported in Europe, particularly Southern Europe, such that by the end of 1991 there were more cases of AIDS among injecting drug users in Europe than in homosexual and bisexual men.

Pattern 2 countries include most of sub-Saharan Africa and areas of the Caribbean. In these regions HIV transmission is predominantly heterosexual and perinatal, with an additional contribution from unscreened blood transfusions and inadequate injection procedures. The overall male-to-female ratio is approximately 1:1 compared with 9:1 in pattern 1 countries. In South America, which would have fitted pattern 1 in the early 1980s, there has been a considerable increase in heterosexual cases (pattern 1–2).

Table 1 *Diseases diagnostic of AIDS without laboratory evidence of HIV (and no other cause of immunodeficiency)*

Candidiasis: oesophageal, pulmonary
Cryptococcosis: extrapulmonary
Cytomegalovirus disease: disseminated
Cryptosporidiosis: diarrhoea persisting for longer than 1 month
Herpes simplex virus infection
Mucocutaneous ulceration lasting for longer than 1 month
Pulmonary or oesophageal infection
Kaposi's sarcoma: patient aged under 60
Primary cerebral lymphoma: patient aged under 60
Lymphoid interstitial pneumonia: child aged under 13
Mycobacterium avium } disseminated
Mycobacterium kansasii } disseminated
Pneumocystis carinii pneumonia
Progressive multifocal leucoencephalopathy
Cerebral toxoplasmosis

Table 2 *Diseases diagnostic of AIDS if laboratory evidence of HIV exists*

Diseases diagnosed definitively
Recurrent/multiple bacterial infections: child aged under 13
Coccidioidomycosis: disseminated
HIV encephalopathy
Histoplasmosis: disseminated
Isosporiasis: diarrhoea persisting for longer than 1 month
Kaposi's sarcoma at any age
Primary cerebral lymphoma at any age
Non-Hodgkin's lymphoma: diffuse undifferentiated B-cell type, or unknown phenotype
Any disseminated mycobacterial disease caused by other than *Mycobacterium tuberculosis*
Mycobacterium tuberculosis: extrapulmonary
Salmonella septicaemia: recurrent
HIV wasting syndrome
Diseases diagnosed presumptively
Candidiasis: oesophageal
Cytomegalovirus retinitis with visual loss
Kaposi's sarcoma
Lymphoid interstitial pneumonia: child aged under 13
Mycobacterial disease (acid-fast bacilli, species not identified by culture): disseminated
Pneumocystis carinii pneumonia
Cerebral toxoplasmosis

Pattern 3 countries include North Africa, the Middle East, Eastern Europe, and most of the countries in Asia and Oceania other than Australia and New Zealand. It would appear that HIV was introduced into these areas late in the global pandemic. Therefore reported cases only represent a small fraction of the world total. However, rapid changes are taking place, particularly in Asia, where there has been a great increase in HIV prevalence, particularly amongst intravenous drug users and prostitutes.

Natural history of infection and classifications of HIV disease stage

NATURAL HISTORY OF HIV INFECTION

At any given time, most people with HIV infection in the world are asymptomatic. Prospective studies of cohorts of infected people with known dates of seroconversion have shown that 50–60 per cent of HIV-infected people will develop symptoms and signs of disease within 10 years of infection (Fig. 1). During this asymptomatic period, many individuals will have abnormal laboratory tests such as low CD4 lymphocyte counts and hypergammaglobulinaemia, and some will develop cutaneous anergy to recall antigens. Most cases of HIV transmission probably occur when the infected person is asymptomatic and neither they nor their sexual partners are aware of the infection risk.

The rate of progression to symptomatic disease varies greatly from person to person. Some studies have shown a correlation between a more rapid progression and an increased age at infection. There is also some evidence that some HLA haplotypes are associated with a worse prognosis. Although there are some individuals who have survived without disease for up to 15 years, more than 90 per cent of HIV-infected patients show some signs of disease progression. Initially, they may have minor problems associated with early symptomatic disease before going on to more obvious opportunistic infections and tumours associated with late symptomatic disease. Eventually, patients develop end-stage disease when they have little immunity and premature death is inevitable.

CLASSIFICATIONS OF HIV DISEASE STAGE

HIV-infected people present with a variety of clinical manifestations which bridge the gap between asymptomatic infection and the later severe immunodeficiency with its life-threatening secondary infectious diseases and tumours. Initially, a large number of different terms were used to describe patients with early and late disease manifestations of HIV infection depending on their symptoms, signs, and laboratory findings. In 1986 the CDC proposed a classification system for HIV infection and disease (Table 3), which has since been widely used.

Table 3 *Centers for Disease Control classification system for HIV infection*

Group I	Acute infection
Group II	Asymptomatic infection
Group III	Persistent generalized lymphadenopathy
Group IV	Other disease
Subgroup A	Constitutional disease (one or more of the following: fever for more than 1 month, weight loss > 10% baseline, diarrhoea for more than 1 month)
Subgroup B	Neurological disease (dementia, myelopathy, peripheral neuropathy attributed to HIV)
Subgroup C	Secondary infectious diseases C1 Those specified in CDC surveillance definition C2 Others: oral hairy leucoplakia, multidermatomal herpes zoster, recurrent salmonella bacteraemia, nocardiosis, tuberculosis, oral candidiasis
Subgroup D	Secondary cancers (Kaposi's sarcoma, non-Hodgkin's lymphoma, primary cerebral lymphoma)
Subgroup E	Other conditions such as lymphoid interstitial pneumonitis

The classification in four principal groups is hierarchical. Those classified in a particular group should not be reclassified in a preceding group if clinical findings resolve, since clinical improvement does not necessarily reflect change in the severity of the underlying disease. Constitutional disease (subgroup IV A) is defined only in the absence of a concurrent illness or condition other than HIV infection to explain the findings. Subgroup E includes clinical findings or diseases not classifiable in the other groups that may be attributed to HIV infection and/or may be indicative of a defect in cell-mediated immunity. This includes patients with chronic lymphocytic interstitial pneumonitis. Also included are those patients whose signs or symptoms could be attributed either to HIV infection or to another coexisting disease not classified elsewhere and patients with other clinical illnesses, the course or management of which may be complicated or altered by HIV infection. Examples include patients with constitutional symptoms not meeting the criteria for subgroup IVA, patients with infectious diseases not listed in subgroup IVC, and patients with neoplasms not listed in subgroup IVD. This classification was not meant to imply any change in the definition of AIDS described previously and used for national and international reporting.

In 1989 the WHO published a proposed staging system based on clinical criteria and lymphocyte counts (Table 4). This has been tested and found to be prognostically valuable and could be applied in areas with limited diagnostic resources, i.e. where the absolute lymphocyte count and not lymphocyte phenotyping was available. This classification relies on two axes. Subjects are characterized into one of four clinical groups and into one of three lymphocyte count strata resulting in 12 cells.

Fig. 1 (a) Incubation period to AIDS from seroconversion. —— all people in the study (n = 1171), ---- those rejected because intervals of seroconversion were ≥25 months. (Modified from Biggar *et al.* (1990), with permission.) (b) Survival of patients with CD4 lymphocytes below 50 × 10^6/l. (Modified from Mills and Jones (1993), with permission.)

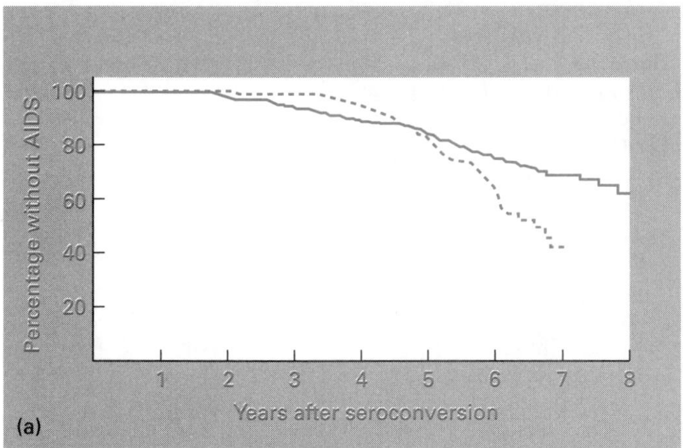

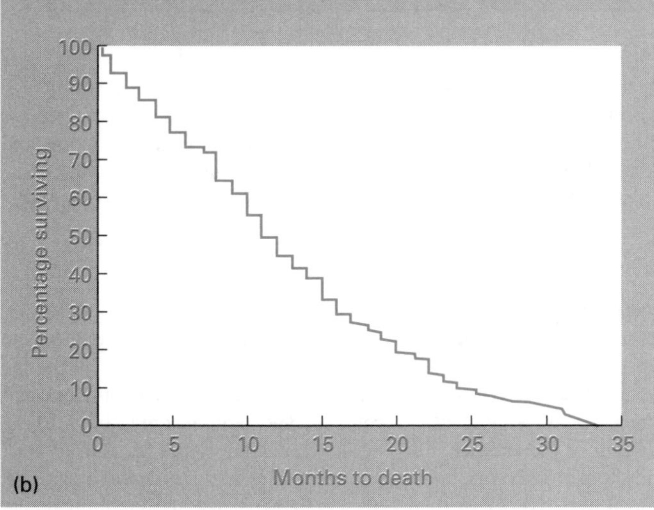

CLINICAL FEATURES OF ACUTE AND CHRONIC INFECTION

Acute infection with HIV may be accompanied by a transient non-specific illness (seroconversion illness) similar to glandular fever, with fever, malaise, myalgia, lymphadenopathy, pharyngitis, and a rash. This has been reported to occur in 10 to 40 per cent of those infected. A

Table 4 *WHO staging system for HIV infection and disease: a clinical/laboratory classification*

Laboratory group			Clinical group			
	Lymphocyte count (× 10⁶/l)	CD4 count (× 10⁶/litre)	1 Asymptomatic	2 Early	3 Intermediate	4 Late
A	>2000	>500	1A	2A	3A	4A
B	1000–2000	200–500	1B	2B	3B	4B
C	<1000	<200	1C	2C	3C	4C

Group 1: asymptomatic or persistent generalized lymphadenopathy—normal activity.

Group 2: early-stage disease—weight loss <10 per cent of body weight, minor mucocutaneous manifestations, herpes zoster within 5 years, recurrent upper respiratory tract infections, symptomatic but normal activity.

Group 3: intermediate stage disease—weight loss >10 per cent of body weight, unexplained chronic diarrhoea for more than 1 month, unexplained prolonged fever for more than 1 month, oral candidiasis, oral hairy leucoplakia, pulmonary tuberculosis within 1 year, severe bacterial infections and/or bedridden less than 50 per cent of the day during the previous month.

Group 4: late-stage disease—definite or presumptive diagnosis of any AIDS-defining illness, according to the Centers for Disease Control (1987) surveillance definition and/or bedridden for more than 50 per cent of the day during the previous month.

transient acute meningoencephalitis, myelopathy, and polyneuropathy have also been described. The meningoencephalitis may present with a prodrome of malaise, fever, and personality change, progressing to severe headache, occasionally convulsions, and loss of consciousness. Acute infection is accompanied by the development of serum antibodies to the core and surface proteins of the virus, usually in 2 to 6 weeks, although seroconversions delayed for up to 3 months have been observed.

Chronic infection then ensues. This is asymptomatic in the early stages. Physical examination may show no abnormality, but about one-third of patients have persistent generalized lymphadenopathy (nodes of 1 cm or more in diameter in two or more non-contiguous extrainguinal sites which cannot be explained by any other infection or condition). Many other patients have lesser degrees of lymphadenopathy. The nodes are symmetrical, mobile, and non-tender. The most common sites of lymphadenopathy are the cervical and axillary lymph nodes, and hilar lymphadenopathy is unusual. It was thought that asymptomatic patients with persistent generalized lymphadenopathy had a more advanced infection that those without. However, prospective studies have shown that asymptomatic anti-HIV-positive patients with and without persistent generalized lymphadenopathy progress to AIDS at the same rate. Biopsy is largely unrewarding in asymptomatic patients, revealing only non-specific follicular hyperplasia. If there are constitutional symptoms such as weight loss or fever, or the nodes are markedly asymmetrical, painful, or rapidly enlarging, or if there is an extranodal mass or coexistent hilar nodes, biopsy is essential. This will exclude tumours, such as lymphoma or Kaposi's sarcoma, or an opportunistic infection such as tuberculosis.

Later in the course of infection non-specific constitutional symptoms develop which may be intermittent or persistent. These include fever with or without nightsweats, diarrhoea, and weight loss (CDC subgroup IVA). Recurrent bacterial chest infections and the constitutional symptoms of fever, weight loss, or diarrhoea which fall short of the CDC IVA classification should also be considered as manifestations of early HIV disease.

Patients may also be affected by a large number of 'minor' opportunistic infections or conditions that tend to affect the mucous membranes and skin (Table 5). Skin conditions encountered include a range of infections: fungal, viral (recalcitrant warts, molluscum contagiosum, herpes simplex, and herpes zoster), and bacterial (folliculitis, impetigo, and furunculosis). The spectrum of other skin disorders ranges from a mere dryness of the skin to severe seborrhoeic dermatitis. Hairy leucoplakia appears typically as greyish-white lesions on the lateral borders of the tongue (Fig. 2). Its histological appearance is characteristic, with keratin projections resembling hairs, koilocytosis, and mild atypia.

Table 5 *Chronic manifestations of HIV infection*

Skin
Viral
Herpes simplex (types 1 and 2): oral and anogenital
Varicella zoster
Human papilloma virus
Molluscum contagiosum
Fungi
Tinea cruris/pedis/corporis/other
Candidiasis
Pityriasis versicolor
Bacterial
Folliculitis: mild, severe, acneiform
Impetigo
Other
Seborrhoeic dermatitis
Psoriasis
Oropharynx
Candidiasis
Hairy leucoplakia
Aphthous ulcers
Herpes simplex
Dental/gum disease
Periodontitis
Abscesses
Necrotizing ulcerative gingivitis

Epstein–Barr virus DNA has been demonstrated in these lesions by hybridization with specific probes, and there have been anecdotal reports of a response to acyclovir therapy. Collections of these symptoms and signs, which are often a prodrome to the development of a major opportunistic infection or tumour, are referred to as AIDS-related complex.

PROGNOSTIC LABORATORY MARKERS

Acute viraemia, detected by the presence of a core protein (p24), by culture, or more recently by the polymerase chain reaction, precedes the appearance of antibodies (IgG and IgM) to the whole virus. While the patient remains asymptomatic, high titres of antibodies to envelope and core proteins persist and p24 remains detectable in only about 10–15 per cent of patients. As immune deficiency develops, the titre of antibody to p24 falls, but the titres of antibodies to the viral envelope proteins (GP41, GP120, and GP160) remain high. p24 antigenaemia recurs with time, and is found in 50 to 60 per cent of patients with symptomatic disease (Chapter 7.10.28).

Prospective cohort studies have identified laboratory markers which predict a more rapid progression to more severe symptomatic disease (Table 6).

Haematological and immunological abnormalities which have been associated with a more rapid progression include anaemia, cytopenias, particularly progressive depletion of CD4-positive (T-helper) lymphocytes, raised CD8-positive (T-suppressor/cytotoxic) lymphocytes, a raised erythrocyte sedimentation rate, raised β_2 microglobulin and IgA, impairment of various non-specific functional assays of cellular immune function, and specific cellular responses to HIV together with viral markers, such as decline in titre or disappearance of anti-p24 and reappearance of p24 in serum, a high viral load, and the appearance of a syncytium-inducing viral phenotype. In the main these are not determinants of disease progression, but reflect the continuing disease process. Currently the length of infection, age at infection, and possible HLA types are the main determinants of disease progression.

An immune neutropenia also occurs which is due in part to antineutrophil antibodies, but counts rarely drop below 1.0×10^9/l. An autoimmune thrombocytopenia also occurs. There is increasing pancytopenia with advancing immunosuppression.

Table 6 *Clinical laboratory abnormalities associated with progression to symptomatic disease*

Lowered CD4-positive lymphocytes
Raised CD8-positive lymphocytes
Anaemia
Cytopenias
Raised erythrocyte sedimentation ratio
Raised β_2-microglobulin
Raised IgA
Lowered cellular immune function
Lowered HIV-specific cytotoxicity
Lowered anti-p24
Raised p24
Raised viral load
Raised syncytium-inducing viral phenotype

Diagnosis of HIV infection

Although the diagnosis of HIV infection can often be made clinically in patients with advanced disease, serological tests are sufficiently reliable to be used as a diagnostic screening test. As shown in Chapter 7.10.28, antibody to envelope protein is found in the serum of all individuals within 3 months of infection. As this antibody persists indefinitely, it forms a highly specific and sensitive test for HIV infection. Modern enzyme-linked immunoabsorbent assay techniques are sensitive to both HIV-1 and HIV-2. False-positive results can occur in infants younger than 18 months old, to whom maternal antibody can be transmitted passively, when some of the older tests are used or blood samples are mistakenly labelled in the laboratory. Therefore many laboratories prefer to confirm positive results by using a different assay and repeating the tests with a fresh blood sample. False-negative results can occur in patients who have recently been exposed to infection or, rarely, in patients who are severely deficient in gammaglobulins. In these cases, or in the neonatal period, detection of p24 antigen, viral culture, or polymerase chain reaction techniques can be used to diagnose infection. However, these techniques have not been validated in the same way as the antibody test, and in the case of p24 antigen false-positive results have been obtained.

Fig. 2 Oral hairy leucoplakia.

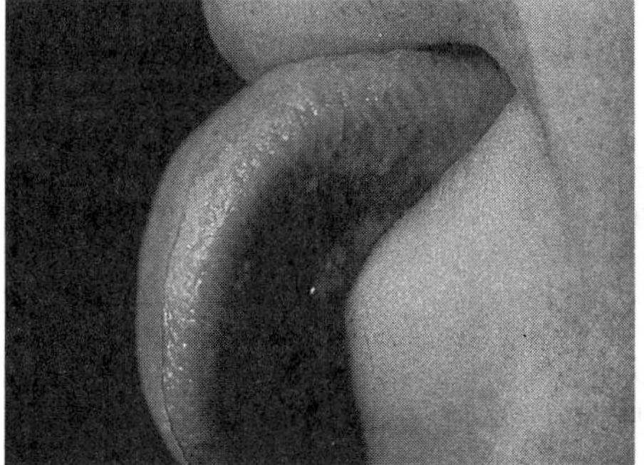

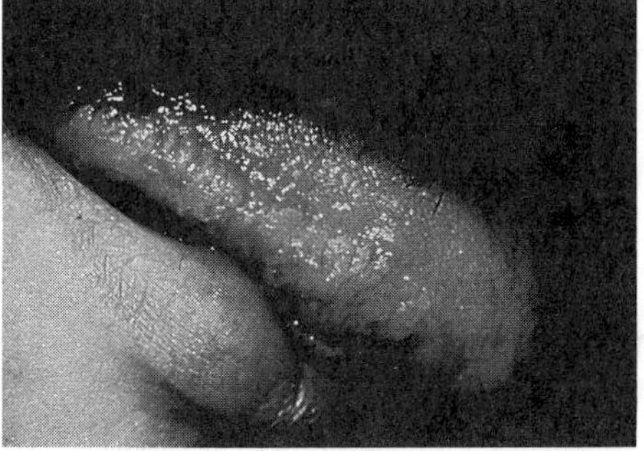

Pretest counselling

In most cases, patients should give informed consent before a HIV test is performed. Clinicians should avoid pressurizing patients to undergo the test simply to reduce their own concerns. Patients should be counselled as to why they want the test, and informed about the benefits and disadvantages of knowing the diagnosis. The main advantages of testing are to reduce patient anxiety in those who are worried about the disease, to reduce the chances of the patient infecting a partner or a future child, and to benefit from the prevention or early treatment of some of the complications of disease. However, the advantage of early diagnosis in terms of mortality is unclear.

The disadvantage of early diagnosis is that some patients, who would otherwise not be anxious about the disease, may become greatly distressed with disruption of their domestic or professional life although they may be free from symptomatic disease for many years. HIV-positive patients find it difficult to travel abroad, gain life or medical insurance, move house, and change job.

In some cases patients who present with severe diseases of uncertain aetiology may benefit medically from an HIV diagnosis because definitive treatment can be initiated. If the patient is too ill to give consent and if it is in the patient's best interest, a test can be performed. However, the result must be kept confidential from all personnel who are not directly involved in the clinical or nursing care of the patient until informed consent about disclosure can be given by the patient.

General management of the asymptomatic patient

There are advantages in the identification of HIV infection at the asymptomatic stage. Infected patients can be educated about common early symptoms and signs so that they can attend the clinic at a stage when new problems are easily dealt with. In addition, routine clinical and laboratory monitoring can aid early detection of waning immunity so that prophylaxis against infections such as pneumocystis pneumonia can be instituted. Serological screening can be carried out to detect past or current infection with toxoplasmosis, cytomegalovirus, hepatitis B, hepatitis C, and syphilis.

Periods of anxiety or depression are not uncommon, given the uncertain prognosis for the individual, and so clinic visits provide an opportunity for the patient to discuss issues with the physician or with a trained counsellor. Such visits can also be used for health education and discussion about safe sex.

Clinic visits also enable discussion about whom the patient has told, or wishes to tell, about his or her HIV status. Patients will discuss telling current or past sexual partners, friends, family, and employers. Infected women will want to consider decisions about contraception and pregnancy. Patients should be encouraged to tell their family doctor their HIV status so that appropriate investigation, treatment, and referral can be made in the event of illness. Dentists should also be informed by patients about their HIV infection. Special dental clinics have been set up to deal with those infected by HIV or hepatitis B as there is still some reluctance to treat such patients in general dental practice.

Currently, an HIV-positive life is uninsurable, in the United Kingdom. The problems that this causes in obtaining mortgages and other types of insurance may need to be discussed. Patients should be given information about the various voluntary organizations that exist to provide support, education, and legal advice.

General management of symptomatic patients

As their HIV infection progresses, patients are at increasing risk of complications. Depletion of CD4 lymphocytes leads to increased susceptibility to infection and tumours, while involvement of macrophages or neuroglial cells leads to 'HIV-specific symptoms' and central nervous system disease. Some of these problems are listed in Tables 1 and 2. The CD4 count of the patient, taken while not acutely ill will allow the patient's disease stage to assessed. The main principle in the management of the ill patient is to strike a balance between invasive diagnostic procedures, which will lead to active treatments and the initiation of palliative measures, and avoidance of overaggressive procedures and treatments. Great care needs to be taken to assess the overall prognosis of the patient and to determine individual needs.

NURSING ISSUES AND NOSOCOMIAL SPREAD OF INFECTION

Patients should be cared for by staff who are familiar with risks of transmission of infection. The risk of infection from a parenteral exposure of blood following a needle-stick inoculation is about 0.25 per cent. There is no need for nursing staff to wear special protective clothing routinely, although gloves should be used, as for all patients, when there is exposure to body fluids. There is no need for patients with HIV to be routinely isolated from other patients. However, isolation rooms are often used because many patients prefer privacy in order to maintain the confidentiality of their disease. In some cases, patients have infections which themselves require isolation. In particular, patients suspected of open tuberculosis should be isolated, and patients with other pathogens (for example cryptosporidium) may be a risk to other immunosuppressed patients.

MANAGEMENT OF FEVER

Patients presenting with fever should be initially investigated, as for any other patient, with a pyrexia of unknown origin as there is an increased susceptibility to pyogenic infections. A full history should be taken, a full examination should be given, cultures of blood, urine, and faeces should be obtained, and chest radiography should be performed. If indicated by the symptoms or signs, occult abscesses (including sinuses and prostate) should be sought. In advanced disease, the most common causes of persistent high swinging fevers are disseminated infection with *Mycobacterium avium-intracellulare* complex (MAC) and lymphoma. MAC is often isolated in the faeces but is not diagnostic of dissemination. Definitive diagnosis of MAC is made by blood cultures using special media. Acid-fast stain of bone marrow or lymph node aspirate may give the diagnosis prior to the culture result. Imaging techniques, in particular CT scanning of the abdomen, are essential to find a suitable site for biopsy to diagnose lymphoma. Rarely, other opportunistic infections such as pneumocystis pneumonia or cryptococcus can present as fever without their typical focal signs.

In some cases, the cause of fever is never found. In early disease the fevers can often resolve spontaneously. In advanced disease fevers can often continue intermittently for many months. Palliative treatment includes non-steroidal anti-inflammatory agents, prednisolone, and therapeutic trials of anti-MAC treatment.

MANAGEMENT OF BREATHLESSNESS

Appropriate treatment of breathlessness is important as the most common cause, pneumocystis pneumonia, can be rapidly progressive. The differential diagnosis includes pneumocystis pneumonia, bacterial pneumonia, pneumothorax, pulmonary Kaposi's sarcoma, other tumours, fungal infections, and heart failure. Routine investigations include chest radiography, arterial blood oxygen saturation and blood cultures. Empirical treatment should include treatment for pneumocystis pneumonia, pneumococcus, and *Haemophilus influenzae* such as a combination of cefuroxime and high dose septrin. Erythromycin should be added if atypical pneumonia is suspected. Corticosteroids should be included if the patient is hypoxic, and continuous positive airway pressure (CPAP) or mechanical ventilation should be considered if necessary to allow diagnosis and time for patients to respond to treatment. Bronchoscopic alveolar lavage should be considered early as sometimes patients progress quickly and become too ill for bronchoscopy without the support of mechanical ventilation. Bronchial biopsy is required if lesions suggestive of tumour or Kaposi's sarcoma are suspected. If the chest radiograph shows diffuse bilateral infiltration and bronchoscopic alveolar lavage fails to reveal any pathogen, presumptive treatment for pneumocystis pneumonia should be continued.

If the patient deteriorates for several days despite definitive or empirical treatment (if no diagnosis is made), the prognosis is poor. Patients unlikely to benefit from mechanical ventilation should be treated palliatively with opiates to reduce anxiety.

MANAGEMENT OF AN ACUTE BRAIN SYNDROME

Patients presenting with focal neurological symptoms or headache need urgent investigation. The most common diagnoses include toxoplasmosis, cryptococcal meningitis, and central nervous system lymphoma, while progressive multifocal leukoencephalopathy is a less common diagnosis. Direct HIV involvement of the central nervous system (encephalopathy) and acute psychosis are less frequent and are diagnosed by exclusion. Toxoplasmosis is less likely if toxoplasmosis antibody has never been detected or if septrin has been given for pneumocystis pneumonia prophylaxis. Similarly, cryptococcal meningitis is less likely if cryptococcal antigen is not detected in the serum or if the patient has been taking continuous fluconazole for Candida. Patients should have CT scans of their brain for focal lesions, and if they are normal, the CSF should be examined under the microscope, cultured, and screened for cryptococcal antigen. Magnetic resonance imaging (MRI) is a more sensitive test for diagnosing toxoplasmosis and should be performed if possible. In the absence of a diagnosis empirical treatment for toxoplasmosis without corticosteroids should be initiated and the brain scan repeated about 2 to 3 weeks later. If the patient deteriorates in the face of treatment a presumptive diagnosis of central nervous system lymphoma can be made and treatment switched to steroids, but the prognosis will be poor. The place of brain biopsy in the management of focal central nervous system lesions remains controversial, since the commonest lesions found following empirical treatment for toxoplasmosis are lymphoma, progressive multifocal leucoencephalopathy, and toxoplasmosis.

MANAGEMENT OF THE WASTING SYNDROME

Weight loss is often one of the more distressing features of progressive HIV infection. Its course fluctuates even in advanced disease. In some cases it can be attributed to specific complications such as diarrhoeal diseases, lymphoma, or disseminated MAC infection. In other cases there appears to be no specific cause other than the advanced HIV infection itself. The use of parenteral feeding, enteral feeding, or anabolic steroids have all proved disappointing. Some patients remain well for many months or even years despite severe weight loss.

MANAGEMENT OF THE DYING PATIENT

In advanced disease, it becomes important for the clinician to decide that the patient has become terminally ill and that the progress of HIV infection and the related complications are essentially irreversible. Patients may become too weak to walk, may become incontinent, and may slowly dement. It is most important to keep the patient comfortable and to control symptoms with antiemetics, antidiarrhoeal agents, analgesics, opiates, and corticosteroids. Good nursing is imperative, and the most important place for nursing (home, hospice, or hospital) should be considered. Unlike cancer, where the terminal phase of the illness can be rapid, some HIV patients remain stable for many weeks or months. Therefore appropriate provision must be made. Patients should be allowed to decide who should be informed of the final diagnosis. Patients are often comforted by the opportunity to discuss their disease with friends or relatives who had not been informed before, and who may need to discuss the implications for their own health.

ROLE OF SURGERY IN HIV

HIV-positive patients tolerate surgery well; there is no special difficulty in wound healing. Those with surgical conditions unrelated to HIV should be offered surgery as indicated. Patients with complications of HIV which may be amenable to surgery (for instance tumours requiring resection) should be offered surgery, but the overall prognosis of their HIV disease should be considered when obtaining their consent.

Although the risk of infection to the surgeon is small and rigorous precautions against infection are recommended in all cases, most surgical staff wish to be informed of the patient's HIV status in planning the operation and time of surgery.

ROLE OF INTENSIVE CARE UNITS

HIV patients rarely require intensive care. Indications are the same as for other patients and there is no particular risk of transmission to intensive care staff. However, intensive care is normally inappropriate in patients with advanced HIV disease whose overall prognosis is currently limited unless recovery from an acute condition is considered to be very likely. The most important role of intensive care is to allow patients presenting with severe pneumocystis pneumonia enough time for antimicrobial agents and corticosteroids to be effective.

Specific complications

PULMONARY COMPLICATIONS (EXCLUDING TUBERCULOSIS AND TUMOURS)

P. carinii remains the most common life-threatening opportunistic infection in patients who progress from chronic HIV infection to AIDS. The presentation is usually subacute, with malaise, fatigue, weight loss, and shortness of breath often developing over several weeks. Clinical suspicion is aroused early in patients who are under regular medical supervision, leading to earlier diagnosis. Typical symptoms include retrosternal or subcostal chest discomfort associated with increasing shortness of breath, a dry cough, and fever. The chest radiograph at presentation may be normal or show fine bilateral perihilar infiltrates (Fig. 3). The arterial oxygen tension is usually depressed. The diagnosis is confirmed by cytological examination of sputum induced with saline, and if this is negative, by fibre optic bronchoscopy with bronchial lavage (Fig. 4). Transbronchial biopsy is now rarely performed because of its complications-haemorrhage and pneumothorax. At the same time other causes of pneumonia or coexistent infection such as mycobacteria, fungi (Cryptococcus and Histoplasma), and cytomegalovirus can be excluded. Cytomegalovirus in the lung is more often a passenger than a pathogen. Exercise oximetry and alternative imaging techniques with radiolabelled compounds are being used in diagnosis. Monoclonal antibodies to pneumocystis proteins may improve diagnostic sensitivity compared with conventional staining techniques. DNA probes for pneumocystis have been developed but are not yet in routine use (see Chapter 7.12.5).

Pyogenic bacterial causes of pneumonia should always be considered, particularly as their presentation may be atypical. As many as 10 per cent of episodes of pneumonia in AIDS patients may be due to bacteria such as *Streptococcus pneumonia, Haemophilus influenzae,* Branhamella, and group B streptococci. Radiological appearances may include diffuse infiltrates, as well as the more typical focal or lobar patterns. Another cause of diffuse abnormality is lymphocytic interstitial pneumonitis, first described in children and now recognized increasingly in adults. The cause is still uncertain.

TUBERCULOSIS AND HIV INFECTION

Introduction and epidemiology

Tuberculosis, which is caused by *Mycobacterium tuberculosis,* is a good model for other 'opportunistic' infections seen in HIV-positive people.

Fig. 3 Pneumocystis pneumonia.

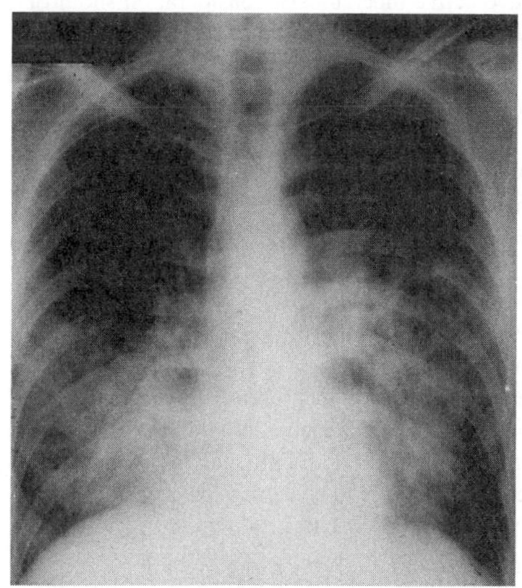

Fig. 4 *P. carinii* cysts from bronchial aspirate.

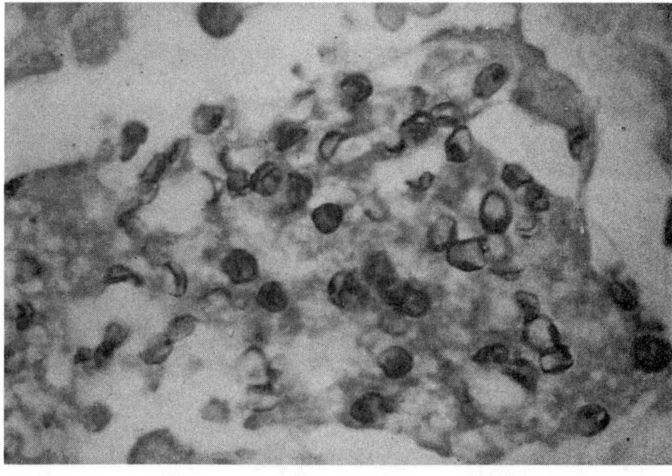

In countries or districts where tuberculosis is a common endemic organism, those who are immunosuppressed by HIV will have had an increased chance of coming into contact with the bacillus at some stage in the past and will have an increased risk of developing disease. Where the background prevalence of tuberculosis is low, dual infection will be uncommon and tuberculosis as a disease in HIV-positive patients will be rare.

The interaction between AIDS and tuberculosis was noted early in the HIV epidemic when many HIV-positive patients from Haiti treated in Florida were found to have active pulmonary tuberculosis. Studies in Central Africa in the mid-1980s showed that more than 60 per cent of newly diagnosed tuberculosis patients were HIV positive at a time when the background seroprevalence of HIV in the population was much lower. In the United States, intravenous drug users were shown to have an increased risk of developing active tuberculosis if they were HIV positive, with the diagnosis of tuberculosis preceding any AIDS-defining event by 6 months. After decades of progressive decline in cases in the United States, notifications of tuberculosis cases started to increase after 1984, soon after the appearance of the HIV epidemic. Similarly, an increase in tuberculosis in association with HIV has been noted in southern Europe, particularly in intravenous drug users.

Most cases of tuberculosis in HIV-positive individuals probably represent reactivation of dormant bacilli. However, as the prevalence of both infections increases in a community, new infections or reinfections may also occur. Studies are currently underway in Africa and elsewhere using molecular techniques to type isolates of *M. tuberculosis* and assess the relative contributions of new infection versus reactivation. When patients are found to have active tuberculosis, consideration should be given to testing for HIV infection and tuberculosis should always be included in the differential diagnosis of patients with HIV-related problems.

Clinical features of tuberculosis in HIV-positive patients

Most cases of tuberculosis in both human immunodeficiency virus-seropositive and HIV-seronegative individuals involve the lungs. The lung parenchyma or the pleura alone may be involved. Patients will usually present with cough, fever, and weight loss, with pulmonary infiltrates on the chest radiograph. There is a wide differential diagnosis in the HIV-infected patient for this presentation, and so it is important to obtain a good sputum specimen to examine for the presence of acid-fast bacilli. Studies in Zambia have shown that the presentation of pulmonary tuberculosis is very similar in HIV-positive and HIV-negative patients. However, HIV-positive cases are less likely to be sputum positive on microscopy, less likely to have cavitation on chest radiography, show more involvement of the lower lobes, and have more extrapulmonary disease. Studies in Africa show that, although the response to anti-tuberculosis treatment in the two groups is similar initially, HIV-positive patients are more likely to die prematurely (often of another bacterial disease) and are more likely to relapse (or be reinfected) after completion of therapy. Pleural effusion is common, with pleural Kaposi's sarcoma being the main differential diagnosis. Miliary tuberculosis occurs but, surprisingly, is relatively rare.

Extrapulmonary tuberculosis is more likely in those with HIV, particularly in southern Europe and the tropics. Tuberculous lymphadenitis is perhaps the most common manifestation, but the gut, and joints, and the genitourinary system may be affected. Tuberculoma in the central nervous system and tuberculous meningitis do not appear to be more common in patients with HIV.

MYCOBACTERIUM AVIUM-INTRACELLULARE COMPLEX (MAC)

People with HIV and AIDS are surviving longer, and many of these severely immunocompromised. With advanced HIV disease and CD4 lymphocyte counts below 50/mm^3, infection with (MAC) has become increasingly common. This organism is ubiquitous in the environment and the route of entry is probably the gastrointestinal tract. MAC usually disseminates in those with HIV and can be cultured from faeces, urine, blood, and bone marrow. About 15–20 per cent of people with AIDS in developed countries acquire MAC infection. These organisms are rarely found in AIDS patients in the tropics, probably because such patients do not survive long enough to be severely immunosuppressed. The usual symptoms associated with MAC are increased weight loss, fever, rigors, night sweats, and diarrhoea.

Other atypical mycobacteria

There are numerous case reports of other non-tuberculosis mycobacteria causing opportunist infection in people with HIV. Perhaps the most interesting is a newly described fastidious organism *Mycobacterium genavese.* This has been found in European patients presenting with fever, diarrhoea and extreme weight loss.

GASTROINTESTINAL MANIFESTATIONS OF HIV

Oral and oesophageal problems

One of the characteristic clinical presentations of HIV disease is a sore mouth and/or dysgusia due to oropharyngeal candidiasis (Fig. 5). Although often an early feature of HIV infection, this problem usually recurs throughout the patient's life. Topical antifungals are usually effective in the early stages, but later systemic antifungal drugs, such as the imidazoles, are required to control the infection. Most cases are caused by *Candida albicans,* but rarely *Candida kreusi* is found.

Oral hairy leucoplakia has been described previously. Periodontal disease is not uncommon in those with HIV. Necrotizing gingivitis may require extensive debridement in addition to antimicrobial therapy. Other patients may be affected by severe ulceration of the oropharynx

Fig. 5 Oral candidiasis.

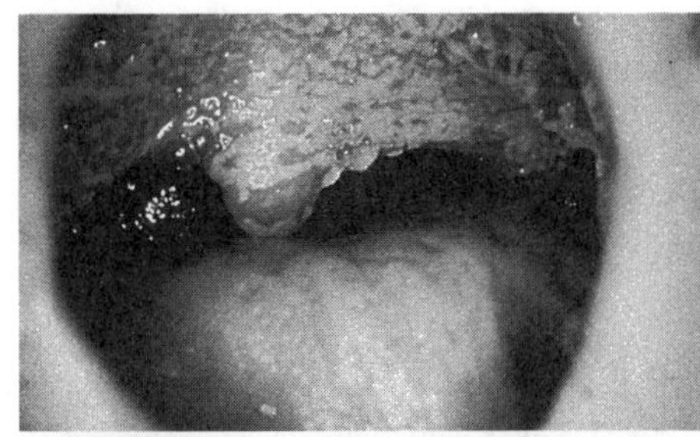

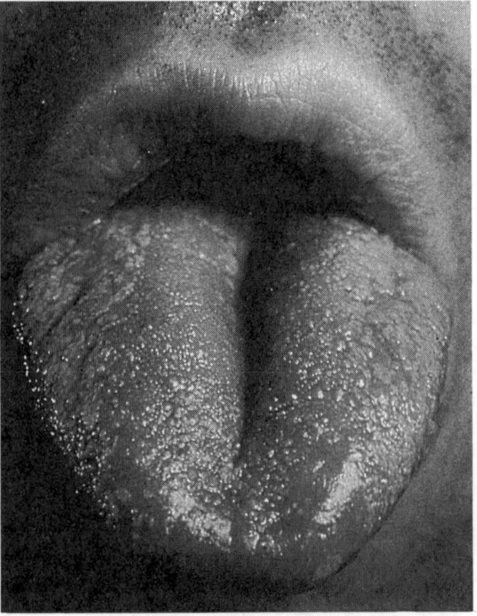

which does not appear to be infective. Ulcers may be solitary or multiple and are usually very painful. They usually regress with local or systemic corticosteroid therapy. Thalidomide has also been found to be beneficial in this condition.

Some patients may present with painful dysphagia due to oesophagitis. The most common cause in patients with HIV is oesophageal candidiasis, an AIDS-defining opportunistic infection. The diagnosis can be confirmed by endoscopy and biopsy, but is usually obvious clinically in a patient with oral Candida and dysphagia. Treatment is with systemic antifungals. Oesophageal candidiasis may recur in late-stage HIV disease and the Candida may become imidazole resistant, requiring treatment with parenteral amphotericin B. Oesophagitis can also be caused by cytomegalovirus and herpes simplex virus. The same type of 'aphthous' ulcers that affect the mouth may occur in the oesophagus and may respond to steroids.

Diarrhoea

Chronic intermittent diarrhoea is a frequent problem in HIV disease. Although sometimes caused by an opportunistic gut infection, no obvious cause can be identified in at least half of the cases. The most common organisms found are *Cryptosporidium parvum* and *Isospora belli.* Microsporidia species have recently been described as new human pathogens in the AIDS era and are frequently associated with diarrhoea.

Although *Giardia intestinalis* and *Entamoeba histolytica* are more commonly found in the faeces of homosexual men than heterosexual men, there is no evidence that these protozoa cause any particular problems in those with HIV. Bacterial infections with enteric pathogens such as Salmonella, Shigella, and Campylobacter do not lead to chronic diarrhoea but may take longer to clear. Salmonella infections in particular may become disseminated and may not be eradicated, even with prolonged antimicrobial therapy.

With advanced disease, MAC infection may lead to diarrhoea among other symptoms. Some patients may develop colitis due to cytomegalovirus. They usually have abdominal pain and tenderness, fever, and bloody diarrhoea. Rectal biopsy reveals evidence of 'owl's eye' inclusion bodies and inflammation. Many patients with HIV develop neuropathy, and some will have symptoms of autonomic neuropathy. These patients may develop diarrhoea which is often troublesome at night. Antidiarrhoeal agents, such as loperamide, and anticholinergics may help to alleviate symptoms.

In at least half of patients with HIV and diarrhoea no cause is found, even with extensive investigation. An enteropathy has been described with reduced villous height. It is likely that HIV is affecting the gut directly or indirectly, possibly by alteration of local cytokines. These patients are best managed by a combination of explanation and antidiarrhoeal drugs, such as loperamide or codeine phosphate.

Some patients may develop diarrhoea or have an exacerbation of existing diarrhoea as a side-effect of medication. Commonly prescribed drugs such as antimicrobial agents, zidovudine, and didanosine may cause diarrhoea.

Liver, gallbladder, and pancreas

The liver may be a site for opportunistic infections and is frequently involved in disseminated MAC infection. Acalculous cholecystitis and cholangitis with strictures and dilatation of the biliary tree (AIDS sclerosing cholangitis) occurs in late-stage disease. Both Cryptosporidium and cytomegalovirus have been implicated as a cause. Drug-induced hepatitis is common with the polypharmacy of late-stage disease. The pancreas is rarely a site for opportunistic infection. However, severe pancreatitis has occurred following treatment with didanosine.

Tumours

The gastrointestinal tract may be involved by one of the two types of tumour associated with HIV infection; Kaposi's sarcoma and non-Hodgkin's lymphoma. These may present with diarrhoea, bleeding, obstruction, and ascites, or as an abdominal mass. There is an increased incidence of squamous-cell carcinoma of the anus in HIV-positive homosexual men.

HIV AND THE NERVOUS SYSTEM

Opportunistic infections

Cerebral toxoplasmosis is the most frequent infection of the central nervous system in AIDS. This disease usually results from reactivation of Toxoplasma cysts in the brain, leading to abscess formation. The abscesses may be single but are usually multiple, presenting with focal neurological signs, fits, or the symptoms of raised intracranial pressure. Radiographically the toxoplasmosis lesions appear as ring-enhancing abscesses on the CT scan with surrounding oedema (Fig. 6). MRI is more sensitive. The only way to make a definite diagnosis is brain biopsy. However, as toxoplasmosis is by far the most common treatable cause of focal cerebral lesions in HIV, it is now standard practice to treat for toxoplasmosis and only consider biopsy if there is no clinical improvement within 7 to 10 days. The differential diagnosis includes cerebral lymphoma, progressive multifocal leucoencephalopathy, cryptococcoma, and gumma.

Although cryptococcal meningitis can occur in immunocompetent people, it accounts for 5 to 10 per cent of opportunistic infections in AIDS. The presentation may be subtle with headache and mild fever, and little in the way of neurological signs. Sometimes fits or cranial nerve palsies occur and occasionally there may be truncal ataxia. Neck stiffness is relatively rare. The diagnosis is made by examination of the cerebrospinal fluid. Usually there are few white cells and the glucose and protein are relatively normal. However, in about 70 per cent of cases India ink staining will show numerous cryptococci which can be cultured on standard Sabouraud's medium, and almost 100 per cent of cases will have detectable cryptococcal antigen in the blood and cerebrospinal fluid.

Progressive multifocal leucoencephalopathy is a progressive demyelinating condition caused by a polyomavirus, usually the JC virus which is cytopathic for oligodendroglia. There can be a variety of clinical manifestations depending on the number and site of demyelinating lesions. There may be focal deficits, personality changes, or ataxia. There is little headache as there is no mass effect. Rapid deterioration over 2 to 4 months is usual. There is no known treatment.

In the later stages of HIV disease, patients may present with cognitive impairment, a decreased level of consciousness, fever, and sometimes seizures. In some cases this may be due to cytomegalovirus infection of the brain and it may respond to ganciclovir or foscarnet. Very rarely, herpes simplex encephalitis may occur.

Fig. 6 Cerebral toxoplasmosis with ring enhancement with contrast and surrounding cerebral oedema (CT scan).

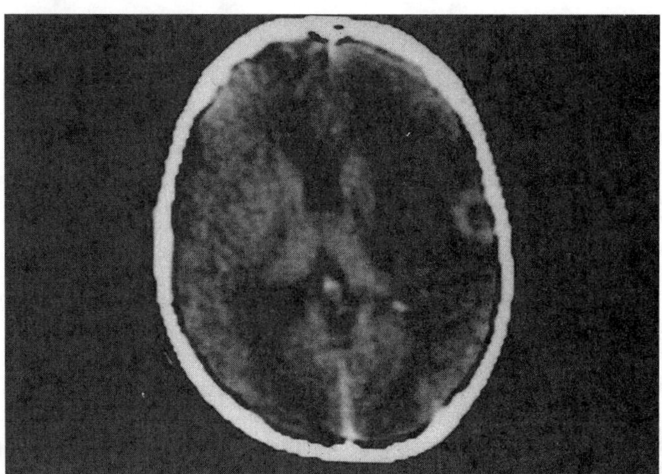

HIV encephalopathy

It has become clear over the past decade that HIV can directly infect the brain, leading to a variety of clinical problems. Up to 80 per cent of patients dying of AIDS show histological evidence of an encephalopathy with neuronal loss, demyelination, and multinucleate giant cells. Particularly in the later stages of HIV disease up to one-third of patients develop cognitive, behavioural and motor dysfunction which was referred to as AIDS dementia complex and is now termed the HIV-1-associated cognitive motor complex. Early on there may be impairment of concentration and memory; later, motor signs appear, such as hyperreflexia, extensor plantar responses, incoordination, and ataxia. This condition may respond to zidovudine treatment.

Myelopathy

A variety of conditions may affect the spinal cord in patients with HIV, but in many cases cord dysfunction is a result of the HIV infection itself. This usually presents as a progressive vacuolar myelopathy with spastic paraparesis, ataxia, loss of sphincter control, and changes in the spinal cord that are pathologically similar to those seen in subacute combined degeneration of the cord (although serum B_{12} levels are normal in HIV myelopathy). Vacuolar myelopathy is often found in association with AIDS dementia complex. Although up to 25 per cent of patients dying with AIDS have a vacuolar myelopathy, only a minority have symptoms and signs before death.

Transverse myelitis may occur, due to HIV itself or varicella-zoster, Herpes simplex, or cytomegalovirus infection. Cytomegalovirus may also cause a polyradiculopathy.

Peripheral neuropathy

Peripheral neuropathy may arise at any stage of HIV infection, even at seroconversion. Mononeuritis multiplex can occur, and patients sometimes present with an acute demyelinating polyneuropathy resembling Guillain–Barré syndrome. However, the most common problem is an axonal peripheral neuropathy, which is seen in 10–15 per cent of patients with AIDS-related complex or AIDS. Sensory symptoms predominate so that pain may limit walking. Autonomic neuropathies are sometimes seen and may lead to postural hypotension or diarrhoea. Finally, some drugs, such as zalcitabine, didanosine, and vincristine, may cause a neuropathy.

Psychiatric problems

In addition to the AIDS dementia complex discussed above, a variety of psychiatric problems occur in those with HIV. Acute psychosis is rare but can occur. Much more common are anxiety or panic attacks and depression. The former may respond best to directed counselling. Depression may require antidepressant medication in addition to counselling and support.

CYTOMEGALOVIRUS RETINITIS

The most common ocular problem is cytomegalovirus retinitis, which is rare in other immunosuppressed patient groups. It is a feature of late-stage HIV disease but, with increasingly prolonged survival of people with AIDS, is becoming more common. Around 5–10 per cent of patients with CD4 counts below 50/μl develop cytomegalovirus retinitis. It usually presents with visual loss, commonly with blurring of vision or sometimes scotoma. Some patients may notice an increase in ocular 'floaters' or flashes of light. The retina has a characteristic appearance with patches of irregular retinal whitening (caused by oedema and necrosis), patches of haemorrhage, and perivascular inflammation (Fig. 7). The retinitis usually starts peripherally and, if unchecked, progresses towards the macula, eventually leading to blindness. Cytomegalovirus retinitis must be distinguished from cotton-wool spots—irregular fluffy retinal lesions that are not associated with haemorrhage or exudate. Cotton-wool spots are common and benign, and often appear and disappear.

The diagnosis is clinical, and is based on retinal appearance and response to treatment. Anti-cytomegalovirus drugs are only virustatic and so treatment aims to halt progression rather than cure disease. As a result, treatment for cytomegalovirus retinitis is lifelong. Viral resistance may be a problem in some long-term survivors. However, if appropriate therapy is used, total blindness is rare.

Although cytomegalovirus retinitis is the most common ocular infection in AIDS, other infections such as acute retinal necrosis, toxoplasma choroidoretinitis, fungi, and bacteria need to be considered.

ACUTE RETINAL NECROSIS

Rarely, acute visual deterioration may occur as a result of varicella-zoster virus infection of the retina, which may or may not be preceded by dermatomal zoster. There may be a necrotizing retinitis that is rapidly progressive and is associated with a vitreal and sometimes an anterior chamber inflammation. In addition, AIDS patients may develop an outer retinal necrosis syndrome. The peripheral retina becomes progressively opacified with little ocular inflammation. There is usually a rapid rate of disease progression with a high rate of retinal detachment. This acute retinal necrosis may go on to affect the other eye, leading to irreversible blindness.

TOXOPLASMA AND CHOROIDORETINITIS

When vision is impaired due to retinitis but inflammatory cells are also seen in the vitreous humour on slit-lamp examination, choroidoretinitis caused by *Toxoplasma gondii* should be considered. Acutely, this may resemble cytomegalovirus retinitis apart from the cells in the vitreous humour. However, the retinal scarring following treatment looks quite different. The disease is more common in countries such as Brazil and France where the background prevalence of toxoplasmosis is much higher than in the United Kingdom.

ACUTE UVEITIS

Uveitis is rare in HIV infection but has recently been reported in patients taking the antimicrobial drug rifabutin in conjunction with clarithromycin. It has been postulated that clarithromycin increases plasma levels of rifabutin to such an extent that an immune-mediated uveitis ensues.

HIV AND TUMOURS

Kaposi's sarcoma

The epidemic of Kaposi's sarcoma in young homosexual men in North America first alerted clinicians to the AIDS epidemic in the early 1980s.

Fig. 7 Cytomegalovirus retinitis.

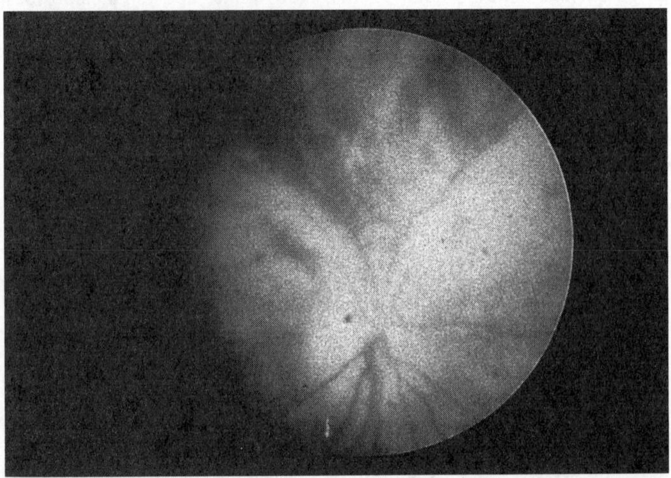

It is still not clear whether it is a true sarcoma. It is mainly a disease of gay and bisexual men and of men and women with HIV in Africa. Kaposi's sarcoma is extremely rare in intravenous drug users, blood transfusion recipients, and haemophiliacs, suggesting that there is a transmissible agent responsible for its development in HIV-positive individuals. Transmission may be sexual or by the faecal–oral route. Recently Kaposi's sarcoma-associated herpes virus-like (KSHV) sequences have been found in the majority of tumourous tissues obtained from patients. This would appear to be a new human herpes virus (human herpes virus 8).

Kaposi's sarcoma characteristically presents as a violaceous skin lesion and is multifocal (Fig. 8). Lesions also occur in mucous membranes, often on the hard palate. Such 'external' lesions may occur in cosmetically unacceptable areas, but in themselves are rarely life-threatening. However, visceral disease also occurs and commonly affects the lungs (Fig. 9) and gastrointestinal tract. Patients may present with dyspnoea, cough, or haemoptysis if the lungs are involved, or can present with abdominal pain, bleeding, or even rarely a protein-losing enteropathy when the gut is affected.

Treatment is never curative. Cutaneous lesions may be left untreated but can be excised if single. Alternatively, local radiotherapy or intralesional chemotherapy are effective. Widespread skin or visceral disease is often treated by systemic chemotherapy, although the lesions frequently relapse unless chemotherapy is given continously. A combination of vincristine and bleomycin is often effective in the short term with relatively mild side-effects. Other agents include etoposide and daunorubicin. Liposomal cytotoxic agents are also being assessed. Whatever therapy is chosen, Kaposi's sarcoma tends to progress relentlessly even after the maximum cumulative doses of chemotherapeutic agents have been employed.

Fig. 8 Disseminated lesions of Kaposi's sarcoma on the trunk.

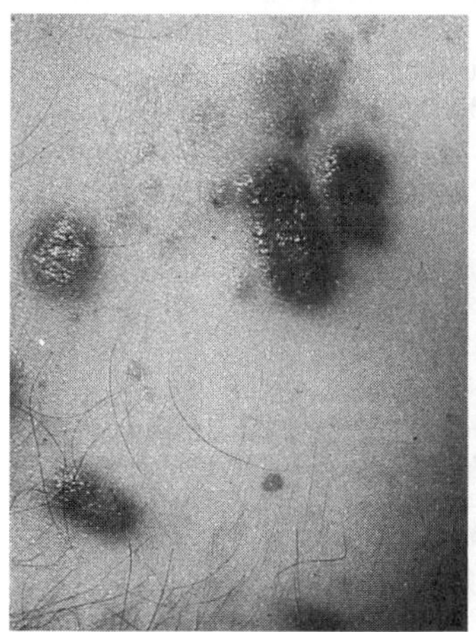

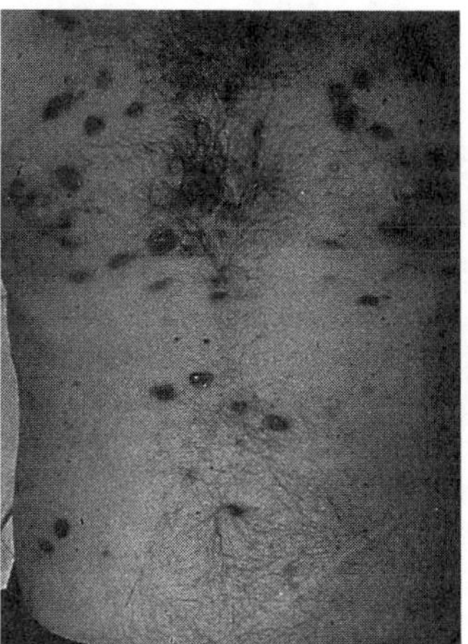

Fig. 9 Pulmonary Kaposi's sarcoma.

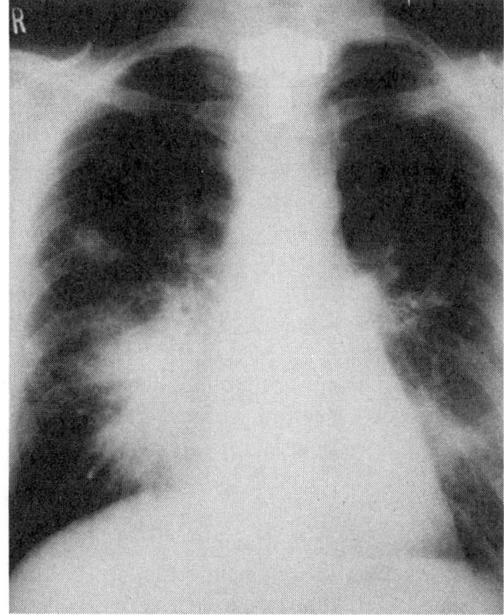

Non-Hodgkin's lymphoma

There is a clear association between HIV infection and the development of B-cell non-Hodgkin's lymphoma. The majority of tumours are extralymphatic and histologically are high grade large cell immunoblastic or non-cleaved small-cell tumours. Many appear to be associated with Epstein–Barr virus infection. Clinical presentation depends on the site and extent of the tumour. However, the central nervous system is a common site of AIDS-related non-Hodgkin's lymphoma. Patients with central nervous system disease usually present with the symptoms and signs of a space-occupying cerebral tumour; the main differential diagnosis is cerebral toxoplasmosis.

The treatment of central nervous system lymphoma in HIV infection is usually unrewarding. Neither chemotherapy nor radiotherapy have much impact on progression. The median survival after diagnosis is about 3 months. AIDS-related lymphoma outside the central nervous system may respond to standard combination chemotherapeutic regimens. Response is better in the less immunosuppressed and generally poor in those who already have an AIDS diagnosis. Many deaths during chemotherapy are due to opportunist infections.

Other tumours in AIDS

Although numerous cases of Hodgkin's disease in association with HIV have been reported, there are no clear epidemiological data that point to a causal link. Recent data suggest that squamous-cell carcinoma of the anus in homosexual men may be more common in those with HIV infection. Cervical carcinoma in women with HIV infection has recently been designated as an AIDS-defining condition, but as yet the epidemiological link between HIV and cervical cancer is unproven.

MISCELLANEOUS HIV-RELATED CONDITIONS

Renal disease

It is now clear that HIV can have a direct effect on the kidneys, leading to a variety of clinical problems. The most common presentation is with nephrotic syndrome and renal failure, although a wide variety of renal presentations occur. Focal and segmental glomerulosclerosis account for most cases of chronic HIV-associated nephropathy, but any type of glomerular lesion is possible. The highest incidence of renal disease in HIV-infected patients seems to be in North America, with most cases occurring in intravenous drug users or the black population (85 per cent of reported cases are in black people).

Renal disease also occurs as a consequence of therapy related to HIV infection. Amphotericin B almost invariably causes renal damage, foscarnet for cytomegalovirus disease has marked renal toxicity, and both pentamidine and co-trimoxazole in the doses used to treat pneumocystis pneumonia can adversely affect renal function.

HIV and the heart

The most common cardiac problem worldwide in patients with HIV is tuberculous pericarditis. In terminal HIV disease, ventricular hypokinesia is common but is probably of little clinical significance, and evidence of myocarditis without a clinical correlate is frequently found at post mortem. Rarely, opportunist infection with *Toxoplasma gondii, Cryptococcus neoformans,* or cytomegalovirus and Kaposi's sarcoma affect the heart.

Children and HIV

In general, children have similar clinical problems to adults when they are infected with HIV. However, there are important differences which deserve comment. The most important problem is how to decide if a child is infected. Most paediatric infections result from vertical transmission of HIV, although some children may be infected by blood products. In Europe, the estimated vertical transmission rate is 14 per cent, while in sub-Saharan Africa the rate appears to be higher (about 30 per cent). The risk of transmission is greater if the mother has advanced HIV disease, if there is vaginal delivery, and if the mother breast feeds. Uninfected children may still have detectable maternal HIV antibody beyond 1 year of age, and conversely children below 6 months of age may have signs and symptoms of HIV disease without detectable antibody. Lymphocyte subsets are also of less value, particularly in very young children, compared with adults.

Failure to thrive, diarrhoea, recurrent bacterial pneumonia, lymphadenopathy, parotitis, and hepatosplenomegaly are all more common in HIV-infected infants. Oesophageal Candida is not uncommon. HIV encephalopathy can occur and other neurological and developmental problems are seen. Lymphoid interstitial pneumonitis occurs more commonly in children than in adults and initially mimics pneumocystis pneumonia or bacterial pneumonia.

Treatment is largely the same as for adults. Zidovudine does appear to be beneficial in symptomatic children and there is evidence that the drug, when taken by pregnant women, may reduce the risk of vertical transmission of HIV. The use of CD4 lymphocyte counts to assess the need for pneumocystis pneumonia prophylaxis is controversial. Survival of perinatally infected children tends to be poor, with one study finding a median survival of 38 months and the highest mortality in the first year.

Overview of treatment of opportunistic infections

The treatment of HIV infection has largely been limited to the treatment of its complications, namely the opportunistic tumours and infections. Most of the infections are due to reactivation of latent organisms in the host or in some cases to ubiquitous organisms to which we are continuously exposed. In general the treatment of these infections suppresses rather than eradicates the organisms, and so relapse is common when treatment is stopped. The side-effects and interactions between many of the drugs used complicate the long-term treatment that is needed.

PROTOZOAL INFECTIONS

Pneumocystis pneumonia

At present pneumocystis pneumonia is treated either by drugs that have become accepted in clinical practice or by investigational drugs. Some doctors regard certain of the investigational drugs as conventional treatment but controlled studies are still in progress to determine their relative efficacy.

High dose intravenous co-trimoxazole for 2 to 3 weeks remains a standard first choice regimen for severe pneumocystis pneumonia, but once fevers and symptoms have settled and blood gas values have improved the drug can be given orally. Side-effects occur in about 30 per cent of patients, typically after 7 to 10 days. Intravenous pentamidine is the treatment of choice if patients are intolerant of co-trimoxazole. Again, side-effects are seen in about 30 per cent of cases; labile blood pressure and labile blood glucose are the most serious. Co-trimoxazole has the advantage of treating bacterial infections that are more common in HIV infection.

Nebulized pentamidine is sometimes used to treat acute pneumocystis pneumonia but should only be used for patients with mild disease. Nebulizers are available which deliver varying amounts of drug with different particle sizes, and so comparison between trials is difficult. The major adverse effect is bronchial irritation leading to cough and wheeze. This can be prevented by keeping particle size small and by using bronchodilators beforehand. Upper-lobe recurrences, extrapulmonary *P. carinii* infections, spontaneous pneumothorax, hypotension, and hypoglycaemia have all been reported in patients receiving inhaled nebulized pentamidine.

Other possibilities for patients who experience side-effects with both sulphonamides and pentamidine are clindamycin with primaquine or dapsone and trimethoprim. Atovaquone, a hydroxy-naphthoquinone, is a more recent addition and, like the other alternative drugs, its efficacy has been established only in mild to moderate pneumocystis pneumonia. Although slightly less effective than co-trimoxazole, atovaquone has significantly fewer side-effects. Its bioavailability is reduced because of its low aqueous solubility and slow and irregular absorption. An improved formulation is being evaluated.

Anecdotal experience, followed by clinical trials, has shown that high dose corticosteroids (equivalent to 40–60 mg prednisolone) are a valuable adjunctive treatment in moderate to severe pneumocystis pneumonia ($po_2 < 60$ mmHg). Treatment is continued for 7 to 10 days.

Prophylaxis for pneumocystis pneumonia is essential after a first attack (secondary prophylaxis) but primary prophylaxis is also recommended for patients with CD4 cell counts below 200/μl or less than 20 per cent of the total lymphocyte count. Co-trimoxazole, 1 tablet once a day or one double strength tablet three times weekly, is the most effective agent. In patients who are unable to tolerate co-trimoxazole, oral dapsone alone, 100 mg daily or dapsone 50 mg daily with pyrimethamine 50 mg weekly, is a good alternative. Nebulized pentamidine is an acceptable choice for patients with CD4 cell counts between 100 and 200/μl. The dose depends on the nebulizer system; with the Respirgard II Nebulizer, the recommended regimen is 300 mg every four weeks. Intravenous pentamidine (250–300 mg every four weeks) can also be used prophylactically.

Toxoplasmosis

In most centres, focal cerebral lesions found on CT or MRI scan are treated empirically as toxoplasmosis because this is the most common cause of such lesions. The condition responds well if treatment is started early, and a combination of sulphadiazine 4–6 g daily and pyrimethamine 50–100 mg daily is the treatment of choice. If sulphonamides are not tolerated, clindamycin 600–1200 mg four times daily can be substituted and has been shown to be an effective alternative in controlled studies. There is no role for corticosteroids in cerebral toxoplasmosis. Lack of clinical response 7 to 10 days into treatment should prompt consideration of brain biopsy to make a definite diagnosis.

Atovaquone 750 mg four times daily and the new macrolides clarithromycin 2 g daily and azithromycin, both given with pyrimethamine 75 mg/daily, have also been used in small uncontrolled studies.

Relapse of cerebral toxoplasmosis is common after treatment is stopped, and maintenance treatment should continue indefinitely. The most appropriate regimen for maintenance treatment or secondary prophylaxis has not been determined, but treatment doses of either sulphadiazine and pyrimethamine or clindamycin and pyrimethamine are usually halved.

It is clear from trials of pneumocystis pneumonia prophylaxis that co-trimoxazole is also an excellent prophylactic for toxoplasmosis whereas inhaled pentamidine is not. Although not proven, dapsone is probably also effective. Similarly, atovaquone, if reliably absorbed, might be expected to provide prophylaxis for both pneumocystis pneumonia and cerebral toxoplasmosis. The new macrolides clarithromycin and azithromycin may provide broad-spectrum prophylaxis for toxoplasmosis, atypical mycobacterial, and bacterial infections.

Cryptosporidiosis and other protozoa

Symptoms of cryptosporidiosis are often intermittent, as is excretion of the oocysts. This has made assessment of treatment difficult. To date, no effective treatment has been found, although a wide variety of for-

Table 7 *Viral opportunistic infections*

Infection	Drug	Duration	Side-effects	Comment
Herpes simplex				
Treatment	Acyclovir 200 mg five times daily orally or 5–10 mg/kg 8 hourly intravenously	5–7 days		Duration may be extended in severe infections
Prophylaxis	Acyclovir 200 mg four times daily	Indefinite		May be possible to reduce frequency
Cytomegalovirus	Ganciclovir 5 mg/kg twice daily intravenously	14–21 days	Neutropenia, anaemia	Marrow suppression potentiated with zidovudine
	Foscarnet (phosphonoformate) 180 mg/kg daily	14–21 days	Renal impairment, hypomagnesaemia, hypercalcaemia, hypocalcaemia, hyperphosphataemia, hypophosphataemia, hypokalaemia, gastrointestinal and genital ulcers	Dose must be adjusted according to renal function
Maintenance	Ganciclovir 6 mg/kg/daily intravenously 5 days a week or 5 mg/kg once daily (indwelling central line required), or 1 g orally thrice daily	Indefinite	As above	
	Foscarnet 90 mg/kg intravenously daily	Indefinite	As above	

mulations have been tried. Symptomatic treatment with codeine phosphate, loperamide, and other drugs, together with fluid, electrolyte, and nutritional support, may be the only effective measure.

Isosporiasis is less common but often responds to co-trimoxazole 960 mg four times a day. However, relapses occur in half of all cases.

There have been no controlled trials of therapy for microsporidiosis. Anecdotal reports of benefit with albendazole are promising, but formal assessment of this drug is lacking.

VIRAL INFECTIONS

Severe mucocutaneous and systemic infections with herpes simplex virus are best treated with acyclovir (Table 7). Prophylaxis is used after severe infection and in patients with chronic HIV infection and increasing severity and frequency of recurrences. These recurrences can be a prelude to the chronic persistent mucocutaneous ulceration characteristic of AIDS.

Varicella zoster virus infections are usually treated with high dose oral acyclovir. However, dissemination of infection from dermatomal varicella zoster is unusual even without treatment. BV-Ara U (1-*B*-D arabinofuranosyl-*E*-5-(2-bromovinyl) uracil) has a 1000-fold greater activity against varicella zoster *in vitro* compared with acyclovir and is being assessed in clinical trials. Acyclovir-resistant herpes simplex and varicella zoster viral infections are emerging as clinically important problems. Both resistant infections have been successfully treated with foscarnet.

Reactivation of cytomegalovirus infection tends to occur when CD4 cell counts are persistently below 50/μl. Ganciclovir (an acyclic analogue of deoxyguanosine) and foscarnet (phosphonoformate, a pyrophosphate analogue which inhibits polymerase enzymes) are both used for the treatment of cytomegalovirus retinopathy (Fig. 7) and gastrointestinal disease (Table 8). Both drugs arrest progression of retinitis in most patients, but maintenance treatment is required to delay the time to further relapse. The role of maintenance treatment in gastrointestinal disease is less clear. The major side-effect of ganciclovir treatment is neutropenia which often precludes the concomitant administration of zidovudine in the treatment period. Foscarnet is not as well tolerated as ganciclovir and may produce reversible renal failure and electrolyte disturbances. Careful and frequent monitoring is required, which complicates out-patient management. A recent study comparing ganciclovir with foscarnet for initial treatment and long-term maintenance in cytomegalovirus retinitis found no difference between the drugs in their ability to prevent progression of disease, but there was a slight survival advantage in those patients treated with foscarnet. The reasons for this are unclear. Ganciclovir is active against herpes simplex and so patients with frequently recurring herpes simplex infections do not require concurrent acyclovir treatment. Both ganciclovir and foscarnet are given intravenously, necessitating indwelling central venous catheters for long-term maintenance therapy. Oral ganciclovir has recently became available for maintenance therapy. It is probably less effective than intravenous therapy but patients are spared the impaired quality of life and risk of infection associated with indwelling catheters. Intravitreal ganciclovir or foscarnet have also been used to avoid the need for long-term intravenous therapy.

FUNGAL INFECTIONS

Dermatophytic fungal infections respond well to imidazole creams. Oral Candida is often asymptomatic in its early stages and may not require treatment. In more severe infections local treatment with frequent nystatin suspension or pastilles or amphotericin lozenges can be used. Systemic treatment with oral imidazoles is required for more severe oropharyngeal and oesophageal candidiasis. Long-term maintenance treatment is sometimes required but can lead to imidazole resistance.

Cryptococcal meningitis is treated with either fluconazole or amphotericin B with or without flucytosine. A large comparative study has shown that the overall mortality was similar in both treatment groups. However, there were more early deaths in the fluconazole group, and

Table 8 *Fungal opportunistic infections*

Infection	Drug	Duration	Side-effects	Comment
Candidiasis				
Local treatment	Nystatin oral suspension pastilles, miconazole oral gel, or amphotericin lozenges, all 4–6 times daily	As required		Relapse common, many patients require systemic treatment
Systemic treatment	Ketoconazole 200 mg daily orally	2–4 weeks	Nausea (less if taken with food), abnormal liver function tests, hepatitis, thrombocytopenia, rash	Relapse common on cessation of treatment
	Fluconazole 50–200 mg daily	2–4 weeks	Nausea, abnormal liver function tests	As above
Maintenance	Ketoconazole 200 mg daily or fluconazole 50 mg daily or alternate days	Indefinite		As above
Cryptococcosis	Amphotericin B at least 0.3 mg/kg/daily ± flucytosine 150 mg/kg/daily in four doses	6 weeks	Nausea, vomiting, rash, bone marrow suppression, renal impairment, hypocalcaemia	Relapse may occur, maintenance needed
	Fluconazole 200–400 mg daily	6 weeks	As above	As above

amphotericin sterilized the cerebrospinal fluid more rapidly. Fluconazole was better tolerated. There was a 20 per cent mortality, and the factors predictive of death were an abnormal mental state, a cryptococcal antigen titre above 1024, and a white-cell count below 0.02×10^9/l in the cerebrospinal fluid. Therefore physicians will probably treat patients with these poor prognostic markers with amphotericin rather than fluconazole. It is likely that flucytosine confers little benefit but increases haematological toxicity, and so increasingly amphotericin B is given alone. With a 20 per cent mortality irrespective of what treatment is used, it is clear that improvements in therapy are required.

Maintenance treatment is required after initial treatment; without it relapse is common. Fluconazole (200 mg/day) was more effective than amphotericin B (1 mg/kg weekly) in a large randomized study. The comparative efficacy of higher doses of amphotericin maintenance therapy is unknown. Liposomal preparations of amphotericin B are being assessed, as are higher doses of fluconazole.

Amphotericin B is still the mainstay of treatment of other systemic fungal infections. Itraconazole has been shown to be effective in the treatment of and secondary prophylaxis for disseminated histoplasmosis.

BACTERIAL INFECTIONS

Tuberculosis

Tuberculosis in HIV infection is treated with standard triple therapy: rifampicin, isoniazid, and pyrazinamide. It is important to obtain material for tuberculosis culture and sensitivity testing so that treatment may be modified in the light of these results. In addition, the usual procedures for isolation of sputum-positive cases and contact tracing should be applied. Rifampicin is a potent enzyme inducer and increases the metabolism of methadone, oral contraceptives, dapsone, fluconazole, ketoconazole, and anticonvulsants among other drugs. Furthermore, ketoconazole inhibits the absorption of rifampicin. If these drugs are given together, blood concentrations of both are reduced. Patients with HIV are more likely than seronegative individuals to have adverse reactions to drugs. Generally, this has not been a problem with anti-tuberculosis drugs. However, in parts of Africa where the sulpha-based drug thiacetazone is used, serious skin reactions, including fatal cases of Stevens–Johnson syndrome, occur much more frequently in those infected with HIV. Although extrapulmonary disease is more common in HIV-seropositive patients than in uninfected controls, the responses to treatment seem to be similar in the developed world if patients are compliant. African studies suggest a higher relapse rate in patients who are HIV positive. Therefore follow-up and defaulter chasing are important. In the past 2 years there have been several outbreaks of tuberculosis resistant to multiple drugs in New York and Florida. Transmission of drug-resistant strains has occurred between patients and from patients to family members, health care workers, and prison guards. Mortality from drug-resistant tuberculosis in this setting is high (around 70–90 per cent).

In HIV-positive American intravenous drug users who are tuberculin positive on skin testing, the risk of developing active tuberculosis increases to about 8 per cent per year compared with a lifetime risk of about 10 per cent in HIV-negative individuals. Studies have shown that isoniazid prophylaxis given for 1 year after skin test conversion in this group significantly reduces the risks of developing clinical tuberculosis. In areas where tuberculosis is highly endemic, such as Haiti and sub-Saharan Africa, similar studies have shown that isoniazid prophylaxis reduces the chances that asymptomatic HIV-infected individuals will develop tuberculosis.

The role of previous BCG vaccination is uncertain but does not appear to be protective for adults with HIV in Africa. However, the administration of BCG to people infected with HIV does not appear to lead to an increased risk of dissemination of the vaccine strain. Chemoprophylaxis in areas of relatively low tuberculosis endemicity, such as Northern Europe, for patients with HIV who have received the BCG vaccine is unclear but is probably not advisable.

Mycobacterium avium-intracellulare complex (MAC)

Most isolates of MAC are resistant to the first- and second-line antituberculosis drugs. If single-drug therapy is used, resistance occurs quickly. In a placebo-controlled study clarithromycin had clear activity alone *in vivo* but resistance occurred within 12 weeks. Various combinations of drugs have been shown to decrease mycobacteraemia and improve symptoms in uncontrolled studies, but the infection is not eliminated. There is little evidence that the treatment of MAC prolongs survival in AIDS. Four-, three-, and even two-drug regimens are being assessed in clinical trials; a typical four-drug regimen consists of ciprofloxacin (500–750 mg twice daily), rifampicin (10 mg/kg daily to a maximum of 600 mg) or rifabutin (450–600 mg daily), clarithromycin

(250–500 mg twice daily), and ethambutol (15 mg/kg to a maximum 1 g daily). Other drugs which are used include clofazimine (100 mg daily) and amikacin (7.5–15 mg/kg daily). Treatment is usually continued for life.

A randomized placebo-controlled study of rifabutin 300 mg daily in over 500 patients with AIDS and CD4 cell counts above 200/μl has shown that there is a significantly longer time lapse before the development of mycobacteraemia and possible a longer period free of symptoms, but no survival advantage has yet been demonstrated.

Antiviral treatment of HIV

Since the discovery of HIV as the cause of AIDS, there has been an extensive search for effective anti-HIV antiviral drugs. All parts of the viral replication cycle have been used as targets for inhibition, and to date the most effective drugs have been the reverse transcriptase enzyme inhibitors (Table 9).

Table 9 *Anti-HIV drugs currently used in clinical trials*

	Examples
Reverse transcriptase inhibitors	
Nucleoside analogues	Zidovudine (ACT) Didanosine (ddI) Zalcitabine (ddC) Lamivudine (3TC)
Non-nucleoside analogues	Neviripine TIBO derivatives
Protease inhibitors	Saquinavar

ZIDOVUDINE

In 1985 zidovudine (3′-azido-3′-deoxythymidine), also known as AZT, was first reported to be active *in vitro* against HIV. The drug is phosphorylated intracellularly to form the triphosphate which is the active metabolite. It inhibits the reverse transcriptase of HIV. Within 6 months it was first administered to patients, and by 1986 the results of the first placebo-controlled clinical trial were reported (Table 10). The efficacy of zidovudine given earlier in the disease has also been studied. The effect of zidovudine in asymptomatic HIV-infected patients (with CD4 counts below 500) was compared with placebo. After treatment for about 12 months, zidovudine slowed the rate progression to symptomatic disease (AIDS-related complex or AIDS) compared with placebo. The success of these trials triggered a wave of optimism that HIV could be treated easily. Anecdotal reports and small studies suggest that, in the short term, zidovudine can increase the patient's weight and their feeling of well-being. It has been reported to have a remarkable effect on HIV-associated thrombocytopenia and on the neurological complications of HIV infection. HIV-related dementia appears to be reversible with zidovudine treatment.

Table 10 *Results of 1986 zidovudine trial*

	Placebo	Zidovudine
Died	19	1
Total	137	145
Median follow-up (days)	120	127

Patients with AIDS-related complex or AIDS were recruited into the study.

Unfortunately it has become clear that the effect of the drug is limited. Uncontrolled studies have shown that, despite zidovudine, the mortality of patients with AIDS is still very high. The Anglo-French study Concorde compared the effects of a policy of 'immediate zidovudine', where asymptomatic patients were given zidovudine immediately after randomization, with 'deferred zidovudine', where patients were given placebo and only received zidovudine when they showed signs of clinical progression. In the deferred arm, about 80 per cent of those who took zidovudine did so either when they developed AIDS-related complex or AIDS or when their CD4 counts dropped below 250/μl. Patients were followed for up to 4 years. As expected from the previous trials, there was a small difference in the rate of progression to AIDS-related complex in the first year of treatment. However, this difference was only transient and, during the 4 years of the trial, there was no overall difference between the groups in rates of progression to AIDS-related complex, AIDS, or death (Fig. 10). Patients in the Concorde trial and in other small long-term trials are being followed to determine whether there are any small differences in overall survival in the longer term.

It thus appears that although zidovudine provides some clinical benefit over the short term (about 1 year), its sustained use as monotherapy does not seem to provide any greater benefit. It is likely that the failure of long-term zidovudine is due to the development of drug resistance. HIV strains isolated from patients taking zidovudine for more than 6 months develop reverse transcriptase mutations conferring zidovudine resistance. These strains are transmissible, with increasing reports of zidovudine-resistant strains being isolated from individuals who have never taken zidovudine.

Zidovudine has important side-effects, but fortunately nearly all of them are reversible. Nausea, myalgia, insomnia, and headaches are common reversible reasons for zidovudine intolerance. Haematological changes are the most common laboratory abnormalities. A macrocytosis usually develops after only a few weeks, but is harmless. The most important adverse event is anaemia which develops in about a third of patients with AIDS. The anaemia is dose dependent and reversible if the drug is stopped. Smaller numbers of patients develop serious neutropenia which again is reversible and dose dependent. The incidence of side-effects increases with disease progression. The Concorde study showed that fewer than 5 per cent stopped zidovudine because of haematological toxicity compared with 0.2 per cent of controls. The incidence of life-threatening or irreversible adverse events is very small and not easily attributable to zidovudine.

The optimum dose of zidovudine is still controversial. Early randomized studies, with short-term clinical outcomes, suggest that there is a U-shaped dose–response curve with 500 mg/day being superior to 1200 or 1500 mg/day. However, the pharmacological basis for this relationship remains unclear. Similarly, the rationale for dosing schedules, which vary from 4 hourly to 12 hourly, is not established. In view of the limited effect of zidovudine on overall survival it is prudent to give a lower dose of zidovudine (for example 200 mg three times daily) to most patients in order to avoid dose-dependent toxicity. Higher doses (1500 mg/day) are often preferred for the treatment of HIV encephalopathy or myelopathy.

DIDANOSINE

Dideoxyinosine (ddI) is subject to acid-mediated hydrolysis and therefore must be administered with a buffer in a sachet or chewable tablet. Because of the long intracellular half-life of the active metabolite (ddI-triphosphate), the drug does not need to be given more frequently than twice a day. Didanosine decreases viral antigenaemia and increases circulating CD4 counts. However, the clinical significance of these changes is unclear. Unfortunately, no large-scale placebo-controlled trials have yet been completed, although the drug has been widely used in patients who are intolerant to zidovudine. The MRC–ANRS European–Australian Alpha trial of didanosine in 1700 symptomatic patients intolerant of zidovudine compared the effect of high dose (750 mg twice daily) with low dose (200 mg twice daily) didanosine. Although the trial was very powerful, there was no difference between the two doses in the rate of development of AIDS, HIV encephalopathy, or mortality. Despite the lack of clinical effect (two-thirds of the patients died), CD4 counts increased more with high dose than with low dose didanosine. Smaller trials have compared the clinical effect of didanosine with zidovudine. In subgroups of patients, particularly those who have taken zidovudine for some time, didanosine appears to be superior to zidovudine. However, the relevance of zidovudine resistance in explaining the differential effect is unclear. *In vitro,* didanosine is effective against zidovudine-resistant strains, although these viruses can also develop resistance to didanosine *in vitro.* More information from clinical trials is required to determine the role of didanosine monotherapy in treatment.

Fig. 10 Results of the Concorde study. (a) Survival by treatment group. (b) AIDS-free survival by treatment group. (c) CDC Group IV disease-free survival.

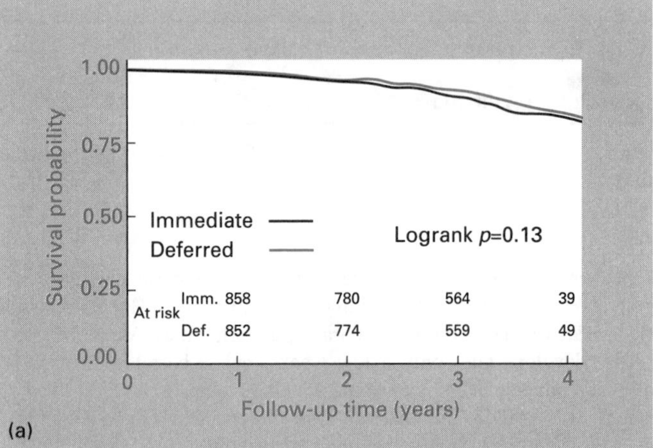

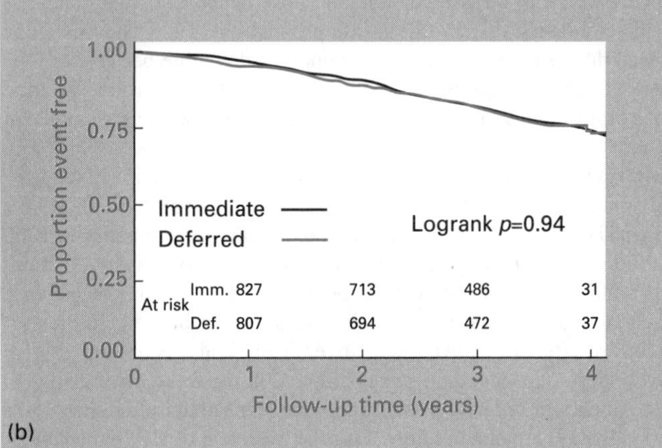

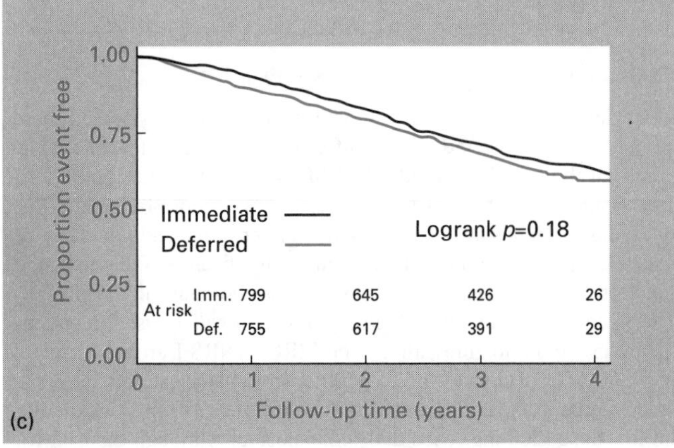

In contrast with efficacy, the toxicity of didanosine is well characterized. Pancreatitis is the most important adverse event. It is dose dependent: about 1 per cent of patients on 750 mg twice daily suffer fatal pancreatitis, but this is much less frequent on lower doses. Diarrhoea is the most common cause of patient intolerance to didanosine, but fortunately it is reversed by stopping treatment.

ZALCITABINE

Dideoxycytidine is well absorbed. Like zidovudine and didanosine it decreases circulating viral antigen and increases CD4 counts. Its main dose-limiting toxicity is peripheral neuropathy. If the drug is not promptly stopped, the neuropathy may not be reversible. There have been no placebo-controlled studies of zalcitabine; comparisons of zalcitabine monotherapy with zidovudine in zidovudine-experienced patients and with didanosine in zidovudine-intolerant patients have not shown any great difference in clinical outcome. It is most likely to be used in combination with other nucleoside analogues.

COMBINATION THERAPY

The development of drug resistance together with the clinical failure of monotherapy has prompted great interest in combination treatments in the hope that they will prevent the development of resistance. The results of one clinical trial comparing zidovudine + zalcitabine, zidovudine monotherapy, and zalcitabine monotherapy in patients who had taken zidovudine for more than 6 months showed no difference in the rate of clinical progression. It is difficult to extrapolate these results to patients who have not taken zidovudine and therefore are likely to be infected with zidovudine-sensitive strains. At present there are a number of clinical trials (the European-Australian Delta trial, the United States trials ACTG 175, and the COPRO trials) comparing zidovudine monotherapy with zidovudine + zalcitabine and zidovudine + didanosine in several thousand patients, some of whom will not have taken zidovudine before. The results of these trials, which are planned to be reported in 1995–1996, will be critical in the evaluation of the efficacy of nucleoside combinations.

EXPERIMENTAL DRUGS

The efficacy of other classes of drugs, such as CD4-receptor-blocking agents, immunomodulators, and immunostimulating agents, has proved disappointing so far (Table 11). At present, different nucleoside analogues, non-nucleoside reverse transcriptase inhibitors (e.g. nevaripine), and the protease inhibitors are being tested in clinical trials. Experimental drugs are screened for their effect on circulating viral load, on circulating CD4 counts, and on the development of viral resistance. Mono and combination therapy with new protease inhibitors and combination therapy with zidovudine and lamivadine (3TC, 2′,3′-dideoxy-3′-thiacytidine) have produced promising changes in these surrogate markers of efficacy. However, the clinical relevance of these changes remains unclear. The results of longer-term trials measuring clinical end-points are needed before the place of these new drugs can be determined.

ANTIVIRAL THERAPY AS PROPHYLAXIS AGAINST HIV INFECTION

The use of antiviral therapy after accidental parenteral exposure to HIV-infected blood is controversial. There is no good clinical evidence that post-exposure zidovudine alters the chances of seroconversion. Anecdotal case reports describe HIV seroconversion after needle-stick injuries despite prompt postexposure treatment with zidovudine. Zidovudine may be useful in reducing the chance of maternal–fetal transmission. A recent randomized controlled study of over 300 pregnant women showed that the zidovudine-treated group had only 16 HIV infected infants compared with 52 in the untreated control group.

Table 11 *Drugs unlikely to be active against HIV*

Suramin
Dextran sulphate
Ribavirin
AL721
CD4 receptor blockers (e.g. modified soluble CD4 receptors)
Immunomodulators
Interferon-α
Dithiocarb (diethyldithiocarbamate, imuthiol)
Isoprinosine (inosine pranobex, imunovir)

CLINICAL TREATMENT OF ESTABLISHED HIV INFECTION

The optimum use of the present anti-HIV antiviral drugs is far from clear. There is a wide range of clinical practice reflecting current uncertainties in treatment; fashions in treatment are likely to change over the next few years as new drugs and combinations and advocated and then tested in clinical trials. At present, treatment decisions focus on the issues of when to start treatment, what drug to give, and what salvage treatment to give.

TREATMENT OF SYMPTOMATIC DISEASE

At present, there is no evidence that any drug or combination is superior to zidovudine monotherapy. The results of Concorde suggest that asymptomatic patients need not be treated immediately. It is not clear at what stage the infection is too advanced for patients to obtain the clinical benefit of zidovudine. The results of the original placebo-controlled study suggest that starting zidovudine in patients with severe AIDS-related complex or AIDS prolongs their survival. Therefore a reasonable policy is to defer routine treatment with zidovudine until patients develop symptomatic disease. The best salvage treatment for patients who are intolerant of zidovudine or who are clinically failing despite zidovudine is unclear. Enthusiastic clinicians will either add or switch to didanosine or zalcitabine. However, there is little evidence that the known toxicity of didanosine or zalcitabine is balanced by any important advantages from treatment.

TREATMENT OF ASYMPTOMATIC INFECTION

In HIV disease the immune system seems to be slowly ablated during the long asymptomatic phase of the infection. If it is assumed that the immune system could never be reconstituted, even with very effective antiviral therapy, early antiviral treatment of HIV disease becomes theoretically attractive. Enthusiasm for pursuing such a policy should be moderated by the disappointing results of early and prolonged treatment with zidovudine. Advocates for early treatment argue that the best hope for asymptomatic patients may be for them to gamble that new treatments, as yet untested, will become available as salvage treatment before their disease progresses on existing therapy. Patients adopting such a policy may suffer the disadvantage of unnecessary toxicity or they may develop resistant viral strains to drugs which would otherwise be more effective as part of combination therapy.

REFERENCES

Biggar, R.J., and the International Registry of seroconverters. (1990). AIDS incubation in 1891 seroconverters from different exposure groups. *AIDS*, **4,** 1959–66.

Broder, S., Merigan, T.C., and Bolognesi, D. (ed.) (1994). *Textbook of AIDS medicine.* Williams and Wilkins, Baltimore, MD.

Chang, Y., *et al.* (1994). Identification of Herpesvirus-like DNA sequences in AIDS-associated Kaposi's sarcoma. *Science,* **266,** 1865–9.

Clumeck, N. (1995). Primary prophylaxis against opportunistic infections in patients with AIDS. *New England Journal of Medicine,* **332,** 739–40.

Concorde Coordinating Committee, Concorde MRC/ANRS (1994). Randomised double blood controlled trial of immediate and deferred zidovudine in symptom free HIV infection. *Lancet,* **343,** 871–81.

Hopkin, J.M. (1991). *Pneumocystis carinii.* Oxford University Press.

Johnston, M. and Hoth, D.F. (1993). Present status and future prospects for HIV therapies. *Science,* **260,** 1286–93.

Mills, G.D., Jones, P.D. (1993). Relationship between CD4 lymphocyte count and AIDS mortality 1986–1991. *AIDS,* **7,** 1383—6.

Neu, H.C., Levy, J.A., and Weiss, R.A. (ed.) (1993). *Focus on HIV.* Churchill Livingstone, Edinburgh.

Piot, P., Kapita, B.M., and Were, J.B.O. (ed.) (1991). *AIDS in Africa.* Current Science, London.

Pizzo, P.A. and Wilfert, C.M. (ed.) (1991). *Paediatric AIDS.* Williams and Wilkins, Baltimore, MD.

Rosen, C.A., Kurth, R., Coutinho, R.A., Schecter, M.T., Shearer, G.M., Wigzell, H., *et al.* (ed.) (1994). *AIDS 1994. A year in review.* Current Science, London.

Scaravilli, F. (ed.) (1993). *The neuropathology of HIV infection.* Springer-Verlag, Berlin.

7.10.30 Human immunodeficiency virus in the developing world

C. F. GILKS

The developing world is now bearing the full brunt of the human immunodeficiency virus (**HIV**) epidemic. More than 90 per cent of new infections are in developing countries and the virus has spread to most areas. In many cities of subSaharan Africa, where infection has been prevalent for a decade or more, HIV has already become the leading (preventable) cause of adult illness and death. Similarly profound changes in patterns of disease and death are likely in those regions of Asia and Latin America where the virus has more recently become epidemic.

In contrast to industrialized countries, where the majority of seropositive adults are asymptomatic for several years and die with an AIDS-defining illness, HIV-related diseases in developing countries appear to start relatively soon after HIV infection and high-grade virulent pathogens predominate; prolonged survival after the first episode of disease is uncommon (Figs 1 and 2). The different spectrum of disease in the developing world seems to relate more to adverse socioeconomic conditions and inadequate health care than to more rapid disease progression or the tropical environment. Unfortunately, many of the clinical data from countries practising advanced medicine are either irrelevant or inapplicable in the developing world.

HIV-1 is the cause of the global epidemic. HIV-2 is restricted geographically to parts of West Africa, although isolated cases have been found elsewhere. It appears to be transmitted less efficiently than HIV-1 but by the same routes. Dual infection can occur and prior infection with one retrovirus does not seem to offer significant protection against the other. Although few data have been published on HIV-2 disease it appears similar to HIV-1 disease but much slower to appear. This chapter deals only with infection and disease caused by HIV-1.

EPIDEMIOLOGY

Distribution

Most parts of the world have reported cases of HIV infection and AIDS. Although subSaharan Africa is the worst affected region, containing perhaps three-quarters of all cases, the virus is now spreading most rapidly in India and South-East Asia. Heterosexual and vertical transmission of the virus have resulted in its wide distribution in the general population, in sexually active adults and young children.

In most areas, HIV infection starts as an urban problem because the virus is first introduced to the larger towns and cities, and social circumstances favour transmission. Initially, infection spreads rapidly in specific core groups such as prostitutes and men who purchase sex frequently. The virus enters the general population and continues to spread. There is much movement of people between town and country. In time the epidemic reaches most rural areas, where transmission is also sustained. Where studies have been done, a clear gradation of HIV seroprevalence can be seen between urban, semiurban, and rural areas.

Regular updates are published, by country and region, by the Global Programme on AIDS (World Health Organization, Geneva), which should be consulted for the most up-to-date information.

Demography

Most infections occur in infants or young children and young, sexually active adults. Women tend to become infected an average of 5 to 10 years earlier than men. Women also have a higher risk of acquiring infection which may, in East Africa, be from 1.2 to 1.5 times greater in females than males. However, because urbanization draws more men than women to the cities, male patients predominate in urban areas. Most adults who die are economically active and have many dependants. Major social and economic problems are emerging: orphans, changes in the dependency ratio, loss of skilled and unskilled labour, and death in the educated élites are the most obvious.

There has been much debate about the demographic impact of HIV infection on Africa. Because most of the population in the developing world is under the age of 15 years and the epidemic is still maturing, it will take several decades for the full impact to emerge. In some areas population growth will slow considerably and in others total population may even decline as the virus becomes endemic.

Fig. 1 The burden of disease caused by HIV infection in the developing and the industrialized worlds. (Reproduced from Gilks 1993, with permission.)

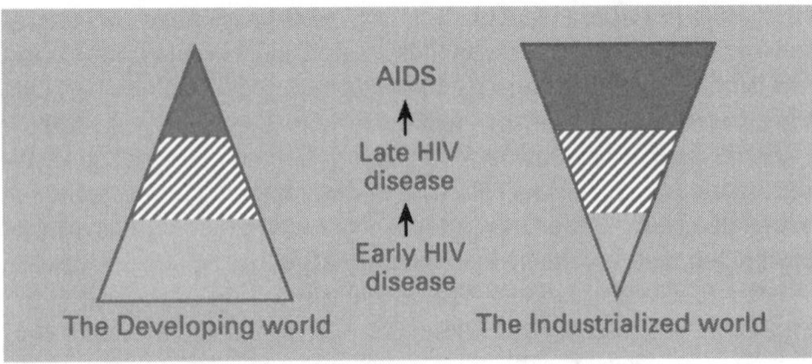

Fig. 2 Early or rapid death in the developing world? The solid line represents the progressive decline in immune function, with AIDS at 7–8 years and death at 10 years, that is typical for affluent male homosexuals living in the United States. In the developing world, HIV-related death seems to be occurring much sooner—perhaps only 5 years after infection. Two distinct biological explanations are possible: (a) early death—normal disease progression (line a) and early death with high-grade pathogen; (b) rapid death—accelerated disease progression (line b) and rapid death with AIDS-defining problem. (Reproduced from Gilks 1993, with permission.)

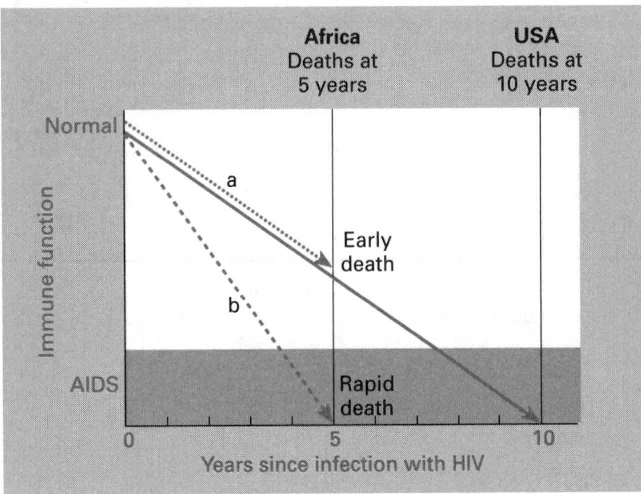

Prevalence

Prevalence is monitored by serological surveys of particular high-risk groups, such as prostitutes or patients with sexually transmitted diseases; or of representative population samples such as military recruits or pregnant women. Surveillance for AIDS is done with a clinical case definition rather than the Centers for Disease Control AIDS definition (many hospitals in the developing world do not have the necessary laboratory facilities to identify specific AIDS indicator diseases). Several definitions, and modifications, have been proposed and the Centers for Disease Control definition was widened in 1993 to include all tuberculosis, recurrent pneumonia, and cervical neoplasia. The role and the usefulness of clinical AIDS surveillance is becoming less clear.

Although the data are of variable quality and often incomplete, several facts are clear. After being introduced to a vulnerable community HIV can spread with great rapidity; in drug users in Bangkok seroprevalence went from 2 to 46 per cent in only 8 months. Extremely high levels of infection can occur through heterosexual transmission. Several African cities including Blantyre, Kampala, Lusaka, and Nairobi have recorded seroprevalence above 20 per cent in antenatal women, and in 1992 in Kigali, Rwanda, 34 per cent of pregnant women were HIV positive. In most cities the epidemic shows so far little sign of levelling off, although in Kinshasa seroprevalence appears to have stabilized below 10 per cent. These differences are not well understood or explained.

The epidemic of HIV disease follows on several years after the epidemic of HIV infection. In many African cities the virus has been established long enough for the majority of medical admissions now to be HIV related; and HIV has become the leading cause of adult illness and death. Although surveillance for clinical AIDS misses much HIV disease and death, particularly the earlier and more treatable problems, it is obvious that the health services are under increasing stress.

Transmission and control

HIV is predominantly transmitted in developing countries by heterosexual intercourse. In most cities there is a preponderance of single men, which encourages prostitution. An early sexual début, particularly for women, and rapid changes of partner are common in some communities. Sexually transmitted diseases are prevalent and are often neglected or incorrectly treated; chancroid and gonorrhoea are important cofactors that facilitate sexual transmission of HIV. In males, being uncircumcised may also be an important risk factor for acquiring infection.

Health information and education to promote safe sex and fewer changes of partner is vital, especially in schoolchildren and other vulnerable groups. Condoms can reduce markedly the transmission of HIV and other sexually transmitted diseases but may be unpopular and unfamiliar in regions where they have not been widely promoted for family planning. Such prejudices can be overcome and social marketing of condoms has been successful, most notably in Zaire. Targeted interventions based around condom distribution and treatment of sexually transmitted diseases in core groups such as female sex workers are effective but expensive. Improving treatment services for sexually transmitted disease has the potential markedly to reduce HIV transmission and is being evaluated in several projects.

Intravenous drug use is widespread in certain areas and can be the vehicle for explosive transmission, as has occurred in Thailand and north-east India. Needles and syringes are shared by many individuals and tragically the epidemic may only be recognized when it is already well established. Education programmes promoting risk reduction, particularly avoiding the sharing of needles or syringes, have been effective in Bangkok.

Blood transfusion has been the easiest route of transmission to control. In many areas, establishing clear and sensible guidelines for the use of blood has reduced dramatically the number of transfusions given, especially to anaemic children with malaria. Widespread provision of facilities for HIV testing has minimized the number of infected units transfused.

Vertical transmission, from mother to infant, is important wherever maternal infection is common. HIV can be transmitted *in utero*, during delivery, and by breast milk. Rates of vertical transmission appear to be much higher in developing countries and may be about 30 per cent. It is unclear how much of the excess can be attributed to breast-feeding, and if breast-feeding is important what advice should be given to seropositive mothers. For infants in poor families the risks of dying through the inappropriate use of formula milks may exceed the risk of acquiring HIV from breast milk.

DIAGNOSIS

Two issues are particularly important in developing countries: the cost of HIV antibody testing, and quality control. Various strategies for reducing costs are suggested by the Global Programme on AIDS: these include using tests appropriate to the existing laboratory capabilities; adoption of cost-effective test strategies; pooling of serum samples before testing; and obtaining the best possible price by bulk purchasing. It is much more difficult to ensure the reliability of test results that come from laboratories without running water or regular electricity, that use test kits which may be difficult to distribute and store correctly, and that have poorly paid staff with low morale and little supervision.

CLINICAL MANIFESTATIONS

The clinical spectrum of HIV disease

Certain conventional or high-grade pathogens (virulent organisms that infect immunocompetent adults) can cause disease in the early stages of HIV infection. *Mycobacterium tuberculosis*, *Streptococcus pneumoniae*, and varicella–zoster virus are the most important. Initially the main abnormality is the high rate of infection; because immune function is relatively well preserved typical pulmonary tuberculosis, lobar pneumonia or dermatomal shingles develop. If the patient is not tested the association with HIV infection may be missed.

With disease progression, clinical features of the underlying immunosuppression such as oral candidiasis, leukoplakia (Plate 1), fungal skin rashes, zoster scar or unexplained weight loss develop; the AIDS-related complex is the preAIDS phase of HIV disease. High-grade pathogens still predominate but a wider range now includes the salmonellae, *Escherichia coli*, shigellae, and *Staphylococcus aureus*. Because immune function is markedly impaired, disease presentation is atypical and the response to therapy may be poor. Extrapulmonary tuberculosis or atypical pulmonary disease is frequent, recurrent pneumococcal infections are common, and non-typhi salmonellae are disseminated and infection may recur. Mixed infections are being increasingly recognized.

Opportunistic pathogens (organisms that do not normally cause disease or reactivate in immunocompetent individuals) become important when immune function is profoundly depressed. The hallmark of AIDS, opportunistic infections such as Pneumocystis, cytomegalovirus or *M. avium*, develop only if the individual has survived long enough for the immune system to become so damaged that it permits infection or reactivation.

High-grade pathogens present earlier and before the opportunistic infections because they are more virulent; if exposure is high they will predominate. Transmission of enteric and respiratory pathogens is intense and unavoidable in the overcrowded and insanitary slums and rural shacks of the developing world, hence tuberculosis, pneumococcal disease, and salmonellosis are very common in HIV infection. In the poorest countries, where access to good health care is very limited, relatively few patients will survive long enough to develop AIDS. In the richer, more rapidly developing countries, which can afford higher per capita spending on health, more will survive and die with AIDS.

There is considerably less exposure to high-grade pathogens in the industrialized world and, overall, much better standards of health care. Such early disease as occurs is promptly diagnosed and treated. Prolonged survival is the rule and AIDS dominates clinical practice. In developing countries only the urban élites have this pattern of disease.

Presentation

In many patients the first indication of underlying HIV disease is respiratory-tract infection. Two presentations predominate: (i) acute cough, fever, and chest pain with abnormal breath sounds and radiological shadowing, which is usually pneumococcal pneumonia; (ii) chronic cough with constitutional disturbances such as weight loss, fever, and night sweats, which is almost always pulmonary tuberculosis. In East African cities such as Nairobi over half the patients with pulmonary tuberculosis or community-acquired lobar pneumonia are now HIV seropositive. Pleural effusions, mostly tuberculous, and acute sinusitis are also important.

Dermatological problems (Plates 2 and 3) are frequent and troublesome but rarely life-threatening. Herpes zoster is another early manifestation, highly predictive of HIV infection in young adults. A chronic, pruritic, generalized maculopapular rash is common in Africa and may be related to scabies. Lack of water for washing makes skin sepsis frequent; extensive local necrosis may develop and infections can occasionally spread, particularly to muscle. Chronic genital ulcers of herpes simplex are seen, especially in patients with a past history of sexually transmitted disease. Kaposi's sarcoma usually presents in the skin.

Gastrointestinal symptoms become increasingly important with more advanced HIV infection and are a frequent cause of hospital admission. 'Slim disease', chronic watery diarrhoea with marked weight loss (Plate 4), is the most common and distressing presentation of AIDS (Fig. 3). Several pathogens have been associated with 'slim', including coccidian parasites, enteric bacteria, disseminated tuberculosis, and HIV itself. Other patients present with a high fever without any focus of infection except the gastrointestinal tract and have a negative malaria smear. Before the HIV epidemic the clinical diagnosis would have been typhoid. In one hospital series in Nairobi, 25 per cent of HIV-positive patients were admitted with this enteric fever-like illness. Most had Gram-negative rod bacteraemia, in particular *Salmonella typhimurium*.

Generalized painless lymphadenopathy, usually symmetrical, occurs in up to 40 per cent of adults as a manifestation of HIV infection with little clinical or prognostic relevance. Asymmetrical involvement of one group may be due to tuberculosis or occasionally Kaposi's sarcoma. Pericardial effusions are seen with increasing frequency and may be either tuberculous or pyogenic. A wide range of neurological symptoms has been reported. The most common presentation is chronic headache with fever and cranial nerve palsies, fungal or tuberculous meningitis. Focal toxoplasma encephalitis is rather infrequently diagnosed clinically.

Fig. 3 Kenyan patient with severe wasting typical of advanced 'slim' disease. (Copyright C.F. Gilks.)

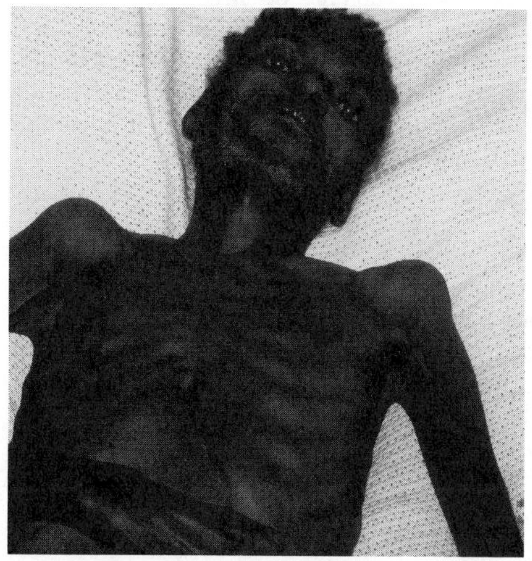

Individual clinical problems

BACTERIAL AND MYCOBACTERIAL INFECTIONS

Tuberculosis

This is an extremely important HIV-associated disease in poor communities. In Abidjan (Ivory Coast) nearly 40 per cent of seropositive adults had evidence of active tuberculosis at autopsy. Because the majority of adults in developing countries are infected with *M. tuberculosis*, and HIV is an important trigger for the reactivation of latent tuberculous infection, it is widely assumed that most active disease develops from prior (childhood) exposure. HIV-infected adults are also highly susceptible to acute primary infection. Given the intense exposure to tuberculosis in most overcrowded populations it seems likely that substantial numbers of cases also arise from acute infection, or reinfection. The underlying mechanisms of the interaction between HIV and tuberculosis are poorly understood (see Chapter 7.10.29).

About three-quarters of cases have pulmonary tuberculosis. Classical, smear-positive, upper-lobe cavitary disease is seen in the early stages of HIV infection and pleural effusions are common. Hilar or paratracheal glands are frequently enlarged. With more advanced immunosuppression, extensive, often bilateral, lower-lobe consolidation is found; sputum microscopy is usually negative but culture is positive. Extrapulmonary disease is frequent, particularly in patients with advanced HIV infection. A broad range of presentations is seen: localized adenopathy with extensive caseation, meningitis, tuberculoma, visceral abscesses, pericardial effusions, peritoneal disease, miliary spread, and disseminated anergic tuberculosis with mycobacteraemia. The clinical features suggest that both acute primary disease and reactivation are occurring.

Diagnosis can be difficult when only radiology and microscopy are available, particularly in paucibacillary pulmonary tuberculosis or extrapulmonary disease. Even if cultures are set up, several weeks are needed to make a positive diagnosis. Most patients will receive empirical therapy pending results or on clinical suspicion alone. Much treatable disease is undoubtedly being missed.

Patients with early HIV infection usually respond well to standard short- or long-course therapy. National treatment guidelines should be followed and all cases notified to the tuberculosis control services. Thiacetazone is associated with high rates of hypersensitivity and should be avoided if possible; if not, close monitoring for skin problems during the first 2 months of therapy will identify most cases early, preventing evolution into Stevens–Johnson syndrome (Plate 5). Patients with disseminated or advanced disease often do poorly, especially if mycobacteraemia is present; 25 to 30 per cent of patients in Africa may die during or soon after completing appropriate therapy. Most deaths are due to community-acquired bacterial infections rather than failure of antituberculosis treatment. Treatment failure because of drug resistance is not a major problem in Africa but will be elsewhere, especially in Asia.

Tuberculosis frequently recurs after therapy. It can be difficult to establish whether relapse or reinfection has occurred; both have been described. Short-course therapy with rifampicin may result in fewer relapses. Several studies are examining whether tuberculosis can be prevented by chemoprophylaxis and, if effective, how such intervention can be implemented. Until there is agreement about this it is vital to concentrate on case detection and follow-up.

Pneumococcal infection

Strep. pneumoniae infection is strongly associated with HIV and the risk of acquiring disease increases progressively after seroconversion. In Abidjan nearly 25 per cent of HIV-seropositive adults had bacterial pneumonia at autopsy. It is unclear why pneumococcal disease is so common in HIV infection as humoral rather than cell-mediated immunity is important in host defence.

Lobar pneumonia accounts for about two-thirds of cases; acute sinusitis, occult bacteraemia, meningitis, pericarditis, skin sepsis, and conjunctivitis is also seen. Most community-acquired pneumonia is pneumococcal but coinfection with *M. tuberculosis*, *Haemophilus influenzae*, or *S. typhimurium* is increasingly being recognized in advanced disease. Extensive disease involving more than one lobe may be more frequent in HIV-immunosuppressed patients. Recurrent disease, primarily reinfection, is extremely common and has been seen in 25 per cent of patients in one cohort in Kenya.

The majority of patients with pneumonia are bacteraemic and Gram-positive diplococci are abundant in sputum. Percutaneous lung aspiration has been safely used in several studies. Where there is no bacteriology laboratory, all cases of lobar pneumonia can be considered pneumococcal and given empirical therapy. Patients respond well to standard penicillin therapy given for 7 days, although fatality rates are consistently higher in seropositive than seronegative patients. Ampicillin, chloramphenicol, and erythromycin are also effective. Lack of response suggests a second or an alternative pathogen.

Although other clinical infections will respond well to penicillin, it can be difficult to establish a diagnosis of pneumococcal disease without culture facilities. Because other pathogens can be responsible, broad-spectrum therapy should be used for suspected septicaemia, sinusitis, meningitis, and pericarditis in the absence of an aetiological diagnosis.

In Nairobi, penicillin resistance appears to be more frequent in pneumococcal isolates derived from HIV-infected patients. As penicillin-resistant pneumococci are already widespread in several parts of sub-Saharan Africa, there is the worrying possibility that HIV will facilitate the appearance and spread of drug resistance. Once therapy is started it is important to complete the full course.

The pneumococcus is the only important HIV-associated pathogen for which a vaccine is available. It is recommended (without efficacy data) in the United States for all HIV-seropositive adults. It seems sensible to wait until the vaccine has been evaluated in developing countries before advocating its widespread use.

The salmonellae

Systemic salmonellosis and probably gastroenteritis are highly associated with HIV infection. *S. typhimurium* and to a lesser extent *S. enteritidis* are the most frequently isolated; other non-typhi salmonellae are less important and HIV does not significantly predispose to or worsen *S. typhi* infection. Gross evidence of bacteraemia was seen in over 15 per cent of HIV-infected adults at autopsy in Abidjan; although not cultured the majority were probably salmonellae. The associated defects in cell-mediated immunity are poorly defined.

Most patients present with an enteric fever-like illness that is clinically indistinguishable from typhoid. In the majority of cases salmonellae can be isolated from blood. *S. typhimurium* coinfection can also occur in patients with tuberculosis or pneumococcal pneumonia. It is unclear if asymptomatic stool carriage and acute gastroenteritis or dysentery are more common in HIV infection. In Nairobi, 10 per cent of patients with chronic diarrhoea and wasting have salmonellae in their stool and often improve with therapy; many have no features of systemic involvement.

Diagnosis requires culture of blood or stool. Drug resistance is widespread, but very heterogeneous, and treatment can be severely compromised if the drug sensitivities are unknown. Many hospitals in developing countries do not have a microbiology laboratory; few cases are identified and there is generally poor recognition of the importance of *S. typhimurium*. In Nairobi, when salmonella bacteraemia was first noted in seropositive patients, mortality was 80 per cent; with better recognition and therapy it is now 30 per cent.

Patients with bacteraemic disease may respond poorly, especially if therapy is delayed, the diagnosis missed or the organism resistant. Antimicrobial resistance is common, especially to the affordable and widely used broad-spectrum antibiotics. Ampicillin with gentamicin is first-line therapy in Nairobi, changing to chloramphenicol if resistance is found. Quinolones are reserved for multiply resistant organisms. Therapy is given for 2 weeks. Recommendations for treatment will vary according to local data on drug resistance and what antimicrobials can be afforded.

Relapses and reinfections occur. Relapses tend to develop in patients with more advanced disease, usually within 6 weeks of stopping therapy, and close follow-up is indicated. There are probably many environmental sources and therefore no obvious ways to prevent exposure. Quinolone maintenance therapy is effective but too costly for most developing countries.

Other pathogenic bacteria

Staph. aureus skin infections are common in HIV-positive patients (Plates 6 and 7); about 10 per cent of lesions also harbour β-haemolytic streptococci or occasionally anaerobes. Extensive local necrosis may develop and infection can be disseminated. Several studies have linked pyomyositis with HIV. Endocarditis appears common only in intravenous drug users. Regular wound cleaning and dressing are important. If the lesion is not healing or is developing atypically, penicillinase-resistant penicillins are necessary.

E. coli is the third most common cause of community-acquired bacteraemia in Nairobi. Most infections are thought to come from the bowel, although urinary-tract infection is more common in HIV-positive patients of both sexes. It usually presents as an enteric fever-like illness. The role of the various pathogenic *E. coli* in chronic diarrhoea is unclear; they were recovered from 15 per cent of 'slim' patients admitted to hospital in Nairobi. Antimicrobial resistance is widespread; chloramphenicol or ampicillin with gentamicin is suitable first-line therapy.

Shigella spp. are frequently isolated from the stool of HIV-positive patients with acute and chronic diarrhoea. They are widely distributed in the community and it has not yet been established if they are important causes of acute or chronic diarrhoea. HIV infection predisposes to bacteraemia. Ampicillin with gentamicin or chloramphenicol is suitable first-line therapy, modified by clinical response and drug sensitivities.

H. influenzae is occasionally isolated from the blood or lung aspirate of patients with acute pneumonia, either as the sole pathogen or with *Strep. pneumoniae*. It is responsible for less than 5 per cent of cases of HIV-related, community-acquired pneumonia and can be treated effectively with ampicillin.

Nocardia spp. may cause a chronic pneumonia that is similar to pulmonary tuberculosis; this is often identified only at autopsy.

There appears to be no important interaction between *M. leprae* and HIV immunosuppression. Neither meningococcal disease nor brucellosis seem to be associated with or exacerbated by HIV infection. There are no data from developing countries on HIV in relation to anaerobic infections, anthrax, bartonellosis, borreliosis, cholera, leptospirosis, listeriosis, melioidosis, mycoplasma diseases, pertussis, plague, group B streptococcal infections, tetanus or any of the rickettsial diseases.

PARASITIC INFECTIONS

Cryptosporidium (see Chapter 7.13.5)

Acute, self-limiting, cryptosporidial infection can occur but infection usually persists, especially in patients with advanced immunosuppression. It causes a chronic, watery diarrhoea which may initially vary in severity but usually becomes unremittent, frequent, and profuse. Patients may have anorexia, nausea, bloating, and abdominal pain and rapidly become debilitated. Fever suggests a secondary bacterial infection.

Although Cryptosporidium is ubiquitous and may be zoonotic, there is marked seasonal and perhaps geographical variation. In African patients with 'slim' disease (chronic diarrhoea and wasting), Cryptosporidium is usually the most frequent pathogen seen; the prevalence of cyst excretion in cross-sectional studies has ranged from 5 to 48 per cent. There is no specific treatment at present. Patients often require rehydration, either with oral rehydration solution or intravenously with saline, dextrose, and potassium. The role of antidiarrhoeal agents in symptom relief has yet to be established.

Isosporiasis

Isospora belli is widespread in the tropics and is an important cause of chronic diarrhoea. In most case series it is identified less frequently than Cryptosporidium and appears absent in some areas of Africa. It is common in the Caribbean, where prevalence in chronic diarrhoea is 15 per cent. Isosporiasis is important to identify because it can be treated effectively with high-dose co-trimoxazole (800 mg sulphamethoxazole and 160 mg trimethoprim, four times daily for 10 days). Recurrences are common and lifelong maintenance therapy is recommended.

Toxoplasma

Toxoplasma gondii occurs throughout the developing world and many adults have latent infection. With advanced immunosuppression (AIDS), latent foci in the brain can reactivate and cause encephalitis. In Nairobi, 20 per cent of HIV-positive hospital patients have serological evidence of reactivation but clinically obvious encephalitis consistent with toxoplasma is uncommon. There are few reports of significant rates of encephalitis, although in Abidjan nearly 20 per cent of patients at autopsy had cerebral toxoplasmosis. The initial reactivation may be clinically silent and the autopsy findings incidental; early disease with non-specific or diffuse signs may be missed; or there may be geographical variation.

Toxoplasma encephalitis is difficult to diagnose definitively, usually requiring a brain biopsy. There are characteristic findings on computerized tomographic scanning but this is not widely available in the developing world. Treatment is expensive: initial therapy with pyrimethamine and sulphadiazine, supplemented with folinic acid, should be followed by lifelong maintenance to prevent relapses. In many developing countries it may not be cost-effective to attempt to diagnose and treat toxoplasma encephalitis.

Microsporidium

Microsporidia have been identified in small bowel biopsies of selected African patients with 'slim', and some species may respond to treatment with albendazole. A systematic evaluation of their overall importance in chronic diarrhoea and advanced HIV disease has yet to be carried out in a tropical environment.

The endemic tropical parasitic diseases

Visceral leishmaniasis is well described in AIDS patients from southern Europe, arising both from acute exposure and reactivation of latent infection. There are few case reports from endemic tropical areas. Seroprevalence is at present low in many of the rural foci, the disease is difficult to diagnose, and patients may die before being immunosuppressed enough to develop visceral leishmaniasis. Any significant interaction would be of great importance in the kala-azar belt of India.

There appears to be no important interaction between malaria and HIV infection in adults; rates of parasitaemia or cerebral malaria are similar and outcome of severe disease is no worse in seropositive than seronegative hospital patients. There is no association between African trypanosomiasis and HIV. Odd case reports have described unusual manifestations of Chagas' disease in seropositive adults. Neither pathogenic amoebae nor giardiae are thought important in 'slim' or are exacerbated by HIV infection.

A few cases of hyperinfection and disseminated disease caused by *Strongyloides stercoralis* have been described but this appears a rare problem. Helminths have not been implicated in 'slim'. There are no data suggesting any important interaction between HIV and schistosomiasis, other flukes, hookworm, ascaris, filariasis, or any of the cestode (tapeworm) infections.

VIRAL INFECTIONS

Herpes zoster

Reactivation of varicella–zoster virus is very common in adult HIV infection (Plate 8). At least 20 per cent of adults will develop shingles and recurrent attacks are common. Although not life-threatening it can be extremely painful. No particular dermatomes are involved but ophthalmic zoster may be seen more frequently in hospital. Extensive necrosis can develop but generalized dissemination is rare. Keloid scars commonly develop in black patients (Plate 9).

High-dose acyclovir will reduce the duration and extent of the eruption but is costly and not widely available. Codeine phosphate, 30 to 60 mg 6-hourly, provides reasonable analgesia. Care is needed to avoid secondary bacterial infection.

Herpes simplex

Persistent or recurrent genital herpetic ulcers are seen, which are often extremely painful. Analgesia can be provided and secondary bacterial infections treated promptly even if acyclovir is not available. Nasolabial 'cold sores' appear no more frequent in HIV-positive adults with pneumonia than in HIV-negative patients.

Enteric viruses

The role of enteric viruses in HIV-associated diarrhoea and enteropathy remains unclear. Limited studies from developing countries have not shown a strong association between acute or chronic diarrhoea, HIV infection, and stool carriage of rotavirus, small, round-structured viruses, coronavirus or adenovirus. There are no data on the novel enteric viruses, such as astrovirus or picobirnavirus, that may be important pathogens in North America.

FUNGAL INFECTIONS

Candidiasis

Oral candidiasis is a common and often painful problem in many patients with moderate or advanced HIV immunosuppression. It may present in several ways; as plaques (pseudomembranous), as flat erythematous lesions (atrophic) or as angular cheilitis. Genital candidiasis is also common, especially in women. It is unclear how many patients develop oesophageal candidiasis. Systemic spread with candidaemia is uncommon.

Infection is relatively easy but expensive to control with amphotericin lozenges, nystatin, or clotrimazole pessaries or daily ketokonazole. Gentian violet is less effective and stigmatizes the patient, although it is much cheaper.

Cryptococcus neoformans

Infection with cryptococcus is highly associated with HIV. Nearly all cases are of variety *neoformans*, although a handful of cases of variety *gattii* have been described. There is wide regional variation in disease prevalence. In Rwanda the cryptococcus accounts for over 20 per cent of pathogens isolated by blood culture but in Nairobi it is less than 5 per cent. In the autopsy series from Abidjan, evidence of infection was seen in only 2.5 per cent.

Most patients present with a subacute or chronic meningitis (Plate 10). A few patients present with high fever and rather non-specific pulmonary symptoms and have fungaemia. Cutaneous nodules are occasionally seen but other manifestations are rare.

Diagnosis can be made without culture by microscopical examination of an Indian ink preparation of cerebrospinal fluid or by a latex agglutination kit. Few centres routinely make blood or sputum cultures so there is an inherent bias towards identifying meningitis rather than pulmonary or generalized disseminated disease.

Both amphotericin B and fluconazole are effective. After initial treatment, lifelong maintenance therapy is recommended. Antifungal drugs are extremely expensive and are not usually stocked in government pharmacies. Most families cannot raise the cost of a full course of treatment. Headaches can be intractable and very difficult to control; sedation may be required in the agitated and confused patient.

Other fungi

Penicillium marneffei infection is emerging as an important systemic mycosis in HIV-positive adults in South-East Asia. *Histoplasma duboisii* (Plate 11) has been reported in seropositive patients in Central Africa and *H. capsulatum* in Central America and the Caribbean. Coccidioidomycosis and paracoccidioidomycosis have been associated with HIV infection in South America. Several other fungal diseases ecologically or geographically restricted to parts of the tropics will probably become recognized as HIV-associated pathogens. They may never be common, as they are usually only seen in advanced immunosuppression.

MALIGNANCIES

Kaposi's sarcoma

Kaposi's sarcoma has always been endemic and relatively common in subSaharan Africa (Plate 12). With HIV infection a different pattern of disease has emerged. Women are more likely to be affected, although there is still a male preponderance. Lesions are more extensive, frequently involve the mucosae (Plates 13 and 14), and often visceralize. Disease is more aggressive and can progress rapidly carrying a poor prognosis (Plates 15 and 16). However, despite being endemic, Kaposi's sarcoma will develop in less than 5 per cent of African patients infected with HIV. Why it is not as prevalent in African adults as it is in North American homosexuals is not well understood. There are few data on Kaposi's sarcoma and HIV from other regions.

Patients are usually diagnosed clinically, although the histological appearances are typical. Many do not receive cytotoxic therapy as it is expensive and not widely available in hospitals in Africa. A relatively cheap regimen using actinomycin D and vincristine has proved effective in HIV-positive patients in Zambia.

Other malignancies

Lymphomas have been recorded in life and at autopsy in Africa but are uncommon and occur much less frequently than in industrialized countries. So far little work has been done on cervical neoplasia and HIV infection; no cases were seen in the Abidjan autopsy series.

OPPORTUNISTIC INFECTIONS

Many African studies have looked carefully for the common AIDS-defining opportunistic infections of the industrialized world. Pneumocystis is rarely diagnosed by bronchoscopy or at autopsy, in perhaps 2 per cent of patients. Although *M. avium* has been isolated from soil samples and colonization was seen in several patients, disseminated disease was only diagnosed once in a 2-year study in Nairobi. It has been seen at autopsy. Overt cytomegalovirus disease is clinically uncommon and, although noted at autopsy, is rarely disseminated. The most likely explanation for the rarity of these opportunistic pathogens in developing countries is that few poor patients survive long enough to develop profound immunosuppression.

Strategies for coping

In many hospitals in Africa over half the medical inpatients are HIV-positive; seroprevalence is even higher in the tuberculosis sanitoria. Health-care budgets are small and inelastic, and the services available to the (seronegative) community are being severely compromised. The greatest initial problem is the volume of new disease rather than a lack of technology or special drugs. In the absence of any clear strategies to cope with the epidemic of HIV disease, health care may collapse in many areas with devastating consequences.

Ways to cope will depend on the finances available; in poorer countries little extra will be available. One strategy is to concentrate on treatable infections in hospital and to develop home-based care for patients with chronic or end-stage problems. Tuberculosis, pneumonia, and enteric fevers are common irrespective of HIV status, so the whole community may benefit from improving the clinical outcome of these infections. Chronically sick patients often prefer being at home if some care and support can be given.

Strategies that have evolved in affluent industrialized countries (focusing on AIDS; modifying disease progression with antiretroviral therapy; developing high-technology diagnosis; preventing disease or recurrence with chemoprophylaxis) are inappropriate in most of the developing world.

REFERENCES

Anderson, R.M., May, R.M., Boily, M.C., Garnett, G.P., and Rowley, J.T. (1991). The spread of HIV-1 in Africa: sexual contact patterns and the predicted demographic impact of AIDS. *Nature*, **352,** 581–9.

Asmuth, D.M. *et al.* (1994). Clinical features of microsporidiosis in patients with AIDS. *Clinical Infectious Diseases*, **18,** 819–25.

De Cock, K.M. *et al.* (1990). AIDS—the leading cause of adult death in the West African city of Abidjan, Ivory Coast. *Science*, **249,** 793–6.

De Cock, K.M., Soro, B., Coulibaly, I.M., and Lucas, S.B. (1992). Tuberculosis and HIV infection in sub-Saharan Africa. *Journal of the American Medical Association*, **268,** 1581–7.

Foster, S.D. (1994). Care and treatment of HIV disease in developing countries from a socioeconomic perspective. *AIDS*, **8** (suppl. 1), S341–347.

Gilks, C.F. (1991). What use is a clinical case definition for AIDS in Africa. *British Medical Journal*, **303,** 1189–90.

Gilks, C.F. (1993). The clinical challenge of the HIV epidemic in the developing world. *Lancet*, **342,** 1037–39.

Gilks, C.F. *et al.* (1990). Life-threatening bacteraemia in HIV-1 seropositive adults admitted to hospital in Nairobi Kenya. *Lancet*, **336,** 545–9.

Gilks, C.F. *et al.* (1992). The presentation and outcome of HIV-related disease in Nairobi. *Quarterly Journal of Medicine*, **82,** 25–32.

Janoff, E.N., Breiman, R.F., Daley, C.L., and Hopewell, P.C. (1992). Pneumococcal disease during HIV infection. *Annals of Internal Medicine*, **117,** 314–24.

Kaldor, J.M., Sittitrai, W., John, T.J., and Kitamura, T. (eds.). (1994). AIDS in Asia and the Pacific. *AIDS*, **8** (suppl. 2), S1–214.

Kamanfu, G., *et al.* (1993). Pulmonary complications of HIV infection in Bujumbura, Burundi. *American Reviews of Respiratory Disease*, **147,** 658–63.

Lucas, S.B. *et al.* (1993). The mortality and pathology of HIV infection in a West African city. *AIDS* **7,** 1569–79.

Mastro, T.D., Satten, G.A., Nopkesoru, T., Sangkhavomya, S., and Longini, I.M. (1994). Probability of female-to-male transmission of HIV-1 in Thailand. *Lancet*, **343,** 204–7.

Mulder, D.W., Nunn, A.J., Kamali, A., Nakiyingi, J., Wagner, H-V., and Kengeya-Kayondo, J. (1994). Two-year HIV-1 associated mortality in a Ugandan rural population. *Lancet*, **343,** 1021–3.

Nunn, P. *et al.* (1991). Thiacetazone commonly causes cutaneous hypersensitivity reactions in HIV-1 seropositive patients treated for tuberculosis. *Lancet*, **337,** 627–30.

Nunn, P. *et al.* (1992). Cohort study of HIV infection in patients with tuberculosis in Nairobi, Kenya. *American Reviews of Respiratory Disease*, **146,** 849–54.

Pape, J.W., Verdier, R.I., and Johnson, W.D. (1989). Treatment and prophylaxis of Isospora belli infection in patients with AIDS. *New England Journal of Medicine*, **320,** 1044–7.

Piot, P., Kapita, B.M., and Were, J.B.O. (eds.). (1991). AIDS in Africa. *AIDS*, **5,** (suppl. 1), s1–208.

Potts, M., Anderson, R., and Boily, M.C. (1991). Slowing the spread of HIV in developing countries. *Lancet*, **338,** 608–13.

Sewankambo, N. *et al.* (1987). Enteropathic AIDS in Uganda. An endoscopic, histological and microbiological study. *AIDS*, **1,** 9–13.

Tamashiro, H., Maskill, W., Emmanuel, J., Fauqueux, A., Sato, P., and Heymann, D. (1993). Reducing the cost of HIV antibody testing. *Lancet*, **342,** 87–90.

World Health Organization. (1994). AIDS—Global data and the current global situation of the HIV/AIDS pandemic. *Weekly Epidemiological Record*, **69,** 5–8.

World Health Organization. (1994). WHO case definitions for AIDS surveillance in adults and adolescents. *Weekly Epidemiological Record*, **69,** 273–5.

7.10.31 HTLV-I and -II and associated diseases

C. R. M. Bangham and S. Nightingale

HTLV-I

Originally isolated from a patient with a cutaneous lymphoma, the human T-cell leukaemia/lymphoma virus type I (**HTLV-I**) was the first pathogenic retrovirus to be discovered in man. In contrast to the human immunodeficiency virus (**HIV**), HTLV-I causes disease in only about 5 per cent of infected people. However, the virus is of special interest and importance because it is associated with two quite different conditions: adult T-cell leukaemia/lymphoma and tropical spastic paraparesis, also known as HTLV-I-associated myelopathy. Associations between HTLV-I infection and other conditions are now being reported (see below); a suggested association with multiple sclerosis has been refuted.

The epidemiology of HTLV-I is unusual. It is endemic in many countries in the tropics, particularly the Caribbean, West Africa, parts of South America, and Papua New Guinea, where the seroprevalence is between 1 and 20 per cent of the population. Elsewhere it is found in certain aboriginal groups in North America, Australia, and northern Japan; however, the largest known area of high endemicity is in southern Japan, on the island of Kyushu, where the seroprevalence in adults aged over 25 years exceeds 20 per cent in certain prefectures. The distribution of the virus, even in highly endemic areas, is uneven, probably because of its poor transmissibility. In the United Kingdom, HTLV-I is found in 1 to 4 per cent of people of Caribbean origin. In North America and Europe, it is also found in some communities of intravenous drug abusers.

There are three important modes of transmission: perinatal and neonatal infection from a seropositive mother, in which breast-feeding is a significant factor; sexual transmission, particularly from males to females; and transmission by infected blood, either by transfusion or by sharing of needles among drug abusers. Transmission of the virus depends on transfer of cells from infected people, for cell-free virus is rare and poorly infectious.

HTLV-I is closely related genetically to leukaemia viruses in monkeys and cattle; its relationship to HIV is distant. It contains the three genes usually found in retroviruses, encoding the core protein Gag, the receptor-binding protein Env, and the polymerase Pol. The polymerase is a reverse transcriptase (RNA-dependent DNA polymerase); this is responsible for converting the viral genome into a double-stranded DNA molecule, called the provirus, which becomes integrated into the host cell DNA. In addition, HTLV-I makes at least two proteins, Tax and Rex, that regulate the transcription of the virus. Tax stimulates the production of new viral RNA, and Rex controls the splicing of viral mRNA.

Although it can infect a wide variety of cell types *in vitro*, HTLV-I replicates efficiently only in CD4+ (helper) T cells; these are the cells that are transformed in adult T-cell leukaemia/lymphoma.

Those infected with HTLV-I, with rare reported exceptions, develop antibodies that recognize the viral proteins. Diagnosis of HTLV-I infection is based on detection of these antibodies in a particle agglutination assay, or the more specific enzyme immunoassay and Western blot. Reliable estimates of the median interval between infection and seroconversion are lacking; this interval can be several years, especially in those infected during childhood. Rare individuals carry HTLV-I nucleic acid but lack antibodies or T cells specific to the virus; the significance of this is not yet understood. Antibody to the Tax protein is present in about half of infected people, and is associated with a higher antibody titre and greater infectivity. About 1 per cent of seronegative individuals in a highly endemic area in Japan were found to have antibody to Tax alone, undetected by the other assays: again, the significance of this awaits clarification. A high proportion of HTLV-I infected individuals have chronically activated cytotoxic T lymphocytes that recognize the

Tax protein; the possible pathogenetic role of these cells in tropical spastic paraparesis is at present under debate.

TROPICAL SPASTIC PARAPARESIS

The association of HTLV-I with tropical spastic paraplegia was first reported in the Caribbean by Gessain in 1985, and in Japan, where it was called HTLV-I-associated myelopathy (HAM), by Osame in 1986. Tropical spastic paraparesis mainly affects those living in, or having emigrated from, areas of endemic HTLV-I infection, but also occurs in others infected by mother–child transmission, sexual activity, intravenous drug abuse, or blood transfusion. The lifetime risk of tropical spastic paraparesis in infected individuals, based on Japanese prevalence data, is about 0.25 per cent. It is more common in women (90 per cent), beginning in the third to sixth decade of life. Progressive spastic paraparesis with gradual onset (rarely rapid) is the major feature, and most patients experience severe difficulty walking or are confined to a wheelchair within 10 years. Minor lower-limb sensory symptoms are common and may precede the onset of weakness by some months, but sensory signs are few. Most patients experience back or leg pain, which may be an early feature. Bladder involvement is common, producing frequency, urgency and incontinence; constipation is also a frequent problem. Other less common features include spastic weakness of the arms, a sensory level on the trunk or Brown–Séquard syndrome, male impotence, sensorineural deafness, and optic atrophy. Rarely, lower motor-neurone signs such as prominent wasting, fasciculation, and areflexia are observed.

The severity of the paraparesis may fluctuate and eventually stabilize, but in contrast to multiple sclerosis, tropical spastic paraparesis does not result in acute relapsing and remitting disease in the spinal cord or elsewhere in the central nervous system.

Patients with tropical spastic paraparesis are seropositive for HTLV-I, usually at titres higher than healthy carriers of the virus. However, progressive paraparesis in an HTLV-I-positive patient should not be assumed to be due to tropical spastic paraparesis, as other spinal disorders may occur in otherwise healthy asymptomatic carriers of HTLV-I. A myelogram or magnetic resonance imaging (**MRI**) scan are usually required to exclude spinal-cord compression, syringomyelia, or intrinsic cord tumour. Serum vitamin B_{12} estimation, and treponema and borrelia serology are needed to exclude metabolic or infective myelopathies. Tropical ataxic myelopathy should be considered in patients who may have suffered cyanide poisoning from poorly prepared cassava. Familial clusters of tropical spastic paraplegia have been reported, but if a patient with a family history has progressive spasticity with little or no weakness and with no sensory level or abnormality of cerebrospinal fluid, a diagnosis of hereditary spastic paraparesis should be considered.

Examination of cerebrospinal fluid usually shows a lymphocytosis of five or more cells/μl, sometimes as high as 50 cells/μl. The cerebrospinal-fluid protein may be elevated to as high as two or three times normal. Positive treponemal serology due to yaws is common among residents of, or emigrants from, the West Indies, but if treponemal serology of cerebrospinal fluid is positive, neurosyphilis should be considered, particularly if there is a history of infection or if other clinical features of syphilis are present. Visual, auditory, and lower-limb somatosensory-evoked potentials may show minor abnormalities, but electromyography and peripheral nerve conduction are usually normal. MRI scanning of the brain may show scattered lesions in the white matter similar to, though usually less extensive than, the lesions seen in multiple sclerosis.

The pathology of the spinal cord consists mainly of perivascular infiltration of mononuclear cells with proliferation of microglia and reactive astrocytic gliosis. There may be demyelination as well as capillary proliferation. The degree of inflammatory response is variable from patient to patient.

There is no specific treatment for tropical spastic paraparesis. Some patients have shown a minor response to corticosteroid treatment, but disease progression cannot be prevented. Physiotherapy and occupational therapy are important in the management of the progressive disability. Urodynamic investigation may help to select appropriate drugs, such as oxybutynine for detrusor instability, or urological surgery, such as an ileal conduit. Spasticity of the legs can be treated with baclofen or dantrolene.

ADULT T-CELL LEUKAEMIA/LYMPHOMA (ATLL)

ATLL was first identified as a syndrome in Japan in the 1970s by Takatsuki and colleagues, and the association with HTLV-I was recognized soon after the discovery of the virus in the 1980s. A person infected with HTLV-I has about a 1 per cent lifetime risk of developing ATLL; the interval between infection and disease is frequently over 20 years. The disease is slightly commoner in males (M:F = 1.2:1), and there is evidence of familial clustering of cases. In highly endemic areas it is an important cause of malignant disease: in Kyushu, Japan, ATLL accounts for 75 per cent of all non-Hodgkin's lymphomas.

The typical clinical features of ATLL are lymphadenopathy, skin infiltrates, and hepatosplenomegaly. Lytic bone lesions and hypercalcaemia are common. The morphology of the leukaemic cells is characteristic: the nucleus is large and lobulated, giving the appearance of a flower. The cells are almost invariably CD4+, and typically the interleukin 2 (**IL-2**) receptor, also known as the Tac antigen or CD25, is strongly expressed on the cell surface. Karyotypic abnormalities are common in the leukaemic cells. Morphologically similar cells are found in small numbers in the peripheral blood in some asymptomatic carriers of the virus. When the proportion of abnormal cells is high, and there is a lymphocytosis, there is a greatly increased risk of development of ATLL. However, in some cases the atypical cells regress spontaneously. Intermediate states between lymphocytosis and frank ATLL are often called 'smouldering' or 'pre'-ATLL.

ATLL results from the malignant proliferation of one or a few clones of cells transformed by HTLV-I. The mechanism of this transformation is not known. The site of provirus integration in the host cell genome is random, indicating that juxtaposition of the provirus to an oncogene is not necessary, and suggesting that the transactivator protein Tax, which can act on any region of the genome, plays a part in oncogenesis. Further indications of a role for Tax come from the demonstration that it induces the expression of several proteins that favour cell proliferation, including IL-2, IL-2 receptor, and the cellular oncogene c-*fos*. However, HTLV-I integration alone is clearly not sufficient to cause leukaemia: several additional events appear to be needed for malignant transformation. The leukaemic cells, cultured *in vitro*, only begin to produce HTLV-I virus particles after about 1 week, suggesting that continuous production of virus is unnecessary for the maintenance of the malignant proliferation.

The syndrome of ATLL has been very refractory to treatment. Sometimes remission can be obtained with cytotoxic regimens, but the disease soon relapses. The mean survival times for acute, lymphomatous, and chronic ('smouldering') ATLL in Japan are 6.2, 10.2, and 24.3 months, respectively.

OTHER DISORDERS ASSOCIATED WITH HTLV-I

Where HTLV-I is endemic, many disorders may occur by chance in asymptomatic carriers of the virus. The aetiological relation of HTLV-I to tropical spastic paraparesis and ATLL is accepted, but the range of disorders for which HTLV-I is responsible is uncertain. A list of disorders that have been associated serologically with HTLV-I is shown in Table 1; the associations are strongest with ATLL and tropical spastic paraparesis. Polymyositis (rarely in combination with tropical spastic paraparesis) has been reported in association with HTLV-I, producing a gradually progressive weakness of proximal muscles, elevated creatine kinase, and a myopathic electromyogram. HTLV-I is sometimes asso-

Table 1 *Disorders associated with HTLV-I*

Adult T-cell leukaemia/lymphoma (ATLL)
Tropical spastic paraparesis or HTLV-I-associated myelopathy (TSP/HAM)
Polymyositis
Chronic arthritis
Uveitis
Motor neurone disease-like disorder
Sicca syndrome
Lymphocytic alveolitis
Chronic infective dermatitis

ciated with predominantly lower motor-neurone features such as weakness, marked wasting, and denervation on electromyography. Rarely, this may result in a clinical picture resembling motor neurone disease. Inflammatory arthropathy and uveitis may be associated with HTLV-I in areas of endemic infection in Japan. Some patients with tropical spastic paraplegia also have sicca syndrome, a rheumatoid-like arthropathy, or a lymphocytic alveolitis. In children, HTLV-I is associated with a chronic infective dermatitis.

Among those at risk of HTLV-I infection, anti-HTLV-I antibodies should therefore be sought in cases of polymyositis, motor neurone disease, and progressive neurological syndromes in which spastic paraparesis is a prominent feature. It is likely that over the next few years the spectrum of HTLV-I-associated disorders will widen.

An association between persistent strongyloidiasis and HTLV-I infection has been suggested but is not proved.

HTLV-II

HTLV-II, a retrovirus closely related to HTLV-I, was first isolated from the tissue of a patient with hairy-cell leukaemia. The virus occurs sporadically in West Africa; in intravenous drug abusers in Europe and North America, infection with HTLV-II is as common as HTLV-I. HTLV-II is common in several native groups in both North and Central America.

Since the early 1980s, HTLV-II has been found in a small number of patients with an atypical form of hairy-cell leukaemia. However, there is not yet sufficient evidence that the virus causes this malignancy. There are case reports of a paralytic syndrome similar to tropical spastic paraplegia in HTLV-II-seropositive individuals; in some cases the paralysis is flaccid rather than spastic.

REFERENCES

Cruickshank, J.K. *et al.* (1989). Tropical spastic paraparesis and human T cell lymphotropic virus type I in the United Kingdom. *Brain*, **112,** 1057–90.

Daenke, S., Parker, C.E., Niewiesk, S., Newsom-Davis, S., Nightingale, S., and Bangham, C.R.M. (1994). Spastic paraparesis in a patient carrying defective HTLV-I proviral sequences but lacking a humoral or cell-mediated immune response to HTLV-I. *Journal of Infectious Diseases*, **169,** 941–3.

Fields, B.N. *et al.* (1990). *Virology*, (2nd edn). Raven Press, New York.

Gessain, A. *et al.* (1985). Antibodies to human T-lymphotropic virus type-I in patients with tropical spastic paraparesis. *Lancet*, **ii,** 407–10.

Jacobson, S., Shida, H., McFarlin, D.E., Fauci, A.S., and Koenig, S. (1990). Circulating CD8+ cytotoxic T lymphocytes specific for HTLV-I pX in patients with HTLV-I associated neurological disease. *Nature*, **348,** 245–8.

Kalyanaraman, V.S. *et al.* (1982). A new subtype of human T-cell leukemia virus (HTLV-II) associated with a T-cell variant of hairy cell leukemia. *Science*, **218,** 571–3.

Kuroda, Y. and Sugihara, H. (1991). Autopsy report of HTLV-I associated myelopathy presenting with ALS-like manifestations. *Journal of Neurological Sciences*, **106,** 199–205.

LaGrenade, L., Hanchard, B., Fletcher, V., Cranston, B., and Blattner, W. (1990). Infective dermatitis of Jamaican children: a marker for HTLV-I infection. *Lancet*, **336,** 1345–7.

Mochizuki, M. *et al.* (1992). HTLV-I uveitis: a distinct clinical entity caused by HTLV-I. *Japan Journal of Cancer Research*, **83,** 236–9.

Morgan, O. StC., Rodgers-Johnson, P., Mora, C., and Char, G. (1989). HTLV-I and polymyositis in Jamaica. *Lancet*, **ii,** 1184–7.

Mowbray, J. *et al.* (1989). Epidemiology of human T-cell leukaemia/lymphoma virus type 1 (HTLV-I) infections in a subpopulation of Afro-Caribbean origin in England. *Journal of Medical Virology*, **29,** 289–95.

Nishioka, K., Maruyama, I., Sato K., Kitajima, I., Nakajima, Y., and Osame, M. (1989). Chronic inflammatory arthropathy associated with HTLV-I. *Lancet*, **i,** 441.

Osame, M. *et al.* (1986). HTLV-I associated myelopathy, a new clinical entity. *Lancet*, **i,** 1031–2.

Parker, C.E., Daenke, S.D., Nightingale, S., and Bangham, C.R.M. (1992). Activated HTLV-I specific cytotoxic T cells are found in healthy seropositives as well as patients with tropical spastic paraparesis. *Virology*, **188,** 628–36.

Poiesz, B.J., Ruscetti, F.W., Gazdar, A.F., Bunn, P.A., Minna, J.D., and Gallo, R.C. (1980). Detection and isolation of type C retrovirus particles from fresh and cultured lymphocytes of a patient with cutaneous T-cell lymphoma. *Proceedings of the National Academy of Sciences* (*USA*), **77,** 7415–19.

Uchiyama, T., Yodoi, J., Sagawa, K., Takatsuki, K., and Uchino, K. (1977). Adult T-cell leukemia: clinical and hematological features of 16 cases. *Blood*, **50,** 481–91.

7.11 Bacteria

7.11.1 Diphtheria

A. B. CHRISTIE* and TRAN TINH HIEN

Diphtheria is an acute infection of the upper respiratory tract and occasionally of other mucous membranes or skin, frequently occurring in children and caused by *Corynebacterium diphtheriae*. The name of the organism is from the Greek and refers to the club-shaped rod, which produces a membrane in the throat of its victim. The disease, diphtheria, may also be of some antiquity and not unknown to the Greeks and the Romans. The 'Egyptian disease' of the Greeks may have been diphtheria and the Romans probably knew the disease as one brought back from North Africa by Scipio's legionnaires in the Hannibalian wars. If so, one aspect of the epidemiology of the disease has not changed in 2000 years, for in the Second World War, the soldiers of Rommel's North Africa Corps certainly carried the disease back into Germany, while on the other side of the world soldiers carried it from the Solomon Islands to civilians in New Zealand. The disease is not, however, characteristically one of military campaigns or of movement. Soldiers in the Second World War had not previously been exposed to the diphtheria bacillus and were highly susceptible to infection when they moved into an area where the bacillus was common. They were Schick positive, whereas most of the natives of the countries they moved into were Schick negative, from early childhood exposure to the bacillus. This difference is at the root of the epidemiology of diphtheria, for it is an infection that illustrates very sharply how the virulence of an organism clashes with the immune status of the host; an infection that causes no symptoms in the highly immune, the carrier state, but an overwhelming, often fatal disease in the patient who has no immunity at all.

C. diphtheriae and diphtheria have been virtually eliminated from Britain, but are still prevalent in many developing countries. There has been a recent increase in incidence in the Russian Federation and the Ukraine.

BACTERIOLOGY

Morphology

C. diphtheriae is a Gram-positive, non-motile, and somewhat pleomorphic organism. The club-shaped forms are long and slender with swollen ends. Some have swellings along their length; these take stains heavily and look like round dots on the body of the bacillus. Sometimes these dots look like a chain of cocci, especially when stained with methylene blue or Neisser's stain. On a slide from a culture of Loeffler's serum several of these forms will be seen, often arranged in pairs, with the pairs grouped to form clusters. Such a slide can be of diagnostic value to a physician who is familiar with diphtheria and has seen the patient from whom the culture was taken. However, one cannot on a slide distinguish between virulent and avirulent *C. diphtheriae*, nor between true diphtheria bacilli and other corynebacteria.

Growth

C. diphtheriae grows readily on ordinary nutrient agar, but much more readily on Loeffler's serum agar, on a slope of which there is a creamy growth within 24 h. A stained slide from these colonies shows many typical bacilli, and during an outbreak this is enough to confirm a clinical diagnosis. On blood tellurite agar the three types of *C. diphtheriae, gravis, mitis*, and *intermedius*, form slightly different colonies and the bacteriologist, if he or she has experience, can often tell one from the other. The three types also differ biochemically. But strains of *C. diphtheriae* may be atypical, and in countries where diphtheria has become a rare disease, microbiologists have difficulty in recognizing *C. diphtheriae* with certainty solely on cultural and biochemical tests.

Toxin production

The serious effects of diphtheria in man are caused by diphtheria toxin, and only by testing the organism for toxigenicity can one finally determine that a corynebacterium is a true *C. diphtheriae* and whether it is pathogenic or not. The ability of an organism to produce bacteriocine or diphthericin corresponds closely with its toxigenicity and such tests may be useful during epidemics, but guinea-pig tests are still the most reliable for toxin production. All strains produce the same toxin, but small changes in the medium, such as the amount of iron, affect the rate of growth and so the amount of toxin produced: the conditions in the throat of a patient may favour the growth of *gravis* and *intermedius* strains more than *mitis* and so lead to the production of more toxin by the first two. There appear to be two factors in diphtheria toxin, factor A the lethal and factor B the spreading factor. Factor A exerts its full lethal effect only when enough B is present, and *gravis* strains always seem to be rich in factor B. Whatever the exact mechanism, very small doses can cause death: it needs only eight times the lethal guinea-pig dose to kill a 5-year-old child. Factor B, not factor A, calls forth protective antibody.

Toxigenic and non-toxigenic *C. diphtheriae*

Toxigenic *C. diphtheriae* carry a tox phage that induces the cell to produce toxin. This phage can pass from a toxigenic to a non-toxigenic strain. This may be important in an outbreak, when the introduction of a toxigenic strain into a community may convert harmless non-toxigenic strains in carriers' throats into dangerous toxigenic strains.

PATHOGENESIS

The action of toxin

Diphtheria exotoxin is a 62-kDa polypeptide, the spreading factor B, which attaches to the cell membrane allowing the lethal factor A to enter the cells, where it catalyses a reaction that inactivates elongation factor 2, the transferase RNA, in eukaryotic cells. This factor is essential for reactions that transfer triplet codes from mRNA to amino acid sequences via tRNA. The inactivation of elongation factor 2 stops synthesis of the polypeptide chains and the most profound effects are on the myocardium, peripheral nerves, and kidneys.

Membrane formation

The typical membrane on the throat or on other parts of the body, the skin for example, is the result of an inflammatory reaction to the presence of multiplying *C. diphtheriae*. Fluid and leucocytes pass from dilated blood vessels on the inflamed surface, where the epithelial cells become necrotic. The fluid clots and grips these dead cells, enmeshing at the same time leucocytes, diphtheria bacilli, cellular debris, and sometimes small blood vessels.

*Dr Barnett Christie died in 1987. Much of his second edition chapter has been retained in this edition.

Effect on nerves

C. diphtheriae does not normally pass beyond the membrane site, but it has occasionally been seen in organs at autopsy, and it has been isolated, though very rarely, from blood taken from contacts before they have developed a membrane in the throat. But there is no doubt that it is toxin that causes the severe damage in diphtheria. It can pass in the bloodstream to the heart and other internal organs and become fixed to cells, but how and where it reaches the nervous system is not so clear. There is evidence to support blood, lymph, and neural spread, and demyelination of peripheral nerves is certainly common. This, and degeneration of sensory and motor fibres, may be seen in the nerves to the eye, the palate, pharynx, larynx, and heart and in the nerves to the muscles of the limbs. Whether the toxin can pass the blood–brain barrier and cause central lesions is not so certain.

Effect on the heart

The lesions in most organs, the liver, spleen, and kidney for example, are non-specific. In the adrenals the changes are usually slight and barely detectable, very different from the congestion and haemorrhage seen in the guinea-pig adrenals. In the heart, changes are common: fatty degeneration of cardiac muscle and infiltration of the interstitium with leucocytes, sometimes affecting the conduction fibres, is seen, but necrosis of the parenchyma is rare. Fibrosis and scarring, if severe, may lead to death in late convalescence, but usually, if the patient survives the acute toxaemic state, the heart recovers completely. Mural endocarditis may occur and embolism may then cause hemiplegia, but valvular endocarditis is a very rare finding. In the late paralytic stage of the disease, neuritic changes may be seen in the nerves to the heart.

Antigenic types

C. diphtheriae can be classified serologically into many subtypes, although it is not clear which antigens are responsible for the differences. There are at least 13 *gravis*, 4 *intermedius*, and 40 *mitis* serological types. The organism may also be classified into types by bacteriophage lysing, and all toxigenic strains are lysogenic. Phage types I to III are *mitis*, IV to V *intermedius*, VII an avirulent *gravis*, and the rest all *gravis* strains. These phage types are stable. Typing based on bacteriocine or diphtheriocin production by *C. diphtheriae* has already been mentioned. One serotype may contain variants that differ both in bacteriocine and bacteriophage characters. Typing is useful, and sometimes essential, in tracing the spread of apparently unconnected outbreaks of the disease.

HOST IMMUNITY AND SPREAD OF INFECTION

The Schick test

The injection of a measured amount of toxin into the skin of the forearm will cause a red reaction (positive Schick test) unless the patient has a sharp enough antibody response to prevent it. This is the basis of the Schick test. A Schick-negative person is very unlikely to get diphtheria or, if he or she does, is likely to have a mild attack. A Schick-positive person may have an attack of any severity, subclinical, mild or fatal. The amount of antibody in a person's serum can be measured by several assay methods but just what level of antitoxin indicates susceptibility is not clear. The antibody response to an antigenic stimulus is more important than the original level of serum antibody. The test measures this response and has stood the test of time.

Schick conversion

The newborn child is often Schick negative, protected by original antibody, but loses this immunity round about the sixth month and becomes Schick positive. The child is then exposed to infection from without, depending on how common *C. diphtheriae* is in the environment. In a highly immunized community, *C. diphtheriae* tends to die out and the child may grow to adult life without meeting the bacillus. Among American soldiers during the Second World War the Schick-positive rate before going overseas was between 35 and 45 per cent. In other parts of the world, *C. diphtheriae* is a common pathogen and the young child meets it early, maybe becoming a faucial, nasal, or aural carrier. Many children suffer severe or fatal attacks before the age of 5 years. This is a pattern that may be seen in large subtropical cities lacking an efficient immunization programme.

Diphtheria in pregnancy

A Sudanese woman in the ninth week of pregnancy developed severe diphtheria with widespread paralysis. She recovered and gave birth at term. The baby was normal, although serological tests suggested that some toxin might have passed through the placenta. This seems to be the only recorded case of diphtheria in pregnancy.

Fomites, dust, and milk

Diphtheria spreads from person to person, from the acute case or the carrier. Fomites and dust are not important, although the organism resists drying and can be isolated from floor dust in a ward or an infected classroom. Diphtheria has been spread by milk contaminated by a human carrier: animals do not suffer from diphtheritic mastitis nor excrete *C. diphtheriae* in their milk, *C. diphtheriae* is a parasite exclusively of man. Pasteurization kills *C. diphtheriae* as does heating at 58°C for 10 min or exposure to most common disinfectants.

CLINICAL FEATURES

Diphtheria is predominantly an infectious disease of children. After an incubation period of 2 to 5 days, it presents in a variety of different forms depending upon the location of the membrane. In clinical practice the disease can be divided into the following types: cutaneous, nasal, faucial, tracheolaryngeal, and malignant diphtheria.

Anterior nasal diphtheria

The main symptom is nasal discharge, thin at first, then thick, purulent, and bloody, with soreness of the nostril and the skin above the lip, and crusting or thin membrane inside the nostril (Fig. 1). Nasal diphtheria is relatively common in infancy. It is often mild except when faucial or nasopharyngeal forms coexist.

Faucial diphtheria

This is the most common form of diphtheria. The onset is slow. The child is off-colour, tired but not acutely ill. He may have no sore throat, very unlike a child with acute streptococcal tonsillitis or early scarlet fever. On the first day of his illness, there may be only a small spot of membrane on his tonsils, a few millimetres wide, yellowish white, and with a crinkled edge (Plate 1). No one is likely to look at the throat at this stage, unless it is a doctor examining contacts. Soon the membrane spreads over most of both tonsils, greyish-yellow, a millimetre thick and all of one piece, not soft and mushy, edged with a rim of redness but confined to the tonsils. The rest of the throat and fauces looks normal. The lymph nodes in the neck are a little enlarged and a little tender.

Fig. 1 Diphtheria: shreds of membrane in the nose.

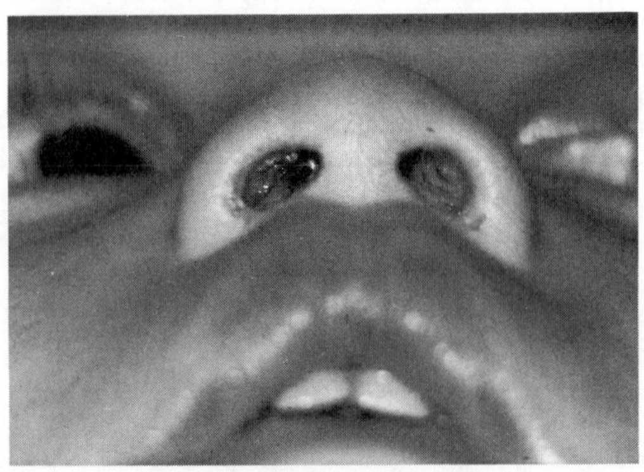

After another day or two the membrane is greenish-black, and later it sloughs off. A typical case of diphtheria is easy to diagnose so long as it is typical, but anyone with experience of diphtheria knows it is dangerous to rely on clinical appearance alone. Tonsillar diphtheria can look very like any other form of tonsillitis.

Tracheolaryngeal diphtheria

Diphtheria of the larynx is usually secondary to faucial diphtheria (85 per cent). Occasionally, there is no membrane on the pharynx at all. The initial symptoms include moderate fever, with hoarseness and unproductive cough. Obstruction to breathing comes on gradually in the course of 24 h or so: the lower intercostal spaces are sucked in as the child breathes in, showing that enough air is not getting in to fill the lungs. Later the fossae above and below the clavicles, the epigastrium, and the sternum itself are sucked in as the child tries to drag air through the narrowed larynx. The child pulls himself up the side of the cot in his struggle for breath, his face congested, and his lips blue. This may bring on a feeble spasm of coughing and he falls back, grey and exhausted from asphyxia. Without tracheostomy the child will soon be dead. Tracheostomy brings rapid relief if the membrane is confined to the larynx and upper part of the trachea. In a few cases the membrane has spread down into the bronchi and bronchioles and then tracheostomy helps very little. In the pure laryngeal case the relief is dramatic and the child falls into a sound sleep.

Malignant diphtheria

The onset is more acute, the patient soon becoming very ill with high fever rapid pulse, low blood pressure, and cyanosis. The membrane spreads from the tonsils to the uvula then creeps forward cross the hard palate (Plate 2), up the nasopharynx, or sometimes down the nostrils. It has a thick edge and as this advances the earlier parts become necrotic. It is now foul, greenish-black, and smelly. The smell, the foetor oris, is not diagnostic, for any foul exudate smells, as, for example in Vincent's angina or infectious mononucleosis. The lymph nodes in the neck are now very swollen, but it is not easy to feel them separately because the surrounding tissues of the neck are swollen too. The whole space between the mandibles and the clavicles is bulging with lymph nodes and oedema; this is the 'bull neck' of malignant diphtheria (Plate 3). The patient may bleed from the mouth, nose, and skin (Plate 4). Cardiac involvement with heart block occurs earlier, within few days from the onset. Such a patient has little hope of recovery.

Skin

In contrast to the severe course of some faucial infections, *C. diphtheriae* often causes chronic but mild infections of the skin. This is especially common in the tropics and has already been mentioned. Perhaps the temperature and the moisture of the skin, and the scanty clothing may have something to do with it. Sores and ulcers are most common on the legs but may occur anywhere. The sores are indolent and slow to heal. Paralysis may occur, usually of the affected limb, or myocarditis, but both are rare. Absorption of toxin is slow from the skin and leads to seroconversion of the patient rather than to any toxic complication.

The eye

Conjunctivitis is not uncommon. Usually this is no more than a slight, catarrhal condition in a patient with faucial diphtheria. Occasionally membrane forms in the lower conjunctiva and spreads over the cornea causing great destruction of tissue.

The gastrointestinal tract

C. diphtheriae may spread to the oesophagus from the fauces causing dysphagia, and there are reports of membrane in the stomach and the intestine; but these are pathological curiosities.

Urogenital tract

Diphtheria may be spread on a child's fingers from the throat to the vulva causing local sores; this is not altogether rare. Occasionally *C. diphtheriae* invades the vagina and even the cervix, when there may be serious absorption of toxin, but this is certainly rare. Diphtheria of the glans or coronal sulcus of the penis has occurred in infants after circumcision. In one case the father was a soldier with unrecognized skin diphtheria. Sores on the penis may also occur on men in conditions where diphtheria of the skin is spreading. A report of diphtheria membrane found on the wall of the bladder at operation is probably unique; the patient developed peripheral neuritis and died of heart failure.

Endocarditis

This must be rare, but cases are on record where *C. diphtheriae* has been isolated from heart blood and valves after death. There is at least one record of a proved case successfully treated with a prolonged course of antimicrobials.

Other corynebacteria

C. ulcerans produces two toxins, one of which seems to be the same as diphtheria toxin. It can cause membranous tonsillitis but rarely seems to cause toxic complications, nor to spread from patient to patient. It has been spread to man in the milk of cows excreting the organism. *C. xerosis* has been isolated from blood of patients with bacterial endocarditis and from prosthetic valves at operation. *C. haemolyticum* has caused outbreaks of tonsillitis with or without a maculopapular rash, and *C. sepsis* caused death in a few patients on immunosuppressive treatment for some other condition. All these, except perhaps *C. haemolyticum*, are uncommon or rare infecting agents. *C. vaginale* (now classified as *Gardnerella vaginalis*) seems to be a common vaginal commensal, and, when present in numbers, a frequent cause of vaginitis. It has also been isolated from the urine of men with cystitis or urethritis and in one from the blood of a patient after prostatectomy.

COMPLICATIONS

Diphtheria is a terrible disease. Even if the patient survives the acute, destructive phase of the infection, he or she is likely to die from the delayed effects of the toxin. The most prominent toxic complications of diphtheria are myocarditis and neuritis. The risk and the severity of toxin damage correlate with the extent of the membrane and the delay in administration of antitoxin.

Cardiovascular changes

Approximately 10 per cent of patients with diphtheria develop myocarditis, although two-thirds of patients with severe infection will have some evidence of cardiac involvement. The frequency of cardiac complications of laryngeal and malignant diphtheria is three- to eightfold higher compared with the faucial form, and two- to threefold higher if antitoxin is given later than 48 h from the onset of disease. The first evidence of cardiac toxicity usually occurs after the first weeks of the illness. The patient complains of pain in the upper abdomen and may vomit; often he becomes apathetic. The pulse is rapid and thready; the blood pressure collapses. The patient is in shock. He may die at this stage or go on to show signs of cardiac failure. The apex beat is displaced downwards and outwards, there are murmurs at all areas, and a triple or gallop rhythm. The liver enlarges; urine is scanty. Electrocardiographic changes are common (Plate 5): a flattening or inversion of the T wave, a lengthening of the PR or QT interval, or in severe cases, bundle-branch or complete block. Atrial or ventricular fibrillation may occur. Death is not inevitable but most deaths from diphtheria do occur at this stage. But if the patient recovers, the recovery is complete.

Paralyses

Paralyses come on late, usually many weeks after the onset of the illness. Palatal paralysis is common, even after tonsillar diphtheria. It comes on about the third week, causes a nasal voice, allows fluids to come down the nose on swallowing, but usually disappears after a week or so—a minor complication with careful management. A little later the child may have blurred vision from paralysis of accommodation or an internal squint from external rectus paralysis—again, a passing inconvenience. About the sixth or seventh week the dangerous paralyses come on: paralysis of the pharynx making swallowing difficult or impossible; paralysis of the larynx adding greatly to the danger; then paralysis of the breathing muscles. The nerves to the heart may be affected, with tachycardia and great irregularity of rhythm. These paralyses are all dangerous to life and many patients die at this stage, often after several weeks when everything seemed to be going well. Sometimes a child is discharged from hospital when all the throat signs have cleared up and he seems well, but dies weeks later in his home from what seems to be a new and unconnected illness. The outlook for a child with late paralysis is not hopeless if skilfully treated; he resembles a child with poliomyelitis, but with this difference, that if he can be kept alive with expert care, the paralyses eventually disappear completely and the child regains normal health, whereas a child with severe poliomyelitis is usually left with some permanent paralysis. Children with late paralyses of diphtheria often suffer from weakness or paralysis of the limbs, especially the legs, but this too always disappears if the child survives the other paralyses.

DIAGNOSIS

Clinical

In many parts of the world diphtheria is still a common disease and there one should always think of diphtheria in a child with exudate on the throat. If the exudate is thick and discoloured, the child should be given antitoxin. Elsewhere the idea of diphtheria is unlikely to enter the mind of doctors who have never seen or heard of a case since qualifying. They know infectious mononucleosis; there is membrane on the patient's throat and the cervical glands are enlarged, but the membrane is white, even after a week, and the neck glands are discrete. It is no great harm to diagnose as diphtheria a case of infectious mononucleosis; but the other way round is a tragic error. Even more tragic is to diagnose a case of bull-neck diphtheria as mumps; always look at the throat. Streptococcal or viral tonsillitis cannot be distinguished from diphtheria with only a few flecks on the tonsils, but it should not be confused with severe membranous diphtheria. Peritonsillar abscess, quinsy, can cause great distortion of the tissues of the throat so that one cannot see the surface of the tonsils and this happen, too, in severe diphtheria, so one must take care. Monilial infection causes soft, white exudate and there are often patches on the cheeks and gums as well. Secondary syphilis in the adult sometimes causes glairy exudate on the tonsils; the patient usually has rash and laryngitis. Leukaemia and other blood dyscrasias cause foul ulceration in the fauces, bleeding into the skin, and great toxicity in the patient, a picture very like severe diphtheria. In such conditions only blood counts and bacteriological investigations can lead to a diagnosis, if they are done. They would be, if the doctor would only think 'Can this be diphtheria?'

Laboratory

Direct stained smears from throat swabs, if positive, can help experienced doctors who have also seen the patient; but only experienced doctors, and only if they look at the smears themselves. Smears from cultures the next day are more helpful during an outbreak and they meet most needs. In isolated cases where there is any bacteriological doubt, full cultural, biochemical, immunological, and guinea-pig tests must be done. Occasionally, with an atypical strain, only a reference laboratory can classify the corynebacterium.

TREATMENT

Only antitoxin can neutralize toxin, and it can do so only before the toxin reaches and damages tissue cells. So it must be given soon as possible after *C. diphtheriae* begins to multiply in a patient's throat; on clinical suspicion and before bacteriological confirmation. Hypertoxic diphtheria is hypertoxic from the start: it is wrong to believe that only in late cases is there danger to life. The dosage depends on the site of primary infection, the extent of membrane, and the delay between the onset and the antitoxin administration: 20 000 to 40 000 units for faucial diphtheria of less than 48-h duration or cutaneous infection; 40 000 to 80 000 units for faucial in excess of 48 h or laryngeal infection; 80 000 to 100 000 units for malignant diphtheria (bull-neck, toxic state).

With highly purified antitoxin the danger from a dangerous serum reaction is much less than the danger of death from hypertoxic diphtheria, but one can over a period of an hour or two give small but increasing doses of antitoxin up to the full intramuscular dose, when the intravenous dose can then be given.

C. diphtheriae is nearly always sensitive to penicillin and it seems logical to give patients a course of the drug, or of erythromycin if the patient is truly sensitive to penicillin. This will get rid of the organisms in the throat or in the skin, but only antitoxin can deal with any toxin that has passed from the organisms into the bloodstream. Most carriers can be cleared with antibiotics. The recommended antibiotic treatment regimens are penicillin G 100 000 u/kg in four divided doses a day until the patient is able to swallow, when oral penicillin V or erythromycin (50 mg/kg) may be substituted for a total treatment period of 10 to 14 days.

For cardiac complications, intensive care is needed. Sedation is essential and often the child needs extra oxygen. Digitalis is useful only when there is congestive failure. A cardiac pacemaker has been used to help a child over temporary conduction failure. Expert assessment is valuable, but perhaps the main requirement, and often the only one available, is skilled nursing. For paralysis, expert nursing is again required; for careful suction of pharyngeal secretions, which the patient cannot swallow or cough out, and for intragastric or intravenous feeding. When breathing fails, assisted ventilation is essential. The work is demanding but rewarding, for even the child with the most severe paralysis can, with care, make a complete recovery.

PREVENTION

Active immunity

Diphtheria is one of the great preventable diseases. With a good immunization programme, there need never be another case. Diphtheria toxoid is usually given, along with tetanus and pertussis vaccine, as DTP to infants between 3 and 6 months old. The usual course is of three doses, the first and second separated by at least 4 weeks, the third after 6 months. In some countries because of geographical and many other difficulties, it may be difficult to arrange three visits to or by the vaccinator, but there is evidence that two doses separated by at least 2 months give protection. This is not to say that two doses are better than three; simply that in difficult conditions two may be enough. A booster dose of diphtheria tetanus (DT) vaccine at school entry, if there is a school, will ensure prolonged immunity. When such a programme is well organized, *C. diphtheriae* finds it hard to spread in the community and diphtheria is no longer a common disease.

The marked increase in numbers of cases of diphtheria in Russian cities, especially Moscow and St Petersburg, and in the Ukraine, over the last few years has prompted a recommendation in Britain that travellers to these areas should have a full course of three injections of vaccine at monthly intervals if they have never been vaccinated and a booster dose of low-dose vaccine if their primary vaccination course was more than 10 years ago.

Passive immunity

Contacts of a patient may be protected for 2 or 3 weeks by 1000 to 2000 u of antitoxin. This may be useful when there is danger of cross-infection in a ward from a missed case, or in home contacts of a patient. However, penicillin given to close contacts may be equally effective. It is certainly the best treatment for carriers.

Control of outbreaks

We have all the tools to control an outbreak in a closed community: the Schick test to detect susceptibles, bacteriology to confirm cases and find the carriers, vaccine to immunize Schick-positive children, and antitoxin or penicillin to protect the children while they are acquiring active immunity. The main need is intelligent application of these measures. Out in the field or in the villages or in wider epidemics, control is not so easy, but the principles are the same. Eradication lies with active immunization.

REFERENCES

Ch'in, K.Y. and Huang, C.H. (1941). Myocardial necrosis in diphtheria with a general review of the lesions of the myocardium in diphtheria. *American Heart Journal*, **22,** 690–701.

Christie, A.B. (1980). *Infectious diseases: epidemiology and clinical practice*, (3rd edn). Churchill Livingstone, Edinburgh.

El Seed, A.M., Dafalla, A.A., and Abboud, O.I. (1982). Intrauterine foetal growth and development and foetal immune response following maternal diphtheria during early pregnancy. *Annals of Tropical Paediatrics*, **1,** 213–19.

Farizo, K.M., Strebel, P.M., Chen, R.T., Kimbler, A., Cleary, T.J., and Cochi, S.L. (1993). Fatal respiratory disease due to *Corynebacterium diphtheriae*: case report and review of guidelines for management, investigation and control. *Clinical Infectious Diseases*, **16,** 59–68.

Gibson, L.F. and Colman, G. (1973). Diphthericin types, bacteriophage types and serotypes of *Corynebacterium diphtheriae* strains isolated in Australia. *Journal of Hygiene (Cambridge)*, **71,** 161–4.

Hart, R.J.C. (1984). *Corynebacterium ulcerans* in humans and cattle in *North Devon. Journal of Hygiene (Cambridge)*, **92,** 161–4.

Helting, T.B. and Zwisler, O. (1976). Breakdown of diphtheria toxin isolation of a stable immunogenic fragment B derivative. *Behring Institut Mitteilungen*, **59,** 92.

Hong, N.T., Phu, V.T., and Hien, T.T. (1985). A study of 2,597 cases of diphtheria treated at Cho Quan Hospital during 10 years (1976–1985). *Annual Scientific Report of Cho Quan Hospital.*

Liebow, A.A. and Bumstead, J.H. (1963). Cutaneous and other aspects of diphtheria. In *History of internal medicine in World War II*, Vol. II, p. 275. Office of the Surgeon General US Army, Washington DC.

Robinson, D.T. and Marshall, F.W. (1934). Investigations on the gravis, mitis and intermedius types of *C. diphtheriae* and their clinical significance. *Journal of Pathology and Bacteriology*, **38,** 73–89.

Simmons, L.E. *et al.* (1980). Diphtheria carriers in Manchester; simultaneous infection with toxigenic and non-toxigenic mitis strains. *Lancet*, **1,** 304–5.

Wilson, S.A.K. (1954). Diphtheria. In *Neurology*, Vol. 11. Butterworth, London.

Streptococci

7.11.2 Pathogenic streptococci

G. COLMAN

The streptococci and related organisms are distributed widely and some species are important pathogens of man or animals. Most, however, are commensals or opportunistic pathogens.

The organisms

Major changes are taking place in the classification and naming of those bacteria formerly brought together in the genus Streptococcus. In the past, species among the streptococci were created because of the need to identify cultures that might cause disease or were of industrial importance. The study of the action of streptococci on blood was the first clue to the identification of the major pathogens and is still reported. The streptococci that lysed erythrocytes in blood agar were called β-haemolytic and included isolates from invasive infections and sore throat. In contrast, strains from illnesses such as bacterial endocarditis, or the normal flora, often caused green discoloration (α-haemolysis), or no apparent change, in the red cells. The description of the Lancefield group antigens provided a workable method for the identification of the pyogenic streptococci—in particular the major human pathogen *S. pyogenes* (Lancefield group A) and also animal pathogens such as *S. agalactiae* (group B) or *S. zooepidemicus* (group C). Greater precision in defining species was achieved with the gradual discovery of appropriate physiological and biochemical tests, such as differences in salt or heat tolerance and species-defining patterns of carbohydrate fermentation and enzymatic activity. This 'classification from below' is being replaced by 'classification from above' in which molecular biologists are creating new genera and species that reflect phylogenetic relationships based, particularly, on the study of sequences of 16*s* ribosomal RNA.

Table 1 gives an outline of the streptococci and related organisms that are handled routinely in medical laboratories. Some of the diseases they cause are listed in Table 2. Six species are aggregates. The species, from two to seven, composing each aggregate have individual names but all those within an aggregate have comparable pathogenicity and reasonable biochemical similarity.

The 'pyogenic streptococci' include species that are almost always β-haemolytic and which have Lancefield group antigens. *S. pyogenes* (group A) is a human commensal and invasive pathogen. *S. agalactiae* (group B) is a major cause of bovine mastitis and an occasional cause of human disease. The Lancefield group C comprises several species including some animal pathogens but one, *S. equisimilis*, is a commensal and occasional pathogen of man. The same is true for the streptococci of group G. Two other species cause purulent disease in man and are properly considered 'pyogenic'. These are the *S. milleri* agg. and *S. pneumoniae* (see Section 7.19).

The so-called oral streptococci are part of the normal flora and seldom cause purulent lesions. Medically they are important as causes of bacterial endocarditis. The organisms brought together in the *S. sanguis* agg. and the *S. oralis* agg. include the 'viridans' streptococci. Mutans and sanguis organisms are involved in the development of dental plaque and members of *S. mutans* agg. are the most likely cause of dental caries (see Chapter 14.5). The tongue is the main site colonized by *S. salivarius* and this organism rarely causes disease. The nutritionally exacting streptococci—*S. adjacens* and *S. defectivus*—will not grow on many of the culture media used routinely unless supplemented with pyridoxal hydrochloride or cysteine. They are consequently one of the causes of 'culture-negative' endocarditis. None of the biotypes of *S. bovis* is present normally in the human mouth but because they have many of the characteristics of the oral streptococci they are considered with them rather than with the enterococci with which they share the group D antigen.

The enterococci are somewhat more resistant to heat and other agents, including antibiotics, than the streptococci. All carry the group D antigen, which is a lipoteichoic acid, in contrast to most other group antigens, which are cell-wall carbohydrates. Among the 18 species in this genus *Enterococcus gallinarum*, *E. casseliflavus*, *E. durans* and *E. hirae* are all organisms that can be isolated from animals or plants but they sometimes cause human infections, for instance urinary tract infection, endocarditis or sepsis in the immunocompromised. Organisms from the environment or food that are related to the streptococci are occasional causes of human disease. They include the aerococci, which have caused urinary tract infection, and also the pediococci and leuconostocs. The last two are vancomycin resistant and have caused endocarditis.

Diseases caused by group A streptococci

S. pyogenes is invasive, but symptomless carriage, particularly in the throat, is more usual and in Europe could be expected in 10 per cent of

Table 1 *The streptococci and related organisms isolated regularly from human sources*

Division	Specific name	Lancefield group	Haemolysis	Main site of carriage
Pyogenic streptococci	*S. pyogenes*	A	β	Throat (vagina)[a]
	S. agalactiae	B	β(−)	Gut (vagina, throat)
	S. equisimilis	C	β	Throat (vagina)
	S. spp.	G	β	Throat (vagina)
	S. pneumoniae	−	α	Throat (vagina)
	S. milleri agg.[b]	−(F,C,G,A)	−(β,α)	Mouth (throat, gut, vagina)
Oral streptococci	*S. sanguis* agg.	−(H)	α	Teeth (throat)
	S. salivarius agg.	−(K)	−	Tongue, throat
	S. mutans agg.	−(E)	−(β,α)	Teeth
	S. oralis agg.	−(O,K,M,)	α	Mouth, throat
	Nutritionally exacting strains	−	−	Mouth
	S. bovis agg.	D	−(α)	Gut
Enterococci	*E. faecalis*	D	−(β)	Gut
	E. faecium	D	α	Gut
	E. avium	D + Q	α	Gut

[a]In parentheses: less common reactions or sites of carriage.

bAggregated species: see text.

Table 2 *Some of the diseases caused in man by streptococci and related organisms*

Organism	Diseases
S. pyogenes	Local sepsis: sore throat, impetigo, pyoderma, wound infection, and others Invasive: lymphangiitis, cellulitis, puerperal sepsis, septicaemia Acute manifestations: scarlet fever, erysipelas Late (non-suppurative) sequelae: rheumatic fever, acute post-streptococcal glomerulonephritis
S. agalactiae	Young babies: early-onset septicaemia with or without meningitis, late-onset meningitis Adults: septicaemia, endocarditis
S. equisimilis and group G spp.	Local sepsis and bacteraemia
S. pneumoniae	Pneumonia, otitis media, meningitis, septicaemia, peritonitis
S. milleri agg.	Abscesses in internal organs—notably in abdominal cavity, brain; pleural empyema
Oral streptococci	Common causes of endocarditis,[a] *S. mutans* associated with dental caries (see Chapter 14.5)
Enterococci	Urinary tract infection, mild wound sepsis, endocarditis, septicaemia

[a]Note almost any streptococcus can cause endocarditis.

children up to 15 years of age, in 2.5 per cent of those aged 15 to 45, and 0.5 per cent of those aged over 45 years. These figures include the healthy, post infection subjects and contacts. Rates are higher in those with crowded living conditions because of respiratory spread. Three-quarters of all haemolytic streptococci isolated from routine throat swabs would be expected to belong to group A, most of the remainder belonging to group B, group C or group G. Away from Europe, in Kuwait or Nigeria for example, carriage of group G can be as common as group A. The receptors for adhesion of *S. pyogenes* are probably lipoteichoic acid or a protein on the bacterial cell surface and fibronectin on mucosal surfaces.

All virulent strains of *S. pyogenes* possess an M protein antigen and so far more than 80 M antigens have been defined. The identification of these proteins provides a laboratory base for epidemiological studies. A streptococcal sore throat probably begins with the formation of a micro-colony of *S. pyogenes*—the clustering of cells being promoted by the M antigen—followed by the release of toxins and proteinases. These inhibit defence mechanisms in the tonsils and pharyngeal mucosa. Pharyngitis is followed by an antibody response to many products of *S. pyogenes* so we know that these products are released during infection. They include: a peptidase, which destroys the complement-derived chemotaxin C5a; the haemolysin activated by thiol compounds (streptolysin O); the scarlet fever toxins A (related to *Staphylococcus aureus* enterotoxin B), B (a variant of streptococcal proteinase), and C; also enzymes that are not known to be directly toxic, including hyaluronidase, several nucleotidases, two streptokinases (fibrinolysins) and diphosphopyridine nucleotidase.

When *S. pyogenes* enters the body through the mucosa of the upper respiratory tract, or a break in the skin, a local lesion may occur or there may be spread along tissue planes or lymphatics. The M antigen is not toxic in itself but it protects the streptococcus from phagocytosis and antibodies to the M protein are opsonic. Upon presentation, patients with serious invasive disease may have fever, shock, and evidence of renal impairment. In two-thirds of these patients the portal of entry is the skin and infection of soft tissue is apparent but in others the site of infection may not be evident. The mortality in patients with group A streptococcal bacteraemia is 25 per cent or more, despite antibiotic therapy. New treatments are therefore needed to control the host response to virulence factors, which induce cytokines including interleukin-6 as well as products that may be directly toxic.

Infections of the upper respiratory tract

STREPTOCOCCAL SORE THROAT

Acute pharyngitis or tonsillitis is one of the most common reasons for seeing a family doctor. A change from illnesses caused mainly by viruses (see Section 7.10) to those often yielding group A streptococci occurs, in Europe, around 5 years of age and the incidence of streptococcal sore throat is highest in those aged 5 to 15 years. In infants and preschool children there may be few definite signs of pharyngitis but fever, nasal discharge, enlarged cervical lymph glands, and otitis media occur. In older children and young adults the fully developed condition exhibits an abrupt onset, with fever (over 38 °C), sore throat and pain on swallowing, headache, swollen bright-red tonsils with discrete white spots on the surface, pharyngeal injection, enlarged anterior cervical lymph nodes, and leucocytosis. Coryza, cough, hoarseness, and laryngitis are not typical manifestations. In any outbreak, gradations are seen from the florid condition just described, through mild sore throat to a symptomless state in which the only evidence of infection is isolation of *S. pyogenes* together with a brisk antibody response. Severe forms of tonsillitis tend to be common during outbreaks in residential institutions housing young people and affects new entrants. The incubation period, at least in outbreaks, is short, usually 1 to 3 days.

After the initial mucosal infection the disease may become localized and this was more common before antibiotics were available. Complications, then, resulted from direct extension from the throat and were otitis media, mastoiditis, and adenitis. It was also found that strains of *S. pyogenes* serotype M1 predominated in these conditions. Otitis media has reappeared in the recent epidemics caused by strains of M-type 1. Infection may also spread into the pharyngeal lymphatic tissue giving rise to peritonsillar or retropharyngeal abscess, or along lymphatics to cervical lymph nodes and less often through fascial planes in the neck. A thin, purulent discharge usually indicates the presence of sinusitis. Invasion of the blood-stream does occur but less often than from cellulitis.

After the acute signs have abated, an untreated patient may continue to feel unwell, fever may persist, the erythrocyte sedimentation rate may be raised, and there may be polyarthritis or arthralgia. This 'post-streptococcal reactive arthritis' is not easily distinguished from mild rheumatic fever, partly because the diagnosis of rheumatic fever is based on the application of a set of guidelines—the Jones criteria.

Scarlet fever

Most cases of scarlet fever are a consequence of streptococcal pharyngitis but the erythematous rash can occur with invasive disease. It is rare with impetigo or pyoderma. At the end of the eighteenth century the London physician Robert Willan observed that sore throat could occur without the rash. Also that different degrees of severity of scarlet fever could occur in the same household and that those who had scarlet fever before could have recurrences of the sore throat but not of the rash. It was only in 1924, however, that *S. pyogenes* was formally demonstrated to be the sole cause of the disease by the development of scarlet fever in one of five volunteers whose throats had been swabbed with a culture isolated from a scarlet fever patient and later by the reproduction of the disease in some susceptibles by the injection of culture filtrates. Injection into the skin of lesser amounts of toxin is followed by local erythema and this was the basis of the Dick test, which used to be used to demonstrate susceptibility to the toxin. The injection of serum from a convalescent case of scarlet fever into the skin of a patient in the acute phase of the disease causes a local blanching of the rash—the Schültz–Charlton reaction. These observations led to the hypothesis that the disease was caused by the direct action of erythrogenic toxin in those that did not have circulating antitoxin—a state analogous to the Schick reaction in relation to diphtheria (see Chapter 7.2). The alternative view, which also has experimental support, is that the scarlet fever toxins, of which three are known, are pyrogenic, erythrogenic, induce lymphocyte proliferation followed by release of cytokines and increase, markedly, susceptibility to endotoxic shock. The rash and the various syndromes such as streptococcal toxic shock are caused, in this view, not by a direct toxic action but by release of substances that have an immunomodulating activity. Thus an adult could be insusceptible to scarlet fever because of circulating antitoxin and a young child might not develop a rash because of lack of prior exposure to toxin.

Production of toxin has been related to patterns of disease. For a generation after 1840, scarlet fever was recorded as the leading cause of death among infectious diseases of childhood. In 1863 the death rate of children under 15 was 4000 per million living. There were 30 000 deaths. A marked decline in mortality began after 1870 and now, although 6000 to 12 000 cases might be notified annually in England and Wales (with a periodicity of about 10 years), they include fewer than 10 recorded deaths. Some cultures of *S. pyogenes* isolated before 1940, from severe cases of scarlet fever, produce up to 15 mg/l of the A toxin but recent isolates yield up to 0.2 mg/l, suggesting there may have been a change in the organism.

The clinical characteristics of scarlet fever include all the signs and symptoms found with a streptococcal sore throat or wound infection. Again, most cases occur in children of school age. The notifications probably include some with viral exanthems while mild infections may escape attention and notification. Cases of moderate severity begin with fever, nausea, and vomiting. Abdominal pain is common. Coughing is notably absent. In addition to acute tonsillitis an enanthem may develop on the palate some hours before the skin rash appears. This appears as bright-red spots superimposed on general redness of the whole pharynx. Early in the disease the tongue is covered with a white fur through which red-tipped papillae appear ('strawberry tongue'). Later, usually after the rash develops, the fur peels off leaving a raw red papillate surface ('raspberry tongue'). The spleen may be palpable and there may be generalized lymphadenopathy.

The rash is usually a diffuse erythema, symmetrical, and blanches on pressure. It is seen most often on the neck, chest, folds of the axilla, elbow, and groin. The rash is commonly punctate and these can be felt ('like sandpaper'). There may be flushing of the cheeks and circumoral pallor. The rash usually appears within the first day of onset and persists for several days. From 2 or 3 days to 3 weeks later, peeling may occur. This takes place most often on the tips of the fingers, toes or ears and less often occurs over large areas of the trunk or limbs.

A streptococcal sore throat is one of the causes of erythema multiforme (see Section 23). The symmetrical, circular lesions of erythema multiforme enlarge to circular plaques ('target lesions'). The face and distal portions of the limbs are affected more often than the trunk.

Streptococcal perianal disease

Streptococcal perianal disease is a superficial, well-demarcated rash, which is not indurated and spreads out from the anus in young children. It is associated with itching, rectal pain on defecation, and blood-stained stools. Perianal cultures from these children yield heavy growths of *S. pyogenes* and pretreatment throat swabs generally contain representatives of the same serotype.

Vulvovaginitis

Among prepubertal girls, vulvovaginitis with a serosanguinous discharge and erythema of the labia and vaginal orifice is often caused by *S. pyogenes*. This condition too is secondary to infection at another site, usually the throat.

Streptococcal impetigo and ecthyma

Virtually any purulent lesion of the skin can yield *S. pyogenes*, including impetigo, infected cuts or lacerations, insect bites, scabies, intertrigo, and ecthyma.

Streptococcal impetigo is superficial and does not affect the dermis. The lesions are heaped up and may be crusted spots or have a red, papular appearance that progresses to a weeping lesion with a serous exudate. These may be localized to a particular part of the body or generalized. They seldom exceed 2 cm in diameter, last for 2 or 3 weeks, unless there is some underlying disorder such as eczema or parasitic infestation, and heal without scarring. In the initial stage there may be small vesicles (Fig. 1), like those seen in the early stage of chickenpox, which soon rupture and become crusted. It can usually be distinguished from staphylococcal impetigo in which the vesicles are typically larger—usually 1 cm in diameter. In Britain it used to be a common disease of childhood ('school sores'), often beginning on the face and scalp and associated with poverty. It remains widespread in rural areas of many developing countries. The lesions generally occur at the site of minor trauma, for instance insect bites or scabies, but can occur on apparently normal skin. Many of the recent reported epidemics have occurred in countries with warm climates but impetigo is in no sense a tropical disease.

Ecthyma is an ulcerated form of impetigo in which the ulceration extends into the dermis (Fig. 2). If untreated it may persist for months and cause scarring. The ulcers have red margins, which develop a purple tinge as they mature. In most the exudate dries and forms large crusts but sometimes there are chronic, weeping ulcers. Cellulitis, abscess formation, lymphangitis, lymphadenitis, and bursitis (if the infection is near a joint) may occur.

In some institutional outbreaks, streptococcal impetigo and sore throat have occurred contemporaneously. The organisms from the skin lesions can, however, often be distinguished by serotyping from those causing tonsillitis. Among the inhabitants of jungles or some Pacific islands *S. pyogenes* and toxigenic strains of *Corynebacterium diphtheriae* frequently coexist in skin sores. The lesions yielding both pathogens cannot be distinguished clinically from those containing *S. pyogenes* as the sole pathogen. The manifestations of diphtheria do not occur in these people because they have circulating antitoxin.

Outbreaks of streptococcal impetigo may occur in adults subject to skin trauma such as members of sports teams or those undergoing initial training for the armed services or police force. Severe forms of ecthyma have occurred among soldiers operating in hot, wet lowlands ('jungle rot'). On the limbs of these men there can be punched out ulcers up to 3 cm in diameter with heaped up edges and bases that are reddish-grey, granular, and covered with exudate. Cuts on the hands and arms are common among workers in the meat trade and occupational infection of cuts with *S. pyogenes* is a problem. In these workers a clean cut that is infected with *S. pyogenes* can become red and swollen within a few hours but the organism can be present in any lesion whether 'clean', 'crusted', or 'septic'. Colonization of lesions with *Staph. aureus* is common but when *S. pyogenes* is present also the lesions may become crusted and persist for several weeks unless treated.

Fig. 1 Streptococcal pyoderma; multiple early lesions.

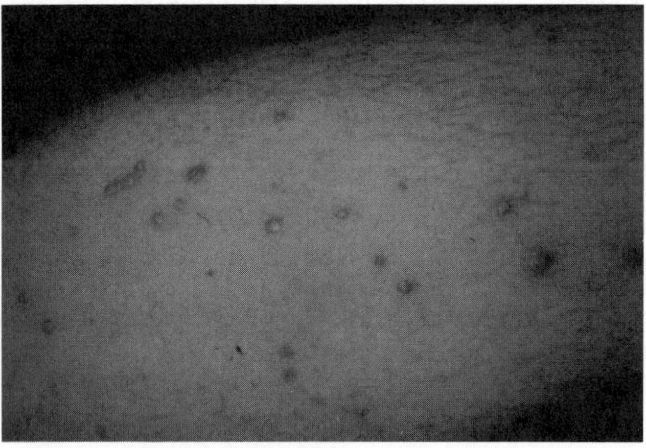

Fig. 2 Streptococcal pyoderma; untreated ecthyma.

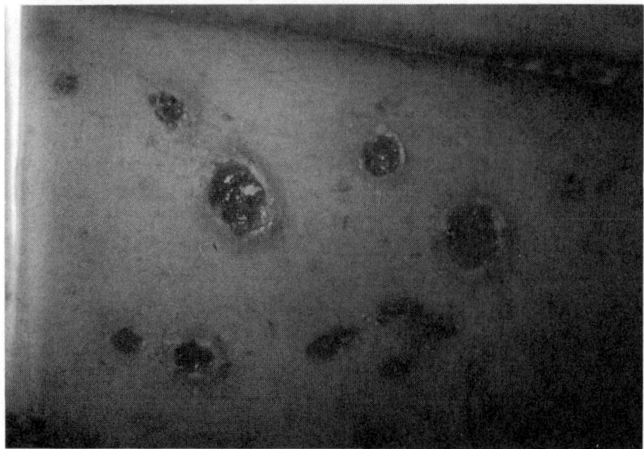

Streptococcal impetigo or ecthyma can be followed by acute glomerulonephritis but not rheumatic fever.

Repeated attacks of impetigo or pyoderma may mean either reinfection or a host defect. In Jamaica, *S. pyogenes* is associated regularly with infective dermatitis. In children with this condition there is severe exudative eczema on the head, axillae, and groins without preceding infantile eczema. There is a fine papular rash and chronic nasal discharge. One or both of *S. pyogenes* and *Staph. aureus* can be isolated from the nasal discharge and skin lesions. The children tested had antibodies to human T-lymphotrophic virus type 1.

Erysipelas

Erysipelas ('the rose' or 'St. Anthony's fire') is one of the streptococcal diseases that affects the elderly more often than the young. In this disease streptococci are localized in the dermis and hypodermis. In many cases there is good evidence, cultural or serological, implicating *S. pyogenes* but the involvement of other organisms, particularly group G streptococci, in some patients seems likely. In the past, two categories of erysipelas were recognized—surgical and idiopathic. The former was common in the nineteenth century and was associated with puerperal sepsis and streptococcal wound infection. Even now erysipelas may occur in one or more of the patients involved in a ward outbreak of streptococcal wound sepsis. The idiopathic form usually affects the face, leg or arm and less often the trunk.

Malaise, headache, and pyrexia often precede the appearance of the local lesion by 12 to 24 h, although in many patients pain, burning, and redness of the skin are the first changes noted. Modes of entry of the organism include skin ulcers, minor trauma, and skin diseases including fungal infections. In some, particularly facial erysipelas, no site of entry is discernible and the patient gives a history of coryza. The lesion has a raised, well-defined margin that extends irregularly. Typically, facial erysipelas begins on the bridge of the nose and spreads rather symmetrically over the cheeks ('butterfly distribution'). It may remain localized or involve the forehead and scalp. Vesicles and bullae containing fluid appear on the surface and when they rupture become crusted. The lesion becomes more oedematous as it spreads and in facial erysipelas one or both eyes may be closed. In the absence of treatment pyrexia (up to 39 °C) continues for a mean of 7 days for facial erysipelas and a mean of 14 days for erysipelas on the leg. Desquamation often occurs as the rash fades.

Bacteraemia develops in 5 per cent of patients. Complications include abscesses or gangrene. Elderly patients may die of intercurrent disease such as pneumonia. Before antibiotics were available the mortality was 10 per cent. Lesions recur in up to 30 per cent of patients at the same site within 3 years of the initial attack.

Wound infections and cellulitis

On admission most burns are free of pathogens but before antibiotics were available and antiseptic procedures were established, infection or colonization of burns with *S. pyogenes* was frequent. Colonization contributes to graft failure and delayed healing. The first sign of infection may be a rise in temperature in a patient previously apyrexial. In some, the main manifestation of infection of burns, and other wounds, is solely an unexpected delay in healing. More often redness and swelling occur, with pus. Cellulitis, lymphangitis, lymphadenitis, bacteraemia, or septicaemia may follow. Sometimes scarlatiniform rashes or glomerulonephritis develop in these patients.

Puerperal fever, a special form of wound infection, develops early in the puerperium. Onset is abrupt and massive invasion of the bloodstream is the rule. Its true incidence is probably masked by the common practice of beginning specific treatment as soon as fever develops and without prior vaginal swabbing.

Cellulitis is an acute, non-purulent, spreading infection of the skin. Group A streptococci are traditionally regarded as the most important cause but staphylococci and, in young children, *Haemophilus influenzae* cause a clinically indistinguishable disease. Cellulitis may develop from a small puncture wound. Late contamination of a healing wound tends to give rise to a more localized inflammation. Pus is not obtained on aspiration. There is often localized tenderness, swelling, increased skin warmth, and local erythema. Sometimes cellulitis caused by *S. pyogenes* has a sharply defined border like erysipelas. Periorbital cellulitis requires specific attention. Streptococcal cellulitis may be followed within hours by bacteraemia or septicaemia.

NECROTIZING FASCIITIS

In the American literature the term necrotizing fasciitis generally comprises any soft-tissue infection spreading along fascial planes, with or without overlying cellulitis. Included are mixed infections caused by bowel organisms, for example, serious wound infections following abdominal surgery and necrotizing infections of the scrotum (Fournier's gangrene) or the vulva or perineum which may develop from perirectal abscesses. Organisms as diverse as gut anaerobes, *S. pyogenes*, *Entamoeba histolytica,* and the marine organism *Vibrio vulnificus* can be responsible. European authors usually focus on infections with a more rapid course from which representatives of *S. pyogenes*, alone or together with *Staph. aureus*, have been isolated. These infections are often community-acquired and usually occur on an arm or leg. At first there is swelling, redness, fever, and pain, followed by purple or bronze discoloration of the skin, then haemorrhagic bullae develop and, around 1 week after onset necrosis of the skin occurs. Lymphangitis and lymphadenitis are uncommon, presumably because the lymphatics are blocked. Biopsy specimens show areas of necrosis in the dermis and subcutaneous fat, there is infiltration with polymorphonuclear leucocytes, vasculitis and thrombosis in vessels in the superficial fascia, and, in lesions of less than 4 days duration, the superficial dermis and epidermis are intact. Blister fluid or the watery reddish discharge contain many streptococci. Antibiotics when combined with surgical removal of infected necrotic tissue are life-saving. The mortality in reported series has reached 40 per cent.

Bacteraemia

Altogether 2 per cent of blood cultures contain *S. pyogenes* and the mortality in these cases approaches 25 per cent despite administration of antibiotics. There are more community-acquired bacteraemias than develop in hospitals. The hospital cases are associated with infection of wounds, decubitus ulcers, the puerperium, erysipelas, and the neonatal period. The probable site of entry of at least half of the community-acquired infections is the skin. In some patients no portal of entry is apparent and streptococcal bacteraemia may not be suspected. Children with a haematological malignancy are one such group. One-half of the patients are admitted in a state of shock, with fever, but sometimes hypothermia, and with involvement of several organs often leading to renal failure. In some there is a history of severe abdominal pain, diarrhoea, and vomiting. Gastroenteritis may be suspected in these patients rather than intra-abdominal sepsis. Some patients may have an erythematous rash. There may be primary pneumonia, or pneumonia secondary to erysipelas or cellulitis. The bacteraemia can occur in elderly patients with diabetes or peripheral vascular disease but also in previously fit younger adults. Small outbreaks have occurred among intravenous drug abusers. Superinfection may follow varicella. The prognosis is poor in malnourished children.

Epidemiology

Longitudinal studies have shown that representatives of various serotypes of *S. pyogenes* can be introduced into a centre but inexplicably only some take hold. They are readily communicable and give rise to epidemics in a variety of circumstances. With rare exceptions the source of infection is human. Particular serotypes, based on detection of M-protein antigens, are associated with certain clinical conditions. For example, serotypes M3 and M6 are common causes of outbreaks of sore throat, while representatives of M55 have caused large outbreaks of pyoderma in the West Indies and strains of M81 are associated with skin sepsis in Britain. The serotypes M1, M3, and M18 are associated with invasive disease. There are three main patterns of transmission, as follows.

Respiratory infections

Streptococcal sore throat is contracted by spread through the air. Infectivity falls off progressively at distances exceeding 2 m, suggesting that the larger salivary droplets generated by sneezing, talking, or coughing are responsible. Patients in the early stage of pharyngitis have many streptococci in the nose and mouth and are very infectious. During convalescence, even if antibiotic treatment was not given, organisms disappear from the saliva, usually also from the nose, over 10 to 21 days. The patient then has little infectivity, even though throat carriage may persist. With adequate treatment with penicillin transmissibility is generally low after 1 to 2 days. Experimentally, insufflation of dust particles containing viable *S. pyogenes* on to the pharynx was not followed by infection.

Spread to wounds and the skin

Direct impact of salivary particles into a wound is an efficient but unusual method of transmission given the exclusion of staff with active infections from duty. The throat carrier who disperses little is also of secondary importance and probably undue significance has been given to the midwife who is a symptomless carrier. Routes of dissemination to wounds resemble those of *Staph. aureus* with nasal carriers and those with septic lesions being important. Particles of dried secretion or infected skin scales may be disseminated the length of a hospital ward. Carriage on healthy skin is unusual but theatre staff who are anal or vaginal carriers have been responsible for outbreaks of infection. Streptococci dispersed in the air or transferred to inanimate objects may remain viable for several weeks but there is reason to believe that the more recently shed organisms are the more infectious.

There is little doubt that the predominant route of spread in pyoderma is from skin to skin, either directly or by way of contaminated objects. There can be passive transfer on insects such as scabies and, in some tropical countries, hippelates flies. Infection of the mother from an infected umbilical stump has been repeatedly demonstrated.

Food-borne spread

Food-borne outbreaks of streptococcal sore throat are not common but the disease is usually severe and vomiting is prominent. Milk, milk products, and egg salads have caused recent outbreaks and probably followed contamination from human cases. In the early part of the twentieth century numerous milk-borne outbreaks were described arising from single herds. In some instances one or more cows were found to have erosive lesions of a teat containing *S. pyogenes*. There had probably been infection from a milker. Such outbreaks are rare following the introduction of pasteurization.

Diagnosis

STREPTOCOCCAL SORE THROAT

In some children with streptococcal pharyngitis the clinical and epidemiological findings are so typical that it is reasonable to treat with oral penicillin after obtaining a culture to confirm the diagnosis. In others this diagnosis cannot be made with certainty on clinical grounds. A throat swab is then taken of the posterior pharynx and tonsils or tonsillar fossae but avoiding the tongue. A record of the number of colonies of *S. pyogenes* that develop is useful. More than 50 colonies are almost always associated with acute infection and fewer than 10 may represent either infection or the carrier state. Kits for the detection of the Lancefield group A antigen directly from throat swabs are available. There are few false-positive reactions with these kits but a positive reaction may not occur with a swab that would yield 10 or fewer colonies. If a negative result is obtained by this method it is generally necessary to continue with a culture. Laboratory confirmation of streptococcal infection helps in the management of contacts who may become ill.

In the past a throat swab was necessary to exclude diphtheria. This is now unlikely in Britain but the possible presence of *C. diphtheriae* should be remembered in those adult cases of sore throat from whom isolation of gonococci may occur. At the same time some uncommon causes of sore throat, namely *C. ovis* and *C. haemolyticum*, will be excluded.

Serological tests play no part in the diagnosis of acute streptococcal sore throat other than, for instance, to exclude infectious mononucleosis (see Chapter 7.10.4). At the onset of a streptococcal sore throat, antibodies are a measure of past exposure and prompt treatment diminishes the response to streptococcal antigens.

SCARLET FEVER

Recognition of the rash is not likely to present difficulties unless the primary streptococcal infection has been missed or the rash is atypical. Some epidermolytic staphylococcal infections and staphylococcal scarlet fever give rise to a rash initially difficult to distinguish from scarlet fever but the epidermolytic infections are followed soon by the separation *en masse* of the outer layers of the epidermis leaving a red, raw surface, or if separation is not complete, Nikolsky's sign appears. Scarlatiniform rashes followed by desquamation and 'strawberry tongue' also occur in staphylococcal toxic shock syndrome and Kawasaki's disease (see Chapter 18.11.9) but in both conditions there is high fever, conjunctival reddening, and severe hypotensive shock. In measles the rash is coarser and more blotchy, appearing after 3 to 4 days of febrile coryza. The rash of rubella may be scarlatiniform on the trunk but usually remains discrete on the limbs and face.

PYODERMA

A clinical diagnosis of streptococcal pyoderma that is unsupported by some form of bacteriological investigation is generally unsafe. If a crusted lesion is present, surface swabbing is inadequate and it is necessary to raise the edge of the crust or scab gently and swab the area beneath.

CELLULITIS AND ERYSIPELAS

Swabbing the skin surface above affected areas in either condition yields *S. pyogenes* in only 20 per cent of cases. More positive results can be obtained by aspiration techniques. A blood culture is indicated in these patients, particularly if they are pyrexial.

STREPTOCOCCAL TOXIC SHOCK-LIKE ILLNESS

This condition has similarities to staphylococcal toxic shock syndrome, notably fever, hypotension, shock, and involvement or failure of several organs. Also, an erythematous rash may be present. It differs from the staphylococcal syndrome, as originally described, because the streptococcal disease is associated additionally with bacteraemia and tissue invasion.

Treatment

Penicillin remains the antibiotic of first choice for treatment of infections with *S. pyogenes*.

There are four possible benefits from treating streptococcal sore throat. First: the illness is shortened. The effects, as measured in controlled trials, are most marked when treatment begins in the first 24 h of illness. Second: the organism is eradicated from the pharynx. This prevents spread and treatment begun on the first or second day of illness reduces by one-half the secondary attack rate in siblings when compared with cases treated after 2 days or more of illness. Patients who have received 7 days of oral penicillin have a significantly higher bacteriological failure rate—defined as persistence or recurrence of the original strain within 21 days—than those receiving ten days of treatment. Third: treatment with penicillin probably has reduced the number of suppurative complications. Fourth: rheumatic fever and possibly also acute glomerulonephritis can be prevented. Although rheumatic fever is now seen rarely in western Europe it remains a major problem in developing countries.

A phenoxypenicillin by mouth is used routinely (Table 3) but if the infection is severe intramuscular benzylpenicillin is used initially, changing to oral administration when the condition improves. Intramuscular repository benzathine benzylpenicillin should be considered when compliance is a problem. From 1980 there have been reports of increasing bacteriological failure rates with oral penicillin in comparison with earlier reports. The presence of penicillinase-producing bacteria in the pharynx and tolerance to penicillin—defined as an increase in the ratio of bactericidal to bacteriostatic concentrations—have been given as causes. This has led some paediatricians in the United States to add rifampin for the last 4 days of a 10-day course of oral penicillin. Others have found fewer bacteriological failures with cephalexin than with a phenoxypenicillin. Erythromycin is often used when allergy to penicillin is suspected or when a decision is made to treat a carrier. This may happen when there are recurrences of tonsillitis despite penicillin treatment. In Britain now, resistance to erythromycin in *S. pyogenes* is of the order of 3 per cent, but outbreaks caused by erythromycin-resistant strains have occurred.

Outbreaks of impetigo and ecthyma can be controlled by widespread use of penicillin combined with topical treatments involving cleansing and the use of disinfectant soaps or creams. Impetigo often occurs as multiple infections within families where the organisms persist and spread, leading to retreatment. The presence of penicillinase-producing organisms may prevent the elimination, by benzylpenicillin, of group A streptococci from severe ecthyma and extensive burns. For this reason some use a β-lactamase-resistant drug for these patients. In burns wards, erythromycin has been used prophylactically and lincomycin or clindamycin used to control outbreaks.

In rapidly spreading septic infections, for example puerperal sepsis, or when septicaemia has appeared, very prompt treatment is essential. Initially, if the infection is known to be caused by *S. pyogenes*, this should be with benzylpenicillin either by intravenous infusion or intramuscular injection. The response to penicillin is sometimes poor in severe infection and has been likened to the apparent insensitivity observed in the laboratory when large inocula are exposed to the drug. Clinically such numbers are likely in overwhelming sepsis, necrotizing fasciitis, or myositis. When infection is well established in the latter conditions, surgical drainage, debridement, fasciotomy, or amputation often saves life. In experimental models of myositis, clindamycin has been more effective than penicillin, perhaps because it inhibits production of protein toxins.

Table 3 *Use of antimicrobial agents for treatment of streptococcal sore throat or mass chemoprophylaxis*

Agent	Dose	Route	Duration (days)
Benzathine benzylpenicillin	1.2×10^6 i.u., $6–9 \times 10^5$ i.u. in children	i.m.	once
Phenoxymethyl or phenoxyethyl penicillin	250 mg, 3 times a day	O	10
Erythromycin	250 mg, 4 times a day (40 mg/kg in children)	O	10
The following agents are effective but are usually not recommended: amoxycillin, flucloxacillin, oral cephalosporins, and clindamycin.			
The following are often ineffective: sulphonamides, trimethoprim, tetracyclines, and chloramphenicol.			

i.u., international units; i.m., intramuscular; O, oral.

For rapidly spreading infections and septicaemia, see text.

Prevention

RESPIRATORY TRACT INFECTION

Infections arise from aerial dispersion over short distances so reduction of overcrowding, when possible, is important. This may be by increasing bed spacing or reducing the number of occupants of a room. Moderate increases in ventilation and dust-suppressive measures have been disappointing in effect. The early treatment of cases eliminates sources but because patients are infectious before symptoms appear, treatment of the symptomatic and carriers may not halt an outbreak. It is, however, worth trying early in an incident. Failure of this form of prevention has occurred when fresh susceptibles enter regularly a community where infection has become established. This has led to the advocacy of mass antibiotic prophylaxis. Epidemics have been halted by giving everyone, except those with penicillin allergy, either oral penicillin for 10 days or a single injection of benzathine penicillin.

Control of streptococcal skin infection is based on the prevention of skin lesions and if they do occur for their protection from *S. pyogenes*. When outbreaks have been associated with physical training, measures like replacement of rough mats or climbing ropes, or substitution of track suits for shorts, have reduced skin damage. The treatment, at the end of each day, of any area of skin damage with a povidone–iodine dry-powder spray has controlled infection in such groups. Epidemics of streptococcal sepsis among meat handlers generally require improvement of local hygiene and 'first aid' in the workplace, use of waterproof, vapour-permeable dressings on all but the most trivial cuts or abrasions, and systemic antibiotic treatment of lesions that are clearly septic.

In developing countries, reduction in the prevalence of impetigo has followed advice on hygiene given in junior schools by teachers. In these children neither medicated soap nor chlorhexidine cream have been effective in reducing either the number of lesions or the proportion that contain *S. pyogenes*. Also, injection of penicillin eradicated the streptococci for some weeks only.

Omphalitis can be prevented by the daily treatment of umbilical stumps with preparations such as chlorhexidine gluconate (0.5 per cent).

Immunization

Synthetic vaccines are being developed composed of polypeptides with the immunodeterminants of the M antigens found, particularly, in strains from rheumatic fever. They are not likely to be available in the near future.

The non-suppurative sequelae of infection with S. pyogenes

Rheumatic fever and acute post-streptococcal glomerulonephritis develop after a latent period in persons who have had an infection with *S. pyogenes*. The latent period tends to be somewhat shorter in glomerulonephritis than acute rheumatic fever. Onset in the latter can occur from 1 to 5 weeks but one manifestation of rheumatic fever, Sydenham's chorea, may occur several months after the streptococcal infection and mitral stenosis may take years to develop. In neither disease are living streptococci present in the specific lesions but they differ in one important respect, rheumatic fever greatly enhances the chances that a subsequent streptococcal infection will be followed by another attack of rheumatic fever but glomerulonephritis shows no such effect. The two diseases rarely follow the same streptococcal infection.

Guttate psoriasis (see Section 23), which appears as eruptive plaques up to 1 cm in diameter, is often preceded by streptococcal infection and may thus be precipitated by immunological mechanisms comparable to the two diseases discussed here.

RHEUMATIC FEVER (SEE ALSO CHAPTER 15.16)

Pathogenesis

By 1889, William Cheadle had fitted together the full syndrome of rheumatic fever: carditis, polyarthritis, tonsillitis, Sydenham's chorea, subcutaneous nodules, and erythema marginatum. Studies in the 1930s using the techniques of epidemiology, bacteriology, and serology provided the link between streptococcal sore throat and rheumatic fever. The pathogenesis of the disease remains unknown. For instance it is not known why the streptococcal infection must occur in the throat, the reason for the apparent susceptibility of some families, why particular serotypes of *S. pyogenes* are more important than others and whether antigenic sites shared by *S. pyogenes* and human tissues are determinative. Strains of the M serotypes 1, 3, 5, 6, and 18 have predominated in the recent resurgence of rheumatic fever in the United States and two-thirds of the isolations from recent sporadic cases in Britain belong to one or other of these serotypes. In outbreaks of sore throat caused by serotypes associated with rheumatic fever up to one-half of previous sufferers will have a recurrence compared with an attack rate of about 2 per cent among untreated subjects who have not had the disease. Candidates for antigenic mimicry include (a) the Lancefield group A antigen and mitral valve glycoprotein, (b) part of the M protein antigen and helical proteins such as myosin, (c) the protoplast membrane and myocardial sarcolemma or neuronal tissue, and (d) the hyaluronate capsule of the bacterium and articular tissues. The HLA-DR alleles 2, 3, and 4 have been found to be somewhat more common in patients with rheumatic fever than in controls.

Clinical features

The latent period between the onset of a streptococcal sore throat and the development of acute rheumatic fever has a mean of 19 days. It is the same length in first attacks and recurrences, unlike serum sickness. The onset may be acute, particularly if arthritis is present, or insidious if the only manifestation is carditis, when fatigue may proceed to congestive cardiac failure. A typical course may last 6 weeks or a remittent course for months and it is difficult to say when the disease ceased to be active because treatment with salicylates or steroids suppresses many of its effects. Nowadays the first attack of rheumatic fever in Britain is almost always milder than in former times, deaths are uncommon, many do not suffer carditis or permanent damage to the heart valves, and

Table 4 *Some of the serological tests that are used in the study of infections with* S. pyogenes

Test	Comment
Extracellular products	
Antistreptolysin O (ASO)	Standard procedure. Antigenically identical haemolysin produced by human pyogenic strains of groups C or G. Response often poor in skin infections. False-positive reactions in patients with hypercholesterolaemia or if serum stored inadequately
Antideoxyribonuclease B (ADB)	Titres raised in infections involving skin. Enzyme formed by nearly all strains of *S. pyogenes*
Antihyaluronidase (AHT)	Antigenically different hyaluronidase in human pyogenic strains of groups C or G
Antistreptokinase (ASK)	Enzyme from group C strain employed routinely in test. Antigenic relation of this enzyme to nephritis-associated protein of *S. pyogenes* not clear
Cell-bound antigens	
M protein	Research procedure. New method needed. Antibody opsonic. More than 80 antigenic forms identified
Group A carbohydrate	Research procedure. Raised titre associated with persistence of rheumatic mitral valve disease

chorea is rare. In many developing countries, and in special groups such as the Aborigines in Australia, Maoris in New Zealand, the Black population of South Africa, the disease can be of a severity and incidence similar to that experienced in Britain before the Second World War.

High recurrence rates are favoured by youth, the clinical severity of the current streptococcal infection, a short interval since the last attack of rheumatic fever, and numerous previous attacks—particularly in those with pre-existing rheumatic heart disease.

Laboratory findings

Detection of raised antibody levels or, better, changes in titres in sequential samples, is often the only reliable evidence of recent infection with *S. pyogenes* because the organism can be isolated from no more than one-quarter of patients by the time the disease has appeared. Antibody titres to several extracellular products are known to rise and fall more quickly than those to cellular components (Table 4) and are thus better indicators of recent streptococcal infection. If reliance is placed on a single determination it is important to know the level of titres that can be found in that community among those who do not have a history of recent streptococcal infection. For example, in Britain the upper limit of titres among teenagers and young adults in the absence of a recent history of infection is antistreptolysin O (**ASO**) 200, antideoxyribonuclease B (**ADB**) 240, and antihyaluronidase (**AHT**) 128. In a comparable population in the West Indies the upper limits can be ASO 300, ADB 400, and AHT 256. If a single determination of one antibody is made, then there is at best an 80 per cent chance of exceeding the normal value for that antibody in subjects who have had recent infection. For that reason laboratories are tending to use two or more tests. There is no titre that is diagnostic of rheumatic fever but antibody levels tend to be higher than among those who have had pharyngitis only and some 80 per cent of children or adults in Britain with acute rheumatic fever will have the following titres or higher: ASO 250, ADB 320, and AHT 300.

Laboratory tests indicating the presence of systemic inflammation are nearly always positive in patients with acute rheumatic fever. The erythrocyte sedimentation rate and C-reactive protein tests commonly used for this purpose are sensitive but are not specific for rheumatic fever. Unlike glomerulonephritis, circulating complement levels are raised. Radiography of the heart, electrocardiography, and echocardiography are used to detect cardiac involvement but are usually not considered laboratory tests. Doppler ultrasonography has been used to identify valvular involvement in patients in whom murmurs cannot be detected during conventional physical examination.

Table 5 *Jones criteria for the diagnosis of acute rheumatic fever (1992 revision)*

Major manifestations	Minor manifestations
Carditis	Clinical:
Polyarthritis	Arthralgia
Chorea	Fever
Erythema marginatum	Laboratory:
Subcutaneous nodules	Acute-phase reactions—erythrocyte sedimentation rate, C-reactive protein
	Electrocardiogram—prolonged PR interval
Plus: Supporting evidence of preceding streptococcal infection: Rising or increased ASO or other streptococcal antibodies, *or* Positive throat culture for *S. pyogenes*, *or* streptococcal antigen test	

Interpretation. The presence of two major criteria, or of one major and two minor criteria, indicates a high probability of the presence of rheumatic fever if supported by evidence of a preceding streptococcal infection.

There are three circumstances in which diagnosis of rheumatic fever can be made without adhering strictly to the Jones criteria. Chorea may occur as the only manifestation of rheumatic fever. Similarly indolent carditis may be the only manifestation in those who come to medical attention months after onset. Finally while most patients with recurrences of rheumatic fever fulfill the Jones criteria it may be difficult, for instance, to establish evidence of acute carditis in someone who has already had rheumatic heart disease.

See: Dajani, A.S. *et al.* (1993). *Circulation*, **87,** 302–7.

Diagnosis

Rheumatic fever may affect several organs or tissues, singly or in combination. No single manifestation, with the exception of Sydenham's chorea, or laboratory test is diagnostic and diagnosis is based on appropriate combinations—the revised Jones criteria given in Table 5. In this guide the term 'major' relates to the diagnostic importance and not to the frequency or severity of the manifestation. The revision of the original Jones criteria was to require evidence of recent streptococcal infection to support the diagnosis of acute rheumatic fever. There are two exceptions to this requirement: in some patients with chorea or carditis of insidious onset the titres of streptococcal antibodies may have all returned to normal when the patient is first seen.

Arthritis is the most common manifestation, occurring in some two-thirds of patients. It is characteristically migratory, commonly affects large joints, is usually not symmetrical, lasts 2 to 3 weeks, and the

Table 6 *Prevention of recurrent attacks of rheumatic fever*

Agent	Dose	Mode
Benzathine benzylpenicillin	1.2×10^6 i.u.	i.m. every 4 weeks[a]
Phenoxymethyl penicillin or phenoxyethyl penicillin	250 mg	O twice daily
Sulphadiazine	1 g (0.5 g in children)	O once daily
(For individuals allergic to penicillin *and* sulphonamides)		
Erythromycin	250 mg	O twice daily

i.u., international units; i.m., intramuscular; O, oral.

[a]If risk is high, administration every 3 weeks is usual.

painful swelling of the joints is reduced within 24 h by the administration of salicylates. Some physicians have suggested that arthritis is less common in tropical countries and that arthralgia, or pain in the absence of objective signs, be added as a 'major' criterion. The difference may, however, be due to the later admission of cases to hospital in poorer countries.

Differential diagnosis includes infective arthritis, infective endocarditis, which can be mistaken for a recurrence of rheumatic fever in those with rheumatic heart disease, and allergic conditions such as drug reactions and serum sickness.

Treatment

The patient should be confined to bed for the duration of the acute attack as measured by raised erythrocyte sedimentation rate and positive test for C-reactive protein. If carditis develops it does so within the first 2 or 3 weeks and close observation is necessary within this time. Salicylates or corticosteroids suppress the acute inflammation. Administration of penicillin does not limit the severity of rheumatic fever but penicillin prophylaxis should begin without delay to prevent the possibility of an early second attack.

Prevention

Primary prevention

Rheumatic fever can be prevented by early and adequate treatment of streptococcal sore throat and associated conditions such as otitis, sinusitis, and mastoiditis. If treatment begins within 6 days of onset of infection, prevention is almost total. The aim is to achieve something like complete elimination of *S. pyogenes* and this requires a full 10-day course of, usually, penicillin, regardless of the time at which signs of infection disappear.

Secondary prevention

The streptococcal sore throat that triggers a recurrence of rheumatic fever need not be symptomatic. Consequently, prevention of recurrences depends on continuous antimicrobial medication rather than diagnosis and treatment of streptococcal sore throat. Patients who have had rheumatic carditis are at greater risk of it recurring and they should receive prophylaxis well into adulthood, perhaps for life. Subjects who have not had carditis are at less risk of cardiac involvement and prophylaxis should continue until at least 5 years have passed since the last attack and perhaps to early adulthood.

Various schedules are given in Table 6. Intramuscular benzathine benzylpenicillin is of particular value in high-risk patients but is painful and may be inconvenient. Most failures of prophylaxis occur in non-compliant patients. Oral prophylaxis is more appropriate for patients at lower risk of recurrence and some physicians change to this method when the patient reaches late adolescence. For prophylaxis, but not treatment, sulphadiazine and oral penicillin are equally effective. Prophylaxis with sulphadiazine is contraindicated in late pregnancy because the drug crosses the placenta and competes with bilirubin for neonatal albumin sites. Allergic reactions to penicillin are more common in adults than children and are less severe with oral penicillin. One form of allergic reaction to this drug is like serum sickness with fever and joint pains. These reactions can be mistaken for rheumatic fever. Patients with rheumatic valvular heart disease require additional short-term antibiotic prophylaxis before some surgical and dental procedures to prevent bacterial endocarditis (see Chapter 15.17).

ACUTE POST-STREPTOCOCCAL GLOMERULONEPHRITIS

Acute post-streptococcal glomerulonephritis (**APSGN**) may follow infection on the throat or skin but only some strains of a limited number of serotypes cause outbreaks. It is characterized by haematuria and oedema with, in more serious cases, renal insufficiency. In many, the disease is symptomless and detected only by finding haematuria on microscopical examination of urine. Often it is mild and persists for a few days only. Rarely strains of group C cause the disease.

Pathogenesis

All glomeruli are involved in APSGN. The disease develops after a latent period of 6 to 10 days after pharyngitis and 14 to 21 days after skin infection. An immunological mechanism is suggested by the latent period between infection and onset, the early decrease in circulating complement, particularly C3, and the finding in biopsy material from the kidney of immune globulins, complement components, and streptococcal proteins. The glomeruli are infiltrated with inflammatory cells, first polymorphonuclear leucocytes then monocytes. The mesangium of the glomerular capillaries is oedematous and infiltrated with inflammatory cells. In the early stages, areas of electron-dense material ('humps') can be seen on the glomerular basement membrane and are generally held to contain IgG and components of complement. The humps generally disappear within 6 weeks. There may be proliferation of endothelial cells as well as epithelial cells of Bowman's capsule, producing crescents. This reaction is to fibrin or fibrin products.

At present, two streptococcal products are the main candidates for the determinant of nephritogenicity. A protein has been found in culture supernates that is unique to strains causing outbreaks of APSGN. It has been identified as a streptokinase (fibrinolysin) and is a plasminogen activator resulting in the production of plasmin, which splits the C3 molecule activating the alternative complement pathway and initiating the inflammatory response in the kidney. This streptokinase has a different amino acid composition to enzyme from strains not associated with APSGN and differs also from the enzyme used in the early treatment of thrombosis. The second candidate is an intracellular protein, endostreptosin, and it too has a remarkable ability to activate the alternative complement pathway. When one or other of these antigens has been studied antibody has been found in almost all patients with APSGN and less often in those with other streptococcal infections. Presumably such antibodies protect against second attacks of APSGN.

Clinical features

The disease occurs most often in young children and young adults but in areas of high incidence, preschool children are most often affected and the frequency falls off with increasing age. In all cases, whether overt or subclinical, haematuria can be detected on microscopic examination. In addition, gross haematuria occurs in less than one-half of patients and may last from a few days to 2 weeks. Proteinuria is present in nearly all patients and other abnormalities of the urine include hyaline, granular, and red blood-cell casts as well as pyuria. Hypertension and oedema are also prominent signs attributed to sodium and water retention. In a minority of patients, hypertension develops with consequent nausea, vomiting, headache, and seizures. The mortality among children admitted to hospital with the condition in developing countries is 5 per cent.

Diagnosis

Evidence should be sought of a prior or current streptococcal infection of the throat or skin. The C3 level is typically decreased for the first 2 weeks of the disease. This is an important confirmatory test. Decreased plasminogen levels and increased plasma fibrinolytic activity has been found in children with APSGN.

The differential diagnosis includes primary disorders of the kidneys and multisystem diseases that can cause haematuria, proteinuria, hypertension, and renal insufficiency. In addition, nephritis associated with other infectious diseases should be considered, although none of the following regularly causes gross haematuria, oedema, and hypertension. Relevant infections include bacterial endocarditis, bacterial sepsis with pneumococci or meningococci, persistent bacteraemia with staphylococci, and viral infections including hepatitis B and human immunodeficiency virus.

Epidemiology

In general, there are two main patterns of disease. APSGN can follow sore throat. Nearly all recent cases in Britain followed pharyngitis and serotypes 1, 4, 12, or 49 predominated. These were the serotypes isolated at about the same time from similar cases in Kuwait. In poor countries, often but not exclusively tropical or subtropical, it follows pyoderma. APSGN in these children is associated particularly with poor hygiene, overcrowded living conditions, and skin diseases such as scabies. Serotypes associated with this form of the disease are 49, 55, 57, and a few others. Post-impetigo nephritis is now rare in Britain but appears to have been common early in the twentieth century and may have been the disease described as 'trench nephritis' in the First World War.

APSGN is uncommon in Britain and is nearly always sporadic. The ratio of subclinical to symptomatic cases may be higher than suspected—in one limited study in the United States this ratio in sporadic cases was approximately 19:1. In some tropical countries where streptococcal infection is common, as many as 1 in 500 of the child population may suffer from nephritis in an epidemic year. In outbreaks in communities where impetigo is common, 20 per cent of streptococcal infections with type 49 can be followed by APSGN but in Britain it occurs in less than 1 per cent of infections with type 49.

Prophylaxis and treatment

If antibiotic treatment of streptococcal infection is to prevent APSGN—and the evidence that it does so is not clear cut—then it seems that treatment must begin within the first 3 days. If a patient with APSGN is still infected with *S. pyogenes*, then antibiotic treatment will help prevent spread of the nephritogenic strain. Once symptoms have appeared, antibiotic treatment does not affect the severity of renal damage. There is no specific treatment for APSGN but control of uraemia and hypertension may be needed in severe cases. Patients may be transferred home when signs subside but periodic examinations of urine and blood pressure are usually done for 6 to 12 months. Antibiotic prophylaxis is not required.

Diseases caused by group C and group G streptococci

Several species of streptococci, two of human origin but more from animals, carry the Lancefield C or G antigen (see Table 1). Further, some strains of *S. milleri* agg. cross-react with A, C, or G sera. The human strains of groups C and G belong to the pyogenic streptococci and may be carried asymptomatically in the throat or vagina of healthy persons. In some parts of Africa, representatives of either group are common in throat swabs.

The pattern of infection with human strains is like that of *S. pyogenes* but the organisms are of lesser virulence. Outbreaks of sore throat, clinically indistinguishable from that caused by group A streptococci, occur from time to time in Britain. In Britain, at least, such outbreaks have not been followed by either rheumatic fever or APSGN. ASO titres were raised in these patients (see Table 4). Other outbreaks have been of skin infections and, when involving pressure sores, cellulitis has sometimes occurred, or if of burns there has been death of applied skin grafts. Outbreaks of puerperal sepsis, not life threatening, have occurred in maternity units. Sporadic cases of all of the above can occur but it is not easy to establish causation. Bacteraemic infections with one or other occur but are less common than with *S. pyogenes*. Underlying causes of the bacteraemias include malignancy, septic arthritis, abdominal infections, and endocarditis. Polymicrobic bacteraemias sometimes occur, with *Staph. aureus* being the most common copathogen. The mortalities in reported bacteraemias have been: group A, 24 per cent (3342 cases); group C, 17 per cent (659 cases); and group G 15 per cent (1470 cases).

Most infections with either organism respond quickly to treatment with benzylpenicillin (see Table 3). Group G infections in cancer patients are a notable exception. Tolerance of penicillin, that is the minimal bactericidal concentration is at least 32 times greater than the minimal bacteriostatic concentration, has been described in some isolates of group G. Combinations of gentamicin with benzylpenicillin were bactericidal for these strains.

S. zooepidemicus, one of the species of group C causing infections in farm animals, sometimes infects man. Outbreaks of infection with this organism have followed consumption of unpasteurized milk or dairy products but acquisition directly from animals has occasionally seemed likely. Infections with this organism have been notable for their severity, causing septicaemia, septic aneurysm, sore throat with lymphadenitis, meningitis or glomerulonephritis. Streptolysin O is not formed by this organism.

Diseases caused by group B streptococci

The group B streptococcus (*S. agalactiae*) has been known for over a century as a cause of mastitis in cattle. It was recognized in the 1930s as a member of the flora of the human vagina, as an occasional cause of puerperal fever, and an uncommon cause of invasive disease in adults. The recent prominence of the organism as a cause of septicaemia and meningitis in and around the neonatal period is due in part to better laboratory procedures and also to the survival of premature babies that would have perished in earlier times. That said, there have been changes in the distribution of pathogens recovered from the bloodstream of infants in the first weeks of life. Before the introduction of antibiotics, *S. pyogenes* and *Staph. aureus* were the most frequently identified pathogens. Gram-negative organisms, especially *Escherichia coli*, became prominent with the introduction of antibiotics and modern nursing procedures. Now the group B streptococcus and *E. coli* make up more than 70 per cent of all isolates from the blood of neonates. There are further differences. In some British and American hospitals the group B streptococcus predominates, salmonellas are important in South America, and more infections with listeria are being diagnosed.

The organism

The chief determinant of virulence appears to be the type polysaccharide. Nearly all human strains carry one or other of six sialic acid-containing polysaccharides that surround the cell wall. In addition a protein antigen(Ic, X, or R) may be carried. Certain combinations are common. Thus representatives of the serotypes III or III/R form one-quarter of all isolates from superficial sites on women but three-quarters of all group B streptococci causing meningitis in infants. The type polysaccharide, like the M protein of *S. pyogenes*, inhibits phagocytosis of the organism. Bovine strains can usually be distinguished in the laboratory from human isolates and rarely cause disease in man.

Clinical features

IN NEONATES

The frequency of serious neonatal disease (septicaemia, meningitis, or both) has been variously quoted as between 0.3 and 5.4 cases/1000 live births but the figures have wide confidence limits. In one British survey, 66 babies among 227 000 developed septicaemia or meningitis due to *S. agalactiae* during the first 8 weeks of life: an attack rate of 0.3/1000. Some participating hospitals, however, had clusters of cases, others none.

Two fairly distinct clinical patterns of serious neonatal infections can be recognized, and predominate, but the clinical spectrum is wide and includes impetigo neonatorum, septic arthritis, osteomyelitis, peritonitis, pyelonephritis, conjunctivitis, and facial cellulitis.

Early-onset disease

Onset is often sudden, frequently within the first 6 to 24 h of life, but it may be present at birth. This indicates, in some at least, an intrauterine onset of infection. The first signs of illness are often abnormal respiratory patterns with tachypnoea and episodes of cyanosis or apnoea. Severe hypoxaemia is due to right-to-left shunting through areas of atelectasis and persistent fetal circulation. The infant's skin is often grey. Septicaemia is always present and one-third of babies develop meningitis as a consequence of this. Some of the mothers whose babies are born septicaemic have evidence of intrauterine infection before delivery, signs of which include fever, foul-smelling and cloudy liquor, and a purulent cervical discharge. The clinical signs in the baby are non-specific. Tachycardia is usually recorded (more than 160 beats/min), the body temperature may be raised or lowered, shock and unexplained respiratory distress are present. Some babies become neutropenic. When respiratory distress is present the idiopathic respiratory distress syndrome may be diagnosed. Areas of atelectasis and hyaline membranes are present in histological sections from autopsy specimens of lungs. The main histological difference from the idiopathic respiratory distress syndrome is the presence of cocci within the membranes. Mortality rates, even with early and intensive treatment, still exceed 25 per cent—half that recorded in the 1970s.

Fig. 3 Distribution by age of bacteraemia and meningitis caused by group B streptococci. Unpublished data of the Communicable Disease Surveillance Centre.

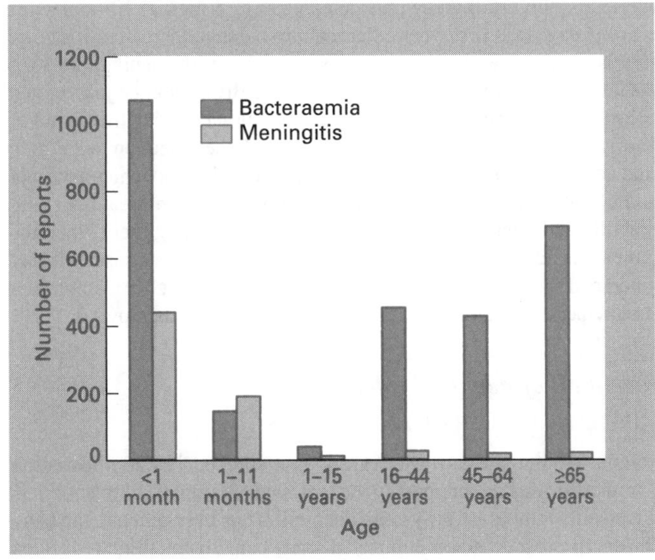

Late-onset disease

This is nearly always a purulent meningitis that cannot be distinguished clinically from other forms of neonatal meningitis. Blood cultures are almost invariably positive. Onset is most common in the second to fourth weeks of life and the incidence falls progressively from the sixth week to the end of the first year (Fig. 3). Late-onset meningitis can occur among babies that have gone home because they were previously healthy, of normal birth weight, and were born after normal labour. Outbreaks have occurred in special-care baby units, for example after the introduction of a baby with early-onset sepsis. Late-onset meningitis forms one-third of all serious, neonatal, group B streptococcal infection. Mortality is 15 to 20 per cent but many survivors suffer sequelae including deafness, mental retardation, or hydrocephalus.

IN ADULTS

Group B streptococcal meningitis is uncommon in adults and 80 per cent of infections are bacteraemic. When meningitis does occur it can usually be associated with previous neurological damage. In general the number of bacteraemic infections increases with age (Fig. 3), apart from a peak in women aged 16 to 44 years, which is associated with childbirth and abortion. Bacteriuria caused by group B streptococci occurs in 1 to 2 per cent of pregnant women and is associated with some cases of intrauterine fetal death and late spontaneous abortion. Patients with post-partum infections develop fever soon after delivery (mean 12 h) and positive blood cultures tend to occur with temperatures of 38.5 °C or greater. In more than one-half of the other bacteraemic adults, one or more predisposing factors can be identified, notably diabetes mellitus, leukaemia or steroid therapy. Endocarditis occurs. Mortality in bacteraemic adults is 15 per cent and is restricted to those with predisposing serious disease or the elderly.

Epidemiology

CARRIAGE

The organism can be recovered from various sites in healthy adults. At first, attention was given to vaginal carriage. Swabs taken from the lower part of the vagina are more often positive than high or cervical swabs and carriage rates of 3 to over 40 per cent have been reported. Higher rates have followed the use of selective media and enrichment techniques. In addition, carriage is, overall, influenced by the sexual activity of the population studied. It is highest in those attending clinics for sexually transmitted diseases—but there is no association of carriage with any particular disease. Families tend to carry the same strain. The urethra, vagina, perineum, and anorectal region have all been suggested as the prime site of carriage. The ratio of anorectal to vaginal carriage is approximately 5:4, both being higher than other sites. The results of swabbing the vagina at successive antenatal visits have led to the suggestion that carriage can be intermittent. If enrichment cultures are made from anorectal and vaginal swabs taken at both 28 and 36 weeks, intrapartum carriage of group B streptococci can be predicted in 90 per cent of cases. In Britain, however, between 20 and 30 per cent of women carry the organism and the neonatal attack rate is 0.3/1000. The cost-effectiveness of mass screening has therefore been questioned.

Some 7 to 10 per cent of normal adults carry group B streptococci in the throat and this appears to be independent of urogenital and anorectal carriage.

EARLY-ONSET NEONATAL DISEASE

This infection is acquired from the genital tract of the mother (Fig. 4). Up to one-half of infants born to carriers are colonized immediately after birth and group B streptococci can be recovered from the external auditory meatus and other sites. Occasionally the organism penetrates the intact fetal membranes and multiplies in the liquor amnii but it is generally believed that the usual mechanism of acquisition is during birth and that the organism enters the lungs with contaminated liquor amnii. If the mother is heavily colonized the baby is more likely to be so too. Heavy colonization of a baby is usually defined as at least 10^5 group B streptococci per culture swab from two or more external skin sites.

No more than 1 in 50 contaminated babies develops early-onset infection. Predisposing factors for babies born to mothers carrying group B streptococci are: prematurity (under 37 weeks gestation), low birth weight (particularly less than 2500 g), in multiple births the presence of sepsis in one of the siblings, intrapartum fever (peak fever in excess of 37.5 °C), prolonged rupture of amniotic membranes (for over 12 h), and chorioamnionitis.

LATE-ONSET DISEASE

The pathogenesis of late-onset disease is not as clear-cut as the early-onset form. Acquisition of the organism from mucosal sites during delivery, with subsequent invasion and bacteraemia, accounts for one-half of cases. Additionally, babies not exposed to the organism at birth may acquire it from hospital sources or family. Exceptionally up to 40 per cent of babies can acquire the organism in hospital nurseries. Prematurity and coexisting lung infection are known predisposing causes for late-onset infections.

ANTIBODY DEFICIENCY AS A DETERMINANT OF NEONATAL DISEASE

Neonatal sepsis caused by group B streptococci of serotype III has not been observed in infants acquiring at least 2 μg/ml of maternally derived IgG to the type polysaccharide. Active placental transfer of maternal IgG is minimal before 32 to 34 weeks of pregnancy. Also, some mothers whose babies developed sepsis had low levels of IgG against a variety of bacterial polysaccharide antigens, including the type-specific polysaccharides of the group B streptococci. None of these mothers suffered from recurrent infections. Some had raised levels of IgM antibody, presumably protecting the mother, but this antibody does not cross the placenta.

Fig. 4 Pattern of colonization and infection with group B streptococci in mothers and babies.

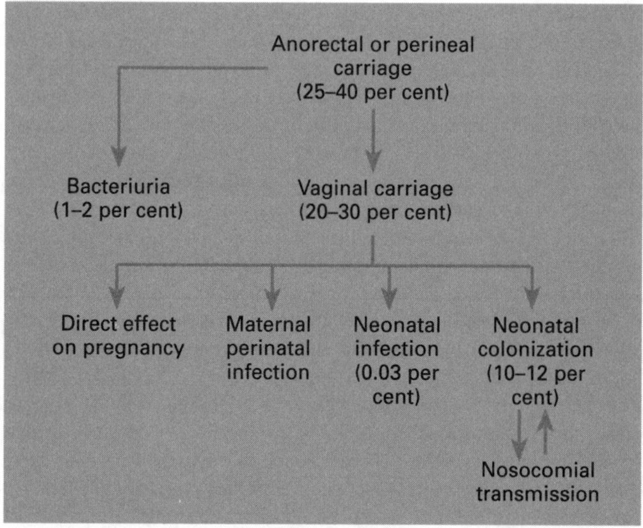

Diagnosis

In cases of suspected septicaemia or meningitis it is seldom possible to predict the nature of the infecting organism from clinical evidence alone. Culture of the blood should be made from a peripheral vessel because if taken from the umbilical vein there may be a false-positive result. Repeated examinations of cerebrospinal fluid are necessary in the newborn with septicaemia because purulent meningitis is a known complication. In the neonate, urinary tract infection with group B streptococci also tends to be associated with septicaemia and meningitis.

Early recognition of early-onset neonatal sepsis can be aided by finding a 5-min Apgar score of less than 7. This occurs in one-quarter of cases of sepsis but one-half of all fatal cases. The finding of pus cells and cocci in gastric aspirates and, perhaps most reliable of all, the detection of the Lancefield group B antigen in urine by latex particle agglutination can provide a provisional diagnosis until the results of cultures are known.

Treatment

Group B streptococci are sensitive to the penicillins and usually also to chloramphenicol and the macrolides. Some strains are resistant to the tetracyclines and, although resistant to the macrolides, there can be synergistic killing of most isolates with suitable mixtures of a penicillin and an aminoglycoside. The minimal inhibitory concentration of penicillin for these organisms is higher than for *S. pyogenes*. In serious infections in adults, larger parenteral doses, given 2-hourly, are necessary and treatment should be continued for a week.

In the newborn, antibiotic therapy of sepsis must begin after specimens have been taken but before results are available. Special problems, familiar to paediatricians, are, first, the small muscle mass, which limits the use of intramuscular injections; in serious infections, antibiotics are usually given intravenously. Second, the newborn is immature in liver and kidney functions; antibiotics such as the penicillins, aminoglycosides, and chloramphenicol may accumulate to toxic levels. Third, sulphonamides may bind to albumin, blocking bilirubin-binding sites and causing hyperbilirubinaemia. Fourth, abnormalities of fluid and electrolyte balance are common and, like the provision of adequate nutrition and ventilation, require careful management. One recommendation for initial treatment of suspected sepsis caused by group B streptococci is benzylpenicillin (15 mg/kg) plus gentamicin (2.5 mg/kg) 12-hourly for the first 3 days (the first week in premature babies), thereafter 8-hourly. There is no consensus on the antibiotic treatment of meningitis in the neonate except that it is difficult to treat. The British source just quoted recommends chloramphenicol for the provisional initial treatment of meningitis in a neonate. Others argue that if the infection were then found to be due to group B streptococci the chloramphenicol present could be antagonistic to ampicillin. They advocate initial treatment with ampicillin and gentamicin (or another aminoglycoside); then, when the organism is identified as a group B streptococcus, its susceptibility defined and the patient is improving rapidly, continuing with ampicillin or benzylpenicillin alone for a total of 10 to 14 days therapy.

Prevention of neonatal infection

PROPHYLACTIC USE OF ANTIBIOTICS

Attempts to eliminate carriage of group B streptococci by administration of ampicillin during pregnancy have failed. Vaginal colonization is reduced only temporarily. Systemic penicillin has been given to the baby at birth. In a randomized controlled trial, benzylpenicillin was given intramuscularly within 1 h of birth to babies weighing less than 2000 g. Neither the incidence nor the mortality from early-onset infection was significantly reduced. This suggests that prevention must begin before delivery. Some two-thirds of cases, and nine-tenths of deaths from early-onset infection occur in babies born to mothers who are carriers of group B streptococci and who have been pregnant for less than 37 weeks, or whose membranes have been ruptured for more than 12 h or who have an intrapartum temperature greater than 37.5 °C. In these mothers, administration of 2 g ampicillin followed by 1 g intravenously every 4 h until delivery eliminated colonization and infection in the neonate. Opinions differ on whether, or not, infants born to mothers receiving this prophylactic treatment should then receive four doses of ampicillin (50 mg/kg) at 12-hourly intervals.

OTHER PROPHYLACTIC MEASURES

As some cases of late-onset disease follow nosocomial transmission of the organism the application of techniques that prevent spread is desirable. In particular, meticulous use of chlorhexidine-containing hand lotions has been shown to reduce transmission by way of the hands. The central problem is the colonized mother–baby pair. Babies dying from septicaemia should be nursed in isolation.

Immunization of all pregnant women with one or more of the group B type polysaccharides has been suggested. The type III polysaccharide is a safe and effective immunogen in normal adults but the proposed recipients are a high-risk group. Moreover, the infrequency of infection and the failure of some women to respond to natural exposure have created further doubts on this procedure.

Passive immunization with hyperimmune globulin preparations is currently not feasible because preparations suitable for intravenous injection contain insufficient type-specific antibody.

Diseases caused by the S. milleri *aggregate*

Members of this group of organisms are found in considerable numbers in the mouth, upper respiratory tract, the gut, and the vagina. The organisms are isolated regularly from deep-seated infections, sometimes in pure culture, sometimes with other members of the normal flora including anaerobes. The organism does cause endocarditis and occasionally septicaemia but more often its presence in blood cultures should prompt a search for a pyogenic focus. It is the organism isolated most frequently from brain abscesses but usually not of the temporal lobe. Some of these abscesses have been associated with frontal sinusitis or dental sepsis. It is a common isolate from serious suppurative lesions in the abdominal cavity, including kidney and subphrenic abscesses. It is often present in suppurative infections in and around the mouth but here, rarely in pure culture. *S. milleri* is a notable cause of liver abscesses, in one-half of which it has been present in pure culture. Some of these patients have a history of abdominal surgery, intestinal perforation, or bowel cancer. It has been isolated more often from inflamed than normal appendices but the significance of this finding is not clear. Other sources have included wounds following appendicectomy, peritonitis and pelvic abscesses, lung abscesses, pleural empyema, and extradural or subdural empyema. It is an uncommon cause of meningitis.

The mechanisms of pathogenicity of *S. milleri* are unknown. Prophylactic use of metronidazole plus gentamicin in patients undergoing colorectal surgery has sometimes been followed by abdominal sepsis caused by *S. milleri*. This has led to the suggestion that an alternative regime that has activity against the organism be used.

Surgical drainage is a necessary part of the management of abscesses. Nearly all strains are fully sensitive to benzylpenicillin, the cephalosporins, erythromycin, and clindamycin but courses of 28 days or longer have been needed for conditions such as liver abscess. *S. milleri* is resistant to the sulphonamides. The choice of antibiotics will be influenced by the presence, or possible presence, of Gram-negative anaerobes.

Diseases caused by the enterococci

The enterococci are part of the saprophytic flora of the gut of man (and animals). *Enterococcus faecalis* represents nine-tenths of the clinical isolates. Next in frequency are representatives of *E. faecium*. There are now more reports of the isolation of *E. avium*, *E. durans*, *E. raffinosus*, *E. gallinarum*, and *E. casseliflavus*, due in part to better laboratory methods. The traditional view has been that some cofactor must exist for the enterococci to sustain a significant infection. This is often still true but is a poor guide to the management of infections in patients with serious underlying disease.

Clinical features

The urinary tract is the most frequent site of enterococcal infection. In men it affects most frequently those aged over 55 years and is associated with instrumentation or structural abnormality. A broader age distribution for urinary tract infection is found in women. The enterococci are often present in wound infections, particularly those associated with intra-abdominal surgery or trauma. In both they are seldom isolated in pure culture.

More cases of enterococcal bacteraemia are being recorded. The source of the organism is often the urinary tract. Many bacteraemias are related to the presence of catheters, either urinary or intravascular, and in some instances simple removal of the invasive device effects cure. Enterococcal bacteraemia can be transient, particularly after procedures such as sigmoidoscopy that involve the gastrointestinal tract. Other bacteraemias arise from wounds, the biliary tract, and in mothers and babies around childbirth. The incidence of neonatal sepsis, both of early and late onset, is one-third of that with the group B streptococci. The predisposing causes are the same with both organisms but the mortality rate in infants with enterococcal sepsis is one-half that found with the group B streptococci. In adults with serious underlying disease the mortality from enterococcal bacteraemia exceeds 50 per cent. Patients at particular risk are those who are granulocytopenic, have renal failure, or malignancy, are immunosuppressed, or if more than half of the body surface is burnt.

An important predisposing cause for enterococcal infection is the prior use of antibiotics. Superinfection has been associated particularly with the use of cephalosporins, ciprofloxacin, or co-trimoxazole. Also, when vancomycin has been used in combination with a cephalosporin for empirical treatment of undiagnosed sepsis, or prophylactically in high-risk patients, vancomycin-resistant enterococci have emerged.

Some enterococci are haemolytic and the haemolysin may be a virulence factor. Again, when enterococci are present in foodstuffs, such as cheeses, pressor amines can be produced, possibly leading to migraine in susceptibles or hypertensive crises in patients receiving monoamine oxidase inhibitors.

Treatment

The treatment of serious enterococcal infection is difficult but is aided by precise identification of the species responsible combined with detailed study of the sensitivity of the organism to potentially useful antibiotics and determination of drug levels in the patient.

Enterococci are more resistant to antibiotics than the streptococci. Ampicillin and amoxycillin, like benzylpenicillin, are bacteriostatic at clinically achievable levels at most sites but are often used for uncomplicated wound or urinary tract infections caused by *E. faecalis*. *E. faecium* has a somewhat higher intrinsic resistance to the penicillins. The enterococci are either insensitive or resistant to all the cephalosporins. β-Lactamase-resistant penicillins are inactive clinically and the currently rare infections caused by *E. faecalis* that forms the enzyme are being treated with ampicillin combined with an inhibitor such as clavulanic acid. Other strains of *E. faecalis* and *E. faecium* are highly resistant to penicillins because of mutations to penicillin-binding proteins.

Many enterococci are resistant to chloramphenicol, clindamycin, erythromycin, and the tetracyclines. Enterococci are normally insensitive to the aminoglycosides but there is often synergistic killing by an aminoglycoside plus an antibiotic that inhibits cell-wall synthesis—such as a penicillin or vancomycin. Combined therapy is necessary to achieve bactericidal activity in the treatment of meningitis, endocarditis, or bacteraemia. One recommendation is for a total daily dosage of ampicillin (150 to 250 mg/kg) or vancomycin (30 mg/kg) and either streptomycin (15 to 30 mg/kg) or gentamicin (3 to 6 mg/kg). Many strains are highly resistant to streptomycin; thus gentamicin must be used for these isolates. However, some 10 per cent of isolates of *E. faecalis* from serious infections in British hospitals are highly resistant to gentamicin and, except for the few that retain normal sensitivity to streptomycin, finding a bactericidal combination is either difficult or impossible. Some cases of bacteraemia caused by gentamicin-resistant strains have been treated adequately with ampicillin alone. High-level resistance to gentamicin is less common among isolates of *E. faecium* but hospital outbreaks with resistant strains have occurred.

A glycopeptide, such as vancomycin, is used when the patient is allergic to penicillin or when the infecting strain is highly resistant to penicillin. Three forms of resistance to the glycopeptide antibiotics occur among the enterococci. 'Van A' strains have inducible, high-level resistance to both vancomycin and teicoplanin. 'Van B' strains have inducible, moderate resistance to vancomycin but retain normal sensitivity to teicoplanin because it does not act as an inducer. The 'A' and 'B' forms of resistance are found in representatives of *E. faecalis* and *E. faecium*. 'Van C' strains have constitutive, low-level resistance to vancomycin only and resistance of this type is a property of virtually all strains of *E. gallinarum* and *E. casseliflavus*. Treatment with vancomycin is ineffective for infections caused by any of the three classes and the efficacy of teicoplanin for infections caused by strains of the classes 'B' and 'C' remains to be established.

Transmission

Enterococcal infection used to be described as almost always endogenous in origin. For example, in prospective studies, strains causing urinary tract infections associated with indwelling catheters had patterns of antibiotic sensitivity similar to rectal or perineal isolates from the same patient but distinguishable from those present on nurses' hands. More recently, clustering of infections caused by strains with new patterns of antibiotic resistance has occurred within centres handling high-risk patients and the strains have spread to other hospitals. The mechanisms of transfer between patients are unknown but control measures that have been found effective in preventing spread of methicillin-resistant staphylococci should be used. These measures include handwashing, careful use of broad-spectrum antibiotics, and barrier precautions for patients infected or colonized with highly resistant strains.

Streptococcal endocarditis

Streptococci remain the largest single group of bacteria causing bacterial endocarditis, constituting at least 60 per cent of the total. Staphylococci, 20 per cent, are the next largest group. This section deals with the special relation of streptococci to the disease process; see Chapter 15.17 for a more general account.

The typical age and sex of those dying from infective endocarditis in England and Wales has changed over the last 60 years. Before antibiotics, 10 per cent of the deaths were in those aged over 65 years, now it is more than 50 per cent. Since the year 1947 more males have died than females. These changes can be explained in part by the occurrence of fewer cases of rheumatic heart disease, which was more common in women, an increasing population of elderly patients treated in hospitals, and the recognition that arteriosclerotic calcific valvular disease in older patients may have an important association with bacterial endocarditis.

The pyogenic streptococci and pneumococci seldom cause endocarditis now. Most cases are caused by streptococci of the oral division. *S. sanguis*, *S. oralis*, and *S. mutans* are the most common causes and are found principally in or around the mouth. *S. bovis* is associated, particularly, with bacterial endocarditis in those aged over 55 years. It is recovered rarely from the human mouth but is present in the bowel. Endocarditis and bacteraemia caused by *S. bovis* are often associated with neoplasms or other ulcerative lesions of the large intestine. In France, an additional association with alcoholic cirrhosis has been noted.

Streptococci may reach the heart valves from septicaemic infection but more often, it is believed, from transient, symptomless bacteraemia. Such bacteraemias are known to arise from dental manipulations that damage periodontal tissues—particularly extraction of teeth, periodontal surgery, and the removal of dental calculus from within the gingival sulcus. Prior dental procedures have been recorded in 15 per cent of cases of bacterial endocarditis. Further, patients who develop bacterial endocarditis caused by one of the oral streptococci and who are permitted to retain apparently healthy teeth are possibly at greater risk of recurrence than those rendered edentulous. Bacteraemias from the gastrointestinal tract, the genitourinary tract, or nosocomial procedures involving access to the bloodstream each account for a further 5 per cent of cases. No portal of entry is evident in 60 per cent of cases. Bacterial endocarditis associated with intravenous drug abuse is usually caused by staphylococci.

Some explanation is needed for the association with endocarditis of streptococci that are not usually thought to be overt pathogens. For example, in procedures involving the gingival sulcus, representatives of many different species enter the bloodstream. Few cases of endocarditis are caused by anaerobes, presumably because conditions on the heart valves are insufficiently reducing to permit growth. In addition, Gram-negative bacteria, because of the nature of their cell wall, are ordinarily killed by the combination of the circulating 'natural' antibodies and complement. The proportion of endocarditis caused by Gram-negative bacteria, even though it is surprisingly small, is probably increasing among severely ill patients. The two factors just mentioned exclude much of the mucosal flora. Some of the oral streptococci involved form a cell-bound polymer, a glucan, during the metabolism of sucrose. This material could increase the size of the seeding mass and limit the diffusion of antibiotics. Another possible virulence factor is a protein that causes platelet agglutination.

Antibiotic prophylaxis of bacterial endocarditis is complex, partly because of the need to identify factors that give, or might give, an increased risk of disease and partly because of the many proposed schedules. Some conditions that commonly predispose to endocarditis include: a history of previous bacterial endocarditis, rheumatic and other acquired valvular lesions, most congenital cardiac defects, prosthetic cardiac valves, and mitral valve prolapse. Most oral streptococci are susceptible to penicillin but administration of the agent leads to selection of resistant strains and also the appearance in the mouth of *S. faecalis*, which cannot usually be isolated from this site. Prophylaxis should therefore be given just before the procedure is begun.

Cases of non-enterococcal endocarditis have been treated effectively with large doses of benzylpenicillin given parenterally for 6 weeks. Many physicians combine this with an aminoglycoside, usually gentamicin, at least for the first 2 weeks. This is said to reduce the chance of relapse and permit a reduction of the total length of treatment to 4 weeks. The difficulties of treatment of enterococcal endocarditis have been mentioned before. A full discussion of the antibiotic prophylaxis and treatment of bacterial endocarditis is given elsewhere (Chapter 15.17).

REFERENCES

Ahrenholz, D.H. (1988). Necrotizing soft-tissue infections. *Surgical Clinics of North America*, **68,** 199–214.

Bisno, A.L. *et al.* (1989). Antimicrobial treatment of infective endocarditis due to viridans streptococci, enterococci, and staphylococci. *Journal of the American Medical Association*, **261,** 1471–7.

Christensen, K.K., Christensen, P., and Ferrieri, P. (ed.) (1985). Neonatal group B streptococcal infections. In *Antibiotics and Chemotherapy*, Vol. 35. Karger, Basel.

Colman, G., Tanna, A., Efstratiou, A., and Gaworzewska, E.T. (1993). The serotypes of *Streptococcus pyogenes* present in Britain 1980–1990 and their association with disease. *Journal of Medical Microbiology* **39,** 465–78.

Colman, G., Efstratiou, A., and Morrison, D. (1992). In *Identification methods in applied and environmental microbiology.* (ed. R.G. Board, D. Jones, and F.A. Skinner), pp. 221–49. Blackwell Scientific, Oxford.

Kaplan, E.L. (ed.) (1994). Understanding group A streptococcal infections in the 1990s: proceedings of a symposium. *Pediatric Infectious Disease Journal*, **13,** 556–83.

Klein, J.O., Feigin, R.D., and McCracken, G.H. (1986). Diagnosis and management of meningitis. *Pediatrics*, **78**(Suppl.), 959–82.

Murray, B.E. (1990). The life and times of the enterococcus. *Clinical Microbiology Reviews*, **3,** 46–65.

Orefici, G. (ed.) (1992). New perspectives on streptococci and streptococcal infections. *Zentralblatt für Bakteriologie*, (suppl. 22).

Simmons, N.A. *et al.* The antibiotic prophylaxis of infective endocarditis. (1982). *Lancet*, **ii.** 1323–6; (1990). *Lancet*, **335,** 88–9; (1992). *Lancet*, **339,** 1292–3.

Stevens, D.L. (1992). Invasive group A streptococcus infections. *Clinical Infectious Diseases*, **14,** 2–13.

Taranta, A. and Markowitz, M. (1990). *Rheumatic fever*, (2nd edn). Kluwer, Dordrecht.

7.11.3 Pneumococcal infection

B. M. GREENWOOD

Streptococcus pneumoniae (the pneumococcus) is a frequent commensal of the upper respiratory tract and an important cause of pneumonia and meningitis. The organism was first identified in saliva by Pasteur and by Sternberg in 1881. In 1886, Weichselbaum showed that the pneumococcus was an important cause of pneumonia. Despite the discovery of antibiotics that are highly effective against the pneumococcus this bacterium still causes many deaths and much illness in industrialized and in developing countries.

The organism

The pneumococcus is a Gram-positive bacterium, which, in clinical specimens, appears as a lanceolate diplococcus. In culture it may form short chains. It grows rapidly on most bacteriological media and on blood agar encapsulated strains form small, shiny colonies that are surrounded by a greenish area of α-haemolysis. Pneumococci grow rapidly in broth but, after some hours of growth, production of autolytic enzymes may lead to death of the culture. Enzymes produced by the pneumococcus include an α-haemolysin (pneumolysin), neuraminidase, hyaluronidase, and leucocidin. The gene for pneumolysin has been cloned and this enzyme has been studied extensively during the past few years as a potential vaccine candidate. Pneumolysin-negative strains show diminished virulence in experimental infections. Pneumococci can be differentiated from other α-haemolytic streptococci by their solubility in bile, and by their sensitivity to ethyl hydrocuprein chloride (Optochin), a compound that was once used in the treatment of pneumococcal infection. Mice are very susceptible to many strains of pneumococci and mouse inoculation has been used to isolate pneumococci from clinical samples.

Virulent strains of pneumococci possess a polysaccharide capsule. At least 83 different serotypes of pneumococci have been identified on the basis of antigenic differences in the composition of their capsular polysaccharides. Pneumococci can be serotyped by the Quellung reaction; exposure to a specific antiserum causes the capsule of the bacterium to swell, or by coagglutination. Characterization of the capsular polysaccharide forms the basis of the main classification system for pneumococci.

Recently, microbiologists have paid more attention to the proteins of the pneumococcus than in the past in the hope that these could provide the basis for a vaccine which would be effective against pneumococci of many capsular serotypes. Pneumococcal surface-protein A (**PspA**) is a membrane protein that can be detected on the surface of the pneumococcus. Typing with monoclonal antibodies has shown that PspA varies antigenically between strains and that pneumococci with the same capsular serotype may have different PspA proteins. Heterogeneity between strains with the same capsular polysaccharide has also been demonstrated by DNA fingerprinting techniques. The gene for another protein (37 kDa) that is partially expressed on the surface of the bacterium has been cloned; this protein is also being studied as a possible vaccine candidate.

Until 25 years ago, nearly all pneumococci were sensitive to all the commonly used antibiotics including penicillin. However, pneumococci with diminished sensitivity to penicillin (minimum inhibitory concentration (**MIC**) 0.1–1.0 μg/ml) and others even more resistant to penicillin (MIC > 1.0 μg) have now been isolated in many parts of the world. In 1967, pneumococci with a diminished sensitivity to penicillin were described in Australia and Papua New Guinea. In 1977, three infants died from meningitis caused by pneumococci that were clinically resistant to penicillin and chloramphenicol in Durban, South Africa; a subsequent outbreak in Johannesburg was caused by pneumococci (type 19A) that were highly resistant to penicillin (MIC > 4 μg/ml) and also resistant to most other antibiotics except rifampicin. Penicillin-resistant pneumococci have continued to cause problems in South Africa and, recently, there have been alarming reports of an increasing prevalence of infections caused by penicillin-insensitive bacteria from several parts of Europe and from other industrialized and developing countries. Thus, in Hungary in 1988/89, 58 per cent of all pneumococcal isolates showed diminished sensitivity to penicillin (MIC > 0.15 μg/ml); many of these bacteria were resistant to tetracycline and co-trimoxazole, and some to chloramphenicol. Similarly, in parts of Spain one-half of all clinical isolates are now penicillin insensitive and most are resistant to other antibiotics also. Penicillin-insensitive pneumococci are generally still infrequent in the United Kingdom and the United States (fewer than 5 per cent of isolates) but much higher levels of resistance were reported recently in Kentucky and Tennessee. Recent experience in Iceland has shown that the situation can change with remarkable rapidity (Fig. 1). The prevalence of penicillin-insensitive pneumococci in many parts of the world is not known with any accuracy but it seems likely that rapid changes are taking place in many developing as well as industrialized

Fig. 1 Increasing prevalence of penicillin-resistant pneumococci in Iceland. The solid bars indicate multiresistant strains. (Reproduced from Kristinsson *et al.* (1992). *Lancet*, **327,** 1606, with permission.)

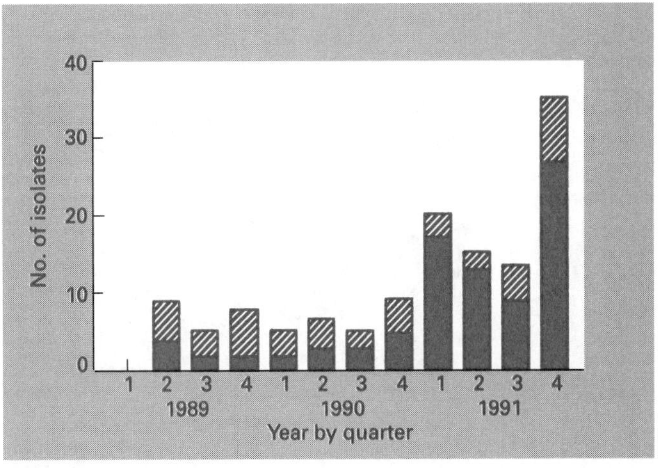

countries. Penicillin-insensitive pneumococci are found most frequently in those with a recent history of hospitalization or antibiotic treatment.

Penicillin resistance is probably acquired in a step-wise fashion as a result of three mutations and it is associated with changes in the penicillin-binding proteins 1 and 2. Resistant strains show heterogeneity in the number and size of their penicillin-binding proteins. Resistance to lysis on exposure to penicillin is sometimes associated with penicillin resistance but the two phenomena are thought to be brought about by different mechanisms. Most penicillin insensitive pneumococci belong to serogroups 6, 14, 19, or 23. Pneumococci do not produce β-lactamase.

Epidemiology

Incidence of pneumococcal infection

The pneumococcus is one of the chief killers of children throughout the developing world. It has been estimated that 4 to 5 million children die from acute respiratory infections each year. Determining the cause of such deaths is difficult, as many of these children die at home and few undergo any laboratory investigations. However, studies in several developing countries have shown that the pneumococcus is the most important cause of pneumonia among children admitted to hospital, accounting for 25 to 50 per cent of cases (Fig. 2). If this applies also to the children who die without investigation, then the pneumococcus is likely to be the cause of at least 1 million deaths a year among the world's children, a similar notoriety to that attributed to malaria.

In industrialized countries, the pneumococcus remains a principal cause of illness and death, and is the most frequent cause of community-acquired pneumonia. Because many cases are treated by primary health-care physicians without laboratory investigation, accurate statistics on the incidence of pneumococcal disease are difficult to obtain. However, in the United States it has been estimated that there are between 150 000 and 500 000 cases of pneumococcal pneumonia each year, with 10 000 to 25 000 deaths, and that 10 to 20 per cent of American children experience at least one attack of pneumococcal otitis media during the first few years of life. Otitis media and its subsequent complications are one of the main causes of childhood illness in most industrialized societies.

Geographical distribution

Pneumococcal disease occurs throughout the world from the Arctic to the tropics. It is most prevalent among communities where crowding and poor living conditions prevail. Some occupational groups, such as South African miners, have a particularly high incidence of the infection. In the United States, the disease is more frequent among blacks than among whites.

Fig. 2 The major causes of pneumonia in children in developing countries as indicated by lung aspiration. The results obtained in 596 children seen during eight studies are shown.

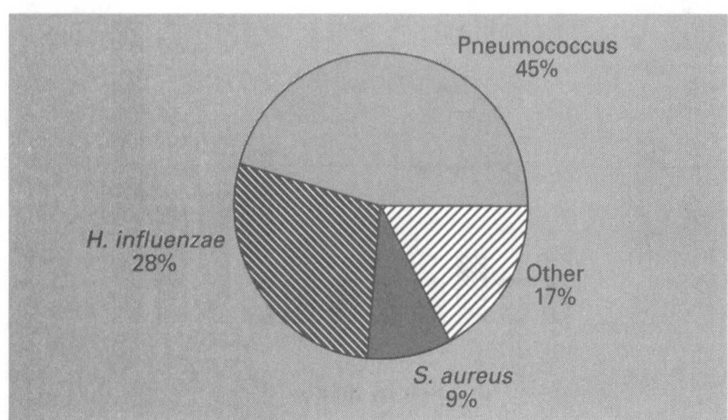

The distribution of pneumococcal serotypes causing clinical disease varies substantially from area to area and, to a lesser extent, from time to time. During the past few years, more data have been acquired on the prevalence of different serotypes in various parts of the world but there are still many areas for which this information is lacking. Collection of this information is essential before vaccination with capsular polysaccharide vaccines is contemplated.

Seasonality

In countries with a temperate climate, pneumococcal pneumonia occurs more frequently in winter than in summer. Winter epidemics of viral respiratory-tract infections, which may be followed by pneumonia, may be one explanation for this seasonal association. In savannah Africa, pneumococcal infection occurs most frequently during the hot, dry time of the year when, as during winter in countries with a temperate climate, absolute humidity is lowest. Perhaps a low absolute humidity impairs local surface defences.

Epidemics

Epidemics of pneumococcal disease are rare but localized outbreaks have been recorded in refugee camps, barracks, and gaols. Pneumococci of several different serotypes have been implicated in these outbreaks.

Age and sex distribution of cases

In industrialized countries, pneumococcal infections are mainly a problem of the young and the old. Pneumococcal meningitis is seen most frequently in the very young and in the elderly, and pneumococcal pneumonia is most frequent in the elderly (Fig. 3). In developing countries, the incidence of pneumococcal pneumonia and meningitis is maximal during the first few years of life but invasive pneumococcal disease is seen more frequently in older children and in young adults than it is in industrialized societies.

Predisposing factors

Several groups of subjects have an increased susceptibility to pneumococcal disease (Table 1). Patients with general debilitating diseases such as diabetes, alcoholism, and drug addiction are at risk; pneumococcal septicaemia is an important cause of death in heroin addicts in some communities. Susceptibility is increased in patients with congenital or

Fig. 3 The age distribution of cases of pneumococcal meningitis and pneumococcal septicaemia in The Netherlands, 1990. (Reproduced from Annual Report, Netherlands Reference Laboratory for Bacterial Meningitis, with permission.)

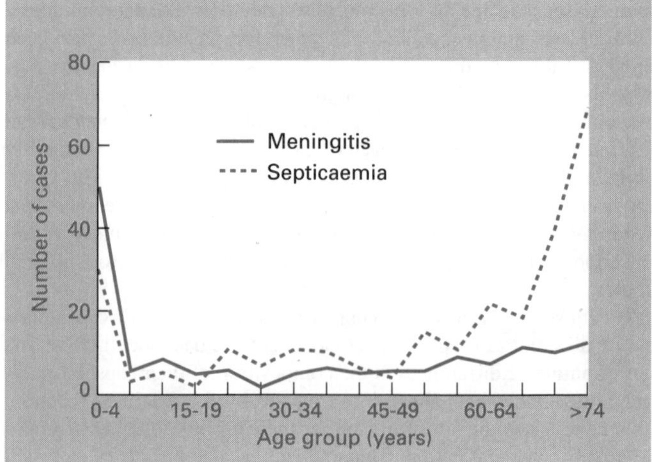

Table 1 *Some important risk factors for pneumococcal pneumonia and septicaemia*

Damage to the respiratory-tract epithelium
Adverse climatic conditions:
Low absolute humidity
Cold
Air pollution:
Respirable particles
Toxic gases
Chemical:
Anaesthetics
Inhaled poisons
Cigarette smoke
Infectious:
Viral infections
Mycoplasma infections
Mechanical:
Bronchial obstruction
Impaired systemic immunity
Hypogammaglobulinaemia:
Congenital
Acquired
Splenic hypofunction:
Traumatic
Sickle-cell disease
Alcoholism and drug addiction
Systemic lupus erythematosus
HIV infection

acquired hypogammaglobulinaemia and in those with an absent or non-functional spleen. Thus, pneumococcal infection is an important complication of sickle-cell disease because many patients with this condition have a malfunctioning spleen as well as a defect in the alternative complement pathway. Patients with congestive cardiac failure or the nephrotic syndrome are also at increased risk of pneumococcal infection. Studies in the United States have shown that subjects with human immunodeficiency virus (**HIV**) infection are about 300 times more at risk from invasive pneumococcal disease than controls, and it has been suggested that the incidence of pneumococcal disease in young and middle-aged adults can be used as an indirect indicator of the prevalence of HIV infection in a community.

Studies in several developing countries have shown an association between exposure to smoke from indoor fires and the incidence of pneumonia in children. Both respirable particles and toxic gases, such as nitrous oxide, probably damage the local defences of the respiratory tract, predisposing to bacterial infections.

Pathogenesis and immunity

Spread of infection

Pneumococci spread from person to person by droplet infection. If local conditions are favourable, inhaled pneumococci become established in the nasopharynx. Nasopharyngeal carriage of pneumococci is extremely common. In industrialized societies, around 25 to 50 per cent of healthy subjects carry pneumococci and carriage rates may reach nearly 100 per cent in developing countries, where a high proportion of babies are colonized within the first few months of life. Longitudinal studies in American children have shown that children may carry a pneumococcus of the same serotype for many months, that acquisition of a new serotype is often associated with an upper respiratory-tract infection, and that circulating type-specific antibody does not prevent acquisition of a new serotype, although it may shorten the duration of carriage.

Local spread of pneumococci from the nasopharynx may cause otitis media and its subsequent complications (Fig. 4). Clinical observations and studies in experimental animals suggest that most cases of pneumococcal pneumonia result from aspiration of the nasopharyngeal secretions containing pneumococci into alveoli but blood-borne spread from the nasopharynx is possible. Pneumolysin impairs the activity of respiratory mucosal cilia. Once established in the lung, pneumococci may spread directly to adjacent pleura or pericardium. From the lung, they may spread through the systemic circulation to reach the meninges, joints, eyes, or other distant sites. Many patients with extrapulmonary pneumococcal disease do not have any signs of pneumonia; whether, in such patients, bacteraemia arises from a subclinical pulmonary focus or directly from the nasopharynx is uncertain.

Pathogenesis of clinical features

Pneumococci produce an acute inflammatory reaction characterized by an increase in vascular permeability, oedema, and an accumulation of polymorphonuclear neutrophil leucocytes (**PMNs**) at the affected site. The endothelium of vessels in affected tissues may be damaged. Several factors contribute to the pathogenesis of this response (Fig. 5). Recent studies in experimental animals have demonstrated that components of the pneumococcal cell wall, in particular techoic acid and peptidoglycan, can induce a powerful inflammatory response. These cell-wall structures stimulate the production by mononuclear cells of the cytokines interleukin (**IL**)-1 and tumour necrosis factor. These cytokines induce the expression by endothelial cells of the receptor molecules CD62, ELAM 1, and ICAM 1, which bind PMNs to the endothelial surface and facilitate their escape into the surrounding tissues. Experimental studies have shown that neutrophils escape through gaps that open up between the endothelial cells of small cerebral vessels and thus gain access to the cerebrospinal fluid. Some pneumococcal capsular polysaccharides activate the alternative complement pathway producing C3a, and C5a, which are chemotactic for PMNs. Activation of the complement pathway may also play a part in initiating the disseminated intravascular coagulation that may occur in patients with fulminating pneumococcal septicaemia.

Although capsular polysaccharide antigens may persist in the serum for many days after an episode of pneumococcal infection, immune-complex disease is a rare complication. A few patients have been

Fig. 4 The pathway of pneumococcal infection.

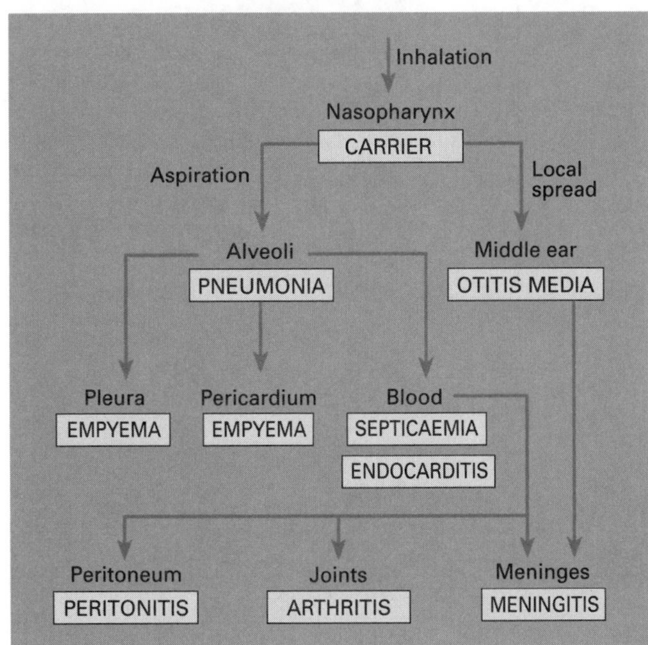

described who developed immune complex-mediated glomerulonephritis after a pneumococcal infection but the allergic arthritis and cutaneous vaculitis that often complicate meningococcal infection are not seen.

The pathogenesis of the jaundice found in some patients with pneumococcal pneumonia is controversial. Some believe that it is due primarily to haemolysis and especially likely to occur in those who are glucose-6-phosphate dehydrogenase deficient. Other believe that it is due mainly to liver-cell damage; liver biopsy may show such damage and cholestasis. Probably both factors are involved in most jaundiced patients.

Immunity

Both local and systemic defence mechanisms are involved in protection against pneumococcal disease. In a healthy subject, nasopharyngeal secretions are prevented from reaching the alveoli by the epiglottis, the sticky mucus that lines the bronchial tree, and by respiratory cilia, which ensure that bacteria trapped in this mucus are carried upwards, away from the alveoli and expectorated or swallowed. Even if pneumococci manage to overcome these mechanical barriers and reach alveoli, they may be destroyed rapidly by alveolar macrophages. Small amounts of antibody and complement are present in alveolar secretions and coating of bacteria with IgG or with C3b promotes their phagocytosis. Surfactant in alveolar secretions may have some protective effect also.

If these initial defence mechanisms are overcome and an acute inflammatory reaction is set in progress, further protective mechanisms come into play at once. PMNs are brought to the site of infection in large numbers and attempt to ingest pneumococci. This they may be unable to achieve unaided. However, complement components are present in acute inflammatory exudates and coating of pneumococci with C3b and C5b, as a result of activation of the alternative complement pathway, may help leucocytes to phagocytose them. Although they may be unable to phagocytose some strains of virulent pneumococci *in vitro*, PMNs may be more successful when they can trap the bacteria against some immobile object such as an alveolar wall. PMNs and non-specific opsonins cannot contain infection with some virulent strains of pneumococci; recovery from infection with these organisms can be achieved only if the untreated patient survives long enough to form specific anticapsular antibodies, which agglutinate pneumococci and which are powerful opsonins. Formation of specific polysaccharide antibodies takes 5 to 7 days. The persistence of capsular polysaccharide antigen in body fluids may suppress antibody production and patients with persistent antigenaemia often have a prolonged and stormy clinical course.

Fig. 5 The pathogenesis of pneumococcal infection.

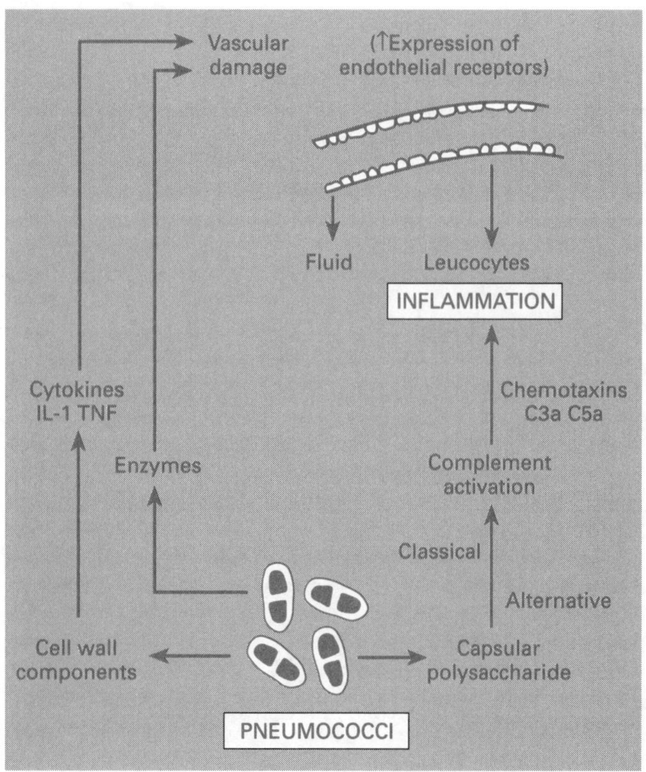

An increase in susceptibility to pneumococcal infection may result from defects in either local or systemic defence mechanisms (Table 1). Factors that impair the cleansing action of the respiratory cilia favour aspiration of infected nasopharyngeal secretions into alveoli. These include cold, anaesthesia, alcohol intoxication, drug overdose, and viral infection of the respiratory tract. Viral infections, such as influenza or measles, increase respiratory-tract secretions, damage the ciliated epithelium of the respiratory tract, and interfere with PMN function. Thus, epidemics of influenza are often followed by an increase in the incidence of pneumonia, especially among elderly people. Infection with *Mycoplasma pneumoniae* also predisposes patients to pneumococcal pneumonia and both organisms are sometimes isolated from patients with lobar pneumonia. Pulmonary oedema favours the growth of any pneumococci that reach the alveoli and predisposes to pneumococcal pneumonia. Mechanical obstruction of a bronchus, for example by carcinoma, has a similar effect.

Systemic immune defects that predispose to invasive pneumococcal disease include congenital or acquired hypogammaglobulinaemia and splenic dysfunction, as seen in patients with sickle-cell disease, emphasizing the importance of splenic phagocytosis as a protective mechanism against pneumococcal infection. Recently, an increase in the incidence and severity of pneumococcal disease has been reported in HIV-positive patients. Which of the many immune defects associated with HIV infection is responsible for this enhanced susceptibility has not been clearly defined.

Pathology

Pneumococcal lobar pneumonia has been used to demonstrate the characteristic features of an acute inflammatory reaction to many generations of medical students, for the sequential features of this response can often be observed in the same pathological specimen. The first response to the presence of pneumococci in alveoli is an exudation of oedema fluid, which helps to carry bacteria into adjacent parts of the lung. PMNs and red blood cells then accumulate in affected alveoli. Finally, the affected part of the lung becomes consolidated with a dense accumulation of PMNs. A remarkable characteristic of pneumococcal lobar pneumonia is the way in which a consolidated lobe can recover completely, both anatomically and functionally. Occasionally, recovery occurs more slowly than usual, and some fibrosis of the lung parenchyma may then occur. Necrosis of lung tissue, resulting in a lung abscess may occur, especially following a type 3 infection, but this complication is rare.

For reasons that are not fully understood, the outcome of the acute inflammatory reaction produced by pneumococci at other sites is rarely as favourable as that observed in the lung. Invasion of the pleura or the pericardium by direct or lymphatic spread frequently results in the formation of pus. The lining walls of the pleural or pericardial cavities become thickened and fibrotic and, even if the accumulated pus is removed, dense fibrous scarring may remain. In the case of the pericardium, this may cause constrictive pericarditis. A similar purulent response is observed when pneumococci lodge in the meninges, the synovium, or other peripheral sites. Arteries and veins may be damaged by this acute inflammatory response.

Clinical features

The clinical features of pneumococcal infection are described most conveniently in relation to the main clinical syndromes that can be caused by pneumococci. However, these syndromes are not mutually exclusive and many patients with pneumococcal disease have more than one clinical manifestation of the infection, for example pneumonia and meningitis.

Pneumonia

Pneumonia is one of the most common manifestations of pneumococcal disease.

SYMPTOMS

In a typical case of pneumococcal pneumonia, the onset of illness is sudden, although there may be a history of a recent upper respiratory-tract infection. Fever is usually the first symptom and it is frequently accompanied by rigors. The patient feels ill, anorexic, and weak. Headache and myalgia may be severe.

Chest pain usually appears during the course of illness. This pain, which results from involvement of the parietal pleura, is sharp and stabbing, and is aggravated by deep inspiration or coughing. The patient may try to obtain relief by splinting the affected side of his chest with his hands or lying on the affected side. If the diaphragmatic pleura is involved, pain may be referred to the shoulder or to the abdomen.

Cough may be absent at the onset of the illness but, in most patients, it becomes a prominent symptom. Cough is initially non-productive and painful. Subsequently it becomes productive of a blood-tinged, 'rusty' sputum. Finally, the sputum becomes frankly purulent.

Among young children and elderly people, pneumococcal pneumonia may present less dramatically. The mothers of young children with pneumonia usually give a history of fever and cough and the mother may have noticed that the child has rapid respiration. Old patients and the immunocompromised may have little or no fever and few respiratory symptoms. In such patients, general malaise and confusion may be the presenting symptoms. The classical features of pneumococcal pneumonia may also be modified by prior antibiotic treatment.

PHYSICAL SIGNS

Adult patients with lobar pneumonia are usually febrile and toxaemic. The rectal temperature may be as high as 40 °C. Oral temperature may be lower because of hyperventilation. When the patient is first examined, no abnormal physical signs may be detected in the respiratory system. Later the classical signs of lobar consolidation may appear. The patient's breathing becomes rapid and distressed, and the nostrils may dilate on inspiration. Cyanosis may be present as a result of diminished alveolar ventilation or shunting of desaturated blood through the consolidated lung. Chest movement is diminished on the affected side. A dull note is obtained on percussion over the affected lobe. On auscultation, bronchial breathing is sometimes detected, fine crepitations are frequent, and a pleural rub may be heard.

General examination usually shows tachycardia and an apical systolic murmur may be detected, as in any patient with a high fever. Examination of the abdomen may show some distension or, when the diaphragmatic pleura has been involved, upper abdominal tenderness and guarding. Jaundice may be present. The patient, especially if elderly, may be confused.

The classical signs of lobar consolidation are found infrequently in infants with pneumococcal pneumonia, although some auscultatory abnormalities, such as crepitations, can usually be detected. In young children, the most prominent features of pneumococcal pneumonia are usually a raised respiratory rate, chest-wall indrawing (Fig. 6) and nasal flaring.

INVESTIGATIONS

A polymorphonuclear neutrophil leucocytosis is usually present; a white-cell count of 15×10^9/l or more is found in about three-quarters of cases and counts as high as 40×10^9/l may occur. A low white-cell count is associated with a poor prognosis. There may be a reticulocytosis. Both conjugated and unconjugated bilirubin levels are raised in jaundiced patients, and serum transaminases may be elevated. The $P\text{O}_2$ is often diminished, and measurement of the degree of hypoxaemia gives an important measure of the severity of the infection, but the $P\text{CO}_2$ is normal unless terminal respiratory failure occurs.

The sputum of untreated patients usually shows large numbers of Gram-positive diplococci, together with PMNs, and culture is frequently positive for pneumococci. However, in industrialized countries, where many patients have received partial treatment before presentation at hospital, sputum microscopy is positive in only about one-quarter of patients and culture positive in about a half. Blood culture is positive in only 10 to 30 per cent of patients.

Radiographs of the chest usually show homogeneous opacification of the affected part of the lung (Fig. 7). Posteroanterior and lateral views

Fig. 6 Severe lower chest indrawing in a child with pneumococcal pneumonia (by courtesy of Dr Alice Greenwood).

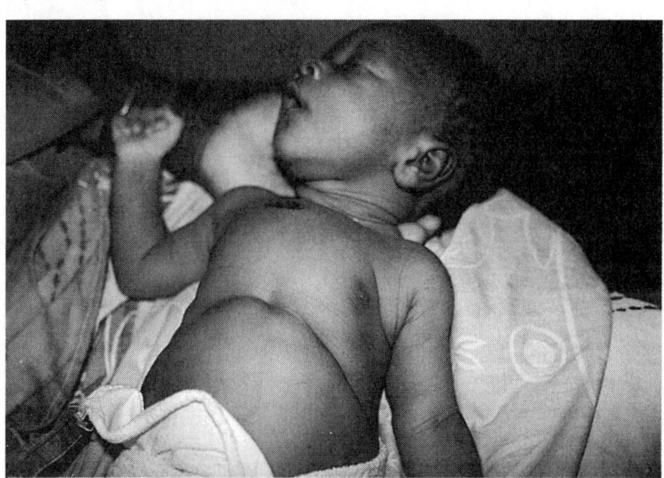

Fig. 7 A lateral chest radiograph showing pneumococcal pneumonia of the right middle lobe (by courtesy of Dr J.T. Macfarlane).

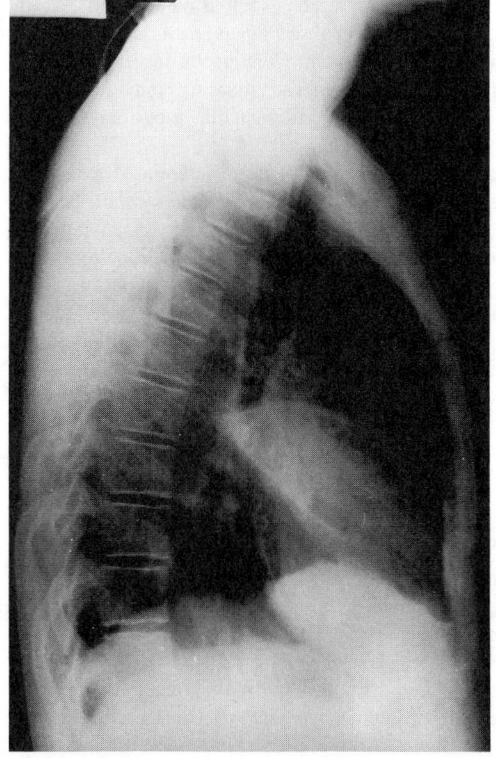

are required to make an accurate anatomical diagnosis of the site of the infection. A small pleural effusion can be seen in some patients. Pneumococci can cause either segmental or lobar consolidation, or patchy shadowing. The latter is encountered more frequently in children. The lower lobes are affected more frequently than the upper. In about one-third of patients, more than one lobe is involved.

DIFFERENTIAL DIAGNOSIS

The initial febrile phase of acute pneumococcal pneumonia cannot be differentiated from that of any other acute febrile illness. Once the characteristic respiratory symptoms and signs have appeared, a diagnosis of acute pneumonia can usually be made on clinical grounds but chest signs may be absent when the patient is first seen. In developing countries, most cases of pneumococcal pneumonia in young children are diagnosed and treated by paramedical primary health-care workers, who may have only limited diagnostic skills.

For this reason the World Health Organization (**WHO**) has devised a simple diagnostic scheme, based predominantly on measurement of the respiratory rate and on observation for lower chest-wall indrawing to help primary health-care workers determine which children with acute respiratory-tract infections probably have pneumonia and require antibiotic treatment (Table 2). This scheme has played an important part in the rationalization of the management of acute respiratory infections in developing countries but other severe infections, including malaria, can give rise to cough and a raised respiratory rate in young children, thus fulfilling the diagnostic criteria for pneumonia. For this reason WHO is now developing an integrated management plan for sick children.

Two important pulmonary conditions that may be confused with acute bacterial pneumonia in adult patients are infarction and atelectasis (Table 3). Rigors and a high fever favour a diagnosis of pneumonia as opposed to one of infarction; a very sudden onset of symptoms and frank haemoptysis favour a diagnosis of infarction. Pulmonary atelectasis, resulting from the aspiration of mucus, may give rise to symptoms and signs that are very similar to those of pneumonia. Fever and signs of toxaemia are usually less marked in patients with atelectasis than in those with pneumonia unless the collapsed area of lung becomes infected. In elderly patients, heart failure with atypical pulmonary oedema may sometimes mimic pneumococcal pneumonia.

Occasionally, subdiaphragmatic lesions such as cholecystitis, a subphrenic abscess, or an amoebic liver abscess cause a clinical picture that mimics that of lower-lobe pneumonia. Conversely, lower-lobe pneumonia, by producing abdominal pain and guarding, may suggest the diagnosis of an acute abdominal condition such as a perforated peptic ulcer, acute cholecystitis, or appendicitis.

Pneumococcal pneumonia can usually be differentiated from viral pneumonias or pneumonia caused by *Mycoplasma pneumoniae* because of its sudden onset, associated severe toxaemia and accompanying polymorphonuclear neutrophil leucocytosis, but differentiation from other forms of acute bacterial pneumonia cannot be made without the aid of microbiological investigations. Klebsiella pneumonia, staphylococcal pneumonia, and legionnaires' disease may all produce a similar clinical picture. Confusion, signs of multisystem damage, lymphopenia, or a low serum sodium should raise the possibility of legionnaire's disease (Chapter 7.11.36).

Table 2 *WHO criteria for the diagnosis of pneumonia in young children who present with cough or difficulty in breathing*

Cough or difficulty with breathing plus Rapid respiration/indrawing
< 2 months > 60 per min
2–11 months > 50 per min
12–59 months > 40 per min
Pneumonia is considered to be severe, requiring admission, if there is chest-wall indrawing and very severe if the child has cyanosis or stops feeding

Table 3 *The differential diagnosis of pneumonia, pulmonary infarction, and atelectasis*

	Pneumococcal pneumonia	Pulmonary infarction	Atelectasis
Sudden onset	+ +	+ + +	+ +
Haemoptysis	+	+ +	–
Fever	+ + +	+	+
Toxaemia	+ + +	+	–
Signs of deep vein thrombosis	+ *	+ +	–

*Found most frequently during the recovery phase of the infection.

COURSE AND PROGNOSIS

Untreated patients who survive long enough to make specific anticapsular polysaccharide antibody recover spontaneously by crisis, or by a more gradual lysis, 7 to 10 days after the onset of their illness. Without treatment the mortality of acute pneumococcal pneumonia is high, especially when bacteraemia is present. Among patients treated promptly with antibiotics, overall mortality is about 5 per cent but mortality remains as high as 30 per cent in patients with bacteraemia despite antibiotic treatment. Mortality is highest among the old and the very young, and among those with an associated underlying illness such as cirrhosis, alcoholism, or heart disease. HIV infection probably enhances mortality but this has not been found in all studies. Infection with certain pneumococcal serotypes, involvement of more than one lobe of the lung, bacteraemia, leucopenia, jaundice, and persistent pneumococcal polysaccharide antigenaemia are all bad prognostic signs. Most deaths from treated pneumococcal pneumonia occur within the first few days of admission to hospital. It is often difficult to establish an exact cause of death in such patients—peripheral circulatory collapse, cardiac arrhythmias, and respiratory failure are some of the contributory factors.

Complications of pneumococcal lobar pneumonia result from local or lymphatic spread of bacteria to adjacent pleura or pericardium, producing pleural or pericardial effusions, or from bacteraemic spread to meninges and other distant foci. The likelihood of one of these infective complications developing is reduced, but not completely abolished, by prompt treatment with antibiotics. Pneumococcal pneumonia may precipitate congestive cardiac failure in elderly patients and can precipitate acute dilatation of the stomach or paralytic ileus. Herpes labialis is a common accompaniment of the infection.

Pleural effusion and empyema

A large pleural effusion or an empyema develops during treatment in a small percentage (2–5 per cent) of patients with established pneumococcal pneumonia. Other patients present with the clinical features of a pleural effusion without preceding symptoms of pneumonia.

SYMPTOMS

Some patients give a history suggestive of a previous parenchymatous lung infection. A history of days or weeks of fever, malaise, anorexia, and marked weight loss is often obtained. Fever may be hectic and accompanied by rigors and episodes of profuse sweating. Patients with a large pleural effusion are breathless and they may complain of dull chest pain on the affected side. A productive cough is unusual unless a bronchopleural fistula is present.

PHYSICAL SIGNS

General examination shows persistent fever and tachycardia. The patient may look toxaemic and there may be signs of recent weight loss. Examination of the chest usually shows the characteristic signs of a pleural effusion—diminished chest movement, dullness on percussion, and diminished breath sounds over the accumulated fluid. The chest wall overlying an empyema may be tender.

INVESTIGATIONS

A persistent polymorphonuclear neutrophil leucocytosis is nearly always present. Radiographs or ultrasonography may be very helpful in localizing a loculated effusion. On aspiration, turbid fluid or thick pus is obtained, which contains pneumococci and degenerate white cells. If antibiotics have been given it may not be possible to culture pneumococci but pneumococcal antigen can usually be detected by immunological assays.

DIFFERENTIAL DIAGNOSIS

Association of persistent pyrexia and leucocytosis with abnormal chest signs indicates a chronic pulmonary infection. Absence of copious, purulent sputum differentiates the condition from a lung abscess. Differentiation from tuberculosis may be difficult on clinical grounds alone. Diagnosis of an empyema is confirmed by the aspiration of pus from the pleural cavity. Repeated needling with a wide-bored needle, preferably under ultrasound control, may be needed to find a loculated empyema.

COURSE AND PROGNOSIS

Untreated, an empyema may rupture through the chest wall (empyema necessitas) or rupture into a bronchus causing a bronchopleural fistula. Even when pus is aspirated and healing achieved, subsequent fibrosis and calcification may seriously restrict expansion of the underlying lung.

Pericardial effusion and empyema

Pneumococci may spread from an infected lower lobe to produce pericarditis. Pericarditis is clinically silent in some patients; in other patients it is manifest only as a transient pericardial rub or as an abnormal electrocardiogram. However, occasionally pericardial involvement is the dominant feature of a pneumococcal infection. Only a proportion of such patients give a history suggestive of an initial acute respiratory-tract infection.

SYMPTOMS

Patients with a pneumococcal pericardial empyema usually give a history of several days, or even weeks, of persistent fever, malaise, anorexia, and weight loss. They may complain of dull, central chest pain and they may have noted swelling of the ankles or of the abdomen.

PHYSICAL SIGNS

Many patients with a pneumococcal pericardial empyema are critically ill by the time that they reach hospital. They are febrile and toxaemic. There may be signs of severe pericardial tamponade—a rapid, small-volume pulse, pulsus paradoxus, a low blood pressure, elevation of the jugular venous pressure, and peripheral oedema and ascites. Percussion of the chest may show some enlargement of the area of cardiac dullness but this is an unreliable clinical sign. The heart sounds are usually faint and, in some patients, a pericardial rub is heard.

INVESTIGATIONS

A peripheral blood polymorphonuclear neutrophil leucocytosis is present and blood culture may be positive for pneumococci. A chest radiograph may show globular enlargement of the heart and there may be radiological evidence of an associated lung infection. An ultrasonographic examination may help to define the best site for drainage. The electrocardiogram shows low-voltage potentials and S–T elevation or depression may be present. On aspiration of the pericardium, turbid fluid or thick pus is obtained from which pneumococci can be isolated or in which pneumococcal antigen can be detected.

DIFFERENTIAL DIAGNOSIS

Detection of the signs of pericardial tamponade in a patient who is febrile and toxaemic should suggest a diagnosis of pericardial empyema. The condition may be confused with tuberculous constrictive pericarditis, but patients with this latter condition usually have a longer history than patients with a pneumococcal pericardial empyema and are less toxic. Staphylococci and, rarely, other pyogenic bacteria can produce a similar clinical picture to that of pneumococcal pericardial empyema. Diagnosis of a pericardial empyema is confirmed by ultrasound and by pericardial aspiration. A pneumococcal pericardial empyema is a medical emergency and, following ultrasonographic examination if this available, pericardial aspiration should be undertaken, if necessary at more than one site, as soon as this diagnosis is seriously suspected.

COURSE AND PROGNOSIS

Pneumococcal pericardial empyema is a serious condition with a high mortality, even in treated patients. Patients who survive the initial episode may develop constrictive pericarditis within weeks or months of their acute illness.

Otitis media

Otitis media is probably the most common form of pneumococcal infection. The condition is seen most frequently in young children but it may also affect adults.

SYMPTOMS

The onset of an attack of acute otitis media is sudden, although there may be a history of a recent upper respiratory-tract infection. Fever and severe pain in the ear are the usual presenting complaints in adults and older children, and patients may complain of deafness and tinnitus. Fever, crying, and extreme irritability are the usual features of the condition in young children, in whom febrile convulsions may occur.

PHYSICAL SIGNS

On examination of the affected ear, the tympanic membrane is seen to be red and swollen, and it may bulge outwards into the external ear. If perforation has occurred, the external ear may be full of pus and a ragged hole may be seen in the tympanic membrane. The affected ear is usually partially deaf. In children, meningism may be present; this must be differentiated from meningitis by lumbar puncture.

LABORATORY FINDINGS

A polymorphonuclear neutrophil leucocytosis is usually found. If the drum has ruptured, pneumococci may be found in the purulent discharge present in the external ear but contaminants are likely to be present also.

DIFFERENTIAL DIAGNOSIS

A clinical diagnosis of otitis media is rarely difficult provided that the ears of all febrile and irritable children are examined carefully. A tympanogram usually shows a characteristic pattern. The aetiology of the condition can be established by examination of fluid obtained from the middle ear with a fine needle. This technique, widely practised in some countries but not in others, may become increasingly useful as determination of the antibiotic sensitivity pattern of pneumococci becomes an essential requirement for optimum treatment of pneumococcal infections.

COURSE AND PROGNOSIS

Prompt treatment is usually followed by a rapid and complete resolution of the infection. However, some patients, especially those in whom rupture of the drum has occurred, are left with partial conductive deafness. When untreated, pneumococcal otitis media can give rise to a chronic discharging ear requiring prolonged and complicated treatment. Spread of the infection posteriorly may result in acute mastoiditis, and spread of the infection upwards can cause pneumococcal meningitis and/or a cerebral abscess.

Pneumococcal meningitis

Pneumococcal meningitis may follow damage to the base of the skull, and it can occur as a complication of pneumococcal otitis media or pneumococcal pneumonia. However, many patients with this condition, the proportion varying from series to series, present with the clinical features of acute pyogenic meningitis and have no features to suggest a primary focus of pneumococcal infection.

SYMPTOMS

Fever and headache are the usual presenting symptoms of pneumococcal meningitis. Headache usually comes on gradually over a few hours; it is generalized and may be very severe. Nausea, backache, and photophobia may develop, and convulsions may occur. Confusion may be the most prominent symptom in elderly patients, and failure to feed the first symptom in infants.

PHYSICAL SIGNS

Patients with pneumococcal meningitis are febrile and toxaemic. Neck stiffness and a positive Kernig sign are usually found in adults and in older children. Impairment of consciousness is often present, which varies in severity from drowsiness and confusion to deep coma. Bradycardia and hypertension may indicate the presence of raised intracranial pressure but papilloedema is rarely seen. Bulging of the anterior fontanelle may be present in infants. Cranial nerve palsies, most frequently of the VIth or of the IIIrd cranial nerve, may be found on presentation and, occasionally, other peripheral localizing neurological signs are present.

An associated pneumococcal lesion, such as otitis media or pneumonia, may be detected. Petechiae are rarely seen. Herpes labialis may be present.

LABORATORY FINDINGS

A peripheral blood polymorphonuclear neutrophil leucocytosis is usually found and a positive blood culture may be obtained.

Examination of the cerebrospinal fluid shows a turbid fluid, which usually contains an increased number of cells and many bacteria. Most of the leucocytes are PMNs. Cerebrospinal-fluid bacterial counts are often very high in patients with pneumococcal meningitis, on average 10 times higher than in patients with meningococcal meningitis. Leucocytes are present in only small numbers in the cerebrospinal fluid of some patients; in such instances the fluid may still be turbid because of the presence of numerous bacteria. The protein level in cerebrospinal fluid is increased and its sugar level decreased below that of blood. Gram stain and culture are usually positive for pneumococci. Many other abnormalities have been detected in the cerebrospinal fluid of patients with pneumococcal meningitis, as in that of patients with other forms of pyogenic meningitis, including an increase in lactic acid concentration, an increase in lactic dehydrogenase level, elevation of IgG and IgM levels, and an increase in levels of fibrin degradation products.

DIFFERENTIAL DIAGNOSIS

It is not usually difficult to establish a clinical diagnosis of pyogenic meningitis in adults and older children with pneumococcal meningitis. However, problems may arise in the very young and in the very old, for signs of meningeal irritation may be absent in both these groups of patients. Fever and irritability may be the only clinical signs of pneumococcal meningitis in an infant. The appearance of confusion may be the only sign indicating involvement of the meninges in an elderly patient with pneumococcal pneumonia. Any adverse change in the psychological or neurological state of an elderly patient with pneumonia is an indication for lumbar puncture.

On clinical grounds, pneumococcal meningitis cannot be differentiated with certainty from other forms of pyogenic meningitis. An associated ear infection or pneumonia favours the diagnosis of pneumococcal infection but is not diagnostic. If petechiae are found, meningococcal meningitis is more likely. Bacteriological diagnosis of pneumococcal meningitis is confirmed by examination of the cerebrospinal fluid.

COURSE AND PROGNOSIS

The prognosis of patients with pneumococcal meningitis is poor. Many patients make no response to treatment, their conscious level deteriorates progressively, and they die within the first 24 to 48 h after their admission to hospital. Other patients make some initial response to treatment but then relapse, their conscious level deteriorates, and new neurological signs appear. This deterioration may be due to the collection of pus in the extradural space or brain but, more usually, follows a vascular occlusion. Patients who deteriorate after an initial clinical improvement must be fully investigated to exclude the presence of a space-occupying lesion. The clinical course of survivors of the early phase of pneumo-

Fig. 8 Mortality from pneumococcal pneumonia by conscious level at the time of presentation. Numbers of patients are shown above the bars. (Reproduced from Baird *et al.* (1976) *Lancet*, **ii,** 1344, with permission.)

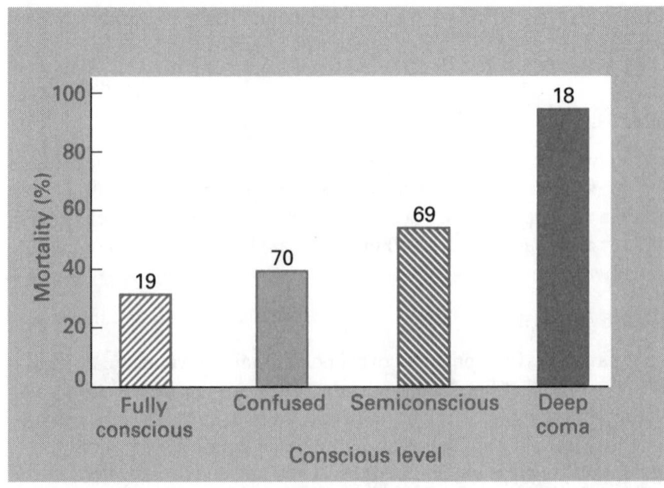

coccal meningitis is often stormy, being complicated by conditions such as bedsores, pneumonia, and venous thrombosis. It has been estimated that over one-half of all survivors from pneumococcal meningitis are left with some intellectual impairment or residual neurological disability such as deafness or partial hemiplegia. Small children who survive may develop hydrocephalus. Relapses may occur when treatment is stopped.

Mortality figures for pneumococcal meningitis vary from series to series but in industrialized countries the true mortality from pneumococcal meningitis is probably around 30 per cent. In developing countries, mortality figures of around 50 per cent have been found consistently. Impairment of consciousness on admission to hospital, associated pneumonia, and a low white-cell count and a high bacterial count in cerebrospinal fluid are all poor prognostic features. Death is almost inevitable in patients who are in deep coma at the time that they are admitted to hospital (Fig. 8).

Why the prognosis of pneumococcal meningitis is so poor is uncertain. Although there is little difference in the clinical features of patients with pneumococcal or meningococcal meningitis on presentation at hospital, death is at least five times more likely in a patient with pneumococcal meningitis than in a patient with meningococcal meningitis regardless of the level of patient care available. Vascular damage, rapid multiplication of bacteria, and defective leucocyte function have all been suggested as possible causes of the poor outcome of patients with pneumococcal meningitis, but the role of these factors has not been clearly documented and the reasons for the very poor prognosis of patients with pneumococcal meningitis remain a mystery.

Other clinical syndromes

Acute, fulminating septicaemia is a rare form of pneumococcal infection that is encountered most frequently in patients without a spleen or who are immunocompromised in some way. A sudden onset of fever, peripheral circulatory collapse, and bleeding (purpura fulminans) are the usual presenting features of this condition, which is clinically indistinguishable from other forms of overwhelming bacterial septicaemia. Leucopenia is usually found. Bleeding is due to disseminated intravascular coagulation. The mortality of this condition is very high, even when treatment is started promptly. A milder form of bacteraemia is sometimes encountered in children who present with fever or febrile convulsions without any obvious focus of pneumococcal infection.

Acute endocarditis may complicate pneumococcal septicaemia but this condition is now encountered only rarely. Healthy heart valves, especially the aortic valve, may be attacked and rupture of the aortic valve may occur, producing severe aortic incompetence. Emboli derived from cardiac vegetations may reach the brain and other organs. Progression of the cardiac lesions may be very rapid and the prognosis of this condition is poor. Valve replacement may be necessary for those who survive the initial episode.

During the course of pneumococcal septicaemia, with or without endocarditis, bacteria may reach many sites where they can multiply to produce a purulent lesion. Pneumococcal arthritis, ophthalmitis, and orchitis may be produced in this way.

Pneumococcal peritonitis is an uncommon condition that is encountered most frequently in patients with the nephrotic syndrome or cirrhosis of the liver, conditions frequently resulting in ascites and generalized impairment in immunity. The condition has been described also in healthy young girls, perhaps as a complication of pelvic infection, and occasionally in neonates. The condition is characterized by a sudden onset of fever, and abdominal pain and tenderness. The ascitic fluid is turbid and contains PMNs and pneumococci. The general features of an acute infection may not be so obvious in patients with cirrhosis, and peritonitis must be considered as a possible diagnosis in any patient with this condition whose clinical state shows a sudden deterioration. The prognosis of pneumococcal peritonitis is poor in patients with a serious underlying illness.

The bacteriological diagnosis of pneumococcal infections

Microbiological confirmation of most forms of invasive pneumococcal disease can usually be made by culture of pneumococci from blood, pus or from pleural, pericardial, peritoneal, or cerebrospinal fluid. However, difficulties arise over the bacteriological diagnosis of pneumococcal pneumonia. Blood culture is positive in only 10 to 30 per cent of cases, and culture of pneumococci from sputum cannot be considered as diagnostic because of the frequent presence of pneumococci in the upper respiratory tract of healthy individuals and the consequent contamination of sputum samples during expectoration. Techniques used to obtain respiratory-tract secretions that are not contaminated by upper respiratory-tract flora include transtracheal aspiration, lung aspiration, and bronchoscopy with the collection of bronchial aspirates or secretions obtained by bronchoalveolar lavage. It is not usually necessary to use these techniques in an uncomplicated case of lobar pneumonia that, on clinical grounds, is thought to be due to a pneumococcal infection. However, invasive investigations may be indicated in patients who are very ill, in those with clinically atypical pneumonia, and in those who have failed to respond to treatment. Transtracheal aspiration is unpleasant for the patient, may cause localized emphysema, and can produce secretions that contain a mixed flora, so this technique is no longer widely used. Lung aspiration with a fine needle is more likely to identify a single pulmonary pathogen. Lung aspiration (Fig. 9) is an easy technique which has provided valuable information on the aetiology of pneumonia in different geographical areas that could not have been obtained in any other way. Lung aspiration may cause haemoptysis or a pneumothorax but, when done by experienced staff and restricted to areas of consolidation, the incidence of significant complications is small. If present, a pleural effusion should be aspirated for microbiological diagnosis.

Treatment with inadequate amounts of an antibiotic may make it impossible to culture pneumococci from clinical samples without preventing progression of the infection. In such circumstances, assays that depend upon the detection of pneumococcal capsular polysaccharide antigens rather than whole bacteria can be diagnostically useful. Capsular polysaccharide antigens can be detected in biological samples by simple immunological assays such as countercurrent immunoelectrophoresis (CIE), latex agglutination, and staphylococcal coagglutination tests but the diversity of capsular polysaccharide antigens makes such assays difficult. Use of pooled antisera reduces sensitivity whilst use of monospecific antisera requires multiple tests for each sample. For this reason assays have been developed based on the C polysaccharide common to all pneumococci. Polysaccharide may be bound *in vivo* to antibody and a new assay that involves dissociation of such complexes has

Fig. 9 Lung aspiration in a patient with pneumonia (by courtesy of Dr Alice Greenwood).

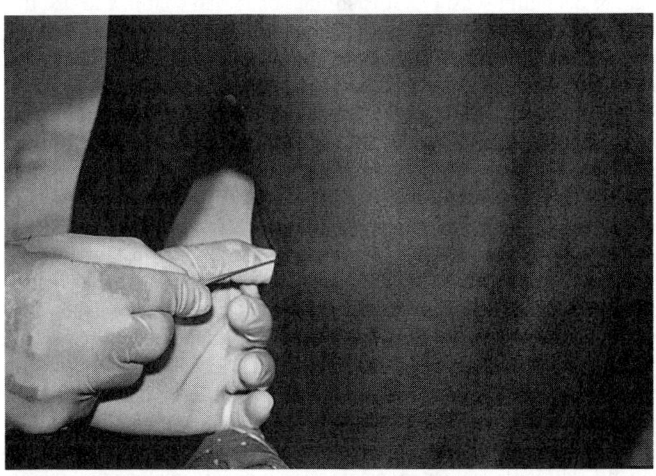

been developed. Pneumococcal polysaccharide antigens have been demonstrated in serum, urine, and cerebrospinal, pleural, peritoneal, synovial, and middle-ear fluids, with a positivity rate comparable to that of culture. Pneumococcal antigen is present in the sputum of nearly all untreated patients with pneumococcal lobar pneumonia, and the specificity of sputum antigen detection is higher than that of sputum culture in differentiating pneumococcal pneumonia from upper respiratory-tract infections.

Antigen detection has the advantage over culture that results are rapid and a positive result may be obtained in partially treated patients in whom culture is negative. However, a positive urine antigen test is not diagnostic of invasive pneumococcal disease and may follow upper respiratory-tract colonization or vaccination. Moreover, antigen detection cannot provide any information on the antibiotic sensitivity of the causative pneumococcus. Thus, antigen detection should be done in parallel with standard microbiological techniques and not as a substitute for them.

Recently, a polymerase chain-reaction assay for the detection of pneumococci has been developed using primers based on part of the autolysin gene but this assay has not yet been subjected to clinical trials.

Antibody assays are of little use in the investigation of individual patients but they can provide useful information about the epidemiological importance of pneumococci as a cause of pneumonia. Because of the multiplicity of capsular serotypes, measuring capsular polysaccharide antibody levels is not a practical approach to diagnosis in an individual patient. However, some success has been achieved by measuring antibodies to pneumolysin in acute and convalescent samples. This assay has proved to be diagnostically more successful in adults than children.

Treatment

Antibiotics

When the last edition of this book was written, penicillin could still be recommended as the usual, first line treatment for patients with pneumococcal disease, with the proviso that physicians should be alert to the possibility of an occasional treatment failure. Because of the dramatic geographical spread of pneumoccocci with diminished sensitivity to penicillin during the past few years this general recommendation can no longer be made. Protocols for the treatment of pneumococcal disease must now take into account the prevalence of penicillin-insensitive pneumococci in the area in question.

Substantial areas remain, for example, parts of the United Kindgom and the United States, where careful surveys have shown that penicillin-insensitive pneumococci are still rare. Because penicillin is such an effective antibiotic for the treatment of infection caused by pneumococci that are penicillin sensitive, it is still reasonable to continue to use this antibiotic as the first line of treatment for pneumococcal infections, including cases of meningitis, in such areas. However, careful watch for possible clinical treatment failures must be kept and antibiotic sensitivity patterns determined for pneumococci isolated from patients with systemic pneumococcal disease. Changes of treatment may be necessary on the basis of these findings.

When used for the treatment of severe pneumococcal infections, penicillin should be given in large doses, for example, an adult dose of 2–4 million units of crystalline penicillin 6-hourly given by intravenous or intramuscular injection. Large doses are particularly important in the treatment of cases of meningitis, as penicillin penetrates relatively poorly into the CSF, and high doses must be maintained throughout the course of treatment (Table 4) so as to compensate for the decrease in the permeability of the blood–brain barrier that occurs as a patient recovers. Ampicillin (500 mg 6-hourly for an adult) or amoxycillin (500 mg 8-hourly for an adult), given by mouth, can be used for the treatment of patients with uncomplicated pneumococcal pneumonia or otitis media.

Table 4 *The duration of antibiotic treatment required in different forms of pneumococcal disease*

5–7 days	10–14 days	4–6 weeks
Otitis media Pneumonia	Meningitis Septicaemia	Endocarditis Empyema Septic arthritis

Co-trimoxazole is a suitable alternative treatment for patients infected with a penicillin sensitive pneumococcus who cannot be given penicillin for any reason and, in developing countries, this antibiotic is used widely for the treatment of children with pneumonia. Chloramphenicol is a better alternative choice than co-trimoxazole for the treatment of patients with pneumococcal meningitis caused by a penicillin sensitive strain because of its ability to diffuse into the CSF.

In areas with an intermediate prevalence of penicillin insensitive pneumococci, and where most penicillin insensitive pneumococci show intermediate rather than high level resistance, penicillin in high dosage can still be used as the first line of treatment for patients with uncomplicated pneumococcal pneumonia or otitis media. Amoxycillin is the preferred treatment for patients with the latter. Should a treatment failure occur, a third-generation cephalosporin such as ceftriaxone (adult dose 2 g per day) is ususally the next choice of antibiotic. In areas with an intermediate prevalence of penicillin-insensitive pneumococci, a third generation cephalosporin, such as ceftriaxone, is usually the first choice of treatment for patients with pneumococcal meningtitis because penicillin may not diffuse into the CSF in sufficient amounts to inhibit pneumococci with an intermediate level of resistance.

In areas where the prevalence of penicillin-insensitive pneumococci is high, and where many insensitive bacteria have high levels of resistance to penicillin, a different strategy is required. In such situations, most experts still recommend high doses of penicillin as the first line of treatment for patients with uncomplicated pneumococcal pneumonia or otitis media, but treatment failures can be expected. However, neither penicillin nor cephalosporins can be used safely for the treatment of patients with pneumococcal meningitis because many pneumococci with high level penicillin resistance are also resistant to cephalosporins. How such patients can best be managed is still a matter of debate. Chloramphenicol, tetracycline, and erythromycin cannot be used as most pneumococci with a high level of penicillin resistance are resistant to these antibiotics also. Alternatives that have been suggested include rifampicin, imipenem, and vancomycin. However, treatment with rifampicin frequently results in the rapid emergence of rifampicin-resistant bacteria and imipenem can cause convulsions. Thus, despite its poor penetration into the CSF and its toxicity, vancomycin is currently recommended as the best treatment for meningitis caused by penicillin-resisitant pneumococci. Because it is poorly absorbed, vanocomycin must be given by intravenous or intramuscular injection (0.5 g 6-hourly for an adult). Some physicians suggest that if meningitis due to a penicillin resistant pneumococcus is suspected then treatment with vancomycin and a cephalosporin should be given until the results of sensitivity tests are known when it may be possible to continue with the cephalosporin alone.

Penicillin-insensitive pneumococci pose particualar problems for developing countries where penicillin, co-trimoxazole, and chloramphenicol are often the only antibiotics widely available. Treatment with a third-generation cephalosporin costs approximately 10 times that of treatment with penicillin and treatment with vancomycin is even more expensive and well beyond the range of most developing countries. Spread of pneumococci resistant to many antibiotics throughout the developing world could result in a major disaster because of the high incidence of infections caused by this bacterium.

The response of patients with pneumococcal lobar pneumonia to treatment with an appropriate antibiotic is usually dramatic. The patient's temperature falls to normal within 24 to 48 h of the start of treatment and the abnormal clinical signs rapidly improve. Within a week or 10 days all abnormal clinical signs have usually disappeared. However, radiological resolution takes several weeks. Patients with pneumococcal meningitis respond more slowly but, if improvement is going to occur, it is usually apparent within the first 5 days after the start of the therapy. Failure of a patient with a pneumococcal infection to respond to treatment suggests that (a) the initial bacteriological diagnosis was incorrect; (b) the infection was caused by a pneumococcus resistant to the antibiotic chosen; (c) a local collection of pus has formed; or (d) that the patient has developed a treatment reaction. Each of these possibilities should be investigated.

Supportive measures

GENERAL NURSING CARE

Patients with acute pneumococcal infections are often extremely ill and require careful nursing, special attention being paid to fluid balance. Patients with fulminating pneumococcal infections require intensive-care facilities. In general, isolation of patients with pneumococcal infection is not necessary but patients with an infection caused by a multiple antibiotic-resistant strain should be isolated.

FLUID THERAPY

Patients with pneumococcal infections are often dehydrated by the time that they reach hospital. Patients with pneumonia may lose large amounts of fluid through the respiratory tract as a result of hyperventilation; patients with pneumococcal meningitis are frequently too confused to drink. For such patients intravenous fluid therapy may be required.

OXYGEN AND PHYSIOTHERAPY

Patients with pneumococcal pneumonia, especially those with more than one lobe of the lung involved, are likely to be hypoxic and require oxygen therapy. If possible the arterial Po_2 should be raised to between 60 and 80 mmHg or the haemoglobin saturation maintained at over 90 per cent as measured by pulse oximetry. When difficulty is experienced in achieving an adequate level of oxygenation, transfer to an intensive-care unit and artificial ventilation may be needed if this is available. Physiotherapy is important in helping the patient to clear tenacious sputum during the recovery phase of the infection.

Careful attention must be paid to the respiratory tract in unconscious patients with pneumococcal meningitis. Intubation and assisted respiration are sometimes employed in patients who have passed into deep coma. The outlook for such patients is so poor that it is doubtful whether these measures are justified.

ANALGESICS

Local pain may be severe in patients with pneumococcal infections and sufficient analgesics should be given to control this symptom. Analgesics with a central depressant action should be avoided whenever possible.

CORTICOSTEROIDS

Several early studies showed that treatment with corticosteroids was of no benefit in patients with pyogenic meningitis. However, recently it has been shown that large doses of dexamethasone for 3 days reduced the incidence of complications, particularly deafness, in American children with pyogenic meningitis, most of whom had a *H. influenzae* type b infection. Furthermore, a study done in Cairo showed a significant reduction in mortality among patients with pneumococcal meningitis given 8 to 10 mg of dexamethasone for 3 days, and a retrospective study of a small group of American children with pneumococcal disease treated with dexamethasone showed that they had a more rapid resolution of fever and a lower overall incidence of neurological sequelae than controls. However, mortality was not reduced. Neither of these studies was a randomized, placebo-controlled trial and so some doubts about the efficacy of dexamethasone in pneumococcal meningitis still remain. Further, larger, well-conducted trials are needed. In the meanwhile, it is probably appropriate to give patients with pneumococcal meningitis, especially children, dexamethasone as the incidence of side-effects related to dexamethasone treatment of meningitis is low.

DRAINAGE OF PUS

Local collections of pus should be removed. Usually, it is possible to remove pus by needle aspiration. If pus is too thick to be removed from the pleural or pericardial space in this way, surgical drainage through a wide-bore tube may be necessary. Even when successful drainage is achieved, scarring may be extensive and decortication of a lung or removal of an adherent pericardium may subsequently be required. Burr holes may be needed to drain extradural or cerebral abscesses complicating pneumococcal meningitis.

Prophylaxis

General improvements in living standards in industrialized countries have probably had a significant impact on the incidence of invasive pneumococcal disease in children but this effect has been less marked in adults. Reduction in air pollution in large urban centres has reduced the incidence of chronic bronchitis and thus probably of some secondary pneumonias. Avoidance of severe overcrowding in barracks, refugee camps, and similar situations may provide some protection against pneumococcal infections.

Chemoprophylaxis

Chemoprophylaxis has been little used in the control of pneumococcal disease because of difficulties in identifying those who are at risk from the infection. Secondary cases are seen only rarely among those who have been in close contact with a patient. Because patients with sickle-cell disease have an increased incidence of pneumococcal infection, children with this condition should be given regular chemoprophylaxis with oral penicillin from the age of 3 months until they have reached at least the age of 2 years, when they should be vaccinated (Fig. 10).

Fig. 10 Protection of children with sickle-cell disease from pneumococcal infection by chemoprophylaxis with oral penicillin. (Reproduced from Gaston *et al.* (1986) *New England Journal of Medicine*, **314,** 1593, with permission.)

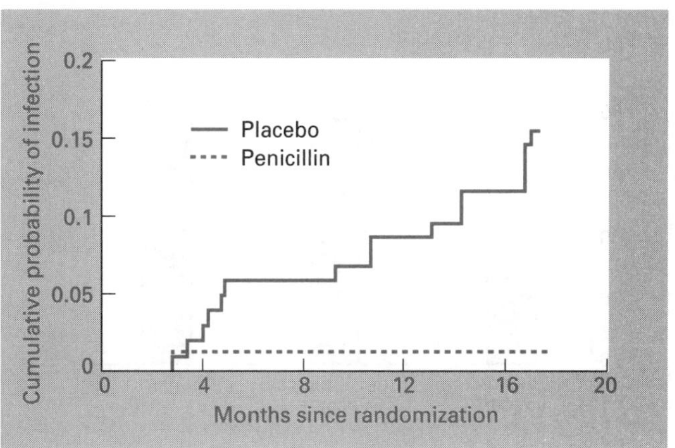

Because vaccine failures have been reported in young children with sickle-cell disease it may be advisable to continue penicillin prophylaxis for several years after vaccination. Some paediatricians also advise penicillin chemoprophylaxis for children with the nephrotic syndrome.

Vaccination

Nearly 50 years ago, McLeod demonstrated clearly that a pneumococcal polysaccharide vaccine protected American airforce recruits against infection with pneumococci of the corresponding serotypes. Two years later, Kauffman reported similar findings in elderly civilians. These promising results evoked surprisingly little interest and serious attempts to produce pneumococcal polysaccharide vaccines commercially were not made until nearly 30 years later, perhaps due in part to a belief that the discovery of penicillin solved the problem of pneumococcal disease. Vaccines comprising purified capsular polysaccharides have been commercially available since the late 1970s. At first, a 14-valent vaccine was used but current vaccines contain 23 capsular polysaccharides representing 80 to 90 per cent of the serotypes responsible for invasive pneumococcal disease in the United States and Western Europe. Initially, there was concern that this vaccine might not be suitable for use in some other parts of the world where the distribution of serotypes differed substantially from that found in the United States. Considerable variations have been demonstrated in the relative importance of different serotypes in different parts of the world, for example type 5 pneumococci are an important cause of invasive disease in West Africa but not in Europe or America, but so far no area has been described in which the 23-valent vaccine would not provide protection against at least 75 per cent of invasive serotypes.

The effectiveness of pneumococcal capsular polysaccharide vaccines in preventing pneumococcal lobar pneumonia has been demonstrated clearly in controlled trials on adults in South Africa and in New Guinea. A trial of a 13-valent vaccine in South African miners showed a 53 per cent reduction in the incidence of radiologically confirmed cases of pneumonia and a 78 per cent reduction in the incidence of radiologically confirmed cases of pneumonia caused by one of the pneumococcal serotypes represented in the vaccine (Fig. 11). A similar reduction in the incidence of bacteriologically proven cases of pneumococcal pneumonia was obtained in a trial made in New Guinea and overall mortality from pneumonia was reduced by 44 per cent in vaccinated subjects. Using a case-control approach it has been estimated that, in the United States, pneumococcal vaccines give about 60 per cent protection against systemic pneumococcal infection in healthy elderly subjects but that they are less effective in those who are immunocompromised in some way (efficacy approximately 20 per cent). However, pneumococcal vaccine does give some protection to patients with sickle-cell disease and to those who have had a splenectomy and such subjects should be vaccinated before splenectomy if this is to be done electively. Studies of the efficacy of pneumococcal vaccines in preventing otitis media have given conflicting results but no clear evidence for sustained protection has been found.

Fig. 11 Protection of South African miners from pneumococcal pneumonia or bacteraemia. The number of cases of infection caused by pneumococci of serotypes represented in the vaccine is shown. There were approximately equal numbers of subjects in each group. (Reproduced from Austrian *et al.* (1976) *Transactions of the Association of African Physicians*, **89,** 184, with permission.)

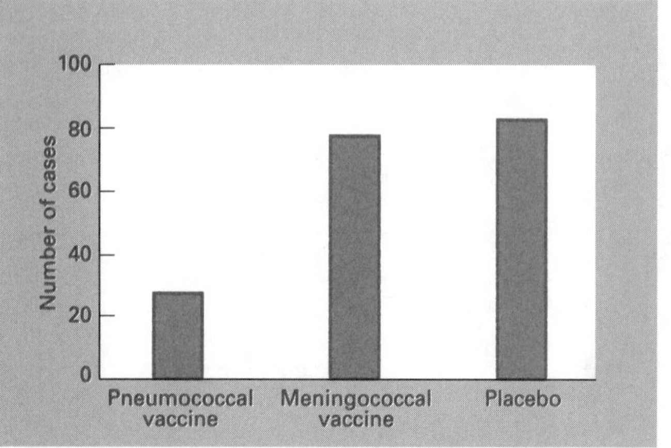

Table 5 *Indications for immunization with pneumococcal capsular polysaccharide vaccine recommended in the United States*

Children over 2 years old
Hyposplenia including sickle-cell disease
Nephrotic syndrome
Cerebrospinal fluid leak
Immunosuppressive disorders including HIV
Other at-risk groups such as Eskimos
Adults
Those over the age of 65 years
Immunocompetent adults with an increased risk of pneumococcal disease such as those with chronic cardiovascular or pulmonary disease, diabetes, alcoholism, and cirrhosis
Immunocompromised subjects with hyposplenia, lymphoma, chronic renal failure, or nephrotic syndrome, and those on immunosuppressive drugs
Subjects with HIV infection

Based on these findings, pneumococcal capsular polysaccharide vaccines are recommended in the United States for several groups of subjects (Table 5). Patients with HIV infection and a CD4 count of less than 500/μl show a diminished response to pneumococcal capsular polysaccharides. Thus, patients with HIV disease should be vaccinated as soon as possible after diagnosis.

Although it has been shown that vaccination of healthy elderly people is cost-effective there has been a reluctance to adopt routine immunization of the elderly in most industrialized countries. Better education on the potential benefits of this vaccine are needed.

In common with other polysaccharide vaccines, pneumococcal polysaccharides are T-independent antigens that are poorly immunogenic in infants and poor at inducing immunological memory. In adults, raised antibody levels have been demonstrated for at least 10 years after vaccination but the duration of clinical protection provided has not been clearly defined. There has been a reluctance to recommend routine reimmunization as second injections can give rise to quite severe local Arthus reactions in those with persistent raised antibody levels but the risks of this side-effect have probably been exaggerated. Infants show a modest response to the most immunogenic polysaccharides, such as the type 1 polysaccharide, but they are unresponsive to the poorly immunogenic polysaccharides such as the type 6. Thus, it was surprising when it was reported that a 23-valent polysaccharide vaccine reduced mortality from pneumonia in children in Papua New Guinea even when vaccination was given as early as 6 months of age. No further trials have been done to substantiate this result and rapid progress with pneumococcal polysaccharide/protein conjugate vaccines (see below) may make such studies unnecessary.

The immunogenicity of polysaccharides in the very young and their ability to induce immunological memory can be enhanced by conjugating the polysaccharide to a protein such as tetanus or diphtheria toxoid. Adoption of this approach has led to the successful development of *H. influenzae* type b vaccines, which are immunogenic when given to infants as young as 2 or 3 months. A similar approach is being followed with the pneumococcus and at least three such vaccines are being developed commercially. There is every reason to believe that these vaccines will be just as effective as their *H. influenzae* counterparts. However, in contrast to invasive *H. influenzae* infections, which are nearly all caused by one capsular serotype, invasive pneumococcal disease may be caused by bacteria of many different serotypes and a complex vaccine will be required containing five to ten conjugates if it is to give protection against a high proportion of pneumococcal infections. Such a vaccine is likely to be expensive and it may be beyond the means of many of the developing countries where such a vaccine is most needed.

It is for these reasons that attempts to develop a vaccine based on a protein antigen common to most pneumococci are of particular importance. This vaccine would be likely to be immunogenic in infants and cheaper than a multivalent conjugate vaccine. So far, animal experiments have been reasonably encouraging and partial protection has been achieved by a recombinant component of the PspA protein and with a detoxified derivative of pneumolysin (pneumolysoid). Pneumolysoid has also been used as the protein carrier component of a pneumococcal polysaccharide conjugate vaccine. Further development of this approach to vaccination against pneumococcal disease should be strongly supported.

REFERENCES

Boulnois, G.J. (1992). Pneumococcal proteins and the pathogenesis of disease caused by *Streptococcus pneumoniae. Journal of General Microbiology*, **138,** 249–59.

Bruyn, G.A., Zegers, B.J., and van Furth, R. (1992). Mechanisms of host defence against infection with *Streptococcus pneumoniae. Clinical Infectious Diseases*, **14,** 251–62.

Farington, M. and Rubinstein, D. (1991). Antigen detection in pneumococcal pneumonia. *Journal of Infection*, **23,** 109–16.

Gaston, M.H. *et al.* (1986). Prophylaxis with oral penicillin in children with sickle cell anaemia. A randomized trial. *New England Journal of Medicine*, **314,** 1593–9.

Girgis, N.I., Farid, Z., Mikhail, I.A., Farrag, I., Sultan, Y., and Kilpatrick, M.E. (1989). Dexamethasone treatment for bacterial meningitis in children and adults. *Pediatric Infectious Diseases Journal*, **8,** 848–51.

Gransden, W.R., Eykyn, S.J., and Phillips, I. (1985). Pneumococcal bacteraemia: 325 episodes diagnosed at St. Thomas's Hospital. *British Medical Journal*, **290,** 505–8.

Jacob, M.R. (1992). Treatment and diagnosis of infections caused by drug-resistant *Streptococcus pneumoniae. Clinical Infectious Diseases*, **15,** 119–27.

Jalonen, E., Paton, J.C., Koskela, M., Kerttula, Y., and Leinonen, M. (1989). Measurement of antibody responses to pneumolysin—a promising method for the presumptive aetiological diagnosis of pneumococcal pneumonia. *Journal of Infection*, **19,** 127–34.

McDaniel, L.S., Sheffield, J.S., Delucchi, P., and Briles, D.E. (1991). PspA, a surface protein of *Streptococcus pneumoniae*, is capable of eliciting protection against pneumococci of more than one capsular type. *Infection and Immunity*, **59,** 222–8.

Markiewicz, Z. and Tomasz, A. (1989). Variation in penicillin-binding protein patterns of penicillin-resistant clinical isolates of pneumococci. *Journal of Clinical Microbiology*, **27,** 405–10.

Marton, A., Gulyas, M., Munoz, R., and Tomasz, A. (1991). Extremely high incidence of antibiotic resistance in clinical isolates of *Streptococcus pneumoniae* in Hungary. *Journal of Infectious Diseases*, **163,** 542–8.

Paton, J.C. *et al.* (1991). Purification and immunogenicity of genetically obtained pneumolysin toxoids and their conjugation to *Streptococcus pneumoniae* type 19 F polysaccharide. *Infection and Immunity*, **59,** 2297–304.

Peltola, H., Anttila, M., and Renkonen, O-V. (1989). Randomised comparison of chloramphenicol, ampicillin, cefotaxime, and ceftriaxone for childhood bacterial meningitis. *Lancet*, **i,** 1281–6.

Pesola, G.R. and Charles, A. (1992). Pneumococcal bacteremia with pneumonia. Mortality in acquired immunodeficiency syndrome. *Chest*, **101,** 150–5.

Quagliarello, V. and Scheld, M.W. (1992). Bacterial meningitis: pathogenesis, pathophysiology and progress. *New England Journal of Medicine*, **327,** 864–72.

Riley, I.D., Lehmann, D., Alpers, M.P., Marshall, T.F. de C., Gratten, H., and Smith, D. (1986). Pneumococcal vaccine prevents death from acute lower-respiratory-tract infections in Papua New Guinean children. *Lancet*, **ii,** 877–81.

Rodriguez Barradas, M.C., Musher, D.M., Hamill, R.J., Dowell, M., Bagwell, J.T., and Sanders, C.V. (1992). Unusual manifestations of pneumococcal infection in human immunodeficiency virus-infected individuals: the past revisited. *Clinical Infectious Diseases*, **14,** 192–9.

Shann, F. (1986). Etiology of severe pneumonia in children in developing countries. *Pediatric Infectious Disease Journal*, **5,** 247–52.

Shapiro, E.D. *et al.* (1991). The protective efficacy of polyvalent pneumococcal polysaccharide vaccine. *New England Journal of Medicine*, **325,** 1453–60.

7.11.4 Staphylococci

S. J. EYKYN

Although others had made observations on coccal organisms, the remarkable polyglot Scottish surgeon, Alexander Ogston, was the first to associate cluster-forming cocci with abscesses, and his classical paper 'Ueber Abscesse' appeared over a century ago. At the suggestion of the Professor of Greek at the University of Aberdeen, he coined the highly appropriate name 'staphylococcus' for the organism (*staphyle*, bunch of grapes; *kokkos*, berry) to distinguish it from the chain-forming streptococci. Ogston's coccus was the organism we now know as *Staphylococcus aureus*, the most important member of the genus Staphylococcus.

Taxonomy

The genus Staphylococcus is classified, along with those of Micrococcus, Stomatococcus, and Planococcus in the family Micrococcaceae. The latter three genera have little in common with the genus Staphylococcus phylogenetically and, with few exceptions, have yet to be shown to be of clinical importance, and they will not be considered further. There are now nearly 30 recognized species of Staphylococcus, but only about half are of human origin (Table 1). Staphylococci are skin commensals of mammals and birds and some species, notably *S. aureus*, are important human pathogens. In the clinical laboratory, *S. aureus* is distinguished from other staphylococci by its ability to coagulate plasma. The slide coagulase test (the method used routinely in clinical laboratories) detects cell-associated clumping factor, sometimes referred to as bound coagulase, which reacts with fibrinogen to cause aggregation of the organisms. Commercial kits, for example Staphaurex (Wellcome) and Staphyslide (bio Mérieux) are now widely used for this test and some of these also detect protein A, present in most strains of *S. aureus*. Occasional strains of *S. aureus* do not produce clumping factor or protein A, and certain other species of staphylococci produce clumping factor, hence the 'gold standard' for the identification of *S. aureus* in the laboratory is the tube coagulase test in which staphylococci are mixed with rabbit or human plasma in a test-tube. This detects extracellular coagulase, sometimes called free coagulase, which activates prothrombin and initiates clot formation in the plasma. The slide coagulase test is used to screen organisms whereas the tube test is confirmatory and is of more taxonomic significance. Other useful screening tests for *S. aureus* are the detection of DNAase activity and growth on mannitol–salt agar with fermentation of mannitol, but neither is as reliable as the tube coagulase test.

Until recently, coagulase-negative staphylococci tended to be classified in most clinical laboratories as *S. epidermidis* (*sensu lato*) or *S.*

Table 1 *Classification of* Staphylococcus *spp. associated with human infection*

Family	Genus	Species
	Staphylococcus	
	Coagulase-positive	*S. aureus*
	Coagulase-negative	*S. auricularis*
		S. capitis
		S. cohnii
		S. epidermidis
		S. haemolyticus
Micrococcaceae:		*S. hominis*
Catalase-positive,		*S. lugdunensis*
Gram-positive		*S. saccharolyticus*
cocci in clusters		*S. saprophyticus*
		S. schleiferi
		S. simulans
		S. warneri
	Micrococcus	
	Stomatococcus	
	Planococcus	

Table 2 *International phage typing scheme for* S. aureus

Phage group	Individual phages
I	29, 52, 52A, 79, 80
II	3A, 3C, 55, 71
III	6, 42E, 47, 53, 54, 75, 77, 83A, 84, 85
V	95, 96
Unclassified	81, 94
Additional phages for MRSA	

saprophyticus or even in more traditional quarters as 'Staph.albus'. The changing taxonomy of this group of organisms has confused microbiologists and clinicians alike. Availability of the ID32 Staph kit (bio Mérieux) has enabled speciation of some (but not all) coagulase-negative staphylococci in the routine laboratory and it is clear that, although most clinical isolates are *S. epidermidis* (*sensu stricto*) or *S. saprophyticus*, several other species can occasionally be important pathogens, as for example, the recently described, *S. lugdunensis*.

Typing

For epidemiological purposes, it is often necessary to differentiate strains of the same species of staphylococcus, and in common with many other organisms, staphylococci are susceptible to bacteriophages. The principal method for typing *S. aureus* involves the use of bacteriophages, and phage typing of *S. aureus* has been organized internationally since 1953. The current international phage set, for use with human strains of *S. aureus*, consists of 23 phages (Table 2). There are four major phage groups, I,II,III, and V, and strains may be lysed by a single phage from one group, more than one phage from a single group, or by phages from more than one group. There are also additional phages for typing methicillin-resistant strains of *S. aureus*. Phage typing of coagulase-negative staphylococci is not organized internationally and interpretation of results is more difficult than for *S. aureus*. Non-typable strains of both *S. aureus* and coagulase-negative staphylococci are found but are much more common with the latter. Molecular typing methods are sometimes useful both for *S. aureus* and coagulase-negative staphylococci; they include plasmid profiling, DNA fingerprinting, and protein patterns.

Staphylococcus aureus

Pathogenicity

S. aureus produces a remarkable variety of extracellular substances; these include general toxic agents, such as catalase, hyaluronidase, lipase, haemolytic toxins, and leucocidin, that may be involved in the pathogenesis of local or systemic inflammation; and specific toxins, such as enterotoxins and epidermolytic toxins, that mediate particular non-suppurative diseases.

Haemolytic toxins

S. aureus produces four substances that disrupt red-cell membranes producing haemolysis, the α-, β-, γ-, and δ-toxins, the most potent of which is α-toxin, which is formed by most strains. It produces impressive biological effects: it is lethal for certain animals and is generally cytotoxic and thus necrotizing, kills leucocytes, lyses platelets, releases catecholamines, and causes renal cortical necrosis, yet remarkably, its role in staphylococcal infection in man remains to be defined. δ-Toxin has similar though less dramatic properties.

Leucocidin

S. aureus also produces a leucocidin, known as the Panton–Valentine leucocidin, that acts selectively on leucocytes and whose activity is distinguishable from the haemolytic toxins.

Enterotoxins

There are seven staphylococcal enterotoxins: types A, B, D, and E, which show major antigenic differences, and type C, which is subdivided into C1, C2, and C3 on the basis of minor antigenic differences. Enterotoxin F is now known to be identical to the toxic shock syndrome toxin. About 40 per cent of strains of *S. aureus* produce enterotoxin, sometimes of more than one type. Staphylococcal food poisoning results from the ingestion of foods containing preformed enterotoxin. Most outbreaks in the United Kingdom are caused by enterotoxin A with or without D (see Table 3), and staphylococci of phage groups III or I and III are most often implicated. Enterotoxins have a wide range of biological activities in addition to their ability to induce vomiting; they are pyrogenic, mitogenic, and can produce thrombocytopenia and hypotension.

Epidermolytic toxins

These toxins cause intraepidermal splitting and are responsible for the scalded skin syndrome as well as for the blistering of impetigo. The production of epidermolytic toxin is particularly associated with (though not confined to) *S. aureus* of phage group II. There are two epidermolytic toxins, ETA, which is heat stable and under chromosomal control, and ETB, which is heat labile and plasmid mediated; most phage-group II staphylococci produce ETA or both ETA and ETB.

Toxic shock syndrome toxin

This toxin, which is responsible for the toxic shock syndrome (see below), was initially investigated by two groups: Bergdoll *et al.* who considered that it was an enterotoxin and called it enterotoxin F, and Schlievert *et al.* who called it pyrogenic exotoxin C. The two independently described toxins appear to be the same and were reclassified in 1984 as toxic shock syndrome toxin 1 (**TSST-1**). Most *S. aureus* isolated from the vagina of patients with toxic shock syndrome associated with menstruation form TSST-1, but only about one-half of strains from the syndrome not associated with menstruation do so. *S. aureus* that produce TSST-1 are usually of phage group I and lysed by phage 29 or 52.

Table 3 *Enterotoxin production by strains of* S. aureus *implicated in 359 outbreaks of food poisoning in the United Kingdom (1969–1990)*

Enterotoxin produced	Strains positive
A	205(57%)
B	6
C	5
D	15
E	3
A and B	12
A and C	9
A and D	55(15%)
A,B and D	4
B and D	1
C and D	28(8%)
None (not A–E)	16

Reproduced from Wieneke, A.A., Roberts, D., and Gilbert, R.J. (1993). Staphylococcal food poisoning in the United Kingdom. *Epidemiology and Infection* (in press), with permission.

Carriage

S. aureus forms part of the normal flora in some individuals; about 25 per cent 'carry' the organism permanently, a similar proportion never do, and the rest do so intermittently. The most common sites for carriage are the nose, axilla, perineum, and toewebs. Nasal carriage rates vary from 10 to 40 per cent in normal adults outside hospital, but higher rates of carriage are often found in patients in hospital, particularly those in hospital for several weeks. High carriage rates are also found in individuals with skin diseases such as eczema, in insulin-dependent diabetics, patients on chronic haemodialysis, and intravenous drug abusers. Some carriers, known as 'shedders', disperse large numbers of staphylococci into the environment on skin squames and the organisms can survive for long periods in the desiccated state. Other carriers contaminate the environment less readily, but activity such as hand scrubbing or showering increases shedding. The carrier state is highly relevant in the epidemiology of *S. aureus* infection, whether this complicates surgery or otherwise; in the majority of cases the source of the pathogen is endogenous.

Host factors in S. aureus *infection*

Intact skin and mucous membranes are one of the host's most important defences against staphylococcal infection. Wounds, whether traumatic or surgical, frequently become colonized with *S. aureus*; this may result in localized infection or in dissemination via the bloodstream to distant sites. Sometimes trivial, even unrecognized, skin trauma precedes such haematogenous spread. Burns and skin diseases are important portals of entry for staphylococci. Certain viral infections such as influenza damage the respiratory epithelium and allow secondary staphylococcal invasion. The presence of foreign material, including intravascular catheters, arteriovenous shunts, and vascular and orthopaedic prostheses, is also relevant to the pathogenesis and perpetuation of staphylococcal infection.

Once *S. aureus* has gained access to the tissues, then the polymorphonuclear leucocyte is the most important line of defence. Phagocytosis involves chemotaxis, opsonization, and intracellular killing of *S. aureus*. Chemotactic defects occur, for example, in Job syndrome (in which patients with recurrent eczema suffer from repeated skin infections and cold abscesses with *S. aureus*), and also in certain other rare syndromes. Opsonic defects tend to predispose to a variety of pyogenic infections, including, but not specifically *S. aureus*, but *S. aureus* is a major pathogen in chronic granulomatous disease producing local and metastatic abscesses. In this disease, intracellular killing by the polymorphs is defective.

Susceptibility of S. aureus *to antibiotics and antiseptics*

Resistance to antibiotics is not an indicator of particular virulence in *S. aureus*. Strains sensitive to all antistaphylococcal antibiotics occasionally cause devastatingly severe community-acquired infections. The majority of isolates of *S. aureus*, however, whether community or hospital acquired, produce β-lactamase and are thus resistant to penicillin itself and a number of related compounds including ampicillin, amoxycillin, piperacillin, and azlocillin. Staphylococcal β-lactamase has a negligible effect on methicillin, nafcillin, and the isoxazolyl penicillins cloxacillin and flucloxacillin, which were introduced specifically for the treatment of staphylococcal infection. A resistance mechanism for these semisynthetic penicillins was soon detected. It is a general mechanism involving all penicillins and most, possibly all, cephalosporins, although it is usually referred to as methicillin resistance. It appears to result from the overproduction of a penicillin-binding protein with a low affinity for β-lactams. Methicillin-resistant strains of *S. aureus* (**MRSA**) were detected soon after the introduction of methicillin in 1960, and reports of their isolation increased until 1971, when they accounted for some 5 per cent of strains submitted to the Staphylococcus Reference Laboratory of the Central Public Health Laboratory in the United Kingdom. MRSA then diminished in frequency in the United Kingdom and some European countries, it is thought possibly as a result of increased prescribing of aminoglycosides. There was then a resurgence in the United Kingdom and elsewhere in the early 1980s, perhaps as a result of the introduction of new penicillin and cephalosporin derivatives. MRSA are usually, but not always, resistant to a variety of other antibiotics in addition to methicillin. This has led to terminological confusion and 'MRSA' has been used to designate both methicillin resistance and multiple resistance. MRSA have been responsible for hospital outbreaks in many countries, and although in many of these outbreaks they have caused colonization rather than infection, genuine infection has also occurred, particularly in vulnerable patients. Colonization with MRSA is a notoriously recalcitrant problem on geriatric wards and spread is difficult to avoid. Worldwide, most MRSAs have been of phage group III or non-typable. Several distinct strains of MRSA have caused epidemics and they are designated E (epidemic) MRSA-1 etc. The control of MRSA within a hospital is an expensive operation, but so too is the cost of treatment and prolonged stay when patients become infected.

S. aureus, whether β-lactamase producing or not, is sensitive to many cephalosporins, though the newer 'third generation' cephalosporins, such as ceftazidime, are much less active against *S. aureus* than are cefuroxime and cephradine.

The incidence of erythromycin resistance is related to use of the antibiotic. It tends to be high (around 20 per cent) in staphylococci isolated from patients with skin diseases; amongst isolates from other patients it is usually about 5 per cent. Staphylococci passaged in the presence of erythromycin or related macrolides may develop a more or less stable resistance not only to the agent tested but to all macrolides. A type of resistance that has been called 'dissociated resistance' emerges in staphylococci during treatment of patients with erythromycin. Most of the staphylococci in populations developing this type of resistance are initially sensitive to erythromycin, but if grown on a medium containing the drug, emerge as highly resistant, not only to erythromycin itself but to the unrelated drug clindamycin as well. In the absence of erythromycin the resistance is lost and the organism appears sensitive.

Among the aminoglycosides, streptomycin was the first agent to which *S. aureus* developed resistance, followed by neomycin, especially when this antibiotic was used topically, and kanamycin. Gentamicin resistance is unusual, except in MRSA, many of which are resistant.

Resistance is attributable either to reduced uptake and binding of the antibiotic or to the production of aminoglycoside-modifying enzymes, or in some strains to both mechanisms.

Resistance of *S. aureus* to fusidic acid is uncommon, but most cultures contain small numbers of resistant mutants and a fully resistant population can emerge both *in vitro* and *in vivo*, the latter being particularly likely after topical use. Resistance of *S. aureus* to vancomycin or teicoplanin has not been reported. Rifampicin is highly active against *S. aureus* but as with fusidic acid, minority populations of resistant cells are found and resistance may emerge during treatment.

The topical antibiotic mupirocin is very active against *S. aureus* and this agent is invaluable in the eradication of staphylococci (especially MRSA) from the nose and other superficial sites. However, resistance has arisen to mupirocin, particularly during prolonged treatment, generally in dermatological patients. As low-level mupirocin resistance has been achieved by training *in vitro*, long-term therapy might be expected to achieve the same result *in vivo*.

Most disinfectants and antiseptics inhibit or kill *S. aureus*. The antiseptics chlorhexidine, hexachlorophane, and iodine or iodine-containing compounds such as povidone iodine are all widely used for skin disinfection and when used correctly are highly effective in removing staphylococci from the skin.

Clinical manifestations

S. aureus usually causes localized infection, sometimes with local spread, but this may result in bacteraemia and haematogenous dissemination of the infection. Thus staphylococcal infection at many sites may arise by either of these mechanisms. Certain staphylococcal syndromes are produced by extracellular toxins rather than local invasion and these will be considered separately, even though the distinction between the different pathogenic mechanisms involved sometimes becomes blurred in the individual patient.

Localized infections

INFECTION OF THE SKIN AND ITS APPENDAGES

Many of these infections arise in association with hair follicles, and minor trauma, maceration, and skin diseases predispose to them. Folliculitis is a superficial infection of the hair follicle commonly, though not exclusively, caused by *S. aureus*; persistent folliculitis of the beard area is known as *sycosis barbae*. Boils (furuncles) are deep-seated infections around a hair follicle; they tend to occur on the neck, axillae, buttocks, and thighs and may be recurrent, sometimes involving more than one member of a family. When several adjacent hair follicles are involved a carbuncle develops, usually on the back of the neck; this consists of a large indurated mass with multiple draining sinuses with associated systemic disturbance. Although boils are very common infections, carbuncles are now rarely seen. Impetigo is a blistering skin lesion with a crusting exudate that affects the exposed areas of the body (often the face), usually in children. Epidermolytic toxin is associated with these infections. Most acute paronychias are caused by *S. aureus*, though these can also be caused by various other bacteria including anaerobes. Mastitis and breast abscess in the puerperium are also caused by *S. aureus*. Newborn babies quite commonly suffer from staphylococcal infection, with septic spots, purulent discharge from the umbilicus, 'sticky eye', and occasionally breast abscess, as well as the much rarer toxin-mediated staphylococcal diseases. Styes, or hordeola, common acute purulent infections of the glands of the eyelid, are also caused by *S. aureus*.

EAR, NOSE AND THROAT INFECTIONS

Staphylococcal infection of the hair follicles or sebaceous glands in the outer half of the external auditory canal gives rise to acute localized otitis externa, a condition characterized by severe pain and itching. Acute otitis media is very seldom caused by *S. aureus*, and staphylococci are only rarely isolated from patients with sinusitis. Although *S. aureus* is commonly grown from throat swabs, the organism behaves as a commensal at this site, and patients from whom it is recovered have usually been taking antibiotics.

WOUND INFECTION

S. aureus remains the most common cause of wound infection after surgery or trauma not involving the mucous membranes with their rich anaerobic commensal flora. The clinical presentation of staphylococcal wound infection varies from minimal erythema and serous discharge, through small abscesses (often in relation to sutures), to marked cellulitis (with deep pus and wound dehiscence) with considerable pain and systemic disturbance. *S. aureus* is an important cause of infection associated with intravascular devices. These infections, which may present as obvious local sepsis or more insidiously, as a pyrexia, often severe, without overt localizing signs, can occur as early as 48 h after insertion of the catheter, but more usually after a longer period. *S. aureus* is also an important pathogen in infections associated with other prosthetic material.

PLEUROPULMONARY INFECTION

Staphylococcal pneumonia arises either from aspiration or from haematogenous spread with metastatic seeding of the lung. Aspiration pneumonia is generally a complication of pre-existing lung disease such as bronchiectasis or bronchial carcinoma, or of a viral respiratory disease, usually influenza. In children, other viral infections of the respiratory tract, including severe measles in developing countries, may be followed by secondary bacterial infection with staphylococci. *S. aureus* from the patient's own carriage sites are presumed to reach the damaged lung tissue via the trachea and bronchi. In contrast to aspiration pneumonia, haematogenous staphylococcal pneumonia characteristically affects a previously normal lung. In some cases there may be an identifiable local infection, often of the skin and usually trivial, that has resulted in haematogenous seeding of *S. aureus*, or there may be evidence of release of infected thrombi via the venous system as, for instance, in tricuspid endocarditis or occasionally when there is an infected intravascular device. Staphylococci can readily be isolated from the blood in haematogenous pneumonia, but bacteraemia seldom accompanies aspiration pneumonia. Whatever its pathogenesis, *S. aureus* pneumonia is a severe disease with high fever and cyanosis. Contrary to what is often thought, when staphylococcal pneumonia is secondary to influenza, it may occur without an obvious influenza-like prodromal illness and with alarming suddenness (Fig. 1(a,b)). It is usually complicated by abscess formation, empyema and, in children, by pneumatoceles and pyopneumothorax, but the radiological findings at presentation vary from local consolidation to multiple, patchy infiltrates, and abscess formation may or may not be detected.

URINARY TRACT INFECTION

S. aureus urinary tract infection is uncommon. Interestingly, the urinary tract is one of the few sites at which coagulase-negative staphylococci are more usual pathogens than *S. aureus*. *S. aureus* infection is unlikely to occur in patients with a normal urinary tract, except in staphylococcal septicaemia, when the organism can often be recovered from the urine, presumably the result of microabscesses in the kidney. Infection sometimes occurs in patients with abnormal bladder function, usually in association with instrumentation or catheterization and presumably from previous urethral colonization with the strain. It may also occur after surgery, such as renal transplantation and open prostatectomy in conjunction with an infected wound.

Bacteraemia and septicaemia

Bacteraemia, in the strict sense, merely implies the presence of bacteria in the blood, that is a positive blood culture in the laboratory; it may or may not be symptomatic in the patient. A symptomatic bacteraemia is usually referred to as a septicaemia. In fact, *S. aureus* in the blood is almost always symptomatic and thus strictly a septicaemia, but the terms tend to be used interchangeably. Most staphylococcal bacteraemias, particularly those acquired in hospital, are secondary to a local site of infection such as a soft tissue lesion, wound, or intravascular access site. It is assumed, though difficult to prove, that *S. aureus* can also gain access to the bloodstream from carrier sites or trivial, unnoticed abrasions that become colonized, as only such a mechanism would explain cases of community-acquired staphylococcal bacteraemia associated with serious, deep-seated infection involving bones, joints, lungs, and heart valves. Such bacteraemias have been called 'primary', and are usually much more severe than those secondary to a defined focus of infection. Primary bacteraemia can occur at any age, and often affects a previously healthy individual. Occasionally, patients with community-acquired *S. aureus* bacteraemia present with profound toxaemia, shock, and dermal evidence of disseminated intravascular coagulation. Such patients often have signs of meningitis, and their cerebrospinal fluid contains polymorphs, often in large numbers, though staphylococci are rarely detected. Not surprisingly, the infection is often thought to be meningococcal (Fig. 2).

Figure 3 shows a fatal case of *S. aureus* septicaemia with disseminated intravascular coagulation. A previously healthy 54-year-old man was febrile and confused, and became hemiplegic within 48 h of admission. Both blood cultures and cerebrospinal fluid (which contained 5000 polymorphs) grew *S. aureus*. Autopsy was refused, but he most probably also had (undiagnosed) endocarditis.

Fig. 1 Chest radiograph of a 24-year-old man with severe staphylococcal pneumonia (a) on admission and (b) 13 days later. The patient was also suffering from influenza B.

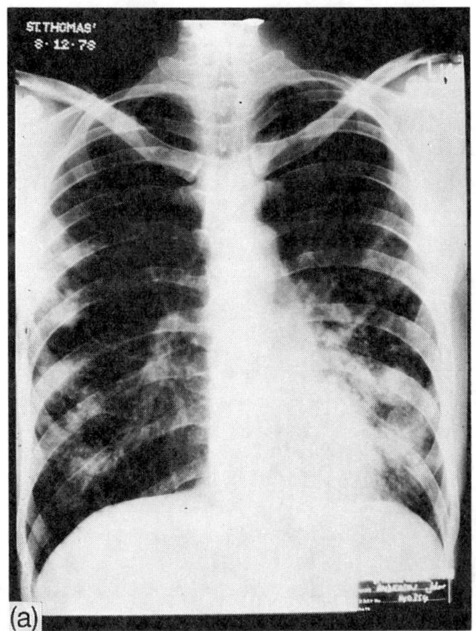

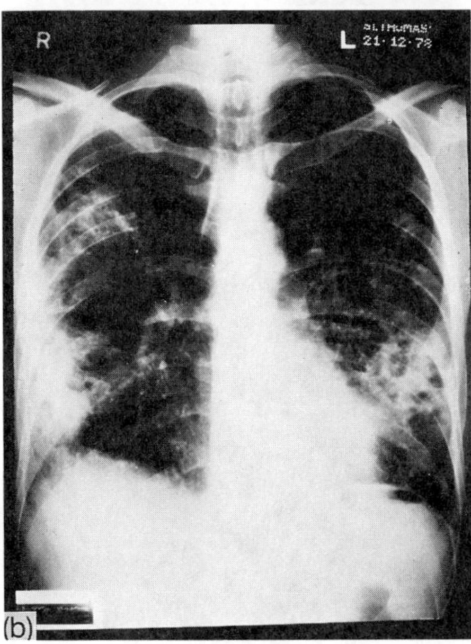

Fig. 2 Meningococcaemic-like infection in a 22-year-old man who died from an aortic-root abscess from *S. aureus* endocarditis on a bicuspid aortic valve. A false-positive meningococcal latex agglutination test on the cerebrospinal fluid (which contained 1500 polymorphs, but no organisms) taken on admission further increased the clinical confusion.

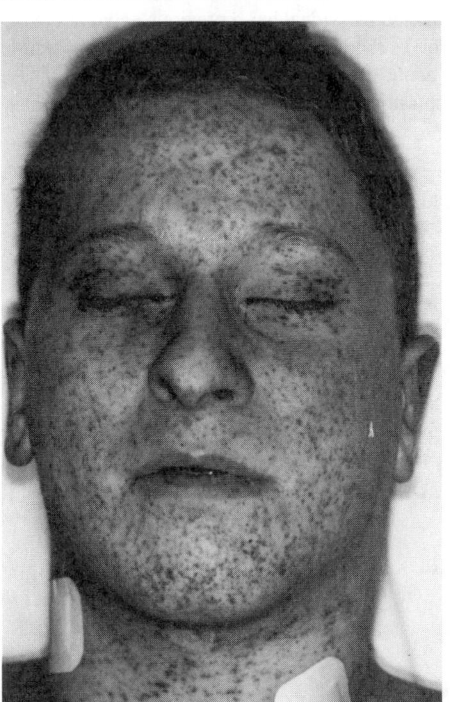

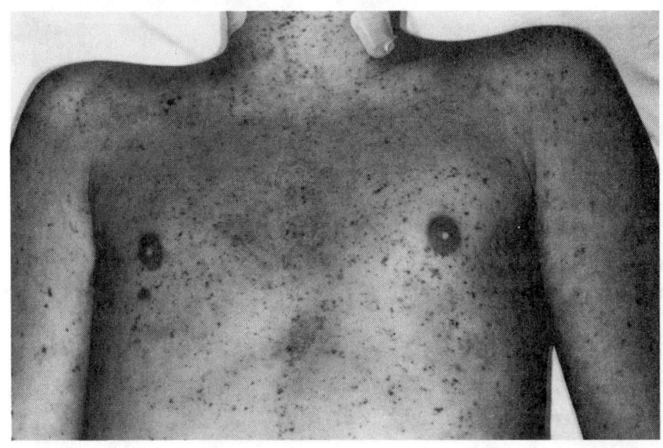

Metastatic (haematogenous) infection

ENDOCARDITIS

As outlined above, *S. aureus* endocarditis usually results from a 'primary', community-acquired bacteraemia with the organism, and is a devastating illness often occurring in a previously healthy individual. An asymptomatic, left-sided valvular abnormality such as a bicuspid aortic valve or mitral leaflet prolapse is sometimes, though not invariably, present. The infection typically presents as an influenza-like illness, often with initial gastrointestinal disturbance. Meningism is seen in about one-quarter of cases and polymorphs but organisms are seldom detected in the cerebrospinal fluid. The patient develops signs of systemic emboli and valvular insufficiency within days, sometimes hours, of admission to hospital. Acute staphylococcal endocarditis is a rapidly destructive disease; there is nothing 'subacute' about *S. aureus* and this infection was called, justifiably, malignant endocarditis by Osler. Emergency valve replacement may be required and should never be delayed; it is this and not further antibiotics that will save the patient's life. Staphylococcal endocarditis is occasionally complicated by splenic abscess (Fig. 4), for which splenectomy is usually required. *S. aureus* endocarditis may also be acquired in hospital as a result of uncontrolled bacteraemia from infected intravascular devices or from sternal wound infection after valve replacement surgery (Fig. 5).

Intravenous drug abusers are at particular risk of staphylococcal endocarditis but unless the affected individual has a previous valvular abnormality, the infection involves the tricuspid valve and presents as a quite different and often less acute illness from that described above. There is fever, malaise, and respiratory signs that result from septic pulmonary emboli.

Fig. 3 Meningococcaemia-like disease. (a) Hand and (b) foot of a man with primary staphylococcal bacteraemia and meningitis who had disseminated intravascular coagulation.

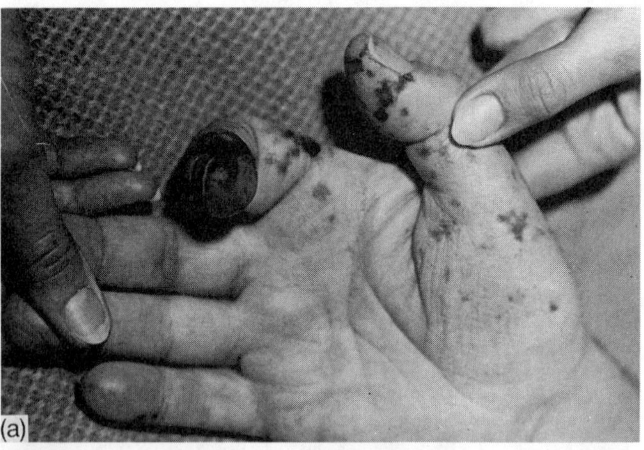

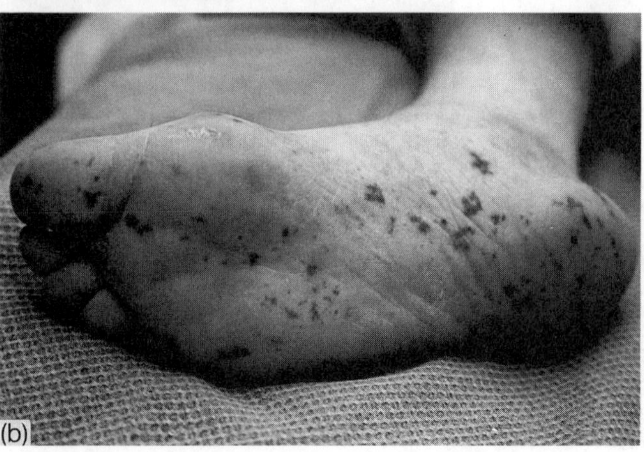

BONE AND JOINT INFECTIONS

Overall, *S. aureus* remains the most common cause of acute bone and joint infection at all ages. Although these infections can result from a 'primary' bacteraemia with *S. aureus*, they can also result from a contiguous focus of infection after trauma or surgery, especially that involving prosthetic implants. During the past decade the incidence of contiguous osteomyelitis and septic arthritis has increased, especially in older patients and particularly in diabetics and those with joint prostheses. The overall incidence of acute haematogenous osteomyelitis has decreased, and there has also been a change in the localization of this infection. Osteomyelitis of the metaphyses of the long bones, an infection seen primarily in children, particularly boys, has decreased and the vertebral column is now the most common site involved. Most patients with staphylococcal vertebral osteomyelitis are middle aged or elderly. The reason for this shift in localization has not been explained. Vertebral osteomyelitis can be a notoriously difficult diagnosis, and pain, not always persistently localized to the spine, the only consistent feature. Fever is not always present, but at least should lead to the taking of blood for culture. Any patient with backache, a high erythrocyte sedimentation rate, and *S. aureus* in the blood should be assumed to have vertebral infection and treated accordingly.

Fig. 4 Splenic abscess complicating staphylococcal endocarditis.

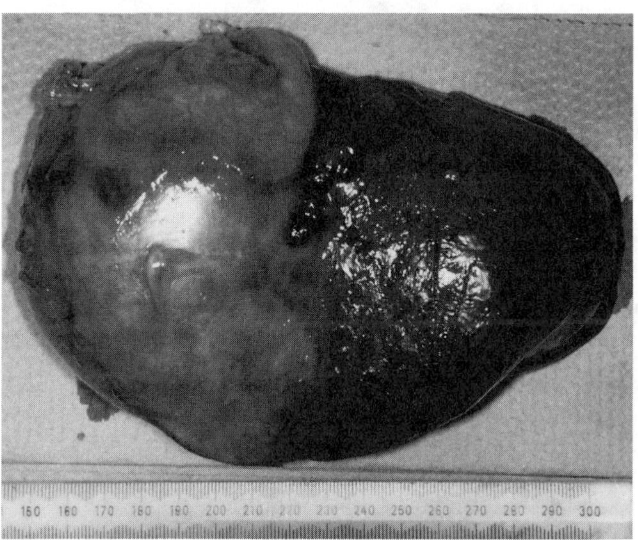

Fig. 5 Huge vegetation on prosthetic mitral valve. Fatal endocarditis resulting from staphylococcal sternal wound infection with dehiscence 4 weeks after mitral valve replacement.

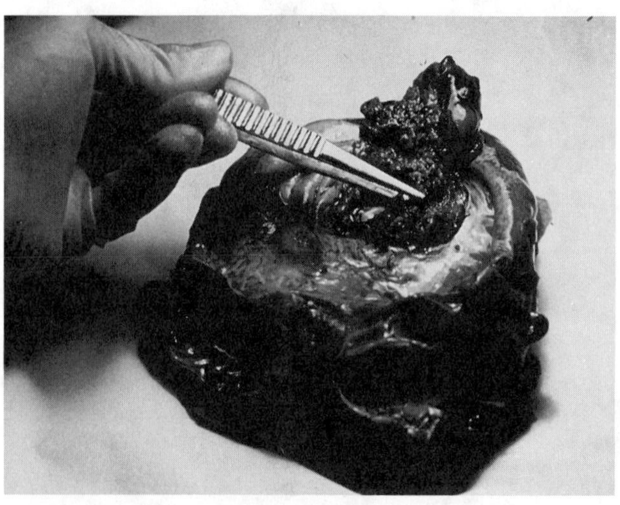

Staphylococcal septic arthritis may occur in previously normal or abnormal joints and at any age. It may involve one or more joints and multiple infection is particularly likely in patients with rheumatoid arthritis, in whom the diagnosis is liable to be delayed as both patient and doctor alike may assume that the symptoms are caused by the underlying disease and the affected joints may not exhibit overt signs of inflammation. The isolation of *S. aureus* from the blood of such a patient should prompt a very careful assessment of all joints, and multiple aspirations may be required to define the extent of the infection. Microscopy and culture of aspirated fluid will rapidly enable the diagnosis to be made.

RENAL CORTICAL ABSCESS (CARBUNCLE) AND PERINEPHRIC ABSCESS

These forms of metastatic staphylococcal infection are rare and usually lead to considerable diagnostic confusion. A renal cortical abscess, also known as a carbuncle, is a multilocular abscess involving the renal parenchyma, the result of the coalescence of cortical microabscesses from haematogenous seeding of the kidney from a previous infection, typically a boil, with *S. aureus*. The patient complains of fevers and loin pain but urinary symptoms are usually absent, and unless the abscess communicates with the excretory system, the urine contains neither pus cells nor *S. aureus*. Although *S. aureus* is by far the most common pathogen in renal carbuncle, perinephric abscesses, that is abscesses external to the renal capsule but within the perinephric fascia, are much more commonly caused by Gram-negative aerobes such as *Escherichia coli* and *Proteus* spp. than by staphylococci. A renal carbuncle may rupture into the perinephric space, thus producing a perinephric abscess. Again, urine cultures are unlikely to be positive, and the signs are similar to those of a renal carbuncle.

Fig. 6 Staphylococcal scalded-skin syndrome in a child. (Reproduced by courtesy of Professor W.C. Noble.)

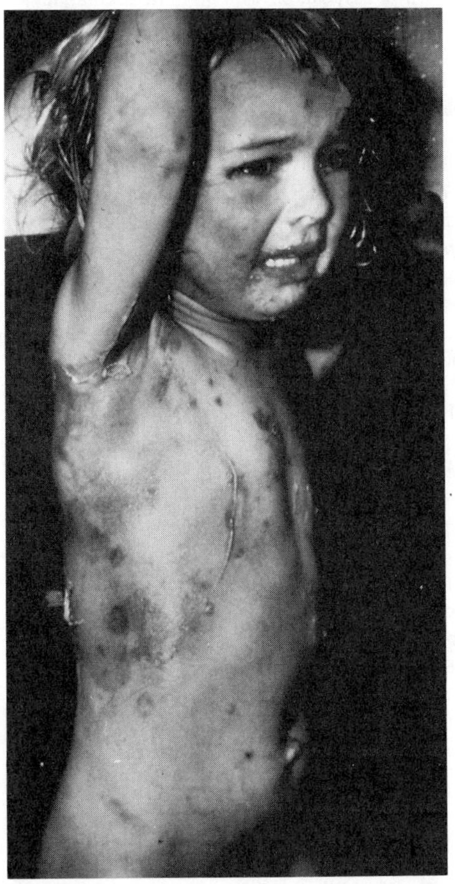

PYOMYOSITIS

Pyomyositis is an acute inflammation of skeletal muscle that is almost unique to the tropics and subtropics, where it is a common infection; it is rarely encountered in temperate climates. Usually a single, large muscle is affected, most commonly the gluteal and quadriceps, but multiple muscle involvement may also occur. The infection predominantly affects males and presents with muscular pain followed by fever, localized pain, induration, and swelling. The infection is almost always caused by *S. aureus* but its aetiology remains obscure and trauma, viral infection, parasitic infection (eosinophilia is common), and malnutrition have all been postulated but none adequately substantiated. If, as seems possible, the infection is haematogenous, the paucity of reports of positive blood cultures would suggest that this probably occurs early in the pathogenesis of the disease. Treatment consists of drainage and antibiotics.

Infections mediated by toxins of S. aureus

STAPHYLOCOCCAL FOOD POISONING

This syndrome, characterized by severe vomiting, nausea, and abdominal cramps and diarrhoea, is caused by the ingestion of staphylococcal enterotoxin preformed in the food. The onset occurs within hours of the ingestion of food that has been contaminated during its preparation by an individual infected with, or shedding, an enterotoxin-producing staphylococcus. Unrefrigerated, protein-rich foods containing meat or milk are particularly likely to support the growth of staphylococci and the subsequent production of enterotoxin, which can survive cooking. Only about 5 per cent of outbreaks of bacterial food poisoning reported to the Communicable Disease Surveillance Centre for which an aetiological agent is identified are caused by *S. aureus*. The diagnosis can be confirmed by culturing the incriminated food, any skin lesions and the nose of food handlers, and (though rarely available) vomitus or stools of the victims. In most outbreaks, both the organism and its toxin can be defined, but occasionally, enterotoxin alone is demonstrated in the food.

STAPHYLOCOCCAL SCALDED SKIN SYNDROME (SSSS)

This rare disease, originally known as Ritter's disease when it was first reported in infants, is more commonly seen in children (Fig. 6) than adults (Fig. 7), and is characterized by the sudden onset of extensive erythema followed by bullous desquamation of large areas of skin. It is caused by the epidermolytic toxins of *S. aureus*. The disease of SSSS must be distinguished from a similar clinical entity that has nothing to do with *S. aureus*, that of toxic epidermal necrolysis (Lyell's syndrome). This disease, which generally occurs in older children and adults, is the result of drug hypersensitivity. Histologically the two entities can readily be distinguished: in SSSS there is intraepithelial splitting at the level of the stratum granulosum, whereas in toxic epidermal neurolysis there is total epidermal loss with separation at the dermal–epidermal junction.

Fig. 7 Staphylococcal scalded-skin syndrome (SSSS) in an adult.

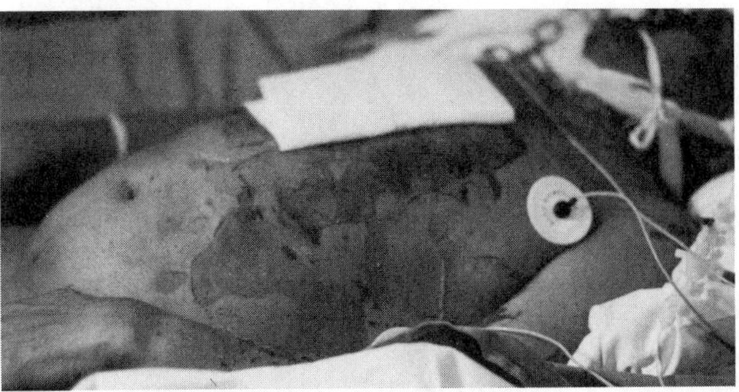

TOXIC SHOCK SYNDROME

This syndrome (Fig. 8), consisting of high fever, mental confusion, erythroderma, diarrhoea, hypotension and renal failure, was first defined by Todd *et al.* in 1978, who reported seven cases, three boys and four girls, aged 8 to 17 years. In five of them, *S. aureus* of phage group I was isolated from the nasopharynx, vagina or a localized abscess, though not from the blood. Although the designation 'toxic shock syndrome' was new, the syndrome was not: it had been recognised 50 years earlier and thought to be staphylococcal scarlet fever. Shortly after Todd's paper appeared there was an epidemic of toxic shock syndrome in women associated with menstruation, initially and predominantly in the United States, but later, though in far fewer numbers, in other countries. It was shown to be associated with the use of tampons, and in the United States with one highly occlusive brand that was then withdrawn from the market, resulting in a decreased incidence of the disease, though not to its disappearance. Such an association had not previously been recognized, and Todd had given no information on menstruation or tampon use for the girls in his series. Toxic shock syndrome has also been described in women who were not menstruating and in men in association with a wide variety of conditions and operations. The diagnostic criteria were refined by the Centers for Disease Control, Atlanta, when investigating the tampon-associated epidemic; these were high fever, erythematous rash, desquamation, marked hypotension, and the failure of three independent organ systems. The syndrome may be fatal and a death rate of around 5 per cent was reported during the 'tampon epidemic'.

Because the syndrome is mediated by toxin, the mainstay of treatment is general supportive measures to combat shock. Antistaphylococcal antibiotics should be given to eradicate the *S. aureus* from the local site and any tampon should be removed. Bacteraemia has rarely been reported in toxic shock syndrome. The staphylococci isolated have usually been resistant only to penicillin. Most cases of menstrually associated toxic shock syndrome are mediated by TSST-1 (see above) produced by phage group I strains of *S. aureus*; the syndrome when not associated with menstruation can occur with strains producing TSST-1, but also with phage group V strains that produce enterotoxin B.

Fig. 8 Toxic shock syndrome. Desquamation of (a) hand and (b) feet in a girl with tampon-associated disease. (Reproduced by courtesy of Dr D. C. Shanson.)

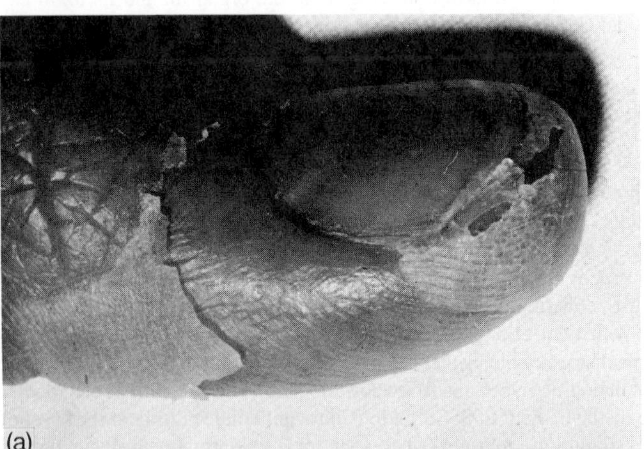

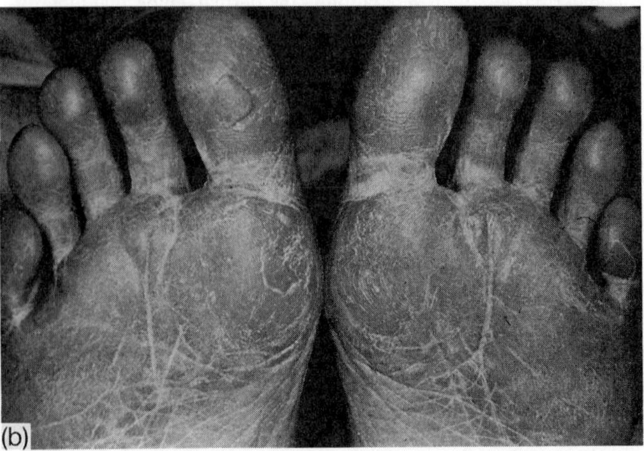

Laboratory diagnosis of S. aureus *infection*

S. aureus is readily isolated in the laboratory from swabs, pus, blood, or other material. A Gram-stained film will often enable a rapid diagnosis of the staphylococcal aetiology to be made: the characteristic clumps of Gram-positive cocci, which may be intracellular as well as extracellular, are readily identifiable. The presumptive microscopic diagnosis can be confirmed by culture within 24 h. Staphylococcal bacteraemia is detected by routine blood culture methods. The isolation of *S. aureus* from a blood culture is almost always indicative of a genuine bacteraemia and the organism should only be dismissed as a contaminant if the patient has extensive skin disease such as eczema. In most cases of staphylococcal bacteraemia, the organism will be isolated from all blood cultures taken, provided that antibiotics have not been given.

Treatment

Drainage of pus, if present, is a prerequisite to the management of infection with *S. aureus*. Drainage may occur spontaneously or with only minor surgical intervention in most superficial infections such as boils, paronychias, styes, and stitch abscesses. Deep abscesses in wounds or organs, and osteomyelitis that has progressed to to the point of pus formation, require definitive surgical drainage, though for lung abscesses postural drainage plus appropriate chemotherapy will usually suffice. Infections that occur in association with an intravascular device or other prosthetic material seldom resolve with antibiotics and removal of the foreign material is nearly always required.

Antibiotic therapy is indicated if the patient is systemically unwell or if the infection shows signs of spreading. Sometimes, antibiotics given early in the course of a potentially localizing pyogenic infection may arrest its progress. Antibiotics are of no benefit in staphylococcal food poisoning but should be given in SSSS and toxic shock syndrome to eradicate the toxin-producing *S. aureus*. The initial choice of agent for staphylococcal infection (before sensitivities become available) depends on the patterns of susceptibility of *S. aureus* in the community from which the patient comes. Penicillin itself is suitable only if the strain does not produce β-lactamase (rarely the case), and should never be used for the initial 'blind' treatment of staphylococcal infection. Similar constraints apply to ampicillin and amoxycillin. For most strains of *S. aureus* there is a wide choice of effective antibiotics. In most instances, a β-lactamase-resistant penicillin (such as flucloxacillin) or cephalosporin (such as cefuroxime) is appropriate but definitive treatment should be based on *in vitro* sensitivity tests. Other appropriate, semisynthetic penicillins include methicillin, cloxacillin, dicloxacillin, oxacillin, nafcillin, and the combination drug co-amoxiclav. Many cephalosporins are effective against *S. aureus* but the 'third generation' agents are less active than the older drugs and should be avoided. Alternative agents to the β-lactams, particularly where the patient is hypersensitive to pencillin penicillin, include the macrolides (of which the most commonly used is erythromycin), and related drugs such as clindamycin and the newer agents clarithromycin and azithromycin. Fusidic acid is an excellent antistaphylococcal agent and most strains of *S. aureus* are initially susceptible to it. It has been used in European countries such as Britain and Germany since the 1960s, and is now marketed in many European countries and in Israel, Canada, and South Africa, but not in the United States. Despite the lack of published evidence there is a wealth of experience of the successful use of fusidic acid, especially for bone and joint infections. Resistance to fusidic acid may arise during treatment, especially when the organism cannot readily be eradicated; this has led to the time-honoured recommendation that fusidic acid should always be given with a second antibiotic. There is scant evidence that this is necessary. The only agents with reliable activity against methicillin- (hence also cephalosporin-) resistant strains are vancomycin and teicoplanin. They should be reserved for the treatment of infections with MRSA, for patients on haemodialysis with staphylococcal infections whatever the susceptibility of the organism (these agents are excreted almost entirely by the kidney and only minimally removed by dialysis, hence can be given at long intervals) and for the treatment of erythromycin-resistant strains in patients hypersensitive to penicillin.

Most staphylococcal infection is satisfactorily treated with a single antibiotic but combination therapy is often used for serious infections, particularly endocarditis and bone or joint infection. Usual combinations include a β-lactam plus fusidic acid or gentamicin, or for MRSA, vancomycin plus rifampicin. There is minimal evidence that any combination is superior to a single agent, although bacteraemia may be cleared more rapidly and defervescence occur sooner with combination therapy. In common with many infections, the length of antibiotic treatment required to treat staphylococcal infection is unknown; what is known is that for serious, community-acquired infections such as endocarditis, bone and joint infections and pneumonia, prolonged treatment is needed, though whether this should be for 4, 5, or 6 weeks is unclear. For most other infections, antibiotics should be given until there is obvious clinical improvement or for about 48 h after fever has resolved. Estimation of teichoic acid antibodies has been recommended as a means of determining the length of treatment required for patients with *S. aureus* bacteraemia and no obvious source for this. Deep-seated or metastatic infection produces a raised antibody response whereas simple bacteraemia does not. These tests are not routinely available and are not consistently reliable.

Persistent positive blood cultures with *S. aureus* despite appropriate antibiotic therapy are seldom an indication for changing the antibiotics, but rather for an assessment of the need for intervention, for example to remove an infected intravascular device, excise an infected heart valve, or aspirate and wash out a joint. Only too frequently the emphasis is on unnecessary *in vitro* tests on the organism and effective management is delayed. Topical antibiotics and antiseptics are useful for the treatment of skin infections such as impetigo. Antiseptics and the antibiotic mupirocin, not used systemically, are preferred to antibiotics that are used systemically because of the risk of resistance. That said, however, topical fusidic acid is widely used with scant evidence of resistance. Topical agents are also used to eliminate the carriage of *S. aureus* either to control the spread of MRSA or in individuals with recurrent superficial staphylococcal infection.

Coagulase-negative staphylococci

Although coagulase-negative staphylococci are the most common contaminants encountered in the laboratory (particularly, though not exclusively, in blood cultures), they can also be important pathogens, whose incidence continues to increase, especially in neonatal intensive care units. The availability of kits for their speciation has served to emphasize that the coagulase-negative staphylococci cannot be regarded as a homogeneous entity; the different species vary not only in their incidence in clinical infections but also in the type and severity of disease produced. Most infections are hospital acquired or associated, but certain species cause severe community-acquired infection.

Pathogenicity

Those coagulase-negative staphylococci (usually *S. epidermidis*) that cause infections associated with plastic prosthetic devices and intravascular catheters produce an exopolysaccharide ('slime'), which is an important factor in enabling the adherence of these organisms to plastic material and probably also in their resistance to phagocytosis and other host defences and to antimicrobial action. Coagulase-negative staphylococci isolated from clinical infections also produce a wide variety of potential toxins including haemolysins, cytotoxins, deoxyribonuclease, fibrinolysin, proteinase, and lipase–esterase, and there are strong similarities between some of these exoproteins and those produced by *S. aureus*. This is of interest as infections caused by, for example, *S. lugdunensis* and *S. simulans* closely mimic that caused by *S. aureus*.

Carriage

The coagulase-negative staphylococci, together with the coryneforms, form the greater part of the human skin flora. They grow in the mouths of hair follicles and on the skin surface, where they form microcolonies. Although many different species are found on the skin, the most common is *S. epidermidis*, and to a lesser extent *S. hominis* and *S. haemolyticus*. Distribution varies on different skin areas, for instance, *S. epidermidis* predominates on the head and trunk whereas *S. hominis* does so on the arms and legs. As its name suggests, *S. capitis* is found mainly on the head. There are also geographical variations.

Host factors in coagulase-negative staphylococcal infection

Most infection with coagulase-negative staphylococci is associated with the presence of prosthetic material both in compromised and non-compromised hosts. Infection of intravascular catheters can arise via the catheter access site or via the catheter hub from frequent disconnections. Prosthetic material can also become infected at the time of percutaneous or surgical implantation. Organisms that had previously entered the bloodstream from an endogenous source might also colonize prosthetic material. Occasionally, as with *S. aureus* infection (only much less frequently than with *S. aureus*), a trivial infection or unnoticed breach in the epithelium allows ingress of coagulase-negative staphylococci to the blood-stream; serious infection, typically endocarditis but occasionally vertebral osteomyelitis, can result.

Antibiotic susceptibility

Coagulase-negative staphylococci from hospital-acquired infections, particularly *S. epidermidis* and *S. haemolyticus*, are usually multiply resistant. The majority of strains are resistant to methicillin (and thus to cephalosporins), and many are also resistant to gentamicin and erythromycin. Thus the usual nosocomial strain of coagulase-negative staphylococcus has an antibiotic susceptibility pattern comparable to many MRSAs. Resistance to vancomycin and teicoplanin has been reported (initially in *S. haemolyticus*), although rarely, amongst coagulase-negative staphylococci. In marked contrast to the multiple resistance of most nosocomial strains, community-acquired infections are likely to be caused by strains sensitive to most antistaphylococcal antibiotics including penicillin. In comparison, community-acquired *S. aureus* infection is seldom caused by penicillin-sensitive strains.

Infections caused by coagulase-negative staphylococci

The majority of infections caused by coagulase-negative staphylococci are acquired in hospital, and these infections are increasingly common. They almost always arise in association with a prosthetic device or implant. Community-acquired infections are rare, though these too seem to be increasing, but are usually severe. In many infections with coagulase-negative staphylococci, isolation of the organism from the blood is essential for the diagnosis, and true bacteraemia must be distinguished from contamination. Repeated cultures should always be taken, preferably from different sites, and only organisms of similar sensitivity and biochemical profile considered the same. Infection with more than one strain is not unusual in nosocomial infections.

Intravascular devices

There has been a marked increase in the incidence of coagulase-negative staphylococcal infection (usually with *S. epidermidis*) of all intravascular devices but particularly in neonates and immunocompromised patients. These organisms are now the most common bacteria involved in such infections. This can only partly be explained by the increased use of these devices. It is prudent to take blood for culture both via the intravascular catheter and from a peripheral site because true bacteraemia is unlikely to be detected only in blood taken from the catheter. The degree of systemic disturbance from these infections varies, and it is this that should determine the approach to treatment. In contrast to infections of intravascular devices caused by *S. aureus*, with those caused by coagulase-negative staphylococci it may be possible to leave the catheter in place and give appropriate antibiotics, usually vancomycin or teicoplanin; sometimes this fails and then the catheter must be removed to control the infection. Very occasionally, as with *S. aureus*, persistent bacteraemia can result in metastatic seeding of heart valve, vertebra, or other site.

Cerebrospinal fluid shunts

Coagulase-negative staphylococci, predominantly *S. epidermidis*, are the most common cause of infection of shunts for hydrocephalus, and these infections can present weeks, months or years after the insertion of the shunt. Coagulase-negative staphylococci also cause infection of cerebrospinal fluid reservoirs used for chemotherapy. Signs of meningitis may be absent and usual findings include low-grade fever, malaise, and shunt malfunction. *S. epidermidis* can be isolated from the blood and the cerebrospinal fluid aspirated from the shunt. Serum antibodies to *S. epidermidis* have been used to monitor treatment and to detect relapse in these infections. Treatment may or may not require removal of the shunt and antibiotics, usually vancomycin with rifampicin, are best given intraventricularly. Occasionally, glomerulonephritis ('shunt nephritis') occurs in patients with colonized shunts; this results from the formation of immune complexes and their deposition on the basement membranes of the glomeruli.

Peritonitis associated with continuous ambulatory peritoneal dialysis (CAPD)

Coagulase-negative staphylococci, predominantly *S. epidermidis*, are the most common cause of peritonitis associated with CAPD; the organisms probably gain access to the peritoneum by manipulation of the catheter connections. Patients have abdominal pain, occasionally nausea, diarrhoea and fever, and abundant polymorphs in the dialysate, in which Gram-positive cocci can sometimes be detected on smear of a spun deposit. If seen they are usually intracellular and scanty. The antibiotic sensitivities of infecting strains vary, and as treatment must always be started before this information is available, vancomycin (preferably intraperitoneally) is the drug of choice. Five days' treatment is usually sufficient.

Endocarditis (see also Chapter 15.17)

Coagulase-negative staphylococci can infect native or prosthetic heart valves and these infections can be acquired in hospital or in the community. Nosocomial native valve infections with coagulase-negative staphylococci (usually *S. epidermidis*) generally result from infected intravascular devices; the affected valve may or may not have been previously abnormal. Nosocomial prosthetic valve endocarditis can be acquired in the theatre (or shortly thereafter) at the time of the original valve replacement and presents within weeks or more often months of surgery ('early onset'). In many series, coagulase-negative staphylococci are the most common cause of early-onset prosthetic valve endocarditis. As with native valves, prosthetic infection can also be acquired from an infected intravascular device; such infections can occur many years after the original valve replacement. Nosocomial staphylococci tend to be multiply resistant.

Community-acquired endocarditis, which may involve native (usually) or prosthetic valves, is increasingly recognized. Most patients with native valve infection have a pre-existing cardiac abnormality. The organisms must come from the patient's skin but predisposing skin lesions are seldom detected. The infection often mimics *S. aureus* endocarditis, with rapidly destructive valvular disease, neurological manifestations, and concomitant vertebral osteomyelitis. The most common pathogen is *S. epidermidis*, but there are increasing reports of other species, particularly *S. lugdunensis* (which seems to be especially virulent), *S. simulans*, and *S. warneri*. These community-acquired strains are frequently penicillin sensitive.

Urinary tract infection

Coagulase-negative staphylococci are urinary pathogens both in the community and in hospital, but different species are involved in these two groups of patients. In the community, the curiously named *S. saprophyticus* is an important urinary pathogen in young, sexually active women, second only to *E. coli*. *S. saprophyticus* is a skin commensal but it is not normally found colonizing the urethra, although it has been isolated from the rectal flora of adult women. It commonly produces cystitis, but may cause upper urinary-tract infection and has also been isolated from infected calculi, and in this context, the ability of many strains of *S. saprophyticus* to split urea rapidly may be significant. Most strains are readily recognized in the laboratory by their resistance to novobiocin. They are sensitive to a wide range of antibiotics and their treatment seldom poses a problem. A small proportion of nosocomial urinary-tract infections are also caused by coagulase-negative staphylococci, predominantly *S. epidermidis*. These infections, which mostly arise after urological surgery, are seldom accompanied by pyuria, and may clear spontaneously on removal of the catheter. Sometimes they are of clinical significance and require treatment, and occasionally they cause bacteraemia, generally the result of instrumentation or catheterization. In contrast with *S. saprophyticus*, nosocomial urinary isolates of coagulase-negative staphylococci are often multiply resistant and antibiotic treatment will be dictated by sensitivity.

Other infections

Coagulase-negative staphylococci are increasingly isolated from the blood of neonates and immunocompromised, neutropenic patients. Distinguishing true bacteraemia from contamination in such groups of patients can be difficult. There is no doubt that, in many cases, bacteraemia is related to the presence of an intravascular catheter. In very low birth-weight neonates, an association between lipid administration and coagulase-negative staphylococcal bacteraemia has been demonstrated. In this population also, colonization of the respiratory tract (generally detected by culture of endotracheal tubes) occurs, and genuine respiratory infection with the organism can arise. In neutropenic patients, especially those who have received broad-spectrum combination therapy with β-lactams and aminoglycosides, sentinel throat and rectal swabs frequently grow coagulase-negative staphylococci, presumably indicative of gastrointestinal colonization with these organisms, and this may well predispose to bacteraemia.

Infection of prosthetic joints and vascular prostheses is sometimes caused by coagulase-negative staphylococci. These organisms, usually multiresistant, are introduced at the time of the surgery, although the clinical signs of infection may not become evident for weeks or months afterwards. Attempts to treat such infections with antibiotics generally fail and removal of the prosthesis is required.

Coagulase-negative staphylococci are the most common cause of postoperative endophthalmitis after cataract and other intraocular surgery. The organisms can be cultured from vitreous washings. Treatment usually involves vitrectomy and intravitreal antibiotics. As with so many nosocomial infections caused by coagulase-negative staphylococci, isolates may be multiply resistant and neither pathogen nor sensitivities are known at the time the intravitreal antibiotics must be given. Hence a combination of vancomycin and gentamicin is recommended; systemic antibiotics are not indicated.

Laboratory diagnosis

It will be clear from much of the foregoing that the laboratory diagnosis of much infection with coagulase-negative staphylococci poses considerably greater difficulties than the diagnosis of *S. aureus* infection. Clinicians should enlist the assistance of a competent microbiologist when assessing culture results of specimens, especially blood cultures, reported to be growing coagulase-negative staphylococci. A further problem with these organisms is the use of broth-enrichment cultures for specimens such as excised tissue; it should be remembered that a single contaminating staphylococcus will multiply in liquid media, thereby misleading unwary clinicians.

Treatment

An integral part of the successful treatment of infections with coagulase-negative staphylococci is a critical clinical assessment of the need for removal of any prosthetic material with which so many infections are associated. That said, most patients will be treated with antibiotics whether the material is removed or not, and often before sensitivity results are available. So many nosocomial infections are caused by resistant strains that the only reliable initial (and often also definitive) therapy is vancomycin or teicoplanin, and there has been a marked increase in the use of these agents over the past decade. The length of treatment in most instances is somewhat arbitrary and the same principles apply to infections with these organisms as to those with *S. aureus*. In contrast, community-acquired infections, usually endocarditis, can often be treated with β-lactam antibiotics, often by penicillin. As with serious *S. aureus* infections, combination therapy is used without evidence of superiority over a single agent.

REFERENCES

Archer, G.L. (1990). Staphylococcus epidermidis and other coagulase-negative staphylococci. In *Principles and practice of infectious diseases* (ed. G.L. Mandell, R.G. Douglas, and J.E. Bennett), pp.1511–18.

Chesney, P.J., Bergdoll, M.S., Davis, J.P., and Vergeront, J.M. (1984). The disease spectrum, epidemiology, and etiology of toxic-shock syndrome. *Annual Review of Microbiology*, **38,** 315–38.

Easmon, C.S.F. and Goodfellow, M. (1990). Staphylococcus and Micrococcus. In *Topley and Wilson's principles of bacteriology, virology and immunity*, Vol. 2, *Systemic bacteriology* (ed. M.T. Parker and B.I. Duerden), pp. 161–86. Edward Arnold, London.

Espersen, F., Fromodt-Moller, N., Rosdahl, V.T., Skinhoj, P., and Bentzon, M.W. (1991). Changing pattern of bone and joint infections due to *Staphylococcus aureus*: study of cases of bacteraemia in Denmark, 1959–1988. *Reviews of Infectious Diseases*, **13,** 347–58.

Etienne, J. and Eykyn, S.J. (1990). Increase in native valve endocarditis caused by coagulase negative staphylococci: an Anglo-French clinical and microbiological study. *British Heart Journal*, **64,** 381–4.

Eykyn, S.J. (1988). Staphylococcal sepsis. The changing pattern of disease and therapy. *Lancet*, **i,** 100–4.

Freney, J. *et al.* (1988). *Staphylococcus lugdunensis* sp. nov. and *Staphylococcus schleiferi* sp. nov., two species from human clinical specimens. *International Journal of Systematic Bacteriology*, **38,** 168–72.

Gemmell, C.G. (ed.) (1986). Coagulase-negative staphylococci. *Journal of Medical Microbiology*, **22,** 285–95.

Kloos, W.E. and Schleifer, K.H. (1975). Isolation and characterisation of staphylococci from human skin. II. Descriptions of four new species: *Staphylococcus warneri, Staphylococcus capitis, Staphylococcus hominis*, and *Staphylococcus simulans*. *International Journal of Systematic Bacteriology*, **25,** 62–79.

Marples, R.R. and Reith, S. (1992). Methicillin-resistant *Staphylococcus aureus* in England and Wales. *Communicable Disease Report*, **3,** R25–9.

Marples, R.R. and Wieneke, A.A. (1991). Toxic shock syndrome in the U.K: 1985–1990. *Communicable Disease Report*, **7,** R91–2.

Macdonald, A. and Smith, G. (ed.) (1981). The staphylococci. In *Proceedings of the Alexander Ogston centennial conference*, Aberdeen University Press.

Pfaller, M.A. and Herwald, L.A. (1988). Laboratory, clinical, and epidemiological aspects of coagulase-negative staphylococci. *Clinical Microbiology Reviews*, **1,** 281–99.

Schleifer, K.H. and Kloos, W.E. (1975). Isolation and characterisation of staphylococci from human skin. I. Amended descriptions of *Staphylococcus epidermidis* and *Staphylococcus saprophyticus* and descriptions of three new species: *Staphylococcus cohnii, Staphylococcus haemolyticus*, and *Staphylococcus xylosus*, *International Journal of Systematic Bacteriology*, **25,** 50–61.

Scully, R.E., Mark, E.J., McNeeley, W.F., and McNeeley, B.U. (1989). Weekly clinicopathological exercises. *New England Journal of Medicine*, **321,** 813–23.

Sheagren, J.N. (1984). *Staphylococcus aureus*. The persistent pathogen. *New England Journal of Medicine*, **310,** 1368–73; 1437–42.

Vandenesch, F., Etienne, J., Reverdy, M.E., and Eykipe, S.J. (1993). Endocarditis due to *Staplylococcus lugdunensis:* report of 11 cases and review. *Clinical Infectious Diseases*, **17,** 871–6.

Waldvogel, F.A. (1990). *Staphylococcus aureus* (including toxic shock syndrome). In *Principles and practice of infectious diseases* (ed. G.L. Mandell, R.G. Douglas and J.E. Bennett), pp.1489–510. Churchill Livingstone, New York.

7.11.5 Meningococcal infection

B. M. Greenwood

Meningococcal disease is caused by infection with a Gram-negative diplococcus, *Neisseria meningitidis*, first identified by Weichselbaum in 1887. It is likely that epidemic meningococcal disease is a relatively new condition. Outbreaks were first recorded in Geneva in 1805 and in New England the following year. Because of the characteristic features of meningococcal disease it seems unlikely that epidemics would have remained unreported had they occurred at an earlier time. Meningococcal disease was reported for the first time in north Africa in 1840 and in subSaharan Africa during the first years of the twentieth century.

The organism

Meningococci usually appear in clinical samples as bean-shaped, Gram-negative diplococci. They are delicate organisms that are sensitive to chilling or drying; therefore samples must be inoculated and cultured as soon as possible after collection. Transport media, such as Stuart's, can be used when this is not possible. Meningococci grow best on enriched media such as Mueller–Hinton, incubated at 37 °C in an atmosphere containing 5 to 10 per cent CO_2. Selective media containing antibiotics such as vancomycin and polymyxin are useful in identifying meningococci at sites with a mixed flora, such as the nasopharynx. Alternatively, swabs can be inoculated directly on to plates containing specific antisera, which results in halo formation around colonies bearing the relevant antigen.

Table 1 *Systems used for the typing of meningococci and for the characterization of individual strains*

Capsular polysaccharide	Eight main capsular types
Outer-membrane proteins	Class based on type 2 or 3 protein; subclass based on type 1 or 5 protein
Lipopolysaccharide	Different types recognized by electrophoresis or immunotyping using monoclonal antibodies
Isoenzyme characterization	Isoenzyme pattern of a panel of several enzymes
Drug sensitivity pattern	Suphonamide sensitivity or resistance
DNA fingerprinting	DNA pattern seen on restriction enzyme digestion.

Meningococci possess an outer polysaccharide capsule, an outer membrane, a cytoplasmic membrane, and an underlying peptidoglycan layer. Some avirulent strains do not have a capsule. Fine pili extend from the outer membrane through the capsule to the outside. On electron microscopy, blebs can be seen in the cell wall, which contain endotoxin.

Structural differences in capsular polysaccharide define eight main serogroups: A, B, C, X, Y, Z, W135, and 29e (Table 1). The composition of each polysaccharide has been defined. The group B polysaccharide, a polymer of *N*-acetyl neuraminic acid, is very similar to that of *Escherichia coli* type K1, an important cause of neonatal meningitis, and shows cross-reactivity with some brain antigens. This latter characteristic may account for its poor immunogenicity.

The outer membrane proteins of the meningococcus can be differentiated by polyacrylamide gel into five main groups. All meningococci have either a class 2 or class 3 principal outer-membrane protein and class 1 and class 5 proteins are found in most strains. Class 5 proteins are variably expressed and a single strain may express one, two, or no class 5 proteins. Lipopolysaccharides present in the cell wall also show considerable structural heterogeneity between strains.

The antigenic variability of various structural components of the meningococcus has been used to develop a number of typing systems. The system currently used most widely is based upon the antigenic characteristics of (a) the capsular polysaccharide, (b) the class 2/3 outer-membrane protein, (c) the class 1 outer-membrane protein, and (d) the organism's sensitivity to sulphonamides. Thus the designation B:2a:P1.1:R indicates a strain with a group B capsular polysaccharide, a type 2a class 2 protein, and a type 1 class 1 protein; and which is resistant to sulphonamides. The development of highly specific monoclonal antibodies has proved of great help in outer-membrane protein typing. Meningococci can also be typed on the basis of the antigenic characteristics of their lipopolysaccharides. Two other systems have been used for characterizing individual strains of meningococci—isoenzyme typing and study of the patterns of DNA produced on digestion with restriction enzymes. Restriction fragments can either be visualized by direct staining or characterized with a DNA probe. Development of a typing system based on DNA patterns is difficult because of the complexity of the patterns produced, but this technique is a good way of demonstrating close similarity between a limited number of isolates (Fig. 1).

Detailed characterization of individual isolates of meningococci has proved useful in two ways. Firstly, it has been possible to show that certain characteristics are associated with virulence. For example, group A meningococci are more likely to produce epidemics than meningococci belonging to other capsular polysaccharide groups and group B subgroup 4:P1.15:R tend to cause invasive disease in teenagers and young adults rather than in children. Secondly, by using combinations of typing techniques, for example isoenzyme characterization and outer-membrane protein typing, it has been possible to identify 'clones' of meningococci responsible for individual outbreaks or epidemics and to study the relation between epidemics. In this way it has been possible to map out the relations between many of the major group A epidemics recorded during the past 30 years and to follow the course of individual epidemics (Fig. 2).

Meningococci are sensitive to most antibiotics. Until 1963, nearly all strains were highly sensitive to sulphonamides, which were very effective in treatment. Sulphonamide resistance is now widespread among bacteria belonging to all the major subgroups. However, in recent years, there has been a decline in the level of sulphonamide resistance in some industrialized countries, perhaps as a consequence of an overall decrease in the use of these drugs. Recently, there have been reports from Southern Africa and from various countries in Europe, particularly Spain, of the emergence of meningococci with a reduced sensitivity to penicillin (mean inhibitory concentration (**MIC**) in the range of 0.1 to 1.0 mg/l). Insensitivity is associated with reduced binding to penicillin.

Fig. 1 DNA fingerprinting of six meningococci showing different staining patterns. Meningococci in lanes 5 and 6 are closely related differing in only one band (by courtesy of Professor B. Bjorvatn).

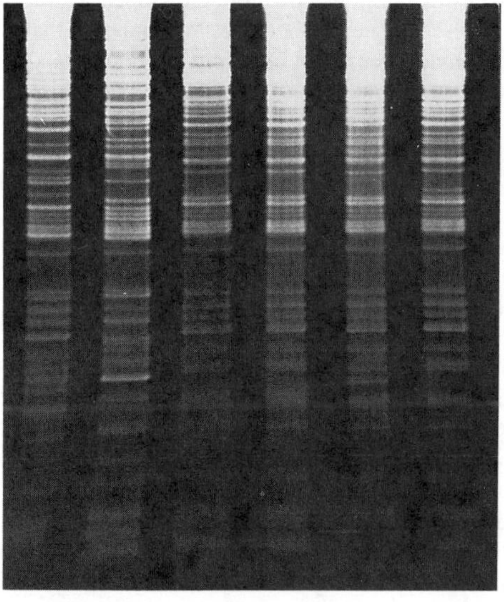

Fig. 2 The spread of the group A meningococcus clone III-I as indicated by molecular epidemiological techniques. From Saudi Arabia the clone was carried to many other countries by pilgrims returning from Mecca. (Reproduced from Achtman (1990) *Reviews of Medical Microbiology*, **1**, 29, with permission.)

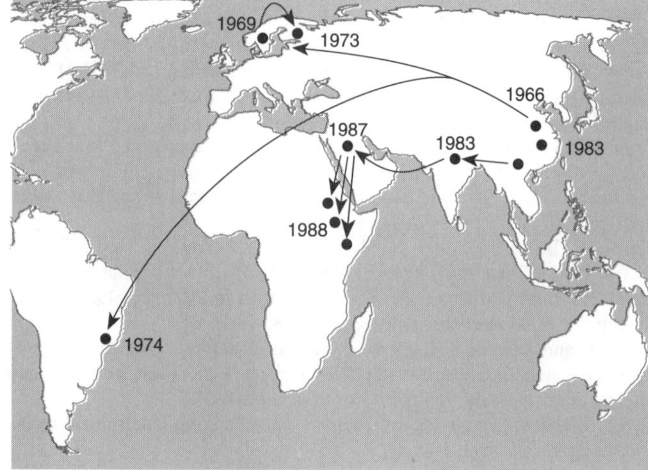

Resistance due to β-lactamase production has been reported in South Africa but is very rare. Penicillin-insensitive isolates are still uncommon in most communities but the emergence of penicillin resistance in the meningococcus is a worrying development.

Epidemiology

Geographical distribution

Meningococcal disease occurs throughout the world, from the Arctic to the edge of the Sahara. In areas with a temperate climate the infection is usually endemic, with an attack rate of around 2 cases/100 000 population per year. However, the collection of national statistics disguises the fact that, even in countries where the infection is endemic, there may be localized areas with a relatively high attack rate. Since the end of the Second World War there have been few large epidemics of meningococcal disease in Europe or North America, but in many industrialized countries there have been periods of several years when the incidence of meningococcal disease has increased substantially over background levels. This phenomenon is well illustrated by data from Norway that show a high incidence of group B disease extending over a period of nearly 20 years. In industrialized societies, most meningococcal disease is caused by bacteria belonging to serogroups B or C, although occasional outbreaks of group A disease occur, as has happened recently in New Zealand.

The main health hazard posed by the meningococcus lies in a belt of subSaharan Africa extending from Ethiopia in the East to The Gambia in the West—the African 'meningitis belt'. Within this area of savannah Africa, important epidemics of meningococcal disease occur every 5 to 10 years. Up to 100 000 people have been affected during individual epidemics and the meningococcus is still responsible for many deaths in this region. Why this geographical area should be so prone to epidemics of meningococcal disease is not known. Within the African 'meningitis belt', epidemics nearly always start in the middle of the dry season, when it is hot and very dry, and end a few months later with the coming of the rains (Fig. 3). Epidemics do not extend into the forest regions of West and Central Africa where conditions of very low absolute humidity are never met, but they may extend occasionally into countries at the eastern end of the belt such as Kenya and Tanzania. The factors responsible for setting off a large epidemic of meningococcal disease are not understood. From the public health point of view it would be very helpful if epidemics could be predicted. No certain way of doing this has yet been found, although recent studies in Burkina Faso suggest that an incidence of more than 15 cases/100 000 population per week over a period of 2 weeks indicates that a local epidemic is likely. Most African epidemics are caused by group A meningococci, although outbreaks of group C meningococcal disease have been reported.

Age

Where meningococcal infection is endemic, most cases of clinical disease are seen among the very young, although in recent years there has been an increase in the number of cases seen in teenagers and young adults in Norway, the United Kingdom, and in other parts of Europe associated with infection with serogroup B15:P1.16:R. When an epidemic occurs, older children and adults are affected more frequently than during periods of endemic infection. In the African 'meningitis belt' the disease is seen most often in children aged 5 to 15 years. In this region, children under the age of 1 year are infected infrequently.

Sex

Susceptibility to meningococcal disease is similar in males and females.

Nasopharyngeal carriers

Most subjects infected with meningococci become asymptomatic nasopharyngeal carriers. The ratio of carriers to cases varies from figures as high as 10 000:1 in situations of endemic transmission to values as low

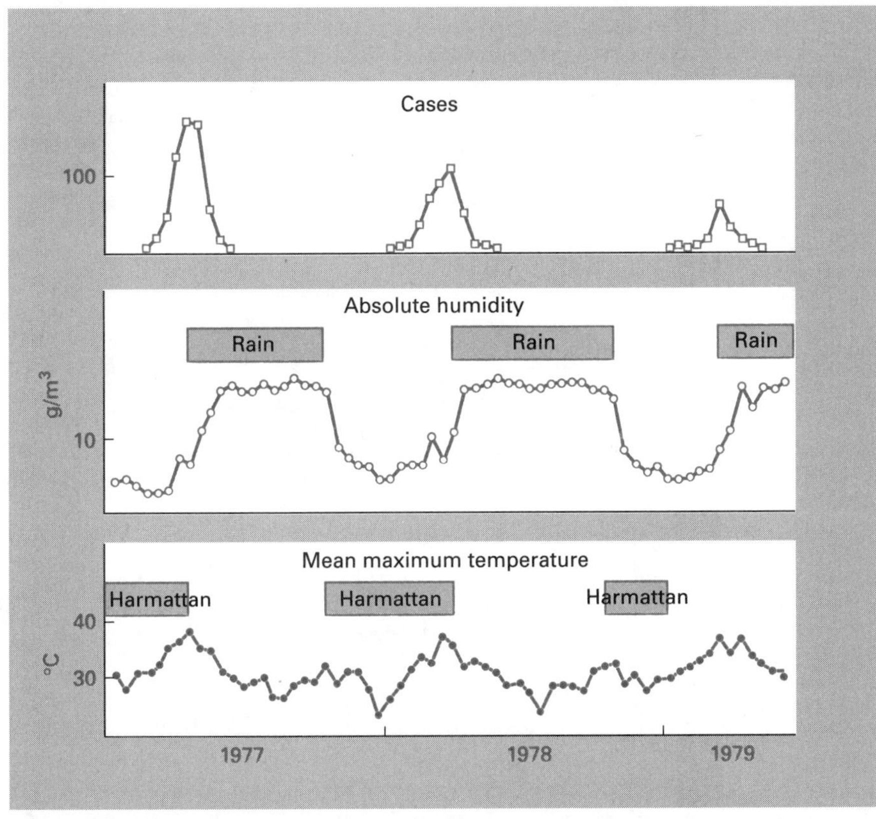

Fig. 3 The seasonality of meningococcal disease in subSaharan Africa. The harmattan is a hot, dusty wind that blows from the Sahara. (Reproduced from Greenwood *et al.* (1984). *Lancet*, **i**, 1339, with permission.)

Table 2 *Risk factors predisposing to the development of meningococcal disease*

Socioeconomic	Poor living conditions—attack rates are highest in deprived sections of a community Overcrowding—outbreaks are frequent in military camps, doss houses, and hostels
Household contact	Subjects in close contact with a case are at risk, especially during epidemics; the risk may be as high as 1 : 20 for siblings of a patient
Damage to respiratory mucosa	Adverse environmental conditions—low absolute humidity may be important in Africa (dry season) and in Europe (winter) Antecedent viral infections—several studies suggest that preceding influenza is a risk factor for meningococcal disease Smoking—both active and passive smoking have been implicated as risk factors in separate studies
Immunological	Deficient levels of IgG or IgM bactericidal antibodies High levels of blocking IgA antibody Hereditary or acquired complement deficiencies, especially late components ABO non-secretor status

Note: So far no evidence has been found that HIV infection predisposes to invasive meningococcal disease.

as 100:1 during epidemics. On the basis of early surveys, it was suggested that outbreaks were likely to occur only when the carrier rate exceeded a certain level. It is now recognized that this relation does not necessarily apply and that epidemics may occur when the carrier rate in the general population is low. Conversely, clinical cases of disease may be rare in populations with a high carriage rate of a potentially pathogenic strain. As an epidemic progresses, the carrier rate of the epidemic strain usually increases.

Risk factors for meningococcal disease

Whether exposure to a meningococcus results in clinical disease or asymptomatic carriage is influenced by a number of factors. Some of the most important are indicated in Table 2. Environmental factors such as adverse climatic conditions or a preceding viral infection, which damage the local defences (Fig. 4), are likely to be very important in determining whether an infection results in asymptomatic carriage or systemic disease.

Pathology

The predominant pathological finding in patients who have died from acute meningococcaemia is vascular damage associated with thrombosis and haemorrhage. There may also be signs of an encephalitis. Haemorrhage into the adrenals is frequently found at autopsy (the Waterhouse–Friderichsen syndrome) and this lesion has been associated with the pathogenesis of meningococcal shock. However, adrenal haemorrhage is probably an unusual cause of this complication as most patients with acute meningococcaemia have elevated plasma cortisol levels and respond normally to stimulation with adrenocorticotrophin.

The meninges of patients with meningococcal meningitis show classical acute inflammatory changes, with oedema, vascular dilatation, fibrin deposition and infiltration with polymorphoneutrophil leucocytes. A vasculitis may be present.

Pathogenesis and immunity

Spread of infection

Meningococci are usually spread by respiratory droplets; occasionally sexual transmission occurs. Most infections are acquired from carriers, who are far more numerous than cases. Asymptomatic carriers may harbour meningococci for many months. In the United States, infection is often introduced into a new household by an asymptomatic carrier father. In Africa, spread from child to child is more important.

To become established in the nasopharynx, meningococci must be able to adhere to nasopharyngeal cells. Pili probably play an important part in adhesion, for encapsulated meningococci with pili adhere strongly to epithelial cells whilst non-piliated encapsulated strains do not. Studies with organ cultures of tonsils have shown that meningococci pass through the mucus barriers, adhere to non-ciliated columnar cells of the nasopharynx, and then pass through these cells by endocytosis to reach the subepithelial tissues (Fig. 5). In contrast, *Haemophilus influenzae* type b usually passes between the epithelial cells. It is likely that in

Fig. 4 The relation between consultations with general practitioners for influenza (per 100 000 population) and the isolation rate for meningococci among samples submitted to a reference laboratory. (Reproduced from Cartwright *et al.* (1991). *Lancet*, **338,** 354, with permission.)

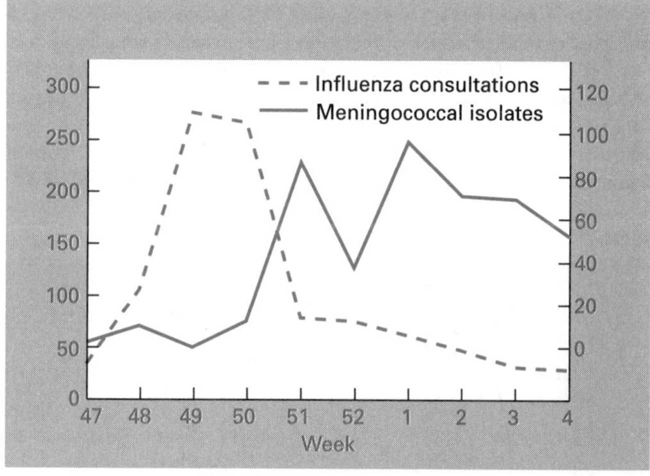

Fig. 5 The pathway by which meningococci reach the circulation (adapted from Stephens and Farley, (1991). *Reviews of Infectious Diseases*, **13,** 22).

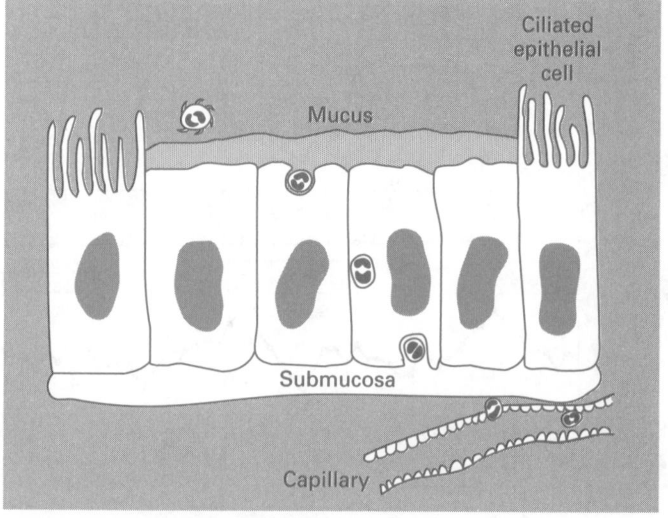

many instances in which bacteria reach the circulation, they are destroyed rapidly by antibody and phagocytic cells before they cause any tissue damage. However, in a few unfortunate individuals, bacteraemia results in the clinical syndrome of acute meningococcaemia. In other subjects, meningococci are cleared from the circulation but lodge in tissues such as the meninges, where they produce local damage. Why some patients develop acute meningococcaemia whilst others develop meningitis is not understood.

Pathogenesis of acute meningoccaemia

Experimental studies have demonstrated clearly the importance of endotoxin released by meningococci in the pathogenesis of the clinical features of acute meningococcaemia, and, in man, prognosis is related to endotoxin levels at the time of presentation as measured by the Limulus lysate assay. The effects of endotoxin are particularly marked on vascular endothelium, leading to an increase in permeability, vaculitis and thrombosis. Endotoxin also activates complement via the alternative pathway with the production of large amounts of C3a and C5a, which probably contribute to the pathophysiological changes seen in acute meningococcaemia. Endotoxin is also a powerful stimulator of the production by monocytes and macrophages of cytokines including interleukin (**IL**)1, IL-6, and tumour necrosis factor. When given to humans, tumour necrosis factor produces many of the symptoms observed in patients with acute meningococcaemia, such a fever, hypotension, thrombocytopenia, clotting abnormalities, and changes in acute-phase proteins. Thus, it seems likely that tumour necrosis factor plays a central part in the pathogenesis of the clinical features of acute meningococcaemia. This view is supported by the results of clinical studies that have shown raised plasma levels of tumour necrosis factor in patients with acute meningococcaemia and a correlation between levels of the factor and prognosis. Tumour necrosis factor induces endothelial cells to secrete nitric oxide, which is a powerful vasodilator, and this may play an important part in producing meningococcal shock. Induced nitric oxide may also contribute to the impaired function of the central nervous system seen frequently in patients with acute meningococcaemia.

Pathogenesis of meningitis

Elevated levels of IL-1, IL-6, and tumour necrosis factor have been demonstrated in the cerebrospinal fluid of patients with meningococcal meningitis and production of these cytokines locally within the central nervous system probably plays an important part in inducing the acute inflammatory reaction that is a characteristic feature of the disease. Enhanced production of tumour necrosis factor occurs before that of IL-1 and IL-6

Pathogenesis of the late complications of meningococcal disease

A proportion of patients with acute meningococcal infections develop arthritis, cutaneous vasculitis, episcleritis, or pericarditis several days after the onset of their illness, at a time when other features of their infection are improving. Skin or synovial biopsies show a vasculitis with inflammatory cells clustered around a damaged, and sometimes occluded, small vessel. Such lesions are sterile and are probably produced by immune complexes. Late complications are seen most frequently in adult patients who are serum meningococcal antigen-positive. They appear at the time when antigen disappears from the circulation and at the time when free antibody can first be detected (Fig. 6); their appearance is associated with a transient fall in serum C3. Deposits of meningococcal polysaccharide antigen, immunoglobulin, and complement can be shown by immunofluorescence around damaged cutaneous vessels and in leucocytes of synovial fluid obtained from inflamed joints. These findings suggest that immune complexes are formed locally at sites, such as the skin and synovium, where antigen is trapped during the bacteraemic phase of the infection.

Local immunity

Little is known about surface immunity to meningococci. It would be anticipated that locally produced secretory IgA antibodies would have a protective role, perhaps by preventing bacterial adherence to epithelial cells, but this has not been proven. Meningococci produce a protease enzyme that splits IgA subclass 1 molecules, destroying many of their antibody properties. Strains isolated from both patients and carriers produce this enzyme, but it is not produced by harmless Neisseria. IgA1 proteases isolated from different strains show considerable heterogeneity at both the protein and gene levels. Cleavage of IgA1 is achieved at one of two sites near the hinge region of the molecule. Isolates from epidemics have been found to give predominantly one cleavage pattern.

Damage to the surface defence mechanisms by an upper respiratory-tract virus infection or by low absolute humidity, causing abrasion of the nasal mucosa, may predispose to systemic meningococcal infection, but this is difficult to prove.

Systemic immunity

The importance of bactericidal antibodies in protection against meningococcal disease has been demonstrated clearly. Among American children of different ages, an inverse relation exists between susceptibility to meningococcal infection and the number of children with bactericidal antibodies (Fig. 7). Furthermore, a study of army recruits showed that

Fig. 6 Serological changes in 13 patients with meningococcal arthritis. (Reproduced from Greenwood *et al.* (1976). *British Medical Journal*, **1,** 797, with permission.)

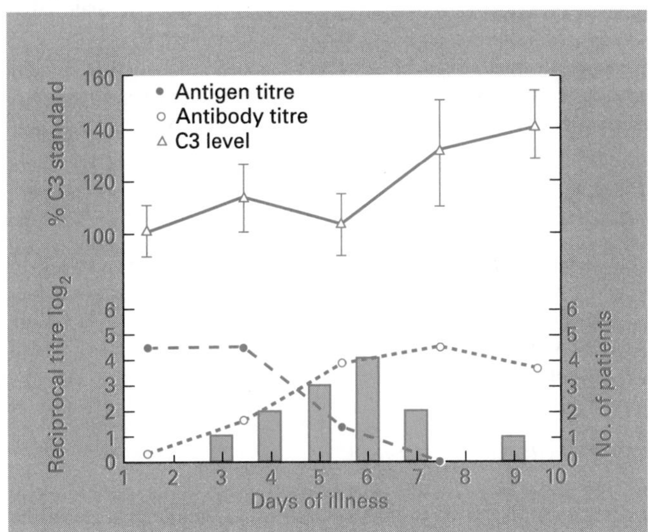

Fig. 7 The relation between the age at onset of meningococcal disease and the prevalence of group C meningococcal antibodies in American subjects of different ages. (Reproduced from Goldschneider *et al.* (1969). *Journal of Experimental Medicine* **129,** 1307, with permission.)

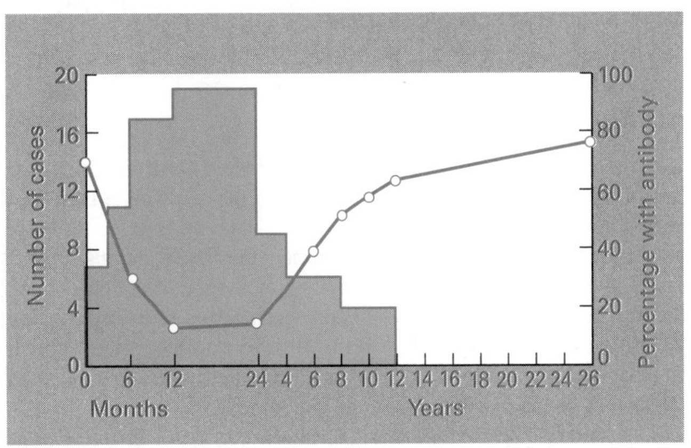

only 3 of 54 recruits who developed group C meningococcal meningitis had a significant titre of anti-group C bactericidal antibody when they entered camp whilst over 80 per cent of recruits who did not develop meningitis had bactericidal antibodies at this time. Why some soldiers had lower initial antibody levels than others was not established. Production of bactericidal antibodies can be induced by nasopharyngeal carriage of a potentially pathogenic meningococcus or by infection with a non-pathogenic organism, such as *N. lactamica*, which shares antigens with meningococci. Antibodies to both the capsular polysaccharide and the outer membrane proteins may be bactericidal.

Both IgG and IgM antibodies can kill meningococci but the action of such antibodies can be blocked by IgA antibodies, which compete for binding sites on the surface of the bacterium. Such blocking antibodies are found frequently in sera obtained from patients with meningococcal disease early in the course of their illness. IgA blocking antibodies, perhaps produced in response to infection with a cross-reactive organism, may be important in inducing susceptibility to systemic meningococcal disease.

Complement plays an important part in antibody-mediated killing of meningococci and patients with congenital or acquired complement deficiencies, especially those with deficiencies of late complement components, show an increased susceptibility to meningococcal disease. However, antibody can kill meningococci in the absence of complement by means of an antibody-dependent cytotoxicity system that involves K cells.

Patients with meningococcal disease develop cell-mediated immune responses to meningococcal components, but whether these reactions have any protective function is not known. Cellular proliferative responses to unrelated antigens are depressed in patients with acute meningococcal disease, as in many other acute infections. This loss of cell-mediated immunity, together with enhanced production of tumour necrosis factor, probably accounts for the activation of herpes simplex infections seen frequently in patients with the infection.

Clinical features

Meningococci can cause a variety of clinical syndromes, varying in severity from a mild sore throat to rapidly fatal acute meningococcaemia. It is convenient to consider these syndromes separately but some overlap may occur; for example, a patient may have features of both acute meningococcaemia and meningitis.

Nasopharyngeal infection

Most nasopharyngeal infections with meningococci are asymptomatic but some subjects develop a mild sore throat at the initial stage of the infection.

Acute meningococcaemia

The proportion of patients with meningococcal disease who develop acute meningococcaemia varies from place to place and from outbreak to outbreak, but it is usually less than 10 per cent.

SYMPTOMS

Acute meningococcaemia is one of the most feared of all infections for it can strike with frightening rapidity; a victim may be well at breakfast time but dead by the same afternoon. Thus, delay in making an early diagnosis and in starting appropriate treatment may be disastrous. Unfortunately, the early clinical features of acute meningococcaemia—fever, general malaise, and headache—are non–specific and indistinguishable from those of many other milder forms of infection. Diarrhoea, which may be severe enough to suggest acute gastroenteritis, is sometimes an early feature of the disease.

PHYSICAL SIGNS

Initial clinical examination may show no abnormalities apart from fever and tachycardia. However, careful examination may show small petechiae in the skin or in the conjunctivae. In dark-skinned subjects, petechiae are seen most readily in the conjunctivae and on the palatal mucosa (Fig. 8). Occasionally, an erythematous rather than a petechial rash is seen. Within hours of the onset of illness more extensive haemorrhagic lesions may appear in the skin and there may be bleeding from mucosae. The blood pressure is often normal initially, but then begins a remorseless fall. The central venous pressure is low and small vessels are usually constricted, giving cold extremities. There may be a gallop rhythm and some patients develop cardiac arrhythmias. The respiratory rate is usually increased. Patients with acute meningococcaemia are often drowsy and confused, and they may rapidly become comatose. Impairment of consciousness can occur in the absence of peripheral circulatory collapse.

LABORATORY FINDINGS

Laboratory investigations usually show a peripheral blood polymorphonuclear neutrophil leucocytosis but leucopenia is found occasionally in fulminating cases. Rarely, meningococci can be seen in peripheral blood leucocytes. There is usually thrombocytopenia and there may be other signs of disseminated intravascular coagulation, such as elevated serum fibrin degradation products and a low plasma fibrinogen. Blood culture is frequently positive and meningococcal polysaccharide antigen can often be detected in the serum. The cerebrospinal fluid is clear and contains a normal, or only slightly elevated, number of white cells. However, culture of cerebrospinal fluid may be positive and meningococcal polysaccharide antigen may be present, even in the absence of an active inflammatory response.

COURSE AND PROGNOSIS

Patients with acute meningococcaemia may die within a few hours of the onset of their illness from irreversible peripheral circulatory collapse,

Fig. 8 Petechiae in the conjunctiva of a patient with meningococcal disease (by courtesy of Professor D.A. Warrell).

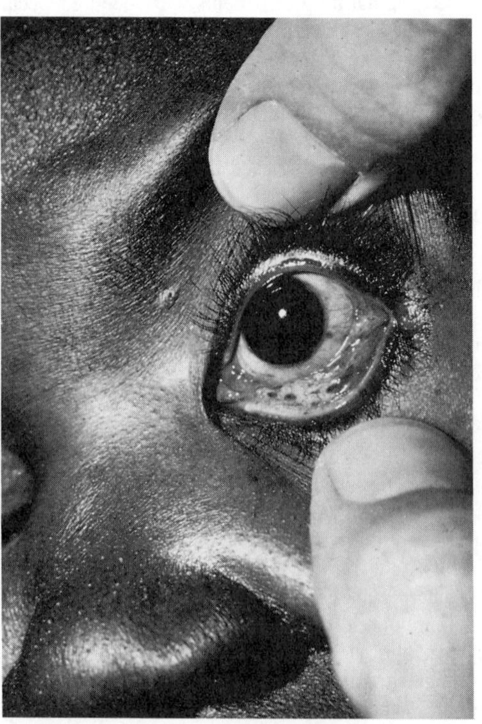

haemorrhage, cardiac arrhythmia, or a combination of all three. Patients with acute meningococcaemia who survive the first few hours of their illness sometimes remain unconscious. They may have convulsions and they may develop a variety of localizing neurological signs such as a hemiplegia. Surviving patients sometimes develop severe pulmonary oedema, which may be complicated by a secondary chest infection, and others develop acute renal failure. Ulceration may occur at the site of haemorrhage into the skin and gangrene of extremities has been recorded. Vascular damage may lead to bone infarction.

About 5 per cent of patients with acute meningococcaemia develop arthritis. This may be caused by direct bacterial invasion of a synovial joint during the initial phase of septicaemia; synovial fluid obtained from such patients contains meningococci. However, arthritis is seen most frequently about 6 days after the onset of illness at a time when other clinical features of the infection are improving, and then it is due to immune-complex formation. Its appearance is associated with a secondary rise in fever and its onset is sometimes accompanied by the appearance of cutaneous vasculitis, episcleritis, or pericarditis. The knee is the joint most frequently affected but any synovial joint or bursa may be affected. Joint signs resolve gradually over a period of days or weeks on symptomatic treatment; progression to a chronic arthritis has not been recorded. The skin lesions of patients with cutaneous vasculitis usually start as blisters; these may rupture to leave extensive superficial ulcers (Fig. 9). Pericarditis is usually asymptomatic, being detected on an electrocardiogram or chest radiograph, but a pericardial effusion can develop and occasionally causes tamponade.

The clinical description given above is one of a classical case of severe acute meningococcaemia. However, acute meningococcaemia may follow a much more benign course characterized by mild fever and petechiae only. Unsuspected meningococcaemia may be revealed only by a routine blood culture. In the African 'meningitis belt' such mild, and sometimes even asymptomatic, cases are seen most frequently at the end of an epidemic.

Death from acute meningococcaemia may occur within a few hours of the first appearance of symptoms or many days later from one of its complications. The overall mortality of acute meningococcaemia varies from outbreak to outbreak, dependent upon the relative proportion of fulminating and mild cases. However, mortality is always high when patients have peripheral circulatory collapse or impairment of consciousness at the time at which they are first seen. Several attempts have been made to develop prognostic scores that can indicate, at the time of presentation, which patients have a poor prognosis, as this information can be helpful in determining management—for example, a decision whether to evacuate a patient to a specialist centre. Use of prognostic scores also allows an assessment to be made of the comparability of different series of patients, for the proportion of cases with severe disease can vary from outbreak to outbreak.

Fig. 9 Cutaneous vasculitis as a complication of meningococcal disease.

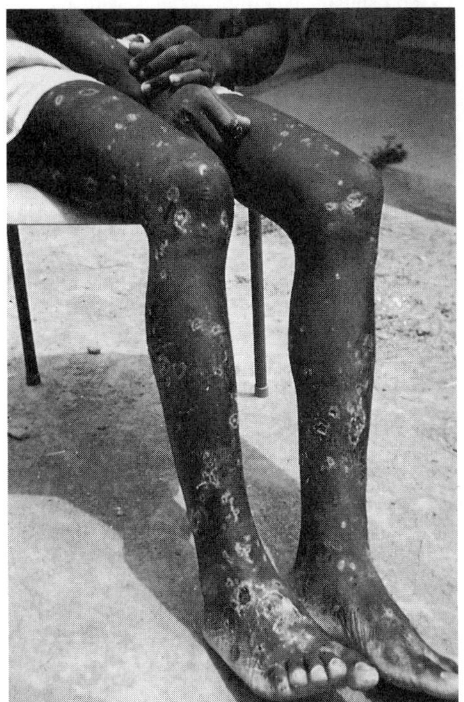

Meningitis

SYMPTOMS

The onset of meningococcal meningitis is generally more gradual than that of acute meningococcaemia. Headache, fever, and general malaise are the usual presenting symptoms. Headache is severe and is usually generalized. Patients may complain also of backache, photophobia, nausea, and vomiting. Convulsions may occur, especially in young children.

PHYSICAL SIGNS

On examination, the patient is found to be febrile and, in older children and in adults, there are usually obvious signs of meningeal irritation such as a stiff neck and a positive Kernig sign. Focal neurological signs may be present; VIth or IIIrd cranial-nerve palsies are the signs found most frequently but occasionally long-tract signs are detected. The presence of raised intracranial pressure may be indicated by bradycardia and hypertension; papilloedema is rarely seen in patients with acute meningococcal meningitis. Petechiae are present in the skin, conjunctivae, or in the palatal mucosa of up to one-half of patients with meningococcal meningitis, a valuable diagnostic sign. Cardiac enlargement, a gallop rhythm, and mild abnormalities on the electrocardiogram are sometimes present, indicating associated myocarditis, but heart failure is rare.

The characteristic clinical abnormalities may be absent in infants with meningococcal meningitis, in whom fever, convulsions, or feeding difficulties may be the only abnormal clinical features. In infants there may be bulging of the anterior fontanelle.

LABORATORY FINDINGS

Laboratory investigation of a patient with acute meningococcal meningitis usually shows a peripheral blood polymorphonuclear neutrophil leucocytosis and raised levels of acute-phase proteins such as C-reactive protein. In a few patients, blood culture is positive and, in about 10 per cent of patients, meningococcal polysaccharide antigen can be detected in the serum. On lumbar puncture a turbid cerebrospinal fluid is usually obtained. The white-cell count in cerebrospinal fluid is increased; nearly all the cells are polymorphonuclear neutrophil leucocytes. The protein is also increased and the sugar is usually low and less than the blood sugar level. Meningococci can often be seen within leucocytes and free within the cerebrospinal fluid, and a positive culture can usually be obtained. Meningococcal polysaccharide antigen can usually be detected in the fluid. Other changes in cerebrospinal fluid that have been described in patients with meningococcal meningitis include an increase in levels of immunoglobulins G and M, lactic acid dehydrogenase, and fibrin degradation products.

COURSE AND PROGNOSIS

Patients with meningococcal meningitis sometimes die suddenly during their first few hours in hospital. It is often difficult to pinpoint an exact cause of death in these patients; inhalation of vomit, coning, or a cardiac arrhythmia are possible causes. Death is rare in patients who survive their first 24 h in hospital. Most surveys have shown an overall mortality for treated meningococcal meningitis of between 5 and 10 percent.

Fortunately, most patients with meningococcal meningitis make an uneventful recovery. About 5 per cent of patients with meningococcal meningitis develop one or more of the allergic complications of meningococcal disease described above. Lesions of herpes simplex may appear during the course of recovery from meningococcal meningitis and are sometimes extensive.

Patients with meningococcal meningitis sometimes develop a secondary spike of fever after making an initial recovery. This may be due to formation of a local collection of pus such as a subdural empyema, to the development of an allergic complication, to the presence of an organism resistant to the antibiotic being used for treatment, to a mistake in the initial bacteriological diagnosis, to a drug reaction, or to a coincidental nosocomial infection. In such patients, a second lumbar puncture should be done and the cerebrospinal fluid obtained recultured. It is doubtful whether it is worthwhile repeating lumbar punctures to monitor the course of treatment in patients who are making an uncomplicated recovery.

The prognosis of patients who survive the initial phase of meningococcal meningitis is better than that for those with peneumococcal or *H. influenzae* meningitis and most make a complete recovery. Some are left with a neurological deficit, in particular deafness, but many of them continue to improve during the following weeks and months. The frequency with which permanent deafness is recorded after meningococcal meningitis varies from series to series and may be related both to the dominant strain of meningococcus and to the quality of treatment available. There is some suggestion that deafness follows a serogroup B infection less frequently than infections caused by other serotypes. In most series, figures for permanent deafness in one or both ears have been in the region of 5 per cent. It has been shown that meningitis is the most important overall cause of deafness in savanna Africa.

Chronic meningococcaemia

This is a rare condition characterized by persistent meningococcaemia. Episodes of fever, urticarial rashes, arthritis, and splenomegaly are the usual clinical features. The pathological basis of these lesions is a vasculitis and it is probable that immune complexes play an important part in the pathogenesis of this syndrome.

Other clinical syndromes

During an episode of meningococcaemia, bacteria may lodge in many tissues, producing an acute inflammatory reaction. Pyogenic arthritis, pericarditis, and panophthalmitis without associated meningitis may be produced in this way. Meningococci have been isolated from patients with urethritis, proctitis, or conjunctivitis. It is likely that in such patients the infection has been transmitted sexually. Meningococci can cause pneumonia. Cases of meningococcal pneumonia were detected first in American military personnel but the condition has now been described in civilians. Most cases of meningococcal pneumonia are caused by meningococci belonging to serogroup Y. Meningococcal pneumonia shows no characteristic clinical features.

Diagnosis

Acute meningococcaemia

Clinical diagnosis of acute meningococcaemia is usually impossible during the earliest stage of the infection, unless suspicion is heightened by the knowledge that the patient has been in close contact with a case of meningococcal disease. During an epidemic, any acute febrile illness must be regarded with suspicion. Meningococcaemia should enter into the differential diagnosis of all patients with fever and petechiae. Once florid haemorrhagic lesions have appeared and shock has intervened, acute meningococcaemia becomes a likely diagnosis. However, other Gram-negative bacteria, rickettsiae, and some viruses such as dengue can produce a similar clinical picture.

Diagnosis of acute meningococcaemia is confirmed by a positive blood culture or by the detection of meningococcal polysaccharide antigen in serum by countercurrent immunoelectrophoresis or other immunological techniques. Immunological assays, which allow a rapid diagnosis to be made, are positive in nearly all patients with severe acute meningococcaemia but may be negative in patients with the mild form of the syndrome. Meningococci can also be isolated frequently from needle aspirates or biopsies of skin lesions.

Meningitis

A clinical diagnosis of acute meningitis is usually made readily in adults and older children on the basis of the characteristic history and abnormal physical signs. Differentiation of acute meningitis from meningism may sometimes be impossible on clinical grounds alone. Signs of meningeal irritation are often absent in infants with acute meningitis. Thus, a possible diagnosis of acute meningitis must be considered in all irritable, febrile infants, especially in those with convulsions. Clinical examination may provide some clue as to the causative organism. Detection of petechiae favours a diagnosis of meningococcal meningitis, whilst detection of an associated middle-ear infection or pneumonia favours a diagnosis of pneumococcal meningitis.

Confirmation of a clinical diagnosis of acute meningitis requires lumbar puncture. Opinion is divided as to whether all infants with febrile convulsions should be lumbar punctured or not; it is wiser to err on the side of doing too many lumbar punctures rather than too few. Lumbar puncture of a patient with meningococcal meningitis, as described above, usually reveals a turbid cerebrospinal fluid under increased pressure. Occasionally the fluid is clear, for approximately 0.2×10^9 cells/l must be present before it appears turbid to the naked eye. Therefore, a cell count in cerebrospinal fluid must be made before a diagnosis of meningitis can be excluded. Nearly all the white cells present in an initial sample of fluid obtained from a patient with meningococcal meningitis are polymorphonuclear neutrophil leucoctyes, thus differentiating the infection from viral meningitis in which lymphocytes predominate. Lymphocytes may be found in the cerebrospinal fluid of patients with meningococcal meningitis after the start of treatment but there is rarely any difficulty in differentiating partially treated bacterial meningitis from viral meningitis. Cerebrospinal fluid from patients with meningococcal meningitis has a high protein and a low sugar content, findings characteristic of all forms of bacterial meningitis.

Meningococci can be demonstrated in the cerebrospinal fluid by Gram stain or culture in up to 80 per cent of patients investigated before the start of treatment. However, culture is often negative in patients who have received antibiotics. In some patients in whom culture is negative, bacterial products can still be demonstrated in cerebrospinal fluid. Endotoxin can be detected in the cerebrospinal fluid of nearly all patients with meningococcal meningitis by the sensitive Limulus assay, but this test cannot differentiate between meningitis caused by the meningococcus and meningitis caused by other types of Gram-negative bacteria such as *H. influenzae* and *E. coli*, which require different treatment. Detection of meningococcal capsular polysaccharide antigen in the cerebrospinal fluid by immunological methods is highly specific. Using simple immunological assays such as latex or staphylococcal coagglutination tests, the sensitivity of antigen detection is comparable to that of culture for group A and group C infections. Immunological tests are less sensitive at detecting group B infections because of the difficulty in producing highly active group B antisera. Slightly higher positivity rates are obtained when more sensitive techniques such as radioimmunoassay and enzyme-linked immunosorbent assays are used, and when serum and urine are examined as well as cerebrospinal fluid. Recently, a sensitive polymerase chain-reaction assay has been developed for the diagnosis of meningococcal infections that uses two oligonucleotides flanking the dihydropteroate synthetase gene as primers.

Collection of a nasopharyngeal swab is a useful investigation in patients with suspected meningococcal meningitis or meningococcaemia. This may yield a meningococcus, even in partially treated patients, which may have been the cause of the patient's illness.

Other syndromes

The presence of meningococci in the nasopharynx is established by culture of a nasopharyngeal swab. Isolation of meningococci is facilitated by use of a selective medium containing antibiotics, such as Thayer–Martin medium, which inhibits normal nasopharyngeal commensals. A diagnosis of chronic meningococcaemia is established by blood culture. Meningococci may be isolated from pus obtained from various metastatic sites. Meningococcal pneumonia is diagnosed by blood culture or by isolation of meningococci from a lung or transtracheal aspirate.

Treatment

Acute meningococcaemia

ANTIBIOTICS

Penicillin remains the antibiotic of choice for the treatment of acute meningococcaemia. Given in high doses by a parenteral route, for example 4 mega units of crystalline penicillin 6-hourly by intravenous injection in adults, it is effective even in infections caused by meningococci which are relatively insensitive to penicillin. Chloramphenicol is an alternative treatment for patients who are known to be sensitive to penicillin or who are at risk of infection with a penicillin-insensitive strain, as most such strains are sensitive to this antibiotic. Because other bacteria that may not respond well to penicillin can cause clinical syndromes identical to acute meningococcaemia, a case can be made for starting treatment initially with a broader-spectrum antibiotic such as a third-generation cephalosporin.

Because of the speed with which meningococcal infections can progress an injection of penicillin should be given immediately a diagnosis of acute meningococcaemia is seriously entertained, even before referral of a patient to hospital and there is some evidence, although this is not conclusive, that this approach can save lives. Antibiotics should be given for 7 days. There is a theoretical risk that administration of penicillin in high dosage could initially worsen the patient's clinical state, as a result of massive destruction of bacteria and the consequent release of endotoxin, but such a Herxheimer reaction has never been clearly demonstrated in patients with this infection.

SUPPORTIVE

A wide variety of supportive measures has been tried in patients with fulminating acute meningococcaemia but none has been particularly successful. Whenever possible, patients with acute meningococcaemia should be nursed in an intensive-care unit. Fluid balance, acid–base status, central venous pressure, and the electrocardiogram should be monitored carefully. Assisted ventilation may be required.

Most such patients have a reduced circulatory volume and require infusion with a plasma expander such as plasma or dextran to maintain their circulation. The central venous pressure should be maintained at between 10 and 15 mmHg if possible. A careful watch must be kept for the development of pulmonary oedema; if pulmonary crepitations appear an intravenous diuretic, such as frusemide, should be given. If the blood pressure cannot be maintained by colloid infusion, it can be increased transitorily by administration of a sympathomimetic amine such as noradrenaline, but giving such a drug increases peripheral vascular constriction and may enhance peripheral tissue damage. A better approach is to use an inotropic agent, such as an infusion of dopamine, which increases tissue perfusion and reduces the afterload on the heart. If a vasodilator is used, then further colloid infusion may be required to maintain the circulation.

The value of corticosteroids in the management of shocked patients with acute meningococcaemia has never been established by a controlled trial. A few patients have adrenocortical insufficiency, which requires replacement therapy. In experimental animals, massive doses of corticosteroids protect against endotoxin-mediated shock by stabilizing platelets, polymorphonuclear neutrophil leucocytes, lysosymes, and endothelial cell membranes. Corticosteroids are most effective when given before endotoxin; their value when given to animals with established shock is doubtful. Thus, if corticosteroids are to be used in patients with acute meningococcaemia to prevent shock, they should be given in large doses, for example 1 g of methylprednisolone, and they should be given as early as possible. However, at present there is insufficient evidence to recommend high-dose steroids as routine therapy.

In the past, digitalis has been used in an attempt to improve myocardial function in patients with acute meningococcaemia but the drug is difficult to control and it has now been superseded by short-acting inotropic agents such as dopamine. If cardiac arrhythmias are detected, they should be treated by conventional means.

Bleeding, associated with disseminated intravascular coagulation, may be an important feature of acute meningococcaemia. A beneficial response to therapy with heparin has been reported in individual cases but a controlled trial showed no overall benefit from this drug. If bleeding is severe, blood transfusion may be required.

Meningococci disappear rapidly from the circulation of patients with acute meningococcaemia treated with high doses of penicillin but for some this may still be too late because they have already been exposed to a potentially lethal dose of endotoxin. Attempts have been made to remove endotoxin by plasmapheresis; successful responses have been reported in small groups of patients but no controlled trials have ever been undertaken and these would now raise substantial ethical difficulties. An alternative approach has been to try to neutralize endotoxin by giving an endotoxin antiserum. The old literature provides support for this approach for, before the introduction of antibiotics, treatment with immune serum reduced mortality from meningococcal infections significantly. Success has been claimed in small numbers of patients but, overall, early experience with this approach has not been encouraging. The recent discovery of the central role of tumour necrosis factor in the pathogenesis of endotoxaemia provides another potential opening for immunotherapy. Antitumour necrosis factor monoclonals suitable for human use have been developed and are now undergoing clinical trials in patients with septicaemia. Analogues of the factor that might be used for treatment are being developed.

Meningitis

ANTIBIOTICS

The conventional antibiotic treatment for acute meningococcal meningitis in adults is 3 to 5 megaunits of crystalline penicillin given intravenously or intramuscularly every 6 h for 5 to 7 days. Parenteral penicillin given in such a dose produces penicillin levels in cerebrospinal fluid well above the MIC for nearly all meningococci and intrathecal antibiotic therapy is unecessary. The recent appearance of penicillin-insensitive strains raises the question of whether penicillin can still be recommended unconditionally as the first choice of treatment for meningococcal meningitis. However, most strains studied so far have proved to be insensitive rather than resistant, with MICs below the level likely to be found in the cerebrospinal fluid following treatment with large doses of parenteral penicillin. Thus, with the exception of areas where the prevalence of insensitive strains is known to be high, it is probably still safe to rely on penicillin as the first line of treatment for this condition. However, physicians should be aware of the possibility of treatment failures with penicillin and be prepared to change antibiotics if necessary. Chloramphenicol, given to adults in a dosage of 750 mg 6-hourly, is an effective alternative to penicillin. It has the advantage that it can be given by mouth as soon as a patient is conscious but, very rarely, it causes marrow depression. Meningococci are very sensitive to cephalosporins and antibiotics such as ceftriaxone and ciprofloxacin are very effective alternative treatments. Sulphonamides should not be used for the treatment of meningococcal meningitis. There is no evidence that combinations of penicillin, chloramphenicol, and sulphonamides are any more effective than penicillin or chloramphenicol given alone.

During epidemics, large numbers of patients with meningococcal disease become ill at the same time, swamping the available medical resources. Under such circumstances, 6-hourly penicillin injections are impracticable and alternative treatments are required. Several studies have demonstrated the efficacy of a single injection of an oily preparation of chloramphenicol (Tifomycine) (adult dose 3 g) and during epidemics this drug has saved many lives. A recent study from Niger and Mali showed that two injections of Tifomycine were as effective as 8 days of intravenous ampicillin in a large series of patients with pyogenic meningitis, 161 of whom had a meningococcal infection. Unfortunately, its continued production is in doubt. A single injection of ceftriaxone would probably be equally effective but the costs of this antibiotic is many times higher than that of Tifomycine, an important consideration for developing countries faced with an epidemic.

The results obtained with Tifomycine suggest that conventional antibiotic regimens for the treatment of meningococcal meningitis are unnecessarily long and that satisfactory results could be obtained with shorter courses of crystalline penicillin or chloramphenicol. However, if new treatment regimens are tried, careful monitoring of patients is essential.

Penicillin and chloramphenicol suppress but do not usually eradicate nasopharyngeal carriage of meningococci and cases have been described when it seems likely that a patient has infected contacts after leaving hospital. Thus, it has been suggested that patients should be given treatment to eradicate carriage (see below) before leaving hospital.

SUPPORTIVE

Unconscious patients with meningitis require careful nursing, particular attention being paid to their airway. Patients with meningitis are often dehydrated, especially in hot countries, because they have a high fever, frequently vomit, and because they may be too confused to drink. Thus, intravenous rehydration may be required. Headache may be very severe and may be an important cause of restlessness. If it cannot be controlled with simple analgesics, pethidine may be needed. Diazepam is of value in quietening restless and violent patients, and in controlling convulsions. If signs of severe raised intracranial pressure are present, dexamethasone should be considered.

The development of arthritis or cutaneous vasculitis during the recovery phase of the infection is not an indication for the continuation of antibiotic therapy. Arthritis responds well to treatment with aspirin. Skin ulcers may require dressings for several weeks and amputation of gangerous extremities is occasionally required.

Recent studies, mainly in the United States, have shown that giving dexamethasone for 4 days to children with pyogenic meningitis reduces the incidence of late complications, especially deafness. These studies contained predominantly children with *H. influenzae* meningitis; there were few with meningococcal disease. Thus no firm recommendations can be made about the efficacy of dexamethasone in meningococcal meningitis. Because of the high incidence of deafness as a result of this form of pyogenic meningitis, a formal trial of dexamethasone is urgently required.

A deterioration in conscious level or the appearance of new focal neurological signs after the start of treatment suggests the development of a subdural effusion or empyema, or of a vascular occlusion. Patients showing these features should be investigated for the presence of a space-occupying lesion by whatever diagnostic means are available. If a filling defect is found, burr holes should be made.

Table 3 *Efficacy of ceftriaxone and rifampicin in eradicating pharyngeal carriage of the meningococcus in family contacts of patients with meningococcal disease in Saudi Arabia*

	Positive cultures Time after treatment	
	6 days	2 weeks
No antibiotic	8/10 (80%)	7/12 (58%)
Ceftriaxone	2/68 (3%)	2/64 (3%)
Rifampicin	9/36 (25%)	5/27 (19%)

Ceftriaxone was given as a single injection of 250 mg for adults and 125 mg for children. Rifampicin was given in a dose of 600 mg for adults and 10 mg/kg for children twice a day for 2 days.

Reproduced From Schwartz *et al.* (1988). *Lancet*, **i**, 1239, with permission.

Prophylaxis

There are two main approaches to the prevention of meningococcal disease, chemoprophylaxis and vaccination. Prevention of overcrowding in barracks and schools probably helps to prevent the spread of meningococcal infection and improved living standards have almost certainly contributed to the decline in the frequency of epidemics of meningococcal disease in industrialized countries during the past 50 years.

Chemoprophylaxis

In the past, chemoprophylaxis with sulphonamides proved very effective in preventing meningococcal infection. Sulphonamides eliminate sulphonamide-sensitive meningococci from nasopharyngeal carriers, thus interrupting transmission in the community for a period. During this time the environmental factors responsible for an outbreak may have disappeared so that stopping chemoprophylaxis does not necessarily result in reactivation of the outbreak.

Unfortunately, many meningococci have become sulphonamide resistant so that sulphonamides can no longer be used routinely for chemoprophylaxis. Some authorities now recommend that they should never be used for prophylaxis. However, if it has been established beyond doubt that an outbreak has been caused by a sulphonamide-sensitive meningococcus, then sulphonamides still provide a cheap and very effective means of prophylaxis. Many antibiotics have been tried as alternative prophylactics. Although penicillin and chloramphenicol are very effective therapeutic agents, they are ineffective prophylactics for reasons that are not completely understood. Minocycline was found to be effective at eliminating carriage but caused an unacceptably high incidence of side-effects in some studies and is no longer used for prophylaxis. Rifampicin has proved to be as effective and less toxic than minocycline, but its use for prophylaxis is associated with the rapid appearance of rifampicin-resistant meningococci and there is a danger that use of the drug for prevention of meningococcal infection in developing countries might favour the appearance of rifampicin-resistant strains of tubercle and leprosy bacilli. Recently, limited studies have shown that a single injection of ceftriaxone or a single dose of oral ciprofloxacillin can eradicate carriage (Table 3). A single dose of ciprofloxacin is cheaper than a course of rifampicin and easier to take.

Recommended antimicrobial doses for chemoprophylaxis are shown in Table 4.

Table 4 *Recommended doses of antimicrobials for chemoprophylaxis against meningococcal disease*

	Sulphadiazine (2 days)	Rifampicin (2 days)	Ceftriaxone (1 day)	Ciprofloxacin (1 day)
Adults	1 g, twice a day	600 mg, twice a day	250 mg, single dose	500 mg, single dose
Children over 1 year	25 mg/kg, twice a day	10 mg/kg, twice a day	125 mg, single dose	125/250 mg, single dose

Vaccination

INTRODUCTION

Attempts to protect against meningococcal infection by vaccination have been made for at least 50 years. Some success was obtained with early vaccines prepared from whole organisms, but other whole-bacteria vaccines were ineffective. Thus, the discovery in 1969 that purified group A and group C meningococcal capsular polysaccharides were immunogenic and that these preparations consistently gave protection against meningococcal disease was a major advance. Bivalent (A + C) and tetravalent (A, C, Y, and W135) capsular polysaccharide vaccines are now widely available.

Meningococcal polysaccharide vaccines, which are T-independent antigens, have a number of unusual characteristics. They are poorly immunogenic in young children and do not activate T memory cells. Booster responses can be induced by reimmunization but the time interval between doses is important and, under certain circumstances, reimmunization fails to give any enhancement of the antibody response.

Several large-scale trials, mainly in Africa but also in Finland and Brazil, have demonstrated clearly that group A and group C capsular polysaccharide vaccines can control epidemics very effectively. Protection is achieved within a week of immunization. How long protection lasts has not been clearly documented. In adults, raised antibody levels persist for many years after vaccination but this is not the case in children. In The Gambia, the antibody levels of children who were 1 to 4 years old at the time of vaccination had fallen to background levels 5 years later. This serological finding supports the clinical observation made in Burkina Faso that vaccine efficacy had fallen to 8 per cent 3 years after vaccination in children immunized at less than 4 years of age. Thus, polysaccharide A and C vaccines are highly effective at halting outbreaks but are less effective at providing sustained protection in children. To try to overcome this problem, polysaccharide–protein conjugate vaccines are being developed, along the lines of the very effective *H. influenzae* type b conjugate vaccines, which will be immunogenic in young children, which will induce immunological memory, and which will provide prolonged protection. One such vaccine has entered the phase of clinical trials. Development of conjugate vaccines that could be given through existing infant Expanded Programmes of Immunization (EPI) and could provide long-lasting protection may finally solve the problem of meningococcal disease in the African 'meningitis belt'.

Whether group A and group C polysaccharide vaccines prevent carriage is controversial; some but not all studies have shown a modest reduction in the prevalence of nasopharyngeal carriage after vaccination. Polysaccharide–protein conjugate vaccines are likely to be more effective in this respect.

The group B capsular polysaccharide is poorly immunogenic and in its native form cannot be used as a vaccine. Attempts have been made to improve its immunogenicity by modifying the structure of the polysaccharide in various ways but clinical vaccines based on this approach have not yet been developed. More success has been achieved with group B vaccines based on outer membrane proteins. A group B vaccine comprising a mixture of outer membrane proteins together with the group C polysaccharide has been developed in Cuba and has proved to be very effective at controlling meningococcal disease in this island, giving protection in two large trials of over 80 per cent. When tried in Brazil the vaccine gave approximately 70 per cent protection in adults but was much less effective in children. Another group B vaccine developed in Norway, which comprises outer membrane proteins of the serogroup B meningococcus together with some lipopolysaccharide, proved to be safe and immunogenic and provided 57 per cent protection against invasive meningococcal disease in a large clinical trial involving nearly 200 000 Norwegian students (Table 5). However, the duration of the protection provided by these group B vaccines is not known. Efforts to develop better group B protein vaccines are continuing.

Table 5 *The results of a group B meningococcal outer-membrane protein vaccine trial undertaken in Norway. Two doses of vaccine were given to schoolchildren aged 14 to 16 years. Randomization was by school.*

	Participants	
	Vaccine	Placebo
Schools	690	645
Pupils	88 800	83 000
Observation	180 600	168 300
Cases	11	24
	Vaccine efficacy 57.2%	

Reproduced from Bjune *et al.* (1991) with permission.

MANAGEMENT OF ENDEMIC MENINGOCOCCAL DISEASE OR SMALL OUTBREAKS

When a single case or a small cluster of cases of meningococcal disease are detected then preventative measures to stop further spread of the infection should be instigated (Fig. 10).

Fig. 10 A scheme for the management of a contact of a patient with meningococcal disease.

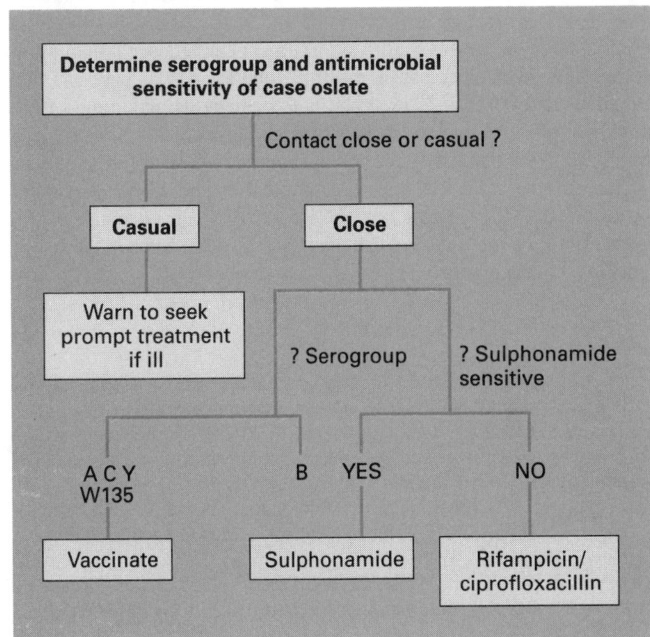

Those most at risk of contracting meningococcal disease are close household contacts of a patient with the infection. During an epidemic, the risk for siblings sleeping in the same room as a patient may be as high as 1 in 20. Such close contacts should receive the full range of prophylactic measures available. If the organism is known to belong to group A, C, W135 or Y, vaccination should be done immediately. However, as many secondary, or perhaps co-primary cases occur within a few days of the onset of illness in the index case, an alternative form of protection is required to cover the period before vaccination induces protective immunity and chemoprophylaxis should be given also.

When a case of meningococcal disease occurs in a residential school, doss house, or barracks, further cases of the infection are likely. Subjects in close contact with the patient, for example those sleeping in the same small dormitory, should be managed in the same way as household contacts. Subjects with less contact with the patient should be vaccinated if the causative meningococcus belongs to serogroup A, C, W135, or Y. Whether such contacts should be given chemoprophylaxis will depend upon the nature of the outbreak—this may be impractical and unecessary if the number of contacts is very large.

It has generally been considered that the risk of spread of infection among pupils in day schools is very low; recently, however there have been a few reports of this, so vaccination and/or chemoprophylaxis for the classmates of a case is probably a wise precaution.

Although the risk of meningococcal disease in hospital personnel is only a little greater than that of the general population there have been fatalities among hospital staff so that vaccination of those who come into regular contact with patients with meningococcal disease or with their laboratory samples is a sensible precaution. Research scientists working with meningococci should also be vaccinated.

MANAGEMENT OF AN EPIDEMIC

The first essential in the management of an epidemic of meningococcal disease is to establish as soon as possible that an epidemic has started. The next essential is to determine as quickly as possible the serogroup and antimicrobial sensitivity pattern of the causative meningococcus. A sound management team must be built up as quickly as possible and, in areas where outbreaks are frequent, an action plan should be in existence that can be activated at short notice. Epidemics of meningococcal meningitis may swamp the routine medical services, a hundred new cases a day is not unusual, so it may be necessary to establish temporary treatment centres. Long-acting chloramphenicol is invaluable in such circumstances. Chemoprophylaxis is of little or no value in the management of epidemics but the effects of vaccination may be dramatic, stopping an epidemic of group A or group C meningococcal meningitis within a few days. Vaccination must be done as soon as possible after an epidemic has been identified if it is to achieve its maximum effect; limited supplies of vaccine should be maintained in areas where epidemics are likely. Unless vaccine is in short supply, when targeted vaccination may be indicated, the whole population should be vaccinated. Too often, lives have been lost unnecessarily when vaccination was delayed until an epidemic was already past its peak. Speed is essential if meningococcal epidemics are to be contained.

REFERENCES

Bjune, G. *et al.* (1991). Effect of outer membrane vesicle vaccine against group B meningococcal disease in Norway. *Lancet*, **338,** 1093–6.

Brandtzaeg, P., Mollnes, T.E., and Kierulf, P. (1989). Complement activation and endotoxin levels in systemic meningococcal disease. *Journal of Infectious Diseases*, **160,** 58–65.

Cartwright, K.A.V., Jones, D.M., Smith, A.J., Stuart, J.M., Kaczmarski, E.B., and Palmer, S.R. (1991). Influenza A and meningococcal disease. *Lancet*, **338,** 554–7.

Cartwright, K., Reilly S., White, D., and Stuart J. (1992). Early treatment with parental penicillin in meningococcal disease. *British Medical Journal*, **305,** 143–7.

Cassio de Moraes, J. *et al.* (1992). Protective efficacy of a serogroup B meningococcal vaccine in Sao Paulo, Brazil. *Lancet*, **340,** 1074–8.

Gedde-Dahl, T.W., Bjark, P., Hoiby, E.A., Host, J.H., and Brun, J.N. (1990). Severity of meningococcal disease: assessment by factors and scores and implications for patient management. *Reviews of Infectious Diseases*, **12,** 973–92.

Kristiansen. B-E., Ask, E., Jenkins, A., Ferner, C., Radstrom, P., and Skold, O. (1991). Rapid diagnosis of meningococcal meningitis by polymerase chain reaction. *Lancet*, **337,** 1568–9.

Kristiansen, B-E., Sorensen, B., and Bjorvatn, B. (1984). Restriction endonuclease fingerprinting of meningococcal DNA. *NIPH Annals*, **7,** 21–8.

Lapeyssonnie, L. (1963). La méningite cérébrospinal en Afrique. *Bulletin of the World Health Organization*, **28,** (suppl.), 3–114.

Moore, P.S. (1992). Meningococcal meningitis in sub-Saharan Africa: a model for the epidemic process. *Clinical Infectious Diseases*, **14,** 515–25.

Olyhoek, T., Crowe, B.A., and Achtman, M. (1987). Clonal population structure of *Neisseria meningitidis* serogroup A isolated from epidemics and pandemics between 1915 and 1983. *Reviews of Infectious Diseases*, **9,** 665–92.

Pecoul, B. *et al.* (1991). Long-acting chloramphenicol versus intravenous ampicillin for treatment of bacterial meningitis. *Lancet*, **338,** 862–6.

Quagliarello, V. and Scheld, W.M. (1992). Bacterial meningitis: pathogenesis, pathophysiology and progress. *New England Journal of Medicine*, **327,** 864–72.

Schwartz, B. *et al.* (1988). Comparative efficacy of ceftriaxone and rifampicin in eradicating pharyngeal carriage of group A *Neisseria meningitidis. Lancet*, **i,** 1239–42.

Sierra, G.V. *et al.* (1991). Vaccine against group B *Neisseria meningitidis*: protection trial and mass vaccination result in Cuba. *NIPH Annals*, **14,** 208–10.

Stephens, D.S. and Farley, M.M. (1991). Pathogenic events during infection of the human nasopharynx with *Neisseria meningitidis* and *Haemophilus influenzae*. *Reviews of Infectious Diseases*, **13,** 22–33.

van Deuren, M., Santman, F.W., Van Dalen, R., Sauerwein, R.W., Span, L.F.R., and van der Meer J.W.M. (1992). Plasma and whole blood exchange in meningococcal sepsis. *Clinical Infectious Diseases*, **15,** 424–30.

Waage, A., Halstensen, A., Shalaby, R., Brandtzaeg, P., Kierulf, P., and Espevik, T. (1989). Local production of tumour necrosis factor, interleukin 1, and interleukin 6 in meningococcal meningitis. Relation to the inflammatory response.*Journal of Experimental Medicine*, **170,** 1859–67.

7.11.6 *Neisseria gonorrhoeae*

D. BARLOW and C. A. ISON

THE ORGANISM

In 1879, Albert Neisser observed the causative agent of gonorrhoea, the first bacterium of the eponymous family of Neisseriaceae. This human pathogen can infect genital sites in non-human primates, and other extragenital animal models have been used to investigate pathogenesis and immunological mechanisms.

PATHOGENESIS

Neisseria gonorrhoeae primarily colonizes the mucosa of the lower genital tract and only occasionally progresses to the upper genital tract or invades to cause systemic disease. For successful colonization, gonococci must avoid being swept away by cervical secretions in women or urine in men; this they do by adhering to the epithelial cell. Both cell surfaces are negatively charged and non-specific factors such as pH, surface charge, and hydrophobicity are important in achieving this association. Attachment to the epithelial surface is then mediated by the specific gonococcal structures of pili and the opa proteins. Gonococci attach preferentially to columnar rather than squamous epithelium. *In vitro* studies using cultures of human fallopian tubes show that gonococci attach to non-ciliated cells and that blebs of the cell envelope are shed that have a toxic effect on adjacent ciliated cells. Lipo-oligosaccharide is the primary mediator of this damage but peptidoglycan may also play some part.

After the gonococci are attached to the epithelial cell, the organisms are taken into the cell and transmitted to the lamina propria, where infection is established. This endocytosis of the gonococcus may be mediated by its major outer-membrane protein, Por (Fig. 1). To multiply in the host, the gonococcus needs a supply of iron and this can be a growth-limiting factor. *N. gonorrhoeae* express receptors on the cell surface for transferrin or lactoferrin to acquire iron from the host, unlike many other bacteria that produce soluble sideropores. For invasion to occur the organism must resist the bactericidal activity of serum. *In vivo*, gonococci are serum resistant as a result of sialylation of lipo-oligosaccharide. *In vitro*, most strains revert to serum sensitivity, although a few remain resistant, suggesting an additional unidentified mechanism.

N. gonorrhoeae is a particularly successful pathogen as it has evolved mechanisms to evade host defences and to cause repeated infection. The main antigens of the outer membrane of the gonococcus that are exposed to the immune response are pili, lipo-oligosaccharide, and three major outer-membrane proteins, Por, Opa, and Rmp. Por (formerly known as protein I or PI) accounts for 60 per cent of the protein of the outer membrane and acts as a porin to allow the passage of hydrophilic molecules. Opa (protein II, PII) consists of a family of heat-modifiable proteins that enhance attachment to epithelial cells, and up to three can be expressed simultaneously. Rmp (protein III, PIII), is closely associated with Por and forms part of the porin.

Of these antigens, pili, opa, and lipo-oligosaccharide are able to alter the surface-exposed part of the molecule and hence present a new antigen to the immune response. In the gonococcus, as in many other organisms, this alteration occurs more frequently than the normal rate of mutation and is known as antigenic variation. On each encounter between organism and host, the gonococcus presents a range of immunologically distinct proteins that are not recognized by the host. Specific antigonococcal antibody is produced during natural infection. Both IgG and IgA directed at surface-exposed antigens can be detected in serum and mucosal secretions. Antigenic heterogeneity of the gonococcal cell surface is probably the chief cause of the lack of any apparently protective antibody. It is also likely that serum antibody has no function in mucosal infection, and immunity afforded by mucosal antibody is short-lived. There is some evidence of serovar-specific immunity, that is antibody produced to Por, in complicated infections in women; repeated episodes of pelvic inflammatory disease occur but women are not reinfected with same Por serotype.

The function of antibody in modifying the course of the infection is unknown. Serum antibodies may limit disseminated infection by activating the complement pathway. *N. gonorrhoeae* isolated from disseminated infection exhibit high levels of resistance to bactericidal effects of serum. Mucosal antibody may interfere with colonization by inhibiting attachment to the mucosa and by enhancing phagocytosis by macrophages. Gonococci are known to be ingested and killed by macrophages and this may be the host's primary mechanism of defence. However, gonococci that are piliated and expressing some opa proteins can survive in phagocytes. The balance between the ability of phagocytes to kill gonococci and survival of bacteria within these cells is a major factor in the pathogenesis of gonorrhoea.

Secretory IgA is the dominant antibody in mucosal secretions and is directed at the major outer-membrane antigens. This antibody would be expected to have a primary role in preventing colonization. However, gonococci produce an extracellular IgA1 protease that cleaves the antibody and renders it inactive.

Protection against gonococcal infection using acquired immunity by vaccination has proved totally unsuccessful. This is due mainly to the antigenic heterogeneity of the antigens chosen as candidate vaccines and because the type or amount of antibody required for protection is unclear. Pilin vaccines have proved unsuccessful, largely because initial trials used whole pili that produced antibody to the homologous strain only. More recent studies have used Por, a more conserved protein, which has the potential to give some protection against complicated or disseminated disease

EPIDEMIOLOGY

The overriding factor influencing endemic levels of gonorrhoea (and other sexually transmitted diseases) is human behaviour (see also Section 21). The availability of effective antimicrobial therapy makes less difference to the number of cases than might be expected. Figure 2 shows the reported cases of gonorrhoea between 1918 and 1991 in England. The sharp decline from 1946 coincided with a more widespread availability of penicillin, appearing to support a causal relationship. However, smaller, but similar, falls occurred after the First World War and in the mid-1930s; and the steady increase between the mid-1950s and the mid-1970s covered a period during which there was a significant increase in the availability of antigonococcal antimicrobials. It is likely that behaviour is at least as important as effective treatment in determining levels of infection, although antimicrobials have significantly reduced the incidence of complications.

Like human immunodeficiency virus (**HIV**) infection, gonorrhoea is not evenly distributed throughout the sexually active population. Sporadic cases are seen in rural areas and small towns but a sizeable population is needed to maintain an endemic of gonorrhoea, the highest incidence being found in larger conurbations and among the young, the socioeconomically deprived, and ethnic minorities. The incidence and prevalence of gonorrhoea serve as the most useful indicators of risky sexual behaviour because diagnosis is speedy and accurate, and the

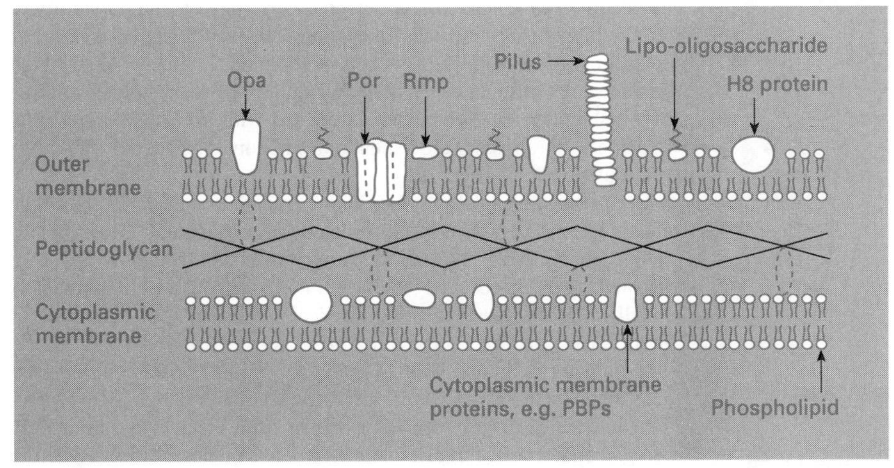

Fig. 1 Schematic representation of the cell envelope of *Neisseria gonorrhoeae*. See text for explanation of symbols.

infection can be treated and reacquired time and time again in the absence of mucosal immunity.

The incidence of neonatal gonococcal ophthalmia and the prevalence of gonorrhoea in antenatal populations measure the success, or otherwise, of control programmes. By both of these criteria gonorrhoea is not a significant problem at present in the United Kingdom.

Gonorrhoea has been shown to be an independent cofactor facilitating acquisition and transmission of HIV infection, presumably by a disruption of normal epithelial protection combined with increased presence of CD4 receptor cells.

The gonococcus has undergone three important adaptations since the Second World War: a decreasing sensitivity to antimicrobials (chromosomally and plasmid mediated); a lengthening of the incubation period; and a lessening of its symptom-producing capabilities. These changes have coincided with (and may well have resulted from) widespread and, in some parts of the world, indiscriminate use of antimicrobials, and they reflect the selective advantage to strains that produce fewer symptoms, at a later stage. The infectivity of the gonococcus is not known but is probably higher for male-to-female transmission (where it may be 80 per cent or more following insertive vaginal intercourse) than in the opposite direction. Condoms reduce transmission of gonorrhoea.

INCUBATION PERIOD, SYMPTOMS, AND SIGNS

The mean incubation period of urethral gonorrhoea in men is increasing, and is now longer than the often quoted (and never referenced) 2 to 5 days. A recent study gave a mean of 7.9 days and a median of 5.6 days (Table 1). The upper limit of the range may be 3 months or more. The classical symptoms of urethral gonorrhoea, discharge and dysuria, have undergone a change in quality and prevalence; urethral discharge with dysuria, as a presentation of gonorrhoea, occurs in less than 60 per cent of cases. The severe, burning discomfort (*chaudepisse*) of yesteryear is rarely reported. Asymptomatic gonococcal infection is seen in up to 5 per cent of cases, some of which will be in the presymptomatic stage. The observed increase, since the 1930s, from 2 to 6 days in the delay between development of symptoms and presentation at a clinic for treatment may be explained by a diminution in severity of symptoms.

In early urethral gonorrhoea, there may simply be a mild meatitis with a minimal mucoid discharge, which later becomes thick, profuse, purulent, and white or off-white. The discharge eventually becomes scanty if the infection is left untreated. Conditions mimicking the classical profuse discharge of gonorrhoea in men are uncommon but the differential diagnosis will include foreign body in the urethra and, rarely, non-gonococcal urethritis.

Table 1 *Historical incubation period (IP) of gonorrhoea in men*

Year of study	No. of patients	Mean IP	Treatment
1932	115	4.9	Topical
1942	220	4.6	Sulphonamides
1952	193	6.0	Penicillin
1954/5	145	6.1	Penicillin
1978	242	6.2	Penicillin
1989	113	7.9	Penicillin

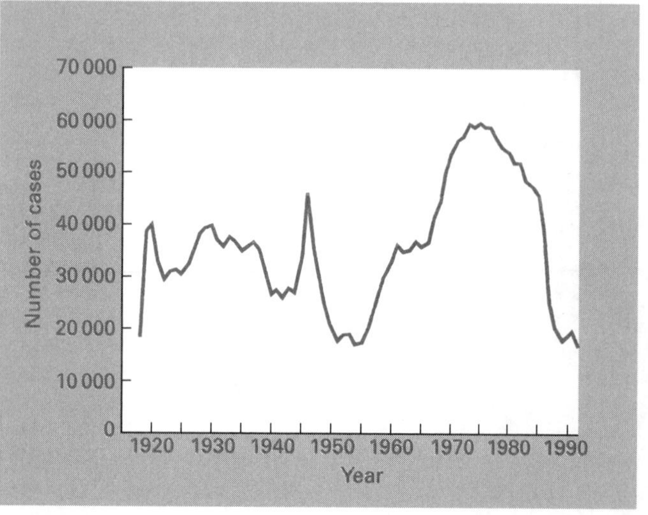

Fig. 2 Reported cases of gonorrhoea in England between 1918 and 1991 (Department of Health).

Oropharyngeal and rectal gonorrhoea in either sex are not often associated with symptoms, apart from the occasional complaint of rectal discharge.

Women with gonorrhoea may have no symptoms until the infection has spread to the pelvis and adnexa. An increase in vaginal discharge (but with no distinguishing features) is noticed by some 40 per cent of infected women, with dysuria occurring in perhaps 12 per cent. The presence of another sexually transmitted disease such as *Trichomonas vaginalis* (found in up to 30 per cent of cases of gonorrhoea in women) may, however, prompt the seeking of medical help.

Diagnostic clinical signs of uncomplicated gonorrhoea in women do not exist, a purulent exudate from the cervical os also being found in other conditions.

COMPLICATIONS

In the Western world, epididymo-orchitis associated with urethral gonorrhoea (usually unilateral) is seen in less than 2 per cent of cases and gonococcal littritis, tysonitis, cowperitis, seminal vesiculitis, and prostatitis constitute but anecdotal case reports today. Likewise, urethral stricture as a late complication is rarely seen. These complications, however, do still occur in countries with less accessible specialist care.

Local complications in women are rare and include bartholinitis, skenitis, and periurethral abscess. Infection may spread to the endometrium, fallopian tubes, and pelvic organs. Commonly, symptomatic pelvic infection first appears towards the end of, or soon after, a menstrual period and probably results from retrograde flow of infected menstrual products. Lower abdominal pain and tenderness (which may be unilateral) and deep dyspareunia occur, with some constitutional upset. Reduced fertility and increased risk of ectopic pregnancy are later sequelae.

The FitzHugh–Curtis syndrome, perihepatitis, is today more often associated with chlamydial than gonococcal infection and has been suggested to result from spread from the pelvis via the right paracolic gutter. Its occurrence in men, although uncommon, suggests the possibility of an alternative route, perhaps lymphatic. This syndrome, like disseminated gonococcal infection, occurs predominantly in women without genital symptoms and the right hypochondrial pain, sometimes referred to the shoulder and sometimes associated with a sympathetic pleural effusion with rub, leads the patient to a surgeon or a general, rather than genitourinary, physician.

Before the development of antibiotics the gonococcus was the single most common organism found in bacterial endocarditis. This complication has not been reported in Britain since the Second World War, although there have been cases in the United States. Meningitis is equally a rarity these days. Gonococcal septicaemia, or disseminated gonococcal infection, occurs in 1 to 2 per cent of cases and affects predominantly skin and joints. Certain auxotypes (those requiring arginine, hypoxanthine and uracil) are associated with disseminated infection and are uniformly sensitive to penicillin. This is a surprisingly benign condition, in contrast to the destructive monoarthritis seen before antibiotics and now more likely to be seen with those few cases caused by penicillinase-producing *N. gonorrhoeae*.

The skin lesions (Plates 1 and 2), found mainly on the extremities, have a reddened surrounding areola and evolve through macular (1–2 mm in diameter), vesiculopustular, haemorrhagic, and necrotic stages. They are virtually pathognomonic of disseminated gonococcal infection, the only other condition with a similar appearance being chronic meningococcal septicaemia. There are usually between four and ten lesions, not particularly painful, and the gonococcus can be cultured from these. Frankly haemorrhagic bullae and erythema nodosum-like lesions have been described.

The involvement of joints may simply be a flitting polyarthralgia, although effusions in larger joints are seen. The shoulder, knee, wrist, and ankle, followed by the small joints of the hands and feet, are commonly involved and an associated tenosynovitis is quite common. Blood culture or examination of effusion may give the diagnosis but, in one large series, 90 per cent were diagnosed by culture of samples from anogenital sites.

Patients who develop this condition tend not to have had genital symptoms and, because women with gonorrhoea are more frequently asymptomatic, they outnumber men with disseminated infection by 5 to 1. The systemic manifestations lead patients to present more often to dermatologists, rheumatologists or general physicians rather than genitourinary physicians.

Prepubertal gonococcal vulvovaginitis should raise the possibility of sexual abuse but there is little doubt that the infection can be transmitted by fomites such as flannels and towels. Gonococcal ophthalmia neonatorum presents with a purulent conjunctival exudate within 48 h of birth and remains important in developing countries; 1 per cent aqueous silver nitrate, applied to the eyes of newborn babies, may be used as a preventive measure. In the United Kingdom, this postnatal prophylaxis is not practised as the prevalence of gonorrhoea in pregnant women is low and neonatal sticky eye is more likely to be due to *Chlamydia trachomatis*.

DIAGNOSIS

Even in a department of genitourinary medicine, the majority of patients will not have gonorrhoea. Much time and effort is spent excluding rather than diagnosing the disease. Investigations therefore need high sensitivity (and specificity). The diagnosis of gonococcal infection in men is easier than in women.

In men, uncomplicated infection affects the anterior urethra. Rectal infection results from insertive anal intercourse or occasionally from digital insertion. Oropharyngeal infection is found in 5 to 20 per cent of cases (the higher figure in homosexual men). Transmission from throat to penis can occur during fellatio. In both sexes the throat may be the source of disseminated gonococcal infection.

In infected women, the organism is found most commonly in the cervix (90 per cent) followed by the urethra (75 per cent), rectum (40 per cent), and oropharynx (15 per cent). Rectal infection in women can result from passive contamination by infected secretions as well as insertive intercourse. In about 5 per cent of cases, the organism will be found only in the rectum or urethra—gonorrhoea has not been excluded unless these two sites have been shown to be free from infection.

Microscopy of a suitably stained specimen is the first line in diagnosis (Plate 3). The organisms must be Gram-negative, intracellular (within the cytoplasm of a leucocyte), and diplococci. In samples from the male urethra, microscopy is highly sensitive (identifying 98 per cent of positives) and highly specific (less than 1 per cent will be found on culture to be *N. meningitidis* or other species).

Microscopy of stained samples from rectum, cervix, and female urethra is much less sensitive, with identification of only 55 per cent, or less, of true positives. Laboratory culture therefore assumes great importance in women. However, microscopy, particularly of samples from the cervix, should still be used because it has the advantage, where positive, of enabling immediate diagnosis and treatment. Because of the preponderance of other neisseriae in the oropharynx, microscopy of samples from this site is not helpful.

Although it may seem unnecessary, in view of the excellent correlation with microscopy, routine culture of samples from the male urethra provides an important means of quality control of the laboratory service, so crucial for diagnosis in women. The culture service may be compromised by a faulty batch of transport/growth media, malfunction of incubators, or new and inexperienced technical assistance. Laboratory culture enables assessment of antimicrobial sensitivities and other characteristics of the organism for epidemiological and management purposes.

A diagnosis of gonorrhoea should prompt search for other sexually transmitted diseases and the initiation of contact tracing.

Culture

Culture of *N. gonorrhoeae* remains the 'gold standard' for the diagnosis of gonorrhoea. Successful isolation depends on good specimen collection, efficient transport to the laboratory, and a suitable culture medium. Specimens can be taken from the urethra, cervix, rectum, and oropharynx with a swab made of material that is not toxic to *N. gonorrhoeae*. Urethra and cervix are often sampled using a disposable loop. The highest isolation rates are obtained if the specimen is inoculated directly on to fresh medium in the clinic, and incubated at 37°C until transported to the laboratory. Where this is impossible, the swab should be immersed in a suitable transport medium such as Stuart's or Amies' and sent to the laboratory as soon as possible.

N. gonorrhoeae colonizes mucosal surfaces and for successful growth *in vitro* an enriched medium and a moist atmosphere are necessary. The media most commonly used are based on Thayer and Martin's original recipe and consist of GC agar base supplemented with lysed horse blood and IsoVitaleX (which contains essential amino acids and glucose). The medium should be selective but non-inhibitory, containing antibiotics to suppress other organisms. This is of particular importance for rectal and pharyngeal specimens (although unusually sensitive strains may occasionally be inhibited). Most media contain a combination of vancomycin, to inhibit Gram-positive organisms, colistin and trimethoprim, to inhibit other Gram-negative organisms, and ampthotericin or nystatin to prevent the growth of yeasts.

Gonococci require moisture for good cultivation and this should be provided by using freshly prepared media (not stored for more than 1 week) and by incubation in high humidity and 7 per cent carbon dioxide. Primary isolation plates should be incubated for at least 48 h before they are discarded as negative. Culture for *N. gonorrhoeae* has a sensitivity approaching 100 per cent in clinics and laboratories with the appropriate experience and skill but it is advisable to repeat full tests at least once when negative results are obtained from gonorrhoea contacts. The isolation rate may be lower in general practice and smaller clinics, primarily because of delay in transporting the specimen.

Other means of detecting gonococci in clinical samples have been developed in recent years, including enzyme-linked assays, immunofluorescence, and DNA probes. It has proved difficult to find a test that is as rapid, simple, and economical as the Gram stain for presumptive diagnosis. Many of the tests have the potential to replace culture (i.e. a high sensitivity and specificity) for confirmation, but are often more expensive and technically demanding. However, at the present time, culture is necessary to provide a viable organism for antimicrobial susceptibility testing and other detection systems are only applicable as adjuncts.

Serological tests lack specificity and sensitivity and should not be used in the diagnosis or exclusion of gonorrhoea.

Identification

The identification of *N. gonorrhoeae* from a primary isolation plate is achieved in two stages: first, screening tests to establish the presence of *Neisseria* spp. and secondly, tests to differentiate *N. gonorrhoeae* from

N. meningitidis and other non-pathogenic species. Colonies that grow on selective gonococcal media, give a positive oxidase reaction (presence of cytochrome *c* oxidase), and are Gram-negative cocci, are considered to be *Neisseria* spp. Identification of *N. gonorrhoeae* has, historically, been achieved with carbohydrate utilization tests; *N. gonorrhoeae* differs from other species in that it produces acid from glucose alone. This was considered the reference method for medicolegal cases for many years.

The development of monoclonal antibodies specific for *N. gonorrhoeae* has broadened the type of tests available. Antibodies raised to epitopes on the two types of the major outer membrane protein, PI, have been linked both to fluorescein (GC Microtrak, Syva Company, USA) or to staphylococcal protein A (Phadebact Monoclonal GC OMNI test, Pharmacia, Sweden). Both tests contain a mixture of antibodies that produce a reagent cross-reactive with strains of *N. gonorrhoeae* but not with other species of *Neisseria*. These tests identify *N. gonorrhoeae* only, whereas carbohydrate utilization tests differentiate between the species of *Neisseria*.

The advantage of immunological reagents is that they can identify colonies direct from the primary isolation medium and a result can be obtained on the same day as the organism is isolated. Both the above reagents have proved highly specific and sensitive, and are widely used. Identification kits incorporating enzyme profiles and carbohydrate utilization are also available commercially and can differentiate between the individual species of *Neisseria*. This approach has not been accepted as readily for two reasons: firstly, the result takes longer to achieve than immunological tests and secondly, this level of identification is seldom required by most laboratories. Confirmation of *N. gonorrhoeae* and exclusion of other *Neisseria* spp. is sufficient for most specimens from the genital tract. Correct identification of *N. gonorrhoeae* is always desirable but is most important in cases of possible sexual or child abuse. In such instances it is sensible to use more than one of the identification tests available to confirm an isolate as *N. gonorrhoeae*.

Typing

The recent development of new typing techniques has allowed the phenotypic characterization of strains of *N. gonorrhoeae*. It has been possible to study reinfection, treatment failure, and coinfection, and to show correlations with pathogenicity and antimicrobial susceptibility patterns. Two methods have been used extensively: auxotyping, determination of nutritional requirement, and serotyping, identifying patterns of reactivity with a panel of monoclonal antibodies.

Auxotyping

The nutritional requirement of different strains of *N. gonorrhoeae* can be determined using a chemically defined medium. A large number of auxotypes has been described but in most studies three or four types predominate: non-requiring (NR) also known as prototrophic (Proto), proline-requiring (Pro), arginine-requiring (Arg) and those requiring arginine, hypoxanthine and uracil (**AHU**). These four auxotypes have been described worldwide, although it is uncommon to find AHU-requiring strains in African studies. AHU strains exhibit particular characteristics: they are hypersensitive to penicillin, serum resistant, and associated with disseminated gonococcal infection. Auxotyping is time-consuming and requires meticulous attention to preparation of the media. It also lacks discrimination in most gonococcal populations.

Serotyping

Classification of *N. gonorrhoeae* using antibodies initially made use of polyvalent antibodies and divided strains into a small number of groups. The development of monoclonal antibodies directed to epitopes on the major outer-membrane protein and porin, PI, has increased the discriminatory power of the technique (Fig. 1). PI is found in two forms, IA and IB, of which only one is normally expressed. A standard panel of 12 antibodies, six specific for PI-A and six for PI-B, are linked to staphylococcal protein A and used in a coagglutination system. The pattern of reactivity with the individual antibodies denotes the serovar. To date a total of 24 IA serovars and 32 IB serovars has been reported.

Since 1986 the serotyping monoclonal antibodies have been shared through a worldwide network that has enhanced the study of the epidemiology of gonorrhoea. Geographical variation in the distribution of serovars has been found in general gonococcal populations; those from large cities are heterogeneous while those from smaller communities are often clonal in nature. Certain serovars, for example IB-2, have been found to be more prevalent in isolates from homosexual men than from heterosexuals. Strong associations between serovar and antimicrobial susceptibility also occur, IB serovars being closely linked to chromosomally mediated resistance.

Auxotyping/serotyping

These are often used in combination to produce auxotype/serovar (A/S) classes. The use of two independent characteristics gives a greater discrimination than when either technique is used alone. This is an advantage in contact tracing and in forensic medicine. Care should be taken when using a phenotypic classification for such purposes because isolates with identical phenotypic characteristics may not be genotypically identical.

ANTIMICROBIAL RESISTANCE

Penicillin has been used as the first-line therapy for gonorrhoea since its introduction. *N. gonorrhoeae* are inherently sensitive to most antibiotics such as penicillin but, with increased usage, both chromosomally mediated and plasmid-mediated resistance has developed. Resistance is most prevalent in the developing world, where the incidence of gonorrhoea is high and appropriate antibiotics are often unavailable or misused. However, in the Western world these strains are usually imported. In 1989 the World Health Organization issued new guidelines for the treatment of gonorrhoea, stating that penicillin should only be used as first line if the gonococcal population is known to be sensitive. If resistance is high or the susceptibility of the gonococcal population is unknown, alternative treatment is recommended: ciprofloxacin (a quinolone), ceftriaxone (a third-generation cephalosporin) or spectinomycin (a macrolide). Of these antibiotics, ciprofloxacin is used increasingly in the United Kingdom because it is taken orally and is highly effective and inexpensive.

Chromosomally mediated resistance

Decreased susceptibility to penicillin was detected as early as 1958 but this could be overcome by increasing the dose of penicillin and by adding probenecid. It was not until the 1970s that strains begun to appear with minimum inhibitory concentrations (**MIC**) to penicillin of more than 1.0 mg/l and posed a therapeutic problem. Chromosomal resistance to penicillin in *N. gonorrhoeae* is the result of the additive effects of multiple loci, *penA*, *mtr*, and *penB*. The locus *penA* confers resistance to penicillin alone and results in a change in the amino acid sequence of penicillin binding protein-2 and a subsequent decreased affinity for penicillin. Mutations at the *mtr* and *penB* loci confer decreased susceptibility to a range of antibiotics including ceftriaxone and ciprofloxacin. The product and function of these two loci are unknown but cell-wall permeability appears to be reduced. A number of modifier loci have also been found, such as *pem* and *tem*, which enhance resistance to penicillin and tetracycline, respectively. *N. gonorrhoeae* with these mutations can exhibit a 120-fold increase in penicillin MIC ($\geqslant$ 1.0 mg/l) and are known as chromosomally mediated resistant *N. gonorrhoeae* (**CMRNG**).

Resistance to the cephalosporins is rare and as yet therapeutic failure with ceftriaxone is undocumented. However, the loci encoding for resistance to penicillin in CMRNG are indistinguishable from those for decreased susceptibility to cephalosporins. If CMRNG continue to increase and are treated inappropriately, it is highly probable that resistance to cephalosporins will emerge.

Therapeutic resistance to spectinomycin has been reported but has not presented a major problem. Mutations on the chromosome affect the ribosome, resulting in a one-step, high-level increase in MIC. Spectinomycin has been an extremely useful antibiotic in treating resistant gonorrhoea and may be important in the future if mechanisms of resistance continue to evolve to newer antibiotics.

Ciprofloxacin has only been used for treatment of gonorrhoea for a short period of time and the relation between therapeutic failures, dosage, and MIC is still unclear. A few treatment failures have been described with MICs of 0.25 to 0.5 mg/l but have resulted mostly from treatment with a single, 250 mg dose. Failure with the higher 500 mg stat dose is uncommon. The mechanism of resistance is unknown but in other organisms results from a mutation in the DNA gyrase A gene and changes in cell wall permeability.

Plasmid-mediated resistance

N. gonorrhoeae exhibiting plasmid-mediated resistance to penicillin were first described in 1976. Simultaneous reports appeared of two strains, one from Africa carrying a plasmid of 3.2 MDa and the second from the Far East carrying a plasmid of 4.4 MDa. Both plasmids encode for the TEM-1 type β-lactamase (penicillinase). The smaller plasmid of 3.2 MDa has a deletion from the 4.4 MDa in a non-functional region. Penicillinase-producing *N. gonorrhoeae* (**PPNG**) carrying the 3.2 and 4.4 MDa plasmids have now spread worldwide, although their prevalence is greatest in countries of the developing world. PPNG carrying plasmids of differing size (2.9, 3.0, and 4.8 MDa) have been described more recently but have not spread in the same manner.

In 1985, plasmid-mediated resistance to tetracycline was first detected. It is high level (MIC $\geqslant$ 16 mg/l) and is due to the acquisition of the *tetM* determinant by the conjugative plasmid of *N. gonorrhoeae*, resulting in a plasmid of 25.2 MDa. Strains carrying this plasmid are known as tetracycline-resistant *N. gonorrhoeae* (TRNG). Tetracycline is not the treatment of choice for gonorrhoea but is commonly used, particularly in African countries, because it is inexpensive and available.

Susceptibility testing

The primary aim of susceptibility testing of *N. gonorrhoeae* is to predict therapeutic failure. However, it is also important to monitor drifts in susceptibility and to detect the emergence of strains resistant to the main, first-line therapies. There is much controversy over the correct method for achieving this for gonoccocci. Determination of zones of inhibition around antibiotic-containing discs has been the method chosen by most clinical laboratories. Gonococci are fastidious organisms that vary in their growth patterns and this method can therefore be difficult to control and interpret. In recent years the breakpoint agar dilution technique, which uses one or two concentrations of antibiotic to estimate the MIC and categorize strains into susceptible, reduced susceptibility, and resistant, has been used increasingly. Determination of the full MIC is not necessary for most laboratories and is best done by reference centres. Plasmid-mediated resistance to penicillin can be easily detected using the chromogenic cephalosporin (nitrocefin) test. Penicillinase-producing strains change the yellow reagent to a pink/red colour within a few seconds and this test can be done directly from the primary isolation plate.

Plasmid-mediated resistance to tetracycline can be detected using either the absence of a zone of inhibition around a 10 μg tetracycline disc or presence of growth on GC agar containing 10 mg/l of tetracycline. Both these screening tests are known to be good predictors of the presence of the 25.2-MDa plasmid and the *tetM* determinant.

TREATMENT

The ideal management of gonorrhoea—diagnosis before treatment—is not universally applied. Problems arise particularly with women who may have been exposed to gonorrhoea, in whom the infection will be present in only some 67 per cent. The 'epidemiological' approach—treatment before (or without) diagnosis—finds favour in many parts of the world and may be without alternative if proper diagnostic facilities are not available. However, this approach leads to unnecessary treatment in a significant number of cases, as does 'cluster' treatment (giving antimicrobials to known contacts, both sexual and social, of an index case) and 'prophylactic' treatment (giving antimicrobials to people before, or after, exposure to potential infection). All of these approaches lead to increased levels of relative resistance to antimicrobials.

Gonococci with plasmid-mediated resistance to penicillin due to production of β-lactamase pose serious therapeutic dilemmas in Third World countries. In the United Kingdom, PPNG remains largely imported, from Africa or the Far East, and such cases can often be predicted by means of travel history or geographical family background.

Many antimicrobials are effective against the gonococcus and penicillin remains the mainstay of treatment, just. Uncomplicated gonorrhoea is ideally treated with a single dose of antimicrobial, either orally or by intramuscular injection. Treatment regimens will depend on the prevailing spectrum of reduced antibiotic sensitivities. In London, in 1994, 2 g of ampicillin with 1 g of probenecid gives a cure rate of well over 95 per cent, as long as patients who may have acquired PPNG are identified and treated appropriately. By contrast, as a measure of reduced sensitivity of organisms in the United States, the Centers for Disease Control in Atlanta advise 3.5 g of amoxycillin with 1 g of probenecid for uncomplicated gonorrhoea. It has been suggested that, when plasmid-mediated resistant strains exceed 5 per cent of the incident gonococcal population, an antimicrobial effective against PPNG, such as ciprofloxacin, should become the standard treatment. However, in the United Kingdom it remains possible to predict the majority of such first- or second-generation imported strains and the simpler penicillin regimen is advised.

Co-trimoxazole, eight tablets, can be used where there is penicillin allergy. Most of the 4-quinolones, for instance ciprofloxacin 500 mg orally, are highly effective against gonorrhoea, including PPNG.

Single intramuscular treatments for uncomplicated gonorrhoea include procaine penicillin 2.4 g, with 1 g of probenecid, third-generation cephalosporins (cefotaxime, 1 g or cephtriaxone, 0.5 g) and spectinomycin, 2 to 4 g. The last three are effective against PPNG.

Oropharyngeal infection responds to a single 500 mg dose of ciprofloxacin.

Complicated infection, such the disseminated type, will require continued treatment for between 1 and 2 weeks with such as 2 g of ampicillin with 1 g of probenecid daily, in divided doses. Response to treatment is very rapid in disseminated gonococcal infection.

There is good evidence that pelvic infection associated with gonorrhoea is likely to be complicated by *Chlamydia trachomatis* and antigonococcal therapy should be changed after 1 or 2 days to oxytetracycline or erythromycin stearate, 2 g daily in divided doses, for 2 weeks. A similar regimen may be used for gonococcal epididymo-orchitis. Rest in bed is advised for both conditions.

Following treatment of gonorrhoea, investigations should be made at 1 to 2 and, say, 10 days to identify relapse and reinfection. Rectal tests of cure in women are important as failure occurs at this site more often than elsewhere. Contact tracing reduces the rate of reinfection.

REFERENCES

Barlow, D. (1977). Disseminated gonococcal infection. In *Advanced medicine 13,* (ed. G.M. Besser) pp. 197–203. Pitman Medical, London.

Barlow, D. and Phillips, I. (1978). Gonorrhoea in women—diagnostic, clinical and therapeutic aspects. *Lancet*, **i,** 761–4.

Barnes, C.B. and Holmes, K.K. (1984). Epidemiology of gonorrhoea: current perspectives. *Epidemiologic Reviews*, **6,** 1–27.

Britigan, B.E., Cohen, M.S., and Sparling, P.F. (1985). Gonococcal infection: a model of molecular pathogenesis. *New England Journal of Medicine*, **312,** 1623–93.

Brooks, G.F. and Donagan, E. (1985) *Gonococcal infection.* Edward Arnold, London.

Easmon, C.S.F. and Ison, C.A. (1987). *Neisseria gonorrhoeae*: a versatile pathogen. *Journal of Clinical Pathology*, **40,** 1088–97.
Easmon, C.S.F. and Ison, C.A. (1991). Current trends in the diagnosis and treatment of gonorrhoea. In *Recent advances in STD and AIDS*, (ed. J.R. Harris and S.M. Forster) pp. 159–82. Churchill Livingstone, Edinburgh.
Holmes, K.K., Counts, G.W., and Mahony, J.D.H. (1971). Disseminated gonococcal infection. *Annals of Internal Medicine*, **74,** 979.
Hook, E.W. and Handsfield, H.H. (1990). Gonococcal infections in the adult. In *Sexually transmitted diseases*, (ed. K.K. Holmes *et al.*). McGraw-Hill, New York.
Ison, C.A. (1990). Methods of diagnosing gonorrhoea. *Genitourinary Medicine*, **66,** 453–9.
Roberts, R.B. (ed.) (1977). *The gonococcus*. Wiley, New York.
Sherrard, J. and Barlow, D. (1993) Gonorrhoea in men. *Lancet*, **341,** 245.
Various authors (1988). Treatment of infections with antimicrobial resistant *N. gonorrhoeae*. (5 papers.) *Sexually Transmitted Diseases*, **15,** 202–43.
Various authors (1989) Perspectives on pathogenic Neisseriae. *Clinical Microbiology Reviews*, Suppl. 2.

Enteropathogenic bacteria

7.11.7 Enterobacteria and miscellaneous enteropathogenic and food-poisoning bacteria

M. B. Skirrow

This chapter describes diseases caused by the large group of intestinal bacteria known as the enterobacteria and specific intestinal infections caused by other groups of bacteria not considered elsewhere in the book. Most of these intestinal infections, whether due to enterobacteria or other bacteria, produce diarrhoea and are a major cause of morbidity and mortality in developing countries, especially among children. Even in technically advanced countries, where such infections are less dangerous, they are nevertheless a substantial drain on economic and health resources.

Among the enterobacterial infections described here are Salmonella enteritis, Shigella dysentery, and enteritis due to various pathogenic types of *Escherichia coli.* Typhoid and paratyphoid fevers are described in Chapter 7.11.8 and Yersinia infections in Chapter 7.11.17. Of the non-enterobacterial infections, enteritis due to Campylobacter, Aeromonas, Plesiomonas, Vibrio parahaemolyticus, and other non-cholera vibrios are included here, as is food poisoning due to *Bacillus cereus.* A general account of infections of the intestinal tract is given in Chapter 14.18.

The enterobacteria

Definition and general description

The term enterobacteria as used here strictly denotes bacteria belonging to the family Enterobacteriaceae. This is a large family of Gram-negative, non-sporing, fermentative bacilli that inhabit the intestinal tracts of man and animals; some exist on plants or in the soil. They are capable of growth in both aerobic and anaerobic conditions, and they are easy to cultivate in the laboratory—indeed they often outgrow and mask more fastidious bacteria. Since they are non-sporing organisms, they are killed by moderate heat (60 °C for 20 min) but they are generally more resistant to chemical disinfectants than are Gram-positive bacteria. They live and multiply in wet conditions but do not readily survive desiccation.

The family Enterobacteriaceae contains over 20 genera. Those most likely to be encountered in medical practice are Salmonella, Shigella, Escherichia, Klebsiella, Enterobacter, Citrobacter, Serratia, Hafnia, Edwardsiella, Erwinia, Kluyvera, Proteus, Providencia, Morganella, and Yersinia. The salmonellae and shigellae are the principal pathogens among these. The others, except for certain strains of *Escherichia coli* and Yersinia, are not intestinal pathogens, but any of them may cause infection elsewhere in the body given the opportunity (see below).

In the laboratory, the inability to ferment lactose is used to distinguish potentially enteropathogenic enterobacteria. Virtually all salmonellae and shigellae are non-lactose fermenters, whereas most of the other enterobacteria—with the exception of Proteus, Providencia, and Morganella—ferment lactose freely. By including lactose and a pH indicator in a culture medium, the colonies of non-lactose fermenters stand out pale against the coloured (acid) colonies of lactose fermenters, hence they can be picked out for further study. 'Coliform bacteria' is a clinically convenient term used to denote lactose-fermenting enterobacteria.

ANTIGENIC STRUCTURE

There are three groups of antigens that are important for the identification of enterobacteria in the laboratory and also for the serological diagnosis of infection, e.g. by the Widal test. First there are the somatic or O antigens present in the main structure of the bacterial cell wall, which consists of complexes of lipopolysaccharide with proteins and lipid. The polysaccharide component of lipopolysaccharide is the O antigen, whereas the lipid component, a complex phosphoglycolipid (lipid A), is the endotoxin that causes circulatory collapse in patients suffering from Gram-negative septicaemia (i.e. endotoxic shock; Chapter 7.19.2). O antigens are often shared between unrelated organisms. Second, there are surface antigens—sometimes in the form of a capsule (e.g. klebsiellae)—which, because of their superficial position, may mask the deeper O antigens unless they are first removed or destroyed by heat. One of the best examples of a surface antigen is the Vi antigen of the typhoid bacillus, so-called because it is associated with virulence. But the designation K (Kauffmann) is used for the surface antigen of other enterobacteria. Third, motile enterobacteria posses flagellar or H antigens that are highly specific within related groups. Salmonellae are almost unique in showing diphasic variation of the H antigen.

This complex antigenic structure makes it possible to serotype many strains within a single species or group, which is of great epidemiological value.

Extraintestinal infections caused by enterobacteria and related organisms

Before proceeding to specific diarrhoeal diseases caused by enterobacteria, a brief account of their infective role elsewhere in the body will be given. It is convenient to include here other non-fastidious Gram-negative bacilli that behave clinically in a similar manner to enterobacteria and are often found in mixed infections with them. Chief among these is *Pseudomonas aeruginosa* (*pyocyanea*), which is notorious as a 'hospital' organism and as a cause of opportunistic and sometimes fatal systemic infection in debilitated or immunosuppressed patients. *Ps. aeruginosa* is naturally resistant to most of the commonly used antimicrobials and also to many antiseptics. Indeed pseudomonads, notably *Ps. cepacia*, are capable of growth in some antiseptic solutions stored at dilute working strengths. Other common opportunistic Gram-negative bacilli are found in the genera Alcaligenes, Acinetobacter, Aeromonas, Flavobacterium, and Chromobacterium.

Gram-negative sepsis has steadily increased over the last few decades, particularly in hospital patients. The widespread use (and abuse) of antibiotics, which are generally more active against Gram-positive bacteria, is one reason, but another is the increasing proportion of susceptible patients that are treated: more are elderly; more receive immunosuppressive or cytotoxic therapy; more have catheters, pacemakers, and prostheses that provide favourable sites for infection; surgery is more complex and adventurous. Enterobacteria, pseudomonads, and similar Gram-negative bacilli easily develop resistance to antimicrobials, which helps them to colonize the hospital environment. Such organisms often replace the normal sensitive bowel flora of patients admitted to hospital, particularly if antibiotics are being given, so the patient's anus then becomes the gateway to colonization and infection elsewhere in the body.

It is against this background that one must consider Gram-negative sepsis, and it is not surprising that these organisms turn up in a wide variety of clinical material. They are frequently found colonizing wounds, sinuses, ulcers, burns, and chronically discharging ears—in fact wherever the body integument is broken. In most cases they are probably of little consequence, but their presence deep in a wound sometimes causes harm by enhancing the growth of anaerobes.

SPECIFIC TYPES OF INFECTION

Urinary tract

This is the most common site for genuine infection as opposed to simple colonization. Such infections range from a simple cystitis to pyelitis, pyelonephritis, and pyonephrosis. Most infections are caused by *E. coli*, but in patients with indwelling catheters or who have undergone genito-urinary surgery, resistant strains of Klebsiella, Enterobacter, Proteus, and *Ps. aeruginosa* are more likely to be the infecting agents. Septicaemia may arise from such infections, particularly after surgery (Chapter 7.19.2); even the simple removal of a urethral catheter from an infected man may cause bacteraemia. *E. coli* strains causing parenteral infection usually belong to one of only a dozen or so serogroups. Proteus infections in male children should alert a clinician to the possibility of a congenital abnormality such as a urethral valve.

Sepsis associated with the intestinal tract

In these infections coliform bacteria are usually found with other bowel flora such as *Bacteroides* spp. and micro-aerophilic streptococci. Peritonitis secondary to a perforated bowel, intraperitoneal abscess (e.g. pelvic, subphrenic, retrocaecal), cholecystitis, cholangitis, and liver abscess are examples of such infections. Remote focal infections such as endocarditis or cerebral abscess may also be caused by coliforms and other bowel flora.

Respiratory tract

Coliform bacteria seldom cause significant respiratory tract infections, but they are often isolated from sputum samples owing to a tendency to colonize the mouths and upper respiratory tract of ill patients, particularly babies. Such colonization is encouraged by antimicrobial chemotherapy. The presence of coliforms in sputum is therefore seldom of any consequence, but a true pneumonia does occasionally occur. The classical type is caused by *Klebsiella pneumoniae* subsp. *pneumoniae* (Friedlaender's bacillus) but this organism accounts for only a tiny proportion of all bacterial pneumonias; most of the klebsiellae isolated from sputum are of the common aerogenes type. Patients with bronchiectasis or cystic fibrosis are especially prone to Gram-negative bronchial infections, notably with capsulated 'mucoid' variants of *Ps. aeruginosa*.

K. ozaenae and *K. rhinoscleromatis* are associated with the uncommon nasal diseases ozaena and rhinoscleroma. In the tropics, *Chromobacterium violaceum* occasionally causes a potentially fatal melioidosis-like disease with septicaemia, pneumonia, and multiple abscess formation.

Neonatal infections

Newborn babies are especially liable to suffer from serious Gram-negative infections. Gram-negative septicaemia, which usually arises from an infected umbilicus, invariably involves the meninges as an incipient if not overt meningitis. Fortunately such events are rare, but coliforms are the most common cause of neonatal meningitis, a fact that contrasts sharply with the scarcity of coliform meningitis after the age of 1 month. *E. coli* is usually responsible, but any of the enterobacteria may be involved. *Proteus mirabilis* infections, which take the form of a meningoencephalitis, are particularly severe, and occasionally this common organism, for reasons that are not understood, has caused disastrous hospital nursery outbreaks.

Salmonella infections

The genus Salmonella takes its name from an American veterinary pathologist D. E. Salmon, who with his colleague Theobald Smith first isolated a member of the group (*Salmonella cholerae-suis*) in 1885. The genus Salmonella is now considered to comprise a single species, *S. enterica*, (syn. *S. cholerae-suis*) and, strictly, the former 'species' such as *S. typhi, S. typhimurium*, and *S. enteritidis* should be referred to as serotype Typhi, Typhimurium, and Enteritidis, respectively (in Roman, not italic type). Pending general acceptance and use of this nomenclature, we retain the established system of referring to salmonellae by their familiar specific names.

S. enterica is divided into seven subspecies, which largely correspond to the old 'subgenera'. Members of subspecies I are predominantly parasites of warm-blooded animals and they include almost all the salmonellae pathogenic for man. The other subspecies comprise organisms that are found mainly in cold-blooded animals or the environment, although they occasionally infect man, notably members of subspecies IIIa and IIIb (the 'Arizona' group). The latter, unlike subspecies-I organisms, ferment lactose, a property that makes their recognition in the laboratory difficult. Clinically it is convenient to divide the subspecies-I salmonellae into those that cause typhoid and paratyphoid fever (*S. typhi; S. paratyphi* A, B, and C, Chapter 7.11.8) and those that cause acute enteritis—usually through food poisoning—such as *S. enteritidis* and *S. typhimurium*.

The food-poisoning group contains about 2250 serotypes. After White and Kauffmann pioneered their antigenic classification in the late 1920s and early 1930s, it became customary to accord a specific Linnean name to each serotype, a policy that may be taxonomically unsound but convenient in practice. It also became customary to name each new serotype after the place at which it was first isolated. Thus salmonella 1,4,12:z:1,7 is *S. indiana* and salmonella 6,8:e,h:1,2 is *S. newport* (antigens are listed in the order O:H phase 1:H phase 2). Strains are divided firstly into some 36 groups according to their main somatic (O) antigens, and then further divided according to their flagellar (H) antigens. Fortunately for the bacteriologist whose task it is to identify salmonellae, most infections are caused by only a small proportion of the 2250 or so known serotypes. In Britain, North America, and many other parts of the world, *S. enteritidis* and *S. typhimurium* together account for at least three-quarters of all salmonella infections. Phage typing is used to recognize strains within these two common 'species'.

Epidemiology

Salmonellae are one of the main causes of foodborne illness throughout the world. In industrialized countries, salmonella infections have steadily increased over the last 20 years, more rapidly since 1985 mainly due to an increase in certain strains of *S. enteritidis*. The incidence of laboratory diagnosed infections is about 50 to 70/100 000 of the population per year; the true incidence is probably at least 10 times higher. The socioeconomic cost is enormous. In the United States it is estimated to be $1.4 billion per annum. In temperate zones, infection rates are highest in late summer.

ANIMAL SOURCES

The food-poisoning salmonellae are enzootic in a wide range of vertebrates, unlike the typhoid and paratyphoid bacilli, which are essentially confined to man. Some salmonellae have a preference for a particular host species; for example, *S. dublin* is primarily a parasite of cattle, *S. pullorum* of poultry, and *S. cholerae-suis* of pigs, but each may infect man given the opportunity. Infection may be acquired from direct contact with infected animals. On the farm the source is often scouring calves and in the home family pets—even terrapins and turtles. But in general, animals are more important as a primary source of infection in the food chain. In developed countries, intensive animal husbandry and mass production methods encourage the spread of salmonellosis. In the case of poultry, modern mechanized plucking and eviscerating methods, which are capable of processing 5000 birds an hour, cause gross cross-contamination.

Animal feeds are often the portal of entry for new salmonella serotypes. The appearance and spread of *S. agona* in Britain and the United States in the early 1970s was traced to its introduction in Peruvian fish meal used in poultry and pig feed. similarly, in the late 1970s, *S. hadar*, formerly unknown in Britain, became well established in turkey stocks after its introduction in feedstuffs from abroad. The prevalence of serotypes is constantly changing. Since 1985, the incidence of *S. enteritidis* infection has risen to unprecedented heights in Europe (mainly phage type 4) and North America (mainly phage types 8 and 13a) and probably elsewhere. The main source is poultry, for which these strains are more than usually invasive (mercifully not for human beings). This caused oviduct infection and contamination of fresh eggs through vertical transmission, a new epidemiological dimension that had far reaching political consequences.

FOOD SOURCES

The net result of the enzootic state is that raw meat and animal products, especially poultry, are commonly contaminated with salmonellae of one sort or another. Unsatisfactory though this is, the consequences are not always as serious as they might appear, for, with certain exceptions, the dose of salmonellae required to cause clinical infection is large and only likely to be reached if multiplication is allowed to occur in the food before consumption. Thus correct handling, preparation, and storage of food can prevent infection. Unfortunately, this ideal is not always attained: failure to handle raw meats separately from cooked foods leads to cross-contamination; incomplete thawing of large frozen carcasses, such as turkeys, results in inadequate cooking and multiplication of surviving bacteria. Raw milk is often contaminated at source and regularly causes infection in those unwise enough to drink it.

Faults in food factories can lead to widespread outbreaks corresponding to the distribution of the product. Major incidents have been caused by failure of heat treatment, or contamination of a food after heat treatment. The list of foods implicated is long, but examples are liquid egg, dried egg, dried-milk infant food, desiccated coconut, bean sprouts, chocolate, and meat pies topped up after cooking with jelly from contaminated dispensing machines.

HUMAN SOURCES

Infection is not readily transmitted from person to person, except among infants, old people, and patients living in closed communities such as nursing homes and asylums. Salmonellae can be especially troublesome in hospital maternity units.

The importance of a salmonella-excreting food handler as a source of infection has been exaggerated. Such a person is more likely to be the victim of handling contaminated animal products at work than a source of infection. It is rarely necessary to suspend an otherwise healthy food handler from duty until clear of salmonellae. However, it is mandatory to suspend a food handler with acute diarrhoea, whatever the apparent cause.

Pathology

The infective dose is governed by many factors, but in general many salmonellae are required to cause symptomatic infection. There are important exceptions. As few as 50 bacteria contained in certain high-fat foods, notably chocolate, cheese, and salami, can cause illness. Anything that reduces gastric acidity, such as atrophic gastritis, treatment with H_2 receptor-blocking agents, and previous gastric surgery, lowers the infective dose; salmonellae cannot withstand exposure to pH below 4.5. Broad-spectrum antibiotics increase susceptibility by suppressing the normal competitive microflora of the gut. The newborn are especially susceptible before the gut becomes normally colonized.

The small intestine is the main site of infection, but the colon may also be affected. Salmonellae are invasive in the bowel mucosa and they can penetrate deep to the lamina propria. Invasion is accompanied by an acute inflammatory response with polymorphonuclear cell infiltration of the submucosa. Flattening or loss of secretory epithelium occurs adjacent to these inflamed areas. Inflammatory cells are usually present in the stools. The mechanism by which salmonellae cause tissue damage is ill understood. Many strains can be made to produce enterotoxin *in vitro*, but its role *in vivo* is far from clear.

Bacteraemia has been reported in 1.5 per cent of all laboratory diagnosed infections, but at much higher rates in patients with *S. choleraesuis* (75 per cent), *S. dublin* (25 per cent), and *S. virchow* phage-type 19 (5.5 per cent) infections. Some of these patients suffer a typhoidal illness and focal infection may arise in almost any organ of the body.

Clinical features

Not everyone who is infected with salmonellae becomes ill. In every food-poisoning outbreak there are unaffected persons who excrete the organism in their faeces. Others suffer a typical attack of acute enteritis lasting 2 or 3 days, and there are usually a few who suffer a more severe, prolonged attack. The proportion of people who become ill is determined by the extent of contamination of the food and the characteristics of the infecting strain. The incubation period is usually 12 to 24 h, but it may range from 6 to 48 h, depending on the size of the infecting dose. The onset is abrupt, with malaise, nausea, headache, abdominal pain, and diarrhoea. Some patients vomit, but seldom more than once or twice. Shivering and fever is common in those that are more than mildly affected. Occasionally there is severe diarrhoea, with fluid, green, offensive stools that may contain mucus and blood. Dehydration, with cramps, oliguria, and uraemia may occur in the more severe type of illness. This is more likely to be seen at the extremes of age, and a fatal outcome is by no means unknown. Patients whose distal colon and rectum are affected may complain of tenesmus and the passage of small, bloody motions; they may also be tender over the sigmoid colon. Salmonella enterocolitis may trigger off an attack of non-specific colitis, acute appendicitis in the young, or mesenteric thrombosis in the elderly.

Reactive arthritis is an occasional late sequel of infection. Estimates of its incidence range from 1.2 to 7.3 per cent of all infections. Patients with HLA-B27 haplotype have a strong predisposition for this troublesome but ultimately benign complication.

CONVALESCENT EXCRETION

Most patients continue to excrete salmonellae in their faeces for a few weeks after infection—about 4 to 8 weeks for adults, and 8 to 24 weeks for infants. The number of organisms present is usually low, but excretors have been found with 10^5 to 10^7 organisms per gram of faeces. Carriage of salmonellae, other than typhoid or paratyphoid bacilli, for more than 6 months is rare.

FOCAL INFECTION

Focal infections may be very difficult to diagnose because they may only manifest themselves long after an episode of enteritis—or the original bowel infection may even have been silent. They have a tendency to chronicity and can mimic tuberculosis, particularly in cases of osteomyelitis of a vertebra or paravertebral abscess. Salmonella osteomyelitis and arthritis are strongly associated with sickle-cell anaemia (see Section 22). Salmonella abscess may develop in the liver, gallbladder, spleen, psoas muscle, uterus (after septic abortion), and in the peritoneal cavity (e.g. subphrenic, pelvic). Patients with deep-seated salmonella infection who remain untreated suffer high mortality.

Laboratory diagnosis

A definitive diagnosis must depend on the isolation of the infecting organism, for salmonella enteritis cannot be distinguished from other forms of enteritis on clinical grounds alone. The culture of salmonellae in the laboratory is a sensitive procedure that allows the detection of small numbers of organisms, even when greatly outnumbered by other bacteria. Identification of serotypes can only be done in specialist reference laboratories possessing a full set of antisera, but most clinical laboratories are able to narrow identification down to a short-list by the use of restricted sets of antisera available commercially. Some reference laboratories offer strain identification of *S. typhimurium, S. enteritidis*, and other common serotypes by phage-typing techniques. Patients produce antibody to their infecting strain during convalescence, but this is seldom of diagnostic value. Strains antigenically related to the typhoid and paratyphoid bacilli will cause the Widal test to become partly positive.

Antimicrobial chemotherapy

Aspects of treatment, in this chapter, are confined to antimicrobial chemotherapy, as fluid and electrolyte replacement, which is the mainstay of treatment for most infective diarrhoeas, is discussed elsewhere (see Chapter 14.2.4).

Antimicrobial therapy of salmonella enteritis should be reserved for more severely affected patients and sometimes patients who are part of an institutional outbreak, in order to reduce the excretion and spread of salmonellae. It is essential for invasive and focal disease, which may require full dosage of the agent to be given for several weeks, as invasive infection due to salmonellae other than typhoid and paratyphoid bacilli tends to be refractory. Laboratory control is necessary, owing to the ever-increasing rates of antimicrobial resistance among salmonellae. Chloramphenicol, cotrimoxazole, tetracyclines, and ampicillin are traditional agents, but fluoroquinolones, notably ciprofloxacin, have proved to be at least as effective and are arguably the agents of choice. Ciprofloxacin has been used with remarkable success to eradicate salmonellae from chronic carriers, including those with *S. typhi*, after other treatments have failed, probably because it is concentrated in bile and mucus. Resistance to ciprofloxacin (and other quinolones) developing during treatment has been reported, which emphasizes the need for close laboratory control.

Prevention and control

The correct hygienic preparation, handling, and storage of food effectively prevents salmonella infection, but lapses are inevitable. The most common fault is a failure to appreciate that the briefest contact between a raw animal product and other foods can be enough to initiate an outbreak of food poisoning; strict separation of the two is the only answer.

Ideally, animal products should be salmonella free, but this is far from the case. Methods of animal husbandry, slaughtering, processing, marketing, and policies for the safe disposal of animal and human waste are all reflected in the incidence of infection in man. Examples of control measures in animals are the compulsory heat treatment of imported and recycled animal feeds, and the competitive exclusion of salmonellae from chicks by dosing with normal gut flora. There should be severe restriction on the use of antimicrobial agents in animal rearing, particularly those that are especially valuable for treating human disease, such as chloramphenicol and the fluoroquinolones. Terminal disinfection of poultry carcasses by irradiation would eliminate all pathogens including salmonellae, but it has a bad public image. This may change, just as there was initial opposition to the pasteurization of milk, a measure of unquestioned value that has prevented countless infections.

Shigella infections: bacillary dysentery

The genus (Shigella) takes its name from a Japanese, Kiyoshi Shiga, who in 1897 was the first to recognize an association between a certain type of Gram-negative bacillus and epidemic dysentery. The organism became known as *Shigella shigae* or Shiga's bacillus (now *Shigella dysenteriae* type 1). This organism remains the most virulent of the shigellae, and it was probably the cause of much of the severe dysentery that ravaged the soldiers of the Crimean war and American civil war. A contemporary writer estimated that in the latter war nearly 2 million American soldiers suffered an attack of dysentery or enteritis and 44 000 died—a mortality rate of 2.5 per cent. After a gradual decline during the early part of this century, this organism re-emerged in the late 1960s as a cause of epidemic dysentery in Central America, Mexico, and the Indian subcontinent. In Nicaragua there were an estimated 13 000 deaths in 1 year, and in Guatemala the monthly death rate reached a peak of 11 000. The situation was aggravated by the appearance in these epidemics of strains with multiple antibiotic resistance, including resistance to chloramphenicol.

Soon after the publication of Shiga's work, Flexner described a similar dysentery bacillus (*Sh. flexneri*), and in 1915 a Dane, Sonne, described a third type (*Sh. sonnei*). The most recently described member of the genus (*Sh. boydii*) is named after Boyd, who published his work in the 1930s. Thus there are four groups of dysentery bacilli, which are differentiated according to biochemical reactions and antigenic structure:

- Group A *Sh. dysenteriae* Does not ferment mannitol. Ten serotypes: only type 1 ('*Sh. shigae*') and type 2 ('*Sh. schmitzi*') are important human pathogens.
- Group B *Sh. flexneri* 13 serotypes and subtypes.
- Group C *Sh. boydii* 15 serotypes.
- Group D *Sh. sonnei* Serologically homogenous, but strains may be differentiated by phage and colicine typing methods.

Most shigellae, like the salmonellae, are non-lactose fermenters (*Sh. sonnei* ferments lactose late), but they are unusual among the enterobacteria in being non-motile and, with one minor exception, they are anaerogenic, that is, they do not produce gas from sugars. *Sh. sonnei* is the least pathogenic and usually causes only minor illness. *Sh. flexneri* and *Sh. boydii* are of intermediate pathogenicity.

Epidemiology

Sh. dysenteriae type 1 is the only shigella capable of causing major epidemics of infection. It thrives under conditions of poverty, overcrowding, and squalor, particularly where there are no proper means of sewage disposal, hence its emergence in times of war and deprivation. It is not endemic in industrialized countries. *Sh. flexneri* occurs worldwide but it is most prevalent in developing countries, as is the less common *Sh. boydii*. Shigellosis differs from other common diarrhoeal diseases of the developing world in that it affects older children and sometimes adults rather than infants.

In Britain and Europe during the 1920s flexner and sonne dysentery were of about equal prevalence, but the former gradually faded and since the Second World War *Sh. sonnei* has accounted for almost all endemic dysentery in these areas. Most infections are in children attending infant and primary schools, but outbreaks in residential institutions such as military barracks also occur. Similar trends have been observed in the United States.

SOURCES AND TRANSMISSION

Unlike salmonellae, shigellae are only found naturally in man and certain non-human primates. Shigellosis is also the most communicable of all bacterial infections of the gut. The infective dose is small. In volunteer studies, dysentery has been produced by as few as 10 to 100 bacteria.

The principal route of transmission is from person to person by the direct faecal–oral spread of bacteria, mainly via the fingers. Apart from the obvious contaminating action of touching or scratching the anal area, or not washing one's hands after defaecation, infective doses of bacteria can be picked up by touching contaminated lavatory seats, flushing handles, taps, door knobs, roller towels, and other objects. Shigellae can survive on the fingers for several hours. Patients are most infectious when their stools are fluid, for not only are organisms present in abundance, but there is greater opportunity for them to be spread by splashing. Non-syphonic water closets containing liquid faeces have been shown to generate bacteria-carrying aerosols that cause widespread contamination of the environment. Cold, dark, damp conditions favour prolonged survival of shigellae deposited on hard surfaces in this way, and under such conditions organisms have been shown to survive for at least 17 days on wooden lavatory seats.

Contaminated fingers easily transfer bacteria to food and drink, which act as a passive vehicles of infection—shigellae do not have to multiply in food to cause infection. Thus the greatest risk is from foods that are most handled during preparation, such as salads, sandwiches, and fruit.

Occasionally, large outbreaks have arisen through the faecal pollution of water supplies. In countries that experience regular flooding, simultaneous increases in dysentery have been observed. Flies can transmit infection from exposed human faeces. The incidence of dysentery tends to parallel fly activity and in one study fly control reduced shigellosis by 85 per cent.

Pathology

The cardinal pathogenic feature of shigellae is their ability to invade and multiply in epithelial cells, which is dependent on the presence of a large plasmid encoding for certain surface proteins. The classic test for invasion is the Sereny test, in which bacteria are instilled into the eye of a guinea-pig, which is then examined for the onset of conjunctivitis, but tissue culture methods have largely replaced it. *Sh. dysenteriae* type 1 produces a powerful exotoxin (Shiga toxin), which is associated with the haemolytic uraemic syndrome, but what other part it plays in the disease process is unclear.

Colonization initially takes place in the jejunum and upper ileum, which usually gives rise to secretory diarrhoea, probably through the action of an enterotoxin. However, the characteristic pathology produced by shigellae is an acute, locally invasive colitis. This ranges from mild, catarrhal inflammation of the mucous membrane of the rectum and sigmoid colon, typical of *Sh. sonnei* infections, to severe, necrotizing lesions affecting the whole colon and sometimes the terminal ileum, such as are seen in the worst forms of *Sh. dysenteriae* type 1 infection. Shigellae penetrate and multiply in the epithelial cells of the colon, invade the mucosa, and may penetrate deep to the lamina propria or even the muscularis mucosae. Yet bacteraemia is rare and virtually limited to patients with immune deficiency. In severe cases the colon may be so damaged that healing can only be effected by fibrosis, which may culminate in stenosis.

Local mucosal changes consist of oedema, capillary engorgement, and leucocyte infiltration. Small haemorrhages are common and the submucous veins may be engorged or thrombosed. The mucous membrane becomes intensely red and blood-stained mucus may be present. In the most severe forms of the disease, areas of mucosa undergo coagulation necrosis, which appear as thickened, semirigid, greyish patches. These eventually separate to leave raw, ulcerated areas that may ultimately fibrose and cause stenosis. Haemorrhage and perforation may also result from such lesions. Extensive lesions lead to much protein loss, which adds to the severe debility that accompanies these infections. The active agent in this process is thought to be the somatic antigen of the organism (i.e., endotoxin).

Clinical features

The incubation period is short, usually 2 to 3 days, but exceptionally it may be as long as a week. The illness usually starts with abdominal colic and watery diarrhoea. In many *Sh. sonnei* infections this is the only feature and there is spontaneous resolution without constitutional symptoms. In the more severe forms of shigellosis, diarrhoea is accompanied by fever, headache, and malaise. After 1 to 3 days the diarrhoea gives way to the passage of small amounts of blood-stained mucus ('redcurrant jelly') and pus, with abdominal cramps and tenesmus—the classic dysenteric syndrome. In severe forms of the disease the sequence is telescoped so that bloody, mucoid stools are passed from the outset. The patient becomes toxic and restless, the pulse rapid and feeble, and there is a risk of death from circulatory failure or haemolytic uraemic syndrome. Recovery in such cases is invariably slow and some patients continue with chronic or relapsing infection resembling ulcerative colitis. Exacerbation of haemorrhoids and rectal prolapse may result from rectal oedema and straining at stool.

Children may show striking meningism, which can be misleading if it occurs before the onset of diarrhoea—and embarrassing if the first liquid stool arrives forcefully in the bed during the performance of a lumbar puncture. Shigellosis in children may also be associated with appendicitis. Occasionally, intussusception is a complication in infants. Shigellae can also cause vaginitis in children and, as the infection may arise without any obvious history of diarrhoea, it can easily pass unrecognized.

Children in developing countries may develop anorexia with nutritional deterioration, protein-losing enteropathy, or intercurrent infection after an attack of dysentery, especially if it follows measles or there is pre-existing malnutrition.

Reactive arthritis, Reiter's syndrome, purulent keratoconjunctivitis, and neuritis are uncommon late complications of infection with any of the shigellae.

Shigellae are usually excreted in the faeces for a few weeks after the illness; about 10 per cent of patients excrete them for more than 10 weeks. Prolonged excretion tends to be common in young children.

Laboratory diagnosis

Isolation in culture remains the standard method for detecting shigellae. They are delicate bacteria that perish in acid conditions, so it is necessary to refrigerate specimens or place them in buffered transport medium if there is to be a delay of more than a few hours before they are delivered to the laboratory.

Antimicrobial chemotherapy

Although antimicrobial therapy is seldom needed for *Sh. sonnei* and other mild forms of shigellosis, it is the mainstay of treatment for severe shigellosis due to *Sh. dysenteriae* type 1 and some *Sh. flexneri* and *Sh. boydii* infections. Laboratory control should always be sought, as strains showing multiple antimicrobial resistance are common, especially in developing countries. Suppression of the normal microbial flora by inappropriate antimicrobial therapy can exacerbate the infection and increase the risk of haemolytic uraemic syndrome.

Co-trimoxazole and ampicillin have for many years been the drugs of choice for shigellosis, but most strains are now resistant; many are also resistant to tetracycline and chloramphenicol. Nalidixic acid is effective and cheap, but high resistance rates have arisen where the drug has been used intensively. Resistance to ciprofloxacin, which is 100 times more active against shigellae than nalidixic acid, is currently uncommon. A single dose of 1 g is effective in adults infected with shigellae other than *Sh. dysenteriae* type 1, but up to 10 doses are required for infections with the latter type. The treatment of children with antibiotic-resistant shigella infection is difficult, as quinolones are potentially toxic for children. A short course of a fluoroquinolone could reasonably be given to severely affected children, but parenteral ceftriaxone (50 mg/kg per day for 5 days) and pivmecillinam are alternatives that have been used successfully.

Table 1 *The major groups of* Escherichia coli *causing diarrhoea in man*

Pathogenicity group	Pathogenicity factor or marker	Commonly found serogroups	Associated disease
Enteroadherent *E. coli* (EAEC)	Locally adherent* (enteropathogenic *E. coli*—EPEC)	O55, O86, O111, O114, O119, O125, O126, O127, O128, O142	Watery diarrhoea, mainly in children
	Diffusely adherent*	Various	Controversial
	Aggregatively adherent*	Various	Acute and persistent diarrhoea in children
Enterotoxigenic *E. coli* (ETEC)	Heat-labile toxin (LT), or heat-stable toxin (ST), or both	O6, O8, O15, O25, O27, O63, O78, O115, O148, O153, O159, O167	Watery diarrhoea in children in developing world; travellers' diarrhoea
Vero cytotoxin-producing *E. coli* (VTEC) (Syn. enterohaemorrhagic *E. coli* (EHEC)	Shiga-like toxins: VT1 (SLTI) VT2 (SLTII)	O157, (O26)	Haemorrhagic colitis; haemolytic uraemic syndrome
Enteroinvasive *E. coli* (EIEC)	Cell invasion like shigellae	O28ac, O112ac, O124, O136, O143, O144, O152, O164	Shigella-like dysentery

*See text.

Prevention and control

The safe disposal of excreta, provision of purified water, and control of flies are fundamental to the control of shigellosis. Where these are lacking, the incidence can be reduced by the promotion of personal and domestic hygiene, notably hand washing after defaecation and before handling food. Unpurified water can be made safe by the addition of hypochlorite tablets; salads and fruit can be disinfected by soaking in water containing 80 parts/10^6 of free chlorine. Breast feeding substantially increases resistance to infection in children, and oral vaccines for use in developing countries are being developed.

Outbreaks of sonne dysentery in schools are difficult to control, but measures should be aimed at preventing spread by the hands. Supervised washing and disinfection of hands after defaecation, and frequent disinfection of lavatory seats, taps, and door knobs are effective if rigorously applied. Only disposable hand towels should be provided. It is impracticable to detect and exclude all children excreting shigellae, so exclusion should be limited to those suffering from diarrhoea, regardless of whether they are known to be infected.

Food handlers who are suffering from dysentery should be excluded from work until they have produced at least three consecutive negative stool samples taken not less than 24 h apart and at least 2 days after cessation of any antimicrobial chemotherapy.

Escherichia coli *infections*

Although most strains of *E. coli* are commensals of the intestinal tract, some have acquired virulence factors that have placed them among the leading causes of diarrhoea, particularly in the developing world. The concept that *E. coli*, the common coliform bacillus, might be capable of causing enteritis is not a recent one. In 1895 the German paediatrician, Escherich, suspected that certain strains of '*Bacterium coli*' caused infantile diarrhoea, but attempts to differentiate pathogenic from non-pathogenic strains were unsuccessful, mainly because adequate serological classification was not available at the time. It was not until the development of Kauffman's serotyping system some 50 years later that progress could be made. It was then noticed that strains of *E. coli* that had been associated with several outbreaks of infantile gastroenteritis studied in Britain between 1945 and 1949 belonged to two serotypes (O111:B4 and O55:B5). Other gastroenteritis-associated serotypes were soon discovered and the group became known as enteropathogenic *E. coli* (**EPEC**). After 1970, several other major pathogenic groups were identified. They are difficult to classify, owing to the complexity of their virulence factors and the tests required to detect them. The following account is necessarily a simplified one.

Enteropathogenic (EPEC) and enteroadherent E. coli *(EAEC)*

We now know that the virulence marker for the classic EPEC strains is the ability to adhere to HEp-2 cells in tissue culture. As they are not the only *E. coli* strains to do this, they form part of a larger group recently named enteroadherent *E. coli* (EAEC). The term EPEC will probably fall into disuse, but its familiarity is such that this will not happen quickly. There are three distinct patterns of adherence to Hep-2 cells:

- locally adherent (bacteria in tight clusters);
- diffusely adherent (bacteria scattered);
- aggregatively adherent (bacteria stacked like bricks).

The locally adherent group is made up of most of the classic EPEC strains (Table 1) but also other strains. Electron microscopy shows that the characteristic lesion of locally adherent *E. coli* in the ileum is an 'attaching and effacing' lesion in the brush-border microvillous membrane. There is intimate contact of the bacterial cell with cup-like projections of enterocytes known as 'pedestals', the formation of dense bundles of microfilaments, and destruction of microvilli. Macroscopically there is nothing to see.

Diffusely adherent *E. coli* are of uncertain pathogenicity. Limited studies have linked aggregatively adherent *E. coli* with acute, sometimes bloody, diarrhoea and persistent diarrhoea in children in developing countries.

EPIDEMIOLOGY

EPEC strains are most important as a cause of endemic diarrhoea in developing countries, where they mainly affect children of 6 to 18 months of age. In developed countries, EPEC infection has declined to low levels over the last 20 or so years. In Britain, EPEC were probably the cause of outbreaks of 'summer diarrhoea' that were common in the nineteenth and early twentieth centuries, and in the 1940s and 1950s they were a major cause of outbreaks in hospitals and day nurseries, in which fatalities of up to 50 per cent were recorded.

CLINICAL FEATURES

The incubation period is usually 1 or 2 days, but with a large inoculating dose it may be as short as 8 h. As with salmonellae the infective dose is high, in the order of 10^5 to 10^{10} organisms. The onset of diarrhoea may be abrupt or gradual, with a tendency for cases with an abrupt onset to be more ill than the others. Stools become loose and green, then orange coloured, and eventually watery. Vomiting is common in more severely affected children and it may be projectile. The combination of watery diarrhoea and vomiting quickly leads to dehydration. The child is at first irritable, may have convulsions, and the temperature rises to 39 to 40 °C. In the absence of prompt fluid replacement, dehydration and metabolic disturbances may become irreversible and the child becomes apathetic and dies. But the disease may be mild and marked only by the passage of a few loose stools without vomiting or general illness; this is the usual pattern in Britain at present. Occasionally the loose stools persist for days or even weeks, but beyond this time it becomes increasingly likely that other factors are involved.

LABORATORY DIAGNOSIS

Cultural methods are currently the only practicable way of detecting EPEC in clinical laboratories. As EPEC colonies look like any other *E. coli* colonies on a culture plate, reliance is placed on testing individual colonies for agglutination in antisera prepared against the common EPEC O serogroups. The method is a blunt one, as not all strains belonging to those serogroups are EPEC, and some EAEC strains belong to serogroups other than the classic ones. Interpretation of cultures is helped by the fact that in EPEC gastroenteritis the infecting strain is predominant and present in almost pure culture. Ideally one would test for adherence, as this is the true marker for pathogenicity. There is a good fluorescence test that detects filamentous actin in the microfilament bundles formed during attachment of EPEC and EAEC to Hep-2 cells (FAS test), but when one has to test several colonies from every culture plate, it becomes impracticable for routine use. As it is, the routine screening of colonies with antisera has to be restricted to samples from children below the age of 2 or 3 years, despite the fact that EPEC diarrhoea occasionally affects adults.

TREATMENT AND PREVENTION

Because the main danger to an infant with EPEC gastroenteritis is dehydration, the most urgent need is to replace fluid and electrolyte loss. Infants may require parenteral fluids. The use of antimicrobial therapy is not generally advocated, but some believe it should be used for children with protracted secretory diarrhoea where there is histological evidence of severe enteropathy.

Measures taken to prevent infection are the same as those for shigellosis. Infection is highly contagious among neonatal infants.

Enterotoxigenic E. coli *(ETEC)*

In 1968 a study of an epidemic of diarrhoea in British troops travelling to South Arabia showed that a single type of *E. coli* (O148:H28) was present in about half the cases. It was later shown to produce a cholera-like enterotoxin. Thus began the story of ETEC—and an important one it is. ETEC are a leading cause of childhood diarrhoea in developing countries and they are the most common cause of traveller's diarrhoea or 'turista'. They are uncommon in temperate regions where hygiene is good, but they have caused outbreaks of infection from contaminated water supplies, including outbreaks on cruise ships. Human beings appear to be the major source of ETEC.

PATHOGENESIS

ETEC are non-invasive, but produce diarrhoea through the action of one or both of two enterotoxins: a heat-labile (**LT**) and heat-stable (**ST**) toxin. LT is a protein related to *Vibrio cholerae* O1 enterotoxin, and like that toxin it causes an outpouring of fluid and electrolytes by activating adenylate cyclase in enterocytes. ST is a peptide that has much the same effect but through activation of guanylate cyclase. These toxins can only exert their effect after the bacteria have adhered to the bowel epithelium by means of host-specific adhesins. For this reason, strains that cause disease in, say, pigs do not do so in man. The dose of bacteria needed to cause disease is large, about 10^8 to 10^{10}.

CLINICAL FEATURES

The incubation period ranges from 1 to 3 days, depending on the size of infecting dose; the period is shorter for strains that only produce ST. The illness consists of watery diarrhoea with abdominal cramps, nausea and sometimes vomiting, seldom lasting for more than 3 days. Severe attacks resemble cholera, with the passage of 'rice-water' stools.

LABORATORY DIAGNOSIS

There is no easy way to detect ETEC in faeces. Standard tests require a search for both LT and ST in the supernatants of broth cultures. LT is usually detected in tissue cultures, ST in suckling mice. There are immunological tests (enzyme-linked immunosorbent assay; radioimmunoassay), mainly for LT, and a simpler precipitin test for LT that can be applied directly to colonies on a culture plate. Although the genetic determinants for enterotoxins are carried on transferable plasmids, ETEC strains fall within a limited range of O serogroups, which are mostly distinct from EAEC serogroups (Table 1). However, the correlation between serogroup and toxigenicity is too imprecise for serogrouping to be of great value. The best approach is to use genetic probes, which can detect genes coding for LT or ST directly in faeces, and even in food and water, but at present the method is too technically complex to be used in clinical laboratories.

Because none of these tests can be made routinely, it is vital that clinicians inform the laboratory if a patient's circumstances make it likely he or she has ETEC infection, so that special tests can be set up.

TREATMENT AND PREVENTION

Fluid and electrolyte replacement is usually all that is required for ETEC diarrhoea as it is of such short duration. Several antimicrobial agents (e.g. co-trimoxazole or trimethoprim), when taken prophylactically, reduce the incidence of ETEC diarrhoea in travellers to endemic areas, but drug toxicity and promotion of drug resistance in other pathogenic organisms are disadvantages. Bismuth subsalicylate inhibits the action of enterotoxins, and travellers taking it prophylactically suffer less diarrhoea than controls. The best way to prevent 'turista' is to avoid uncooked foods, especially salads, untreated water, and ice in drinks.

Vero cytotoxin-producing E. coli *(VTEC)*

These strains, so called because they produce irreversible cytopathic changes in African vervet monkey kidney (Vero) cells, were first described in Canada in 1977. A few years later they were linked unequivocally with human disease: toxigenic strains were found in two groups of people in the United States who developed haemorrhagic colitis after eating a specific brand of beef 'patty', and in 8 of 15 children with haemolytic uraemic syndrome in Canada, two of whom died. VTEC are now the chief single cause of acute renal failure in children in the United Kingdom and North America. Because of their association with haemorrhagic colitis they are also known as enterohaemorrhagic *E. coli* (EHEC).

VTEC produce two sorts of Vero cytotoxin (**VT**): VT1 is closely similar to Shiga toxin of *Sh. dysenteriae* type 1 and is neutralized by antiShiga toxin; VT2 is not neutralized by the antitoxin. These toxins are also known as Shiga-like toxins (SLTI and SLTII). At least three-quarters of the VTEC strains causing human disease belong to serogroup O157, mostly O157:H7.

The incidence of human VTEC infection is highest in summer

months. In North America the main identified source of VTEC is dairy cattle, but VTEC have also been found in pigs. Elsewhere information is incomplete. Beef products, raw milk, and an unchlorinated water supply have been incriminated as sources in outbreaks, but infection can also be passed from person to person.

CLINICAL FEATURES

The clinical picture of VTEC infection is one of crampy abdominal pain and bloody diarrhoea with little or no fever. The diarrhoea is usually watery at first and in mild cases remains so. Haemolytic uraemic syndrome may set in anything from 2 to 14 days (mean 7 days) after onset of illness, particularly in children and old patients. In the United Kingdom the mortality from haemolytic uraemic syndrome in children has been placed at 2 to 10 per cent and the rate of permanent sequelae 15 per cent. Rarely, the syndrome arises without the prodromal haemorrhagic colitis.

LABORATORY DIAGNOSIS

The ideal approach is to use DNA probes to detect genes encoding for VT1 and VT2 in faeces and isolated colonies, but this is too complex and costly for use in clinical laboratories. A compromise is to culture faeces on sorbitol MacConkey agar, on which *E. coli* O157 colonies appear pale because of their inability to ferment sorbitol, unlike conventional strains of *E. coli*. Pale colonies are then tested for agglutination in O157 antiserum. The disadvantages are that the proportion of VTEC in faecal flora may be low and the method does not detect VTEC of other serogroups, but it is currently the only practicable front line test.

Another feature of VTEC infection is that the bacteria disappear from the stools rapidly; they can be found in only about one-third of patients one week after onset of illness. Serological tests that detect antibody to either VT or the lipopolysaccharide of O157 are valuable, especially for retrospective diagnosis in patients who present late with haemolytic uraemic syndrome.

TREATMENT

The most important element in treatment is to watch for signs of haemolytic uraemic syndrome, so that the patient can be given the necessary supportive treatment at the earliest opportunity should the complication arise. There is no clear evidence of the efficacy of antimicrobial agents, either to reduce acute symptoms or reduce the risk of the syndrome arising. However, there is convincing evidence that the risk of haemolytic uraemic syndrome is increased by taking antimotility agents.

Enteroinvasive E. coli *(EIEC)*

These strains are similar to shigellae both culturally and in their pathogenicity. They give a positive Sereny test, invade HeLa cells, and cause bacillary dysentery. It is estimated that about 5 per cent of all diarrhoea in areas with poor hygiene is due to EIEC. As with shigellae, most infections are in older children and adults. Occasional foodborne outbreaks have arisen in developed countries, mainly in residential institutions. EIEC belong to a limited number of serogroups, the most common being O124 (Table 1). In the laboratory they tend to be provisionally identified as shigellae (they ferment lactose late) until more detailed tests show their true identity.

Miscellaneous enteropathogenic and food poisoning bacteria

Campylobacter infections

The name Campylobacter (Greek, curved rod) was coined by French workers in 1963 for a group of small, curved or spiral, microaerophilic Gram-negative bacteria formerly classified as vibrios. They now form part of a unique superfamily of spiral bacteria comprising Campylobacter, Arcobacter, Wolinella, Helicobacter, and 'Flexispira'. Campylobacters have a single flagellum at one or both poles of the bacterial cell, which gives them a characteristic, rapid darting motility (Fig. 1). The type species, *Campylobacter fetus* (originally *Vibrio fetus*), was first isolated in England in 1906 from aborted sheep fetuses. Soon afterwards it was recognized as a major cause of infectious abortion in cattle and sheep, but it was not until the 1970s that *C. jejuni* and *C. coli* (collectively *C. fetus* subsp. *jejuni* in obsolete American nomenclature) were recognized as a common cause of acute enteritis in man. Special selective techniques are required for their isolation from faeces and this is why they went undetected for so long. *C. fetus* occasionally infects man, but only as an uncommon opportunist causing systemic infection, sometimes with diarrhoea, in patients with immune deficiency or a serious underlying disease.

Well over 100 serotypes of *C. jejuni* and *C. coli* have been defined according to two classes of antigen: heat-stable O (lipopolysaccharide) antigens, and heat-labile surface and flagellar protein antigens. The most widely used typing schemes for these two classes of antigen are, respectively, those of Penner and Lior.

Several other campylobacters and related bacteria are associated with infection of the human intestinal tract. *C. lari* (*laridis*) accounts for about 0.1 per cent of all cases of campylobacter enteritis. *C. upsaliensis*, *C. hyointestinalis*, and *Arcobacter butzleri* are only isolated regularly from children with diarrhoea in developing countries, although *A. butzleri* was implicated in an outbreak of abdominal pain, without diarrhoea, in an Italian school. *Helicobacter cinaedi* and *H. fennelliae* are associated with proctitis in homosexual men.

Epidemiology

Campylobacter enteritis is the most common bacterial infection of the gut in industrialized countries. In the United Kingdom some 44 000 infections were reported in 1993, representing an incidence of 80/100 000. In temperate zones there is a remarkably consistent and unexplained rise of incidence in early summer. In developed countries, campylobacter enteritis affects people of all ages, especially young adults, but in developing countries the infection is almost entirely confined to children below the age of 2 to 3 years, for by this time they have become immune through repeated exposure.

Like salmonellosis, campylobacter enteritis is a zoonosis. Campylobacters are found in a wide variety of warm-blooded animals, especially birds, in which they form part of the normal intestinal flora. Pigs are the main host of *C. coli*. Infection may be acquired by direct contact with infected animals. This may be occupational, as in the case of farmers, slaughtermen, and poultry processors, or domestic, where the usual source is a pet puppy or kitten with campylobacter diarrhoea. But more often infection is transmitted indirectly via contaminated meat, milk, and water. The consumption of raw or barbecued meats, especially chicken, carries a distinct risk of infection.

Broiler chickens are the most prolific source of campylobacters. Retailed chicken carcasses are almost universally contaminated, so self-infection when handling them in the kitchen, or cross-contamination to

Fig. 1 Electron micrograph of a campylobacter (× 6650). (By courtesy of Mr D.R. Purdham.)

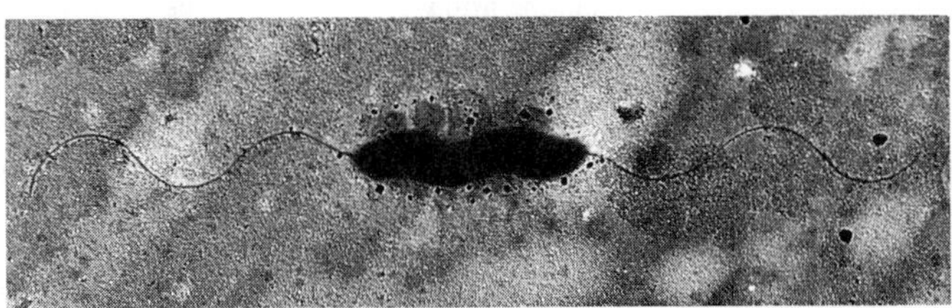

other foods readily occurs if good hygienic practice is not observed. Campylobacters do not multiply in food like salmonellae; the infective dose is small enough for the food to act as a simple vehicle, just as it does for shigellae. Cases of foodborne infection therefore tend to be sporadic, or in small family outbreaks, rather than in the form of explosive outbreaks as in salmonella food poisoning. However, major outbreaks affecting as many as 3000 people have been caused by the consumption of contaminated raw milk or untreated water.

The ubiquitous nature of campylobacters makes it difficult to pinpoint the sources of sporadic infections. There are probably many routes of infection still to be discovered. For example, it was recently found that in certain areas of Britain in early summer, infection was caused by wild birds (magpies and jackdaws) pecking the caps and contaminating the contents of doorstep-delivered milk bottles.

In general the infectivity of campylobacters is low, probably because they cannot withstand drying. Secondary cases are unusual in common-source outbreaks. The only human sources of consequence are toddlers with diarrhoea. Food handlers who are healthy excreters are a negligible risk provided they wash their hands after defaecation.

Pathology

The spiral nature of campylobacters enables them to penetrate, colonize, and migrate in the mucus covering the intestinal epithelium in a way that conventional bacteria cannot. Infection starts in the upper small intestine, but it progresses distally to affect the terminal ileum and the colon in most cases. There is an acute inflammatory response, with crypt abscess formation in the mucosa indistinguishable from that caused by salmonellae. This, and the presence of mesenteric adenitis, suggest that campylobacters invade the mucosa.

Bacteraemia is detected in only 0.1 to 0.2 per cent of infections, but this figure probably underestimates the true incidence, as blood cultures are seldom taken from patients with acute diarrhoea, particularly early in the disease.

Many strains produce a cholera-like enterotoxin and/or a Vero cytotoxin *in vitro*, but their role in the pathogenesis of the disease is unclear.

Specific antibodies to the infecting strain appear in patients' blood from about the fifth day and remain detectable for several months.

Clinical features

After an incubation period of 2 to 7 days (mean 3 days) the illness starts either with abdominal pain and diarrhoea, or with a prodromal period of fever, headache, and other influenza-like symptoms that precedes the diarrhoea by a few hours to a few days. A fever of 40 °C or more is not unusual and it may be associated with convulsions in children and delirium in adults. Vomiting is not a conspicuous feature of the disease, though nausea is usual. Abdominal pain tends to be more severe than in other forms of acute infective diarrhoea and it can be of a type and severity that suggests acute appendicitis (see below). Inflammatory cellular exudate can be detected microscopically in the stools of most patients and after a day or two frank blood may appear. Severe diarrhoea seldom lasts more than 2 or 3 days, but loose stools and abdominal pain may persist for a while and patients feel washed out and wretched. A brief relapse is not uncommon at this point. Death is rare and usually due to some associated disorder. Chronic disease or carriage of the bacteria in immunocompetent subjects has not been reported; most patients are culture negative by about the fifth week.

MISLEADING PRESENTATIONS AND COMPLICATIONS

Suspected appendicitis, particularly in older children and young adults, is the main reason for the admission of patients with campylobacter enteritis to hospital. If laparotomy is done, the usual findings are an inflamed, oedematous ileum and enlarged, fleshy mesenteric lymph nodes, but occasionally there is genuine appendicitis. In uncomplicated enteritis, abdominal tenderness may be present, but not the true signs of acute peritonitis.

Some patients may present with the symptoms and sigmoidoscopic appearances of acute ulcerative colitis. The danger here is that they might be given steroids rather than antibiotics. On the other hand, campylobacter infection sometimes exacerbates pre-existing inflammatory bowel disease and both conditions have to be treated.

Campylobacter infection can also mimic intussusception in infants, who tend to pass bloodstained motions without obvious diarrhoea. Several cases of cholecystitis have been reported and biliary tract infection has probably been the cause of rare instances of pancreatitis and hepatitis. Other rare complications are gastrointestinal haemorrhage, haemolytic uraemic syndrome, glomerulonephritis, and rashes in the form of urticaria and erythema nodosum.

There are two important late complications that arise 1 to 3 weeks after the onset of enteritis: reactive arthritis and Guillain–Barré syndrome (acute idiopathic polyneuropathy). The reactive arthritis is no different from that seen after other forms of acute bacterial diarrhoea. Its incidence has been estimated at about 1 per cent of all cases. Guillain–Barré syndrome is much less frequent but more serious. Measurements of the proportion of Guillain–Barré syndrome associated with campylobacter infection range from 14 to 38 per cent—the largest known 'cause'. Moreover, recent Japanese studies have shown a striking preponderance of strains of *C. jejuni* serogroup O19 (Penner) among cases of Guillain–Barré syndrome associated with campylobacters, which is all the more significant as strains of this serogroup are found in less than 2 per cent of intestinal infections.

Laboratory diagnosis

A definitive diagnosis can only be made in the laboratory, as the disease cannot be distinguished clinically from other forms of bacterial diarrhoea. The isolation of campylobacters is not difficult but it requires special media and atmospheric conditions. The precautions taken to preserve the viability of shigellae in faecal samples apply equally to campylobacters, for they are at least as perishable. Campylobacters are sufficiently abundant in freshly voided diarrhoea stools to be seen microscopically in wet or stained smears. Although not as sensitive as culture, the method can give a quick answer in cases where, for example, surgery is contemplated.

A retrospective diagnosis can be made serologically in culture-negative patients who have a suspected late complication such as reactive arthritis.

Antimicrobial chemotherapy

Although several commonly used antibiotics, notably erythromycin, are active against campylobacters, they are of limited value because patients are usually recovering by the time a bacteriological diagnosis is made, which is usually 5 to 6 days into the illness. Thus, in trials of antibiotic treatment, campylobacters have been cleared from the stools, but patients have only shown clinical benefit if treatment was started when they first sought medical help, that is, before bacteriological diagnosis. A reasonable policy is to give a short course of an appropriate antimicrobial agent is a patient is still acutely ill when the diagnosis is made.

Erythromycin is the drug of first choice. A suitable regimen is erythromycin stearate, 500 mg twice daily for 5 days for adults, or erythromycin ethyl succinate, 40 mg/kg per day for children. In most places, erythromycin resistance rates have remained at less than 5 per cent; most erythromycin-resistant strains are *C. coli.* Tetracycline is an alternative but resistance rates of 5 to 25 per cent have been reported. Ciprofloxacin is very effective against campylobacters, but resistance can develop during treatment. Ciprofloxacin resistance of 11 to 50 per cent has been reported in countries where enrofloxacin has been extensively used in poultry. Gentamicin is recommended for rare, life-threatening infections. It should be noted that campylobacters are naturally resistant to almost all cephalosporins and partially resistant to ampicillin.

Prevention and control

As campylobacters and salmonellae share the same food-producing animal hosts, the measures taken to control salmonellosis also apply to campylobacters. Much remains to be done to unravel the epidemiology of campylobacter carriage in broilers, so that measures can be devised for reducing the present excessively high contamination rates. In the meantime, reliance must be placed on promoting good hygienic practice in food handling and preparation. Raw milk and untreated water should not be consumed.

Non-cholera vibrios and vibrio-like organisms

Vibrios are curved, non-sporing, Gram-negative bacilli possessing a single polar flagellum, which gives them a characteristic rapid darting or oscillating motility—hence the derivation of their name from the Latin, *vibrare*, to shake. Most vibrios live harmlessly in fresh, brackish, or salt water, but a few are pathogenic, notably *Vibrio cholerae* (see Chapter 7.11.11), which is medically by far the most important of the group. Next in importance is *V. parahaemolyticus*, which is described below. *V. fluvialis* is occasionally isolated from patients with watery diarrhoea and vomiting and there are other species of doubtful pathogenicity. *V. vulnificus* is a rare cause of severe septicaemia arising from intestinal infection acquired by eating raw oysters or other sea food. Some vibrios, notably *V. alginolyticus*, cause external otitis in swimmers and infection of wounds exposed to sea or brackish water.

Vibrio parahaemolyticus

This marine organism was first associated with human disease in Japan in 1963, since when it has come to be recognized as the most common cause of food poisoning in that country. Seafood is the main source of the organism, and the high incidence of infection in the Far East is doubtless due to the popularity of raw fish. *V. parahaemolyticus* is most plentiful in warm waters of the world, but it has been isolated from North Atlantic and Pacific coastlines. Food poisoning has been reported from Europe, America, Africa, South-East Asia, and Australia, and in these regions most of the reported infections have followed the consumption of crabs and prawns. The vibrios can survive inside crabs that have been boiled. With shellfish, poisoning is most likely to arise through contamination after cooking, for a few organisms picked up from a working surface contaminated by the raw product can multiply at atmospheric temperatures. This is one reason why the incidence of infection in temperate regions is higher in summer than in winter.

After ingestion, *V. parahaemolyticus* multiplies in the gut and produces an enterotoxin. It is not invasive, nor is toxin preformed in the food before consumption. The incubation period is usually 10 to 20 h but it spans 2 to 48 h. The number of organisms required to cause illness is large and infections are almost always foodborne. Symptoms consist of abdominal colic with watery diarrhoea, sometimes vomiting, and often a mild fever. The illness seldom lasts for more than 1 or 2 days and excretion of the organisms generally ceases within 10 days. Tetracycline shortens the period of excretion, but it is hardly justifiable to use antibiotics for a short, self-limiting disease. Infected patients are not an important source of infection despite the fact that organisms are excreted in enormous numbers while the patient has diarrhoea.

LABORATORY DIAGNOSIS

The marine vibrios grow poorly or not at all on media that are not supplemented with extra salt. Therefore, if the clinician suspects marine food poisoning, the laboratory must be informed so that appropriate methods can be used. The Kanagawa test (β-haemolysis on medium containing human blood) is sometimes done as an indication of pathogenicity: most of the strains associated with diarrhoea are Kanagawa-positive whereas many strains isolated from sea water give a negative test.

Aeromonas and Plesiomonas infection

Aeromonads are ubiquitous in water, soil, and cold-blooded animals; some are major pathogens in fish. Three species are associated with diarrhoeal disease in man, *Aeromonas hydrophila*, *A. sobria*, and *A. caviae*, but probably only a few strains are capable of causing diarrhoea. Several pathogenicity factors, including the production of toxins, have been described. In temperate climates the incidence of aeromonad-associated diarrhoea is 50 to 100 times less than that of salmonella or campylobacter diarrhoea, but infections are more frequent in hot climates and in hot seasons. Thus, most aeromonad infections are encountered in travellers returning from tropical and subtropical regions. Water is thought to be the main vehicle of infection. Lack of evidence of common-source outbreaks or conclusive evidence that aeromonads by themselves cause severe disease lessens their status as enteric pathogens. However, in Western Australia, persistent aeromonad-associated diarrhoea with blood and mucus mimicking ulcerative colitis has been described; these patients were treated successfully with trimethoprim.

Plesiomonas shigelloides is another aquatic vibrio-like organism that is occasionally associated with diarrhoea, usually of a mild nature. It has been implicated in outbreaks of diarrhoea in the Far East and has been isolated from sporadic cases throughout the world. Fewer than 100 cases a year are reported the United Kingdom.

Bacillus cereus

This organism is a member of a large group of Gram-positive, aerobic, spore-forming bacilli of universal distribution. Most of them are of no medical importance, other than as a common cause of food spoilage, but exceptions are the anthrax bacillus (Chapter 7.11.18) and *B. cereus*, which is a closely related species. Under certain circumstances *B. cereus* can cause food poisoning; it can also cause wound sepsis. The fact that it is a sporulating organism means that it can survive harsh physical conditions, which include the temperatures reached in many cooking procedures.

Two patterns of food poisoning are caused by *B. cereus*: one, first described in Norway in 1950, is like clostridial food poisoning (see Chapter 7.11.21) with an incubation period of 8 to 16 h and symptoms of abdominal pain and diarrhoea; the other is like staphylococcal food poisoning with a sudden onset of nausea and vomiting within 1 to 5 h of eating the infected food. The former diarrhoeal type is associated with a wide variety of foods ranging from meat and vegetables to dessert dishes and ice-cream. By contrast, the vomiting type, first recognized in Britain in 1971, is almost exclusively associated with boiled or fried rice from Chinese restaurants or 'take-away' shops. In these cases the rice usually yields counts of *B. cereus* in the range 10^6 to 10^9/g. Such astronomically high counts can arise only if the rice is left for long periods at high ambient temperatures after soaking or boiling. Unfortunately, it is convenient for such establishments to prepare rice in bulk in advance of demand, so that a batch may be kept for 24 h or more before it is used up. Refrigeration is unpopular because chilling tends to cause the rice grains to stick together.

The two patterns of food poisoning are usually caused by different serotypes and the toxins are distinct. The 'diarrhoeal' enterotoxin is an unstable protein with a relative molecular mass of 38 to 46 kDa; it is probably the pyogenic and pyrogenic factor in *B. cereus* wound infections. The 'emetic' toxin is a heat-stable compound, probably a peptide, with M_r of about 10 kDa.

As *B. cereus* food poisoning is an intoxication rather than an infection,

Table 2 *Principal microbial causes of food poisoning outbreaks*

Organism	Mechanism	Incubation period in hours (extreme range)	Main symptom
Salmonella	Infection	12–24 (6–48)	Diarrhoea, 1–7 days
Staphylococcus aureus	Toxin, preformed in food	2–6	Vomiting, 6–24 h
Clostridium perfringens	Toxin, preformed in food, also in gut	8–22	Diarrhoea, 1–2 days
Clostridium botulinum	Toxin, preformed in food	12–36 (2–192)	Neurological
Vibrio parahaemolyticus	Infection	12–18 (2–48)	Diarrhoea, 1–2 days
Bacillus cereus	Toxin, preformed in food	1–5	Vomiting, 6–24 h
	Toxin, preformed in food, also in gut	8–16	Diarrhoea, 12–24 h
Norwalk and small round-structured viruses (SRSV)	Infection	15–50	Vomiting and diarrhoea, 12–72 h

symptoms are short-lived. Diagnosis depends on finding counts of *B. cereus* in excess of 10^5/g in the suspect food and its detection in vomitus or faeces of victims. As *B. cereus* is ubiquitous, prevention depends on the observance of correct procedures in food preparation.

Similar patterns of food poisoning have occasionally been attributed to *B. subtilis* and *B. licheniformis.*

Food poisoning: a summary

Nowadays it is customary to talk of foodborne infection rather than food poisoning in order to unify the approach to the control of the many agents known to be transmitted via food, which include protozoa (e.g. amoebae, Giardia, Cryptosporidium) and helminths (e.g. *Trichinella spiralis*) as well as bacteria and viruses. This is logical enough, but it is wise to retain a sharp awareness of the few agents capable of causing sudden, explosive outbreaks of illness requiring immediate intervention. In this context, the dissonance embodied in the term 'food poisoning' gives it emotive overtones that are not misplaced. Table 2 summarizes the main forms of microbial food poisoning and intoxication commonly presenting as sudden outbreaks. Page references are given for the organisms not included in this chapter.

REFERENCES

Bennish, M.L. and Salam, M.A. (1992). Rethinking options for the treatment of shigellosis. *Journal of Antimicrobial Chemotherapy*, **30,** 243–7.

Bennish, M.L. (1991). Potentially lethal complications of shigellosis. *Reviews in Infectious Diseases*, **13** (suppl. 4), S319–S324.

Carpenter, C.C.J. (1990). Other pathogenic vibrios. In *Principles and practice of infectious diseases*, (3rd edn), (ed. G.L. Mandell, R.G. Douglas, and J.E. Bennett), pp. 1646–9. Churchill Livingstone, New York.

Doyle, M.P. (ed.) (1989). *Foodborne bacterial pathogens*, Dekker, New York.

Gilbert R.J. and Roberts, D. (1990). Foodborne gastroenteritis. In *Topley and Wilson's principles of bacteriology, virology and immunity*, (8th edn), Vol. 3, (ed. M.T. Parker and L.H. Collier), pp. 489–512. Arnold, London.

Glynn, J.R. and Bradley, D.J. (1992). The relationship between infecting dose and severity of disease in reported outbreaks of salmonella infections. *Epidemiology and Infection*, **109,** 371–8.

Griffin, P.M. and Tauxe, R.V. (1991). The epidemiology of infections caused by *Escherichia coli* O157:H7, other enterohemorrhagic *E. coli*, and the associated hemolytic uremic syndrome. *Epidemiologic Reviews*, **13,** 60–98.

Gross, R.J. (1991). The pathogenesis of *Escherichia coli* diarrhoea. *Reviews in Medical Microbiology*, **2,** 37–44.

Healing, T.D., Greenwood, M.H., and Pearson A.D. (1992). Campylobacters and enteritis. *Reviews in Medical Microbiology*, **3,** 159–67.

Kain, K.C., and Kelly, M.T. (1989). Clinical features, epidemiology, and treatment of *Plesiomonas shigelloides* diarrhea. *Journal of Clinical Microbiology*, **27,** 998–1001.

Law, D. (1994). Adhesion and its role in the virulence of enteropathogenic *Escherichia coli. Clinical Microbiology Reviews*, **7,** 152–73.

Maloney, W.J. and Guerrant, R.L. (1992). Epidemiology, therapy, and prevention of infection with *Salmonella* organisms. *Current Opinion in Infectious Diseases*, **5,** 74–9.

Mathewson, J.J. and DuPont H.L. (1992). *Aeromonas* species: role as human pathogens. *Current Clinical Topics in Infectious Diseases*, **12,** 26–36.

Mishu, B. and Blaser, M.J. (1995). Other *Campylobacter* and *Campylobacter*-like species. In *Infections of the gastrointestinal tract*, (ed. M.J. Blaser, P.D. Smith, J.I. Radvin, H.B. Greenberg, and R.L. Guerrant), in press. Raven Press, New York.

Parker, M.T. (1990). Bacillary dysentery. In *Topley and Wilson's Principles of bacteriology, virology and immunity*, (8th edn), Vol. 3, (ed. M.T. Parker and L.H. Collier), pp. 447–457. Arnold, London.

Skirrow, M.B. and Blaser, M.J. (1995). *Campylobacter jejuni*. In *Infections of the gastrointestinal tract*, (ed. M.J. Blaser, P.D. Smith, J.I. Radvin, H.B. Greenberg, and R.L. Guerrant), in press. Raven Press, New York.

7.11.8 Typhoid and paratyphoid fevers

J. RICHENS

Typhoid

Typhoid means 'like typhus', a disease whose name means 'smoke' in Greek. The smoke refers to the mental clouding that characterizes advanced cases of both diseases. The term enteric fever is a convenient collective term for the small group of salmonelloses lacking an animal reservoir and known as typhoid and paratyphoid fevers. Typhoid fever is a prime example of an infectious disease that used to be a leading cause of death in the cities of Europe and America but was brought under control long before the introduction of antibiotics by vigorous public health measures. In much of the world, prevention has proved elusive and, despite large advances, typhoid causes 5 per cent or more of deaths in areas of high transmission.

Epidemiology

Typhoid has been described throughout the globe. In affluent countries the great majority of cases are seen in returned travellers. On rare occasions, point-source outbreaks occur when there is a breakdown of one of the many measures taken to ensure the provision to the public of safe drinking water and food free of contamination by pathogenic bacteria. In poorer countries, typhoid is associated particularly with bad sanitation, poverty, crowding, and war. The epidemiological pattern is one of continuous transmission with a tendency to peak in hot, dry weather and, sometimes, at the onset of rains. Epidemic outbreaks may be superimposed on this underlying pattern. A recent (1986) estimate of global typhoid suggested 33 million cases annually with half a million deaths. Areas of notably high incidence, estimated to have 100 to 1000 cases/100 000 population per year include parts of Chile, Nepal, South Africa, Indonesia, and India. The proportion of people carrying *Salmonella typhi* in Santiago has been estimated at 0.7 per cent. In poorer countries, case-fatality rates in patients admitted to hospital are typically about 10 per cent, a figure close to the overall mortality of untreated typhoid. More severe forms of typhoid appear to be less frequent in Central and South America. Case-fatality rates rarely exceed 1 per cent in patients treated promptly with antibiotics.

Pathogenesis

AETIOLOGY

The agent of typhoid, strictly, *S. enterica* subsp. *enterica*, serotype Typhi, popularly known as *S. typhi*, is a robust, Gram-negative bacillus that infects only man (and possibly the occasional fruit-bat) but is capable of survival in hostile environments such as ice, dust, clothes, and water. The polysaccharide envelope antigen known as Vi has no intrinsic virulence but appears to confer virulence by masking the oligosaccharide somatic O antigen from immunological attack. The organism possesses flagella that contain the protein flagellar or H antigen. *S. typhi* can acquire R plasmids, which endow it with resistance to chloramphenicol, amoxycillin, and co-trimoxazole. Extensive studies of *S. typhimurium* in recent years have identified a variety of genes (*phoP/phoQ*, *ompR*, *envZ*) that enable the organism to adapt to changes in the environment, such as shifts of pH, osmolality, and calcium concentrations, and to withstand the effects of microbicidal proteins (defensins) present in the phagosomes of phagocytic cells. Similar genes are believed to exist in *S. typhi* and various mutants are being examined for vaccine potential.

TRANSMISSION

Typhoid is transmitted mainly by the faecal–oral route. The ultimate source in most cases is an asymptomatic or recently symptomatic individual who carries the organism. Patients with acute typhoid are a relatively infrequent source of transmission, even in unsanitary conditions. Less commonly, typhoid infection is transmitted by infected urine, sputum, vomit, or pus. The organism may be conveyed directly to food or drink by the contaminated fingers of a carrier or indirectly by flies or through contamination of water supplies by infected sewage. The first is exemplified by the tale of 'Typhoid Mary', an Irish cook who was clearly identified as the source of infection in 53 cases of typhoid, three of them fatal, in the United States a century ago. The famous tin of Argentinian corned beef responsible for the more recent Aberdeen outbreak was cooled in river water polluted by untreated effluent. *S. typhi* thrives in milk products and cold meats. It can be concentrated several hundredfold by shellfish reared in contaminated sea water. Occasional transmission by contaminated hospital instruments, laboratory mishaps, and by anal intercourse has been recorded.

Fig. 1 Typhoid at autopsy, showing transmural ulceration of Peyer's patches in the distal ileum.

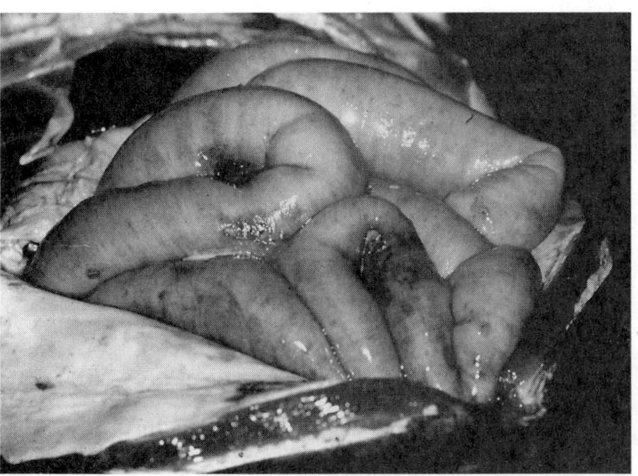

Infective dose

Hornick's studies on the inmates of the Jessup House of Correction established that 10^7 organisms of the Quailes strain would infect 50 per cent of healthy volunteers. The infective dose is smaller with more virulent strains or when gastric acidity is reduced by antacids or vagotomy. There is evidence in both man and from animal models of genetic influences on the response to Salmonella infections; with an inoculum of given size and strain, individuals will show varying responses; for example, some may develop acute disease, others may develop transient pyrexia and bacteraemia, and others still may become symptomless excreters without any symptoms.

MULTIPLICATION AND DISSEMINATION

Bacteria reaching the gut multiply and, without causing damage, pass through both normal enterocytes and the M cells that overlie gut-associated lymphoid tissue to reach the lamina propria. They continue through the mesenteric nodes and thoracic duct to reach the blood stream. Isolation of *S. typhi* from both blood and stool at this very early stage of infection has occasionally been recorded in man. For the remainder of the incubation period the bacteria multiply silently and blood cultures are sterile. A secondary bacteraemia then follows and the patient begins to experience symptoms.

The infection now disseminates widely to the liver, gallbladder, spleen, and bone marrow, and back, via the bile, to Peyer's patches. The precise site of multiplication of *S. typhi* is debated. Most authorities consider *S. typhi* to be a facultatively intracellular organism that multiplies chiefly within macrophages but substantial recent data indicate that it may multiply in parenchymal cells of the liver and, extracellularly, in the liver sinusoids and amongst tissue debris. Hsu has argued that ability to resist phagocytosis may be more important for virulence than ability to survive intracellularly. Histopathological examination of infected tissue shows an initial influx of polymorphs, followed by the development of 'typhoid nodules', clusters of lymphocytes and macrophages with ingested bacteria, erythrocytes, and other debris concentrated in principal organs of the reticuloendothelial system but also to be found in sites such as the kidney, testis, and parotid glands. Observation of this process in Peyer's patches shows an initial marked hypertrophy that makes the lymphoid tissue stand out prominently from the surrounding mucosa. The tissue then becomes ischaemic and necrotic, forming a dark slough (Figs. 1 and 2); haemorrhage and perforation are

Fig. 2 Distal ileum from patient with fatal perforation showing black, necrotic slough overlying ulcerated Peyer's patch and 1.5 cm perforation admitting pathologist's fingertip.

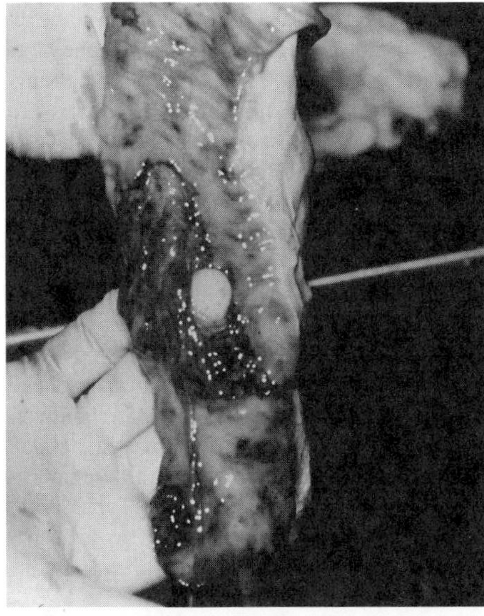

potential consequences. In addition to the typhoid nodules, various non-specific pathological alterations associated with sepsis are seen in skeletal muscle (Zenker's degeneration), the myocardium, kidneys, lungs, and brain.

The pathogenetic mechanisms underlying these events remain poorly understood. For many years, interest focused on endotoxin (lipo-oligosaccharide components of the bacterial cell wall) released by dying bacteria and demonstrable in the blood of patients with typhoid. Endotoxin is capable of inducing both symptoms and pathological changes characteristic of typhoid but experimental work by Hornick and others demonstrated that it was possible to reproduce all the essential features of typhoid in volunteers desensitized to the effects of endotoxin. More recently, it has been suggested that the pathogenesis of typhoid can be more readily attributed to a cytokine cascade induced by the host immune response, together with inflammatory damage mediated by neutrophil proteases, free oxygen radicals, and arachidonic acid metabolites. The benefits of high-dose steroids in severe typhoid (see below) have been attributed to inhibition of this inflammatory damage. The role of tumour necrosis factor, whose release is triggered by endotoxin and which appears to play an important part in the genesis of other forms of Gram-negative septic shock, remains unknown in typhoid. The correlation between high levels of tumour necrosis factor and poor outcome observed in infections such as malaria and meningitis has not so far been demonstrated in typhoid. In mouse models of salmonella infection, antibodies to tumour necrosis factor-α appear to convert a sublethal to a lethal infection by inhibiting macrophage function.

IMMUNE RESPONSE

Studies of the immune response in typhoid patients have shown that there is a cell-mediated response that lasts around 16 weeks. There is a specific mucosal immune response that lasts up to 48 weeks, while circulating anti-O and -H agglutinins persist for up to 2 years. Volunteers given a standard inoculum of *S. typhi* at a mean of 20 months after their initial infection had a 75 per cent reduction of clinical typhoid. The serum antibody titres observed in typhoid have no correlation with the clinical outcome or relapse rates, except for the strong association between persistently elevated titres to Vi and chronic carriage.

Suppression of cell-mediated immunity by human immunodeficiency virus (**HIV**) or in transplant patients is associated with recurrent salmonellosis, though for reasons, so far unexplained, this is seldom *S. typhi* salmonellosis.

Clinical features

Typhoid is predominantly an infection of children and young adults. It affects both sexes equally. Despite the huge diversity of clinical features there are often few specific findings to assist clinical diagnosis in the early stages. The incubation is dictated by the infecting strain, the number of organisms ingested, and host factors. The extremes of the range are 3 to 60 days, but most infections occur 7 to 14 days after exposure.

Typhoid is, above all, a fever. In the past much has been made of stepwise contour of the temperature chart in cases observed during the first week of illness. Of more value to the clinician is the knowledge that this fever rarely shows an abrupt onset, that rigors are uncommon, and that, when fully developed, the fever of typhoid reaches a high plateau of 39 to 40 °C, which shows strikingly little diurnal variation compared to other fevers. Exceptions to this are seen in late or complicated typhoid and in patients treated with aspirin.

The most constant accompaniment of the fever in typhoid is headache. Along with this go non-specific symptoms to be expected of a significant infection—malaise, lassitude, myalgia, arthralgia, anorexia. In classical typhoid, constipation is a frequent early symptom though the majority of patients will experience loose motions at some time. Typhoid can occasionally present like the zoonotic salmonelloses as an acute gastroenteritis and in some patients a transient episode of diarrhoea and vomiting occurs at the time of infection. AIDS patients contracting typhoid or paratyphoid reportedly present with fulminant diarrhoea or colitis. The so-called pea-soup stools are not particularly common and may have been a result of the bland, milk-based diets that were once in vogue. Bloody diarrhoea may be seen. The presence of ileal ulceration and mesenteric lymphadenopathy is predictably associated with varying degrees of abdominal pain, usually diffuse and poorly localized but occasionally sufficiently intense in the left iliac fossa to suggest appendicitis. Nausea and vomiting are relatively infrequent in uncomplicated typhoid but are seen with abdominal distention in more severe cases. Other symptoms of early typhoid are cough, sore throat, and a tendency to epistaxes.

With the majority of typhoid patients, especially those who have access to prompt diagnosis and treatment, the disease does not progress beyond the symptoms already outlined. In poorer countries, clinicians are much more likely to be familiar with typhoid in its second, third, or fourth week of evolution. Untreated typhoid usually runs its course over a period of about 4 weeks. The fever makes its gradual ascent in the first week, remains on a high plateau during the second, and then makes a gentle descent in the third and fourth. The most notable clinical developments in the later stages of typhoid are accelerating weight loss, weakness, the alteration of the patient's mental state that gives typhoid its name, and the development of the principal complications such as haemorrhage, perforation, and refractory hypotension. In poorer countries, substantial numbers of patients do not present until such complications develop and thus typhoid will be encountered with widely varying presentations as acute abdomen, intestinal haemorrhage, pneumonia (so-called pneumotyphoid), nephritis (nephrotyphoid), and acute psychosis. While an altered mental state may be a prominent, early presenting feature, in the majority of patients it only develops after some days of sustained high fever. Typically it manifests initially as mental apathy and progresses to an agitated delirium. It is frequently accompanied by tremor of the hands, tremulous speech, and gait ataxia.

Physical examination in early typhoid is frequently unrewarding, revealing nothing beyond an elevated temperature. Careful, repeated examinations are required to avoid missing minor degrees of splenomegaly or to catch the rash, which has special diagnostic value but may amount to no more than half a dozen spots for 2 or 3 days. By the end of the first week, the patient's skin is characteristically hot and dry. A tachycardia is found in most patients notwithstanding the well-known capacity typhoid has for producing temperature pulse-dissociation (relative bradycardia). The blood pressure must be recorded regularly, as hypotension has important prognostic and therapeutic implications. A coated tongue is often observed. The lenticular rose spots appear at the end of the first week. In their most characteristic form they consist of a sparse collection of pink, maculopapular lesions on the abdominal wall,

Fig. 3 Typhoid rash in Melanesian patient; in this case, sparse, purpuric (non-blanching) macules centred round the umbilicus.

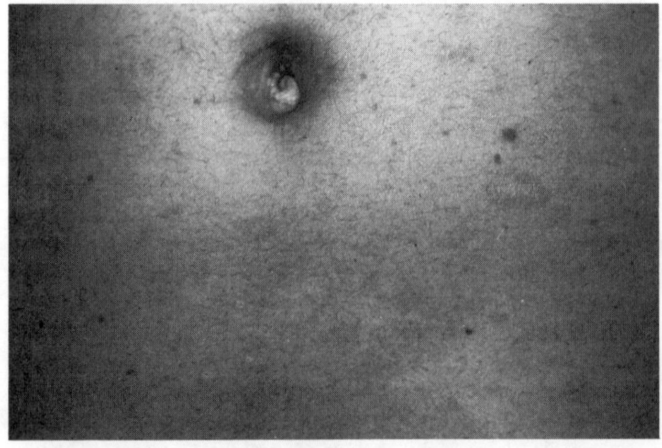

which blanch with pressure and fade after 2 or 3 days. The frequency of their occurrence was put by Osler at 90 per cent in whites and 20 per cent in blacks. Less commonly the rash may be seen to extend on to the rest of the trunk and arms. Melanesian typhoid patients develop purpuric macules that do not blanch (Fig. 3). Oral herpetic lesions are said to occur less frequently in typhoid than during malaria or pneumonia.

It is common to hear adventitious sounds, mostly scattered wheezes, when examining the chest of typhoid patients. On occasions the respiratory symptoms and signs may so prominent as to suggest a diagnosis of pneumonia. These findings with a normal chest radiograph in patient with high fever should always alert the clinician to the possibility of typhoid.

Inspection of the abdomen may reveal the typhoid rash, or distension. The most frequent finding on palpation is a diffuse tenderness, which is occasionally localized to the area of the terminal ileum. Intra-abdominal inflammation of sufficient extent to induce retention of urine is well recognized in typhoid (Fig. 4). A moderate degree of soft, tender hepatosplenomegaly is the rule in later cases of typhoid but it much less likely to be found in the early period of the illness.

One of the most striking features of typhoid in patients progressing into the third week of illness is the facial appearance, which is distinctive enough to merit the term 'typhoid facies'. Typically this face is thin, flushed, with bright eyes and a dull, heavy, staring, apathetic expression (Fig. 5). Further neurological examination of the patient is likely to reveal a fine tremor of the outstretched hands, tremor of tongue and speech, and possibly some degree of gait ataxia. If the patient's condition deteriorates further the features so ably described in the writings of Louis and Osler make their appearance—muttering delirium, twitchings of the fingers and wrists (subsultus tendinum), agitated plucking at the bedclothes (carphology), and a staring, unrousable stupor (coma vigil).

Fig. 4 Retention of urine in confused 30-year-old female patient admitted with typhoid.

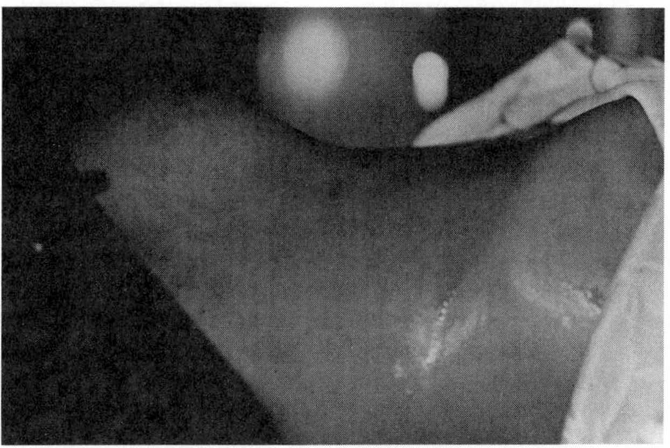

Fig. 5 Typhoid facies: 18-year-old male with severe typhoid.

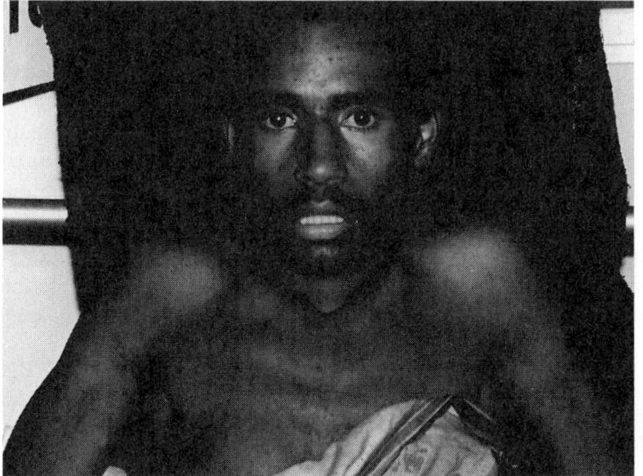

TYPHOID IN CHILDREN

Typhoid can develop in neonates born to infected mothers. The disease tends to take a milder course in children but age-specific case-fatality rates for cases admitted to hospital are higher in under-fives. The main points of difference with adult typhoid are a greater frequency of presentations with diarrhoea and vomiting, jaundice, febrile convulsions or typhoid meningitis. Nephritis was reported in 3 per cent of one large paediatric series. Blood-culture studies of children under the age of 2 years presenting to outpatient clinics with fever in Chile have revealed that typhoid (and paratyphoid) in young children can behave like a mild respiratory illness. Relative bradycardia may carry greater diagnostic significance for typhoid in febrile children.

Diagnosis

The definitive diagnosis of typhoid rests on demonstrating, by means of culture, that a patient with symptoms of the disease is infected with *S. typhi* and that this infection does not represent subclinical urinary or faecal carriage of the organism. The differential diagnosis of typhoid centres on innumerable other conditions that present with an influenza-like illness. These are mainly viral, bacterial, or protozoal infections but include many other conditions that present with unexplained fever such as lymphoproliferative disorders and vasculitis. Typhoid should figure high on the list of possible diagnoses of unexplained fever in travellers and patients in whom suspected malaria has not been confirmed or has not responded to antimalarial therapy.

CULTURE

Published comparisons of different methods of culture for *S. typhi* consistently report that the best yields are to be had from bone marrow aspirates. This method has the added advantage of providing cultures that are often positive for some days after the start of antibiotic therapy. A convenient way to obtain the requisite 1 to 2 ml of aspirate, with minimal inconvenience to patient and operator, is to employ the fine-needle technique described by Hedley *et al.* (1982) (*Lancet,* **ii,** 415–16). It is standard practice to culture blood, urine, and faeces also but such samples will only exceptionally provide a positive culture when marrow culture is negative.

The yield of positive blood cultures can reach 80 per cent. It is maximized by taking generous volumes, by repeat cultures, and by careful attention to providing the optimum ratio of blood to broth (1:10). There are conflicting data as to whether higher yields can be obtained by culturing blood clots to which streptokinase (100 u/ml) has been added. Culture of the mononuclear fraction of blood has recently been shown to concentrate organisms (which may be as few as one per ml) and to speed identification. In view of the high concentration of organisms in the bile in typhoid, culture of intestinal fluid obtained by duodenal string capsule is theoretically attractive and has been shown to have comparable sensitivity to blood culture, particularly if the string is left in place overnight. The procedure is more cumbersome than other methods and not recommended for routine use, except possibly for children and in the search for carriers.

The number of organisms recoverable from faeces increases through the course of the illness. Rectal swabs are less satisfactory than faecal samples. The results must be interpreted with caution in endemic areas with many carriers. Isolation from urine is more common in areas endemic for schistosomiasis. Rose spots, when present, can give a positive culture in 70 per cent of patients.

When specimens are sent for culture, it is important that a suitable variety of selective and enrichment media is employed. A number of different species of Salmonella give rise to typhoid-like illnesses and each has slightly differing requirements. Most positive cultures come up in the first week but 2, or even 3 weeks of culture are needed to maximize the yield.

SEROLOGY

The role of serology in the diagnosis of typhoid is contentious. To some extent, improvements in culture diagnosis have obviated the need for serology but, more recently, serological methods have found new applications in the field of rapid diagnosis. The disadvantages of the traditional tube Widal test are the time taken to demonstrate a rise in titre, the delay or absence of antibody responses in some patients, high titres of antibody present in certain populations, the difficulties of interpretation of results in those previously infected, vaccinated or started on antibiotic treatment, and cross-reactions between salmonellae and related organisms. Studies of the Widal in South America, Sudan, and West Africa have suggested it is of limited value, whereas very high predictive values for a single titre of O antibody in excess of 1:40 have been reported in Indonesia and Papua New Guinea. What emerges from these various studies is that Widal serology is only of value when accurate and up-to-date information is available about the predictive values of positive serology for the population where the test is to be used. In Malaysia, Rose and Abraham have shown that it is possible to diagnose typhoid with 80 per cent specificity and 92 per cent sensitivity on the basis of six simple clinical and laboratory findings (including the Widal test) in a setting where culture cannot be done.

RAPID DIAGNOSIS OF TYPHOID

Antibodies to commercially available O and H antigens can be demonstrated rapidly using a slide agglutination technique. *S. typhi* antigens in body fluids can be demonstrated by agglutination of *Staph. aureus* coated with specific antisera or, more recently, using monoclonal antibodies.

OTHER TESTS FOR TYPHOID

Many alternative methods (passive haemagglutination, latex agglutination, counterimmune electrophoresis, radioimmunoassay, enzyme immunoassay, indirect fluorescent antibody tests, monoclonal antibodies, IgM capture, DNA probes) for detection of antibodies to O, H, and Vi as well as to an array of newly defined *S. typhi* antigens, and for the direct detection of these antigens and salmonella DNA in body fluids, have been described with promising results. Many of these are more sensitive than conventional Widal testing, but doubts remain about specificity and cost in field conditions. Few have so far been adopted for routine use.

OTHER LABORATORY FINDINGS IN TYPHOID

Common haematological findings include a mild normochromic anaemia, mild thrombocytopenia, and an increased erythrocyte sedimentation rate. The frequency of true leucopenia has been overstated in the past; most patients have a total white-cell count within the normal range. Leucocytosis suggests either perforation or an incorrect diagnosis. Laboratory evidence of mild disseminated intravascular coagulation is common but rarely of clinical significance. Common biochemical findings include hyponatraemia, hypokalaemia, and elevation of liver enzymes. The urine often contains some protein and white cells.

Management

The aims of management are to eliminate the infection with antibiotics swiftly, to restore fluid and nutritional deficits, and to monitor the patient for dangerous complications.

ANTIBIOTICS (SEE TABLE 1 FOR DOSES)

Effective antibiotic therapy in typhoid shortens the duration of illness and reduces illness and deaths from complications. This response does not indicate wholesale elimination of *S. typhi*, which is liable to re-emerge to cause relapse and asymptomatic carriage in a significant proportion of patients. Management of mild typhoid without recourse to antibiotics has been described from Hong Kong. *S. typhi* is often cultured from blood in the presence of concentrations of antibiotics that are highly bactericidal to the same isolate *in vitro* and from work in tissue-culture systems it appears that many normally bactericidal antibiotics do no more than impede its replication. So far, no antibiotic has been found to prevent patients wholly from relapsing or becoming carriers, but there is currently much interest in reports that the fluorinated quinolones and newer cephalosporins perform better in this respect than chloramphenicol.

Chloramphenicol is also being displaced from its long-held position as the treatment of choice for typhoid because of the extent of R plasmid-mediated resistance. Although the drug-resistant strains that first emerged in Mexico, Vietnam, and Thailand in the 1970s have now given way to drug-sensitive isolates again, multiresistant *S. typhi* is currently causing substantial problems in India, Pakistan, and Bangladesh. Despite this, in much of the world, chloramphenicol remains a valuable drug for the management of typhoid. The optimum dosage schedule has never been agreed upon. Lower dosages and shorter courses are more likely to lead to relapse and asymptomatic carriage, whilst higher dosages run the risks of reversible, dose-related, bone marrow suppression. The extent to which irreversible marrow aplasia follows chloramphenicol treatment for typhoid in endemic countries is unknown but many physicians believe it may be substantially lower than in Caucasian populations. Chloramphenicol can induce haemolytic crises in patients with more severe forms of glucose 6-phosphate dehydrogenase deficiency. The use of loading dosages and complicated reducing dosage schedules has no documented advantage.

The chief rivals to chloramphenicol among the cheaper antibiotics are co-trimoxazole, amoxycillin (not ampicillin), and furazolidone. Numerous comparative trials have examined end-points such as clearance rates, days to defervescence, days to clinical improvement, mortality, and various complications. Unfortunately, small sample sizes and differences in the types of patients recruited, length of follow-up, and definitions of end-points make it impossible to make a useful meta-analysis of these trials. The clinical efficacy of each is roughly comparable and to choose between them is largely a matter of taking into account local data on antibiotic susceptibility and weighing up the various adverse reactions associated with each.

Preliminary data on the use of fluorinated quinolones (ciprofloxacin, fleroxacin, norfloxacin, pefloxacin, and ofloxacin) and cephalosporins (cefoperazone, cefixime, and ceftriaxone) suggest that these drugs, when compared with chloramphenicol or co-trimoxazole, produce lower mortality in mouse models, and, in man, higher cure rates, faster defervescence and resolution of symptoms, lower relapse rates, and lower rates of asymptomatic carriage after recovery. These are good grounds to recommend these drugs where resources permit and particularly for patients from regions with significant amounts of multiresistant *S. typhi*. Fluorinated quinolones remain relatively contraindicated for pregnant women and children although favourable results have been reported from the use of ciprofloxacin in children with severe typhoid. Optimum dosage schedules remain to be established. Some investigators are examining courses as short as 3 days with these drugs but while success rates are encouraging the advantages are likely to be offset by increases in relapse and carriage rates and by the emergence of resistant organisms.

SUPPORTIVE CARE

The patient's principal symptoms will be fever and headache. Cooling measures are preferred to antipyretics for relief of fever. Simple anal-

Table 1 *Guidelines for drug dosages in typhoid*

Antibiotic	Daily dose	Route[a]	Doses/day	Duration
Chloramphenicol	50–75 mg/kg	O/IM/IV[b]	4	14 days
Co-trimoxazole	6.5–10 mg/kg trimethoprim; 40 mg/kg sulphamethoxazole	O/IM/IV	2–3	14 days
Amoxycillin	75–100 mg/kg	O/IM/IV	3	14 days
Furazolidone	7.5 mg/kg	O	4	14 days
Cefoperazone	100 mg/kg until defervescence, then 50 mg/kg	IM	2	14 days
Ceftriaxone	50–60 mg/kg	IM	2	7–10 days
Cefixime	20 mg/kg	O	2	14
Ciprofloxacin	0.5–1 g	O/IV	2	14 days
Norfloxacin, ofloxacin	800 mg	O/IV	2	10 days
Pefloxacin	800 mg	O/IV	2	14 days
Enoxacin	400 mg	O/IV	2	14 days
Fleroxacin	400 mg	O/IV	1	7–14 days
Treatment of carriers				
Ampicillin or amoxycillin with probenecid	100 mg/kg 30 mg/kg	O	3–4	3 months[c]
Co-trimoxazole	6.5–10 mg trimethoprim	O	2	3 months
Ciprofloxacin	1500 mg	O	2	28 days
Norfloxacin	800 mg	O	2	28 days

[a]Oral therapy is satisfactory for most patients. Parenteral therapy is generally reserved for severely ill patients.

[b]The oral route is preferred; there are reports of lower blood levels of chloramphenicol in patients given parenteral therapy.

[c]The duration of treatment can be shortened if parenteral therapy is given, e.g. 8-hourly intravenous ampicillin for 2 weeks.

O, oral; IM, intramuscular; IV, intravenous.

gesics may be used to relieve the headache until the antibiotics take effect (usually within 48 h), though it should be remembered that paracetamol can lengthen the half-life of chloramphenicol five-fold and antipyretics have been blamed for triggering hypotension in severely ill patients. Most patients can eat and drink normally. Bland diets are not required and there is no evidence that they protect the bowel from perforation. Patients may require antifungal therapy for oral candidiasis whilst taking antibiotics. The daily ward-round should include assessment of the patient's mental state and circulatory status, and repeated examination of the patient's abdomen for hints of impending perforation and to detect splenomegaly and rose spots, if these were not observed on admission.

Severe cases of typhoid (see below), particularly those with impairment of consciousness or hypotension, are best managed in an intensive care unit. Parenteral fluids may be required to make up fluid, sodium, and potassium deficits in patients dehydrated by poor oral intake, large insensible fluid loss, diarrhoea, vomiting, or sequestration of fluids in the bowel. Sedation will be required for disturbed patients.

Complications

Table 2 gives an extensive, though not exhaustive, list of the complications of typhoid. Most of them are rare and only likely to be encountered in patients who present with untreated disease of 2 or more weeks' duration. Occasionally, a complication dominates the clinical picture and deflects attention from the underlying diagnosis of typhoid. The more common and important complications of typhoid are discussed below.

SEVERE TYPHOID

Studies from Indonesia and Papua New Guinea have indicated that an important subgroup of typhoid patients can be identified, on the basis of mental state or cardiovascular status, who have a 50 per cent mortality and who account for the great majority of typhoid cases with a fatal outcome. The treatment of such patients with high doses of dexamethasone substantially reduced the mortality in trials reported from Jakarta. The criteria for severe typhoid were marked mental confusion or shock, defined as a systolic blood pressure of less than 90 mmHg in adults or less than 80 mmHg in children, with evidence of decreased skin, cerebral, or renal perfusion. In adults, dexamethasone, 3 mg/kg infused intravenously over half an hour, followed by eight doses of 1 mg/kg 6-hourly, resulted in a 10 per cent case-fatality rate compared to one of 55.6 per cent in controls. There is no place for the use of steroids in cases of typhoid not meeting these criteria and there is evidence that the use of more modest dosages (e.g. up to 1.6 g hydrocortisone daily) is not beneficial, even in severe typhoid. It has been suggested that steroid use may predispose to perforation and haemorrhage and higher relapse rates in India but no association was noted in the Jakarta studies. If steroids are given, there are theoretical grounds for administering the first dose before starting antibiotics in order to dampen the cytokine burst induced by dying bacteria. Results of adopting this approach in typhoid have not been reported.

INTESTINAL PERFORATION

This most feared complication of typhoid occurs in less than 5 per cent of patients. The usual site is the terminal ileum (Figs. 1 and 2). Three-quarters of cases are single perforations and occur after about 20 days of illness. The clinical presentation of perforation is rarely abrupt. More often there is a subtle transition from vague abdominal pain and tenderness to rather more definite pain and restlessness with a rise in pulse rate and fall of blood pressure. Distension and guarding increase gradually. Rigidity, absent bowel sounds, and loss of resonance over the liver due to pneumoperitoneum may take several hours to appear. A chest radiograph may confirm free gas under the diaphragm; ultrasonography is useful for demonstrating and aspirating pockets of faeculent fluid in the peritoneal cavity.

The most favourable outcome after perforation occurs in those who, after adequate resuscitation, proceed to operation as quickly as possible. Conservative management of perforation is rarely advocated these days except where surgical expertise is lacking or moribund patients present several days after perforation. Simple closure of perforations is often

Table 2 *Complications of typhoid*

Abdominal
Intestinal perforation
Intestinal haemorrhage
Hepatitis
Cholecystitis (usually subclinical)
Spontaneous splenic rupture
Rupture and haemorrhage from mesenteric nodes
Pancreatitis
Genitourinary
Retention of urine
Glomerulonephritis
Pyelonephritis
Cystitis
Orchitis
Cardiovascular
Myocarditis
Pericarditis
Endocarditis
Asymptomatic ECG changes
Phlebitis and arteritis
Deep venous thrombosis
Gangrene
Shock
Sudden death
Respiratory
Bronchitis
Laryngeal ulceration
Glottal oedema
Pneumonia (*S. typhi*, *Strep. pneumoniae*)
Neuropsychiatric
Delirium
Psychotic states
Depression
Deafness
Meningitis
Encephalomyelitis
Transverse myelitis
Signs of upper motor-neurone lesions
Signs of extrapyramidal disorder
Impairment of coordination
Optic neuritis
Peripheral and cranial neuropathy
Guillain–Barré syndrome
Pseudotumor cerebri
Haematological
Disseminated intravascular coagulation (usually subclinical)
Anaemia
Haemolysis
Haemolytic uraemic syndrome
Focal infections
Abscesses of brain, liver, spleen, breast, thyroid, muscles, lymph nodes
Parotitis
Pharyngitis
Osteitis, especially tibia, ribs, spine
Arthritis
Other
Myopathy
Hypercalcaemia
Decubitus ulceration
Abortion
Relapse

adequate but more experienced surgeons state that more complex procedures designed to bypass the worst-affected sections of the ileum reduce postoperative morbidity, which can be substantial. Closure of the perforation should be accompanied by vigorous peritoneal toilet and administration of metronidazole. The overall survival of patients undergoing surgery for perforation is 70 to 75 per cent, but is as high as 97 per cent in the best series. This compares with survival rates of around 30 per cent in conservatively managed patients.

INTESTINAL HAEMORRHAGE

Testing for occult blood is often positive in typhoid. Silent bleeding may be signalled by sudden collapse of a patient or a steadily falling haematocrit. Frank bleeding is an infrequent complication seen mostly in the third week and only very rarely fatal. Most episodes of bleeding are self-limiting and only a few require transfusion or, in exceptional circumstances, surgical intervention. Intra-arterial vasopressin has been used successfully to halt haemorrhage.

RELAPSE

Relapse in typhoid is a second episode of illness, usually somewhat milder than the first, generally occurring a week or two after the recovery of an otherwise healthy individual from a first attack. It should be distinguished from the multiple recurrences of septicaemic salmonellosis with metastatic foci described in association with schistosomiasis, opisthorchiasis, sickle-cell disease, and HIV infection. Isolates obtained from relapsing patients are generally identical to those obtained during the first episode. Before antibiotics were introduced they were seen in about 10 per cent of patients and sometimes occurred more than once. The management of relapse is the same as that for the initial episode. Isolates are generally still sensitive to the antibiotics used in the first episode. Some physicians give a shorter course of treatment in view of the milder illness and extreme rarity of further relapses.

Carriers

Most patients with typhoid continue to excrete *S. typhi* in their stools or urine for some days after starting antibiotic treatment. Among fully recovered patients a proportion, labelled convalescent carriers, continue to excrete for periods up to 3 months. The 3 per cent or so of patients still excreting at 3 months are unlikely to cease and at 1 year meet the formal definition of 'chronic carrier'. When carriers are detected by screening about 25 per cent may give no history of acute typhoid. Faecal carriage is more likely to develop in individuals with gallbladder disease and is thus most common in women over the age of 40; in the Far East there is an association with opisthorchiasis. Urinary carriage is particularly associated with schistosomiasis but is also found with conditions such as nephrolithiasis. Carriers rarely experience symptoms but acute typhoid can supervene and an increased risk of carcinoma of the gallbladder has been reported.

Carrier screening employs a combination of culture and serological methods. Patients discharged after treatment for typhoid with six negative stool and three negative urine specimens and negative Vi serology are considered free of infection. The majority of patients with positive stools at the completion of treatment will only excrete temporarily and can be safely followed up. The time to consider antibiotic eradication of carriage comes in those still excreting at 3 months, or possibly earlier in patients considered to be at particular risk of communicating the infection to others. The patient with a persistently elevated or rising Vi antibody titre is likely to be a carrier. Repeated checks of urine and faeces should be made and consideration given to obtaining bile cultures if these are negative. In Egypt, demonstration of H antibody in urine has been useful in identifying carriers.

Eradication of carriage requires prolonged high-dose antibiotics (Table 1). In the past, ampicillin, amoxycillin, and co-trimoxazole have all been used with success. More recently, good results have been reported with norfloxacin and ciprofloxacin. Cholecystectomy and nephrectomy, once widely used to eliminate carriage (and not without some operative mortality) are hard to justify on public health grounds alone, but can be considered if antibiotic methods fail and there are indications for operation beyond the elimination of carriage. The success rates of surgery are increased by giving antibiotics as well.

Prevention

The virtual elimination of typhoid from industrialized countries can be attributed largely to the provision of safe drinking water, the safe disposal of human sewage, legal enforcement of high standards of food hygiene, care in detecting and monitoring chronic carriers, and prompt investigation and intervention on the occasions when these safeguards are breached. Useful tools in tracing the source of outbreaks are phage typing of isolates, DNA fingerprinting, registers of known carriers and their phage types, and the use of sewer swabs to trace back isolates to their source.

In poorer parts of the world, many of these measures have not been instituted. Studies have shown that provision of lavatories and clean water can halve exposure. In Bangkok, mass annual vaccination of children has produced a marked reduction in typhoid in children. For those that live in or travel to such areas the options are to kill *S. typhi* in water by heating to 57 °C, iodination or chlorination, to be particularly careful with food prepared outside the home and to be immunized. Patients and convalescents with typhoid should be advised to wash their hands after using the toilet and before preparing food and to use separate towels.

VACCINES

Three different types of vaccine for typhoid are currently marketed. None offers more than partial protection against paratyphoid infection and the protection afforded by each can be overcome by large inocula of bacteria. Efficacy figures are broadly comparable for all vaccines but derive largely from trials conducted in heavily exposed populations and show a tendency to overestimate benefit in persons without prior exposure. The new live oral Ty21a vaccine is a mutant lacking galactose epimerase, which undergoes four to five cell divisions in the gut, penetrates the wall, and then fades out. This vaccine has few side-effects but is expensive. Four capsules are reconstituted immediately before ingestion and taken with sodium bicarbonate on two occasions at least 2 days apart. The new Vi vaccine is a stable one with low production costs and few side-effects, given as a single intramuscular dose of 25 μg providing 70 to 80 per cent protection for 3 years. The heat-inactivated, phenol-preserved vaccine is the most widely used of the older, killed vaccines (51–65 per cent protection). Two doses of 0.5 ml are given 4 to 6 weeks apart, the first dose intramuscularly, the second intradermally to limit the frequent side-effects of fever, local pain, and malaise. Three-yearly boosters are recommended. Very severe reactions are occasionally reported and there is a handful of reports that suggest that breakthrough typhoid in persons vaccinated with the outer, parenteral vaccines can be more dangerous. The need for vaccination is greatest amongst schoolchildren in endemic areas. Travellers, particularly those to the Indian subcontinent and parts of South America, should consider vaccination but should be aware that the risks are low (105–118 cases per million travellers to India) and that the efficacy of currently recommended doses in previously unexposed adults remains unproven.

Paratyphoid fever

Of the three forms of paratyphoid, type B has the widest distribution and resembles typhoid most closely. Paratyphoid A occurs chiefly in Asia and Africa and paratyphoid C in Asia and the Middle East. Paratyphoid A and C are more likely to present with a gastroenteritic than a typhoidal type of illness. *S. paratyphi* causes more asymptomatic infections than *S. typhi*. Outbreaks of paratyphoid are much more often food-borne than water-borne, probably because larger inocula are needed to establish infection. In comparison with typhoid the incubation period is shorter (4–5 days), the illness is shorter, and the incidence of complications including relapse and long-term carriage is lower. A fatal outcome is rare. A notable clinical difference is that the rash of paratyphoid is often much more florid, with more and larger lesions extending much further over the trunk. The management of paratyphoid is essentially the same as that of typhoid. Paratyphoid organisms may display multidrug resistance like *S. typhi*. Eradication of carriage with quinolones has been less successful in paratyphoid than in typhoid.

REFERENCES

General

Bhutta, Z.A., Naqvi, S.H., Razzaq, R.A., and Farooqui, B.J. (1991). Multidrug-resistant typhoid in children: presentation and clinical features. *Reviews of Infectious Diseases*, **13,** 832–6.

Butler, T., Islam, A., Kabir, I., and Jones, P.K. (1991). Patterns of morbidity and mortality in typhoid fever dependent on age and gender: review of 552 hospitalized patient with diarrhea. *Reviews of Infectious Diseases*, **13,** 85–90.

Edelman, R. and Levine, M.M. (1986). Summary of an international workshop on typhoid fever. *Reviews of Infectious Diseases*, **8,** 329–49.

Gotuzzo, E. *et al.* (1991). Association between the acquired immunodeficiency syndrome and infection with *Salmonella typhi* or *Salmonella paratyphi* in an endemic typhoid area. *Archives of Internal Medicine*, **151,** 381–2.

Hsu, H.S. (1989). Pathogenesis and immunity in murine salmonellosis. *Microbiological Review*, **53,** 390–409.

Mastroeni, P., Arena, A., Costa, G.B., Liberto, M.C., Bonina, L., and Hormaeche, C.E. (1991). Serum TNF alpha in mouse typhoid and enhancement of a Salmonella infection by anti-TNF alpha antibodies. *Microbial Pathogenesis*, **11,** 33–8.

Miller, S.I., Kurral, A.M., and Mekalanos, J.J. (1989). A two-component regulatory system (phoP phoQ) controls *Salmonella typhimurium* virulence. *Proceedings of the National Academy of Sciences (USA)*, **86,** 5054–8.

Osuntokun, B.O., Bademosi, O., Ogunremi, K., and Wright S.G. (1972). Neuropsychiatric manifestations of typhoid fever in 959 patients. *Archives of Neurology*, **27,** 7–13.

Antibiotics

Dutta, P. *et al.* (1993). Ciprofloxacin for treatment of severe typhoid fever in children. *Antimicrobial Agents and Chemotherapy*, **37,** 1197–9.

Islam, A. *et al.* (1988). Randomized treatment of patients with typhoid fever by using ceftriaxone or chloramphenicol. *Journal of Infectious Diseases*, **158,** 742–7.

Sarma, P.S.A. and Durairaj, P. (1991). Randomized treatment of patients with typhoid and paratyphoid fevers using norfloxacin or chloramphenicol. *Transactions of the Royal Society of Tropical Medicine and Hygiene*, **85,** 670–1.

Soe, G.B. and Overturf, G.D. (1987). Treatment of typhoid fever and other systemic salmonellosis with cefotaxime, ceftriaxone, cefoperazone and other newer cephalosporins. *Reviews of Infectious Diseases*, **9,** 719–36.

Wallace, M.R., *et al.* (1993). Ciprofloxacin versus ceftriaxone in the treatment of multiresistant typhoid fever. *European Journal of Clinical Microbiology and Infectious Diseases,* **12,** 907–10.

Carriers

Caygill, C.P., Hill, M.J., Braddick, M., and Sharp, J.C. (1994). Cancer mortality in chronic typhoid and paratyphoid carriers. *Lancet*, **343,** 83–4.

Gotuzzo, E. *et al.* (1988). Use of norfloxacin to treat chronic typhoid carriers. *Journal of Infectious Diseases*, **157,** 1221–5.

Lanata, C.F., Tafur, C., Benavente, L., Gotuzzo, E., and Carillo, C. (1990). Detection of *Salmonella typhi* carriers in food handlers by Vi serology in Lima, Peru. *Bulletin of the Panamerican Health Organization*, **24,** 177–82.

Diagnosis

Gilman, R.H., Terminel, M., Levine, M.M., Hernandez-Mendoza P., and Hornick, R.B. (1975). Relative efficacy of blood, urine, rectal swab, bone-marrow and rose-spot cultures for recovery of *Salmonella typhi* in typhoid fever. *Lancet*, **i,** 1211–13.

Hoffman, S.L. *et al.* (1986). The Widal slide agglutination test, a valuable rapid diagnostic test in typhoid fever patients at the Infectious Diseases Hospital of Jakarta. *American Journal of Epidemiology*, **123,** 869–75.

Rose, I.N. and Abraham, T. (1987). Predicting enteric fever without bacteriological culture results. *Transactions of the Royal Society of Tropical Medicine and Hygiene*, **81,** 1022–6.

Rubin, F.A. *et al.* (1990). Rapid diagnosis of typhoid fever through identification of *Salmonella typhi* within 18 hours of specimen acquisition by culture of mononuclear cell/platelet fraction of blood. *Journal of Clinical Microbiology*, **28,** 825–7.

West B., Richens, J.E., and Howard, P.F. (1989). Evaluation in Papua New Guinea of a urine coagglutination test and a Widal slide agglutination test for rapid diagnosis of typhoid fever *Transactions of the Royal Society of Tropical Medicine and Hygiene*, **83,** 715–17.

Perforation

Bitar, R. and Tarpley, J. (1985). Intestinal perforation in typhoid fever: a historical and state-of-the-art review. *Reviews of Infectious Diseases*, **7,** 257–71.

Butler, T., Knight, J., Nath, S.K., Speelman, P., Roy, S.K., and Azad, M.A.K. (1985). Typhoid fever complicated by intestinal perforation: a persisting fatal disease requiring surgical management. *Reviews of Infectious Diseases*, **7,** 244–56.

Steroids

Hoffman, S.L. *et al.* (1984). Reduction of mortality in chloramphenicol-treated severe typhoid fever by high-dose dexamethasone. *New England Journal of Medicine*, **310,** 82–8.

Punjabi N.H. *et al.* (1988). Treatment of severe typhoid fever in children with high dose dexamethasone.*Pediatric Infectious Diseases Journal*, **7,** 598–600.

Rogerson, S.J., Spooner V.J., Smith, T.A., and Richens J. (1991). Hydrocortisone in the treatment of severe typhoid fever. *Transactions of the Royal Society of Tropical Medicine and Hygiene*, **85,** 113–16.

Vaccines

Forrest, B.D., LaBrooy, J.T., Dearlove, C.E., and Shearman, D.J. (1992). Effect of parenteral immunization on the intestinal immune response to *Salmonella typhi* Ty21a. *Infection and Immunity*, **60,** 465–71.

Ivanoff, B., Levine, M.M., and Lambert, P.H. (1994). Vaccination against typhoid fever: present status. *Bulletin of the World Health Organization*, **72,** 957–71.

Further reading

Christie, A.B. (1987). Typhoid and paratyphoid fevers. In Christie, A.B. *Infectious diseases: epidemiology and clinical practice*, (4th edn) Vol. 1 (ed. A.B. Christie), pp. 100–646. Churchill Livingstone, Edinburgh. An outstanding, detailed and generously referenced monograph on typhoid.

Parker, M.T. (1990). Enteric infections: typhoid and paratyphoid fever. In *Topley and Wilson's principles of bacteriology, virology and immunity* (8th edn) Vol. 3, pp. 423–46. Arnold, London. 1990. A useful chapter covering microbiological aspects of typhoid in depth.

7.11.9 Rhinoscleroma

J. RICHENS

Rhinoscleroma or scleroma is a chronic infection of the upper respiratory tract, characterized by inflammatory growths and caused by *Klebsiella rhinoscleromatis*. The disease has an unusual and unexplained distribution, being found in small, concentrated pockets around the world, particularly in poor rural communities. Africa has foci in the north and east; the Asia–Pacific region has foci in Siberia, Turkestan, the Middle East, India, Pakistan, China, the Philippines, Indonesia, and Papua New Guinea. There are many foci in South and Central America; it remains common in Guatemala, where it has been tentatively identified in terracotta Maya heads of AD 300 to 600. The disease has now largely disappeared from previously important foci in Eastern and Central Europe, where it was initially described by Hebra and Kaposi in 1870.

Aetiology

K. rhinoscleromatis can be isolated from 60 per cent of lesions and is widely, though not universally, believed to be the intracellular organism that is observed in smears and sections. Patients with the disease show high titres of antibody specific for somatic and capsular antigens of this organism and the intracellular bacteria have been shown to have a high affinity for antisera specific for Klebsiella capsular antigen III. *K. rhinoscleromatis* can induce and be recovered from histologically similar lesions in the lungs but not the nose of albino mice.

Pathogenesis

Transmission is believed to be from person to person in endemic areas. The incubation period is unknown. Three stages are recognized in the pathogenesis of rhinoscleroma, all of which may be present at different sites in the same patient. Stage one has all the features of an atrophic rhinitis, with squamous metaplasia, hyperkeratosis, and atrophy. The nodular second stage consists of a granulomatous inflammatory reaction to the presence of *K. rhinoscleromatis* within macrophages, which appear to be unable to kill the organism. This reaction leads to the formation of bulky, soft-tissue masses in the respiratory mucosa. The process can extend into and destroy neighbouring soft tissues, cartilage, bone, and skin. Systemic spread does not occur but local spread may convey the infection to any point from the nares down to the lung hila. Histopathological examination shows a dense infiltrate of plasma cells amongst which are scattered the pathognomonic foam cells of Mikulicz, large histiocytes containing Gram-negative bacilli. In addition, Russell bodies, which originate from effete plasma cells, are often observed within macrophages. In the third stage of the disease, the infiltrates of early rhinoscleroma give way to increasing amounts of fibrosis and the organisms ultimately disappear.

Fig. 1 Rhinoscleroma in a 30-year-old man from Papua New Guinea causing characteristic nasal splaying (Hebra nose) and obstruction of the left nostril. (Reproduced from Cooke, R. (1987). *Colour Atlas of Anatomical Pathology*, p. 31. Churchill Livingstone, Edinburgh, with permission.)

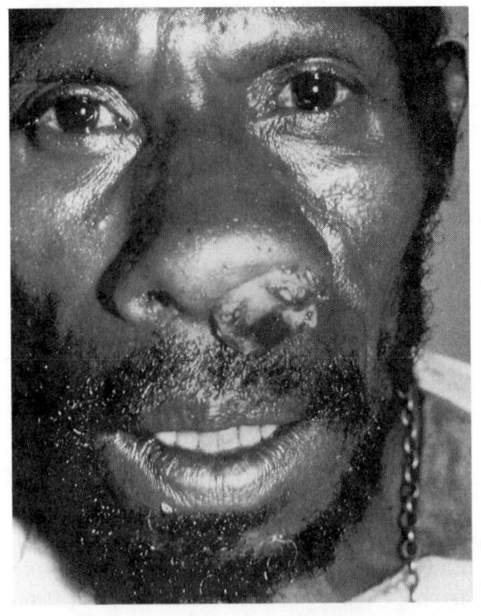

Clinical

Rhinoscleroma runs a very slow, fluctuating course over many years, progressing through atrophic, nodular, and fibrotic stages. Patients' general health is not affected. Most present with various combinations of nasal obstruction, nasal deformity (splaying of the lower nose, often with a visible growth extending down to the upper lip and around the alae nasi, known as Hebra nose), or bleeding (Fig. 1). Some patients present with symptoms indistinguishable from an atrophic rhinitis, with a foul-smelling nasal discharge and crust formation. An important subgroup of patients presents with stridor. Spread of nodular disease into neighbouring structures such as the paranasal sinuses, lacrymal apparatus, orbits, anterior cranial fossa, middle ear, nasopharynx, skin of the upper lip, and cervical glands may occur and has been increasingly recognized since the introduction of computerized tomographic (**CT**) scanning and sinus endoscopy. The most dangerous complication of rhinoscleroma is severe upper-airway obstruction; among other complications and sequelae reported are subglottic laryngeal stenosis, empyema of the maxillary sinus, and squamous carcinoma. Unusual oropharyngeal lesions of rhinoscleroma have recently been reported in a patient with HIV infection.

Diagnosis

The diagnosis is best made by smear or biopsy combined with culture. The intracellular organisms stain well with Giemsa or silver stains and poorly with haematoxylin and eosin. Periodic acid–Schiff staining and specific demonstration of Klebsiella antigens in tissue are helpful. Sensitive and specific haemagglutination tests for capsular antibody in serum have been described. Involvement of the trachea can be recognized on lateral neck radiographs or on CT scans, where concentric, irregular narrowing of the airway and crypt-like irregularities may be seen. Laryngoscopy, bronchoscopy, and endoscopy of the sinuses and nasopharynx may reveal additional sites of involvement.

Treatment

The traditional treatment for rhinoscleroma has been a combination of broad spectrum antibiotics, monitored by repeat cultures, regular nasal lavage with saline, and surgery for obstruction. Monotherapy with streptomycin, tetracyclines, ampicillin, or cotrimoxazole given for 4 to 8 weeks may work for patients with early disease but failure rates are high for more advanced cases. Improved results have been reported with clofazimine (100 mg twice daily for 3 months) and rifampicin (450 mg daily for 6 weeks). A recent trial reported substantially better results with ciprofloxacin 250 mg twice daily for 4 weeks compared with rifampicin 300 mg twice daily and cotrimoxazole for 6 months. The best topical therapies reported include 20 per cent tetracycline ointment, 23 per cent acriflavine, and intralesional rifampicin.

Debulking operations and nasal dilatation with temporary insertion of polythene tubes have been used to deal with obstructing nasal lesions. Such operations carry the risk of leaving an atrophic rhinitis and should always be carried out after antibiotic therapy or with antibiotic cover to minimize the risk of spread. The carbon dioxide surgical laser has recently been introduced with encouraging results in the management of rhinoscleroma. Late cases with fibrotic stenoses may require reconstructive surgery.

Poor understanding of the transmission and epidemiology of rhinoscleroma has so far made it impossible to design practical interventions to prevent the disease. Where the disease has declined in incidence, this has been generally attributed to improved standards of living.

REFERENCES

Borgstein, J., Sada, E. and Cortes, R. (1993) Ciprofloxacin for rhinoscleroma and ozena. *Lancet*, **342,** 122.

Gamea, A.M. (1988). Local rifampicin in treatment of rhinoscleroma *Journal of Laryngology and Otology*, **102,** 319–21.

Gamea, A.M. (1990). Role of endoscopy in diagnosing scleroma in its uncommon sites. *Journal of Laryngology and Otology*, **104,** 619–21.

Maher, A.I., el-Khashlan, H.K., Soliman, Y., and Galal, R. (1990). Rhinoscleroma management by carbon dioxide surgical laser. *Laryngoscope*, **100,** 783–8.

Meyer, P.R., Shum, T.K., Becker, T.S., and Taylor, C.R. (1983). Scleroma (rhinoscleroma). A histologic immunohistochemical study with bacteriologic correlates. *Archives of Pathology and Laboratory Medicine*, **107,** 377–83.

Paul, C., *et al.* (1993). Infection due to *Klebsiella rhinoscleromatis* in two patients infected with human immunodeficiency virus. *Clinical Infectious Disease*, 16, 441–20.

Shehata, M.A. and Salama, A.M. (1989). Clofazimin in the treatment of scleroma. *Journal of Laryngology and Otology*, **103,** 856–60.

Ssali, C.L.K. (1975). The management of rhinoscleroma. *Journal of Laryngology and Otology*, **89,** 91–9.

7.11.10 Anaerobic bacteria

S. J. EYKYN

Although anaerobic infection theoretically includes all infections associated with anaerobic bacteria, those infections mediated by clostridial toxins constitute a clinically distinct group and are considered elsewhere (clostridia), as is actinomycosis. Anaerobes that produce infections unassociated with toxins are sometimes referred to as the 'non-sporing' anaerobes or the 'non-clostridial' anaerobes, but such terms are rather misleading as they exclude members of the genus *Clostridium.* Clostridia, including sometimes *Cl. perfringens*, occur with non-sporing anaerobes in a variety of infections in which they do not declare their toxic potential, and in these infections, their presence or absence makes no difference to the course of the disease.

Anaerobic infections are very common, even if not always recognized as such, and may affect any tissue or organ. They may thus present to all clinicians regardless of speciality. Remarkably, these infections were intensively studied in Europe at the turn of the century but then largely ignored, other than by a few enlightened souls, for many years. Anaerobic bacteria (with the exception of *Clostridium* spp. and the occasional *Bacteroides fragilis*) were seldom isolated in clinical laboratories until the mid-1970s when an 'anaerobic renaissance' was initiated by American researchers and the anaerobes were 'rediscovered' as common and important human pathogens. Since then, enormous advances have been made in the isolation, taxonomy, clinical diagnosis, management, and prevention of anaerobic infection.

Taxonomy

The classification and characterization of many anaerobic bacteria present considerable difficulties and only dedicated anaerobists can hope (or need) to be abreast of current taxonomy. The many synonyms for some of these organisms bear witness to these difficulties: for example, Finegold quoted over 50 for the organism now classified as *Fusobacterium necrophorum.* Such taxonomic confusion is further increased by the many reports that refer to any Gram-negative anaerobic bacillus as a 'Bacteroides' and to those resistant to ampicillin and penicillin as *B. fragilis.* Other difficulties arise when differentiating fastidious micro-aerophilic or capnophilic (carbon dioxide-requiring) bacteria from true anaerobes; this is particularly true of certain streptococci including *Streptococcus milleri.* Such differentiation has therapeutic as well as taxonomic implications because metronidazole, which is so effective against anaerobes, is inactive against most micro-aerophilic and capnophilic bacteria.

Recently, the development of chemotaxonomic methods, particularly those of DNA base composition, DNA homology, and RNA sequencing, has resulted in the reclassification of many anaerobes. The genus Bacteroides is now limited to the *B. fragilis* group of organisms. The saccharolytic species that were previously included in the *B. melaninogenicus-oralis-ruminicola* group have been assigned to the new genus Prevotella and this genus includes both pigmented and non-pigmented species. Asaccharolytic pigmented Gram-negative rods are now known as Porphyromonas. Other taxonomic changes have affected the anaerobic Gram-positive cocci: the genus Peptococcus retains only the species *P. niger*, all the others have become *Peptostreptococcus* spp. As these taxonomic changes affect some clinically important anaerobes, the new nomenclature will be used in this chapter. Table 1 lists some of the clinically important anaerobes together with their old and new names where appropriate.

Table 1 *Some clinically important anaerobic bacteria including taxonomic changes where relevant*

Anaerobic bacilli
Gram-positive bacilli
Spore-forming:
Clostridium perfringens
Other *Clostridium* spp.
Non-spore-forming:
Actinomyces spp.
Bifidobacterium spp.
Eubacterium spp.
Propionibacterium spp.
Gram-negative bacilli
Bacteroides fragilis
Bacteroides spp. (*fragilis*-like)
Prevotella melaninogenica[a]
Other *Prevotella* spp.[a]
Porphyromonas asaccharolytica[a]
Fusobacterium necrophorum
Other *Fusobacterium* spp.
Anaerobic cocci
Gram-positive cocci
Peptostreptococcus spp.[b]
Gram-negative cocci
Veillonella spp.
Spirochaetes
Treponema vincentii[c]

[a]Previously Bacteroides; [b]now includes most *Peptococcus* spp:; [c]previously Borrelia.

Anaerobic commensal flora of man

The normal commensal flora of man consists largely of anaerobes; they are found on all mucosal surfaces and also on the skin.

Skin

It is surprising that, although the skin is constantly exposed to air, it still supports a considerable anaerobic microflora, the main components of which are the 'anaerobic diphtheroids', that is, the propionibacteria, including the lipolytic species *Propionibacterium acnes* associated with acne.

Mouth

Anaerobes are found in the tonsillar crypts, the crypts of the tongue, the gingival crevices, and in dental plaque. Although some anaerobic species are found in young infants, the variety and number of anaerobes increases markedly with the eruption of the teeth. Predominant members of the oral anaerobic flora include *Prevotella* spp., *Fusobacterium* spp., *Peptostreptococcus* spp., *Veillonella* spp., and various anaerobic Gram-positive rods. The *B. fragilis* group of anaerobes are rarely found in the mouth, and *Porphyromonas* spp. only in small numbers if at all.

Intestine

The stomach and upper small intestine are normally either sterile or contain only small numbers of transient organisms, including anaerobes that come from food, saliva, and nasopharyngeal secretions. The flora of the terminal ileum, on the other hand, resembles that of the colon and contains a vast and diverse anaerobic flora, which becomes established by the second year of life. Anaerobic bacteria constitute about 99 per cent of the bacterial faecal mass. *Bacteroides* spp. account for 20 to 30 per cent of the various species isolated. *B. vulgatus* is the most abundant anaerobe in faeces, while *B. fragilis*, clinically the most important isolate, is a relatively minor component. However, recent studies have shown that the occurrence of *B. fragilis* in the colonic flora has been underestimated, and when colonic flora (in specimens obtained by lavage and biopsy of the colonic mucosa) rather than faecal flora was investigated, the proportion of *B. fragilis* in it was 44 per cent compared with only approximately 4 per cent in the faecal flora. By comparison, *B. vulgatus* accounted for only 30 per cent of the colonic flora but 45 per cent of the faecal flora. *Clostridium* spp. are also found in large numbers and most of the other anaerobic genera occur in the colon.

Genitourinary tract

The normal flora of the vagina is predominantly anaerobic, consisting mostly of lactobacilli, but also small numbers of *Prevotella* spp., fusobacteria, and peptostreptococci. The urethral anaerobic flora has been less extensively studied but peptostreptococci are found in small numbers.

Pathogenesis

The anaerobic bacteria that cause human infection are almost always derived endogenously from the host's own commensal flora; exceptions to this include bite and punch injuries, in which the anaerobic oral flora of another is inoculated into the victim, and neonatal sepsis, in which the vaginal anaerobes are pathogenic in the baby. Anaerobic infections are usually polymicrobial, with not only several different anaerobic species involved but usually aerobic species as well. The anaerobic component of these mixed infections seems to be the more important. Predisposing factors include disruption of the normally intact cutaneous or mucosal barriers, tissue injury and necrosis, impaired blood supply, and obstruction of a hollow viscus. Although the normal flora of man consists of several hundred different anaerobic species, only a limited number are commonly found causing clinical infection and these are not necessarily the most numerous species in the normal flora. This suggests that virulence factors must be involved in these infections. Such factors include adhesins, capsules, lipopolysaccharide, hydrolytic and other enzymes, soluble metabolites and products, and growth factors. Precise virulence determinants for most anaerobic infections have not been established.

Adhesins

Surface attachment structures such as fimbriae have been described in some strains of *B. fragilis* and in other anaerobic species and may enable adherence to epithelial cells, an important factor in the initiation of colonization and infection.

Capsules

Capsule formation has been described in *B. fragilis*, some other *Bacteroides* spp., peptostreptococci, and *Fusobacterium* spp. Capsules confer resistance to phagocytosis, inhibit the migration of macrophages, and potentiate abscess formation.

Lipopolysaccharide

The lipid A component of the *B. fragilis* lipopolysaccharide differs chemically in certain respects from enterobacterial lipid A and this may account for its low endotoxic activity. *F. necrophorum* and *F. nucleatum*, interestingly, have conventional endotoxic lipopolysaccharide.

Enzymes

Most anaerobic pathogens produce a wide variety of enzymes including immunoglobulin proteases, enzymes capable of inactivating plasma proteins of importance in the initiation and control of the inflammatory response, and enzymes capable of degrading tissue components. A definitive role for each has not been established.

Diagnosis of anaerobic infection

Clinical

A working knowledge of the nature and whereabouts of the normal human commensal anaerobic flora is invaluable to the clinician, whatever his or her speciality. Much, though not all, anaerobic infection arises in obvious association with this commensal flora. The most helpful clinical indication of some common anaerobic infections is their putrid pus or discharge, the result of the metabolic products of anaerobic bacteria. No other group of organisms gives rise to such a foul, nauseating smell. But not all anaerobic infections produce putrid pus. Anaerobic infections, particularly necrotizing ones, are sometimes associated with cellulitis and this may be mistaken for streptococcal cellulitis. Gas formation in infected tissues is highly suggestive of anaerobes. Such a finding is readily confused by the inexperienced with clostridial gas gangrene, but this is very rare in the developed world, and is accompanied by profound toxaemia and prostration, whereas non-clostridial anaerobic infections with gas formation are common and usually far less dramatic. Gas formation is not, however, the prerogative of anaerobes; it can occasionally occur with aerobic infections. Another useful clue to the presence of anaerobes is a laboratory report of 'sterile pus' despite the detection of definite organisms on a Gram-stained film of the specimen. Lastly, for any patient who is receiving antibiotics that are inactive against anaerobes, such as aminoglycosides or (in the case of the *B. fragilis* group) penicillin, ampicillin, or most other β-lactams, and who still appears septic, an anaerobic infection should be considered.

Collection and transport of specimens for anaerobic bacteriology

Although all anaerobic bacteria are sensitive to oxygen, they cannot be considered as a homogeneous group in their aerotolerance. Some anaerobes, such as *B. fragilis* and *Cl. perfringens* for example, will tolerate 2 to 4 per cent oxygen, whereas other clinically important organisms, such as *Fusobacterium* spp. and some *Peptostreptococcus* spp., are much more sensitive to air or oxygen and thus more difficult to grow in the laboratory and also much less likely to survive the journey from patient to culture medium.

Until the renewed interest in the 1970s, few laboratories ever isolated the more fastidious anaerobes. The best specimens for the isolation of anaerobes are aspirates, pus (in a universal container) or excised tissue; although rapid delivery of such specimens to the laboratory is desirable, in practice, anaerobes (even fastidious species) survive remarkably well in pus and tissue. Swabs are less satisfactory for recovery of anaerobes, but are often all that is available, and for them an efficient transport medium such as Stuart's is ideal. It must be said, however, that clinical laboratories frequently recover anaerobes from swabs that are not received in transport media. Various rather complex commercial systems for the collection and transport of specimens for anaerobic bacteriology have been devised; they are unlikely to appeal to any busy clinician. Many clinical specimens will be routinely cultured for anaerobes and no specific directive will be required from the clinician. Expectorated sputum is an exception and clinicians should be aware that the diagnosis of an anaerobic pleuropulmonary infection is best made from an invasive specimen; occasionally copious putrid sputum is produced and such a specimen is worth culturing anaerobically, but liaison with the laboratory is required to ensure that this is done.

Laboratory

The putrid smell of the pus in many anaerobic infections has already been mentioned, and in such cases, even swabs will be noticeably foul when they are processed in the laboratory. There are also certain useful direct examinations of clinical material that will indicate the presence of anaerobes. The Gram-stained smear is often diagnostic to the experienced microscopist; it characteristically contains a variety of different bacteria, Gram-negative and Gram-positive, rods and cocci. Filamentous or spindle-shaped Gram-negative rods (often hard to see) confirm the presence of fusobacteria. Gas liquid chromatography (**GLC**) has been extensively used in the past on anaerobic specimens to detect the volatile fatty acids produced by many anaerobes. It is an expensive, sophisticated technique that is only rarely capable of detecting the presence of unsuspected anaerobes; more usually, it merely confirms a diagnosis already made from the smell of the specimen and its Gram stain. Many GLC machines now lie idle in clinical laboratories, a monument to past enthusiasms! Ultraviolet light will produce bright red fluorescence of pus or tissue containing some species of *Prevotella* and *Porphyromonas*, thereby confirming their presence in the specimen, but this too has been largely abandoned as a diagnostic tool.

Successful culture of anaerobes requires fresh media and a reliable system for maintaining an anaerobic atmosphere, which should include 10 per cent carbon dioxide. Most laboratories now have special anaerobic cabinets and no longer rely on old-fashioned anaerobic jars. While the relatively aerotolerant anaerobes such as *B. fragilis* and *Cl. perfringens* will usually grow in 24 h, many anaerobes take much longer. Fastidious anaerobes require undisturbed anaerobiosis and leaving inoculated culture plates out on the bench is likely to result in failure. The definitive identification of many anaerobes is a lengthy and technically demanding process and taxonomic exactitude has minimal appeal to clinicians, especially when it has taken weeks to produce. Commercially available, anaerobe identification kits using enzyme profiles enable rapid identification of the commonly isolated species but they require practice both in setting up and in interpreting the results. Minimal skill is required to identify the *B. fragilis* group and *Cl. perfringens*, and that is really sufficient for most clinical purposes. However, it is clearly important that a limited number of laboratories retain sufficient skill to advise on the more unusual species and to define the patterns of infection associated with different sites.

Clinical spectrum of anaerobic infection

Infections of the head and neck

ACUTE NECROTIZING ULCERATIVE GINGIVITIS

This condition, also known as Vincent's disease, Vincent's gingivostomatitis, trench mouth, and fusospirochaetosis, affects the gingiva and buccal mucosa and was one of the earliest anaerobic infections to be described. The characteristic symptoms of painful, bleeding gums, sometimes with a pseudomembrane, and with accompanying foul breath, readily suggest the diagnosis, which can be confirmed in the laboratory on a Gram-stained smear in which large numbers of spirochaetes (mostly the organism now known as *Treponema vincentii*), fusiforms, and other bacteria are seen.

DENTAL SEPSIS

The anaerobic oral commensal flora is found together with various aerobic and micro-aerophilic oral commensal bacteria in periodontal infection, dental abscesses, and other oral infections and in postoperative infections associated with maxillofacial surgery.

INFECTIONS OF THE NECK AND JAW

These unusual necrotizing infections are frequently anaerobic and may be accompanied by marked cellulitis and oedema, and cause respiratory embarrassment. Ludwig's angina is the name given to infection involving the main anterior compartment of the neck, the submandibular space. The source of the infection is usually the lower molar teeth, but it can also arise from tonsillar infection as in the patient shown in Fig. 1. It may spread to involve the chest, with mediastinal abscess and empyema. Infection of branchial cysts is usually anaerobic.

EAR, NOSE, AND THROAT INFECTIONS

Anaerobes are frequently isolated from excised tonsillar tissue from patients with recurrent streptococcal tonsillitis and it seems likely that these organisms are relevant in tonsillitis. They are also involved in peritonsillar abscesses (quinsy). Anaerobes, particularly fusobacteria, but also other oral commensals, are commonly found in infections (usually chronic) involving sinuses, middle ear, and mastoid. This predilection of anaerobes (often with *Streptococcus milleri*) for chronic sinus and middle-ear infection is important in the consideration of the bacterial aetiology of cerebral abscesses arising from such underlying sepsis. Chronic sinus infection occasionally also results in acute orbital cellulitis.

Infections of the central nervous system

Anaerobic bacteria are the principal pathogens in cerebral abscesses other than those that follow surgery or trauma. Otogenic cerebral abscesses are the most common and usually involve the temporal lobe or cerebellum. *B. fragilis* is usually isolated and aerobes, particularly *Proteus* spp. are often also present. In contrast, frontal-lobe abscesses of sinusitic or dental origin are most likely to be caused by *S. milleri*, although oral anaerobes may also be found. *B. fragilis* is not associated with frontal-lobe abscesses. Anaerobes very rarely cause meningitis and such cases are associated with underlying anaerobic infection with direct extension of this.

Fig. 1 Spreading cellulitis of the neck resulting from tonsillar sepsis (fatal)—'anaerobic neck'.

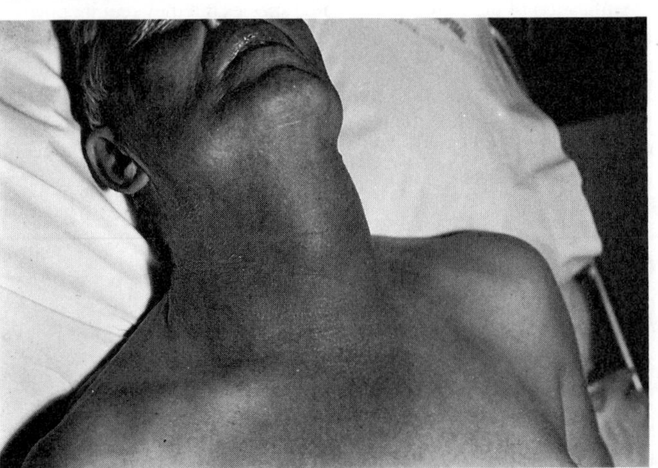

Pleuropulmonary infection

Most anaerobic pleuropulmonary infection is the result of aspiration of oropharyngeal secretions. It can also result from haematogenous seeding from an anaerobic bacteraemia, particularly with fusobacteria (see Necrobacillosis below). Anaerobic pleuropulmonary infections include aspiration pneumonia, necrotizing pneumonitis, lung abscess, and empyema, as well as secondary infection in underlying conditions such as bronchiectasis and bronchial carcinoma. The anaerobes involved are the oral commensals and *B. fragilis* is only likely to be found in metastatic infection from an intestinal source. Patients with an anaerobic lung abscess will usually admit to the revolting taste (as well as the smell) of their sputum and this is a useful clue to the diagnosis. Definitive bacteriological diagnosis of anaerobic pleuropulmonary infection can seldom be made by culture of expectorated sputum, and invasive procedures are usually required. Transtracheal aspiration, advocated in the United States, is seldom done elsewhere, and satisfactory specimens can often be obtained by fibreoptic bronchoscopy. In lung abscess, percutaneous transthoracic aspiration can be useful, not only to obtain a specimen for bacteriological diagnosis, but also to assist in drainage of the abscess. Such specimens should preferably be obtained before antibiotics are given; in practice they seldom are.

Intra-abdominal infections

These are common anaerobic infections, hardly surprising in view of the rich anaerobic microflora of the colon. They are usually associated with intra-abdominal pathology such as perforated gastric or duodenal ulcers, appendicitis, diverticulitis, inflammatory bowel disease, or malignancy, and produce peritonitis or frank abscess formation. Primary anaerobic peritonitis has only rarely been reported, usually in patients with underlying ascites. Most infections are polymicrobial and the predominant anaerobes are those of the *B. fragilis* group. Before the advent of antianaerobic prophylaxis for intestinal surgery, postoperative anaerobic wound infection, abscess formation, and even septicaemia were commonly seen on surgical wards. Such infections are much less common now, but despite prophylaxis, they do occasionally occur.

Hepatic and biliary-tract infection

Although hepatic abscesses are rare, they are quite likely to be caused by anaerobic bacteria as well as by *S. milleri*; sometimes both types of bacteria are found. The most common anaerobes are the *Fusobacterium* spp. and *B. fragilis*. Such abscesses arise from biliary-tract infection, haematogenous spread from an intestinal source, or the direct extension of contiguous infection. Although aerobes are the predominant pathogens in biliary infection, anaerobes can also be grown from the bile, particularly where there is obstructive disease and stasis. Anaerobes, especially *B. fragilis* and *Clostridium* spp., are also sometimes cultured from the blood (usually with aerobes) in biliary sepsis. Cholangitis in patients who have had previous enterobiliary anastomoses may also be caused by anaerobes.

Infections of the female genital tract and neonatal infection

Anaerobic bacteria are, with *Gardnerella vaginalis*, the cause of the malodorous vaginal discharge in the common condition now known as bacterial vaginosis (Chapter 21.4). They also cause tubo-ovarian sepsis,

Bartholin's abscess, endometritis, septic abortion, and infection associated with intrauterine contraceptive devices. Vaginal hysterectomy carries a high risk of postoperative anaerobic infection, but wound infection after abdominal hysterectomy is more likely to be caused by *Staphylococcus aureus* than anaerobes and should be uncommon with good operative technique. In pregnancy, prolonged rupture of the membranes is associated with anaerobic infection and foul-smelling liquor is often noted, although in the past this was not attributed to the presence of anaerobes. In such cases, anaerobes, of vaginal origin, can be cultured not only from the liquor but also from the placenta (which also smells) and frequently from the nasogastric aspirate, ear, and other surface swabs of the newborn baby, which may develop anaerobic pneumonitis. Anaerobic bacteria are an important, if underemphasized, cause of neonatal sepsis. Anaerobic infections of the female genital tract and neonatal infections are usually caused by *Prevotella* spp., *Porphyromonas* spp., *Fusobacterium* spp., and *Peptostreptococcus* spp., very rarely by *B. fragilis*.

Infections of the male genitalia and prostate

The commensal anaerobic flora of the male urethra is found in a variety of genital infections including balanoposthitis, and the foul odour of anaerobic balanoposthitis is well known to genitourinary physicians. Anaerobes also cause secondary infection of penile lesions such as syphilitic ulcers, condylomata acuminata, and malignancies. Scrotal abscesses are usually caused by anaerobes unless they follow acute epididymo-orchitis with an associated urinary-tract infection. Anaerobic scrotal abscesses arise either *de novo*, when they probably result from secondary infection of blocked apocrine glands and are characteristically recurrent, or after surgery to the genitalia or urethra.

The rare condition known as Fournier's gangrene, so vividly described over a century ago, is a synergistic, necrotizing infection involving the scrotum, but also often extending into the perineum, thighs, and abdominal wall. It is characterized by the sudden onset of intense pain and swelling with foul discharge and gas in the tissues as well as marked systemic disturbance. In fact, the condition originally described by Fournier differs from that seen today. His disease occurred in previous healthy young men, whereas the infection that bears his name is now seen in middle-aged or elderly men, particularly diabetics and alcoholics, and there is a cutaneous, anorectal, or genitourinary source for the anaerobes, which usually include *B. fragilis*.

Acute prostatic abscesses are now rarely seen, but they are sometimes caused by anaerobes. Anaerobes may also be relevant in the diagnostically ill-defined entity we know as chronic prostatitis, and they can sometimes be cultured from expressed prostatic secretion. However, the difficulties of sampling prostatic fluid that has not been contaminated with the normal urethral anaerobic flora make interpretation of such culture results very difficult.

Infection of the urinary tract

Genuine urinary infection caused by anaerobes is very rare, so much so that urine is not routinely cultured anaerobically. Anaerobes can be recovered from the urine in heavy growth when there are abnormalities within the urinary tract such as vesicocolic fistulae, tumours, pyonephrosis, and perinephric abscess. Conduit specimens of urine may also sometimes grow anaerobes.

Bone and joint infection

Anaerobes are very uncommon but occasionally important pathogens in acute osteomyelitis and septic arthritis. These infections are likely to be misdiagnosed because few orthopaedic surgeons and rheumatologists are aware of them. Acute anaerobic osteomyelitis affecting long bones is likely to be caused by *Fusobacterium* spp. whereas acute vertebral osteomyelitis, a infection occurring mainly in elderly patients, is more likely to be caused by *B. fragilis*. Acute anaerobic septic arthritis is most likely to be encountered in patients with underlying rheumatoid arthritis or other joint pathology and again is likely to be caused by *B. fragilis*. Numerous organisms, including anaerobes, can usually be isolated from cases of chronic osteomyelitis where there are bone sequestra and necrosis.

A special mention should be made of human bite and closed fist injuries of the hand. These may penetrate the synovium and give rise to joint infection. Such infections have a well-deserved evil reputation and are invariably anaerobic.

Skin and soft tissue infection

DIABETIC FOOT ULCERS

Diabetic foot ulcers yield a variety of organisms, including anaerobes, on culture. Anaerobic infections may be associated with underlying chronic osteomyelitis and sometimes with cellulitis, necrotizing fasciitis, and gas formation. This condition (for which surgery is the only remedy) is readily confused by the inexperienced with clostridial gas gangrene; it is, however, seldom accompanied by the prostration and toxaemia that characterize clostridial infection.

VENOUS ULCERS

Anaerobes, particularly *Peptostreptococcus* spp. are often isolated from swabs taken from venous ulcers and these are frequently offensive, though whether from the anaerobes or the occlusive dressings is unclear. Anaerobes are secondary invaders and play no proven part in the aetiology or perpetuation of the ulcer.

DECUBITUS ULCERS

These are frequently infected with anaerobes, particularly *B. fragilis*, and anaerobic bacteraemia may occasionally result.

SEBACEOUS CYSTS

Anaerobes, notably *Peptostreptococcus* spp., are often isolated from infected sebaceous cysts, but many clinically infected cysts prove sterile on culture even with adequate techniques for anaerobic culture.

AXILLARY ABSCESS AND HIDRADENITIS SUPPURATIVA

Whilst most axillary abscesses are caused by *Staph. aureus*, some are anaerobic. These abscesses tend to be more indolent than staphylococcal abscesses, they have satellite lesions adjacent to the main abscess, and they always recur. These recurrences ultimately can result in the distressing condition of hidradenitis suppurativa. (Fig. 2). Anaerobic axillary abscesses and hidradenitis suppurativa result from apocrine blockage and the anaerobic infection is secondary to this. A variety of anaerobes is involved but seldom *B. fragilis*. Despite the foul odour characteristically complained of by these patients, their infection is generally assumed to be staphylococcal and they are condemned to endless courses of flucloxacillin. How the anaerobes reach the blocked apocrine glands is not known. Hidradenitis suppurativa is not confined to the axilla; it can occur at any site where these glands occur—perineum, groins, buttocks, and back.

PERIRECTAL ABSCESS

These abscesses are frequently caused by anaerobes but they cannot be considered as a bacteriologically homogeneous group. Those abscesses that are associated with an underlying fistula yield gut-specific anaerobes of the *B. fragilis* group as well as coliforms. Perirectal abscesses without an associated fistula are usually anaerobic but are not infected with gut-specific organisms; these abscesses may well result from secondary infection of blocked apocrine glands.

BREAST ABSCESS

Although breast abscesses are usually assumed to be staphylococcal, those occurring in the non-puerperal woman are just as likely to be anaerobic. Anaerobic breast abscesses are secondary infections of an underlying blocked duct, a situation akin to that described for hidradentitis suppurativa. They are usually recurrent, subareolar, and associated with inverted nipples. Various anaerobes are responsible, though rarely *B. fragilis*.

HUMAN AND ANIMAL BITES

Human bites have already been mentioned with reference to infection of the joints of the hand, but they may involve other parts of the body. Although animal bites can also give rise to anaerobic infection, they are more likely to become infected with *Pasteurella* spp. (see Chapter 7.11.17).

PARONYCHIA

About a third of paronychias are caused by anaerobes, usually though not invariably occurring with aerobes. The anaerobes are oral commensals and are probably transferred to the fingers by licking or biting. Anaerobic paronychias are usually less acute than those caused by *Staph. aureus* or *Strep. pyogenes* but are otherwise indistinguishable.

Synergistic necrotizing infections

Anaerobic bacteria, usually with aerobes as well, cause a range of so-called synergistic infections. These are spreading, necrotizing infections that can involve skin, fascia, and sometimes muscle. The bacteriology in the earlier reports of these conditions was rather incomplete but it is clear that many species can be involved. The eponymous conditions of Fournier's gangrene (see above) and Meleney's synergistic infection are examples of synergistic necrotizing infections and they are probably just examples of a whole range of synergistic infections of similar pathogenesis. These infections, which can affect many areas of the body, can occur spontaneously, or after trauma or surgery (Fig. 3), but why remains a mystery.

Bacteraemia and endocarditis

Anaerobic infection at any site, but particularly intra-abdominal infection, can be accompanied by bacteraemia, sometimes with shock. Anaerobes account for only around 5 per cent of positive blood cultures, with those of the *B. fragilis* group isolated most frequently. They are also found in polymicrobial bacteraemia. By the time the laboratory reports the presence of an anaerobe in a blood culture, the type and site of the infection has already been established. In a few cases, and particularly with the isolation of *F. necrophorum* from the blood, the finding may be crucial in determining the diagnosis. Here the use of GLC directly on the blood culture bottle can sometimes enable much more rapid detection of an anaerobe than conventional methods. Anaerobic endocarditis has been reported, but is very rare.

Fusobacterial bacteraemia, necrobacillosis, and Lemierre's postanginal septicaemia

From the foregoing it will have been readily apparent that the anaerobic infections so far described have been characteristically polymicrobial with not only several anaerobic species but also several aerobic species frequently isolated. Fusobacteria (that is *F. necrophorum*, probably also *F. nucleatum*, and perhaps other species as well) are able to act as sole (and very virulent) pathogens to produce severe infections. Their virulence is probably attributable to their different lipopolysaccharide, which is similar to that of Gram-negative aerobic bacteria. Although these serious infections are rare, they were well described in the preantibiotic era. They are now constantly being 'rediscovered' by different clinicians and microbiologists, each convinced that they are describing a new disease. The species most often isolated from septicaemic disease is *F. necrophorum* and it is to this species that the term necrobacillosis refers.

NECROBACILLOSIS

The term necrobacillosis has been used by veterinarians for many years to describe infections at various sites in animals (such as calf diphtheria, liver abscesses, and foot rot) that are characterised by tissue necrosis, abscess formation, and putrid smell. The main pathogen in these animal infections is *F. necrophorum*, but in many cases it forms part of a mixed culture. These infections seem to follow injury to the skin or mucous membranes. The earliest reports of necrobacillosis in man were of zoonotic skin infections, but in 1930, two fatal cases that presented 'hitherto undescribed clinical and pathological features of systemic infection' were described. One was a girl of 19 years who died of lung abscesses, septic arthritis of the hip, and jaundice 6 days after developing a sore throat with rigors, and the other was a 64-year-old man who died of a retropharyngeal abscess with gangrene and extension into the peritracheal and subcutaneous tissues. The former case conforms exactly to those described in 1936 as 'post-anginal septicaemia' by Lemierre (see below). The latter sounds more like necrotizing fasciitis. Further clarification of the entity of necrobacillosis was provided in 1955 by the

Fig. 2 Hidradenitis suppurativa of axilla.

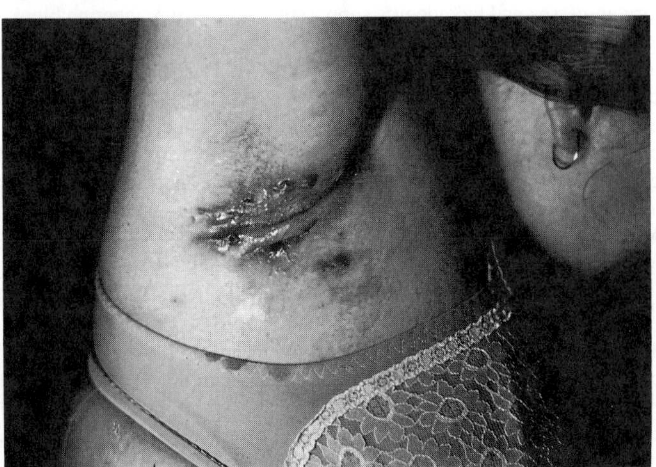

Fig. 3 Necrotizing fasciitis involving perineum, buttock, and thigh 3 weeks after gastrectomy for carcinoma.

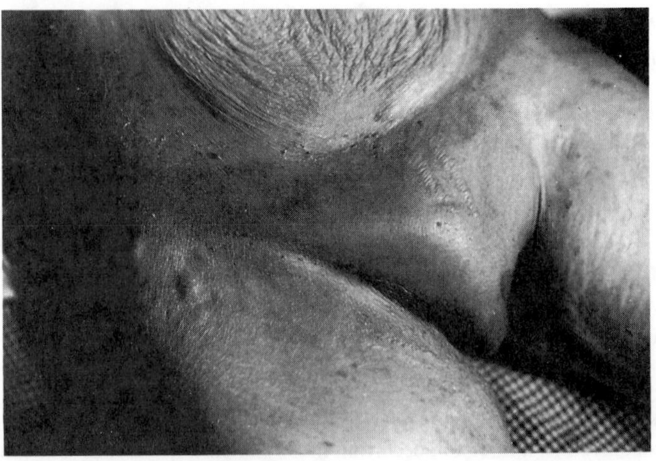

British physician Alston, who recognized four different types of infection caused by *F. necrophorum*: those involving the skin and subcutaneous tissues, a large group in which the infection started with a sore throat or with otitis media, a third group associated with the female genital tract, the alimentary tract or the urinary tract, and a fourth group with empyema. Pyaemia and abscesses were very common in the last three groups. Alston's second group corresponds to Lemierre's postanginal septicaemia, although Lemierre considered that septicaemias arising from otitis media and mastoiditis were a separate group and I would agree with this. Since Alston's study there have been sporadic case reports of necrobacillosis and, in 1989, a series of 45 cases culled from over 20 hospitals throughout the United Kingdom was published. There is no doubt that these severe fusobacterial septicaemic infections continue to occur, even if they are often misdiagnosed. The term necrobacillosis is best used to describe any septicaemic infection with *F. necrophorum* and those cases with postanginal septicaemic infection should be designated as Lemierre's disease because they constitute a distinct entity.

LEMIERRE'S POSTANGINAL SEPTICAEMIA (LEMIERRE'S DISEASE)

This unique manifestation of necrobacillosis occurs in young previously healthy people, usually in their teens or early twenties; although Lemierre suggested that the infection affected both sexes equally, the recent series in the United Kingdom contained a male predominance. There is always an antecedent sore throat, which may be particularly severe; sometimes there is acute tonsillitis. Painful cervical lympadenopathy is usual and sometimes septic jugular thrombophlebitis occurs. Within days, sometimes only hours, of the onset of the sore throat, rigors develop, with marked systemic upset and often evidence of impaired renal and hepatic function. Disseminated intravascular coagulation may also occur. Metastatic spread is characteristic and this most commonly involves the lung, but also bone, joint, liver, and brain. The 'pneumonia' is often severe and extensive (Fig. 4) and mechanical ventilation may be required; cavitation of the septic infarcts and empyema may occur. Unless the relevance of an antecedent sore throat is appreciated in such patients, the diagnosis will be missed. Although *F. necrophorum* is readily isolated from blood cultures (as in the case mentioned), its identification can pose problems. It is usually mistaken for a Bacteroides and as such can lead to a spurious search for some gut pathology.

F. necrophorum is very sensitive to both penicillin and metronidazole (though usually resistant to erythromycin), yet the infection responds only very slowly to antibiotic treatment and this slow response is akin to that seen with other severe community-acquired infections caused by both Gram-negative and Gram-positive organisms. It reflects the innate virulence of the organism.

Fig. 4 Chest radiograph taken on admission to hospital of a 21-year-old heating engineer who had developed rigors and severe shortness of breath about a week after a sore throat. He was thought to have possible legionnaire's disease, hence given erythromycin (to which fusobacteria are usually resistant); *F. necrophorum* was isolated from blood cultures.

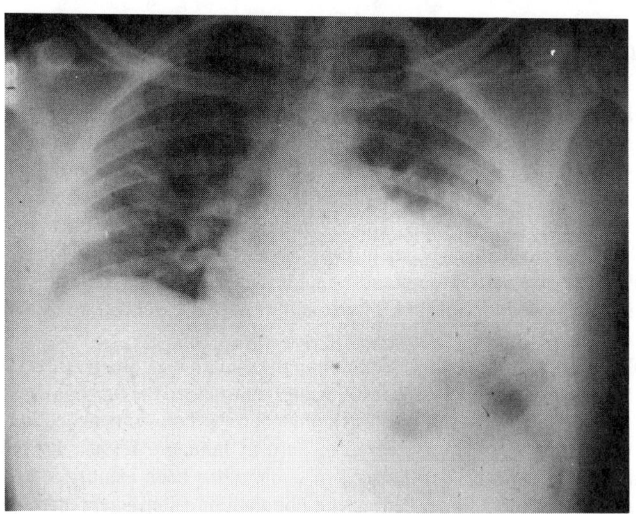

Sensitivity of anaerobic bacteria to antimicrobial agents

Metronidazole (and other nitroimidazoles)

The susceptibility of most anaerobic bacteria to antimicrobial agents is remarkably uniform. Intrinsic resistance is often predictable and acquired resistance is uncommon. Metronidazole and other nitroimidazoles such as tinidazole, are unique amongst the antimicrobial agents that are active against anaerobic bacteria in that they are only active against anaerobes and have no activity against aerobic organisms. Although metronidazole has been used to treat anaerobic infections for about 30 years, most clinically important anaerobes remain extremely sensitive to it and resistance has only rarely been reported during treatment. There is little to choose between the activity of the different nitroimidazoles.

β-Lactam antibiotics

Contrary to popular belief, many anaerobes are still very sensitive to benzylpenicillin; these include many strains of *Prevotella* spp., *Porphyromonas* spp., and *Fusobacterium* spp. as well as clostridia, peptostreptococci, and spirochaetes. The *B. fragilis* group are almost uniformly resistant to penicillin, and resistance is also increasing amongst Prevotella and Porphyromonas. These penicillin-resistant anaerobes are also resistant to ampicillin, amoxycillin, the acylureidopenicillins (e.g. azlocillin and piperacillin), the carboxypenicillins (e.g. carbenicillin and ticarcillin), and most cephalosporins; only those cephalosporins of the cephamycin type (e.g. cefoxitin) have any useful activity and it is not uniform within the *B. fragilis* group. This resistance to β-lactams results from a constitutive β-lactamase possessed by these strains. The addition of the β-lactam inhibitor clavulanic acid in the antimicrobial co-amoxiclav renders the *B. fragilis* group susceptible to the amoxycillin in the combination. The new carbapenem imipenem is also active against most strains.

Other agents

Almost all anaerobes remain very sensitive to the lincosamide clindamycin, and its antianaerobic activity is similar to that of metronidazole. Chloramphenicol is also highly active against anaerobes. Other agents with useful activity include erythromycin, co-trimoxazole (but both these agents are technically difficult to test in the laboratory), and tetracyclines. The glycopeptides vancomycin and teicoplanin, whilst inactive against most Gram-negative anaerobes, possess useful activity against clostridia and peptostreptococci. Neither the aminoglycosides nor the quinolones are active against anaerobes.

Treatment of anaerobic infection

Surgical intervention, particularly drainage of pus and excision of necrotic tissue, is of paramount importance in anaerobic infections and in many of these infections it will be all that is required. Indeed, a failure to carry out effective surgery will result in the persistence or even spread of the infection whatever antibiotic is given. Certain infections will respond to antibiotics alone and examples include necrobacillosis (though non-pulmonary metastatic lesions may require surgery) and lung abscess (though drainage of the pus, usually by effective physiotherapy, sometimes also with bronchoscopy, is essential). As has been already mentioned, most anaerobic infection is polymicrobial, with aerobes as well as anaerobes involved. Thus in devising antimicrobial therapy for such infections, it must not only be decided which agent to use for the anaerobes, but also whether it is necessary to give an agent for the aerobes as well. It is of interest that there is *in vitro* evidence that anaerobes impair phagocytosis in mixed infections and this might well be relevant in the undoubted success of the selectivity antianaerobic drug metronidazole alone in many of these mixed infections. It has, nevertheless, become universally accepted practice to cover both groups of bacteria.

For anaerobic infections other than those caused by the *B. fragilis* group there is a wide choice of agent, but few clinicians think of anaerobes in distinct groups, and it is easier to recommend overall anaerobic cover; this is best provided by metronidazole. It is illogical to give metronidazole with drugs such as co-amoxiclav, which themselves have excellent antianaerobic activity. Until the mid-1970s, lincomycin, and then clindamycin, was widely used to treat anaerobic infection but then it was realized that they were particularly likely to cause antibiotic-associated diarrhoea and pseudomembranous colitis, although these side-effects were not unique to this group of antibiotics. Serendipitously with this discovery of the unwanted side-effects of clindamycin came the belated rediscovery of the antianaerobic activity of metronidazole, which had already been on the market as an oral preparation since the end of the 1950s. The rapid introduction of the intravenous preparation meant that anaerobic infection soon became (and has remained) synonymous with metronidazole in the United Kingdom. In the United States particularly, warnings of the potential genotoxicity of metronidazole predicted from animal and bacterial test systems (which has never been substantiated) meant that other agents have often been preferred. It is unlikely that any comparative therapeutic trial would be able to differentiate between the efficacy of the various regimens that are used to treat anaerobic infection.

Prevention of anaerobic infection

It seems remarkable that surgical prophylaxis for operations likely to be followed by postoperative anaerobic wound infection did not become routine until the mid-1970s. Incredible though it might appear today, there were no ethical objections to our undertaking a double-blind trial of intravenous metronidazole versus placebo (saline) in elective colorectal surgery in 1976! Many trials bear witness to the efficacy of such prophylaxis in surgery involving sites with an anaerobic commensal flora and the putrid wound infections so familiar to gastrointestinal surgeons in the past (Fig. 5) are rarely seen today. In the same way that the treatment of anaerobic infection now routinely includes an antiaerobe drug, most regimens for surgical prophylaxis likewise include cover for both groups of bacteria. This may well not be necessary but it has become routine. Antianaerobic prophylaxis is thus given for many different types of surgery, but particularly for that involving the gastrointestinal tract and the genital tract. What has emerged from the multiplicity of trials is a consensus that such prophylaxis should be perioperative and of short duration, and this generally means from one to three doses given intravenously, the first with the induction of anaesthesia. The number of possible regimens is enormous.

Fig. 5 Wound sepsis following elective colorectal surgery.

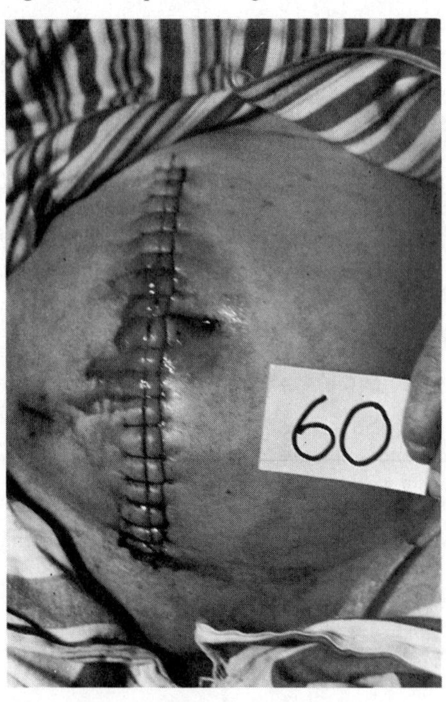

REFERENCES

Alston, J.M. (1955). Necrobacillosis in Great Britain. *British Medical Journal*, **ii**, 1524–1528. Old paper providing insight into various clinical presentations of fusobacterial septicaemia.

Duerden, B.I. and Drasar, B.S. (ed.) (1991). *Anaerobes in human disease*. Arnold, London.

Eykyn, S.J. (1989). Necrobacillosis. *Scandinavian Journal of Infectious Diseases* (suppl. 62), 41–6.

Finegold, S.M. and George, W.L. (ed.) (1989). *Anaerobic infections in humans*. Academic Press, New York.

Hofstad, T. (1992). Virulence factors in anaerobic bacteria. *European Journal of Microbiology and Infectious Diseases*, **11**, 1044–8.

Lemierre, A. (1936). On certain septicaemias due to anaerobic organisms. *Lancet*, **i**, 701–3. This paper contains the classic description of post-anginal septicaemia.

Patrick, S. (1993). The virulence of *Bacteroides fragilis*. *Reviews in Medical Microbiology*, **4**, 40–9.

Unattributed (1984). International symposium on anaerobic bacteria and their role in disease. *Reviews of Infectious Diseases*, **6**, (suppl. 1).

7.11.11 Cholera

C. C. J. Carpenter

Cholera is an acute illness caused by an enterotoxin elaborated by *Vibrio cholerae* that have colonized the small bowel. In the more severely ill patients, fluid and electrolytes are rapidly lost from the gastrointestinal tract, resulting in hypovolaemic shock, metabolic acidosis, and, if untreated, death.

Aetiology and epidemiology

V. cholerae are short (0.2–0.4 × 1.5–4.0 μm), slightly curved, Gram-negative rods that are readily seen in the excreta of patients with cholera.

Cholera has been endemic for two centuries in the Ganges delta of West Bengal and Bangladesh, has caused multiple epidemics throughout the Indian subcontinent, and has been responsible for seven global pandemics in the past 170 years. The seventh pandemic, the only pandemic of the twentieth century, began in 1961, rapidly extended from Indonesia (Sulawesi) westward throughout Asia, ultimately involved the whole of Africa and Mediterranean Europe, and in 1991 extended to South America.

The introduction of the seventh cholera pandemic to South America in 1991 occurred in explosive fashion, and represented the first epidemic outbreak of cholera in the Western hemisphere in the twentieth century. Cholera cases were first observed in Peru in January of 1991; by the end of the year over 300 000 cases of cholera had been identified. It is estimated that over 20 per cent of the population of Peru were infected by *V. cholerae* during 1991. Infection rapidly spread to the adjoining South American countries, and to Central America. By the end of 1992, cholera cases had been recognized in all except four of the South and Central American nations (Fig. 1).

Man is the only known mammalian host and natural victim of *V. cholerae*. Most major epidemics of this disease have been waterborne, and water plays a large part in the transmission of *V. cholerae* in the endemic rural areas in the Ganges delta. During large pandemics, however, the direct contamination of food as well as water with infectious excreta is important. Contaminated fresh vegetables appeared to have been an influential factor in transmission of cholera in Israel in the 1970 outbreak, and shellfish in the spread of cholera in Naples in 1973. Shellfish clearly have the capacity to harbour *V. cholerae* in high concentration for long periods without obvious damage to the host; they were initially a principal vehicle in the transmission of the outbreak of cholera in the coastal cities of Peru in 1991. Contaminated water appears, however, to have played the significant role in the explosive spread of cholera throughout South and Central America in 1991 to 1993.

People with mild or asymptomatic infections (contact carriers) may also help to disseminate epidemic disease. The clinical case:infection ratio with the classical *V. cholerae* biotype is about 1:6; with infection by the el Tor biotype, this ratio may be as low as 1:50. A prolonged gallbladder carrier state occasionally develops in adults convalescing from cholera caused by the el Tor biotype. The role of such convalescent carriers in the transmission of the disease, if any, has not been clarified. *V. cholerae* does not survive well in fresh water, but may survive for long periods in seawater; this observation was confirmed in association with the 1973 outbreak of cholera in Portugal.

In the endemic areas of Bangladesh and West Bengal, cholera is predominantly a disease of children. Attack rates are 10 times greater in the 1- to 5-year age group than in those over 20 years of age. When the disease spreads to previously uninvolved areas, the attack rates are initially at least as high in adults as in children. This has been the case in the current epidemic in South and Central America, with complications being more severe in elderly individuals. As the disease becomes endemic in new locations, as has occurred in the Philippines over the past 25 years and in Africa over the past 15 years, the endemic epidemiological pattern develops, with the disease becoming far more common in young children.

Fig. 1 Rapid spread of epidemic cholera across South and Central America, 1991–1992. (Reprinted from *Morbidity and Mortality Weekly Reports*, (1992) **42,** 89, with permission.)

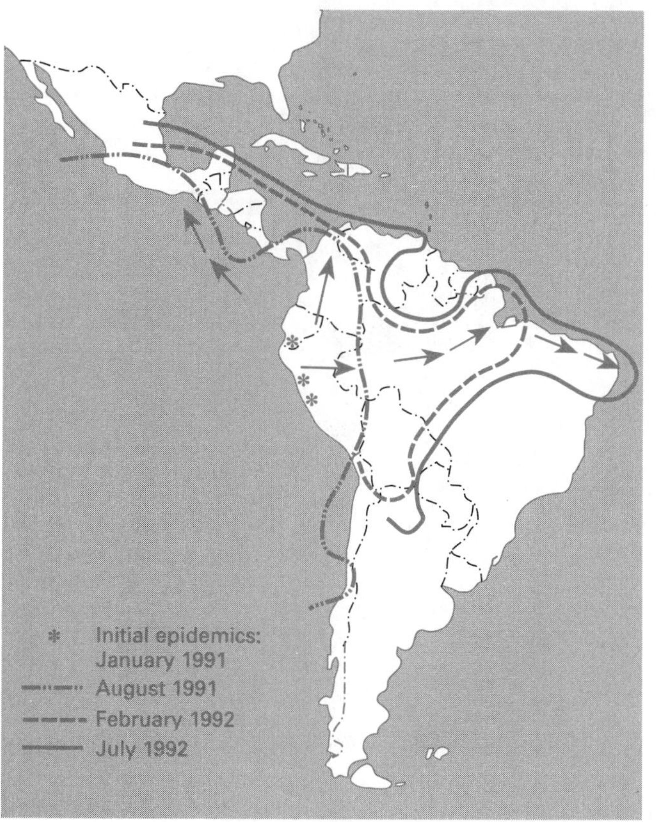

Pathogenesis

V. cholerae cause disease when a large number of viable organisms are ingested, survive passage through the stomach, colonize the small bowel, and produce enterotoxin. The incubation period may vary from 12 h to as long as 6 days, but is usually between 24 and 72 h. Because of the remarkable susceptibility of *V. cholerae* to gastric acid, an enormous number of micro-organisms must be ingested to cause illness in previously healthy individuals. Volunteer studies have indicated that the ingestion of even a thousand million organisms will not consistently produce disease in fasting healthy adults. If, however, gastric acid is neutralized by sodium bicarbonate, or by a high-protein meal, ingestion of a million viable organisms may produce clinical disease in roughly 50 per cent of normal individuals. The individual with relative or absolute achlorhydria is, therefore, abnormally susceptible to cholera; this susceptibility has been emphasized by the very high relative incidence of cholera in individuals with total or subtotal gastrectomy in the outbreaks of cholera in Israel and Italy during the last two decades.

Once vibrios have colonized the small bowel, a well-defined enterotoxin is produced. This is a protein of 84 000 Da consisting of two well-defined moieties. The B, or binding, moiety has five identical subunits, each of roughly 11 500 Da; each subunit is capable of combining to a GM-1 monosialoganglioside molecule in the gut mucosal cell wall. The A, or activating, moiety is divided into two unequal subunits: a larger, or A-1, subunit of roughly 23 000 Da, and a smaller, or A-2, subunit of roughly 6000 Da. The binding subunits of the enterotoxin combine extraordinarily rapidly to the monosialogangliosides in the small-bowel epithelial cell wall, and, at body temperature, binding becomes irreversible within minutes after the initial contact of the binding subunits with the GM-1 monosialogangliosides. This irreversibility suggests that the binding subunits become incorporated into the cell membrane. Following this rapid binding, the A-1 subunit migrates through to the inner surface to the epithelial cell membrane, where it stimulates ADP ribosylation of a 41 000-Da adenylate cyclase component bearing the guanyl nucleotide site. This results in a modification of the guanosine triphosphate-binding protein, inhibits the guanosine triphosphate 'turn-off' reaction, and thus increases the activity of adenylate cyclase. The resultant increase in intracellular levels of cyclic AMP leads to rapid excretion of electrolytes into the small-bowel lumen.

The net secretion of fluid and electrolytes by gut mucosal cells in cholera reflects a dual effect on two different intestinal ion-transport sites. In the villous cells the absorption of sodium chloride via the neutral sodium chloride cotransport system is inhibited. In the crypt cells the increased intracellular AMP results in active stimulation of chloride secretion. The net effect of inhibition of sodium absorption and stimulation of chloride secretion is the rapid outpouring of isotonic fluid into the intestinal lumen at a rate that exceeds the absorptive capacity of the colon, thus resulting in the loss of an isotonic fluid with the electrolyte pattern described in Table 1. In adults with voluminous diarrhoea the electrolyte in cholera stool is remarkably consistent, being nearly isotonic with plasma, with sodium and chloride concentrations slightly less than those of plasma, bicarbonate concentration twice that of plasma, and potassium concentration three to five times that of plasma. In very young children with cholera the mean sodium and chloride concentrations are 15 to 20 mmol/l less than those observed in older patients.

All signs, symptoms, and metabolic derangements in cholera result directly from the rapid loss of these fluids from the gut. All segments of the small bowel participate in the increased secretion of isotonic fluid,

Table 1 *Electrolyte concentrations in cholera stool of adults (mmol/l)*

	Admission	48 h after admission
Sodium	116	126
Chloride	100	90
Potassium	30	16
Bicarbonate	40	50

Mean values, 38 patients.

and the resultant fluid lost represents the sum of the contributions of each of the small-bowel segments, slightly modified during passage through the colon.

Clinical features

The clinical onset of cholera is generally abrupt, with painless, watery diarrhoea. Stool volumes vary greatly, and in all epidemics there are large numbers of mild cases in which the fluid loss is not severe enough to require admission to hospital. In the more severe cases, however, the initial stool volume may exceed 1500 ml. At variable intervals after the onset of diarrhoea, vomiting ensues; this is also characteristically effortless and productive of rice-watery material. In fulminant cases, severe muscle cramps, most commonly involving the calf muscles, almost invariably develop. Prostration occurs at varying intervals after the onset of symptoms, in direct relation to the magnitude of fluid loss.

When first seen by the physician, the severely ill cholera patient presents a characteristic appearance (Fig. 2(a)). He is collapsed, cyanotic, with no palpable peripheral pulses, pinched facies, and scaphoid abdomen. The skin turgor is remarkably diminished. The voice is weak, high-pitched, and often nearly inaudible. Vital signs include tachycardia, varying degrees of tachypnoea, hypopyrexia, and hypotension, often with no obtainable blood pressure. Heart sounds are faint or inaudible, and bowel sounds are hypoactive or entirely absent. Large alterations in mental status are not common in adults; the adult usually remains well oriented, although apathetic, even in the face of severe hypovolaemic shock. As many as 10 per cent of small children, however, may have central nervous abnormalities that range from stupor to convulsions.

Laboratory abnormalities are those that would be expected to result from massive gastrointestinal loss of an isotonic, alkaline, virtually protein-free fluid (Table 2). They include increased plasma and whole-blood specific gravity, elevated plasma protein, decreased plasma bicarbonate, low arterial pH, normal plasma sodium, slightly increased plasma chloride, and moderately elevated plasma potassium. Because the bicarbonate loss is proportional to stool volume, the decrease in whole-blood pH is roughly proportional to the increase in plasma protein concentration at all stages of the untreated disease. The abnormal blood chemical findings are rapidly corrected with appropriate fluid therapy (Table 2).

The illness may last from 12 h to 7 days, and later clinical manifestations depend on the adequacy of therapy. With adequate fluid and electrolyte repletion, recovery is remarkably rapid (Fig. 2(b,c)). If therapy is inadequate, the case mortality rate may exceed 50 per cent. The important causes of death are hypovolaemic shock, uncompensated metabolic acidosis, and renal failure. When renal failure occurs, the characteristic pathological findings are those of acute tubular necrosis secondary to prolonged hypotension.

Diagnosis

The working diagnosis of cholera should be made on the basis of the clinical picture; appropriate fluid and electrolyte replacement therapy, as indicated by the physical findings, should be initiated immediately. Although a cholera-like illness may be caused by micro-organisms other than *V. cholerae*, most frequently by enterotoxigenic *Escherichia coli*, the resulting physiological and metabolic abnormalities are the same, so that identical intravenous and oral electrolyte therapy may be used in all such cases.

After appropriate therapy has been started, a travel history should be obtained. The diagnosis of cholera is unlikely if the patient has not recently been in a known endemic or epidemic area. Stool examination should then be made. As the cholera enterotoxin causes neither inflammation nor destruction of intestinal mucosa, neither leucocytes nor erythrocytes are usually seen on microscopical examination of fresh

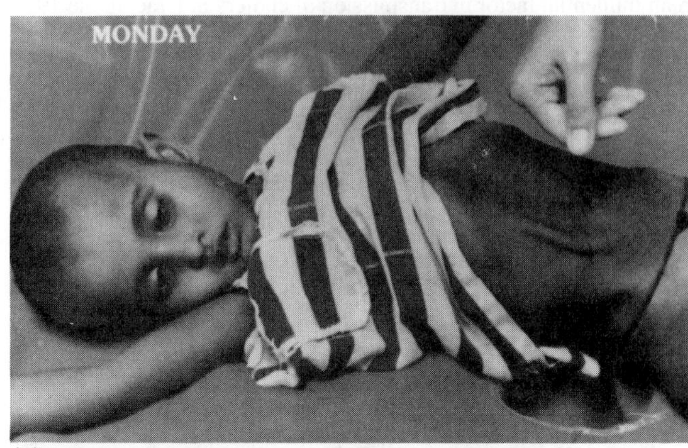

(a)

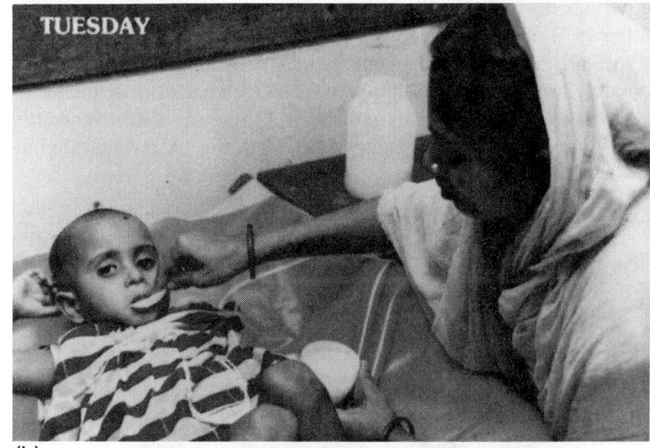

(b)

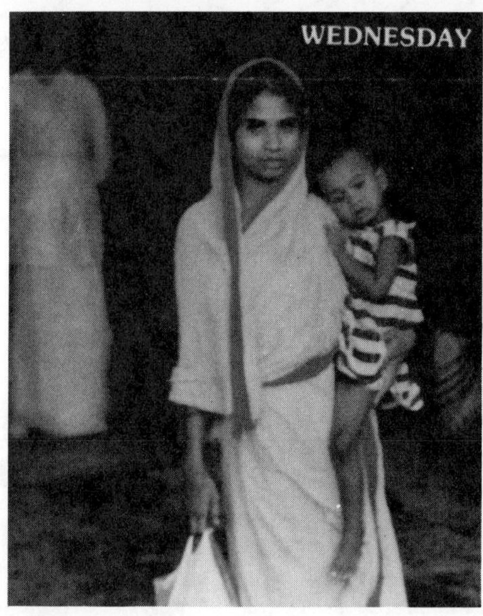

(c)

Fig. 2 Oral rehydration therapy (ORT) in cholera: (a) Before treatment; (b) after 24 h of ORT; (c) asymptomatic after 48 h of ORT.

Table 2 *Blood chemical determinations in 38 adult cholera patients before and hours after intravenous fluid therapy*

	Mean values ± SD	
	Admission	4 h after admission
Arterial blood pH	7.17 ± 0.06	7.40 ± 0.05
Plasma bicarbonate (mmol/l)	7.0 ± 4.0	20.0 ± 3.0
Plasma potassium (mmol/l)	5.6 ± 0.4	3.2 ± 0.3
Total plasma protein (g/dl)	14.2 ± 0.8	7.5 ± 0.6

cholera stool stained with methylene blue. This, however, is not absolute, as cholera may occasionally be superimposed on other acute or chronic inflammatory bowel disease. With dark-field microscopy, rapid tentative diagnosis can be made by direct observation of the characteristic rapid motility of the comma-shaped bacilli in fresh stool. Group- and type-specific antisera immobilize homologous strains and clearly distinguish them from other vibrios. *V. cholerae*, which are slow lactose fermenters, grow rapidly on a number of selective media, including bile-salt agar, glycerine–taurocholate–tellurite agar, and thiosulphate–citrate–bile-salt–sucrose (**TCBS**) agar. Of these, TCBS agar has the distinct advantage of not requiring sterilization before use. On TCBS agar, *V. cholerae* can be distinguished from other enteric micro-organisms by a distinct, opaque yellow, colonial appearance. Distinction between the two major serotypes—Inaba and Ogawa—is made by slide agglutination with type-specific antisera.

Distinction between the two major *V. cholerae* biotypes, classical and el Tor, is important for epidemiological purposes. The el Tor is distinguished from the classical biotype by its resistance to polymyxin B, as well as its resistance to Mukerjee's choleraphage type IV.

Management

Successful therapy demands only prompt replacement of gastrointestinal losses of fluid and electrolytes.

INTRAVENOUS FLUIDS

A diarrhoea treatment solution, recommended for intravenous therapy by the World Health Organization, may simply be prepared by adding 4 g sodium chloride, 6.5 g sodium acetate, and 1 g potassium chloride to a litre of sterile, pyrogen-free, distilled water. Alternatively, Ringer's lactate solution may be administered. Either of these preparations should be infused intravenously and rapidly, 50 to 100 ml/min in adults, until a strong radial pulse has been restored. Subsequently the same fluid should be infused in quantities equal to gastrointestinal losses. If these losses cannot be measured accurately, intravenous fluid should be given at a rate sufficient to maintain a normal pulse volume and normal skin turgor. Overhydration can be avoided by careful observation of the neck veins and by auscultation of the lungs. Close observation of the patient is mandatory during the acute phase of the illness, as an adult patient can lose as much as 1 litre of isotonic fluid per hour during the first 24 h of the disease. Inadequate or delayed restoration of electrolyte losses results in a very high incidence of acute renal insufficiency.

In children, complications are both more frequent and more severe. The most serious include stupor, coma, and convulsions (unique to child patients), pulmonary oedema, and cardiac arrhythmias. The central nervous complications may be due to hypoglycaemia (observed only in child patients), hypernatraemia resulting from the administration of isotonic fluid to the young patient (who, unlike the adult, produces stool with a sodium concentration significantly less than that of plasma), or cerebral oedema, presumably secondary to rapid fluid shifts during the administration of intravenous fluids. Pulmonary oedema may result if fluids are given intravenously at too rapid a rate before the correction of the metabolic acidosis. Cardiac arrhythmias may result from potassium depletion in children, but rarely occur in adults with cholera. Each of these complications can be avoided by the careful administration of intravenous fluids that are designed to replace the faecal electrolyte losses. The diarrhoea treatment solution, recommended by the World Health Organization for cholera as well as for other acute diarrhoeal diseases, has been used successfully to correct the acidosis, hypokalaemia, and hypoglycaemia without provoking hypernatraemia. If Ringer's lactate solution is used in the child patient, peroral supplementation of potassium and glucose is needed. The outcome in childhood cholera should be essentially as favourable as that in the adult disease, with an overall mortality rate of less than 1 per cent.

ORAL REPLACEMENT FLUIDS

Oral replacement of water and electrolytes is remarkably effective in both adults and children, especially if initiated immediately after onset of watery diarrhoea. An oral glucose–electrolyte solution (prepared by the addition of 20 g glucose, 3.5 g sodium chloride, 2.5 g sodium bicarbonate, and 1.5 g potassium chloride to 1 litre of drinking water) can be given in mild cholera cases throughout the course of illness, and is also satisfactory in more severe cases once the hypovolaemic shock has been corrected by the initial rapid intravenous fluid therapy. When oral therapy is employed, about 1.5 volumes of oral solution must be given to replace each volume of stool loss. Glucose is an essential component of this solution, in that the success of oral therapy in cholera depends upon enhanced intestinal absorption of sodium in the presence of intraluminal glucose. Although the cholera enterotoxin inhibits neutral sodium-chloride absorption by the intestinal mucosal brush border, it does not impair the glucose-facilitated sodium transport across the same membrane. Because in many rural areas glucose is not available, sucrose–electrolyte solutions have been evaluated and have been shown to be equally effective. When sucrose is used, 40 g sucrose must be added to each litre of fluid given, as sucrose is rapidly broken down into equal amounts of glucose and fructose, and only the glucose metabolite is effective in enhancing the sodium absorption. In addition, cereals and other starchy foods can also replace glucose. The starch is rapidly broken down in the gut, providing both glucose and amino acids to facilitate sodium absorption. This increase in substrate at low osmolarity leads to more rapid volume replacement and may result in up to 40 per cent reduction in fluid loss in severe cholera.

ANTIMICROBIALS

Although adequate fluid therapy results in rapid recovery in virtually all cholera patients, the required volume of replacement fluid may be enormous, and in extreme cases, may exceed twice the weight of the patient (Fig. 3). Adjunctive therapy with antimicrobials dramatically reduces the duration and volume of diarrhoea and results in rapid eradication of vibrios from the faeces. Tetracycline in a dose of 40 to 50 mg/kg body weight daily, given in four equal portions perorally every 6 h for 2 days, was uniformly successful in this regard until 1980, when tetracycline-resistant vibrio strains were first isolated. Furazolidone and trimethoprim/sulphamethoxazole are also effective, and may be used in the case of tetracycline resistance, but are less desirable than tetracycline because of relatively more frequent adverse side-effects. Fortunately, most *V. cholerae* strains remain highly sensitive to tetracycline.

Results with current management

When the current cholera epidemic reached Peru in January of 1991, the medical community was quickly mobilized to deliver effective therapy. With the early use of oral rehydration therapy, supplemented by intravenous fluids in the most seriously ill patients, a survival rate greater than 99 per cent has been achieved in over 400 000 cholera patients in Peru. Similar survival rates have been achieved in adjacent South American countries, albeit with fewer cases. This magnificent achievement is unprecedented, and provides the most convincing demonstration to date of the effectiveness of oral rehydration therapy properly administered by well-prepared medical and paramedical personnel.

Immunization and prevention

Immunization using two injections of standard commercial vaccine (containing 1000 million killed vibrios per ml) provides 60 to 80 per cent protection for 3 to 6 months to adults in cholera endemic areas. The short duration and relative lack of efficacy of the standard vaccines has led to intense study of immunological mechanisms in cholera over the past few years. As both the vibrios and the enterotoxin are confined to the intestinal lumen, effective antibodies must be present within the lumen. Patients convalescent from cholera develop high levels of both agglutinating and vibriocidal antibodies against cell-wall constituents of the vibrio; presumably the short-term protection that follows infection with *V. cholerae* results from the leakage of such IgG antibodies into the intestinal lumen. Current vaccine research is focused on peroral immunization by antigens that result in production of IgA antibodies within the intestinal lumen. A vaccine that combines killed whole vibrios with the B subunit of choleratoxin provides moderate (roughly 60 per cent) protection for at least 3 years. In addition, live attenuated *V. cholerae* vaccines with genetic deletions of the active subunit of choleratoxin have also proved effective in studies in volunteers. Intensive studies directed toward the improvement of peroral vaccines continue. At the present time, careful hygiene provides the only certain protection against cholera.

Immunization has not proved to be effective in altering the transmission of cholera or in altering the convalescent carriage of *V. cholerae*. Administration of cholera vaccine is therefore not recommended by the World Health Organization for travellers who visit endemic areas.

Fig. 3 A convalescent cholera patient, surrounded by the bottles of intravenous fluids that were required to ensure his survival, demonstrates the major logistics problem in treating large numbers of patients, in the absence of adjuvant antimicrobial therapy. (From Carpenter, C.C.J. in Field *et. al.* (1980), with permission.)

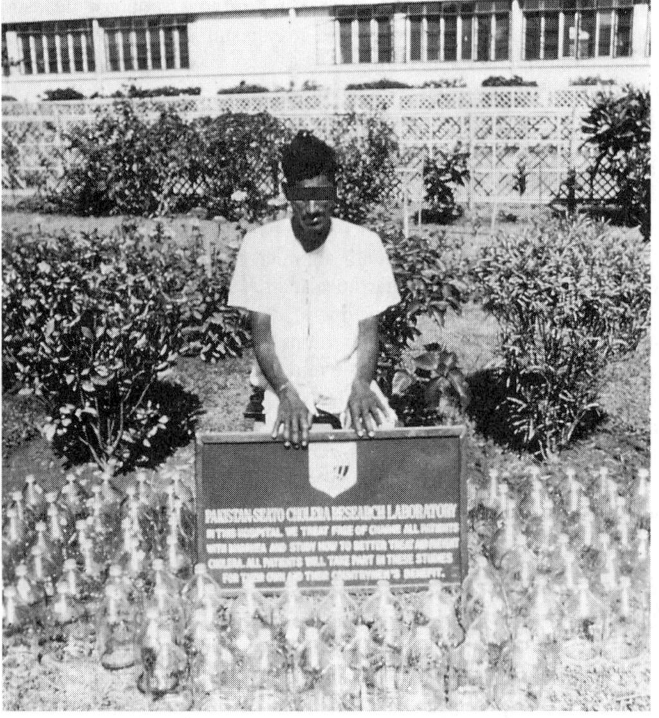

REFERENCES

Barua, D. and Greenough, W.B. (ed.) (1992). *Cholera*. Plenum, London.

Carpenter, C.C.J. (1992). The treatment of cholera: clinical science at the bedside. *Journal of Infectious Diseases*, **166,** 2–14.

Clemens, J.D. *et. al.* (1990). Field trial of oral cholera vaccines in Bangladesh: results from three-year follow-up. *Lancet*, **335,** 270–3.

Current Trends, Updates (1992). Cholera—Western hemisphere. *CDC Morbidity and Mortality Weekly Reports*, **4,** 666–8.

Field, M. (1971). Intestinal secretion: effect of cyclic AMP and its role in cholera. *New England Journal of Medicine*, **284,** 1137–45.

Field, M., Fordtran, J.S., and Schultz, S.G. (ed.) (1980). *Secretory diarrhea*. American Physiological Society, Bethesda MD.

Holmgren, J. and Lonroth, I. (1975). Oligometric structure of cholera toxin: characteristic of H and L subunits. *Journal of General Microbiology*, **86,** 49–57.

Pierce, N.F., Greenough, W.B., and Carpenter, C.C.J. (1971). *Vibrio cholerae* enterotoxin and its mode of action. *Bacteriological Reviews*, **35,** 1–13.

7.11.12 *Haemophilus influenzae*

E. R. Moxon

General

The genus Haemophilus comprises many Gram-negative bacilli that share certain growth-factor requirements for haemin and/or NAD. These are commensals, usually found in the mouth or nasopharynx of many species of animals, that also exhibit pathogenic behaviour. In man, the most important species is *Haemophilus influenzae*, first reported by Pfeiffer in 1892. The sensational claim that it was the primary agent of epidemic influenza proved fallacious. None the less, this heterogeneous species causes a wide range of diseases. It is indigenous to man; no other natural host is known. It is among the bacteria normally found in the pharynx (not the mouth) and, to a lesser extent, also in the mucosae of the conjunctiva and the genital tract. Spread from one individual to another occurs by airborne droplets, or by direct contagion with secretion. Exposure to *H. influenzae* occurs perinatally; the organisms are often not eliminated by antibiotics, and carriage of one or more strains for periods of days to months is common. Up to 80 per cent of the population are carriers and, as a consequence, the presence of *H. influenzae* in cultures obtained from the upper (but not the lower) respiratory tract is a normal finding. Most people are colonized with unencapsulated (non-typable strains), but in 3 to 5 per cent of individuals, the isolates make a capsule—most commonly that of serotype b. In general, carriers of *H. influenzae* remain healthy, but occasionally disease occurs. Two contrasting patterns of *H. influenzae* disease can be identified (Table 1). The first, and most serious in its consequences, is invasive infection, associated with bacteraemia, such as meningitis, epiglottitis, cellulitis, and septic arthritis. These infections are usually caused by virulent type b strains, rarely by strains having the other capsular serotypes. Characteristically, they occur in young children. The second category includes less serious but more common infections that occur as a result of contiguous spread of *H. influenzae* within the respiratory tract; for example, otitis media, sinusitis, conjunctivitis, and bronchopneumonia. These infections are usually, but not invariably, caused by unencapsulated strains, and their occurrence is usually conditioned by obvious impairment of the normal host clearance mechanisms that act to eliminate *H. influenzae* from the respiratory tract.

The above generalizations are not hard and fast; in particular, unencapsulated strains are an important cause of severe pneumonia, often associated with bacteraemia, among young children in the Third World and they are a well recognized cause of bacteraemic infections in adults.

Table 1 *Carriage and pathogenicity of* Haemophilus influenzae

Strains	Common upper respiratory-tract carriage rates (%)	Principal manifestations of pathogenicity
Non-encapsulated	50–80	Exacerbations of chronic bronchitis, otitis media, sinusitis, conjunctivitis; bacteraemic infections rare; patients commonly adults
Encapsulated, type b	2–4	Meningitis, epiglottitis, pneumonia and empyema, septic arthritis, cellulitis, osteomyelitis, pericarditis, bacteraemia; rarer manifestations include glossitis, tenosynovitis, peritonitis, endocarditis, ventriculitis, associated with infected shunt tubing
Encapsulated types a, c–f	1–2	Rarely incriminated as pathogens

Reproduced from Turk (1982), with permission.

Epidemiology, pathogenesis, and immunology

The factors underlying colonization by *H. influenzae* are poorly understood, as are the reasons for its tropism in man. In explants of human respiratory-tract epithelial tissues, *H. influenzae* shows marked tropism for mucus. Attachment to epithelial cells is facilitated by inhibition of ciliary clearance mechanisms by cell-wall glycopeptides and by specific bacterial adhesins, such as pili. The importance of type b capsule as a crucial factor in the pathogenesis of systemic infections has been well established in animal models. Lipopolysaccharide plays a dual role; it facilitates survival in the blood, and is a key molecule in the pathophysiology of damage to tissues such as the blood–brain barrier. Prior virus infections (e.g. influenza) potentiate infection and appear to facilitate both contiguous spread within the respiratory tract, as in otitis media or sinusitis, and the probability of dissemination into the blood to cause bacteraemia. In a rat model of type b meningitis, *H. influenzae* invades the epithelial cells of the nasopharynx, enters the submucosal vessels and reaches the meninges and the cerebrospinal fluid by bloodstream dissemination. The occurrence of meningitis correlates strikingly with the intensity of bacteraemia; impaired function of early complement components, antibody, or the fixed cells of the macrophage/monocyte series increase susceptibility to bacteraemia and meningitis.

Among the host factors governing susceptibility to invasive type b infection, the role of serum antibodies to the type b capsule (polyribosylribitol phosphate) are critical. Serum anticapsular antibodies activate complement-mediated bactericidal and opsonic activity and mediate protective immunity against systemic infections in man. The serum of neonates and young infants, up to 3 months old, generally has sufficient amounts of passively acquired antibody to afford protection. Thereafter, the natural decline of these maternally derived antibodies is followed by a period lasting until the age of 2 to 4 years when antibody is absent, or inadequate in amount to provide protection. The delay of acquisition of serum anticapsular antibodies is characteristic of children less than 2 years old and is a major reason for the high attack rates of *H. influenzae* type b invasive disease in early infancy. Apparently, many infants are not exposed to type b in infancy and the antigenic stimulus for these antibodies may often be through exposure to commensal bacteria or ingested foods, which induce immunity through their cross-reacting antigens. In contrast to systemic type b infections where deficiencies in opsonophagocytic mechanisms are paramount, impairment of non-specific host defence mechanisms is the most obvious feature of individuals who have disease caused by unencapsulated *H. influenzae*. Predisposing factors that impair ciliary clearance and/or the integrity of respiratory epithelium include smoking, virus infections, immunodeficiency, or chronic lung disease (e.g. cystic fibrosis). The role of local (secretory) and systemic antibodies to unencapsulated *H. influenzae* is poorly understood; polymorphisms of key microbial targets, outer-membrane proteins and lipopolysaccharide limit the effectiveness of these clearance mechanisms.

Haemophilus influenzae *type b*

MENINGITIS

Despite the availability of antibiotics and more recently an effective vaccine, type b meningitis is the most common cause of purulent meningitis in childhood worldwide, and the cause of substantial numbers of deaths and permanent brain damage in survivors. Accurate epidemiological data upon which to gauge the magnitude of the global problem are lacking. Before the introduction of routine immunization in the United States, a child's overall risk of developing this disease in the first 5 years of life was about 1:500, and in Europe 1:800. However, 10-fold or greater attack rates (1:50) are typical of Alaskan Eskimos, and similar data have been noted in Australian aborigines. The majority of the cases occur in young children of less than 5 years old, the peak incidence being from about 3 months to 2 years of age. Reported risk factors include male sex, black rather than white race, absence of breast feeding, socioeconomic deprivation, winter months, siblings (often asymptomatic carriers), and attendance at day-care or preschool nurseries. Although *H. influenzae* meningitis does not occur in true epidemics, small outbreaks have been described in children attending preschool nurseries or day-care centres.

Meningitis is the most common and serious manifestation of systemic infection by *H. influenzae*. A typical presentation is of a few days' antecedent symptoms of upper respiratory-tract infection, typically in a young child; an associated or preceding otitis media is common. None of the clinical features distinguishes it from other forms of purulent meningitis. The most common signs are fever and altered nervous-system function ranging from irritability to coma, but young babies may be afebrile and have a few of the specific symptoms and signs, such as headache, nuchal rigidity, or photophobia, that result from meningeal inflammation. Raised intracranial pressure produces headache and vomiting and may cause a bulging fontanelle in young infants. Papilloedema is rare. Seizures are a common feature in children (about 25 per cent) either before admission or early in the acute phase. In about 5 per cent of infants the signs of systemic sepsis are severe and, rarely, these are the predominant clinical feature; such children may have a fulminating course and die within in a few hours. The insidious development over several weeks, reminiscent of tuberculous meningitis, has been well described and may result in partial treatment in the early stages. Associated findings due to bacteraemia include painful swelling of one or more joints, facial cellulitis, endopthalmitis, and pericarditis. Petechial rashes similar to those typical of the meningococcal infection do occur but are very uncommon. Subdural effusions are present in about one-third of children and occur most frequently in the younger babies.

The key to diagnosis is examination of the cerebrospinal fluid after lumbar puncture and/or blood cultures. An increase in the number of white cells in the spinal fluid, usually in excess of 100 mm^2, most of which are polymorphs, is typical. In early cases, organisms may be cultured from the fluid despite the absence of a pleocytosis. In approximately 70 per cent of instances where prior treatment has not been given, stained smears reveal pleomorphic Gram-negative coccobacilli, which are mainly extracellular. Filamentous organisms are common and prior antibiotic treatment can result in altered morphology. The staining technique is particularly important; *H. influenzae* is more easily missed than meningococci or pneumococci, and may be confused with the latter if the Gram stain is under-decolorized, as the poles of *H. influenzae* bacilli take up stain more avidly and may be mistaken for Gram-positive diplococci. Methylene blue is more sensitive for detecting organisms than Gram stain but less specific. Use of antiserum (commercially available) allows identification of type b *H. influenzae* by causing apparent capsular swelling (Quellung reaction) of organisms in cerebrospinal fluid, or through the detection of the soluble polysaccharide antigen using counterimmunoelectrophoresis, latex agglutination, or enzyme immunoassay. For these, testing of blood and urine, as well as cerebrospinal fluid, may be useful. Because *H. influenzae* type b is found as a commensal in the nasopharynx of healthy individuals, upper respiratory-tract swabs are of limited value.

EPIGLOTTITIS

Acute respiratory obstruction caused by a cellulitis of the supraglottic tissues is a potentially lethal disease with a characteristically fulminating onset. Swelling of the epiglottis and aryepiglottic folds with complete obliteration of the vallecula and pyriform sinus is typical. The patient is usually a child aged 2 to 7 years, more rarely an infant, but its occurrence in older children and adults is well known. The onset is often explosive, initial features being sore throat, fever, and dyspnoea progressing rapidly to dysphagia, pooling of oral secretions, and drooling of saliva from the mouth. The child is restless and anxious, and adopts a sitting position with neck extended and chin protruding in order to reduce airway obstruction. Abrupt deterioration commonly occurs within a few hours, resulting in death in the absence of adequate treatment. Although sudden death is usually due to airway obstruction, it may also result from less well-defined mechanisms associated with sepsis. In some cases, the course may be less dramatic, with a prodromal illness of sore throat and hoarseness from one to several days preceding the onset of acute symptoms. The characteristic findings are that the epiglottis is red and swollen, and has a striking resemblance to a bright-red cherry obstructing the pharynx at the base of the tongue. This disorder can produce considerable local oedema as a result of the loose texture of the submucosa on the lingual aspect of the epiglottis. The trachea appears normal. Examination of the larynx should be done only in a setting in which an airway can be placed, as this examination, if injudiciously performed, may lead to fatal respiratory obstruction. The most important aspect of management of acute epiglottitis is the provision of an adequate airway and ventilation, preferably through nasotracheal intubation.

PNEUMONIA AND EMPYEMA

This occurs most often in children under 5 years of age and presents with a lobar pneumonia, often with pleural involvement, and an effusion that is often sterile. The only clinical feature that tends to distinguish it from bacterial pneumonia due to *Staphylococcus aureus* or *Streptococcus pneumoniae* is the more insidious onset. Progressive and particularly severe dyspnoea, together with tachycardia and evidence of cardiovascular failure, suggest pericarditis, an uncommon but important complication. Many observers stress the frequency with which primary pneumonia is accompanied by evidence of infection elsewhere, for example meningitis or epiglottitis. *H. influenzae* pneumonia in adults with primary lung disease or alcoholism has been recognized increasingly in recent years. Irrespective of age, radiographic findings are typically those of a segmented, lobar, bronchopneumonic or interstitial pattern, but cavitation is rare.

CELLULITIS

This important complication of type b infection occurs in young children, who present with fever and a raised, warm, tender area of distinctive reddish-blue hue most often located on one cheek, or in the periorbital region, that progresses rapidly over a few hours. The distinctive colour, its location, and the age of the child (rarely older than 2 years) should help in making the diagnosis. Its recognition is important as there is invariably an accompanying bacteraemia; some of these children have, or develop, evidence of other septic foci, including meningitis.

SYNDROME OF OCCULT BACTERAEMIA

Children, particularly those aged 6 to 36 months, may develop bacteraemia without evidence of local disease. Although *Strep. pneumoniae* is the most common cause of this syndrome, *H. influenzae* is the second most common aetiological agent. High fever and lethargy, a raised white count with immature polymorphonuclear neutrophils and an absence of localizing signs of infection in a young child are typical, and make it an extremely difficult but important diagnostic dilemma, especially in children with sickle-cell disease, or with a previous splenectomy. These individuals may worsen rapidly and develop septic shock or a localized purulent focus.

SEPTIC ARTHRITIS

H. influenzae type b is one of the most common causes of septic arthritis in children under 2 years of age. Typically, there is involvement of a single, large, weight-bearing joint, without osteomyelitis. However, the signs and symptoms may be more subtle and synovial involvement of large joints is an important cause of prolonged fever and irritability. Culture-negative, antigen-positive joint fluid is common. Response to drainage and appropriate systemic antibiotics is usually dramatic and apparently curative, but long-term follow-up is important because residual joint dysfunction occurs in a proportion of children. Septic arthritis due to type b strains is well documented in adults, many of whom have predisposing factors such as trauma, rheumatoid arthritis, systemic lupus erythematosus, diabetes mellitus, splenectomy, multiple myeloma, lymphoma, or common variable hypogammaglobulinaemia.

TREATMENT OF DISEASES CAUSED BY TYPE B STRAINS

Before the availability of antibiotic treatment, *H. influenzae* meningitis was invariably fatal. With the introduction of chloramphenicol in 1950, survival rates of 95 per cent or more have been possible. Overall, chloramphenicol remains an excellent drug for treating *H. influenzae* meningitis, but isolates showing resistance have emerged. These are still rare in most countries, but in certain geographical locations, for example Spain, the prevalence of strains resistant to chloramphenicol can exceed 50 per cent. Chloramphenicol carries a dose-related, reversible, bone-marrow toxicity, but this is rarely a problem and can be completely avoided if serum concentrations are monitored. Idiosyncratic bone-marrow aplasia has been reported but is extremely rare. Ampicillin, formerly considered an ideal treatment for *H. influenzae* meningitis, is no longer favoured because of the relatively high prevalence of β-lactamase-producing strains. In the United Kingdom, this form of antibiotic resistance occurs in approximately 13 per cent of isolates; the prevalence is higher (20 per cent) in the United States. There is now a trend to use parenteral third-generation cephalosporins as initial treatment of suspected bacterial meningitis. Ceftriaxone or cefotaxime have been shown to be highly effective, but these drugs have not been shown to sterilize cerebrospinal fluid more rapidly, or improve prognosis, when compared to chloramphenicol.

Antibiotic treatment is only one facet of the management of a child with *H. influenzae* meningitis. Critical attention must be given to supportive management (see Chapter 24.15.1). Adequate ventilation must be ensured, especially in individuals with coma or seizures. Fluid management must be judicious so as to maintain adequate perfusion of tissues, especially where disease is complicated by hypovolaemia and acidosis. On the other hand, inappropriate secretion of antidiuretic hormone is the rule, and may be sufficiently severe to cause or worsen cerebral oedema. For this reason, as long as adequate perfusion is ensured, fluid restriction (approximately two-thirds of maintenance) is recommended for about 72 h into treatment. Although controversial, corticosteroid therapy to reduce inflammation is now recommended by many. A trial has demonstrated that dexamethasone (0.15 mg/kg every 6 h for the first 4 days) reduces the incidence of sensorineural hearing loss in *H. influenzae* meningitis.

The outlook for *H. influenzae* meningitis is that approximately 95 per cent will survive but that about 8 per cent of survivors have central nervous sequelae, the most common problem being sensorineural deafness. Routine immunization with conjugate vaccines, begun in 1992 in the United Kingdom, should prevent more than 90 per cent of the 1000 or more cases of type b disease that occur each year.

Mortality from meningitis has remained constant at about 5 to 10 per cent for four decades and, despite effective antibiotics, children surviving serious type b infections sustain an unacceptably high frequency of serious sequelae.

CHEMOPROPHYLAXIS

Young children in the same household are at significantly increased risk of secondary invasive infection by *H. influenzae* type b.

Before the introduction of routine immunization, estimates of the secondary attack rates in household contacts in the United States were 2 to 4 per cent and in day-care centres as high as 1.3 per cent. Comparable data for the United Kingdom, and indeed other countries in Europe, are not available. It was suggested that antibiotic treatment of age-susceptible contacts for children with invasive *H. influenzae* disease could decrease this secondary attack rate. Rifampicin given orally once daily for 4 days is effective in eradicating nasopharyngeal carriage, and is currently recommended for all household contacts (children and adults) where there are children (other than the index case) less than 4 years old. Nursery, playschool and day-care centre contacts should be considered household contacts. None the less, several instances of apparent failure of rifampicin to prevent secondary cases have been reported, including cases in which the disease isolate was resistant to rifampicin. This, together with the expected fall in type b disease that is expected as a result of routine immunization, indicates that chemoprophylaxis will cease to be a significant public health measure, especially as even before the availability of immunization, only a small proportion (under 5 per cent) of the total number of systemic type b infections could be prevented through this strategy.

ACTIVE IMMUNIZATION

Several considerations stimulated research to develop an effective vaccine to prevent diseases caused by *H. influenzae* type b. In the late 1960s it was recognized that stimulation of serum antibodies specific for the type b capsule, a polymer of ribose and ribotol phosphate (designated **PRP**) could prevent type b infection. Subsequently, clinical trials of PRP indicated its poor immunogenicity and inability to protect infants and children under 2 years of age, and as PRP vaccine offered protection to only a minority of those contracting serious type b infections, further research was directed towards developing conjugate vaccines, whose immunogenicity for young children was much improved. Conjugate vaccines involve chemical linking of PRP to a carrier protein, such as tetanus toxoid. Currently, at least four different conjugate vaccines have been developed commercially and all have proved to be very safe and capable of affording high levels (in excess of 90 per cent) of protection to children immunized as early as 2 months. Conjugate vaccines are given by subcutaneous injection, most conveniently at the same time as routine immunization with diphtheria/pertussis/tetanus vaccine. Although the vaccines have been in routine use for only a short time, the number of cases of serious type b disease among immunized populations has fallen dramatically.

Diseases caused by non-typable H. influenzae

PNEUMONIA

Unencapsulated *H. influenzae* is an important cause of pneumonia in children and adults, especially the elderly, and in individuals with established lung disease such as chronic bronchitis. The clinical features are indistinguishable from other forms of bacterial pneumonia; fever, cough and purulent sputum. Because non-typable (unencapsulated) *H. influenzae* is part of the normal upper respiratory-tract flora, diagnosis depends on critical evaluation of sputum samples, or invasive procedures such as transtracheal aspirates. The early blood cultures may be positive. For the above reasons, the true incidence of pneumonia due to these organisms is not known, but after the pneumococcus, they are probably the next most common cause of bacterial pneumonia acquired in the community in industrialized countries.

In many countries where adverse socioeconomic circumstances are prevalent, acute pneumonia in infants caused by non-typable *H. influenzae* is a major cause of illness and death. The importance of acute respiratory-tract infections as an important global health problem has deservedly, and perhaps belatedly, resulted in the establishment of large international programmes (for example, such as that sponsored by the World Health Organization) with the aim of increasing its recognition, appropriate management, and prevention.

It has been recognized for many years that exacerbations of chronic bronchitis correlate with an increase in the production of purulent sputum from which non-typable *H. influenzae* are cultured. Such episodes are often precipitated by prior viral infection. This common clinical presentation, together with serological studies and the benefits of antibiotic therapy, indicate a likely, but unproven, role for non-typable forms. A current view holds that the progressive damage in chronic lung disease of individuals with conditions such as chronic bronchitis, cystic fibrosis, and hypogammaglobulinaemia occurs through the heightened and protracted inflammatory response to a variety of bacteria, including non-typable *H. influenzae*, in individuals whose respiratory tract lacks the appropriate clearance mechanisms.

MATERNAL AND NEONATAL SEPSIS

Non-typable *H. influenzae* is a well-documented cause of tubo-ovarian abscess or chronic salpingitis. Diagnosis is established by tubal cultures at laparoscopy or cultures of peritoneal fluid. Also, endometritis and amniotitis are well described, especially following premature rupture of membranes, and occasionally result in an associated septicaemia. More ominous, the infant born to such mothers, often prematurely, may develop life-threatening neonatal septicaemia, meningitis, and a form of acute respiratory-distress syndrome that is indistinguishable from that caused by early-onset, group B streptococci.

ACUTE OTITIS MEDIA AND SINUSITIS

H. influenzae accounts for about one-fifth of all cases of acute bacterial otitis media and more than 90 per cent of the strains isolated from middle-ear fluid are non-typable. Although such episodes occur at any age, they are most common in children aged 6 months to 5 years. Because more than two-thirds of children have had one or more episodes of otitis media by the age of 3 years, a conservative estimate would indicate that more 100 000 cases of otitis media associated with non-typable *H. influenzae* occur each year in the United Kingdom. These are also a common cause of sinusitis in both adults and children.

CONJUNCTIVITIS

H. influenzae is an important cause of purulent conjunctivitis and, in contrast to the sporadic nature of other *Haemophilus* infections, can occur in outbreaks. Most of the strains are non-typable and many have particular phenotypic characteristics that, until recently, were considered sufficiently distinctive to merit separate speciation as *H. aegyptius*. However, analysis of these strains by modern genetic techniques indicates that *H. aegyptius* belongs to the same species as *H. influenzae*; these strains are now referred to as *H. influenzae* biogroup *aegyptius*. Interest in these strains was heightened when, in 1984, an apparently new and serious disease was described in Brazilian children who developed life-threatening infections caused by biogroup *aegyptius*, now known as Brazilian purpuric fever. Its peak age incidence is 1 to 4 years; purulent conjunctivitis, high fever, vomiting, purpura, vascular collapse, and a high mortality are characteristic. Blood cultures are positive for biogroup *aegyptius* strains but the cerebrospinal fluid is sterile.

OTHER INFECTIONS

All of the diseases that are commonly caused by type b strains are, on rare occasions, caused by strains of capsular serotypes a, c, d, e, and f as well as non-typable strains. In addition, there are a number of unusual infections documented in small series and case reports: these include endocarditis, cholecystitis, peritonitis, mastoiditis, epididymo-orchitis, and urinary-tract infection. Two other members of the genus, *H. parainfluenzae* and *H. aphrophilus*, are causes of disease, especially endocarditis. *H. ducreyi* is dealt with in Chapter 7.11.13.

TREATMENT

Serious infections caused by non-typable *H. influenzae*, such as meningitis, lower respiratory-tract infections, tubal abscess, and neonatal sepsis, require systemic treatment with a third-generation β-lactam (e.g. cefuroxime) or co-trimoxazole. Chloramphenicol is also highly effective but its serum concentrations would need to be monitored carefully, especially in premature infants. Sinusitis and otitis media caused by non-typable strains are often treated effectively with oral amoxycillin, but Augmentin (amoxycillin with clavulanic acid) would be preferable given the relatively high incidence of strains producing β-lactamase. Oral co-trimoxazole would be an equally sound or alternative choice for trimethoprim-susceptible strains. The use of antibiotics as prophylaxis or treatment of exacerbations of chronic bronchitis is controversial but many advocate their use either to reduce the number of haemophili in the lower respiratory tract or to eradicate them. Drugs of the tetracycline group are effective, but are contraindicated in pregnancy, impaired renal function, or children less than 10 years of age; amoxycillin and co-trimoxazole have also proved useful.

PASSIVE IMMUNIZATION

An important group of individuals with increased susceptibility to infection with *H. influenzae*, but particularly non-typable strains, is that of immunodeficiency, especially primary deficiency of antibody synthesis. These persons benefit from infusion of immunoglobulin preparations either intramuscularly or intravenously. This form of immunoglobulin replacement undoubtedly decreases the incidence of systemic infections in these individuals and the number of episodes of both upper and lower respiratory-tract infections caused by *H. influenzae*.

REFERENCES

Booy, R. and Moxon, E.R. (1991). Immunisation of infants against *Haemophilus influenzae* type b in the UK. *Archives of Disease in Childhood*, **66,** 1251–4.

Daum, R.S., Granoff, D.M., Mäkelä, P.H., Moxon, E.R., and van Alphen, L. (ed.) (1992). Epidemiology, pathogenesis, and prevention of *Haemophilus influenzae* disease. *Journal of Infectious Diseases*, **165**(suppl. 1).

Hoiseth, S.K. (1991). The genus *Haemophilus*. In *The prokaryotes*, a handbook on the biology of bacteria: ecophysiology, isolation, identification, applications, (ed. A. Balows, H.G. Trüper, M. Dworkin, W. Harder, and K.H. Schleifer), pp. 3304–30. Springer-Verlag, New York.

Moxon, E.R. (1986). The carrier state: *Haemophilus influenzae*. *Journal of Antimicrobial Chemotherapy*, **18,** S17–24.

Moxon, E.R. and Wilson, R. (1991). The role of *Haemophilus influenzae* in the pathogenesis of pneumonia. *Reviews of Infectious Diseases*, **13,** S518–27.

Murphy, T.F. and Apicella, M.A. (1987). Nontypable *Haemophilus influenzae*: a review of clinical aspects, surface antigens, and the human immune response to infection. *Reviews of Infectious Diseases*, **9,** 1–15.

Turk, D.C. (1982). Clinical importance of *Haemophilus influenzae*. In Haemophilus influenzae, *epidemiology, immunology and prevention of disease*, (ed. S.H. Sell and P.F. Wright), pp. 3–9. Elsevier Biomedical, New York.

7.11.13 *Haemophilus ducreyi* and chancroid

A. R. RONALD

Introduction

Genital ulceration is the presenting feature of sexually transmitted diseases in about 2 per cent of patients in Western societies whereas in the developing world, 10 to 50 per cent of patients with sexually transmitted diseases have genital ulcers. In Western societies, genital herpes and primary syphilis are the most common aetiological agents. In the developing world, *Haemophilus ducreyi* accounts for most ulcers. Granuloma inguinale and lymphogranuloma venereum are only occasionally imported into Western society and few endemic foci exist.

The epidemiological association between genital ulcers, particularly chancroid, and the increased risk of transmission of human immunodeficiency viruses (**HIV**) 1 and 2 have created renewed interest in strategies to control genital ulcer disease.

Soft chancre or ulcus molle was differentiated from the hard, indurated chancre of syphilis by Philippe Ricord in 1838. In 1889, the Neopolitan dermatologist Augosto Ducrey identified short chains of streptobacillary rods in exudate in ulcers following inoculation with chancroid pus. Although he could not culture the organism, he concluded that the chains of bacilli were responsible for chancroid.

Aetiology

Haemophilus ducreyi is a small, faintly staining, Gram-negative, non-motile rod. Occasionally it will show bipolar staining. Due to extracellular linkage of the bacterial cells, the organism frequently forms chains and can classically be seen as a 'school of fish' arrangement on Gram stain from infected tissue. The organism is fastidious, requires haemin, and is difficult to isolate unless cultured on supplemented selective media in a special environment. *H. ducreyi* colonies are usually apparent only after 48 h of incubation, yellow-grey in colour, dome shaped, and varying in size and opacity. They are extremely cohesive and the entire colony can be nudged with a straight wire across the culture plate.

The organism is oxidase positive, has a broad range of phosphatase activity, but does not ferment carbohydrates and appears to be enzymatically inert. Recent DNA hybridization studies suggest that, although it belongs to the family Pasteurellaceae, it is not closely related to *Haemophilus* spp. and perhaps should be placed in a new genus.

Epidemiology

Chancroid is endemic in many developing countries particularly in Eastern and Southern Africa, Thailand, India, and the Caribbean. The annual incidence in adult males exceeds 1/1000 in most of these countries. It occurs sporadically in industrialized countries, most frequently at major ports. During the last two decades, there have been about 15 separate outbreaks in North America. In most outbreaks, prostitutes were the reservoir for continuing dissemination of *H. ducreyi*. The male to female ratio was usually 5:1 or higher. The age patterns are those of other sexually transmitted diseases. Male circumcision decreases susceptibility to infection with *H. ducreyi* by about threefold.

The epidemiology of *H. ducreyi* is controversial and the possible role of asymptomatic carriage is uncertain. In a study in Kenya, all the source contacts of 10 men with culture-positive chancroid had genital ulcers. Among 29 secondary contacts, 17 had ulcers and 3 had positive cervical cultures for *H. ducreyi*; that is, a man with chancroid had a 50 per cent or greater likelihood of infecting his sexual partner. At present there is no evidence for a large asymptomatic reservoir of *H. ducreyi*.

H. ducreyi is rarely transmitted non-sexually. Occasionally, chancroid lesions on the fingers or breasts may reflect direct contact from a genital lesion on the sexual partner or autoinoculation. Although some investigators have reported the isolation of *H. ducreyi* from herpetic ulcers or from non-ulcerated oral or genital mucosa, these observations have not been confirmed.

Pathogenesis and pathology

H. ducreyi presumably gains access through a break in the epithelium. The size of inoculum required to initiate infection is unknown. The role of virulence factors such as adhesin, cytotoxins, or haemolysins is unknown. After an incubation period that varies from 3 to 10 days, an inflammatory papule develops, which rapidly ulcerates. Inguinal adenitis develops in about 40 per cent of the patients. A proportion of these nodes suppurate, with coalescence and bubo formation. The pathogenesis of these changes is not understood. Infection does not progress further and *H. ducreyi* is not known to spread from mothers to their newborn. Although both humoral and cell-mediated responses to *H. ducreyi* are described, their role in preventing or modifying infection is unknown.

The histological appearances of the chancroid ulcer have only recently been described. Perivascular and interstitial mononuclear-cell infiltrates predominate, with occasional giant-cell granulomas. There is endothelial swelling and proliferation with invasion of neutrophils. *H. ducreyi* can be seen extracellularly and also within keratinocytes, endothelial cells, and histiocytes. Immunohistological studies demonstrate that the lymphocytes are primarily T cells and the histiocytes are predominantly of Langerhans-cell lineage.

Clinical features

The chancroidal ulcer begins as a tender papule, which ulcerates and enlarges. It is painful, irregular, and sharply demarcated, but is rarely indurated and usually lacks surrounding cutaneous inflammation. The base of the ulcer is uneven with a greyish-yellow purulent exudate that bleeds during sampling. About 50 per cent of men and 70 per cent of women have multiple ulcers.

Numerous variants of chancroid have been described, including giant ulcers formed when several smaller ulcers merge, dwarf chancroid with shallow, round, tiny ulcers resembling herpes, follicular chancroid, which mimics pyogenic infection and is usually limited to hairy regions, transient ulceration associated with acute regional lymphadenitis similar to lymphogranuloma venereum, a painless, single ulcer often misdiagnosed as primary syphilis, and raised, indurated, 'beefy' lesions not unlike granuloma inguinale. Rarely, superinfection with necrotizing anaerobic bacteria will produce a rapidly progressive, destructive, even gangrenous, lesion. In men as many as 25 per cent, and in women at least 50 per cent of ulcers could be attributed to aetiological agents other than *H. ducreyi* in the absence of laboratory investigation. The index of suspicion for chancroid increases in populations in which the disease is endemic.

Chancroidal lesions occur anywhere on the genitalia. However, in uncircumcised men over 50 per cent of ulcers occur on the prepuce, with about three-quarters of these on the external skin as single or multiple ulcers. The coronal sulcus is the second most common site (Fig. 1), often with ulcers around its entire circumference. The skin of the shaft, the glans, and in about 15 per cent of patients, the scrotum or the skin surrounding the genitalia are the site of ulcers. Some men present with a 'septic sore', usually on the prepuce but occasionally on the shaft of the penis. Several millilitres of pus can be trapped in the skin without an obvious ulcer. Kissing lesions are common on adjacent cutaneous surfaces. In women, lesions occur in decreasing frequency on the fourchette, labia majora and minora, perianal area, and medial aspects of the thighs. Cervical ulcers are uncommon and vaginal-wall ulcers are rare.

Inguinal lymphadenopathy appears in about 40 per cent of men and 20 per cent of women within 7 to 10 days of ulceration. The lymph nodes are initially discrete, very tender, and bilateral in one-half of affected patients. If untreated, lymphadenopathy progresses within a week to a suppurative bubo that may rupture and form an inguinal abscess. Abscesses may drain copious quantities of pus and penetrate deeply in the groin.

Laboratory diagnosis

Primary syphilis must be suspected in all patients who present with genital ulceration. Although the classical features of syphilis and chancroid appear to place them at opposite ends of a spectrum of genital ulceration, in at least 15 per cent of patients the presentations are indistinguishable.

Definitive diagnosis of chancroid requires culture of *H. ducreyi*. The Gram stain is not sufficiently sensitive or specific for diagnosis, although the appearance of Gram-negative rods in a 'school of fish' arrangement with intracellular organisms suggests *H. ducreyi*. A serological test is not available. Diagnostic nucleic-acid probes, the polymerase chain reaction, and antigen-capture procedures are currently under investigation and may shortly become commercially available. Due to technical difficulties the sensitivity of *H. ducreyi* culture in most studies is in the range of 60 to 80 per cent. However, specificity is very high, perhaps

Fig. 1 Chancroid: multiple penile ulcerations and a broken-down inguinal bubo (by courtesy of P. L. Perine, Seattle).

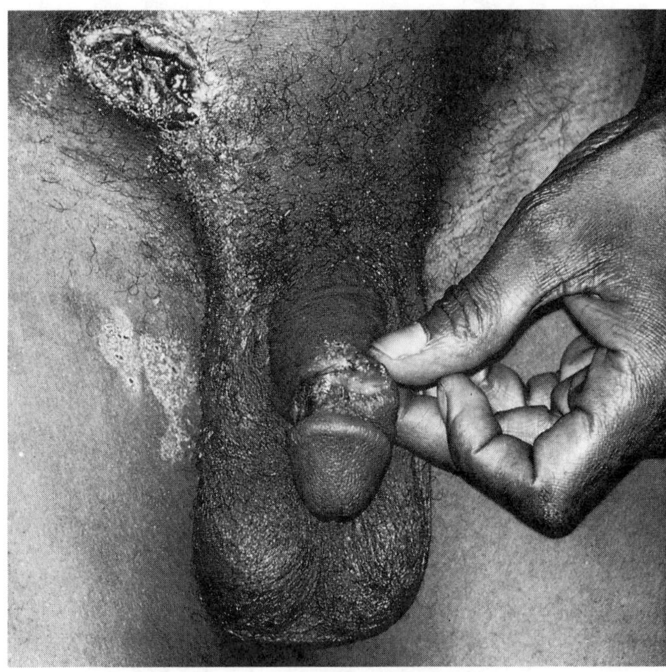

100 per cent, as asymptomatic carriage of *H. ducreyi* is rare. Two or more sexually transmitted pathogens may be present in 5 to 10 per cent of patients presenting with genital ulcers. Concomitantly with positive cultures for *H. ducreyi*, cultures may be positive for *Herpes simplex* or dark-field positive for *T. pallidum*.

No transport medium has been developed for *H. ducreyi* but on a swab the organism will survive longer at 4°C than at room temperature. If possible, exudate from the ulcer or bubo should be inoculated directly on to the primary selective medium. Recent studies have shown that gonococcal agar with added vancomycin (3 mg/l) to inhibit growth of Gram-positive bacteria, vitamin supplement and 0.25 per cent activated charcoal, supports the growth of *H. ducreyi* very well. This medium has replaced gonococcal and Mueller–Hinton agar with fetal calf serum as primary culture medium for *H. ducreyi*.

Cultures for *H. ducreyi* should be incubated at 33°C in an environment with 5 per cent CO_2 and maximum humidity. A candle extinction jar with a moist paper towel is adequate. Distinct colonies usually appear within 48 h but the cultures should be held for at least 72 h before being discarded as negative. *H. ducreyi* is further identified by its Gram stain and its ability to use nitrate, a positive oxidase test, and a requirement for X factor.

Antimicrobial susceptibility for *H. ducreyi* has not been standardized. Agar dilution tests correlate with the clinical response. Before 1960, isolates were susceptible *in vitro* to tetracycline, streptomycin, chloramphenicol, sulphonamides, and penicillin. Plasmid-mediated resistance appeared during the 1970s. Four different plasmids are known to encode for β-lactamase production, two for sulphonamide resistance, two for tetracycline resistance, and others for chloramphenicol, kanamycin, and streptomycin resistance. Perhaps in response to antimicrobial pressure, these plasmids have spread rapidly throughout the world. They are closely related to those in *Neisseria gonorrhoeae* and in *Haemophilus influenzae*.

Fortunately, all isolates remain susceptible to the third-generation cephalosporins, fluoroquinolones, and macrolide antimicrobial agents.

Natural history

In the absence of specific treatment, chancroid is a prolonged illness with slow resolution and frequent recurrence. During the First World War, soldiers with chancroid were off duty for a mean of 25 days. Genital ulcers and inguinal abscesses have been reported to persist for years.

Treatment

Circumcision, cleanliness, and saline soaks were routinely used to promote healing before sulphonamides became available. In 1938, sulphonamides were discovered to be an effective treatment with an average time to healing of about 10 days, and later ampicillin, streptomycin, and tetracycline were also shown to be effective. However, during the 1970s, treatment failures to tetracycline, chloramphenicol, and ampicillin were usual among soldiers in Vietnam. Parenteral cephalothin became the routine therapy.

The studies in Kenya were the first to demonstrate a correlation between *in vitro* resistance and the clinical response to treatment. Isolates with plasmids encoding for β-lactamase were not cured with ampicillin. Tetracycline and sulphonamide failures correlated with *in vitro* resistance. However, in several studies trimethoprim/sulphamethoxazole proved very effective. A single large dose was as effective as more prolonged courses of therapy. During the 1980s this regimen became standard therapy in much of the world.

Other regimens have been investigated. Ceftriaxone in a single dose of 250 mg intramuscularly, ciprofloxacin in a dose of 500 mg once daily for 3 days, fleroxacin as a single dose of 400 mg, erythromycin as a dose of 250 mg three times a day for 7 days, and azithromycin as a single 1-g dose all cure over 95 per cent of HIV-seronegative men with chancroid. No resistance has yet been reported to any of the quinolones or macrolides. However, the emergence and spread of trimethoprim resistance has largely curtailed the usefulness of this agent, which is no longer recommended either in combination with sulphonamides or alone.

Recent studies have shown that, both in men and women, treatment failures are much more likely if there is concurrent infection with HIV, particularly if short courses of therapy are prescribed. In a recent study, only 2 of 11 uncircumcised men with chancroid and HIV infection were cured with a single-dose of 250 mg of ceftriaxone. This observation is important as HIV-1 is commonly present in *H. ducreyi*-infected individuals. In Kenya over 30 per cent of men and women with chancroid are HIV-1 seropositive and in Zambia over 50 per cent are concurrently infected. As a result, at least a week of therapy should probably be prescribed routinely and patients should be followed to ensure complete resolution of their chancroid.

Epidemiological associations between HIV-1 and H. ducreyi

Numerous studies during the past 5 years have confirmed that chancroid is a risk factor for the heterosexual spread of HIV-1 and HIV-2. Genital ulcers in women increases two- to eightfold their susceptibility to HIV-1 infection following heterosexual contact with HIV-1-infected men. The presence of genital ulcers in HIV-1-infected women increases the excretion of HIV-1 into vaginal secretions and dramatically increases the probability that their partners will become HIV-1 infected. In one study, 1 per cent of circumcised men exposed to presumed HIV-infected prostitutes acquired HIV-1 concomitantly with gonococcal infection, whereas almost 30 per cent of uncircumcised men who acquired genital ulcer disease also acquired HIV-1.

HIV infection alters the clinical appearance of the ulcer. There is more extensive local disease and less lymphadenitis. Presumably because of a less effective host response, treatment failures have become commonplace.

A mathematical model suggests that control of chancroid may substantially reduce heterosexual transmission of HIV—perhaps by 50 per cent or more.

Prevention and control

In Western societies, chancroid has been effectively controlled on numerous occasions by effective treatment regimens for men with genital ulcers and by widespread follow-up and treatment of their sexual contacts, particularly prostitutes. Most women who are the source of chancroid in men are asymptomatic, despite the presence of ulcers, and they continue to be sexually active. Contact tracing is necessary as these women may not seek treatment.

The use of condoms by clients dramatically reduces the acquisition of ulcers from prostitutes. Programmes to reduce prostitution, to treat infections in women who sell sex, and to ensure the use of condoms by all clients will rapidly reduce and perhaps eradicate chancroid from some populations. Control measures targeted to selected populations can be very effective. Interventions currently under way in developing countries suggest that this may be the most cost-effective way rapidly to slow the transmission of HIV-1 and perhaps HIV-2.

REFERENCES

Albritton, W.L. (1989). Biology of *Haemophilus ducreyi*. *Microbiological Reviews*, **53**, 377–89.

Cameron, D.W. *et al.* (1989). Female to male transmission of human immunodeficiency virus type 1: risk factors for seroconversion in men. *Lancet*, **ii**, 403–7.

Hammond, G.W., Slutchuk, M., Scatliff, J., Sherman, E., Wilt, J.C., and Ronald, A.R. (1980). Epidemiologic, clinical, laboratory and therapeutic

features of an urban outbreak of chancroid in North America. *Reviews of Infectious Diseases*, **2,** 867–79.
Kreiss, J.K. *et al.* (1989). Isolation of human immunodeficiency virus from genital ulcers in Nairobi prostitutes. *Journal of Infectious Diseases*, **160,** 380–4.
Morse, S.A. (1989). Chancroid and *Haemophilus ducreyi. Clinical Microbiology Review*, **2,** 137–57.
Pepin, J. *et al.* (1992). Association between HIV-2 infection and genital ulcer diseases among male sexually transmitted disease patients in The Gambia. *AIDS*, **6,** 489–93.
Plourde, P.J. *et al.* (1992). A randomized, double-blind study of the efficacy of fleroxacin versus trimethoprim-sulfamethoxazole in men with culture-proven chancroid. *Journal of Infectious Diseases*, **165,** 949–52.
Plourde, P.J. *et al.* (1994). Human immunodeficiency virus type 1 seroconversion in women with genital ulcers. *Journal of Infectious Diseases* (in press).
Plummer, F.A. *et al.* (1983). Single-dose therapy of chancroid with trimethoprim-sulfametrole. *New England Journal of Medicine*, **309,** 67–71.
Simonsen, J.N. *et al.* (1988). Human immunodeficiency virus infection in men with sexually transmitted diseases. *New England Journal of Medicine*, **319,** 274–8.
Tyndall, M.W. (1993). Ceftriaxone no longer predictably cures chancroid in Kenya. *Journal of Infectious Diseases*, **167,** 469–71.

7.11.14 Bordetella

C. C. LINNEMANN, JR.

Bacteria of the genus Bordetella are primarily pathogens of the respiratory tract of man and animals because of their propensity for adhering to ciliated epithelial cells. The only distinctive presentation of Bordetella infections is the whooping cough syndrome or pertussis, which is characterized by paroxysmal coughing, an inspiratory whoop, and lymphocytosis. This syndrome is usually caused by *B. pertussis*, although the other two species that cause disease in man, *B. parapertussis* and *B. bronchiseptica*, have occasionally been reported to produce the same syndrome. In the past, pertussis also has been attributed to viral infections. This misconception resulted from two factors—the difficulty of isolating *B. pertussis* from infected patients, and the frequent excretion of adenoviruses by patients infected with *B. pertussis*.

Bordetella infections should be suspected when the clinician is confronted either by a patient with a persistent lower respiratory tract infection manifested by paroxysmal coughing, with or without an inspiratory whoop; or by a patient with any respiratory symptoms who has been in close contact with a documented infection. Even with a high index of suspicion, most Bordetella infections will go unrecognized because the symptoms are indistinguishable from other respiratory tract infections, and because appropriate diagnostic tests usually are made only in patients with typical pertussis. *B. bronchiseptica* is a common pathogen in animals and should be considered in animal handlers with respiratory tract infections. However, most *B. bronchiseptica* infections will not be diagnosed from Bordetella cultures, but from routine cultures collected to evaluate infections in immunosuppressed patients.

The causative agent

Bordetella are small, aerobic, Gram-negative coccobacillary organisms. *B. pertussis* is a fastidious bacterium that is inhibited by a variety of media constituents such as fatty acids. For this reason, cultures must be made on special media containing additives that will inactivate these inhibitors. This organism grows slowly in culture, requiring 2 to 5 days to produce recognizable colonies. *B. parapertussis* and *B. bronchiseptica* are less fastidious and faster growing. These organisms will grow on a simple infusion agar or blood agar within 1 or 2 days.

Bordetella pertussis adheres to ciliated epithelial cells in the respiratory tract. Attachment is followed by ciliostasis and subsequent loss of the ciliated cells. A similar sequence has been observed in dogs infected with *B. bronchiseptica.* Numerous biologically active components and properties have been identified in the Bordetella, including filamentous haemagglutinin, agglutinogens, pertussis toxin (lymphocytosis-promoting factor), adenylate cyclase, and haemolysin; but there is no direct evidence for the role of these in the pathogenesis of disease in man. New vaccines are being studied that contain selected components such as the filamentous haemagglutinin and pertussis toxin, and appear to offer some protection. Although these organisms are not invasive and usually remain on the surface of the respiratory tract, there are isolated reports of bacteraemia with *B. parapertussis* and *B. bronchiseptica.*

Epidemiology

Man is the only known reservoir of *B. pertussis* and *B. parapertussis*, in contrast to *B. bronchiseptica*, which is found in dogs, rabbits, guinea-pigs, swine, and other animals. *B. pertussis* is transmitted by droplets from symptomatic patients. Occasionally, asymptomatic infections have been identified, but there is no evidence that these are important in the spread of disease, and there are no chronic carriers. It is assumed that the transmission of *B. parapertussis* is similar to that of *B. pertussis. B. bronchiseptica* infections are reportedly acquired from contact with animals, but infections have also been reported in hospital patients with no obvious exposure to animals, suggesting that man may be a reservoir for *B. bronchiseptica.*

In the era before vaccine was available, epidemics of *B. pertussis* spread through schools, and the schoolchildren carried the infection into their homes. The secondary attack rates in susceptible children were 25 to 50 per cent in schools, and 70 to 100 per cent in homes. The high secondary attack rates at home reflected the intense and prolonged exposure to the organism. Most children developed clinically recognizable disease. Mild infections or reinfections occurred in adults caring for sick children; these illnesses were known as 'grandmother's cough' or 'nurses' cough'.

In the vaccine and antibiotic era, major epidemics have disappeared in most developed countries. Mortality from *B. pertussis* was decreasing before the introduction of vaccine, but the number of cases was not. The case rate did not decrease significantly until after the vaccines were introduced. This was demonstrated clearly in the United States and Canada, where effective vaccines were widely used, and the incidence of pertussis decreased to 1 to 2/100 000 per year (Fig. 1). The effect of vaccine was not as dramatic in the United Kingdom, which may have been related to early problems with vaccine efficacy and lower levels of vaccine usage. Pertussis did decrease in the United Kingdom, and the resurgence of *B. pertussis* in the late 1970s, following a decrease in vaccine usage, provided a natural experiment demonstrating the effect of vaccine on the epidemiology of the disease.

In a highly vaccinated population, adults may play a more important part in the transmission of disease. Before vaccine was available, the source of infection could be identified in most cases as another child. It has now become more difficult to trace the source, and, in very young infants, an adult family member frequently appears to be the source. Hospital epidemics have also demonstrated the part adults play in transmission. Physicians or nurses may acquire infection from a patient and then transmit it to other hospital staff and to patients.

The epidemiology of *B. parapertussis* is similar to that of *B. pertussis* except that is has not been modified by vaccine usage. *B. parapertussis* is widespread in many countries, but it is seldom recognized because of the mildness of the disease. Studies in Denmark have reported that epidemics occur in that country every 4 years and alternate with epidemics of *B. pertussis.* There is only limited information on the epidemiology of *B. bronchiseptica.* In the small surveys of animal handlers and hospital patients that have been reported, *B. bronchiseptica* was rarely found.

Clinical manifestations

After infection with *B. pertussis*, clinical illness begins in 7 to 10 days with non-specific upper respiratory symptoms, malaise, anorexia, and sometimes a low-grade fever. Traditionally, this is called the catarrhal stage and is indistinguishable from any other mild respiratory infection. Towards the end of this stage a dry, hacking cough appears and becomes progressively worse. Older and presumably partially immune patients may not progress beyond the catarrhal stage. After 1 to 2 weeks, the paroxysmal stage begins and continues for several weeks. The cough is now paroxysmal, and prolonged coughing episodes may be followed by the characteristic 'whoop', which is produced by forced inspiration through a partially closed glottis. In severe cases, the paroxysms of coughing may be followed by vomiting, and may be associated with epistaxis, petechiae, conjunctival or scleral haemorrhages, haemorrhagic myringitis, or periorbital oedema. Young infants may not have the whoop, and their paroxysms of coughing may be followed by cyanosis and apnoea. Fever is uncommon at this stage in uncomplicated infections. The convalescent stage begins after 2 to 4 weeks, with gradually resolving paroxysms of coughing. The coughing may persist for weeks to months, and exacerbations with whooping may occur with subsequent respiratory viral infections.

The most characteristic laboratory finding is a leucocytosis with lymphocytosis that appears toward the end of the catarrhal stage and continues in the paroxysmal stage. The lymphocytosis is most marked at the time of the most severe coughing and represents a proportional increase in both T and B lymphocytes. The lymphocytosis may not occur in either very young infants or older children and adults.

The appearance of fever suggests a secondary bacterial infection complicating the *B. pertussis* infection. Otitis media and pneumonia are the most common infectious complications, but these seem to have been less frequent in recent years. Atelectasis still occurs as a result of bronchial obstruction by the thick mucus, but bronchiectasis is uncommon. The pressures developed during the paroxysmal coughing probably contribute to the pulmonary, haemorrhagic, and gastrointestinal complications that may include mediastinal and subcutaneous emphysema, pneumothorax, inguinal hernias, and rectal prolapse. The most serious non-infectious complications are neurological, usually convulsions, but also paralysis, coma, blindness, deafness, and movement disorders. There are no good data on the exact incidence of these complications, but they are extremely rare.

Fig. 1 The effect of pertussis vaccine on the incidence and mortality of pertussis in the United States. The lines superimposed on the graph indicate the trends prior to the vaccine and as projected if vaccine had not been introduced.

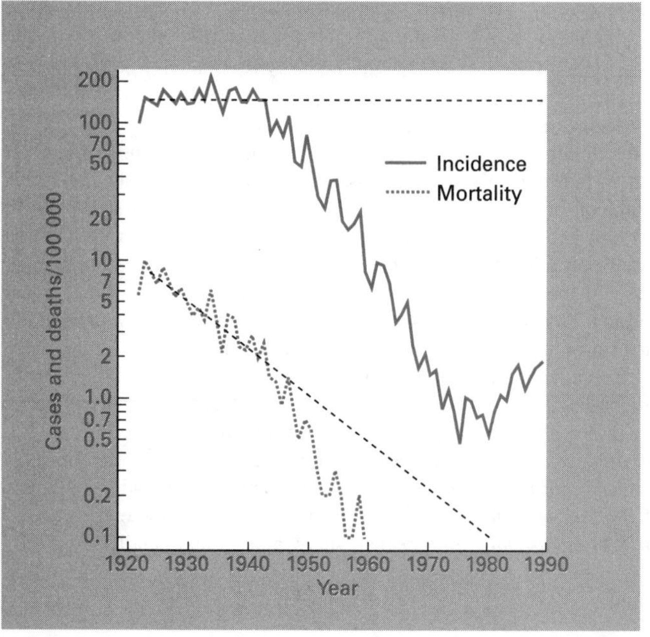

B. parapertussis produces the same respiratory illness as *B. pertussis*, except that most infections are associated with milder clinical manifestations. Twenty per cent or less of children will develop the whooping cough syndrome. This syndrome is even rarer with *B. bronchiseptica* infections. A non-descript bronchitis is probably the most common clinical presentation, although findings in one series of hospital-acquired *B. bronchiseptica* infections suggested that this organism was usually a non-pathogen in the respiratory tract. However, *B. bronchiseptica* can cause sinusitis, tracheobronchitis, and pneumonia in immunosuppressed patients, and bacteraemia, endocarditis, peritonitis, and meningitis have been reported.

Diagnosis

Bordetella infections are diagnosed by isolation of the organism. Fluorescent-antibody staining of material obtained by nasopharyngeal swabs from patients with *B. pertussis* infections will provide a presumptive, but not a definitive, diagnosis. There may be considerable observer variation in interpretation of such stains, and good reagents are difficult to obtain. Infections can be diagnosed by antibody responses as measured by assays such as enzyme immunoassay, but few laboratories provide these as routine diagnostic tests, and the available enzyme immunoassays have not been useful for diagnosing acute infections. Therefore, the diagnosis depends on recovering the organism from appropriate specimens.

B. pertussis cultures used to be obtained by the cough plate technique, where an open agar plate was held in front of a patient, coughing induced, and the plate sprayed with respiratory secretions. Fortunately, this has been replaced by the nasopharyngeal culture technique. A wire calcium alginate swab is passed through the nose until it touches the posterior nasopharynx, allowed to remain for a few seconds, and removed. Cotton swabs may be used if the cotton is proved to be non-bacteriostatic for *B. pertussis*. The swabs are streaked on to Bordet–Gengou agar plates, both with and without an antibiotic such as cephalexin. Multiple cultures may be useful in increasing the number of patients from whom *B. pertussis* can be recovered. The organism has not been recovered from blood or sites other than the respiratory tract. Because *B. pertussis* is a slow-growing bacterium, cultures must be held for 6 days before being discarded.

B. parapertussis and *B. bronchiseptica* can be recovered on Bordet–Gengou medium from patients in whom these organisms were the cause of pertussis, and they also grow on routine media used for recovery of Gram-negative bacteria. There are case reports of both of these organisms being recovered in blood cultures, and *B. bronchiseptica* has been cultured from urine.

Treatment

Most patients with pertussis can be managed at home, but very young children may need to be in hospital to ensure good nursing care. Cough medicines are of no value, nor is passive immunization with the currently available immunoglobulin preparations. Salbutamol has been suggested but not proven to be of use. Some physicians sedate young children, but this should be done carefully, if at all. Steroids have been reported in two studies to shorten the clinical course. In one study, children received betamethasone orally in a dose of 0.075 mg/kg per day, and in another, hydrocortisone sodium succinate intramuscularly in a dose of 30 mg/kg per day for 2 days, followed by tapering doses for 7 to 8 days. This may be useful in severe cases in young infants, but more experience with steroid treatment is needed before a general recommendation can be made.

B. pertussis and *B. parapertussis* are sensitive to a variety of antimicrobials, including erythromycin, tetracycline, chloramphenicol, and trimethoprim–sulphamethoxazole. Early treatment during the catarrhal stage will shorten the course of the clinical illness, but, if treatment is not started until the paroxysmal stage, antimicrobials will have only a limited effect. Thus, the best chance that physicians have to alter the clinical disease with antimicrobial therapy is when they treat symptomatic contacts of patients with diagnosed infections. Even though there is little clinical benefit, patients in the paroxysmal stage should receive antimicrobials to render them non-infectious to others. Erythromycin is the drug of choice. Children should receive 40 to 50 mg/kg a day, and adults, 1.5 to 2 g a day, for 14 days. Nasopharyngeal cultures will become negative in the first few days of treatment, but the erythromycin should be continued to prevent bacteriological relapses (Fig. 2). Trimethoprim–sulphamethoxazole has been used in children who do not tolerate erythromycin, although its efficacy has not been proven.

B. bronchiseptica is sensitive to tetracycline and chloramphenicol like the other *Bordetella*, but not to erythromycin. Antipseudomonal penicillins and aminoglycosides have been used successfully to treat serious infections, although the optimal treatment regimen has not been determined.

Prevention

The patient with *B. pertussis* infection should avoid close contact with susceptible individuals to prevent droplet transmission. The untreated patient will remain contagious for weeks, but communicability will decrease rapidly after the initiation of erythromycin therapy, with nasopharyngeal cultures becoming negative within 48 to 72 h. Patients admitted to hospital are usually isolated for the first 5 days of treatment.

Although there are no definitive studies, clinical experience suggests that chemoprophylaxis with erythromycin may be effective. Therefore, close contacts of patients with *B. pertussis* infection should be treated with erythromycin, just like children with disease. If unimmunized, vaccination should continue according to routine schedules. Some recommend that in addition to erythromycin, a booster dose of vaccine should be given to preschool children who have not received a booster within six months. For exposures with a lower risk of transmission, such as those that occur outside the home or day-care centre, contacts should be treated with erythromycin only if they develop respiratory symptoms.

Prevention of *B. pertussis* infections relies on the use of vaccine. Pertussis vaccine has been clearly shown to prevent disease, but is associated with frequent local reactions, with or without fever, and rare neurological complications. There are only limited data on serious reactions, but these occur less frequently after vaccination than with clinical disease. The available vaccine is a killed whole-bacterial preparation that can be given with diphtheria and tetanus toxoids. An effective immunizing schedule includes three injections at 1- to 2-month intervals beginning at 6 to 12 weeks of age, and a fourth dose given 1 year after the third. A booster dose is given before entry to school. New acellular vaccines containing several bacterial components, including filamentous haemagglutinin and pertussis toxin, have replaced whole-cell vaccines

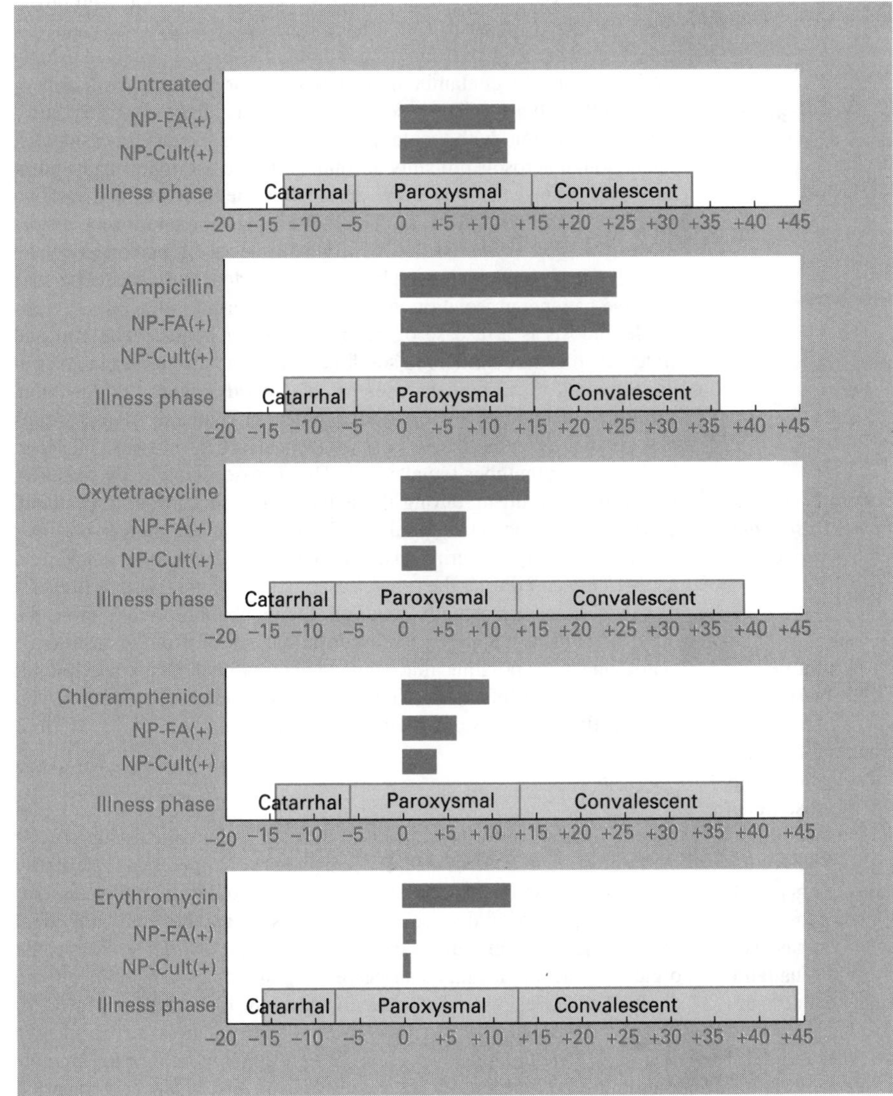

Fig. 2 Duration of excretion of *B. pertussis* as detected by fluorescent antibody staining and culture, and the effect of antimicrobial treatment. The graphs show comparison (group means) of patients treated with antimicrobial agents with untreated control patients. (Reproduced from Bass, J. W. *et al.* (1969). *Journal of Pediatrics*, **75**, 768, with permission.)

in Japan, and have been licensed in the United States for the fourth and fifth doses. To date, there are no studies directly comparing the two types of vaccine for efficacy.

Pertussis vaccines usually are not given after 6 years of age because of the local reactions, although vaccine has been given to adults to control an institutional outbreak. Immunity after pertussis vaccine is neither complete nor lifelong. In one study, protection against infection was lost by 12 years after vaccination. However, re-exposure to *B. pertussis* may induce continuing immunity in previously vaccinated patients. There are no vaccines generally available for *B. parapertussis* or *B. bronchiseptica.*

REFERENCES

Bass, J.W., Klenk, E.L., Kotheimer, J.B., Linnemann, C.C., and Smith, M.H.D. (1969). Antimicrobial treatment of pertussis. *Journal of Pediatrics*, **73,** 768–81.

Broomhall, J. and Herxheimer, A. (1984). Treatment of whooping cough: the facts. *Archives of Disease in Childhood*, **59,** 185–7.

Gilchrist, M.J.R. and Linnemann, C.C., Jr. (1988) Pertussis. In *The laboratory diagnosis of infectious diseases: principles and practice* (ed. A. Balows, W.J. Hausler, Jr., and E.H. Lennette), pp. 403–10. Springer-Verlag, New York.

Keller, M.A., Aftandelians, R., and Connor, J.D. (1980). Etiology of pertussis syndrome. *Pediatrics*, **66,** 50–5.

Linnemann, C.C., Jr. (1979). Host–parasite interactions in pertussis. In *International symposium on pertussis* (ed. C. Manclark and J. Hill), pp. 3–18, US Government Printing Office, Washington, DC.

Linnemann, C.C., Jr. and Nasenbeny, J. (1977). Pertussis in the adult. *Annual Review of Medicine*, **28,** 179–85.

Thomas, M.G. (1989). Epidemiology of pertussis. *Review of Infectious Diseases*, **11,** 255–62.

Woolfrey, B.F. and Moody, J.A. (1991). Human infections associated with *Bordetella bronchiseptica. Clinical Microbiology Reviews*, **4,** 243–55.

7.11.15 Melioidosis and glanders

D. A. B. DANCE

Melioidosis

DEFINITION

Melioidosis is the name given to any infection of man or animal caused by the saprophytic bacterium *Burkholderia (Pseudomonas) pseudomallei.* The clinical manifestations of infection are extremely varied.

HISTORY AND GEOGRAPHICAL DISTRIBUTION

The disease was first recognized in Burma in 1911 by Whitmore and Krishnaswami, who commented on the similarity of both the clinical features and the causative organism to those of glanders, and proposed the name *Bacillus pseudomallei.* The term melioidosis, derived from the Greek $\mu\eta\lambda\iota\sigma$ (glanders or distemper of asses), was subsequently suggested in 1921 by Stanton and Fletcher, who studied the disease in Malaysia. Further cases were observed in the French and Dutch colonies in South-East Asia (now Vietnam, Cambodia, and Indonesia) before the Second World War, and over 400 French and American soldiers developed the disease whilst fighting in Vietnam. In 1949, melioidosis was found to be endemic in northern Australia, and more recently it has been recognized as an important public health problem in north-east Thailand.

The true distribution of melioidosis apparently extends beyond tropical south-east Asia and Australia, as sporadic cases have been reported from the Indian subcontinent, the Pacific Islands, Central Africa, Central and South America, and the Caribbean. The disease is probably under diagnosed in many of these regions, as relatively sophisticated laboratory facilities are necessary to confirm the diagnosis. Reports of cases in Iran and an epizootic that occurred in France during the 1970s have indicated that the disease is not confined to the tropics.

AETIOLOGY

B. pseudomallei is an ovoid, oxidase-positive, motile, Gram-negative bacillus that often exhibits 'safety-pin' bipolarity. In the past it has been placed in several genera, including Malleomyces, Loefflerella, and Pfeifferella, but since the 1960s it has been classified in the genus Pseudomonas, comprising RNA group II along with *P. mallei*, *P. pickettii*, and *P. cepacia*, with which it may be confused in culture. This group has recently been assigned to a new genera, Burkholderia.

It grows well on most standard culture media, giving rise to rough or wrinkled and smooth colony types and producing a sweet, earthy smell. It has often been overlooked or discarded as a contaminant by bacteriologists unfamiliar with its characteristics, but is easy to identify using modern biochemical test kits such as the API 20NE. Only a minority of strains is pigmented, and it should rarely be confused with *P. aeruginosa.* Intrinsic resistance to aminoglycosides and polymyxins is a useful clue to its identity.

TRANSMISSION AND EPIDEMIOLOGY

Melioidosis was long thought to be a zoonosis, but French workers in Vietnam proved that *B. pseudomallei* was an environmental saprophyte, readily isolated from soil and surface water, particularly rice paddy, in endemic areas. Man and animals are thought to become infected usually by inoculation or contamination of wounds or mucosae with soil or water, although a specific episode of exposure is rarely identified. Iatrogenic inoculation with contaminated solutions occurs occasionally. Inhalation of aerosols probably accounted for the disproportionate number of cases in helicopter crew during the Vietnam war and for two laboratory-acquired infections. The role of ingestion and insect vectors in transmission is doubtful. Only two instances of person-to-person spread, one probably venereal, have been reported, but it would be wise to nurse patients in isolation where facilities permit.

Melioidosis is a disease of people in regular contact with soil and water, such as rice farmers in south-east Asia and aborigines in Australia. Some 20 to 50 human cases are diagnosed annually in Australia, while several hundred are reported each year in Thailand. All age groups may be affected, although the peak incidence occurs from 40 to 60 years. Male cases outnumber females 3:2. The disease is markedly seasonal, with a peak occurring during the annual rains: in north-east Thailand, *B. pseudomallei* accounts for almost 20 per cent of community-acquired septicaemias, outnumbering cases caused by *Staphylococcus aureus* and *Escherichia coli* during the rainy season. Although this pattern suggests that most cases are recently acquired, the incubation period before the onset of clinically apparent melioidosis has varied from 2 days to 26 years, and it is possible that some other seasonal factor precipitates relapses of latent infections. The proportion of seropositive people who are latently infected is unknown.

CLINICAL FEATURES

Several attempts have been made to develop a clinical classification of melioidosis, but none is entirely satisfactory. While *B. pseudomallei* may cause infections that are acute or chronic and localized or disseminated, one form of disease may progress to another and individual patients are often difficult to categorize. *B. pseudomallei* is a pyogenic organism, causing localized abscesses or granulomas, depending on the duration of the lesion, and septicaemia when the bloodstream is invaded. As up to 49 per cent of the population in endemic areas has antibodies to *B. pseudomallei*, most infections are presumably mild or asymptomatic; a flu-like illness associated with seroconversion has been reported from Australia. In addition, the infection may remain latent for over 20 years, causing relapses at times of intercurrent stress ('Vietnam time-bomb'). The most common manifestations of culture-positive melioidosis seen in patients admitted to hospital are described below.

Septicaemic melioidosis

Sixty per cent of cases of culture-positive melioidosis have positive blood cultures. Most of these are clinically septicaemic, although *B. pseudomallei* may sometimes be isolated from the blood of patients with a relatively mild febrile illness, presumably reflecting overspill from occult or apparent localized foci. There is usually a short history (median 6 days; range 1 day to 2 months) of high fever and rigors. Approximately half have evidence of a primary focus of infection, usually pulmonary or cutaneous. Confusion and stupor, jaundice and diarrhoea may also be prominent features. Initial investigations usually reveal anaemia, a neutrophil leucocytosis, coagulopathy, and evidence of renal and hepatic impairment. Such patients often deteriorate rapidly, developing widespread metastatic abscesses, particularly in the lungs, liver and spleen, and metabolic acidosis with Kussmaul's breathing. Once septic shock has supervened, fatality approaches 95 per cent, many patients dying within 48 h of admission. Other poor prognostic features include absence of fever, leucopaenia, azotaemia, and abnormal liver function tests.

If the patient survives this acute phase, the manifestations of the multiple foci that result from dissemination become prominent. The organism may seed to any site. Cutaneous pustules or subcutaneous abscesses occur in approximately 10 per cent of cases and an abnormal chest radiograph is found in 80 per cent of patients, the most common pattern being widespread, nodular shadowing ('blood-borne pneumonia'; Fig. 1). Other common sites for secondary lesions include the liver and spleen, kidneys and urinary tract, and bones and joints. Involvement of the central nervous system (e.g. brain abscess or a recently described syndrome comprising peripheral motor weakness, brain-stem encephalitis, aseptic meningitis, and respiratory failure) may also occur.

Localized melioidosis

The lung is the most frequent site of localized melioidosis. Acute bronchitis or pneumonia may occur, but the most common manifestation is a subacute, cavitating pneumonia accompanied by profound weight loss, which is often confused with tuberculosis or lung abscess (Fig. 2). Relative sparing of the apices and the infrequency of hilar adenopathy may help to distinguish melioidosis from tuberculosis. Any lung zone may be affected, although there is a predilection for the upper lobes. Complications include pneumothorax, empyema and purulent pericarditis, and ultimately progression to septicaemia.

Acute suppurative parotitis is a characteristic manifestation of melioidosis in children, accounting for approximately one-third of childhood cases in north-east Thailand (Fig. 3). The reason for this strong age–site association is obscure. Most cases are unilateral and result in parotid abscesses that require surgical drainage, although they may rupture spontaneously into the auditory canal. Facial nerve palsy and septicaemia are rare complications.

Localized *B. pseudomallei* infection may affect any other organ. Well-described examples include cutaneous and subcutaneous abscesses, lymphadenitis, osteomyelitis and septic arthritis, liver and/or splenic abscesses, cystitis, pyelonephritis, prostatic abscesses, epididymo-orchitis, keratitis, and, rarely, brain abscesses.

PATHOGENESIS AND VIRULENCE

The outcome of contact with *B. pseudomallei* depends on the host's immune system, the virulence of the infecting strain, and the size of the inoculum. Melioidosis that is severe enough to be seen in hospital is an opportunistic disease, as over 70 per cent of patients have underlying predisposition to infection. Little is known about the specific immunological mechanisms responsible for protection, although cell-mediated immunity is probably of particular importance. In Thailand, the most common precipitating factors are diabetes and chronic renal disease. Other associated conditions include malignancy, immunosuppressive treatment (particularly steroids), liver disease, alcohol or drug abuse, and pregnancy. Relapse of latent infection usually occurs at times of intercurrent stress (trauma or burns, onset of malignancy or diabetes, other acute infections), and it is thus possible that infection with the human immunodeficiency virus will unmask further cases of latent melioidosis.

Fig. 1 Septicaemic melioidosis: widespread nodular shadowing—'bloodborne pneumonia' (by courtesy of Professor Sornchai Looareesuwan).

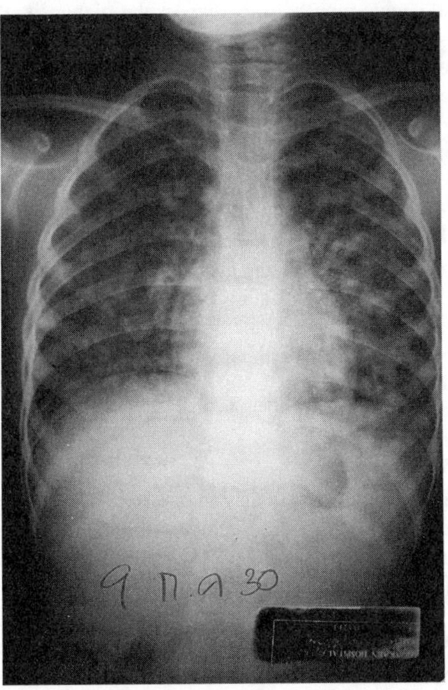

Fig. 2 Necrotizing *P. pseudomallei* pneumonia with central cavitation and fluid level in a rice farmer in north-eastern Thailand being treated with corticosteroids for nephrotic syndrome. Such patients are often misdiagnosed as having smear-negative tuberculosis, but fail to respond to antituberculosis chemotherapy. (By courtesy of Professor Sornchai Looareesuwan.)

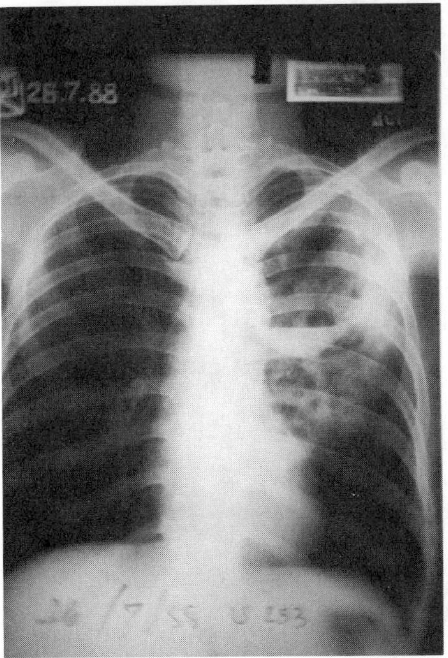

Virulence factors of *B. pseudomallei* are poorly understood, although interstrain differences in virulence undoubtedly occur. A heat-labile exotoxin and lipopolysaccharide are probably important during the septicaemic phase, the latter through the production of host-derived cytokines (tumour necrosis factor, interleukins). Haemolysins, proteases, lecithinase, and lipase probably contribute to local tissue damage. *B. pseudomallei* is able to survive inside phagocytic cells *in vitro*, and intracellular survival *in vivo* may contribute to the refractory and persistent nature of melioidosis.

DIAGNOSIS

The protean manifestations of melioidosis make it difficult to diagnose on clinical grounds alone. Because of the propensity for latency, the diagnosis should be considered in any patient who has ever visited an endemic area and presents with septicaemia, abscesses or, chronic suppuration, particularly if there is evidence of an underlying disease such as diabetes mellitus. Specific diagnosis depends on the detection of *B. pseudomallei* or of corresponding antibodies. The laboratory should always be warned if melioidosis is suspected, both to enable appropriate methods and media to be employed, and to alert staff to the risk of infection ('category 3' organism).

Fig. 3 (a) Acute suppurative parotitis—a common manifestation of childhood melioidosis in north-east Thailand. This child had parotid abscesses that required drainage despite having already ruptured into the auditory canal, extensive overlying ulceration, facial nerve palsy, and septicaemia. (b) Ulceration over healing parotid abscess. (By courtesy of Professor Sornchai Looareesuwan.)

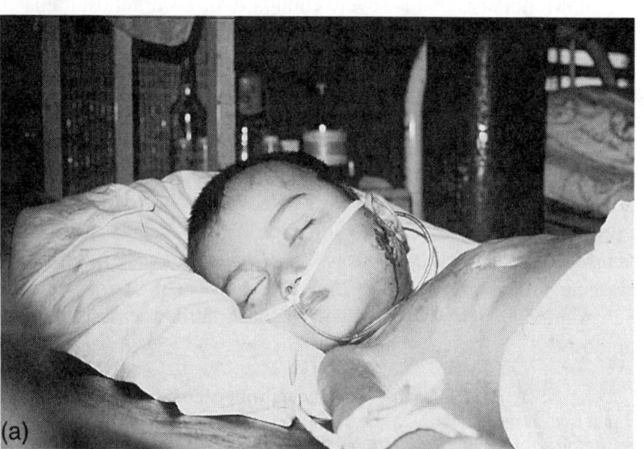

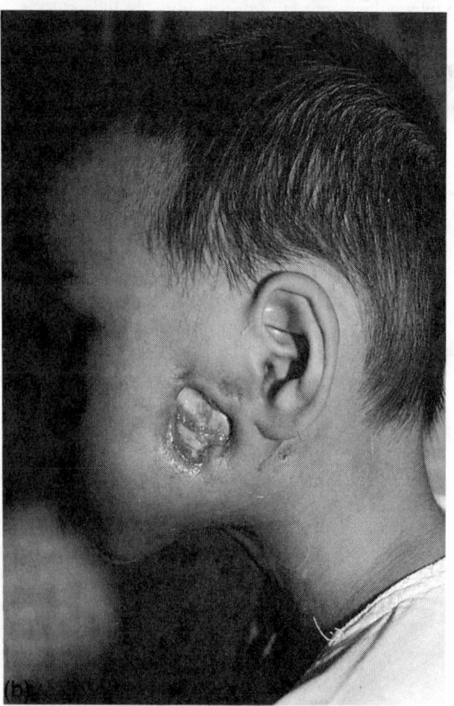

Microscopy of pus or secretions may reveal bipolar or unevenly staining Gram-negative rods, but this is neither specific nor sensitive. Several rapid diagnostic techniques are under development but are not yet routinely available. The mainstay of diagnosis is isolation and identification of *B. pseudomallei*, which takes at least 48 h. The organism should be sought in blood, pus, urine, sputum, or any other appropriate specimen. In children or others unable to produce sputum, culture of a throat swab using selective techniques has a sensitivity approaching that of sputum culture.

The indirect haemagglutination test, which detects antibodies to heat-stable antigens (probably lipopolysaccharide), is widely used for the detection of *B. pseudomallei* antibodies, and IgG enzyme-linked immunosorbent assays appear to give similar results. These tests are useful in patients from non-endemic areas in whom a single indirect haemagglutination titre in excess of 1:40 at presentation is highly suggestive of melioidosis. In populations continually exposed to *B. pseudomallei*, the high background seropositivity reduces the predictive value of the test, and in such patients only a rising or very high titre suggests active melioidosis. Alternatively, assays that detect specific IgM (indirect immunofluorescence, enzyme-linked immunosorbent) correlate better with disease activity. Unfortunately, such tests are not widely available.

TREATMENT, PROGNOSIS, AND PREVENTION

Treatment—general

Patients with septicaemic melioidosis require intensive supportive treatment and should ideally be managed in an intensive care unit. Particular attention should be paid to correction of volume depletion and septic shock, respiratory and renal failure, and hyperglycaemia or ketoacidosis, and abscesses should be drained whenever possible. Corticosteroids are of doubtful benefit, but antiendotoxin and anticytokine antibodies remain to be evaluated.

Treatment—specific

B. pseudomallei is intrinsically resistant to many antibiotics, including aminoglycosides and early β-lactams. Indeed, failure to defervesce during treatment with these agents may help to suggest the diagnosis of melioidosis. The organism is usually sensitive *in vitro* to extended-spectrum cephalosporins (e.g. ceftazidime), imipenem, ureidopenicillins (e.g. piperacillin), β-lactam/β-lactamase combinations (e.g. co-amoxiclav), chloramphenicol, and tetracyclines, with variable results for folate antagonists (e.g. co-trimoxazole). The fluoroquinolones (e.g. ciprofloxacin) are relatively inactive.

Two recent studies have shown that ceftazidime reduces the mortality of acute severe melioidosis compared with conventional combination regimens (chloramphenicol plus doxycycline plus co-trimoxazole). Co-trimoxazole was given concurrently in one study on the basis of its better intracellular penetration, but it is unclear whether this improves the long-term outcome. Co-amoxiclav has also given promising preliminary results, both parenterally in severe disease and orally for mild cases. Until further data are available, the following are recommended:

Initial treatment (severe disease)

Ceftazidime (120 mg/kg per day intravenously in divided doses, or an equivalent dose adjusted for renal function), with or without co-trimoxazole (10/50 mg/kg per day), for at least 2 weeks or until fever has subsided. In β-lactam allergic patients, chloramphenicol, 100 mg/kg per day, and doxycycline, 4 mg/kg per day, with or without co-trimoxazole, 10/50 mg/kg per day) should be used. Following these regimens, oral maintenance is needed to reduce the risk of relapse.

Maintenance treatment (or mild disease)

Oral agents (co-amoxiclav, approx. 30/15 mg/kg per day, possibly combined with extra amoxycillin, 30 mg/kg per day), or the conventional combination regimen as above, should be given for between 6 weeks and 6 months according to clinical progress. The optimal doses and duration of oral treatment remain to be determined.

Prognosis

Even with optimal treatment, fatality from acute severe melioidosis is high (25–40 per cent). In patients who survive, there is often chronic illness resulting both from the disease itself and the underlying conditions. Furthermore, over 20 per cent of patients may relapse after apparent recovery, often years after their initial infection, despite long courses of antibiotics. Long-term follow-up should therefore be arranged. Monitoring of IgM titres or C-reactive protein may assist in the early detection of relapse. Patients should also be carefully monitored bacteriologically both during and after treatment in order to detect the development of antibiotic resistance, which occurs in 5 to 10 per cent of cases.

Prevention

No *B. pseudomallei* vaccine has been developed for human use, although experimental vaccines have been used in animals. Prevention is thus limited to the avoidance of contact with *B. pseudomallei* in the environment, hospital or laboratory, particularly by 'at-risk' individuals such as diabetics. Whilst this is feasible in developed countries, it is often impractical for the inhabitants of regions where melioidosis is most prevalent.

Glanders

DEFINITION

Glanders is a disease of equines caused by the bacterium *Burkholderia (Pseudomonas) mallei*, which may occasionally be transmitted to man or other animals. Traditionally, glanders, a systemic disease involving the respiratory tract (Fig. 4), has been distinguished from farcy, a cutaneous infection also caused by *B. mallei* (Fig. 5).

HISTORY AND GEOGRAPHICAL DISTRIBUTION

Glanders of horses is a disease of antiquity, identifiable in the writings of Aristotle in the fourth century AD. Its communicability to man was recognized in the early nineteenth century and the causative agent was first isolated nearly 30 years earlier than that of melioidosis. In the early part of the twentieth century, equine glanders was present worldwide and was still relatively common in Europe and the United States. Over 200 000 horses were destroyed as a result of glanders during the First World War. However, no naturally acquired case has been reported in the United States or the United Kingdom since 1938, although occasional laboratory-acquired infections have occurred. This remarkable decline has been attributed variously to the compulsory slaughter of infected or seropositive animals, the decreasing use of the horse, and the removal of communal water troughs.

Currently, glanders is still known to occur in parts of the Middle East, Africa, and Asia, although the true incidence is uncertain. Occasional cases have arisen amongst carnivora in non-endemic areas, probably through the ingestion of contaminated imported meat. The most recent such outbreak affected lions in Istanbul Zoo.

Fig. 4 Glanders of the respiratory tract in a horse, showing profuse nasal discharge (by courtesy of Dr P. Nicoletti).

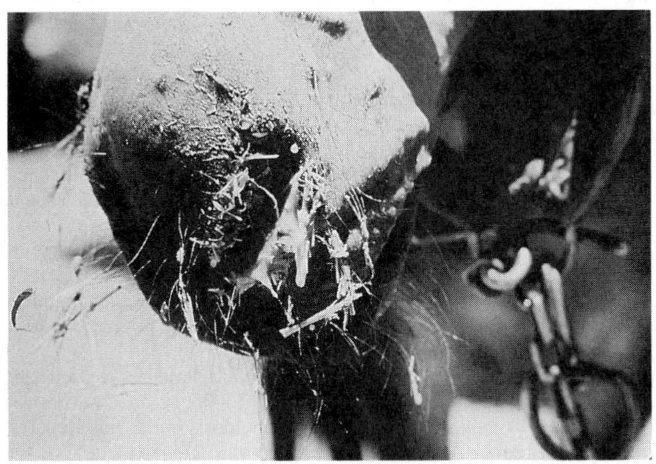

AETIOLOGY

B. mallei is an irregularly staining, Gram-negative bacillus that is atypical for a pseudomonad in giving a variable oxidase reaction and being non-motile. It cross-reacts serologically with *B. pseudomallei*, and grows readily, although less luxuriantly than *B. pseudomallei*, on most culture media. Its rarity means that most microbiologists are unfamiliar with its characteristics, and it might easily be overlooked unless sought specifically.

TRANSMISSION

Human glanders, which was rare even when equine glanders was common, is primarily an occupational disease of those in close contact with infected animals. Infection is thought usually to result from contamination of wounds, abrasions, or mucous membranes. The organism is

Fig. 5 Cutaneous glanders ('farcy') in horses: (a) dilated lymphatics; (b) dilated lymphatics with discharge (by courtesy of Dr P. Nicoletti).

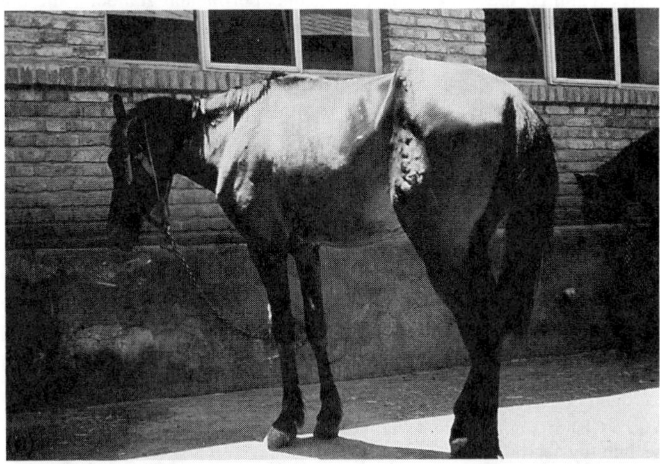

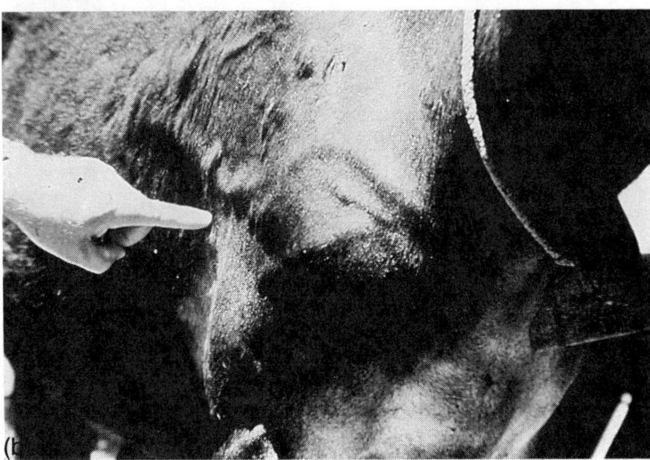

particularly hazardous to laboratory workers, who probably acquire infection by inhalation, and this route may also account for some naturally acquired cases. Person-to-person spread has occurred, so patients require isolation. The role of ingestion in human infections is uncertain. *B. mallei* is more delicate than *B. pseudomallei* and is usually considered to be an obligate parasite. It may, however, survive for up to 4 weeks in water, so infection from the inanimate environment is also a possibility.

CLINICAL FEATURES

The manifestations of glanders are similar to those of melioidosis, as originally observed by Whitmore. A spectrum of presentations is seen, ranging from occult infections, which are probably under-reported, to overwhelming sepsis resulting in severe toxaemia and widespread abscesses, culminating in delirium, shock, and death. Untreated, glanders may be fatal within days or may persist for many years with remissions and relapses. Distinctions between acute and chronic infections and between glanders and farcy are artificial, as an acute phase may precede or follow chronic disease and localized cutaneous infection may disseminate or may result from metastatic infection. Commonly reported manifestations have included wound infection and ulceration, lymphangitis with abscesses along the course of lymphatic drainage ('farcy buds'), ulceration of the respiratory (especially nasal) mucosa (Fig. 6), polyarthritis, pneumonia and lung abscesses, and nodular abscesses in any site, particularly muscle and subcutaneous tissue. A widespread, necrotizing skin eruption has been described as a terminal and relatively characteristic feature of disseminated glanders. Fatality in reported cases has been high (over 90 per cent), but this is probably an overestimate.

PATHOGENESIS AND VIRULENCE

Several animal species are susceptible to experimental glanders, and the pathogenesis of infection in these models has been described. However, although interstrain differences in virulence have been reported, the specific virulence factors of *B. mallei* have been little studied. Animal species also vary in their susceptibility to infection, with cattle, pigs, rats, and fowl being intrinsically resistant, but it is not clear whether underlying diseases render man susceptible to glanders.

DIAGNOSIS

As with melioidosis, the clinical manifestations of glanders are rarely pathognomonic. The diagnosis thus hinges on an appropriate history (contact with animals in an endemic area or laboratory exposure) and on isolation and identification of *B. mallei* from an appropriate clinical specimen (e.g. blood, wound swab or pus, sputum), the detection of specific antibodies or, possibly, cutaneous hypersensitivity. Although *B. mallei* will grow on orthodox media, the laboratory should be alerted if the diagnosis is suspected, both to increase the chances of detection and because, like *B. pseudomallei*, *B. mallei* is a category 3 pathogen. Selective techniques have been described, but recent experience of these is limited, and no rapid diagnostic tests have been developed.

Serological tests (complement fixation, bacterial agglutination or haemagglutination, or enzyme-linked immunosorbent assays), may be available through reference or veterinary laboratories, but are of little use in acute cases and may give cross-reactions in patients exposed to *B. pseudomallei*. Skin testing with a crude extract of *B. mallei* (mallein) has been used for screening animals and has been reported to be useful in human glanders, but cannot be recommended because of its unreliability, the risk of adverse reactions, and problems in obtaining mallein.

Fig. 6 Glanders in a horse: stellar ulcerative lesions on the mucosa of the nasal septum (by courtesy of Dr P. Nicoletti).

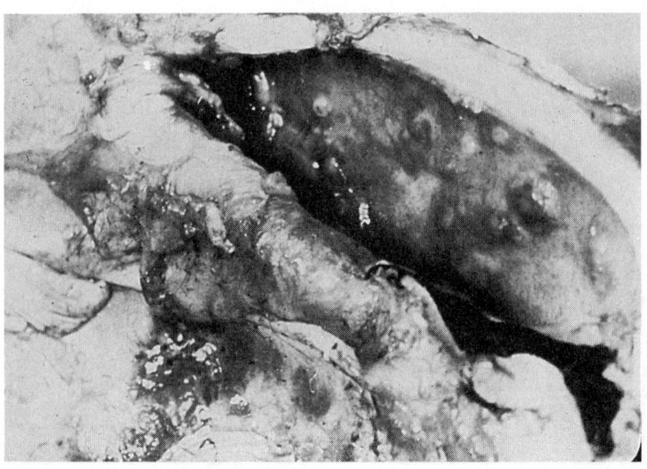

TREATMENT AND PREVENTION

As most human infections occurred in the pre-antibiotic era, data on treatment are scarce. The organism is sensitive *in vitro* to aminoglycosides, tetracyclines, sulphonamides, and trimethoprim, but resistant to early β-lactams and colistin. Sulphonamides in full doses for at least 20 days were effective in curing experimental infections and have been used successfully to treat human cases. Until further data are available, initial treatment for severe glanders should comprise an aminoglycoside, possibly in combination with co-trimoxazole, in doses appropriate to renal function and with monitoring of the serum levels. Mild infections can probably be treated with co-trimoxazole or a tetracycline. Treatment should be continued for at least 3 weeks and probably longer, depending on the patient's response. Long-term follow-up to detect relapse should be arranged.

There is no effective vaccine for either human or animal use, and prevention in those countries where glanders persists will depend on veterinary public-health measures and the continued reduction of reliance on the horse as a means of transport.

REFERENCES

Melioidosis

Ashdown, L.R. (1981). Relationship and significance of specific immunoglobulin M antibody response in clinical and subclinical melioidosis. *Journal of Clinical Microbiology*, **14**, 361–4.

Chaowagul, W. *et al.* (1989). Melioidosis: a major cause of community-acquired septicemia in Northeastern Thailand. *Journal of Infectious Diseases*, **159**, 890–9.

Dance, D.A.B. (1990). Melioidosis. *Reviews in Medical Microbiology*, **1**, 143–50.

Dance, D.A.B. (1991). Melioidosis: the tip of the iceberg? *Clinical Microbiology Reviews*, **4**, 52–60.

Dance, D.A.B. *et al.* (1989). Acute suppurative parotitis caused by *Pseudomonas pseudomallei* in children.*Journal of Infectious Diseases*, **159**, 654–60.

Dhiensiri, T., Puapairoj, S., and Susaengrat, W. (1988). Pulmonary melioidosis: clinical-radiologic correlation in 183 cases from northeastern Thailand. *Radiology*, **166**, 711–15.

Guard, R.W., Khafagi, F.A., Brigden, M.C., and Ashdown, L.R. (1984). Melioidosis in Far North Queensland. A clinical and epidemiological review of twenty cases. *American Journal of Tropical Medicine and Hygiene*, **33**, 467–73.

Howe, C., Sampath, A., and Spotnitz, M. (1971). The pseudomallei group: a review. *Journal of Infectious Diseases*, **124**, 598–606.

Kanai, K. and Dejsirilert, K. (1988). *Pseudomonas pseudomallei* and melioidosis, with special reference to the status in Thailand. *Japanese Journal of Medical Science and Biology*, **41**, 123–57.

Leelarasamee, A. and Bovornkitti, S. (1989). Melioidosis: review and update. *Reviews of Infectious Diseases*, **11**, 413–25.

Rode, J.W. and Webling, D.D'A. (1981). Melioidosis in the Northern Territory of Australia. *Medical Journal of Australia*, **21**, 181–4.

Sookpranee, T., Sookpranee, M., Mellencamp, M.A., and Preheim, L.C. (1991). *Pseudomonas pseudomallei*, a common pathogen in Thailand that is resistant to the bactericidal effects of many antibiotics. *Antimicrobial Agents and Chemotherapy*, **35,** 484–9.

Sookpranee, M., Boonma, P., Susaengrat, W., Bhuripanyo, K., and Punyagupta, S. (1992). Multicenter prospective randomized trial comparing ceftazidime plus co-trimoxazole with chloramphenicol plus doxycycline and co-trimoxazole for treatment of severe melioidosis. *Antimicrobial Agents and Chemotherapy*, **36,** 158–62.

Suputtamongkol, Y., Dance, D.A.B., Chaowagul, W., Wattanagoon, Y., and Wuthiekanun, V. (1991). Amoxycillin-clavulanic acid treatment of melioidosis. *Transactions of the Royal Society of Tropical Medicine and Hygiene*, **85,** 672–5.

Vatcharapreechasakul, T., Suputtamongkol, Y., Dance, D.A.B., Chaowagul, W., and White, N.J. (1992). *Pseudomonas pseudomallei* liver abscess: a clinical, laboratory and ultrasonographic study. *Clinical Infectious Diseases*, **14,** 412–17.

White, N.J., Dance, D.A.B., Chaowagul, W., Wuthiekanun, V., and Pitakwatchara, N. (1989). Halving of mortality of severe melioidosis by ceftazidime. *Lancet*, **ii,** 697–700.

Woods, M.L. *et al.* (1992). Neurological melioidosis: seven cases from the Northern Territory of Australia. *Clinical Infectious Diseases*, **15,** 163–9.

Glanders

Howe, C. (1950). Glanders. In *Oxford system of medicine*, Vol. 5, pp. 185–202. Oxford University Press.

Howe, C. and Miller, W.R. (1947). Human glanders: report of six cases. *Annals of Internal Medicine*, **26,** 93–115.

7.11.16 Plague

T. Butler

History

As a disease of antiquity and a zoonotic infection of rodents, plague doubtless made its debut on earth millions of years before man evolved. Epidemic bubonic plague was vividly described in biblical and in medieval times, with ravaging effects. Plague may have caused more deaths than most other diseases and warfare combined; it was estimated to have killed a fourth of Europe's population in the Middle Ages. The present pandemic of plague began in China in the 1860s and spread to Hong Kong in the 1890s. The genus of the plague bacillus is called Yersinia because Alexandre Yersin (1863–1943) went to Hong Kong in 1894 and successfully isolated the causative organism in pure culture. This pandemic was subsequently spread by rats transported on ships to California and to ports in South America, Africa, and Asia. Urban plague transmitted by rats was brought under control in most affected cities but the infection was transferred to sylvatic rodents, which allowed it to become entrenched in rural areas of these countries. In the first half of the twentieth century, India was severely affected by plague epidemics and suffered more than 10 million deaths. In the 1960s and 1970s, Vietnam during its war became the leading country for plague, reporting more than 10 000 cases a year. Before 1970, *Yersinia pestis* was called by its earlier name *Pasteurella pestis*.

Bacteriology

Y. pestis is a Gram-negative, bipolar-staining bacillus that belongs to the bacterial family Enterobacteriaceae. It grows aerobically on most culture media, including blood agar and MacConkey agar. It does not ferment lactose and forms small colonies on MacConkey agar after 24-h incubation at 35°C. On triple–sugar–iron agar, *Y. pestis* produces an alkaline slant and acid butt because it ferments glucose. It is non-motile and negative for citrate utilization, urease, and indole.

Like the other yersiniae, the plague bacillus produces V and W antigens, which confer a requirement for calcium to grow at 37°C. This property, mediated by a 45 MDa plasmid, is essential for virulence and plays a part in adapting the organism for intracellular survival and growth. Other important virulence factors include the production of lipopolysaccharide endotoxin, a capsular envelope containing the antiphagocytic principle fraction I antigen, the ability to absorb organic iron in the form of a haemin, and the presence of the temperature-dependent enzymes coagulase and fibrinolysin.

Epidemiology

Plague occurs worldwide, with most of the human cases reported from developing countries of Asia and Africa. During the decade of the 1980s there were 8554 cases of human plague reported to the World Health Organization. Of these, 981 died. The countries that reported more than 100 cases during the 1980s were in the order from greatest to least: Tanzania, Vietnam, Zaire, Brazil, Madagascar, Peru, Uganda, Burma, Bolivia, United States of America, and Botswana. In the United States, all the plague cases occurred in the south-western states of New Mexico, Arizona, Colorado, Utah, and California. Most of the American cases occur during the months of May to October, when people are outdoors coming into contact with rodents and their fleas. Each endemic region has a specific season when plague tends to occur.

Plague is primarily a zoonotic infection. It is transmitted among the natural animal reservoirs, which are predominantly urban and sylvatic rodents, by flea bites, or by ingestion of contaminated animal tissues. Throughout the world, the urban and domestic rats *Rattus rattus* and *R. norvegicus* are the most important reservoirs of the plague bacillus. These and other rodent reservoirs tolerate plague infection and develop prolonged bacteraemia, giving their fleas ample opportunity to transmit infection. However, during epizootics, when human cases are likely to be reported, intensity of infection in susceptible rodents is increased, leading to 'die-offs' of sometimes massive numbers of rodents. The timing of epizootics is dependent on seasonal factors, density of non-immune rodents, and proliferation of fleas on rodent hosts. The most efficient vector for transmission is the oriental rat flea *Xenopsylla cheopis*. In sylvatic foci of plague, such as occur in the United States, the important reservoirs are the ground squirrel, rock squirrel, and prairie dog. Each of these rodents harbours its own species of fleas. Man is an accidental host in the natural cycle of plague, when he is bitten by an infected rodent flea, and appears to play no part in the maintenance of plague in nature. Only rarely, during epidemics of pneumonic plague, is the infection passed directly from person to person. Rarely, hunters can develop infection by handling contaminated animal tissues.

In the United States, males and females have been equally affected. Sixty per cent of cases occur in those less than 20 years old. Although most cases occur in whites, the attack rate among American Indians living in endemic areas such as Arizona, New Mexico, and Utah is 10 times the rate among non-Indians living in the same states (1.4 cases/100 000 population and 0.1/100 000 population, respectively). Within endemic areas, risk factors associated with acquiring plague include direct contact with rodents or carnivores, the presence of refuges and food sources for wild rodents in the immediate vicinity of the home, and possibly failure to control fleas on pet dogs and cats.

Pathogenesis

When a flea ingests a blood meal from a bacteraemic animal infected with *Y. pestis*, the coagulase of the organism causes the blood to clot in the foregut leading to blockage of the flea's swallowing. *Y. pestis* multiplies in the clotted blood. During attempts to ingest a blood meal, a blocked flea may regurgitate thousands of organisms into a patient's skin. The inoculated bacteria migrate by cutaneous lymphatics to the regional lymph nodes. The flea-borne bacilli possess a small amount of envelope antigen (fraction I) and are readily phagocytosed by the host's

Table 1 *Plague syndromes*

Syndrome	Features
Bubonic	Fever, painful lymphadenopathy (bubo)
Septicaemic	Fever, hypotension without bubo
Pneumonic	Cough, haemoptysis, with or without bubo
Cutaneous	Pustule, eschar, carbuncle, or ecthyma gangrenosum, usually with bubo
Meningitis	Fever, nuchal rigidity, usually with bubo

polymorphonuclear leucocytes and mononuclear phagocytes. *Y. pestis* resists destruction within mononuclear phagocytes and may multiply intracellularly with elaboration of envelope antigen. If lysis of the mononuclear cell occurs, the bacilli released are relatively resistant to further phagocytosis. The involved lymph nodes show polymorphonuclear leucocytes, destruction of normal architecture, haemorrhagic necrosis, and dense concentrations of extracellular plague bacilli. Transient bacteraemia is common in bubonic plague, and, in the absence of specific therapy, purulent, necrotic, and haemorrhagic lesions may develop in many organs. Hypotension, oliguria, altered mental status, and subclinical disseminated intravascular coagulation may be noted and are attributable to endotoxaemia.

Clinical manifestations

BUBONIC PLAGUE

Although plague infection of man can assume many and protean clinical forms, the most common presentation is bubonic plague, which has a distinctive clinical picture (Table 1). The people of plague endemic regions know the disease and have local names, such as *dich hach* in Vietnamese, that conjure up the horror of recalled fatalities during previous seasons. During an incubation period of 2 to 8 days following the bite of an infected flea, bacterial proliferate in the regional lymph nodes. Patients are typically affected by the sudden onset of fever, chills, weakness, and headache. Usually, at the same time, after a few hours, or on the next day, they notice the bubo, which is signalled by intense pain in one anatomical region of lymph nodes, usually the groin, axilla, or neck. A swelling evolves in this area, which is so tender that the patients typically avoid any motion that might provoke discomfort. For example, if the bubo is in the femoral area, the patient will characteristically flex, abduct, and externally rotate the hip to relieve pressure on the area and will walk with a limp. When the bubo is in an axilla, the patient will abduct the shoulder or hold the arm in a splint. When a bubo is in the neck, patients will tilt their heads to the opposite side.

The buboes are oval swellings that vary from 1 to 10 cm in length and elevate the overlying skin, which may appear stretched or erythematous. They may appear either as a smooth, uniform, ovoid mass or as an irregular cluster of several nodes with intervening and surrounding oedema. Palpation will typically elicit extreme tenderness. There is warmth of the overlying skin and an underlying, firm, non-fluctuant mass. Around the lymph nodes there is usually considerable oedema, which can be either gelatinous or pitting in nature. Occasionally, there is a large area of oedema extending from the bubo into the region drained by the affected lymph nodes. Although infections other than plague can produce acute lymphadenitis, plague is virtually unique for the suddenness of onset of the fever and bubo, the rapid development of intense inflammation in the bubo, and the fulminant clinical course that can produce death as quickly as 2 to 4 days after the onset of symptoms. The bubo of plague is also distinctive for the usual absence of a detectable skin lesion in the anatomical region where it is located as well as for the absence of an ascending lymphangitis near it (Fig. 1).

The groin is the most common site of the buboes in plague. In clinical reports that have distinguished femoral from inguinal locations, the femoral site was found to be the more common. Other common sites are the axillae and neck. The reason for a given distribution of buboes is presumed to be the distribution of flea bites, which inoculate the bacteria into the skin to migrate to the regional lymph nodes.

In uncomplicated bubonic plague the patients are typically prostrate and lethargic, and often exhibit restlessness or agitation. Occasionally, they are delirious with high fever, and seizures are common in children. Temperatures are usually elevated in the range 38.5 to 40.0°C, and the pulse rates are increased to 110 to 140/min. Blood pressures are characteristically low, in the range of 100/60 mmHg, owing to extreme vasodilatation. Lower pressures that are unobtainable may occur if shock ensues. The liver and spleen are often palpable and tender.

Most patients with bubonic plague do not have skin lesions; however, about one-quarter of patients in Vietnam did show varied skin findings. The most common were pustules, vesicles, eschars, or papules near the bubo or in the anatomical region of skin that is lymphatically drained by the affected lymph nodes, and they presumably represent sites of the flea bites (Fig. 2). When these lesions are opened they usually contain white cells and plague bacilli. Rarely, these skin lesions progress to extensive cellulitis or abscesses. Ulceration, however, may lead to a larger plague carbuncle.

Another kind of skin lesion in plague is purpura, which is a result of the systemic disease. The purpuric lesions may become necrotic, resulting in gangrene of distal extremities, the probable basis of the epithet 'Black Death' attributed to plague through the ages. These purpuric

Fig. 1 A right femoral bubo consists of an enlarged, tender lymph node with surrounding oedema.

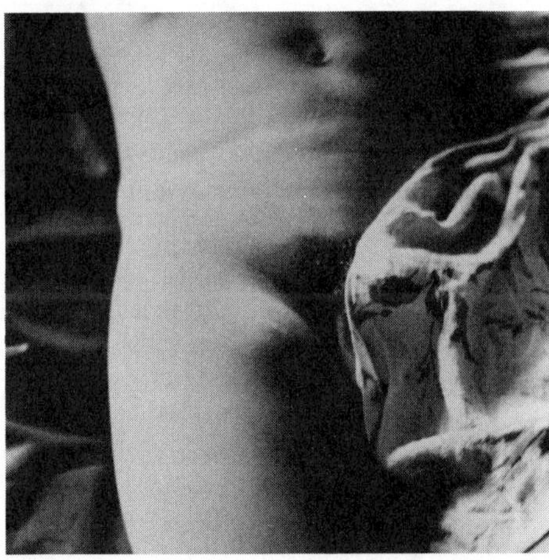

Fig. 2 A right axillary bubo was accompanied by a purulent ulcer on the abdomen, which was the presumed site of the flea bite.

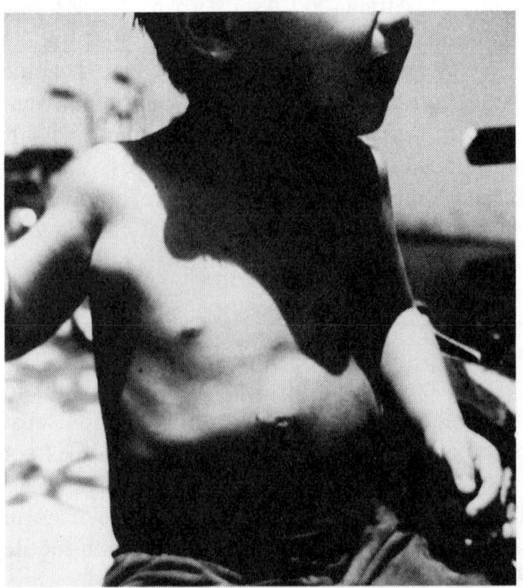

lesions contain blood vessels affected by vasculitis and occlusion by fibrin thrombi, resulting in haemorrhage and necrosis.

SEPTICAEMIC PLAGUE

A distinctive feature of plague, in addition to the bubo, is the propensity of the disease to overwhelm patients with a massive growth of bacteria in the blood. In the early acute stages of bubonic plague, all patients probably have intermittent bacteraemia. Single blood cultures obtained at the time of hospital admission in Vietnamese patients were positive in 27 per cent of cases. A hallmark of moribund patients with plague is high-density bacteraemia, so that a blood smear revealing characteristic bacilli has been used as a prognostic indicator in this disease. Occasionally in the pathogenesis of plague infection, bacteria are inoculated and proliferate in the body without producing a bubo. Patients may become ill with fever and actually die with bacteraemia but without detectable lymphadenitis. This syndrome has been termed 'septicaemic plague' to denote plague without a bubo. In New Mexico, 25 per cent of plague was septicaemic in 1980 to 1984 and the case fatality rate of 33 per cent in these instances was three times higher than in bubonic plague because of delays in diagnosis and treatment.

PNEUMONIC PLAGUE

One of the feared complications of bubonic plague is secondary pneumonia. The infection reaches the lungs by haematogenous spread of bacteria from the bubo. In addition to the high mortality, plague pneumonia is highly contagious by airborne transmission. It presents in the setting of fever and lymphadenopathy as cough, chest pain, and often haemoptysis. Radiographically, there is patchy bronchopneumonia, cavities, or confluent consolidation. The sputum is usually purulent and contains plague bacilli.

Primary inhalation pneumonia is rare now but is a potential threat following exposure to a patient with plague who has a cough. It can be so rapidly fatal that persons reportedly have been exposed, become ill, and died on the same day. Plague pneumonia is invariably fatal when antibiotic therapy is delayed more than a day after the onset of illness.

OTHER SYNDROMES

Plague meningitis is a rarer complication and typically occurs more than a week after inadequately treated bubonic plague. It results from a haematogenous spread from a bubo and carries a higher mortality rate than uncomplicated bubonic plague. There appears to be an association between buboes located in the axilla and the development of meningitis. Less commonly, plague meningitis presents as a primary infection of the meninges without antecedent lymphadenitis. Plague meningitis is characterized by fever, headache, meningism, and pleocytosis with a predominance of polymorphonuclear leucocytes. Bacteria are frequently demonstrable with a Gram stain of spinal-fluid sediment, and endotoxin has been demonstrated by the limulus test in spinal fluid.

Plague can produce pharyngitis that may resemble acute tonsillitis. The anterior cervical lymph nodes are usually inflamed, and *Y. pestis* may be recovered from a throat culture or by aspiration of a cervical bubo. This is a rare clinical form of plague that is presumed to follow the inhalation or ingestion of plague bacilli.

Plague presents sometimes with prominent gastrointestinal symptoms of nausea, vomiting, diarrhoea, and abdominal pain. These symptoms may precede the bubo or, in septicaemic plague, occur without a bubo; they commonly result in diagnostic delay.

Laboratory findings

The white blood-cell count is typically elevated in the range of 10 000 to 20 000 cells/mm^3, with a predominance of immature and mature neutrophils. Severely ill patients tend to have the higher white blood-cell counts. Occasionally, some patients, especially children, may develop myelocytic leukaemoid reactions with white-cell counts as high as 100 000/mm^3. Examination of the white blood cells in the peripheral blood smear typically reveals cytoplasmic vacuolations, toxic granulations, and Dohle bodies that are characteristic of acute bacterial infections. Blood eosinophils are characteristically diminished or absent in the acute stage of infection but return to normal or elevated levels during convalescence. Blood platelets may be normal or low in the early stages of bubonic plague. Although patients with plague rarely develop a generalized bleeding tendency from profound thrombocytopenia, disseminated intravascular coagulation is common in this infection. Fibrin(-ogen) degradation products in the sera indicative of disseminated intravascular coagulation were detected in elevated titres in most patients tested in Vietnam. 'Liver function tests', including serum aminotransferases and bilirubin, are frequently abnormally high. Renal function tests may be abnormal in hypotensive patients.

Diagnosis

Plague should be suspected in febrile patients who have been exposed to rodents or other mammals in the known endemic areas of the world. A bacteriological diagnosis is readily made in most patients by smear and culture of a bubo aspirate. The aspirate is obtained by inserting a 20-gauge needle on a 10-ml syringe containing 1 ml of sterile saline into the bubo and withdrawing it several times until the saline becomes blood-tinged. Because the bubo does not contain liquid pus, it may be necessary to inject some of the saline and immediately reaspirate it. Drops of the aspirate should be placed on to microscopic slides and air-dried for both Gram and Wayson's stains. The Gram stain will reveal polymorphonuclear leucocytes and Gram-negative coccobacilli and bacilli ranging from 1 to 2 μm in length. Wayson's stain is prepared by mixing 0.2 g of basic fuchsin (90 per cent dye content) with 0.75 g of methylene blue (90 per cent dye content) in 20 ml of 95 per cent ethyl alcohol. This mixture is then poured slowly into 200 ml of 5 per cent phenol. A smear, after being fixed for 2 min in absolute methanol, is stained for 10 to 20 s in Wayson's stain, washed with water, and dried. *Y. pestis* appears as light-blue bacilli with dark-blue polar bodies and the remainder of the slide has a contrasting pink counterstain (Fig. 3). Smears of blood, sputum, or spinal fluid can be handled similarly (Fig. 4).

The aspirate, blood, and other appropriate fluids should be inoculated on to blood and MacConkey agar plates and into infusion broth for bacteriological identification. At some reference laboratories, a serological test, the passive haemagglutination test utilizing fraction I of *Y. pestis*, is available for testing acute- and convalescent-phase serum. In patients with negative cultures, a fourfold or greater increase in titre

Fig. 3 Wayson's stain of a bubo aspirate shows bipolar bacilli.

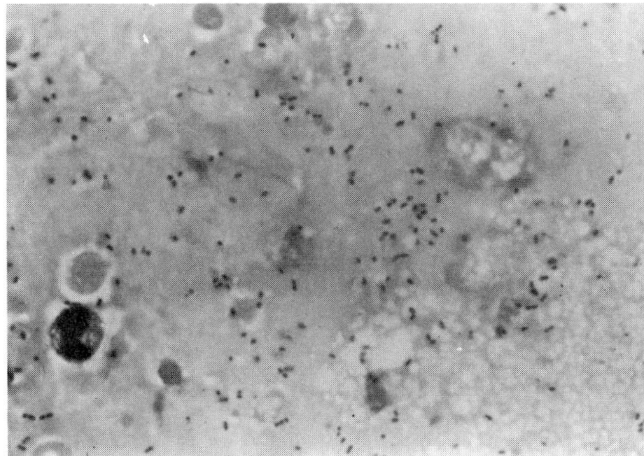

or a single titre of 1:16 or higher is presumptive evidence of plague infection.

Treatment and prevention

ANTIMICROBIALS

Untreated plague has an estimated mortality rate of greater than 50 per cent and can evolve into a fulminant illness complicated by septic shock. Therefore, the early institution of effective antimicrobial therapy is mandatory following appropriate cultures. In 1948, streptomycin was identified as the drug of choice for the treatment of plague by reducing the mortality rate to less than 5 per cent. No other drug has been demonstrated to be more efficacious or less toxic. Streptomycin should be given intramuscularly in two divided doses daily, totalling 30 mg/kg body weight per day for 10 days. Most patients improve rapidly and become afebrile in about 3 days. The 10-day course of streptomycin is recommended to prevent relapses because viable bacteria have been isolated from buboes of patients with plague during convalescence. The risk of vestibular damage and hearing loss due to streptomycin is minimal. This antibiotic should be used cautiously, however, in pregnant women, in older patients who would have trouble adapting to vestibular damage, and in patients with previous hearing difficulty. In such patients, the course of streptomycin can be shortened to 3 days following the disappearance of fever. Renal injury as a result of streptomycin therapy is rare with this regimen; however, renal function should be monitored. If the serum creatinine rises significantly, the dose of streptomycin should be reduced. In mild renal failure, the recommended dose is about 20 mg/kg per day, and in advanced renal failure, it is 8 mg/kg every 3 days.

For patients allergic to streptomycin or in whom an oral drug is strongly preferred, tetracycline is a satisfactory alternative. It is given orally in a dose of 2 to 4 g/day in four divided doses for 10 days. Tetracycline is contraindicated in children younger than 7 years of age and in pregnant women because it stains developing teeth. It is also contraindicated in renal failure.

For patients with meningitis who require a drug with good penetration into the cerebrospinal fluid and for patients with profound hypotension in whom an intramuscular injection may be poorly absorbed, chloramphenicol should be given intravenously, a loading dose of 25 mg/kg of body weight followed by 60 mg/kg per day in four divided doses. After clinical improvement, chloramphenicol should be continued orally to complete a total course of 10 days. The dosage may be reduced to 30 mg/kg per day to lessen the magnitude of bone marrow suppression, which is reversible after completion of therapy. The irreversible bone-marrow aplasia associated with chloramphenicol is so rare (estimated to occur in 1 in 40 000 patients) that its consideration should not deter the use of chloramphenicol in patients seriously ill with plague infection.

Fig. 4 Gram stain of spinal fluid in plague meningitis shows numerous Gram-negative bacilli.

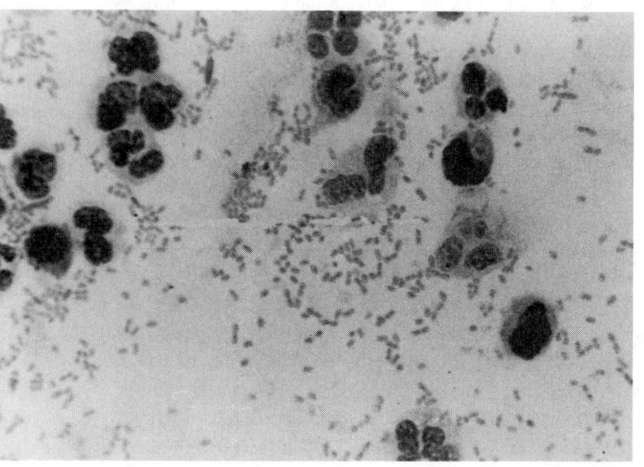

Other antimicrobial drugs have been used in plague with varying success. These include sulphonamides, trimethoprim-sulphamethoxazole, kanamycin, gentamicin, and ampicillin. These drugs either are less effective than streptomycin or have not been subjected to adequate clinical studies and, therefore, should not be chosen.

Antimicrobial resistance in human isolates of *Y. pestis* has never been reported, nor has resistance emerged during antibiotic therapy. Streptomycin, tetracycline, and chloramphenicol given alone are clinically very effective, and relapses are exceedingly rare. Therefore, there is no rationale for using multiple antimicrobial agents to treat plague.

SUPPORTIVE THERAPY

Most patients are febrile, with constitutional symptoms including nausea and vomiting. Hypotension and dehydration are common. Therefore, intravenous 0.9 per cent saline solution should be given to most patients for the first few days of the illness or until improvement occurs. Patients in shock will require additional quantities of fluid, with haemodynamic monitoring and the judicious use of adrenaline or dopamine. There is no evidence that corticosteroids are beneficial in plague. Although disseminated intravascular coagulation is commonly present and purpura occasionally develops in severely ill patients, therapy with heparin has no proven benefit in plague infections.

The buboes usually recede without local therapy. Occasionally, however, they may enlarge or become fluctuant during the first week of treatment, requiring incision and drainage. The aspirated fluid should be cultured for evidence of superinfection with other bacteria, but this material is usually sterile.

Precautions

Plague is an internationally quarantinable disease. Accordingly, all patients with suspected plague should be reported to the appropriate health department and to the World Health Organization. Patients with uncomplicated infections who are promptly treated present no health hazards to other people. Those with cough or other signs of pneumonia must be placed in strict respiratory isolation for at least 48 h after starting antimicrobial therapy or until the sputum culture is negative. The bubo aspirate and blood must be handled with gloves and with care to avoid aerosolization of these infected fluids. Laboratory workers who process the cultures should be alerted to exercise precautions; however, standard bacteriological techniques that safeguard against skin contact with, and aerosolization of, cultures should be adequate.

Vaccine

A formalin-killed vaccine, Plague Vaccine U.S.P. (Cutter Laboratories, Berkeley, California 94710), is available for travellers to epidemic or hyperendemic areas (e.g. Madagascar), for individuals who must live and work in close contact with rodents in these areas, and for laboratory workers who must handle live *Y. pestis* cultures. A primary series of two injections is recommended with a 1- to 3-month interval between them. Booster injections are given every 6 months for as long as exposure continues. In Britain, vaccine is obtainable, for named patients only, from Geer Laboratories, PO Box 800, Lenoir, North Carolina 28645, USA, but experience over recent years indicates a high rate of unpleasant reactions. Early antimicrobial therapy after suspected exposure is an alternative policy. In addition to vaccination, people living in endemic areas should provide themselves with as much personal protection against rodents and fleas as possible, including living in rat-proof houses, wearing shoes and garments to cover the legs, and dusting houses with insecticide.

Reservoir and vector control

The control of plague by health departments requires knowledge of the epidemiology of infected animals, vectors, and the contact of man with these animals in any particular area. In the United States, the Plague Branch of the Centers for Disease Control in Fort Collins, Colorado, has a field team of entomologists, mammalogists, and epidemiologists to investigate cases of plague. A specific approach to each case should be chosen and usually consists of using insecticides around homes, trapping of animals, and educating people to avoid contact with certain animals. Urban plague has been successfully controlled in many cities around the world by quarantine, rat control, and the use of insecticides. Sylvatic plague, however, defies definitive control because the wild rodent reservoirs are so widespread and diverse.

REFERENCES

Butler, T. (1983). *Plague and other Yersinia infections*. Plenum Medical, New York.

Craven, R.B. and Barnes A.M. (1991). Plague and tularemia. *Infectious Diseases Clinics of North America*, **5,** 165–75.

Crook, L.D. and Tempest, B. (1992). Plague. A clinical review of 27 cases. *Archives of Internal Medicine*, **152,** 1253–6.

Ferber, D.M. and Brubaker, R.R. (1981). Plasmids in *Yersinia pestis. Infection and Immunity*, **31,** 839–41.

Hull, H.F., Montes, J.M., and Mann, J.M. (1986). Plague masquerading as gastrointestinal illness. *Western Journal of Medicine*, **145,** 485–7.

Hull, H.F., Montes, J.M., and Mann, J.M. (1987). Septicemic plague in New Mexico. *Journal of Infectious Diseases*, **155,** 113–18.

Kaufmann, A.F., Boyce, J.M., and Martone, W.J. (1980). Trends in human plague in the United States. *Journal of Infectious Diseases*, **141,** 522–4.

Mann, J.M., Martone, W.J., Boyce, J.M., Kaufman, A.F., Barnes, A.M., and Weber, N.S. (1979). Endemic human plague in New Mexico: risk factors associated with infection. *Journal of Infectious Diseases*, **140,** 397–401.

Rosquist, R., Skurnik, M., and Wolf-Watz, H. (1988). Increased virulence of *Yersinia pseudotuberculosis* by two independent mutations. *Nature*, **334,** 522–5.

Welty, T.K. *et al.* (1985). Nineteen cases of plague in Arizona. A spectrum including ecthyma gangrenosum due to plague and plague in pregnancy. *Western Journal of Medicine*, **142,** 641–6.

7.11.17 Yersiniosis, pasteurellosis, and tularaemia

(a) Tularaemia

A. D. PEARSON

DEFINITION

Tularaemia is a zoonotic, arthropod- and water-borne disease caused by *Francisella tularensis,* a small, Gram-negative bacterium that has a complex maintenance system in ticks, wildlife, and aquatic ecosystems. Human infections occur in many countries, predominantly in the Northern Hemisphere. Within the species *F. tularensis* there are several subspecies (Table 1) identified by their virulence, epidemiology and ecology, and by minor differences in biochemical characters.

History of F. tularensis and its geographical distribution

The discovery of tularaemia is attributed to McCoy who, in 1911, reported a plague-like illness in Californian ground squirrels *(Citellus beecheyi)* and who with Chapin isolated a new agent, which they called *Bacterium tularens.* A similar agent had been observed in Europe in 1896 and 1903 by Horne, who saw tiny, plague-like, bipolar-staining coccobacilli in Scandinavian lemmings *(Lemmus lemmus)* and transferred the agent to guinea-pigs.

Wherry and Lamb described the first human case in North America, diagnosed by isolation of the causative organism, in 1914. The possible extent of human infection in America was not realized until an investigation of 'deerfly fever' by Francis in the Pahvant valley of Utah. In the United States, between 1924 and 1950, 23 309 cases were recognized, with 9.5 per cent case fatality. Streptomycin was introduced in 1949, after which there was a reduction to 0.89 per cent case fatality between 1960 and 1968 (2594 cases with 23 deaths). Published reports from the former USSR and Europe, as well as North America, describe more than a million cases of human tularaemia during the last 70 years. Tularaemia foci occur throughout the world but the majority of cases have been diagnosed in the Northern Hemisphere. Two types of infection have been described in man: *F. tularenis* subspecies *tularensis* or type A (referred to in the text as subsp. *tularensis*) and *F. tularensis* subspecies *holarctica* or type B (referred in text as subsp. *holarctica*). Subsp. *tularensis* primarily affects ticks and lagomorphs (hares and rabbits) and is more virulent for man and rabbits than subsp. *holarctica.* Since, in North America, 95 per cent of the recognized human infections are thought to be due to subsp. *tularensis,* most Western textbooks of medicine and microbiology describe only the clinical presentations and epidemiology associated with this subspecies. In Europe, infection is by the less virulent subsp. *holarctica,* which has a greater variety of reservoirs and vectors than subsp. *tularensis* causing even greater diversity of symptoms and presentations than in America. The clinician needs to understand these differences in epidemiology when diagnosing tularaemia in people who may have acquired infection while travelling in endemic areas.

Clinical presentations of tularaemia (rabbit fever, deerfly fever, Ohara disease)

The clinical types and presentations of tularaemia depend on the route of transmission of the organism and its virulence. In all but the mildest infections the patient suffers from fever, chills and prostration, and has a relapsing, protracted illness unless treated or vaccinated. Infections resulting from skin contact with animals or insect bites are the most frequent recognized clinical presentations of tularaemia in the western part of the Northern Hemisphere. Infection by the airborne route usually causes pulmonary disease while ingestion causes abdominal or oropharyngeal tularaemia.

Case histories

CLINICAL INFECTIONS WITH *F. TULARENSIS* SUBSP. *TULARENSIS* (TYPE A)

American workers have based their classification of the human types of tularaemia on the illnesses produced by subsp. *tularensis* (type A) organisms (Fig. 1).

Ulceroglandular tularaemia

Most cases reported in North America are ulceroglandular. They present with sudden chills, fever, and often severe headache. At the site of the initial entry of the organism there is an indurated and ragged ulcer, often quite small and usually causing little pain, but associated with a local, tender lymphadenopathy that may steadily increase in size and frequently suppurates. Ulceroglandular tularaemia may present with lymphadenopathy without a visible skin ulcer. There may be a protracted and relapsing illness, especially if diagnosis and treatment are delayed.

Cases 1–3: ulceroglandular tularaemia acquired during 1985 in the United States

An 18-year-old man (case 1) had shot two rabbits behind his home in Gloucester County, New Jersey, on 9 November 1985. After eviscer-

Table 1 *Designation of genus Francisella*

Subspecies and synonyms	Distribution and reference strains
F. tularensis subsp. *tularensis*[a] (synonyms: type A; *F. tularensis* subsp. *nearctica*)	Type strain is ATCC 6223 (avirulent) Virulent typical strain is GIEM strain Schu, which was first isolated in 1941 from man in the United States Distributed predominantly in N. America
F. tularensis subsp. *holarctica*[a] biovar I (erythromycin sensitive) (synonyms: type B; *F. tularensis* subsp. *palaearctica*)	Reference strain GIEM c/a7 isolated from man in 1976 in the Moscow region of former USSR Distributed primarily from western and northern regions of Europe and eastern Siberia, the Far East and Kazakhstan, and occasionally from N. America
F. tularensis subsp. *holarctica*[a] biovar II (erythromycin resistant) (synonyms: type B; *F. tularensis* subsp. *palaearctica*)	Reference strain GIEM 503 is the type strain of this subspecies This biovar is distributed only in Eurasia, Central and Eastern Europe, the Caucasus, and predominantly in western Siberia and Kazakhstan
F. tularensis subsp. *holarctica*[a] biovar japonica (synonym: *F. tularensis* var. *palaearctica japonica*)	Reference strain GIEM Miura was isolated from man in 1975 Originally isolated in Japan in 1926 from a human lymph node This biovar is distributed only on the Japanese islands
F. tularensis subsp. *mediasiatica*[a]	Isolated in the middle Asian region of the USSR (Alma-Ata) in 1965 from a gerbil Distributed only in central Asian USSR and mediated only by ticks and strains of Lepus and Gerbillinae
F. tularensis biogroup novicida[b] (synonym: *F. novicida*)	First isolated from water in Utah in 1951 and later from human cases in USA
F. philomiragia[b] (synonym: *Yersinia philomiragia*)	First isolated in 1959 from a dying muskrat in Utah, USA. Type strain is ATCC 25015 other strains isolated from water and human cases

[a]Validly described by Olsufiev and Meshcheryakova (1983), who revised their previous nomenclature of these subspecies.

[b]Validly described by Hollis *et al.*(1989).

Fig. 1 Clinical presentations of human tularaemia caused by *F. tularensis* subsp. *tularensis* (type A, *nearctica*) and classification of clinical forms caused by subsp. *holarctica* (type B, *palaearctica*).

Clinical presentations subsp. *tularensis* (type A, *nearctica*)

American classification
Ulceroglandular
Pulmonary
Typhoidal (enteric or cryptogenic)
Oculoglandular

Classification of clinical forms, subsp. *holarctica* (type B, *palaearctica*)

Primary stage with primary complex
External
Ulcero-oculo-oral-tonsillar glandular forms

Generalized infection with septicaemia
Internal
Influenzal/pulmonary forms

Secondary generalization
Erythema nodosum
General glandular swelling
Multiple lung infiltrations
Abdominal organs
Central nervous system

ating them, he gave them to a woman aged 67 (case 2) and her husband, aged 64 (case 3), who skinned and froze the rabbits, from which *F. tularensis* was subsequently isolated. Two days after dressing the rabbits the young man became ill with an ulcerated hand lesion, axillary lymphadenopathy, and fever but no diagnosis was made at the time. On 23 November the two neighbours were admitted to hospital with sepsis and hand lesions. The woman was treated with gentamicin, cefazolin, and insulin for late-onset diabetes. After 3 days the treatment was changed to streptomycin. Despite these measures, disseminated intravascular coagulation, respiratory failure, and hypotension developed, and she died 7 days after admission. Tularaemia was diagnosed by serology in all three cases. Case 1 had an antibody titre of 1280 on 29 November; case 2 had an eight-fold rise in titre to 1:160 and case 3 had a titre of 1:320 on 3 December rising to 1280 after 14 days.

Oculoglandular tularaemia

Oculoglandular tularaemia presents with the primary lesion in the conjunctiva or cornea, accompanied by conjunctivitis with congestion, oedema, and a characteristic unilateral preauricular lymphadenopathy. This uncommon form of tularaemia is usually associated with a history of splashing the face while cleaning infected animals, swimming in contaminated water, or from laboratory accidents.

Case 4: oculoglandular tularaemia in the United States

A 9½-year-old American boy presented to a local hospital with a weeping right eye, right facial swelling and tenderness, and a low-grade fever. Therapy was begun with intravenous oxacillin and topical gentamicin. On the third hospital day his temperature was 40 °C and he was transferred to another hospital where a copious exudate from the right conjunctiva and a 5-mm bulbar conjunctival ulcer were noted. The preauricular and submandibular lymph nodes were large, tender, and oedematous. Slit-lamp examination of the right eye revealed multiple, yellow nodules with shallow necrotic ulcers on both the upper and lower conjunctivae. The white blood-cell count was 7300/mm^3, (72 per cent neutrophils, 20 per cent lymphocytes, and 8 per cent monocytes). Specimens from the conjunctivae and preauricular node yielded a pure culture of *F. tularensis*. The agglutination titre against *F. tularensis* showed a rise from less than 1:20 on the fifth day of illness to 1:80 by the third week. The patient was afebrile within 24 h of starting therapy with intravenous chloramphenicol and gentamicin. The swelling and lymph node tenderness had regressed by the end of his 10-day course of therapy.

Pulmonary tularaemia

Pulmonary disease results from the inhalation of infected aerosols. The LD_{50} of some strains of *F. tularensis* by this route is one bacterium. In the pulmonary form there are multiple areas of lung consolidation that tend to coalesce, sometimes with hilar lymphadenopathy. This form is often clinically severe, with marked toxaemia, but sometimes there is extensive lung consolidation with few symptoms.

Case 5: pulmonary tularaemia acquired in the United States during 1982

On 31 December a 50-year-old, previously healthy man was admitted to a hospital with a 2-week history of fever, chills, and productive cough. On admission, he had bilateral pneumonia with a white blood-cell count of 28 400, and therapy was begun with ampicillin. His condition worsened, with respiratory failure requiring mechanical ventilation and acute renal failure necessitating dialysis. The patient's wife said he had skinned a rabbit 1 week before onset of symptoms. Gentamicin was begun on 2 January. Although blood cultures and the lung biopsy were subsequently reported positive for *F. tularensis,* the diagnosis was initially confirmed by a fourfold rise in *F. tularensis* titres from 1:8 to 1 in 32 between the third and eleventh days of admission. The agglutination titre subsequently rose to 1:16 000 on 18 January. The patient eventually recovered normal renal and respiratory function.

Abdominal tularaemia (typhoidal, cryptogenic)

Abdominal tularaemia presents with a variety of symptoms and signs, sometimes with severe toxaemia whose appearances suggest septicaemia and apparent endotoxic shock, either with signs referable to the abdomen or on occasion without any signs. Typhoidal tularaemia is seen in people who have eaten improperly cooked, infected meat, drunk contaminated water, or in laboratory workers.

Case 6: typhoidal tularaemia—laboratory-acquired infection in the United States in 1958

A 43-year-old black man was admitted with a 5-day history of severe sweats, fever, sore throat, productive cough, nausea, vomiting, fatigue, weakness, and retrobulbar pain. Dyspnoea, blood-tinged sputum, and moderate diarrhoea were present, with an oral temperature ranging between 104 ° and 106 °F. There was moderate oedema of the nasal mucosa and diffuse hyperaemia of the pharynx. Examination of the chest revealed dullness to percussion, crepitant râles, and a pleural friction rub over the upper two-thirds of the left side, but the right side was clear. The chest film revealed a diffuse, mottled infiltrate in the upper lobe of the left lung, a left hilar prominence, and an early, reticulated infiltrate in the right cardiophrenic angle. The abdomen was normal. The patient was treated with tetracycline orally (1 g loading dose followed by 0.5 g every 6 h) but whilst the temperature fell from 106 °F in the next 24 h the respiratory rate rose to 60 with accompanying cyanosis and a tracheal rattle. Chest films on the seventh day of illness revealed multiple, 0.5-cm lesions throughout the right and left lung fields. Oxytetracycline (1.5 g daily) was given intravenously for the next 5 days, with intravenous fluids, oxygen, intermittent nebulization of a bronchodilator, and intravenous aminophylline in an attempt to decrease the respiratory distress. Despite control of the fever and absence of vascular collapse, the patient's condition remained critical. A tracheotomy was done on the fourth hospital day to reduce dead air space and to permit more direct aspiration and intermittent removal of the thick, tenacious, yellow, bloody secretions. On the eighth day, paraldehyde was needed to control delirium. Within the next 48 h the patient improved and oral administration of tetracycline, 3 g/day, continued for the remainder of a 21-day course of therapy. By the thirteenth hospital day the patient was afebrile and the respiratory rate was normal. The patient recovered after a 2-month illness. Streptomycin-resistant *F. tularensis* was isolated from the sputum, blood culture, and gastric and pharyngeal washings. The agglutinin titre increased from 1:150 during the second week of illness to 1:1280 and 1:2560 by the third and fourth weeks.

CLINICAL INFECTIONS WITH *F. TULARENSIS* SUBSP. *HOLARCTICA* (TYPE B)

The organisms causing tularaemia in Asia and Europe appear to have the same characteristics as the less virulent American subsp. *holarctica* bacteria such as caused an outbreak of 72 cases in Vermont in 1968. The clinical types of tularaemia resulting from infections with subsp. *holarctica* (see Table 2) need to be distinguished from the classical American tuleraemia and may be differentiated in terms of localization and lesser severity by the system introduced in the former USSR, which distinguishes primary and internal complexes from secondary spread of infection. Clinicians in Western Europe have continued to classify European cases using the American system, but the Eastern European approach is more informative.

Ulcero-cutano-oculo-oral-tonsillar glandular forms

Ulceroglandular tularaemia presents in European acquired cases with either induration or an ulcer at the site of a mosquito bite or single or multiple lesions (Plate 1) after skinning an infected area. The lymphadenopathy (Plate 2) in the drainage area of the primary ulcer or indurated area will be accompanied by the sudden onset of chills, fever, and, frequently, a severe headache. Later in the course of ulceroglandular disease hyposensitivity reactions, such as erythema nodosum, may develop (Plate 3).

Case 7: ulcero-cutanoglandular tularaemia in Norway in 1934

A 57-year-old man, whilst fishing in northern Norway during August 1934, was bitten on his neck by mosquitoes. The area became very swollen and irritated. The patient had not been in contact with hares or other rodents. The patient felt unwell on 20 August, but had no localized pain until the evening, when his throat became painful, and he had an axillary temperature of 38.5 °C. The following day the doctor found very tender glands on both sides of the neck. Later, on 21 August, the patient became semiconscious and had a severe headache and fever above 39 °C.

Between 25 August and 15 September an egg-sized, glandular abscess developed on the right side of his neck. On 15 September it was incised. The patient was discharged from the hospital fully recovered after an illness lasting 6 weeks. A sample of the pus from the abscess appeared to be sterile. The pus was inoculated into a guinea-pig, which died 3 weeks later. A second guinea-pig was inoculated from the first and died after 8 days. A small, Gram-negative rod isolated from the second guinea-pig was agglutinated by tularaemia serum (from an epidemic in Prague) to a dilution of 1 in 1280. Mosquito-borne tularaemia was the most common source of reported infections in North Sweden in the 1970s.

Case 8: oral-tonsillar tularaemia—Norway 1970 (Plate 4)

A 62-year-old farmer felt ill on 20 March with high fever and difficulties in swallowing because of swelling in the throat. One week later he developed an elongated, very tender swelling on the left side of the neck. On 3 April he was admitted to hospital with an axillary temperature of 38.5 °C, a white blood-cell count of 7200, and an erythrocyte sedimentation rate of 84 mm. On examination he had a lingual tonsillitis with necrosis of the lymphoid tissue at the base of the tongue. Anterior to

Table 2 *Comparison of contact and airborne outbreaks of tularaemia*

Symptoms and signs	Contact outbreak No. cases	%	Airborne outbreak No. cases	%
Fever	38	97	343	85
Ulceration (cutaneous)	29	74		
Lymphadenitis	31	79	65	16
Chills	23	59	285	70
Myalgia	22	56		
Malaise	20	51	179	44
Diapheresis	11	28		
Headache	9	23	230	57
Nausea and/or vomiting	3	8	73	18
Fatigue			350	86
Exanthem			142	35
Sore throat			129	32
Chest pain (pleuritic)	2	5		
Cough (non-productive)	2	5		
Infected ulcers/oral ulcers			81	20
Conjunctivitis			107	26
Muscle/joint pains			136	34
Symptoms of pneumonia			46	11

[a]Young *et al.* (1969): Vermont epidemic in 1968 of 39 symptomatic cases.

[b]Dahlstrand *et al.* (1971): Jamtland epidemic between 1966–67 of 405 serologically verified cases.

the left sternomastoid there was a 12 × 6 cm swelling that was very tender. He was treated with penicillin and erythromycin after a throat swab produced pneumococci and staphylococci. There was a rapid improvement in the throat but the neck tumour increased in size. The tularaemia agglutination test was 1:2000. He was treated with tetracycline but had a long drawn-out illness, with persistent neck swelling 2 months later.

Generalized tularaemia

Case 9: tularaemia with septicaemia

A 79-year-old woman who lived 200 miles north of Stockholm was admitted to hospital having become acutely ill with headache, vertigo, prostration, and fever. On examination, her temperature was 38.5 °C, there was no lymphadenopathy, and no ulcerated skin lesions. Her white blood-cell count was 8800/mm^3 and her erythrocyte sedimentation rate 35 mm. A chest radiograph on the day of admission was normal. Five days later, however, a right dorsal infiltrate was seen. During the first five hospital days her temperature varied between 39 and 40 °C, and she suffered from malaise, backache, and vomiting. *F. tularensis* subsp. *holarctica* was isolated from two blood cultures. Gentamicin therapy was instituted on the seventh day of admission. Thereafter, the temperature slowly returned to normal and the patient was discharged 2 weeks later. Follow-up 5 weeks after discharge showed remission. There was a rise in the titre of agglutinating antibodies against *F. tularensis* from less than 1:40 on the third day of illness to 1:320 2 months later.

Case 10: travel-associated tularaemia diagnosed May 1971, Berkshire, England

A 68-year-old English man, after walking in the Allegehny mountains on 1 and 2 May, removed a flat, hard tick about 3 mm in diameter from his right buttock. The next afternoon he felt unwell and by evening had a temperature of 38.3 °C. On 4 May he noticed a swelling in the right groin. He felt better after a 3-day course of antibiotics, but on 11 May he relapsed, and 2 days later, in Canada, a doctor found a small (15 mm) ulcer on the right buttock and a plum-sized swelling in the groin. After treatment with tetracycline, 1.5 g daily for 4 days, and bacitracin ointment, the ulcer began to heal but the swelling in the groin increased. The patient returned to England but still felt unwell. The buttock ulcer had a hard, red edge, and the gland in the right groin persisted. He was given tetracycline-nystatin for 5 weeks. The patient's general condition improved slowly, but the inguinal swelling began to fluctuate; by 8 June it had started to discharge so it was evacuated and the surrounding tissues infiltrated with chloramphenicol. By 23 July the cavity had healed completely and thereafter the patient remained well. Blood samples taken on 26 May and 4 June showed titres of 1:640 and 1:5120, respectively. Fluorescent antibody tests indicated the presence of *F. tularensis* antigen.

CLINICAL PRESENTATION OF *F. TULARENSIS* BIOGROUP NOVICIDA INFECTIONS

Infections with *F. tularensis* biogroup novicida strains are rare but tularaemia-like illnesses have been described.

Case 11: ulceroglandular presentation in North America

A 26-year-old man from Louisiana presented with a 3-week history of a tender, enlarging lump on the left side of his neck. He had no underlying diseases. Physical examination revealed a large lymph node on the left side of his neck. A biopsy of the lymph node showed necrotizing granulomas, and a *F. 'novicida'*-like bacterium was grown from the tissue. The patient was given a 2-week course of tetracycline after excision of the lymph node and made an uneventful recovery.

Case 12: septicaemia in a patient with presenting illness

A 52-year-old man with a history of alcoholism and chronic peptic ulcer disease was admitted to hospital after 3 days of dizziness, nausea, vomiting, and fever (39.7 °C). Six blood cultures collected from different sites over a 24-h period grew an *F. 'novicida'*-like bacterium. The patient was begun on intravenous cefoxitin and the fever subsided over 3 days. He was discharged after 6 days in a fair condition.

CLINICAL PRESENTATIONS OF *F. PHILOMIRAGIA* INFECTIONS

The first isolations of *F. philomiragia* were from a moribund muskrat and from water samples in Utah. In a report of 14 patients between 1974 and 1986 with *F. philomiragia* infection, 13 of them came from scattered locations in the United States and one from Switzerland, and all but one had pre-existing illnesses. The organism had been isolated from the blood of nine patients, from the lung or pleura of three, and from the peritoneum and the meninges in single cases. The 13 patients for whom records were available had fever, and in five there was evidence of pneumonia. Five cases had chronic granulomatous disease, two had myeloproliferative disorders, and one had recurrent pleural effusions. Five other patients had recently suffered from a near-drowning incident in sea or estuarine water (*F. philomiragia* is a halophile). All of the organisms tested formed β-lactamase and were ampicillin resistant; all were sensitive to quinolones, aminoglycosides, chloramphenicol, and cefoxitin.

Clinical diagnosis

In a known endemic region for *F. tularensis,* a provisional diagnosis can often be made on clinical evidence supported by information about the patient's possible exposure, occupation, and recent activities, particularly when a primary lesion is present. When there is no local ulcer, and if the patient has left the area in which the infection was acquired, the illness presents simply as a persistent and debilitating case of 'fever', pneumonitis or tonsillitis in which a detailed travel and epidemiological history and laboratory investigations are essential for diagnosis (see Table 3).

CHEMOTHERAPY

Aminoglycosides are bactericidal for *F. tularensis* and should be used for the treatment of subsp. *tularensis* (type A) and severe infections with subsp. *holarctica* (type B). Streptomycin is generally considered to be the drug of choice by many physicians experienced in treating tularaemia, and usually produces a dramatic clinical response. Chloramphenicol and tetracycline are less effective in patients with systemic infection. The organism survives intracellularly and may give rise to a protracted and relapsing illness, which requires treatment for at least 7 to 14 days and frequently 1 to 2 months. Tetracyclines are adequate for mild infections with subsp. *holarctica* if given in an oral dose of 2 g/day for 2 weeks. Oral tetracycline may be used for chemoprophylaxis.

Table 3 *Detection and typing methods for* F. tularensis

Method
A. *Evidence of antigen*
Isolation of organism:[a]
1. Direct culture on glucose cysteine blood agar (GCBA)
(a) Peptone cysteine agar
(b) Tryptose broth medium
(c) Animal inoculation[b]
(i) guinea-pigs
(ii) infant white mice
(iii) adult white mice
2. Fluorescent antibody detection of antigen
B. Evidence of antibody
1. Agglutination reactions:
(a) Rapid slide microagglutination
(b) Microagglutination test (MAT)
(c) Tube agglutination
(d) Microtitre plate agglutination
2. Haemagglutination inhibition
3. Gel diffusion
4. ELISA:
(a) Using lipopolysaccharide
(b) Using sonicated extract
5. Radiometric assay
6. Monoclonal antibody
C. *Evidence of delayed hypersensitivity*
1. Intradermal skin test
2. Lymphocyte stimulation
3. Interleukin-2 production
D. *Genomic methods*
1. 16*s* RNA hybridization

[a]Refer samples to laboratory handling dangerous pathogens if *F. tularensis* subsp. *tularensis* (type A) is suspected. Refer to a reference of special pathogen laboratory if subsp. *holarctica* (type B).

[b]Seek advice of a reference facility before requesting laboratory confirmation by animal inoculation.

DETECTING THE CAUSATIVE ORGANISM

Attempts should be made to isolate *F. tularensis* only in laboratories with safety cabinets approved for working with dangerous pathogens. Swabs or aspirates from local lesions and lymph glands should be transported in approved containers. Strains of *F. tularensis* may grow slowly on primary culture and may only be isolated by subcutaneous injection of material into white mice. Attempts to isolate subsp. *tularensis* strains (type A) should be made only when suitable containment facilities are available and laboratory staff are aware of the possible diagnosis and of the hazards of handling the organism. These risks may be reduced by using an immunofluorescence method to identify organisms in tissue smears.

MORPHOLOGY

Strains from the different subspecies of *F. tularensis* are morphologically indistinguishable. *In vivo,* the organism occurs as tiny coccobacilli (0.2–0.7 μm) surrounded by a capsule. Older cultures are frequently pleomorphic, with ovoid, bacillary, bean-shaped, dumb-bell, and filamentous forms occurring. The organism is Gram-negative, non-motile, and does not form spores (Fig. 2).

ISOLATION AND CULTURAL CHARACTERS

F. tularensis colonies on glucose cysteine blood agar are 1 to 3 mm in diameter after 48 to 72 h, greyish, and usually viscous with a greenish discoloration of the surrounding medium. Colonial characteristics may differ markedly on other media. The optimum temperature for growth is 37 °C. Carbon dioxide is beneficial for growth but the organism will not grow under full anaerobic conditions. *F. tularensis* is cytotrophic and grows well in the developing chick embryo, in which it causes death in 3 to 4 days when inoculated on to the chorioallantoic membrane. Animal passage is the optimal method for isolation of wild strains. Subcutaneous inoculation of strains of subsp. *tularensis* into the guinea-pig leads to death in 5 to 8 days. Subscapular injection into white mice is the preferred method for the isolation of subsp. *holarctica* (type B).

BIOCHEMICAL PROPERTIES AND SERODIAGNOSIS

F. tularensis gives a weak catalase reaction and, under optimal conditions, forms acid but no gas in glucose and usually in maltose, mannose and laevulose, but not in sucrose. Its oxidase reaction is negative but it forms H_2S. Differentiation between the *tularensis* and *holarctica* subspp. relies on the ability of the former to ferment glycerol and a positive citrulline ureidase test.

The organism is killed by exposure to 0.1 per cent formaldehyde for 10 min, and to moist heat at 55 °C for 10 min. *F. tularensis* strains are indistinguishable by agglutination, haemagglutination, and immunofluescence tests. Subspp. *tularensis* and *holarctica* cannot be distinguished by agglutination tests. A fourfold rise in titre or a titre of 1:320 in a single sample by the end of the third week of illness are diagnostic of tularaemia. Antibody may persist for years after infection. Enzyme-linked immunosorbent assay techniques are available for the early detection of tularaemia, with the advantage that class-specific immunoglobulins can be detected. Delayed hypersensitivity can be detected by means of an intradermal test (Table 3). This is a sensitive method of diagnosis but has the disadvantage of interfering with subsequent *in vitro* tests.

Epidemiology

GEOGRAPHICAL DISTRIBUTION AND INCIDENCE

The distribution of foci of *F. tularensis* throughout the Northern Hemisphere is shown in Fig. 3. The distribution of tularaemia foci in Europe is shown in Fig. 4. The geographical variations in incidence of the disease is poorly documented because of highly variable ascertainment. A peak occurred between the two World Wars but incidence rates have fallen since the recognition of occupational hazards and the development of effective vaccines. It is reported that, in the former USSR, mass vaccination reduced the number of reported cases from 100 000 of subsp. *holarctica* per year between 1926 and 1942 to a few hundred per year at the present time. The year of peak incidence in North America was 1939, with 2291 cases giving a rate of 17.5/1 million population. This had fallen to 291 cases in 1984 (1–2/million).

ECOLOGY

Subsp. *tularensis* in the United States is carried by ground squirrels, cotton-tail rabbits, hares and jack-rabbits, and it can be found from time to time in other wild and domestic animals. Human infections are in the main sporadic and occur in two seasonal peaks, one in the summer, associated with tick bites, and the other in the winter attributed to hunting, mainly of rabbits. Various ticks of the genera Dermacentor, Amblyomma, Haemaphysalis, and Ixodes transmit the organism. Infections have also been attributed to dog ticks and contact with sick dogs. Human

Fig. 2 Electron micrograph of *F. tularensis* subsp. *holarctica.*

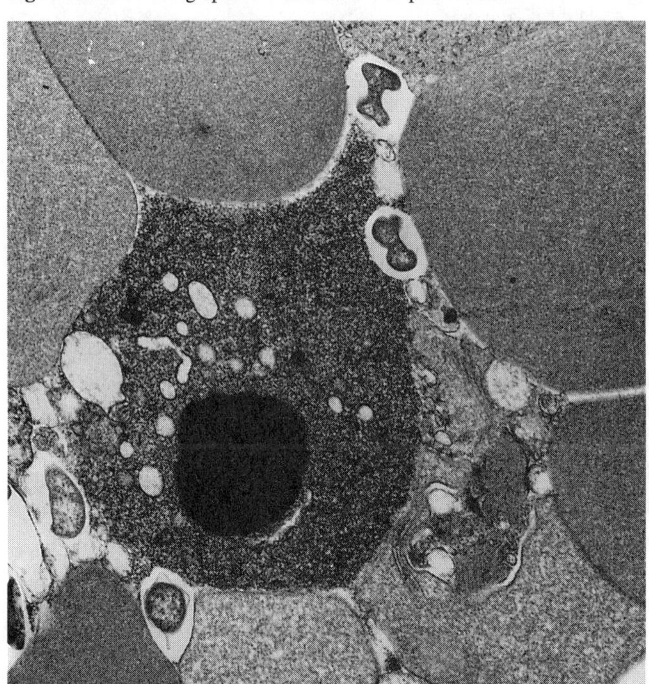

Fig. 4 Tularaemia foci in Europe.

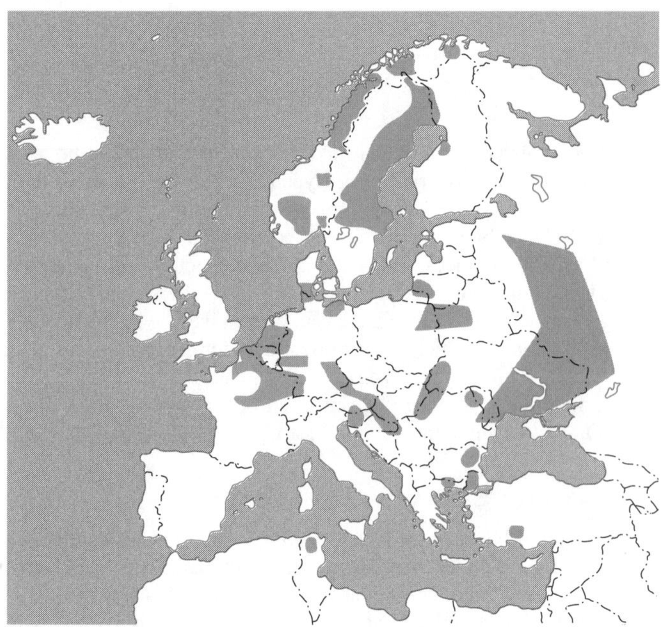

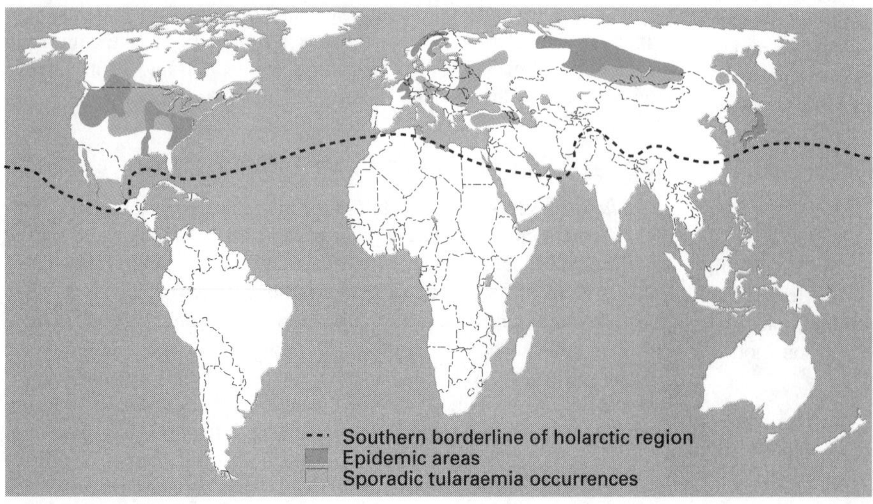

Fig. 3 Tularaemia foci around the world.

infection with subsp. *holarctica* (type B) has been much less frequently described in the United States. Strains of this type have been isolated from muskrats, in which they cause epizootics.

In the republics of the former USSR, subsp. *holarctica* strains are harboured in a wide variety of ecological situations: in meadow, steppe, forest, swamp, foothills and taiga, and in a variety of mammals, mainly rodents, including mice, voles, water-rats, muskrats, and gerbils, as well as hares. The main tick vectors are of the genera Dermacentor, Ixodes, and Rhipicephalus. The susceptibility and sensitivity of animals have been used to categorize subsp. *holarctica* into three groups: rodents and hares are the most susceptible; cats and dogs are moderately susceptible, while primates and cattle are relatively resistant but nevertheless develop an immune response. Human infection occurs under a variety of circumstances, largely depending upon the nature of the contact—residential or occupational—within the endemic focus. In the former USSR, four epidemic types are recognized: type I contact epidemics, resulting from touching infected animals, for example, by hunters and butchers; type II epidemics spread by the bites of arthropods, ticks, and mosquitoes; type III outbreaks are water or foodborne—water is usually contaminated by the dead bodies or excreta of infected animals (subsp. *holarctica* can survive in water at 4 °C for at least 5 months); and type IV outbreaks, resulting from airborne dissemination of infection acquired by the inhalation of contaminated particles, such as dust from rodent-infested hay. Similar conditions have been described in adjacent parts of Europe; in Norway, infections have been attributed to lemmings and hares, in Sweden to hares and voles, and in Germany and south-eastern Europe to field mice. In contrast to the United States, epidemics of tularaemia are well recognized in tularaemia foci.

PREVENTION

The main objective is to reduce, as much as possible, human contact with the species of animals, their ectoparasites, and the arthropods known to be the principal vectors in endemic areas. Public-health physicians need to assess the risk and give appropriate advice. Immunization may be considered when contact with potentially infected material is inevitable. Since the Second World War, preventive measures in endemic areas have been based on the dual processes of education, and vaccination for selected high-risk groups. Live, attenuated strains of subsp. *holarctica* have been used extensively as vaccines since the 1940s and have been shown to be effective. The preferred method of vaccination at that time was by the inhalation of dried viable vaccine. Subsequently, an attenuated strain of *F. tularensis* (live vaccine strain, **LVS**) was selected for study in the United States. It was shown to be superior to a killed vaccine in immunizing humans and in experimental animals. Exposure of human volunteers to LVS vaccine by inhalation led at most to a mild, self-limiting illness, as demonstrated by subsequent airborne challenge with a virulent strain of *F. tularensis,* indicating a substantial though not total immunity. The routine use of LVS vaccine in laboratory workers who regularly handle *F. tularensis* led to a reduction in the number of laboratory-acquired tularaemia infections but cases still occurred. An extensive literature exists about the detection, prevention, and cure of infections with *F. tularensis* in the event of its use as an agent for biological warfare.

It is important for clinicians to inform the laboratory if they suspect specimens for isolation of *F. tularensis* subsp. *tularensis* (type A) as laboratory aerosols cause serious and occasionally fatal laboratory acquired infection. Untreated subsp. *tularensis* infection presenting as pulmonary or abdominal tularaemia has a high mortality.

REFERENCES

Anthony, L.S.D., Burke, R.D., and Nano, F.E. (1991). Growth of *Francisella* spp. in rodent macrophages. *Infection and Immunity,* **59,** 3291–6.

Behan, K.A. and Klein, G.C. (1982). Reduction of *Brucella* species and *Francisella tularensis* cross-reacting agglutinins by dithiothreitol. *Journal of Clinical Microbiology,* **16,** 756–7.

Buchanan, T.M., Brooks, G.F., and Brachman, P.S. (1971). The tularemia skin test. 325 skin tests in 210 persons: serologic correlation and review of the literature. *Annals of Internal Medicine,* **74,** 336–43.

Burke, D.S. (1977). Immunization against tularaemia: analysis of the effectiveness of live *Francisella tularensis* vaccine in prevention of laboratory-acquired tularemia. *Journal of Infectious Diseases,* **135,** 55–60.

Canonico, P.G., McManus, A.T., Mangiafico, J.A., Sammons, L.S., McGann, V.G., and Dangerfield, H.G. (1975). Temporal appearance of opsonizing antibody to *Francisella tularensis:* detection by a radiometabolic assay. *Infection and Immunity,* **11,** 466–9.

Dahlstrand, S., Ringertz, O., and Zetterberg, B. (1971). Airborne tularemia in Sweden. *Scandinavian Journal of Infectious Diseases,* **3,** 7–16.

Eigelsbach, H.T. and McGann, V.G. (1984). Gram-negative aerobic cocci. In *Bergey's manual of systematic bacteriology,* Vol. 1, (ed. N.R. Krieg and J.G. Holt), pp. 394–9. Williams & Wilkins, Baltimore.

Forsman, M., Juoppa, K., Sjostedt, A., and Tarnvik, A. (1990). Use of RNA hybridization in the diagnosis of a case of ulceroglandular tularemia. *European Journal of Clinical Microbiology and Infectious Diseases,* **9,** 784–5.

Fulop, M.J., Webber, T., Manchee, R.J., and Kelly, D.C. (1991). Production and characterization of monoclonal antibodies directed against the lipopolysaccharide of *Francisella tularensis. Journal of Clinical Microbiology,* **29,** 1407–12.

Hollis, D.G., Weaver, R.E., Steigerwalt, A.G., Wenger, J.D., Moss, C.W., and Brenner, D.J. (1989). *Francisella philomiragia* comb. nov. (formerly *Yersinia philomiragia*) and *Francisella tularensis* biogroup novicida (formerly *Francisella novicida*) associated with human disease. *Journal of Clinical Microbiology,* **27,** 1601–8.

Hopla, C.E. (1974). The ecology of tularemia. *Advances in Veterinary Science,* **18,** 25–53.

Ito, M., Nishiyama, K., Hyodo, S., Shigeta, S., and Ito, T. (1985). Weight reduction of thymus and depletion of lymphocytes of T-dependent areas in peripheral lymphoid tissues of mice infected with *Francisella tularensis. Infection and Immunity,* **49,** 812–18.

Jusatz, H.J. (1960). The geographical distribution of tularemia throughout the world, 1911–1959. In *World atlas of infectious disease,* Pt. III, (ed. E. Rodenwaldt), pp. 1–12. Falk-Verlag, Hamburg.

Osulfiev, N.G. (1958). *Problems of epidemiology and prophylaxis of tularaemia.* Medgiz, Moscow.

Osulfiev, N.G. and Meshcheryakova, I.S. (1983). Subspecific taxonomy of *Francisella tularensis* McCoy and Chapin 1912. *International Journal of Systematic Bacteriology,* **33,** 872–4.

Overholt, E.L. *et al.* (1961). Analysis of 42 cases of laboratory acquired tularemia. Treatment with broad spectrum antibiotics. *American Journal of Medicine,* **30,** 785–806.

Pollitzer, R. (1967). *History and incidence of tularemia in the Soviet Union. A review.* Institute of Contemporary Russian Studies, Fordham University, New York.

Ringertz, O. and Dahlstrand, S. (1968). Culture of *P. tularensis* in the 1966–67 outbreaks of tularemia in Sweden. Laboratory methods and precautions against laboratory infections. *Acta Pathologica et Microbiologica Scandinavica,* **72,** 464.

Saslaw, S., Eigelsbach, H.T., Wilson, H.R., Prior, J.A., and Carhart, S. (1961). Tularemia vaccine study. II. Respiratory challenge. *Archives of Internal Medicine,* **107,** 702–14.

Sawyer, W.D. and Dangerfield, H.G. (1966). Antibiotic prophylaxis and therapy of airborne tularemia. *Bacteriological Reviews,* **30,** 542–50.

Viljanen, M.K., Nurmi, T., and Salminen, A. (1983). Enzyme-linked immunosorbent assay (ELISA) with bacterial sonicate antigen for IgM, and IgG antibodies to *Francisella tularensis:* comparison with bacterial agglutination test and ELISA with lipopolysaccharide antigen. *Journal of Infectious Diseases,* **148,** 715–20.

Young, L.S. *et al.* (1969). Tularemia epidemic, Vermont 1968: 47 cases linked to contact with muskrats. *New England Journal of Medicine,* **280,** 1253–60.

Zuerlein, J. and Smith, P.W. (1985). Diagnostic utility of the sterile agglutinin tests. *Journal of the American Medical Association,* **254,** 1211–14.

7.11.17(b) Pasteurellosis

A. D. PEARSON

Definition

Pasteurellosis in man is a spectrum of disease, caused principally by *Pasteurella multocida,* which ranges from localized, infected cat or dog bites, abscesses, cellulitis, lymphadenopathy and osteomyelitis to systemic infection with septicaemia, septic arthritis, and respiratory and central nervous involvement. Asymptomatic carriage and overt infection with *Pasteurella* spp. are common occurrences in animals but are less frequently recognized as a cause of zoonotic human disease. The genus *Pasteurella* formerly comprised 20 taxa, of which 10 were known to be associated with human disease, but five of the 10 species found in man are no longer classified as members of the Pasteurella group (Table 1). Textbook accounts of pasteurellosis continue to describe human infections in association with the previously recognized species *P. ureae, P. pneumotropica,* and *P. aerogenes.* The first two of these are more closely related to the Actinobacillus group. This account of pasteurellosis summarizes the diagnostic and clinical literature relevant to human infections with *P. multocida* subsp. *multocida* and subsp. *septica,* and lists the association of human disease with *P. canis, P. dagmatis,* and *P. bettyae* (Table 1).

Epidemiology

P. multocida is both common and widely distributed in animals and birds, and should therefore always be considered when treating animal bites and in the differential diagnosis of a wide variety of clinical conditions, several of which are potentially fatal. It is a commensal of domestic and wild animals and some avian species, yet is capable of causing serious epizootic infection. Reported isolation rates from the nose, oral cavity, and throat are between 7 and 90 per cent in cats, 50 to 70 per cent in dogs, and 51 per cent in pigs. The organism has also been isolated from rodents, rabbits, cattle, sheep and horses, and a variety of zoo animals ranging from lions, panthers, lynx, and cougars to buffalos and monkeys. *P. multocida* causes snuffles in rabbits (a source of human infection in animal-house staff), avian cholera in waterfowl, pneumonia in sheep and goats, and shipping fever in cattle, which is a haemorrhagic septicaemia following a primary infection with myxovirus. It is in laboratory colonies of rabbits, or in cattle during shipping, that epizootics occur; these can be a serious cause of illness and death in animals, and may lead to occupational contact with human colonization or overt infection.

P. multocida is transmitted to man by direct contact, usually by cat or dog bites, and less commonly by the airborne route, which results in colonization of the upper respiratory tract, occasionally leads to chest infection or, rarely, to secondary invasive disease. The bacteria can remain viable in soil and water for up to a month and persist for 1 to 3 months in dead carcasses. Non-culturable but viable forms have not been reported but if they exist would prolong infectivity of environmental sources. Surveillance in the United Kingdom under-reports pasteurellosis, with laboratory isolations listed by the Communicable Disease Surveillance Centre varying from 118 in 1971 to 387 in 1986 and 262 in 1992. Animal bites account for 1 per cent of Accident and Emergency consultations in North America and so represent an important public-health problem. Of these bites, 1 in 10 requires stitching and 1 to 2 per cent of those bitten are admitted to hospital. The reported morbidity in North America due to pasteurella infection is 6.7/100 million population per year. Cat bites and scratches (and, rarely, just contact in patients with human immunodeficiency virus infection) are more likely to become infected than dog bites but account for only 5 to 15 per cent of those who present in casualty with wounds caused by animals. Almost all the other bites reported in North America (75–90 per cent) are due to dogs. The infection rate from penetrating dog bites varies from 2 to 29 per cent (usually 5–15 per cent).

Human infection has resulted from the bites of wild cougars and wolves, and from caged or penned animals of an immense variety from rabbits to lions and rats to pigs. Infection in man has also been reported from a variety of less obvious animal exposures, including being kicked by a horse and clearing out turkeys. There is a single report of an outbreak involving seven debilitated patients in a hospital. This outbreak was of interest because it involved just 7 of 143 patients on two wards during a 6-month period, with an overall attack rate of 4.9 per cent. The results of a detailed epidemiological investigation, together with microbiological typing of *P. multocida* strains, suggested that the possible source was a cat belonging to a therapist and that transmission might be by hand contact or via clothing. No further cases occurred after the resignation of the therapist. No other such outbreaks have been reported in the literature and there are no reports of case-to-case spread.

Clinical features

WOUNDS AND SOFT TISSUE INFECTIONS AFTER ANIMAL BITES

Wound infections from cat and dog bites are the main cause of pasteurellosis and, while culture of such wounds yields a variety of bacterial species (2.8–3.6 bacterial species per wound), *P. multocida* is isolated from up to 25 per cent of infected dog bites and in most cases does not cause serious local inflammation. A small proportion of patients with *P. multocida*-infected bites progress, sometimes rapidly, to a severe infection with cellulitis and bone necrosis, some cases having a protracted course despite appropriate intensive antibiotic therapy. When symptoms develop, in about 50 per cent of cases they appear within a day of being bitten: there is a local reddening of the site with throbbing pain; a third of patients have a purulent discharge, 15–20 per cent cellulitis, and 10 per cent develop regional lymphadenopathy. The complications of local infections are listed in Table 2. Occasionally, pasteurellosis from an animal bite can be fatal in a patient with underlying disease.

Case 1: cellulitis

A 54-year-old man was bitten by a cat on his forearm and was treated 9 h later with tetanus toxoid and with flucloxacillin, 250 mg four times a day. The patient was admitted to hospital in a collapsed state 40 h after having been bitten and died 2 h later despite treatment with 1.5 g cefuroxime and 1 g methyl prednisolone. Blood cultures yielded *P. multocida* resistant to flucloxacillin but susceptible to penicillin and cefuroxime. The patient had a history of ischaemic heart disease, non-insulin dependent diabetes mellitus, and a 13-year history of rheumatoid arthritis treated with steroids for that time. Autopsy examination revealed necrotizing cellulitis around the bite, with lung conjestion and alveolar haemorrhages. Both the soft tissue and lung sites contained Gram-negative coccobacilli.

Five of fifteen reported deaths from pasteurellosis followed bites or scratches by animals. This underlines the importance of treating patients with animal bites or scratches with appropriate antibiotics as soon as possible after the injury has been sustained.

ORAL AND RESPIRATORY INFECTION

P. multocida has been isolated from patients with tonsillitis, otitis media, sinusitis, and pneumonia but the pathogenic significance is unclear because most of these patients also suffered from chronic bronchitis or bronchiectasis (Table 2). In these cases, there may be long-term colonization of the respiratory tract.

Table 1 *Designation of pathogens from Pasteurella*

Subspecies and synonyms	Distribution
P. aerogenes[a]	Found in human infections following pig bites
P. anatis	Found in the intestinal tract of ducks
P. avium	Hearts and infraorbital sinuses of chickens; lungs from calves with pneumonia
P. bettyae (*'P. bettii'*)	Bartholin gland abscesses and finger infections in man
P. canis	Oral cavities of dogs and bites in man
P. dagmatis (*P. pneumotropica* type Henriksen; *Pasteurella* 'gas'; *Pasteurella* group I)	Isolated from dogs and cats Found in human local and systemic infections resulting from animal bites
P. gallinarum	Found in chickens
P. haemolytica[a] (*P. haemolytica* type A)	Cattle, farm and domestic animals
P. langaa	Found in respiratory tracts of healthy chickens
P. lymphangitidis (BL bacterium)	Lymphangitis in cattle in southern India
P. mairii	Abortion in sows, septic infections in piglets
P. multocida subsp. *gallicida*	Pathogenic for poultry
P. multocida subsp. *multocida*	Isolated from birds and most mammals Pathogenic in man, causing cutaneous infections and abscesses following bites or scratches from various animals
P. multocida subsp. *septica (P. septica)*	Causes septic infections in animals and man
P. pneumotropica biotypes Jawetz/Heyl[a]	Laboratory animals and dogs, and bites in man
P. stomatis	Found in the respiratory tracts of cats and dogs
P. testudinis[a]	Found only in tortoises
P. trehalosi (*P. haemolytica* type T)	Associated with septicaemia in older lambs
P. ureae[a]	Human respiratory tract and meningitis
P. volantium	Found in the wattles of domestic poultry

[a]No longer considered to be members of genus Pasteurella (Mutters *et al.* 1985).

Table 2 *Infections caused by Pasteurella multocida:* presentations and complications

Skin and soft tissue infections
Cellulitis; subcutaneous abscess; infected decubitus or stasis ulcer; wound infection
Oral and respiratory infections
Tonsillitis or peritonsillar abscess; sinusitis, pharyngitis, epiglottitis; otitis media, mastoiditis and submandibular abscess; lung abscess; tracheobronchitis, pneumonia and empyema
Serious invasive infections
Cardiovascular:
Endocarditis; bacteraemia; mycotic aneurysm; purulent pericarditis; infected vascular graft
Bone and joint:
Septic arthritis; osteomyelitis; septic arthritis with osteomyelitis; bursitis; prosthetic joints
Central nervous system:
Meningitis; brain abscess; subdural empyema
Gastrointestinal tract:
Liver abscess; spontaneous bacterial peritonitis; omental or appendiceal abscess; peritonitis due to ruptured viscus; gastroenteritis
Genitourinary tract:
Cystitis or pyelonephritis; infected ileal loop and renal abscess; uterine infection; vaginitis, cervicitis; bartholin gland abscess; chorioamnionitis; epididymitis
Eyes:
Conjunctivitis; corneal ulcer; endophthalmitis

INVASIVE INFECTION

Meningitis, brain abscesses, septic arthritis (Table 2) pyelonephritis, endocarditis, and septicaemia may be caused by *P. multocida.*

Case 2: peritonitis

A 12-year-old boy was admitted with fever, abdominal pain, and vomiting of 24-h duration. Acute appendicitis with perforation was suspected. During appendectomy the surgeon unexpectedly found a nodose liver and an excess of pale to purulent ascitic fluid. Intravenous therapy with netilmicin and metronidazole was started during the operation and continued for 3 days. After the operation the patient developed jaundice and oozing of ascitic fluid from the abdominal wound. Culture of peritoneal fluid taken during surgery revealed *P. multocida,* which was also cultured three times from the oozing ascitic fluid after the operation. Therapy with penicillin was started and continued for 10 days, *P. multocida* no longer being isolated from the ascitic fluid 3 days after treatment with penicillin.

Biopsy of the liver showed cirrhosis and signs of acute active hepatitis, but tests for hepatitis A and B were negative. Questioning of the parents and the patient revealed that the patient had had symptoms compatible with liver disease for the last 6 months and had suffered from two attacks of pneumonia in the previous year. Recovery took 4 weeks before discharge from hospital; the patient remained with a newly discovered cirrhosis of unknown aetiology.

Case 3: meningitis

An 89-year-old woman presented with a 12-h history of headache and drowsiness. A neighbour's cat had bitten her calf 12 days earlier and she had developed cellulitis, which, after treatment with erythromycin (250 mg, three times a day), had resolved over the next 8 days. The woman had preorbital ecchymoses the day before admission. Focal neurological signs were absent and a CT scan of the head was normal. The patient was put on i.v. ceftazidime (2 g, three times a day) and i.v. ampicillin (2 g every 4 h) until culture of *P. multocida* at 36 h revealed an organism resistant to erythromycin and sensitive to penicillin. Peni-

Table 3 *Detection and typing methods for Pasteurella multocida*

Method
A. *Diagnosis and culture*
1. Isolation and identification
2. Selective medium
B. *Biotyping*
1. Staphylococcal hyaluronidase
2. Acriflavin
3. Biochemical
C. *Serotyping*
1. Capsular antigen haemagglutination
(a) Indirect passive (PHA)
(b) Counterimmunoelectrophoresis (CIE)
2. Somatic-antigen gel diffusion
3. ELISA
4. Classification
D. *Phage typing*
E. *Evidence of pathogenicity*
1. Mouse virulence
F. *Genome*
1. DNA probes for *tox*A gene
2. Ribotyping

cillin (2 million units 4-hourly) was given and within 24 h the patient was afebrile and had improved neurologically. Treatment was discontinued at day 17 when the lumbar puncture was normal. Isolates of *P. multocida* from the patient's cerebrospinal fluid and from the mouth of the cat were shown to be similar by serotyping and restriction enzyme analysis.

Diagnosis and treatment

The methods for isolation, characterization, and typing of *P. multocida* are summarized and referenced in Table 3. It is important to check the antimicrobial susceptibility of any isolates as the preceding case histories indicate that there may be an unsatisfactory outcome when erythromycin and flucloxacillin had been used to treat animal bites. Penicillin G, ampicillin, third-generation cephalosporins, carbenicillin, and tetracyline are active against *P. multocida.*

REFERENCES

Bisgaard, M. (1993). Ecology and significance of Pasteurellaceae in animals. *International Journal of Medical Microbiology, Virology, Parasitology and Infectious Diseases,* **279,** 7–26.

Chapple, C.R. and Fraser, A.N. (1986). *Pasteurella multocida* wound infections—a commonly unrecognized problem in the casualty department. *Injury,* **17,** 410–11.

Drabick, J.J. *et al.* (1993). *Pasteurella multocida* pneumonia in a man with AIDS and nontraumatic feline exposure. *Chest,* **103,** 7–11.

Frederiksen, W. (1993). Ecology and significance of Pasteurellaceae in man—an update. *International Journal of Medical Microbiology, Virology, Parasitology and Infectious Diseases,* **279,** 27–34.

Mutters, R., Ihm, P., Pohl, S., Frederiksen, W., and Mannheim, W. (1985). Reclassification of the genus *Pasteurella* Trevisan 1887 on the basis of deoxyribonucleic acid homology, with proposals for the new species *Pasteurella dagmatis, Pasteurella canis, Pasteurella stomatis, Pasteurella anatis,* and *Pasteurella langaa. International Journal of Systematic Bacteriology,* **35,** 309–22.

Weber, D.J., Wolfson, J.S., Swartz, M.N., and Hooper, D.C. (1984). *Pasteurella multocida* infections. Report of 34 cases and review of the literature. *Medicine,* **63,** 133–53.

7.11.17(c) Yersiniosis

A. D. PEARSON

Definition

Yersiniosis is a bacterial disease with a wide spectrum of clinical and immunological manifestations caused mainly by two enteric pathogens *Yersinia enterocolitica* and *Yersinia pseudotuberculosis* (Table 1). The disease ranges from acute watery diarrhoea in young children to acute mesenteric adenitis mimicking appendicitis in older children to extra-intestinal infection and potentially fatal septicaemia or a mild primary illness with *Y. enterocolitica* infection presenting with arthritis or erythema nodosum as post-infectious sequelae.

Occurrence

Y. enterocolitica has been recognized as a cause of diarrhoea throughout the world and in some areas is reported to cause up to 1 to 3 per cent of all cases of acute enteritis. Two thirds of cases of *Y. enterocolitica* occur in infants and children while the majority of *Y. pseudotuberculosis* infections are in people aged 5 to 20 years. An important source of *Y. enterocolitica* for man is the pig, where the pharynx may be heavily colonized. More than 50 serotypes have been recovered from a wide variety of asymptomatic animals, as well as from environmental sources. *Y. pseudotuberculosis* is a zoonotic disease of wild and domesticated mammals and birds with man as an incidental host.

Aetiology

Y. enterocolitica isolates comprise an heterogeneous species divided biochemically into four biotypes and immunologically into fifty types, based on the somatic lipopolysaccharide antigen, of which serotypes O:3, O:8, O:9 and 5,27 cause infection in man. Serotype 3 strains are found in Europe, Canada, Africa, and Asia; serotype 8 is the predominant type in the United States; serotype 9 has been reported frequently from Finland and other European countries; serotype 5,27 is reported in association with bacteraemic complications in compromised patients. *Y. pseudotuberculosis* strains comprise a homogenous species characterized by six serological types (I to VI). In Europe serotype I strains are most frequently recognized in man and animals; types II and III are less common. Serotypes IV and V are rarely isolated while serotype VI has been isolated only from rabbits in Japan.

A common virulence factor for *Y. enterocoliticia, Y. pseudotuberculosis,* and *Y. pestis* is a 40–50 megadalton plasmid not found in other commensal members of the genus.

Clinical features and diagnosis

The clinical manifestations of yersiniosis are well documented as a variety of acute presentations with or without secondary immunological complications. The most commonly recognized form of yersiniosis is an acute enteritis due to *Y. enterocolitica* which is indistinguishable from enteric infections with Salmonella or Campylobacter illness with diarrhoea, abdominal pain, nausea and vomiting. This contrasts with the pseudoappendicitis syndrome of abdominal pain caused by acute mesenteric lymphadenitis. The majority of patients diagnosed as having *Y. pseudotuberculosis* infection present with mesenteric lymphadenitis while only 15 to 20 per cent of *Y. enterocolitica* infections present with this syndrome. The clinical picture is that of acute or subacute appendicitis with pain in the middle or lower right quadrant of the abdomen and a temperature of 35 to 40°C. Signs of peritoneal irritation are observed but at laparotomy the appendix usually appears normal or is

Table 1 *Designation of genus Yersina*[a]

Subspecies and synonyms	Distribution
Y. enterocolitica (synonym: Pasteurella X). Currently five biotypes are distinguishable	Distributed widely in water, pigs, and other animals including man. Biotypes 1–4 are pathogenic for man causing a broad range of yersiniosis infections. Biotype 5 are found predominantly in hares. Originally isolated in 1933 but not aetiologically incriminated until the 1960s
Y. pseudotuberculosis (synonym: *'Pasteurella pseudotuberculosis'*)	Distributed widely in birds and animals. Pathogenic for man. Originally isolated in 1883 from guinea pigs. Confirmed as human pathogen in 1954 when recovered from mesenteric lymph nodes
Y. fredericksenii	Distributed in aquatic ecosystems and soil. Possible opportunistic pathogen for man
Y. intermedia	Distributed in aquatic ecosystems, soil, frogs, and snails. Possible opportunistic pathogen for man
Y. kristensenii	Distributed in aquatic ecosystems and soil. Not known to be pathogenic for man
Y. aldovae (synonym: *Y. enterocolitica*-like group X2)	Distributed in aquatic ecosystems and soil. Not known to be pathogenic for man
Y. bercovieri (synonym: *Y. enterocolitica* biogroup 3B)	Distributed in aquatic ecosystems, soil and vegetables. No evidence of pathogenicity for man
Y. mollaretti (synonym: *Y. enterocolitica* biogroup 3A)	Distributed in aquatic ecosystems, soil, animals, and vegetables. Not known to be pathogenic for man
Y. rohdei	Isolated from dog and human faeces and water. Clinical significance as a diarrhoeal agent in humans is uncertain
Y. ruckeri[b] (synonym: Red mouth or RM bacterium)	Causative agent of red mouth disease of trout
Y. pestis (synonym: *Pasteurella pestis*)	Causative agent for plague (see Chapter 7.11.16)

[a]Biochemical characteristics from Barrow and Feltham, eds. (1993). *Cowan and Steel's Manual for the Identification of Medical Bacteria* (3rd edn). Cambridge University Press.

[b]Phylogenetically unlikely to be a member of Yersinia.

mildly congested with some clear fluid in the peritoneal cavity. Pathognomonic is the finding of enlarged mesenteric lymph nodes in the ileocaecal angle with a hyperaemic mesentery in the region of the affected nodes with or without swelling of the terminal ileum and caecum. These clinical presentations must be distinguished from Crohn's disease, tuberculosis, and neoplasia. Most cases are self limiting but complications include diffuse ulceration of the small intestine and colon, perforation, intussusception, toxic megacolon, cholangitis, and mesenteric vein thrombosis.

Patients with *Y. enterocolitica* may present with focal infection in a variety of extraintestinal sites in the absence of bacteraemia: pharyngitis with cervical lymphadenopathy, cutaneous manifestations varying from cellulitis, wound infections and abscess formation, pyomyositis, osteomyelitis, conjunctivitis, urinary tract infections, renal disease, pneumonia, and lung abscesses. Bacteraemia with *Y. enterocolitica* is most often recognized in compromised patients or in people overloaded with iron. There is a case fatality rate of 34 to 50 per cent when bacteraemic infection with *Y. enterocolitica* is associated with cirrhosis and alcoholism, therapy with immunosuppressive drugs or desferrioxamine, cirrhosis, haemochromatosis, acute iron poisoning, transfusion dependent blood dyscrasia, and diabetes. Metastatic infection resulting from bacteraemia may lead to a variety of complications of which the case literature reports endocarditis, infection of intravenous catheters, rupture of vascular protheses, meningitis, and septic arthritis.

Secondary immunological implications occur 1 or 2 weeks after the onset of gastrointestinal symptoms and are typically a polyarticular arthritis or erythema nodosum; less common are Reiter's syndrome, glomerulonephritis, or myocarditis.

The incubation period for primary yersiniosis is probably 3 to 7 days and generally under 10 days; secondary arthritis and erythema nodosum follow 4 to 14 days after the prodromal illness. The inflammatory arthri-

Table 2 *Detection and typing methods*
(a) **Yersinia enterocolitica**

Method
A. Evidence of pathogenicity
1. Calcium dependency
2. Animal inoculation: mouse virulence
3. Autoagglutination
4. HeLa cell infection
5. Plasmid presence
6. Outer membrane proteins
7. Enzyme immunoassay
8. Production of V and W antigens
9. Cell surface hydrophobicity
B. Detection
1. Cold enrichment
2. Selective media
C. Serotyping
1. Agglutination reactions
(a) Tube agglutination
(b) Indirect haemagglutination
(c) Microtitre agglutination
2. ELISA
3. Radioimmunoassay
4. Immunofluorescent antibody assay
D. Biotyping
1. Electrophoresis
2. Biochemical characterization
3. Polymerase chain reaction

Table 2 (*cont.*)
(*b*) **Yersinia pseudotuberculosis**

Method
A. Evidence of pathogenicity
1. Calcium dependency
2. Outer membrane proteins
3. Autoagglutination
4. Enzyme immunoassay
5. Plasmid presence
B. Detection
1. KOH enrichment
C. Serotyping
1. Tube agglutination
2. Microagglutination
D. Biotyping
1. Electrophoresis
2. Polymerase chain reaction

tis may persist for 1 to 4 months followed by a prolonged period of stiffness and arthralgia.

Diagnosis

Consideration of yersiniosis in the differential diagnosis of enteritis, appendicitis, metastatic focal infection, and bacteraemia is essential if the microbiologist is to confirm diagnosis by culture or changes in serology. The methods available to the laboratory and clinician are summarized in Table 2. A comparison of the laboratory findings in *Y. enterocolitica* and *Y. pseudotuberculosis* is given in Table 3.

Treatment

Antimicrobical therapy is not indicated in uncomplicated enterocolitis or pseudoappendicitis syndrome resulting from yersiniosis. A double blind placebo controlled trial of antimicrobial treatment of *Y. enterocolitica* enterocolitis infection in children failed to demonstrate any shortening in the course of the illness. Localized infection in the gastrointestinal tract, septicaemia, and enterocolitis in compromised patients requires appropriate antimicrobial treatment with third generation cephalosporins, quinolones, or aminoglycosides. *Y. enterocolitica* isolates are usually resistant to most penicillins and first generation cephalosporins. *Y. pseudotuberculosis* isolates are usually sensitive to benzylpenicillin and ampicillin, while both species are sensitive to tetracyclines.

Table 3 *A comparison of laboratory findings in* **Y. enterocolitica** *and* **Y. pseudotuberculosis** *infection*

	Y. enterocolitica	*Y. pseudotuberculosis*
Culture:		
Stools	Positive 2–8 weeks from onset of symptoms	Seldom positive
Lymph nodes	Ileocaecal angle usually positive: other lymph nodes rarely positive	Ileocaecal angle usually positive: other lymph nodes rarely positive
Appendix	Occasionally positive (4%)	Seldom positive
Serology:		
Antibody titres		
Acute	Low or absent	High at onset (160–640)
Convalescent	High especially with arthritis or erythema nodosum	Decline rapidly if no complications
Histopathology		
Macroscopic		
Appendix	Usually normal	Usually normal
Mesenteric lymph-nodes	Enlarged, soft, inflamed, may form retroperitoneal mass	Multiple, frequently matted, enlarged 1–4 cm diameter; cut surface, fleshy reddish gray containing yellowish microabscesses
Ileum	Ileitis: oedematous, congested serosa, hypertrophied Peyer's patches, mucosal ulceration	Ileitis infrequent
Microscopic		
Appendix	Focal ulceration	Mild inflammation; occasional microabscess
Mesenteric lymph nodes	Proliferation of large pyroninophilic cells (basophilic stem cell hyperplasia) correlating with antibody response; no characteristic microabscesses or giant cells	Characteristic 4-stage microabscess formation: (i) lymphoid tissue hyperplasia (ii) diffuse reticulocyte hyperplasia (iii) multiple epitheloid granulomata with giant cells (iv) central coagulative necrosis of granulomas with PMN
Intradermal test	None available	Positive: raised, indurated, erythematous zone 1–2 cm

Table 4 *Outbreaks of yersiniosis*
(a) **Y. enterocolitica** *(1972–1990)*

Location	Seasonality month	No. of cases	Attack rate primary (%)	Common vehicle or source	Predominant serotype
Finland	April	7	N/A	Hospital patient	9
North Carolina, USA	April	16	76	Puppies‡	8
Canada	April	138	16	? Raw milk	5,27
Saskatchewan, Canada	February–April	3	75	Possibly water‡	21
New York, USA	September	38	10	Chocolate milk	8
Japan	April	1051	12	Milk	3
Newfoundland, Canada	July	9	N/A	Hospital patient	5
New York, USA	July	159	35	Powdered milk, chow mein	8
Washington, USA	December	50	N/A	Tofu, spring water	8
Pennsylvania, USA	February	16	48	Bean sprouts immersed in well water	8
Southern USA	June	172	N/A	Pasteurized milk‡	13a,13b
New York, USA	May	4	N/A	Water most likely	3
Czechoslovakia	September	15	10	Not identified	3
Japan	January	189	43	Not identified	3
Japan	July	544	52	Not identified	3
Japan	July	198	18	Not identified	3
Japan	April	296	36	Not identified	3
Japan	June	145	30	Not identified	3
Japan	January	6	7	Not identified	3
Japan	November	184	19	Not identified	3
Japan	May	641	35	Not identified	3
Japan	June	102	11	Not identified	3
Georgia, USA	December–January	15	N/A	Pork chitterlings	3

‡Epidemiologically implicated as the common vehicle or source, but material was not available for culture.

(b) **Y. pseudotuberculosis** *(1954–1984)*

Location	Seasonality month	No. of cases	Attack rate primary (%)	Common vehicle or source	Predominant serotype
Vladivostok, Former Soviet Union	Extended	300	N/A	Rodents	-
Kent, England	January	4	N/A	Pet dog possibly	1a
Finland	December–March	19	N/A	Not identified	3
Japan	June	35	69	Meat products, vegetables, rice‡	5a
Japan	June	4	57	Meat products, vegetables, rice‡	5a

‡Epidemiologically implicated as the common vehicle or source, but material was not available for culture.

Epidemiology

There are marked differences in the reported frequency and distribution of *Y. enterocolitica* infections. Ascertainment biases, variation in clinical awareness, and incomplete reporting of Yersinia as an enteric pathogen make interpretation of the literature both difficult and imprecise. There is general agreement that in Europe, especially in Scandinavia and Belgium, sporadic infection with *Y. enterocolitica* serotypes O:3 and O:9 are common while outbreaks with these or other serotypes are rare. The most important sources of these infections are thought to be pork, especially when tongues are eaten undercooked or raw, and contact with household pets, especially sick puppies and kittens.

In North America numerous outbreaks of *Y. enterocolitica* have been recognized, (Table 4(a)) of which several have been caused by serotype 8. Epidemics have usually been caused by contamination of a food vehicle from a meat source or water; three such outbreaks were traced to chocolate milk, tofu (soybean cake), and pork chitterlings. Sporadic cases in the United States are less common than in England and associated with multiple serotypes. Transmission is by the faecal–oral route

Fig. 1 All Yersinia isolations in England and Wales reported to CDSC, 1980-1993. (Provisional source: 1980-88 Annual Tables, 1989-93 CDR Comptuter reports.)

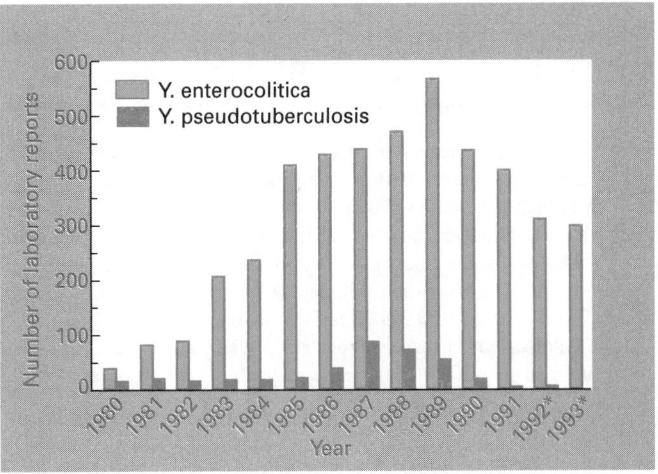

after eating or drinking food or water contaminated by colonized or infected animals or people. Hospital acquired infection occurs by nosocomial transmission and by the use of stored blood from asymptomatic donors or individuals who had gastrointestinal illness within 2 weeks of their blood donation. Because of the ability of *Y. enterocolitica* to multiply both in food products under refrigeration and in aerophilic conditions, at-risk products are raw or undercooked pork or any uncooked meat stored in evacuated plastic bags.

Cases and outbreaks of yersiniosis due to *Y. pseudotuberculosis* are less commonly recognized. Figure 1 shows the comparison of laboratory diagnosed cases of yersiniosis in England and Wales between 1980 and 1993 and Table 4(b) lists the few rare reports of outbreaks of *Y. pseudotuberculosis.* Not unexpectedly this zoonotic infection results from contact with animals or birds and there has been no evidence of person to person transmission.

REFERENCES

Black, R.E., Jackson, R.J., Tsai, T., *et al.* (1978). Epidemic *Yersinia enterocolitica* infection due to contaminated chocolate milk. *New England Journal of Medicine*, **298,** 76–79.

Bottone, E.J. (1977). *Yersinia enterocolitica*: a panoramic view of a charismatic microorganism. *Critical Reviews in Microbiology*, 211–241.

Cover, T.L. and Aber, R.C. (1989). *Yersinia enterocolitica. New England Journal of Medicine*, **321,** 16–24.

Greenwood, M.H. (1993). *Yersinia enterocolitica*, detection and treatment. *Encyclopaedia of Food Science, Food Technology and Nutrition*, **7,** 4962–67.

Gutman, L.T., Ottesen, E.A., Quan, T.J., Noce, P.S., and Katz, S.L. (1973). An inter-familial outbreak of *Yersinia enterocolitica* enteritis. *New England Journal of Medicine*, 1372–77.

Hoogkamp-Korstanje, J.A.A. (1987). Antibiotics in *Yersinia enterocolitica* infections. *Journal of Antimicrobial Chemotherapy*, **20,** 123–31.

Larson, J.H. (1979). The spectrum of clinical manifestations of infections with *Yersinia enterocolitica* and their pathogenesis. *Contributions to Microbiology and Immunology*, **5,** 257–69.

Lee, L.A., Taylor, J., Carter, G.P., Quinn, B., Farmer, J.J., and Tauxe, R.B. (1991). *Yersinia enterocolitica* O:3: an emerging cause of pediatric gastroenteritis in the United States. *Journal of Infectious Diseases*, **163,** 660–3.

Nakano, T., Kawaguchi, H., Nakao, K., Maruyama, T., Kamiya, H., and Sakurai, M. (1989). Two outbreaks of *Yersinia pseudotuberculosis* 5a infection in Japan. *Scandinavian Journal of Infectious Diseases*, **21,** 175–9.

Vantrappen, G., *et al.* (1977). Yersinia enteritis and enterocolitis: gastroenterological aspects. *Gastroenterology*, **72,** 220–7.

7.11.18 Anthrax

A. B. Christie and P. C. B. Turnbull

The word 'anthrax' derives from the Greek *anthrakos*, meaning coal, and alludes to the characteristic sore or 'eschar' with its coal-black centre. The French and Italian names for the disease, *carbon* and *carbonchio*, similarly allude to this typical lesion. The disease has names in many other languages referring to various of its dramatic signs and symptoms, such as *Milzbrand* (German) or *miltvuur* (Dutch), meaning 'spleen fire'; *pustula maligna* (Spanish); or to its source of infection, such as woolsorters' disease, ragpickers disease, and Siberian plague. Local or tribal names for the disease may often be encountered while travelling through endemic countries.

Dr. A.B. Christie died in 1987. Much of his second edition chapter has been retained in this edition.

Anthrax is primarily a disease of herbivores, although few mammals or birds are thought to be totally resistant to it. Man generally acquires anthrax directly or indirectly from animals. Human anthrax remains common in anthrax endemic countries, principally Africa and Asia, where owners still skin and eat animals that have died of the disease; the value of the carcass as meat in such places still greatly outweighs the perceived hazard from cutting it up and eating it. In non-endemic regions far away from Africa and Asia, occasional cases still occur as a result of the handling of wool, hair, hides, or bones imported from endemic areas.

Bacteriology

ANTHRAX BACILLUS

Bacillus anthracis, as a member of the genus Bacillus, is a Gram-positive, aerobic, spore-forming, rod-shaped bacterium of approximately 3–8 × 1–2 μm, characteristically square-ended in appearance. It is one of the few species within the genus that is non-motile. In the presence of oxygen, spores are formed, one per bacillary (vegetative) cell (the sporangium) in the centre of the cell and not causing it to swell (in other species the spores may be laterally placed or may swell the sporangium).

In the animal body, the bacilli occur in pairs or short chains, but in laboratory culture they form long, filamentous chains. In the absence of oxygen and in the presence of HCO_3^-, the bacilli surround themselves with a polypeptide capsule. These conditions are met in the body and the presence of capsulated, square-ended bacilli in short chains on polychrome methylene blue-stained (M'Fadyean stain) smears of vesicular fluid from the eschar or of blood at death is a reliable diagnostic test.

Bacillus and spore

The vegetative bacillus is not a hardy organism and finds it difficult to survive in nature in competition with saprophytes, especially the organisms of putrefaction. If an animal dies of anthrax and its body is left lying in summer heat at a temperature greater than about 25°C, anthrax bacilli may not be found in it after 3 to 4 days, having been overwhelmed by the putrefactive organisms. At lower temperatures, putrefaction will take place more slowly and the anthrax bacilli will persist for longer periods.

If the bacilli escape from a carcass and the outside temperature is greater than about 20°C with high humidity, they form spores quickly and have a greater chance of surviving in pasture. At lower temperatures, spore formation is slower and fewer may survive the delay. The ecology of anthrax, and the environmental and climatic factors affecting survival of the bacterium and seasonal cycles of infection of animals, are complex and still poorly understood even though the disease has been known for a very long time.

The spore is resistant to levels of heat, cold, pH, desiccation, and chemicals that would kill most other living things; once formed following the death of an animal from anthrax the spores can survive in the environment to infect other animals years or even decades later. Their survival probably depends on their inclination to germinate (i.e. to produce the vegetative form again) and this is affected by seasonal changes of temperature and moisture, and possibly by competition with other organisms.

Breaking the cycle of infection depends on applying good animal husbandry. As seen in Fig. 1, the best approaches to this are destruction of the carcass by incineration (without opening for autopsy or butchery) or, as preferred in parts of Europe, or taking it without delay for rendering. Any spillage or exudation of blood should be decontaminated with 5 to 10 per cent formalin (best option), 4 per cent glutaraldehyde, or 3 to 4 per cent hydrogen peroxide.

As well as being able to survive for long periods on dry soil, *B. anthracis* spores can also survive on animal hair, wool, hides, bones, or any other contaminated material, and in this way can be transported from one part of the world to another, causing disease in animals and man far away in time and place.

Effect of heat and disinfectants

Dry heat at 150°C for 1 h, or boiling for 10 min, will normally destroy spores, but the most reliable treatment is autoclaving at 121°C for 15 min; even then, penetration of bulky wool, hair, and bedding must be complete. Spores may survive freezing and thawing. They are also resistant to certain disinfectants, particularly the phenolics and quarternary ammonium compounds. Formaldehyde is probably the most universally useful fumigant or, in solutions as formalin, the best disinfectant (usually used at 5 to 10 per cent solutions equivalent to 1.5 to 3 per cent dissolved formaldehyde (saturated formalin = approx. 37 per cent formaldehyde solution)). Glutaraldehyde (4 per cent) is also effective. Oxidizing agents potassium permanganate (4 per cent) or hydrogen peroxide (4 per cent) are also sporicidal. Exposure times vary with the conditions under which decontamination or disinfection are being carried out but generally should exceed 1 h following full penetration of the item concerned with the oxidizing agents and 4 h with the aldehydes. Hypochlorites are not reliably effective.

An alternative, non-damaging approach to decontamination of bulk materials such as bales of wool is irradiation to reach 25 kGy or more at the lowest dose position (i.e. the most dense point at depth in the bale, usually its core).

Pathogenesis and transmission

Herbivores are the most susceptible species and generally acquire anthrax when grazing from ground where anthrax spores are lingering. *B. anthracis* is not an invasive organism and requires a lesion through which to establish its infection. In grazing or browsing herbivores such lesions probably result from uptake of sharp soil particles or thorns, spiky leaves or grass.

On entry into the lesion, the spores germinate to set up a local infection or get carried to the regional lymph nodes where the systemic infection is initiated with involvement of the spleen soon after (see Fig. 1). In the lymph nodes and spleen the bacteria multiply and produce toxin more or less silently (i.e. without the appearance of symptoms) until, at some point, the organs break down releasing, in a burst, the toxin and large numbers of the bacilli. This leads to sudden onset of hyperacute illness. Fever starts a few hours before disorientation sets in, with shock, coma, and death occurring in the space of about 1 h. In livestock, antimicrobial treatment can still save the animal's life if given immediately upon onset of fever. In untreated herbivores, the mortality rate is estimated as being 70 to 100 per cent.

The course of the disease is generally slower in the more resistant omnivorous or carnivorous species, with lower mortality rates. Local oedema and swollen lymph nodes, particularly mandibular and pharyngeal, are early pathognomonic signs. Oedema in the neck, if severe enough, may result in death from asphyxiation rather than from the disease itself.

Human resistance to anthrax is considered intermediate between that of herbivores and carnivores. Although human beings occasionally contract the disease by eating contaminated meat (intestinal anthrax), by far the most common form is cutaneous anthrax acquired from skinning or butchering carcasses or handling products from animals that have died of the disease. The organism gains entry through cuts or abrasions in the skin, predominantly at exposed sites such as the hands, arms, or head and neck. Occasionally, pulmonary anthrax is contracted from breathing spore-laden dust in industries that process animal products from endemic regions.

Numerous reports and personal accounts testify to the relative resistance of man to anthrax. In the United States, before the availability of vaccines, studies in high-risk industries (e.g. wool, hair, hides, bonemeal) showed that workers 'chronically exposed to anthrax' had annual case rates of only about 1 per cent. In one mill, the outcome of air sampling suggested that the workers inhaled 600 to 1300 anthrax spores during an 8 h shift without ill effect.

In the cutaneous form, the infection usually remains localized, pro-

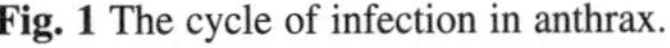

Fig. 1 The cycle of infection in anthrax.

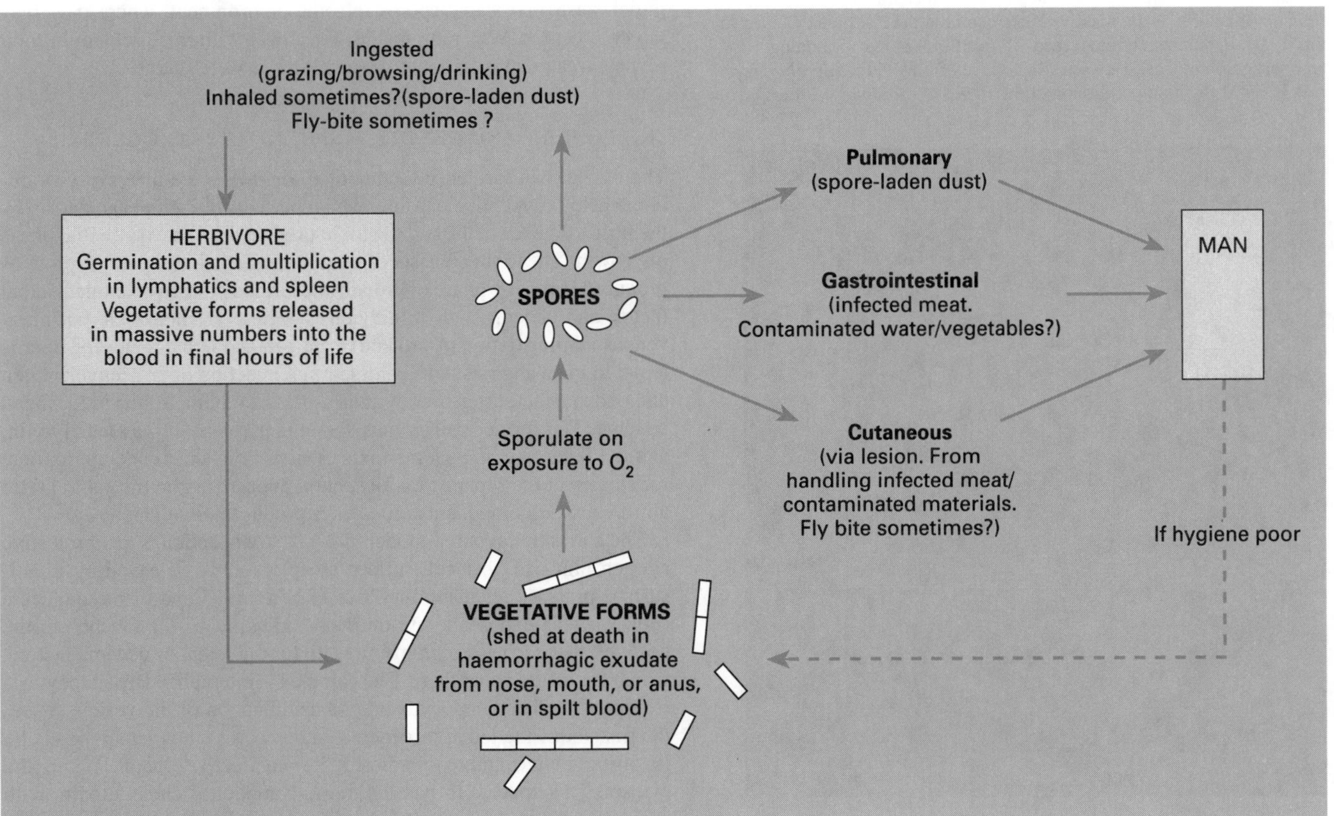

ducing the characteristic eschar and oedema at the site of infection, but occasionally it can spread systemically as described above. In pulmonary infections, some germination occurs in the lungs but studies in monkeys in the 1950s indicated that the spores can apparently persist in the alveoli for long periods and are slowly taken up by alveolar macrophages to the lymph nodes where, if the infection 'takes', they germinate and multiply.

In some countries, biting flies transmit the disease to man, giving rise to cutaneous anthrax on exposed areas such as the face; this may also occur in animals but skin lesions are rarely reported. In herbivores, this is presumably because the animal succumbs before the local lesion has had the opportunity to develop.

SPREAD FROM ANIMALS—CYCLE OF INFECTION

An animal dying of anthrax excretes anthrax bacilli in enormous numbers in bloody discharges from the nose, mouth, and anus. At death the blood contains 10^7 to 10^9 bacilli/ml (Fig. 2). A proportion of these, falling on the ground, will sporulate to produce persisting contamination from which other animals may become infected (see Fig. 1). If the carcass is opened, spillage of more blood increases the contamination of the surroundings, and the *B. anthracis* may then find its way into pools, ditches, and ponds. An animal dying in a cowshed or other building can grossly contaminate straw and manure.

Infection in livestock normally occurs by uptake of the organism from the environment and is not transmitted directly from animal to animal. The cycle of infection can be broken by disinfection of soil, ground, or bedding contaminated by the terminal bloody discharges and disposal of the carcass as described above.

Among wild animals, herbivores usually acquire anthrax by ingesting spores deposited on the soil or in water by an infected animal. Occasionally they may acquire it by osteophagia (licking bones to supplement mineral intake). Carnivores (e.g. dogs, lions, cheetahs) contract the disease directly by feeding on anthrax carcasses.

Fig. 2 Anthrax bacilli occluding the lumen of a blood capillary. A characteristic of anthrax is the massive bacteraemia in the last hours of life. At the point of death, numbers often exceed 10^8 bacilli/ml blood. (Scanning electron micrograph by A.B. Dowsett. Reproduced from *PHLS Microbiology Digest*, **9**(3), 1992, by kind permission of the *PHLS Microbiology Digest*.) (× 1250)

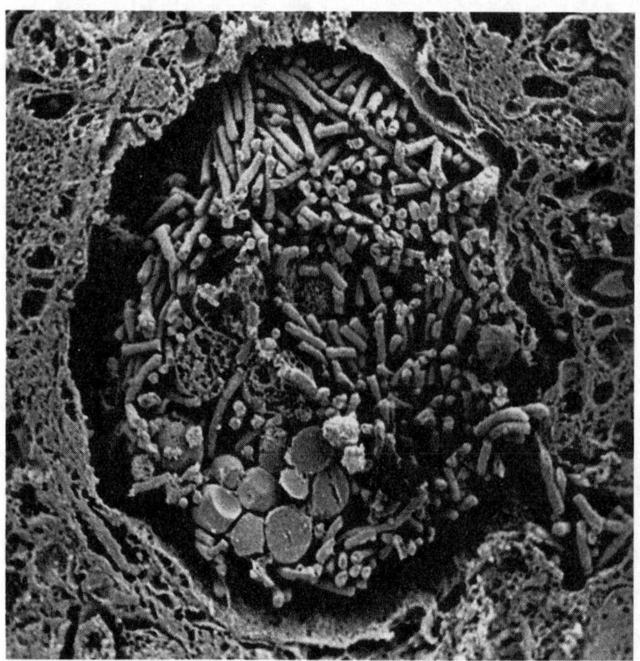

Person-to-person spread has been documented in the Gambia. Apart from close physical contact, such as children playing together, transmission was promoted by the communal use within families of palm-fibre loofahs (back-scrubbing implements), which were found to be infected with *B. anthracis* spores. Antibodies were found in healthy close contacts of the clinical cases.

NON-INDUSTRIAL AND INDUSTRIAL ANTHRAX

Human anthrax is traditionally classified as either non-industrial or industrial depending on whether the disease is acquired directly from animals or indirectly during handling and processing of contaminated animal products. Non-industrial anthrax usually affects people who work with animals or animal carcasses, such as farmers, abattoir workers, knackers, butchers, and veterinary personnel, and is almost always cutaneous, though occasionally intestinal if, as occurs in developing countries, the owners skin, butcher, and eat the meat. Industrial anthrax, occurring as a result of handling and processing contaminated hair, wool, hides, bones, or other animal products, is usually cutaneous but has a higher chance of being pulmonary through inhalation of spore-laden dust.

The trade in hides, wool, hair, and, to a lesser extent, bones between developing, anthrax-endemic countries and developed non-endemic countries has decreased since the first half of the twentieth century, largely as a result of man-made alternatives. However, specialized leather and woollen industries continue to depend on hides and wool from particular species or breeds that can only be raised in countries which are still endemic; similarly, 'sun-dried' bones from animals that die naturally in tropical or subtropical Asia or Africa have qualities for gelatin, glue, and charcoal production that cannot be reproduced in temperate Europe or North America. Demand in developed countries for bonemeal for feeds and fertilizers continues to exceed domestic availability and remains dependent on extensive importation.

Most industrial processes kill anthrax spores, so final products such as processed wool and woollen goods, leather, and charcoal are free of spores. However, effluent from early stages of processing such as the initial wash may carry spores into the environment, where they may infect livestock. Water companies must deal with this problem in their sewage treatment works and the resulting sewage sludge.

MOLECULAR AND GENETIC ASPECTS OF PATHOGENESIS

The two known virulence factors of *B. anthracis* are the poly-γ-D-glutamic acid polypeptide capsule, which protects it from phagocytosis by the host's defence cells, and the toxin produced in the exponential phase of growth. The toxin consists of three synergistic but separable proteins produced in the log phase of growth and termed protective antigen, lethal factor, and oedema factor. Individually, these are non-toxic but intravenous administration of protective antigen and lethal factor together is lethal to mice and rats, while intradermal injection of protective antigen and oedema factor together in guinea-pigs or rabbits results in localized oedema. The former pair is thus sometimes referred to as lethal toxin, and the latter pair as oedema toxin. This is convenient and appropriate for studies of the separate entities, but it appears that in the natural state all three toxin components are always produced simultaneously.

The currently favoured model of *in vivo* toxin action is that protective antigen binds to host cell-surface receptors and is cleaved by a cell-surface protease releasing the 20-kDa N-terminal end of the molecule (Fig. 3). This exposes a site on the 63-kDa piece still attached to the host cell that carries a high-affinity site for the lethal or oedema factors, which compete to bind there. The complex is internalized by endocytosis (receptor-mediated endocytosis) and acidification of the vesicle causes the transfer of the lethal or oedema factors across the membrane via 63 (kDa)-protective antigen-mediated, ion-conductive channels into the cytosol. This appears to parallel the A-B model of cholera toxin, with lethal and oedema factors acting as competing 'A' moieties and the 63-protective antigen as the 'B' moiety.

Oedema factor is a calmodulin-dependent adenylate cyclase, which, by catalysing the abnormal production of cAMP, produces the altered water and ion movements that lead to the characteristic oedema of anthrax. Calmodulin is the major eukaryotic intracellular calcium receptor, indicating that the action of oedema factor is targeted at the eukaryotic host cell. High intracellular cAMP concentrations are cytostatic but not lethal in most cell types. The role of oedema factor in the anthrax infection may be to prevent mobilization and activation of the polymorphonuclear leucocytes and thereby the phagocytosis of the bacteria.

Fig. 3 The mode of action of anthrax toxin (model of Leppla (1991)). Protective antigen (PA) binds to host cell-surface receptors (1) and is cleaved by a cell-surface protease releasing a 20-kDa piece (2). This exposes a secondary receptor for the lethal factor (LF) and (o)edema factor (EF) components of the toxin, which compete to bind to it (2). The complex is internalized by receptor-mediated endocytosis (3) and acidification of the resulting vesicle leads to the transfer of the LF or EF across the vesicular membrane into the cytosol where they effect their catalytic actions (4).

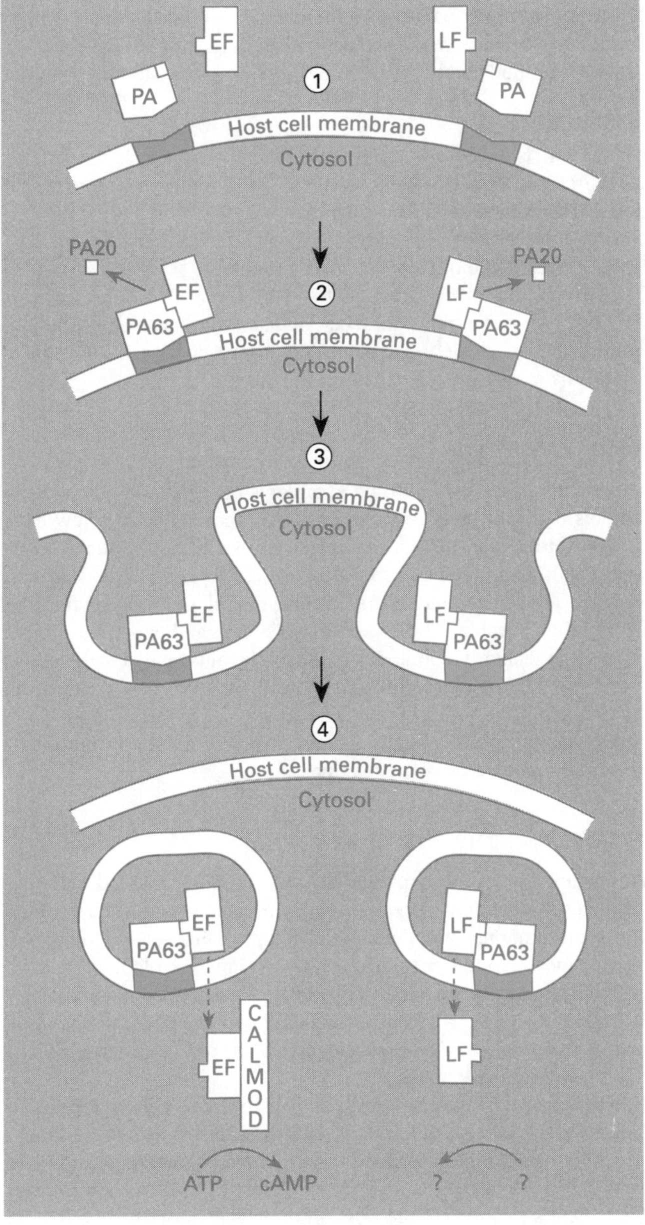

Lethal factor is also probably an enzyme and there is evidence that it too is calmodulin dependent, but its substrate, products, and mode of action are as yet unknown. However, the effects of lethal toxin (lethal factor + protective antigen) administration match those observed in animals dying from anthrax and it is accepted that the complex of these two is the main cause of tissue damage and death.

The genes for the virulence factors, capsule and toxin, lie on two large plasmids. The three toxin genes, *pag, lef,* and *cya,* encoding protective antigen, lethal factor, and oedema factor, respectively, are located on the 170–185 kbp (119 MDa) plasmid, pXO1, and have all been cloned and sequenced revealing secreted proteins of 735 amino acids (protective antigen; equivalent to 82.7 kDa), 776 amino acids (lethal factor, 90.2 kDa), and 767 amino acids (oedema factor, 88.8 kDa). Similarly, cloning and sequencing of the genes involved in capsule synthesis, which reside on a 90–95 kbp (60 MDa) plasmid, pXO2, have revealed three cistrons designated *capA, capB,* and *capC,* which code for three membrane-associated enzymes mediating the polymerization of D-glutamic acid via the *B. anthracis* cell membrane. Coding for elaboration of both toxin proteins and capsule is under bicarbonate or CO_2 regulation; in the case of the toxin, bicarbonate control is through activation of gene transcription.

Comparison of DNA sequences has revealed extensive nucleotide homology in the regions coding for the N-terminal 300 amino acids of the lethal and oedema factors, strongly indicating that the protective antigen-binding sites of these proteins reside here. Extensive protease cleavage studies on protective antigen, together with site mutagenesis of such sites (rendering them resistant to proteases) and monoclonal antibody studies of binding and toxic activities of epitopes, have elucidated the interrelations and actions of protective antigen, lethal factor and oedema factor together and with each other, and of protective antigen with eukaryotic host cells. Very recently (1992), furin, an endoprotease predominantly localized in the Golgi membrane, has been identified by implication as the enzyme principally responsible for cleaving and activating the native protective antigen.

Loss of either pXO1 or pXO2 and consequent loss of the ability to produce toxin or capsule lead to loss of virulence. This evidently can occur naturally. $pXO1^+/pXO2^-$ strains form the basis of anthrax vaccines (see 'Prevention' below).

As the only readily obtainable or identifiable entities truly specific to *B. anthracis* and not shared by other *Bacillus* species, the toxin antigens form the best basis for enzyme immunoassays for anti-anthrax antibodies. Antibodies to the purified toxin antigens are the basis for new diagnostic systems on the principle that the presence of the toxin indicates the presence of the bacterium. Similarly, gene probes under development for rapid anthrax detection systems are based on sequences within the genes encoding the toxin antigens or the capsule precursors.

The improved understanding of anthrax toxin at the molecular level in the last few years has led to a number of alternative ideas and approaches for improving anthrax vaccines in the future (see below).

Clinical manifestations and diagnosis

CUTANEOUS ANTHRAX

The anthrax sore begins like an ordinary pimple, which grows rapidly in 2 to 3 days. Its centre ulcerates, but by about day 4 or 5 becomes a dry, black, firmly adherent scab surrounded by a circle of purplish vesicles (Fig. 4). This is the typical anthrax sore or eschar, at one time often referred to as 'malignant pustule', although it is neither malignant nor pustular. Pus develops only if the lesion is secondarily infected; alternatively, the presence of pus may indicate that the cause is not anthrax. Differential diagnosis includes boil, orf, plague, primary syphilitic chancre, erysipelas, glanders, and tropical ulcer.

Most anthrax sores are about 2 to 3 cm across, but some may be up to 6 to 7 cm, occasionally even larger. In contrast, sometimes they may not exceed a pin-head in size; there may be massive oedema around a tiny sore. Substantial to massive oedema is a primary characteristic of anthrax. From a sore in the neck, the oedema may spread down over the chest and abdomen or, from a lesion on the arm or wrist, up the arm and down the trunk (Fig. 5). There is always swelling around the sore. Sometimes the vesicles around the sore are large and bullous; on occasion there are vesicles but no eschar or, alternatively, an eschar but no vesicles. In the partially immune patient, the lesion may look like an innocent pimple. The typical sore looks angry and tender but usually there is little local pain.

Fig. 4 Anthrax sore showing central eschar and ring of vesicles.

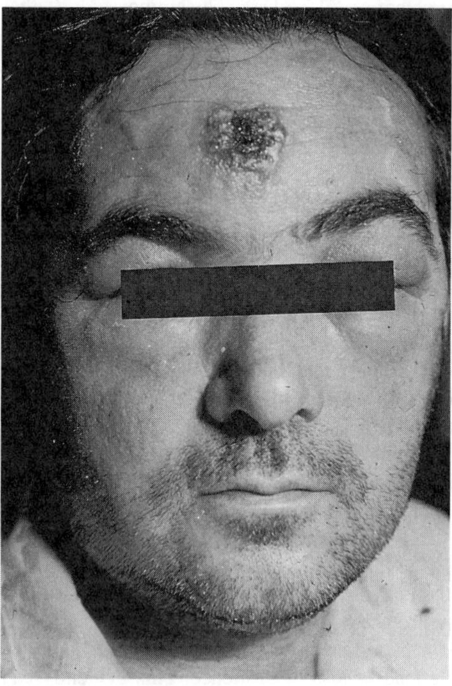

Fig. 5 Anthrax: healing eschar of chest wall. The primary sore was on the back of the patient's neck. Oedema spread from the neck over the chest and abdomen into the scrotum.

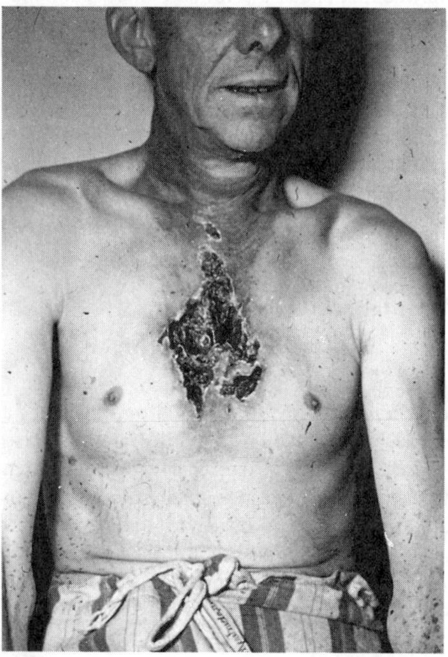

The oedema is non-pitting, and the skin is usually neither hot nor red. There is no pus beneath the swelling, no abscess to open: the urge to incise it must be resisted as this will lead only to an intractable sinus and scarring. Lymph nodes usually enlarge and may be tender, but here again there is no abscess formation.

In uncomplicated cases, the eschar begins to resolve about 10 days after the appearance of the initial papule. Resolution is slow—2 to 6 weeks regardless of treatment—but usually complete. Most sores heal and leave little trace, but over the jaw or the eye, scarring may be serious and require surgical repair, especially when the eyelid is damaged. The oedema is often very slow to resolve, even when the sore has healed: again the impulse to incise must be resisted. The same is true of the lymphadenitis, which may also last a long time.

General symptoms

The amount of illness varies. Occasionally the patient continues to feel well but chill, headache, anorexia and nausea are common. The temperature may be normal, but more often is around 38.3 to 38.8°C. In severe cases the patient may have rigors and the temperature reaches 40°C. A fall to subnormal level in these patients is an ominous sign, as is vomiting, weakness, and a thready pulse. In most cases the illness is not more than moderately severe and responds rapidly to treatment.

Complications

When the sore is on the lower part of the face or on the neck, the oedema may encircle the neck and press on the trachea. Sometimes there is also oedema of the larynx, and these two may make breathing difficult. Tracheotomy must be done without delay; once the oedema has become extensive, finding the trachea becomes a problem.

In cases coming late to treatment and in the rare case that is overwhelming from onset, there may be circulatory collapse and bleeding. There may be petechiae on the mesentery and elsewhere, haemorrhagic mediastinitis or massive intestinal haemorrhage.

PULMONARY ANTHRAX

Illness begins insidiously with no symptoms or with mild non-specific symptoms of slight fever and malaise. This phase (two to a few days after exposure) ends with the abrupt onset of chills and often blood-stained vomit. In an hour or two the patient is dyspnoeic, cyanosed, and acutely ill. The temperature soars, the chest is full of moist sounds, the pulse rapid and feeble. The spleen may be enlarged and tender, there may be some tender lymph nodes in the axilla, but there is nothing else to point to the diagnosis except perhaps the patient's occupation. Untreated, the patient dies in 2 to 3 days.

Milder cases probably occur as bronchitis in which the diagnosis of anthrax is not considered or recognized.

INTESTINAL ANTHRAX

This is analogous to cutaneous anthrax with the anthrax sore developing on the intestinal mucosa instead of the skin, most often in the terminal ileum or caecum; the upper ileum, duodenum, stomach, and oropharynx are sometimes affected in the same way. Symptoms of mild to acute gastroenteritis may occur but are sometimes absent. As with pulmonary anthrax, sudden onset of severe malaise follows the benign incubation period of two to a few days, with fever, shock, collapse, and death all occurring within a few hours.

The occurrence of intestinal anthrax in temperate regions appears to be unrecorded. As with pulmonary anthrax, it is responsive to timely treatment but the problem is that it may go unrecognized until too late to treat effectively. Effective treatment is likely to depend on awareness of the patient's history and the possibility or likelihood that it could be anthrax. Like pulmonary anthrax, it is probable that there are subclinical or undiagnosed mild cases with spontaneous recovery; there is some serological evidence for this.

ANTHRAX MENINGITIS

This is a rare complication usually of cutaneous anthrax, but it can arise from any of the forms of the disease. The meninges are inflamed and in some parts haemorrhagic. Cerebrospinal fluid may be bloodstained and contain anthrax bacilli. The outlook is poor, though with immediate treatment recovery is possible.

PATHOLOGY

In most countries, autopsies of animals or human beings known or suspected to have died of anthrax are forbidden. Inadvertent autopsies reveal a consistent picture of dark, unclotted blood, markedly enlarged haemorrhagic spleen and affected lymph nodes, and petechial haemorrhages of the other viscera. In intestinal anthrax, the intestinal mucosa is dark red with glassy oedema and areas of necrosis at the site of the eschar. At laparotomy in one patient with intestinal anthrax who recovered, the mesentery was covered with petechiae and there was a typical anthrax sore in the duodenum.

SECOND ATTACKS AND INFECTION IN VACCINATED PEOPLE

These can occur although sometimes the lesion is very small and there are no vesicles, no eschar, and no oedema. Anthrax bacilli can be isolated from scrapings of the lesion, but unless anthrax is suspected, it is unlikely that such examination of a small pimple will be made, and the sore will probably heal undiagnosed.

LABORATORY DIAGNOSIS

The clinical diagnosis of anthrax is confirmed by directly seeing or isolating the infecting *B. anthracis* from cutaneous lesions, or from blood or affected organs after death. These procedures are straightforward provided that antimicrobial treatment has not already been started.

In cutaneous anthrax, fresh smears are made of vesicular fluid or, in later lesions, fluid from under the eschar (obtained by holding the edge of the eschar up with tweezers and applying a capillary tube under the raised edge). In fatal cases, smears are made of blood, or lymph node or spleen aspirates; in meningitic cases, smears are made of cerebrospinal fluid. The ethanol- or heat-fixed smears, stained for 30 to 60 s with polychrome methylene blue (M'Fadyean stain) reveal the bacilli (blue-black, frequently square-ended in short chains) surrounded by the pink capsule.

In bacteriological confirmation, an isolate with typical colonial morphology that is non-haemolytic, non-motile, sensitive to the γ-phage and penicillin, and which produces the capsule is *B. anthracis*.

The approach to diagnosis is essentially the same for animals except that specimens will usually be from the dead animal. Traditionally an ear clipping is taken (to minimize spilling blood) and smears and culture are made on fluid from the soft tissue of these. However, the non-clotting blood characteristic of the disease usually makes it possible for blood to be aspirated into a syringe from some vein and, for the purposes of smears and culture, this is the approach to be recommended for herbivorous animals. In more resistant species such as pigs, dogs, and cats, the blood may not carry large numbers of *B. anthracis* at death and fluid from enlarged mandibular or suprapharyngeal lymph nodes may be required to confirm diagnosis.

Selective approaches are available for isolation of *B. anthracis* from environmental samples, materials of animal origin or specimens from old carcasses, but these are not highly sensitive and, depending on how important it is to detect *B. anthracis* if present, it may be necessary to resort to isolation of the bacterium by injecting homogenized specimen into mice or guinea-pigs and re-isolating the *B. anthracis* when they succumb to anthrax. Injection in guinea-pigs remains the most sensitive method of detection and isolation of *B. anthracis* from difficult specimens, although, for ethical reasons, it is an approach of last resort to be taken only when absolutely essential or unavoidable.

Treatment

Penicillin or its relatives are the best antimicrobials. Isolates resistant to penicillin have only been reported on two or three occasions and there is no evidence that resistance, when it does occur, is readily transmissible.

A suitable course of treatment is benzylpenicillin, 250 000 units 6-hourly for 3 to 5 days: the sore becomes sterile within 24 to 48 h. In severely toxic or late cases, the first doses may be given intravenously. *B. anthracis* is sensitive to many other broad-spectrum antibiotics; these include tetracyclines, chloramphenicol, gentamicin, and erythromycin, but there is no need to use these drugs unless the organism is reported as resistant to penicillin or the patient is truly sensitive to it. It is the experience of some veterinarians that treatment with tetracylines is not always fully effective.

Despite the rapid effect of antibiotics on the infecting *B. anthracis*, the eschar takes a long time, sometimes several weeks, to pass through its cycle of development and resolution and there is no way of hurrying this (Fig. 6). As emphasized above, the urge to incise must be resisted. There are no live anthrax bacilli in the lesion after the course of treatment and no need to keep the patient in hospital until the scab separates.

On resolution, there is usually a pale scar left on the skin. Very occasionally there is damage to the underlying tissue sufficient to require surgical repair. This is especially so where the eyelid has been affected.

In pulmonary, intestinal, or hypertoxic cases, penicillin is still the best drug but the patient needs intensive care as well. In late stages of infection, even if treatment overcomes the bacteraemia, toxin-induced shock may still lead to death. With the availability of modern plasmaphoresis techniques, plasmaphoresed serum or gammaglobulin from a vaccinated person could well be of life-saving value in an emergency.

As indicated earlier, when there is much oedema in the neck region and breathing is threatened, it is wise to do tracheotomy early.

Prevention

In highly developed countries, anthrax is not an epizootic disease. Well-supervised disposal of carcasses from the occasional cases of anthrax that occur in cattle, sheep, pigs, or horses and of materials contaminated from these carcasses, and disinfection of affected premises, backed up by immediate vaccination of other members of the affected herd ensure

Fig. 6 Anthrax: healing eschar.

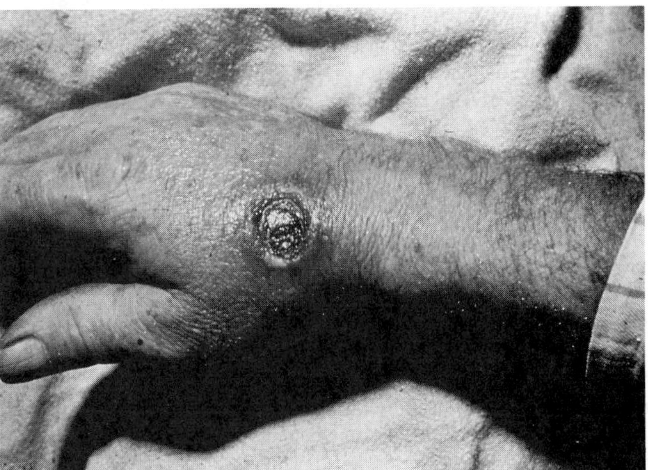

good containment and control of the disease. In Britain, when a case of anthrax occurs in a herd, the herd is kept under close observation; antimicrobial therapy is administered at the first sign of fever in any of the animals. (As the livestock vaccine is a live vaccine, vaccination and antimicrobial therapy cannot be carried out simultaneously.)

In less developed countries, where shepherds and herdsmen roam over miles of arid country with their animals, these approaches are often impossible. Animals may die in large numbers in some areas. The only realistic approach is mass vaccination of animals against anthrax. However, this currently involves annual inoculation with the live spore vaccine (see below), and is, for logistical and economic reasons, frequently easier said than done. In many endemic regions, the animals graze over vast tracts of land beyond the reach of roads or vehicles and the limited resources of the veterinary services place severe limitations on everything from transport to syringes.

VACCINES

Credit for design of the vaccine that turned anthrax from the major scourge it once was throughout the world to an effectively controlled disease goes to Dr M. Sterne, whose live spore vaccine for livestock developed in the 1930s is still used in most countries where anthrax is still encountered. The vaccine consists of approximately 10^7 spores/ml of his strain $34F_2$ in 50 per cent glycerine–saline with about 0.5 per cent saponin, which acts as an adjuvant by causing irritation and inflammation at the vaccination site. The strain $34F_2$ was a rough avirulent dissociant derived from an isolate from a case of bovine anthrax. It was subsequently shown that this strain had lost plasmid pXO2 and, in being unable to produce the capsule, was more or less avirulent (see below). The strain still produces the toxin and protects by inducing antibody to protective antigen.

Although theoretically avirulent in being acapsular, the Sterne strain does retain a residual virulence and occasional casualties in sheep and laboratory animals are encountered with its use; goats seem to be especially susceptible to ill effects of live spore vaccination. As a result of this, the live vaccine was not considered suitable for human use in Western countries and acellular vaccines were developed in the United Kingdom in the 1950s and in the United States in the 1960s. The British vaccine consists of an alum-precipitated cell-free filtrate of Sterne strain cultures grown in such a way as to maximize the content of protective antigen.

From an understanding of the cycle of infection of anthrax (see Fig. 1) it is clear that control of anthrax depends on control of the disease in herbivorous animals, which, for most human purposes, means livestock. Administration of the human vaccine is therefore only indicated for persons in at-risk occupations such as wool, hide, meat and bonemeal processing, certain veterinarians, and laboratory workers.

With the unfortunate association that has developed between anthrax and biological aggression, military concerns about protection against the disease have provided the main impetus behind research into the pathogenesis of, and protection against, anthrax in recent years. Doubts about the rather crude human vaccines of the 1950s and 1960s, together with the recent rapid advances in the understanding of the pathogenesis of the disease, have led to the design of novel putative alternatives based on the newly acquired abilities to purify the toxin antigens and to engineer their production in alternative hosts to the original Sterne strain.

It has now been satisfactorily demonstrated that protective antigen is the essential single component for an effective anthrax vaccine but that a stimulant of cellular immunity is also necessary. In live vaccines, the host organism itself serves this purpose and one category of novel putative vaccines involves recombinants consisting of a host (the Sterne strain fully cured so that it produces no toxin or capsule, other *Bacillus* species or an invasive virus such as the vaccinia virus) carrying the protective antigen gene and the mechanism for expressing it.

Perhaps the greatest appeal of the recombinant approach is that, with an appropriate vector, it offers the potential for development of oral vaccines for both human and animal use. Salmonella-protective antigen recombinants, for example, are under development for this purpose. Apart from the general desirability of orally over parenterally administered preparations, such vaccines would be of considerable value in poorly developed areas or in outbreaks threatening endangered susceptible wildlife species where administration of large numbers of doses by syringe and needle is impossible. For animals at least, however, the obstacles to development of a vaccine that is effective in the target species and of a delivery system that guarantees uptake by the majority of targeted animals are formidable and will take many years to overcome.

In the meantime, as far as improved human vaccines are concerned, probably the best way to go in the more immediate future is towards a subunit vaccine consisting of purified protective antigen and a suitable adjuvant to produce the necessary cellular immune stimulus.

IN INDUSTRY

The graph of the decline in the incidence of human anthrax in Britain since the early part of the twentieth century (Fig. 7) is probably more attributable to improved industrial hygiene than any other reason. Part of this amounted to good ventilation, dust control measures, and so on; another part resulted from pretreatment of imported materials that could be so treated, such as wool and hair, which, from the 1930s to the 1960s, were disinfected by the Duckering process involving sequential soaks in 0.25 per cent soda liquor, soap liquor, and 2 per cent formaldehyde solution followed by rinsing and drying. Since 1970 it would appear that the contamination rates of imported wool and hair have decreased and only consignments found to be positive when tested for the presence of anthrax spores are now treated, this being by irradiation.

No process has been derived for the disinfection of hides and skins that does not damage them and association of anthrax with tanneries has remained stronger than it has with the wool and hair industries. Nevertheless, the marked reduction in the number of tanneries in recent years (presumably from the increased use of man-made alternatives) and the increasing tendency for the first stage of tanning to be done before hides or skins leave the exporting country have reduced the extent of imported anthrax from this source also.

Meal of imported bone, hoof, or horn origin for feeds and fertilizers remains a source of anthrax entering this country. However, although

Fig. 7 Graph showing the declining incidence of human anthrax in Britain in the twentieth century (kindly supplied by the PHLS Communicable Disease Surveillance Centre and reproduced with permission).

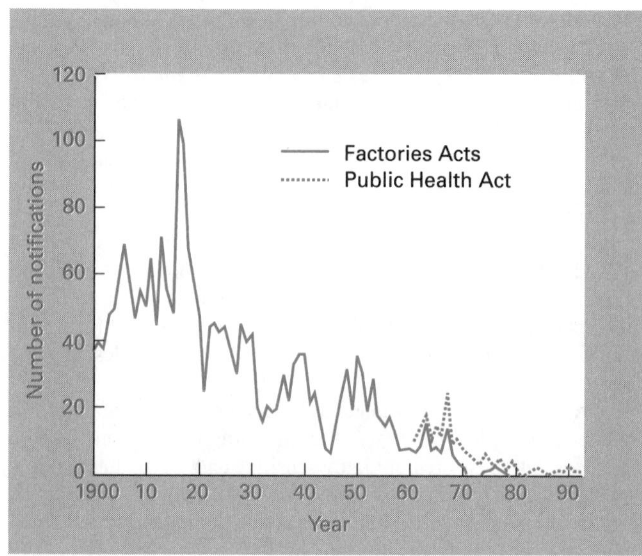

statutory requirements for sterilization of bonemeal do not exist, many manufacturers regard sterilization as good practice, thereby again reducing the likelihood of transmission of the disease through this type of product.

Most companies concerned with processing materials that may carry anthrax spores add the offer of vaccination to employees (see above) in addition to high standards of industrial hygiene. The result is that human anthrax is exceedingly rare in Britain today.

REFERENCES

Dahlgren, C.M., Buchanan L.M., Decker, H.M., Freed, S.W., Phillips, C.R., and Brachman, P.S. (1960) *Bacillus anthracis* aerosols in goat hair processing mills. *American Journal of Hygiene*, **72,** 24–31.

Heyworth, B. *et al.* (1975). Anthrax in the Gambia: an epidemiological study. *British Medical Journal*, **iv,** 79–82.

Leppla, S.H. (1991). The anthrax toxin complex. In *Sourcebook of bacterial protein toxins*, (ed. J.E. Alouf and J.H. Freer), pp. 277–302. Academic Press, New York.

Molloy, S.S., Bresnahan, P.A., Leppla, S.H., Klimpel, K.R., and Thomas, G. (1992). Human furin is a calcium-dependent serine endoprotease that recognizes the sequence Arg-X-X-Arg and efficiently cleaves anthrax toxin protective antigen. *Journal of Biological Chemistry*, **267,** 16396–402.

Turnbull, P.C.B. (1991). Anthrax vaccines: past, present and future. *Vaccine*, **9,** 533–9.

Turnbull, P.C.B., Doganay, M., Lindeque, P.M., Aygen, B., and McLaughlin, J. (1992). Serology and anthrax in humans, livestock and Etosha National Park wildlife. *Epidemiology and Infection*, **108,** 299–313.

Turnbull, P.C.B. *et al.* (1992). *Bacillus anthracis* but not always anthrax. *Journal of Applied Bacteriology*, **72,** 21–8.

Turnbull, P.C.B., Bohm, R., Chizyuka, H.G.B., Fujikura, T., Hugh-Jones, M.E., and Melling, J. (1993). *Guidelines for the surveillance and control of anthrax in humans and animals*. World Health Organization, WHO/Zoon, 93 107.

7.11.19 Brucellosis

M. M. MADKOUR

Brucellosis is a common, classical zoonotic disease of worldwide distribution. It is transmitted to man from infected animal reservoirs. Human brucellosis may be caused by one of four species: *Brucella melitensis* (the most common cause) from goats, sheep, and camels; *B. abortus* from cattle; *B. suis* from hogs; and *B. canis* from dogs. Brucella organisms are small, non-encapsulated, non-motile, non-sporing, Gram-negative, aerobic bacilli, which are facultative intracellular parasites. They can survive for up to 8 weeks in unpasteurized, white, soft goat's cheese. They tend to die within 60 to 90 days in cheese that has undergone lactic acid fermentation during the period of maturity. Freezing milk or its products does not destroy the organisms, but they are killed by boiling or pasteurization. Brucella organisms are shed in urine, stools, vaginal discharge, and products of conception. They remain viable in dried soil for up to 40 days and for longer if the soil is damp.

Epidemiology

There are only 17 countries in the world that are brucellosis free: Norway, Sweden, Finland, Denmark, Switzerland, the former Czechoslovakia, Romania, the United Kingdom including the Channel Islands, The Netherlands, Japan, Luxembourg, Cyprus, Bulgaria, Iceland, and the Virgin Islands of the United States. Canada and New Zealand are about to be declared brucellosis-free countries. However, the overall incidence of brucellosis in the world is increasing. With the ease of modern travel, patients may contract the disease while visiting endemic countries.

The true global incidence of human brucellosis is difficult to determine, because of the lack of essential statistics, disease reporting, and notification systems in many countries. Even in developed countries there are reports indicating that the incidence of human brucellosis is estimated to be 3 to 26 times higher than official figures.

THE RISK TO PUBLIC HEALTH

In endemic areas of developing countries, brucellosis affects predominantly males and younger age groups. Farm animals such as goats, sheep, camels, and cattle are kept in the backyards of houses and considered as pets. Children frequently come into close contact with them (Fig. 1) and may contract the disease. Childhood brucellosis indicates endemicity of the disease in that area. Serious human maternal morbidity and fetal loss through abortion, intrauterine death, and premature delivery, or active disease in neonates, are public health risks in endemic areas of developing countries. Where brucellosis is controlled in animals, human brucellosis is mostly an occupational disease, particularly among workers in meat-processing industries and in farmers, veterinarians, and laboratory workers.

MODES OF TRANSMISSION

In endemic areas, animal contact through inhalation of organisms is the most frequent cause of infection, particularly among children (Fig. 1), herdsmen, dairy-farm workers, and laboratory workers. Ingestion of untreated milk or its products, or raw meat, liver or bone marrow, is a common route of infection through the gastrointestinal tract, particularly among those taking antacids. Penetration of intact or abraded skin is a common route of infection among abattoir workers in developing and developed countries. Accidental autoinoculation or conjunctival splashing of live brucella vaccine during animal vaccination are well-recognized routes of infection among veterinarians. Transplacental transmission of infection from mother to fetus may occur. Brucella organisms have been isolated from human breast-milk, and nursing mothers may infect their infants through breastfeeding. Sexual transmission in man, similar to that in animals, has recently been reported, with isolation of the organisms from human semen. Other uncommon routes of transmission include blood transfusion and bone marrow transplants.

Pathogenesis

Polymorphonuclear leucocytes migrate to the site of entry and phagocytosis of the organism occurs. Activated macrophages play a similar

Fig. 1 In endemic areas the most common source of infection is animal contact. Farm animals are kept in the backyards of houses and are considered as pets. They are a risk to public health.

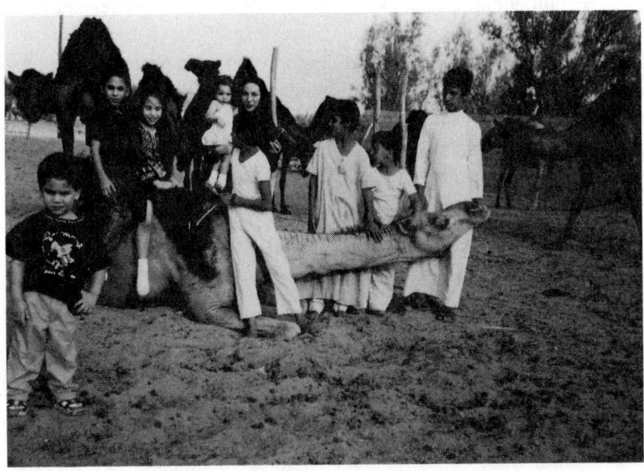

Table 1 *History and symptoms in 500 patients with brucellosis due to* B. melitensis

History/symptoms	Number	%
Animal contact	368	73.6
Raw milk/cheese	350	70.0
Raw liver ingestion	147	29.4
Family history	188	37.6
Fever	464	92.8
Chills	410	82.0
Sweating	437	87.4
Body aches	457	91.4
Lack of energy	473	94.6
Joint pain	431	86.2
Back pain	431	86.2
Headaches	403	80.6
Loss of appetite	388	77.6
Weight loss	326	65.2
Constipation	234	46.9
Abdominal pain	225	45.0
Diarrhoea	34	6.8
Cough	122	24.4
Testicular pain (of 290 males)	62	21.3
Skin rash	72	14.4
Sleep disturbances	185	37.0

Table 2 *Signs in 500 patients with brucellosis due to* B. melitensis

Signs	*N*	%
Ill looking	127	25.4
Pallor	110	22.0
Lymphadenopathy	160	32.0
Splenomegaly	125	25.0
Hepatomegaly	97	19.4
Arthritis	202	40.4
Spinal tenderness	241	48.0
Epididymo-orchitis	62	21.3
Skin rash	72	14.4
Jaundice	6	1.2
CNS abnormalities	20	4.0
Cardiac murmur	17	3.4
Pneumonia	7	1.4

role. The interaction between host and bacteria determines the outcome of the infection. Intracellular multiplication of the organisms may occur. They then pass through lymphatics to regional lymph nodes and organs rich in reticuloendothelial tissue. Other organs and tissues may be invaded through the bloodstream.

Cell-mediated immunity plays an important part in protection against brucella infection. Non-specific inflammatory-cell infiltrates or granulomas may develop. Caseation, necrosis, and abscess formation may also occur. Production of specific antibodies is important. IgM is the first to appear, followed a few days later by IgG. After a few months, the IgM level tends to fall while IgG remains high.

Clinical features

The incubation period is about 1 to 3 weeks but may extend up to several months. Brucellosis is a disease of protean manifestations that may simulate other febrile illnesses. Its clinical features are not specific. In endemic areas, diagnosis is relatively easy. However, in non-endemic areas of developed countries, clinicians should remember brucellosis in the differential diagnosis of a febrile illness. A history of travel to endemic areas should be obtained, as well as the patient's occupational history. The clinical features of brucellosis largely depend on the species of the organism and may vary widely. *B. melitensis* has a high pathogenicity, producing more intense symptoms. The onset may be sudden (1–2 days) or gradual (1 week or more). It presents as a febrile illness, with or without localization to particular organs. Brucellosis has been arbitrarily classified into acute, subacute, chronic, bacteraemic, serological, localized, or mixed types, which does not serve any purpose. The term 'active brucellosis with or without localization' may be more useful for the purpose of diagnosis and treatment. The most frequent symptoms are given in Table 1. The fever has no distinctive pattern that could differentiate it from other febrile illnesses, despite the old name 'undulant fever'. It usually shows diurnal variation, being normal in the morning and high in the afternoon and evening. Chills or rigors with profuse sweating may simulate malaria. Patients with brucellosis commonly look deceptively well and, less frequently, may look acutely ill. Physical signs may be lacking despite the multiplicity of symptoms, which may be labelled as psychological. The frequency of physical signs is shown in Table 2.

Complications

BONES AND JOINTS

Pathogenesis

Reactive arthritis may occur in brucellosis. Septic arthritis may result from blood-borne spread to the synovium or from extension of brucella osteomyelitis in a neighbouring long bone (Fig. 2). Brucella spondylitis starts in the superior end-plate, an area of rich blood supply. The infection may either regress and heal or progress to involve the entire vertebra, disc space, and adjacent vertebrae (Figs 3, 4, and 5). Early lesions are localized in the anterior aspect of the superior end-plate at the disc–vertebral junction, leading to a small area of bone destruction. Bone healing takes place at the same time, leading to sclerosis (Figs 3, 4, and 5).

Arthritis is commonly polyarticular and migratory, affecting mainly the large joints including the knee, hip, sacroiliac (Fig. 4), shoulder, sternoclavicular, wrist, ankle, and interphalangeal joints in decreasing order of frequency. Septic monoarthritis may lead to destruction of the affected joint if undiagnosed. Joints affected include the knee, hip, sternoclavicular and sacroiliac joints, and the shoulder. Spondylitis may involve single or less frequently multiple sites. The lumbar spine, particularly L4, is the most frequent site. The average age of onset of brucella spondylitis is 40 years; it is extremely rare during childhood.

Fig. 2 Brucella septic arthritis and osteomyelitis in a 22-year-old man with brucellosis. Scintigram showing increased uptake in the left knee and the distal half of the left femur.

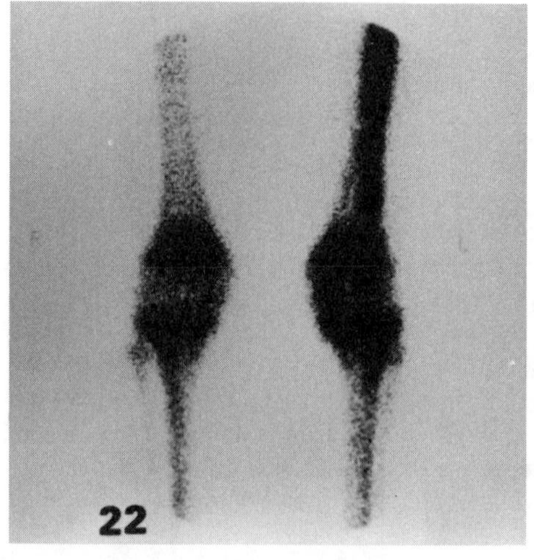

Extrasponal brucella osteomyelitis is rare. Long bones, particularly the femur (Fig. 2), tibia, humerus or manubrium sterni, may be affected. Bursitis, tenosynovitis, and subcutaneous nodules may also occur. Unlike with septic arthritis and osteomyelitis due to other organisms the peripheral white-cell count is normal and the erythrocyte sedimentation rate is normal or accelerated. The total white-cell count in synovial fluid ranges from 4000 to 40 000/mm^3 with 60 per cent polymorphonuclear cells. Glucose in synovial fluid may be reduced, but protein is usually raised and culture is positive in about 50 per cent of the cases.

Fig. 3 Advanced brucella spondylitis in a 51-year-old man. Lateral radiograph showing bone destruction of the superior end-plate of L4 and healing with osteophyte formation associated with reduction of the L3/4 disc space.

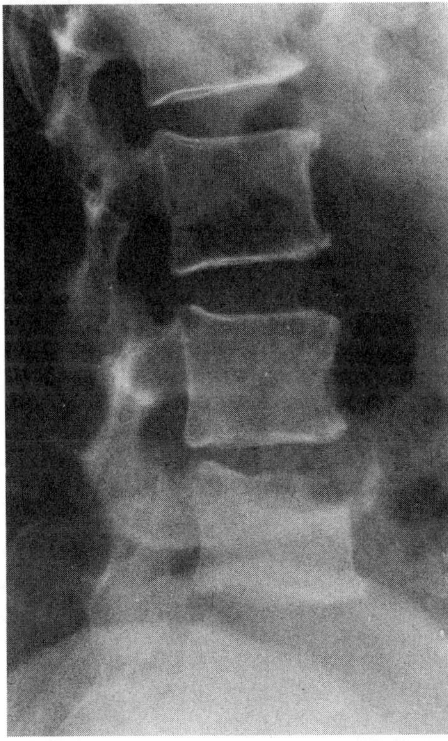

Fig. 4 Brucella spondylitis and sacroiliitis in a 38-year-old man with brucellosis. Posterior view of the scintigram showing diffuse increased uptake in the body of L3 and L4. Note the increased uptake in the left sacroiliac joint.

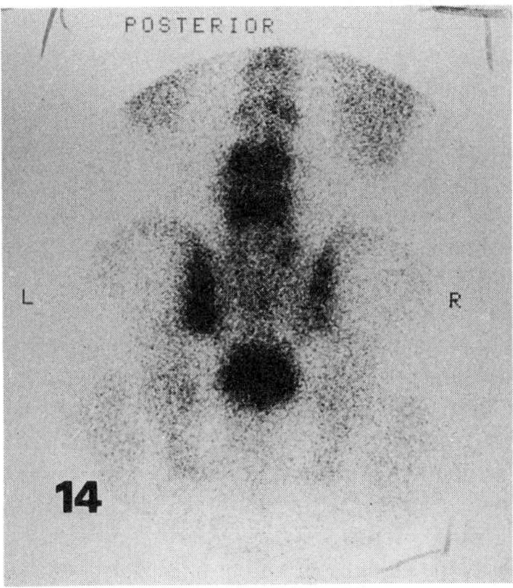

CARDIOVASCULAR

These complications may include endocarditis, myocarditis, pericarditis, aortic-root abscess, mycotic aneurysms, thrombophlebitis, and pulmonary embolism. The most frequent of these is endocarditis, which used to be the leading cause of death. The outcome is now more favourable with recent advances in diagnosis, cardiac surgery, and treatment. Brucella endocarditis usually occurs on a previously damaged valve or a congenital malformation (Fig. 6), but can occur even on normal valves. The clinical features are similar to those caused by other organisms. Patients who live in endemic areas and have what has been labelled as 'sterile infective endocarditis' should have their blood culture extended for a period of up to 6 weeks.

RESPIRATORY

Respiratory complications are common but, because they are usually mild, clinicians tend to overlook them. A flu-like illness with sore throat and mild dry cough is a common feature. Rarely, other complications may include hilar and paratracheal lymphadenopathy, pneumonia, solitary or multiple nodular lung shadowing, even with abscess formation,

Fig. 5 Brucella spondylitis: midsagittal magnetic resonance image with long *TR/TE* showing diffuse, high signal intensity in L3 and L4. Note the diffuse narrowing of the spinal canal at this level and the loss of definition of the posterior aspect of the vertebrae.

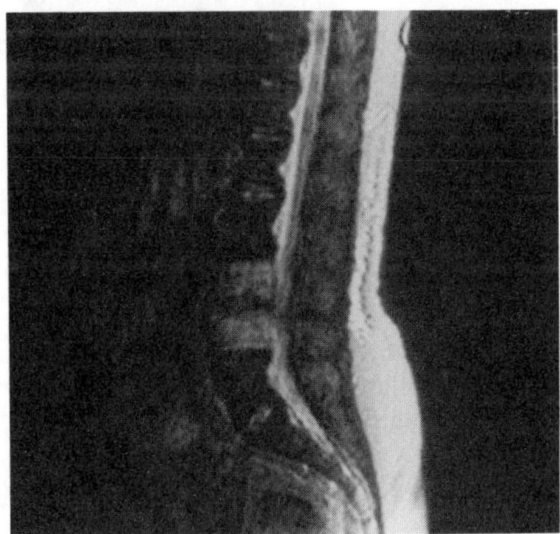

Fig. 6 Two-dimensional echocardiogram, parasternal long axis in a 6-year-old boy who had had tetralogy of Fallot and cardiac surgery 2 years earlier. He presented with fever and congestive cardiac failure and was found to have brucella endocarditis. The echocardiogram shows the presence of a vegetation on the Dacron patch in the ventriculoseptal defect. *Brucella melitensis* was grown from the blood and vegetations.

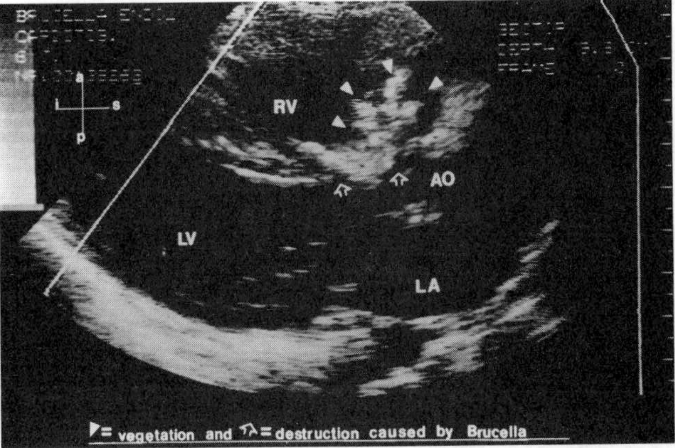

soft-tissue miliary shadowing, pleural effusion, empyema, or mediastinitis.

GASTROINTESTINAL

Gastrointestinal complications are usually mild and are rarely a presenting feature of the disease. They include tonsillitis, hepatitis with mild jaundice (either non-specific or granulomatous) (Fig. 7), with suppuration and abscess formation. Actual cirrhosis is rare. Deep jaundice is not a feature of brucellosis. Splenic enlargement with abscess formation is rarely reported. Mesenteric lymphadenopathy with abscess formation, cholecystitis, peritonitis, pancreatitis, and ulcerative colitis are described. The liver transaminases, alkaline phosphatase, and serum bilirubin may be mildly raised. The clinical and biochemical evidence of liver involvement is far less frequent than liver biopsies have indicated. The diagnostic significance of splenomegaly becomes doubtful in countries where malaria and bilharzia are also common.

GENITOURINARY

Genitourinary complications may be the presenting feature of brucellosis. They include unilateral or bilateral epididymo-orchitis in children and in adults, prostatitis, seminal vesiculitis, dysmenorrhoea, amenorrhoea, tubo-ovarian abscesses, chronic salpingitis, and cervicitis. Acute nephritis or acute pyelonephritis-like features, renal calcifications, and calyceal deformities may occur. Renal granulomatous lesions with abscess formation, with caseation and necrosis, may occur, as may cystitis and posterior urethritis.

Urine culture may be positive in about 50 per cent of patients with brucellosis. Brucella organisms have recently been isolated from human semen during investigation of possible sexual transmission.

NEUROBRUCELLOSIS

Neurobrucellosis is an uncommon but serious complication. Despite the multiplicity of symptoms, abnormal neurological findings may be lacking. They include meningoencephalitis, multiple cerebral or cerebellar abscesses, ruptured mycotic aneurysm, cranial-nerve lesions, transient ischaemic attacks, hemiplegia, myelitis, radiculoneuropathy and neuritis, Guillain–Barré syndrome, a multiple sclerosis-like picture, paraplegia, sciatica, granulomatous myositis, and rhabdomyolysis. The psychiatric features of brucellosis are no greater than those caused by other infections. Neurobrucellosis may be caused by direct blood-borne invasion by brucella organisms, pressure from destructive spinal lesions, vasculitis, or an immune-related process. In meningoencephalitis the cerebrospinal fluid pressure is usually elevated and the fluid may look clear, turbid, or, rarely, haemorrhagic; the protein, cells (predominantly lymphocytes), and oligoclonal immunoglobulin are raised, while glucose may be reduced or normal. Brucella organisms may be cultured from cerebrospinal fluid.

Fig. 7 Photomicrograph of a liver biopsy from a patient with brucellosis showing a macrogranuloma composed of epithelioid cells and giant cells. Haematoxylin and eosin; × 120.

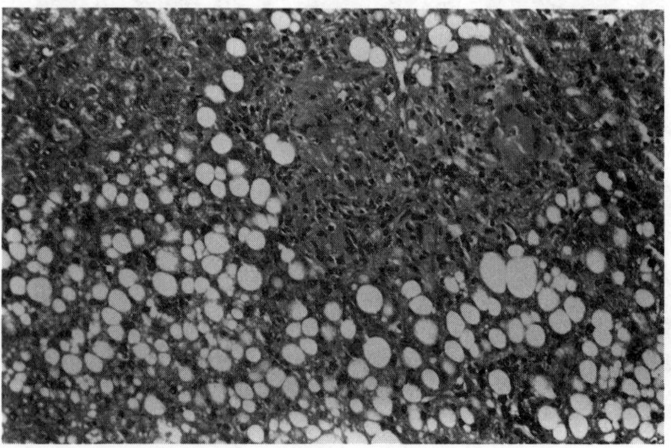

PREGNANCY

In endemic areas the outcome of pregnancy in man is similar to that in animals: normal delivery, abortion, intrauterine fetal death, premature delivery, or retention of the placenta and other products of conception.

SKIN

Skin complications are uncommon. They include maculopapular eruptions and contact dermatitis, particularly among veterinarians and farmers assisting animal parturition. Other dermatological manifestations include erythema nodosum, purpura and petechiae, chronic ulcerations, multiple cutaneous and subcutaneous abscesses, vasculitis, superficial thrombophlebitis, discharging sinuses, and (rarely) pemphigus.

OCULAR

Direct splashing of live brucella vaccine into the eyes may cause conjunctivitis. Keratitis, corneal ulcers, uveitis, retinopathies, subconjunctival and retinal haemorrhages, retinal detachment, and endogenous endophthalmitis with positive vitreous cultures are well documented. Neuro-ophthalmic complications of brucella meningitis may lead to papilloedema, papillitis, retrobulbar neuritis, optic atrophy, and ophthalmoplegia due to lesions of the IIIrd, IVth and VIth cranial nerves.

OTHER RARE COMPLICATIONS

Thyroiditis, adrenal insufficiency, and the syndrome of inappropriate secretion of antidiuretic hormone have been reported.

Diagnosis

The diagnosis of brucellosis depends on the presence of clinical features together with a positive blood culture or tissue culture and/or the detection of raised brucella agglutinins in the patient's serum. Most authorities will consider a agglutination titre of 1/160 or higher to be significant in a symptomatic patient living in a non-endemic area. However, in endemic areas only titres of 1/320 to 1/640 or higher are considered significant. In endemic areas, otherwise asymptomatic individuals offering to donate blood may be found to have high brucella titres and should not be considered to be suffering from brucellosis. Follow-up 2 to 4 weeks later is necessary in such individuals to exclude subclinical infection.

The presence of brucella antibodies in the patient's serum can be detected by the the standard tube test, rose bengal plate test, 2-mercaptoethanol test, antihuman globulin test (Coombs), radioimmunoassay, and enzyme immunoassay. The antigens commonly used for serological screening are prepared from *B. abortus*, which cross-reacts with *B. melitensis* and *B. suis* antibodies as well. However, they do not cross-react with *B. canis* antibodies. To detect these antibodies, antigen prepared from *B. canis* organisms is needed, but they are not available commercially. A cross-reaction with tularaemia and cholera may occur. This can be distinguished by testing simultaneously for brucella, tularaemia, and cholera antibodies. Occasionally, brucella agglutination tests are negative in patients with positive tissue cultures. The prozone phenomenon is a false-negative standard tube test caused by the presence of blocking antibodies in the α-globulin (IgG) and in the α_2-globulin (IgA) fractions. This phenomenon can be avoided by screening sera at low and high titres. An elevated IgM antibody indicates recent infection, while low titres indicate previous contact with the organism. An elevated IgG indicates active disease.

Extended incubation of blood cultures (for up to 6 weeks) should be requested if brucellosis is suspected. At least 10 ml of blood should be used, incubated at 37°C and subcultured on duplicate blood agar plates (with and without an atmosphere of 10 per cent CO_2). Blood or bone marrow cultures may be positive in 50 to 70 per cent of patients.

HAEMATOLOGICAL CHANGES

The total white-cell count is usually normal and leucopenia with relative lymphocytosis does not always occur. Thrombocytopenia is less common and haematological features of disseminated intravascular coagulation are rare. The erythrocyte sedimentation rate is of no diagnostic value. 'Liver function tests', liver biopsies, and cerebrospinal and synovial fluid changes have been discussed under pathogenesis and complications.

Treatment

Control and prevention of brucellosis should be directed primarily towards eradication of the disease in animals. The brucella organism is intracellular and therefore relatively inaccessible to antimicrobials. A combination of a tetracycline and an aminoglycoside remains the most effective regimen because of its synergistic effect. Oral doxycyline (100 mg, twice daily) is preferred to other tetracylines (500 mg, 6-hourly) because of its rapid and complete absorption from the duodenum, longer half-life (18–22 h), and more efficient tissue penetration (it is more lipid soluble). Suitable aminoglycosides are streptomycin, netilmicin or gentamicin. Streptomycin is given intramuscularly in a dose of 1 g/day for patients under 45 years of age and 0.5 to 0.75 g/day for older patients. The plasma trough concentration should be 1 to 2 μg/ml. Netilmicin, 4 to 6 mg/kg a day intramuscularly in two divided doses, can be used for outpatient treatment. The plasma trough concentration should be 2 to 4 μg/ml. Gentamicin is only used for patients in hospital as it is usually given as an intravenous infusion of 2 to 5 mg/kg daily, in divided doses, 8-hourly. The plasma trough should be 1 to 2 μg/ml. Combined therapy with a tetracycline and an aminoglycoside should be given for 1 month, followed by a tetracycline and rifampicin (600–900 mg/day as a single oral dose) or a tetracycline and co-trimoxazole (two tablets, 480 mg each, twice daily) for a further 1 to 2 months. This regimen has a relapse rate of 7 per cent. Shorter periods of treatment have a higher relapse rate. Most patients with brucellosis are treated as outpatients and only those with complications (e.g. endocarditis, neurobrucellosis, osteomyelitis, septic arthritis, and renal impairment), or who are pregnant or are infants, require admission to hospital.

Ciprofloxacin (750 mg, 8-hourly, oral) and other fluoroquinolones are synthetic broad-spectrum antibiotics with intracellular penetration used by some for treatment of brucellosis. There are reports of the development of resistance and cross-resistance with other quinolones and high relapse rates. Quinolones showed no synergism with other agents.

CHILDREN

Infants and children under 7 years of age should be treated with a combination of rifampicin and co-trimoxazole for 2 to 3 months. However, in those with serious complications in endemic areas where some discoloration of the teeth is of secondary importance, doxycycline can be used, in combination, as described above: doxycycline, 50 to 100 mg/day orally; gentamicin, infants aged up to 2 weeks, 3 mg/kg every 12 h—aged 2 weeks to 12 years, 2 mg/kg every 8 h intramuscularly or by slow intravenous injection or intravenous infusion; netilmicin, infants aged up to 1 week, 3 mg/kg every 12 h—aged over 1 week, 2.5 to 3 mg/kg every 8 h intramuscularly, or by intravenous injections or infusions; rifampicin, 10 to 20 mg/kg a day, either orally or by slow intravenous injection as a single daily dose; co-trimoxazole, infants and children up to 6 months of age, 8 to 10 mg/kg a day in two to four equally divided doses intravenously, or 200 mg/day sulphamethoxazole and 40 mg/day trimethoprim in two divided doses orally (5-ml suspension in two equally divided doses)—children under 40 kg in weight should be given 8 mg/kg every 12 h.

ENDOCARDITIS

Most patients with brucella endocarditis respond to antimicrobials alone and may require elective surgery at a later date for a pre-existing valve disease or congenital abnormalities. In a minority of patients, urgent surgery under the cover of antimicrobials may be required if the patient develops cardiac failure or aortic-root abscess.

PREGNANCY

The combination of co-trimoxazole and rifampicin for 2 to 3 months is the most suitable regimen.

RENAL IMPAIRMENT

Doxycycline can be used safely in patients with renal impairment and will not cause further deterioration of renal function. Aminoglycosides can be used only if there are facilities for measuring plasma drug concentrations and testing renal function. Otherwise, patients should be given doxycycline and rifampicin or doxycycline and co-trimoxazole for 2 to 3 months.

MENINGITIS

Rifampicin, 600 to 900 mg/day, should be added to the combination therapy for the whole duration of treatment.

Response to treatment

In acute brucellosis, patients become afebrile and other constitutional symptoms greatly improve within 4 to 14 days. The liver and spleen become impalpable within 2 to 4 weeks. Patients may experience an acute, intense flare-up of symptoms—the Jarisch–Herxheimer reaction—shortly after starting treatment, particularly with tetracyclines. This reaction is only transient and does not necessitate discontinuation of therapy. Follow-up of clinical, blood culture, and serological tests should be every 3 to 6 months for 2 years.

Human vaccine

Human vaccine for brucellosis, used in the former Soviet Union, China, and France, was found to be effective in reducing markedly the rate of infection. Two injections, each of 1 mg of phenol-insoluble fraction, were given 2 weeks apart. It provides effective but short-lived immunity and should be repeated every 2 years. Vaccination is indicated in workers with an occupational risk of developing brucellosis.

REFERENCES

Al-Jubair, K., Al-Fagih, M., Ashmeg, A., Belhaj, M., and Sawyer, W. (1992). Cardiac operation during active endocarditis. *Journal of Thoracic and Cardiovascular Surgery*, **104**, 487–90.

Al-Sibai, M.B., Halim, M.A., El-Shaker, M.M., Kahn, B.A., and Qadri, S.M. (1992). Efficacy of ciprofloxacin for treatment of brucella melitensis infections. *Antimicrobial Agents and Chemotherapy*, **36**, 150–2.

Madkour, M.M. (1989). *Brucellosis*. Butterworths, London. A complete up-to-date monograph on brucellosis which is enhanced by a large number of high-resolution, CT scans, scintigrams and magnetic resonance images.

Madkour, M.M. (1989). Occupation-related infectious arthritis. In *Baillière's Clinical Rheumatology*, Vol. 3, (ed. G. Balint), pp. 157–92. Baillière Tindall/Saunders, London.

Sharif, H.S. *et al.* (1989). Brucellar and tuberculous spondylitis: comparative imaging features. *Radiology*, **17**, 419–25.

Vanderam, B., Zech, F., de Cooman, S.I., Bughin, C., Gigi, J., and Wauters, G. (1990). Isolation of brucella melitensis from human sperm. *European Journal of Clinical Microbiology and Infectious Diseases*, **9**, 303–4.

7.11.20 Tetanus

F. E. Udwadia

Tetanus is an acute, often fatal disease, resulting from the contamination of a wound by *Clostridium tetani*, a spore-forming, Gram-positive, motile, rod-shaped, obligate anaerobic organism. Under anaerobic conditions the vegetative form of the organism produces a powerful exotoxin, which on reaching the central nervous system causes the increased muscle tone and spasms that characterize the disease.

EPIDEMIOLOGY

The spores of *C. tetani* are ubiquitous but the natural habitat is soil, particularly cultivated soil rich in manure. Spores are commonly found in animal faeces, may also be detected in human faeces, and can occasionally be recovered from house dust or from the air of occupied buildings, slums, and even hospitals and operating theatres.

Tetanus is a killer disease chiefly afflicting the poor, uneducated, and underprivileged people of the world. It is thus widely prevalent in India, Bangladesh, Pakistan, parts of South-East Asia, Africa, the eastern Mediterranean region, and South America. In these countries, where immunization programmes are inadequate, the disease is most common in the young and newborn. A recent survey in Uganda identified 15 neonatal tetanus deaths per 1000 live births. Worldwide, about 800 000 neonates die of tetanus each year. In the West, the disease is now increasingly rare. Even so, in the United States, 60 to 80 cases have been reported each year since 1980. The decline is related to effective immunization programmes, and also to richer economies, better medical services, education, and mechanization of agriculture. The disease in the West is more frequent in people older than 50 years, in whom effects of immunization have worn off, in the unimmunized, in the impoverished, and in drug addicts.

Neonatal tetanus (NT) has for all practical purposes been eradicated in Western countries and in North America. Current epidemiologic studies done by the WHO in 1992 have established that neonatal tetanus accounts for 50 per cent of neonatal mortality and 25 per cent of infant mortality in most developing countries. The majority of deaths occurred in the poorest countries of the world, with three WHO Regions accounting for 80 per cent of all deaths from neonatal tetanus—40 per cent of deaths in the South-East Asia Region [SEAR], and 20 per cent each in the African Region [AFR] and the Western Pacific Region [WPR] (Fig. 1). Even so, as compared to 1988, there has been a 20 per cent reduction in the neonatal tetanus mortality rate (NTMR), amounting to an estimated fall in global NTMR from 6.5 to 4.5 neonatal tetanus deaths/1000 live births.

Fig. 1 Estimated deaths from neonatal tetanus occuring by region, 1992.

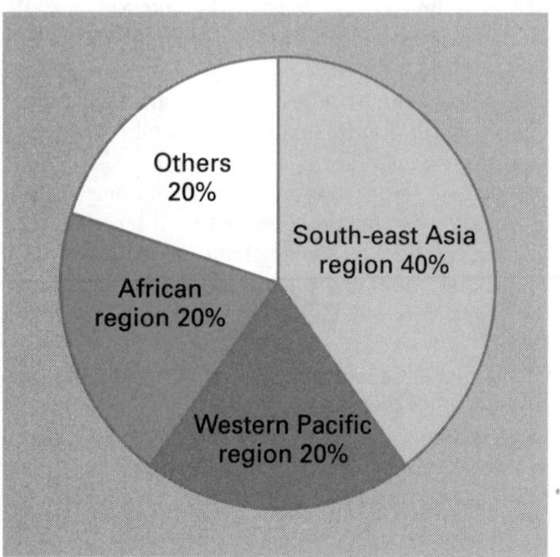

PHYSIOPATHOLOGY

Under anaerobic conditions (e.g. presence of necrotic tissue, active infection, foreign body), the tetanus bacillus within a wound produces two toxins—tetanospasmin and tetanolysin. Only tetanospasmin has clinical effects. The mechanism of spread of tetanospasmin is illustrated in Fig. 2. The released toxin spreads to underlying muscles and is bound to receptors containing gangliosides on the neuronal membranes of presynaptic nerve terminals. Unknown receptors other than gangliosides can also bind toxin. The toxin is then internalized and transported intra-axonally and retrogradely within peripheral nerves to cells of motor neurones of that segment of the cord supplying those muscles. The toxin almost always also enters, and circulates in the blood-stream. It does not cross the blood–brain barrier, but diffuses through the blood to bind to nerve terminals in muscles throughout the body. It is then transported retrogradely within numerous axonal pathways of all peripheral nerves to reach the α motor-neurone cell bodies of the whole spinal cord and brainstem. It thereby also reaches the sympathetic chain, the preganglionic sympathetic neurones in the lateral horns of the spinal cord, and the parasympathetic centres. After reaching the cell bodies in the spinal cord and brain-stem, the toxin, by an unknown mechanism, passes retrogradely across the presynaptic cleft to bind to ganglioside receptors on presynaptic nerve terminals of inhibitory interneurones. The main action of the toxin within the central nervous system is to block the release of inhibitory neurotransmitters, chiefly glycine and γ-aminobutyric acid, from nerve terminals of inhibiting neurones. This blockage releases motor and autonomic neurones from inhibitory control. The

Fig. 2 Retrograde intra-axonal transport of tetanospasmin and its main site of action in the CNS.

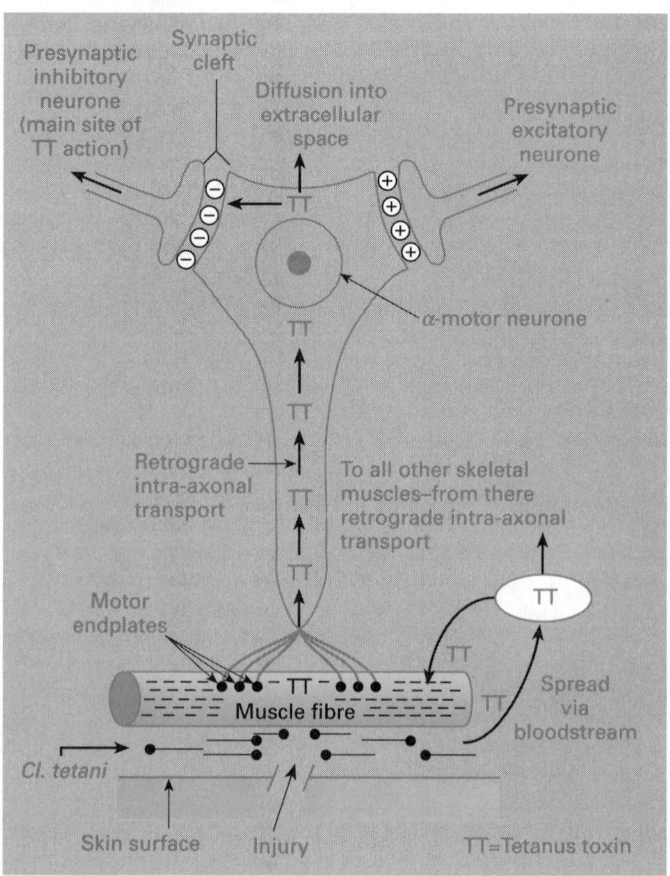

molecular mechanism behind this action is unknown. The toxin may well alter a calcium-dependent process necessary for neurotransmitter release. The uncontrolled, excessive, disinhibited efferent discharge from motor neurones in the cord and brainstem to both agonist and antagonist muscles leads to widespread muscle rigidity and to reflex spasms characteristic of generalized tetanus. Muscles of the jaw, face, and head are involved first because the toxin has to travel along shorter axonal pathways to reach their controlling motor neurones in the brainstem. Muscles of the trunk and limbs are involved a little later because the toxin travels longer axonal pathways to their controlling motor cells in the cord. Disinhibited autonomic discharge leads to disturbances in autonomic control, particularly to sympathetic overactivity with excessive catecholamines in the blood. Medullary centres and hypothalamic centres may also be affected by tetanus toxin.

When, rarely, tetanus toxin does not reach the bloodstream but spreads from the site of the wound along regional axonal pathways to motor neurones in a localized segment of the cord, local tetanus results. Rigidity and spasms are restricted to a group of muscles.

Tetanus toxin can also produce a peripheral neuromuscular blockade by preventing release of acetylcholine, similar to the effect of botulinum toxin. This peripheral paralytic effect is observed in cephalic tetanus.

Altered respiratory physiology

Hypoxia and hypocapnia are frequently observed. Hypoxia is due to ventilation–perfusion inequalities and to increase in venous admixture. Hypocapnia is related to tachypnoea. There is also an increase in the V_D/V_T ratio. Uncontrolled continuous seizures worsen hypoxia and cause mild to moderate hypercapnia. Pulmonary complications accentuate disturbances in respiratory physiology.

Altered haemodynamics

Severe tetanus without complications is characterized by a high-output, hyperkinetic circulatory state with marked tachycardia, increased stroke-volume index, increased cardiac index, and a normal, left ventricular stroke-work index (Fig. 3). There is also an increase in the compliance of the vascular system due to arteriolar, capillary, and venous dilatation, chiefly in skeletal muscle. These changes have been attributed to increased muscle contractions, increased sympathetic tone, and a rise in core temperature.

Disturbances in the autonomic nervous system can affect the circulatory state profoundly and are discussed under ‘Complications’. Specially interesting are occasional ‘autonomic storms’ characterized by wild fluctuations in sympathetic activity with corresponding changes in systemic vascular resistance, arterial blood pressure, and cardiac rate. These lead to cardiovascular instability and are dangerous for the patient.

Myocardial function after volume challenge is also suspect in severe tetanus. Whether this is related to tetanus toxin, to increased catecholamine levels in blood, or to unknown factors incidental to any critical illness remains uncertain.

Fig. 3 Haemodynamic observations in 19 patients with severe uncomplicated tetanus (means ± SD). Stippled areas are range of normal values. HR, heart rate; PCWP, pulmonary capillary-wedge pressure; CI, cardiac index; LVSWI, left ventricular stroke-work index; SVRI, systemic vascular-resistance index; PVRI, pulmonary vascular-resistance index.

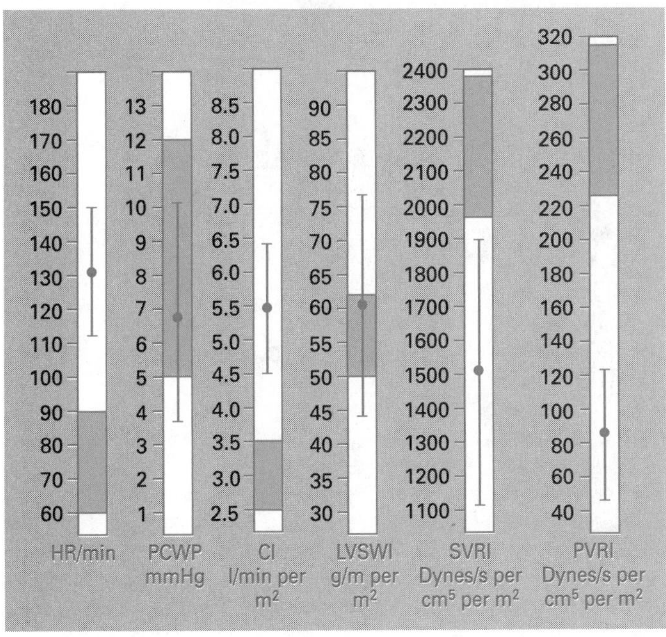

Other dysfunctions

Severe tetanus is associated with dysfunction of several other organ systems related to the management of the severe illness by prolonged ventilatory support, but the possibility of a direct action of tetanus toxin on other organ systems cannot be excluded.

CLINICAL FEATURES

Some 15 to 25 per cent of patients with tetanus have no evidence of a recent wound, for the disease can result from the most trivial of wounds; in fact it is more often seen with minor wounds, which are more likely to be neglected, than with major injuries. Contamination of the wound with garden soil or manure, or injury by rusty metals, are particularly dangerous. Tetanus can complicate burns, ulcers, gangrene, necrotic snake bites, discharging middle-ear infections, septic abortions, and childbirth. It can occur after intramuscular injections, particularly of drugs producing tissue necrosis (such as quinine), and after surgery. Tetanus neonatorum is most often due to non-sterile obstetric techniques, and in India to the dreadful practice of applying cowdung to the cut surface of the umbilical cord.

The clinical features of tetanus are rigidity, muscle spasms, and seizures. Severe tetanus is invariably associated with autonomic disturbances.

Muscle stiffness or rigidity

Stiffness of the masseters is often the first manifestation of the disease, resulting in difficulty in opening the mouth—trismus or lockjaw. In very mild cases this may be the main feature with, perhaps, just a hint of stiffness in other groups of muscles. Ordinarily, stiffness extends to muscles of the face, all skeletal muscles, and often involves muscles of swallowing causing dysphagia. The facial expression in tetanus is quite diagnostic. The eyes appear partially closed, the forehead is furrowed, the corrugator muscle contracted, the nostrils flared, nasolabial folds prominent, and the lips pursed, thinned and stretched, with the angles of the mouth extending outwards and often turned slightly down, producing a‘risus sardonicus’ (Fig. 4). This smile is perhaps more pathetic than sardonic. The expression is one of pain, anguish, and fear. Stiffness of the neck muscles results in retraction of the head. The muscles of the chest are stiff and the breathing movements are restricted. The abdomen often shows board-like rigidity. The arms and legs are often ramrod stiff and in children marked stiffness in the muscles of the back can lead to opisthotonos similar to that observed in meningitis (Fig. 5).

Muscle spasms

Mild cases of tetanus exhibit only stiffness without spasms. Spasms or seizures are characterized by a marked reflex exaggeration of the underlying rigidity, producing tonic contractions of the stiff muscles. They are frequently brought on by touch but may also be triggered by visual, auditory, or emotional stimuli. Seizures vary in severity and frequency. They may be mild, infrequent, and brief (lasting a few seconds) or severe, protracted, excruciatingly painful, and spontaneous, the patient appearing to be in a state of perpetual convulsion. Protracted severe spasms render breathing impossible or shallow, irregular and ineffective, so that the patient becomes very hypoxic and even cyanosed. Spasm of pharyngeal muscles prevents swallowing of saliva, so that pharyngeal secretions accumulate and are often aspirated into the lungs, causing atelectasis and aspiration pneumonia. Laryngeal spasm may occur by itself; it may accompany generalized spasms and can produce unexpected sudden death from asphyxia.

Patients with severe tetanus have fever, tachycardia, and, often, an unstable cardiovascular system. Unless expertly managed, they usually die of respiratory complications, circulatory failure, or cardiac arrest.

Autonomic nervous-system disturbances

In severe tetanus there is invariably involvement of the sympathetic and parasympathetic nervous systems. Features include tachycardia exceeding 150 beats/min despite curarization and without an undue increase in core temperature, drenching sweats for no apparent reason, frequent modest elevations in systolic and/or diastolic arterial blood pressure, increase in salivary and tracheobronchial secretions, and evidence of increased reflex vagal tone and activity.

Severity of tetanus

Grading the severity of tetanus is not just an academic exercise; it is useful both in prognosis and in the management of the disease. The criteria listed below are subjective and arbitrary but have stood the test of time in our unit.

Grade I (mild)

Mild to moderate trismus; general spasticity; no respiratory embarrassment; no spasms; little or no dysphagia.

Grade II (moderate)

Moderate trismus; well-marked rigidity; mild to moderate but short-lasting spasms; moderate respiratory embarrassment with tachypnoea in excess of 30 to 35/min; mild dysphagia.

Grade III (severe)

Severe trismus; generalized spasticity; reflex and often spontaneous prolonged spasms; respiratory embarrassment with tachypnoea in excess of 40/min; apnoeic spells; severe dysphagia; tachycardia in excess of 120/min.

Grade IV (very severe)

Features of grade III plus violent autonomic disturbances involving the cardiovascular system. These include episodes of severe hypertension and tachycardia alternating with relative hypotension and bradycardia, or severe persistent hypertension (diastolic pressure of more than 110 mmHg), or severe persistent hypotension (systolic pressure under 90 mmHg).

Cephalic tetanus

This occurs after an injury to the head and is confined to muscles innervated by the cranial nerves. It is characterized by unilateral facial palsy, trismus, facial stiffness of the unparalysed half, nuchal rigidity, pharyngeal spasms causing dysphagia, and frequent laryngeal spasms with danger of death from asphyxia. Rarely, facial palsy is bilateral (Fig. 6). Paresis of the glossopharyngeal, vagus, and rarely of the oculomotor

Fig. 4 Facies in tetanus.

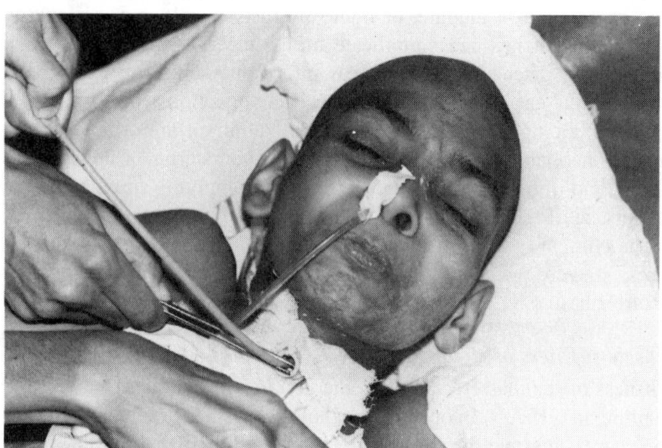

Fig. 5 Opisthotonos in severe tetanus during seizures.

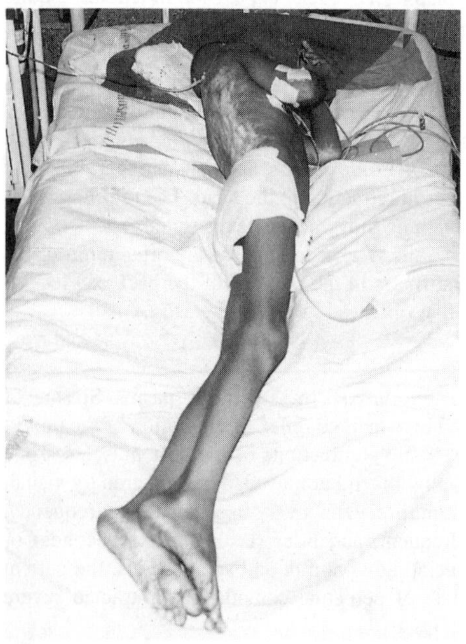

Fig. 6 Cephalic tetanus: patient with injury to left forehead presenting as bilateral VIIth lower motor neurone palsy (Photograph 1). Photographs 2–4 show stages in recovery and are taken at weekly intervals. It is important to note that the part of the face nearest the lesion recovers last. It is also noteworthy that during recovery the muscles become overactive as demonstrated by narrowed palpebral fissures (By courtesy of Dr F.D. Dastury.)

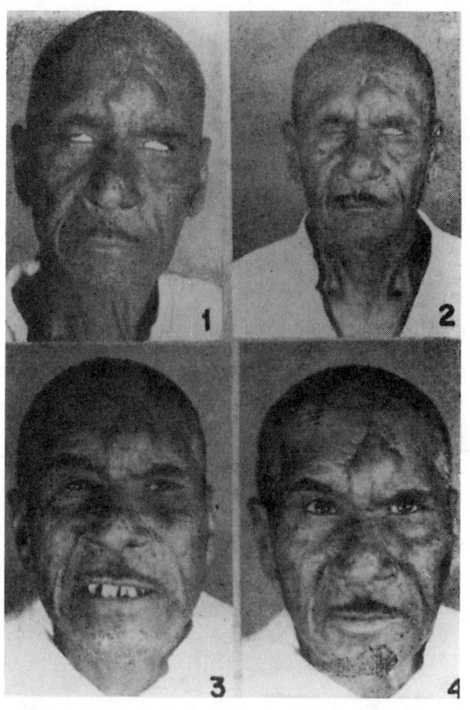

nerves may also occur. Cephalic tetanus may graduate to generalized tetanus.

Tetanus neonatorum

The earliest symptom is a difficulty and inability to suckle and swallow due to stiffness of muscles of the jaw and pharynx. There is increasing stiffness, with the classical tetanus facies (Fig. 7), flexion at the elbows with the fists clenched and drawn to the thorax, extension of the knees with plantar flexion of the ankles and toes, and opisthotonos. Muscle spasms make breathing difficult; autonomic disturbances are frequent and death results from cardiorespiratory failure.

Local tetanus

Rarely, rigidity and spasms may be localized to muscles adjacent to the wound or confined to a limb.

NATURAL HISTORY

The incubation period of tetanus (time between the injury and the first symptom) averages 7 to 10 days but may range from 1 to 2 days to 2 months. The period of onset is the time between the first symptom and the onset of spasms, and ranges from 1 to 7 days. The shorter the incubation period and the period of onset, the greater the severity of the disease. The period of onset is more reliable than the incubation period in gauging the severity of tetanus, as 20 per cent of patients give no history of injury and in these the incubation period is undetermined. The severity of tetanus increases to its maximum over a period of 7 to 10 days, remains at a plateau for the next 1 to 2 weeks, and then gradually declines over another 10 to 15 days. Muscle stiffness, painful myostatic contractions, and ankle clonus may persist for weeks after recovery. The natural history of tetanus is punctuated by numerous complications, as discussed later. Severe tetanus is a markedly catabolic process and significant weight loss is always observed, even in patients who recover.

COMPLICATIONS

The course and management of moderate and in particular severe tetanus is bedevilled by complications that can involve almost any organ in the body. Some of these complications, chiefly those involving the respiratory and cardiovascular systems, are inherent to tetanus. Others are related to the prolonged management of critically ill individuals paralysed by curare and on tracheostomy and ventilator support for 3 to 6 weeks.

Fig. 7 Characteristic facies in neonatal tetanus.

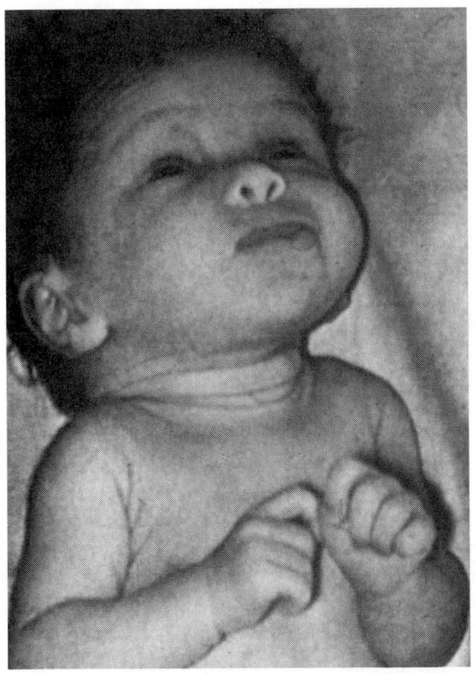

Respiratory

Respiratory complications include collapse, aspiration pneumonia, pneumonia, and bronchopneumonia. They are more frequent in patients treated conservatively but also occur in those treated with tracheostomy and ventilator support. Bronchopulmonary infections are generally due to Gram-negative organisms—chiefly klebsiellae, *Pseudomonas aeruginosa*, and Enterobacter. Prolonged laryngeal spasm if unrelieved can cause death. In fulminant tetanus, severe hypoxia and respiratory failure due to incessant spasms is inevitable if these patients are not curarized and ventilated. An unusual respiratory complication in moderate and severe tetanus is sudden episodes of severe respiratory distress with tachypnoea, not associated with an increase in hypoxia, hypercapnia or bronchospasm. These attacks are inexplicable but suggestive of a form of release of inhibitory control over the respiratory centre, probably due to the action of tetanus toxin. The adult respiratory distress syndrome may occur as a feature of complicating sepsis, but can also be caused by tetanus *per se.* Complications related to tracheostomy (particularly stomal infection) and to prolonged ventilator support (chiefly pneumothorax, pneumomediastinum, and pulmonary infection) are also observed.

Cardiovascular and autonomic

Cardiovascular complications in severe tetanus are chiefly mediated through the autonomic nervous system. Tachycardia, often as high as 170 to 180 beats/min, can persist for days. Persistent hypotension, labile hypertension, moderately severe persistent systolic and diastolic hypertension, and severe peripheral vasoconstriction with a shock-like state are all observed. Hypertensive patients are often exquisitely sensitive to β-blockers. 'Autonomic storms' are characterized by episodes of sudden sinus tachycardia (more than 150/min) with severe hypertension (blood pressure often 180–220/110–130 mmHg), followed within hours by a sudden slowing of the heart (50–90/min) with a fall in blood pressure (below 100 mmHg systolic). Such cardiovascular instability may be a forewarning of cardiac arrest and death. Increased vagal tone is evident at times by sudden, severe bradycardia and patients may arrest when the trachea is sucked out. Cardiac arrhythmias include supraventricular tachycardia, junctional rhythms, supraventricular and ventricular extrasystoles, and short bursts of spontaneously reverting ventricular tachycardia. Hyperthermia (over 41°C rectal) sometimes occurs abruptly; very rarely hypothermia is observed, suggesting involvement of the hypothalamus.

Sudden death

Sudden cardiac arrest causing death remains the single most dreaded complication of moderate and severe tetanus. It occurs under the following circumstances:

- marked cardiovascular instability due to fluctuating sympathetic tone;
- excessive vagal activity causing reflexly induced bradycardia and arrest, as during suctioning of the pharynx and trachea;
- severe hypoxia due to unrelenting seizures or prolonged laryngeal spasm;
- abrupt rise in core temperature (to in excess of 41°C) causing cardiovascular collapse;
- impaired infranodal conduction, perhaps due to tetanus toxin *per se*;
- massive pulmonary embolism;
- for no obvious reason.

Other complications

These are generally incidental to the prolonged and difficult management of critically ill individuals on ventilator support. The most dreaded complication is septicaemia, with the evolution of the sepsis syndrome with multiple organ failure. Sepsis is iatrogenic and is usually due to Gram-negative organisms—chiefly klebsiellae and *Ps. aeruginosa*. The potential sources of sepsis are the tracheostomy wound, central venous lines, urinary catheters, ventilator tubings, pulmonary infection, infected bedsores, and septic peripheral thrombophlebitis. Gastrointestinal complications are very common and include upper gastrointestinal bleeds, ileus, and diarrhoea. Renal insufficiency can result from sepsis or the use of aminoglycosides, from prerenal factors, or from multiple causes. Fluid and electrolyte disturbances (in particular hypokalaemia and hyponatraemia) are common and are aggravated by profuse sweating. Fractures, generally of one or more midthoracic vertebrae, may occur during severe spasms, particularly when these are poorly controlled. They produce no neurological sequelae, little or no pain, and generally heal without any significant deformity. Miscellaneous complications include tendon injuries, thrombophlebitis, peripheral neuropathy, bedsores, and corneal ulcers. Anaemia and hypoproteinaemia are frequently observed in long critical illnesses. Deep-vein thromboses are a complication of immobility and hypovolaemia; massive pulmonary embolism may result.

DIAGNOSIS

The diagnosis is based solely on the clinical features. Absence of a wound does not exclude tetanus. Trismus produced by tetanus should be distinguished from masseteric spasm due to an alveolar or peritonsillar abscess. Dystonic reactions caused by phenothiazines and metoclopramide, and spasms due to hypocalcaemic tetany may mimic the disease superficially. Meningitis and meningoencephalitis can also produce trismus, rigidity, seizures, and opisthotonos, but can be differentiated by examination of the cerebrospinal fluid, which is normal in tetanus. Cephalic tetanus can be mistaken for rabies because of severe dysphagia. However, hydrophobia never occurs in tetanus.

MORTALITY

The prognosis and mortality depend upon the severity of tetanus. A short incubation period (under 4 days) and a short period of onset (under 2 days) signal the rapid evolution of severe disease and are associated with a high mortality (over 50 per cent). Tetanus neonatorum carries a mortality of 60 to 80 per cent. The mortality rate in various reported series from different countries ranges between 20 and 60 per cent, and is higher in the older age group. Until recently the overall mortality from tetanus in Bombay was around 30 per cent, and from severe tetanus in patients admitted to a large teaching hospital in Bombay over 70 per cent, often approaching 100 per cent. This high mortality was related to the failure to grasp the importance of critical care and ventilatory support in severe tetanus. The introduction of these features in management reduced the overall mortality to 12 per cent and the mortality in severe tetanus to 23 per cent. Again, out of 34 adult patients with very severe tetanus admitted to a well-equipped intensive care unit at a private hospital in Bombay, there were just two deaths (mortality 6 per cent). Thus, despite adverse prognostic factors, the mortality of severe tetanus in adults is drastically reduced with the effective use of the management principles outlined below.

MANAGEMENT

Mild tetanus (grade I) poses no serious problems except when complicated by a serious septic wound, which can itself cause death. However, it is important to stress that grade I (mild) tetanus can progress over a period of days to grade II (moderate) or even grade III and grade IV (severe) tetanus. Such cases therefore merit close observation. Wherever possible, all patients with tetanus should be admitted to an intensive care unit. In the larger cities of India, patients with tetanus, who are almost always from the poorer strata of society, are admitted to special tetanus wards in government or municipal hospitals. Unfortunately, through lack of funds and through a strange apathy, these wards are generally ill-equipped and poorly staffed. Motivation and training for better patient care, coupled with basic equipment for respiratory care and support, can work wonders in reducing mortality even in the absence of full intensive-care facilities.

The use of antiserum

All patients should be given antiserum on admission to hospital. Equine antiserum is the only one generally available in poor developing tropical countries. Ten thousand units are given by slow intravenous injection after first doing a sensitivity test. However, fatal anaphylaxis can occur even when no skin hypersensitivity is demonstrable (see also rabies and snake bite). Human tetanus immunoglobulin, which is superior to the equine antiserum, produces no hypersensitivity reaction and, if available, should be given in preference to the equine in a dose of 3000 to 5000 units intravenously or intramuscularly. The intrathecal use of tetanus antiserum is best avoided as claims for its efficacy remain unproven. Local infiltration of 3000 units of tetanus antitoxin around an obvious wound is still practised in some units, though again its efficacy is difficult to prove. Antitoxin has no action on toxin that has already been fixed to nervous tissue; at best one can hope that it serves to neutralize any newly liberated or unbound tetanus toxin. Antiserum should be given before local manipulation of the wound, which is treated according to usual surgical principles with debridement of necrotic tissue and delayed primary suturing.

Antibiotics

Two mega units of crystalline penicillin are given intravenously 6-hourly for 8 days. Though effective against *C. tetani in vitro*, its use in this disease is disappointing. Other antimicrobials may be necessary to counter secondary complicating infections. Metronidazole, 500 mg intravenously 8-hourly for 10 days, has also been currently recommended.

Management strategies

Mild or grade I tetanus should be treated conservatively with the use of sedatives and muscle relaxants. Patients with grade II or moderate tetanus should, in addition to sedatives and relaxants, have a tracheostomy. Patients with grade III or IV (severe) tetanus require sedation, tracheostomy and continuous ventilatory support after they have been paralysed with curare-like drugs, until spasms relent and recovery ensues.

Use of sedatives and muscle relaxants

This forms the traditional conservative management of tetanus. Its aim is to reduce rigidity and control spasms without significantly depressing respiration. It remains the cornerstone of management of mild (grade I) and moderate (grade II) tetanus. Drugs used include diazepam, chlorpromazine, phenobarbitone, paraldehyde, mephenesin, and meprobamate. Diazepam is most frequently used; the dosage in children and adults is 5 to 20 mg thrice daily and in neonates 2 mg thrice daily. In mild tetanus it is given orally; in moderately severe tetanus it is best given by slow intravenous infusion over 24 h. It is best not to exceed a dose of 80 to 100 mg/24 h in adults, even in the presence of marked rigidity. Higher doses will inevitably depress respiration. Some units prefer the use of chlorpromazine, 50 mg four times a day intramuscularly in adults, 25 mg in children, and 12.5 mg in neonates. Combinations of diazepam and chlorpromazine, or diazepam, chlorpromazine, and phenobarbitone, can be used if there is no alternative. The dose of phenobarbitone is 200 mg in adults, 100 mg in children and 30 mg in neonates, given intramuscularly every 8 or 12 h. The ideal sedative and muscle-relaxant schedule for each patient should be tailored to ensure continuous sedation at a level that ensures sleep, but that still allows the patient to be aroused to obey commands. An objective guide, particularly in moderately severe tetanus, is relaxation of the abdominal muscles, which feel much less stiff to palpation. Laryngeal spasm should be countered by the prompt intravenous injection of 50 mg chlorpromazine, 10 to 20 mg diazepam, or succinylcholine.

Tracheostomy

This is mandatory for severe (grade III, IV) tetanus. It should also be done in moderate tetanus, simply because even in an intensive care unit the most important preventable cause of death is a sudden, prolonged laryngeal spasm leading to asphyxia. The patient's inability to swallow secretions and the use of heavier sedation in many cases of moderately severe tetanus are both indications for elective tracheostomy.

Induced paralysis with ventilator support

Severe tetanus (grade III, IV) has an appallingly high mortality when managed conservatively with high doses of sedatives and muscle relaxants. These patients not only require prompt elective tracheostomy but also ventilatory support after neuromuscular blockade and paralysis by curare-like drugs (gallamine, pancuronium, vecuronium). These are essential when good intensive-care facilities are available, and can be used even when good monitoring facilities are lacking, provided that the unit or ward has trained medical and nursing staff and the basic equipment for respiratory care. Results in such units may not be as good as in well-staffed and -equipped intensive care units, but are still far superior to those obtained with conservative management alone. Pancuronium or gallamine are generally available in poor countries; the former is to be preferred, as it has little or no effect on the cardiovascular system. Pancuronium, 2 to 4 mg, or gallamine, 20 to 40 mg, are given intravenously. The dose and frequency of administration are titrated for each patient, so that the ensuing neuromuscular blockade and paralysis allows efficient ventilator support. This is checked by periodic measurements of arterial $Pa\text{O}_2$, $Pa\text{CO}_2$, and pH. Initially the curare-like drug may be needed every 0.5 to 1 h for 1 to 2 weeks; as the patient improves the interval may be extended to 2, 4, or 6 h. Patients with fulminant tetanus with incessant spasms may be virtually impossible to paralyse completely. Twitches invariably break through within half an hour of the use of the drug, but these do not interfere with efficient ventilatory support. The average period of ventilatory support in severe tetanus is around 3 to 4 weeks, but may vary from 10 days to 6 weeks. Once spasms cease, pancuronium is stopped; ventilator support is continued until the patient is deemed fit to be weaned. The tracheostomy tube is removed only when patients can handle their upper respiratory secretions by coughing and swallowing effectively.

Many units continue to use high doses of sedatives and muscle relaxants (most commonly diazepam, 120 to 150 mg a day intravenously) even during the period of induced paralysis and ventilator support. This is unnecessary, unwise, and probably dangerous. Excellent results are obtained with not more than 30 to 40 mg diazepam given intravenously over 24 h. This schedule dulls the edge of anxiety without depressing vital centres.

In poor countries the management of severe tetanus is often constrained by paucity of trained nursing staff and material resources (in particular of ventilators). Ethical considerations then restrict the use of ventilator support to (a) patients with grade IV tetanus; (b) patients with grade III tetanus whose spasms are uncontrolled on a conservative regimen and whose $Pa\text{O}_2$ is below 55 mmHg on 6 to 8 l oxygen/min; (c) patients who develop lung collapse, pneumonia or any other serious complication that itself merits ventilatory support.

Treatment of autonomic circulatory disturbances

A number of drugs have been tried to control autonomic cardiovascular disturbances and 'autonomic storms' in severe tetanus. These include β-blockers, heavy sedation, intravenous morphine, intravenous labetalol, intravenous infusion of magnesium sulphate, and intravenous clonidine. These do not significantly alter the high mortality. It is best to rely on good overall care, efficient cardiorespiratory support, and to avoid drugs that strongly depress the central or autonomic nervous systems. Drugs acting on the cardiovascular system should be used sparingly, with constant monitoring, and only when they are deemed absolutely essential to alter grossly deranged haemodynamics. Hypotensive spells are treated with a volume load and if this is ineffective or contraindicated, by inotropic support with dopamine or dobutamine titrated to maintain a systolic pressure just above 100 mmHg. Hypertensive episodes with a systolic blood pressure in excess of 200 mmHg or a diastolic in excess of 100 mmHg are treated with a small oral dose of propranolol (5–10 mg) or 5 mg of sublingual nifedipine. Bradyarrhythmias are treated with intravenous atropine and persistent sinus tachyarrhythmias of more than 170/min with oral verapamil, 40 mg twice or thrice daily. In this situation it is best not to use more than 30 to 40 mg of diazepam intravenously per day. Sedatives and drugs used in a dose that strongly depress the central or autonomic nervous systems probably contribute to a high mortality by predisposing to cardiac arrest (particularly after acute hypotensive spells and sudden bradyarrhythmias) and by preventing successful resuscitation. These management principles have achieved a very low mortality (6 per cent) in severe tetanus.

Treatment of other complications

Prompt and correct diagnosis will allow appropriate treatment of complications arising during the natural course and management of severe tetanus. These complications may involve almost every system in the body.

Critical care and nursing

Critical care of the whole patient and expert nursing play a vital part in reducing complications and preventing death. External stimuli should be reduced to a minimum and physical examination should be gentle, as even touch easily triggers spasms in tetanus. The airway should be kept patent by gentle suction of pooled saliva and secretions at the back of the throat. Care of the tracheostomy in all its minutest detail is of great importance. Gentle, frequent change of posture and expert physiotherapy to the chest to open up collapsed lobes or segments are vital. A small intravenous bolus dose of diazepam should be given before physiotherapy, and in those on neuromuscular blockade, physiotherapy should be done while the patient is under the maximal influence of pancuronium or gallamine. The following are particularly important:

- Maintaining adequate arterial $Pa\text{O}_2$, oxygen saturation, and oxygen transport to the tissues.
- Maintaining fluid, electrolyte, and acid–base balance.
- Maintaining circulatory support in critically ill hypotensive patients—either by using a volume load or a slow intravenous infusion of dopamine at 5 to 10 μg/kg per min. A central venous line with monitoring of central venous pressure is very useful. Haemodynamic monitoring of pulmonary arterial pressure, pulmonary capillary-wedge pressure, and cardiac output often helps management.
- Prevention, early detection, and prompt control of infection and sepsis with appropriate antibiotics.
- Detecting (by frequent monitoring) and treatment (by physical methods and by paracetamol) of hyperpyrexia—a surreptitious killer in tetanus.

Nutrition

Tetanus is a dreadfully catabolic disease and so good nutrition is important for survival. A caloric intake of 3500 to 4000 calories with at least 100 g of protein is given in the form of semiliquid and liquid food through a nasogastric tube. A nasogastric tube can precipitate severe laryngeal spasms and should be passed only after elective tracheostomy or appropriate sedation. Intravenous alimentation is necessary if ileus or severe diarrhoea develop.

PREVENTION

Tetanus is an easily preventable disease. Prevention is through active immunization with adsorbed tetanus toxoid (**ATT**) and through proper management of wounds and injuries.

Active immunization

Good immunization in infancy is achieved by the use of the triple vaccine (tetanus, diphtheria, whooping cough) in three doses at monthly intervals. Protection is absolute for 1 year, but partial protection remains without further booster doses for many years. A compulsory and well-implemented vaccination programme against tetanus in infants, with a booster dose at 4 to 6 years of age, would go a long way to reducing sharply the incidence of the disease in developing countries. All unimmunized individuals over 7 years old should also be given ATT or tetanus–diptheria toxoid in three doses—the first and second are given 6 weeks apart and the third 6 months after the second. Booster doses every 10 years are advocated, but would be practically impossible in the teeming populations of Third World countries. An attack of tetanus does not confer immunity, and so the patient needs to be actively immunized after recovery. The first dose of toxoid should be given during convalescence and the next two doses at the recommended intervals.

Immunization after minor uninfected wounds

ATT (0.5 ml) should be administered promptly if the immunization status is unknown, in unimmunized or partially immunized individuals, and in patients who have been adequately immunized by ATT if more than 10 years have elapsed since the last dose of the toxoid. In these circumstances, especially in poor countries, ATT is also given before emergency surgery, deliveries, and obstetric procedures. Passive immunization with equine tetanus antitoxin or with human tetanus immunoglobulin is not indicated for clean minor wounds.

Immunization after infected or major wounds

The indications for the administration of ATT in infected or major wounds are the same except that it would be safer to use a booster dose even in well-immunized individuals if more than 5 years have elapsed since the last dose of ATT. Passive immunization is recommended in all individuals who have not been immunized, who are partially immunized, or whose immunization status is unknown. Human tetanus immunoglobulin should be given in a dose of 250 to 500 units intramuscularly. If this is not available, equine antitoxin should be given in a dose of 5000 units intramuscularly.

Prevention of tetanus neonatorum

The incidence of neonatal tetanus is now considerably reduced but still remains horrendous in all developing countries of the world. In 1989, the World Health Assembly adopted the goal of elimination of neonatal tetanus by 1995, and the Expanded Programme on Immunization promoted a three-pronged strategy comprising: (i) immunization of all women in the childbearing age group with at least two doses of tetanus toxoid (preferably in the last two trimesters); (ii) provision of clean deliveries; (iii) strengthening of surveillance of neonatal tetanus to identify high risk areas. Implementation of the above-mentioned strategies has achieved gratifying results, but it is highly unlikely that the aim of eliminating neonatal tetanus by 1995 will be realized.

REFERENCES

Adams, E.B., Laurence, D.R., and Smith, J.W.G. (1969). *Tetanus*. Blackwell Scientific, Oxford.

Sutton, D.N., Trenlitt, M.B., Woodcock, T.E., and Nielsen, M.S. (1990). Management of autonomic dysfunction in severe tetanus: the use of magnesium sulphate and clonidine. *Intensive Care Medicine*, **16,** 75–80.

Trujillo, M.H., Castillo, A., Espana, J., Menzo, H., and Zefra, R. (1987). Import of intensive care management in the prognosis of tetanus: analysis of 641 patients. *Chest*, **92,** 63–5.

Udwadia, F.E., Lall, A., Udwadia, Z.F., Sekhar, M., and Vora, A. (1987). Tetanus and its complications: intensive care and management experience in 150 Indian patients. *Epidemiology and Infection*, **99,** 675–84.

Udwadia, F.E. *et al.* (1992). Haemodynamic studies during the management of severe tetanus. *Quarterly Journal of Medicine*, **83,** 449–60.

Udwadia, F.E. (1994). *Tetanus*. Oxford University Press, Bombay.

7.11.21 Botulism, gas gangrene, and clostridial gastrointestinal infections

H. E. LARSON

Botulism

DEFINITION

Botulism is an acute, symmetrical, descending paralysis of cranial and autonomic nerves produced by the exotoxin of *Clostridium botulinum*. Intoxication usually results from the ingestion of canned, smoked, or fermented foods contaminated by *C. botulinum* spores. Rarely *C. botulinum* infects wounds or colonizes the intestinal tract of infants and adults; symptoms can be produced by toxin absorbed from these sites.

OCCURRENCE

C. botulinum is an anaerobic, spore-forming micro-organism, widely distributed in soil and mud. Food is easily contaminated with spores, which survive brief periods of heating at 100°C. Subsequently, the anaerobic conditions required for food preservation also suit proliferation of the organism and release of toxin during storage. The occurrence of botulism reflects eccentricities in food preparation and use among different countries and ethnic groups. Cases have been associated with sausage preparation in Europe (Latin *botulus*, a sausage), fermented milk in Africa, home-canned vegetables in North America, fermented stew in Japan, and imported fish in the United Kingdom. Typically, outbreaks involve small groups of individuals, reflecting the domestic origin and use of the incriminated food product. However, home-canned peppers served in restaurants in the United States caused two large outbreaks. Botulism is rare in the United Kingdom, there having been nine outbreaks between 1922 and 1989 involving a total of 46 persons. This is probably because home canning is discouraged and people of British origin are disinclined to eat exotic fermented dishes.

Outbreaks caused by commercially processed foods are infrequent, but there is the potential for correspondingly greater impact where ingredients from several suppliers are blended and foods widely distributed. Some outbreaks have involved only single contaminated items, such as in the Loch Maree episode in 1922 where eight people died after eating duck paste, the 1978 outbreak in Birmingham involving four people who ate tinned Alaskan salmon, and one case in 1989 following a meal on a commercial airliner. Blown cans call attention to the possibility of spoilage, but in the Birmingham case spoilage may not have been noted because gas resulting from bacterial fermentation leaked out of a small defect in the can. Contamination of hazelnut purée added to commercially produced yogurt caused 27 cases of botulism in Wales and north-west England in June 1989, the largest recorded outbreak of food-borne botulism in the United Kingdom. Most of the potentially contaminated cartons could not be accounted for, suggesting variability in attack rate or failure to diagnose mild symptoms. Commercially prepared chopped garlic in soybean oil was responsible for 36 cases in North America. Cases were dispersed over at least eight provinces and states in three countries. Uneviscerated fresh fish has recently been associated with botulism, usually where there have been deficiencies in refrigeration.

AETIOLOGY

Seven types of *C. botulinum* are distinguished (A–G), depending on the serological specificity of the toxin produced. Types A, B, and E account for nearly all human cases; types F and G are rare. Types C and D are chiefly responsible for botulism in domestic and wild fowl, and may cause economically significant losses. Toxin production by types C and D depends on the presence of specific prophages. The serotypes implicated in outbreaks of botulism generally parallel the geographical distribution of spores in soil. Type E is nearly always associated with fish, but because outbreaks caused by fish products involve types A and B as well as E, a serotype cannot be inferred from the clinical history.

Spores of *C. botulinum* are more resistant to heating than those of other pathogenic clostridia. They can survive up to 2 h of boiling (100°C), but are killed rapidly at autoclave temperatures (120°C).

THE TOXIN

C. botulinum produces a heat-labile, protein neurotoxin, which is one of the most potent substances known. The lethal dose for mice is in the range of 10 pg. The molecule (150 kDa) is composed of two peptide chains connected by disulphide bonds. The biological activity appears to be dependent upon the dichain structure. Botulinum toxin can be detoxified by treatment with formalin with retention of its ability to elicit antibody formation. In cultures the toxin first appears as a protoxin, which is subsequently activated by a trypsin-like enzyme. Botulinum toxin is rapidly inactivated by heating at ordinary cooking temperatures. For example, it loses activity at 80°C in 5 min and at temperatures above 85°C in 1 min or less. Botulinum toxin is used to produce temporary muscle weakness in the treatment of strabismus, blepharospasm, and torticollis.

PATHOGENESIS

Botulinum toxin is absorbed directly across mucous membranes; tissue invasion by replicating organisms does not regularly occur. Locally acting toxin may produce some symptoms but cranial-nerve paralysis results from bloodstream distribution. Cranial nerves are preferentially affected because botulinum toxin binds more rapidly to sites where the cycles of depolarization and repolarization are frequent. Binding is irreversible and the toxin cannot thereafter be neutralized by antitoxin. Recovery occurs when nerve terminals sprout from the axon to form new motor end-plates.

Botulinum toxin blocks impulse transmission mediated by acetylcholine, such as at myoneural junctions, at autonomic ganglia, and at parasympathetic nerve terminals. Impulse conduction within peripheral nerves and muscle contraction is not affected. Transmission is blocked because the toxin prevents release of acetylcholine from the presynaptic membrane. Synthesis of acetylcholine and impulse transmission within terminal nerve fibrils remain intact. On the other hand, the miniature end-plate potentials spontaneously generated by release of acetylcholine in a resting nerve decrease and eventually disappear in the presence of toxin. If a poisoned nerve is stimulated repetitively, temporary summation of acetylcholine release occurs, producing an augmented response (Fig. 1). Labelled toxin is localized at the neuromuscular junction. Its specificity for acetylcholine transmitter sites has been used to identify cholinergic nerves in the small intestine, salivary gland, sinoatrial node, and nerve ganglia.

C. botulinum can replicate within the human gastrointestinal tract and release toxin, resulting in the development of botulism. The syndrome originally recognized as infant botulism has now been extended by finding the same pathogenesis in a few adults.

Fig. 1 Electromyography in botulism. The muscle action potential is markedly reduced, but following tetanic stimulation, it is augmented. (Redrawn from Gutmann, L. and Pratt, L. (1976). Pathophysiologic aspects of human botulism. *Archives of Neurology*, **33**, 177, by permission. Copyright 1976, American Medical Association.)

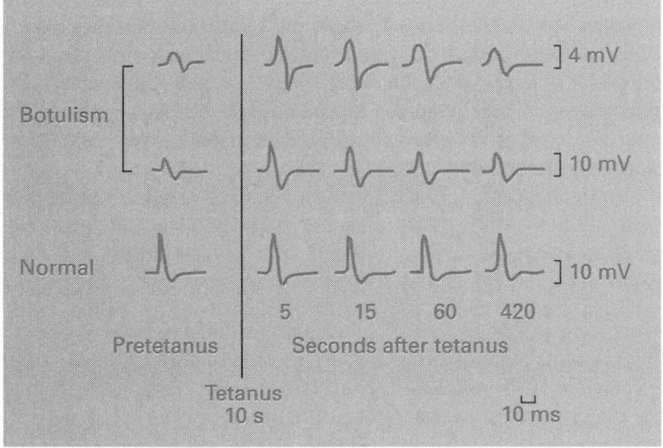

HISTORY

The symptoms of botulism vary from mild fatigue to severe weakness and collapse leading to death within a day. It has been a cause of sudden, unexpected death in previously healthy individuals. The first symptoms may suggest gastrointestinal-tract illness: nausea, vomiting, abdominal bloating, and dryness in the mouth and throat. Some patients have nervous complaints initially, such as dizziness, unsteadiness on standing, diplopia, and blurred vision. Subsequently the difficulties progress to include difficulty with speech or swallowing, weakness or paralysis in the limbs, and generalized weakness and lassitude. The dryness of the mouth may become so severe as to cause pain in the tongue and throat. Eventually there may be difficulty holding up the head, constipation, urinary hesitancy, and progressive difficulty in breathing. Symptoms are noted between 12 and 72 h after eating poisoned food. Patients with short incubation periods are likely to have ingested large amounts of toxin. However, clinical attack rates in botulism vary and individuals are known to have ingested large amounts of contaminated food without developing symptoms.

PHYSICAL EXAMINATION

Negative findings in botulism are pertinent. Higher mental functions are preserved, although sometimes patients have been drowsy. Sensation is intact. Fever is unusual. Clinical signs reflect involvement of the autonomic and motor nervous systems. The mouth is dry and the tongue is furrowed. Lateral rectus weakness in the eyes produces internal strabismus. Failure of accommodation is common and the pupils may be fixed in mid position or dilated and unresponsive to light. Ptosis, weakness of other extraocular muscles, and inability to protrude the tongue or to raise the shoulders are other early findings. Weakness in the limbs is of the flaccid, lower motor-neurone type and deep tendon reflexes are initially preserved. Facial muscles may be spared; gag and corneal reflexes are not lost. Even if not present initially, weakness of the respiratory muscles can develop later and deterioration can be very rapid. Hypotension without compensatory tachycardia, intestinal ileus, and urinary retention are evidence of the widespread autonomic paralysis. Patients are described whose symptoms and signs are virtually confined to the autonomic nervous system.

DIAGNOSIS

The diagnosis in the first case of an outbreak is often missed because cranial-nerve symptoms and signs may be ignored in what is apparently a gastrointestinal disturbance. Clinical findings are characteristic and the differential diagnosis usually lies between botulism and the descending form of acute inflammatory polyneuropathy or Guillain–Barré syndrome. Other diagnoses that may come to mind include diphtheria, intoxication with atropine or organophosphorus compounds, myasthenia gravis, cerebrovascular disease involving the brain-stem and producing bulbar palsy, paralytic rabies, tick paralysis, and neurotoxic snake bite. Botulism has been incorrectly diagnosed as pharyngitis and at least once a patient was subjected to exploratory laparotomy because of severe intestinal ileus.

Sometimes patients with other types of poisoning are thought to have botulism. This concern most often arises with an outbreak of staphylococcal food poisoning. Individuals with carbon monoxide poisoning have been mistakenly been thought to be poisoned by food, but they invariably have headaches and altered consciousness. Poisoning from chemicals or fish produces rapid onset of symptoms. Mushroom poisoning is characterized by severe abdominal pain.

The diagnosis of botulism can be confirmed by testing for botulinum toxin in the patient's serum, urine, or stomach contents. Mice are inoculated intraperitoneally with 0.5 ml of sample, with and without mixing with polyvalent botulinum antitoxin. The mice are then observed for signs of botulism. The specific toxin serotype can be identified by repeating the tests using monospecific antitoxins. Free toxin in patient's serum may be detected for as long as 28 days after the onset of symptoms if antitoxin has not been given.

Electromyography can be helpful in confirming a diagnosis of botulism. Single or low-frequency stimuli evoke muscle action potentials that are reduced in amplitude. In contrast, tetanic or rapid stimuli produce an enhanced response. Nerve conduction velocities are normal. This result readily differentiates botulism from the Guillain–Barré syndrome. Although the Eaton–Lambert syndrome also shows facilitation after repetitive stimuli, that disorder is more easily differentiated from botulism on clinical grounds. Patients with botulism may show slight improvement when given edrophonium chloride with or without 3,4-diaminopyridine, but the response is very much less than in patients with myasthenia gravis.

TREATMENT

The priorities in management are assessment of respiratory function followed by administration of antitoxin. Survival from botulism may depend upon successful management of respiration; in modern times most deaths occur from complications of respiratory support. Initially, respiratory effort should be monitored carefully by means of vital capacity or peak flow measurements; deterioration may occur rapidly. Subsequent provision of 3 to 4 weeks of respiratory support may be a severe test of the resources of even a specialized unit, potentially requiring tracheostomy, repeated bronchoscopy with bronchial lavage, parenteral nutrition, and early treatment of infections with appropriate antimicrobials. Note that some aminoglycoside antimicrobials can potentiate neuromuscular blockade. A breathing circuit incorporating intermittent mandatory ventilation can be used to assist breathing in partially paralysed patients.

Some patients with botulism become profoundly hypotensive; this can be secondary to hypoxaemia, acidosis, and accumulated fluid deficits or be a feature of the autonomic paralysis. The best approach for treatment of autonomic paralysis is to expand the intravascular volume using whole blood, protein, and/or saline. The venous pressure should be monitored centrally and kept at +10 to 15 cmH_2O. If this approach fails, dopamine infusion can be tried. Initially it should be given cautiously at a rate of 2.5 to 3.0 μg/kg per min and titrated to the patient's blood pressure, pulse, and urine output.

Trivalent (types A, B, and E) antitoxin should be given, as there is evidence that it reduces case fatality and shortens the course of the illness. The earlier it can be given, the more useful its effect. Multivalent antitoxin is employed as the toxin type cannot be specified from the clinical history, and treatment is initiated before the diagnosis is confirmed by animal tests. Antitoxin is available from designated regional hospitals in the United Kingdom: half the dose is given intramuscularly and half intravenously. The antitoxin available is horse serum. It is customary to give 0.1 ml intradermally as a test dose in case of hypersensitivity, but most serum reactions are not the result of type I hypersensitivity and are not predicted by this test. For patients known to be sensitive to horse serum, human botulism immune plasma can be obtained from the Center for Disease Control, Atlanta, Georgia, USA.

Some physicians treat with penicillin to eliminate the possibility that toxin might be formed endogenously. Many years ago it was shown that patients dying of botulism carried bacilli in their intestine. The discovery that clinical disease could result from toxin formed within the gastrointestinal tract of both infants and adults makes antimicrobial treatment a more reasonable idea than was formerly thought. Drugs capable of reversing neuromuscular blockade have been used to treat patients with botulism. However, neither hydrochloride nor guanidine 3,4-diaminopyridine has had any noticeable effect on respiratory muscle weakness or tidal volume. Gastric lavage, repeated high enemas, and cathartics have been given to attempt to remove unabsorbed toxin from the gastrointestinal tract. Nasogastric suction may be indicated in cases with severe ileus and catheter drainage for urinary retention.

The mortality from botulism in the early part of the twentieth century was 60 to 70 per cent, but this improved to 23 per cent for cases reported between 1960 and 1970 since the use of respiratory support. In a single large outbreak in 1977 there were no deaths among 59 cases. Recovery from botulism depends upon the formation of new neuromuscular junctions; clinical improvement thus takes weeks or months. One severe case required respiratory support for 173 days with eventual recovery. Very prolonged fatigue and dyspnoea on exertion can be due to factors other than the neuromuscular blockade.

WOUND BOTULISM

Rarely, symptoms and signs of botulism develop in individuals who are injured. Recognition may be complicated by the presence of fever from septic wound complications, from frank gas gangrene, or by the absence of gastrointestinal symptoms. Respiratory failure may occur in a patient receiving aminoglycosides. The diagnosis is confirmed by electromyography; botulinum toxin is detected in serum in about half of the reported cases. *C. botulinum* can be recovered from wounds in the absence of clinical botulism. The incubation period averages 7 days with a range of 4 to 17 days. Clinical findings and management are the same as for patients with food-borne botulism.

INFANT BOTULISM

Since 1976, botulism has been recognized in infants under 6 months of age. The cases have been sporadic and not connected with ingestion of spoiled food. Previously healthy babies develop constipation, which may then progress over 3 to 10 days to poor feeding, irritability, a hoarse cry, and weakness in head control. Examination shows a generally weak, hypotonic, afebrile infant, with cranial-nerve paralysis. Abnormalities in eye movements and pupillary reactions are sometimes present and deep tendon reflexes are reduced or absent. The range in severity is considerable, but respiratory failure can develop and there have been several deaths. Most recover completely. The diagnosis can be confirmed by finding *C. botulinum* and toxin in the faeces, and by electromyography. Botulinum toxin is not present in the serum.

The disease is thought to follow ingestion of *C. botulinum* spores, which then become established in the infant's gastrointestinal tract, multiplying and producing toxin. Excretion of *C. botulinum* and toxin may continue for as long as 3 months after clinical recovery. Honey has been implicated as a source of spores for some cases. Other than supportive measures, no consistent pattern in treatment using antitoxin, antibiotics, cathartics, or enemas has been established.

Gas gangrene

DEFINITION

Gas gangrene is a rapidly developing and spreading infection of muscle by toxin-producing clostridial species, especially *C. perfringens* (formerly known as *C. welchii*). It is accompanied by profound constitutional toxicity and is invariably fatal if untreated.

AETIOLOGY

Although mention of gas gangrene inevitably conjures up visions of battlefield injury, cases occur after civilian and iatrogenic trauma. High-velocity missiles and impacts now regularly feature in war and peace. The actual incidence of the disease depends upon the conjunction of a number of factors. Viable forms of the causative clostridial species must be present and the local environment of the wound must be conducive to their growth. Proximity to faecal sources of the bacteria is a risk factor, as in hip surgery, in adrenaline injections into the buttock, and in amputation of the leg for ischaemic vascular disease. Wound contamination with dirt, shrapnel or bits of clothing reduces local oxygen concentrations. Similarly, wounds involving large muscle masses in the shoulder, hip, thigh, and calf, wounds produced by high-velocity projectiles, damage to major arteries, crush injuries, open fractures, and burns carry a higher risk. The incidence of gas gangrene after trauma reflects the speed at which injured people are evacuated and receive appropriate treatment. During the Vietnam and Falklands conflicts there were very few cases of gas gangrene among American and British wounded cared for by highly organized surgical teams. In comparison, when a jet airliner crashed in the Florida everglades, 8 of the 77 injured survivors developed the disease.

Gas gangrene is caused by certain anaerobic, Gram-positive, spore-forming bacilli capable of producing exotoxins that damage living tissues. Most cases are caused by *C. perfringens* type A, but in some series 30 to 60 per cent have been due to *C. novyi* and 5 to 20 per cent to *C. septicum*. In small numbers of cases *C. histolyticum*, *C. sordellii*, and *C. fallax* have been found. Not uncommonly more that one species is isolated from a case. Clostridia occur naturally in the soil and in the gastrointestinal tracts of man and animals. Even toxin-producing species are mainly saprophytes and strict conditions for their growth must be met. Oxygen directly inhibits the growth of gas-gangrene bacteria and prevents toxin production. However, possession of the enzyme superoxide dismutase can permit the organisms to survive in the presence of small amounts of oxygen. Necrotic tissue, foreign bodies, and ischaemia in a wound all reduce the locally available oxygen.

Infrequently, gas gangrene occurs without preceding trauma. It can be a primary infection of the perineum or scrotum, or present in a limb, secondary to seeding from clostridial colonization of a colonic neoplasm. *C. septicum* is found in a higher percentage of these cases than where there is a history of trauma. This organism is more aerotolerant than other clostridial species, which may allow infection of previously healthy tissue.

TOXINS

The clostridia responsible for gas gangrene elaborate a wide range of toxin activities with from 4 to more than 12 separate toxins described for *C. septicum*, *C. novyi*, and *C. perfringens*. Subtypes of these organisms can be defined according to which toxins are found in culture supernatants. The enzyme targets of many of the toxins have been characterized, although the toxic and enzyme activities are not always perfectly correlated. Experimental inoculation of culture filtrates reproduces the histological findings of gas gangrene except for oedema and gas. Examination by electron microscopy shows gaps of 7.5 to 18 nm appearing in the plasma membrane as early as 1 h after injection. These plasma-membrane defects increase with time and can be visualized adjacent to toxin molecules that have been labelled with ferritin. Toxin is not detected in the tissues or serum of patients with gas gangrene, possibly because the toxin binds rapidly and irreversibly.

HISTORY

The incubation period of gas gangrene is usually less than 4 days, often less than 24 h, and occasionally as short as 1 to 6 h. The most characteristic symptom is pain at the site of the wound. Patients will describe this as severe or excruciating and sudden in onset. Subsequent evolution of symptoms and signs can be very rapid. The patient may be prevented from giving an adequate history by toxicity.

PHYSICAL EXAMINATION

Very early it may be difficult to account for the patient's pain by objective physical findings. Swelling, bluish discoloration, or darkening of the skin at the affected site may then be noted. The traumatic or surgical wound becomes oedematous and a thin, serous ooze emerges. Pain steadily increases in severity: the overlying skin becomes stretched and develops a brown or 'bronzed' discoloration. Haemorrhagic vesicles and finally areas of frank necrosis may then appear. A sweet odour from the wound has been described. In spite of the name, gas is not invariably present, especially early in the disease. Later, crepitus can be felt and the wound becomes exquisitely tender.

Concomitantly, profound constitutional symptoms develop. Patients become sweaty and febrile, and though alert and oriented, very distressed by their condition. The pulse is elevated out of proportion to the fever, which is not necessarily high. Death may occur within 48 h of onset.

At operation, infected muscle appears dark red with purple discoloration; frank gangrene and liquefaction may be seen. Involved muscle is devitalized and does not contract after direct stimulation.

True clostridial myonecrosis must be differentiated from anaerobic cellulitis and from anaerobic streptococcal myositis. Anaerobic cellulitis is a purulent wound infection where putrifying anaerobic clostridia have colonized muscle and other tissues made necrotic by trauma. Streptococcal myositis is a spreading muscle infection with anaerobic streptococci and either *Streptococcus pyogenes* or *Staphylococcus aureus*. Neither is necessarily associated with the pronounced constitutional toxicity characteristic of gas gangrene and neither requires as radical excision. Diabetic patients develop gas gangrene but this is due to their predisposition to ischaemic vascular disease. Numerous micro-organisms, both aerobic and anaerobic, can produce gas in tissues.

DIAGNOSIS

The diagnosis of gas gangrene has to be made on clinical grounds as treatment must be initiated urgently. Sudden deterioration in a post-operative patient or following trauma requires examination of the wound and surrounding tissue or removal or windowing of the plaster cast. Prompt recognition and treatment improves the prognosis. Cases of primary gas gangrene and cases following elective surgery may have a higher fatality because the disease is unexpected and recognition delayed.

Gram stain of the wound discharge, of an aspirate, or of a needle biopsy may aid diagnosis. In gas gangrene there are many large, plump, Gram-positive bacilli, usually without spores because *C. perfringens* in clinical lesions often does not sporulate. Few, if any, polymorphonuclear leucocytes are present. On the other hand, anaerobic streptococcal myositis and anaerobic cellulitis both show many leucocytes and the former long chains of Gram-positive cocci. Radiology has been used to detect small amounts of intramuscular gas in early lesions, but the absence of gas does not exclude the diagnosis. Culture of clostridia does not confirm a diagnosis of gas gangrene, as simple colonization without clinical disease occurs in up to 30 per cent of wounds.

TREATMENT

Surgical removal of all affected muscle is essential. The decision to remove only muscle tissue or to amputate is a finely balanced surgical judgement, best when informed by previous experience.

Although not substitutes for surgery, antimicrobials, hyperbaric oxygen, and administration of antitoxin have been thought to be helpful adjunctive therapies. Penicillin is the drug of choice, in doses that offer hope of obtaining diffusion into relatively avascular areas (i.e. 20–30 million units daily). If the patient has a history of angio-oedema or anaphylaxis following administration of penicillin, clindamycin can be substituted at a dose of 900 mg every 6 h. There is experimental evidence but no clinical confirmation that clindamycin and metronidazole might be superior to penicillin, perhaps by reducing toxin production.

Hyperbaric oxygen is widely used to treat gas gangrene. Although an effect on mortality has never been shown by controlled trials, its application is well supported by experimental evidence. Proponents claim dramatic relief from the constitutional toxicity and clearer demarcation between involved and uninvolved muscle at operation, which may permit a more conservative resection. One hundred per cent oxygen is given at 303 kPa for 60 to 120 min, two to three times daily. With this schedule toxicity is minimal. Comparable mortality rates have been achieved without using hyperbaric oxygen.

Therapeutic administration of gas-gangrene antitoxin is also controversial. Some authorities report abandoning its use many years ago or are cautious of possible reactions to horse serum. On the other hand, its use in very toxic cases may be justified and during the Second World War it was said to have reduced mortality.

Patients with gas gangrene need supportive measures to combat shock, blood loss, and dehydration. *C. perfringens* septicaemia in association with gas gangrene is not common. It is heralded by massive haemolytic anaemia and jaundice. Septicaemia with micro-organisms such as *Escherichia coli* can occur and should be treated with intravenous gentamicin or as guided by antibiotic susceptibility testing. Acute renal failure may complicate gas gangrene, a result of the renal tubular toxicity of free haemoglobin or myoglobin.

PREVENTION

Gas gangrene is worth preventing; the mortality of established disease, even in specialized centres, still ranges between 11 and 31 per cent. For elective operations associated with an increased risk, such as amputation for ischaemic vascular disease, the principle is to achieve antimicrobial levels in tissues before surgery. Conventionally, penicillin is given intravenously before surgery and postoperatively for 5 days. Metronidazole may be useful in patients who are hypersensitive to penicillin.

The principle in traumatic wounds is to eliminate the conditions that allow gas-gangrene bacilli to proliferate. The kinetic energy of the wounding device should be assessed. High-velocity missiles distribute energy radially from their path, producing more extensive tissue damage than missiles at low speeds or with a small mass. Wounds should be excised widely by resection back to healthy, viable muscle and skin. Closure is delayed for 5 to 6 days until it is certain that the wound is free of infection. Military surgeons usually give penicillin in high dosage over this period.

Experiments with gas gangrene in sheep have shown that both passive and active immunization can confer protection. Antitoxin gave best results when given up to 9 h after wounding but some protection could be seen as late as 18 h. Active immunization protects, but in man this requires the clear definition of risk categories. It is helpful to know that, if needed, potent toxoids can be prepared for each of the causative species.

Clostridial infections of the gastrointestinal tract

Pseudomembranous colitis

DEFINITION

Pseudomembranous colitis is an acute exudative infection of the colon caused by *C. difficile*. The name derives from plaques of necrotic membrane that adhere to the mucosal surface in the clinically most severe form of the disease (Fig. 2).

AETIOLOGY

The clostridial aetiology of pseudomembranous colitis became known in 1977. *C. difficile* is an anaerobic, spore-forming, Gram-positive bacillus. Strains from patients with colitis produce at least two potent exotoxins capable of eliciting an inflammatory response in animal tissues. The organism and free toxin can regularly be detected in the faeces of patients with pseudomembranous colitis but not in patients with other established causes for diarrhoea. The toxins are lethal when inoculated into small laboratory animals. A gram of liquid stool from a patient with pseudomembranous colitis may contain thousands of animal lethal doses.

Antimicrobial treatment plays an accessory part in the development of the colitis by reducing native resistance to colonization with *C. difficile*. Healthy adults rarely carry *C. difficile*. Infants and young children do so more often, but these strains may not produce toxin. Because colonization and antimicrobial treatment may occur at different times, antibiotic-susceptible strains of *C. difficile* are able to produce disease. In this sense, pseudomembranous colitis is an opportunistic infection. Resistance to colonization requires viable intestinal bacteria, but it is not known which species or combination of species determines this resistance. Usually resistance to colonization will spontaneously reconstitute itself unless an antimicrobial effect persists within the gut.

CLINICAL HISTORY

The single most pertinent detail of the medical history is previous antimicrobial treatment, which is the most common occasion for pseudomembranous colitis. Suspicion of *C. difficile* colitis is therefore heightened by such a history; it is fortuitous for patients with Campylobacter or Salmonella infection to have been given antibiotics. Direct questioning may be needed to elicit this history; antimicrobials may have been

Fig. 2 Pseudomembranes on the rectal mucosa in a patient with *C. difficile* colitis.

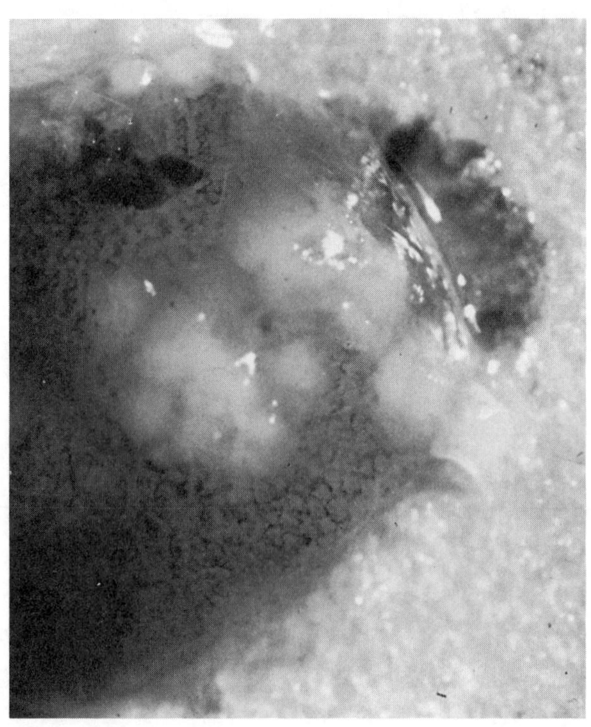

self-administered, taken for trivial complaints, or used as long as 3 or 4 weeks before the start of diarrhoea. Pseudomembranous colitis has been reported to follow the use of every antimicrobial in common medical practice, but its association with lincomycin, clindamycin, ampicillin, amoxycillin, and cephalosporins is strongest. However, it occasionally occurs in individuals with no previous medical history or is secondary to conditions like chronic colonic obstruction, colonic carcinoma, leukaemia, or uraemia. Pseudomembranous colitis was identified as a pathological entity in the last century, before any understanding of antimicrobials and their clinical use. Community-acquired cases are sporadic but there may be a history of other hospital-or nursing home-associated cases. The disease is more common in older patients but the typical syndrome has been described in people of all ages including infants.

The start of symptoms varies from mild, self-limiting diarrhoea, or debilitating, prolonged diarrhoea, to acute fulminating toxic megacolon, which may be difficult to distinguish from acute obstruction or peritonitis (Fig. 3). The illness may start surreptitiously; persistent diarrhoea may have resisted all attempts at symptomatic relief. Community-acquired cases tend to have a longer history of diarrhoea, perhaps a week or more before seeking medical attention, than patients with Campylobacter or Salmonella infection. Stools are described as watery or porridge-like, although occasionally obstipated patients with apparently spurious diarrhoea may actually have colitis. Patients may develop sudden chills, fever, and signs of an abdominal catastrophe, and those with acute findings have been subjected to exploratory laparotomy. Elderly patients may have diarrhoea that resolves and then recurs at intervals of one to several days. Severe abdominal pain is not common and patients do not often report frank blood in the stools.

PHYSICAL EXAMINATION

Elderly patients appear tired, toxic, and ill. Low fever, a dry furred tongue, and abdominal tenderness, sometimes with peritonism, are the most common clinical signs. Signs of dehydration may be present, but hypotension attributable to hypovolaemia is not common. Spiking temperatures may also be seen and a distended, tense, abdomen can suggest colonic obstruction.

Fig. 3 Acute toxic dilatation of the colon in an elderly patient with pseudomembranous colitis.

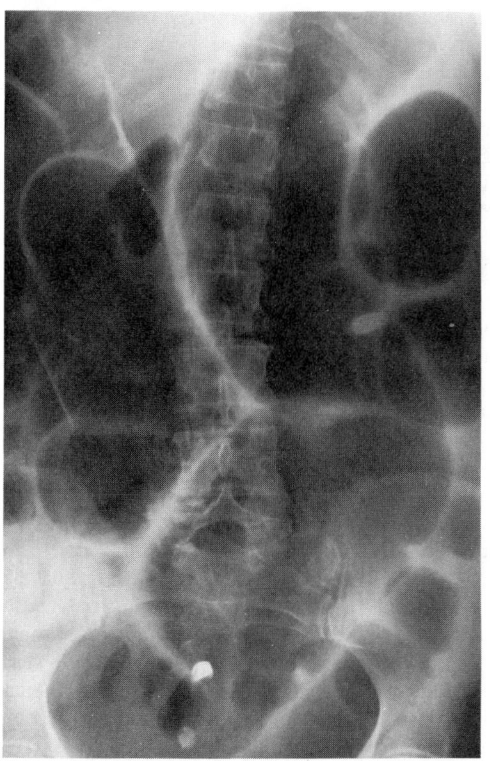

DIAGNOSIS

Many patients show polymorphonuclear leucocytosis, sometimes with counts of 30 000/μl or more. Leucocytes are present in the faeces. Chemical findings in patients with prolonged diarrhoea include azotaemia and hypoalbuminaemia; the azotaemia may appear to be out of proportion to the dehydration. If clinical findings suggest acute colitis, every attempt should be made to establish a specific and aetiological diagnosis. Faeces should be examined for the presence of *C. difficile* toxin, as this establishes a mechanism for the diarrhoea. Sigmoidoscopy with rectal biopsy is also helpful because the raised, mucoid to opaque yellow plaques (0.2–2 mm across) are diagnostic. Even if the mucosa appears normal, multiple sectioning of a biopsy may reveal microscopic lesions (Fig. 4). Some patients with *C. difficile* colitis do not have visible pseudomembranes, either because lesions are distributed unevenly in the colon or because the illness is mild and short. In these cases the diagnosis can only be confirmed by testing for toxin and *C. difficile*. Rarely, patients with pseudomembranes on sigmoidoscopy or rectal biopsy may fail to yield *C. difficile* even when optimal techniques are used for culture or toxin detection. Histological examination of such lesions usually fails to reveal focal areas of mucosal necrosis. Confluent pseudomembrane formation appears to be the end result of several types of colonic mucosal injury and not a finding specific to *C. difficile* infection. Although sigmoidoscopy would not appear to be necessary routinely for diagnosis, the differential diagnostic possibilities such as inflammatory bowel disease or colonic obstruction can make it useful.

The differential diagnosis of pseudomembranous colitis includes other forms of antimicrobial-associated colitis, diarrhoea due to *Salmonella*, *Shigella*, and *Campylobacter* species, intestinal amoebiasis, Crohn's disease, and non-specific ulcerative colitis. These can be differentiated by sigmoidoscopy and rectal biopsy, or by microscopy and culture of the faeces. Two-thirds or more of patients with simple antimicrobial-associated diarrhoea do not have infection with *C. difficile*. Often they complain of sudden abdominal pain and bloody diarrhoea that subsides within a day or two of stopping antimicrobial treatment. Occasionally, patients may be infected with *C. difficile* in addition to another micro-organism capable of causing diarrhoea. Infection with *C.*

Fig. 4 A rectal biopsy diagnostic of pseudomembranous colitis. There is a flame-like eruption of fibrin and polymorphonuclear leucocytes from a focal area of mucosal necrosis.

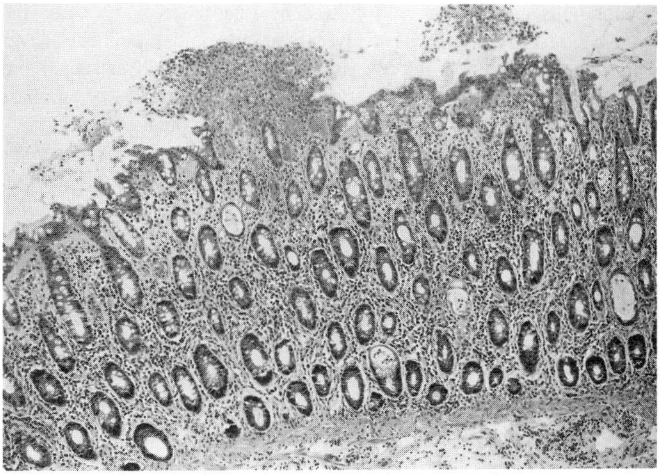

difficile may exacerbate symptoms in some patients with inflammatory bowel disease.

In the laboratory, culture of *C. difficile* from stools and from environmental sites requires differential methods. For this reason and because toxin-negative strains are found that are unrelated to diarrhoeal illness, it is not widely used for diagnosis. Toxin is usually assayed by means of its ability to produce characteristic cytopathic changes in tissue-culture cells. The identity of the toxin in unknown specimens is established by the cytopathic effect and by neutralization with either specific antitoxin or cross-reacting *C. sordellii* antitoxin. Diagnostic toxin tests are also available using antibody-linked detectors; these are less sensitive than tissue culture assay, but rapid.

TREATMENT

Stopping the causative antimicrobial may allow *C. difficile* colitis to resolve spontaneously. If clinical circumstances dictate active intervention, however, specific treatment to eradicate *C. difficile* and its toxin from the stools has been shown to produce clinical improvement in a randomly allocated, placebo-controlled trial. The antimicrobial of choice is one to which *C. difficile* is susceptible and which is not absorbed following oral administration. Vancomycin fulfils both criteria and may be given in a dose of 125 mg every 6 h. Severe cases usually show improvement after 48 h of treatment and signs and symptoms rapidly return to normal. Metronidazole, 250 mg four times a day, also appears to be effective, although it is absorbed. Some physicians regard it as less effective than vancomycin. Bacitracin may also be useful. Failure to respond to vancomycin suggests that the diagnosis is incorrect or that an additional condition or complication may be present. Parenteral administration of either vancomycin or metronidazole may fail to cure the infection. Patients who are dehydrated need fluid resuscitation, but if the principal findings are constitutional toxicity and peritonism, direct treatment against the source of the toxin should be the chief objective. Cholestyramine resins bind *C. difficile* toxin *in vitro*, but have no effect on the clinical course of the colitis.

Pseudomembranous colitis has been successfully treated by colectomy. Patients may be subjected to exploratory laparotomy when the abdominal signs suggest peritonitis. However, the disease is completely reversible by appropriate antimicrobial treatment. If a diagnosis of pseudomembranous colitis has been established, it is appropriate to wait for medical treatment to have an effect unless there is an absolute surgical indication like free abdominal air or complete intestinal obstruction. In patients who are unable to take vancomycin orally, some physicians have attempted to instill it into the colon via a caecostomy tube; others combine intragastric vancomycin, intermittent clamping of the nasogastric tube, and parenteral metronidazole. No *C. difficile* antitoxin is available in the United Kingdom.

Any of the suggested antimicrobial treatment regimens for pseudomembranous colitis may be followed by relapse. In some cases the relapse illness is clinically more severe than the original. There has never been any evidence that relapse is due to antimicrobial resistance and patients continue to respond to treatment with the original or an alternative drug. Patients relapse both because antimicrobial treatment may not completely clear them of *C. difficile* and because a new exposure to environmental strains has occurred. There is evidence from animal experiments that vancomycin and metronidazole themselves can induce susceptibility to the disease and prolonged treatment may produce prolonged susceptibility. On the other hand, patients whose *C. difficile* colitis resolves without specific treatment do not relapse. There may be multiple relapses and many regimens have been suggested for their management. These include tapering doses of vancomycin, a Lactobacillus preparation three times a day, or cholestyramine three times a day after a therapeutic course of vancomycin. Cholestyramine can be combined with Lactobacillus but not with vancomycin. Normal flora may be reconstituted by giving a suspension of normal faeces as an enema.

It may be necessary under certain circumstances to continue an antimicrobial when a patient has developed pseudomembranous colitis. There is no evidence to suggest that concurrent therapy with vancomycin will not be successful, although some authorities believe that clinical improvement occurs more slowly. It would be reasonable to replace a drug commonly associated with pseudomembranous colitis by one which is not, such as a quinolone, aminoglycoside, tetracycline, or sulphonamide. Repeat treatment with an inducing antimicrobial at some later time is not contraindicated in a patient who has recovered from pseudomembranous colitis.

PREVENTION

Clusters of cases of pseudomembranous colitis were reported from particular medical and surgical units before its infectious aetiology was understood. Now it is known that *C. difficile* may contaminate the environment of a patient with diarrhoea, that prospective culture shows that patients may acquire the organism, and that cross-infection between patients can be demonstrated by typing the isolated strains of *C. difficile*. The chain of infection for isolated cases may be difficult to trace because spores can persist for weeks to months. As many patients receiving antimicrobial treatments are potentially at risk, those with pseudomembranous colitis ought to be nursed in barrier isolation. Patients with diarrhoea, especially those who are incontinent, are more important sources of cross-contamination than those with formed stools. Physical cleanliness, enteric precautions, confinement to a single room, and reduced use of the most frequent inducing antimicrobials are the approaches most often used to reduce institutional cross-infection. There is no proven value in retesting patients until they are free of toxin nor in treating asymptomatic toxin excretors.

Necrotizing enterocolitis

DEFINITION

Necrotizing enterocolitis is a fulminating clinical illness characterized by extensive necrosis of the intestinal mucosa and sometimes the entire gut wall. Numerous terms have been used to describe geographical variants of the condition such as darmbrand (Germany), enteritis necroticans, pig bel (Papua New Guinea), or gas gangrene of the bowel, depending upon whether the cases are sporadic in adults or epidemic in people of all ages.

Necrotizing enterocolitis occurs in infants, especially those with an associated medical condition such as birth asphyxia, respiratory-distress syndrome, or catheterization of the umbilical artery. Cases of neonatal necrotizing enterocolitis have sometimes occurred in clusters.

AETIOLOGY

In most adult patients in whom appropriate pathological and bacteriological investigations have been done, *C. perfringens* (*C. welchii*) has been implicated. In sporadic cases this is usually *C. perfringens* type A. Gram stain of the necrotic mucosa and the bowel wall shows many Gram-positive bacilli whose morphology and immunofluorescent staining suggest *C. perfringens*.

However, in the German and especially in the Papua New Guinean outbreaks, there is substantial evidence implicating *C. perfringens* type C. This type produces large amounts of β-toxin, which has lethal and necrotizing effects on tissues. Papua New Guinean highlanders have a high prevalence of β-antitoxin, but antibodies are rare in people who have lived where the disease is uncommon. Patients with pig bel show rising β-antitoxin titres, and specific passive or active immunization has been shown to prevent disease. *C. perfringens* type C causes a similar disease in piglets, but it is not clear whether exogenous human infection with these organisms occurs or whether the lesions are produced by the overgrowth of endogenous clostridia. Sweet potato, a local dietary staple, contains an inhibitor of trypsin. Combined with a low-protein diet this may impair the ability of the intestine to inactivate endogenously produced β-toxin. However, the methods used for roasting the pigs offer many opportunities for clostridial contamination.

It has not been proved that clostridia are the cause of neonatal necrotizing enterocolitis.

HISTORY AND PHYSICAL EXAMINATION

The patient may be an isolated case, over 50 years of age or recovering from gastric surgery. Such sporadic cases are regularly reported from Scandinavia, Europe, the United States, Australia, and the Middle East. Or the patient may be one in an epidemic outbreak as was described in postwar Germany and among the highlanders of Papua New Guinea. These follow ingestion of contaminated food or a dramatic change in eating habits, such as occurs when the highlanders engage in pig feasting. Symptoms develop suddenly in someone who was previously well. There is severe abdominal pain, which is colicky at first and afterwards becomes continuous. Bloody diarrhoea and vomiting may occur. The patient may be extremely toxic and go into shock. On examination there is fever, with abdominal distension, localized or diffuse tenderness, and reduced bowel sounds. A tender mass may be palpated. Later, intestinal malabsorption or chronic partial obstruction may develop because of scarring.

TREATMENT AND PREVENTION

Patients with suspected pig bel should be treated by aspirating gastric contents through a large nasogastric tube and by administering intravenous fluids. Pyrantel is given by mouth and the bowel rested by fasting. One megaunit of benzylpenicillin is given intravenously every 4 h and the patient observed for surgical complications. Mild cases recover without surgical intervention, but if surgical indications are present, the mortality ranges from 35 to 100 per cent. As pig bel continues to be a common disease in Papua New Guinea, consideration should be given to the use of a *C. perfringens* type C toxoid vaccine in local areas. Two doses spaced 3 to 4 months apart have been shown to prevent the disease.

Clostridium perfringens food poisoning

OCCURRENCE AND CLINICAL FINDINGS

In the United Kingdom and the United States, food poisoning caused by *C. perfringens* is the third most common type of food-borne illness. Meat and poultry are responsible for at least 90 per cent of the outbreaks, which occur where food is prepared in large quantities. Two-thirds of the reported outbreaks are in schools, hospitals, factories, restaurants, or catering establishments, and in a typical outbreak 35 to 40 people are affected. An estimated 12 000 cases were associated with a single outbreak in 1969.

The circumstances surrounding an outbreak repeat themselves with monotonous regularity. A meat dish is prepared by stewing, braising, boiling, or steaming and this is allowed to stand at ambient temperatures for a period of 4 to 24 h. The food is served cold or after desultory rewarming. Six to 12 h after eating the meal, the victims complain of crampy abdominal pain and then diarrhoea. Vomiting is unusual and fever inconsequential. Twelve to 24 h later the diarrhoea and pain have subsided. Fatal cases occur rarely; at autopsy they show severe enterocolitis.

Undoubtedly many cases of *C. perfringens* food poisoning occur at home but are not reported because symptoms are self-limiting and because confirmation requires special bacteriological methods. However, antibodies to the toxin mediating the symptoms are very common and it is likely that nearly everyone has experienced this disease once or more in their lifetime.

AETIOLOGY

C. perfringens is an ubiquitous, sporulating anaerobe with an unparalleled virtuosity for production of biologically significant toxins. The clinical effects of infection with any particular strain may depend largely on its toxin-producing capacity. Strains associated with food poisoning have a number of special characteristics. They are type A, although their production of α-toxin is variable; they are often heat resistant. Eighty-six per cent of food-poisoning strains produce a specific, heat-labile enterotoxin. Toxin production *in vitro* is closely associated with sporulation rather than with the multiplication of vegetative cells. *In vivo*, toxin probably acts by damaging enterocyte membranes. Free enterotoxin has been detected in diarrhoeal stool after *C. perfringens* food poisoning, antibody to enterotoxin increases after such episodes, and ingestion of 8 to 12 mg of enterotoxin by volunteers produces abdominal pain and diarrhoea.

C. perfringens is a normal human faecal organism, is regularly found in the intestinal tract of domestic animals, often contaminates raw meat, and can be carried by flies. The distribution of enterotoxin-producing strains may be more restricted. However, surface contamination of meat with *C. perfringens* is more common and subsequent rolling or grinding will distribute these organisms throughout. Heat-resistant strains survive cooking at maximum temperatures of 100°C. Spores then germinate and multiply to 10^6 to 10^7 cells/g in the highly advantageous, anaerobic environment created when meat cools slowly or stands at ambient temperature. Reheating may not kill these cells; when ingested they will multiply still further, sporulate, and release their toxin.

Enterotoxin-producing strains of *C. perfringens* may sometimes cause diarrhoea by means of overgrowth in the gut. Patients, usually elderly, begin to experience diarrhoea without known contact with contaminated food. The diarrhoea may be short lived or persist intermittently for several months. Colony counts of 10^8 to 10^{10}/g of faeces are associated with the presence of high titres of free toxin. Previous antimicrobial treatment may encourage the overgrowth and the same strain has been found to cross infect patients.

REFERENCES

Botulism

Case records of the Massachusetts General Hospital No. 48 (1980). *New England Journal of Medicine*, **303,** 1347–55.

Critchley, E.M.R., Hayes, P.J., and Isaacs, P.E.T. (1989). Outbreak of botulism in north west England and Wales, June, 1989. *Lancet*, **ii,** 849–53.

Das Gupta, B.R. and Sugiyama, H. (1977). Biochemistry and pharmacology of botulinum and tetanus neurotoxins. In *Perspectives in toxicology*, (ed. A.W. Bernheimer), pp. 88–119. Wiley, New York.

McCroskey, L.M. and Hatheway, C.L. (1988). Laboratory findings in four cases of adult botulism suggest colonization of the intestinal tract. *Journal of Clinical Microbiology*, **26,** 1052–54.

Schreiner, M.S., Field, E., and Ruddy, R. (1991). Infant botulism: a review of 12 years' experience at the Children's Hospital of Philadelphia. *Pediatrics*, **87,** 159–65.

Gas gangrene

Darke, S.G., King, A.M., and Slack, W.K. (1977). Gas gangrene and related infection: classification, clinical features and aetiology, management and mortality. A report of 88 cases. *British Journal of Surgery*, **64,** 104–12.

Freer, J.H. and Arbuthnott, J.P. (1976). Biochemical and morphologic alterations of membranes by bacterial toxins. In *Mechanisms in bacterial toxins*, (ed. A.W. Bernheimer), pp. 169–93. Wiley, New York.

MacLennan, J.D. (1962). The histotoxic clostridial infections of man. *Bacteriology Reviews*, **26,** 177–276.

Shouler, P.J. (1983). The management of missile injuries. *Journal of the Royal Navy Medical Service*, **69,** 80–4.

Stevens, D.L. *et al.* (1990). Spontaneous, nontraumatic gangrene due to *Clostridium septicum. Reviews of Infectious Diseases*, **12,** 286–96.

Gastrointestinal infections

Bartlett, J.G. (1992). The 10 most common questions about *Clostridium difficile*-associated diarrhea/colitis. *Infectious Diseases in Clinical Practice*, **1,** 254–9.

Hobbs, B.C. (1974). *Clostridium welchii* and *Bacillus cereus* infection and intoxication. *Postgraduate Medical Journal*, **50,** 597–602.

Larson, H.E., Price, A.B., Honour, P., and Borriello, S.P. (1978). *Clostridium difficile* and the aetiology of pseudomembranous colitis. *Lancet*, **i,** 1063–6.

Lawrence, G.W., Murrell, T.G.C., and Walker, P.D. (1979). Pigbel. *Papua New Guinea Medical Journal*, **22.**

Tuberculosis and its problems in developing countries

7.11.22 Tuberculosis

P. D. O. Davies, D. J. Girling and J. M. Grange

The causative organism

The tubercle bacillus was discovered by Robert Koch in 1882 and, together with the leprosy bacillus, was included in the genus Mycobacterium in 1898. There are four species, or perhaps variants of a single species, of mammalian tubercle bacilli: *Mycobacterium tuberculosis*, the human tubercle bacillus; *M. bovis*, the bovine tubercle bacillus; *M. africanum*, a rather heterogeneous type found in Equatorial Africa and having properties intermediate between the former two species; and *M. microti*, a very rarely encountered pathogen of voles and other small mammals.

M. tuberculosis is divisible into the classical type discovered by Koch and the South Indian (or Asian) type, which is also found among immigrants in countries outside Asia. The South Indian type has low virulence in guinea-pigs, contains certain unique cell-wall lipids and, in common with *M. bovis*, is usually susceptible to the isoniazid analogue thiophene-2 carboxylic acid hydrazide (TCH).

The vaccine strain, bacillus Calmette–Guérin (**BCG**), was supposedly derived from a strain of *M. bovis*, although it is now distinguishable from this and other tubercle bacilli.

There are three main phage types of *M. tuberculosis*: A, I (intermediate), and B. Type I corresponds to the South Indian type, although this is more easily identifiable by cultural characteristics. As an epidemiological tool, phage typing has been superseded by restriction fragment length polymorphism.

Like *M. leprae*, the mammalian tubercle bacilli are obligate pathogens but, unlike *M. leprae*, they may replicate outside as well as inside living cells and may be cultivated *in vitro*. The genus Mycobacterium contains about 50 species that are normally environmental saprophytes, although some species cause opportunist disease of animals and man (see Chapter 7.11.24).

Morphology and staining

Tubercle bacilli are rods, usually slightly curved, about 4 μm long and 0.5 μm in diameter. In clinical specimens they often occur in small clumps and in early cultures they usually appear as rope-like microcolonies termed 'serpentine cords' (Fig. 1). Cord formation was once, erroneously, regarded as a marker of virulence. Mycobacteria are Gram-positive, although they are not easily stained by this method. They are resistant to decolorization by mineral acids after staining with arylmethane dyes such as carbol fuchsin, hence the term acid-fast bacilli. They are also resistant to decolorization by alcohol though, contrary to some reports, this property does not differentiate tubercle bacilli from saprophytic mycobacteria.

Biological effects of mycobacterial cell components

The cell wall (Fig. 2) is more complex than in any other bacterium. It is characterized by a very high content of lipids, many of which have important biological functions.

Surface peptidoglycolipids (mycosides) are analogous structurally and functionally to the O antigens of Gram-negative bacteria; they determine colony morphology, and bacteriophage and seroagglutination type. Some glycolipids, especially cord factor (trehalose dimycolate) and sulpholipids, are toxic but their role in virulence is uncertain. These lipids, together with peptidoglycan, are powerful adjuvants involved in granuloma formation. Lipoarabinomannan interferes with the processing of antigen and its presentation to T cells, and may therefore suppress protective immune responses. It also triggers release of tumour necrosis factor from activated macrophages (see below).

Virulence and host range

Virulence factors in *M. tuberculosis* and other mycobacteria have proved elusive. Except perhaps in the case of *M. ulcerans*, toxic substances are not primary determinants of mycobacterial virulence. Virulence is probably a result of resistance to the innate, non-specific defence mechanisms in the tissues and within macrophages, and of the ability to induce inappropriate immune reactions.

Mammalian tubercle bacilli cause disease in a wide range of mammals—*M. bovis* in cattle and badgers and, less frequently, in deer and other wild or feral mammals. Experimentally, *M. bovis* is highly virulent in rabbits, although natural disease is rare. Man is an incidental host,

Fig. 1 Microcolonies of *Mycobacterium tuberculosis* showing serpentine cords (by courtesy of Mr Bryan Allen).

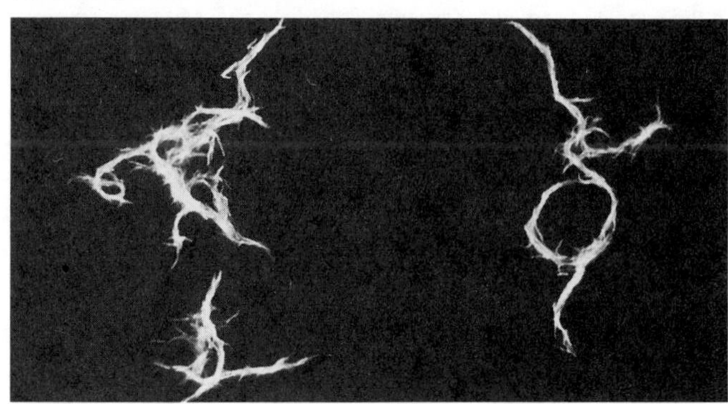

Fig. 2 A diagrammatic representation of the structure of the mycobacterial cell wall.

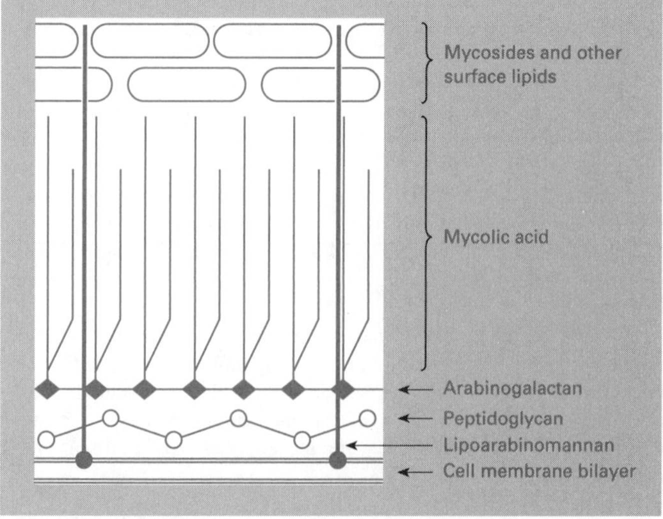

usually acquiring infection by drinking contaminated milk, although infection of farm workers may occur by the aerogenous route. People with *M. bovis* pulmonary disease may infect cattle but evidence for person-to-person transmission is limited and anecdotal.

M. tuberculosis rarely causes overt disease in cattle but contact with infectious human beings may result in tuberculin conversion. Although the South Indian variant and some isoniazid-resistant strains are of low virulence for the guinea-pig, human disease due to these bacilli is indistinguishable from that caused by guinea-pig virulent strains. *M. microti* is attenuated for man. It has been used as a vaccine strain in some clinical trials and afforded a degree of protection similar to BCG, but was abandoned in favour of BCG as some recipients developed local lupus-like lesions.

Pathology and immunology

Immune responses in tuberculosis may be either protective, leading to resolution of disease, or tissue destroying, leading to the pathological characteristics of active disease. Both types of response are cell-mediated and there has been considerable controversy about whether protective and immunopathological responses are manifestations of the same mechanism, differing only in degree, or whether they represent different mechanisms. There is evidence that protective immune responses are induced by antigens that are common to all mycobacterial species while antigens restricted to tubercle bacilli are responsible for immunopathological reactions, for BCG vaccine protects against leprosy and lymphadenopathy caused by environmental ('atypical') mycobacteria.

Fig. 3 A granuloma of tuberculosis, showing a central area of caseation, epithelioid cells, lymphocytes, and multinucleate giant cells (by courtesy of Dr William Taylor).

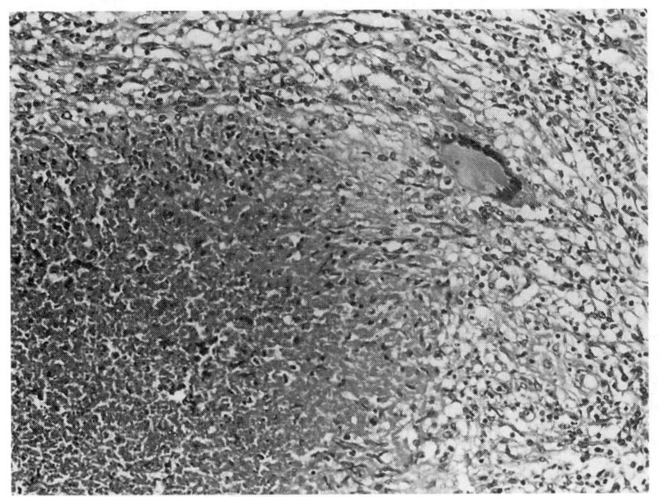

The varied clinical and pathological features of human tuberculosis are either primary or post primary.

The initial lesion of tuberculosis occurs at the site of implantation of the bacillus, usually the lung, skin or alimentary tract including the tonsil. Implanted bacilli are ingested by polymorphs and macrophages, some of which migrate to the draining lymph nodes where secondary lesions develop, causing nodal enlargement. The initial pulmonary lesion, the Ghon focus, together with the hilar lymphadenopathy, forms the primary complex of Ranke. Some bacilli are disseminated through lymphatics and blood, leading in some cases to meningeal, bone, and renal involvement.

The characteristic histological lesion of tuberculosis is the granuloma, which consists of a chronic, compact aggregate of activated macrophages (epithelioid cells), some of which fuse to form multinucleate giant cells (Fig. 3). Granulomas develop very soon after infection as a result of non-specific chemotaxis and activation of macrophages by various mycobacterial components. The primary complex often heals with calcification.

Specific immune responses

Mycobacterial antigens are processed by antigen-presenting cells such as the dendritic cells in the lymph nodes and presented to antigen-specific T cells. These T cells undergo clonal expansion and, by means of interferon-γ and other cytokines, are able to recruit and activate macrophages (Fig. 4) more effectively and to enhance the formation of granulomas. Once activated by interferon-γ, the macrophages are further activated by endogenous conversion of inactive 25-OH vitamin D_3 to the active $1,25(OH)_2$ vitamin D_3 (calcitriol).

In mouse macrophages, mycobacteria are killed by oxygen-dependent mechanisms, especially by the generation of hydrogen peroxide and nitric oxide. While human macrophages are certainly able to inhibit

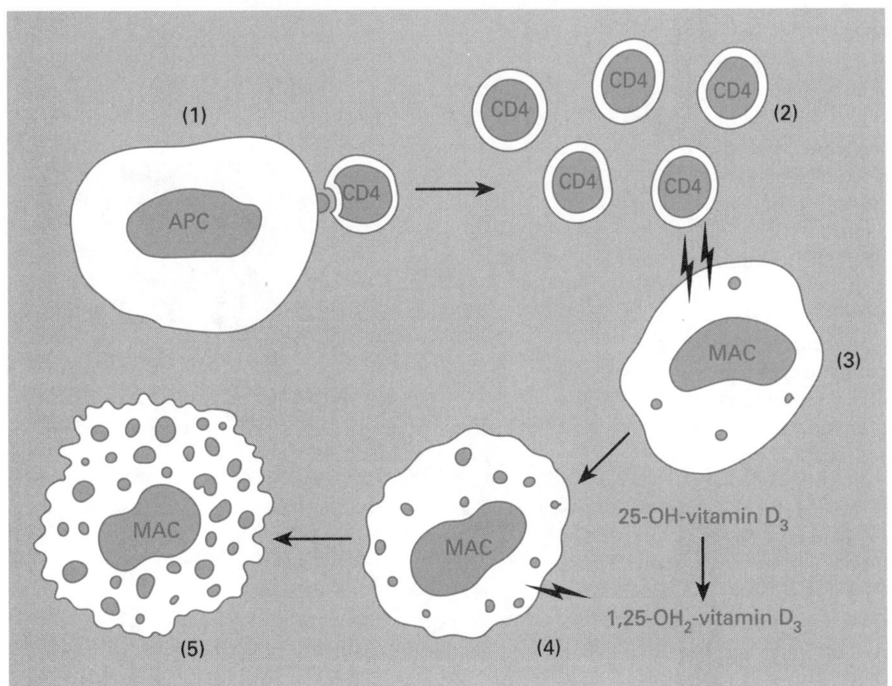

Fig. 4 The steps involved in macrophage activation. (1) Mycobacterial antigen is presented to T helper/inducer (CD4) lymphocytes by the antigen-presenting cell (APC). (2) The activated T cells undergo clonal proliferation. (3) Interferon-γ and other cytokines activate the macrophage (MAC). (4) This activation induces a hydrolase that converts inactive 25-OH-vitamin D_3 to its active metabolite 1,25 $(OH)_2$-vitamin D_3. (5) This metabolite further activates the macrophage.

growth of virulent tubercle bacilli, attempts to demonstrate killing *in vitro* have been unconvincing. Thus the exact role of the human macrophage in the killing of tubercle bacilli *in vivo* is uncertain. Protective immunity in tuberculosis is probably the property of the granuloma *in toto* rather than the isolated macrophage. Being composed of metabolically active cells, the centre of the granuloma is anoxic and acidic and leads to tissue necrosis, which, from its cheese-like appearance, is termed caseation. The anoxia, acidosis, and free fatty acids in the necrotic caseous material provide an environment that is very unfavourable for mycobacterial growth or survival. As a result, most of the bacteria die, the lesions become quiescent, and are subsequently sealed off by fibrous scar tissue. However, a few bacilli may survive and may give rise to postprimary tuberculosis years or decades later.

Delayed hypersensitivity

Three to eight weeks after the primary infection delayed hypersensitivity develops, shown by a skin reaction to injected mycobacterial antigen, usually purified protein derivative of tuberculin. The exact mechanism of this necrotic reaction, originally described by Robert Koch in the guinea-pig, is poorly understood. It has two elements: first, a non-specific inflammatory reaction characterized by the accumulation of many blood-derived white cells in the pericapillary spaces and, secondly, a more specific reaction leading to oedema and induration of the overlying skin. In larger tuberculin reactions there is a distinct slowing of the blood flow centrally so that there is insufficient oxygen for the many metabolically active inflammatory cells at the test site. This results in anoxia, acidosis, and, in some cases, overt necrosis.

A positive tuberculin test indicates previous exposure to mycobacterial antigens through infection with one of the tubercle bacilli or to BCG vaccination. Exposure to environmental mycobacteria may, in some instances, lead to cross-reactivity. Tuberculin reactivity does not correlate with protective immunity.

Postprimary tuberculosis

This results from reactivation of quiescent, endogenous, primary infection or from exogenous reinfection. Reactivation usually occurs in the upper lobes of the lung, perhaps because of the higher oxygen tension at this site. In contrast to primary disease, extensive caseous necrosis occurs in the lesions, due in part to the release of tumour necrosis factor from activated macrophages and may lead to the development of large tumour-like masses termed tuberculomas (Fig. 5). Tumour necrosis factor is identical to cachectin, the substance responsible for the wasting (previously termed consumption or phthisis) characteristic of advanced untreated tuberculosis. It has been shown that sequential activation of macrophages by interferon-γ and calcitriol prime them for release of tumour necrosis factor and that a potent trigger for such release is lipoarabinomannan, a mycobacterial cell-wall component. In necrotizing reactions, T-cell factors render tissue cells exquisitely sensitive to killing by tumour necrosis factor through an unknown mechanism. There is assumed to be a causal relation between the positive tuberculin reaction and this extensive necrosis.

Being anoxic and acidic, the tuberculoma contains very few acid-fast bacilli. Release of proteases by macrophages softens or liquefies the caseous material so that if the lesion erodes into a bronchus, the liquefied material is discharged and a cavity is formed (Fig. 6). As oxygen and carbon dioxide may freely enter the cavity, the bacilli are now able to replicate; enormous numbers are found in the cavity wall and expectorated sputum so that the patient is said to have open or infectious tuberculosis. Before chemotherapy, the only beneficial treatments for pulmonary tuberculosis were surgical procedures designed to close the cavity and to prevent such free replication of the bacilli.

Dissemination of bacilli to regional lymph nodes and more distant organs is uncommon in postprimary disease, but bacilli may spread directly via the air passages from cavities to other parts of the lungs and

Fig. 5 (a) A tuberculoma in the excised right upper pulmonary lobe of a 34-year-old woman. The preoperative (b) anteroposterior and (c) lateral chest radiographs.

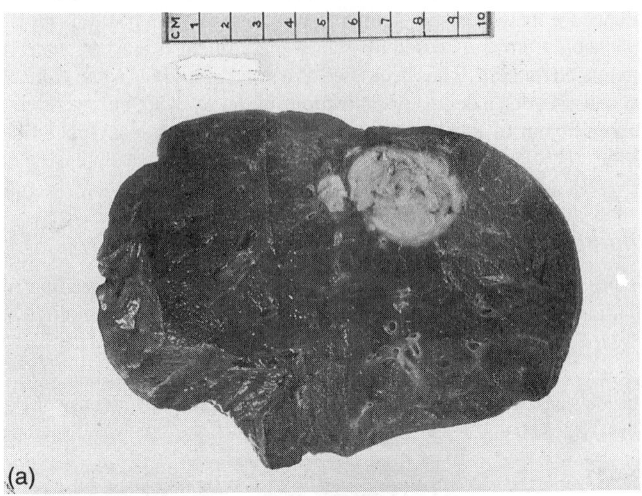

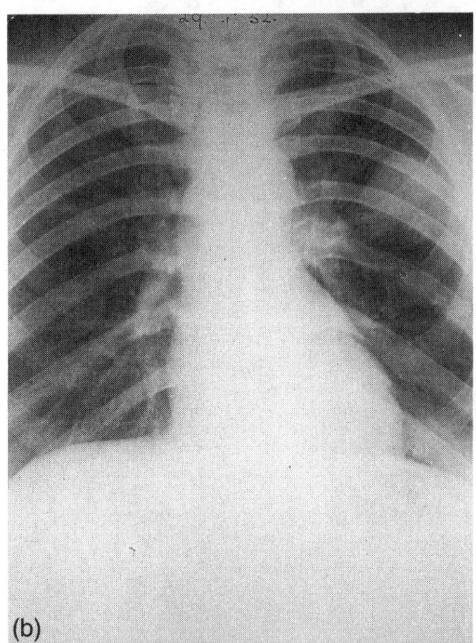

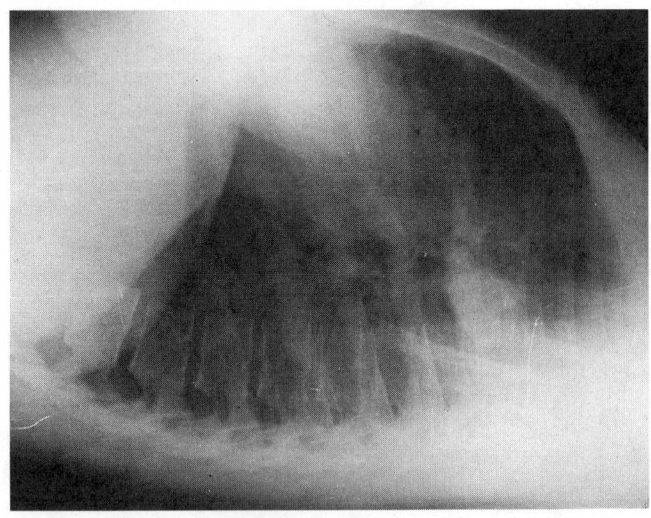

to the larynx. Bacilli in swallowed sputum may cause indurating lesions in the alimentary tract.

Tuberculosis and immunosuppression

A degree of non-specific immunosuppression is found in active tuberculosis but is rectified by effective antituberculous therapy. The tuberculin test may be negative in advanced tuberculosis; in early studies this led to the false assumption that tuberculin reactivity was a correlate of protective immunity.

Patients with congenital or acquired immunosuppression are particularly prone to tuberculosis. Worldwide, the most important predisposing cause of immunosuppression leading to tuberculosis is human immunodeficiency virus (**HIV**) infection. As cavity formation is the result of an active immune response, many immunosuppressed patients do not have cavities but develop spreading lesions of rather indeterminate radiological appearance. Non-pulmonary lesions and disseminated disease are frequently encountered.

Infection by HIV considerably enhances the reactivation rate of tuberculosis in the infected (tuberculin-positive) person: about 10 per cent of doubly infected people develop active tuberculosis each year. Although HIV-related tuberculosis usually responds to standard antituberculosis therapy, tumour necrosis factor and other immunological mediators generated by the immune response to tuberculosis trigger the replication of HIV. Thus active tuberculosis, even if effectively treated, may result in an earlier onset of AIDS. Accordingly, preventive antituberculous therapy of doubly infected persons is indicated whenever possible.

Clinical bacteriology

Collection of specimens

The collection of adequate specimens is essential for reliable bacteriological examination. All containers for specimen collection and transport must be sterilized, as 'pseudoepidemics' of mycobacterial disease due to environmental mycobacteria have resulted from the use of unsterile containers.

Sputum should be collected into wide-mouthed, screw-capped glass or plastic pots. As such containers are easily contaminated on the outside, they should be placed in plastic bags for transport to the laboratory. At least three sputum samples, preferably early-morning samples, should be collected. A suitable quantity for bacteriological examination is from 2 to 5 ml. If the patient fails to produce sputum, secretions may be stimulated by the inhalation of ultrasonically nebulized hypertonic saline. Alternatively, the larynx may be swabbed, but the diagnostic yield is low; this should only be done by trained personnel, who should wear masks or visors as the patient may cough violently when the specimen is taken.

In children or other patients who cannot produce sputum, gastric contents may be aspirated through a nasogastric tube in the early morning before food or drink are taken. The patient should be asked to cough and swallow several times before aspiration. The acidic aspirate must either be neutralized or sent at once to the laboratory. Such material is suitable for culture but, owing to the presence of environmental mycobacteria in water and food, microscopical detection of acid-fast bacilli may be misleading.

Fibreoptic bronchoscopy enables specimens to be obtained from abnormal areas of the lung by brushing, bronchoalveolar washing, and by bronchial or transbronchial biopsy.

For examination of urine, three early-morning specimens should be obtained. Pleural, peritoneal, and pericardial fluids should be collected into bottles containing citrate to prevent clotting. When possible, biopsies of the pleural, peritoneal, and pericardial membranes, as well as the corresponding fluids, should be obtained. An alternative technique, which gives a significantly higher yield of positive cultures, is to add aspirated fluids directly to an equal quantity of double-strength Kirschner medium, which is then incubated.

Biopsy specimens should be divided in half. One half should be fixed in formalin for histological examination and one half sent unfixed for bacteriology. (It is surprising how often formalin-fixed specimens are sent to the bacteriology laboratory.) Pus and necrotic tissue contain very few viable mycobacteria, so biopsies of tissue adjacent to necrotic areas should be obtained if possible.

Fig. 6 The right upper and middle pulmonary lobes of a 46-year-old man showing tuberculomas and cavities in the upper lobe and caseous aspiration foci in the middle lobe.

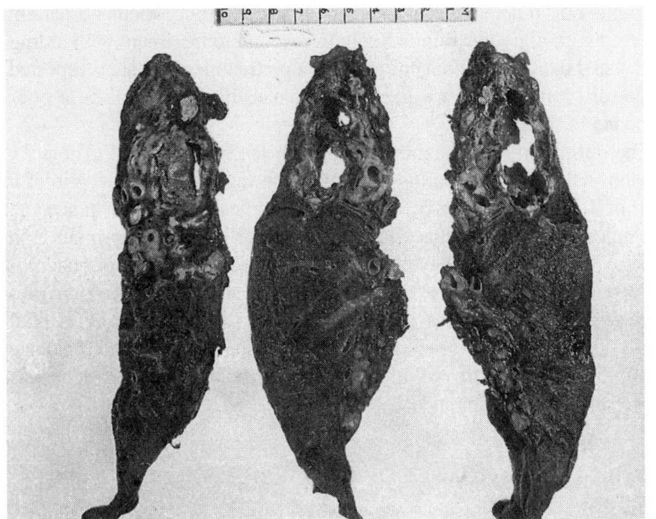

Microscopical examination

Sputum smears are prepared by spreading purulent portions of the sputum specimen or the centrifuged deposit after decontamination (see below) on a glass slide with a wire or plastic loop or a swab stick. After drying and heat fixing, the smear is stained with an arylmethane dye, decolorized by acid (or acid and alcohol) and counterstained. In the Ziehl–Neelsen method, slides are stained with carbol fuchsin and examined by light microscopy. Alternatively, if facilities are available, smears may be stained with auramine O or rhodamine, or both, and examined by fluorescence microscopy. Both methods depend on the acid-fastness of mycobacteria but the use of fluorescence microscopy is far less tiring to the technical staff.

Sputum microscopy is the mainstay of diagnosis in the developing nations on account of its simplicity and rapidity. It is, however, relatively insensitive and bacilli are only seen in about half the patients with active pulmonary tuberculosis. Sputum must contain at least 5000 bacilli/ml for them to be detectable by microscopy. Epidemiological studies have revealed a close correlation between sputum smear positivity and the infectiousness of the patients.

Microscopy is also used to detect acid-fast bacilli in urine, pleural, peritoneal, and cerebrospinal fluid after centrifugation, and in homogenates or histological sections of tissue.

Culture

Cultural techniques are more sensitive than microscopy and permit identification and drug susceptibility tests to be made. They are, however, much more time-consuming and costly, and require a high standard of technical competence.

As tubercle bacilli grow very slowly, they are readily overgrown by fungi or other bacteria in the specimen. This may be avoided by treating the specimen with an agent, usually an acid or alkali, that will prefer-

Table 1 *Subdivision of the mammalian tubercle bacilli isolated from human beings*

Type of tubercle bacillus	Oxygen preference	Nitratase	Susceptibility to TCH*	Susceptibility to pyrazinamide
M. tuberculosis classical	Aerobic	Positive	Resistant	Susceptible
M. tuberculosis South Indian	Aerobic	Positive	Susceptible	Susceptible
M. africanum type I	Microaerophilic	Negative	Susceptible	Susceptible
M. africanum type II	Microaerophilic	Positive	Susceptible	Susceptible
M. bovis	Microaerophilic	Negative	Susceptible	Resistant
BCG	Aerobic	Variable	Susceptible	Resistant

*Thiophene-2-carboxylic acid hydrazide (5 mg/l).

entially kill organisms other than mycobacteria. Sputum samples are usually treated with sodium hydroxide (Petroff method), sometimes with the addition of a mucolytic agent that facilitates the concentration of tubercle bacilli by centrifugation. Alternatively, specimens may be inoculated into media containing a 'cocktail' of antimicrobial agents that permit only mycobacteria to replicate.

Lowenstein–Jensen medium is the most widely used. It contains eggs, glycerol, and mineral salts, and is solidified by heating. The glycerol may be replaced by pyruvate to stimulate growth of *M. bovis*. Clear agar-based media are used for special purposes.

Specimens, decontaminated if necessary, are inoculated on to at least two slopes of media, one containing glycerol and the other pyruvate, and incubated at 35°C for 8 weeks, or 12 weeks if incubator space is available. Specimens from skin lesions are incubated at 32°C.

The radiometric method of culture, which depends on production of $^{14}CO_2$ in antibiotic-supplemented selective broth, permits mycobacteria to be detected rapidly, usually within 2 to 10 days, so that drug susceptibility tests can be done rapidly. It is too expensive for routine use in developing countries.

Culture in liquid media (Middlebrook or Kirschner broth) or on slides immersed in liquid media permits more rapid detection of mycobacterial growth than standard solid media, although detection is less rapid than by radiometry. A combined antimicrobial-supplemented selective broth and slide culture system is commercially available (MB Check, Roche). Pericardial, pleural, and peritoneal fluids may be inoculated, at the bedside, into double-strength Kirschner broth.

Mycobacteria are detectable in clinical specimens by polymerase chain reaction and by the demonstration of tuberculostearic acid by mass spectroscopy but these techniques are not yet widely available.

Identification tests

Most mycobacteria isolated in clinical laboratories are members of the tuberculosis complex. The first step in identification is to distinguish members of this complex from the environmental mycobacteria by their slow rate of growth, lack of pigment production in light or dark, growth at 35°C but not at 25°C, and failure to grow in media containing 500 mg of *p*-nitrobenzoic acid per litre.

Four tests allow division of the tuberculosis complex into individual species (*M. tuberculosis, M. bovis*, and *M. africanum* and BCG): reduction of nitrate to nitrite (nitratase test), oxygen preference (aerobic strains grow on the surface of semisolid agar media while micro-aerophilic strains form a band deep in the medium), susceptibility to 5 mg thiophene-2-carboxylic acid hydrazide (**TCH**) per litre, and susceptibility to pyrazinamide (Table 1). Classical and South Indian types of *M. tuberculosis* are separable by TCH susceptibility. *M. africanum* type 1, usually from West Africa, and type 2, more frequent in East Africa, are also distinguishable. On glycerol-containing media, colonies of *M. tuberculosis* are usually large and heaped up (eugonic) and produce nicotinamide while those of *M. bovis* are small and flat (dysgonic).

Other mycobacterial species can be identified by specialist reference laboratories using a range of cultural and biochemical tests, supplemented by lipid chromatography, specific antibodies, and DNA probes.

Drug susceptibility tests

There are four main types: absolute concentration, resistance ratio, proportion, and radiometric. In the absolute concentration method, standard amounts of bacilli are inoculated on media containing a range of concentrations of drug to estimate the minimal inhibitory concentration. However, the concentration of active drug in the medium is affected by various factors. In the resistance ratio method, which is very similar in principle, this problem is overcome by expressing the ratio of the mean inhibitory concentration of the test strain to that of a set of known susceptible strains, irrespective of the absolute drug concentration.

In the proportion method, the percentage of resistant mutants in the culture at given drug concentrations is estimated by comparison of colony counts on drug-free and drug-containing media. If more than 1 per cent of bacterial cells grow on the drug-containing medium, the strain is regarded as being resistant.

Results of these tests may not be available for 6 to 8 weeks because of the slow growth of tubercle bacilli. Rapid radiometric methods are reliable and their high cost is justified in areas where multidrug-resistant bacilli are prevalent.

Susceptibility tests should be done only if the reliability and consistency of their results can be guaranteed by careful standardization and quality control.

Drug resistance

There is no absolute definition of drug resistance. Cultures of 'susceptible' tubercle bacilli contain bacteria with a range of drug susceptibilities, including a few drug-resistant mutants. The aim of susceptibility testing is not to detect these mutants but to determine whether a patient infected with a given strain is likely to respond to treatment with a drug at its usual therapeutic concentration. If a pretreatment isolate is reported to be resistant, it does not necessarily mean that there will be a poor response to treatment.

The definition of resistance depends on the method used (Table 2). Strains with resistance ratios of 1 or 2 are regarded as susceptible; a ratio of 4 implies resistance, and one of 8 indicates high resistance.

Clinically, drug resistance is divisible into 'initial' or 'primary', in patients who claim that they have never received antituberculous chemotherapy, and 'acquired' or 'secondary', when it occurs during chemotherapy and is due to the selection of drug-resistant mutants. Initial resistance may be due to infection with a resistant strain or to resistance acquired as a result of previous medication of which the patient was unaware or wished to conceal.

CLINICAL SIGNIFICANCE OF INITIAL RESISTANCE

The incidence of initial resistance varies greatly from country to country. For example, initial resistance to isoniazid, streptomycin or to both these

Table 2 *Definitions of resistance to the main antituberculosis drugs with the mean inhibitory concentration (MIC) and proportion methods*

Drug	MIC (mg/l)	Proportion method: Drug concentration (mg/l)	Proportion method: Minimal proportion of resistant bacilli (%)
Isoniazid	1.0	0.2	1
Streptomycin	32.0	4.0	10
Rifampicin	64.0	40.0	1
Pyrazinamide	100.0*	100.0	10
Thiacetazone	2.0	2.0	10
PAS	8.0	0.5	1
Ethambutol	5.6	2.0	10
Ethionamide	80.0	20.0	10

*The test is set up at pH 4.75, 4.85, and 4.95. The MIC on the most acid medium on which heavy growth occurs on drug-free medium is used. On reading the MIC, the 10-colony endpoint is used.

drugs is found in about 4 per cent of isolates from patients in the United Kingdom, 8 per cent in the United States, 10 per cent in France, and 28 per cent in Hong Kong. In most countries, initial resistance to rifampicin, pyrazinamide, and ethambutol is rare, but a high incidence of rifampicin resistance is being reported in some regions.

Sometimes it is wrongly assumed that if a patient is found to have bacilli initially resistant to one or more component drugs of the prescribed regimen, those drugs should be replaced. This policy is unjustified as treatment is usually successful in patients with initial resistance. A change of regimen should be considered only if the patient fails to respond to treatment. Poor compliance is a far more important reason for failure of chemotherapy than is drug resistance. The only clinical value of pretreatment susceptibility testing is for selection of the best regimen for a patient who is not responding to primary chemotherapy.

CLINICAL SIGNIFICANCE OF ACQUIRED RESISTANCE

Most bacteriological relapses after the completion of chemotherapy are due to drug-susceptible organisms. If such relapse occurs during the course of therapy it is almost certain that the patient is not taking the drugs. Persistence or recurrence of positive cultures in patients known to be taking their drugs is much more likely to be associated with the emergence of drug resistance. This can occur if an inadequate regimen has been prescribed or the patient fails to take all the drugs regularly, thereby allowing the number of viable resistant mutants to increase while numbers of susceptible organisms decrease (Fig. 7). The regimen must be changed if acquired resistance emerges and drug susceptibility testing has enabled suitable retreatment regimens to be selected.

Susceptibility testing is useful:

(1) in research, to elucidate the mechanisms of drug action;
(2) to study the epidemiology of drug resistance in a community so that antituberculosis programmes can be planned;
(3) to determine the pattern of acquired resistance to guide retreatment of patients whose primary chemotherapy has failed.

Epidemiology

The global pattern of tuberculosis was radically transformed during the 1980s. Up until about 1985, global patterns of tuberculosis had been steady and almost predictable. In the industrialized world, where reliable records are available, case rates had declined progressively, except during the war years, from the first half of the nineteenth century. In the developing world, the picture has not been so clear, but rates were either declining or remaining fairly constant. From the mid-1980s, however, there was a dramatic change. In most developed countries, the rate of decline slowed and, particularly in the United States, in Great Britain, and in some other countries has begun to climb. In the developing world, particularly in subSaharan Africa, the number of cases has begun to rise, at an alarming rate in some areas. This change seems to be largely attributable to HIV infection, though migration and social deprivation have probably contributed.

Tuberculosis services, including methods of assessing the impact of tuberculosis in a population, are undergoing extensive revision. In many parts of the developed world, both clinical and public health services for tuberculosis had virtually ceased to exist, as demand had declined. With the present resurgence, a radical rethink of tuberculosis control strategy and relearning of old skills has been needed.

In most developed countries, tuberculosis is predominantly a disease of elderly people, recent immigrants from Third World countries, members of ethnic minorities, and the immunocompromised. HIV is expanding this last group. In the developing world, tuberculosis remains predominantly a disease of young adults.

The relation between disease and infection

An estimated one-third of the world's population is infected with the tubercle bacillus (Fig. 8). Every year approximately 8 million cases of tuberculosis arise from this infected pool and 3 million die. Those with disease infect approximately 100 million each year. Once infected, the likelihood of developing tuberculosis is 10 per cent in a lifetime; approximately 5 per cent within a year of infection, and a further 5 per cent later, some as long as 50 years or more after initial infection.

The impact of HIV on disease

In an individual infected with *M. tuberculosis*, HIV increases substantially the risk and shortens the time of developing disease. Those with double infection have an estimated 10 per cent risk of developing active tuberculosis each year, and those with HIV infection alone a greatly

Fig. 7 Diagrammatic representation of the emergence of resistance in the lungs of a patient treated with isoniazid alone. As treatment proceeds, the susceptible organisms are killed and replaced by the growth of resistant mutants. As soon as the proportion of resistant to susceptible organisms changes from its usual value of about 1 in 10^6 to about 1 in 10^4, the strain can be shown to be resistant in a susceptibility test. (Reproduced from Mitchison (1968), with permission.)

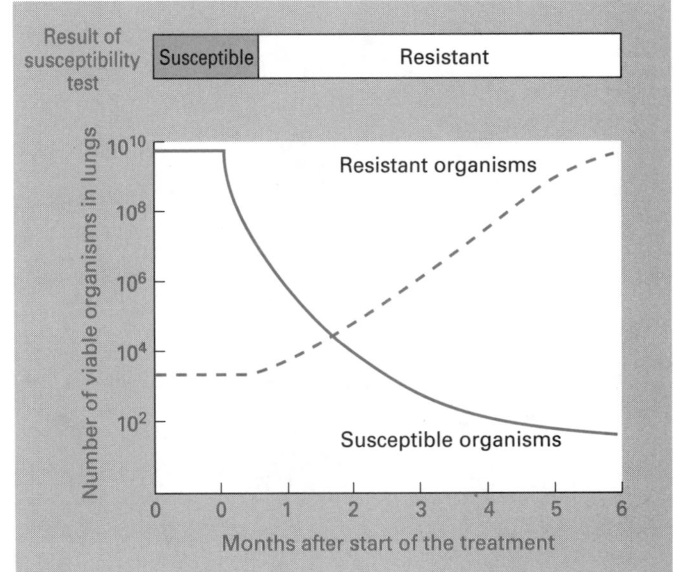

increased risk of contracting tuberculosis. In 1992, the World Health Organization estimated that there were 12 million HIV-positive people worldwide, of whom 4 million were also infected with *M. tuberculosis*: 78 per cent of those with double infection live in subSaharan Africa.

Methods of assessing the impact of tuberculosis in a population

Epidemiological studies are used to monitor both infection by the tubercle bacillus and overt tuberculosis. Infection is a state in which the tubercle bacillus is present in the body without producing symptoms or detectable evidence of disease. In overt tuberculosis, one or more organs shows evidence of an active pathological process by symptoms, signs, bacteriologically, or radiographically. There are four main epidemiological methods for assessing the impact of infection or disease on a population: mortality, morbidity, prevalence of sputum smear-positive cases, and annual risk of infection.

MORTALITY

Historically, mortality has been the most reliable method of assessing the impact of tuberculosis in a population, but it has become less accurate since the introduction of effective chemotherapy.

Some statistics on deaths from tuberculosis have been available in England since the London Bills of Mortality in the sixteenth century. Continuous records giving a cause of death are available from 1629, but the total population was not enumerated accurately before the National Census of 1801 and so only the proportion of deaths from tuberculosis can be given. These approached a peak of about 26 per cent around 1800 and declined to 12 per cent in 1850 and 9 per cent in 1910. Since the start of compulsory death certification in 1840, an accurate estimate of the death rate from tuberculosis could be made using population data from decennial censuses. Between 1860 and 1900 there was a reduction of 20 per cent in deaths from respiratory tuberculosis and 30 per cent in deaths from other forms of the disease, rates being highest in early adult life. The decline in tuberculosis mortality continued throughout the twentieth century except during the First World War and, to a lesser extent, the Second World War. Between 1930 and 1950, death rates were highest for females aged 25 to 34 years and males aged 55 to 64. Since 1950, mortality has been highest in patients aged 75 years and over, and deaths in males have exceeded those in females by 2 to 1. A typical example of the changing impact of tuberculosis mortality on different age groups through the decades in a developed country (Japan) is shown in Fig. 9.

Fig. 8 A schematic diagram to show the dynamic changes in tuberculosis infection worldwide.

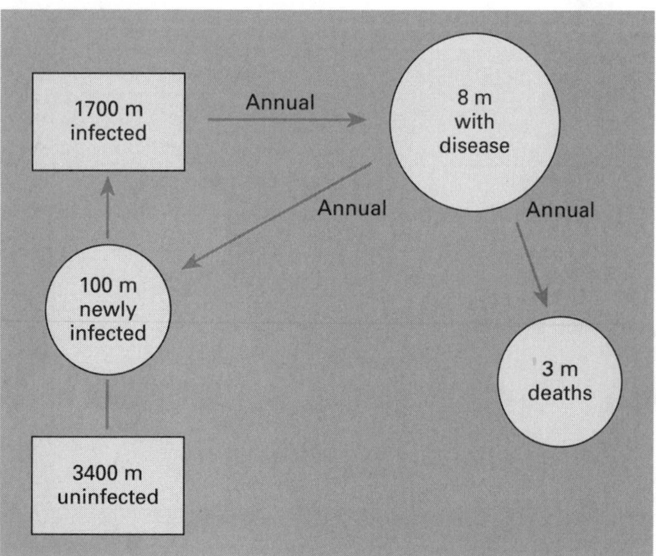

MORBIDITY—NOTIFICATION

Notification by a clinician 'who believes a patient is suffering from tuberculosis' has been compulsory in Great Britain since 1912. Any clinician diagnosing a case of tuberculosis, whether infectious or not, must complete a notification form and send it to the proper officer for the district in which the patient is normally resident. Contact tracing can then be instigated. Notification is the basis for national statistics. Most other developed countries have similar systems but they were stopped during the 1970s in some. Since effective chemotherapy was introduced in the 1950s, notification has probably provided the best guide to the impact of tuberculosis in a population, but its accuracy depends on the patient's presenting to the clinician, and on the clinician's making the diagnosis and notifying the authorities. Notification, where efficiently applied, indicates the number of new cases over a period of time. If the total population is known, the rate or incidence can be derived.

In Great Britain the annual notification rate declined throughout the twentieth century, except during the wars. However, the rate of decline slowed during the 1960s and 1970s, mainly as a result of immigration from the Indian subcontinent. From 1985, there was further slowing in decline and, in 1987, incidence began to increase for reasons that are less clear (Fig. 10). In 1988 the incidence among the white, Indian, and Pakistani/Bangladeshi populations in Great Britain was 4.7, 134.6, and 100.5/100 000, respectively.

In the white population of Great Britain, incidence in males is nearly double that of females (6.2 compared with 3.3/100 000). The incidence is lowest among children and teenagers (1.5/100 000) and highest among males aged 65 or more (18.3/100 000). For the 35 years up to 1993, however, there was an annual decline in incidence in all age groups of 8.5 per cent for females and 7.6 per cent for males, being greatest in the 15 to 24-year age group (12.6 per cent) and least in those over 64 years (2.7 per cent for females and 3.7 per cent for males.)

Fig. 9 Change in the age distribution curve of tuberculosis mortality rate for Japan, 1940 to 1985. It can be seen that as the disease becomes less frequent it affects the elderly rather than the young. (Reproduced from *Vital statistics*, Ministry of Health and Welfare, Japan, with permission.)

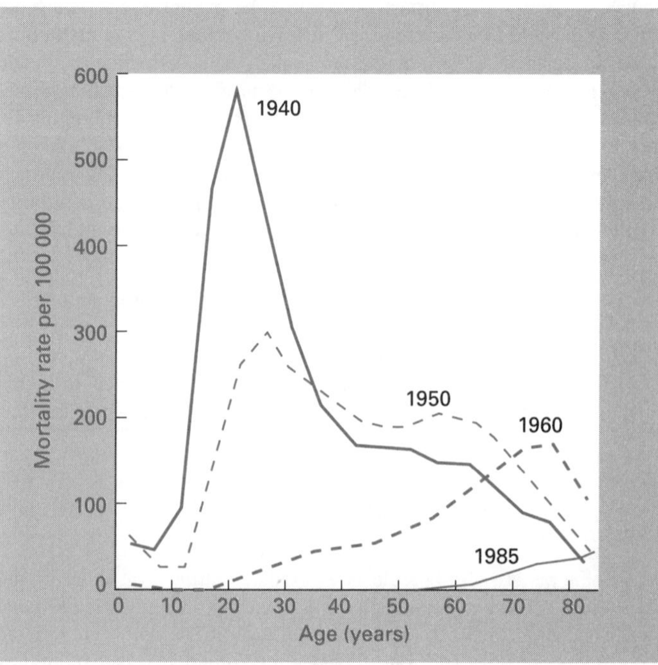

The incidence of tuberculosis in immigrants declines with increasing length of residence in Great Britain, but remains higher than in the indigenous population. There is also a higher incidence among individuals from ethnic minority groups who were born in Great Britain. High incidences of tuberculosis are found in other developed countries among ethnic minority groups and recent immigrants from developing countries.

Morbidity in other Westernized industrial countries

Other developed countries such as the United States, Japan, Switzerland, and Scandinavia have also experienced an increase in cases of tuberculosis since the mid-1980s. This was first observed in the United States in 1985, when a deviation from the expected exponential decline in tuberculosis occurred. The relative increase in the United States since 1987 was very similar to that seen in England and Wales. While HIV-related disease was undoubtedly a factor, the increase in inner cities such as New York predated the likely impact of HIV and was probably related to increasing social deprivation and a reduction in community services for disease control. Immigration from poorer countries is likely to be the principal cause of disease increase in European countries.

PREVALENCE

The point prevalence of tuberculosis is defined as the number of cases in a numerically defined population at a specified point in time. As tuberculosis is a chronic disease, the prevalence of the disease is higher than the annual incidence of new cases. The prevalence may be determined by conducting a survey of an indicator of active tuberculosis, such as sputum smear positivity or characteristic radiological abnormalities. Prevalence surveys are of the greatest value in developing countries where notification schemes may be difficult to set up and operate efficiently. Estimates of changes in the prevalence of tuberculosis can be made by sputum smear and radiological surveys of a random sample of a population at two points in time.

Prevalence surveys often give underestimates of the impact of tuberculosis on a community. During the 1950s and 1960s, mass miniature chest radiography surveys were made in Great Britain and some other countries but they detected only about 15 per cent of cases of active disease. The coverage, or case-detection ratio, is the fraction or percentage of diagnosed and notified cases to the number of cases predicted from the annual risk of infection (see below).

Fig. 10 Graph of notifications (all forms) of tuberculosis by year for England and Wales from 1954 to 1991. The slowing of the decline from the mid-1960s to 1980 was due to immigration, largely from the Indian subcontinent. The reasons for the increase since 1987 are not yet clear.

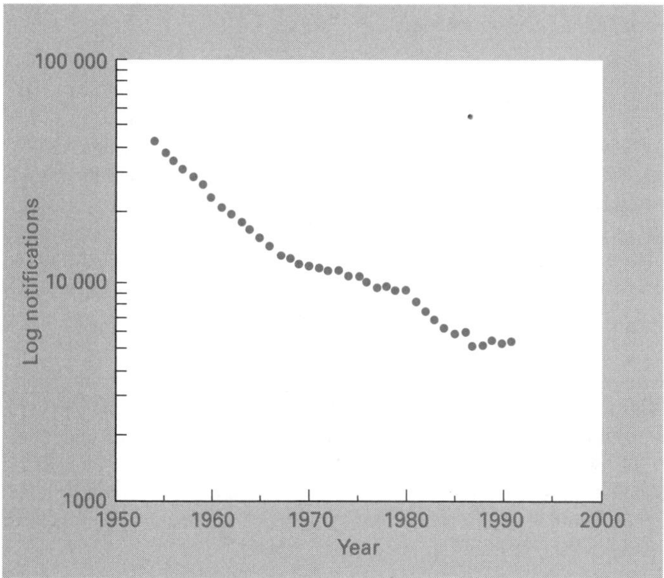

ANNUAL RISK OF INFECTION

Most infected people develop a delayed hypersensitivity reaction when challenged with an intradermal injection of tuberculin (see below). This reactivity usually develops about 3 to 8 weeks after the initial infection. The tuberculin test is the standard method for detecting infected people. It aids tuberculosis control programmes by allowing those infected by a source case to be traced.

The annual risk of infection is calculated by skin testing members of an appropriate age group, such as schoolchildren or military recruits, over several years. The annual risk of infection gives an indirect measurement of the number of open or infectious cases of tuberculosis in the community and provides one of the best means of estimating the efficacy of tuberculosis control measures.

An approximation of the true prevalence of tuberculosis in a high-prevalence country may be determined by assuming that a 1 per cent annual risk of infection implies a prevalence of between 39 and 59 infectious (smear-positive) cases of pulmonary tuberculosis per 100 000 population and that for every smear-positive case there are 1.22 cases of smear-negative and non-pulmonary tuberculosis.

Tuberculin testing

The three principal methods for tuberculin testing are the Mantoux, Heaf, and tine tests.

Mantoux test

In the Mantoux test, 0.1 ml of solution containing a known number of international units (**TU**) of purified protein derivative (**PPD**) of tuberculin is injected intradermally. The diameter of the induration is read 48 to 72 h later. Induration of 5 mm or more is usually regarded as positive. In Great Britain, PPD is supplied in three dilutions:

1 in 100 = (1000 TU/ml) = 100 TU/0.1 ml;
1 in 1000 = (100 TU/ml) = 10 TU/0.1 ml;
1 in 10 000 = (10 TU/ml) = 1 TU/0.1 ml.

In other countries, 5 TU is usually used for standard Mantoux testing. If tuberculosis is suspected, testing should be started at the lowest dilution to prevent a severe reaction.

Heaf test

The Heaf test is made on the volar surface of the forearm using a spring-loaded, six-needled gun, which introduces a drop of undiluted PPD (100 000 TU/ml) into the dermis.

The reaction is read 3 to 10 days later:

Grade I: four or more discrete papules;
Grade II: confluent papules forming a ring;
Grade III: a disc of induration;
Grade IV: a disc of induration greater than 10 mm in diameter or vesiculation of the disc.

Because of the risk of transmission of hepatitis, HIV, and other viruses, formal sterilization of the Heaf gun is mandatory. Detachable magnetic heads are now available.

Tine test

The tine test is similar in principle to the Heaf test but uses a disposable device with four prongs (tines) coated with freeze-dried PPD. It is very convenient for single tests, but is not recommended because variable coating and absorption of PPD into the skin leads to a high incidence of false results.

Interpretation of the tuberculin test

Approximate equivalence of the Heaf test to 10 TU PPD by the Mantoux test is shown in Table 3. Heaf (or Mantoux) testing a population can be

Table 3 *Equivalence of Heaf test to Mantoux (10 TU PPD)*

Heaf grade	Mantoux (mm induration)
0	0–4
I	5–9
II	10–14
III	15–19
IV	20+

expected to provide a series of reactions as shown in Fig. 11, 87 per cent having a grade 0 or I reaction (up to 9 mm of induration to 10 TU PPD by the Mantoux test). Only 6 per cent will have grade III or IV Heaf (greater than 15 mm of induration to 10 TU), regarded in the United Kingdom as indicating infection by *M. tuberculosis*. BCG will convert 80 per cent of individuals to grade I or II. Those with grade III or IV should still be regarded as having infection by *M. tuberculosis* but 11 per cent in these categories are attributable to BCG.

The cut-off point for a positive test (i.e. indicating infection with *M. tuberculosis*) may vary from country to country as tuberculin reactions are affected by exposure to environmental mycobacteria.

In the United States, where 5 TU of PPD is used in the standard Mantoux test, a cut-off point of 10 mm of induration is accepted for the country as a whole, though this may be varied according to locality and the particular risk of the individual being tested.

A grade III or IV Heaf test probably denotes infection and should be followed up. Grade II reactions require follow-up only if they come from a high-risk group, such as an immigrant group, or if they are close contacts of a case of tuberculosis (see next section).

Tuberculosis control

Successful control of tuberculosis demands correct assessment of disease, infection and risk of infection, and appropriate action.

The principal methods and actions are as shown in Table 4.

Fig. 11 Histogram showing percentages of children aged approximately 13 years with various grades of Heaf reactivity. Two populations are shown, one unvaccinated and the other vaccinated.

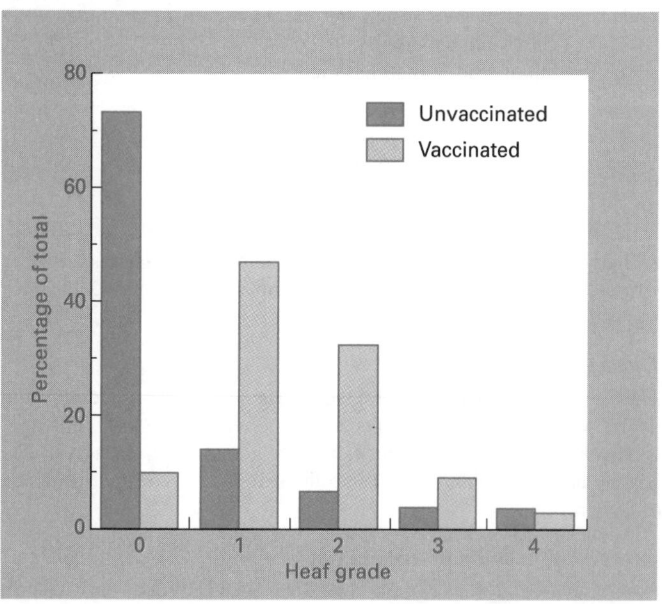

Table 4 *Method and action in tuberculosis control*

Method	Action
Case finding	
Passive: patient presents to clinic Active: survey high-risk groups	Treatment of patient with disease
Detection of infected individuals at risk of developing disease	Chemoprophylaxis
Prevention of established infection in individuals not yet infected	BCG or chemoprophylaxis

Case finding (active)

CONTACTS

Close contacts of patients with smear-positive tuberculosis should be screened, particularly those in the same household, as about 10 per cent will develop the disease. A scheme for examination and management of close contacts is shown in Fig. 12.

Screening of casual contacts of sputum smear-positive cases will yield less than 1 per cent of further cases. Contacts of adults with smear-negative or extrapulmonary disease need not be screened but close contacts of children with primary tuberculosis (pulmonary, pleural, meningeal or erythema nodosum) should be screened, as infection is likely to be recent, and a source case should be identified and treated to prevent further spread of disease to the community.

Close contacts of children found to have a strong tuberculin reaction on routine school testing should be screened to identify the source of infection, if infection is thought to be recent or if the child is from a high risk group.

IMMIGRANTS

Recent immigrants from countries with high prevalence rates of tuberculosis (e.g. Africa, Indian subcontinent, South-East Asia) should be screened by chest radiography. It is suggested that immigrants should be screened if they come from a country with an annual incidence of tuberculosis of 40 or more per 100 000. In the absence of radiological evidence of tuberculosis, a tuberculin test should be made. If this is strongly positive, preventive chemotherapy should be recommended for children and young adults (up to 35 years of age). If it is negative, BCG vaccination is recommended.

HIV-POSITIVITY

At least 30 per cent of those with concurrent HIV and *M. tuberculosis* infections will develop overt tuberculosis. Preventive chemotherapy is strongly recommended.

HEALTH WORKERS

Health and hospital workers vary in their risk of contracting and disseminating tuberculosis. Staff working with children or immunocompromised patients should have a chest radiograph before starting work. Mortuary workers, microbiology staff, and those caring for patients with tuberculosis should have a pre-employment chest radiograph and tuberculin test. Those who are tuberculin negative should be given BCG. Routine chest radiography during employment is not recommended. Other health workers should be given BCG vaccination, if indicated. Other specific precautions need not be taken.

OTHERS AT RISK

Tuberculin-positive intravenous drug users and those whose chest radiographs suggest healed tuberculosis but who have never had a full course of chemotherapy should be considered for preventive chemotherapy.

Chemoprophylaxis

There are two types: primary prophylaxis is given to uninfected people at high risk of infection (e.g. small children in close household contact with a smear-positive patient); secondary prophylaxis, more properly termed preventive therapy, is given to healthy but infected people to prevent overt tuberculosis. The usual regimens are isoniazid alone for 6 to 12 months or isoniazid with rifampicin for 3 months. Preventive therapy (secondary prophylaxis) is recommended for the following:

1. Recent tuberculin converters (i.e. those recently infected). command.
2. Tuberculin-positive children under the age of 5 years.
3. Strongly positive reactors (Heaf grade III or IV) in high-risk groups such as immigrants from countries with a high prevalence of tuberculosis.
4. Children found to have strong tuberculin reactions (grade III or IV) on routine school testing, even though the risk of disease is low. Some countries, especially the United States, where BCG vaccination is not given, have more aggressive policies of preventive chemotherapy, recommending it for any

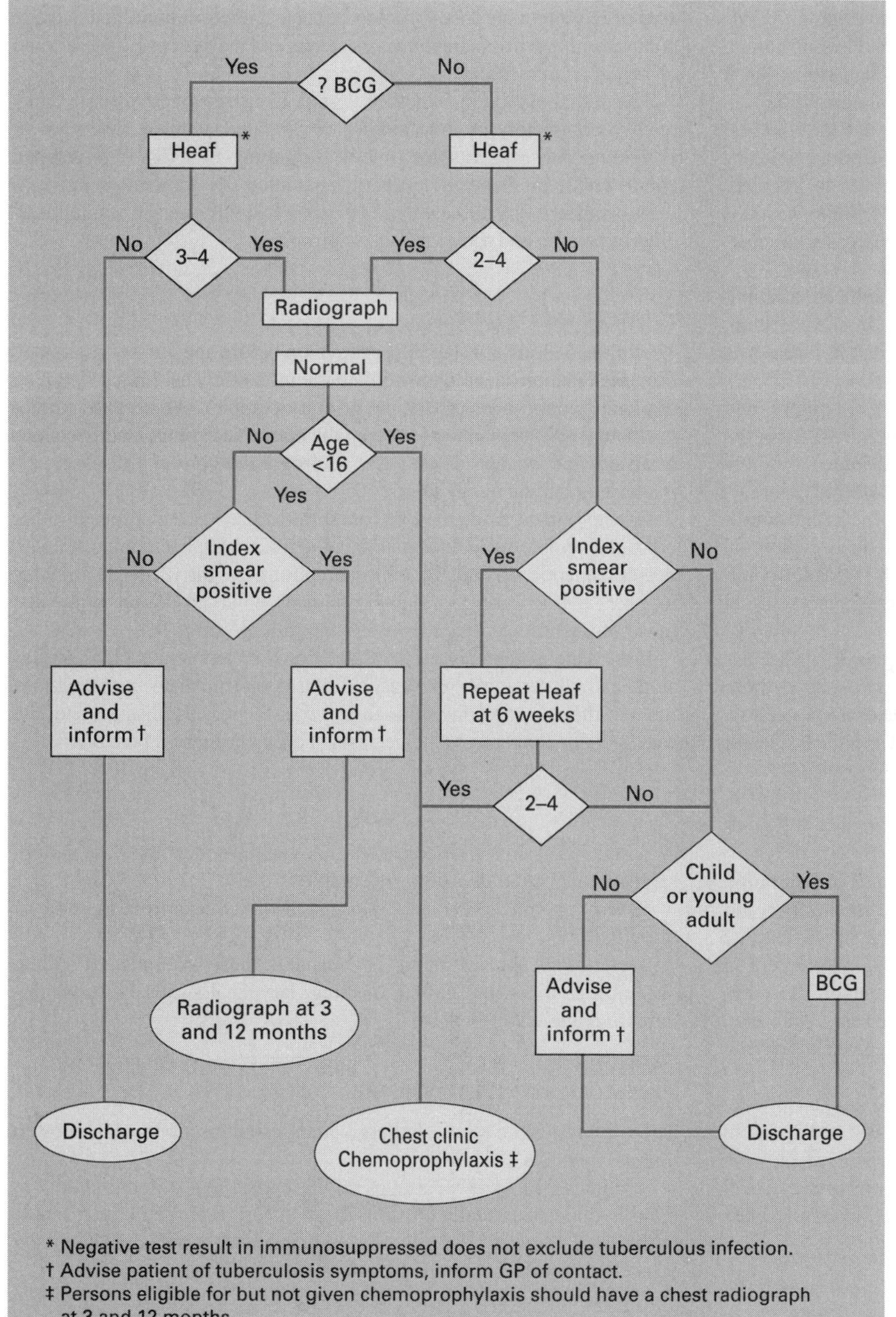

Fig. 12 Examination of close contacts of tuberculosis. *Note*: children under 2 years who are close contacts of an adult index patient with positive sputum smears should be given chemoprophylaxis irrespective of tuberculin status plus BCG later if applicable. (Reproduced from *Thorax*, with permission.)

infected (tuberculin-positive) person under the age of 35 years. The possible benefits must be balanced against the risk of side-effects.

5. Patients with evidence of old, healed tuberculosis who are about to be treated with corticosteroids or other immunosuppressive agents.
6. HIV-positive people with positive tuberculin reactions.
7. Close contacts of smear-positive cases with a Heaf grade III or IV and who are under 16 years, or under 35 if they are in a high-risk group. Prophylaxis is indicated for some close contacts who are grade II, and have not had previous BCG (Fig. 12).

BCG vaccination

Originally BCG was given orally to neonates to mimic natural infection by *M. bovis* because self-healing tuberculosis of bovine origin in childhood was thought to protect against pulmonary tuberculosis of human origin (Marfan's law), but for reasons of safety and standardization, it is now prepared as a freeze-dried vaccine for intradermal injection.

The mode of action of BCG is poorly understood but its principal benefit is the prevention of serious non-pulmonary forms of primary tuberculosis. It affords no appreciable protection if given to infected, tuberculin-positive people. Thus, unless used widely for many years, it has little impact on the numbers of open or infectious cases of postprimary tuberculosis in a community.

The efficacy of BCG vaccination shows wide geographical variation, as revealed by a number of major BCG trials (Table 5). In Great Britain, the protective efficacy, irrespective of the incidence of the disease, is about 75 per cent when given to children aged 13 years.

Vaccination policies vary considerably from country to country, and even between health authorities in a given country. In Great Britain the national policy is still that schoolchildren should be vaccinated routinely at the age of 11 to 13 years. Vaccination should also be offered to infants born into communities where the risk of infection is high (e.g. immigrants from the Indian subcontinent). Those exposed to occupational risk (e.g. health workers), those about to travel to high-incidence countries, and tuberculin-negative contacts of smear-positive patients should also be vaccinated (Fig. 12).

Mass BCG vaccination of neonates may be valuable. There is evidence that vaccination at a very early age is beneficial even in those countries where later vaccination seems to confer little or no protection. Further trials are required to determine efficacy and the ideal age for vaccination (directly at birth or after a few weeks).

TECHNIQUE

Only those negative on tuberculin testing (under 10 mm of induration to 10 TU by the Mantoux or grade 0 or I by the Heaf method) should be vaccinated; 0.1 ml (0.05 ml for neonates) of freeze-dried vaccine suspended in a dilutent is injected intradermally over the lower insertion of the deltoid in the left arm. Consistency of the vaccination site facilitates subsequent surveys based on the presence of BCG scars. A nodule, which usually ulcerates, develops and persists for about 6 weeks, leaving a small scar.

Adverse reactions are rare and are usually caused by faulty technique. They include local abscess formation with, occasionally, enlargement or suppuration of the regional lymph nodes. Generalized infection is extremely rare and usually occurs only in the immunosuppressed. Local abscesses should be drained. Isoniazid or erythromycin may hasten recovery.

BCG VACCINATION AND HIV INFECTION

The World Health Organization recommends that, in high-prevalence countries, children with clinical signs of AIDS should not be given BCG vaccine but asymptomatic HIV-positive children should be vaccinated. In low-prevalence countries, BCG is not recommended for children born to HIV-positive mothers unless, after the age of 12 to 15 months (when maternal antibodies have been eliminated) they are found to be HIV-negative. HIV-positive adults should not be given BCG but may be given primary chemoprophylaxis if they are at high risk of infection.

The clinical course of tuberculosis

Tuberculosis is spread principally by inhalation of expectorated droplet nuclei containing bacilli. Rarely, infection is acquired by drinking milk containing *M. bovis* or by traumatic inoculation into the skin. Only a small proportion of those infected develop overt tuberculosis. Determinants of the outcome of primary infection are poorly understood but probably include various non-specific immune defence mechanisms, the size of the infecting dose, priming of the specific immune defences by contact with environmental mycobacteria, and the patient's general state of health and nutrition.

The initial infection, whether or not it causes overt disease, may resolve completely or may merely be contained, with progression to postprimary disease at some time in the future (Fig. 13). In developed countries the incidence of primary tuberculosis is declining relative to that of postprimary disease, which is increasingly seen in immigrants, elderly people, and the immunocompromised.

Primary tuberculosis

The initial lesions of tuberculosis develop before specific cell-mediated immune reactions develop to contain the infection. Dissemination to the regional lymph nodes causes the primary complex and there is further haematogenous spread to all parts of the body. Necrosis is inconspicuous or absent and, except in rare cases of progressive primary disease, pulmonary cavitation is not seen.

Asymptomatic cases may be found on routine examination. In other cases the symptoms include cough, sometimes with haemoptysis, fever, decreased appetite and, in children, failure to thrive. Signs include wheezes due to bronchial compression by enlarged lymph nodes and those of pneumonia secondary to lobar collapse (Fig. 14).

Immediate complications include bronchopneumonia, pleural effusion, and disseminated (miliary) disease. Intermediate complications include the various non-pulmonary forms of primary disease and late complications include bronchiectasis and postprimary tuberculosis.

DIAGNOSIS

A peripheral lesion with enlarged hilar lymph nodes on chest radiography is diagnostic of a primary complex.

Tuberculin conversion usually occurs 3 to 8 weeks from the time of infection.

Bacteriological confirmation is unusual because sputum is difficult to obtain in children, but gastric washing, laryngeal swabs, or bronchoscopy may yield the diagnosis.

ALLERGIC MANIFESTATIONS

There are two main types of allergic manifestations, erythema nodosum and phlyctenular conjunctivitis.

Erythema nodosum consists of raised tender areas of induration, 2 to 5 cm in diameter, usually on shins or on knees, thighs, and the extensor surfaces of forearms and elbows, associated with arthralgia of larger joints and fever. The tuberculin test is almost invariably positive.

Phlyctenular conjunctivitis, which may occur in some children within 1 year of the primary infection, consists of small, multiple, yellow or grey conjunctival nodules near the limbus, with a sheaf of dilated vessels.

Table 5 *The protective efficacy of BCG vaccination found in nine major trials*

Population studied	Date of commencement	Duration (years)	Age range	Protection conferred (%)
North American Indian	1935–38	9–11	0–20 months	80
Chicago, USA	1937–48	12–23	3 months	75
Georgia, USA	1947	20	6–17 years	0
Illinois, USA	1947–48	19–20	Young adults	0
Puerto Rico	1949–51	5–7.5	1–18 years	31
Georgia/Alabama, USA	1950	14	Over 5 years	14
United Kingdom	1950–52	15	14–15 years	78
South India (Bangalore)	1950–55	9–14	All ages	30
South India (Madras)	1969–71	7.5	All ages	0*

*A 15-year follow-up revealed a low level of protection (17 per cent) in those aged 0–14 years at vaccination and no protection in older age groups.

TREATMENT AND OUTCOME

Standard chemotherapy is used. Most primary infections pass unnoticed and may be detected only by tuberculin conversion or if a subsequent radiological examination reveals a calcified focus. Non-pulmonary disease, such as tuberculous meningitis or miliary tuberculosis, may result from haematogenous dissemination. In many cases the infection lies dormant for many years.

Postprimary tuberculosis

Postprimary tuberculosis occurs in the previously infected, usually tuberculin-positive, person as a result of endogenous reactivation of a dormant infection or of exogenous reinfection. For unknown reasons, lesions usually develop in the upper parts of the lungs. Necrosis is prominent, resulting in large solid lesions (tuberculomas) and cavities (see Figs 5 and 6). The local lymph nodes are not usually involved and haematogenous dissemination is rare, except in the immunocompromised. Infection can spread to other parts of the lungs and the larynx through the bronchial tree. Bacilli may be swallowed in sputum, causing indurated lesions of the alimentary tract.

The course of postprimary tuberculosis is very variable. Some patients progress from being completely well to having extensive disease within a few weeks or even days while others have chronic symptoms for several years before seeking medical attention. In the prechemotherapeutic era, about one-third of patients died, one-third apparently achieved a spontaneous cure, and one-third developed chronic disease with gradual healing by fibrosis over many years.

PRESENTATION

Postprimary tuberculosis can range clinically from absence of symptoms to extreme prostration. Patients may be slightly unwell for several months before seeking medical attention, during which time extensive disease may develop. Most cases are pulmonary (about 85 per cent of cases among white patients in Great Britain) but involvement of non-

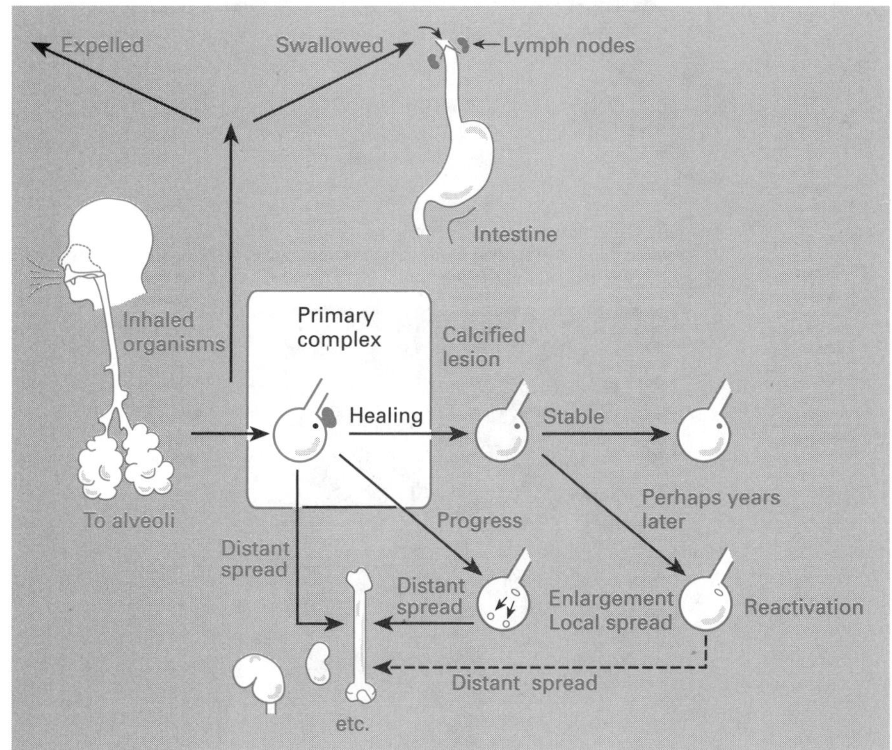

Fig. 13 Diagramatic representation of the ways in which tuberculosis may spread through the body.

respiratory sites is common in immigrants and in the immunocompromised.

Some symptom-free patients are detected on routine screening; others present with malaise, weight loss, fever, night sweats, and anorexia. Those with pulmonary disease may present with cough (worse in the morning and sometimes with haemoptysis), chest pain, breathlessness, and signs of pneumonia. Patients with advanced disease may have severe weight loss. On examination, the lung signs are variable and usually less evident than the radiological signs would suggest. They include crackles, diminished breath sounds, and bronchial breathing. Patients with chronic disease may have tracheal deviation and coarse crackles over the area of disease due to fibrosis. A pleural effusion may be present.

DIAGNOSIS

Given adequate facilities, the diagnosis of postprimary pulmonary tuberculosis usually poses few problems. Occasionally, diagnosis may prove very difficult and is made retrospectively after a successful trial of chemotherapy. The most important diagnostic tools are bacteriological and radiological but some cases are diagnosed by histological appearances and tuberculin reactivity.

Sputum (and other specimens) for bacteriological examination should be obtained as outlined above. Microscopical demonstration of acid-fast bacilli in sputum smears provides a rapid presumptive diagnosis, although the technique is not very sensitive and fails to distinguish between tubercle bacilli and environmental mycobacteria. The more sensitive cultural methods, including rapid radiometric ones, prove the diagnosis. In principle, the polymerase chain reaction should provide an extremely specific, sensitive, and rapid diagnosis but more research is required before it is suitable for routine diagnosis.

Radiological changes, though sensitive, are rather non-specific. Tuberculosis may cause virtually any radiological abnormality and atypical pictures are not uncommon, especially in HIV-positive and other immunocompromised persons. Thus bacteriological confirmation should always be sought. The following radiological features are characteristic of postprimary pulmonary tuberculosis:

(1) soft, floccular, unilateral or bilateral, nodular shadowing in the upper lobes, particularly in the posterior and apical segments (Fig. 15);

Fig. 14 Anteroposterior chest radiograph of a 2-year-old child showing right hilar and paratracheal lymph-node enlargement and lobar collapse due to primary tuberculosis.

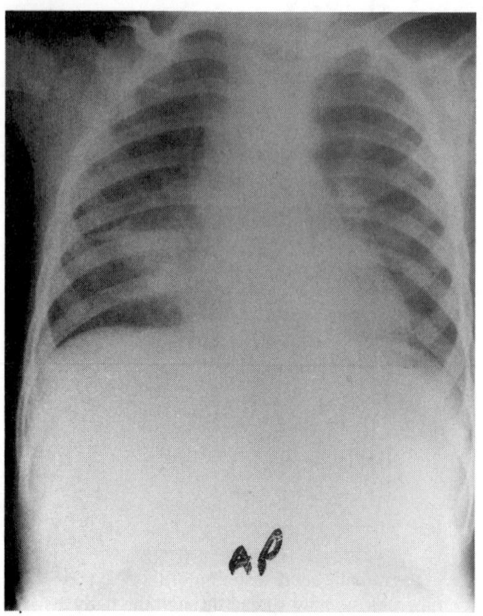

(2) cavitation, usually in the upper posterior parts of the lung (Fig. 16);

(3) calcification due to old, healed disease;

(4) linear shadowing indicative of fibrosis in the upper zones;

(5) a combination of (3) and (4) and soft shadowing—this is highly suggestive of reactivation of old, healed, postprimary disease;

(6) small ($<$ 1 cm diameter) nodules throughout the lung fields, indicative of miliary disease (Fig. 17);

(7) pleural effusion or mediastinal enlargement;

(8) extensive patchy shadowing throughout the lung fields indicative of widespread tuberculous bronchopneumonia (Fig. 18).

Granulomas, with caseation and giant cells, in lung biopsies obtained by fibreoptic bronchoscopy or in non-pulmonary lesions, are virtually diagnostic of tuberculosis. If caseation is not present, the differential diagnosis includes sarcoidosis, lymphomas, and foreign-body granulomas.

A strongly positive Mantoux test ($>$ 15 mm induration to 10 TU PPD)

Fig. 15 Anteroposterior chest radiograph of a 43-year-old man showing extensive bilateral tuberculosis.

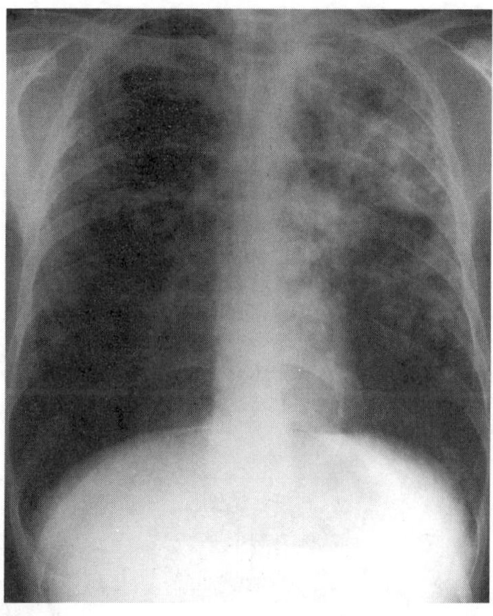

Fig. 16 Anteroposterior chest radiograph of 67-year-old woman with chronic active disease suggested by deviation of the trachea to the left. There is a large cavity in the left upper zone.

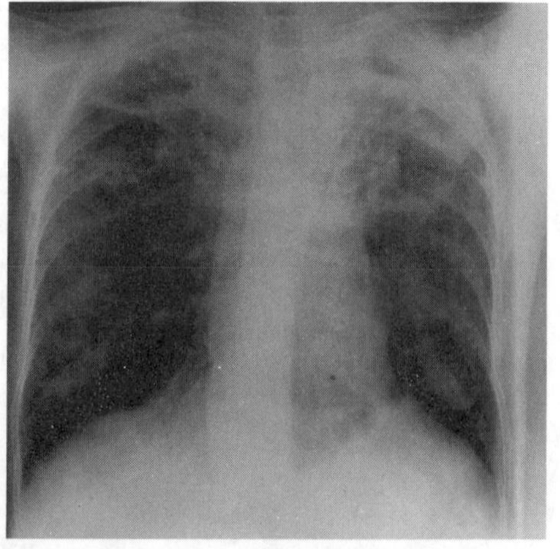

in a patient with other evidence of active tuberculosis strongly supports the diagnosis. Strong reactions may, however, occur in healthy people with repeated occupational exposure to infectious tuberculosis patients and in those with old, healed disease.

The results of other laboratory tests are not specific. Often there is a normal white-cell count or a slight lymphocytosis, a high erythrocyte sedimentation rate, and an iron-deficiency anaemia.

Despite a huge amount of research, there is no reliable serological test. Detection of chemical structures unique to *M. tuberculosis*, such as tuberculostearic acid, by gas chromatography or mass spectroscopy provides a rapid, sensitive, and specific diagnosis but the complex and costly equipment is seldom available.

COMPLICATIONS

Postprimary pulmonary tuberculosis may present with a complication due to the direct spread of bacilli or with an indirect complication. Direct complications include:

1. Pleural effusion due to direct spread of the disease from the lung to the visceral pleura. Diagnosis may be made by biopsy. Addition of corticosteroids to antituberculous chemotherapy reduces the volume of the effusion and may limit subsequent scarring.

Fig. 17 Miliary disease in a 70-year-old woman (by courtesy of Dr P. Ormerod).

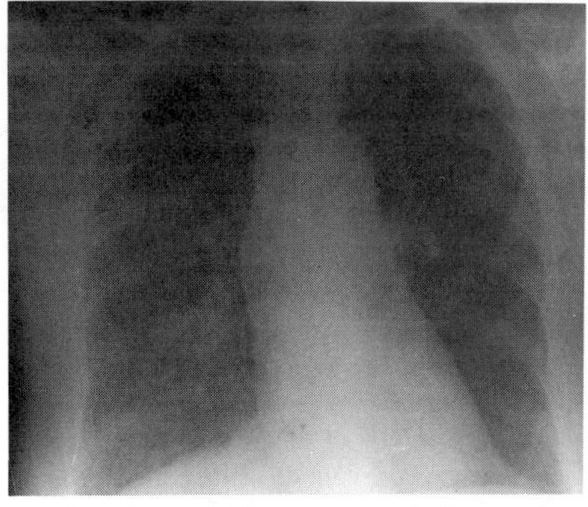

Fig. 18 Patchy consolidation of tuberculous bronchopneumonia in a 28-year-old Chinese woman. Bronchoscopy revealed tuberculomas studding the left main and left lower-lobe bronchi.

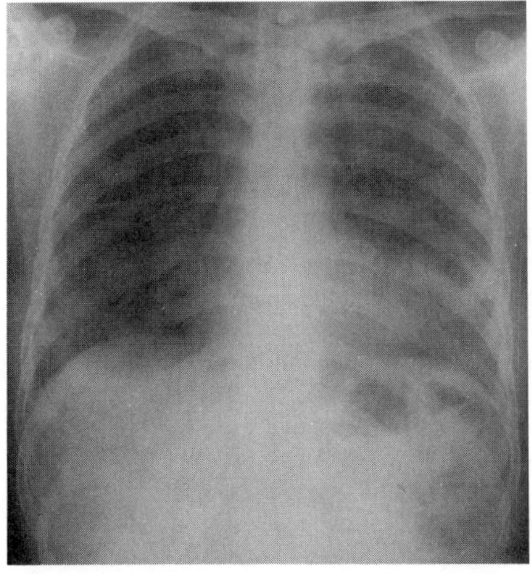

2. Empyema: a pleural effusion may progress to empyema, characterized by purulent, 'sterile', pleural fluid. Surgical drainage may be required towards the end of a course of chemotherapy.
3. Laryngeal disease caused by secondary infection of the vocal chords by bacilli in sputum and leading to pain and dysphonia.
4. More distant spread of disease.

Indirect complications include:

(1) airflow obstruction due to a swelling of bronchial lymphatics which may cause partial or complete bronchial obstruction;
(2) aspergilloma due to the colonization of old cavities resulting in a ball of fungal hyphae;
(3) haemoptysis, which may occur during active disease or many years later due to a breakdown of fibrous scarring or invasion by an aspergilloma and which may be fatal.

Differential diagnosis

Tuberculosis has been called the great mimic as its signs and symptoms are extremely variable. It must be differentiated from a wide range of other diseases including:

1. Carcinoma of the lung, particularly in middle-aged or elderly smokers. Squamous-cell carcinoma frequently cavitates and so may be confused with postprimary tuberculosis. The absence of acid-fast bacilli in the sputum of patients with a cavity should lead to a suspicion of carcinoma, although tuberculosis and carcinoma may coexist. When there is doubt, tissue for histological examination should be obtained by transbronchial, percutaneous, or open lung biopsy.
2. Pneumonia: unresolved pneumonia, especially if due to staphylococci or *Klebsiella* spp. may proceed to cavitation and resemble tuberculosis on radiography.
3. Allergic bronchopulmonary aspergillosis: this is confirmed by tests for antibody to Aspergillus.
4. Fibrotic lung disease due to sarcoidosis, extrinsic allergic alveolitis, pneumoconiosis, and silicosis: a biopsy and negative tuberculin test aid the diagnosis of sarcoidosis and immunological screening aids that of extrinsic allergic alveolitis. Pneumoconiosis and silicosis are suggested by occupational histories. Silicosis predisposes to tuberculosis so the two diseases may coexist.
5. The chronic malaise and cachexia of tuberculosis resembles that due to anorexia nervosa, diabetes mellitus, and hyperthyroidism.
6. Tuberculosis may present as pyrexia of unknown origin. Other causes, particularly malignancies, must be considered.
7. Mediastinal lymphadenopathy, which in Great Britain is a common presentation of tuberculosis in immigrants from Africa and the Indian subcontinent, may also be a presenting feature of lymphoma. Biopsies should be obtained whenever possible.

Outcome

The overall mortality for all forms of tuberculosis in Great Britain is about 8 per cent, varying from under 1 per cent for children and young adults to over 30 per cent in those aged 75 years or more. Mortality is higher for patients with extensive disease, smear positivity and cavitation. Mortality appears to be the same in both sexes, even though males are twice as likely to develop pulmonary disease. Most deaths occur early in treatment: a recent study showed that over two-thirds of deaths due to pulmonary tuberculosis occurred within 4 weeks of starting chemotherapy.

Even when chemotherapy is successful, long-term sequelae due to scarring may occur, especially if disease was extensive before treatment.

Tuberculosis in the HIV-positive patient

HIV testing should be considered in all cases of tuberculosis. HIV considerably accelerates the progression of infection by the tubercle bacillus to overt disease by reducing the host's cell-mediated immunity. In Africa, tuberculosis is common in HIV-infected people and is often the earliest sign of immunosuppression because the tubercle bacillus is relatively more virulent than other pathogens associated with HIV infection and overcomes host immunity at a higher CD4 count.

Non-respiratory disease, particularly lymph-node disease, is much more common in the HIV-infected host. Pulmonary disease is less often cavitating and smear-positive. For this reason, tuberculosis may be more difficult to diagnose. Induced sputa, using nebulized hypertonic saline, may be helpful in providing specimens for bacteriological testing. Bronchoalveolar washings may be required.

Chemotherapy is usually effective but relapse, perhaps due to a subsequent infection, is more common than in HIV-negative patients.

Multidrug-resistant tuberculosis

There have been a number of reports recently, from the United States, of outbreaks of multidrug-resistant tuberculosis. These differ from previously described outbreaks in that they have spread rapidly, involved larger numbers of patients, and occurred in institutions.

A total of 253 cases in seven such outbreaks had been reported by the end of 1992. The number of cases in each outbreak ranged from 7 to 70. All involved the transmission of multidrug-resistant tuberculosis from patient to patient or from patient to health-care worker. In four outbreaks the strain was resistant to seven drugs (isoniazid, rifampicin, streptomycin, ethambutol, ethionamide, kanamycin, and rifabutin). Because many patients were HIV-positive, mortality was high (60–89 per cent) and the disease progressed rapidly from diagnosis to death (median interval, 4–16 weeks). At least five health-care workers died in these outbreaks, four of whom were known to be HIV-seropositive.

Though the causes of multidrug-resistance are not yet clear there is an association with a history of previous treatment, HIV-seropositivity, homelessness, and drug abuse. Patients who are homeless and/or drug abusers are more likely to have been in contact with source cases who may have been poorly compliant with therapy, thus increasing the chance that they will develop secondary resistance and infect others with drug-resistant strains.

Multidrug-resistant strains have also been reported from other parts of the world, particularly the non-industrialized countries. Strains resistant to at least one drug may also be becoming more common, being reported in immigrants to the United States from Vietnam (33 per cent), Philippines (35 per cent), Mexico (15 per cent), China (39 per cent), and South Korea (45 per cent).

The emergence of multidrug resistance has brought with it enormous ethical and administrative problems. These include the social consequences of isolating and treating patients against their wishes, the cost of therapy with alternative drugs, amounting to US $200 000 or more per patient in order to achieve a 50 per cent cure rate, and the problem of long-term isolation of those who do not respond to such therapy. Surgical procedures may be required as an adjunct to chemotherapy.

Management of the patient with tuberculosis

Most patients with tuberculosis, whether pulmonary or extrapulmonary, are well enough to be managed as outpatients. Hospital admission to obtain specimens such as bronchoalveolar washings to confirm the diagnosis for sputum smear-negative pulmonary tuberculosis may be required. Where day-case facilities are available, admissions may be unnecessary.

For the particularly ill patient or the elderly, admission for observation during the first days of treatment may be advisable as adverse reactions to treatment are more common and severe in these groups. As noted above, for reasons not fully understood, mortality tends to be highest in the few weeks immediately after treatment has started. The strongly smear-positive patient is rendered non-infectious very soon after the beginning of treatment so that isolation is not necessary beyond 2 weeks of treatment. Segregation may be necessary where HIV-positive patients are being nursed on the same ward. Often bacilli can be detected microscopically in sputum for some months after treatment has begun because dead bacilli may continue to be expectorated. After 2 to 3 months of treatment, cultures are almost always negative. A full 6 months of treatment is required to prevent relapse.

Severely ill patients may present with hypoxia and hyponatraemia and require the necessary supportive measures. Addison's disease is now uncommon in the developed world, but it should be considered in the ill, prostrate, or comatose patient. Mineralocorticoid and corticosteroid supplements are required. Hypercalcaemia is rare. Long-term admission may be necessary for a few non-compliant patients, such as those who are alcoholic or mentally defective, to ensure that they receive a full course of supervised chemotherapy. In New York, increasing numbers of patients are defaulting from outpatient regimens. An intermittent supervised form of chemotherapy, in which the patient attends an outpatient clinic two or three times a week, is used in a number of countries. It is suitable for urbanized communities, such as Hong Kong. If necessary, therapy may be directly administered by district nurses, or specialist tuberculosis nurses, in the home of patients unable to take medication on their own. This relieves hospital beds.

After treatment has started, initial follow-up should be monthly for two visits. Sputum may be obtained for culture to ensure there is conversion. Follow-up chest radiographs are usually unnecessary. Jaundice, sickness, and cutaneous side-effects usually occur in the first month, forcing the patient to stop therapy, which is why an early appointment is essential.

With good compliance, relapse is rare so that once a course of treatment is completed routine follow-up is unnecessary. A chest radiograph at the completion of treatment is probably of value for comparison should relapse occur.

Non-respiratory tuberculosis

A substantial minority of cases of tuberculosis, particularly in immigrants, ethnic minorities, and immunocompromised patients, occur at sites other than the lung. A recent survey of tuberculosis notifications in England and Wales showed that 20 per cent of white patients and 47 per cent of patients of Indian subcontinent ethnic origin presented with non-pulmonary disease (Table 6).

LYMPH-NODE TUBERCULOSIS

Cervical nodes are the most frequently involved extrathoracic lymph nodes. Formerly lymph-node tuberculosis was a common affliction, termed scrofula or the King's evil from the belief that it could be cured by the monarch's touch. Cervical lymphadenopathy may be part of a primary complex, usually involving the tonsillar nodes. It may also result from haematogenous dissemination or lymphatic spread from intrathoracic disease, in which case the supraclavicular nodes are usually involved and mediastinal or paratracheal lymphadenopathy may be seen on chest radiography. In countries with a high prevalence of tuberculosis children and young adults are most frequently affected whereas in low-prevalence countries the disease is more common in older adults, particularly women.

Lymph-node swelling is usually slow and insidious. A single node or a number in a particular chain may be affected. They feel rubbery or hard and may be tender. They may suppurate to form abscesses and sinuses that result in a chronic discharge of pus. Spread of disease from the sinuses may cause chronic skin tuberculosis (scrofuloderma). One- to two-thirds of patients have fever, night sweats, weight loss, and malaise.

Table 6 *Non-respiratory disease sites by ethnic origin in a survey of tuberculosis notifications in England and Wales*

	Ethnic origin	
Disease site	White *N* (%)	Indian subcontinent *N* (%)
Lymph node	86 (37)	205 (52)
Bone and joint	31 (13)	51 (13)
Genitourinary tract	65 (28)	16 (4)
Abdomen	14 (6)	57 (14)
Central nervous system	10 (4)	21 (5)
Miliary	19 (8)	27 (7)
Abscess	10 (4)	14 (4)
Other	18 (8)	32 (8)
Total number of patients*	233 (100)	345 (100)

*Some patients had lesions at more than one site.

Histological and microscopical confirmation of the diagnosis should be attempted. Because of the small numbers of bacteria present, microscopical examination is usually negative and culture is positive in only 70 per cent of cases. Surgical intervention may lead to chronically discharging sinuses, which may take months to heal.

Standard chemotherapy is effective. The nodes may enlarge during or after chemotherapy, perhaps as a result of hypersensitivity reactions. Corticosteroids are often used to reduce such enlargement but are of unproven efficacy. Surgery may, on rare occasions, be required for cosmetic reasons. The treatment of mediastinal lymphadenitis, which in Great Britain is particularly common in immigrants from Asia, is the same as for pulmonary tuberculosis.

Lymphadenitis in children and, to an increasing extent, young adults may be caused by environmental mycobacteria (see Chapter 7.11.24).

The differential diagnosis includes sarcoidosis, lymphoma, and carcinoma.

GENITOURINARY TUBERCULOSIS

Genitourinary tuberculosis is usually a late manifestation of infection and therefore tends to affect older patients. Lesions first appear in the renal cortex, perhaps because higher oxygen tension favours bacterial growth. Disease may then extend into the renal pelvis with spread to ureter, bladder, and genitalia. Ureteric obstruction with hydronephrosis is the most common complication. Tuberculosis of the female genitalia (fallopian tubes and uterus) is usually the result of haematogenous spread from a focus of disease elsewhere.

Urinary-tract disease

Clinical features include frequency and dysuria, ureteric colic, loin pain, backache, loin swelling due to a cold abscess, and symptoms of renal failure. Constitutional symptoms are uncommon unless other organs are affected.

Tuberculosis should be suspected in the presence of 'sterile' pyuria. At least three early-morning urine specimens should be taken for culture, as environmental mycobacteria often contaminate the genital tract. Acid-fast bacilli are rarely seen on direct smear.

It is important to assess renal function and to watch for the development of anatomical abnormalities during and after treatment.

Standard chemotherapy is used. Drugs excreted unchanged by the kidney, such as streptomycin and ethambutol, should be avoided when there is renal impairment. Ureteric obstruction may be avoided by giving corticosteroids at a dose of 20 to 40 mg daily for the initial 3 months of chemotherapy. Surgical intervention may be required for ureteric obstruction.

Genital tuberculosis

In males the epididymis is the most common site of genital tuberculosis, causing scrotal pain and swelling. Nodularity of the epididymis, vas deferens, and seminal vesicles may be felt. Sinus formation with skin involvement may occur.

In the female the fallopian tubes and endometrium are the usual sites of disease. Pain, menstrual disorder, dyspareunia, and vaginal discharge may occur. Infertility is usual. Diagnosis may be made by histological or bacteriological examination of appropriate biopsies and endometrial curettings.

BONE AND JOINT DISEASE

Orthopaedic tuberculosis remains a potentially crippling disease in the developing world, particularly as it usually affects children and young adults. In the developed world it is becoming increasingly rare. The spine is involved in about half the cases. The knee, hip, ankle, wrist, and elbow are involved in decreasing frequency, but any bony site may be affected and multiple sites are frequent. Infection of long bones tends to begin at the ends. The lesion may rupture through bone into the soft tissues causing a cold abscess. This is common in spinal disease and a paravertebral abscess may develop. Such abscesses may track along fascial planes in soft tissue and present at distant sites.

Spinal tuberculosis (Pott's disease)

The usual presenting symptom is back pain. A tracking abscess may present as a fluctuant mass on the chest wall or, in the case of a psoas abscess, in the groin. Late cases may present with kyphosis, paraesthesia or paraplegia. Examination may show local tenderness, muscular spasm or kyphosis.

Disease usually starts in the anterior aspect of the intervertebral disc and spreads to adjacent vertebrae along the anterior longitudinal ligaments, resulting in erosion of the anterior edges of the superior and inferior vertebral borders. Progressive destruction results in loss of volume of vertebral bodies anteriorly, with loss of height and kyphosis. More than one disc space may be involved and lesions may 'skip' with healthy vertebrae in between. Lower thoracic and lumbar vertebrae are those most commonly affected.

Lateral radiography often shows a characteristic appearance (Fig. 19) with loss of volume anteriorly. A computerized tomographic scan my show anterior erosion (Fig. 20). An attempt to obtain tissue for culture should be made, but a wide excision is required to ensure adequate specimens. The differential diagnosis includes pyogenic infections and malignant metastases; the latter more commonly involve the pedicles and spinal bodies leaving the discs intact.

Treatment is by standard chemotherapy. In the absence of severe deformity and spinal-cord compression, operative procedures afford little benefit, although in skilled hands radical excision and bone grafting ('Hong Kong operation') results in more rapid bony fusion and less residual spinal deformity.

TUBERCULOUS MENINGITIS

Tuberculous meningitis is an uncommon disease in developed countries, accounting for only 2 per cent of tuberculosis in England and Wales. It is more common among immunosuppressed patients and in immigrants from developing nations, among whom children and young adults are most often affected. It is also prevalent in some developing countries, such as India and China. Tuberculous meningitis is fully discussed in Chapter 24.15.1.

ABDOMINAL TUBERCULOSIS

Tuberculosis of the gastrointestinal tract may be a manifestation of primary tuberculosis caused by consuming milk containing *M. bovis*. More commonly it occurs in patients with postprimary pulmonary tuberculosis who have swallowed infected sputum. Tuberculous peritonitis, however, is rarely associated with pulmonary disease. The usual symptoms are those of subacute intestinal obstruction—recurrent abdominal pain and constipation—together with constitutional symptoms and weight loss. A plain abdominal radiograph may show fluid levels. The 'doughy abdomen' said to be characteristic of tuberculous peritonitis is an uncommon late manifestation.

The diagnosis is made by histological and bacteriological examination of specimens obtained at laparotomy or laparoscopy, or by needle biopsy.

Standard chemotherapy is used. The use of corticosteroids to prevent obstructions and adhesions due to scarring remains controversial.

TUBERCULOUS PERICARDITIS

Tuberculous pericarditis is rare in developed countries, accounting for less than 1 per cent of cases of tuberculosis in Great Britain. It is more common among immunosuppressed patients and in some African and Asian populations, notably the Xhosa people of Transkei in southern Africa.

Disease is usually due to the erosion of adjacent infected lymph nodes into the pericardial space. It presents as pericardial effusion, subacute or chronic constrictive pericarditis, or a combination of the two. Subacute constriction is typically associated with the presence of fibrocaseous material within the pericardial space, chronic constriction with fibrosis, and calcification.

The onset of effusion or subacute constriction is usually insidious, with fever, malaise, substernal pain, and dyspnoea on exertion. The signs include sinus tachycardia, arterial pulsus paradoxus, raised jugular venous pressure, hepatomegaly and ascites, the last three being particularly prominent in the presence of constriction. A pericardial rub may be heard. Effusion, especially if it develops rapidly, may cause tamponade. The electrocardiogram commonly shows non-specific but widespread T-wave abnormalities and low-voltage QRS complexes. On radiography, the heart shadow is enlarged, particularly when an effusion is present. Ultrasonography, computerized tomography, and magnetic resonance imaging may be useful in some cases.

Chronic constriction may develop weeks to years after the subacute stage, despite therapy. The cardiac silhouette may be normal in size but a ring of pericardial calcification may be seen.

The diagnosis of tuberculous pericarditis may be confirmed by histological examination of a pericardial biopsy. Conventional cultures of pericardial aspirates are positive in about 60 per cent of cases of effusion but the yield may be improved to 75 per cent by direct 'bedside' inoculation of pericardial fluid into double-strength liquid Kirschner medium.

Treatment is with standard antituberculosis chemotherapy. Pericardiectomy may be required for the relief of constriction. The addition to antituberculosis chemotherapy of prednisolone, 60 mg daily then in tapering doses over 11 weeks, has been shown to increase the rate of clinical improvement and reduce the risk of death. In cases of effusion it reduces the need for repeated pericardiocentesis and in cases of constriction the need for pericardiectomy.

LUPUS VULGARIS

Lupus vulgaris is a manifestation of tuberculosis of the skin, usually of the head and neck. Jelly-like nodules first appear, which may go on to ulcerate and cause extensive scarring. Standard chemotherapy is usually effective.

Fig. 19 Lateral radiograph of tuberculosis of the spine (Pott's disease) showing collapse of the L2 and L3 vertebrae and of the intervertebral disc (by courtesy of Professor Alan Scher, University of Stellenbosch, South Africa).

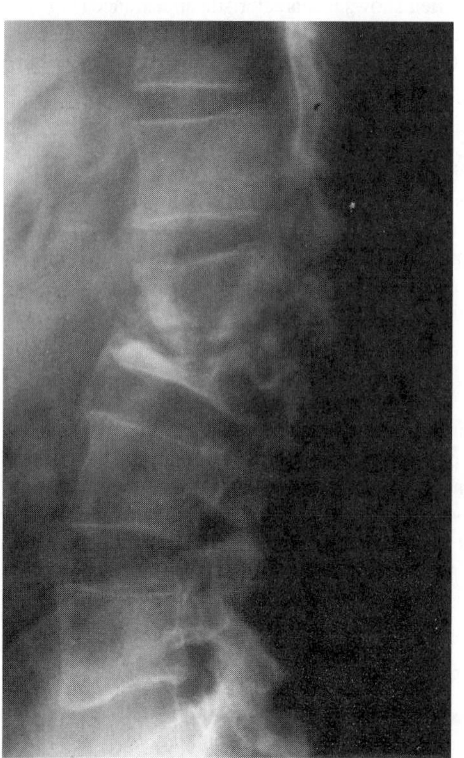

Fig. 20 (a) and (b) Two consecutive computerized tomographic scans of a vertebra taken at an interval of several months showing progressive erosion. Note the body of the vertebra is affected from anterior backwards.

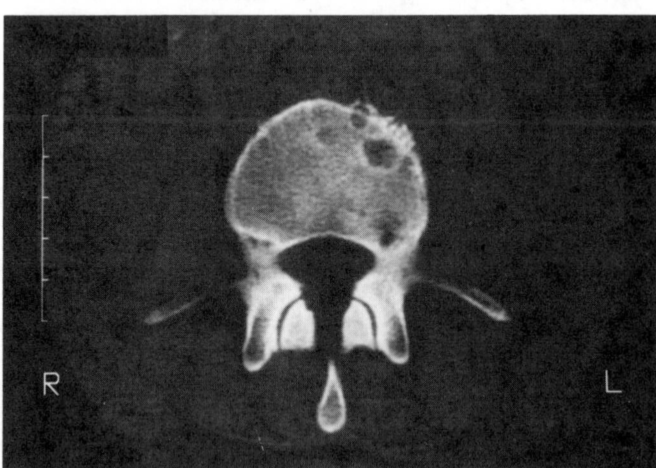

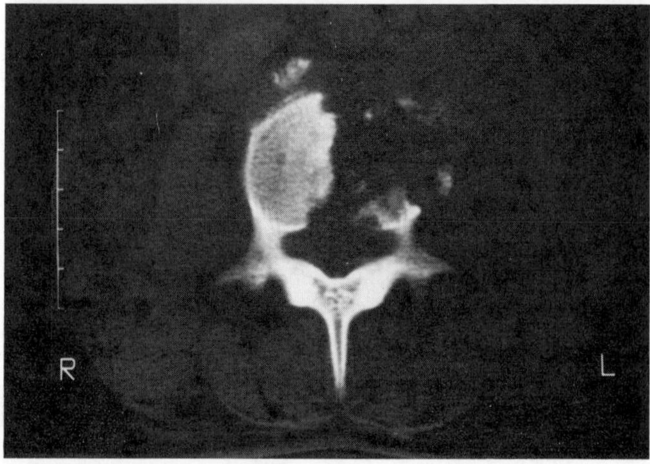

The antituberculosis drugs

The three key first-line drugs used for previously untreated patients are isoniazid, rifampicin, and pyrazinamide. Ethambutol and streptomycin are valuable additional drugs, and in some countries thiacetazone and *p*-aminosalicylic acid are still used. Reserve drugs, which may be used when first-line treatment has failed, are ethionamide or prothionamide, kanamycin, capreomycin, viomycin, cycloserine, and quinolones such as ofloxacin.

All strains of *M. tuberculosis* contain drug-resistant mutants; active tuberculosis, however limited in its extent, should therefore never be treated with a single drug because of the risk that acquired resistance will emerge.

The clinically important characteristics of the drugs are summarized in Table 7 and their dosages are shown in Table 8.

ISONIAZID

Isoniazid (isonicotinic acid hydrazide) is the main drug used in the treatment of all forms of tuberculosis. After a single oral dose, similar peak serum concentrations are seen in all patients, but 4 to 6 h after administration the serum concentrations differ according to the rate at which individuals metabolize the drug. There is a genetically determined bimodal distribution of slow and rapid acetylators, giving mean serum half-lives of about 3 and 1.4 h, respectively. The half-life may be prolonged in those with grossly impaired hepatic function.

Isoniazid inhibits the metabolism of phenytoin, carbamazepine, and ethosuximide, so that the dosages of these drugs may have to be reduced during its administration, particularly in slow acetylators. It forms a hydrazone with pyridoxine and can inhibit enzymes involved in the synthesis of nicotinamide from tryptophan; it can thereby cause or exacerbate pyridoxine and, more rarely, nicotinic acid deficiency (see also 'Patients with HIV infection or AIDS' below).

RIFAMPICIN

Rifampicin is an excellent combination drug for isoniazid, and is also useful in reserve regimens when it has not already been used. It is usual to give the drug half an hour before a meal, although this is not essential if inconvenient. A high proportion is bound to plasma proteins. Desacetylrifampicin, its main metabolite, is also biologically active.

Rifampicin induces hepatic microsomal enzymes, and hence reduces the serum half-lives and clinical efficacy of a number of drugs, including corticosteroids (the dosages of which should be doubled during rifampicin administration), digitoxin, coumarin anticoagulants, oral contraceptives, the antidiabetic sulphonylureas and biguanides, and dapsone, if given concurrently. Patients should be told that it may turn their urine, and occasionally other body fluids, red (see also 'Patients with HIV Infection or AIDS' below).

PYRAZINAMIDE

The main metabolite of pyrazinamide, pyrazinoic acid, inhibits the renal tubular secretion of uric acid, causing the serum uric acid concentration to rise; this is much more marked during daily than intermittent administration of the drug. Exceptionally, high serum uric acid concentrations may precipitate acute gout in patients with this disease. The drug is not active against *M. bovis*.

ETHAMBUTOL

Ethambutol is bacteriostatic for *M. tuberculosis* in the dosages that can safely be given, and is used to prevent the emergence of strains resistant to other drugs. It should be avoided in the treatment of patients with impaired renal function as it may accumulate and cause serious ocular toxicity. It should not be given to young children or any patient unable to report early symptoms of ocular toxicity. The British Thoracic Society recommends that renal function and visual acuity should be assessed before the drug is prescribed, the recommended dosage should not be exceeded, any history of eye disease should be recorded, the patient should be told that the drug may rarely affect vision and drugs should be stopped immediately should vision become impaired, patients complaining of visual disturbance during chemotherapy should be referred to an ophthalmologist for detailed examination, and the family practitioner should be told what information and instructions have been given to the patient. All these precautions and pieces of advice to the patient should, of course, be recorded in the case notes.

STREPTOMYCIN

After parenteral administration, the serum half-life of streptomycin, an aminoglycoside, may be greatly prolonged if renal function is impaired. Its half-life is considerably longer in newborn babies and in adults over about 40 years of age than in older children and young adults, thereby increasing the risks of toxicity. The drug should be avoided in patients with conditions affecting the VIIIth cranial nerve because of its ototoxicity, in pregnant women because it crosses the placenta and can damage the fetal VIIIth nerve, in patients with myasthenia because it is a weak neuromuscular blocker, and in those known to be hypersensitive to the drug because of the risk of a severe reaction.

THIACETAZONE

Thiacetazone, a thiosemicarbazone, is bacteriostatic for *M. tuberculosis* but is widely used in developing countries as a combination drug with isoniazid because of its cheapness. It should not be given to patients with liver disease because of its hepatotoxicity.

p-AMINOSALICYLIC ACID (PAS)

PAS (*p*-aminosalicylic acid and its salts) is bacteriostatic for *M. tuberculosis* and is used either as a companion drug with isoniazid or as a reserve drug when it has not already been used. Because it frequently causes gastrointestinal reactions and is bulky and unpleasant to take, it has now largely been replaced by other drugs. It should not be given to patients with impaired renal function and its sodium salt should not be given when a restricted sodium intake is necessary.

ETHIONAMIDE AND PROTHIONAMIDE

The use of ethionamide or prothionamide (propyl ethionamide) is limited by their adverse effects, notably gastrointestinal irritation. However, this tends to be less severe in children than in adults and less severe with prothionamide than with ethionamide.

OTHER AMINOGLYCOSIDES

Kanamycin, capreomycin, and viomycin can be used either as alternatives to the more active streptomycin in patients hypersensitive to that drug, or as reserve drugs. There is cross-resistance between the three, and between kanamycin, viomycin, and streptomycin.

CYCLOSERINE

Cycloserine has a low level of activity and is only used as a reserve drug. Its use is limited by the mental disturbances it not infrequently causes. It should not be given to patients with a history of epilepsy or psychiatric disturbance.

OFLOXACIN

A number of the quinolone antibiotics have antimycobacterial activity. Ofloxacin, one such drug, is a valuable reserve antituberculosis drug. If

Table 7 *The clinically important characteristics of the antituberculosis drugs*

Drug	Activity against non-mycobacterial pathogens	Cross-resistance with other antituberculosis drugs	Absorption from the gastrointestinal tract	Penetration into cerebrospinal fluid	Main route of elimination
Isoniazid	Inactive	None	Good	Good	Acetylation in the liver
Rifampicin	Active	Other rifamycins	Delayed by fatty food	Poor	Excreted as desacetylrifampicin in the bile
Pyrazinamide	Inactive	None	Good	Good	Metabolized to pyrazinoic acid
Ethambutol	Inactive	None	Good	Poor	Excreted unchanged in urine
Streptomycin*	Active	Kanamycin Viomycin	None	Poor	Excreted unchanged in urine
Thiacetazone	Inactive	Ethionamide Prothionamide	Good		Partly metabolized, partly excreted unchanged in urine
PAS	Inactive	None	Good	Poor	Partly metabolized, partly excreted unchanged in urine
Ethionamide or prothionamide	Inactive	Thiacetazone	Good	Good	Metabolized in the liver
Other aminoglycosides*	Active	Aminoglycosides	Poor	Poor	Excreted unchanged in urine
Cycloserine	Inactive	None	Good	Poor	Partly metabolized, partly excreted unchanged in urine
Ofloxacin	Active	None	Good	Moderate	Excreted unchanged in urine

*The aminoglycosides should not be given to pregnant women.

Table 8 *Dosages of the antituberculosis drugs*

Drug	Daily dosage: Adults and children (mg/kg)	Daily dosage: Adults: Weight (kg)	Daily dosage: Adults: Dose	Intermittent dosage: Adults and children (mg/kg)	Intermittent dosage: Adults: Weight (kg)	Intermittent dosage: Adults: Dose
Isoniazid	5		300 mg	15		
Rifampicin	10	<50	450 mg	15		600–900 mg
		≥50	600 mg			
Pyrazinamide	35	<50	1.5 g	50, three times a week	<50	2.0 g
		≥50	2.0 g		≥50	2.5 g
				75, twice a week	<50	3.0 g
					≥50	3.5 g
Ethambutol[1]	25 for 2 months, then 15*			30, three times a week 45, twice a week		
Streptomycin	15–20	<50	750 mg	15–20	<50	750 mg
		≥50	1.0 g		≥50	1.0 g
Thiacetazone	4 (for children)		150 mg			
PAS (sodium salt)	300		10–15 g			
Ethionamide and prothionamide	15–20	<50	750 mg			
		≥50	1.0 g			
Kanamycin[2]	10–15		500 mg–1.0 g			
Capreomycin[2]	15		1.0 g			
Viomycin[2]	15		1.0 g	30, twice a week		2.0 g
Cycloserine[2]	15	<50	750 mg			
		≥50	1.0 g			
Ofloxacin[2]	15		800 mg			

[1]It is important to calculate the dose accurately to ensure efficacy and avoid toxicity.

[2]Adults only.

*Most clinicians use 15 mg/kg for the initial 2 months.

Table 9 *Adverse reactions to the antituberculosis drugs*

Isoniazid	
Uncommon:	Hepatitis, cutaneous hypersensitivity, peripheral neuropathy
Rare:	Giddiness, convulsions, optic neuritis, mental symptoms, haemolytic anaemia, aplastic anaemia, agranulocytosis, lupoid reactions, arthralgia, gynaecomastia
Rifampicin	
Uncommon:	Hepatitis, cutaneous reactions, gastrointestinal reactions, thrombocytopenic purpura; febrile reactions during intermittent or irregular administration
Rare:	During intermittent or irregular administration—shortness of breath, shock, haemolytic anaemia, acute renal failure
Pyrazinamide	
Common:	Anorexia, nausea, flushing
Uncommon:	Hepatitis (dose-related), vomiting, arthralgia, cutaneous hypersensitivity
Rare:	Sideroblastic anaemia, photosensitization
Ethambutol	
Uncommon:	Retrobulbar neuritis (dose-related), arthralgia
Rare:	Hepatitis, cutaneous hypersensitivity, peripheral neuropathy
Streptomycin	
Common:	Cutaneous hypersensitivity, giddiness, numbness, tinnitus
Uncommon:	Vertigo, ataxia, deafness
Rare:	Renal damage, aplastic anaemia, agranulocytosis
Thiacetazone	
Common:	Gastrointestinal reactions, cutaneous hypersensitivity, vertigo, conjuctivitis
Uncommon:	Hepatitis, erythema multiforme, exfoliative dermatitis, haemolytic anaemia
Rare:	Agranulocytosis
PAS	
Common:	Gastrointestinal reactions
Uncommon:	Cutaneous hypersensitivity, hepatitis, hypokalaemia
Rare:	Acute renal failure, haemolytic anaemia, thrombocytopenia, hypothyroidism
Ethionamide and prothionamide	
Common:	Gastrointestinal reactions, salivation, metallic taste
Uncommon:	Cutaneous hypersensitivity, hepatitis
Rare:	Alopecia, convulsions, deafness, diplopia, gynaecomastia, hypotension, impotence, mental symptoms, menstrual irregularity, hypoglycaemia, peripheral neuropathy
Other aminoglycosides	
Common:	Cutaneous hypersensitivity
Uncommon:	Deafness (kanamycin, viomycin), vertigo (capreomycin, viomycin)
Rare:	Renal damage, hypokalaemia, hypocalcaemia
Cycloserine	
Common:	Dizziness, headache, slurred speech, confusion, tremor, insomnia, convulsions, depression (suicide risk), psychosis
Uncommon:	Cutaneous hypersensitivity, hepatitis, memory loss
Ofloxacin	
Uncommon:	Gastrointestinal reactions, headache, dizziness, insomnia
Rare:	Convulsions, hallucinations

possible, it should be avoided in patients with renal failure, and it should not be given to those with known allergy to quinolones.

Adverse effects of the antituberculosis drugs (Table 9)

The standard recommended combination of isoniazid, rifampicin, and pyrazinamide is usually well tolerated and rarely causes serious toxicity. Neurological reactions to isoniazid probably result from pyridoxine deficiency and can usually be prevented by giving 10 mg pyridoxine daily to those patients who may be pyridoxine deficient; these include alcoholics, pregnant women, the old, and the malnourished. These reactions are rare among rapid acetylators and well-nourished patients. Convulsions respond to anticonvulsants together with pyridoxine 100 mg intravenously. Gastrointestinal reactions to rifampicin can usually be alleviated by giving the drug during or directly after a meal.

Thrombocytopenic purpura, shock, acute haemolytic anaemia, and acute renal failure are rare reactions to rifampicin, but may occur for the first time when treatment is resumed after an interval. If one of these reactions occurs, the drug should be withdrawn immediately and never given again. All these potentially serious rare reactions are usually reversible.

Pyrazinamide-induced arthralgia usually responds well to symptomatic treatment, for example with aspirin.

Ethambutol can cause a dose-related retrobulbar neuritis with a reduction in visual acuity, central scotoma, impaired red–green colour vision, and peripheral-field defects. These are reversible if administration of the drug is stopped as soon as they are detected, but they can progress to optic atrophy and permanent blindness if the drug is continued.

The effects of streptomycin-induced ototoxicity can become permanent. If severe and persistent symptoms occur, the drug should be withdrawn. The risk of ototoxicity is especially high in patients aged more than 40 years in whom, also, recovery is slower and less often complete than in younger patients. Ototoxicity can occur in the fetus of a pregnant woman given the drug.

Thiacetazone is well tolerated in some communities but not in others, for reasons that are not understood. It is poorly tolerated in patients of Asian ethnic origin but there are large geographical as well as racial variations in the frequency and severity of its adverse effects. Severe cutaneous reactions to thiacetazone are so common in HIV-positive subjects that this drug should be avoided in these patients.

In general, adverse reactions tend to be more frequent and more severe with second-line than with first-line drugs.

CUTANEOUS AND GENERALIZED HYPERSENSITIVITY REACTIONS

Mild cutaneous reactions to an antituberculosis regimen may be self-limiting and require only symptomatic treatment without interrupting or altering the regimen.

Generalized reactions usually occur during the first 1 or 2 months of chemotherapy. They consist of a rash, sometimes accompanied by periorbital swelling and conjunctivitis, and by systemic symptoms and signs such as fever, malaise, vomiting, aching limbs, headache, generalized lymphadenopathy, hepatosplenomegaly, and occasionally jaundice.

The principles of management are:

(1) stop all chemotherapy until the reaction has subsided;
(2) identify the drug or drugs responsible;
(3) resume adequate chemotherapy as soon as possible, using at least two drugs to which the patient is not hypersensitive.

The patient should be desensitized to the drug or drugs responsible only if this is necessary for the resumption of adequate chemotherapy.

Once the reaction has subsided, daily challenge doses of the drugs should be given, starting with the drugs that are least likely to have caused the reaction, so that administration of these can be resumed with the minimum of delay while, if necessary, challenge doses and desensitizing doses of other drugs are given. Challenge doses of each drug of the regimen should be given in the sequence in which they are shown in Table 10, until a reaction occurs. If there is no reaction to either of the challenge doses shown in the table, administration of that drug should be continued in full dosage. If the reaction was severe, smaller initial challenge doses, approximately one-tenth of those shown under day 1, should be used.

It is important to desensitize under cover of at least two drugs to which the patient is not hypersensitive, to prevent the emergence of drug resistance. If the reaction was severe or involved more than one drug, desensitization should be done under corticosteroid cover, but no attempt should be made to desensitize a patient with severe exfoliative dermatitis or renal reactions.

If the patient had a reaction to the second challenge dose but not to the first, desensitization should be started with a dose equal to the first challenge dose. If there was a reaction to the first challenge dose, desensitization should be started with a dose approximately one-tenth that of the first challenge dose. Desensitizing doses should be given, on an inpatient basis if possible, twice a day in steadily increasing amounts until the full dose is reached. It is usually possible to make each dose double the previous one. If a reaction occurs during desensitization, the dose should be reduced again and thereafter increased more gradually.

Cutaneous and generalized hypersensitivity reactions tend to be more common and more severe in HIV-positive patients than in others (see also 'Patients with HIV Infection or AIDS' below).

HEPATITIS

It is unnecessary to test for liver-cell damage routinely during antituberculosis chemotherapy, unless the patient has liver disease. Small, transient, and symptomless increases in serum hepatic enzyme concentrations are usual during the early weeks of treatment, which should not therefore be interrupted or altered because of them. If clinically evident hepatitis occurs, all drugs should be stopped while liver damage is confirmed by appropriate tests. If the hepatitis has been caused by the drug regimen, it usually resolves rapidly. Treatment with the same drugs can often be resumed uneventfully, but tests for liver-cell damage should be made regularly. The aim should be to resume treatment, with either the original or an alternative regimen, as soon as possible.

The risk of drug-induced hepatitis is about 1 per cent, but increases with age. Deaths from presumed drug-induced hepatitis are rare.

Table 10 *Challenge doses for detecting cutaneous or generalized hypersensitivity*

Drug	Challenge doses: Day 1	Day 2
Isoniazid	50 mg	300 mg
Rifampicin	75 mg	300 mg
Pyrazinamide	250 mg	1.0 g
Ethionamide, prothionamide	125 mg	375 mg
Cycloserine	125 mg	250 mg
Ethambutol	100 mg	500 mg
PAS	1.0 g	5.0 g
Thiacetazone	25 mg	50 mg
Streptomycin or other aminoglycoside	125 mg	500 mg

Challenge doses of the drugs of the regimen should be given in the sequence in which they are shown. The drugs near the bottom of the list are the ones most likely to cause a reaction. If the reaction was a severe one, smaller initial challenge doses should be given (approximately one-tenth the doses shown for day 1).

Scientific basis of chemotherapy

In the lesions of untreated patients with pulmonary tuberculosis (Fig. 21), there are likely to be large numbers of bacilli in open cavities with a plentiful supply of oxygen, isolated from the host's acquired immune defences, growing continuously and multiplying rapidly (population A in Fig. 21). At the other extreme there will be small numbers of dormant bacilli, such as those deprived of oxygen in closed lesions (population D). Between these extremes there will be semidormant bacilli. These include organisms in a low environmental pH, which can occur in early acute inflammatory lesions or within the phagolysosomes of macrophages (population B), and those in an unstable part of a lesion and therefore metabolizing only briefly and intermittently (population C).

The antituberculosis drugs vary in their bactericidal action, defined as their ability to kill large numbers of actively metabolizing bacilli rapidly; their sterilizing action, defined as their capacity to kill semidormant bacilli; their ability to prevent the emergence of acquired resistance by suppressing the growth of drug-resistant mutants; and their suitability for intermittent use.

BACTERICIDAL ACTION

Isoniazid is the most powerful bactericidal drug. It probably kills some 90 per cent of the bacillary population during the first few days of chemotherapy. Rifampicin is also important in this respect.

STERILIZING ACTION

Rifampicin and pyrazinamide are the most important sterilizing drugs because of their unique ability to kill semidormant bacilli capable of surviving the bactericidal action of isoniazid and so of giving rise to relapse after treatment.

The bacilli specifically killed by pyrazinamide are those with their metabolism partly inhibited by an acid environment. The antibacterial activity of the drug has been shown to increase markedly with increasing bacterial inhibition by acid. The bacilli specifically killed by rifampicin are probably those that are dormant but subject to transient favourable changes in their environment and so to short periods of active metabolism. It has been shown that rifampicin begins to kill bacilli within an hour of exposure of a culture to the drug; this compares with more than a day for isoniazid.

Completely dormant bacilli are unlikely to be killed by any drug.

PREVENTING THE EMERGENCE OF ACQUIRED RESISTANCE

Drug resistance emerges by mutation and so even populations of bacilli that have not been exposed to antituberculosis drugs contain small numbers of resistant mutants. If inadequate drug combinations are used, these mutants are likely to replace killed, susceptible bacilli and give rise to drug-resistant disease.

The effectiveness of drugs in preventing the emergence of acquired resistance depends on the extent to which they can inhibit bacilli continuously, whatever their rate of metabolism, even when there is some irregularity in drug taking. Among the first-line drugs, isoniazid and rifampicin are the most effective in preventing the emergence of resistance to other drugs, and streptomycin and ethambutol are only slightly less so. Pyrazinamide is less effective, and thiacetazone and PAS are the least effective.

COMBINED DRUG ACTION

The combination of isoniazid, rifampicin, and pyrazinamide has proved to be highly effective, containing as it does the most powerful bactericidal drug, isoniazid, the two uniquely active sterilizing drugs, rifampicin and pyrazinamide, and the two drugs most effective in preventing the emergence of acquired resistance, isoniazid and rifampicin.

SUITABILITY FOR INTERMITTENT USE

The finding that 400 mg of isoniazid given as a single dose each day was more effective than 200 mg given twice a day led to a number of clinical trials of thrice-weekly, twice-weekly and once-weekly chemotherapy. These have shown that isoniazid, rifampicin, pyrazinamide, streptomycin, and ethambutol are all effective when given intermittently in the dosages shown in Table 8. The dose size of intermittent streptomycin cannot be raised above the daily dose size because of the risk of acute toxicity. The effective dose size of rifampicin is similar whether it is given daily or intermittently. Thiacetazone is less effective when given intermittently than when given daily.

Fig. 21 A diagrammatic representation of the hypothesis of special components of the bacterial population in lesions and the drugs that kill them (adapted from Mitchison (1979), with permission).

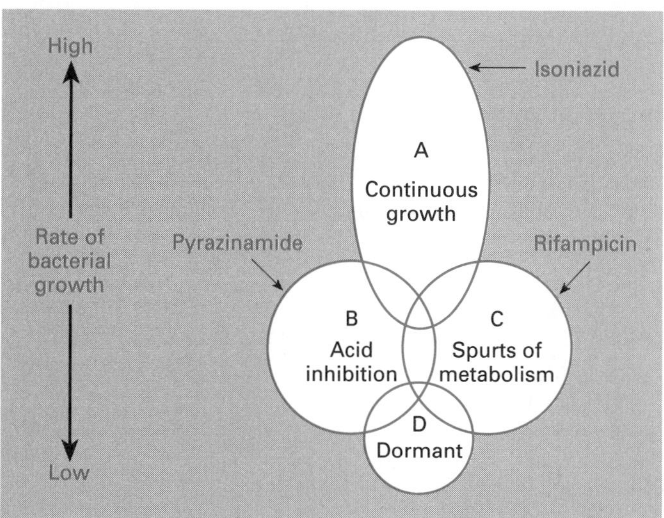

Table 11 *Regimens of chemotherapy*

Standard 6-month regimen
2HRZ/4HR

Variants of standard 6-month regimen
1. When fully supervised, intermittent chemotherapy can be organized:
   - $2HRZ/4H_3R_3$
   - $2HRZ/4H_2R_2$
   - $2E_3H_3R_3Z_3/4H_3R_3$
   - $2S_3H_3R_3Z_3/4H_3R_3$
2. When there is a high level of initial resistance:
   - 2EHRZ/4HR
   - 2SHRZ/4HR

Or add E (or S), where appropriate, to the initial phase of one of the variants

Alternative less active regimens of longer duration
1. With a highly active initial 4-drug phase:
   - 2SHRZ/6HT
   - $2SHRZ/6S_2H_2Z_2$
2. With a less active or no initial phase:
   - 2SHR/7HR
   - 2EHR/7HR
   - 9HR
   - 2SHT/10HT
   - 2SHE/10HE
   - 2SHP/10HP
   - $2SHT/10S_2H_2$
   - $2SHP/10S_2H_2$

H, isoniazid; R, rifampicin; Z, pyrazinamide; E, ethambutol; S, streptomycin; T, thiacetazone; P, PAS. Prefix number, months' duration of that phase of chemotherapy; subscript number, number of doses per week in intermittent phases of chemotherapy.

Antituberculosis regimens

RECOMMENDED REGIMEN FOR NEWLY DIAGNOSED PATIENTS

The regimen recommended by the International Union Against Tuberculosis and Lung Disease for newly diagnosed patients (Table 11) is a 6-month regimen of isoniazid (**H**), rifampicin (**R**), and pyrazinamide (**Z**), given daily for 2 months or 8 weeks (2HRZ), followed by isoniazid and rifampicin for 4 months (4HR); the standard abbreviation for this regimen is 2HRZ/4HR.

Fixed-dose combination preparations of all three drugs and of the first two should be used when available to aid compliance and to reduce the risk of incorrect dosage, but it is essential that only those preparations are used for which studies have shown that bioavailability of the component drugs is not adversely affected by combining them.

This standard regimen should be used in the treatment of pulmonary and extrapulmonary disease in adults and children. It has the ability (i) to cure patients rapidly, even the majority of those who default after 2 to 3 months of treatment; (ii) to cure the great majority of patients with bacilli initially resistant to isoniazid; and (iii) to prevent therapeutic failure due to the emergence of acquired resistance. The regimen need be given for no longer than 4 months (2HRZ/2HR) in the treatment of patients considered to have active pulmonary tuberculosis requiring chemotherapy, but in whom the radiographic lesion is small and all of at least two adequately examined sputum smears are negative.

There are variants of this regimen that have advantages in some circumstances, as follows.

1. Intermittent administration

The continuation phase may be given three times or twice a week: $2HRZ/4H_3R_3$ or $2HRZ/4H_2R_2$. Every dose of the continuation phase can then be given under the direct observation of outpatient health staff, paramedical staff, or lay people taught to supervise chemotherapy. In this way the level of compliance is known and a high level can be encouraged.

In programmes in which chemotherapy is administered throughout under full supervision to outpatients, the regimen may be given three times a week from the start. When this is done, either ethambutol (**E**) or streptomycin (**S**) should be added to the initial phase:

$$2E_3H_3R_3Z_3 \text{ or } 2S_3H_3R_3Z_3/4H_3R_3.$$

2. Populations with a high level of initial drug resistance

When there is a high level of initial drug resistance, or if the patient's strain is suspected to be resistant to isoniazid, a fourth drug, ethambutol or streptomycin, should be added to the initial phase.

ALTERNATIVE, LESS ACTIVE REGIMENS

When optimal chemotherapy is not available in a population (as in developing countries) or cannot be used in individual patients, one of the alternative regimens shown in Table 11 may be used. However, these drug combinations are weaker than those in the recommended regimen and therefore need to be given for longer than 6 months. Although the drugs are cheaper the total cost of these regimens per patient cured is unlikely to be reduced. Priority should be given to the first two, both of which have a highly active initial four-drug phase (SHRZ) daily for the first 2 months.

In countries or populations with a high prevalence of HIV infection, streptomycin is best avoided because of the risk of spreading HIV with contaminated needles or syringes. If this drug is used, disposable needles and syringes must be used.

PATIENTS WHOSE PRIMARY CHEMOTHERAPY HAS FAILED

When there is no response to chemotherapy in a patient who has been fully compliant it is probable that the initial strain was multiply drug resistant. When there is bacteriological response at first, followed by bacteriological failure while chemotherapy is still being given, this is probably because acquired drug resistance or additional resistance has emerged. In either case the regimen must be changed but it is first necessary to try to establish whether apparent failure was really due to the patient's failure to take chemotherapy. Once it is clear that the patient is no longer responding to the prescribed regimen, a careful assessment is necessary. A detailed drug history should be compiled, including the compliance of the patient in treatment. Susceptibility tests on cultures taken after treatment failure may be helpful, but only if they have been done by a laboratory practising good quality control.

Whenever possible, the patient should be retreated for at least 12 months from the time the sputum smears become negative, using a regimen containing, for the first 3 to 4 months, at least three drugs to which the organisms are likely to be susceptible; preferably three that have not been used before and for which there is no cross-resistance with any that have. Chemotherapy should then be continued with at least two drugs. A single drug should not be added to a regimen that has failed, except as a last resort when resistance to all other available drugs is likely to have emerged.

Retreatment should be fully supervised, in hospital if necessary, especially if the patient has been uncooperative in the past. Careful bacteriological monitoring is essential.

PATIENTS IN WHOM RELAPSE HAS OCCURRED AFTER CHEMOTHERAPY

Relapse after chemotherapy is rare if the recommended regimen or one of its variants has been administered regularly by an efficient service and the patient has complied and responded well during treatment. If relapse occurs in these circumstances, or in a patient who defaulted after only a short period of regular chemotherapy, resistance is unlikely to have emerged, and the patient should be retreated with the same drug combination, but for 9 rather than 6 months and under stricter supervision.

If an inferior regimen has been used, or if relapse has occurred in a patient whose chemotherapy was poorly supervised and who has taken the drugs irregularly for much of the time, resistance is much more likely to have emerged and the patient should be managed as one whose primary chemotherapy has failed.

PATIENTS WITH IMPAIRED RENAL FUNCTION

In patients with impaired renal function, drugs such as isoniazid, rifampicin, pyrazinamide and ethionamide or prothionamide, which are eliminated by metabolism or biliary excretion, should be given in their usual dosage, whatever the degree of renal impairment. Such patients should be treated with the recommended regimen (2HRZ/4HR) without modification. If possible, drugs such as ethambutol, aminoglycosides and ofloxacin, which are excreted unchanged in the urine, should be avoided.

PATIENTS WITH IMPAIRED HEPATIC FUNCTION

It should not be assumed that patients with impaired hepatic function are more at risk than others for hepatic toxicity, although this may be so. The rate of metabolism of both isoniazid and rifampicin is reduced when liver function is grossly impaired. In treating such patients, many clinicians prefer to use daily isoniazid and ethambutol for 12 months, giving streptomycin as well for the first 2 months. Whatever regimen is used, tests for liver-cell damage should be made regularly during treatment.

PREGNANT WOMEN

None of the antituberculosis drugs has been shown to have teratogenic effects in the human fetus. If a woman is known to be pregnant when tuberculosis is diagnosed, the pregnancy is likely to have advanced beyond 12 weeks, by which time there is little risk.

Streptomycin should never be given at any stage of the pregnancy because of the risk of damaging the VIIIth cranial nerve of the fetus.

BREAST-FEEDING WOMEN

Women receiving antituberculosis drugs can safely breast-feed their infants. Such an infant ingests at most 20 per cent of the usual therapeutic dose of isoniazid daily from the milk, and a much lower proportion of the other drugs. The risk of toxic reactions in the infant is thus very low.

PATIENTS WITH HIV INFECTION OR AIDS

Response to the recommended antituberculosis regimen (2HRZ/4HR) is usually good in tuberculous patients with HIV infection or AIDS, and this is the regimen that should be used, being given for the standard 6-month duration. Nevertheless, successful antituberculosis treatment should be followed by lifelong prophylaxis with daily isoniazid because relapse is more likely to occur than in patients with an intact cell-mediated immune mechanism and because there is evidence that recurrence of tuberculosis can itself accelerate the progression of HIV disease.

Compliance is likely to be poor in some groups of patients, particularly intravenous drug users; treatment should be given to such patients under full supervision. Adverse reactions to the antituberculosis drugs are common in HIV-positive patients, particularly cutaneous and hypersensitivity reactions, haematological reactions, and hepatic toxicity. Anaphylactic reactions to rifampicin may occur. Rifampicin and isoniazid may interact with ketoconazole and fluconazole, making antifungal treatment ineffective. Also, ketoconazole can inhibit the gastrointestinal absorption of rifampicin, thereby reducing the efficacy of the antituberculosis regimen. Whenever possible, these drugs should not be given together.

REFERENCES

Brewis, A.L., Gibson, G.J., and Geddes, D.M. (1990) (Chapter 24 of) *Respiratory medicine.* Baillière Tindall, London.

British Thoracic Society Joint Tuberculosis Committee (1990). Chemotherapy and management of tuberculosis in the United Kingdom: recommendations of the Joint Tuberculosis Committee of the British Thoracic Society. *Thorax*, **45,** 403–8.

British Thoracic Society Joint Tuberculosis Committee (1990). Control and prevention of tuberculosis in Britain: an updated code of practice. *British Medical Journal*, **300,** 995–9.

British Thoracic Society Joint Tuberculosis Committee (1992). Guidelines on the management of tuberculosis and HIV infection in the United Kingdom. *British Medical Journal*, **304,** 1231–3.

Collins, C.H., Grange, J.M., and Yates, M.D. (1985) *Organization and practice in tuberculosis bacteriology.* Butterworths, London.

Committee on Treatment of the International Union Against Tuberculosis and Lung Disease (1988). Antituberculosis regimens of chemotherapy: recommendations of the committee. *Bulletin of the International Union Against Tuberculosis and Lung Disease*, **63,** 60–4.

Crofton, J., Horne, N., and Miller, F. (1992) *Clinical tuberculosis.* MacMillan, London.

Davies, P.D.O. (ed.) (1994). *Clinical Tuberculosis.* Chapman & Hall, London.

Department of Health (1992). *Immunisation against infectious disease.* pp. 76–94. HMSO, London.

Girling, D.J. (1989). The chemotherapy of tuberculosis. *In The biology of the mycobacteria. Vol. 3: clinical aspects of mycobacterial disease*, (ed. C. Ratledge, J.L. Stanford, and J.M. Grange.), pp. 285–323. Academic Press, London.

Grange, J.M. (1988). *Mycobacteria and human disease.* Arnold, London.

Humphries, M. (1992). The management of tuberculous meningitis. *Thorax*, **47,** 577–81.

Mitchell, D.M. and Miller, R.F. (1992). Recent developments in the management of the pulmonary complications of HIV disease. *Thorax*, **47,** 381–90.

Mitchison, D.A. (1979). Basic mechanisms of chemotherapy. *Chest*, **76,** 771–81.

Seaton, A., Seaton, D., and Leitch, A.G. (1989). (Chs 13–15 of) *Crofton and Douglas' respiratory diseases.* Blackwell Scientific, Oxford.

7.11.23 Particular problems of tuberculosis in developing countries

C. G. Uragoda

Developing countries are not uniformly poor. At one extreme there are the impoverished nations struggling to provide a basic health service, while at the other extreme are the nearly developed countries, such as the newly industrialized south-east Asian states, with well-developed tuberculosis control programmes. This section mainly concerns the economically backward nations.

Measures for the control of tuberculosis are the same for developed and developing countries, but constraints to their application in the latter have resulted in a tremendous disparity in the problem of tuberculosis in the two areas. In developing countries, which are faced with a shortage of resources, both monetary and trained manpower, a large proportion of patients with tuberculosis remain undiagnosed due to the limited availability of diagnostic facilities, especially radiography. The inclusion of the two potent but costly drugs rifampicin and pyrazinamide in treatment schedules is beyond the capacity of many of these countries. A sound health-care infrastructure through which control measures could be channelled is lacking in several of them. A poor transport system or the high cost of travel is a disincentive to prospective patients seeking treatment. A shortage of trained personnel, including doctors, nurses, and technicians, may hamper the programme. Some countries are handicapped by their own natural barriers: for example the mountainous terrain in Nepal or the archipelagos in Indonesia and the Maldives pose a serious challenge to health workers in delivering care to the isolated communities living in these areas. In some countries such as India, large tracts of land are sparsely provided with health centres, and therefore the long distances that patients are obliged to travel deter them from seeking treatment. Many developing countries are saddled with other health problems, which are equally or more pressing, and consequently a low priority is given to tuberculosis control by some governments.

Many Western countries are now considering eradication of tuberculosis, but the disease remains a major health problem to many developing countries where eradication is but a distant dream. The World Health Organization (**WHO**) estimates that 8 million new cases of tuberculosis occur every year in the world, and of these 95 per cent are in developing countries, which also account for 99 per cent of the 3 million annual deaths.

Developing countries must constantly attempt to improve their national control programmes. This obviously cannot be achieved in a short time. It is therefore desirable for each country to formulate a long-term national plan, which would envisage progressive upgrading of the programme, phase by phase, over a period of years. Such improvements, depending on the country, may include an increase in the number of chest clinics, radiographic units and microscopes, and the introduction of short-course chemotherapy. It may not always be possible strictly to adhere to such a time schedule, but some progress can be achieved each year, within the framework of a previously agreed plan. A plan of this sort was drawn up for Sri Lanka with the locally available skill and experience. It appears to be working satisfactorily. It covers the period 1988 to 2000, and some of the targets, such as the establishment of additional chest clinics in some areas, introduction of short-course chemotherapy, and delegation of responsibility for health education to the national tuberculosis association, have already been met.

International organizations, notably the WHO, have helped developing countries in the fight against tuberculosis. Without this assistance many of these countries would have been in a worse plight. Over the years, the WHO has offered drugs, equipment, advisers, and training facilities, while the United Nations Childrens Fund has donated BCG vaccine. The International Union Against Tuberculosis and Lung Disease (**IUATLD**) is responsible for successful programmes in some African and South American countries. The World Bank, too, has recently shown an interest in tuberculosis (for example in Bangladesh).

At the national level, non-governmental organizations have a part to play. Many countries have their own national tuberculosis associations. Generally there is more scope for their activities in countries where governmental programmes are weak. Some national associations in developed countries have, like international agencies, helped Third World countries. An example is Japan, which conducts regular training programmes for doctors and other health workers engaged in the control of tuberculosis.

The increasing tendency towards permanent and temporary migration from poor countries to the rich has posed tuberculosis-related problems for the host country as well as to the immigrants themselves. In developed countries, the incidence of tuberculosis among Asian immigrants is considerably higher than the national average in the host country. It matches that in their home country and may create sociological problems in the country of adoption.

There is currently an exodus of workers, usually of the lower and middle classes, from Asian and African countries to the oil-rich Middle East on short-term contracts. Workers are given a medical examination soon after arrival. The discovery of radiographic lesions suggestive of tuberculosis usually results in their repatriation, which is both psychologically and financially traumatic. A prerecruitment medical examination, as is done in Sri Lanka, could avert much of this unnecessary suffering.

Diagnosis

In developing countries, detection of as many cases as possible and their successful treatment are of vital importance in the control of the disease. Unlike in developed countries, many cases go undetected, especially in remote areas where health facilities are poor. The stigma of tuberculosis interfered with its diagnosis in some developing countries, but this has decreased.

In developing countries, tuberculosis is invariably diagnosed by passive case finding where patients who present with respiratory symptoms at health centres are examined. In order to increase the number of cases detected, as many patients with respiratory symptoms as possible should be encouraged to seek treatment at these centres. One method of encouragement is public health education. The impact of a programme directed at small groups of the community, as is done in some countries, is difficult to assess and may take years to show results. An effective means would be to address the public at large through television or radio but such programmes may be expensive. In Sri Lanka, a series of television advertisements about leprosy has resulted in a sharp rise in the number of patients detected, but for tuberculosis the high cost of television time has prevented the launching of such a programme. The authorities have, instead, opted for the next best medium, the radio, where talks on tuberculosis are broadcast from time to time.

Another method of increasing the yield of cases is through community health workers, both governmental and voluntary. They can persuade patients with suggestive symptoms to attend health centres. Some governments that have subscribed to the WHO goal of 'Health for all by the year 2000' have created an infrastructure of workers to deliver primary health care at the grass roots. They are well placed, during their regular house-to-house visits, to advise any likely patients they come across to seek treatment. Voluntary health workers may play a similar role. The national tuberculosis association in Sri Lanka, through its several branches in the provinces, has trained a large number of volunteers who can help in the detection of new cases in their community.

In many developing countries, diagnosis of pulmonary tuberculosis in peripheral centres is based on sputum microscopy alone, while radiography is available only in the larger centres. Some countries cannot afford to treat sputum-negative, radiographically diagnosed patients. Wherever possible, smear-positive patients should be referred to the nearest radiographic centre for confirmation of diagnosis. This is especially important in areas of high prevalence of atypical mycobacterial sensitivity such as south India and Sri Lanka. In a study of the differential tuberculin test in Sri Lanka, in which a battery of antigens from different species of mycobacteria was used, the proportion of reactors to the 'Gause' strain of scotochromogens was significantly greater than to tuberculin from *Mycobacterium tuberculosis*. As the microscopical appearance of these atypical forms is similar to that of *M. tuberculosis*, the diagnosis of tuberculosis solely by sputum microscopy in such high-prevalence areas may lead to false positives. It is important that developing countries should diagnose tuberculosis correctly, for apart from ethical considerations, false positives would place an extra burden on the cost of treatment. The significance of this point was demonstrated in a WHO-sponsored baseline survey of tuberculosis conducted in Sri Lanka in 1970–71. In a randomly selected sample of 1307 symptomatic persons, 123 individuals excreted atypical mycobacteria, while *M. tuberculosis* was cultured in only 64.

False positives may also arise through incorrect laboratory methods. In some developing countries, laboratory practice involves recycling, after cleaning, of microscope slides, including smear-positive ones. Acid-fast bacilli from the previous examination may remain fixed despite cleaning, leading to false positives. All smear-positive slides must be discarded. The extra expense to the national programme for replacements is negligible compared to the expense of unnecessary treatment. Routine sputum culture is too expensive for developing countries, and the time it takes to yield results makes it an unsuitable routine diagnostic tool for these countries. However, culture facilities should be available for selected cases, specially for detection and management of relapses and identification of atypical mycobacteria. Depending on the size of the country, there should be one or more laboratories with culture facilities to serve as referral centres. Where such centres do not exist in a country, provision for the establishment of one should be incorporated in the national plan. At present Sri Lanka has only one such laboratory, but a few more are planned for the provinces.

Radiographic facilities at a reasonable distance from one another are necessary for the diagnosis of smear-negative cases in countries that can afford to treat such patients. In addition to the capital outlay to be incurred in installing these machines, the regular supply of films and chemicals requires budgetary provision. Some countries such as Sri Lanka use miniature radiography as a screening procedure in chest clinics where large numbers are served. The machine, which has a camera attachment fitted to it, serves as a dual-purpose unit where either miniature or standard film could be used as required. The initial cost of such a unit is somewhat higher than that of a standard one, but running costs are less and the turnover of patients more rapid. Preferably all miniature units in the country should be of a uniform type using the same size of roll film. Shortage of film is less likely to occur than if several sizes have to be imported. Film 70 mm wide strikes a reasonable balance between economy and accuracy; 45-mm films are too small for accurate reading, while 100-mm films are too expensive. As miniature radiography exposes the subject to a slightly higher dose of radiation than standard chest radiography, it should be avoided in children and pregnant women.

Active case finding where populations at large are radiographically screened for tuberculosis by mobile units is no longer adopted in developing countries, and is not recommended for developed countries either. The cost per case detected is unduly high, while lesions may develop rapidly in between rounds of radiographic examination. It still has a place for special groups, such as miners, in whom the incidence of pulmonary tuberculosis is several times higher than in the general population. Radiography in miners has the advantage of detecting pneumoconiosis as well. In Sri Lanka, graphite miners, in whom the prevalence of tuberculosis is five times that in the general population, are regularly submitted to radiography at static units in clinics situated near the mines. It is not necessary to maintain expensive mobile units for this purpose. New cases of pulmonary tuberculosis and graphite pneumoconiosis are detected at each round.

In developing countries where radiographic facilities are inadequate, diagnosis of tuberculosis in children is unreliable, for this depends more on radiography than sputum microscopy and culture examination. Many affected children in these countries go undiagnosed. As 95 per cent of reported cases of childhood tuberculosis are smear negative and therefore non-infectious, their impact on the epidemiological situation in a country is minimal.

The tuberculin test has limited diagnostic value in developing countries where BCG vaccination at birth is widespread. The WHO-recommended intradermal test using PPD RT-23 has been adopted in many of these countries. Some clinicians attach diagnostic importance to a large tuberculin reaction in a suspected case of primary tuberculosis, or to its complications such as pleural effusion, but the level at which it becomes significant has not been determined.

New methods of diagnosis may be available in the future. Unless they are cost-effective, they are unlikely to be of much benefit to developing countries.

Treatment

Appropriate strategies for the successful treatment of tuberculosis are clearly defined, but their application in some developing countries is beset with seemingly insurmountable problems. The overall cure rate in some of these countries is less than 50 per cent, though the standard drug regimens they adopt are capable of yielding much better results. One of the main reasons for this unduly high failure rate is poor compliance on the part of patients. They tend to discontinue treatment more often with longer regimens than with short-course chemotherapy.

The significant advance in treatment in recent times was the introduction of 6- to 8-month short-course chemotherapy where four drugs, including rifampicin and pyrazinamide, are used during the first 2 months. It has a special advantage for developing countries despite the high cost of these two drugs. Even if patients default after 2 months of treatment, 90 per cent would become smear negative, and the remaining 10 per cent would also convert if a further 2 to 4 weeks of treatment were given. Many of the patients who have had 3 or 4 months of treatment will not relapse. Rifampicin and pyrazinamide are very effective against dormant tubercle bacilli and therefore help in reducing relapses.

Short-course chemotherapy is expensive but for averting deaths it has been found to be more cost-effective than a standard 12-month regimen consisting of isoniazid and thiacetazone supplemented with streptomycin in the first 2 months. Short-course chemotherapy has now been introduced in many developing countries in Latin America, East Africa, South Asia and the Middle East. Its use in IUATLD-assisted national programmes in several subSaharan countries has shown that it can be successfully deployed despite enormous difficulties.

The inexpensive thiacetazone, which is a WHO- and IUATLD-recommended drug, is widely used in Africa, but is tolerated much less well by Asian populations. Sri Lanka, for example, abandoned its use a couple of decades ago due to the high level of side-effects, which interfered with compliance. Nearly 25 per cent of patients developed nausea, vomiting, diarrhoea, and rashes.

Hospital beds are not essential for the management of the average case, but some should be reserved for use in special situations. In some countries, as in Sri Lanka, separate wards in general hospitals have been set apart for use of patients with tuberculosis.

Both short-course and standard chemotherapy may be given to outpatients. However, in some countries treatment is started in hospital to ensure supervision, and therefore compliance. This was the strategy used by the IUATLD in subSaharan countries when short-course chemotherapy was introduced. It prevented the waste of costly drugs, while patients from rural areas who had no ready access to health care were given the opportunity of getting effective treatment. Excellent sputum conversion rates were achieved at the end of 2 months when short-course chemotherapy was well supervised. Admission to hospital, despite its advantages, is a costly exercise that developing countries can ill afford.

Short-course chemotherapy has had an unexpected advantage in Sri Lanka. Patients with pulmonary tuberculosis were, for over 20 years, routinely offered initial admission to hospital. Introduction of short-course chemotherapy, which meant a shorter stay in hospital, has resulted in redundancy of many hospital beds, and therefore a considerable saving in expenses. The total bed strength, which stood at 2056 in 1988 just before introduction of short-course chemotherapy, has now been reduced to 1477.

The efficacy of standard chemotherapy is adversely affected by the level of drug resistance in the community. This is high in developing countries. The incidence of primary isoniazid resistance between 1976 and 1978 was 10.6 per cent in India, 22.9 per cent in Thailand, and 32.6 per cent in Bolivia; it was 10.0 per cent in Sri Lanka in 1982. In some of these countries, it was largely due to the inappropriate use of drugs in the past: a combination of just two drugs was used in some national programmes; large-scale treatment by general practitioners using inadequate regimens was another reason in some countries. However, it is most unlikely that primary resistance as it now occurs in developing countries will interfere with the efficacy of four-drug, short-course chemotherapy.

In many developing countries there are other factors that may interfere with proper chemotherapy. Drugs may be ordered from the cheapest sources, where bioavailability of drugs, specially rifampicin and isoniazid, is not tested. Treatment in national programmes is usually given free of charge, but in countries where private treatment is readily available for tuberculosis, patients may discontinue drugs if they run short of money. It is important for the national programme to ensure a steady flow of drugs to treatment centres. Some countries may import adequate stocks, but fail to distribute them when they are needed. Such interruptions of supply may have a serious impact if drugs in reduced dosage or inadequate combinations are issued to patients.

BCG vaccination

Surveys in different countries on the effectiveness of BCG show a wide variation, ranging from 0 to 80 per cent. In some parts of the developing world, as in south India, the high prevalence of atypical mycobacterial infection has been incriminated as a cause for its low effectiveness.

Some developed countries are considering discontinuation of routine BCG vaccination because of their favourable epidemiological situation. On the other hand, it continues to be part of the strategy for the control of tuberculosis in developing countries, where it is usually given at birth. There is no evidence, particularly from the developing countries, that it would protect children beyond 15 years of age.

The practice in some countries of giving a second BCG vaccination has been largely abandoned now. In Sri Lanka, the second BCG vaccination, which was given in school at 10 years of age, was discontinued several years ago.

The epidemiological impact of BCG vaccination in developing countries was overrated until the mid-1970s. As more than 95 per cent of reported cases among children are smear negative and therefore non-infectious, preventing childhood tuberculosis by BCG vaccination has little overall epidemiological influence. The realization of this fact was a blow to developing countries that had banked heavily on BCG as a cheap but effective means of controlling tuberculosis.

In many developing countries, BCG vaccination is done as part of the Expanded Programme of Immunization and the coverage in many of these is very high, reaching almost 100 per cent of the eligible population in Sri Lanka. It has been estimated that even with total coverage and assuming the protection to be 40 to 70 per cent, BCG will prevent only about 6 per cent of deaths. It is imperative, therefore, that developing countries, while continuing with BCG vaccination of newborns, should strengthen case finding and treatment, which are the most powerful means of controlling tuberculosis.

Chemoprophylaxis

Policy on chemoprophylaxis varies among developing countries. It is not adopted at all in some countries, for their tuberculosis control programmes are already overwhelmed with large numbers of patients who have to be accorded priority in treatment. Treatment with isoniazid for 6 months is inexpensive, but if the intake is not done selectively from the large infected population, the infrastructure may not be able to cope with the influx.

A reasonable policy would be to offer chemoprophylaxis to unvaccinated but tuberculin-reactive children who are household contacts of patients with tuberculosis. The younger the child the stronger is the indication. In order to increase compliance it is necessary to explain to the parents the rationale of treating an asymptomatic child.

Tuberculosis and human immunodeficiency virus (HIV) infection

The outlook for the control of tuberculosis in some developing countries, specially in subSaharan Africa, has been adversely affected by the high prevalence of HIV infection. HIV infection is the greatest known risk factor for the development of tuberculosis, so progression from mycobacterial infection to disease is common in those developing countries with a high level of dual infection. It is estimated that about 30 per cent of those with dual infection would progress to active tuberculosis. A sharp increase in the number of cases of tuberculosis has already occurred in some African countries such as Tanzania and Malawi. Studies in the subSaharan countries and the Caribbean have shown that 20 to 60 per cent of patients with tuberculosis are HIV seropositive.

While 80 per cent of tuberculosis-infected individuals in developed countries are in the age group of 50 years and over, 75 per cent in developing countries are below the age of 50 years. As HIV infection, too, is concentrated in the under-50 year age group, there is greater chance of dual infection in developing countries.

HIV infection has placed an enormous extra burden on tuberculosis control programmes in some African countries that have limited resources. Apart from the additional load of new cases that has to be managed, the unusual pattern of their clinical manifestations may present difficulties in diagnosis, specially if paramedical personnel are employed in case finding. Cavitation may be absent and sputum smear negative. Extrapulmonary involvement is common. There is a higher mortality among tubercular patients who are also HIV infected, as is the case in some subSaharan countries.

In Asia, the prevalence of HIV infection is still relatively low, but this may change. Already Thailand is experiencing an epidemic of HIV infection, and there are indications that this is happening in India, too. If this trend continues, Asia will also have to contend with the HIV-related problems in tuberculosis control that confront Africa.

Streptomycin is a commonly used drug in these countries, and when administered with improperly sterilized glass syringes and non-disposable needles may be a means of transmitting HIV infection, specially in endemic areas. The alternative of using disposable syringes and needles is costly, but with a little more expense the orally administered rifampicin, which is a much superior drug, could be substituted for streptomycin. A similar problem arises in the case of tuberculin testing when syringes and needles are recycled.

In some developing countries where BCG is routinely given at birth, the high prevalence of HIV-infected mothers is a matter for concern. It is known that immunodeficient children born to HIV-infected women may develop disseminated BCG disease when vaccinated at birth. The issue has been brought into focus in Uganda where there is a higher prevalence of HIV-infected children than in the United States. The current WHO recommendation is to continue the present practice of BCG vaccination of newborns in these countries and to withhold it only from symptomatic HIV-infected children.

Tuberculosis when diagnosed early in the course of HIV infection usually responds to regimens containing rifampicin. Adverse reactions to thiacetazone, an inexpensive drug commonly used in Africa, are more common in HIV-infected patients.

In the United States and some other developed countries, an alarming multiple drug resistance has recently arisen. In a few outbreaks, usually associated with HIV-infected individuals, *M. tuberculosis* was found to be resistant to the two important drugs, rifampicin and pyrazinamide, and in some instances to other drugs as well. Poor compliance in this category of patients, for various reasons such as drug abuse, has been blamed for this. Transmission of these resistant bacilli to other HIV-infected people has been reported in settings where there is close contact as in prisons and hospitals, and to family members and health workers. If this were to occur in developing countries with high levels of HIV infection, the outcome would be potentially disastrous. Patients with AIDS if found in large numbers in the community, as in subSaharan Africa, would form a group highly susceptible to the acquisition of drug-resistant tuberculosis and likely to transmit it to others. A chain reaction of this nature would be difficult to control. Treatment will require the use of expensive drugs for long periods, as well as other resources such as hospital beds for prolonged stay. Such facilities are usually beyond the means of developing countries.

REFERENCES

Global Programme on AIDS and Tuberculosis Programme (1989). *Statement on AIDS and tuberculosis.* World Health Organization in collaboration with International Union Against Tuberculosis and Lung Disease, Geneva.

Murray, C.J.L., Styblo, K., and Rouillon, A. (1990). Tuberculosis in developing countries: burden, intervention and cost. *Bulletin IUATLD*, **65**, 6–24.

Pinto, M.R.M., Arseculeratne, S.N., Uragoda, C.G., and Hemawardene, D.M. (1972). Differential tuberculin testing in rural populations in Ceylon. *Tubercle*, **53**, 182–97.

Scientific Committees of the IUATLD (1991). Tuberculosis in children. *Bulletin IUATLD*, **66**, 61–7.

Snider D.E. and Roper, W.L. (1992). The new tuberculosis. *New England Journal of Medicine*, **326**, 703–5.

Styblo, K. (1988). The potential impact of AIDS on the tuberculosis situation in developed and developing countries. *Bulletin IUATLD*, **63**, 25–8.

Styblo, K. (1988). Overview and epidemiological assessment of the current global tuberculosis situation: with an emphasis on tuberculosis control in developing countries. *Bulletin IUATLD*, **63**, 39–44.

ten Dam, H.G. (1990). BCG vaccination and HIV infection. *Bulletin IUATLD*, **65**, 38–9.

7.11.24 Disease caused by environmental mycobacteria

J. M. Grange, D. J. Girling, and P. D. O. Davies

Introduction

In addition to the tubercle and leprosy bacilli, the genus Mycobacterium contains about 50 species that exist naturally as environmental saprophytes. Some of these species of environmental mycobacteria occasionally cause opportunistic disease in man and animals. The environmental mycobacteria are divisible into two main groups, the slow and rapid growers, according to their rate of growth on subculture. (Rapid growers may, paradoxically, require prolonged incubation for their primary isolation.) Originally allocated to broad groups according to pigmentation and other cultural characteristics, almost all environmental mycobacteria are now readily identified at species level. Some species are closely related, notably *M. avium* and *M. intracellulare*, which are usually referred to as *M. avium-intracellulare* or the MAI complex.

Most of the slow growers are able to cause human disease but, with

Table 1 *The principal environmental mycobacteria causing opportunistic disease in man*

Slow growers	
M. avium[a]	'Avian tubercle bacillus'
M. intracellulare[a]	
M. scrofulaceum[b]	'Scrofula scotochromogen'[c]
M. kansasii	
M. xenopi	
M. szulgai	
M. malmoense	
M. simiae	
M. marinum	Cause of swimming-pool granuloma
M. ulcerans	Cause of Buruli ulcer
M. haemophilum	Rare cause of skin granulomas in transplant recipients
M. gordonae	'Tap-water scotochromogen'[c] Common in the environment but a rare cause of disease
M. terrae	Extremely rare cause of infection of wounds contaminated by soil
Rapid growers	
M. chelonae[d]	'Turtle tubercle bacillus'
M. fortuitum	'Frog tubercle bacillus'

[a]Usually grouped together as *M. avium-intracellulare* or MAI complex.

[b]Sometimes grouped with the above in the MAIS complex.

[c]Scotochromogens form yellow pigments in the dark.

[d]Previously spelt *M. chelonei*.

rare exceptions, the only pathogenic rapid growers are *M. chelonae* and *M. fortuitum*. The principal pathogenic environmental mycobacteria are listed in Table 1.

The environmental mycobacteria cause two named diseases with characteristic features: swimming-pool granuloma caused by *M. marinum* and Buruli ulcer caused by *M. ulcerans*. The other mycobacterioses are much less specific, often resembling tuberculosis, and require identification of the causative organism for diagnosis.

Ecology and epidemiology

Environmental mycobacteria are particularly associated with water and are found in swamps, ponds, rivers, and estuaries. Some species, including *M. marinum* and *M. gordonae*, prefer free water, while *M. terrae* is found in wet soil. Others, especially *M. kansasii* and *M. xenopi*, have colonized piped water supplies. They are also found in compost and on plants. They are readily transmissible to man in potable water, by inhalation of aerosols, or by traumatic inoculation. Infection of man by environmental mycobacteria is widespread and common but overt disease is rare. Such infection may result in immunologically effective contact, manifesting as cross-reactions on tuberculin testing. It has been postulated that exposure to environmental mycobacteria modifies the protective efficacy of subsequent BCG vaccination, thereby explaining the diversity of protection seen in the major BCG trials.

The population of mycobacterial species in the environment varies from region to region and is affected by many factors including temperature and the pH and mineral content of soil and water. The incidence of overt disease is related to the species and numbers of mycobacteria in the environment, the opportunities for infection, and the susceptibility of the human population. Person-to-person transmission of overt disease very rarely, if ever, occurs.

As they are of environmental origin, the prevalence of disease caused by these mycobacteria in man is unaffected by tuberculosis control measures designed to break the cycle of person-to-person transmission. Thus, although the incidence of such disease remains fairly constant, it is rising relative to tuberculosis in those countries where the incidence of tuberculosis is declining. In recent years, however, there has also been an absolute increase in the incidence of disease due to environmental mycobacteria in many countries because of immunosuppression, notably by AIDS.

The types of environmental mycobacterial disease in man

The environmental mycobacteria cause four main types of disease: chronic pulmonary, lymphadenitis, post-inoculation, and disseminated.

CHRONIC PULMONARY DISEASE

This form of environmental mycobacterial disease usually, but not always, occurs in patients with predisposing local lung lesions such as industrial dust disease, old tuberculous cavities, cancer, cystic fibrosis and bronchiectasis, or generalized autoimmune or immunosuppressive disorders. However, a substantial minority of cases occur in people who are apparently healthy. Most patients are middle aged or elderly and men are much more frequently affected than women.

The most frequent causes worldwide are *M. avium-intracellulare* and *M. kansasii*. *M. xenopi* is more restricted geographically but frequently occurs in southern England. Rare causes include *M. scrofulaceum*, *M. szulgai*, *M. malmoense*, and *M. chelonae*.

M. avium-intracellulare and *M. chelonae* are particularly likely to cause severe, progressive and, if not treated successfully, fatal disease. *M. kansasii* and *M. xenopi* appear to be less virulent.

There are no diagnostically reliable clinical differences between pulmonary environmental mycobacterial disease and tuberculosis, although the onset of the former may be more insidious. Radiologically, the lesions show certain differences from those of tuberculosis. These include thin-walled cavities with limited surrounding exudate, clustering opacities around a central translucent area, less prominent soft shadowing, and a tendency for the disease to be localized and unilateral. Although these appearances may raise the index of suspicion, none of them permits a reliable differentiation from pulmonary tuberculosis. Diagnosis therefore depends on the isolation and identification of the causative organism. In contrast to *M. tuberculosis*, environmental mycobacteria isolated from sputum may not be the primary cause of disease; they may be transitory contaminants of the pharynx or secondary saprophytes of diseased tissue. There are no certain criteria for defining environmental mycobacterial lung disease, but diagnosis generally requires at least two pure cultures from specimens taken at least 1 week apart from patients with compatible symptoms and clinical and radiological signs in whom other causes, including tuberculosis, have been rigorously excluded.

LYMPHADENITIS

This is principally a disease of young people, with about half the cases occurring in children under the age of 5 years. It usually affects the cervical nodes but other lymph nodes, such as the axillary or inguinal, may be involved, especially in older patients. Many mycobacterial species cause lymphadenitis, most commonly *M. avium-intracellulare* and *M. scrofulaceum*. Most cases occur in otherwise healthy children with no obvious predisposing cause but some cases in older age groups are associated with human immunodeficiency virus (**HIV**).

In most cases without predisposing causes, a single node is involved and surgical excision, which is often done for diagnostic purposes, is curative. More limited treatment, such as incision and drainage, may lead to sinus formation and should be avoided. Disseminated disease may develop in a few children, particularly those with some form of congenital immune deficiency, and in HIV-positive people.

POST-INOCULATION MYCOBACTERIOSES

Buruli ulcer (*M. ulcerans* infection) is characterized by large skin ulcers and occurs in certain localized regions, mostly in the tropics. This disease is thought to result from inoculation of *M. ulcerans* into the skin by spiky vegetation.

The natural habitat of *M. marinum*, the cause of swimming-pool granuloma or fish-tank granuloma, is water; it enters cuts and abrasions acquired whilst indulging in aquatic activities such as swimming and tending to tropical fish-tanks. The cutaneous lesions are usually warty, although pustules and ulcers may develop. There may be a 'sporotrichoid' spread of lesions along the draining lymphatics (Fig. 1.) The lesions usually heal spontaneously after a few months, but treatment with minocycline, trimethoprim with sulphamethoxazole, or a combination of rifampicin and ethambutol accelerates resolution. There have been occasional reports of tenosynovitis, carpal tunnel syndrome, osteomyelitis, and disseminated disease due to *M. marinum*.

Most other cases of post-inoculation disease are caused by the rapid growers *M. chelonae* and *M. fortuitum*. The most common lesions are post-injection abscesses, which may occur sporadically or in mini-epidemics due to use of contaminated multidose vaccines or other injectable materials. Abscesses develop from 1 to 12 months after injection and may enlarge to 7 cm or more in diameter. They tend to be very chronic and to remain localized, but multiple abscesses with spreading cellulitis may develop in insulin-dependent diabetics. Localized abscesses usually respond well to excision or curettage, but chemotherapy (see below) may be required for multiple or spreading lesions.

Trauma to the cornea predisposes to infection by *M. chelonae* and *M. fortuitum*. Treatment with amikacin drops and erythromycin ointment may lead to a temporary resolution but relapse is common, especially in cases due to *M. chelonae*, and corneal grafting is usually required.

More serious infections have followed accidental inoculation during surgical operations, especially when contaminated materials, including heart-valve xenografts, have been inserted. Contamination during cardiac-valve surgery has resulted in mycobacterial endocarditis with septicaemia and osteomyelitis of the sternum requiring extensive débridement.

DISSEMINATED DISEASE

Before HIV, disseminated environmental mycobacterioses were extremely uncommon. Some cases, usually due to *M. avium-intracellulare* or *M. chelonae*, occur in young people with congenital immune deficiencies (Fig. 2) and others, due principally to *M. chelonae*, occur in renal transplant recipients. Disease due to *M. haemophilum* is very rare and usually manifests as multiple skin lesions in transplant recipients. As suggested by the name, this mycobacterium requires the addition of blood or other sources of iron to the medium for its *in vitro* cultivation.

Since 1981, the situation has changed dramatically. There are now many AIDS-related cases of disseminated infection by environmental mycobacteria. For reasons that are not clear, the great majority of such infections (96 per cent in the United States) are due to members of the *M. avium-intracellulare* complex and, furthermore, usually due to strains of those serotypes shown by DNA homology to belong to *M. avium* rather than *M. intracellulare*. The incidence of AIDS-related *M. avium-intracellulare* infection shows geographical variations. In the United States about 50 per cent of AIDS patients develop *M. avium-intracellulare* disease; a similarly high incidence is found in Holland, but this condition is not so prevalent in England and Sweden and is very uncommon in Africa. Such infection is usually a late event in the course of AIDS, almost always occurring after the patient has suffered from other AIDS-defining infections.

The diagnosis of AIDS-related *M. avium-intracellulare* disease is made by culture of sputum and blood or of biopsies of liver, lymph nodes or bone marrow. The bacilli may be isolated from faeces in disseminated disease but they may also be present in the intestinal tract of healthy persons.

The mechanism of establishment of this disease in man is poorly understood. Some workers consider it to be the result of recent infection while others postulate that the disease emerges from dormant foci of infection in the lymphatic tissue of the alimentary or respiratory tracts acquired many years previously.

The average life expectancy of AIDS patients with *M. avium-intracellulare* disease is less than that of those with other AIDS-defining infections. This may reflect the later onset of the mycobacterial infection. It is an important cause of complications and death. Treatment, though difficult (see below), is worthwhile as it improves the quality of the remaining months of the patient's life. The symptoms—fever, night sweats, weight loss, those of anaemia and general malaise—are rather non-specific and may be caused by other AIDS-related infections. Involvement of the intestine may lead to malabsorbtion and chronic diarrhoea.

Fig. 1 *Mycobacterium marinum* infection. A small lesion at the base of the thumb (arrowed) and secondary lesions on the wrist and forearm due to 'sporotrichoid' spread (by courtesy of Dr G. Haase).

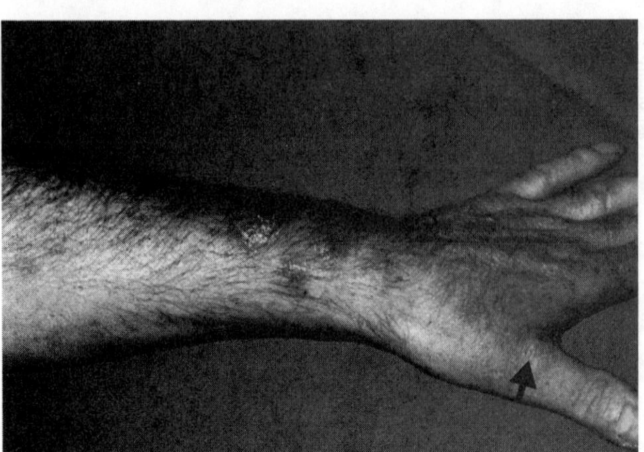

Fig. 2 Ulcers of the lower lip as the initial manifestation of disseminated *Mycobacterium chelonae* infection in a 4-year-old girl with autosomal IgA deficiency (by courtesy of Dr K. Schopfer).

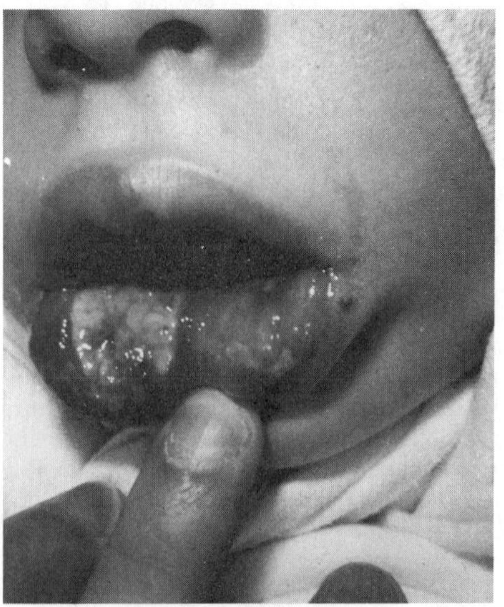

Table 2 *Recommended regimens for treatment of pulmonary infections due to the more usually encountered, slow-growing environmental mycobacteria*

M. avium-intracellulare, M. xenopi, M. malmoense in non-AIDS patients:
24 months' rifampicin, ethambutol, and isoniazid
or
24 months' rifampicin and ethambutol
M. kansasii:
9 months' rifampicin, ethambutol, and isoniazid
or
3 months' rifampicin, ethambutol, and isoniazid followed by 6 months' rifampicin and ethambutol
or
9 months' rifampicin and ethambutol
M. avium-intracellulare in AIDS patients:
Clarithromycin or azithromycin and two companion drugs selected from rifabutin, clofazimine, ciprofloxacin, and ethambutol

Table 3 *Antibacterial agents used for the therapy of disease due to the rapidly growing species* M. chelonae *and* M. fortuitum

Erythromycin
Trimethoprim
Sulphamethoxazole plus trimethoprim (co-trimoxazole)
Doxycycline
Cephalosporins: cefoxitin
Amikacin
Gentamicin
Ethionamide
Quinolones:[a] ofloxacin, ciprofloxacin
Imipenem[b]

[a]*M. chelonae* is resistant to quinolones *in vitro*.

[b]*In vitro* tests may falsely indicate resistance owing to the instability of imipenem in the culture media.

Therapy

This depends on the site and severity of the infection, the presence of predisposing conditions such as congenital or acquired immune suppression, the species of mycobacterium and, in some cases, the result of *in vitro* drug-susceptibility tests.

As indicated above, skin lesions may be cured by excision, curettage or drainage, and isolated lymph-node involvement by excision of the node. Surgical excision of pulmonary lesions, rarely employed in tuberculosis, is useful in the treatment of localized disease due to environmental mycobacteria, especially when there is an underlying localized abnormality of the lung, such as an old tuberculous cavity.

Despite *in vitro* resistance to most of the antituberculosis drugs, most cases of pulmonary disease due to *M. avium-intracellulare* and other slow-growing environmental mycobacteria respond to prolonged courses of five or six of these drugs, provided that these regimens could be tolerated. Three-drug regimens containing rifampicin, ethambutol, and isoniazid are equally effective. Unlike in tuberculosis, ethambutol appears to be more effective than isoniazid and should be continued for the full duration of therapy, provided that ocular toxicity does not occur. In some cases, standard antituberculosis therapy with rifampicin, isoniazid, and pyrazinamide may have been prescribed on the basis of a positive Ziehl–Neelsen smear or a preliminary culture report. In this case, pyrazinamide should be replaced by ethambutol.

Treatment for 18 or 24 months produces up to 80 per cent cure rate in disease due to *M. avium-intracellulare, M. xenopi*, and *M. malmoense*. Shorter regimens are effective for treatment of *M. kansasii* infections. Recommended regimens are summarized in Table 2. Pulmonary disease in HIV-positive patients is either a manifestation of, or likely to proceed to, disseminated disease and should be treated as such (see below).

The older second-line antituberculosis drugs such as ethionamide, cycloserine, and capreomycin have proved effective in some cases that were unresponsive to the above regimens. There is some evidence that quinolones or macrolides are useful in such infections, particularly in those due to rifampicin-resistant strains.

There have been no comparative trials of drug regimens for disease due to the rapidly growing species *M. chelonae* and *M. fortuitum*. Therapy is therefore based on anecdotal experience and the results of *in vitro* susceptibility tests. The duration of therapy depends on clinical response. Drugs for which efficacy has been demonstrated are listed in Table 3. Localized disease often responds to erythromycin with trimethoprim, while spreading or disseminated disease may require the addition of amikacin, gentamicin, or a cephalosporin. Other effective drugs include the quinolones for *M. fortuitum* and imipenem for *M. chelonae* infections, although clinical experience with these antimicrobials is limited.

Disseminated *M. avium-intracellulare* infection in patients with AIDS responds, at least to some extent, to orally administered multidrug regimens containing rifabutin, ethambutol, clofazimine, and either ciprofloxacin or isoniazid (Table 2). The US Task Force on *M. avium* infections recommends that clarithromycin or azithromycin should be included in all regimens. Amikacin is also effective but, as it must be given intravenously, it is usually given only for a short initial period or if the oral regimen proves ineffective. No recommendations on duration of therapy have been made. In many cases, it is necessary to continue the therapy for the rest of the patient's life.

REFERENCES

Collins, C.H., Grange, J.M., Noble, W.C., and Yates, M.D. (1985). *Mycobacterium marinum* infections in man. *Journal of Hygiene (Cambridge)*, **94,** 135–49.

Grange, J.M. (1988). *Mycobacteria and human disease*. Arnold, London.

Grange, J.M., Noble, W.C., Yates, M.D., and Collins, C.H. (1988). Inoculation mycobacterioses. *Clinical and Experimental Dermatology*, **13,** 211–20.

Horsburgh, C.R. and Selik, R.M. (1989). The epidemiology of disseminated mycobacterial infection in the acquired immunodeficiency syndrome (AIDS). *American Reviews of Respiratory Diseases*, **139,** 4–7.

Jenkins, P.A. and Banks, J. (1994). In *Clinical Tuberculosis*, (ed. P.D.O. Davies), Ch. 3 and 13. Chapman & Hall, London.

Mitchell, D.M. and Miller, R.F. (1992). Recent developments in the management of the pulmonary complications of HIV disease. *Thorax*, **47,** 381–90.

Pitchenik, A.E. and Fertel, D. (1992). Medical management of AIDS patients: tuberculosis and nontuberculous mycobacterial disease. *Medical Clinics of North America*, **76,** 121–71.

Ratledge, C., Stanford, J.L., and Grange, J.M. eds. (1989). *The biology of the Mycobacteria.* Vol. 3 Academic Press, New York. Contains excellent chapters on skin lesions and deep tissue lesions due to environmental mycobacteria.

7.11.25 Leprosy (Hansen's disease, hanseniasis)

M. F. R. Waters

Definition

Leprosy is a chronic inflammatory disease of man caused by *Mycobacterium leprae*, which displays a wide clinical 'spectrum' related to host ability to develop and to maintain specific cell-mediated immunity. In high-resistant 'tuberculoid' leprosy, localized signs are restricted to skin and peripheral nerve, whereas low-resistant 'lepromatous' leprosy is a generalized bacteraemic disease involving many systems, with widespread lesions of the skin, peripheral nerves, upper respiratory tract, the reticuloendothelial system, eyes, bone, and testes. Common complications include immunologically mediated inflammatory episodes ('reactions'), secondary inflammation in the anaesthetic areas that result from nerve damage, and deformity of face, hands, and feet.

Aetiology

M. leprae, discovered by Hansen in Norway in 1873, is an intracellular, rod-shaped organism, 1 to 7 μm long and 0.25 μm in width, more acid- and less alcohol-fast than *M. tuberculosis*, which it resembles. Despite repeated claims to have grown *M. leprae in vitro*, none has been confirmed to date, although incorporation of tritiated thymidine and of palmitic acid by bacilli in short-term culture, without multiplication, has been obtained. Successful experimental transmission was not achieved until 1960, when Shepard reported limited infection in mouse foot-pads, and subsequently similar infections have been claimed in hamster and rat foot-pads and the ears of hamsters and mice. A foot-pad inoculation of 5000 or 10 000 bacilli yields 10^6 after 6 to 8 months, but in normal mice no subsequent increase occurs. During the log phase of multiplication, the generation time is 12 to 13 days, the longest of any known bacterium. In thymectomized–irradiated mice multiplication continues, yields of 10^9 per foot-pad being not uncommon with lepromatous histology, and systemic spread occurs; this enhancement can be prevented by transfusions of syngeneic lymphocytes. Lepromatous leprosy may also be obtained in nude mice and in a proportion (about three-quarters) of immunologically normal, nine-banded armadillos inoculated with leprosy bacilli. Such armadillos are now the main source of *M. leprae* for immunological and biochemical studies and for the preparation of a possible vaccine. Recently, several species of monkey have also been reported susceptible.

M. leprae is detected in the skin lesions of patients by Wade's 'scraped incision' method. After being cleaned, the skin is pinched to exclude blood, and a small cut made in the skin fold some 5 mm long and 2 to 3 mm deep. One side of the cut is then scraped with the back of the scalpel point. The tissue pulp collected on the blade is spread on a glass slide, dried, fixed, and stained by the Ziehl–Neelsen method, care being taken never to overheat the carbofuchsin. Leprosy bacilli are very scanty in tuberculoid lesions and are often not detected by routine methods. They become more numerous as the spectrum is crossed and are present in huge numbers in lepromatous lesions. A lepromatous patient may have as many as 10^{12} bacilli in the body. Many untreated lepromatous patients excrete leprosy bacilli in their nasal secretions. Therefore 'nose-blows', collected in polythene handkerchiefs, can be smeared and examined for acid-fast bacilli, although it should be remembered that saprophytic mycobacteria may occasionally be present in the upper respiratory tracts of healthy people. The density of bacilli in smears or tissues is termed the bacterial index, which is best scored on Ridley's logarithmic scale, at one end of which the finding of one to nine leprosy bacilli in 100 oil-immersion fields is graded 1+ and at the other end the finding of over 1000 bacilli in a single oil-immersion field is graded at 6+.

In lepromatous tissues, the bacilli are characteristically in 'cigar-bundle' groups, and in large aggregates or 'globi', the latter situated in multinucleate Virchow giant cells derived from histiocytes. The cytoplasm of many bacilli is fragmented; such bacilli are dead. Dead bacilli are very slowly broken down, and may remain in tissues for many months or years, only slowly releasing their antigens. The percentage of solid-staining, presumed viable, bacilli in smears or tissues is termed the morphological index.

A standardized, autoclaved suspension of *M. leprae*, extracted either from human or from armadillo lepromatous tissue, is used as an intradermal skin test, the 'lepromin' test, which gives an assessment of specific sensitization in leprosy patients. The early (Fernandez) reaction is similar to a tuberculin reaction and is read at 48 h. The late (Mitsuda) reaction is read at 3 to 5 weeks and gives an accurate assessment of specific cell-mediated immunity; it is negative in lepromatous and strongly positive in tuberculoid patients. The test is not, however, diagnostic as it is often positive in patients who do not have leprosy, including those who have never visited leprosy-endemic areas, and shows some cross-reactivity with tuberculin.

There is no known animal reservoir of leprosy, although infection of wild armadillos in a limited area of the United States of America has been discovered, and naturally occurring infections in a captive chimpanzee and in mangabey monkeys have been reported.

Although *M. leprae* cannot yet be grown *in vitro*, mapping of its genome is far advanced, and a complete gene 'library' held in *Escherichia coli*.

Epidemiology

Past governmental returns submitted to the World Health Organization produced a conservative estimate of a world total of 10.6 million leprosy patients. Following the introduction of limited duration (albeit for months or years) multidrug therapy in 1982, and a change in definition of a 'registered case' as one requiring or receiving specific chemotherapy, the current estimate is around 5.5 million leprosy patients. Perhaps more helpful is the detection rate of around 600 000 new patients per year. In addition, there are 2 to 3 million patients who have completed chemotherapy, but are left with significant deformity, who may require ancillary treatment for the rest of their lives. For the importance of leprosy lies not only in numbers, but also in the chronicity of the disease, which frequently disables, but now seldom kills. Therefore it makes disproportionate demands on the health services and economies of developing countries. Leprosy occurs in almost all tropical and warm-temperate climate regions, including Japan and Korea, parts of southern Europe, and several states of the United States. It has only recently died out in northern Europe and Canada and, perhaps surprisingly, does not appear to have become re-established as an endemic disease despite the widespread immigration from the tropics that has occurred over the last 40 years. Leprosy is associated particularly with overcrowding, and as living standards rise, the disease becomes less common.

The main source of infection in the community consists of untreated or relapsed lepromatous patients, who may shed 10^8 leprosy bacilli in 24 h in their nasal secretions. *M. leprae* is also secreted in the breast milk of untreated lepromatous mothers, although few bacilli are excreted through intact skin. Bacilli from dried nasal secretions remain viable after being kept in the dark or in shade for at least 24 h and sometimes for more than 7 days, and thus could be largely responsible for the spread of leprosy, which appears to have many similarities to the spread of tuberculosis. Never the less, the exact mode of infection remains unknown. Entry via the upper respiratory tract, the most likely route, is supported by the finding of microlesions in nasal-biopsy specimens obtained from healthy contacts and by animal studies. Entry through contaminated skin remains a possibility, as it does via the gastrointestinal tract in babies. Insects are known to carry bacilli, but in such small numbers that significant spread by bites appears unlikely. Transplacental infection is unproven, although antigen may cross the placenta.

Unfortunately, hitherto there has been no simple, specific skin test, comparable to the Mantoux test in tuberculosis, which could be used for studying the spread of subclinical infection in the community. Small-scale studies employing specific lymphocyte transformation tests have confirmed sensitization due to subclinical infection. An enzyme-linked immunosorbent assay for antibody to a specific phenolic glycolipid (PGL-1)-secreted antigen is positive in virtually all untreated lepromatous and around 20 to 50 per cent of untreated tuberculoid patients. In endemic areas, the proportion positive of the general population is variable, but is usually 5 to 10 per cent, with perhaps 15 to 20 per cent of close contacts positive; yet only subjects with high antibody titres are at high risk and some negative subjects may subsequently develop clinical leprosy.

Opportunity for contact with the disease, especially in childhood, appears important in the spread of leprosy. The incidence of disease among household contacts of lepromatous leprosy is 5 to 10 times, and among those of tuberculoid leprosy about twice as high as in the general population: this does not necessarily indicate that tuberculoid leprosy is infectious, it may merely reflect the tuberculoid family's contact with an unidentified lepromatous case. Only perhaps 5 per cent of spouses of lepromatous patients acquire the disease.

Studies of genetic markers, especially HLA, have produced no firm evidence that genetic factors account for the susceptibility of a minority of the exposed population to develop clinical leprosy. But recent work indicates that certain HLA-DR phenotypes correlate with the type of leprosy developed by an infected contact.

The incubation period is measured in years, being longer in lepromatous than tuberculoid leprosy. In leprosy-endemic areas, the overall peak incidence occurs in the 20 to 35-year-old group, although that for tuberculoid leprosy usually occurs in the 5 to 19-year-old group; nevertheless leprosy is not uncommon in old age, presumably associated with declining cell-mediated immunity. In a group of American servicemen sent to the tropics the tuberculoid incubation period averaged 4 years and the lepromatous 10 years, although the range was wide in both types of leprosy. The incidence of tuberculoid leprosy is higher than for lepromatous leprosy. In most races, at least from puberty onwards, the incidence of leprosy is higher in males than in females.

Pathology and clinical manifestations

Whatever the portal of entry of *M. leprae*, the target organ for the invading bacilli is probably the endoneurium, an immunologically protected site. Once leprosy bacilli have been engulfed by Schwann cells, their subsequent fate and the type of disease that ensues is decided by the speed and degree of resistance developed, and maintained, by the infected individual. This in turn may be related to the route (and frequency) of antigen presentation and load of antigen presented to the immune system, to variations in non-specific cell-mediated immunity, and to past exposure to other, especially environmental, mycobacteria and to BCG.

INDETERMINATE LEPROSY

Child contacts may develop a single (rarely two or three) hypopigmented macule, 2 to 5 cm in diameter, which when fully developed shows hypoaesthesia and decreased sweating. The majority of such lesions are self-limiting, fading after some months, but about a quarter may evolve to one of the determinate 'spectrum' types of leprosy to be described. Histological changes are slight and non-specific, consisting of lymphocytic cuffing around the dermal appendages and neurovascular bundles. After careful searching, an acid-fast bacillus may eventually be found within a dermal nerve.

THE SPECTRUM OF LEPROSY

Apart from its extreme chronicity, leprosy has two special features. One is the invasion by *M. leprae* of certain superficial nerves, which may become thickened and firm. The other is the wide range of clinical and histological manifestations, reflecting the intricacies of the host–parasite relationship. The spectrum of leprosy was first defined by Ridley and Jopling (1966) who proposed a 5-group system of classification according to certain immunological features. These included the cytology of the host cells of the monocyte–macrophage series (whether histiocytic or epithelioid), the degree of infiltration by lymphocytes, and the bacterial density. The five groups are, in order across the spectrum, tuberculoid (**TT**), borderline-tuberculoid (**BT**), (mid-) borderline (**BB**), borderline-lepromatous (**BL**), and lepromatous (**LL**). This classification enables most patients to be diagnosed accurately from their clinical features, although the intermediate 'borderline' (dimorphous) BT, BB, and BL groups are relatively unstable; they tend to move towards lepromatous in the absence of treatment and toward tuberculoid after the institution of effective chemotherapy.

Skin lesions, which are best seen in good oblique light, may occur anywhere, although they only very rarely involve the hairy scalp, axillae, and perineum. The nerves of predilection, which should always be palpated, include the ulnars at and above the medical epicondyle of the humerus, the superficial radials and medians at the wrist, the great auriculars at the posterior edge of the sternocleidomastoid muscle, usually running about 1 cm above the external jugular vein, the lateral popliteals at the neck of the fibula, and the posterior tibials posterior to the medial malleolus. The surals, the superficial peroneals, and the supraorbitals are sometimes palpably enlarged. When nerves of predilection are affected, appropriate regional anaesthesia may develop, and appropriate muscle weakness and wasting may occur, resulting in claw hand (ulnar and/or median), foot drop, and claw toes. Branches of the facial and trigeminal nerves, although not palpable, may also be involved, leading respectively to lagophthalmos and to corneal anaesthesia. Wrist drop from radial-nerve involvement is comparatively rare. In the sensory nerves, it is the small-calibre fibres that are principally affected, so that temperature, light touch, and superficial pain sensation, together with sweating, are routinely lost. Pressure and deep pain are lost late, and vibration sense and proprioception are normally preserved. Tendon reflexes are also preserved.

TUBERCULOID LEPROSY (TT)

When a high degree of cell-mediated immunity is developed, the infection remains very localized and asymmetrical. Only a small number of skin lesions develop, usually one to three, although the cutaneous sensory nerve supplying the skin of the lesion is frequently thickened.

Typically, a tuberculoid skin lesion is large and annular, with a sharply raised outer edge and thin, erythematous rim that slopes gradually to a hypopigmented, flattened centre. In profile, it resembles a saucer the right way up. The surface is dry with loss of sweating, sometimes scaly, and usually with a diminished number of hairs; established lesions are always markedly anaesthetic, save for some situated in the midline of the face or forehead. Sometimes the lesion is a plaque or a hypopigmented macule. The nerves of predilection are little involved, either none or only one being enlarged; rarely, however, symptoms and signs may be purely neural, related to a single thickened nerve. Histological examination of the active edge of the skin lesion reveals a tuberculoid granuloma, consisting of whorls of epithelioid cells enclosed by lymphocytes, surrounding neurovascular elements and extending up to the epidermis without leaving the papillary zone clear. The epidermis may be eroded; acid-fast bacilli are so scanty as to be seldom found, and dermal nerves within the granuloma are unrecognizable. Caseation is absent in the skin, but may occur in nerve. The lepromin test and the specific lymphocyte transformation test are strongly positive. The lymph node draining the skin-lesion area is free from paracortical infiltrate, but immunoblasts may be present.

BORDERLINE TUBERCULOID LEPROSY (BT)

The skin lesions, which may be very few to moderate in number, resemble those of TT leprosy, although they are usually smaller in size, or else small 'satellite' lesions may be present near the periphery of the larger lesions (Fig. 1). Sharp-edged papules may also occasionally appear. Cutaneous sensory nerves are occasionally enlarged (Fig. 2), whereas asymmetrical enlargement of the peripheral nerves of predilection is common, although caseation only rarely occurs; sometimes the symptoms and signs may be purely neural, related to one or more thickened nerves, although such patients occasionally develop visible skin lesions after commencing on effective chemotherapy. Therefore BT leprosy is often associated with deformity of one or both hands and/or feet. A patient may present with burns or infection of anaesthetic fingers or with a plantar ulcer in an anaesthetic foot. Lagophthalmos may result in exposure keratitis. Although the histological appearances in skin resemble those of TT leprosy, the tuberculoid granuloma tends to be more diffuse and there is usually a clear, though narrow, subepidermal zone and no epidermal erosion; although many dermal nerves are destroyed, some may still be seen, swollen and infiltrated, and small numbers of leprosy bacilli may be detected, usually in Schwann cells or in the erectores pilae muscle. Draining lymph nodes often have an epithelioid-cell, sarcoid-like, paracortical infiltrate. The lymphocyte transformation and lepromin tests are moderately positive.

Fig. 1 Active tuberculoid annular lesions showing the sharp outer edge, thin, raised, erythematous, dry rim, and the broad, hypopigmented, dry centre with slight hair loss. The 'satellite' lesion at the lower outer edge indicates that this is borderline-tuberculoid leprosy. As shown, biopsies and smears should be taken from the raised, active rim.

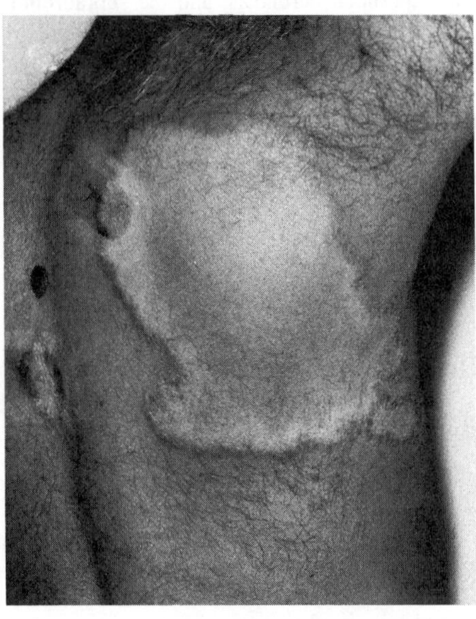

BORDERLINE LEPROSY (BB)

The skin lesions are rather numerous, though asymmetrical, vary markedly in size, and are erythematous or hypo- or hyperpigmented. Papules and plaques may occur, but the most characteristic lesion is annular with a broad rim (Fig. 3). The outer edge is often flattish and irregular; it rises to a thick inner edge overlooking a sharply 'punched-out', hypopigmented, anaesthetic centre. In profile, the lesion resembles a saucer the wrong way up, save that where the cup should sit is a deep central depression. Satellite lesions are common. Widespread, usually moderate, enlargement of the nerves of predilection may occur, with or without associated muscle weakness and wasting. Histologically, the skin lesion consists of a diffuse epithelioid infiltrate with small numbers of scattered lymphocytes; some dermal nerves are visible; bacilli are present in moderate numbers, especially in Schwann cells and epithelioid cells; there is a subepidermal clear zone. Lymph nodes show a diffuse, epithelioid-cell, paracortical infiltrate. The specific lymphocyte transformation and lepromin tests are usually negative.

BORDERLINE LEPROMATOUS LEPROSY (BL)

The skin lesions are moderate to many in number, although still usually somewhat asymmetrical in distribution, and the intervening skin appears normal. They consist of erythematous or hyperpigmented papules, often dimpled in outline, nodules or plaques that are moist and succulent, and that possess normal or near-normal sensation. Hypopigmented macules with indefinite edges may also be present, somewhat asymmetrical and, in particular, variable in size (Fig. 4). Often the first one or two lesions to develop have the characteristic appearance of punched-out BB annu-

Fig. 2 The lateral supraclavicular nerve is clearly visible and enlarged as it crosses the clavicle and runs towards the proximal edge of the large, borderline–tuberculoid, annular lesion. Nerve biopsy confirmed the presence of epithelioid-cell granuloma.

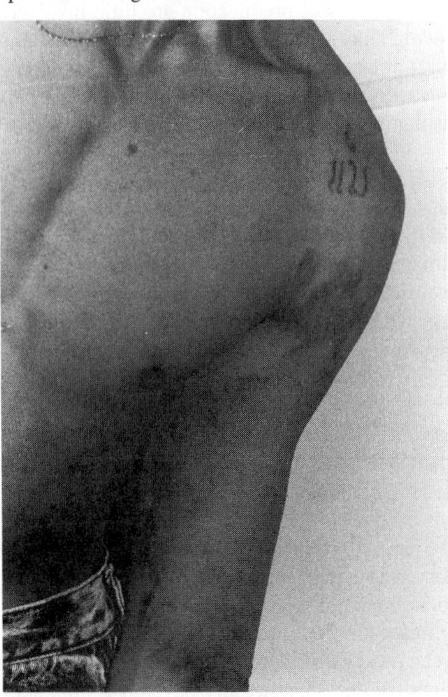

Fig. 3 Borderline annular lesions on the shoulder and back: the rim is broad, the edge irregular, and the 'punched-out' centre is hypopigmented and anaesthetized.

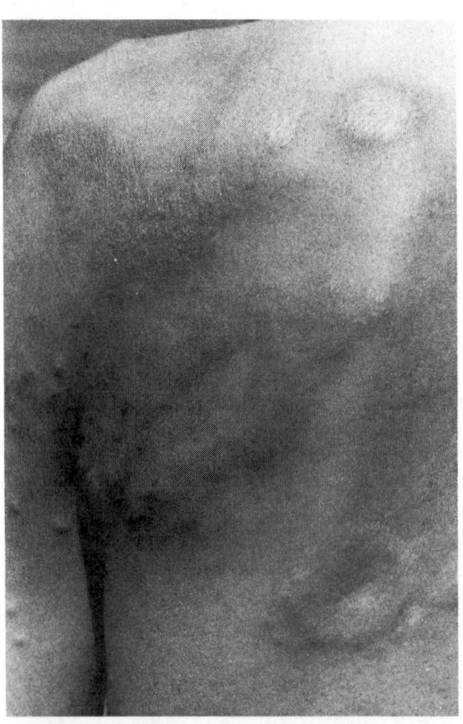

lar lesions, indicating progression (downgrading) from BB leprosy. Nerves of predilection close to the latter may be markedly enlarged; elsewhere they may be only slightly enlarged. Ear lobes may appear normal, or may be asymmetrically or, more rarely, symmetrically enlarged. The eyebrows and nasal cartilage and bones are unaffected. Although bacilli are very numerous in the lesions, they are often undetected in the normal-looking skin. Histological examination of a skin lesion reveals a diffuse histiocytic granuloma, dermal nerves are visible with an 'onion-skin' perineurium, and there are many bacilli present both in the histiocytes and in Schwann and perineurial cells. Lymphocytes are either rather scanty or else present in considerable numbers in some segments of the granuloma; in the latter case, they are CD8+, T-suppressor lymphocytes. Lymph nodes show diffuse histiocytic infiltrate in the paracortical region, with some hypertrophy of the germinal centres. The specific lymphocyte transformation and lepromin tests are negative.

LEPROMATOUS LEPROSY (LL)

The early manifestations are dermal, never neural. At this stage the skin lesions consist of very numerous, small, symmetrical, vague-edged, hypopigmented macules with erythematous, smooth, shiny surfaces that are neither anaesthetic nor anhydrotic, and small papules with indefinite edges. The nerves of predilection may show little thickening, though in more advanced cases they are symmetrically enlarged. Thickening of the nasal mucosa often occurs early, eventually giving rise to nasal blockage and blood-streaked discharge. With time, plaques and nodules develop, and the skin progressively thickens as the lepromatous infiltrate increases; the lines on the face coarsen and deepen, giving a 'leonine facies', and the ear lobes enlarge. Nodules may occur in the mucosa of the palate, and on the nasal septum, and even on the sclera. The lips often swell, and the eyebrows and eyelashes become scanty and are lost (Figs. 5 and 6). Iritis and keratitis are common. The nasal cartilage and bones may be gradually destroyed, resulting in saddle-nose deformity. Lepromatous laryngitis may cause hoarseness or stridor. Oedema of the extremities sometimes occurs, and the skin of the lower part of the legs often becomes firm and waxy in appearance and ulcerates easily. The lymph nodes are often enlarged, especially the epitrochlear and axillary, and testicular involvement may lead to atrophy and occasionally to gynaecomastia. In the absence of treatment, the dermal nerves are gradually destroyed, leading to a progressive pseudo 'glove-and-stocking' anaesthesia; light touch, pain and temperature sensation are eventually

Fig. 4 Borderline lepromatous leprosy: there are numerous moist, shiny plaques on the face, neck, and over the right nipple, typical of BL leprosy, although large, broad-rimmed BB lesions were present on the limbs indicating recent 'downgrading' from BB to BL.

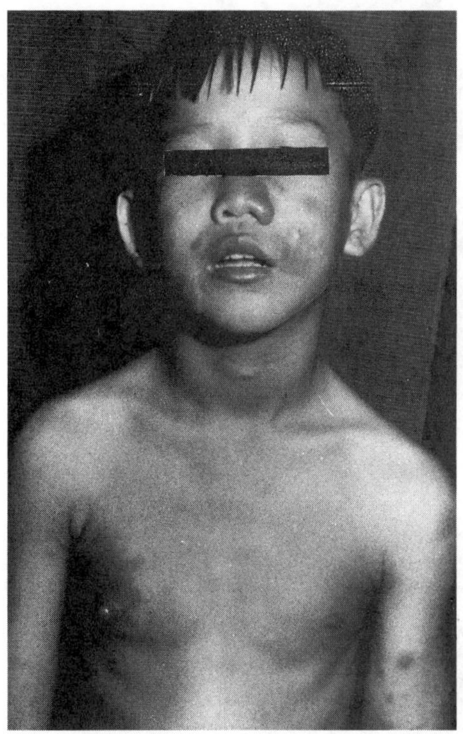

Fig. 5 Active, untreated lepromatous leprosy, showing generalized infiltration of the skin, swelling of fingers and lips, and thinning of eyebrows and eyelashes. The residual annular lesions visible in both pectoral regions indicate that this patient has 'downgraded' from borderline.

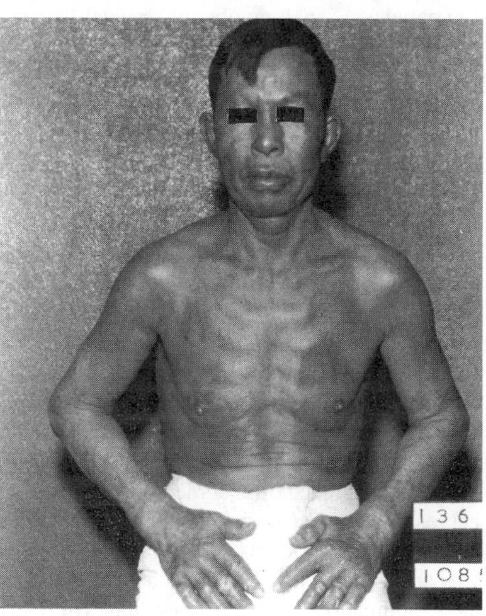

Fig. 6 Leonine facies in advanced untreated lepromatous leprosy, with gross thickening of the ear lobes. The skin of the trunk and limbs is infiltrated and mildly erythematous, and small papules are present on some knuckles.

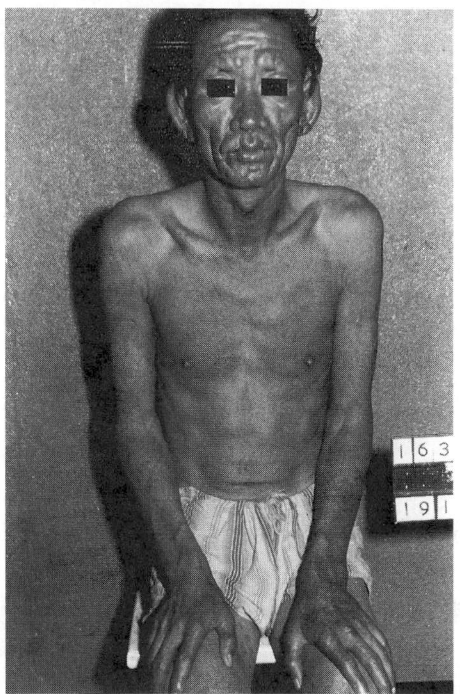

lost over most of the body except the hairy scalp, axillae, perineum, and groins, but position sense is well preserved. Therefore, patients can continue to use their hands almost normally (unless there is motor weakness), but because of the peripheral anaesthesia, some patients repeatedly traumatize their fingers and toes; as a result, the digits progressively shorten and, in addition, secondary infection may occur, leading to local osteitis and tissue damage. Radiographs of the hands of untreated LL patients may, rarely, reveal asymmetrical phalangeal 'cysts', presumed to be due to lepromatous infiltrate. In some long-standing cases, whether treated or untreated, there is absorption of the terminal phalanges, and typical 'pencilling' of the heads and shafts of the metatarsals. Radiographs of the face may reveal atrophy of the nasal spine and of the maxillary alveolar process, the latter often being associated with loss of the upper central incisors.

Many lepromatous cases originate as borderline, and in these 'subpolar lepromatous' (LLs) patients, a small number of residual BB-type or, more rarely, BT-type lesions with central anaesthesia may be found, with associated increased enlargement of the neighbouring nerve of predilection. In Central America, some lepromatous patients develop diffuse infiltrate with no nodules, plaques or papules (primary diffuse lepromatous leprosy). Should an LL patient relapse, whether from failure to take treatment or from developing drug resistance, his new lesions are initially usually asymmetrical; in addition, they are often more rounded and more discrete from the surrounding skin than typical lepromatous papules and nodules, and such relapse lesions are described as 'histoid'.

Histologically, the dermis is massively and diffusely infiltrated with foamy histiocytes full of leprosy bacilli and globi-containing Virchow giant cells. In contrast, bacilli are only rarely found either in the epidermis, which is thinned with flattening of the rete ridges, or in the 'clear zone' immediately below the epidermis. In polar lepromatous (LLp) leprosy, which has not downgraded from borderline, lymphocytes are very scanty, and nerves appear near normal in the infiltrate apart from the bacilli within them. In LLs patients, small numbers of lymphocytes and plasma cells are scattered in the lepromatous infiltrate and dermal nerves may show lamination of the perineurium. Untreated lepromatous patients suffer from bacteraemia and bacilli are present often in large numbers in the reticuloendothelial system, especially in the spleen, the Kupffer cells of the liver, and the lymph nodes draining the skin. These are frequently enlarged, with hypertrophy of the germinal centres, numerous plasma cells at the corticomedullary junction, and almost complete replacement of the paracortical area with histiocytes laden with acid-fast bacilli. Bacilli are also present in the testes in large numbers, although they are scanty in the kidneys, and the central nervous system, heart, and lungs appear to be unaffected.

Reactions

The active multiplication and spread of *M. leprae* clinically causes usually no more than a mild erythema of skin lesions. Nevertheless, episodes of acute or chronic inflammation, known as 'reactions', may occur in any type of leprosy except indeterminate. The majority of reactions occur in patients receiving effective chemotherapy, and there is evidence that they are immunologically mediated. Unless they are adequately treated, they may result in crippling deformity. Although terminology has not yet been standardized, nearly all reactions can be classified into two main groups.

NON-LEPROMATOUS LEPRA REACTIONS (REVERSAL, UPGRADING, OR JOPLING TYPE I REACTIONS)

These occur very frequently in treated BT, BB, and BL, and more rarely in LLs leprosy, the reactions usually commencing within a few weeks of the start of treatment in BT, but often only after several months of treatment in BL and LLs patients. They may also occur in untreated BT patients. Over the course of a few days or weeks, the leprous lesions themselves become markedly swollen, erythematous and often scaly, new skin lesions may appear, and the hands and feet and sometimes the face may become oedematous (Fig. 7). The friable skin lesions may ulcerate, leading to unsightly scarring. Painful (or sometimes painless) neuritis may develop, with or without signs of reaction in the skin, in one or more nerves of predilection, especially in those already enlarged, and may rapidly result in (further) functional nerve damage (Fig. 8). The reaction usually lasts for several months before gradually fading. By then, most but by no means all patients are found to have changed in

Fig. 7 Reversal or upgrading reaction: this BL patient developed new, sharp-edged, well-defined, erythematous plaques with desquamating surfaces about 6 months after changing chemotherapy for drug resistance.

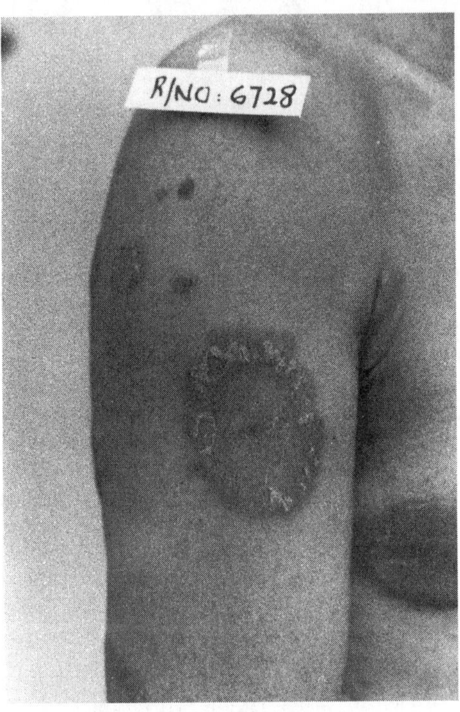

Fig. 8 Reversal-reaction plaque on the left cheek and ear: the edge of this BT lesion has become very sharply defined, more raised, and erythematous, dry, and scaly. Treatment with corticosteroids is imperative, as the patient is at grave risk of rapidly developing lagophthalmos due to associated involvement of branches of the facial nerve.

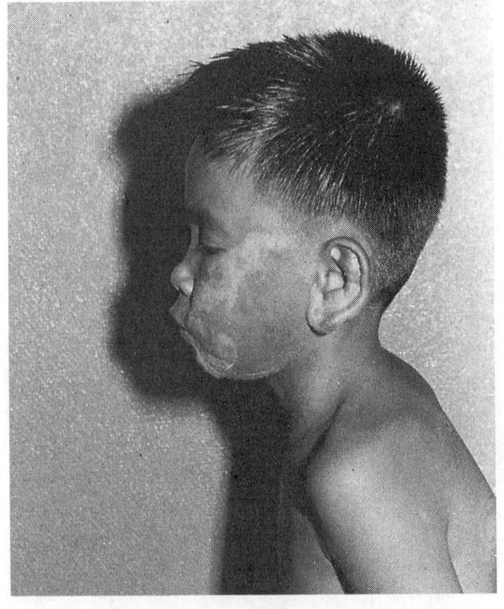

classification towards tuberculoid. The histological picture is variable, but usually shows oedema and disruption of the granuloma, proliferation of fibroblasts, and the presence of giant cells of the Langhans or foreign-body type. In those patients who become more tuberculoid, the granuloma eventually reforms, with characteristics appropriate to the new classification.

Clinically similar reactions may rarely occur in untreated or ineffectually treated (for example, as the result of the development of drug resistance), BT, BB or BL patients, which, when they subside, lead to a change of classification towards lepromatous. Such reactions are known as 'downgrading reactions'.

ERYTHEMA NODOSUM LEPROSUM (LEPROMATOUS LEPRA OR JOPLING TYPE 2 REACTIONS)

Erythema nodosum leprosum occurs only at the lepromatous end of the leprosy spectrum, and up to 50 per cent of treated LL patients, and the occasional untreated LL or treated BL, suffer from one or more episodes of this type of reaction. Over the course of a few hours, a crop of painful, erythematous papules develops, typically on the extensor surfaces of the limbs, but in severe attacks over much of the body except the scalp (Fig. 9). In BL patients, most papules erupt in juicy plaques or nodules in which the concentration of leprosy bacilli is highest. The papules become more purple over 2 or 3 days and then gradually subside, leaving dark staining of the skin. The episodes are usually associated with general malaise, often with high afternoon fever (the temperature on waking being subnormal), and sometimes with bone pain. They may be of all degrees of severity, in some patients being isolated and almost unnoticed and in others occurring continuously over months or years, leading, if untreated, to gross prostration, weakness, and occasionally death. In severe erythema nodosum leprosum, the papules may form sterile pustules and ulcers (Fig. 10). Other systems may also be involved: the most frequent complication is painful neuritis, usually of the ulnar, median, or lateral popliteal nerves, which may result in increasing muscle weakness and anaesthesia of appropriate distribution, but acute lymphadenitis, iridocyclitis, and epididymo-orchitis may also occur, and more rarely nephritis and large-joint arthritis. Episodes of erythema nodosum leprosum usually commence a few months after the start of effective treatment and are sometimes precipitated by intercurrent infection or by physical or mental stress. Histologically, erythema nodosum leprosum resembles the Arthus phenomenon, with polymorphonuclear infiltrate, some vasculitis, and breaking-down foam cells on a background of resolving lepromatous granuloma with fragmented leprosy bacilli.

Fig. 9 Erythema nodosum leprosum (ENL) on the forehead of a patient with early lepromatous leprosy. The papules (and nodules) are firm and tender, with rather indefinite edges. In dark-skinned patients the ENL lesions are often easier to feel than to see, especially over the extensor surfaces of the arms and thighs.

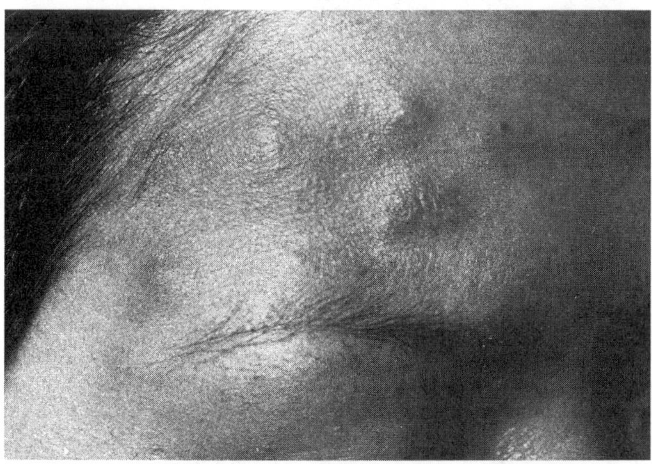

Fig. 10 Pustular and ulcerating erythema nodosum leprosum in a debilitated lepromatous patient. (Patient of Dr William Jopling.)

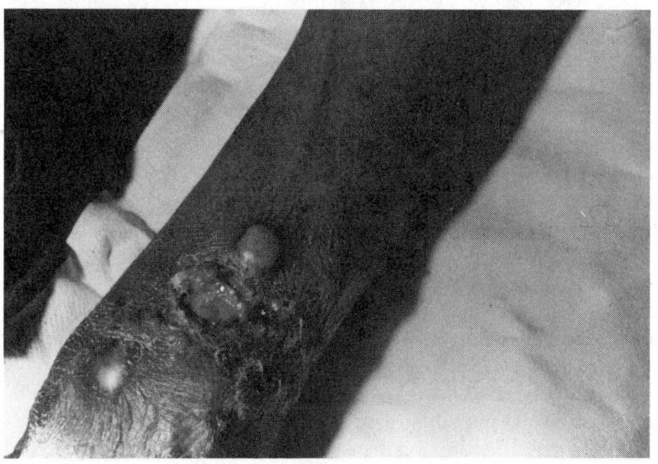

THE LUCIO REACTION

Untreated Central American patients suffering from diffuse lepromatous leprosy may develop irregularly edged, erythematous lesions of the skin, especially on the lower limbs, which scab and ulcerate, eventually healing with typical ragged scars. Histologically, there is vasculitis leading to small infarcts of the skin. Unlike erythema nodosum leprosum, the condition usually subsides once effective antileprosy treatment has been commenced.

Haematology and immunology

In LL and BL leprosy, mild normochromic anaemia may occur. This may become more marked in chronic erythema nodosum leprosum, during episodes of which a polymorphonuclear leucocytosis is also usually present.

Reversal of the albumin:globulin ratio occurs in many LL and some BL patients, and IgG is almost always raised, although IgM and IgA are more variable. Such patients often give false-positive tests for syphilis, and long-standing LL patients may also give positive tests for thyroglobulin antibodies, LE cells, antinuclear factor, and cryoglobulin.

In untreated LL and BL patients, there is gross specific depression of cell-mediated immunity for *M. leprae*, as evidenced by the negative specific lymphocyte transformation and lepromin tests. In addition, there is variable, non-specific depression of cell-mediated immunity, which gradually improves with treatment. There is a relative and absolute depression in the number of circulating T lymphocytes in the blood of untreated LL patients with depression of the T-helper: T-suppressor cell ratio. What factor or factors initiate the gross depression of cell-mediated immunity in lepromatous leprosy still remains uncertain, although possible failure of secretion of interleukin 2 and the role of suppressor cells are being investigated. Recent evidence suggests that T-helper cells in lepromatous skin lesions predominantly belong to subset 2 (Th2), and secrete interleukin 4. Shepard has shown that the pre-priming of experimental mice with intravenous *M. leprae*, 1 week before the intradermal inoculation of *M. leprae*, prevented the subsequent development of specific sensitization. Early lepromatous leprosy was also obtained in a single experimental gibbon, whose infecting dose of *M. leprae*, given 15 years earlier, was administered largely, although not entirely, intravenously; armadillos are also most easily infected by this route.

The depression of specific cell-mediated immunity very rarely alters in LL patients in under 20 to 25 years of effective chemotherapy; up to 20 years almost all remain lepromin negative, and should they relapse at this stage, do so with lepromatous or histoid lesions. After around 25 years without any evidence of relapse, many LL patients become weakly positive on lepromin testing, presumably because it takes this length of time for the bulk of the leprosy antigens to be removed from the skin, and a few such patients have been reported to have relapsed with BT-type lesions.

From lymphocyte transformation studies, reversal reactions are thought to be due to an increase in delayed-type hypersensitivity, usually associated with an increase in cell-mediated immunity, even though the protective antigens of *M. leprae* have not yet been identified. Such reactions may be produced experimentally in thymectomized–irradiated or nude mice that have already developed lepromatous leprosy, by the administration of syngeneic lymphocytes. There is no experimental model for erythema nodosum leprosum. This type of reaction is believed to be due to immune-complex formation, the antigen being derived from the cytoplasm of dead leprosy bacilli and the antibody from the markedly elevated serum immunoglobulin levels that occur in LL leprosy, although at the time of an episode of erythema nodosum leprosum, the circulating T-helper: T-suppressor cell ratio returns towards normal. Most of the manifestations of the erythema nodosum leprosum syndrome could be explained by the local formation of immune complexes, although the glomerulonephritis is presumed to be due to circulating immune complexes and the systemic manifestations (e.g. fever) to the secretion of tumour necrosis factor alpha. Intradermal immune complexes have been detected in the lesions of the Lucio reaction.

Diagnosis and differential diagnosis

The diagnosis of leprosy should always be considered in any patient with skin or peripheral-nerve lesions who has resided in an endemic area. It should especially be suspected when skin or nasal symptoms persist despite routine treatment, in idiopathic foot drop, in unusual presentations of arthritis and erythema nodosum, in chronic plantar ulceration, and in painless burns or injuries to the hands and feet. The discovery of one or more of the following three findings is almost pathognomonic for spectrum leprosy: (i) anaesthetic skin lesions, which are present in almost all TT, BT, and BB patients and in many BL and LLs patients; (ii) the thickening of one or more nerves, either of predilection or cutaneous sensory, as nerve enlargement is found in some TT, many BT, and the great majority of BB, BL, and LL patients; and (iii) the presence of acid-fast bacilli in skin smears, which are positive in some BT and in all untreated BB, BL, and LL patients. Therefore skin lesions should be tested for anaesthesia, peripheral nerves systematically palpated for thickening, and skin smears taken from both ear lobes and up to four typical skin lesions. The diagnosis should be confirmed by biopsy of the skin, the whole depth of the dermis being included in the specimen. In pure neural leprosy, a thickened sensory nerve can be safely biopsied, for example the superficial radial at the wrist, the superficial peroneal in front of the ankle, or the great auricular in the neck. The diagnosis of indeterminate leprosy is especially difficult; biopsy examination may not be possible, especially if the single lesion is on the face, and sensory testing may be difficult to interpret in children, although most cooperate with hot and cold testing. The finding of lack of sweating in the lesion is particularly helpful; alternatively, a histamine test may be done as the flare is often impaired or absent in a leprosy macule, due to damage to the dermal sympathetic nerves.

Leprosy is the only common cause of peripheral-nerve thickening and its finding will exclude almost all other neurological conditions; it may, however, occur in direct peripheral-nerve injury, in which there will be an appropriate history and residual signs of trauma, primary systemic and, rarely, secondary amyloidosis, in which amyloid may be detected in an appropriate organ biopsy, and in hereditary motor and sensory neuropathy types I and III (Déjérine–Sottas disease), which can be differentiated from leprosy by the familial history, and by the absence of skin lesions and of acid-fast bacilli. The anaesthesia of TT and BT leprosy differentiates tuberculoid lesions from vitiligo, mycotic skin infections, lupus erythematosus, and psoriasis, as well as from lupus vulgaris and sarcoidosis; histological examination of the two last conditions will reveal the presence of normal cutaneous nerves in the otherwise very similar granuloma. Certain conditions bear a superficial resemblance to lepromatous leprosy, including diffuse cutaneous leishmaniasis, secondary syphilis, neurofibromatosis, mycosis fungoides, and dermal deposits in Hodgkin's disease, but may be easily differentiated by the absence of nerve thickening and the failure to find acid-fast bacilli in the skin smears.

Treatment

In leprosy as much as in any other disease it is necessary to treat the 'whole patient'. This is because of the strong sense of stigma still persisting needlessly in many cultures, the extreme chronicity of the infection and the liability to relapse after many years, the high incidence of reactions occurring in patients receiving correct chemotherapy, and the continuing possibility of damage to anaesthetized hands and feet even after the infection with *M. leprae* has been cured.

TREATMENT OF THE INFECTION—CHEMOTHERAPY

Effective chemotherapy with the sulphone drugs was introduced in 1943, and dapsone, slowly effective but cheap and usually non-toxic, became the drug of choice by 1951. For the next 25 years monotherapy was generally prescribed, for, unlike tuberculosis, drug resistance was very slow to make its appearance. But relapse off treatment, following the ending of prolonged bacteriostasis or due to microbial persistence, was quickly recognized. Therefore the duration of treatment recommended by successive Expert Committees of the World Health Organization (**WHO**) became more and more prolonged, eventually becoming at least 2 years for TT leprosy ('to clinical inactivity plus 18 months') and about 20 years ('to smear negativity plus 10 years') in LL leprosy, though many gave it 'for life'. But secondary dapsone resistance, first proven in 1964, increased steadily in incidence in LL and BL patients, and from 1977, primary dapsone resistance began to be detected in any type of leprosy. Therefore, drugs known to be of value in the treatment of leprosy and tuberculosis were carefully studied under experimental conditions, and the principal ones found to be bactericidal for *M. leprae* on mouse foot-pad testing are listed in Table 1. Moreover, many patients receiving monotherapy became increasingly poorly compliant after about 3 to 4 years because they failed to detect any further clinical improvement. Therefore attention was directed to the possibility of multidrug therapy of limited duration, and two regimens very suitable for general use were recommended by the WHO Study Group on Chemotherapy of Leprosy for Control Programmes (1982). These regimens were designed to be as effective, cheap, acceptable, and supervisable as possible, to be cost-effective, and to lessen the burden on both patients and leprosy control schemes.

Over the past decade about 55 per cent of all registered leprosy patients have received WHO multidrug therapy or very similar regimens. Compliance rates have been excellent, and relapse rates to date extraordinarily low, although perhaps a further decade of follow-up is required for full evaluation. New drug resistances appear to have been virtually completely prevented, although the minimum duration of treatment required to keep relapses due to microbial 'persisters' in LL and BL leprosy to an acceptably low level is not yet known—that is, whether it is safe to stop after 2 years, or whether treatment should be continued until smear negativity is reached. It is the current aim of WHO to extend multidrug therapy to all known (registered) cases of leprosy worldwide, so that the prevalence rate can everywhere reach below 1 in 10 000 inhabitants by the year AD 2000—which is a realistic objective and would reduce the status of leprosy to that of a minor public health problem—and the incidence to less than 1 per 100 000 per annum, a far more problematic objective in view of the long incubation period of the disease. With WHO multidrug therapy plus the recently discovered bactericidal drugs, it is possible to envisage the complete eradication of

Table 1 *Minimum inhibitory concentrations (MIC) against* M. leprae, *peak serum concentrations, durations of coverage, and bactericidal activities of standard antileprosy drugs*

Drug	Human dosage (mg)	MIC in mice (ng/ml)	Ratio peak serum concentrations[a] to MIC	Duration for which serum concentrations exceed MIC (days)[b]	Bactericidal activity[c]
Rifampicin	600	300	30	1	++++
Dapsone	100	3	500	10	+
Ethionamide	375	50	40	1	++[d]
Prothionamide	375	50	40	1	++[d]
Clofazimine[e]	50–100	?	?	?	+
Ofloxacin	400				+++
Minocycline	100	200		10–20	+++
Clarithromycin	500				+++

[a]Ratio of peak serum concentrations in man after a single dose to MIC determined in the mouse.

[b]Serum concentrations in man after a single dose.

[c]Relative degrees of bactericidal activity (+, ++, ++++).

[d]Not yet assessed clinically in this dosage.

[e]Because clofazimine is deposited in cells, the significance of serum concentrations is uncertain.

Adapted from Ellard, G. A. (1980). *Leprosy Review*, **51,** 200 and WHO Study Group (1994).

leprosy, though this could well take 150 years, provided that the medico-political will prevails. Time alone will tell.

Dapsone (4-4′-diaminodiphenyl-sulphone, DDS)

This drug is as cheap as aspirin and may be given by mouth or parenterally. Clinical improvement is detected from about 3 months after starting dapsone in LL and BL patients (often earlier in TT, BT, and BB leprosy) and from around this time bacilli from nose and skin will no longer infect normal mice; the morphological index (**MI**) reaches zero by 6 months, although the bacterial index (**BI**) takes many years (2 in BB, 4–5 in BL, and 8–11 in LL) to become smear negative. Small numbers of viable, presumed physiologically dormant, bacilli have been detected persisting in a number of tissue sites in LL patients treated continuously for at least 10 years, and it is thought that these 'persisters' could cause a patient to relapse if treatment is stopped. The relapse rate, however, among 362 LL and BL patients treated for around 20 years with supervised dapsone therapy only totalled 8.6 per cent (1.04/100 person years) for the succeeding 9 years off treatment.

The recommended standard adult dose is 100 mg/day (1–2 mg/kg body weight) by mouth. This dosage gives a peak blood level about 500 times the serum minimal inhibitory concentration (**MIC**), which explains why drug resistance was seldom seen in the early days of dapsone chemotherapy. Dapsone resistance, which develops in a step-wise manner, has been detected 2 to 37 years after the start of treatment, sometimes long after the patient had become smear negative. New, active, usually asymmetrical lesions, typically histoid, or else papules and small plaques with high BI and MI, are found on a background of resolving or resolved lepromatous leprosy. Bacilli from the relapse lesions will grow in the foot-pads of mice treated with dapsone mixed in their diet. Low-dosage dapsone and irregular treatment predispose to the development of secondary dapsone resistance. Estimates of its prevalence in various countries and areas range between 2 and 36 per cent; in West Malaysia it rose from 0.2 per cent in 1966 to 10 per cent of all registered LL and BL patients in 1981. Proven primary dapsone resistance has now been widely reported.

The important toxic side-effect of dapsone is allergy, which may occur in one of several hundred patients. Three to seven weeks after starting dapsone, the patient develops fever, pruritus and dermatitis, and sometimes also jaundice and psychosis; the dapsone must be stopped immediately and prednisolone given for several weeks. Other rare side-effects include dose-related methaemoglobinaemia, and haemolytic anaemia in glucose 6-phosphate dehydrogenase-deficient patients.

Rifampicin (rifampin)

This is so rapidly bactericidal that a single dose of 600 to 1200 mg renders an LL patient a minimal public health risk within a few days, bacilli obtained from the skin 3 days after the dose usually failing to multiply in the foot-pads of mice.

Clinical improvement begins within 7 to 14 days of starting rifampicin and the MI falls to zero within 6 weeks. Nevertheless, the BI falls no faster than with dapsone and persisting viable bacilli have been detected after 5 years of treatment in the dosage of 600 mg daily. The recommended dosage is 10 to 15 mg per kg body weight, that is 600 mg to those weighing 35 kg or over, preferably given on an empty stomach. Rifampicin may be given daily or, because of the prolonged generation time of *M. leprae*, monthly; monthly rifampicin (600 mg originally given on two consecutive days every 4 weeks) has been used safely for 20 years and has proved as effective as daily dosage. Under field conditions, once-monthly rifampicin is not only much cheaper but also easier to supervise than daily rifampicin; weekly rifampicin is not recommended because of the high incidence of toxic side-effects that have been reported in tuberculosis patients. A single dose of 600 mg gives a peak blood level about 30 times the MIC. As rifampicin resistance develops relatively rapidly and easily in lepromatous leprosy, this drug should always be used in combination with at least one other effective antileprosy drug.

Rifampicin is a potent microsomal enzyme inducer when given daily, and its possible effect on the metabolism of other drugs given concurrently should always be remembered.

Clofazimine

This is a riminophenazine dye, which is fat soluble and deposited in fat and other cells; therefore its MIC cannot be measured, although the minimum effective dose preventing multiplication of *M. leprae* in mice is very low, of the order of 0.0001 per cent in the diet. In the dosage of 100 to 200 mg daily it kills leprosy bacilli at about the same speed as dapsone. Various intermittent dosages, from 100 mg three times a week to 600 mg on two consecutive days every 4 weeks, are also effective but give a slightly slower rate of kill. In high dosage, the drug is also anti-inflammatory and has been widely used in dark-skinned races in a dose of 100 mg three times a day to control erythema nodosum leprosum reactions, though several weeks elapse before its full anti-inflammatory effect is produced. As prolonged high dosage may cause serious diarrhoea, the dose should be reduced after about 3 months. In the dose of 50 mg daily (best given after the main meal), the drug is relatively non-toxic, its chief disadvantage being that it causes a reddish-brown pigmentation of the skin with increased melanin production, especially in areas exposed to sunlight, which is objectionable to many light-skinned patients. Surprisingly, after 30 years of use, no fully confirmed case of clofazimine resistance has to date been reported.

Prothionamide and ethionamide

These are interchangeable and give cross-resistance with each other and also with the bacteriostatic drug thiacetazone. Ethionamide probably kills *M. leprae* slightly faster than dapsone and certainly more slowly than rifampicin, but has been studied in relatively few lepromatous patients. The dosage of 500 mg daily gave a 10 to 20 per cent incidence of dose-related gastric intolerance and nausea, and a smaller but significant incidence of jaundice. A dose of 375 mg of either drug gives a peak blood concentration about 40 times the MIC. Resistance to ethionamide has been reported after 5 to 8 years of monotherapy. Prothionamide has been more widely used, usually in the dosage of 350 mg daily, but only in combined chemotherapy. Ethionamide, or prothionamide, in the dosage 5 mg/kg body weight, was the only standard alternative to clofazimine in those patients requiring triple-drug therapy who will not accept clofazimine pigmentation, but is now being replaced by one or other of the newly identified antileprosy drugs, such as ofloxacin or minocycline.

RECOMMENDED REGIMENS

Multibacillary leprosy

(All LL, BL, and BB patients and those BT and indeterminate patients who are skin-smear positive for AFB at diagnosis): because in the past dapsone monotherapy was used worldwide, three groups of patients have to be considered, namely, those newly diagnosed with active untreated leprosy who may or may not be suffering from primary dapsone resistance; those who have undergone active relapse either from failure to take treatment with the resulting multiplication of persisters or because of the emergence of secondary dapsone resistance; and those who appear to be responding normally to treatment with dapsone monotherapy, but who could well relapse in the future from the development of dapsone resistance. Therefore the chemotherapeutic aims are to treat effectively all newly diagnosed patients whether or not they are suffering from primary dapsone resistance, to treat effectively and immediately any patients who have relapsed from secondary dapsone resistance, to prevent the emergence of secondary dapsone resistance both in the newly-diagnosed patients and in those now under apparently successful treatment with dapsone monotherapy, and to prevent the emergence of secondary resistance to any other antileprosy drug used in each regimen, especially rifampicin. Therefore it is essential to give a minimum of three drugs, assuming one of the three is dapsone, to prevent the emergence of resistance to a second drug should dapsone resistance, whether primary or secondary, be present.

As mouse foot-pad diagnosis of dapsone resistance is only available in a limited number of centres and takes 6 to 12 months to complete, the WHO Study Group (1982) designed a single regimen to cover all types of multibacillary patients. It is equally effective in both treated and untreated, and in dapsone-sensitive and dapsone-resistant patients, and provides basic supervision of the more expensive drugs, particularly rifampicin. The regimen consists of:

- rifampicin, 600 mg once monthly (or every 4 weeks), supervised;
- clofazimine, 50 mg daily, unsupervised, plus 300 mg (supervised) every month or 4 weeks;
- dapsone, 100 mg daily, unsupervised.

The WHO regimen was designed for field conditions. Where regular monthly supervision is not possible, but when compliance is known to be good, it may be preferred to double the dose of rifampicin, the patient being given 600 mg on two consecutive days each month or ever 4 weeks. (Under these conditions, the 'supervised' 300 mg dose of clofazimine may be omitted.) Alternatively, in remote areas, or during the rainy season, several months' supply of blister packs of the drugs may be given to the patient or to the village health-care worker or headman.

Although this regimen has been recommended for all three main groups of patients already enumerated, its duration depends upon the individual patient's group and leprosy classification. It is recommended that the regimen should always be given for a minimum period of 2 years, and that it should normally be continued until a patient reaches smear negativity. Therefore untreated LL patients may receive 8 to 10 years' triple-drug treatment before all therapy is stopped when smear negativity is achieved, whereas, for example, smear-negative patients treated hitherto with dapsone monotherapy would receive 2 years' treatment. Relapse rates after stopping triple-drug therapy are surprisingly low to date, of the order of 0.12/100 person years of follow-up, although further long-term follow-up is still required for full evaluation in this very chronic infection. The possibility that 2 years' treatment alone for all MBL patients might be sufficient is under investigation, and is tentatively recommended in high prevalence field situations (WHO, 1994), but long-term results are still awaited. Those few patients who have relapsed after multidrug therapy and have been investigated have not been found to have acquired any new drug resistances.

Patients who find clofazimine completely unacceptable may be given 250 to 375 mg (5 mg/kg body weight) of prothionamide or ethionamide. However, in view of the toxicity of the last two drugs, the alternatives of minocycline or ofloxacin are now preferred (WHO, 1994).

Paucibacillary leprosy

It is important to treat effectively and in the shortest possible time, all skin-smear negative tuberculoid and indeterminate patients, whether suffering from dapsone-sensitive or primary dapsone-resistant leprosy, even though the latter could only normally be diagnosed by failure to improve after a period of treatment with dapsone monotherapy. Short-course chemotherapy with rifampicin (either eight weekly doses of 900 mg or 14 to 21 daily doses of 600 mg) was known to provide a fully effective treatment in tuberculoid leprosy on a 2- to 3-year follow-up. Therefore short-course rifampicin therapy in paucibacillary leprosy is both practical and acceptable. The recommended regimen consists of rifampicin 600 mg monthly for six doses, each dose being carefully supervised, plus dapsone 100 mg daily unsupervised for 6 months. Because the bacterial load is usually so tiny in paucibacillary leprosy, resistance to rifampicin is unlikely to develop should the patient be suffering from primary dapsone resistance. It is the aim of WHO that all patients should complete the 6 months' treatment within 9 months; therefore, when a brief interruption in treatment occurs, the patient should continue his course where he left off; when the interruption is prolonged (say, more than 4 months), then the patient should recommence a full 6 months' course. In those tuberculoid patients receiving steroid therapy for reversal reaction beyond 6 months after commencing treatment, it is recommended that chemotherapy should be continued until steroid therapy is stopped.

Some authorities have been unhappy to stop treatment at 6 months if the skin lesions are still at all erythematous and raised ('active'). However, most of the signs of tuberculoid leprosy result from antigen recognition rather than bacterial multiplication. 'Active' skin lesions may sometimes appear about 2 months after starting treatment in pure neural leprosy, and, even more strikingly, tuberculoid leprosy has been noted to develop in tuberculosis patients treated for around 2 months with daily rifampicin, when virtually all leprosy bacilli must have been killed.

So far, crude relapse rates have been very satisfactorily low, of the order of 0.13/100 person years of follow-up. It is probable that this is a considerable overestimate, as late reversal reactions are known to occur, if rarely, up to the fourth year in BT leprosy because mycobacterial antigen is so slowly destroyed, and it is often impossible to distinguish them from tuberculoid relapse due to very limited bacterial multiplication. A few cases of undoubted multibacillary relapse have been reported, which raise doubts over the correctness of the original paucibacillary classification. Further long-term studies are required.

Should a patient be unable to come every month for his supervised dose of rifampicin, the rifampicin may either be given unsupervised, preferably in a blister pack, if the compliance record is good, or else should be given whenever the patient is able to attend, at intervals of not less than 1 month, until six doses have been given, sufficient unsupervised dapsone being provided to cover the whole period of treatment.

NEW ANTILEPROSY DRUGS

Although the two WHO regimens have proved both very acceptable and highly effective with remarkably low relapse rates and with a very low incidence of toxic side-effects, certain difficulties have been identified. The total duration of treatment remains prolonged, if much shorter than in the dapsone era. It is not yet known if 2 years (as opposed to until achievement of smear negativity) is sufficient in untreated LL and BL disease, and from currently available evidence there is little hope that less than 2 years using standard drugs will prove adequate. Many light-skinned patients experience social and psychological stress from the increase in skin pigmentation caused by clofazimine, fearing that neighbours will thereby detect their diagnosis and stigmatize them; therefore their compliance may become very poor. But the current alternative to clofazimine, prothionamide, has proved too hepatotoxic for widespread use in certain areas, including China and South-East Asia, and is no longer recommended. Thirdly, some centres, especially those with poor-quality skin-smear laboratories, have difficulty in distinguishing pauci- from multibacillary leprosy. Therefore a single short-course regimen incorporating two or more highly bactericidal drugs might justifiably be used for all types of leprosy, and would also be of value for those patients unable to attend a clinic every month, as required for standard WHO multidrug therapy. The new drugs used would have to achieve a 10^4 kill of leprosy bacilli, the size of kill estimated as necessary to eliminate naturally occurring rifampicin-resistant bacilli in lepromatous patients, within the limited period, rather than the 2 years allowed with dapsone plus clofazimine or prothionamide.

Fortunately, three new drugs, or groups of drugs, have been identified, which achieve a 10^4 kill of *M. leprae* within 1 to 3 months. Among the 4-fluoroquinolones, ofloxacin has been shown to give such a kill in 3 months in mice, and ofloxacin (400 mg daily) and pefloxacin (800 mg daily) have given a similar kill in 1 month in a pilot study in man. Sparfloxacin is likely to be as least as effective, but ciprofloxacin is ineffective against *M. leprae*.

Minocycline, the only fat-soluble tetracycline, has also been shown to be highly bactericidal in mice, and in the dosage of 100 mg daily in a pilot study in man, achieved a 10^4 kill within 3 months. There is increasing evidence that the erythromycin derivative, clarithromycin, in the dosage 500 mg daily in man, is also highly bactericidal, and from its mode of action on ribosomal enzymes it may be synergistic with minocycline. Therefore there are a number of potentially excellent alternatives to standard multidrug therapy that, combined with monthly rifampicin, are likely to achieve a kill of all actively metabolizing and intermittently metabolizing *M. leprae* within 1 to 6 months. But their effect on microbial persisters is unknown; therefore relapse rates remain the only final test of efficacy, and require a full 5 years, and preferably 10 years of follow-up for adequate assessment. Careful long-term research is now required, and various regimens (including a courageous 1 month regimen) are under study, but the outstanding requirement remains to reach all diagnosed leprosy patients worldwide, with standard WHO multidrug therapy. It should also be noted that ultra-short-course regimens, although highly desirable from the point of view of public health and compliance, could in the absence of careful patient education lead to delay in the diagnosis of reactions in individual patients off chemotherapy, and result in preventable permanent nerve damage.

TREATMENT OF REACTIONS

It is essential to continue the course of antileprosy chemotherapy unchanged in patients suffering from reactions.

Erythema nodosum leprosum

The symptoms of mild erythema nodosum leprosum may usually be controlled with paracetamol or soluble aspirin, supported when necessary by a course of stibophen, 2 ml daily parenterally for 5 days. The treatment of severe erythema nodosum leprosum is best commenced in hospital. Erythema nodosum leprosum is graded severe if there is high fever and severe general malaise or if moderate fever lasts more than 4 weeks, if the papules become pustular and/or ulcerate or if they coalesce, if there is lymphadenitis, if the nerves become painful or if there is any loss of nerve function, if there is iridocyclitis, orchitis, or arthritis, or if urine examinations reveal persistent albuminuria with red cells present on microscopy. There are three alternative regimens. Prednisolone usually suppresses erythema nodosum leprosum rapidly in an initial dose of 30 to 40 mg daily, which can often subsequently be lowered. But not infrequently steroid therapy proves to be prolonged, and severe steroid toxicity may occur. Therefore steroids are best reserved for short courses to control episodic erythema nodosum leprosum or for short-term cover for operations, childbirth, and similar situations. The drug thalidomide is equally effective in controlling erythema nodosum leprosum and in general is safer than steroids, but its use is contraindicated in women of child-bearing age because of its teratogenic properties. Nevertheless, it is the drug of choice in males and postmenopausal females. The initial dosage is 200 mg twice daily; subsequently it is progressively lowered to a maintenance dose, usually of 50 to 100 mg nightly, which may be continued for years. Thalidomide peripheral neuropathy has not yet been reported in patients with erythema nodosum leprosum, although regular neurological checks are indicated in those receiving long-term therapy. The third alternative is clofazimine, 300 mg daily for an initial period of about 3 months, the dosage being subsequently progressively lowered. Clofazimine is the safest drug for premenopausal women, but it is not as powerful as thalidomide or prednisolone and it takes 4 to 6 weeks to achieve its full erythema nodosum leprosum-suppressive action; therefore, if a very rapid action is required, it may need to be combined initially with prednisolone. In iridocyclitis, local treatment with steroid and homatropine eye drops is also recommended.

Severe chronic erythema nodosum leprosum may last for years, only dying out as a patient's bacterial load as measured by the BI approaches zero. Recent work suggests that the rate of fall of the BI can be accelerated by cytokine immunotherapy, particularly with recombinant interleukin 2, but research is needed to see if this also shortens the duration of chronic erythema nodosum leprosum.

Reversal reactions

Mild reactions can usually be controlled with paracetamol or soluble aspirin, with or without stibophen. In severe reactions, the signs of inflammation should be suppressed with prednisolone. Reactions are graded severe if there is marked fever and malaise, if there is oedema of the hands and feet, if the skin lesions ulcerate, or if there is nerve pain and tenderness or loss of nerve function. The initial dose of prednisolone required is usually 30 to 40 mg daily; this may be reduced during the subsequent 3 to 4 weeks, but maintenance therapy with dosage of the order of 15 to 20 mg daily may be required for several months before the prednisolone can be finally tailed off and stopped. An acutely painful nerve should be rested by splinting of the appropriate limb. Serial voluntary-muscle and sensory-nerve tests are essential in assessing whether successful control of neuritis has been achieved.

TREATMENT OF NEURITIS

Untreated patients with a recent history (less than 3–6 months) of increasing nerve damage, or found to have one or more tender nerves, should be given steroids for several months, commencing with the specific chemotherapy. Neuritis occurring during treatment should be treated as for the appropriate reaction, whether erythema nodosum leprosum or reversal.

ANCILLARY TREATMENT

It is essential to educate patients to protect their anaesthetized limbs, which they should inspect daily for injuries and secondary infection. Callosities over pressure points should be regularly softened by soaking in water, and trimmed. Well-fitting, socially acceptable shoes with microcellular rubber insoles help to prevent plantar ulceration. A plantar ulcer requires rest or the application of a below-knee walking-plaster splint and appropriate treatment of secondary infection. Injured or infected anaesthetized hands may also require splinting to prevent the patient from using the inflamed but pain-free limb. Patients suffering from lagophthalmos or paralysis of hands or feet require physiotherapy and may be helped by reconstructive surgery. Facial deformity may be improved by plastic surgery.

Prognosis

Before the advent of specific chemotherapy, LL patients used to die from intercurrent infection, laryngeal obstruction, or amyloid nephritis; blindness was common. Some BT and most BB and BL patients tended to lose cell-mediated immunity so that their disease became more lepromatous. Patients with TT leprosy, however, and about three-quarters of those with indeterminate leprosy, eventually cured themselves. With early diagnosis and correct treatment, the prognosis is now excellent. Death from LL leprosy is rare, although secondary amyloidosis still occasionally occurs, especially in inadequately treated erythema nodosum leprosum, where the diagnosis must be made in the prenephrotic stage and the causative erythema nodosum leprosum completely suppressed long term with thalidomide if death from renal failure is to be prevented. Widespread nerve damage may still develop in BT and BB patients, either if diagnosis is delayed or if reversal reactions are inadequately treated. Patients who fail to care for anaesthetic limbs may develop increasing deformity, and amputation may become necessary for chronic osteomyelitis. Iridocyclitis may cause impairment of vision or blindness and cataract is common in LL patients.

Prophylaxis

The strategy of leprosy control still relies on early case finding and treatment of infectious LL and BL patients. Vaccination with BCG gives some protection, both in children and in whole populations, although no attempt was made in these studies to distinguish naive subjects from those already infected with *M. leprae*. In Ugandan children it gave 80 per cent protection, whereas in a highly endemic area in Myanmar it gave only 20 per cent protection overall, and significant protection only in the 0 to 4 years age group. This would suggest that preference should be given to vaccinate young, presumed naive subjects, and that BCG given to neonates and infants for protection against tuberculosis may also be protective against leprosy; indeed, in a study in South India, protection was better against leprosy than against tuberculosis.

Vaccination with several other culturable mycobacteria is being investigated. A vaccine consisting of irradiated-killed *M. leprae* derived from armadillos combined with live BCG has been developed by the IMMLEP Committee of WHO. This vaccine is able to protect animals against infections with leprosy, but its evaluation in human populations may take another decade. In all these larger current studies, as in the past, no attempt has been made to identify naive (non-infected) subjects. The use of the WHO vaccine for immunotherapy as an adjunct to chemotherapy of multibacillary leprosy is also being studied, with the objective of attempting to overcome both specific anergy and microbial persistence.

Contact tracing, especially of child contacts of LL and BL patients, remains important. Such children could be offered (further) BCG vaccinations and their sera tested for PGL-1 antibody (which, if present in high titre, would suggest significant risk of developing leprosy and would indicate further investigation with skin-smear testing and careful follow-up). In areas of low endemicity, with few sources of infection, and in non-endemic countries, child contacts could also be offered chemoprophylaxis with rifampicin, probably best given monthly for six doses.

The protective antigens of *M. leprae* have not yet been identified. Once they are, the corresponding genes could be extracted from the *M. leprae* gene library, and the technology is already well advanced for their insertion into a suitable vector, probably BCG, to produce a second-generation vaccine.

REFERENCES

Bloom, B.R. and Jacobs, W.R., Jr. (1989). New strategies for leprosy and tuberculosis and for development of Bacillus Calmette–Guerin into a multivaccine vehicle. *Annals of the New York Academy of Sciences (USA)*, **569,** 155–73.

Convit, J., Aranzazu N., Ulrich, M., Pinardi, M.E., Reyes, O., and Alvarado, J. (1982). Immunotherapy with a mixture of *Mycobacterium leprae* and BCG in different forms of leprosy and in Mitsuda-negative contacts. *International Journal of Leprosy*, **50,** 415–24.

Ellard, G.A. (1990). Editorial. The chemotherapy of leprosy. Part 1. *International Journal of Leprosy*, **58,** 704–16.

Ellard, G.A. (1991). Editorial. The chemotherapy of leprosy. Part 2. *International Journal of Leprosy*, **59,** 82–94.

Fine, P.E.M. (1985). The Kellersberger Memorial Lecture, 1985. The role of BCG in the control of leprosy. *Ethiopian Medical Journal*, **23,** 179–91.

Gelber, R.H. *et al.* (1992). A clinical trial of minocycline in lepromatous leprosy. *British Medical Journal*, **304,** 91–2.

Grosset, J.-H., Ji, B., Guelpa-Lauras, C.C., Perani, E.G., and N'Deli, L.N. (1990). Clinical trial of pefloxacin and ofloxacin in the treatment of lepromatous leprosy. *International Journal of Leprosy*, **58,** 281–95.

Ji, B. and Grosset, J.-H. (1990). Recent advances in the chemotherapy of leprosy. *Leprosy Review*, **61,** 313–29.

Jopling, W.H., Ridley, M.J., Bonnici, E. and Depasquale, G. (1984). A follow-up investigation of the Malta-Project. *Leprosy Review*, **55,** 247–53.

Kaplan, G. *et al.* (1991). The systemic influence of recombinant interleukin 2 on the manifestations of lepromatous leprosy. *Journal of Experimental Medicine*, **173,** 993–1006.

Kirchheimer, W.F. and Storrs, E.H. (1971). Attempts to establish the armadillo (*Dasypus novemcinctus* Linn.) as a model for the study of leprosy. *International Journal of Leprosy*, **39,** 693–702.

Noordeen, S.K., Lopez Bravo, L., and Sundaresan, T.K. (1992). Estimated number of leprosy cases in the world. *Bulletin of the World Health Organization*, **70,** 7–10.

Rees, R.J.W., Waters, M.F.R., Weddell, A.G.M., and Palmer, E. (1967). Experimental lepromatous leprosy. *Nature*, **215,** 599–602.

Ridley, D.S. (1974). Histological classification and the immunological spectrum in leprosy. *Bulletin of the World Health Organization*, **51,** 451–65.

Ridley, D.S. and Jopling, W.H. (1966). Classification of leprosy according to immunity: a five-group system. *International Journal of Leprosy*, **34,** 255–73.

Shepard, C.C. (1960). The experimental disease that follows the injection of human leprosy bacilli into foot pads of mice. *Journal of Experimental Medicine*, **112,** 445–54.

Shepard, C.C. (1981). A brief review of experiences with short-term clinical trials monitored by mouse-foot-pad inoculation. *Leprosy Review*, **52,** 299–308.

Waters, M.F.R., Rees, R.J.W., Pearson, J.M.H., Laing, A.B.G., Helmy, H.S., and Gelber, R.H. (1978). Rifampicin for lepromatous leprosy: nine years' experience. *British Medical Journal*, **i,** 133–6.

WHO Study Group on Chemotherapy of Leprosy for Control Programmes (1982). *World Health Organization Technical Report Series*, No. 67. WHO, Geneva.

WHO Expert Committee on Leprosy: Sixth Report (1988). *World Health Organization Technical Report Series*, No. 768. WHO, Geneva.

WHO Study Group on Chemotherapy of Leprosy. (1994). *World Health Organization Technical Report Series*, No. 847. WHO, Geneva.
Yamamura, M. *et al.* (1992). Cytokine patterns of immunologically mediated tissue damage. *Journal of Immunology*, **149**, 1470–5.

7.11.26 *Mycobacterium ulcerans* infection

M. F. R. Waters

Synonyms

Bairnsdale ulcer, Buruli ulcer.

Definition

A skin disease caused by *Mycobacterium ulcerans*, which usually starts as an indurated nodule that breaks down to form a chronic expanding ulcer with a necrotic base and a deeply undermined edge; the lesion may heal spontaneously, often with extensive scarring.

Aetiology

M. ulcerans, first described by MacCullum and his colleagues in 1948, is a rod-shaped, acid-fast bacillus, 3 to 6 μm long and 0.2 to 0.35 μm in width, with rounded ends and parallel sides, which occurs singly and in groups in the necrotic base and undermined edge of the ulcer (not in the growing, outer edge of the lesion). Many bacilli are extracellular; some are intracellular in macrophages. *M. ulcerans* grows best at 33 °C. On primary isolation, usually rather poor growth occurs at 30 or 33 °C, and none at 37 °C, on solid media such as Lowenstein–Jensen's and Petragnani's. Growth usually improves on passage, when the cream or pale-yellow colonies take 3 to 4 weeks to appear, the generation time being about 24 h. Primary isolation is often more easily achieved by the inoculation of infected material into the hind feet of mice. After 4 to 6 weeks the footpads swell and may ulcerate; at 8 to 10 weeks some mice develop a spreading, generalized oedema, due to the secretion of a soluble exotoxin. On intravenous inoculation of *M. ulcerans* in mice, lesions develop on the cold extremities, namely, the nose, tail, ears, feet, and scrotum.

In vitro, *M. ulcerans* is able to degrade hydroxyproline. It is usually sensitive to streptomycin, and often to rifampicin (rifampin) and clofazimine, but resistant to isoniazid, thiacetazone, and PAS.

Immunodiffusion studies reveal at least 12 antigenic compounds, of which five are species specific.

An extract of sonicated *M. ulcerans*, standardized for protein content, known as 'Burulin' is used for a specific skin test; it is negative in patients while the ulcer is actively spreading and expanding, but becomes positive once the reactive, self-healing phase commences. As the exotoxin causes both tissue necrosis (resulting in the only mycobacterial disease in which a bacterial toxin rather than host response causes tissue destruction), and immunosuppression of cell-mediated immunity, it is tempting to speculate that healing is related to the production by the host of antitoxin antibodies, but this has apparently never been investigated.

Epidemiology

Although first identified in Bairnsdale, Victoria, Australia, most known centres of *M. ulcerans* infection are in tropical rural areas near rivers, including the Congo in Zaire, the Buruli district (upper Nile and Lake Kyoga) in Uganda, the river Nyong in the Cameroons, the Kumasi and Sepik rivers in Papua New Guinea, and near lowland swamp jungle in Malaysia. Several cases have been reported from Central and tropical South America. There is a strong association, direct or indirect, with tropical rain forest, or in Australia with residual warm-temperate riverine forest.

The incidence is usually higher in children than in adults, and in some areas women are more affected than men; tuberculin-negative individuals may be more liable to the disease than tuberculin-positive reactors.

The method of transmission is unknown, although it is assumed that the infection is introduced through a skin abrasion or by an insect bite. *M. ulcerans* has been found in chronically infected bone following a snake bite. No vector has been detected, nor has *M. ulcerans* as yet been isolated from the environment. A small focus of infection in koala bears has recently been reported. Subclinical infections are thought to occur, and Burulin is being used in epidemiological studies.

The incubation period is usually probably around 3 to 13 weeks, but undoubtedly may sometimes be as long as 1 to 2 years.

Pathology

In early, non-ulcerated lesions, there is a vague-edged, indurated, opaque area of necrotic fat with no functional capillaries situated in the lower dermis and subcutaneous adipose tissue. Microscopically, the faint outline of the dead fat cells may be made out in some places, swollen, lacking in nuclei, and separated from each other by amorphous eosinophilic material. Inflammatory cells are not conspicuous and, at the junction of the viable and necrotic tissue, there is also a lack of any significant vascular or inflammatory cell response, although a few macrophages, lymphocytes, and plasma cells may be present. Colonies, clumps, and individual *M. ulcerans* are found concentrated in the centre of the necrotic zone, in which scattered calcification may occur. As the area of non-inflammatory necrosis expands, the corium is undermined and ulcerates, and secondary infection may develop. In self-healing ulcers, the induration eventually softens, the necrotic tissue separates, non-caseating epithelioid granulomas are laid down, and acid-fast organisms become very scanty, and are usually intracellular.

Clinical features

Initially, a painless, small, well-demarcated, indurated, subcutaneous swelling develops, attached to the skin, but not to the deep tissues. The lesion is almost always single, and most occur on the limbs, often near joints, although the site is more variable in young children. There is little or no systemic upset or fever, and the regional lymph node is not enlarged. In most cases, the lesion increases steadily in size, the overlying skin desquamating and becoming hyperpigmented before eventually ulcerating at the centre (Fig. 1). The ulcer edge is characteristically overhanging, and may be undermined to a distance of 5 to 15 cm (Fig. 2). Satellite ulcers or lesions may also appear, but metastatic spread is rare. Once ulceration has occurred, secondary pyogenic infection may take place, and a foul-smelling slough forms. Some lesions remain unchanged for months; others grow rapidly in size, within a few weeks covering much of a limb or the trunk. Even so, there is little pain or tenderness or, save for slight fever, evidence of systemic upset, presumably due to exotoxin immunosuppression. In the absence of treatment, healing slowly occurs, resulting in widespread scarring and often contractures and deformities.

The diagnosis is suggested by the characteristic appearance of the swelling and ulcer, the absence of pain or lymph-node enlargement, and the failure to respond to standard tropical-ulcer therapy. It is confirmed by the finding of acid-fast bacilli in the necrotic ulcer base, the isolation of *M. ulcerans* in culture at 33 °C or in mice, and by the histological appearance of the lesions.

The differential diagnosis at the pre-ulceration stage includes boils, foreign-body granuloma, infected sebaceous cyst, low-grade fibrosarcoma, and tumours of the skin appendages; at the ulcerating stage, tropical, mycotic, parasitic, and malignant ulcers and yaws.

Fig. 1 *Mycobacterium ulcerans* ulceration of the knee, showing the necrotic sloughing ulcer base and the indurated, desquamating, undermined surrounding skin (patient of Drs A.B.G. Laing and A.H. Smelt).

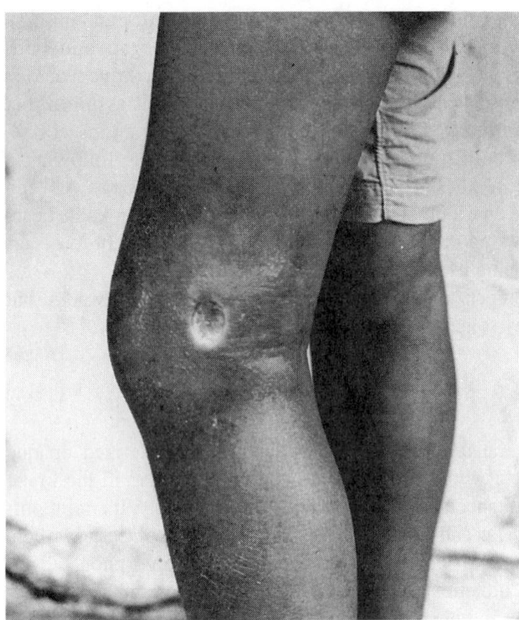

Fig. 2 Ulcer of the arm, showing the overhanging edge. The lesion had stopped increasing in size and was starting to heal.

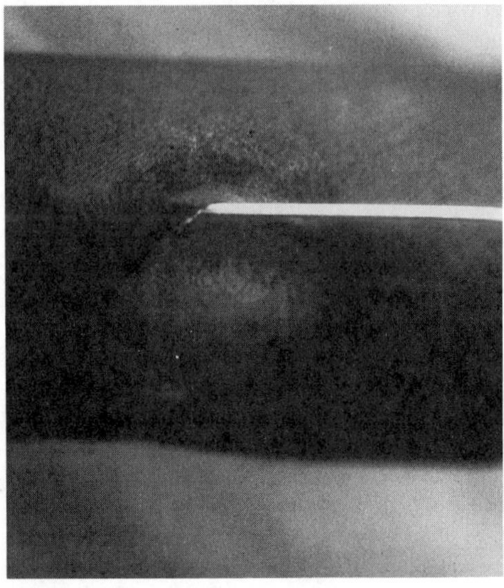

Treatment

Treatment with antibiotics such as streptomycin, clofazimine or rifampicin, to which sensitivity of the strain of *M. ulcerans* has been confirmed, has little healing effect by itself, although it is usually given to cover surgery. Early nodular lesions should be totally excised, followed, if possible, by primary closure of the incision. In ulcerated lesions, all diseased tissue is best excised, followed by skin grafting; all dead tissue must be removed, otherwise grafting will fail with delayed healing and increased scarring. Before surgery, secondary pyogenic infection should be controlled with antibiotics, and the ulcer irrigated with saline. The value of the application of local heat is being investigated.

Prognosis

The severity of resulting scarring is greatly improved by early diagnosis and adequate surgical treatment.

Prevention

In areas of high risk, health education should lead to early presentation and diagnosis; BCG vaccination of children may afford some protection.

REFERENCES

Connor, D.H. and Lunn, H.F. (1965). *Mycobacterium ulcerans* infection (with comments on pathogenesis). *International Journal of Leprosy*, **33,** 698–705.

Hayman, J.A. (1985). Clinical features of *Mycobacterium ulcerans* infection. *Australian Journal of Dermatology*, **26,** 67–73.

Hayman, J.A. (1991). Postulated epidemiology of *Mycobacterium ulcerans* infection. *International Journal of Epidemiology*, **20,** 1093–8.

MacCullum, P., Tolhurst, J.C., Buckle, G., and Sissons, H.A. (1948). A new mycobacterial infection in man. *Journal of Pathology and Bacteriology*, **60,** 93–122.

Pimsler, M., Sponsler, T.A., and Meyers, W.M. (1988). Immunosuppressive properties of the soluble toxin from *Mycobacterium ulcerans*. *Journal of Infectious Diseases*, **157,** 577–80.

Ravisse, P. (1977). Skin ulcer due to *Mycobacterium ulcerans* in Cameroon. I. A clinical, epidemiological and histological study. *Bulletin de la Société de Pathologie Exotique*, **70,** 109–24.

7.11.27 Actinomycoses

K. P. SCHAAL

DEFINITION

Actinomycosis is a subacute to chronic, granulomatous, and suppurative inflammatory disease that tends to progress slowly and usually gives a rise to multiple abscesses and draining sinus tracts. These features may be caused by a variety of different fermentative actinomycetes usually of the genera Actinomyces and Propionibacterium, but sometimes of the genus Bifidobacterium. Because 'actinomycosis' does not denote a disease attributable to a single pathogen, the term 'actinomycoses' is preferable.

Aetiology of human actinomycoses

Actinomyces israelii and *A. gerencseriae* are by far the most frequent and most characteristic causative agents of human actinomycoses. *A. gerencseriae* emerged from the former sero- and biovariety 2 of *A. israelii* in 1990. A third species of filamentous fermentative Gram-positive bacterium, *Propioni-bacterium propionicum*, is a much less common cause of actinomycotic lesions (Table 1).

Several other fermentative actinomycetes are occasionally isolated from actinomycosis-like inflammatory processes (Table 1). In a given case, it is often difficult to decide whether these actinomycetes are causative primary pathogens or merely contaminants, especially when the specimen has had contact with mucosal secretions. However, *A. naeslundii*, *A. odontolyticus*, *A. viscosus*, *A. meyeri*, and *Bifidobacterium dentium* are thought to be capable of producing human infections clinically identical to those caused by *A. israelii*, *A. gerencseriae*, or *P. propionicum* (Table 1).

SOME BASIC PROPERTIES OF PATHOGENIC FERMENTATIVE ACTINOMYCETES

Microscopic appearance

The cellular morphology of typical fermentative actinomycetes that cause human disease is remarkably variable. In the host tissue as well as in early cultural stages, these actinomycetes usually produce Gram-positive, wavy, slender filaments of up to 1 μm in diameter, which may show true branching. However, in smears of pus or older cultures the

Table 1 *Fermentative actinomycetes isolated from human abscess, empyema or sinus discharge at the Institute for Medical Microbiology and Immunology, University of Bonn, between 1984 and 1991*

Species identified	*n*	%
Actinomyces israelii	588	56.4
A. gerencseriae	259	24.9
A. naeslundii	79	7.6
A. odontolyticus	12	1.2
A. viscosus	43	4.1
A. meyeri	3	0.3
Bifidobacterium dentium	5	0.5
Propionibacterium propionicum	36	3.5
Corynebacterium matruchotii	12	1.6
Rothia dentocariosa	5	0.5
TOTAL NUMBER OF ISOLATES	1042	100.0

Modified from Schaal and Lee (1992).

organisms may appear as shorter or longer rods; these may have clubbed or clavate ends and may occur in diphtheroidal arrangements (Y-, V-, T-forms). Although Gram-positive, the uptake of the dye is often irregular, giving rise to a beaded or barred appearance. None of the fermentative actinomycetes is acid-fast.

Culture

The common pathogenic species prefer a marked reduction of the atmospheric oxygen tension and an increased carbon dioxide concentration. However, not all of these actinomycetes are strict anaerobes but facultatively anaerobic carboxiphilic (capnophilic) bacteria with considerable inter- and intraspecific variation in oxygen tolerance.

Colony morphology

Characteristic mycelial, 'spider-like' colonies are produced by only a few species and often merely during the first days of incubation. Because of the comparatively low growth rate of the fermentative actinomycetes and the small size of their filaments, these diagnostically important structures usually become visible only under the microscope at low magnifications. Upon further incubation, the mycelia frequently begin to disintegrate, giving rise to shorter or longer rods or short filaments. The degree of disintegration differs from species to species and even from strain to strain within one species, so that the mature colonies after 7 to 14 days of incubation vary from highly mycelial to rough (molar-tooth colony) to smooth (without any filamentous structures left). Certain pathogenic species such as *A. meyeri* do not form filaments initially.

Identification

The identification of unknown isolates of fermentative actinomycetes is still not easy and requires considerable experience. Under routine conditions, a species diagnosis of acceptable certainty is achieved most easily and quickly by direct or indirect immunofluorescence techniques because all species possess species-specific surface antigens. However, more reliable results are obtained by a combination of chemotaxonomic tests and the determination of the acid end-products of the fermentative carbohydrate metabolism by gas chromatography, with the examination of certain physiological properties. Gene probes or other molecular techniques for identifying unknown actinomycete isolates have not yet been widely used.

Pathogenesis and pathology

All the fermentative actinomycetes pathogenic to man are found regularly and abundantly in the mouths of healthy adults. In the digestive, respiratory, and genital tracts, however, these microbes occur only sporadically or in low numbers. The same is true for the mouths of babies before teething and of adults after loss of all natural teeth. Therefore, these actinomycetes may be considered facultatively pathogenic commensals of the human mucous membranes, which, apart from the very rare actinomycotic wound infections after human bites or fist fights, produce disease exclusively as endogenous pathogens.

For active invasion of the tissue, fermentative actinomycetes apparently require more complex conditions than a simple epithelial defect of the skin or the mucous membranes. Prerequisite is a negative redox potential, on which the pathogenic species are dependent for optimal growth. This may be caused by insufficient blood supply (resulting from circulatory or vascular diseases, crush injuries, or foreign bodies) or by the reducing and necrotizing capacity of other microbes in the lesion.

Synergistic polymicrobial infection

These so-called concomitant bacteria may act primarily as the trigger to the actinomycotic process and may strengthen the relatively low invasive power of the pathogenic fermentative actinomycetes by providing aggressive enzymes (e.g. hyaluronidases) and toxins. Thus, true actinomycoses are essentially always mixed infections. In this polymicrobial inflammatory process, the actinomycetes act as the specific component, the so-called 'guiding organisms', which are responsible for the characteristic course and the late symptoms of the disease. In contrast, the synergistic concomitant flora, which may vary considerably in species composition and number of species from case to case, is often responsible for the clinical picture at the beginning of the infection and for certain complications.

Most of the concomitant micro-organisms are part of the resident or transient surface flora of the mucous membranes of man. In more than 50 per cent of the actinomycoses examined in our laboratory, the concomitant flora consisted exclusively of anaerobes; the remaining cases were caused by a mixture of strict anaerobes and aerobically growing facultative anaerobes or aerobes (Table 2). In addition to the pathogenic actinomycetes, up to 10 different bacterial species have been identified in a single actinomycotic lesion. Altogether, the spectrum of the concomitant organisms comprises about 100 species, the most important of which are shown in Table 2, together with their relative incidences.

Particularly pronounced synergistic interactions appear to exist between pathogenic fermentative actinomycetes, especially *A. israelii* and *A. gerencseriae*, and *Actinobacillus* (*Haemophilus*) *actinomycetemcomitans*. The last organism, the name of which refers to its characteristic association with actinomycetes, is also the most important concomitant bacterium that may sustain the inflammatory process under similar clinical symptoms even after chemotherapeutic elimination of the causative actinomycete. Furthermore, most characteristic and very common companions of the actinomycetes are black-pigmented *Bacteroidaceae* (*Prevotella* spp., *Porphyromonas* spp.), fusobacteria, so-called microaerophilic streptococci, and coagulase-negative staphylococci.

Histopathology

Initially, inflammatory granulation tissue develops and either breaks down to form an acute abscess or chronic, multiple abscesses with connective tissue proliferation. The pathognomonic sulphur granules are found in about 25 per cent of the cases in the suppurative foci, in abscess contents, or in sinus discharge. They are of the highest diagnostic importance.

These sulphur granules, which were originally designated 'Drusen' in Harz's first description of *Actinomyces bovis* (1877), are macroscopically visible (up to 1 mm in diameter), yellowish, reddish to brownish particles, which, when derived from human cases, exhibit a cauliflower-like appearance under the microscope at low magnifications (Fig. 1). At slightly higher magnifications (100 ×) and when the particle has been gently pressed between slide and cover slip, it becomes apparent that

Table 2 *Concomitant actinomycotic flora (predominantly cervicofacial infections)*

Species/group identified	*n*	%
Aerobically growing organisms		
Coagulase-negative staphylococci	891	27.9
Staphylococcus aureus	405	12.7
α-Haemolytic streptococci	357	11.2
β-Haemolytic streptococci	157	4.0
Haemophilus influenzae/parainfluenzae	3	0.1
Enterobacteriaceae	81	2.5
Neisseria spp.	47	1.5
Non-fermenters	6	0.2
Yeasts	3	0.1
No aerobic growth	1509	47.2
Anaerobes and capnophils		
Actinobacillus (*Haemophilus*) *actinomycetemcomitans*	731	22.9
'Microaerophilic' streptococci	937	29.3
Peptostreptococcus spp.	583	18.2
Black-pigmented Bacteroidaceae	1204	37.7
Non-pigmented *Bacteroides/Prevotella* spp.	446	14.0
Fusobacterium spp.	1040	32.5
Leptotrichia buccalis	653	20.4
Eikenella corrodens	527	16.5
Capnocytophaga spp.	14	0.4
Propionibacterium spp.[a]	974	30.5
Lactobacillus spp.	17	0.5
TOTAL NUMBER OF CASES EXAMINED	3197	100.0

[a]Other than *P. propionicum*.

Modified from Schaal and Lee (1992).

these granules consist of a conglomerate of filamentous actinomycete microcolonies formed *in vivo* and surrounded by tissue reaction material, especially polymorphonuclear granulocytes. At high magnification a Gram-stained smear of the completely crushed granule reveals that the microcolonies consist of clusters of Gram-positive, interwoven branching filaments with radially arranged, peripheral hyphae. The Gram stain always shows the presence of a variety of other Gram-positive and Gram-negative rods and cocci, which represent the concomitant flora. In tissue sections and also in purulent discharge, the sulphur granules often show a club-shaped layer of hyaline material on the tips of peripheral filaments, which, in addition to the size of the filaments and to the presence of the concomitant organisms, can aid in the differentiation of actinomycotic sulphur granules from macroscopically similar particles of various other microbial and non-microbial origins. If tissue sections are stained with haemotoxylin–eosin and examined at high magnifications (700–1000 ×) using oil immersion, the clubs appear eosinophilic and reveal a basically stained filament in their centres when properly in focus. The name 'sulphur granules' relates solely to their yellow colour.

Clinical manifestations

The primary actinomycotic lesion usually develops in tissue adjacent to a mucous membrane at sites such as cervicofacial, thoracic, and abdominal. The infection tends to progress slowly and to penetrate without regard to natural organ borders, or to spread haematogenously even to distant sites such as the central nervous system. Remission and exacerbation of symptoms with and without antibiotic treatment is characteristic. As in other endogenous microbial diseases, the incubation period of actinomycoses is not defined; it is assumed that it usually takes 4 weeks until the first symptoms appear, but the incubation period may also be much longer or considerably shorter.

CERVICOFACIAL ACTINOMYCOSES

In the vast majority of cases, the primary actinomycotic lesion involves the face or neck. In a series of 3266 cases of human actinomycoses diagnosed in our laboratories during the past 20 years there was face and neck involvement in 97.9 per cent, but other figures differ considerably from these, especially those from the United States.

Conditions predisposing to cervicofacial actinomycotic infections include tooth extractions, fractures of the jaw, periodontal abscesses, foreign bodies penetrating the mucosal barrier (bone splinters, fish bones, seeds), and suppurating tonsillar crypts. Seeds found accidentally in a few actinomycotic abscesses during the early days of actinomycosis research led to the wrong assumption that the causative agents were acquired from the environment by chewing contaminated vegetable material. The belief that actinomycosis was an exogenous infection persisted for decades, although it was soon shown that the pathogenic fermentative actinomycetes exclusively exist as commensals or parasites of man and other animals and are not able to survive outside their hosts.

The primary actinomycotic lesion in the cervicofacial area either presents as an acute, usually odontogenic, abscess or cellulitis of the floor of the mouth, or as a slowly developing, chronic, hard, painless, reddish or livid swelling. Small acute actinomycotic abscesses may heal after surgical drainage alone. More often, however, the acute initial stage follows a subacute to chronic course if no specific antimicrobial treatment is given, thereby imitating the primarily chronic form, which exhibits regression and cicatrization of central suppurative foci while the infection progresses peripherally producing hard, painless, livid infiltrations. Chronic infiltrative lesions produce multiple, new areas of liquefaction, fistulae (Fig. 2), which often discharge pus containing sulphur granules and which may develop spontaneously or after surgical incision, and multilocular cavities with poor healing and a tendency to recur after temporary regression of the inflammatory symptoms.

With inappropriate or no treatment, cervicofacial actinomycoses extend slowly, even across organ borders, and may become life threatening by invasion of the cranial cavity or the bloodstream.

THORACIC ACTINOMYCOSES

In all parts of the world, thoracic actinomycoses are much less common than the cervicofacial form (Table 3). Thoracic actinomycoses usually

Fig. 1 Actinomycotic sulphur granule. Micrograph of a particle embedded in 1 per cent methylene blue solution, original diameter 0.8 mm. Note the cauliflower-like structure in the centre of the particle and the partially blue-stained granulocytes in the periphery.

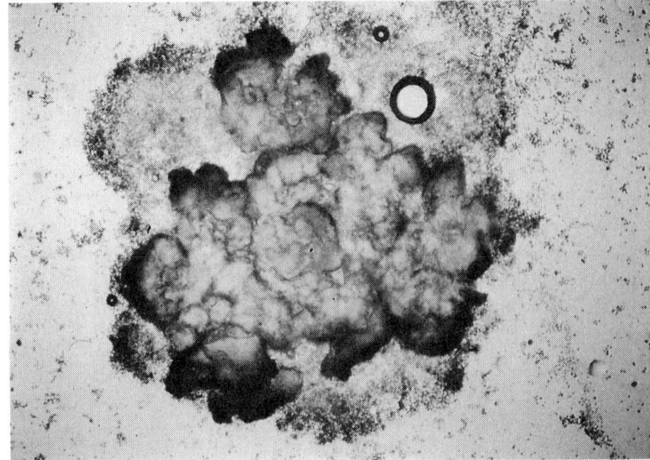

develop after aspiration or inhalation of material from the mouth (dental plaque and calculus, tonsillar crypt contents) or a foreign body that contains or is contaminated with the causative agents. Occasionally, it may result from extension of an actinomycotic process of the neck, from an abdominal infection perforating the diaphragm, or from a distant focus by haematogenous spread.

Primary pulmonary actinomycoses present as bronchopneumonic infiltrations that may imitate tuberculosis or bronchial carcinoma radiographically. There may be single dense or multiple spotted shadows in which cavitations may develop (Fig. 3). If not diagnosed and treated properly, pulmonary infection may extend through to the pleural cavity producing empyema, to the pericardium, or to the chest wall; it may even appear as a paravertebral (psoas) abscess tracking down to the groin.

ABDOMINAL ACTINOMYCOSES

Actinomycoses of the abdomen and pelvis are rare (Table 3). They originate either from acute perforating gastrointestinal diseases (appendicitis, diverticulitis, various ulcerative diseases), from surgical or accidental trauma including injuries caused by ingested bone splinters or fish bones, or from inflammations of the female internal reproductive organs.

The uterus and the cervical canal have only recently begun to attract attention as possible sources of actinomycoses of the pelvic cavity and abdominal organs. Women who wear intrauterine contraceptive devices or vaginal pessaries for long periods often show a characteristic colonization of the cervical canal and the uterine cavity by various fermentative actinomycetes and other anaerobes. This collection of microbes, which is particularly abundant along the thread of the intrauterine contraceptive device within the cervical canal, closely resembles the synergistic actinomycotic flora, although the presence of these organisms is not necessarily accompanied by symptoms. Only a minority of these women develops symptoms such as fever, pain, or vaginal discharge. Usually, the symptoms disappear within 4 to 8 weeks after the intrauterine device has been removed. Occasionally, however, an invasive actinomycotic process may develop, which is difficult to diagnose because it closely resembles cervical carcinoma.

Most of the abdominal actinomycoses present as slowly growing tumours, which, in the absence of sinus tracts discharging pus containing sulphur granules, are difficult to differentiate from malignant processes (e.g. carcinoma of the rectum or the cervix). By direct extension, any abdominal tissue or organ may be involved, including muscle, liver, spleen, kidney, fallopian tubes, ovaries, testes, bladder, or rectum. Haematogenous liver abscesses have been seen, especially from genital actinomycoses.

Fig. 2 Primarily chronic cervicofacial actinomycoses with several draining sinus tracts and livid discoloration of the skin in a 42-year-old man.

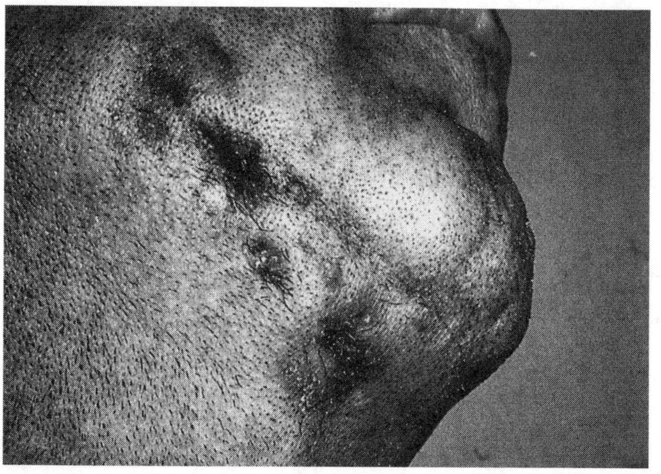

Table 3 *Localization of human actinomycotic infections*

Body site involved	*n*	%
Cervicofacial area	3197	97.9
Thoracic organs	41	1.3
Abdominal organs including pelvis	20	0.6
Extremities	4	0.1
Central nervous system	4	0.1
TOTAL NUMBER OF CASES	3266	100.0

Modified from Schaal and Pulverer (1984).

ACTINOMYCOTIC INFECTIONS OF THE CENTRAL NERVOUS SYSTEM

Actinomycoses of the brain and the spinal cord are now very rare. They arise from direct extension of cervicofacial infections. Haematogenous spread is also possible, particularly from primary lesions in the lungs or abdomen. The spinal canal may be directly involved from these sites. Brain abscess is much more common than meningitis.

ACTINOMYCOSES OF BONE

In contrast to animal actinomycoses, bone involvement is very rare in man. It usually develops by direct extension from soft tissue infection. This may result in a periostitis with new bone formation visible upon radiography. If the bone itself is invaded, localized areas of bone destruction surrounded by increased bone density usually develop. Mandible, ribs, and spine are most frequently involved.

Fig. 3 Chest radiograph of pulmonary actinomycoses of the right upper lobe in a 62-year-old man. The disease was only diagnosed after a huge subcutaneous abscess had developed covering the whole right shoulder blade.

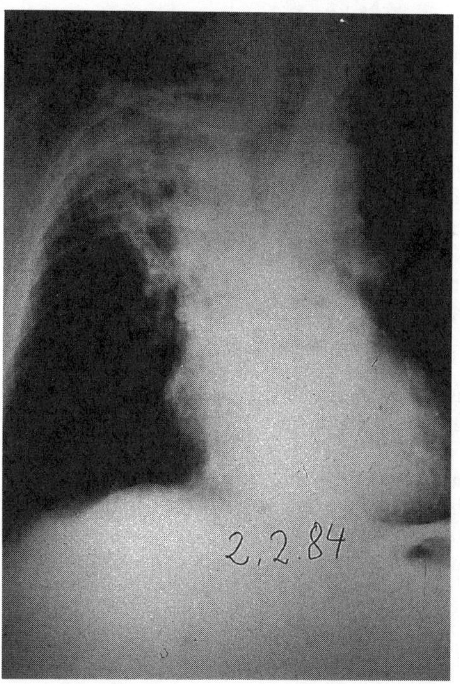

CUTANEOUS ACTINOMYCOSES

Actinomycotic lesions of the skin are extremely rare. Usually, they originate from wounds that were contaminated with saliva or dental plaque following human bites or fist fights, but they may also result from haematogenous spread. Symptoms are similar to those of cervicofacial actinomycoses.

Diagnosis

Clinical symptoms are often misleading, especially in the early stages of the disease, histopathological appearances are unreliable, and diagnosis primarily rests on bacteriological methods.

RADIOGRAPHY

In cervicofacial cases, radiography is useful only for detecting bone involvement. In thoracic actinomycoses, radiographic changes are not diagnostic. However, a pulmonary infiltrate associated with a proliferative lesion or destruction of ribs is highly suggestive of either actinomycosis or a tumour. In abdominal actinomycoses, radiography may help to locate the process and to identify the involvement of organs such as liver, kidney, urinary bladder, or ureter. Distinction between actinomycosis and a tumour is usually not possible until abscesses and sinus tracts can be identified. Radiographs are also inclusive in cases of central nervous actinomycoses or bone involvement.

LABORATORY DIAGNOSIS

Clinical chemistry and haematology

Small, localized actinomycotic lesions are not associated with abnormalities. In advanced cases, however, especially those in the thoracic or the abdominal area, a raised erythrocyte sedimentation rate and pronounced leucocytosis may be found.

When the central nervous system is involved, a polymorphonuclear or mononuclear pleocytosis is commonly found. The protein content is frequently elevated and the sugar content is usually moderately depressed.

Bacteriology

Pus specimens containing sulphur granules and looking like semolina should prompt the clinician to ask and the bacteriologist to look specifically for actinomycetes, using suitable culture techniques and other methods.

Collection and transport of specimens for the bacteriological diagnosis

Pus, sinus discharge, bronchial secretions, granulation tissue, or biopsy specimens are suitable. Precautions must be taken to prevent contamination of the specimen by indigenous mucosal flora. In cases of cervicofacial actinomycoses, pus should therefore be obtained only by transcutaneous puncture of the abscesses or by transcutaneous needle biopsy. When abscesses have already been incised, a sufficient amount of pus should be collected instead of using only a swab.

Sputum always contains oral actinomycetes including the characteristic pathogenic species *A. israelii*, *A. gerencseriae*, or *Propionibacterium propionicum*. Therefore, bronchial secretions should be obtained by transtracheal aspiration, or by transthoracic, percutaneous needle biopsy. Percutaneous puncture of suspected abscesses is often the only way of obtaining suitable specimens for diagnosing abdominal actinomycosis.

The transport of specimens to the bacteriological laboratory should be as fast as possible, preferably by messenger. Alternatively, a reducing transport medium such as one of the modifications of Stewart's medium should be used. When a suitable transport medium is used, the specimen should still arrive in the laboratory within 24 h, although it has occasionally proved possible to isolate actinomycetes from specimens that took 7 days or more to get to the diagnostic laboratory by post.

Microscopic examination of specimens

A quick and comparatively reliable tentative diagnosis is possible when sulphur granules are present. Suspected particles are removed from the specimen by a platinum loop or needle and transferred to a glass slide with a drop of 1 per cent methylene blue solution. The material is covered with a cover slip, which is gently pressed down, and the suspected granule is then observed at low magnification (100 ×). The sulphur granules appear as cauliflower-like particles with an unstained centre and a blue-stained periphery that consists of leucocytes and short filaments radiating from the centre (Fig. 1). The particle is then crushed between two slides and Gram stained. Characteristic filamentous, branched, Gram-positive structures and a variety of other Gram-negative and Gram-positive bacteria together with partially damaged leucocytes are demonstrable under high magnification with oil immersion. The presence of concomitant bacteria is necessary for the identification of an actinomycotic sulphur granule. If only Gram-positive filamentous structures are visible, the granule may consist of Nocardia, Actinomadura, or Streptomyces, indicating a diagnosis of actinomycetoma rather than actinomycosis, with considerable therapeutic implications.

Isolation and identification of the causative agents

Use of transparent culture media and careful microscopic examination of the cultures (on Fortner plates) after at least 2, 7 and 14 days of incubation allows a specialized laboratory to detect possible actinomycete colonies and to subculture them for identification. After 2 to 3 days of incubation, characteristic spider-like microcolonies of *A. israelii*, *A. gerencseriae* or *P. propionicum* may be visible under the microscope. In most cases, however, it takes 7 to 14 days for filamentous colonies characteristic of a pathogenic actinomycete species to become visible. Isolation and definite identification to the species level may require a further 1 to 2 weeks.

Aetiologically relevant fermentative actinomycetes must be distinguished from morphologically similar and taxonomically related contaminants derived from the mucous membranes or from equally similar aerobic actinomycetes of the genera *Nocardia, Actinomadura*, or *Streptomyces*. A detailed bacteriological analysis of the concomitant flora may be helpful in choosing the most appropriate antimicrobial treatment. Techniques such as gene probes or the polymerase chain reaction for detecting pathogenic fermentative actinomycetes are being developed.

Serological diagnosis

None of the routine serological methods has yet provided satisfactory results. However, an indirect immunofluorescence test and an immunoassay with cytoplasmic antigens have been used in the diagnosis of human actinomycoses. Their sensitivity appeared low, but specific antibodies to *A. israelii*, *A. gerencseriae*, and *P. propionicum*, when present, are highly indicative of an invasive actinomycotic infection, active or cured. Antibodies to *A. naeslundii* and *A. viscosus* are often present and can usually be ascribed to a preceding periodontal disease or similar condition. Thus, the rare invasive infections due to these actinomycetes cannot be diagnosed serologically.

Treatment

Before the antimicrobial era, incision and drainage of pus was the basic treatment for human actinomycosis, but relapses were common. A dramatic change in the treatment, and in the prognosis, of human actinomycosis occurred with the advent of penicillins. Penicillin G was found to be active *in vitro* against the pathogenic actinomycetes and *in vivo* against the disease, but there have been many reports on relapses or incomplete cure even after long courses of high-dose treatment. The efficacy of penicillin G is limited by the presence of various concomitant bacteria with different patterns of antibiotic sensitivity. β-Lactamase production by some of the synergistic polymicrobial flora such as *Bacteroides* spp. or staphylococci may protect others that are susceptible to penicillins. *Actinobacillus* (*Haemophilus*) *actinomycetemcomitans* is also usually resistant to penicillin G, although this organism does not produce β-lactamase. Chronic cases often require higher doses and, rarely, prolonged courses of the drugs because their tissue concentrations remain lower than in acute cases.

The current basis for antimicrobial treatment of actinomycoses is the aminopenicillins. These are slightly more active against the pathogenic actinomycetes than is penicillin G. They are also able to inhibit *Act. actinomycetemcomitans*, which is usually resistant to narrow-spectrum penicillins. However, aminopenicillins are not β-lactamase resistant, so that the presence of β-lactamase producers may impair their therapeutic efficacy. β-Lactamase producers, such as *Bacteroides fragilis*, *B. thetaiotaomicron*, or *Staphylococcus aureus* (β-lactamase-producing), are uncommon in cervicofacial actinomycoses. In thoracic and especially in abdominal actinomycoses, however, β-lactamase-producing concomitant organisms are usually present.

For cervicofacial actinomycoses, amoxicillin plus clavulanic acid has proved to be the treatment of choice. Three doses of 2.2 g amoxicillin plus clavulanic acid per day for 1 week and three doses of 1.1 g of the combination for an additional 7 days usually result in complete cure. Very rarely, chronic cervicofacial actinomycotic infections require an additional week of antimicrobial treatment.

Thoracic actinomycoses usually respond to the same regimen. However, it is advisable to maintain a dose of 2.2 g, three times per day for 2 weeks, and to continue treatment for 3 to 4 weeks. Advanced pulmonary cases may require the addition of 2 g of ampicillin three times a day in order to increase the aminopenicillin tissue concentration and, depending on the composition of the concomitant flora, possibly also the addition of an antimicrobial specifically active against strict anaerobes (metronidazole, clindamycin) or resistant Enterobacteriaceae such as *Klebsiella* spp. or *Enterobacter* spp. Enterobacteriaceae and β-lactamase-producing *Bacteroides* spp. must be considered in cases of abdominal actinomycoses. Suitable antimicrobial combinations for these cases are amoxicillin plus clavulanic acid plus metronidazole plus tobramycin (gentamicin) or ampicillin plus clindamycin plus an aminoglycoside. Imipenem could also be a good choice, but this drug has not yet been used very often for treating actinomycotic infections. Neither clindamycin nor metronidazole should be used alone for clindamycin is nearly completely ineffective against *Act. actinomycetemcomitans* and metronidazole shows no activity at all against pathogenic actinomycetes. The use of other combinations, including additional aminoglycosides, cephalosporins, or β-lactamase-stable penicillins, may be necessary depending on the presence of unusual aerobic organisms. In patients allergic to penicillins, tetracyclines or possibly cephalosporins may be tried instead of aminopenicillins.

Prognosis

The prognosis of cervicofacial and cutaneous actinomycoses is good provided that the diagnosis is established early and the antimicrobial treatment is adequate. However, thoracic, abdominal, and systemic infections remain serious conditions that require all possible diagnostic and therapeutic efforts. Even late diagnosis of these forms usually results in complete cure, when proper treatment measures are taken. Without these the prognosis is grave.

Epidemiology

Actinomycoses are not transmissible and cannot be brought under control by vaccination or measures that prevent spread. Sporadically, they occur worldwide. In Germany, the incidence of the disease was estimated to range from 1 : 40 000 (acute and chronic cases together) to 1 : 80 000 (chronic cases alone) per year, which is higher than usually assumed.

It has long been recognized that males are affected about two to four times more frequently than are females. According to our observations, this predisposition is restricted to the cervicofacial form in mature males. This could indicate that hormonal influences play a part in the development of the infection. Actinomycoses may affect patients of any age. However, men are predominantly affected between the 20th and 40th year of life, and women are mostly ill in the second and third decade. Before puberty and in old age, actinomycoses occur sporadically, but lack the preferential involvement of males.

The high incidence of cervicofacial actinomycoses—or the relatively infrequent occurrence of the thoracic and abdominal forms—in Germany as compared to other countries, in particular the United States, may reflect different patterns of use of antimicrobials particularly penicillins, in dentistry. In addition, differences in procedures for, and the intensity of, oral hygiene, as well as differing diagnostic techniques and experience may contribute to differences in the distribution of the disease.

Other diseases caused by fermentative actinomycetes

Actinomycetes play some part in dental caries and periodontal disease but are clearly not the most important microbes that contribute to the development of these important health problems.

Lacrimal canaliculitis with and without conjunctivitis is commonly caused by fermentative actinomycetes. The most important actinomycete species that may cause canaliculitis are *P. propionicum*, *A. viscosus*, and *A. israelii*. Occasionally, *A. naeslundii*, *A. gerensceriae* or *A. odontolyticus* may also be isolated from these conditions. The concomitant flora, when present, is usually less complex than that of typical actinomycoses. Apart from *Streptococcus pneumoniae* or *Haemophilus influenzae*, the species composition of this polymicrobial flora is similar to that of classical actinomycotic lesions. Removal of the lacrimal concretions that are usually present and local application of antibiotics always results in prompt cure.

A. pyogenes, which has been known for many years as 'Corynebacterium pyogenes', is primarily the causative agent of various suppurative infections of domestic animals (mastitis in cows and peritonitis and pleuritis in swine). In man, this organism may cause acute pharyngitis or urethritis, or cutaneous or subcutaneous suppurations.

A. multifermentans, until recently known as CDC group 1 coryneform bacteria, as well as *A. anitratus* (CDC group 1-like coryneform bacteria) have been isolated from abscesses in association with mixed anaerobic flora or from human blood cultures.

REFERENCES

Eibach, H.W., Neuhaus, W., Günther, W., Bolte, A., Pulverer, G., and Schaal, K.P. (1992). Clinical relevance and pathognomonic significance of actinomycotic colonization of intrauterine pessaries. *International Journal of Feto-Maternal Medicine*, **5**, 40–2.

Herzog, M., Pape, H-D., Schaal, K.P., and Beck, R. (1984). Metastasierende Aktinomykose. In *Fortschritte der Kiefer- und Gesichts-Chirurgie*, Vol. XXIX, *Septische Mund-Kiefer-Gesichts-Chirurgie*, (ed. G. Pfeifer and N. Schwenzer), pp. 157–8. Thieme Verlag, Stuttgart.

Niederau, W., Pape, W., Schaal, K.P., Höffler, U., and Pulverer, G. (1982). Zur Antibiotikabehandlung der menschlichen Aktinomykosen. *Deutsche Medizinische Wosenschrift*, **107**, 1279–83.

Pulverer, G., and Schaal, K.P. (1984). Medical and microbiological problems in human actinomycoses. In *Biological, biochemical, and biomedical aspects of actinomycetes*, (ed. L. Ortiz-Ortiz, L.F. Bojalil, and V. Yakoleff), pp. 161–70. Academic Press, New York.

Schaal, K.P. (1986). Genus *Arachnia* Pine and Georg 1969, 269. In *Bergey's manual of systematic bacteriology*, Vol. 2, (ed. P.H.A. Sneath, N.S. Mair, M.E. Sharpe, and J.G. Holt), pp. 1332–42. Williams & Wilkins, Baltimore.

Schaal, K.P. (1986). Genus *Actinomyces* Harz 1877, 133. In *Bergey's manual of systematic bacteriology*, Vol. 2, (ed. P.H.A. Sneath, N.S. Mair, M.E. Sharpe, and J.G. Holt) pp. 1383–1418. Williams & Wilkins, Baltimore.

Schaal, K.P. (1992). The genera *Actinomyces, Arcanobacterium*, and *Rothia*. In *The Prokaryotes*, (2nd edn), *A handbook on the biology of bacteria: ecophysiology, isolation, identification, applications*, Vol. I,(ed. A. Balows, H.G. Trüper, M. Dworkin, W. Harder, and K.H. Schleifer), pp. 850–905. Springer-Verlag, New York.

Schaal, K.P. and Lee, H-J. (1992). Actinomycete infections in humans—a review. *Gene*, **115,** 201–11.

Schaal, K.P. and Pulverer, G. (1984). Epidemiologic, etiologic, diagnostic, and therapeutic aspects of endogenous actinomycete infections. In *Biological, biochemical, and biomedical aspects of actinomycetes*, (ed. L. Ortiz-Ortiz, L.F. Bojalil, and V. Yakoleff), pp. 13–32. Academic Press, New York.

Schaal, K.P., Herzog, M., Pape, H-D., Pulverer, G., and Herzog, S. (1984). Kölner Therapiekonzepte zur Behandlung der menschlichen Aktinomykosen von 1952–1982. In *Fortschritte der Kiefer- und Gesichts-Chirurgie*, Vol. XXIX, *Septische Mund-Kiefer-Gesichts-Chirurgie*, (ed. G. Pfeifer and N. Schwenzer), pp. 151–6. Thieme, Verlag, Stuttgart.

Slack, J.M. and Gerencser, M.A. (1975). *Actinomyces, filamentous bacteria. Biology and pathogenicity*. Burgess, Minneapolis.

7.11.28 Nocardiosis

R. J. HAY

Nocardiosis (nocardiasis) is the infection caused by *Nocardia* species, usually *Nocardia asteroides* but, less commonly, *N. brasiliensis, N. caviae*, and *N. transvaliensis*. The term is most commonly applied to systemic infection due to these organisms but can also be used to describe cutaneous disease that follows the implantation of infection. These organisms are also important causes of actinomycetoma, particularly in Mexico and Central America.

The nocardiae are Gram-positive, filamentous, branching bacteria that ramify in infected tissues. They can also break up into bacillary forms and, in some conditions, aggregate into grains typical of mycetomas. These organisms are aerobic and partially acid fast. They grow readily on ordinary laboratory media.

Pathogenesis

Nocardia species are found in soil, particularly where there is decaying vegetation. They can also be isolated from the air and, in most cases, infection is by the airborne route; rarely nocardiosis can be acquired after inoculation into the skin. The characteristic histopathological response to infection is the production of polymorphonuclear leucocyte abscesses without extensive fibrosis. Caseation and palisading granulomas are not generally seen. Metastases can occur in other organs. Dissemination of infection to the skin can occur in such systemic infections. By contrast, in primary cutaneous infections the lesion is usually localized to an abscess containing filaments at the site of inoculation and is accompanied by local lymphadenopathy. Mycetoma grain formation may occur in some of these infections that follow inoculation. It is not known why, in some patients, transcutaneous infection with nocardia results in the development of a mycetoma whereas in others a subcutaneous abscess containing filaments is formed. The tendency to develop into mycetomas appears to be more common with *Nocardia brasiliensis* infections.

Epidemiology

Otherwise healthy patients may be infected by nocardia, although the frequency of subclinical exposure and sensitization in normal populations is unknown. However, the majority of patients with systemic nocardiosis are immunocompromised, most commonly with a condition that affects the expression of T lymphocyte-mediated immune responses. The list of underlying conditions includes:

(1) malignancies, including cancer and lymphoma;
(2) AIDS and other immunodeficiency states such as chronic granulomatous disease;
(3) solid-organ transplantation;
(4) other conditions that require high doses of corticosteroids, such as collagen-vascular disease and rheumatoid arthritis;
(5) pre-existing pulmonary disease—alveolar proteinosis, in particular, seems to predispose to nocardiosis.

The usual site of primary infection is the lung and the disease may remain restricted to this site. It may also be disseminated to other organs, particularly to the brain and skin. Nocardiosis can occur at any age, although it is rare, particularly in childhood.

Clinical features

PRIMARY CUTANEOUS NOCARDIOSIS

This is an uncommon infection that appears to follow traumatic inoculation of organisms in a superficial abrasion. The usual primary lesion is a small nodule, ulcer or abscess at the site of inoculation. There may be a small chain of secondary nodules (cf. sporotrichosis) along the course of a lymphatic and local lymphadenopathy is common. Some such cases resolve spontaneously. This form of disease is usually caused by *Nocardia asteroides*.

NOCARDIA MYCETOMA

This is discussed in Chapter 7.12.1. *Nocardia brasiliensis* is the usual cause.

PULMONARY NOCARDIOSIS

Pulmonary infection is seen in about 75 per cent of cases of systemic nocardiosis, even where there are disseminated lesions elsewhere. Symptoms of pulmonary nocardiosis are variable, with cough, fever, and leucocytosis. In otherwise healthy individuals the changes and signs may be very similar to pulmonary tuberculosis, whereas in the immunocompromised patient the lesions present as rapidly developing, single or multiple lung lesions. In AIDS patients, symptoms are often minimal, even in the presence of extensive disease. These changes are reflected by the course of the disease. In some patients, progression is rapid, in others chronic.

Chest radiographs may show segmental or lobar infiltrates, cavitation, nodules, or diffuse miliary infiltrates. Calcification is not common. The infection may spread locally to involve adjacent structures such as the pleural space and diaphragm or may spread to other sites. Very occasionally, nocardiae can be isolated from sputum of otherwise healthy patients. Whether this reflects the process of asymptomatic sensitization is not known. Most cases of pulmonary nocardiosis are caused by *N. asteroides*.

DISSEMINATED NOCARDIOSIS

Haematogenous spread is common in the immunocompromised patient and may occur without evidence of pulmonary infection. The most common site for dissemination is the brain, where it presents with localized abscesses without meningeal involvement. The signs are those due to an intracerebral space-occupying lesion. Spread to other sites is less common, although dissemination to skin, liver, kidneys, and bone may occur.

The acute disseminated forms and those with involvement of the central nervous system have the worst prognosis. Continued therapy with corticosteroids also appears to have bad prognostic significance. Infection in AIDS patients may not be recognized before death. Rapid diagnosis is therefore a key to successful management. By contrast, pulmonary infection in otherwise healthy patients is usually a chronic process and has to be distinguished from tuberculosis.

Laboratory diagnosis

The infection is often recognized initially by direct microscopy of pus, bronchial washings or tissue. In Gram stains the organisms can be shown as fine, branching filaments, although distinction from other bacteria may be difficult if short, rod-like forms predominate. A modified acid-fast stain using weak acid can be used to demonstrate filaments.

Nocardia species grow on ordinary media aerobically. Colonies may take 2 to 3 weeks to appear and cultures need prolonged incubation. Growth is generally more rapid on Lowenstein–Jensen medium.

Histopathological examination is useful in some cases. Filaments stain with modified acid-fast stains using an aqueous solution of a weak acid for decolorization but can also be highlighted with the methenamine-silver stain (Grocott modification). The branching nature of the organism is best appreciated in histopathological material. Other pathogens such as pneumocystis may also be present in histopathological material.

Serological tests (usually counterimmunoelectrophoresis or enzyme immunoassay) can be obtained in reference centres and are generally used to monitor the progress of therapy rather than establish the diagnosis.

Therapy

The mainstays of therapy are sulphonamides such as sulphadiazine and sulphafurazole, given in doses of 4 to 6 g daily. Co-trimoxazole is also effective, particularly in pulmonary forms, although the ratio of the trimethoprim to sulphonamide components is not ideal for intracerebral infections. In many cases, drainage of abscesses may hasten recovery. Unfortunately, there have been no multicentre clinical studies aimed at reaching a consensus on the most appropriate therapy for this uncommon infection. Thus, much of the recommended drug therapy is derived from the personal experiences of few cases. It is, for instance, the general practice to use two antibiotics.

Other drugs that have been used include amikacin, ampicillin, and minocycline—although testing is necessary before using these. Experience of newer drugs is similarly limited. For instance, ciprofloxacin, cefotaxime, and imipenem are all active *in vitro* but clinical experience with them is limited at present.

Clustering of cases may occur occasionally, suggesting exposure to a common source of infection. In two such episodes there had been extensive construction work in the vicinity of the hospital involved. At present, no methods of prevention are known, although the existence of more than two cases in a single or adjacent wards should alert clinicians to the possibility of environmentally acquired infection.

REFERENCES

Arroyo, J.C., Nichols, S., and Carroll, G.F. (1977). Disseminated *Nocardia caviae* infection. *American Journal of Medicine*, **62,** 409–12.

Beaman, B.L., Burnside, J., Edwards, B., and Causey, W. (1976). Nocardial infections in the United States, 1972–1974. *Journal of Infectious Diseases*, **134,** 286–92.

Boiron, P., Provost, F., Chevrier, G., and Dupont, B. (1992). Review of nocardial infections in France, 1987–1990. *European Journal of Clinical Microbiology and Infectious Diseases*, **11,** 709–14.

Curry, W.A. (1980). Human nocardiosis. *Archives of Internal Medicine*, **140,** 818–24.

Georghiou, P.R. and Blacklock, Z.M. (1992). Infection with Nocardia species in Queensland. A review of 102 clinical isolates. *Medical Journal of Australia*, **156,** 692–7.

Gorevic, P.D., Katler, E.I., and Angus, B. (1980). Pulmonary nocardiosis. Occurrence in men with systemic lupus erythematosus. *Archives of Internal Medicine*, **140,** 361–70.

Hay, R.J. (1983). Nocardial infections of the skin. *Journal of Hygiene*, **91,** 385–91.

Houang, E.T., Lovett, I.S., Thompson, F.D., Harrison, A.R., Joeckes, A.M., and Goodfellow, M. (1980). Nocardia asteroides infection—a transmissible disease. *Journal of Hospital Infection*, **1,** 31–6.

Javaly, K., Horowitz, H.W., and Wormser, G.P. (1992). Nocardiosis in patients with human immunodeficiency virus infection. Report of 2 cases and review of the literature. *Medicine*, **71,** 128–38.

7.11.29 Rat bite fevers

D. A. Warrell

INTRODUCTION

Between 1948 and 1952, 322 rat bites were reported in Baltimore, United States, in a population of 900 000 people. Fifty per cent of the victims were less than 6 years old and 25 per cent were less than 1 year old. Eighty per cent were bitten while asleep. Patients with diabetic or leprous neuropathy are particularly vulnerable. Rodent bites have been responsible for transmitting a number of infections including lymphocytic choriomeningitis and other arenaviruses (Chapter 7.10.22), rabies, leptospirosis, melioidosis, tularaemia, plague, murine typhus, trench fever, *Pasteurella multocida*, and the two rat bite fevers caused by *Streptobacillus moniliformis* and *Spirillum minus*.

Streptobacillus moniliformis *infection*

(streptobacillary rat bite fever and haverhill fever)

Obsolete synonyms for *Streptobacillus moniliformis* include *Actinomyces muris*, *Actinobacillus muris*, *Actinobacillus putorii*, *Streptomyces muris ratti*, *Haverhillia multiformis*, and *Streptobacillus actinoides*. It is part of the normal pharyngeal flora of up to 50 per cent of wild and laboratory rats and can be recovered from the nasopharynx, middle ear, saliva, and urine. However, it can also produce severe illnesses in rodents, such as septicaemia, pneumonia, conjunctivitis, polyarthritis, and abortion. The organism has been isolated from rats, mice, guinea-pigs, gerbils, squirrels and turkeys, and from animals that feed on rodents such as cats, dogs, pigs, ferrets, and weasels.

S. moniliformis derives its name from the filaments and chains with yeast-like swellings seen in mature cultures on solid media. It is a non-motile, pleomorphic, filamentous, Gram-negative rod, 1 to 5 μm long, and is micro-aerophilic. It can be grown in ordinary blood culture media, but thrives only when blood, serum or ascitic fluid are added (for example, trypticase soy agar with 20 per cent horse or rabbit serum added under 8 per cent CO_2). In liquid media, 'puff ball' colonies appear in 1 to 6 days. In concentrations exceeding 0.0125 per cent, sodium polyanethol sulphonate ('Liquoid'), a laboratory anticoagulant often added to blood culture broths for isolating aerobic bacteria, inhibits growth of *S. moniliformis*. In culture, L-phase variants occur spontaneously. These lack a cell wall and are therefore resistant to penicillin. The organism has been cultured from patients' bite wounds, blood, synovial and pericardial fluid, and from abscesses.

EPIDEMIOLOGY

The infection occurs worldwide in two forms. Rat bite fever is caused by bites or scratches by rodents or their predators, or mere contact with these mammals, living or dead. In some countries, 10 per cent of those bitten by wild rats will be infected. Most of those bitten by rats are children of poor families living in urban areas. A rat bite may not be suspected, as many are inflicted while the patient is asleep. Laboratory staff who work with rats are also at special risk. Haverhill fever, named after a town in Massachusetts, follows ingestion of raw milk, food, or water contaminated by rats. An outbreak in a boarding school in England in 1983 affected 304 people, 43 per cent of the school's population, and was attributed to contamination of the water supply by rats.

CLINICAL FEATURES

After an incubation period of usually less than 10 days and often as little as 1 to 3 days, there is a sudden high fever with rigors, vomiting, severe headache, myalgia, and muscle tenderness. Evidence of the bite has usually disappeared by this stage. Seventy-five per cent of patients develop a rash 1 to 8 days later. Discrete erythematous macules, 1 to 4 mm in diameter, appear symmetrically on the lateral and extensor surfaces and over the joints. They are often most marked on the hands and feet (palms and soles), with associated petechiae, but also occur on the face. Papules, vesicles, and pustules with scabs have also been described. About half the patients develop an asymmetrical migratory polyarthralgia or arthritis, usually involving the knees, ankles, elbows, shoulders, and hips, and often associated with effusions. Joint pains may be the dominant symptom in patients with rat bite fever. Diarrhoea and loss of weight are described in young children. Fever and other symptoms subside in a few days in treated cases, but fever may persist for 1 to 2 weeks, or relapse over several months, and arthritis for many months in those untreated. Severe infections can lead to bronchitis, pneumonia, metastatic abscess formation (including cerebral abscess), myocarditis, pericarditis with effusion, subacute glomerulonephritis, interstitial nephritis, splenitis or splenic abscess, amnionitis, and anaemia. Infective endocarditis, usually with underlying rheumatic or other valve disease, has been described in 17 cases.

Haverhill fever (erythema arthriticum epidemicum) follows a similar clinical course after the patient has drunk unpasteurized milk or contaminated water. Vomiting, stomatitis, and upper respiratory-tract symptoms such as sore throat are said to be more prominent than in rat bite fever.

DIAGNOSIS

Unlike *Spirillum minus* infection (*sodoku*), the incubation period is short, the bite wound heals permanently with little local lymphadenopathy, the rash is morbilliform or petechial, and arthritis is common.

The diagnosis can be confirmed by culturing the organism from blood, joint fluid, or pus. In patients with infective endocarditis the differential diagnosis of the slow-growing micro-aerophilic organism will include *Haemophilus aphrophilus* (Chapter 15.17), *Cardiobacterium hominis*, *Actinomyces actinomycetencomitans*, and *Eikenella corrodens*. A high or rising titre of agglutinins and complement-fixing or fluorescent antibodies may be detected in 2 to 3 weeks. A peripheral leucocytosis of 10 000 to 30 000/μl is usual and false-positive serological tests for syphilis are found in 15 to 25 per cent of cases.

TREATMENT

S. moniliformis is sensitive to penicillin and can be treated with procaine benzylpenicillin (adult dose, 600 mg or 600 000 units) by intramuscular injection 12-hourly for 7 to 14 days, or by penicillin V, 2 g a day by mouth. Penicillin-resistant L-variants are susceptible to streptomycin, tetracycline, and probably erythromycin. For patients hypersensitive to penicillin, erythromycin, chloramphenicol, tetracycline or cephalosporins can be used. Erythromycin was used successfully in the boarding-school outbreak of Haverhill fever in England in 1983.

Patients with endocarditis should be treated with intravenous benzylpenicillin, 4.8 to 14.4 g (8 000 000–24 000 000 units) each day for 4 to 6 weeks, or procaine benzylpenicillin, 4.8 mega units daily by intramuscular injection for 4 weeks if the cultured organism has a sensitivity of 0.1 μg/ml. Addition of streptomycin improves bactericidal activity and eliminates L-forms.

PROGNOSIS

The untreated mortality was 10 to 13 per cent. Overall mortality in patients with endocarditis has been 53 per cent. Residual arthralgia, persisting for as long as 10 years, has been described.

Spirillum minus *infection* (sodoku, sokosha)

Spirillum minus was formerly known as *Spirochaeta* or *Spirillum morsus muris* and *Spirillum minor*. It may be found in the blood of up to 25 per cent of apparently healthy rodents and in eye discharge and mouths of rats with interstitial keratitis and conjunctivitis. *S. minus* is a relatively thick, tightly coiled, Gram-negative spirillum (not a spirochaete), 2.5 to 5.0 μm long, with two to six (commonly three) spirals, resembling campylobacters. It darts about under the power of its terminal flagella. Continuous culture on artificial media has not been achieved, but the organism can be demonstrated by inoculating material from the bite wound, regional lymph nodes, or blood intraperitoneally into mice or guinea-pigs. Organisms usually appear in the rodent's blood within 5 to 15 days of inoculation.

EPIDEMIOLOGY

Sodoku is found worldwide but is particularly common in Japan. It results from bites, scratches or mere contact with rodents or their predators including dogs, cats, and pigs.

CLINICAL FEATURES

The initial bite wound usually heals without signs of local inflammation. After an incubation period of 5 to 30 days, usually 7 days or more, there is sudden fever, which, in untreated cases, reaches its height in 3 days and resolves by crisis after a further 3 days. Other acute symptoms include rigors, myalgia, and prostration. At the start of the illness the healed bite wound becomes inflamed and swollen; it may break down to become necrotic or suppurative. Regional lymph nodes are usually enlarged and tender. The exanthem often starts at the site of the bite and spreads from there. It consists of angry, purplish or reddish-brown, indurated papules, plaques or macules with urticarial lesions. Arthralgia may be severe but there are no joint effusions. Severe manifestations including meningitis, cerebral abscess, encephalitis, endocarditis, myocarditis, myocardial abscess, pleural effusion, chorioamnionitis, subcutaneous abscesses, and involvement of liver, kidney, and other organs are seen in about 10 per cent of cases. Relapses of fever, rash, and other symptoms lasting 3 to 6 days may occur between remissions of a week or so for 2 to 4 months and occasionally up to a year in untreated patients.

DIAGNOSIS

Clinically, *sodoku* is distinguishable from streptobacillary rat-bite fever by its longer incubation period, by the marked reaction at the bite site with local lymphadenopathy at the start of symptoms, by the different rash (dark papular rather than morbilliform and petechial), and by the rarity of arthritis. The diagnosis can be confirmed by examining aspirate from the bite wound, lymph nodes, exanthem or blood by dark-field microscopy or by staining with Wright's or Giemsa stain. Spirochaetes can be detected in the blood, peritoneal fluid or heart muscle of inoculated rodents but cannot be cultured on artificial media. No specific serological tests are available. False-positive serological tests for syphilis are found in 50 to 60 per cent of cases and reactions with Proteus OXK are also common.

DIFFERENTIAL DIAGNOSIS OF RAT BITE FEVERS

An acute, severe, febrile illness following a rat bite, or other contact with rodents or their predators, should raise the possibility of other rodent-related infections such as *Pasteurella multocida*, which produces local pain and erythema within a few hours of the bite, plague, tularaemia, leptospirosis, murine typhus and arenaviruses such as lymphocytic choriomeningitis and, in Africa, Lassa viruses. In the cases where rodent contact is unlikely the differential diagnosis is broadened to include other rickettsial diseases such as Rocky Mountain spotted fever, meningococcaemia, erythema multiforme, and chlamydial and viral (especially coxsackie) infections. Ingestion of raw milk should also raise the possibility of brucellosis.

TREATMENT

Penicillin is the drug of choice. For adults, procaine benzylpenicillin, 600 mg (600 000 units), should be given 12-hourly for 7 to 14 days. Penicillin V, 2 g/day by mouth, is also said to be effective. A Jarisch–Herxheimer reaction complicated treatment with arsenicals in the old days and may also follow penicillin treatment.

PROGNOSIS

Untreated mortality is about 2 to 10 per cent.

Prevention of rat bite fevers

These infections can be prevented by rodent control, by encouraging laboratory workers to wear gloves and use correct techniques when handling rodents, to clean all rodent bite wounds, and to take prophylactic penicillin when bitten. Haverhill fever is prevented by avoiding consumption of raw milk, by monitoring water supplies, especially those not derived from the mains, and by controlling rat populations.

REFERENCES

Brown, R.McP. and Nunemaker, J.C. (1942). Rat-bite fever. A review of the American cases with reevaluation of etiology; report of caes. *Bulletin of the Johns Hopkins Hospital*, **70,** 201–327.

Lambe, D.W., McPhedran, A.M., Mertz, J.A., and Stewart, P. (1973). *Streptobacillus moniliformis* isolated from a case of Haverhill Fever: biochemical characterisation and inhibitory effect of sodium polyanethol sulfonate. *American Journal of Clinical Pathology*, **60,** 854–60.

McEvoy, M.B., Noah, N.D., and Pilsworth, R. (1987). Outbreak of fever caused by *Streptobacillus moniliformis*. *Lancet*, **ii,** 1361–3.

Parker, F. and Hudson, N.P. (1926). The etiology of Haverhill fever (erythema arthriticum epidemicum). *American Journal of Pathology*, **2,** 357–79.

Raffin, B.J. and Freemark, M. (1979). Streptobacillary rat bite fever: a pediatric problem. *Pediatrics*, **64,** 214–17.

Roughgarden, J.W. (1965). Antimicrobial therapy of rat bite fever: a review. *Archives of Internal Medicine*, **116,** 39–54.

Rupp, M.E. (1992). *Streptobacillus moniliformis* endocarditis: case report and review. *Clinics in Infectious Diseases*, **14,** 769–72.

Spirochaetes

7.11.30 Lyme disease

W. BURGDORFER and T. G. SCHWAN

Definition

Lyme disease is a tick-borne spirochaetosis with clinical manifestations in several organ systems, such as the skin, joints, central nervous system, and heart. It is caused by *Borrelia burgdorferi*, a recently discovered spirochaete associated with various tick vectors, primarily those of the *Ixodes ricinus–I. persulcatus* complex. Although other blood-sucking arthropods such as mosquitoes, deer flies, and fleas have proved capable of mechanical transmission, there is no evidence that these are of importance in the epidemiology of this disease.

Lyme disease was first described in 1977 as a new clinical entity following investigations of outbreaks of arthritis among children and adults in East Haddam, Lyme, and Old Lyme in Connecticut, United States. Although 13 of 51 patients had the characteristic erythema chronicum migrans preceding arthritis, the disease was considered to be distinct from previously reported cases with erythema chronicum migrans in Wisconsin and Connecticut, and from those in Europe where, since the beginning of the century, erythema migrans had been reported to be associated with the ixodid tick, *I. ricinus*.

The recent discovery of *B. burgdorferi* as the causative agent of Lyme disease in the United States and the detection in *I. ricinus* of spirochaetes indistinguishable from the Lyme disease agent have led to investigations that not only confirmed the spirochaetal aetiology of European erythema migrans but also showed that this entity, like Lyme disease, represents a complex syndrome with the diagnostic skin lesion often followed by neurological, arthritic, and even cardiac complications. Lymphocytic meningoradiculitis (Bannwarth's syndrome), acrodermatitis chronica atrophicans, and lymphocytoma (lymphadenitis benigna cutis) are now known to be associated with erythema migrans. Patients who have recovered from these ailments have been shown to have high titres of antibodies to *B. burgdorferi*. Spirochaetes similar, if not identical, to this agent have been recovered from the spinal fluid of a patient suffering from lymphocytic meningoradiculitis and from the skin lesion of a patient with acrodermatitis chronica atrophicans.

Clinical manifestations

The early disease is usually characterized by an expanding annular skin lesion erythema chronicum migrans (Fig. 1), which may be accompanied by fever, headache, stiff neck, myalgia, arthralgia, malaise, and enlargement of lymph nodes. These early clinical manifestations may last for several weeks and may be followed by recurrent or chronic arthritis and neurological and cardiac sequelae, although not necessarily in that order. Patients may experience a mild disease with erythema migrans but without other manifestations; or they may show skin, nerve, heart, and joint involvement at the same time; others lack the annular skin lesions.

Maternal–fetal transmission of the Lyme disease spirochaete has been documented in a woman who contracted Lyme disease during the first trimester of pregnancy. The premature child died of congenital heart disease during the first week of life. Although spirochaetes were detected in the infant's spleen, kidney, and bone marrow, an association between the intrauterine infection and the infant's death could not be established. Among another 19 patients with Lyme disease during pregnancy, 14 were completely normal but in the remainder there were cases of intrauterine fetal death, prematurity, and developmental delay with cortical blindness. It is important to diagnose and treat Lyme disease as early as possible during pregnancy.

Development of erythema chronicum migrans is a unique clinical marker. It is characterized by a small, red papule or macule, often considered to be the site of the tick bite, which 3 to 23 days later spreads centrifugally with indurated, usually flat, borders up to 2 cm wide. The centres of early lesions are usually erythematous and indurated, but may also be vesicular or necrotic. As the lesions expand, their centres clear. Common sites for these itching, burning, and painful lesions are the thigh, groin, and axilla. In some patients, secondary annular lesions may appear within several days after onset of the initial lesions; they are generally smaller, less migratory, and lack the indurated centres. During or soon after resolution of the initial and secondary lesions, new lesions may develop in the form of red circles and blotches (2–3 cm in diameter) that do not migrate but may persist for several weeks.

Early signs of nervous involvement are meningeal irritation and attacks of headache, neck pain, and stiffness. After several weeks to months, about 15 per cent of patients develop neurological abnormalities, such as meningitis, cranial nerve lesions such as Bell's palsy, and peripheral radiculoneuropathy.

In Europe, lymphocytic meningoradiculitis (Bannwarth's syndrome) is the most common manifestation of infection of the central nervous system. These manifestations may last for months but usually resolve completely.

Within a few weeks to 2 years after onset of illness, about 60 per cent of patients develop brief (a few weeks to months) but recurrent attacks of mono- or oligoarticular arthritis in the form of migratory musculoskeletal pains in joints, tendons, bursae, muscles, or bone. Arthritis with joint swelling usually begins months after onset and is characterized by intermittent attacks of swelling and pain, especially in the knee. Large and small joints may become affected, with a few patients showing symmetrical polyarthritis. In about 10 per cent of patients, involvement of large joints becomes chronic and leads to the erosion of cartilage and bone.

From as early as 4 days to 3 months after onset, about 10 per cent of patients experience fluctuating degrees of atrioventricular block and acute myopericarditis, ventricular dysfunction, and cardiomegaly. Usually preceded by erythema chronicum migrans, these cardiac complications may be accompanied by neurological manifestations, such as meningoencephalitis, cranial as well as peripheral neuropathy, and arthritis. Accompanying symptoms include syncope or dizziness, shortness of breath, and substernal chest pain lasting from 3 days to about 6 weeks.

The aetiological agent

The causative agent of erythema migrans in Europe and of Lyme disease in the United States, although long suspected to be bacterial, possibly spirochaetal, remained elusive until 1981. Then, during a survey of rickettsiae in the ixodid tick, *I. scapularis* (= *I. dammini*) (Fig. 2) from Shelter Island, New York, a spirochaete was discovered that reacted strongly in the indirect immunofluorescence test with convalescent sera from patients with Lyme disease. Of 126 adult *I. scapularis*, 77, (61 per cent) were infected with spirochaetes that could readily be isolated in modified Kelly's medium, a medium suitable for culturing certain relapsing-fever spirochaetes. Similar spirochaetes were subsequently discovered in the European tick vector, *I. ricinus*.

That these micro-organisms cause Lyme disease and erythema migrans has since been confirmed serologically as well by their recovery from blood, cerebrospinal fluid, myocardium, and skin lesions of patients.

Investigations into the genetic and phenotypic characteristics of Lyme disease spirochetes have shown that these micro-organisms represent a new species, *Borrelia burgdorferi*. Recent work by some European investigators has shown that genetic differences among the Lyme disease spirochaetes warrants the distinction of three genomic groups or species, currently designated as *B. burgdorferi sensu stricto*, *B. garinii*, and *B. afzelii*. The current nomenclature for these spirochaetes is not entirely satisfactory and will probably undergo further changes in the near future.

B. burgdorferi is a helical bacterium, 0.18 to 0.25 × 4 to 30 μm (Fig. 3a). An outer membrane surrounds the protoplasmic cylinder consisting of the peptidoglycan layer, cytoplasmic membrane, and the enclosed cytoplasmic contents. Seven periplasmic flagella (axial filaments or axial fibrils) are attached subterminally at each end in a row parallel to the organisms's long axis and overlap at the central region of the cell (Fig. 3(b)). These flagella are responsible for the organism's rotational and translational movements, which provide motility. *B. burgdorferi*, which stains moderately well with Giemsa, uses carbohydrates such as glucose as sources of energy and carbon. Like certain tick-borne spirochaetes of relapsing fever, it grows well in modified Kelly's medium (also referred to as BSK-II medium) between 34 and 37 °C and has a generation time of 11 to 12 h at 35 °C.

Geographical distribution

Human cases of Lyme disease have been reported in most of the 48 contiguous United States. However, most have been reported from three geographical areas: the north-east and midwest, where *I. scapularis* is the principal vector; and the west where *I. pacificus* carries the spirochaete. Between 1975 and 1979, a total of 512 cases of Lyme disease were diagnosed. Of these, 503 occurred in north-eastern, 5 in midwest-

Fig. 1 Typical erythema migrans lesion on the arm of a Lyme disease patient.

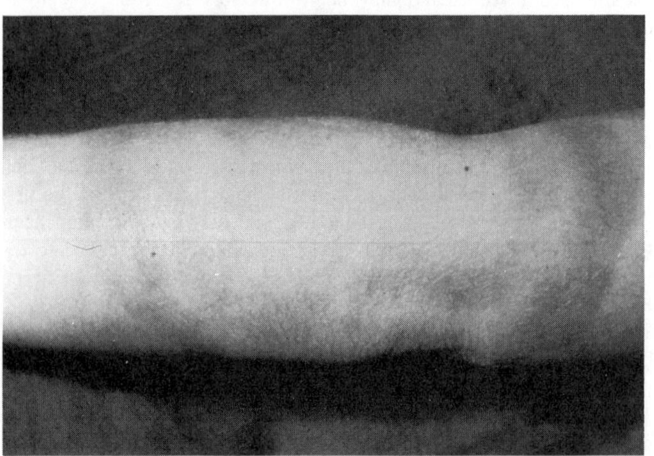

Fig. 2 *Ixodes scapularis*. Female on the left, male on the right (× 15).

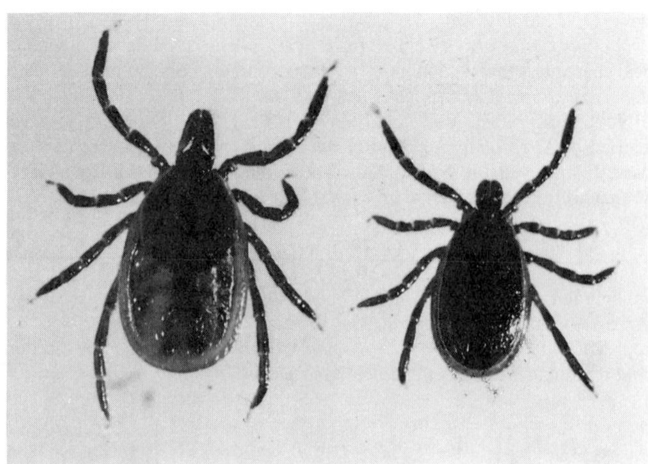

ern, and 4 in western states. In 1980, 226 cases of Lyme disease came to the attention of the Centers for Disease Control in Atlanta. In 1982, after the discovery of the causative agent of Lyme disease, surveillance was intensified and it has become a reportable disease. Since then, the number of reported cases in the United States has increased, and from 1982 to 1992, 50 000 human cases were reported with the highest incidence in Connecticut, New York, Rhode Island, and New Jersey.

In Europe, Lyme disease and related disorders have been reported from practically all countries within the distributional area of *I. ricinus*, which includes Scandinavia, middle, eastern, and most of southern Europe. Although hundreds of cases are recorded in the European literature, their distribution and total numbers have not been reviewed. Cases have also been reported from England where *I. ricinus* is abundant, and from Australia where the arthropod vector has not yet been identified. Lyme disease spirochaetes have been isolated from *I. persulcatus* ticks in several parts of Asia, including Russia, China, Japan, and Korea, although the number of human cases from these areas is not known.

Epidemiology

The prevalence of infected ticks varies. On Shelter Island, New York, the source of the first isolate of *B. burgdorferi*, up to 100 per cent of *I. scapularis* (= *I. dammini*) were found to carry spirochaetes. In California, on the other hand, not more than 2 per cent of *I. pacificus* were infected, and in Switzerland, up to 36 per cent of *I. ricinus* harboured spirochaetes. Spirochaetes indistinguishable from *B. burgdorferi* have also been detected in *Amblyomma americanum*, *Dermacentor variabilis*, *Rhipicephalus sanguineus*, and *Haemaphysalis leporispalustris*.

Mammalian reservoirs for the spirochaete are also suitable hosts for the immature stages of the ticks that also transmit spirochaetes to man. Throughout the north-east and northern midwest United States, white-footed mice, *Peromyscus leucopus*, serve both as hosts for Ixodes ticks and sources of spirochaetes. In California, woodrats (Neotoma) and kangaroo rats (Dipodomys) maintain the spirochaete in enzootic cycles with the tick *I. neotomae*; however, most people are probably infected when bitten by infective *I. pacificus*. In Europe and Asia, little is known about the rodent reservoirs for Lyme spirochaetes; however, the genera Clethrionomys and Apodemus appear to be good candidates and hosts for immature *I. ricinus* and *I. persulcatus*.

Fig. 3 (a) Scanning electron micrograph of *B. burgdorferi* associated with midgut epithelium of infected tick (scale bar: 1.0 μm). (b) Transmission electron micrograph of *B. burgdorferi*. Inset represents a cross-section with arrows pointing towards flagella (scale bar: 0.2 μm; scale bar in inset: 0.2 μm). (By Mr S. F. Hayes, Rocky Mountain Laboratories.)

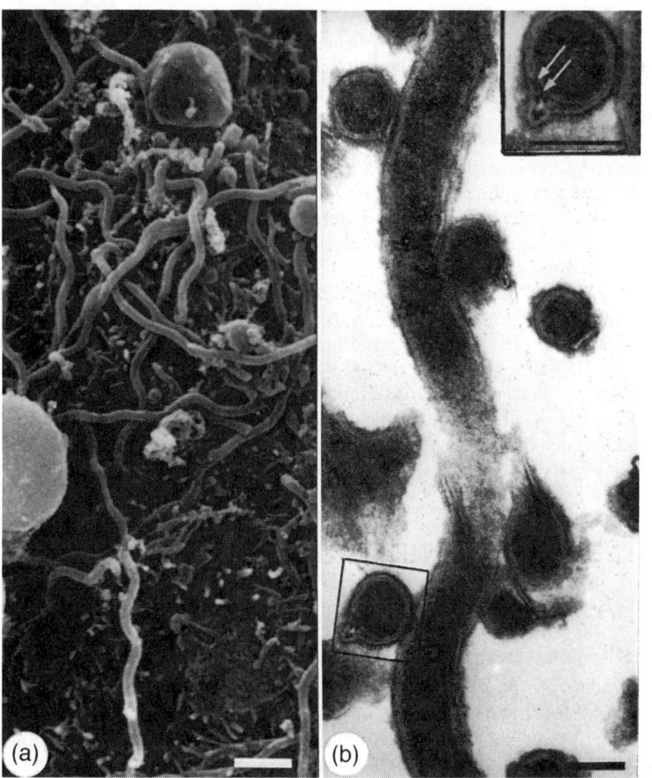

In the United States as well as in Europe, domestic dogs may be heavily infested with tick vectors and represent important means by which ticks are brought into the immediate environment of man. Dogs are also susceptible to *B. burgdorferi* and suffer intermittent, oligoarticular arthritis similar to that in human Lyme disease.

Little is known about the development of *B. burgdorferi* in ticks and the mechanisms by which this spirochaete is transmitted to host animals and to man. In most ticks, development of the spirochaete is confined to the midgut, where the organisms are closely associated with the microvillous brush border whence they invade the intercellular spaces of the gut lining. In a few ticks, the spirochaetes seem to be capable of penetrating the gut epithelium and then by way of the haemocele they invade various tissues, particularly the central ganglion. Ticks with a generalized infection undoubtedly transmit disease spirochaetes via saliva. They have also proved capable of passing spirochaetes transovarially, but this occurs very infrequently and infected small mammals are necessary to maintain the spirochaetes in nature and infect new generations of ticks. There is also evidence that the distribution of spirochaetal infection in filial ticks decreases and becomes limited to the central ganglion as the ticks develop to nymphs and adults. Although still unproved, transmission of *B. burgdorferi* probably occurs also by regurgitation of spirochaete-containing gut content.

Diagnosis

Currently, a diagnosis of Lyme disease is based primarily on the clinical picture, especially if it includes the development of lesions following tick bite and exposure in an area where the disease is endemic. Histological demonstration of silver-stained spirochaetes in skin biopsy specimens, and cultivation of the organisms from blood, cerebrospinal fluid, and skin also are useful diagnostic methods but of low sensitivity and seldom used in clinical laboratories. In the absence of erythema chronicum migrans, the diagnosis may be confirmed serologically by the indirect immunofluorescence or enzyme immunoassay with cultured spirochaetes. Because of the close relationship of *B. burgdorferi* to other spirochaetes, particularly those causing relapsing fever and syphilis, cross-reactions do occur leading to false-positive serological tests when using whole spirochaetes for the antigen in the test. Patients who are treated early in the illness with appropriate antibiotics may not develop a detectable serological response to *B. burgdorferi*. Intrathecal synthesis of specific IgG antibodies to *B. burgdorferi* has been demonstrated in patients with lymphocytic meningoradiculitis. Detection of these antibodies may be helpful in diagnosing infection of the central nervous system. The polymerase chain reaction offers the potential for detecting a very small number of spirochaetes in clinical samples, but many practical problems with this assay make it unlikely to become widely used in the clinical laboratory in the immediate future. Recombinant DNA technology has also been used to clone and express specific, individual proteins of the Lyme disease spirochaete to be used in serological assays with greater specificity.

Treatment

Antimicrobials are effective but dosage and duration of course are not yet agreed upon for more chronic forms of the disease. For early disease (skin lesions), treatment with oral tetracycline, 250 mg four times a day for at least 10 days and again for up to 20 days if symptoms persist and recur, is recommended. In children, phenoxymethylpenicillin, 50 mg/kg body weight per day (not less than 1 g/day or more than 2 g/day) in divided doses for the same duration is effective. Erythromycin, 30 mg/kg body weight per day in divided doses for 15 to 20 days, should be given to patients who are allergic to penicillin. High-dose intravenous benzylpenicillin, 20 million units a day in divided doses, or ceftriaxone, are recommended for the treatment of neurological abnormalities. However, despite this therapy, patients may continue to have frequent arthralgias and musculoskeletal pain. One placebo-controlled double-blind trial indicated that intramuscular benzathine penicillin (2.4 million units weekly for 3 weeks) was effective for established arthritis. Intravenous benzylpenicillin, 20 million units a day in divided doses for 10 days, also cured some patients. Intra-articular corticosteroids should be avoided. Regardless of the antibiotic given for Lyme disease, recurrent episodes of headache, or pain in joints, tendons, bursae, or muscles occur in about half of the patients. For some cases, treatment failure suggests that an alternative diagnosis should be considered.

Vaccines

Immunization with a whole-cell vaccine of inactivated *B. burgdorferi* that protected against experimental infection in Syrian hamsters has led to the commercial development of a vaccine for dogs. A recombinant vaccine prepared from the spirochaetes's outer-surface protein A (OspA) is being evaluated for human use.

REFERENCES

Ackermann, R. *et al.* (1984). Spirochäten-Aetiologie der Erythema-chronicum-migrans Krankheit. *Deutsche Medizin Wochenschrift*, **109**, 92–7.

Afzelius, A. (1921). Erythema chronicum migrans. *Acta Dermato-Venereologia*, **2**, 120–5.

Anderson, J.F. and Magnarelli, L.A. (1984). Avian and mammalian hosts for spirochete-infected ticks and insects in a Lyme disease focus in Connecticut. *Yale Journal of Biology and Medicine*, **57**, 627–41.

Anderson, J.F., Magnarelli, L.A., Burgdorfer, W., and Barbour, A.G. (1983). Spirochetes in *Ixodes dammini* and mammals from Connecticut. *American Journal of Tropical Medicine and Hygiene*, **32**, 818–24.

Åsbrink, E., Hederstedt, B., and Hovmark, A. (1984). The spirochetal etiology of Acrodermatitis chronica atrophicans, Herxheimer. *Acta Dermato-Venerologica*, **64**, 506–12.

Barbour, A.G. (1984). Isolation and cultivation of Lyme disease spirochetes. *Yale Journal of Biology and Medicine*, **57**, 521–5.

Bosler, E.M., *et al.* (1983). Natural distribution of the *Ixodes dammini* spirochete. *Science*, **220**, 321–2.

Brown, R.N. and Lane, R.S. (1992). Lyme disease in California: a novel enzootic transmission cycle of *Borrelia burgdorferi*. *Science*, **256**, 1439–42.

Burgdorfer, W., Barbour, A.G., Hayes, S.F., Benach, J.L., Grunwaldt, E., and Davis, J.P. (1982). Lyme disease—a tick-borne spirochetosis? *Science*, **216**, 1317–19.

Burgdorfer, W., Barbour, A.G., Hayes, S.F., Péter, O., and Aeschlimann, A. (1983). Erythema chronicum migrans—a tick-borne spirochetosis. *Acta Tropica*, **40**, 79–83.

Burgdorfer, W., Lane, R.S., Barbour, A.G., Gresbrink, R.A., and Anderson, J.R. (1985). The Western black-legged tick, *Ixodes pacificus*: a vector of *Borrelia burgdorferi*. *American Journal of Tropical Medicine and Hygiene*, **34**, 496–7.

Centers for Disease Control (1985). Update: Lyme disease and cases occurring during pregnancy. *Morbidity and Mortality Weekly Reports*, **34**, 375–84.

Johnson, R.C., Kodner, C., and Russell, M. (1986). Active immunization of hamsters against experimental infection with the Lyme disease spirochete. *Infection and Immunity*, **54**, 897–8.

Kohls, G.M., Hoogstraal, H., and Clifford, C.M. (1961). Observations on the subgenus *Argas* (Ixodoidea, Argasidae, *Argas*). 5. Study of *A. brevipes* Banks, 1908, from birds in Arizona and California, U.S.A., and Baja California, Mexico. *Annals of the Entomological Society of America*, **54**, 869–77.

Kornblatt, A.N., Urband, P.H., and Steere, A.C. (1985). Arthritis caused by *Borrelia burgdorferi* in dogs. *Journal of the American Veterinary Medical Association*, **186**, 960–4.

Muhlemann, M.F. (1984). Thirteen British cases of erythema chronicum migrans, a spirochaetal disease. *British Journal of Dermatology*, **111**, 335–9.

Pfister, H.W., Einhäupl, K., Preac-Mursic, V., Wilske, B., and Schierz, G. (1984). The spirochetal etiology of lymphocytic meningoradiculitis of Bannwarth (Bannwarth's syndrome). *Journal of Neurology*, **231**, 141–4.

Rosa, P.A., and Schwan, T.G. (1989). A specific and sensitive assay for the Lyme disease spirochete, *Borrelia burgdorferi*, using the polymerase chain reaction. *Journal of Infectious Diseases*, **160**, 1018–29.

Rosa, P.A., Hogan, D., and Schwan, T.G. (1991). Polymerase chain reaction analyses identify two distinct classes of *Borrelia burgdorferi*. *Journal of Clinical Microbiology*, **29**, 524–32.

Russell, H., Sampson, J.S., Smith, G.P., Wilkinson, H.W., and Plikaytis, B. (1984). Enzyme-linked immunosorbent assay and indirect immunofluorescence assay for Lyme disease. *Journal of Infectious Diseases*, **149**, 465–70.

Schlesinger, P.A., Duray, P.H., Burke, B.A., Steere, A.C., and Stillman, T. (1985). Maternal-fetal transmission of the Lyme disease spirochete, *Borrelia burgdorferi*. *Annals of Internal Medicine*, **103**, 67–8.

Schulze, T.L. *et al.* (1984). *Amblyomma americanum*: a potential vector of Lyme disease in New Jersey. *Science*, **224**, 601–3.

Simpson, W.J., Burgdorfer, W., Schrumpf, M.E., Karstens, R.H., and Schwan, T.G. (1991). Antibody to a 39 kDa *Borrelia burgdorferi* antigen (P39) as a marker for infection in experimentally and naturally inoculated animals. *Journal of Clinical Microbiology*, **29**, 236–43.

Simpson, W.J., Schrumpf, M.E., and Schwan, T.G. (1990). Reactivity of human Lyme borreliosis sera with a 39-kilodalton antigen specific to *Borrelia burgdorferi*. *Journal of Clinical Microbiology*, **28**, 1329–37.

Stanek, G., Wewalka, G., Groh, V., Neumann, R., and Kristoferitsch, W. (1985). Differences between Lyme disease and European arthropod-borne borrelia infections. *Lancet*, **i**, 401.

Steere, A.C. and Malawista, S.E. (1979). Cases of Lyme disease in the United States: locations correlated with distribution of *Ixodes dammini*. *Annals of Internal Medicine*, **91**, 730–3.

Steere, A.C., Pachner, A.R., and Malawista, S.E. (1983). Neurologic abnormalities of Lyme disease: successful treatment with high-dose intravenous penicillin. *Annals of Internal Medicine*, **99**, 767–72.

Steere, A.C. *et al.* (1983). The spirochetal etiology of Lyme disease. *New England Journal of Medicine*, **308**, 733–40.

Steere, A.C. *et al.* (1984). The clinical spectrum and treatment of Lyme disease. *Yale Journal of Biology and Medicine*, **57**, 453–61.

Steere, A.C. *et al.* (1985). Successful parenteral penicillin therapy of established Lyme arthritis. *New England Journal of Medicine*, **312**, 864–74.

Weber, K., Schierz, G., Wilske, B., and Preac-Mursic, V. (1984). European erythema migrans disease and related disorders. *Yale Journal of Biology and Medicine*, **57**, 463–71.

Wilske, B. and Schierz, G. (1986). Intrathecal production of specific antibodies against *Borrelia burgdorferi* in patients with lymphocytic meningoradiculitis (Bannwarth's syndrome). *Journal of Infectious Diseases*, **153**, 304–14.

Wilske, B., Schierz, G., Preac-Mursic, V., Weber, K., Pfister, H.W., and Einhäupl, K. (1984). Serological diagnosis of erythema migrans disease and related disorders. *Infection*, **12**, 331–7.

7.11.31 Other Borrelia infections

D. A. WARRELL

The borreliae are large, loosely coiled, motile spirochaetes. *Borrelia recurrentis* is the cause of louse-borne relapsing fever, while tick-borne relapsing fever is caused by *B. duttoni* and a number of other species or groups of Borrelia. The recently discovered *B. burgdorferi* is the cause of Lyme disease. *B. vincenti*, now renamed *Treponema vincentii*, has, with *Fusobacterium* (*Bacteroides*) *fusiforme*, been implicated in acute necrotizing ulcerative gingivitis and Vincent's angina but it is now regarded as part of the normal flora of the mouth.

Relapsing fevers

The borreliae that cause relapsing fevers are spirochaetes 8 to 20 μm long and 0.2 to 0.6 μm thick, with 3 to 15 coils and 15 to 30 axial filaments or flagella in some strains. These motile organisms divide by transverse binary fission. They can be stained in blood films (Fig. 1) by a wide variety of routine methods including Giemsa, Leishman, and Romanovsky stains; Wright's stain is rapid and convenient. Dark-ground examination and the acridine orange fluorescent (QBC®) method can also be used. Several species of Borrelia including *B. recurrentis* have now been cultured in Kelly's BSKII artificial media. Borrelia can also be cultured on chick chorioallantoic membrane and perpetuated in rodents and ticks. Plasmid DNA has been detected in at least three Borrelia species.

EPIDEMIOLOGY

Louse-borne (epidemic) relapsing fever

The human body louse, *Pedunculus humanus corporis*, and to a lesser extent the head louse (*P.h. capitis*) are the sole vectors, which become infected while feeding on blood from a human patient. The louse's infected haemolymph may be inoculated through the skin when it is crushed by scratching, but spirochaetes can also penetrate intact skin: in this way a new infection can arise. Lice move from person to person when there is crowding and poor hygiene. When the host's surface body temperature deviates far from 37°C, as a result of death, fever, or exposure, or if infested clothing is discarded, the louse is forced to find a new host. The chaos of war, famine, and other disasters favours the spread of lice and epidemic louse-borne infections such as relapsing fever and typhus. The yellow plague in Europe in AD 550 and the famine fevers of the seventeenth and eighteenth centuries were probably relapsing fever. During the first half of the twentieth century it is estimated that there were at least 50 million cases, with a 10 per cent mortality. Epidemics occurred in Europe, the Middle East, and the northern third of Africa, starting in 1903, 1923, and 1943. The major endemic focus of the disease persists in the highlands of Ethiopia, where there is an annual epidemic coinciding with the cool, rainy season when people are forced to wear lice-infested clothes and crowd together into shelters. An annual incidence of 10 000 cases in Ethiopia seems likely. Recent outbreaks have occurred in the Sudan, Somalia, West Africa, and Vietnam.

Fig. 1 *Borrelia recurrentis* spirochaetes in a Giemsa-stained, thin blood film from a patient with louse-borne relapsing fever. (Copyright D. A. Warrell.)

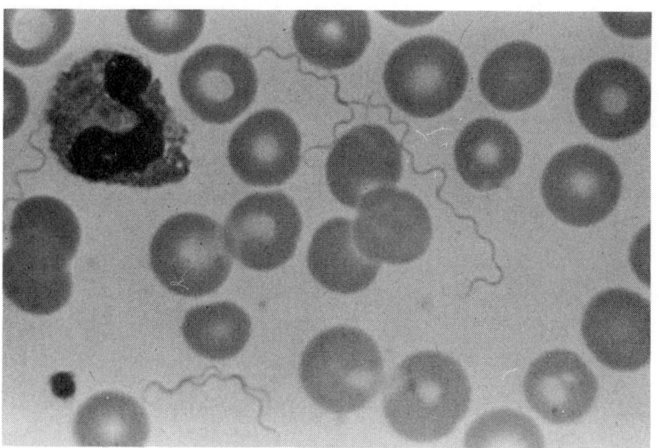

Other endemic foci may exist in the Balkans, the Peruvian and Bolivian Andes, and China. There is no known animal reservoir. Between epidemics, the infection persists in man in mild or asymptomatic form.

Tick-borne (endemic) relapsing fever

There is a close, but not exclusive, relationship between the species of Borrelia, their soft (argasid) tick vectors and reservoirs (genus Ornithodoros), and mammal reservoir species. For example, in East and Central Africa, the domestic tick *O. moubata* transmits *B. duttoni* between humans; there is no known animal reservoir. In western North Africa and the Middle East, however, various small rodents have burrows in or near human dwellings, and borreliae of the Crocidurae group may be transmitted to man by the rodent tick *Alectrobius sonrai* (formerly *O. erraticus sonrai*). In the western United States, *O. hermsi*, a parasite of chipmunks and other tree squirrels, transmits *B. hermsii* to man, especially to individuals who sleep in tick-infested log cabins near the Grand Canyon, Arizona. Other important borreliae causing tick-borne relapsing fever (and their tick vectors) include: *B. hispanica* (*A. sonrai*) in Africa; *B. persica* (*O. tholozani*) in the Middle East; *B. venezuelensis* (*O. venezuelensis*) in Central and South America; and *B. turicatae* (*O. turicatae*), *B. parkeri* (*O. parkeri*), and *B. mazzotti* (*O. mazzotti*) in North America. When night-feeding ticks have access to man, tick-borne relapsing fever may result.

Tick-borne relapsing fever has occurred in most continents except Australasia and the Pacific region. It is particularly common in West Africa, where a recent survey revealed a prevalence of 1 per cent among children (in western Senegal). At one health centre in Rwanda, 1650 proven cases are treated each year (6 per cent of all patients). In North America, cases are usually isolated and sporadic but in 1968, 11 out of a group of 42 boy scouts were infected on Browne Mountain, Washington, while camping in rodent-infested cabins, and in 1973 there were 62 cases among people staying in the log cabins along the north rim of the Grand Canyon. Two hundred and eighty cases of tick-borne relapsing fever have been identified in the United States during the past 25 years. In Colorado the incidence is increasing (23 confirmed cases since 1977). In Jordan, from 1959 to 1969, there were 723 cases of tick-borne relapsing fever, with four deaths.

Spirochaetes enter the tick in its blood meal from infected humans or animals. Unlike *B. recurrentis*, they invade the tick's salivary and coccal glands, and genital apparatus, and so can be transmitted when the tick feeds on a new host and transovarially to the tick's progeny. Thus ticks are reservoirs of borreliae while lice are not. Ticks infest the burrows, caves, tree stumps, and roughly built shacks that shelter their mammal hosts—rodents, insectivores, lagomorphs, bats, and small carnivores. In Western countries, tick-borne relapsing fever may occasionally be diagnosed in travellers, in intravenous drug abusers, and in recipients of blood transfusions.

PATHOPHYSIOLOGY

The physiological changes during the spontaneous crisis and the Jarisch–Herxheimer reaction induced by antimicrobial treatment in louse-borne relapsing fever are typical of an 'endotoxin reaction'. Although endotoxin or endotoxin-like activity has been described for other spirochaetes: *B. burgdorferi*, *Treponema hyodysenteriae*, *B. vincenti* and *B. buccalis*, and *Leptospira canicola*, it has not been detected consistently in patients nor found by gas–liquid chromatography or Limulus assay in sonicates of *B. recurrentis*, *B. hispanica* or *T. pallidum*. In patients with louse-borne relapsing fever who were treated with procaine penicillin, symptoms of the severe Jarisch–Herxheimer reaction were associated with a transient marked elevation in plasma concentrations of tumour necrosis factor, interleukin 6, and interleukin 8. The stimulus for cytokine release seems to be phagocytosis of spirochaetes made susceptible by the action of penicillin. Benzylpenicillin attaches to penicillin-binding protein I in *B. hermsii* spirochaetes. Large surface blebs are produced and the damaged spirochaetes are phagocytosed rapidly by neutrophils in the blood and by the spleen.

Complement may enhance phagocytosis of spirochaetes, especially in the non-immune host, but the complement system is not essential for elimination of spirochaetes, whether or not specific immunoglobulins are present. *In vitro*, surface contact with spirochaetes induces mononuclear leucocytes to produce pyrogen and thromboplastin, which could be responsible for the fever and disseminated intravascular coagulation in louse-borne relapsing fever. There is some evidence to suggest that kinins are released during the Jarisch–Herxheimer reaction of syphilis and louse-borne relapsing fever. The marked peripheral leucopenia that develops during the reaction is more likely to be the result of sequestration, perhaps in the pulmonary blood vessels, than to destruction of leucocytes. Spirochaetes may be found in the organs that bear the brunt of the infection (liver, spleen, myocardium, and brain), but it is not clear how their pathological effects are produced. The petechial rash results simply from thrombocytopenia and is not a vasculitis. The cardiorespiratory and metabolic disturbances in relapsing fever are principally the result of persistent high fever, dramatically accentuated by the Jarisch–Herxheimer reaction or spontaneous crisis.

IMMUNITY AND THE RELAPSE PHENOMENON

Studies of the relapse phenomenon in mice infected with *B. hermsii* have demonstrated spontaneous variation of protein antigens resulting in a mixed population of up to 26 new serotypes. The mechanism that alters the expression of variable major protein (**VMP**) antigens has been partly elucidated. Extrachromasomal DNA on linear plasmids recombines to activate the genes controlling VMP synthesis. Between attacks, spirochaetaemia may persist, even though it is undetectable by microscopy and is insufficient to produce symptoms. Spirochaetes may retreat to immunologically compromised sites such as the brain and eye. Antibody destroys the population of spirochaetes to which it is specific and selects out antigenic variants, but does not affect the rate of antigenic variation.

PATHOLOGY

Spirochaetes are usually confined to the lumen of blood vessels but tangled masses are also found in the characteristic splenic miliary abscesses (Fig. 2) and infarcts, and within the central nervous system adjacent to haemorrhages. A perivascular, histiocytic, interstitial myocarditis is found in the majority of cases and may be responsible for conduction defects, arrhythmias, and myocardial failure resulting in sudden death. Splenic rupture with massive haemorrhage, cerebral haemorrhage, and hepatic failure are other causes of death. The liver shows hepatitis with patchy mid-zonal haemorrhages and necrosis (Fig. 3). There is meningitis and perisplenitis; most serosal cavities and surfaces of viscera are studded with petechial haemorrhages (Fig. 4). Thrombi are occasionally found occluding small vessels, but the peripheral gangrene sometimes found in patients recovering from louse-borne typhus is not seen.

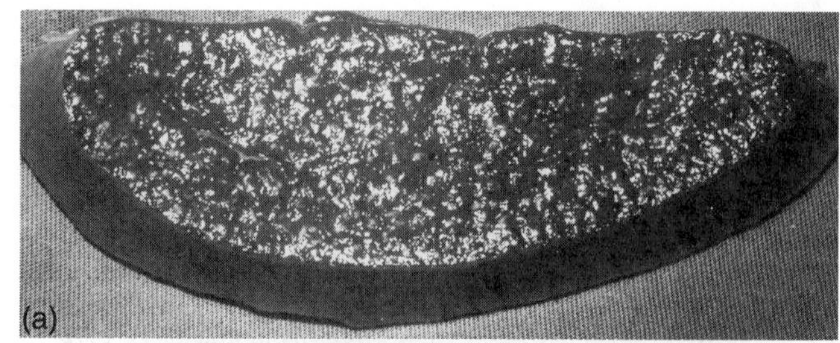

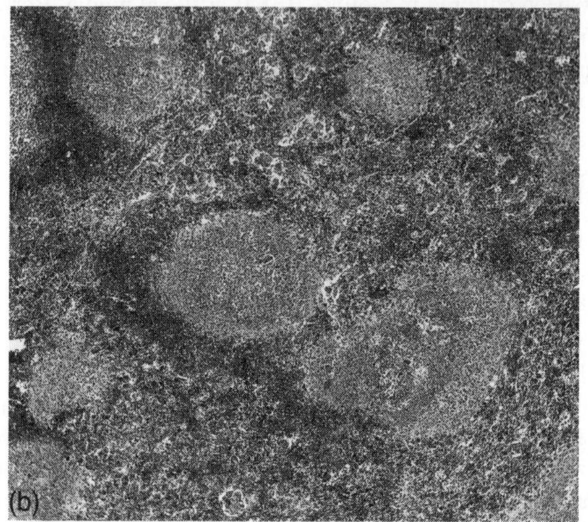

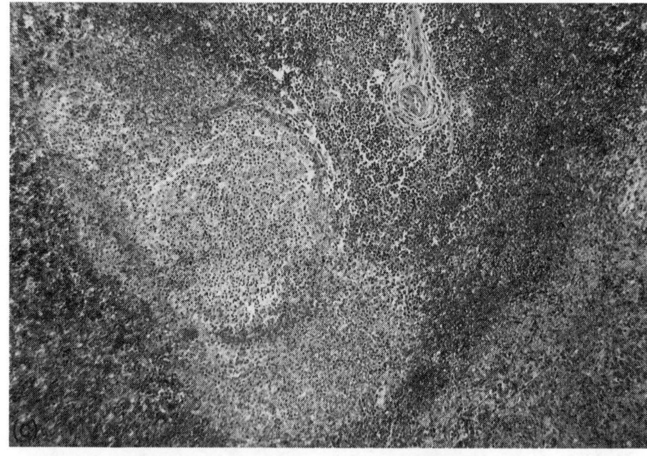

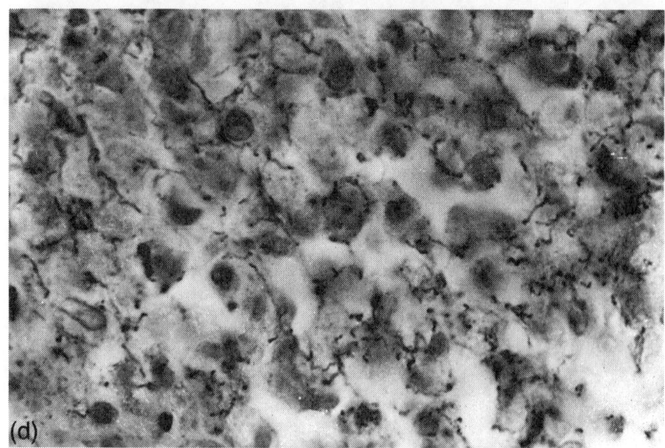

Fig. 2 Splenic miliary abscesses in louse-borne relapsing fever: (a) section of spleen at autopsy (Copyright D. A. Warrell.); (b) miliary microbscesses as seen under the microscope (× 38) (Armed Forces Institute of Pathology photograph, negative number 75-8838); (c) microabscesses involve both follicles and extrafollicular areas of the spleen—the pale area of extrafollicular necrosis is clearly demarcated from the surrounding pulp (× 78) (Armed Forces Institute of Pathology photograph, negative number 77326); (d) Warthin–Starry stain showing tangled masses of spirochaetes at the periphery of an abscess (× 1186) (Armed Forces Institute of Pathology photograph, negative number 77317).

CLINICAL FEATURES

The illness starts suddenly with rigors and a fever that mounts to nearly 40°C in a few days. Early symptoms are headache, dizziness, nightmares, generalized aches and pains often focused in the lower back, knees and elbows, anorexia, nausea, vomiting, and diarrhoea. Later there is upper abdominal pain, cough, and epistaxis. Patients are usually prostrated; most are confused. Hepatic tenderness is the most common sign (about 60 per cent). The liver is palpably enlarged in about half of cases. Splenic tenderness and enlargement are slightly less common. Jaundice has been reported in between 10 and 80 per cent of patients. A petechial or ecchymotic rash is seen in between 10 and 60 per cent; the lesions occur particularly on the trunk (Fig. 5). Other sites of spontaneous bleeding include the nose in 25 per cent, and less commonly the lungs, gastrointestinal tract, conjunctivae (Fig. 6), and retinae. Many patients have tender muscles. Meningism occurs in about 40 per cent of cases; other neurological features include cranial-nerve lesions, monoplegias, flaccid paraplegia, and focal convulsions attributable, perhaps, to cerebral haemorrhages.

Time course and relapses

The incubation period is 4 to 18 (average 7) days. In untreated cases of the louse-borne disease, the first attack of fever resolves by crisis in 4 to 10 (average 5) days whereas in tick-borne disease initial fever lasts only about 3 days. There follows an afebrile remission of 5 to 9 days and then a series of up to five relapses in louse-borne disease and up to 13 in tick-borne disease (Fig. 7). No petechial rash occurs during the relapses, which are generally less severe than the initial attack, but may be associated with iritis or iridocyclitis and severe epistaxis.

Differences between louse-borne and tick-borne relapsing fever

The tick-borne disease is generally milder and less drawn out. The incidence of some symptoms and signs in the two diseases appears strikingly different. For example, in some series of cases, only 7 per cent of patients with tick-borne relapsing fever were jaundiced and neurological signs were more common than in the louse-borne disease.

Severe manifestations

These include myocarditis, which presents as acute pulmonary oedema, liver failure and severe bleeding attributable to thrombocytopenia, liver damage, and disseminated intravascular coagulation. Dysentery, salmonellosis, typhoid, typhus, malaria, and tuberculosis have been described in association with relapsing fever.

Fig. 3 Liver in louse-borne relapsing fever: congestion with prominent Küpffer cells and lymphocytic and neutrophil infiltrate predominantly in the central and mid-zonal areas (× 500) (Armed Forces Institute of Pathology photograph, negative number 75-6523).

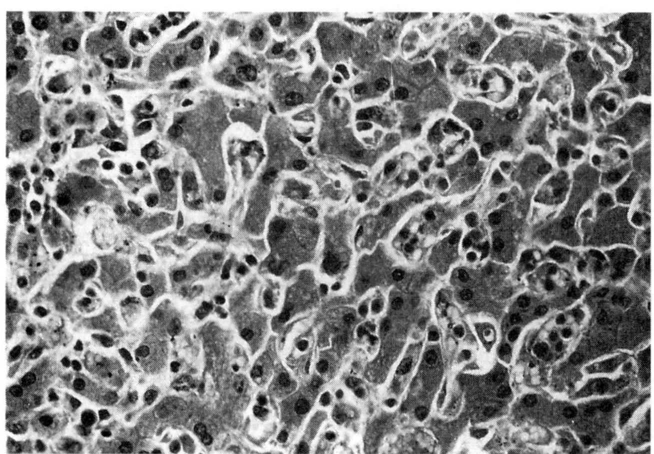

Fig. 4 Epicardial and endocardial haemorrhages in a victim of louse-borne relapsing fever. (Copyright D. A. Warrell.)

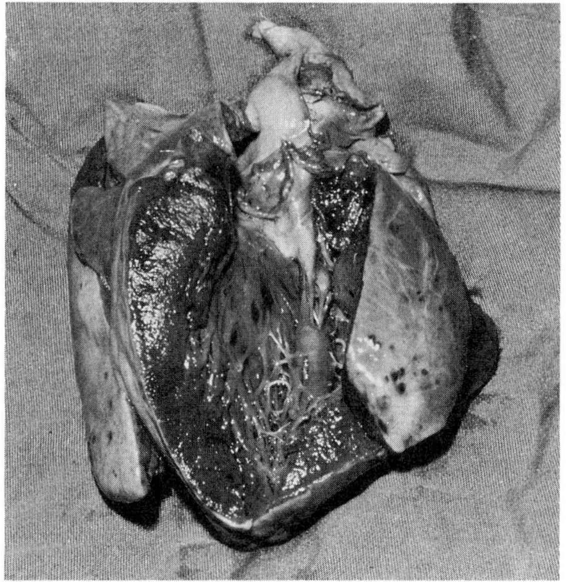

Fig. 5 Ethiopian patient with severe louse-borne relapsing fever; note emaciation and petechial rash. (Copyright D. A. Warrell.)

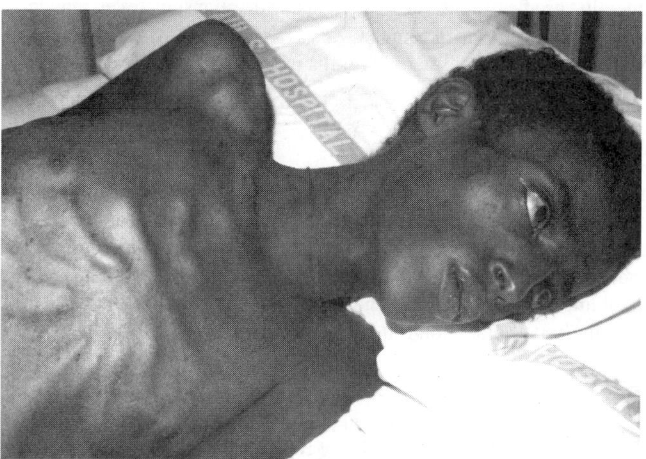

Fig. 6 Subconjunctival haemorrhages in louse-borne relapsing fever. (Copyright D. A. Warrell.)

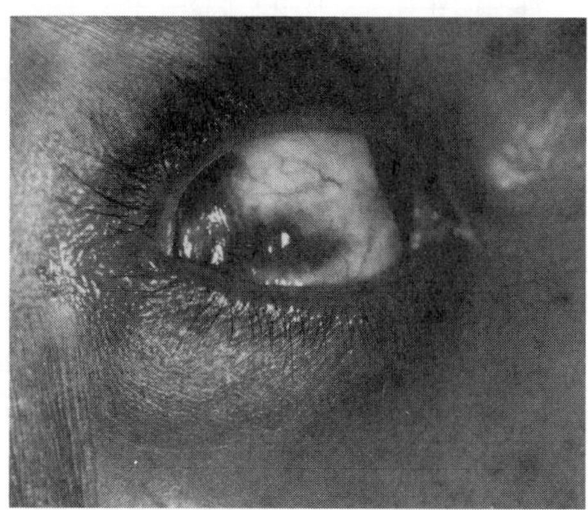

The spontaneous crisis and Jarisch–Herxheimer reaction

Whether or not treatment is given, an attack of relapsing fever usually ends dramatically. About 1 h after intravenous tetracycline, or on about the fifth day of the untreated illness, the patient becomes restless and apprehensive, and suddenly begins to have distressingly intense rigors, which last 10 to 30 min. The ensuing phenomena have features of a classical endotoxin reaction. During the chill phase, temperature, respiratory and pulse rates, and blood pressure rise sharply. Delirium, gastrointestinal symptoms, cough, and limb pains are associated. Some patients die of hyperpyrexia at the peak of fever. The flush phase, which lasts several hours, is characterized by profuse sweating, a fall in blood pressure, and slow decline in temperature. Deaths during this phase follow intractable hypotension or the development of acute pulmonary oedema and are attributable to myocarditis. The classical Jarisch–Herxheimer reaction is in syphilis (Chapter 7.11.34). Similar reactions have been described in Lyme disease and leptospirosis (treated with penicillin), sodoku (arsenicals), *Brucella melitensis* (tetracycline), and even in meningococcal infections.

DIAGNOSIS

In the febrile patient, spirochaetes can usually be demonstrated in thin or thick blood films stained with Giemsa or Wright's stain and counterstained for 10 to 30 min with 1 per cent crystal violet, or by dark-field examination (see Fig. 1). Towards the end of the attack, during remissions, and particularly in children with tick-borne disease, spirochaetaemia may not be detectable. In these cases, blood or cerebrospinal fluid can be injected intraperitoneally into young mice, which will develop spirochaetaemia within 14 days. Serological methods are not generally used. The serum of patients with relapsing fever may give positive reactions with Proteus OXK, OX19, and OX2, and false-positive serological responses for syphilis in 5 to 10 per cent of cases.

DIFFERENTIAL DIAGNOSIS

In a febrile patient with jaundice, petechial rash, bleeding, and hepatosplenomegaly, the differential diagnosis will include falciparum malaria, yellow fever, viral hepatitis, rickettsial infections, especially louse-borne typhus, and leptospirosis. The diagnosis can be quickly confirmed by examining a blood smear, but the possibility of a complicating infection, particularly typhoid, should not be forgotten.

PROGNOSIS

The mortality in treated cases is less than 5 per cent. During major epidemics of louse-borne relapsing fever, mortalities of 40 per cent or higher have been reported. Deaths during relapses are most unusual; they occur only in the tick-borne disease.

TREATMENT

Antimicrobials

Although tick-borne relapsing fever is usually milder than the louse-borne variety, it is more difficult to treat because spirochaetes persist in tissues such as the central nervous system and eye, and produce relapses. Oral tetracycline, 500 mg 6-hourly for 10 days, is, however, effective. Oral erythromycin can be given to pregnant women (500 mg 6-hourly for 10 days) and children (125–250 mg 6-hourly for 10 days). In patients unable to swallow tablets, treatment can be initiated with intravenous tetracycline hydrochloride, 250 mg, or erythromycin lactobionate, 300 mg.

Louse-borne relapsing fever is readily cured with a single oral dose of 500 mg of tetracycline or 500 mg of erythromycin stearate. Few patients with severe louse-borne relapsing fever are able to swallow the tablets without vomiting them up: a more reliable treatment is a single intravenous dose of tetracycline hydrochloride, 250 mg, or, for pregnant women and children, a single intravenous dose of erythromycin lactobionate, 300 mg (children, 10 mg/kg body weight). In mixed epidemics of louse-borne relapsing fever and louse-borne typhus a single oral dose of 100 mg of doxycycline has been effective.

Benzylpenicillin (300 000 u), procaine penicillin with benzylpenicillin (600 000 u), and procaine penicillin with aluminium monostearate (600 000 u), all by intramuscular injection, have been used but they may fail to prevent relapses, and the long-acting preparations produce only slow clearance of spirochaetaemia. Chloramphenicol is effective in tick-borne relapsing fever in a dose of 500 mg 6-hourly for 10 days in adults and 250 mg 6-hourly for 10 days in older children; and in louse-borne relapsing fever in a single dose of 500 mg by mouth or intravenous injection in adults.

Jarisch–Herxheimer reaction

Antimicrobials have reduced the mortality of relapsing fevers from 30 to 70 per cent to less than 5 per cent, but drugs such as tetracycline, which usually eliminate spirochaetes rapidly from the blood and prevent

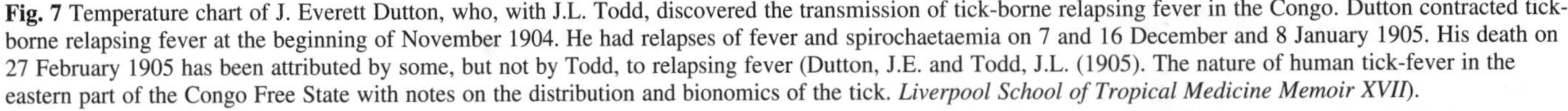

Fig. 7 Temperature chart of J. Everett Dutton, who, with J.L. Todd, discovered the transmission of tick-borne relapsing fever in the Congo. Dutton contracted tick-borne relapsing fever at the beginning of November 1904. He had relapses of fever and spirochaetaemia on 7 and 16 December and 8 January 1905. His death on 27 February 1905 has been attributed by some, but not by Todd, to relapsing fever (Dutton, J.E. and Todd, J.L. (1905). The nature of human tick-fever in the eastern part of the Congo Free State with notes on the distribution and bionomics of the tick. *Liverpool School of Tropical Medicine Memoir XVII*).

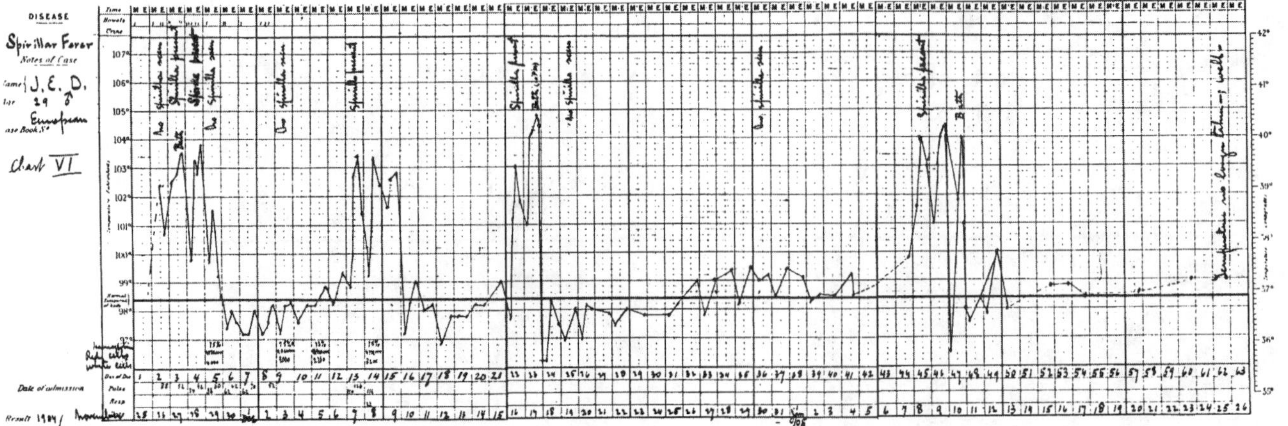

relapses, often induce a severe Jarisch–Herxheimer type of reaction that may occasionally prove fatal. Clearly, in a disease with such a high natural mortality, treatment cannot be withheld, especially as severe spontaneous crises, which may also prove fatal, occur in a large proportion of louse-borne cases after the fifth day of fever. There is no evidence, however, that the shorter and more intense reaction following tetracycline is more dangerous than the more prolonged but apparently milder reaction following slow-release penicillin. Hydrocortisone, in doses up to 20 mg/kg, and paracetamol do not prevent the reaction but reduce peak temperatures, hasten the fall in temperature, and lessen the fall in blood pressure during the flush phase. Pretreatment with oral prednisolone can prevent the Jarisch–Herxheimer reaction of early syphilis, but in louse-borne relapsing fever, an oral dose of prednisolone, 3 mg/kg, given 18 h before tetracycline treatment and infusion of betamethasone, 3.75 mg/kg, do not prevent the reaction. However, meptazinol, an opioid antagonist with agonist properties, diminishes the reaction when given in a dose of 100 mg by intravenous injection. The discovery of an explosive release of tumour necrosis factor, interleukin 6 and interleukin 8 just before the start of the Jarisch–Herxheimer reaction prompted the testing of a polyclonal, ovine, Fab, antitumour necrosis factor antibody. Infused for 30 min before treatment with intramuscular penicillin this antibody suppressed the reaction.

Supportive treatment

Patients must be nursed in bed for at least 24 h after treatment to prevent postural hypotensive collapse and the precipitation of fatal cardiac arrhythmias. Hyperpyrexia should be prevented with antipyretics and vigorous fanning with tepid sponging. Although patients with acute louse-borne relapsing fever have an expanded plasma volume, most are dehydrated and relatively hypovolaemic. Adults may need four or more litres of isotonic saline intravenously during the first 24 h. Infusion should be controlled by monitoring of jugular venous, central venous, or pulmonary artery-wedge pressures. Particularly during the flush phase of the Jarisch–Herxheimer reaction or spontaneous crisis, acute myocardial failure may develop. This is signalled by a rise in central venous pressure above 15 cmH_2O; 1 mg digoxin should be given intravenously over 5 to 10 min. Because of the intense vasodilatation, diuretics may accentuate the circulatory failure by causing relative hypovolaemia. Oxygen should be given during the reaction, particularly in severe cases. Vitamin K should be given in all cases with prolonged prothrombin times. Heparin is not effective in controlling coagulopathy and should not be used. Complicating infections—typhoid, salmonellosis, bacillary dysentery, tuberculosis, typhus and malaria—must be treated appropriately.

Fig. 8 Shaving heavily-infested hair in an Ethiopian patient with louse-borne relapsing fever. (Copyright D. A. Warrell.)

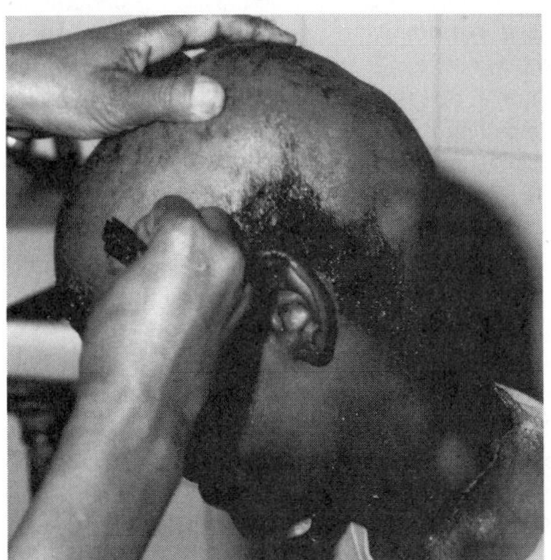

Delousing

Patients with louse-borne relapsing fever are infectious until they have been thoroughly deloused by shaving off infested hair (Fig. 8), washing with soap or 1 per cent lysol solution, and dusting with 10 per cent DDT, 1 per cent malathion or 0.5 per cent permethrin. Their clothes, instinct with infected lice, are disinfected by heat. Ticks should be searched for and removed but they usually feed for a short time and then detach and so are rarely found by the time the patient presents with tick-borne relapsing fever. A recent study in Ethiopia demonstrated that treatment of cases of louse-borne relapsing fever with antimicrobials was not effective in controlling an epidemic without the addition of vigorous delousing measures.

PREVENTION

Tick control can be attempted by spraying buildings with insecticides such as 2 per cent benzene hexachloride or 0.5 per cent malathion, and by reducing the number of rodent vectors. Lousiness is prevented by improved hygiene and use of DDT or other insecticide powders.

REFERENCES

Anderson, T.R. and Zimmerman, L.E. (1955). Relapsing fever in Korea. A clinicopathologic study of eleven fatal cases with special attention to association with salmonella infections. *American Journal of Pathology*, **31,** 1083–109.

Barbour, A.G. (1987). Immunobiology of relapsing fever. *Contributions to Microbiological Immunology*, **8,** 125–37.

Bryceson, A.D.M., Parry, E.H.O., Perine, P.L., Warrell, D.A., Vucotich, D., and Leithead, C.S. (1970). Louse-borne relapsing fever. A clinical and laboratory study of 62 cases in Ethiopia and a reconsideration of the literature. *Quarterly Journal of Medicine*, **39,** 129–70.

Butler, T., Aikawa, M., Habte-Michael, A., and Wallace, C. (1980). Phagocytosis of *Borrelia recurrentis* by blood polymorphonuclear leukocytes is enhanced by antibiotic treatment. *Infection and Immunity*, **28,** 1009–13.

Felsenfeld, O. (1965). Borrelia, human relapsing fever and parasite-vector-host relationships. *Bacteriology Reviews*, **29,** 46–74.

Felsendfeld, O. (1971). *Borrelia: strains, vectors, human and animal borreliosis.* Green, St Louis.

Goubau, P.F. (1984). Relapsing fevers. A review. *Annales de la Societé Belge de Médicine Tropicale*, **40,** 335–64.

Horton, J.M. and Blaser, M.J. (1985). The spectrum of relapsing fever in the Rocky Mountains. *Archives of Internal Medicine*, **145,** 871–5.

Negussie, Y. *et al.* (1992). Detection of plasma tumor necrosis factor, interleukins-6 and -8 during the Jarisch–Herxheimer reaction of relapsing fever. *Journal of Experimental Medicine*, **175,** 1207–12.

Plasterk, R.H.A., Simon, M.I., and Barbour, A.G. (1985). Transposition of structural genes to an expression sequence on a linear plasmid causes antigenic variation in the bacterium *Borrelia hermsii. Nature*, **318,** 257–63.

Sundnes, K.O. and Teklehaimanot, A. (1993). Epidemic of louse-borne relapsing fever in Ethiopia. *Lancet*, **342,** 1213–15.

Teklu, B., Habte-Michael, A., Warrell, D.A., White, N.J., and Wright, D.J.M. (1983). Meptazinol diminishes the Jarisch–Herxheimer reaction of relapsing fever. *Lancet*, **i,** 835–9.

Trape, J.F. *et al.* (1991). Tick-borne borreliosis in West Africa. *Lancet*, **337,** 473–5.

Warrell, D.A., Perine, P.L., Krause, D.W., Bing, D.H., and MacDougal, S.J. (1983). Pathophysiology and immunology of the Jarisch–Herxheimer like reaction in louse-borne relapsing fever: comparison of tetracycline and slow-release penicillin. *Journal of Infectious Diseases*, **147,** 898–909.

Warrell, D.A., Pope, H.M., Parry, E.H.O., Perine, P.L., and Bryceson, A.D.M. (1970). Cardiorespiratory disturbance associated with infective fever in man: studies of Ethiopian louse-borne relapsing fever. *Clinical Science*, **39,** 123–45.

7.11.32 Leptospirosis

V. Sitprija

Leptospirosis is an infectious disease caused by the *Leptospira interrogans* complex. The disease is characterized by a broad spectrum of clinical manifestations including fever, chills, headache, conjunctivitis, and muscular pains. In mild cases the disease may be subclinical. Jaundice and renal failure are seen in the severe infection known as Weil's disease.

Aetiology

Leptospires are spirochaetes belonging to the order Spirochaetales and family Treponemataceae. The organism is tightly coiled, thin, and flexible, 5 to 20 μm long and 0.1 to 0.2 μm wide with a bend at one end. It is highly motile with a corkscrew motion. The outer membrane is multilayered, which is essential for the viability of the organism. The cytoplasmic membrane–peptidoglycan complex is located beneath the outer membrane. The flagella are wound around the protoplasmic cylinder. Leptospires are demonstrable by dark-field examination and silver impregnation stain. The organisms are easily cultivated aerobically at 28 to 30 °C in buffered alkaline 2 per cent nutrient agar containing peptone or serum enrichment. Other media also used for culture include Noguchi's ascitic-fluid medium, membranes of developing chick embryo, and synthetic media containing inorganic salts.

L. interrogans is the only species of leptospire. It is divided into two complexes: the interrogans complex, which is pathogenic, and the biflexa complex, which is saprophytic. Definite antigenic differences are noted between the two complexes. The interrogans complex has 30 serogroups and approximately 240 serotypes or serovars. All serotypes are serologically related with cross-reactivity in serological tests, indicating overlapping in the antigenic structure. An important development has been the classification to genospecies based on the results of studies of DNA hybridization and RNA gene restriction mapping. Two kinds of antigens have been identified. The surface antigen contains protein polysaccharide and is serotype specific, while the somatic antigen contains lipopolysaccharide and is genus specific. The outer membrane of the organism is a potent immunogen and is the target for the immunoglobulin–complement bactericidal reaction. The organisms possess haemolysin, which is soluble, non-dialysable, thermolabile, and oxygen stable. Various enzymes including catalase, transamidase, lipase, hyaluronidase, and oxidase are present. The presence of endotoxin has been shown in certain serotypes.

Epidemiology

Rodents, especially rats, are the most important reservoir. *Rattus norvegicus* and *Mus musculus* carry a broad spectrum of serotypes. Other mammalian hosts include cattle, pigs, goats, hamsters, mice, voles, gerbils, coypus, hedgehogs, shrews, dogs, jackals, foxes, mongooses, civets, skunks, raccoons, and marsupials. Leptospires have also been isolated from birds and reptiles. The organisms may exist in the animal host without causing pathological damage. Leptospires may be isolated from urine, blood, and brain of seronegative rats. Rodents usually do not succumb to the infection. Their alkaline urine pH and renal tissue pH are favourable for the organism's survival, permitting permanent colonization and urinary shedding. On the other hand, animals susceptible to infection are only temporary urine shedders.

The major vectors to man are rodents. Transmission occurs by direct contact with blood, tissue, or urine of infected animals or exposure to an environment contaminated by leptospires. The moisture, warmth, and optimum pH of soil or surface water in tropical and temperate climates are suitable for the organisms, and they may survive for weeks. Dry climate, excessive sunlight, and chemical pollution tend to kill the organisms.

Leptospires enter a host through abrasions in the skin or through intact mucous membranes including conjunctiva, vagina, and nasopharynx. Entrance through the intact skin is unlikely, although prolonged exposure of the skin to contaminated water may provide an opportunity for invasion. Infection via the intestinal mucosa can occur when leptospiral-contaminated food is ingested in quantity.

People working in an environment infested by rats or other animals, or where there is infected material or water, are prone to infection. For example, 11 to 13 per cent of Britain's 65 000 dairy farmers show serological evidence of past infection. In the tropics, leptospirosis may account for 15 per cent of fever of unknown origin with high incidence during the rainy season. Some serotypes may be traced to certain animal hosts. Icterohaemorrhagiae can be traced to rat exposure, gryppotyphosa to vole contact, seroje to pig, canicola to dog, and pomona and hardjo to cattle exposure. *L. hardjo* is prevalent among cattle in Wales and Australia and gives rise to many human infections. Leptospirosis can be found almost anywhere in the world if it is searched for.

Pathogenesis

Once they have gained entry, leptospires spread through the bloodstream to all organs. Multiplication occurs in both blood and tissues. Within 24 h the organisms can be isolated in most tissues except brain, skeletal muscles, and aqueous humour. After 48 h they are recoverable from all tissues. Multisystem involvement results from bacterial invasion and toxic reactions. Clearance of the organisms is accomplished by phagocytosis and humoral mechanisms. Leptospires rapidly disappear from the blood after the appearance of agglutinins. After the spirochaetaemic phase, which lasts from 4 to 7 days, the organisms can be recovered only from renal and ocular tissues. Leptospiruria continues for 1 to 4 weeks.

Three mechanisms are involved in the pathogenesis of leptospirosis: direct bacterial invasion, non-specific inflammatory factors, and immunological reactions.

DIRECT BACTERIAL INVASION

Tissue damage in the acute phase of infection is related to bacterial multiplication. The presence of leptospires is necessary for the development of the lesions in the early stage of the disease. It is not clear whether the lesions are caused by bacterial migration *per se* or by factors inherent in bacterial virulence such as bacterial enzymes, metabolites, or toxins. Hyaluronidase, which may assist in bacterial penetration, cytotoxic factor, and haemolysin have been identified. Vascular endothelial damage with haemorrhage is attributed to cytotoxic factor derived either from bacteria or interaction between leptospires and the host cells. The role of haemolysin in human disease is not clear. Haemolysis is not an important feature in human leptospirosis, although it may occur in some cases. Haemolytic anaemia results from cell-membrane injury characterized by reductions in sphingomyelin and phosphatidylethanolamine. The red blood cells appear thorny and spiculated in peripheral smears. Leptospiral infection is interesting in that in the early stages multiplication of organisms is very rapid, resulting in acute and intense organ dysfunction. The fact that there is marked peripheral leucocytosis in the absence of neutrophilic infiltration in the tissue is worth pointing out, and suggests the role of toxins in the pathogenesis of the disease. Several clinical features in leptospiral infection resemble endotoxaemia. Human patients may have a positive limulus lysate test; those with a positive test have a higher serum creatinine, bilirubin, and leucocyte count than those with a negative test. Yet, endotoxin is present only in certain serotypes. The role of endotoxin of intestinal bacteria had been considered, but was later excluded by the observation that infection of germ-free animals produced lesions similar to those seen in control animals. Serum C3 may be decreased in the early stage of the disease, presumably because of complement activation through the alternative pathway by either leptospires or endotoxin.

The kidney and the liver are most affected by leptospires. In the kidney, leptospires initially cause glomerular injury, and by haematogenous spread, the organisms reach peritubular capillaries (Fig. 1) and migrate to the interstitium (Fig. 2), renal tubules, and tubular lumen causing interstitial nephritis and tubular necrosis. Cellular infiltration is predominantly mononuclear. Polymorphonuclear cells may appear in the early stage of glomerular injury. In the liver, there is centrilobular necrosis with the proliferation of Kupffer cells being responsible for jaundice. As severe pathological changes occur at a time when leptospires are rarely found in the lesion, it seems plausible that the toxin released by the organisms is responsible for liver injury. It remains puzzling, however, that leptospires are present in the cerebrospinal fluid and the aqueous humour early in the course of the disease without causing damage.

NON-SPECIFIC INFLAMMATORY FACTORS

Certain pathophysiological changes that occur in infection also contribute to causing organ dysfunction. These changes include hypovolaemia, blood hyperviscosity, and intravascular coagulation. Cytokines (especially tumour necrosis factor), complement activation, and free radicals are also involved in tissue injury. Hypovolaemia in leptospirosis is attributed to decreased fluid intake, increased insensible fluid loss, and increased vascular permeability caused by chemical mediators released during inflammation. Increased blood viscosity is accounted for by increased plasma fibrinogen and hypovolaemia. A low-grade intravascular coagulation is also observed, shown by the presence of fibrin degradation products in the serum. These factors can compromise the microcirculation, leading to capillary stasis and tissue anoxia. Capillary permeability is therefore further increased, resulting in fluid leakage, haemoconcentration, and a further rise in blood viscosity, creating a vicious cycle. Hypoperfusion in severe infection may also be the result of cardiac dysfunction. Although these non-specific factors do not play the primary role in the development of the lesions, they contribute to organ dysfunction. In fact, they are important in the pathogenesis of renal failure in leptospirosis. Impaired renal function is both toxic and ischaemic in origin.

Fig. 1 Demonstration of leptospires (arrowed) in the peritubular capillary of a hamster 3 h after inoculation (by courtesy of Dr V. Boonpucknavig).

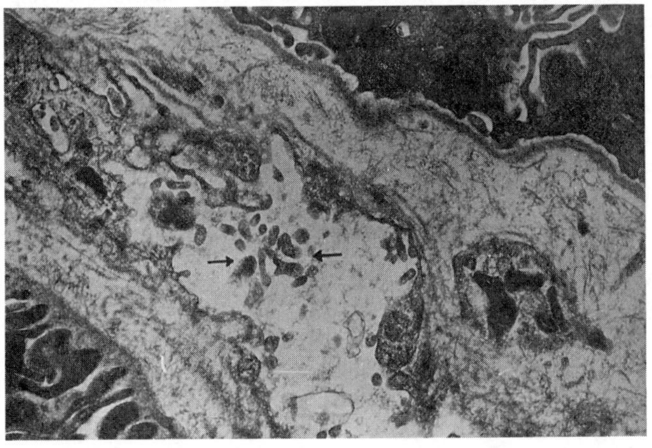

Fig. 2 Demonstration of leptospires (arrowed) in the renal interstitium of a hamster 6 h after inoculation (by courtesy of Dr V. Boonpucknavig).

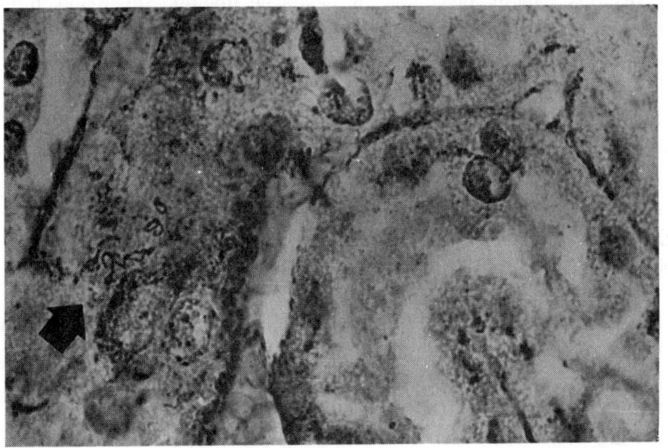

IMMUNOLOGICAL MECHANISM

In leptospiral infection, IgM antibodies are produced first, followed by the appearance of IgG, which persists for a longer period of time. The average curves of IgM and agglutinating antibodies are similar. The IgM response is usually higher than the IgG response, and may last for several months. IgG and complement are required for leptospiricidal activity of macrophages. IgA response is irregular and usually delayed. The immune response is effective in clearing the organisms, but may also produce inflammatory reactions. The role of antibodies in the pathogenesis of renal lesions is convincing in certain animal species. In canine leptospirosis, renal lesions with immunoglobulin deposition have been shown, and the disease runs a chronic course and may lead to chronic renal failure. This has not been observed in man. Both non-specific host reactions and cell-mediated immunity participate in the cellular response to leptospiral invasion. Initial interstitial and glomerular changes are non-specific inflammatory reactions to leptospires, and in hamsters these changes occur a few hours after inoculation of organisms. Cell-mediated immunity plays a part in the later stages. Lymphocytes may be involved in eliminating leptospires from the renal interstitium. It is interesting that the rise in antibody titre coincides with inflammatory lesions such as meningitis and uveitis. Many authorities agree that meningeal inflammation is not caused by leptospiral invasion. The fact that leptospires are isolated consistently from the cerebrospinal fluid but disappear during the onset of meningeal signs following antibody formation suggests that immunological mechanism is responsible for the development of meningitis. An immunological basis for uveitis is suggested by the prolonged persistence of leptospires in the ocular fluid and the demonstration of agglutinins in the aqueous humour.

Pathology

Leptospires cause primarily vascular changes. The cytotoxic factor produces damage to the vascular endothelium causing haemorrhage in the mucous membranes, skin, lungs, kidneys, and other organs. Haemorrhage occurs early in the acute stage during the febrile period.

LIVER

Hepatic lesions consist of focal centrilobular necrosis with focal lymphocytic infiltration and disorganization of liver-cell plates, but seldom with fatal results. Proliferation of Kupffer cells, with cholestasis associated with scanty round cell infiltration in the periportal areas, is often noted. Histological changes in the liver are in general not diagnostic and correlate poorly with the degree of functional impairment. Electron microscopy reveals mitochondrial destruction. Histochemically, the activity of succinic, isocitric, glutamic, and lactic dehydrogenases is reduced in association with functional changes. Jaundice is cholestatic in type with elevation of alkaline phosphatase out of proportion to the mild rise in transaminases. In animals, liver lesions are noted within 24 h of inoculation of leptospires because the liver is the primary site of leptospire multiplication. However, in man it is of interest that severe pathological changes occur at the time when it is hard to find leptospires in the tissue.

KIDNEY

Renal changes occur early in the course of the disease before functional changes are noticeable. The kidneys are grossly swollen with pale cortex and congested medulla. Mesangial proliferation with polymorphonuclear cell infiltration is noted early during bacterial invasion. Focal thickening of the basement membrane and fusion of foot processes are shown by electron microscopy. There is deposition of C3 in the arteriolar wall and in the glomeruli. C1q and IgM deposition may be noted occasionally in the mesangial area. By electron microscopy, dense deposits may be demonstrated in the basement membrane and subepithelial area. Vascular changes in the kidney consist of endothelial swelling and necrosis with platelet aggregation especially in the corticomedullary region. Interstitial nephritis may be observed without any alteration of renal function and forms the basic renal lesion in human leptospirosis (Fig. 3). Cellular infiltration consists of mononuclear cells and a few eosinophils. Tubular necrosis is seen in cases with acute renal failure. Proximal tubular degeneration is common, and distal tubules are affected when the disease progresses. Basement membrane disruption may be noted. Although tubular necrosis and interstitial nephritis are observed in renal failure, interstitial nephritis chronologically precedes tubular necrosis because leptospires migrate through the peritubular capillaries to the interstitium and thence to the renal tubules. Renal tubular enzymuria may precede the development of histological lesions.

HEART

Epicardium, endocardium, and myocardium may be involved. Myocardial changes may be focal or diffuse, characterized by interstitial oedema with infiltration of mononuclear cells and plasma cells. Necrosis may be associated with neutrophil infiltration. There may be focal haemorrhages in the myocardium, and endocarditis.

STRIATED MUSCLE

Vacuolation of myofibril cytoplasm is noted early in the course of the disease. The other changes consist of loss of cellular detail and fragmentation resulting in homogeneous or irregular acidophilic masses. Polymorphonuclear cell infiltration is minimal. Leptospiral antigen is demonstrable in the muscle. In most cases myopathy resolves completely within 2 weeks, as leptospiral antibodies develop.

Fig. 3 Interstitial nephritis with mononuclear cell infiltration in a patient with leptospirosis.

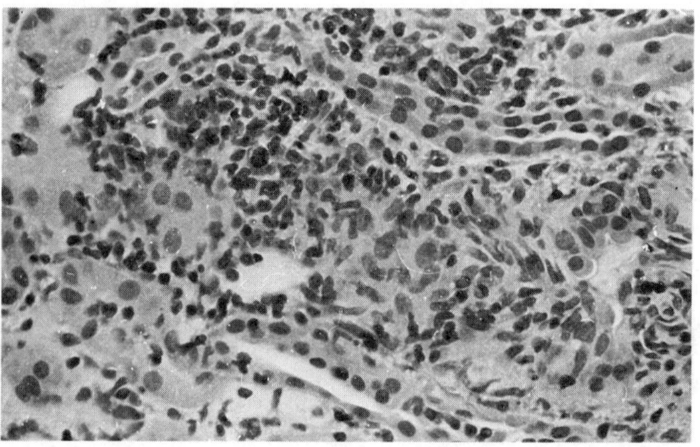

CENTRAL NERVOUS SYSTEM

The meninges show some thickening with a slight increase in the number of arachnoid mononuclear cells. Although leptospires can be isolated from cerebrospinal fluid and meninges, they disappear rapidly following the onset of meningeal irritation, which occurs during the second week. It is believed that meningitis is immunological in mechanism and not caused by the invasion of the meninges by leptospires. Encephalitis, myelitis, radiculitis, and peripheral neuritis are uncommon. Perivascular infiltration of blood vessels in the spinal cord, basal ganglia, hippocampus, and white matter of the cerebellum has been described.

OTHER ORGANS

Haemorrhage in the gastrointestinal tract attributable to endothelial damage may occur. Haemorrhage is also found in the lungs, pleura, and tracheobronchial tree. Pulmonary oedema caused by increased capillary permeability may occur. Adrenal haemorrhage is rare. Interstitial oedema and monoculear cell infiltration may occur. Persistence of leptospires in the aqueous humour may be responsible for chronic, recurrent, and latent uveitis. Haemorrhage in the pancreas has also been shown.

Clinical manifestations

The incubation period varies from 7 to 12 days, but may range from 2 to 20 days; it has no prognostic significance. The variability of symptoms reflects the dose of the organisms and the host factors. In its mild form the disease may present as a non-specific fever, and can be diagnosed only by serological tests. Leptospirosis may present as Weil's disease with jaundice and multiorgan involvement or as an acute but anicteric form with milder clinical symptoms. Ninety per cent of cases are anicteric. In general, both anicteric and icteric cases follow a biphasic course.

SEPTICAEMIC PHASE

The initial septicaemic phase is characterized by fever with chills, myalgia, headache, abdominal pain, skin rash, vomiting, and conjunctival injection lasting from 4 to 7 days. Because leptospires are present in all tissues, the symptoms are systemic. Renal involvement is invariably present, ranging from urinary sediment changes and mild proteinuria to renal failure. Leucocyturia, more than 5 cells/high-power field, haematuria, and granular casts are often noted. Total urinary protein excretion is often less than 1 g/24 h. Renal failure occurs in 44 to 67 per cent of cases. Jaundice with impairment of liver function may be present in severe cases. Among the symptoms, headache, myalgia, fever, and chills are most common, occurring in over 85 per cent of cases. The other symptoms include diarrhoea, arthralgia, cough, sore throat, bone pain, splenomegaly, lymphadenopathy, and hepatomegaly.

Headache is usually intense, sometimes throbbing, and is often not controlled by analgesics. It is commonly frontal, and may be associated with retrobulbar pain. Persistent headache may indicate meningitis. On occasions, mental disturbances including delirium, hallucination, and psychotic behaviour may be observed. Tachycardia is common, but relative bradycardia may occur. Cardiac arrhythmias are found in 18 per cent of cases.

Myalgia, either localized or generalized, is one of the hallmarks in leptospiral infection. Calf, abdominal, and lumbosacral muscles are often affected. After the septicaemic period, myalgia disappears. Conjunctival suffusion, photophobia, ocular pain, and conjunctival haemorrhage are frequently observed. Abdominal pain, especially when associated with nausea and vomiting, presents a difficult problem in differential diagnosis, and may even lead to abdominal exploration. Splenomegaly is noted in 15 to 25 per cent of cases. Pulmonary involvement occurs frequently and is manifested by a dry cough, occasionally with blood-stained sputum. There may be rales on physical examination. Pleural rub and pericardial rub are rare. A variety of patterns shown by a chest radiograph includes small patchy lesions, confluent infiltration or even consolidation (Fig. 4). The lesions are prevalent in the periphery of the lung. Acute respiratory distress syndrome may occur in severe infection, and has grave prognostic significance. Skin rashes may be macular, maculopapular, erythematous, urticarial, or haemorrhagic (Fig. 5). and are confined largely to the trunk, but any area may be involved. A pretibial erythematous eruption has been noted in patients with autumnalis infection. Pharyngitis occurs in 23 per cent of anicteric cases. Lymphadenopathy is seen in 15 to 15 per cent of cases. Parotitis, orchitis, epididymitis, prostatitis, otitis media, and arthritis occur rarely. Mild bleeding may be seen in leptospirosis, especially in icteric cases, and epistaxis may occur. Hypotension and congestive heart failure may be observed in severe cases.

Fig. 4 Gross bilateral radiographic changes attributable to pulmonary oedema and haemorrhage in a Brazilian man with leptospirosis (copyright D. A. Warrell).

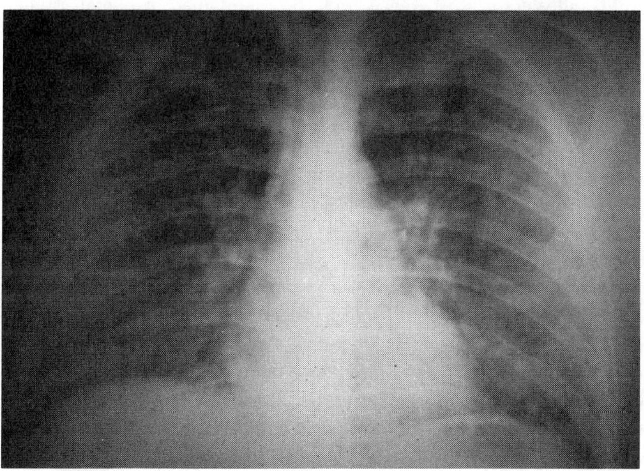

Fig. 5 Subconjunctival haemorrhage, epistaxis, and petechiae (right axilla) in an English patient with Weil's disease (copyright D. A. Warrell).

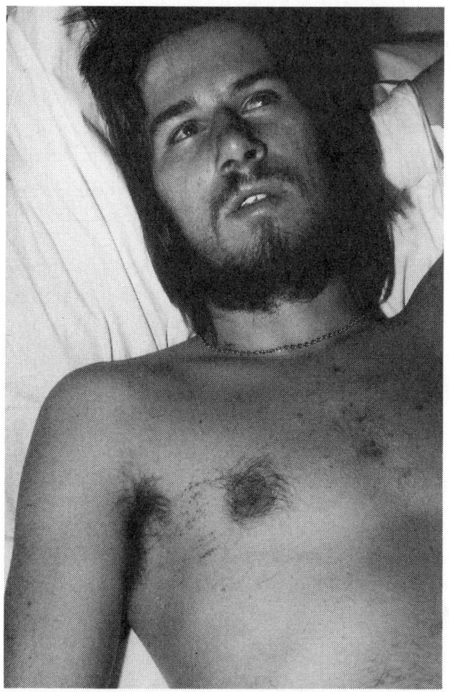

IMMUNE PHASE

The second or immune phase varies from 4 to 30 days. Fever has already subsided with the disappearance of leptospires from most tissues except for the kidney and aqueous humour. This period coincides with the rise in circulating antibody titres. There may be no symptoms in 35 per cent of cases. Meningitis, uveitis, rash, and secondary fever may occur. Hepatic and renal manifestations that continue from the first phase are still present and may even be more severe in some patients. Meningeal reactions are found in 80 to 92 per cent of cases, but less than 50 per cent are symptomatic. Meningeal symptoms disappear within a few days, but rarely may persist for 2 weeks. Cerebrospinal-fluid pleocytosis may last as long as 80 days, but usually disappear within 2 weeks. Cerebrospinal-fluid pressure is usually less than 200 mmH$_2$O. In the early stage, polymorphonuclear cells predominate, but later mononuclear cells account for most of the cells. Encephalitis, focal weakness, spasticity, paralysis, nystagmus, seizures, visual disturbances, peripheral neuritis, cranial nerve palsies, radiculitis, myelitis, and Guillain-Barré syndrome are rare findings.

The anterior uveal tract may be affected by the third week of illness. It is characterized by iritis, iridocyclitis, and choroido retinitis. Uveitis may be unilateral or bilateral.

Jaundice, impaired renal function, changes in consciousness, and sometimes vascular collapse occur in Weil's disease. Any leptospiral infection, irrespective of serotype, can in its severe form produce the syndrome. Jaundice, cholestatic in type, occurs without significant hepatocellular destruction. The serum bilirubin is often less than 20 mg/dl, but may be as high as 80 mg/dl. Jaundice may last from a few days to several weeks. Renal dysfunction, haemorrhagic complications, and cardiovascular collapse occur more frequently in patients with severe jaundice.

Renal manifestations are common in Weil's disease, although they also occur in anicteric leptospirosis. Renal failure is hypercatabolic in type. Hyperuricaemia and hyperphosphataemia are occasionally observed. Severe oliguria or even anuria may be seen in the patient with hyperbilirubinaemia. Rarely, haemolytic–uraemic syndrome, evidenced by the presence of fragmented or distorted erythrocytes, reticulocytosis, thrombocytopenia, haemolysis, and intravascular coagulation, may be noted. Hypokalaemia may develop secondary to kaliuresis.

Diagnosis

Leptospirosis should be differentiated from other febrile illnesses such as malaria, enteric fever, rickettsial diseases, glandular fever, brucellosis, viral hepatitis, influenza, dengue fever, relapsing fever, atypical pneumonia, and aseptic meningitis.

Leucocytosis with neutrophilia is usual, but leucopenia can occur. The erythrocyte sedimentation rate is elevated along with a rise in plasma fibrinogen, which is often noted early in the course of the disease. Plasma fibrinogen of over 1000 mg/dl has been reported. Blood viscosity is increased. Thrombocytopenia is observed in occasional cases. Increased serum fibrin degradation products are often observed. Mild intravascular haemolysis may occur but is uncommon. There may be mild anaemia. Serum C3 may be decreased during, the early stage of the disease, presumably due to complement activation through the alternative pathway.

Urinalysis shows abnormalities. Mild proteinuria and cellular elements in the urinary sediment are often observed. Elevation of blood urea nitrogen and serum creatinine is noted in 67 per cent of cases. In severe renal failure there may be hyperuricaemia and hyperphosphataemia.

Jaundice is cholestatic in type with increased serum alkaline phosphatase and serum bilirubin accompanied by modest elevations of serum transaminases. Transaminases may be markedly elevated in hypotensive patients. Serum creatine phosphokinase is often increased due to muscular involvement.

Pleocytosis is observed in cerebrospinal fluid, with an early rise in polymorphonuclear cells that is later followed by mononuclear cells. Cerebrospinal-fluid sugar is normal, and protein is very slightly raised.

CULTURE

Isolation of leptospires from blood or cerebrospinal fluid can be made only during the first 10 days of clinical illness. Urine culture becomes positive after the second week until 1 month. For routine use, Fletcher's semisolid medium and Stuart's medium are recommended. The EMJH (Ellinghausen, McCullough, Johnson, and Harris) medium is now often used. Multiple cultures should be obtained. Blood specimens should be collected during the leptospiraemic stage before antimicrobial treatment. Growth of leptospires in Fletcher's semisolid medium usually does not occur until several weeks after inoculation. Animal inoculation may be used, especially when the specimen is contaminated. Dark-field microscopy of body fluids for leptospires can be made by experienced clinicians, yet it is difficult to see the organism. Fluorescent antibody techniques may be applied to detect leptospires in the urine and tissue preparation. Immunoperoxidase procedure is specific and convenient for detecting leptospiral antigens in the lesion.

SEROLOGY

Serological diagnosis is very helpful during the second week of the disease. Diagnostic antigens appropriate to the local serogroups of leptospires must be selected. In macroscopic slide-agglutination tests killed or formalinized antigens are used, but in microagglutination tests live antigens are used. Macroscopic slide agglutination is often done as a screening test. The test is rapid and easy, and is designed to provide serogroup specificity. When positive results are obtained, the titre and specific serotype are determined by microscopic agglutination. Other serological tests include complement fixation, an erythrocyte sensitizing substance test, a haemolytic test, and an indirect immunofluorescent test. These tests may become positive earlier than the agglutination tests. They also revert to negative earlier, and therefore are of limited value in the diagnosis. The haemagglutination test offers the advantage of detecting antibodies as early as 4 days after the onset of illness. It is genus specific and is less time consuming than the microscopic agglutination test. The microcapsular agglutination test, in which leptospiral antigens are adsorbed on synthetic carrier capsules, can detect antileptospiral antibodies in the early stage of the disease when the microagglutination test is negative. Diffusion in gel enzyme-linked immunosorbent assay detects antibodies to both surface and cytoplasmic antigens, while a microscopic agglutination test detects only antibodies to surface antigen. Enzyme immunoassay is used as an additional test or alternative to microagglutination. It is sensitive and can be used for early diagnosis.

Polymerase chain reaction is a powerful tool in the diagnosis of leptospirosis. It is sensitive and reliable for detection of leptospires in clinical specimens.

The microagglutination test is still the most widely used. It should employ representative strains of all serogroups known to exist in the area. The serological criteria for diagnosis include a fourfold or greater rise in titre during the course of the disease. Elevated microscopic agglutination titres are commonly noted by the tenth day of illness. A slow rise in antibody titre has been observed in patients with severe infection and in severe uraemia. In leptospirosis a single microscopic agglutination titre of 1:100 is sufficient to warrant a diagnosis of previous infection.

Treatment

Penicillin, streptomycin, tetracycline, and erythromycin are among the antimicrobials capable of killing leptospires. Although the beneficial role of the antimicrobial agents in human leptospirosis is controversial, most investigators agree that, to be effective, penicillin or tetracycline should be given within 4 to 7 days of the onset of the disease. A Jarisch-Herxheimer reaction may occur when penicillin is given early in the course of the disease. Early institution of antimicrobial treatment may prevent some complications. The duration of leptospiruria may be reduced. Parenteral aqueous benzylpenicillin in a dosage of 1 mega unit at 6-hourly intervals for a period of 1 week is recommended in adults. In severe infection intravenous administration of penicillin, 1.5 mega units, or ampicillin, 1 g, is advised. Recent work indicates that antimicrobial administration is effective even when treatment is started late in the course of the disease. The dose may be modified when there is renal failure. For patients with penicillin hypersensitivity, tetracycline at a dosage of 2 g daily is recommended provided renal function is normal. Doxycycline (200 mg daily) can also be used.

Fluid and electrolyte balance must be maintained, especially when the patient is febrile. In renal failure this problem is even more critical. Haemodialysis or peritoneal dialysis may be needed when renal failure is severe. As renal failure is catabolic in type, dialysis may have to be done frequently. In hyperbilirubinaemic renal failure, exchange blood transfusion is fruitful in reducing the serum bilirubin and chemical mediators and improving the renal function.

Prognosis

Most patients recover. Mortality is greater in elderly patients and in those with severe jaundice, thrombocytopenia, acute respiratory failure, and renal failure. However, dialysis has much reduced fatality in such cases. The long-term follow-up of those with renal failure shows good recovery of renal function. Interstitial fibrosis with permanent renal tubular dysfunction is rare, and this is in contrast to canine leptospirosis in which chronic renal failure may occur. Iridocyclitis may persist for several years. Fetal mortality is high when leptospirosis is associated with pregnancy.

Prevention

Vaccines are effective in preventing the disease in animals. The outer-membrane vaccine is more effective than the whole-cell and protoplasmic-cylinder vaccines. Its use in man is impracticable due to the presence of many serotypes. However, vaccination against a specific serotype prevalent in the area has been shown to be effective. The other methods include surface decontamination, the wearing of protective clothing, and the eradication of the animal reservoir. Chemoprophylaxis with doxycycline, 200 mg weekly, prevents infection but is recommended only for short-term use in high-risk individuals.

Prophylactic injection of penicillin is a reasonable precaution in people who fall into waterways known to be contaminated with leptospires.

REFERENCES

Adler, B. and Faine, S. (1978). The antibodies involved in the human immune response to leptospiral infection. *Journal of Medical Microbiology*, **11,** 387.

Banfi, E., Cinco, M., Bellini, M., and Soranzo, M.R. (1982). The role of antibodies and serum complement in the interaction between macrophages and leptospires. *Journal of General Microbiology*. **128,** 813–16.

Berman, S.J., Tsai, C., Holmes, K., Fresh, J.W., and Walten, R.H. (1973). Sporadic anicteric leptospirosis in South Vietnam. A study in 150 patients. *Anuals of Internal Medicine*, **79,** 167–73.

Bey, R.F. and Johnson, R.C. (1982). Immunogenicity and humoral and cell-mediated immune responses to leptospiral whole cell, outer envelope, and protoplasmic cylinder vaccines in hamsters and dogs. *American Journal of Veterinary Research*, **43,** 835–40.

Bhamarapravati, N., Boonyapaknavig, V., Viranuvatti, V., Tuchinda, U., Bunnag, D., and Nye, S. (1966). Liver changes in leptospirosis: a study of needle biopsies in 22 cases. *American Journal of Proctology*, **17,** 480–87.

Edelweiss, E.L. and Mailloux, L. (1982). The curve of immunoglobulins in human leptospirosis. *International Journal of Zoonoses*, **9,** 51–6.

Feigin, R.D., and Anderson, D.C. (1975). Human leptospirosis. *CRC Critical Reviews of Clinical Laboratory Sciences* **5,** 413–67.

Finco, D.R. and Low, D.G. (1967). Endotoxin properties of *Leptospira canicola. British Medical Journal. American Journal of Veterinary Research*, **128,** 1863–1872.

Friedland, J.S. and Warrell, D.A. (1991). The Jarisch-Herxheimer reaction in leptospirosis: possible pathogenesis and review. Rev. Infect. Dis. **13,** 207–210.

Knight, L.L., Miller, N.G., and White, R.J. (1973). Cytotoxic factor in the blood and plasma of animals during leptospirosis. *Infection and Immunity*, **8,** 401–5.

Leptospirosis on the African Continent (1992). Proceedings of a CEC/STD3 Research Meeting. University of Zimbabwe and Royal Tropical Institute, N.H. Swellengrebel Laboratory of Tropical Hygiene, Amsterdam, The Netherlands.

Mackay-Dick, J. and Robinson, J.F. (1957). Penicillin in the treatment of 84 cases of leptospirosis in Malaya *Journal of the Royal Army Medical Corps*, **103,** 186–97.

Morrison, M.I., and Wright, N.G. (1976). Canine leptospirosis: an immunological study of interstitial nephritis due to *Leptospira canicola, Journal of Pathology*, **120,** 83–9.

Ramadass, P., Jarvis, B.D.W., Corner, R.J., Penny, D. and Marshall, R.B. (1992). Genetic characterisation of pathogenic Leptospira species by DNA hybridization. *International Journal of Systematic Bacteriology*, **42,** 215–19.

Seguro, A.C. Lomar, A.V., and Rocha, A.S. (1990). Acute renal failure of leptospirosis: nonoliguric and hypokalemic form. *Nephron*, **55,** 146–51

Sitprija, V. (1984). Renal involvement in leptospirosis. In: *Proceedings of the 9th International Congress of Nephrology*, pp. 1041–52. Springer Verlag, New York.

Sitprija, V., Pipatanagul, V., Mertowidjojo, K., Boonpucknavig, V., and Boonpucknavig, S. (1980). Pathogenesis of renal disease in leptospirosis: clinical and experimental studies. *Kidney International*, **17,** 827–36.

Takafuji, E.T. *et al.* (1984). An efficacy trial of dexycycline Chemoprophylaxis against Leptosirosis. *New England Journal of Medicine*, **310,** 497–500.

Turner, L.H. (1973). Leptospirosis. *British Medical Journal* **1,** 537–40.

Watt, G. *et al.* (1988). Placebo-controlled trial of intravenous penicillin for severe and late leptospirosis. *Lancet*, i, 433–5.

7.11.33 Non-venereal treponemes: yaws, endemic syphilis, and pinta

P. L. Perine

Yaws is one of the endemic treponematoses, a group of chronic, granulomatous diseases caused by spirochaetes belonging to the genus Treponema. Yaws occurs mainly in children living in rural areas in warm, humid climates between the Tropics of Cancer and Capricorn. About 10 per cent of untreated cases develop late, disfiguring or crippling lesions of skin, bone, and cartilage.

Aetiology

Yaws is caused by *Treponema pertenue*, a spirochaete that is morphologically identical to *T. pallidum*, the cause of venereal and non-venereal syphilis, and to *T. carateum*, the cause of pinta. These treponemes share common antigens so that infection by one species produces varying degrees of cross-immunity to the others. No serological test exists that differentiates the antibodies produced, and none of these organisms grows *in vitro*. The only means of differentiating yaws, syphilis, and pinta is their epidemiological characteristics and the pattern of infection produced by the respective treponemes in man and experimentally infected laboratory animals (Table 1).

The treponemes of yaws, syphilis, and pinta are fragile and readily killed by exposure to atmospheric oxygen, drying, mild detergents, or antiseptics. They prefer temperatures below 37 °C, which may explain their predilection for the skin and bones of the extremities. These organisms cannot penetrate intact skin, and gain entry to the body through small abrasions and lacerations.

The pathogenic treponemes are small, corkscrew-shaped organisms measuring 0.5 μm in width and 7 to 20 μm in length. Because of their small mass, they cannot be seen by the ordinary microscope unless the dark-ground technique is used.

Epidemiology

Yaws is transmitted by direct contact with an infectious lesion or by fingers contaminated with lesion exudate. Yaws transmission is enhanced by a crowded environment with poor sanitation and personal hygiene. The disease is usually acquired in childhood between the ages of 5 and 15. Statistically, there are no racial or sex differences that distinguish those who become infected, and in endemic areas more than 80 per cent of the population are infected.

Climatic conditions influence the type of yaws lesion and its transmission. In humid, warm environments the early lesion tends to proliferate and teems with spirochaetes, thus increasing the infectious reservoir; whereas in dry, arid climates or seasons the reverse is true.

Yaws and other endemic treponematoses have undergone dramatic changes in prevalence over the past three decades. The first change was a precipitous decrease in cases brought about by mass penicillin treatment campaigns in the 1950s and 1960s sponsored by the World Health Organization. An estimated 152 million people were examined and 46.1 million clinical cases, latent infections, and contacts were treated. The yaws reservoir was greatly reduced in West and Central Africa, Central and South America, and Oceania. However, over the past decade, yaws has been resurgent in the rural populations of Ecuador, the Ivory Coast, Ghana, Togo, Benin, Zaire, the Central African Republic and Ethiopia in Africa, and in the island nations in the pacific. This is because of limited surveillance and premature dismantling of the yaws control programmes. To cope with this resurgence, several nations initiated new campaigns of mass treatment in the 1980s.

Some African nations, like Nigeria, previously rendered yaws-free by mass treatment campaigns, have also experienced a sharp rise in the incidence of venereal syphilis. This increase in venereal syphilis may represent a decline of herd immunity to yaws, and thereby to syphilis.

Endemic syphilis is also transmitted by non-venereal contact among children. In contrast to yaws, transmission of infection by contaminated drinking vessels may be more common than by direct contact with infectious lesions, and the disease tends to be familial with spread of infection from children to adults rather than to the community in general. Endemic syphilis lesions are virtually indistinguishable from early yaws, and the two diseases may occur at different times in the same population but not in the same person. Venereal syphilis can be acquired by children through social contact with adults suffering from venereal syphilis and then be spread by non-venereal, person-to-person contact if the level of sanitation and personal hygiene are low.

The Sahelian nations of Mali, Niger, Burkina Faso, and Senegal have reported dramatic increases in the number of cases of endemic syphilis. The disease is also prevalent among the nomadic tribes of the Arabian peninsula, where late complications such as osteoperiostitis predominate.

Several variants of endemic syphilis are recognized by their geographical distribution. Although each is caused by the same organism, different strains of endemic *T. pallidum* and different factors modify dis-

Table 1 *Major features of the treponematoses*

Feature	Venereal syphilis	Endemic syphilis	Yaws	Pinta
Organism*	*T. pallidum*	*T. pallidum*	*T. pertenue*	*T. carateum*
Age of infection	15–10	2–10	5–15	10–30
Occurrence	Worldwide	Africa; Middle East	Africa, South America, Oceania, Asia	Central and South America
Climate	All	Dry, arid	Warm, humid	Warm, rural
Transmission				
Direct:				
Venereal	Common	Rare	No	No
Non-venereal	Rare	Rare	Common	Common
Congenital	Yes	Unproven	No	No
Indirect:				
Contaminated utensils	Rare	Common	Rare	No
Insects	No	No	Rare	No
Reservoir of infection	Adults	Infectious and latent cases	Infectious and latent cases; ?non-human primates	Infectious cases
Ratio infectious:latent cases	1:3	1:2	1:3–5	?
Late complications				
Skin	+	+	+	+
Bone, cartilage	+	+	+	No
Neurological	+	Unproven	No	No
Cardiovascular	+	Unproven	No	No

*DNA homology tests detect no difference between strains of *T. pallidum* and *T. pentenue*.

ease expression. Examples are *bejel* of the Eastern Mediterranean and North Africa; *njovera* or *dichuchwa* of Africa; and the now extinct *sibbens* of Scotland, *radesyge* of Norway, and *skerjevo* of Yugoslavia. *Bejel* is the only type of endemic syphilis still prevalent. It is found in mainly seminomadic people living in the Saharan regions of Africa. Improved standards of living, better medical care, and mass penicillin treatment campaigns have greatly reduced disease prevalence.

Pinta is restricted to the Western hemisphere and is found today only in remote parts of Central and South America, principally in the semiarid region of the Tepalcatepec Basin of southern Mexico and focal areas of Columbia, Peru, Ecuador, and Venezuela. Active surveillance and treatment programmes greatly decreased the prevalence of pinta.

Pathenogenesis

The lesion of yaws and the other treponematoses are largely due to the immune response of the host to the treponeme. As far as can be determined, none of these treponemes carries or produces toxic substances. They have the ability to invade living cells without causing apparent injury. Cell destruction and tissue damage are probably due to the action of immune cells that injure normal tissue in the process of killing treponemes.

Host immunity reaches its highest level after several months of infection, just before disseminated lesions heal and latency begins. Thereafter the host is immune to reinfection and is not contagious, but since not all treponemes are killed, infectious lesions may reappear as immunity wanes over time. Most yaws patients experience two or three infectious relapses during the first 5 years of infection.

In venereal and possibly endemic syphilis, infection is systemic and late lesions may develop in any organ or tissue of the body. In yaws, *T. pertenue* produce lesions only in skin and osseous tissue, although it is certain that periodically the organism spread systemically; *T. carateum* resides only in the skin. This peculiar tissue tropism is unexplained. It is probably an inherent property of the treponeme, acting in concert with climatic factors.

Clinical features

The clinical course of yaws and endemic syphilis resembles that of venereal syphilis with division of infection into primary, secondary, and tertiary or late stages, each stage separated by a quiescent or latent period. None of the endemic treponematoses, however, progresses by these clearly defined stages of infection as does venereal syphilis. In yaws, lesions are described as early, comprising those of the primary (initial) and secondary (disseminated) stage, and late, which correspond to the tertiary stage.

The initial lesion in yaws usually appears on the extremities after an incubation period of 3 to 5 weeks. Characteristically it is a papule; a painless lesion which appears at the site of infection, enlarges, forming a raspberry-like, vegetative lesion called a papilloma. The papilloma is round to oval, elevated and not indurated, ranging in size from 1 to 3 cm in diameter. The surface teems with spirochaetes and is often covered by a thin yellow crust, which is easily removed. The papilloma may ulcerate as it enlarges and becomes secondarily infected with other microorganisms. Lymph nodes draining the initial lesion may enlarge and become tender but systemic symptoms are rare.

Secondary or disseminated papillomata appear after 2 to 6 months, often without an intervening latent period, on the skin of moist areas such as the axillae, joint flexures, genitalia, and the gluteal cleft (Fig. 1). They also occur on the soles and palms and, because they are tender, may interfere with gait and use of the hands. Papillomata in different stages of development persist for 6 to 8 months and heal without scar formation unless they become secondarily infected. Despite the size and number of lesions, children with generalized papillomata experience little discomfort or other constitutional symptoms.

Slightly raised, scaly, pigmented, macular yaws lesions measuring from 1 to 4 cm in diameter commonly occur when the climate is dry and arid. These lesions have the same distribution as papillomata and may appear together with lesions of different morphology in the same patient (maculopapular yaws).

The periosteum and osseous tissue of the bones of the extremities are frequently inflamed during early yaws, causing swelling, night-pain, and tenderness. Painful osteoperiostitis of the legs affecting mainly the tibia and fibula is especially common. Scaly, tender, hyperkeratotic lesions of the palms and soles also occur and may be incapacitating. Hyperkeratotic and bone lesions are not contagious, and macular lesions are only minimally so.

One or more relapses of secondary-type lesions usually occur during the first 5 years of infection, each separated by a period of latency. Late yaws lesions occur thereafter in about 10 per cent of untreated cases.

Late yaws lesions are not infectious because they contain few treponemes. Cutaneous plaques produce atrophic scars; subcutaneous, granulomatous nodules erode skin and produce deep ulcers that destroy underlying tissue and disfigure. Hyperkeratotic palmar and plantar yaws are incapacitating and often prevent the use of hands, or the ability to walk normally. The weight is placed on the sides of the feet, which produces a gait much like that of a crab ('crab' yaws; Fig. 2).

The granulomas of late yaws have a histological appearance like the gumma of syphilis. These proliferative lesions may involve the palate and destroy the soft tissues of the nose, causing a terrible disfiguration called gangosa (Fig. 3). Gummatous periostitis of the skull, fingers, and long bones is erosive and often retards or stops growth. Active periostitis is occasionally found in young and middle-aged adults who had yaws in childhood.

The clinical differentiation of yaws from endemic syphilis may not be possible. The initial lesions of endemic syphilis usually appear at the mucocutaneous borders of the mouth or on the oral mucous membranes (mucous patches) as the result of transmission by contaminated drinking vessels. Although mucous patches are very rare in yaws, ulceropapillomata around the mouth are common, and the axillary and anogenital papillomata of yaws are indistinguishable from the condylomata lata of venereal and endemic syphilis. Late ulceronodules and osteoperiostitis are seen in late endemic syphilis, but cardiovascular and neurologic complications do not occur or are extremely rare.

The lesions of pinta are easily differentiated from yaws and syphilis. The initial papule appears on the skin of the extremities and enlarges slowly over a period of several weeks or months to form an erythematous plaque. Satellite papules form at the edge of the lesion and undergo a similar type of evolution. The plaques coalesce to form violaceous, pigmented plaques that, in several years, slowly dispigment from lighter shades of blue to white, leaving atrophic depigmented scars.

Fig. 1 Early ulceropapillomatous yaws.

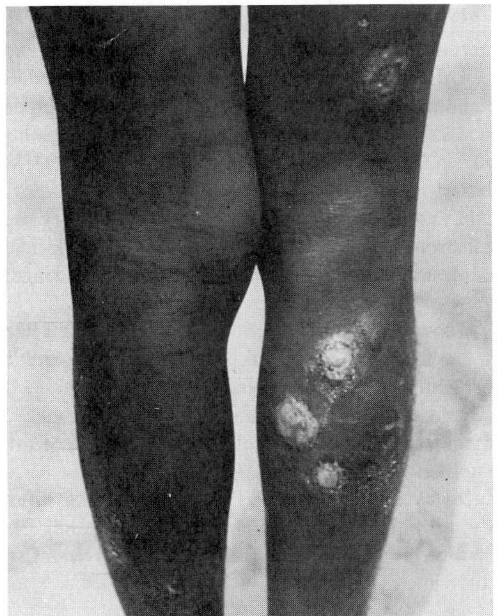

Ulceronodular skin lesions of yaws and endemic syphilis resemble tropical ulcers. Yaws lesions are not as painful, necrotic, nor as deep as tropical ulcers, which are usually singular and restricted to the lower one-third of the leg.

Plantar warts are frequently confused with plantar papillomata of yaws and both conditions may occur in the same patient.

Diagnosis

The diagnosis of yaws is made by a combination of clinical assessment, of positive dark-ground examination of lesions, and of reactive serological tests for syphilis. Early and late yaws should be diagnosed with

Fig. 2 Planter papillomata with hyperkeratotic, macular, early plantar yaws ('crab' yaws); these lesions are painful.

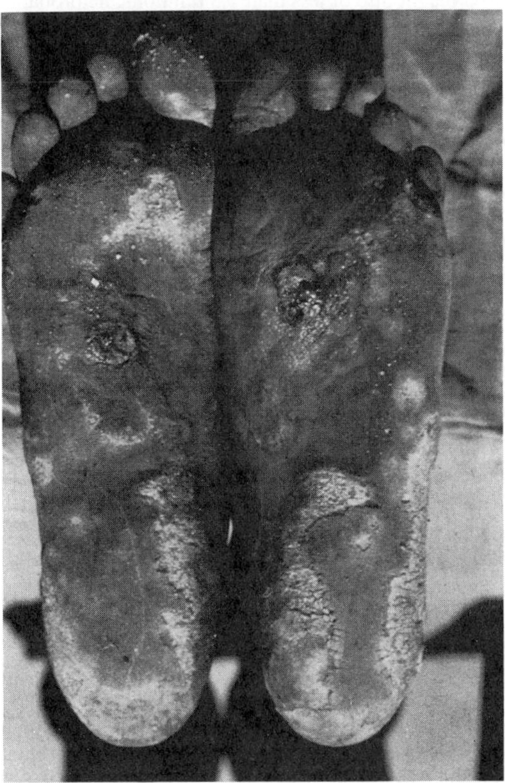

Fig. 3 Gangosa (rhinopharyngitis mutilans) of endemic syphilis and yaws in an adolescent child.

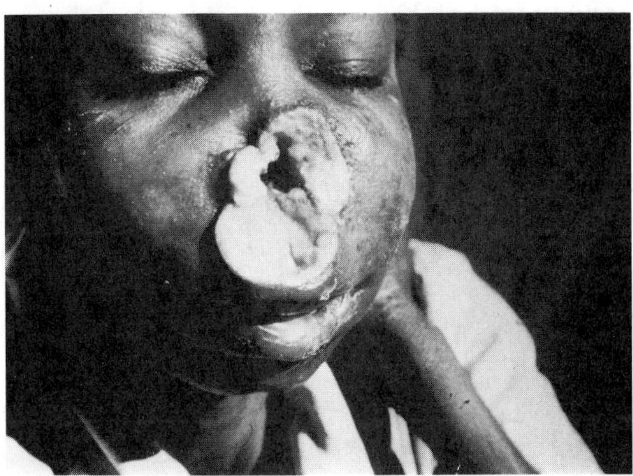

caution unless there is evidence that the patient resides or has lived in a yaws-endemic area.

The diagnosis of early yaws, or endemic syphilis, is not difficult in endemic areas where the disease has existed for centuries. The local population in such areas is usually well informed about the different types and characteristics of yaws lesions. The most difficult diagnostic problem arises when a person who had yaws as a child emigrates to an area of the world where the disease never existed. Such a person usually has reactive serological tests for syphilis and may have a few atrophic scars suggestive of earlier infection. What are the chances that this patient has or has had venereal syphilis? Should he be treated for latent yaws or syphilis?

The patient's social and medical history should be carefully reviewed. Clinical findings suggestive of old yaws (scars, inactive tibial periostitis), and the absence of stigmata of congenital and venereal syphilis support the diagnosis of inactive or treated yaws.

If the patient has a reagin titre of less than 1:8 dilutions, he probably does not have active latent yaws or syphilis. If he received at least one therapeutic dose of long-acting penicillin in his native country during a yaws campaign, he requires no further treatment. On the other hand, if the patient is a contact of a case of infectious venereal syphilis, he should be treated as potentially infected with syphilis, because *T. pallidum* occasionally superinfects people who have had yaws as children. If treatment is given, the patient should receive a certificate stating the drug and dosage used and the results of his serological tests for future reference. Otherwise, some of these patients will be retreated unnecessarily by each new physician they consult.

Treatment and prevention

Long-acting benzylpenicillin given by intramuscular injection is the recommended treatment for all the endemic treponematoses. The preparation used in previous mass treatment campaigns was penicillin aluminimum monostearate (**PAM**), but benzathine penicillin is currently recommended because it is longer acting and more readily available than is PAM. Active infections and non-infectious cases should be given 1.2 mega units in a single intramuscular injection; children under 10 years of age receive 0.6 mega units. Patients allergic to penicillin may be given tetracycline or erythromycin, 500 mg by mouth four times daily for 2 weeks; children under 10 years of age should be given erythromycin in dosages adjusted for their age.

Prevention of yaws in a community requires elimination of the reservoir of infection by penicillin treatment. This reservoir comprises both incubating and early latent cases, the latter being the more important because of their tendency to relapse with infectious lesions. The experience of the yaws mass-treatment campaigns indicated that the entire population should receive penicillin when the prevalence of clinically active yaws was over 10 per cent in the community (total mass treatment); that active cases, all children under 15, and obvious adult contacts of infectious cases should be treated when the prevalence of clinically active yaws was between 5 to 10 per cent (juvenile mass treatment); and that only active cases, household, and other obvious contacts need be treated when less than 4 per cent of the population has clinically active yaws. Contacts receive the same dose of penicillin as active cases.

The yaws control programme sponsored by the World Health Organization attempted to create an ever-enlarging yaws-free area by carefully planned and conducted mass-treatment campaigns. The consolidation phase of these campaigns required long-term, expensive, active surveillance for yaws to prevent its reintroduction or resurgence in a community. The costs of maintaining these programmes increased enormously, and the resulting curtailment of control campaigns permitted a resurgence of the disease in many parts of the world. Control programmes should now be fully integrated into the primary health-care system.

REFERENCES

Guthe, T. (1969). Clinical, serological and epidemiological features of framboesia tropica (yaws) and its control in rural communities. *Acta Dermatologica-Venerologia, Stockholm*, **49,** 343–68.

Hackett, C.J. and Loewenthal, L.J.A. (1960). *Differential diagnosis of yaws*, World Health Organization, Geneva.

Meheus, A. and Antal, G.M. (1992). The endemic treponematoses: not yet eradicated. *World Health Statistical Quarterly*, **45,** 228–37.

Noordhock, G.T. and van Embden, J.D.A. (1991). Yaws, an endemic treponematosis reconsidered in the HIV era. *European Journal of Clinical Microbiology and Infectious Diseases*, **10,** 4–5.

Perine, P.L., Hopkins, D.R., Niemel, P.L.A., St. John, R.K., Causse, C., and Antal, G.M. (1984). *Handbook of endemic treponematoses.* World Health Organization, Geneva.

7.11.34 Syphilis

D.J.M. WRIGHT and G. W. CSONKA

Definition

Venereal syphilis is a systemic contagious disease of great chronicity caused by *Treponema pallidum* and capable of being congenitally transmitted. The natural host is man. It has an incubation period of around 3 weeks at the end of which a primary sore develops at the site of inoculation; usually on the genitalia, associated with regional lymphadenitis. In most patients this is followed by the secondary bacteraemic stage characterized by a symmetrical rash, generalized lymphadenopathy, and other lesions. After a latent period of many years this is terminated in 40 per cent by a destructive and potentially dangerous late stage which may involve the skin, mucous membranes, skeleton, CNS, eyes, hearing, and above all the aorta. Occasionally other organs are also affected. Any of these stages may be absent or so unapparent as to be overlooked.

The introduction of penicillin has profoundly changed the course and prognosis of syphilis and has made it the most curable of all sexually transmitted diseases if treated early.

Distribution

Venereal syphilis, unlike non-venereal syphilis has a worldwide distribution and knows no climatic, racial, or geographical barriers.

Bacterial taxonomy

T. pallidum is a bacterium which belongs to the Treponema family and causes not only venereal syphilis but the non-venereal endemic childhood syphilis, bejel and njovera. Other pathogenic treponemes include *T. pertenue* (yaws) and *T. carateum* (pinta), *T. cuniculi* found in rabbits and *T. fribourg-blanc* (in monkeys).

There are a number of non-pathogenic treponemes such as *T. denticola, T. microdentium* and *T. macrodentium* in the mouth. They are difficult to distinguish from *T. pallidum* and for that reason dark-field examination of mouth lesions should be avoided because of the danger of misdiagnosis.

Other treponemes of low pathogenicity reside in the genital tract like *T. balanitides* which can together with fusiform bacili under anaerobic conditions superinfect genital lesions producing 'fusospirochaetosis'. It is likely that Reiter's spirochaete *(T. phagedenis),* originally thought to cause syphilis, is a member of this group. These treponemes differ from *T. pallidum* and are unlikely to be confused.

Molecular differences have now separated the gut spirochaetes from the treponema family, forming a variety of new species including the Brachyspira and Serpulina group. The latter includes *S. hyodysenteriae,* the causative agent of swine dysentery.

Table 1 *Borrelia and treponema compared*

Characteristic	Borrelia	Treponema
Length (mm)	7–24	4–19
Width (mm)	0.2–0.5	0.15–0.3
Wavelength (mm)	1.7–3.3	0.5–1.8
Number of flagella	7–30*	1–9
Cytoplasmic tubules	–	+
Mode of division	septum	constriction
Romanowsky stain	+	–
Arthropod borne	+	–

*Seven flagella have been found in isolates of *Borrelia burgdorferi*.

T. pallidum is a delicate, motile spiral organism, 6 to 15 μm long and 0.15 μm wide which renders it below the level of resolution of light microscopy and hence the need for dark-field or phase contrast illumination. It has an outer membrane, an electron-dense layer, and a cytoplasmic membrane. As with other bacteria, the cell wall has a trilaminar structure, the inner membrane constituting a cytoplasmic membrane, while between the outer two layers there are axial filaments, structurally analogous to bacterial flagella, which wind around the axis of the organism and may be responsible for the motility of *T. pallidum.* All treponemes have not more than nine axial filaments, which distinguishes treponemes from borrelia (Table 1). *T. pallidum* has the unique ability to bend in the middle to form a V-shape, if suspended in a medium of low viscosity. Motility does not necessarily indicate viability as mobile *T. pallidum* have been observed after they have been retained for 90 days in capillary tubes. *T. pallidum* may remain infective for up to a week in 'survival media' and depending on the nature of the media, show limited multiplication; however, attempts at reproducible subculture of the microbe have to date been signally unsuccessful. Low concentrations of oxygen (between 3 and 5 per cent) may enhance survival. In practice, *T. pallidum* is propagated by infecting rabbits intratesticularly, harvesting the spirochaetes from the resulting lesions, and then maintaining the strains by further reinoculation. Strains may also be preserved for many years by holding them in liquid nitrogen or at −70 °C. In this way, a supply of spirochaetes is available for use in serological tests and for research.

Experimental inoculation of *T. pallidum* into man or animals, show that the organism divides every 30 to 32 h. This multiplication rate indicates that the approximate infective dose of bacteria lies between 10^6 and 10^7 organisms, giving an average incubation period of 3 weeks. The cell wall contains peptidoglycan in the inner layer of the bacterial membrane accounting for the microbes susceptibility to penicillin. The phospholipids in the outer membrane, of which cardiolipin is the most prominent hapten, provides the antigenic basis for the synthetically substituted VDRL used as a serological test for syphilis. Extracts of other components of the cell wall, probably other surface membrane proteins, have not yielded more specific tests than those currently available. A particular disappointment has been the flagella antigen, which non-specifically, react with antibodies found in most known sera. The antibodies have been raised presumably against flagella antigens of commensal spirochaetes as well as other bacteria. The flagella antigen has not only failed to protect against re-infection but does not even inhibit motility possibly because the bacteria tend to be covered by an amorphous mucopolysaccharide outer layer which is immunologically inert.

Origin of syphilis

Clinical differences between treponematosis have been explained as an adaptation of the organism to changing climatic factors, especially humidity and temperature and improvement in hygiene, with wearing of clothes and less frequent intimate contacts between children. Yaws is found throughout the tropical belt, while pinta was forced to retreat into remote indigenous communities in South and Central America. The non-venereal childhood syphilis such as bejel and similar conditions was found in more temperate climes such as in the Middle East, Yugoslavia, British Isles, Scandinavia, and South Africa. The lack of congenital transmission of these venereal treponematoses arose because they were essentially childhood infections and by the time these children were old enough to have their own offspring, the disease had become non-infectious. The treponeme which caused venereal syphilis was perhaps an adaptation to wearing clothes and was therefore obliged to seek shelter in the protected, warm, and moist regions of the genitalia and so became a sexually transmitted infection. It spread throughout the world as an adult disease and because there appears to be no solid cross-immunity, may exist side by side with the non-venereal treponematoses.

The principal objection is that the adaptive theory fails to explain why *T. pallidum sensu stricto,* unlike the other treponematoses, involves the central nervous system, aorta, and visceral organs and why, at the end of the fifteenth century the virulent venereal form swept through Europe and Asia and eventually became the milder modern syphilis. The alternative idea that Columbus introduced this new disease from the Caribbean islands, is usually termed the Columbian theory. In this theory, venereal syphilis is considered a disease apart from other treponematoses. If the Columbian theory is rejected, the sudden emergence of virulent syphilis still remains to be explained.

What is certain is that there are no certain descriptions of syphilis before this time. The finding of skeletons, with long bone lesions compatible with syphilis, centuries before the 15th century epidemic of syphilis, is at the best speculative, while the lack of such skeletons from America makes the relationship with the coincidental discovery of America and the advent of 'new world' syphilis even more doubtful.

Until genomic differences in the variety of known treponemes are identified which in turn will lead to molecular dating, based on natural mutation rates of these differences, the flood of ink on how syphilis began, will continue to flow. What can be said is that morphologically, serologically, and metabolically indistinguishable treponemes have been isolated from monkeys *(T. fribourg blanc)* and those that progressively cause a more visceral forms of human diseases—Pinta *(T. carateum),* Yaws *(T. pallidum* subs. *pertenue)* and endemic syphilis *(T. pallidum* subs. *endemicans).*

The recognition of the contagious nature of the disease was recorded in 1530 by Fracastro. His poem *syphilis sive morbus gallicus,* was an advertising 'puff' for the syphilis nostrum, gum guaicum and was rewarded with a medical professorship. Klebs ultimately proved the infectivity of syphilis by reproducing syphilic lesions following the inoculation of syphilitic tissue into rabbits. The use of a prolonged Giemsa stain, allowed Hoffman finally to identify the treponemes in 1905. Clinically, the pervading idea of infectivity has been extended to divide the disease into infectious and non-infectious phases, rather than Ricord's older classification, which staged the progressive complications of syphilis.

Epidemiology

TRANSMISSION, EFFECT OF HIV EPIDEMIC

Sexual transmission is the rule in adult patients. The untreated patient remains infective for 4 years after acquiring the infection. Asexual transmission by close contact with an open lesion of early acquired or congenital syphilis is rare. Other unusual modes of transmission are by direct blood transfusion with blood from an infectious individual and contact with infected fomites. Congenital syphilis still remains a problem, except in Northern Europe.

INCIDENCE

There has been a steady decline in the incidence of syphilis in the West since the 1850s, interrupted only by major wars (Fig. 1). Since 1940 there has been a 99 per cent drop in admissions of general paresis of the insane (GPI) and congenital syphilis in the United States, and the trend is similar in the United Kingdom and Europe. There has also been a sharp reduction in all other forms of late syphilis. Gumma have almost disappeared. Early syphilis has not declined to the same degree since the Second World War. In the United States, syphilis reached a low in 1956, with 6576 reported cases but by 1992 had risen to 83 902 infectious acquired cases. A similar pattern is also found in most European countries. During the 1970s and 1980s there was a steady increase in the number of cases of early syphilis. This had been largely due to homosexual practices. In 1980, 58 per cent of cases of syphilis in the United Kingdom were in homosexuals.

Since that time the United Kingdom and American rates have diverged. The appearance of AIDS and the national programmes for 'safe sex' has resulted in the annual number of cases of infectious syphilis falling to 337 in the United Kingdom in 1993, most of the recent infections being acquired heterosexually abroad. In the United States, however, despite the fall in the number of homosexual males infected, the number of cases of syphilis have continued to rise, especially in the underprivileged Afro-American and Hispanic community and among the HIV infected drug abusers. By 1992, there were approximately 34 000 cases of primary and secondary syphilis and 3850 cases of congenital syphilis in children under the age of 2 years, compared with 1986, when only 57 such cases were recorded in the United States. The failure of the Public Health Service in the United States to cope is reflected in the resurgence of congenital syphilis. In other parts of the world, notably in the Far East, infected prostitutes may play a central role in the spread of early syphilis. Estimates by WHO suggest that there are 10 to 20 million cases of syphilis each year.

A fashion for use of spectinomycin, an antibiotic which has no effect on incubating syphilis, for the primary treatment of penicillinase producing *Neisseria gonorrhoea* is unlikely to have made a major contribution to the rising incidence of syphilis. It could be argued that a reduced number of cases of syphilis might be seen, because a shorter follow-up might be required, than if the conventional penicillin treatment had been given.

THE CHANGING CLINICAL PRESENTATION OF SYPHILIS

There is some clinical evidence that syphilis is becoming milder and less typical. This has been especially noted in neurosyphilis and the virtual disappearance of the gumma. The widespread use of antibiotics for unrelated conditions may be responsible. This is supported by finding that meningovascular syphilis has not shown the dramatic decrease of GPI and tabes dorsalis, possibly because the last two conditions take many more years to develop, giving cumulative chances of antibiotics being given. It is also possible that the disease is tending to become milder and less typical as a result of 'natural' changes which appear to have started long before the antibiotic era. For whatever reasons, syphilis is apparently becoming clinically less clear-cut. Its exclusion by serology and other tests becomes more important in patients attending the dermatologist, neurologist, ophthalmologist, the ENT specialist, or cardiologist with conditions of uncertain pedigree.

The advent of AIDS has led to a re-examination of the progression and manifestations of concomitant syphilis. Although a variety of unusual syphilitic rashes have been described in association with HIV infections, all of them are recorded in the older literature. The suggestions that there might be an increase in syphilitic meningovascular relapse in patients with HIV infections, again may reflect the natural history of syphilis, since approximately 20 per cent of patients with early syphilis have a pleocytosis in the CSF. If these patients are untreated, about one-fifth develop neurosyphilis. The high prevalence of syphilis in HIV patients leads to an apparent rather than a real increase in syphilis complications. Holtom, in California found that in patients partially treated for syphilis with concomitant HIV infections, about 9 per cent developed a pleocytosis and 1 per cent then developed neurological disease. Unlike mycobacterial infections where unusual presentations of tuberculosis occur in patients with AIDS, the presentation of early neurosyphilis seems to be characteristic of the disease. This is possibly because the vasculitis of syphilis is not due to the cellular immune response but to the adherence of the spirochaete to the endothelial layer of the blood vessel. The blood vessel first becomes more permeable and subsequently there is proliferation of this layer. Simultaneously, the spirochaete induces a cellular infiltrate. These changes lead to endarteritis, which is the hallmark of the disease. What is true is that syphilitic relapses do not occur despite the potential for the persistence of spirochaetes (see below) and that benzathine penicillin G is less effective in eliminating spirochaetes (see below) in patients with altered immunity. However, doubt has been cast as to whether eradication of spirochaetes always occurs in the non-immunecompromised patient. Wilner and Brody found that one third of the patients with a syphilitic encephalitis (GPI) who had been followed for 30 years, developed neurological signs at the end of the period, despite having had 'adequate' penicillin therapy. Only 7 per cent of the non-syphilitic control group of demented patients, evinced new neurological signs. These were presumably due to cerebrovascular degenerative disease. Even in the pre-AIDS era, Rothenberg, when he reviewed the efficacy of penicillin in the treatment of neurosyphilis, found that it was not always effective. Lastly, laboratory experiments show that it is more likely that syphilis has a deleterious effect on the progression of AIDS rather than the reverse.

Fig. 1 Incidence rhythms of venereal diseases (1850–1970). The peaks tend to relate to the aftermaths of wars: (1850) Crimea, (1880) Afghan campaigns, (1900) Boer War, (1918) First World War—gap, (1946) Second World War. Figures for venereal disease relate mainly to syphilis until 1915; thereafter figures relate to gonorrhoea to show underlying 20–25-year generation cycles of upsurge in sexually-transmitted diseases.

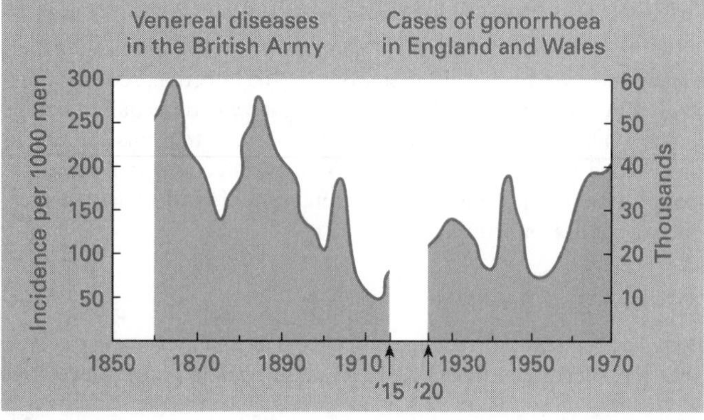

SEX AND RACE

Early syphilis is less florid in women than men and is almost asymptomatic during pregnancy. Cardiovascular syphilis is at least twice as common in men than women where it is more severe and appears earlier. Neurosyphilis is always more common in men than women. The reasons for these differences are not known.

Caucasians suffer more commonly from neurosyphilis than Negroes and they in turn are much more prone to develop cardiovascular syphilis than Caucasians.

INFECTIVITY

The estimated figure for infectivity varies but is commonly assumed to be around 50 per cent for both homosexual and heterosexual patients. After a single exposure the figure is nearer 25 per cent.

SOME CONTROL MEASURES

The main reason for increased case identification is the more intensive use of serological tests for syphilis. Another valuable control measure is contact tracing, which varies greatly in different countries, but should be standard practice everywhere. Its use across international borders should be developed with proper safeguards to preserve confidentiality. Other measures which should prove valuable are the education of the young without inducing anxiety, the education of doctors, and the encouragement of regular check-ups of high-risk individuals, such as homosexual men and prostitutes. A more controversial suggestion is to treat contacts of infectious syphilis epidemiologically in certain situations, e.g. promiscuous individuals, known defaulters, and those who may infect their regular consort if not treated.

These measures can be expected to uncover up to 75 per cent of all cases of syphilis.

Persistence of treponemal forms

Persistence of *T. pallidum*-like forms in the CSF, aqueous humour, lymph nodes, and other tissues in penicillin-treated patients with late or late latent syphilis has been reported from several centres. The same phenomenon is the basis for relapses after penicillin treatment in borreliosis (see Chapters 7.11.30, 7.11.31). In some cases, the forms may have been non-pathogenic treponemes or artifacts, but in others rabbit inoculation confirmed them to be pathogenic *T. pallidum.* These treponemes appeared to be fully sensitive to penicillin in animal experiments. The survival *in vitro* of *T. pallidum* in media containing high concentrations of penicillin, probably relates to the poor quality of the media which prevented replication rather than a lack of bactericidal activity on the part of penicillin. The first report of persistence of *T. pallidum* after treatment deemed to be adequate, appeared in France and subsequently in the United States, yet more than 30 years later, many authorities do not believe that the finding has been fully proven. As these cases are very infrequently reported there appears to be no need to change our ideas about treatment or prognosis.

The central paradox of untreated syphilis is how the treponeme survives despite the strong cellular and humoral response. However syphilis progresses, reinfection or reinoculation produces a lesion depending on the clinical stage of the disease the patient has reached. If the patient has passed into the secondary stage with a maculopapular rash, the reinoculation lesion is a papule, whereas, if the patient had advanced to the tertiary phase, a gumma would appear at the inoculation site. Whether, in the Tuskegee study, the absence of any complication of syphilis in approximately half the patients after 40 years follow-up represents immunity with eradication of the treponeme, remains unknown.

THE NATURAL COURSE OF UNTREATED SYPHILIS

T. pallidum penetrates the abraded skin and intact mucous membrane. Within hours it becomes disseminated via the bloodstream and lymphatics and is beyond any effective local treatment. The incubation period is traditionally given as 9 to 90 days but in practice it is around 3 weeks (range, 2 to 6 weeks). The time depends on the size of the inoculum, sexual practice, and hygienic measures. A single treponeme leads to the longest incubation period. The primary lesion develops at the site of contact and heals in 2 to 6 weeks. In a proportion of patients a secondary stage appears 6 weeks after the primary lesion has healed but there may be an overlap of the healing primary and the onset of the secondary stage. In some cases the period between these stages can be prolonged to several months. The main characteristic of the secondary stage is a generalized, symmetrical, painless, and non-irritating rash. In about 20 per cent of cases infectious relapses occur during the following year (range, 1 to 4 years). In the rest, the latent symptomatic period follows and may persist for life in at least 60 per cent. In 30 to 40 per cent a third late destructive stage develops. Its more benign form involves only the skin, mucous membranes, and bones. In the serious form the CNS, aorta, and other internal organs are affected. The major events are shown in Figs 2 and 3.

The course of untreated syphilis has been investigated in the now famous Oslo study (1891–1951) in which 1978 patients with early syphilis were left untreated and studied. Approximately 1000 patients were finally analysed with the following results: relapsing secondary syphilis was observed in 25 per cent; cardiovascular syphilis was diagnosed in 10.4 per cent; CNS lesions in 6.5 per cent; and gumma of the skin, mucous membranes, or bone in 16 per cent. A total of 23 per cent died as a direct result of syphilis. Serious late syphilitic complications were twice as common in men that women.

This study is open to several criticisms. The study was completed before all the patients had died and there was an insufficient number of autopsies (24 per cent). Thus some late complications may have escaped inclusion. The study took place at a time when many patients died young, mainly due to tuberculosis, and once again late complications may have been underestimated. Furthermore, some of the patients are now thought to have suffered from non-venereal endemic syphilis which was not uncommon in Norway at that period, and finally some of the patients were apparently reinfected, so that the study is not the natural history of one infection. Lastly, there was a non-randomized selection of patients and a lack of controls. The Oslo study is therefore of greater historical interest than of practical value in predicting the fate of patients with untreated syphilis.

In the more recent Tuskegee study of Negro males with latent syphilis (1932–72), it was found that one-third died of late syphilis, mostly due to cardiovascular lesions. In postmortem investigations, aortitis was present in 40 to 60 per cent, far in excess of the clinical diagnosis, supporting the view that the cardiovascular lesion is the most important

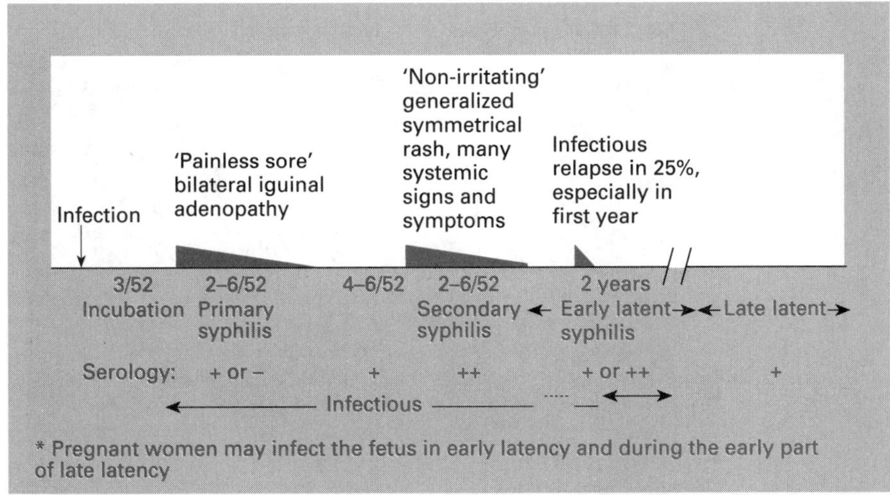

Fig. 2 The course of untreated early acquired syphilis.

and lethal late syphilitic complication. Though the death rate directly attributed to late syphilis is round 30 per cent in several studies, the incidence may be higher as there is some evidence that the patients are more prone to other diseases including hypertension. In all the more recent reports the incidence of CNS syphilis and gumma is much lower than in the Oslo study, suggesting that a change is taking place in the evolution of the disease.

Clinical features

PRIMARY SYPHILIS

The first sign is a small, painless papule which rapidly ulcerates. The ulcer (chancre) is usually solitary, round or oval, painless, and often indurated (Fig. 4). It is surrounded by a bright red margin. It is not usually secondarily infected, a feature of all open syphilitic lesions of any stage. The reason for this might repay investigation. *T. pallidum* can be demonstrated in the serum from the sore which is easily obtained after slightly abraiding the base. In heterosexual men the common sites are the coronal sulcus, the glans, and inner surface of the prepuce but may be found on the shaft of the penis and beyond. In homosexual men the ulcer is usually present in the anal canal, less commonly in the mouth (Fig. 5) and genitalia. In women most chancres occur on the vulva, the labia, and more rarely the cervix where they are liable to be overlooked.

Extragenital chancres usually involve the lips where they become large and associated with some oedema. Other sites are the mouth, buttocks, and fingers. The regional lymph nodes are invariably enlarged a few days after the appearance of the chancre and with genital sores they are bilaterally involved. The lymph nodes are painless, discrete, firm, and not fixed to surrounding tissues.

Atypical primary sores are not uncommon and depend on the size of the inoculum and the immunological status of the patient; thus a small inoculum usually produces a small atypical ulcer or papule and looks trivial. This may also be the case in patients who had previously treated syphilis and the lesion may be dark-field negative.

Histologically the chancre shows perivascular infiltration with plasma cells and histiocytes, capillary proliferation, and obliterative endarteritis

Fig. 3 The course of untreated late acquired syphilis. Asymptomatic neurosyphilis is present in 20 per cent and 20 per cent of these develop clinical neurosyphilis. Cardiovascular syphilis starts subclinically many years earlier and when clinically apparent, it is in fact in an advanced state. Prognosis: gumma heals spontaneously in a few years. Cardiovascular syphilis is usually fatal without treatment. Neurosyphilis: general paresis has a poor prognosis without treatment, meningovascular syphilis commonly responds well to penicillin, tabes progresses slowly but penicillin has no obvious influence. Overall mortality of untreated syphilis: 20 to 30 per cent.

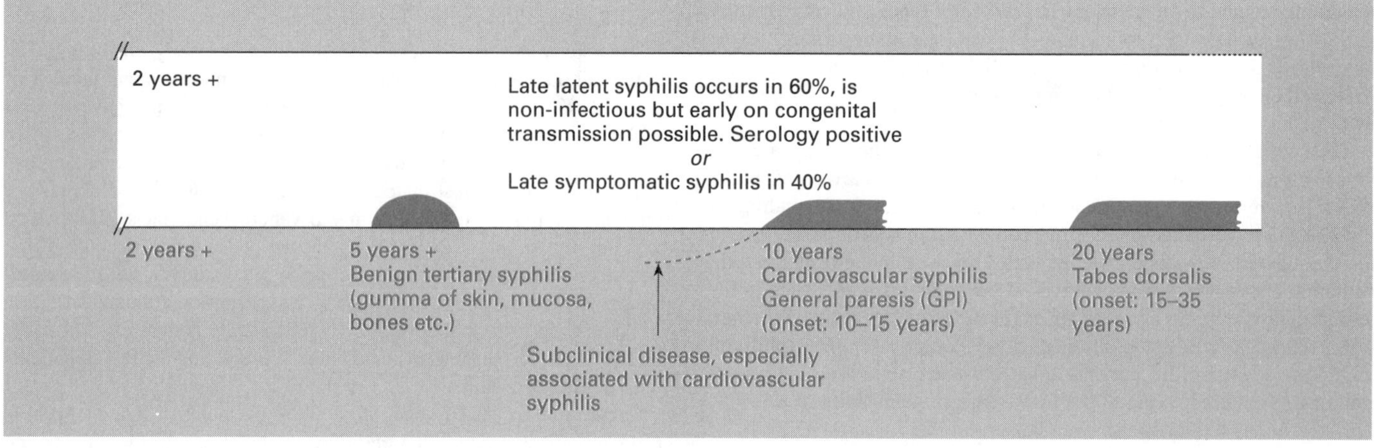

Fig. 4 Large primary sore. Note the even shape and the absence of secondary infection.

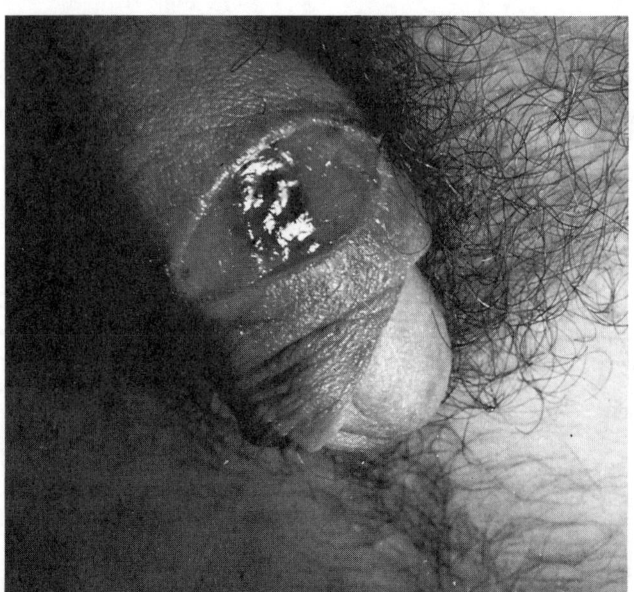

Fig. 5 Healing primary sore of the lip with some induration around it.

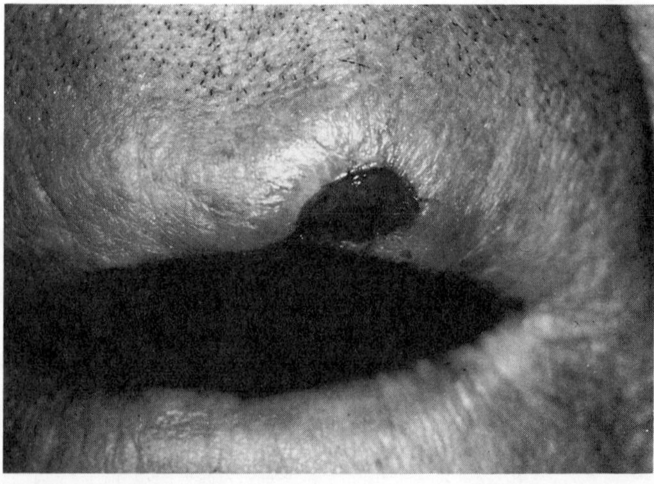

and periarteritis. The affected lymph nodes contain numerous treponemes, a depletion of lymphocytes, follicular hyperplasia, and histiocytic infiltration. If *T. pallidum* cannot be recovered from the primary sore, it may be possible to demonstrate it from the needle aspirate of the regional lymph node.

DIFFERENTIAL DIAGNOSIS

All genital sores must be regarded as syphilitic until proven otherwise, especially when they are solitary and painless.

Genital lesions which must be differentiated from primary syphilis are:

1. Genital herpes (see Chapter 21.3), which is much more common than syphilis in either sex. It is characterized by a crop of painful or irritating vesicles which develop into shallow erosions. In the first attack there is also painful inguinal adenitis.
2. Traumatic sores. These are painful, irregular erosions which may become secondarily infected.
3. Erosive balanitis. These are inflammatory, irregular erosions which may become purulent in the uncircumcised.
4. Fixed drug eruptions. These are macules or occasionally ulcers following various drugs, especially tetracyclines.
5. Chancroid. This is mostly seen in the tropics and presents as painful, superficial, 'soft chancre', which is often multiple with painful suppurative regional adenitis.

Other conditions which may have to be considered are scabies, Behçet's syndrome, donovanosis, and lymphogranuloma venereum.

Secondary syphilis

The lesions are numerous, variable, and affect many systems. Inevitably there is a symmetrical, non-irritating rash and generalized painless lymphadenopathy. Constitutional symptoms are mild or absent; they include headaches, which are often nocturnal, malaise, slight fever, and aches in joints and muscles. The rash is commonly macular, pale red, and sometimes so faint as to be appreciated only in tangential light. It may be papular and sometimes squamous (Fig. 6). Pustular and necrotic rashes are rarely seen in temperate climates but still occur in tropical regions. The later the secondary rash develops, the more exuberant it becomes. The distribution of the rash can be of great diagnostic help. It usually covers the trunk and proximal limbs, but when it is seen on the palms, soles, and the face, syphilis should always be high on the list of probable causes (Figs. 7 and 8). In warm and moist areas such as the perineum, external female genitalia, perianal region, axillae, and under pendulous breasts, the papules enlarge into pink or grey discs, the condylomata lata, which are highly infectious (Fig. 9). Mucous patches in the mouth and genitalia are painless greyish-white erosions forming circles and arcs ('snail-track ulcers'). They too are very infectious.

Meningism and headache especially at night are due to low-grade meningitis which can be confirmed by a raised cell count and raised protein in the CSF.

Less common lesions include alopecia and laryngitis. Syphilitic hepatitis is usually associated with a marked rise in serum phosphatase. There are non-specific inflammatory changes in liver biopsy material which are quite unlike those found in viral hepatitis. A nephrotic syndrome may develop and glomerular immune-complex deposits have been observed. Pain in the bones, often worse at night, is usually due to periostitis. Uveitis may be seen both in secondary and tertiary syphilis. In about one-fifth of patients recurrent infectious episodes occur especially during the first year after the secondary stage.

All these lesions disappear spontaneously and leave no evidence behind. It was repeatedly suggested in the older literature that extensive skin lesions had a protective effect and that late lesions of the CNS or aorta were less likely in such cases. It was believed that this was due to elaboration of significant amounts of protective antibodies by the skin lesions but no formal proof of this interesting idea has been presented. If true, one might further speculate that the extensive and prolonged skin lesions so prominent in all types of non-venereal syphilis may be a factor protecting these patients from the severe complications of the late stages.

Latent syphilis

By definition the patient is asymptomatic with normal CSF findings but positive serology for syphilis. It is arbitrarily divided into early (<2 years) and late latent (>2 years) syphilis. Infectiousness does not stop

Fig. 6 (a, b) Secondary papular syphilitic rashes. (c) Late secondary/early tertiary papulosquamous lesions.

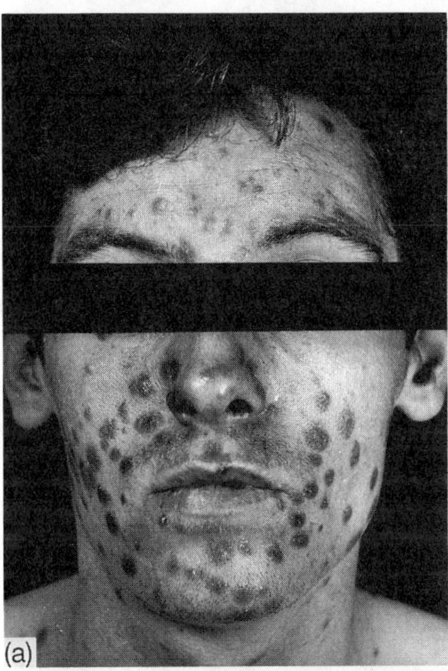

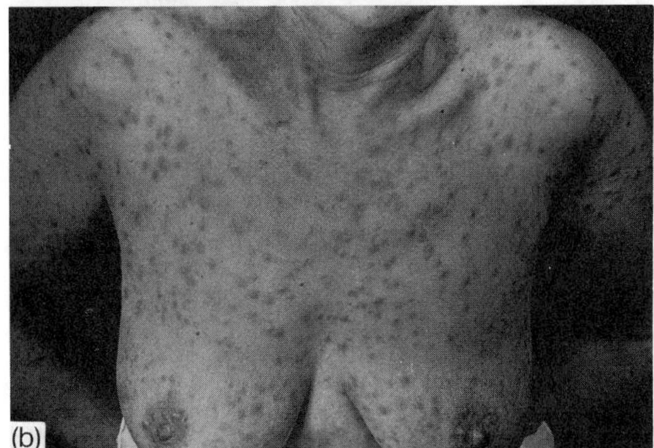

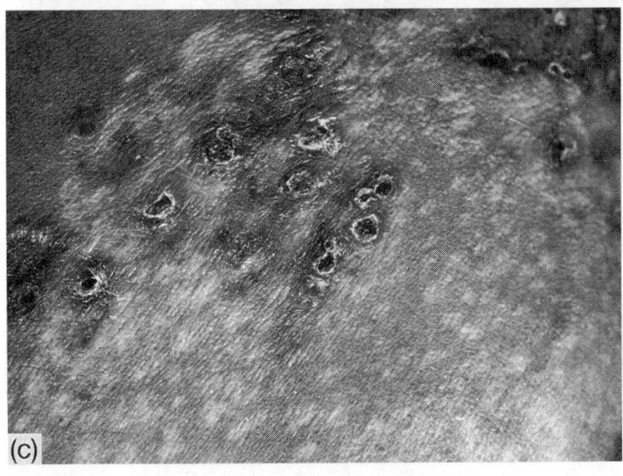

Fig. 7 Secondary papulosquamous rash of the soles.

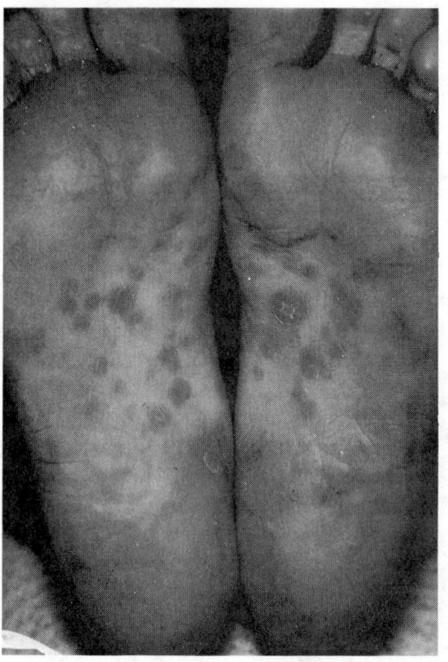

Fig. 8 Secondary rash of the palms.

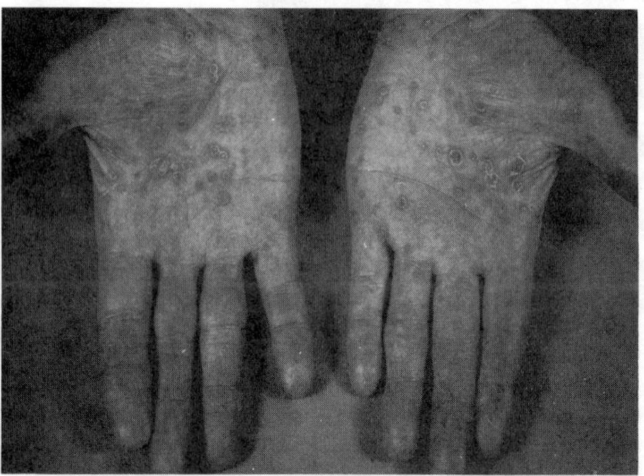

Fig. 9 Condylomata lata.

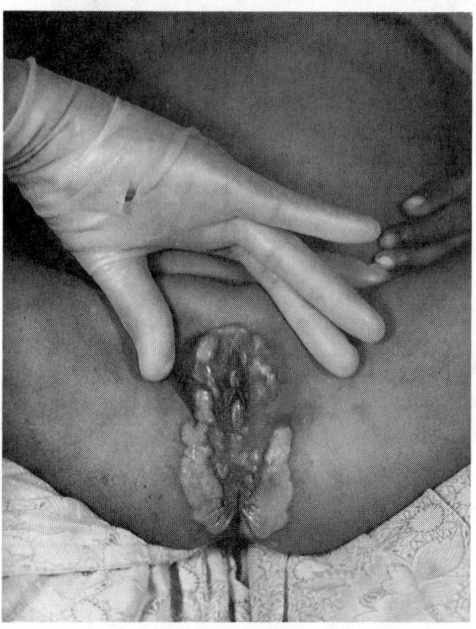

with the advent of latency, as women may continue to give birth to congenitally infected infants during the early latent stage and for at least 2 years into the late latent stage. Approximately 60 per cent of patients remain latent for the rest of their lives, the only evidence of syphilis being positive serology with a usually low titre. The rest develop clinical late syphilis but autopsy studies indicate that a higher proportion has subclinical infection especially of the cardiovascular system.

LATE SYPHILIS (TERTIARY SYPHILIS)

This includes late latent syphilis already referred to, benign tertiary syphilis, involvement of viscera, the CNS, and the aorta.

Pathogenesis of late benign syphilis

The gumma is a chronic granulomatous lesion which is an intense inflammatory response to a few treponemes. Histologically there is central necrosis with peripheral cellular infiltration of lymphocytes, mononuclear cells, and occasional giant cells with perivasculitis and obliterating endarteritis. *T. pallidum* is present and can be demonstrated by rabbit inoculation. Grin in Yugoslavia proposed two hypotheses to explain gumma formation: (1) reactivation of treponemes in a sensitized host who is untreated or inadequately treated (see Fig. 10), or (2) superinfection in a patient hypersensitized with the passage of time to *T. pallidum;* this appeared to be a common occurrence in endemic nonvenereal syphilis.

Clinical manifestations

1. *Cutaneous gumma.* The gumma is a chronic granulomatous lesion which is usually single but may be multiple or diffuse (Fig. 11). Histologically there is central necrosis with peripheral cellular infiltration of lymphocytes, plasma cells, and

Fig. 10 (a, b) Homosexual male allergic to penicillin treated for early syphilis with erythromycin six years ago. Now recurrence of penile lesions with a high VDRL titre. Dark-field negative for *T. pallidum* and biopsy suggests gummata. Reinfection cannot be excluded. Responded to tetracycline. Thus could be reinfection or treatment failure. (By courtesy of Dr Adam Lawrence.)

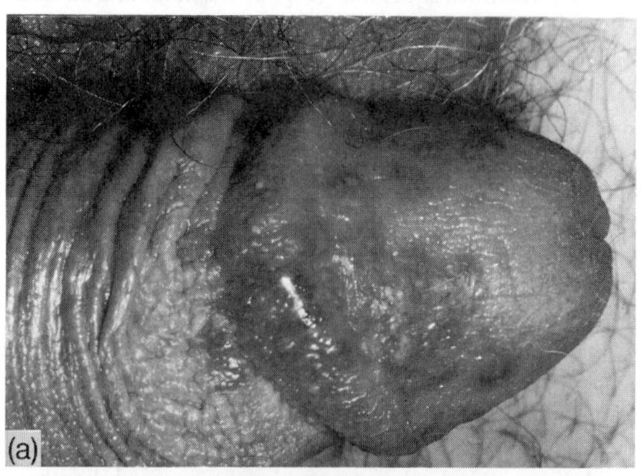

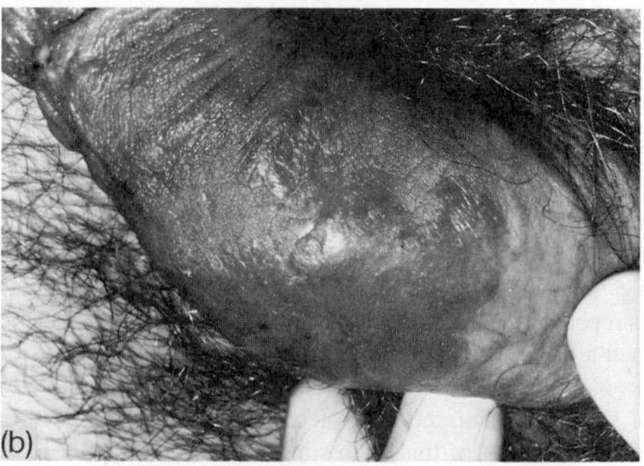

occasional giant cells with perivasculitis and obliterating endarteritis. *T. pallidum* is present and can be demonstrated by rabbit inoculation. Clinically it starts as a slowly progressive painless nodule which becomes dull red and breaks down into one or several indolent punched-out ulcers. The base has a 'wash-leather' appearance and is remarkably free from secondary infection (Fig. 12) and often resembles other granulomatous conditions. It heals slowly from the centre which may become depigmented, whilst the periphery shows hyperpigmentation. Eventually a paper-thin scar forms. This combination of pigmentation, depigmentation, and atrophic scars can be of considerable retrospective diagnostic help. The sites preferentially involved are the face, legs, buttocks, upper trunk, and scalp. The process may be more superficial, producing papulosquamous lesions which include the palms and soles. It too heals with the typical scars already described.

2. *Mucosal gumma.* These are most commonly seen in the oropharynx and involve the palate, pharynx, and the nasal septum. They tend to be destructive, causing perforation of the hard palate and the nasal septum. In the pharynx and the larynx they tend to lead to severe scarring. The most serious lesion is the diffuse gummatous infiltration of the tongue leading first to a general swelling of the organ, then due to loss of papillae to a smooth red surface (Fig. 12). After a while the poor blood supply produces necrotic white patches on the dorsum of the tongue and this leucoplakia has a strong tendency to become malignant; thus regular checkups with biopsy are necessary (Fig. 13). Penicillin has no effect on the progress of syphilitic glossitis at this late stage.
3. *Late syphilis of bones.* Osteoperiostitis of long bones such as the tibia and fibula causes thickening and irregularities which may be diffuse as in the 'sabre tibia' or localized and evident as a circumscribed bony swelling. Unlike most other syphilitic lesions, those of the bone are often painful, the pain being worse at night. Very rarely the process breaks through the skin producing a chronic 'syphilitic osteomyelitis'. Lesions of the palate, nasal septum, and the skull are destructive, leading to bone defects of the hard palate and nasal septum, and multiple osteolytic lesions of the skull.

Fig. 11 Multiple gummatous ulcers. This is a typical site.

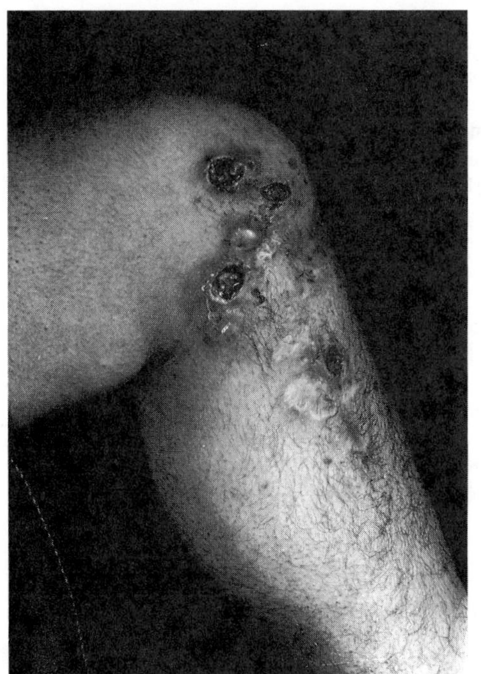

Differential diagnosis

1. *Mucocutaneous gumma.* The superficial skin lesions may have to be differentiated from fungal skin lesions, psoriasis, Kaposi's sarcoma, and iodide rashes. The deep gummata may resemble deep mycoses, sarcoidosis, tuberculosis, leprosy, donovanosis, lymphogranuloma venereum, reticulosis, and epithelioma of the skin.

   Serological tests for syphilis, which must include specific reactions such as the FTA-ABS, prompt response to penicillin, and

Fig. 12 Single gumma. Note the punched-out ulcer and absence of secondary infection.

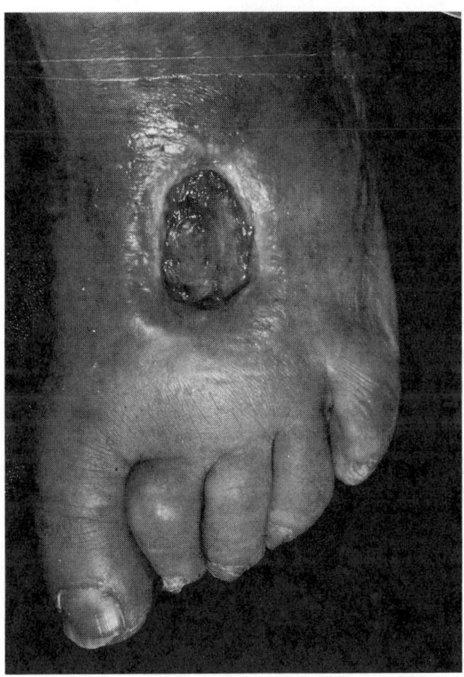

Fig. 13 Late syphilitic glossitis, early stage.

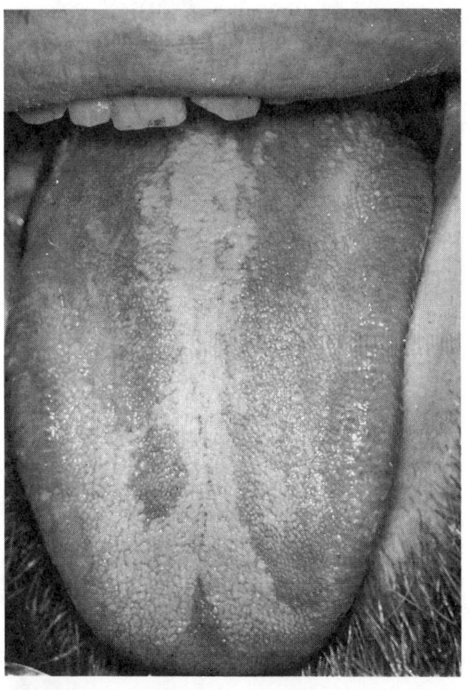

possibly evidence of syphilis elsewhere should clarify the diagnosis.

It is not uncommon to see patients with ulcers or nodes of the skin or various organs and a positive serology for syphilis. A diagnosis of syphilis is made, treatment is given, and only after obvious therapeutic failure is the diagnosis reconsidered and malignancy found. Positive blood tests for syphilis may be coincidental and, as late symptomatic syphilis is rare whereas malignancy is not, this differential diagnosis should always be taken into account.

2. *Late syphilis of bones.* Conditions to be considered include primary and secondary carcinoma, Paget's disease, chronic osteomyelitis, tuberculosis, and leprosy. All forms of non-venereal syphilis except pinta give rise to similar lesions.

Visceral syphilis

This is not common and response to treatment is variable. Late syphilis may involve the liver, eyes, stomach, lungs, and testes.

1. *Liver.* Multiple gummata of the liver give rise to irregular hepatomegaly ('hepar lobatum'), which may be asymptomatic. Symptoms may result from pressure on bile ducts or blood vessels or destruction of liver parenchyma. Antisyphilitic treatment is reported to lead to accelerated fibrosis with distortion of the liver architecture and an increase in symptoms ('therapeutic paradox'), but the available data are too scanty to confirm this.
2. *Eyes.* Uveitis, choroidoretinitis, or optic atrophy may sometimes be the sole feature of late syphilis. Uveitis can also develop during early syphilis. Response of the late form to penicillin is poor. Optic atrophy is further discussed under neurosyphilis.
3. *Stomach.* Single or diffuse gummatous infiltrations of the stomach have been described and are said to respond to antisyphilitic treatment.
4. *Lungs.* Single or multiple gummata are rare and respond to treatment.
5. *Testis.* Gummatous infiltration and dense fibrosis may produce smooth painless enlargement of a testis. Testicular sensation is lost. In the only case seen by us penicillin had no effect.
6. *Paroxysmal cold haemoglobinuria.* Syphilis is a rare cause of this haemolytic anaemia.

It is often claimed by patients who had recent treatment for late latent syphilis that it improved their well-being. This may be a psychological reaction but it is also possible that it is due to an effect on subclinical visceral lesions. The warning given earlier against undue delay in the diagnosis of malignant disease because of misleading positive serology for syphilis which is coincidental, applies even more strongly in this section.

Asymptomatic neurosyphilis

There are no neurological manifestations but the CSF shows abnormalities such as a raised cell count (5 or more cells/ml), raised protein (over 40 mg/ml), and commonly a positive FTA-ABS test. The VDRL is less reliable and if it is the sole abnormality, it is probably due to passive transfer and not due to intrinsic production of antibodies in the CNS. However, if there are atypical neurological signs as well, it is safest to treat as neurosyphilis.

Neurosyphilis of any kind is more common in Caucasians than Negroes and at least twice as common in men than women.

Experience shows that if the CSF is normal 2 years after untreated infection, neurosyphilis will not develop. If the serology for syphilis becomes negative, that too effectively rules out neurosyphilis. If neurosyphilis is present, the Dattner criteria of cure is a normal cell count and protein level in CSF, 6 months after treatment.

Symptomatic neurosyphilis (see Chapter 24.15.5)

Syphilitic deafness and vertigo

The eighth nerve may be involved in basal meningovascular syphilis resulting in vertigo and deafness. The prognosis for hearing loss is uncertain but it appears that when it is advanced it becomes permanent. Syphilitic nerve deafness may also develop in congenital and late syphilis as a single lesion and in our experience the prognosis is poor despite use of corticosteroids in addition to penicillin.

Laboratory diagnosis of syphilis

DARK-FIELD MICROSCOPY

The organism is seen in the wet preparation by dark-field microscopy and shows a steady 'deliberate' linear progression (translation). It can be detected from fluid taken from open lesions in early syphilis and failing that in the needle aspirate from affected lymph nodes. In late lesions the organism is not readily demonstratable by microscopy but occasionally can be isolated by xenodiagnosis. The pathogenic treponemes which cause syphilis, non-venereal syphilis, yaws, and pinta cannot be morphologically differentiated from each other, give rise to the same serological reactions, and are susceptible to penicillin but give rise to dissimilar lesions both in man and in laboratory animals.

Dark-field microscopy of wet-mounted material from the chancre or open lesions of early acquired or early congenital syphilis should show *T. pallidum* without difficulty. Sometimes it is negative in the presence of lesions. This may be due to recent use of antiseptics on the lesion, to a small number of treponemes being present, or with reinfection. In any case, the examination should be repeated two or three times before accepting a negative result. Needle aspirates from regional lymph nodes may be successful when direct examination of the sore is difficult or when the sore has healed. In view of the excellent serological tests available, this procedure is now rarely used. Immunostaining directly with monoclonal antibody or by indirect fluorescent antibody staining of air-dried smears or tissue specimen has recently been reported to show numerous *T. pallidum* in a cutaneous gumma but not by dark-field microscopy or silver staining. Handsfield *et al.* suggest that this finding might explain the histologically vigorous reaction in tertiary syphilis. This novel and surprising result will need further study, as its implications are considerable.

SEROLOGY

As yet no laboratory test is available to distinguish one treponematosis from another. The preliminary finding of a base pair change in the TpN19 sequence in the yaws treponeme, has not been confirmed.

Two classes of antibody tests are available: (a) those that measure non-specific antibodies (IgG and IgM) against lipoidal antigens (lipoidal antibody tests formerly called reagin tests), and (b) those that measure specific antibodies stimulated by antigenic components of the treponeme and further divided into those stimulated by antigens found in pathogenic treponemes only and those shared with non-pathogenic treponemes.

The non-specific cardiolipin antibodies act on lipoidal antigen which results from action of *T. pallidum* on host tissue. It mirrors disease activity.

The specific antigen is derived from *T. pallidum* and does not differentiate between past or present infection and is therefore of no value in assessing activity.

The interpretation of the tests is given in Table 2.

ANIMAL INOCULATION

Animal inoculation with material from late lesions or in cases of 'persistent *T. pallidum*—like forms' is usually reserved for research pur-

Table 2 *Interpretation of serological tests in syphilis*

Diagnosis	VDRL	Titre	TPHA	FTA-ABS IgG	FTA-ABS IgM	Comment
Early untreated primary syphilis	+ or −	Rising	+ or −	+	+	FTA-ABS is the first test to become +. VDRL − in 30%
Untreated late primary *or* secondary syphilis *or* reinfection *or* untreated or recently treated late syphilis	+	High or rising	+	+	+	
Untreated latent syphilis	+ or −	Moderate	+	+	+	
Treated early syphilis	−		+ or −	−	−	
Treated latent syphilis	+ or −	Low	+ or −	−	−	
Neurosyphilis any type, treated or untreated *or* cardiovascular syphilis	+ or −	Varies	+ or −	+	+	CSF: FTA-ABS often +. VDRL − in 30%
Active gumma (skin, mucosa, bone)	+	Varies	+	+	+	
Early congenital syphilis	+	Rising	+	+	+	In some infants, tests may be negative for weeks until immunologically more mature
Passive transfer of maternal antibodies	+	Same or lower than mother	−	+	−	FTA-ABS IgM
Late congenital syphilis	+	Low or moderate	+	+	+	
Biological false-positive reaction	+	Low	−	−	−	FTA-ABS may be weakly positive

False positive reaction: VDRL will be of low titre. TPHA may give false positive results in 2 per cent. FTA-ABS may give borderline positive in pregnancy and systemic lupus. TPI negative in such problem sera.

poses. In recent years, tests utilizing the polymerase chain reaction to detect treponemal nucleotides in amniotic or cerebrospinal fluid, have been found to be no more sensitive than the detection of live spirochaetes by animal inoculation of these fluids. Removal of inhibitors in serum, even if DNA is extracted with diatoms, fails to improve sensitivity of the polymerase chain reaction but the technique may be useful in detecting treponemal nucleotides in biopsy specimens.

CURRENTLY USED SEROLOGICAL TESTS FOR SYPHILIS

Lipoidal antigen tests

1. *Rapid plasma reagin (RPR) test.* This can be automated and is useful for screening purposes. It is least technically demanding (no microscope needed). It uses carbon-containing cardiolipin antigen and needs a minimal amount of blood. Filter paper and glass fibre discs can be used to post samples to laboratories; they are therefore mainly for use by primary health centres in outlying rural areas.
2. *VDRL test.* This is the preferred test and as it is used worldwide there is a good chance of it becoming standardized. It is simple and inexpensive. It is above all a quantitative test and as the titres reflect activity, it is of great value for this purpose. It may, for example, be the only evidence of re-infection in a patient with previous syphilis whose VDRL was either negative or weakly positive after treatment. A sharp sustained rise of the titre four-fold or higher even in the absence of clinical signs is good evidence of active infection. False positive VDRL is usually of a low titre (1:8 or less). The VDRL test becomes positive during the primary stage and rises to its maximum during the secondary stage (1:32 or more). After successful treatment, the titre declines (1:4 or less), and if treatment was given early in the disease it often becomes negative. An occasional small and transient rise in titre (two tubes) is of no significance. It is worth remembering that the immunofluorescent test which detects cardiolipin F levels tends to be positive only in active infections.

Specific antitreponemal tests

1. *The T. pallidum haemagglutination (TPHA) test.* This is a very valuable and simple test using an indirect haemagglutination method with red cells sensitized by sonicated *T. pallidum* extract. It is almost as specific as the almost obsolescent TPI reaction but is less sensitive than the FTA-ABS. False positive reactions occur in up to 2 per cent. The micromethod is particularly suitable for screening purposes. Together with the VDRL, it is probably the best combination for routine use. In cases of doubt the FTA-ABS test is added. TPHA can be adapted for automation. There is no standard 'cut off' for the TPHA in the CSF.
2. *The FTA-ABS test.* This uses the indirect fluorescent technique with killed *T. pallidum* as antigen. The organisms are fixed on a slide to which the serum is added. The antibody in the serum will unite with the treponemes and this can be made visible by adding antihuman globulin conjugated with a fluorescent stain which attaches itself and produces fluorescence of the treponemes seen by fluorescent microscope. The test has been made more specific by absorbing the group antibodies with a sonicate derived from Reiter's treponemes. The test is then called FTA-ABS. The FTA-ABS is the most sensitive test available and is also specific. It becomes positive earlier during the primary stage of syphilis than other procedures. It is not suitable for assessing activity, as it persists long after successful treatment. When the routine serology includes the VDRL and TPHA tests, the FTA-ABS test should be added in cases of problem sera.
3. *The FTA-ABS-IgM test.* In the search for a specific test to differentiate active infection which has to be treated from adequately treated or 'burnt-out' inactive disease, the FTA-ABS-IgM is being evaluated to test for specific IgM which develops in the course of syphilis. This test sometimes gives false-positive reactions owing to the presence of anti-IgG globulins (e.g. rheumatoid factor) and false-negative reactions have also occurred; thus there are problems in the use of this test in the

elderly. Its use in the rapid early diagnosis of congenital syphilis was considered some years ago as a great advance. The basis for its use is that IgG is a small molecule and passes through the placenta; thus the baby may inherit maternal IgG but not necessarily the infection. Tests such as the VDRL may therefore be positive in the newborn by passive transfer and may take 3 months to disappear. IgM is a large molecule and does not pass through the placenta; thus if it is found in the neonate, it must be assumed that it is produced by the infected infant.

New tests

A variety of EIA tests have been devised and some are commercially available, such as the CAPTIA IgG, IgM. However, they have no practical advantage over current tests. Attempts with purified antigens from *T. pallidum* may be specific, although they tend to lose sensitivity, for example, those employing the TpN19 or Tp44.5 antigens. The problem is that early cases may not always have antibodies to a specific antigen. It would be better, therefore, to screen with as many antigens as possible. This is achieved by Western blotting, which allows the separation by gel-electrophoresis of all the major stable antigens of the spirochaete (Table 3), and enables a distinction to be made between the non-specific and specific antibody reactions with given bands. The need for designating specific bands is exemplified by the observation of finding on average, at least five stained bands, in sera from post-primary syphilis. It is therefore better to choose specific bands for the diagnosis of syphilis. Usually, the 14 000 and 44–46 000 molecular weight bands are regarded as specific, although the diagnosis would be very uncertain if they were the only bands stained. The technique has been miniaturized and is commercially available but it is unlikely to come into routine use because of expense. It may still have special application in seronegative syphilis (perhaps syphilis occurring with HIV infection) but not in primary syphilis, where up to half the cases show no reaction in this test. The real value of identifying these bands is to find a candidate for a potential vaccine to protect against syphilis. If such a vaccine was to be developed using just one of these proteins or a component of the protein, immunoblots would come into their own, as they would distinguish an antibody response to vaccine from that produced in the natural infection.

Diagnosis of neurosyphilis by examination of the CSF

The traditional tests include the VDRL, cell count, total protein globulin, and goldsol curve. The last two tests are now obsolete. The CSF VDRL is unreliable as it can be negative in up to 50 per cent of samples from patients with active neurosyphilis. Cell counts exceeding 5/mm^3 (but usually not above 50/mm^3) and protein above 40 mg/ml are non-specific signs of inflammation.

The specific FTA-ABS and TPHA tests in the CSF may be positive due to passive transfer of serum IgG from adequately treated patients. If they are negative, active neurosyphilis can almost certainly be excluded. There are several newer tests being investigated, some of which are based on the presence of specific IgM antibodies in the CSF especially if a capture technique is used which would indicate active neurosyphilis. Others use quantitative estimation of the CSF TPHA titre in relation to measures of the blood/CSF barrier over a period of time as a reflection of response to treatment. The combined use of specific serology with either differential CSF/serum immunoglobulin or albumin (TPHA index) or immunoglobulin estimations, is under study. The aim of these tests is to demonstrate fresh synthesis of intrathecal antibody. The detection of IgM oligoclonal antibodies or the presence of light chains in the CSF has not been persued. The tests have not yet been fully evaluated but it appears probable that one of several of these will be used in the future to determine the presence or absence of active neurosyphilis.

Biological false-positive test for syphilis

These concern mainly the cardiolipin tests and are classified as acute if they occur in drug addicts, autoimmune disease (when they may precede the symptoms by years), leprosy, and in a small proportion of people over 70. Particular mention should be made of the thrombotic antiphospholipid syndrome. The confirmatory TPHA and FTA-ABS are always negative. A biological false-positive test may occur acutely in the CSF in aseptic meningitis or in a seropositive patient, when a traumatic tap may give a false impression of a positive cardiolipin test in the CSF, following transfer of plasma antibody.

Table 3 *Major antigens of* Treponema pallidum (adapted from C. Penn)

Designation*	Molecular weight	Description and comments
TpN83	82 000	Major component of cytoplasmic filaments or fibronectin binding protein
TpN60	59 000	Homologue of Hsp60 or GroEL heat shock protein. Cross-reactive antigen
TpN47	45 000	Lipoprotein. The most abundant polypeptide and dominant antigen
TpN44.5 (TmpA)	42 000	Lipoprotein. Also abundant. Recombinant form purified and experimental diagnostic reagent
TpN41	39 500	Lipoprotein. Homologue of the MglB periplasmic sugar binding protein of *Escherichia coli*
TpN37	37 000	FlaA flagellin. Abundant, dominant antigen. Member of class of spirochaetal flagellar "sheath" proteins
TpN35	35 500	Lipoprotein. Less abundant and dominant antigen
TpN34.5	34 500	FlaB flagellins, homologues of other bacterial flagellins
TpN33	33 000	
TpN30	32 000	Form flagellar core
TpN29–35 (TpD)	30–38 000	Lipoprotein, moderately antigenic
TpN24–28 (TpE)	24–29 000	Lipoprotein, moderately antigenic
TpN19 (4D) (Tp1–1)	19 000	Subunit of a large, heat labile complex which in recombinant *E. coli* is a ring structure
TpN17	17 000	Lipoprotein, strongly antigenic
TpN15	15 000	Lipoprotein, strongly antigenic

*TpN designations are those of Norris *et al.* (1993).

Serological tests for syphilis in HIV infection

The report by Hicks and colleagues in 1987, of a patient whose secondary syphilis, proven by biopsy but with negative VDRL and FTA-ABS test was a landmark in syphilis serology. If such a case had been seen earlier in this century, it would have been diagnosed as 'malignant' syphilis which by definition tended to be seronegative.* This case also indicates that a clinical diagnosis had to be made without the benefit of

*The presence of enhanced delayed sensitivity, as reflected by skin test reactions, is a further feature of malignant syphilis. It is unlikely that the occasional syphilitic skin manifestations seen in concurrent HIV infections are related to these older descriptions of 'florid syphilis'. It has been suggested that the histological necrosis seen in these skin lesions are associated with immune-complex formation.

Table 4 *Treatment for syphilis based on WHO draft recommendations 1993*

	Aqueous procaine penicillin G[b]		Benzathine penicillin G	
Type of syphilis	Daily dose single IM injection	Total number of days	Total dose IM (mg)	Total number of days
Early syphilis (primary, secondary, early latent, early re-infection)	1200	10	2360	1
Late latent syphilis (more than 2 years) and late benign syphilis[a]	1200	15	7080	3
Cardiovascular syphilis	1200	20	Not to be given	
Neurosyphilis	1200 + Probenecid 500 mg by mouth q.d.s.	10–14	Aqueous crystalline penicillin G[c] (12–24 megaunit) daily given as 1.2–24 megaunits every 4 h IV for 14 days	
Optic atrophy (congenital or acquired)	As for neurosyphilis			
Eighth nerve deafness and vertigo	As for neurosyphilis *plus* corticosteroids			
Syphilis of the tongue	As for late syphilis and consult ENT specialist for regular follow-up			
Early congenital syphilis including *suspected* early congenital syphilis	Crystalline penicillin G 50 mg/kg IM in 2 divided doses × 10 days		Aqueous procaine penicillin G 37.5 mg/kg IM single daily dose × 10 days	
Late congenital syphilis (over 2 years duration)	As for late latent syphilis (dose adjusted for age)			
Interstitial keratitis 2 years duration)	Procaine penicillin as for neurosyphilis (*plus* 0.5% prednisolone eye drops hourly until controlled)			
Patients allergic to penicillin: acquired syphilis of less than 2 years' duration	Tetracycline: 500 mg by mouth q.d.s. × 15 days		*If pregnant* erythromycin: 500 mg by mouth q.d.s. × 15 days	
acquired syphilis of more than 2 years' duration	Tetracycline: 500 my by mouth q.d.s. × 30 days		Erythromycin 500 mg by mouth q.d.s. × 30 days	
Patients with HIV and syphilis	As for stage of syphilis but not benzathine penicillin			

[a]In patients with gumma of the larynx, late neurosyphilis, especially general paresis, and cardiovascular syphilis, especially with angina try to minimize any Herxheimer reaction by covering the first injection of penicillin with corticosteroid started the day before injection.

In patients diagnosed as symptomatic cardiovascular syphilis consult cardiac surgeon from the start with a view to possible cardiac surgery (removal of coronary ostial stenosis, aortic valve replacement, repair or replacement of aneurysmal aortic segment). If there is congestive heart failure treat it before giving penicillin.

[b]Procaine penicillin G: 300 mg = 300 000 units

Benzathine penicillin G: 900 mg = 1.2 megaunits

[c]Aqueous crystalline penicillin G = 0.5 megaunits

serology. Further work showed that persistent seronegative syphilis did not exist. There seemed to be a delay in the untreated patient, in developing positive tests both in the serum and CSF, if HIV infection was present. The serology tended also to become negative a shorter time after treatment. Rarely, a negative VDRL was obtained, because of a prozone phenomenon (i.e. the optimal proportions of the antigen: antibody reaction were not met). The higher titres of cardiolipin antibodies in HIV infections may be a reflection of the B-cell dysgammaglobulinaemia seen in this condition.

The management of syphilis

Suggestions for drug treatment of syphilis are given in Table 4. As soon as a diagnosis of infectious syphilis has been made, the patient should be interviewed by the social worker regarding all sexual contacts. In the case of primary syphilis this should cover the previous 3 months; in patients with secondary syphilis this should be extended to 1 year, and in patients with early latent syphilis to 2 years because of the possibility of infectious relapses during that period. The patient is warned against intercourse during treatment and for a further 2 weeks. Experience suggests that advice for longer abstinence will be disregarded in many cases and is almost certainly unnecessary.

If the patient gives no history of penicillin allergy, it is the first choice for the treatment of all stages of the disease. Sir Alexander Fleming predicted that penicillin would continue to be effective against syphilis even if not necessarily for other infections and he has proved to be right. Penicillin is as effective now as it was more than 40 years ago when it was first introduced. If there is penicillin allergy, the alternative drugs are tetracycline/doxycycline and erythromycin. The recent finding of a wild strain of *T. pallidum* resistant to erythromycin has led to an extensive investigation into the use of newer cephalosporins. Cephalosporins are effective but there is cross-allergy with penicillin in 5 to 7 per cent of patients and they are therefore not advised. These alternative drugs have not been fully evaluated or compared with penicillin to assess their value and some of their drawbacks, notably the poor concentration in the brain and in the fetus.

The optimal dose or duration of treatment with penicillin or the other drugs has not been established and therefore a great variety of treatment schemes have been put forward, although the results appear to be similar, suggesting that a fair degree of variation is permissible. The general tendency is to treat with larger doses and over a longer period of time in the later stages of syphilis; some prefer to repeat the course. There is no convincing evidence that large, much extended, or repeated courses give any added benefit.

There is good experimental evidence that serum concentrations of penicillin should be at least 0.03 g/ml, should be maintained for 8 to 10 days, and that troughs in the concentration should not exceed 15 h.

Some physicians prefer a single injection of the long-acting benzathine penicillin (2.4 million units) for the sake of simplicity, but the concentration reached is low and does not give a useful level in the CSF; also the injection is quite painful. Others repeat this dose weekly, for 3 weeks. We prefer not to use this preparation; in exceptional circumstances where a patient cannot to attend more than once and is unable to continue treatment elsewhere, it may be justified but as an alternative the full course of erythromycin or tetracycline could be given. In patients with neurosyphilis and HIV infections, treponemes have been demonstrated in the CSF after benzathine penicillin G treatments and in these patients, the expected decline in VDRL CSF titres after treatment occurred less often than in those without concurrent HIV infection. All treponemal infections are unaffected by sulphonamides, rifampicin, and quinolones in clinical dosage.

Procaine penicillin has several advantages over other penicillin preparations and is preferred by many. In some centres the course is 1 million units/day for 10 days; in others it is given for 20 days though evidence that such a prolonged course gives better results, is lacking. Procaine penicillin in 2 per cent aluminium monostearate (PAM) has a prolonged action and was used extensively by the World Health Organization in their mass campaign against non-venereal syphilis in a few centres.

PENICILLIN REACTIONS

All patients receiving penicillin injections should be kept in the clinic for 15 to 20 min as severe reactions needing immediate treatment will develop well within this period. An emergency tray to deal with anaphylactic penicillin reaction must be readily available wherever penicillin is given. It should contain ampoules of 1:1000 adrenaline solution, syringes and needles, intravenous hydrocortisone, injectable antihistamine, aminophylline, an airway, respirator (Ambu bag or Brooke's respirator), and oxygen with face mask or nasal catheter.

PREVENTION OF PENICILLIN REACTIONS

Some 3 to 5 per cent of the population in the United Kingdom are allergic to penicillin and it is essential to enquire about this; if there is a history, penicillin must not be given. This fact should be displayed prominently on the cover of the medical notes and the patient told to inform any doctor who may wish to give this antibiotic. Careful history taking may, however, show that the 'allergy' to penicillin is doubtful, e.g. the rash antedated the giving of penicillin and may have been due to one of the childhood infections. It is quite common to be told that patients who apparently did have a penicillin reaction, had no problems when the antibiotic was inadvertently given subsequently as penicillin allergy is a transient phenomenon. In such cases we still prefer to avoid giving penicillin.

CLINICAL FEATURES

The most serious reaction is anaphylactic shock appearing immediately or within a minute or two after the injection. The more immediate the onset, the more severe the attack. The patient becomes unconscious, stops breathing, and becomes pulseless. Very rarely the patient dies immediately. A fatal outcome is estimated to occur one or two times per 100 000 injections. In the more moderate reaction the patient feels faint with acute anxiety and a feeling of impending death; there may be oedema of the face, possibly with an asthmatic attack, soon followed by urticaria. Arthralgia and some pyrexia may develop. The urticaria is liable to last 1 to 2 weeks.

The commonest form is the delayed reaction when urticaria appears days after injection or oral penicillin. Arthralgia and fever may develop.

Sometimes a local reaction around the injection site is seen. It can be urticarial but is more commonly a painful red swelling and usually responds to rest. It is best to discontinue the course, as recurrences are otherwise common.

In some patients a hysterical episode follows an injection and may be due to procaine or possibly inadvertent intravenous injection. It passes off spontaneously.

TREATMENT OF THE ANAPHYLACTIC REACTION

The patient is laid flat with feet up and head down. Blood pressure and pulse are monitored throughout. Adrenaline 1:1000 (0.5–1.0 ml) is given intramuscularly without delay. If bronchospasm develops, 250 mg aminophylline in 10 ml water is administered by slow intravenous injection. Intravenous hydrocortisone (100 mg) may also be tried and may be repeated. Some prefer intravenous antihistamine (chlorpheniramine injection 10–20 mg). Adrenaline, nevertheless, is the mainstay of treatment. If there is no response, the cardiac arrest team is summoned. If recovery is slow, the patient should be admitted as recurrences may occur occasionally. In any case the patient must be kept under observation for several hours. Later, urticaria develops in most patients and prophylactic antihistamines by mouth are indicated.

TREATMENT OF THE DELAYED REACTION

The leading feature is urticaria, possibly with oedema of the face, arthralgia, and some fever. Such patients respond to oral antihistamines such as chlorpheniramine 4 mg four times daily or terfenadine 60 mg twice daily until the condition is controlled. If it is very severe, prednisolone 10 mg four times daily may be added for a few days, reducing it as soon as possible. Penicillinase is not recommended as it may produce reactions of its own.

PROCAINE REACTION

Two types of reaction are recognized. (1) The patient shows extreme anxiety with a feeling of impending death. Sometimes there are hallucinations, disorientation, and depersonalization. The reaction is self-limited. It may be due to reduced procaine esterase leading to high procaine blood levels. Patients should be restrained and reassured. (2) The reaction is similar but associated with hyperventilation, hypertension, tachycardia, and vomiting. Rarely cardiovascular collapse has been reported but without fatalities. The reaction is thought to follow accidental intravenous administration of procaine penicillin leading to microemboli of the lungs and brain. Supportive treatment is usually sufficient.

VASOVAGAL ATTACKS

This occurs most commonly in young men following intramuscular injection or after having blood taken. The patient looks very pale and may faint. He may slump to the floor and occasionally go stiff and have jerky movements. The most important diagnostic sign is a slow pulse. Recovery is rapid once he is laid flat on a couch. There is a tendency for recurrence in the same individual under similar circumstances and this can usually be prevented by giving injections or taking blood whilst the patient is lying down.

THE JARISCH–HERXHEIMER REACTION

This systemic reaction is believed to be due to the release of endotoxin-like substances when large numbers of *T. pallidum* are killed by antibiotics. It is mainly associated with early syphilis. The incidence of the reaction appears to be related to the total number of the organism in the body. The mechanism may not be straightforward as it is not a feature of neonatal syphilis or non-venereal syphilis in childhood. The reaction can be expected in 50 per cent of primary syphilis, 90 per cent of secondary syphilis, and in 25 per cent of early latent infection, but is very rare in late syphilis.

The reaction begins 4 to 12 h after the first injection, lasts for a few hours or up to a day, and is not seen with subsequent treatment. There is malaise, slight to moderate pyrexia, a flush due to vasodilation, tachycardia, and leucocytosis, and existing lesions become more prominent. In some patients with early syphilis, a secondary rash may become visible which was absent before treatment. Rarely, syphilis may be suspected by the appearance of the febrile reaction of the Jarisch–Herxheimer, perhaps with a fleeting rash, when treating another infection with a treponemocidal antibiotic (e.g. penicillin in gonorrhoea).

In early syphilis the reaction is only a minor nuisance. In late syphilis it can on very rare occasions be more serious. Thus in neurosyphilis it may lead to a rapid irreversible progression, and in general paresis it can cause exacerbation amounting to temporary psychosis. Sudden death has been reported in cardiovascular syphilis. In laryngeal gumma, local oedema may necessitate tracheotomy.

It is customary to give corticosteroids in late symptomatic syphilis starting a day before the first penicillin injection and tailing it off the day after the first injection. This does not prevent the Herxheimer reaction but is said to ameliorate it. The analogous reactions in relapsing fever have been modified by meptazinol.

We never withhold penicillin in late syphilis because of the remote chance of a reaction, nor do we give small initial doses as it is not dose-related. The patient with early syphilis should be warned about the possibility of mild indisposition on the day of the first injection and be advised to go to bed and take aspirin.

FOLLOW-UP

It is generally sufficient to perform blood tests 1, 3, 6, and 12 months after treatment of early syphilis. In late symptomatic syphilis, surveillance is for life. The frequency of attendance must be adapted to the condition; thus in patients with leucoplakia of the tongue (Fig. 14), a regular check-up every 3 months is recommended or at any time between, should the lesions increase. In symptomatic cardiovascular syphilis regular radiological and clinical examination is essential to determine any change which might suggest the need for cardiac surgery. In neurosyphilis the follow-up varies with individual needs and an annual review might be adequate. There is no consensus of opinion about the follow-up in latent syphilis.

However, if there is a satisfactory serological response, a period of 2 to 3 years seems reasonable. In early congenital syphilis the observation time should be similar to that of early acquired syphilis. In late latent congenital syphilis no further attendance is necessary unless symptoms of interstitial keratitis or other lesions not prevented by penicillin develop.

In high-risk patients such as male homosexuals and prostitutes a regular check-up every 3 months for syphilis and other sexually transmitted diseases is advised. In special circumstances the interval may have to be much shorter. If such patients have had syphilis, the VDRL should have become negative or of a low titre after treatment. If the titre suddenly rises fourfold or more, reinfection must be assumed and treated accordingly.

Fig. 14 Syphilitic leucoplakia of the tongue; premalignant.

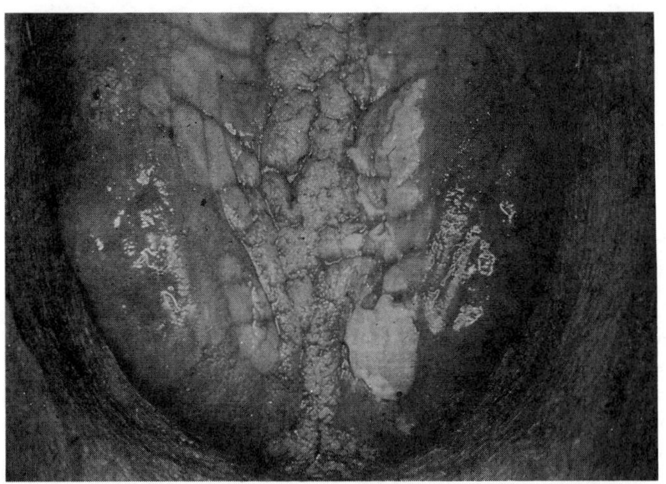

PROPHYLAXIS AND ABORTIVE TREATMENT

In the United States it is recommended to treat asymptomatic contacts of early syphilis as there is a 50 per cent chance of infection. Such preemptive treatment is likely to reduce the spread of infection in the promiscuous or in those likely to infect their spouses or regular sexual partners and is also indicated in persons known to be unreliable attenders. Such patients, however, should be encouraged to keep to the simple follow-up schedule of early syphilis. We follow this practice and believe that this is an important measure in certain communities in reducing the spread of infection. It is only fair to state that opinion in the United Kingdom is divided and some feel strongly that treatment before diagnosis is 'second-rate medicine'.

The proper use of condoms will do much to prevent infection of all forms of sexually transmitted diseases and should be recommended to all those most likely to become infected. It is, unfortunately, these very people who often find this advice unacceptable. Various vaginal chemical spermicidal creams give a small degree of protection but are quite unreliable in this respect.

REFERENCES

Byrne, R.E., Laska, S., Bell, M., Larson, D., Phillips, J. and Todd, J. (1992). Evaluation of a *Treponema pallidum* western immunoblot assay as a confirmatory test for syphilis. *Journal of Clinical Microbiology,* **30,** 115–22.

Goldmeier. D. and Hay, P. (1993). A review and update on adult *Sexually-transmitted* syphilis, with particular reference to its treatment. *International Journal of Disease and AIDS,* **4,** 70–82.

Gordon, S.M., Eaton, M.E., George, R., *et al.* (1994). A response of symptomatic neurosyphilis to high dose intravenous penicillin G, with human immunodeficiency virus infection. *New England Journal of Medicine* **331,** 1469–73.

Gourevitch, M.N., Selwyn, P.A., Davenny, K., *et al.* (1993). Affects of HIV infection on the serologic manifestations and response to treatment of syphilis in intravenous drug users. *Annals of Internal Medicine,* **118,** 350–5.

Grimble, A.S. (1971). Venereal disease in the young patient: a perspective. *Guy's Hospital Reports,* **120,** 323–6.

Grimpel, E., Sanchez, P.J., Wendel, G.D., *et al.* (1991). Use of polymerase chain reaction and rabbit infectivity testing to detect *Treponema pallidum* in amniotic fluid, fetal and neonatal sera and cerebrospinal fluid. *Journal of Clinical Microbiology,* **29,** 1711–18.

Haas, J.S., Bolan, G., Larsen, S.A., Clement, M.J., Bacchetti, P., and Moss, A.R. (1990). Sensitivity of treponemal tests for detecting prior treated syphilis during human immunodeficiency virus infection. *Journal of Infections Diseases,* **162,** 862–6.

Handsfield, H.H., Lukehart, S.A., Sell, S., Norris, S.J., and Holmes, K.K. (1993). Demonstration of *Treponema pallidum* in a cutaneous gumma by indirect immunoflourescence. *Archives of Dermatology,* **119,** 677–80.

Hicks, C.B., Benson, P.M., Lupton, G.C., and Tramont, E.C. (1987). Seronegative secondary syphilis in patients infected with human immunodeficiency virus and Kaposi sarcoma. *Annals of Internal Medicine,* **107,** 492–7.

Holtom, P.D., Larsen, R.A., Leal, M.E., and Leedom, J.M. (1992). Prevalence of neurosyphilis in HIV infected patients with latent syphilis. *American Journal of Medicine,* **93,** 9–12.

Hookey, J.V., Barrett, S.P., Reed, C.S., and Barber, P. (1994). Phylogeny of human intestinal spirochaetes inferred from 16s rDNA sequence comparisons. *FEMS Microbiology Letters,* **117,** 345–9.

Johns, D.R., Tierney, M., and Felsenstein, D. (1987). Alterations in the natural history of neurosyphilis by concurrent infection with human immunodeficiency virus. *New England Journal of Medicine,* **316,** 1569–72.

Keir, G. (1994). Cerebrospinal fluid proteins in neurosyphilis and HIV infections. *International Journal of Sexually-transmitted Disease and AIDS* **5,** 310–17.

Lukehart, S.A., Hook, E.W., Baker-Zander, S.A., Colker, A.C., Critchlow, C.W., and Handsfield H.H. (1988). Invasion of the central nervous system by *Treponema pallidum.* Implications for diagnosis and treatment. *Annals of Internal Medicine,* **109,** 855–62.

McCracken, G.H. and Kaplan, J.M. (1974). Penicillin treatment for congenital syphilis. A critical reappraisal. *Journal of the American Medical Association,* **228,** 855–8.

Norris, S.J. (1989). Syphilis. In *Immunology of sexually transmitted diseases* (Ed. D.J.M. Wright. pp. 1–31. Kluwer, Dordrecht.

Norris, S.J. (1993). Polypeptides of *Treponema pallidum:* progress towards understanding their structural, functional and immunologic roles. *Microbiology Reviews,* **57,** 750–79.

Oriel, J.D. (1994). *Scars of Venus: a history of venereology.* p. 1–181. Springer Verlag. London.

Rothenburg, R. (1976). Treatment of neurosyphilis, *Journal of the American Medical Association,* **3,** 153–8.

Schouls, L.M. (1992). Molecular Biology of *Treponema pallidum.* In *Molecular and cell biology of sexually transmitted diseases* (Eds. D.J.M. Wright and L. Archard) pp. 85–129. Chapman and Hall, London.

Tomberlin, M.G., Holton, P.P., Owens, J.L., and Larsen, R.A. (1994). Evaluation of neurosyphilis in human immunodeficiency virus-infected individuals. *Clinics in Infectious Diseases,* **18,** 288–94.

US Department of Health and Human Services, Public Health Services: Centers for disease control. (1993). *Sexually transmitted disease surveillance, 1992.* pp. 6–11, 139–148, (definitions: 185–187). Atlanta, GA.

WHO. *Draft recommendations for the management of sexually transmitted diseases.* WHO advisory group meeting. (1993). pp. 24–31. WHO, Geneva. WHO/GPA/STD/93.1.

Wicher. K., Noordhoek G.T., Abbruscatto, F., and Wicher, V. (1992). Detection of *Treponema pallidum* in early syphilis by DNA amplification. *Journal of Clinical Microbiology,* **30,** 497–500.

Wilner, E . and Brady, J.A. (1968). Prognosis of general paresis after treatment. *Lancet,* **ii,** 1370–1.

Wright, D.J.M. and Doniach, D. (1971). The significance of cardiolpin immunofluorescence (CLF). *Proceedings of the Royal Society of Medicine,* **64,** 419–22.

7.11.35 Listeria and listeriosis

P. J. Wilkinson

Listeria monocytogenes

Listeria monocytogenes is a non-sporing, Gram-positive bacillus that can be cultivated under aerobic and anaerobic conditions on a range of laboratory media between pH 6 and pH 9, and at temperatures between 1 and 45 °C, although optimum growth occurs between 30 and 37 °C. Morphologically, *L. monocytogenes* resembles a diphtheroid, from which it is distinguishable in a hanging-drop preparation by its characteristic 'tumbling' motility. Colonies on blood agar are β-haemolytic and have a bluish-grey colour. Growth is enhanced in an atmosphere enriched with carbon dioxide, and *Listeria* spp. are catalase-positive, oxidase-negative, methyl red-positive, and Voges–Proskauer (VP) positive.

The genus listeria

The definition of the genus Listeria includes the property, demonstrated by *L. monocytogenes,* of producing a monocytosis in rodents, keratoconjunctivitis in rabbits, and septic lesions in various organs of warm-blooded animals. The disease as described in rabbits in 1926 was characterized by large-celled mononucleosis. Although *L. monocytogenes* is the only human pathogen in the genus, six other species of Listeria have been described, namely *L. innocua, L. ivanovii, L. seeligeri, L. welshimeri, L. grayi,* and *L. murrayi.*

Isolation and culture of listeria *spp.*

Whereas *L. monocytogenes* is the only species likely to be isolated from blood, cerebrospinal fluid, pus or tissues, other *Listeria* spp. may be found in faeces, food, soil, water, sewage sludge, and decaying vegetation. Cold enrichment (4 °C) in a non-selective broth medium has been used to enhance the isolation of *Listeria* spp. but is now superseded by the use of new selective media. Some food-processing methods (heating, chilling, freezing, chemical treatment) may cause sublethal injury to the microbial flora, and new approaches leading to the efficient recovery of sublethally injured *Listeria* spp. from foods are currently being investigated.

Typing and subtyping L. monocytogenes

L. monocytogenes is subdivided into serotypes on the basis of somatic (O) and flagellar (H) antigens. Eleven serotypes (1/2a, 1/2b, 1/2c, 3a, 3b, 4a, 4b, 4c, 4d, and 4e) are currently recognized. Because the majority of human infections are caused by serotypes 4b and, to a lesser extent, 1/2a and 1/2b, serotyping is of limited value in epidemiological investigations. Subtyping systems currently under development and evaluation include phage typing, multilocus enzyme electrophoresis, plasmid analysis, restriction fragment length polymorphism, and ribosomal DNA fingerprinting (ribotyping). Most subtyping methods available at present are laborious and do not easily permit the rapid screening of large numbers of isolates.

Rapid detection of Listeria *spp.*

Methods are becoming available for the rapid detection of *Listeria* spp. in clinical specimens and in food. These include immunoassays, DNA probe assays, and a two-step, nested polymerase chain reaction that may offer a means of detecting *L. monocytogenes* DNA retrospectively in preserved clinical specimens.

Pathogenesis of L. monocytogenes

The factors that influence whether invasive disease will occur include the virulence of the infecting organism, the susceptibility of the host, and the size of the infecting dose of bacteria.

The transmission of *L. monocytogenes* infection In food, this requires penetration of the organism through the intestine. Multiplication can then occur in various types of cells including non-immune phagocytes and cells of Peyer's patches. The production of listeriolysin O is thought to permit pathogenic *Listeria* spp. to disrupt vacuolar membranes and pass from the phagosome into the cytoplasm, where conditions for multiplication may be more favourable.

The virulence of *L. monocytogenes* This is related to the production of specific toxins, including listeriolysin O and haemolysin.

Host susceptibility This is related to cell-mediated immunity and most listeriosis occurs in people in whom this is depressed by pregnancy, disease, or immunosuppressive or cytotoxic therapy. Although reports of listeriosis in patients with AIDS may seem infrequent, listeriosis occurs at least 300 times more often in such patients, although other opportunistic infections are more common. In experimental mice, susceptibility to listeria infection can be genetically linked.

Listeriosis

ANIMALS

Listeriosis in mammals causes abortions and meningoencephalitis. Epizootics of listeriosis were observed in herds of cattle and sheep long before outbreaks of listeriosis were recognized in man. Healthy animals can be gastrointestinal carriers of *L. monocytogenes.* Silage is a source of infection with *L. monocytogenes* in domestic ruminants. Listeriosis was therefore regarded as a zoonosis; human disease was thought to result from illness in animals and the animal host was considered to be the primary reservoir for the organism. However, most cases of human listeriosis occur in town dwellers with no history of direct contact with animals, and the disease is rare in rural areas. Since 1980, epidemiological evidence has accumulated that shows human listeriosis to be predominantly a food-borne infection.

HUMANS

Despite increasing public awareness and concern, listeriosis remains a rare, although serious, infection in industrialized countries. For example, only 100 to 150 cases of culture-confirmed listeriosis are notified annually from Britain and Ireland. This contrasts with some 30 000 cases of salmonellosis and campylobacter infection.

Between 1987 and 1989, there was a sharp rise in cases of listeriosis notified in Britain and Ireland, from 108 (1986) to 248 (1987), 309 (1988) and 266 (1989). Most cases were due to *L. monocytogenes* serotype 4b, and the majority of the excess cases were associated with two particular subtypes of serotype 4b, namely 4bX and 4b phage type 6, 7, which were also found in high counts in a brand of meat paté that was widely sold in the United Kingdom. A warning in July 1989 by the Chief Medical Officer to pregnant women and vulnerable (immunocompromised) persons not to eat meat paté was followed by a decline in cases to pre-1987 levels (130 in 1991) and the virtual disappearance from human cases of subtypes 4bX and 4b phage type 6, 7. In 1993, an outbreak in France with *L. monocytogenes* serovar 4b, lysovar 2671/108/312 was associated with the consumption of pork rillettes.

Epidemiological patterns of human listeriosis

There are two main epidemiological patterns for human listeriosis.

1. Epidemic disease:
   (a) community-acquired outbreaks of common-source, food-borne listeriosis;
   (b) hospital-acquired outbreaks, spread by cross-infection.
2. Sporadic infections:
   (a) isolated cases of community-acquired, food-borne listeriosis;
   (b) sporadic, localized skin and eye infections acquired occupationally by workers with animals or their products.

Food-borne listeriosis

An outbreak in 1981 in Nova Scotia provided the first reported evidence for the transmission of listeriosis by food. Forty-one cases (7 adult, 34 maternofetal) had eaten coleslaw produced by one manufacturer. Unopened packages of coleslaw contained the serotype (4b) and phage type of *L. monocytogenes* implicated in the outbreak. Cabbages incorporated without heat treatment into coleslaw had been obtained from fields that were manured from a flock of sheep known to have had cases of listeriosis.

Other outbreaks of food-borne listeriosis have been associated with vegetables, raw fish, fresh cream, pasteurized milk, fruit, Mexican-style soft cheese, Swiss soft cheese (Vacheron Mont d'Or), salami, Brie cheese, pork rillettes, and meat paté.

Sporadic cases of food-borne listeriosis have been attributed to the consumption of undercooked chicken, undercooked hot-dogs, turkey franks, ice-cream, and other dairy products. A large case-control study of dietary risk factors in sporadic listeriosis by the Listeria Study Group, United States Centers for Disease Control showed that cases were more likely than matched controls to have eaten soft cheeses or food purchased from store delicatessen counters. In immunosuppressed patients, eating undercooked chicken also increased the risk of listeriosis.

As a result of the evidence to date, the United Kingdom Department of Health advises pregnant women and the immunocompromised to avoid eating foods that are liable to be contaminated with high levels of *Listeria* spp., in particular:

- soft ripened cheeses such as Brie, Camembert, and blue-vein types;
- all types of paté;
- cook-chill meals and ready-to-eat poultry unless thoroughly reheated until piping hot before they are eaten.

Hospital-acquired listeriosis

Clusters of cases of late-onset neonatal listeriosis have been reported from a number of countries. Poor hand hygiene, close contact between infected patients and their mothers, and fomites such as rectal thermometers, contaminated resuscitation equipment, and contaminated mineral oil used to bathe newborn infants have all been implicated. Both person-to-person and food-borne spread have been suspected in outbreaks amongst adult immunosuppressed patients in hospital.

Occupationally acquired listeriosis

Eye and skin infections without systemic involvement have occasionally been reported in agricultural, veterinary, and laboratory workers who have been directly exposed to infected animals or culture material.

Clinical features

L. monocytogenes can cause a wide range of clinical presentations from asymptomatic carriage or a mild, influenza-like illness to fatal septicaemia and meningoencephalitis. The following syndromes are recognized:

(1) maternofetal listeriosis;
(2) neonatal listeriosis;
(3) listeriosis in children and adults:
   (a) septicaemia,
   (b) meningoencephalitis,
   (c) other localized infections.

Maternofetal listeriosis This syndrome can occur at any time during pregnancy. The mother may develop a fever, with headache, myalgia, and back pain, associated with the bacteraemic phase of the disease. Lower back pain may mimic urinary-tract infection. Transplacental infection causes amnionitis, usually leading to either spontaneous septic abortion or premature labour with the delivery of an infected fetus or baby.

Neonatal listeriosis When of early onset, neonatal listeriosis has a high mortality and results from intrauterine infection. Usually, the mother has had an influenza-like illness before the onset of labour. The liquor is meconium-stained and the baby septic and jaundiced, with signs of purulent conjunctivitis, bronchopneumonia, meningitis, or encephalitis. Granulomas affecting many organs are a unique feature of this disease, which is therefore also termed granulomatosis infantisepticum. Late-onset disease occurs after several days to weeks in a baby who is initially healthy. Although the mother's genital tract is the usual source of infection, spread in nurseries and labour suites has also been described.

Listeria septicaemia This occurs mainly in patients with malignancies, in transplant recipients, and in immunosuppressed and elderly people. Most present with fever, hypotension, and shock but a third to a half develop meningitis, which may be the presenting feature.

Listeria meningoencephalitis This may start abruptly but in adults it can also develop insidiously, with progressive focal neurological signs even in the absence of a brain abscess. Most patients have meningism, but fever may not be marked, particularly in elderly or immunosuppressed people. Listeriosis should be considered in any patient with an acute brain-stem disorder associated with fever, particularly if there are no risk factors for cerebrovascular disease.

Other localized infections These are rare and occur mainly in immunosuppressed people. They include osteomyelitis, septic arthritis, cholecystitis, abscesses, and peritonitis. They usually result from seeding during an initial bacteraemic phase, but can also result from direct, occupational exposure.

Diagnosis

Microbiological diagnosis

Definitive microbiological diagnosis of invasive listeriosis is made by blood culture. This diagnosis may be supported by the microscopic demonstration of Gram-positive bacilli in a stained smear, and by culture of the organism from meconium, nose or eye swabs, urine, cerebrospinal fluid, blood, tracheal aspirate, placental tissue, and/or lochia.

Cultures from sites such as the vagina or faeces have the disadvantage that a positive result is not diagnostic of listeriosis and may show carriage of *L. monocytogenes* only. Moreover, antenatal vaginal examination to obtain a high vaginal or endocervical swab is not without risk to the pregnancy.

Serological tests

Tests for listeria antibodies in maternal and cord blood samples are unhelpful. They are unsuitable for screening either symptomatic patients or asymptomatic pregnant women who are worried that they could have become infected from eating a high-risk food.

Acute-phase markers

The common markers of bacterial infection, such as assays of C-reactive protein, may support a clinical diagnosis of listeriosis while the results of bacterial culture are awaited. Serial, quantitative estimations of C-reactive protein may be helpful in monitoring the efficacy of antimicrobial chemotherapy.

Antibiotic treatment

There have been no controlled clinical trials of antibiotic treatments for listeriosis, and views about the optimal antibiotic regimen are generally based on small series, historical comparisons, and clinical experience.

L. monocytogenes is generally susceptible *in vitro* to the aminoglycosides (e.g. gentamicin), ampicillin, benzylpenicillin, chloramphenicol, ciprofloxacin, erythromycin, imipenem, mezlocillin, rifampicin, some sulphonamides, tetracyclines, trimethoprim, and vancomycin. The organism is only moderately susceptible to some cephalosporins (cefazolin, cefotaxime, ceftriaxone) and resistant to most others, including the oral cephalosporins and ceftazidime. Some strains are partly resistant to penicillin, but synergy can be demonstrated *in vitro* between ampicillin and gentamicin, and between mezlocillin and gentamicin, combinations that are bactericidal, as is gentamicin alone.

The current consensus favours a combination of ampicillin and gentamicin as the treatment of choice for listeriosis. Because of its potential for fetal toxicity, gentamicin is best avoided in pregnancy, when ampicillin or amoxycillin may be used alone. Successful treatment has also been reported with intravenous chloramphenicol and with co-trimoxazole.

Treatment failures have been reported with penicillin alone and with cephalosporins, despite apparent *in vitro* susceptibility. Rifampicin has not been evaluated in human listeriosis, but it is theoretically attractive because of its ability to cross the blood–brain barrier, enter polymorphonuclear leucocytes, and kill intracellular bacteria. However, rifampicin is bacteriostatic against *L. monocytogenes in vitro* and, like chloramphenicol, may be antagonistic when used with ampicillin or penicillin. Ciprofloxacin has *in vitro* activity against *Listeria* spp. but it has not yet been evaluated in listeriosis.

The appropriate duration of therapy also remains unsettled. A period of 2 weeks has been sufficient in some series, but recurrence after 14 days of treatment has been noted, particularly in immunosuppressed patients, so 3 to 6 weeks of treatment is probably safer. This longer course, which should also be considered in neonatal listeriosis, is likely to improve the outcome when organisms are sequestered in deep granulomatous tissues.

Neonatal listeriosis should be treated with ampicillin or amoxycillin, 200 to 400 mg/kg a day in four divided doses given intravenously or intramuscularly for at least 3 weeks (up to 6 weeks in meningitis), and combined with gentamicin in conventional doses for the first 14 days. Adults should be given intravenous ampicillin or amoxycillin, 6 to 12 g daily in three or four divided doses, combined with gentamicin for the first 14 days in a dosage of 5 mg/kg per day, adjusted according to renal function with the help of plasma concentration measurement. Focal listeriosis may be treated with ampicillin or amoxycillin, 3 to 6 g daily or 100 mg/kg daily, until clinical resolution.

In cases of genuine penicillin allergy, effective treatment is difficult. A tetracycline such as minocycline, which penetrates the cerebrospinal fluid relatively well, may be considered in combination with gentamicin. Some success has been reported with co-trimoxazole and with chloramphenicol. Vancomycin has also been proposed, but there is at present insufficient information to recommend it.

Prognosis

Despite antibiotic therapy, the mortality of septicaemia and meningoencephalitis with *L. monocytogenes* remains high (20–50 per cent). There is significant long-term morbidity in the survivors. Efforts should therefore continue to be focused on the prevention of this infection by improvement in the microbiological safety of methods of food production and preparation, and by education of the public so that vulnerable people can avoid high-risk foods.

REFERENCES

Department of Health (1991). *While you are pregnant: safe eating and how to avoid infection from food and animals.* HMSO, London.

Gellin, B.G. and Broome, C.V. (1989). Listeriosis. *Journal of the American Medical Association*, **261**, 1313–20.

House of Commons Social Services Committee (1989). *Food poisoning: listeria and listeriosis.* HMSO, London.

McLauchlin, J., Hall, S.M., Velani, S.K., and Gilbert, R.J. (1991). Human listeriosis and paté: a possible association. *British Medical Journal*, **303,** 773–5.

Murray, E.G.D., Webb, R.A., and Swann, M.B.R. (1926). A disease of rabbits characterized by a large mononuclear leucocytosis, caused by a hitherto undescribed bacillus, *Bacterium monocytogenes. Journal of Pathological Biology*, **29,** 407–39.

Réseau national de la Santé publique. (1994). Epidémie de listériose à lysovar 2671-108-312 en France. *Bulletin Épidémiologique Hebdomadaire*, **34,** 157–8.

Schlech III, W.F. (1991). Listeriosis: epidemiology, virulence and the significance of contaminated foodstuffs. *Journal of Hospital Infection*, **19,** 211–24.

Schuchat, A., Swaminathan, B., and Broome, C.V. (1991). Epidemiology of Human Listeriosis. *Clinical Microbiology Reviews*, **4,** 169–83.

Schuchat, A. *et al.* (1992). Role of foods in sporadic listeriosis: 1. Case-control study of dietary risk factors. *Journal of the American Medical Association*, **267,** 2041–5.

Wilkinson, P.J. (1989). Ignorance about listeria. *British Medical Journal*, **299,** 276–7.

Wilkinson, P.J. (1992). Uncommon infections: 2. Listeriosis. *Prescribers' Journal*, **32,** 26–31.

7.11.36 Legionellosis and legionnaires' disease

J. B. KURTZ and J. T. MACFARLANE

In 1976 an outbreak of pneumonia occurred among American legionnaires who had attended a convention in a Philadelphia hotel. A total of 221 people developed pneumonia, 'legionnaires' disease', of whom 34 died. Initially there was some difficulty in determining the cause but subsequently it was shown by workers at the Centers for Disease Control, Atlanta, that a newly identified organism, named after this outbreak,

Legionella pneumophila, was responsible. Since this discovery, other outbreaks and sporadic cases have been recognized both retrospectively and prospectively. The first known epidemic, diagnosed retrospectively by serological studies, occurred in 1965 at a psychiatric hospital in Washington DC and involved 81 patients (15 deaths).

More recently, other *L. pneumophila* serotypes (14) have been identified and other species of legionella besides *L. pneumophila* have been isolated from clinical and environmental samples. There are now 43 recognized species in the Legionellaceae family and more continue to be added to the list. Clinical illness caused by members of the family Legionellaceae is referred to as legionellosis. Legionnaires' disease is pneumonia caused by *L. pneumophila.* Non-pneumonic legionellosis ('Pontiac fever') is a self-limiting, 'flu-like illness, without radiographic changes in the lung, caused by many different legionella species. What determines the type of illness that will follow infection is unknown. Although, in a given outbreak, disease of both pneumonic and non-pneumonic types occurs, usually either one or other form predominates. *L. pneumophila* is responsible for over 80 per cent of legionellosis and of the 14 serogroups, serogroup 1 is the most frequently encountered as human infections. Other legionella species appear to be less pathogenic and are more frequently found as opportunist pathogens in immunocompromised people. Some have caused disease, others have only been isolated from the environment and have yet to be implicated as human pathogens (Fig. 1).

The organism

The Legionellaceae are aerobic, non-sporing bacilli whose cell walls contain distinctive branched-chain fatty acids. This permits species identification by gas–liquid chromatography. The closeness of the relationship of 18 different legionellae species as determined by variations in the sequence of the highly conserved 16*s* ribosomal RNA between the species is shown in the dendrogram in Fig. 1. Those species in bold print have caused human illness.

Legionellae appear as slender rods of variable lengths from coccal to filamentous forms, 20 μm or longer. They stain red with Gram stain. In the laboratory, legionellae are fastidious in their growth requirements and will not grow on standard bacteriological media. Aces buffered charcoal yeast-extract (**BCYE**) agar, pH 6.9, supplemented with L-cysteine, α-ketoglutarate and iron, is a very satisfactory medium and is made semiselective by the addition of antibacterial and antifungal agents that suppress other microflora in specimens from contaminated sites. On BCYE agar, incubated at 35 to 37 °C, typical colonies usually appear in 3 to 5 days; occasional slow-growing strains require the plates to be incubated for 10 days. Some legionella species, grown on BCYE agar, autofluoresce when exposed to long-wave ultraviolet light (approx. 365 nm). The family Legionellaceae can be divided into three groups by this observation: the majority, including *L. pneumophila*, which do not fluoresce; blue/white fluorescent species (*L. bozemanii, L. dumoffii, L. gormanii, L. anisa, L. cherrii, L. parisiensis, L. stegerwaltii* and *L. Tusonensis*); and *L. erythra* and *L. rubilucens* that fluoresce red.

Suspected colonies are checked for their inability to grow on BCYE agar from which L-cysteine has been omitted. Immunofluorescence, using a panel of antisera is then usually sufficient for the routine identification of legionella species (and serogroups). When isolates from a patient and a suspected environmental source (see below) have been made, an accurate comparison of the strains should be undertaken. Both genotypic (e.g. restriction fragment length polymorphism) and phenotopic (e.g. monoclonal antibody reaction pattern) methods of identification should be used in parallel to see whether the two isolates are indistinguishable or different.

Epidemiology

The natural habitat of legionellae is fresh water of streams, lakes and thermal springs, moist soil, and mud. They have been found worldwide in waters with temperatures varying from 5 to 62 °C and pH of 5.4 to 8.2. These organisms are inhibited by sodium chloride and are not found

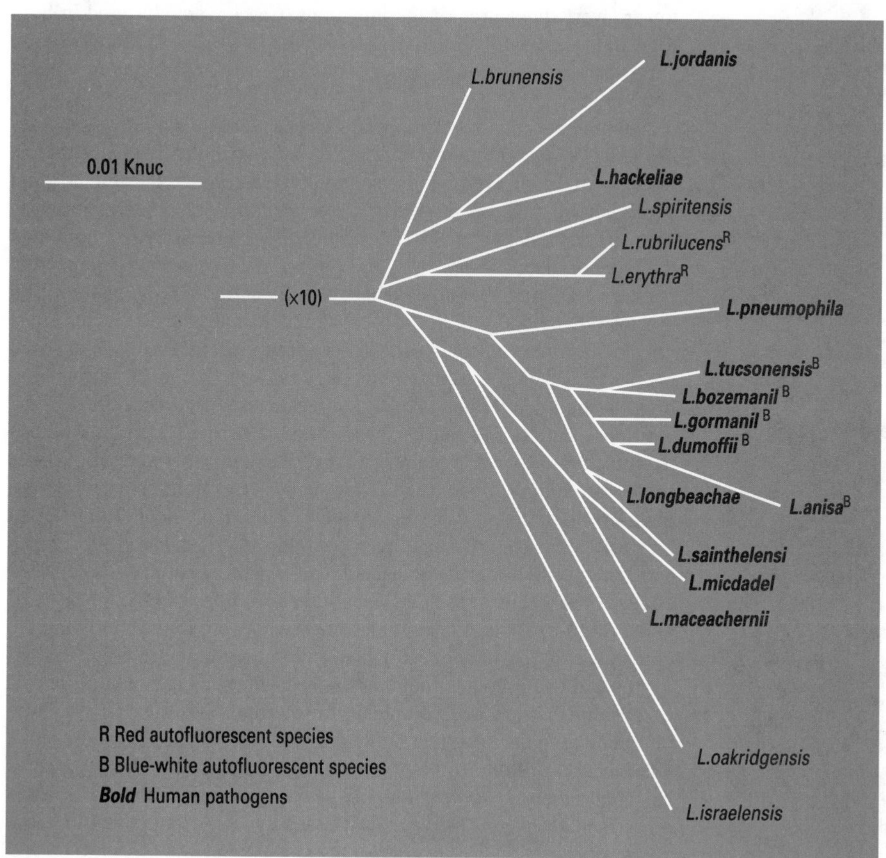

Fig. 1 Phylogenetic tree showing the relationships within the family Legionellaceae. The tree is rooted by reference to *Coxiella burnetii*. (By courtesy of N.K. Fry, Central Public Health Laboratory, London.)

in sea water. In natural habitats they are found in only small numbers, forming part of the consortium of micro-organisms that makes up the biofilm. This includes amoebae and other protozoa, in certain of which it has been shown legionellae can multiply and survive. Inside these protozoa the bacteria form microcolonies (Fig. 2(a)), which are protected from adverse conditions (for example, in amoebic cysts from desiccation and up to 50 parts/10^6 free chlorine). This association might therefore help the bacteria to disseminate widely.

Legionellae have been found in small numbers in water distribution systems, through which they can colonize man-made habitats, again as part of the biofilm from which they are shed into the water. Factors that encourage colonization and multiplication are temperature (20–45 °C) and stagnation. The most common sites in buildings in which legionellae have been found are hot-water calorifiers and storage tanks, where there are temperature strata often providing ideal conditions for growth at the bottom. Piped water, especially hot water from the calorifiers in large buildings and industrial complexes with long runs of pipework, is a potential source of infection. The classical example was the endemic of legionnaires' disease in the Wadsworth Medical Center in California, where there was an average of 4.5 cases per month between May 1977 and February 1980. Control was finally achieved by continuous chlorination (1–2 parts/10^6) of the incoming water (see Prevention below). Other well-recognized sources include:

- recirculating water in air-conditioning and cooling systems;
- whirlpool spas and other warm-water baths;
- decorative fountains;
- nebulizers and humidifier reservoirs of hospital ventilation machines if topped up with contaminated tap water.

Potting compost was the source of one outbreak of pneumonia caused by *L. longbeachae* serogroup 1 in South Australia.

Dissemination of infection is by contaminated water droplets (aerosol), which are inhaled. In order to cause infection the droplets must be of a size (less than 5 μm diameter) that can reach the alveoli of the lungs. Taps and shower heads produce very localized aerosols whereas the water droplets (drift) contained in the airstream released from a cooling tower may be carried a considerable distance in suitable weather conditions and expose a greater number of people to risk. Large, explosive outbreaks affecting people not only in a building but also in the vicinity are typical of a cooling-tower source. For example, in the 1976 Philadelphia outbreak, those infected in the street developed 'Broad Street pneumonia' and passers-by were infected in both the Stafford Hospital outbreak in 1985 (101 cases, 28 deaths) and near the BBC building, London, in 1988 (79 cases, 2 deaths). Person-to-person spread of legionellosis has never been recorded.

Although most studies of legionnaires' disease have been of outbreaks, sporadic cases account for about three-quarters of those reported in England and Wales. A source is only exceptionally found for them. Some of these sporadic events become part of an outbreak when other cases can be linked to them epidemiologically in time and space, as when patients from different geographic areas give a history of visiting a common site within the incubation period of their illnesses. An association with overseas travel was found in one-third of the sporadic cases in England and Wales for the 3 years 1979 to 1986. Apart from travel, an analysis of sporadic (better called non-travel, non-outbreak) cases in Glasgow between 1978 and 1986 supported the hypothesis that cooling towers were the source of the infections. Cases were clustered in both time and space, with a relative risk three times greater for people living within 500 m of a cooling tower compared with those living more than 1000 m away.

In temperate countries legionellosis has a seasonal pattern, most cases occurring in the summer and autumn. A multicentre British Thoracic Society study of community-acquired pneumonia requiring hospital admission in 1982–83 showed that 2 per cent had legionnaires' disease. This suggests that about 1500 cases occur per year in Britain, although the number of confirmed cases in England and Wales notified annually between 1979 and 1986 ranged between 129 and 211. Obviously, within this overall incidence there are local variations in frequency, as the Glasgow experience indicates. The susceptibility to infection of exposed people varies. For non-pneumonic legionellosis the attack rate is very high. In the Lochgoilhead Hotel outbreak caused by *L. micdadei* in the whirlpool spa, 91 per cent of those exposed were affected. In contrast, the attack rate for legionnaires' disease is about 1 per cent and illness is more common in men than in women (2–3:1). Immunosuppression, pre-existing chronic disease, smoking, and high alcohol intake all increase vulnerability. Subclinical or mild infections can follow exposure, as indicated by serological surveys of workers (nurses, hotel staff, etc.) at sites where there have been outbreaks. For example, of the staff at the Stafford District General Hospital who were tested following the outbreak in 1985, 42 per cent had an antibody titre of 1 in 16 or greater.

Hospital-acquired legionellosis has been a particular problem. This is because of the size and complexity of the buildings and the difficulty of maintaining the hot water hot (storage at 60 °C and 50 °C at the taps), either because of the length of pipework or for fear of scalding patients. Hospital patients, too, are a highly susceptible population and species other than *L. pneumophila* more frequently cause infections in these circumstances.

Fig. 2 The intracellular situation of legionella. (a) A microcolony of *L. pneumophila* within the amoeba *Acanthamoeba palestinensis*. (b) A neutrophil containing numerous legionellae intact within vacuoles (reproduced from Macfarlane, J.T. (1990). Acute respiratory infections in adults. *Respiratory Medicine* (ed. R.A.L. Brewis, G.J. Gibson, and D.M. Geddes). Balliere Tindall, London, by permission from the editors, and by courtesy of T.S.J. Elliott.)

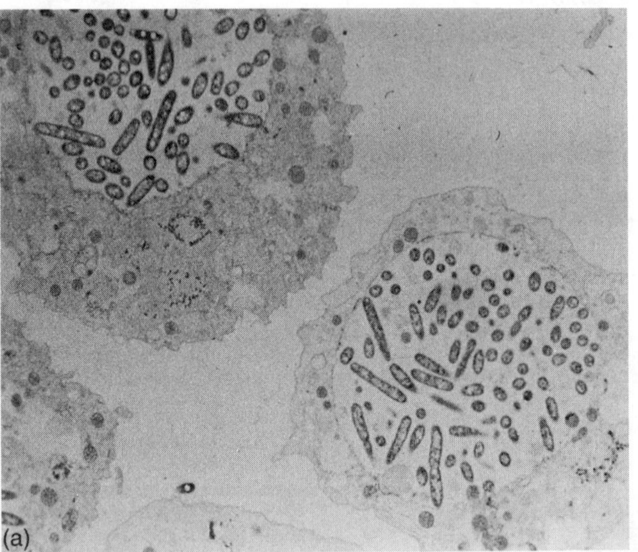

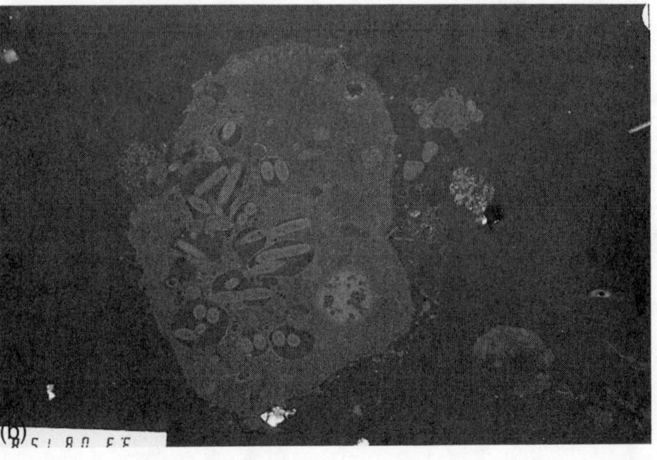

Table 1 *Clinical features of 739 patients with legionella pneumonia*

Respiratory symptoms (%)	
Cough	75
New sputum production	45
Dyspnoea	50
Chest pain	36
Haemoptysis	21
Bronchial breathing in lung	16
Crepitations in lung	74
General symptoms (%)	
Rigors	59
Headaches	32
Confusion	45
Diarrhoea	33
Fever over 39 °C	70

Data adapted from Table 3.2: Bartlett, C.R., Macrae, A.D., and Macfarlane, J.T. (1986). *Legionella infections*. Edward Arnold, London, with permission of the publishers.

Clinical manifestations

Over 80 per cent of infections are caused by *L. pneumophila* species, most commonly serogroup 1. *L. micdadei* is the second most common pathogen, more often affecting immunocompromised individuals.

As noted before, legionella infections manifest in two main forms, pneumonia or Pontiac fever. It is not clear why people similarly exposed may develop either one or the other form of the disease although differing virulence of legionella strains and also host factors are likely to be important.

Legionella pneumonia

A broad range of clinical presentation exists, varying from asymptomatic or mild infection (shown only by seroconversion) through to the rapidly progressive severe pneumonia that is more commonly equated with legionnaires' disease. Large studies have suggested that legionella infection is the cause of around 2 to 5 per cent of cases of community-acquired pneumonia admitted to hospital, although there is wider geographical and seasonal variation. Unlike most other bacterial respiratory pathogens, infection tends to lead to moderate or severe infection rather than mild illness, and most patients require hospital admission within 5 to 7 days of the start of symptoms.

The incubation period is usually 2 to 10 days, with a mean of 7 days; males are two to three times more frequently affected than females. Infection at the extremes of age is rare and the highest incidence is in 40 to 70-year-old people, with a mean of 53 years. People particularly at risk include cigarette smokers, alcoholics, diabetics, and those with chronic illness or who are receiving corticosteroids or immunosuppressive therapy. Consequently, the type of patient who requires admission to hospital is particularly at risk from a nosocomial source.

CLINICAL FEATURES (TABLE 1)

Typically, the illness starts fairly abruptly with high fevers, shivers, bad headache, and muscle pains. Upper respiratory tract symptoms, herpes labialis, and skin rashes are uncommon. The cough that follows may be insignificant and dry initially but dyspnoea is common and the illness often progresses quickly. Sometimes there may be a history of a recent hotel holiday abroad or a stay in hospital, which can alert the clinician to the possible diagnosis.

The patient commonly looks toxic and ill, with a high fever over 39 °C in three-quarters of cases. Sometimes non-respiratory features, such as confusion and delirium or diarrhoea, which occur in more than one-half of the patients, can dominate the clinical picture, masking the true diagnosis of pneumonia although localizing signs can invariably be detected in the chest. Focal neurological signs, particularly of a cerebellar type, are well described but meningitis does not occur. Amnesia on recovery is common.

LABORATORY FINDINGS

The total white count is usually only moderately raised, to 15 000 × 10^6/l in two-thirds of cases, often with a lymphopenia. Hyponatraemia, hypoalbuminaemia, and abnormality of liver function tests are detected in over one-half of the cases. Other features may include raised blood urea and muscle enzymes, hypoxaemia, haematuria, and proteinuria but none of these is unique for legionella pneumonia. Gram stain of sputum stain typically shows few pus cells and no predominant pathogen; initial blood and sputum cultures are negative unless dual infection is present.

RADIOGRAPHIC FEATURES

Radiographic shadowing is usually homogeneous and commonly confined to one of the lower lobes on presentation. Characteristically, radiographic deterioration occurs with spread of shadows both within the same lung and to the opposite side. (Fig. 3). A small pleural effusion can occur in one-quarter of cases; lung cavitation is rare except in immunosuppressed patients.

Clearance of pulmonary shadows in survivors is particularly slow, with only two-thirds of radiographs being clear within 3 months and some taking more than 6 months to clear.

COMPLICATIONS

A wide variety of complications has been reported, affecting nearly every system of the body. These probably arise more commonly from a multisystem toxic effect rather than from direct spread of the bacteria, which appears rare.

The most important, immediate pulmonary complication is acute respiratory failure requiring assisted ventilation, which occurs in up to 20 per cent of cases. Cardiac complications including pericardial and myocardial involvement are well recognized. A wide variety of neurological complications has been reported, leading to the suggestion of a specific neurotoxin. Acute, but usually reversible, renal failure may be seen in severe disease. There is anecdotal evidence that full clinical recovery

Fig. 3 The chest radiograph of a 58-year-old man who returned from a hotel holiday by the Mediterranean with legionella pneumonia. There is extensive, bilateral, homogeneous consolidation. He required assisted ventilation for worsening respiratory failure.

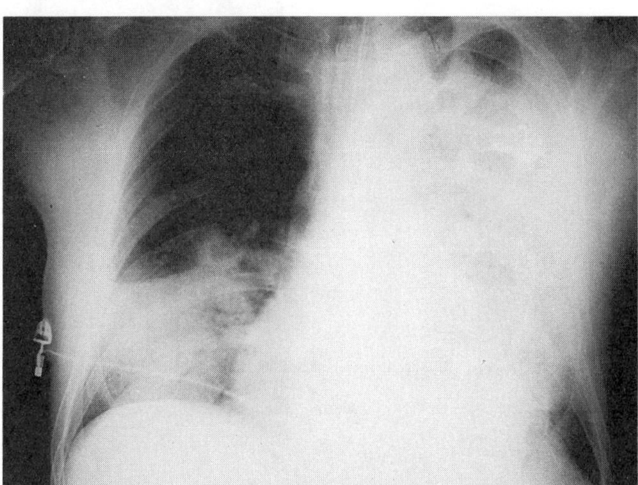

may be very slow but properly controlled follow-up studies of the rate of recovery and incidence of prolonged sequelae in survivors are required.

Pontiac fever

This is the acute non-pneumonic form of legionella infection and presents as a short-lived, self-limiting, flu-like illness. The attack rate is extremely high, with an incubation period of usually 36 to 48 h. Previously healthy people are usually affected, with high fever, shivers, headache, myalgia, malaise and dizziness, some dry cough but no localizing signs in the chest (Fig. 4). Investigations and chest radiograph are normal, and illness improves spontaneously, usually within 5 days. The diagnosis is usually made retrospectively by serological testing and treatment is symptomatic. Deaths have not been reported, although non-specific symptoms and lassitude may be experienced following recovery. It is possible that Pontiac fever is a reaction to inhaling amounts of legionella antigen from large numbers of predominantly dead bacteria.

Laboratory diagnosis

There is a range of laboratory procedures that can be used to diagnose legionellosis:

(1) culture on a permissive medium, e.g. BCYE agar;
(2) direct detection of bacteria or their nucleic acid;
(3) urinary antigen detection;
(4) serological response.

Suitable specimens from which legionellae can be isolated are expectorated sputum, endotracheal aspirates, bronchoalveolar lavage fluid, pleural aspirates, and lung. Culture must be done on suitable medium with added antimicrobials to make it semiselective. Isolation is the method of choice; it allows the causative strain to be typed and compared with those from the environment. A quicker diagnosis can be made by examining these samples directly for evidence of legionellae. With specific monoclonal antisera the bacteria can be visualized by immunofluorescence or immunoperoxidase techniques. Alternatively DNA hybridization to legionella ribosomal RNA or the use of the polymerase chain reaction can detect the bacterial nucleic acid directly in a specimen.

Soluble antigen is excreted in the urine for 1 to 3 weeks during the acute pneumonia and longer in immunocompromised infected patients. Tests to detect *L. pneumophila* serogroup 1 urinary antigen have a high specificity and sensitivity. For other *L. pneumophila* serogroups and legionella species there is concern about specificity and these tests have not yet been validated.

Serology is the most widely used diagnostic approach, especially with the indirect fluorescent antibody assay using formalinized yolk sac or heat-killed preparations of legionella bacteria as antigens. The microagglutination technique is also used. The major problem with serodiagnosis is the delay due to the slow production of antibodies, peak titres appearing 2 to 4 weeks after the onset of illness.

In Britain the serological criteria for diagnosis of *L. pneumophila* serogroup 1 are either a fourfold rise in indirect fluorescent antibody titre to more than 64 or a single titre in excess of 128 (or microagglutination titre of greater than 32). The single titre that gives a presumptive diagnosis must be determined locally and be higher than a cut-off level of antibody in that population. Only 20 per cent of patients with legionnaires' disease have diagnostic titres of antibody within 3 days of hospital admission, although about 40 per cent will have lesser but suggestive antibody levels by that time. Approximately 20 per cent of those infected appear not to respond serologically.

Background antibody titres to non-serogroup 1 *L. pneumophila* and other legionella species have not been as closely studied and the significance of antibodies to them is less clearly understood. Although some heterologous cross-reacting antibodies may be produced, infections with legionellae other than *L. pneumophila* serogroup 1 do not necessarily give rise to antibody to the latter, which is the commonly used antigen. Reference laboratories therefore use a battery of antigens to increase their ability to diagnose legionellosis. In Denmark, for example, 13 antigens are used and, in 1990, of 171 serologically diagnosed cases, 93 were *L. pneumophila* serogroup 1 to 6 while 78 were non-*L. pneumophila* legionellosis caused by other species. Occasionally patients with Q fever, leptospirosis, *Citrobacter freundii*, and more commonly with campylobacter infections make antibodies that cross-react with *L. pneumophila* serogroup 1. As diarrhoea can be an early feature of legionnaires' disease as well as the major consequence of campylobacter enteritis, it is important to culture stool samples and interpret with caution the legionella serology from such patients.

Fig. 4 Clinical features of 314 patients with non-pneumonic legionellosis (Pontiac fever). (Data adapted from Glick *et al.* (1978) and Goldberg *et al.* (1989).)

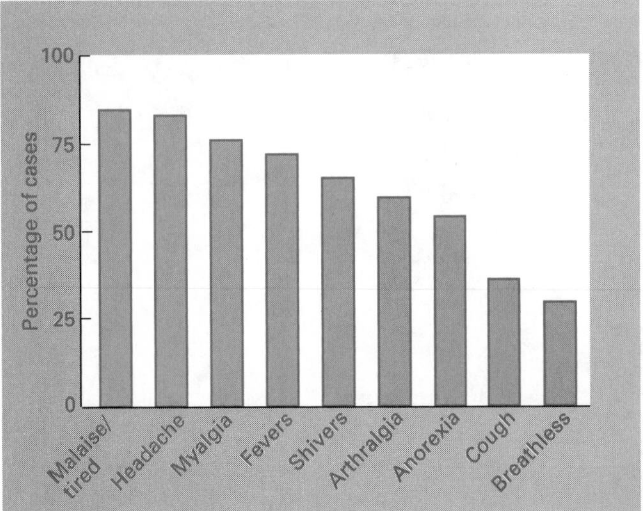

Differential diagnosis

Unfortunately there is no distinctive clinical, laboratory, or radiographic pattern that allows the early differentiation of legionella infection from other, more common causes of pneumonia. Epidemiological clues such as recent foreign travel or infection occurring during the summer months can be valuable pointers, as well, of course, as knowledge of a local epidemic. Important clues suggesting legionella pneumonia in this context include high fever, confusion, multisystem involvement, absence of a predominant bacterial pathogen on sputum examination, and lack of response to β-lactam antibiotics such as amoxycillin.

Such clinical features can also be seen with mycoplasma infection, psittacosis, and Q fever. Mycoplasma pneumonia tends to affect younger people, who give a longer history of illness and are usually less ill.

Therapy

There are no clinical trials on the efficacy of different antimicrobials for legionella infection and recommendations are based on retrospective case studies, as well as *in vitro* and animal experiments. Although the organism is susceptible to a wide range of antimicrobials *in vitro*, the most relevant factor is their ability to penetrate intracellularly into alveolar macrophages where the legionella organism hides and divides (see Fig. 2(b)). Erythromycin is at present recommended as the drug of first choice, in dosages of 500 to 1000 mg every 6 h, being given intravenously if required. Treatment is generally recommended for up to 2 to 3 weeks to prevent relapse, although shorter courses are often effective.

In vitro and animal experiments support the efficacy of rifampicin, quinolones, and newer macrolides. Rifampicin is often recommended as additional therapy to erythromycin, in a dose of 600 mg once or twice daily in patients who are deteriorating. Anecdotal reports also support the use of doxycycline and ciprofloxacin.

General supportive measures are particularly important, with attention to adequate hydration and correction of hypoxaemia with the early use of assisted ventilation for advancing respiratory failure.

Prognosis and mortality

The two most important factors affecting outcome include the prior health of the patient and appropriate, early therapy. The fatality rate in previously fit patients is low, in the order of 5 to 15 per cent, but in immunosuppressed individuals can approach 75 per cent.

Pathology

The lungs are usually the only organs affected in fatal cases and reveal lobar consolidation. Affected lung tissue on section characteristically shows a severe inflammatory response, with alveoli and terminal bronchioles distended by fibrin-rich debris, macrophages, and neutrophils (Fig. 5). In survivors, alveolar and interstitial fibrotic changes can result from the organization of fibrin and hyaline membranes. During the acute phase, organisms can be demonstrated within alveolar spaces by silver or immunofluorescence stains.

Prevention

Legionellosis is acquired from environmental water sources by the inhalation of water droplets. At first all the cases were attributed to exposure to the drift escaping from cooling towers of recirculating cooling systems. Now it is known that domestic and industrial piped water is the source of many cases. As legionellae are ubiquitous in natural waters there are three aspects to consider in reducing the risk of legionellosis:

(1) measures to minimize colonization, growth, and release of legionellae into the atmosphere;
(2) physical or chemical treatment of water to kill the bacteria;
(3) the protection of maintenance personnel who work on contaminated systems.

Fig. 5 Photomicrograph of an alveolus of a patient who died of legionella pneumonia. Note that the alveolar space is packed with mononuclear cells and fibrin. (Reproduced with permission from Macfarlane, J.T., Finch, R.G., and Cotton, R.E. (in press). *Colour Atlas of Respiratory Infections*. Chapman and Hall, London.)

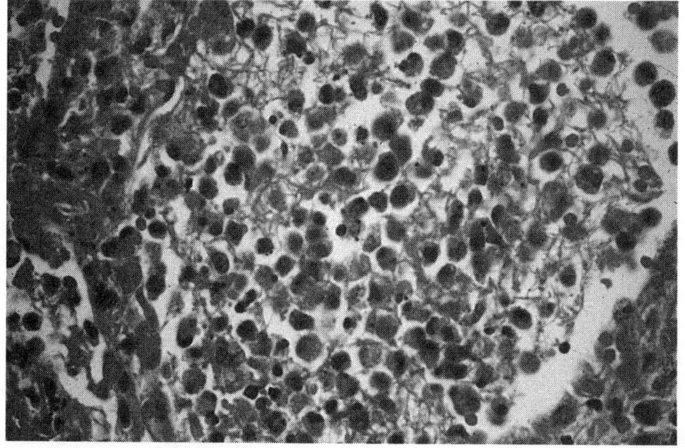

In Britain, particularly following the Stafford Hospital outbreak, a large number of publications aimed at minimizing the risk of legionellosis have appeared. In 1991 in Britain an Approved Code of Practice, *The Prevention or Control of Legionellosis (including Legionnaires' Disease)*, sets out statutory requirements for dealing with this risk. Together with the Health and Safety guidance booklet HS(G)70, which was published with it and should be consulted for more details, the Code applies wherever water is stored or used in a way that may create 'a reasonably foreseeable risk of legionellosis'. Examples are:

- recirculating water systems incorporating a cooling tower or evaporative condenser;
- hot-water systems with a volume greater than 300 l;
- hot- and cold-water systems of any size, serving a particularly susceptible population;
- water systems that create a spray and are likely to exceed a water temperature of 20 °C;
- whirlpool baths.

In any building or environment, systems that could be colonized by legionellae must be identified and their potential risks assessed. Then a scheme is prepared for prevention or control. The most important principle to follow is to avoid holding water at temperatures between 20 and 45 °C, which is the range in which legionella multiplication occurs. Other general precautions include:

- prevention of water stagnation and the elimination of 'dead legs';
- avoidance of plumbing and engineering materials that can provide nutrients for bacterial growth;
- preventing the concentration of sediments in the water by cleaning and good maintenance;
- the use of chemical or other water treatment, where appropriate and safe, to prevent bacterial growth;
- reduction or prevention of aerosol dispersion.

The implementation of the control scheme and maintenance programme must be monitored and records kept of all procedures, treatments, and test results. Above all, a senior manager must be appointed to have overall responsibility.

The Second Report of the Committee of Inquiry into the outbreak of Legionnaires' disease in Stafford in April 1985 recommended dry cooling equipment for air-conditioning plants. Although this may be preferred in some circumstances, dry cooling brings problems of weight, noise, high running costs, fouling by air pollution, and above all the inability to cool sufficiently in hot weather. Recent improvements in wet cooling-system designs have made them easier to clean. Improved drift eliminators have reduced water droplets discharged into the atmosphere from cooling towers from 2 to 0.001 per cent of the circulating water. The number of bacteria released has consequently fallen. Biocidal treatment of the recirculating water in cooling systems is also essential. This will not only kill bacteria in the water but also prevent the build up of biofilm throughout the system. If well designed, correctly installed and properly maintained, wet cooling systems do not pose a risk of infection.

The design and construction of hot- and cold-water services is equally important. The layout should ensure that hot water is kept hot and cold water remains at less than 20 °C. Where cold water is being supplied to a susceptible population, for example patients in hospital, and cannot be kept adequately cool, additional chlorination may be necessary. The design of calorifiers should prevent temperature stratification of the water inside. Hot water must be stored at 60 °C and reach 50 °C at taps within 1 min. Warm, recirculating water in whirlpool baths is filtered and chemically treated; regular maintenance and monitoring are essential to ensure these systems are safe. Routine bacterial tests of water quality (total viable counts and detection of faecal coliforms) will not give any indication of the presence or absence of legionellae in a water system. Water sampling specifically for legionella is necessary to monitor the efficacy of maintenance and precautionary measures and in the event of an associated human infection, to trace the source.

REFERENCES

Bartlett, C.R., Macrae, A.D., and MacFarlane, J.T. (1986). *Legionella infections*. Arnold, London.

Bhopal, R.S., Fallon, R.J., Buist, E.C., Black, R.J., and Urqhart, J.D. (1991). Proximity of the home to a cooling tower and the risk of non-outbreak Legionnaires' disease. *British Medical Journal*, **302,** 378–83.

Boswell, T.C.J. and Kudesia, G. (1992). Seropositivity for legionella in campylobacter infection. *Lancet*, **339,** 191.

Committee of Inquiry (1986). *First report of the Committee of Inquiry into the outbreak of Legionnaires' disease in Stafford in April 1985*, Cmnd 9772. HMSO, London.

Committee of Inquiry (1987). *Second report of the Committee of Inquiry into the outbreak of Legionnaires' disease in Stafford in April 1985*, Cmnd 256. HMSO, London.

Edelstein, P.H. and Meyer, R.D. (1988). Legionella pneumonias. In *Respiratory infections: diagnosis and management*, (2nd edn) (ed. J.E. Pennington). Raven Press, New York.

Fields, B.S. (1991). The role of amoebae in legionellosis. *Clinical Microbiology Newsletter*, **13,** 92–3.

Glick, T.H. *et al.* (1978). Pontiac fever: an epidemic of unknown aetiology in a health department. *American Journal of Epidemiology*, **107,** 149–60.

Goldberg, D.J. *et al.* (1989). Lochgoilhead fever: an outbreak of non-pneumonic Legionellosis due to *Legionella micdadei*. *Lancet*, **i,** 316–18.

Harrison, T.G. and Taylor, A.G. (ed.) (1988). *A laboratory manual for* Legionella. Wiley, Chichester.

Health and Safety Commission (1991). *Approved Code of Practice—The prevention or control of legionellosis (including Legionnaires' disease)*. HMSO, London.

Health and Safety Executive (1991). *The control of legionellosis including Legionnaires' disease*, HS(G)70. HMSO, London.

Research sub-committee of the British Thoracic Association (1987). Commonly-acquired pneumonia in British hospitals 1982–3: a survey of aetiology, mortality, prognostic factors and outcome. *Quarterly Journal of Medicine*, **62,** 195–200.

Shands, K.N. *et al.* (1985). Potable water as a source of Legionnaires' disease. *Journal of the American Medical Association*, **253,** 1412–16.

Woodhead, M.A. and Macfarlane, J.T. (1985). The protean manifestations of Legionnaires' disease. *Journal of the Royal College Physicians (London)*, **19,** 224–230.

Rickettsial diseases

7.11.37 Rickettsial diseases including ehrlichioses

D. H. Walker

Introduction

Rickettsial diseases comprise a heterogeneous group of infections. Considering the diversity of organisms categorized as rickettsiae, this is not surprising (Table 1). Rickettsiae are obligate intracellular bacteria, which, during at least a part of their existence, occupy specific arthropods as their environmental niche. Genera of rickettsiae that cause human illness include Rickettsia, Ehrlichia, and Coxiella. Organisms of the genus Rickettsia are transmitted to man by their arthropod hosts and invade the cells of the blood vessel; consequently, these vasculotropic diseases have epidemiological and clinical similarities. In contrast, organisms of the genus Ehrlichia invade mononuclear phagocytes, lymphocytes, or polymorphonuclear leucocytes and do not cause primary vascular injury. Nevertheless, infection with *E. chaffeensis* is transmitted by tick bite and is known to cause a disease resembling Rocky Mountain spotted fever. *Coxiella burnetii* is the most disparate rickettsial organism in its evolutionary relations, its ecological niche both in the environment and at the subcellular level, and in its clinical manifestations. Man acquires *C. burnetii* mainly by inhalation of aerosols from birth products of infected animals. The organisms proliferate within the acidic phagolysosome of host macrophages and cause an illness that ranges from acute atypical pneumonia to chronic endocarditis.

The public health importance of rickettsioses remains incompletely defined. They are considerably more difficult to diagnose clinically and epidemiologically than is generally appreciated, and effective, specific laboratory diagnostic methods are not available in many geographical areas. When physicians routinely consider rickettsial diagnoses for febrile illnesses and specific diagnostic and epidemiological investigations are made, rickettsioses are found to be endemic in many areas throughout the world. Active surveillance detects a much higher incidence of rickettsial diseases than is depicted by routine public-health reporting. Serological surveys suggest that there is significant, unrecognized exposure of many populations to rickettsial organisms. It is particularly important to consider a rickettsial diagnosis when caring for the neglected poor of developing countries and travellers returning from areas endemic for rickettsial diseases. It is probable that there are very high incidences of murine typhus, scrub typhus, boutonneuse fever, some other spotted fevers, and Q fever in many human populations. The incidence of some spotted fevers and human ehrlichioses is at present undefined. Rickettsiae cause infections of previously healthy, active persons, and if undiagnosed, diagnosed late, or untreated, some rickettsioses, particularly Rocky Mountain spotted fever, epidemic typhus, scrub typhus, and Q fever endocarditis, are life threatening. Deaths also occur in patients with boutonneuse fever, Israeli spotted fever, human ehrlichioses, and murine typhus.

Early treatment with antimicrobial agents active against rickettsiae shortens the course of illness and is potentially life saving (Table 2). Unfortunately, many commonly prescribed antibiotics, including the penicillins, cephalosporins, and aminoglycosides, have no effect on the course of rickettsial diseases. Lack of a generally available laboratory test that is diagnostic during the acute, treatable stage of illness challenges the physician's clinical acumen and knowledge of rickettsial diseases.

The most dramatic rickettsial disease is louse-borne epidemic typhus fever. There are compelling arguments that *R. prowazekii* has strongly influenced the outcome of many wars between the 1500s and the 1930s. During the Thirty Years War, between 50 and 75 per cent of the population of what is now Germany died primarily of typhus fever and bubonic plague. Napoleon's invasion of Russia with 550 000 troops in 1812 was defeated by typhus fever, cold winter weather, and starvation. The 3000 surviving soldiers brought home the rickettsiae, which spread through Europe killing 2 million persons. During the First World War, the Russian revolution, and its aftermath, 30 million persons suffered typhus fever and 3 million died. Wherever there are war, famine, floods, and other massive disasters leading to widespread louse infestation of a population, the threat of epidemic typhus exists. Famine-stricken parts of Africa, war-torn areas of Eastern Europe, and economically devastated republics of the former USSR are currently at risk of epidemic louse-borne typhus.

The scientific concept of a rickettsia emerged and was clarified during the development of our general understanding of infectious diseases and microbiology. The concept of a rickettsia is beginning to seem outmoded as the contemporary view of these micro-organisms places them clearly in the framework of bacterial evolution. Between 1906 and 1909, Howard Ricketts showed that Rocky Mountain spotted fever is an infectious disease transmissible to guinea-pigs and monkeys and that the tick now known as *Dermacentor andersoni* is the vector and reservoir. The agent was retained by a filter as are bacteria. The concept of a virus as we know it did not exist, and rickettsiae were sometimes referred to as viruses. In 1909, Charles Nicolle demonstrated the transmission of epidemic typhus by the human body louse. Between 1916 and 1922, S. Burt Wolbach showed that in the characteristic vascular lesions the

Table 1 *Aetiology, epidemiology, and ecology of rickettsial diseases*

Disease	Agent	Geographical distribution	Natural history	Transmission to man
Spotted fevers				
Rocky Mountain spotted fever	*R. rickettsii*	North, Central, and South America	Transovarial maintenance in ticks: less extensive horizontal transmission from tick to mammal to tick	Tick bite
Boutonneuse fever	*R. conorii*	Mediterranean basin, Africa, Asia	Transovarial maintenance in ticks; role of horizontal transmission is not clear	Tick bite
North Asian tick typhus	*R. sibirica*	Russia, China, Mongolia, Pakistan, Kazakhstan, Kirgiziya, Tadzhikistan	Transovarial maintenance in ticks; horizontal transmission from tick to mammal to tick	Tick bite
Oriental spotted fever	*R. japonica*	Japan	Presumably a transovarial tick host; the role of horizontal transmission is not clear	Tick bite
Queensland tick typhus	*R. australis*	Eastern Australia	Transovarial transmission in Ixodes ticks; the role of horizontal transmission is not clear	Tick bite
Rickettsialpox	*R. akari*	USA, Ukraine, Croatia, possibly worldwide	Transovarian transmission in *Liponyssoides sanguineus* mites; horizontal transmission from mite to mouse to mite	Mite bite
Typhus fevers				
Epidemic typhus	*R. prowazekii*	South America, Africa, Asia, Central America, Mexico	Man to louse to man	Louse faeces scratched into skin
Sylvatic typhus	*R. prowazekii*	United States	Flying squirrel to louse and flea ectoparasites to flying squirrel	Presumably flea of flying squirrels to man
Recrudescent typhus	*R. prowazekii*	Worldwide	Reactivation of latent human infection years after acute illness	None
Murine typhus	*R. typhi*	Worldwide, predominantly tropical and subtropical	Rat to rat flea to rat; opossum to cat flea to opossum	Flea faeces scratched into skin, rubbed into conjunctiva, or inhaled
Scrub typhus	*R. tsutsugamushi*	Japan, southern and eastern Asia, northern Australia, islands of the western and south-western Pacific	Transovarial transmission in Leptothrombidium chiggers	Chigger bite
Ehrlichioses				
Human ehrlichiosis	*E. chaffeensis*	USA, Portugal, Spain, Mali	Unknown	Tick bite
Sennetsu ehrlichiosis	*E. sennetsu*	Japan, Malaysia	Unknown	Unknown
Q fever	*C. burnetii*	Worldwide	Mammals including sheep, goats, cattle, rabbits and cats; ticks	Aerosol of infected mammalian birth products
Rochalimaea infections				
Trench fever	*R. quintana*	Europe, North America	Louse to man to louse	Louse faeces
Bacillary angiomatosis, peliosis, and cat-scratch disease	*R. henselae*	United States	Unknown	Unknown

aetiological agents of Rocky Mountain spotted fever and epidemic typhus had the morphology of intracellular bacteria. However, unlike most bacteria, rickettsiae could not be cultivated in broth or on nutrient agar. Rickettsiae require isolation and propagation in eukaryotic cells of laboratory animals, embryonated eggs, or cell culture, conditions similar to those required by viruses and chlamydiae. When electron microscopy became available, rickettsiae were observed to resemble Gram-negative bacteria. Contemporary molecular analyses reveal that the spotted-fever and typhus groups of the genus Rickettsia are very closely related to one another and not to *R. tsutsugamushi*. They are relatively close relatives of Ehrlichia and Rochalimaea (an extracellular bacterium recently reclassified to the genus Bartonella) and are evolutionarily distant from Coxiella and Chlamydia. Tradition maintains the concept of rickettsiae as obligate intracellular bacteria associated with ticks, fleas, lice, mites, and chiggers; however, this text will present the rickettsial diseases according to the logic determined by taxonomy and pathogenesis, with separate sections for the spotted fever/typhus rickettsioses, ehrlichioses, scrub typhus, and Q fever.

Table 2 *Effect of specific antibiotics on the course of rickettsial disease*

Disease	Mean duration of fever (days)	Average mortality (%)	Mean duration of fever after treatment (days)	Mortality (%)
Rocky Mountain spotted fever	16 (8–20)	20[a]	3	4[c]
Rickettsialpox	7 (3–12)	0	2	0
Other tick-borne rickettsioses	16 (7–16)	2	3	1[c]
Epidemic typhus	14 (8–20)	20	2	2
Brill–Zinsser disease	9 (7–12)	0[b]	2	0[b]
Murine typhus	12 (8–18)	2	2	0[c]
Human ehrlichiosis	11 (2–19)	2	2	1
Sennetsu ehrlichiosis	14	0	2	0
Q fever	10 (3–20)	1[b]	3	1[d]

[a]Fatality varies with age, sex and race.

[b]Fatal cases unusual.

[c]Occasional fatality with delay of treatment.

[d]Rare fatality with chronic types such as endocarditis.

Vasculopathic rickettsial diseases of the spotted fever and typhus groups

Aetiological agents

These bacteria measure approximately 0.3 × 1.0 μm and have a cell wall typical of Gram-negative bacteria. Components of the outer membrane include a 120-kDa surface protein, a 17-kDa lipoprotein, and lipopolysaccharides. Differences in the lipopolysaccharide antigens are the principal basis for the traditional antigenic separation of the spotted-fever and typhus groups. Spotted-fever group rickettsiae possess another important cell-wall protein often designated as the 190-kDa protein. Conformation-dependent epitopes on the 120- and 190-kDa proteins form the basis of serotyping, the accepted method for determining the species of Rickettsia. Many of these rickettsiae have such genetic similarity that if judged by the criteria applied to most extracellular bacteria they would be consolidated into a much smaller number of species. Ecological separation and reduced selective pressure, owing to their intracellular location in arthropods lacking immune systems, may explain their genetic conservatism. Indeed, these organisms are highly adapted to their intracellular niche with specific carrier-mediated membrane transport systems for ATP, ADP, AMP, nicotinamide adenine dinucleotide, lysine, proline, other amino acids, potassium ions, and uridine 5′-diphosphoglucose, which are readily available in the cytosol of the host cell.

Epidemiology

The epidemiology of these rickettsioses is determined by the encounter between man and the infected arthropod vectors. The seasonal incidence and geographical distribution are determined by the vector's activity. Spotted-fever group rickettsiae are maintained in nature principally by transovarial and transtadial transmission in their tick or mite hosts. The most virulent rickettsiae are capable of killing their arthropod hosts; For example, *R. prowazekii* routinely kills the human body louse vector, and *R. rickettsii* occasionally kills its tick host. Those rickettsiae that are pathogenic for their arthropod hosts require horizontal transmission to initiate infection of new arthropod hosts. Thus, ticks sometimes become infected with *R. rickettsii* when feeding as larvae or nymphs on rickettsaemic, small feral mammals, and all infected lice acquire *R. prowazekii* from rickettsaemic people. Thus, for each rickettsiosis there is a balance between the rickettsia and its natural host. Some apparently non-pathogenic rickettsiae are maintained totally by transovarial transmission. Reactivation of latent *R. prowazekii* infection in man is the source for infection of lice that initiates epidemics of typhus fever.

Spotted-fever group rickettsiae are transmitted to man by secretion of infected tick saliva into the blood pooled at the site of the bite. Typhus-group rickettsiae are transmitted to man by infected louse or flea faeces deposited on human skin during arthropod feeding, with subsequent scratching of the organisms into the skin. It is possible that fluid or faeces of infected ticks crushed between the fingers could enter a cutaneous wound or be rubbed into the conjunctival membrane. Although aerosols of rickettsiae are highly infectious, it seems unlikely that inhalation of infected, dried flea or louse faeces could be an important mode of transmission.

Pathogenesis

Rickettsiae of some species of the spotted-fever group frequently invade endothelial cells at the cutaneous portal of entry, proliferate, and cause a focus of dermal and epidermal necrosis, an eschar. Rickettsiae spread via the bloodstream to all parts of the body, where they come in contact with the endothelial cells lining the blood vessels. After their attachment to the endothelial cell membrane, phagocytosis is induced and rickettsiae escape from the phagosome into the cytosol, where they proliferate by binary fission (Fig. 1). Epidemic typhus rickettsiae reach massive numbers intracellularly until the endothelial cell bursts, a dramatic pathogenic event, with further spread of the rickettsiae to other cells. Spotted-fever group rickettsiae leave earlier and continuously from the host cell via filopodia, long host-cell processes. The ultrastructural cytopathic effect of spotted-fever group rickettsiae on the host cell suggests injury to the cell membrane with consequent influx of water. The pathogenic mechanism appears to be an effect of the physiological growth of rickettsiae and to involve lipid peroxidation of host cell membranes by free radicals, protease activity, and a rickettsial phospholipase A_2. Rickettsial lipopolysaccharides are essentially non-endotoxic in the quantities present during human infections, and there is no evidence of any rickettsial exotoxin.

Host immune, inflammatory, and coagulation systems are activated with apparent overall benefit to the patient. It has been suggested that some cytokines and inflammatory mediators, such as interferon-γ, tumour necrosis factor-α, kallikrein, kinin, prostacyclin, thromboxane, and leukotrienes, cause some of the pathological manifestations of rickettsial diseases. It is very likely that host factors such as interleukin (**IL**)-1, tumor necrosis factor-α, and IL-6 are involved in fever and the acute-phase response. Injury to endothelium results in multifocal deposition of platelet plugs, which minimize the formation of petechiae. This utilization of platelets in more extensive disease results in thrombocytopenia, but very rarely hypofibrinogenaemic disseminated intravascular coagulation. The haemostatic thrombi are usually non-occlusive and thus seldom cause microinfarcts (Fig. 2).

Progressive, disseminated infection and injury to endothelial cells cause increased vascular permeability, oedema, hypovolaemia, and signs and symptoms resulting from multifocal vascular injury in affected organs (Fig. 3). Infection of the pulmonary microcirculation and the resulting increase in vascular permeability produce non-cardiogenic pulmonary oedema or adult respiratory distress syndrome, a life-threatening condition that may require supplemental oxygen and mechanical ventilation. Although the host immune lymphohistiocytic response to rickettsial infection of the myocardial microcirculation is often described histologically as interstitial myocarditis, cardiac dynamics indicate that myocardial function is preserved. Arrhythmias may, at least in part, result from vascular lesions affecting the conduction system. The local effects of the vascular lesions in the brain, coupled with hypoperfusion, are associated with coma and seizures in severe cases (Fig. 4), and the multifocal infectious lesions in the dermis are the basis for the maculopapular, sometimes petechial, rash. Acute renal failure occurs in severe cases, usually as prerenal azotaemia or less frequently as acute tubular necrosis associated with severe hypotension. Rickettsial vascular lesions also are observed in the wall of the gastrointestinal tract, pancreas, liver, skeletal muscle, and other organs; these seem to be the basis for frequent nausea, vomiting, abdominal pain, and mild-to-moderate elevations in serum aminotransferases and variable elevations in serum creatine kinase.

Fig. 1 Electron photomicrograph of spotted fever rickettsiae in the cytosol of a pulmonary vascular endothelial cell (generously provided by Vsevolod L. Popov). Bar = 1 μm

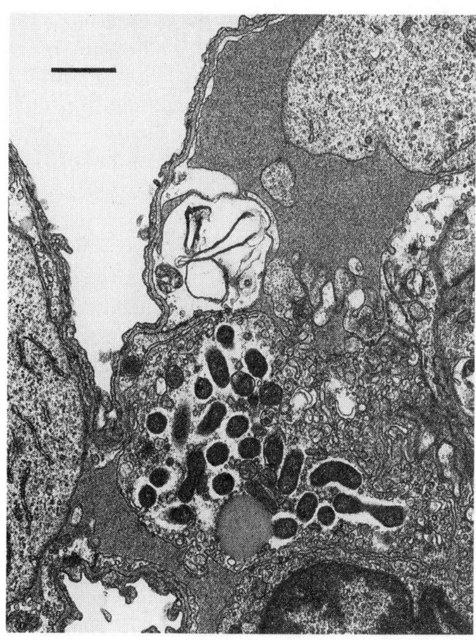

Fig. 2 Severe rickettsial injury to two adjacent blood vessels with intramural and perivascular infiltration by host immune and phagocytic cells and non-occlusive mural thrombi that are not causing distal ischaemia but are plugging foci of severe damage to the vessel wall.

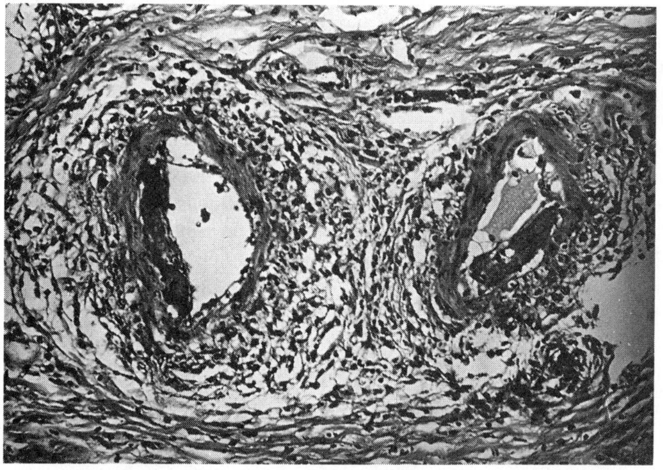

Fig. 3 Immunoperoxidase-stained *Rickettsia rickettsii* appear as dark bacilli in endothelial cells of a cerebral blood vessel with perivascular oedema but no host immune-cell infiltration.

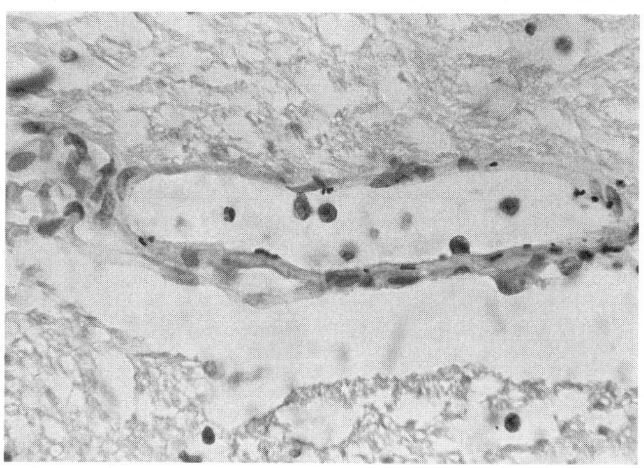

Fig. 4 Epidemic typhus fever. The typical lesion of rickettsial encephalitis is exemplified by the typhus nodule in the brain of a patient (death about 12th day) showing perivascular infiltration by macrophages and lymphocytes. (Reproduced from *Medical Clinics of North America* (1959), **43,** 1512, by permission.)

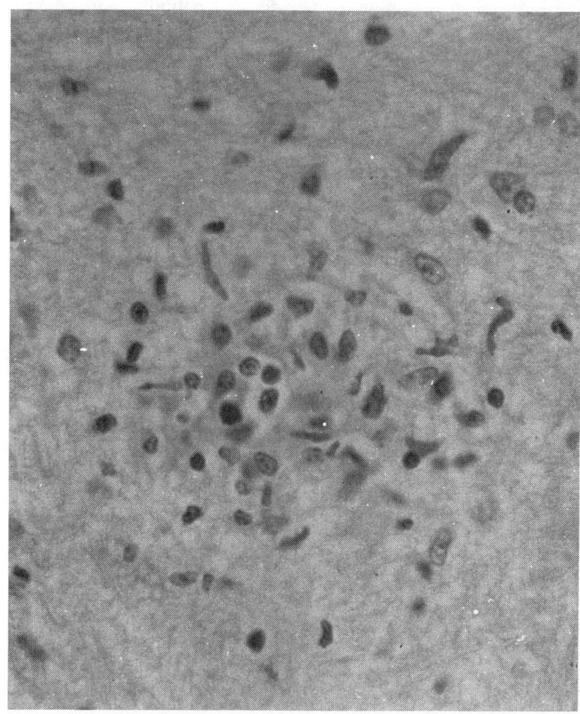

Clinical manifestations

The incubation period of rickettsial diseases generally ranges from a few days to 2 weeks with an average of 1 week after cutaneous inoculation or deposition of the organisms by the tick, mite, louse, or flea. The incubation time appears to be related inversely to the dose of inoculum. The clinical picture frequently observed in patients admitted to hospital a week or more into the course of their illness is that of a late, severe stage, often owing to delay in diagnosis and treatment. A more accurate image of rickettsioses recognizes the variability of clinical manifestations: some rickettsial species are more virulent, some individuals develop more severe disease, and severity increases progressively during the first week or two of illness.

The onset of rickettsioses is clinically non-specific, with malaise, chills, fever, myalgia, and headache that is often severe. The next few days' symptoms—anorexia, nausea, vomiting, abdominal pain, photophobia, and cough—suggest systemic involvement. A rash usually appears after 3 to 5 days of illness, is often absent at the time of presentation for medical care, and does not appear at all in a substantial portion of patients. The rash is frequently difficult to detect in patients with darkly pigmented skin. Initially, it consists of macular or maculopapular lesions, 1 to 5 mm in diameter, representing foci of numerous contiguous endothelial cells infected by rickettsiae and a surrounding zone of varying degrees of vasodilatation and dermal oedema. When compressed, these erythematous lesions blanch. In later stages of more severe disease, the intensely infected blood vessels in the centre of the maculopapule are breached and a petechia appears. At this stage, compression of the rash does not blanch the haemorrhagic focus.

Pulmonary endothelial infection often results in cough and may cause pulmonary oedema, radiographic infiltrates, hypoxaemia, dyspnoea, and pleural effusions in severe cases. Neurological manifestations parallel the severity of illness, being absent in mild cases, consisting of lethargy in moderate cases, and, in severe cases, developing early and progressing to confusion, delirium, stupor, ataxia, coma, focal neurological signs, and seizures. Rickettsial infection of the blood vessels in the meninges, brain, and spinal cord may cause pleocytosis of the cerebrospinal fluid, usually 10 to 100 cells/μl with variable proportions of mononuclear and polymorphonuclear leucocytes, and/or an increased protein concentration; the glucose concentration is usually normal.

Although serum aminotransferases and bilirubin may be elevated, jaundice is observed in less than 10 per cent of patients, and hepatic failure does not occur. The white blood-cell count is usually normal, but an increased proportion of immature myeloid cells may be present. Mild anaemia may develop during the course of illness. The acute-phase reaction occurs in many patients, with increased concentrations of some plasma proteins, including C-reactive protein, haptoglobin, α_1-antitrypsin, fibrinogen, factor VIII, and the third and fourth components of complement, and a decrease in transferrin. Hypoalbuminaemia is probably the result of leakage of this plasma protein into the interstitial space because of increased permeability of the microcirculation. Hyponatraemia occurs in many patients with rickettsial diseases and is rarely caused by the syndrome of inappropriate secretion of antidiuretic hormone. Actually, hyponatraemia is most often the result of the appropriate secretion of antidiuretic hormone in response to the hypovolaemic state. Immune clearance of rickettsiae, repair of injured blood vessels, and regeneration of the endothelial lining are associated with defervescence, correction of capillary permeability, restoration of blood volume, and finally resolution of oedema.

Diagnosis

DIFFERENTIAL DIAGNOSIS

In the early days of illness before the rash appears, the clinical differential diagnosis is extensive and includes influenza, typhoid fever, enteroviral infection, and infectious diseases suggested by geographical exposure (e.g. malaria, Lassa fever). Nausea, vomiting, and abdominal pain may suggest infectious enterocolitis. Prominent abdominal tenderness has occasionally led to the differential diagnosis of acute surgical abdomen and to exploratory laparotomy. Cough and abnormalities of physical and radiographic examination of the chest may suggest bronchitis or pneumonia. Fever, seizures, coma, neurological signs, and abnormalities of the cerebrospinal fluid may lead to consideration of meningitis and arboviral or herpes simplex viral encephalitis. If an eschar is detected, the differential diagnosis may include cutaneous anthrax, tularaemia, syphilis, and chancroid. Although the onset of rash should add rickettsial diseases to the list of diagnostic possibilities, if they had not already been considered, the differential diagnosis of similar febrile exanthems would also include meningococcaemia, Gram-negative bacterial sepsis, toxic-shock syndrome, leptospirosis, disseminated gonococcal infection, secondary syphilis, measles, rubella, enteroviral exanthem, infectious mononucleosis, dengue or arenaviral haemorrhagic fevers, idiopathic or thrombotic thrombocytopenic purpura, and immune-complex vasculitides (e.g. systemic lupus erythematosus). Reliance upon the recognition of a typical rash may result in delayed or missed diagnosis because the rash usually does not appear until day 3 to 5 of illness and does not appear at all in at least 10 per cent of patients. Although it is important to enquire about exposure to ticks, fleas, mites, and lice and to consider the seasonal occurrence of rickettsial diseases in the geographical location of exposure, it should be clearly understood that a large number of people are unaware of their exposure to arthropods and that cases may occur outside of the seasonal peak in the summer months.

LABORATORY DIAGNOSIS

With rare exceptions, clinical microbiology laboratories render little or no assistance to the diagnosis of rickettsial diseases in the acute stage of illness. The most widely available diagnostic assays are serological, and while very useful in confirming the diagnosis in the convalescent stage, they seldom detect specific antibodies to rickettsial antigens during the first week of illness. At present, the best serological assays generally available are an indirect immunofluorescent antibody test, indirect immunoperoxidase antibody test, and latex agglutination test. These tests detect antibodies that are cross-reactive within the spotted-fever or typhus group and thus cannot distinguish murine typhus from epidemic typhus or boutonneuse fever from rickettsialpox. The indirect immunofluorescent antibody assay has the best combination of sensitivity (94–100 per cent) and specificity (100 per cent). The indirect immunoperoxidase antibody assay performs similarly. Because these tests detect long persistence of IgG as well as the relatively early appearance of IgM, it is important to determine the most efficient cut-off titre in a particular population, based upon the seroprevalence rate. Usually the diagnostic threshold is set at a titre of 64 to 128; however, some geographical areas require a higher threshold titre. Definitive diagnosis should be established by demonstration of a fourfold or greater rise in titre between acute and convalescent serum samples. The latex agglutination test detects IgM most effectively and has good sensitivity (71–98 per cent) and specificity (93–100 per cent). Because disappearance of IgM antibody results in a fall in titre after the rise in titre, a single titre of 128 or greater is considered diagnostic. Future developments in serological diagnosis may include enzyme immunoassays, possibly with standardized recombinant antigens or synthetic peptides. Disease-specific assays for antibodies to species-specific rickettsial epitopes have been reported. The classical complement fixation test has fallen into disuse because of its low sensitivity, and the Weil–Felix tests of agglutination of *Proteus* OX-19 and OX-2, although still used in some places, should be discarded and replaced because of poor sensitivity and specificity.

Isolation of the aetiological organism, the definitive diagnosis of an infectious disease, is seldom attempted for rickettsiae because of the biohazard. Recovery of rickettsiae by inoculation of animals has been employed since Ricketts' investigations of 1906; however, the classical propagation of rickettsiae in animals and embryonated eggs is cumbersome. The contemporary approach to isolation of rickettsiae utilizes cell culture with detection of rickettsiae after 48 to 72 h in antibiotic-free, shell-vial cultures.

The timely detection of rickettsiae at the point in the course of illness when the patient presents for medical care and the initial diagnostic and therapeutic decisions are being made has been achieved by visualization of the rickettsial organisms and by amplification of specific sequences of rickettsial DNA by the polymerase chain reaction (**PCR**). Identification of rickettsiae by immunofluorescence or immunoperoxidase in skin requires the presence of a rash to determine the site for biopsy. This immunohistological approach has a sensitivity of approximately 70 per cent and a specificity of 100 per cent in the hands of an experienced microscopist. A novel approach to the identification of rickettsial organisms that can be employed even during the period of illness before the onset of rash is immunofluorescent staining of rickettsiae in circulating endothelial cells. Immunomagnetic beads coated with a monoclonal antibody to a plasma membrane antigen of endothelial cells captures injured cells that have become detached from the basement membrane. Examination of these circulating endothelial cells revealed diagnostic rickettsiae in the earliest evaluated specimen in more than half of patients in the first report of this method. In contrast, detection of rickettsial DNA after amplification by the PCR has not been very successful in the timely diagnosis of rickettsial infections early in the course of illness. For most circumstances, empirical treatment based upon clinical suspicion of a rickettsiosis is followed by a specific laboratory confirmation of the diagnosis. Treatment should not be withheld while awaiting the results of diagnostic serology, rickettsial isolation, or PCR.

Treatment

Spotted-fever and typhus-group rickettsioses respond favourably to treatment with doxycycline (200 mg/day for adults and children greater than 45 kg, and 4.4 mg/kg body weight per day day for smaller children), tetracycline (2 gm/day in four divided doses for adults and 25 mg/kg body weight per day in four divided doses for children), or chloramphenicol (2 g/day in four divided doses for adults and 50 mg/kg body weight per day day in four divided doses for children). Fluoroquinolones are active against rickettsiae, and ciprofloxacin (200 mg, intravenously every 12 h or 750 mg orally every 12 h), ofloxacin (200 mg orally every 12 h), and pefloxacin (400 mg intravenously or orally every 12 h) have been used successfully to treat boutonneuse fever. Epidemic typhus fever has been treated effectively under field conditions with a single, 200 mg dose of doxycycline. Treatment is generally continued for 2 or 3 days after defervescence to avoid relapse of the infection.

Intravenously administered doxycycline or chloramphenicol is employed when oral treatment cannot be used because of vomiting or coma. Chloramphenicol and josamycin (3 g/day for 8 days)have been used to treat rickettsioses during pregnancy when the tetracyclines are contraindicated.

Supportive treatment includes careful replacement of intravenous fluid volume to correct hypotension, hypoperfusion, and prerenal azotaemia; this may require monitoring of pulmonary capillary-wedge pressures to lessen the possibility of precipitating or exacerbating pulmonary oedema. Hyponatraemia is rarely severe enough to be life threatening, and homeostasis of serum sodium usually occurs within 48 h of initiation of antirickettsial treatment and fluid replacement. Severely ill patients may suffer seizures and should then be given anticonvulsants. Severe thrombocytopenia may warrant platelet transfusions, but heparin should not be given. Renal failure associated with acute tubular necrosis is frequently managed by haemodialysis, and hypoxaemia associated with interstitial pneumonitis and non-cardiogenic pulmonary oedema may necessitate supplemental oxygen and mechanical ventilation. Excellent nursing care, particularly for patients in the intensive care unit, is a critical factor.

Prevention

IMMUNIZATION

Immunity to reinfection with spotted-fever or typhus-group rickettsiae is quite strong, although some patients with epidemic typhus fever will develop recrudescence of latent *R. prowazekii* infection many years after their acute infection. Immunity to rickettsiae is mediated mainly by T lymphocytes. Interferon-γ and tumour necrosis factor-α appear to be key effectors. Once rickettsiae leave the host cell for the extracellular environment, opsonizing antibodies and activated macrophages play an adjunctive part in clearing them from the body.

Vaccines containing whole, killed organisms do not confer complete protective immunity, although some reduction of severity of illness and mortality has been observed. A live, attenuated vaccine against *R. prowazekii* confers protection. However, some patients develop mild typhus fever, and reversion of the vaccine strain to a pathogenic state has been demonstrated after *in vivo* passage of the organisms. Thus, there are at present no vaccines in general use against rickettsial diseases. Contemporary research suggests that the 120-kDa surface protein of typhus group rickettsiae and the 190-kDa cell-wall protein of spotted-fever group rickettsiae contain epitopes recognized by T lymphocytes and are candidates for the development of molecularly based subunit vaccines.

VECTOR CONTROL

Because rickettsial diseases are zoonoses with reservoirs in nature, eradication is not a possibility with current knowledge of the vector biology of the hosts. Reduction of vector and reservoir populations has been used to control epidemic typhus, murine typhus, and rickettsialpox. Delousing measures, including the use of insecticides and washing of clothing in hot water, reduce the spread of louse-borne epidemic typhus. Rodent control and application of insecticides can remarkably decrease the incidence of murine typhus and is an approach to control of rickettsialpox.

Avoidance of exposure to tick-borne rickettsiae is virtually the only preventive approach available. Tick repellents and protective clothing are theoretically useful but are seldom employed effectively. Regular daily or twice-daily inspection of the entire body, especially the scalp and groin, and prompt removal of ticks prevents inoculation of rickettsiae. The best method for tick removal is to grasp the anterior parts of the tick firmly with pointed forceps flush with the skin and to exert steady traction until the intact tick is removed, frequently with a bit of attached skin. Care should be taken to avoid introduction of potentially infected tick fluids into the wound or mucous membranes. The tick bite wound should be thoroughly cleaned.

REFERENCES

Hechemy, K.E., Paretsky, D., Walker, D.H., and Mallavia, L.P. (ed.) (1990). *Rickettsiology: current issues and perspectives.* Vol. 590 of the *Annals of the New York Academy of Sciences*, New York.

Kaplan, J.E. and Schonberger, L.B. (1986). The sensitivity of various serologic tests in the diagnosis of Rocky Mountain spotted fever. *American Journal of Tropical Medicine and Hygiene*, **35,** 840–4.

Rehacek, J. and Tarasevich, I.V. (1988). *Acari-borne rickettsiae & rickettsioses in Eurasia.* Publishing House of the Slovak Academy of Sciences, Bratislava.

Walker, D.H. (1988). *Biology of rickettsial Diseases*, Vols. I and II. CRC Press, Boca Raton, FA.

Walker, D.H. and Fishbein, D.B. (1991). Epidemiology of rickettsial diseases. *European Journal of Epidemiology*, **7,** 237–45.

Winkler, H.H. (1990). *Rickettsia* species (as organisms). *Annual Review of Microbiology*, **44,** 131–53.

Spotted fevers

Boutonneuse fever

AETIOLOGY

The most prevalent spotted-fever rickettsiosis in Europe and Africa is boutonneuse fever, which frequently goes by the synonym Mediterranean spotted fever. Emphasis in this chapter will be placed on this disease as an excellent example of a spotted-fever rickettsiosis. For many years, all spotted-fever rickettsiosis occurring in southern Europe, Africa, and southern Asia was considered to be boutonneuse fever. This conclusion was based upon the effective cross-neutralization of the lethal effect of intravenously inoculated high doses of viable rickettsiae from South Africa, Kenya, Morocco, and India by antisera to all these strains. *Rickettsia conorii* has also been isolated in Spain, France, Croatia, Georgia, Russia, Ukraine, Pakistan, and Ethiopia. Recent investigations reveal that *R. conorii* has more antigenic diversity than the other carefully analysed spotted-fever group rickettsia, *R. rickettsii*, and that there are probably at least two other new spotted-fever rickettsial species pathogenic for man in Africa and western Asia.

EPIDEMIOLOGY

The incidence of boutonneuse fever has increased dramatically in Spain, France, Italy, and Portugal during the last 15 years. The changes in the ecology of *R. conorii*, which is particularly associated with the tick *Rhipicephalus sanguineus*, that might explain the upsurge in cases have not been elucidated. *R. conorii* is maintained in *Rh. sanguineus* transovarially and is transmitted to humans by tick bite. The peak of cases along the Mediterranean coast of southern Europe occurs in July and August when immature stages of the tick predominate. The incidence of boutonneuse fever correlates with prevalence of spotted-fever group rickettsiae in ticks and the prevalence of antibodies to such rickettsiae in dogs and man. Boutonneuse fever occurs in urban, suburban, and rural environments, owing largely to the carriage of *Rh. sanguineus* by dogs in each of these settings.

Among patients ill enough to be admitted to hospital, mortality rates of 1.4 to 5.6 per cent have been observed. A severe form of the disease with 33 per cent mortality occurs in persons who are elderly or have underlying diseases, alcoholism, or glucose-6-phosphate dehydrogenase deficiency.

PATHOGENESIS

The pathological basis for tissue injury in boutonneuse fever is illustrated by the *tache noire* (black spot) or eschar at the site of the infective tick bite. Endothelial infection and injury by *R. conorii* causes perivascular oedema and dermal and epidermal necrosis. The necrosis is apparently not secondary to thrombosis, which is usually absent or inconsequential. Reduction in the number of rickettsiae in the eschar is associated with a perivascular influx of lymphocytes and macrophages. The lymphocytic infiltrate is virtually all T lymphocytes with more T-helper/inducer cells than T-cytotoxic/suppressor cells. It is suspected that these perivascular cells elaborate interferon-γ and tumour necrosis factor-α, which may have a paracrine antirickettsial effect on intraendothelial organisms. Cytotoxic T lymphocytes and natural killer cells recognize rickettsial antigens expressed on the surface of infected cells and might destroy both rickettsiae and their host cell. Autopsies of fatal cases of boutonneuse fever show systemic vascular infection and injury by *R. conorii*, with lesions in the brain, meninges, lungs, kidney, gastrointestinal tract, liver, pancreas, heart, spleen, and skin including sites of peripheral gangrene. Clinical and experimental studies support the premise that direct rickettsial injury of infected endothelial cells is the major pathogenic event. Hepatic biopsies taken during the course of non-fatal boutonneuse fever contain multifocal hepatocellular necrosis with a predominantly mononuclear cellular response.

CLINICAL MANIFESTATIONS

During the incubation period of boutonneuse fever, a red papule appears at the site of the tick bite and progresses to develop into an eschar in approximately 70 per cent of diagnosed cases. It is often associated with regional lymphadenopathy. Subsequently, onset of illness is marked by fever, sometimes accompanied by headache and myalgias. The rash most often appears on the fourth day of illness but may be delayed, is maculopapular, and involves the palms and soles. It is petechial in only 10 per cent of patients and fails to appear at all in some patients. Other signs and symptoms may include nausea, vomiting, cough, dyspnoea, conjunctivitis, stupor, meningism, lymphadenopathy, and hepatomegaly. Increased vascular permeability manifested as mild oedema, hypoalbuminaemia, and arterial hypotension characterizes the pathophysiology of boutonneuse fever. Clinical laboratory evaluation (aggregate data) reveals anaemia in one-third of patients, with blood haemoglobin concentration of less than 100 g/l in 11 per cent of patients occurring particularly in severe cases. The white blood-cell count is usually normal, with leucopenia in 18 per cent and leucocytosis in 28 per cent of patients. Platelet counts less than 100×10^9/l are detected in 12.5 per cent of the patients. Hyponatraemia of less than 130 mmol/l occurs in 23 per cent; hypocalcaemia of less than 2.1 mmol/l in 38 per cent is presumably related to the hypoalbuminaemia. Hypoproteinaemia is observed in 23 per cent of patients.

Serum urea and creatinine concentrations are elevated in 25 and 17 per cent of patients, respectively. Serum concentrations of aspartate and alanine aminotransferases are increased in 39 and 37 per cent, respectively, and serum bilirubin is greater than 20 μmol/l in 9 per cent. Severe illness occurs in 6 per cent of patients and may be manifested by cutaneous purpura and other haemorrhagic phenomena, neurological signs, altered mental status, respiratory symptoms and hypoxaemia, acute renal failure, thrombocytopenia, and often even death.

DIAGNOSIS

Reliance upon the detection of the complete triad of fever, rash, and eschar will result in delayed diagnosis in many patients and misdiagnosis in some. A relatively small proportion of patients can recall exposure to ticks.

In the acute stage of illness, laboratory diagnosis can be established by immunohistological demonstration of *R. conorii* in a biopsy of the *tache noire* or rash, or in circulating endothelial cells separated from the peripheral blood by magnetic beads coated with a monoclonal antibody to an endothelial cell-membrane antigen, as described above. *R. conorii* can be isolated by intraperitoneal inoculation in guinea-pigs or in shell-vial cell culture. Diagnostic serological methods currently used include the indirect immunofluorescent antibody assay and latex agglutination test, both of which have commercially available reagents, as well as the indirect immunoperoxidase assay and complement fixation test. Western immunoblots have demonstrated that antibodies are directed mainly at the major 120- and 190-kDa surface proteins and lipopolysaccharides.

TREATMENT

See under 'Vasculopathic rickettsial diseases' above.

PREVENTION

There is no vaccine to protect against *R. conorii.* A crude lysate containing the recombinant *R. conorii* 190-kDa protein antigen confers strong protection against experimental infection of vaccinated guinea-pigs.

Rocky Mountain spotted fever

The pathogenic basis for differences between the most virulent strains of *R. rickettsii* and distinctly less pathogenic strains is not known.

Remarkably close genetic relationships have been demonstrated between *R. rickettsii* and other spotted-fever and typhus-group rickettsiae including *R. conorii* (91–94 per cent), *R. sibirica* (70–74 per cent), *R. montana*, a non-pathogenic rickettsia (73 per cent), *R. australis* (53 per cent), *R. akari* (46 per cent), *R. prowazekii* (47 per cent), and *R. typhi* (42 per cent).

Understanding of the ecology of *R. rickettsii* requires an explanation of the tick–rickettsia relationship and the competition among different rickettsial species for the ecological niche in the tick. *R. rickettsii* is somewhat pathogenic for Dermacentor ticks, perhaps explaining why fewer than 1 in 1000 ticks in endemic areas contains *R. rickettsii*. In most areas studied, less than 10 per cent of ticks contain any rickettsiae. The most prevalent rickettsial species are *R. bellii, R. montana*, and *R. rhipicephali*, which are generally considered as non-pathogenic. The evidence suggests that prior infection of ticks with some prevalent non-pathogenic spotted-fever group rickettsiae interferes with the establishment of transovarian transmission of *R. rickettsii*. The explanation for the dramatic, asynchronous, geographical fluctuations in the incidence of Rocky Mountain spotted fever that occur over periods of 5 to 20 years or longer is not known. Early in the century, Rocky Mountain spotted fever had a high incidence in the western United States; at present few cases are diagnosed in the Rocky Mountains. A rise in incidence, particularly in the south-eastern states during the 1970s, to a peak of 1192 cases in 1981, was followed by a decrease in the annual occurrence to approximately 600 cases in recent years.

R. rickettsii, the most virulent rickettsial species of the spotted-fever

Fig. 5 The early rash of Rocky Mountain spotted fever consists of pink macules in this 4-year-old boy on the fourth day of illness.

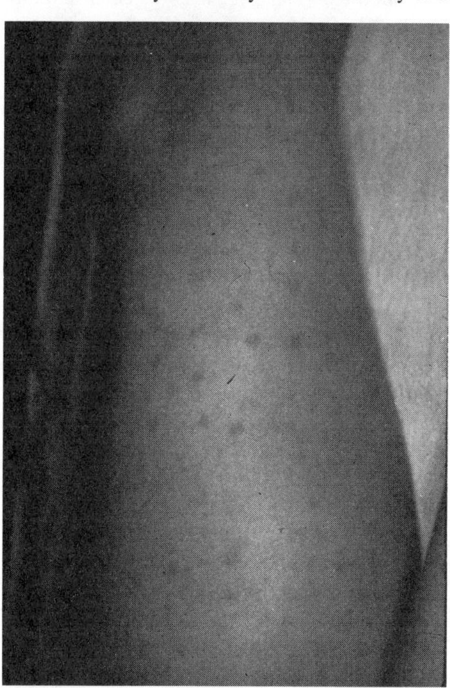

Fig. 6 Rocky Mountain spotted fever. Series showing haemorrhagic exanthem in a 4-year-old boy on about the eighth day of illness. Note oedema of face, hands, arms, and feet, and bleeding from mouth. There was evidence of disseminated intravascular coagulation (DIC). Specific therapy with chloramphenicol, glucocorticoids for several days, and no heparin was used. Recovery was complete.

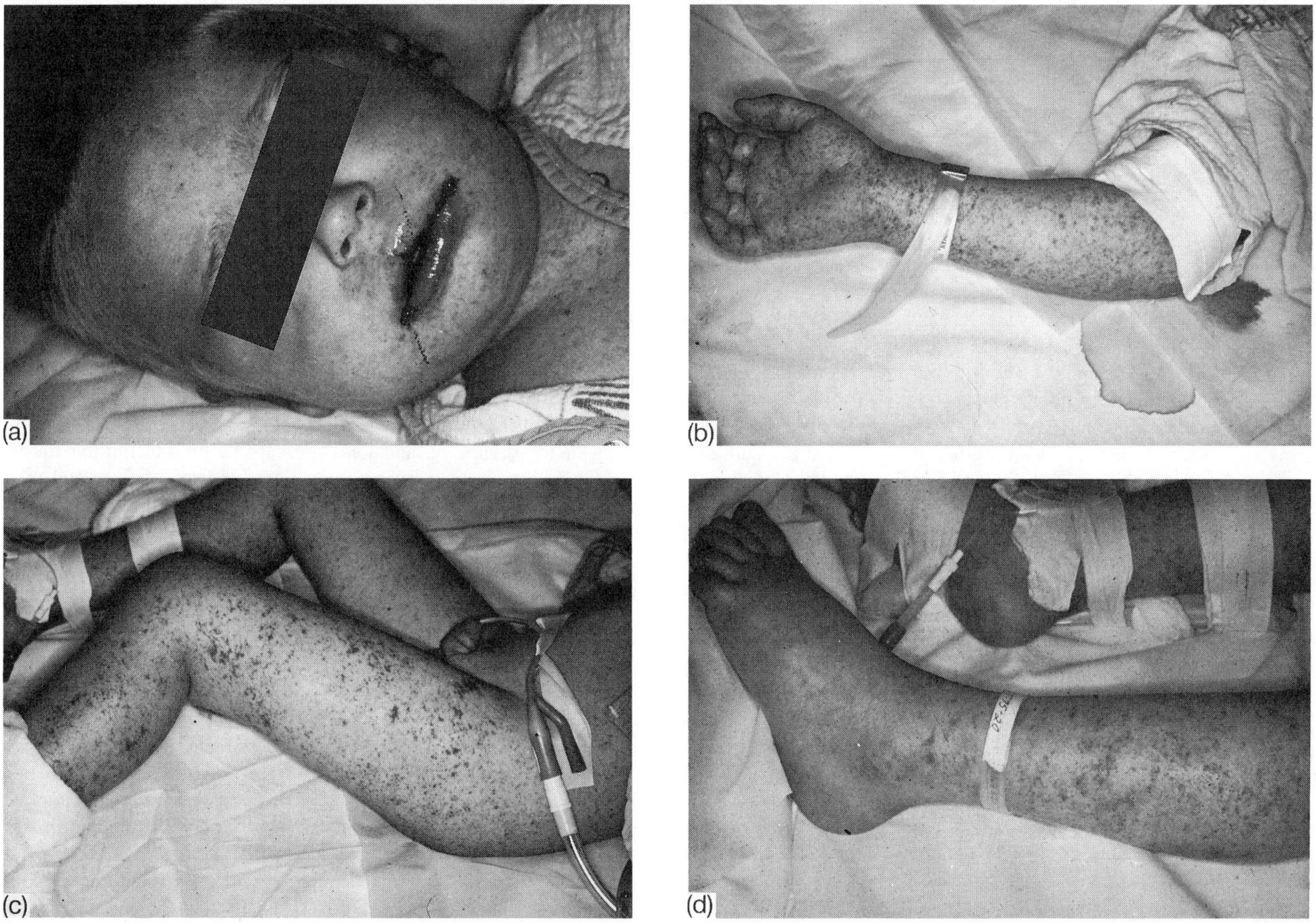

(a)

(b)

(c)

(d)

group, is also more invasive for man than other rickettsial species, causing infection not only of endothelial cells but also vascular smooth-muscle cells. Host factors also play a part in severity of illness. Fatality rates are higher in older patients, males, and blacks. Fulminant Rocky Mountain spotted fever with death occurring within 5 days after onset is associated with haemolysis, particularly in black males with glucose-6-phosphate dehydrogenase deficiency.

Clinically, Rocky Mountain spotted fever illustrates vividly the most severe manifestations of rickettsial disease and the often confusing multisystem symptoms. Untreated, Rocky Mountain spotted fever has a 20 per cent fatality rate. In recent series, the death rate has been 3 to 4 per cent, with respiratory failure in 12 per cent, acute renal failure in 14 per cent, and anaemia requiring red-cell transfusion in 11 per cent. Thrombocytopenia occurs in 32 to 52 per cent of patients. Coma is highly associated with a fatal outcome, occurring in 86 per cent of fatal cases and only 6 per cent of non-fatal.

Early in the illness, nausea or vomiting occurs in 38 to 56 per cent of cases and abdominal pain in 30 to 34 per cent. Jaundice is present in 8 to 9 per cent of cases, and the serum bilirubin concentration is elevated in 18 to 30 per cent. Even the rash must not be expected to have a set picture; it usually appears on the third day of illness, but can appear on or after day 6 in 20 per cent (Fig. 5). In 10 per cent of patients, a rash never appears. While classical teachings emphasize that the rash is petechial and involves the palms and soles, petechiae occur in only 41 to 59 per cent of cases and appear late in the course, only on or after day 6 in 74 per cent, and the palms and soles have rash lesions in 36 to 82 per cent with involvement occurring after day 5 in 43 per cent (Fig. 6).

The gastrointestinal, neurological, and respiratory signs and symptoms often are diagnostically confusing. Moreover, the expected triad of fever, rash, and history of tick bite is observed in only 3 per cent of patients during the first 3 days of illness when patients frequently seek medical attention. A history of tick exposure is obtained from only 60 per cent of patients. In addition to the indirect immunofluorescent antibody assay and the latex agglutination test, the reagents for a solid-phase enzyme immunoassay for antibodies to *R. rickettsii* are commercially available.

Other tick-borne spotted-fever rickettsioses

Although *R. sibirica*, *R. australis*, and *R. japonica* have distinct antigenic differences in their surface proteins, DNA sequences, tick hosts, and known geographical distribution, the clinical diseases are very similar to one another and to boutonneuse fever. The spotted-fever rickettsiosis of south-eastern Australia and Queensland tick typhus are clinically similar, although their aetiological rickettsiae have not been shown to be identical. Israeli spotted fever differs from boutonneuse fever in that eschar formation is usually lacking; the Israeli spotted-fever rickettsia appears to differ antigenically and genetically from *R. conorii*. Many rickettsiae of the spotted-fever group isolated from ticks are distinct species, but their relation to human disease is undetermined. It is conceivable that the high prevalence of antibodies to such rickettsiae and asymptomatic seroconversions might be explained, at least in part, by exposure to these rickettsiae of indeterminate pathogenicity.

Rickettsialpox

R. akari has been isolated in the United States, Ukraine, Croatia, and Korea, and is the only rickettsia that has a gamasid mite as its natural host. *R. akari* is maintained by transovarian transmission in *Liponyssoides sanguineus*, which has the domestic mouse, *Mus musculus*, as its host. It would seem likely that rickettsialpox has a wider distribution and greater incidence worldwide than is now recognized.

A cutaneous papule appears during the incubation period at the site where the mite has fed and evolves into an eschar over the next 2 to 7 days. About 10 days after the mite bite, onset is characterized by malaise, fever, chills, severe headache, and myalgia. A macular rash consisting of discrete erythematous lesions, 2 to 3 mm in diameter, appears 2 to 6 days later and evolves into maculopapules and then papules that develop central, deep-seated vesicles in some, but not all, patients. The vesicular rash introduces chickenpox and herpes simplex viral infection into the differential diagnosis.

REFERENCES

Brettman, L.R. *et al.* (1981). Rickettsialpox: report of an outbreak and a contemporary review. *Medicine*, **60,** 363–82.

Gross, E.M. and Yagupsky, P. (1987). Israeli rickettsial spotted fever in children. A review of 54 cases. *Acta Tropica*, **44,** 91–6.

Helmick, C.G., Bernard, K.W., and D'Angelo, L.J. (1984). Rocky Mountain spotted fever: clinical, laboratory, and epidemiological features of 262 cases. *Journal of Infectious Diseases*, **150,** 480–8.

Kaplowitz, L.G., Fischer, J.J., and Sparling, P.F. (1981). Rocky Mountain spotted fever: a clinical dilemma. *Current Clinical Topics in Infectious Diseases*, **2,** 89–108.

McDade, J.E. and Newhouse, V.F. (1986). Natural history of *Rickettsia rickettsii. Annual Review of Microbiology*, **40,** 287–309.

Raoult, D., Weiller, P.J., Chagnon, A., Chaudet, H., Gallais, H., and Casanova, P. (1986). Mediterranean spotted fever: clinical, laboratory and epidemiological features of 199 cases. *American Journal of Tropical Medicine and Hygiene*, **35,** 845–50.

Sexton, D.J., Dwyer, B., Kemp, R., and Graves, S. (1991). Spotted fever group rickettsial infections in Australia. *Review of Infectious Disease*, **13,** 876–86.

Uchida, T., Uchiyama, T., Kumano, K., and Walker, D.H. (1992). *Rickettsia japonica* sp. nov., the etiological agent of spotted fever group rickettsiosis in Japan. *International Journal of Systematic Bacteriology*, **42,** 303–5.

Walker, D.H. and Gear, J.H.S. (1985). Correlation of the distribution of *Rickettsia conorii*, microscopic lesions, and clinical features in South African tick bite fever. *American Journal of Tropical Medicine and Hygiene*, **34,** 361–71.

Walker, D.H., Occhino, C., Tringali, G.R., Di Rosa. S., and Mansueto, S. (1988). Pathogenesis of rickettsial eschars: the tache noire of boutonneuse fever. *Human Pathology*, **19,** 1449–54.

Typhus fevers

Murine typhus

Endemic flea-borne typhus fever caused by *R. typhi* is prevalent on all continents except Antarctica. It occurs most often in warm, coastal ports where it is maintained in a commensal cycle involving rat fleas, *Xenopsylla cheopis*, and rats, *Rattus rattus* and *Rattus norvegicus*. Highly infectious *R. typhi* organisms deposited on the skin in infected flea faeces cause rickettsaemia of 1 to 2 weeks' duration in rats when uninfected fleas acquire the rickettsiae by taking a blood meal. The fleas remain infected for life. A relatively small proportion of infected fleas transmit *R. typhi* transovarially, and fleas are capable of transmitting murine typhus by bite as well as in faeces. Other species of fleas and other mammals can also maintain an infectious cycle of *R. typhi*. For example, the cat flea, *Ctenocephalides felis*, which feeds on opossums, racoons, skunks, and humans as well as cats, is a natural and experimental host for *R. typhi*. Recently, a new typhus-group rickettsial species was discovered in cat fleas, which maintain the agent by transovarial transmission. This rickettsia, currently designated the ELB agent, differs genetically from *R. typhi* at least as much as *R. canada* (a presumed non-pathogenic, tick-borne, typhus-group rickettsia) differs from *R. typhi* and *R. prowazekii*. This agent, which has yet to be isolated and propagated even in cell culture, was characterized genetically by sequence analysis of DNA amplified in the polymerase chain reaction. Scientists engaged in the application of this emerging technology are discovering more new organisms that may be agents of human illness.

Murine typhus is a neglected disease that is very frequently misdiagnosed. The triad of fever, headache, and rash is present in only some 13 per cent of patients when first examined by a physician. In a recently reported series from a known endemic area, murine typhus was the initial diagnosis in only 11 per cent of the patients. A rash is detected in 80 per cent of fair-skinned persons and in 20 per cent of blacks. The rash appears an average of 2 days after the initial physician contact. Multisystem vascular infection is suggested by nausea (48 per cent), vomiting (40 per cent), abdominal pain (23 per cent), diarrhoea (26 per cent), cough (35 per cent), abnormal chest radiographs (23 per cent), thrombocytopenia (48 per cent), elevated serum hepatic transaminases (90 per cent), and central nervous abnormalities (8 per cent) including confusion, stupor, and hallucinations. Murine typhus rickettsiae have been demonstrated in the lungs, brain, kidneys, liver, and heart. Although mortality from murine typhus is only 1 to 2 per cent, the illness frequently incapacitates the patient for 2 weeks or so. Nearly 10 per cent of patients admitted to hospital are admitted to an intensive care with acute renal failure, respiratory failure, or severe abnormalities of the central nervous system including seizures. Older age, a prolonged interval before specific antimicrobial treatment, and prior treatment with a sulpha-containing drug are risk factors for severe disease.

Epidemic typhus, recrudescent typhus, and sylvatic typhus

There are three conditions when patients suffer illness caused by *R. prowazekii*: epidemic louse-borne typhus fever, recrudescence of latent infection years after acute epidemic typhus, and zoonotic infection acquired from the ectoparasites of infected flying squirrels. Typical cases are characterized by intense headache, prostration, continuous high fever, a macular rash usually appearing on the fourth or fifth day of illness, myalgia, and neurological abnormalities. A pink, erythematous rash that blanches on pressure appears first in the axillary folds and trunk. Within 24 to 48 h the rash becomes red, petechial, and does not blanch on pressure (Fig. 7). Its development is centrifugal from the trunk to the extremities, the opposite of Rocky Mountain spotted fever. In Wolbach's series of epidemic typhus in Poland at the end of the Second World War, he studied patients who were more ill than most, and whose mortality was 13.3 per cent as compared with approximately 7 per cent overall in that epidemic. These patients, on admission, had cough (nearly all), rales (71 per cent), and mental dullness (14 per cent). During their course, which was in the pre-antibiotic era, they developed delirium (48 per cent), rales (80 per cent), coma (6 per cent), seizures (1 per cent), and gangrene (3 per cent). A more recent series reported nausea (30 per cent) and abdominal pain (30 per cent).

In poor, remote populations, particularly in cold, highland areas, louse-borne typhus may smoulder uncontrolled in susceptible populations over a 3-year period that is curtailed by the development of immunity in the population. The incidence declines in summer months because of louse control through bathing and washing of clothes. The infection is now restricted to a few foci of sporadic occurrence in eastern Europe, central Africa, Ethiopia, southern Africa, Afghanistan, northern India, China, Mexico, Central America, and the Andes Mountains of South America. However, the danger of spread still exists. Mixed epidemics of louse-borne typhus and louse-borne relapsing fever (Chapter 7.11.31) have been described.

Recrudescent typhus (Brill–Zinsser disease) is the most important reservoir for initiation of epidemic louse-borne typhus in a susceptible population. The clinical manifestations are similar to the primary illness, epidemic typhus, although generally somewhat milder (Fig. 8).

Natural infections of flying squirrels, *Glaucomys volans*, by *R. prowazekii* in the eastern United States are maintained in a cycle involving the squirrels' lice and fleas. The infection has been transmitted to man most probably by the squirrel flea. Clinical manifestations include fever (100 per cent), headache (81 per cent), centrifugal maculopapular rash (66 per cent), confusion (44 per cent), myalgia (42 per cent), gastrointestinal symptoms (43 per cent), and coma (28 per cent). There have been no reported deaths.

REFERENCES

Azad, A.F. (1990). Epidemiology of murine typhus. *Annual Review of Entomology*, **35**, 553–69.

Dumler, J.S., Taylor, J.P., and Walker, D.H. (1991). Clinical and laboratory features of murine typhus in South Texas, 1980 through 1987. *Journal of the American Medical Association*, **266**, 1365–70.

Perine, X.X., (1992). *Communicable Infectious Diseases*, **14**, 1149–58.

Walker, D.H., Parks, F.M., Betz, T.G., Taylor, J.P., and Muehlberger, J.W. (1989). Histopathology and immunohistologic demonstration of the distribution of *Rickettsia typhi* in fatal murine typhus. *American Journal of Clinical Pathology*, **91**, 720–4.

Ehrlichial diseases

Aetiological agents

The obligate intracellular bacteria that cause animal and human ehrlichioses are cultivated with great difficulty, if at all, in cell culture. Ehrlichiae are related to spotted-fever and typhus rickettsiae at the level of

Fig. 7 Epidemic typhus fever. Typical truncal rash in louse-borne typhus on about the eighth day of illness showing many discrete haemorrhagic lesions.

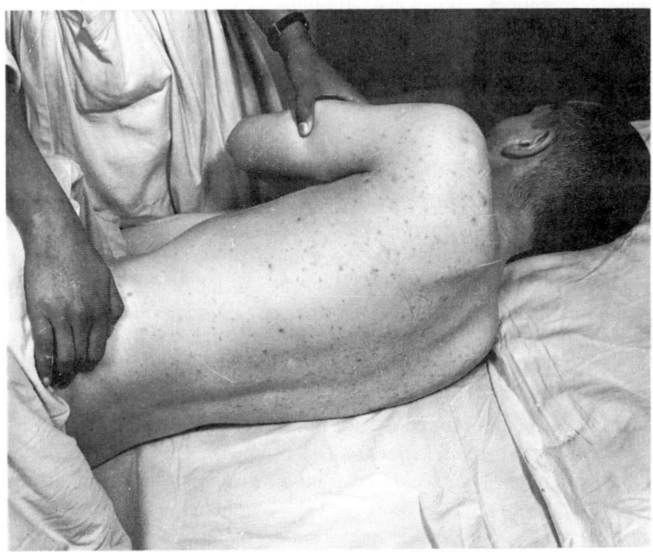

Fig. 8 Recrudescent typhus (Brill–Zinsser disease). Note the erythematous macular rash on the trunk. Illness is in an adult whose initial infection with typhus was 30 years earlier in Poland; second attack was a week after appendectomy—full recovery.

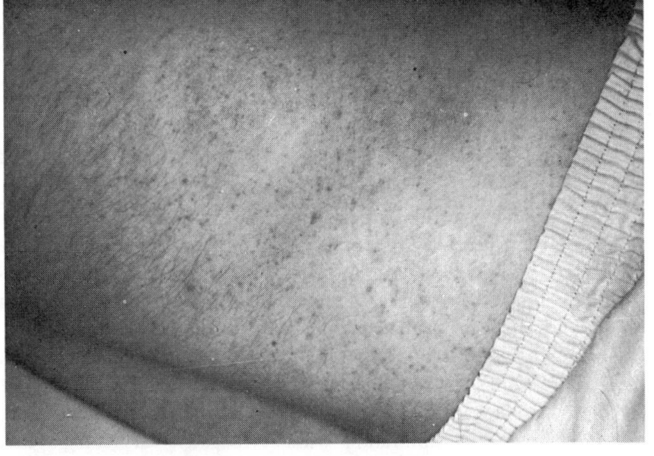

85 per cent sequence similarity of the highly conserved 16*S* rRNA gene, indicating the existence of a common ancestor. However, ehrlichiae differ from these rickettsiae in that they lack lipopolysaccharide in their cell walls, reside within a cytoplasmic phagosomal vacuole, and invade phagocytic blood cells as their target in the host. Ehrlichiae are quite distinct from the chlamydiae. The three ehrlichiae that have been implicated as human pathogens are *E. chaffeensis*, *E. sennetsu* and a granulocytic ehrlichia, closely related to *E. phagocytophila*. Genetic and antigenic analysis of the members of the genus *Ehrlichia* reveals three distinct clusters. *E. chaffeensis* is quite similar to *E. canis* and *E. ewingii*, which cause infections of dogs. *E. sennetsu* is similar to *E. risticii*, an equine pathogen. *E. phagocytophila*, an infectious agent of sheep, cattle and bison, seems to be identical by DNA sequence comparison to *E. equi*, an infectious agent of horses, although neither organism has been cultivated successfully.

Ehrlichial organisms are sometimes considered on the basis of whether their target cells are monocytes–macrophages or granulocytes. Both *E. chaffeensis* and *E. sennetsu* are primarily found in monocytes and macrophages. A most unusual canine ehrlichia, *E. platys*, infects platelets.

Ehrlichiae presumably enter the host cell via phagocytosis, and they actively inhibit fusion of lysosomes with the phagosome. They undergo binary fission to form clusters of organisms contained within the host vacuolar membrane. When stained by the Wright–Giemsa method, the cluster of organisms appears dark violet-blue and stippled and is called a morula from the Latin word for mulberry. Ultrastructurally, ehrlichiae are small (0.2–1.0 μm), Gram-negative bacteria.

Epidemiology

Ehrlichioses for which the ecology and transmission are known are maintained in a cycle involving a mammalian host and a tick vector. The ticks acquire the ehrlichial infection while, as larvae or nymphs, they feed on infected mammalian hosts. Although the ticks remain infected as they moult from stage to stage, transovarian transmission does not occur.

The epidemiology is related to the seasons of tick activity, and most patients recall a recent tick bite. *E. chaffeensis* infections peak between May and July, are acquired mostly in rural areas, and occur mainly in males (78 per cent). *E. chaffeensis* DNA sequences have been detected in the American dog tick, *Dermacentor variabilis*, and antigenically reactive organisms have been detected by immunofluorescence in the Lone Star tick, *Amblyomma americanum*. Infections reportedly have been acquired in at least 20 states of the United States, mostly in the south-east and south-central regions, but cases have also been diagnosed in Europe (Portugal and Spain) and Africa (Mali).

Sennetsu ehrlichiosis has been recognized in Japan and Malaysia. The vector of *E. sennetsu* is not known. Tick bite and ingestion of seafood infested with ehrlichia-containing helminths are possible modes of transmission.

Human granulocytic ehrlichiosis, apparently transmitted by tick bite, has been recognized recently in the United States.

Human ehrlichioses

Haemopoietic cells, including lymphoid, mononuclear, and polymorphonuclear leucocytes, are the primary targets of infection by *E. chaffeensis*. The bone marrow is most often hyperplastic, although hypocellular and normocellular marrow has been observed. Macrophages are observed to form granulomas or histiocytic infiltrations in the bone marrow of three-quarters of patients. Leucopenia (1300–4000 cells /μl) with diminution of both neutrophils and lymphocytes and concurrent thrombocytopenia (usually 50 000–140 000 platelets/μl, but occasionally less than 20 000 is most probably caused by peripheral sequestration. The characteristic histopathological lesion is a mild-to-moderate perivascular lymphohistiocytic infiltration without the vascular damage that would be apparent in a rickettsial infection. The perivasculitis is observed in virtually any organ, including meninges, brain, kidney, and heart. Hepatic involvement may include focal hepatocellular necrosis, intrasinusoidal, foamy histiocytes, periportal and perivascular lymphohistiocytic infiltrates, and granulomas. Interstitial mononuclear pneumonitis has been observed, as well as diffuse alveolar damage leading to a macrophage-rich organizing pneumonia. *E. chaffeensis* has been demonstrated by immunohistological means in the bone marrow, liver, spleen, lymph nodes, lung, kidney, and epicardium and by immunocytological means in mononuclear cells in the cerebrospinal fluid.

Growth of *E. chaffeensis* in cell culture results in the eventual destruction of the host cell. However, the paucity of infected cells in autopsy studies raises the question whether indirect effects such as those exerted by various cytokines might be involved in the pathogenesis of human ehrlichiosis.

Clinically, human ehrlichiosis ranges from asymptomatic seroconversion to fatal infection. Most patients have a fever, headache, chills, malaise, nausea, myalgias, and anorexia. A rash is observed in only about one-third of patients overall, but occurs in a large proportion of infected children. Adults are more likely to have cough, diarrhoea, and lymphadenopathy; children more often develop oedema of the hands or feet. Pulmonary infiltrates occur frequently, and respiratory insufficiency required incubation and mechanical ventilation in 18 per cent of patients in one series. Acute renal insufficiency and abnormalities of the central nervous system have been reported. Cerebrospinal fluid pleocytosis was documented in one-quarter of a series of moderately to severely ill patients. Leucopenia (67 per cent), thrombocytopenia (58 per cent), and mild-to-moderate elevations in serum hepatic aminotransferases (80 per cent) are the most often demonstrated clinical laboratory abnormalities.

The differential diagnosis includes Rocky Mountain spotted fever, meningococcaemia, bacterial sepsis, infective endocarditis, toxic-shock syndrome, influenza, typhoid fever, Q fever, Kawasaki disease, infectious mononucleosis, enteroviral infections, hepatitis, idiopathic or thrombotic thrombocytopenic purpura, pneumonia, aleukaemic leukaemia, lymphoma, Colorado tick fever and other tick-borne infections including Lyme borreliosis, tularaemia, babesiosis, and relapsing fever.

Laboratory diagnosis is not widely available. Only two isolates of *E. chaffeensis* have been obtained, and the fastidious nature of these organisms required prolonged culture in a dog histiocytoma cell line (DH82) before detection of ehrlichial morulae. Visualization of *E. chaffeensis* in peripheral white blood cells is rarely achieved. The standard diagnostic test is indirect immunofluorescent antibody assay utilizing DH82 cell-cultivated *E. chaffeensis* as antigen. A fourfold rise or fall in titre with a peak of 80 or greater is considered diagnostic. Human ehrlichiosis can also be diagnosed by detection of specific sequences of *E. chaffeensis* DNA amplified from the patient's peripheral blood by the PCR and by immunohistological demonstration of *E. chaffeensis* in tissue samples.

E. chaffeensis is susceptible to tetracyclines but not chloramphenicol *in vitro*, and human ehrlichiosis responds favourably to treatment with tetracycline (25 mg/kg body weight per day in four divided doses) or doxycycline (200 mg/day in two divided doses).

Prevention would follow the precautions to avoid tick bite as described above.

Human granulocytic ehrlichiosis may be recognized clinically by the presence of ehrlichiae-filled morulae in peripheral blood neutrophils of patients with fever, headache, myalgia, and malaise. Among 12 documented cases, two patients died. Doxycycline appears to provide effective antiehrlichial therapy when given sufficiently early in the course.

Sennetsu ehrlichiosis

E. sennetsu was isolated in 1953 from the blood, bone marrow, and lymph node of a 25-year-old Japanese man who had an illness resembling infectious mononucleosis. The disease was reproduced by inoculation of ehrlichiae into human volunteers from whose blood *E. sennetsu* was again recovered. After a mean incubation period of 2 weeks, patients suffer sudden onset of chills and a fever that persists for 2 weeks. Other frequent symptoms are headache and myalgia. Enlargement of the post-auricular and posterior cervical lymph nodes is noted 5 to 7 days after onset. Hepatosplenomegaly occurs in one-third to one-half of patients, aseptic meningitis only occasionally, and rash very rarely. Leucopenia early in the course is followed by absolute lymphocytosis with greater than 10 per cent atypical lymphocytes in the late febrile and convalescent stages. Serum hepatic aminotransferases are elevated to a mild-to-moderate degree. Laboratory diagnosis can be achieved by isolation of *E. sennetsu* in mice and by detection of specific serum antibody by indirect fluorescent antibody assay or complement fixation test. Treatment with tetracycline results in defervescence after 24 to 48 h.

REFERENCES

Anderson, B.E., Dawson, J.E., Jones, D.C., and Wilson, K.H. (1991). *Ehrlichia chaffeensis*, a new species associated with human ehrlichiosis. *Journal of Clinical Microbiology*, **29,** 2838–42.

Anderson, B.E. *et al.* (1992). Detection of the etiologic agent of human ehrlichiosis by polymerase chain reaction. *Journal of Clinical Microbiology*, **30,** 775–80.

Chen, S.-M., Dumler, J.S., Bakken, J.S., and Walker, D.H. (1994). Identification of a granulocytotropic *Ehrlichia* species as the etiologic agent of human disease. *Journal of Clinical Microbiology*, **32,** 589–95.

Dumler, J.S. and Walker, D.H. (1991). Human ehrlichiosis. *Current Opinion in Infectious Diseases*, **4,** 597–602.

Eng, T.R. *et al.* (1990). Epidemiologic, clinical, and laboratory findings of human ehrlichiosis in the United States, 1988. *Journal of the American Medical Association*, **264,** 2251–8.

Rikihisa, Y. (1991). The tribe *Ehrlichieae* and ehrlichial diseases. *Clinical Microbiology Review*, **4,** 286–308.

Tachibana, N. (1986). Sennetsu fever: the disease, diagnosis, and treatment. In *Microbiology 1986*, (ed. L. Leive), pp. 205–8. *American Society of Microbiology*, Washington, DC.

7.11.38 Scrub typhus

KYAW WIN and G. WATT

Scrub typhus or Tsutsugamushi fever is an acute, febrile disease of rural Asia. The causative organism, *Rickettsia tsutsugamushi*, is transmitted to man by the bite of a larval mite (chigger). An eschar and regional lymphadenopathy often develop at the site of infection, and may be followed by a systemic illness ranging in severity from inapparent to fatal. Untreated scrub typhus is associated with case fatality rates varying from 0 to 50 per cent. Many cases go undiagnosed, particularly those in which an eschar cannot be found. Unfortunately, serological confirmation is available only in specialized reference centres and there is no satisfactory, commercially available diagnostic test.

AETIOLOGY AND EPIDEMIOLOGY

R. tsutsugamushi is morphologically indistinguishable from other rickettsiae but differs from them antigenically. There are multiple serotypes of *R. tsutsugamushi*: infection with one type confers only transient cross-immunity to another.

Scrub typhus is a zoonosis. Larval mites of the *Leptotrombidium deliense* group become infected with *R. tsutsugamushi* during blood feeds on their usual hosts—small rodents, particularly wild rats of the subgenus Rattus. Man becomes infected when he accidentally encroaches on a zone where the chigger–rodent cycle is taking place. Typically such zones are made up of transitional or secondary vegetation, hence the term scrub typhus. Infected chiggers are generally found in only very circumscribed foci within these zones. Large numbers of cases can occur when man enters these so-called 'mite islands'. During the Second World War, for example, 1255 allied soldiers became ill

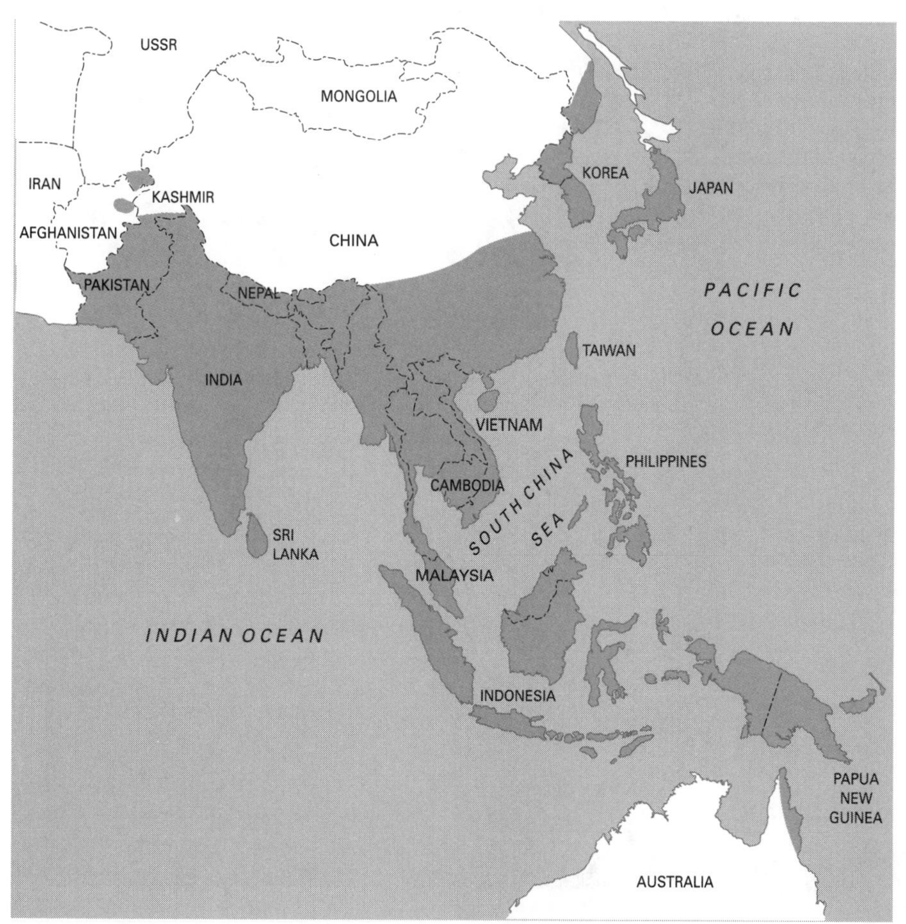

Fig. 1 Geographical distribution of scrub typhus. (Redrawn from Oaks *et al.*, 1983, *Scrub typhus*. Bull, No. 21, Institute for Medical Research, Malaysia, Fig. 2 p. 25, with permission.)

with *R. tsutsugamushi* infection on two small islands off the coast of New Guinea during a period of only 4 months.

The endemic area for scrub typhus forms a triangle bounded by northern Japan and south-eastern Siberia to the north, Queensland, Australia, to the south, and Pakistan to the west (Fig. 1). This triangle contains a diverse range of habitats suitable for the vector, including alpine meadows, cleared rain forests, seashores, semideserts, and even subarctic scree in the Himalayas.

PATHOGENESIS AND CLINICAL FEATURES

Scrub typhus is a disseminated, multiorgan vasculitis and perivasculitis of the small blood vessels. This helps to explain the great diversity of clinical manifestations. Clinical severity is very variable: the mortality of untreated *R. tsutsugamushi* infection ranged from 0 to 50 per cent before the advent of antimicrobial. The diagnostic difficulties created by the protean symptoms and signs of this disease are increased by the lack of a rapid, sensitive, and specific laboratory method of confirming *R. tsutsugamushi* infection.

The chigger bite can occur on any part of the body and is usually unnoticed. An eschar (Fig. 2) forms at the bite site in about 60 per cent of primary infections and in considerably fewer secondary infections. The eschar begins as a small, painless papule, which develops during the 6- to 18- (usually 9–12-) day incubation period. It enlarges, undergoes central necrosis, and acquires a blackened scab to form a lesion resembling a cigarette burn. Regional lymph nodes are enlarged and tender. The eschar is generally well developed and healing by the time symptoms begin.

Fever and headache begin abruptly, and are frequently accompanied by myalgias, malaise, and weakness. More specific clues to the presence of scrub typhus are deafness and tinnitus, which occur in up to a third of cases, as well as conjunctival suffusion and lymphadenopathy (Fig. 3), which are common. A macular rash is a helpful sign, but is difficult to see on dark-skinned individuals. The rash appears on the trunk late in the first week of illness and then spreads peripherally and becomes maculopapular.

Pulmonary involvement (Fig. 4) frequently dominates the clinical picture in mild cases and, with encephalitis, (Fig. 5) and myocardinitis (Fig. 6), is the principal cause of death in patients with severe disease. Cough, tachypnoea, and infiltrates on the chest radiograph are one of the most common presentations of scrub typhus, but the radiographic appearances are not pathognomonic. In severe cases, tachypnoea progresses to

Fig. 2 Eschar of scrub typhus. (Copyright D. A. Warrell.)

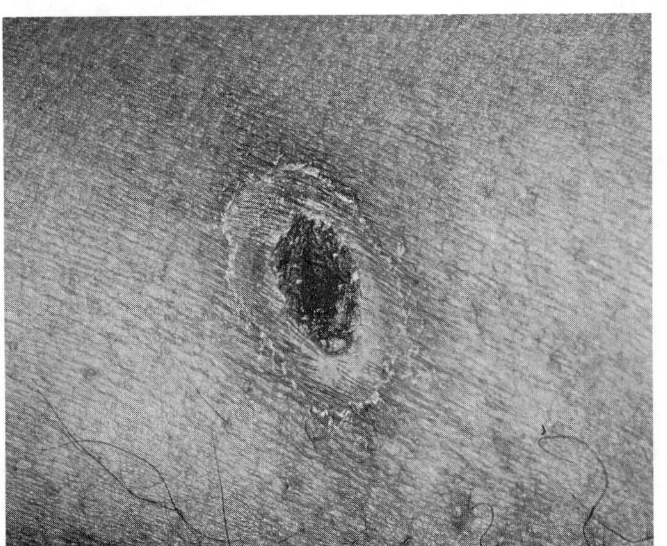

Fig. 3 Lymph node draining eschar in scrub typhus. There is a large area of necrosis near the medulla and smaller areas in the cortex (Armed Forces Institute of Pathology photograph no. 77483).

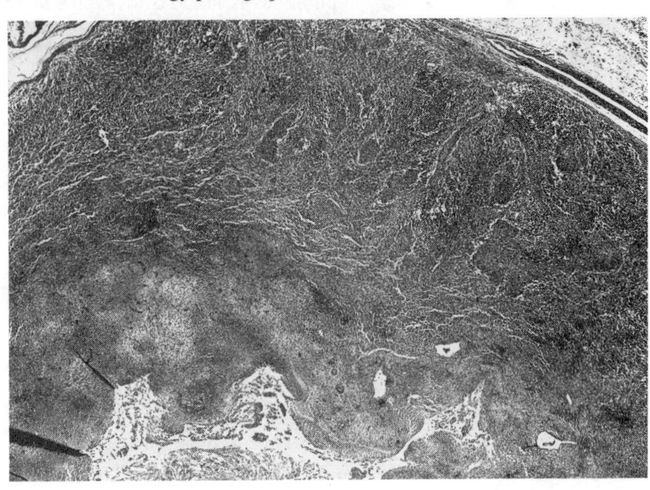

Fig. 4 Interstitial pneumonitis in scrub typhus, with oedema, mononuclear infiltrate, and hyaline membrane lining the alveoli (Armed Forces Institute of Pathology photograph no. 82718).

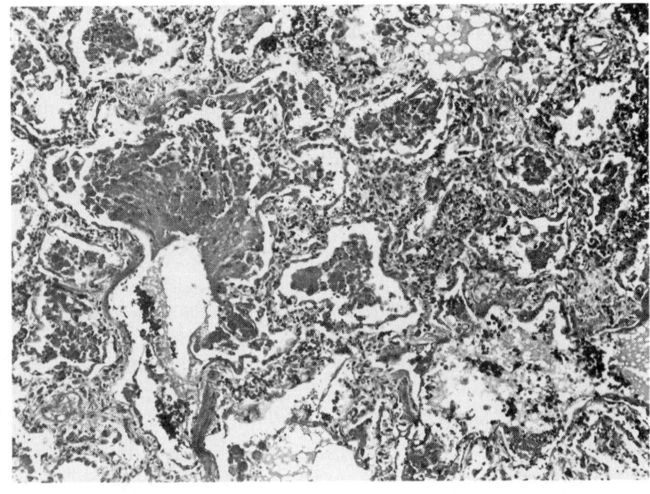

Fig. 5 'Typhus nodule' in the cerebral cortex in scrub typhus (Armed Forces Institute of Pathology photograph no. 78187).

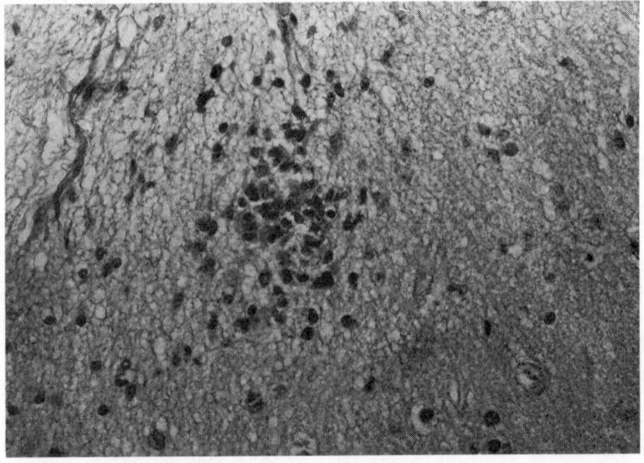

dyspnoea, the patient becomes cyanosed and a syndrome resembling acute respiratory distress syndrome may ensue. Apathy, confusion, and personality changes in moderate cases of scrub typhus may give way to stupor, convulsions, and coma in severe cases. In non-fatal cases, abnormalities resolve completely, although deafness and personality changes may persist for months.

Laboratory findings

There is no cluster of laboratory results that is helpful in indicating *R. tsutsugamushi* infection. Slight elevations of the total white—cell count are typical and mild rises in liver transminases also occur. Laboratory findings are chiefly useful to rule out other infections (see below).

DIAGNOSIS

The diagnosis is straightforward in a patient who lives in or has visited an endemic area and who has an eschar, rash and generalized lymphadenopathy. Unfortunately, this presentation is rare. Many patients present with no specific clinical features; in parts of Malaysia 23 per cent of cases of pyrexia of unknown origin had serological evidence of acute scrub typhus. The single most useful diagnostic clue is the eschar, which is pathognomonic when seen by a physician experienced in scrub typhus. However, even a typical eschar can be overlooked or misdiagnosed. The number of potential differential diagnoses is enormous in patients without an eschar. Malaria, dengue fever, and leptospirosis are just some tropical infections that can mimic scrub typhus.

Laboratory confirmation of *R. tsutsugamushi* infection is difficult. The Weil–Felix test with Proteus OX-K is the only commercially available serodiagnostic method, but is extremely insensitive. The immunofluorescent antibody and immunoperoxidase tests are currently the serodiagnostic methods of choice but are not available outside a few reference centres.

TREATMENT

Prompt antimicrobial therapy is the single most important factor in shortening the disease, reducing mortality, and speeding convalescence. Treatment must often be presumptive, however, because laboratory confirmation of diagnosis is rarely available early enough to influence management. The benefits of avoiding severe scrub typhus by early treatment generally far outweigh the risks of a 1-week course of antimicrobials. Either tetracycline (500 mg, four times a day) or doxycycline (100 mg, twice a day) for 7 days can be used. Shorter treatment courses are curative, but associated with a high rate of recrudescence. Chloramphenicol (50–75 mg/kg a day) is also effective. Parenteral therapy should be used in patients who are vomiting or have severe disease. Scrub typhus is said to be even more susceptible to antimicrobials than other rickettsioses; patients generally become afebrile within 24 to 36 h of beginning therapy. Recent (unpublished) observations have identified a focus of scrub typhus in Chiang Rai, Northern Thailand with diminished susceptibility to doxycycline and chloramphenicol. Its geographical boundaries have not yet been defined, nor has a mechanism of resistance been identified.

Good supportive care and early detection of complications are important in severe cases if a good outcome is to be obtained. Fluid management is particularly difficult because patients are often hypotensive but have increased vascular permeability due to vasculitis. There is a high risk, therefore, of iatrogenic pulmonary oedema, which may be difficult to diagnose early because of concomitant scrub-typhus pneumonitis. Fluid management is best accomplished in an intensive care unit whenever possible, with careful monitoring of pulmonary capillary wedge pressure or central venous pressure.

Fig. 6 Interstitial myocarditis in scrub typhus showing separation of muscle bundels (Armed Forces Institute of Pathology photograph no. 76879).

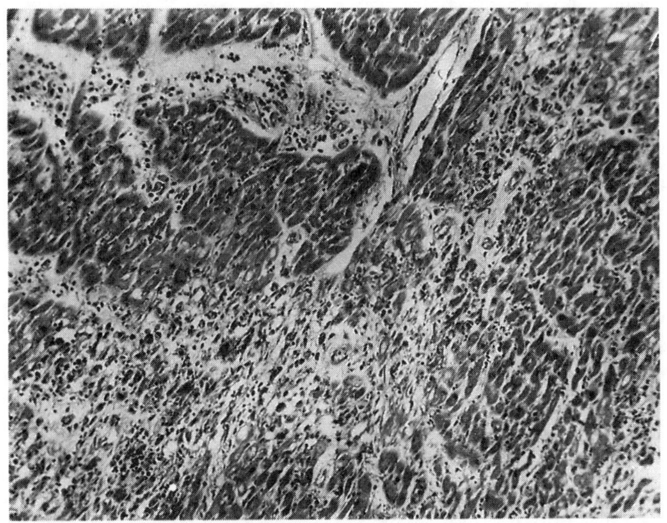

CONTROL

Weekly doses of 200 mg of doxycycline can prevent *R. tsutsugamushi* infection. Non-immune populations occupationally exposed would benefit most from scrub typhus protection, but chemoprophylaxis should also be considered in high-risk travellers, such as those backpacking or trekking in endemic areas. Daily doxycycline is often recommended for the prevention of the drug-resistant strains of falciparum malaria, which are particularly prevalent in parts of Asia, but it is not known whether this regimen will prevent scrub typhus. Contact with chiggers can be reduced by not sitting or lying directly on the ground and by applying repellant to the tops of boots, socks, and on the lower trousers. Effective killed vaccines have not yet been developed to prevent scrub typhus.

REFERENCES

Anderson, D.R., Hopps, M.E., Barile, M.F., and Bernheim, B.S. (1965). Comparison of the ultrastructure of several rickettsiae, ornithosis virus and mycoplasma in tissue culture. *Journal of Bacteriology*, **90,** 1387–404.

Anon. (1988). Scrub typhus pneumonia. *Lancet*, **ii,** 1062.

Anon. (1991). Bitten, hot and mostly spotty. *Lancet*, **i,** 143–4.

Brown, G.W., Robinson, D.M., Huxsoll, D.L., Na, T.S., Lim, K.J., and Sannasey, G. (1976) Scrub typhus: a common cause of illness in indigenous populations. *Transactions of the Royal Society of Tropical Medicine and Hygiene*, **70,** 444–8.

Chayakul, P., Panich, V., and Silpapojakul, K. (1988). Scrub typhus pneumonitis: an entity which is frequently missed. *Quarterly Journal of Medicine*, **256,** 595–602.

Furuya, Y. *et al.* (1991). Use of monoclonal antibodies against *Rickettsia tsutsugamushi Kawasaki* for serodiagnosis by enzyme-linked immunosorbent assay. *Journal of Clinical Microbiology*, **29,** 340–5.

Johnson, D.E., Crum, J.W., Hanchalay, S., and Saengruchi, C. (1982). Seroepidemiological survey of *Rickettsia tsutsugamushi* infection in a rural Thai village. *Transactions of the Royal Society of Tropical Medicine and Hygiene*, **76,** 1–3.

McClain, J.B., Joshi, B., and Rice, R. (1988). Chloramphenicol, gentamicin, and ciprofloxacin against murine scrub typhus. *Antimicrobial Agents and Chemotherapy*, **32,** 285–6.

Oaks, S.C., Ridgway, R.L., Shirai, A., and Twartz, J.C. (1983). Scrub typhus. In *Bulletin 21*. Institute for Medical Research, Malaysia.

Rapmund, G. (1984). Rickettsial diseases of the Far East: new perspectives. *Journal of Infectious Diseases*, **149,** 330–8.

Sayen, J.J., Pond, H.S., Forrester, J.S., and Wood, F.C. (1946). Scrub typhus in Assam and Burma. *Medicine*, **25,** 155–214.

Silpapojakul, K., Ukkachoke, C., Krisanapan, S., and Silpapojakul, K. (1991). Rickettsial meningitis and encephalitis. *Archives of Internal Medicine*, **9,** 1753–7.

Silpapojakul, K. *et al.* (1991). Scrub and murine typhus in children with obscure fever in the tropics. *Pediatric Infectious Diseases Journal*, **10,** 200–3.

Smadel, J.E. and Jackson, E.B. (1947). Chloromycetin, an antibiotic with chemotherapeutic activity in experimental rickettsial and viral infectious. *Science*, **106,** 418–19.
Twartz, J.C., Shirai, A., Selvaraju, G., Saunders, J.P., Huxsoll, D.L., and Groves, M.G. Doxycycline prophylaxis for human scrub typhus. *Journal of Infectious Diseases*, **146,** 811–18.
Weiss, E. (1992). Rickettsias. In *Encyclopedia of microbiology*, Vol. **3,** pp. 585–610. Academic Press, San Diego.
Woodward, T.E. (1990). Rickettsial infection. In *Current therapy in infectious disease 3*, (ed. E.H. Kass, and R. Platt), pp. 305–8. Decker, Toronto.

7.11.39 *Coxiella burnetii* infections (Q fever)

T. J. Marrie

History

In August 1935, Dr. Edward Holbrook Derrick, director of the Laboratory of Microbiology and Pathology of the Queensland Health Department at Brisbane was asked to investigate an outbreak of undiagnosed febrile illness among workers at the Cannon Hill abattoir. It became apparent to Derrick that he was dealing with a type of fever that had not been previously described—he named it Q (for query) fever. A couple of years later, Sir Frank Macfarlane Burnet in Australia and Herald Rea Cox in the United States isolated the micro-organism responsible for Q fever. In 1948 the name *Coxiella burnetii* was proposed for this micro-organism. Cox and Burnet both died in 1986.

Coxiella burnetii *(Fig. 1)*

This micro-organism has a Gram-negative cell wall and measures $0.3 \times 1 \mu m$. It is the sole species of its genus and, while it is a member of the family Rickettsiaceae, comparisons of 16*S* rRNA sequences shows that *C. burnetii* and *Wolbachia pecsica* are members of the γ-subdivision of purple bacteria while rickettsiae belong to the α-subdivision. *C. burnetii* is an obligate phagolysosomal parasite of eukaryotes. The low pH of the phagolysosome is necessary for optimal functioning of *C. burnetii* enzymes. It multiplies by transverse binary fison and undergoes sporulation. It stains well by Gimenez stain. The cell envelope contains outer membrane protein, lipopolysaccharide, and peptidoglycan. The genome is 1.04×10^9 Da in size. Six strains of *C. burnetii* (Hamilton, Vacca, Rasche, Biotzere, Corazon, Dod) have been described and all but the Corazon strain have been shown to contain a plasmid.

Fig. 1 Transmission electron micrograph showing *Coxiella burnetii* cells within a macrophage in the heart valve of a patient with Q fever endocarditis. The dark material in the centre of each cell is condensed DNA. × 15 000.

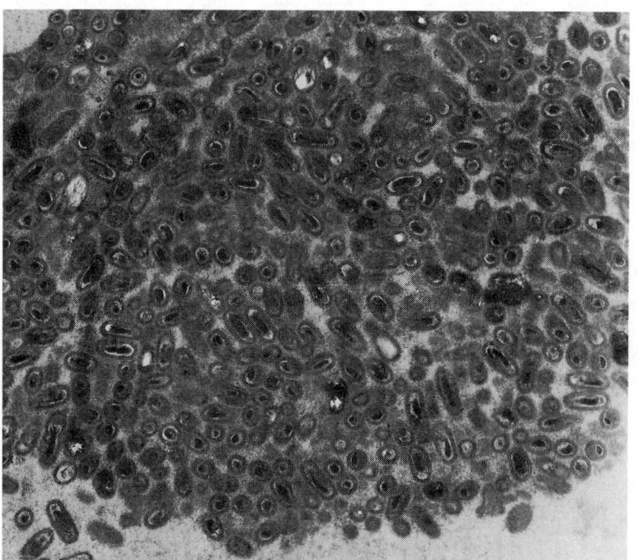

Strains Biotzere and Corazon have been associated with chronic Q fever; the Dod strain is avirulent. *C. burnetii* undergoes phase variation akin to the smooth to rough transition in some enteric Gram-negative bacilli. In nature and laboratory animals it exists in the phase-1 state. Repeated passage of phase-I virulent organisms in embryonated chicken eggs led to conversion to phase-II avirulent forms. These two antigenic phases differ in the sugar composition of their polysaccharides, in their buoyant density in caesium chloride, and in their affinity for haematoxylin and basic fuchsin dyes. Antibodies to phase-I antigens predominate in chronic Q fever while the reverse is true for acute Q fever.

C. burnetii has survived for 586 days in tick faeces at room temperature, 160 days or more in water, in dried cheese made from contaminated milk for 30 to 40 days, and for up to 150 days in soil.

Epidemiology

Q fever is a zoonosis. There is an extensive wild-life and arthropod (mainly ticks) reservoir of *C. burnetii*. Domestic animals are infected through inhalation of contaminated aerosols or by ingestion of infected material. These animals rarely become ill but abortion and stillbirths may occur. *C. burnetii* localizes in the uterus and mammary glands of infected animals. During pregnancy there is reactivation of *C. burnetii* and it multiplies in the placenta, reaching 10^9 hamster infective doses per gram of tissue. The organisms are shed into the environment at the time of parturition. Man becomes infected after inhaling organisms aerosolized at the time of parturition or later when organisms in dust are stirred up on a windy day. Infected cows have shed *C. burnetii* in milk for up to 32 months while sheep shed the organism in faeces for 11 to 18 days postpartum.

Infected cattle, sheep, and goats are the animals primarily responsible for transmitting *C. burnetii* to man. In Atlantic Canada, infected parturient cats spread this micro-organism to man.

Given the above facts the epidemiology of *C. burnetii* infections is usually predictable. Thus, those individuals who are prone to develop Q fever are farmers, abattoir workers, and those in related occupations. There are many interesting facets to the epidemiology of Q fever: an outbreak of Q fever affected 415 residents of a Swiss valley, who lived along a road over which sheep travelled to and from mountain pastures. From May to July 1989, more than 100 cases of Q fever occurred in the West Midlands of England, chiefly the Birmingham area. No common source was found but, as the outbreak coincided with lambing season and as the summer was early and dry that year, it was postulated that wind-borne contaminated dust resulted in the outbreak. A group of poker players in Halifax, Nova Scotia played in a room where a cat gave birth to kittens. They all developed Q fever pneumonia—poker players' pneumonia. *C. burnetii* was isolated from the cat's uterus.

There have been several outbreaks of Q fever in hospitals and research institutes due to transportation of infected sheep to research laboratories. Individuals whose offices or laboratories were along the transportation route have developed Q fever as well as those involved in research.

Some studies have suggested that ingestion of contaminated milk is a risk factor for acquisition of Q fever; volunteers seroconverted but did not become ill after ingesting such milk.

Percutaneous infection, such as when an infected tick is crushed between the fingers, may occur but is rare and accounts for very few cases of Q fever worldwide. Transmission via a contaminated blood transfusion has rarely occurred.

Vertical transmission from mother to child has been infrequently reported. It is likely that this is much more common than we realize. It is also likely that reactivation of latent Q fever occurs during pregnancy in the human female as it does in other animals.

Person-to-person transmission has been documented on a few occasions. Twelve cases of Q fever occurred at the Institute of Pathology at Tubingen University; person-to-person transmission is assumed to have occurred. There is no need to isolate patients admitted to hospital with this illness; however, precautions should be taken during the examination of infected cadavers.

Sexual transmission of *C. burnetii* has been demonstrated in mice under laboratory conditions. Whether such transmission occurs in man or other animals is unknown.

A most peculiar aspect of the epidemiology of Q fever is that in some areas where *C. burnetii* is present in wild and domestic animals there are frequently cases of Q fever in man, while in other areas with the same rate of *C. burnetii* infection among wildlife and domestic animals Q fever is rare in man.

The following countries should be considered major areas for *C. burnetii* infection: Australia, United Kingdom, the South of France, Germany, the People's Republic of China, Nova Scotia Province of Canada, Portugal, Spain, The Netherlands, and Uruguay. Forty-five countries on five continents have reported cases of Q fever.

Q fever

CLINICAL FEATURES

Man is the only animal known almost always to develop illness following infection with *C. burnetii*. There is an incubation period of about 2 weeks (range 2–29 days) following inhalation of *C. burnetii*. A dose-response effect has been demonstrated experimentally and clinically. In cat-related outbreaks of Q fever those who cleaned up the products of conception had the shortest incubation period and the most severe illness. *C. burnetii* is one of the most infectious agents known to man; a single micro-organism is able to initiate infection. The resulting illness in man can be divided into acute and chronic varieties.

Acute Q fever

Self-limiting febrile illness

The most common manifestation of acute Q fever is a self-limiting febrile illness. In areas where Q fever is endemic, 12 per cent or more of the population have antibodies to *C. burnetii*—most of these infections are subclinical.

Pneumonia (Figs. 2 and 3)

This is the most commonly recognized manifestation of Q fever. The onset is non-specific with fever, fatigue, and headache. The headache may be very severe, occasionally so severe that it prompts a lumbar puncture. A dry cough of mild to moderate intensity is present in 24 to 90 per cent of patients. About one-third have pleuritic chest pain. Nausea, vomiting, and diarrhoea do occur in 10 to 30 per cent of patients. Most cases of *C. burnetii* pneumonia are mild; however, about 10 per cent of cases are severe enough to require admission to hospital; rarely, assisted ventilation is necessary. Death is rare in Q fever pneumonia and is usually due to comorbid illness. Examination of the chest reveals crackles but frequently there are no abnormal findings. The physical findings of consolidation are present in 30 per cent of cases. The white blood-cell count is usually normal; it is elevated in one-third of patients. There may be mild elevation of liver enzymes, two to three times normal. Reactive thrombocytosis is surprisingly common, occurring in 60 per cent of patients and often reaching values of 700 to 800 $\times$ 10^9/l. Microscopic haematuria is a common finding.

The chest radiographic manifestations of Q fever pneumonia are usually indistinguishable from those of any bacterial pneumonia (Fig. 3). However, rounded opacities are suggestive of this infection (Fig. 2). Some investigators have reported delayed clearing of the pneumonia; however, in our experience resolution is usually complete within 3 weeks.

Hepatitis

The liver is probably involved in all patients with acute Q fever. There are three clinical pictures

(i) pyrexia of unknown origin with mild to moderate elevation of liver function tests;
(ii) a hepatitis-like picture;
(iii) 'incidental hepatitis'.

In incidental hepatitis the chief manifestation of Q fever is infection of another organ system with mild elevation of liver function tests. Liver biopsy reveals the distinctive 'doughnut' granuloma, consisting of a granuloma with a central lipid vacuole and fibrin deposits

Neurological manifestations

Encephalitis, encephalomyelitis, toxic confusional states, optic neuritis, and demyelinating polyradiculoneuritis are uncommon manifestations of Q fever.

Rare manifestations

These include myocarditis, pericarditis, bone marrow necrosis, lymphadenopathy, pancreatitis, mesenteric paniculitis, erythema nodosum, epididymitis, orchitis, priapism, and erythema annular centrifugum.

Chronic Q fever

The usual manifestation of chronic Q fever is that of culture-negative endocarditis. Seventy per cent of these patients have fever and nearly

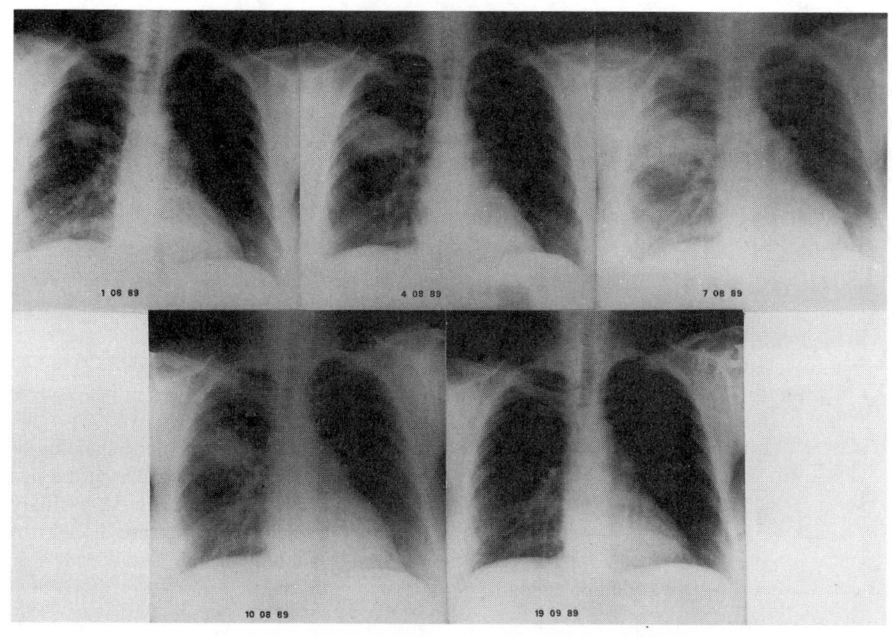

Fig. 2 Serial chest radiograph of a 35-year-old patient with Q fever pneumonia. The first radiograph (1 August 1989) shows a right upper-lobe, round opacity that increases in size over the next 6 days. The pneumonia has completely cleared by 19 September 1989.

all have abnormal native or prosthetic heart valves. Hepatomegaly and or splenomegaly occur in about half of these patients and one-third have marked clubbing of the digits A purpuric rash due to immune complex-induced leucocytoclastic vasculitis and arterial embolism occur in about 20 per cent of patients. Hyperglobulinaemia (up to 60 g/l) is common and is a useful clue to chronic Q fever in a patient with the clinical picture of culture-negative endocarditis.

Other manifestations of chronic Q fever include osteomyelitis, infection of aortic aneurysm, and infection of vascular prosthetic grafts.

The strains of *C. burnetii* that cause chronic Q fever are different from those that cause acute Q fever. Only isolates of the Biotzere and Corazon strain have been recovered from cases of chronic infection. The QpRS plasmid and chromosomally integrated sequences with homology to QpRS are found in endocarditis isolates. Peripheral blood lymphocytes from patients with Q fever endocarditis are unresponsive to *C. burnetii* antigens *in vitro* while responding normally to other antigens.

DIAGNOSIS

A strong clinical suspicion based on the epidemiology and clinical features as outlined above is the cornerstone of the diagnosis of Q fever. This suspicion is confirmed by determining a fourfold or greater increase in antibody titre between acute and 2- to 3-week convalescent serum samples. A variety of serological tests is available: complement fixation, microimmunofluorescence, and enzyme immunoassay. The immunofluorescent antibody test is easiest to use. In acute Q fever the antibody titre to phase-II antigen is higher than that to phase-I while the reverse occurs in chronic Q fever. In chronic Q fever, antibody titres are extremely high, in the order of 1:8192 and higher to phase-I antigen. In acute Q fever, antibody titres to phase-I antigen are rarely in excess of 1:512, while peak antibody titres to phase-II antigen are 1:1024 to 1:2048.

TREATMENT

Quinolones and rifampicin are the most active agents *in vitro* against *C. burnetii.* Tetracyclines, and trimethoprim–sulphamethoxazole have been used successfully to treat this infection. Acute Q fever is treated with a 2-week course of tetracycline, doxycycline, or trimethoprim–sulphamethoxazole. Chronic Q fever should be treated with two antimicrobial agents for at least 2 years. Some authorities recommend lifelong therapy for chronic Q fever. We use rifampicin, 300 mg twice a day, and ciprofloxacin, 750 mg twice a day, as agents of first choice.

Fig. 3 Portable anteroposterior chest radiograph of a 72-year-old male with Q fever pneumonia. Note the bilateral lower-lobe opacities. This radiographic picture is indistinguishable from pneumonia due to any other microbial agent.

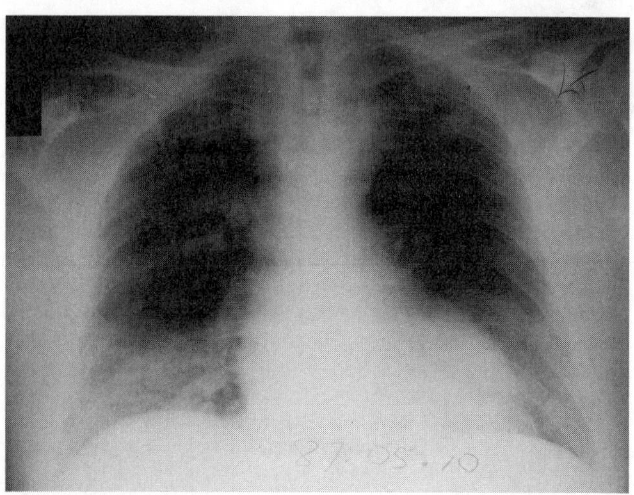

Rifampicin and doxycycline or tetracycline and trimethoprim–sulphamethoxazole have also been used to treat chronic Q fever. Antibody titres should be measured every 6 months for the first 2 years. A progressive decline in antibody titre reflects successful treatment of chronic Q fever. Cardiac valve replacement may be necessary as part of the management of chronic Q fever. The decision to replace a valve is made for haemodynamic reasons. Prosthetic valve endocarditis due to *C. burnetii* has been successfully treated without valve replacement.

PREVENTION

A formalin-inactivated *C. burnetii*, whole-cell vaccine is protective against infection and has a low rate of side-effects; 1 per cent of vaccinees developed an abscess at the inoculation site and another 1 per cent had a lump at this site 2 months after vaccination.

Other measures to reduce Q fever infection are the use of only seronegative pregnant sheep in research facilities and control of ectoparasites on livestock.

REFERENCES

Babudieri, B. (1959). Q fever: a zoonosis. *Advances in Veterinary Science*, **5,** 81–181.

Derrick, E.H. (1937). 'Q' fever, new fever entity: clinical features, diagnosis and laboratory investigation. *Medicine Journal of Australia*, **2,** 281–99.

Ellis, M.E., Smith, C-C., and Moffatt, M.A.J. (1983). Chronic or fatal Q fever infection: a review of 16 patients seen in northeast Scotland (1967–1980). *Quarterly Journal of Medicine*, **205,** 54–66.

Marrie, T.J., Durant, H., Williams, J.C., Mintz, E., and Waag, D.M. (1988). Exposure to parturient cats is a risk factor for acquisition of Q fever in Maritime Canada. *Journal of Infectious Diseases*, **158,** 101–8.

Marrie, T.J. (ed.) [1990], *Q fever, the disease*. CRC Press, Boca Raton, Fa.

Qizilbash, A-H. (1983). The pathology of Q fever as seen on liver biopsy. *Archives Pathology and Laboratory Medicine*, **107,** 364–7.

Samuel, J.E., Frazier, M.E., and Mallavia, L.P. (1985). Correlation of plasmid type and disease caused by *Coxiella burnetii. Infection and Immunity*, **48,** 359–65.

Sawyer, L.A., Fishbein, D.B., and McDade, J.E., (1987). Q fever: current concepts. *Reviews of Infectious Diseases*, **9,** 935–46.

Turck, W.P.G. *et al.* (1976). Chronic Q fever. *Quarterly Journal of Medicine*, **45,** 193–217.

Welsh, H.H., Lennette, E.H., Abinanti, F.R., and Win, J.F. (1958). Air-borne transmission of Q fever: the role of parturition in the generation of infective aerosols. *Annals New York Academy Sciences*, **70,** 528–40.

Williams, J.C. and Thompson, H.A. (1991), *Q fever: the biology of Coxiella burnetii*. CRC Press, Boca Raton, FL.

7.11.40 Cat scratch disease, bacillary angiomatosis, and trench fever

B. A. PERKINS

You have raised the veil which for centuries had covered infectious diseases; you have discovered and demonstrated their microbian nature.

Joseph Lister speaking of Louis Pasteur at a celebration of his 70th birthday, in Paris, December 27, 1892.

Introduction

And over a century later, we continue to expand our understanding of the 'microbian nature' of diseases, both old and new. During the last decade, the aetiology of cat scratch disease was discovered, bacillary angiomatosis was recognized, and the relationship of these diseases to trench fever, an epidemic scourge of soldiers in the First World War, was demonstrated.

Recent progress in understanding of these diseases was stimulated by two observations in 1983. First, bacilli were seen in lymph nodes of patients with cat scratch disease. Second, what is now known to be bacillary angiomatosis was described in a human immunodeficiency virus (**HIV**)-infected patient; cultures of affected tissues were negative but bacilli could be seen. The staining characteristics and morphological appearances of the bacilli and the histories of cat scratches given by patients with both diseases suggested that cat scratch disease and bacillary angiomatosis might be caused by the same agent.

In 1988, investigators at the Armed Forces Institute of Pathology in Washington, DC reported isolation of a bacterium from lymph nodes of patients with cat scratch disease and suggested that it was the cause of the disease. The bacterium was initially called the 'cat scratch disease bacillus' and later classified as *Afipia felis*. However, its role as the principal cause of cat scratch disease was questioned by results of a revolutionary technique used to identify the aetiology of bacillary angiomatosis in the absence of positive cultures. Researchers at Stanford University used eubacterial primers in a polymerase chain reaction (**PCR**) to amplify bacterial 16*s* ribosomal gene fragments directly from tissue biopsies in bacillary angiomatosis. Specimens from several unrelated patients yielded a unique 16*s* gene sequence belonging to a previously uncharacterized micro-organism most closely related to *Rochalimaea quintana*, the aetiological agent of trench fever, identified in 1969. Simultaneously, another group reported isolation, after lysis–centrifugation, of a Gram-negative bacterium from the blood of febrile patients. The 16*s* ribosomal gene sequences identified in the tissue biopsies from patients with bacillary angiomatosis were found to be identical or closely related to the 16*s* ribosomal gene sequence of this bacterium. The organism was classified as a new species of rochalimaea and named *Rochalimaea henselae. R. henselae*, while closely related to *R. quintana*, is not related to *A. felis*. Recently, *R. henselae* and *R. quintana* have been placed in the same genus as *Bartonella baciliformis* (Chapter 7.11.44).

A *Bartonella henselae*-based, indirect immunofluorescent antibody test developed for the diagnosis of bacillary angiomatosis was strongly positive in sera from patients with suspected cat scratch disease, but these were negative when tested with an *A. felis*-based immunofluorescent assay. The association between cat scratch disease and *B. henselae* was further strengthened by a study in which sera from cases of cat scratch disease and case-associated cats were found to be positive with the *B. henselae* immunofluorescent antibody, whereas sera from asymptomatic family members and control cats were negative. *B. henselae* has now also been isolated from patients with apparent cat scratch disease as well as from domestic cats.

Recent studies of bacillary angiomatosis have shown that owning a cat is a risk factor for the disease and have provided additional serological, PCR-based sequence, and cultural data supporting an aetiological role for both *B. henselae* and *B. quintana*.

There has been substantial progress in our understanding of these diseases but many questions remain unanswered. The most difficult problem is to explain how cat scratch disease can be caused by *B. henselae*, bacillary angiomatosis by *B. henselae* and *B. quintana*, and trench fever by *B. quintana* when each of these diseases has such different clinical features. Host factors are one possible explanation but more research is needed.

Cat scratch disease

INTRODUCTION

Cat scratch disease is characterized by the development of regional lymphadenopathy after a cat scratch. Its first description appeared in France in 1950. Since then, there have been numerous publications about its possible cause, epidemiology, clinical features, and therapy. Although it has long been considered an infectious disease, the aetiological agent had, until recently, remained elusive.

EPIDEMIOLOGY

Cat scratch disease has been reported most often from North America, Europe, and Asia but its true distribution may be worldwide. Most epidemiological information has been based on case series but some attempts have been made to develop population-based estimates for the incidence of cat scratch disease. A recent case-control study of potential risk factors has confirmed some traditionally held beliefs and raised additional questions, the most provocative of which is whether fleas might be involved in transmission.

In the United States, the estimated incidence of cat scratch disease in ambulatory patients is 9 cases/100 000 population. Some 0.8 cases/100 000 population are discharged from hospital with a diagnosis of cat scratch disease. These data support earlier estimates and suggest that cat scratch disease affects about 22 000 persons each year in the United States, resulting in approximately 2000 hospital admissions.

Some important epidemiological aspects of cat scratch disease have been reported consistently. First, most cases of cat scratch disease are children. Depending on the study, estimates of the proportion of cases occurring in people less than 18 years of age range from 55 to 87 per cent. Secondly, in temperate areas, cat scratch disease has a distinct seasonal variation in occurrence with an autumn/winter peak. Thirdly, males and females appear to be affected equally.

The association between cats and the development of cat scratch disease was the basis for recognition of this disease. Over 90 per cent of reported cases have a history of contact with a cat, usually involving a scratch or bite and most often by a kitten under 12 months of age. Cats implicated in transmission of cat scratch disease usually show no overt signs of illness. There have been occasional reports suggesting that injuries from other animals or inanimate objects may also result in cat scratch disease.

Multiple cases of cat scratch disease are often seen within a family, presumably related to exposure to the same cat. When this occurs, family members usually become unwell within a few weeks of each other, suggesting that cats may be infectious for only a short period.

In the United States, risk factors for the development of cat scratch disease including owning or being scratched or bitten by a kitten but not by an adult cat. Compared to cat-owning controls, patients with cat scratch disease were more likely to have at least one pet kitten with fleas. This suggests that fleas may be involved in transmission of cat scratch disease.

AETIOLOGY

Recent findings suggest that *B. henselae* is responsible for most cases of cat scratch disease. The best evidence is serological, epidemiological, and from use of molecular probes rather than culture, but *B. henselae* has been isolated from patients with cat scratch disease and from domestic cats. *Afipia felis*, formerly known as the 'cat scratch bacillus', has also been isolated from lymph nodes of patients with cat scratch disease. Defining the precise roles of *B. henselae* and *A. felis* in cat scratch disease will require additional studies.

B. henselae is a small, curved, pleomorphic, Gram-negative rod that is oxidase and catalase negative, X-factor dependent, and sensitive to a broad range of commonly used antimicrobials including ampicillin, tetracycline, trimethoprim-sulphamethoxazole, and aminoglycosides. It is most closely related to *B. quintana*, the louse-borne agent of trench fever. There are three other known species in the genus Bartonella; *B. vinsoni*, which was isolated from voles and is not known to cause human disease, *B. elizabethae*, which was isolated from a patient with endocarditis, and *B. baciliformis* (see Chapter 7.11.44).

Bartonella currently belongs to the order Rickettsiales and is the only rickettsial genus to grow on artificial media. Based on recent DNA studies, the genera Bartonella and Rochalimaea have been unified and the family Bartonellaceae may be removed from the order Rickettsiales.

CLINICAL PRESENTATION

Regional lymphadenopathy is the most common clinical feature of cat scratch disease (Fig. 1). The most common sites of lymphadenopathy are axillary, cervical, and submandibular, but this may be generalized. Affected nodes are often tender and occasionally suppurate. About one-half of patients have 'primary inoculation lesions' manifested by skin papules, pustules, or other evidence of abnormal healing (Fig. 1). These lesions typically develop at the site of a cat scratch or bite 3 to 10 days after injury and precede the onset of lymphadenopathy by 1 to 2 weeks. Mild systemic complaints are common. About one-third of patients complain of fever and one-quarter have malaise or fatigue. Other non-specific clinical features associated with cat scratch disease include headache, anorexia, weight loss, vomiting, sore throat, rashes (especially erythema nodusum or multiforme, papulovesicular or maculopapular eruptions, or thrombocytopenic purpura), and splenomegaly. Although considered to be a self-limiting illness, signs and symptoms of cat scratch disease often persist for 2 to 4 months.

Atypical manifestations of cat scratch disease occur in less than 10 per cent of cases. Among these manifestations, Parinaud's oculoglandular syndrome is the most common. Patients present with a granuloma of the eyelid or conjunctiva and ipsilateral preauricular lymphadenitis. Recovery is usually complete without sequelae. Encephalopathy or other neurological disease, occasionally complicates cat scratch disease. Onset is sudden and usually follows the development of lymphadenopathy by 1 to 6 weeks. Although neurological signs are often dramatic and frequently include seizures and coma, patients recover completely over periods ranging from days to months. The cerebrospinal fluid is usually unremarkable. Hepatic granulomas, osteomyelitis, and pulmonary involvement have also been reported as rare complications of cat scratch disease. All parts of the respiratory tract may be affected; bilateral hilar lymphadenopathy and primary atypical pneumonia have been reported. Severe manifestations have been described in an immunocompromised patient. Fatalities are extremely rare.

Fig. 1 Crusted erythematous papules at the site of a cat scratch above the umbilicus with bilateral inguinal lymphadenopathy, which developed 10 days later, in a 7-year-old boy (Copyright D. A. Warrell).

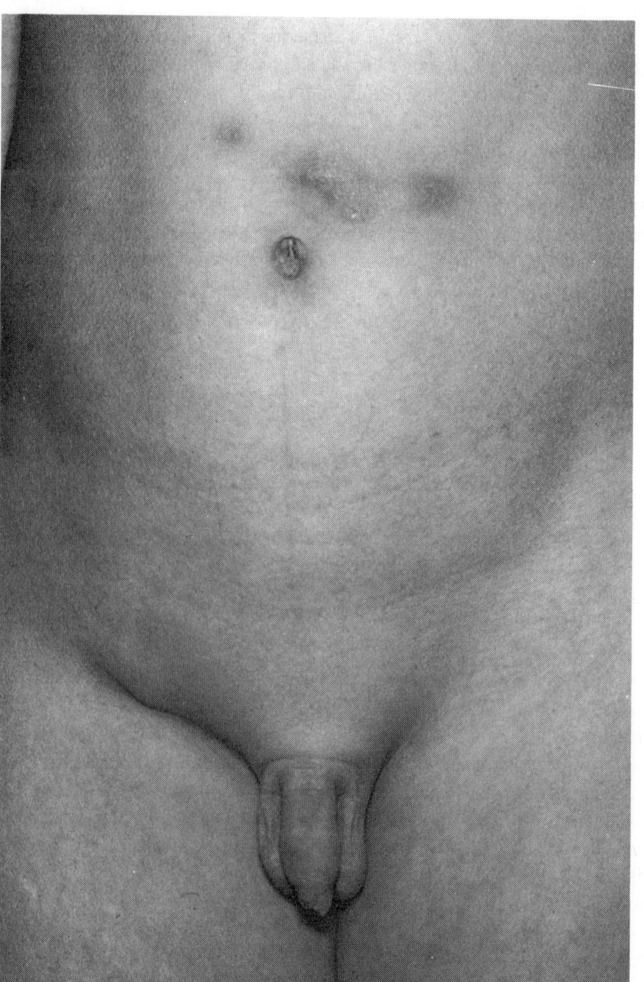

DIAGNOSIS

The diagnosis of cat scratch disease has been made when three of the following four criteria are met in a patient with lymphadenopathy: (i) history of cat contact, with presence of a scratch or primary inoculation lesion; (ii) positive cat scratch disease skin-test antigen response; (iii) negative laboratory results for other causes of lymphadenopathy; and (iv) characteristic histopathological appearances (microabcesses or granulomas) in a lymph node.

The cat scratch disease skin-test antigen is prepared from pus (aspirated from lymph nodes of patients with cat scratch disease) by pasteurization but there have been concerns about its safety. Although its use is still advocated by some for diagnosis of cat scratch disease, this material is generally unlicensed and is difficult to standardize.

New serological assays based on measurement of antibodies to *B. henselae* appear to be sensitive and specific for diagnosis of cat scratch

Fig. 2 Bacilli in tissue. Photomicrograph of Warthin—Starry silver impregnation stained section of an inguinal lymph-node from a patient with a skin test positive for cat scratch disease. A vessel containing erythrocytes is cut in cross-section, bacilli are seen singly and in chains outlining the vessel (× 630). (Reproduced from Wear *et al.* (1983). *Science*, **221,** 1403–5, Armed Forces Institute of Pathology negative 82-11271, with permission.)

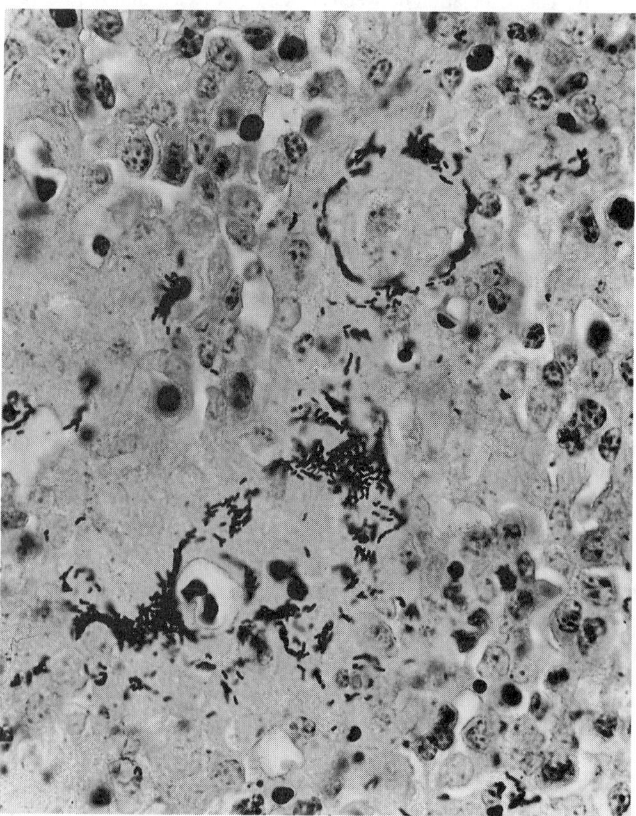

disease. Once standardized and made widely available, these tests should eliminate the need for skin-test antigen preparations, reliance on clinical diagnosis alone, and need for surgical biopsy.

If biopsy is undertaken, the Warthin-Starry silver stain can be used to visualize characteristic bacteria in affected tissues (Fig. 2). *B. henselae* can be isolated from lymph nodes in routine clinical microbiology laboratories if special efforts are made. Biopsy material should be placed on saline-soaked gauze and transported immediately to the laboratory, ground in a tissue grinder and directly plated on to fresh chocolate, CDC, anaerobic blood (sheep blood with added hemin and L-cysteine), and human blood agar. Cultures should be incubated at 35 °C in 5 per cent CO_2, with the plates kept upright for 24 h and then inverted. Plates must be observed for up to 6 weeks. Desiccation of plates has been a problem in some laboratories. This can be prevented by storing cultures in a gas-permeable, moisture-retaining envelope. Plating a relatively large inoculum may be important for isolation of *B. henselae* and will help prevent desiccation.

DNA probes are available for detection of Bartonella species in tissue samples, but are not yet sensitive enough to be useful for diagnosis of cat scratch disease.

TREATMENT

Antimicrobials have not yet been shown to be effective in the treatment of cat scratch disease. There are reports that rifampin, ciprofloxacin, trimethoprim-sulphamethoxazole, and gentamicin may benefit some patients. Antimicrobials should be considered for severe cases of cat scratch disease but for the vast majority treatment should be directed toward relief of discomfort with analgesics. Spontaneous resolution of the infected node is common, but aspiration or surgical removal may be necessary. Healing is usually rapid.

PREVENTION

Avoid cat scratches and bites. Cats implicated in transmission need not be destroyed.

Bacillary angiomatosis

INTRODUCTION

Bacillary angiomatosis was described in 1983 in an HIV-infected patient with fever and skin nodules. Since then it has been seen in many other HIV-infected patients (affecting skin and other organs) as well as in a few apparently immunocompetent individuals.

EPIDEMIOLOGY

Most cases of bacillary angiomatosis have been reported from the United States but its incidence and global distribution are unknown. Epidemiological information is based on case reports, small case series and a single case-control study. In the largest reported series of cases ($n = 48$), 42 (88 per cent) were HIV infected, 1 was HIV negative and immunodeficient, and 5 (10 per cent) were HIV negative and apparently immunocompetent.

The possible association between cats and bacillary angiomatosis was recognized soon after its description. Risk factors for bacillary angiomatosis include owning a cat and a history of a recent cat lick, scratch, or bite. In addition to animal contact (cats in four of five, and bird in one), all five cases of bacillary angiomatosis who were HIV negative and apparently immunocompetent reported being bitten by insects, including mites, chiggers, fleas, and fire ants.

AETIOLOGY

B. quintana (three patients) and *B. henselae* (one patient) have recently been isolated from cutaneous lesions of bacillary angiomatosis. The aetiological role of rochalimaea species in bacillary angiomatosis is also supported by serological and molecular probe data.

The morphological and staining characteristics, biochemical and antimicrobial sensitivity profiles, as well as phylogenetic caveats for *B. quintana* are similar to those described for *B. henselae* in cat scratch disease.

CLINICAL PRESENTATION

Bacillary angiomatosis derives its name from the vascular proliferation and presence of numerous bacillary organisms in affected tissues. It has been reported to involve numerous tissues including skin, lymph node, muscle, bone, bone marrow, brain, liver, and spleen. Bacillary angiomatosis affecting the liver (also 'bacillary peliosis hepatis') and spleen has been referred to as 'bacillary peliosis' but is more accurately termed parenchymal bacillary angiomatosis.

The most commonly recognized clinical presentation of bacillary angiomatosis is cutaneous or subcutaneous skin lesions in an HIV-infected individual, often with a low CD4 cell count. The skin lesions often mimic Kaposi's sarcoma. The presence of fever is variable and lesions may be diffuse or isolated, and slowly or rapidly progressive. Elevated liver enzymes and alkaline phosphatase are often seen in those with involvement liver or bone.

DIAGNOSIS

Biopsy and histological examination of affected tissue is needed for diagnosis of bacillary angiomatosis. It is not possible to distinguish bacillary angiomatosis clinically from Kaposi's sarcoma or other diseases that may affect the skin, spleen, liver, and other tissues, especially in HIV-infected or other immunocompromised persons. Histological criteria for the diagnosis of bacillary angiomatosis include characteristic vascular proliferation on routine haematoxylin- and -eosin staining, and of demonstration of bacillary organisms by silver staining (Warthin-Starry, Steiner, or Dieterle) or electron microscopy.

B. henselae and *B. quintana* have been isolated from cutaneous lesions of bacillary angiomatosis after cultivation of tissue homogenates with endothelial-cell monolayers, followed by plating of the supernatants on to solid agar. These organisms can also be isolated from the blood using a lysis–centrifugation method.

Preliminary data suggest that DNA probes may be useful for detection of *Bartonella* species in tissue samples. Serological assays based on measurement of antibodies to *Bartonella* species may be useful but further studies are needed.

TREATMENT

Numerous reports suggest that antimicrobials are effective against bacillary angiomatosis. Erythromycin or doxycycline appear to be the best agents. Cutaneous and subcutaneous bacillary angiomatosis should be treated for at least 4 weeks. Treatment of parenchymal bacillary angiomatosis should be continued for a minimum of 6 weeks. Resolution of lesions is often complete but recurrence is common and longer courses of therapy may be warranted.

PREVENTION

See cat scratch disease trench fever.

Trench fever

INTRODUCTION

Trench fever, also called His–Werner disease, Quintan fever, shin-bone fever, and Volhynian fever, is a febrile illness first described among British soldiers in 1915. From 1915 to 1918 it was thought to account from 40 to 60 per cent of all illnesses among soldiers. There were no deaths but morbidity was significant. By 1918 it was concluded that trench fever was an infectious disease and that the aetiological agent was transmitted by the human body louse. In 1961, *B. quintana* was isolated from the blood of a patient with trench fever and Koch's postulates for the causation of trench fever by *B. quintana* were fulfilled in 1969. Since the end of the Second World War, reports of trench fever have been rare but recent data suggest that cases may have escaped recognition; clusters of cases in homeless alcoholic men have been identified in Seattle and France.

EPIDEMIOLOGY

Endemic foci of trench fever have been identified in Poland, the former Soviet Republics, Mexico, Bolivia, North Africa, Ethiopia, and Burundi but its true incidence and geographical distribution are unknown.

B. quintana is transmitted by inoculation of contaminated louse faeces through a break in the skin from a louse bite or other injury. The incubation period is 7 to 30 days. Trench fever is not transmitted directly from person to person. The human body louse becomes infected by ingesting infected human blood.

CLINICAL PRESENTATION

High fever is the most common clinical feature of trench fever. Headache and myalgia are common prodromal symptoms. Onset of fever is acute or insidious and is often associated with headache, dizziness, and pains in the back, eyes, and legs, especially in the shins. Splenomegaly is common and a red macular rash (lesions 2–4 mm in diameter) may appear transiently. Complete recovery usually occurs within 5 to 6 weeks without antimicrobial therapy. Trench fever is not fatal but about half of the patients will have relapse of illness with fever and myalgia. Endocarditis has been described in recent reports.

DIAGNOSIS

Blood culture using blood agar plates incubated at 37 °C under 5 per cent CO_2 should yield growth of *B. quintana* within 2 weeks. Lysis–centrifugation methods for blood culture may also be useful. Serological assays may be valuable in the absence of positive cultures.

TREATMENT

Clinical response to tetracycline or chloramphenicol is prompt. It is not known whether extended therapy will prevent relapses.

PREVENTION

Control of the human body louse will prevent transmission of trench fever.

REFERENCES

Brenner, D.J. *et al.* (1991). Proposal of Afipia gen. nov. with *Afipia felis* sp. nov. (formerly the cat scratch bacillus), *Afipia clevelandis* sp. nov. (formerly the Cleveland Clinic Foundation strain), *Afipia broomeae* sp. nov., and three unnamed genospecies. *Journal of Clinical Microbiology*, **29,** 2450–60.

Brenner, D.J., O'Connor, S.P., Winkler, H.H., and Steigerwalt, A.G. (1993). Proposals to unify the genera *Bartonella* and *Rochalimaea*, with descriptions of *Bartonella quintana* comb. nov., Bartonella vinsonii comb. nov., Bartonella henselae comb. nov., and Bartonella *elizabethae* comb. nov., and to remove the family *Bartonellaceae* from the order *Rickettsiales. International Journal of Systematic Bacteriology*, **43,** 777–86.

Carithers, H.A. (1985). Cat-scratch disease: an overview based on a study of 1,200 patients. *American Journal of Diseases of Children*, **139,** 1124–33.

Debre, R., Lamy, M., Jammet, M-L., Costil, L., and Mozziconacci, P. (1950). La maladie des griffes de chat. *Bulletin et Memoires de la Societé Medicale de Hôpital Paris*, **66,** 76–9.

Dolan, M.J. *et al.* (1993). Syndrome of *Rochalimaea henselae* adenitis suggesting cat scratch disease. *Annals of Internal Medicine*, **118,** 331–6.

Jackson, L.A., Perkins, B.A., and Wenger, J.D. (1993). Cat scratch disease in the United States: an analysis of three national databases. *American Journal of Public Health*, **83,** 1707–11.

Koehler, J.A., Quinn, F.D., Berger, T.G., LeBoit, P.E., and Tappero, J.W. (1992). Isolation of rochalimaea species from cutaneous and osseous lesions of bacillary angiomatosis. *New England Journal of Medicine*, **327,** 1625–31.

Koehler, J.E., Glaser, C.A., and Tappero, J.W. (1994). *Rochalimaea henselae* infection. A new zoonosis with the domestic cat as reservoir. *Journal of the American Medical Association*, **271,** 531–5.

Leboit, P.E. *et al.* (1988). Epithelioid hemangioma-like vascular proliferation in AIDS: manifestation of cat scratch disease bacillus infection? *Lancet*, **i,** 960–3.

Margileth, A.M. (1992). Antibiotic therapy for cat-scratch disease: clinical study of therapeutic outcome in 268 patients and a review of the literature. *Pediatric Infectious Diseases Journal*, **11,** 474–8.

Regnery, R.L., Anderson, B.E., Clarridge III, J.E., Rodriquez-Barradas, M.C., Jones, D.C., and Carr, J.H. (1992). Characterization of a novel rochalimaea species, *R. henselae* sp. nov., isolated from blood of a febrile, human immunodeficiency virus-positive patient. *Journal of Clinical Microbiology*, **30,** 265–74.

Regnery, R.L., Olson, J.G., Perkins, B.A., and Bibb, W. (1992). Serologic response to 'Rochalimaea henselae' antigen in suspected cat-scratch disease. *Lancet*, **339,** 1443–5.

Relman, D. A. (1995). Has trench fever returned? *New England Journal of Medicine*, **332,** 463–4.

Relman, D.A., Loutit, J.S., Schmidt, T.M., Falkow, S., and Tompkins, L.S. (1990). The agent of bacillary angiomatosis. *New England Journal of Medicine*, **323,** 1573–80.

Schwartzman, W.A. (1992). Infections due to Rochalimaea: the expanding clinical spectrum. *Communicable Infectious Diseases*, **15,** 893–900.

Slater, L.N., Welch, D.F., Hensel, D., and Coody, D.W. (1990). A newly recognized fastidious gram-negative pathogen as a cause of fever and bacteremia. *New England Journal of Medicine*, **323,** 1587–93.

Stoler, M.H., Bonfiglio, T.A., Steigbigel, R.T., and Pereira, M. (1983). An atypical subcutaneous infection associated with acquired immune deficiency syndrome. *American Journal of Clinical Pathology*, **80,** 714–18.

Tappero, J.W. *et al.* (1993). The epidemiology of bacillary angiomatosis and bacillary peliosis. *Journal of the American Medical Association*, **269,** 770–5.

Wear, D.J., Margileth, A.M., Hadfield, T.L., Fischer, G.W., Schlagel, C.J., and King, F.M. (1983). Cat scratch disease: a bacterial infection. *Science*, **221,** 1403–5.

Zangwill, K.M. *et al.* (1993). Cat scratch disease in Connecticut: epidemiology, risk factors, and evaluation of a new diagnostic test. *New England Journal of Medicine*, **329,** 8–13.

Chlamydial infections and lymphogranuloma venereum

7.11.41 Chlamydial infections

D. TAYLOR-ROBINSON, D. C. W. MABEY, AND J. D. TREHARNE

Ancient writings identify chlamydial disease as one of the major scourges of man. Thus, trachoma is discernible as a cause of blindness in ancient Chinese and Egyptian writings. It was, however, L. Halberstaedter and S. von Prowazek who, in 1907, first described intracytoplasmic inclusions in conjunctival scrapings from trachoma patients and recognized the involvement of an infectious agent. Four years later, K. Lindner reported similar inclusions in ophthalmia of newborn infants and in urethral and cervical material from their mothers, infections that became known as 'inclusion blenorrhoea' or 'paratrachoma'. In 1930, the first isolation of a chlamydial agent (*Chlamydia psittaci*) from psittacosis was made in laboratory animals by S.P. Bedson and colleagues, that is about 27 years before T'ang and coworkers isolated in fertile hens' eggs the genomically and biologically different agent, *Chlamydia trachomatis*, from trachoma. Two years later, B.R. Jones and colleagues were successful in attempts to isolate the same agent from the genital tract and the eye in paratrachoma. The advent of the cell-culture technique about this time paved the way for the isolation of *C. trachomatis* in 1965 by this much more sensitive means. This, together with the development of ways of measuring immunological responses, made it possible to explore the nature, range, prevalence, and pathogenesis of clinical conditions associated with chlamydial infection.

In this chapter, diseases caused by the four chlamydial species outlined below are discussed. In the case of *C. psittaci*, attention is drawn more to human infection than to infection in other mammalian or avian species. In considering the various clinical conditions, diagnosis and treatment are not always discussed for each, but these aspects are brought into focus separately where features applicable to all clinical settings are outlined.

CLASSIFICATION

Chlamydial organisms, or chlamydiae, are ubiquitous pathogens infecting many species of mammals and birds. The genus Chlamydia now comprises four species: *C. trachomatis*, *C. psittaci*, *C. pneumoniae*, and the recently speciated *C. pecorum*. *C. trachomatis* is pathogenic for man and causes ocular, genital, and systemic infections that affect millions of people worldwide. Infections caused by *C. psittaci* are not confined to birds but extend to a variety of animals, resulting in major economic losses in animal husbandry. In addition, *C. psittaci* may be transmitted occasionally to man. *C. pneumoniae* also causes human disease and does not appear to have any animal reservoir; it has been associated with outbreaks of respiratory infection in North America, Europe, and Asia. The fourth chlamydial species, *C. pecorum*, appears to cause pneumonia, polyarthritis, encephalomyelitis, and diarrhoea in cattle and sheep.

GROWTH CYCLE

Chlamydiae have probably evolved from host-independent, Gram-negative ancestors that originally contained peptidoglycan in their cell wall. The chlamydial envelope is similar to that of Gram-negative bacteria, having both an inner and outer membrane; chlamydiae are best considered as bacteria that are specialized for an intracellular existence. The infectious chlamydial organism, the elementary body, is electron dense, deoxyribonucleic acid rich, and approximately 300 to 400 nm in diameter. The elementary bodies of *C. pneumoniae* often, but not always, have a wide periplasmic space and appear pear shaped. Those of the other chlamydial species have a narrow periplasmic space and are spherical. These obligate prokaryotic parasites of eukaryotic cells begin their intracellular life cycle after binding to the host cell (see below). They enter the cell by 'parasite-specified' endocytosis. Whether this mechanism is phagocytic or pinocytic is not known. Inside the host cell, fusion of the chlamydia-containing endocytic vesicle with lysosomes is inhibited by some unknown mechanism; the elementary body then begins its unique developmental cycle. It first loses its rigidity and this leads to an increase in porin activity, which facilitates the exchange of nutrients between the newly developing reticulate body and the host cell. Intense ribosomal activity occurs within the cytoplasm and after approximately 10 h the elementary bodies have differentiated into the larger (800–1000 nm), non-infectious, metabolically active, reticulate bodies. These divide by binary fission and by 20 h they begin to reorganize into a new generation of elementary bodies (Fig. 1), which reach maturation 20 to 30 h after entry into the cell: their rapid accumulation within the endocytic vacuole precedes their release into the extracellular environment between 30 and 48 h after the start of the cycle.

CELL ATTACHMENT

Specific regions of the chlamydial 40-kDa major outer-membrane protein (**MOMP**) may function as adhesins by promoting electrostatic and hydrophobic reactions with eukaryotic host cells. A more likely mechanism of binding to cells seems to involve glycosaminoglycan on the surface of chlamydiae. Chlamydial outer-membrane proteins of 18 and 30 kDa have also been shown to attach to eukaryotic cells but their true importance in this role is questionable.

SEROVARS AND PROTEIN PROFILE

All species within the genus Chlamydia contain a common, heat-stable, lipopolysaccharide antigen, which has a low molecular mass. Although it is demonstrated easily on the surface of the reticulate body, it does not appear to be immunoaccessible on the surface of the elementary body. The MOMP is the immunodominant protein of the elementary body and this contains epitopes that exhibit genus, species, and serovar

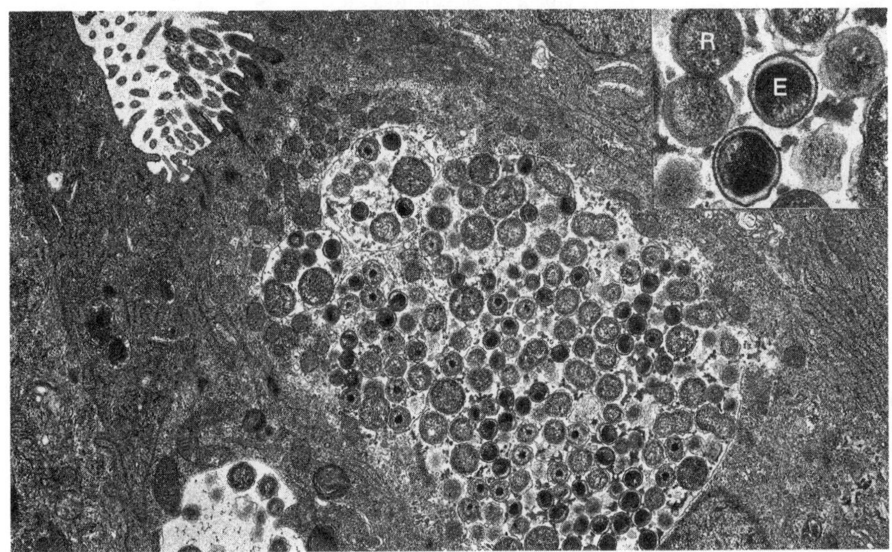

Fig. 1 Elementary bodies (E) and reticulate bodies (R) of *C. trachomatis* forming an inclusion in oviduct cell shown by transmission electron microscopy. × 000.

specificity. The epitope that exhibits serovar specificity is the basis of the microimmunofluorescence test by which the *C. trachomatis* species has been separated into 15 serovars. Those designated A, B, Ba, and C are responsible mainly for endemic trachoma of eye-to-eye transmission, while serovars D to K are responsible for chlamydial oculogenital infections. There are also three *C. trachomatis* serovars, L1, L2 and L3, that cause the genital disease, lymphogranuloma venereum. At present, there is only one serovar within the *C. pneumoniae* species, although minor geographical serovar variations have been described. The loosely defined *C. psittaci* species is likely to contain a wide variety of host-related serovars and it is possible that what is currently defined as *C. psittaci* will be redefined as more than one species. Amino acid sequences of the MOMPs of all *C. trachomatis* serovars are now known and epitope maps of different antigenic domains have been elucidated. It appears that the MOMP genes consist of five highly conserved regions punctuated by four short variable sequences. Serovar-specific epitopes have been demonstrated in variable sequence in I and II, while species-specific epitopes have been found in variable sequence IV. It is also probable that these variable sequences have some role in chlamydial pathogenesis. *C. trachomatis*, *C. psittaci*, and *C. pneumoniae* species have been compared and, although there is only 10 per cent DNA homology between each of them, MOMP gene analysis of the respective species reveals up to 65 per cent amino acid homology, indicating a probable common ancestor.

A common chlamydial 57-kDa protein has been described that has homology with the GroEL heat-shock protein of *Escherichia coli*. It is thought that the damaging sequelae of chlamydial infections, such as scarring in trachoma, tubal adhesions following pelvic inflammatory disease, and reactive arthritis consequent to urethritis, may result from the release of soluble mediators of inflammation in response to the 57-kDa protein. Apart from the 57-, 40-, 30-, and 18-kDa proteins mentioned already, others described are the 12/15-kDa cysteine-rich polypeptides, which, like MOMP, are probably required for the structural rigidity of the chlamydial outer membrane, and a 35-kDa protein synthesized during the reorganization of elementary to reticulate bodies, which may be implicated in the transformation of reticulate to elementary bodies. Other less well-defined chlamydial proteins have been observed, but any role they might have in the pathogenesis and immunobiology of chlamydial infections must await further study.

Trachoma

Trachoma is a chronic keratoconjunctivitis caused by serotypes A, B, Ba, and C of *C. trachomatis*. It is believed to affect some 500 million people, of whom 7 million are blind and 10 million have visual impairment as a consequence. After cataract, it is the most common cause of blindness worldwide.

Trachoma is now confined largely to developing countries, but this was not always the case. Moorfields Eye Hospital in London was founded in the nineteenth century specifically as a trachoma hospital, so great was the burden of the disease among the poor population there. Trachoma is a disease rather of poverty than of hot climates, and in some respects the relation between genital and ocular chlamydial infections resembles that between syphilis and non-venereal treponematoses. In poor communities where hygienic standards are low, there is direct transfer of chlamydiae from eye to eye (cf. skin to skin for non-venereal treponematoses), and trachoma is endemic. As standards of hygiene improve, this mode of transmission is no longer possible and trachoma becomes less of a problem. The oculogenital serovars (D–K) continue to be transmitted through sexual contact or from mother to infant.

CLINICAL FEATURES

The active (inflammatory) stage of the disease, a follicular conjunctivitis (Plates 1 and 2), affects chiefly the subtarsal conjunctiva, but follicles occur elsewhere on the conjunctiva and at the limbus, where on resolution they leave characteristic shallow depressions known as Herbert's pits. New vessels (pannus) may be seen at this stage of the disease in the cornea (Plate 3), usually at the superior margin, and punctate keratitis may also be a feature. Symptoms are mild or non-existent, so that the disease may not be suspected until the upper eyelid is everted. Active trachoma is seen primarily among children in endemic areas. Among older children and adults in such areas, conjunctival fibrosis often develops as the follicles resolve (Plate 4). If this scarring is severe it may distort the upper lid margin, leading to entropion (Plate 5). The lashes rub against the globe (trichiasis), causing continuous discomfort and eventually, in some cases, blindness due to corneal damage.

The World Health Organization has proposed criteria for the clinical diagnosis of active trachoma and its potentially blinding sequelae and for grading their severity as follows.

- *Trachomatous inflammation—follicular (TF)*: five or more follicles, each at least 0.5 mm in diameter, in the upper tarsal conjunctiva (Plate 1);
- *Trachomatous inflammation—intense (TI)*: pronounced inflammatory thickening of the tarsal conjunctiva that obscures more than half the normal deep tarsal blood vessels (Plate 2);
- *Trachomatous conjunctival scarring (TS)*: easily visible scarring in the tarsal conjunctiva (Plate 4);
- *Trachomatous trichiasis (TT)*: at least one eyelash rubbing on the eyeball (Plate 5)—evidence of recent removal of inturned eyelashes also graded as trichiasis;
- *Corneal opacity (CO)*: easily visible corneal opacity over the pupil, so dense that at least part of the pupil margin is blurred when viewed through the opacity.

Communities with a high prevalence of intense inflammatory disease (TI) are likely to have high rates of trachoma-related blindness in the future unless measures to intervene are introduced.

EPIDEMIOLOGY

The reservoir of infection in communities with endemic trachoma is the eye and possibly the nasopharynx of children with active disease. The higher prevalence of active disease and scarring found among women than among men in most endemic settings is probably due to the closer contact between women and children. The exact means by which *C. trachomatis* is transferred from one individual to another has not been established unequivocally, but the following routes of transmission, not mutually exclusive, have been suggested:

(1) direct spread from eye to eye, for example by children sharing a bed, or playing together;
(2) spread via fingers;
(3) indirect spread by means of fomites, for example cloths used to wipe the eyes, bed sheets, eye make-up;
(4) spread from the nasopharynx by coughing or sneezing, or from the gastrointestinal or genital tracts;
(5) transmission by eye-seeking flies.

The importance of flies in the transmission of trachoma probably varies with season and from one locality to another.

The blinding sequelae of trachoma seldom occur among those with oculogenital chlamydial infections outside trachoma endemic areas, and conjunctival scarring was found to occur less often and to be less severe among emigrants who moved to Canada from a trachoma endemic region of India than among those who remained. Severe conjunctival scarring probably occurs only among individuals repeatedly exposed to reinfection.

Clustering

Trachoma is a focal disease, the prevalence of which may vary considerably from one village community to the next. Active cases tend to cluster by household, and the increased prevalence observed among siblings of active cases implies that transmission often occurs within the family; this suggests that prolonged intimate contact is required for the transmission of chlamydiae and the subsequent development of trachoma. Seroepidemiological studies have shown that members of an infected household generally share the same serovar, lending further support to the concept of intrafamilial transmission.

Social factors

Trachoma has disappeared from large regions of the world as living conditions have improved, but remains prevalent among poor communities in developing countries. Socioenvironmental variables associated with trachoma, in addition to indicators of poverty, include distance to and type of water supply, crowding, absence of latrines, and the presence of animal excreta and flies. Behavioural factors include the amount of water used, the frequency of washing, nose-blowing and eye-wiping practices, and sharing of eye make-up. A difficulty in identifying specific risk factors for trachoma is the close relation that is frequently found between many of these variables, but the availability and use of water are important.

DIAGNOSIS

In trachoma endemic areas the diagnosis is generally made on clinical grounds, as most cases of follicular conjunctivitis are due to trachoma and laboratory facilities are usually lacking. The giant papillae of vernal conjunctivitis may be mistaken for trachomatous follicles, and pannus may also be seen in vernal conjunctivitis. A number of viral infections can cause follicular conjunctivitis, adenovirus infection being the most common. Intense cases of trachoma (TI), in which follicles may not be visible, should be distinguished from bacterial conjunctivitis. The diagnosis of trachomatous scarring is usually obvious, as few other conditions cause conjunctival scarring of the upper lid.

Laboratory diagnosis depends on the detection of *C. trachomatis*, which may be found in about 50 per cent of cases of active disease (TF or TI), but in only a minority of cases of scarring disease (TS). The diagnostic methods used are discussed later in this chapter.

TREATMENT

Inflammatory trachoma (TF and TI) responds to treatment with antimicrobial agents active against *C. trachomatis*. In the treatment of individual cases it is advisable to combine systemic therapy with topical (see Table 4), in order to eradicate nasopharyngeal carriage. Because of the rapid rate of reinfection in endemic areas, treatment of individuals is ineffective and the World Health Organization has recommended regimens for mass treatment with topical 1 per cent tetracycline ointment. This should be applied twice daily for at least 6 weeks or for five consecutive days each month for 5 months.

Trichiasis and entropion require surgical correction. Numerous lid operations have been described, but few have been evaluated prospectively. It seems that tarsal rotation may be the operation of choice; in addition to reducing discomfort and preventing visual deterioration, it leads to an improvement in visual acuity.

PREVENTION

The importance of water has been mentioned. In Mexico, children who washed their faces seven or more times per week were found to be less likely to have trachoma than those who washed less often. Although disputed by some, this finding has aroused considerable interest because it suggests that face washing could be a simple intervention that might easily be the target of health education campaigns. Preliminary results of an intervention trial in Tanzania suggest that health education, in which rural villagers are taught to wash their faces regularly, may be effective in the control of trachoma.

Genital-tract infections

Infections of the genital tract due to *C. trachomatis*, summarized in Table 1, are found worldwide and are common, occurring, at least in developed countries, much more often than gonococcal infections. In Sweden, widespread and effective diagnostic testing, coupled with aggressive contact tracing and treatment, have greatly reduced chlamydial genital infections. This has not been achieved in other developed countries, although the relentless increase in such infections may have reached a plateau in some. The economic burden on health services is enormous. In the United States, for example, it was estimated that for the period 1980 to 1985 the annual incidence of chlamydial cervicitis was about 2 million cases and that of pelvic inflammatory disease and its sequelae 300 000 cases, the former costing about 180 million dollars and the latter more than 900 million dollars.

Non-gonococcal urethritis

C. trachomatis may be detected far more frequently in the urethra of men with non-gonococcal urethritis than in those without; in other words, there is fulfilment of the first of Koch's postulates, but it is unusual to detect chlamydiae in more than 50 per cent of cases of non-gonococcal urethritis. They have also been reported in about 10 to 25 per cent of young men with asymptomatic urethral infections. If sought assiduously by the use of sensitive methods (see below), inapparent infections may be found to occur much more frequently than is generally believed. While it is likely that chlamydiae are a cause of chronic non-gonococcal urethritis, the mechanism of disease is a matter of debate (see below).

In women, there is no doubt that chlamydial urethral infection may cause urethritis but, in contrast to men, infection and inflammation are almost always asymptomatic. Thus, the dysuria and frequency of the urethral syndrome are rarely of chlamydial origin. Furthermore, chlamydiae would seem to have no part to play in chronic urological complaints in women.

Prostatitis

There is no evidence that chlamydiae cause acute symptomatic prostatitis. Claims to have recovered chlamydiae from expressed prostatic fluids of patients with chronic abacterial prostatitis or to have detected them in prostatic tissue have been criticized, because chlamydiae in the urethra have been mistakenly regarded as being in the prostate, or because the diagnosis of disease did not follow the classical Stamey approach, and some claims defied rational belief. In one study of 50 patients in which a diagnosis of chronic abacterial prostatitis was established by the Stamey procedure, abnormal areas of echogenicity were defined by transrectal prostatic ultrasonography and biopsy specimens were taken from them, the needle being introduced transperineally to avoid the urethra. Histological and immunological examination of the tissues confirmed their chronic inflammatory nature, but chlamydiae were not detected in any of them by culture and direct immunofluorescence techniques, although 2 of 18 tested proved positive by a polymerase chain-reaction assay. These largely negative observations, together with the failure to detect chlamydial antibody, support the belief that chlamydiae are not often implicated directly in the chronic phase of the disease. However, detection of chlamydiae in the chronic phase in a few patients, together with the inability to exclude an active role for them at an earlier stage, may mean that a portion, at least, of chronic disease is chlamydial in origin and is maintained possibly by immunological means. A predominance of CD8 cells in the tissues is consistent with this notion.

Epididymo-orchitis

C. trachomatis is responsible primarily for this condition in young men (35 years of age or less) in developed countries, as it has been detected

Table 1 *Assessment of the extent to which* C. trachomatis *is involved in various oculogenital and associated diseases*

Disease	Evidence that *C. trachomatis* is a cause*	Proportion of disease due to *C. trachomatis*
In men		
Acute non-gonococcal urethritis (NGU)	++++	Up to 50%
Postgonococcal urethritis	++++	Up to 50%
Persistent and recurrent NGU	+	?
Acute and chronic prostatitis	+	?
Acute epididymo-orchitis	++++	Up to 50%
Infertility	−	
In women		
Urethritis	+++	?
Bartholinitis	+	?
Vaginitis	−	
Bacterial vaginosis	−	
Cervicitis	++++	About 50%
Cervical dysplasia	+	
Endometritis	+++	?
Salpingitis	++++	40–60%
Periappendicitis	++	?
Perihepatitis	+++	?
Infertility	+++	⩾ 8% due to chlamydial salpingitis
Ectopic pregnancy	+++	?
Abortion	−	
In men or women		
Conjunctivitis	++++	?
Otitis media	++	?
Arthritis (Reiter's syndrome)	+++	About 40%
Endocarditis	++	?
Pharyngitis	−	
Proctitis	++	?
Lymphogranuloma venereum	++++	100% (by definition)
In infants		
Conjunctivitis	++++	Up to 50%
Pneumonia	++++	30%?
Chronic lung disease	++	?
Gastroenteritis	−	

* ++++, overwhelming; +++, good; ++, moderate; +, weak; −, none

in at least one-third of epididymal aspirates in studies in the United States and the United Kingdom. A strong correlation has been shown between the presence of IgM and IgG chlamydial antibodies, measured by microimmunofluorescence, and the occurrence of such chlamydia-positive disease. In developing countries, however, *Neisseria gonorrhoeae* is still a major cause of acute epididymitis, although chlamydiae are important too. In patients older than 35 years, an age boundary that is only a guideline and not strict, epididymo-orchitis tends to be caused by urinary-tract pathogens.

Convincing evidence that chlamydiae have been detected in the testes or that a previous chlamydial urethral infection or asymptomatic chlamydial infection causes male infertility has not been forthcoming.

Cervicitis

Chlamydiae do not have any discernible role in causing bartholinitis, bacterial vaginosis, or vaginitis. They have been found occasionally in the vagina after hysterectomy, but probably as 'contaminants', the cervix being the primary target for chlamydial infection. *C. trachomatis* is well known to cause mucopurulent/follicular cervicitis (Plate 6 (a, b)), although infection may often be asymptomatic. Postmenopausal chlamydial cervicitis has been purported to occur, but women less than 25 years of age, unmarried, using oral contraceptives, and who have signs of cervicitis are the most likely to have a chlamydial infection.

Chlamydiae have been found more frequently in women with cervical intraepithelial neoplasia than in those without, but it is likely that the association is related to their sexual behaviour and does not reflect any causal link.

Pelvic inflammatory disease

On clinical grounds, it is impossible to distinguish chlamydial from gonococcal pelvic inflammatory disease in an individual case, although break-through vaginal bleeding, current use of an oral contraceptive, and an elevated erythrocyte sedimentation rate have been related more often to chlamydial than gonococcal disease. Canalicular spread of chlamydiae to the upper genital tract leads to endometritis, which is often plasma-cell associated and sometimes intensely lymphoid. Further spread causes salpingitis (Plate 7), perihepatitis (the Curtis Fitz-Hugh syndrome) (Plate 8) sometimes confused with acute cholecystitis in young women, in addition to periappendicitis and other abdominal complaints. The fundamental reason for dissemination of the organisms from the source of infection may be impossible to identify, but surgical trauma, for example termination of pregnancy, or insertion or removal of an intrauterine contraceptive device, are obvious predisposing factors.

Chlamydial infection is the major cause of salpingitis in developed countries. Sometimes the diagnosis is missed and infertility is the first indication of tubal disease. Infertility may be the outcome in about 10 per cent of cases of chlamydial pelvic inflammatory disease. Other consequences are ectopic pregnancy, which also may arise as a result of a subclinical chlamydial tubal infection, and chronic pelvic pain. What factors determine precisely the development of such sequelae in chlamydial pelvic inflammatory disease are unclear, although there is evidence that the number and severity of the infections influence subsequent fertility rates. Infertility could be due to endometritis or blocked or damaged tubes resulting from cellular infiltrates, or perhaps abnormalities of ovum transportation.

Other diseases associated with *C. trachomatis*

The diseases mentioned below are mainly caused by or associated with *C. trachomatis*, but as they do not involve the genital tract directly there is a possibility that other chlamydial species might be involved.

Adult paratrachoma (inclusion conjunctivitis)

Adult chlamydial ophthalmia is distinguished from trachoma because it is caused by serovars D to K of *C. trachomatis* and commonly results from the accidental transfer of infected genital discharge to the eye rather than by eye-to-eye transmission. It is seen in patients who often have a concomitant genital chlamydial infection. Chlamydiae can be detected in conjunctival specimens and in this respect the condition is different from the 'reactive' conjunctivitis seen in Reiter's syndrome (see below), where isolation from the conjunctivae is extremely unusual. Adult chlamydial ophthalmia usually presents as a unilateral follicular conjunctivitis of acute or subacute onset, the incubation period ranging from 2 to 21 days. The features are swollen lids, mucopurulent discharge, papillary hyperplasia due to congestion and neovascularization and, after a week or more, follicular hypertrophy. Punctate keratitis may develop 2 to 3 weeks after the onset of conjunctivitis. Pannus formation, similar to that in trachoma, may be seen, but iritis is rare. Although the disease is generally regarded as benign and self-limiting, it is in the untreated cases that pannus and scarring are apt to occur, but impairment of vision is rare. Treatment, mentioned elsewhere, should be systemic rather than topical, and patients and their sexual contacts should be investigated for the existence of genital chlamydial infections and managed accordingly.

Otitis media

Apart from being associated with inflamed eardrums in infants who have conjunctivitis and/or pneumonia (see below), *C. trachomatis* has been isolated from or detected in aural discharges from adolescent or adult patients with chlamydial ophthalmia. About one-third have otitis media, complaining of blocked ears and hearing loss. To what extent otitis media *per se* might be due to *C. trachomatis*, or perhaps more appropriately to *C. pneumoniae*, is unknown.

Arthritis

Arthritis occurring together with or soon after non-gonococcal urethritis has been termed sexually acquired reactive arthritis (**SARA**); in about one-third of cases, conjunctivitis and other features characteristic of Reiter's syndrome are seen. The notion that at least one-third of cases of SARA or Reiter's syndrome are initiated by chlamydial infection was based originally on serological evidence. Finding *C. trachomatis* elementary bodies by direct immunofluorescence, chlamydial DNA by a polymerase chain reaction, together with chlamydial antigen by an immunoperoxidase technique and chlamydial particles by electron microscopy in the joints of such patients leaves no doubt as to the validity of this concept. *C. trachomatis* elementary bodies have also been found in the joints of women with 'seronegative' arthritis. The failure to detect viable chlamydiae in the joints of patients with SARA may be due to their rapid disappearance, the pathogenesis having an immunological basis. If this is the case, it is not encouraging for an antibiotic therapeutic approach. Despite this, there are suggestions that early tetracycline therapy is worth trying.

It is feasible that *C. pneumoniae*, even more than *C. psittaci*, could have a role in the pathogenesis of arthritis. In particular, the occurrence of *C. pneumoniae* as a respiratory pathogen in children raises the possibility of its contribution to the initiation and/or perpetuation of chronic juvenile arthritis, a notion worthy of exploration.

Immunocompromised states

C. trachomatis has been isolated from the lower respiratory tract of a few immunocompromised adults with pneumonia, some after renal transplantation, but its role in pathogenesis is uncertain because other agents were recovered from some. *C. pneumoniae* would seem to be a more likely candidate for respiratory involvement. In contrast, large studies have shown that *C. trachomatis* is not an important respiratory-tract pathogen in patients with AIDS and the same probably applies to *C. pneumoniae*. Genital chlamydial disease does not seem to be more widely prevalent, or severe in such immunodeficient individuals. Finally, there is no evidence that hypogammaglobulinaemic patients are especially prone to infection with any of the chlamydial species.

Lymphogranuloma venereum *(see Chapter 7.11.42)*

Neonatal infections

Chlamydial infection of infants delivered by caesarean section and/or signs of chlamydial infection at the time of birth indicate that intrauterine infection can occur, but the major risk of infection to the infant is from passing through an infected cervix. Whether or not chlamydial conjunctivitis and pneumonia of the newborn constitute a problem depends on the prevalence of maternal cervical infection, which varies widely.

Neonatal conjunctivitis

Various observations have led to the conclusion that between one-fifth and one-half of infants exposed to *C. trachomatis* infecting the cervix at the time of birth develop conjunctivitis. The disease usually occurs 1 to 3 weeks after birth and is characterized by a mucopurulent discharge (Plate 9) and occasionally by pseudomembrane formation. Although it may be quite severe, corneal ulceration and follicle formation are rare and the disease is usually self-limiting, resolution occurring without visual impairment. If complications do arise, however, they tend to be in infants that have not been treated.

Neonatal respiratory-tract infection

The realization that *C. trachomatis* could cause neonatal pneumonia lagged behind its recognition as a cause of conjunctivitis. The association with pneumonia was first suggested by the development of the disease in an infant that had been treated successfully for conjunctivitis and from whom *C. trachomatis* was recovered from the respiratory tract. Overall, about 10 to 20 per cent of exposed infants develop pneumonia, that is about half of those who develop conjunctivitis, but pneumonia is not always preceded by conjunctivitis. A history of recent conjunctivitis and bulging eardrums is found in only about half of the cases. Chlamydial pneumonia occurs usually between the fourth and eleventh week of life, preceded by upper respiratory symptoms. The disease is characterized by an afebrile, protracted course in which there is tachypnoea and a prominent, stacatto cough. Generalized hyperinflation of the lungs with bilateral, diffuse, and symmetrical interstitial infiltration and scattered areas of atelectasis are the radiographic findings.

Evidence that *C. trachomatis* is a cause of pneumonia in the newborn includes recovery of the micro-organism from neonatal lung specimens; its association with the well-defined clinical features; the occurrence of IgM antibody to *C. trachomatis* in the serum of infants with pneumonia; and the production of lesions similar histologically to those seen in human infants in the lungs of infant baboons after experimental infection with *C. trachomatis*. A relative eosinophilia in some cases suggests hypersensitivity but, whatever the mechanism, permanent lung damage may ensue. Thus, children who have experienced a chlamydial infection during infancy are more likely to develop obstructive lung disease and asthma than are those who have had pneumonia due to other causes.

Infection at other sites in the newborn

Apart from the eyes and respiratory tract, the vagina and rectum may be colonized by *C. trachomatis* at birth. Vaginal colonization has not been associated with clinical disease, nor has there been evidence for chlamydial gastroenteritis in infants, although the possibility has been considered.

Chlamydia pneumoniae infections

In 1989, *C. pneumoniae* was defined as the third species of the genus Chlamydia, although prototype strains of this novel species were isolated from conjunctival material collected in the mid-1960s from patients in trachoma endemic areas. The two original isolates (TW-183 and IOL-207) were found to be identical serologically and distinctly different from isolates of *C. trachomatis* and *C. psittaci*. Extensive serological surveys established that *C. pneumoniae* infections have a worldwide prevalence and that specific antibody may be detected in a wide variety of population groups. The difficulty of isolation is suggested by the fact that it was not until 1983 that a third *C. pneumoniae* strain was isolated, this time from the throat of a patient with acute pharyngitis. Since then, most isolations of the organism have been made from patients with respiratory infections.

CLINICAL FEATURES

Although the broad spectrum of clinical disease associated with cultural and/or serological evidence of infection with *C. pneumoniae* differs with age, the observations reported in several studies in both North America and Scandinavia provide an eclectic clinical picture. At the outset of acute disease, pharyngitis is often present, although a cough may take some time to develop; fever is uncommon. In mild cases, chest radiographs usually reveal a unilateral pneumonia, whereas in patients needing hospital care bilateral pneumonia is quite common. Bronchitis is associated with some infections and more than 80 per cent of patients with lower respiratory-tract disease develop a sore throat. In young adults, approximately 5 per cent of primary sinusitis is associated with *C. pneumoniae*. Overall, pneumonia has been the most common feature of *C. pneumoniae* infection, although it is often difficult to distinguish clinically from pneumonia caused by other micro-organisms, for example *Mycoplasma pneumoniae*.

A serological association of chronic *C. pneumoniae* infection with chronic coronary heart disease and acute myocardial infarction, noted by Finnish investigators, has provided a possible further and more contentious role for *C. pneumoniae* in human disease. While patients in both these groups have been found to have antibody to *C. pneumoniae* significantly more often than age-matched controls, it has been suggested that smoking status was not sufficiently taken into account and that this may confound the association between *C. pneumoniae* and coronary heart disease. The possibility that *C. pneumoniae* infection is a significant risk factor for the development of such disease is supported by detection of the organisms in atheromatous plaques of coronary arteries.

EPIDEMIOLOGY

C. pneumoniae organisms appear to be transmitted from person-to-person without any intermediate host. In a study of community-acquired pneumonia in Halifax, Nova Scotia between 1981 and 1984, current infection with *C. pneumoniae* was detected in 6 per cent of 301 consecutive patients, a proportion similar to that attributed to infection with *Haemophilus influenzae*, and more than that caused by influenza A virus, *Legionella* spp. and *M. pneumoniae*. The chlamydial aetiology of these infections could not have been deduced from the clinical findings alone. *C. pneumoniae* appears also to be a significant cause of nosocomial pneumonia in patients in hospital with underlying, pre-existing chronic disease and possibly may play a part in chronic obstructive pulmonary disease. Serological evidence would seem to indicate that *C. pneumoniae* is endemic in many areas and many populations, although localized epidemics of infection have been recorded in both military and civilian groups in Scandinavia, the United States, and the United Kingdom. Further epidemiological data suggest that transmission in families, schools, and other institutions is not uncommon.

Whatever the role that *C. pneumoniae* plays in disease, infection appears to be far more widespread than is indicated by the number of patients presenting with overt respiratory signs and symptoms. It probably causes many mild respiratory infections that were previously thought to be viral in origin. It is also likely that a large proportion of infections previously labelled 'human psittacosis/ornithosis' were mistakenly regarded as such, in reality being due to *C. pneumoniae*. The full extent and spectrum of disease caused by, or associated with, this ubiquitous chlamydial species is only just beginning to be unravelled.

Chlamydia psittaci infections

The *C. psittaci* species comprises a widely diverse group of organisms that cause disease in a variety of animals and birds and occasionally may be transmitted to man. The spectrum of disease in animals includes overt clinical conditions such as enteritis, placental and fetal infections, abortion, sterility, pneumonia, and encephalitis, all of which cause significant economic losses in the animal husbandry industry. These chlamydial infections may cause human disease through transmission of the organisms either as a result of contact with infected animals or birds or from contact with faecal materials from an infected source. Psittacosis may be a hazard to those who keep pet birds or who work in poultry processing plants, or in animal husbandry. There are many species of birds known to harbour the organisms, but psittacine bird species, poultry, and pigeons are probably the major sources of human infection.

CLINICAL FEATURES

Human respiratory infection with *C. psittaci* (psittacosis) is equally common in either sex. It is uncommon and mild in childhood and usually affects adults, particularly those in the 30- to 60-year age group. After an incubation period of 1 to 2 weeks, the clinical presentation can vary quite widely from a mild influenza-like illness to a fulminating toxic

Table 2 *Advantages and disadvantages of chlamydial detection procedures*

Factor considered	Culture	Direct fluorescent antibody	Enzyme immunoassay	Polymerase chain reaction
Condition of specimen transport	Rapid or at low temperature	Unimportant if fixed	Unimportant if in buffer	Speed not crucial if at low temperature; may use fixed specimens
Storage requirements	4 °C if overnight; liquid nitrogen if long term	4 °C if short term; −20 °C and fixed if long term	4 °C if 3–5 days; freezing if longer	4 °C if short term; −70 °C if long term
Evaluation of adequacy of specimen	Not practical	Evaluate during test	Not practical	Determine whether DNA present
Special equipment or procedure	Centrifuge	Fluorescence microscope	ELISA reader	Thermocycling machine and electrophoresis equipment
Processing of specimen	Tedious	Simple	Relatively simple	Lengthy and requires precautions against DNA contamination
Reading of test	Subjective and moderately tedious	Subjective and tedious	Objective and simple	Objective and simple
Duration of test	48–72 h	30 min	3 h	12–24 h
Sensitivity of test	70–80%	Up to 100%	Usually 60–70%	Up to 100%

state with multiple organ involvement. The disease may be insidious in onset over a few days or start abruptly with high fever, rigors, and anorexia. Headache occurs in most, a cough, often dry, in over two-thirds, and arthralgia and myalgia in over one-third. Inspiratory crepitations are more common than classical signs of consolidation. Chest radiographs usually show patchy shadowing, most often in the lower lobes. Homogeneous lobar shadowing is less common, and miliary and nodular patterns even less so. Hilar lymphadenopathy has been reported in up to two-thirds of patients and a pleural reaction in more than half, but significant pleural effusions are infrequent. Extrapulmonary complications, mostly rare, ascribed to *C. psittaci* include endocarditis, myocarditis, pericarditis, a toxic confusional state, encephalitis, meningitis, tender hepatomegaly, splenomegaly, pancreatitis, haemolysis, and disseminated intravascular coagulation. It is likely that some mild respiratory disease has been mistaken in the past for that caused by *C. pneumoniae*, particularly if the diagnosis was based entirely on the complement fixation test. Perhaps only now, with the advent of superior laboratory tests, will the true pattern of respiratory disease due to *C. psittaci*, and of the extrapulmonary complications, unfold.

In addition to respiratory disease, ovine *C. psittaci* strains have been shown to cause abortion, albeit rarely, in pregnant women after exposure to sheep suffering from enzootic abortion during the lambing season. The strains isolated from the human fetuses and placentae were definitely of ovine origin and usually were from sheep farmers' wives who had been in contact with aborting ewes. Ocular disease in man has been reported following contact with cats infected with the feline keratoconjunctivitis (**FKC**) agent. This organism may cause a follicular conjunctivitis similar to that caused by *C. trachomatis* serovars D to K. The FKC agent has been isolated from the genital tract of female cats, suggesting a parallel with human *C. trachomatis* infection.

The diverse *C. psittaci* species comprises chlamydial strains that have been isolated from animal species such as cattle, sheep, goats, swine, horses, rabbits, guinea-pigs, cats, dogs, opossums, koala bears, and frogs, as well as many avian species. There are no doubt significant biological and pathogenic differences between all these strains and the microimmunofluorescence serotyping test has provided a useful tool for their immunological differentiation. In addition, genetic analysis using DNA hybridization techniques, restriction endonuclease analysis of chlamydial genomic DNA, and MOMP gene sequence analysis have usually confirmed the groupings defined by the microimmunofluorescence test. To date, the following groupings of *C. psittaci* strains have been proposed: nine serovars from mammalian species, seven serovars from avian species, and two biovars from koala bears. In general, these serovar groupings tend to reflect the host species from which the *C. psittaci* strain originated. The *C. psittaci* species is undoubtedly a diverse group of organisms in which the relatively low degree of homology between serovars exhibited in DNA–DNA hybridization analyses signals the possibility of further speciation among organisms currently assigned to the species. This is exemplified by the recent proposal of a fourth chlamydial species, *C. pecorum* sp. nov., causing pneumonia, polyarthritis, encephalomyelitis, and diarrhoea in cattle and sheep.

Diagnosis of chlamydial infections

The laboratory diagnosis of chlamydial infection depends on detection of the organisms or their antigens and to a much lesser extent on serology. The procedures mentioned, with some of their advantages and disadvantages, are summarized in Table 2. Several aspects of specimen collection are worth emphasizing. Certain swabs, for example those that are cotton tipped, are superior to others, and swabs provided in commercial enzyme immunoassay kits may be toxic if used for collecting specimens for culture. Examination of two or more consecutive swabs from patients rather than one improves the chlamydial detection rate. This may be achieved when examining the genital tract in women by pooling cervical and urethral specimens or taking three cervical specimens and culturing them individually. The advantage of a marginally superior detection rate has to be weighed against the burden imposed on the patient, clinician, and laboratory staff. Thus, another approach to increasing sensitivity, apart from using multiple specimens, is to use an instrument that increases the number of chlamydia-infected cells collected. A 'cytobrush' has been used for this purpose but is likely to be successful only if used without causing bleeding and if cells do not remain trapped within it, limitations that may reduce its value in routine practice. 'First-catch' urine specimens, ignored for years because they were found not to be suitable for chlamydial culture, are unquestionably valuable samples in men and to a lesser extent in women, provided that the centrifuged deposits are tested by sensitive, non-cultural methods.

CULTURE OF CHLAMYDIAE

The growth of chlamydiae more than 25 years ago in cultured cells, rather than in embryonated eggs, revolutionized both their detection and chlamydial research. Many cell lines, such as McCoy and Buffalo green monkey kidney, are suitable for the growth of *C. trachomatis*; *C. pneumoniae* is particularly difficult to isolate and this may be facilitated by using a line of human lung cells. The method of detection used widely for *C. trachomatis* involves the centrifugation of specimens (not required for *C. psittaci*) on to McCoy cell monolayers that are treated with cycloheximide, and less often on to HeLa 229 cells treated with diethylaminoethyl (**DEAE**)–dextran. Lymphogranuloma venereum strains are more likely to grow in cells that have not been treated with DEAE–dextran than are other *C. trachomatis* serovars, a property that has been exploited to identify such strains. Inoculation of the cell cultures is followed by incubation and immunofluorescence staining with a monoclonal antibody or with a vital dye, usually Giemsa, to detect inclusions; one blind passage may increase sensitivity. In competent hands, detection of inclusions in cell cultures, especially by immunofluorescence, provides the specificity that imbues this technique with high legal standing and the rationale for regarding it as the 'gold standard' against which non-cultural methods should be compared. In practice, the cell-culture technique is no more than 70 to 80 per cent sensitive and is slow and labour intensive, drawbacks that have hastened the development of non-cultural methods.

STAINING OF CHLAMYDIAE

Staining of cells in ocular and genital specimens with vital dyes was used first to detect chlamydial inclusions, but the method is insensitive and often non-specific. Papanicolaou-stained cervical smears provide an excellent example of these drawbacks. In contrast, tests in which elementary bodies are detected directly by using species-specific fluorescent monoclonal antibodies are rapid, and for *C. trachomatis* oculogenital infections have sensitivities ranging from 70 to 100 per cent and specificities from 80 to 100 per cent; the tests require skilled microscopy but if read by competent observers who are capable of detecting a few elementary bodies, the values are at the top of these ranges.

ENZYME IMMUNOASSAYS

Skilled microscopy with its associated fatigue, and the labour involved in culture, are not required for enzyme immunoassays that detect chlamydial antigens and this accounts for their popularity. The recorded sensitivities of various enzyme immunoassays range from 60 to 100 per cent and the specificities from 90 to 100 per cent. However, comparisons against poor reference tests account for most of the higher values and the clinician should not be beguiled by false claims; the lower values in the ranges are closer to reality, and it is not possible to detect small numbers of chlamydial organisms of whatever species by means of the enzyme immunoassays.

DNA PROBES AND THE POLYMERASE CHAIN REACTION (PCR)

DNA probes are about as sensitive as the most sensitive enzyme immunoassays and some probes are available commercially, but they have been superseded by the PCR. By enabling enormous amplification of a DNA sequence specific to the chlamydial species, PCR has overcome the problem of poor sensitivity. It is only a little more sensitive than the most sensitive cell culture and no more so than direct immunofluorescence, although it may provide evidence for the existence of chlamydiae in chronic or treated disease when viable or intact organisms no longer exist. Unquestionably, PCRs have a place in research, but the ease of DNA contamination has so far prevented their wide application for routine diagnosis, although this is likely to change with commercial interest and input.

SEROLOGICAL TESTS

Complement fixation tests and enzyme immunoassays, among others, have been used to measure chlamydial antibodies, but most of the pertinent information has come through the use of the microimmunofluorescence test by which class-specific antibodies (IgM, IgG, IgA or secretory) may be measured. A fourfold or greater increase in the titre of antibody (IgM and/or IgG) detected by this more specific test, accompanied by suggestive clinical findings, may be regarded as diagnostic. Nevertheless, appropriately spaced sera are often not available and the value of serology in the diagnosis of chlamydial infections in individual patients is limited. A good correlation has been found between the presence of IgG and/or IgA antibody in tear fluids and the isolation of *C. trachomatis* from the conjunctiva in endemic trachoma and adult ocular paratrachoma. In genital infections, serum antibodies in women occur frequently in the absence of a current chlamydial infection of the cervix. When cervical chlamydial infections occur, although the antibody titres are greater than those in men with non-gonococcal urethritis, a rising titre is seen rarely and even the presence of antibody in local secretions is unreliable for diagnosis. In pelvic inflammatory disease, pre-existing antibody or delay in clinical diagnosis usually prevent diagnosis by a rising antibody titre, but the titres tend to be higher, especially in the Curtis Fitz-Hugh syndrome, than in uncomplicated cervical infections. A very high IgG antibody titre, for example in excess of 512, is suggestive of an aetiological association in pelvic disease, but caution should be exercised because high titres do not always correlate with detection of chlamydiae and are associated more with chronic or recurrent disease. It has been alleged that a distinction can be made between current and past genital chlamydial infections by measuring specific IgA antibody in a single serum sample, but it would be unwise to place any diagnostic reliance on this, since chlamydial IgA antibody has been noted to persist for several years in some patients who have had pelvic inflammatory disease. In distinct contrast, the detection of specific *C. trachomatis* IgM antibody in babies with pneumonia is pathognomonic of chlamydia-induced disease.

In primary infections with *C. pneumoniae*, IgM antibody is considered to develop within a few weeks and IgG antibody by 2 months. In repeat infections, IgM antibody does not develop but the development of IgG is more rapid and to a greater titre than in a primary infection. If only single and not paired sera are available, it may be difficult to interpret information in which there may be cross-reacting antibodies to the other species. Only in children is the finding of *C. pneumoniae* antibody in a single serum sample an assurance of infection with this species. It is no longer sensible to base the diagnosis of psittacosis solely on the complement fixation test as this will not distinguish between *C. psittaci* and *C. pneumoniae* infections.

Overall conclusions

Culture techniques are not used in most laboratories, but they still have the greatest force in cases of litigation. The enzyme immunoassays vary widely in sensitivity and clinicians should put pressure on laboratory staff to use the most sensitive, knowing that even these will fail to detect infection in some patients. Laboratory staff who receive few samples and are thus able to use direct immunofluorescence tests, should be known to be skilled in reading them, otherwise both sensitivity and specificity will suffer. The PCR has the potential for overcoming both these problems and is the test of the future. Great care should be taken not to misinterpret serological results, which, with a few exceptions, have limited value.

Treatment of chlamydial infections

Chlamydiae are particularly sensitive to drugs that interfere with protein synthesis, for example tetracyclines and macrolides, but are sensitive also to a variety of other drugs, some of which have been tested both *in vitro* and *in vivo* in the last few years. The minimum inhibitory concentrations of a wide range of antibiotics are presented in Table 3; the antibiotics are listed in order of diminishing *in vitro* activity. The range of concentrations reflects observations made by different investigators

Table 3 *Susceptibility of* Chlamydia trachomatis *to various antibiotics**

Antibiotic	Minimum inhibitory concentration (μg/ml)	Minimum bactericidal concentration (μg/ml)
Rifampicin	0.005–0.25	0.015–0.25
Rosaramicin	0.015–0.25	0.05–0.25
Minocycline	0.015–0.5	
Tetracycline	0.02–0.5	0.02–2.0
Doxycycline	0.025–0.5	
Oxytetracycline	0.03–0.25	0.5
Erythromycin	0.03–0.5	0.1–4.0
Josamycin	0.03	
Roxithromycin	0.03	0.06
Miocamycin	0.06–0.125	
Chlortetracycline	0.125–2.5	0.125–2.5
Azithromycin	0.125	
Clindamycin	0.25–2.0	
Spiramycin	0.5	
Ofloxacin	0.5–1.0	0.5–1.0
Ciprofloxacin	1.0–2.0	1.0–2.0
Benzylpenicillin	0.25–50.0	1.0–> 100.0
Ampicillin	0.25–50.0	> 100.0
Sulphamethoxazole	0.5–50.0	
Chloramphenicol	1.0–10.0	> 8.0–10.0
Augmentin	2.0	
Lomefloxacin	2.0–4.0	
Amoxycillin	2.0–> 4.0	
Rosoxacin	4.0–8.0	4.0–8.0
Sulphisoxazole	2.0–200.0	2.0–500.0

* In addition, the following antibiotics with minimum inhibitory concentrations (MIC) in excess of 8 μg/ml have been tested and are shown more or less in order of increasing MIC: amifloxacin, enoxacin, pefloxacin, trospectomycin, sulphamethiazole, cloxacillin, norfloxacin, cephaloridine, trimethoprim, spectinomycin, flumequine, novobiocin, nalidixic acid, kanamycin, lincomycin, colistin, gentamicin, vancomycin, metronidazole, streptomycin.

more than differences between chlamydial strains, particularly as testing procedures are not standardized. The exact order in which the antibiotics are placed is arguable, but the overall pattern is likely to be correct. Antibiotics with a minimum inhibitory concentration of 2.0 or more μg/ml are of no therapeutic value and will not be considered further. At the top of the list, the rifampicins are probably more active than the tetracyclines *in vitro* but are usually reserved for mycobacterial infections. If considered in cases of chronic disease, it should be remembered that there is evidence for the emergence of chlamydial resistance to rifampicin, a drawback that is negligible with rifabutin.

Tetracyclines remain the drugs given most widely for chlamydial infections. Although tetracycline resistance has been reported, resistant strains do not seem to have accounted for the occasional anecdotal reports of failure to respond to tetracyclines or of recovery of chlamydiae following such therapy. Vigilance should still be kept for tetracycline-resistant strains that could jeopardize clinical practice, particularly as the move away from non-cultural procedures has made their detection less easy. Of the macrolides, erythromycin is the one most often used as an alternative to tetracyclines and is the drug of choice for the treatment of chlamydial infections in infants, young children, and in pregnant and lactating women. Azithromycin in a single dose remains expensive but is gaining favour because it is effective and enhances compliance. Other alternatives, such as some of the quinolones, particularly ofloxacin, are effective but have not found regular use.

More detailed recommendations for dose and duration of antibiotic treatment are presented in Table 4, and several aspects are worth emphasizing further. The principle of giving systemic treatment as well as topical to eradicate nasopharyngeal carriage in trachoma applies also in neonatal chlamydial conjunctivitis, where topical treatment provides no additional benefit. Oral erythromycin should be given to treat the conjunctivitis and to prevent the development of pneumonia. Recently, azithromycin in a single oral dose (20 mg/kg) was shown to be as effective as 6 weeks of topical tetracycline in treating active trachoma and may well become the drug of choice. Azithromycin has also been shown to be effective, as a single 1-g oral dose, in the treatment of non-gonococcal urethritis although expense has so far excluded its routine use. In complicated genital-tract infections such as epididymo-orchitis and pelvic inflammatory disease, treatment may need to be given before a microbiological diagnosis can be established, and additional broad-spectrum antibiotic cover is required. Treatment for complicated, deep-seated disease of the genital tract is usually extended. In the case of *C. pneumoniae* and *C. psittaci* infections, treatment follows the same principles as for *C. trachomatis* infections, as they are susceptible to the same types of antibiotic. Finally, whatever the virtue of a particular drug, treatment is likely to be most effective when the duration of administration is long rather than short, suboptimal doses are avoided, compliance is strict, and when, in the case of genital infections, patients and partners are found and treated by active contact tracing.

Pathogenesis and immune response

The immune response to chlamydial infections may be protective or damaging, and contribute to the pathogenesis of disease.

HISTOPATHOLOGY

The clinical and pathological hallmark of chlamydial infection, whatever the anatomical site, is the lymphoid follicle. Follicles contain typical germinal centres (Plate 10), consisting predominantly of B lymphocytes, with T cells in the parafollicular region, which has been shown in a non-human primate model of trachoma to contain a majority of CD8 cells. Between follicles the inflammatory infiltrate contains plasma cells, dendritic cells, macrophages, and polymorphonuclear leucocytes in addition to T and B lymphocytes.

Late stages of chlamydial infection are characterized by fibrosis, seen typically in trachoma and pelvic inflammatory disease. T lymphocytes are also present and outnumber B cells and macrophages. Biopsies taken from patients with cicatricial trachoma and persisting inflammatory changes show a predominance of CD4 cells, but those from patients in whom inflammation has subsided contain mainly CD8 cells.

IMMUNOPATHOLOGY

In cell cultures, *C. trachomatis* causes lysis of infected cells about 48 h after infection, but *in vivo* it is unusual to find more than a small proportion of cells containing chlamydial inclusions; and 50 per cent or more of cases of active trachoma may be chlamydia-isolation negative. Chlamydiae have little effect on the ciliated epithelium of oviducts in organ culture, and so it seems unlikely that cell damage caused directly by *C. trachomatis* is responsible for the pathology of chlamydial infection. In view of the histopathological features that have been mentioned, the fact that chlamydiae cause immense damage to oviducts in the intact host and that vaccination has sometimes caused more damage than protection, it is reasonable to suppose that much of the pathology might be immunologically mediated.

Repeated ocular infection by chlamydiae induces progressively worse disease with a diminished ability to isolate the organisms, features noted both naturally and experimentally. There is also experimental evidence that such events occur in the genital tract. For example, primary inoculation of the oviducts of pig-tailed macaques with *C. trachomatis* pro-

Table 4 *Recommended treatment schedules for chlamydial infections and associated diseases*

Disease/infection	Antibiotic	Dose schedule[a]	Duration (days)
Trachoma	Topical tetracycline	1% ointment twice daily for 5 days each month	6 months
	together with		
	Tetracycline HCl	500 mg 4 times daily	21
	or		
	Doxycycline	100 mg twice daily	21
	or		
	Erythromycin sortearate	500 mg 4 times daily	21
	or		
	Azithromycin alone	20 mg/kg	Single dose
Adult inclusion conjunctivitis	Antibiotics and regimens as for trachoma but without topical treatment		14
Non-gonococcal urethritis (NGU)	Antibiotics and regimens as for oral treatment of trachoma[b]		7
Epididymo-orchitis	Ampicillin	3.5 g	
	Then antibiotics as for NGU		10
Cervicitis/urethritis	Antibiotics and regimens as for NGU		7
Pelvic inflammatory disease			
For ambulatory patient:	Ampicillin	3.5 g	
	Then doxycycline	100 mg twice daily	10
For hospitalized patient:	(a) Doxycycline	100 mg twice daily (i.v.)	⩾4
	Then doxycycline	100 mg twice daily	10[b]
	or		
	(b) Clindamycin	600 mg 4 times daily (i.v.)	⩾4
	and gentamicin	2 mg/kg (i.v.)	⩾4
	and then	1.5 mg/kg 3 times daily	
	Clindamycin	450 mg 4 times daily	10[c]
Lymphogranuloma venereum	Antibiotics and regimens as for trachoma but usually without topical eye treatment		⩾14
	or		
	Trimethoprim-sulphamethoxazole[d]	80 mg twice daily	⩾14
Neonatal infections	Erythromycin syrup	50 mg/kg daily in 4 divided doses	14
C. pneumoniae infections	Antibiotics and regimens as for NGU except doxycycline twice daily		7–21[e]
C. psittaci infections	Antibiotics and regimes as for NGU except doxycycline twice daily		⩾14

[a]All antibiotics orally unless otherwise indicated.

[b]For NGU, azithromycin given in a single 1g dose.

[c]Total duration of therapy 14 days.

[d]Less successful but does not mask concomitant syphilis.

[e]Relapse more often with short course.

duced a self-limiting salpingitis with minimal residual damage, whereas repeated tubal inoculation caused hydrosalpinx formation with adnexal adhesions. The exaggerated response of inflammatory trachoma was also induced by the ocular instillation of a Triton X-100 extract of surface antigens of the guinea-pig inclusion conjunctivitis agent in previously infected, but not naive, guinea-pigs. The time-course and histopathology of the response showed it to be due to delayed hypersensitivity. In the cynomolgus monkey model, a similar phenomenon was effected by a genus-specific protein of 57 kDa that has sequence homology with the GroEL heat-shock protein of *E. coli*. While there seems no doubt about the importance of this antigen, the exact role that it may have in chronic non-gonococcal urethritis and pelvic inflammatory disease is unknown. Longitudinal studies of trachoma have shown that certain individuals appear predisposed to persistent severe inflammatory disease, perhaps reflecting genetically determined differences in the immune response to sensitizing chlamydial antigens.

PATHOGENESIS OF SCARRING

Fibrosis or scarring is a late sequel of chlamydial infection. Long-term follow-up of trachoma in Tunisia showed that children with severe papillary hypertrophy were more likely to develop scarring in later life, and the formation of adhesions is a complication of chlamydial pelvic inflammatory disease. The pathogenesis is, however, unclear. Epidemiological and experimental studies of trachoma show that fibrosis occurs only after repeated reinfection, but it appears to progress in the absence of viable chlamydiae, as trachoma patients with scarring are generally chlamydia-isolation negative. Two hypotheses have been suggested to explain this. First, such patients may be 'latently' infected with non-infectious, possibly non-replicating organisms, because chlamydial antigen and DNA can be detected in a proportion of isolation-negative cases of scarring trachoma. Second, an autoimmune mechanism could be involved because expression of class II antigens of the major histocompatibility complex has been demonstrated on conjunctival epithelial cells in trachoma.

It is possible that interferon-γ may be responsible for both these putative phenomena. This cytokine is secreted by lymphocytes from immune subjects on incubation with chlamydial antigen, and has been shown to inhibit the intracellular growth of *C. trachomatis in vitro*, arresting development at the non-infectious, reticulate-body stage. It has also been shown to induce class II expression in a variety of cell types, both *in vitro* and *in vivo*. It is feasible that other cytokines, particularly those that stimulate fibroblast activity, such as interleukin 1 and tumour necrosis factor-β, may participate in the pathogenesis of scarring due to chlamydial infection.

PROTECTIVE IMMUNITY AND PROSPECTS FOR A VACCINE

Recovery from ocular *C. trachomatis* infection involves cell-mediated immunity in the owl monkey, and both cell-mediated and humoral immunity play a part in the resolution of genital *C. psittaci* infection in the guinea-pig. The mechanism is not clear because there is little to suggest that cytotoxic T cells play a major role in the control of such intracellular pathogens, as might be expected.

The epidemiology of trachoma suggests that protective immunity follows natural infection, as active disease is uncommon in adults in endemic areas, and *C. trachomatis* can rarely be isolated from them. Similarly, the chlamydial isolation rate for men with non-gonococcal urethritis is lower in those who have had previous episodes. Women who had cervical chlamydial infections accompanied by IgM and IgG antibodies to *C. trachomatis* were less likely to develop salpingitis than those without such antibodies. Animal experiments suggest that protective immunity to ocular infection with *C. trachomatis* is mediated by local secretory IgA antibody. Antibodies in the tears of children with trachoma will partially neutralize chlamydial infectivity for the owl monkey eye, but as a positive correlation has been found between local antibody levels and the presence of *C. trachomatis* in the eye in trachoma endemic communities, not all local antibody is protective. An explanation may come from the fact that monoclonal antibodies which neutralize *C. trachomatis* infection *in vitro* bind to surface-exposed epitopes in the variable domains of the MOMP and are, in general, serovar specific.

Overall, some, but certainly not all, data based on natural observations and animal experiments indicate that chlamydial infection in the eye, respiratory or genital tract provides a degree of resistance to reinfection, although the mechanisms may differ. Despite the fact that evidence for protection against a repeat infection is sparse, it has been sufficient to encourage continued attempts to develop a vaccine.

Hypersensitivity seems to have contributed to the relatively unsuccessful attempts to vaccinate against trachoma, and in some instances the disease was made worse. The failure of *C. trachomatis* vaccines containing whole organisms emphasizes the need to concentrate on the development of subunit vaccines containing antigens that provide protective immunity rather than those that evoke damaging hypersensitivity. The molecular strategy to achieve this depends on identifying relevant protective surface antigens, defining the structure of the epitopes on these antigens that generate protective immunity, and then engineering a maximum immune response to the selected region. The most likely vaccine candidate identified so far is the 40 kDa MOMP. High-level expression of MOMP in *E. coli* (**rMOMP**) has made it possible to produce large quantities of antigen required for vaccine production. Studies in a mouse model of salpingitis induced by *C. trachomatis* showed that parenteral vaccination with rMOMP reduced the severity of salpingitis in three-quarters of the animals compared with mock-immunized controls and slightly reduced the duration of chlamydial colonization in the lower genital tract. Mice vaccinated via the gut shed fewer chlamydiae but had little reduction of oviduct damage. Such modest signs of protection suggest that vaccine development is worthwhile. A vaccine of limited protective efficacy might prove adequate for the control of trachoma by reducing the frequency of reinfection, and hence the severity of disease, without eliciting sterilizing immunity.

REFERENCES

Barron, A.L. (1988). *Microbiology of chlamydia.* CRC Press, Boca Raton FA.

Beem, M.O. and Saxon, E.M. (1977). Respiratory-tract colonization and destinctive pneumonia syndrome in infants infected with *Chlamydia trachomatis. New England Journal of Medicine*, **296,** 306–10.

Darougar, S. (ed.) (1983). Chlamydial disease. *British Medical Bulletin*, **39.**

Dawson, C.R., Jones, B.R., and Tarizzo, M.L. (1981). *Guide to trachoma control in programmes for the prevention of blindness.* World Health Organization, Geneva.

De Schryver, A. and Meheus, A. (1990). Epidemiology of sexually transmitted diseases. *Bulletin of the World Health Organization*, **68,** 639–54.

Grayston, J.T. *et al.* (1990). A new respiratory tract pathogen: *Chlamydia pneumoniae* strain TWAR. *Journal of Infectious Diseases*, **161,** 618–25.

Mabey, D.C.W., Bailey, R.L., and Hutin, Y.J.F. (1992). The epidemiology and pathogenesis of trachoma. *Review of Medical Microbiology*, **3,** 1–8.

Mårdh, P-A., Paavonen, J., and Puolakkainen, M. (ed.) (1989). *Chlamydia.* Plenum, New York.

Martin, D.H. *et al.* (1992). A controlled trial of a single dose of azithromycin for the treatment of chlamydial urethritis and cervicitis. *New England Journal of Medicine*, **327,** 921–5.

Monnickendam, M.A. (1988). Chlamydial genital infections. In *Immunology of sexually transmitted diseases*, (ed D.J.M. Wright), pp. 117–61. Kluwer, Dordrecht.

Morrison, R.P., Lyng, K., and Caldwell, H.D. (1989). Chlamydial disease pathogenesis. Ocular delayed hypersensitivity elicited by a genus specific 57 kD protein. *Journal of Experimental Medicine*, **169,** 663–75.

Reacher, M.H., Muñoz, B., Alghassany, A., Daar, A.S., Elbualy, M., and Taylor, H.R. (1992). A controlled trial of surgery for trachomatous trichiasis of the upper lid. *Archives of Ophthalmology*, **110,** 667–74.

Taylor-Robinson D. (1991). Genital chlamydial infections: clinical aspects, diagnosis, treatment and prevention. In *Recent advances in sexually transmitted diseases and AIDS*, (ed. J.R.W. Harris and S.M. Forster), pp. 219–62. Churchill Livingstone, Edinburgh.

Taylor-Robinson, D. and Thomas, B.J.(1991). Laboratory techniques for the diagnosis of chlamydial infections. *Genitourinary Medicine*, **67,** 256–66.

Taylor-Robinson, D. and Ward, M.E. (1989). Immunity to chlamydial infections and the outlook for vaccination. In *Vaccines for sexually transmitted diseases*, (ed. A. Meheus and R.E. Spier), pp. 67–85. Butterworth, London.

Thylefors, B., Dawson, C.R., Jones, B.R., West, S.K., and Taylor, H.R. (1987). A simple system for the assessment of trachoma and its complications. *Bulletin of the World Health Organization*, **65,** 477–83.

Treharne, J.D. (1991). Recent developments in the biology of the *Chlamydiae. Reviews of Medical Microbiology*, **2,** 45–9.

Ward, M.E. and Clarke, I.N. (1990). New perspectives in chlamydial biology and development. In *Chlamydial infections*, (ed. W.R. Bowie *et al.*), pp. 3–14. Cambridge University Press.

Washington, A.E., Johnson, R.E., and Sanders, L.L. (1987). *Chlamydia trachomatis* infections in the United States. What are they costing us? *Journal of the American Medical Association*, **257,** 2070–2.

7.11.42 Lymphogranuloma venereum

P. L. Perine

Lymphogranuloma venereum is a systemic, sexually transmitted disease caused by serovars L1, L2, L2a, and L3 of *Chlamydia trachomatis*. Serological cross-reaction is observed with other types of *C. trachomatis*. The chlamydiae of lymphogranuloma venereum are more invasive than the other serotypes and cause disease primarily in lymphatic tissue. Acute manifestations include an inguinal syndrome with painful swelling of inguinal, femoral, and deep iliac lymph nodes, and an anorectal syndrome characterized by an ulcerative proctitis. Late complications include genital elephantiasis, rectal stricture, and penile and rectovaginal fistula.

EPIDEMIOLOGY

Lymphogranuloma venereum is found worldwide, but its major incidence is limited to endemic foci in subSaharan Africa, South-East Asia, South America, and the Caribbean. All races are equally susceptible to infection, but the reported sex ratio is usually greater than 5:1 in favour of men. This is because early clinical lymphogranuloma venereum is recognized much more frequently in men than in women, who may not be diagnosed until late complications develop.

In North America and Europe, lymphogranuloma venereum is usually diagnosed in travellers, seamen, and military personnel returning from endemic areas, and in male homosexuals. The reservoir of infection is presumed to be asymptomatically infected women and male homosexuals. The frequency of infection following exposure is not known, but the coincidence of lymphogranuloma venereum in sexual partners indicates that transmission occurs much less often than is the case in gonorrhoea and syphilis.

PATHOGENESIS

The chlamydiae of lymphogranuloma venereum invade the host by attachment to and invasion of epithelial cells in the urogenital tract and rectosigmoid colon. Chlamydiae multiply, destroy cells and are carried to regional lymph nodes, whence they may spread systemically. Host immunity presumably limits chlamydial multiplication, cell destruction, and the progression of disease in the majority of cases, but it may not eliminate organisms from the body. Latent infection occurs, but its mechanism is poorly understood.

Although a small papule or necrotic genital lesion may be the first sign of infection, the pathology is largely restricted to the regional lymph nodes. These rapidly enlarge. Inflammation of the capsule causes the nodes to mat together. Multiple minute abscesses form in the parenchyma; in the absence of treatment they may coalesce and form sinus tracts, which rupture through the overlying skin.

Scar tissue may obstruct lymphatic flow causing lymphoedema and elephantiasis of the genitalia. Patients become sensitized to chlamydial antigens, and the chronic inflammatory response to their presence in tissue causes hyperplasia and necrosis. The end-result may be strictures, ulceration, and fistula.

CLINICAL FEATURES

Three stages of infection, designated primary, secondary, and tertiary, are usually recognized. Following an incubation period of 3 to 21 days, the primary lesion appears on or within the genital tract. It occurs in fewer than 25 per cent of cases and may escape notice. It is a small, painless, papular, vesicular, or ulcerative lesion that disappears spontaneously within a few days and leaves no scar. In men the lesion is on the penis, in women most commonly on the fourchette. These lesions, and especially rectal lesions in homosexual men, may go unnoticed. Extragenital primary lesions on fingers or tongue are rare. A small ulcerative lesion usually appears at the site of infection and invariably causes regional lymphadenitis.

The manifestations of the secondary stage are conventionally separated into inguinal and genitoanorectal syndromes. The more common inguinal syndrome is usually seen in men and is manifested by acute, painful bubo formation of the inguinal lymph nodes. The skin overlying the bubo is stretched taut and has a bluish discoloration. The lymphadenopathy is unilateral in two-thirds of cases, and in rare instances it may be so extensive that the inguinal mass is cleaved by the inelastic Poupart's ligament—the almost pathognomonic 'groove sign' of lymphogranuloma venereum. Buboes are accompanied by fever, malaise, chills, arthralgia, and headache. About 75 per cent of buboes suppurate and form cutaneous sinus tracts. Sinus drainage may persist for several weeks or months and, occasionally, an indurated inguinal mass forms which may persist for a lifetime.

In women, the external and internal iliac lymph nodes and the sacral lymphatics are involved more frequently than are the inguinal lymph nodes. Fever, chills, and malaise occur and may not be associated with lymphogranuloma venereum unless the pelvis is examined. Signs include a hypertrophic cervicitis with discharge of pus from the cervical os, backache, and adnexal tenderness due to enlarged retroperitoneal lymph nodes. None of these findings, however, is specific for lymphogranuloma venereum.

In both sexes, a genitoanorectal syndrome characterized by a haemorrhagic proctitis or protocolitis may occur, a result of chlamydial invasion of epithelial cells lining the lower intestinal tract. It is found more frequently in women, probably as the result of contamination of the anal area with infectious vaginal secretions or by spread of infection by the pelvic lymphatics. The rectal mucosa may be directly infected by chlamydiae in women or homosexual men during receptive rectal intercourse. The mucosa is friable and hyperaemic. Scattered ulcerations 1 to 2 cm in diameter with granular bases are seen by proctosigmoidoscopic examination. The inflammatory process is limited to the rectosigmoid colon and is accompanied by fever, a mucopurulent or bloody anal discharge, tenesmus, and diarrhoea. Histopathological changes in such cases may mimic Crohn's disease. The process usually resolves spontaneously after a period of several weeks.

Early proctocolitis is rarely complicated by rectal abscesses, fistula in ano, rectovaginal, rectovesical, and ischiorectal fistulas. Late in the course of the disease, a rectal stricture located 2 to 6 cm from the anal orifice and extending proximally for several centimetres may develop.

Rare manifestations of the secondary stage of lymphogranuloma venereum are acute meningoencephalitis, papillary-follicular conjunctivitis, synovitis, pneumonia, and cardiac involvement. Conjunctivitis is usually the result of autoinoculation of infected material from buboes, the vagina, or rectum to one or both eyes. Although it may cause enlargement of the maxillary and postauricular lymph nodes (Parinaud's oculoglandular syndrome), the follicular conjunctivitis is self-limiting.

The lesions of the tertiary stage appear after a period of latency of several years, during which the only evidence of infection is scars from secondary lesions and positive serological tests for lymphogranuloma venereum. Late complications are rarely seen today because they can be prevented by treatment with a variety of broad-spectrum antibiotics, which may coincidentally cure lymphogranuloma venereum when given to the patient for other infections.

Genital elephantiasis caused from a combination of lymphoedema, hyperplasia, and necrosis is the most common tertiary complication. It occurs predominantly in women as a sequel to the genitoanorectal syndrome and is very rare in men. Gross ulceration and granulomatous hypertrophy of the vulva ('esthiomene') is now rare. The elephantiasis may be accompanied by polypoid growths, which, when they occur in the perianal area, resemble haemorrhoids ('lymphorrhoids'). Fistulae occur frequently in association with elephantiasis. These lesions are often very painful and interfere with normal functions of the affected parts. Secondary bacterial infection is usual and accelerates tissue necrosis.

Rectal stricture is the most serious tertiary lesion and is found almost exclusively in women or homosexual men. Symptoms include constipation, tenderness, and pain. Complete obstruction may lead to bowel perforation. Rectovaginal fistula is common in women.

DIAGNOSIS

Three different categories of diagnostic tests are used to diagnose lymphogranuloma venereum. They are the Frei skin test, the identification of lymphogranuloma chlamydiae from infected tissue, and serological tests. The classical Frei skin test for lymphogranuloma venereum has fallen into disfavour because it is neither highly sensitive nor specific for lymphogranuloma venereum. As a result, Frei antigen is no longer commercially produced.

Chlamydiae of lymphogranuloma can be identified in infected tissue when special stains and microscopical techniques are used, by isolation in the yolk sac of embryonated hen eggs, in tissue culture, or by nucleic-acid hybridization techniques. Chlamydial tissue culture is more sensitive than is microscopical examination of infected tissue, but only 25 to 40 per cent of patients with lymphogranuloma venereum have positive cultures of bubo aspirate, endourethral or endocervical scrapings, or of other infected material. Yield can be improved by culturing specimens from a variety of sites.

Several serological tests detect chlamydial antibody in serum. The oldest and most widely used is the complement fixation test, which uses an antigen common to all chlamydiae and is, therefore, not specific for lymphogranuloma venereum. However, the titre of complement-fixing antibody in acute lymphogranuloma venereum infections is usually greater than 1:64. Although a fourfold or greater increase in titre between acute and convalescent sera renders the diagnosis of lymphogranuloma venereum more certain, this is rarely observed. The complement-fixation titre usually declines rapidly after adequate treatment.

The different serovars of *C. trachomatis* can be distinguished by the microimmunofluorescent test. In this test, the different strains of *C. trachomatis* are placed separately or in groups on microscope slides and reacted with varying dilutions of the patient's serum in an indirect fluorescent antibody assay. Microimmunofluorescent antibody titres are frequently greater than 1:256 in acute sera from patients with lymphogranuloma venereum. Because of the broad cross-reactivity seen in the microimmunofluorescent test between different strains, it may not be possible to determine which of the serovars of lymphogranuloma venereum is responsible for a given infection.

When possible, a serum specimen should be tested first by complement fixation and then, if strongly positive, by microimmunofluorescence. The combination of a positive complement fixation and microimmunofluorescence in high-titre in a patient with typical signs and symptoms is diagnostic of lymphogranuloma venereum.

A fluorescein-conjugated monoclonal antibody, an antigen capture immunoassay, and nucleic-acid hybridization techniques can be used to detect elementary bodies of *C. trachomatis* in infected tissues. The monoclonal antibody test has been used to diagnose ocular and other anogenital chlamydial infections and may prove to be useful in the diagnosis of lymphogranuloma venereum.

Other diseases that must be considered in the differential diagnosis of the inguinal lymphogranuloma venereum syndrome are genital herpes, syphilis, chancroid, donovanosis, extrapulmonary tuberculosis, cat-scratch disease, plague, filariasis, lymphoma, and other malignant diseases. Lymphadenitis of the deep iliac nodes may mimic appendicitis or pelvic inflammatory disease. Many surgeons, ignorant of lymphogranuloma venereum, have mistaken a bubo for an incarcerated inguinal hernia and realize their error only at the time of surgery.

Primary genital herpes (see Chapter 21.3) provides the greatest diagnostic confusion. Constitutional symptoms are similar in both infections, and anogenital herpetic lesions with inguinal lymphadenitis mimic primary lymphogranuloma venereum. Herpetic patients often have tender, discretely enlarged, inguinal lymph nodes, but these seldom reach the size seen in lymphogranuloma venereum. The inguinal lymphadenitis common in primary syphilis and the suppurative inguinal buboes characteristic of chancroid occur at the same time as genital chancres or ulcers, but the combination is seldom found in lymphogranuloma venereum. Nevertheless, dark-ground examination and serological tests for syphilis, as well as cultures of genital ulcers and bubo aspirates for *Haemophilus ducreyi* and *Neisseria gonorrhoeae*, should be part of the diagnostic evaluation of any patient with genital lesions and lymphadenitis. One or more of these diseases may occur simultaneously in the same patient. The proctitis of the genitoanorectal syndrome of lymphogranuloma venereum may be indistinguishable from that seen at the onset of chronic ulcerative, acute amoebic, or antibiotic-associated colitis. Every patient with haemorrhagic proctitis should, therefore, be carefully evaluated by proctosigmoidoscopical and radiological examination, rectal biopsy, culture, and other tests of stool for both bacterial and parasitic pathogens.

Patients with ulcerative colitis and regional ileitis may have positive complement-fixing chlamydial serological tests in high titre and a positive microimmunofluorescent test. Only in rare instances, however, have chlamydiae of lymphogranuloma been isolated from an inflamed bowel, and, despite circumstantial evidence, no causal relation has been proved to exist between lymphogranuloma venereum and these diseases. Positive chlamydial tests are also seen occasionally in patients with cat-scratch fever.

Tuberculosis and certain parasitic and fungal infections of the genital tract cause lymphoedema and elephantiasis of the genitalia. Tissue biopsy and special culture techniques may differentiate elephantiasis due to lymphogranuloma venereum from other causes.

TREATMENT

Of the several antimicrobial drugs active against lymphogranuloma chlamydiae in tissue culture, only a few are used to treat patients with lymphogranuloma venereum. Oral tetracycline, 1 to 2 g daily, or a sulphonamide such as sulphadiazine, 4 g daily, are usually recommended. There is little evidence to support the choice of one drug rather than another, and only marginal evidence that antimicrobial treatment is better than symptomatic treatment alone in acute inguinal lymphogranuloma venereum. Fever and bubo pain rapidly subside after antimicrobials are started, but buboes may take several weeks to resolve. Suppuration and rupture of buboes with sinus formation are usually prevented by antimicrobials. It is not known how long treatment need be continued to prevent relapse and progression of disease. A minimum of 2 weeks is recommended. The patient's sexual partner should be treated at the same time, to prevent reinfection. Unruptured, fluctuant buboes should be aspirated by syringe through a large-bore needle. This prevents sinus formation. Surgical incision and drainage is neither necessary nor recommended. Buboes that are draining should be covered with dressings soaked in antiseptic solution until dry, in order to prevent autoinoculation and nosocomial infection.

The fistulae, strictures and elephantiasis of chronic lymphogranuloma venereum may require plastic repair. Surgery should not be attempted until the patient has achieved weeks or months of antimicrobial treatment, which often reduces the degree of inflammation and necrosis so that healing proceeds normally and only limited surgical repair is necessary.

PROGNOSIS

The early manifestations of lymphogranuloma venereum are self-limiting. Late sequelae are rarely seen today, even in areas of the world where the disease is still common. At one time, rectal fibrosis was thought to predispose to carcinoma, but there is little supporting evidence. In the pre-antibiotic era, rectal stricture causing complete bowel obstruction, perforation, and death was reported.

Genital elephantiasis, and rectovaginal and other types of fistula are important social and medical problems in several lesser developed nations in Africa and Asia. Whether or not lymphogranuloma venereum is aetiologically significant in these problems is unknown.

REFERENCES

Barnes, R.C. (1989). Laboratory diagnosis of human chlamydial infections. *Clinical Microbiology Reviews*, **2,** 119–36.

Greaves, A.B., Hilleman, M.R., Taggart, S.R., Bankhead, A.B., and Feld, M. (1957). Chemotherapy in bubonic lymphogranuloma venereum. *Bulletin of the World Health Organization*, **16,** 227–289.

Martin, D.H. *et al.* (1992). A controlled trial of a single dose of azithromycin for the treatment of chlamydial urethritis and cervicitis. *New England Journal of Medicine*, **327,** 921–5.

Perine, P.L. *et al.* (1980). Diagnosis and treatment of lymphogranuloma venereum in Ethiopia. In *Current chemotherapy and infectious disease*, pp. 1280–2. American Society of Microbiology. Washington DC.

Quinn, T.C. *et al.* (1981). Chlamydia trachomatis proctitis. *LYMPHOGRANULOMA VENEREUMNew England Journal of Medicine*, **305,** 195–200.

Schachter, J. (1977). Lymphogranuloma venereum and other nonocular *Chlamydia trachomatis* infections. In *Nongonococcal urethritis and related infections* (ed. D. Hobson and K.K. Holmes), pp. 91–7. American Society of Microbiology, Washington DC.

7.11.43 Mycoplasmas

D. TAYLOR-ROBINSON

Characteristics of mycoplasmas

Mycoplasmas, originally called pleuropneumonia-like organisms (**PPLO**), are the smallest free-living micro-organisms. They lack a cell wall so that they are resistant to penicillins and other antimicrobials which act on this structure. Instead, they are bounded by a pliable unit membrane (Fig. 1), which encloses the cytoplasm, DNA, RNA, and other metabolic components necessary for propagation in cell-free media. Mycoplasmas have a number of other characteristics that also distinguish them from bacteria, chlamydiae, and viruses (Table 1). Furthermore, they are not related to the L-phase variants of bacteria.

Despite the general similarity among mycoplasmas, they comprise a heterogenous group of micro-organisms that differ from one another in DNA composition, nutritional requirements, metabolic reactions, antigenic composition, and host specificity. Taxonomically, the mycoplasmas are divided into three orders (Table 2), the Mycoplasmatales, of which the families Mycoplasmataceae and Spiroplasmataceae (helical organisms) both require sterol for growth, the Acholeplasmatales, which do not, and the oxygen-sensitive, strictly anaerobic Anaeroplasmatales, one genus of which also does not need sterol. The mycoplasmas isolated commonly from man belong to the family Mycoplasmataceae. This comprises the genus Mycoplasma, which contains organisms that do not hydrolyse urea, and the genus Ureaplasma, the organisms of which do hydrolyse this substrate. The latter originally were termed T-strains or T-mycoplasmas because of the tiny (T) colonies they form on agar medium, in contrast to the larger characteristic 'fried-egg'-like colonies produced by most other mycoplasmas (Fig. 2).

The small size of the mycoplasma genome restricts their metabolic capabilities. Nevertheless, apart from their importance in man, certain mycoplama species are of economic importance because of the pneumonia, arthritis, keratoconjunctivitis, and mastitis they cause among livestock and poultry in Africa, Australia, and other parts of the world. Furthermore, a number of mycoplasma species are a laboratory nuisance as occult contaminants of cell cultures.

Fig. 1 Electron micrograph of *M. pulmonis* (murine origin), illustrating that the organism does not have a bacterial cell wall but has a trilaminar unit membrane (arrow); also note what appears to be a terminal structure (T). × 66 000.

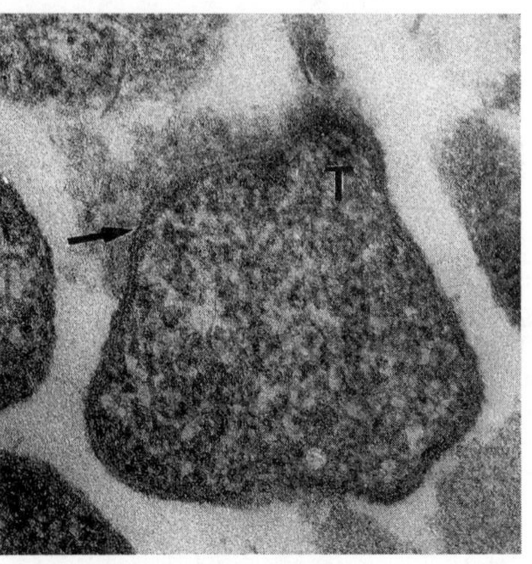

OCCURRENCE OF MYCOPLASMAS IN MAN

Fourteen mycoplasma species constitute the normal flora or are pathogens of humans (Table 3). Most of them are found in the oropharynx. There is little information, as yet, about the distribution or significance of *M. penetrans* and none about that of *M. spermatophilum*, both of which have been discovered in the genitourinary tract.

Respiratory infections

The relation between mycoplasmas and respiratory disease

Evidence that mycoplasmas, apart from *M. pneumoniae*, are implicated aetiologically in acute respiratory disease is accruing. *M. genitalium* was found originally in the male genitourinary tract but it was subsequently isolated from a small proportion of respiratory specimens, which also contained *M. pneumoniae*. The significance of *M. genitalium* in the respiratory tract remains to be determined, as does that of *M. fermentans*. The latter mycoplasma has been detected in the throat more often than hitherto by means of the polymerase chain reaction (**PCR**) (see later) and has been recovered from adults presenting with an acute influenza-like illness, sometimes deteriorating rapidly with development of an often fatal respiratory-distress syndrome. *M. hominis*, on the other hand, is far less virulent. Although adult male volunteers given large numbers of *M. hominis* organisms orally developed a mild exudative pharyngitis accompanied by an antibody response, attempts to demonstrate that this mycoplasma is a cause of naturally occurring sore throats in children and adults have been unsuccessful.

In the late 1930s, non-bacterial pneumonias were first recognized and brought under the heading of primary atypical pneumonia to distinguish them from typical lobar pneumonia. Gradually, primary atypical pneumonia was recognized to be aetiologically heterogeneous and, in one variety, cold agglutinins often developed. It was from this form of disease that an infectious agent was isolated in embryonated eggs. This micro-organism, the 'Eaton agent', produced pneumonia in cotton rats and hamsters, and for a number of years was thought to be a virus. However, serious doubts about this arose when it was found to be affected by chlortetracycline and gold salts, and its mycoplasmal nature was established finally by cultivation on a cell-free agar medium. The agent was subsequently called *M. pneumoniae* and its ability to cause respiratory disease was established fully by studies based on isolation, serology, volunteer inoculation, and vaccine protection.

M. pneumoniae *disease manifestations*

M. pneumoniae produces a spectrum of effects from inapparent infection to mild, afebrile, upper respiratory-tract disease to severe pneumonia. Clinical manifestations are often not sufficiently distinctive to permit an early definitive diagnosis of mycoplasmal pneumonia. Indeed, this shares the features of other non-bacterial pneumonias in that general symptoms, such as malaise and headache, often precede chest symptoms by 1 to 5 days, and radiographic examination frequently reveals evidence of pneumonia before physical signs, such as râles, become apparent. Usually, only one of the lower lobes is involved and the radiograph most often shows patchy opacities. About 20 per cent of patients suffer bilateral pneumonia, but pleurisy and pleural effusions are unusual. The course of the disease is variable but often protracted. Thus, cough, abnormal chest signs, and changes in the radiograph may persist for several weeks and relapse is a feature. The organisms also may persist in respiratory secretions despite antibiotic therapy, and this is particularly so in hypogammaglobulinaemic patients, where excretion may continue for months or years rather than weeks. Although a few very severe infections have been reported, occurring usually in patients with immunodeficiency or sickle-cell anaemia, death has been rare. In chil-

Table 1 *Characteristics of mycoplasmas compared to those of bacteria, chlamydiae, and viruses*

Characteristic	Mycoplasmas	Bacteria	Chlamydiae	Viruses
Size (diameter)	0.3μm[1]	1–2μm	0.3 μm	< 0.5 μm
Lack of a cell wall	Yes	No	No	Yes
Contain both DNA and RNA	Yes	Yes	Yes	No
Multiplication on cell-free medium	Yes	Yes	No	No
Multiplication dependent on host-cell nucleic acid	No	No	No	Yes
Usually require sterol and native protein for propagation	Yes	No	No	No
Intrinsic energy metabolism	Yes	Yes	Yes	No
Usually narrow range of host specificity	Yes	No	No	Yes
Growth inhibited by specific antibody alone	Yes	No	Yes	Yes
Resistant to cell-wall active antibiotics (e.g. penicillins)	Yes	No	No	Yes
Resistant to antibiotics that inhibit metabolism (e.g. tetracycline)	No	No	No	Yes

[1] Smallest organisms capable of propagation.

Table 2 *Classification, and some distinguishing features, of mycoplasmas (class Mollicutes)*

Classification		Distinguishing features			
		Sterol required	Genome size (kbp)	Mol% G + C of DNA	Other characteristics
CLASS:	Mollicutes				
Order I:	Mycoplasmatales				
FAMILY I:	Mycoplasmataceae	Yes	580–1380	23–41	
Genus I:	*Mycoplasma* About 100 species				
Genus II:	*Ureaplasma* Five species; *U. urealyticum* has at least 14 serotypes		730–1160	27–30	Urea metabolized
FAMILY II:	Spiroplasmataceae	Yes	970–1970	25–31	Helical structure
Genus I:	*Spiroplasma* Eleven or more species including *S. citri*				
Order II:	Acholeplasmatales				
FAMILY I:	Acholeplasmataceae	No	1230–1690	27–36	
Genus I:	*Acholeplasma* Twelve species				
Genus II:	*Mesoplasma*		825–1100		Requires 0.04% Tween 80
Order III:	Anaeroplasmatales				
FAMILY I:	Anaeroplasmataceae				Obligate anaerobes
Genus I:	*Anaeroplasma* Four species	Yes	About 1600	29–33	
Genus II:	*Asteroleplasma* One species	No	About 1600	40	

dren, infection has been characterized occasionally by a prolonged illness with paroxysmal cough followed by vomiting, thus simulating the features of whooping cough.

Extrapulmonary manifestations

Illness caused by *M. pneumoniae* is limited usually to the respiratory tract, but a wide variety of extrapulmonary clinical conditions may occur during the course of the respiratory illness or as a sequel to it. These complications and an estimation of the frequency of their occurrence are shown in Table 4. Whether any of them might be due to *M. genitalium* is a moot point. Haemolytic anaemia with crisis is brought about by the development and action of cold agglutinins (anti-I antibodies). There is dispute about the mechanism of their production but the organisms may alter the I antigen on erythrocytes sufficiently to stimulate an autoimmune response. It is possible that some of the other clinical conditions, such as the neurological complications, may arise in a similar way. However, invasion of the central nervous system cannot be discounted as there is one report of the isolation of *M. pneumoniae* from cerebrospinal fluid.

DIAGNOSIS

Mycoplasmas are Gram negative but are not recognizable in Gram-stained smears. The diagnosis depends, therefore, on culturing specimens and/or performing a specific (complement fixation) or non-specific (cold agglutinin) serological test. The usual medium employed for isolation of *M. pneumoniae* consists of PPLO broth, 20 per cent horse serum and 10% (v/v) fresh yeast extract (25 per cent w/v). However, it seems that a more sensitive medium is that used for the isolation of spiroplasmas, comprising essentially a conventional mycoplasma broth medium with fetal calf serum and a tissue-culture supplement. Either medium is supplemented with thallium acetate, penicillin, and glucose, with phenol red as a pH indicator. The fluid medium, inoculated with sputum, throat washing, pharyngeal swab, or other specimen, is incubated at 37°C and a colour change (red to yellow), which occurs usually within 4 to 21 days, signals the fermentation of glucose (Table 3), with production of acid, owing to multiplication of the organisms. This preliminary identification may be confirmed after subculturing to agar medium. Erythrocytes of various species adsorb to colonies of many different mycoplasmas (haemadsorption) (Fig. 3) Because erythrocytes, other than those of chicken origin, adsorb only to colonies of *M. pneumoniae* and *M. genitalium* of human origin (Table 3), haemadsorption reduces the diagnostic options, identification being confirmed usually by demonstrating inhibition of colony development around discs impregnated with specific antiserum (Fig. 4).

Fig. 2 (a) 'Fried-egg'-like mycoplasma colonies (one not well formed) and a larger bacterial colony. Transmission light microscopy, × 43. (b) Section through mycoplasma colonies illustrating growth in the depth of the agar. × 78.

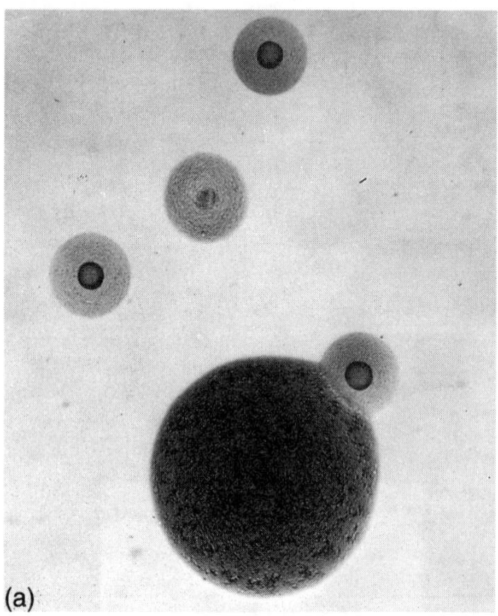

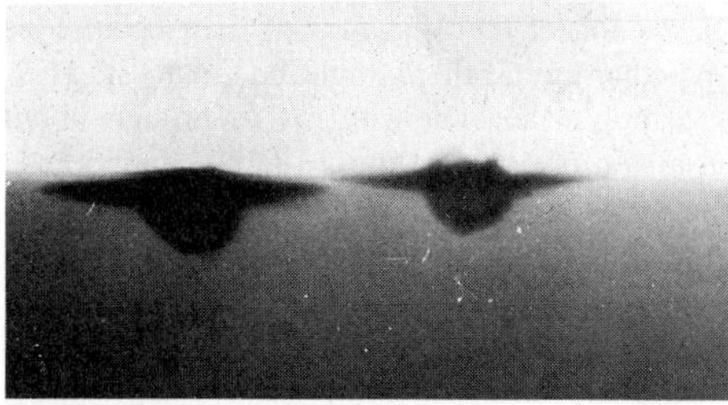

Culture and identification are slow but PCR technology provides the opportunity for a different strategy. Rapid determination of *M. pneumoniae* positivity and then continued culture of only those specimens that are PCR-positive should make for a speedier diagnosis. However, currently the PCR is used only as a research tool or in special circumstances; in routine practice, reliance is placed on serology for diagnosis. Antibody is detectable by a variety of procedures but many are not practical. However, a complement-fixation test is undertaken in many laboratories and a fourfold or greater rise in antibody titre with a peak at about 3 to 4 weeks after the onset of disease is said to occur in about 80 per cent of cases and be indicative of a recent infection. An antibody titre of 1 : 128 or greater in a single serum is suggestive of an infection in the previous few weeks or months; a fourfold or greater fall in antibody titre, perhaps over 6 months, may be helpful but, sometimes, it may be difficult to relate it to a particular prior illness. More difficult, however, is the problem of specificity because it is now realized that the complement-fixation test does not distinguish between *M. pneumoniae* and *M. genitalium.* Until the frequency of occurrence of *M. genitalium* in the respiratory tract and its capacity to cause disease there has been resolved, the diagnosis of *M. pneumoniae* infections based on the complement-fixation test will remain obscure. Diagnosis based on a single serum sample is always difficult whatever the test; an antibody titre of 1 : 128 (or 1 : 160) in an indirect haemagglutination test, for which kits are available commercially, may be regarded as suggestive in an appropriate clinical setting but specificity is again open to question. More specific perhaps is the microimmunofluorescence test in which IgM antibody is sought; its presence provides some confidence in making an accurate diagnosis of a current infection or one within the previous few weeks. Cold agglutinins, detected by agglutination of O Rh-negative erythrocytes at 4°C, develop in about half the patients. Although they are occasionally induced by a number of other conditions, a titre of 1 : 128 or greater is suggestive of a recent *M. pneumoniae* infection. This assumes that *M. genitalium* is not able to stimulate cold agglutinins. When the test is negative, it should be repeated perhaps after a week because a rise in the titre of cold agglutinins is meaningful.

EPIDEMIOLOGY

Relation to age

M. pneumoniae affects children and adults, the consequence of infection depending upon age. Thus, about a quarter of infections in persons 5 to 15 years old result in pneumonia, while about 7 per cent of infections in young adults do so. Thereafter, pneumonia is even less frequent, but generally is more severe the older the patient.

Relative importance of *M. pneumoniae*

Although *M. pneumoniae* causes inapparent and mild upper respiratory-tract infections more commonly than severe disease, it is responsible for only a small proportion of all upper respiratory-tract disease, most of it being of viral aetiology. Acute pharyngitis, occurring mostly in adolescents and younger persons, is due mainly to group A streptococci and rarely to *M. pneumoniae*, which plays a relatively greater part in producing lower respiratory-tract disease. *Chlamydia pneumoniae* is now recognized as an important respiratory pathogen and this micro-organism, as well as various bacteria, cause most cases of pneumonia. However, in certain groups of people, pneumonia caused by *M. pneumoniae* is more frequent than that caused by respiratory viruses. Thus, in the United States, it has been calculated that in a large general population, the proportion of all pneumonias due to *M. pneumoniae* is about 15 to 20 per cent, and in certain populations, for example military recruits, it has been responsible for as much as 40 per cent of acute pneumonic illness. There is very little evidence that other infections predispose to infection by *M. pneumoniae* or vice versa. The occurrence of *Haemophilus influenzae* pneumonia soon after infection by *M. pneumoniae* seems to be a rare event.

Table 3 *The biological features, occurrence, and disease association of mycoplasmas isolated from humans*

Mycoplasma	Metabolism of:	Preferred atmosphere	Haemadsorption	Frequency of isolation from the: Respiratory tract	Genitourinary tract	Rectum	Eye	Blood	Cause of disease
M. buccale	Arginine	Anaerobic[1]	No	Rare	-[2]	-	-	-	No
M. faucium	Arginine	Anaerobic	Yes[3]	Rare	-	-	-	-	No
M. fermentans	Glucose, arginine	Anaerobic	No	Common	Rare	-	-	Rare	?Yes
M. hominis	Arginine	Aerobic	No	Rare	Common	Common	Rare	Very rare	Yes
M. genitalium	Glucose	Anaerobic	Yes	?	Common	?	?	?	Yes
A. laidlawii	Glucose	Anaerobic	No	Rare	-	-	-	-	No
M. lipophilum	Arginine	Anaerobic	No	Rare	-	-	-	-	No
M. orale	Arginine	Anaerobic	Yes[3]	Common	-	-	-	-	No
M. penetrans	Glucose, arginine	Anaerobic	Yes	-	?Rare	?	?	?	?
M. pneumoniae	Glucose	Aerobic	Yes	Rare[4]	Very rare	-	-	-	Yes
M. primatum	Arginine	Anaerobic	No	-	Rare	-	-	-	No
M. salivarium	Arginine	Anaerobic	No	Common	Rare	-	-	-	No
M. spermatophilum	Arginine	Anaerobic	No	-	?Rare	?	?	?	?
U. urealyticum	Urea	Anaerobic	Serotype 3 only	Rare	Common	Common	Rare	Very rare	Yes

[1] 5% CO_2, 95% nitrogen; [2] no reports of isolation; [3] with chick erythrocytes only; [4] Except in disease outbreaks.

Table 4 *Extrapulmonary manifestations of* M. pneumoniae *infections*

System	Manifestations	Estimated frequency
Cardiovascular	Myocarditis, pericarditis	< 5%
Dermatological	Erythema multiforme; Stevens-Johnson syndrome; other rashes	Some skin involvement in about 25%
Gastrointestinal	Anorexia, nausea, vomiting, and transient diarrhoea;	14–44%
	hepatitis;	?
	pancreatitis	?
Genitourinary	Tubo-ovarian abscess;	Insignificant
	acute glomerulonephritis	?
Haematological	Cold agglutinin production;	About 50%
	haemolytic anaemia;	?
	thrombocytopenia;	?
	intravascular coagulation	50 reported cases
Musculoskeletal	Myalgia, arthralgia,	14–45%
	arthritis	?
Neurological	Meningitis, meningoencephalitis, ascending paralysis, transient myelitis, cranial-nerve palsy, poliomyelitis-like illness	6–7%

Fig. 3 Colony of *M. agalactiae* (caprine origin) with guinea-pig erythrocytes adherent to the surface. This phenomenon of haemadsorption shown after addition of a 1 per cent suspension of erythrocytes, incubation at 37°C for 30 min, removal of cells, and gentle washing of the agar surface.

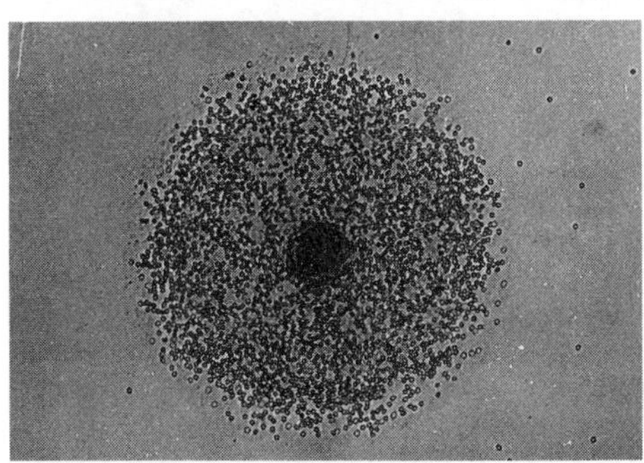

Fig. 4 Mycoplasma identification by agar growth inhibition. Colony development inhibited around a filter-paper disc impregnated with specific antiserum. Note also antibody–antigen precipitation at edge of inhibition zone.

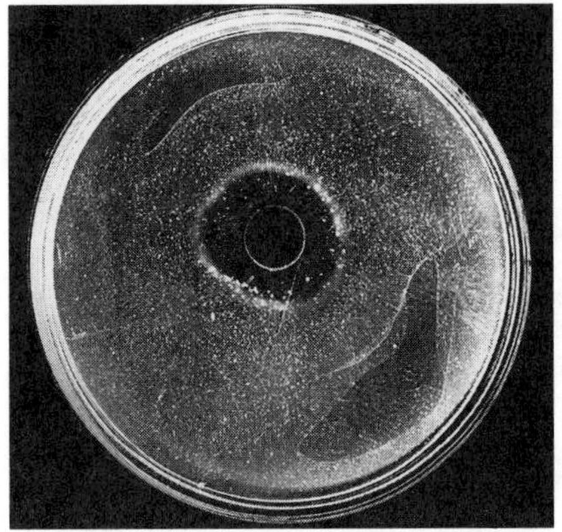

Distribution and spread of infection

M. pneumoniae infections have been reported from every country where appropriate diagnostic tests have been undertaken. Infection is endemic in most areas and occurs during all months of the year, with a predilection for late summer and early autumn. However, epidemic peaks have been observed about every 4 to 7 years in some countries. The incubation period ranges from 2 to 3 weeks and spread from person to person occurs slowly, usually where there is continual or repeated close contact, for example in a family, rather than where there is only casual contact.

IMMUNOPATHOLOGICAL FACTORS IN THE DEVELOPMENT OF *M. PNEUMONIAE* PNEUMONIA

Initial adherence of *M. pneumoniae* organisms to respiratory mucosal epithelial cells (Fig. 5) is a crucial factor in the pathogenesis of disease. After cytadsorption, mediated by P1, P30 and possibly up to seven other proteins on the surface of the organisms, immune mechanisms play an important part in the development of *M. pneumoniae* pneumonia in man, as indicated by several observations. Death due to this pneumonia has rarely been reported so that the histopathological picture is derived mainly from experimental infection of hamsters and natural mycoplasmal disease in other animals. The pneumonic infiltrate is predominantly a peribronchiolar and perivascular cuffing by lymphocytes, most of which are thymus dependent (Fig. 6). The importance of cell-mediated immune mechanisms in the pathogenesis of *M. pneumoniae* pneumonia is indicated by the fact that immunosuppression of hamsters, in a variety of ways, results in ablation of the pneumonia or a decrease in its severity. The development of a cell-mediated immune response to *M. pneumoniae* has been shown further by positive lymphocyte transformation, macrophage migration inhibition and delayed-hypersensitivity skin tests. A polysaccharide–protein fraction of the organisms is involved in this response rather than the glycolipid that is the main antigenic determinant in complement fixation and other serological reactions. The initial lymphocyte response is followed by a change in the character of the bronchiolar exudate, with polymorphonuclear leucocytes and macrophages predominating. The rather slow development of these events on primary infection contrasts with an accelerated and often more intense host response seen on reinfection. To at least some extent, therefore, the pneumonia caused by *M. pneumoniae* is an immunopathological process. Children of 2 to 5 years of age often possess mycoplasmacidal antibody, suggesting infection at an early age, although it is not clear whether the antibody is induced entirely by *M. pneumoniae* infection. Nevertheless, it is tempting to suggest that the pneumonia which occurs in older persons is an immunological over-response to reinfection, the lung being infiltrated by previously sensitized lymphocytes.

Fig. 5 Electron micrograph of ciliated epithelial cells in the tracheal mucosa of a hamster infected with *M. pneumoniae*. Note cilia (c) and individual organisms (m), some with specialized terminal structure oriented towards the membrane of the host cell (arrows). × 9880.

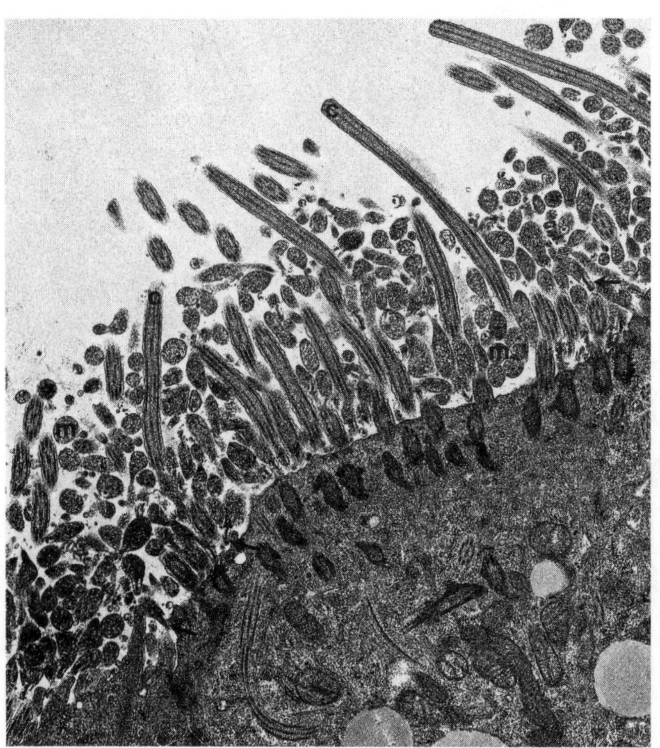

TREATMENT

Mycoplasmas are indifferent to the penicillins, cephalosporins, and other antimicrobials that affect cell-wall synthesis, but they are generally sensitive to those antimicrobials that inhibit protein synthesis. Thus, *M. pneumoniae*, like other mycoplasmas, is sensitive to the tetracyclines and apparently more sensitive to erythromycin than the other mycoplasmas of human origin. It is also inhibited by the newer macrolides, such as clarithromycin and azithromycin, and the newer quinolones, such as sparfloxacin. The value of tetracyclines was shown first in a controlled trial of dimethylchlortetracycline in United States marine recruits, a dose of 300 mg three times daily for 6 days significantly reducing the duration of fever, pulmonary infiltration, and other signs and symptoms. Since then other trials have also provided evidence for the effectiveness of various tetracyclines, as well as erythromycin and other macrolides. Planned trials provide the most favourable conditions for determining the value of antimicrobials but in civilian practice they have proved less effective, probably because disease is often well established before treatment is instituted. Despite this, it is worthwhile treating with an antimicrobial. For pregnant women and children it is advisable to use erythromycin rather than a tetracycline, and the former has sometimes proved more effective than a tetracycline in adults. Successful treatment of clinical disease, however, is not always accompanied by early eradication of the organisms from the respiratory tract, probably because the drugs only inhibit their multiplication and do not kill them. This is a possible reason for relapse in some patients and a plausible reason for recommending a 2- to 3-week course of antimicrobial treatment. It is a moot point whether early treatment would prevent some of the complications but, nevertheless, it should commence as soon as possible. As laboratory confirmation of *M. pneumoniae* infection may be slow, it would seem wise to start antimicrobial treatment on the basis of the clinical evidence and a cold agglutinin and/or suggestive sero-

Fig. 6 Pneumonia 2 weeks after intranasal inoculation of a hamster with *M. pneumoniae*. Note peribronchiolar and perivascular infiltration of mononuclear cells, predominantly lymphocytes. Haematoxylin and eosin, × 98.

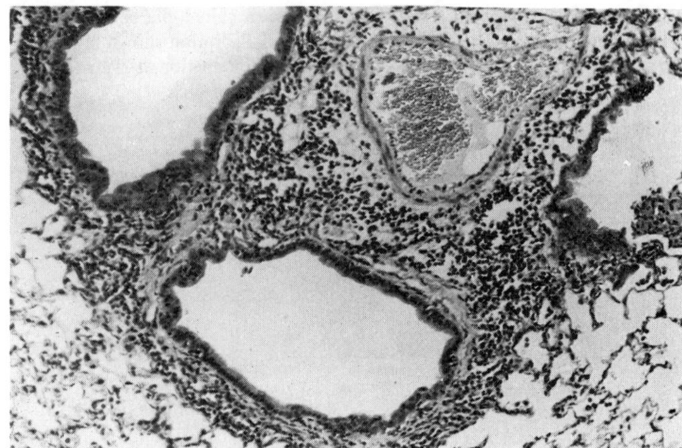

logical antibody titre in a single serum sample, despite the drawbacks, mentioned previously, of attempting to make a serological diagnosis.

The true value of corticosteroids is in doubt, although, in conjunction with antimicrobials, they appear to have been helpful in patients with severe pneumonia and erythema multiforme.

PREVENTION

Resistance to disease

One of the best ways of assessing the relative importance of cell-mediated and humoral immune mechanisms in resistance is to determine the ability of lymphocytes and of serum from immune animals to confer immunity when they are transferred to recipient, non-immune animals. Most of the information on the protective capacity of 'immune' cells and serum has been obtained not from the *M. pneumoniae* hamster model but from another mycoplasmal pneumonia model, the *M. pulmonis* infection of mice. Serum from mice infected up to 5 weeks previously protects recipient syngeneic mice against respiratory disease, whereas spleen cells do not. This suggests that humoral immune mechanisms are relatively more important than cell-mediated ones in resistance. However, serum antibody to *M. pneumoniae* does not confer complete protection against infection or disease, as they may occur despite high titres of, for example, serum mycoplasmacidal antibody. Furthermore, mycoplasmal infection of the respiratory tract of laboratory animals may stimulate only a weak antibody response and yet induce greater resistance to reinfection and disease than parenteral inoculation with organisms that stimulate much higher titres of serum antibodies. Such observations have led to the belief that local immune factors are crucial in resistance. The correlation between the resistance of adult volunteers to *M. pneumoniae* disease and the presence of IgA antibody in respiratory secretions is consistent with this contention. This antibody could provide the first line of defence by preventing attachment of the organisms to respiratory epithelial cells.

Vaccination

The efficacy of formalin-inactivated *M. pneumoniae* vaccines in preventing pneumonia caused by this mycoplasma has ranged from 28 to 67 per cent in field trials. The failure of some killed *M. pneumoniae* vaccines to protect fully may have been due to poor antigenicity, but others induced serum antibody levels similar to those that develop after natural infection. This suggests that the relatively poor protection afforded by the killed vaccines may have been due to their inability to stimulate cell-mediated immunity and/or local antibody and they are no longer produced commercially. With local antibodies in mind, live attenuated vaccines, particularly those based on temperature-sensitive mutants of *M. pneumoniae*, were developed. They could multiply at the temperature of the upper, but not the lower, respiratory tract and some produced pulmonary infection in hamsters without causing pathological changes, and induced significant resistance to subsequent challenge with virulent wild strains of *M. pneumoniae*. However, because the same mutants produced some disease in human volunteers they were considered unacceptable for general human use and this approach to vaccination was abandoned. Currently, recombinant DNA vaccines involving P1 and other proteins, and a live adenovirus recombinant vaccine developed by cloning a component of the *M. pneumoniae* P1 gene into an adenovirus vector, are being explored.

Chronic respiratory disease

As mycoplasmas of animals are frequently involved in chronic illnesses, the possible role of mycoplasmas in human chronic respiratory disease, particularly chronic bronchitis, is worthy of consideration.

M. PNEUMONIAE INFECTIONS

The isolation of *M. pneumoniae* from some patients experiencing an acute exacerbation of chronic bronchitis, in addition to a serological response, suggests that this mycoplasma apart from viruses, is sometimes responsible for the exacerbation. In addition, complement-fixing antibody to *M. pneumoniae* occurs more frequently in the serum of patients suffering from chronic bronchitis than in that of normal subjects. However, the real contribution of *M. pneumoniae* in this situation is difficult to assess because it is also evident that patients with chronic bronchitis sometimes acquire mycoplasmal infections without an apparent worsening of this disease.

M. pneumoniae frequently persists in the respiratory tract long after clinical recovery and occasionally the respiratory disease it causes has a protracted course. Furthermore, tracheobronchial clearance is very much reduced soon after infection and there is a tendency for slower clearance, in comparison with that in healthy subjects, even 1 year later. Despite this there is no evidence that *M. pneumoniae* is a primary cause of chronic bronchitis, or that it is responsible for maintaining chronic disease other than by possibly causing some acute exacerbations.

OTHER MYCOPLASMAL INFECTIONS

There is no doubt that *M. salivarium*, *M. orale*, and perhaps other mycoplasmas present in the oropharynxes of healthy persons spread to the lower respiratory tracts of some patients suffering from chronic bronchitis. While there is no evidence that these mycoplasmas are a cause of acute exacerbations, antibody responses to them occur in association with such exacerbations more frequently than at other times, which suggests that the organisms, normally associated with silent infections, are more antigenic during exacerbations. This is probably due to increased mycoplasmal multiplication and participation in tissue damage brought about primarily by viruses and bacteria, and it is tempting to conjecture that in this way the mycoplasmas play some part in perpetuating a chronic condition.

Mycoplasmas in the vagina are rarely transmitted to the infant *in utero*, but they are often transmitted during birth and *U. urealyticum* organisms (ureaplasmas), in particular, may be isolated from the throats and tracheal aspirates of newborns. Ureaplasmas occasionally seem to be the cause of respiratory disease, particularly in very low birth-weight infants (under 1000 g), which have died or have developed chronic lung disease twice as often as uninfected infants of similar birth weight or those of over 1000 g. *M. hominis* has also been implicated in pneumonia soon after birth, albeit even more rarely. Whether *M. genitalium* might be involved is unknown, but the possibility exists because it has been detected in the vagina.

Genitourinary and related infections

Clinical conditions in which there is evidence strongly suggesting that mycoplasmas have an aetiological role, at least in part, will be considered in some detail. Other diseases in which the role of mycoplasmas is minimal, or the evidence for a mycoplasmal cause is weak and/or contentious are mentioned briefly. All are summarized in Table 5.

DIAGNOSIS

Swabs from the urethra or vagina provide a slightly more sensitive means of collecting specimens for mycoplasmal isolation than urine specimens. The basic medium is similar to that described for the isolation of *M. pneumoniae*, the formulation for the isolation of spiroplasmas, mentioned previously, but without thallium acetate, being best for the isolation of *M. genitalium*. Advantage is taken of the metabolic activity of the mycoplasmas (Table 3) in order to detect their growth. Clinical material is added to separate vials of liquid medium containing phenol red and 0.1 per cent glucose, arginine, or urea. *M. genitalium* metabolizes glucose and changes the colour of the medium from red to yellow. *M. fermentans* does this also but, in addition, it converts arginine to ammonia, as do *M. hominis* and *M. primatum*. Ureaplasmas possess a urease that breaks down urea to ammonia too. In each case, the pH of

Table 5 *The association of genital mycoplasmas with human genitourinary, reproductive, and perinatal disease*

Disease	Evidence suggesting a causal relation of: *M. hominis*	*U. urealyticum*	Comments on the relation and proportion of disease attributable to mycoplasmas
Non-gonococcal urethritis (NGU)	None	Strong	The proportion of NGU caused by ureaplasmas may be 10–30%
Urethroprostatitis	None	Some	Ureaplasmas may cause some acute but not chronic disease; *M. hominis* appears not to cause either acute or chronic disease
Epididymitis	None	Some	Ureaplasmas involved in one case of acute disease
Urinary calculi	None	Weak	Experimentally, ureaplasmas cause bladder calculi in male rats but so far little evidence for a cause of natural human disease
Pyelonephritis	Strong	None	*M. hominis* causes some cases of acute pyelonephritis and exacerbations
Reiter's disease	None	Some	Relation based on lymphocytic proliferative response to specific ureaplasmal antigen
Abscess of Bartholin's gland	Very weak	None	Doubtful whether *M. hominis* involved
Vaginitis, vaginosis, and cervicitis	None	None	*M. hominis* and to a lesser extent ureaplasmas associated with bacterial vaginosis, but a causal relation is unproven
Pelvic inflammatory disease	Strong	Weak	*M. hominis* causes a small proportion of cases, but very doubtful that ureaplasmas do
Postabortal fever	Strong	None	*M. hominis* is responsible for some cases, but the proportion is unknown
Postpartum fever	Strong	Some	*M. hominis* and to a much lesser extent ureaplasmas cause some cases
Involuntary infertility	None	None	Ureaplasmas are associated with reduced sperm motility, but a causal relation is unproven
Premature labour	Some	None	*M. hominis* involved, possibly as part of bacterial vaginosis
Spontaneous abortion and stillbirth	None	None	Maternal and fetal infections associated with spontaneous abortion, but a causal relation is unproven
Chorioamnionitis	None	Some	An association exists, but a causal relation is unproven
Low birth weight	None	Some	An association exists in some studies, but a causal relation is unproven

the medium increases and there is a colour change from yellow to red. The colour change produced by ureaplasmas occurs usually within 1 to 2 days, while that for *M. genitalium* may take 50 days or longer. Indeed, it has become clear that attempts to culture this mycoplasma and *M. fermentans* often fail and that they may be detected much more reliably by using PCR technology. When colour changes have occurred in liquid medium, subculture to agar medium results in the formation of colonies of about 200 to 300 μm diameter by most genital mycoplasmas; those of *M. genitalium* are usually smaller but vary in size up to 200 μm. Ureaplasma colonies are small (15–60 μm) (Fig. 7(a)) and, on medium containing manganous sulphate, are brown in colour and, therefore, are detected more easily (Fig. 7(b)). On ordinary blood agar, *M. hominis*, but not ureaplasmas, produces non-haemolytic pinpoint colonies, the nature of which can be established by the methods outlined above. The metabolism-inhibition technique is often used to detect antibodies to *M. hominis* and the ureaplasmas. Specific metabolites (arginine for *M. hominis* and urea for ureaplasmas) are incorporated in liquid medium containing phenol red, organisms, and antibody. The antibody inhibits multiplication and metabolism of homologous organisms, thus preventing a change in colour of the pH indicator. The indirect haemagglutination technique is useful for detecting antibody to *M. hominis*. In addition, a microimmunofluorescence procedure is valuable for measuring antibodies to *M. hominis* and *M. genitalium* but this and other tests such as the enzyme immunoassay tend to be used as research tools only.

Fig. 7 (a) Colony of *Ureaplasma urealyticum* (15 μm diameter) (arrow) adjacent to colonies of *M. hominis* (90 μm dia.) grown from urethral exudate. Oblique light, × 68. (b) Dark colonies of *U. urealyticum* with colonies of *M. hominis* on agar containing manganous sulphate. × 136.

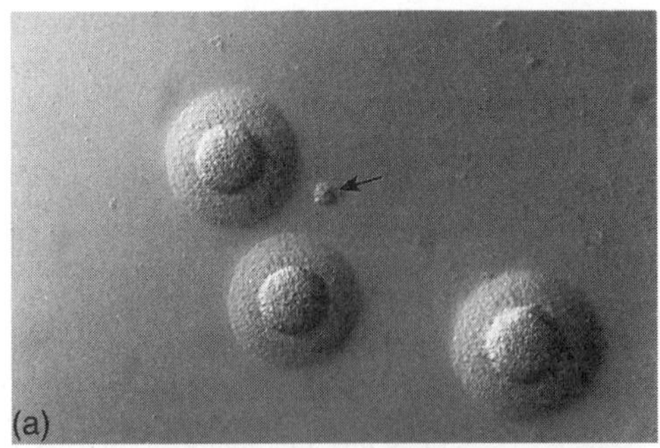

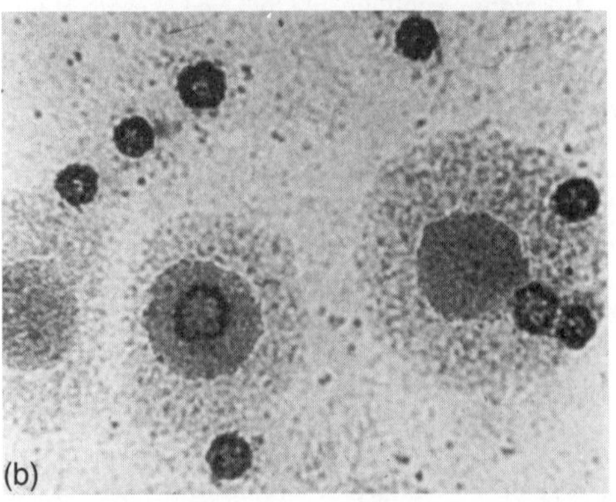

Non-gonococcal urethritis and complications

There have been many studies concerned with the role of large-colony-forming mycoplasmas. It is clear that most of them cannot be considered as significant causes of non-gonococcal urethritis because they are isolated so rarely from the genitourinary tract either in health or disease (Table 3). However, *M. genitalium* (Fig. 8(a)) has now been associated strongly with acute non-gonococcal urethritis, being detected by the PCR in about 20 per cent of such cases but in only 6 per cent of healthy controls. This mycoplasma, like *M. pneumoniae*, adheres to epithelial cells (Fig. 8(b)); it has been detected by a DNA probe and by a PCR in about one-quarter of men with persistent or recurrent non-gonococcal urethritis, and may account for some of these cases. Although *M. hominis* may be isolated from about 20 per cent of patients with acute non-gonococcal urethritis, the results of numerous studies have failed to implicate this mycoplasma as a cause. Nevertheless, the possibility that some cases of non-gonococcal urethritis are associated with bacterial vaginosis in sexual partners in whom *M. hominis* organisms are to be found in large numbers should not be overlooked. Contentious for many years has been the role of ureaplasmas in non-gonococcal urethritis. However, the results of several lines of investigation, discussed below, indicate that they are one of the causes.

ISOLATION STUDIES

One of the difficulties in assessing the significance of ureaplasmas in non-gonococcal urethritis is that they are only one of the potential causes and they need to be evaluated in relation to other micro-organisms, such as chlamydiae, a complex situation of which earlier workers were unaware. Furthermore, the selection of inappropriate controls has probably contributed most to the difference between the result of one investigation and another. Ureaplasmas have been isolated significantly more frequently from patients suffering from non-gonococcal urethritis than from subjects apparently free of disease in about half the investigations, whereas the rate of isolation for these two groups has been about the same in the other studies. Certainly, their failure to provide a clear-cut answer to the problem of ureaplasmal pathogenicity should deter future investigators from pursuing studies that are not quantitative in nature. If ureaplasmas are involved in the pathogenic process, it would be reasonable to expect them to be present in larger numbers than if they were behaving only as commensals; a few workers have provided quantitative data to support this idea.

Fig. 8 (a) Electron micrograph of *M. genitalium*, negatively stained, to show flask-shaped appearance and terminal specialized structure (arrow). × 90 000. (b) *M. genitalium* adhering to Vero cell by the terminal structure. × 60 000. (Figures 8(a) and 8(b) reproduced from Tully *et al.* (1983). *International Journal of Systematic Bacteriology*, **33**, 387, with permission.)

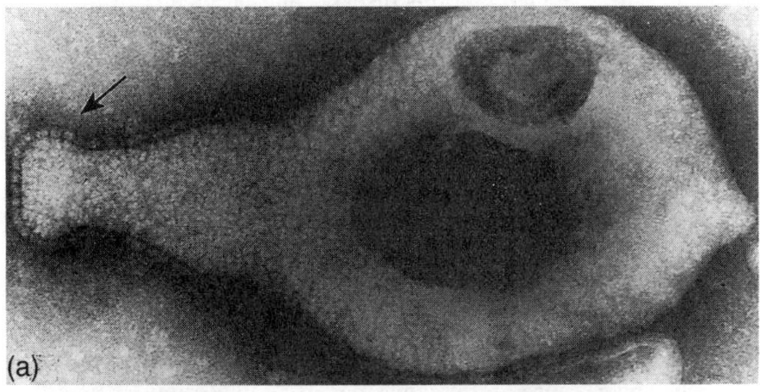

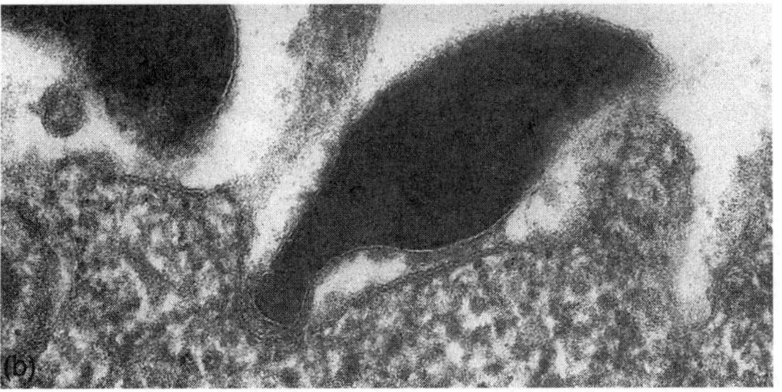

ANTIMICROBIAL THERAPY

Antimicrobials have been used in several ways to assess the role of ureaplasmas in non-gonococcal urethritis. Suboptimal doses of doxycycline have caused a temporary disappearance of both symptoms and ureaplasmas from the urine, the return of symptoms being accompanied by reappearance of the organisms in numbers similar to those found before treatment. Placebo-controlled trials of tetracycline in conjunction with comprehensive microbiological investigations have been few, but in one such trial there was a significant association between minocycline therapy and the resolution of symptoms and signs in patients from whom only ureaplasmas had been isolated. The association was only a little less convincing than that seen between therapy and resolution of disease in patients from whom only chlamydiae had been isolated. Antimicrobials that differentiate between ureaplasmas and other potentially pathogenic micro-organisms have been used. Thus, urethritis in men who harboured chlamydiae and ureaplasmas was unaffected by treatment with aminocyclitols (streptomycin and spectinomycin), which eradicated ureaplasmas only, and, similarly, treatment with sulphafurazole, which eliminated chlamydiae only, was ineffective. Patients have been treated also with minocycline or rifampicin, the former being active against both micro-organisms but the latter against chlamydiae only. A larger proportion of patients responded to minocycline than to rifampicin, and those infected with ureaplasmas failed to respond to rifampicin significantly more often than those who were not infected. These findings would be difficult to explain if ureaplasmas had no involvement in non-gonococcal urethritis. About 10 per cent of ureaplasmas are resistant to tetracyclines and the urethritis of some patients infected by them responds only to treatment with antimicrobials, such as erythromycin, to which the organisms are susceptible.

ANIMAL MODELS AND HUMAN EXPERIMENTATION

Some ureaplasma strains, unpassaged in the laboratory, have produced urethritis and an antibody response in male chimpanzees inoculated intraurethrally. Furthermore, three investigators who inoculated themselves intraurethrally each developed urethritis. In one detailed study, two of them received 5×10^4 ureaplasma organisms, of serotype 5, which had been isolated from a patient with non-gonococcal urethritis in whom no other potentially pathogenic micro-organisms could be detected, although *M. genitalium* was not sought at that time. The first subject developed urethritis characterized by dysuria, frequency, urethral discomfort, and pyuria. Ureaplasmas were isolated consistently from urine, but they and the associated symptoms and signs disappeared during treatment with minocycline. The second subject had evidence of mild urethritis, and, like the first, a transient antibody response, but also urinary threads, containing polymorphonuclear leucocytes, which persisted for at least 6 months after treatment with minocycline had eliminated the organisms from meatal, urine, and semen samples. Before treatment, ureaplasmas were found mostly in fractionated semen samples of prostatic origin, pointing to infection of that organ. These results indicate that some ureaplasmas are likely to be pathogenic under natural conditions and that they may be capable of initiating chronic disease. In this regard, it should be noted that some hypogammaglobulinaemic patients develop a chronic urethrocystitis in which persistent ureaplasmal and/or *M. hominis* infections seem to be responsible.

INTERPRETATION OF THE FINDINGS IN NON-GONOCOCCAL URETHRITIS

C. trachomatis infection (see Chapter 7.11.41) accounts for probably no more than 50 per cent of cases of non-gonococcal urethritis and the question arises of whether ureaplasmal infection fills part of the remaining gap. It would seem unreasonable to take the view that all the results of the studies outlined above are entirely spurious. It seems more rational to believe that these cumulative data are indicative of a pathogenic role for ureaplasmas in the male genital tract. However, if ureaplasmas are a cause of non-gonococcal urethritis, why are they found so often in men without urethritis; and, as they exist so frequently in the female genital tract, why is non-gonococcal urethritis not even more common? Possible explanations may be that: (a) only certain ureaplasma serotypes and/or only a certain number of ureaplasma organisms are pathogenic; (b) ureaplasmas involve only the prepuce and meatus in men without disease but under some circumstances invade the urethra to cause non-gonococcal urethritis, procedures used so far not having distinguished between the different sites of colonization; (c) ureaplasmas produce non-gonococcal urethritis that resolves spontaneously but the organisms then persist; (d) ureaplasmas produce non-gonococcal urethritis but those within the prostate and paraurethral glands are not always eliminated by treatment and are sometimes detected in the urethra; and (e) ureaplasmas cause only the first or early episodes of non-gonococcal urethritis, later encounters resulting in colonization without urethritis. These suggestions may not be mutually exclusive. It is not clear how much the newly suggested role for *M. genitalium* confuses the picture but studies designed to resolve the part played by ureaplasmas in non-gonococcal urethritis should take into account all potential pathogenic micro-organisms and be quantitative rather than qualitative in nature. Meanwhile, it should be emphasized that testing for ureaplasmas on a routine basis is not profitable, as positive results, so easy to obtain, are difficult for the clinician to interpret and use in patient management.

Ureaplasmas are a rare cause of acute non-chlamydial epididymitis, the organisms having been recovered from the urethra and directly from epididymal aspirate fluid, accompanied by a specific antibody response. Information suggesting that the prostate becomes infected during the course of an acute ureaplasmal infection of the urethra is scanty, although ureaplasmas have been isolated more frequently and in greater numbers from patients with acute urethroprostatitis than from controls, and most of those with more than 10^3 organisms in expressed prostatic fluid responded to tetracycline therapy. In contrast, ureaplasmas have not been found in prostatic biopsy specimens from patients with chronic abacterial prostatitis, and, in most studies, *M. hominis* has not been associated with prostatitis of any kind.

Pyelonephritis

M. hominis has been isolated, sometimes in pure culture, from the upper urinary tract of almost 10 per cent of patients with acute pyelonephritis. In addition, antibody to *M. hominis*, measured by the indirect haemagglutination technique, has been demonstrated in the serum and urine of some of these patients. In contrast, the mycoplasma has not been found in the upper urinary tract of patients with non-infectious urinary-tract diseases nor has antibody been detected in their urine. The data suggest that *M. hominis* causes a few cases of acute pyelonephritis or acute exacerbations of chronic pyelonephritis and that ureaplasmas are involved less often if at all.

Pelvic inflammatory disease

Micro-organisms present in the vagina and lower cervix may ascend to the normally sterile upper-genital tract and cause inflammation of the fallopian tubes and adjacent pelvic structures. Like non-gonococcal urethritis, non-gonococcal pelvic inflammatory disease does not have a single cause and the possibility that infection by genital mycoplasmas might be one cause has engaged the attention of numerous investigators. Three sorts of evidence indicate that this is so.

M. hominis has figured prominently among more than a dozen reports of the isolation of large-colony-forming mycoplasmas from inflamed fallopian tubes, tubo-ovarian abscesses, and pelvic abscesses or fluid. Swedish workers collected specimens by laparoscopy and found *M. hominis* in the tubes of about 10 per cent of women with salpingitis but not in those of women without signs of the disease, an observation that has found some support with investigators in the United Kingdom. In addition, *M. hominis* has been isolated significantly more often from the cervix and urethra of patients with salpingitis than from those without disease. Hysterosalpingography may occasionally stimulate inflammation of the fallopian tubes in women who carry *M. hominis* in the lower genital tract. Whether this is apt to occur particularly in women who have large numbers of *M. hominis* organisms in the vagina as a consequence of bacterial vaginosis and, indeed, whether the latter is, in general, a stimulus to the development of pelvic inflammatory disease are moot points.

Ureaplasmas have been studied less intensively, but they have been isolated directly from the fallopian tubes of a very small proportion of patients with acute salpingitis, from pelvic fluid, and from a tubo-ovarian abscess. *M. pneumoniae* is reported to have been isolated also from such an abscess. The significance of these findings is unclear but it would seem that ureaplasmas are of little consequence and certainly likely to be of far less importance than *M. hominis*. The availability of a PCR for *M. genitalium* should now make it possible to establish whether this mycoplasma is involved in pelvic inflammatory disease.

SEROLOGICAL STUDIES

Several workers have found *M. hominis* complement-fixing antibody titres to be greater in the serum of some patients with salpingitis than in that of other women serving as controls. Antibody to this mycoplasma was found by Swedish workers, who used the more sensitive indirect haemagglutination technique, in about half the patients with salpingitis but in only 10 per cent of healthy women. Furthermore, a significant rise or fall in antibody titre occurred during the course of disease in more than half of the women who had *M. hominis* in the lower genital tract. Others found that patients with gonococcal pelvic inflammatory disease were more likely to respond to *M. hominis* than those without such disease; they suggested that damage incurred by the gonococci was a factor in the serological response and questioned the primary role of *M. hominis*. However, a response to *M. hominis* has been seen quite often in women in whom gonococci were not the cause of pelvic inflammation. In addition, a significant antibody response to *M. genitalium* has been detected in about one-third of women with pelvic inflammatory disease in whom antibody responses to *M. hominis* and chlamydiae could not be detected.

Antibody responses to *U. urealyticum* have been detected less often than responses to *M. hominis* in patients with pelvic inflammatory disease. This is consistent with the impression that ureaplasmas are less important than *M. hominis* in this disease, but the greater difficulty of detecting antibody responses to ureaplasmas has to be recognized.

ORGAN CULTURE AND ANIMAL MODELS

Organ cultures, in which tissues can be maintained in a condition similar to that *in vivo*, provide a tool for examining the relation between micro-organisms and the epithelial cell surface. Fallopian-tube organ cultures are particularly useful in this respect because ciliary activity may be assessed and used as an index of cell viability. In such cultures, gonococci destroy the epithelium, whereas *M. hominis* organisms, although multiplying, produce no more than swelling of some of the cilia. No damage has been caused by ureaplasmas of human origin. This differential effect may be a true reflection of the pathogenic potential of these micro-organisms *in vivo*. However, failure to demonstrate damage does not mean necessarily that the organisms are avirulent, because organ-culture studies are not able to account for the part that the host immune system may play in pathogenesis. Studies in intact animals may be helpful in elucidating this aspect. It is of interest, therefore, that the introduction of *M. hominis* into the oviducts of grivet monkeys and *M. genitalium* into the oviducts of these monkeys, as well as those of marmosets, resulted in a self-limited acute salpingitis and parametritis with an antibody response, whereas ureaplasmas had no effect.

These various data indicate that *M. hominis* and perhaps *M. genitalium* have a primary pathogenic role in some cases of acute pelvic inflammatory disease.

Postabortal fever

The results of various studies suggest a role for *M. hominis* in fever after abortion (see Section 13). Thus, this mycoplasma has been isolated from the blood of about 10 per cent of women who had such fever but not from afebrile women who had abortions, nor from normal pregnant women. In addition, a rise in the titre of antibody to *M. hominis* has been detected in half the women who become febrile but in only a small proportion of those who have abortions and remain afebrile. Thus, the evidence indicates that *M. hominis* causes some cases of postabortal fever but there is none to suggest that ureaplasmas do likewise, possibly because studies have not been focused on this micro-organism. Patients recover whether or not they receive appropriate antimicrobial treatment.

Postpartum fever

Like other micro-organisms in the vagina, genital mycoplasmas have been found transiently in the blood after normal vaginal delivery. In one study, the blood of about 8 per cent of women contained mycoplasmas, mostly ureaplasmas, a few minutes after delivery, but the organisms did not persist and were not associated with postpartum fever. However, there have been many reports of individual patients with postpartum fever from whose blood *M. hominis* has been isolated a day or more after delivery, and in whom an antibody response has been detected. In fact the organisms have been isolated from the blood of 5 to 10 per cent of such women and, as they are seldom recovered from the blood of afebrile postpartum women, the inference is that *M. hominis* induces postpartum fever. The patients have a low-grade fever for a day or two after delivery, are not severely ill, and recover uneventfully without antibiotic therapy. Whether fever occurs predominantly in women who have bacterial vaginosis in which there is proliferation of *M. hominis* together with various bacteria in the vagina has not been resolved, nor has the contribution of *M. hominis* relative to that of the other micro-organisms.

Joint infections

Rheumatoid arthritis

The knowledge that mycoplasmas cause several animal arthritides, and that gold salts inactivate mycoplasmas and have a beneficial effect on rheumatoid arthritis, provided the impetus to search for mycoplasmas in the joints of persons suffering from this disease. However, attempts over almost 40 years by more than 20 investigators to detect mycoplasmas in rheumatoid synovial fluids or tissues either failed or produced inconsistent and unrepeatable results. There seems no doubt that the rheumatoid joint is not the source of those mycoplasmas (*M. hyorhinis, M. hominis*) that were recovered by means of tissue-culture techniques, these being nothing more than culture contaminants. The case made in the late 1960s and early 1970s, based on apparent isolation and immunological observations, that *M. fermentans* was important in the pathogenesis of rheumatoid arthritis has not been substantiated. However, the advent of PCR technology would appear to offer a further and perhaps more definitive approach to resolving any possible association between mycoplasmas and rheumatoid arthritis.

M. pneumoniae *and other mycoplasmal infections*

A feature of the mycoplasmal arthritides of animals is that the mycoplasmas isolated from the joints are found also in the respiratory tract. The question must arise, therefore, of whether the known respiratory pathogenic mycoplasma of man, namely *M. pneumoniae*, causes arthritis. In this regard, there is no doubt that infection is often accompanied by non-specific arthralgia or myalgia (Table 4) during the acute phase, and occasionally it leads to migratory polyarthritis affecting middle-sized joints in adults. This mycoplasma may be implicated also in some cases of Still's disease, either as an initiating factor or in exacerbations of existing disease; this notion is based on the demonstration of a fourfold or greater rise in antibody titre or a single high titre and not on isolation of *M. pneumoniae* organisms from joints, although in immunologically deficient patients isolation has been successful (see below).

M. hominis has been isolated from septic hip joints that have developed in patients after childbirth. The arthritis responds to tetracycline therapy and the diagnosis should be considered in a postpartum arthritis which is unaffected by penicillin.

Reiter's disease (see also Section 21)

Several investigators have considered the possibility that arthritis following or concomitant with sexually transmissible, non-gonococcal urethritis (sexually acquired reactive arthritis; **SARA**) or arthritis, conjunctivitis and urethritis (Reiter's disease) might be due to mycoplasmal infection. It is clear, however, that the problems encountered in defining the role of mycoplasmas in non-gonococcal urethritis are no less apparent when considering these complications. An important difficulty in investigating such patients is that often they have been treated with antimicrobials before microbiological investigations can be attempted. Despite this, several workers have isolated *M. hominis* and/or ureaplasmas from the genital tract of patients with reactive arthritis as frequently as from those suffering from uncomplicated non-gonococcal urethritis, although this does not indicate that the organisms are a cause of the complications. A further problem is the involvement of *C. trachomatis*, which is capable of initiating the pathological events in about 50 per cent of genetically predisposed men and a proportion of women who develop SARA or Reiter's disease, that is in those who are HLA-B27 positive. The initiating factor in the others is unknown but the possible role of ureaplasmas should not be ignored in view of their implication in uncomplicated non-gonococcal urethritis. In this respect, arthritis has been seen to develop in untreated patients with non-gonococcal urethritis from whom ureaplasmas, but not chlamydiae, were isolated from the urethra. The organisms have not been isolated from synovial fluids or tissues but synovial lymphocytes from some patients have been shown to proliferate *in vitro* in response to ureaplasmal antigens. Although such data are provocative, further evidence is required to establish convincingly a link between ureaplasmas and SARA or Reiter's disease.

Arthritis in hypogammaglobulinaemic patients

Arthritis of mycoplasmal aetiology (Fig. 9) should be considered in hypogammaglobulinaemic patients (see Section 4) who develop an abacterial septic arthritis. Thus, *M. pneumoniae* (in one instance together with *M. genitalium*), *M. hominis*, *M. salivarium*, and, in particular, ureaplasmas have been isolated from synovial fluids of a small proportion of these patients. The organisms were recovered in such a way as to indicate that they were derived from the inflamed joints and were not spurious laboratory contaminants. The arthritis usually responds to tetracyclines or other antimicrobials to which the organisms are sensitive, an indication that they are a cause of the disease. Intravenous therapy may be required and administration of antiserum prepared specifically against the organism in question may be helpful in the few patients whose disease does not respond to antimicrobial therapy.

Conditions of rare or equivocal mycoplasmal aetiology

The occurrence of *M. hominis* or ureaplasmas in cerebrospinal fluid from cases of neonatal meningitis or brain abscess is due presumably to infection *in utero* or to colonization at birth with subsequent infection. This is a rare event but should be considered in cases of neonatal disease of the central nervous system in which the results of bacteriological staining and culture are negative.

M. hominis organisms, apart from inducing fever after abortion or normal childbirth, have been associated with fever attributed to burns and trauma, and have been implicated in some wound infections. These organisms are found in large numbers in the vaginas of women who have bacterial vaginosis. If they have any role in the pathogenesis of this condition, it is only together with a variety of bacteria, which are found also in profusion. *M. hominis* has been associated with premature labour but in view of the fact that this pregnancy outcome has been associated strongly with bacterial vaginosis, the involvement of this mycoplasma would seem to be as part of the bacterial vaginosis syndrome.

Fig. 9 (a) Damage to the knee joint of a hypogammaglobulinaemic patient caused by *U. urealyticum* infection. (b) Sinus connected with the shoulder joint of a hypogammaglobulinaemic patient; ureaplasmas were isolated repeatedly from the sinus exudate. (By courtesy of A.D.B. Webster.)

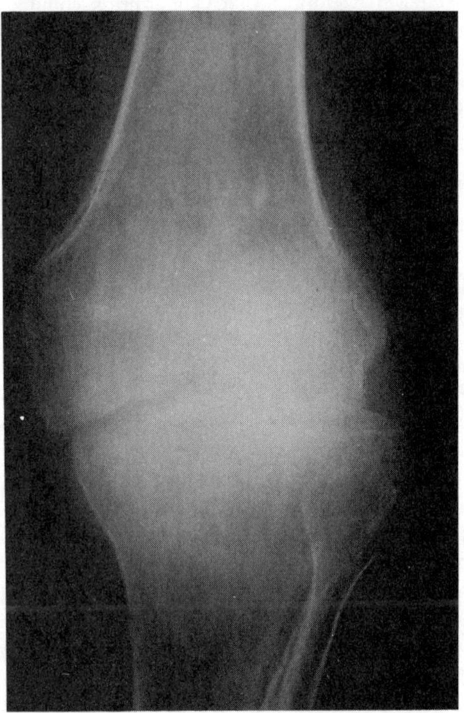

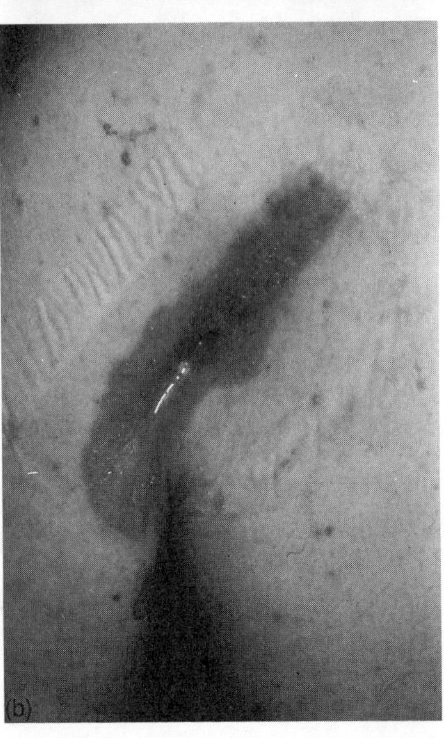

The results of studies on the role of ureaplasmas in urinary calculi and in infertility, particularly among a subgroup of women whose problem is associated with a male factor, are provocative, and ureaplasmas have been associated also with chorioamnionitis, spontaneous abortion, and low birth weight. It is noteworthy, however, that like *M. hominis* organisms, ureaplasmas are found in larger numbers in the vagina of women with bacterial vaginosis than in those without disease. Thus, it is worthy of consideration that, in the reproductive problems referred to, ureaplasmas are involved only or predominantly as part of the bacterial vaginosis syndrome and that to consider them alone may be misleading.

Association of mycoplasmas with AIDS

Differences in the interval between acquiring the human immunodeficiency virus, type 1 (**HIV-1**) and developing symptoms and further disease, together with the low frequency of HIV-infected lymphocytes in the peripheral blood, led to the proposal that additional factors are required to bring about the profound loss of CD4+ T cells inherent in the pathogenesis of AIDS. Irrespective of whether this notion has validity or not, the idea that mycoplasmas might act as a cofactor, enhancing virus replication and accelerating disease progression, was fuelled by studies *in vitro*. In these, treatment of HIV-infected cell cultures with tetracyclines or fluoroquinolones, active against mycoplasmas, inhibited cell killing without affecting virus replication. In other studies, certain mycoplasmas (*M. fermentans*, *A. laidlawii*) enhanced cytopathic changes by HIV-1. Such *in vitro* observations were preceded by those on *M. fermentans in vivo*. Attempts to indicate a virus in Kaposi's sarcoma tissue culminated in the recovery of a mycoplasma in cell culture, possibly a cell-culture contaminant, which was termed initially '*M. incognitus*', but identified later as *M. fermentans*. Antibody prepared against this mycoplasma, together with observations by electron microscopy, were instrumental in demonstrating that *M. fermentans* was distributed widely in tissues taken at autopsy from AIDS patients. Subsequently, it was shown to be linked strongly with AIDS-associated nephropathy and, more recently, was found by some workers, who used PCR technology, in blood leucocyte preparations from HIV-positive but not HIV-negative individuals and in urine samples from HIV-positive patients exclusively. Other workers claimed to have cultured not only *M. fermentans* from the blood of a few HIV-positive men, but also *M. pirum*, hitherto detected only as a contaminant in cell cultures; in addition, they detected *M. genitalium* by means of a PCR.

More recent events in a rapidly developing field of investigation have been as follows. Some investigators, who used a PCR, detected *M. fermentans* in the blood, throat, and urine of 10, 23, and 8 per cent of HIV-seropositive patients, respectively, almost all of whom were homosexual men. These patients probably had the mycoplasma before they acquired the virus because the mycoplasma was detected with similar frequency in samples taken from HIV-seronegative patients, a large proportion of whom were homosexual men, attending a sexually transmitted disease clinic (9, 20, and 6 per cent for blood, throat, and urine, respectively). The existence of mycoplasmas in the blood increases the chance of interaction with the immune system; cytokines so induced could enhance HIV replication with increased loss of CD4+ cells, in this way the mycoplasma acting as a cofactor. However, no association was found between infection by *M. fermentans* and the stage of the disease, the patients' CD4+ count or the viral load. This does not eliminate the possibility that a mycoplasmal infection could influence the speed of disease progression. Whether this is so or not will be addressed best by longitudinal studies of HIV-positive patients with and without concurrent mycoplasmal infection.

A further finding of interest has been the isolation of a previously unknown mycoplasma, now termed *M. penetrans*, from urine sediments of a small number of homosexual men infected with HIV-1, most of whom had AIDS. This mycoplasma is highly invasive of eukaryotic cells, and antibody to it, detected by an enzyme-linked immunosorbent assay, was found in the sera of 40 per cent of AIDS patients, but in only 0.3 per cent of HIV-seronegative subjects, 0.9 per cent of subjects attending sexually transmitted disease clinics, and in none of a group of patients with other immune dysfunctions. The apparent association of *M. penetrans* with HIV infection and AIDS, and the significance of this association, undoubtedly warrant continued investigation.

REFERENCES

Cassell, G.H. and Cole, B.C. (1981). Mycoplasmas as agents of human disease. *New England Journal of Medicine*, **304**, 80–9.

Maniloff, J. (ed.) (1992). *Mycoplasmas. Molecular biology and pathogenesis*. American Society for Microbiology, Washington, DC.

Murray, H.W., Masur, H., Senterfit, L.B., and Roberts, R.B. (1975). The protean manifestations of *Mycoplasma pneumoniae* infections in adults. *American Journal of Medicine*, **58**, 229–42.

Taylor-Robinson, D. (1989). Genital mycoplasma infections. In *Clinics in laboratory medicine. Sexually transmitted diseases*, (ed. F.N. Judson), Vol. 9, pp. 501–23. Saunders, Philadelphia.

Taylor-Robinson, D., and McCormack, W.M. (1980). The genital mycoplasmas. *New England Journal of Medicine*, **302**, 1003–10; 1063–7.

Taylor-Robinson, D., and Taylor, G. (1976) Do mycoplasmas cause rheumatic disease? In *Infection and immunology in the rheumatic diseases*, (ed. D.C. Dumonde), pp. 177–86. Blackwell Scientific, Oxford.

Tully, J.G., and Whitcomb, R.F. (ed.) (1979) *The mycoplasmas*, Vol. 2, *Human and animal mycoplasmas*. Academic Press, London.

Tully, J.G., Rose, D.L., Whitcomb, R.F., and Wenzel, R.P. (1979). Enhanced isolation of *Mycoplasma pneumoniae* from throat washings with a newly modified culture medium. *Journal of Infectious Diseases*, **139**, 478–82.

7.11.44 Bartonellosis

E. A. Llanos-Cuentas, C. Maguiña-Vargas, and D. A. Warrell

Definition

Bartonellosis (Carrión's disease, verruga peruana, Oroya fever, Guaitará fever) is a non-contagious infectious disease, which is endemic in the western Andes and interAndean valleys of Peru and occasionally has been reported in Colombia and Ecuador. The acute stage is characterized by infection of red blood cells leading to anaemia; in the late stage the patients develop dermal nodules, which are called 'verrugas'. This disease produces a temporary, reversible immunosuppression in the host, which explains why secondary opportunistic infections are common.

Aetiological agent

Barton, a Peruvian physician, described the causative organism in 1905. *Bartonella bacilliformis* is a small, motile, aerobic, Gram-negative bacillus that stains deep red or purple with Giemsa (Fig. 1). This haemotropic bacterium varies in morphology and quantity during various stages of the disease. In spite of being a pleomorphic organism, two essential types are distinguishable: bacilli or rod-shaped forms and coccoid forms. Rod-shaped forms predominate in the acute stage of the disease and coccoid in the convalescent stage. *B. bacilliformis* may occur in or on erythrocytes (Fig. 2) or in endothelial cells of infected human beings. The organism is 2 to 3 μm long and 0.2 to 2.5 μm thick. In cultures, 1 to 10 flagella 3 to 10 μm long may originate from one end of the organism. Bartonella can be cultured in blood-containing semisolid medium, or protease peptone containing rabbit serum and haemoglobin at 28 °C under aerobic conditions.

Epidemiology

The disease has occurred since preColumbian times, as proven by artistic representations in preInca potteries. Bartonellosis is an endemic disease mainly in narrow river valleys and canyons usually in west Andean and sometimes in interAndean valleys of the central and east Andes of Peru (Fig. 3). Outbreaks have been described in similar areas in Colombia (in 1939) and in Zumba, Ecuador (Fig. 4). It occurs between 500 and 3200 m above sea level. There are high and low transmission seasons yearly and interepidemic periods occur every 10 to 15 years. Transmission is greatest towards the end of the rainy season (March to May). In recent years, human infections by haemotropic bacteria have been described in Thailand, Sudan, the United States, and Niger. A human case of infection by rickettsial Eperythrozoon has been reported from the former Yugoslavia. Although the organisms are clearly distinct from *B. bacilliformis*, these diseases showed intriguing clinical parallels, with extra- or intraerythrocytic bacteria.

In endemic areas the disease appears in childhood and usually produces few symptoms. Outsiders generally develop acute, severe forms

Fig. 1 Smear of peripheral blood with red blood cells parasitized by coccoid forms of *Bartonella bacilliformis* (Wright's stain: × 1048). (Reproduced by courtesy of Professor Juan Takano Moron.)

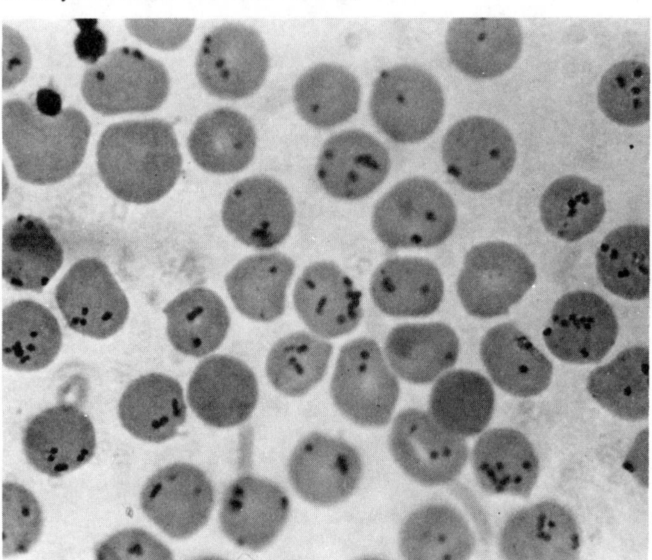

Fig. 2 Ultrastructure of coccobacillary form of *B. bacilliformis* in a red blood cell (× 31 915): mc, cell membrane; N, nucleus; C, cytoplasm; pb, bacterial cell wall. (Reproduced by courtesy of Professor Juan Takano Moron.)

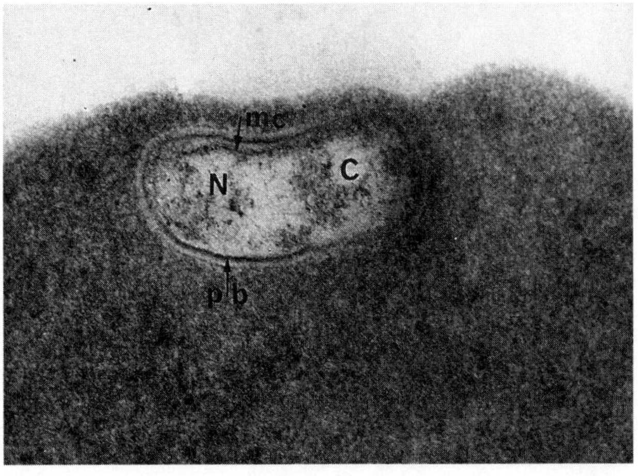

of the disease (Oroya fever). Large epidemics have occurred when large groups of non-residents enter endemic areas. In 1870 an epidemic involved the personnel engaged in building the railroad from Lima to Oroya (Fig. 5); estimated mortality was 7000. Infection results from the bite of female sandflies, *Lutzomyia verrucarum* and other species. The vectors are closely associated with human dwellings and, because they are active during twilight hours, man acquires bartonellosis in the hours near sunrise and sunset. The reservoir is unknown. Herrer isolated *B. bacilliformis* from a *Phyllotis andinum* and donkeys in the endemic area. Horses and mules with 'verrugas' have been reported. In endemic areas some healthy people have positive blood cultures.

Fig. 3 Endemic area for bartonellosis, Rimac Valley, Peru (by courtesy of Professor David H. Molyneux, Liverpool).

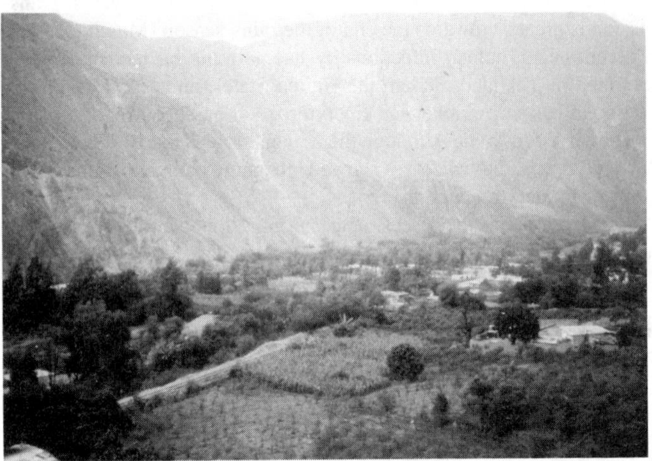

Fig. 4 Geographical distribution of bartonellosis.

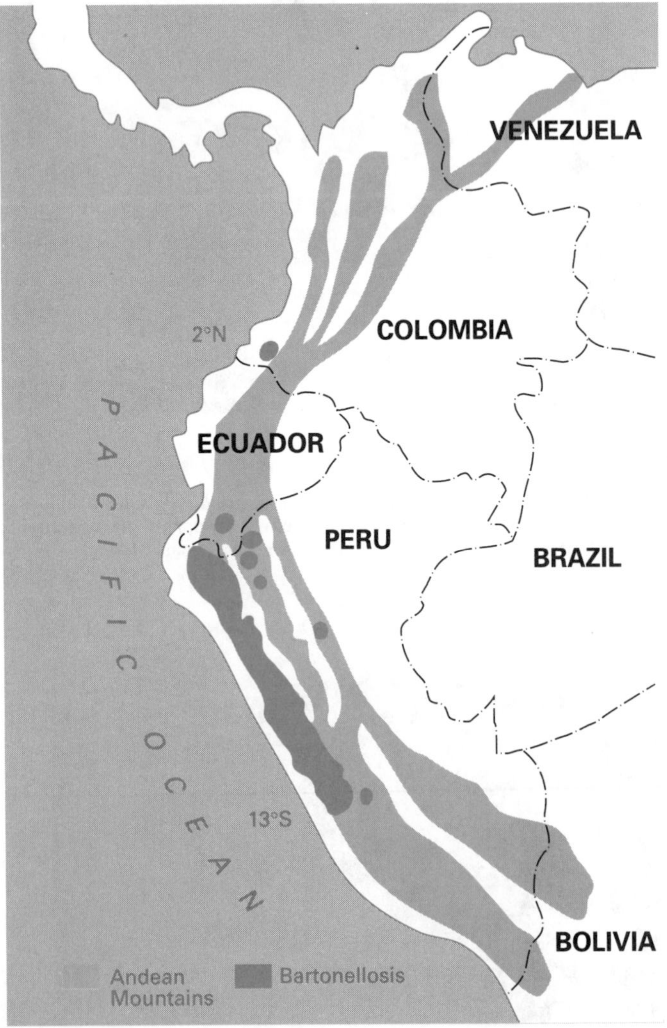

Pathogenesis

After inoculation of *B. bacilliformis* through a sandfly bite, the bacteria multiply in endothelial cells of small vessels, and phagocytic cells near the skin. Systemic invasion and multiplication in endothelial cells and red blood cells follows. In the most serious cases, 95 to 100 per cent of red cells are infected with numerous bacteria. The hallmark of the disease is the severe anaemia caused by massive infection of red blood cells and subsequent erythrophagocytosis. Several mechanisms contribute to anaemia: increased fragility, form and size alterations, reduced half-life of infected and non-infected red cells. Some inhibition of haemoglobin synthesis, probably induced by toxic factors, has also been invoked, since red-cell production increases dramatically with reduction of bacteraemia. Erythrophagocytosis contributes to lymphadenopathy and hepatosplenomegaly. 'Blockade' of the mononuclear phagocytic system and the presence of free circulating iron leads to superinfection, usually by enterobacteria, during the anaemia stage or early recovery from it. Recently, transient depression of cellular immunity has been reported. During the anaemic phase, mild lymphopenia with a reduction of OKT4, a mild increase of OKT8, and decrease of the polyclonal stimulation of the lymphocytes occurs.

A few weeks to months after the acute illness has subsided, the cutaneous form, 'verruga peruana' may develop (Fig. 6). The vascular skin lesions show endothelial proliferation and histiocytic hyperplasia (the cells contain degenerate organisms; Fig. 7) and later show fibrosis and necrosis. Electron microscopy of verrucous tissue shows *B. bacilliformis* in the interstitial tissues, indicating that the presence of the bacteria is important for this unusual vascular response to occur. 'Verruga peruana' results from persistent infection, a probably insufficient immune response, and a peculiar vascular reaction, which could be caused by bacterial products as an angiogenic factor.

In 1885, D.A. Carrión, a Peruvian medical student, linked both phases of the disease by self-experimentation and died.

Clinical features

The disease has two stages, anaemic and eruptive, with an asymptomatic intermediate period. After an incubation period of around 60 days (range 10 to 210 days), non-specific prodromal symptoms appear: onset is usually gradual with malaise, mild chills, fever, and headache. Occasion-

Fig. 5 'Puente verrugas' at an altitude of 1800 m above sea level near Lima, Peru (by courtesy of Mr E. J. Perez).

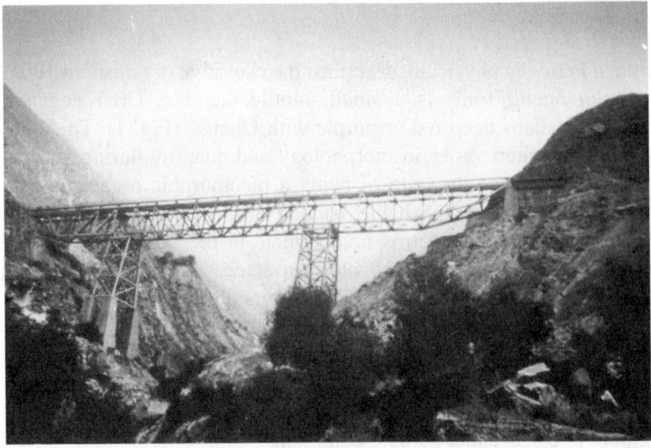

ally, high fever may develop rapidly or build up over a few days. It is accompanied by sweating and rigors. Common symptoms include weakness, aching of the head, back, and extremities, prostration, and depression. The clinical picture is dominated by severe (haemolytic) anaemia: the patients rapidly become pale, dyspnoeic, and jaundiced. There may be hepatosplenomegaly, generalized lymphadenopathy, pericardial effusion, exudates, and retinal haemorrhages in the fundus; and sometimes generalized oedema, a fine vesicular or petechial rash, and exceptionally meningoencephalomyelitis. The duration of this state is variable (generally 2–4 weeks). In pregnant women, the disease in this phase may cause abortion, fetal death, and transplacental transmission of the disease; maternal death is common.

In the intermediate period the patients are asymptomatic and recover from the anaemia through great bone marrow activity. This pre-eruptive period varies from weeks to months.

In the eruptive stage, many nodular lesions of varying size appear on the face, trunk, and limbs, during a period of one or more months and usually persist for 3 to 4 months. There is accompanying mild arthralgia, myalgia, and sometimes fever. The red or purplish skin lesions vary from papules a few millimetres in diameter to pedunculated or plaque-like lesions a few centimetres across. Most often the eruption is miliary (miliary form) with many haemangioma-like lesions of the dermis (Plate 1). Nodular lesions (nodular form) are larger but fewer and more prominent on the extensor surfaces of arms and legs (Plate 2). They are painless and prone to bleeding, secondary infection, and ulceration. The appearance may resemble haemangioma, granuloma pyogenicum, Kaposi's or fibrosarcoma, leprosy (hystioid form), or yaws. Occasionally one to a few, large, deep-seated lesions that often ulcerate (mular form) develop. These tend to appear near joints, where they may be painful and limit motion. Apart from skin, the mucous membranes of the mouth, conjunctiva and nose, serous cavities, and the gastrointestinal and genitourinary tracts may be involved. The eruptive phase tends to heal spontaneously, although the course is often prolonged. Inhabitants of endemic areas usually develop the eruptive stage as the sole manifestation of the disease.

Fig. 6 Histological section of miliary skin lesion of 'verruga peruana', a sessile or partly pedunculated molluscum-like lesion (Armed Forces Institute of Pathology photograph negative no. 77355).

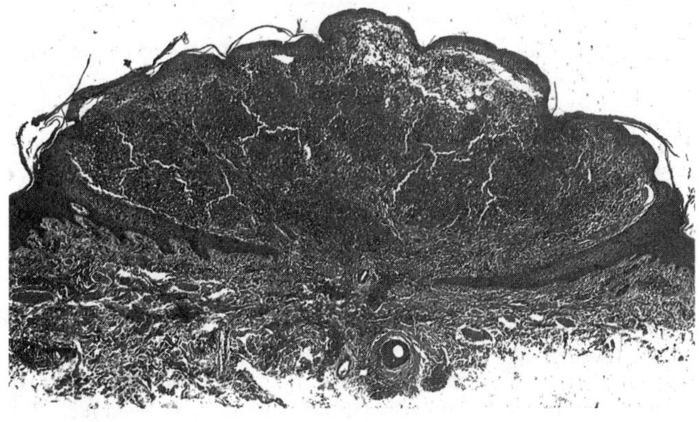

Fig. 7 Electron micrograph of a vascular skin lesion (verruga peruana) showing six *B. bacilliformis* in the fibrillar intertitial matrix (FIM). The bacteria show their cell wall, cell membrane, and internal structure. The clear cytoplasm of a histiocyte (H) is also seen. (Reproduced by courtesy of Professor Sixto Pecavarren, Department of Pathology, UPCH and HBCH.)

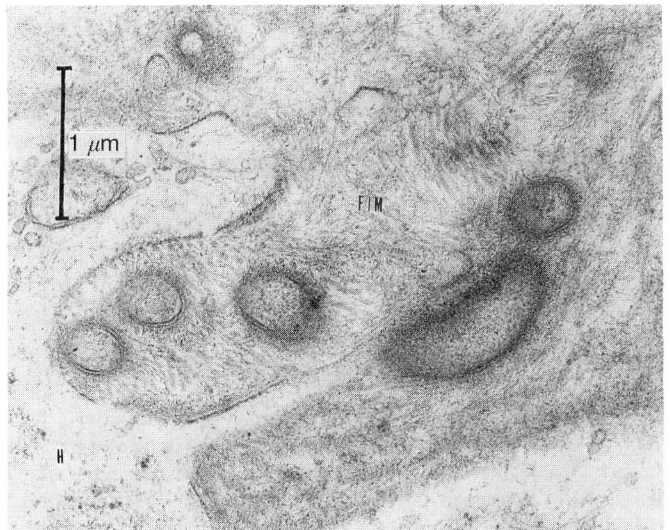

The principal complication is superinfection, leading to septicaemia, which occurs at different stages of the disease but generally in the later part of the anaemic stage and during the intermediate stage. Formerly, *Salmonella typhi*, *S. typhimurium*, *S. dublin*, *Mycobacterium tuberculosis*, and Enterobacter were the most frequent pathogens. Reactivation of tuberculosis, toxoplasmosis, histoplasmosis, pneumonia, and staphylococcal infections are some of the other infections that are now frequent.

Diagnosis

Two elements must be considered: residence in an endemic area and a compatible clinical picture with demonstration of the bacteria in the blood film. Enzyme immunoassay, indirect immunofluorescence, and Western blot are new serological tests that are not generally available.

LABORATORY FEATURES

Bartonella can be isolated from the blood during the anaemic stage and sometimes during the eruptive stage. The enriched media may be positive in 4 to 28 days at 25 to 28 °C. As fever develops, intraerythrocytic bacteria are visible in thick and thin films stained with Giemsa, Wright, or other variants of the Romanovsky stain. Organisms can also be seen and cultivated in the skin lesions of verrucous tissue. The haemolytic anaemia is Coombs' test negative. The blood picture is a macrocytic and hypochromic anaemia with polychromasia, anisocytosis, and poikilocytosis. The reticulocytosis is marked (average 11 per cent). The marrow is hyperactive and megaloblastic with erythrophagocytosis. The white-cell count is not markedly elevated unless there is secondary infection. Thrombocytopenia is quite common. After the crisis the intracellular organisms become coccoid and later disappear, the white-cell count rises, and there is lymphocytosis. Eosinophils, which are usually absent during the acute stage, reappear in peripheral blood differential counts.

Prognosis and treatment

Death is usually during the anaemic phase, and in the preantibiotic era varied between 20 and 95 per cent. At present it is around 8 per cent in patients admitted to hospital. Alterations of consciousness (excitement, stupor, and coma) and progressive or focal neurological features, biochemical evidence of hepatic dysfunction (increased serum glutamic-oxalacetic and -pyruvic transaminases and alkaline phosphatase), pulmonary complications (non-cardiogenic pulmonary oedema), anasarca (severe hypoalbuminaemia), and pregnancy are associated with a higher mortality.

Chloramphenicol, penicillin, erythromycin, co-trimoxazole, norfloxacin, and tetracycline are dramatically effective, usually eliminating the fever in less than 48 h. Because of the common association with salmonellosis, chloramphenicol is the treatment of choice in a dose of 50 mg/kg a day for 7 days. Supportive treatment includes transfusion of packed red cells and dexamethasone (if there is severe neurological involvement). Rifampicin (10 mg/kg a day for 10 days) or streptomycin (15 mg/kg a day for 10 days) are the drugs indicated for treatment of the verrucous form.

Prevention

When transmission is around dwellings, sandflies can be temporarily eliminated by spraying inside and outside with DDT or pyrethroids. Bites usually occur after dusk. They can be prevented by insect repellents, sleeping inside fine-mesh nets, or by avoiding sleeping in highly endemic areas.

REFERENCES

Cuadra, M. (1981). *Bartonella bacilliformis*. In *Medical microbiology and infectious diseases*, (ed. A.I. Braude), p. 510. Saunders, Philadelphia.

Cuadra, M. and Takano, J. (1969). The relationship of *Bartonella bacilliformis* to the red blood cells as revealed by electron microscopy. *Blood*, **33,** 708–16.

Kreier, J.P. and Ristic, M. (1981). The biology of hemotropic bacteria. *Annual Reviews of Microbiology*, **35,** 325–38.

Lumbreras, H. and Guerra, H. (1988). Bartonellosis. In *Tropical medicine and medical parasitology*, (ed. R. Golsmith and D. Heyneman), p. 172–4. Lange Medical, Los Altos CA.

Maguiña, C. and Gotuzzo, E. (1988). La enfermedad de Carrión. *Revista de Enfermedades Infecciosas y de Microbiologia Clínica*, **6,** 432–5.

Puntaric, V. *et al.* (1986). Eperythozoonosis in man. *Lancet*, **ii,** 868–9.

Recavarren, S. and Lumbreras, H. (1972). Pathogenesis of the verruga of Carrion's disease. *American Journal of Pathology*, **66,** 461–4.

7.11.45 Donovanosis (granuloma inguinale)

J. RICHENS

Donovanosis is a sexually transmitted infection characterized chiefly by anogenital and inguinal ulceration. It is rarely encountered outside a handful of endemic foci in the tropics. The cause is an intracellular Gram-negative bacillus called *Calymmatobacterium granulomatis*. The disease was first described in India in 1882 as an 'ulcerating granuloma of the pudenda'. In 1950, Marmell introduced the term donovanosis to replace the older names granuloma venereum and granuloma inguinale, which are often confused with lymphogranuloma venereum. The same Charles Donovan lent his name to both the intracellular amastigotes of lieshmaniasis (Leishman–Donovan bodies) and to the intracellular Gram-negative bacteria that are the pathognomonic feature of donovanosis (Donovan bodies).

Aetiology

Two basic assumptions are made about the aetiology of donovanosis by most authorities. The first is that it is an infectious disease caused by the organisms visualized as intracellular Donovan bodies within lesions. The second is that the organism isolated from donovanosis patients in chick embryo yolk sac initially by Anderson in 1942 and subsequently by others, and currently termed *C. granulomatis*, is identical with those Donovan bodies. The strongest grounds for the first assumption are experimental transmission of the disease from patient to volunteer, the consistent relation between typical clinical lesions and the presence of Donovan bodies, and the disappearance of these bodies with successful antibiotic treatment. Evidence for the identity of *C. granulomatis* with Donovan bodies rests on the close morphological similarity between the two; the isolation of *C. granulomatis* from typical and otherwise sterile lesions of donovanosis, and the demonstration, by complement fixation tests and immunofluorescence, respectively, that patients have high titres of specific antibody that react with both.

Only 14 isolates of *C. granulomatis* have been described in the published literature, the last in 1962. Studies of these isolates have established little beyond the fact that it is a Gram-negative organism which will not grow on solid media, that it is sensitive to many broad-spectrum antibiotics *in vitro*, that it produces a capsule, and that it appears to share antigens with *Klebsiella* spp. Experimental inoculations with these bacteria are non-pathogenic to animals and, in a human subject, produced only subclinical infection.

Epidemiology

The main endemic areas for donovanosis are currently Papua New Guinea, India, particularly in the south-east, South Africa, and Brazil. Even in these countries it rarely accounts for more than 5 per cent of genital ulcers, exceptions being Papua New Guinea (50 per cent of genital ulcers in some areas) and Durban (10–20 per cent). Smaller foci have been reported in Central America, the Caribbean, the Guianas, Argentina, Zambia, Zimbabwe, Malaysia, Vietnam, China, and among Australian aboriginals. With the notable exception of South Africa, donovanosis appears to be retreating in many parts of the world. The most striking example of this is the southern United States, where thousands of cases used to occur every year. This decline been largely attributed to improved living conditions and the availability of antibiotics.

The likelihood of being infected with donovanosis appears to depend on a combination of social, environmental, and genetic factors. The disease is particularly associated with low socioeconomic status, poor hygiene, and prostitution. Dark-skinned races appear to show increased susceptibility, though this may simply reflect socioeconomic status. Many individuals do not develop the infection in spite of repeated and prolonged exposure to an infected, untreated, regular partner. The highest reported rates of infection in partners of donovanosis patients have been just over 50 per cent; many studies report much lower figures. In the exceptional circumstances of the donovanosis epidemic that affected Marind-Anim of Dutch New Guinea in the 1920s up to 30 per cent of adults became infected through ritual homosexual and heterosexual promiscuity. It has not been established whether any form of carrier state exists. The predilection of donovanosis for the genitalia of sexually active persons and its association with other sexually transmitted disease argue strongly for a sexual mode of transmission but patients may transfer the infection to extragenital sites by autoinoculation and rare instances of non-sexual and perinatal transmission have been recorded. Goldberg has isolated *C. granulomatis* from faeces on a single occasion and put forward arguments for non-sexual transmission.

Pathogenesis

Human experimental data suggest that transmission requires direct contact with an infected lesion and cannot occur through intact skin. The organism appears to have a special tropism for dermal macrophages, in which it seems able to avoid damage by lysosomal enzymes and toxic oxygen metabolites. The response to infection is characterized by vigorous granulomatous inflammation that damages the skin and subcutaneous tissues. Extension of the infection is predominantly a local process of spreading ulceration. The frequent inguinal lesions are probably seeded by lymphatic spread but, in general, involvement of lymphatics and lymph nodes in donovanosis is much less prominent than in lymphogranuloma venereum. Haematogenous dissemination and spread to the upper genital tract of women occur exceptionally and demonstrate the organism's ability to survive in deeper tissues. Lesions in women tend to be more extensive and may progress rapidly during pregnancy.

Clinical features

The best estimates of the incubation period range from 3 to 40 days. The first sign of infection is the development of a small papule, which then ulcerates. The small early lesion, like other forms of genital ulcer, is most common on the distal penis in men and near the introitus in women, and is not easily differentiated from other genital lesions. If the lesion is allowed to progress, certain distinctive features may become apparent. These are a deep red colour, contact bleeding, low levels of pain and tenderness unless secondary infection is present, a well-defined, rolled edge, and, quite frequently, elevation above the level of the surrounding skin. Lesions, even of short duration, are often accompanied by local oedema, particularly in women. Many variants of donovanosis have been described. These include dry, warty, hypertrophic lesions with a cobblestone appearance; painful, excavated ulcers; lesions with an ill-defined edge showing diffuse subcutaneous infiltration. Chronic lesions tend to expand gradually along skin folds and across to apposed skin surfaces forming a large, continuous area of ulceration, with a characteristic serpiginous outline (Fig. 1). Inguinal lesions are common, especially in men. They start as a firm, subcutaneous swellings and often go on to ulcerate. The term 'pseudobubo' was originally coined to describe a subcutaneous inguinal abscess in donovanosis but is now frequently used loosely to describe the other varieties of inguinal lesion. Primary lesions of the cervix occur and are notorious for simulating carcinoma of the cervix. The uterus, fallopian tubes, ovaries, and adnexae may all be involved, simulating other forms of pelvic inflammatory disease with abscess formation or simulating malignancy with development of a frozen pelvis, large, hard masses or hydronephrosis. Anal lesions in women commonly spread directly from the introitus; in men they are associated with anal intercourse. Involvement of the rectum very seldom occurs.

Extragenital lesions of donovanosis occur most often in and around the mouth and sometimes on the neck. Haematogenous dissemination of donovanosis is associated especially with the trauma to an infected uterine cervix during pregnancy. The usual presentation is with one or more lytic bone lesions, which may break out through overlying skin. Spread to liver, spleen, and lung occurs exceptionally.

Complications of donovanosis include extensive scar formation, lymphoedema of the genitalia, penile autoamputation, and the development of squamous carcinoma in active or healed lesions. Secondary infection with fusospirochaetal organisms can cause rapid, extensive, and sometimes fatal tissue destruction.

Diagnosis

The diagnosis of donovanosis requires the demonstration of Donovan bodies within large histiocytes in material taken from a lesion (Fig. 2). Such cells may be present in profusion or extremely scanty. The best chance in making a diagnosis lies in combining a biopsy from the base or leading edge of a lesion with a series of dabs from the cut surface of the specimen. Where Donovan bodies are numerous a simple scraping or rolled cotton-wool swab from the cleaned surface of a lesion may suffice. Cytological material is best stained with Giemsa, Wright's or Leishman stains. For histological material, Giemsa and silver stains are the most helpful. Donovan bodies are easily missed in sections stained with haematoxylin and eosin. The characteristic histological picture of donovanosis comprises some degree of epithelial hyperplasia at the margins of the lesion, a dense plasma-cell infiltrate, and scattered histiocytes containing Donovan bodies. Successful isolation of *C. granulomatis* has not been reported for over 30 years. It is only likely to succeed when material, rich in Donovan bodies, is taken from an unruptured or minimally contaminated lesion and inoculated into the yolk sac of chick embryos. Serological and skin tests for donovanosis have been described in the past but are not currently in routine use. All patients should be screened for concomitant infections; syphilis is frequently cotransmitted with donovanosis. Patients with donovanosis are more likely to acquire and transmit human immunodeficiency virus (**HIV**).

Donovanosis is readily confused with other sexually transmitted genital infections, particularly chancroid (a variant of chancroid, dubbed 'pseudogranuloma inguinale' has recently been described), syphilis, and anogenital cutaneous amoebiasis. Elevated lesions of donovanosis can resemble condylomata lata, genital warts, and squamous carcinoma. Lymphoedema and inguinal lesions, prior to ulceration, may suggest lymphogranuloma venereum or filariasis. The most common misdiagnoses are of squamous carcinoma of penis, vulva or cervix, an error that may be compounded by misinterpretation of the epithelial hyperplasia as neoplastic and failure to identify Donovan bodies in haematoxylin and eosin-stained sections. The disease that shows the closest histological similarity to donovanosis is rhinoscleroma.

Treatment and prevention

A wide selection of antibiotics is available for the treatment of donovanosis. Tetracyclines or co-trimoxazole are the most widely favoured at present. Good results have also been obtained with erythromycin and lincomycin, which are safer for use in pregnant women. Chloramphenicol has been the preferred drug in Papua New Guinea for many years. More recently, norfloxacin, thiamphenicol, and ceftriaxone have been shown to work well. All drugs are given by mouth in standard doses and treatment should be continued until lesions have re-epithelialized and possibly longer, as relapse occurs quite commonly. Clinical resistance to most of these antibiotics has been reported; such cases may respond to a change of antibiotic. Surgical extirpation of lesions is some-

Fig. 1 Characteristic serpiginous ulcer in female patients with long-standing donovanosis.

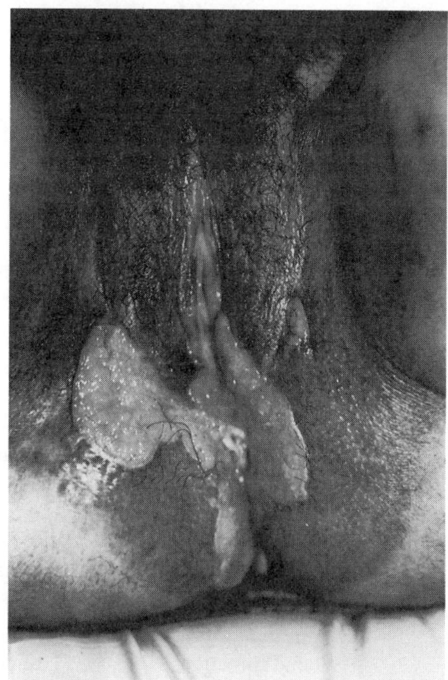

Fig. 2 Donovan bodies: Giemsa-stained smear from donovanosis lesion demonstrating the characteristic 'closed safety pin' appearance of encapsulated organisms within a large histiocyte.

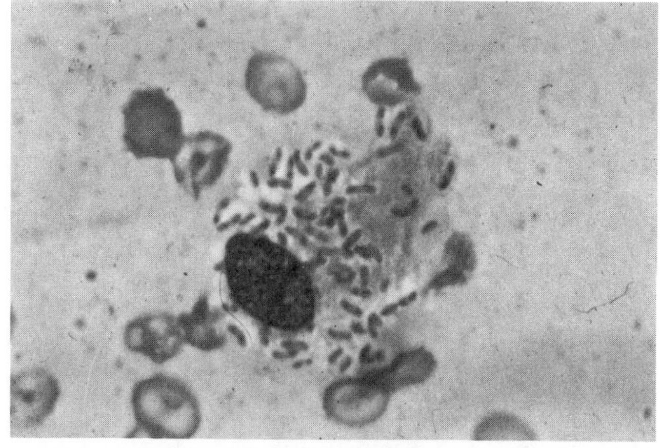

times undertaken in refractory cases but carries the risk of disseminating the disease if effective antibiotic cover is not given. Combined antibiotic therapy (e.g. erythromycin with lincomycin) should be considered in patients with HIV infection, severe disease, and resistant cases. Lesions in pregnant women may respond poorly to monotherapy. Caesarian section is indicated in pregnant women with incompletely treated lesions of the uterine cervix. Plastic surgical procedures can do much to help patients with elephantiasis and strictures resulting from donovanosis.

Partners of patients should be examined and treated if infected. Epidemiological treatment of contacts is not generally advocated because of low transmission rates. The main hopes for the control of donovanosis lie in health education, condom promotion, and interventions targeted at prostitutes and their partners.

REFERENCES

Goldberg, J. (1959). Studies on granuloma inguinale. IV. Growth requirements of *D. granulomatis* and its relationship to the habitat of the organism. *British Journal of Venereal Diseases*, **35**, 266–8.

Kuberski, T. (1980). Granuloma inguinale (Donovanosis). *Sexually Transmitted Diseases*, **7**, 29–36.

Merianos, A., Gilles M., and Chuah, J. (1994). Ceftriaxone in the treatment of chronic donovanosis in central Australia. *Genitourinary Medicine*, **70**, 84–9.

Rajam, R.V. and Rangiah, P.N. (1954). Donovanosis (granuloma inguinale, granuloma venereum). *WHO Monograph Series*, **24**, 1–72.

Ramanan, C., Sarma, P.S.A., Ghorpade, A., and Das, M. (1990). Treatment of donovanosis with norfloxacin. *International Journal of Dermatology*, **29**, 298–9.

Richens, J. (1992). The diagnosis and treatment of donovanosis (granuloma inguinale). *Genitourinary Medicine*, **32**, 441–52.

Sehgal, V.N. and Prasad, A.L. (1986). Donovanosis. Current concepts. *International Journal of Dermatology*, **24**, 8–16.

Vogel, L.C. and Richens, J. (1989). Donovanosis in Dutch South New Guinea: history, evolution of the epidemic and control. *Papua New Guinea Medical Journal*, **32**, 203–18.

7.11.46 'Newer' and lesser known bacteria causing infection in humans

J. PAUL

The list of rare bacterial pathogens is growing quite rapidly, mainly because of the recognition by microbiologists of new species among already familiar groups of organisms and because of the increasing opportunities presented to relatively non-pathogenic commensal and environmental bacteria to cause infection by immunocompromised patients, invasive devices, and prostheses. The hospital environment has become a special habitat for a set of species prone to cause nosocomial infection such as *Acinetobacter* spp., coryneforms, and *Pseudomonas* spp. Sophisticated laboratory methods have allowed the characterizing of fastidious organisms, such as the newly described agents of cat scratch disease, and the bacterium associated with Whipple's disease has been described but remains uncultured. Some bacteria were recognized as pathogens long ago but have remained unfamiliar rarities, many of them being causes of rare zoonoses, such as *Erysipelothrix rhusiopathiae* (the cause of erysipeloid) and *Burkholderia mallei* (formerly in the genus Pseudomonas and the cause of glanders), or with limited geographical distributions, such as *Burkholderia pseudomallei* (formerly in the genus Pseudomonas and the cause of melioidosis) associated with rice paddies in South-East Asia. Newly recognized zoonotic agents include *Helicobacter cinaedi*, associated with hamsters, and a number of animal oral commensals causing bite infections, including *Neisseria canis*, *Capnocytophaga canimorsus*, *Pasteurella stomatis*, and *Weeksella zoohelcum.* Some well-known bacteria acquire temporary obscurity through changes in nomenclature, a notable recent example being the *Bacteroides melaninogenicus* group, now correctly referred to the genus Prevotella, where naturally there will be some time lag before the new name becomes universal in the literature and on laboratory reports.

Table 1

Organism	Infections	Treatment	Notes	References
Achromobacter (see *Alcaligenes*)			Not in approved lists of bacterial names	
Acidaminococcus fermentans	Abdominal and lung abscesses	Drainage Metronidazole	As part of mixed anaerobic flora	1
Acinetobacter *baumannii* *calcoaceticus* *haemolyticus* *johnsonii* *junii* *lwoffi*	Septicaemia, UTI Wound infections Abscesses, endocarditis Meningitis Osteomyelitis Catheter cellulitis	Aminoglycosides Ureidopenicillins Ceftazidime Imipenem	Recently split into six species; often causing nosocomial infection in debilitated patients; outbreaks occur; often a colonist or contaminant	2–9
Actinobacillus actinomycetemcomitans	Periodontitis Endocarditis Abscesses Pericarditis Meningitis	Penicillin (and gentamicin for endocarditis)	Sometimes associated with actinomycosis	10–12
Actinobacillus *equuli* *lignieresii* *suis*	Wound infection Abscesses Endocarditis Meningitis	Ampicillin (and gentamicin for endocarditis)	Animal contact and bites	13–14
Actinobacillus ureae (formerly *Pasteurella ureae*)	Meningitis, pneumonia Endocarditis Hepatitis Peritonitis	Ampicillin (and gentamicin for endocarditis), chloramphenicol	Respiratory tract colonist	15–16

Organism	Infections	Treatment	Notes	References
Aerococcus *urinae* *viridans*	Endocarditis UTI, wounds Abscesses	Penicillin (and gentamicin for endocarditis)		17–19
Aeromonas *caviae* *hydrophila* *jandaei* *media* *schubertii* *veronii*	Wound infection Septicaemia Meningitis Abscesses Acute diarrhoea	Aminoglycosides Chloramphenicol Ceftazidime Co-trimoxazole	Infection often related to aquatic exposure Leech bites	20–34
Afipia *felis*	Wound infection Lymphadenopathy	Aminoglycosides Imipenem Ceftriaxone	Cat scratch disease (CSD) *Bartonella henselae* is the other CSD agent CSD therapy poorly evaluated	35
Afipia *broomeae*	Bone marrow Synovial fluid	Imipenem Ceftriaxone		35
Afipia *clevelandensis*	Tibial biopsy	Imipenem Ceftriaxone		35
Agrobacterium *radiobacter*	Endocarditis, CAPD peritonitis UTI	Co-trimoxazole Gentamicin		36–38
Alcaligenes *dentrificans* *dentrificans* *dentrificans* *xylosoxidans* (formerly *Achromobacter xylosoxidans*) *eutrophus* *faecalis* *latus* *piechaudii* *ruhlandii*	Septicaemia, CAPD peritonitis, pneumonia, ear infection	Ureidopenicillins Ceftazidime	Often in debilitated patients Nosocomial infections	39–43
Alloiococcus *otitis*	Otitis media		Role as pathogen poorly defined	44–46
Arachnia *propionica*	Actinomycosis Brain abscess	Penicillin		47–48
Arcanobacterium *haemolyticum* (formerly *Corynebacterium haemolyticum*)	Tonsillitis Lymphadenopathy Cellulitis Brain abscess Septicaemia Osteomyelitis	Penicillin Erythromycin		49–51
Arcobacter (formerly *Campylobacter*) *butzleri* *cryaerophilus* *nitrofigilis*	Abdominal cramps Diarrhoea	Self-limiting		52–54
Bacillus spp.	See under species group	Vancomycin Clindamycin Aminoglycosides Imipenem Penicillin	Other than the well-known known *B. anthracis* and *B. cereus*, *Bacillus* spp. cause a variety of eye and general infections.	55–57
Bacillus *alvei*	Pneumonia Septicaemia Meningitis		Most spp. are incriminated by only a few reports Correct speciation is difficult outside reference laboratories	58

Continued

Table 1 (*cont.*)

Organism	Infections	Treatment	Notes	References
			Vancomycin is usual empiric treatment for septicaemia Some strains are vancomycin resistant *Bacillus* spp. are common colonists and contaminants	
Bacillus brevis coagulans	Corneal infections Bacteraemia			
Bacillus circulans megaterium	Meningitis			
Bacillus laterosporus macerans	Septicaemia			
Bacillus licheniformis	Septicaemia Eye infection Food poisoning			
Bacillus pumilus	Meningitis Bacteraemia			
Bacillus sphaericus	Lung infection Bacteraemia			59
Bacillus subtilis	Meningitis, UTI Endocarditis Eye infections Pneumonia			60
Bacillus thuringiensis	Corneal infection		*B. thuringiensis* is a biological insecticide	61–62
Bartonella (see Chapter 7.11.40 and 7.11.44)				283
Bilophila wadsworthia	Appendicitis, hepatic abscess	Metronidazole	Role in appendicitis undefined	63–64
Branhamella catarrhalis (see *Moraxella catarrhalis*)				
Brevibacterium casei epidermidis	CAPD peritonitis Meningitis	Erythromycin Vancomycin Gentamicin	Often contaminant from skin flora	65–66
Burkholderia cepacia (formerly *Pseudomonas cepacia*)	Bacteraemia, UTI, endocarditis, lung infections in cystic fibrosis Septic arthritis	Ureidopenicillins Ceftazidime Co-trimoxazole	*Burkholderia* spp. (formerly *Pseudomonas* RNA group II) are resistant to aminoglycosides Serious infection in cystic fibrosis has poor prognosis regardless of susceptibilities	67–69
Burkholderia mallei (formerly *Ps. mallei*)	Glanders	Sulphadiazine	Recently developed cephalosporins and penicillins need to be evaluated	70

Organism	Infections	Treatment	Notes	References
Burkholderia pickettii (formerly *Ps. pickettii*)	Bacteraemia, UTI, meningitis	Piperacillin Cephalosporins Tetracycline		71–72
Burkholderia pseudomallei (formerly *Ps. pseudomallei*)	Melioidosis	Ceftazidime Chloramphenicol	Ceftazidime for serious infections Co-trimoxazole	73–74
Campylobacter fetus fetus	Fever, diarrhoea Meningoencephalitis Endocarditis, abscesses	Erythromycin Ampicillin Gentamicin Chloramphenicol		75
Campylobacter fetus venerealis	Bacterial vaginosis		Role as human pathogen poorly defined Faeces of homosexual men	76
Campylobacter hyointestinalis lari (formerly *C. laridis*) *upsalensis*	Diarrhoea Bacteraemia Abscess	Erythromycin Ampicillin Gentamicin		77–81
Campylobacter concisus curvus (formerly *Wolinella curva*) *sputorum rectus*(formerly *W. recta*			From the human gingival flora Role as pathogens poorly defined	
Campylobacter mucosalis	Enteritis	Self-limiting		82
Campylobacter butzleri (see *Arcobacter butzleri*) *cinaedi* (see *Helicobacter cinaedi*) *fennelliae* (see *H. fennelliae*)				
Campylobacter pyloridis (see *H. pylori*)				
Capnocytophaga canimorsus (formerly DF-2) *cynodegmi*	Wound infection, septicaemia Abscesses Meningitis	Penicillin	Dog bites Splenectomy	83–85
Capnocytophaga gingivalis ochracea sputigena	Periodontitis Septicaemia	Penicillins Tetracycline Chloramphenicol Ciprofloxacin	Infections in granulocytopenic patients	86–87
Cardiobacterium hominis	Endocarditis, meningitis	Penicillin and gentamicin		88–89
CDC group DF-3	Diarrhoea Bacteraemia	Tetracycline	Immunocompromised	90–93
CDC group IV c-2	Bacteraemia Wound infection	Ureidopenicillins Ceftazidime Imipenem		94–96
Cedecea davisae lapagei neterii	Bacteraemia	Chloramphenicol Cefamandole Gentamicin		97–98

Continued

Table 1 (*cont.*)

Organism	Infections	Treatment	Notes	References
Cellulomonas turbata (formerly *Oerskovia turbata*)	Bacteraemia Endocarditis	Amikacin Co-trimoxazole Chloramphenicol		99–100
Chromobacterium violaceum	Septicaemia Abscesses Osteomyelitis Eye infection	Erythromycin Chloramphenicol Tetracycline Gentamicin	Associated with soil and water exposure	102–103
Chryseomonas luteola (formerly *Ps. luteola*)	Bacteraemia Endocarditis CAPD peritonitis	Ampicillin, cefotaxime Aminoglycosides		104
Comamonas (formerly *Pseudomonas* RNA group III) *acidovorans* *terrigena* *testosteroni*	Bacteraemia Conjunctivitis UTI	Ureidopenicillins Ceftazidime Ciprofloxacin Imipenem Aminoglycosides	Infections in neutropenic patients	104–107
Corynebacterium spp.		Empiric therapy is poorly defined for most species Unless otherwise stated, vancomycin is likely to be an effective treatment for serious systemic infection pending susceptibility results Corynebacteria (diphtheroids) are common colonists and contaminants. Speciation may be difficult		108
Corynebacterium 'aquaticum'	UTI, endocarditis, meningitis, CAPD peritonitis	Ampicillin Chloramphenicol Gentamicin	Not in approved lists of bacterial names	109–111
Corynebacterium bovis	Septicaemia, eye infection, peritonitis	Erythromycin and rifampicin		112
Corynebacterium jeikeium (JK diphtheroids)	Wounds, UTI, meningitis, peritonitis, osteomyelitis, endocarditis	Vancomycin	Nosocomial skin colonist Outbreaks reported among debilitated patients	113–115
Corynebacterium kutscheri	Septic arthritis			116
Corynebacterium matruchotii	Eye infection			117
Corynebacterium minutissimum	Erythrasma Bacteraemia, endocarditis			118
Corynebacterium mycetoides	Tropical ulcer Septicaemia			
Corynebacterium pseudodiphtheriticum	UTI, endocarditis Lymphadenopathy Necrotizing tracheitis	Penicillin		119
Corynebacterium pseudotuberculosis	Lymphadenitis Pulmonary infection	Drainage, excision Penicillin and erythromycin	Sheep contact	120
Corynebacterium renale	Abscesses			
Corynebacterium striatum	Lung abscess	Cefuroxime Ampicillin		121
Corynebacterium 'ulcerans'	Diphtheria-like disease, pharyngitis	Erythromycin	Not in approved lists of bacterial names	122
Corynebacterium urealiticum (formerly D2)	UTI, septicaemia Peritonitis Pneumonia	Vancomycin		123–125

Organism	Infections	Treatment	Notes	References
Corynebacterium xerosis	Endocarditis Osteomyelitis	Penicillins, cephalosporins Vancomycin		126–128
Corynebacterium group A-4	Endophthalmitis			129
Corynebacterium group E	Septicaemia	Penicillin Chloramphenicol		130
Corynebacterium group F1	UTI	Amoxycillin Erythromycin Vancomycin		124
Corynebacterium group G2	Endocarditis	Ampicillin Cephalosporins Gentamicin Vancomycin		131
Corynebacterium group I1	Endocarditis			132
Corynebacterium group 1	Endophthalmitis			129
Corynebacterium group 2	Bacteraemia Wounds		Significance undefined	129
Edwardsiella tarda	Wound infection, abscesses Gastroenteritis	Penicillins Aminoglycosides	Aquatic exposure, penetrating fish injury	133–136
Ehrlichia chaffeensis	Fever Lymphopenia	Tetracycline	Human ehrlichiosis Tick bites, USA	137–138
Ehrlichia sennetsu	Infectious mononucleosis-like illness		Sennetsu ehrlichiosis in Japan	137
Eikenella corrodens	Septicaemia, endocarditis, abscesses, joint infection	Penicillin (and gentamicin for endocarditis)	Human and animal bites	139–142
Erysipelothrix rhusiopathiae	Erysipeloid, septicaemia, endocarditis	Penicillin	Animal contact	143–144
Escherichia adecarboxylata (see *Leclercia adecarboxylata*)				
Escherichia fergusonii	Bacteraemia Wound, UTI	Chloramphenicol Gentamicin	Ampicillin resistant	145
Escherichia hermanii	Wounds	Chloramphenicol Cephalosporins Gentamicin		146
Escherichia vulneris	Wounds	Ampicillin Cephalosporins Gentamicin		147
Eubacterium spp.	Wounds, abscesses Septicaemia	Penicillin		148
Ewingella americana	Septicaemia, wounds, UTI	Ampicillin Cefuroxime		149
Flavimonas (formerly *Pseudomonas*) *oryzihabitans*	Septicaemia CAPD peritonitis Eye infection	Ampicillin Tetracycline Gentamicin Cefotaxime		150–152
Flavobacterium breve capsulatum	Bacteraemia Meningitis Eye infection	Susceptibility varies Ciprofloxacin Rifampicin	Nosocomial infections in debilitated patients and neonates	153–156

Continued

Table 1 (*cont.*)

Organism	Infections	Treatment	Notes	References
gleum *heparinum* *indologenes* *meningosepticum* *mizutae* formerly *Sphingobacterium* *mizutae*) *multivorum* formerly *Sph.* *multivorum*) *spiritivorum* (formerly *Sph.* *spiritivorum*) *thalpophilum* *abunchiae*	Endocarditis	Vancomycin Imipenem Erythromycin Pefloxacin		
Fusobacterium *fusiforme* *gonidiaformans* *mortiferum* *naviforme* *necrophorum* *nucleatum* *ulcerans*	Lung abscess Other abscesses Bacteraemia Endocarditis	Penicillin and metronidazole Drainage	Necrobacillosis	157–158
Gemella *haemolysans* *morbillorum* (formerly *Strep.* *morbillorum*)	Penicillin or Vancomycin (and gentamicin for endocarditis) Bacteraemia Endocarditis		159–160	
Haemophilus *aegyptius*	Conjunctivitis Septicaemia Meningitis	Ampicillin Chloramphenicol Cephalosporins	Often considered as biogroup of *H. influenzae*. Brazilian purpuric fever	161–162
Haemophilus *aphrophilus* *paraphrophilus* *parainfluenzae* *segnis*	Sinusitis Pneumonia Otitis media Endocarditis Abscesses	Cefuroxime Cefotaxime Chloramphenicol Ampicillin Aminoglycosides	Ampicillin and gentamicin used to treat endocarditis	163–168
Hafnia *alvei*	Bacteraemia	Susceptibility variable	May cause diarrhoea	169
Helicobacter *pylori* (formerly *Campylobacter* *pyloridis*)	Gastritis	Ampicillin Bismuth salts		170
Helicobacter *cinaedi* (formerly *Campylobacter* *cinaedi*)	Proctitis in homosexual men. Septicaemia.	Ampicillin Gentamicin	Contact with hamsters	171–173
Helicobacter *fennelliae*-like (formerly *Campylobacter* *fennelliae*)	Gastroenteritis		Contact with dogs	174
Kingella *denitrificans* *kingae*	Septic arthritis in children, meningitis Endocarditis	Penicillins	Penicillin and gentamicin for endocarditis	175–178
Kingella *indologenes* (see *Suttonella* *indologenes*)				

Organism	Infections	Treatment	Notes	References
Kluyvera *ascorbata* *cryocrescens*	Bacteraemia UTI, bile Intravascular devices Mediastinitis	Aminoglycosides Ceftazidime Ciprofloxacin Imipenem		179–180
Koserella *trabulsii*	Wounds, UTI Knee fluid	Chloramphenicol Gentamicin		181
Kurthia *gibsonii* *sibirica* *zopfii*	Bacteraemia Endocarditis	Penicillin		182–183
Lactobacillus *acidophilus* *casei alactosus* *casei casei* *casei rhamnosus* *confusus* *plantarum* *salivarius salicinius*	Abscesses Bacteraemia Endometritis Endocarditis Lung infection UTI	Cephalosporins Vancomycin Penicillins Aminoglycosides Clindamycin	May be resistant to vancomycin	184–187
Lactococcus (formerly *Streptococcus*) *garviae* *lactis*	Bacteraemia, endocarditis, UTI	Penicillin and gentamicin		188
Leclercia *adecarboxylata* (formerly *Escherichia adecarboxylata*)	Bacteraemia Wounds	Ampicillin Cefuroxime Gentamicin		189
Leminorella *grimontii* *richardii*	UTI	Chloramphenicol Tetracycline Gentamicin	Isolated from stools but significance unknown	190
Leuconostoc *citreum* *lactis* *mesenteroides* *paramesenteroides*	Meningitis Bacteraemia	Penicillin and gentamicin	Vancomycin resistant	191–193
Listonella damsela (formerly *Vibrio damsela*, see *Photobacterium damselum*)				
Megasphaera *elsdenii*	Endocarditis	Metronidazole		194
Methylobacterium *extorquens* *mesophilicum* (formerly *Ps. mesophilica*)	Bacteraemia CAPD peritonitis	Ureidopenicillins Imipenem Aminoglycosides Chloramphenicol		195–198
Mobiluncus *mulieris* *curtisii*	Bacterial vaginosis Chorioamnionitis Endometritis	Ampicillin Cephalosporins Clindamycin		199–201
Moraxella *atlantae* *lacunata* *nonliquefaciens* *osloensis* *phenylpyruvica*	Conjunctivitis Wound infection Endocarditis Abscesses Osteomyelitis	Penicillin	Penicillin resistance is rare	202–205
Moraxella *catarrhalis* (formerly *Branhamella*)	Respiratory infections Endocarditis Bacteraemia	Cefuroxime	Some authors retain *Branhamella catarrhalis*	206–207

Continued

Table 1 (*cont.*)

Organism	Infections	Treatment	Notes	References
Moraxella urethralis (see *Oligella urethralis*)				
Neisseria cinerea elongata elongata e. nitroreductens flavescens lactamica mucosa perflava polysaccharea sicca subflava	Meningitis Bacteraemia Endocarditis Osteomyelitis	Penicillin Cephalosporins	Bacteraemia in AIDS reported for several species Penicillin resistance rarely reported in commensal *Neisseria* spp.	208–212
Neisseria canis	Wounds	Amoxicillin	Cat bites	213
Ochrobactrum anthropi (formerly *Achromobacter* group Vd)	Bacteraemia	Imipenem Ceftazidime	Nosocomial infections in debilitated patients	214
Oerskovia turbata (see *Cellulomonas turbata*)				
Oerskovia xanthineolytica	Meningitis Pyonephrosis Endophthalmitis CAPD peritonitis	Vancomycin and gentamicin		215–219
Oligella urethralis (formerly *Moraxella urethralis*)	UTI, septicaemia	Aminoglycosides Cephalosporins	Associated with urinary catheters	220–221
Pasteurella aerogenes bettii caballi canis dagmatis haemolytica multocida multocida m. septica pneumotropica stomatis	Wound infection Septicaemia Abscesses Pneumonia Endocarditis Meningitis	Penicillin Tetracycline Ciprofloxacin	Pasteurella infections in man relate to species associated with animals, although there may be no history of a bite or contact Identification may be difficult outside a reference laboratory	222–227
Pasteurella (see *Actinobacillus ureae*) *ureae*				
Pediococcus acidilactici	Bacteraemia	Imipenem Gentamicin Chloramphenicol	Debilitated hospital patients Vancomycin resistant	228–230
Photobacterium damselum (formerly *Listonella damsela* and *Vibrio damsela*)	Necrotizing wound infection	Debridement Penicillins Tetracycline Chloramphenicol	Some recent authors retain *Vibrio damsela* Penetrating fish injury	231
Plesiomonas shigelloides	Gastroenteritis, septicaemia, meningitis, endophthalmitis	Ciprofloxacin Trimethoprim Cephalosporins	Associated with contaminated food and water	232–234

Organism	Infections	Treatment	Notes	References
Porphyrimonas (formerly *Bacteroides*) *asaccharolytica* *endodontalis* *gingivalis*	Mixed anaerobic infections at various sites	Metronidazole Drainage	A recently described genus to include some pigmenting, oral, former *Bacteroides* spp.	235
Prevotella (formerly *Bacteroides*) *bivia* *buccae* *corporis* *denticola* *disiens* *heparinolytica* *intermedia* *loeschii* *melaninogenica* *oralis* *oris* *oulora* *ruminicola* *veroralis*	Abscesses, often above the diaphragm (lung, dental), often in mixed anaerobic flora Wounds, bacteraemia Bite infections Genital tract infections	Metronidazole Drainage	A recently described genus to include the well-known former *Bacteroides melaninogenicus* and allied species	236
Pseudomonas		Often multiresistant	*Pseudomonas* spp. are referred to five RNA groups that imply differences in their phylogenies; groups II, III, and V have been placed in new genera and group IV is likely to follow	237–239
RNA group I, fluorescent *Pseudomonas* *aeruginosa* *fluorescens* *putida*	Bacteraemia, UTI Wound infection	Ureidopenicillins Aminoglycosides Ceftazidime Ciprofloxacin Imipenem	Groups are shown here to aid understanding of taxonomic changes and because the RNA groups relate to differences in medical importance	
RNA group I, non-fluorescent *Pseudomonas* *alcaligenes* *avenae avenae* *avenae citrulli* (formerly *Ps. pseudalcaligenes citrulli*) *avenae konjac* (formerly *Ps. pseudalcaligenes konjac*) *mendocina* *pseudalcaligenes pseudalcaligenes* *pseudalcaligenes citrulli* (see *Ps. avenae citrulli*) *pseudalcaligenes konjac* (see *Ps. avenae konjac*) *stutzeri*	Wound infections Abscesses, septic arthritis, conjunctivitis Endocarditis, meningitis	Ureidopenicillins Aminoglycosides Cephalosporins Ciprofloxacin Imipenem	Pseudomonads are important causes of nosocomial infection, often in association with vascular cannulae and urinary catheters and in debilitated patients	

Continued

Table 1 (*cont.*)

Organism	Infections	Treatment	Notes	References
RNA group II *Pseudomonas* *cepacia* (see *Burkholderia cepacia*) *mallei* (see *Bu. mallei*) *pickettii* (see *Bu. pickettii*) *pseudomallei* (see *Bu. pseudomallei*)			*Burkholderia* is the recently validated generic name for RNA homology group II *Pseudomonas* spp.	
RNA group III *Pseudomonas* *acidivorans* (see *Comamonas acidivorans*) *terrigena* (see *Co. terrigena*) *testosteroni* (see *Co. testosteroni*)				
RNA group IV *Pseudomonas* *diminuta* *vesicularis*	Septicaemia		Hospital environment Rare opportunistic infections	239
RNA group V *Pseudomonas* *maltophilia* (see *Xanthomonas maltophilia*)				
Pseudomonas mesophilica (see *Methylobacterium mesophilicum*)			*M. mesophilicum* and the two following spp. were formerly placed in the genus *Pseudomonas* but outside the system of the five RNA homology groups.	
Pseudomonas paucimobilis (see *Sphingomonas paucimobilis*)				
Pseudomonas putrefaciens (see *Shewanella putrefaciens*)				
Psychrobacter immobilis	Meningitis Bacteraemia Eye infection	Penicillins, aminoglycosides Chloramphenicol		240–241
Rahnella aquatilis	UTI, septicaemia	Ciprofloxacin	Immunocompromised patients	242–243
Rhodococcus equi (formerly *Corynebacterium equi*)	Bacteraemia Lung abscesses Osteomyelitis	Vancomycin Aminoglycosides Erythromycin	Especially AIDS and the immunocompromised	244–246
Rochalimaea henselae	Lymphadenopathy Skin lesions	Tetracycline Erythromycin	It has recently been proposed that Rochalimaea be transfered to the genus Bartonella Cat scratch disease (*Afipia felis* is also a CSD agent; CSD therapy poorly evaluated) Bacillary angiomatosis	247–252

Organism	Infections	Treatment	Notes	References
Rochalimaea elizabethae	Endocarditis	Flucloxacillin and gentamicin		253
Rochalimaea quintana	Fever, bacteraemia Skin lesions	Tetracycline Erythromycin	Trench fever Bacillary angiomatosis	247–248
Roseomonas gilardii cervicalis fauriae	Bacteraemia Wound infection Eye infection Urogenital infection	Aminoglycosides Imipenem Tetracycline	Formerly CDC 'pink coccoid' groups I-IV	282
Rothia dentocariosa	Endocarditis Abscesses	Penicillin and gentamicin		254
Serratia fonticola marcescens plymuthica proteamaculans (formerly *S. liquefaciens*)	Septicaemia Burn sites Osteomyelitis Abscesses	Imipenem Ceftazidime Ciprofloxacin	Nosocomial outbreaks reported. Sometimes multiresistant	255–260
Shewanella alga putrefaciens (formerly *Alteromonas putrefaciens* and *Ps. putrefaciens*)	Abdominal sepsis Meningitis Bacteraemia UTI	Ampicillin Cefotaxime Chloramphenicol Gentamicin	Debilitated patients	261–63
Sphingobacterium (see *Flavobacterium*)				
Sphingomonas paucimobilis (formerly *Ps. paucimobilis*)	Septicaemia, UTI, wound infections, CAPD peritonitis	Ureidopenicillins Ceftazidime Aminoglycosides	Nosocomial infections	264
Stenotrophomonas maltophilia (see Xanthomonas)				
Stomatococcus mucilaginosus (formerly *Micrococcus mucilaginosus*)	Endocarditis	Vancomycin and gentamicin (rifampicin)		265
Suttonella indologenes (formerly *Kingella indologenes*)	Endocarditis Eye infection	Penicillin	Penicillin and gentamicin for endocarditis	266
Tatumella ptyseos	Bacteraemia UTI	Ampicillin Tetracycline Chloramphenicol Gentamicin	Isolated mainly from sputum, where its significance is unknown	267
Tropheryma whippelii	Whipple's disease		Uncultured organism	268
Veillonella atypica dipsar parvula	Mixed anerobic infections Abscesses Bacteraemia	Metronidazole		269
Vibrio alginolyticus	Wound infection Ear infection	Chloramphenicol Tetracycline	Aquatic exposure Septicaemia in the immunocompromised	270–71
Vibrio carchariae	Wound infection	Debridement Cephalosporins Chloramphenicol Gentamicin	Shark bite	272
Vibrio cincinnatiensis	Bacteraemia	Moxalactam Chloramphenicol Cephalosporins	No defined risk factor	273

Continued

Table 1 (*cont.*)

Organism	Infections	Treatment	Notes	References
Vibrio damsela (see *Photobacterium damselum*)				
Vibrio fluvialis furnissii hollisae mimicus	Diarrhoea	Self-limiting Tetracycline Chloramphenicol	Contaminated water or shellfish	270,274
Vibrio metschnikovii	Septicaemia Diarrhoea	Tetracycline Chloramphenicol		275
Vibrio vulnificus	Wound infection Septicaemia Meningitis Endometritis	Debridement Tetracycline Penicillins Gentamicin Chloramphenicol	Aquatic exposure, penetrating fish injury	276–277
Weeksella zoohelcum (formerly Group IIj)	Wound infection Septicaemia Meningitis	Cefotaxime Penicillins Ciprofloxacin Tetracycline	Dog and cat bites	278
Yersinia aldovae frederiksenii intermedia kristensenii	Enterocolitis Soft tissue infections	Tetracycline Chloramphenicol Aminoglycosides	Medical importance of *Yersinia* spp. other than the well-known *Y. pestis*, *Y. pseudotuberculos* and *Y. enterocolitica* is poorly defined	279
Yokenella regensburgei (see *Koserella trabulsii*)				
Xanthomonas campestris maltophilia (formerly *Ps. maltophilia*)	Bacteraemia Wound infection	Ureidopenicillins Cephalosporins Ciprofloxacin Aminoglycosides	Often multiresistant Nosocomial infections *X. maltophilia* has recently been transferred to *Stenotrophomonas*	280–81

CAPD, continuous ambulatory peritoneal dialysis; CDC, Centers for Disease Control; CSD, cat scratch disease; UTI, urinary tract infection.

Bacterial taxonomy and its attendant system of nomenclature aim to provide a logical classification of these organisms, ideally to include all species arranged according to their relatedness and phylogeny. Such a system allows orderly study of the species and maximizes progress in medically relevant fields such as virulence and the action of antibiotics. Unfortunately the process is at an early stage and the revision of known groups may irritate the clinician with name changes and the splitting of species. The correct nomenclature is given in the *Approved lists of bacterial names* (1989) (ed. V.B.D. Skerman, V. McGowan, and P.H.A. Sneath) and the *Index of the bacterial and yeast nomenclature changes* (1992) by W.E.C. Moore and L.V.H. Moore. Newly approved names are listed in the *International Journal of Systematic Bacteriology*. Pending formal description, medically important bacteria are sometimes referred to in clinical literature by alphanumeric groups of the Centers for Disease Control, Atlanta (CDC groups). Two of the most useful textbooks giving information on obscure medically important bacteria are *Manual of clinical microbiology*, 5th edn (1991) (ed. A. Balows, W.J. Hausler, Jr., K. Herrman, H.D. Isenberg, and H.J. Shadomy) and *Cowan and Steel's manual for the identification of medical bacteria*, 3rd edn (1993) (ed. G.I. Barrow and R.K.A. Feltham).

Table 1 lists genera in alphabetical order with a rough guide to described infections and treatment with key references. Many of the organisms listed are readily found in the general or hospital environment or are human commensals rarely causing infection other than in debilitated or immunosuppressed patients or in association with intravascular cannulae, prostheses, penetrating injury or surgery. Hence, caution must be exercised in interpreting whether or not such organisms are causing infection. Antibiotics are listed as a guide only: there is no substitute for susceptibility data derived from the isolate causing the infection. Some of the organisms are described in greater detail in other parts of this section.

REFERENCES

1. Sugihara, P.T., Sutter, V.L., Attebery, H.R., Bricknell, K.S., and Finegold, S.M. (1974). Isolation of *Acidaminococcus fermentans* and *Megasphaera elsdenii* from normal human feces. *Applied Microbiology* **27,** 274–5.
2. Bouvet, P.J.M. and Grimont, P.A.D. (1986). Taxonomy of the genus *Acinetobacter* with recognition of *Acinetobacter baumanni* sp. nov. *Acinetobacter haemolyticus* sp. nov., *Acinetobacter johnsonii* sp. nov., and *Aci-*

netobacter junii sp. nov. and emended descriptions of *Acinetobacter calcoaceticus* and *Acinetobacter lwoffii*. *International Journal of Systematic Bacteriology*, **36,** 238–40.

3. Bergogne-Bérézine, E. and Joly-Guillou, M.L. (1991). Hospital infection with *Acinetobacter* spp.: an increasing problem. *Journal of Hospital Infection*, **18A,** 250–255.
4. Urban, C. *et al.* (1993). Effect of sublactam on infections caused by imipenem-resistant *Acinetobacter calcoaceticus* biotype *anitratus*. *Journal of Infectious Diseases*, **167,** 448–51.
5. Towner, K.J. and Chopade, B.A. (1987). Biotyping of *Acinetobacter calcoaceticus* using the API 20NE system. *Journal of Hospital Infection*, **10,** 145–51.
6. French, G.L., Casewell, M.W., Roncoroni, A.J., Knight, S., and Phillips, I. (1980). A hospital outbreak of antibiotic-resistant *Acinetobacter anitratus*: epidemiology and control. *Journal of Hospital Infection*, **1,** 125–31.
7. Haley, S., Paul, J., Crook, D.W. and White, S.H. (1990). *Acinetobacter* sp. L-form infection of a cemented Charnley total hip replacement. *Journal of Clinical Pathology*, **43,** 781.
8. Rosenthal, S.L. and Freundlich, L.F. (1977). The clinical significance of *Acinetobacter* species. *Health Laboratory Sciences*, **14,** 194–8.
9. Kropec, A., Hübner, J., and Daschner, F.D. (1993). Comparison of three typing methods in hospital outbreaks of *Acinetobacter calcoaceticus* infection. *Journal of Hospital Infection*, **23,** 133–41.
10. Ellner, J.J., Rosenthal, M.S., Lerner, P.I. and McHenry, M.C. (1979). Infective endocarditis caused by slow-growing, fastidious, Gram-negative bacteria. *Medicine* (Balt.) **58,** 145–58.
11. Geraci, J.E., Wilson, W.R. and Washington II, J.A. (1980). Infective endocarditis caused by *Actinobacillus actinomycetemcomitans*. Report of four cases. *Mayo Clinic Proceedings*, **55,** 415–19.
12. Kristinsson, K.G., Thorgeirsson, G. and Holbrook, W.P. (1988). *Actinobacillus actinomycetemcomitans* and endocarditis. *Journal of Infectious Diseases*, **157,** 599.
13. Peel, M.M., Hornidge, K.A., Luppino, M., Stacpoole, A.M., and Weaver, R.E. (1991). *Actinobacillus* spp. and related bacteria in infected wounds of humans bitten by horses and sheep. *Journal of Clinical Microbiology*, **29,** 2535–8.
14. Dibb, W.L., Digranes, A., and Tønjum, S. (1981). *Actinobacillus lignieresii* infection after a horse bite. *British Medical Journal*, **283,** 583.
15. Marriot, D.J. and Brady, L.M. (1983). *Pasteurella ureae* meningitis. *Medical Journal of Australia*, **2,** 455–6.
16. Noble, R.C., Marek, B.J., and Overman, S.B. (1987). Spontaneous peritonitis caused by *Pasteurella ureae*, *Journal of Clinical Microbiology*, **25,** 442–4.
17. Aguirre, M. and Collins, M.D. (1992). Phylogenetic analysis of some *Aerococcus*-like organisms from urinary tract infections: description of *Aerococcus urinae* sp. nov. *Journal of General Microbiology*, **138,** 401–5.
18. Colman, G. (1967). *Aerococcus*-like organisms isolated from human infections. *Journal of Clinical Pathology*, **20,** 294–7.
19. Nathavitharana, K.A. *et al.* (1983). Acute meningitis in early childhood caused by *Aerococcus viridans*. *British Medical Journal*, **286,** 1248.
20. Davis, W.A., Kane, J.G., and Garagusi, V.F. (1978). Human *Aeromonas* infections: a review of the literature and a case report of endocarditis. *Medicine* (Baltimore), **57,** 267–77.
21. Whitlock, M.R., O'Hare, P.M., Sanders, R., and Morrow, N.C. (1983). The medicinal leech and its use in plastic surgery: a possible cause of infection. *British Journal of Plastic Surgery*, **36,** 240–4.
22. Mercer, N.S.G., Beere, D.M., Bornemisza, A.J., and Thomas, P. (1987). Medicinal leeches as sources of wound infection. *British Medical Journal*, **294,** 937.
23. Gluski, I., Batash, D., Shoseyov, D., Mor, A., Kazak, K., Azizi, E., and Boldur, I. (1992). A 15-year study of the role of *Aeromonas* spp. in gastroenteritis in hospitalised children. *Journal of Medical Microbiology*, **37,** 315–8.
24. Joseph, S.W. *et al.* (1991). *Aeromonas jandaei* and *Aeromonas veronii* duel infection of a human wound following aquatic exposure. *Journal of Clinical Microbiology*, **29,** 565–9.
25. Ong, K.R., Sordillo, E., and Frankel, E. (1991). Unusual case of *Aeromonas hydrophila* endocarditis. *Journal of Clinical Microbiology*, **29,** 1056–7.
26. Janda, J.M. and Duffey, P.S. (1988). Mesophilic aeromonads in human disease: current taxonomy, laboratory identification, and infectious disease spectrum. *Reviews of Infectious Diseases*, **10,** 980–97.
27. Agger, W.A., McCormick, J.D., and Gurwith, M.J. (1985). Clinical and microbiological features of *Aeromonas hydrophila*-associated diarrhea. *Journal of Clinical Microbiology*, **21,** 909–13.
28. Hickman-Brenner, F.W., Fanning, G.R., Arduino, M.J., Brenner, D.J., and Farmer III, J.J. (1988). *Aeromonas schubertii*, a new mannitol-negative species found in human clinical specimens. *Journal of Clinical Microbiology*, **26,** 1561–4.
29. Hickman-Brenner, MacDonald, K.W., Steigerwalt, A.G., F.W., Fanning, M.J., Brenner, D.J., and Farmer III, J.J. (1987). *Aeromonas veronii*, a new ornithine decarboxylase-positive species that may cause diarrhea. *Journal of Clinical Microbiology*, **25,** 900–6.
30. Wolff, R.L., Wiseman, S.L., and Kitchens, C.S. (1980). *Aeromonas hydrophila* bacteremia in ambulatory immunocompromised hosts. *American Journal of Medicine*, **68,** 238–40.
31. Young, D.G., and Barr, R.J. (1981). *Aeromonas hydrophila* infection of the skin. *Archives of Dermatology*, **117,** 244.
32. Champsaur, H., Andremont, A., Matthieu, D., Rottman, E., and Auzepy, P. (1982). Cholera-like illness due to *Aeromonas sobria*. *Journal of Infectious Diseases*, **145,** 248–254.
33. Janda, J.M. and Brenda, R. (1987). Importance of *Aeromonas sobria* in aeromonas bacteremia. *Journal of Infectious Diseases*, **155,** 589–91.
34. Motyl, M.R., McKinley, G., and Janda, J.M. (1985). *In vitro* susceptibilities of *Aeromonas hydrophila*, *Aeromonas sobria*, and *Aeromonas caviae* to 22 antimicrobial agents. *Antimicrobial Agents and Chemotherapy*, **28,** 151–3.
35. Brenner, D.J. *et al.* (1991). Proposal of *Afipia* gen. nov., with *Afipia felis* sp. nov. (formerly the Cat scratch Disease Bacillus), Afipia clevelandensis sp. nov. (formerly the Cleveland Clinic Foundation Strain), *Afipia broomeae* sp. nov., and three unnamed genospecies. *Journal of Clinical Microbiology*, **29,** 2450–2460.
36. Plotkin, G.R. (1980). *Agrobacterium radiobacter* prosthetic valve endocarditis. *Annals of Internal Medicine*, **93,** 839–40.
37. Hammerberg, O., Bialowska-Hobrzanska, H., and Gopaul, D. (1991). Isolation of *Agrobacterium radiobacter* from a central venous catheter. *European Journal of Clinical Microbiology and Infectious Diseases*, **10,** 450.
38. Freney, J. *et al.* (1985). Septicemia caused by *Agrobacterium* sp. *Journal of Clinical Microbiology*, **22,** 683–5.
39. Rolston, K.V.I. and Messer, M. (1990). The *in-vitro* susceptibility of *Alcaligenes denitrificans* subsp. *xylosoxidans* to 40 antimicrobial agents. *Journal of Antimicrobial Chemotherapy*, **26,** 857–60.
40. Peel, M.M., Hibberd, A.J., King, B.M., and Williamson, H.G. (1988). *Alcaligenes piechaudii* from chronic ear discharge. *Journal of Clinical Microbiology*, **26,** 1580–1.
41. Igra-Siegman, Y., Chmel, H., and Cobbs, C. (1980). Clinical and laboratory characteristics of *Achromobacter xylosoxidans* infection. *Journal of Clinical Microbiology*, **11,** 141–5.
42. Holmes, B., Snell, J.J.S., and Lapage, S.P. (1977). Strains of *Achromobacter xylosoxidans* from clinical material. *Journal of Clinical Pathology*, **30,** 595–601.
43. Reverdy, M.E. *et al.* (1984). Nosocomial colonisation and infection by *Achromobacter xylosoxidans*. *Journal of Clinical Microbiology*. **19,** 140–3.
44. Faden, H. and Dryja, D. (1989). Recovery of a unique bacterial organism in human middle ear fluid and its possible role in chronic otitis media. *Journal of Clinical Microbiology*, **27,** 2488–91.
45. Aguirre, M. and Collins, M.D. (1992). Development of a polymerase chain reaction-probe test for identification of *Alliococcus otitis*. *Journal of Clinical Microbiology*, **30,** 2177–80.
46. von Graevenitz, A. (1993). Erratum: revised nomenclature of *Alloiococcus otitis*. *Journal of Clinical Microbiology*, **31,** 1402.
47. Riley, T.V. and Ott, A.K. (1981). Brain abscess due to *Arachnia propionica*. *British Medical Journal*, **i,** 1035.
48. Brock, D.W., George, L.K., Brown, J.M., and Hicklin, M.D. (1973). Actinomycosis caused by *Arachnia propionica*. *American Journal of Clinical Pathology*, **59,** 66–77.
49. Fell, H.W.K., Nagington, J., Nayler, G.R.E., and Olds, R.J. (1977). *Corynebacterium haemolyticum* infections in Cambridgeshire. *Journal of Hygiene (Cambridge)*, **79,** 269–74.
50. Jobantputra, R.S. and Swain, C.P. (1975). Septicaemia due to *Corynebacterium haemolyticum*. *Journal of Clinical Pathology*, **28,** 798–800.
51. Greenman, J.L. (1987). *Corynebacterium hemolyticum* and pharyngitis. *Annals of Internal Medicine*, **106,** 633.

52. Vandamme, P. *et al.* (1992). Outbreak of recurrent abdominal cramps associated with *Arcobacter butzleri* in an Italian school. *Journal of Clinical Microbiology*, **30,** 2335–2337.
53. Tee, W., Baird, R., Dyall-Smith, M., and Dwyer, B. (1988). *Campylobacter cryaerophila* isolated from a human. *Journal of Clinical Microbiology*, **26,** 2469–2473.
54. Vandamme, P., Falsen, E., Rossau, R., Hoste, B., Seegers, P., Tygat, R., and DeLey, J. (1991). Revision of *Campylobacter. Helicobacter* and *Wolinella* taxonomy: emendation of generic descriptions and proposal of *Arcobacter* gen. nov. *International Journal of Systematic Bacteriology*, **41,** 88–103.
55. Ihde, D.C. and Armstrong, D. (1973). Clinical spectrum of infection due to bacillus species. *American Journal of Medicine*, **55,** 839–45.
56. Slimans, R., Rehm, S., and Shlaes, D.M. (1987). Serious infections caused by *Bacillus* species. *Medicine* (Baltimore), **66,** 218–23.
57. Weber, D.J., Saviteer, S.M., Rutala, W.A., and Thomann, C.A. (1988). *In vitro* susceptibility of *Bacillus* spp. to selected antimicrobial agents. *Antimicrobial Agents and Chemotherapy*, **32,** 642–5.
58. Coundron, P.E., Payne, J.M., and Markowitz, S.M. (1991). Pneumonia and empyema infection associated with a *Bacillus* species that resembles *B. alvei. Journal of Clinical Microbiology*, **29,** 1777–9.
59. Isaacson, P., Jacobs, P.H., MacKenzie, A.M.R., and Mathew, J.A.W. (1976). Pseudotumour of the lung caused by infection with *Bacillus sphaericus. Journal of Clinical Pathology*, **29,** 806–11.
60. Reller, L.B. (1973). Endocarditis caused by *Bacillus subtilis. American Journal of Clinical Pathology*, **60,** 714–18.
61. Samples, J.R. and Buettner, H. (1983). Corneal ulcer caused by a biological insecticide (*Bacillus thuringiensis*), *American* Journal of *Ophthalmology*, **95,** 258–60.
62. Samples, J.R and Buettner, H. (1983). Ocular infection caused by a biological insecticide. *Journal of Infectious Diseases*, **148,** 614.
63. Kasten, M.J., Rosenblatt, J.E., and Gustafson, D.R. (1992). *Bilophila wadsworthia* bacteremia in two patients with hepatic abscesses. *Journal of Clinical Microbiology*, **30,** 2502–3.
64. Summanen, P., Downes, J., Roberts, M.C., Wexler, H., and Finegold, S.M. (1989). *Bilophila wadsworthia*, gen. nov. and sp. nov., a unique gram-negative anaerobic rod recovered from appendicitis specimens and human faeces. *Journal of General Microbiology*, **135,** 3405–11.
65. Pitcher, D.G. and Malnick, H. (1984). Identification of *Brevibacterium* from clinical sources. *Journal of Clinical Pathology*, **37,** 1395–8.
66. Gruner, E., Pfyffer, G.E., and von Graevenitz, A. (1993). Characterization of *Brevibacterium* from clinical sources. *Journal of Clinical Microbiology*, **31,** 1408–12.
67. Yabuuchi, E. *et. al.*, (1993). Proposal of *Burkholderia* gen. nov. and transfer of seven species of the genus *Pseudomonas* homology group II to the new genus, with the type species *Burkholderia cepacia* (Palleroni and Holmes 1981) comb. nov. *International Journal of Systematic Bacteriology*, **36,** 1251–75.
68. Gessner, A.R. and Mortensen, J.E. (1990). Pathogenic factors of *Pseudomonas cepacia* isolates from patients with cystic fibrosis. *Journal of Medical Microbiology*, **33,** 115–20.
69. Glass, S. and Govan, J.R.W. (1986). *Pseudomonas cepacid*—fatal pulmonary infection in a patient with cystic fibrosis. *Journal of Infection*, **13,** 157–8.
70. Miller, R., Pannell, L., and Ingalls, M.S. (1948). Experimental chemotherapy in glanders and melioidosis. *American Journal of Hygiene*, **47,** 205–13.
71. Lacey, S. and Want, S.V. (1991). *Pseudomonas pickettii* infections in a paediatric oncology unit. *Journal of Hospital Infection*, **17,** 45–51.
72. Fujita, S., Yoshida, T., and Matsubara, F. (1981). *Pseudomonas pickettii* bacteremia. *Journal of Clinical Microbiology*, **13,** 781–782.
73. Dance, D.A.B. (1990). Melioidosis. *Reviews of Medical Microbiology* **1,** 143–50.
74. Dance, D.A.B. (1991). Melioidosis: the tip of the iceberg? *Clinical Microbiology Reviews*, **4,** 52–60.
75. Francioli, P., Herzstein, J., Grob, J-P., Vallotton, J-R., Mombelli, G., and Glauser, M.P. (1985). *Campylobacter fetus* subspecies *fetus* bacteremia. *Archives of Internal Medicine*, **145,** 289–92.
76. Blazer, M.J. (1990). *Campylobacter* species. In *Principles and practice of infectious diseases*, (3rd edn), (ed. G.L. Mandell, R.G. Douglas, and J.E. Bennett). Churchill Livingstone, New York.
77. Edmonds, P. *et al.* (1987). *Campylobacter hyointestinalis* associated with human gastrointestinal disease in the United States. *Journal of Clinical Microbiology*, **25,** 685–91.
78. Simon, A.E. and Wilcox, L. (1987). Enteritis associated with *Campylobacter laridis. Journal of Clinical Microbiology*, **25,** 10–12.
79. von Graevenitz, A. (1990). Revised nomenclature of *Campylobacter laridis, Enterobacter intermedium,* and *'Flavobacterium branchiophila.' International Journal of Systematic Bacteriology*, **40,** 211.
80. Gaudreau, C. and Lamothe, F. (1992). *Campylobacter upsalensis* isolated from a breast abscess. *Journal of Clinical Microbiology*, **30,** 1354–6.
81. Walmsley, S.L. and Karmali, M.A. (1989). Direct isolation of atypical thermophilic *Campylobacter* species form human feces on selective agar medium. *Journal of Clinical Microbiology*, **27,** 668–70.
82. Figura, N. *et al.* (1993). Two cases of *Campylobacter mucosalis* enteritis in children. *Journal of Clinical Microbiology*, **31,** 727–8.
83. Decoster, H., Snoeck, J., and Pattyn, S. (1992). *Capnocytophaga canimorsus* endocarditis. *European heart Journal*, **13,** 140–2.
84. Brenner, D.J., Hollis, D.G., Fanning, G.R., and Weaver, R.E. (1989). *Capnocytophaga canimorsus* sp. nov. (formerly CDC group DF-2), a cause of septicemia following dog bite, and *C. cynodegmi* sp. nov., a cause of localised wound infection following dog bite. *Journal of Clinical Microbiology*, **27,** 231–5.
85. Anderson, H.K. and Pedersen, M. (1992). Infective endocarditis with involvement of the tricuspid valve due to *Capnocytophaga canimorsus. European Journal of Clinical Microbiology and Infectious Diseases*, **11,** 831–2.
86. Bilgrami, S. *et al.* (1992). *Capnocytophaga* bacteremia in a patient with Hodgkin's disease following bone marrow transplantation: case report and review. *Clinics in Infectious Diseases* **14,** 1045–9.
87. Bernard, K., Cooper, C., Tessier, S., and Ewan, E.P. (1991). Use of chemotaxonomy as an aid to differentiate among *Capnocytophaga* species, CDC group DF-3, and aerotolerant strains of *Leptotrichia buccalis. Journal of Clinical Microbiology*, **29,** 2263–5.
88. Savage, D.D., Kagan, R.L., Young, N.A., and Horvah, A.E. (1977). *Cardiobacterium hominis* endocarditis: description of two patients and characterization of the organism. *Journal of Clinical Microbiology*, **27,** 75–80.
89. Wormser, G.P. and Bottone, E.J. (1983). *Cardiobacterium hominis*: review of microbiologic and clinical features. *Reviews of Infectious Diseases*, **5,** 680–91.
90. Gill, V.J., Travis, L.B., and Williams, D.Y. (1991). Clinical and microbiological observations on CDC group DF-3, a Gram-negative coccobacillus. *Journal of Clinical Microbiology*, **29,** 1589–92.
91. Blum, R.N., Berry, C.D., Phillips, M.G., Hamilos, D.L., and Koneman, E.W. (1992). Clinical illness associated with isolation of dysgonic fermenter 3 from stool samples. *Journal of Clinical Microbiology*, **30,** 396–400.
92. Aronson, N. and Zbick, C.J. (1988). Dysgonic fermenter 3 bacteremia in a neutropenic patient with acute lymphocytic leukemia. *Journal of Clinical Microbiology*, **26,** 2213–15.
93. Bangsborg, J.M., Frederiksen, W., and Bruun, B. (1990). Dysgonic fermenter 3-associated abscess in a diabetic patient. *Journal of Infection*, **20,** 237–40.
94. Zapardiel, J. *et al.* (1991). Peritonitis with CDC group IVc-2 bacteria in a patient on continuous ambulatory peritoneal dialysis. *European Journal of Clinical Microbiology and Infectious Diseases*, **10,** 509–11.
95. Dan, M., Berger, S.A., Adeska, D., and Levo, Y. (1986). Septicemia caused by the Gram-negative baceria CDC IVc-2 in an immunocompromised human. *Journal of Clinical Microbiology*, **23,** 803.
96. Crowe, H.M. and Brecher, S.M. (1987). Septicemia with CDC group IVc-2, an unusual gram-negative bacillus. *Journal of Clinical Microbiology*, **25,** 2225–6.
97. Farmer III, J.J., Sheth, N.K., Hudzinski, J.A., Rose, H.D., Asbury, M.A. (1982). Bacteremia due to *Cedecea neteri* sp. nov. *Journal of Clinical Microbiology*, **16,** 775–8.
98. Grimont, P.A.D., Gimont, F., Farmer III, J.J., and Asbury, M.A. (1981). *Cedecea davisae* gen. nov., sp. nov. and *Cedecea lapagei* sp. nov., new Enterobacteriaceae from clinical specimens. *International Journal of Systematic Bacteriology*, **31,** 317–26.
99. Le Prowse, C., McNeil, M.M., and McCarty, J.M. (1989). Catheter-related bacteremia caused by *Oerskovia turbata. Journal of Clinical Microbiology*, **27,** 571–2.
100. Reller, L.B., Maddoux, G.L., Eckman, M.R., and Pappas, G. (1975). Bacterial endocarditis caused by *Oerskovia turbata. Annals of Internal Medicine*, **83,** 664–6.
101. Tucker, R.E., Winter, W.G., and Wilson, H.D. (1979). Osteomyelitis

associated with *Chromobacterium violaceum* sepsis: a case report. *Journal of Bone and Joint Surgery*, **61,** 949–51.

102. Feldman, R.B. (1984). *Chromobacterium violaceum* infection of the eye: a report of two cases. *Archives of Ophthalmology*, **102,** 711–13.

103. Sorensen, R.U., Jacobns, M.R., and Shurin, S.B. (1985). *Chromobacterium violaceum* adenitis acquired in the northern United States as a complication of chronic granulomatous disease. *Pediatric Infectious Diseases Journal*, **4,** 701–2.

104. Holmes, B., Steigerwalt, A.G., Weaver, R.E., and Brenner, D.J. (1987). *Chryseomonas luteola* comb. nov. and *Flavimonas oryzihabitans* gen. nov. comb. nov. *Pseudomonas*-like species from human clinical specimens and formerly known respectively as groups Ve-1 and Ve-2. *International Journal of Systematic Bacteriology*, **37,** 245–50.

105. Horowitz, H., Gilroy, S., Feinstein, S., and Gilardi, G. (1990). Endocarditis associated with *Comamonas acidovorans*. *Journal of Clinical Microbiology*, **28,** 143–5.

106. Atkinson, B.E., Smith, D.L., and Lockwood, W.R. (1975). *Pseudomonas testosteroni* septicemia. *Annals of Internal Medicine*, **83,** 369–70.

107. Tamaoka, J., Ha, D-M., and Komagata, K. (1987). Reclassification of *Pseudomonas acidovorans* den Dooren de Jong 1926 and *Pseudomonas testosteroni* Marcus and Talalay 1956 as *Comamonas acidovorans* comb, nov. and *Comamonas testosteroni* comb. nov., with an emended description of the genus *Comamonas*. *International Journal of Systematic Bacteriology*, **37,** 52–9.

108. Lipsky, B.A., Goldberger, A.C., Tompkins, L.S., and Plorde, J.J. (1982). Infections caused by non-diphtheria corynebacteria. *Reviews of Infectious Diseases*, **4,** 1220–35.

109. Morris, A.J., Henderson, G.K., Bremner, D.A., and Collins, J.F. (1986). Relapsing peritonitis in a patient undergoing continuous ambulatory peritoneal dialysis due to *Corynebacterium aquaticum*. *Journal of Infection*, **13,** 151–6.

110. Weiner, M. and Werthamer, S. (1975). *Corynebacterium aquaticum* septicemia. *American Journal of Clinical Pathology*, **64,** 378–81.

111. Tendler, C. and Bottone, E.J. (1989). *Corynebacterium aquaticum* urinary tract infection in a neonate and concepts regarding the role of the organism as a neonatal pathogen. *Journal of Clinical Microbiology*, **27,** 343–5.

112. Vale, J.A. and Scott, G.W. (1977). *Corynebacterium bovis* as a cause of human disease. *Lancet*, **ii,** 682–4.

113. Philippon, A., and Bimet, F. (1990). *In vitro* susceptibility of *Corynebacterium* Group D2 and *Corynebacterium jeiceium* to twelve antibiotics. *European Journal of Microbiology and Infectious Diseases*, **9,** 892–5.

114. Gill, V.L., Manning, C., Lamson, M., Woltering, P., and Pizzo, P.A. (1981). Antibiotic-resistant group JK bacteria in hospitals. *Journal of Clinical Microbiology*, **13,** 472–7.

115. Quinn, J.P., Arnow, P.M., Weil, D., and Rosenblath, J. (1984). Outbreak of JK diphtheroid infections associated with environmental contamination. *Journal of Clinical Microbiology*, **19,** 668–71.

116. Messina, O.D., Maldonado-Cocco, J.A., Pescio, A., Farinati, A., and Garcia-Morteo, O. (1989). *Corynebacterium kutscheri* septic arthritis. *Arthritis and Rheumatism*, **32,** 1053.

117. Wilhelmus, K.R., Robinson, N.M., and Jones, D.B. (1979). *Bacterionema matruchotii* ocular infections. *American Journal of Ophthalmology*, **87,** 143–7.

118. Golledge, C.L. and Phillips, G. (1991). *Corynebacterium minutissimum* infection. *Journal of Infection*, **23,** 73–6.

119. Colt, H.G., Morris, J.F., Marston, B.J., and Sewell, D.L. (1991). Necrotizing tracheitis caused by *Corynebacterium pseudodiphtheriticum*: unique case and review. *Reviews of Infectious Diseases*, **13,** 73–6.

120. Goldberger, A.C., Lipsky, B.A., and Plorde, J.J. (1981). Suppurative granulomatous lymphadenitis caused by *Corynebacterium ovis (pseudotuberculosis)*. *American Journal of Clinical Pathology*, **76,** 486–90.

121. Barr, J.G., and Murphy, P.G. (1986). *Corynebacterium striatum*: an unusual organism isolated in pure culture from sputum. *Journal of Infection*, **13,** 297–8.

122. Meers, P.D. (1979). A case of classical diphtheria, and other infections due to *Corynebacterium ulcerans*. *Journal of Infection*, **1,** 139–42.

123. Chomarat, M, Breton, P., and Dubost, J. (1991). Osteomyelitis due to *Corynebacterium* group D2. *European Journal of Clinical Microbiology and Infectious Diseases*, **10,** 43.

124. Soriano, F., and Ponte, C. (1992). A case of urinary tract infection caused by *Corynebacterium urealyticum* and coryneform group F1. *European Journal of Clinical Microbiology and Infectious Diseases*, **11,** 626–8.

125. Soriano, F., and Fernandez-Roblas, R. (1988). Infections caused by antibiotic-resistant *Corynebacterium* group D2. *European Journal of Clinical Microbiology and Infectious Diseases*, **7,** 337–41.

126. Porschen, R.K., Goodman, Z., and Rafai, B. (1977). Isolation of *Corynebacterium xerosis* form clinical specimens. *American Journal of Clinical Pathology*, **68,** 290–3.

127. Liakim, and R., Silkoff, P., Lugassy, G., and Michel, J. (1983). *Corynebacterium xerosis* endocarditis. *Archives of Internal Medicine*, **143,** 1995.

128. Krish, G., Beaver, W., Sarubbi, F., Verghese, A. (1989). *Corynebacterium xerosis* as cause of vertebral osteomyelitis. *Journal of Clinical Microbiology*, **27,** 2869–70.

129. Na'was, T.E., Hollis, D.G., Moss, C.W., and Weaver, R.E. (1987). Comparison of biochemical, morphologic, and chemical characteristics of Centers for disease Control fermentative coryneform groups 1,2, and A-4. *Journal of Clinical Microbiology*, **25,** 1354–8.

130. Guillard, F., Appelbaum, P.C., and Sparrow, F.B. (1980). Pyelonephritis and septicemia due to Gram-positive rods similar to *Corynebacterium* Group E (aerotolerant *Bifidobacterium adolescentis*). *Annals of Internal Medicine*, **92,** 635–6.

131. Austin, G.E., Hill, E.O. (1983). Endocarditis due to *Corynebacterium* CDC group G2. *Journal of Infectious Diseases*, **147,** 1106.

132. Malanoski, G.J., Parker, R., and Eliopoulos, G.M. (1992). Antimicrobial susceptibilities of a *Corynebacterium* CDC group II strain isolated from a patient with endocarditis. *Southern Medical Journal*, **80,** 923.

133. Maskell, R. and Pead, L. (1990). A cluster of *Edwardsiella tarda* infection in a day-care center in Florida. *Journal of Infectious Diseases*, **162,** 282.

134. Hargreaves, J.E., and Lucey, D.R. (1990). Life-threatening *Edwardsiella tarda* soft tissue infection associated with catfish puncture wound. *Journal of Infectious Diseases*, **162,** 1416.

135. Janda, J.M. *et al.* (1991). Pathogenic properties of *Edwardsiella* species. *Journal of Clinical Microbiology*, **29,** 1997–2001.

136. Murphey, D.K., Septimus, E.J., and Waagner, D.C. (1990). Catfish-related injury and infection: report of two cases and review of the literature. *Clinics in Infectious Diseases*, **14,** 689–93.

137. McDade, J.E. (1990). Ehrlichiosis—disease of animals and humans. *Journal of Infectious Diseases*, **161,** 609–17.

138. Anderson, B.E, Dawson, J.E., Jones, D.C. and Wilson, K.H. (1991). *Ehrlichia chaffeensis*, a new species associated with human ehrlichiosis. *Journal of Clinical Microbiology*,**29,** 2838–42.

139. Dupon, M., d'Ivernois, C., Malou, M., Tauzin-Fin, P., Boineau, F., and Lacut, J.Y. (1991). Sacro-iliac joint infection caused by *Eikenella corrodens*. *European Journal of Clinical Microbiology and Infectious Diseases*, **10,** 529–30.

140. Stoloff, A.L. and Gillies, M.L. (1986). Infections with *Eikenella corrodens* in a general hospital: a report of 33 cases. *Reviews of Infectious Diseases*, **8,** 50–3.

141. Suwangol, S., Rothkopf, M., Smith, S.M., Le Blanc, D., and Eng, R. (1983). Pathogenicity of *Eikenella corrodens* in humans *Archives of Internal Medicine*, **143,** 2265–8.

142. Pérez-Pomata, M.T., Domínguez, J., Horcajo, P., Santidrián, F., and Bisquert, J. (1992). Spleen abscess caused by *Eikenella corrodens*. *European Journal of Clinical Microbiology and Infectious Diseases*, **11,** 162–3.

143. MacGowan, A.P. and Reeves, D.S. (1991). Tricuspid valve infective endocarditis and pulmonary sepsis due to *Erysipelothrix rhusiopathiae* successfully treated with high doses of ciprofiaxacin but complicated by gynaecomastia. *Journal of Infection*, **22,** 100–1.

144. Venditti, M., Gelfusa, V., Tarasi, A., Brandimarte, C., and Serra, P. (1990). Antimicrobial susceptibilities of *Erysipelothrix rhusiopathiae*. *Antimicrobial Agents and Chemotherapy*, **34,** 2038–40.

145. Farmer, III, J.J. *et al.* (1985). *Escherichia fergusonii* and *Enterobacter taylorae*, two new species of Enterobacteriaceae isolated from clinical specimens. *Journal of Clinical Microbiology*, **21,** 77–81.

146. Brenner, D.J. *et al.* (1982). Atypical biogroups of *Escherichia coli* found in clinical specimens and description of *Escherichia hermanii* sp. nov. *Journal of Clinical Microbiology*, **15,** 703–13.

147. Brenner, D.J., McWhorter, A.C., Leete Knutson, J.K., and Steigerwalt, A.G. (1982). *Escherichia vulneris*: a new species of Enterobacteriaceae associated with human wounds. *Journal of Clinical Microbiology*, **15,** 1133–40.

148. Sans, M.D. and Crowder, J.G. (1973). Subacute bacterial endocarditis

caused by *Eubacterium aerofaciens*: report of a case *American Journal of Clinical Pathology*, **59,** 576–80.

149. Devreese, K., Claeys, G., and Verschraegen, G. (1992). Septicaemia with *Ewingella americana. Journal of Clinical Microbiology*, **30,** 2746–7.

150. Podbielski, A., Mertens, R., Ziebold, C., and Kaufhold, A. (1990). *Flavimonas oryzihabitans* septicaemia in a T-cell leukaemic child: a case report and review of the literature. *Journal of Infection*, **20,** 135–41.

151. Bendig, J.W.A., Mays, P.J., Eyers, D.E., Holmes, B., and Chin, T. (1989). *Flavimonas oryzihabitans (Pseudomonas oryzihabitans*; CDC group Ve-2): an emerging pathogen in peritonitis related to continuous ambulatory peritoneal dialysis? *Journal of Clinical Microbiology*, **27,** 217–18.

152. Levett, P.N., Garrett, D.A., and Wickramasuriya, T. (1991). *Flavimonas oryzihabitans* as a cause of ocular infection. *European Journal of Clinical Microbiology and Infectious Diseases*, **10,** 594–5.

153. Reina, J., Borrell, N., and Figuerola, J. (1992). *Sphingobacterium multivorum* isolated from a patient with cystic fibrosis. *European Journal of Clinical Microbiology and Infectious Diseases*, **11,** 81–2.

154. Holmes, B., Hollis, D.G., Steigerwalt, A.G., Pickett, M., and Brenner, D.J. (1983). *Flavobacterium thalpophilum*, a new species recovered from human clinical material. *International Journal of Systematic Bacteriology*, **33,** 677–82.

155. Freney, J. *et al.* (1987). Septicemia caused by *Sphingobacterium multivorum. Journal of Clinical Microbiology*, **25,** 1126–8.

156. Thong, M.L., Puthucheary, S.D., and Lee, E.L. (1981). *Flavobacterium meningosepticum* infection: an epidemiological study in a newborn nursery. *Journal of Clinical Pathology*, **34,** 429–33.

157. Moore-Gillon, J., Lee, T.H., Eykyn, S.J., and Phillips, I. (1984). Necrobacillosis: a forgotten disease. *British Medical Journal*, **288,** 1526–7.

158. George, W.L., Kirby, B.D., and Sutter, V.L. (1981). Gram-negative anaerobic bacilli: their role in infection and patterns of susceptibility to antibiotic agents. II Little-known *Fusobacterium* species with miscellaneous genera. *Reviews of Infectious Diseases*, **3,** 599–626.

159. Chatelain, R. *et al.* (1982). Isolement de *Gemella haemolysans* dans trois cas d'endocardites bacteriennes. *Médecine et Maladies Infectieuses*, 12, 25–30.

160. Kilpper-Bälz, R. and Schleifer, K.H. (1988). Transfer of *Streptoccocus morbillorum* to the *Gemella* genus, *Gemella morbillorum* comb. nov. *International Journal of Systematic Bacteriology*, **38,** 442–443.

161. Brenner, D.J. *et al.* (1988). Biochemical, genetic, and epidemiologic characterization of *Haemophilus influenzae* biogroup aegyptius (*Haemophilus aegyptius*) strains associated with Brazilian purpuric fever. *Journal of Clinical Microbiology*, **26,** 1524–34.

162. Brazilian Purpuric Fever Study Group (1987). *Haemophilus aegyptius* bacteremia in Brazilian purpuric fever. *Lancet*, **ii,** 761–3.

163. Bieger, R.C., Brewer, N.S., and Washington II, J.A. (1978). *Haemophilus aphrophilus*: a microbiologic and clinical review and report of 42 cases. *Medicine* (Baltimore), **57,** 345–55.

164. Defèbvre, L., Ghawche, F., Muller, J.P., Savage, C., and Destée, A. (1992). Abcès cérébral à *Haemophilus aphrophilus* et cardiopathie congénitale cyanogène. *Médecine et Maladies Infectieuses*, **22,** 751–2.

165. Goldberg, R. and Washington II, J.A. (1978). The taxonomy and antimicrobial susceptibility of *Haemophilus* species in clinical specimens. *American Journal of Clinical Pathology*, **70,** 899–904.

166. Julander, L., Lindberg, A.A., and Swanbom, M. (1980). *Haemophilus parainfluenzae*: an uncommon cause of septicemia and endocarditis. *Scandinavian Journal of Infectious Diseases*, **12,** 85–9.

167. Jones, R.N., Slepack, J., and Bigelow, J. (1976). Ampicillin-resistant *Haemophilis paraphrophilus* laryngo-epiglottitis. *Journal of Clinical Microbiology*, **4,** 405–7.

168. Visvanathan, K. and Jones, P.D. (1991). Ciprofloxacin treatment of *Haemophilus paraphrophilus* brain abscess. *Journal of Infection*, **22,** 306–7.

169. Washington III, J.A., Birk, R.J., and Ritts, R.E. (1971). Bacteriologic and epidemiologic characteristics of *Enterobacter hafniae* and *Enterobacter liquefaciens. Journal of Infectious Diseases*, **124,** 379.

170. Marshall, B.J. (1986). *Campylobacter pyloridis* and gastritis. *Journal of Infectious Diseases*, **153,** 650–7.

171. Orlicek, S.L., Welch, D.F., and Kuhls, T.L. (1993). Septicemia caused by *Helicobacter cinaedi* in a neonate. *Journal of Clinical Microbiology*, **31,** 569–71.

172. Vandamme, P., Falsen, E., Pot, B., Kersters, K., and De Ley, J. (1990). Identification of *Campylobacter cinaedi* isolated from blood and faeces of children and adult females. *Journal of Clinical Microbiology*, **28,** 1016–20.

173. Totten, P.A. *et al.* (1985). *Campylobacter cinaedi* (sp. nov.) and *Campylobacter fennelliae* (sp. nov.): two new campylobacter species associated with enteric disease in homosexual men. *Journal of Infectious Diseases*, **151,** 131–139.

174. Burnens, A.P., Stanley, U.B., and Nicolet, J. (1993). Novel *Campylobacter*-like organisms resembling *Helicobacter fennelliae* isolated from a boy with gastroenteritis and from dogs. *Journal of Clinical Microbiology*, **31,** 1916–17.

175. Yagupsky, P. *et al.* (1992). High prevalence of *Kingella kingae* in joint fluid from children with septic arthritis revealed by the BACTEC blood culture system. *Journal of Clinical Microbiology*, **30,** 1278–81.

176. Goldman, I.S., Ellner, P.D., Francke, E.L., Garvey, G., and Squilla, A. (1980). Infective endocarditis due to *Kingella denitrificans. Annals of Internal Medicine*, **93,** 152–3.

177. Jenny, D.B., Letendre, P.W., and Iverson, G. (1988). Endocarditis due to *Kingella* species. *Reviews of Infectious Diseases*, **10,** 1065–6.

178. Namnyak, S.S., Quinn, R.J.M., and Ferguson, J.D.M. (1991). *Kingella kingae* meningitis in an infant. *Journal of Infection*, **23,** 104–6.

179. Farmer III, J.J. *et al.* (1981). *Kluyvera*, a new (redefined) genus in the family Entrobacteriaceae: identification of *Kluyvera ascorbata* sp. nov. and *Kluyvera cryocrescens* sp. nov. in clinical specimens. *Journal of Clinical Microbiology*, **13,** 919–33.

180. Sierra-Madero, J., Pratt, K., Hall, G.S., Stewart, R.W., Scerbo, J.J. and Longworth, D.L. (1990). *Kluyvera* mediastinitis following open-heart surgery: a case report. *Journal of Clinical Microbiology*, **28,** 2848–9.

181. Hickman-Brenner, F.W., Huntley-Carter, G.P., Fanning, G.R., Brenner, D.J., and Farmer III, J.J. (1985). *Koserella trabulsi*, a new genus and species of *Enterobacteriaceae* formerly known as enteric group 45. *Journal of Clinical Microbiology*, **21,** 39–42.

182. Elston, H.R. (1961). *Kurthia bessonii* isolated from clinical material. *Journal of Pathology and Bacteriology*, **81,** 245–7.

183. Pancoast, S.J., Ellner, P.D., Jahre, J.A., and Neu, H.C. (1979). Endocarditis due to *Kurthia bessonii. Annals of Internal Medicine*, **90,** 936–7.

184. Chomarat, M., and Espinouse, D. (1991). *Lactobacillus rhamnosus* septicemia in patients with prolonged aplasia receiving ceftazidime-vancomycin. *European Journal of Clinical Microbiology and Infectious Diseases*, **10,** 44.

185. Rahman, M. (1982). Chest infection caused by *Lactobacillus casei ss rhamnosus. British Medical Journal*, **284,** 471–2.

186. Sussman, J.I., Baron, E.J., Goldberg, S.M., Kaplan, M.H., and Pizzarello, R.A. (1986). Clinical manifestation and therapy of *Lactobacillus* endocarditis: report of a case and review of the literature. *Reviews of Infectious Diseases*, **8,** 771–776.

187. Bantar, C.E., Relloso, S., Rodriguez Castell, F., Smayevsky, J., and Bianchini, H.M. (1991). Abscess caused by vancomycin-resistant *Lactobacillus confusus. Journal of Clinical Microbiology*, **29,** 2063–4.

188. Elliott, J.A., Collins, M.D., Pigott, N.E., and Facklam, R.R. (1991). Differentiation of *Lactococcus lactis* and *Lactococcus garviae* from humans by comparison of whole-cell protein patterns. *Journal of Clinical Microbiology*, **29, 2731–4.**

189. Tamura, K., Sakazaki, R., Kosako, Y., and Yoshizaki, E. (1986). *Leclercia adecarboxylata* gen. nov., comb. nov., formerly known as *Escherichia adecarboxylata. Current Microbiology*, **13,** 179–82.

190. Hickman-Brenner, F. *et al.* (1985). *Leminorella*, a new genus of Enterobacteriaceae: identification of *Leminorella grimontii* sp. nov. and *Leminorella ricchardii* sp. nov. found in clinical specimens. *Journal of Clinical Microbiology*, **21,** 234–9.

191. Friedland, I.R., Snipelisky, M., and Khoosal, M. (1990). Meningitis in a neonate caused by *Leuconostoc* sp. *Journal of Clinical Microbiology*, **28,** 2125–6.

192. Bernaldo de Quirós, J.C.L. *et al.* (1991). *Leuconostoc* species as a cause of bacteremia: two case reports and a literature review. *European Journal of Clinical Microbiology and Infectious Diseases*, **10,** 505–9.

193. Horowitz, H.W., Handwerger, S., and van Horn, K.G. (1987). *Leuconostoc*, and emerging vancomycin-resistant pathogen. *Lancet*, **i,** 1329–30.

194. Brancaccio, M. and Legendri, G.G. (1979). *Megasphaera eldenii* endocarditis. *Journal of Clinical Microbiology*, **10,** 72–4.

195. Kaye, K.M., Macone, A., and Kazanjian, P.H. (1992). Catheter infection caused by *Methylobacterium* in immunocompromised hosts: report

of three cases and review of the literature. *Clinics in Infectious Diseases*, **14,** 1010–14.

196. Gould, F.K., Venning, M.C., and Ford, M. (1990). Successful treatment with chloramphenicol of *Pseudomonas mesophilica* peritonitis not responding to aztreonam and gentamicin. *Journal of Antimicrobial Chemotherapy*, **26,** 458–9.

197. Rutherford, P.C., Narkowicz, J.E., Wood, C.J., and Peel, M.M. (1988). Peritonitis caused by *Pseudomonas mesophilica* in a patient undergoing continuous ambulatory peritoneal dialysis. *Journal of Clinical Microbiology*, **26,** 2441–3.

198. Smith, S.M., Eng, R.H.K., and Forrester, C. (1985). *Pseudomonas mesophilica* infections in humans. *Journal of Clinical Microbiology*, **21, 314–17.**

199. Schwebke, J.R., Lukehart, S.A., Roberts, M.C., and Hillier, S.L. (1991). Identification of two new antigenic subgroups within the genus *Mobiluncus. Journal of Clinical Microbiology*, **29,** 2204–8.

200. Glupczynski, T. *et al.* (1984). Isolation of *Mobiluncus* in four cases of extragenital infection in adult women. *European Journal of Clinical Microbiology*,**3,** 433–5.

201. Spiegel, C.A. (1987). Susceptibility of *Mobiluncus* species to 23 antimicrobial agents and 15 other compounds. *Antimicrobial Agents and Chemotherapy*, **31,** 249–52.

202. Silverfarb, P.M. and Lawe, J.E. (1968). Endocarditis due to *Moraxella liquefaciens. Archives of Internal Medicine*, **122,** 512–13.

203. Ebright, J.R., Lentino, J.R., and Juni, E. (1982). Endophthalmitis caused by *Moraxella nonliquefaciens. American Journal of Clinical Pathology*, **77,** 362–3.

204. Bøvre, K., Henriksen, S.D. (1967). A new *Moraxella* speceies, *Moraxella osloensis*, and a revised description of *Moraxella nonliquefaciens International Journal of Systematic Bacteriology*, **17,** 127–35.

205. Bøvre, K., Fuglesang, J.E. and Hagen, N. (1976). *Moraxella atlantae* sp. nov. and its distinction from *Moraxella phenylpyruvica. International Journal of Systematic Bacteriology*, **26,** 511–21.

206. Percival, A. *et al.* (1977). Pathogenicity of and beta-lactamase production by *Branhamella (Neisseria) catarrhalis. Lancet*, **ii,** 1175.

207. Catlin, B.W. (1991). *Branhamaceae* fam. nov., a proposed family to accommodate the genera *Branhamella and Moraxella. International Journal of Systematic Bacteriology*, **41,** 320–3.

208. Herbert, D.A., and Ruskin, J. (1981). Are the 'non-pathogenic' neisseriae pathogenic? *American Journal of Clinical Pathology*, **75,** 739–43.

209. Morla, N., Guibourdenche, M., and Riou, J-Y. (1992). *Neiseria* spp. and AIDS. *Journal of Clinical Microbiology*, **30,** 2290–4.

210. Wong, J.D. and Janda, J.M. (1992). *Neisseria* species, *Neisseria elongata* subsp. *nitroreductens*, with bacteremia, endocarditis, and osteomyelitis. *Journal of Clinical Microbiology*, **30,** 719–20.

211. Berger, S.A., Gorea, A., Peyser, M.R., and Edberg, S.C. (1988). Bartholin's gland abscess caused by *Neisseria sicca. Journal of Clinical Microbiology*, **26,** 1589.

212. Gay, R.M. and Sevier, R.E. (1978). *Neisseria sicca* endocarditis: report of a case and review of the literature. *Journal of Clinical Microbiology*, **8,** 729–732.

213. Guibourdenche, M., Lambert, T., and Riou, J.Y. (1989). Isolation of *Neisseria canis* in mixed culture from a patient after a cat bite. *Journal of Clinical Microbiology*, **27,** 1673–4.

214. Holmes, B., Popoff, M., Kiridjian, M., and Kersters, K. (1988). *Ochrobactrum anthropi* gen. nov., sp. nov. from human clinical specimens and previously known as group Vd. *International Journal of Systematic Bacteriology*, **38,** 406–16.

215. Rihs, J.D., McNeil, M.M., Brown, J.M., and Yu, V.L. (1990). *Oerskovia xanthineolytica* implicated in peritonitis associated with peritoneal dialysis: case report and review of *Oerskovia* infections in humans. *Journal of Clinical Microbiology*, **28,** 1934–7.

216. Cruikshank, S.J., Gawler, A.H., and Shaldon, G. (1979). *Oerskovia* species: rare opportunistic pathogens. *Journal of Medical Microbiology*, **12,** 513–15.

217. Truant, A.L., Satishchandran, V., Eisenstaedt, R., Richman, P., and McNeil, M.M. (1992). *Oerskovia xanthineolytica* and methicillin-resistant *Staphylococcus aureus* in a patient with cirrhosis and variceal hemorrhage. *European Journal of Clinical Microbiology and Infectious Diseases*, **11,** 950–951.

218. Kailath, E.J., Goldstein, E., and Wagner, F.H. (1988). Case report: meningitis caused by *Oerskovia xanthineolytica. American Journal of Medical Sciences*, **295,** 216–17.

219. Hussain, Z., Gonder, J.R., Lannigan, R., Stoakes, L. (1987). Endophthalmitis due to *Oerskovia xanthineolytica. Canadian Journal of Ophthalmology*, **22,** 234–6.

220. Mesnard, R., Sire, J.M., Donnio, P.Y., Riou, S.Y., and Avril, J.L. (1992). Septic arthritis due to *Oligella urethralis. European Journal of Clinical Microbiology and Infectious Diseases*, **11,** 195–6.

221. Rossau, R. *et al.* (1987). *Oligella*, a new genus including *Oligella urethralis* comb. nov. (formerly *Moraxella urethralis*) and *Oligella ureolytica* sp. nov. (formerly CDC group IVe): relationship to *Taylorella equigenitalis* and related taxa. *International Journal of Systematic Bacteriology*, **37,** 198–210.

222. Sneath, P.H.A. and Stevens, M. (1990). *Actinobacillus rossii* sp. nov., *Actinobacillus seminis* sp. nov., nom. rev., *Pasteurella bettii* sp. nov., *Pasteurella lymphangitidis* sp. nov., *Pasteurella mairi* sp. nov., and *Pasteurella trehalosi* sp. nov. *International Journal of Systematic Bacteriology*, **40,** 148–53.

223. Johnson, R.H. and Rumans, L.W. (1977). Unusual infections caused by *Pasteurella multocida. Journal of the American Medical Association*, **237,** 146–7.

224. Rogers, B.T., Anderson, J.C., Palmer, C.A., and Henderson, W.G. (1973). Septicaemia due to *Pasteurella pneumotropica. Journal of Clinical Pathology*, **26,** 396–8.

225. Pouëdras, P., Donnio, P.Y., Le Tulzo, Y., and Avril, J.L. (1993). *Pasteurella stomatis* infection following dog bite. *European Journal of Clinical Microbiology and Infectious Diseases*, **12,** 65.

226. Yaneza, A.L., Jivan, H., Kumari, P., and Togoo, M.S. (1991). *Pasteurella haemolytica* endocarditis. *Journal of Infection*, **23,** 65–7.

227. Holst, E., Rollo, J., Larsson, L., and Nielsen, J.P. (1992). Characterization and distribution of *Pasteurella* species recovered from infected humans. *Journal of Clinical Microbiology*, **30,** 2984–7.

228. Mastro, T.D., Spika, J.S., Lozano, P., Appel, J., and Facklam, R.R. (1990). Vancomycin-resistant *Pediococcus acidilactici*: nine cases of bacteremia. *Journal of Infectious Diseases*, **161,** 956–960.

229. Sire, J.M., Donnio, P.Y., Mesnard, R., Pouëdras, P., and Avril, J.L. (1992). Septicaemia and hepatic abscess caused by *Pediococcus acidilactici. European Journal of Clinical Microbiology and Infectious Diseases*, **11,** 623–5.

230. Colman, G. and Efstratiou, A. (1987). Vancomycin-resistant leuconostocs, lactobacilli and now pediococci. *Journal of Hospital Infection*, **2,** 1–3.

231. Coffey, J.A., Harris, R.L., Bradshaw, M.W., and Williams, T.W. (1986). *Vibrio damsela*: another potentially virulent marine vibrio. *Journal of Infectious Diseases*, **153,** 800–2.

232. Clark, R.B., Lister, P.D., Arneson-Rotert, L., and Janda, J.M. (1990). *In vitro* susceptibilities of *Plesiomonas shigelloides* to 24 antibiotics and antibiotic-β-lactamase-inhibitor combinations. *Antimicrobial Agents and Chemotherapy*, **34,** 159–60.

233. Kain, K.C. and Kelly, M.T. (1989). Antimicrobial susceptibility of *Plesiomonas shigelloides* from patients with diarrhea. *Antimicrobial Agents and Chemotherapy*, **33,** 1609–10.

234. Brenden, R.A., Miller, M.A., and Janda, J.M. (1988). Clinical disease spectrum and pathogenic factors associated with *Plesiomonas shigelloides* in humans. *Clinics in Infectious Diseases*, **10,** 303–16.

235. Shah, H.N. and Collins, M.D. (1988). Proposal for reclassification of *Bacteroides asaccharolyticus, Bacteroides gingivalis*, and *Bacteroides endodontalis* in a new genus, *Porphyromonas. International Journal of Systematic Bacteriology*, **38,** 128–31.

236. Shah, H.N. and Collins, D.M. (1990). *Prevotella*, a new genus to include *Bacteroides melaninogenicus* and related species formerly classified in the genus *Bacteroides. International Journal of Systematic Bacteriology*, **40,** 205–8.

237. Palleroni, N.J. (1984). Family 1. Pseudomonadaceae. In *Bergey's manual of systematic bacteriology*, Vol. 1, (ed. N.R. Krieg and J.G. Holt). Williams & Willkins, Baltimore.

238. Woese, C.R. (1987). Bacterial evolution. *Microbial Reviews*, **51,** 221–71.

239. Elting, L.S. and Bodey, G.P. (1990). Septicemia due to *Xanthomonas* species and non-aeruginosa *Pseudomonas* species: increasing incidence of catheter-related infections. *Medicine* (Baltimore), **69,** 296–306.

240. Lloyd-Puryear, M., Wallace, D., Baldwin, T., and Hollis, D.G. (1991). Meningitis caused by *Psychrobacter immobolis* in an infant. *Journal of Clinical Microbiology*, **29,** 2041–2.

241. Gini, G.A. (1990). Ocular infection caused by *Psychrobacter immobilis* acquired in a hospital. *Journal of Clinical Microbiology*, **28,** 400–1.
242. Alballaa, S.R., Qadri, H.S.M., Al-Furayh, O., and Al-Qatary, K. (1992). Urinary tract infection due to *Rahnella aquatilis* in a renal transplant patient. *Journal of Clinical Microbiology*, **30,** 2948–50.
243. Goubau, P., Van Aelst, F., Verhaegen, J., and Boogaerts, M. (1988). Septicaemia caused by *Rahnella aquatilis* in an immunocompromised patient. *European Journal of Clinical Microbiology and Infectious Diseases*, **7,** 697–9.
244. Sane, D.C. and Durack, D.T. (1986). Infection with *Rhodococcus equi* in AIDS. *New England Journal of Medicine*, **314,** 56–7.
245. Berg, R., Chmel, H., Mayo, J., and Armstrong, D. (1977). *Corynebacterium equi* infection complicating neoplastic disease. *American Journal of Clinical Pathology*, **68,** 73–7.
246. Van Etta, L.L. (1983). *Corynebacterium equi*: a review of twelve cases of human infection. *Reviews of Infectious Diseases*, **5,** 1012–18.
247. Slater, L.N., Welch, D.F., Hensel, D., and Coody, D.W. (1990). A newly recognised fastidious Gram-negative pathogen as a cause of fever and bacteremia. *New England Journal of Medicine*, **323,** 1587–93.
248. Relman, D.A., Loutit, J.S., Schmidt, T.M., Falkow, S., and Tompkins, L.S. (1990). The agent of bacillary angiomatosis: an approach to the identification of uncultured pathogens. *New England Journal of Medicine*, **323,** 1573–80.
249. Regnery, R.L., Olson, J.G., Perkins, B.A., and Bibb, W. (1992). Serological response to '*Rochalimaea henselae*' antigen in suspected cat-scratch disease. *Lancet*, **339,** 1443–5.
250. Patnaik, M., Scwartzman, W.A., Barka, N.E., and Peter, J.B. (1992). Possible role of *Rochalimaea henselae* in pathogenesis of AIDS encephalopathy. *Lancet*, **340,** 971–2.
251. Koeler, J.E., Quinn, F.D., Berger, T., LeBoit, P.E., and Tappero, J.W. (1992). Isolation of *Rochalimaea* species from cutaneous and osseous lesions of bacillary angiomatosis. *New England Journal of Medicine*, **327,** 1625–31.
252. Tompkins, D.C. and Steigbigel, R.T. (1993). Rochalimaea's role in cat scratch disease and bacillary angiomatosis. *Annals of Internal Medicine*, **118,** 388–9.
253. Daly, J.S. *et al.* (1993). *Rochalimaea elizabethae* sp. nov. isolated from a patient with endocarditis. *Journal of Clinical Microbiology*, **31,** 872–81.
254. Broeren, S.A. and Peel, M.M. (1984). Endocarditis caused by *Rothia dentocariosa. Journal of Clinical Pathology*, **37,** 1298–92.
255. Yu, V.L. (1979). *Serratia marcescens*: historical perspective and clinical review. *New England Journal of Medicine*, **300,** 887–92.
256. Pfyffer, G.E. (1991). *Serratia fonticola* as an infectious agent. *European Journal of Clinical Microbiology and Infectious Diseases*, **11,** 199–200.
257. Zbinden, R. and Blass, R. (1988). *Serratia plymuthica* osteomyelitis following a motorcycle accident. *Journal of Clinical Microbiology*,**26,** 1409–10.
258. Clark, R.B. and Janda, J.M. (1985). Isolation of *Serratia plymuthica* from a human burn site. *Journal of Clinical Microbiology*, **21,** 656–7.
259. Horowitz, H.W., Naelman, K.G., Van Horn, S.E., Weekes, L., Goyburu, L., and Wormser, G.P. (1987). *Serratia plymuthica* sepsis associated with infection of central venous catheter. *Journal of Clinical Microbiology*, **25,** 1562–3.
260. Bollet, C., Gainnier, M., Sainly, J-M., Orhesser, P., and de Micco, P. (1991). *Serratia fonticola* isolated from a leg abscess. *Journal of Clinical Microbiology*, **29,** 834–5.
261. Nozue, H. *et al.* (1992). Isolation and characterization of *Shewanella alga* from human clinical specimens and emendation of the description of *S. alga* Simidu *et al.*, 1990, **335,** *International Journal of Systematic Bacteriology*, **42,** 628–34.
262. Marne, C., Pallarés, R., and Sitges-Sera, A. (1983). Isolation of *Pseudomonas putrefaciens* in intraabdominal sepsis. *Journal of Clinical Microbiology*, **17,** 1173–4.
263. Laudat, P., Audurier, A., Loulergue, J., Legros, B., and Lapierre, F. (1983). *Pseudomonas putrefaciens* meningitis. *Journal of Infection*, **7,** 281–3.
264. Southern, P.M. and Kutscher, A.E. (1981). *Pseudomonas paucimobilis* bacteremia. *Journal of Clinical Microbiology*, **13,** 1070–3.
265. Condron, P.E., Markowitz, S.M., Moharty, L.B., Schatzki, P.F., and Payne, J.M. (1987). Isolation of *Stomatococcus mucilaginosus* from drug user with endocarditis. *Journal of Clinical Microbiology*, **25,** 1359–63.
266. Jenny, D.B., Letendre, P.W., and Iverson, G. (1987). Endocarditis caused by *Kingella indologenes*. *Reviews of Infectious Diseases*, **9,** 787.
267. Hollis, D.G., Hickman, F.W., Fanning, G.R., Farmer III, J.J., Weaver, R.E., and Brenner, D.J. (1981). *Tatumella ptyseos* gen. nov., sp. nov., a member of the family *Enterobacteriaceae* found in clinical specimens. *Journal of Clinical Microbiology*, **14,** 79–88.
268. Relman, D.A., Schmidt, T.M., MacDermott, R.P., and Falkow, S. (1992). Identification of the uncultured bacillus of Whipple's disease. *New England Journal of Medicine*, **327,** 293–301.
269. Rogosa, M. (1984). Family I. Veillonellaceae Rogosa 1971, 232. In *Bergey's manual of systematic bacteriology*, Vol. 1, (ed. N.R. Krieg and J.G. Holt). Williams & Wilkins, Baltimore.
270. West, P.A. (1989). The human pathogenic vibrios—a public health update with environmental perspectives. *Epidemiology and Infection*, **103,** 1–34.
271. Darbas, H., Boyer, G., Jean-Pierre, H., and Riviere, M. (1992). *Vibrio alginolyticus*: isolement chez trois patients. Revue de la littérature. *Medecine et Maladies Infectieuses*, **22,** 643–647.
272. Pavia, A.T., Bryan, J.A., Maher, K.L., Hester, T.R., and Farmer, J.J. *Vibrio carchariae* infection after a shark bite. *Annals of Internal Medicine*, **111,** 85–6.
273. Bode, R.B., Brayton, P.R., Colwell, R.R., Russo, F.M., and Bullock, W.E. (1986). *Vibrio cincinnatiensis* causing meningitis: successful treatment in an adult. *Annals of Internal Medicine*, **104,** 55–6.
274. Hickman-Brenner, F.W. *et al.* (1982). Identification of *Vibrio hollisae* sp. nov. from patients with diarrhea. *Journal of Clinical Microbiology*, **15,** 395–400.
275. Jean-Jacques, W., Rajashekaraiah, K.R., Farmer III, J.J., Hickman, F.W., Morris, J.G., and Kallick, C.A. (1981). *Vibrio metschnikovii* bacteremia in a patient with cholecystitis. *Journal of Clinical Microbiology*, **14,** 711–12.
276. Bonner, J.R., Coher, A.S., Berryman, C.R., and Pollock, H.M. (1983). Spectrum of *Vibrio* infections in a Gulf coast community. *Annals of Internal Medicine*, **99,** 464–9.
277. Levine, W.C., Griffin, P.M., and the Gulf Coast *Vibrio* Working Group (1993). *Vibrio* infections on the Gulf Coast: results of first year of regional surveillance. *Journal of Infectious Diseases*, **167,** 479–83.
278. Reina, J. and Borrell, N. (1992). Leg abscess caused by *Weeksella zoohelcum* following a dog bite. *Clinics in Infectious Diseases*, **14,** 1162–3.
279. Bercovier, H. and Mollaret, H.H. (1984). Genus XIV Yersinia Van Loghem 1944, 15. In *Bergey's manual of systematic bacteriology*, Vol. **1,** (ed. N.R. Krieg and J.G. Holt) Williams & Wilkins, Baltimore.
280. Zuravleff, J.J. and Yu, V.L. (1982). Infections caused by *Pseudomonas maltophilia* with emphasis on bacteremia: case reports and a review of the literature. *Reviews of Infectious Diseases*, **4,** 1236–46.
281. Palleroni, N.J. and Bradbury, J.F. (1993). *Stenotrophomonas*, a new bacterial genus for *Xanthomonas maltophilia* (Hugh 1980) Swings *et al.* 1983. *International Journal of Systematic Bacteriology*, **43,** 606–9.
282. Rihs, J.D., Brenner, D.J., Weaver, R.E., Steigerwalt, A.G., Hollis, D.G., and Yu, V.L. (1993). *Roseomonas*, a new genus associated with bacteremia and other human infections. *Journal of Clinical Microbiology*, **31,** 3275–83.
283. Brenner, D.J., O'Connor, S.P., Winkler, H.H. and Steigerwalt, A.G. (1993). Proposals to unify the genera *Bartonella* and *Rochalimaea* with descriptions of *Bartonella quintana* comb. nov., *Bartonella vinsonii* comb. nov., *Bartonella henselae* comb. nov., and *Bartonella elizabethae* comb. nov., and to remove the family *Bartonellaceae* from the order Rickettsiales. *International Journal of Systematic Bacteriology*, **43,** 777–86.

7.12 Fungal infections (mycoses)

7.12.1 Fungal infections

R. J. HAY AND D. W. R. MACKENZIE

Introduction

Fungi are saprophytic or parasitic organisms that are normally assigned to a distinct Kingdom. As eukaryotes, they have the complex subcellular organization and highly organized genetic material seen in both animal and plant cells. The cell wall is a distinctive feature of fungi and contains complex macromolecules such as chitin. The arrangement and reproduction of individual cells is also characteristic. Most fungi form new cells terminally, which remain connected to form long, branching filaments or hyphae (the mould fungi). Some reproduce in a similar manner but each new cell separates from the parent by a process of budding (the yeast fungi). It is a feature of certain fungi to be yeast-like during one phase of their life history but hyphal at another, a phenomenon known as dimorphism. In culture, mould fungi usually form a cottony growth on laboratory media while yeasts normally have a smooth, shiny appearance.

Fungi adversely affect man in a number of ways. They cause disease indirectly by spoilage and destruction of food crops with subsequent malnutrition and starvation. Many of the common moulds produce and release spores, which may act as airborne allergens to produce asthma or hypersensitivity pneumonitis. Fungi elaborate complex metabolic by-products, some of which are useful to man, such as the penicillins. However, others are toxic. Disease caused by the ingestion of fungal toxins includes both poisoning by eating certain mushrooms (mycetism) and damage caused by the ingestion of minute quantities of toxin (mycotoxicosis), for instance in contaminated grain. The contribution of the latter mechanism to human disease remains largely unexplored. Finally, fungi may invade human tissue. Medical mycology is largely concerned with this last group. Invasive fungal diseases are normally divided into three groups: the superficial, subcutaneous, and deep mycoses. In superficial infections, such as ringworm or thrush, fungi are confined to the skin and mucous membranes. Extension deeper than the surface epithelium is rare. Subcutaneous infections are usually tropical: the main site of involvement is within subcutaneous tissue, although secondary invasion of adjacent structures such as bone or skin may occur. In deep or systemic infections, deep viscera such as lung, spleen or brain are invaded. This classification of mycoses is based on the main 'sphere of involvement' by the causal organisms, but there are rare exceptions. For instance, brain involvement has been recorded in patients with chromoblastomycosis, which is normally a subcutaneous infection.

The fungi causing systemic mycoses are often classified in two groups: the opportunists and the pathogens. The former cause disease in overtly compromised individuals. These contrast with the true pathogens, which cause infection in all subjects inhaling airborne spores.

REFERENCES

General

Evans, E.G.V. and Richardson, M.D. (ed.) (1989). *Medical mycology—a practical approach*, pp. 17–45. IRL Press, Oxford.

Hay, R.J. (ed.) (1989). Tropical fungal infections. In *Tropical medicine and communicable diseases*, Vol. 4. Ballière Tindall, London.

Hay, R.J. (1992). *Fungi and the skin*. Gower, London.

Rebell, G. and Taplin, D. (1970). *Dermatophytes—their recognition and identification*. University of Miami Press.

Warnock, D.W. and Richardson, M.D. (ed.) (1990). *Fungal infection in the compromised patient*. Wiley, Chichester.

Superficial fungal infections

The main superficial mycoses are the dermatophyte infections, superficial candidosis, and tinea versicolor (Section 23). These are both common and widespread. Rare superficial infections include tinea nigra, and black or white piedra.

Dermatophyte infections (dermatophytoses)

Aetiology

The dermatophyte or ringworm infections are caused by a group of organisms capable of existing in keratinized tissue such as stratum corneum, nail or hair. Mechanisms of pathogenicity are thought to be linked to production of extracellular enzymes, such as the three distinct keratinases produced by *Trichophyton mentagrophytes*, but other proteases may also be involved.

Epidemiology

Some dermatophyte fungi have a worldwide distribution; others are more restricted. The most common and most widely distributed is *Trichophyton rubrum*, which causes different types of infection in different parts of the world. It is commonly associated with athlete's foot (tinea pedis) in temperate areas and tinea corporis (body ringworm) in the tropics. This distinction is not based solely on climatic factors, as immigrants from tropical countries, particularly the Far East, may still have tinea corporis caused by *T. rubrum* when living in northern Europe. Certain dermatophytes are limited to defined areas. For instance, tinea imbricata caused by *T. concentricum*, is found in hot, humid areas of the Far East, Polynesia, and South America. Scalp ringworm tends to occur in well-defined endemic areas in Africa. In different regions, different species of dermatophytes may predominate. Thus, in North Africa, the most common cause of tinea capitis is *T. violaceum*; in southern parts of the continent, the major agents may be *Microsporum audouinii*, *M. ferrugineum*, and *T. soudanense*. Not all dermatophyte infections are endemic and dominant species may disappear to be replaced by others. *M. audouinii*, once endemic and common in the United Kingdom, has largely disappeared as a cause of scalp ringworm, probably because of improved treatment and detection of carriers. Conversely, dermatophytes common to an immigrant group may be introduced into their new society.

Dermatophytes may be passed from person to person (anthropophilic infections), from animal to man (zoophilic) or soil to man (geophilic). Sources of zoophilic organisms in Europe include cats and dogs, cattle, hedgehogs, and small rodents. Rarer sources include horses, monkeys, and chickens. Lesions produced by zoophilic species may be highly inflammatory.

Factors governing the invasion of stratum corneum are largely unknown, but heat, humidity, and occlusion have all been implicated. Recently, it has been suggested that the carbon dioxide tension at the skin surface may be a critical factor.

Clinical features

The clinical features of dermatophyte infections are best considered in relation to the site involved. Often the term tinea, followed by the Latin name of the appropriate part (e.g. *corporis*—body) is used to describe the clinical site of infection.

TINEA PEDIS

Scaling or maceration between the toes particularly in the fourth interspace, is the most common form of dermatophytosis seen in temperate countries. Itching is variable, but may be severe. Sometimes blisters may form both between the toes and on the soles of the feet. The causative organisms are commonly *T. rubrum* and *T. interdigitale*, the latter being responsible for the vesicular forms. Similar appearances can be caused by *Candida albicans* and in the bacterial infection, erythrasma.

'DRY TYPE' INFECTIONS OF THE SOLES AND PALMS

These are normally caused by *T. rubrum*. Palms or soles have a dry, scaly appearance, which in the soles may encroach on to the lateral or dorsal surfaces of the foot. The palmar involvement is often unilateral, an important diagnostic feature (Plate 1). Nail invasion is often seen (see below). Itching is not prominent, and infections are usually chronic.

TINEA CRURIS

Infections of the groin, most often caused by *T. rubrum* or *Epidermophyton floccosum*, are relatively common. They occur in both tropical and temperate climates, although in the former the infection may spread to involve the whole waist area in both males and females. Tinea cruris in females is uncommon in Europe. An erythematous and scaly rash with a distinct margin extends from the groin to the upper thighs or scrotum. Itching may be severe. Coincident tinea pedis is common, and patients should be examined for this.

ONYCHOMYCOSIS (CAUSED BY DERMATOPHYTES)

Invasion of the nail plate is most often seen with *T. rubrum* infections. The plate is invaded distally and becomes thickened and friable. Onycholysis may be seen. More rarely, and most often with *T. interdigitale*, the dorsal surface of the plate is invaded, causing superficial white onychomycosis.

TINEA CORPORIS (BODY RINGWORM)

Dermatophyte or ringworm infection on the trunk or limbs may produce the characteristic annular plaque with a raised edge and central clearing (Plate 2). Scaling and itching is variable. Lesions caused by zoophilic organisms may be highly inflammatory and in certain cases, particularly those caused by *T. verrucosum*, intense itching, oedema, and pustule formation (kerion) may develop. This reaction is seldom secondarily infected by bacteria but is a response to the fungus on hairy skin. Infections of the beard, tinea barbae, are often highly refractory to treatment.

On the legs, an unusual variant, nodular folliculitis may superficially resemble erythema nodosum. A hot, tender, dermal nodule is formed on the shin or lower leg. However, close inspection usually reveals its relation to a hair follicle and some scaling. *T. rubrum* is the usual cause.

Facial dermatophyte infections may mimic a variety of non-fungal skin diseases, including acne, rosacea, and discoid lupus erythematosus. However, the underlying annular configuration can usually be distinguished. The term tinea incognito is used to describe such atypical lesions.

TINEA CAPITIS (SCALP RINGWORM)

In the United Kingdom, the most common cause of scalp ringworm is *Microsporum canis*, originating from an infected cat or dog. Scalp ringworm is mainly a disease of childhood, with rare infections occurring in adult women. Spontaneous clearance at puberty is the rule. *M. canis* causes an 'ectothrix' infection where spores form on the outside of the hair shaft and the scalp hair breaks above the skin surface. Scaling, itching, and loss of hair occur. Other causes of ectothrix infection include *M. audouinii*, which is now rare in Europe, but still seen in the tropics. This infection can be spread from child to child and cause serious social handicap. The infection may occur in epidemic form, particularly in schools. By contrast, infections with *M. canis* are acquired from a primary animal source rather than by spread from human lesions.

In endothrix infections where sporulation is within the hair shaft, scaling is less pronounced and hairs break at scalp level (black dot ringworm). Examples include *T. tonsurans* and *T. violaceum*, the latter being most prevalent in the Middle East, parts of Africa and India, although it is being recognized with increasing frequency in Europe.

Favus, now most often seen in the tropics, is a particularly chronic form of ringworm where hair shafts become surrounded by a necrotic crust or scutulum. Individual crusts coalesce to form a pale, unpleasant-smelling mat over parts of the scalp. Such infections may cause extensive and permanent hair loss.

TINEA IMBRICATA (TOKELAU)

This infection in endemic in parts of the Far East, West Pacific, Central and South America, and is caused by *T. concentricum*. In many cases the trunk is covered with scales laid down in concentric rings producing a 'ripple' effect. Alternatively, large, loose scales (tiled, Latin—*imbricata*) may form. The infection is often chronic, and may constitute a serious social handicap. There is some evidence that susceptibility of this disease in Papua New Guinea may be inherited as an autosomal recessive trait.

Laboratory diagnosis

The mainstays of diagnosis are direct microscopy of skin scales mounted in potassium hydroxide (20 per cent) to demonstrate hyphae, and culture. Scalp hairs may also be examined in a similar way, and the site of arthrospore formation, inside or outside the shaft, determined. Further tests, such as the ability to penetrate hair, may be used to separate similar cultures. Identification of organisms is important, as it will indicate the source of infection in scalp ringworm for example.

When large numbers of children are involved, screening of scalp infections with a filtered ultraviolet (Wood's light) lamp is useful. Certain species, including *M. canis* and *M. audouinii*, cause infected hair to fluoresce with a vivid greenish light. Scalps can also be screened for infection by passing a sterile brush or scalp massager through the hair and plating this directly on to an agar plate.

Treatment

The treatment of dermatophyte infections depends to an extent on the nature and severity of infection. Topical therapy is reserved for circumscribed infections such as athlete's foot and tinea corporis, not involving hair or nail keratin. Scalp and nail infections, severe or widespread ringworm, and failures of topical therapy are usually treated orally with griseofulvin, itraconazole, or terbinafine.

Older treatments such as Castellani's paint, which contains magenta and resorcinol, are still employed with some patients. However, the most common and cheapest preparation is Whitfields ointment (benzoic acid compound). The half-strength preparation is well tolerated and can be applied twice daily to localized lesions. More specific antifungal drugs in topical form are more expensive and there is no clear evidence that they are more effective, although they are better tolerated and may be quicker in action than Whitfield's ointment. The important compounds in this group are miconazole, clotrimazole, ketoconazole, and econazole, which are imidazole derivatives, undecenoic acid, and tolnaftate. They are all very similar in their clinical efficacy but topical terbinafine is particularly rapid. Adverse reactions are rare.

Griseofulvin is an orally effective antifungal used against dermatophytosis, including scalp ringworm and nail infections. It is normally given in doses of 0.5 to 1.0 g daily in adults or 10 mg/kg daily in children. Treatment should be continued for at least 6 weeks in tinea capitis. The griseofulvin tablets are prepared in a microcrystalline form and are probably best absorbed when given with a meal. Side-effects are not common, but include headache, nausea, and urticaria. The drug can also precipitate acute intermittent porphyria in predisposed subjects. Griseofulvin is effective in most forms of dermatophytosis, although responses in 'dry type' infections and onychomycosis are generally poor. Toe-nail infections, in particular, often fail to respond or relapse rapidly after treatment.

Newer alternatives include terbinafine, ketoconazole, and itraconazole. Terbinafine (250 mg daily) is rapidly effective in most forms of dermatophytosis that require oral therapy and also produces rapid responses in toe-nail and sole infections, without a high rate of relapse. Itraconazole is somewhat similar in its profile. For most infections it is given in doses of 100 mg daily but for nail infections 200 mg is used. Terbinafine and itraconazole have largely replaced griseofulvin for oral of treatment dermatophytosis.

REFERENCES

Dermatophytosis

Cox, F.W., Stiller, R.I., and South, D.A. (1982). Oral ketoconazole for dermatophyte infections. *Journal of the American Academy of Dermatology*, **6,** 455–62.

de Vroey, C., (1985). Epidemiology of ringworm (dermatophytosis). *Seminars in Dermatology*, **4,** 185–200.

Goodfield, M.J.D., Rowell, N.R., Forster, R.A., Evans, E.G.V., and Raven, A. (1989). Treatment of dermatophyte infections of the finger or toe nails with terbinafine (SFG 86–327, Lamisil) an orally active fungicidal agent. *British Journal of Dermatology*, **121,** 753–8.

Gugnani, H.C. and Njoku-Obi, A.N.U. (1986). Tinea capitis in school children in East Nigeria. *Mykosen*, **29,** 132–44.

Hay, R.J. (1982). Chronic dermatophyte infections I. Clinical and mycological features. *British Journal of Dermatology*, **106,** 1–6.

Torssander, J. *et al.* (1988). Dermatophytosis and HIV infection—study in homosexual men. Acta *Dermatologica et Venereologica*, **68,** 53–9.

Scytalidium infections

The organisms, *Scytalidium dimidiatum* (*Hendersonula toruloidea*), and *S. hyalinum*, can cause a superficial scaly condition that resembles 'dry type' of dermatophyte infection on the palms or soles. Nail-plate destruction may also occur, the lateral border of the nail being the initial site of invasion. The disease has been seen in Europe, almost invariably in immigrants from the tropics, particularly the Caribbean, West Africa, and India or Pakistan. Its prevalence in the tropics is unknown, although in some surveys it has been shown to be relatively common. In skin scrapings the tortuous hyphae may resemble those of a dermatophyte but the organisms do not grow on media containing cycloheximide, which is often incorporated into agar for routine dermatophyte isolation.

Treatment is difficult, but some improvement may follow the use of keratolytic compounds such as salicylic acid. The organisms do not respond to griseofulvin, azoles or tolnaftate.

REFERENCES

Scytalidium

Gentles, J.C. and Evans, E.G.V. (1970). Infection of the feet and nails with *Hendersonula toruloidea. Sabouraudia*, **8,** 72.

Gugnani, H.C., Nzelibe, F.K., and Osunkwo, I.C. (1986). Onychomycosis due to *Hendersonula toruloidea* in Nigeria. *Journal of Medical and Veterinary Mycology*, **24,** 239–41.

Hay, R.J. and Moore, M.K. (1984). Clinical features of superficial fungal infections caused by *Hendersonula toruloidea* and *Scytalidium hyalinum. British Journal of Dermatology*, **110,** 677–83.

Miscellaneous nail infections

Occasionally, fungi other than dermatophytes, Hendersonula or Scytalidium are isolated from dystrophic nails. These include *Scopulariopsis brevicaulis*, *Acremonium* (*Cephalosporium*) species, and certain types of Aspergillus. These infections are usually seen in the elderly. It is often difficult, particularly with *Aspergillus* species, to establish that the organism is playing a pathogenic role.

Pityriasis versicolor (tinea versicolor)

Aetiology

Pityriasis versicolor is a superficial infection caused by *Malassezia furfur*. Although most common in tropical countries, it has a worldwide distribution. Dermal penetration does not occur.

M. furfur is probably the parasitic form of a common saprophytic yeast, often called *Pityrosporum orbiculare*, which can be found on normal skin. Conversion of this yeast from a saphrophytic to a parasitic phase has been observed following renal transplantation. It is likely that the state of host immunity plays some part in pathogenesis and depression; for instance, endogenous or exogenous corticosteroids potentiate the disease in some individuals. However, it is also commonly seen in normal individuals, and climatic factors or sun exposure are believed to trigger the infection in many cases. There is no effective animal model for studies of this disease.

Epidemiology

Pityriasis versicolor is very common in the tropics, where it may be widespread on the body. Its incidence in temperate climates has increased over the last 20 to 30 years.

Clinical features

The rash of pityriasis versicolor is asymptomatic or mildly pruritic. Its presents with scaling, confluent macules on the trunk, upper arms or neck. These may be hypopigmented or hyperpigmented. In some individuals and in the tropics, other areas including face, forearms, and thighs may be involved.

The diagnosis is rarely confused with other complaints, although eczema or ringworm infections are sometimes considered. Patients are often anxious to exclude leprosy, but the two are unlikely to be mistaken. In vitiligo, depigmentation is complete and there is no scaling.

Laboratory diagnosis

The diagnosis is made by demonstration of the yeasts and hyphae of *M. furfur* in skin scales removed by scraping. Culture is difficult and unnecessary.

Treatment

Treatment with keratolytics, including sulphur or Whitfield's ointment, may be effective. More usually, 2 per cent selenium sulphide or 20 per cent sodium hyposulphate lotions are used. Topical miconazole, clotrimazole or econazole are also effective. Oral itraconazole may be used in recalcitrant cases. Whatever the treatment, relapse is common.

Other pityrosporum infections

Pityrosporum yeasts have been implicated in the pathogenesis of a number of other skin diseases such as seborrhoeic dermatitis and a form of itchy folliculitis, Pityrosporum folliculitis. The evidence connecting seborrhoeic dermatitis, one of the most common of skin diseases, and Pityrosporum is largely concerned with the response of antifungal drugs and the observation that improvements in the rash mirror disappearance of organisms from the skin. Severity of the skin condition does not appear to reflect the numbers of yeasts on the skin surface.

REFERENCE

Pityrosporum

Mathes, B.M. and Douglas, M.C. (1985). Seborrheic dermatitis in patients with acquired immunodeficiency syndrome. *Journal of the American Academy of Dermatology*, **13,** 947–51.

Superficial candidosis (candidiasis)

Aetiology

Superficial candidosis is a term used to describe a group of infections of skin or mucous membranes caused by species of the genus Candida. They range in severity from oral thrush to chronic mucocutaneous candidosis, a chronic infection refractory to conventional treatment.

Candida albicans is the species most frequently involved. It is a saprophytic yeast often found as a commensal in the mouth and gastrointestinal tract, and is commonly present in the vagina. Several factors may influence the incidence of carriage. For instance, oral colonization is more common in hospital staff than in equivalent non-hospital subjects. Vaginal carriage is more common in pregnancy. Other factors (Table 1) are known that predispose to conversion from a commensal to a parasitic role with the causation of disease—candidosis. The list includes factors that influence host immunological response, such as carcinoma, AIDS, or cytotoxic therapy, those that disturb the population of other microorganisms (e.g. antibiotics), and those that affect the character of the epithelium, e.g. dentures.

Other species of Candida may also cause superficial infections, but are less common. They include *C. tropicalis, C. parapsilosis, C. guilliermondii*, and *C. pseudotropicalis.*

Epidemiology

Superficial Candida infections are seen in all countries.

Clinical features

There are a number of clinically distinct types of superficial infection caused by *Candida* species, as follows.

ORAL CANDIDOSIS (THRUSH)

Oral infection by Candida is fairly common, particularly in infancy and old age, or in association with antibiotic or cytotoxic therapy, or in diseases where the immune response may be impaired. In the older age group, the wearing of dentures is a predisposing factor. The lesions present with discomfort both in the mouth and at the corners of the lips. The mouth and buccal mucosa show patchy or confluent, white adherent plaques. Angular cheilitis usually accompanies the oral lesions. In longstanding cases, the plaque may become hypertrophic, with oedema of the mucosal surfaces, or the mucosa may appear glazed and raw.

There is a significant correlation between leukoplakia and oral candidosis, and it has been suggested that the infection may lead to epithelial dysplasia.

The diagnosis is made by the demonstration of yeasts and hyphae of Candida in smears, and by culture.

Table 1 *Predisposing factors in superficial candidosis*

1. Local epithelial defects, occlusion, constant immersion in water etc. e.g. damaged nail folds, beneath dentures
2. Defects of immunity (primarily T cell or phagocytosis)
   (*a*) primary immunological disease, e.g. chronic granulomatous disease
   (*b*) immunodefects secondary to intercurrent illness, e.g. leukaemia
   (*c*) immunodefects secondary to therapy, e.g. cytotoxic therapy in organ transplantation
3. Drug therapy, e.g. antibiotics
4. Carcinoma or leukaemia
5. Endocrine disease
   (*a*) diabetes mellitus
   (*b*) hypothyroidism, hypoparathyroidism, hypoadrenalism (in chronic mucocutaneous candidosis)
6. Physiological changes, e.g. infancy, pregnancy, old age
7. Miscellaneous disorders, e.g.
   (*a*) iron deficiency
   (*b*) zinc deficiency
   (*c*) Malabsorption

VAGINAL CANDIDOSIS (THRUSH)

A similar infection can occur in the vagina with secondary spread to the vulva. This is seen in normal women, as well as in pregnancy or in association with diabetes mellitus. Vaginal candidosis has been diagnosed increasingly in recent years, and this may reflect a genuine upsurge of the disease. It has been suggested that some of this increase may be due to the use of the contraceptive pill, to changes of sexual habits, or to a modification of the normal bacterial flora.

As with oral candidosis, soreness is the main symptom, although irritation may occur. A creamy discharge is also common, and white plaques may form on the vaginal wall. In chronic infections, the mucosa is inflamed, but plaques are often absent. The diagnosis is confirmed principally by direct microscopy and secondarily by culture.

Secondary spread of the infection to the vulva is common, with the development of a red, scaling rash. Beyond its edge, small satellite scales and pustules are seen, features typical of superficial Candida infections.

PARONYCHIA

Infection around the nail fold is seen in people whose occupations involve frequent wetting of the hands (e.g. cooks) or in those with eczema or psoriasis. In some cases, the inflammation is caused by bacterial infection, but Candida may also be a primary cause. The condition presents with painful, red swelling of the nail fold. Pus may be discharged. Secondary invasion of the lateral border of the nail plate by Candida may occur from this site.

CANDIDA INTERTRIGO

Infection of the moist folds of the skin in the groin or under the breasts causes itching and discomfort. The area becomes macerated and erythematous. Candida may contribute to this condition, but is certainly not the only factor. It may also superinfect the napkin area in infants. The presence of satellite pustules (see above) is a useful indicator of involvement by Candida in the disease process.

Direct invasion of toe-web folds by Candida closely resembles 'athlete's foot' caused by dermatophytes. A similar erosive infection may occur in the finger webs, and is seen most commonly in the tropics.

Laboratory diagnosis

All these infections are diagnosed by microscopy and culture. When associated with the condition, Candida cells are always evident on microscopy. Culture establishes the specific identity but as a rule, is of less value than direct microscopy. Serology is unhelpful in superficial candida infections.

Chronic superficial candidosis

Chronic Candida infections of the mouth, vagina, and nail present problems in management. Chronic oral candidosis, for instance, is associated with leukoplakia. Predisposing causes should be searched for. The most serious of this group of infections is chronic mucocutaneous candidosis, a rare condition in which chronic skin, nail, and mucosal infection coexist (Plate 3). A series of underlying genetic, endocrine (hypoparathyroidism, hypoadrenalism or hypothyroidism) and immunological abnormalities has been found. Other superficial viral or fungal infections may also be present in these patients, whose condition is normally diagnosed in childhood.

Oral candidosis is one of the earliest signs of AIDS, occurring in a high proportion of patients. The appearances are similar to those seen with other groups, although plaque formation may be very extensive. In addition, an erythematous form without plaques may also occur.

Treatment

Two groups of drugs are effective in superficial candidosis. The polyenes such as nystatin and amphotericin B are topically active in many forms of candidosis. They are often less effective in oral candidosis in immunodeficient patients including those with AIDS. Likewise, topical azole drugs such as miconazole and clotrimazole are usually effective in superficial candidosis. For resistant cases, oral therapy with fluconazole, itraconazole or ketoconazole may be necessary.

For vaginal infections topical creams or vaginal preparations should be used—many requiring only a single treatment. In recalcitrant cases it may be necessary to use oral therapy such as fluconazole or itraconazole. Longer courses may be necessary with these drugs.

REFERENCES

Candidosis

Birse, C., Fonzi, W.A., Saporito, S., Irwin, M., and Sypherd, P.S. (1992). Molecular genetics of dimorphism in *Candida albicans*. In *New strategies in fungal disease*, (ed. J.E. Bennett, R.J. Hay, and P.K. Peterson), pp. 133–52. Churchill Livingstone, Edinburgh.

Bodey, G.P. (ed.) (1993). *Candidiasis. Pathogenesis, diagnosis and treatment*. Raven Press, New York.

Dwyer, J.M. (1981). Chronic mucocutaneous candidiasis. *Annual Reviews of Medicine*, **32,** 491–7.

Gough, P.M. *et al.* (1985). Candidosis of the genital tract in non-pregnant women. *European Journal of Obstetrics Gynecology and Reproductive Biology*, **19,** 237–46.

Greenspan, D. and Greenspan, J.S. (1987). Oral mucosal manifestations of AIDS. *Dermatologic Clinics*, **5,** 733–7.

Horn, R., Wong, B., Kiehn, T.E., and Armstrong, D. (1981). Fungemia in a cancer hospital: changing frequency, earlier onset and results of therapy. *Reviews of Infectious Diseases*, **7,** 646–55.

Meunier, F. (1989). Candidiasis. *European Journal of Clinical Microbiology and Infectious Diseases*, **8,** 438–47.

Torssander, J. *et al.* (1987). Oral *Candida albicans* in HIV infection. *Scandinavian Journal of Infection*, **189,** 291–5.

Wey, S.B., Mori, M., Pfaller, M.A., Woolson, R.F., and Wenzel, R.P. (1989). Risk factors for hospital acquired candidemia. *Archives of Internal Medicine*, **149,** 2349–53.

Miscellaneous superficial mycoses

There are a number of relatively rare, superficial fungal infections such as tinea nigra, and black or white piedra. They never cause invasive disease, and are mainly confined to the tropics.

Tinea nigra

Tinea nigra is a superficial infection confined to the epidermis of the palms or soles, and more rarely elsewhere. The initial lesion is a dark macule without scaling, which resembles a brown stain on the skin and spreads slowly over the palmar or plantar surface. The disease is normally asymptomatic.

On scraping the skin, brown pigmented hyphae can be seen by direct microscopy, and the causative organism, *Phaeoanellomyces werneckii*, isolated.

The lesion responds to Whitfield's ointment.

Black piedra

Black piedra is a disease of the tropics in which small, dark nodules form on hair shafts in the scalp or, less commonly, elsewhere. There are no symptoms. Each nodule consists of a dense mat of hyphae containing the sexual spores (ascospores) of the fungus.

The diagnosis is made by direct microscopy of infected hair, and the isolation of *Piedraia hortae*. Treatment using formalin solution or amphotericin B lotion is usually effective.

White piedra

White piedra occurs in both temperate and tropical climates, and is rare. It produces pale nodules on the hair of the beard, groin or scalp. The hair shaft may fracture. The nodule consists of hyphae, arthrospores (spores formed by fragmentation of hyphae), and blastospores (budding yeast cells). The organism *Trichosporon beigelii* can be readily cultured. The treatment is similar to that for black piedra.

The subcutaneous mycoses

Subcutaneous infections caused by fungi are rare, and are mainly seen in the tropics. It is usually assumed that the organisms gain entry via the skin, although there is good evidence for this only in the case of mycetoma. However, the majority of the causative organisms in this group of infections can be isolated from vegetation or soil. Involvement of deep viscera is rare. Attempts to establish experimental infections that resemble the human disease have been largely unsuccessful. A clearer understanding of the pathogenesis therefore awaits such a model system. These infections tend to be chronic, and chemotherapy is quite lengthy and frequently unsuccessful.

Mycetoma (Madura foot)

Aetiology

Mycetoma is a chronic infection involving subcutaneous tissue, bone, and skin, in which colonies of infecting fungi or actinomycetes (grains) are found within a network of burrowing abscesses and sinuses.

A list of the more common organisms that cause mycetoma is shown in Table 2. By tradition, the organisms are divided into two groups, the actinomycetomas and the eumycetomas, caused by actinomycetes and fungi, respectively. The size and colour of the grain (red, pale, or dark) are important clues to their identification. The organisms can be found in the natural environment, and some have even been identified in association with Acacia thorns in an endemic area. The infection is initiated when an infected thorn is left implanted in deep tissue. However, many years may elapse before the formation of a mycetoma.

Epidemiology

The disease is seen primarily in the tropics, although rare cases, apart from imported ones, may occur in temperate areas. Countries with the

Table 2 *Causes of mycetoma*

1. Fungi, e.g.	*Madurella mycetomatis*
	M. grisea
	Pseudallescheria boydii
	Exophiala jeanselmei
	Leptosphaeria senegalensis
	Species of *Acremonium, Aspergillus, Fusarium*
2. Actinomycetes, e.g.	*Nocardia brasiliensis*
	Actinomadura madurae
	A. pelletieri
	Streptomyces somaliensis

most reported cases include Sudan, India, Senegal, Mexico, and Venezuela. However, the disease is widely distributed in the tropics, particularly to the south and east of the Sahara Desert in Africa.

The pattern of prevalence of infections caused by certain organisms differs strikingly in different parts of the world. For instance, *Streptomyces somaliensis* is the most common in the Sudan and Middle East. *Madurella grisea* is mainly found in the New World. Altogether about 60 per cent of reported infections are caused by actinomycetes, of which *Nocardia brasiliensis* is the most common (Chapter 7.11.28).

Clinical features

Early mycetomas may present as a circumscribed area of hard subcutaneous swelling. Later, sinus tracts open on to the skin surface and visible grains may be discharged, along with serosanguinous fluid (Plate 4). Bone erosion and destruction, leading to deformity, may occur. However, severe pain is rarely a problem. Local lymph node invasion may occur, but more widespread involvement is very rare.

Feet and lower legs are the most common areas involved, but the arms, buttocks, chest, and head may all be sites of infection. Mycetoma cause by *N. brasiliensis* may occur in any site, but one favoured area is the chest wall.

The radiological features of mycetoma are cortical erosion, followed by the development of lytic deposits in bone. Periosteal proliferation and destruction, leading to deformity, may follow. The periosteal reaction may be pronounced in actinomycete infection.

Laboratory diagnosis

The diagnosis is made by the demonstration and identification of grains obtained from the sinus openings by gentle pressure or curettage. If these measures are not successful, tissue should be obtained by deep surgical biopsy. Grains can be mounted in potassium hydroxide and examined microscopically. Those containing filaments 3 to 4 μm in diameter or more are caused by true fungi (eumycetomas), and those with filaments less than 1 μm by actinomycetes (actinomycetomas). These features can usually be distinguished by direct microscopy.

The morphology of grains fixed, sectioned, and stained with haematoxylin and eosin is typical. Special stains are less helpful. Grains can be used for culture, although several attempts at isolation may have to be made. Serology (e.g. immunodiffusion) can also be helpful, particularly when cultures are difficult to obtain.

Treatment

Actinomycetomas may respond to sulphones such as dapsone (50–100 mg daily) or sulphonamides such as sulphadiazine. The treatment of choice for many is long-term co-trimoxazole (two to three tablets twice daily) with an initial 2 to 3 months of streptomycin or rifampicin. Treatment may have to be continued for many months or years. Dapsone is an effective and cheaper alternative to co-trimoxazole. Extensive actinomycetomas may respond poorly, although generally marked improvement is obtained, even when lytic bone lesions are well established.

The eumycetomas seldom respond to antifungal therapy. On rare occasions griseofulvin, amphotericin B, ketoconazole, and itraconazole have produced remission or cure. A trial of therapy may be attempted, where the patient can be monitored closely in outpatient departments. Otherwise, radical surgery or amputation is usually necessary. Small, local excisions are rarely successful.

Mycetoma is slowly progressive and increasingly disabling. However, wider dissemination is very rare, and therefore cases are seldom fatal, except where the skull is involved. However, the deformity caused by the disease may be severely disabling.

REFERENCES

Mycetoma

Mahgoub, E.S. (1976). Medical management of mycetoma. *WHO Bulletin*, **54,** 303–10.

Mahgoub, E.S. and Murray, I.G. (1973). Mycetoma. *Heinemann Medical*, London.

Mariat, F., Destombes, P., and Segretain, G. (1977). The mycetomas: clinical features, pathology, etiology and epidemiology. *Contributions to Microbiology and Immunology*, **4,** 1–39.

Chromoblastomycosis

See Chapter 7.12.3 and Plate 5.

Sporotrichosis

Aetiology

The most common clinical form of sporotrichosis is a subcutaneous infection, which may spread proximally from its initial site in a series of nodules along the course of a lymphatic. More rarely, systemic involvement is seen, for example in the lung (see under systemic mycoses).

The causative organism *Sporothrix schenckii* can be found in soil, vegetation, or in association with plants or bark. People who develop the subcutaneous infection may have had contact with material that harbours the organism, such as moss or flowers (e.g. florists). It is assumed that the pathogen gains entry via an abrasion and in some endemic areas there is often a preceding history of a scratch or insect bite.

Epidemiology

Although sporotrichosis was once prevalent in Europe, particularly France, non-imported cases are now very rare in this area. However, the disease is seen in the United States, Mexico, Central and South America, and Africa. In the late 1930s, there was a remarkable epidemic of sporotrichosis in workers in the Witwatersrand gold mines. The source of infection was a large number of wooden pit props contaminated with the organism. Other, smaller 'epidemics' have been described in certain groups, such as Mexican pottery workers packing ceramics in straw. Normally, however, cases are sporadic in incidence.

Systemic sporotrichosis is much rarer, and cases have mainly been described from the United States.

Clinical features

There are two main clinical types of subcutaneous sporotrichosis.

The first, the fixed type, presents with a solitary cutaneous ulcer or nodule. In this form of the disease, infection does not spread along lymphatics. It has been suggested that it is most common in children, and it has been described most frequently in Central and South America.

In the lymphangitic form, an initial nodule forms on a limb or extremity, such as a finger. This may break down and ulcerate. Subsequently, one or more secondary nodules develop along the draining lymphatic channel, which may ulcerate through the skin. Other variants include the psoriasiform or verrucous types or a superficial granuloma that resembles lupus vulgaris. These usually represent chronic infection.

Rarer forms include secondary spread via scratching, which may present with multiple widespread ulcers or multiple cutaneous lesions secondary to systemic disease.

Fixed-type sporotrichosis may resemble many other forms of cutaneous ulceration. However, in endemic areas a major source of confusion is cutaneous leishmaniasis. The lymphangitic variety may also resemble other infections, notably atypical mycobacterial infections, particularly fish-tank granuloma, or 'sporotrichoid' leishmaniasis.

Treatment

Some cases of sporotrichosis may heal spontaneously. However, treatment is usually advised to prevent scar formation. The treatment of choice is potassium iodide administered in a saturated aqueous solution. The starting dose is 0.5 to 1 ml, given three times daily, and this is increased drop by drop per dose to 3 to 6 ml, three times daily. The mixture is more palatable if given with milk. Treatment should be given for a month after clinical resolution. Itraconazole is an alternative.

REFERENCES

Sporotrichosis

Bibler, M.R. *et al.* (1986). Disseminated sporotrichosis in a patient with HIV infection after treatment for acquired factor VIII inhibitor. *Journal of the American Medical Association*, **256,** 3125–6.

de Albornoz, M.C.B. (1989). Sporotrichosis. In *Tropical fungal infections*, (ed. R.J. Hay), *Baillière's clinical tropical medicine and communicable diseases*, Vol. **4,** pp. 71–96. Baillière Tindall, London.

Itoh, M., Okamoto, S., and Kanya, H. (1986). Survey of 260 cases of sporotrichosis. *Dermatologica*, **172,** 203–13.

Subcutaneous zygomycosis (basidiobolomycosis)

Subcutaneous zygomycosis is an infection primarily seen in children in Africa or the Far East (Indonesia). It is characterized by the development of localized woody swellings on the limbs or trunk. The swelling is rarely inflammatory, but has a well-defined leading edge, and is hard. Progression is slow. The causative organism *Basidiobolus haptosporus* can be cultured or demonstrated histologically in biopsy material.

Although resolution has been recorded without treatment, therapy is normally given. Potassium iodide solution is the treatment of choice, and is given in as high a dose as possible (cf. sporotrichosis).

Conidiobolomycosis (rhinoentomophthoromycosis)

Conidiobolomycosis is a similar infection confined to subcutaneous tissue and presenting with painless swelling. The infection is mainly seen in West Africa, but a case has been seen in the Caribbean. There are important differences from subcutaneous zygomycosis. The disease is most common in young adults, and is confined to facial tissues around the nose, the forehead, and the upper lip. The initial site of infection is in the region of the inferior turbinate in the nose. The diagnosis is established by biopsy or culture. The causative organism is *Conidiobolus coronatus*. The treatment of choice is high-dose potassium iodide and co-trimoxazole. Relapse after treatment is common, and residual fibrosis may be severely disfiguring. Ketoconazole has been reported to be effective.

Lobo's disease (lobomycosis)

Lobo's disease is a subcutaneous infection. The organism, in tissue, appears to be a yeast. It has a tendency to form chains of four to six yeast cells with prominent nucleoli, joined by a narrow, intercellular bridge. However, the organism has never been cultured from human cases and can only be identified by biopsy and histology. The disease is seen in countries of South America around, and north of, the Amazon basin, and cases are also seen in Central America. Often, exposed sites (e.g. ear lobes) are invaded and small nodules containing the organisms develop. These may resemble keloids. More diffuse plaques may also be seen. Deep invasion has not been documented. The treatment is excision, and there is no effective chemotherapy.

Systemic mycoses

The systemic or deep visceral mycoses include some of the rare and more serious of the fungal infections. There are two main types of infection in this group, those caused by organisms which invade normal hosts, the pathogens, and those which only cause disease in compromised patients, the opportunists. The fungi associated with these two types of infection differ in their innate levels of pathogenicity, but an element of opportunism, depending on host susceptibility, is usually recognizable in all cases of systemic mycoses.

The systemic pathogens cause infections such as histoplasmosis or coccidioidomycosis. These diseases have well-defined endemic zones and the majority of those exposed remain symptomless but develop positive skin tests. However, in certain patients, chronic local or disseminated disease may occur. In the systemic infections caused by opportunistic fungi, there is usually a serious underlying abnormality in the patient, such as carcinoma or lymphoma. Such infections are worldwide in occurrence: where tissue invasion occurs the mortality is high. Cryptococcosis, a systemic yeast infection, has features of both types of systemic disease and occurs in both normal and immunosuppressed subjects.

The systemic pathogen infections are histoplasmosis, coccidioidomycosis, blastomycosis and paracoccidioidomycosis. The significance of various laboratory tests in these infections is shown in Table 3.

Histoplasmosis (see also Section 17)

There are two forms of histoplasmosis. In both types, the organism is present in tissue in its yeast phase. In small-form or classical histoplasmosis, the diameter of the yeast cells is between 3 and 4 μm. Infections are most common in the United States, but sporadic cases are reported widely from the New World, Africa, and the Far East. By contrast, large-form or African histoplasmosis is most common in Central Africa, south of the Sahara and north of the Zambezi river. Yeast forms in infected tissue are much larger, 10 to 15 μm in diameter. Both infections are clinically distinct (see below), but cultural isolates are indistinguishable.

Classical or small-form histoplasmosis (histoplasmosis capsulati)

AETIOLOGY

Histoplasmosis is a systemic infection caused by *Histoplasma capsulatum*. The main route of infection is pulmonary. The majority of those exposed are sensitized without overt signs of infection, but more rarely chronic pulmonary or disseminated forms of the disease are seen.

The organism, *H. capsulatum*, can be found in soil in endemic areas. Its growth is facilitated by the presence of bird excreta, for instance, in old chicken houses, bird roosts, and barns. In tropical and some temperate areas, bat guano plays a similar role, although there is evidence

Table 3 *Laboratory tests in systemic mycoses*

	Direct microscopy	Significance of positive culture	Serology	Histology
Histoplasmosis				
1. Classical (small form)	Sometimes positive	Significant	ID, CIE, CFT	Yeasts (3–4 μm)
2. African	Positive in pus (valuable)	Significant	ID, CFT	Yeasts (10–15 μm)
Coccidioidomycosis	Positive in pus, sputum etc. (valuable)	Significant NB Handle with caution	ID, CFT, TP, CIE	Spherules (50–150 μm)
Blastomycosis	Positive in pus, sputum etc. (valuable)	Significant	ID, CFT, CIE (unreliable)	Yeasts (4–10 μm) Broad-based buds
Paracoccidioidomycosis	Positive in pus, sputum etc. (valuable)	Significant	ID, CFT, TP	Yeasts (5–15 μm) Multiple buds
Cryptococcosis	Often positive in CSF (rare in urine, pus) NB Indian ink	Significant	ID, CFT, WCA, IF Latex agglutination (antigen)	Encapsulated yeasts (5–10 μm) Mucicarmine positive
Systemic candidosis	Positive in oral smears, sputum etc. (interpret with caution)	Significance depends on site and presence of positive microscopy	ID, CFT, WCA, CIE ? Role of antigen detection	Yeasts (5–10 μm) and hyphae
Invasive aspergillosis	Rarely positive	Depends on site Positive sputum cultures not always significant	ID, CIE Rarely positive	Hyphae—dichotomous branching
Invasive zygomycosis	Rarely positive	Depends on site Rarely positive	ID, CIE	Hyphae—broad and aseptate

Abbreviations: CFT, complement fixation test; CIE, counterimmunoelectrophoresis; ID, immunodiffusion; IF, immunofluorescence; RIA, radioimmunoassay; TP, tube precipitation; WCA, whole-cell agglutination.

that the bat, unlike birds, may carry and be infected by the organism. Exposure to a suitable source, such as a cave containing bats, is often recorded in acute epidemic histoplasmosis (see below). It is rarely identified in more slowly evolving cases.

The disease was first diagnosed in Panama in 1904 by Darling, who thought that the organism was a protozoa. It was subsequently shown to be a fungus in 1934 by De Monbreun. Up to 1945, all reported cases were examples of disseminated disease. However, in later years it was recognized that *H. capsulatum* could also be asymptomatic or cause chronic lung disease similar to tuberculosis. The condition of the host is extremely important in determining the clinical course and manifestations of histoplasmosis. Slowly evolving (chronic), disseminated disease may occur in normal individuals. However, infants, elderly people, or those with certain neoplastic disorders appear to be more likely to develop the more rapidly progressive forms of disseminated infection.

EPIDEMIOLOGY

The major endemic area, as shown by skin testing, is in the central region of the United States around the Ohio and Mississippi valley basins. Prevalence is highest in the states of Tennessee, Kentucky, and Ohio. Up to 95 per cent of those skin tested in certain parts of these areas have positive delayed reactions to intradermal histoplasmin (cf Mantoux test). Scattered cases of active disease, healed calcified foci in chest radiographs, and foci found at autopsy representing inactive histoplasmosis also provide evidence of spread within this area. However, the disease also occurs in other parts of the United States, Mexico, Central and South America, Africa, the Far East, and Australia. The organism has been recovered from soil in central Italy, but no human cases have been diagnosed there. Outside the major endemic areas in the United States, human cases are often extremely rare, and much of the evidence of the endemicity comes from positive skin tests or the presence of the organism in selected sites, such as caves.

Although there has been considerable discussion on the nature of soil factors responsible for the growth of *H. capsulatum*, the conditions limiting its occurrence to certain areas are largely unknown.

CLINICAL FEATURES

The clinical forms of histoplasmosis can be placed in several clinical groups:

(1) asymptomatic;
(2) acute symptomatic pulmonary
(a) acute epidemic,
(b) acute reinfection;
(3) chronic pulmonary;
(4) disseminated (acute, subacute and chronic);
(5) primary cutaneous (by inoculation).

Asymptomatic infection

Over 99 per cent of patients becoming infected in endemic areas record no overt symptoms but develop a positive skin test. The incidence of positive skin tests declines in individuals above the age of 60 years.

Acute (symptomatic) pulmonary histoplasmosis

Acute epidemic histoplasmosis

Groups of individuals exposed to a source of infection, for instance, during cave exploration, or those who may have inhaled a large infecting dose, often develop a symptomatic illness 12 to 21 days after exposure. The main features are pyrexia, cough, chest pain, and malaise. Flitting arthralgia and, less commonly, erythema nodosum or multiforme may occur. The radiological appearances may be much more severe than would be supposed from the symptoms, and hilar lymph-node enlargement and diffuse, patchy consolidation suggesting pneumonitis may occur (Plate 6).

These patients develop precipitating or complement-fixing antibody, but this often follows the peak of illness. About 50 per cent of those with symptoms do not develop positive antibody responses. Likewise, skin test conversion is often too late to be of diagnostic value, and its use is normally contraindicated, as a single histoplasmin test may cause the development of false-positive serological results. Cultures are often negative. The symptoms and history of exposure to a suitable source, combined with a rising antibody titre, are often the best evidence of infection.

The majority of cases require no specific therapy apart from rest. Those with severe or prolonged symptoms or impaired gas exchange require intravenous amphotericin B or itraconazole. The lung lesions often heal to leave multiple scattered pulmonary calcifications.

Acute reinfection histoplasmosis

Massive acute exposure to *H. capsulatum* in sensitized individuals is believed by some physicians to cause a less severe infection associated with bilateral pulmonary infiltrates. The incubation period is shorter than with acute epidemic histoplasmosis, namely 5 to 10 days.

Chronic pulmonary histoplasmosis

Chronic pulmonary disease caused by *H. capsulatum* is mainly seen in the United States. It is more common in males and smokers, and there is often underlying pulmonary emphysema. Early cases may present with pyrexia and cough, but malaise and weight loss occur later. Lesions may heal initially, but relapse is common, leading to established consolidation and cavitation. The most common radiological appearance of early lesions is of unilateral, wedge-shaped, segmental shadows in the apical zones. Subsequently, the disease may become bilateral, with fibrosis and cavitation. In some cases, extensive and progressive destruction of lung tissue may occur.

Culture and serology are both helpful methods of diagnosis in this form of histoplasmosis, but repeated attempts may be required before positive results are obtained.

In early cases, resolution may occur on rest alone. However, relapse occurs in at least 25 per cent of cases, and these patients may require amphotericin B therapy or itraconazole. Although chemotherapy may virtually sterilize lesions, fibrosis persists and relapse may occur. Surgical excision or lobectomy is sometimes effective.

Solid lung tumours may persist after the primary infection. These may be single (coin lesions) or multiple, and have to be distinguished from carcinomas. The diagnosis is normally made at surgery, although the presence of calcification may give a clue to the nature of the lesion (histoplasmoma). The organisms can be demonstrated by histopathology, but they are seldom viable.

Disseminated histoplasmosis

There is considerable variation in the rate of progression of histoplasmosis that has spread beyond the initial focus in the lung. In rapid or acutely disseminated cases, widespread infiltration of reticuloendothelial cells of bone marrow, spleen, and liver may occur. Gastrointestinal lesions, endocarditis, and meningitis are less common, and meningitis is more usually associated with a slower course of disseminated disease. Infants, elderly people or immunosuppressed patients are more susceptible to acute dissemination. The most prominent symptoms are fever and weight loss, with accompanying hepatosplenomegaly. Extensive purpura and bruising secondary to thrombocytopenia may occur. The blood picture may reflect marrow infiltration with organisms, leading to pancytopenia. Disseminated histoplasmosis is also seen in AIDS patients. The clinical manifestations are not significantly different, although skin papules and ulcers have been reported in many; isolation of Histoplasma from blood has also been reported more frequently in these patients. It is particularly important to consider histoplasmosis in such patients and not to ascribe the clinical features to any underlying disease. Cultures, including sputum or bone marrow, should be taken. Serology is often positive, with high titres of complement-fixing antibodies occurring in some patients.

A much more slowly progressive form of disseminated histoplasmosis may present with persistent oral ulcers, chronic laryngitis or adrenal insufficiency. Granulomata, few of which contain organisms, can be found in the liver in some patients. Such cases may present up to 30 years after the patient has left an endemic area. In the United Kingdom, this form is the most widely recognized presentation of histoplasmosis, often occurring in Europeans who have worked in Africa or the Far East. Such imported cases are, nevertheless, very rare.

The diagnosis of disseminated histoplasmosis is made on culture or biopsy of affected areas. Sera may only be positive in low titres and in all cases adrenal involvement should be looked for.

Treatment is required in all forms of disseminated histoplasmosis. Itraconazole is preferred by most physicians, although amphotericin B may be necessary in some patients. Oral ketoconazole is an alternative.

Primary cutaneous histoplasmosis

Primary infection sometimes follows accidental inoculation of viable organisms in a laboratory or autopsy room. This type of infection is normally associated with a chancre at the site of inoculation and regional lymphadenopathy. The condition is self-limiting.

African histoplasmosis

Overt pulmonary involvement is rare in this form of histoplasmosis, and the normal portal of entry of the pathogen not known. The most common presenting features are skin lesions (papules, nodules, abscesses or ulcers) or lytic bone deposits. Solitary or multiple foci may be present, and in the latter instances rapid progression and death may occur. In such cases, gastrointestinal and lung lesions may develop.

The diagnosis is normally made by culture, smear or biopsy. The organism *H. capsulatum* var. *duboisii* is identical to that causing classical histoplasmosis in culture, but in lesions the yeast forms are considerably larger (10–15 μm).

While local excision of skin nodules have been reported to be curative, treatment with itraconazole, ketoconazole, or amphotericin B is usual. Some patients will respond to cotrimoxazole. A skeletal scan should be made to detect occult foci of infection.

REFERENCES

Histoplasmosis

Drouhet, E. (1989). African histoplasmosis. In *Tropical fungal infections*, (ed. R.J. Hay), *Baillières clinical tropical medicine and communicable diseases*, pp.221–47. Baillière Tindall, London.

Goodwin, R.A., Shapiro, J.L., Thurman, G.H., Thurman, S.S., and DesPrez, R.M. (1980). Disseminated histoplasmosis: clinical and pathologic correlations. *Medicine*, **59,** 1–33.

Goodwin, R.A., Loyd, J.E., and DesPrez, R.M. (1981). Histoplasmosis in normal hosts. *Medicine*, **60,** 231–66.

Mandell, W., Goldberg, D.M., and Neu, H.C. (1986). Histoplasmosis in patients with the acquired immune deficiency syndrome (AIDS). *Annals of Internal Medicine*, **111,** 655–9.

Wheat, L.J., Slama, T.G., Norton, J.A., and Zeckel, M.L. (1985). Histoplasmosis in the acquired immune deficiency syndrome. *American Journal of Medicine*, **78,** 203–10.

Wheat, L.J., Kohler, R.B., and Tewari, R.P. (1986). Diagnosis of disseminated histoplasmosis by detection of *Histoplasma capsulatum* antigen in serum and urine specimens. *New England Journal of Medicine*, **314,** 83–8.

Blastomycosis (see also Section 23)

Blastomycosis (North American blastomycosis) caused by *Blastomyces dermatitidis* is a systemic fungal infection in which skin and lung involvement are common features.

The infective organism, *B. dermatitidis*, has only been isolated from the environment on rare occasions. Positive sites have included soil and rotten timbers. The organism infects man and domestic animals, particularly the dog.

Epidemiology

Blastomycosis was originally thought to be confined to North America where it occurs sporadically throughout the south and east-central area and in areas of central Canada. 'Epidemics' of acute disease are rare, and where these occur a source of infection is rarely demonstrated.

More recently, cases have been found in Africa. Again, these are widely scattered from the north coast to the southern parts of the continent, and are rare in all areas. Patients with the disease have also been reported from the Middle East and Central Europe.

Clinical features

The clinical forms of blastomycosis differ from histoplasmosis in a number of important aspects. The existence of an asymptomatic form has not been proved conclusively, because there is no reliable skin test. Acute infections or infections in groups are rare, and the features are often similar to histoplasmosis (acute pulmonary). However, specific serological tests may be negative in 30 to 50 per cent of cases. The demonstration of the organisms in sputum and positive cultures are more reliable diagnostic criteria. Although some cases undoubtedly resolve without sequelae, some physicians advise chemotherapy, with a short course of amphotericin B in acute cases of blastomycosis.

CHRONIC PULMONARY BLASTOMYCOSIS

Chronic consolidation or cavitation of the upper or mid zones occur with chronic pulmonary infections. Fever, malaise, and cough with sputum are seen. Weight loss may be prominent. Culture is again the most reliable method of diagnosis.

The mainstay of treatment is amphotericin B, given in a total dose of 2 g or more.

DISSEMINATED BLASTOMYCOSIS

Although generalized infiltration in skin, lungs, and liver may occur over a short period, leading to rapid death, signs of chronic extrapulmonary dissemination are more usual.

The skin is an area that is frequently involved (chronic cutaneous blastomycosis). The face or forearms and hands are common sites for skin lesions. These are slow, spreading, verrucose plaques with central scarring. The initial lesion is often a dermal nodule. Many such cases have underlying pulmonary consolidation, or cavities. The diagnosis is established by biopsy and culture.

Bone deposits in the form of lytic lesions, and involvement of the genitourinary tract, particularly the epididymis, are also seen in chronic disseminated blastomycosis. Unlike tuberculosis, the kidneys are often spared.

It is interesting that only a few cases of blastomycosis have been reported in AIDS patients.

In slowly progressive forms of blastomycosis, itraconazole (200–400 mg daily) has proved to be very effective. Alternatively, amphotericin B can be given intravenously and is indicated where there is rapidly progressive disease.

REFERENCES

Blastomycosis

Emerson, P.A., Higgins, E., and Branfoot, A. (1984). North American blastomycosis in Africans. *British Journal of Diseases of the Chest*, **78,** 286–91.

Sarosi, G.A. and Davies, S.F. (1979). Blastomycosis. *American Reviews of Respiratory Diseases*, **120,** 911–38.

Coccidioidomycosis

See Chapter 7.12.2 and Plate 7.

Paracoccidioidomycosis

See Chapter 7.12.4.

Systemic sporotrichosis

In addition to causing cutaneous disease, *Sporothrix schenckii* may be responsible for a systemic mycosis. The infection is rare and has been mainly reported from the United States. Involvement may be confined to a single site such as a lung or a joint, or it may be multifocal. Cavitation in the lung associated with weight loss and pyrexia is probably the most common variety of systemic sporotrichosis. Unlike cutaneous forms of the disease, systemic sporotrichosis responds poorly to potassium iodide, and amphotericin B is the treatment of choice.

Infections due to Penicillium marneffei

Penicillium marneffei is a mould fungus that is a natural pathogen of the bamboo rat in South Asia. Cases in man behave rather like disseminated histoplasmosis, with which this infection is easily confused. Infiltration of the liver, spleen, bone marrow, lungs, and skin all occur in this infection. Such cases have mainly been described from southern China and South-East Asia. The growth of a red mould and the presence of non-budding, divided, intracellular yeast-like fungi is characteristic. This infection has been reported in a number of AIDS patients: it is one of the most common opportunistic infections in AIDS patients in Chiang Mai, Thailand. Amphotericin B or itraconazole are the main treatments.

REFERENCES

Penicilliosis

Deng, Z., Ribas, J.L., Gibson, D.W., and Connor, D.H. (1988). Infections caused by *Penicillium marneffei* in China and South East Asia: review of eighteen published cases and report of four more cases. *Review of Infectious Diseases*, **10,** 640–52.

Rare systemic infections

These include pulmonary invasion by *Geotrichum candidum* (geotrichosis) and adiaspiromycosis, a respiratory infection caused by *Emmonsia crescens* or *E. parva*. Isolated examples of human disease caused by fungi are consistently reported and almost always occur in the immunosuppressed host. In these patients many fungi that are normally saprophytes in the environment may invade and cause disease.

Systemic mycoses caused by opportunistic fungi

The opportunistic mycoses are a worldwide problem, although fortunately rare in most countries. In recent years they have been recognized more frequently with the increase in the use of transplantation of organs such as heart or bone marrow and in the more effective but immunocompromising regimes of cancer chemotherapy. Opportunistic invasion by organisms such as Candida or zygomycetes (Mucor, Absidia) may also occur in cases of malnutrition. One of the recent trends in the management of the severely immunocompromised patient has been the emergence of new pathogens such as non-*albicans* species of *Candida* or other organisms such as *Fusarium, Trichosporon,* or *Hansenula* species.

The opportunists present particular problems in diagnosis and management. Because many of the organisms are normally saprophytic, it has to be positively established that they have assumed an invasive role. Mere isolation may not provide sufficient evidence and in some instances low titres of antibody may be present even in normal hosts. The significance of various laboratory tests in these infections is shown in Table 3. Treatment is also difficult and it is important in most cases to attempt to reverse the process that led to the establishment of the infection. This may mean interrupting courses of cytotoxic therapy or risking loss of a transplant by reducing immunosuppressive therapy.

Systemic candidosis

Aetiology

In addition to their role in superficial infections, yeasts of the genus Candida may also cause invasive systemic disease. The clinical forms described range from a temporary candidaemia to disseminated invasive disease, sometimes with involvement of a single organ, site or body cavity (deep focal candidosis) as may occur in peritonitis or meningitis. Urinary tract infections may also be caused by *Candida* species.

The factors underlying systemic Candida infections are shown in Table 4. All these factors are important in disrupting the balance by which Candida is maintained as a saprophyte. Intravenous or central venous pressure lines may serve as a portal of entry or as a nidus for circulating yeasts in a candidaemia. Antibiotic therapy may upset the balance by inhibiting a potentially competitive bacterial flora.

C. albicans is the most common species involved but other species may be isolated, particularly in cases of endocarditis, for example, *C. parapsilosis*. *C. tropicalis* has been implicated in infections of neutropenic patients. Portals of entry include the gastrointestinal tract (common), skin, and urinary tract (rare). However, superficial candidosis or saprophytic colonization of mouth, skin or airways may also occur in compromised patients and does not necessarily indicate systemic invasion.

Epidemiology

Systemic infections caused by *Candida* species are worldwide in distribution.

Clinical features

CANDIDAEMIA

The isolation of Candida in blood culture may be linked to any of the factors listed in Table 4. Common predisposing features are the presence of intravenous lines, previous surgery (mainly gastrointestinal), antibiotic therapy or neutropenia. Patients develop a swinging fever and feel generally unwell. Clinical shock may occur.

Many such cases resolve following removal of predisposing factors, particularly the intravenous lines. However, a careful watch should be kept to exclude the presence of established invasive disease. Other sites should be searched for evidence of infection; for example, egg, urine by culture or the presence of white cells. Signs of muscle invasion (tenderness) or metastatic skin nodules should be excluded. Other signs of invasion include the development of new cardiac murmurs or of soft, white, retinal plaques caused by Candida. Persistently positive blood cultures or high antibody titres may also indicate possible deep invasion.

DISSEMINATED CANDIDOSIS

Although multiorgan invasive candidosis may follow candidaemia, at least 50 per cent of disseminated infections develop in patients without

Table 4 *Predisposing factors in deep Candida infections*

1. Local defects, foreign bodies, e.g. prosthetic heart valves, intravenous lines
2. Defects of immunity (primarily T cell or phagocytosis), e.g. cytotoxic therapy or SLE
3. Drug therapy, e.g. antibiotics
4. Carcinoma or leukaemia
5. Endocrine disease, e.g. diabetes mellitus in urinary tract candidosis
6. Physiological changes, e.g. infancy, old age and pregnancy (urinary tract)
7. Miscellaneous disorders, e.g.
   (*a*) malnutrition
   (*b*) surgery such as gastrointestinal resections
   (*c*) drug addiction

initially positive blood cultures. The features of some forms of invasive candidosis are listed above (under Candidaemia). Although Candida may be isolated from the sputum in these patients, there is rarely objective evidence of lung invasion. Moreover, there is no radiological appearance that is diagnostic of pulmonary candidosis and, indeed, chest radiographs may even appear normal. General localizing signs may be a late feature of disseminated candidosis.

Laboratory diagnosis of disseminated candidosis

The diagnosis may be made by culture and repeated attempts to isolate should be made where cultures are initially negative. Numerous techniques have been used to detect antibody in disseminated candidosis. However, ideally more than one procedure should be used, for example whole-cell agglutination combined with counterimmunoelectrophoresis. Changes of titre are often more significant than single values, particularly where antibody levels are low. None the less, 20 per cent or more of genuine cases may not have detectable antibody. Few antigen detection methods have stood the test of time and there are no commercially available antigen detection systems that significantly improve the detection rate.

By themselves, positive cultures, particularly from sputum, or the presence of antibodies do not necessarily prove the existence of deep-seated candidosis. A positive isolation may simply indicate the presence of colonization and normal individuals may have low titres of antibody to Candida. If there is a readily accessible lesion to biopsy, such as a skin nodule or even a pulmonary infiltrate, this may provide the best evidence of invasion, although such procedures may carry their own risk (Plate 8).

Treatment of disseminated candidosis

Untreated disseminated candidosis is normally progressive and fatal. The signs must be separated from, for instance, bacterial septicaemia, which may coexist with the Candida infection.

The treatment of invasive candidosis is intravenous amphotericin B given until there is a clinical and mycological response. This may take between 2 and 20 weeks depending on the site of infection and the underlying state of the patient. Although there is objective evidence as yet to support the addition of flucytosine in doses of 150 to 200 mg/kg body weight daily, it may give additional advantage in serious infections or where cure may hampered by poor penetration of amphotericin B such as in the eye. Fluconazole in doses of 200 to 800 mg daily can also be used.

DEEP FOCAL CANDIDOSIS

Candida infections in the peritoneum or meninges most often follow direct implantation after dialysis or surgery. Alternatively, secondary invasion from the middle ear or a perforated bowel is also possible. The signs and symptoms are similar to bacterial meningitis or peritonitis but Candida is isolated. Sometimes these infections clear spontaneously but normally treatment is instituted with amphotericin B. Once again fluconazole is an alternative approach.

CANDIDA ENDOCARDITIS

Invasion of heart valves, mainly the mitral or aortic valves, most commonly follows homograft replacement, but it may occur also in leukaemic patients or drug addicts. The symptoms are similar to bacterial endocarditis. However, Candida vegetations may reach considerable size. Embolic phenomena may involve obstruction of large vessels including the femoral artery or large cerebral vessels. The detection of large vegetations using an echo scanning device, particularly in cases with negative blood cultures, should raise the possibility of fungal endocarditis. Blood cultures are usually positive at some stage in the illness but repeated sampling may be necessary. High antibody titres are usually seen in such cases and serological tests are therefore of considerable value.

Untreated Candida endocarditis is uniformly fatal. There is also a high mortality associated with cases in which early surgical intervention is precipitated by impending heart failure. Normally, treatment consists of amphotericin B given intravenously and, where possible, valve replacement. There is no evidence to suggest that the addition of flucytosine to the regimen increases the effectiveness of treatment. However, the relapse rate is high and combination therapy may therefore be a reasonable approach on theoretical grounds.

URINARY TRACT CANDIDOSIS

Candida species may be isolated from the urine particularly in conditions associated with urinary stasis such as neurogenic bladder or where there is an indwelling catheter. Maturity-onset diabetes mellitus is another predisposing factor. There is no value in using the presence of pyuria or quantitative yeast-colony counts to assess the significance of infection. Treatment is normally given where there are symptoms such as dysuria or frequency or where there is a potential risk of invasion such as in immunosuppressed patients.

Trial of conservative therapy such as the removal of a urinary catheter should be attempted before chemotherapy with fluconazole is started.

Aspergillosis

Aetiology

There are a number of different disease states caused by the fungal genus Aspergillus. These range from allergic disorders to invasive disease. As a rule the organism affects predisposed hosts.

Most diseases associated with Aspergillus are caused by *A. fumigatus*. *A. flavus* may cause invasive disease primarily in the United States or an erosive paranasal granuloma in tropical countries. Both these species, together with *A. niger*, may also cause an intracavitary fungus ball or aspergilloma. On rare occasions other species are involved. Otomycosis, an infection of the external ear, may be caused by several species of *Aspergillus*, but *A. niger* is the most common organism isolated. *Aspergillus* species are common in the environment in dust, soil or vegetable material. They are common laboratory contaminants. They may also be isolated from sputum in patients with diseased airways (e.g. chronic bronchitis), although in the United Kingdom they are not often cultured from this source in other patients including leukaemics. The significance of the isolation of the organism in sputum may therefore vary with the nature of the underlying disease.

Epidemiology

Aspergillus infections are sporadic but ubiquitous. Invasive disease and aspergillomas are found in all countries. The former is more common in patients receiving transplantation and intensive cytotoxic therapy. There are other regional trends in aspergillosis. The destructive paranasal granuloma normally caused by *A. flavus* is most often seen in the tropics or in patients who originate from these areas. *A. nidulans* has been found to be a rare cause of mycetoma in the Sudan. Otomycosis appears to be more common in the tropics.

Clinical features

COLONIZATION BY ASPERGILLUS

Aspergillus species are not infrequently isolated from patients with chronic obstructive airways disease. Such positive cultures can rarely be correlated with clinical symptoms except in certain specific conditions, described below.

ALLERGIC BRONCHOPULMONARY ASPERGILLOSIS

Allergic bronchopulmonary aspergillosis is associated with persistent endobronchial growth of Aspergillus, usually *A. fumigatus*. In predisposed subjects, such as atopics, an immunological response to the organism probably involving both type I and type III hypersensitivity may contribute to the disease. The condition may start in childhood or early adult life.

Symptoms of reversible airways obstruction (e.g. asthma) are seen in early cases. However, where extensive bronchial damage has occurred, patients may present with breathlessness and a chronic productive cough. Mucoid plugs containing hyphal elements may be expectorated.

In many cases the chest radiograph shows scattered linear shadows in the peripheral lung fields. In order to establish the diagnosis a positive Aspergillus prick test, eosinophilia, the presence of Aspergillus in sputum, and weakly positive precipitins in serum are all helpful.

Treatment is difficult particularly in late cases. Attempts to remove the organism from the airways using antifungal therapy, if successful, are normally of only temporary benefit. Therapy is therefore aimed at the inflammatory response rather than the organism, and bronchodilators where appropriate, or inhaled corticosteroids are given.

ASPERGILLOMA

The development of a fungal ball in an existing pulmonary cavity is most commonly associated with aspergilli, although other organisms including *Pseudallescheria boydii, Coccidioides immitis*, and *Candida albicans* may also produce this condition. Frequently there are no symptoms apart from intermittent cough. However, haemoptysis of varying severity may develop. The condition is diagnosed by positive cultures and the presence of high titres of specific antibody in serum. Radiologically an opacity can be demonstrated in a cavity and this can usually be shown to move with changes of posture.

In some cases the fungal mass is expectorated and no action is required. However, where a decision to treat is reached the most reliable approach is surgical excision. Recurrent or severe haemoptysis would be an indication for intervention. Parenteral antifungal therapy is rarely successful. Local instillation of antifungal drugs is attended by a high frequency of relapse, and to be effective, they have to be delivered into the cavity by cannula under radiological control.

INVASIVE ASPERGILLOSIS

In severely compromised individuals particularly patients with leukemia, neutropenia, AIDS, collagen disorders or those on immunosuppressive regimens, *A. fumigatus*, and less commonly, *A. flavus*, may invade tissue. The initial site is normally lung, but extrapulmonary dissemination may occur, particularly to brain, kidney, liver, and skin. Symptoms such as pyrexia and cough are often masked by the patient's poor general state and other fungal or bacterial infections often coexist. Although a variety of radiographic appearances may be seen, rapid development of a discrete focus of pulmonary consolidation, which may appear to cavitate, should arouse suspicions, particularly in the presence of a positive Aspergillus culture. Often, however, both culture and serology are negative and biopsy offers the best chance of establishing the diagnosis.

Treatment should not be delayed. Intravenous amphotericin B in full dosage (1 mg/kg body weight daily) is the recommended treatment. Itraconazole is also active, although there is less information at present on its use in the neutropenic patient. Liposomal amphotericin B is an alternative. Combined therapy using amphotericin and flucytosine has also not been fully evaluated in invasive aspergillosis and is probably best reserved for patients who have not responded to amphotericin B alone. If possible, predisposing factors such as neutropenia should be corrected by temporary interruption of cytotoxic therapy.

There are two rarer types of invasive disease caused by Aspergillus. Endocarditis is uncommon but usually follows homograft valve replacement and may be accompanied by myocardial invasion. Secondly, an erosive granuloma containing aspergilli within the paranasal sinuses (paranasal aspergilloma) may invade the orbit or brain.

The mortality of all invasive forms of aspergillosis, even with treatment, is high.

REFERENCES

Aspergillosis

Karam, G.H. and Griffin, F.M. (1986). Invasive pulmonary aspergillosis in non-immunocompromised, non-neutropenic hosts. *Reviews of Infectious Diseases*, **8**, 357–62.

Patterson, R., Greenberger, P.A., and Radcin, R.C. (1982). Allergic bronchopulmonary aspergillosis: staging as an aid to management. *Annals of Internal Medicine*, **96**, 286–91.

Rinaldi, M.G. (1983). Invasive aspergillosis. *Reviews of Infectious Diseases*, **5**, 1061–77.

Weber, D.J. and Rutala, W.A. (1989). Epidemiology of hospital acquired fungal infections. In *Diagnosis and therapy of systemic fungal infections*, (ed. K. Holmberg and R. Meyer), pp. 1–24. Raven Press, New York.

Cryptococcosis

Aetiology

Cryptococcosis is a systemic infection caused by *Cryptococcus neoformans*. Its most common clinical feature is meningitis, but pulmonary, cutaneous, and widely disseminated forms of the infection are also recognized. There are two varieties of *C. neoformans* called *C. neoformans neoformans* and *C neoformans gattii*. They differ in their geographic range and ecology. The *neoformans* variety dominates in AIDS patients.

C. neoformans neoformans is a yeast that can be isolated from the environment, although it is most often found in pigeon excreta. Its growth from soil appears to be enhanced by certain nitrogenous compounds such as creatinine in the pigeon droppings. The birds are not infected, although their crops may be heavily colonized. Very large numbers of organisms (e.g. 1×10^7 yeasts/g of droppings) may be found in densely populated urban areas. *C. neoformans* var. *gattii* has recently been detected in leaf and bark debris of certain eucalyptus species.

The portal of entry is usually the lung, from where the organism spreads to involve other organs or sites such as the meninges. Although many isolates from natural sources have small cells, one sequel to tissue invasion is the development of a large, mucoid capsule *in vivo*, a feature that may confer some protection to the organism. Infections with *C. neoformans* are seen in both normal and immunocompromised hosts. The main underlying processes are sarcoidosis, Hodgkin's disease, collagen disease, carcinoma, the administration of systemic corticosteroid therapy, or AIDS, the commonest predisposition.

Epidemiology

Cryptococcosis has been recorded from most countries, although it is most prevalent in the United States and Australia. Before the AIDS epidemic in the United States approximately 50 per cent of cases were said to occur in normal persons. By contrast, in the United Kingdom 85 per cent of cases were found in patients with underlying disorders. There is no skin-test reagent widely available, but some pilot studies in the United States suggest that workers exposed to the organism (e.g. in laboratories) are more likely than other groups to have a positive skin test without any overt sign of infection. It is probably, therefore, that there is an asymptomatic form of cryptococcosis (cf. histoplasmosis). Additional evidence for the existence of subclinical infection is provided by the repeated isolation of *C. neoformans* in sputum from individuals without evidence of disease.

Clinical features

PULMONARY CRYPTOCOCCOSIS

Acute or subacute respiratory disease caused by *C. neoformans* rare in most parts of the world, but is well recognized in the United States. The disease consists of a chest infection with fever and cough and scattered, often well-circumscribed, areas of pulmonary infiltration seen on radiographs. In some patients no treatment is required, and the whole process resolves, although it is probably advisable to give chemotherapy to those with prolonged disease or underlying abnormalities. The laboratory diagnosis is made by biopsy or culture. Serological tests for antibody or capsular polysaccharide antigen (latex test) are often negative. In treated cases a course of amphotericin B or fluconazole is advised, depending on the clinical response.

Isolated cryptococcal granulomas (cryptococcoma) may present as coin lesions and are removed surgically to exclude carcinoma. Once the correct diagnosis is made, many workers advise a short course of amphotericin B or fluconazole as there is a small risk of dissemination to other organs following surgery.

DISSEMINATED CRYPTOCOCCOSIS

The best-recognized form of extrapulmonary cryptococcosis is meningitis. This may present with signs of acute meningism. However, more usually the features are less specific. Pyrexia, headache, and mental changes such as confusion or drowsiness occur. The mental changes probably follow the development of hydrocephalus. Blurring of vision and papilloedema may also occur. Cranial nerve involvement is less common. AIDS patients present with disseminated disease. The signs of meningeal involvement may be very subtle and the infection has often spread to other sites such as liver and spleen as well as skin (Plate 9).

The cerebrospinal fluid shows pleocytosis that is highly variable. Often there are excessive numbers of lymphocytes, but sometimes polymorphonuclear leucocytes abound. In some cases only small numbers of white cells (4–10) are seen. Characteristically, but not invariably, the glucose concentration falls and protein rises. Cryptococci can be seen in some cases in an India ink or nigrosin preparation, which is used to highlight the capsule. A spun sediment is best for this purpose. The organism can also be cultured from the cerebrospinal fluid. The latex test for antigen is usually positive for cerebrospinal fluid, but on rare occasions this is negative. The antigen titre has both diagnostic and prognostic value. Initial high (> 100) titres are likely to correlate with relapse following therapy and with a poor prognosis. In AIDS patients, antigen titres over 1:1000 convey poor prognosis and blood cultures are often positive. Extrameningeal disease should be looked for by sputum or urine culture and serology in patients presenting with meningitis.

OTHER SITES

Cryptococci may disseminate to other sites including liver and spleen, kidney, skin, or bone. Infection in skin and bone are most often seen in patients with sarcoidisis. In every case, underlying deep disseminated lesions (e.g. meningitis) may be found. The methods of diagnosis and treatment are similar to those seen with meningitis. Only a small proportion of cases of cryptococcosis may have detectable antibody (15–30 per cent), and this may occur late in the course of therapy.

It is important in all cases where cryptococcosis presents with lesions in an extrameningeal site to exclude occult meningitis by lumbar puncture.

Therapy

In the non-AIDS patient the combination of flucytosine (150–180 mg/kg daily) and intravenous amphotericin B (0.3–0.6 mg/kg daily) is the most widely used treatment. It is possible to induce recovery with this approach and treatment is generally continued for at least 6 weeks or longer if necessary. The clinical response and antigen levels are useful for monitoring progress.

The situation is different in AIDS patients because it is seemingly impossible to achieve complete recovery and residual antigen titres are commonplace. The object of therapy is to induce the most rapid remission possible, followed by long-term suppressive therapy. There are various regimens used for induction of remission. The use of amphotericin B with or without flucytosine is favoured by many. This is given for 2 weeks and is then followed by indefinite treatment with fluconazole or itraconazole to prevent relapse.

REFERENCES

Cryptococcosis

Clark, R.A., Greet, D., Atkinson, W., Valainis, G.T., and Hyslop, N. (1990). Spectrum of *Cryptococcus neoformans* infection in 68 patients infected with acquired immunodeficiency virus. *Reviews of Infectious Diseases*, **12,** 768–77.

Dismukes, W.E. (1988). Cryptococcal meningitis in patients with AIDS. *Journal of Infectious Diseases*, **157,** 624–7.

Kovacs, J.A. *et al.* (1985). Cryptococcosis in the acquired immunodeficiency syndrome. *Annals of Internal Medicine*, **103,** 533–8.

Stevens, D.A. (1990). Fungal infections in AIDS patients. *British Journal of Clinical Practice*, **44** (suppl. 71), 11–22.

Swinne-Desgain, D. and de Vroey, C. (1987). Epidémiologie de la cryptoccose. *Revista Iberica de Micologia*, **4,** 77–83.

Invasive zygomycosis (mucormycosis, phycomycosis)

Aetiology

Invasive disease caused by mucor-like (zygomycete) fungi is rare. In the compromised host it may lead to paranasal destruction, necrotic lung or skin lesions, and disseminated disease.

The causative organisms commonly belong to three genera, Absidia, Rhizopus, and Rhizomucor. More rarely other organisms such as Cunninghamella or Saksenaea have been implicated. Most of the agents are associated with decaying vegetable matter and are common airborne moulds. The route of infection is highly variable: they may invade via the lungs, paranasal sinuses, gastrointestinal tract or damaged skin. The predisposing illness may in some way determine the site of clinical invasion. Underlying factors include diabetic ketoacidosis (rhinocerebral involvement), leukemia and immunosuppressive therapy (lung and disseminated infection), malnutrition (gastrointestinal infection), and burns or wounds (cutaneous invasion). These patterns are not always strictly followed.

Epidemiology

Invasive zygomycosis is rare but has a worldwide distribution. Its invasive nature, particularly the tendency to involve blood vessels and its selection of compromised hosts, distinguish this form of infection from subcutaneous zygomycosis, which is also caused by zygomycete species.

Clinical features

The most characteristic features of this type of infection are the extensive necrosis and infarction that may follow blood vessel invasion leading to thrombosis. A similar type of invasion may occur with invasive aspergillosis but is usually less prominent. Invasive zygomycosis follows a number of different patterns.

The infection may initially localize in one of several sites. The most common is in the paranasal sinuses and this is most often seen in diabetic patients with ketoacidosis. The patient presents with fever and unilateral facial pain. Subsequently there may be facial swelling with nasal obstruction and proptosis. There may be invasion into the orbit leading to blindness, into the brain, and the palate. Palatal ulceration should be searched for. Widespread dissemination with infarction of major organs or limbs may occur subsequently. A similar pattern of invasion of surgical wounds or burns may occur and has on occasions been associated with contamination of dressing packs. Infections are initially localized causing extensive necrosis around the original wound. Gastrointestinal invasion may be heralded by perforation of viscera, and diarrhoea or haematemesis or melaena.

Alternatively a patient may present with established pulmonary or widespread dissemination. Such patients are usually leukaemics or are severely immunosuppressed. Neutropenia is often seen.

Once infection has spread beyond the original site, invasive zygomycosis is almost invariably fatal with or without treatment.

Laboratory diagnosis

The diagnosis is suggested by the combination of infection and extensive infarction, particularly if it occurs in any of the sites mentioned. The organisms may be difficult to culture even from biopsy and histology is often the quickest way of establishing the diagnosis. Serology is frequently negative.

Treatment

Treatment should be initiated as soon as possible and extensive surgical debridement combined with intravenous amphotericin B in maximum daily dosage offers the best chance of success. Local instillations of amphotericin B may also be used where appropriate (e.g. nasal sinuses). Some physicians also recommend anticoagulation with heparin to forestall thrombosis. Despite therapy the mortality remains high. Liposomal amphotericin B also has been used with some success.

Rhinosporidiosis

Rhinosporidiosis is an infection found in India, Sri Lanka, parts of East Africa, and South America. It is characterized by polypoid growth from the nose or conjunctiva. The causative organism can be demonstrated in tissue and consists of aggregates of large sporangia containing spores in various phases of development. However, they have never been successfully cultured and their fungal nature has only been assumed from their morphological appearance in histology.

The treatment is surgical excision.

Otomycosis and oculomycosis

External otitis is often multifactorial but in some cases dense fungal colonization can contribute to the picture. In severe cases, the external ear may be plugged by a dense mat of mycelium. *Aspergillus* species are the most common organisms cultured, particularly *A. niger*, but Candida, Penicillium, and Mucor may all contribute. Intensive ear toilet may eradicate the infection without recourse to antifungal agents.

Infections of the eye, particularly the cornea, caused by fungi (oculomycosis) are rare. They often follow penetrating injuries to the globe or contamination of lacerations. An opacity develops within the cornea with associated pain and chemosis. An exudate is usually present in the aqueous humour. Prompt treatment with intensive topical instillation of drugs containing an antifungal drug such as miconazole or econazole is necessary every 2 to 4 h. Perforation of the eye may occur in advanced cases.

Approaches to management of fungal infections

The main antifungal agents can be considered in four main groups: the polyenes, azoles, morpholines and allylamines, and an assortment of drugs of specific activity that are not related.

The polyene antifungals are macrolide substances derived originally from species of *Streptomyces*. They include amphotericin B, natamycin, and nystatin. More recent additions to this group are partricin and mepartricin. Polyenes are poorly soluble in water and amphotericin B is the only one widely used as a parenterally administered drug. Nystatin and natamycin are purely topical. Amphotericin B is metabolized in the liver and penetrates body cavities, cerebrospinal fluid, and urine poorly. The polyenes have broad activity against a wide range of fungi; however, natamycin is the only one that is reasonably effective in dermatophytosis. The mode of action of the polyenes appears to involve inhibition of sterol synthesis in the fungal cell membrane.

The imidazoles are synthetic antifungal agents. They include miconazole, clotrimazole, econazole, isoconazole, ketoconazole, tioconazole, and bifonazole. The triazole series contains two potent oral agents, fluconazole and itraconazole. Most are used topically except for ketoconazole (oral), itraconazole (oral), and miconazole (intravenous). These are metabolized in the liver and, like amphotericin B, affect fungal cell-membrane synthesis and penetrate cerebrospinal fluid and urine in low concentrations. The imidazoles have a broad spectrum of activity against many fungi, although neither miconazole nor ketoconazole are useful for aspergillus infections. By contrast, itraconazole is active *in vitro* against aspergilli. Fluconazole is less active against moulds and there are instances of both primary (*C. krusei*, *C. glabrata*) and secondary resistance to this compound. The allylamines such as terbinafine are primarily active against superficial fungi but *in vitro* appear to have fungicidal activity at low concentrations.

Other antifungal drugs include flucytosine, which is a synthetic pyrimidine analogue. Given either intravenously or orally it is mainly useful for chromomycosis and certain yeast infections. Drug resistance is a major problem with flucytosine, particularly with cryptococcus. The drug shows a number of modes of action including disruption of RNA transcription following uptake by the cell. Griseofulvin is derived from a species of *Penicillium*. It can be given orally and is only useful against dermatophytes. It is best absorbed when given with a meal and selectively accumulates in stratum corneum in concentrations approximately 10 times greater than serum levels. Griseofulvin acts by inhibiting intracellular microtubule formation. There are a large number of unrelated antifungal drugs, such as tolnaftate, haloprogin, and chlorphenesin, that are only used topically.

Table 5 *Topical antifungals*

Benzoic acid compound (Whitfield's ointment)
Benzoyl peroxide
Clotrimazole
Econazole
Ketoconazole
Miconazole
Natamycin
Nystatin
Salicyclic/tannic/boric acid cream
Sulconazole
Terbinafine
Tolnaftate
Undecenoate mixtures

Management of superficial infections

Specific details of therapy are included under the separate diseases. The topical agents that can be used for different superficial mycoses are shown in Table 5. Benzoic acid compound (Whitfield's ointment), which contains 2 per cent salicylic acid and 2 per cent benzoic acid, acts as a keratolytic agent by causing exfoliation of the superficial layers of the stratum corneum. Other topical agents with only weak antifungal activity include gentian violet (candidosis or dermatophytosis), Castellani's paint, which contains magenta and resorcinol (candidosis or dermatophytosis), and brilliant green (dermatophytosis). Two per cent selenium sulphide remains a highly effective method of treating pityriasis versicolor by application once daily for 2 weeks. Twenty per cent sodium hyposulphite is an alternative.

The more specific antifungals such as the polyenes, amphotericin B, nystatin, and natamycin (candidosis) or the imidazoles (candidosis, dermatophytosis, and pityriasis versicolor) are highly effective and probably quicker, although more expensive, than the keratolytics or dyes. Local irritancy can be a problem particularly with Whitfield's ointment, which is usually given as a half-strength preparation. Allergic contact dermatitis is rare but has been recorded from some imidazoles (miconazole, clotrimazole, tioconazole) and tolnaftate.

Terbinafine or itraconazole are in some ways more active in many forms of dermatophytosis requiring oral therapy than griseofulvin. In onychomycosis they are preferred. Terbinafine has occasional side-effects, mainly related to gastrointestinal intolerance, although it may also cause transient loss of taste. Itraconazole likewise can cause gastrofjintestinal discomfort and nausea. Both drugs rarely cause hepatic injury, with a frequency of less than 1:120 000. This is in contrast with ketoconazole, which also causes hepatitis but in around 1:8000 cases. Liver function tests should be monitored if ketoconazole is used extensively over any length of time. In high doses ketoconazole may block human androgen biosynthesis causing side-effects such as gynaecomastia.

The overall cure rate of onychomycosis caused by dermatophytes was poor. Using griseofulvin alone only 40 per cent of toe-nail infections will remain free from reinfection after 1 year to 18 months of therapy. Both terbinafine and itraconazole lead to remission of toe-nail infections in only 3 months. Amorolfine, a morpholine drug, is used in the topical treatment of nail disease where there is less than complete involvement of the nails.

Management of deep mycoses

There are very few drugs that are effective in systemic fungal infections and those that are used should always be accompanied by supportive measures and, if possible, an attempt to eliminate any predisposing conditions. For instance, if their condition permits, a patient who has developed a candidaemia while a central venous line is in place should be managed by removal of the line. However, most physicians would also use 7 days of fluconazole as well. In the neutropenic patient a positive blood culture would be regarded as evidence of septicaemia and all would be required to have antifungal therapy.

The polyene group of antifungal antibiotics, which includes natamycin and nystatin, is normally used most frequently in topical preparations. Amphotericin B is the only drug in this group that is given parenterally. It forms a fine colloidal suspension and must be freshly made up. The drug is given in a 5 per cent dextrose infusion not containing additional drugs, if possible. A test dose of 1 to 5 mg is given over 2 h and this is followed by gradually increasing doses over the next 3 to 9 days to the normal maximum of 0.6 to 1.0 mg/kg body weight daily depending on the infection. In some cases this slow approach may help the patient to tolerate the drug better or may define the dose at which side-effects such as pyrexia start. In severely ill cases, half of the full dose may be given 4 h after a test dose of 5 mg, usually under hydrocortisone cover. The full dose is given 24 h later. Side-effects include thrombophlebitis, nausea, hypotension, and pyrexia. Renal clearance may fall in the initial period but this usually returns to normal after a temporary halt in therapy. More permanent renal tubular damage may follow a total dose of 4 g or more. Amphotericin B does not enter urine, cerebrospinal fluid or peritoneal fluid in significant concentrations. So, for instance, in cases of fungal meningitis, local instillations of 0.5 to 1.0 mg of amphotericin B dissolved in cerebrospinal fluid may be given in addition to intravenous therapy, although a maximum of 15 mg (*in toto*) is normally not exceeded. Arachnoiditis and sensory or motor disturbances may follow intrathecal injection of amphotericin B. An indwelling (Ommaya) reservoir is sometimes used for instillation of the drugs into the cerebral ventricle but its insertion carries serious perioperative and postoperative complications, particularly secondary infection.

Amphotericin B is normally given until clinical or mycological cure is induced. This is often difficult to judge accurately and in many of the mycoses caused by the systemic pathogens a course of at least 2 g is often used on an empirical basis. In the opportunistic infections, lower total doses are probably effective and the length of treatment should depend on the clinician's judgement.

Flucytosine (5-fluorocytosine) is an effective antifungal agent that is primarily active against yeasts such as Candida and Cryptococcus. It is well absorbed after oral administration and is given in four divided doses totalling 150 to 200 mg/kg body weight daily. It enters urine, cerebrospinal fluid, and peritoneal fluid. Its excretion is reduced in renal failure and the daily dose should be reduced accordingly and blood levels monitored. The drug can also be given intravenously.

The main disadvantage of flucytosine is the development of either primary or secondary drug resistance in a significant number of isolates, and when given in toxic doses it may cause bone marrow depression. The serum level should not be allowed to rise above 100 to 120 μg/ml. The drug is mainly used in urinary or peritoneal candidosis or chromomycosis. An important use is its combination with amphotericin B (see below).

Combination amphotericin B and flucytosine therapy may offer a highly effective method of treatment. Theoretically as the drugs synergize, the dose of amphotericin B may be reduced. In cryptococcal meningitis, combination therapy using a dose of 0.3 to 0.6 mg/kg body weight of amphotericin B with the normal dose of flucytosine is more effective at sterilizing the cerebrospinal fluid and preventing relapse. In other forms of systemic infection such as candidosis there is little evidence that it is more effective than amphotericin B alone, although this may in time prove to be the case.

The azole drugs are also used in systemic mycoses. Fluconazole is given in systemic candidosis, urinary tract infections, and as a long-term suppressive, in addition to primary therapy, in cryptococcosis in AIDS patients. Side-effects are uncommon, although it can cause nausea and vomiting. Fluconazole can be given orally or intravenously. Itraconazole has been evaluated in a variety of systemic mycoses from aspergillosis to cryptococcosis. Its active range includes histoplasmosis, sporotrichosis, chromoblastomycosis, blastomycosis, coccidioidomycosis, and paracoccidioidomycosis. Itraconazole is only used as an oral preparation. Its absorption is often defective in AIDS and bone marrow-transplant patients and in these groups the mean daily dosage is doubled (200 mg).

The use of leucocyte growth factors has been reported to improve the recovery from fungal infections. The most effective combination has been a mixture of granulocyte and granulocyte–monocyte colony-stimulating factors. Further studies of these compounds in the neutropenic patients are warranted.

Liposomal or lipid-complexed forms of amphotericin B are now either available or in development. The potential advantage of these drugs is that the frequency of renal side-effects is considerably reduced, thus allowing the physician to use higher daily doses (2–4 mg/kg daily).

REFERENCES

Therapy

Davies, R.R. (1980). Griseofulvin. In *Antifungal chemotherapy*, (ed. D.C.E. Speller), p. 149–82. Wiley, Chichester.

Davies, R.R., Everall, J.D., and Hamilton, E. (1967). Mycological and clinical evaluation of griseofulvin for chronic onychomycosis. *British Medical Journal*, **iii**, 464.

Fromtling, R.A. (1980). Overview of medically important antifungal azole derivatives. *Clinical Microbiology Reviews*, **1**, 187–17.

Medoff, G. and Kobayashi, G.A. (1980). The polyenes. In *Antifungal Chemotherapy*, (ed. D.C.E. Speller), pp. 3–34. Wiley, Chichester.

Petranyi, G., Meingassner, J.G., and Mieth, H. (1987). Antifungal activity of the allylamine derivative, terbinafine, *in vitro*. *Antimicrobial Agents and Chemotherapy*, **31**, 1365–8.

Polak, A. (1992). Preclinical data and mode of action of amorolfine. *Dermatology*, **184** (suppl.), 3–7.

Powderly, W.B., and Van't Wout, J.W. (1992). *Fluconazole*. Marius Press, Lancs.

Strauss, J.S. (1982). Ketoconazole and the liver. *Journal of the American Academy of Dermatology*, **6**, 546.

7.12.2 Coccidioidomycosis

J. R. GRAYBILL

This is a systemic fungus infection caused by the dimorphic fungus *Coccidioides immitis*. *C. immitis* resides in rather arid, temperate climates of the Americas, ranging from the pampas of Argentina up through the Texas and Arizona deserts to southern California. The fungus grows in a mycelial form characterized by barrel-shaped arthroconidia alternating with ghost cells. The ability to grow on most media in 7 to 10 days, and the extreme fragility of the mycelium, make this one of the most dangerous pathogens for accidental laboratory inhalation.

The conidium is small enough to penetrate to the distal airways, where it rounds up, enlarges over several days, and subdivides into many cells divided by septa and surrounded by a thick outer wall. This spherule is more than 20 μm in diameter, much larger than a leucocyte, and the thick wall is highly characteristic and can be readily identified in a standard haematoxylin/eosin stain as well as the silver stains commonly used.

Clinical features

The normal course of coccidioidomycosis is either lack of symptoms (up to 40 per cent of patients) or the development of a pneumonitic process that may resolve in several weeks, may cavitate promptly and then heal by scarring, may persist for months, or may progressively enlarge or spread to other lobes, and, in 1 to 2 per cent of patients, may disseminate. Concurrent diabetes mellitus is associated with cavitary pulmonary disease. Factors associated with progression and dissemination outside the lungs include immunosuppression (including, but only rarely, AIDS), black or Amerindian race, and negative fungal-antigen skin tests.

Persistent pulmonary coccidioidomycosis includes infiltrative and cavitary disease that has been present for more than 3 months. Extrapulmonary dissemination generally involves skin, bone, and joint, causes meningitis in up to 20 per cent of patients, and, less commonly, is widespread.

Dissemination is probably much more frequent than we appreciate. Widespread dissemination is less common, but may be associated with AIDS and a CD4 cell count below 100/mm^3. Disseminated disease in the immunologically intact host is milder, and is associated with nodules and a focal inflammatory process in the bone and joints. In patients with remarkably depressed cell-mediated immunity, there may be abscesses discharging pus laden with polymorphonuclear leucocytes and spherules. In meningeal involvement, the clinical presentation resembles tuberculous or cryptococcal meningitis. However, in coccidioidal meningitis there may be eosinophilia in the cerebrospinal fluid. The course of meningitis may end with cerebrovascular accidents from vascular involvement, cranial neuropathies from basilar meningitis, or obstructive or communicating hydrocephalus.

Diagnosis

Coccidioidomycosis is diagnosed through a history of exposure 2 to 3 weeks before onset of disease, appropriate clinical symptoms, a cerebrospinal fluid consistent with chronic meningitis, pathognomonic appearances of biopsies, sputum samples yielding the organism in cultures, and serology. Two serological techniques are widely used. Precipitating antibodies are IgM, and rise within 2 weeks of infection in 90 per cent of patients. These antibodies decline after several weeks, even if the infection continues to be aggressive. The other antibody is used in a complement-fixation test (IgG). Because some antibodies consume complement, an immunodiffusion method has been used. Complement-fixation titres rise usually 3 to 6 weeks after infection. Unlike the precipitating antibodies, the others are titred, and in general the higher the titre the worse the disease. A titre of 1:16 in serum suggests disseminated disease. These antibodies often do not rise until 4 to 6 weeks have passed, and then remain high for years. They were thought to decline on clinical improvement but recent studies have found that complement-fixing antibodies often remain elevated throughout the course of illness. Finally, there is an antigen test that is promising, particularly in patients such as those with AIDS who may have false-negative serology.

Treatment

Coccidioidomycosis is among the most difficult diseases to treat. Traditionally, amphotericin B has been used at 50 mg, three times a week, for non-meningeal disease. Treatment continues for 2 to 3 g total dose, or until the patient clinically improves. Failures and relapses are common, as in renal failure from repeated courses of amphoterin B. Treatment of meningitis has required that amphotericin be given intrathecally. Even when delivered via an Ommaya reservoir, via cisternal puncture, and with corticosteroids, treatment has been toxic, with severe arachnoiditis and transverse myelitis. The dose is raised gradually from 0.05 to 0.5 mg, three times weekly, and continues on a gradually decreasing frequency of dose until the titres decline and the cerebrospinal fluid becomes normal.

Because of these difficulties, ketoconazole was evaluated in coccidioidomycosis soon after it became available. Initial reports of 60 to 80 per cent success were later tempered in multicentre studies in which fewer than 40 per cent of patients with non-meningeal disease achieved remission. Relapses were also frequent after treatment was completed (more than 40 per cent of patients. Ketoconazole was useful in as many as 70 per cent of meningitis patients who could tolerate the doses of 1200 to 2000 mg/day. Unfortunately, the majority of patients could not take these high doses, usually because of gastrointestinal intolerance. Nevertheless, ketoconazole pointed the way to azole therapy.

Both fluconazole and itraconazole have been used in large multicentre studies, with uniform criteria for improvement. Response rates to either drug, even at 400 mg/day for 9 to 14 months, have been 50 to 60 per cent, and relapses seem less frequent than with ketoconazole. Both drugs are in a comparative study at this time. For meningitis, fluconazole is clearly the drug of choice at 400 mg/day given indefinitely. More than 75 per cent of patients responded remarkably to this well-tolerated regimen. Unfortunately, many patients with AIDS and coccidioidomycosis do not respond well to treatment, and eventually appear to escape from whatever drug is used.

REFERENCES

Bronniman, D.A. *et al.* (1987). Coccidioidomycosis in the acquired immunodeficiency syndrome. *Annals of Internal Medicine*, **106,** 373–9.

Drutz, D.J. and Catanzaro, A. (1978). Coccidioidomycosis. Parts I and II. *American Reviews of Respiratory Diseases*, **117,** 559–85; 727–71.

Galgiani, J.N. and Ampel, N.M. (1990). Coccidioidomycosis in human immunodeficiency virus-infected patients. *Journal of Infectious Diseases*, **162,** 1165–9.

Stevens, D.A. (1980). *Coccidioidomycosis: a text.* Plenum Press, New York.

7.12.3 Chromomycosis

M. A. H. Bayles

Aetiology

Chromomycosis, one of the intermediate subcutaneous mycoses, is a chronic granulomatous fungal infection characterized histologically by the presence of brown, spherical fungal cells known as sclerotic cells or fumagoid bodies. In most cases, the lesions are confined to the skin and subcutaneous tissues. In the past there has been great confusion over nomenclature of the aetiological agents of chromomycosis. At present, five agents assigned to four genera are recognized as causing chromomycosis. They are:

(1) *Fonsecaea pedrosoi*, which occurs in high rainfall areas and is found worldwide;
(2) *Cladosporium carrionii*, the sole cause of chromomycosis in arid areas;
(3) *Phialophora verrucosa*, the first agent to be described;
(4) *Fonsecaea compactum*, an uncommon cause and isolated only a few times;
(5) *Rhinocladiella aquaspersa*, the rarest cause.

Sporadic cases caused by other dematiaceous fungi such as *Cladosporium trichoides* and *Taeniolélla boppii* have been reported from Uganda and Brazil.

Epidemiology

The principal endemic areas for chromomycosis are the tropical and subtropical countries including Central and South America, Costa Rica, Africa, Japan, Australia, Malagasy, and Indonesia. Curiously, sporadic cases have been reported from Finland and Russia.

Although soil itself does not seem to be a particularly good substrate, the various agents of chromomycosis occur as saprobic fungi in the environment and have been isolated from soil, decaying vegetation and rotting wood. Strains of *F. pedrosoi* and *P. verrucosa* have been isolated from the atmosphere but proved less virulent than those isolated from human lesions or organic material.

Infection occurs as a result of trauma, however minor, the fungi gaining entrance through a cut, abrasion, or thorn prick. Farmers and labourers in agricultural areas are most likely to be exposed to contaminated material. Although lesions on exposed areas may be accounted for in this way it was suggested by Wilson in 1958 that lesions on non-exposed areas may result from a previously unrecognized pulmonary focus. Bacquero later demonstrated the presence of *F. pedrosoi* in bronchial washings and subsequently proved their pathogenicity by inoculating those strains into normal skin of human volunteers and recovering the fungus from the ensuing skin lesions. Other methods of transmission have included metal particles from automobiles, and acupuncture. Person-to-person and animal-to-man transmission have not so far been reported. Chromomycosis has rarely been reported in children and it may be that factors other than trauma and exposure to contaminated material are necessary for its development.

Pathogenesis

Host resistance and virulence of the organism are the two main factors associated with the pathogenesis of this disease. Chromomycosis occurs mainly in healthy individuals. However, it has been found in patients where immunosuppression has occurred either from underlying disabling disease or from chemotherapy. Although the mechanism of granuloma formation is not well understood, it appears that lipids extracted from these fungi and cell-wall constituents may be responsible for this reaction.

Clinical features

The initial lesion of chromomycosis is a small papule at the site of trauma, which gradually enlarges. Nodules and tumours develop, producing a malodorous discharge; eventually, over a period of years, a wide variety of morphological patterns may emerge including dry, hyperkeratotic plaques, verrucose lesions, and large, cauliflower-like masses. Extensive cicatricial plaques, surrounded by peripherally spreading vegetative lesions, may also be present. Evolution is slow and lesions usually involve the lower limb. However, any part of the body may be involved and the sites may be multiple.

Dissemination occurs by (i) surface spread, (ii) the lymphatics, the most common method, (iii) autoinoculation from scratching, and (iv) haematogenously, resulting in subcutaneous lesions at sites distant from the primary. Visceral metastases are known to occur and involvement of the central nervous system, respiratory system, larynx, and vocal chords has been recorded. Therapeutically, therefore, early diagnosis is important.

Complications of long-standing chromomycosis include lymphoedema, flexion deformity of joints, and development of squamous carcinoma.

Diagnosis

Although the history and clinical presentation may suggest the diagnosis, the varied clinical presentation of chromomycosis necessitates consideration of other granulomatous diseases such as sporotrichosis, cutaneous tuberculosis, Hansen's disease, blastomycosis, candidosis, leishmaniasis, paracoccidioidomycosis, rhinosporidiosis, tertiary syphylis, squamous carcinoma, and even psoriasis, sarcoidosis, and discoid lupus erythematosus.

Therefore, to establish a definitive diagnosis, histological and mycological investigations are essential. Diagnosis is confirmed by the presence of the characteristic brown, sclerotic bodies in histological sections. From both epidemiological and therapeutic points of view, culture is necessary as *F. pedrosoi* is the most difficult of the causative fungi to eradicate whereas *C. carrionii* responds rapidly to treatment.

Treatment

Small, single, localized lesions are satisfactorily eradicated by cryosurgery, but long-term follow-up is needed to assess accurately the success of this treatment. Thermotherapy has been found effective by some, again principally in the management of small, single lesions, but here the possibility of a burn must be borne in mind. Rapid spread of the disease has been associated with inadequate surgery, curettage, and electrodesiccation.

Oral monotherapy has been unsuccessful in the majority of cases and drug resistance remains a problem. The most effective treatment at present is a combination of 5-flucytosine with either thiabendazole or itraconazole. Ketoconazole, either alone or combined with 5-flucytosine, produces only a moderate response. Of the newer drugs, saperconazole (at the time of writing withdrawn by the manufacturers) is reportedly effective in treating infections caused by *F. pedrosoi* and terbinafine, as demonstrated by *in vitro* testing, has the potential to be effective.

Whatever method of treatment is used, chromomycosis although clinically healed, should be followed-up for at least 2 years before its total eradication can be assumed.

REFERENCES

Bayles, M.A.H. (1989). Chromomycosis. In *Tropical fungal* infections, Vol. 4 of *Baillière's clinical* tropical medicine and communicable diseases, pp. 45–70. Baillière Tindall, London.

Bacquero, G.F., Lopez, B.P., and Lescay, B.R. (1961). Cromoblastomicosis experimental: cromoblastomicosis producida experimentalmente con cepas de *Hormodendrum pedrosoi* obtenida por lavado bronquial de enfermos que padecen la affecion. *Boletin de la Sociedad Cubana de Dermatologia y Sifilografia*, **18,** 19–28.

Grigoriu, D., Delacretaz, J., and Borelli, D. (1987). In *Medical mycology*, (English edn), pp. 333–42. Hans Huber, Toronto.

McGinnis, M.R., Ajello, L., and Schell, W.A. (1985). Mycotic diseases: a proposed nomenclature. *International Journal of Dermatology*, **24,** 9–15.

Silva, C.L. and Ekizlerian, S.M. (1985). Granulomatous reaction induced by lipids extracted from *Fonsecaea pedrosoi*, *Fonsecaea compactum*, *Cladosporium carrionii* and *Phialophora verrucosum. Journal of General Microbiology*, **131,** 187–94.

Silva, C.L. and Fazioli, R.A. (1985). Role of the fungal cell wall in the granulomatous response of mice to the agents of chromomycosis. *Journal of Medical Microbiology*, **20,** 299–305.

Wilson, J.W. (1958). Importancia de las enfermedades fungosas en imunologia. *Boletin de la Sociedad Cubana de Dermatologia y Sifilografia*, **15,** 115–24.

7.12.4 Paracoccidioidomycosis

M. A. S. Yasuda

Definition

Paracoccidioidomycosis is a systemic granulomatous disease that involves mainly the lungs, phagocytic mononuclear system, mucous membranes, skin, and adrenals. The only aetiological agent is a dimorphic fungus, *Paracoccidioides brasiliensis*. This mycosis is geographically restricted to Central and South America, ranging from Mexico to Argentina.

History

The disease was first described in 1908 by Lutz, a Brazilian scientist, and in 1912, Splendore classified the organism as a yeast of the genus

Zymonema. In 1928, Almeida and Lacaz suggested the name Paracoccidioides and in 1930, Almeida named the fungus *Paracoccidioides brasiliensis*. Until 1977, the disease was known as South American blastomycosis, Lutz–Splendore–Almeida's disease, paracoccidioidal granuloma or Brazilian blastomycosis. In that year it was renamed paracoccidioidomycosis.

Epidemiology

Paracoccidioidomycosis is the most common endemic human mycosis in Latin America. The majority of clinically diagnosed cases have been reported in Brazil. Highly endemic areas in Brazil include the states of São Paulo, Rio de Janeiro, Rio Grande do Sul, Goiás, Mato Grosso, Minas Gerais, and Paraná. The disease is also prevalent in Colombia, Venezuela, Argentina, Uruguay, Paraguay, Guatemala, Equador, Peru, and Mexico. No cases have been reported in Chile, Peru, Belize, Nicaragua, Guyana, Surinam and French Guyana. It was estimated that 10 per cent of both the Colombian and Brazilian populations were infected (3 million and 14.5 million, respectively, in 1989). As notification of this disease is not compulsory in these countries, and many cases may go undiagnosed, it is likely that incidence, prevalence, and morbidity are underestimated. Imported cases have been recorded in the United States, Europe, and Asia.

The infection rate, indicated by the intradermal paracoccidioidin test, ranges from 6.0 to 60.6 per cent among rural and urban populations of endemic and non-endemic areas. Rates of infection are higher in rural than urban areas. It is most prevalent among people in their teens in highly endemic regions and among people in their twenties in low endemic areas. Infection is observed with the same frequency in both sexes.

The disease is found primarily among individuals from 30 to 50 years old, who are agricultural workers or have lived in endemic areas. The sex ratio of clinical cases is 10 or more males to each female among adults, while it is equally distributed among prepubescent boys and girls. This may be explained by the ability of the oestrogens to inhibit the transformation of mycelium or conidia to yeast. Spouses of patients are rarely affected by the disease, which suggests that hormonal and genetic factors play a part in the distribution of this mycosis. Transmission from one person to another has not been shown.

Ecology

The geographical regions in which paracoccidioidomycosis is most commonly found are humid areas where the soil is more frequently acidic and the temperature ranges from 15 to 30 °C. The fungus seems to thrive in these areas, while excessive humidity, dry weather, and frequent winds adversely affect it.

P. brasiliensis has rarely been found in its natural habitat. It has been isolated from soil, animals such as armadillos and bats, dog food, and penguin faeces. It has also been isolated from the intestinal contents of bats and there is an unconfirmed report of isolation from the tissue of a squirrel monkey. Efforts to maintain the fungus in bat intestines have been unsuccessful. The saprophytic habitat of *P. brasiliensis* has yet to be discovered.

Aetiology

MYCOLOGY

P. brasiliensis is a dimorphic fungus, which can be cultivated either as a mould or a yeast. When cultured at 25 °C it appears after 15 to 30 days as white, tufted colonies, which later became velvety and cracked or glabrous, leathery, and brownish. When Sabouraud dextrose agar is used the mycelium shows hyaline septate hyphae with branches. It rarely produces conidia in this medium. Arthroconidia, aleuroconidia, and arthroaleurioconidia measuring 2 to 5 μm in diameter have been cultured in carbohydrate-free media containing natural substrates.

P. brasiliensis also grows as a yeast in human and animal tissues (Fig. 1) and in cultures maintained at 37 °C. It grows slowly. Wrinkled, folded, whitish, glabrous colonies can be observed after 7 to 20 days. Under direct microscopy, yeast forms can be observed as oval, spherical, or elliptical cells with doubly refractile walls; the cells vary in size from buds of 2 to 10 μm in diameter to mature cells of 20 to 30 μm (Fig. 2). Mother cells may produce 10 to 12 uniform or variably sized buds, forming the characteristic 'pilot wheel' shape observed in biological samples or in infected tissues.

VIRULENCE

Virulence is defined as the ability to produce disseminated infection in experimental animals. Variation in the virulence of different fungal isolates has been documented but little is understood of the biochemical basis for these differences.

The presence of higher levels of α-1,3 glucan in virulent strains of *P. brasiliensis* compared with avirulent strains was initially related with virulence, but no correlation has been shown between glucans or other lipids and virulence in experimentally-induced infections.

Pathogenesis

Several observations provide evidence that the respiratory route is the main portal of entry and the lung is the primary site of infection:

1. The fungus is found in the lungs of patients who died of paracoccidioidomycosis.

Fig. 1 Small and large yeast forms of *Paracoccidioides brasiliensis* in the lung of a transplant recipient. Methenamine silver.

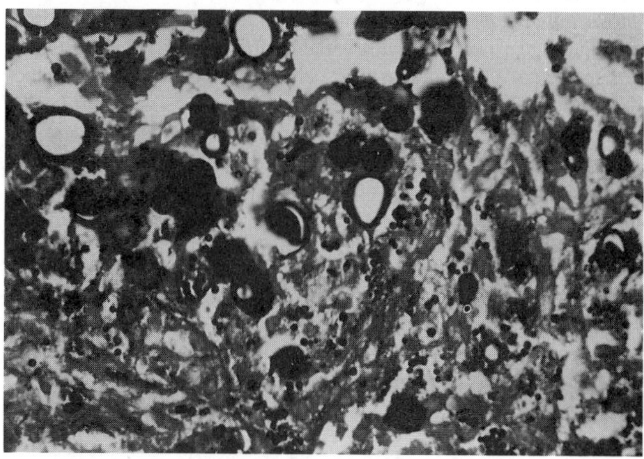

Fig. 2 Scanning election micrograph of multiple budding yeast cell of *Paracoccidioides brasiliensis* (by courtesy of C.S. Lacaz).

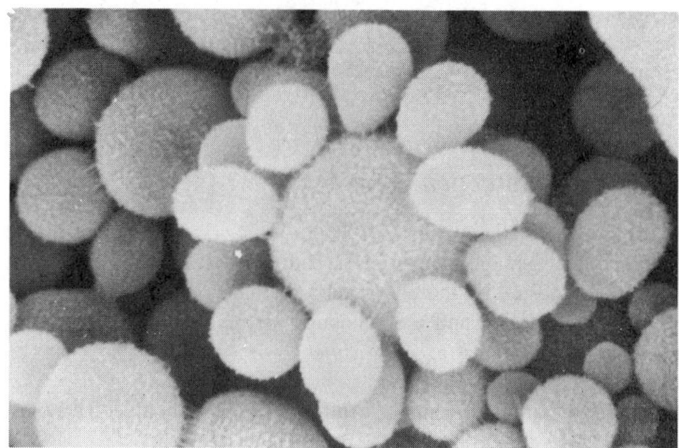

2. A primary lymph-node complex is found in infected children.
3. Pulmonary radiographic lesions are found in healthy people showing a positive paracoccidioidin test.
4. The fungus can be isolated from soil, and may be inhaled as aerosolized infective conidia. Accidental inoculation of the skin has been followed by the development of a cutaneous lesion in a laboratory worker.

The first fungus–host contact occurs through inhalation of airborne conidia. When mice are experimentally infected through the respiratory route, conidia have been observed in the alveoli soon after inoculation. Some 12 to 18 h after the exposure, yeast forms can be observed in the alveoli. There is an initial inflammatory response, which is mediated by polymorphonuclear cells, followed by granuloma formation.

The primary infective complex develops at the inoculation site and involves the surrounding lymphatic vessels and regional lymph nodes. The fungus spreads to other parts of the lung through peribronchial lymphatic vessels and drains into regional lymph nodes. Haematogenous dissemination to a variety of organs and tissues may occur at this time. The lesions usually undergo involution and the fungi remain dormant if the host's immune response can control their proliferation.

A balanced host–fungus relationship is associated with the absence of symptoms, although in some children or young adults, acute disease may arise, primarily affecting the phagocytic mononuclear system.

In adult life, previously quiescent lesions may become reactivated, especially in the lungs, leading to the adult or chronic form of the disease. The mechanism of reactivation is not understood.

Pathology

The characteristic lesion is a granuloma containing *P. brasiliensis* cells. The infected tissue may exhibit a predominantly proliferative, granulomatous inflammatory response, and/or an exudative reaction, sometimes resulting in necrosis, with variable numbers of neutrophils and large numbers of extracellular yeast cells, leading to a chronic epithelioid granuloma.

There is some relation between immunological responses and the observed pattern of granulomas. A strong late-hypersensitivity response to fungal antigens has been associated with the presence of epithelioid granulomata, while an exudative inflammatory response has been associated with a poor late-hypersensitivity response to fungal antigens. The presence of lymph-node fistulae has been correlated with the disseminated forms of the disease, and consequently, to a deficient late-hypersensitivity response.

The inflammatory process of paracoccidioidomycosis leads to fibrosis, causing stenosis of the larynx or trachea, pulmonary fibrosis, and lymph-node blockade, which are important causes of death in these patients.

Autopsy studies, mainly of adult patients, indicate that the organs most frequently involved are the lungs (42.0–96.0 per cent), adrenals (44.0–80.0 per cent), lymph nodes (28.0–72.0 per cent), pharynx/larynx (18.0–60.0 per cent), and skin/other mucosal surfaces (2.7–64.0 per cent). Central nervous involvement was reported in 2.2 to 36.0 per cent of the autopsy cases, bowel in 2.7 to 28.4 per cent, liver in 21.0 to 37.5 per cent, bones in 4.7 to 8.35 per cent, and kidney in 6.2 to 12.6 per cent.

Host–fungus interaction

NON-SPECIFIC IMMUNE RESPONSE

The influence of genetic factors on the individual susceptibility to this mycosis is suggested by the observation of higher rates of HLA phenotypes Ag B13, B40, and Cw3 among patients than in controls. In isogenic mice, resistance to *P. brasiliensis* is controlled by a single autosomal gene.

The ability of circulating human neutrophils or bronchoalveolar washing human cells to digest the yeast forms of fungi was impaired in severe cases, while this defect was absent in uninfected family members of patients. As this deficiency has not been shown *in vitro* against *Candida albicans*, it might represent an evasive mechanism of *P. brasiliensis*. In addition, the greater ability of polymorphonuclear cells from conidia infected mice to kill the fungus in relationship with normal mice suggests the activation of these cells by substances released through specific immune response.

SPECIFIC IMMUNE RESPONSE

The relation of the severity of the human disease to deficient late hypersensitivity was established through intradermal tests for ubiquitous antigens and paracoccidioidin, or through lymphoblastic transformation tests to mitogens and *P. brasiliensis* antigen. Many factors seem to be related to this deficient T-cell response, including deficient antigen presentation, antigen excess circulating immune complexes, and deficiency of receptors to interleukin 2. The different distribution of T-lymphocyte subpopulations according to the clinical form of the disease (decreased CD4 in chronic form and increased CD8 in acute form) suggests that different mechanisms might be involved in each form. The patient with the chronic form has been sensitized and has been able to control the fungal multiplication for many years, in contrast to the patient with the acute form of the disease.

The deficient T-cell response is followed by a decreased ability of macrophages to control fungal multiplication and to kill the fungus. This capacity of murine pulmonary macrophages is increased *in vivo* and *in vitro* by treatment with interferon-γ. The importance of late hypersensitivity in protection has been observed recently in patients receiving cytotoxic therapy for associated neoplasm and in those with AIDS.

Recently, production of IL 4, but not interferon suggests a predominant TH2 type of response to *P. brasiliensis* in an acute model of this mycosis. Antibodies may enhance phagocytosis through opsonization of the fungus but their role in the resistance is not established.

Clinical features

The clinical picture ranges from an asymptomatic course to severe disseminated disease, which can lead to death. The incubation period is unknown except in a laboratory worker, who developed a skin lesion some days after an accidental inoculation. The disease has been reported in children 3 years of age or older, who had lived for some years in the endemic area. Even though a long incubation period might be supposed in these cases, the exact moment of the first host–fungus contact was not known.

The following classification of clinical forms of paracoccidioidomycosis has been proposed:

(1) paracoccidioidomycosis infection;
(2) regressive (self-healing) paracoccidioidomycosis;
(3) paracoccidioidomycosis disease
  (a) acute form (juvenile type)
    (i) moderate,
    (ii) severe;
  (b) chronic form (adult type)
    (i) mild,
    (ii) moderate,
    (iii) severe;
(4) sequelae.

Localization of the affected tissue or organ and the characterization of severity of the disease according to established criteria contribute to make this classification easily and uniformly appliable. Impairment of general and nutritional conditions, and impairment of functions (lung, brain, adrenals, bone marrow) are employed to classify the patients according to the severity of the disease. Deficient response to skin test (paracoccidioidin) occurs in more severe cases.

ACUTE FORM (JUVENILE TYPE)

Children, adolescents, and younger adults (under 30 years old) are affected, males and females in equal numbers. Only 1.0 to 20.0 per cent of the patients fall into this group. There is progression for 2 to 3 months or more, characterized by involvement of the phagocytic mononuclear system. Cervical, axillary, and inguinal nodes are the most commonly enlarged (Fig. 3). Nodes are initially hard but are sometimes fluctuant and drain pus rich in fungi. Less frequently, deep-seated lymph nodes may also be affected. Involvement of mesenteric nodes may be accompanied by an acute clinical picture, similar to appendicitis. When the hepatic perihilar lymph nodes are enlarged, they may produce symptoms of obstructive jaundice. Abdominal ultrasonographic and tomographic studies have been employed to detect such lymph-node involvement.

The liver and spleen are usually moderately enlarged. Bones (clavicle, scapulae, ribs, skull, long, and flat bones) and, rarely, the bone marrow may be involved. Radiographs show lytic lesions without periosteal reaction. Small-bowel involvement may be asymptomatic or produce abdominal pain, diarrhoea, constipation, and even intestinal obstruction. Radiological studies of the digestive tract reveal hypersecretion, dystonia, decreased or increased intestinal transit time, and thickening of mucous membrane folds in about 50 per cent of clinical cases.

Fever and weight loss are common. Mucocutaneous lesions are more frequent in some geographical areas. Generally there are multiple lesions as a result of haematogenous or lymphatic dissemination. Highly transitory levels of eosinophils (up to 30 000/mm^3) have been uncommonly described.

Clinical lung involvement is rarely described in this form of paracoccidioidomycosis. In some case reports either bronchopneumonia or primary complex-like disease was observed. Direct microscopy or sputum culture in the absence of clinical or radiological signs have shown the presence of *P. brasiliensis* in such acute cases, and tomography or radioisotopic studies have been able to detect pulmonary involvement in patients without signs and symptoms. In some series, hilar and perihilar adenopathy, pleural effusion, and even parenchymal lesions have been shown by chest radiography in a small percentage of patients, sometimes in the absence of clinical features.

The differential diagnosis includes hematological diseases such as lymphoma and leukaemia. Hodgkin's disease in a patient with acute paracoccidioidomycosis and even in the same lymph node affected by *P. brasiliensis* has been described. Other infections such as tuberculous lymphadenitis and, in endemic areas, visceral leishmaniasis may also simulate the acute form of paracoccidioidomycosis.

Fig. 3 Lymph-node and skin involvement in a patient with the acute form of paracoccidioidomycosis (by courtesy of C.S. Lacaz).

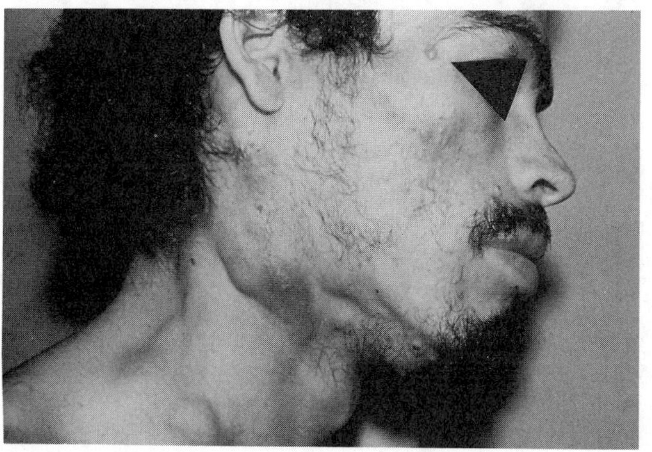

CHRONIC FORM

Usually 30- to 50-year-old men, who have worked in agricultural areas, are affected. The male:female ratio is 10 to 25:1. The evolution is insidious and in many cases clinically mild.

The organ most frequently involved is the lung, followed by skin and mucous membranes, mainly pharynx, larynx, and trachea. Lymph nodes and adrenals may be compromised. More than one organ or tissue is usually involved such as lung plus mucous membranes, lung plus lymph nodes, or lung plus lymph nodes plus mucous membranes. Less frequently, intestine, spleen, bones, central nervous system (brain, cerebellum, meninges), eyes, genitourinary system, myocardium, pericardium and arteries are involved.

The patients may be asymptomatic or complain of dyspnoea, cough, sometimes purulent sputum, and rarely haemoptysis. Fever is unusual. Physical examination is frequently normal or there may be scattered râles. In contrast, chest radiography commonly reveals bilateral, asymmetrical, reticulonodular infiltrates in the middle and lower parts of the lungs (Figs. 4, 5). Apical cavities and pleural effusions are less fre-

Fig. 4 Predominantly interstitial infiltrate in both lungs in a patient with chronic paracoccidioidomycosis.

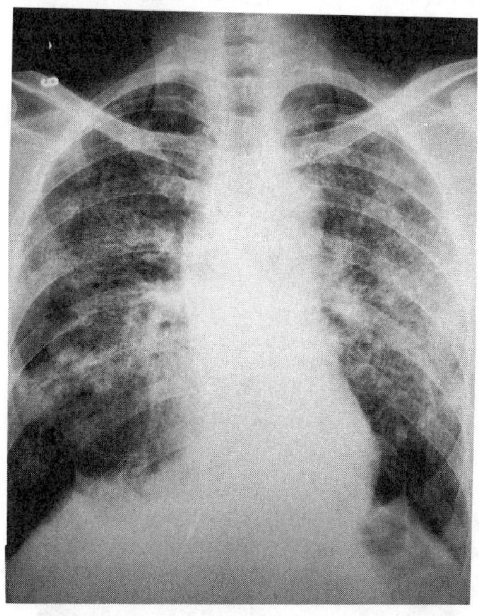

Fig. 5 Alveolar and interstitial infiltrates in both lungs in a patient with chronic paracoccidioidomycosis.

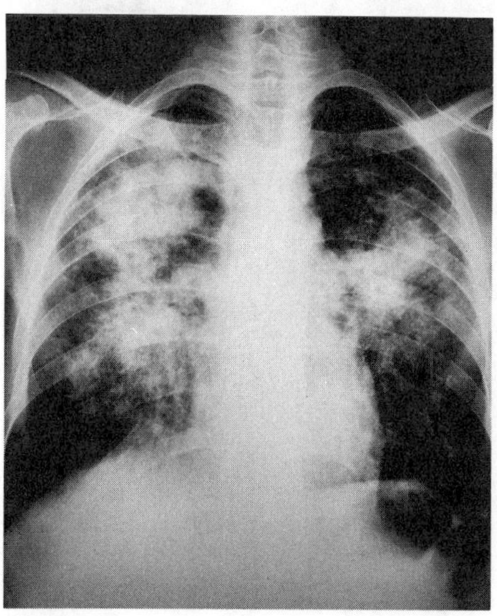

quently observed. Lung tomography (1 mm/slices) and gallium-67 radioisotopic studies are more sensitive.

Cutaneous lesions include papules, pustules, ulcers, crusted ulcers, vegetations, tuberculoids, verrucoids or acneiform lesions mainly on the face (Fig. 6) or limbs. Multiple, scattered lesions result from haematogenous dissemination. Subcutaneous cold abscesses, more commonly associated with bone lesions, can occur.

Mucosal lesions are usually in the mouth and/or oropharynx, including palate, uvula, and tonsils, or in the respiratory tract, involving mainly larynx (vocal cords, glottis and epiglottis) and trachea. Pain is usually intense, and may hamper mastication and swallowing. Consequently, there may be intense weight loss of about 20 kg in few months, suggesting malignant disease. Hoarseness and dysphonia result from laryngeal lesions, and may lead to obstruction of the upper respiratory tract. Examination shows ulcerative, verrucous, vegetant, and infiltrative 'moriform' stomatitis. The last is characteristic of this mycosis and appears as shallow ulcers, with a granular surface showing multiple, fine, haemorrhagic points.

Few lymph nodes may be involved, in contrast to the acute form of the disease.

Uni-or bilateral lesions in the adrenal glands (Fig. 7) were found in about one-half of patients coming to autopsy. Partial adrenal insufficiency has been documented in about 40 per cent of the cases but only 7.4 per cent were symptomatic. In some endemic areas of Brazil, this mycosis represents the most important cause of adrenal insufficiency.

Many diseases may simulate chronic paracoccidioidomycosis, for example tuberculosis and neoplasia, when the respiratory tract, adrenals or the skin are affected. Cutaneous involvement may simulate leishmaniasis and other mycosis. Concomitant tuberculosis is observed in about 10 to 15 per cent of cases of pulmonary paracoccidioidomycosis and has also been described in cases of lymph-node involvement by *P. brasiliensis*. Bronchitis may simulate active paracoccidioidomycosis in the cases with chronic pulmonary obstructive disease or cor pulmonale (see under Sequelae). Carcinomas may arise in pulmonary or mucosal mycotic lesions and, less frequently, lymphoma in pulmonary lesions.

SEQUELAE

Nowadays these constitute one of the most important problems in the management of paracoccidioidomycosis. Although fungal multiplication has been controlled by chemotherapy, involvement of vital functions might cause the patient's death.

Acute form

Lesions in the small intestine and mesenteric lymph nodes may fibrose causing lymphatic obstruction, intestinal malabsorption or protein-losing enteropathy. A clinical picture of severe malnutrition and immunodeficiency has been reported (Fig. 8). Lack of late hypersensitivity to mitogens and fungal antigen, and hypogammaglobulinaemia have been documented. Chilous ascites and oedema may develop, and active clinical paracoccidioidomycosis may not be detected by routine mycological and serological tests. However, at autopsy, multiple budding of the fungi in focal areas of lymph nodes, bone marrow or adrenals, sometimes

Fig. 6 Mucocutaneous lesions in a patient with chronic paracoccidioidomycosis (by courtesy of C.S. Lacaz).

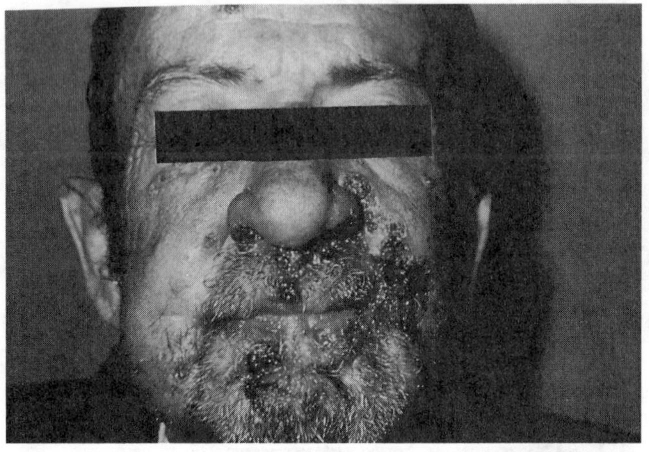

Fig. 7 Bilateral adrenal lesions in a patient with chronic paracoccidioidomycosis (by courtesy of the Department of Pathology, Faculdade de Medicina da Universidade de São Paulo).

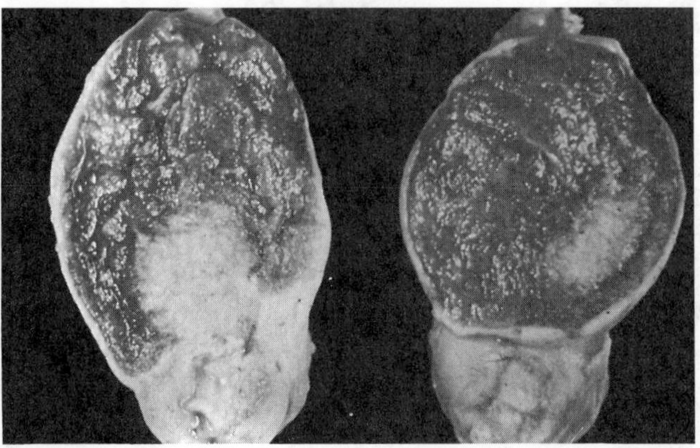

Fig. 8 Ascites, cachexia, and immunodeficiency due to malabsorption and protein-losing enteropathy as a sequelae of acute paracoccidioidomycosis (by courtesy of M. Shiroma).

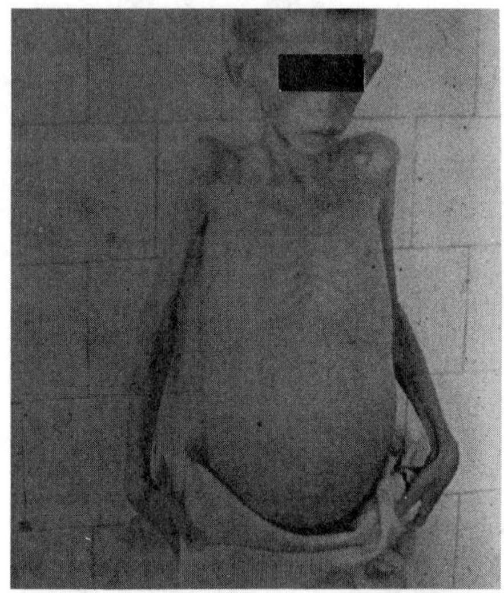

Fig. 9 Extensive interstitial involvement and large areas of emphysema in a patient with chronic paracoccidioidomycosis (chest computerized tomography—1-mm slices).

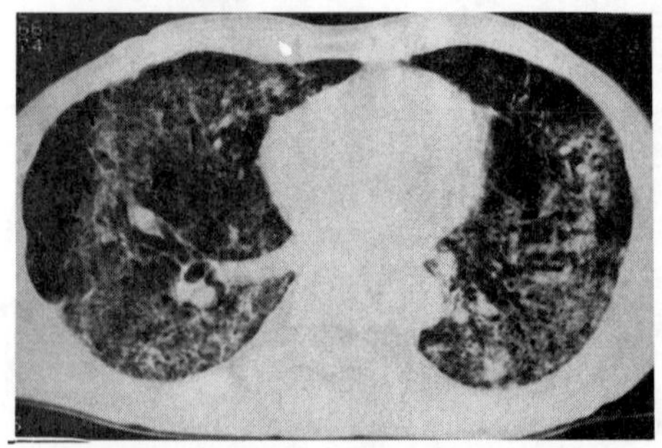

Table 1 *Correlation between the immunological and histopathological findings and the clinical forms of paracoccidioidomycosis*

Severity	Severe	Moderate	Mild
Clinical forms	Acute/chronic	Chronic/acute	Chronic
Intradermal tests			
Paracoccidioidin	–	+/–	+
Ubiquitous Ag/PHA[a]	–	+/–	+
'In vitro' tests[b]			
PHA	–	+/–	+
Suppressive factor (patient's serum/plasma)	+	–/+	–
Increased T-cell subpopulation	CD8 (acute)	CD8 (acute)	
Decreased T-cell subpopulation	CD4 (chronic)	CD4 (chronic)	CD4 (chronic)
Histopathology			
Epithelioid granuloma	–	+/–	+
Loosening granuloma	++	+	–
Fungi	+++	++	+/–
Antibodies			
Immunoglobulins (IgG/E)	+++	++	+
Specific antibodies	+++	++	+
Immune complexes	++	+/–	–

[a]Ag, antigen; PHA, phytohaemagglutinin.

[b]Lymphoblastic transformation test.

circumscribed by fibrosis has been found. The most frequent and severe development is severe intra- or extracellular superinfection. Systemic *Mycobacterium tuberculosis* infections, systemic or pulmonary *Cryptococcus neoformans* infections, staphylococcal or streptococcal sepsis and/or cellulitis, and recurrent Neisseria meningitis have been reported.

Chronic form

As the lesions usually tend to heal by fibrosis, sequelae such as microstomy, and laryngeal, tracheal, or even bronchial stenosis may be observed. Corrective surgery is indicated.

Pulmonary emphysema, fibrosis, respiratory insufficiency, and finally, cor pulmonale are frequent sequelae (Fig. 9). Obstructive and restrictive patterns of ventilatory defect have been found in about 36 and 16 per cent of patients. As many as 30 per cent of these patients may die as a result of respiratory or cardiorespiratory failure.

Diagnosis

MICROBIOLOGICAL IDENTIFICATION

Direct examination

Sputum, pus from lymph nodes, and material from the skin or mucous membrane lesions are placed on a slide with a drop of 10 per cent potassium hydroxide for microscopy. Isolated or budding (single or multiple) mother cells are observed. The mucocutaneous lesions and the pus from lymph nodes are commonly rich in yeast forms, but there are few in the sputum. As the yeast may either grow in chains or appear as single buds, the differential diagnosis includes *C. neoformans*, candidal species, and *H. capsulatum.*

Culture

Specimens are cultured at 37 °C on blood, chocolate, or yeast-extract agar. The colonies are produced after 7 days, usually in 10 to 20 days. Cultures can be maintained, at 25 °C, on Sabouraud's dextrose agar, where the colonies may be noticed after 15 to 30 days.

HISTOPATHOLOGY

Silver or periodic acid–Schiff staining is required to detect the fungus in sputum. Diagnostic features are the variable size (1–30 μm) of the yeast cells, and their multiple budding. Proliferative or exudative reaction as described (Pathology) may be observed.

IMMUNOLOGICAL TESTS

Serological reactions

Immunodiffusion (Ouchterlony) and counterimmunoelectrophoresis are the best techniques initially. Sensitivities and specificities are as high as 95.0 per cent. Cross-reactions were mainly with other deep mycoses such as histoplasmosis, aspergillosis, cryptococcosis, and candidiasis.

Complement fixation and indirect immunofluorescence are less reliable tests for diagnosis, but they can be employed in patients under treatment.

Recently, enzyme immunoassays employing a 43-kDa glycoprotein have shown high sensitivity and specificity.

Antibody titres tend to decrease about 3 months after starting specific therapy and to disappear after 6 months to 5 years or more.

Antigenaemia has been considered as a useful indication in an immunocompromised host presenting undetectable or low level of antibodies in the sera.

Correlation between immunological–histopathological findings and clinical forms

This is outlined in Table 1.

Therapy

Clinical active disease is treated for 3 to 6 months, followed by maintenance therapy with sulphametoxipiridazine after the resolution of clinical signs and symptoms, continued for many months or until 1 to 2 years after antibody levels have fallen to normal.

Severe cases of acute or chronic disease should be treated with intravenous infusion of amphotericin B. The daily dose begins at 0.1 to 0.2 mg/kg, increasing up to 1.0 mg/kg. The total dose depends on the clinical form and on the patient's progress. It often ranges from 1 to 3 g or more. As soon as the patient improves, sulpha or imidazole drugs can be substituted. Toxic reactions to amphotericin B include fever, chills, headache, anaemia, and nephrotoxicity characterized by hypokalaemia and azotaemia. In most cases, these reactions can be controlled until the end of the course of therapy. Itraconazole has produced good results in a few severe cases, especially in cases of histoplasmosis associated with AIDS. However, this drug has not been formally compared to amphotericin B in the most severe cases of paracoccidioidomycosis.

In milder cases, sulpha or imidazole drugs have been shown to be effective. In a randomized trial, sulphadiazine (150 mg/kg per day), itraconazole (50–100 mg/day), and ketoconazole (200–400 mg/day) were equally effective in patients with moderately severe disease. Sulphadiazine is the best sulphonamide, employed in daily doses of 150 mg/kg for children and up to 6 g for adults. Hypersensitivity reactions and crystaluria have rarely been reported mainly in the absence of urine alkalinization. The combination of 160 mg of trimethoprim and 800 mg of sulphamethoxazole also appears to be effective.

Ketoconazole, in one daily dose of 200 to 400 mg for adults and 5 to 8 mg/kg a day for children, given by mouth, gave good results. Itraconazole is effective in one daily dose of 50 to 300 mg, given by mouth, and causes fewer side-effects than ketoconazole. Fluconazole has been used in a few cases and achieves high levels in the cerebrospinal fluid.

Prognosis

The drugs in current use can control paracoccidioidomycosis in most cases, but management is difficult in some patients. Normalization of cellular specific responses, particularly of skin test (paracoccidioidin) is indicative of a good prognosis.

Some disseminated and severe cases of the acute form and less frequently of the chronic form of the disease, with or without immunosupressive conditions, cannot be controlled by available drugs or drug combinations. The use of immunostimulants has not been subjected to randomized studies. Patients with sequelae present some difficulties.

In acute cases with recurrent infections and cellular and humoral immunodeficiency secondary to lymphatic blockade and protein-losing enteropathy, special diets have been employed to improve immunity and nutritional state. Unfortunately, most of these patients have died from severe systemic infections. Pulmonary fibrosis, respiratory insufficiency, and cor pulmonale are frequent causes of death.

Finally, even though the disease is easily controlled in the majority of cases, the treatment course is long. In Brazil, the abandonment of treatment is the most important cause of therapeutic failure.

REFERENCES

Brummer, E., Hanson, L.H., Restrepo, A., and Stevens, D.A. (1988). *In vivo* and *in vitro* activation of pulmonary macrophages by IFN-gamma enhanced killing of *Paracoccidioides brasiliensis* or *Blastomyces dermatitidis*. *Journal of Immunology* **140,** 2786–9.

Brummer, E., Hanson, L.H., and Stevens, D.A. (1991). Kinetics and requirements for activation of macrophages for fungicidal activity: effect of protein synthesis inhibitors and immunosupressants on activation and fungicidal mechanisms. *Cellular Immunology* **132,** 236–45.

Calich, V.L.G., *et al.* (1985). Susceptibility and resistance of inbred mice to *P. brasiliensis*. *British Journal of Experimental Pathology*, **66,** 585–94.

Del Negro, G., Melo, E.H.L., Rodbard, D., Melo, M.R., Layton, J., and Wachslicht-Rodbard, H. (1980). Limited adrenal reserve in paracoccidioidomycosis: cortisol and aldosterone responses to 1–24 ACTH. *Clinical Endocrinology*, **13,** 553–9.

Hostetler, J.S., *et al.* (1993). Effect of an anti-IL4, interferon-gamma and an antifungal triazole (SCH 42427) in paracoccidioidomycosis: correlation of IgE levels with outcome. *Clinical Experimental Immunology*, **94,** 11–16.

Lemle, A., Wanke, B., Miranda, J.L., Kropf, G.L., Mandel, M.B., and Mandel, S. (1983). Pulmonary function in paracoccidioidomycosis (South American blastomycosis): an analysis of the obstructive defect. *Chest*, **83,** 827–8.

Lutz, A. (1908) Uma mycose pseudococcidica localizada na boca e observada no Brasil. Contribuição ao conhecimento das hyphomicoses americanas. *Brasil médica*, **22,** 121–4.

Marques, S.A. *et al.* (1985). Paracoccidioidomycosis: a comparative study of the evolutionary serologic, clinical and radiologic results for patients treated with ketoconazole or amphotericin B plus sulfonamides. *Mycopathologia*, **89,** 19–23.

Mendes-Giannini, M.J.S.M., *et al.* (1989). Detection of 43 000 molecular weight glycoprotein in sera of patients with paracoccidioidomycosis. *Journal of Clinical Microbiology*, **27,** 2842–5.

Mota, N.G.S. *et al.* (1985). Correlation between cell-mediated immunity and clinical forms of paracoccidioidomycosis. *Transactions of the Royal Society of Tropical Medicine Hygiene*, **79,** 765–72.

Musatti, C.C., Rezkallah, M.T., Mendes, E., and Mendes, N.F. (1976). 'In vivo' and in 'vitro' evaluation of cell mediated immunity in patients with paracoccidioidomycosis. *Cellular Immunology*, **24,**365–78.

Naranjo, M.S., Trujillo, M., Munera, M.I., Restrepo, P., Gomez, I., and Restrepo, A. (1990). Treatment of paracoccidioidomycosis with itraconazole. *Journal of Medical and Veterinary Mycology*, **28,** 57–76.

Negroni, R., Palmieri, O., Koren, F., Tiraboschi, I.N., and Galimberti, R.I. (1987). Oral treatment of paracoccidioidomycosis and histoplasmosis with itraconazole in humans. *Reviews of Infectious Diseases*, **9,** (suppl. 1), 47–50.

Ratto, O.R. (1982). Lesões pulmonares. Aspectos clínicos e funcionais. In *Paracoccidioidomicose. Blastomicose Sul-Americana*, (ed. G. Del Negro, C.S. Lacaz, and A.M. Fiorillo), pp. 161–9. Sarvier ED USP, São Paulo.

Restrepo, A. (1985). The ecology of *Paracoccdioides brasiliensis*: a puzzle still unsolved. *Journal of Medical Mycology*, **23,** 323–34.

Restrepo, A. *et al.* (1976). The gamut of paracoccidioidomycosis. *American Journal of Medicine*, **61,** 33–42.

San-Blas, G. (1982). Cell wall of fungal human pathogens: its possible role in host-parasite relationships. A review. *Mycopathologia*, **79,** 159–84.

San Blas, G., San Blas, F., Ordaz, D., Centeno, S., and Albornoz, M.C. (1984) Chemical changes in cell wall structure of five strains of *Paracoccidioides brasiliensis*. *Sabouraudia*, **22,** 255–7.

Shikanai-Yasuda, M.A. *et al.* (1991). Randomized therapeutic trial with itraconazole, ketoconazole and sulfadiazine in paracoccidioidomycosis. In *Proceedings*, Congress of the International Society for Human and Animal Mycology, Montreal, Canada. Abstracts, p. 148.

Shikanai-Yasuda, M.A. *et al.* (1992). Immunodeficiency secondary to juvenile paracoccidioidomycosis: associated infections. *Mycopathologia*, **117,** 139–44.

Silva, G.F. and Roque-Barreira, M.C. (1992). Antigenemia in paracoccidioidomycosis. *Journal of Clinical Microbiology* **30,** 381–385.

Sugar, A.M., Restrepo, A., and Stevens, D.A. (1984). Paracoccidioidomycosis in the immunosupressed host; report of a case and review of the literature. *American Reviews of Respiratory Diseases*, **128,** 340–2.

Tuder, R., Ibrahim, R., Godoy, C.E., and Brito, T. (1985). Pathology of the human pulmonary paracoccidioidomycosis. *Mycopathologia*, **92,** 179–88.

7.12.5 Pneumocystis carinii

J. M. HOPKIN

Pneumocystis carinii is a fungal organism that is the leading cause of potentially fatal opportunistic pneumonia in the immunosuppressed. Effective culture of pneumocystis has not been achieved and its environmental source is unknown.

Epidemiology of disease and infection

Pneumocystis pneumonia occurs exclusively in the immunosuppressed, notably those with depression of T-lymphocyte immunity and less commonly severe hypogammaglobulinaemia. It was first recognized as a cause of human disease as an epidemic pneumonia in marasmic institutionalized infants in Europe and the Middle East from 1940 to 1960. As this epidemic subsided, it was found to complicate the use of immunosuppressive drug regimens in childhood leukaemia and organ transplantation. The annual attack rate for pneumocystis pneumonia was 20 per cent in each of these groups before chemoprophylaxis became a regular part of treatment schedules. Patients with AIDS are especially susceptible, suffering an attack rate of 70 per cent annually without chemoprophylaxis; in the United States the annual number of reported cases of pneumocystis pneumonia rose from approximately 70 in 1970 to 60 000 in 1990.

The occurrence of IgG antibodies to purified pneumocystis antigen in up to 80 per cent of European and American populations by 10 years of age suggests regular exposure to the organism, but the virtual absence of the organism in samplings from normal lungs, assayed by monoclonal antibody or DNA amplification, implies that clearance is highly effective in the normal human. As a corollary, it is likely that pneumonia in the immunosuppressed is the result of freshly acquired infection. Though horizontal transmission between immunosuppressed subjects is possible, the demonstration of pneumocystis-like organisms in ambient air and its fungal classification suggests that acquisition from an environmental source, as yet unidentified, is more important. Though cases occur through the year, there is some predominance in the autumn months. Pneumocystis can infect the lungs of a range of mammals but the organisms infecting different hosts are shown to be genetically distinct.

The parasite: interaction with lung

Comparative DNA analysis has established that *P. carinii* is a fungal organism. Though disseminated infection is documented in AIDS, pneumocystis is generally confined to the alveolar space of the lung. There, it shows two morphological forms, the trophozoite and the cyst, each of 4 to 6 μm diameter (Fig. 1). The trophozoite is an amoeboid, thin-walled structure with a single nucleus and cellular organelles typical of a lower eukaryote; it displays close apposition to the cell surface of the flat, type I pneumocyte but cell penetration and destruction do not occur. The cyst is a rounded, more thick-walled structure containing up to eight daughter cells or sporozoites, destined to be released as trophozoites. The cyst lies free within the alveolar space associated with a good deal of foamy debris. The number of organisms may rise to 10^9/g of tissue, and the apposition of the trophozoites to the type I pneumocyte and the presence of debris and cysts in the alveolar space produce profound disturbance of oxygen exchange and, untreated, fatal hypoxaemia. In the interstitium of the infected lung, there is a variable degree of lymphocyte and plasma-cell infiltration; pneumocystis pneumonia was once known as interstitial plasma-cell pneumonia.

The cell surface of pneumocystis contains heavily glycosylated proteins and carbohydrate polymers including chitin. Its biochemical pathways are typical of a lower eukaryote; studies of its folate pathway have demonstrated that pyrimethamine and trimethoprim have greater avidity for pneumocystis dihydrofolate reductase than for host mammalian enzymes.

Clinical features

The clinical features of *P. carinii* infection are consistent but not reliably diagnostic under different clinical circumstances because the syndrome can be mimicked by other infections—including cytomegalovirus, tuberculosis, and other fungi—and by non-infectious pulmonary complications in the immunosuppressed, including drug-induced disease or pulmonary oedema.

The onset of disease ranges between acute and insidious (over 2–4 weeks); the latter is a more regular feature in AIDS. The principal symptom is breathlessness, which is initially exertional but ultimately is present at rest though not accompanied by orthopnoea. Cough occurs in approximately half the cases but results in sputum production in few. Mild chilling or a sensation of fever is present in half the cases, significant pyrexia (in excess of 38 °C) is documented in the great majority at presentation. Chest pain and wheeze are not features of pneumocystis pneumonia.

On examination, the absence of chest signs is typical, though sparse crepitations may be heard in up to a third of cases. The presence of tachypnoea and cyanosis depends on the severity of disease, which may be quite variable at presentation.

Untreated, the disease progresses with mounting tachypnoea and intense hypoxaemia and cyanosis.

In the AIDS group, rare cases of disseminated pneumocystis infection are well documented. Tissues involved variably include lymph nodes, spleen, liver, bone marrow, the choroid, and retina. Clinical features associated with such spread include general malaise, fever, painless lymphadenopathy and splenomegaly, anaemia, and visual disturbance.

Investigations

The plain chest radiograph and arterial blood gas estimates are the essential investigations for preliminary assessment. Together with recording of temperature and respiratory rate, they are used also for the monitoring of progress.

The chest radiograph shows diffuse bilateral change, in the great

Fig. 1 Electron micrograph of *Pneumocystis carinii* showing (a) the trophozoite phase adherent to the surface of a type I pneumocyte and (b) the cyst phase of the organism.

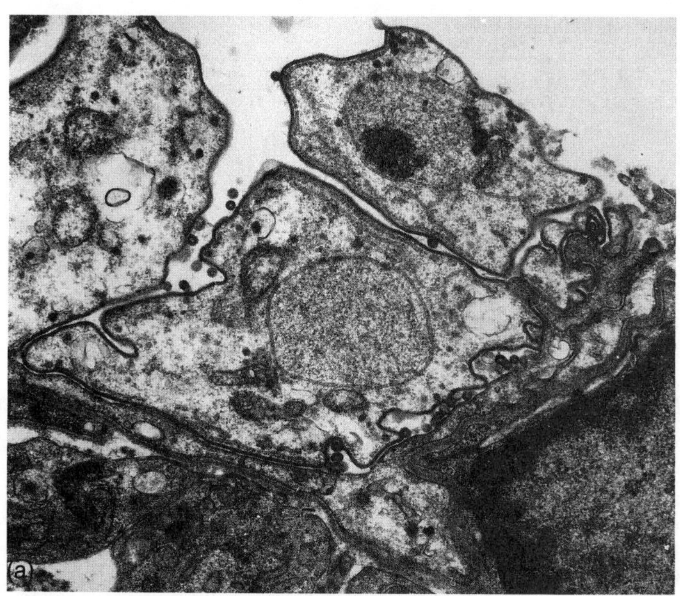

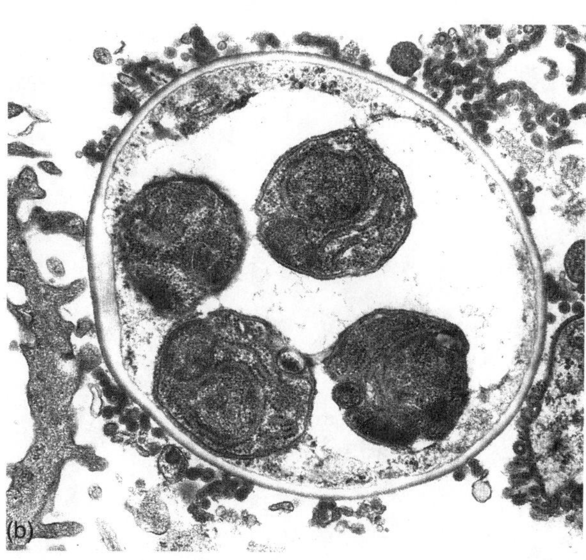

majority, which may appear granular, nodular or reticular (Fig. 2). Cystic spaces may be seen in a minority. Pleural effusion is not a feature but pneumothorax is a rare complication. Blood gas analysis shows varying degrees of hypoxaemia and disease tends to be consistently more severe in the non-AIDS group. Case series studies have shown median blood-gas disturbance values as follows: in non-AIDS, Po_2 6.5 kPa (50 mmHg equivalent to oxygen saturation of 80 per cent) with Pco_2 4 kPa (30 mmHg); in AIDS, 8.6 kPa (65 mmHg equivalent to oxygen saturation of 91 per cent) and Pco_2 4 kPa at presentation. The advent of reliable percutaneous oximetry offers an effective and simple alternative to arterial blood gas measurement in the assessment of initial hypoxaemia and response to treatment.

The diagnosis of pneumocystis pneumonia is established by identification of the organism in lung samplings. Sputum is produced in few cases and the samplings most commonly used are saline lavage samples taken at fibreoptic bronchoscopy or sputum induced by inhaled, nebulized, hypertonic (2.7 per cent) saline. The organism may be identified on microscopy after (a) methenamine silver staining for the cyst phase of the organism (Fig. 3);(b) Giemsa staining that demonstrates the small, punctate nuclei of the trophozoites and intracystic sporozoites; or (c) fluorescence-tagged monoclonal antibody. Application of any of these stains to bronchoscopic lavage offers a highly sensitive and specific technique for the diagnosis of the pneumonia; application to induced sputum may allow diagnostic rates ranging from 40 to 80 per cent in laboratories with great expertise. More recently, DNA amplification has been developed as a highly effective diagnostic technique offering a greater than 95 per cent sensitivity with both induced sputum and bronchoscopic lavage; the presence of a positive polymerase chain-reaction signal equivalent to 10^4 organisms/ml of clinical sample is highly predictive of pneumocystis pneumonia but lesser signals, consistent with subclinical infection, may be found up to 20 per cent of individuals with severe immunosuppression (Fig. 4).

Treatment

Pneumocystis pneumonia in patients with leukaemia, organ transplants, and AIDS is fatal if untreated. With prompt diagnosis, specific treatment results in a cure rate of 70 to 80 per cent. The treatment of first choice is the combination of trimethoprim and sulphamethoxazole given orally (20 mg trimethoprim, 100 mg sulphamethoxazole/kg body weight daily

Fig. 2 Chest radiograph of two AIDS subjects with *Pneumocystis carinii* pneumonia showing (a) ground glass and (b) nodular diffuse changes.

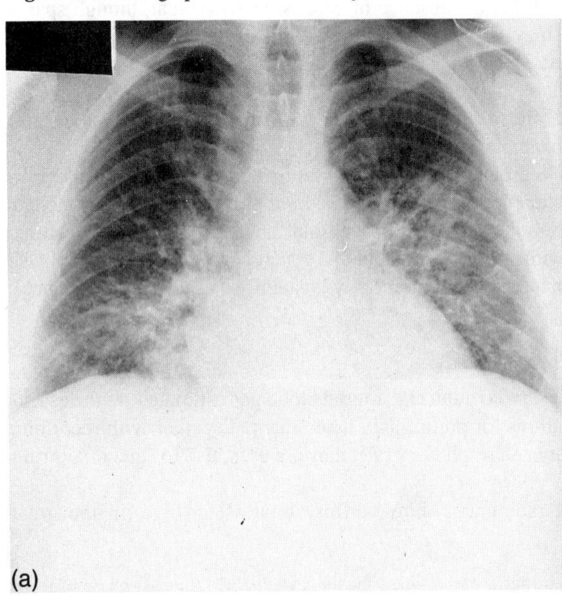

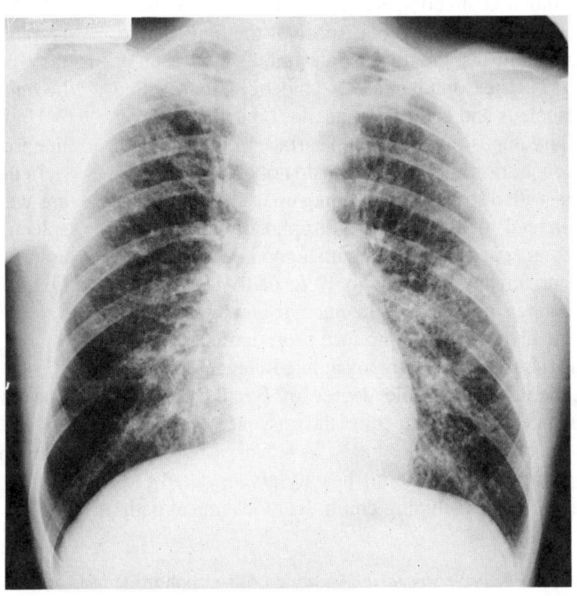

Fig. 3 The cyst phase of the organism demonstrated on microscopy of alveolar lavage after methenamine silver staining. (a) Low power, (b) higher power.

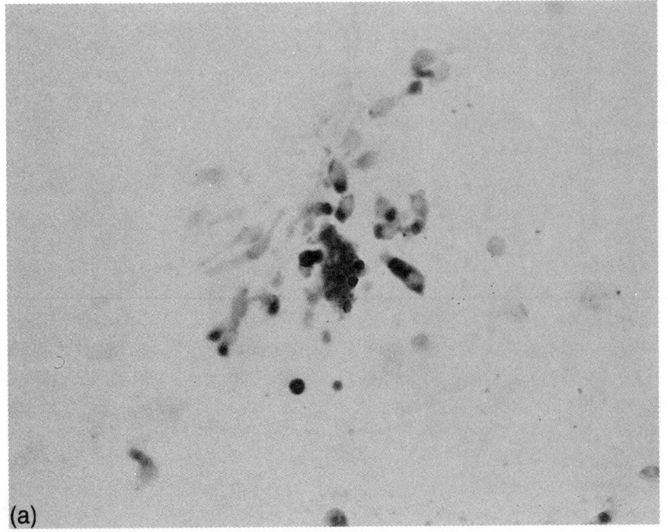

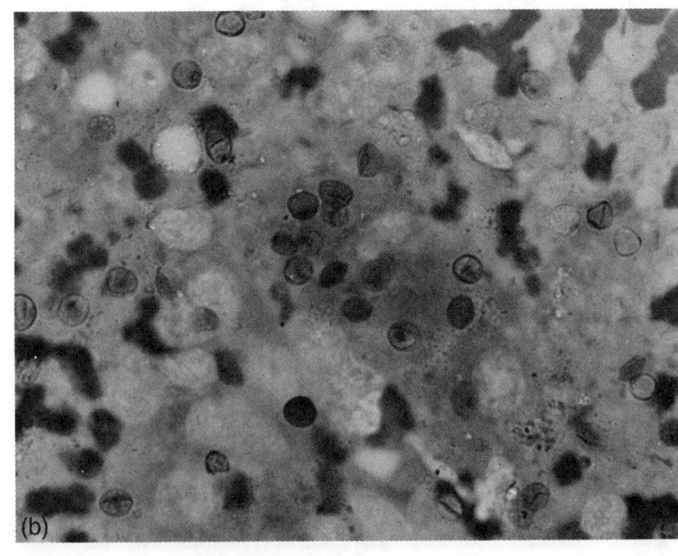

in three to four divided doses) or intravenously (trimethoprim 15 mg, sulphamethoxazole 75 mg/kg daily, again as three to four divided doses). Doses need to be adjusted when significant renal failure is present, aiming for trimethoprim concentrations of 5 to 8 μg/ml at 2 h after dosage.

In the leukaemic and organ transplantation groups, fever usually resolves within 4 days and hypoxaemia within 1 week in survivors; treatment should be continued for 2 weeks. The drug is well tolerated but if hypersensitivity develops, change to the alternative agent, pentamidine isethionate, is appropriate. Pentamidine is administered as 4 mg/kg daily as a slow intravenous infusion over 2 h, again over 14 days. Slow administration minimizes the risk of toxic reactions seen more frequently when pentamidine was given as a bolus intramuscular injection; hypotension, hypoglycaemia, and impaired renal function were regularly encountered. Both co-trimoxazole and pentamidine achieve the same response rates and there is little evidence suggesting that change from one drug to the other, because of lack of response, improves outlook.

In the AIDS group the disturbed immunological state, including high levels of IgE, results in a very high rate (up to 60 per cent) of adverse reactions to both co-trimoxazole and pentamidine. Reactions can include fever, rash and pruritus, headache, vomiting, and marrow suppression. If reactions to co-trimoxazole are relatively mild, it is currently recommended to continue with therapy but to control side-effects with antihistamines and antiemetics as required. Pentamidine remains the second choice agent in the AIDS group and for cases of pneumocystis pneumonia of mild severity (Po_2 above 7.5 kPa) pentamidine can be used at reduced dosage 3 mg/kg daily intravenously or as a nebulized preparation (600 mg dissolved in 6 ml water) daily. It must be delivered via an effective nebulizer such as the Respigard II system (Marquest, Englewood, Colorado), guaranteed to produce particle size of 1.5 μm and thereby ensure effective alveolar delivery. When side-effects are intolerable in the AIDS group, then other agents such as combination trimethoprim and dapsone, combination clindamycin/primaquine, or atovaquone are required. In clinical trials, regimens based on such drugs have produced good response rates in patients with pneumocystis pneumonia of mild to moderate severity. Pneumocystis pneumonia in AIDS requires treatment for 3 weeks to prevent early relapse.

Adjunctive therapy with corticosteroid has been found useful in AIDS patients with severe pneumocystis pneumonia, when the start of anti-pneumocystis therapy often results in a decline in arterial Po_2 of 1 to 2 kPa in the first 3 days. Treatment should generally be given as prednisolone, 40 mg daily for 5 days.

In non-AIDS patients, for example the transplant population, survival from pneumocystis pneumonia may depend upon temporary withdrawal of immunosuppressive agents such as cyclosporin and azathioprine.

In all patients, supportive treatment for hypoxaemia is required. Supplementation of inspired oxygen via a nasal cannula (flow 3–4 l/min) is simple and often effective. If not, an oxygen mask capable of delivering 60 per cent inspired oxygen may be required. In unrelieved hypoxaemia, temporary artificial ventilation may be considered, although it is not currently recommended for patients with AIDS because of the greater than 90 per cent mortality for such patients with pneumocystis pneumonia requiring ventilation and because of the currently unrescueable immune deficiency of that disease.

Fig. 4 DNA amplification for *P. carinii* shows a specific, 346-bp band visible after ethidium staining (a) and confirmed by oligohybridization (b).

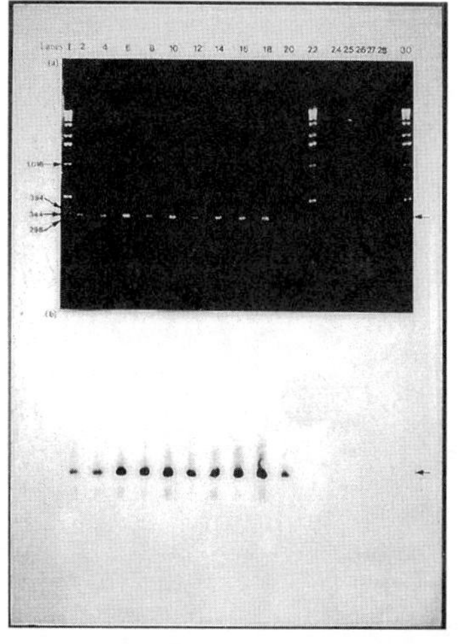

Prevention

The only proven form of prevention for pneumocystis pneumonia is chemoprophylaxis administered as periodic oral co-trimoxazole or inhaled nebulized pentamidine.

In non-AIDS patients, for example children who are being treated for acute lymphoblastic leukaemia or organ transplant recipients, routine chemoprophylaxis with co-trimoxazole is recommended from the initiation of immunosuppressive treatment and to last for a minimum of 6 to 12 months in a dosage of trimethoprim, 5 mg/kg a day, sulphamethoxazole, 25 mg/kg a day, in two divided doses on 3 days a week. Half the dose is equally effective in renal transplant recipients.

In AIDS subjects, chemoprophylaxis may be initiated when CD4 lymphocyte counts fall to 150 and should always be maintained after a proven episode of successfully treated pneumocystis pneumonia. Toxicity to low-dosage co-trimoxazole, usually 160/800 mg (two tabs) daily is less than with full-dosage treatment but side-effects may demand a change of schedule to the less effective but less toxic inhaled pentamidine as 300 mg monthly delivered by a Respigard II nebulizer. Recurrence rate in the first year is approximately 18 per cent for nebulized pentamidine compared with 4 per cent for the oral co-trimoxazole regimen.

REFERENCES

Conte, J.E., Chernoff, D., Feigal, D.W., Jr., Joseph, P., McDonald, C., and Golden, J.A. (1990). Intravenous or inhaled pentamidine for treatment *Pneumocystis carinii* pneumonia in AIDS: a randomized trial. *Annals of Internal Medicine*, **113**, 203–9.

Gagnon, S., Boota, A.M., Fischl, M.A., Baier, H., Kirksey, O.W., and La Voie, L. (1990). Corticosteroids as adjunctive therapy for severe *Pneumocystis carinii* pneumonia in the acquired immunodeficiency syndrome—a double-blind, placebo-controlled trial. *New England Journal of Medicine*, **323**, 1444–20.

Hopkin, J.M. (1991) *Pneumocystis carinii*. Oxford University Press.

Hughes, W.T. (1992). A new drug (hydroxynaphthoquinone, 566C80) for treatment of *Pneumocystis carinii* pneumonia. *Annals of Internal Medicine*, **116,** 953.

Hughes, W.T., Rivera, G.K., Schell, M.J., Thornton, D., and Lott, L. (1987). Successful intermittent chemoprophylaxis for *Pneumocystis carinii* pneumonia. *New England Journal of Medicine*, **316,** 1627–32.

Hughes, W.T., *et al.* (1993). Comparison of atovaquone with cotrimoxazole in pneumocystis pneumonia in AIDS. *New England Journal of Medicine,* **328,** 1521–7.

Lipschik, G.Y. *et al.* (1992). Improved diagnosis of *P. carinii* infection by polymerase chain reaction on induced sputum and blood. *Lancet*, **340,** 203–6.

Masur, H. (1992). Prevention and treatment of pneumocystis pneumonia. *New England Journal of Medicine*, **327,** 1853–60.

Post, C., Dutz, W., and Nasarian, I. (1964). Endemic *Pneumocystis carinii* pneumonia in South Iran. *Archives of Disease in Childhood*, **39,** 35–40.

Ruf, B. and Pohle, H.D. (1989). Clindamycin/primaquinine for *Pneumocystis carinii* pneumonia. *Lancet*, **ii,** 626–7.

Sattler, F.R., Cowan, R., Nielsen, D.M., and Ruskin, J. (1988). Trimethoprim-sulfamethoxazole compared with pentamidine for treatment of *Pneumocystis carinii* noncrossover study. *Annals of Internal Medicine*, **109,** 280–7.

Schneider, M.M.E. *et al.* (1992). A controlled trial of aerosolized pentamidine or trimethoprim-sulfamethoxazole as primary prophylaxis against *Pneumocystis carinii* pneumonia in patients with human immunodeficiency virus infection. *New England Journal of Medicine*, **327,** 1836–41.

Telzak, E.E. and Armstrong, D. (1994). *Extrapulmonary infection and other unusual manifestations of* Pneumocystis carinii *in* Pneumocystis carinii *Pneumonia* (ed. P. D. Walzer). Marcel Dekker, New York.

Wachter, R.M., Luce, J.M., and Hopewell, P.C. (1992). Critical care of patients with AIDS. *Journal of the American Medical Association*, **267,** 541–7.

Wakefield, A.E. *et al.* (1990). Detection of *Pneumocystis carinii* with DNA amplification. *Lancet*, **336,** 451–3.

Wakefield, A.E., Miller, R.M., Guiver, L., and Hopkin, J.M. (1991). DNA amplification for the diagnosis of pneumocystis pneumonia from induced sputum. *Lancet*, **i,** 1378.

7.13 Protozoa

7.13.1 Amoebiasis

R. Knight

INTRODUCTION

The amoebic species infecting man belong to two very different groups: the obligate parasitic species of the gut including the major pathogen *Entamoeba histolytica*; and the normally free-living, water and soil amoebae, which can become facultative tissue parasites. All motile feeding amoebae are called trophozoites; they move with pseudopodia and divide by binary fission. The hyaline external cytoplasm, the ectoplasm, is a contractile gel that surrounds the sol endoplasm containing numerous phagocytic and pinocytic vacuoles. Most species can form environmentally resistant cysts by rounding up and secreting a relatively rigid, chitinous cyst wall. Nuclei are not visible in the living organism but their structure, after staining, is very important in classification and identification. Part of the nuclear chromatin is concentrated centrally as the endosome, while the remainder lines the nuclear membrane as the 'peripheral chromatin'.

The parasitic gut amoebae

These are anaerobes that normally live as commensals close to mucosal surfaces. Bacteria in the same environment generate the necessary physicochemical conditions and act as a food source. These amoebae grow readily in bacteria-associated liquid cultures. Apart from *E. gingivalis*, all species occur in the colon. The cytoplasm contains no mitochondria or other membrane-bound organelles. Cysts contain refractile rods called chromatoid bodies, which are a ribosome store, and a glycogen vacuole; both types of structure slowly disappear as cysts age in the environment.

Five of the eight species infecting man belong to the genus Entamoeba, having a nucleus with a small endosome and abundant peripheral chromatin. The genus is grouped according to the number of nuclei in the spherical mature cyst. In the first group, with eight nuclei, is *E. coli*; this is a non-pathogen and the most common species in most surveys. In the second group, with four-nucleated cysts, are *E. histolytica* and *E. hartmanni*; the latter is a non-pathogen and was formerly referred to as 'small race *E. histolytica*'. Size is the only simple diagnostic criterion. *E. hartmanni* cysts are less than 10 μm in diameter. The third group contains the non-pathogen *E. polecki*, which is primarily a pig parasite; the cyst has one nucleus and an 'inclusion body'. Human infections are common in highland Papua New Guinea where man and pig may share a peridomestic environment; elsewhere it is rare. Lastly there is *E. gingivalis*, which has no cystic stage; it lives in the mouth within gingival pockets and tonsillar crypts. It is spread by kissing or more indirect oral contact. Its possible role in periodontal disease was formerly dismissed but there is now renewed interest following recognition of its high prevalence in individual lesions in people with this condition; it may act as a bacterial vector within the lesions. It has been found on intrauterine devices removed because of symptoms. Both in the uterus and in the mouth this amoeba occurs in association with the bacterium *Actinomyces israeli*.

Endolimax nana and *Iodamoeba buetchlii* both have nuclei with large endosomes and no visible peripheral chromatin. Cysts of the former are oval in shape with four nuclei; those of the latter are somewhat irregular in shape with a single nucleus and a large glycogen vacuole that stains prominently with iodine. Neither species is pathogenic.

Dientamoeba fragilis is unique in several ways. It has no cystic stage and about 60 per cent of trophozoites have two nuclei; the endosome is large and lobulated without peripheral chromatin. Transmission is within the eggs of the threadworm Enterobius. It causes a relatively mild diarrhoeal illness and may be common in institutional contexts; it is also found within some resected appendices. Electron micrographs suggest that it is a trichomonad rather than a true amoeba; binucleate forms are in arrested telophase. Mechanisms of pathogenicity are not defined but response to amoebicides is good.

Free-living amoeba

Several species produce cytopathic changes in cultured cell monolayers and cerebral invasion after intranasal inoculation into mice and other animals. They grow readily on *Escherichia coli* grown upon agar, producing clear plaques resembling those due to lytic phage. One isolate was initially named the 'Ryan virus' when throat swabs were inoculated on to monkey kidney monolayers—a classical example of failure to use the microscope. These amoebae are aerobic and their cytoplasm contains mitochondria, Golgi complexes, and a contractile vacuole; their natural food is bacteria.

Several hundred human infections are now documented. The human pathogens are thermophilic and can be isolated from hot springs, the warm water of health spas, air-conditioning systems and humidifiers, and much more rarely from tap water. In natural waters they proliferate in the summer months and where there is thermal pollution. Under dry conditions, trophozoites form resistant cysts that permit survival and also airborne dispersal; cysts can resist chlorination.

Most human disease is caused by *Naegleria fowleri* and two species of *Acanthamoeba*; their biology and clinical effects differ and they will be considered separately. A shared feature is the very large central nuclear endosome, quite different from that of *E. histolytica*, from which differentiation may be necessary in tissue sections. *N. fowleri* and related organisms are also one of the causes of 'humidifier fever', a form of extrinsic allergic alveolitis presenting with fever, cough, and sometimes progressive pulmonary fibrosis and dyspnoea. The amoebae grow readily in the warm water of the cooling units of air-conditioning systems. In these environments bacteria of the genera Legionella and Listeria may live symbiotically within the amoebae. They can persist within the phagosome of the amoebae, being resistant to lyzosomal enzymes. Surprisingly, Legionella can survive encystment: the amoebae provide a refuge for these bacteria when chlorination or other antibacterial measures are applied.

These organisms also account for the 'coprozoic amoebae' sometimes found in faecal specimens, especially when they are not fresh. Their presence results either from contamination of the specimen or the excystation of cysts that have passed through the gut following ingestion or inhalation.

Entamoeba histolytica infection

Biology and pathogenicity

Within the host *E. histolytica* trophozoites occur in two forms: as an intraluminal commensal of the caecum and proximal colon; or as an invasive pathogen. In the majority of infected people *E. histolytica* is entirely commensal. Live commensal amoebae measure 10 to 20 μm in diameter, the endoplasm is granular and contains bacteria; the pseudopodia are relatively blunt and movement is rather sluggish. The transmissive, cystic form of the parasite is derived entirely from this commensal population. Encystment occurs within the colonic lumen and never outside the body, but cyst maturation can continue in the environment. Intestinal hurry from any cause, including the use of laxatives, can lead to the appearance of commensal trophozoites in the faeces.

Invasive trophozoites may reach 30 to 40 μm in diameter; they are usually very active with apparently purposeful, unidirectional movements during which they become considerably elongated. Their most important diagnostic characteristic is the presence of host erythrocytes within the endoplasm, which otherwise appears clear and contains no bacteria. Trophozoites containing red blood cells are described as haematophagous. Damage to host cells occurs during cell-to-cell contact; cytolytic enzymes are released and also amoebopore, a complement-like protein, which can puncture cell membranes. Progression through tissues is by active movement, facilitated by secreted collagenase; leucocytes are drawn chemotactically towards the amoebae but most are rapidly destroyed on contact.

Strain characterization has shown that isolates belong to two groups. Pathogenic strains show a number of correlated features: enhanced erythrophagocytosis; reduced surface charge; agglutination by concanavalin A; resistance to complement-mediated lysis; greater cytopathic effect on cell monolayers; greater pathogenicity when inoculated into rat caecum or hamster liver; and an ability to grow in semisolid media, and in axenic culture—that is without living associates. Characterization by isoenzyme electrophoresis enables zymodemes to be identified; these are populations defined by electrophoretic patterns using a standard set of enzymes (Fig. 1). Of the naturally occurring zymodemes so far identified 10 are pathogenic and 12 non-pathogenic. This distinction is very striking; all isolates from symptomatic bowel disease and liver abscess have been pathogenic zymodemes and follow-up studies indicate that all those infected with these strains become seropositive. Zymodeme status is a stable character, and, although virulence can be temporarily modified *in vitro* or by animal passage, there is no change in zymodeme. Some non-pathogenic zymodemes do have mild cytopathic effects *in vitro* and in experimental animals but there is currently no evidence that they cause significant disease in humans, although they may induce low-titre seropositivity. It has now been formally proposed that these two groups of amoebae justify specific designations, with the name *E. dispar* used for the non-pathogen, which is always a commensal. In contrast, true *E. histolytica* trophozoites may be commensal or invasive. A small number of atypical strains have been isolated; these grow at room temperature and can survive in hypotonic media. They belong to non-pathogenic zymodemes and may be identical to *E. moschkovskii*, a free-living species that has been found in sewage in several parts of the world.

Host factors may increase susceptibility among patients infected with pathogenic strains. Thus steroid therapy given systemically or locally into the rectum carries great risk, as may cytotoxic therapy. Severe bowel disease is particularly common in late pregnancy and the puerperium. Before puberty both sexes are equally susceptible to hepatic amoebiasis but in adults this condition is at least seven times more common in males. Local disease can also favour tissue invasion; thus amoebic ulceration may be superimposed upon colonic and rectal cancers, or those of the uterine cervix. Colonic invasion is favoured by concurrent helminthic infection with Trichuris and intestinal schistosomiasis, and by overt or latent, non-specific colitis. Hepatic lesions are more common in the presence of liver-cell damage, including that due to alcohol. Infection with human immunodeficiency-virus appears to have little effect on outcome; infection by non-pathogenic zymodemes does not lead to amoebic disease, even in patients with AIDS. The role of protein energy malnutrition is uncertain.

Epidemiology

Amoebic disease must be distinguished from amoebic infection. The estimated annual global mortality due to this parasite is 40 000 to 110 000. The incidence of disease is particularly high in Mexico, parts of South America, Natal, the west coast of Africa, and parts of South-East Asia; crowded poor urban communities are often the worst affected. However, even in tropical countries the proportion of pathogenic strains does not exceed 10 per cent, and in many temperate countries this proportion, among residents, is now virtually nil. Nearly all cases now seen in temperate countries will have acquired their infection elsewhere, although indigenous outbreaks do still occur, for instance in northern Canada and in Japan. Pathogenic zymodemes introduced into temperate

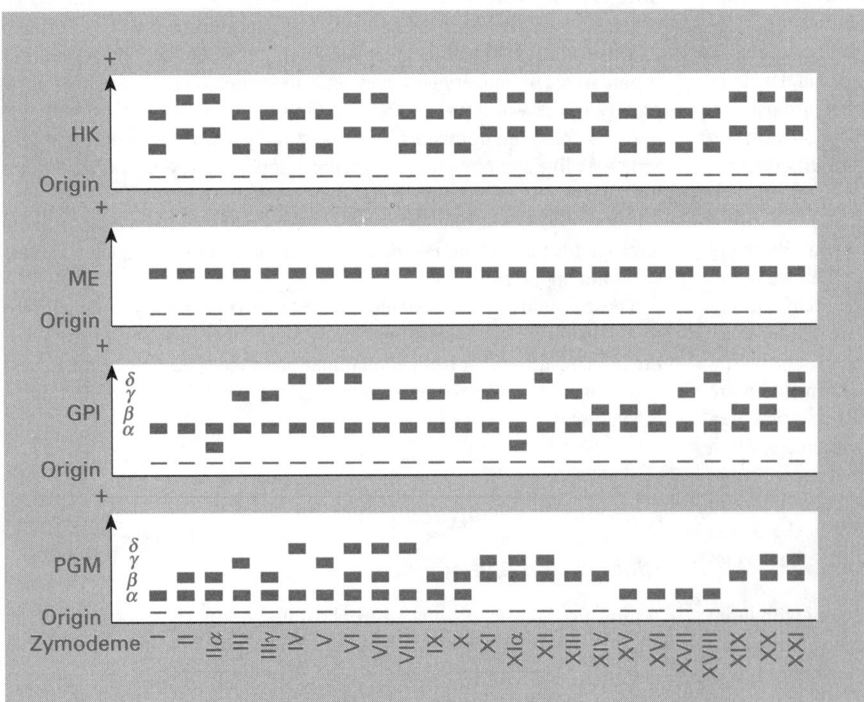

Fig. 1 Zymodemes of *Entamoeba histolytica* identified using EC 5319 glucose phosphate isomerase (GPI); EC 11140 L-malate: $NADP^+$ oxidoreductase (oxaloacetate decarboxylating) (ME); EC 2751 phosphoglucomutase (PGM); and EC 2711 hexokinase (HK). A zymodeme is a population of amoebae differing from similar populations in the electrophoretic mobility of certain enzymes. The markers for pathogenicity are the absence of the α band together with the presence of the β band in PGM. Advanced bands in HK confirm the PGM results. The only exception is zymodeme XIII which lacks advanced HK bands. (Reproduced from Sargeaunt, P.G. (1990). *Mitteilungen der Österreichischen Gesellschaft für Tropenmedizin und Parasitologie*, **12,** 1–4, with permission.) Zymodemes XIα and XXI are laboratory 'hybrids.'

countries rarely become established, although non-pathogenic strains persist; the reason is unknown. In some tropical countries the disease may be rare, although infection is common.

Apart from the very rare transfer of trophozoites during sexual contact or when colonic irrigation equipment is shared, transmission is exclusively by ingestion of cysts. Excystment occurs in the lower ileum and caecum. Symptomless or convalescent carriers are the main source of infection; patients with dysentery normally pass only trophozoites in their stool, and therefore are non-infectious. Under optimal environmental conditions, cysts remain viable for 2 months. The number of cysts passed by a carrier varies from day to day. When low it may be undetectable; some people have persistently high counts, which may reach 45 million/day. The minimal infective dose is unknown. The prepatent period is 4 to 8 days. The infection is eventually self-limiting but can exceed 10 years. The mean duration is 2 to 3 years. Tissue invasion can occur at any time during an infection with a pathogenic strain, but is much more common during the first 4 months; the incubation period may be as short as 7 to 10 days.

The global prevalence of *E. histolytica* infection is about 10 per cent, and in some tropical countries it may exceed 30 per cent. In most of Western Europe and temperate North America, prevalence is now generally below 1 per cent, but it can be high in institutions and among male homosexuals. The shape of age–prevalence curves give clues to modes of transmission. A steady rise with age until a plateau is reached in adolescence or early adult life suggests that infection rates are independent of age. All the modes of faeco-oral transmission occur in amoebiasis; of special importance is the infected food handler. Vegetables may be contaminated when human faeces are used as fertilizer, or when faeces-polluted water is used for irrigation or for 'freshening' vegetables before sale in the market place; fly-borne transmission is important in some contexts. Direct spread occurs within institutions for children and the mentally handicapped, and can produce outbreaks. Household clustering is common; hand-fed infants are frequently infected from the fingers of their mother. Cyst ingestion also occurs in sexual contexts. Drinking water can be contaminated in the home or at surface-water sources. Contamination of piped water supplies can lead to disease outbreaks when a pathogenic zymodeme is involved, as happened in the Chicago hotels epidemic in 1933.

Both wild and captive monkeys may show high prevalence and they can develop symptomatic or asymptomatic bowel-wall invasion. Limited studies of colony non-human primates in the United States and Britain have shown non-pathogenic zymodemes. Both dogs and rats may be infected from human sources; amoebic dysentery is described in dogs but is very rare.

Pathology (Fig. 1)

The basic lesion is cell lysis and tissue necrosis, which, by creating locally anoxic and acidic conditions, favours further penetration of the parasite into the tissues. Most amoebae are seen at the advancing edge of the lesion, with very few in the healthy tissue beyond. Pathogenic strains have an oxygen tolerance up to 5 per cent and can detoxify oxygen radicals, partly by scavenging catalase from host erythrocytes. The inflammatory-cell response comprises a mild, or moderate, local accumulation of lymphocytes and polymorphs; local tissue oedema and capillary dilatation may be prominent. In tissue sections, amoebae are often surrounded by a clear space due to cell shrinkage. They stain indistinctly with haematoxylin and eosin but they appear bright red with periodic acid–Schiff stain; iron haematoxylin is necessary to show nuclear detail. Cysts of *E. histolytica* are never seen in tissue.

Amoebic lesions of the gut are most common in the rectosigmoid and caecum but can occur anywhere in the large bowel—involvement may be patchy or continuous; less commonly the appendix or terminal ileum are affected. The initial lesions are either small, discrete erosions of the interglandular mucosa, or crypt lesions that begin as colonocyte lysis within the confines of the basement membrane and then extend to form a microabscess at the crypt base. Unrestrained, the lesions extend through the mucosa, across the muscularis mucosa and into the submucosa, where they expand laterally to produce lesions that are typically flask shaped in cross-section, with normal intervening mucosa. Further lateral spread of the submucosal lesions leads to their coalescence, and later, to denudation of overlying mucosa. The bowel wall may become appreciably thickened. Blood vessels involved in the disease may thrombose, bleed into the gut lumen or, in the case of portal-vein radicles, provide a vehicle for the dissemination of amoebae to the liver. Secondary bacterial infection is often minimal and confined to areas of ulcerated mucosa. In very severe lesions, and usually in association with toxic megacolon, there is an irreversible coagulative necrosis of the bowel wall.

Amoebomas are tumour-like lesions of the colonic wall measuring up to several centimetres in length; they are most common in the caecum and may be multiple. Histologically there is tissue oedema, with a mixed picture of healing, and new areas of epithelial loss and tissue destruction; round-cell infiltration is patchy. Lesions may be annular and rarely an amoeboma initiates an intussusception; narrow, stricture-like amoebomas may occur in the anorectal region.

Amoebae reach the liver passively in the portal vein from the gut. Probably very few become established and a nidus of tissue necrosis may be necessary; a result, for example, of local venous thrombosis or embolism. Once initiated, however, the amoebic lesion extends progressively in all directions to produce the liver-cell necrosis and liquefaction that constitute an 'amoebic liver abscess'. The lesions are most common in the upper part of the right lobe of the liver; multiple lesions are common in patients with coexistent amoebic bowel ulceration, and in children. Liver abscesses are more or less spherical and well demarcated from surrounding liver tissue, which show considerable local compression in macroscopic specimens. On microscopy the liquefactive lesion is surrounded by hyperaemia and a moderate inflammatory-cell response; a fibroblastic reaction occurs only in long-standing lesions. Untreated, nearly all liver abscesses eventually extend into adjacent structures and most complications are produced in this way. Secondary bacterial infection is rare and usually follows rupture or aspiration; however, Salmonella infections of amoebic liver abscess are reported.

Patients with uncomplicated amoebic dysentery may develop mild, or even moderate, hepatomegaly. Its pathogenesis is similar to that seen in other inflammatory bowel diseases; microscopy shows periportal leucocytes. There is no pathological basis for a diffuse form of invasive amoebic hepatitis.

Immunological responses

Invasive amoebiasis evokes both humoral and cellular immune responses. Most detectable amoebic antibody is IgG, which may persist for several years after successful therapy. In active disease, IgM antibody may be found. Immediate skin sensitivity to amoebic antigen, presumably mediated by IgE antibody, is demonstrable in some patients with active disease. Coproantibodies may be detectable. Lymphoblast transformation to amoebic antigen can be shown in most patients after recovery but an antigen-specific depression is common in active disease, especially liver abscess.

Bowel disease may remit spontaneously, although the mechanisms, which involve T cells and macrophages, are not fully defined. Some host risk factors are mediated by failure of these mechanisms. *E. histolytica* can evade antibody in several ways: capping of antibody–antigen complexes, membrane resistance to complement, and shedding of surface antigen. When incubated with fluorescein-labelled antibody, live amoebae initially round up, but soon there is reactivation as the dye passes to the uroid—the tail end of the amoeba—prior to its shedding. Extraintestinal lesions, including those of the liver, progress inexorably without any immunological restraint. Protective immunity has been achieved in animal models; in man, clinical relapse from persisting intraluminal infection can occur after therapy, but is less common than might be expected, suggesting some immune protection.

Reactive arthritis, uveitis, and other immunologically mediated complications of colitis are extremely rare in amoebiasis.

All infections by pathogenic zymodemes, symptomatic or not, induce seropositivity. Very low antibody titres can occur in people carrying non-pathogenic zymodemes and these responses are presumed to derive from intraluminal amoebae.

Clinical manifestations

Invasive intestinal amoebiasis

The clinical features show a wide spectrum from minimal changes in bowel habit to severe dysentery. Lesions may be limited to a small part of the large bowel or extend throughout its length. A relapsing course is common.

AMOEBIC COLITIS WITH DYSENTERY

Dysentery, the passage of loose or diarrhoeal stools containing fresh blood, occurs when there is generalized colonic ulceration, or when more localized lesions occur in the rectum or rectosigmoid. Onset may be gradual, intermittent, or much less commonly, acute. Typically, constitutional upset is initially mild and the patient remains ambulant; mild or moderate abdominal pain is common, and is often colicky and maximal over affected parts of the gut. Tenesmus can occur but is rarely severe. Stools vary in consistency from semiformed to watery; they are foul-smelling and always contain some visible blood, together, usually, with some mucus; even when watery, some faecal matter is nearly always present. Symptoms frequently wax and wane over a period of weeks or even months and such patients can become debilitated and wasted. In a few patients the disease runs a fulminating course.

The most frequent physical sign is abdominal tenderness in one or both iliac fossae; but tenderness may be generalized. Affected gut may be palpably thickened. A low fever is common, but dehydration is uncommon. There may be some diffuse, non-tender hepatomegaly, especially when the colonic lesions are widespread. Abdominal distension occurs in the more severely ill patients, who sometimes pass relatively small amounts of stool.

When stool microscopy reveals no haematophagous trophozoites a careful proctoscopy or sigmoidoscopy should be done. The endoscopic appearances may be non-specific in early, acute, or very severe colitis; the findings are hyperaemia, contact bleeding, or confluent ulceration. In more chronic cases the presence of normal-looking intervening mucosa is highly suggestive of amoebiasis; early lesions are often elevated, with a pouting opening only 1 to 2 mm in diameter; later, ulcers may reach 1 cm or more in diameter, with an irregular outline and often a loosely adherent, yellowish or grey exudate. Mucosal scrapings or superficial biopsies taken at endoscopy should be examined immediately by wet-preparation microscopy.

AMOEBIC COLITIS WITHOUT DYSENTERY

When ulceration is limited to the caecum or ascending colon, it rarely produces dysentery; similarly early, mild, or localized lesions elsewhere in the colon may give rise to no dysenteric symptoms. Patients complain of frequent changes in bowel habit and may notice occasional blood-staining of the stool that may wrongly be attributed to haemorrhoids; flatulence is common and may be associated with colicky pains. Often the only physical sign is tenderness in the right iliac fossa, or elsewhere along the course of the colon. Some patients will eventually go into complete remission; others progress to a dysenteric illness.

The most important diagnostic measure is repeated stool examination for haematophagous amoebae; the finding of cysts or commensal trophozoites is of little diagnostic value, especially in endemic areas. Sigmoidoscopy is often normal when the distal bowel is not involved. But, when available, colonoscopy may reveal typical lesions in the proximal colon.

SPECIAL FORMS OF AMOEBIC COLITIS

Fulminant colitis

This may arise *de novo*, for example in pregnant women or during steroid therapy, or it may evolve during a dysenteric illness. Patients show progressive abdominal distension, vomiting, and watery diarrhoea; they become shocked. Bowel sounds are absent and there may be little or no abdominal tenderness, guarding, or rigidity. Plain radiographs may reveal free peritoneal gas, together with acute gaseous dilatation of the colon; affected segments of bowel may appear relatively narrow and show visible musosal pathology. Barium enema and full sigmoidoscopy are contraindicated. Stools will contain haematophagous trophozoites.

Amoeboma

These present as an abdominal mass, most frequently in the right iliac fossa. The lesion may be painful, tender, and associated with fever. Bowel habit is altered and some patients have intermittent dysentery, especially if lesions are multiple or distal. Evidence of partial or intermittent bowel obstruction may be present, particularly when lesions are distal and annular.

Localized perforation and amoebic appendicitis

Sudden perforation with peritonitis can occur from any deep amoebic ulcer; alternatively, leakage may lead to a pericolic abscess or retroperitoneal cellulitis. Amoebic appendicitis is an uncommon but important condition that occurs when amoebic lesions are confined to the appendix and caecum. The clinical presentation can resemble that of simple appendicitis, although there may be some clinical evidence of dysentery. When the condition is unrecognized at appendicectomy the outcome can be disastrous with gut perforation. Whenever this condition is suspected, fresh smears should be made from the resected appendix, and examined immediately.

Rectal bleeding

Some patients with amoebiasis present with rectal bleeding, with or without tenesmus; this occurs particularly in children. Massive bleeding into the gut lumen can occur in any form of amoebic colitis but is rare.

Postdysenteric syndromes

After successful therapy a few patients continue to have dysenteric symptoms. Sigmoidoscopy shows a reddened, oedematous mucosa with superficial erosions, and amoebic antibody titres remain high. The condition only occurs in persons who have had extensive amoebic colitis; it is usually self-limiting over a period of months. Strictures in the rectosigmoid are another late sequel to severe amoebic colitis, although most patients make a full recovery.

DIFFERENTIAL DIAGNOSIS

Amoebic colitis must be differentiated from other causes of infective colitis, especially that due to Shigellae, non-typhoidal Salmonellae, and Campylobacter. High-volume diarrhoea, copious mucus, and severe tenesmus are all uncommon in amoebiasis. In temperate countries, non-specific ulcerative colitis and colorectal carcinoma create the greatest diagnostic problems. Parasitic conditions to be considered are intestinal schistosomiasis, heavy Trichuris infection, and balantidiasis. More chronic amoebic pathology may clinically resemble diverticulitis, Crohn's disease, ileocaecal tuberculosis, and anorectal lymphogranuloma venereum.

E. histolytica can invade carcinomas, so the finding of this parasite should not necessarily defer the search for other possible diagnoses; therapeutic trials may be difficult to interpret in this situation and may cause unnecessary delay.

Clostridium difficile colitis may resemble amoebiasis and should be considered especially in patients who have received antibiotics.

Hepatic amoebiasis

Less than half of all patients give any convincing history of dysentery. Of those that do, most develop liver lesions within a few weeks while a few have concurrent dysentery. In those with no dysenteric history the interval between presumed infection and presentation may be as short as 3 weeks, or as long as 15 years; for most it is between 8 weeks and a year.

The dominant symptoms are fever and sweating, liver or diaphragmatic pain, and weight loss. Onset of constitutional symptoms is often insidious; but pain may begin abruptly. Most patients seek medical help within 1 to 4 weeks. Fever is typically remittent, with a prominent evening rise, brief rigors, and very profuse sweating. Liver pain may be poorly localized initially and later become pleuritic, referred to the right shoulder tip, or localized to the abdominal wall. Within a few weeks, patients lose much weight and often become anaemic; a painful dry cough is common.

Fig. 2 Amoebic liver abscess. Hepatic enlargement with focal tenderness in a Thai woman (by courtesy of Professor S. Looareesuwan).

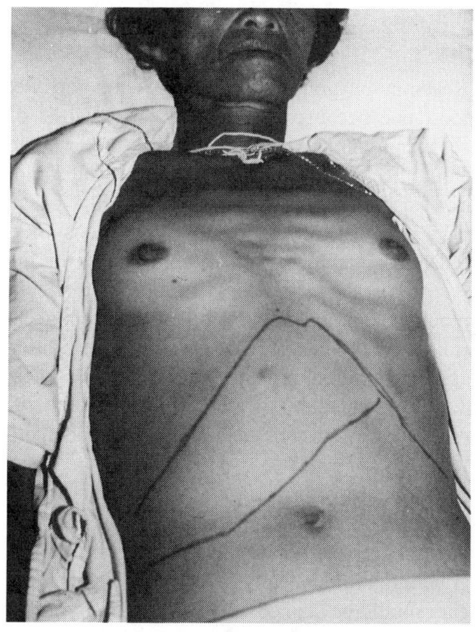

The most important clinical finding is liver enlargement (Fig. 2). with localized tenderness, which should be searched for in the right hypochondrium, the epigastrium, and along all the intercostal spaces overlying the liver. Liver pain, on compression or heavy digital percussion, is a less useful sign. Left-sided lesions can present as an epigastric mass. Hepatomegaly may be difficult to detect by abdominal palpation when enlargement is mainly upwards, but bulging of the right chest wall may be noted, together with a raised upper level of liver dullness on percussion. Reduced breath sounds or crepitations may be heard at the right lung base. Jaundice is rare unless lesions are multiple, very large, or encroach on the porta hepatis.

Important radiological findings are a raised, or locally upward-bulging, right diaphragm (Fig. 3) with immobility on screening, areas of lung collapse or consolidation, and sometimes a pleural effusion. A neutrophil leucocytosis is almost invariably present, the erythrocyte sedimentation rate is raised, and there is commonly normochromic normocytic anaemia. 'Liver function tests' are frequently completely normal, or there may be a raised alkaline phosphatase; less commonly the serum transaminase, lactic dehydrogenase or bilirubin is elevated. Liver scanning to demonstrate a filling defect is of great value; about 70 per cent of lesions are solitary, but multiple lesions are common in children and those with concurrent dysentery. Ultrasonographic scans and computerized tomography are the most useful; the findings on isotope scans do not always correspond. Lesions appear round or oval, and are usually 4 to 10 cm in diameter at the time of presentation. On ultrasonography most are hypoechoic with well-defined walls without enhanced echoes. Margins are sometimes less well defined initially and a few lesions appear solid or show a heterogeneous echo pattern.

Stool microscopy is of very little diagnostic value except when there is current dysentery. Many patients show no evidence of *E. histolytica* in their stool, even after repeated examinations.

COMPLICATIONS

Most complications involve extension of hepatic lesions into adjacent structures: most commonly the right chest, the peritoneum, and the pericardium. Upward extension usually produces adhesions between the liver, the diaphragm, and the lung; in consequence, subphrenic rupture and amoebic empyema are rare, although a right serous pleural effusion

Fig. 3 Amoebic liver abscess, radiographic changes: (a) elevated right diaphragm; (b) enormous abscess in the right lobe of the liver outlined with air (fluid level) and contrast medium introduced during the aspiration of more than 1 l of pus; (c) lateral view, same patient as (b). (By courtesy of Professor Sornchai Looareesuwan.)

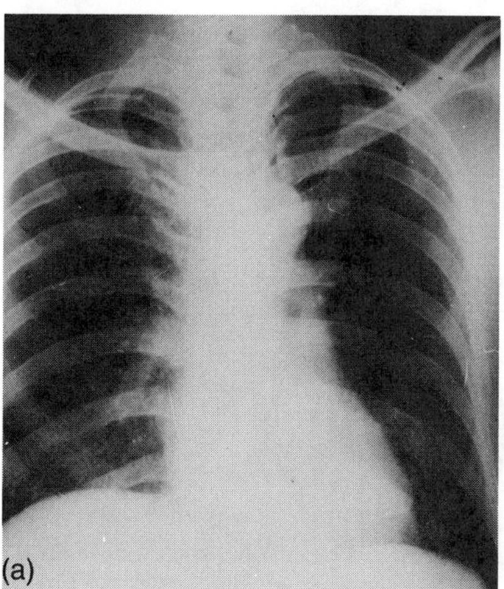

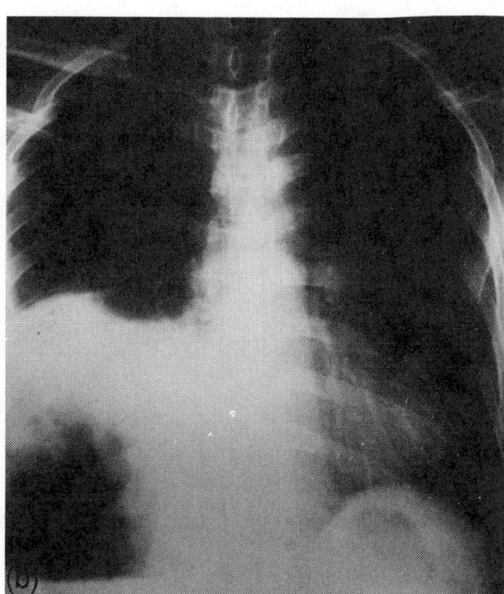

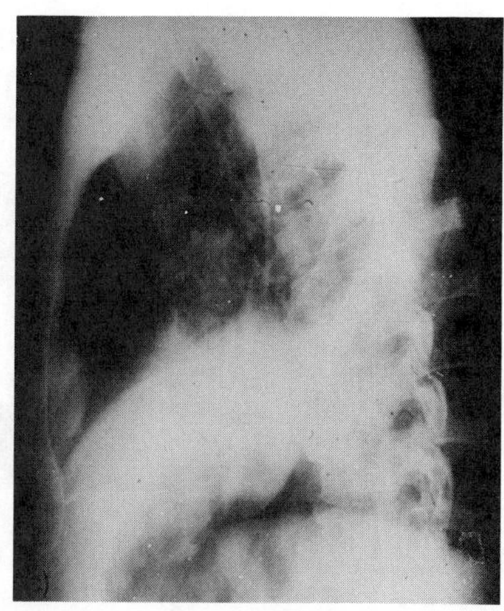

is not uncommon. Untreated, the disease process advances upwards through lung tissue until a bronchus is reached. A hepatobroncial fistula results and the patient may cough up large quantities of brownish, necrotic liver tissue, the so-called 'anchovy sauce' sputum. Rupture into the peritoneum can occur at any time; it is sometimes the mode of presentation of an amoebic liver abscess, the cause of peritonitis being discovered only at laparotomy. Amoebic pericarditis usually results from upward extension of a left-lobe liver lesion, or less commonly, one in the right lobe or lung. Patients have retrosternal pain, a pericardial friction rub, or a serous effusion. When rupture occurs, cardiac tamponade and shock can develop rapidly. The diagnosis is most difficult when an underlying liver abscess was not suspected.

Less commonly the lesion extends through the skin producing a sinus and cutaneous lesion. The gut, stomach, vena cava, spleen, and kidney are occasionally involved by direct spread. Blood-borne spread to the lung produces a lesion resembling an isolated, pyogenic lung abscess, but this is rare. Amoebic brain abscesses due to *E. histolytica* are rare: they may be suspected during life but most are discovered post-mortem; all such patients have an amoebic liver abscess (Fig. 4).

Jaundice may occur when a large lesion compresses the common bile duct or when multiple lesions compress several intrahepatic bile ducts. Rupture into a major bile duct is rare but can cause haemobilia. Portal-vein compression occasionally produces portal hypertension and congestive splenomegaly.

DIFFERENTIAL DIAGNOSIS

Amoebic serology and scanning have now greatly simplified diagnosis. However, a few patients, generally less than 5 per cent, are initially seronegative; scanning patterns may be atypical before lesions have liquefied. When these diagnostic resources are not available, many conditions must be considered. The most frequent in tropical countries is primary hepatocellular carcinoma, but malignant secondary deposits in the liver cause similar problems. Pyogenic abscess, especially when cryptogenic, may be clinically indistinguishable and this condition is quite common in some Asian countries. Other conditions to be distinguished are lesions of the right lung base and right pleura, subphrenic abscess, cholecystitis, septic cholangitis including that resulting from aberrant Ascaris worms, and liver hydatid cysts.

Needle aspiration of the liver (Fig. 5) may be necessary for diagnostic or therapeutic purposes (see below). Suspected pyogenic abscess is the main indication for the former; blood cultures should also be taken. Whenever possible, liver scanning should precede the procedure, which should be monitored by ultrasound. A therapeutic amoebicide trial is generally preferable to diagnostic needling of the liver. For example, attempted aspiration of a hepatoma commonly produces a brisk haemorrhage. Typically the aspirate in hepatic amoebiasis is pinkish-brown, odourless, and bacteriologically sterile; less commonly it is yellow or whitish. A thinner, malodorous, or frothy aspirate suggests bacterial infection.

Cutaneous and genital amoebiasis

Skin ulceration due to *E. histolytica* produces deep, painful, and foul-smelling lesions that spread rapidly. Secondary bacterial infection is common and may mask the amoebic pathology. Lesions are most frequent in the perianal area, but also occur at colostomy stomas, laparotomy scars, and at the site of skin rupture by a hepatic lesion.

In the female, genital involvement results from faecal contamination, the extension of perianal lesions, or by the formation of internal fistulae from the gut, which can involve the bladder. Lesions of the vulva and uterine cervix may resemble carcinoma, but it must be remembered that amoebiasis may be superimposed on a carcinoma. In the male, genital lesions follow rectal coitus, the lesion beginning as a balanoposthitis and progressing rapidly.

Laboratory diagnosis

Microscopy and culture

The identification of live haematophagous trophozoites in temporary wet mounts is of prime importance because it confirms the diagnosis of invasive amoebic disease. Examinations are best made in ward or clinic side-rooms. Amoebae should be sought in dysenteric bowel-wall scrapings, in the last portion of aspirate from a liver abscess (Fig. 6), in sputum, and in the material obtained from suspected skin lesions. Skin lesions should be incised and scrapings taken from the sides of the incision. In non-dysenteric stools, flecks of pus, blood or mucus should be looked for and examined. The amoebae remain active for about 30 min at room temperature. If necessary the material should be diluted with normal saline, preferably buffered to pH 6.8. Other microscopical features of faeces in invasive gut amoebiasis are scanty or absent leucocytes, clumped or degenerating red cells, and sometimes Charcot–Leyden crystals.

If wet preparations are not made, or are negative, either a portion of the specimen should be preserved in polyvinyl alcohol or SAF (sodium acetate–acetic acid–formalin) fixative for later smear preparation, or drying faecal smears should be fixed immediately in Schaudinn's solution. In either case, fixed smears should be stained with Gomori trichrome or Heidenhain's iron haematoxylin. Recognition of an *Entamoeba* nucleus

Fig. 4 Metastatic brain abscess in a patient with an amoebic liver abscess. (By courtesy of Professor Sornchai Looareesuwan.)

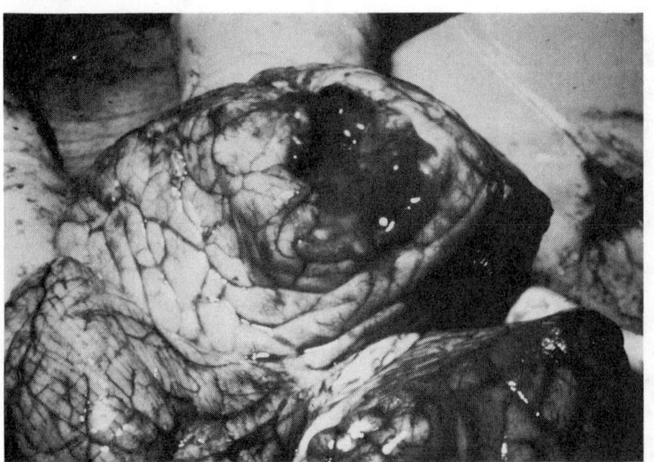

Fig. 5 Diagnostic/therapeutic aspiration of 'anchovy sauce pus' from a patient with amoebic liver abscess (copyright Professor D.A. Warrell).

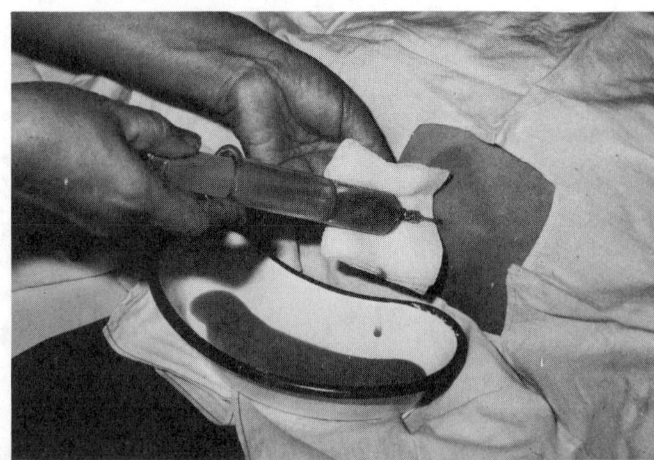

is relatively easy but, unless erythrocytes are present, identification as *E. histolytica* requires considerable expertise and is based upon details of nuclear structure. Amoebae remain alive in unfixed specimens kept at 4 °C for up to 4 h, and are sometimes identifiable on rewarming.

Cysts of *E. histolytica* are quite easy to recognize in wet mounts made from faecal specimens. However, an eyepiece micrometer is essential to differentiate this species from the smaller *E. hartmanni*. Direct mounts are made by emulsifying a small portion of stool in 1 per cent eosin, and in Lugol's iodine. Provided the eosin preparations are thin enough, cysts stand out as round or oval, white objects against a pink background. Nuclear structure cannot be seen but the refractile chromatoids bodies can. The iodine preparation stains the nuclei and the glycogen vacuole. Using direct mounts for cysts the diagnostic sensitivity, per specimen, is only about 30 per cent, hence concentration using the formol–ether sedimentation method is normally used, giving a 70 per cent sensitivity. Concentrates are examined as a wet mount in Lugol's iodine. Three negative stool-concentrate examinations on different days will miss only about 3 per cent of infections.

Cultivation of intestinal amoebae with bacterial associates in Robinson's medium is relatively easy. Lysates of such cultures, at 48 or 72 h, provide material for zymodeme assay. Stained, fixed smears from cultures can be made for specific identification but this is difficult unless *E. histolytica* antibody and indirect immunofluorescent staining is used. Monoclonal antibody to pathogenic *E. histolytica* is particularly useful in this context and can also be applied to smears made directly from faecal specimens. DNA probes have also been used to identify pathogenic and non-pathogenic isolates. Positive cultures from extraintestinal sites are useful because they must be pathogenic *E. histolytica*; in liver aspirates, particularly, amoebae are often difficult to find microscopically.

Immunological tests

Many serodiagnostic methods have been applied to amoebiasis. However, seropositivity cannot distinguish current and past tissue invasion. The more sensitive methods are indirect haemagglutination, enzyme immunoassay, indirect immunofluorescence, and countercurrent immunoelectrophoresis. Latex agglutination and gel-diffusion precipitation are also used, the former being commercially available as a slide test, taking only minutes to perform. When titres are low, complete agreement between tests is not obtained and it is useful for laboratories to do more than one test. Using sensitive tests, over 95 per cent of patients with liver abscess are seropositive, as are about 60 per cent of those with invasive bowel disease; patients with amoeboma are nearly all seropositive. All patients with tissue invasion eventually become seropositive, as do those with apparently symptomless infections by pathogenic zymodemes. Titres decline after therapy but may remain positive for 2 years or more with the more sensitive tests. Protein antigens specific for pathogenicity are now becoming available for use in serological testing.

New methods for detection of amoebic antigen in faeces or serum hold promise especially when the recognized antigen is specific for pathogenic status.

Fig. 6 Aspirate from amoebic liver abscess showing margin of hepatocytes and haematophagous trophozoites of *E. histolytica*. (By courtesy of Professor Sornchai Looareesuwan.)

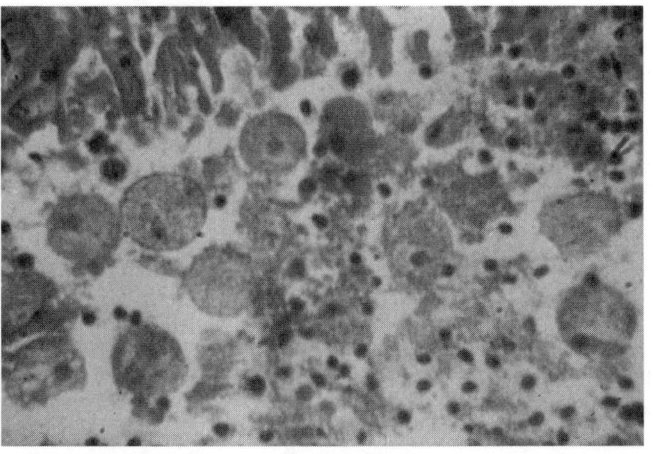

Treatment

Amoebicidal drugs

Some drugs destroy invasive amoebae in the tissues, others act upon those in the bowel lumen; they are known as tissue and luminal amoebicides, respectively. Parasitological cure implies that both tissue and intraluminal infections have been eliminated.

METRONIDAZOLE, TINIDAZOLE, AND OTHER NITROIMIDAZOLE COMPOUNDS

These are very potent tissue amoebicides, whose activity within the gut lumen is relatively poor. The greatest clinical experience has been obtained with metronidazole. Tinidazole is at least as effective as metronidazole in amoebic liver abscess and is usually less toxic. None of the other compounds, which include ornidazole, nimorazole and nitrimidazine, has shown greater efficacy than metronidazole, which remains the favoured drug in this group.

Oral metronidazole is rapidly and completely absorbed and reaches all tissues. There is an enterohepatic circulation but most of the drug is excreted by the kidney; concentrations in the colonic lumen are low unless there is mucosal inflammation. Within *E. histolytica*, as within other anaerobic organisms, the nitro group is reduced to a toxic compound that binds to DNA and blocks its replication. In short courses, metronidazole is very safe but some patients complain of nausea, a metallic taste in the mouth, weakness or dizziness; a few develop urticaria and other rashes, or transient ataxia. A brownish-red discoloration of the urine may occur and there is a disulphiram-like interaction with alcohol. Prolonged courses can cause leucopenia and peripheral neuropathy. Evidence of oncogenicity in animals and mutagenicity in bacteria has caused concern, but the risks in man appear to be very small. Caution is necessary in the first trimester of pregnancy.

The usual adult dose of metronidazole is 800 mg, thrice daily for 5 or 8 days; the paediatric dose is 35 to 50 mg/kg in three divided doses. Lower doses, such as 400 mg thrice daily in adults, are frequently effective in invasive disease but may fail to eliminate the intraluminal infection and so clinical relapse can occur. Single daily doses of 2 or 2.4 g have been used in adults but effectiveness in severe disease is poorly documented and there is no advantage in non-ambulant patients. The parenteral preparation, 500 mg as a 0.5 per cent aqueous infusion, is invaluable in severely ill patients. It is given 8-hourly at a rate of 5 ml/min.

Tinidazole has the advantage of a single daily dose, 2 g in adults and 50 to 60 mg/kg in children. A 5- or even a 3-day course may be sufficient for tissue amoebae but rates of parasitological cure may be low. A parenteral preparation is sometimes available.

EMETINE

The alkaloid emetine hydrochloride is a tissue amoebicide. It is obtained from ipecacuanha, the powdered root of the Brazilian plant *Cephaelis ipecacuanha*, which was brought to Europe in 1658. Use of the purified alkaloid was introduced into medicine in 1912; it is now considered obsolete by most Western practitioners. Nevertheless, where appropriate nitroimidazoles are unavailable, as continues to be the case in many tropical contexts, this drug will continue to be life saving, especially when a parenteral drug is needed. Emetine hydrochloride is given by daily intramuscular or deep subcutaneous injection (1 mg/kg daily, maximum 60 mg) for a maximum of 10 days. The drug is cumulative and cardiotoxic, especially after the sixth day; electrocardiographic monitoring is recommended and bedrest is essential.

The synthetic derivative, racemic 2-dehydroemetine hydrochloride, was introduced in 1959. It is excreted more rapidly in the urine and appears to be less toxic; it is used at a daily dose of 1.25 mg/kg (maximum 90 mg).

CHLOROQUINE

This drug binds strongly to tissue protein, especially that of the liver. It continues to be a reserve drug in hepatic amoebiasis. It has very little amoebicidal activity in the gut wall and none within the gut lumen. The standard course of treatment in adults is chloroquine base, 150 mg four times daily for 2 days, followed by 150 mg twice daily for 19 days (paediatric dose 10 mg/kg daily). Side-effects are exceptional at this dosage, and unless the patient has been taking long-term chloroquine previously there is no risk of retinopathy.

ANTIMICROBIALS

Tetracycline, erythromycin, and the oral aminoglycoside paromomycin (aminosidine) have potential uses in amoebiasis. Besides their intentional use in therapy, their effects upon amoebic disease should not be overlooked in other contexts. Tetracycline was once widely used, orally or parenterally, in severe amoebic dysentery with or without bowel perforation; its activity is mainly indirect and a consequence of its antibacterial activity. Erythromycin has a greater direct amoebicidal action and can be used in non-severe invasive intestinal disease. It is very safe and is especially useful in infants and young children; it is a poor luminal amoebicide. Paromomycin can be used for mild invasive bowel disease, and as a luminal amoebicide.

DILOXANIDE FUROATE

This dichloroacetanilide derivative is marketed as Furamide; it has strong amoebicidal activity *in vitro*. Absorption from the gut is poor and side-effects are minimal, flatulence being the most significant. It is used only as a luminal amoebicide, the standard dosage in adults being 500 mg thrice daily for 10 days (paediatric dose, 20 mg/kg daily in three divided doses). Other drugs in this group are clefamide, quifamide, and etofamide.

DI-IODOHYDROXYQUIN

This 5-hydroxyquinoline compound is a luminal amoebicide; it has been very widely used—activity relates to its chelation of ferrous iron. Only about 5 per cent of an oral dose is absorbed. Side-effects are usually mild and include headache, nausea, rashes, and pruritus ani; they are partly attributable to iodine sensitivity. Very occasional cases of optic neuritis are reported. The usual dosage schedule in adults is 650 mg thrice daily for 20 days (paediatric dose, 30 mg/kg in three divided doses to a maximum of 2 g daily).

The related compound iodochlorhydroxyquine (Clioquinol) has been associated with subacute myelo-optic neuropathy in Japan, with a few cases elsewhere. Most instances resulted from prolonged, unsupervised use between 1967 and 1970; genetic factors may also be involved. There is no evidence that di-iodohydroxyquin (Diodoquin) causes this syndrome.

Patient management

INVASIVE INTESTINAL AMOEBIASIS

Metronidazole for 5 days will be the first choice in most patients. If follow-up stool examination cannot be done to assess parasitological cure, it is wise to extend treatment to 8 or 10 days; alternatively, a 5-day course of metronidazole can be followed by diloxanide.

Supportive management plays a major role in patients with complicated amoebic colitis, with emphasis on fluid and electrolyte replacement, gastric suction, and blood transfusion as necessary. Gut perforation in the context of extensive colitis carries a very poor prognosis; management may have to be medical. Parenteral metronidazole is invaluable in these contexts because of its activity against anaerobic bacteria in the peritoneum and blood stream. Gentamicin plus a cephalosporin will normally be given as well.

Amoebomas respond well to metronidazole; a slow response should arouse suspicion that the amoebic lesion is superimposed upon other pathology, particularly a carcinoma.

Surgical management is important in several situations. Acute colonic perforation in the absence of diffuse colitis, or ruptured amoebic appendicitis may be amenable to local repair. In the case of diffuse colitis, local repair, or end-to-end anastomosis, may not be possible because of the poor condition of the gut wall: temporary exteriorization with an ileostomy may be necessary. In fulminant colitis with multiple perforation the viability of the gut wall is uncertain and the only options may be medical management or total colectomy; in a few patients a more local excision, such as right hemicolectomy, may be possible.

When nitroimidazoles are contraindicated, or not available, then erythromycin is useful in non-severe colitis. If emetine is used then 5 days may be sufficient and the risks of cardiotoxicity will be minimized; it should be followed by diloxanide.

NON-INVASIVE CARRIER STATE

Convalescent carriers should always be treated as if they carry a pathogenic zymodeme; the same applies to family contacts of cases. Infections acquired in temperate countries, including those in male homosexuals or in institutional residents or staff, need not be treated unless there are grounds for suspecting that a pathogenic strain is involved. It continues to be wise to treat people infected with *E. histolytica* who come to temperate countries from the tropics, especially when gut symptoms are present.

Diloxanide is currently the drug of choice. Metronidazole is also effective, but an 8-day course may be necessary and side-effects troublesome; concurrent giardial infection is an indication for this drug. Unfortunately cure rates with tinidazole are very low when followed up at 1 month.

Alternatives are di-iodohydroxyquin and paromomycin.

HEPATIC AMOEBIASIS

Metronidazole or tinidazole are the drugs of choice; more data are available on the former and parenteral metronidazole can be used in patients who undergo laparotomy. A favourable response to medical treatment alone can be expected in about 85 per cent of patients. Liver abscesses may rupture before, during or after chemotherapy. Intra-abdominal rupture will always require laparotomy. Extension into the pleural or pericardial cavities necessitates drainage of these structures, together with aspiration of the liver lesion; pericardial drainage is most urgent when tamponade is present. Hepatopulmonary lesions generally require drainage of the liver lesion but medical treatment alone has been successful in some cases. Antimicrobials will always be needed when the abscess ruptures into the peritoneum or lung.

The most common management problem is slow response to the amoebicide. Patients whose pain and fever do not subside by 72 h are at significantly greater risk of rupture or therapeutic failure, and aspiration is generally to be recommended. A change to emetine plus chloroquine has been proposed in this context, but this is difficult to justify as clinically significant drug resistance has not yet been reported. A likely explanation of poor initial response is a tense lesion that restricts drug entry. Regular ultrasonographic monitoring is of great value in such patients as localization will indicate the risk of rupture and also guide the aspiration procedure. No change in lesion size on ultrasound can be expected during the first 2 weeks, although its outline may become clearer. Percutaneous aspiration with a wide-bore needle will be possible in most patients; if unsuccessful or anatomically contraindicated, then surgical help should be sought. Left-lobe lesions should be aspirated percutaneously only if they are superficial. Resolution of lesions on scans may take many months but is normally complete; the resolution time is difficult to predict and in small or moderate lesions it is apparently unaffected by aspiration.

The combination of emetine with chloroquine is as effective as metronidazole or tinidazole, and should be used when nitroimidazoles are not available. In non-critical situations, chloroquine alone can be used, although some would recommend therapy for 10 weeks in this circumstance.

Even though not detected, an infection of the gut lumen must always be assumed to be present and diloxanide given.

Therapeutic failures can occur with metronidazole or tinidazole. In some instances, hepatic reinvasion from the gut appears to be responsible; in others, poor drug entry into the lesion.

INVASIVE AMOEBIASIS AT OTHER SITES

Cutaneous and genital amoebiasis respond well to metronidazole, partly perhaps, because these lesions often contain anaerobic bacteria. Amoebiasis at other sites is nearly always secondary to hepatic lesions and the chemotherapy will be the same. Metronidazole crosses the blood–brain barrier and should be used in the desperate situation of amoebic brain abscess due to *E. histolytica*.

Prognosis

Uncomplicated invasive intestinal disease and uncomplicated hepatic amoebiasis should normally have a mortality rate of less than 1 per cent. In complicated disease the mortality is much greater and may reach 40 per cent for amoebic peritonitis with multiple gut perforation. Prognosis is usually better in centres where the disease is common and more likely to be recognized early. Late diagnosis increases the probability of complicated disease and mortality rises accordingly.

Unless parasitological cure is achieved, and the gut completely freed of *E. histolytica*, clinical relapse is quite common, especially when certain host factors, such as non-specific colitis, are present. There is so far no evidence of naturally occurring strains of *E. histolytica* resistant to normally used drugs. Hepatic scans show that nearly all liver abscesses completely disappear within 2 years; the median resolution time is 8 months. In secondarily infected lesions, bizarre hepatic calcification may be seen years afterwards. Healing of the bowel is remarkably rapid and complete; occasionally after severe dysentery, partial fibrous strictures persist.

Prevention

In less-developed countries the incidence of amoebiasis will fall as sanitary measures are introduced to combat other faeco-orally transmitted infections. Chlorination of water supplies does not destroy amoebic cysts, but adequate filtration will remove them. Regular stool screening of food handlers and domestic staffs is of questionable value because most detected infections will be non-pathogenic; health education is important with encouragement to have a medical check if diarrhoea occurs. Repeated mass chemotherapy with metronidazole or diloxanide has been used in Mexico and elsewhere where invasive disease is common; it may be justified in temperate countries when pathogenic strains enter a high-risk population—single-dose metronidazole, 2 g at monthly intervals, may be appropriate.

Visitors to the tropics should not attempt chemoprophylaxis; in particular, long-term unsupervised use of hydroxyquinoline drugs must be strongly deprecated. Simple hygienic measures provide considerable protection. Boiling water for 5 min kills cysts. Cooked foods should not be purchased from markets or street vendors, or from places where flies are prevalent. Fruit that can be peeled should be safe. Salad vegetables can be soaked in a dilute solution of sodium hypochlorite and then rinsed in boiled water. A weak solution of iodine is a more potent cysticide than chlorine.

In temperate countries, routine stool examinations are recommended for returning visitors from the tropics, and for new residents coming from such countries. In those with gut symptoms or a history of dysentery, several specimens should be examined and amoebic serology is helpful.

Naegleria fowleri infection

Biology and epidemiology

N. fowleri causes primary amoebic meningoencephalitis. It is an amoeboflagellate with two trophozoite forms in the free-living state; an amoeba that moves rapidly with a single pseudopodium, and a non-feeding, non-dividing flagellate with four to six flagella. Transformation to the latter occurs in water and hypotonic media and these free-swimming forms facilitate dispersal. Nearly all patients give a history of swimming or diving in warm fresh water, or spa water, between 2 and 14 days before the illness began. Several small common-source outbreaks have occurred, especially during warm summer months in temperate countries. Amoebic trophozoites are presumed to cross the human cribriform plate from the nasal mucosa to the olfactory bulbs and subarachnoid space, as they do experimentally in mice after nasal insufflation.

Pathology

The basic lesion is an acute necrotizing meningoencephalitis; at autopsy the brain is oedematous and there is a blood-stained purulent exudate in the subarachnoid space, especially within the basal cisterns. Areas of cerebral softening are located in the midbrain, pons, medulla, and inferior surfaces of the frontal lobes; the olfactory bulbs are grossly damaged. Microscopically, amoebae are seen at the advancing edge of the necrotic lesion and extending into healthy tissue, particularly along perivascular routes. Inflammatory reaction near the amoebae is minimal, but neutrophils often extend from the subarachnoid space into grey matter. The necrotic tissue shows petechial haemorrhages, demyelination, and neuronal degeneration. As a terminal event amoebae may disseminate throughout the body. Cysts are never formed in the tissues.

Clinical features and diagnosis

Nearly all patients have previously been in good health; many are young adults and children. Initially, nasal symptoms and headache are common but within a few days patients become seriously ill with fever, neck rigidity, coma, and later, convulsions; localizing neurological signs are uncommon. Many patients die within a few days of the onset of the meningitic illness but some have been kept alive for long periods on a ventilator. In some patients the nasal and faucial mucosa is oedematous and congested. Possibly some patients experience a mild, self-limiting illness.

Lumbar puncture reveals a purulent, turbid, and frequently blood-stained cerebrospinal fluid. The protein level is very high and the glucose generally low; neutrophils, red cells, and amoebae are seen on microscopy. Counts of several hundred amoebae per cubic millimetre are common but they may be mistaken for macrophages. When not seen initially, they must be urgently looked for in wet cerebrospinal-fluid specimens; phase-contrast microscopy is preferred and activity is greatest between 25 and 37 °C. Unless amoebae are seen, bacterial meningitis will be suspected; on Gram staining amoebae appear as indistinct smudges. Fixed preparations stained with iron haematoxylin will show full details of nuclear structure. Confirmation is by aerobic culture, at 37 and at 45 °C, on a confluent growth of *Escherichia coli* on an agar plate.

Although so far only about 200 cases have been documented since the first human case was reported in 1965, it is likely that some are missed. Some are discovered at autopsy, and at least three cases have been diagnosed retrospectively from preserved pathological material. Specific antisera can be raised in rabbits, and after incubation with tissue sections, the amoebae can be recognized with fluorescein-tagged antiglobulin.

Treatment

Amphotericin B is the only effective drug. It should be given by daily intravenous infusion, and intrathecally, with the dosage regimens used for cryptococcal meningitis. So far, very few patients have survived but this may partly be due to diagnostic delays. Drugs used for *E. histolytica* are of no value in this condition. Miconazole and other imidazoles are active against this organism *in vitro* and could be tried in humans.

Acanthamoeba infections

Biology and epidemiology

Most human cases have shown either a granulomatous amoebic encephalitis, or an amoebic keratitis. These soil amoebae have no flagellate form; the pseudopodia are called acanthopodia, being multiple, small and thin. Cysts are thick walled, angulated and buoyant; their dispersal may be wind-borne. Man becomes infected by swallowing or inhaling cysts or amoebae, or they may contaminate wounds or corneal abrasions.

Acanthamoeba species are sometimes isolated from throat or nasal swabs. They may also be cultured from stool specimens, the cysts having passed harmlessly through the gut. Because clinically evident infections occur mainly in predisposed persons, Acanthamoeba should be regarded as an opportunistic parasite as well as a facultative one.

Pathology, clinical features, and diagnosis

Lesions are granulomatous, and progress slowly unless a body space such as the subarachnoid or aqueous humour is reached. Some patients have a local predisposing lesion, such as craniofacial trauma or vascular brain infarct. Others have a systemic disorder such as lymphoma, other malignancy, or diabetes mellitus; relatively acute cerebral lesions are described in a few patients with AIDS. Cerebral lesions arise by haematogenous spread or by direct spread from adjacent cranial tissues; clinically and pathologically they resemble chronic bacterial brain abscesses. Primary lesions have been described from the lung, orbit, scalp and underlying skull, maxillary sinuses, middle ear, and the gastric wall. A few patients are infected from the nasal mucosa in a manner identical to that of Naegleria.

Corneal lesions present as indolent ulcers unresponsive to antibiotics or corticosteroids. Infection may be by wind-borne cysts upon a damaged epithelium or from contact lenses. Solutions used to store, or wash, lenses can be contaminated by these amoebae, many of which are resistant to some antiseptics, especially as cysts.

Unless these amoebae are found in wet preparations from corneal lesions, or in cerebrospinal fluid, the diagnosis of the diverse pathology caused by these organisms will be based upon histological examination. Cysts may be seen in tissue, but trophozoites may be missed unless stained with iron haematoxylin to show the large central endosome. Indirect immunofluorescence, using specific antisera, can also be used to locate amoebae in tissue and establish their specific identity. Cultural diagnosis from fresh biopsy material is as for Naegleria. Most non-ocular infections appear to be due to *A. culbertsoni*, but corneal lesions are usually due to *A. polyphaga*. Serodiagnosis may help in diagnosis, but low titres occur in some normal persons.

Recently, meningoencephalitic infections with leptomyxid amoebae have been described with a pathology, including antecedent skin lesions, similar to that of Acanthamoeba; reports are from Latin America, Canada, and Australia.

Treatment and prevention

The *in vitro* drug sensitivities of isolates differ greatly and should be urgently tested; a wide spectrum of resistance is common. Amphotericin B or flucytosine will be the initial choice for systemic use. Eye lesions have sometimes responded to local propamidine and neomycin, but the latter is not cysticidal; combinations of topical propamidine with chlorhexidine or polyhexamethylene have recently been successful. Corneal grafting may be necessary.

Wearers of contact lenses must take especial care to avoid contamination especially when storage cases are used; raw tap water may contain Acanthamoeba. The most appropriate disinfectants are chlorhexidine and hydrogen peroxide.

REFERENCES

Gut amoebae

Ahmed, L., Salama, Z.A., El Rooby, A., and Strickland, G.T. (1989). Ultrasonographic resolution time for amebic liver abscess. *American Journal of Tropical Medicine and Hygiene*, **41,** 406–10.

Allason-Jones, E., Mindel, A., Sargeaunt, P.G., and Williams, P. (1986). *Entamoeba histolytica* as a commensal parasite in homosexual men. *New England Journal of Medicine*, **315,** 353–6.

Barnes, P.F., De Cock, K., Reynolds, T.N., and Ralls, P.W. (1987). A comparison of amebic and pyogenic abscess of the liver. *Medicine*, **66,** 472–83.

Diamond, L.S. and Clark, C. G. (1993). A redescription of *Entamoeba histolytica* Schandinn, 1903 (emended Walker 1911) separating it from *Entamoeba dispar* Brumpt, 1925. *Journal of Eukaryote Microbiology,* **40,** 340–4.

Freeman, O., Akamaguna, A., and Jarikre, L.N. (1990). Amoebic liver abscess: effect of aspiration on the resolution or healing time. *Annals of Tropical Medicine and Parasitology*, **84,** 281–7.

Irusen, E.M., Jackson, T.F.H.G., and Sinjee, A.E. (1992). Asymptomatic intestinal colonization by pathogenic *Entamoeba histolytica* in amoebic liver abscess prevalence response to therapy and pathogenic potential. *Clinical Infectious Diseases,* **14,** 889–93.

Luaces, A.L., Osono, L.M., and Barrett, A.J. (1993) A new test for infection by *Entamoeba histolytica. Parasitology Today,* **9,** 69–71.

Martinez-Palomo, A. (ed.) (1986). *Amoebiasis*. Elsevier, New York.

Ravdin, J.I. (ed.) (1988). *Amebiasis. Human infection by* Entamoeba histolytica. Wiley, New York.

Ravdin, J.I. (1989). Amebiasis now. *American Journal of Tropical Medicine and Hygiene*, **41,** (suppl.), 40–8.

Ravdin, J.I. (1994). Diagnosis of invasive amoebiasis—time to end the morphology era. *Gut,* **35,** 1018–21.

Sargeaunt, P.G. (1987). The reliability of *Entamoeba histolytica* zymodemes in clinical diagnosis. *Parasitology Today*, **3,** 40–4 and 156.

Seal, D.V. (1994). *Acanthamoeba keratitis. British Medical Journal,* **308,** 1116–7.

Sharma, M.P., Rai, R.R., Acharya, S.K., Ray, J.C., and Tandon, B.N. (1989). Needle aspiration of amoebic liver abscess. *British Medical Journal*, **299,** 1308–9.

Spencer, M.J., Garcia, L.S., and Chapin, M.R. (1979). *Dientamoeba fragilis.* An intestinal pathogen in children? *American Journal of Diseases of Childhood*, **133,** 390–3.

Thompson, J.E., Forlenza, S., and Verma, R. (1985). Amebic liver abscess: a therapeutic approach. *Reviews of Infectious Diseases*, **7,** 171–9.

Walsh, J.A. (1986). Problems in the recognition and diagnosis of amoebasis:

estimation of the global magnitude of morbidity and mortality. *Reviews of Infectious Diseases*, **8,** 228–38.

Yang, J. and Scholten, T. (1977). *Dientamoeba fragilis*: a review with notes on its epidemiology, pathogenicity, mode of transmission, and diagnosis. *American Journal of Tropical Medicine and Hygiene*, **26,** 16–22.

Free-living amoebae

Carter, R.F. (1972). Primary amoebic meningo-encephalitis. *Transactions of the Royal Society of Tropical Medicine and Hygiene*, **66,** 193–208.

Martinez, A.J. (1985). *Free-living amoebas: natural history, prevention, diagnosis, pathology and treatment of disease*. CRC Press, Boca Raton, FA.

Seal, D.V. (1994). Acanthamoeba keratitis. *British Medical Journal*, **308,** 1116–7.

Taratuto, A.L., Monges, J., Acefe, J.C., Meli, F., Paredes, A., and Martinez, A.J. (1991). Leptomyxid amoeba encephalitis: report of the first case in Argentina. *Transactions of the Royal Society of Tropical Medicine and Hygiene*, **85,** 77.

Warhurst, D.C. (1985). Pathogenic free-living amoebae. *Parasitology Today*, **1,** 24–8.

Wiley, C.A. *et al.* (1987). *Acanthamoeba* meningoencephalitis in a patient with AIDS. *Journal of Infectious Diseases*, **155,** 130–3.

7.13.2 Malaria

D. Bradley, C.I. Newbold, and D.A. Warrell

Introduction

Malaria remains the most important human parasitic disease globally, causing over 170 million clinical cases annually, of whom over a million die, mostly in Africa. It has had large effects on the course of history and settlement in tropical regions, and it is currently responsible for the loss of some 35 million disability-adjusted life years each year, about 2.6 per cent of the total disease burden of the world. In recent years malaria has been subject to massive control efforts, with varying degrees of success, and the disease has been resurgent for the last two decades. The recent history of health care in the Third World can only be understood in the light of malaria eradication programmes. The nomination of malaria as the pre-eminent tropical disease is thus well deserved, and the problems of both treatment and control today are more complex and intractable then ever before.

Parasitology

Whereas there are over a hundred species of malarial parasite *(Plasmodium),* there are only four species that have man as their natural vertebrate host. These are *P. falciparum, P. malariae, P. vivax, and P. ovale.* In addition, rare zoonotic infections have been recorded from non-human primate malarias such as *P. knowlesi, P. simium,* and *P. cynomolgi.*

Each of the human malarias has biological, morphological, and clinical characteristics (Table 1) that distinguish them from each other. Despite these differences, the overall biology of the life cycle is similar for the various species. This is summarized schematically in Fig. 1.

In both the mosquito and mammalian hosts the life cycle of *Plasmodium* spp. can be seen to consist alternately of invasive stages and stages capable of intracellular asexual division. There is also a sexual stage of the life cycle, which, by facilitating the exchange of genetic information between different parasite strains or genotypes, assists in the generation of genetic diversity within the parasitic population.

Infection is initiated when sporozoites from the salivary glands of a female *Anopheles* mosquito are inoculated during a blood meal into the human bloodstream. How these organisms target and invade hepatic parenchymal cells is still unclear. The process is extremely rapid, probably starting within a few minutes and being largely complete within 30 min. Entry into the hepatocyte may be direct or may possibly occur after passage of the parasite through Kuppfer cells. Once inside the liver cell, two alternative pathways of differentiation are possible.

In all species the parasites initiate a round of intracellular asexual multiplication. However, in addition, in *P. vivax* and *P. ovale* infections a proportion of them enter a cryptobiotic phase in which they are termed hypnozoites. These may lie dormant for months or even years before starting to divide and giving rise to the late relapses characteristic of infections with these species. In *P. falciparum* and *P. malariae* infections there is no cryptobiotic phase and so relapses from the liver do not occur. Nevertheless, both of these infections are of a chronic nature and, if untreated, blood infections may persist for a few years in the case of *P. falciparum* or decades in the case of *P. malariae.*

Once initiated, the time required to complete the intrahepatic multiplication is again dependent on the parasite species (Table 1). The products of the liver stage (the extraerythrocytic merozoites) are liberated in their thousands from each parenchymal cell into the bloodstream. Here they attach to and invade circulating erythrocytes. Inside the erythrocyte, asexual division begins and, over a period of 48 h *(P. falciparum, P. vivax, P. ovale)* or 72 *(P. malariae),* the parasites develop through a well-defined series of morphological changes from 'ring' forms to trophozoites and finally to schizonts containing daughter erythrocytic merozoites. These are liberated by red-cell lysis and immediately invade uninfected erythrocytes producing a repetitive cycle of invasion and multiplication. Because the intraerythrocytic division cycle is, in general, fairly synchronous (particularly in *P. vivax* and *P. ovale* infections) and also tied to the diurnal cycle of the host, red-cell lysis and merozoite release occur at approximately the same time of day for the duration of the infection for a given individual. Some of the components of the infected cell that are released at this time induce the release of cytokines such as tumour necrosis factor and interleukin 1, which give rise to the periodic 'agues' that have long been a diagnostic feature of malaria infection. The asexual blood forms are, in fact, the only forms of the parasite that give rise to clinical symptoms.

A small proportion of the merozoites within red cells can undergo a different pathway of development into male and female gametocytes. The development and morphology of these sexual stages is another feature that varies considerably between different parasite species. Once fully matured, the gametocytes may return to the mosquito if ingested during a blood meal.

Inside the mosquito's midgut, male and female gametes are liberated from their host red cells and fuse to form a zygote. This develops into an ookinete, which is able to penetrate the gut wall and form an oocyst. At this point a further series of asexual divisions takes place, giving rise to sporozoites that migrate to the insect salivary glands and thus complete the life cycle.

Genetics of the parasite

For technical reasons the performance and analysis of a single cross takes several months and so the available classical genetic data are extremely limited. In order to carry out genetic analysis, the first requirement is the availability of genetically homogeneous (i.e. cloned) material. The necessity of establishing clones of parasites has revealed the tremendous diversity that exists in populations of organisms in the wild. Variation has been found in isoenzyme types, in antigenic markers, in drug-resistance markers, and also in the virulence of different isolates. Such genetic diversity has an important bearing on the disease, for an individual infection may consist of different parasite genotypes of varying drug resistance. It is also relevant when considering the variety of antigenic types that a human host may need to experience before becoming clinically immune. The first major conclusion from genetic analysis

Table 1 *Developmental characteristics of human malaria parasites*

Species	*P. falciparum*	*P. vivax*	*P. ovale*	*P. malariae*
Prepatent period[a]	8–25 days	8–27 days	9–17 days	15–30 days
Length of asexual erythrocytic cycle	48 h	48 h	48 h	72 h
Red cells parasitized	All	Reticulocytes	Reticulocytes	Mature erythrocytes
Merozoites per schizont	8–32	12–24	4–16	6–12
Relapse from persistent liver infection	No	Yes	Yes	No, but persistent red-cell infection up to 30 years
Drug resistance	Yes	Yes	No	No

[a]Time from infective mosquito bite to appearance of parasites in the blood.

of *Plasmodium* spp. was that during the intraerythrocytic cycle in the blood, the parasites were haploid. The diploid phase of the life cycle occurs after gamete fusion in the mosquito and meiosis takes place in the invertebrate host. Following this observation, crosses have been done using isoenzyme, drug-resistance, and antigenic markers in both rodent malarias and using *P. falciparum in vitro.*

Detailed studies of the segregation of resistance to chloroquine and pyrimethamine first demonstrated that genes for these phenotypes segregated in typically Mendelian fashion consistent with mutations at unlinked loci. However, in the case of resistance to chloroquine alone, some evidence was obtained that multiple mutations at independent loci may give rise to resistance and that in some cases resistance was stable in the absence of drug pressure. More recently, analysis of crosses between chloroquine sensitive and resistant clones of *P. falciparum* have resulted in the identification of a locus, on chromosome 7, that segregates with the resistant phenotype, but the genetics of chloroquine resistance is still the subject of lively debate.

The difficulty in making large numbers of crosses has meant that most of the genetic data have been obtained with molecular biological rather than genetic techniques. Pulsed-field gel electrophoresis has shown that

Fig. 1 Development cycle of Plasmodium (redrawn by permission of F. Hoffman-la-Roche Ltd, Basel).

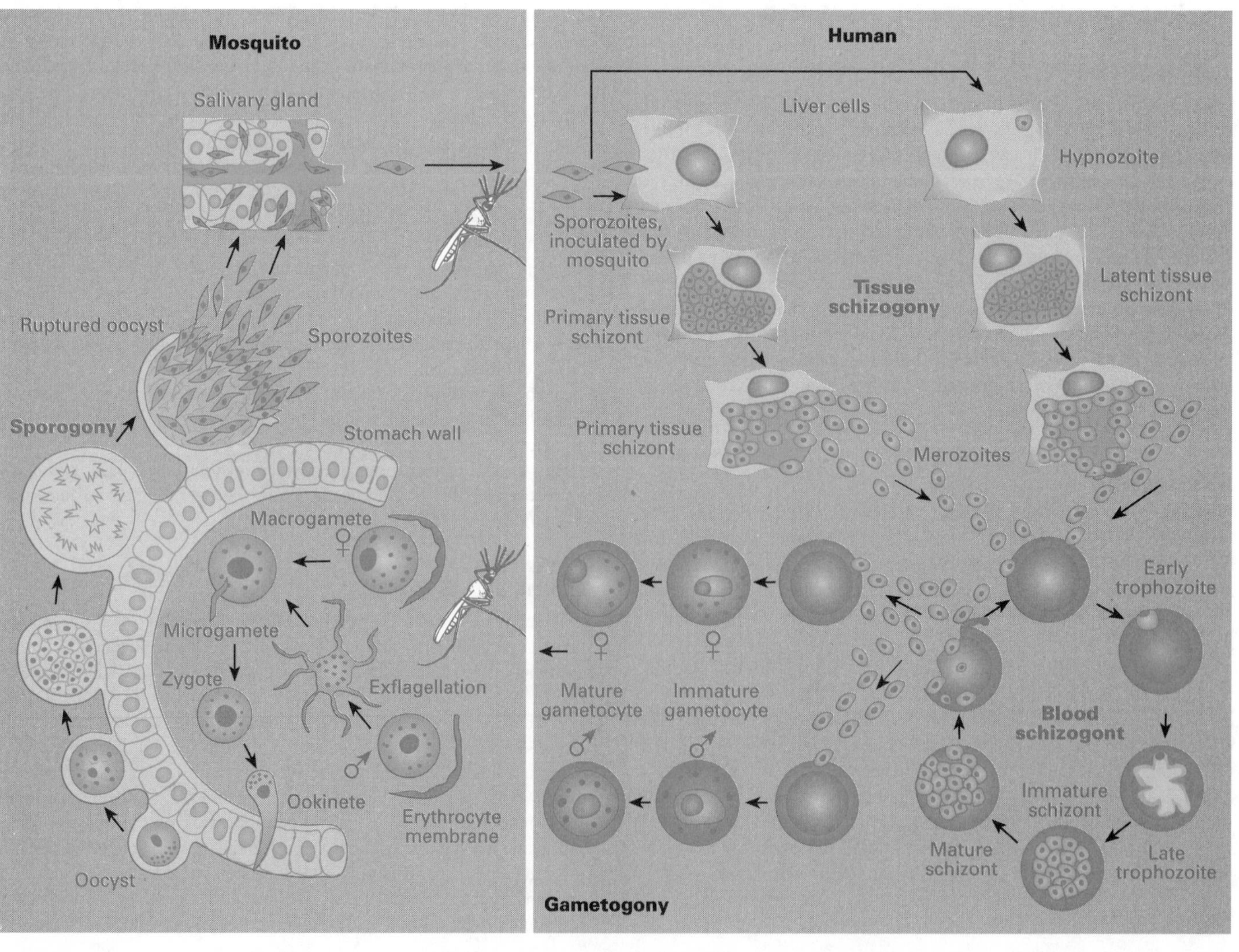

the parasite has 14 chromosomes, which can be uniquely identified by the presence of a number of defined markers on each. The central regions of the chromosomes are stable but the telomeric and subtelomeric regions diversify rapidly, giving rise to large size differences in homologous chromosomes from different isolates. Genes close to these regions can undergo partial or complete deletion in cultured parasites but as some of these genes appear to be essential for growth *in vivo,* these aberrant genotypes are not found in field isolates.

Biochemistry

Although the biochemistry of the asexual intraerythrocytic stages of mammalian malarias has not been studied in great detail, some of the features of the metabolic biochemistry of human malarias appear to be of clinical significance and these will be discussed below.

GENERAL BIOCHEMISTRY

Energy metabolism

As they appear to lack a complete citric-acid cycle, parasitized erythrocytes are unable to oxidize glucose completely. They do, however, accumulate greatly increased amounts of glucose compared to uninfected control red cells. This increased glucose uptake is associated with both increased transport and metabolism. Incomplete oxidation of glucose results in the secretion of large amounts of lactate, particularly towards the end of the asexual cycle. This may have some relevance to the pathology of acute infection.

One area of the biochemistry of the human malarias that was, for many years, controversial is the presence or absence of a parasite-specific glucose-6-phosphate dehydrogenase **(G6PD).** This question relates not only to parasite metabolism but also to the observed epidemiological correlation between host G6PD deficiency and malarial endemicity. It is now clear that *P. falciparum* has the capacity to synthesize its own G6PD but it seems that the enzyme is only induced in G6PD-deficient red cells. Because induction is reported to take place over a few cycles of growth, this has generated a hypothesis to explain the observation that heterozygote females may be the main protected group. G6PD is located on the X chromosome so that parasite growth in deficient males or homozygous females can be supported by the induced parasite enzyme. As heterozygote females are genetic mosaics as a result of X inactivation, parasites spend half of their time in normal cells and half in deficient cells. Induction of the parasite enzyme is thus incomplete and parasite growth is adversely affected.

Nucleotide metabolism

Despite their lack of a complete citric-acid cycle, parasites do consume low levels of oxygen and posses small amounts of cytochromes. This is due in part to the oxidation of dihydroorotate to orotate during the biosynthesis of pyrimidines. Parasites are able to synthesize pyrimidines *de novo* but require an exogenous source of purines, which they are able to metabolize via salvage pathways to generate precursors for nucleic acid synthesis. This pathway is the target of a new class of antimalarial drug, the hydroxynaphthoquinones, currently being evaluated in clinical trials.

Because the parasites rely on the *de novo* synthesis of folic acid for their supply of folates, they are susceptible to inhibitors of folate biosynthesis such as the sulphonamides. These have consequently been used as antimalarial drugs. The parasite dihydrofolate reductase is an additional target for malaria chemotherapy because the enzyme has a much higher substrate affinity than its host counterpart. Inhibition of this enzyme indirectly blocks DNA synthesis by blocking the recycling of dihydrofolate to tetrahydrofolate and hence preventing the methylation of uridine to produce thymidine. Appropriate doses of drugs such as pyrimethamine are, therefore, far more inhibitory to the parasite dihydrofolate reductase than to the human enzyme.

Lipid metabolism

The parasitized erythrocyte has an increased ratio of phospholipid to cholesterol and elevated amounts of saturated fatty acids. There is no evidence for *de novo* fatty acid biosynthesis in malarial parasites, so these changes must arise from selective accumulation and modification of lipids derived from the host. Severe or moderate infections with *P. falciparum* also lead to significantly elevated plasma lipid concentrations in the host.

Molecular biology

Despite the advances in *in vitro* culture and so in the means to purify specific parasite proteins, the quantities of material involved are extremely small. The most straightforward way to overcome this problem and rapidly to obtain primary-sequence data from malarial polypeptides of interest is to clone and sequence the relevant genes. Most of the data available have been obtained on clones selected by their reaction either with immune sera or with defined monoclonal antibodies. There are two particularly striking observations that result from these approaches. First, DNA from *P. falciparum* has proved to have an unusual base composition with an average A + T content of approximately 80 per cent. This is slightly lower in coding sequence and higher in the intergenic regions. One result of this is an abnormal codon usage, heavily biased to those codons containing A and T. Secondly, a very high proportion of genes studied are characterized by the presence of large blocks of tandemly repeated amino acid sequences. The fact that these repeat structures are found in some 'housekeeping genes' as well as in most genes identified by antibody screening suggests that they reflect a fundamental process specific to these organisms. It has been proposed, as yet without any direct supporting evidence, that these sequences may act as immunological decoys. The only convincing explanations offered for such a hypothesis are that they may act as T-independent antigens, or that the presence of multiple, low-affinity cross-reactivities between different repeats serves to prevent the affinity maturation of specific B cells. The repeat sequences themselves frequently show great diversity between different parasite isolates, making it unlikely that they have a structural role.

Comparison of rRNA sequences of different species of *Plasmodium* somewhat surprisingly shows that *P. falciparum* is more closely related to avian malarias than to other mammalian species. Sequence data from extrachromosomal elements suggest that these circular DNA molecules may be of plant rather than animal origin.

PROTEINS/ANTIGENS

Many of the genes cloned to date have been expressed in a variety of bacterial, viral, or eukaryotic expression systems. The proteins (or defined fragments of them) have been used mainly in immunochemical or vaccination studies. This is discussed in more detail below. As a result of their original identification with antibody, structure/function information for these proteins is relatively sparse. A small number of enzymes have been cloned and these in general show conservation of sequence in the important functional regions.

Considerable interest has been focused on molecules expressed on the surface of the different lifecycle stages. The surface proteins of sporozoite and sexual stages are dealt with in the section on vaccination. In the asexual stages, molecules expressed on the surface of the merozoite, the invasive free-living form, and on the surface of infected red cells have attracted particular interest. Several merozoite surface proteins have been identified, cloned, and sequenced; at least some of these appear to be involved in the process of invasion of new erythrocytes. Other proteins have been implicated in invasion by virtue of their ability to bind specifically to the surface of normal red cells, but not to cells rendered refractory to invasion. Because red-cell invasion is an essential step in asexual parasite multiplication, understanding the molecular basis of it could lead to new forms of therapy.

Molecules on the surface of the infected red cell have been studied because of their involvement in the adherence of infected cells to vascular endothelium and because they appear to be a target of the protective immune response. Biochemical, immunochemical, and cell biological data reveal that a family of high molecular-weight molecules undergo a process of rapid, clonal, antigenic variation. The genes for this group of proteins (PFEMP), have recently been cloned.

Many other parasite-derived proteins are secreted into the host red cell, but do not find their way to the cell surface. Some of these interact specifically with the red-cell cytoskeleton and so are presumably important in modifying the host-cell environment in favour of the parasite.

In vitro culture

Since 1975 it has been possible to grow asexual forms of *P. falciparum* in long-term culture. All that is required is to incubate parasitized erythrocytes in a suitable growth medium with uninfected red cells in an atmosphere of low oxygen and high carbon dioxide tension. Such cultures can be maintained indefinitely, provided that parasites are removed and fresh erythrocytes added at appropriate intervals. The availability of large numbers of *P. falciparum* parasites without recourse to patients or experimental non-human primates has speeded up considerably much of the basic research on malaria and also permitted the development of *in vitro* tests for sensitivity to certain antimalarial drugs. Cultured parasites can also be used as a source of blood films or crude antigen for antimalarial antibody screening tests, which may be used epidemiologically or for screening blood donors for potential activity. More recently it has been reported that the complete development of the hepatic stage of *P. falciparum* has been achieved *in vitro*. As gametocytes can also be produced from *in vitro* culture of asexual blood forms, all of the parasite stages that grow in man can now be cultured in the laboratory. This important development allows the direct study of intrahepatic parasites both from an immunological standpoint and for the development of new drugs against this stage.

The other human malarias have not yet been maintained successfully in long-term culture.

Biology of the mosquito vector

Human malarial parasites are transmitted by a single mosquito genus, Anopheles, but there are many species and these vary in their habits and breeding places, and in their effectiveness as malaria vectors. Detailed identification is a specialist matter, but Anopheles can be distinguished from other mosquitoes in the adult stage by the way that the female, when taking a blood feed, inclines her whole body at an angle to her victim while the other, culicine, mosquitoes have the body parallel to the skin surface (Fig. 2). In the larval stages, the anopheline larva has a small breathing siphon and its body rests parallel to the surface film, whereas that of the culicine hangs downwards from the tip of its longer siphon, which ends at the surface film (Fig. 3).

The female Anopheles needs a blood meal before egg laying so that adult life consists of finding a suitable blood meal, resting while it is digested, flying off to lay eggs at a suitable water body, and then repeating this cycle every few days. The eggs, larvae, and pupae develop in water and the winged adults emerge. There are around 400 species in the genus Anopheles, but only a limited number will be present in any region. Moreover, only a few species in a given locality are likely to be important malaria vectors, for ecological reasons, because to transmit malaria the mosquitoes need to be sufficiently abundant, to bite people rather than only some other vertebrate host, and to live long enough for ingested gametocytes to develop through to sporozoites. Identification of the main vector species in an area is the basis for the design of specific control measures. Most anophelines are selective in their breeding sites, so knowledge of the larval ecology permits engineering and other measures to be directed at selective removal of the vector habitat, a process called 'species sanitation'.

The behaviour of the adult mosquito will dictate which insecticidal strategies are most likely to succeed. Anophelines vary in their preferred feeding and resting locations, though the majority bite in the evening and night. They may bite indoors (endophagic) or outside (exophagic). This determines whether the use of bednets and screened doors and windows will protect, or whether long sleeves and protective footwear when outside the house are more relevant. Of greater importance is where the female rests overnight to digest the blood meal. Endophilic mosquitoes, which rest on the inside walls of houses and in the roof, are thereby exposed to residual insecticides previously sprayed on the walls, whereas exophilic mosquitoes, resting outside houses, may escape the effects of insecticidal attack. The success of many antimalarial efforts has depended on the major vectors in several continents being endophilic, and failures of attempted eradication have sometimes resulted from exophilic vector species being present, as in many forested areas of South-East Asia. Anopheline mosquitoes extend into temperate countries, and in the United Kingdom several species exist capable of transmitting some imported malaria strains.

Epidemiology

Malaria is widely distributed throughout the tropics (Fig. 4) except for the south-central Pacific islands. *P. falciparum* is the predominant species in the highly endemic areas of Africa, New Guinea, and Haiti, while *P. vivax* is more common in Central America, North Africa, and southern and western Asia. Both species are prevalent in South America, the rest of Asia, and Oceania. *P. malariae* is widespread but often overlooked, and in West Africa *P. ovale* largely replaces *P. vivax,* to which the indigenous inhabitants are resistant.

The epidemiological features of human malaria differ markedly even between endemic areas. At one extreme, as in West Africa, everyone is infected shortly after birth, parasitaemia is almost universal throughout childhood, and the brunt of mortality falls in early childhood; epidemics do not occur. By contrast, as in parts of North India, malaria is an epidemic disease affecting all ages and causing temporary dislocation of community life due to the concurrent illness of the people. These

Fig. 2 Feeding posture of different types of adult mosquito. (a) Culicine, (b) Anopheline.

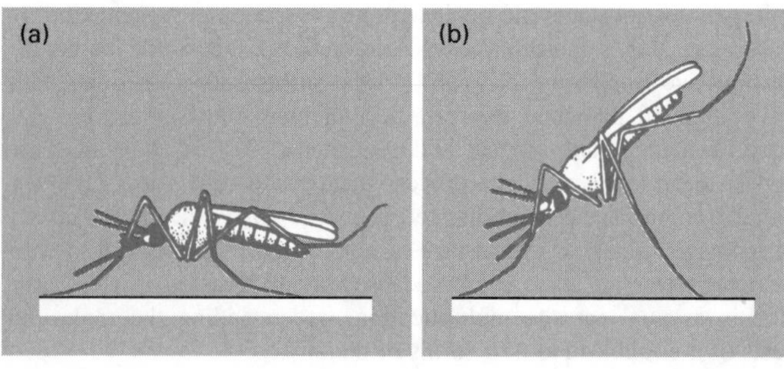

Fig. 3 Resting posture of different types of mosquito larva. (a) Culicine, (b) Anopheline.

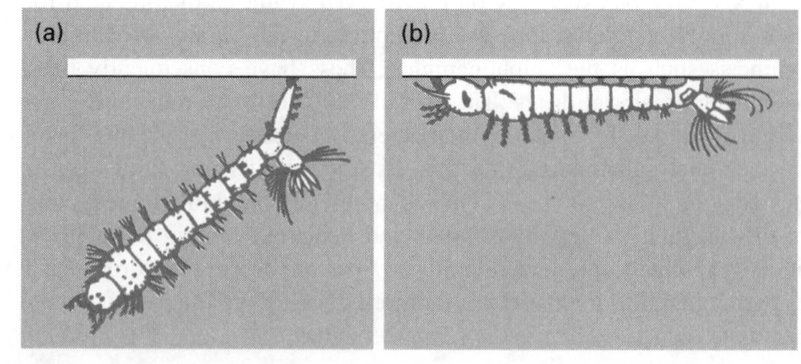

differences result from differing levels of malaria transmission affecting the pattern of immunity in the human population, so that to understand even the clinical spectrum of malaria seen in patients from a given locality it is essential to understand the local epidemiological situation. The epidemiology of malaria is complex but relatively well understood. Attempts at control in recent years have changed the epidemiological pattern in many areas.

Climate and mosquito ecology are the primary determinants of malarial epidemiology. Once the biology of the relevant mosquito is understood, much of the complex epidemiology of malaria falls into place. Transmission of the parasites is, as described earlier, by bite of the female anopheline mosquito. There is some variation in susceptibility to malaria within the anophelines, so that *P. falciparum* from Africa may fail to develop in some European anophelines even under optimal conditions, but usually in a given locality the indigenous anopheline mosquitoes will be capable of transmitting the local malaria strains, so that variation in the importance of species as vectors depends mainly on their behaviour and ecology.

Three characteristics mainly determine the differences in epidemiology that are seen. They are the density, man-biting habit, and longevity of the mosquito. Density is the number of vectors present in a place relative to the human population. Malaria transmission will tend to be proportional to mosquito density, as might be expected. The man-biting habit combines two features: the frequency with which the female mosquito feeds and the choice of host. A mosquito that feeds frequently will clearly have a greater chance both of picking up and passing on the parasite, while a mosquito that feeds, as many do, on animals other than man, will be less able to transmit human malaria: only meals taken from people are relevant to transmission. The man-biting frequency may be as high as 0.5/day in *A. gambiae,* an African mosquito that feeds on alternate days and preferentially on people; while *A. culicifacies,* a vector in South Asia, may feed only every third day and as few as 10 per cent of its meals may be from people, giving a man-biting habit of 0.033/day. Because malaria transmission is proportional to the square of the man-biting habit, as transmission involves both parasite uptake by bite and subsequent inoculation to man by a second bite, this factor has a large effect on malaria transmission.

Mosquito longevity has an even greater effect. The duration of the extrinsic cycle, that is the interval between a mosquito ingesting infective gametocytes and the first day on which sporozoites are present in the salivary glands ready for transmission, depends on the ambient temperature as shown in Fig. 5, but will rarely be less than 10 days. Thus, only mosquitoes that become infected and then survive for longer than the duration of the extrinsic cycle (say 10 days) can pass on the infection. As mosquitoes of a given species have a relatively constant probability of dying during a day, regardless of age, the longevity may be described by the probability of surviving through one day, and it varies greatly between mosquito species and environments. It will affect transmission very greatly indeed: if the chance of survival through one day is p and the duration of the extrinsic cycle n days, then transmission is proportional to p^n, that is, something like the tenth power of p. Thus the most effective transmission of malaria will be by a long-lived mosquito that occurs at high density and frequently bites people. *A. gambiae* and its sister species *A. arabiensis* best fit this description and are the predominant African malaria vectors.

Malaria transmission is most conveniently measured in terms of the basic case reproduction rate **(BCRR).** This is the average number of new cases of malaria that will result from one human case of malaria in a place, assuming all the other people are non-immune and uninfected. The BCRR may vary from over 1000 in some areas of Africa to below 1. Where the BCRR is less than 1, the infection will not replace itself and the disease will die out. In the 'real world,' the BCRR will vary

Fig. 4 Malarious areas of the world. Epidemiological assessment of the status of malaria, 1991 (WHO 93 460) (reproduced, by permission of the World Health Organization, from World Malaria Situation in 1991. *Weekly Epidemiological Record* (1993). **68,** 246).

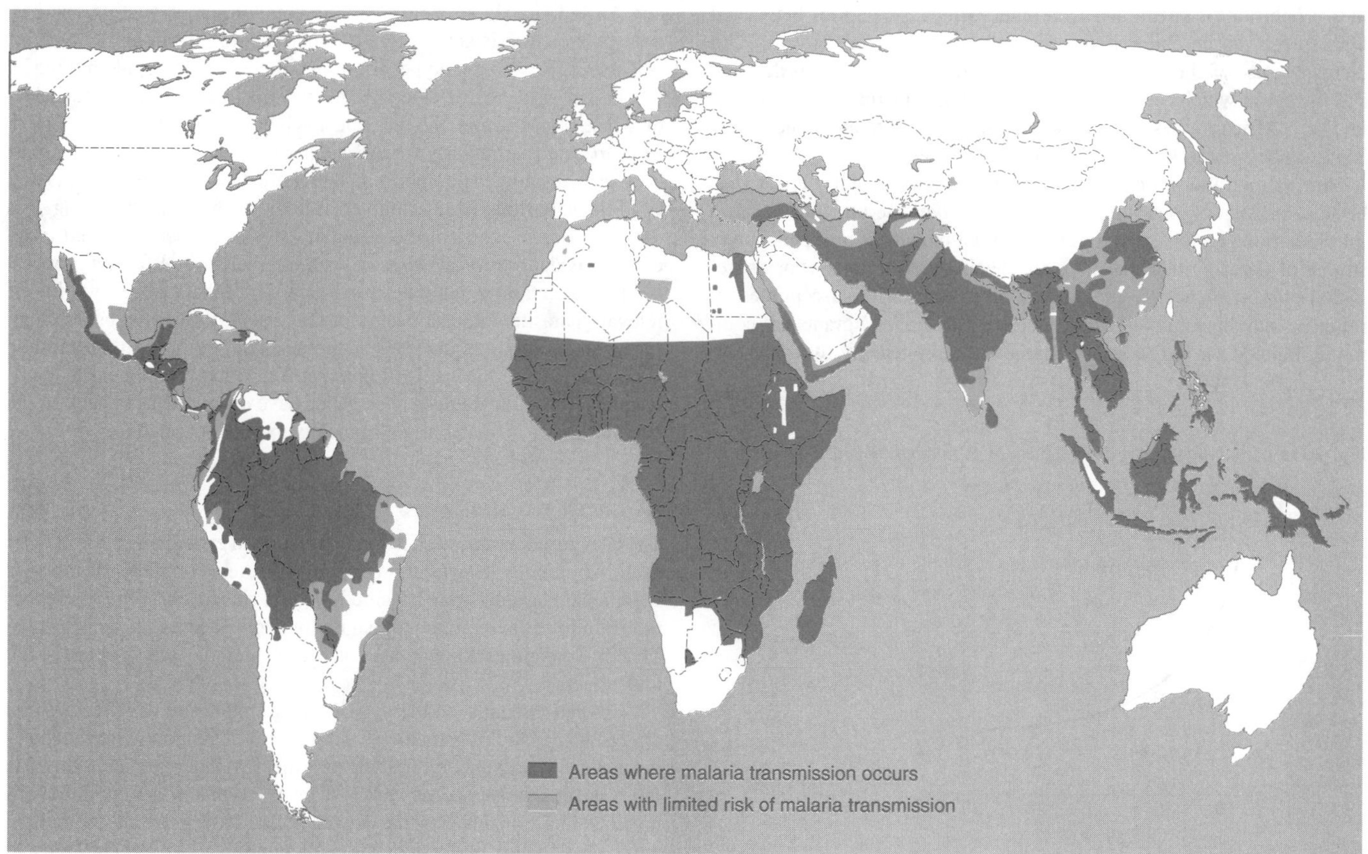

considerably about a mean value. In areas with a very high BCRR everyone will become infected, the variation will be immaterial, and the amount of malaria seen will be determined by acquired human immunity. This is the situation called stable malaria (Table 2) and is seen in subSaharan Africa and New Guinea particularly. Because the BCRR is so high, control methods aiming to break transmission have to reduce it by a factor of perhaps 1000 to bring the BCRR below 1. By contrast, in places where the BCRR is, say, 3, natural variations will cause the BCRR to be below 1 for much of the time. There will be intermittent periods of transmission, and epidemics will occur from time to time. This is called unstable malaria. Because human immunity will be much less, people of all ages will get ill during the epidemics, but the transmission will be much easier to control. Unstable malaria is dramatically evident but kills fewer people than stable malaria, in which the brunt of the mortality falls on young children.

Even in stable malaria, seasonal variation may occur. In the African savannah, no mosquitoes may bite during the hot dry season and in more temperate zones it may be too cold for transmission for part of the year, but the annual peaks will be comparable, with all children infected each year. While the division between stable and unstable malaria is the most useful (Table 2), an earlier classification of areas by the parasite prevalence in children or by the proportion of children aged 2 to 9 years with enlarged spleens is often still used (Table 3). The prevalence of splenic enlargement gives a better cumulative picture of the amount of malaria than does the parasite prevalence, which is influenced by casual chemotherapy.

Under endemic conditions there is still a great deal of variation in risk to a non-immune visitor. At one extreme, in rural Tanzania an unprotected person is likely to be bitten on average by more than one infective mosquito nightly, whilst in a highly malarious part of India the corresponding rate is perhaps five times yearly or less. Yet both will be perceived as highly malarious places by the local inhabitants.

The epidemiological background to clinical malaria is never again likely to be steady. The widespread availability of chloroquine and other effective chemotherapy in endemic areas has resulted in early treatment of a proportion of infections. This often leads to disparities between a high spleen rate in children and an artificially low parasite rate. With increasing use of chemotherapy, the acquisition of immunity is deferred and the age at which cerebral malaria is seen may increase; for example, in West African areas of intense transmission, cerebral malaria has begun to be seen in late childhood in urban areas.

Human migration is commonly associated with malaria epidemics, because population pressure in hilly areas drives the inhabitants down into malarious regions, or migrants between malarious areas encounter strains of parasite to which they are incompletely immune, or aggregation of workers at new sites mixes the infected with susceptibles, or refugees may have impaired resistance to infection. Migrants are commonly blamed for introducing malaria, but more usually they are non-immunes suffering from the disease acquired from the indigenous inhabitants.

Fig. 5 The period of extrinsic development of *P. falciparum* and *P. vivax*.

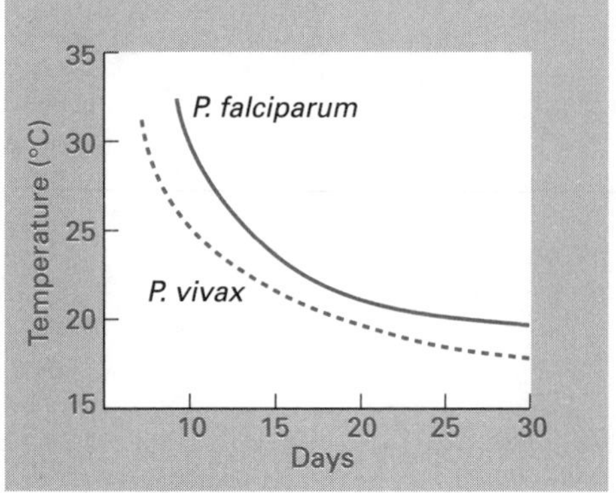

Susceptibility to infection and innate resistance

For practical purposes, all four human plasmodia are confined to people, though experimentally they are transmissible to *Aotus* and other neotropical monkeys and some higher apes, and exceptionally, zoonotic strains have been reported, while simian malaria parasites can very rarely infect man in nature. People of West African origin are strikingly insusceptible to *P. vivax* infection. This correlates with extreme rarity of the Duffy blood-group antigen alleles Fy^a and Fy^b, which appear to act as receptors for penetration of the red cell by the merzoites.

Other genetic determinants affect the course and outcome of infection. Although *P. falciparum* is responsible for around 1 million deaths annually in African children, mortality would be much greater but for a number of inherited resistance factors, and for the processes of acquired resistance discussed in the next section.

The high mortality associated with malaria is perhaps best illustrated by the way in which a number of otherwise disadvantageous genes have been selected in chronically exposed populations because of the resistance to malaria that they confer. J.B.S. Haldane was the first to suggest that the high frequencies of haemoglobinopathies seen in many tropical and subtropical regions may have arisen through the positive selection of heterozygotes by malaria. It has since become clear for several mutations affecting haemoglobin production or structure that these have reached their present frequencies by this selective mechanism. The best-known example is sickle-cell disease, due to a point mutation in position six of the β-globin chain. Here the mutant-gene frequency is stabilized because the enhanced survival of heterozygotes is counterbalanced by the lethal consequences of homozyosity in developing countries. Protection afforded to heterozygotes is seen most dramatically in case-control studies, which show that the relative risk of severe malaria between heterozygotes and controls is about 1 to 10. Perhaps surprisingly, parasite rates and densities at the population level are very similar in normal and AS individuals, except in very young children, indicating that heterozygotes are resistant to disease rather than to infection.

Table 4 lists the genotypes for which there is either epidemiological or clinical evidence of selection by malaria. Despite this often clear evidence of protection, the mechanisms involved are still controversial. *In vitro* data (particularly for AS heterozygote cells) indicate that parasite growth and development can be retarded under some experimental conditions, but this is not a universal finding. One hypothesis suggests that parasites in many of these mutant cells are under increased intracellular oxidant stress and so have decreased survival. A further proposal is that protection is immune based and that enhanced recognition of relevant parasite antigens occurs in the variant host cells, but no consensus exists and it is unclear whether a single mechanism, or multiple genotype-specific mechanisms operate. It is, however, evident that collectively, these innate resistance genes have a significant impact on the natural history of malaria in chronically exposed populations.

Acquired resistance

Those exposed to repeated malarial infection in endemic areas gradually acquire immunity in several stages, but it is rarely complete. It is species specific and largely strain specific. The first change observed is a reduction in clinical symptoms and signs for a given level of parasitaemia. This is sometimes known as 'tolerance' and the mechanism is not understood.

Acquired resistance to the parasites takes months to develop and first affects the density of gametocytes in the peripheral blood. Subsequently the density of asexual erythrocytic parasites, trophozoites, and schizonts falls and gradually reaches very low levels so that under conditions of holoendemic transmission the prevalence of infection falls by half in those aged 15 years compared with children. Infected older children and

Table 2 *The major differences between stable and unstable malaria*

	Unstable	Stable
Basic case reproduction rate (BCRR)	Lowish, variable	High
Endemicity	Usually low	Usually high
Epidemics	Likely	Not seen except in migrants
Seasonal changes	Marked	Fall only in cold or dry season
Predominant parasite	*P. vivax*	*P. falciparum*
Incidence changes	Uneven and large	Small and only seasonal
Immunity population	Variable	High
Clinical effects most in	All ages	Young children
Determinants:		
Mosquito life	Short	Long
Man-biting habit	Low	High
Climate suitable	Short periods	Long periods
Anopheline density for transmission	High	Low is sufficient
Control	Feasible	Extremely difficult

Table 3 *The traditional terminology for levels of malaria endemicity*

Term	Spleen rate in children (%)
Hypoendemic	<10
Mesoendemic	11–50
Hyperendemic	51–75, >25 in adults
Holoendemic	>75, low in adults

Table 4 *Human genetic polymorphisms associated with resistance to malaria*

α-Thalassaemia	Haemoglobin C	Class 1 MHC[a]
β-Thalassaemia	Ovalocytosis	Class 2 MHC
Haemoglobin S	G6PDH[b] deficiency	Duffy blood group
Haemoglobin E	ABO blood groups	S-s U blood group

[a]MHC, major histocompatibility complex; [b]G6PDH, glucose 6-phosphate dehydrogenase.

adults from highly endemic areas often have very low-level, persistent, asymptomatic parasitaemias combined with relative resistance to superinfection.

It is clear that in a highly endemic area for *P. falciparum* there are several parasite strains circulating, and concepts of why resistance is so slowly acquired may either emphasize a balance in immune responses or the successive infection with various strains combined with a largely strain-specific response. The latter is favoured at present. Severe malaria in very young children is ascribed to multiple infections over a short time, and the cerebral malaria that predominates in slightly older children is possibly due to some more virulent strains.

Infants born to immune mothers are partially protected against severe malaria attacks by transplacental antibodies and those acquired from breast milk, for a few months, after which the infant suffers from severe malaria attacks with only gradual acquisition of resistance. Adult non-immunes, including visitors to the tropics from non-malarious areas, are equally susceptible to high mortality in their first few attacks, while women from an endemic area become more susceptible during pregnancy (second trimester), especially the first pregnancy. Splenectomy, whether for a complication of malaria or otherwise, also increases susceptibility to malaria, which may have a fatal outcome.

The mechanisms central to the development of acquired resistance are not understood in detail. Indeed the host/parasite interaction is sufficiently complex that the dominant factors vary dramatically with the choice of model system. It is clear that a variety of different effector mechanisms operates and that the most important of these differs with the stage of infection. Generally, immunity is stage specific, in that immunity to either sporozoite challenge or to gametocyte transmission does not protect against asexual parasites. It also has components that are specific for the parasite species, strain, and antigenic variant within a strain. Thus protection against infection by sporozoites appears to be mediated largely by cytotoxic T cells, which can kill infected hepatocytes, although antibody to the repeat regions of the circumsporozoite protein may also have a role. Specific T and B cells in addition to non-antigen-specific mechanisms are involved in the control of asexual parasitaemia. The central role of antibody has been demonstrated by a variety of passive transfer experiments in people and experimental animals. Pooled immunoglobulin from highly immune donors is extremely effective in rapidly reducing parasitaemia, but not in the long-term control of infection. Maintaining parasite numbers below subclinical levels requires the involvement of T cells, as shown by adoptive transfer experiments in animals. Work in rodents suggests that early in infection, Th1 cells are critical but that later in the course of infection cells of a Th2 phenotype are more important. High levels of cytokines such as tumour necrosis factors **(TNF)** during acute infection are a feature of severe malaria and are associated with a poor outcome. The acute response in non- or semi-immune individuals, while vital to the control of parasitaemia, may also contribute to the pathogenesis of disease by triggering a variety of non-specific effector mechanisms.

Clinical immunity takes many years and several infections to be effectively induced. It is also a non-sterilizing response, as immune adults are constantly and demonstrably reinfected. Several explanations have been put forward for these observations. Generalized, parasite-induced immunosuppression certainly does occur and may be clinically relevant in the response to certain non-malarial antigens such as meningococcal vaccine. It is not clear, however, whether overall it is any more severe than in other acute viral or bacterial infections. One area where it does seem to play a definite part is in the development of Burkitt's lymphoma, in which case it has been shown that individuals with acute *P. falciparum* infection have impaired T-cell control of endogenous, Epstein–Barr virus-infected, B-cell proliferation. Other explanations for the difficulty in inducing effective immunity have involved interference by the parasite in the development of specific responses. This could either be by the presence of important T-independent antigens, which induce a relatively poor response with no memory, or by the effect of cross-reactive, tandem-repeat elements in inhibiting affinity maturation of specific B cells. Perhaps the most likely explanation is the extreme polymorphism or clonal variation of immunologically relevant antigens such that the host requires exposure to a variety of 'strains' before a broadly effective response can develop. If the latter is true, then it presents formidable problems to vaccine development.

Molecular pathology

All the pathology associated with malaria infection is attributable to asexual parasite multiplication in the bloodstream. No adverse effects are caused by the quantitatively small degree of parasite invasion and multiplication within hepatocytes, nor by the presence of relatively small numbers of circulating gametocytes. The consequences to the host of the intraerythrocytic multiplication of parasites range from a variety of severe, but not life-threatening symptoms common to all the species that infect man, to the potentially lethal complications associated with acute *P. falciparum* infection and the chronic renal damage caused by some infections with *P. malariae.* The relative severity of *P. falciparum* infections, as well as the ability to culture this parasite *in vitro,* has meant that it has been the focus of most experimental effort.

It had been noted for centuries that malaria was characterized by periodic fevers. Once the causative organism was identified, it was clear that the bouts of fever in general followed the synchronous release of new merozoites into the bloodstream as each cycle of erythrocytic multiplication was completed. While it was assumed that the release of infected cell contents that occurs at this time was responsible for fever induction, it was not until very recently that it was proven that components of the infected cell such as the lipid, glycosyl phosphatidyl inositol anchor of a parasite membrane protein (perhaps MSP-1) could directly induce the release of cytokines such as TNF and interleukin 1 from macrophages. Moreover, it was demonstrated that older stages of parasites within erythrocytes were differentially sensitive to physiological increases in temperature, so that the effect of fever was both to limit parasite multiplication and to maintain synchronous development. Measurements of TNF in children suffering from severe malaria also demonstrated that very high levels of this cytokine were associated with a lethal outcome, although the correlation was not sufficient to be a useful prognostic indicator.

The principal life-threatening complications of *P. falciparum* in African children are cerebral malaria and severe anaemia often associated with metabolic acidosis and respiratory distress. The clinical picture in non-immune adults is more complex and can include single or multiple organ failure. Mechanisms responsible for severe malarial anaemia are poorly understood but include parasite-induced dyserythropoiesis and accelerated red-cell clearance of both normal and infected cells by both immune and non-immune mechanisms (see below). However, the central event underlying the pathology of most other manifestations of severe falciparum malaria is the cytoadherence and resulting sequestration of infected cells, which is unique to this organism (Fig. 6–9 and Plates 1 and 2). Only the younger developmental stages of the parasite circulate, as the more mature forms adhere to specific receptors on venular endothelium. The distribution of infected cells found in tissue sections suggests that the chief sites of infected cell sequestration correlate with specific organ dysfunction. It is assumed, but not formally proven, that the reduction in, or obstruction of, local blood flow associated with the partial occlusion of small vessels with infected cells results in reduced perfusion and tissue damage. Some have suggested that the sequestered cells may induce local release of a number of potentially toxic or pharmacologically active compounds (such as reactive oxygen species or nitric oxide) from macrophages, neutrophils or endothelium, and that these may affect tissues locally.

While the detailed mechanisms by which sequestered cells result in the specific symptoms seen in cases of severe falciparum malaria remain largely unresolved, much more progress has been made in understanding the molecular interactions that lead to sequestration. Several endothelial receptors have been identified, including CD36 (formerly platelet glycoprotein IV), thrombospondin, intercellular adhesion molecule 1 **(ICAM-1),** and more recently, vascular cell adhesion molecule **(VCAM)** and E-selectin. Most field isolates bind to CD36 and thrombospondin and the majority bind to ICAM-1; to date there are insufficient data on VCAM and E-selectin. *In vitro* assays of purified proteins reveal great variability in absolute levels of adhesion between isolates. No good correlation has yet emerged between the ability of parasites to bind to individual receptors and disease pattern. These studies are, however, fraught with difficulty and many more data are needed to resolve this point. The parasite molecules involved in adhesion are well characterized biochemically but have not yet been cloned, so that primary-sequence data are not available. They form a family of red-cell surface proteins that undergo clonal antigenic variation during a single infection and that also appear to be targets of a host-protective antibody response.

Recent studies have revealed two further properties of some parasite isolates: the rosetting of uninfected erythrocytes around red cells containing mature developmental forms of the parasite and autoagglutination of infected erythrocytes in the absence of immune serum. The mechanisms of these interactions are unknown, but rosetting has been linked

Fig. 6 Cytoadherence of parasitized red blood corpuscles as studied *in vitro.* (a) Transmission electron micrograph showing a cross-section through a human umbilical vein endothelial-cell monolayer and attached parasitized red blood corpuscle. En endothelial cell; K knobs; P = parasite. *Insert,* detail showing the close apposition of the two cell membranes particularly at the sites of knobs (arrowheads) (by courtesy of Dr D. Ferguson, Oxford). (b) Scanning electron micrograph of an infected red cell with numerous knobs (K), adhering to a C32 amelanotic melanoma cell. Note the numerous microvilli (Mv) apparently anchoring the parasitized red blood corpuscle (by courtesy of Dr D. Ferguson, Oxford).

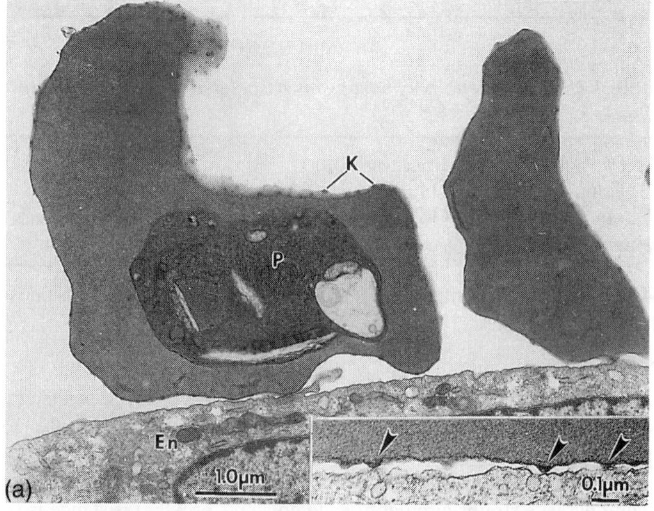

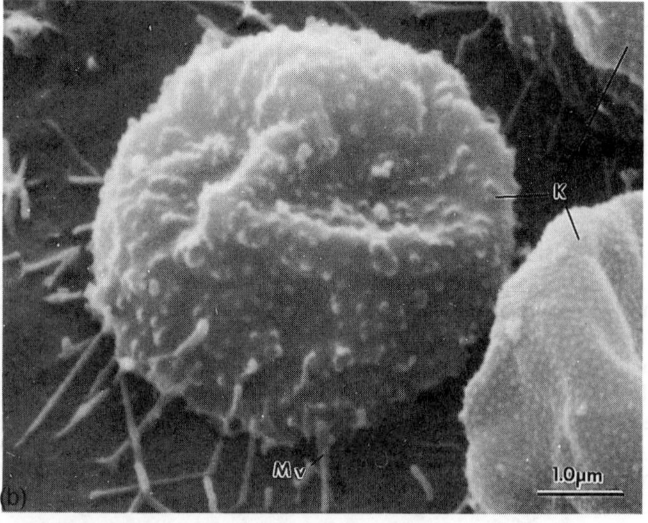

to cerebral malaria in some, but not all, studies. It is presumed that the multicellular aggregates, if they occur *in vivo,* may exacerbate vascular obstruction caused by sequestration.

Despite the life-threatening nature of severe falciparum malaria, and the enormous number of childhood deaths that it causes in subSaharan Africa, the mortality rate of all malaria infections is extremely low. In holoendemic areas, infections in children are universal and constant yet only a small proportion of those infected show clinical symptoms at any one time and only a fraction of these go on to develop severe illness. This is probably only partially explained by the known innate resistance factors and acquired immunity, and so it is likely that unidentified factors are also important in determining how far individual infections progress from parasitaemia to clinical illness and finally to severe disease.

Pathology

BRAIN

Only falciparum malaria causes cerebral pathology. At autopsy, the brain is sometimes oedematous but evidence of cerebral, cerebellar, or medullary herniation is rarely seen. The small blood vessels, including those of the leptomeninges, are congested with parasitized red blood cells containing malaria pigment (Figs 7 and 8). This gives the surface of the brain its characteristic leaden or plum-coloured appearance and the cut surface a slatey-grey hue. Many of the parasites are schizonts and other mature forms. In larger vessels, parasitized red cells form a layer along the endothelium ('margination') (Fig. 9). Up to 70 per cent of erythrocytes in the cerebral vessels are parasitized and these are more tightly packed than in other organs. The cerebrovascular endothelium shows pseudopodial projections, which may be in close apposition to electron-dense, knob-like protruberances on the surface of parasitized

Fig. 7 Brain section of a patient who died of cerebral malaria, showing a blood vessel packed with red blood corpuscles, the majority of which were identified as being infected by the presence of parasites (P), or, at higher magnification, the presence of knobs (by courtesy of Dr D. Ferguson, Oxford).

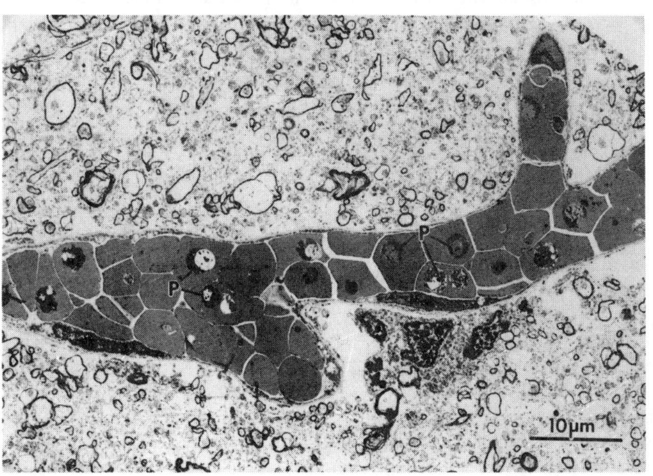

Fig. 8 Cerebral malaria. A parasitized erythrocyte within a cerebral venule. The parasites are undergoing schizogony (P), and membranes appear to be attached to the parasitophorous vacuole at one point. Dense fibrillar material is present within the lumen of the vessel (F). Numerous finger-like endothelial pseudopodia are present (→). Astrocyte footpads are swollen (FP). (Reproduced from MacPherson, *et al.,* (1985). *American Journal of Pathology,* **119,** 385–401, with permission.)

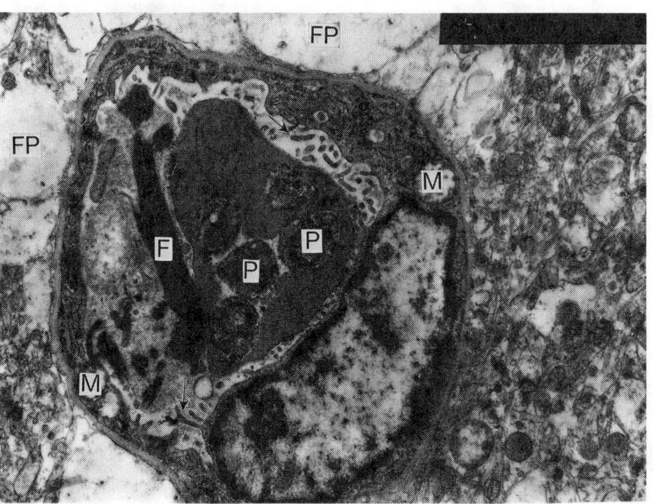

Fig. 9 (a) Section through a blood vessel located in adipose tissue from a patient suffering from multiorgan failure due to *P. falciparum* infection, showing a number of parasitized red blood corpuscles (P) adhering to endothelial cells (En) (by courtesy of Dr D. Ferguson, Oxford). (b) Detail of part of a blood vessel, from the same patient as in (a), showing a parasitized red blood corpuscle with numerous knobs (arrowheads) adhering to an endothelial cell (En). P parasite. (By courtesy of Dr D. Ferguson, Oxford.)

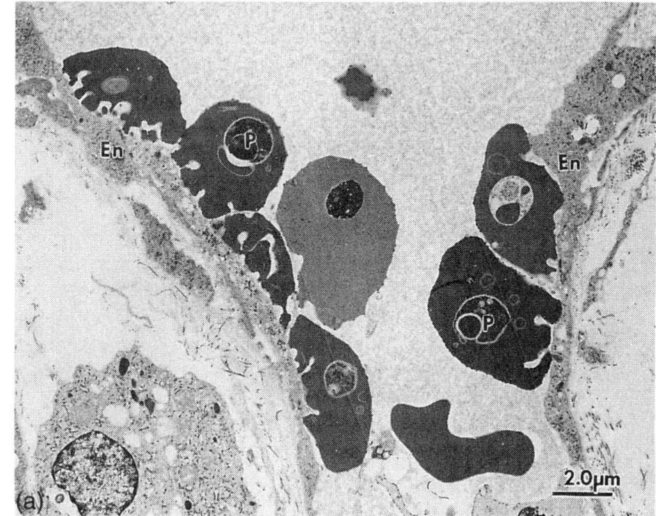

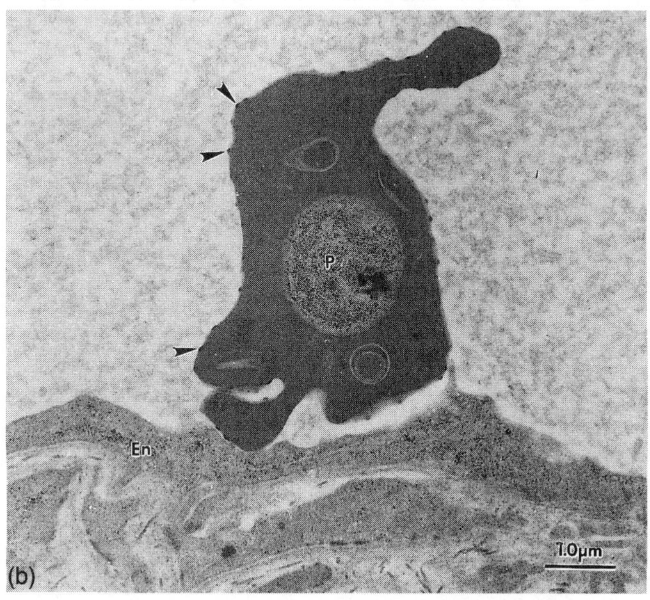

red cells (Figs 10 and 11). Numerous petechial haemorrhages are seen in the white matter, resulting from haemorrhages from end arterioles, proximal to occlusive plugs of parasitized red cells and fibrin. Focal ring haemorrhages can be found centred on small subcortical vessels (Plate 3). Dürck's granulomata (Plate 4), small collections of microglial cells surrounding an area of demyelination, may develop at the site of these haemorrhages, but an inflammatory cell response is generally lacking.

BONE MARROW

There is evidence of iron sequestration, erythrophagocytosis, and dyserythropoiesis (Fig. 10) in the acute phase of falciparum malaria, but maturation defects were present in the marrow for at least 3 weeks after clearance of parasitaemia. Increased numbers of large, abnormal-looking megakaryocytes have been found in the marrow and the circulating platelets may also be enlarged, suggesting dyspoietic thrombopoiesis. Malaria pigment and parasites can be found in monocytes and phagocytes in the marrow, even when they are not detectable in peripheral blood.

LIVER

The liver is affected by all four species of human malaria parasites, but changes are most severe in falciparum malaria. The liver is enlarged and oedematous, and coloured brown, grey or even black as a result of deposition of malaria pigment. Hepatic sinusoids are dilated, containing hypertrophied Kupffer cells and parasitized red cells that appear to obstruct the circulation. Parasitized and uninfected red cells are phagocytosed by Kupffer cells, endothelial cells, and sinusoidal macrophages. Small areas of centrilobular necrosis, which are occasionally seen in severe cases, may be attributable to shock or disseminated intravascular coagulation. Hepatocytes usually show only mild abnormalities but may be depleted of glycogen in some patients who are hypoglycaemic. Lymphocytic infiltration of portal tracts has been described (see also Tropical splenomegaly syndrome).

GASTROINTESTINAL TRACT

Cytoadherent, sequestered, parasitized red cells may be found in the small and large bowel, especially in capillaries of the lamina propria and larger submucosal vessels. The bowel may appear congested, with mucosal ulceration and haemorrhage.

KIDNEY

Glomerular lesions range from the acute transient glomerular nephritis of falciparum malaria to the chronic lesions of quartan malarial nephrosis. In severe falciparum malaria, with or without 'blackwater fever', acute renal failure is associated with the histopathological changes of acute tubular necrosis. Parasitized red cells may be found in glomerular

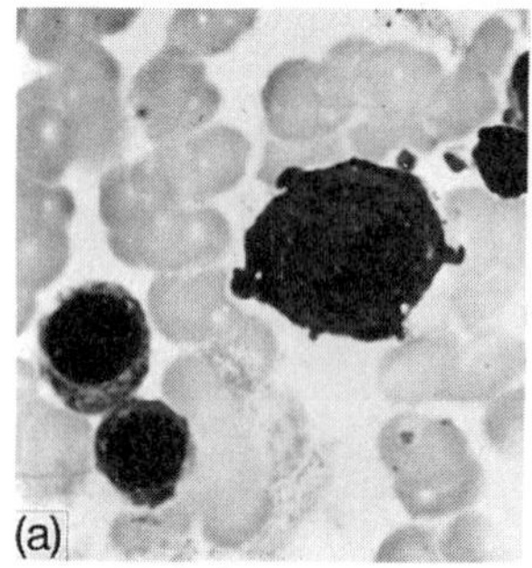

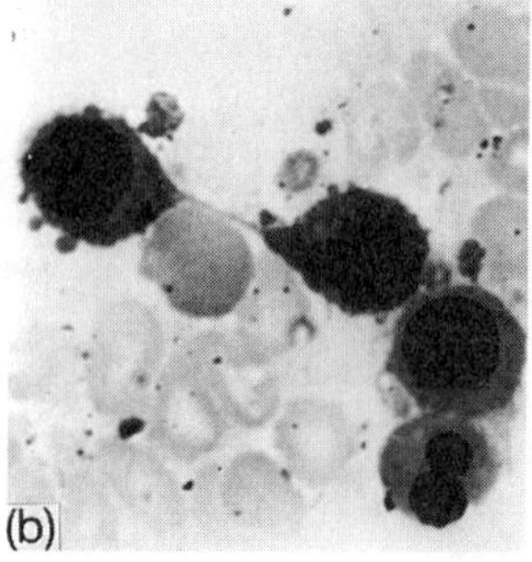

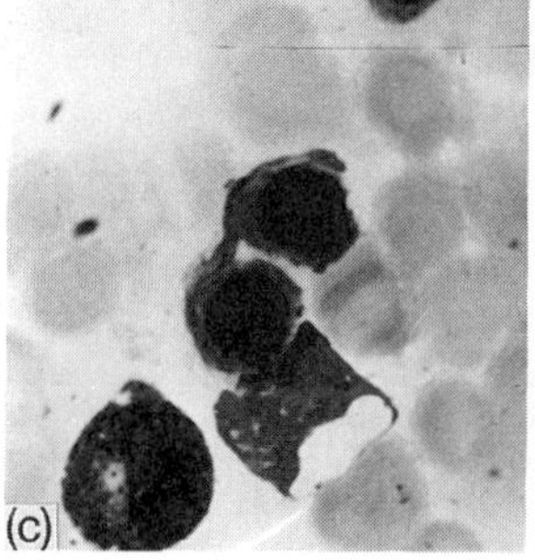

Fig. 10 Bone marrow smears from patients with falciparum malaria, showing dyserythropoiesis. Normoblasts show intercytoplasmic bridging (a, b, c,) and multinuclearity (b). (Reproduced from Phillips, *et al.* (1986). *Quarterly Journal of Medicine,* **58,** 305–23 with permission.)

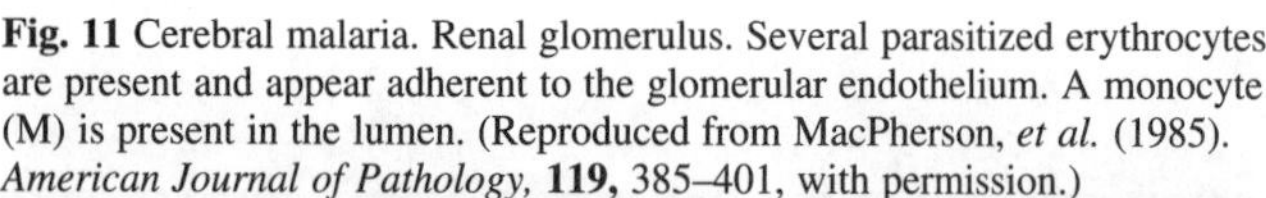
Fig. 11 Cerebral malaria. Renal glomerulus. Several parasitized erythrocytes are present and appear adherent to the glomerular endothelium. A monocyte (M) is present in the lumen. (Reproduced from MacPherson, *et al.* (1985). *American Journal of Pathology,* **119,** 385–401, with permission.)

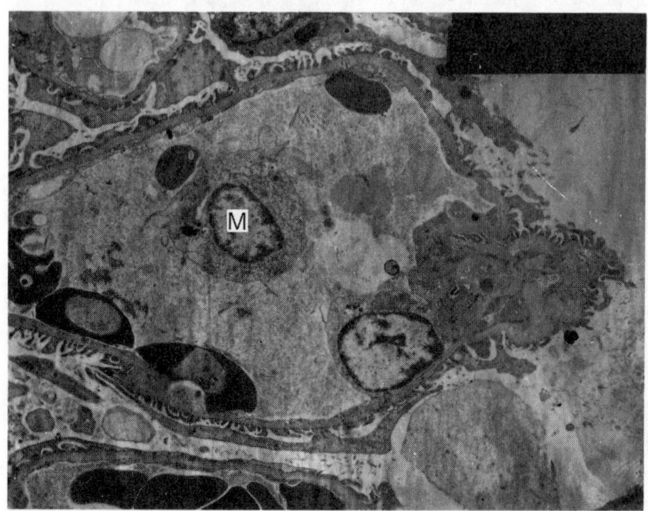

Fig. 12 Cerebral malaria. Lung. Venules (V) close to alveolus (Alv) are packed with large numbers of inflammatory cells, including neutrophil polymorphs (P), monocytes (M) and lymphocytes (L). (Reproduced from MacPherson, *et al.* (1985). *American Journal of Pathology,* **119,** 385–401, with permission.)

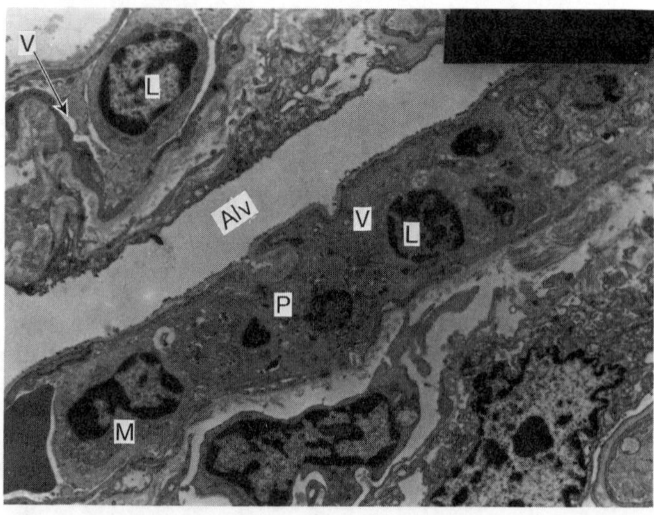

and peritubular capillaries (Fig. 11), with fibrin thrombi and pigment-laden macrophages. Tubular pigment casts are prominent in cases of blackwater fever.

LUNG

The lungs are oedematous in almost all patients dying of malaria. Pulmonary capillaries and venules are packed with inflammatory cells (Fig. 12) including neutrophils, plasma cells and pigment-laden macrophages, and with parasitized red cells. The vascular endothelium is oedematous, causing narrowing of the capillary lumen, and there is interstitial oedema and hyaline-membrane formation. Secondary bronchopneumonia is a common finding.

SPLEEN

The spleen is large, engorged, and dark-red or greyish-black in colour. The red and white pulp is congested and hyperplastic, and the splenic cords and sinuses are filled with phagocytic cells containing pigment, parasitized red cells, and non-infected red cells. Tropical splenomegaly syndrome is described below.

HEART

There is no evidence of myocarditis. Subendocardial and epicardial petechial haemorrhages are unusual. The myocardial capillaries are congested with parasitized red cells, pigment-laden macrophages, lymphocytes, and plasma cells. However, the parasitized cells are not tightly packed and there is no evidence of cytoadherence.

Pathophysiology

ANAEMIA

This is attributable mainly to the destruction or phagocytosis of parasitized red cells, but other mechanisms contribute. The bone marrow shows dyserythropoietic changes (Fig. 10). Initial iron sequestration and hypoferraemia may be explained by the very marked hyperferritinaemia, an acute-phase reaction. There is evidence of immune-mediated haemolysis in some populations. Erythrocyte survival is reduced even after the disappearance of parasitaemia. Increased splenic clearance of non-parasitized as well as parasitized red cells has been demonstrated.

Intravascular haemolysis occurs in patients whose erythrocytes are congenitally deficient in enzymes such as G6PD in response to oxidant drugs such as primaquine. However, in classical blackwater fever, G6PD levels are, by definition, normal and the mechanism is unknown, although quinine-mediated haemolysis has been suspected.

THROMBOCYTOPENIA

This is attributable to sequestration in the spleen rather than to failure of production by the marrow or immune-mediated lysis.

CEREBRAL MALARIA

Mechanical obstruction to the microcirculation of the brain by cytoadherent, parasitized red cells and perhaps 'rosettes' of uninfected red cells stuck around a parasitized red cells, is now thought to be the principal mechanism leading to coma. Red blood cells infected with some strains of *P. falciparum* develop adhesive properties as they mature. Parasite-derived protein such as PfEMP-1 expressed on the surface of the parasitized red cell may act as a ligand that binds to receptors such as ICAM-1 on cerebral venular endothelium. The expression of ICAM-1, and some other receptors involved in cytoadherence of parasitized red cells, may be increased by TNF and other cytokines. Obstruction to cerebral blood flow could result in 'stagnant anoxaemia', leading to coma. In Thai adults with cerebral malaria, global cerebral blood flow was inappropriately low and there was evidence of cerebral anaerobic glycolysis with increased lactate concentrations in the cerebrospinal fluid. In African children with cerebral malaria, plasma concentrations of TNFα, interleukin 1α and other cytokines correlate closely with disease severity as judged by parasitaemia, hypoglycaemia, case fatality, and the incidence of neurological sequelae. As well as enhancing cytoadherence, cytokines may have other effects on cerebral function, perhaps by releasing nitric oxide, which interferes with neurotransmission, or by leading to generation of free oxygen radicals. Cytokines may also be responsible for fever, hypoglycaemia, coagulopathy, dyserythropoiesis, and leucocytosis in falciparum malaria.

In South-East Asian adults, the opening pressure of cerebrospinal fluid at lumbar puncture was usually normal and cerebral oedema was demonstrable (by computerized tomographic (CT) scan) during life in only a small minority and usually as an agonal phenomenon. In these patients there was little evidence that brain swelling contributed to coma. However, in African children with cerebral malaria, intracranial pressure is usually elevated and there is evidence of brain swelling in the majority of those examined by CT scan. Ischaemic damage resulting from a critical reduction in cerebral perfusion pressure and other factors such as hypoglycaemia and status epilepticus are thought to be important in the mechanism of brain damage in these children.

PULMONARY OEDEMA

This may develop in patients who have been overloaded with fluid in hospital and have elevated central venous and pulmonary-artery wedge pressures. More commonly, the clinical picture is of adult respiratory distress syndrome, with normal or low hydrostatic pressures in the pulmonary vascular bed. In these cases, the mechanism is likely to be increased pulmonary capillary permeability resulting from leucocyte products and cytokines. The histological appearances of neutrophil sequestration in the pulmonary capillaries (Fig. 16), increased permeability, and hyaline membrane formation are consistent with this hypothesis.

HYPOGLYCAEMIA

This can be caused by cinchona alkaloids (quinine or quinidine), which are potent stimulators of insulin secretion by the pancreatic β-cells. The resulting reduction in hepatic gluconeogenesis and increased peripheral glucose uptake by tissues results in hypoglycaemia. In malaria, glucose consumption is increased by fever, infection, anaerobic glycolysis, and the metabolic demands of the malaria parasites. Glycogen reserves may be depleted, especially in children and pregnant women, as a result of fasting and 'accelerated starvation'. In African children with severe malaria, adult patients with severe disease and pregnant women, hypoglycaemia develops spontaneously (without treatment with cinchona alkaloids) and is associated with appropriately low plasma insulin concentrations. Plasma lactate and alanine concentrations are elevated and ketone bodies are moderately increased. Counter-regulatory hormone levels are usually very high. The mechanism of hypoglycaemia in these cases may be inhibition of hepatic gluconeogenesis by TNF and other cytokines.

ACUTE RENAL FAILURE

Hypovolaemia, from dehydration, is responsible in the majority of patients whose acute olguria and renal dysfunction is reversible by fluid replacement. Hyperparasitaemia, jaundice, and haemoglobinuria are associated with a high risk of acute tubular necrosis. Renal cortical perfusion is reduced during the acute stage of the disease. Renal cortical necrosis must be rare, as survivors rarely show evidence of chronic renal impairment. Cytoadherence of parasitized red blood cells in the renal microvasculature (Fig. 11), deposition of fibrin microthrombi, and prolonged hypotension ('algid malaria') may contribute to acute renal failure. Quartan malarial nephrosis is discussed below.

HYPONATRAEMIA

In patients with relatively normal plasma osmolalities, this has been attributed to inappropriate secretion of antidiuretic hormone triggered by fever or reduced effective plasma volume, but in Thai patients the levels of that hormone were appropriately high in patients who were proved to be grossly hypovolaemic by carefully monitored fluid-repletion studies. Sodium depletion may be responsible for some cases of hyponatraemia.

HYPOVOLAEMIA AND 'SHOCK' ('ALGID MALARIA')

This may result from hypovolaemia (dehydration and, rarely, haemorrhagic shock following splenic rupture or gastrointestinal haemorrhage) but is most often associated with a secondary Gram-negative bacteraemia. The source may be intravenous cannulae, urethral catheter or aspiration pneumonia. Transient immunosuppression, impaired macrophage function or 'blockade' of the reticuloendothelial system may increase the susceptibility of patients to severe secondary bacterial infections.

Clinical features

The pathogenic species of *Plasmodium* cause acute febrile illnesses characterized by periodic febrile paroxysms occurring every 48 or 72 h with afebrile asymptomatic intervals and a tendency to recrudesce or relapse over periods of months or even years. The severity of the attack is determined by the species and strain, and hence the geographical origin, of the infecting parasite; on the age, genetic constitution, state of immunity, general health and nutritional state of the patients, and on their use of antimalarial drugs.

FALCIPARUM MALARIA ('MALIGNANT' TERTIAN OR SUBTERTIAN MALARIA)

The shortest interval between infecting mosquito bite and parasitaemia is 5 days, but this prepatent period is usually 9 to 10 days. The incubation period (the interval between infection and the first symptom) usually ranges from 7 to 14 days (mean 12 days) but may be prolonged further by immunity, chemoprophylaxis or partial chemotherapy. In Europe and North America, 98 per cent of patients with imported falciparum malaria present within 3 months of arriving back from the malarious area. A few present up to 1 year later, but none after more than 4 years.

Several days of prodromal symptoms such as malaise, headache, myalgia, anorexia, and mild fever are interrupted by the first paroxysm. Suddenly the patient feels inexplicably cold (in a hot climate) and apprehensive. Mild shivering quickly turns into violent shaking with teeth chattering. There is intense peripheral vasoconstriction and gooseflesh. Some patients vomit. The rapid increase in core temperature may trigger febrile convulsions in young children. The rigor lasts up to 1 h and is followed by a hot flush with throbbing headache, palpitations, tachypnoea, prostration, postural syncope, and further vomiting while the temperature reaches its peak. Finally, a drenching sweat breaks out and the fever defervesces over the next few hours. The exhausted patient sleeps. The whole paroxysm is over in 8 to 12 h, after which the patient may feel remarkably well. These symptoms are typical of a classical 'endotoxin reaction' produced by typhoid vaccine, infection with Gram-negative bacteria, or release of TNF and other cytokines by other agents. Classical tertian or subtertian periodicity (48 and 36 h between fever spikes) is rarely seen with falciparum malaria. A high irregularly spiking, continuous or remittent fever, or daily (quotidian) paroxysm, is more usual. Other common symptoms are headache, backache, myalgias, dizziness, postural hypotension, nausea, dry cough, abdominal discomfort, diarrhoea, and vomiting. The non-immune patient with falciparum malaria usually looks severely ill, with 'typhoid' facies and, in dark-skinned races, a curious greenish complexion. Commonly there is anaemia and a tinge of jaundice, with moderate tender enlargement of the spleen and liver. Useful negative findings are the lack of lymphadenopathy and rash (apart from herpes simplex 'cold sores') and focal signs.

Cerebral malaria and other severe manifestations and complications

The global case fatality of falciparum malaria is probably around 1 per cent or 1 to 3 million deaths per year. Cerebral malaria is the most important of the severe manifestations of *P. falciparum* infection, accounting for 80 per cent of these deaths. Patients who have been feverish and ill for a few days may have a generalized convulsion from which they do not recover consciousness or their level of consciousness may decline gradually over several hours. High fever alone can impair cerebral function causing drowsiness, delirium, obtundation, confusion, irritability, psychosis, and, in children, febrile convulsions. The term cerebral malaria, implying encephalopathy specifically related to *P. falciparum* infection, should be restricted to patients with unrousable coma (no appropriate verbal response and no purposive motor response to noxious stimuli—Glasgow Coma Scale ≤7/11) and evidence of acute *P. falciparum* infection, in whom other encephalopathies, including hypoglycaemia and transient postictal coma, have been excluded. Patients with cerebral malaria may have mild meningism but neck rigidity and photophobia are rare. Retinal haemorrhages (Plate 5) are present in about 15 per cent of African and South-East Asian cases, but exudates are rare. (In Papua New Guinea these changes are not confined to patients with severe falciparum malaria.) Papilloedema is very rare (0.5 per cent of cases). Dysconjugate gaze is common. In adult patients the pupillary, corneal, oculocephalic, and oculovestibular reflexes are normal. Muscle tone and tendon reflexes are usually increased and there is ankle clonus. The plantar responses are extensor and abdominal reflexes are absent. In African children, brain-stem reflexes may be abnormal and there may be neurological evidence of severe intracranial hypertension with rostrocaudal progression suggesting cerebral, cerebellar, and medullary herniation. Hypotonia (Plate 6) is more common than in adults. In patients of all ages, extensor posturing (decerebrate or decorticate rigidity), associated with sustained upward deviation of the eyes (not the transient upward gaze of oculogyric crisis), pouting and stertorous breathing, is sometimes, but not always, associated with hypoglycaemia (Plates 7 and 8). About half of adult patients and more children have generalized convulsions. Focal seizures and localizing neurological signs are uncommon in patients with strictly defined cerebral malaria. Less than 5 per cent of adult survivors have persisting neurological sequelae; these include cranial-nerve lesions, extrapyramidal tremor, and transient paranoid psychosis. However, more than 10 per cent of African children who survive an attack of cerebral malaria suffer from sequelae such as hemiplegia (Plate 9), cortical blindness, epilepsy, ataxia, and mental retardation.

Anaemia (see above) is an inevitable consequence of all but the mildest infections. It is most common and severe in pregnant women, children (Plate 10), and in patients with high parasitaemia, schizontaemia, secondary bacterial infections and renal failure.

Spontaneous bleeding, from the gums (Plate 11) and gastrointestinal tract, is seen in less than 5 per cent of adult patients with severe malaria. It is rare in children.

Jaundice (Plate 12) is common in adults but rare in children. Biochemical evidence of severe hepatic dysfunction is unusual. Hepatic failure suggests concomitant viral hepatitis or another diagnosis.

Hypoglycaemia is being recognized increasingly in patients with malaria. Pregnant women with severe or uncomplicated falciparum malaria and other patients with severe disease may become hypoglycaemic from a few hours to 6 days after starting quinine or quinidine, even after the parasitaemia has cleared. Pregnant women and children with malaria, and other patients with hyperparasitaemia and complicating bacteraemias, may all become hypoglycaemic early in their illness and without quinine therapy. The symptoms and signs of hypoglycaemia—anxiety, tachycardia, breathlessness, feeling cold, confusion, sweating, lightheadedness, restlessness, fetal bradycardia, other signs of fetal distress, coma, convulsions and extensor posturing—may be misinterpreted as merely manifestations of malaria.

Hypotension and shock ('algid malaria') is seen in patients who develop pulmonary oedema, metabolic acidosis, complicating bacteraemias, and massive gastrointestinal haemorrhage. Mild supine hypotension with a marked postural drop in blood pressure is usually attributable to vasodilatation and relative hypovolaemia. Cardiac arrhythmias are rare but may be precipitated by rapid infusion or excessive doses of antimalarial drugs such as chloroquine, quinine or quinidine. Patients with coronary insufficiency may develop angina during febrile crises of malaria. Patients with severe malaria sometimes develop complicating bacterial infections such as aspiration pneumonia, urinary-tract infections, infected bedsores, and phlebitis at intravenous drip sites.

Oliguria, with increased blood urea and serum creatinine concentrations, is seen in about a third of patients with severe malaria. Most of these respond to cautious rehydration, but 10 per cent develop renal failure requiring dialysis.

In patients whose red blood cells are deficient in G6PD (and other enzymes), intravascular haemolysis and haemoglobinuria (Plate 13) may be precipitated by oxidant antimalarial drugs, especially primaquine, whether or not they have malaria. Classical blackwater fever is the association of haemoglobinuria with severe manifestations of falciparum malaria including renal failure, hypotension and coma, in a non-immune patient who is not G6PD deficient.

Metabolic acidosis is seen in association with hyperparasitaemia, hypoglycaemia, and renal failure. Usually it results from lactic acidosis, even in patients with renal failure. In African children, respiratory distress, associated with severe anaemia and metabolic acidosis, is emerging as a syndrome, which carries a higher mortality than cerebral malaria. Mild hyponatraemia with reduced plasma osmolality is often attributable to intravenous therapy with 5 per cent dextrose alone in patients who are salt depleted and dehydrated.

Pulmonary oedema (Plate 14) appears to be the terminal event in most fatal adult cases of falciparum malaria. It may develop late in the clinical course as a result of fluid overload or in patients with severe disease in the absence of fluid overload. It may also appear suddenly after delivery in pregnant women who are in positive fluid balance. The earliest sign is an increase in respiratory rate. Pulmonary oedema may be difficult to differentiate from aspiration pneumonia, a common complication in comatose patients, and metabolic acidosis. Radiography may be needed to make this distinction with confidence. The patients who are not fluid overloaded resemble those with adult respiratory distress syndrome with a normal jugular venous, central venous or pulmonary-artery wedge pressure.

Cerebellar dysfunction

A rare presentation of falciparum malaria is cerebellar ataxia with unimpaired consciousness. Similar signs may be seen in patients recovering from cerebral malaria and, in Sri Lanka, delayed cerebellar ataxia has been described 3 to 4 weeks after an attack of fever attributable to falciparum malaria. Complete recovery is the rule.

Malarial psychosis

Acute psychiatric symptoms in patients with malaria may be attributable to their drug treatment, including antimalarial drugs such as chloroquine, mefloquine, and the obsolete mepacrine, and exacerbation of pre-existing functional psychoses. However, in some patients, organic mental disturbances associated with malaria infection have been the presenting feature or, more often, have developed during convalescence after attacks of otherwise uncomplicated malaria or cerebral malaria. Depression, paranoia, delusions, and personality changes should probably be classified as brief reactive psychoses. These symptoms rarely last for more than a few days.

VIVAX, OVALE, AND MALARIAE MALARIAS

The prepatent and incubation periods for *P. vivax* are 8 to 13 and 12 to 17 days, respectively; for *P. ovale* 9 to 14 and 15 to 18 days; and for *P. malariae* 15 to 16 and 18 to 40 days. Some strains of *P. vivax,* especially those from temperate regions (*P. v. hibernans* from Russia, *P. v. multinucleatum* from China) may have very long incubation periods (250–637 days). Only about one-third of imported cases of vivax malaria present within a month of returning from the malarious area; 5 to 10 per cent will present more than a year later.

The 'benign' malarias cause paroxysmal, feverish symptoms no less hectic and distressing than those of falciparum malaria. Prodromal symptoms are said to be more severe with *P. malariae* infection. In untreated cases, the characteristic tertian (48–50 h) interval between fever spikes may be seen with vivax and ovale and the quartan (72 h) pattern in *P. malariae* infections.

This periodicity is established after several days of irregular fever. Vivax and ovale malarias have a persistent hepatic cycle, which may give rise to relapses every 2 to 3 months for 5 to 8 years in untreated cases. *P. malariae* does not relapse but a persisting, undetectable parasitaemia may cause recrudescences for more than 50 years.

Although symptoms may be severe and temporarily incapacitating, especially in non-immunes, the acute mortality is very low. For example, there were no deaths during the 1969 Sri Lankan epidemic of half a million cases of vivax malaria. Only in immunocompromised, splenectomized or debilitated patients are the 'benign' malarias likely to prove life-threatening.

An important practical point is that indigenous West Africans are very rarely infected with *P. vivax.* Patients suffering from vivax malaria may become anaemic, thrombocytopenic, and mildly jaundiced with tender hepatosplenomegaly. Splenomegaly may be particularly gross in areas of *P. malariae* infection (see also Tropical splenomegaly syndrome). In debilitated patients with vivax malaria, anaemia rarely may be severe enough to be life-threatening. Splenic rupture, which carries a mortality of 80 per cent, is more common with vivax than falciparum malaria. It results from acute, rapid enlargement of the spleen, with or without trauma; chronically enlarged spleens are less vulnerable. Ruptured spleen presents with abdominal pain and guarding, haemorrhagic shock (tachycardia, postural hypotension and prostration), fever, and a rapidly falling haematocrit. These features may be misattributed to malaria itself.

Cerebral vivax malaria has occasionally been reported especially with the long incubation period *P. v. multinucleatum* in China. In none of the published cases was mixed falciparum infection or another encephalopathy adequately excluded. The same strictures apply to cerebral *P. malariae* malaria, especially as this parasite coexists with *P. falciparum* throughout most of its range. The acute symptoms of ovale and malariae malarias may be as severe as those of vivax infection, but anaemia is less severe and the risk of splenic rupture is lower. *P. ovale* causes negligible mortality, but *P. malariae* causes many deaths from nephrotic syndrome (see below).

MALARIA IN PREGNANCY AND THE PUERPERIUM

Malaria is a major cause of maternal death, abortion, stillbirth, premature delivery, and low birthweight in those areas of the tropics where malaria transmission is unstable and women of child-bearing age have little acquired immunity. Even in some hyperendemic areas, clinical symptoms and parasitaemia are worse in primiparous than in multiparous women and other patients. In non-immunes, cerebral and other forms of severe falciparum malaria are more common in pregnancy. In the great epidemic in Sri Lanka in 1934–5 the mortality among pregnant women was 13 per cent, twice that in non-pregnant women, and in Thailand, where malaria has been the most important cause of maternal mortality, cerebral malaria in late pregnancy has a mortality of 50 per cent. In some parts of Africa, a quarter to a half of all placentae are parasitized. The incidence is highest in primiparae. In the malaria endemic region, the susceptibility of pregnant women to malaria has been attributed to temporary immunosuppression caused by increased corticosteroid secretion and other mechanisms. However, this would not explain the particular vulnerability of primiparae.

In most endemic regions, birth weights of neonates born to women with malaria are significantly less than those of controls. Fetal distress was observed in 6 out of 12 Thai women with malaria who were beyond the twenty-ninth week of pregnancy. Painless uterine contractions were detected in seven out of eight who were not in labour. This uterine activity subsided as the patients' temperatures were reduced by simple cooling.

Severe anaemia, exacerbated by malaria, is an important complication of pregnancy in many tropical countries. Especially in communities where chronic hookworm anaemia is prevalent, cardiac failure may develop in late pregnancy.

Asymptomatic hypoglycaemia may occur in pregnant women with malaria before antimalarial treatment, and pregnant women with severe uncomplicated malaria are particularly vulnerable to quinine-induced hypoglycaemia (see above).

There is an increased risk of pulmonary oedema precipitated by fluid overload or by the sudden increase in peripheral resistance, or autotransfusion of hyperparasitaemic blood from the placenta, which occurs just after delivery (Plate 14).

Prevention

Malaria is so dangerous in pregnancy that pregnant women who cannot leave the area of transmission must be given antimalarial prophylaxis extending into the early puerperium. This is a most important part of antenatal care.

CONGENITAL AND NEONATAL MALARIA

Vertical transmission of malaria can be diagnosed by detecting parasitaemia in the neonate within 7 days of birth, or later if there is no possibility of postpartum, mosquito-borne infection. Save for a few discordant reports, most evidence from malarious parts of the world indicates that congenital malaria is extremely rare, despite the high prevalence of placental infection. This confirms the adequacy of the placental barrier and the protection provided by IgG from the immune mother, which crosses the placenta. Congenital malaria is, however, much more common in infants born to non-immune mothers, and there is an increased incidence during malaria epidemics. All four species can produce congenital infection, but because of its very long persistence *P. malariae* causes a disproportionate number of cases in non-endemic countries. Fetal plasma quinine and chloroquine concentrations are about one-third of the simultaneous maternal levels. Thus, antimalarial concentrations adequate to cure the mother might result in subtherapeutic concentrations in the fetus. Quinine and chloroquine are excreted in breast milk, but the suckling neonate would receive only a few mg/day. Maternal hypoglycaemia, a common complication of malaria or its treatment with quinine, may produce marked fetal bradycardia and other signs of fetal distress.

Differential diagnosis

The clinical features of congenital malaria include fever, irritability, feeding problems, hepatosplenomegaly, anaemia, and jaundice. Unless parasites are found in the smear from a heel prick or cord blood, the patient may be misdiagnosed as having rhesus incompatibility or another congenital infection such as cytomegalovirus, herpes simplex, rubella, toxoplasmosis, or syphilis.

TRANSFUSION MALARIA AND 'NEEDLESTICK' MALARIA

Malaria, like trypanosomiasis, Colorado tick fever, human immunodeficiency viruses, hepatitis viruses and some other pathogens can be transmitted in blood from apparently healthy donors. Exceptionally, donors may remain infective for up to 5 years with *P. falciparum* and *P. vivax,* 7 years for *P. ovale,* and 46 years for *P. malariae.* Because the infecting forms are erythrocytic (not sporozoites), no exoerythrocytic (hepatic) cycle will be established and so vivax and ovale malarias will not relapse. Theoretically, parasitaemia might be detectable immediately and the incubation period should be shorter than with mosquito-transmitted malaria. However, the incubation period tends to be longer because of the time needed to build up parasitaemias sufficient to cause symptoms. Mean incubation periods are 12 (range 7–29) days for *P. falciparum,* 12 (range 8–30) days for *P. vivax* and 35 (range 6–106) days for *P. malariae.* Whole blood, packed cells, leucocyte or platelet concentrates, fresh plasma, marrow transplants, and haemodialysis have been responsible for transfusion malaria. As patients requiring transfusion are likely to be debilitated and may be immunosuppressed, and there may be a long delay before making the diagnosis because malaria is not suspected, unusually high parasitaemias may develop with *P. falciparum* and *P. malariae.* With *P. ovale* and *P. vivax* infections, the parasitaemia is usually limited to 2 per cent because only reticulocytes are invaded. Severe manifestations are common, mortality may be high, for example, 8 out of 11 in a group of heroin addicts, and even acute *P. malariae* infections may prove fatal.

Prevention

Outside the malaria endemic area, donors who have been in the tropics during the previous 5 years should be screened for malarial antibodies (indirect fluorescent antibody) (see below). In the endemic area, recipients of blood transfusions can be given antimalarial chemotherapy, or at least should be watched carefully for evidence of infection.

MONKEY MALARIAS

Human erythrocytes can be infected with at least six species of simian plasmodia. There have been rare cases of natural infections or accidental laboratory infections by *P. brazilianum, P. cynomolgi, P. inui, P. knowlesi, P. schwetzi,* and *P. simium.* Severe feverish and systemic symptoms have been described but no cerebral or other severe complications. No patient has died. Parasitaemia may remain undetectable for 2 to 6 days after the start of symptoms. Periodicity is quotidian *(P. knowlesi)* or tertian (*P. simium* and *P. cynomolgi*). Infectivity and virulence may be enhanced by repeated passage in man. Chloroquine is the treatment of choice.

Diagnosis

Malaria can present with a wide range of symptoms and signs, none of them diagnostic. **It must be excluded by repeated thick and thin blood smears in any patient with acute fever and an appropriate history of exposure.** Outside the malaria endemic area, patients should be asked about travel during the previous year. The possibility of malaria must not be dismissed because the patient took prophylactic drugs, for none is completely protective. Short airport stopovers, even on the runway, or working in or living near an international airport, may allow exposure to an imported, infected mosquito. Transmission by blood transfusion or 'needlestick' should be borne in mind. Those who grew up in an endemic area will lose their immunity after living for a few years in the temperate zone and become vulnerable when they return to their homeland on holiday. In malaria endemic regions, a large proportion of the immune population may have asymptomatic parasitaemia and it cannot be assumed that malaria is the cause of the patient's symptoms. The diagnosis of malaria may be missed, even in the endemic zone, during an epidemic of some other infection (e.g. meningitis, pneumonia, cholera).

Table 5 *Differential diagnosis of malaria*

Symptom	Diagnosis
Acute fever	Heat stroke, hyperpyrexia of other causes, other infections, other causes of fever
Fever and impaired consciousness (cerebral malaria)	Viral, bacterial, fungal, protozoal (e.g. African trypanosomiasis) or helminthic meningoencephalitis, cerebral abscess Head injury, cerebrovascular accident, intoxications (e.g. insecticides), poisonings (e.g. antimalarial drugs), metabolic (diabetes, hypoglycaemia, uraemia, hepatic failure, hyponatraemia) Septicaemias
Fever and convulsions	Encephalitides, metabolic encephalopathies, hyperpyrexia, cerebrovascular accidents, epilepsy, drug and alcohol intoxications, poisoning, eclampsia, febrile convulsions, and Reye's syndrome (children)
Fever and haemostatic disturbances	Septicaemias (e.g. meningococcaemia), viral haemorrhagic fever, rickettsial infection, relapsing fevers, leptospirosis
Fever and jaundice	Viral hepatitis, yellow fever, leptospirosis, relapsing fevers, septicaemias, haemolysis, biliary obstruction, hepatic necrosis (drugs, poisons)
Fever with gastrointestinal symptoms	Travellers' diarrhoea, dysentery, enteric fever, other bacterial infections, inflammatory bowel disease
Fever with haemoglobinuria ('blackwater fever')	Drug-induced haemolysis (e.g. oxidant antimalarials in glucose 6-phosphate-dehydrogenase-deficient patient), favism, transfusion reaction, dark urine of other causes (e.g. myoglobinuria, urobilinogen, porphobilinogen)
Fever with acute renal failure	Septicaemias, yellow fever, leptospirosis, drug intoxications, poisonings, prolonged hypotension
Fever with shock ('algid malaria')	Septicaemic shock, haemorrhagic shock (e.g. massive gastrointestinal bleed, ruptured spleen), perforated bowel, dehydration, hypovolaemia, myocarditis

Differential diagnosis (Table 5)

Malaria should be considered in the differential diagnosis of any acute febrile illness until it can be excluded by a definite lack of exposure, by repeated examination of blood smears, or by a therapeutic trial of antimalarial chemotherapy. In Europe and North America, imported malaria has been misdiagnosed as influenza, viral hepatitis, viral encephalitis or travellers' diarrhoea, sometimes with fatal consequences. Cerebral malaria must be distinguished from other infective meningoencephalitides. Cerebrospinal-fluid examination will identify most of these infective causes (see Chapter 24.15.2). Abdominal reflexes are brisk in patients with psychotic stupor and hysteria but absent in cerebral malaria. Recognition of poisoning will depend largely on the history or the clinical circumstances. Overdose of antimalarial drugs (chloroquine and quinine) can be confused with cerebral malaria. Intravenous drug abusers are at risk both from severe malaria and drug overdose. Alcoholism may be confused with cerebral malaria, whether the patient presents simply as 'drunk' or with delirium tremens or encephalopathy.

Misdiagnosis of a viral haemorrhagic fever in a case of imported malaria is potentially dangerous as the patient may be placed in a high-containment unit where basic investigations such as examination of a blood smear may not be possible because of fear of infection. Jaundice is not a common feature of viral haemorrhagic fevers except yellow fever.

Malaria in pregnancy may be confused with viral hepatitis, acute fatty liver with liver failure or eclampsia, and in the puerperium with puerperal sepsis or psychosis.

Laboratory diagnosis

MICROSCOPY

It is most important to confirm the diagnosis by examining thick and thin blood films on several occasions (Plate 15). Parasites may be found in blood taken by venepuncture, finger-pulp or ear-lobe stabs, and from the umbilical cord and impression smears of the placenta. In fatal cases, cerebral malaria can be confirmed rapidly as the cause of death by making a smear from cerebral grey matter (see Plate 1) obtained by needle necropsy through the foramen magnum, superior orbital fissure, ethmoid sinus via the nose, or through a fontanelle in young children. Sometimes no parasites can be found in peripheral blood smears from patients with malaria, even in severe infections. This may be explained by partial antimalarial treatment or by sequestration of parasitized cells in deep vascular beds. In these cases parasites or malarial pigment may be found in bone marrow aspirate. Pigment may be seen in circulating neutrophils. A number of Romanowski stains, including Field's, Giemsa, Wright's and Leishman's, are suitable for malaria diagnosis. The rapid Field's technique, which can yield a result in minutes, and Giemsa are recommended. Smears may be unsatisfactory because the slides are not clean; stains are unfiltered, old or infected; buffer pH is incorrect (it should be 7.0–7.4); drying is too slow, especially in a humid climate (producing heavily crenated erythrocytes); or the blood has been stored in anticoagulant causing lysis of parasitized erythrocytes. It is difficult to make a good smear if the patient is very anaemic. Common artefacts resembling malaria parasites are superimposed platelets, particles of stain and other debris, and pits in the slide. Other erythrocyte infections such as bartonellosis and babesiosis may be misdiagnosed as malaria. Parasites should be counted in relation to the total white-cell count (on thick films when the parasitaemia is relatively low) or erythrocytes (on thin films).

NEWER DIAGNOSTIC METHODS

An experienced microscopist can detect as few as 5 parasites/μl (0.0001 per cent parasitaemia) in a thick film and 200/μl (0.004 per cent parasitaemia) in a thin film. Becton-Dickinson's QBC (quantitative buffy coat) method involves spinning blood in special capillary tubes in which parasite DNA is stained with acridine orange and a small float presses the parasitized red blood cells against the wall of the tube where they can be viewed by ultraviolet microscopy. In expert hands, the sensitivity of this method can be as good as with conventional microscopy of thick blood films but species diagnosis is difficult, and the method is much more expensive. Becton-Dickinson's 'Para Sight F' dipstick antigen-capture assay employs a monoclonal antibody detecting *P. falciparum* histidine-rich protein-2 (PfHRP-2) antigen. It is rapid (taking about 20 min), sensitive, and specific for *P. falciparum.* Enzyme and radioimmunoassays, DNA probes (using chemoluminescence for detection), and polymerase chain-reaction (PCR) methods now approach the sensitivity of classical microscopy. They take much longer (up to 72 h), are much more expensive, and are unlikely to replace microscopy for routine diagnosis. However, some of these newer methods could be automated for screening blood donors or for use in epidemiological surveys and, in the case of PCR, identification of parasite strains as well as species is possible.

SEROLOGICAL TECHNIQUES

Malarial antibodies can be detected by immunofluorescence or enzyme immunoassay for epidemiological surveys, for screening potential blood donors, and occasionally for providing evidence of recent infection in non-immunes. In future, detection of protective antibodies will be important in assessing the response to malaria vaccines (see below).

Other laboratory investigations

Anaemia is usual, with evidence of haemolysis. Serum haptoglobins may be undetectable. The direct antiglobulin (Coombs') test is usually negative. Neutrophil leucocytosis is common in severe infections whether or not there is a complicating bacterial infection, but the white count can also be normal or low. Thrombocytopenia is common in *P. falciparum* and *P. vivax* infections; it does not correlate with severity. Prothrombin and partial thromboplastin times are prolonged in up to one-fifth of patients with cerebral malaria. Concentrations of plasma fibrinogen and other clotting factors are normal or increased, and serum levels of fibrin(ogen) degradation products are normal in most cases. Fewer than 10 per cent of patients with cerebral malaria have evidence of disseminated intravascular coagulation. However, antithrombin III concentrations are often moderately reduced and have prognostic significance. Total and direct (unconjugated) plasma bilirubin concentrations are usually increased, consistent with haemolysis, but in some patients with very high total bilirubin concentrations there is a predominance of conjugated bilirubin, indicating hepatocyte dysfunction. Some patients have cholestasis. Serum albumin concentrations are usually reduced, often grossly. Serum aminotransferases, 5′-nucleotidase, and especially lactic dehydrogenase are moderately elevated, but not into the range seen in viral hepatitis. Hyponatraemia is the most common electrolyte disturbance. Mild hypocalcaemia (after correction for hypoalbuminaemia) and hypophosphataemia have been described, especially when the patient has been given blood or a glucose infusion. Biochemical evidence of generalized rhabdomyolysis (elevated serum creatine phosphokinase concentration, myoglobinaemia and myoglobinuria) has been found in some patients. In about a third of patients with cerebral malaria, blood urea is increased above 80 mg/dl (13 mmol/l) and serum creatinine above 2 mg/dl (176 μmol/l). Lactic acidosis occurs in severely ill patients, especially those with hypoglycaemia and renal failure. It may be suspected if there is a wide 'anion gap'. Blood glucose must be checked frequently, especially in children, pregnant women and severely ill patients, even if the patient is not receiving quinine treatment and is fully conscious. A 'stix' method, with or without photometric quantification, is rapid and convenient. Microscopy and culture of cerebrospinal fluid is important in patients with cerebral malaria to exclude other treatable encephalopathies. In cerebral malaria the cerebrospinal fluid may contain up to 15 lymphocytes/μl and increased protein concentration. Pleocytosis of up to 80 cells/μl, mainly leucocytes, may be found in patients who have had repeated generalized convulsions. The cerebrospinal-fluid glucose will be low in hypoglycaemic patients and this result may be the first hint of hypoglycaemia. In view of the finding of cerebral compression and high opening pressures in many African children with cerebral malaria, some paediatricians prefer to delay lumbar puncture, while covering the possibility of bacterial meningoencephalitis with empirical antimicrobial treatment. Blood cultures should be done in patients with a high white count, shock, persistent fever or an obvious focus of secondary bacterial infection. Gram-negative rod bacteria (*E. coli, Pseudomonas aeruginosa* etc.) have been cultured from the blood of adult patients with 'algid' malaria. In Gambian children there was an association between malaria and non-typhoid Salmonella septicaemia.

Urine should be examined by microscope and dipstix. Common abnormalities are proteinuria, microscopic haematuria, haemoglobinuria, and red-cell casts. The urine is literally black in patients with severe intravascular haemolysis. Urine specific gravity should be measured: the optical method is most convenient when urine output is small. Rapid measurement of plasma quinine or quinidine concentrations is possible in some hospitals. This is a valuable way of monitoring chemotherapy.

Treatment

ANTIMALARIAL DRUGS

Antimalarial drugs can be grouped as follows:

1. Arylaminoalcohols, comprising quinoline methanols such as the cinchona alkaloids, quinine and quinidine (extracted from the bark of the cinchona tree), and mefloquine and the phenanthrene methanol, halofantrine.
2. 4-Aminoquinolines, such as chloroquine and amodiaquine.
3. Folate-synthesis inhibitors, including type 1 antifolate drugs, which compete for dihydropteroate synthase (e.g. sulphones and sulphonamides), and type 2 antifolate drugs, which inhibit malarial dihydrofolate reductase (e.g. the biguanides, proguanil and chlorproguanil, and the diaminopyrimidine, pyrimethamine).
4. 8-aminoquinolines, such as primaquine and WR238,605.
5. Antibiotics, such as tetracycline, doxycycline, clindamycin, azithromycin, and fluoroquinolones.
6. Peroxides (sesquiterpene lactones)—artemisinin (qinghaosu) derivatives from the Chinese medicinal plant, *Artemisia annua,* and its semisynthetic analogues (artemether, arteether, artesunate and artelinic acid).
7. Naphthoquinones, such as atovaquone (BW566C80).
8. Iron-chelating agents, such as desferrioxamine.

The stages of the lifecycle sensitive to some of the principal antimalarial drugs are shown in Fig. 13. Among blood schizonticides, artemisinin derivatives can prevent the development of rings or trophozoites, but quinine and mefloquine cannot stop development before the stage

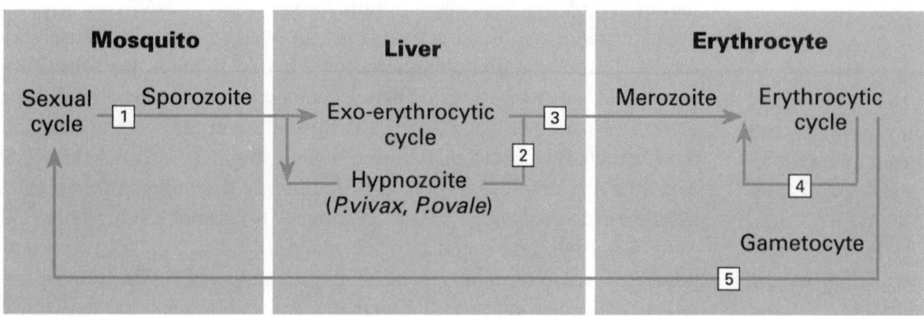

Fig. 13 Stage specificity of antimalarial drugs. 1. Sporontocidal (e.g. proguanil, pyrimethamine, atovaquone); 2. Hypnozoitocidal (e.g. primaquine WR-238, 605); 3. Tissue schizontocidal (e.g. proguanil, pyrimethamine); 4. Blood schizontocidal (e.g. chloroquine, quinine, artemisinin); 5. Gametocytocidal (e.g. primaquine, WR-238, 605; chloroquine for *P. vivax, P. malariae,* and *P. ovale*).

of mature trophozoites, and pyrimethamine–sulphadoxine combinations do not prevent the development of schizonts.

Mechanism of action of antimalarial drugs

The mode of action of the antifolate drugs is well understood and described above. Chloroquine is concentrated in the parasite's lysosomes, where haemoglobin is digested, and may act by inhibiting the haempolymerase that converts toxic haemin into insoluble haemozoin (malarial pigment). Alternatively, the drug may interfere with parasite feeding by disrupting its food vacuole. Antimalarial antibiotics are all inhibitors of ribosomal protein synthesis and probably act on the parasite's mitochondria. In the case of artemisinin derivatives, iron within the parasite probably catalyses the cleavage of the endoperoxide bridge leading to the generation of free radicals, which then form covalent bonds with parasite proteins (alkylation). Naphthoquinones, such as atovaquone, act on the electron-transport chain in malarial mitochondria through their structural similarity to coenzyme Q. No satisfactory explanation of the mode of action of the other antimalarial drugs is yet available.

The alarming spread of drug resistance has prompted great experimental effort to reveal the mechanism of resistance. The observation that chloroquine resistance could be reversed *in vitro* by high concentrations of drugs such as the calcium-channel blocker verapamil, which in other situations could reverse the multidrug resistance *(mdr)* phenotype acquired by some tumour cells, focused attention on a malarial homologue of the human *mdr* gene. Recent work suggests involvement of the *P. falciparum mdr1* gene early in the development of resistance, but segregation of resistance in the cloned progeny of a cross showed that the product of a second, uncharacterized gene product from chromosome 7 was also required.

Chloroquine

Despite the widespread resistance of *P. falciparum* to this drug, and the recent emergence of chloroquine-resistant *P. vivax* in New Guinea and adjacent areas of Indonesia, chloroquine is still the most widely used antimalarial drug. It remains the treatment of choice for most vivax and all ovale and malariae infections, and for uncomplicated falciparum malaria acquired in the few areas where the parasite remains sensitive to this drug (Central America north-west of the Panama Canal, Haiti and the Dominican Republic, and parts of the Middle East). After oral administration, it is rapidly and almost completely absorbed, peak plasma concentrations being reached in about 2 h. Absorption after intramuscular or subcutaneous injection is very rapid, which can produce dangerously high plasma concentrations unless small doses are given frequently. This probably explained the deaths of some children soon after they had received intramuscular injections of chloroquine. About half the absorbed dose is excreted unchanged by the kidney, the remainder being converted to active metabolites in the liver. Therapeutic blood concentrations persist for 6 to 10 days after a single dose and the terminal elimination half-time is 1 to 2 months. Plasma concentrations above about 250 ng/ml produce unpleasant symptoms such as dizziness, headache, diplopia, disturbed visual accommodation, dysphagia, nausea, and malaise. Chloroquine, even in small doses, may cause pruritus of the palms, soles, and scalp in dark-skinned Africans, Haitians, and Asians. Chloroquine may exacerbate epilepsy and photosensitive psoriasis. Cumulative, irreversible retinal toxicity from chloroquine has been reported after lifetime prophylactic doses of 50 to 100 g base (i.e. after 3–6 years of taking 300 mg of base per week) although this is most unusual. Chloroquine overdose is described in Chapter 8.2.9. Chloroquine is safe during pregnancy and lactation.

Amodiaquine, a 4-aminoquinoline structurally similar to chloroquine, retains activity against chloroquine-resistant strains of *P. falciparum* in some geographical areas. Unlike chloroquine, it is metabolized to a toxic quinoneimine that can produce a toxic hepatitis and potentially lethal agranulocytosis (which occurred in up to 1 in 2000 people taking amodiaquine prophylactically). Amodiaquine is still quite widely used but because of its risks and the limited therapeutic advantage over chloroquine, its use for prophylaxis and repeated treatment is now discouraged by the World Health Organization.

Quinine

With the spread of chloroquine-resistant *P. falciparum,* quinine again became the treatment of choice for falciparum malaria. Given by mouth it is rapidly and almost completely absorbed, producing peak plasma concentrations within 1 to 3 h. One-fifth is excreted in the urine and the rest is metabolized in the liver. The elimination half-time in healthy people is approximately 11 h and in patients with malaria approximately 16 h. Intravenous injection of quinine is dangerous as high plasma concentrations may result during the distribution phase, causing fatal hypotension or arrhythmias. However, quinine can be given safely if it is diluted and infused intravenously over 2 to 4 h. When intravenous infusion is not possible, but parenteral treatment is needed, quinine may be given by intramuscular injection divided between the anterior part of the thighs. For intramuscular injection, the stock solution of quinine dihydrochloride (300 mg/ml) should be diluted to 60 mg/ml. It is well absorbed from this site and complications are rare provided that strict sterile precautions are observed. Because most deaths from severe falciparum malaria occur within the first 96 h of starting treatment, it is important to achieve parasiticidal plasma concentrations of quinine as quickly as possible. This can be accomplished safely by giving a loading dose of twice the maintenance dose. A loading dose of 20 mg of the salt per kg and an 8 to 12-hourly maintenance dose of 10 mg/kg have proved safe and effective in children and adults in many tropical countries. The initial dose of quinine should not be reduced in patients who are severely ill with renal or hepatic impairment, but in these cases the maintenance dose should be reduced to 3 to 5 mg/kg if parenteral treatment is required for longer than 48 h. Little is known about optimal and safe quinine dosage in elderly and obese patients outside malaria endemic areas.

The minimum inhibitory concentration of quinine for *P. falciparum* in South-East Asia and other areas of the tropics has risen steadily. Longer courses of quinine and combination with other drugs, such as Fansidar, tetracycline or clindamycin, have been required for complete cure. Recently, cases of RII and RIII resistance (failure to clear or failure to reduce parasitaemia in the first 7 days of treatment) to quinine have been documented in Thailand and Vietnam. Quinine should not be withheld or stopped in patients who are pregnant or haemolysing. In the doses used to treat malaria it does not stimulate uterine contraction or cause fetal distress. Hypoglycaemia is the most important complication of quinine treatment (see above). Plasma quinine concentrations above 5 mg/l produce a characteristic group of symptoms—'cinchonism'—transient high-tone deafness, giddiness, tinnitus, nausea, vomiting, tremors, blurred vision, and malaise. Rarely, quinine may give rise to haemolysis, thrombocytopenia, disseminated intravascular coagulation, hypersensitivity reactions, vasculitis, and granulomatous hepatitis. Blindness, deafness, and central nervous depression are commonly observed in patients who have attempted suicide by taking overdoses of quinine. These features are rarely seen in patients being treated for malaria, even though their plasma quinine concentrations may exceed 20 mg/l. This discrepancy may be explained by the increased binding of quinine to α-1 acid glycoprotein (orosomucoid) and to other acute-phase reactive serum proteins in patients with malaria.

Quinidine, the *d*-diastereomer of quinine, is more effective against resistant strains of *P. falciparum* but is more cardiotoxic. Because of its use for cardiac arrhythmias, it is more generally available (as quinidine gluconate injection) than parenteral quinine in continental Europe and North America, and in the United States has replaced quinine for the parenteral treatment of malaria. It must be infused slowly while the electrocardiogram and blood pressure are monitored. Infusion should be slowed if the blood pressure falls, the plasma concentration exceeds 22 μmol/1 (7 mg/ml), or if the QT_c interval increases by more than 25 per cent.

Mefloquine

This synthetic drug is effective against some *P. falciparum* strains resistant to chloroquine, pyrimethamine–sulphonamide combinations, and quinine. It is too irritant to be given parenterally, but is well absorbed when given by mouth, reaching peak plasma concentrations in 6 to 24 h. The elimination half-time is 14 to 28 days. The drug can be given as a single dose but, to reduce the risk of vomiting and other gastrointestinal side-effects, the dose is best divided into two halves given 6 to 8 h apart. Gastrointestinal symptoms occur in 10 to 15 per cent of patients but are usually mild. Less frequent side-effects include nightmares and sleeping disturbances, dizziness, ataxia, sinus bradycardia, sinus arrhythmia, postural hypotension, and an 'acute brain syndrome' consisting of fatigue, asthenia, seizures, and psychosis. Mefloquine treatment should be avoided in pregnant women, especially during the first trimester, and pregnancy should be avoided within 3 months of stopping mefloquine. People taking β-blockers and those with a past history of epilepsy or psychiatric disease should also avoid the drug. Unfortunately, *in vitro* resistance to mefloquine and treatment failures have now been reported in South-East Asia, Africa, and South America.

Halofantrine

This synthetic antimalarial compound is active against multiresistant, including mefloquine-resistant, *P. falciparum.* Only an oral preparation is available. Bioavailability is low, variable, but perhaps doubled if the drug is taken with a fatty meal. The recommended dose for adults and children weighing more than 37 kg is 500 mg (two tablets) taken every 6 h for three doses. The manufacturers recommend that this course should be repeated 1 week later in non-immune subjects. Maximum plasma concentrations are reached 3 h after the last of the three doses and the elimination half-time is 1 to 3 days for the parent drug, 3 to 7 days for the principal active metabolite. There is some evidence of cross-resistance with mefloquine and the emergence of resistance in Africa, South America, and South-East Asia. Side-effects are generally less than with mefloquine, consisting of abdominal pain and diarrhoea. However, it has been shown recently that halofantrine prolongs the QT_c interval and may induce fatal arrhythmias in susceptible individuals. It is therefore contraindicated in patients with a family history of QT_c prolongation, those with a clinical condition associated with prolonged QT_c interval (for example, electrolyte disorders, thiamine deficiency, myocardial disease), and in those with known or suspected cardiac abnormalities. It is also contraindicated in pregnancy and during breast feeding.

Artemisinin

Artemisinin or qinghaosu (pronounced 'ching-how-soo') is the active principal of the Chinese medicinal herb *Artemisia annua—Compositae* (sweet wormwood), which has been used as a treatment for fevers in China for more than 1000 years. Antimalarial activity resides in the endoperoxide structure. It destroys young trophozoites as well as other blood stages of *P. falciparum,* including chloroquine-resistant strains, and clears parasitaemia more rapidly than any other antimalarial drug. Dihydroartemisinin, the active metabolite, is cleared rapidly. In China, clinical trials with intravenous artesunate (a water-soluble hemisuccinate), intramuscular artemether (the methyl ether suspended in peanut oil), and oral and suppository preparations of artemisinin produced very encouraging results in the treatment of multiresistant *P. falciparum* infections, suggesting perhaps a halving of mortality in cerebral malaria compared to quinine. More recently, studies in South-East Asia, Africa, and South America in cerebral and other severe forms of falciparum malaria have provided evidence of a rapid effect judged by fever and parasite clearance, suggestion of a reduction of mortality, and negligible toxicity. The high recrudescence rates reported in earlier trials were attributed to inadequate dosage. In animal toxicity studies, there has been evidence of neurotoxicity, brainstem neuronal damage, and QT_c prolongation but these effects have not been seen in human patients. In severe falciparum malaria, most experience has been gained with intramuscular artemether, given in a loading dose of 3.2 mg/kg on the first day (as a single dose or divided, 12 h apart) followed by 1.6 mg/kg per day until the patient is able to take an oral drug such as mefloquine. Artesunate, although inherently unstable in aqueous solution, can be made up with 5 per cent bicarbonate just before injection and given by intravenous or intramuscular injection (2 mg/kg on the first day followed by 1 mg/kg until the patient can take oral treatment). An extra dose of 1 mg/kg can be given 4 to 6 h after the initial loading dose in hyperparasitaemic patients. Suppository formulations of artemisinin have proved effective in severe falciparum malaria in China and Vietnam, and could prove particularly valuable in treating children at peripheral levels of the health service. Oral preparations of artemisinin and artesunate are effective for uncomplicated falciparum malaria and vivax malaria but they are not yet needed in most parts of the malaria endemic area and it is generally felt that their distribution should be strictly controlled.

Primaquine

This is the only available drug effective against exoerythrocytic (hepatic) forms of *P. vivax* and *P. ovale,* and is essential for the radical cure of these infections. It is also gametocytocidal for all species of malaria. Mass treatment of patients with *P. falciparum* infection could eliminate the sexual cycle in mosquitoes by sterilizing gametocytes. Its elimination half-time is 7 h. The principal drawback of primaquine is that it causes haemolysis in patients with congenital deficiencies of erythrocyte enzymes, notably G6PD. However, severe intravascular haemolysis is unusual even in G6PD-deficient patients, except in certain areas of the world such as the Mediterranean (e.g. Sardinia) and Sri Lanka. Primaquine can cross the placenta and cause severe haemolysis in a G6PD-deficient fetus, most commonly a boy. It is also excreted in breast milk. It should not be used during pregnancy or lactation in areas where G6PD deficiency is prevalent. Primaquine, like sulphonamides and sulphones (e.g. dapsone) can produce severe haemolysis and methaemoglobinaemia in patients with congenital deficiency of NADH methaemoglobin reductase. The patient quickly develops dusky cyanosis, noticed first in the nail beds. In patients with G6PD deficiency, weekly dosage with 45 mg of primaquine is better tolerated than the usual daily dose of 15 mg. In the Solomon Islands, Indonesia, Thailand, and Papua New Guinea a total dose of 6.0 mg/kg (twice the usual dose) or even more may be needed to eliminate the primaquine-resistant Chesson-type strain of *P. vivax.* This is usually given as 15 mg base/day for 28 days. WR238,605, a new 8-aminoquinoline, is now in clinical trials. It is more than 10 times more active a hypnozoiticide than primaquine.

Sulphonamide–pyrimethamine combinations (Fansidar, Metakelfin etc.)

These synergistic combinations were once valuable in the treatment of chloroquine-resistant falciparum infections worldwide. A single adult dose of three Fansidar tablets (1500 mg sulfadoxine, 75 mg pyrimethamine) proved safe and effective, and is useful as an emergency standby for travellers out of the reach of medical facilities and as an adjunct to quinine in the treatment of *P. falciparum* infections in areas of increasing quinine resistance. However, in most of South-East Asia, China, Oceanea, Latin America, and Africa already troubled by chloroquine resistance, resistance to pyrimethamine–sulphonamide combinations is also spreading. An intramuscular formulation has proved effective against *P. falciparum* in southern Africa. Pyrimethamine is a folate inhibitor and so may cause folic acid deficiency in pregnant women and others unless folinic acid supplements are given. The sulphonamide components of these combinations are potentially dangerous. In patients who are hypersensitive to sulphonamide they may cause systemic vasculitis, Stevens–Johnson syndrome or toxic epidermal necrolysis. In the United States the risk of fatal reactions has been calculated as 1 in 18 000–26 000 prophylactic courses. Aplastic anaemia and agranulocytosis can also occur. Pyrimethamine and sulphonamide cross the placenta and are excreted in milk. In the fetus and neonate, sulphonamides can displace bilirubin from plasma protein-binding sites causing kernicterus. For these reasons, sulphonamide–pyrimethamine combinations are not recommended for treatment during pregnancy or lactation unless no alternative drug is available, nor for prophylaxis at all.

P. vivax and *P. malariae* parasitaemias are generally cleared by all the drugs effective against *P. falciparum.* However, in some scattered areas, sulphonamide–pyrimethamine combinations may not be effective because of pyrimethamine resistance.

Hydroxynaphthoquinones

Atovaquone (BW566C80) is the most promising of these compounds. Against multiresistant *P. falciparum* there was initial clearance of parasitaemia but a high incidence of recrudescences resulting from the rapid development of resistance. Fortunately, combination with proguanil or tetracycline appears to prevent this problem and atovaquone–proguanil is now undergoing clinical trials. Atovaquone is also of value in patients with toxoplasmosis and *Pneumocystis pneumoniae* infection.

Iron chelators

Desferrioxamine can eliminate parasitaemia when used alone in uncomplicated falciparum malaria. Studies in Zambian children with cerebral malaria demonstrated a reduction in duration of coma and parasite clearance times when desferrioxamine was added to conventional quinine therapy. As well as its antimalarial activity, which may be due to depriving the parasite of iron, desferrioxamine is also a free oxygen radical scavenger, which may be beneficial in severe falciparum malaria.

Other antimalarial compounds

Several antimicrobial drugs, including tetracycline, clindamycin and sulphonamides such as co-trimoxazole, have some antimalarial activity and have been used, usually in combination with a quinoline compound. Generally, they kill parasites too slowly to be used alone. In an emergency, in the absence of quinoline antimalarials, they could be used to treat malaria. In Africa, co-trimoxazole has been advocated as a first-line treatment for febrile illnesses in children, where it is not possible to distinguish clinically between malaria and an acute respiratory-tract infection.

PRACTICAL ANTIMALARIAL CHEMOTHERAPY

Prescribing quinoline antimalarial drugs

The various salts of quinoline compounds contain greatly differing amounts of base. If the prescription fails to specify salt or base, or which particular salt is intended, serious problems can arise. Where possible, the dose of base should be prescribed. This is generally accepted for chloroquine, amodiaquine, mefloquine and primaquine, but, in the case of quinine and quinidine, weights of salts are usually quoted. Conversions are given in Table 6.

Table 6 *Salt base equivalents of common quinoline antimalarial drugs*

Antimalarial drug	Salt (mg)	Base (mg)
Amodiaquine sulphate	130	100
Chloroquine sulphate	136	100
Chloroquine phosphate	161	100
Chloroquine hydrochloride	123	100
Halofantrine hydrochloride	107	100
Mefloquine hydrochloride	110	100
Primaquine phosphate	18	10
Quinidine gluconate	145	100
Quinidine sulphate	108	100
Quinine bisulphate	145	100
Quinine dihydrochloride	105	100
Quinine hydrochloride	105	100
Quinine sulphate	103	100

Treatment of uncomplicated malaria (Table 7)

Patients suffering from vivax, ovale, and malariae malarias, and those with uncomplicated falciparum malaria, can usually be given antimalarial drugs by mouth. However, feverish patients may vomit the tablets. The risk of vomiting can be reduced if the patient lies down quietly for a while after taking an antipyretic such as paracetamol. The initial dose of antimalarial drug may have to be given by injection in those who vomit persistently.

Treatment of severe falciparum malaria (Table 8)

Appropriate chemotherapy should be started as soon as possible as there is a highly significant relation between delay in chemotherapy and mortality. Whenever possible, dosage should be calculated according to body weight. The parenteral administration of drugs is the rule for patients with severe and complicated falciparum malaria. In the case of cinchona alkaloids, this is most safely and effectively achieved by infusing the drug, diluted in isotonic fluid, intravenously over a period of 2 to 4 h. The aims of chemotherapy are different in severe and uncomplicated malaria. In severe malaria, parasiticidal plasma concentrations must be achieved as quickly as possible and sustained for long enough to ensure rapid clearance of parasitaemia. In these patients, the use of single-dose regimens to ensure compliance, the prevention of recrudescences (RI resistance), and the killing of gametocytes are of secondary importance, while symptoms that are troublesome to the fully conscious patient with uncomplicated malaria, such as cinchonism or pruritus, are acceptable in the treatment of a life-threatening illness and should not limit dosage.

The therapeutic response must be carefully monitored by repeated clinical assessment, measurement of temperature, pulse, blood pressure, and examination of blood films. Patients should be switched to oral treatment as soon as they are able to swallow and retain tablets. They must be watched carefully for signs of drug toxicity. In the case of cinchona alkaloids, the most common toxicity during antimalarial treatment is the development of hypoglycaemia. The blood sugar should, therefore, be checked frequently.

General management

Patients with severe malaria should be transferred to the highest level of care available, preferably the intensive care unit. They must be nursed in bed because of their postural hypotension. Body temperatures above 38.5°C are associated with febrile convulsions, especially in children, and between 39.5 and 42°C with coma and permanent neurological sequelae. In pregnant women, hyperpyrexia contributes to fetal distress. Temperature should therefore be controlled by fanning, tepid sponging, cooling blanket or antipyretic drugs such as paracetamol (15 mg/kg in tablets by mouth, or powder washed down a nasogastric tube, or as suppositories). Pyrazolones such as metamizole sodium (Dipyrone) are widely used in tropical countries but carry an unacceptable risk of inducing agranulocytosis.

CEREBRAL MALARIA

Convulsions, vomiting, and aspiration pneumonia are common, so patients should be nursed in the lateral position with a rigid oral airway or endotracheal tube in place. They should be turned at least every 2 h to avoid bed sores. Vital signs, Glasgow coma score, and occurrence of convulsions should be recorded frequently. Convulsions can be controlled with diazepam given by slow intravenous injection (adults 10 mg, children 0.15 mg/kg) or intrarectally (0.5–1.0 mg/kg), or with paraldehyde drawn in a glass syringe and given by intramuscular injection (0.1 ml/kg). A single dose of phenobarbital (15 mg/kg by intramuscular

Table 7 *Antimalarial chemotherapy in adults or children with uncomplicated malaria who can swallow tablets*

Chloroquine-resistant *P. falciparum* or species or origin unknown	Chloroquine-sensitive *P. falciparum* or *P. vivax, P. ovale, P. malariae* or monkey malarias
1. *Quinine* Adults: 600 mg of the salt 3 times each day for 7 days and, if quinine resistance is known or suspected, followed by *either* Fansidar 3 tablets (sulfadoxine 500 mg per tablet, pyrimethamine 25 mg tablet)[d] *or* tetracycline 250 mg 4 times each day for 7 days when renal function has returned to normal[c] Children: approximately 10 mg of the salt/kg 3 times each day for 7 days and, if quinine resistance is known or suspected, followed by Fansidar (dose see 3 below) **OR**	1. *Chloroquine* Adults: 600 mg of the base on the 1st and 2nd days; 300 mg on the 3rd day. Children: approximately 10 mg base/kg on the 1st and 2nd days; 5 mg/kg on the 3rd day
2. *Mefloquine* Adults: 15–25 mg of the base/kg[b] (maximum 1500 mg) given as 2 doses 6–8 h apart Children: 25 mg of the base/kg given as 2 doses 6–8 h apart **OR**	For radical cure of vivax/ovale add 2. *Primaquine* Adults (except pregnant and lactating women and G6PD-deficient patients): 15 mg base/day on days 4–17 *or* 45 mg/week for 8 weeks[a] Children: 0.25 mg base/kg/day on days 4–17 *or* 0.75 mg/kg/week for 8 weeks[a]
3. *Fansidar* Sulfadoxine (500 mg per tablet) plus pyrimethamine (25 mg)[d] Adults: 3 tablets as a single dose Children: <1 year ¼ tablet, <5 years ½ tablet, <9 years 1 tablet, <15 years 2 tablets	

For salt/base equivalents see Table 6.

[a]For Chesson-type strains (SE Asia, W Pacific) use double dose or double duration up to a total dose of 6 mg/kg in daily doses of 15–22.5 mg in adults.

[b]Depending on geographical area and presumed immunity.

[c]Alternative to tetracycline is doxycycline 100 mg daily for 7 days. Tetracycline and doxycycline are contraindicated in pregnancy.

[d]Sulfadoxine + pyrimethamine (Fansidar) and other sulphonamide–pyrimethamine combinations are contraindicated if the patient is hypersensitive to sulphonamide or is pregnant or lactating.

injection) can be given on admission to prevent convulsions. Stomach contents should be aspirated through a nasogastric tube to reduce the risk of aspiration pneumonia. Elective endotracheal intubation is indicated if coma deepens and the airway is jeopardised. Deepening coma with signs of cerebral herniation is an indication for CT or magnetic resonance imaging, or a trial of treatment to lower intracranial pressure, such as intravenous infusion of mannitol (1.0–1.5 g/kg of 10–20 per cent solution over 30 min) or mechanical hyperventilation to reduce the arterial $p\mathrm{CO}_2$ to below 4.0 kPa (30 mmHg).

A number of potentially harmful remedies of unproven value have been recommended for the treatment of cerebral malaria. Two double-blind trials of dexamethasone (2 mg/kg and 11 mg/kg intravenously over 48 h) in adults and children in Thailand and Indonesia showed no reduction in mortality but prolongation of coma and an increased incidence of infection and gastrointestinal bleeding. Low molecular-weight dextrans, osmotic agents, heparin, adrenaline, cyclosporin A, prostacyclin, and oxpentifylline have been advocated for the treatment of cerebral malaria without adequate evidence and in some cases despite obvious toxicity.

The most interesting future prospects for the treatment of cerebral malaria involve the use of soluble receptor-peptide sequences or antibodies to reverse cytoadherence and sequestration in the brain, antirosetting agents, and antibodies directed against TNFα and other relevant cytokines (see Pathophysiology above).

ANAEMIA

Indications for transfusion with preferably fresh, compatible whole blood or packed cells include a low (less than 20 per cent or rapidly falling) haematocrit, severe bleeding or predicted blood loss (for example, imminent parturition or surgery), hyperparasitaemia, and failure to respond to conservative treatment with oxygen and plasma expanders. When screening of transfused blood is inadequate and infections such as human immunodeficiency virus, human T-lymphotrophic virus, and hepatitis viruses are prevalent in the community, criteria for blood transfusion must be even more rigorous. Exchange transfusion is a safe way of correcting the anaemia without precipitating pulmonary oedema in those who are fluid overloaded or chronically and severely anaemic. The volume of transfused blood must be included in the fluid-balance chart. Diuretics such as furosamide can be given intravenously in a dose of 1 to 2 mg/kg body weight to promote diuresis during the transfusion, and in all cases transfusion must be cautious with frequent observations of the jugular or central venous pressure and auscultation for pulmonary crepitations. Survival of compatible donor red cells is greatly reduced during the acute and convalescent phases of falciparum malaria.

DISTURBANCES OF FLUID AND ELECTROLYTE BALANCE

Fluid and electrolyte requirements must be assessed individually in patients with malaria. Circulatory overload with intravenous fluids or blood transfusion may precipitate fatal pulmonary oedema, but untreated hypovolaemia is dangerous as it may lead to shock, lactic acidosis, and renal failure. Hypovolaemia may result from salt and water depletion through fever, diarrhoea, vomiting, insensible losses, and poor intake. The state of hydration is assessed clinically from the ocular tensions, skin turgor, peripheral circulation, postural change in blood pressure, peripheral venous filling, and jugular or central venous pressure. The history of recent urine output and measurement of urine volume and specific gravity may be useful. Adult patients with severe falciparum malaria usually require between 1000 and 3000 ml of intravenous fluid during the first 24 h of hospital admission. Fluid replacement should be controlled by observations of jugular, central venous or pulmonary-

Table 8 *Antimalarial chemotherapy in adults or children with severe malaria or in those who cannot swallow tablets*

Chloroquine-resistant *P. falciparum* or origin unknown	Chloroquine-sensitive *P. falciparum*[a] or *P. vivax, P. ovale, P. malariae* or monkey malarias
1. *Quinine* Adults: 20 mg of the salt/kg (loading dose)[c] diluted in 10 ml/kg isotonic fluid by i.v. infusion over 4 h, then 10 mg/kg over 4 h, 8–12-hourly until patients can swallow Children: 15 mg of the salt/kg (loading dose)[c] diluted in 10 ml/kg isotonic fluid by i.v. infusion over 2 h, then 10 mg/kg over 2 h, 12-hourly until patients can swallow The 7-day course should be completed with quinine tablets approximately 10 mg salt/kg 8-hourly[d,e] **OR** 2. *Quinine* (in intensive care unit) 7 mg of the salt/kg (loading dose)[c] i.v. by infusion pump over 30 min followed immediately by 10 mg/kg (maintenance dose) diluted in 10 ml/kg isotonic fluid by i.v. infusion over 4 h, repeated 8–12-hourly until patient can swallow etc[d,e] **OR** 3. *Quinidine* (in intensive care unit) 6.2 mg of the base/kg (loading dose)[c] i.v. by infusion over 1–2 h, followed by 0.012 mg/kg per min by infusion pump for 72 h or until the patient can swallow, then quinine tablets to complete 7 days treatment[d] **OR** 4. *Artemether* or *Artesunate* (when licensed and available) (See text for details)	1. *Chloroquine*[b] 10 mg base/kg (maximum 600 mg) diluted in isotonic fluid by continuous i.v. infusion over 8 h, followed by 15 mg base/kg (maximum 900 mg) by continuous i.v. infusion over 24 h **OR** 2. *Quinine* (see above, left-hand column)
If it is not possible to give drugs by intravenous infusion 1. *Quinine* 20 mg of the salt/kg (loading dose)[c] diluted to 60 mg/ml, by deep i.m. injection (half dose into each anterior thigh) with strict sterile precautions, then 10 mg/kg 8–12-hourly until patient can swallow etc[d,e] 2. *Artemether, Artesunate,* or *Artemisinin* (when licensed and available) by i.m. injection or suppository	1. *Chloroquine*[b] Total dose 25 mg base/kg given either (a) i.m. or s.c. 2.5 mg/kg 4-hourly; *or* (b) i.m. or s.c. 3.5 mg/kg 6-hourly. **OR** 2. *Quinine* i.m. (see above, left-hand column)

For salt/base equivalents see Table 6.

[a]Currently restricted to Haiti, Dominican Republic, Central America, and parts of Middle East.

[b]Parenteral chloroquine should be used with great caution in young children.

[c]Loading dose must not be used if patient started quinine, quinidine, or mefloquine treatment within preceding 12–24 h.

[d]In areas of known or suspected quinine resistance add tetracycline 250 mg 4 time each day or doxycycline 200 mg daily for 7 days except for children under 8 years and pregnant women *or* add Fansidar (doses in Table 7) except in patients known to be sulphonamide hypersensitive or in pregnant or lactating women.

[e]In patients requiring more than 48 h of parenteral therapy reduce the dose by one-third to a half to 6.7–6 mg of the salt per kg 8–12-hourly.

artery wedge pressures. Hyponatraemia (plasma sodium concentration 120–130 mmol/l) usually requires no treatment and these patients should be cautiously rehydrated with isotonic saline if they are clinically dehydrated, have low central venous pressures, high urinary specific gravity, and low urine sodium concentration (below 25 mmol/l).

RENAL FAILURE

Patients with falling urine output and elevated blood urea nitrogen and serum creatinine concentrations can be treated conservatively at first but established acute renal failure must be treated with dialysis. Hypovolaemia is corrected by cautious infusion of isotonic saline until the central venous pressure is in the range +5 to +15 cmH_2O. If urine output remains low after rehydration, increasing doses of slowly infused intravenous frusemide (up to a total dose of 1 g) and finally intravenous infusion of dopamine (2.5–5 μg/kg per min) can be tried. If these measures fail to achieve a sustained increase in urine output, strict fluid balance should be enforced with particular emphasis on fluid restriction. Indications for dialysis include a rapid increase in serum creatinine level, hyperkalaemia, fluid overload, metabolic acidosis, and clinical manifestations of uraemia (diarrhoea and vomiting, encephalopathy, gastrointestinal bleeding, and pericarditis). Haemofiltration or haemodialysis are theoretically preferable in malaria but peritoneal dialysis has proved effective in tropical countries. The initial doses of antimalarial drug should not be reduced in patients with renal failure but, after 48 h of parenteral treatment, the maintenance dose should be reduced by one-third to one-half.

METABOLIC ACIDOSIS

This is usually attributable to lactic acidosis or renal failure. It should be treated by improving perfusion and oxygenation by correcting hypovolaemia, clearing the airway, increasing the inspired oxygen concentration, and by treating septicaemia, a frequently associated complication. Severe acidosis (pH less than 7.20) can be treated by cautious infusion of sodium bicarbonate, tris (hydroxymethyl)-aminomethan or dichloroacetate (which stimulates muscle pyruvate dehydrogenase) but, if the patient is uraemic, early dialysis is the treatment of choice.

PULMONARY OEDEMA

This must be prevented by propping the patient up at 45° and controlling fluid intake so that the jugular or central venous pressure is kept below +5 cmH_2O. Those who develop pulmonary oedema should be propped upright and given oxygen to breathe. In a well-equipped intensive care unit, the judicious use of vasodilator drugs can be controlled by monitoring haemodynamic variables, fluid overload can be corrected by haemoperfusion, and oxygenation can be improved by mechanical ventilation with positive end-expiratory pressure.

HYPOTENSION AND 'SHOCK' ('ALGID MALARIA')

This should be treated as for bacteraemic shock. The circulatory problems should be corrected with plasma expanders, dopamine, and broad-spectrum antimicrobial treatment (e.g. gentamicin with ceftazidime or cefuroxime plus metronidazole) should be started immediately, bearing in mind that likely routes of infection include the urinary tract, lungs, and the gut. Other causes of shock in patients with malaria include dehydration, blood loss (e.g. following splenic rupture), and pulmonary oedema.

HYPOGLYCAEMIA

This may be asymptomatic, especially in pregnancy, and its clinical manifestations may be confused with those of malaria. Blood sugar must be checked every few hours, especially in patients being treated with cinchona alkaloids. It may arise despite continuous intravenous infusions of 5 or even 10 per cent dextrose. A therapeutic trial of dextrose (1 ml/kg by intravenous bolus injection) should be given if hypoglycaemia is proved or suspected. This should be followed by a continuous infusion of 10 per cent dextrose. Glucose may be given by nasogastric tube to unconscious patients or by peritoneal dialysis in those undergoing this treatment for renal failure. Among agents that block insulin release, diazoxide was ineffective, but octreotide (Sandostatin), a synthetic somatostatin analogue, proved effective in some severe cases of quinine-induced hypoglycaemia.

HYPERPARASITAEMIA

In non-immune patients, mortality increases with parasitaemia, exceeding 50 per cent with parasitaemias above 500 000/μl. Exchange transfusion might be expected to reduce the parasitaemia more rapidly than optimal chemotherapy alone and could have the added advantages of removing harmful metabolites, toxins, cytokines and other mediators, and restoring normal red-cell mass, platelets, clotting, factors, albumin, and other depleted substances. Potential dangers of the procedure include electrolyte disturbances (for example hypocalcaemia), cardiovascular complications, and introduction of infectious agents in the blood and through infection of intravascular lines. The use of exchange transfusion, haemopheresis, and plasmapheresis has been reported in more than 80 patients, the vast majority of whom survived. There was undoubtedly some reporting bias. Some patients showed clinical improvement, such as recovery of consciousness, and restoration of urine flow, soon after the procedure. However, there have been a few recent reports of adult respiratory distress syndrome developing during the procedure. Efficacy of exchange transfusion is never likely to be put to the test of a randomized comparative study but, where facilities allow and screening of donor blood is adequate, the procedure should be considered in non-immune patients who are severely ill, who have deteriorated on conventional treatment, and who have parasitaemias in excess of 10 per cent. The introduction of antimalarials, such as artemisinin derivatives, which clear parasitaemia very rapidly, may obviate the need for exchange transfusion.

SPLENIC RUPTURE

Acute adbominal pain and tenderness with left shoulder-tip pain and shock in patients with vivax and falciparum malaria should suggest the possibility of splenic rupture, especially if there is a history of abdominal trauma. Free blood in the peritoneal cavity and a torn splenic capsule can be detected by ultrasound or CT and confirmed by needle aspiration of the peritoneal cavity, laparoscopy or laparotomy. Conservative management with blood transfusion and close observation in an intensive care unit is sometimes successful but access to surgical help is essential in case there is a sudden deterioration.

DISSEMINATED INTRAVASCULAR COAGULATION

Patients with evidence of a coagulopathy should be given vitamin K (adult dose 10 mg by slow intravenous injection). Cryoprecipitates, platelet transfusions, and fresh-frozen plasma should be considered.

MANAGEMENT OF THE PREGNANT WOMAN WITH MALARIA

Malaria must be diagnosed and treated rapidly in pregnant women. Unwarranted fears of abortifacient and fetus-damaging effects of antimalarial drugs have led to delay or even withdrawal of treatment, but experience since the nineteenth century has confirmed the safety of quinine in pregnancy. Chloroquine has been used extensively without ill effect to mother or fetus. However, sulphonamide–pyrimethamines, tetracycline, primaquine, and aspirin (but not paracetamol) are contraindicated in late pregnancy, mefloquine should be avoided if possible, especially during the first trimester, and halofantrine is contraindicated throughout pregnancy. In pregnant women, the total apparent volume of distribution of quinine is reduced and the drug is eliminated more rapidly. Initial dosage is the same as in non-pregnant patients, but in severe cases requiring prolonged parenteral treatment, the dose, but not the frequency of administration, should be reduced. The main danger of quinine in pregnancy is its stimulation of insulin secretion with resulting hypoglycaemia (see above). Blood glucose must be checked at least once a day in pregnant women with malaria, whether or not they are receiving quinine. Maternal fever should be reduced as soon as possible. Induction of labour, caesarean section, or speeding up of the second stage of labour with forceps or vacuum extractor should be considered in patients with severe falciparum malaria. Fluid balance is particularly critical in these patients. If possible, central venous pressure should be monitored. Exchange transfusion of 1000 to 1500 ml of blood in late pregnancy proved an effective way of managing severe anaemia with high-output cardiac failure in Nigeria. Circulating volume could be reduced and the risk of postpartum pulmonary oedema lessened by replacing exfused blood with a smaller volume of packed cells.

Prognosis

The mortality of acute vivax, ovale, and malariae malarias is negligible. Strictly defined cerebral malaria has a mortality of about 10 to 15 per cent when medical facilities are good, and may be less than 5 per cent in Western intensive care units. Antecedent factors that predispose to severe falciparum malaria include lack of acquired immunity or lapsed immunity, splenectomy, pregnancy, and immunosuppression. There is a strong correlation between density of parasitaemia and severity. Severe clinical manifestations, such as impaired consciousness, retinal haemorrhages, renal failure, hypoglycaemia, haemoglobinuria, metabolic acidosis and pulmonary oedema, carry a bad prognosis. The case mortality of pregnant women with cerebral malaria, especially primiparae in the third trimester, is approximately 10 times greater than in non-pregnant patients. The following laboratory findings carry a poor prognosis: peripheral schizontaemia, peripheral leucocytosis exceeding 12 000/μl, high cerebrospinal-fluid lactate or low glucose, low plasma antithrombin III, serum creatinine exceeding 265 μmol/l, or blood urea nitrogen more than 21.4 mmol/l, haematocrit less than 20 per cent, blood glucose less than 2.2 mmol/l, and elevated serum enzyme concentrations (for example, aspartate and alanine aminotransferases, lactate dehydrogenase).

Chronic immunological complications of malaria

QUARTAN MALARIAL NEPHROSIS

In parts of East and West Africa, South America, India, South-East Asia and Papua New Guinea, there is epidemiological evidence linking *P. malariae* infection to immune-complex glomerulonephritis, leading to nephrotic syndrome. Few of those exposed to repeated *P. malariae* infections develop nephrosis, suggesting that additional factors are involved. The histological changes, which are not entirely specific, are of a progressive focal and segmental glomerulosclerosis with fibrillary splitting or flaking of the capillary basement membrane, producing characteristic lacunae. Electron-dense deposits beneath the endothelium can be seen by electron microscopy. Immunofluorescence reveals glomerular deposits of immunoglobulins and C3, and *P. malariae* antigen, in about 25 per cent of cases. More than half the patients present by the age of 15 years with typical features of nephrotic syndrome. *P. malariae* is frequently found in blood smears and *P. malariae* antigen in renal biopsies in children but not in adults. The renal lesions may be perpetuated by autoimmune mechanisms. The pattern of immunofluorescent staining has some prognostic significance. Few patients respond to corticosteroids, but some are helped by azathioprine and cyclophosphamide, especially those whose renal biopsies show the coarse or mixed patterns of immunofluorescence. Antimalarial treatment is not effective. This condition could be prevented by antimalarial prophylaxis and has disappeared in countries such as Guyana during a period of malaria eradication.

TROPICAL SPLENOMEGALY SYNDROME (HYPER-REACTIVE MALARIAL SPLENOMEGALY)

Transient splenomegaly is a feature of acute attacks of malaria in non-immune or partially immune patients, while progressive splenomegaly is seen in children resident in malarious areas during the process of their acquiring immunity to the infection. However, a separate entity has been described in Africa (especially Nigeria, Uganda, and Zambia), the Indian subcontinent (Bengal, Sri Lanka), South-East Asia (Vietnam, Thailand, and Indonesia), South America (Amazon region), Papua New Guinea, and the Middle East (Aden). The defining features are residence in a malarious area, chronic splenomegaly, elevated serum IgM and malarial antibody levels, hepatic sinusoidal lymphocytosis, and a clinical and immunological response to antimalarial prophylaxis. This condition is thought to result from an aberrant immunological response to repeated infection by any of the species of malaria parasite.

Pathophysiology

In Flores, Indonesia, the mechanism has been worked out in some detail. The interaction of repeated malarial infections, in this case perhaps with *P. vivax,* with unknown host factors leads to the production of IgM lymphocytotoxic antibodies specific for activated, suppressor T lymphocytes, which normally regulate IgM production. The resulting disinhibition of B lymphocytes leads to their overproduction of IgM, forming immune complexes or, more likely, macromolecular aggregates of IgM (cryoglobulins). The need to clear these aggregates stimulates the reticuloendothelial system and causes the progressive and eventually massive splenomegaly and hepatomegaly. The decrease in suppressor/cytotoxic (CD8) lymphocytes increases the helper:suppressor (CD4:CD8) ratio. Antimalarial chemoprophylaxis, by removing the antigenic stimulus provided by repeated malarial infections, allows the patient's immune system to return to normal. There are some differences between tropical splenomegaly syndrome in Africa, Flores, and Papua New Guinea. In Africa, but not in Flores or Papua New Guinea, there is a peripheral lymphocytosis resulting from an increase in B lymphocytes, and distinction from chronic lymphatic leukaemia may be difficult. In Ghana, clonal rearrangements of the JH region of the immunoglobulin gene were found in patients with tropical splenomegaly who failed to respond to proguanil chemoprophylaxis, suggesting that the syndrome may evolve into a malignant lymphoproliferative disorder. Some of these patients had features of splenic lymphoma with villous (hairy) lymphocytes. In Africa and Papua New Guinea, IgG levels were significantly increased, but not in Flores. In Flores only the titres of *P. vivax* IgM antibodies were higher in patients with the splenomegaly syndrome, but in Papua New Guinea titres of *P. falciparum, P. vivax,* and *P. malariae* were increased, and in Africa *P. falciparum* and *P. malariae* are the species involved. The familial tendency of the tropical splenomegaly syndrome in Africa and Papua New Guinea suggests a genetically determined predisposition.

Clinical features

In malaria endemic areas, patients with tropical splenomegaly syndrome are distinguishable by their progressive splenic enlargement persisting beyond childhood. The spleen may be enormous, filling the left iliac fossa, extending across the midline, and anteriorly producing a visible mass with an obvious notch. The liver is usually enlarged, especially its left lobe. Symptoms attributable to the spleen include a vague dragging sensation and occasional episodes of severe pain with peritonism, suggesting perisplenitis or splenic infarction. Anaemia may become severe enough to cause the features of high-output cardiac failure. Acute haemolytic episodes are described. These patients are vulnerable to infections, especially of the skin and respiratory system, and most deaths are attributable to overwhelming infection. Chronic hypersplenic neutropenia or failure to mobilize neutrophils in response to acute bacterial infections may be the cause. The prognosis is poor: among Crane's patients in Papua New Guinea, 57 per cent of those with massive splenomegaly were dead within 7 years.

Patients with splenic lymphoma with villous lymphocytes (Ghana) had splenic discomfort, anorexia and hepatosplenomegaly, with infiltration of the bone marrow with villous lymphocytes.

Laboratory findings

Severe chronic anaemia is the result of destruction and pooling in the spleen and dilution in an increased plasma volume. Thrombocytopenia may also be caused by splenic sequestration; it rarely causes bleeding. There is neutropenia and, in Africa patients, peripheral lymphocytosis and lymphocytic infiltration of the bone marrow. Serum IgM is greatly elevated.

The essential histopathological feature is lymphocytosis of the hepatic sinusoids with Kupffer-cell hyperplasia. In some cases, round-cell infiltration of the portal tracts is associated with fibrosis, leading to portal hypertension. In the spleen there is dilation of the sinusoids, hyperplasia of the phagocytic cells with evident erythrophagocytosis, and infiltration with lymphocytes and plasma cells. No histopathological explanation has been found for the episodes of acute splenic pain.

In patients with splenic lymphoma and villous lymphocytes, more than 30 per cent of circulating lymphocytes are villous. These cells can be distinguished from hairy-cell leukaemia by their lack of CD_{25}, CD11c, and tartrate-resistant acid phosphatase markers.

Differential diagnosis

Tropical splenomegaly syndrome must be distinguished from other causes of chronic, painless, massive splenomegaly, including leukaemias, lymphomas, myelofibrosis, thalassaemias, haemoglobinopathies, visceral leishmaniasis (by examination of bone marrow or splenic aspirates), and schistosomiasis (by liver biopsy, rectal snip, and stool examination). Lymphomas (especially chronic lymphatic leukaemia and follicular lymphoma—see above) and even leukaemias may develop in patients with the splenomegaly syndrome. Non-tropical idiopathic splenomegaly (normal serum IgM) and Felty's syndrome produce a similar histological picture in the liver. Many cases of splenomegaly in the tropics remain undiagnosed.

Treatment

Prolonged antimalarial chemoprophylaxis is the most important element of treatment. Seventy per cent of Crane's patients showed marked improvement after 12 months of chemotherapy. The choice of drug will depend on the local sensitivity of whichever species or group of species of malaria parasite are thought to be responsible for this syndrome (see Chemoprophylaxis below). The short- and long-term dangers of splenectomy rule out this procedure in the rural tropics. Similarly, splenic irradiation and antimitotic agents are dangerous and unnecessary. Folic acid may be needed. Diagnosis of patients with splenic lymphoma with villous lymphocytes (Ghana) is important as, in this condition, the risks of splenectomy are outweighed by the benefits.

ENDEMIC BURKITT'S LYMPHOMA (SEE CHAPTER 7.10.4)

Endemic Burkitt's lymphoma, a tumour of the jaw, abdomen, and other areas that spreads to the bone marrow or meninges, is the most common type of childhood malignant disease in many parts of East and West Africa and Papua New Guinea. It has also been reported from Brazil, Malaysia, and the Middle East. Burkitt noticed that its distribution (by altitude, temperature, and rainfall) and even its seasonal incidence followed that of holoendemic falciparum malaria. Outside the malaria endemic area, Burkitt's lymphoma occurs sporadically. There is a suggestion that the B-cell line in Caucasian cases comes from lymphoid tissue whereas in African cases it comes from the bone marrow. Epstein–Barr virus **(EBV)** produces a lifelong infection of B lymphocytes. In normal individuals this is controlled by specific, HLA-restricted, cytotoxic T cells, which recognize a virus-induced, lymphocyte-detected membrane antigen (LYDMA) on B cells. Immunosuppression, as in recipients of renal allografts, allows uncontrolled proliferation of the EBV-infected B-cell line, which may give rise to one of the three chromosomal translocations [t(8;14), t(2;8), t(8;22)] that activate the c-*myc* oncogene on chromosome 8 responsible for malignant transformation. Acute *P. falciparum* infection leads to a reduction in numbers of suppressor T (CD8) lymphocytes and a decrease in helper:suppressor (CD4:CD8) ratio, allowing proliferation and increased immunoglobulin secretion by EBV-infected B cells. No lymphocytotoxic antibody is found in acute plasma samples to explain the decrease in suppressor T cells. These tumours may grow so rapidly that massive local tissue destruction results in urate nephropathy and acute renal failure. Cyclophosphamide, vincristine, methotrexate, and prednisolone are used in chemotherapy, producing remissions in 80 to 90 per cent of patients and long-term survival of 20 to 70 per cent. Breakdown of large tumours during the first week of chemotherapy may be so dramatic that acute tumour lysis syndrome may be precipitated. This consists of metabolic acidosis, hyperuricaemia, hyperphosphaturia, hyperphosphataemia, hyperproteinaemia and hyperkalaemia, which may result in fatal cardiac arrhythmia and acute uric-acid nephropathy with renal failure.

Malaria control

The rational control of malaria dates from the discovery of mosquito transmission of the infection and since then has mainly relied on breaking the chain of transmission, often by attacks on the vector. As insecticide resistance of mosquitoes and drug resistance of parasites increase, the environmental methods previously used to control anopheline breeding are being revived. Currently a change of emphasis is taking place, from reliance on insecticidal control of vectors to viewing early diagnosis and prompt treatment of human cases as being more feasible and affordable. There is also greater stress on breaking the person/mosquito interface, and hopes of an effective vaccine are cautiously rising.

TRANSMISSION CONTROL

Mosquitoes may be controlled in two ways: by removing, poisoning or otherwise changing their larval habitats and so reducing their numbers; or by killing the adult mosquitoes by means of insecticides. These may be sprayed into the air for a transient effect or put on to the surfaces where mosquitoes rest to obtain a persistent or residual effect. Other methods may simply deter mosquitoes from biting people. Combination methods whereby insecticide is put on a mechanical barrier such as a bednet are currently much favoured and are discussed separately. For the future, there is also much interest in finding ways to transfect mosquitoes with genes that may render them unable to transmit malaria, by incorporating them into an appropriate agent that will spread through mosquito populations. Although killing the adult mosquitoes or their larvae will reduce mosquito numbers, and lower malaria transmission proportionately, residual insecticides have a greater effect on the expectation of life of the adults, preventing them from surviving many days, and thereby reducing malaria transmission much more than might otherwise be expected.

Mosquito species are highly selective in their choice of larval habitat, and there are usually few major vector species in a given locality. The selective destruction of vector breeding sites, called species sanitation, is a long-term method of mosquito control. Sites can be rendered unsuitable for vector breeding by drainage, changing the rate of water flow, and adding or removing shade, cutting emergent vegetation, and altering margins of water bodies. Near the sea, salinity changes may be relevant. For small reservoirs and irrigation canals, cyclical changes in water level by means of a large siphon may control larvae by alternately stranding and flushing. Intermittent drying out of irrigation channels may be of value. No generalizations are possible as, for example, water fluctuations that control vectors in the southern United States would increase breeding in subSaharan Africa. Enough local information is available to guide public-health engineering interventions in most endemic areas. As these and other measures against breeding reduce mosquito density, and transmission is proportional to density, environmental control is most effective in areas of unstable malaria. Because costs of environmental measures are related to the area of land and water involved, and the benefits are related to the human population, efficient environmental control of malaria is most likely to be economically feasible in areas of high population density. In towns and cities it needs to extend beyond the periurban fringe where the poor are concentrated. Control of mosquitoes such as *A. gambiae,* that utilize temporary pools as small as hoof prints, is very difficult by environmental means without ruthless discipline.

Where habitats cannot be drained or rendered structurally unsuitable, chemical larvicides may be used. Diesel oil at 40 1/hectare of water surface with or without the addition of insecticides will prevent the larvae breathing when it is spread on the water surface with the addition of a spreading agent. In the correct formulation, 1 kg/hectare of Paris green is effective, but 2 to 20 kg/hectare of temephos (Abate) granules is a safer alternative, usually needing to be repeated weekly or fortnightly.

The use of residual insecticides applied to walls and other indoor surfaces gives a far more persistent effect, so that DDT at 2 g/m^2 will remain toxic to endophilic anophelines for 6 months or more on a non-absorbent wall material as may λ-cyhalothrin at a much lower dosage, while organophosphorus insecticides such as malathion, propoxur, and fenitrothion at the same dosage last about 3 months. This approach is a community one, requiring coverage of all houses and shelters, as it relies on killing the mosquito after it has fed. Where the aim is individual or family protection, a knock-down insecticide used before evening in a screened house is more relevant.

Prudent behaviour can greatly reduce the risk of an infective mosquito bite, especially for the visitor to an endemic area. As anophelines bite mostly in the evening, remaining in a screened area from dusk, wearing long sleeves and leg coverings, and sleeping beneath a mosquito net are of real, if underestimated, benefit. Recently, use of bednets impregnated with synthetic pyrethroids such as permethrin or λ-cyhalothrin has been found to give substantial malaria protection in endemic areas, even reducing the number of clinical attacks in areas of high transmission. The effect is due to a combination of reduced access of mosquitoes to people because of the net, a repellent and lethal effect of the insecticide on the mosquitoes trying to bite, and sometimes an effect on mosquito density so that even those outside the nets may get some protection. Nets are most effective when mosquito biting is concentrated late at night, and they can give good protection to babies in cots. The large-scale operational use of impregnated bednets in endemic areas is being explored at present, as it is the most hopeful means of control pending development of an operational vaccine.

As engineering methods are costly, though long lasting, and insecticides can be viewed as polluting the environment, other methods of mosquito control have been sought, with variable success. Genetic control of anophelines is not feasible at present; biological control is often a useful accessory method and usually relies on small fish, especially of such genera as *Gambusia* and *Lebistes* that preferentially feed on mosquito larvae. Species of fish that survive drying out of the habitat as eggs are now of interest. The micro-organism *Bacillus thuringiensis* is used in control, but it effectively functions as a biological insecticide because it produces a toxin.

CONTROL POLICY AND MALARIA ERADICATION

The present status of malaria control needs to be understood in a historical context, especially as it is important in the evolution of health policy in the Third World.

During the Second World War, synthetic antimalarials became available and the enormous potential of DDT for malaria control became apparent. Because DDT, and other residual insecticides, remain on treated surfaces for months, act by poisoning resting mosquitoes after their blood meals, and thereby reduce mosquito longevity even more than density, they appeared to have an almost miraculous effect on malaria transmission. When they were used for control purposes on Mediterranean islands after the war and supplies were interrupted after several years, it was found that, although the mosquito populations returned rapidly, the malaria parasite reservoir had in some cases died out so that the disease had permanently gone away, or been eradicated. This was then undertaken as a deliberate policy in other countries and eradication programmes were launched against malaria in most parts of the world except subSaharan Africa. The then recently established World Health Organization encouraged and coordinated this effort as its largest single activity. Eradication is completely different from control of a disease. Eradication is an all-or-none removal of the parasite from a country or other large area, conceived of as a time-limited capital project. Before it can be attempted, funds must be available to carry it through to completion as all the investment will be lost if success is not attained. To achieve these demanding goals, malaria eradication in most countries was set up as a largely autonomous, 'vertical', disease-specific programme. Great success was achieved throughout the 1950s and 1960s. Malaria was eradicated from the United States and Europe, while even in countries such as India there was a 500-fold reduction in incidence.

The approach to eradication became relatively rigid, in view of the stringent requirements for success. An initial phase of survey, planning, raising finance, and training staff was followed by the 'attack phase', which aimed to stop malaria transmission by residual insecticide spraying (Fig. 14). After 4 years, when few parasites remained in the population, spraying ceased, the mosquitoes returned, and in this phase of consolidation the remaining cases and microfoci of transmission were treated. In the resulting malaria-free maintenance phase of the programme there was a continuing need to prevent cases of malaria from being imported, and to deal with any immediate secondary cases resulting from local transmission, called 'introduced' cases.

Once malaria eradication as a global policy got under way, it had great momentum. If a country eradicated malaria, it became enthusiastic for its neighbours to do likewise and so reduce the hazard of reimportation of the infection. Moreover, as a capital investment programme it was initially easy to obtain funding when success was slow in coming. An added urgency was provided by the emergence and spread of DDT resistance. It was felt that global eradication had to be achieved before insecticide resistance became widespread, as alternatives to DDT were more expensive and required more frequent application. By the 1970s, in many countries, eradication had already been attained or efforts began to falter. Moreover, the capital investment nature of eradication meant that when programmes finally collapsed they tended to do so dramatically, and the transition back to the recurrent activities that comprise malaria control has not been easy so that the world malaria situation then deteriorated.

Countries may now be grouped into four broad categories. First are those from which malaria has been eradicated or has died out. They may have a substantial problem of imported malaria cases; more than 2000 such cases per year are reported in the United Kingdom, with 5 to 10 deaths, and about 1000 per year in the United States, with 10 deaths. They may also have occasional secondary cases, 'introduced malaria' if the local conditions and anophelines are suitable, the odd case of congenital malaria, and a problem of transfusion malaria if the blood donor panel is not either screened for malaria antibodies or overseas travellers excluded (the last is increasingly impracticable). Lastly, these normally malaria-free countries may rarely have locally transmitted cases occurring in the vicinity of their major international airports, due to the accidental importation of infective mosquitoes on incoming aircraft that have been inadequately disinsectized. Returning travellers are the main but not the only source of malaria in countries following eradication.

The second group of countries, those of subSaharan Africa with *A. gambiae*-transmitted malaria, have been substantially unaffected by the eradication programmes. Malaria risk is extremely high and always has been, visitors not taking chemoprophylaxis are very liable to contract malaria, and the local inhabitants are subject to holoendemic stable malaria, though the picture is confused by large-scale casual chemotherapy. Mortality in children from malaria remains high.

In the third group of countries, which includes India, Indonesia, Pakistan, and many smaller countries of Asia and Oceania, eradication attempts had remarkable success in the attack phase, with over a 100-fold reduction in case incidence, but the programme has since collapsed. Malaria is both resurgent and often chloroquine resistant, and the risk in any locality may be high but is often ill defined and changing. Local

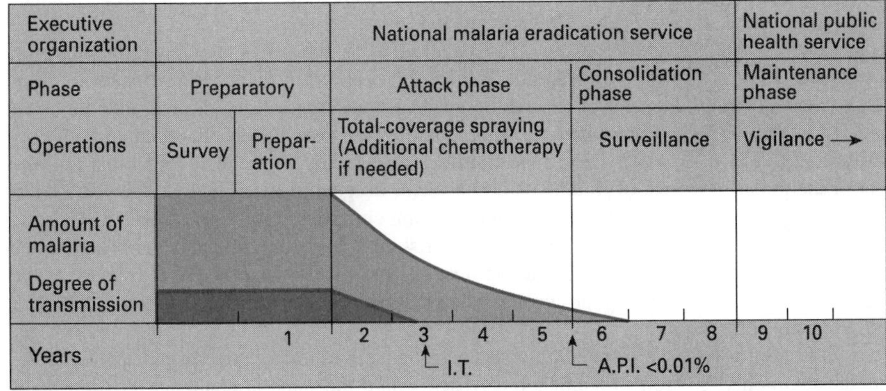

Fig. 14 Diagram of a standard plan and time-scale for a national malaria eradication programme. (By courtesy of the late Professor L. J. Bruce-Chwatt.)

residents have limited acquired immunity. There is a particular risk for former inhabitants who have migrated elsewhere in the 1960s and early 1970s and return as visitors—this applies, for example, to many Asians settled in the United Kingdom. They left, at the peak of eradication efforts, an almost malaria-free area and now are revisiting a place that may have become highly malarious without their knowledge.

Control programmes in South and South-East Asia have continued to be based on the organizations set up for the eradication campaigns and have gone on relying heavily on house spraying with residual insecticides, particularly DDT where resistance to it is absent. Household compliance with having their houses sprayed has fallen, often to below 50 per cent, and morale is low in many countries. Often malaria has been banished from the less endemic plains, but malaria along the forest fringes and international borders, which often coincide along the hills, remains a major hazard, sometimes fuelling epidemics in other areas. The forest-fringe vectors *A. dirus* and *A. minimus* tend to be exophilic (they rest outdoors) and sometimes also feed outdoors.

The fourth group of countries have had incomplete success with eradication but have successfully achieved a transition to control so that malaria risk may be very low over large parts of the country but there are also persisting malarious zones. This makes any advice on malaria risk for the country as a whole difficult to give and will explain the diverse opinions given to intending visitors to such countries.

Views on how malaria should be controlled today are changing steadily, but the current view was crystallized in late 1992 at an international meeting of Ministers of Health convened by the World Health Organization in Amsterdam. It comes closer to a counsel of despair than of promise, and can only really be viewed as a holding operation until new and more effective tools become available; it contains a good deal of ambiguity. The four elements are (i) early diagnosis and prompt treatment, (ii) selective and sustainable preventive measures, (iii) early detection and containment of epidemics, and (iv) regular reassessment of the malaria situation and especially its ecological, social, and economic determinants. It is—or at the least is seen as—a change of focus from stopping transmission to preventing death and reducing morbidity. The first component accepts that, for much of subSaharan Africa, it is not technically possible, and for many other places it is not economically feasible, to stop malaria transmission but that even then much can be done to limit the damage done by the parasite. There is much evidence that childhood mortality from malaria has fallen considerably from the level of 5 to 10 per cent of all children born that was needed to maintain the observed frequency of the sickle-cell gene in African countries and was observed in the early, population-based studies. It is at a much lower level today, as a result of treatment of febrile children, but is still very high and can be reduced by practicable and affordable chemotherapy. The second element, of preventive measures directed against transmission, is feasible in some areas of unstable malaria, in cities where the population density per unit area is high, and in areas of organized industrial or plantation agricultural activity. Malaria epidemics occur not only in areas of highly unstable malaria but also as a result of refugee and transmigration situations bringing susceptibles into endemic areas, and as a result of long-term climatic changes (whether or not they are due to global warming) that allow malaria transmission to ascend tropical mountains. Increasing political instability in countries of Central Asia may lead to the reintroduction of malaria due to deterioration of surveillance, while water-resource development projects in developing countries may also be associated with increased transmission. With so many ecological and other changes currently taking place, the need for a flexible approach to control and frequent reassessment of the malariological situation is clear.

PREVENTION OF MALARIA IN TRAVELLERS

The prevention of malaria in travellers, particularly those usually resident in non-malarious areas but visiting endemic regions, is becoming increasingly difficult, owing to the spread of resistance to the commonly available antimalarials, which means that prevention cannot be completely successful. The three components of advice to travellers must therefore be: (i) awareness of risk; (ii) reduction of exposure to being bitten by anopheline mosquitoes; (iii) chemoprophylaxis where appropriate. The first two of these are even more important than the third in preventing malaria mortality.

Preventive advice is subject to uncertainty. This is because unequivocal data on efficacy are often unavailable, published studies are conflicting, and the degree of resistance to many prophylactics is not well mapped. The balance between risk of malaria and risk of side-effects involves value judgements on which experts differ. Moreover, prospective travellers consult several sources of advice, obtain different opinions, and compliance with any regimen falls. Published advice is usually by country (the World Health Organization annually produces the most useful list of risk areas) and is inevitably directed towards prophylaxis for the areas of greatest transmission. Consultation with someone who knows the country and the travellers' itinerary may well lead to good advice that differs and is more specific. The intelligent traveller needs to be made aware of these issues but also requires clear advice that must include the general points in the following paragraph.

For any traveller to an endemic area there is a risk of malaria. No prophylactic regimen will give total protection, but many will reduce the risk of a malaria attack substantially. In the event of a fever while travelling, or afterwards, malaria must be considered as a diagnosis. Strict compliance, even with a suboptimal prophylactic regimen, is more important than vacillation over finding the optimal one. There are many additional ways to reduce the risk of malaria. Bednets impregnated with a pyrethroid insecticide (permethrin, deltamethrin, or λ-cyhalothrin) should be used, properly tucked in, and without tears or other holes through which mosquitoes might enter. A well-screened bedroom and other accommodation, combined with use of a knock-down insecticide when the doors are closed, will give substantial protection. Clothes that deter mosquito bites, repellent sprays and soaps (containing *N, N*-diethyl-*m*-toluamide (DEET) or permethrin) and avoiding exposure to bites in the evenings will also help.

In malarious areas from which chloroquine-resistant *P. falciparum* is absent, mainly in Western Asia, North Africa and Central America, chloroquine 300 mg (base), usually two tablets taken once a week, will give good protection except that since it acts as a suppressive of the blood forms of *Plasmodium* it will not prevent late attacks of *P. vivax* or *P. ovale*. Proguanil, 100 mg daily, or 200 mg daily in areas of intense transmission, will act as a true causal prophylactic but is poorly protective against *P. vivax* in these doses. The extremely low incidence of adverse side-effects from proguanil makes it acceptable to long-term residents in endemic areas. Chloroquine is suitable for up to 6 years of use, but beyond this proguanil may be substituted. Recommendations are summarized in Tables 9 and 10.

By 1993, chloroquine-resistant *P. falciparum* had been reported from most malarious countries, and it constitutes a massive and increasing problem in subSaharan Africa and in South-East Asia (where multiple drug resistance is common). Newer drugs and the more effective drug combinations for prophylaxis against chloroquine-resistant *P. falciparum* carry a significant risk of severe toxic side-effects that has to be balanced against the malaria risk, which varies greatly within countries, especially in Asia. Where the proportion of malaria resistant to chloroquine is low or the degree of resistance limited, the combination of chloroquine and proguanil [b(1), Table 9] has the advantage of low toxicity and appears effective in many areas, including India and the rest of South Asia. These two drugs also have a good safety record in pregnant women and in young children. Long-term use of prophylactic chloroquine only carries a risk of retinopathy (probably very small) once the total cumulative dose exceeds 100 g of base (over 6 years at the standard prophylactic dose). Pruritis can be a problem in those with dark skins.

However, chloroquine/proguanil no longer provides adequate protection in subSaharan Africa where the malaria challenge in rural areas

Table 9 *Recommended malaria prophylaxis (adult dose) in addition to general measures specified in text*

(a) Where chloroquine-resistant *P. falciparum* is absent:
1. Chloroquine 300 mg base weekly (best for short-term visitors)
2. Proguanil 200 mg daily (best for long-term residents)

(b) Where chloroquine-resistant *P. falciparum* is not widespread and is predominantly of low degree:
1. Chloroquine 300 mg base weekly *plus* proguanil 200 mg daily

(c) Where highly chloroquine-resistant *P. falciparum* occurs:[a]
1. Mefloquine 250 mg weekly
or
2. Chloroquine 300 mg base weekly *plus* proguanil 200 mg daily
or
3. Doxycycline 100 mg daily
or
4. Chloroquine 300 mg base weekly *plus* Maloprim 1 tablet weekly (pyrimethamine-dapsone fixed combination)

[a](c)1 and (c)3 are more effective in some areas of SE Asia, Africa and South America, but there is a low but significant risk of severe side-effects. (c)2 is the safest of the four (c) regimens so far as toxic side-effects are concerned and is preferred for pregnant women and, with reduced dose, for young children (Table 10). (c)4 is still an acceptable alternative for New Guinea and the Western Pacific, but its efficacy is declining.

may exceed one infective bite per night and resistance is common, nor in South-East Asia with a much lower transmission rate but a greater range of drugs to which *P. falciparum* is resistant.

Alternative prophylactic regimens involve the use of mefloquine, doxycycline, or Maloprim (a fixed drug combination of 12.5 mg pyrimethamine and 100 mg dapsone per tablet). Mefloquine (see above) has become by far the most widely used of these as it gives very substantial protection and requires a dose of one tablet weekly. In 1993, resistance to mefloquine outside Thailand and Cambodia was rarely reported. The drug has a long half-life and until recently was only recommended for journeys of 3 months or less, but data from the United States Peace Corps in Africa suggests that no late adverse reactions are encountered in the first year or two. The main serious early side-effects of mefloquine are neuropsychiatric, and include anxiety, depression, delusions, fits, and psychotic attacks. The frequency of these is disputed. Airline passenger surveys have shown a frequency of 1:10 000, but experienced doctors in the United Kingdom assert a much higher frequency and further data are needed. If such side-effects are going to occur, they are usually manifest within 3 weeks of commencing chemoprophylaxis and often earlier. Mefloquine is only slowly cleared from the body. As its safety during early pregnancy is uncertain, it is not recommended for those in the first trimester of pregnancy or at risk of pregnancy during the 3 months after the end of chemoprophylaxis. It is contraindicated in people with a history of epilepsy or psychiatric disease. Mefloquine is currently the most appropriate chemoprophylaxis for subSaharan Africa, the Amazonas region of Brazil, and areas of South-East Asia with high levels of malaria transmission. Sporadic cases of mefloquine resistance are already reported from Africa, and on the border between Thailand and Cambodia up to 40 per cent of cases of falciparum malaria are mefloquine resistant. Under these circumstances, for adults (except pregnant women) doxycycline is an appropriate chemoprophylactic. An alternative for travellers to such areas as Papua New Guinea is the use of the fixed drug combination Maloprim (12.5 mg pyrimethamine and 100 mg dapsone per tablet).

Maloprim alone gives poor protection against *P. vivax* and chloroquine may be given concurrently [c(2), Table 9]. The dose of Maloprim must not exceed one tablet a week or the incidence of the otherwise uncommon side-effect, agranulocytosis, rises. Methaemoglobinaemia occasionally occurs under Maloprim chemoprophylaxis.

In patients with epilepsy, proguanil or Maloprim or doxycycline do not increase the risk of fits and can be used for prophylaxis, depending on the particular geographical area and level of risk.

The following drugs are unsuitable for chemoprophylaxis (but Fansidar has a role in treatment): amodiaquine because of the high risk of agranulocytosis, Fansidar (25 mg pyrimethamine and 100 mg sulphadoxine per tablet) because of the frequency of severe skin reactions, and pyrimethamine on its own, because it is ineffective in most areas.

The risk of malaria is much higher in subSaharan Africa than elsewhere and it would be folly not to take prophylactics except where the altitude is too great for transmission to occur or in the non-endemic southern parts of the continent (see Fig. 4). In Asia, the risk is usually much lower. Visitors to the air-conditioned hotels of the larger cities of South-East Asia do not need prophylaxis but elsewhere in Asia there may be urban malaria. Proguanil does not protect adequately against malaria in South-East Asia, and travellers to the areas of higher transmission will need regimens c(2) or c(3). Those residing for long periods of time may prefer vigilance and early treatment of fevers, but awareness of the risk is essential. Freedom from malaria in Asia by travellers does not mean that they will escape infection in Africa!

Because no prophylactic is completely effective in chloroquine-resistant *P. falciparum* areas, travellers who may be in remote areas and away from prompt medical assistance should carry a therapeutic dose of Fansidar (three tablets), quinine (see above), or mefloquine. Resistance to Fansidar has been reported from many countries with highly chloroquine-resistant malaria.

Whatever the prophylactic regimen used, it should be continued for at least 4 weeks after returning to a non-endemic area. Compliance is hard to achieve, but 4 weeks of continued prophylaxis will prevent most cases of imported malaria. Whatever precautions are taken, the possibility of malaria must, however, be borne in mind by the traveller and pointed out to any medical adviser, whom he or she must seek in case of a fever.

MALARIAL VACCINES

Present tools for malaria control are inadequate, and are becoming less effective due to increasing resistance of *P. falciparum* to more drugs and the spread of insecticide resistance among anopheline mosquitoes. Moreover, new drugs and insecticides tend to be more expensive and beyond the reach of many severely affected countries. Many inhabitants of endemic areas will have inadequate access to health care when the disease strikes. For all these reasons an effective vaccine against malaria, and especially falciparum malaria, is desperately needed.

Considerable experimental effort has therefore been directed in recent years to the development of immunoprophylaxis for malaria. Because immunity to the disease is specific both for the parasite species and the stage of the life cycle, the goals have been to investigate independently means of developing vaccines against sporozoites, asexual blood forms, and gametocytes of *P. falciparum.*

For experimental convenience a variety of non-human primate or rodent model systems have also been used, as immunization and challenge studies are far easier to perform. Parallels have subsequently been sought in *P. falciparum* grown in culture, in non-human primate hosts, and ultimately in man. These animal models are, however, often inappropriate for the human infection and this is reflected in the unsuccessful outcome of most human vaccine trials.

In animal model systems with laboratory strains of parasites, some early results were very encouraging. For example, immunization of rodents with irradiated sporozoites or passive transfer of monoclonal antibodies to the sporozoite surface induced up to 100 per cent protection against challenge infection. Similarly, in rodents, immunization with gamete preparations induced complete transmission-blocking

Table 10 *Doses of prophylactic antimalarial drugs for children*[a]

Age	Weight (kg)	Fraction of adult dose: Chloroquine with proguanil	Maloprim (pyrimethamine and dapsone)	Mefloquine
0–5 weeks		1/8	Not recommended	Not recommended
6 weeks–11 months		1/4	1/8[b]	Not recommended
1–5 years	10–19	1/2	1/4	Not recommended under age 2 years
	15–19			1/4 (2–5 years)
6–11 years	20–39	3/4	1/2	1/2 (6–8 years); 3/4 (9–11 years)
⩾ 12 years	>40	Adult dose	Adult dose	Adult dose

When both are available, weight is a better guide than age for children over 6 months old.

[a]For children aged under 2 years in areas of chloroquine resistance the appropriate medication is chloroquine plus proguanil. Chloroquine is available as a syrup but the proguanil has to be powdered on to jam or food. Measures against mosquito bites are specially important.

[b]Not feasible to prepare unless a paediatric formulation is available.

immunity. By using recombinant DNA techniques it has, however, proved possible to produce large quantities of defined parasite antigens, so that current strategies centre around the use of such parasite proteins or portions of them rather than whole organisms. In the case of the sporozoites, where most effort has been focused, DNA sequencing has generated the entire sequence of a protein covering the surface of the organism (circumsporozoite protein or **CSP**) from a variety of species and strains. Because the molecule has a region consisting of a tandemly repeated amino-acid sequence that is both immunodominant and species specific, this region has been synthesized and coupled to a carrier polypeptide. In experimental monkeys such material induces antibodies of the appropriate specificity that can neutralize sporozoite infectivity *in vitro*. Unfortunately, human trials with such vaccines have been disappointing. Only a small proportion of volunteers were protected, and a poor and variable antibody response was generated. Further animal studies revealed that antibody production is probably not the most important host-protective immune response to sporozoites and that cytotoxic or cytokine releasing CD8+ T cells, which kill infected hepatocytes directly, are necessary for sterilizing immunity. A second sporozoite surface protein has recently been identified, which can enhance the protective effect of CSP in rodents, probably via similar mechanisms. In view of the fact that even in endemic areas, high levels of antiCSP antibodies are insufficient to prevent reinfection, more attention is now being focused on the induction of appropriate major histocompatibility complex class 1-restricted responses. These are more difficult to induce experimentally and the situation is further complicated by considerable sequence diversity in *CSP* genes in those regions of the molecule that can act as T-cell epitopes. Recent case-control studies have identified a human class 1 allele that is associated with protection from severe malaria. Peptides from an antigen specific to the liver stage have now been found that interact specifically with this allele, and cells responding to this peptide can be found in residents of endemic areas. This is an exciting new approach, but it has yet to be demonstrated directly that these particular peptide-specific responses are protective in people.

In general, vaccination with asexual blood stages or with purified blood-stage antigens has had much more variable results. Many different recombinant antigens have been used to vaccinate experimental rodents and non-human primates, with varied outcomes. Protection is rarely if ever complete and usually required the use of Freund's complete adjuvant (which is unacceptable in man) for optimum results. Because many different proteins had some protective activity, the next steps were uncertain. Only a small number of candidates could realistically be followed through to human trials, so that an arbitrary choice has to be made.

Promising results have been obtained with a different approach. Patarroyo used a wide variety of peptides derived from sequence data from numerous malarial proteins initially to vaccinate monkeys in order to identify relevant protective peptides. The most active of these were then used to immunize monkeys, resulting in complete protection in some cases. The same peptides, after polymerization, were subsequently used in human trials. A significant proportion of volunteers were resistant to blood-transmitted infection and much larger field studies were then undertaken. Although the early trials that gave protection had design limitations, a subsequent randomized trial in Latin America showed approximately 50 per cent protection and in Tanzania gave 31 per cent protection. Trials of the Patarroyo vaccine are now under way in Thailand and The Gambia, with results due in 1995, that should define the efficacy and promise of this vaccine.

Searching for an asexual-stage vaccine is made more difficult because there is no *in vitro* test for protective immunity. At present, the only way to determine the immune status of a person is by monitoring the outcome of infection.

Many antigens currently under study have been identified because they were recognized by serum from endemic-area adults, who have an extremely diverse response to malarial antigens, much of which is irrelevant to protection. One of the only antigens for which a role in host protection has been suggested in field studies is a highly variable antigen on the infected cell surface. This protein has yet to be cloned and is a difficult target for vaccines because of its enormous diversity.

In the sexual stages, several antigens on the surface of gametocytes, zygotes, and ookinetes have been identified and cloned. Antibodies to these can significantly reduce or abolish transmission. They act by being taken up with the blood meal and preventing the development of the parasite within the mosquito. While these will form an important component of an overall vaccination strategy, two problems are apparent. First, in some experiments, transmission has been found to be enhanced when antibody levels are low, suggesting that it will be necessary to maintain high antibody titres. Second, because of the stage specificity of immunity, such a vaccine would not directly benefit the recipient because it would only affect the sexual stages and these do not cause disease. It would therefore be used in combination with a vaccine against sporozoites or asexual stages.

An alternative strategy to eliminating the parasite is to attempt protection against disease. This could either be directed against parasite molecules that induce the release of cytokines or at those molecules involved in binding to particular endothelial receptors, so preventing cerebral malaria. Antibodies that prevent binding have been extensively studied in experimental systems.

The criteria for successful vaccination will vary with different groups. Travellers or the military would expect close to 100 per cent protection from clinical disease, whereas in Africa a reduction in morbidity and mortality alone would be a large step.

In either case the vaccine would need to be stable, effective after one or two doses, provide immunity of sufficiently long duration, and be easy to administer. For real utility in Africa it would need to be effective in young infants.

Because the first malaria prototype vaccine to be tried out in people on a large scale has been the polymerized synthetic peptides developed by Patarroyo on the basis of the SPf66 antigen of *P. falciparum*, the results are awaited with much interest. It is still premature to predict the effectiveness of this vaccine globally, but its development will encourage further progress in a field that has repeatedly been characterized by raised and then dashed hopes.

REFERENCES

Alonso, P.L. *et al.* (1994). Randomised trial of efficacy of SPf66 vaccine against *Plasmodium falciparum* malaria in southern Tanzania. *Lancet,* **344,** 1175–81.

Bates, I., Bedu-Addo, G., Bevan, D.H., and Rutherford, T.R. (1991). Use of immunoglobulin gene rearrangements to show clonal lymphoproliferation in hyper-reactive malarial splenomegaly. *Lancet,* **337,** 505–7.

Beadle, C. *et al.* (1994). Diagnosis of malaria by detection of *Plasmodium falciparum* HRP-2 antigen with a rapid dipstick antigen-capture assay. *Lancet,* **343,** 564–8.

Berendt, A.R., *et al.* (1994). Molecular mechanisms of sequestration in malaria. *Parasitology,* **108,** S19–28.

Bradley, D.J. and Warhurst, D.C. (1995). Malaria prophylaxis: guidelines for travellers from Britain. *British Medical Journal* **310,** 709–714.

Field, J.W., Sandosham, A.A., and Fong, Y.L. (1963). *The microscopical diagnosis of human malaria: 1. A morphological study of the erythrocytic parasites in thick blood films,* (2nd edn). Studies of the Institute for Medical Research, Federation of Malaya, No. 30.

Field, J. and Shute, P.G. (1956). *The microscopic diagnosis of human malaria,* Part II A, *Morphological study of the erythrocytic parasites,* (2nd edn), pp. 22–52. Government Press, Kuala Lumpur.

Garnham, P.C.C. (1966). *Malaria parasites and other Haemosporidia.* Blackwell Scientific, Oxford.

Gilles, H.M. and Warrell, D.A. (1993). *Bruce Chwatt's essential malariology,* (3rd edn). Arnold, London.

Hill, A.V. (1992). Malaria resistance genes: a natural selection. *Transactions of the Royal Society of Tropical Medicine and Hygiene,* **86,** 225–6; 232.

Kwiatkowski, D. *et al.* (1990). TNF concentration in fatal cerebral, non-fatal cerebral, and uncomplicated *Plasmodium falciparum* malaria. *Lancet,* **336,** 1201–4.

Lawson, J.B. (1967). Malaria in pregnancy. In *Obstetrics and gynaecology in the tropics,* (ed. J.B. Lawson and D.B. Stewart), pp. 59–72. Arnold, London.

Looareesuwan, S. *et al.* (1985). Quinine and severe falciparum malaria in late pregnancy. *Lancet,* **ii,** 4–8.

Luzzi, G.A. and Peto, T.E.A. (1993). Adverse effects of antimalarials. An update. *Drug Safety,* **8,** 295–311.

McGuire, W., *et al.* (1994). Variation in the TNF-α promoter region associated with susceptibility for cerebral malaria. *Nature,* **371,** 508–11.

MacPherson, G.G., Warrell, M.J., White, N.J., Looareeesuwan, S., and Warrell, D.A. (1985). Human cerebral malaria: a quantitative ultrastructural analysis of parasitized erythrocyte sequestration. *American Journal of Pathology,* **119,** 385–401.

Miller, L.H. (1994). Impact of malaria on genetic polymorphism and genetic diseases in Africans and African Americans. *Proceedings of the National Academy of Sciences (USA),* **91,** 2415–19.

Nardin, E.H. and Nussenzweig, R.S. (1993). T cell responses to pre-erythrocytic stages of malaria: role in protection and vaccine development against pre-erythrocytic stages. *Annual Reviews of Immunology,* **11,** 687–727.

Newton, C.R.J.C. *et al.* (1991). Intracranial pressure in African children with cerebral malaria. *Lancet,* **337,** 573–6.

Newton, C.R.J.C. *et al.* (1994). Brain swelling and ischaemia in Kenyans with cerebral malaria. *Archives of Disease in Childhood,* **70,** 281–7.

Ockenhouse, C.F. (1993). The molecular basis for the cytoadherence of *Plasmodium falciparum*-infected eryrthrocytes to endothelium. *Seminars in Cell Biology,* **4,** 297–303.

Patarroyo, M.E. *et al.* (1988). A synthetic vaccine protects humans against challenge with asexual blood stages of *Plasmodium falciparum* malaria. *Nature,* **332,** 158–61.

Phillips, R.S. (1992). Vaccination against malaria. *Immunobiology,* **184,** 240–62.

Roberts, D.J. *et al.* (1992). Rapid switching to multiple antigenic and adhesive phenotypes in malaria. *Nature,* **357,** 689–92.

Roberts, D.J., Biggs, B.A., Brown, G., and Newbold C.I. (1993). Protection, pathogenesis and phenotypic plasticity in malaria. *Parasitology Today,* **9,** 281–6.

Saul, A. (1992). Towards a malaria vaccine: riding the rollercoaster between unrealistic optimism and lethal pessimism. *South East Asian Journal of Tropical Medicine and Public Health,* **23,** 656–71.

Targett, G.A.T. (Ed.) (1991). *Malaria: Waiting for the vaccine.* John Wiley, Chichester.

Turner, G.D.H., *et al.* (1994). An immunohistochemical study of the pathology of fatal malaria. *American Journal of Pathology,* **145,** 1057–69.

Valero, M.V. *et al.* (1993). Vaccination with SPf66, a chemically synthesised vaccine, against *Plasmodium falciparum* malaria in Colombia. *Lancet,* **341,** 705–10.

Warrell, D.A., Molyneux, M.E., and Beales, P.F. (ed.) (1990). Severe and complicated malaria (2nd edn) World Health Organization Malaria Action Programme. *Transactions of the Royal Society of Tropical Medicine and Hygiene,* **84** (suppl.).

Warrell, D.A. *et al.* (1982). Dexamethasone proves deleterious in cerebral malaria. A double-blind trial in 100 comatose patients. *New England Journal of Medicine,* **306,** 313–19.

Warrell, D.A., Phillips, R.E., and Garrard, C.S. (1991). Intensive care unit management of severe malaria. *Clinical Intensive Care,* **2,** 86–96.

Wellcome Trust (1994). Artemisinin. Proceedings of a meeting convened by the Wellcome Trust on 25–27 April 1993. *Transactions of the Royal Society of Tropical Medicine and Hygiene,* **88** (suppl.), S11-65.

Wernsdorfer, W.H. and McGregor, I.A. (1988). *Malaria. Principles and practice of malariology.* Churchill Livingston, Edinburgh.

White, N.J. and Ho, M. (1992). The pathophysiology of malaria. *Advances in Parasitology,* **31,** 83–173.

White, N.J. *et al.* (1983). Severe hypoglycemia and hyperinsulinaemia in falciparum malaria. *New England Journal of Medicine,* **309,** 61–6.

World Health Organization (1990). *Practical chemotherapy of malaria: report of a WHO scientific group,* Technical Report Series No. 805. WHO, Geneva.

World Health Organization (1993). *A global strategy for malaria control.* WHO, Geneva.

World Health Organization (1992). *Implementation of the global malaria control strategy. Report of a WHO strategy group on the implementation of the global plan of action for malaria control 1993–2000,* WHO Technical Report Series No. 839. WHO, Geneva.

World Health Organization (1995). *International travel and health.* WHO, Geneva.

7.13.3 Babesia

T. K. RUEBUSH

Definition

Babesia are tick-borne intraerythrocytic protozoan parasites of wild and domestic animals that occasionally infect man. The disease caused by these organisms is known as babesiosis or piroplasmosis, and ranges from asymptomatic infections to severe, fatal illnesses characterized by fever, haemolytic anaemia, jaundice, haemoglobinuria, and renal failure. Babesiosis is of historical interest because *Babesia bigemina* was the first organism shown to be transmitted by an arthropod.

Epidemiology

Although Babesia infections are uncommon in man, they are widespread in both wild and domestic animals, particularly in the tropics and subtropics. In some areas these infections are responsible for serious economic losses in livestock. More than 70 different species of Babesia have been described in a variety of vertebrate hosts, for example, *B. divergens* (probably identical to *B. bovis*) and *B. bigemina* (cattle), *B. caballi* (horses), *B. canis* (dogs), and *B. microti* (rodents).

Ixodid, or hard-bodied ticks, are the only known vectors of *Babesia* spp. Parasites are ingested by the tick when it feeds on an infected host; the organisms then divide and spread throughout the body of the tick. In some species of ticks, Babesia organisms enter the ovaries and are passed transovarially through the egg to the developing larval stage. The parasite is then transmitted to its vertebrate host during the next blood meal. Other tick species ingest the organisms during one stage and then transmit the infection after they have moulted to the subsequent stage (transtadial passage).

Babesiosis is a zoonotic disease. Humans are infected accidentally when they intrude on the natural cycle of transmission between the tick and its domestic or wild animal host.

Cases of human babesiosis have been reported from former Yugoslavia, France, the former Soviet Union, Ireland, Scotland, Spain, Mexico, and the United States. Epidemiologically, several differences exist between the European and North American cases. The infections acquired in Europe have been sporadic in occurrence and widely distributed geographically. The causative organism is *B. divergens*, a parasite of cattle. Nearly all occurred in people who had had splenectomies, a factor that may have increased their susceptibility to the parasite. In contrast, most of the infections from North America have been acquired in a circumscribed area along the north-east coast of the United States. These were caused by *B. microti*, a parasite of rodents, which has a much broader host range than *B. divergens* and is capable of infecting people with functioning spleens. Recently a Babesia-like organism has been implicated in infections in splenectomized patients in northern California.

The vector in the European cases is probably *Ixodes ricinus*, the tick responsible for transmission of the parasite among cattle. *Ixodes dammini*, a tick that feeds on rodents during its larval and nymphal stages and on deer as an adult, is the vector of *B. microti*. These are the same tick species responsible for the transmission of Lyme disease in Europe and the north-eastern United States.

Only *B. microti* has been transmitted by blood transfusion, perhaps because of its tendency to cause prolonged asymptomatic parasitaemia and its ability to survive in banked blood.

Pathogenesis

When infected ticks feed on a vertebrate host, the parasites apparently enter red blood cells directly, without the preliminary exoerythrocytic stage that occurs in malaria. Within the red cell the organisms multiply by budding, forming two or four daughter cells. When the infected cell ruptures, the parasites are liberated and invade other erythrocytes, repeating the cycle.

The spleen plays an important part in resistance to Babesia infections. Infections in splenectomized animals are more severe than in animals with intact spleens, and splenectomy months or even years after the initial infection may lead to a recurrence of parasitaemia. A similar association between splenectomy and severity of illness has been observed in man.

The age of the host can also influence its response to a Babesia infection. In animals, infections acquired early in life tend to be mild or asymptomatic, with much lower mortality rates than in older animals. An association between age and severity of illness has also been noted in many of the cases of human *B. microti* infection. Symptomatic infections are most common in individuals over 40 years of age, while young persons usually have mild or subclinical infections. No such relation has been observed in splenectomized individuals infected with *B. microti* or in human *B. divergens* infections.

Symptoms

Patients infected with *B. divergens* usually have a 1- to 3-day history of fatigue, malaise and occasional nausea, vomiting and diarrhoea. This is rapidly followed by high fever, shaking chills, jaundice, and the production of small amounts of dark or blood-stained urine. Before becoming infected, most of the reported patients had undergone splenectomy for conditions that included trauma, surgical accidents, portal hypertension, and Hodgkin's disease.

The major findings on physical examination are fever, hypotension and jaundice. Anaemia is generally severe, with elevated reticulocyte counts and nucleated red cells on blood smear. Leucocyte counts range from normal to more than 40 000/mm^3, with an increase in juvenile and mature polymorphonuclear neutrophils. Marked elevations in levels of bilirubin, liver enzymes, blood urea nitrogen, and creatinine are common. The course of illness is generally characterized by progressive haemolytic anaemia, haemoglobinaemia, haemoglobinuria, jaundice, and renal insufficiency, leading to death in the majority of cases.

Human *B. microti* infections range from asymptomatic infections to prolonged severe illnesses. In patients with intact spleens the illness usually begins 1 to 4 weeks after a tick bite, with gradual onset of anorexia, fatigue, fever, chills, and generalized myalgia. Findings on physical examination are usually limited to fever and occasional mild hepatosplenomegaly. Most patients have a mild to moderately severe haemolytic anaemia, with low to normal white blood-cell counts. Slight elevations of liver enzymes and bilirubin are noted in about half the patients. The acute illness usually lasts a few weeks to a month, but asymptomatic *B. microti* parasitaemia may persist for many months after clinical recovery. Asplenic patients infected with *B. microti* usually have higher levels of parasitaemia and more severe haemolytic anaemia than those with functioning spleens and several fatal cases have been reported.

Fig. 1 *Babesia microti* trophozoites in a blood film. × 1000. (By courtesy of V. Zaman.)

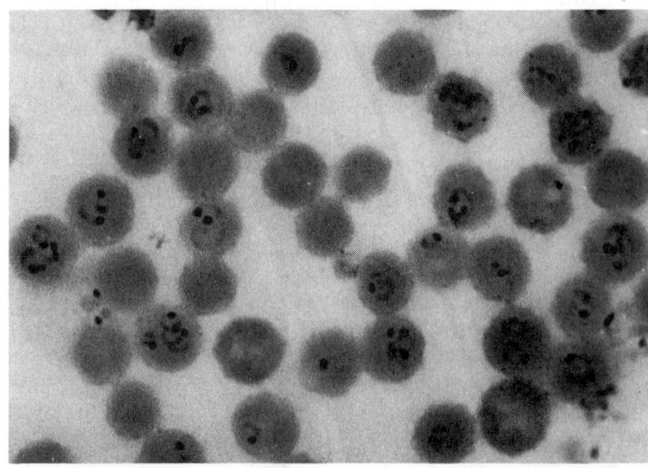

Diagnosis

The diagnosis of babesiosis should be considered in any patient with fever and a history of tick bite. Although cases of human babesiosis have been reported only from Europe and North America, the diagnosis cannot be ruled out in persons from other areas, since Babesia infections in animals have a worldwide distribution. With *B. divergens* infections, the rapid onset of haemolytic anaemia, jaundice, haemoglobinuria, and renal insufficiency should suggest the diagnosis. In contrast, human *B. microti* infections can easily be mistaken for a variety of viral or bacterial illnesses due to their non-specific clinical presentation.

Babesia parasites are most easily recognized in thin or thick blood smears stained with Giemsa. The organisms are variable in morphology and are frequently mistaken for malaria parasites. *Babesia divergens* ranges from round, oval, or piriform in shape to small ring forms. Dividing forms usually consist of two daughter cells held together by a thin strand of cytoplasm. *Babesia microti* parasites resemble *Plasmodium falciparum* rings (Fig. 1). Babesia can be distinguished from malaria parasites by the absence of pigment in erythrocytes infected with the older stages of Babesia.

In cases in which organisms are not detected in blood smears, intraperitoneal or intravenous inoculation of susceptible laboratory animals with blood from the patient has been helpful in the diagnosis. *Babesia microti* parasitaemia usually appears in hamsters within 2 to 4 weeks after inoculation. Although *B. divergens* seems to have a narrower host range than *B. microti*, the organism has been successfully isolated in gerbils.

Serological tests for babesiosis may aid in diagnosis, but should not be considered a substitute for parasitological diagnosis. Although cross-reactions between Babesia and malaria occur, titres are generally highest to the infecting organism.

Treatment and prevention

No generally effective drugs are available for the treatment of human babesiosis. In the case of *B. divergens* infections, therapy is complicated by the rapidly progressive course of the disease, and most patients who have recovered have been aggressively managed with blood transfusions and renal dialysis. Combinations of pentamidine plus co-trimoxazole and quinine plus clindamycin have been reported to reduce parasitaemia, but experience with these drugs is very limited.

Human *B. microti* infections in patients with intact spleens are usually self-limiting, although symptoms and parasitaemia may persist for several months. Symptomatic treatment is probably sufficient in most cases. In asplenic patients, more aggressive therapy is required. Recent experience with several severely ill patients who recovered after treatment with a combination of quinine and clindamycin (25 mg/kg per day of each for 7 to 10 days) suggests that this may be the best available treatment. Exchange transfusions have also been used successfully in several patients with very high levels of parasitaemia.

The only effective means of preventing Babesia infections is by avoiding areas infested with ticks. Insect repellents are probably of little value.

REFERENCES

Fernandez Villar, B., White, D.J., and Benach, J.L. (1991). Human babesiosis. *Progress in Clinical Parasitology*, **2**, 129–43.

Golightly, L.M., Hirschhorn, L.R., and Weller, P.F. (1989). Fever and headache in a splenectomized woman. *Reviews of Infectious Diseases*, **11**, 629–37.

Persing, D.H., *et al.* (1995). Infection with a Babesia-like organism in northern California. *New England Journal of Medicine*, **332**, 298–303.

Rosner, F., Zarrabi, M.H., Benach, J.L., and Habicht, G.S. (1984). Babesiosis in splenectomized adults: review of 22 reported cases. *American Journal of Medicine*, **76**, 696–701.

7.13.4 Toxoplasmosis

J. Couvreur and Ph. Thulliez

Parasitology, epidemiology, transmission

Toxoplasma gondii is an ubiquitous coccidian parasite. Its definitive host is the cat. It exists in three forms: the oocyst excreted with the cat faeces can stay in the soil for months under certain conditions of temperature and humidity; the tachyzoite multiplies intracellularly (Fig. 1); cysts, the result of this intracellular multiplication, can persist as viable parasites in brain and striated muscle tissues throughout the life of the host.

The prevalence of Toxoplasma antibodies is high in most populations. Their presence depends mostly upon eating habits in a given community; it is well defined in fertile women—for instance 72 per cent seropositive in Paris, 36 per cent in Stuttgart, 54 per cent in Padua, and 21 per cent in London.

Transmission in acquired toxoplasmosis occurs mainly after the ingestion of cysts. Infection is in four stages: acute, subacute, chronic, and relapses. Organisms spread from the gut by lymphatics and the bloodstream throughout the body, reaching every organ, where they multiply intracellularly (acute stage). Termination of this stage depends upon the development of both cell-mediated and humoral immunity. Whenever the host is immunocompetent, the parasite encysts and will persist in host tissues without any inflammatory process as long as the cyst is not disrupted (chronic stage). If the host is or becomes immunocompromised, there is a tendency for the cysts to release bradyzoites and Toxoplasma becomes an opportunistic infective agent.

Congenital infection occurs transplacentally by transmission of tachy-

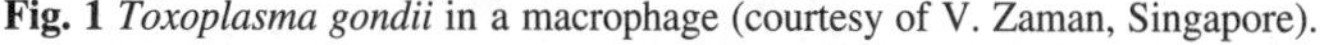

Fig. 1 *Toxoplasma gondii* in a macrophage (courtesy of V. Zaman, Singapore).

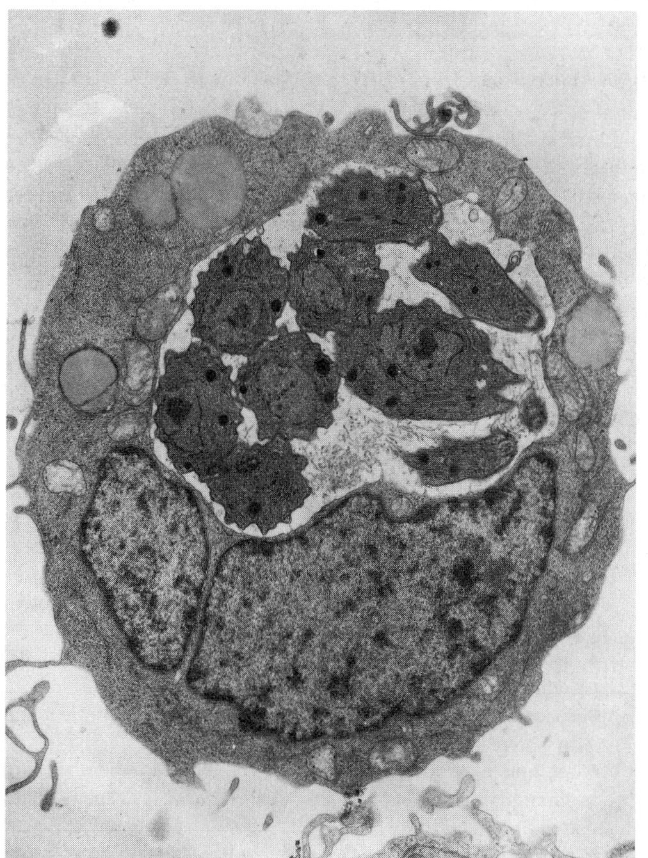

zoites when a previously uninfected woman acquires the infection during pregnancy.

Acute acquired toxoplasmosis

Acquired toxoplasmosis is usually subclinical. Clinical presentation, when it occurs, consists of lymphadenopathy. The most characteristic sites of the affected nodes are posterior cervical, suboccipital, retro-auricular, and submental. Supraclavicular, axillary, pectoral, epitrochlear, and inguinal locations are less frequent. Most often lymphadenopathy is localized to a few nodes in one area but it can be generalized. Nodes can be painful and tender for 1 or 2 weeks. They are rarely larger than walnuts, smooth, well defined, mobile, and never suppurate; they can persist for months or even a year. Mesenteric lymphadenopathy has been observed. Other clinical signs and symptoms are fatigue for several weeks, headache, myalgias, low-grade fever for one or several weeks, and, rarely, a transient rash. Hepatomegaly and splenomegaly are rare. Neurological or ocular involvement and myocarditis are exceptional in normal, immunocompetent patients.

The peripheral leucocyte count is variable. There is a relative neutropenia with lymphocytosis. Atypical lymphocytes indistinguishable from those in infectious mononucleosis may be seen. Inversion of the CD4/CD8 ratio has been noticed more often in clinical toxoplasmosis than in subclinical forms. Some features suggest toxoplasmosis rather than infectious mononucleosis: there is no pharyngitis, oral petechiae, or splenomegaly; lymphadenopathy is less marked but persists longer. Atypical lymphocytes are less numerous and disappear sooner. Eosinophilia may be seen.

The histological appearance is characteristic when there are groups of epithelioid cells scattered throughout the node, or immature sinus histiocytosis and follicular hyperplasia with phagocytosis and nuclear debris. Inflammatory infiltrates may sometimes extend into perinodal tissues and be misinterpreted as lymphogranuloma, lymphoma or sarcoidosis.

Toxoplasmosis of the central nervous system

Central nervous involvement can be observed in any form of acquired toxoplasmosis. The selectivity of Toxoplasma for brain tissue has been ascribed to low local immunity. In animal experiments, tachyzoites are demonstrated in brain 5 days after intraperitoneal inoculation, with ensuing perivascular inflammation with mononuclear cells. Tachyzoite-infected cells provoke multiple foci of micronecrosis. Mononuclear cells gather into microglial nodules associated with Toxoplasma antigen. Cysts appear apart from the inflammatory process. Intermediate appearances are observed between disseminated foci of macroglial nodules, and more or less numerous large necrotic areas and large space-occupying masses.

Clinical features of central nervous damage are of subtle onset and very protean:

- generalized encephalitis with meningeal involvement and localizing signs with fever, headache, progressive drowsiness progressing to coma and death within a few days or weeks;
- encephalitis with meningeal involvement shown by mild lymphocytic pleocytosis and moderate elevation of protein content;
- 'pseudotumour cerebri' syndrome with transient intracranial hypertension;
- space-occupying mass with focal signs and/or intracranial hypertension mimicking a tumour or a brain abscess;
- multiple mass lesions, which can be the cause of hemisensory abnormalities, hemiparesis, cranial nerve palsy, aphasia and tremors;
- miscellaneous patterns, which include confusion, psychiatric features, seizures, and signs of brain-stem or spinal cord injury.

The above patterns can progress to death within 2 weeks as a fulminant disease or persist for several months or even years with or without therapy. Such cases show a pattern of chronic relapsing encephalitis.

The diagnosis of toxoplasmosis of the nervous system can be difficult. Computerized tomography (**CT**) and magnetic resonance imaging (**MRI**) are useful for evaluation of cerebral injury. However, the lack of specificity of the clinical signs and imaging of central nervous injury can be misleading. Serological data can also be perplexing. Biopsy is advocated whenever the diagnosis is uncertain. It is mandatory to look for an underlying disease or an immunodeficiency.

Ocular toxoplasmosis

Toxoplasma infection is the most common cause of retinochoroiditis and posterior uveitis. It causes a focal necrotizing retinitis. In the acute or subacute stage it appears as cottonwool-like, patchy areas of the fundus with more or less vitreous exudate. The lesion heals within 3 to 6 weeks, leaving a punched-out scar with central atrophy and a progressing peripheral black pigmentation. The lesion can be macular or peripheral, single or multiple. It can reach the size of the disc in diameter. Atypical patterns are possible, such as retinal detachment, haemorrhage, and injury of the optic nerve. In congenital toxoplasmosis, the lesion is often bilateral. Presenting signs may be microphthalmia and strabismus.

The natural history of ocular toxoplasmosis suggests that the first retinal lesion can occur during the subacute stage, weeks or a few months after the beginning of the infection, more often than later during the chronic stage of the infection. It is the result of a previous colonization of the retina and its immediate cause is the rupture of a cyst. The pathophysiology of the inflammation associated with the flare-up of retinochoroiditis is controversial: either delayed sensitivity to Toxoplasma antigens, secondary proliferation of parasites or more likely both.

The major cause of toxoplasmic retinochoroiditis is congenital toxoplasmosis. Ocular injury is observed in 76 per cent of clinical cases. Ninety per cent of cases of retinochoroiditis discovered in infants and young children and at least 20 per cent in adults are attributable to congenital toxoplasmosis. It can be seen at birth or occurs much later, even in a previously normal retina, as in the case of 35 to 85 per cent of children with congenital toxoplasmosis. There is a peak frequency of new lesions during puberty and adolescence. There is some evidence that early treatment of even subclinical congenital toxoplasmosis decreases this risk.

Ocular disease is seldom the result of acquired toxoplasmosis, probably less than 1 per 1000 of postnatal infections.

The diagnosis of ocular toxoplasmosis should never rely on ophthalmic examination alone. The fact that it occurs mainly during the chronic stage of the infection, while the antibody titre is low, is a major problem. This can be solved by the demonstration of a local synthesis of antibodies in the aqueous humour.

Toxoplasmosis and immunodeficiency

Impaired cell-mediated immunity is important in determining the severity of the infectious process in acquired toxoplasmosis. In more than half of the cases, cerebral toxoplasmosis occurs in patients with underlying systemic disease and/or immune deficiency either spontaneous or drug induced. Any patient with severe toxoplasmosis should be investigated for an immune defect, even subtle, and for an underlying disease. Conversely, patients with known immune deficiency must be followed clinically and serologically for the potential development of a Toxoplasma infection.

Severe toxoplasmosis in immunodeficiency is usually related to the relapse of a chronic infection. It has been assumed that the long persistence of unruptured cysts in brain tissue is due to the low tissue levels of enzymes, which do not affect the cyst wall. That this equilibrium can be disrupted whenever the immunity of the host is altered is demonstrable experimentally and clinically. In animals with chronic infection, corticosteroids and irradiation can induce proliferation of Toxoplasma in the nervous tissue. The occurrence of an immunodeficiency either spontaneously or iatrogenically in man can be complicated by severe toxoplasmosis.

Among malignancies, the most common condition associated with toxoplasmic encephalitis is Hodgkin's disease. Other associated lymphoproliferative disorders are lymphosarcoma, non-Hodgkin's lymphoma, and angioimmunoblastic lymphadenopathy. All types of leukaemias are involved. Five per cent of cerebral infections in patients treated in cancer centres are caused by Toxoplasma.

Severe toxoplasmosis has been reported in organ transplant recipients. It is rare in renal, liver, and bone marrow transplantations but more frequent in heart and heart–lung transplantations in which the risk can reach 57 per cent in mismatched transplantation: serological positive donor/negative recipient. This risk is mainly related to the infected heart-tissue transplant. It is increased by the use of steroids for graft rejection. Conversely, cyclosporin has antiparasitic activity. The risk is reduced with pyrimethamine as 'blanket therapy' in recipients.

Patients with AIDS are the most frequent victims of toxoplasmosis of the central nervous system, lungs, and heart. The risk of central nervous involvement is 6 to 12 per cent in seropositive patients. Toxoplasmic encephalitis was observed in 25 to 80 per cent of patients with AIDS and evidence of cerebral infection. Serological investigation in large series of patients with AIDS revealed that the prevalence of Toxoplasma antibodies was the same as in the community but that IgG antibody titres of more than 200 i.u. were more frequently encountered in AIDS patients, particularly in those with less than 200 CD4 lymphocytes per μl, which can be considered as a risk factor that requires chemoprophylaxis.

The toxoplasmic origin of clinical manifestations encountered in immunocompromised patients is often difficult to confirm. Significant abnormalities of antibody titres may be absent. Attempts to isolate Toxoplasma from cerebrospinal fluid, from myocardial and cerebral biopsies, or from bonchoalveolar lavage may be necessary.

Congenital toxoplasmosis (Fig. 2)

MATERNOFETAL TRANSMISSION

Following seroconversion during pregnancy, 31 per cent of infants are infected, 2 per cent suffer intrauterine death, and 67 per cent are uninfected. These overall data vary according to the date of maternal infection: before pregnancy, 0 per cent; during the first month, 1 per cent; during the second and third month, 17 per cent; in the second trimester, 45 per cent; during the ninth month, 90 per cent. The date of maternal infection is also important for the clinical pattern of the fetopathy: 83 per cent of fetuses are infected, often severely, after infections in the first trimester compared with 10 per cent of mild infections when maternal infection is in the ninth month. The risk of fetopathy is reduced by more than 50 per cent if spiramycin is given to the mother. Very rare cases of transmission following chronic infection for years before pregnancy were observed in immunocompromised mothers.

Placental infection is synonymous with fetopathy. The placenta is a transmitting organ of great importance. If maternofetal transmission occurs early after maternal infection, fetopathy will be severe. If it is delayed, the fetus will be protected by passively transmitted maternal antibodies and Toxoplasma will have a tendency to encyst in fetal tissues without causing major pathology. Serological and clinical progression may thus be delayed for months after birth.

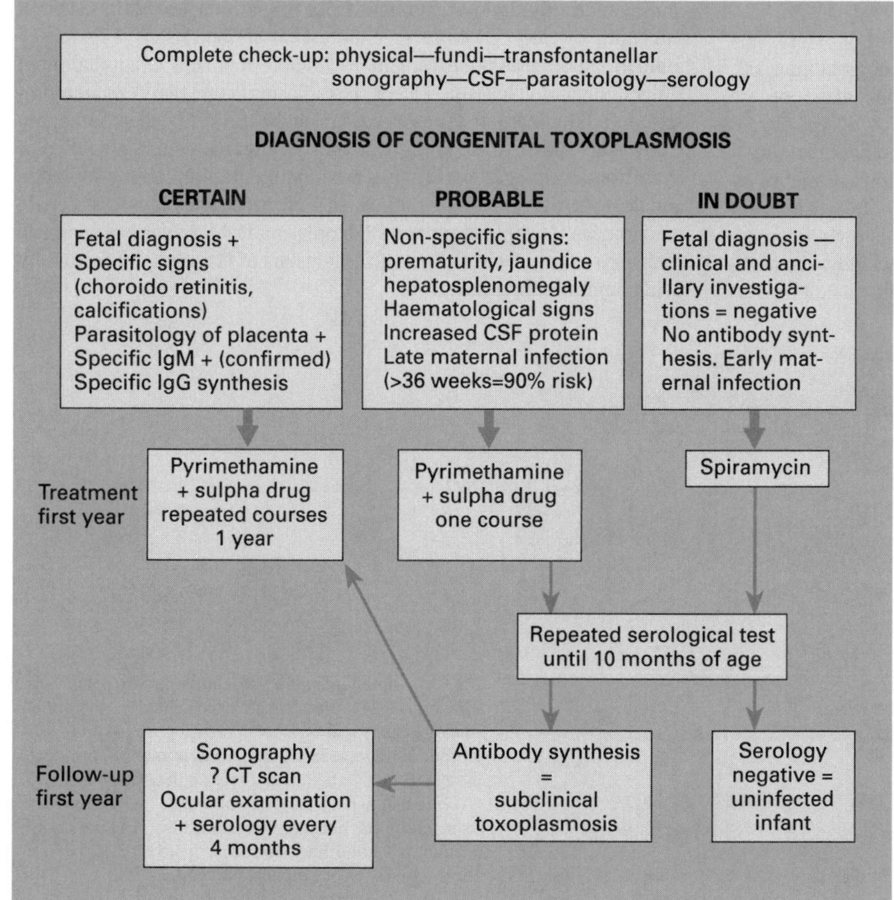

Fig. 2 Algorithm for neonates at risk of toxoplasmic fetopathy.

CLINICAL PATTERNS

Presentation of congenital toxoplasmosis is very protean, as follows:

1. Systemic disease of the newborn with rash, jaundice, thrombocytopenic purpura, hepatosplenomegaly, pneumonia and progressive uveitis, high cerebrospinal-fluid protein, cerebral ventricular dilatation, and encephalomyelitis.
2. Neurological disease of the infant: hydrocephalus or microcephaly, microphthalmia, retinochoroiditis, and cerebral calcification. Hydrocephaly, always related to a stenosis of the duct of Sylvius, can often be discovered several months after birth in an infant initially considered to be normal. A shunt is required.
3. Mild disease with isolated retinochoroiditis or mild cerebral calcification without any sign of cerebral injury.
4. Subclinical disease: prospective studies of acquired infection in pregnant women revealed that this is the most common pattern seen in more than 50 per cent of cases of congenital toxoplasmosis. To differentiate between subclinical toxoplasmosis and absence of infection is a common challenge for the paediatrician.
5. Relapses: flare-ups of retinochoroiditis can develop in infants, children and adolescents, even in a previously intact retina, in up to 85 per cent of cases (see Ocular toxoplasmosis). The possibility of late relapses in cerebral tissue is confirmed by the frequency of increased local synthesis of antibodies in cerebrospinal fluid (see Laboratory diagnosis). Complete work-up, especially examination of cerebrospinal fluid is mandatory in any form of congenital toxoplasmosis, even when subclinical.

LABORATORY DIAGNOSIS

Serology (Fig. 3)

Antibodies formed in response to the different membrane or cytoplasma antigens differ in their specificity and in their immunoglobulin class. These differences are very helpful in diagnosing the stage of the infection.

IgG antibodies detected by the dye test and the indirect immunofluorescent test appear some 2 weeks after the acquisition of the infection and reach a maximum titre of 300 to 3000 i.u. within 2 months, form a plateau for months and sometimes years, and slowly decrease but persist for the life of the host. IgG antibodies detected by the high-sensitivity agglutination test in the presence of mercaptoethanol (**AGG-HS**) initially parallel those of the dye test but frequently rise for a longer time and persist often at a higher level for years. With the AGG test using methanol-treated antigen (AGG-AC), IgG antibodies show the same initial progress but their titre declines to 50 i.u. or less after 3 to 6 months. IgG antibodies detected by the indirect haemagglutination test lag a few weeks behind those in the dye test and rise more slowly. Their maximum titre is reached in 4 to 6 months. They stay at a higher level than those of the dye test.

IgM antibodies appear first within a few days. They reach a maximum titre within 4 weeks. The indirect fluorescent test can turn negative within 4 to 12 weeks but IgM can be detected, usually at a low titre, for months and even years in a minority of patients, particularly when enzyme immunoassays are used.

Synthesis of Toxoplasma IgG antibodies can be demonstrated in the infant suspected of congenital infection by comparing the ratio of the concentration of specific IgG and total IgG of a recent sample with that of previous ones. In the absence of infection, this ratio decreases as the infant produces IgG that does not contain specific Toxoplasma antibodies. If the ratio remains the same or increases, the diagnosis is established.

Intrathecal or intraocular production of specific IgG antibodies can be determined by comparing the ratio of specific to total IgG in cerebrospinal fluid or aqueous humour with that of the serum specimen.

It must be borne in mind that the dye test and AGG-HS are more sensitive methods (2 i.u.) than indirect fluorescence (8 to 12 i.u.). Serological investigation requires paired samples of serum taken at 3-week intervals. A fourfold rise in titre of specific IgG indicates a recent (less than 2 months old) infection. The diagnosis can be very difficult in patients with immunodeficiency who, very often, have low titres or no significant derangement of antibodies.

Detection of *Toxoplasma gondii*

Toxoplasma can be isolated from blood, cerebrospinal, bronchoalveolar and amniotic fluids, placenta, and from tissue biopsies by inoculation into mice or into cell cultures. Fluorescent antibody and peroxidase–antiperoxidase techniques are more reliable than the examination of stained smears. The isolation of Toxoplasma from blood or cerebrospinal fluid indicates the presence of an active, probably acute infection. Conversely, positive isolation from muscle after enzymatic digestion or even from brain and heart tissues are possible in old, chronic infection and do not prove a recent or progressing infection. The polymerase chain reaction can be applied to detect Toxoplasma DNA in various samples; it has proved useful in the prenatal diagnosis of congenital infection by using amniotic fluid only.

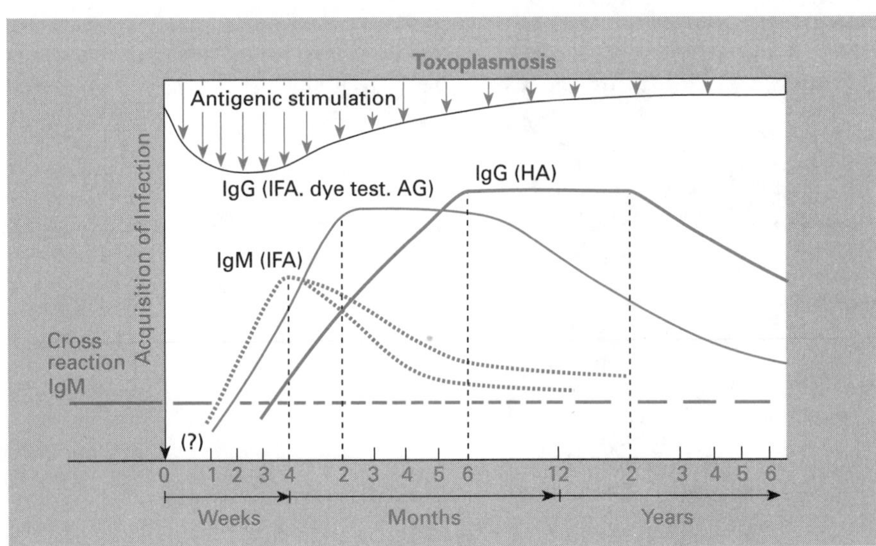

Fig. 3 Antibody response to acquired toxoplasma infection. IgM antibodies are represented by the dotted lines—either rapid or slow decreasing titre—IgG antibodies detected by the indirect immunofluorescent assay (IFA), dye test, and direct agglutination test (AG) are shown by the thin solid line; IgG antibodies detected by the haemagglutination test (HA) are shown by the thick solid line. (Modified from the Symposium Bio Merieux, Lyon, France, November 1982.)

TREATMENT

Drugs

The combination of pyrimethamine-sulpha drugs is the best treatment. Pyrimethamine is given orally in a daily dose of 0.5 to 1 mg/kg or 50 mg in adults. A loading dose can be given every 2 to 3 days (mean half-life, 4.5 days). The dosage of sulphadiazine, the drug currently used, is 50 to 80 mg/kg per day, 2 to 4 g in two to three divided doses in adults.

The combination of pyrimethamine, 25 mg, and sulphadoxine (a long-acting sulpha drug), 500 mg, in a tablet (Fansidar) is given orally at a dosage of one tablet/20 kg body weight every 7 to 10 days.

It is necessary to monitor the blood count in any treatment with pyrimethamine-sulpha because of the possibility of bone marrow depression resulting in anaemia, thrombocytopenia, and leucopenia with pyrimethamine and leucopenia and granulopenia with sulpha drugs. Folinic acid, 50 mg by the oral or intramuscular route every 3 to 6 days, can prevent pyrimethamine side-effects. Spiramycin, oral dose 50 to 100 mg/kg in infants and 3 g/day in adults, proved active in experimental infection and can prevent maternal–fetal transmission, but its activity in overt progressive disease remains questionable.

Indications

Acquired toxoplasmosis.

The common lymphadenopathy can be treated with spiramycin for 1 or 2 months. Any case with involvement of the central nervous system requires pyrimethamine-sulpha treatment until the signs have subsided and signs on CT imaging have improved. Long-term treatment with pyrimethamine-sulphadoxine is then recommended. In immunocompetent patients, the therapeutic response occurs within 7 to 10 days. Resolution of clinical features and abnormalities on CT and MRI can be very good. In immunocompromised patients the lesions cannot be totally suppressed. Long-term treatment with pyrimethamine alone can be used in AIDS patients who cannot tolerate sulpha drugs and as 'blanket therapy' in patients with AIDS or organ transplants. The use of interferon-γ, which is considered to be a major defence against Toxoplasma, might be proposed in the future.

Congenital toxoplasmosis.

In any case with a suspicion of this diagnosis, even subclinical, treatment should be given. Three to five 21-day courses of the pyrimethamine-sulpha combination during the first year proved effective in reducing the risk of secondary choroidoretinitis. More intensive treatment with continuous pyremethamine-sulpha for 6 months or even longer is under evaluation.

In patients less than 1 year old, maturation of cellular immunity of the host is theoretically sufficient for protection and allows discontinuation of the treatment. However, if a relapse occurs, pyrimethamine-sulphadoxine can be given for months.

Prevention of congenital taxoplasmosis includes serological screening of pregnant women, recommendations for prophylaxis, and serological follow-up for those who proved seronegative. The risk of fetopathy is reduced by a half by spiramycin. The recognition of fetopathy by intrauterine diagnosis and serial ultrasonography either allows elective termination or is a guide to the efficacy of treatment *in utero.*

REFERENCES

Couvreur, J. and Desmonts, G. (1962). Congenital and maternal toxoplasmosis: a review of 300 congenital cases. *Developmental Medicine and Child Neurology*, **4,** 519–30.

Couvreur, J. and Desmonts, G. (1988). Toxoplasmosis. In *Parasitic infections in pregnancy and the newborn*, (ed. C. MacLeod), pp. 112–47. Oxford Medical, Oxford.

Couvreur, J. and Desmonts, G. (1988). Acquired and congenital toxoplasmosis. In *Handbook of clinical neurology*, Vol. 8(52), Microbial disease, (ed. A.A. Harris), pp. 351–3. Elsevier, Amsterdam.

Couvreur, J., Desmonts, G., Tournier, G., and Collin, E. (1984). La production locale accrue d'anticorps dans le liquide cephalo-rachidien au cours de la toxoplasmose congenitale. *Annales de Pediatrie (Paris)*, **3,** 839–5.

Couvreur, J. *et al.* (1991). Foetopathie toxoplasmique: Traitement in utero par l'association pyrimethamine sulfamides. *Archives Françaises de Pediatrie*, **48,** 397–403.

Daffos, F., Forestier, F., Capella-Pavlosky, M., Thulliez, P., and Aufrant, C. (1988). Prenatal management of 746 pregnancies at risk for congenital toxoplasmosis. *New England Journal of Medicine*, **318,** 271–5.

Desmonts, G. and Couvreur, J. (1974). Congenital toxoplasmosis: a prospective study of 378 pregnancies. *New England Journal of Medicine*, **290,** 1111–16.

Desmonts, G., and Couvreur, J. (1985). Toxoplasmosis. In *Current diagnosis*, (ed. R. Conn), pp. 274–87. Saunders, Philadelphia.

Frenkel, J.K. (1971). Toxoplasmosis. In *Pathology of protozoal and helminthic diseases*, (ed. R.A. Marcial-Rojas), pp. 254–90. William & Wilkins, Baltimore.

Grant, P.H., Gold, J.W.M., Roseblum, M., Niedzwieck, D., and Armstrong, D. (1990). Toxoplasma gondii serology in H.I.V. infected patients: the development of central nervous system toxoplasmosis in AIDS. *Acquired Immunodeficiency Syndrome*, **4,** 519–21.

Leport, C., Raffi, F., and Matheron, S. (1988). Treatment of central nervous system toxoplasmosis with pyrimethamine-sulfadiazine combination in 35 A.I.D.S. patients. Efficacy of long term continuous therapy. *American Journal of Medicine*, **84,** 94–100.

Luft, B.J. and Remington, J.S. (1985). Toxoplasmosis of the central nervous system. In *Current clinical topics in infectious diseases*, Vol. 6, (ed. J.S. Remington and M.N. Swartz), pp. 315–58. McGraw-Hill, New York.

Remington, J.S. (1974). Toxoplasmosis in the adult. *Bulletin of the New York Academy of Medicine*, **50,** 211–27.

Remington, J.S. and Desmonts, G. (1990). Toxoplasmosis. In *Infectious diseases of the fetus and newborn infant*, (3rd edn), (ed. J.S. Remington and J.O. Klein.) Saunders, Philadelphia.

7.13.5 Cryptosporidium and cryptosporidiosis

D. P. CASEMORE and D. A. WARRELL

INTRODUCTION

The cryptosporidia are obligate intracellular parasites infecting a wide variety of vertebrate host species. There are several well-defined species, although it appears that infection in man is usually with one species, *Cryptosporidium parvum.* First described in mice, by Tyzzer in 1912, *C. parvum* was recognized as a cause of scours in calves in the early 1970s but was not described in man until 1976. In the 1980s it emerged worldwide as a common cause of acute, self-limiting gastroenteritis in otherwise healthy subjects, especially children, and of severe or life-threatening infection in the severely immunocompromised, especially those with AIDS.

Biology

Cryptosporidium spp. are members of the coccidia (phylum Apicomplexa) having an oocyst stage containing four motile, naked sporozoites (i.e. not within an inner sporocyst). The sporozoites have a characteristic apical complex that helps attachment to and penetration of host cells and then appears to reform into the attachment/feeder organelle. Cryptosporidia are monoxenous, that is they complete their life-cycle (Figs. 1–9) in a single host. Oocysts, the transmissible stage, result from sexual union.

Different species are found in mammals (e.g. *C. muris, C. parvum*), birds (e.g. *C. meleagridis, C. baileyi*), reptiles (e.g. *C. serpentis*), and fish (*C. nasorum*). A number of other species have been described, some of which were shown subsequently not to be cryptosporidia, some are

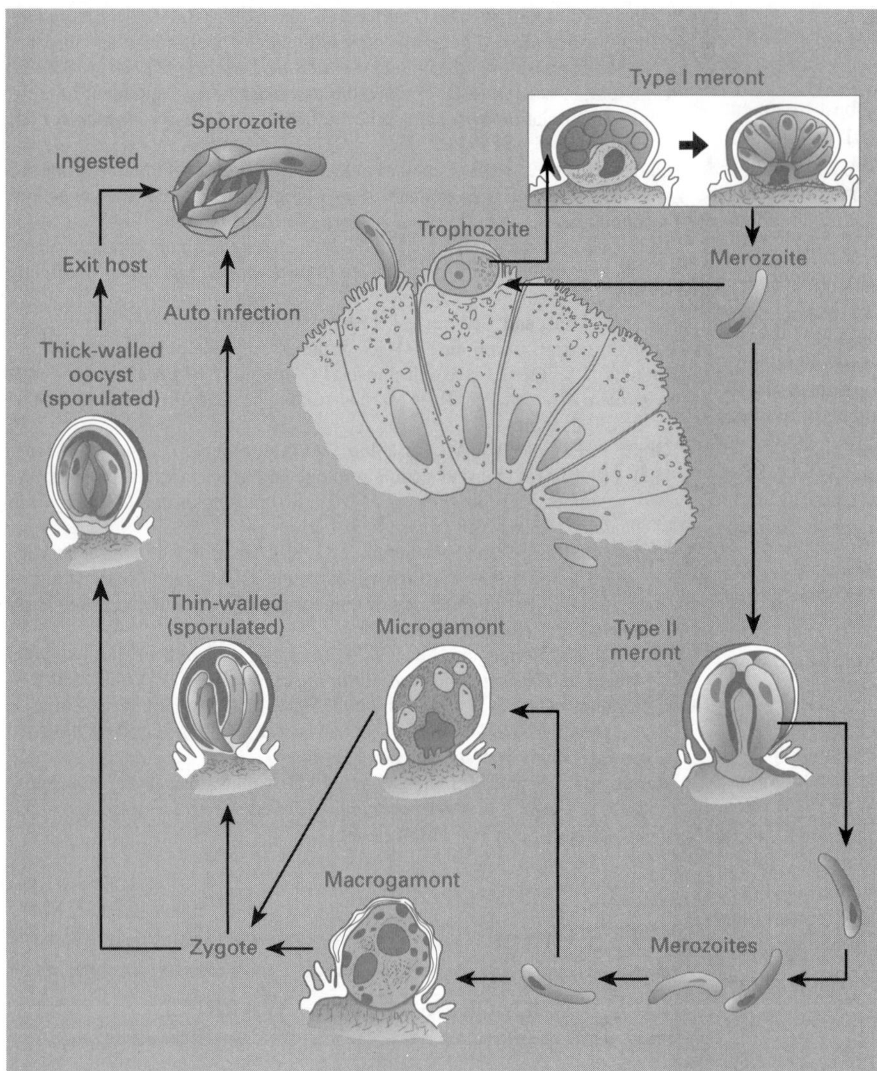

Fig. 1 Diagrammatic representation of the lifecycle of *C. parvum* as it occurs in the mucosal epithelium of an infected mammalian host. Infection follows ingestion of the oocyst, which releases four motile sporozoites. These each take up an intracellular but extracytoplasmic location and develop into trophozoites (uninucleate meronts), which, on maturation, undergo schizogony (asexual multiple budding). The first-stage meronts appear to produce eight merozoites, some of which recycle to form further type I meronts. The second stage, or type II meronts, produce four merozoites, which form gamonts (sexual stages) that mature as either macrogametes, or as microgamonts containing 16 motile microgametes. Most (around 80 per cent) of the zygotes formed after fertilization of the macrogametes by the microgametes develop into thick-walled oocysts, which then sporulate, usually by the time they are excreted. These environmentally resistant oocysts are the form that transmit the infection. The rest have only a thin unit membrane, which ruptures to release the sporozoites in situ to produce an autoinfective cycle. (Adapted from a drawing by Kip Carter, University of Georgia, shown by courtesy of Dr W.L. Current and CRC Press, Inc, Boca Raton.)

Fig. 2 Light micrograph of a semithin section showing the apparently superficial (pseudo-external) location of the parasite along the edge of the epithelium. (Toluidine blue-stained, semithin section.) Figures 2 to 9 provided from photographs by A. Curry and D.P. Casemore.

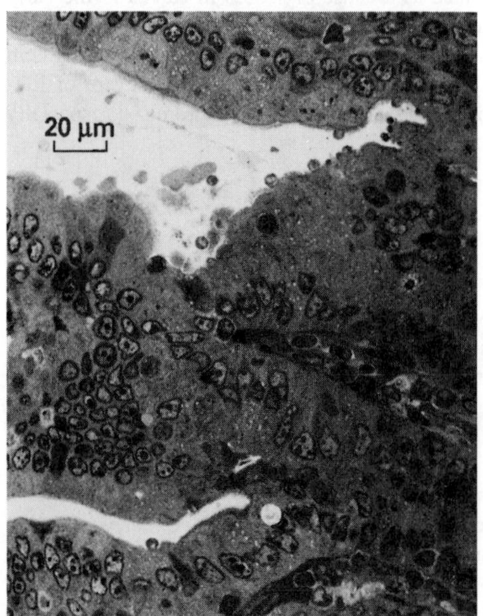

synonyms (usually for *C. parvum*), and some are inadequately characterized. The species can be distinguished morphometrically, by tissue location, host range, and increasingly by molecular biological techniques.

C. parvum, and to a lesser degree the other species, are readily cross-transmissible to a variety of hosts. *C. parvum* is not tissue specific, being capable of infecting the entire enteric tract and associated organs; it may also infect the respiratory tract, but shows a predilection for the lower ileum during the primary stages of infection. *C. muris* is restricted to the glands of the stomach. Avian species may produce asymptomatic infection in birds, particularly of the bursa, or clinical infection, especially of the respiratory tract. *C. serpentis* has been associated with gastritis in snakes.

Infection follows the ingestion of oocysts, the environmentally hardy, transmissible stage that contains the infective sporozoites. These motile bodies are released through a suture in the oocyst wall and quickly attach superficially to cells and round up to form a trophozoite, which develops beneath the host cell's outer membrane. The site of infection is usually the brush border of enterocytes in the small bowel, but the parasite is able to infect other epithelial and parenchymal cells. It can be grown in culture, but it has not yet proved possible to produce large numbers of parasites this way. The complex lifecycle includes both asexual and sexual stages of replication (merogony or schizogony, gametogony, sporogony) (Figs 1–9). Some stages recycle, producing very large numbers of parasites. The endogenous (tissue) stages are uniquely located within a parasitophorous vacuole, the outer layers of which are derived from the host cell's outer membranes. They are thus intracellular but extra-cytoplasmic. During the acute stage of infection, many millions of oocysts are produced each day, most of which are fully sporulated and infectious.

MOLECULAR BIOLOGY

Much of the current information seems conflicting or contradictory because of differences in methods and interpretation. Even the number of chromosomes varies in different reports. Protein and non-protein antigens and some enzymes have been characterized, and some of the genes that encode them have been cloned and sequenced. Some genes coding for structural proteins have also been characterized, including actin and tubulin, both of which are important for parasite motility, and hence invasion. These may prove useful target molecules for the development of anticryptosporidial compounds.

Nucleic acid sequences, isoenzymes, and other molecular structures have helped to differentiate isolates and species. Differences between isolates of *C. parvum* from various sources suggest that those derived from different animals hosts and humans may differ. These findings, which contradict epidemiological evidence, have not yet been explained.

Techniques have been developed for the detection and characterization of cryptosporidial components, such as sodium dodecyl sulphate–polyacrylamide gel electrophoresis and Western blotting for proteins, and the polymerase chain reaction for nucleic acid sequences. Sensitive, genetically based probes may be applied to the detection of the parasite in clinical and environmental samples. Some of these techniques may be developed for epidemiological use.

Fig. 3 Electron micrograph of a transverse section of small bowel of a mouse infected with *C. parvum*. The section shows numerous developmental stages: uninucleate meronts (trophozoites); type I meronts (schizonts) containing merozoites in which may be seen the darker granules of the apical complex organelles; the degenerate remains of a schizont and a free-swimming merozoite within the lumen; macrogamonts showing dark wall-forming granules and electron-lucent polysaccharide (amylopectin) food-storage granules. The parasitophorous vacuole can be clearly seen surrounding the parasite stages. Some of the intracellular stages appear to be free within the lumen because of the plane of sectioning.

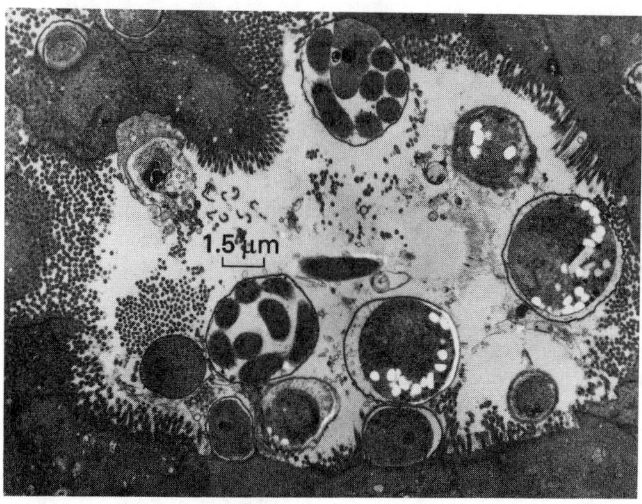

Fig. 4 Electron micrograph of a vertical section of *C. parvum* in murine bowel. The section shows a uninucleate meront (trophozoite) and a type I meront (schizont). The complex lamellar attachment zone or feeder organelle with its electron-dense layer, and the apical complex structures within the merozoites are clearly seen. There is some evidence of elongation of adjacent microvilli.

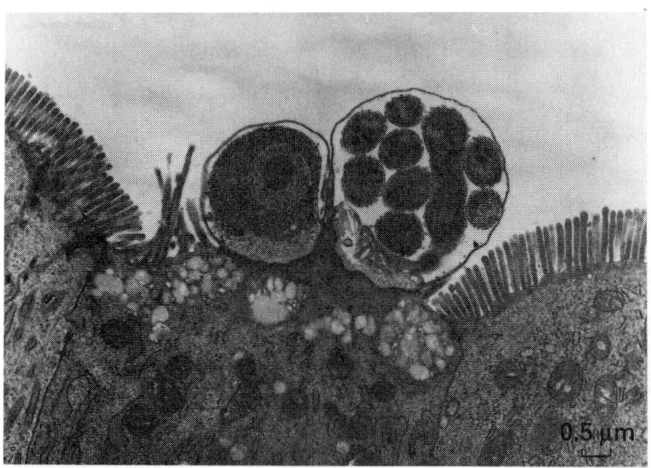

Epidemiology

C. parvum has been reported worldwide and is common in man and in livestock animals, especially lambs and calves. Because of the diversity

Fig. 5 Electron micrograph of a vertical section of a developing *C. parvum* asexual stage in murine bowel tissue. The section shows a meront (schizont) that has undergone nuclear division. The parasitophorous vacuolar membrane, the attachment zone or feeder organelle with its electron-dense layer, and extensive endoplasmic reticulum can be seen.

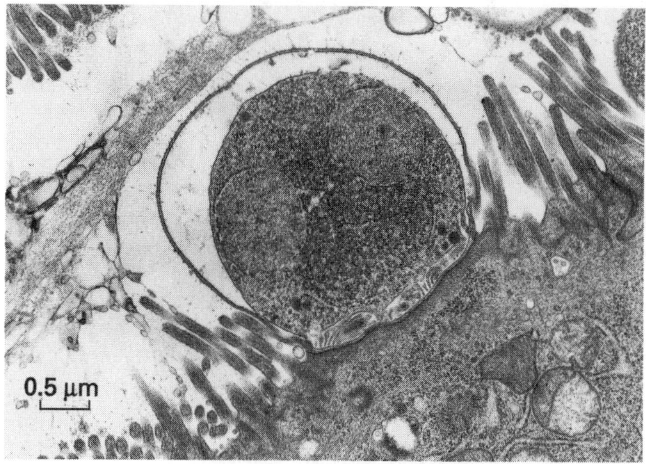

Fig. 6 Electron micrograph of a vertical section of *C. parvum* in murine bowel tissue. The section shows a type II meront that has undergone nuclear division and is budding to form merozoites (two of four can be seen) in which the nuclei and apical organelles can be seen. Prominent endoplasmic reticulum, can be seen in the parent cytoplasm.

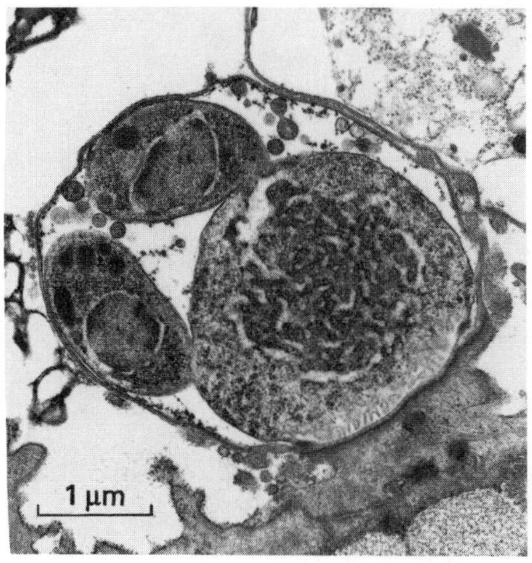

of host species, the epidemiology of the human infection is complex, involving both direct and indirect routes of transmission from animals to man and from person to person. Zoonotic infection by direct contact with livestock, especially lambs and calves, is common, particularly in children, including those from urban homes and schools visiting educational farms.

In the United Kingdom and the United States there have been a number of well-documented outbreaks resulting from contamination of public drinking-water supplies, some involving thousands of cases (403 000 in Milwaukee). Such outbreaks usually result in secondary transmission from person to person and are thus, strictly speaking, community-propagated outbreaks initiated by water, rather than water-borne outbreaks in the classical sense.

Infection is common in children attending playgroups and day-care centres, and results mainly from direct faecal–oral transmission, although the infection may be introduced, in the first instance, through zoonotic contact. Domestic pets are an uncommon source of infection. Cryptosporidium is a common cause of travellers' diarrhoea. Avian cryptosporidia do not seem to be transmissible readily to mammals, including man, but opportunistic infection with an organism resembling *C. baileyi* has been reported in an AIDS patient.

Fig. 7 Electron micrograph of an oblique section of a parasite in murine bowel tissue. The section shows a mature microgamont that has formed microgametes in which the typical elongated nucleus and unusual shape can be seen. The surrounding membrane appears to be intact prior to release of the motile gametes.

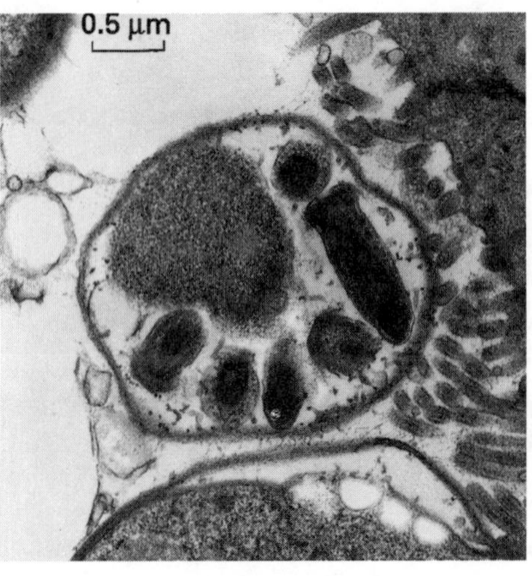

Fig. 8 Electron micrograph of a vertical section of *C. parvum* in murine bowel tissue. The section shows a thin-walled oocyst containing fully developed sporozoites. The remains of the attachment zone can be seen on the host cell.

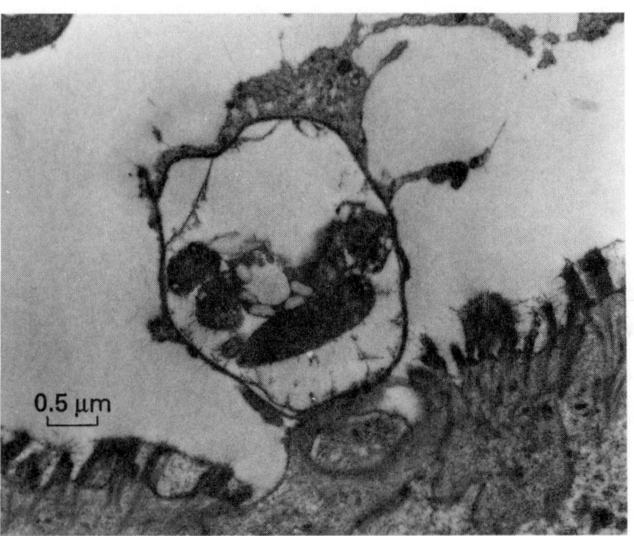

DEMOGRAPHY

Age and sex distribution

In some developing countries, infection is common in infants aged less than 1 year. In developed countries, infection is uncommon in such infants and is most common in children aged from 1 to 5 years. In a large, 2-year survey in the United Kingdom (of more than 60 000 patients) in which all diagnostic specimens submitted were screened, nearly a third of cases were found in young adults; the infection was uncommon in adults over 45 years, including the elderly. Because of the dynamics of transmission, a relative increase in adult cases is often seen in water-borne outbreaks. Therefore adults must not be excluded from screening. In Finland there are differences in age-specific incidence; infection occurs mainly in adults who have travelled abroad. The relative absence of symptomatic infections among young children there is unexplained. Distribution appears to be the same in both sexes.

Temporal distribution

There is evidence of seasonal peaks in several studies worldwide. In the United Kingdom there is a clear pattern of peaks in the spring and in late autumn or early winter, which do not necessarily both occur in any one locality, nor recur year by year. They coincide generally with lambing and calving, with other farming events such as muck spreading, and with maximal rainfall. Temporal peaks are seen in some other countries and are often associated with similar factors, which emphasizes the importance of water as a vehicle and livestock as reservoirs of human infection.

Frequency of occurrence

Laboratory rates of detection in non-immunocompromised subjects average about 2 per cent (range < 1–5 per cent) in developed countries and about 8 per cent in developing countries (range 2–30 per cent). Published reports show that the infection ranks about fourth in the list of pathogens detected in stools submitted to the laboratory, and in the United Kingdom represents about 6 to 8 per cent of the positive findings, somewhat less frequent, generally, than giardiasis. Among young children in the United Kingdom, cryptosporidiosis is more common than salmonella infection and during peak periods detection rates may exceed 20 per cent. This varies, however, from year to year and from district to district, depending on the population sampled and on the criteria used for selection of specimens for screening. It is difficult to be certain how these figures reflect true incidence and prevalence.

Fig. 9 Electron micrograph of a section of pelleted faecal material containing *C. parvum*. The section shows a thick-walled oocyst containing four developing sporozoites and a residual cytoplasmic body.

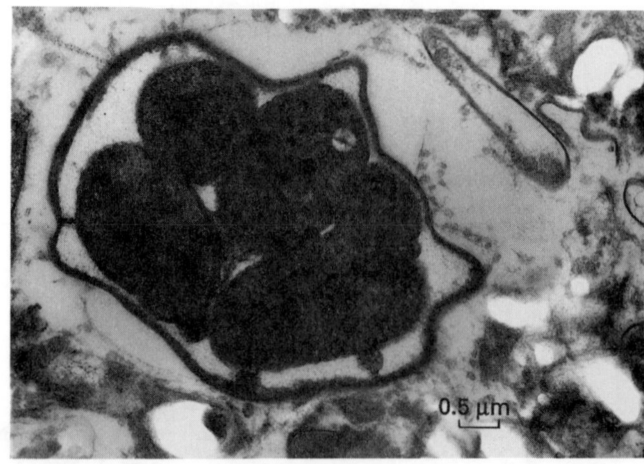

Cryptosporidiosis is one of the most common causes of diarrhoea in AIDS patients and, in some studies, prevalence exceeded 50 per cent. Infection rates are not generally increased for other immunocompromised groups, although in some such the infection may be of increased severity, especially if their immunological deficit is profound.

Clinical aspects

PATHOLOGY

Histopathology

There is mucosal involvement of the small bowel, other parts of the gastroenteric tract, and sometimes beyond. Moderate to severe abnormalities of villous architecture occur, with stunting and fusion of villi and lengthening of crypts. There may be evidence of mild inflammation, with cellular infiltration into the lamina propria.

The endogenous stages of the parasite are generally inconspicuous and appear as small (2–8 μm) bodies, apparently superficially attached to the brush border, unevenly distributed over the apical cells and within the crypts of the villi (Fig. 2 *et seq.*). Although the infection is usually mucosal, submucosal infection has been occasionally reported, suggesting the possibility of haematogenous dissemination. Peaking and apoptosis of infected cells have also been reported. There is usually little intracellular change at the ultrastructural level beyond the attachment zone of the parasite.

Rectal biopsy may reveal mild, non-specific proctitis. Extensive and chronic involvement of the bile duct and gallbladder is seen in some AIDS patients.

In AIDS patients, respiratory-tract involvement is not uncommon. Cough and other respiratory symptoms are common in immunocompetent individuals with cryptosporidiosis but the reason for this is not clear.

Immunological response

An immune response has been demonstrated in each of the four main immunoglobulin classes. The limited studies of seroprevalence indicate that the infection is common, even in developed countries. The variety of immunodeficient conditions in which cryptosporidiosis has been reported to show increased severity or persistence suggests that both humoral and cellular factors have a role in limiting infection. Reports differ on the effect of breast feeding on incidence in infancy but some studies suggest a protective effect; it is not possible to say whether this is due to immunological factors or to protection from the environment, or both.

A number of antigenic molecules, conserved and variable, have been identified, some of which have been shown to induce protective antibodies in laboratory studies and may, thus, be of potential value in immunotherapy. Hyperimmune bovine colostrum has been used therapeutically, apparently with some benefit. Conversely, the presence of specific antibodies in colostrum fails to protect young livestock from acquiring infection. Small-animal models have been used to study the immune response and pathogenesis. These, however, differ from man in their response. As with the molecular genetic studies, some of the results are contradictory.

Although functioning humoral and cellular immunity seem to be important in limiting or controlling infection, it currently appears that, in animal models, CD4+ and CD8+ T lymphocytes and interferon-γ are especially important in limiting infection. In humans, CD4 cell counts of fewer than 200 cells/mm^3 probably indicate the need to take special care to avoid exposure to Cryptosporidium and a poor prognosis if infection occurs.

Possible pathogenic mechanisms

The watery diarrhoea is characteristic of non-inflammatory infection of the small bowel, especially that associated with toxin-producing organisms and enteric viruses. It is possible that there may be production of a secretagogue, neurotoxin, or other toxin, although none has so far been identified. The unique location of the parasite would provide a direct pathway for such substances to the host cell. Several mechanisms have been suggested to explain the symptoms: reduction in absorptive capacity, particularly for water and electrolytes; increase in secretory capacity from crypt hypertrophy; osmotic effects from loss of brush-border enzymes (e.g. disaccharidases) resulting in malabsorption of sugars, increased osmolality of chyme, and subsequent microbial fermentation of sugars in the colon (which may account for the characteristic offensive smell).

CLINICAL PRESENTATION IN OTHERWISE HEALTHY (IMMUNOCOMPETENT) PEOPLE

Cryptosporidiosis in the immunocompetent is a self-limiting, acute gastroenteritis with a variety of presenting symptoms. The incubation period is difficult to define accurately given the wide range of possible reservoirs and routes of infection, but in cases where the time of infection can be assessed (for example, contact with an infected calf) it is about 5 to 7 days (range probably 2–14 days but wider limits have been suggested). There may be a prodrome of one to a few days, with malaise, abdominal pain, nausea, and loss of appetite.

Gastrointestinal and sometimes systemic ''flu-like' symptoms start suddenly. Diarrhoea is the most common symptom, the stools being described as watery, greenish with mucus in some cases, and 'very offensive'. Patients may open their bowels more than 20 times a day but more usually 3 to 6 times. Other symptoms include colicky, abdominal pain, especially after meals, anorexia, nausea, vomiting, abdominal distension, and marked weight loss (sometimes more than 10 per cent). In patients who have blood and pus in the stool, a mixed infection with Campylobacter should be suspected. Systemic symptoms, including malaise, headache, myalgias, and fever, occur in about 20 to 40 per cent of patients. Gastrointestinal symptoms usually last about 7 to 14 days, occasionally 5 or 6 weeks, but weakness, lethargy, mild abdominal pain, and intermittent loose bowels may persist for a month. Oocyst excretion can continue for 2 to 3 weeks after the disappearance of symptoms, which may create problems in the control of outbreaks.

Asymptomatic infection appears to be common in some developing countries, probably reflecting hyperendemicity. Such cases appear to be uncommon in developed countries. The severity of cryptosporidiosis in otherwise healthy subjects is illustrated by a study of 85 patients in an outbreak reported by the PHLS Communicable Diseases Surveillance Centre (unpublished data): 93 per cent had diarrhoea, more than 80 per cent had loss of appetite and abdominal pain; for 12 symptoms listed, 72 (85 per cent) complained of five to nine symptoms (mode, 18 cases complained of seven symptoms); median duration of illness was 13 days (range 1 to >35 days); nine were admitted to hospital with a mean stay of 3 days; and there was a mean of 2.14 general practitioner consultations. Those who have some immunity resulting from a previous infection, for example an adult family member or occupational contacts of acute cases, may have very mild symptoms limited to a few loose stools and perhaps some nausea and loss of appetite, or may be asymptomatic.

There is no evidence of transplacental transmission but infection during late pregnancy may cause metabolic disturbances in the mother, leading to the infant's failure to thrive. Failure to thrive has also been observed in older infants and children, and may be associated with persistent infection and enteropathy.

Severe abdominal pain may be associated with evidence of pancreatitis. Sequelae include toxic megacolon and reactive arthritis. In immunocompetent patients, deaths are rarely attributable to cryptosporidiosis.

CLINICAL PRESENTATION IN IMMUNOCOMPROMISED PATIENTS

Susceptibility to cryptosporidiosis and the severity of the disease is increased in patients who are immunocompromised as a result of AIDS, hypo- or agammaglobulinaemia, severe combined immunodeficiency, leukaemia, malignant disease, bullous pemphigoid, during immunosuppressive treatment with cyclophosphamide and corticosteroids as in patients undergoing bone marrow transplantation, and in children immunosuppressed by measles and chickenpox, especially where there is associated malnutrition.

Infection in leukaemic patients may be unusually severe, particularly when associated with aplastic crises, and may then require modification of chemotherapy to control the infection.

Symptoms of cryptosporidiosis usually develop insidiously in immunocompromised patients. Diarrhoea may be frequent, profuse, and watery, like cholera. Patients may open their bowels up to 25 times, passing up to 20 litres of infected fluid stool per day but usually less profuse. Associated symptoms include colicky, upper abdominal pain often associated with meals, severe weight loss (averaging 18 kg during the 4- to 6-month period in one series of patients), weakness, malaise, anorexia, and low-grade fever. Physical examination may reveal other features of HIV infection such as lymphadenopathy, oral candidiasis, wasting, dehydration, and diffuse abdominal tenderness. Infection with Cryptosporidium in immunocompromised patients may involve the pharynx, oesophagus, stomach, duodenum, jejunum, ileum, appendix, colon, rectum, gallbladder, bile duct, pancreatic duct, and the bronchial tree (in association with other pathogens such as cytomegalovirus and *Pneumocystis carinii*). Cholecystitis, sclerosing cholangitis, pancreatitis, hepatitis, and respiratory-tract symptoms may occur, with or without diarrhoea. Cryptosporidial cholecystitis, which presents with right upper-quadrant abdominal pain and persistent nausea and vomiting is usually associated with severe diarrhoea. About 10 per cent of AIDS patients with cryptosporidiosis have biliary involvement.

Except in those patients in whom the suppression of the immune system can be relieved by stopping immunosuppressant drugs, severe symptoms are likely to persist until the patient dies either from some other opportunistic infection or malignant disease or as a result of dehydration, acid–base or electrolyte disturbances, and cachexia.

NOSOCOMIAL INFECTION

There are a number of reports of transmission to health-care staff from patients, and between patients. In several nosocomial outbreaks there appeared to have been transmission of Cryptosporidium to staff caring for infected, immunocompromised patients. In one of these, serological studies suggested increased exposure among the staff involved in the care of an AIDS patient with confirmed cryptosporidiosis, although this was not confirmed by finding oocysts in their stools. In another episode, one nurse acquired infection following exposure to a bone-marrow transplant recipient with cryptosporidiosis. Five nurses contracted cryptosporidiosis from a terminally ill AIDS patient despite supervision by an experienced infection-control nurse. The patient was suffering from several infections, including cryptosporidiosis, and had early dementia. He had profuse, watery diarrhoea and vomiting, both of which proved difficult to control. Large numbers of cryptosporidia were persistently present in the stool, and were also found in his vomit. He was producing over 6 l of watery stool, which, together with the intractable vomiting and dementia, probably led to significant environmental contamination. The importance of aerosol spread is uncertain.

In an outbreak among patients in a bone-marrow transplant unit, contamination of the environment was demonstrated. Three of six leukaemic children with cryptosporidiosis were thought to have acquired their infection while in hospital. In an outbreak among child patients, poor hand-washing practice was identified as an important factor, and nasogastric feeding tubes were thought to have been the vehicle of transmission. In an outbreak with high mortality in a ward of immunocompromised patients in Denmark, transmission was probably by patients' hands via a ward ice-making machine.

LABORATORY INVESTIGATIONS

Usually, the stool from patients with cryptosporidiosis does not contain blood, pus, cells, or Charcot–Leyden crystals. This may be helpful in distinguishing cryptosporidiosis from acute diarrhoeas caused by amoebiasis, bacillary dysentery, and isosporiasis. Microscopic and serological diagnosis of cryptosporidiosis is discussed below. Cryptosporidiosis may be associated with other bowel pathogens, both in presumed immunocompetent people in tropical countries and in immunocompromised patients. In AIDS patients, common associated infections are with cytomegalovirus and *Isospora belli*. Campylobacters and giardia may also be found in immunocompetent patients. Peripheral leucocytosis and eosinophilia are found rarely. Serum electrolyte abnormalities will develop in patients who become severely dehydrated. In immunocompromised patients with cryptosporidial cholecystitis, serum alkaline phosphatase and γ-glutamyl transpeptidase levels are raised, while aminotransferases and bilirubin may remain normal.

Radiographic abnormalities include dilatation of the small bowel, mucosal thickening, prominent mucosal folds and abnormal motility, and in the biliary system, dilated distal biliary ducts, stenosis with an irregular lumen, and other changes reminiscent of primary sclerosing cholangitis. In the bowel mucosa there is histological evidence of enterocyte damage, villous blunting, and inflammatory-cell infiltration of the lamina propria. Histopathological appearances of the biliary tract resemble primary sclerosing cholangitis.

DIFFERENTIAL DIAGNOSIS

In immunocompetent patients, cryptosporidiosis should be considered in any acute diarrhoeal illness with abdominal pain and other gastrointestinal symptoms with or without systemic ''flu-like' symptoms. The diagnosis is particularly likely in patients with travellers' diarrhoea, those who work with farm animals, in children from day-care centres and institutions, and in health care personnel, who may have acquired the infection from patients. In immunocompetent patients, the symptoms of cryptosporidiosis resemble those of giardiasis, but they last longer. Intense abdominal pain and cramps are more common but bloating, anorexia, and weakness are less common in cryptosporidiosis.

In immunocompromised patients, especially in those with AIDS, isosporiasis is clinically indistinguishable, but can be diagnosed by finding the organisms in the stool. The discovery of Charcot–Leyden crystals in the stool suggests isosporiasis. This infection responds to treatment with trimethoprim and sulphamethoxazole.

TREATMENT

In immunocompetent patients, the illness is self-limiting, but they may become dehydrated and require intravenous fluids, electrolytes, and symptomatic treatment for their vomiting and diarrhoea.

Immunocompromised patients with persistent severe diarrhoea, malabsorption, and other complications may require prolonged palliative treatment. They should avoid excess milk, as lactose intolerance may develop. Parenteral feeding and fluid, electrolyte, and nutrient replacement may be needed. Antiperistaltic agents such as loperamide, diphenoxylate or opiates may increase abdominal pain and bloating. Antiemetics may be needed for symptomatic relief. Temporary relief of biliary obstruction has been achieved by endoscopic papillotomy and of cholecystitis by cholecystectomy.

Many antimicrobials have been tried, both *in vivo* and *in vitro*, without any real success, although some reports suggest possible activity with paromomycin (Humatin), letrazuril/diclazuril, somatostatin, azidothymidine, diloxanide furoate, furazolidone, amprolium, and the macrolides. Immunotherapy (e.g. bovine colostrum, hyperimmune immunoglobulin and transfer factor, and interleukin 2) has been attempted, also with variable results. The macrolide spiramycin showed early promise that has not been confirmed; the drug, as with some others reported to have a therapeutic effect, appears to have little or no direct effect on the parasite itself, although some patients may have amelioration of their symptoms. Zydovudine (Retrovir) therapy may also result in remission or amelioration of symptoms. It is difficult in this case, as with some of the above, to separate the effect of drugs from that of fluctuations in immune competence, including those resulting from antiviral therapy. There is some indication that AIDS patients with multiple gut infections may gain some remission through successful eradication of coinfection.

Laboratory detection and diagnosis

Diagnosis of cases may be made by finding the characteristic endogenous stages (Figs 2–8) in histological sections, using light and electron microscopy, but depends primarily upon the detection of oocysts in stools (Plates 1–10), as part of a planned screening process. The oocysts of *C. parvum* are spherical or slightly ovoid, about 4 to 6 μm, and appear refractile in wet preparations with a highly refractile inner body, the cytoplasmic residuum; the four sporozoites are difficult to distinguish even with special optical systems. The four nuclei can be demonstrated by staining with diamidinophenylindole (DAPI). Several conventional stains have been adapted for diagnostic purposes, such as the modified Ziehl–Neelsen method and phenol–auramine fluorescent stain. Indirect immunofluorescent antibody and enzyme immunoassay methods, using monoclonal antibodies, are commercially available. Screening practice and the selection criteria used vary, and have been the subject of recommendations in the United Kingdom to improve standardization of approach to screening and of reporting for epidemiological purposes.

Concentration of stool specimens is not usually required for diagnosis in acute cases, although oocyst excretion does fluctuate as the infection progresses. Patients may continue to excrete oocysts, usually in low numbers, for a variable period after resolution of symptoms. Detection of low-level excretion is difficult with the diagnostic laboratory methods currently in use.

The diagnosis and control of cryptosporidial infection requires a knowledge of the biology of the organism and accurate identification with adequate quality control. A variety of microscopical structures may readily be mistaken for oocysts. These may include fungal spores (moulds and mushrooms), yeasts, and other parasite forms such as cysts of *Balantidium*, sporocysts of *Isospora*, or oocysts of *Cyclospora* spp. Such misidentification may lead to delay in reaching a correct diagnosis and even to pseudo-outbreaks with consequent unnecessary investigation and concern.

Serological methods have little value in individual cases and are generally reserved for seroepidemiological studies, including the investigation of nosocomial outbreaks.

Environmental detection methods have been developed but the lack of enrichment culture techniques, because of the obligate parasitism of the organism, limits detection. Molecular methods, such as the polymerase chain reaction and gene probes, may yield useful information about speciation and the typing of isolates for epidemiology, and will allow the development of ultrasensitive detection systems.

Infectivity, resistance, and control

INFECTIVITY

Human volunteer studies are now in progress in United States. The data suggest a minimum infective dose of some 30 oocysts and an ID_{50} of 214, for the single isolate tested. Animal studies and volunteer studies with other enteric protozoa suggest a low infective dose. In monkeys the infective dose was fewer than 10 oocysts: in gnotobiotic lambs the minimum infective dose was 1 to 5 oocysts.

RESISTANCE AND DISINFECTION

The oocyst stage can survive for many months in a cool, moist environment. Oocysts are, however, highly susceptible to desiccation, freezing, and moderate heat (e.g. pasteurization temperatures). They are remarkably resistant to most disinfectants and antiseptics, including chlorine at concentrations far greater than those used in water treatment. Some disinfectants may be more effective if used at elevated temperature (≥37°C). Oocysts are sensitive to 10 vol (3 per cent) hydrogen peroxide, and to ozone. Reduction of faecal contamination and of oocyst numbers by physical cleaning are thus essential for control.

The adequate disinfection of instruments such as endoscopes is difficult. Prolonged immersion in glutaraldehyde at elevated temperature, after thorough cleaning, may be required.

CONTROL OF TRANSMISSION

Primary control is by limiting the opportunity for faecal–oral transmission. With faecally incontinent patients, this may prove difficult. Infectivity of asymptomatic cases is unknown but symptom-free subjects not in contact with immunocompromised patients can normally be permitted to work if they use good hygiene. The multiple reservoirs and routes of transmission of Cryptosporidium, and the heavy output of oocysts in infected hosts, can make control difficult in practice, particularly as the infective dose appears to be low. Contamination of water supplies is inevitable from time to time, even in developed countries, and may be the source of some sporadic cases and outbreaks. Spread via fomites is possible but this route is limited by the effect on oocysts of desiccation. In male homosexual patients, transmission may result from sexual practices. There is evidence, however, of temporal peaks suggesting that, as with the general population, zoonotic exposure and water are sources of their infections.

When a public advisory notice is issued to boil water, the practicability of boiling for long periods may be questioned. However, water that has simply been raised to the boil is likely to be safe. Bottled water and water from point-of-use filters are unlikely to contain parasites but may carry an increased bacterial load, the health significance of which is low for normal subjects but which is uncertain for the immunocompromised. AIDS patients should be advised never to drink water that has not been boiled.

As more hospitals become involved in the care of the increasing numbers of AIDS patients, the staff of infectious disease units, and those of other wards to which such patients may be admitted, need to be particularly vigilant in the management of patients with cryptosporidiosis. Staff involved with the care of such cases should report even minor gastrointestinal symptoms and be investigated to minimize risk of spread to other patients or to staff or their families.

REFERENCES

Anon (1990). *Cryptosporidium in water supplies*, Dept. of Health/Dept. of Environment, (Report of the Group of Experts, Chairman, Sir John Badenoch). HMSO, London.

Blanshard, C., Jackson, A.M., Shanson, D.C., Francis, N., and Gazzard, B.G. (1992). Cryptosporidiosis in HIV-seropositive patients. *Quarterly Journal of Medicine*, **85,** 813–23.

Casemore, D.P. (1990). Cryptosporidiosis. In *Recent advances in infection* **3,** (ed. D.S. Reeves and A.M. Geddes), pp. 209–36. Churchill-Livingstone, Edinburgh.

Casemore, D.P. (1991). Broadsheet No. 128: The laboratory diagnosis of human cryptosporidiosis. *Journal of Clinical Pathology*, **44,** 445–51.

Casemore, D.P., and Roberts, C. (1993). Guidelines for screening for Cryptosporidium in stools: report of a joint working group. *Journal of Clinical Pathology*, **46,** 2–4.

Connolly, G.M. (1990). Clinical aspects of cryptosporidiosis. *Baillière's Clinical Gastroenterology*, **4,** 443–54.

Current, W.L. and Bick, P.H. (1989). Immunobiology of *Cryptosporidium* spp. *Pathology and Immunopathology*, **8,** 141–60.

Dubey, J.P., Speer, C.A., and Fayer, R. (ed.) (1990). *Cryptosporidiosis of man and animals.* CRC Press, Boca Raton, FA.

Foot, A.B.M., Oakhill, A., and Mott, M.G. (1990). Cryptosporidiosis and acute leukaemia. *Archives of Disease in Childhood*, **65,** 236–7.

Hart, C.A. and Baxby, D. (1987). Cryptosporidiosis in children. *Pediatric Review Communications*, **1,** 311–41.

Palmer, S.R. and Biffin, A. (1990). Cryptosporidiosis in England and Wales: prevalence and clinical and epidemiological features. *British Medical Journal*, **300,** 774–7.

Petersen, C. (1992). Cryptosporidiosis in patients infected with the human immunodeficiency virus. *Clinics in Infectious Diseases*, **15,** 903–9.

Soave, R. and Armstrong, D. (1986). *Cryptosporidium* and cryptosporidiosis. *Reviews of Infectious Diseases*, **8,** 1012–23.

7.13.6 Cyclospora

D. P. CASEMORE

INTRODUCTION

Organisms producing large, acid-fast, spore-like forms have been recognized in faecal specimens from patients with diarrhoea examined by modified Ziehl–Neelsen stain for the detection of cryptosporidium. They have been described variously as cryptosporidium-like bodies, fungal spores, and cyanobacteria (blue-green algae-like), but have more recently been definitively identified as oocysts of a protozoan parasites belonging to the genus Cyclospora. They have been detected worldwide, most often in residents of, or travellers returning from, developing countries. There is some evidence, including the peak incidence in the rainy season, for water-borne transmission.

NATURAL HISTORY

Cyclospora are coccidia and have many features typical of apicomplexans with a life-cycle similar to the cryptosporidia; they have an oocyst stage, which, when sporulated, produces two sporocysts, each containing two sporozoites (1.2 × 9.0μm in those identified so far in human infection). The oocysts require an extrinsic period for sporulation following excretion. When first excreted they have a characteristic morular inner structure (see below). The reservoir of infection has not currently been identified but could well be a small rodent or insectivore (such as moles), or possibly birds, species of all of which are known to harbour members of the genus. The species infecting man has not been found in other hosts and may, like many other species of coccidia, be restricted to a single host species. It has tentatively been named *C. cayetanensis* n.sp. The importance of secondary transmission is currently unclear. The requirement for an extrinsic period of sporulation implies that transmission must therefore be indirect.

Infection occurs in people of all ages; it has been detected most commonly in those from developing countries and among adults who have travelled to Nepal, Indonesia, Southern and Central America, and other underdeveloped areas, but cases have also been identified in the United States and the United Kingdom.

Fig. 1 Longitudinal section through jejunal biopsy specimen to show single intracellular parasite (transmission electron microscopy). (Reproduced from Bendall, R.P., Lucas, S., Moody, A., Tovey, G., and Chiodini, P.L. (1993). Diarrhoea associated with cyanobacterium-like bodies: a new coccidian enteritis of man. *Lancet*, **341,** 590–2, with permission. © The Lancet Ltd.)

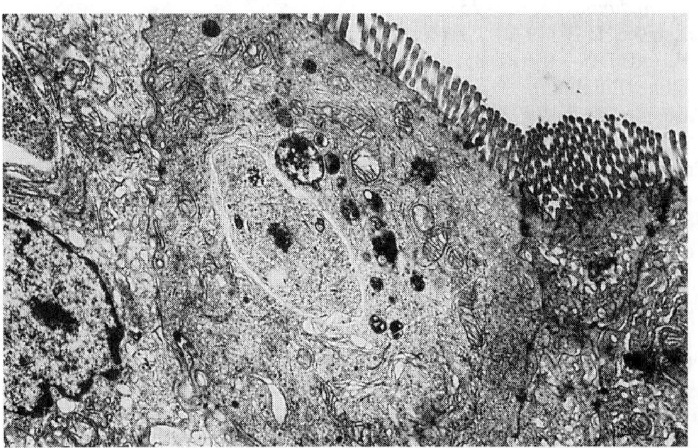

CLINICAL PRESENTATION

Symptoms include protracted, watery diarrhoea with a mean duration of about 6 (range 1–8) weeks, flatulence, bloating, dyspepsia, malaise, and marked weight loss. Asymptomatic infection has been described in indigenous people in developing countries, probably reflecting endemicity and recurrent infection in the immune. The site of infection is primarily the small intestine, where the parasite is found intracytoplasmically midway between the nucleus and the cell membrane at the luminal side.

TREATMENT

Co-trimoxazole (1 tablet twice a day for 7 days) has proved effective in eradicating the infection.

DIAGNOSIS

The oocysts are excreted in stools in large numbers during the acute stage and variably thereafter; they can be detected by modified Ziehl–Neelsen staining, although the acid-fast staining is variable (Plates 1, 2). They are 8 to 10μm in size, and have visible surface and internal structure. Phase-contrast microscopy reveals the internal morula, a collection of refractile, membrane-bound, spherical bodies, 1 to 2μm in size, within an outer wall. By fluorescence microscopy they may show characteristic blue autofluorescence.

Endogenous stages may be detected intracellularly beneath the brush border of enterocytes in jejunal biopsy specimens, and possibly other tissues, by light and electron microscopy (Plate 3, Fig. 1). Transmission electron microscopy should reveal typical apicomplexan structures within an intracellular parasitophorous vacuole.

CONTROL

As the source of the parasite is currently unknown, specific recommendations to limit the reservoir cannot be made. Transmission is almost certainly primarily by an indirect faecal–oral route and hence can be limited by the usual hygienic precautions including avoidance of unboiled water, water-washed, unpeeled fruit, salads, uncooked vegetables etc. in endemic areas.

REFERENCES

Bendall, R.P., Lucas, S., Moody, A., Tovey, G., and Chiodini, P.L. (1993). Diarrhoea associated with cyanobacterium-like bodies: a new coccidian enteritis of man. *Lancet*, **341,** 590–2.

Casemore, D.P. (1994). Cyclospora: another ''new'' pathogen. *Journal of Medical Microbiology,* **41,** 217–9.

Casemore, D.P., Gardner, C.A., and Mahoney, C.O. (1994). Cryptosporidial infection with special reference to nosocomial transmission of *Cryptosporidium parvum:* a review. *Folia Parasitologica,* **41,** 17–21.

Hoge, C.W. *et al.* (1993). Epidemiology of diarrhoeal illness associated with coccidian-like organism among travellers and foreign residents in Nepal. *Lancet*, **341,** 1175–9.

Hoge, C.W. *et al.* (1995). Placebo-controlled trial of co-trimoxazole for cyclospora infections among travellers and foreign residents in Nepal. *Lancet,* **345,** 691–3.

Ortega, Y.R., Sterling, C.R., Gilman, R.H., Cama, V.A., and Diaz, F. (1993). Cyclospora species—a new protozoan pathogen of humans. *New England Journal of Medicine*, **328,** 1308–12.

7.13.7 Sarcocystosis

V. Zaman

Humans can act as both the final and intermediate host of the parasites belonging to the genus Sarcocystis. In their lifecycle there is an alternation of sexual generation of the parasite in the intestinal tissues of a predator host (carnivores including snakes, omnivores, and scavenger animals) and asexual generation in the tissues of a prey animal (herbivores and omnivores including rodents). The predator animals act as the final hosts and excrete oocysts or sporocysts in the faeces. The animal eaten by a predator acts as an intermediate host because cysts are present in the muscles and other tissues (Fig. 1).

Sarcocystis hominis (syn. **Isospora hominis***)*

The intermediate host is cattle. Human infection results from eating uncooked beef. Prevalence in human populations is not known but the lifecycle has been studied in human volunteers.

CLINICAL ASPECTS

The majority of patients passing oocysts are asymptomatic and the development of the sporogonic stage in human intestine is either non-pathogenic or only slightly pathogenic, resulting in mild gastrointestinal upset. However, the symptoms may vary, depending on the number of parasites ingested, and severe symptoms may occur after ingestion of heavily infected beef. This probably happened in six patients from Bangkok who developed symptoms suggestive of segmental necrotizing enteritis.

DIAGNOSIS

This is based on the detection of oocysts or sporocysts in the faeces of infected individuals (Fig. 2). The size of sporocysts ranges from 13.6 to 16.4 μm by 8.3 to 10.6 μm. Occasionally, sporocysts may be seen attached in pairs and covered by a thin, transparent cyst wall (Fig. 3).

TREATMENT

No chemotherapeutic agents are available. Prevention consists of not eating uncooked beef.

Fig. 1 Sarcocyst in muscle: the thickness of the cyst wall varies in different species; in this species a thick, striated wall is visible and the elongated structures inside the cyst are cystozoites. (× 400).

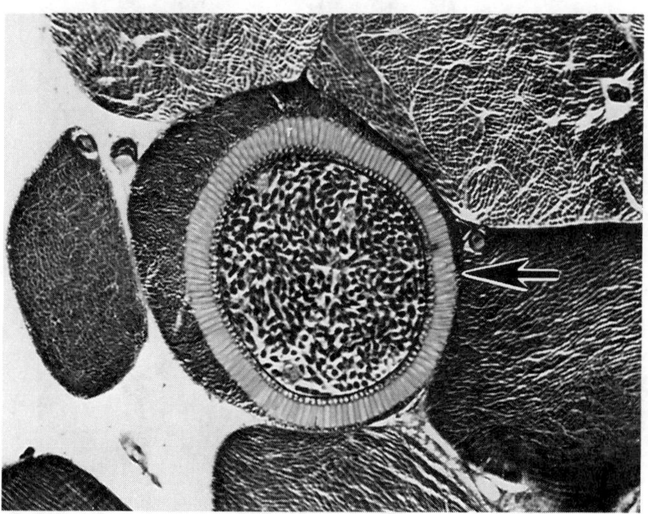

Sarcocystis suihominis

The lifecycle is similar to that of *S. hominis*, except that the intermediate host is the pig.

CLINICAL ASPECTS

Human volunteers given infected tissues have experienced diarrhoea and mild fever.

As in the case of *S. hominis* the intensity of symptoms probably varies with the size of the infective dose. If large amounts of heavily infected pork are ingested, symptoms could be quite severe. As this rarely happens, the majority of patients have only mild or no symptoms.

DIAGNOSIS

This is based on the detection of oocysts or sporocysts in faeces; these are almost identical to those of *S. hominis*.

TREATMENT

No chemotherapeutic agents are available. Prevention consists of not eating raw pork.

Fig. 2 Sarcocystis hominis: sporocyst with sporozoites; residium (food store) can be seen at one end. × 1000.

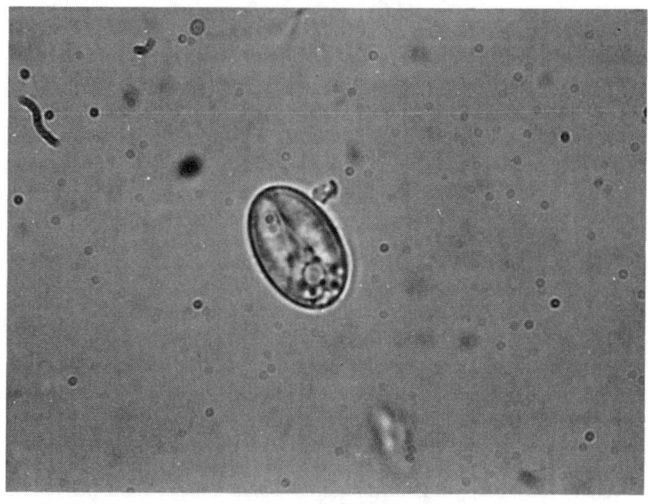

Fig. 3 Sarcocystis hominis: sporocysts attached in a pair. × 1000.

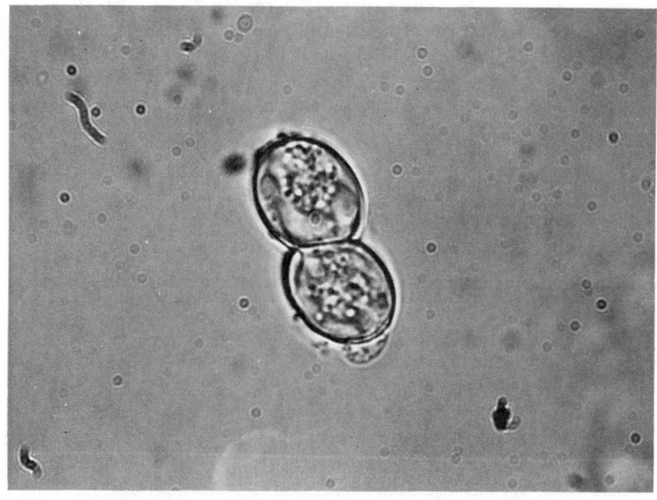

Sarcocystis spp.

These produce sarcocystis in human muscles. There is probably more than one species involved. Infection is acquired by the ingestion of oocysts or sporocysts passed in the final hosts. The final hosts are unknown but could be carnivores, such as dogs or cats.

CLINICAL ASPECTS

The majority of cases are asymptomatic. The infection is diagnosed from a muscle biopsy for other diseases or at autopsy. It appears that the cysts of some species are found only in skeletal muscles while others occur in cardiac and skeletal muscles. On the basis of morphology it is possible to differentiate the cysts into four types.

DIAGNOSIS

In tissue sections, Sarcocystis can be easily diagnosed and it is generally not difficult to differentiate it from Toxoplasma tissue cysts. In the case of Sarcocystis the cyst wall is distinct and the cystozoites are larger. Toxoplasma cystozoites are PAS positive while Sarcocystis cystozoites are PAS negative.

TREATMENT

None is available.

REFERENCES

Aryeetey, M.E. and Piekarski, G. (1976). Serologische Sarcocystis—Studien an Menschen und Ratten. *Zeitschrift fur Parasitenkunde*, **50,** 109–24.

Beaver, P.C., Gadgil, R.K., and Morera, P. (1979). *Sarcocystis* in man: a review and report of five cases. *American Journal of Tropical Medicine and Hygiene*, **28,** 819–44.

Bunyaratvej, S., Bunyawongwiroj, P., and Nitiyanant, P. (1982). Human intestinal sarcosporidiosis: report of six cases. *American Journal of Tropical Medicine and Hygiene*, **31,** 36–41.

Häfner, U. and Frank, W. (1984). Host specificity and host range of the Genus Sarcocystis in three snake-rodent life cycles. *Zentralblatt für Bakteriologie Parasitenkunde, Infektionskrankheiten und Hygiene A*, **256,** 296–9.

Heydorn, A.O. (1977). Beitrage zum Lebenszyklus der Sarkosporidien. IX. Entwicklungszyklus von *Sarcocystis suihominis* n. spec. *Berliner und Münchener Tierärztliche Wochenschrift*, **99,** 218–24.

Mehlhorn, H. and Heydorn, A.O. (1977). Light and electron microscopic studies of *Sarcocystis suihominis*. I. The development of cysts in experimentally infected pigs. *Zentralblatt für Bakteriologie, Parasitenkunde, Infektionskankheiten und Hygiene*, Abteilung 1: Originale Reihe B *A*, **239,** 124–39.

Rommell, M. and Heydorn, A.O. (1972). Beitrage zum Lebendszyklus der Sarkosporidien. III. *Isospora hominis* (Railliet und Lucet, 1891) Wenyon, 1928, eine Dauerform der Sarkosporidien des Rindes und des Schweins. *Berliner und Münchener Tierärztliche Wochenschrift*, **85,** 143–5.

7.13.8 Giardiasis, balantidiasis, isosporiasis, and microsporidiosis

M. F. HEYWORTH

Giardiasis

CAUSATIVE ORGANISM

Giardiasis is caused by *Giardia lamblia*, a protozoan parasite that colonizes the human small-intestinal lumen. The parasite's lifecycle comprises two stages: motile trophozoites (Fig. 1) and thick walled, ellipsoidal cysts that are excreted in the faeces. *G. lamblia* trophozoites are dorsoventrally flattened organisms with eight flagella and a ventral adhesive disc that enables them to become attached to the luminal surface of intestinal epithelial cells. Trophozoites absorb nutrients from the contents of the small-intestinal lumen. New hosts acquire the infection by ingesting *G. lamblia* cysts; exposure of cysts to gastric acid leads to emergence of trophozoites from the cysts. Trophozoites encyst in the small-intestinal lumen, and the resulting cysts are excreted from the host. Giardia trophozoites have two nuclei and no mitochondria; they generate energy by anaerobic metabolism.

Besides *G. lamblia*, other species of *Giardia* are recognized. These include *G. muris*, a rodent parasite, and *G. agilis*, which infects amphibians. *G. lamblia* (synonymous with *G. intestinalis* and *G. duodenalis*) can infect other mammals in addition to man.

EPIDEMIOLOGY

G. lamblia infection is usually acquired by drinking water that contains cysts. Other modes of spread include direct faecal–oral transmission of cysts, as in day-care centres for infants and small children, and occasional food-borne transmission of cysts. Water-borne giardiasis occurs in hikers drinking from mountain streams and lakes contaminated by *G. lamblia* cysts, and has occurred as a result of contamination of municipal water supplies by sewage. Dogs, cats, beavers, and muskrats can harbour infections with Giardia trophozoites that are morphologically similar or identical to those that infect man. Each of these non-human mammals can be infected by oral administration of *G. lamblia* cysts obtained from human faeces. It is, however, still unclear whether giardiasis is a zoonosis, that is, an infection spread from animals to man.

Immunodeficiency predisposes to the occurrence of severe and persistent giardiasis (Table 1). Human immunodeficiency states that are associated with giardiasis include conditions that impair host antibody responses ('common variable' hypogammaglobulinaemia and X-linked immunoglobulin deficiency). Some patients with common variable hypogammaglobulinaemia and chronic giardiasis also have abnormally enlarged lymphoid follicles in the small intestine (nodular lymphoid

Fig. 1 Scanning electron micrograph of three *Giardia lamblia* trophozoites on a jejunal biopsy specimen from a patient with giardiasis. The dorsal surfaces of two trophozoites are visible (D), and the ventral adhesive disc of the other trophozoite is shown (V). Illustration by courtesy of Dr. Robert L. Owen; modified from Carlson, J.R., Heyworth, M.F., and Owen, R.L. (1984). Giardiasis: Immunology, diagnosis and treatment. *Survey of Digestive Diseases*, **2,** 201–13, S. Karger AG, Basel, and used by permission.

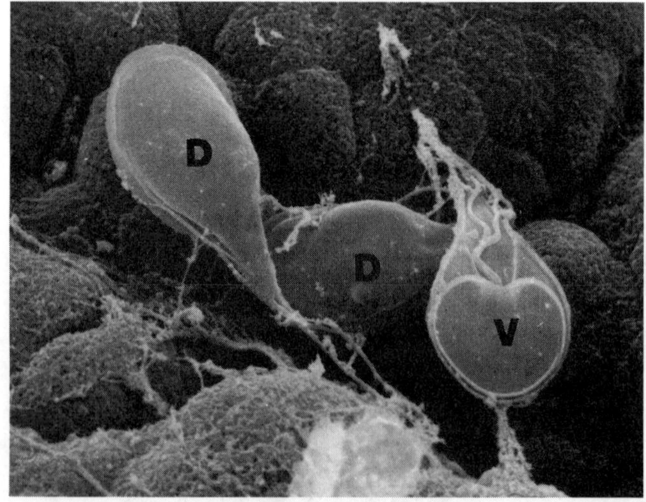

Table 1 *Immunodeficiency states associated with Giardia lamblia infection*

Example or cause of immunodeficiency	Comments
'Common variable' hypogammaglobulinaemia (deficiency of IgG, IgA, ± IgM)	Intestinal plasma cells reduced in number or absent; associated with chronic giardiasis
X-linked immunoglobulin deficiency	Associated with chronic giardiasis
Radiation therapy/cytotoxic chemotherapy	Bone marrow transplant recipients and/or patients with malignancy
AIDS due to human immunodeficiency virus (HIV)	Giardia-specific serum antibody levels lower than in HIV-negative Giardia-infected persons

Modified, with permission, from Heyworth, M.F. (1992). The immunology of giardiasis. In *Immunology of gastrointestinal disease*, (ed. T.T. MacDonald), pp. 263–82. Kluwer, Lancaster.

hyperplasia), which contain numerous immature B lymphocytes that express IgM on their surfaces. Another abnormal feature in patients with nodular lymphoid hyperplasia is that the intestinal mucosa does not contain any detectable IgA-producing plasma cells. The underlying abnormality in such individuals is thought to be a failure of intestinal B lymphocytes to switch from expression of surface IgM to expression of surface IgA. Chronic giardiasis in patients with nodular lymphoid hyperplasia is believed to result from absence of IgA (including anti-Giardia IgA) in intestinal secretions, consequent to the absence of IgA-producing plasma cells in the intestinal mucosa of such individuals.

As noted in Table 1, there is evidence that individuals infected by the human immunodeficiency virus (**HIV**) with giardiasis have an impaired serum antibody response to *G. lamblia*. Whether they also have an impaired intestinal antibody response to the parasite is unknown. In HIV-infected persons, the prevalence of giardiasis appears to be lower than that of cryptosporidiosis or *Pneumocystis carinii* infection. The reason for this apparent difference in prevalence is not known.

CLINICAL FEATURES

G. lamblia infections can be asymptomatic (as shown by cyst excretion in the absence of symptoms), and can also cause a variety of clinical problems. These include watery diarrhoea, steatorrhoea (due to fat malabsorption), and weight loss (reflecting impaired absorption of nutrients). Other clinical features include nausea, abdominal cramps and borborygmi, diminished appetite, abdominal distension, eructation of foul-tasting gas ('purple burps'), and passage per rectum of foul-smelling flatus. Giardiasis does not lead to gastrointestinal bleeding. In immunologically normal persons, untreated giardiasis typically lasts for several weeks, with symptoms that fluctuate in severity. Clinical sequelae that have occasionally been reported in giardiasis include megaloblastic anaemia resulting from impaired absorption of vitamin B_{12} or folic acid, and psychiatric symptoms that were apparently due, in some cases, to deficiency of the same vitamins.

PATHOPHYSIOLOGY

The mechanisms responsible for diarrhoea and malabsorption in giardiasis are not completely understood. In some individuals with giardiasis, villi in the small intestine are reduced in length. This abnormality can be reversed by eradicating the infection, and is of unknown pathogenesis. Shortening of microvilli on the luminal surface of intestinal epithelial cells has been observed in mice with *G. muris* infection, in gerbils infected with *G. lamblia*, and in small-intestinal biopsies from human subjects with giardiasis. Reduced activity of intestinal disaccharidases has been reported in Giardia-infected human subjects, gerbils, and mice. In the light of this information, it is conceivable that the diarrhoea that occurs in human giardiasis is partly osmotic in origin (resulting from undigested disaccharides in the intestinal lumen).

G. lamblia trophozoites cultured in the presence of sodium glycocholate take up this bile salt from the culture medium. Uptake of bile salts by trophozoites in the intestinal lumen may, therefore, contribute to the fat malabsorption that occurs in some patients with giardiasis.

IMMUNOLOGY

Immunocompetent individuals with giardiasis develop serum IgM, IgA, and IgG antibody responses against *G. lamblia* trophozoites. As with antibody responses to other infectious organisms, the serum IgM response to trophozoites is transient, but serum antitrophozoite IgG appears to persist for years after clearance of giardiasis. For protection against intestinal infections, such as giardiasis, intestinal antibody is more important than serum antibody. In human volunteers who were deliberately infected with *G. lamblia*, an intestinal IgA response to the parasite was documented. Similarly, *G. muris*-infected mice develop an intestinal IgA response to *G. muris* trophozoites. In mice at least, production of intestinal antitrophozoite IgA and clearance of *G. muris* infection appear to be dependent on CD4+ (helper) T lymphocytes.

Studies with rodents have provided direct evidence that antitrophozoite IgA has a protective effect against Giardia infections. For example, incubation of *G. muris* trophozoites with antitrophozoite IgA reduces the ability of these organisms to infect mice. Furthermore, the number of cysts excreted by Giardia-infected rats is diminished by intraduodenal administration of antitrophozoite IgA. Other work suggests that antitrophozoite IgA in human and mouse milk helps to protect neonates of these species against Giardia infections. Antitrophozoite IgA does not kill Giardia trophozoites in the presence or absence of complement. Instead, currently available evidence suggests that this antibody coats trophozoites, inhibiting their capacity to become attached to the intestinal epithelium, and leading to their peristaltic expulsion from the host intestine.

DIAGNOSIS

Traditional methods for diagnosing giardiasis include stool microscopy to look for *G. lamblia* cysts; this can be done on unstained faecal specimens, or on specimens incubated with Lugol's iodine, which stains the cysts brown. If faecal microscopy for cysts is negative, but there is a high clinical suspicion of giardiasis, potentially informative additional diagnostic tests include microscopic examination of duodenal fluid or duodenal biopsies for *G. lamblia* trophozoites. Duodenal fluid can be obtained by aspiration at endoscopy, or by means of an 'Enterotest' capsule, a device consisting of a coiled thread inside a gelatin capsule; one end of the thread protrudes from the capsule. After an overnight fast, individuals to be tested are asked to swallow the capsule, and the free end of the protruding thread is taped to the face. If technically successful, in a patient with giardiasis, the capsule enters the duodenum, where the gelatin is digested and the previously encapsulated thread adsorbs duodenal secretions and trophozoites. Approximately 4 h after the capsule has been swallowed, the thread is pulled out of the patient's

Table 2 *Various drug regimens for treating giardiasis*

Drug	Daily dose	Treatment duration	Comments
Quinacrine	6 mg/kg body weight	7 days	Divided in 3 doses/day
Metronidazole	15 mg/kg	7 days	Divided in 3 doses/day
Tinidazole	50 mg/kg	Single dose	
Ornidazole	1 g (total dose)	Single dose	
Furazolidone	8 mg/kg (adult)	7–10 days	Divided in 3 or 4 doses/day
	5 mg/kg (paediatric)		Liquid preparation available for paediatric use
Paromomycin	30 mg/kg	10 days	Divided in 3 doses/day
			Poorly absorbed from the gastrointestinal tract lumen
			Has been used for treating giardiasis during pregnancy

mouth, and fluid squeezed from the thread is examined microscopically for trophozoites.

In recent years, these diagnostic approaches have been supplemented by enzyme immunoassays for detecting *G. lamblia* antigens in faecal specimens. In diagnosing giardiasis, enzyme immunoassay for antigen(s) is more sensitive than stool microscopy (i.e. there is a smaller percentage of false-negative results than with stool microscopy for *G. lamblia* cysts). In one study, 22 faecal samples from individuals with presumptive giardiasis were examined microscopically for cysts, and tested by enzyme immunoassay for a 65-kDa glycoprotein of *G. lamblia*. Only 16 of the samples were found to be positive by microscopy, but all 22 samples were positive by immunoassay.

Testing of human sera for antibodies against *G. lamblia* trophozoites is not a useful method for diagnosing current infection. The presence or absence of serum IgG antitrophozoite antibody correlates poorly with the presence or absence of current infection (as judged by faecal microscopy for *G. lamblia* cysts). Some investigators have reported a strong positive correlation between serum IgM antitrophozoite antibody and current infection with *G. lamblia*. However, in one study of individuals with microscopically documented giardiasis, IgM antitrophozoite antibody was found in sera from only 33 per cent of such individuals (24 IgM antibody-positive sera out of 73 sera tested).

Although unreliable as a diagnostic criterion for current *G. lamblia* infection, the presence of anti-*Giardia* antibodies in human sera may be a guide to the prevalence of former giardiasis in a population.

PREVENTION

Filtration of municipal water supplies removes *G. lamblia* cysts. Water can be filtered through sand or diatomaceous earth. The cysts can also be removed from water by membrane filters that have a pore diameter of less than 5 μm. *Giardia* cysts in water are killed by boiling.

Water intended for human consumption can be screened for *G. lamblia* cysts by microscopic examination of any particulate material obtained by filtration. This examination can include fluorescence microscopy of particulate material incubated with fluorescent antibodies directed against *G. lamblia* cysts. A sensitive method that has recently been developed for detecting cysts involves polymerase chain reaction (**PCR**) amplification of *G. lamblia* DNA. Using oligonucleotide primers that anneal specifically to short regions of *G. lamblia* DNA, in conjunction with PCR amplification of DNA flanked by sequences complementary to the primers, the technique can detect DNA from a single *G. lamblia* cyst, and can distinguish *G. lamblia* and *G. muris* cysts. This sensitive and specific technique is likely to facilitate the detection of *G. lamblia* cysts in water samples.

TREATMENT

Table 2 summarizes various drug regimens for the treatment of giardiasis; the mode of action of several agents listed is not entirely clear. In the 1970s, it was shown that metronidazole inhibited nucleic acid synthesis in protozoa. Paromomycin is an aminoglycoside antibiotic. Drugs of this type bind to ribosomal RNA and block protein synthesis, in micro-organisms that are sensitive to the drugs.

The question of whether or not to treat asymptomatic *G. lamblia* infection (detected by finding cysts in faecal specimens) has generated some controversy. The current consensus is that treatment of asymptomatic cyst excretors, with one or other of the drugs listed in Table 2, is warranted. Elimination of Giardia infection in asymptomatic individuals reduces the opportunity for transmission of the parasite to other persons.

REFERENCES

Adam, R.D. (1991). The biology of *Giardia* spp. *Microbiological Reviews*, **55,** 706–32.

Buret, A., Hardin, J.A., Olson, M.E., and Gall, D.G. (1992). Pathophysiology of small intestinal malabsorption in gerbils infected with *Giardia lamblia*. *Gastroenterology*, **103,** 506–13.

Davidson, R.A. (1984). Issues in clinical parasitology: the treatment of giardiasis. *American Journal of Gastroenterology*, **79,** 256–61.

Gillin, F.D. *et al.* (1990). Isolation and expression of the gene for a major surface protein of *Giardia lamblia*. *Proceedings of the National Academy of Sciences (USA)*, **87,** 4463–7.

Heyworth, M.F. (1992). Immunology of *Giardia* and *Cryptosporidium* infections. *Journal of Infectious Diseases*, **166,** 465–72.

Isaac-Renton, J.L. (1991). Laboratory diagnosis of giardiasis. *Clinics in Laboratory Medicine*, **11,** 811–27.

Mahbubani, M.H., Bej, A.K., Perlin, M.H., Schaefer, F.W., Jakubowski, W., and Atlas, R.M. (1992). Differentiation of *Giardia duodenalis* from other *Giardia* spp. by using polymerase chain reaction and gene probes. *Journal of Clinical Microbiology*, **30,** 74–8.

Nash, T.E., Herrington, D.A., Losonsky, G.A., and Levine, M.M. (1987). Experimental human infections with *Giardia lamblia*. *Journal of Infectious Diseases*, **156,** 974–84.

The Medical Letter on Drugs and Therapeutics (1993), Vol. 35 (Issue 911), pp. 111–22. Drugs for parasitic infections. The Medical Letter, Inc., New Rochelle, NY.

Balantidiasis

CAUSATIVE ORGANISM

This infection is caused by *Balantidium coli*. The organism is a ciliate protozoan, and is the largest protozoan parasite of man. *B. coli* has a two-stage lifecycle comprising motile ciliated trophozoites that parasitize the colon (Fig. 2), and non-motile cysts. Spread of the infection to new hosts occurs by ingestion of the parasite. A study in the Philippines (published in 1913) showed that monkeys fed with *B. coli* cysts subsequently developed *B. coli* infection of the gastrointestinal tract.

CLINICAL FEATURES

Human subjects with *B. coli* infection can be asymptomatic, or can develop diarrhoea with stools that are either watery or that consist of blood and mucus. In severe *B. coli* infection, patients can develop colonic ulceration, colonic perforation, peritonitis, gangrene of the appendix (resulting from the presence of *B. coli* in the appendiceal wall), and spread of the parasite to the liver or lungs. Balantidiasis is a rare cause of liver abscess. As is evident from the spectrum of clinical features that occur in severe balantidiasis, this infection can be fatal. Balantidiasis may be clinically indistinguishable from amoebiasis, bacillary dysentery, and ulcerative colitis.

Fig. 2 Light micrograph of *Balantidium coli* trophozoite (arrow) in colonic tissue. Cilia are visible on the surface of the organism. Arrowheads indicate tissue plasma cells. × 705. Modified from Neafie, R.C. (1976). Balantidiasis. In *Pathology of tropical and extraordinary diseases*, Vol. 1 (ed. C.H. Binford and D.H. Connor), pp. 325–7. Armed Forces Institute of Pathology, Washington DC, and used by permission.

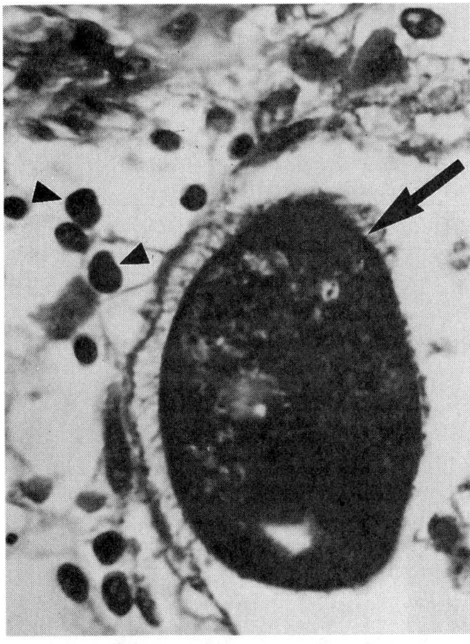

Fig. 3 Light micrograph of *Balantidium coli* trophozoites in ulcerated colonic mucosa of a patient with balantidiasis. The trophozoites are visible as large cells in the right-hand half of the illustration. Photomicrograph by Zane Price, by courtesy of Dr Edward K. Markell. From Markell, E.K., Voge, M., and John, D.T. (1992). *Medical parasitology* (7th edn). Saunders, Philadelphia, and used by permission.

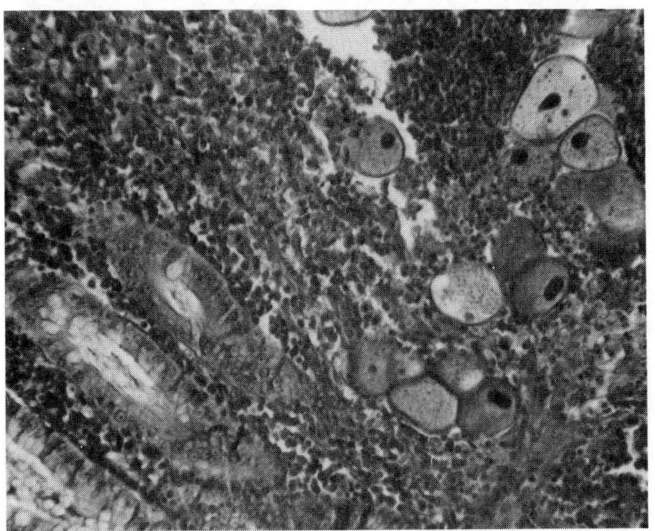

EPIDEMIOLOGY

Balantidiasis has been seen in temperate and tropical countries. The epidemiology is poorly understood, but there is circumstantial evidence that man can acquire the infection from animals. A high prevalence of *B. coli* infection has been seen in human communities that live in close proximity to *B. coli*-infected pigs (for example, in New Guinea). Consequently, there has been speculation that pigs are a reservoir for spread of the infection to man. However, balantidiasis has also occurred in human subjects who had no known contact with pigs or other animals. Clusters of cases of balantidiasis have been seen in long-stay psychiatric hospitals.

PATHOPHYSIOLOGY

The mechanism by which *B. coli* produces disease has not been identified. *B. coli* trophozoites ingest erythrocytes and bacteria, and it is justifiable to speculate that their ability to penetrate host tissues results from the production of one or more proteases. This suggestion, however, awaits verification. In the 1950s, it was reported that *B. coli* trophozoites produce hyaluronidase, but there is no recent confirmation or refutation of this report.

DIAGNOSIS

Balantidiasis can be diagnosed by microscopic examination of diarrhoeal stools, or of colonic mucus obtained at sigmoidoscopy. Examination may show motile trophozoites or, less frequently, cysts of *B. coli*. In persons with balantidial colitis, rectal inflammation, ulceration, and bleeding may be visible at sigmoidoscopy. Histological examination of rectal biopsies may reveal *B. coli* trophozoites in the mucosa (Fig. 3).

TREATMENT

Patients with balantidiasis have been treated empirically with various antimicrobial agents. The existing literature contains little interpretable information about the effectiveness of such treatment, although eradication of the parasite has been reported in some individuals treated with metronidazole or tetracycline. Surgical intervention may be necessary in patients with liver abscess or clinical evidence of appendicitis or colonic perforation.

REFERENCES

Dorfman, S., Rangel, O., and Bravo, L.G. (1984). Balantidiasis: report of a fatal case with appendicular and pulmonary involvement. *Transactions of the Royal Society of Tropical Medicine and Hygiene*, **78,** 833–4.

Ladas, S.D., Savva, S., Frydas, A., Kaloviduris, A., Hatzioannou, J., and Raptis, S. (1989). Invasive balantidiasis presented as chronic colitis and lung involvement. *Digestive Diseases and Sciences*, **34,** 1621–3.

Lee, R.V., Prowten, A.W., Anthone, S., Satchidanand, S.K., Fisher, J.E., and Anthone, R. (1990). Typhlitis due to *Balantidium coli* in captive lowland gorillas. *Reviews of Infectious Diseases*, **12,** 1052–9.

Walzer, P.D., Judson, F.N., Murphy, K.B., Healy, G.R., English, D.K., and Schultz, M.G. (1973). Balantidiasis outbreak in Truk. *American Journal of Tropical Medicine and Hygiene*, **22,** 33–41.

Isosporiasis

CAUSATIVE ORGANISM

Isospora belli, the cause of isosporiasis, is a coccidian parasite of the human small intestine. Other coccidian protozoa that infect man include

Sarcocystis spp., *Cryptosporidium parvum*, and *Toxoplasma gondii*. Coccidia of the genus Isospora infect many species of vertebrate, and are relatively or absolutely host-specific. There is no evidence that, under natural conditions, *I. belli* infects any vertebrate species other than man. Experimental transmission of *I. belli* to gibbons was, however, reported in 1967.

The lifecycle of *I. belli* has not been completely delineated. Oocysts of this organism are ellipsoidal structures that are excreted in the stools of infected individuals (Figs. 4 and 5). This stage of the parasite initially contains a single mass of chromatin (sporoblast), which divides once. Still surrounded by the oocyst wall, each daughter sporoblast then matures into a sporocyst, which contains four banana-shaped sporozoites. Studies with *Isospora* spp. that infect non-human hosts strongly suggest that new hosts become infected by ingesting mature oocysts. *In vitro* experiments have shown that sodium taurocholate induces sporozoites to emerge from sporocysts of *Isospora* spp. (the experimental conditions for this work mimic the environment in the small intestinal lumen of potential hosts). It is believed that, *in vivo*, Isospora sporozoites penetrate epithelial cells of the host small intestine. Subsequent development comprises an asexual pathway (production of merozoites, which infect additional epithelial cells) as well as a sexual pathway, which leads to production of oocysts (Fig. 6).

EPIDEMIOLOGY

The specific name *Isospora belli* reflects the fact that infection with this organism was seen in military personnel during the First World War. At that time, and subsequently, *I. belli* oocysts were noted in faecal specimens from individuals with diarrhoea. Many of these individuals, however, were simultaneously infected with enteric organisms that are known to be pathogenic (including *Giardia lamblia, Entamoeba histolytica*, and *Shigella* spp.), and it was difficult to show unambiguously that *I. belli* infection causes symptoms. Various developmental stages of *I. belli* have been seen by light-microscopic examination of jejunal biopsies from persons infected with this organism (Fig. 7). It is likely that transmission of *I. belli* infection occurs via ingestion of oocysts, although the possible vehicles for such transmission (for example, food or water contaminated by oocysts) have not been identified.

I. belli oocysts have been found in faecal specimens from patients with AIDS who had persistent diarrhoea. Whether HIV infection actually increases the susceptibility of human subjects to *I. belli* infection is not, however, known. The existing literature contains case reports of individuals with various types of leukaemia or lymphoma who also had *I. belli* infection, possibly as a result of immunosuppression attributable to the haematological malignancy. The types of leukaemia and lymphoma seen in such individuals have included adult T-cell leukaemia (caused by human T-cell leukaemia virus type 1), acute lymphoblastic leukaemia, and Hodgkin's disease.

Fig. 4 Light micrograph of *Isospora belli* oocysts, each containing one sporoblast. × 1650. Illustration by courtesy of Dr. William L. Current. From Garcia, L.S. and Bruckner, D.A. (1993). *Diagnostic medical parasitology* (2nd edn). American Society for Microbiology, Washington DC, and used by permission.

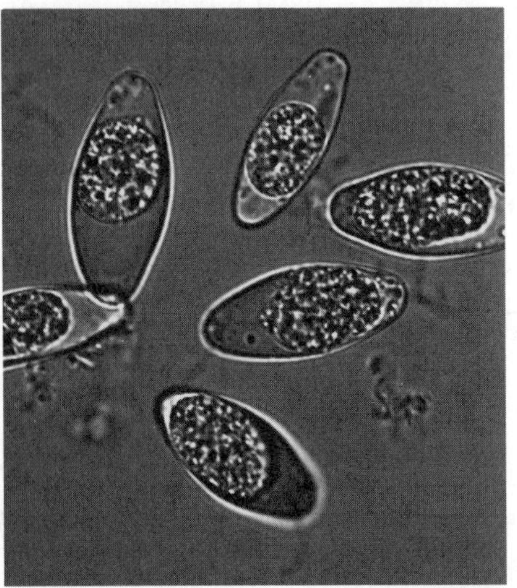

Fig. 5 Light micrograph of an *Isospora belli* oocyst containing two sporoblasts. × 2500. Illustration by courtesy of Dr. William L. Current. From Garcia, L.S. and Bruckner D.A. (1993). *Diagnostic medical parasitology* (2nd edn). American Society for Microbiology, Washington DC, and used by permission.

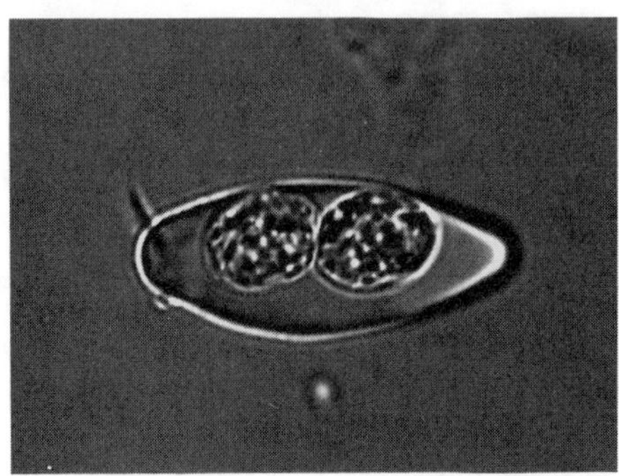

Fig. 6 Lifecycle of Isospora, based partly on studies of *Isospora* spp. that parasitize non-human hosts. Illustration by Gwen Gloege, by courtesy of Lynne S. Garcia. From Garcia, L.S. and Bruckner, D.A. (1993). *Diagnostic medical parasitology* (2nd edn). American Society for Microbiology, Washington DC, and used by permission.

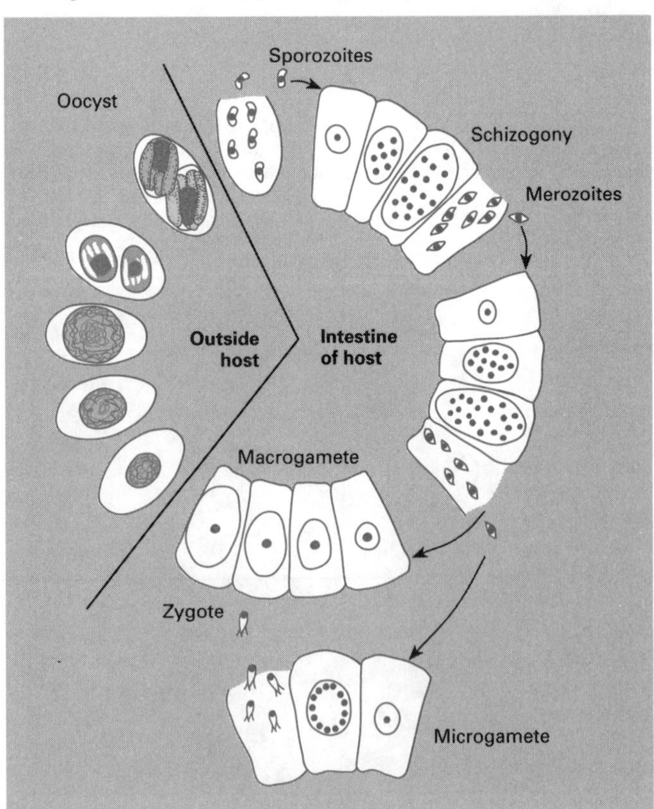

CLINICAL FEATURES

Watery diarrhoea, abdominal cramps, and fat malabsorption have been reported in persons with *I. belli* infection. In at least some of the reported cases it is likely that *I. belli* was responsible for the diarrhoea and malabsorption that were documented. Two pieces of evidence support this contention. First, in some individuals with diarrhoea, *I. belli* was the only potentially or actually pathogenic organism seen in faecal specimens or in jejunal biopsies. Secondly, treatment of some *I. belli*-infected patients with trimethoprim-sulphamethoxazole or pyrimethamine was rapidly followed by resolution of gastrointestinal symptoms and cessation of oocyst excretion.

Clinical case reports suggest that HIV infection increases the chronicity of diarrhoea that results from *I. belli* infection. Although the pathogenesis of diarrhoea in anyone with HIV infection can be multifactorial, chronic watery diarrhoea in HIV-infected individuals has been convincingly ascribed to *I. belli* infection. Several of the *I. belli*-infected patients who responded to trimethoprim-sulphamethoxazole or pyrimethamine treatment were HIV infected. Diarrhoea attributable to *I. belli* infection in HIV-infected people can lead to life-threatening dehydration.

DIAGNOSIS

Isosporiasis can be diagnosed by microscopic examination of faecal specimens for *I. belli* oocysts. These structures are translucent, and may be difficult to see in unstained specimens. Their visibility is increased by incubation with carbol-fuchsin, which stains sporoblasts and sporocysts red.

TREATMENT

I. belli infection is rare (or, at least, rarely diagnosed), and most of the documentation of its treatment consists of anecdotal case reports. In 1986, diarrhoea attributed to *I. belli* infection was reported in 15 HIV-infected individuals in Haiti. These patients were treated with trimethoprim-sulphamethoxazole and, in each case, diarrhoea stopped within 2 days of the start of this treatment. Diarrhoea recurred in several of the patients after trimethoprim-sulphamethoxazole treatment had been stopped. The suggestion that pyrimethamine may be effective in treating *I. belli* infection is based on anecdotal case reports.

Fig. 7 Light micrograph of jejunal biopsy from a patient with isosporiasis. *Isospora belli* merozoites are present (arrow). × 1100. Illustration by courtesy of Dr. Robert L. Owen; modified from Garcia, L.S., Owen, R.L., and Current, W.L. (1988). Isosporiasis. In *Laboratory diagnosis of Infectious diseases, principles and practice*, Vol. 1, *Bacterial, mycotic, and parasitic diseases* (ed. A. Balows, W.J. Hausler, M. Ohashi, and A. Turano), pp. 897–903. Springer-Verlag, New York, and used by permission.

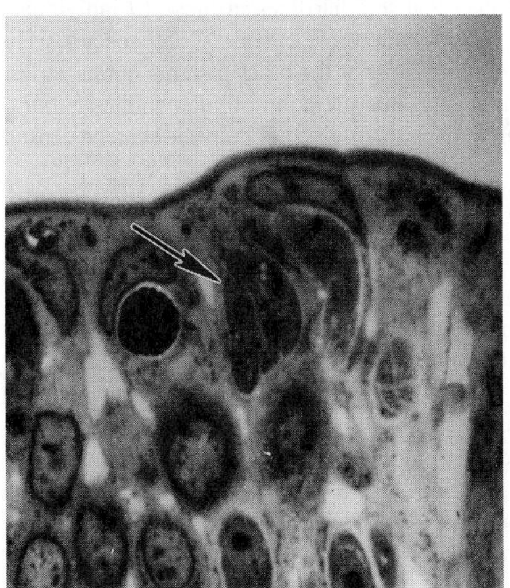

REFERENCES

DeHovitz, J.A., Pape, J.W., Boncy, M., and Johnson, W.D. (1986). Clinical manifestations and therapy of *Isospora belli* infection in patients with the acquired immunodeficiency syndrome. *New England Journal of Medicine*, **315,** 87–90.

Garcia, L.S., Owen, R.L., and Current, W.L. (1988). Isosporiasis. In *Laboratory diagnosis of Infectious diseases, principles and practice*, Vol. 1, *Bacterial, mycotic, and parasitic diseases*, (ed. A. Balows, W.J. Hausler, M. Ohashi, and A. Turano), pp. 897–903. Springer-Verlag, New York.

Greenberg, S.J., Davey, M.P., Zierdt, W.S., and Waldmann, T.A. (1988). *Isospora belli* enteric infection in patients with human T-cell leukemia virus type I-associated adult T-cell leukemia. *American Journal of Medicine*, **85,** 435–8.

Lindsay, D.S. (1990). *Isospora*: infections of intestine: biology. In *Coccidiosis of man and domestic animals*, (ed. P.L. Long), pp. 77–89. CRC Press, Boca Raton FL.

Pape, J.W., Verdier. R-I., and Johnson, W.D. (1989). Treatment and prophylaxis of *Isospora belli* infection in patients with the acquired immunodeficiency syndrome. *New England Journal of Medicine*, **320,** 1044–7.

Weiss, L.M., Perlman, D.C., Sherman, J., Tanowitz, H., and Wittner, M. (1988). *Isospora belli* infection: treatment with pyrimethamine. *Annals of Internal Medicine*, **109,** 474–5.

Whiteside, M.E., Barkin, J.S., May, R.G., Weiss, S.D., Fischl, M.A., and MacLeod, C.L. (1984). Enteric coccidiosis among patients with the acquired immunodeficiency syndrome. *American Journal of Tropical Medicine and Hygiene*, **33,** 1065–72.

Microsporidiosis

CAUSATIVE ORGANISMS

Microsporidia are protozoa with features that are sufficiently distinctive for the organisms to be classified as a separate phylum (Microspora). Several hundred species of microsporidia have been described. Microsporidia are obligate intracellular parasites of hosts that include other protozoa, insects, crustaeceans, fish, amphibians, reptiles, birds, and mammals. Economically important diseases of honey-bees and silkworms are caused by microsporidia of the genus Nosema. Microsporidia are eukaryotic organisms (as defined by the possession of a discrete nucleus surrounded by a nuclear membrane), but have primitive features that they share with bacteria. These features include the absence of mitochondria, and the presence of ribosomes that have a sedimentation coefficient identical to that of bacterial ribosomes (70S). Furthermore, microsporidian ribosomal RNA has little sequence homology with ribosomal RNA of other eukaryotes. Because of these structural and genetic features, it has been suggested that microsporidia are evolutionarily ancient organisms.

The lifecycle of microsporidia comprises an extracellular stage (spore) and various stages that occur in the cytoplasm of host cells. Spores (Fig. 8) are shed into the environment by infected hosts, and infect other members of the host species. It is not known how spores of microsporidia enter human hosts, but plausible routes include ingestion in food or water, and inhalation of spores. *In vitro* studies have shown that spores infect host cells by extruding a hollow tube, which remains attached to one pole of the spore and forms a channel from the interior of the spore to the tip of the tube. Extrusion of this polar tube occurs with explosive speed; the tip of the tube penetrates a host cell, and sporoplasm (spore contents) passes along the lumen of the tube into this cell. Replication of the parasite and subsequent development of spores occur in host cells. It is unclear how microsporidia spread within infected vertebrate hosts. However, some species of microsporidia infect macrophages, and migration of infected macrophages within the host is one conceivable mechanism by which microsporidia reach organs that are distant from the site of initial infection.

Microsporidia that infect man are listed in Table 3 and indicated diagrammatically in Fig. 9. When it has been sought, *Enterocytozoon bieneusi* has been found in approximately one-third of patients with diarrhoea, weight loss, and human immunodeficiency virus (HIV) infection. Each of the other species of microsporidia listed in Table 3 has so far been documented in fewer than 5 to 10 patients. Several of these species have been reported from only one patient each. In the case of such rarely diagnosed infections, it seems reasonable to question the taxonomic validity of some of the 'species' listed in Table 3. Indeed, the species designated *Microsporidium ceylonensis* and *Microsporidium africanum* were placed in a genus (Microsporidium) created for microsporidia of unclear identity. Within the genus Encephalitozoon, however, there is evidence that *E. cuniculi* and *E. hellem* are distinct species. These organisms differ biochemically and antigenically, as judged by gel electrophoresis of their proteins, and by immunoblotting of these proteins with anti-Encephalitozoon antisera.

Besides the species of microsporidia listed in Table 3, at least one unnamed, apparently distinct, microsporidian species has been seen in intestinal epithelial cells and macrophages of patients infected with HIV.

Table 3 *Species of microsporidia that infect man*

Species	Site of infection
**Enterocytozoon bieneusi*	Small intestinal epithelium (enterocytes), bile duct epithelium
**Encephalitozoon cuniculi*	Corneal epithelium, conjunctiva, nasal mucosa, peritoneum, liver, urinary tract
**Encephalitozoon hellem*	Corneal epithelium, conjunctiva, respiratory tract, urinary tract
Encephalitozoon species	Organisms isolated from urine and cerebrospinal fluid
Nosema connori	Generalized
Nosema corneum	Corneal stroma
Nosema ocularum	Corneal stroma
Pleistophora species	Muscle
'*Microsporidium ceylonensis*'	Corneal stroma
'*Microsporidium africanum*'	Corneal stroma
**Septata intestinalis*	Duodenal epithelium, kidney

*Described in patients with HIV infection

EPIDEMIOLOGY

To date, the only patients known to be infected with *Enterocytozoon bieneusi* were also infected with HIV. As noted in Table 3, additional species of microsporidia have been shown to infect HIV-positive individuals. These clinical observations suggest that HIV infection predisposes to infection with *Enterocytozoon bieneusi*, and with other species of microsporidia listed in Table 3. However, the prevalence of microsporidian infections in persons who are not infected with HIV is unknown. One plausible possibility is that HIV infection impairs protective immunity against microsporidia, with the result that these organisms cannot be cleared from the host. This possibility is supported by studies with mice. *Encephalitozoon cuniculi* infection is lethal in athymic nude mice (which lack functional T lymphocytes), but not in immunocompetent mice. Furthermore, nude mice can be protected against lethal *E. cuniculi* infection by injection with lymphocytes from immunocompetent mice that have been infected with the parasite.

The only known case of *Nosema connori* infection (Table 3) occurred in a human infant with a hypoplastic thymus.

Antibodies against microsporidia have been detected in human sera by various methods, including enzyme-linked immunosorbent assay (ELISA) procedures and immunoblotting on microsporidian proteins separated by gel electrophoresis. Since the early 1980s, there have been several epidemiological surveys of human sera, to determine the prevalence of antimicrosporidian antibodies in various populations. In one such study, antibodies against *Encephalitozoon* species were detected in sera from 14 of 115 Swedes who had visited tropical areas. In the same study, anti-Encephalitozoon antibodies were found in 38 of 100 sera from patients with malaria. These observations raise the intriguing, though untested, possibility that arthropod vectors transmit some species of microsporidia to human hosts. In a paper published in 1991, anti-Encephalitozoon antibodies were reported in 1.2 to 13 per cent of sera from various diseased human populations (including patients with malaria, schistosomiasis, and unspecified renal diseases), but in only 0.2 per cent of 1003 sera from allegedly healthy blood donors.

Because *Enterocytozoon bieneusi* infects intestinal epithelial cells (Table 3), it seems reasonable to assume that these cells are infected by *E. bieneusi* spores that are ingested by the host. Direct evidence that mammals can be infected with microsporidia by ingestion of spores comes from studies with rabbits and mice. These animals can be infected with *Encephalitozoon hellem* and HIV. This patient's tracheal and bronchial epithelial cells were heavily infected with *E. hellem.*

Fig. 8 Diagram of a microsporidian spore, showing internal structure. Illustration by courtesy of Professor Elizabeth U. Canning. Modified from Canning, E.U. and Hollister, W.S. (1992). Human infections with microsporidia. *Reviews in Medical Microbiology*, **3**, 35–42, and used by permission.

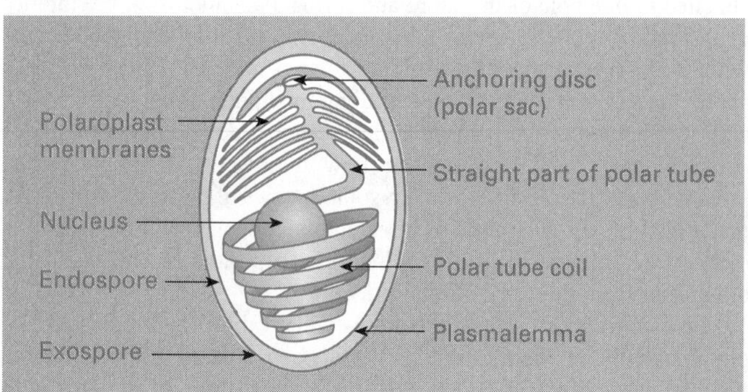

CLINICAL FEATURES

From 1985 onwards, *Enterocytozoon bieneusi* has been reported in small intestinal biopsy specimens from patients with HIV infection, persistent watery diarrhoea, and weight loss. It is not clear whether *E. bieneusi* was the cause of diarrhoea in these patients; several of them were simultaneously infected with other intestinal parasites, including *Cryptosporidium parvum* and *Giardia lamblia.* In one study, *E. bieneusi* was the only micro-organism seen on electron microscopy of intestinal biopsies from 19 of 67 HIV-infected patients who had diarrhoea. This finding does not, however, establish that the diarrhoea in these 19 individuals was caused by *E. bieneusi.* No micro-organisms of any species were seen in intestinal biopsies from most of the other patients in this series, all of whom had diarrhoea. The interpretation of such studies is complicated by the unanswered question of whether diarrhoea can be caused by HIV *per se.*

Enterocytozoon bieneusi infection of the biliary tract has occasionally been described in HIV-infected patients, at least one of whom had sclerosing cholangitis. Case-reports of other microsporidian infections in HIV-infected patients include rare descriptions of hepatitis, peritoneal infection, paranasal sinusitis, conjunctivitis, and superficial corneal inflammation, attributed to organisms of the genus Encephalitozoon. Muscle biopsies from a patient who had muscle weakness and contractures showed inflammation, fibrosis, and spores of a microsporidian regarded as belonging to the genus Pleistophora (Table 3). This patient was immunodeficient, but lacked detectable circulating antibodies against HIV, and was presumed not to be infected with this retrovirus. The prognosis in patients with microsporidiosis and HIV infection is determined by the stage of HIV infection.

Infection of the corneal stroma by microsporidia classified as *Nosema* species has been described occasionally. The affected patients were immunocompetent and had reduced visual acuity, with or without corneal ulceration. Encephalitozoon infections have been described in two children with epileptic seizures. Spores of *Encephalitozoon* species were present in urine from both of these children, and in cerebrospinal fluid from one of them.

DIAGNOSIS

Human microsporidian infections have been documented by histological examination (including electron microscopy) of tissue specimens. For example, *Enterocytozoon bieneusi* infection has been diagnosed by electron microscopy or light microscopy of fixed, sectioned intestinal biopsies that were obtained at endoscopy. This parasite occupies the supra-

Fig. 9 Lifecycles of microsporidian genera that infect man. The elliptical structure at the top of the diagram represents an empty spore, from which sporoplasm has been discharged through an extruded polar tube. Illustration by courtesy of Professor Elizabeth U. Canning. Modified from Canning, E.U. and Hollister, W.S. (1992). Human infections with microsporidia. *Reviews in Medical Microbiology*, **3**, 35–42, and used by permission.

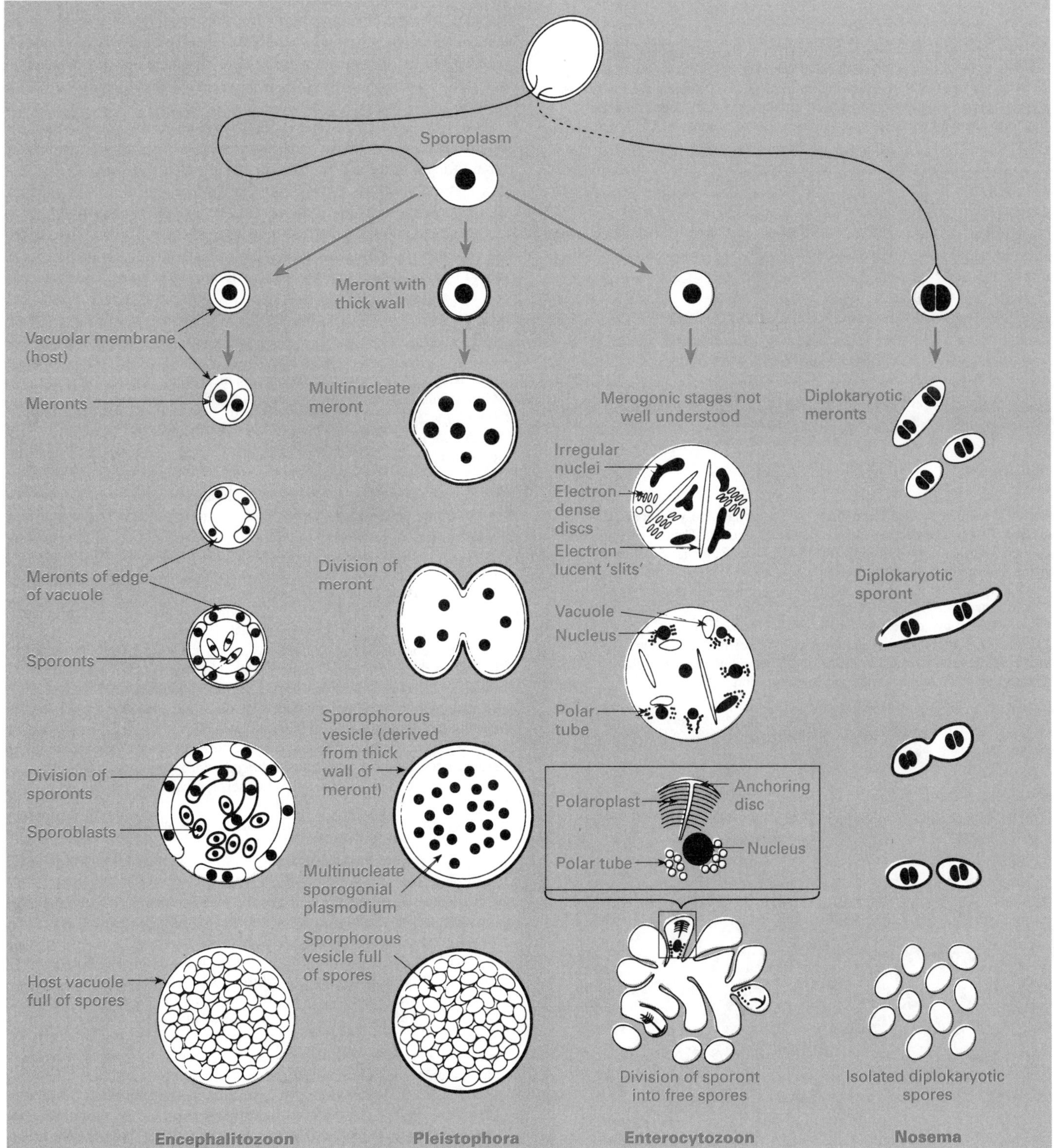

nuclear cytoplasm of enterocytes (Figs. 10 and 11). *E bieneusi* infection has also been diagnosed by light microscopic examination of Giemsa-stained smears prepared from unfixed intestinal biopsies. Another diagnostic approach involves light microscopic examination of faecal filtrates or duodenal aspirates for *E. bieneusi* spores. Cytospin centrifugation of such specimens on to microscope slides, followed by Giemsa staining, enables the spores to be recognized. Spores of *E. bieneusi* are ovoid, with dimensions of approximately 1.5 μm in length and 0.9 μm in width. As noted above, there have been rare instances in which Encephalitozoon spores were seen in human urine and cerebrospinal fluid.

Fig. 10 Light micrograph of jejunal biopsy from an HIV-infected patient with *Enterocytozoon bieneusi* infection (toluidine blue stain). Spores of *E. bieneusi* are indicated by arrows; these spores are present in the supranuclear cytoplasm of an enterocyte (right-hand arrow), and in the intestinal lumen and a space where the epithelium has sloughed. Illustration by courtesy of Dr Robert L. Owen.

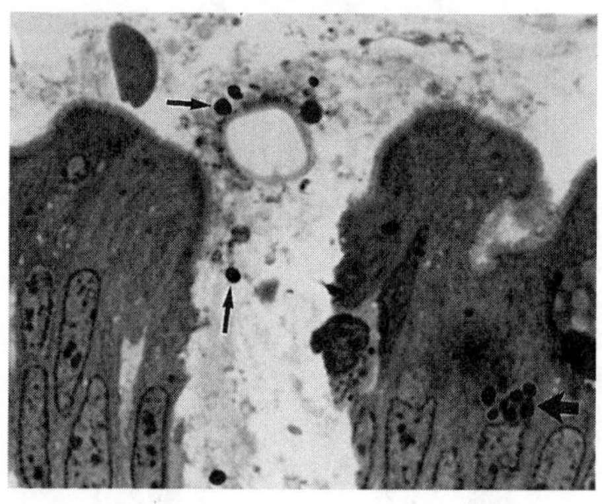

Fig. 11 Transmission electron micrograph of jejunal biopsy from an HIV-infected patient with *Enterocytozoon bieneusi* infection. The microvillus border (epithelial surface) is at the top of the photograph. *E.. bieneusi* stages in enterocytes are as follows: proliferative plasmodia (1), early sporogonial plasmodia (2), late sporogonial plasmodia (3), and spores (4). A spore in a necrotic enterocyte is indicated by the arrow. Bar (lower left quadrant) = 1 μm. Illustration by courtesy of Dr Robert L. Owen. From Cali, A. and Owen, R.L. (1990). Intracellular development of *Enterocytozoon*, a unique microsporidian found in the intestine of AIDS patients. *Journal of Protozoology*, **37**, 145–55, and used by permission.

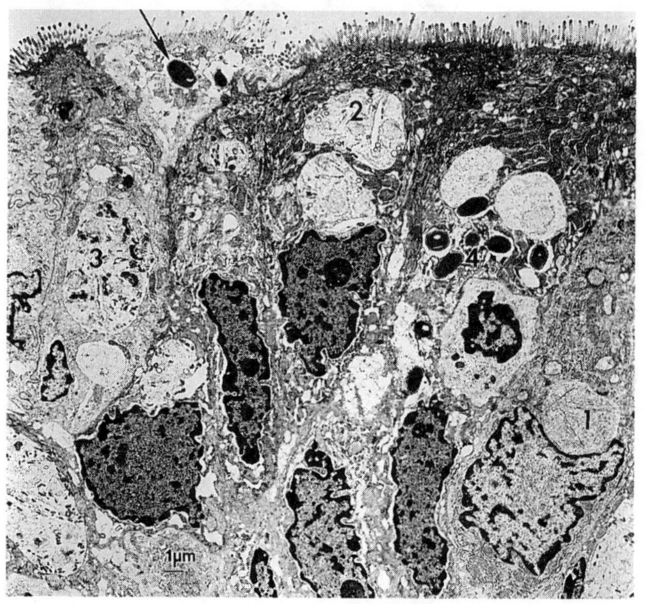

Human Encephalitozoon infections have been confirmed by transmission of infection from human specimens to mammalian cell lines grown *in vitro*.

TREATMENT

No drug treatment has been shown to eliminate human microsporidian infections. Patients with *E. bieneusi*-associated diarrhoea have been treated with metronidazole, albendazole, or octreotide. A few such patients were symptomatically improved (as judged by reduced stool frequency) after treatment with one or other of these drugs. However, it is unclear whether this improvement was the result of the drug treatment. Controlled therapeutic trials of the drugs mentioned above have not yet been carried out in patients with *E. bieneusi*-associated diarrhoea. *Septata intestinalis* seems more responsive to albendazole than does *E. bieneusi*.

Two HIV-infected patients with Encephalitozoon infection of the superficial cornea were respectively treated with systemic itraconazole (an antifungal drug) and propamidine isethionate eye-drops. Treatment was reportedly followed by symptomatic improvement in both patients. Microsporidian infection of the corneal stroma has been treated by corneal transplantation in at least two patients, with results that have ranged from failure (opacification of the transplant) to apparent success, as judged by transparency of the graft 6 months after transplantation.

REFERENCES

Bryan, R.T., Cali, A., Owen, R.L., and Spencer, H.C. (1991). Microsporidia: Opportunistic pathogens in patients with AIDS. *Progress in Clinical Parasitology*, **2,** 1–26.

Cali, A., Meisler, D.M., Lowder, C.Y., *et al.* (1991). Corneal microsporidioses: characterization and identification. *Journal of Protozoology*, **38,** 215S–217S.

Cali, A. and Owen, R.L. (1990). Intracellular development of *Enterocytozoon*, a unique microsporidian found in the intestine of AIDS patients. *Journal of Protozoology*, **37,** 145–55.

Canning, E.U. and Hollister, W.S. (1990). *Enterocytozoon bieneusi* (Microspora): prevalence and pathogenicity in AIDS patients. *Transactions of the Royal Society of Tropical Medicine and Hygiene*, **84,** 181–6.

Canning, E.U. and Lom, J. (1986). *The Microsporidia of Vertebrates*. Academic Press, London. A comprehensive survey of microsporidia that infect vertebrates. Human infections are covered for the period up to and including the initial years of the AIDS epidemic.

Didier, P.J., Didier, E.S., Orenstein, J.M., and Shadduck, J.A. (1991). Fine structure of a new human microsporidian, *Encephalitozoon hellem*, in culture. *Journal of Protozoology*, **38,** 502–7.

Hollister, W.S., Canning, E.U., and Willcox, A. (1991). Evidence for widespread occurrence of antibodies to *Encephalitozoon cuniculi* (Microspora) in man provided by ELISA and other serological tests. *Parasitology*, **102,** 33–43.

Kelly, P. *et al.* (1994). *Septata intestinalis*: a new microsporidian in Africa. *Lancet*, **344,** 271–2.

Orenstein, J.M. (1991). Microsporiiosis in the acquired immunodeficiency syndrome. *Journal of Parasitology*, **77,** 843–64.

Pol, S., Romana, C., Richard, S., *et al.* (1992). *Enterocytozoon bieneusi* infection in acquired immunodeficiency syndrome-related sclerosing cholangitis. *Gastroenterology*, **102,** 1778–81.

Schwartz, D.A., Bryan, R.T., Hewan-Lowe, K.O., *et al.* (1992). Disseminated microsporidiosis (*Encephalitozoon hellem*) and acquired immunodeficiency syndrome: autopsy evidence for respiratory acquisition. *Archives of Pathology and Laboratory Medicine*, **116,** 660–8.

Vossbrinck, C.R., Maddox, J.V., Friedman, S., Debrunner-Vossbrinck, B.A., and Woese, C.R. (1987). Ribosomal RNA sequence suggests microsporidia are extremely ancient eukaryotes. *Nature*, **326,** 411–14.

Weber, R., Bryan, R.T., Owen, R.L., Wilcox, C.M., Gorelkin, L., and Visvesvara, G.S. (1992). Improved light-microscopical detection of microsporidia spores in stoool and duodenal aspirates. *New England Journal of Medicine*, **326,** 161–6.

7.13.9 *Blastocystis hominis*

V. Zaman

This is now regarded as a member of the subkingdom Protozoa, but its srRNA is not closely related to any known protozoan genus. It does not belong to the family Sporozoa or Sarcodina, as was previously thought.

Fig. 1 *B. hominis* from culture showing binary fission; the cytoplasm is lying at the periphery. v, vacuole. Phase contrast, × 400.

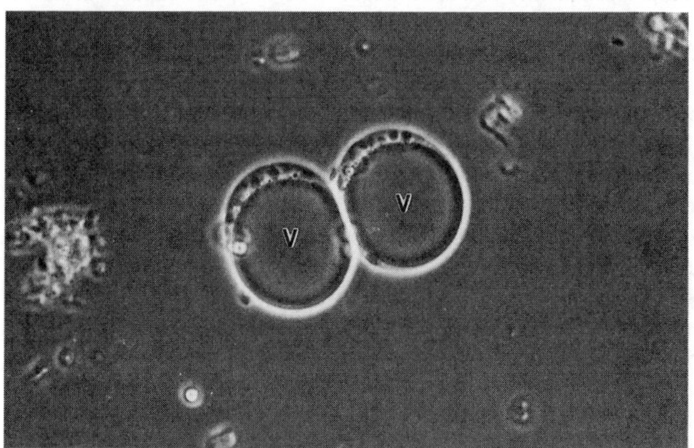

Fig. 2 *B. hominis* from culture showing the great variation in size. v, vacuole. Dark field, × 400.

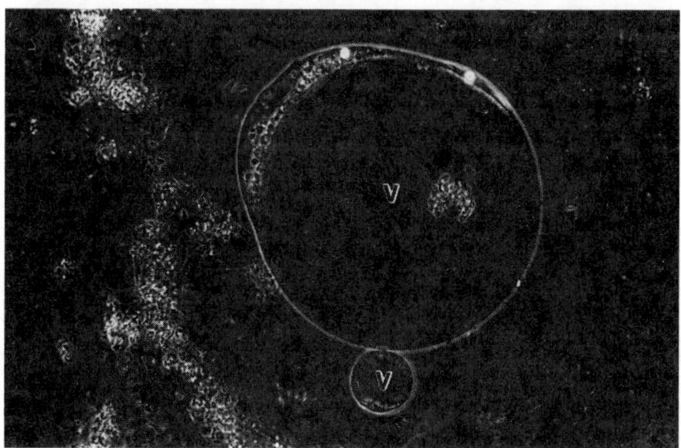

Fig. 3 *B. hominis*. Electron micrograph showing the peripheral cytoplasm (c) and the central vacuole (v); the inclusions in the cytoplasm are mitochondria. × 5000.

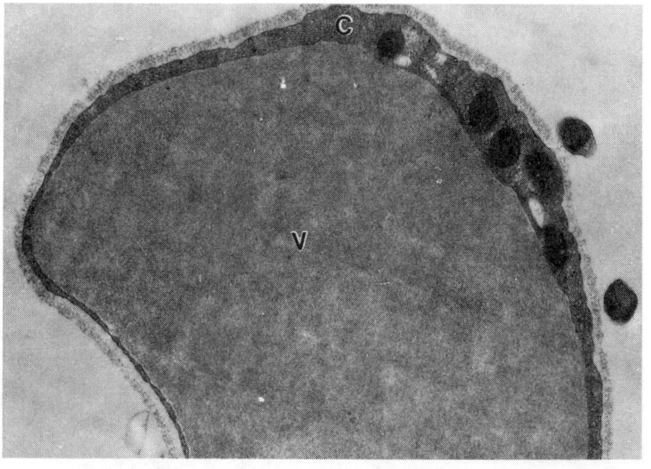

Its life-cycle also remains mostly unknown and a cyst-like stage has only recently been observed, indicating that transmission probably occurs by the faecal–oral route.

Morphologically similar organisms have been isolated from a wide range of animals including rodents, birds, primates, reptiles, and insects. It is not known whether man gets infected from animals or whether human Blastocystis is a distinct species. A recent study has shown that human strains can be divided into two separate groups based on protein and DNA analyses. It is possible that, like *Entamoeba histolytica*, there may be pathogenic and non-pathogenic strains, which may explain why some individuals get symptoms and many others do not. Host factors may also be important but the parasite does not seem to give rise to any special problem in AIDS. The only report in which the parasite was shown to 'invade' intestinal tissues is not convincing.

Morphology (figs. 1, 2, 3)

They are generally spherical in shape but their size and internal contents are very variable. The size ranges from 5 to 40 μm with occasional giant cells reaching 200 μm. In cultures they can be divided into three groups: (i) vacuolated, (ii) granular, and (iii) amoeboid.

The vacuolated form predominates in faecal specimens and is characterized by a large central 'vacuole' with the cytoplasm lying at the periphery of the cell. Nuclei and mitochondria are found in this peripheral part. The central 'vacuole' does not stain for lipid, starch, cellulose, or glycogen and its function is unknown. Division of the vacuolated form is by binary fission. It is claimed that in the granular form division occurs by endodyogeny and endosporulation.

Clinical aspects

According to one school of thought this parasite is a pathogen and can cause various gastrointestinal problems including diarrhoea, anorexia, flatus, and abdominal discomfort. Symptoms usually last about 3 to 10 days, but may persist for months. Eosinophilia occurs in some cases. There appears to be a favourable response to metronidazole therapy.

Diagnosis

This is based mainly on stool examination. It has been claimed that patients having problems attributable to Blastocystis pass a large number of parasites (mostly vacuolated forms) in their stools. Because of their spherical shape they could be easily mistaken for Entamoeba cysts and vice versa. The best method of microscopic examination is phase contrast, which shows the contents of the parasite and the peripheral cytoplasm clearly. Blastocystis grows easily in media used for culturing *E. histolytica* and this is a much more sensitive method than microscopy.

Treatment

As its pathogenicity is in doubt, no clear guidelines exist. *In vitro* studies have shown that the parasites are killed by emetine, metronidazole, furazolidone, trimethoprim-sulphamethoxazole, di-iodohydroxyquin, and pentamidine. The most widely accepted drug is metronidazole, which is given in a dose of 750 mg, three times daily for 5 days (for children 35–50 mg/kg in three divided doses for 5 days).

REFERENCES

Boreham, P.F.L., Upcroft, J.A., and Dunn, L.A. (1992). Protein and DNA evidence for two demes of *Blastocystis hominis* from humans. *International Journal of Parasitology*, **22**,: 49–53.

Editorial (1991). *Blastocystis hominis*: commensal or pathogen. *Lancet*, **337**, 521.

Miller, R.A. and Minshew, B.H. (1988). *Blastocystis hominis*: an organism in search of a disease. *Reviews of Infectious Diseases*, **10**, 930–8.

Stenzel, D.J. and Boreham, P.F.L. (1991). A cyst-like stage of *Blastocystis hominis*. *International Journal of Parasitology*, **21**, 613–15.

7.13.10 Human African trypanosomiasis

D. H. SMITH

Human African trypanosomiasis (sleeping sickness) is caused by subspecies of the protozoan haemoflagellate *Trypanosoma brucei* (subgenus Trypanozoon) and transmitted by tsetse flies (*Glossina*). *T. brucei* is widely distributed in wild and domestic animals, and man, in Africa between 15°N and 20°S in 36 countries extending from the subSaharan region in the north to the deserts of Botswana and Namibia in the south. Human disease exists in more than 200 foci and occurs in two main forms known as *T.brucei gambiense* and *T.b.rhodesiense*. *T.b.gambiense* usually produces a chronic infection occurring focally through areas of West and Central Africa and *T.b.rhodesiense* causes more acute, severe disease occurring in East and southern Africa (Fig. 1).

Human trypanosomiasis has caused massive epidemics in the past. At the turn of the century, in Zaire and around Lake Victoria, large epidemics caused at least three-quarters of a million deaths. Although only approximately 20 000 cases are reported each year to the World Health Organization, gross under-reporting, reduced surveillance, and recent epidemics in Zaire, Uganda, Tanzania, Mozambique, and Sudan underline the continuing importance of human trypanosomiasis in public health. Trypanosomiasis of domestic animals and man remains an important deterrent to development in endemic areas and shows increased prevalence associated with war, civil disturbance, and refugee groups as well as deteriorating health services and disease-specific control programmes.

Aetiology

In the vertebrate host, trypanosomes range from 25 × 2.5 μm (long slender forms) to 19 × 3.5 μm (short stumpy forms) (Fig. 2). The undulating membrane is prominent and continues as a free flagellum. In addition to a centrally placed nucleus, trypanosomes also possess a kinetoplast, composed of DNA and sited at the base of the undulating membrane.

Fig. 1 The geographical distribution of African trypanosomiasis.

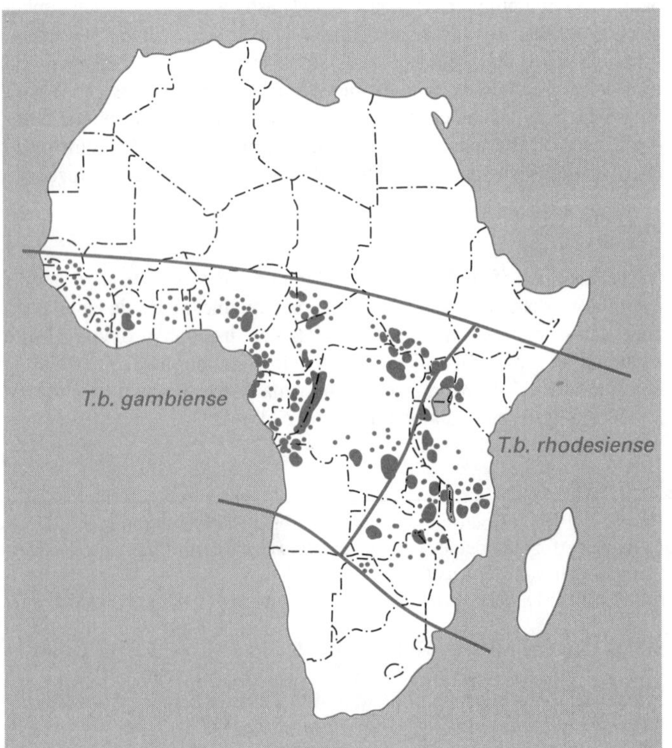

Trypanosomes are taken up during tsetse feeding into the fly's midgut, where they develop into procyclic forms and multiply. They lack the surface glycoprotein coat and are non-infective to vertebrates. After 2 weeks the parasites migrate to the salivary glands and develop into epimastigotes and then non-dividing metacyclic forms, which are infective to mammalian hosts. In the human host there is rapid development into long, slender, rapidly dividing forms coated by variant surface glycoprotein, which, by extensive and regular antigenic variation, allows trypanosomes to evade host immune responses. Short stumpy forms develop subsequently and are thought to be the stage capable of developing in tsetse.

There are no morphological differences between *T.b.gambiense*, *T.b.rhodesiense*, and human non-infective *T.b.brucei*. Biochemical techniques, especially isoenzyme electrophoresis, have shown the diversity of *T.brucei* populations (zymodemes) and identified more clearly the role of animal reservoirs of human infection. *T.b.rhodesiense* comprises at least two distinct groups, 'busoga' and 'zambezi', both with extensive animal reservoirs but with distinct geographical ranges and clinical effects. 'Zambezi' group parasites occur predominantly in the southern range of *T.b.rhodesiense*, and cause less severe infections and possibly asymptomatic infections; the 'Busoga' group is prevalent in foci in East Africa and associated with more acute, severe disease presenting more often with chancres. Other *T.brucei* groups occurring in animals appear to be non-infective to man; these zymodemes are not found in human infection and trypanosomes are inactivated by incubation with human serum (the blood incubation inoculation test) due to parasite lysis by high-density lipoproteins. *T.b.gambiense* appears to be a distinct subspecies without an important animal reservoir. The 'Bouaflé' group, also occurring in West and Central Africa and found in wild and domestic animal hosts, also causes human infection.

Transmission and epidemiology

Sleeping sickness is usually transmitted biologically from infected tsetse flies (Fig. 3) although mechanical transmission via Glossina or other biting flies may occur, as well as transmission from blood transfusion. Congenital transmission occurs in *T.b.gambiense* and the clinical importance of this may have been underestimated. *Glossina* spp. are long lived and require shade and humidity for resting and larviposition. Females produce a single larva, which rapidly pupates in moist, shaded soil. Both sexes take blood meals every 3 or 4 days. Infection rates in tsetse flies are usually low.

Fig. 2 Trypanosomes in human blood film (stained with Field's stain). Polymorphic trypanosomes, with both short stumpy and long slender forms from a patient with *T.b.rhodesiense* infection (copyright D.H. Smith).

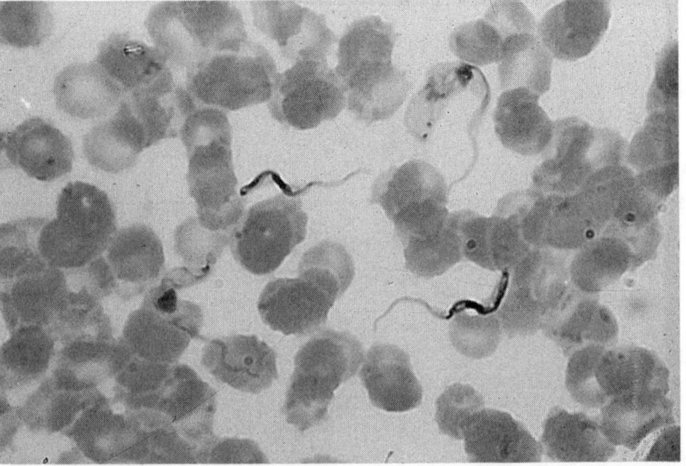

Human sleeping sickness is transmitted by two groups of *Glossina* spp. *T.b.gambiense* is transmitted by Glossina 'palpalis' group flies and *T.b.rhodesiense* by Glossina 'morsitans' group. 'Palpalis' group flies, *G.palpalis*, *G.tachinoides*, and *G.fuscipes*, inhabit forest, riverine or lacustrine situations and feed on man readily, leading to high man–fly contact notably at river margins during washing and water collection. 'Morsitans' group flies, *G.morsitans*, *G.pallidipes*, and *G.swynnertoni* are less dependent on shade and humidity and inhabit more open woodland savannah. Many have feeding preferences for larger animals and feed more readily on man when preferred hosts are unavailable. The important vectors and animal reservoirs of human trypanosomiasis are shown in Table 1.

T.B.GAMBIENSE

In most endemic areas, man is the only important reservoir of infection. In many endemic, riverine habitats, the disease is focal and prevalence rates in foci may rise to high levels. High and rising endemicity is favoured by the prolonged, relatively mild, haemolymphatic stage and the feeding preferences of the transmitting *Glossina* spp.; it is highest at focal points of intense man–fly contact. Transmission in forest habitats is usually lower.

T.B.RHODESIENSE

Throughout most of the range, infection is maintained in wild animal reservoirs, especially wild game animals such as bushbuck. Infection in domestic animals, including bovids and pigs, brings the parasite into closer contact with human populations, increasing the potential for outbreaks. Both wild and domestic reservoir hosts usually develop low-grade, sustained parasitaemia with few clinical manifestations, although dogs suffer severe, usually fatal, infection. Man is infected sporadically and particular occupational groups are predominantly at risk: hunters, poachers, game wardens, tourists, cattle herders and others, such as fishermen, who pass through tsetse-infested areas.

EPIDEMIC T.B.RHODESIENSE

More recently it has been recognized that epidemic *T.b.rhodesiense* occurs in settled areas, especially around Lake Victoria. Recent epidemics have occurred in Busoga, south-eastern Uganda, since 1976, with a peak monthly incidence in excess of 1000 cases. Under these circumstances, *T.b.rhodesiense* is transmitted by *G.f.fuscipes*, a 'palpalis' group fly that has extended its range from existing riverine and lacustrine to more peridomestic habitats as a result of diminished land use during a period of civil disturbance and subsequent invasion of agricultural land with *Lantana camara*, which provides dense thicket close to settled populations.

Fig. 3 Adult tsetse fly (*Glossina* spp.) probing on a crocodile (by courtesy of J. McNamara).

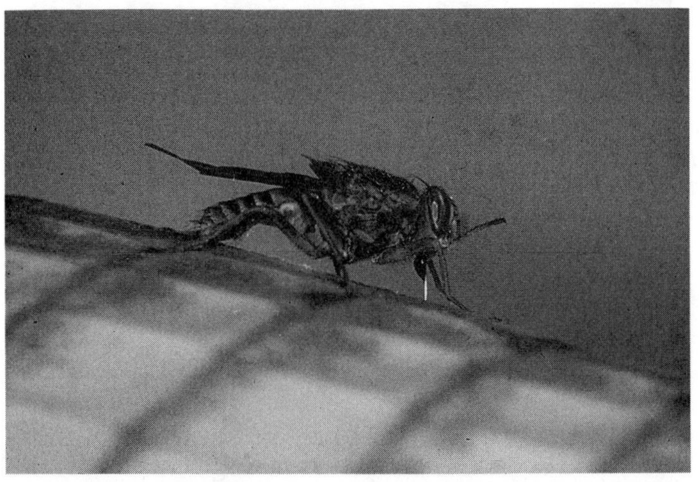

Under epidemic conditions in East Africa, reservoir hosts include domestic animals (cattle, pigs, and possibly dogs) as well as transmission from person to person, especially where infection rates are high and treatment delayed. The close proximity of tsetse fly populations to human communities has caused large outbreaks and epidemics affecting all age groups.

Pathogenesis

Trypanosomes divide rapidly at the site of inoculation and may induce the typical 'chancre', with marked tissue response characterized by a cellular reaction—vasculitis with perivascular mononuclear-cell infiltration, oedema, tissue damage, and local lymphadenopathy. Trypanosomes then circulate through the blood and lymphatic system. Frequent antigenic variation of the surface glycoproteins, with an antigen repertoire of some 1000 variants, leads to fluctuating waves of parasitaemia, the predominantly IgM antibody response, and the relapsing nature of the early haemolymphatic stage.

Parasites eventually invade the central nervous system from the choroid plexus, spreading throughout the cerebrospinal fluid and Virchow–Robin spaces, and producing perivascular infiltration and the characteristic meningoencephalitis (Fig. 4). The brain-stem is mainly involved, although cortical areas are also affected. The brain is oedematous and intracranial pressure elevated. The inflammatory response includes vasculitis, lymphocytic and plasma-cell infiltration, and characteristic foamy, IgM-laden plasma cells, the 'morular cells of Mott'. Neuronal destruction and focal demyelination occur late in the course of the meningoencephalitis. The neuropsychiatric manifestations of late-stage trypanosomiasis may in part be biochemically mediated through neurotransmitters and cytokines from activated astrocytes. Raised concentrations of prostaglandin D_2, associated both with febrile responses and sleep disturbances, have recently been demonstrated in late-stage *T.b.gambiense*. Pathological lesions also occur in the heart (pancarditis), kidneys, serous membranes, and the endocrine system.

The immunological response is characterized by polyclonal B-lymphocyte activation accompanied by immunosuppression, disturbance of cytokines and other mediators, immune-complex formation, and autoantibody production, all of which may contribute to the pathological processes. Antibody production is predominantly IgM. A haemolytic anaemia occurs in early human trypanosomiasis but is usually mild compared to that found in infections in animals. In endemic areas, other associated causes of anaemia are also common. Thrombocytopenia is a common finding. Myocardial, renal, and hepatic involvement, jaundice, and disseminated intravascular coagulation also occur in severe infections.

Clinical features

A trypanosomal chancre (Fig. 5) develops at the site of inoculation in *T.b.rhodesiense* but the frequency of this varies markedly. Trypanosomes multiply in the extracellular tissue fluid in the chancre and rapidly invade lymphatics and gain access to the blood. A patent parasitaemia arises within days of the development of the chancre—haemolymphatic stage (stage I). After a variable period, parasites invade the central nervous system and cerebrospinal fluid leading to a meningoencephalitis—meningoencephalitic stage (stage II).

There is considerable variation in the severity of disease and the progression to meningoencephalitis. In *T.b.gambiense* infections the early symptoms are mild and meningoencephalitis develops late and runs a protracted course over months or years. In *T.b.rhodesiense* the initial stage is acute and severe, with early progress to, and rapid progression of, meningoencephalitis leading to death within 3 to 6 months. However, in any geographical focus a wide range of disease is usually observed, partly explained by the heterogeneity of circulating strains of parasites in many foci of infection.

Table 1 *The epidemiological features of human African trypanosomiasis*

	Vector	Main reservoir and transmission	Animal reservoir	
			Wild	Domestic
T.b.gambiense	'Palpalis' group tsetse:	Man	Kob	Cattle
West and Central Africa	*G.palpalis*	High focal endemicity	Hartebeest	Pig
	G.tachinoides	Riverine: water collection and washing points		
		Forest		
T.b.rhodesiense	'Morsitans' group tsetse:	Wild game animals		
Endemic sporadic	*G.morsitans*	Sporadic infection	Bushbuck	Cattle
East and southern Africa	*G.pallidipes*	High-risk groups and activities	Reedbuck	Pig
			Waterbuck	Dog
T.b.rhodesiense	'Palpalis' group tsetse	Domestic animals	Hartebeest	Sheep
Epidemic	*G.fuscipes*	Man	Lion	Goat
East Africa, Kenya, Uganda		Outbreaks and epidemics	Hyena	
		Both sexes all age groups	Kob	
		Peridomestic transmission		

Bushbuck, *Tragelaphus scriptus*; reedbuck, *Redunca redunca*; waterbuck, *Kobus ellipsiprymnus*; hartebeest, *Alcephalus scriptus*; kob, *Kobus kob*; lion, *Panthera leo*; hyena, *Crocuta crocuta.*

THE TRYPANOSOMAL CHANCRE

The chancre develops within a few days of an infected bite. It starts as a small, raised, oedematous papule, which rapidly increases in size. It varies from a raised, circumscribed, oedematous disc several centimetres in diameter with surrounding erythema to an acute inflammatory lesion with marked local oedema, erythema, and local lymphadenopathy. Chancres are tender, painful, and may ulcerate. They increase in size during the first week and then subside during the subsequent 2 or 3 weeks leaving a scar with changes in pigmentation (Fig. 5). In *T.b.gambiense* infection, chancres are rarely seen; in *T.b.rhodesiense* they may be present in 10 to 50 per cent of infections.

HAEMOLYMPHATIC TRYPANOSOMIASIS (STAGE I)

The clinical features of haemolymphatic trypanosomiasis are mostly non-specific. Episodes of fever occur, with chills, rigors, prostration, headache, general malaise, and joint pains. In *T.b.gambiense* infections, the early stage is often mild and may be asymptomatic. Febrile episodes become less severe as the disease progresses. Lymphadenopathy is common, especially in *gambiense* infections where enlargement of the posterior cervical glands is characteristic (Winterbottom's sign). Hepatosplenomegaly occurs in up to 30 per cent of patients. A transient erythematous rash, 'circinate erythema', occurs on the trunk or extremities but is visible only in fair skins. Myocarditis with cardiac arrhythmia or cardiac failure occurs in *T.b.rhodesiense* infections and may lead to early death. Patchy oedema is common, especially periorbital oedema and facial puffiness. Anaemia occurs in the early stages, especially in *T.b.rhodesiense.* In severe infections there is hepatic and renal involvement, and a coagulopathy with haemorrhagic features.

Fig. 4 Section of brain in African trypanosomiasis—perivascular infiltration and morular cell.

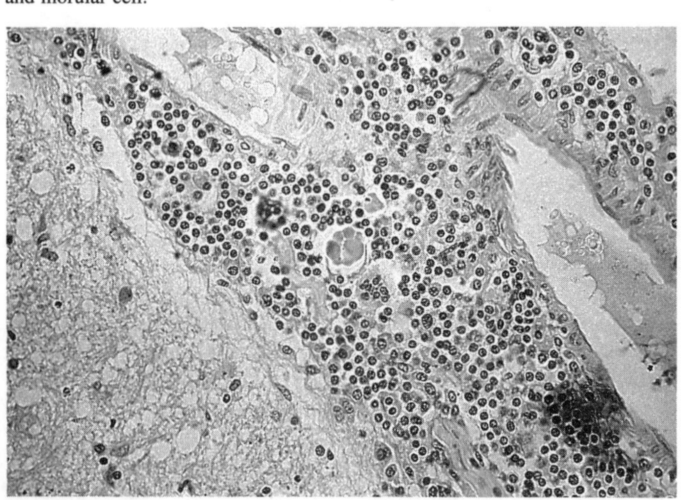

Fig. 5 An 9-month-old infant with a healing chancre with increased pigmentation (*T.b.rhodesiense*)

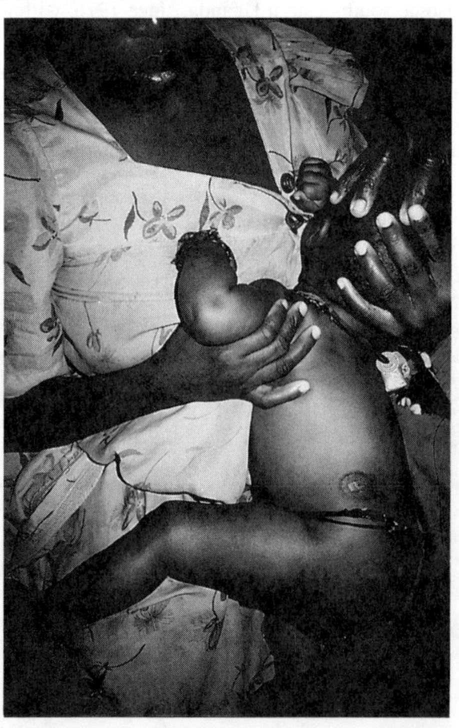

MENINGOENCEPHALITIC TRYPANOSOMIASIS (STAGE II)

Meningoencephalitis is an inevitable consequence of infection. In *T.b.rhodesiense* infections, cerebral involvement occurs within weeks of initial infection; in *T.b.gambiense* it is delayed for months or years. The onset is insidious and early involvement of the central nervous system cannot be determined clinically. Headache increases and becomes more protracted, and there may be neck stiffness. Changes in behaviour and personality occur early, before the objective development of meningoencephalitis. Features include apathy, loss of interest, lack of attention, agitation, and paranoid and delusional states. Individuals lose interest in their surroundings and their own well-being, and may exhibit inappropriate or uncharacteristic behaviour. Circadian rhythms are disturbed; abnormalities of sleep including diurnal and inappropriate somnolence are characteristic (Fig. 6). At night there is insomnia, often with agitation. The facies are blank and expressionless. Speech becomes slow, slurred, and incoherent. Extrapyramidal and cerebellar features are the characteristic neurological features.

Tremors, muscle fasciculation, and choreo-athetotic movements may occur. The gait becomes slow, unsteady, and then grossly ataxic. There may be abnormal, 'parkinsonian' features with shuffling gait and rigidity. Primitive reflexes such as the cheiro–chin reflex occur and indicate frontal-lobe involvement. Kerandel's sign refers to the delayed but intensified response to painful stimuli. Intractable pruritus is common and increases as the disease progresses. Pyramidal signs and focal cranial-nerve lesions are less common. Reflexes are usually exaggerated early but may be lost later.

The meningoencephalitis advances relentlessly with progressive stupor. Convulsions are common in advanced disease and indicate a poor prognosis. There is progressive wasting and cachexia, and sleeping sickness usually terminates in deepening coma and death. In the later stages, intercurrent infection may supervene, notably bronchopneumonia. Endocrine abnormalities include amenorrhoea, impotence, female fat distribution and gynaecomastia in men, and abortion. Testosterone or oestrogen levels are reduced. Other endocrine abnormalities described include hypothyroid states, low-T_3 syndrome, and adrenal insufficiency.

The clinical course of infection in children is more severe and may present atypically. Progression to meningoencephalitis is rapid and convulsions occur more frequently. Trypanosomiasis in tourists and visitors is also more severe and acute. In some endemic areas, very mild or asymptomatic infections have been described. There is evidence that some patients are parasitaemic for long periods but appear to remain in good health.

Fig. 6 Late-stage meningoencephalitic trypanosomiasis due to *T.b.gambiense*.

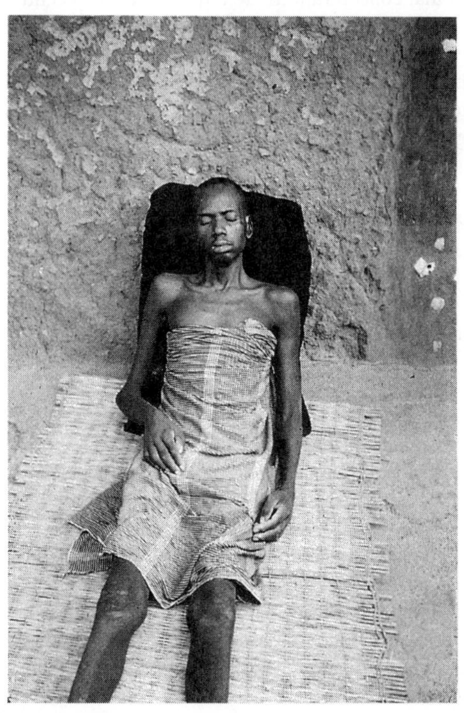

REINFECTION

Infection with African trypanosomes does not protect from reinfection. Although uncommon, in highly endemic areas and especially in occupationally exposed individuals, repeated infections may occur. Reinfection presents in the same way as a primary infection, with an haemolymphatic stage that may include a chancre. Reinfection cannot be differentiated from relapse with certainty.

Diagnosis

The clinical diagnosis of trypanosomiasis is difficult. The features of early disease are non-specific and resemble malaria and other common endemic febrile disease. In *T.b.gambiense* the early stages of infection may be subclinical. Routine laboratory tests show a normal total white-cell count with a normal or increased lymphocyte count, elevated erythrocyte sedimentation rate, anaemia, thrombocytopenia, elevated IgM, and coagulation abnormalities but these findings are non-specific. In severe infections, tests of renal and hepatic function (notably liver enzymes) may be abnormal. The serum albumin is low and there may be hypocomplementaemia, circulating immune complexes, and rheumatoid factor. Spurious hypoglycaemia is found if blood sugar estimation is not done immediately.

A parasitological diagnosis provides the only certain proof of infection. This includes examination of blood, lymph-gland needle aspirates (especially in *T.b.gambiense*), chancre aspirates, and cerebrospinal fluid for trypanosomes. Repeated examination of the blood may be required, especially in *T.b.gambiense* and late-stage infections. Trypanosomes may also be seen in marrow smears (a sensitive method, although not used routinely) and various serous effusions. Examination of material for motile trypanosomes must be done as soon after sample collection as possible. Animal inoculation is a very sensitive technique in *T.b.rhodesiense* infections.

Wet-film examination for motile trypanosomes is simple but insensitive. Thick blood films, stained with Giemsa or Field's stain, improve the sensitivity. Sensitivity is further improved in microhaematocrit centrifugation with examination of the area above the buffy coat. Examination of multiple haematocrit tubes further improves the sensitivity. The quantitative buffy-coat technique (QBC®), a modification of microhaematocrit centrifugation where motile trypanosomes are stained with acridine orange and examined by fluorescent microscopy of the expanded buffy coat (Fig. 7), has recently been shown to be a very sensitive and rapid diagnostic technique (Fig. 7). The mini anion-exchange column, using a DEAE–cellulose anion-exchange column, allows larger volumes of blood to be examined but is technically difficult except in special centres.

Immunological tests provide presumptive evidence of infection and are of particular use in population surveys, especially in *T.b.gambiense* infections. Tests used include indirect immunofluorescence, enzyme-linked immunosorbent assay, indirect haemagglutination, IgM levels in blood and cerebrospinal fluid, and the 'card agglutination test for trypanosomiasis' (**CATT**). The CATT test, which utilizes a commonly occurring variant surface antigen of *T.b.gambiense* (LiTat 1.3) has been used as a field test for the preliminary screening of populations in areas of Gambian sleeping sickness. A particular advantage of the CATT test is that the result is available rapidly and individuals can be investigated further without the difficulties associated with follow-up. The specificity and sensitivity vary with disease endemicity as well as geographically; in some foci the specificity is low due to the absence of LiTat 1.3 antigens in locally circulating *T.b.gambiense*. Antigen detection tests are being developed but are not yet available for routine use.

CEREBROSPINAL-FLUID FINDINGS IN LATE-STAGE TRYPANOSOMIASIS

In view of the limitations of chemotherapy, a confirmed infection with African trypanosomes requires examination of the cerebrospinal fluid to determine the presence of meningoencephalitis. The clinical features of early cerebral involvement are non-specific and unreliable. Meningoencephalitis is therefore defined by the presence of abnormalities in cerebrospinal fluid: cell count above 5/mm^3 (commonly between 50 and 500 cells/mm^3), elevated protein level, raised IgM, or the presence of trypanosomes. Double centrifugation techniques improve the sensitivity for detecting trypanosomes. The most sensitive indicator of meningoencephalitis is elevation of the cell count (predominantly lymphocytes); counts increase with advancing meningoencephalitis and are usually less than 1000/mm^3.

Differential diagnosis

The differential diagnosis of trypanosomiasis includes a wide range of clinical syndromes. In endemic areas a knowledge of local endemicity is essential in alerting the clinician to the diagnosis (Table 2). As outlined above, in *T.b.rhodesiense* the majority present early in the course of infection, whilst *T.b.gambiense* infections may present months or even years after infection, usually with meningoencephalitis.

In non-endemic areas, trypanosomiasis due to *T.b.rhodesiense* should be considered in travellers from East and southern Africa who have visited game parks. The infection is usually acute and severe, commonly presenting as a severe febrile illness often with high parasitaemia, hepatic and renal involvement, myocarditis, and coagulopathy. *T.b.gambiense* infections may present months or years after exposure, with a febrile illness, meningoencephalitis or neuropsychiatric features.

The chancre is almost pathognomonic but may be confused with other insect bites, skin infections, an 'eschar' or cutaneous anthrax. The early haemolymphatic stage is readily confused with many other febrile illnesses, especially malaria, relapsing fevers, typhoid, brucellosis, arboviral fevers including viral haemorrhagic fever, tuberculosis, and visceral leishmaniasis. The fever may be relapsing or low grade, especially in *T.b.gambiense* infections. Myocarditis may dominate the clinical picture.

The meningoencephalitis of trypanosomiasis may be confused with a wide range of inflammatory cerebral infections. Cerebral malaria and pyogenic meningitis are usually of rapid onset. The clinical features of AIDS and the associated opportunistic infections including tuberculosis and cryptococcal meningitis closely resemble trypanosomiasis. In geographical areas where both infections occur, exclusion of trypanosomiasis is important. Trypanosomiasis may also be confused with a variety of psychiatric syndromes and may mimic focal neurological disorders, parkinsonism, and space-occupying cerebral lesions.

Fig. 7 Fluorescing trypanosomes in the quantitative buffy-coat (QBC) test. The technique concentrates parasites stained with acridine orange in the QBC test.

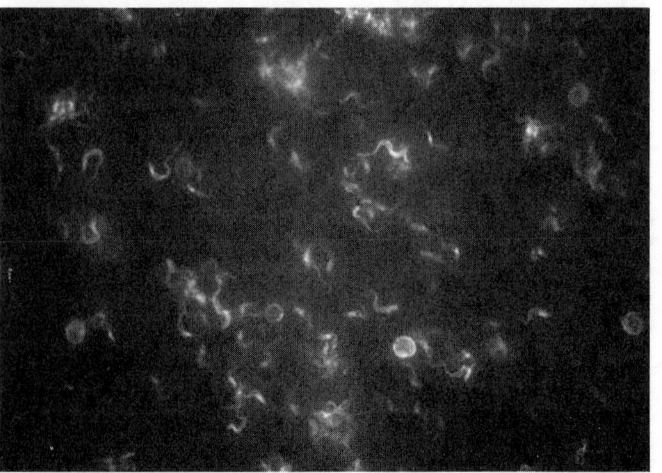

Table 2 *The differential diagnosis of human African trypanosomiasis*

Chancre
Pyogenic skin infections
Insect bites
Eschar
Cutaneous anthrax
Haemolymphatic trypanosomiasis
Malaria
Typhoid
Relapsing fever
Arbovirus infections
Viral haemorrhagic fevers
Leishmaniasis
Tuberculosis
Brucellosis
Myocarditis
Meningoencephalitic trypanosomiasis
Bacterial meningitis
Cerebral malaria
HIV/AIDS and associated infections
Tuberculous meningitis
Cryptococcal meningitis
Viral encephalitis
Syphilis
Focal neurological disease
Space-occupying lesions
Psychiatric illness

Treatment

The specific treatment of trypanosomiasis is determined by the stage of infection. In early infection, before involvement of the central nervous system, suramin is the drug of choice for both forms of infection and pentamidine is also effective in *T.b.gambiense*. Once trypanosomal meningoencephalitis is present, more toxic drugs that cross the blood–brain barrier in trypanocidal concentrations are required. Until recently, melarsoprol has been the only effective treatment for late-stage trypanosomiasis. Recently, Ornidyl (difluoromethylornithine; **DFMO**) has been developed for late-stage *T.b.gambiense* infections. The observed synergism between drugs used for the treatment of sleeping sickness has promoted the investigation of drug combinations, especially in the absence of novel trypanocidal compounds.

Early stage I trypanosomiasis

Suramin (Antrypol, Germanin, Bayer 205 sodium suramin) is the treatment of choice in the early stages of both *T.b.rhodesiense* and *T.b.gambiense* infections. Suramin is a bitter white powder, soluble in water. It is dissolved in sterile water to give a 10 per cent solution (1 g to 10 ml water), which should be used within 30 min of preparation. An initial test dose of 2 to 5 mg/kg is given, followed by 20 mg/kg weekly (maximum dose 1 g) to a total dose of 5 g.

Idiosyncratic reactions occur infrequently (approx 1:2000) with the sudden onset soon after injection of vomiting, shock, and collapse, which may prove fatal; 1/1000 adrenaline, hydrocortisone, and antihistamines should be available. Severe reactions occur more frequently with concurrent onchocerciasis. An important side-effect is renal toxicity: proteinuria is frequent but does not require cessation of suramin unless heavy or accompanied by casts. Other side-effects include skin reactions, exfoliative dermatitis, tenderness of palms and soles, bone marrow depression, haemolytic anaemia, hepatitis and jaundice, diarrhoea, and adrenocortical insufficiency.

Pentamidine (pentamidine isethionate or pentamidine methanesulphonate (Lomidine)) is available as a powder or a 10 per cent solution. The dose is 3 to 4 mg/kg (calculated as base), usually given by intramuscular injection daily or on alternate days for 7 to 10 days. Intravenous injection is associated with acute hypotension more frequently than intramuscular. Pentamidine is effective in early-stage *T.b.gambiense* infection.

Side-effects after injection include acute hypotension and syncope, ventricular tachycardia, and cardiac arrest. Hypoglycaemia due to hyperinsulinaemia occurs and diabetes may develop after prolonged administration. Pentamidine may also cause vomiting and abdominal pain, nephrotoxicity, and peripheral neuritis.

Late-stage (stage II) trypanosomiasis

Melarsoprol (Arsobal, MelB), a trivalent arsenical (melarsen oxide with British antiLewisite), is produced as a sterile solution in propylene glycol in 5-ml ampoules (36 mg/ml). It enters the cerebrospinal fluid in low but effective concentration in late-stage trypanosomiasis due to both *T.b.gambiense* and *T.b.rhodesiense*. A water-soluble arsenical, melarsonyl potassium (Trimelarsen, MelW) can be given intramuscularly. It is said to be more toxic than melarsoprol but has been used rarely.

Melarsoprol is given empirically in a series of short courses by slow intravenous injection. Treatment schedules provide courses of intravenous injections with 'rest' periods, providing a total dose of melarsoprol of 35 to 37.5 ml over a 3- or 4-week period. Regimens in *T.b.rhodesiense* start with low doses that increase slowly throughout the course of treatment; in *T.b.gambiense*, initial doses are higher and treatment courses shorter.

Melarsoprol is extremely toxic. It must be given by slow, careful, intravenous injection. It is irritant and thrombophlebitis is common, whilst extravasation leads to severe cellulitis. During injection, nausea, abdominal or retrosternal pain, and vomiting may occur. The most important toxicity is a reactive arsenical encephalopathy, which occurs in 2 to 10 per cent of patients. This encephalopathy arises more frequently in advanced, late-stage trypanosomiasis and is thought to be immunologically mediated. It is characterized by sudden neurological deterioration, commonly in the first week of treatment between the first two courses of melarsoprol. There is a sudden deterioration in conscious level, often heralded by convulsions and a variety of neuropsychiatric manifestations. The condition may prove fatal in up to 50 per cent of patients. Management includes sedation and anticonvulsants, cessation of melarsoprol, and measures to reduce cerebral oedema. The role of dimercaprol (British antiLewisite) is uncertain. Melarsoprol can be reintroduced after recovery. Although corticosteroids have proved of little benefit in the treatment of established reactive arsenical encephalopathy, prophylactic prednisolone (1 mg/kg) significantly reduced its incidence in *T.b.gambiense* infection in one study. A less common, usually fatal haemorrhagic encephalopathy also occurs with melarsoprol therapy. Other toxicity includes arthralgia, limb pains, nausea and vomiting, severe diarrhoea, peripheral neuropathy, skin reactions, hepatic and renal toxicity, and 'Herxheimer-like' reactions. Haemopoietic toxicity includes agranulocytosis, aplastic anaemia, and thrombocytopenia, as well as haemolysis in the presence of glucose 6-phosphate dehydrogenase deficiency.

α-Difluormethylornithine (Ornidyl, Eflornithine, DFMO) is an inhibitor or ornithine decarboxylase and limits polyamine biosynthesis. It is effective in the treatment of melarsoprol-resistant, late-stage trypanosomiasis caused by *T.b.gambiense*. It has also been used in initial treatment of both early and meningoencephalitic *T.b.gambiense*. Limited experience in arsenical-unresponsive *T.b.rhodesiense* infections indicates that Ornidyl is ineffective. The present dose advocated is 100 mg/kg (400 mg/kg daily), 6-hourly for 14 days intravenously (in 250-ml drip). It can also be given orally but is less effective. It is expensive and difficult to administer due to its insolubility in water but reported side-effects are less than with melarsoprol. They include diarrhoea, abdominal pain, anaemia, neutropenia, thrombocytopenia, and hair loss.

Table 3 *Treatment of late-stage trypanosomiasis: schedule for melarsoprol therapy* for adult after initial treatment with suramin or pentamidine and examination of cerebrospinal fluid*

Day	1	2	3
	0.5 0.36	1.0 0.72	1.5 (ml) 1.1 (mg/kg)
Day	10	11	12
	2.0 1.4	2.5 1.8	3.0 (ml) 2.2 (mg/kg)
Day	19	20	21
	3.0 2.2	4.0 2.9	5.0 (ml) 3.6 (mg/kg)
Day	28	29	30
	5.0 3.6	5.0 3.6	5.0 (ml) 3.6 (mg/kg)

*Melarsoprol by slow intravenous injection.

MANAGEMENT REGIMENS AND TREATMENT SCHEDULES

After the parasitological confirmation of diagnosis, suramin (or pentamidine in *T.b.gambiense*) should be given initially. Lumbar puncture is then done and further therapy determined by the results. Early (stage I) infections are treated by completing treatment courses with suramin or pentamidine and late-stage (stage II) infection is treated with melarsoprol or Ornidyl in *T.b.gambiense* infections. Treatment schedules for late-stage trypanosomiasis vary regionally but usually provide a total dose of 35 to 37.5 ml melarsoprol. Severely debilitated patients and advanced late-stage disease should be treated cautiously at first. Nutritional deficiencies and anaemia should be corrected. Drug toxicity emphasizes the need for accurate diagnosis.

The prognosis is excellent in early infection but becomes increasingly poor with advancing meningoencephalitis. Residual neurological, psychological, and behavioural abnormalities increase in frequency with the severity of meningoencephalitis. The main causes of death are severe meningoencephalitis with coma, reactive arsenical encephalopathy and other drug toxicity, myocarditis, and intercurrent infections. Relapse occurs after treatment of both early and late-stage disease.

A widely used melarsoprol regimen used in East Africa gives four 3-day courses of melarsoprol, each course separated by a 7-day interval (Table 3).

In West Africa, the modified Neujan regimen uses daily injections of 5 ml melarsoprol for 4 days and the number of courses is determined by the initial cell count in cerebrospinal fluid. Patients with fewer than 20 cells/mm^3 receive one series of injections, those with 21 to 100 cells/mm^3 receive two courses, and those with more than 100 cells/mm^3 three courses. Courses are separated by 1-week intervals. Patients in relapse are treated with four courses. An alternative regimen used in *T.b.gambiense* gives a rising dose in each course: 1.7 ml on day 1, 3.3 ml on day 2 and 5 ml on day 3 over three, spaced courses. An additional 5 ml is given on day 4 during courses two and three.

FOLLOW-UP AND RELAPSE

After treatment all patients must be followed up for 2 years. Relapse may be difficult to identify clinically and cannot be differentiated from reinfection. Examination of cerebrospinal fluid should be repeated after treatment and at subsequent follow-up, ideally at 3 months initially and 6-monthly thereafter. The features of relapse include a return of meningoencephalitic symptoms with prominent behavioural changes. A patent parasitaemia is unusual. Abnormalities of cerebrospinal fluid improve slowly after treatment and may not return to normal for many months. The earliest feature of relapse, in the cerebrospinal fluid, is a comparative increase in cells; protein levels increase and trypanosomes may be identified, especially by the double centrifugation technique; immunodiagnostic tests are also of value in identifying relapse in cerebrospinal fluid.

Relapse after treatment of stage I infections occurs more frequently where initial treatment has either been inappropriate or inadequate. In one series of patients treated without examination of cerebrospinal fluid but with no clinical features of meningoencephalitis with *T.b.rhodesiense*, the relapse rate was 50 per cent. Relapse after melarsoprol therapy may be due either to individual variations in handling arsenicals or true parasite resistance. Relapse after treatment of early infection should be treated with melarsoprol. In *T.b.gambiense* infections, relapse after melarsoprol should be treated with Ornidyl. Relapse in *T.b.rhodesiense* infection is usually treated with further melarsoprol. Other drugs of potential value in relapse include nifurtimox (Lampit R) and nitrofurazone (Furacin R).

Prevention and control

In the past, heroic attempts to control transmission included mass resettlement of human populations away from areas of transmission, destruction of wild game reservoir populations, and extensive destruction of tsetse habitats. Large-scale aerial and ground spraying with insecticides has been used in the control of trypanosome infections in domestic animals, and also in outbreaks of human disease, for example in the Llambwe Valley in Kenya and in Busoga in Uganda. Control efforts are now focused increasingly on the development of cost-effective strategies that operate within existing health facilities and include community participation. Control of sleeping sickness requires an integrated approach.

Control in endemic areas requires effective systems for the identification and management of disease. The non-specificity of the infection demands adequate laboratory resources and trained personnel. In areas of *T.b.rhodesiense*, passive surveillance is usually sufficient as the disease is severe and patients will present early for medical attention. A diagnosis of parasitism is possible with simple techniques, especially in early infection. In epidemics, especially when the disease is not recognized by the community, active surveillance and health education measures become more important. Effective surveillance with identification of early infections simplifies the therapy and improves the mortality. In *T.b.gambiense*, passive surveillance is not enough. The early stage is mild and persistent and may be asymptomatic; active surveillance and population screening are then required to identify infection and control transmission. This includes clinical examination, screening for lymphnode enlargement, gland aspiration, and parasite identification. Peripheral parasitaemia is often lower than in *T.b.rhodesiense* and immunodiagnostic tests play a more important part in population screening. The CATT has been used in *T.b.gambiense* areas for the initial screening of populations, followed by the investigation of CATT-positive individuals. The specificity can be improved by testing plasma (and diluted plasma) rather than whole blood.

There are few circumstances where eradication of vectors is feasible. Vector control therefore aims at reducing or eliminating contact between man and tsetse fly. Both ground spraying of tsetse-infested thicket with dieldrin and aerial spraying with endosulphan have been used in control programmes. Tsetse traps and targets have more recently been used extensively to control fly populations (Fig. 8). Traps can be impregnated with insecticides (synthetic pyrethroids) and the attractiveness of traps and targets can be enhanced by the use of attractant odours, especially for 'morsitans' group tsetse. Control of infection in animal reservoir populations has been attempted by restricting the range and movements of domestic cattle, treatment of domestic stock with trypanocidal drugs, and the use of 'pour ons' (the external application of synthetic pyrethroids).

The importance of man–fly contact in human trypanosomiasis suggests that environmental methods, the development of effective systems of land use that restrict tsetse habitats, and good agricultural and animal husbandry practices are all important long-term measures in the control of disease. The movements of refugee groups, as in Uganda, Sudan, and Zaire, have promoted the introduction and spread of infection in new areas. Settlement programmes and development projects must include an assessment of the risks of sleeping sickness and, where appropriate, identify strategies to mitigate the adverse effects.

REFERENCES

Bailey, J.W. and Smith, D.H. (1992). The use of acridine orange QBC technique in the diagnosis of African trypanosomiasis. *Transactions of the Royal Society of Tropical Medicine and Hygiene*, **86,** 630.

Godfrey, D., Baker, R.D., Rickman, L.R., and Mehlitz, D. (1990). The distribution, relationship and identification of enzymic variants in the subgenus *Trypanozoon*. *Advances in Parasitology*, **29,** 1–74.

Greenwood, B.M. and Whittle, H.C. (1980). The pathogenesis of sleeping sickness. *Transaction of the Royal Society of Tropical Medicine and Hygiene*, **74,** 716–25.

Haller, L., Adams, H., Meruvze, F., and Dago, A. (1986). Clinical and pathological aspects of human African trypanosomiasis (*T.b.gambiense*) with particular reference to reactive arsenical encephalopathy. *American Journal of Tropical Medicine and Hygiene*, **35,** 94–9.

Molyneux, D.H., deRaat, P., and Seed, J.R. (1984). African human trypanosomiasis. In *Recent advances in tropical medicine 1*, (ed. H.M. Gilles), pp. 39–62. Churchill Livingstone, Edinburgh.

Mulligan, H.W. (ed.) (1970). *The African trypanosomiases*. George Allen and Unwin, London.

Pentreath, V.W. (1991). The search for primary events causing the pathology in African trypanosomiasis. *Transactions of the Royal Society of Tropical Medicine and Hygiene*, **85,** 145–7.

Pepin, J., Guern, C., Ethier, L., Milord, F., Mpia, B., and Mansinsa, D. (1989). Trial of prednisolone prevention of melarsoprol-induced encephalopathy in gambiense sleeping sickness. *Lancet*, **i,** 1246–9.

Poltera, A.A. (1985). Pathology of human African trypanosomiasis with reference to experimental African trypanosomiasis and infections of the central nervous system. *Medical Bulletin*, **14,** 169–74.

Triolo, N., Trove, P., Fusco, C., and leBras, J. (1985). Report on 227 cases of human African trypanosomiasis (*Trypanosoma gambiense*) in children between 0 and 6 years. Results of 17 years observations. *Médicine Tropicale*, **45,** 251–7.

Van Nieuwenhove, S. (1992). Advances in sleeping sickness therapy. *Annales de la Société Belge de Médecine Tropicale*, **72** (suppl. 1), 39–51.

Wellde, B.T. (1989). Trypanosomiasis in the Llambwe Valley, Kenya *Annals of Tropical Medicine and Parasitology*, **83** (suppl. 1).

World Health Organization (1986). *Epidemiology and control of African trypanosomiasis*, Technical Report Series 739. WHO, Geneva.

Fig. 8 Pyramidal traps (insecticide impregnated) placed at points of high man–fly contact can be effective in the control of trypanosomiasis (copyright D.H. Smith).

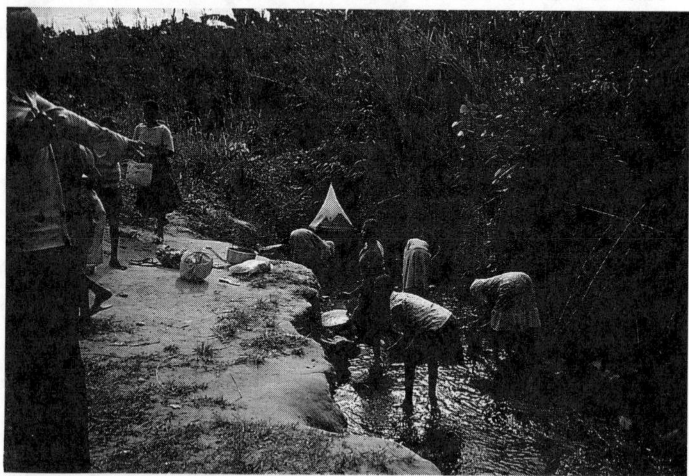

7.13.11 American trypanosomiasis

P. D. Marsden

Chagas' disease

No eponym is more richly deserved, for Carlos Chagas in the decades after his discovery was announced in 1909 described the lifecycle and the principal manifestations in man of *Trypanosoma cruzi* infection.

Restricted to North and South America the cycle of transmission of *T. cruzi* between blood-sucking triatomine bugs (Fig. 1) and mammals is long-standing in evolutionary time. This is reflected in documentation of more than 100 mammalian reservoirs. *T. cruzi* does not infect birds or reptiles. The majority of vector bugs are linked with these sylvatic cycles but several species have adapted to life with man, possibly because blood meal sources became scarce and man is a large blood reservoir. Bug-infested houses are of poor quality with cracks in the mud walls providing hiding places for the bugs (Fig. 2). Bugs tend to localize in the house fabric near blood-meal sources (e.g. the beds). They are nocturnal feeders and, once having ingested an infected blood meal, can remain infected for their natural life (2 years). Transmission is by contamination with bug faeces containing infective trypanosomes. With a rise in intra-abdominal pressure during feeding, many bugs defaecate while on the skin. Like African trypanosomiasis, Chagas' disease transmission usually occurs in remote rural communities. Although many bug species are vectors, the three important ones are *Triatoma infestans* (Argentina, Chile, Brazil, Bolivia, Paraguay, Uruguay, Peru), *Rhodnius prolixus* (Venezuela and Colombia), and *Panstrongylus megistus* (north-east Brazil). Transmission of *T. cruzi* to man has occurred in all South and Central American countries, Mexico, and in the state of Texas in the United States. Countries where it constitutes a big public health problem are Brazil, Argentina, Venezuela, Chile, Peru, and Bolivia. In Brazil, transmission to man is almost unknown in the Amazon basin because the bug species present are sylvatic, and an Indian house, having no walls, is unsuitable for bug colonization.

Different geographical regions show differences in the pathogenicity to man of the *T. cruzi* strains present in the area. Examples are the high prevalence of symptomatic acute cases in northern Argentina. Megasyndromes are common on the Brazilian Central Plateau but absent in Venezuela. Cardiomyopathy is common in both these countries but relatively rare in Chile. Positive seroreactors in central Brazil have more electrocardiographic changes than those in the extreme south of that country. *T. cruzi* strains from Argentina and Chile respond better to antitrypanosomal drug therapy than those of Brazil.

The great majority of new infections occurring yearly are in children in the first decade of life living in bug-infested houses. Interest is now being shown in transmission by blood transfusion and congenital infections but together they do not account for more than 5 per cent of new infections. In general, documentation of the size of the problem of American trypanosomiasis in each country is improving. For instance, Venezuela estimates 1 million infected people and Brazil has recently completed a nationwide serological survey giving an estimate of 6 million human infections. In some states of Brazil up to 20 per cent of the population has positive serology. A distinction must be made, however, between positive serology, indicating *T. cruzi* infection, and Chagas' disease where there is clinical evidence of organ damage. To establish the prevalence of Chagas' disease a nationwide electrocardiographic survey in positive seroreactors is in progress in Brazil. An attempt to control *Triatoma infestans* in Cone Sul countries is being organized at the time of writing.

Pathogenesis

T. cruzi can be seen directly in the peripheral blood only in the acute phase of the disease. In fact its presence is the best definition of the acute phase as all other signs are variable (Fig. 3). It is a trypanomastigote with a very large kinetoplast (a DNA organelle characteristic of this family). Multiplication only occurs in the amastigote phase, which grows in a variety of tissue cells especially muscle. Chronic inflam-

Fig. 1 (a) *Rhodnius prolixus* adult (approximately three times natural size) (by courtesy of the Wellcome Museum of Medical Science). (b) The Mexican bug *Dipetalogaster maximus* on a human hand—the largest triatomine known.

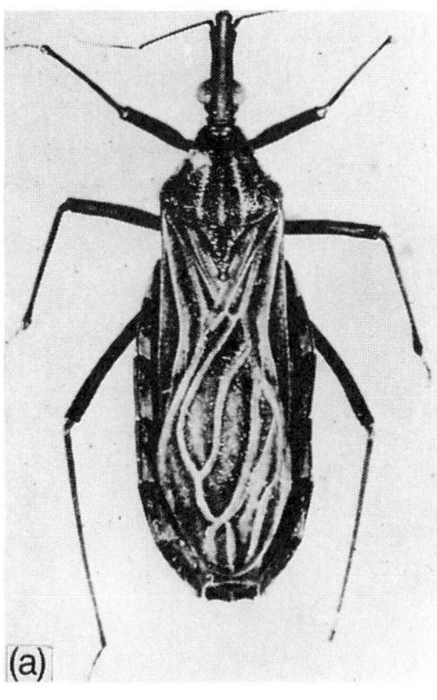

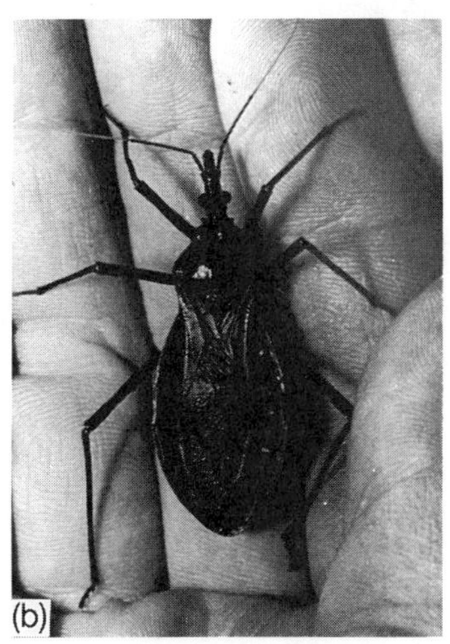

Fig. 2 (a) Wall made of lath and mud, an ideal bug habitat (by courtesy of the Wellcome Museum of Medical Science). (b) House demolition to study triatomine ecology. Note the complexity of fabric: bark and Portugese tiles on the roof, and wood or cracked mud walls.

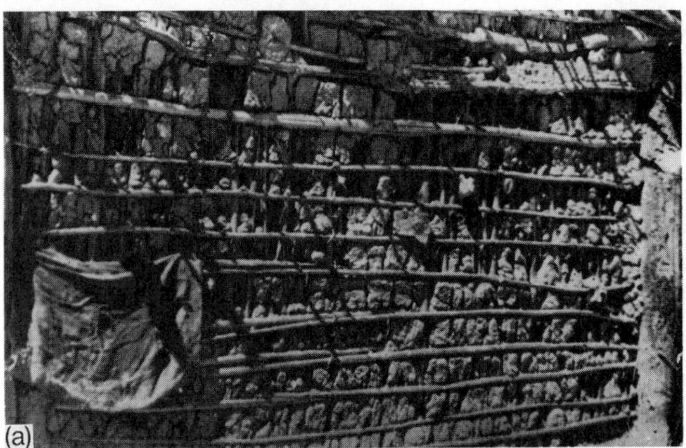

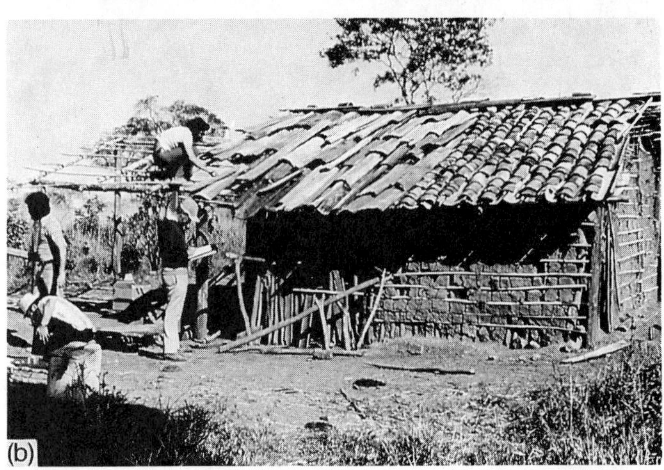

mation of the heart muscle and the smooth muscle of the gut is the basis of the pathology, the infiltrate being mainly of lymphocytes and plasma cells. Early in the infection such infiltrates in the heart muscle are associated with amastigote nests but in chronic cases parasites cannot be found (Fig. 4). An autoimmune process has been suggested to explain this finding. There is some evidence that *T. cruzi* shares a common antigen with heart muscle, stimulating sensitized lymphocytes to destroy non-parasitized muscle fibres. A circulating autoantibody (endothelial-vascular-interstitial antibody or EVI) has been detected in Chagasic patients but the titre of this antibody does not correlate well with the presence of cardiomyopathy.

The Chagasic heart at autopsy shows a thinning of the ventricular muscle and frequently an apical aneurysm. Many muscle fibres are fragmented and the infiltration of lymphocytes and plasma cells is associated with areas of oedema, degeneration, and haemorrhage (Fig. 5).

After the initial wave of parasitaemia the number of circulating trypanosomes falls below detectable levels. IgM and IgG antibodies, however, usually appear within a month. The presence of IgM antibodies assists in confirming congenital Chagas' disease in the neonate. However, as in the treponematoses, small numbers of viable organisms persist in the tissues, probably for life. One site where multiplication persists is in the smooth-muscle wall of the suprarenal vein. Decades after the childhood infection the chronic cardiomyopathy may result in heart muscle failure or conduction disturbances due to inflammation of the Purkinje fibres. A similar inflammation around parasympathetic ganglia in the smooth muscle of the gut wall leads to incoordinated peristalsis. Solid residues accumulating in the oesophagus and colon give rise to megasyndromes.

Fig. 3 *T. cruzi* in peripheral blood; note the large kinetoplast.

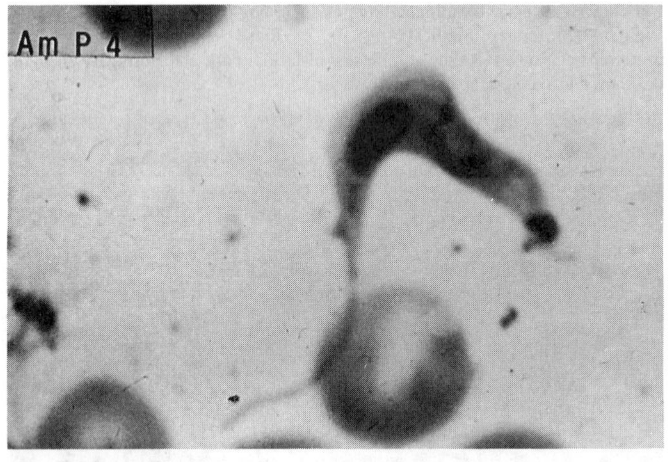

Fig. 4 Amastigotes in cardiac (left) and smooth (right) muscle.

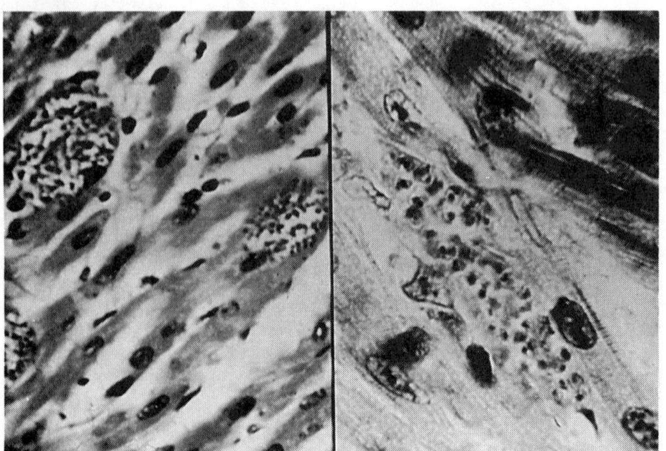

Clinical presentation and diagnosis

Patients usually know the triatomine bugs well. It is very important to ask for a past history of living in a bug-infested house and to have a specimen of the bugs to show the patient available in the outpatient department.

There are three phases of the infection. The acute phase usually passes unnoticed but there may be an inflamed swelling or chagoma at the site of entry of the trypanosomes (Fig. 6). Romañas' sign is when this swelling involves the eyelids (Fig. 7). Such clinical evidence of local parasitic multiplication occurs in about half of the detected cases. Reticulo-endothelial activation is evidenced by hepatosplenomegaly and lymphadenopathy. There is less than a 5 per cent mortality in this phase, either from acute heart failure or meningoencephalitis. Congenital Chagas' disease is acute Chagas' disease in the neonate and clinically can closely resemble other neonatal infections such as toxoplasmosis, cytomegalic inclusion disease, and syphilis. Abortions are more frequent in infected pregnant women. Laboratory investigation detects the circulating trypanosomes in fresh blood smears. Failing this the Strout technique, where the supernatant from clotted blood is examined, is usually posi-

Fig. 5 Chronic chagasic cardiomyopathy showing destruction of muscle fibres and areas of haemorrhage.

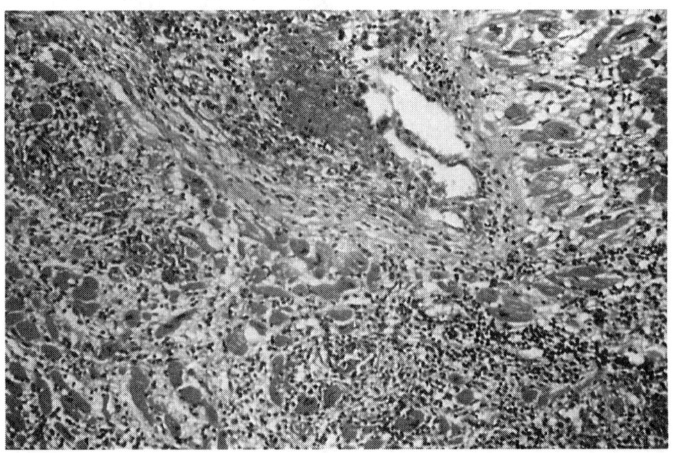

Fig. 6 Chagoma: the baby trapped an infected bug under its chin; *T. cruzi* recovered by needling the trypanosomal chancre.

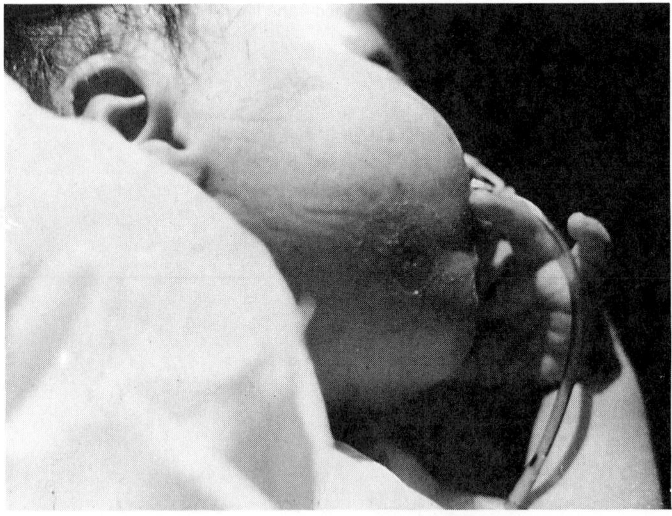

tive. There is a lymphocytosis and often a false positive unabsorbed Paul Bunnel test. Blood cultures, mouse inoculation, and xenodiagnosis all reveal circulating *T. cruzi*.

The term intermediate phase is useful to emphasize that, after infection in early life, decades may pass before clinical syndromes appear. During this time the patient has evidence of infection but not disease, the definition of this phase. Detection is based on serology which has improved greatly in recent years. Ideally complement fixation, indirect fluorescent antibody, and indirect haemagglutination tests should all be done on the same sera and usually there is close concordance. Fifty per cent of these patients have small numbers of circulating trypanosomes detectable by xenodiagnosis, a technique where uninfected bugs are fed on the patient and subsequently examined 30 days later for infection. Xenodiagnosis tends to be more frequently positive in younger patients in this phase.

From the field study in São Felipe, Bahia, comes information on the outcome of this phase. In 10 years follow-up of 400 patients 96 (24 per cent) developed electrocardiographic abnormalities and 5 clinically detectable mega-oesophagus. In many patients with positive serology disease never appears. The most famous case is Berenice who at age 2 was diagnosed in the acute phase by Carlos Chagas himself. As an old woman she had no detectable heart or gut pathology.

The chronic phase of Chagas' disease appears decades after infection but a rare subacute form has been described where heart muscle failure supervened months after the acute phase. Chagasic cardiomyopathy has two principal manifestations: heart muscle failure and conduction defects. Bilateral ventricular failure is the rule since a panmyocarditis is the pathology. Therefore patients usually have little pulmonary oedema but marked congestive failure. Intraventricular thrombi are common, and systemic or pulmonary emboli may be the initial sign of this disease. Heart size is variable but it is frequently greatly enlarged with feeble pulsation on screening (Fig. 8). There are no organic valvular lesions, only functional mitral or tricuspid incompetence. Complete right bundle branch block with left anterior hemiblock is a very characteristic electrocardiographic finding but extrasystoles and any form of AV conduction defect may be present. Left bundle branch block and atrial fibrillation are rare. Complete heart block with Stokes-Adams attacks may cause the patient's admission to hospital. Repeated heart failure, massive embolus, or cardiac arrest are common causes of death. Severe heart disease is commoner in males 30 to 50 years old (possibly due to increased cardiac work in this sex).

Mega-oesophagus has been classified into four degrees of severity depending mainly on oesophageal diameter on barium swallow. In the most severe grades (III and IV) difficulty in swallowing may lead to wasting and parotid gland hypertrophy (the 'cat face') (Fig. 9). Food residue overspill may produce lung infections and bronchiectasis. The patient gives a clear history of swallowing difficulty and with each mouthful may need water to accomplish deglutition. Likewise megacolon is associated with abnormal constipation (weeks). Faecal impaction, sigmoid volvulus, and toxic megacolon with *E. coli* septicaemia are side-effects of megacolon.

The role of parasympathetic denervation producing other gastrointestinal, endocrine, and renal abnormalities has to be further defined. Absence of patellar reflexes in seropositive patients suggests peripheral neuropathy.

Laboratory diagnosis relies heavily on positive serology as in the treponematoses. Serological reference laboratories are located in Washington, Rio de Janeiro, Belo Horizonte, Goiânia, São Paulo, and Buenos Aires. Serology should be checked by one of the central reference laboratories if the local laboratory concerned has little experience with the tests.

Indirect immunofluorescence, indirect haemagglutination, and enzyme immunoassay are all over 95 per cent reliable if positive and

Fig. 7 Romañas' sign: bipalpebral unilateral oedema, usually lasting several weeks.

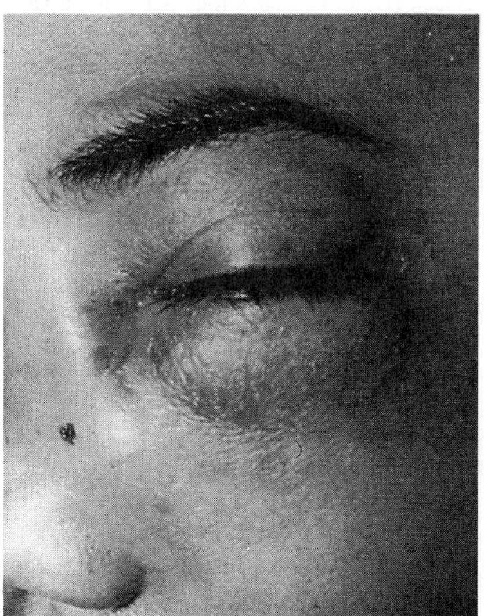

Fig. 8 Posteroanterior chest radiograph showing enlarged heart level in mega-oesophagus.

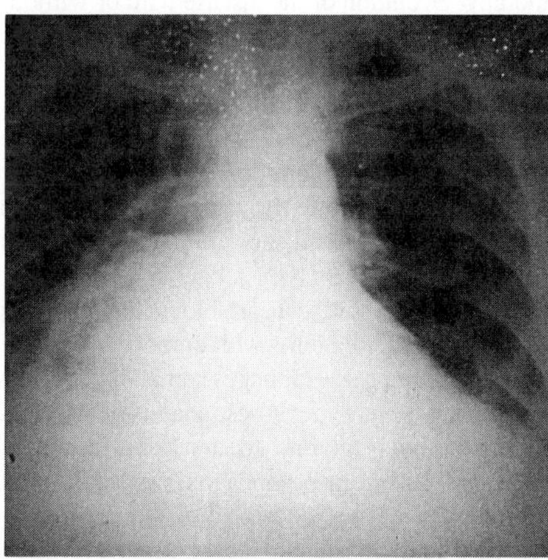

Fig. 9 Parotid gland enlargement in a Brazilian child with advanced mega-oesophagus (the 'cat face').

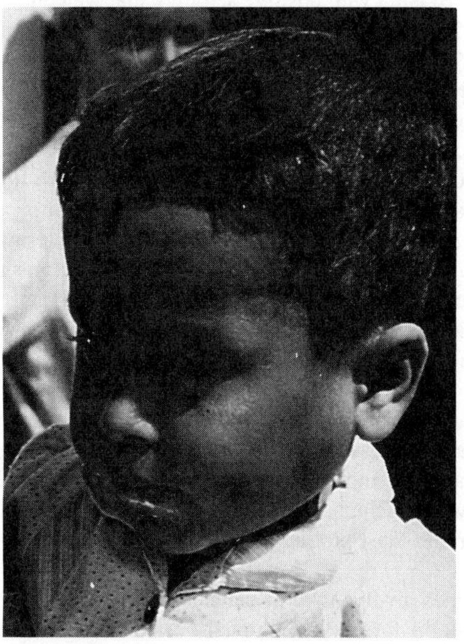

negative control sera are run. False-positive reactions can occur with conditions of abnormal immunoglobulin production such as lepromatous leprosy, visceral and mucocutaneous leishmaniasis, treponematoses, hyperimmune malarious splenomegaly, collagenoses, autoimmune disorders, multiple myeloma, and the hereditary macroglobulinaemias. *T. rangeli* is especially important above the Amazon basin as a cause of false-positive routine serology.

Treatment and prevention

It is generally agreed that the acute stage should be treated with an antitrypanocidal drug because damage to parasympathetic ganglia is thought to occur in the acute stage and theoretically the parasitaemia reduction achieved with such drugs should be advantageous. Two drugs are in common use. Nifurtimox (Lampit) is given in an oral dose of 8 mg/kg body weight for 60 or 90 days. The longer course of 120 days shows no better results on follow-up and is prone to more side-effects, especially convulsions and psychosis. Production of this drug was discontinued in 1991. Benzidazole (Rochagan) is given in an oral dose of 6 mg/kg body weight for 30 or 60 days. It is now the drug of choice. A serious side-effect, fortunately rare, is an exfoliative dermatitis. Both drugs produce anorexia, weight loss, headache and dizziness, gastric irritation, and, in 12 to 30 per cent, peripheral neuritis.

There is no evidence that patients in the intermediate or chronic phase benefit from such drug therapy. Evolution of the disease with or without these drugs in such studies as are available at the present time appears to be the same. Control of heart failure with digitalis and diuretics is of benefit but the response is frequently not good. Digitalis sensitivity is common, especially in the presence of hypokalaemia. Antiarrhythmic drugs must be used with caution. Procaine amide and lignocaine may help in ventricular tachycardia or multiple extrasystoles. β-Adrenergic blocking agents may produce bradycardia and shock, and propranalol is contraindicated.

Pacemaker implantation to relieve severe heart block has a better prognosis if the heart is of normal size. Patients with embolization may benefit from anticoagulation. Early mega-oesophagus can be relieved by balloon dilatation but established, severe mega-oesophagus and megacolon require surgery. Cardiotomy is giving good results in mega-oesophagus. Half the patients with mega-oesophagus have abnormal electrocardiograms.

Congenital Chagas' disease and transfusion acute disease require Lampit or Rochagan therapy. Transfusion infection can be prevented by either rejecting seropositive potential donors or, failing this mixing the blood with gentian violet for 24 h (dilution 1:4000). We have so many donors in our hospital in Brasilia with positive serology that we cannot afford to reject them. Using gentian violet we have never had a case of transfusion infection.

The effectiveness of residual insecticides in controlling domestic bug population was first reported in the 1940s. Since then widespread campaigns have been conducted in many South American countries. Obviously, fresh infections occurring yearly in children pose a problem for hospital medical services in the future. Although the economic impact of this disease cannot be calculated, it must be considerable both in terms of morbidity and mortality in farming communities and in the strain it poses on hospital services. Chagas' disease is the most common cause of admission to our medical service in Brasilia. Half our patients admitted for the first time with congestive heart failure are dead within 2 years.

Few endemic infections respond as well to domiciliary insecticide spraying as *T. cruzi*. This is because the vector bug is vulnerable, living in poor housing materials that modern insecticides easily penetrate. Also, because of the slow lifecycle, insecticide resistance emerges late, although it is recorded in the most prolific bug species (*Rhodnius prolixus*) in Venezuela.

Field control programmes involve total insecticide cover of all domiciles and peridomiciles in the farm where domicilary vector bugs have been found. Today, pyrethroids are favoured by users for their long-term residual action and by the householders for the lack of smell and low mortality rate among domestic animals compared to benezene hexachloride (BHC), which was previously used.

It is the vigilance required to detect reinvasion of houses by vector bugs that usually weakens as the years pass. We have 13 years' observations in Mambaĩ, Goiãs-Brazil of the same rural community in 50 farms. We have devised simple longitudinal vigilance methods applicable to national campaigns, where the family plays an active part in recording bug presence and calling the team to arrange respraying. Improvement of buildings is much more costly and should be reserved for problematical, persistently bug-infested houses.

Certainly in Brazil, the country with the largest infected population, the situation will continue to improve as a result of Ministry of Health control programmes. However, for decades a large number of patients with cardiomyopathy and megasyndromes will continue to be seen in the hospital outpatient service due to the long period of evolution of a *T. cruzi* infection acquired in childhood.

REFERENCES

Anonymous (1988). Pyrethroids. *Parasitology Today*, **4,** 51–317.

Brener, Z. and Andrade, Z. (1979). *Trypanosoma cruzi e doença de Chagas*. Ed. Guanabara Koogan, Rio de Janeiro.

Dias, J.C.P. (1987). Control of Chagas' disease in Brazil. *Parasitology Today*, **3,** 336–41.

Garcia-Zapata, M.T.A. and Marsden, P.D. (1992). Control of the transmission of Chagas' disease in Mambaĩ, Goiãs-Brazil (1980–1988). *American Journal of Tropical Medicine and Hygiene*, **46,** 400–43.

Garcia-Zapata, M.T.A., McGreevy, P.B., and Marsden, P.D. (1991). American trypanosomiasis. In *Hunters tropical medicine*, (7th edn) (ed. T. Strickland) pp. 628–37. Saunders, Philadelphia.

Garcia-Zapata, M.T.A., Marsden, P.D., Soares, V.A., and Castro, C.N. (1992). The effect of plastering a house persistently infested with *Triatoma infestans* (Klug 1934). *Journal of Tropical Medicine and Hygiene*, **95,** 420–3.

Garcia Zapata, M.T.A. and Marsden, P.D. (1993). Chagas' disease: control and surveillance through use of insecticides and community participation in Mambai Goias Brazil. *Bulletin of The Panamerican Health Organization*, **27,** 265–79.

Koberle, F. (1968). Chagas' disease and Chagas' syndromes: the pathology of American trypanosomiasis. *Advances in Parasitology*, **6,** 63–116.

Marsden, P.D. (1983). The transmission of Trypanosoma cruzi to man and its control. In *Human ecology and infectious disease* (ed. N.A. Croll and J.M. Cross), pp. 253–89. Academic Press, New York.

Marsden, P.D. (1984). Chagas' disease, clinical aspects. In *Recent advances in tropical medicine*, Vol. 1, (ed. H.M. Gilles), p. 63–87. Churchill Livingstone, Edinburgh.

PAHO (1975). *American trypanosomiasis research*, PAHO Scientific Publication. No. 318. Pan-American Health Organization, Washington DC.

Fig. 10 *T. rangeli* in peripheral blood; note small kinetoplast.

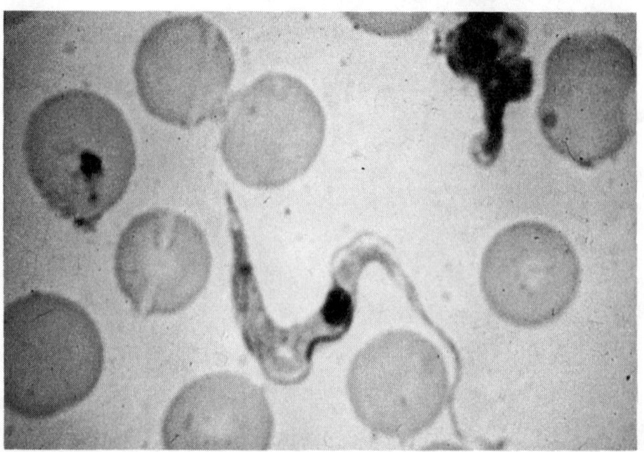

Trypanosoma rangeli

This second species of New World mammalian trypanosome infecting man is also found in many sylvatic animals. The trypomastigote can be distinguished easily from *Trypanosoma cruzi* by the small size of the kinetoplast and this morphological feature helps to identify the epimastigotes present in the triatomine vector (Fig. 10). Members of the genus Rhodnius are mainly responsible for *T. rangeli* transmission. This occurs mainly in central and northern South America (Venezuela, Colombia, Ecuador), although there have been at least three reports of *T. rangeli* in Brazil. The parasite is a severe, sometimes lethal, infection of triatomine bugs but a benign infection of mammals including man. In an infected bug, epimastigotes are found not only in the intestinal tract but in the haemolymph and salivary glands as well and transmission is effected either by bite (infected saliva) or faecal contamination. The main medical importance is the estimation of infection in wild-caught bugs in epidemiological surveys, and indeed *T. cruzi* and *T. rangeli* may exist in the same bug. For this reason, haemolymph and salivary gland examinations of such bugs are necessary in endemic areas. *T. rangeli* is rare below the Amazon basin and such detailed bug examination is unnecessary as a routine in Central Brazil.

In man the trypomastigote may be seen in peripheral blood smears for weeks. No apparent symptoms or pathology occur. It can be detected for years by xenodiagnosis and appears to divide by binary fission in the peripheral blood. The absence of a tissue phase may account for its non-pathogenicity. *T. rangeli* cross-reacts with *T. cruzi* on serological testing as one would expect because Leishmania cross-react. Serological ways of differentiating between the two infections have been reported but are rarely used routinely in the relevant laboratories.

REFERENCE

D'Alessandro-Bacigalupo, A. and Saravia, N.G. (1992). Trypanosoma rangeli. In *Parasitic Protozoa* (eds. J.P. Kreier and J.R. Baker) (2nd edn) Vol. 2, pp. 1–54. Academic Press, San Diego.

7.13.12 Leishmaniasis

A. D. M. BRYCESON

INTRODUCTION

Leishmaniasis is caused by parasites of the genus Leishmania. The infection is normally zoonotic, in wild or peridomestic canines or rodents, among which it is transmitted by phlebotomine sandflies. The disease in man is usually either cutaneous or visceral. Within these broad categories there are variations in disease patterns that reflect differences in pathogenicity between species of Leishmania and differences in response between individual patients. The most important variant is mucosal leishmaniasis of South and Central America.

Although the mode of transmission in several natural foci is known, human leishmaniasis has seldom been eradicated and its distribution and prevalence appear to be increasing, especially in Latin America and Africa. In certain places the disease is common and important but there are few accurate statistics.

AETIOLOGICAL AGENT

In its vertebrate host the amastigote form of the parasite is found in cells of the reticuloendothelial system. It is round or oval, about 2 to 3 μm in diameter, with no protruding flagellum. The nucleus and kinetoplast stain deeply with the Romanovsky stains and give the organism its characteristic appearance (Fig. 1). In the sandfly or in culture medium it is in the elongated, motile, promastigote form with an anterior flagellum.

At least 15 species of Leishmania cause disease in man. The most important are shown in Table 1. Unnamed species cause cutaneous disease in Namibia and the Dominican Republic. Genetic markers are used to distinguish species; isoenzyme patterns and DNA hybridization are the most popular. These techniques have confirmed the distinctions accorded on epidemiological and clinical grounds. Monoclonal antibodies raised against known species are proving useful in identifying unknown isolates.

LIFECYCLE

The main reservoir hosts and vectors are given in Table 2. Sandflies require a precise microclimate that is provided in precise locations in each endemic focus at certain seasons of the year. Sandfly populations fluctuate widely, depending on climate and competing species.

Amastigotes are ingested from blood or tissues of the mammalian host by the female fly, and transform into promastigotes in the midgut where they develop before migrating to the pharynx and proboscis, rendering the fly infective after about 10 days. Transmission is often seasonal.

Cutaneous leishmaniasis

EPIDEMIOLOGY (SEE ALSO TABLE 1)

Leishmania major causes cutaneous leishmaniasis in the hot, dry lands of the Old World. Gerbils are the usual reservoirs. The vectors live in rodent burrows, where the infection rate is high, and bite man readily. Hunters, travellers, tourists, and dwellers at oases or in new settlements are affected. The disease may be sporadic or epidemic.

L. tropica causes cutaneous leishmaniasis in towns. *Phlebotomus sergenti* lives in crevices in buildings and banks. Better building techniques, antimalarial spraying, case finding, and treatment have removed this scourge from many towns, where previously every citizen bore the scar.

L. aethiopica is a highland parasite. Hyraxes live in holes in rock faces and large trees. The vector bites people sleeping in their huts. The disease is endemic and most people are affected by early adulthood.

L. donovani causes post-kala-azar dermal leishmaniasis in India. *L. infantum* causes simple, self-healing skin lesions and rarely mucosal lesions in some parts of southern Europe and North Africa. The epidemiology is described later.

In the New World, epidemiological patterns are emerging slowly

Fig. 1 Amastigotes of *L. donovani* in a reticuloendothelial cell from the splenic aspirate of a patient with visceral leishmaniasis.

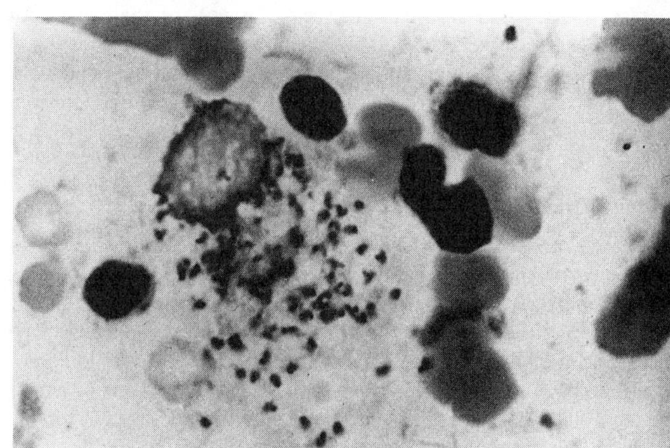

Table 1 *Epidemology of leishmaniasis*

Organism	Geography	Reservoir	Vector
Old World			
L. donovani	North-east India, Bangladesh, Burma	Man	*Phlebotomus argentipes*
L. infantum	Mediterranean basin, Middle East, China, central Asia	Dogs, foxes, jackals	*P. perniciosus, P. major, P. chinensis et al.*
L. donovani (Africa)	Sudan, Kenya, Horn of Africa, ?Senegambia	?Rodents in Sudan, ?canines ?man	*P. orientalis, P. martini*
L. major	Semideserts in Middle East, north India, Pakistan, North Africa, Central Asia	Gerbils (especially *Rhombomys, Meriones et al.*)	*P. papatasi*
L. major	SubSaharan savanna, Sudan	Rodents (especially *Arvicanthus, Tatera*)	*P. duboscqi*
L. tropica	Towns in Middle East, Mediterranean basin, Central Asia	Man, ?dogs	*P. sergenti*
L. aethiopica	Highlands of Kenya, Ethiopia	Hyraxes (*Procavia, Heterohyrax*)	*P. longipes, P. pedifer*
New World			
L. chagasi	Central America, northern South America, esp. Brazil, Venezuela	Foxes, dogs, opossums (*Didelphys*)	*Lutzomyia longipalpis*
L. mexicana	Yucatan, Belize, Guatemala	Forest rodents (especially *Ototylomys*)	*Lu. olmeca*
L. amazonensis	Tropical forests of South America	Forest rodents (especially *Proechimys, Oryzomys*)	*Lu. flaviscutellata*
L. brasiliensis	Tropical forests of South and Central America	?Forest rodents, peridomestic animals	*Psychodopygus wellcomei et al., Lutzomyia* spp
L. guyanensis	Guyanas, Surinam into Brazil, Colombia	Sloths (*Choleopus*) arboreal anteaters (*Tamandua*)	*Lu. umbratilis*
L. panamensis	Panama, Costa Rica, Colombia	Sloths (*Choleopus*)	*Lu. trapidoi et al.*
L. peruviana	West Andes of Peru, Argentine highlands	Dogs	*Lu. verrucarum, Lu. peruensis*

because the distributions of parasites overlap and some species are difficult to culture. Transmission is usually in the forest, where there are many species of rodents and sandflies. The vector of *L. mexicana* bites man reluctantly, but those who spend a long time in the forest during the rainy season, such as the collectors of chicle or chewing-gum latex, are bitten. *L. amazonensis* has a wide distribution throughout the rain forests in several species of common rodents. *Lutzomyia flaviscutellata* is, however a zoophilic night biter and human disease is relatively rare.

L. brasiliensis, the major cause of American cutaneous and mucosal leishmaniasis, is the most widely distributed of the New World Leishmania from Belize to Paraguay. The epidemiology is still poorly understood but infections have been found in many different wild and domestic animals. The vectors are highly anthropophilic and human infection is common in all who enter the forests. Periurban foci of infection are increasing. *L. guyanensis* and *L. panamensis* are less widely distributed. The reservoir hosts are arboreal. The vectors oviposit on the forest floor and may bite forest workers and hunters in the early morning.

L. peruviana causes high-altitude endemic cutaneous leishmaniasis. In some villages over 90 per cent of children acquire the infection from domestic dogs.

PATHOGENESIS

Leishmania inoculated by the sandfly invade and multiply in macrophages in the skin. After a period, which experimentally is determined by the size of the inoculum, the parasitized macrophage granuloma is recognized immunologically and becomes clinically apparent. The lesion is infiltrated by lymphocytes and plasma cells. When the appropriate ratio of cells to parasites is reached, piecemeal necrosis or extensive focal necrosis of parasitized cells begins. The basal layer of the epidermis is damaged: hyperkeratosis and ulceration occur, the ulcer being filled with a crust of hyperkeratotic debris, dried exudate, dead cells and parasites. This activity may continue for many months before the infection is eliminated, while the clinical lesion remains static. Antibody-dependent, cell-mediated responses are thought to be important. The classical response of macrophage activation is less common and less efficient, and occurs especially in chronic lesions when parasites are scanty: epithelioid cells and Langhans' giant cells produce a picture similar to that of non-caseous tuberculosis. Rarely, the parasite mass and antigen load suppress the cellular immune response, producing a histological picture of vacuolated, parasitized macrophages, with little or no lymphocytic infiltrate, a normal or attenuated epidermis, and the clinical picture of diffuse cutaneous leishmaniasis (**DCL**).

Variations of the basic pattern reflect on the one hand the ability of a given species of Leishmania to induce or suppress the immune response, to metastasize or to invade cartilage, and on the other hand the speed and efficiency with which the patient can mount an immune response. Circumstantial factors, such as inoculum size and site of infection, also affect the clinical picture.

L. major is the most immunogenic and allergenic of the Old World Leishmania, causing most necrosis. *L. tropica* is less immunogenic and causes less inflamed, slow-healing sores. It is also associated with chronic relapsing or recidivans lesions that have a tuberculoid histology. *L. aethiopica* and *L. amazonensis* are able to suppress cell-mediated immunity specifically and may cause DCL. In the Dominican Republic this anergy is associated with the presence of circulating suppressor monocytes. *L. aethiopica* shares with *L. mexicana* and *L. brasiliensis* the ability to invade cartilage. Cartilaginous lesions are extremely chronic. *L. brasiliensis* is capable of metastasizing through the bloodstream early in the course of infection to sites deep in the mucosa of the nose or mouth, commonly against the nasal cartilage, where it may lie dormant. After months or years the parasite multiplies and the response

Table 2 *Clinical features of cutaneous leishmaniasis*

Parasite and lesion	Natural outcome	Treatment
L. major		
Self-healing rural sores	3–5 months Disabling scars	Physical/topical/nil Sb 10–20 mg/kg/day × 3 weeks (?some unresponsive)
L. tropica		
1. Self-healing urban sores	10–14 months	Physical/topical/nil Sb 10–20 mg/kg/day × 3 weeks
2. Leishmaniasis recidivans	> 10 years, destructive	Sb 10–20 mg/kg/day × 3–6 weeks
L. infantum		
1. Self-healing, nodular	1–3 years	Physical/topical/nil Sb 10–20 mg/kg/day × 3 weeks
2. Mucosal	Persists	Sb 10–20 mg/kg/day × 3 weeks.
L. aethiopica		
1. Self-healing, nodular	2–5 years	Physical/topical/nil (Sb 20 mg/kg/12hrs × 8 weeks)
2. Mucocutaneous	> 10 years, destructive	Pentamidine 4 mg/kg/week × 8
3. Diffuse CL	Persists, disfiguring	Pentamidine 4 mg/kg/week or aminosidine 15 mg/kg/day × months
L. mexicana		
1. Self-healing	6–8 months	Physical/topical/nil Sb 10–20 mg/kg/day × 3 weeks
2. Chiclero ear	> 10 years, destructive	Sb 10–20 mg/kg/day × ?
L. amazonensis		
1. Self-healing	?Duration	?Sb 10–20 mg/kg/day × 3 weeks
2. DCL	Persists, relapses disfiguring	Sb 10–20 mg/kg/12 hourly × months
L. brasiliensis		
1. Self-healing	6–24 months, later mucosal	Sb 10–20 mg/kg/day × 3–6 weeks
2. Mucosal	Persists, destructive	Sb 20 mg/kg/day × 4–6 weeks
L. guyanensis		
1. Self-healing,	?6–8 months, rare later mucosal	Sb 10–20 mg/kg/day × 3 weeks
2. Lymphatic nodules 'pian bois'		If poorly responsive to Sb, use pentamidine
L. panamensis		
Self-healing	?Duration, rare later mucosal	Sb 20 mg/kg/day × 3 weeks
L. b. peruviana		
Self-healing	?Duration	Physical/topical/nil Sb 10–20 mg/kg/day × 3 weeks

it elicits is characterized by necrosis, vasculitis, and tissue destruction. Occasionally, *L. panamensis* or *L. guyanensis* cause mucosal leishmaniasis.

Inbred strains of mice show distinct, genetically determined differences in susceptibility and immune response to leishmanial infection. Two haplotypes, HLA-BW22 and -DQW3, are associated with susceptibility to cutaneous leishmaniasis in Venezuela. Amerindians mount a less destructive response to *L. brasiliensis* than do negroes. Immunity to reinfection with a given species of leishmania is usually lifelong. Second infections have been reported, especially in the elderly or immunosuppressed.

CLINICAL FEATURES

A nodule, erythematous in pale skins, develops at the site of the infected sandfly bite after an incubation period of a few days to several months. A thin, golden crust forms. The nodule reaches its final size, usually 1 to 5 cm diameter, over weeks or months. The crust may remain superficial, or thicken to replace the nodule, or may fall away leaving an ulcer with a raised edge (Fig. 2). Satellited papules are common. After months or years (Table 2) the lesion starts to heal slowly, leaving a depressed, mottled scar. Secondary infection is unimportant. The lesion is not normally painful, but may disfigure or disable if scarring is severe or over a joint.

There are many deviations from this classical pattern, some of which tend to be associated with a particular species of Leishmania. Sores due to *L. major* occur on any exposed site (Fig. 3). They form and heal most rapidly and may be greatly inflamed and exudative: the so-called wet or rural sore. By contrast, sores due to *L. tropica* tend to be less inflamed: the so-called dry or urban sore. Lesions due to *L. infantum* have an incubation period of many months, and are usually small, nodular, and persistent over several years. Most *L. aethiopica* lesions are central on the face and single. Satellite papules accumulate to produce a slowly growing, shiny tumour, or plaque that may not crust nor ulcerate (Fig. 4). If the site is at the mucocutaneous border, primary mucocutaneous leishmaniasis may develop, producing swelling of the lips and expansion and elongation of the nose, though little destruction of tissue, and last for many years.

L. brasiliensis often causes deep, usually single, ulcers with a granulomatous base. Up to 15 per cent of patients will relapse after spontaneous or therapeutic cure. Sores due to *L. guyanensis* are fleshy and protuberant, and tend to be multiple on the limbs, resembling yaws, 'pian bois'. This parasite and *L. panamensis* are more commonly associated with metastatic lesion along the draining lymphatics than are the other species. *L. mexicana* lesions, 'chiclero ulcer', are commonly on

Fig. 2 'Punched out' ulcer with nodular edge, characteristic of *L. brasiliensis*, Brazil (by courtesy of Professor Alfredo Pons).

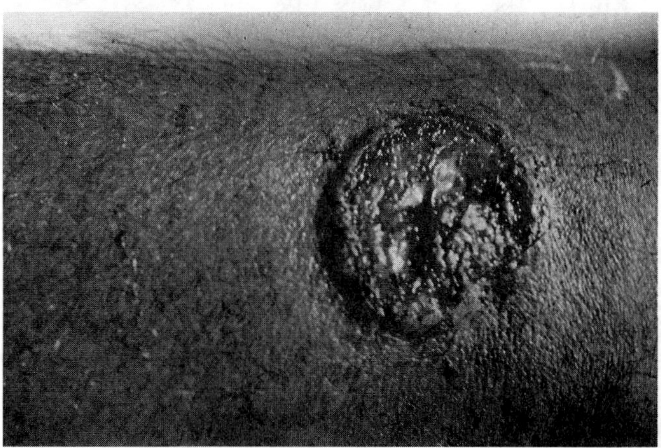

the side of the face or behind the ears. Many are on the pinna of the ear. These take years to heal and may destroy the pinna.

Three forms of cutaneous leishmaniasis do not heal spontaneously: DCL, leishmaniasis recidivans, and American mucosal leishmaniasis.

Diffuse cutaneous leishmaniasis

This occurs in about 1 per 10 000 infections with *L. aethiopica*, a much greater proportion of infections with *L. amazonensis*, and is the rule with infection with the unnamed parasite of the Dominican Republic. The primary nodule spreads locally without ulceration, and secondary blood-borne lesions appear on other sites in the skin, often symmetrically, affecting especially the face and the cooler extensor surfaces of the limbs (Fig. 5). External genitalia may be affected, but the eye, mucosae, viscera, and peripheral nerves are spared, in contrast with lepromatous leprosy, which DCL superficially resembles. The infection proceeds gradually over many years.

Leishmaniasis recidivans or lupoid leishmaniasis

This is a rare complication especially of *L. tropica* infection. The sore heals, but despite the presence of well-established cellular immunity, papules recrudesce in the edge of the scar and the lesion spreads slowly over many years. It is most common on the face and may be destructive.

American mucosal leishmaniasis, espundia

Up to 40 per cent of patients with cutaneous ulcers due to *L. brasiliensis* may develop mucosal lesions, half of them within 2 years of the appearance of the original lesion, and 90 per cent within 10 years. Delays of up to 35 years have been reported. About one in six cases of mucosal leishmaniasis give no history of a previous primary skin lesion. In almost all cases the nasal mucosa is affected, and in a third another site is also involved: the pharynx, palate, larynx, and upper lip, in order of frequency. The initial lesion is a nodule or polyp, usually on the inferior

Fig. 3 Multiple crusted and nodular sores of cutaneous leishmaniasis due to *L. major*, Nigeria.

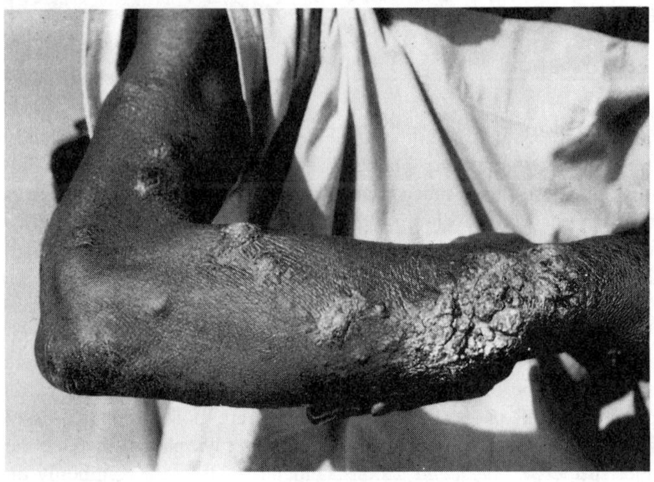

Fig. 4 Spreading nodular lesion, typical of *L. aethiopica*, Kenya.

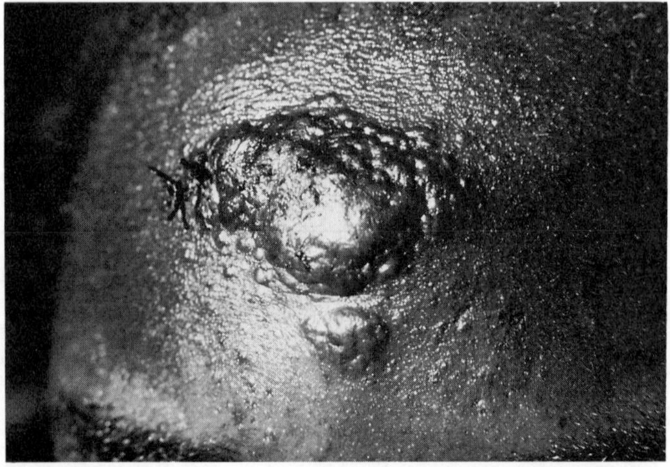

Fig. 5 Diffuse cutaneous leishmaniasis, caused by *L. aethiopica*, Ethiopia.

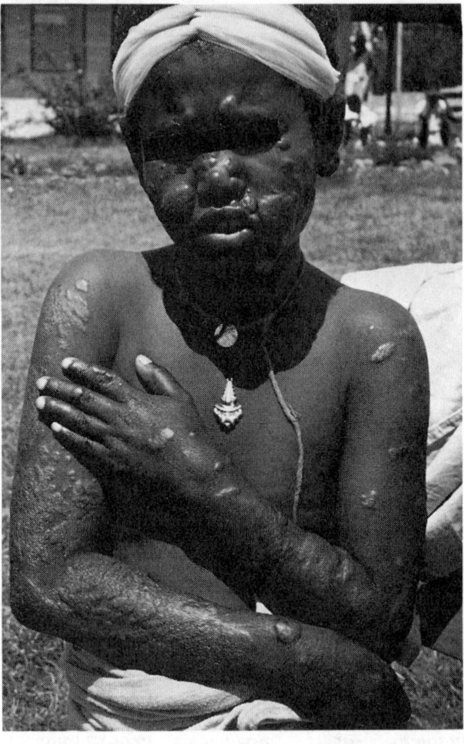

Fig. 6 Severe mutilation of mouth and nose in a Brazilian mucosal leishmaniasis due to *L. brasiliensis* (by courtesy of Professor Philip Marsden).

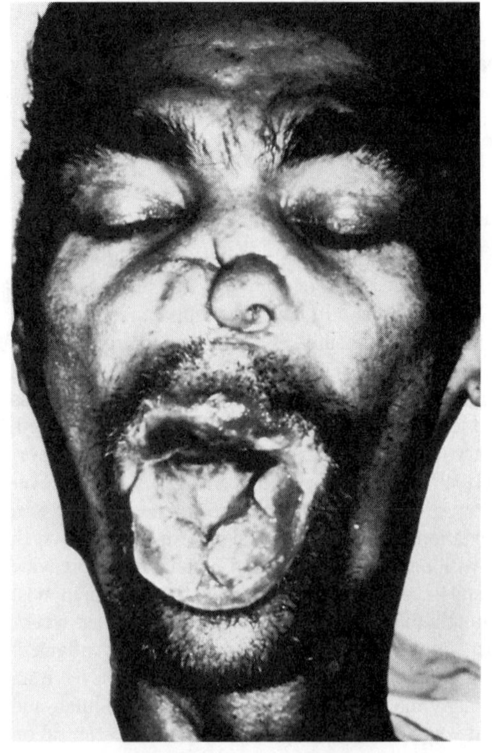

turbinate, and the initial symptom is of nasal obstruction. Mucosal leishmaniasis is slowly destructive, the septum perforates, and eventually the whole nose and mouth may be destroyed (Fig. 6). It commonly presents as protuberant overgrowth of the nose, or cicatrization, which causes an elongated 'tapir' nose. Death may result from secondary sepsis, starvation or laryngeal obstruction. *L. peruviana* does not cause mucosal leishmaniasis. The risk with *L. panamensis* and *L. guyanensis* is less than with *L. brasiliensis*.

LABORATORY FINDINGS

Parasitological diagnosis

Leishmania may normally be isolated from 80 per cent of sores during the first half of their natural course. After that, parasitological diagnosis becomes more difficult. The nodule, or the nodular edge of the ulcer, is grasped firmly between finger and thumb till it blanches. An incision is made a few millimetres long into the dermis with the point of a scalpel, which is used to scrape dermal tissue and juice, not blood. Material obtained may be used to inoculate special diphasic culture medium and to prepare smears for staining with Giemsa, Wright's, or Leishman's stain (Fig. 1). Occasionally it is necessary to remove the crust and obtain material from the base of the ulcer.

Biopsy material may be used to make impression smears and be ground for culture. Histological examination is less likely to reveal identifiable parasites, but sensitivity may be improved by immunological staining.

Species diagnosis is desirable for American parasites, to assess the risk of mucosal leishmaniasis. Isoenzyme techniques are the best developed but are too slow to be of immediate use in taking a decision on treatment. DNA hybridization and monoclonal antibody methods are suited to rapid diagnosis on a few smeared or cultured parasites, but are not yet generally available.

Diagnosis of mucosal leishmaniasis presents special problems because the lesion is often inaccessible and the parasites lie deeply in it. Deep-punch biopsy is usually necessary. If biopsy material is used and hamster inoculation is added to the isolation techniques, about 70 per cent of cases may be diagnosed parasitologically.

Immunological diagnosis

The leishmanin test is a test of delayed hypersensitivity which becomes positive in over 90 per cent of cases of cutaneous and mucosal leishmaniasis by the time of crusting or ulceration, and is 95 per cent specific. It may not be positive in all cases of *L. aethiopica* infection and is negative in DCL.

The antigen is a suspension of 10^5 washed promastigotes in 0.1 ml of 0.5 per cent phenol saline. The test should be standardized for each geographical area and parasite species. Clinical evaluation of a positive test must take into account naturally acquired positivity in the population at risk. Antibodies are not consistently produced in detectable titres, except in mucosal leishmaniasis, where enzyme immunoassay and immunofluorescence are useful for diagnosis and the latter for assessment of treatment.

TREATMENT

Old World sores or those due to *L. mexicana*, *L. amazonensis*, and *L. peruviana* that are not troublesome may be left to heal naturally. But those that are disfiguring, potentially disabling, inconvenient or around the ankle, where they heal slowly, should be treated either locally or systemically. Systemic treatment is required when there is risk that the sore may be due to *L. brasiliensis*, *L. panamensis*, or *L. guyanensis*, also when the sore is too large or badly sited for local treatment, if it is severely inflamed or ulcerated, if cartilage is invaded, or if there is lymphatic spread. Mucosal leishmaniasis, DCL, and recidivans leishmaniasis require systemic treatment (see also Tables 2 and 3.)

Table 3 *Simplified dosage regimens for pentavalent antimonials based on body surface area (BSA) according to the formula bsa* $m^2 = 0.1\sqrt[3]{kg^2}$*, whereby a 20 kg child receives 20 mg Sb/kg at 542 mg Sb/m²*

Nearest weight of patient (kg)	Calculated dose mg Sb	Recommended dose as ml of	
		Pentostam (mg Sb)	Glucantime (mg Sb)
90	1088	11.0 (1100)	13.0 (1105)
80	1006	10.0 (1000)	12.0 (1220)
70	925	9.5 (950)	11.0 (935)
60	832	8.5 (850)	10.0 (850)
50	737	7.5 (750)	9.0 (765)
40	635	6.5 (650)	7.5 (637)
30	524	5.0 (500)	6.0 (510)
20	400	4.0 (400)	5.0 (425)
10	252	2.5 (250)	3.0 (255)
5	159	2.0 (200)	2.5 (212)

Pentostam (Wellcome Foundation) = sodium stibogluconate solution, containing 100 mg Sb/ml. Glucantime (Specia) = meglumine antimoniate solution containing 85 mg Sb/ml.

Adapted from Anabwani and Bryceson, A.D.M. (1982). *Indian Paediatrics*, **19**, 819–22.

Local treatment

Surgery, curettage, and cryotherapy are methods of removing small sores. Temperatures above 37 °C kill cutaneous species of *Leishmania* and promote efficient lymphocyte and macrophage activity. Lesions accurately heated for several days at 40 to 42 °C with a thermostatically controlled electric pad or water sack will heal quickly. In my experience, local infiltration of drugs is difficult, painful, and unreliable, although others have reported success using pentavalent antimonials. Leishmanicidal ointments are under evaluation.

Systemic treatment

All cutaneous species of Leishmania are sensitive to pentavalent antimonials in conventional dosage (Table 2) except *L. aethiopica*, but there are special considerations in cutaneous disease. Pentavalent antimonials are poorly concentrated in the skin, and are less efficient than in visceral disease. Natural healing is disadvantaged because of low temperature, and lesions on the limbs often respond poorly to systemic treatment. The local application of heat is a useful adjunct. Acquired resistance to antimonials has been induced in *L. brasiliensis* in patients with mucosal leishmaniasis, and *L. amazonensis* in patients with DCL, because of the old practice of fixed, short courses of treatment and use of an excessive (28 mg Sb/kg) single daily dose, which was toxic and required the use of rest periods. It is essential to use an adequate dose for long enough and not to interrupt treatment. Most simple infections respond to pentavalent antimonial in a single daily dose of 10 to 20 mg Sb/kg once daily within 3 weeks. (See Tables 2 and 3). *L. panamensis* requires a full 20 mg Sb/kg daily. *L. brasiliensis* sores should be treated for a week beyond parasitological cure, usually about 3 weeks, to prevent mucosal leishmaniasis. *L. aethiopica* will respond slowly to a dose of 20 mg Sb/kg given every 12 h; but in cases of DCL or primary mucocutaneous disease due to this parasite pentamidine should be given in a dose of 4 mg/kg once *weekly*. Aminosidine is a useful alternative. Patients with DCL should be treated for at least 3 months longer than it takes to clear parasites from the skin, and relapses should be retreated promptly. Most cases of American mucosal leishmaniasis and of leishmaniasis recidivans may be cured by daily antimonial (20 mg Sb/kg if tolerated, and given for 4 to 6 weeks). Relapsed cases of mucosal leishmaniasis have usually become unresponsive to antimonials and should be treated with amphotericin B for at least 2 months. In addition, severe cases of mucosal leishmaniasis may require antibiotics for secondary sepsis, attention to nutrition, and later plastic surgery.

The antifungal azole drugs interfere with the synthesis of ergosterol, the essential sterol of leishmanial cell membranes. Ketocomazole, 600 mg orally for 30 days, shows promise in infections due to *L. major* and *L. panamensis.*

Visceral leishmaniasis

EPIDEMIOLOGY

Visceral leishmaniasis is found in four main zoogeographical zones (Table 1). In the belt that embraces the Mediterranean littoral and stretches across the Middle East and Central Asia, appearing again in Northern and Eastern China, *L. donovani* causes a zoonosis among domestic dogs, foxes, and jackals. Human disease is endemic in many places and children under 5 years of age are especially affected: hence this parasite is also named *L. infantum.* In other places the disease is sporadic. Non-immune adults such as tourists, hunters, and soldiers are susceptible. The Ganges and Brahmaputra river valleys of India and Bangladesh are the home of epidemic visceral leishmaniasis, or kala-azar, which returns approximately every 15 to 20 years and has spread into Burma, Assam, and other parts of the subcontinent. Humans are the reservoir. *P. argentipes* rests in cattle sheds and bites in the houses at night. In the interepidemic period the parasite survives in patients with post-kala-azar dermal leishmaniasis. The majority of cases are under 15 years old and mortality may be high.

Visceral leishmaniasis is endemic in large parts of rural Sudan and Kenya. The Nile rat, *Arvicanthus niloticus*, was incriminated as the reservoir in Sudan, but in Kenya this and other rodents harbour *L. major*, not *L. donovani.* The infection may be endemic, when older children and teenagers are most commonly affected. Sporadic cases also occur in nomads and visitors. An epidemic that began in southern Sudan in the late 1980s is still raging, and has caused over 40 000 deaths. It has been especially severe among refugees from the civil war. The disease is absent in subSaharan West Africa, but occasional cases have been reported from Sene-Gambia and from central and southern Africa.

In South America the disease is most common in north-eastern Brazil, where older children are affected. Foxes bring the infection to the homesteads while raiding chicken houses.

Visceral leishmaniasis may be transmitted by blood transfusion from subclinical cases and appear unexpectedly in immunosuppressed patients, for example after renal transplantation, or as a coinfection with the human immunodeficiency virus (HIV).

PATHOGENESIS

For every case of classical visceral leishmaniasis, there are about 30 subclinical infections. In these the infection is arrested either in the skin or in the viscera, with the formation of tuberculoid granulomata and the acquisition of leishmanian positivity and life-long immunity to *L. donovani.* A third of these cases develops a low transient titre of antileishmanial antibodies. In an endemic area of Brazil, severely malnourished children were eight times more likely to develop overt disease than were well-nourished children.

Established visceral infections are characterized by the failure of specific cell-mediated immunity. The leishmanin test is negative and lymphocytes do not respond *in vitro* to leishmanial antigens. The parasite multiplies freely in macrophages in the spleen, bone marrow, lymphoid tissues, and jejunal submucosa. In the liver Kupffer cells and occasionally hepatocytes are parasitized. Histological examination shows a variable degree of granuloma formation, and of interstitial inflammation that may lead to fibrosis. Parasites may also be found in dermal histiocytes and circulating monocytes. In the spleen especially there is massive reticuloendothelial hyperplasia and infiltration with plasma cells and Russell bodies. Small splenic infarcts may develop. The parasites themselves are not toxic.

Globulins are overproduced, especially IgG, some of which is antileishmanial antibody and some autoantibody, especially rheumatoid factor. Complement is activated and immune complexes, commonly containing IgM, circulate in high titre. Surprisingly these events seldom cause much anatomical damage or physiological disorder. Immune complex-mediated nephritis is rare. At autopsy, kidneys show tubular cloudy swelling and sometimes thickening of the glomerular mesangium, or amyloid deposition. Biochemical tests of hepatic function usually are virtually normal. The low plasma albumin probably reflects the intestinal lesion. About half the patients have mild malabsorption of xylose and vitamin A, but seldom diarrhoea. The cause of jaundice in visceral leishmaniasis is obscure: in my experience it is more usually due to intercurrent viral hepatitis than the disease itself or drugs. Spontaneous bleeding is unusual and is associated with hypoprothrombinaemia. Cardiopulmonary function, though never measured, seems unimpaired unless anaemia is very severe, but autopsy studies have shown a specific interstitial pneumonitis.

In adults, visceral leishmaniasis is characterized by anaemia, often associated with leucopenia and thrombocytopenia. The anaemia results mainly from shortened red-cell survival with destruction of cells in the spleen, together with splenic pooling and sequestration (hypersplenism). In young children, profound anaemia may develop rapidly as a result of severe haemolysis. Again, the red cells are destroyed largely in the spleen but the reason for the very short red-cell survival is not clear. Ferrokinetic studies indicate a mild degree of ineffective erythropoiesis, but the predominant defect is haemolysis. In a small proportion of cases Coombs' test is positive, but the significance of the finding is uncertain.

There is also a general suppression of cell-mediated immune responses, characterized by cutaneous anergy to intradermal antigens. *In vitro*, lymphocytes fail to respond to these antigens and their response to phytohaemagglutinin is reduced. Presumably this suppression, the leucopenia, and the hypoalbuminaemic malnutrition underlie the susceptibility to secondary infection that so often kills the patient with visceral leishmaniasis.

CLINICAL FEATURES

Although it is known that *L. infantum* may cause typical cutaneous leishmaniasis in parts of the Mediterranean basin, elsewhere skin lesions are not detectable in self-healing *L. donovani* infections, and patients with visceral leishmaniasis rarely show a primary or intercurrent skin lesion. In Sudan, marked lymphadenopathy with minor skin lesions may be due to *L. donovani.*

Males get visceral leishmaniasis three or four times more often than females. For age patterns see under Epidemiology. The incubation period is usually between 2 and 8 months. In endemic areas the onset is usually ill defined, and several months elapse before the patient seeks help because of fever, discomfort from an enlarged spleen, abdominal swelling, weight loss, cough, or diarrhoea. Classically the fever spikes twice daily, usually without rigors, but daily, irregular or undulant fevers are common. Europeans and Americans who have acquired the disease while visiting an endemic area more commonly experience an abrupt onset, with high fever and rapid progression of illness with toxaemia, weakness, dyspnoea, and acute anaemia.

Physical signs depend to some extent on the duration of the disease, the pre-existing nutritional state of the patient, and the presence of complications. Early cases, detected during field surveys, have only symptomless splenomegaly. Late cases are thin with wasted muscles. One-third show hair changes and pedal oedema typical of hypoalbuminaemia, but ascites is rare. Hyperpigmentation of face, hands, feet, and abdomen is characteristic of visceral leishmaniasis in India (kala-azar means black sickness). Occasionally, in Africa, leishmanial nodules may be found in the palate or nares. The spleen is massively enlarged, often reaching the left or even right iliac fossa. It is smooth and non-tender unless there has been a recent infarct. The liver is moderately enlarged in one-third of cases. Generalized lymphadenopathy is present in half the African patients, but is less common in India or Europe. Jaundice, mucosal and retinal haemorrhage, uveitis, and episcleritis are found occasionally.

COURSE AND COMPLICATIONS

Gradually over months or years the patient becomes emaciated and exhausted with a huge, protuberant abdomen (Fig. 7). Intercurrent infections are common, especially pneumococcal otitis, pneumonia and septicaemia, tuberculosis, measles, and other locally important infections such as brucellosis, bacillary dysentery, amoebic dysentery, and rarely, cancrum oris. Untreated, 80 to 90 per cent of patients die.

Post kala-azar dermal leishmaniasis (PKDL)

Twenty per cent of Indian patients and 5 per cent of African patients develop a rash on the face and extensor surfaces of the arms and legs after spontaneous or natural recovery. In India the rash begins after an interval of 1 or 2 years and progresses over many years: pale macules become erythematous plaques or nodules resembling lepromatous leprosy, and almost all the body surface may be involved (Fig. 8). Histology shows macrophages with a variable degree of parasitization, and a structureless infiltrate of lymphocytes and plasma cells. In Africa the rash appears while the patient is recovering, often before leaving hospital, as discrete nodules which show a tuberculoid histology. It heals spontaneously within 6 months. PKDL very rarely visceralizes, yet the parasite is enzymatically indistinguishable from its viscerotropic parent.

Visceral leishmaniasis and the acquired immune deficiency syndrome (AIDS)

Since 1986, visceral leishmaniasis has been recognized as a complication of infection with the human immunodeficiency virus (**HIV**). Visceral leishmaniasis is thought to represent reactivation of latent infection with Leishmania. The problem is greatest in southern Europe, where HIV and *L. infantum* are both endemic. In Spain, 50 per cent of adults with visceral leishmaniasis are HIV positive, and it is estimated that 3 per cent of HIV-infected individuals will acquire visceral leishmaniasis. The cardinal signs of visceral leishmaniasis in this situation are unexplained fever, splenomegaly, and leucopenia but the presentation may not be typical. Often the parasite is found by chance, for example in a rectal or skin biopsy taken for other purposes, or in broncheolar lavage. The bone marrow is teeming with parasites, but two-thirds of cases have no detectable antileishmanial antibodies. In 90 per cent of cases the CD4 count is under 0.3×10^6/l, and the CD4:CD8 ratio is under 1.

Fig. 7 Visceral leishmaniasis in a Kenyan child. Note the wasting and massive enlargement of spleen and liver.

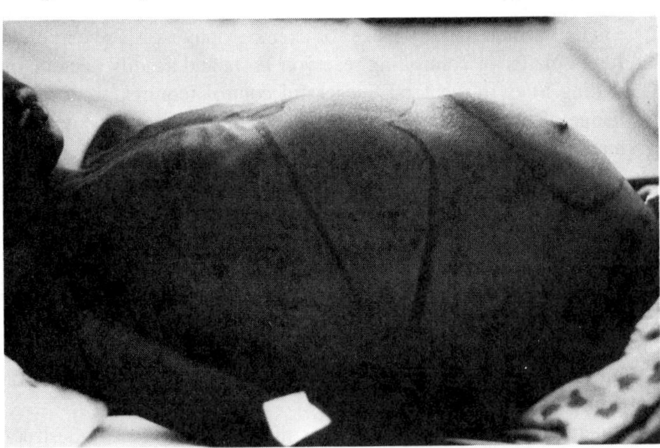

LABORATORY FINDINGS

Parasitological diagnosis

Leishmania may be isolated using the techniques described earlier from material taken from reticuloendothelial tissue. Positive yields are of the order: spleen over 95 per cent, bone marrow or liver 85 per cent, African lymph node 65 per cent, buffy coat 70 per cent. Bone marrow aspiration is most commonly used, but the technique is painful, requires special needles, and is insensitive in early cases. Splenic aspiration is simple, painless and safe if the prothrombin time is normal and the platelet count above 40×10^9/l. Palpate the spleen and mark its outline. Using a 1¼ inch × 21-gauge needle attached to a 5-ml disposable syringe, penetrate the skin over the spleen, pull the plunger back 1 ml and plunge the needle into the spleen upwards at an angle of 45 ° and withdraw instantly, maintaining suction. The tiny amount of material obtained is adequate to inoculate two culture tubes and make two to four smears. Afterwards, pulse and blood pressure are monitored for 8 h. Parasites in smears are usually extracellular, and if scanty demand a long, patient search. For research or in the management of difficult cases it is useful to quantitate the parasites on a logarithmic scale.

Culture is 1 log more sensitive than smears, and is seldom needed. Occasionally the diagnosis is made accidentally on biopsy of bone marrow, liver, lymph node, or jejunal mucosa.

Immunological diagnosis

Antibodies are present in high titre and detectable by all the usual techniques. Indirect immunofluorescence is suitable for individual cases, using amastigotes or promastigotes as antigen. There is some cross-reactivity, but at low titre, with antinuclear antibodies. Complement fixation was popular in the past, but sera are often anticomplementary. Enzyme-linked immunosorbent assay is the technique of choice for field diagnosis; it is over 95 per cent specific and sensitive. The direct agglu-

Fig. 8 Post-kala azar dermal leishmaniasis in an Indian child, showing the typical hypopigmented macular rash. Note also the nodules on the lower lip.

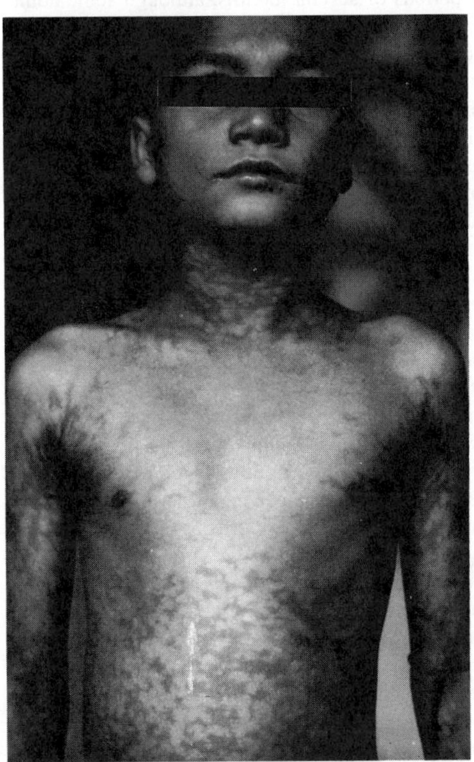

tination test is easier to do, but less specific. The leishmanin test is negative.

Other findings

The haemoglobin concentration is low (under 7 g/dl in half the patients) with a normochromic, normocytic picture in the absence of iron or folate deficiency. The anaemia usually reflects the chronicity of the infection, but sometimes develops rapidly. Often there is no reticulocytosis. Serum iron and total iron-binding capacity are reduced. Leucopenia (under 3×10^6/l) reflects neutropenia and eosinopenia. Lymphocyte counts are normal. The platelet count is usually around 100×10^9/l. Serum albumin is low (20 g/l) and globulin high (70 g/l), IgG and IgM being approximately thrice and twice the normal population values. Complement levels C4 and C3 are usually normal, but Clq and circulating immune complexes are high. Serum levels of tumour necrosis factor are raised 10 to 20-fold. Hepatic enzymes are normal or slightly elevated. Prothrombin and partial thromboplastin times are usually normal until late in the disease. There are no characteristic findings in the urine.

TREATMENT

Chemotherapy

Liposomal amphotericin B is the best drug for visceral leishmaniasis. It is concentrated and retained in reticuloendothelial cells and is not toxic. The optimal dosage has not yet been established, but is likely to be of the order of 2–3 mg/kg body weight daily for 10 days. All patients respond promptly, but immunosuppressed patients relapse. At the moment it is far too costly for most countries where visceral leishmaniasis is endemic.

A pentavalent antimonial remains the drug of choice. Two preparations are available: sodium stibogluconate containing 100 mg antimony (Sb) per ml and meglumine antimoniate containing 85 mg Sb/ml. When used in equivalent Sb doses they are of equal efficacy and toxicity. The elimination half-life of the major component is 2.5 h and 90 per cent of the drug is excreted in the urine in 8 h. The drug is preferentially concentrated in the liver and spleen.

In doses of 10 to 20 mg Sb/kg body weight daily, the drug is virtually non-toxic, even over periods of several months, although some adults become anorexic at the higher dose. Routine electrocardiograms are unnecessary using conventional dosage. Children require and tolerate more Sb/kg than adults.

Doses in excess of 20 mg Sb/kg body weight are usually toxic, causing malaise, anorexia, nausea, vomiting, and muscle pains. Hepatic enzyme levels may rise and haemoglobin levels fall, but return to normal when treatment is stopped. The electrocardiogram develops unimportant T-wave changes and occasionally prolongation of the corrected QT interval, which may herald the development of a serious arrhythmia. Table 3 recommends dosage based on body surface area, and thus takes into account the difference in requirements between children and adults. Using this regimen, adults do not receive the full 20 mg Sb/kg and are less likely to experience side-effects. Treatment is given for 3 to 4 weeks, according to the geographical area. If it is essential, for example during an epidemic, to give a shorter course of treatment, 10 mg Sb/kg may be given every 8 h for 10 days in complete safety.

The drug is given by intramuscular injection, which may be painful, or by intravenous injection through a fine-gauge needle, slowly to reduce the risk of venous thrombosis. Should toxic effects develop, rest for 1 day and reduce each dose by 2 mg Sb/kg.

The aminoglycoside antibiotic aminosidine (Gabbromycina, Carlo Erba Farmitalia) is equally effective and well tolerated, in a dose of 15 mg/kg body weight daily for 21 days by intramuscular injection or intravenous infusion over 90 min.

Patients who are immunoincompetent as a result of HIV coinfection or immunosuppressive drugs respond slowly, require longer treatment, and are more liable to relapse than immunocompetent patients. Ideally, treatment should be monitored by splenic aspirate counts of parasites, and continued to an extrapolated − 2 logs, usually about 2 to 3 weeks beyond parasitological curve. Aminosidine is the drug of choice, as it is well tolerated and not prohibitively expensive. Renal function and hearing should be monitored.

Supportive treatment

Intercurrent infection must be sought and treated. Patients with tuberculosis should be given 2 weeks extra antimony as they are more likely to relapse. The stool should be examined for parasitic cysts and ova, and cultured if there is diarrhoea. Haemorrhage is usually associated with hypoprothrombinaemia, which may be correctable by vitamin K. Blood transfusion is rarely needed. A protein-rich diet should be provided and specific nutritional deficiencies corrected.

Response to treatment

Patients usually feel better, and fever stops within a few days. Haemoglobin levels start to rise in the second week. Fever, splenic size, haemoglobin, serum albumin, and body weight are the most useful monitors of progress. Proof of parasitological cure is not usually necessary once the optimum duration of treatment has been established in that area.

Reassessment at 6 weeks and 6 months will detect over 90 per cent of relapses, except in eastern Africa where a further examination at 1 year is advised. Serum albumin level becomes normal within 6 weeks, haemoglobin and globulin levels within 6 months. The spleen normally becomes impalpable within 1 year. Persistent splenomegaly may be due to relapse or to other endemic diseases such as malaria or schistosomiasis. Normally there are no sequelae, though in some countries cirrhosis has been attributed to visceral leishmaniasis. About 80 per cent of patients acquire cellular hypersensitivity to leishmanial antigens gradually between 3 and 12 months. The 20 per cent that remain anergic are not especially liable to relapse, but are presumed non-immune.

Using the regimens above, relapse rates should be almost zero in Mediterranean and Indian disease and about 2 per cent in African disease. Relapsed patients are slower to respond, and run a 40 per cent chance of further relapse(s) and of becoming unresponsive to antimony. Relapsed patients should be treated with 20 mg Sb/kg daily for at least 8 weeks, monitored by quantitative weekly splenic aspirates.

About 1 per cent of previously untreated patients will fail to respond to antimony. Primary resistance is increasing in India. Unresponsiveness is, however, usually secondary to previous courses of antimony, often inadequate in dose or duration, or interrupted, and is due to parasite resistance to the drug. The options are: (i) aminosidine; (ii) amphotericin B in a dose of 0.5 to 1 mg/kg by intravenous infusion on alternate days for 2 to 4 weeks; (iii) AmBisome.

PREVENTION AND CONTROL OF CUTANEOUS AND VISCERAL LEISHMANIASIS

There is no vaccine nor any place for chemoprophylaxis. Prevention is therefore a matter of controlling reservoir hosts and sandfly vectors, or of avoiding bites by vectors. Successful control requires an accurate knowledge of transmission for each parasite or ecological focus. Such information is not always available.

In the Old World, urban cutaneous leishmaniasis is controlled by case-finding and treatment, better housing, and domestic spraying with residual insecticides, while rural leishmaniasis is controlled in the Middle East and North Africa by destruction of gerbil colonies. Traditionally in the Middle East, and currently in Israel, live virulent *L. major* is inoculated to cause an immunizing infection under controlled conditions. In the New World, cutaneous leishmaniasis of the forest cannot be controlled, but *L. peruviana* infections may be, by treatment or destruction of infected dogs.

Mediterranean visceral leishmaniasis may be controlled by destruction or treatment of dogs, but the reservoir in foxes persists. In India, mass campaigns to spray houses and cattle sheds are needed, supplemented during epidemics by early diagnosis and treatment. In the inter-epidemic period, cases of PKDL should be sought and treated.

Individuals may take precautions to prevent infection during the season of transmission. Against day-biting sandflies long sleeves and trousers should be worn, and insect repellent creams applied to exposed skin. At night, individuals should sleep under fine mesh nets that have been impregnated with permethrin.

REFERENCES

Altes, J. *et al.* (1991). Visceral leishmaniasis: another HIV-associated opportunistic infection? Report of eight cases and review of the literature. *AIDS*, **5,** 201–7.

Cerf, B.J., Jones, T.C., Badaro, R., Sampaio, D., Teixeira R. and Johnson, W.D., Jr. (1987). Malnutrition as a risk factor for severe visceral leishmaniasis. *Journal of Infectious Diseases*, **156,** 1030–3.

Davidson, R.N., Di Martino, L., Gradoni, L., *et al.* (1994). Liposomal amphotericin B (Ambisome) in Mediterranean visceral leishmaniasis. *Quarterly Journal of Medicine*, **87,** 75–81.

Duarte, M.I.S. and Corbett, C.E.P. (1987). Histopathological patterns of the liver involvement in visceral leishmaniasis. *Revista do Instituto de Medicina Tropical de São Paolo*, **29,** 131–6.

Grimaldi, G., Jr., Tesh, R.B., and McMahon-Pratt D. (1989). A review of the distribution and epidemiology of leishmaniasis in the New World. *American Journal of Tropical Medicine and Hygiene*, **41,** 687–725.

Grogl, M., Thomason, T.N., and Franke, E.D. (1992). Drug resistance in leishmaniasis: its implication in systemic chemotherapy of cutaneous and mucocutaneous disease. *American Journal of Tropical Medicine and Hygiene*, **47,** 117–26.

Ho, M., Keoch, D.K., Iha, D.W., and Bryceson A.D.M. (1983). Immunosuppression in Kenyan visceral leishmaniasis. *Clinical and Experimental Immunology*, **51,** 207–14.

Hommel, M. (1978). The genus *Leishmania*: biology of the parasites and clinical aspects. *Bulletin of the Institut Pasteur*, **76,** (the whole volume).

Jahn, A. and Diesfeld, H.J. (1983). Evaluation of a visually read ELISA for serodiagnosis and sero-epidemiological studies of kala-azar in the Baringo District, Kenya. *Transactions of the Royal Society of Tropical Medicine and Hygiene*, **32,** 451–8.

Kozevnikov, P.K. (1963). Two nosological forms of cutaneous leishmaniasis. *American Journal of Tropical Medicine and Hygiene*, **12,** 719–24.

Lara, M.L. *et al.* (1991). Immunogenetics of human American cutaneous leishmaniasis: study of HLA haplotypes in 24 families from Venezuela. *Human Immunology*, **30,** 129–35.

Lightner, L.K., Chulay, J.D., and Bryceson, A.D.M. (1983). Comparison of microscopy and culture in the detection of *Leishmania donovani* from splenic aspirates. *American Journal of Tropical Medicine and Hygiene*, **32,** 296–9.

Llanos Cuentas, E.A., Cuba, C.C., Barreto, A.C., and Marsden P.D. (1984). Clinical characteristics of human *Leishmania brasiliensis brasiliensis* infection. *Transaction of the Royal Society of Tropical Medicine and Hygiene*, **78,** 845–6.

Muigai, R., Gatei, D.G., Shaunak, S., Wozniak, A., and Bryceson, A.D.M. (1983). Jejunal function and pathology in visceral leishmaniasis. *Lancet*, **ii,** 476–9.

Netto, E.M. *et al.* (1990). Long-term follow-up of patients with *Leishmania (Vianna) braziliensis* infection and treated with Glucantime. *Transactions of the Royal Society of Tropical Medicine and Hygiene*, **84,** 367–70.

Olliaro, P. and Bryceson, A.D.M. (1993). Practical progress and new drugs for changing patterns of leishmaniasis. *Parasitology Today*, **9,** 323–8.

Pampiglione, S., Manson-Bahr, P.E.C., La Placa, M., Borgatti, M.A., and Musumeci, S. (1975). Studies in Mediterranean leishmaniasis 3: the leishmanin skin test in kala-azar. *Transactions of the Royal Society of Tropical Medicine and Hygiene*, **69,** 60–8.

Ridley, D.S. and Ridley, M.J. (1983). The evolution of the lesion in cutaneous leishmaniasis. *Journal of Pathology*, **141,** 83–96.

Rodgers, M.R., Popper, S.J., and Wirth D.F. (1990). Amplification of kinetoplast DNA as a tool in the detection and diagnosis of *Leishmania. Experimental Parasitology*, **71,** 267–75.

Walton, B.C. (1980). Evaluation of chemotherapy of American Leishmaniasis by the indirect fluorescent antibody test. *American Journal of Tropical Medicine and Hygiene*, **29,** 747–52.

Weigle K.A., de Davalos M., Heredia, H., Molineros, R., Saravia N.G., and d'Alessandro, A.D. (1987). Diagnosis of cutaneous and mucocutaneous leishmaniasis in Colombia: a comparison of seven methods. *American Journal of Tropical Medicine and Hygiene*,**36,** 489–96.

World Health Organization (1990). *Control of the leishmaniases, Technical Report Series* 793. No. WHO, Geneva.

7.13.13 Trichomoniasis

J. P. Ackers

Trichomoniasis is caused by infection with the protozoan parasite *Trichomonas vaginalis*; an important cause of vaginal discharge and other symptoms in women, it is much less often diagnosed in men.

T. vaginalis is a motile, round or oval flagellate, approximately 10 to 13 μm long and 8 to 10 μm wide when living; fixed and stained it is about 25 per cent smaller. Diagnostic features include the jerky motility, induced by four anterior flagella and the undulating membrane, and a rigid, microtubular rod (the axostyle), which runs through the body and projects as a long, thin spine from the posterior end. Staining reveals a nucleus, a prominent Golgi-like organelle (the parabasal body), and a large number of dense granules. *T. vaginalis* is both phagocytic and pinocytotic but will grow happily in complex but particle-free media. Its metabolism is basically anaerobic and fermentative, although it tolerates oxygen. The dense granules have been named hydrogenosomes; otherwise found only in a few anaerobic protozoa and fungi, they are unrelated but functionally equivalent to mitochondria (which are not found in trichomonads). They are the site of the oxidation of pyruvate to acetate and hydrogen, while the earlier glycolytic enzymes are cytosolic. Otherwise *T. vaginalis* is, biochemically, fairly limited, relying upon external sources for many amino acids, purines, pyrimidines, and lipids. The life-cycle is simple, multiplication being by binary fission. No resistant cysts are formed and no intermediate or reservoir hosts involved in transmission.

Two other trichomonads are rare human parasites—*T. tenax*, which is normally found in the periodontal crevices but which may possibly, very rarely, spread to the respiratory tract, and *Pentatrichomonas hominis*, which is an uncommon and probably commensal inhabitant of the large bowel. All three species appear to be site specific and urogenital trichomoniasis is not due to contamination from other sites.

Pathology

In women, *T. vaginalis* may be found in the vagina and the exterior cervix in over 95 per cent of infections, but is only recovered from the endocervix in 13 per cent. The urethra and Skene's glands are also very commonly infected. Dissemination beyond the lower urogenital tract is extremely rare and is not found even in severely immunocompromised patients. There is a definite predilection for squamous epithelium under the influence of oestrogen. It is possible that female trichomoniasis may slightly increase the probability of HIV virus transmission via heterosexual intercourse. In men, the urethra is the most common site of infection, but the organism has also been recovered from epididymal aspirates. Prostatic involvement has been reported, but its frequency and significance are not clear.

In vitro T. vaginalis has a well-defined, contact-mediated, cytotoxic effect, but the relation of this to pathogenesis *in vivo* is not known. The organism activates complement and thus attracts neutrophils several of which can cooperate to kill the parasite, but their presence in large numbers may be responsible for much of the pathology observed.

Epidemiology

Despite the difficulty often experienced in isolating the organism from male contacts of infected women, all epidemiological evidence suggests that the vast majority of infections are sexually acquired. As cultured *T. vaginalis* have been shown to survive for many hours if kept damp (for example on sponges or face-cloths) the theoretical possibility of non-venereal transmission exists. It is also known that a small proportion (5 per cent or less) of female babies of infected mothers will themselves be infected during birth, but there is no real evidence that the infection can persist until puberty and any infection discovered in a child should immediately raise the suspicion of sexual abuse.

Few, if any, studies have been made of genuinely unselected populations, but it has been estimated that in the United States 3 million, and world-wide 180 million, women contract the infection each year. Most surveys have examined either pregnant women or those attending sexually transmitted disease clinics; there are wide national variations, but most report 10 to 25 per cent infected, although the full range is 0 to 63 per cent. The highest incidence coincides with the years of maximum sexual activity. In most clinic surveys, female cases outnumber male by 5 or 10 to 1, partly because the number of parasites in males is usually much lower than in females and because the proportion of male partners of infected women who are diagnosed positive declines quite rapidly with time after exposure. In several developed countries there has been a sharp decline in the incidence of trichomoniasis in the past decade; it is not known why this has occurred, nor whether it is a world-wide phenomenon.

Symptoms

Multiple infections are common in patients with trichomoniasis, which makes it difficult to extract the symptoms specifically due to *T. vaginalis*. A recent study eliminated confounding effects and showed that trichomoniasis remained significantly associated with symptoms of yellow vaginal discharge and vulvar itching, and signs of colpitis macularis ('strawberry cervix'), purulent vaginal discharge, and vulval and vaginal erythema. Colpitis was seen frequently if colposcopy was undertaken, but hardly ever found by naked-eye examination. Dyspareunia, mild dysuria, and lower abdominal pain are also described, although less frequently than the above, and in most series 10 to 50 per cent of women are asymptomatic. Vaginal pH is usually elevated.

The majority of men with trichomoniasis are asymptomatic, but the parasite is clearly responsible for a small but significant proportion (5–15 per cent) of non-gonococcal urethritis. The discharge is usually only present in very small amounts, but the condition is not clinically distinguishable from other types of non-gonococcal urethritis.

Diagnosis

The symptoms and signs described above are in no case sufficient to establish the diagnosis, which must be made by detecting the parasite. This is most frequently (and most cheaply) done by wet-film microscopic examination of vaginal (not endocervical) secretions, urethral scrapings mixed with a drop of saline, centrifuged urine sediment or prostate fluid. The specimen should be examined as soon as possible: a motile trichomonad is unmistakable, while a rounded up or dead one is nearly unrecognizable. Size and jerky motility are all but diagnostic; identification is confirmed by observing the flagella (in healthy organisms they will be moving too quickly to be counted) and the undulating membrane. Phase-contrast dark-field or bright-field illumination with the substage condenser almost closed should be used. This procedure will detect about half to three-quarters of infected women, but only 10 to 20 per cent of infected men; staining procedures (acridine orange, Giemsa) do not seem to help. Papanicolaou-stained cervical smears detect *T. vaginalis* with about the same sensitivity as wet films, but the specificity is low and false positives common. The inflammatory response to the parasite makes examining cervical smears from infected women unreliable, but there is no evidence that *T. vaginalis* can induce premalignant changes.

At present, culture is the only technique with significantly greater sensitivity; media vary in efficiency but several very good ones are described (see References). Most will be positive within 48 h but should be kept for 7 to 10 days before being finally discarded. A number of new immunological tests, some available in kit form, are coming into use; although still experimental and expensive, they can combine the speed of the wet film with the sensitivity of culture methods.

Treatment

The 5-nitroimidazole drugs were introduced in 1960 and provided the first and so far only group of effective chemotherapeutic agents. All these drugs have similar potencies and success rates but differ somewhat in their pharmacokinetics. Doses given here are for metronidazole and should be adjusted to give the equivalent amount of other compounds. Two regimens are used—the original one of 250 mg, three times a day for 7 days; or alternatively a single 2-g dose. The advantages of the single-dose regimen include better compliance and less interference with the normal flora, but side-effects (nausea, metallic taste, disulphiram-like reaction to alcohol) may be more noticeable. Cure rates in women are similar (about 95 per cent) with both regimens if male sexual partners are also treated, but appear to be lower with the single-dose regimen if they are not. Only the 7-day regimen has been extensively evaluated in males, where it is equally effective. The acute toxicity of metronidazole is low, but it is a mutagen and long-term, high-dose administration to mice can produce lung tumours. Follow-up of treated women has failed to show any excess malignancies and any risk from short-term treatment appears to be very small. Similarly, there is no evidence that the drug is teratogenic, but it does cross the placenta and it seems only prudent to avoid its use during the first trimester if at all possible. Local treatments (such as 100 mg of clotrimazole intravaginally, or simple douching) have very disappointing long-term cure rates but may be of value in controlling symptoms during pregnancy until metronidazole can be used. In considering whether or not to treat it should be borne in mind that there is a small amount of evidence linking trichomoniasis with preterm delivery and low birthweight.

Treatment failures with any of the 5-nitromidazole drugs are rare, but a small but slowly growing proportion is due to resistant isolates. Careful measurement of sensitivity *in vitro* under controlled oxygen tension is necessary to obtain consistent results, but a high level of resistance can be shown in some isolates. Although still a minor anxiety, the literature before 1960 shows clearly the misery caused by untreatable female trichmoniasis, and it is alarming that no alternative therapy is available.

REFERENCES

Ackers, J.P. and Yule, A. (1988). Immunological diagnosis of Trichomoniasis. In *Immunological diagnosis of sexually transmitted diseases*, (ed. H. Young and A. McMillan), pp. 275–302. Dekker, New York.

Borchardt, K.A. and Smith, R.F. (1991). An evaluation of an InPouch TV culture method for diagnosing *Trichomonas vaginalis* infection. *Genitourinary Medicine*, **67**, 149–52.

Bramley, M. (1976). Study of female babies of women entering confinement with vaginal trichomoniasis. *British Journal of Venereal Diseases*, **52,** 58–62.

British Co-operative Clinical Group (1992). An investigation, by questionnaire, of cases of recalcitrant vaginal trichomoniasis seen in genitourinary medicine clinics in the United Kingdom. *International Journal of STD and AIDS*, **3,** 24–7.

Gardner, W.A., Jr., Culberson, D.E., and Bennett, B.D. (1986). *Trichomonas vaginalis* in the prostate gland. *Archives of Pathology and Laboratory Medicine*, **110,** 430–2.

Honigberg, B.M. (ed.) (1989). *Trichomonads parasitic in humans*. Springer-Verlag, New York.

Laga, M., *et al.* (1993). Non-ulcerative sexually transmitted diseases as risk factors for HIV-1 transmission in women: results from a cohort study. *AIDS*, **7,** 95–102.

Langley, J.G., Goldsmid, J.M., and Davies, N. (1987). Venereal trichomoniasis: role of men. *Genitourinary Medicine*, **63,** 264–7.

Lossick, J.G. (1990). Treatment of sexually transmitted vaginosis/vaginitis. *Reviews of Infectious Diseases*, **12,(suppl. 6),** S665–81.

Lossick, J.G. and Kent, H.L. (1991). Trichomoniasis: trends in diagnosis and management. *American Journal of Obstetrics And Gynecology*, **165,** 1217–22.

Saxena, S.B. and Jenkins, R.R. (1991). Prevalence of *Trichomonas vaginalis* in men at high risk for sexually transmitted diseases. *Sexually Transmitted Diseases*, **18,** 138–42.

Wolner Hanssen, P. *et al.* (1989). Clinical manifestations of vaginal trichomoniasis. Journal of the American Medical Association, **261,** 571–6.

7.14 Nematodes

7.14.1 Filiariasis

B. O. L. DUKE

General principles of filarial infections and diseases

THE PARASITES AND THE DISEASES THEY CAUSE

Clinicians called upon to diagnose and treat patients with filarial infections need to be aware of the general features of this group of diseases.

It is estimated that well over 100 million people living in tropical countries have detectable infections with one or more of the pathogenic human filarial parasites. Perhaps 10 times that number live in areas where these parasites are endemic and are therefore at risk of infection. Filarial parasites thus present an enormous public health problem.

There are nine recognized filarial species for which man is the normal definitive host. Six commonly cause disease, namely *Wuchereria bancrofti*, *Brugia malayi*, and *B. timori*, the widespread lymphatic-dwelling filarial worms causing filarial fever, adenolymphangitis, and elephantiasis; *Onchocerca volvulus* causing cutaneous onchocerciasis and river blindness; *Loa loa*, which produces Calabar swellings; and *Mansonella streptocerca*, which causes minor itching and depigmented skin lesions that may be confused with early leprosy. The three others, *M. perstans, M. semiclarum*, and *M. ozzardi* are, with rare exceptions, non-pathogenic and may be regarded as common but incidental parasitoses.

Some *Dirofilaria* spp., which normally parasitize dogs or other animals, are occasionally transmitted to man, in whom they may undergo partial or aberrant development and thus cause disease.

GEOGRAPHICAL DISTRIBUTION

In the tropics the clinician must know which parasites occur in the country where he or she is practising. In non-tropical practice it must be ascertained which filarial parasites are endemic in the area from which the patient comes or to which he has paid a visit.

LIFE HISTORY OF THE PARASITE AND ITS VECTORS

As aids to diagnosis and prognosis, the clinician should know the probable duration of life of the various stages of the parasite, and should appreciate which stage(s) of each parasite cause the manifestations of disease. The clinician also needs to know which insects are vectors of the various parasites so that the patient can be warned of the dangers of re-exposure and given advice on simple measures to avoid reinfection.

Adult filarial worms live in the lymphatic vessels, the subcutaneous and deep connective tissues, or the serous cavities, according to species. Their life-spans extend for many years. The fertilized females produce a continuous supply of living motile embryos, known as microfilariae, which find their way to the blood or skin according to species. The life-span of microfilariae is of the order of 6 to 24 months and they do not develop further unless they are ingested by a blood-feeding female insect capable of acting as a vector or intermediate host of the parasite concerned. The microfilariae of some species living in the blood exhibit periodicity, that is, they are only found in the peripheral blood at a certain period of the 24 h, which coincides with the biting activity of the vector. The rest of the time they lie hidden in the pulmonary circulation.

Inside the vector the microfilariae develop, without multiplying, for 6 to 15 days when, after moulting three times, they become infective (third-stage) larvae or L_3, lying mainly in the head and proboscis of the insect. When the insect again bites man they burst out and enter the human host through the wound made by the proboscis. The L_3 moults within a few days to the L_4 stage, which then migrates to the adult sites and moults again to form an immature adult. In man, development from the L_3 to the adult worm, with production of detectable microfilariae, takes some 3 to 18 months according to species.

INTENSITY OF INFECTION

One L_3 inoculated into a human remains as one worm, male or female and, when adult, it needs to find and mate with another worm of the opposite sex before microfilariae can be produced. Although one (re) fertilized and fecund female can produce large numbers of microfilariae, either continuously or intermittently, throughout her life, those microfilariae that are not ingested by a vector will eventually die in the body. It follows that repeated exposure to L_3 over a period of years is necessary before infections of high intensity (whether in terms of adult worms or microfilariae) can build up in the human host.

INFECTION VERSUS DISEASE

In areas where filarial parasites are endemic it is very likely that a large proportion of the human population will be infected. A smaller proportion will have infections that are detectable parasitologically, and a smaller proportion still will show signs and symptoms of filarial disease. Not everyone who harbours a filarial infection is in need of treatment and often it is only those who have manifest disease, or who are at high risk of developing disease, that need treatment.

In endemic areas usually it is heavily infected persons who are most likely to show severe signs and symptoms of filarial disease. Unfortunately such patients are often the most difficult to treat for they may suffer severe reactions when large numbers of parasites die in their tissues as a result of treatment. On the other hand, it may not be necessary to get rid of all the filarial parasites in a heavily infected patient in order to reduce the risk of disease developing. A light residual infection may be well tolerated in place of a heavy disease-producing infection.

IMMUNOLOGICAL FACTORS AND EXPOSURE IN EARLY LIFE

The immunological response of the patient to a filarial parasite may also be of great importance in the production of disease. People who are first exposed in adult life frequently suffer severely from relatively light infections, whereas those who have been exposed to filarial antigens *in utero* or to transmission from early childhood may develop a good degree of tolerance to their parasites. However, there are also certain individuals who mount excessive immunological responses to their parasites and this may lead to the appearance of severe disease syndromes.

NUTRITIONAL STATUS AND CONCOMITANT DISEASE

Patients born, bred, and living in the rural tropics are often malnourished, heavily infected, and harbour a number of other helminthic, protozoal, or bacterial infections. Treatment of their filarial disease may present a much more difficult clinical problem than does the treatment of an otherwise healthy and well-nourished expatriate who has acquired a light infection during a short spell in the tropics.

MULTIPLE INFECTIONS WITH FILARIAL PARASITES

In some tropical countries, multiple infections with filarial infections are common. In parts of Africa, *O. volvulus*, *L. Loa*, *W. bancrofti*, *M. perstans*, and *M. streptocerca* may be found in the same patient. Reactions to a concomitant infection may complicate the treatment of the parasite that is causing clinical disease, especially if both are susceptible to the same drug.

DIAGNOSIS

The diagnosis of filariasis has to be made largely on clinical or parasitological grounds. Immunological tests, although improving in their specificity and sensitivity, still have a limited role to play. However, in puzzling cases, if all the available immunological tests are negative, the diagnosis of filariasis (*sensu lato*) becomes unlikely. By contrast, a positive result, while consistent with the diagnosis of filariasis, does not necessarily prove that the clinical picture is due to such an infection.

CHEMOTHERAPY

Many of the adverse reactions to chemotherapy are due to the death of parasites in the tissues, and much of the skill in treatment consists in damping down these reactions, either by the use of anti-inflammatory compounds or by giving low doses of the filaricide at the outset.

Specific filaricides are few and by no means entirely satisfactory in their actions. However, the advent of ivermectin (Mectizan®) in 1987 has greatly improved the prospects of large-scale control and suppression of onchocerciasis, and it may well also improve some aspects of the treatment of lymphatic filarial infections and of loiasis.

Diethylcarbamazine citrate has been replaced by Mectizan as the microfilaricide for treatment of onchocerciasis, but it is still widely used for its macrofilaricidal action against Wuchereria and Brugia infections. It is believed to act mainly by 'unmasking' filarial parasites so that they are suddenly recognized as foreign bodies to be destroyed by the host's defence system.

Suramin remains as an effective but potentially toxic macrofilaricide for *O. volvulus*. It has recently been joined by amocarzine, which has similar actions but is also potentially toxic. Melarsonyl potassium and other arsenicals should never be used on account of the dangers of arsenical encephalopathy; antimonials should be avoided as being too toxic and uncertain in their action; mebendazole, levamisole, metrifonate, and sundry other partial microfilaricides now have little or no place in the treatment of filarial diseases.

REFERENCES

Denham, D.A. (1978). *Counting and identifying microfilariae*, pp. 1–24. London School of Hygiene and Tropical Medicine.

Meyers, W.M., Neafie, R.C., Connor, D.H., Anderson, J., and Font, R.L. (1976). Diseases caused by filarial nematodes. In *Pathology of tropical and extraordinary diseases*, (ed. C.H. Binford and D.H. Connor), pp. 340–96. Armed Forces Institute of Pathology, Washington DC.

Sasa, M. (1976). *Human filariasis—a global survey of epidemiology and control*, pp. 1–819. University Park Press, Baltimore.

Onchocerciasis

GEOGRAPHICAL DISTRIBUTION AND VECTORS

Transmission of *Onchocerca volvulus* occurs mainly near the fast-flowing watercourses where the Simulium vectors (black-flies) breed (Fig. 1). In Africa, infection may be acquired from members of the *S. damnosum* complex across the tropical subSaharan belt, reading from west to east, in Senegal, Mali, Burkina Faso, Niger, Guinea Bissau, Guinea, Sierra Leone, Liberia, Côte d'Ivoire, Ghana, Togo, Benin, Nigeria, Cameroon, Chad, Central African Republic, Gabon, Congo, Zaire, Equatorial Guinea, Burundi, Angola, Sudan, Ethiopia, Uganda, Tanzania, and Malawi. There is also a focus in Yemen. Species of the *S. neavei* complex are important vectors locally in parts of East and Central Africa.

In America, *S. ochraceum* is the main vector in Guatemala and Mexico. Smaller foci occur in Venezuela (*S. metallicum* and *S. pintoi*), Brazil (*S. amazonicum/sanguineum* group), Ecuador (*S. exiguum* and *S. quadrivittatum*), and Colombia (*S. exiguum*).

LIFE-CYCLE OF THE PARASITE AND PATHOLOGY

The adult worms (males 5 cm × 0.2 mm; females 50 cm × 0.4 mm) live in fibrous nodules (Fig. 2). They have an average life-span of 9 to 10 years but may live up to 15 years. Some nodules are subcutaneous and palpable; others, probably more numerous, lie deep and impalpable, between the muscles, and against the capsules of joints (especially the hip joint) or the periosteum of the long bones. Very occasionally a nodule may suppurate, but usually they cause no clinical manifestations *per se*.

The microfilariae are large (220–350 × 5–9 mm). They can live for 12 to 24 months, and they cause almost all the pathology of onchocerciasis. In the skin, their presence, and especially their death, provokes small granulomatous reactions infiltrated with eosinophils, which lead to itching and a rash. Prolonged and heavy infection of the skin leads to fibrosis, scarring of the papillae, replacement of dermal collagen by hyalinized scar, and atrophic changes. When microfilariae invade the eye, either directly from the skin to the conjunctiva and cornea, or via the sheaths of the posterior ciliary vessels to reach the interior of the globe, they give rise to all the ocular lesions of the disease. The pathology of the anterior-segment lesions centres on microfilarial granulomata; that of the posterior-segment lesions is not so well understood. Although microfilariae have been found in the retina and optic nerve, there may

Fig. 1 Simulium (black-fly) vector of onchocerciasis.

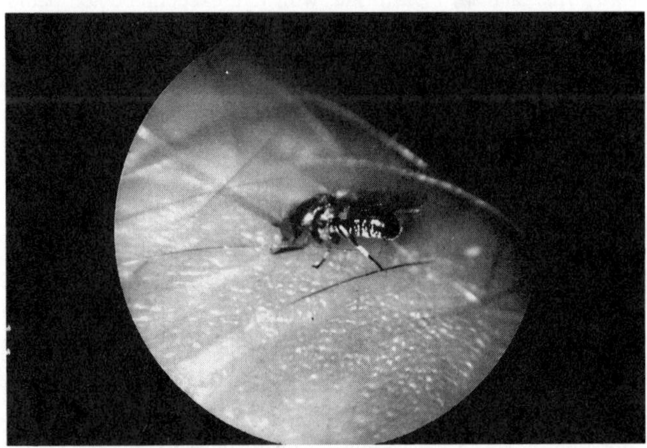

Fig. 2 Adult worms in excised nodules.

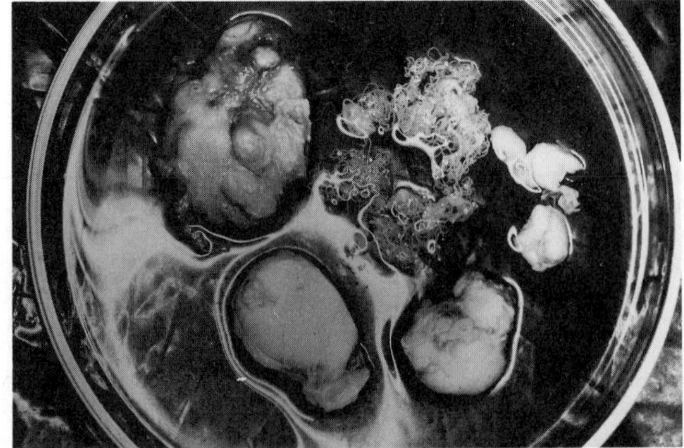

also be an autoimmune response to retinal proteins incited by the presence of parasites.

The prepatent interval between the inoculation of infective larvae by Simulium and the first appearance of microfilariae in the skin is usually 9 to 18 months.

CLINICAL PICTURE

The clinical picture in heavily infected patients varies from one geographical area to another. In the hot Sudan–savanna zones of West and Central Africa, severe eye lesions (especially sclerosing keratitis) are common and the overall blindness rate in the worst-affected villages may reach 15 per cent. In the forest zones of West and Central Africa, blindness rates are generally lower but skin changes and lymphatic lesions may be marked. In Mexico and Guatemala, head nodules are common and, if untreated, may be associated with blindness; but skin lesions are generally mild. In South America, skin disease may be severe but there are few serious eye lesions. In Yemen, an exaggerated cutaneous and lymphatic form of the disease is common. It usually affects one limb and is known as *sowda* (the Arabic word for black) (Fig. 3). There is considerable evidence that there are different forms or strains of *O. volvulus* associated with the different clinical patterns of the disease in various geographical or bioclimatic zones.

Palpable nodules

Subcutaneous, palpable nodules normally lie over bony prominences, especially the knees, trochanters, iliac crests, ribs, and scapulae (Fig. 4). Those on the head must be searched for carefully and removed. The patient should be asked to help in locating them, and it is sometimes necessary to shave the head in order to find them. A common site for small nodules is behind the ear.

Skin lesions

'Acute' lesions

Those who most commonly present for treatment are lightly and recently infected individuals, including expatriates and some indigenous people, who become infected for the first time in later childhood or adult life during temporary residence in an area of transmission. They present on account of the pruritic cutaneous lesions of onchocerciasis (*gâle filarienne*).

Typically such individuals harbour an adult worm or worms (often impalpable) in the subcutaneous or deep tissues on one side of the limb girdle concerned. Microfilariae then invade the skin, predominantly over the same anatomical quarter, and give rise to a persistent and variously itchy rash of typically lop-sided distribution (Fig. 5). It usually involves the buttock, thigh, and leg on one side, with extensions to the opposite buttock and up the back; or the shoulder and arm on one side, with extensions down the back, across to the other shoulder or up the same

Fig. 3 A case of sowda affecting the left leg of a boy from the Yemen (photograph by Dr D. H. Connor, U.S.A.F.I.P.).

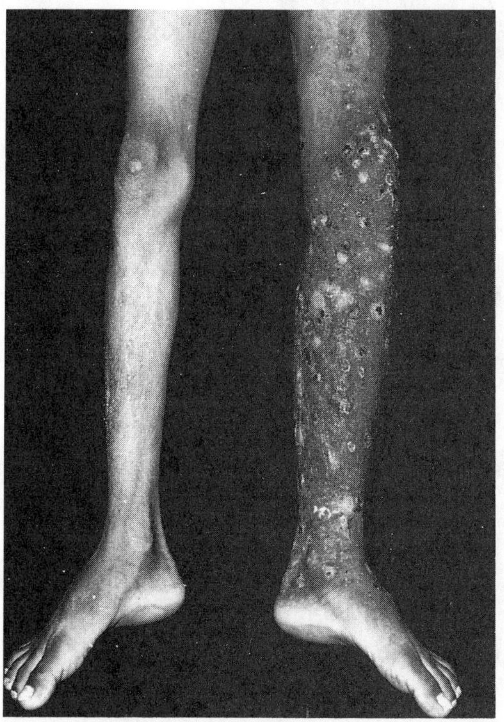

Fig. 4 Prominent subcutaneous nodules.

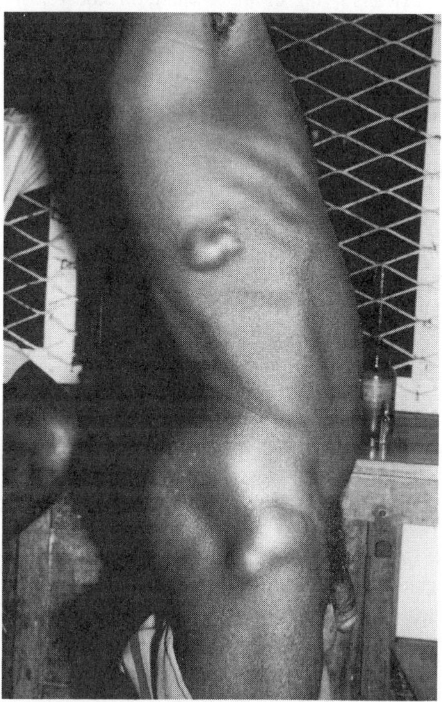

Fig. 5 Papular pruritic rash of onchocerciasis.

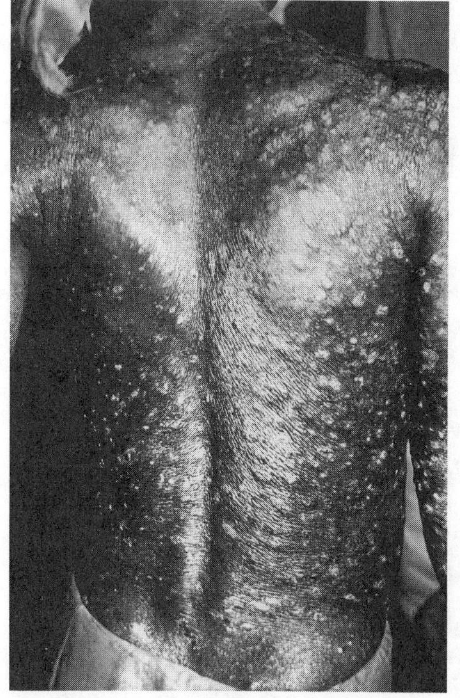

side of the neck. The rash comprises numerous small, discrete papules, 1 to 3 mm in diameter, which show red on a white skin. Wheals, vesicles, scratch marks, and secondary skin infection may be superimposed. The skin fold is thickened on the affected side, and the skin may be blacker than normal in black individuals or reddened in white. Sometimes a slightly thickened and lichenified skin is seen, without accompanying pruritus or rash. Usually there is some enlargement of the inguinal or axillary lymph nodes on the affected side. Deep-seated aches and pains may be felt in the limb concerned.

Chronic lesions of the skin and lymph glands

Chronic, disfiguring and sometimes disabling skin lesions, resulting from long-standing, heavy infection with *O. volvulus* microfilariae, are most often seen in adult Africans living in areas where onchocerciasis is endemic. The lower limbs, where the highest concentrations of microfilariae are found, are usually worst affected. There is gross lichenification and thickening of the skin with hyperpigmentation, giving way later to the atrophy and slackness of 'lizard' skin; and a mottled depigmentation, especially common over the shins (Fig. 6). The skin is poorly nourished, and heals badly. Indolent tropical ulcers often develop following minor abrasions. The femoral and inguinal lymph glands enlarge (Fig. 7) and may hang in pockets of loose skin (hanging groins) (Fig. 8), a condition that may predispose to herniae. Elephantiasis of the lower limbs or of the scrotum may develop. Microfilariae are usually abundant in the skin, unless the infection has 'burnt out'; there may be many nodules.

Ocular lesions

Microfilariae (not the adult worms) can invade all tissues of the eye except the lens. The main ocular lesions can be divided according to the seriousness of their import.

Lesions of less serious import

Punctate keratitis. This is composed of so-called snowflake opacities, which are cellular aggregates around dead microfilariae in the cornea. They vary in number from 1 to 100 or more, tend to be peripheral and/or interpalpebral in distribution, and are up to 0.5 mm in diameter. Usually they are symptomless but sometimes there is associated photophobia and watering. They are characteristic of light and recent infections. They resolve spontaneously, usually without vascularization, but may be succeeded by new lesions, and are not *per se* of serious import.

Fig. 6 Mottled depigmentation of shins.

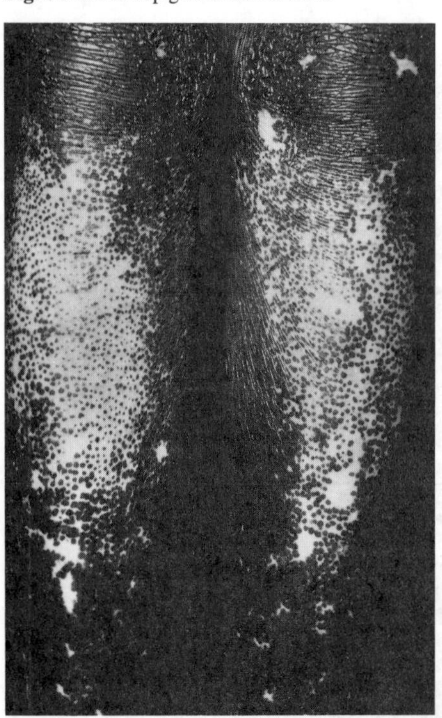

Lesions of serious import

The ocular lesions of serious import usually develop in heavy and often long-standing infection, particularly in children with head nodules.

Sclerosing keratitis. This lesion is characteristic of heavy infection with abundant microfilariae in the cornea, and is particularly common in the Sudan–savanna belt of Africa. The limbus is often swollen (limbitis) and a chronic interstitial keratitis develops from the sides and below. It is headed by a slowly advancing zone of milky opacification in the corneal stroma, behind which develops a scantily vascularized and usually pigmented 'pannus'. The clear segment above may contain many hundreds of visible microfilariae, both living and dead. The affected area of the cornea becomes opaque (Fig. 9(a)) and finally the pupillary area may be obscured.

Fig. 7 Inguinal and femoral lymphadenopathy.

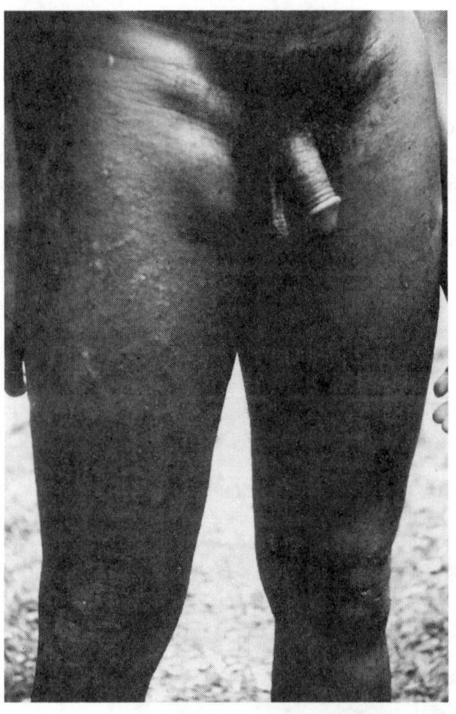

Fig. 8 'Hanging groins'.

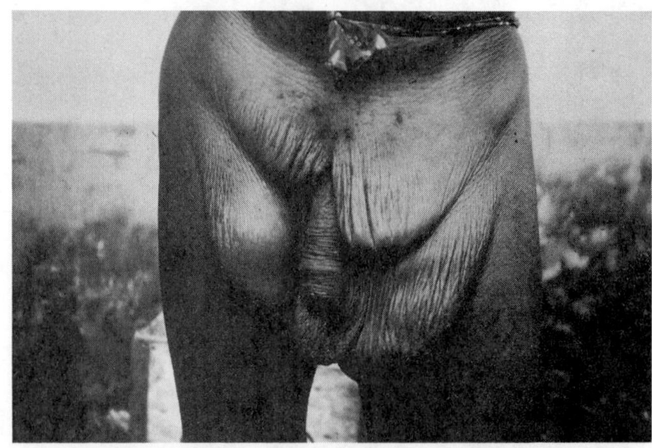

Anterior uveitis. Acute episodes of uveitis are superimposed on a chronic inflammatory process. The pigment ruff of the pupil is lost and the pupil becomes distorted (Fig. 9(a)), often pear shaped, with or without posterior synechiae. Secondary glaucoma and cataract may follow and are commonly the causes of ultimate blindness.

Fundus lesions. Choroidoretinal lesions may develop, sometimes terminating in the classical Hissette–Ridley fundus. Typically the lesions are bilateral. They start temporal to the macula and involve primarily the retinal pigment epithelium. Large, well-defined patches of choroidoretinal degeneration develop, involving much of the posterior fundus (Fig.9(b)). Within these areas the retinal elements (excluding the retinal vessels) and the choriocapillaris disappear, and the choroidal vessels appear bright orange, pink or white, according to the degree of their sclerosis. Irregular pigment masses are seen and the optic disc often shows a consecutive atrophy (Fig.9(b)). The surrounding retina appears healthy.

Optic neuritis. In other instances a postneuritic optic atrophy is seen. There is sheathing of the retinal vessels for a varying distance from the optic disc and narrowing of the retinal arteries. The visual fields are greatly reduced, with only tubular vision remaining. Loss of twilight and night vision is a common, early diagnostic symptom.

Generalized signs and symptoms

Extreme wasting, dwarfism with delayed sexual development, epilepsy, and a failure to react immunologically to antigenic, stimuli have all been associated with heavy *O. volvulus* infection.

DIAGNOSIS

Firm diagnosis depends on seeing *O. volvulus* microfilariae in a skin snip or in the eye, or finding a nodule containing adult worms. Skin snips are usually positive in patients with advanced lesions. They are best taken from the iliac crests or the lateral calf in Africa, or from the scapula in Latin America. In patients with acute pruritic skin lesions, a presumptive diagnosis can be made on clinical grounds, especially if the rash is predominantly unilateral. There is usually some degree of eosinophilia.

Skin snips

To take a skin snip the skin is cleaned with spirit, a suitable needle is inserted horizontally into the epidermis to raise up a small, cone-shaped fold of skin, and the top of this fold is sliced off with a safety razor blade to remove a piece of skin 2 to 3 mm in diameter and 0.5 to 1.0 mm deep, which should be bloodless on removal. Alternatively the snip can be taken using a much more expensive scleral punch of the Holth (2 mm) or Walser type. The snip is placed in a drop of normal saline on a slide and is examined at intervals over 30 min, using a × 10–50 magnification, for the presence of motile microfilariae of *O. volvulus*. If negative after 30 min, it may be kept in a moist chamber overnight and then re-examined. *O. volvulus* microfilariae are relatively large and sturdy organisms, 220 to 350 mm in length, without a sheath. They have a slightly bulbous head and a pointed tail, and they exhibit vigorous lashing and wriggling movements. In practice, they have only to be distinguished in Africa from those of the much rarer *Mansonella streptocerca*, which are thinner, have shepherd's-crook tails, and make shivering and stretching movements; and in South America from the shorter and smaller blood-dwelling microfilariae of *M. ozzardi*, which are occasionally found in skin snips. If there is doubt as to the identity of living microfilariae, the slide should be dried, fixed, stained (Mayer's haemalum or Giemsa), and compared with the illustrations in standard works on parasitology.

Fig. 9 (a) Onchocerciasis of the anterior segment of the eye, showing sclerosing keratitis and distorted eccentric pupil from anterior uveitis—patient blind. (b) Onchocerciasis of the posterior segment of the eye showing Hissette-Ridley fundus and optic atrophy—patient still had central keyhole vision.

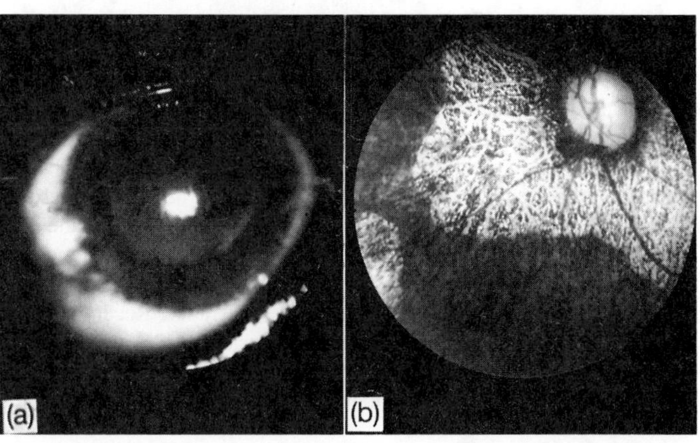

Microfilariae in the eye and elsewhere

In the eye, microfilariae can be seen with a slit lamp at a magnification of × 20–25. In the cornea they may be either alive (visible in the reflected beam as translucent and slowly motile bodies) or dead (straight and opaque, often with cellular reaction around them, seen in the direct beam). In the anterior chamber, they can be seen as shining bodies floating and wriggling in the aqueous humour, and the numbers visible can often be increased by making the patient sit for 1 min with the head inverted between the knees before the examination is made. With the aid of a slit lamp and a Goldman three-way mirror, living microfilariae can sometimes be seen as bright, apple-green bodies moving slowly within the retina.

Microfilariae are sometimes also found in urine, blood, sputum, cerebrospinal fluid, and hydrocele fluid, especially in heavily infected patients.

Mazzotti test

In lightly infected patients, microfilariae are often very hard to find. If two to six snips and an adequate eye examination fail to reveal microfilariae then, rather than continuing to take more snips, it is better to do a Mazzotti test. For this, 50 mg of diethylcarbamazine citrate is given by mouth. The test is positive if, within 30 min to 24 h, there develops an acute exacerbation of the itching and of the rash, centred on the previously affected parts but extending also further afield. Sometimes the affected area of skin becomes swollen, hot, and itchy without a papular rash appearing. These changes are due to inflammatory reactions around microfilariae that have been 'unmasked' and are being destroyed in the skin. As there is always a risk, however slight, of doing damage to the posterior segment in patients with onchocerciasis, the Mazzotti test should only be done on symptomatic subjects who are suspected of being lightly infected and in whom microfilariae cannot be demonstrated in the skin or eye by normal means.

Differential diagnosis

The differential diagnosis of early pruritic cutaneous onchocerciasis is from (*a*) scabies, which often coexists in Africans; (*b*) streptocerciasis, by identification of the microfilariae of *M. streptocerca*; (*c*) prickly heat; (*d*) contact dermatitis; and (*e*) insect bites, especially those of Culicoides or Simulium, which may cause great irritation to persons newly arrived in the tropics.

TREATMENT

Aims and indications

The aims of treatment are to get rid of the microfilariae without doing further damage to specialized tissues in the process, and to kill or permanently sterilize the adult worms. To be fully effective in preventing visual loss, treatment must therefore be given before the delicate ocular tissues have been irreparably damaged. Chemotherapy is the usual method but it may be supplemented by nodulectomy.

Now that ivermectin is freely available, anyone with onchocerciasis can be provided with safe and effective suppressive therapy. Nevertheless there are three groups of sufferers who are in special need of treatment.

'Acute' pruritic skin eruptions

This group includes (*a*) most expatriate patients presenting to physicians in temperate climates; (*b*) patients of the *sowda* type, with scanty microfilariae but maximum skin reaction, most of whom are resident in endemic areas.

Threat of severe eye lesions and blindness

Such patients will mainly be heavily infected natives of the endemic area. Danger signs are:

(1) presence of a head nodule;
(2) more than five microfilariae in a skin snip taken at the outer canthus of the eye;
(3) more than five microfilariae in the anterior chamber;
(4) more than 20 microfilariae in the cornea;
(5) evidence of night blindness or peripheral-field loss;
(6) presence of any serious lesion of ocular onchocerciasis at an early stage.

Individuals with any of these signs are at increased risk of developing severe eye lesions and blindness, even though their eyes may still be clear at the time of examination.

Disabling skin and lymph-node lesions

People with disabling skin and lymph-node lesions (hanging groins, herniae, elephantiasis of the scrotum or lower limbs, etc.) may require surgical treatment for these conditions in addition to specific therapy for onchocerciasis.

Methods of treatment

Treatment may be considered under the headings of microfilaricides, macrofilaricides, and nodulectomy.

Microfilaricides

The advent of ivermectin has revolutionized the treatment of onchocerciasis. In 1987, this drug, already widely used in veterinary medicine as a gastrointestinal anthelminthic cum ectoparasiticide, was registered in France for the treatment of human onchocerciasis under the name of Mectizan®. Shortly afterwards, the manufacturers (Merck) set up a Mectizan Donation Program to provide the drug free of charge to individuals or organizations considered by a newly established Mectizan Expert Committee to be capable of distributing it in a safe and reliable manner to persons living in areas endemic for onchocerciasis.

Ivermectin is the first drug that can be used safely for the mass treatment of onchocerciasis. Supplies of Mectizan for large-scale distribution programmes may be requested on application forms, which are available from The Executive Secretary, The Mectizan Expert Committee, One Copenhill, Atlanta, Georgia 30307, USA. Small quantities of the drug for compassionate use by physicians may be obtained by writing to Dr Philippe Gaxotte, Directeur Médical, Laboratoires Merck, Sharp and Dohme—Interpharma, 106 Avenue Jean-Moulin, 78170 La Celle St Cloud, France.

Ivermectin is a macrocyclic lactone. For onchocerciasis patients it constitutes a non-toxic, single-dose (150 μg/kg), oral treatment given, according to the patient's weight, as one-half to two 6-mg tablets of Mectizan. The drug clears almost all the microfilariae from the skin within 2 to 3 days and is remarkable in that the clearance is accompanied by little or no Mazzotti reaction. For this reason it should now be used exclusively, instead of diethylcarbamazine citrate, as the microfilaricide for *O. volvulus*.

Microfilariae in the eye are not killed directly, probably because the drug does not penetrate into the aqueous or the cornea; but within a few weeks those that were in the eye move out and are not replaced. Thus, treatment with ivermectin does not damage either the anterior or the posterior segment of the eye in patients with onchocerciasis but it does improve lesions of the anterior segment and prevent their further development. It is also very probable, but not yet proven with statistical significance, that the further development of posterior segment lesions will be arrested.

Ivermectin is not directly macrofilaricidal at a single dose, but it has various actions on adult *O. volvulus*. The exodus of intrauterine microfilariae from the female is blocked for periods of 3 to 12 months after a single dose; the number of male worms in nodules is reduced and higher proportions of female worms are not inseminated; and there is some evidence that repeated doses given over periods of 3 years or more have a slow action of attrition on the adult female worms.

Ivermectin is now widely used for the large-scale control of onchocerciasis and several million doses have been given, without mishap, in mass distribution programmes designed to control morbidity and reduce transmission. The practising physician now has available a drug that can suppress the symptoms of onchocerciasis for periods of up to a year, and a treatment that can safely be given to almost anyone suffering from the disease.

For individual treatment, Mectizan should be given at least once a year, but the best clinical results will probably follow from giving this suppressive treatment every 3 months. Ivermectin should not be given to children under 5 years old, to pregnant women, to mothers in the first week of lactation, to persons who are otherwise severely ill or in whom the blood–brain barrier may be deficient, or during outbreaks of cerebrospinal meningitis. If significant Mazzotti or other adverse reactions (including severe postural hypotension) occur in the 24 to 72 h following treatment, palliative symptomatic medication (antipyretics, antihistamines, oral fluids, and possibly corticosteroids) should be given.

Macrofilaricides

An effective macrofilaricide can bring about a radical cure of onchocerciasis. Until recently, the only usable macrofilaricide was suramin, a potentially toxic compound given by intravenous injection. This drug has recently been joined by amocarzine, the first oral macrofilaricide, which is still undergoing clinical trials for individual treatment. Although the need for radical macrofilaricidal treatment in expatriate patients may be considerably less since the arrival of ivermectin, the demand for an effective, easily administered, non-toxic macrofilaricide, for use in large-scale treatment aimed at eliminating onchocerciasis, is still great. Unfortunately, suramin cannot be used for this purpose, and it is also doubtful whether amocarzine will ever meet the need. Nevertheless, a description of treatment with each of these drugs is given here as either may still be needed for individual treatment.

Suramin treatment. This should begin within 1 to 2 weeks of a treatment with Mectizan given to eliminate most of the microfilariae from the body, for unpleasant reactions to suramin will be greatly reduced if the basic microfilarial load has been eliminated before starting treatment. Immediately before injection the white suramin powder, which should have been stored in the dark, is dissolved in pyrogen-free distilled water to form a 10 per cent solution. The solution should be given slowly by intravenous injection. The standard macrofilaricidal course in the past has been to give an initial dose of 0.1 g to test for very rare idiosyncrasy, and to follow this by 1.0 g weekly, for adults of 60 kg or more, to a total of 4 to 7 g, depending on the patient's tolerance. Recent trials in Africans indicate that a course of weekly doses at 0.2, 0.4, 0.6, 0.8, 1.0, 1.0 g for an adult of 60 kg or more may be better tolerated and will permanently sterilize or kill the majority of the adult worms. Doses for children and adults under 60 kg should be reduced in proportion to their weight.

Patients with disease of the liver or kidneys should not be treated with suramin, nor should pregnant women, or the old and weak. The urine should be examined for albumin and casts before each injection. Suramin excretion is almost invariably accompanied by some albuminuria; and in low degrees this may be ignored, but a heavy albuminuria and the presence of many granular casts, especially in a patient who has begun to feel and look unwell, are indications to interrupt treatment for a week or to stop it altogether.

Minor manifestations of the drug itself may be *(a)* tenderness of the soles and palms; *(b)* polyuria and increased thirst; *(c)* tiredness, anorexia, and malaise. More severe toxic signs, which indicate stopping treatment, are *(a)* severe prostration; *(b)* ulceration of the mouth and tongue; *(c)* exfoliative dermatitis; *(d)* chronic diarrhoea; *(e)* high fever and bronchitis; *(f)* swelling, pain, and immobilization of limb joints.

Reactions to the effect of suramin on the adult worms include *(a)* tenderness, swelling, and even abscess formation in subcutaneous nodules; *(b)* deep abscesses centred round worms lying between the muscles; *(c)* painful immobilization of the hip in a semiflexed position, presumably due to reaction around deep nodules near the capsule of the hip joint.

Reactions due to the effect of suramin on any remaining microfilariae include *(a)* itching and inflammation of the skin, with or without papular or vesicular eruptions and desquamation; *(b)* iridocyclitis and/or the development or exacerbation of an optic neuritis. Betamethasone may be necessary to prevent or to reduce any of the above reactions.

At the end of a course of suramin, the adult *O. volvulus* are likely to have been sterilized and most will be moribund; but they may take some weeks to die, and living microfilariae may continue to escape from their uteri for 3 to 4 months. Further treatment with ivermectin is likely to be needed to deal with these.

Amocarzine treatment. This Ciba-Geigy drug, recently developed for use in man, was formerly known as CGP 6140. Chemically it is 4-nitro-4-(*N*-methyl-piperazynl-thiocarbonyl-amino)-diphenylamine, and it has now been tested on some hundreds of patients. The drug is absorbed better and in a more constant manner if given after a meal, and the optimal dosage schedule is 3 mg/kg given twice daily, after food, for three consecutive days. This dosage may be expected to kill some 80 per cent of the adult worms, but it is also microfilaricidal, reducing skin counts of microfilariae to about 10 per cent of pretreatment levels within a week. Some Mazzotti-type reactions have been reported in association with the latter property. Microfilarial concentrations in the eye fall more slowly and there are no reports of adverse effects on the eye. The main toxic manifestations appear to affect the central nervous system. Dizziness, disorientation, and a positive Romberg sign have been reported in patients treated with this drug but all these complications have been reversible.

Nodulectomy

Head nodules, especially common in Mexico and Guatemala, should always be removed as early as possible. Other nodules may be removed if they are a nuisance to the patient. Nodulectomy is done under local anaesthesia (2 per cent lignocaine), preferably without adrenaline. After incising the skin and fascial layers, the nodule is shelled out using curved, blunt-pointed scissors. Bleeding points must be carefully secured, for the nodule has a rich blood supply and formation of a haematoma is a common postoperative complication. Before suturing, the operator should feel in the wound for 'seed' nodules not felt from the surface. Removal of nodules deep in the chest wall or around the knee joint requires special care lest damage be done to the pleura, joint capsule, or communicating bursae.

Entire adult worms may be obtained alive from excised nodules by digesting the surrounding host tissue with collagenase (Fig. 2)

Symptomatic treatment of reactions in the eye during chemotherapy

The development of a red eye during treatment with any micro- or macrofilaricidal drug usually indicates an onchocercal iridocyclitis. This requires immediate recognition and careful treatment to avoid the development of synechiae. Atropine sulphate drops (1 per cent) should be instilled, with due regard to the possibility of provoking mydriatic glaucoma; and corticosteroid drops or ointment should be instilled at least three-hourly until the inflammation is controlled. In patients showing temporarily increased intraocular pressure, acetazolamide (250 mg, four times a day) may be helpful until the crisis is past.

PROPHYLAXIS

There is no practically effective chemoprophylactic for *O. volvulus* infection. Personal exposure to Simulium can be reduced by wearing clothing that protects those body areas that are most exposed to their bites, that is, long trousers, stockings, and closed footwear help against *S. damnosum*, *S. neavei*, *S. metallicum*, and some other South American vectors; long-sleeved shirts, and a hat and veil help against *S. ochraceum*.

REFERENCES

Anderson, J. and Fuglsang, H. (1977). Ocular onchocerciasis. *Tropical Diseases Bulletin*, **74,** 257.

Buck, A.A. (ed.) (1974). *Onchocerciasis—symptomatology, pathology, diagnosis* pp. 1–80. World Health Organization, Geneva.

Duke, B.O.L. (1990). Human onchocerciasis—an overview. *Acta Eidensia*, **59,** 9–24.

Taylor, H.R. and Greene, B.M. (1989) The status of ivermectin in the treatment of onchocerciasis. *American Journal of Tropical Medicine and Hygiene*, **41,** 460–6.

World Health Organization (1987). *Third Report of the WHO Expert Committee on Onchocerciasis*, WHO Technical Report Series No. 752, pp. 1–167. World Health Organization, Geneva.

Loiasis

GEOGRAPHICAL DISTRIBUTION AND VECTORS

Transmission of *Loa loa* is confined to the West African forest block east of the Dahomey (Benin) gap; and to the Central African equatorial forest block and its fringes. Infections are commonly acquired in southern Nigeria, Cameroon, Gabon, Equatorial Guinea, Congo, and Zaire; they occur less frequently in southern Chad, the Central African Republic, Sudan and Uganda, and Angola. *L. loa* is spread by tabanid flies of the genus *Chrysops*, known as 'red flies' or 'mangrove flies'.

LIFECYCLE OF THE PARASITE AND PATHOLOGY

Development from infective larvae to fertile adult worms takes about 5 months. The adult worms (males 3–4 cm × 0.35 mm; females 5–7 cm × 0.5 mm) are freely motile in the subcutaneous tissue and along the fascial planes, and they may live for up to 15 years. They cause the fugitive Calabar swellings that are characteristic of loiasis and may be reactions to the discharge of uterine contents or pheromones. An adult worm may occasionally be seen traversing the bulbar conjunctiva and the death of a worm under the skin may cause an inflammatory reaction.

The sheathed microfilariae (225–300 × 10 mm) are relatively large and show a diurnal periodicity in the blood. They probably live for about a year and are non-pathogenic except that, when present in high densities, their death under treatment with diethylcarbamazine citrate may block the capillaries of the brain or retina.

CLINICAL PICTURE

Infective Chrysops bites may cause very severe swelling and itching. The infective larvae of *L. loa* are large (2 mm long) and often very numerous (100–200) in a single fly. Discrete papules may develop in the skin in association with the L_3 or L_4 larvae as they move away from the site of entry over the ensuing 1 to 4 weeks.

Adult worms moving under the skin may cause prickling and itching sensations; those moving deeper in the fascial planes cause shifting aches and pains, and paraesthesiae. Allergic, oedematous, subcutaneous Calabar or 'fugitive' swellings, 5 to 10 cm or more in diameter, may develop anywhere but are common on the back of the hand or on the arm. They last from some hours to several days and are often brought on by local muscular activity. The overlying skin may be red, hot, and painful, resembling cellulitis; and it may also itch. The swellings can be very large and temporarily incapacitating. Sometimes an adult worm can be seen moving under the skin.

The adult worm may also cross the conjunctiva (Fig. 10)—a dramatic experience for the patient. The worm becomes visible for a matter of 5 to 30 min and may be removed by prompt surgical intervention under local conjunctival anaesthesia. Its passage is accompanied by reddening, swelling of the eyelids and conjunctiva, watering, and photophobia; the periorbital tissues may swell so as to close the eye.

It is often lightly and recently infected individuals who suffer most from Calabar swellings and who seek treatment. The swellings may cause a significant loss of working time in labour forces (for example on rubber plantations) in endemic areas and this is a good reason for treatment. People with infections of long standing may be entirely asymptomatic and, if so, are probably best left untreated.

An association between loiasis and endomyocardial fibrosis has been suspected, possibly attributable to the high eosinophilia that is sometimes encountered.

DIAGNOSIS

The diagnosis is made on the clinical picture, which has only to be distinguished from the effects of insect bites and stings, and septic cellulitis. Marked eosinophilia (up to 10 000/mm^3) is almost invariable and may help to distinguish a Calabar swelling from cellulitis. Finding the microfilariae in day blood, or the sight of an adult worm, will confirm the diagnosis, but in many patients with Calabar swellings no microfilariae can be found.

TREATMENT

Diethylcarbamazine citrate is effective against the microfilariae, the L_3 and L_4 stages and a good proportion of the adult worms of *L. loa*. The standard course for killing the adult worms is 6 mg/kg daily, in three divided doses after food, continued for 3 weeks. Courses of 7 days duration, at the same daily dosage and repeated at intervals of a month, may sometimes be more effective, but in some infected people some of the adult worms remain resistant to the drug even after repeated courses. The adult worms often surface and become visible under the skin when they die under treatment.

Fig. 10 Adult *L. loa* crossing the bulbar conjunctiva (photograph by Dr J. Anderson).

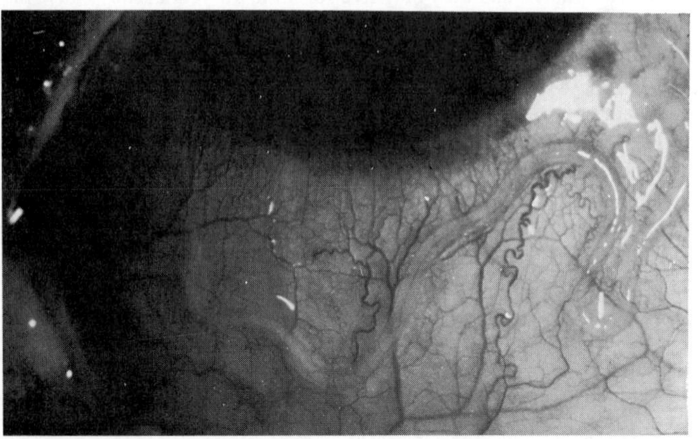

The dangers of treatment with diethylcarbamazine in patients infected with *L. loa* are two. First, many such patients may also harbour infections with *O. volvulus*, which can give rise to severe Mazzotti reactions when this drug is used. Second, in patients with a daytime *L. loa* microfilaraemia in excess of 100 mf/50 mm^3, there is always some risk that the sudden destruction of microfilariae under the action of diethylcarbamazine may, in addition to producing a febrile reaction, give rise to capillary blockage by dead and dying microfilariae in the brain, meninges, and retina (leading to a meningoencephalitic syndrome, which can be fatal). The risk of this happening becomes greater as the pretreatment concentration of microfilariae in the blood increases.

If coincident infection with *O. volvulus* is found or suspected, the patient should be treated first with a dose of ivermectin (150 μg/kg Mectizan) to eliminate temporarily, and with minimum reaction, the microfilariae of that species. The ivermectin itself may also serve to reduce the *L. loa* microfilariae for some weeks or months so that treatment with diethylcarbamazine, aimed at the adult Loa worms, can proceed. In any case, it is wise to start diethylcarbamazine treatment with a low dose (25–50 mg on the first day) and, depending on the patient's response, to increase this by doubling the dose each day until the level of 6 mg/kg per day is reached. This dosage can then be continued for 1 to 3 weeks, as desired. Adverse reactions in the course of this schedule may require corticosteroid therapy to control them.

In patients with very high microfilaraemia (in excess of 500 mf/50 mm^3) the risk of capillary blockage in the central nervous system must be taken very seriously. In extreme cases, cytophoresis has been used to extract most of the microfilariae from the patient's blood before giving diethylcarbamazine cautiously under steroid cover. Alternatively, mebendazole (100–500 mg, thrice daily, continued for 4 to 6 weeks) may gradually reduce the microfilaraemia without complications. Although this drug does not kill adult Loa, it may make it safe to use diethylcarbamazine for this purpose.

PROPHYLAXIS

Diethylcarbamazine citrate has a chemoprophylactic action against *L. loa*. For an adult, courses of 200 mg twice daily for three consecutive days once each month will probably kill all infective larvae and immature worms inoculated during the previous month, and this at the expense of a minor papular reaction in the skin around dead parasites. Prophylaxis may also be achieved by taking 300 mg diethylcarbamazine once a week during periods of exposure. Prevention of Chrysops bites depends in large measure on wearing long trousers, fly-screening of houses, and clearance of the forest around dwelling places.

REFERENCES

Editorial (1986). *Loa loa*—a pathogenic parasite. *Lancet*, **ii,** 554

Fain, A. (1978). Les problèmes actuels de la loase. *Bulletin of the World Health Organization*, **56,** 155.

Nutman, T.B. *et al.* (1988). Diethylcarbamazine prophylaxis for human loiasis: results of a double blind study. *New England Journal of Medicine*, **319,** 752–6.

Other filarial infections

STREPTOCERCIASIS

Mansonella streptocerca, causing streptocerciasis, occurs in the more humid parts of Ghana, Togo, Nigeria, Cameroon, Gabon, Congo, Equatorial Guinea, and Zaire. Transmission is by *Culicoides* (especially *C. grahamii*), commonly but erroneously known as 'sandflies'.

The adult worms and microfilariae are found in the skin, mainly on the torso. Diagnosis is by finding the characteristic crook-tailed microfilariae in skin snips. Infections are usually asymptomatic but sometimes give rise to a chronic itching rash composed of very small, urticarial papules, not unlike the acute rash of onchocerciasis. Hypopigmented macules, probably associated with the adult worms, which lie very near the surface, may be seen in dark-skinned patients and these may often be taken for early tuberculoid leprosy. The differential diagnosis can only be made by biopsy and it is always possible that both infectious agents may occur together.

Diethylcarbamazine citrate kills both microfilariae and adult worms, but the reactions are never so violent as in onchocerciasis. A course of diethylcarbamazine at 2 mg/kg three times a day for 7 to 10 days should suffice for an adult, but if coincidental infection with *O. volvulus* exists it would be advisable initially to give a dose of ivermectin to eliminate the microfilariae of the latter species.

PERSTANS FILARIASIS

Mansonella perstans (formerly known as *Dipetalonema* or *Acanthocheilonema perstans*) is common and widespread in tropical Africa south of the Sahara, in parts of South America, and in Algeria, Tunisia and New Guinea. Transmission is by *Culicoides* spp. *M. semiclarum*, described from Zaire, is a similar parasite.

The adult worms live in serous cavities, in the mesentery and retroperitioneal tissues. The microfilariae are found in the blood and they are non-periodic. High proportions of persons living in endemic areas are infected.

M. perstans may produce an eosinophilia but is generally considered to be non-pathogenic. Normally no treatment is necessary. However, patients infected with microfilariae closely resembling those of *M. perstans* have been found in Zimbabwe suffering from meningeal symptoms (with microfilariae in the cerebrospinal fluid) and general malaise. Such infections may be a virulent form of *M. perstans*, but it has also been suggested that they were caused by the monkey parasite *Meningonema peruzzi*. Diethylcarbamazine is ineffective but some success in treatment has been reported following combined dosage with mebendazole (100 mg, thrice daily after meals) and levamisole (100 mg, twice daily).

MANSONELLIASIS OZZARDI

Mansonella ozzardi is confined to South and Central America and the West Indies. Transmission is by *Simulium* spp. in South America and by Culicoides in the Caribbean. The morphology of the adult worms, described for the first time from experimentally infected Patas monkeys, has led to a reclassification of *perstans*, *semiclarum*, and *streptocerca* into the genus *Mansonella*. The microfilariae occur in the blood and are non-periodic. They may also be found in skin snips, where they have to be distinguished from those of *O. volvulus*.

In the West Indies, infections are considered to be non-pathogenic. In the Amazon region, joint pains, fever, lymphadenopathy and headache have been attributed to this parasite. Treatment with diethylcarbamazine citrate is variously reported as being ineffective against the parasite but effective in reducing the allegedly associated symptoms.

DIROFILARIASIS

Infections with *Dirofilaria immitis*, the dog heart-worm, with *D. repens* (from dogs or cats), or with *D. tenuis* or *D. ursi* (from the racoon and bear, respectively) are occasionally transmitted by their mosquito vectors to man. Case reports come from the United States, Japan, Australia, Europe, Africa, Asia, and South America.

In man, *D. immitis* never reaches maturity and the immature worm usually ends up in the lung giving rise to infarction vasculitis and the formation of a granuloma. This may be discovered as a 'silent' coin lesion on a chest radiograph, or it may be associated with chest pain, cough, haemoptysis, and fever. There is no certain way to make a prospective diagnosis, for there is never any microfilaraemia and immunological tests cannot be taken as conclusive. Hence the differential diagnosis from bronchial carcinoma, secondary neoplasms, or systemic fungal infections in the lung can only be made with certainty after removal (by lobectomy) and histopathological examination.

D. tenuis, *D. repens*, and *D. ursi* can give rise to a subcutaneous granuloma anywhere in the body or under the conjunctiva. Surgical removal is the only treatment and subsequent histopathological examination makes the diagnosis.

REFERENCES

Adolphi, P.E., Kagan, I.G., and McQuay, R.M. (1962) Diagnosis and treatment of *Acanthocheilonema perstans* filariasis. *American Journal of Tropical Medicine and Hygiene*, **11,** 76–88.

Dayal, Y. and Neafie, R.C. (1975). Human pulmonary dirofilariasis: a case report and review of the literature. *American Review of Respiratory Diseases*, **112,** 437.

Marinkelle, C.J. and German, E. (1970). Mansonelliasis in the Comisaria del Vaupes of Colombia. *Tropical Geographic Medicine* **22,** 101–11.

Meyers, W.M. *et al.* (1972). Human streptocerciasis. A clinicopathologic study of 40 Africans (Zairians) including identification of the adult filaria. *American Journal of Tropical Medicine and Hygiene*, **21,** 528–45.

Meyers, W.M. *et al.* (1978). Streptocerciasis: degeneration of adult *Dipetalonema streptocerca* in man following diethylcarbamazine therapy. *American Journal of Tropical Medicine and Hygiene*, **27,** 1137–47.

7.14.2 Lymphatic filariasis

B. A. SOUTHGATE

Introduction

General principles of filarial infections

Lymphatic filarial parasites are nematode round worms whose site of pathogenesis is the lymphatic vascular system, where adult worms live. Three species produce infection and disease: *Wuchereria bancrofti* causes Bancroftian filariasis; *Brugia malayi* and *B. timori* cause Brugian filariasis (Malayan and Timorian filariasis, respectively). These diseases are widespread in warm-climate areas and show much local clinical variation due to parasite strain differences, heterogeneity of immune responses, and variations in intensity of infective challenge and incidence rates of infection. Some 770 million persons live in endemic areas, 65 to 70 per cent of them in China, India, and Indonesia; 73 million are infected with *W. bancrofti* and 6 million with *B. malayi* or *B. timori*. These are relatively crude estimates, and true figures must be higher; in particular, subSaharan Africa must have many unidentified foci of infection.

Definition

Lymphatic filariasis is a disease resulting from infection with one of the three specified parasites; pathology results from the direct effects of adult worms and their excretory/secretory products on lymphatic vessels, and the immune response to helminthic antigens by the human host. Microfilariae play no part in causing lymphatic pathology; disease due to unmated adult worms can occur in their absence. Microfilariae are responsible for the syndrome of tropical pulmonary eosinophilia.

Aetiology—the lifecycle of the parasites

Adult worms are smooth, thread-like, and creamy-white; their life-span is 2 to 5 years, with over 40 years recorded on one occasion. Males are

40 mm long and 0.1 mm in diameter; females are 80 to 100 mm × 0.25 to 0.30 mm. They live in lymphatic vessels and nodes. After mating, sexually mature females produce embryos known as microfilariae, which are shed from the uterus and migrate into lymph and blood. Microfilariae of all three species are sheathed, range from 180 to 290 μm in length and 7.5 to 10.0 μm in diameter; their characteristic species morphology in stained blood films is the diagnostic feature of filariasis. Microfilariae may be found in peripheral blood by day and night, with a small peak in concentration by day (diurnally subperiodic form) or night (nocturnally subperiodic form); in most endemic regions, microfilariae are nocturnally periodic with a peak concentration between 22.00 and 02.00 h, and periodicity must be considered by the physician taking blood samples for parasitological diagnosis. Microfilariae have a short life-span of up to 12 months, and their further development is totally dependent on ingestion by a compatible mosquito vector. After uptake, microfilariae penetrate the gut wall, settle in the thoracic flight muscles, and develop for 9 to 15 days. The resultant infective larva migrates to the head and enters the human body at the next blood meal. Following a moult, the immature juvenile filaria enters the peripheral lymphatic system and moves centrally to settle in a major vessel just distal to a lymph node. Here it moults again, becoming adult and mating if an adult of the opposite sex is available. The time from infective larval entry to sexual maturity in the body can be as little as 3 months, but the usual time from exposure to patent microfilaraemia is 8 to 24 months.

Epidemiology of lymphatic filariasis

Transmission and spread of infection

Transmission involves obligatory development in a mosquito vector specific to a particular geographical area, and no other mode of spread occurs except rare instances of transplacental passage of microfilariae. The vectors of *W. bancrofti* belong to the genera Culex, Aedes, and Anopheles; those of *B. malayi* and *B. timori* to Mansonia and Anopheles. This is important because the anatomical pattern of disease may be affected by the biting habits of the local vector species, and because vector control may offer the most cost-effective means of disease prevention in organized public health programmes.

Geographical distribution and vectors

W. BANCROFTI INFECTIONS

There are three clinicoepidemiological types of Bancroftian filariasis, each associated with one vector genus, Culex, Anopheles, or Aedes. The bioecology of vectors has two interactions with the parasites and man significant in determining epidemiological patterns, clinical features, diagnostic methods, and approaches to community control.

Culex transmission

This accounts for more than 70 per cent of filariasis infections; most of the areas involved are urban or semiurban due to the breeding habits of Culex, and occur in India, Sri Lanka, parts of China, Egypt, Central and South America, some Caribbean Islands, and urban areas of East Africa. Culex bites mainly on the legs, thus clinical lesions predominantly affect the legs and genitalia; microfilariae are nocturnally periodic. The mosquito/filaria host/parasite relationship is limitation, the success rate of parasites developing in the vector from ingested microfilariae to infective larvae increasing as microfilarial density in ingested blood declines; this implies that community control will require high efficiency and resurgence of transmission will always be a danger, even from conditions of near eradication.

Anopheles transmission

Endemic areas and anopheline breeding sites are rural and occur in East and West Africa, Papua New Guinea, Vanuatu, parts of China, and limited areas of tropical America. Like Culex, Anopheles is mainly a leg biter and thus disease is largely in the legs and genitalia; microfilariae are nocturnally periodic. The mosquito/filaria host/parasite relationship is facilitation, the success rate from ingested microfilariae to infective larvae decreasing as microfilarial concentration in ingested blood declines; this implies that community control could be successful in eradicating infection, as has been achieved in the Solomon Islands and parts of southern Togo, with little danger of recrudescence of transmission or disease.

Aedes transmission

This is the least frequent type of Bancroftian filariasis. Endemic areas are rural and occur in the South Pacific islands including Fiji, Western Samoa, American Samoa, Tahiti and the French Polynesian Islands, Tonga, the Cook Islands, and New Caledonia; patchily in Thailand, the Philippines, Vietnam, and the Nicobar Islands. *Aedes* spp. feed throughout the 24 h with a slight daytime peak. They feed on the upper as well as the lower half of the body. Consequently, microfilariae are diurnally subperiodic and clinical lesions are seen in the arms and breasts more frequently than in other endemic areas of the world. The mosquito/filarial host/parasite relationship for Aedes is limitation, as for Culex, with the same implications for community control activities.

B. MALAYI INFECTIONS: CLINICOEPIDEMIOLOGICAL TYPES

Swamp forest

Infection is a rural zoonosis, with monkeys and carnivores as reservoirs and Mansonia as vectors. The mosquito/filaria host/parasite relationship is proportionality, the success rate of ingested microfilariae in developing to infective larvae remaining constant as ingested microfilarial densities decline; no predictions can be made for the success of community control programmes. Biting can occur by day, but is mainly by night and microfilariae are nocturnally subperiodic. It is found in Malaysia, Indonesia (west, north Indonesia (north, west, and east Sumatra, east and south-east Kalimantan)), and southern Thailand. Leg biting by Mansonia causes virtually all disease to be confined to those limbs, and indeed to below the knees.

Transitional zones

Infection is rural and is a mixed anthroponosis and zoonosis, with monkeys and domestic cats as reservoirs, Mansonia and Anopheles as vectors; both proportionality and facilitation occur. Microfilariae are intermediate between nocturnally subperiodic and nocturnally periodic; pathology is found below the knees. Endemic areas occur in Malaysia, Indonesia (Buru), and southern Thailand.

Established agricultural areas

Infection is a pure anthroponosis with Anopheles as the main vector and Mansonia an accessory vector; microfilariae show full nocturnal periodicity. This is found in India (mainly Kerala), Malaysia, Indonesia (Sulawesi), China, Korea, Vietnam, and southern Thailand. Mass administration of diethylcarbamazine in salt has led to virtual eradication of infection in some areas of China where *An. sinensis* is the vector, with no recrudescence after cessation of control measures, owing to the facilitation mechanism.

B. TIMORI INFECTIONS

This least common of the filariases is a human infection transmitted only by *An. barbirostris* in the Indonesian islands of Timor, Flores, Rote, and Alor.

Clinicoepidemiological patterns of filariasis

Five patterns describe the vast majority of foci; their distinctive features are summarized in Table 1. Explanations for these characteristic features are as follow.

Table 1 *The five main clinicoepidemiological patterns of lymphatic filariasis in endemic areas*

Pattern*	Microfilarial prevalence	Microfilarial density	Transmission intensity	Filarial fever	Acute lymphatic disease	Hydrocele	Obstructive lymphopathy of limbs
A	++++	++++	++++	++++	++++	++++	++++
B	++++	+++	+++	++++	++++	+	+
C	+	+	+++	++++	++++		
D	+	+	+++	+	+	++++	++++
E	+	+	+	+	+	+	+

* See text.

Pattern A

Long-standing, intense transmission in a population subject to little immigration or emigration: many people are prenatally sensitized by filarial antigens, due to high prevalence rates of infection and high intensities of transmission.

Pattern B

Recent introduction of transmission or recent increase in intensity of transmission, due to natural or man-made ecological changes, such as dam construction or the adoption of large-scale, irrigated rice growing.

Pattern C

Mass immigration of susceptible, uninfected, and unsensitized populations into endemic areas, as in agricultural resettlement schemes (Indonesia—Sulawesi) and military operations (United States Armed Forces in the South Pacific during the Second World War). Few people are prenatally sensitized by filarial antigens.

Pattern D

Recent emigration of young, microfilaraemic but clinically unaffected people, usually in search of employment. Older, diseased amicrofilaraemic persons remain behind. Many residents are prenatally sensitized by filarial antigens.

Pattern E

Long-standing, low-intensity transmission in a stable population with little immigration or emigration; few people are prenatally sensitized by filarial antigens due to low prevalence rates of maternal infection resulting from low intensity of transmission.

Clinical aspects of lymphatic filariasis

The clinical syndromes seen in those who have lived their whole lives (including life *in utero*) in endemic areas differ from those seen in people exposed for the first time after reaching the age of full immunological competence. Maternal infection predisposes to the development of immune tolerance or extreme hyporesponsiveness in offspring, thus increasing susceptibility to infection and microfilaraemia, but paradoxically reducing the incidence and severity of immunologically mediated clinical disease. Adult immigrants to endemic areas experience much higher rates of disease than the indigenous inhabitants, or children who migrate before the age of 5 years. Women have lower rates and densities of microfilarial infection and lower rates of clinical disease than men; age of peak prevalence of infection and disease is higher than for men. The filariases have an exceptionally wide clinical spectrum, and the relative abundance of different symptoms and signs differs from one endemic area to another (see Table 1 above). The categories of infection/disease status common to all endemic areas are illustrated diagrammatically with their immunological correlates in Fig. 1.

ASYMPTOMATIC AMICROFILARAEMIA

A proportion of the population in all endemic areas shows no microfilaraemia or clinical disease. These individuals are referred to as 'endemic normals' and have the same exposure as infected and diseased persons. Some are truly uninfected; others have natural or acquired immunity to infection; some harbour subclinical infections with unpaired or infertile worms, or have microfilarial densities too low to be detected using any practicable volume of blood. This state has long been recognized from observations but has only been confirmed and categorized since the development of methods for detecting circulating filarial antigens and ultra-low-density microfilarial concentrations in blood.

Fig. 1 The clinical categories of lymphatic filariasis with their immunological correlates (TPE, tropical pulmonary eosinophilia).

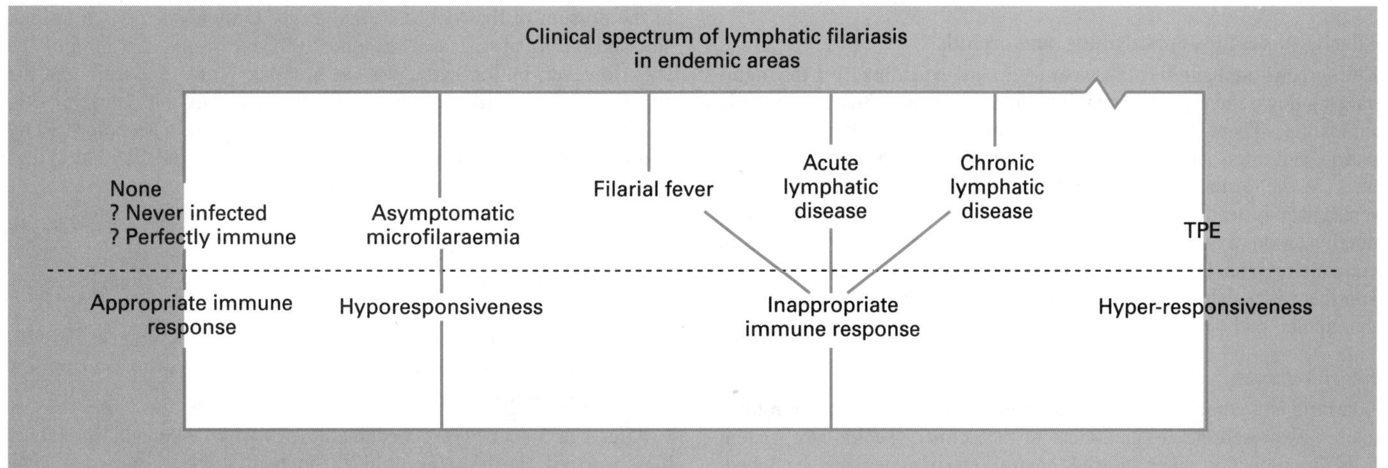

ASYMPTOMATIC MICROFILARAEMIA

Many people are microfilaraemic in endemic areas—sometimes with very high densities—and yet completely free from disease. Some remain in this state for many years, others revert to the amicrofilaraemic condition while remaining asymptomatic; still others develop disease either with or without losing their microfilaraemia.

ACUTE LYMPHATIC FILARIASIS

In immigrants to endemic areas the clinical incubation period can be as short as 2 months for *B. malayi* and just under 4 months for *W. bancrofti*. There are differences in the relative frequencies of acute lesions in Brugian and Bancroftian disease; lymphadenitis and lymphangitis of the legs are characteristic of Brugian infections, while lesions of the male genitalia predominate in Bancroftian disease, legs and arms being less affected.

Filarial fever

Some clinicians warn against diagnosing filarial fever in the absence of specific evidence of filarial infection, but in some endemic areas a syndrome in known infected persons is well recognized by local inhabitants. It consists of recurrent episodes of fever with chills, rigors, and sweating, accompanied by headache, bone and joint pains, general malaise, anorexia, vomiting, and even delirium. The cause of fever is controversial, but some episodes appear to be due to secondary bacterial (usually streptococcal) infection and respond rapidly to antibiotics, while others are relieved by specific microfilaricidal therapy. Often typical signs of acute filariasis will supervene during the course of an attack of fever. In regions where filariasis and malaria coexist, filarial fever is an important differential diagnosis. Attacks last 3 to 7 days, may recur at irregular intervals over many years, and can persist long after the patient has left an endemic area; initial attacks of fever have been seen in expatriates as long as 20 years after the last possible exposure.

Filarial lymphadenitis and lymphangitis of the limbs

The onset is abrupt, affecting the inguinal nodes in Brugian disease, the inguinal, popliteal, axillary, and epitrochlear nodes in Bancroftian disease. Attacks are accompanied by filarial fever, and are precipitated by physical activity or intercurrent infections; they can be crippling in severity and confine patients to bed. Lymph node inflammation resolves within a few days but is sometimes followed by severe retrograde, painful lymphangitis; typically this spreads peripherally but rarely centripetally from the affected node. Cellulitis of the whole limb may supervene, and the node may form an abscess or suppurate to form an ulcer. Oedema occurs during severe attacks and acute disease may pass gradually into chronic lymphatic obstruction; in some patients acute episodes recur at intervals of once yearly to as many as 50 times yearly but others may only experience one or two attacks before complete resolution.

Filarial funiculitis, epididymitis, and orchitis

Retrograde lymphangitis of the spermatic cord extending from the inguinal ring down the inguinal canal into the scrotum is known as 'endemic funiculitis'. There is acute pain, fever, malaise and tenderness on palpation, and often acute epididymo-orchitis with scrotal oedema and redness and the formation of fluid in the tunica vaginalis. Attacks are recurrent and may lead to chronic disease; funiculitis is the most common manifestation of acute Bancroftian filariasis seen in adult immigrants to endemic regions. Genital involvement is very rare in Brugian filariasis, and there is usually a suspicion that Bancroftian infection coexists, or that genital pathology is non-filarial.

Filarial abscess

Filariasis is a controversial cause of abscess, but the incidence rate of abscesses presenting for treatment to the primary health-care system falls dramatically when filarial control programmes are launched. Abscesses are often sterile, may be situated in nodes or along the path of vessels, and if they suppurate leave a clean ulcer discharging serosanguineous fluid. Sterile abscesses in muscles are reported from areas of diurnally subperiodic *W. bancrofti* infection. The scars of healed abscesses may provide evidence in cases of difficult differential diagnosis.

CHRONIC LYMPHATIC FILARIASIS

Not all those developing chronic filariasis have a history of previous acute disease; long exposure to repeated infection is required, and chronic disease appears 10 to 20 years after first exposure. Chronic filariasis increases in frequency and severity with increasing age, being progressive and cumulative in nature, and only rarely resolves without treatment. Patients with chronic disease are often amicrofilaraemic, or have very low densities of microfilariae; New Guinea seems to be an exception to this rule. The mechanism of chronic lesions is retardation and eventual failure of lymph flow from progressive lymph-vessel dilatation and obstruction, and the formation of varices in fibrosed and incompetent vessels. The most common features of chronic Bancroftian filariasis are hydrocele; lymphoedema and elephantiasis of (in order of decreasing frequency) the legs, the scrotum, the arms, the penis, the breasts, and the vulva; and chyluria. There are geographical variations in this pattern and a few detailed studies suggest that involvement of the female external genitalia is underestimated. The characteristic signs of chronic *B. malayi* and *B. timori* infections are lymphoedema followed by elephantiasis of the legs below the knee, or less commonly of the arm below the elbow; genital involvement and chyluria do not occur. The onset of chronic filariasis does not coincide with the cessation of acute episodes, which may continue for many years and indeed may become more frequent and more severe.

Hydrocele

Filarial hydroceles are fluid swellings of the tunica vaginalis; the fluid is clear and straw-coloured. Hydroceles follow repeated attacks of funiculitis and are seldom painful. Bleeding and extravasation of lymph cause fluid to appear bloodstained or turbid and milky. Hydroceles are commonly unilateral at first but soon become bilateral, although there are often remarkable differences in size. Repeated tapping may lead to their conversion into a hard, fibrotic mass and cause abscess formation. Hydrocele fluid may contain microfilariae when examination of blood proves negative, but absence of microfilariae does not refute a filarial aetiology for the hydrocele.

Lymphoedema and elephantiasis

The most common site is the leg. Lymphoedema in patients with Brugian filariasis is preceded by an history of several years of attacks of lymphadenitis and lymphangitis; this is less often obtained in Bancroftian filariasis. The onset is most frequently around the ankles, spreading to the dorsum of the foot, calf, and thigh. Lymphoedema is transient, soft and pitting at first, and responds well to rest and elevation of the leg. However, pitting oedema soon becomes brawny oedema and the swelling is then hard and permanent; subcutaneous thickening of skin and hyperkeratosis occur, and there is fissuring of skin accompanied by nodular, warty, papillomatous changes, especially in the feet. The World Health Organization has classified lymphoedema as follows:

- *grade I lymphoedema*: mostly pitting oedema; spontaneously reversible on elevation;
- *grade II lymphoedema*: mostly non-pitting oedema; not spontaneously reversible on elevation;
- *grade III lymphoedema (elephantiasis)*: gross increase in volume in a grade II lymphoedema, with dermatosclerosis and papillomatous lesions.

After 1 to 3 years, lymphoedema develops into elephantiasis. Fibroblastic activity in the lymph fluid of interstitial spaces in oedematous limbs leads to subcutaneous fibrotic tissue; the maximum size of the affected limb may not be attained for many years. Elephantiasis is mostly unilateral, and starts in middle age, but affected children and young adults are occasionally seen, as is bilateral disease.

Chyluria and lymphuria

The rupture of abdominal lymphatic varices into the renal pelvis or bladder gives rise to chyluria when the lymphatic vessel is draining the intestine, or lymphuria when not. Chylous urine is opaque and milky due to suspended fat globules, whereas lymphuria has a normal appearance; blood is frequently present and the condition is then termed haematochyluria or haematolymphuria. Prolonged attacks of chyluria lead to a syndrome resembling malabsorption, and lymphuria can produce a state of protein loss resembling the nephrotic syndrome. Urine containing chyle or lymph will coagulate, and the condition may present as retention of urine due to coagula, but aching in the back, pelvis, and groins from the distended lymph varices is a more common mode of presentation.

OCCULT FILARIASIS

Occult filariasis is infection in which microfilariae are destroyed at an accelerated rate by hyper-responsiveness of the host immune system, and are almost never seen in peripheral blood. Pathophysiologically it is quite distinct from other forms, being due to microfilariae and not adults. It is preferable to call those forms of filariasis (such as acute lesions in immigrants to endemic areas and late-stage elephantiasis) that are often associated with amicrofilaraemia, 'filariasis without microfilaraemia', reserving 'occult filariasis' for true immunological hyper-responsiveness.

Tropical pulmonary eosinophilia

The main form of occult filariasis is tropical pulmonary eosinophilia; very few people in an endemic area develop this; the male:female ratio is 2:1 and children are rarely affected. There is persistent, paroxysmal night cough, wheezing, and dyspnoea, as in bronchial asthma; hypereosinophilia (absolute counts from 3000 to 50 000/mm^3 of blood); reduction in vital capacity, total lung capacity, and residual volume; and radiographic signs of diffuse miliary lesions and enhanced bronchovascular markings. There are exceptionally high titres of filarial antibodies and low-grade fever. If untreated, tropical pulmonary eosinophilia progresses to chronic pulmonary fibrosis and emphysema. It can result from Bancroftian or Brugian infection and occurs in Indonesia, India, Malaysia, Singapore, Vietnam and rarely the Caribbean, Latin America, and the Pacific Islands; it seems to be absent from Africa.

Other possible syndromes of occult filariasis

Arthritis of the knee joint, endomyocardial fibrosis, skin rashes, thrombophlebitis, and nerve palsies have all been attributed to occult filariasis.

Diagnosis of filarial infections

Clinical

Careful history taking, including a geographical history of residence and travel, and full clinical examination are essential. Because lesions of the limbs and genitals can cause serious feelings of 'being dirty', and being 'ashamed and rejected by society', full psychological assessment is also important.

Parasitological

Definitive species diagnosis is parasitological; measured capillary or venous blood specimens taken at peak microfilarial density times are processed into stained blood films or filtered through membrane filters, using standard techniques. For individual diagnosis, 100 μl or 1 ml of blood are used.

Immunodiagnosis

These tests are the subject of intensive research at present. The species and stage sensitivity and specificity of antigen- and antibody-detection assays are being improved. Their use in practice should be as a supplement to parasitological tests and clinical judgement. Immunodiagnosis gives valuable confirmation in tropical pulmonary eosinophilia.

Lymphoscintigraphy

Using radiolabelled albumin or dextran, lymphoscintigraphy allows monitoring of damaged lymphatics during treatment.

Treatment of lymphatic filariasis

CHEMOTHERAPY

Diethylcarbamazine citrate (DEC)

This is the drug of choice for the treatment of individual patients. Treatment kills most microfilariae but only some adults. As the objectives of treatment are to eliminate parasites and to cure, reduce or prevent morbidity, most patients will need repeated courses. The dose schedule for Bancroftian filariasis is 6 mg of DEC per kg body weight/day for 12 consecutive days, given orally in tablet form in two or three divided doses after food; for Brugian filariasis this is reduced to 3 or 4 mg/kg body weight daily. This course will usually have to be repeated three or four times at monthly intervals if maximum effects are to be achieved. DEC will clear microfilaraemia, prevent recurrences of acute manifestations, and produce improvement in lymphoedema and early elephantiasis.

Tropical pulmonary eosinophilia and other forms of occult filariasis are treated with DEC at 6 mg/kg body weight daily for 21 days, but relapses are common and retreatment should be at 12 mg/kg body weight daily for 30 days.

The direct toxic effects of DEC in therapeutic doses are negligible. Reactions to the destruction of parasites may be systemic, including headache, bone and joint pains, anorexia, nausea and vomiting, dizziness, and sleepiness. Local effects are mainly acute exacerbations of pre-existing lesions, including asthmatic attacks in patients with tropical pulmonary eosinophilia. Adverse reactions are more common and more severe in Brugian than in Bancroftian infections, usually occur in the first 12 h of treatment, and can be reduced by initiating treatment with low doses of DEC for a few days. Patients should always be warned of the possibility of reactions; antipyretics and analgesics are helpful. Caution should be observed in treating patients from Africa with DEC, in view of the possibility of infection with *Onchocerca volvulus* or *Loa loa*; fatal reactions can occur with DEC in these infections and expert advice should always be sought.

DEC has been used in millions of patients in numerous community programmes aimed at control or eradication of infection. Many dosage regimens and formulations have been tried, including incorporation of DEC in salt, annual single-dose treatment of whole populations, and selective therapy of proved parasite positives. Much success has been achieved, and remarkably, no fatalities have been reported.

Ivermectin and other drugs

Following its success in the community treatment of onchocerciasis, ivermectin has undergone field trials at eight sites around the world for Bancroftian filariasis and at three sites for Brugian filariasis. So far, good microfilaricidal effects have been observed particularly at high single oral dosages of 200 to 400 μg/kg body weight. Effects on adult worms and signs and symptoms of disease are not yet clear. Further research is needed.

Albendazole at a dose of 400 mg twice daily for 21 days showed less microfilaricidal effect than DEC but appeared to have a good macrofilaricidal action, and could be a useful drug for treating clinical disease; again, further research is needed.

In clinical trials in India and China, coumarin produced significant reductions in oedema and in symptoms and complications of elephantiasis; the improvements were present 1 year after treatment and adverse reactions were few and trivial. Further trials of this drug are urgently needed.

SURGICAL MANAGEMENT OF LYMPHATIC FILARIASIS

Conservative treatment such as nocturnal leg elevation, firm pressure bandaging and elastic stockings, scrupulous attention to local foot care and infections, and the judicious use of diuretics can be invaluable in preventing deterioration in cases of lymphoedema and elephantiasis. In carefully selected cases more radical surgical procedures such as lymphnodovenous shunt and lymphovenous shunt, combined with the removal of excess skin and fibrous and fatty tissue, produce significant improvement lasting for years.

Hydroceles can be managed by repeated tapping but usually need radical excision. Chyluria has been successfully treated by a variety of procedures including stripping the lymphatics from the pelvis of the kidney and cystoscopic fulguration of leaking varices in the bladder mucosa. Diagnostic lymphangiography itself often seems to stop the flow of chyle into urine.

REFERENCES

Addiss, D.G., Eberhard, M.L., Lammie, P.J., Hitch, W.L., and Spencer, H.C. (1991). Tolerance of single high-dose ivermectin for treatment of lymphatic filariasis. *Transactions of the Royal Society of Tropical Medicine and Hygiene*, **85,** 265–6.

Bundy, D.A.P., Grenfell, B.T., and Rajagopalan, P.K. (1991). Immunoepidemiology of lymphatic filariasis: the relationship between infection and disease. *Parasitology Today*, **7,** A71–75 and *Immunology Today*, **12,** A71–75.

Eberhard, M.L. and Lammie, P.J. (1991). Laboratory diagnosis of filariasis. *Clinical and Laboratory Medicine*, **11,** 977–1010.

Eberhard, M.L., Hightower, A.W., McNeeley, D.F., and Lammie, P.J. (1992). Long-term suppression of microfilaraemia following ivermectin treatment. *Transactions of the Royal Society of Tropical Medicine and Hygiene*, **86,** 287–8.

Mackenzie, C.D. and Kron, M.A. (1985). Diethylcarbamazine: a review of its action in onchocerciasis, lymphatic filariasis and inflammation. *Tropical Diseases Bulletin*, **82,** R1–37.

Ottesen, E.A. (1985). Efficacy of diethylcarbamazine in eradicating infection with lymphatic-dwelling filariae in humans. *Review of Infectious Diseases*, **7,** 341–56.

Ottesen, E.A. (1987). Description, mechanisms and control of reactions to treatment in the human filariases. In *Filariasis*, Ciba Foundation Symposium 127, (ed. D. Evered and S. Clark), pp. 265–83. Wiley, Chichester.

Ottesen, E.A. *et al.* (1990). A controlled trial of ivermectin and diethylcarbamazine in lymphatic filariasis. *New England Journal of Medicine*, **322,** 1113–17.

Partono, F. (1987). The spectrum of disease in lymphatic filariasis. In *Filariasis*, Ciba Foundation Symposium 127, (ed. D. Evered and S. Clark), pp. 15–31. Wiley, Chichester.

Sasa, M. (1976). *Human filariasis*. University Park Press, Baltimore and London.

Southgate, B.A. (1992). Intensity and efficiency of transmission and the development of microfilaraemia and disease: their relationship in lymphatic filariasis. *Journal of Tropical Medicine and Hygiene*, **94,** 1–12.

Southgate, B.A. (1992). The significance of low density microfilaraemia in the transmission of lymphatic filarial parasites. *Journal of Tropical Medicine and Hygiene*, **94,** 79–86.

Southgate, B.A. and Bryan, J.H. (1992). Factors affecting transmission of *Wuchereria bancrofti* by anopheline mosquitoes. 4. Facilitation, limitation, proportionality and their epidemiological significance. *Transactions of the Royal Society of Tropical Medicine and Hygiene*, **86,** 523–30.

Srividya, A., Pani, S.P., Rajagopalan, P.K., Bundy, D.A.P., and Grenfell, B.T. (1991). The dynamics of infection and disease in bancroftian filariasis. *Transactions of the Royal Society of Tropical Medicine and Hygiene*, **85,** 255–9.

Taylor, A.E.R. and Denham, D.A. (1992). Diagnosis of filarial infections including a review of recent abstracts from *Tropical Diseases Bulletin* (May 1986–December 1990). *Tropical Diseases Bulletin*, **89,** R1–33.

World Health Organization (1984). *Lymphatic filariasis. Fourth report of the WHO Expert Committee on Filariasis*, World Health Organization Technical Report Series No. 702, pp. 48–66. WHO, Geneva.

World Health Organization (1992). *Lymphatic filariasis: the disease and its control. Fifth report of the WHO Expert Committee on Filariasis*, World Health Organization Technical Report Series No. 821, pp. 8–13 and 42–53. WHO, Geneva.

7.14.3 Guinea-worm disease: human dracunculiasis

M. M. KLIKS

The aetiological agent of human dracunculiasis, *Dracunculus medinensis*, is the largest nematode to infect man. Owing to its size, spectacular appearance at the skin surface, and exquisitely painful emergence, early observers believed it to be a snake, hence its biblical title, 'the fiery serpent'.

GEOGRAPHICAL DISTRIBUTION

Human guinea-worm disease was once endemic throughout Africa, the Arabian peninsula, the Middle East, Central and South Asia and, for a brief period, the Caribbean region. In the remaining endemic countries of South Asia and West and Central Africa (Fig. 1), perhaps 1 million cases occur focally among the poorest and most remote populations. Elsewhere, diagnoses of human dracunculiasis are very rare and occur almost exclusively in immigrant workers and students or tourists from those areas. Dracunculiasis probably no longer exists as a human disease in countries of the Arabian peninsula, Egypt, Iraq, Iran, Afghanistan, and the Central Asian republics. Single cases of indigenous transmission to man have been reported from Japan and Korea, and infections in domestic animals are known from China, Kazakhstan, and Uzbekistan.

Infection with *D. medinensis* can occur only in people who drink water from unprotected ground-water sources contaminated with infective third-stage larvae contained in its minute crustacean vector. Hence, this disease has not been reported in casual visitors, tourists or even long-term expatriate residents of endemic regions who generally live in urban areas with piped water-supply systems. However, the growing popularity of 'ecotourism' may bring large numbers of outsiders deep into the endemic areas, which, not unexpectedly, are some of the most 'primitive' places on earth.

Human dracunculiasis is an example of a politico-economic disease. It occurs only among segments of a nation's population that are on the fringe of modernization, generally excluded from benefits of basic education, clean water, and minimal primary health care, and are denied any effective access to democratic political processes.

LIFE HISTORY OF THE PARASITE AND EPIDEMIOLOGY

Infection is acquired when copepod crustaceans, 0.5 to 1.5 mm long, containing infective third-stage larvae of *D. medinensis* are ingested in drinking water (Fig. 2) and is associated with an absence of protected household water supplies. Immature worms migrate to the body cavities where they mature and mate, after which the males disappear. Between 9 and 14 months later gravid females, 70 to 120 cm long, migrate within the subdermal and subcutaneous connective tissues, usually reaching the extremities. There the female produces a chemical that causes the formation of a blister adjacent to its vulva. An ulcer soon forms at the site (Fig. 3) through which the worm protrudes, releasing up to 1 million rhabditiform larvae, particularly when stimulated by the immersion of

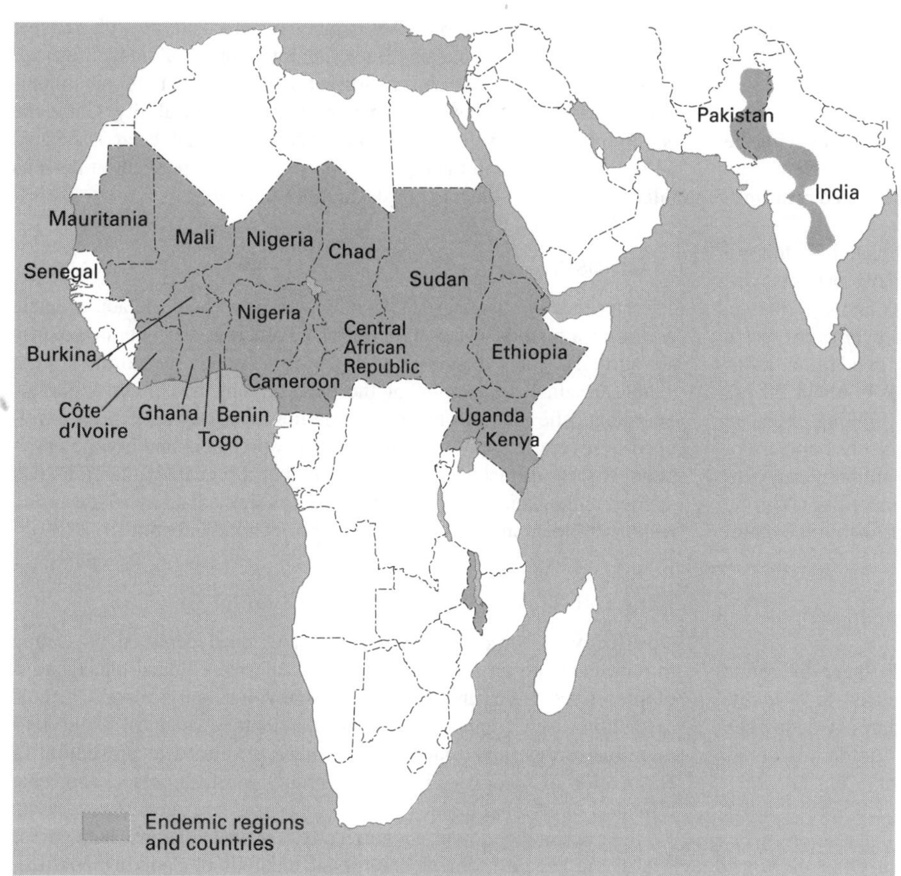

Fig. 1 Geographical distribution of dracunculiasis in 1993. There remain a few foci in eastern Pakistan. In the adjacent hyperendemic areas of Rajasthan State in India and in large foci in Maharashra and Madhya Pradesh States thousands of cases occur annually despite a decade of national control efforts. Small foci in Yemen and Saudi Arabia spontaneously disappeared during the 1980s. The disease was eradicated in the Central Asian Republics (1926–33) and Iran (1970s) by intensive, task-dedicated campaigns. The majority of cases now occur in Nigeria, Sudan, Uganda, and Burkina Faso, all of which have military dictators and suffer from social, economic, and political unrest.

Fig. 2 Lifecycle of guinea-worm in man. (a) Copepods infected with third stage larvae are ingested in drinking water; larvae are released in the intestine, migrate to the body cavity, mature and mate. (b) After 12 to 15 months gravid female worms migrate to the limbs, cause a blister to form and release first stage larvae into water. (c) First stage larvae survive in water for 3 to 5 days until ingested by copepods. (d) Larvae undergo two moults in the copepod and are infective in 2 to 3 weeks.

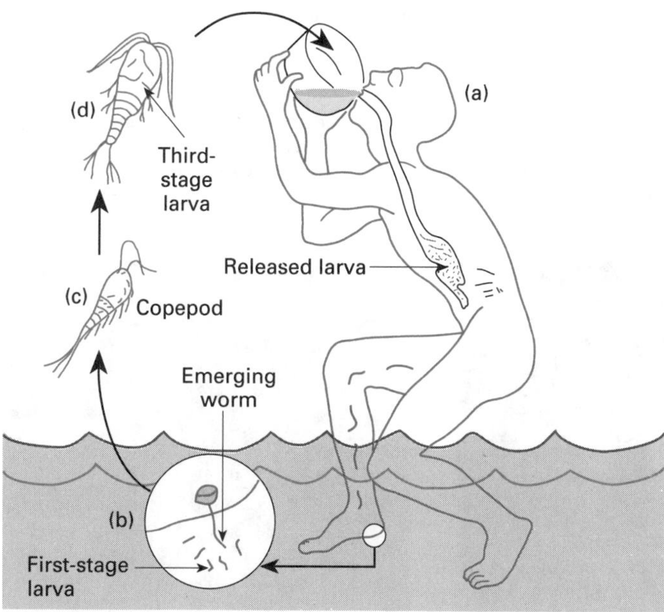

Fig. 3 Surgically-assisted manual extraction of prepatent guinea-worm before formation of blister or abscess. (a) The extent of the worm is determined by palpation. Firm massage is used to loosen worm from surrounding connective tissues. When available, local anaesthetic is injected and a small (5–10 mm) incision made adjacent to a coil of the worm, near its midpoint if possible. (b) A blunt probe is used to separate the worm from connective tissues and to lift out a section of worm sufficiently long to grasp with the fingers. Gentle traction and firm massage along the limb toward the incision facilitates removal. When the entire worm cannot be removed at once it should be ligated, rolled on to a piece of gauze, and taped down and the wound dressed until the next session. Photographs by Malissa C. Kliks, CTS Foundation, Gouera village, Burkina Faso, August 1989.

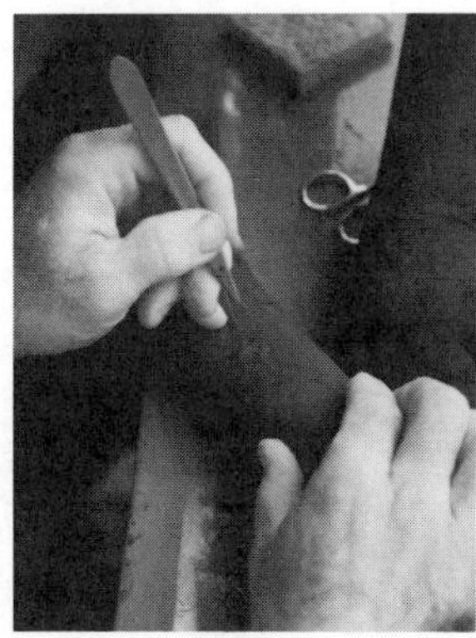

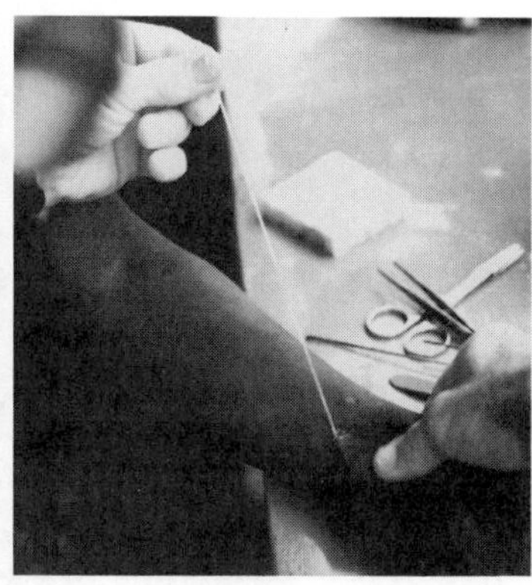

the lesion into water, as when the patient enters a pond to fetch drinking water. Larvae are actively ingested by the copepod and become infective to the human definitive host in about 2 weeks.

Thus, the onset of acute symptoms and transmission for the next year's infections are simultaneous and tend to be synchronous with the advent of the rains and the planting season. A dry-season cycle occurs in some areas when the copepod vectors become concentrated in shrinking, ephemeral drinking-water sources.

There is abundant evidence of both partial and complete immunity to dracunculiasis. In any hyperendemic community most patients will experience the emergence of only one or two worms annually (some, usually the same individuals, will have many more emerge), even though all residents ingest dozens of infective larvae. In addition, it has been observed often that part of the population, usually about 20 per cent, has never experienced patent infection despite lifelong exposure and the repeated annual occurrence of clinical disease in members of their immediate household. The presence of specific antibody can generally be demonstrated in all residents of such endemic villages during the season of transmission/emergence, whether or not worm(s) eventually emerge.

CLINICAL PICTURE

Detection of prepatent dracunculiasis is occasionally made by astute recognition of the distinct prodromal symptoms related to systemic hypersensitivity. Usually, however, the infection becomes evident when a migrating mature female worm is seen just under the dermis of the trunk and limbs (Fig. 3(a)) or by the appearance of a blister which becomes an ulcer (Fig. 4(a)) and leads to abscess formation (Fig. 4(b)). Gravid worms usually emerge on the extremities, but also from the scrotum (Fig. 4(c)), nipple, sublingual gland, and vulva. Often the worm is no longer visible, having been broken during attempted extraction and/or having retracted into the lesion or disintegrated (Fig. 4(b)) after discharging its larvae.

Under conditions of intense transmission in hyperendemic areas, many infective larvae are ingested annually. Of these, only a few survive ultimately to emerge and expel their larvae; however the simultaneous emergence of several worms is not unusual. Cryptic infections are probably common; numerous larvae are killed and encapsulated by host tissue responses and can be seen radiographically. Not infrequently, larvae lodge in sensitive ectopic sites, most often in joints, the orbit, or the central and peripheral nervous systems, leading to severe arthritic changes, blindness, and septic subdural abscesses.

Uncomplicated cases with emergent worms resolve in 2 to 3 weeks, but most victims are incapacitated for at least 6 weeks. The destruction of worms in host tissues provokes delayed hypersensitivity with massive swelling and exquisite pain. Bacterial infection is almost universal, resulting in cellulitis and abscess formation. Repeated or chronic inflammation leads to ankylosis of joints and permanent disability. Gangrene is common in severe untreated cases and tetanus has been associated with dracunculiasis in many areas: approximately 1 per cent of persons infected dies from dracunculiasis and its sequelae.

DIAGNOSIS

The presence of characteristic lesions with or without the adult female worm, or a history of having lived or travelled in an endemic country are sufficient for a diagnosis of dracunculiasis. Where worms are not visible a saline preparation of the exudate may reveal active larvae. Serodiagnostic methods using enzyme immunoassay have been developed in several laboratories and can detect prepatent and cryptic infections. A skin test using worm body fluids or a prepared antigen extract applied to the patient's forearm provokes an immediate hypersensitivity response in persons with pre-emergent or ectopic infections.

TREATMENT AND PATIENT MANAGEMENT

No effective, specific anthelminthic agent has been identified, but testing in both man and an animal model is under way. Clinical management of prepatent, acute, and chronic cases involves surgical and manual extraction, use of appropriate anti-inflammatory, analgesic, and antimicrobial drugs, and supportive nursing care aimed at prevention or elimination of secondary infections, reduction of abscesses, and rehabilitation of effected limbs.

However, in the remote, economically deprived villages where guinea worm is a severe problem, traditional methods of applying poultices made of leaves, charcoal, and mud, and attempts at manual extraction often lead to exacerbation of symptoms. Under these unhygienic conditions, soaking or applying hot, moist compresses at the affected site and gentle massage toward the opening can promote drainage of the abscess and facilitate removal of worms using light traction. Between treatments the lesions should be carefully bandaged to prevent infection and escape of infective larvae should the patient enter a drinking-water source.

Where possible, migrating worms appearing in the dermis (Fig. 3(a)) should be removed by making a small incision adjacent to the worm near its midpoint, lifting out a loop of the worm using a blunt curved probe and applying gentle traction to it while firmly massaging the affected limb along the tract of the worm toward the opening (Fig. 3(b)). Should the worm rupture, or should it be necessary to ligate it before

Fig. 4 (a) Acute inflammation, two blisters; right one opened to reveal intact adult guinea-worm and ulcer beneath; left one spontaneously exuding fluid containing first stage larvae. After hot water soaking both worms were removed with gentle traction and massage. (b) Chronic inflammation, multiple ulcers, and abscesses on foot and ankle containing disintegrating guinea worms; over a 3-week period the patient had broken off parts of three worms. After hot water soaking and massage the remaining worm fragments emerged. (c) Acute inflammation; an adult worm emerging from ulcer on scrotum was removed intact with gentle traction. Photographs by M. M. Kliks, CTS Foundation; (a) Rajasthan, India, (b) (c) Gouera village, Burkina Faso.

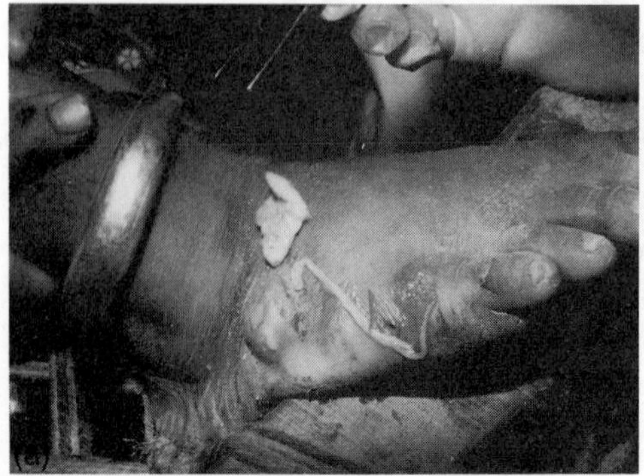

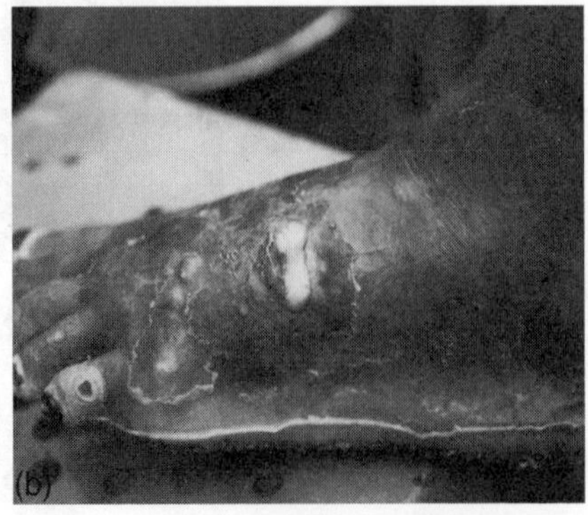

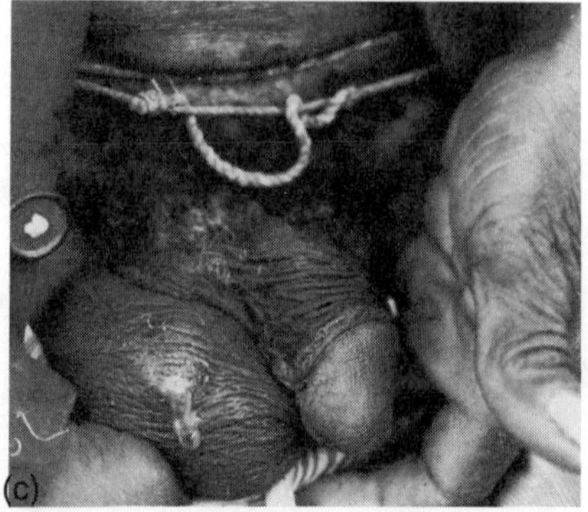

complete removal, care must be taken to prevent its body fluids from coming into contact with the patient's tissues.

After blister formation and emergence of the worm, extraction is complicated by inflammatory processes and patients' unwillingness to cooperate owing to severe pain. Anti-inflammatory, antimicrobial, and analgesic drugs should be administered and hot, moist packs applied to the lesion for some hours before trying to remove worms. During removal the area around the lesion should be firmly massaged toward the opening while applying gentle traction to the worm. Surgical enlargement of the opening may be useful. In this manner, intact and fragmented worms can usually be removed in one or two sessions of 5 to 10 min each.

PROPHYLAXIS, PREVENTION, AND CONTROL

Personal prophylaxis is by avoiding contaminated drinking water or by brief boiling or filtering through cloth to retain copepods: monofiliment nylon, 100 to 200 μm mesh, is ideal, but even cotton shirt cloth is quite effective. Temporary prevention can be achieved in relatively small drinking-water sources by application of temephos (Abate) granules, which eliminates copepod vectors for several weeks to months. At the village level, medical education programmes demonstrating the role of copepods in the lifecycle (Fig. 5(a)), cloth filtration of drinking water (Fig. 5(b)), prohibiting infected persons from entering the community drinking-water supply to fetch water, and the use of occlusive bandaging over active lesions are inexpensive and effective control measures that should be promoted by local public-health officials.

Fig. 5 Health education activities. Local health workers using Centre Muraz's *Eliminon le Ver de Guinea* cartoon booklet to teach mode of transmission and control. (a) Demonstration of copepods in drinking water. (b) Demonstration of use of any finely woven cloth to filter household and field workers' drinking water to remove copepod vectors. Photographs by M. M. Kliks, and colleagues, CTS Foundation, Birnin Gwari village, Kaduna State, Nigeria, September 1989.

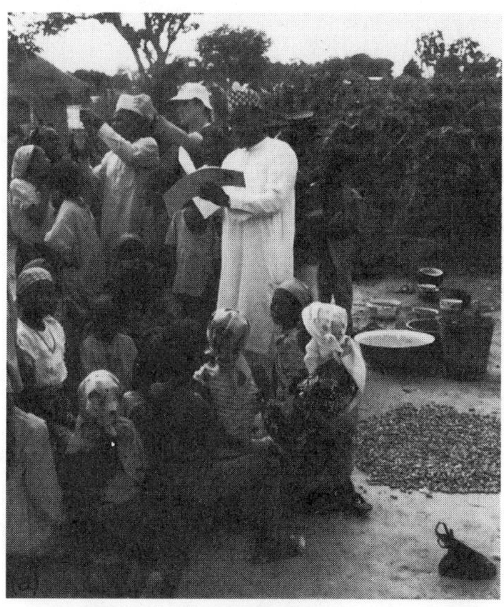

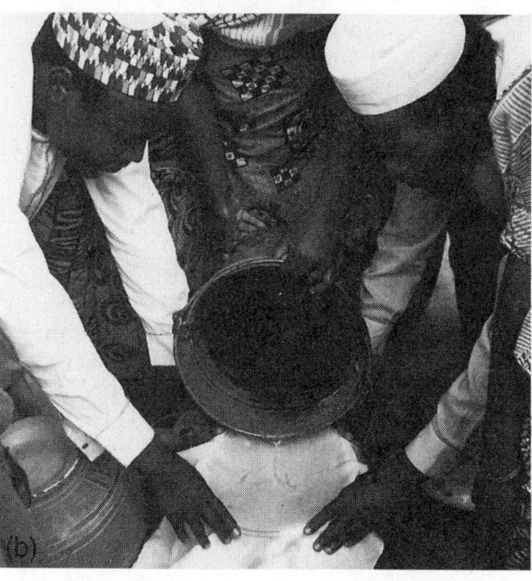

The installation and use of a convenient and reliable, safe water supply such as a covered tube-well with hand pump or even a hand-dug well protected by a parapet will immediately eliminate the disease. Most endemic villages lack the resources and knowledge to make significant improvements in their water supplies and many governments are reluctant to expend scarce developmental funds on such impoverished, unproductive populations, even when international assistance agencies request that they do so.

THE GLOBAL ERADICATION EFFORT

Since the mid-1980s, national programmes for control and eradication of Guinea-worm disease have been developed in almost all endemic countries. In the strategy adopted in most countries, central governmental authorities directed that case-detection surveys and intervention efforts be integrated into existing primary health-care systems, which were already severely stressed. Survey coverage was often poor, interventions ineffective, and data often not reliable because of shortages of funds, poorly trained and insufficiently motivated health personnel, and a lack of political will.

Admirable progress has been made, however, in greatly reducing the global toll of dracunculiasis: up until 1980 it was estimated that there were between 5 and 50 million cases worldwide annually; in 1991 the United States Centers for Disease Control estimated annual incidence to be just under 3 million cases; by March of 1993 it reported that about 375 000 had been detected in some 20 000 villages in national search efforts. It is probable that these figures seriously underestimate the true status of dracunculiasis. Local control and eradication has been achieved in those regions and isolated villages where funds were made available to install safe drinking-water sources and/or where thorough medical education and cloth filtration of drinking water were introduced.

Although 'scheduled' for global eradication by 1995, it is likely that thousands, if not hundreds of thousands, of cases will continue to appear in this decade in the most hyperendemic areas of India and in Nigeria, Burkina Faso, Sudan, Uganda, and other West and Central African countries. Given the deteriorating social, economic, and political conditions in the endemic areas and the failure of wealthier nations to provide the required capital resources, Guinea-worm disease will persist, and perhaps even expand its range.

It has been evident for several years that the original strategy of central government agencies aiming to provide safe or protected water supplies to every endemic village would not be feasible because of the lack of funds available from international and national sources to meet the huge capital expenditures required. During 1992 there was a notable, if overdue, shift away from expensive hydrological interventions to community action strategies using task-dedicated cadres (rather than existing primary health-care workers) as 'trained, village-based' workers who educate villagers using standardized visual aids, document, treat and manage cases, protect and improve water sources, and distribute cloth filters. At the same time, many central government public-health authorities have begun to permit, and even encourage, private-sector initiatives, including those by civic clubs, citizens' and business groups, and even commercial enterprises to contribute to the elimination of this terrible disease through 'adopt-a-village' programmes.

Tragically, in many of the worst affected African countries, civil unrest creating masses of refugees, the political attitudes of the ruling élite, the scarcity of health-care resources, and the lack of democratic institutions, apart from poverty and ignorance, make it highly probable that human dracunculiasis will persist well into the next millennium.

REFERENCES

Hopkins, D.R., and Hopkins, E.M. (1992). Guinea worm: the end is in sight. In *Medical and health annual*, pp. 11–26. Encyclopedia Britannica, Chicago.

Kliks, M.M., and Rao, C.K. (1984). Development of a rapid ELISA for early serodiagnosis of dracunculiasis. *Journal of Communicable Diseases*, **16,** 287–94.

Rhode, J.E., Sharma, B.L., Patton, H., Deggan, C., and Sherry, J.M. (1993). Surgical extraction of Guinea worm: disability reduction and contribution to disease control. *American Journal of Tropical Medicine and Hygiene*, **48,** 71–6.

Muller, R. (1971), *Dracunculus* and dracunculiasis. *Advances in Parasitology*, **9,** 73–151.

7.14.4. Strongyloidiasis, hookworm, and other gut strongyloid nematodes

R. KNIGHT

Strongyloidiasis

The parasitic female worms of the genus Strongyloides are parthenogenic. They measure 2 to 2.5 mm in length and normally live in tunnels between the enterocytes of the crypts of Lieberkühn in the duodenum and jejunum. In the external environment larvae may develop directly, through two moults, into infective larvae, in a manner similar to that of hookworm (Fig. 1). Or alternatively, by the indirect cycle, into free-living male and female adult worms, about 1 mm in length, that produce a second generation of infective larvae. In either case the cycle is completed when infective larvae penetrate the skin and are carried in the venous circulation to the lungs, whence they ascend the bronchi to be swallowed and so reach the upper small bowel, where they mature.

Strongyloides stercoralis

BIOLOGY AND EPIDEMIOLOGY

Eggs hatch immediately on reaching the gut lumen, and the first-stage larvae (Fig. 2) then normally pass down the gut without moulting. Direct development in faecally contaminated soil takes 24 to 48 h; free-living adults mature in 72 to 96 h, and live for up to 10 days. Infective larvae can persist in the soil for 3 weeks. There is no second generation of free-living adults.

In addition to these cycles there are two types of autoinfection; these are important because they enable infection to persist in the host for long periods. In external autoinfection, infective larvae penetrate the perianal skin after rapid direct development on soiled skin. In internal autoinfection, larvae mature to the infective stage within the lumen of the gut and invade the mucosa of the small intestine or colon, and then pass via the gut lymphatics and portal vein to the lungs and back to the gut. In some patients, uncontrolled internal autoinfection leads to hyperinfection with massive worm loads and severe pathology.

S. stercoralis is widely distributed in the tropics, where prevalence may be 5 to 10 per cent or higher in humid lowlands. It remains endemic in the southern United States, Japan, and in parts of Southern Europe, for example, among Swiss and Italian horticulturalists. It also occurs in institutions when soil temperatures are high enough. Transmission among male homosexuals is very rare. Transmammary transmission is postulated but unproven.

Host risk factors are of great importance for internal autoinfection. Steroid and cytotoxic therapy are the most important, but also at risk are those with lymphomas and some other malignancies, hypochlorhydria, diabetic ketosis, hypogammaglobulinaemia, and malnutrition. In the tropics, hyperinfection may occur without evident host factors. Despite coprevalence with human immunodeficiency virus type 1 over much of its range, it now appears that this viral infection does not predispose significantly to *S. stercoralis* hyperinfection, except in a very few patients with advanced AIDS.

Servicemen in the Second World War became infected in Thailand and other parts of South-East Asia, mostly as prisoners of war. Many of these infections still persist and such people are at risk of hyperinfection if given steroids.

PATHOLOGY

In most persistent infections the parasite load is very low, evokes little or no pathological response, and the patient is free of symptoms. In some primary infections and when worm intensities are higher there is villous blunting with oedema and cellular infiltration of the mucosa, leading to malabsorption and protein-losing enteropathy. In more severe infections and in hyperinfection the small-gut wall becomes oedematous and thickened with impaired motility, and the mesenteric lymph nodes are enlarged. In massive autoinfection there is patchy mucosal loss and some adult worms are found deep in the mucosa from where larvae may invade directly without entering the gut lumen. Invading infective larvae can produce a diffuse or haemorrhagic colitis; migrating or ectopic larvae may be found in any organ of the body. Peritoneal and pleural effusions occur and the lungs show pneumonitis and terminally alveolar haemorrhages. Rarely, adult female worms develop ectopically in the

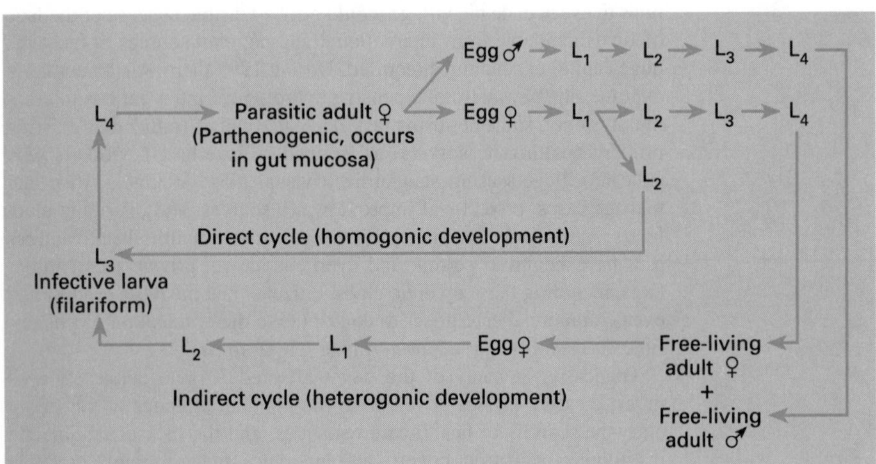

Fig. 1 Basic lifecycle in the genus Strongyloides; L_1, L_2, L_3, and L_4 are the larval stages. The indirect cycle occurs in the soil or faecal mass. Eggs of the parasitic female *S. stercoralis* hatch in the gut lumen and direct development may occur not only in the external environment but also on the perianal skin to produce external autoinfection, or in the gut lumen to produce internal autoinfection. The eggs of the parasitic female *S. fuelleborni* appear in the faeces and internal autoinfection is not possible.

lungs, and these account for the occasional presence of eggs and rhabditiform larvae in sputum.

CLINICAL

Light persistent infections

Symptoms, if any, are usually intermittent, with episodes of upper abdominal pain, wheezy cough, and pruritus ani. Blood eosinophilia is common, and may be the only clinical finding. A pathognomonic sign is a rapidly migrating urticaria known as 'larva currens' that occurs on the buttocks, thighs, and lower trunk; it is a form of cutaneous larva migrans, arising from external autoinfection.

Moderate infections

Gut symptoms predominate, with diarrhoea and malabsorption. Weight loss and anorexia are prominent and not infrequently there is leg oedema. Pulmonary and skin lesions are not common. In primary infections a Loeffler's pneumonitis can occur, with high eosinophilia.

Hyperinfection

Diarrhoea is often severe, and sometimes bloody if there is colitis. Vomiting and abdominal distension may progress to pseudo-obstruction. Lung symptoms are common. Patients are often afebrile and without blood eosinophilia; they can deteriorate rapidly and develop Gram-negative septicaemia, shock or meningitis, especially if they are immunosuppressed. Hypoglycaemia is a feature of autoinfection in malnourished children.

DIAGNOSIS

Rhabditiform larvae should be sought in the stool (Fig. 2). They may be scanty and numbers do not necessarily correlate with symptoms. Live larvae are seen in fresh, wet, microscopical preparations or Baermann concentrates. Using agar-plate coprocultures a result is obtainable in 48 h, earlier than with conventional charcoal cultures. Formol–ether concentrates are also useful but sensitivity can be low. When stool specimens are not fresh, filariform Strongyloides larvae may be found, and also rhabditiform hookworm larvae from hatched eggs. Duodenal aspiration is another useful technique. In hyperinfection, larvae may be found in sputum and in pleural, peritoneal, or cerebrospinal fluids.

Serodiagnosis is useful, especially as a screening test in non-endemic areas. In heavy infections, small-bowel barium studies show segmental dilatation, narrowing, and abnormal motility; in hyperinfection, plain abdominal films may show fluid levels.

Fig. 2 First stage larvae of *S. stercoralis* in stool.

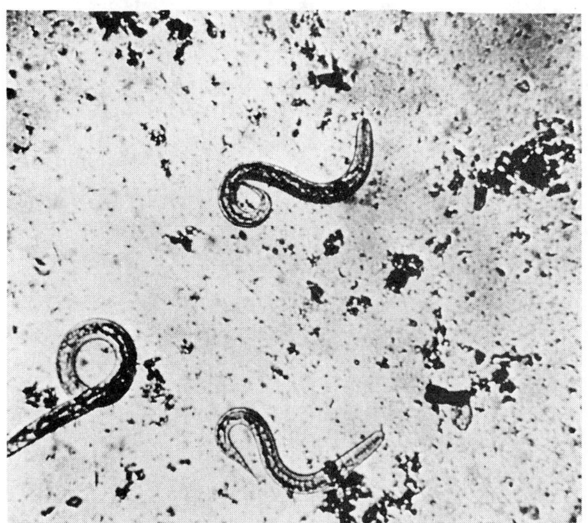

TREATMENT

Thiabendazole remains the drug of choice; 25 mg/kg is given twice daily (maximum 3 g per day), usually for 3 days. Intolerance is common and drug-induced hepatitis is reported. Treatment may fail in hyperinfection, which continues to have a high mortality. Such patients need supportive care and parenteral antimicrobials. Albendazole is an alternative in non-urgent cases but cure rates are rather low. Invermectin appears to be effective for this infection, using a single oral dose of 200 μg/kg, repeated after 1 week or 200 μg/kg daily for 3 days, but experience is so far limited. The risks of corticosteroid and cytotoxic therapy are so high in transplant patients, for example, that empirical therapy may be justifiable in those likely to be infected.

Strongyloides fuelleborni

This species differs from *S. stercoralis* in that eggs do not hatch in the gut lumen; thus there can be no internal autoinfection. In faeces the eggs are thin-walled and contain a larva; hatching occurs within a few hours. In Africa this parasite is common in most non-human primates. In the forests of West and Central Africa, particularly Zaire, people are commonly infected, mainly from zoonotic sources. Elsewhere, for instance in Zambia and adjacent countries, there appears to be person-to-person transmission. Infected volunteers have developed wheezing, upper abdominal pain, and loose stools, but symptomatology in natural human infections is poorly defined.

In Papua New Guinea a subspecies of this parasite, *S. f. kellyi*, is common in several communities, with high prevalence in both children and adults. In a few endemic foci a distinctive 'swollen belly syndrome' is associated with enormously high faecal egg counts and protein-losing enteropathy. Infants aged 2 weeks to 6 months are affected and show abdominal distension, diarrhoea, breathing difficulties, weight loss, hypoproteinaemia, and peripheral oedema; untreated, the mortality is high. There are no non-human primates in Papua New Guinea and no animal reservoir for this parasite is known. In infants, external autoinfection occurs when they are nursed in soiled string-bag cradles; transmammary transmission is suspected but not so far proven.

S. fuelleborni infection should be treated with thiabendazole. Supportive care including plasma infusion or blood transfusion, plus antibiotic cover, is needed for 'swollen belly syndrome' in Papua New Guinea.

Hookworm and other gut strongyloid nematodes

Adult nematodes of the order Strongylida have a muscular pharynx, and the males have a caudal copulatory bursa, supported by muscular rays. Three superfamilies infect man. The true hookworms belong to the Ancylostomatoidea, which have a well-developed, globular buccal capsule, and a mouth armed ventrally by prominent teeth or cutting plates. The genus Trichostrongylus belongs to the Trichostrongyloidea, which have a greatly reduced buccal capsule. The Strongyloidea include two genera infecting man, Ternidens and Oesophagostomum; the buccal capsule is well developed but bears no prominent oral armature.

The adult worms of all these parasites live attached to, or buried within, the bowel mucosa. The ovoid eggs of all genera are very similar in appearance, with thin, transparent shells that reveal the segmented embryo within; commonly an 8- to 16-cell morula. Eggs hatch in the soil and development proceeds through three stages with two moults. The first and second larval stages feed upon bacteria. They are described as rhabditiform, because of resemblance to the unrelated soil nematode Rhabditis; the pharynx is short, muscular, and constricted in the posterior third, just anterior to a posterior bulb. The third stage, the infective filariform larva, does not feed and may retain the cuticle of the second stage; the pharynx is long and slender, without any constriction. Species identification of adults depends on several cuticular structures—the buccal capsule and its oral armature, and the bursa and copulatory spicules of the male. Generic identification is possible using filariform larvae from cultures. Hosts are usually infected percutaneously or orally.

The hookworms

BIOLOGY AND EPIDEMIOLOGY

Most infections by adult worms are due to *Ancyostoma duodenale* and *Necator americanus*, although in parts of Asia a feline species, *A. ceylanicum*, also matures in man. Several other carnivore species accidentally infect human beings by the percutaneous route and produce zoonotic cutaneous larva migrans.

Adult worms are greyish-white and measure 8 to 13 mm in length; they taper at both ends. Anteriorly the worms are flexed dorsally, giving them their hooked appearance. They attach themselves to the wall of the jejunum by drawing mucosa into the buccal cavity, whose oral armature assists anchorage (Fig. 3). By means of lytic enzymes, anticoagulants, and a vigorous pharyngeal pump, blood and tissue fluids are ingested. Worms move to new locations quite frequently, partly in response to host immunological responses. Females produce 5000 to 20 000 eggs per day, but output per worm declines as worm load rises. In the soil, development is temperature dependent. Under optimum conditions eggs hatch within 2 days and larvae develop to the infective stage in 5 days; they can persist in sandy soil for up to a month. Larvae penetrate host skin after soil contact, most commonly between the toes. After entry into dermal venules and lymphatics they are carried to the lung, where they penetrate the alveoli, ascend the bronchi and trachea, and after being swallowed, re-enter the gut where the final moult occurs. Eggs (Fig. 4) can appear in the faeces 50 to 60 days after cutaneous exposure.

N. americanus is found in the warm, moist tropics where transmission is more or less perennial. Its introduction to the Americas dates from the transatlantic slave trade. It is a smaller worm than *A. duodenale* and the mouth is guarded by two cutting plates. The mean egg output, per female, is 8000 per day and the life-span may exceed 5 years; transmission is exclusively by the percutaneous route.

A. duodenale is primarily a subtropical and temperate species. Soil development can occur at lower temperatures. It is widely distributed in North Africa, the Middle East, the Indian subcontinent, central and northern China, and in parts of South and Central America. Formerly it occured widely in southern Europe and Japan, but here it has declined greatly. In the past it was responsible for 'miner's anaemia'; in the Gotthard tunnel and Cornish tin mines the lack of sanitation and warmth favoured larval development and transmission rates were very high. Worms measure 9 to 13 mm in length. The mouth is guarded by two pairs of sharp teeth. Females produce 15 000 eggs per day. The worms live for about 1 year. In addition to the percutaneous route, infection may be oral on contaminated vegetables; larvae can penetrate the buccal mucosa and undergo transpulmonary migration, or can be swallowed and develop directly within the gut mucosa. Infection may also be transplacental; in China severe hookworm disease is reported in very young infants. Another feature of the lifecycle is arrested development. Larval maturation is delayed at the third or fourth stage within skeletal muscle, or more commonly, in the gut mucosa. This postpones the onset of patent infection and is an adaptive mechanism to irregular or seasonal transmission.

The prevalence of hookworm in the tropics is commonly 20 to 50 per cent, with higher figures in rural agricultural communities. Aridity and coolness at higher altitudes limit transmission, but irrigation schemes usually favour it by raising the water table. In most endemic populations the prevalence of infection and the worm load both rise with age to reach a plateau in adults. Children commonly acquire clinically significant infections between the ages of 5 and 10 years. Within communities, individuals differ greatly in worm load; susceptibility to new infections is determined by immunological, behavioural, and genetic factors.

Hookworms evoke immunological responses, including IgE antibody and eosinophilia, which limit the proportion of larval worms that mature to adults, the adult life-span, and also female fecundity. It is uncertain whether treatment leads to diminution of these protective responses.

PATHOLOGY

Hookworms damage the mucosa mechanically and by the inflammatory response they evoke; bleeding continues at former attachment sites. Gut motility is affected, especially in primary infections and in children, and

Fig. 3 Adult worm of *N. americanus* showing relationships of its pharynx to a jejunal villus.

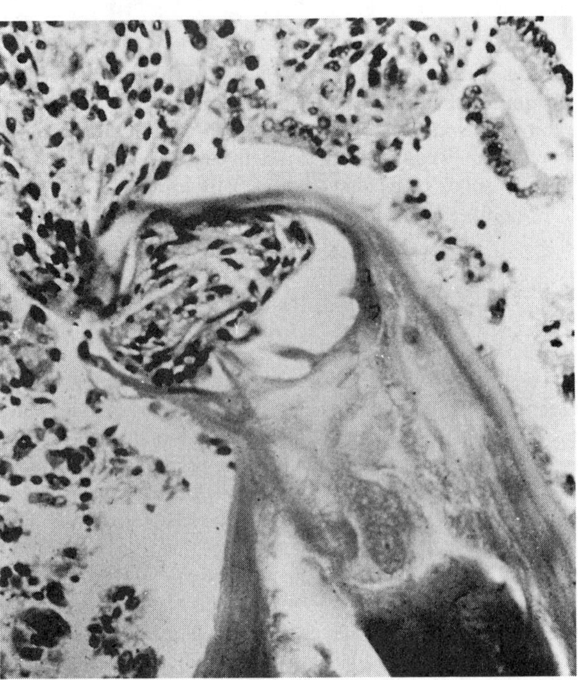

Fig. 4 Egg of *N. americanus*.

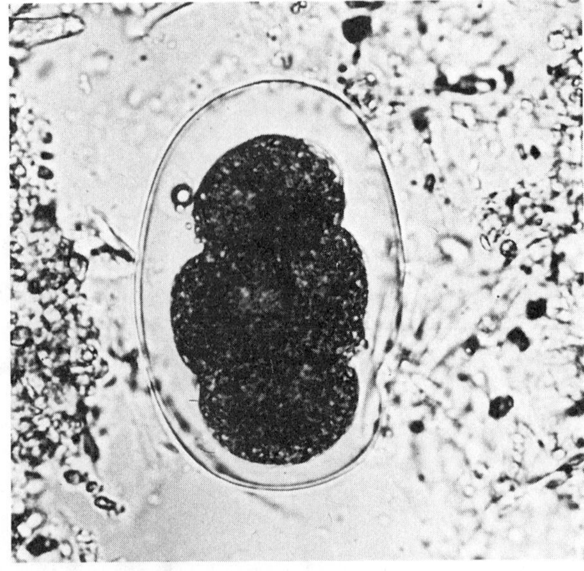

this may affect digestive and absorptive function. Diffuse enterocyte changes leading to malabsorption have been reported, but they are indistinguishable from non-specific tropical enteropathy and of doubtful significance. The major pathogenic mechanism is ingestion of plasma, interstitial fluid, and red cells by the adult worms. *A. duodenale* ingests about 0.15 ml of blood daily, and *N. americanus* 0.05 ml. Most red cells pass through the worm's gut and a proportion of the iron content, variously estimated at 10 to 50 per cent, is reabsorbed by the host. Because worm loads are commonly above 50, and may reach 500 or more, the cumulative effect can be serious. The main nutritional effects are iron deficiency and hypoproteinaemia. The rate at which blood loss leads to anaemia is determined by worm load, the duration of infection, iron stores, other blood loss, and dietary iron. Children, and pregnant or lactating women, with little reserve iron, can become anaemic in a few months; in a previously healthy adult male it can take 2 years or more. Loss of albumin into the gut may exceed the capacity of the liver to replace it; synthesis is depressed by low dietary protein, and by the anaemia. Hypoproteinaemia has important haemodynamic consequences because it limits the normal, compensatory expansion of plasma volume that occurs in chronic anaemia. While the risk of pulmonary oedema is less, transition to a state of low cardiac output is made more likely. Gastric hypochlorhydria is common in hookworm anaemia and increases susceptibility to other gut infections.

Cutaneous lesions are due to hypersensitivity and damage by the enzymes released by migrating larvae. Pulmonary lesions arise when larvae escape from pulmonary capillaries and enter the alveoli; both trauma and hypersensitivity are involved, and the interstitial pneumonitis is of the Loeffler type.

CLINICAL FEATURES ATTRIBUTABLE TO ADULT WORMS

In acute primary infections and in children, epigastric pain is common and may be associated with poor appetite and sometimes diarrhoea. Anorexia is an important mechanism leading to nutritional deficit in children. A few patients develop overt gut bleeding, and melaena is reported in transplacentally infected infants in China.

Most patients present with slowly progressive iron-deficiency anaemia; such patients typically have no gut symptoms. Exertional dyspnoea may begin at haemoglobin levels of 8 g/dl, but may not be noted until it falls to 5 g/dl. Palpitations, weakness, and faintness on exertion are common; sometimes there is precordial pain or leg claudication. Tinnitus is common, and some patients are aware of their jugular vascular bruit. A puffy oedema of the face, arms, and hands is typical, and often unaccompanied by dependent oedema. In severe cases, mental apathy and depression are common, and in adults, amenorrhoea or impotence. Pica is common, especially in pregnancy, and geophagy can lead to acquisition of other soil-transmitted nematodes.

Milder degrees of anaemia cause reduced physical-work performance in adults. In children, growth and development may be slowed and cognitive impairment can lead to reduced scholastic achievement.

Assessment of cardiovascular status is essential in anaemic patients, to differentiate a well-compensated, high-output state from a dangerous low-output one.

CLINICAL FEATURES ATTRIBUTABLE TO LARVAL WORMS

Cutaneous lesions take the form of migrating, itchy, red, serpiginous papules, known as creeping eruption or cutaneous larva migrans. They commonly become vesiculated and excoriated, and this leads to bacterial pyoderma. In many endemic populations, lesions attributable to *A. duodenale* or *N. americanus* are either unnoticed or transient. Among estate workers the condition is known as 'ground itch'; prominent lesions occur in laboratory infections.

Zoonotic hookworms produce more vigorous lesions that may continue to move for several months. Most infections are due to *A. braziliense*, which is common in dogs throughout the tropics, subtropics, and warmer temperate regions. Less common are infections by two other dog parasites, *A. caninum* and *Uncinaria stenocephala*, and the cattle hookworm *Bunostomum phlebotomum*. Infections occur on sandy bathing beaches, in children's play areas, and by contact with pet sandboxes. Lesions are most common on the lower legs and buttocks, but also occur on the arms and face. They must be distinguished from those due to Strongyloides, Gnathostoma, and dermal myiasis.

Wheezy cough due to pneumonitis is more common with *A. duodenale*; symptoms can continue for many months after one exposure, owing to remobilization of larvae arrested in muscle. Lung symptoms are most prominent in heavy primary infections.

DIAGNOSIS

Stool microscopy will reveal eggs (Fig. 4), except in patients with prepatent infections; examination of stool concentrates is rarely necessary. It is useful to estimate the faecal egg count as this provides some measure of the intensity of infection. The simplest method is a semiquantitative wet smear, using 2 mg of stool. For more precise results the use of the McMaster counting chamber is recommended. An alternative is the modified Kato technique, but this requires special care as hookworm eggs can overclear and become invisible. Egg counts are expressed per gram of stool; account must be taken of sampling variation, the day-to-day variation in egg output, and the density-dependent depression of egg output with higher worm loads. Isotope studies indicate that, with either species, 1000 eggs per gram is equivalent to 2.2 ml of blood loss per day. Culture to the infective larval stage, using the Harada Mori technique, will differentiate the two major species and the other genera of gut strongyloid nematodes. About 500 mg of stool is smeared on a strip of filter paper, which is placed in a test tube containing 3 ml of water; tubes are incubated upright, unsealed, at about 25°C; larvae appear in the water after the fifth day.

Haematological findings are microcytic hypochromic anaemia, eosinophilia, low serum ferritin and iron, raised serum transferrin, and reduced bone-marrow haemosiderin. Where there is endemic malaria a mixed blood picture is common.

TREATMENT

Safe and effective anthelminthics are now available. A single 400-mg dose of albendazole, or mebendazole, 100 mg twice daily for 3 days, are both very effective. Alternatives are pyrantel, 10 mg/kg daily for three or four doses, or bephenium, 5 g daily for three doses, the latter being less effective for *N. americanus*.

To replace iron reserves, oral ferrous sulphate will suffice in most patients, but several weeks of medication may be necessary. When compliance is doubted, consideration should be given to intramuscular iron dextran or iron sorbitol. When adequate precautions can be taken it is sometimes appropriate to use total-dose intravenous infusion of iron dextran.

Blood transfusion may be necessary in pregnancy, and when cardiac output is compromised. Packed, or sedimented, red cells should be used and normally only one or two units will be required. Frusemide may be necessary to cover the transfusion, but in other circumstances diuretics should be used with caution. Depletion of plasma volume in hookworm anaemia patients with hypoproteinaemia can compromise cardiac output. Even bedrest in formerly ambulant patients can lead to significant diuresis. Oral fluids must not be restricted.

Chemotherapy should generally be avoided in pregnancy; such patients should be managed with iron replacement or iron supplements only.

Cutaneous lesions can be treated with thiabendazole, 25 mg/kg in two divided doses, for 2 days, or locally with thiabendazole in a dimethylsulphoxide base. Alternatively, albendazole 400 mg or ivermectin 200 μg/kg, as a single dose will be effective for many patients.

CONTROL

Population-based measures are necessary when endemicity and morbidity are high. Latrines are generally beneficial, but can create foci for transmission. Peridomestic drainage lowers the water table, and reduces risk of transmission around latrines. Provision of piped water limits the need to walk to surface-water sources and so reduces contact with soil polluted by promiscuous defaecation. Washing and cooking vegetables will reduce oral *A. duodenale* transmission. Where human excreta is used as fertilizer, composting and chemical ovicides are needed.

Cash-crop estates, plantations, and irrigation schemes provide opportunities for managed control. Safe latrines should be provided, together with subsidized footwear.

Anthelminthic drugs can be deployed in several ways. Even when laboratory stool tests are not done, certain target groups can be treated empirically because of their likelihood of infection. Examples are: agricultural and sewage workers; clinic outpatients with pallor; anaemic blood donors; and children with protein-calorie malnutrition. Alternatively, communities may be treated, either without individual tests—mass chemotherapy; or those with positive stool tests—selective chemotherapy. Population chemotherapy aims to reduce both prevalence and mean worm load. The relative costs of drugs and diagnosis must be considered, and will change during the course of a programme. Single-dose medication is best and possible with albendazole, 400 mg, or mebendazole, 600 mg. Using either pyrantel, 10 mg/kg, or mebendazole, 100 mg twice daily, it is necessary to give 3 days' medication. The ascaricides levamisole and piperazine have little action against hookworm. Chemotherapy should be repeated two or four times yearly; timing at the end of the dry season is most efficient. Both metrifonate, used for *Schistosoma haematobium* control, and ivermectin, used for onchocerciasis control, will have significant activity against hookworm.

In all interventions, community participation is essential and health education is necessary to reinforce the measures used.

Other gut strongyloids

TRICHOSTRONGYLUS SPP.

These are common and economically important gut parasites of domestic ungulates. Infection is by ingestion of filariform larvae on vegetation. Development in the gut is direct, without lung migration. Adults are reddish-brown, 5 to 10 mm in length, and live with their anterior ends embedded in the jejunal mucosa where they feed on tissue fluid, not blood.

Human infection has been recorded with eight species; *T. colubriformis* and *T. orientalis* are the most important. Prevalence rates, which may exceed 25 or even 50 per cent, are highest in Iran, Iraq, Egypt, and Japan. Most infection is derived from sheep, goats, cattle, and camels, but in Iran *T. orientalis* is non-zoonotic. Worms cause mucosal damage, and loss of protein and some blood; clinical features include abdominal pain, eosinophilia, and sometimes anaemia. The eggs are longer and narrower than those of hookworm, which they closely resemble; larval culture is required for reliable differentiation. Infections respond to drugs used for hookworm.

TERNIDENS AND OESOPHAGOSTOMUM

Human infection with *Ternidens deminutus* is locally common in parts of Central and Southern Africa, in particular Zimbabwe, where a 40 per cent prevalence is reported in Harare, and in Zambia and South Africa, with reports from Zaire and Tanzania. Infection is direct following oral ingestion of larvae; adult worms are 8 to 16 mm long. They live partly embedded in the colonic mucosa, where they produce superficial ulceration and cystic nodules. The worm is sometimes referred to as 'false hookworm', because of the similarity of their eggs in faeces; differentiation is important both clinically and epidemiologically. Non-human primates are infected in much of Africa, but most human infections are non-zoonotic; it responds to drugs used for hookworm.

Species of the genus Oesophagostomum are important parasites of primates and ungulates. Fourth-stage larvae and immature adults live in the colonic wall, often deeply situated or in the subserosa; lesions may become bacterially infected or perforate. Normally, adult worms return to the gut lumen. Most human infections are reported from forested parts of West and Central Africa; in particular Ivory Coast, Togo, Ghana, Zaire, and Uganda. Other records are from Kenya, Brazil, and Indonesia. Most cases have presented surgically with masses, or abscesses, located in the caecum or other parts of the colon; or with bowel obstruction, or ectopic lesions in the peritoneum or abdominal wall. Clinically the lesions simulate carcinoma, tuberculosis, appendicitis, and amoeboma; they have been described as 'helminthomas' or 'helminthic pseudotumours'. Diagnosis in such cases has been histological.

The eggs are indistinguishable from those of hookworm and they may be absent in prepatent surgical cases. In some remote villages of north Togo and Ghana the condition has several local names, and faecal surveys, using larval culture, have shown that prevalence in human beings may reach 30 per cent. It is likely that many human infections are overlooked; chemotherapy has been little studied in man, but benzimidazoles are used in veterinary practice where the parasites are known as 'nodular worms'. In Africa most human infections are with the monkey parasite *O. bifurcatum*, or *O. stephanostomum*, a parasite of anthropoid apes; in Asia, *O. aculeatum* is the likely cause. The ungulate species do not appear to infect man.

REFERENCES

Strongyloidiasis

Ashford, R.W., Barnish, G., and Viney, M.E. (1992). *Strongyloides fuelleborni kellyi*: infection and disease in Papua New Guinea. *Parasitology Today*, **8**, 314–18.

Cook, G.C. (1987). *Strongyloides stercoralis* hyperinfection syndrome: how often is it missed? *Quarterly Journal of Medicine* (New Series), **64**, 625–9.

Gam, A.A., Neva, F.A., and Krotoski, W.A. (1987). Comparative sensitivity and specificity of ELISA and IHA for serodiagnosis of strongyloidiasis with larval antigens. *American Journal of Tropical Medicine and Hygiene*, **37**, 157–61.

Genta, R.M. (1986). *Strongyloides stercoralis*: immunobiological considerations on an unusual worm. *Parasitology Today*, **2**, 241–6.

Genta, R.M. (1989). Global prevalence of strongyloidiasis: critical review with epidemiologic insights into the prevention of disseminated disease. *Reviews of Infectious Diseases*, **11**, 755–67.

Genta, R.M., Weesner, R., Douce, R.W., Huitger-O'Connor, T., and Waltzer, P.D. (1987). Strongyloidiasis in United States veterans of the Vietnam and other wars. *Journal of the American Medical Association*, **258**, 49–52.

Gill, G.V. and Bailey, J.W. (1989). Eosinophilia as a marker for chronic strongyloidiasis: use of a serum ELISA test to detect asymptomatic cases. *Annals of Tropical Medicine and Parasitology*, **83**, 249–52.

Gompels, M.M., Todd, J., Peters, B.S., Main, J., and Pinching, A.J. (1991). Disseminated strongyloidiasis in Aids: uncommon but important. *AIDS*, **5**, 329–32.

Grove, D.I. (ed.) (1989). *Strongyloidiasis: a major roundworm infection in man*. Taylor and Francis, London.

Grove, D.I. (1994). Strongyloidiasis: a conundrum for gastroenterologists. *Gut*, **35**, 437–40.

Igra-Siegman, Y., Kapila, R., Sen, P., Kaminski, Z.C., and Louria, D.B. (1981). Syndrome of hyperinfection with *Strongyloides stercoralis*. *Reviews of Infectious Diseases*, **3**, 397–407.

Koga, K. *et al.* (1991). A modified agar plate method for detection of *Strongyloides stercoralis*. *American Journal of Tropical Medicine and Hygiene*, **45**, 518–21.

Neva, F.A. (1986). Biology and immunology of human strongyloidiasis. *Journal of Infectious Diseases*, **153**, 397–406.

Hookworm

Anderson, R.M. and Medley, G.F. (1985). Community control of helminth infections of man by mass and selective chemotherapy. *Parasitology*, **90**, 629–30.

Anderson, R.M. and Schad, G.A. (1985). Hookworm burdens and faecal egg counts: an analysis of the biological basis of variation. *Transactions of the Royal Society of Tropical Medicine and Hygiene*, **79**, 812–25.

Caumes, E., Carriere, J., Datry, A., Gaxotte, P., Davis, M., and Gentilini, M. (1993). A randomized trial of ivermectin versus albendazole for the treatment of cutaneous larva migrans. *American Journal of Tropical Medicine and Hygiene*, **49**, 641–4.

Gilles, H.M. and Ball, P.A.J (ed.) (1991). *Human parasitic diseases*, Vol. 4, *Hookworm infections*. Elsevier, Amsterdam

Pawlowski, Z.S., Schad, G.A., and Stott, G.J. (1991). *Hookworm infection and anaemia. Approaches to prevention and control*. World Health Organization, Geneva.

Roche, M. and Layrisse, M. (1966). The nature and causes of hookworm anaemia. *American Journal of Tropical Medicine and Hygiene*, **15**, 1029–1102.

Schad, G.A. and Warren, K.S. (ed.) (1990). *Hookworm disease: current status and new directions*. Taylor and Francis, London.

OTHER STRONGYLOIDS

Anthony, P.P. and McAdam, I.W.J. (1972). Helminthic pseudotumours of the bowel: thirty four cases of helminthoma. *Gut*, **13**, 8–16.

Barrowclough, H. and Crome, L. (1979). Oesophagostomiasis in man. *Tropical and Geographic Medicine*, **31**, 133–8.

Bundy, D.A.P., Terry, S.I., Murphy, C.P., and Harris, E.A. (1985). First record of *Trichostrongylus axei* infection of man in the Caribbean Region. *Transactions of the Royal Society of Tropical Medicine and Hygiene*, **79**, 562–3.

Kilala, C.P. (1971). *Ternidens deminutus* infecting man in Southern Tanzania. *East African Medical Journal*, **48**, 636–45.

Polderman, A.M., Krepel, H.P., Baeta, S., Blotkamp, P., and Gigasse, P. (1991). Oesophagostomiasis, a common infection in man in northern Togo and Ghana. *American Journal of Tropical Medicine and Hygiene*, **44**, 336–344.

Ross, R.A., Gibson, G.I., and Harris, E.A. (1989). Cutaneous oesophagostomiasis in man. *Transactions of the Royal Society of Tropical Medicine and Hygiene*, **83**, 394.

Stewart, T.B. and Gasbarre, L.C. (1989) The veterinary importance of nodular worms (*Oesophagostomum* spp). *Parasitology Today*, **5**, 209–13.

7.14.5 Nematode infections of lesser importance

D. I. Grove

From time to time, a patient may be encountered who harbours an unusual nematode. Some of these organisms are free-living parasites and the patient has a spurious infection, usually as the result of ingestion of the worm or following the *in vitro* contamination of a clinical specimen such as faeces or urine. Other individuals may have true infections with worms being found either in the gastrointestinal tract or in the tissues. Many of these infections are with parasites of animals that are adapted poorly to the human host and are unable to complete their development in man. Thus, worms in varying stages of development including larvae, adults, and eggs may be found in specimens. Some parasites may be recovered from fluids and are viewed intact, whereas others are seen only in histological sections. If there is uncertainty in identifying the intact worm, help may often be obtained from a veterinary parasitologist who may be more used to dealing with the species concerned. Histologically, definitive diagnosis may be very difficult. Nematode infections of the eye are especially hard to diagnose and sometimes no satisfactory conclusion is reached (see references 2, 3, 43). A summary of rarely reported nematodes is shown in Table 1.

Nematodes found in the gastrointestinal tract may respond to a benzimidazole agent such as mebendazole (100 mg orally, twice daily for up to 3 days). Thiabendazole (25 mg/kg, twice daily for several days) has been used traditionally for the treatment of systemic larval infections but its effectiveness is very variable. The related compound, albendazole (10 mg/kg orally, daily for up to 1 week), may be more active than thiabendazole and is absorbed better from the gut than mebendazole. If these drugs fail, ivermectin (0.15 mg/kg orally, daily for several days) may be tried. Other drugs that have been used in these unusual nematode infections include levamisole and diethylcarbamazine. Unfortunately, some infections are refractory all to anthelmintics. Nevertheless, these worms generally cannot multiply in man and the parasites will die spontaneously after months or years.

REFERENCES

1. Africa C.M. and Garcia, E.Y. (1936). A new nematode parasite (*Cheilospirura* sp.) of the eye of man in the Philippines. *Journal of the Philippine Islands Medical Association*, **16**, 603–7.
2. Ashton, N. and Cook, C. (1979). Allergic granulomatous nodules of the eyelid and conjunctiva. *American Journal of Ophthalmology*, **87**, 1–28.
3. Beaver, P.C. and Bowman, D.D. (1984). Ascaridoid larva (Nematoda) from the eye of a child in Uganda. *American Journal of Tropical Medicine and Hygiene*, **33**, 1272–4.
4. Beaver, P.C., Jung, R.C., and Cupp, W.E. (1984). *Clinical Parasitology*, (9th edn), pp. 825. Lea and Febiger, Philadelphia.
5. Beaver, P.C., Horner, G.S., and Bilos, J.Z. (1974). Zoonotic onchocerciasis in a resident of Illinois and observations on the identification of *Onchocerca* species. *American Journal of Tropical Medicine and Hygiene*, **23**, 595–607.
6. Beer, R.J. (1971). Experimental infection of man with pig whipworm. *British Medical Journal*, **i**, 44.
7. Bhaibulaya, M. and Indrangarm, S. (1975). Man, as an accidental host of *Cyclodontostomum purvisi* (Adams, 1933), and the occurrence in rats in Thailand. *Southeast Asian Journal of Tropical Medicine and Public Health*, **6**, 391–4.
8. Biocca, E. (1959). Infestazione umana prenatale da *Spirocerca lupi* (Rud, 1809). *Parassitologia*, **1**, 137–42.
9. Botero, D. and Little, M.D. (1984). Two cases of human *Lagochilascaris* infection in Colombia. *American Journal of Tropical Medicine and Hygiene*, **33**, 381–6.
10. Buckley, J.J. (1933). *Necator suillis* as a human infection. *British Medical Journal*, **i**, 699–700.
11. Chandler, A.C. (1938). *Diploscapter coronata* as a facultative parasite of man, with a general review of vertebrate parasitism by rhabditoid worms. *Parasitology*, **30**, 40–5.
12. Deardorff, T.L., Overstreet, R.M., Okihiro, M., and Tam, R. (1986). Piscine adult nematode invading an open lesion in a human hand. *American Journal of Tropical Medicine and Hygiene*, **35**, 827–30.
13. Eberhard, M.L., Hurwitz, H., Sun, A.M., and Coletta, D. (1989). Intestinal perforation caused by larval *Eustrongylides* (Nematoda: Dioctophymatoidae) in New Jersey. *American Journal of Tropical Medicine and Hygiene*, **40**, 648–50.
14. Evans, A.C., Markus, M.B., and Steyne, E. (1990). A survey of the intestinal nematodes of bushmen in Namibia. *American Journal of Tropical Medicine and Hygiene*, **42**, 243–7.
15. Fox, A.S., Kazacos, K.R., Gould, N.S., Heydemann, P.T., Thomas, C., and Boyer, K.M. (1985). Fatal eosinophilic meningoencephalitis and visceral larva migrans caused by the raccoon ascarid *Baylisascaris procyonis*. *New England Journal of Medicine*, **312**, 1619–23.
16. Fülleborn, F. (1927). Durch Hakenwurmlarven des Hundes (*Uncinaria stenocephala*) beim Menschen erzeugte 'Creeping Eruption'. *Abhandlungen aus dem Gebiet der Auslandskunde, Hamburg Universität (Fetschrift Nocht)*, **26**, 121–33.
17. Gardiner, C.H., Koh, D.S., and Cardella, T.A. (1981). *Micronema* in man: third fatal infection. *American Journal of Tropical Medicine and Hygiene*, **30**, 586–589.
18. Gardiner, C.H. and Schantz, P.M. (1983). *Mammomonogamus* infection in a human: report of a case. *American Journal of Tropical Medicine and Hygiene*, **32**, 995–7.
19. Ginsburg, B., Beaver, P.C., Wilson, E.R., and Whitley, R.J. (1984). Dermatitis due to larvae of a soil nematode, *Pelodera strongyloides*. *Pediatric Dermatology*, **2**, 33–7.
20. Gutierrez, Y., Cohen, M., and Machiaco, C.N. (1989). *Dioctophyme* [*sic*] larva in the subcutaneous tissues of a woman in Ohio. *American Journal of Surgical Pathology*, **13**, 800–2.
21. Hunter, G.W. and Worth, C.B. (1945). Variations in response to filari-

Table 1

Nematode	Geographical distribution	Usual host	Mode of transmission	Stage of development	Clinical features	Suggested treatment	References
Agamomermis spp.	?	Free-living, grasshoppers	? ingestion	Larvae, adults	Spurious; worms in mouth, faeces, urethra	Manual removal if necessary	4
Anatrichosoma cutanea	Asia, Africa	Monkeys	?	Larvae	Cutaneous larva migrans	Thiabendazole, albendazole	30
Ancylostoma caninum	Widespread	Dogs	Cutaneous penetration	Larvae, ? adults	Cutaneous larva migrans, myositis, pulmonary infiltrates, eosinophilic enteritis	Mebendazole (enteritis), thiabendazole (other)	21,32,39
Ancylostoma malayanum	Asia	Bear	?	?	?	Mebendazole	49
Ascaris suum	Widespread	Pigs	Ingestion of eggs	Larvae, ? adults	Pneumonitis, abdominal discomfort	Albendazole	37
Baylisascaris procyonis	North America	Racoons	Ingestion of eggs in soil	Larvae	Visceral and ocular larva migrans, eosinophilic meningoencephalitis	Albendazole	15
Bunostomum trigonocephalum	Widespread	Sheep	Cutaneous penetration	Larvae	Cutaneous larva migrans	Albendazole	33
Cheilospirura spp.	Widespread	Birds	? ingestion of arthropods	Larvae	Conjunctival nodule	Excision	1
Contracaecum spp.	Widespread	Fish, birds	Ingestion of undercooked fish	Larvae	See anisakiasis	See anisakiasis	42
Cyclodontostomum purvisi	Asia	Rats	?	Adults	Worms in faeces	Mebendazole	7
Dioctophyma renale	Widespread	Mammals	Ingestion of aquatic annelids, amphibia, crustacea, fish	Larvae, adults	Haematuria, retroperitoneal mass, subcutaneous nodule	Excision	20
Diploscapter coronata	Widespread	Free-living	Ingestion in vegetation	Adults	Spurious; worms in stomach contents, urine	Unnecessary	11,47
Eustrongylides spp.	Widespread	Fish, birds	Ingestion of undercooked fish	Larvae	Peritonitis	Laparotomy and surgical removal	13,48
Gongylonema pulchrum	Worldwide	Ruminants, swine	Ingestion of beetles, cockroaches etc.	Adult	Migrating worm, especially in the oral cavity	Surgical removal	22
Haemonchus contortus	Widespread	Sheep, cattle	? ingestion of larvae on vegetation	Adults	?	Mebendazole	44
Lagochilascaris minor	Central and South America	?	?	Adults, eggs, larvae	Subcutaneous abscess in head and neck; nasopharyngeal or sinus lesions, encephalitis	Surgical removal; levamisole, diethylcarbamazine, thiabendazole	9,41
Mammomonogamus (= *Syngamus*) *laryngeus*	Central and South America	Cattle, felines	?	Adults	Cough, pharyngeal lesion	Endoscopic removal	18,45
Meloidogyne (= *Heterodera*) spp.	Widespread	Plant parasite	Ingestion of vegetation; contamination of faecal specimen	Eggs, larvae	Spurious; eggs and larvae in faeces	Unnecessary	25

Meningonema peruzzii	Africa	Monkeys	?	Larvae	Meningoencephalitis	Albendazole	36
Mermis nigrescens	North America	Grasshoppers	? ingestion of adult worm	Adult	Worm in mouth	Manual removal	38
Metastrongylus elongatus	Widespread	Pigs	Ingestion of earthworms	Adult	Worm in gut or respiratory tract	Albendazole	4,33
Micronema deletrix	Widespread	Free-living; horses	Trauma or skin lesions	Adults, larvae, eggs	Meningoencephalitis; generalized spread	Albendazole	17
Necator suillis	Central America	Pigs	Percutaneous	Adults	?	Mebendazole	10
Onchocerca spp. (not *volvulus*)	Widespread	Cattle, horses	Insect-borne	Adults,	Subcutaneous nodule; eye lesions	Surgical excision	5
Ostertagia spp.	Widespread	Cattle, sheep	? ingestion of adult worms in undercooked abomasum	Adults	? spurious; worms in gut	Mebendazole	23
Parastrongylus spp.	Africa	Rodents	Ingestion of snails	Larvae, adults	Eosinophilic meningitis	Albendazole	35
Pelodera (= Rhabditis) strongyloides	Widespread	Free-living	Cutaneous	Larvae	Papular dermatitis	Albendazole, topical corticosteroid	19
Philometra spp.	Widespread	Fish	Cutaneous injury	Adults	Worms in laceration	Manual removal	12
Phocanema spp.	Widespread	Fish	Ingestion of undercooked fish	Larvae	See anisakiasis	See anisakiasis	24
Physaloptera caucasica	Europe, Africa	Primates	? ingestion of beetles, cockroaches	Adults, eggs	Sometimes spurious; abdominal pain; small-bowel gangrene	Mebendazole; surgical removal	14,34
Rhabditis spp.	Widespread	Free-living	Ingestion	Adults	Spurious; worms in faeces, urine, skin	Unnecessary	4
Rictularia spp.	Widespread	Mammals, birds	? ingestion	Adult	Found in an appendix		27
Spirocerca lupi	Widespread	Dogs, wolves	? ingestion of beetles	Adults	Intestinal obstruction and peritonitis in a baby	Surgery	8
Syphacia spp.	Widespread	Mice	Ingestion	Eggs, adults	? spurious; worms in faeces	Mebendazole if necessary	40
Terranova spp.	Widespread	Fish	Ingestion of undercooked fish	Larvae	See anisakiasis	See anisakiasis	29
Tetrameres fissispina	Widespread	Birds	? ingestion of grasshoppers, cockroaches	Adults	? spurious; worms in gut	Mebendazole	33
Thelazia californiensis	North America	Mammals	Deposition on eye by fly	Adults	Conjunctivitis	Manual removal	31
Thelazia callipaeda	Asia	Dogs, rabbits	Deposition on eye by fly	Adults	Conjunctivitis	Manual removal	28,50
Trichuris suis	Widespread	Pigs	Ingestion of eggs	Eggs, larvae, adults	Usually asymptomatic	Mebendazole	6
Trichuris vulpis	Widespread	Dogs	Ingestion of eggs	Eggs, larvae, adults	Usually asymptomatic	Mebendazole	26
Turbatrix (= Anguillula) aceti	Widespread	Free-living (including vinegar, acetic acid)	Accidental inoculation	Larvae, adults	Spurious; urine, vaginal discharge, blood smears (in stains)	Unnecessary	46
Uncinaria stenocephala	Widespread	Dogs, cats	Cutaneous penetration	Larvae	Cutaneous larva migrans	Thiabendazole, albendazole	16

form larvae of *Ancylostoma caninum* in the skin of man. *Journal of Parasitology*, **31**, 366–72.
22. Illescas-Gómez, M.P., Osorio M.R., Garcia, V.G., and Morales, M.A.G. (1988). Human *Gongylonema* infection in Spain. *American Journal of Tropical Medicine and Hygiene*, **38**, 363–5.
23. Kasimov, G.B. (1941). (The first case of ostertagiasis in man). *Meditsinskaya Parazitologiya i Parazitarnÿe Bolezni*, **10**, 121–3, (in Russian). Abstracted in *Tropical Diseases Bulletin*, (1943), **40**, 326.
24. Kates, S., Wright, K.A., and Wright, R. (1973). A case of human infection with the cod nematode *Phocanema* sp. *American Journal of Tropical Medicine and Hygiene*, **32**, 606–8.
25. Keller, A.E. (1935). The occurrence of eggs of *Heterodera radicicola* in human feces. *Journal of Laboratory and Clinical Medicine*, **20**, 390–2.
26. Kenney, Y. and Yermakov, V. (1980). Infection of man with *Trichuris vulpis*, the whipworm of dogs. *American Journal of Tropical Medicine and Hygiene*, **29**, 1206–8.
27. Kenney, M., Eveland, L.K., Yermakov, V., and Kassouny, D.Y. (1975). A case of *Rictularia* infection of man in New York. *American Journal of Tropical Medicine and Hygiene*, **24**, 596–9.
28. Kosin, E., Kosman, M.L., and Depary, A.A. (1989). First case of human thelaziasis in Indonesia. *Southeast Asian Journal of Tropical Medicine and Public Health*, **20**, 233–6.
29. Koyama, T. *et al.* (1973). *Terranova* (Nematoda: Anisakidae) infection in man. II. Morphological features of *Terranova* sp. larva found in human stomach wall. *Japanese Journal of Parasitology*, **21**, 257–61.
30. Le V.H., Duong, H.M., and Nguyen, L.V. (1963). Premier cas de capillariose cutanée humaine. *Bulletin de la Société de Pathologie Exotique*, **56**, 121–6.
31. Lee, R.D. and Parmelee, W.D. (1958). Thelaziasis in man. *American Journal of Tropical Medicine and Hygiene*, **7**, 427–8.
32. Little, M.D., Halsey, N.A., Cline, B.L., and Katz, S.P. (1983). *Ancylostoma* larva in a muscle fiber of man following cutaneous larva migrans. *American Journal of Tropical Medicine and Hygiene*, **32**, 1285–8.
33. Mao, S.P. (1991). Protozoan and helminth parasites of humans in mainland China. *International Journal for Parasitology*, **21**, 347–51.
34. Nicolaides, N.J., Musgrave, J., McGuckin, D., and Moorhouse, D.E. (1977). Nematode larvae (Spirurida: Physalopteridae) causing infarction of the bowel in an infant. *Pathology*, **9**, 129–35.
35. Nozais, J.P., Moreau, J., Morlier, G., Kouame, J., and Doucet, J. (1980). Premier cas de méningite a éosinophiles en Cote-d'Ivoire avec présence d'un *Parastrongylus* sp. dans le liquide céphalo-rachidien. *Bulletin de la Société de Pathologie Exotique*, **73**, 179–82.
36. Orihel, T.C. and Esslinger, J.H. (1973). *Meningonema peruzzii* gen. et sp. n. (Nematoda: Filarioidea) from the central nervous system of African monkeys. *Journal of Parasitology*, **59**, 437–41.
37. Phills, J.A., Harrold, A.J., Whiteman, G.V., and Perelmutter, L. (1972). Pulmonary infiltrates, asthma and eosinophilia due to *Ascaris suum* infestation in man. *New England Journal of Medicine*, **286**, 965–70.
38. Poinar, G.O. Jr., and Hoberg, E.P. (1988). *Mermis nigrescens* (Mermithidae: Nematoda) recovered from the mouth of a child. *American Journal of Tropical Medicine and Hygiene*, **39**, 478–9.
39. Prociv, P., and Croese, J. (1990). Human eosinophilic enteritis caused by the dog hookworm, *Ancylostoma caninum. Lancet*, **355**, 1299–302.
40. Riley, W.A. (1920). A mouse oxyurid, *Syphacia obvelata*, as a parasite of man. *Journal of Parasitology*, **6**, 89–92.
41. Rosemberg, S., Lopes, M.B.S., Masuda, Z., Campos, R., and Vieira Bressan M.C.R. (1986). Fatal encephalopathy due to *Lagochilascaris minor* infection. *American Journal of Tropical Medicine and Hygiene*, **35**, 575–8.
42. Schaum, E., and Müller W. (1967). Die Heterocheilidiasis. Eine Infektion des Menschen mit Larven von Fisch-Ascariden. *Deutsche Medizinische Wochenschrift*, **92**, 2230–3.
43. Sivalingam, A., Goldberg, R.E., Augsburger, J., and Frank, P. (1991). Diffuse unilateral subacute neuroretinitis. *Archives of Ophthalmology*, **109**, 1028.
44. Sweet, W.C. (1924). The intestinal parasites of man in Australia and its dependencies as found by the Australian Hookworm Campaign. *Medical Journal of Australia*, **i**, 405–7.
45. Timmons, R.F., Bowers, R.E., and Price, D.L. (1983). Infection of the respiratory tract with *Mammomanogamus* [*sic*] (*Syngamus*) *laryngeus*: a new case in Largo, Florida, and a summary of previously reported cases. *American Review of Respiratory Diseases*, **128**, 566–9.
46. Todd, J.C. and Sanford, A.H. (1943). *Clinical diagnosis by laboratory methods*. Saunders, Philadelphia.
47. Witenberg, G. (1951). Some unusual observations on helminthiasis in Israel. *Harefuah*, **41**, 178–80.
48. Wittner, M., Turner, J.W., Jacquette, G., Ash, L.R., Salgo, M.P., and Tanowitz, H.S. (1989). Eustrongylidiasis—a parasitic infection acquired by eating sushi. *New England Journal of Medicine*, **320**, 1124–6.
49. Yorke, W., and Maplestone, R.A. (1926). *The nematode parasites of vertebrates*. Churchill, London.
50. Yospaiboon, Y., Sithithavorn, P., Maleewong, V., Ukosanakarn, U., and Bhaibulaya, M. (1989). Ocular thelaziasis in Thailand: a case report. *Journal of the Medical Association of Thailand*, **72**, 469–73.

7.14.6 OTHER GUT NEMATODES

V. Zaman

Ascariasis

Ascariasis is an infection caused by *Ascaris lumbricoides*. Normally, the adult worms are located in the small intestine. In unusual circumstances, such as fever, irritation due to drugs, anaesthesia, and bowel manipulation during surgery, the worms may migrate to ectopic sites where they may give rise to severe disease.

GEOGRAPHICAL DISTRIBUTION

The distribution is cosmopolitan but the parasite occurs more frequently in moist and warm climates. In some rural tropical areas, the entire population may be infected. It is relatively more common in children, who also carry higher worm loads.

MORPHOLOGY

A mature worm is cylindrical with tapering ends. It is creamy white to light brown in colour. The female measures 20 to 35 cm in length and 3 to 6 mm in breadth. The male measures 12 to 31 cm in length and 2 to 4 mm in breadth and has a curved tail. The head has three lips at the anterior end, which carry minute teeth or denticles along their margins. The lips can be closed or extended, allowing the worm to ingest food. In cross-section, the worm reveals a thick cuticle, adjacent to which is the hypodermis which projects into the body cavity in the form of lateral

Fig. 1 (a) *Ascaris lumbricoides* in the bile duct (× 125). (b) Anisakis larva in cross-section in human stomach showing large bulbous lateral chords

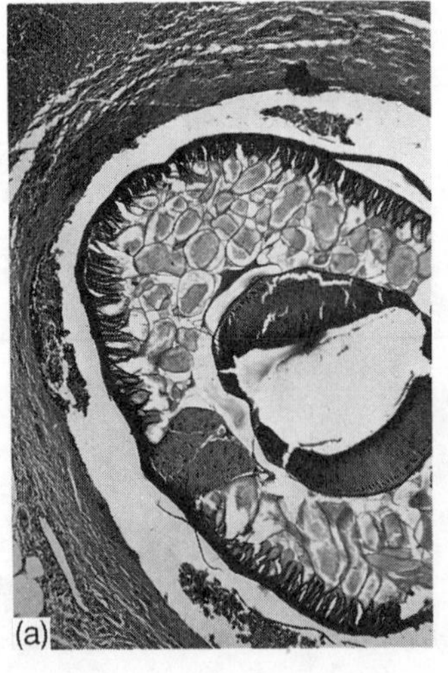

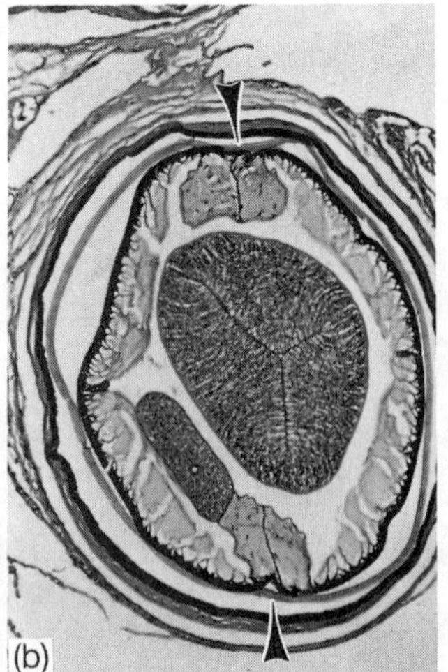

chords (Fig. 1(a)). The somatic muscle cells are large and elongated and lie adjacent to the hypodermis. The worm is able to maintain its position in the small intestine by the activity of these muscles. If the somatic muscles are paralysed by anthelminthics, it is expelled by peristalsis.

The fertilized eggs are ovoidal and measure 60–70 × 30–50 μm. When freshly passed they are not infective and contain a single cell. In the soil, the larva becomes infective. The cell is surrounded by a thin vitelline membrane. Around the membrane is a thick, translucent shell, which in turn is surrounded by an irregular, albuminous coat. The albuminous coat is sometimes lost or can be removed by chemical treatment, resulting in a decorticated egg. Until recently, it was assumed that the brown coloration of the egg was due to bile pigment, but tannins in the egg shell are probably responsible. The unfertilized eggs are 88–94 × 40–44 μm and have disorganized contents. The larvae of *A. lumbricoides* may be seen in infected lungs and measure up to 2 mm in length, and 75 μm in diameter. They have a central intestine, paired excretory columns, and prominent lateral alae.

LIFECYCLE (SEE FIG. 2)

The gravid female produces 200 000 to 250 000 eggs daily. These take 3 or 4 weeks to develop into the infective stage, which is probably the third-stage rather than the second-stage larva as was previously thought. The eggs are resistant to chemicals and low temperature and may remain viable for years in moist soil. On ingestion, the infective larva hatches out in the small intestine and penetrates the intestinal wall to enter the portal circulation. From the liver it is carried to the heart and via the pulmonary artery to the lungs. In the lungs, it breaks out of the capillaries into the alveoli and undergoes another moult to become a fourth-stage larva. From the lungs the larva moves up to the bronchi and then crawls over the epiglottis to enter the digestive tract. In the intestine, it moults again to become a sexually mature worm. The lifespan of an adult worm is approximately 1 year, after which it is spontaneously expelled. In hyperendemic areas, children are being continuously infected so that as some worms are being expelled, others are maturing to take their place.

CLINICAL ASPECTS

In the majority of cases, the infected individual remains asymptomatic. However, there is much evidence to indicate that the presence of Ascaris causes nutritional problems and hinders the normal development of children. Occasionally, patients may develop fever, malaise, urticaria, intestinal colic, nausea, vomiting, diarrhoea, and central nervous disorders.

The migration of larval Ascaris through the lungs may produce varying degrees of pneumonitis and bronchospasm known as Loeffler's syndrome. Chest radiographs may show diffuse mottling and increased prominence of peribronchial markings. There is generally high eosinophilia and the condition subsides after 7 to 10 days unless reinfection occurs. The larvae of *A. suum* (pig Ascaris) may also produce sever pneumonitis and bronchospasm in areas where pig farming is common.

Occasionally, ascariasis can cause severe, life-threatening disease. This could happen in the following situations.

1. When large numbers of worms get entangled to form a bolus and block the intestinal lumen producing signs and symptoms of acute intestinal obstruction.
2. When ectopic migration results in the entry of the worm into the appendix, common bile duct, or pancreatic duct. When the

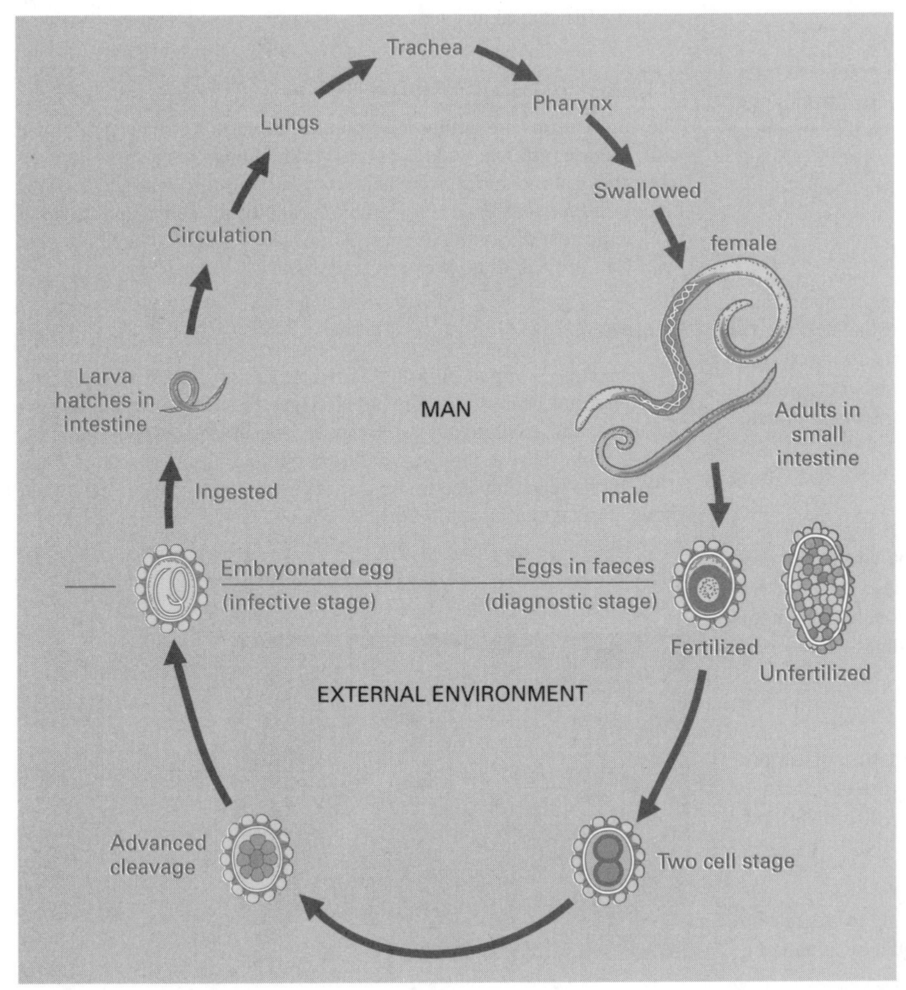

Fig. 2 Lifecycle of *Ascaris lumbricoides*. (Adapted from Center for Disease Control, Atlanta, Georgia, USA.)

biliary tract is invaded, there is severe colic, often followed by suppurative cholangitis and multiple liver abscesses resulting from the disintegration of the trapped worm and secondary bacterial infection. Disintegration of the female worm releases a large number of eggs in the liver that can be recognized on histological examination.

3. When the worm impacts in the ampulla of Vater causing acute pancreatitis and pancreatic necrosis.

DIAGNOSIS

This is usually made by detecting Ascaris eggs in the faeces. Sometimes, the patient brings developing or adult worms that have been passed in the faeces or have emerged from the anus or the nose in a sick child. They are roughly the size and have the appearance of earthworms. Occasionally, adult worms are outlined in the intestines during barium-meal examination.

TREATMENT

Whenever possible, all positive cases, irrespective of the worm load, should be treated as even a few worms can undergo ectopic migration with dangerous consequences.

Pyrantel pamoate

A single dose of 10 mg/kg body weight is effective in curing over 90 per cent of cases. Side-effects are mild, if any, and the drug is well tolerated. It has the advantage of also being active against *Enterobius vermicularis* and hookworms. This broad-spectrum activity is useful in endemic areas where multiple nematode infections are common.

Mebendazole

This drug is also a broad-spectrum anthelminthic with good host tolerance. It is given as 100 mg twice daily for 3 days, irrespective of age. Unfortunately, there are a few reported cases of ectopic migration induced by the drug. The manufacturers now advise against this drug in children under 2 years of age as there is a report of severe neurological toxicity in a young child.

Levamisole hydrochloride

This is probably the most effective antiascaris agent and produces rapid paralysis of the worm. It is administered as a single dose of 150 mg for adults and 50 mg for persons under 10 kg. Side-effects are more common than with pyrantel and mebendazole. This drug has occasionally resulted in blood dyscrasias when used in prolonged treatment of autoimmune diseases and rheumatoid arthritis.

Piperazine salts

These are widely used because of their low cost and high degree of efficacy which includes *E. vermicularis*, but not hookworm. The dose is 75 mg/kg (maximum of 3.5 g) given as a single dose daily for two consecutive days. Prior fasting is not required. Occasionally, symptoms involving the central nervous system such as unsteadiness and vertigo have been reported.

Oxantel plus pyrantel

This preparation contains 100 mg of each drug per tablet. It is commercially available and is superior to pyrantel when antitrichuris activity is also needed. It is given as a single dose of 10 to 20 mg/kg body weight.

If signs of intestinal obstruction develop in a child living in an endemic area, ascariasis is a distinct possibility. The child should be admitted to hospital and prepared for surgical intervention. To start with the measures should be:

(1) decompression of the bowel through an intestinal tube with constant suction;
(2) rehydration and restoration of electrolyte balance by intravenous drip;
(3) antipyretics if fever is present;
(4) introduction of an appropriate dose of piperazine citrate through the intestinal tube.

In most cases this conservative therapy will relieve the obstruction and the child will rapidly recover. If, however, the signs of obstruction persist and the general condition of the child worsens, laparotomy is required. Acute obstructive jaundice or pancreatitis due to obstruction of the common bile duct by Ascaris also requires urgent surgical intervention.

PREVENTION AND CONTROL

As Ascaris eggs can survive in the soil for many years, prevention and control in the endemic areas is difficult. Mass chemotherapy given at intervals of 6 months along with environmental sanitation can break the cycle. Prevalence rates of ascariasis and other soil-transmitted helminths are greatly reduced by improvement in housing. At a personal level, infection is prevented by eating only cooked food and by avoiding green vegetables and salads in countries where human faeces are used as a fertilizer and where this parasite is endemic.

Anisakiasis

Anisakiasis is an infection caused by the larvae of nematodes belonging to the family Anisakidae.

GEOGRAPHICAL DISTRIBUTION

The adult worms are commonly found in cetaceans (whales, dolphins, and porpoises) in many parts of the world. Human beings are infected when they eat raw or improperly cooked fish or squid. The incidence is highest in Japan, followed by Holland, Scandinavia, and countries along the Pacific cost of South America. A few cases have also been reported from California and the Western United States.

MORPHOLOGY

This is a large group of parasites and complete speciation of adults and larvae has not been done. The larval stages found in man can be recognized as those belonging to the family, Anisakidae only, by the presence of large lateral chords, which are bulbous in cross-section (Fig. 1(b)). In the scanning electron microscope the ventral side of the mouth shows a triangular boring tooth (Fig. 3).

Fig. 3 Anisakis larva: third-stage larva of *A. simplex* showing the tip of the boring tooth (arrow). (× 400).

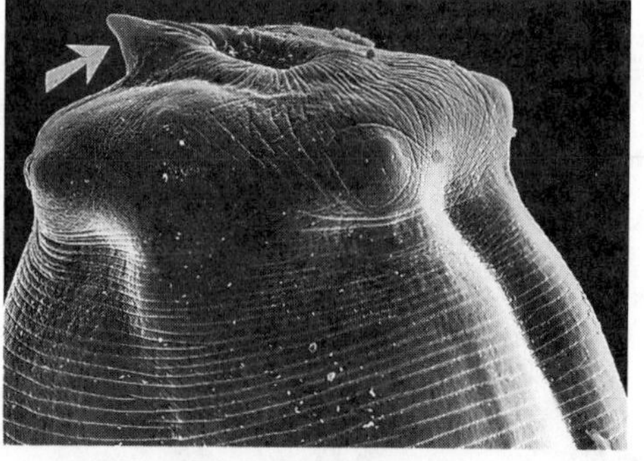

LIFECYCLE

Adults live in the lumen of the intestine of cetaceans, eggs are passed in water, second-stage larvae are ingested by crustaceans, which are then ingested by fish or squid where they enter the muscles; cetaceans and man get infected by eating fish or squid. In man, larvae do not develop to maturity but attach themselves to the mucosa of stomach or intestine.

CLINICAL ASPECTS

The majority of patients present with gastric symptoms that develop within 4 to 24 h of eating infected fish. The symptoms are due to ulceration produced by the larvae as they burrow into the mucous membrane. In addition to epigastric pain, nausea and vomiting, there may be haematemesis during the acute stage of the disease. If there is mild pain and the patient is left untreated, the infection can proceed to a chronic stage with tumour formation. The small intestine may be involved, resulting in severe pain in the lower abdomen, which may be misdiagnosed as appendicitis.

DIAGNOSIS

Gastroscopy often reveals the lesion and the presence of larvae attached to the mucous membrane. Radiographs with a barium meal may show the presence of single or multiple ulcers and outline the worm. Serological tests are now available in some specialized centres.

TREATMENT

In acute infection an attempt should be made to remove all the larvae through a gastroscope. In chronic cases, surgical removal of the ulcerated areas or the tumor may be required. No effective chemotherapy is available. Infection is prevented by avoiding ingestion of raw fish and squid.

Capillariasis

Capillariasis is an infection by parasites belonging to the genus Capillaria. Two species infect man, *C. philippinensis*, which produces intestinal capillariasis, and *C. hepatica*, which produces hepatic capillariasis.

GEOGRAPHICAL DISTRIBUTION

C. philippinensis has been described from the Philippines and Thailand. In the Philippines, the distribution of the disease includes the western and northern coastal areas of Luzon and the north-east of Mindanao. In Thailand, the infection is mostly sporadic and widely scattered. Infection has also been reported from Japan and recently from Dubai in the Middle East. *C. hepatica* is a rare human parasite but is commonly found in rodents in many parts of the world.

MORPHOLOGY

Adult *C. philippinensis* are thin, small worms measuring 2.5 to 4.3 mm in length. They have a row of stichocytes at the anterior end, as in Trichuris. The eggs measure 36 to 45 μm in length and 19–21 μm in breadth, and have bipolar plugs, also like Trichuris (Fig. 4). However, unlike Trichuris, the eggs are not barrel shaped and the plugs do not protrude from the lateral ends. The adults of *C. hepatica* measure 52 to 104 mm in length and the anterior region contains the stichocytes. The eggs measure 48–66 × 28–36 μm and have bipolar plugs. The eggshell is thick and distinctly striated.

LIFECYCLE

The lifecycle of *C. philippinensis* has not been completely worked out, but man is infected by eating freshwater fish and especially their succus entericus containing the infective larvae. Fish-eating birds act as natural or reservoir host. In nature, therefore, there is a fish–bird cycle with man becoming involved accidentally. The main danger with this parasite lies in the possibility of autoinfection, which leads to very heavy worm loads.

C. hepatica is found in the liver of rodents and other mammals. The eggs are discharged in the liver tissue and remain there until the animal dies (Fig. 5). They eventually reach the soil by the decay of the carcass. Human beings are infected by accidentally swallowing embryonated eggs from the soil.

CLINICAL ASPECTS

C. philippinensis can produce severe and even fatal disease. Patients often present with abdominal pain, diarrhoea, and borborygmi or gurgling stomach. As the worm load increases due to autoinfection, diarrhoea becomes more severe, with anorexia, nausea, and vomiting. Prolonged diarrhoea leads to cachexia and muscular wasting. There may also be signs of hypotension and cardiac failure. In untreated cases, the mortality rate is close to 20 per cent.

In *C. hepatica* infection, symptoms of visceral larva migrans may be present. The patient may have an enlarged tender liver with low-grade fever and eosinophilia.

Fig. 4 *Capillaria philippinensis* egg (× 1400).

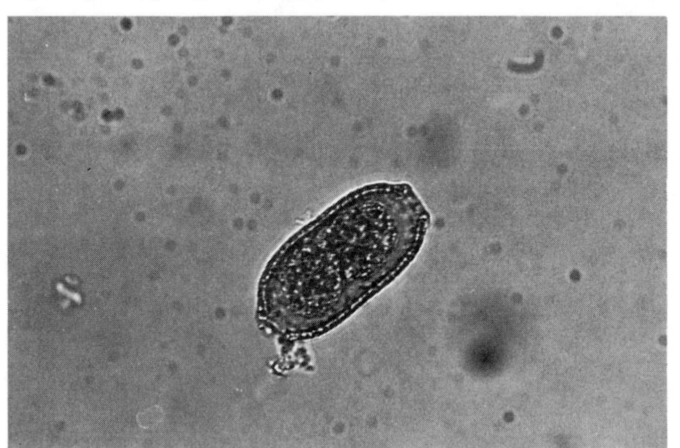

Fig. 5 *Capillaria hepatica* eggs in the liver (× 250).

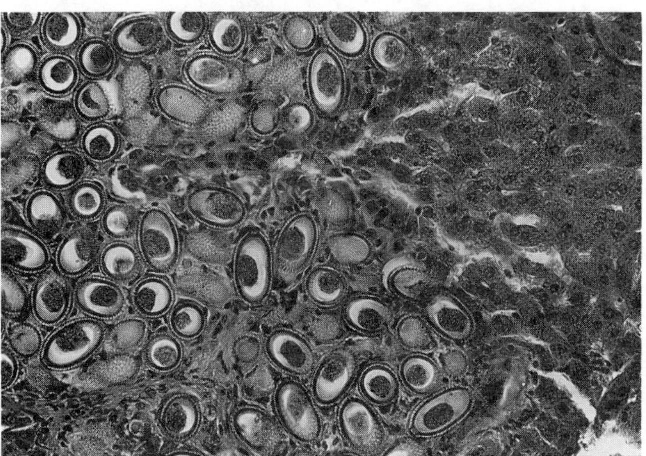

DIAGNOSIS

With *C. philippinensis*, diagnosis is made by finding the typical eggs in the faeces. Larvae or adult worms may also be present and repeated stool examination may be required in some cases. The parasite may also be found in jejunal aspirate or biopsy. With *C. hepatica*, diagnosis is made by identifying the parasite or eggs in a liver biopsy.

TREATMENT

All cases of *C. philippinensis* should be treated with mebendazole in a dose of 200 mg, twice daily, until the symptoms subside and the eggs completely disappear from the faeces after repeated stool examination. This may take up to 20 days or more. Supportive measures to overcome malnutrition and diarrhoea will be required in severely ill patients. There is no specific treatment of *C. hepatica* infection. Infection with *C. philippinensis* is prevented by not eating raw fish in the endemic regions of South-East Asia.

Trichinosis

Trichinosis is an infection caused by *Trichinella spiralis*.

GEOGRAPHICAL DISTRIBUTION

The infection is endemic in many parts of the world where pork is consumed. These areas include Central and Eastern Europe, Central, South, and North America, and parts of Africa and Asia. Infection is also endemic in the Arctic regions resulting from eating polar bear meat.

MORPHOLOGY

The adult males are small nematodes measuring 1.4 to 1.6 mm. The female is viviparous and about twice as long as the male. The anterior part contains a row of glandular cells (stichocytes) as in *Trichuris trichiura*. The male worm lacks a spicule but has two copulatory papillae on the sides of the cloacal opening.

LIFECYCLE (SEE FIG. 6)

Human beings become infected by eating improperly cooked pork or pork products such as sausages. In some parts of the world, wild boars are heavily infected. After ingestion, the larvae are liberated in the small intestine and mature into adults. The female deposits larvae in the intestinal tissues from where they find their way into the bloodstream and then into the striated muscles of the body (Fig. 7). The most heavily parasitized muscles are the diaphragm, tongue, laryngeal, and abdominal muscles. After penetration, the larva undergoes three moults and coils into a spiral, which eventually becomes enclosed in a thick-walled cyst. In this form, the larva may remain viable for many years.

Pigs become infected by eating infected scrap and garbage from slaughterhouses or farms. Occasionally, they become infected by eating carcasses of infected rats.

CLINICAL ASPECTS

The majority of individuals with light infection remain asymptomatic. In cases of heavy infection, the disease manifests itself in three clinical stages.

1. The invasion stage

This is seen during the first week of infection and is due to juveniles and adults burrowing into the intestinal tissues. The patient complains of abdominal pain, nausea and vomiting, and diarrhoea of varying intensity. There may be fever, profuse sweating, and tachycardia.

2. The migration stage

This usually begins after the first week of infection. During this period, the larvae are liberated into the circulation by the gravid female and find their way to the muscles. Symptoms are attributable to toxic effects of

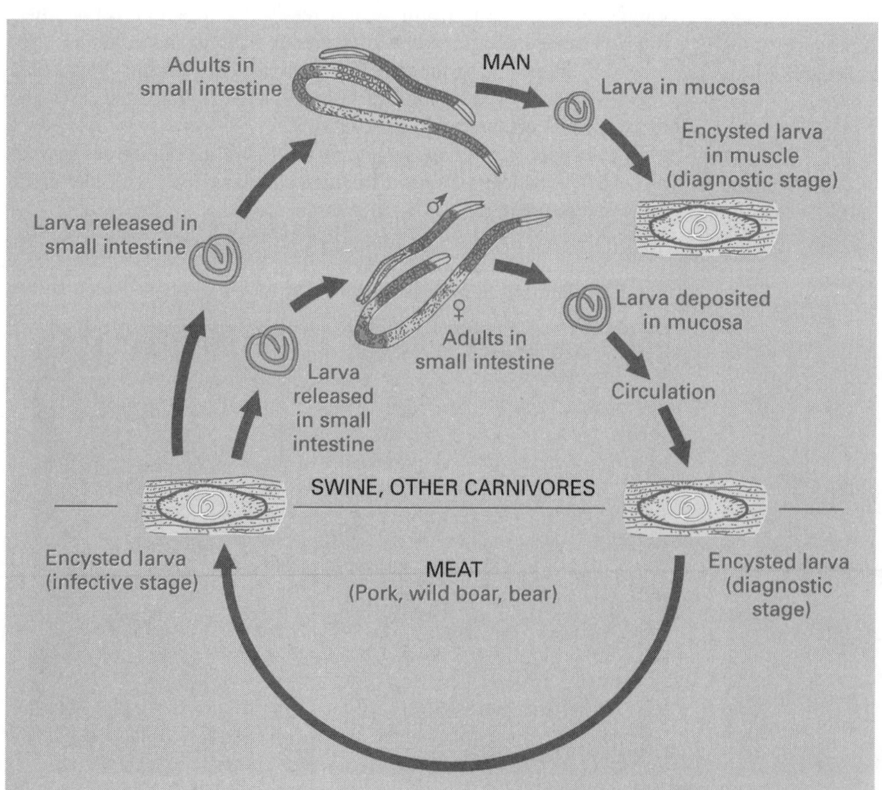

Fig. 6 Lifecycle of *Trichinella spiralis*. (Adapted from Center for Disease Control, Atlanta, Georgia, USA.)

the larvae and hypersensitivity reactions triggered by the liberation of parasite antigens. There is oedema of the face and periorbital tissues, fever, muscular tenderness, and hypereosinophilia. Complications involving the myocardium, lungs, and the central nervous system may occur due to the migrating larvae. However, the larvae do not encyst in the myocardium. A fine, macular skin rash, particularly on the trunk, may appear and last for a few days.

3. The encystment stage

This usually begins after the third week of infection. There is usually a gradual recovery from the symptoms. In a few cases with heavy infection, the symptoms may get worse and death may occur due to myocardiac failure, and respiratory and central nervous involvement. All serological tests become positive during this stage.

DIAGNOSIS

This is based on a combination of clinical and epidemiological evidence. In a characteristic case, the patient will give a history of gastrointestinal disturbances (invasion stage) within 48 h of eating pork products, wild boar, or bear meat. If the patient comes in the later stage (migration stage), there is periorbital oedema, myositis, irregular fever, and hyperosinophilia.

Among the various serological test that become positive during the encystment stage, the two most commonly used are the skin test and the slide flocculation test. Recently, enzyme immunoassay has also been used. The skin-test antigen is made from larvae and gives an immediate-type reaction in positive cases. The test is very good for surveys but unsuitable for the detection of acute disease as it remains positive for many years after infection. The slide flocculation test is also prepared from larval antigen, which is attached to cholesterol particles. In a positive reaction, flocculation is seen under the microscopes. The test remains positive for about 10 months after infection. Serum enzymes such as aminotransferases are elevated. Muscle biopsy is positive in approximately 90 per cent of clinically positive cases.

TREATMENT

The prognosis is good and most patients recover after the larvae have encysted. The mainstays of treatment are bedrest and salicylates. In myocarditis and severe myalgia, oral prednisone for 3 to 5 days (0.5–1.0 mg/kg per day) is useful and provides symptomatic relief. In experimental animals, thiabendazole is able to kill encysted larvae. In man, its efficacy against larvae is doubtful but it provides symptomatic relief. The dosage of 25 to 50 mg/kg per day for 2 to 5 days is given and this usually brings down the fever and eosinophilia. Mebendazole appears to be a good alternative to thiabendazole as it has fewer side-effects, and is given at a dosage of 300 mg daily for 7 days. A higher dose of 1000 mg daily for 10 to 14 days is recommended by some authorities to ensure complete killing of larvae. Even with this high dosage, side-effects appear not to be serious, consisting of mild Jarisch-Herxheimer type reactions at the start of therapy. The manufacturer does not recommend giving mebendazole to children under 2 years of age.

Fig. 7 Trichinella spiralis in human muscle (× 100).

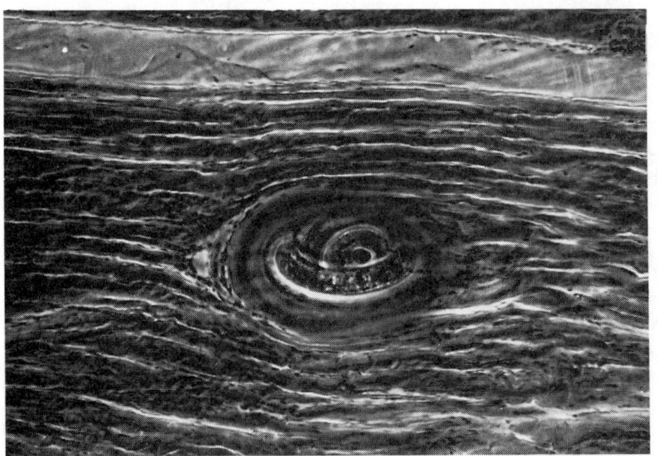

CONTROL AND PREVENTION

Trichonosis in the pig population can be greatly reduced or eliminated by hygienic rearing methods. Larvae in pork can be killed by freezing at −18°C for 24 h. Thorough cooking of pork is the best safeguard against infection in all endemic areas.

Enterobiasis

Enterobiasis is an infection caused by *Enterobius vermicularis*.

GEOGRAPHICAL DISTRIBUTION

This is one of the few parasites that is more prevalent in the temperate regions of the world than in the tropics. Children are more often involved than adults. It occurs in groups such as families living together, inmates of hostels, and in army camps.

MORPHOLOGY

The male is approximately 5 mm long with a diameter of 0.1 to 0.2 mm. The female is approximately 13 mm long with a diameter of 0.3 to 0.5 mm. The gravid female has two distended uteri that practically fill the whole body. The male has a single spicule and a curved tail. The cuticle has cervical alae, which enable its easy recognition. The eggs are generally flattened on one side and measure approximately 50 to 60 μm in length and 20 to 30 μm in breadth. They have a thick, transparent shell. The eggs are unembryonated when passed but become infective within a few hours.

LIFECYCLE

The adults are mainly located in the caecal region (Fig. 8), and the female deposits its eggs on the anus and perianal skin. Direct person-to-person infection occurs by inhalation and swallowing of the eggs. In addition, autoinfection occurs by contamination of fingers. It may occur as a sexually transmitted disease among male homosexuals. There is no visceral migration and the larva matures into an adult in the lumen of the intestinal tract. The lifecycle of the parasite is completed in about 6 weeks. Unlike Ascaris and Trichuris eggs, which need many days of development in soil before becoming embryonated, Enterobius eggs are embryonated when passed, hence there is rapid transmission from person to person.

CLINICAL ASPECTS

The most common presenting symptom is pruritus ani. This can be very troublesome and occurs more often during the night. Persistent itching may lead to inflammation and secondary bacterial infection of the perianal region. Infected children may suffer from insomnia, emotional disturbance, anorexia, weight loss, and enuresis. Occasionally, adult worms may migrate, entering the female genital tract. Inside the uterus or the Fallopian tube they may get encapsulated and produce symptoms of salpingitis. In adolescents and children it is an important cause of vulvovaginitis. The parasite may also get lodged in the lumen of the appendix, leading to appendicitis (Fig. 9). The lifespan of the parasite is 3 to 6 weeks.

DIAGNOSIS

The eggs are not usually found in the faeces. They are most easily found around the anus, by swabbing or using cellulose adhesive tape. The anal examination for eggs should be done before defecation or bathing. Sometimes intact worms are passed in the faeces and can be easily recognized by their size and shape.

TREATMENT

Attention to personal hygiene is an important part of treatment and prevention. The patient should be instructed to keep nails short and wash hands with soap and water after defaecating. The bed cover and sleeping garments should be changed every day and the floor in the bedroom kept clean. With these simple hygienic measures, infection will disappear on its own, due to the short lifespan of the parasite.

Many drugs are available to treat the infection and it is advisable to treat all the children and adults in the same household at the same time. Piperazine citrate is given in a dose of 65 mg/kg for 7 days. The course is repeated after 2 weeks. Piperazine is contraindicated in renal and liver disease and epilepsy. Pyrantel pamoate is equally effective in a single dose of 10 mg/kg (maximum 1 g) and its side-effect profile is better than piperazine. The drug is repeated after 2 weeks. Mebendazole is effective in a single dose of 100 mg, repeated after 2 weeks. This drug is contraindicated in pregnancy. Pyrvinium pamoate is specific for *E. vermicularis* and is given in a single dose of 5 mg/kg (maximum 350 mg), repeated after 2 weeks. The main disadvantage of this drug is that it can stain garments and skin with a bright red colour.

Trichuriasis

Trichuriasis is an infection caused by *Trichuris trichiura*.

GEOGRAPHICAL DISTRIBUTION

It has a worldwide distribution and is the most common intestinal nematode in some tropical regions such as South-East Asia.

MORPHOLOGY

The adult male measures 30 to 45 mm and the female 35 to 50 mm in length. The parasite is commonly known as the whip-worm because the anterior three-fifths is thin and elongated and the posterior two-fifths is bulbous and fleshy. One important feature of this group of worms is the possession of a thin, elongated oesophagus that is surrounded by gland

Fig. 9 *Enterobius vermicularis* in the lumen of the appendix (× 250).

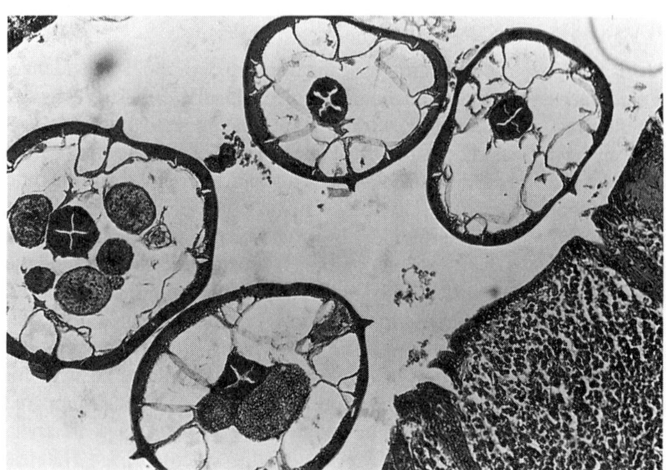

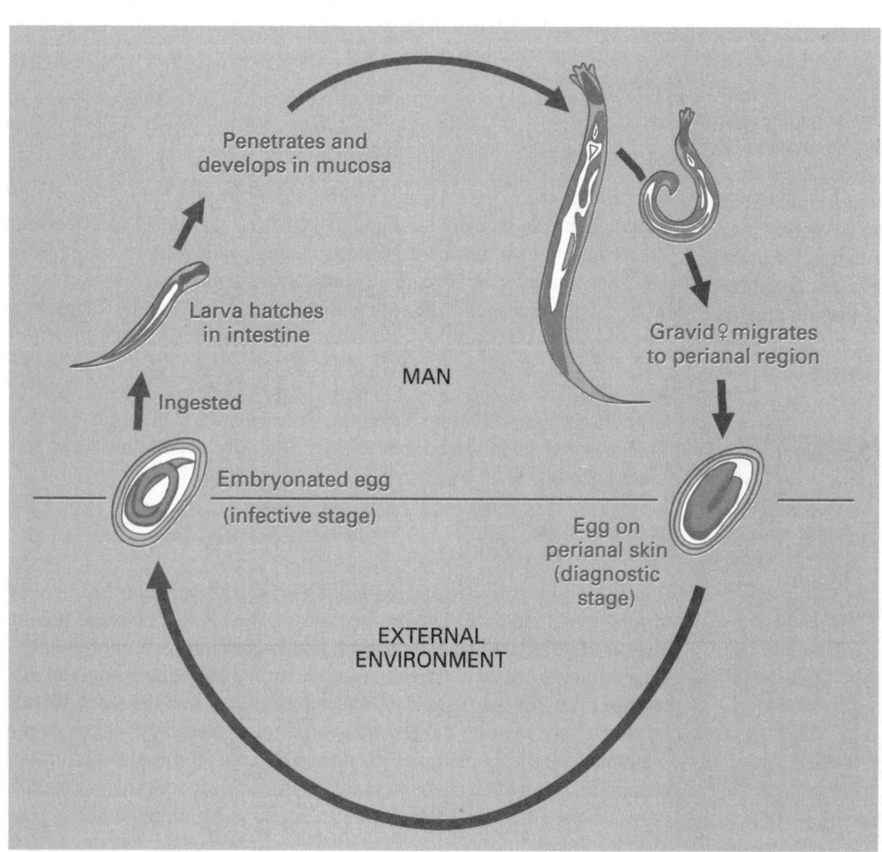

Fig. 8 Lifecycle of *Enterobius vermicularis*. (Adapted from Center for Disease Control, Atlanta, Georgia, USA.)

cells known as stichocytes. The adults are mainly located in the caecum and produce barrel-shape eggs, 22 to 50 µm long. At the lateral ends, they have transparent, blister-like plugs, which are single celled when freshly passed. In the soil the eggs become infective in about 3 weeks.

LIFECYCLE (SEE FIG. 10)

Infection occurs by the ingestion of the embryonated egg. The larva does not undergo visceral migration but penetrates the gut for a short period before returning to the lumen to mature into adult stage. The worms attach themselves to the large intestine by threading their anterior end into the epithelium (Fig. 11). The posterior end hangs free in the lumen of the bowel. The whole period of development in the host takes about 3 months to complete.

CLINICAL ASPECTS

Light infections are generally asymptomatic. In heavy infections, there is colitis with the passage of blood and mucus in faeces. The clinical picture is often similar to that of amoebic dysentery. Heavy infection in children leads to anaemia resulting in oedema, and cardiac failure. There may be marked clubbing of fingers. The anaemia is probably due to bleeding from the damaged and inflamed mucous membrane rather than sucking of blood by the parasite itself. In some cases, prolapse of the rectum occurs, probably due to constant irritation produced by the worms and the weakness of the levator ani muscle. Occasionally, the worm may lodge itself in the lumen of the appendix and cause acute appendicitis. The subtler form of trichuriasis is associated with long-term failure of children to grown in height, although they may not appear emaciated.

Fig. 11 *Trichuris trichiura*: anterior end embedded in the superficial layer of intestine epithelium (× 250).

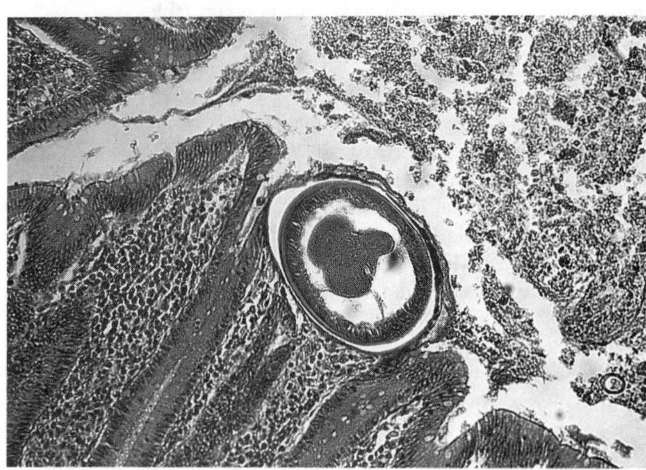

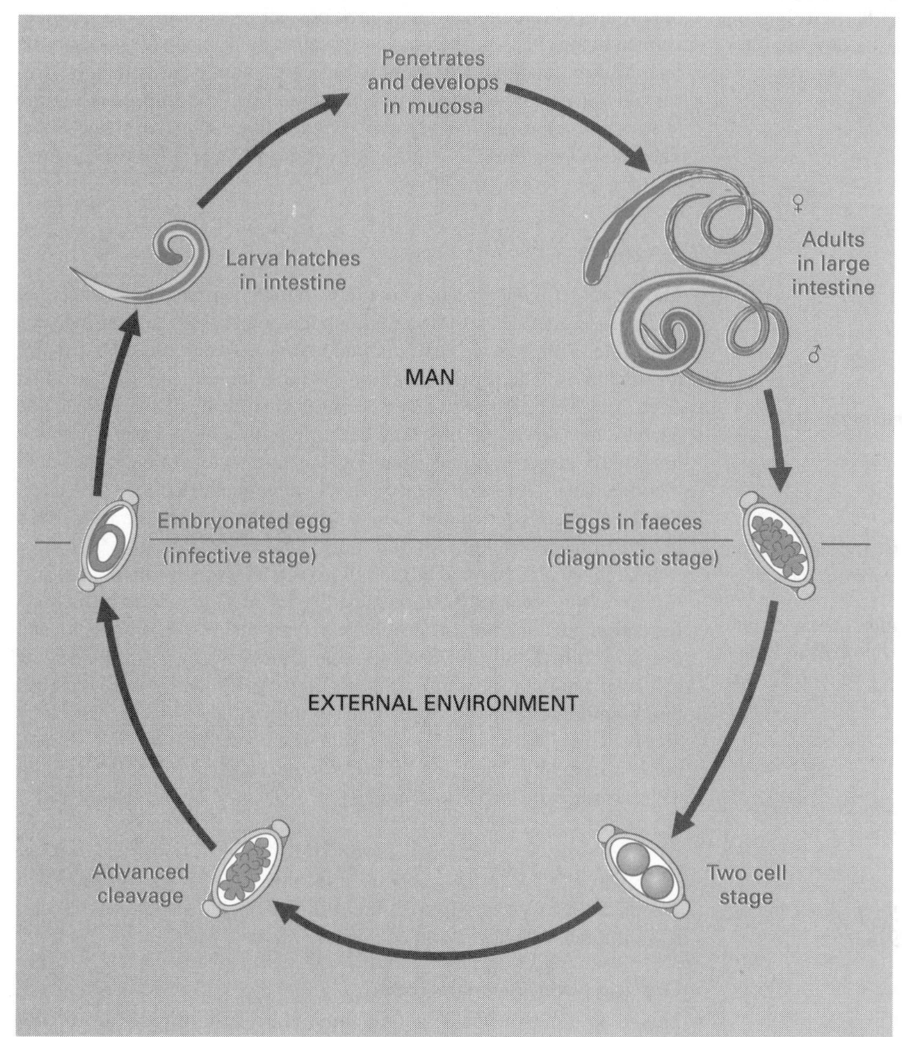

Fig. 10 Lifecycle of *Trichuris trichiura*. (Adapted from Center for Disease Control, Atlanta, Georgia, USA.)

DIAGNOSIS

This is based on finding characteristic barrel-shaped eggs in the faeces. Eosinophils and Charcot–Leyden crystals are often present. Sigmoidoscopy or proctoscopy may show worms attached to the mucous membrane and sometimes intact worms may be passed out in the faeces.

TREATMENT

Three useful chemotherapeutic agents are now available.

Mebendazole

A synthetic benzimidazole derivative active against other intestinal nematodes in addition to Trichuris. During therapy, abnormal Trichuris eggs are produced as the drug interferes with embryogenesis. Side-effects are few and it is well tolerated. Dosage is 100 mg, twice daily for 3 days, irrespective of the age of the patient. However, the manufacturers now advise against this drug in children under 2 years of age and it is contraindicated in pregnancy. A closely related compound, flubendazole, is also available and is given in the same dose as mebendazole.

Albendazole

This, another synthetic benzimidazole derivative, is effective in a single dose of 4 mg/kg. As with mebendazole, abnormal eggs are produced, which do not embryonate. It is contraindicated in pregnancy.

Oxantel plus pyrantel pamoate

This combination is effective against *A. lumbricoides*, *E. vermicularis*, hookworm, and *T. trichiura*. Dosage is 10 to 20 mg/kg body weight of each component as a single dose. In heavy infections, the drug may be repeated two or three times.

Preventive measures are the same as in ascariasis.

REFERENCES

Ascariasis

Crompton, D.W.T., Nesheim, M.C., and Pawlowski, Z.S. (ed.) (1989). *Ascariasis and its prevention.* Taylor & Francis, London.

Anisakiasis

Kliks, M.H. (1986). Human anisakiasis: an update. *Journal of the American Medical Association*, **255,** 2605.

Capillariasis

Cross, J.H. and Basaca-Sevilla, V. (1983). Experimental transmission of *Capillaria philippinensis* to birds. *Transactions of the Royal Society of Tropical Medicine and Hygiene*, **77,** 511–14.

El Hassan S.E.H. and Mikhail, W.E. (1991). Malabsorption due to *Capillaria philippinensis* in an Egyptian woman in Dubai, United Arab Emirates. *Transactions of the Royal Society of Tropical Medicine and Hygiene*, **86,** 79.

Trichinosis

Campbell, W.C. (1983) Trichenella *and trichinosis. Plenum*, New York.

Trichuriasis

Cooper, E.S. and Bundy, D.A.P. (1987). Trichuriasis. *Baillière's Clinical Tropical Medicine and Communicable Disease*, **2,** 629–43.

7.14.7 Toxocariasis and visceral larva migrans

V. Zaman

Visceral larva migrans is the name given to a syndrome characterized by hepatomegaly, fever, respiratory symptoms, and high eosinophilia. It is mainly caused by migrating larvae of *Toxocara canis* and *T. cati*. Other parasites that may cause this syndrome are *Ancylostoma* spp., Spirometra, Gnathostoma, and Alaria.

GEOGRAPHICAL DISTRIBUTION

Toxocarial infection occurs wherever there is a significant dog and cat population. Many cases have been reported from the United States and other Western countries apparently resulting from close association between these animals and man. Surveys in Great Britain have shown that approximately 2 to 3 per cent of the population possess antibodies to this parasite.

LIFE-CYCLE

The infection of *T. canis* is maintained in the dog population by direct transmission from the soil containing embryonated eggs, from transplacental transmission from bitch to puppies, through the maternal milk to puppies, and by dogs eating infected meat containing larvae. These multiple routes of infection ensure that almost all puppies are born infected. Human beings become infected by ingesting embryonated eggs from the soil. Mainly toddlers and young children are involved as they tend to eat soil and dirt. The larvae hatch out in the small intestine and migrate to various organs of the body including the liver, lungs, eye, and brain. They do not mature into adult worms in man. After some time a granuloma forms around the larvae.

MORPHOLOGY

The larva of *T. canis* is approximately 18 to 20 μm in diameter and that of *T. cati* is about 15 to 17 μm in diameter, otherwise they are indistinguishable. Both species have pointed lateral alae and two lateral excretory columns. The posterior region of the larva contains the intestinal tract. The *Toxocara* spp. larva is much smaller in diameter than the *Ascaris* spp. larva and this may be the reason why Ascaris larvae are not widely dispersed in the tissues as they are unable to enter the small blood vessels. *Toxocara* spp. eggs are similar in size to those of Ascaris but the surface is pitted and identification is easy. Eggs are never seen in human faeces as adults mature only in dogs and cats.

In animals and man the migrating toxocara larvae eventually get surrounded by a granuloma. Various cell types are involved in granuloma formation and include macrophages, lymphocytes, eosinophils, and fibroblasts. In a fully formed granuloma the larvae get surrounded by layers of fibrous tissue and inflammation subsides. It is now accepted that granuloma formation is caused by the immune system, especially T cells. Granuloma formation is an attempt by the host to limit disease, but it also favours the larva by ensuring its survival for a long time in a circumscribed area (Figs. 1 and 2).

CLINICAL ASPECTS

Toxocariasis may cause two different clinical pictures: classical visceral larva migrans syndrome and ocular toxocariasis.

Classical visceral larva migrans

This is seen most often in young children because of pica (dirt or soil eating). The majority remain asymptomatic. In a minority symptoms develop consisting of muscular pain, lassitude, anorexia, cough, and urticarial rashes. Physical signs include rhonchi, hepatomegaly, splenomegaly, and lymph-gland enlargement. The acute phase generally lasts for 2 to 3 weeks after which recovery occurs. Sometimes the resolution of all the signs may take up to 18 months. Rarely the infection may end fatally if a massive dose of parasites has been ingested.

Ocular larva migrans

This is caused by granuloma formation in the eye. If this is near to the macula, impairment of vision or even blindness may occur. The patient may come with the complaint of visual difficulty in one eye, with or without strabismus. As the generalized manifestation of visceral larva migrans may not be present, diagnosis is often difficult. Unlike in visceral larva migrans, eosinophilia may be absent. On fundoscopy a rounded swelling, often near the optic disc, may be detected.

DIAGNOSIS

1. In classical visceral larva migrans there is leucocytosis with marked eosinophilia (20–80 per cent). In ocular larva migrans there may be no peripheral eosinophilia.
2. Serological tests are useful. An enzyme immunoassay using extracts of excretory–secretory products of *T. canis* larvae is positive in the majority of patients with visceral larva migrans. In ocular larva migrans the vitreous fluid is shown to have antibodies to the parasite.
3. Biopsy of the liver may show larvae with granulomas and eosinophilic infiltration. However, biopsy is rarely done because the chances of obtaining the appropriate specimen are remote, unless it is a massive infection. If facilities are available, laparoscopy may permit direct biopsy of a granuloma, which appears as a white dot on the liver surface.

Fig. 1 Granuloma formation in an experimentally infected monkey showing a large number of giant cells and some fibroblastic reaction. Arrow marks the larva. Haematoxylin and eosin, ×400.

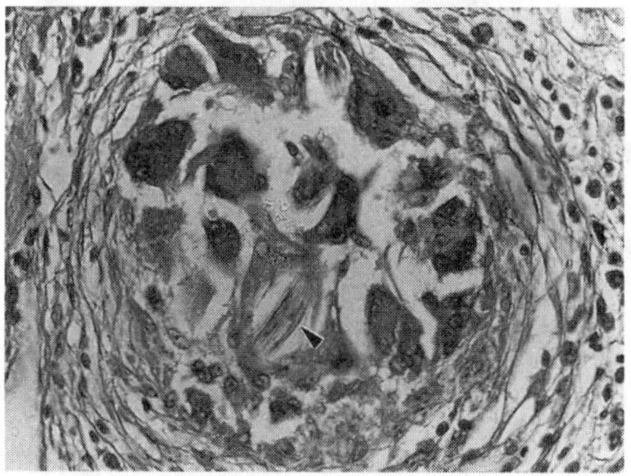

Fig. 2 Granuloma formation in the same animal as in Fig. 1 at a later stage, when the larva is completely surrounded by fibroblasts. Haematoxylin and eosin, ×400.

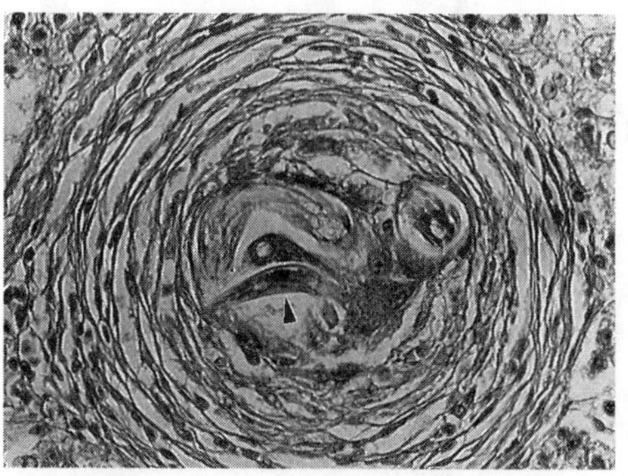

TREATMENT

No antihelminthic drug is completely effective in killing the larvae and most patients recover without specific therapy. Thiabendazole has been tried in a dosage of 25 mg/kg twice daily for 5 days and diethylcarbamazine in a dosage of 6 mg/kg a day in three divided doses for 2 to 3 weeks with indefinite results. There is a possibility that the use of antihelminthics may sometimes provoke a greater inflammatory response, with worsening of the clinical picture, due to injury of the parasite. In severe cases, corticosteroids have been used with reports of improvement.

In ocular larva migrans, visible larvae can be photocoagulated by laser. Vitrectomy has been used in some cases, and local and intraocular steroids also appear to be of same value.

REFERENCES

Shields J.A. (1984). Ocular toxocariasis. A review. *Surveys of Ophthalmology*, **28,** 361–81.

Soulsby, E.J. (1983). Toxocariasis. *British Veterinary Journal*, **139,** 471–5.

7.14.8 Angiostrongyliasis

SOMPONE PUNYAGUPTA

Cerebrospinal and abdominal angiostrongyliasis are the two clinical diseases caused by accidental human infections with two species of rat nematode, *Angiostrongylus cantonensis* and *Angiostrongylus costaricensis*, respectively. *A. costaricensis* is also known as *Morerastrongylus costaricensis.*

Cerebrospinal angiostrongyliasis, also known as eosinophilic meningitis, is prevalent in many Asian–Pacific countries including Hawaii, Tahiti, Cook Island, Caroline Island, New Hebrides, Guam, American Samoa, New Caledonia, the Philippines, Indonesia, Malaysia, Thailand, Vietnam, Taiwan, Hong Kong, Japan, India, East New Britain (Papua New Guinea), and Australia. The disease has also been reported from Cuba, Egypt, Ivory Coast, and Madagascar. Abdominal angiostrongyliasis, characterized as eosinophilic enteritis, is an important disease in Central and South America, from Mexico, Costa Rica, El Salvador, Panama, Honduras, Venezuela, Columbia, and Brazil.

Angiostrongyliasis cantonensis

Eosinophilic meningitis is a clinical entity characterized by involvement of the central nervous system associated with eosinophilic pleocytosis. It was rarely recognized until the major South Pacific outbreaks during the Second World War. Since the discovery of *A. cantonensis* in a human brain by Rosen and colleagues in 1962, there have been at least 50 parasitologically proven cases, and thousands of clinically diagnosed cases.

Adult *A. cantonensis* reside in the pulmonary arteries of rats; the first-stage larvae hatch from the eggs lodged in terminal vessels, and migrate along the air passages and intestine. Various slugs, snails, and crustacea serve as intermediate as well as transporting hosts by picking up the larvae from the soil. The infective third-stage larvae then develops. Human beings are infected when they eat apple snails (*Pila* spp.), giant African snails (*Achatina fulica*), and possibly shrimps, fish, and vegetables contaminated with larvae (Fig. 1). Recently there was a report of infection following ingestion of monitor lizard (*Varanus bengalensis*).

PATHOGENESIS

A. cantonensis is a neurotropic parasite both in man and rat. In the rat, after being ingested the larvae migrate to the brain and thereafter moult twice to become fifth-stage larvae, after which they leave the brain and reach the adult stage in the pulmonary arteries. The fate of larvae after involvement of the human brain is uncertain. Most of them leave the brain but some die in there or in the spinal cord, some reach the eyes, and a very few are found in the lungs. The period of central-nervous involvement covers roughly 4 weeks.

The disease is induced by an immunoallergic reaction to the 'toxic' substances from this unnatural parasite of man. Mononuclear and eosinophilic infiltrations are observed along the migration tracks, around vessels, and in the meninges (Fig. 2). Tissue reaction around a dead worm is much more severe than around a living one (Fig. 3). Scattered areas of minute haemorrhages are evidence of mechanical injury (Fig. 4). At autopsy, worms may be found in the spinal cord, eye chambers, and lungs. The degree of clinical severity depends upon the numbers of infecting worms in each patient, varying from a few to hundreds. The disease is usually benign, sometimes subclinical and self-limiting, with complete recovery in most cases. Yet it may be severe, resulting in acute cerebral dysfunction, permanent neurological deficits, or even death. The incubation period varies from 3 to 36 days with an average of 2 weeks but tends to be shorter in severe cases.

CLINICAL FEATURES

Most patients present with a history of acute, intermittent, unbearable, occipital and bitemporal headache, which lasts through the clinical course. The most useful clinical clue is the absence of significant fever except in patients with severe disease, who may present with deteriorating cerebral symptoms. Patients may experience neck stiffness: meningism can be elicited in only about 15 per cent of mild cases but more in severe cases. Nausea and vomiting are frequent during the first week. Varying degrees of disturbed consciousness are uncommon except in

Fig. 2 Tracks in the human brain showing disruption of nervous tissue and cellular infiltration.

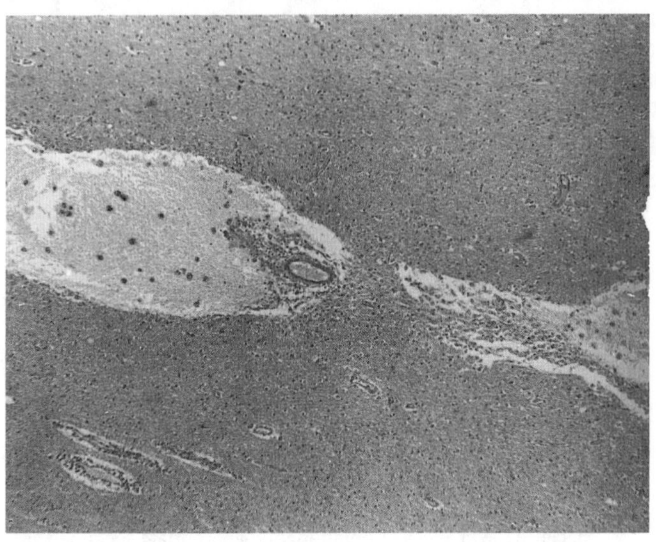

Fig. 1 Important food sources of human infection: (a) pila snails, (b) *A. fulica*, (c) shrimps, (d) vegetables contaminated with land snails.

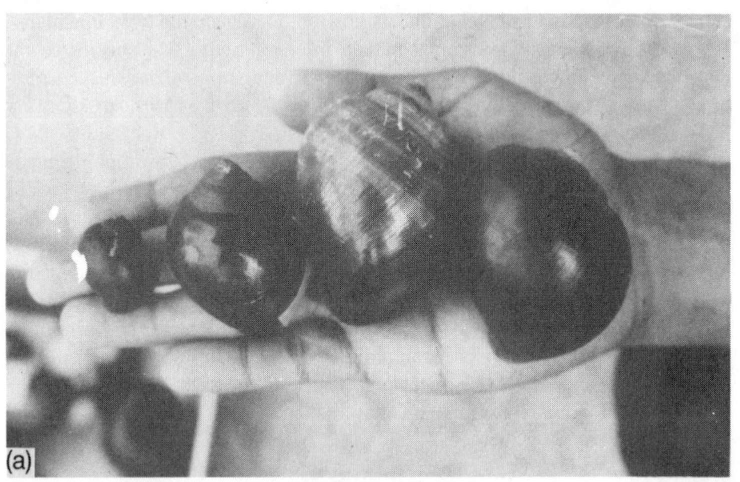

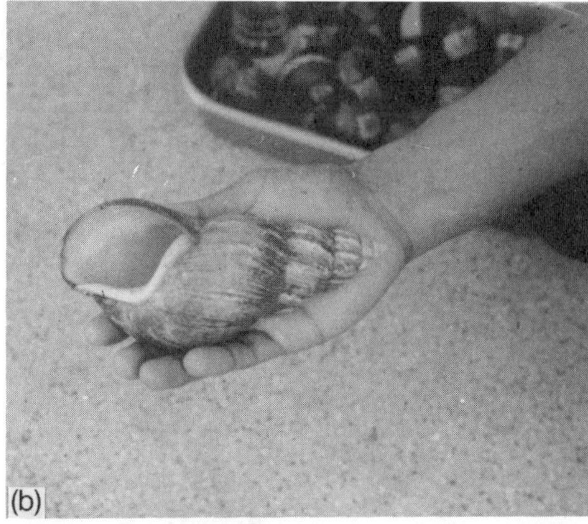

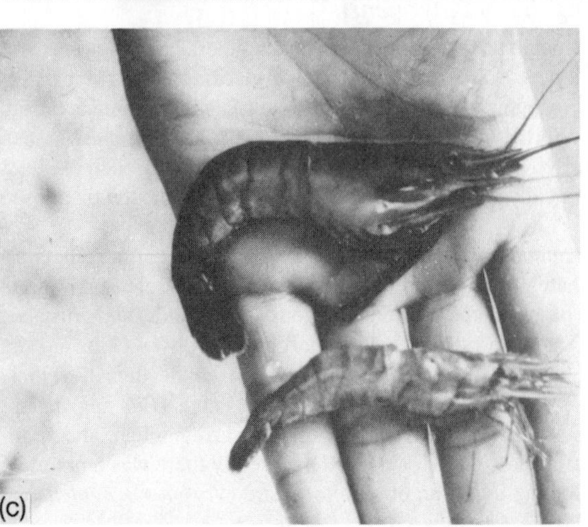

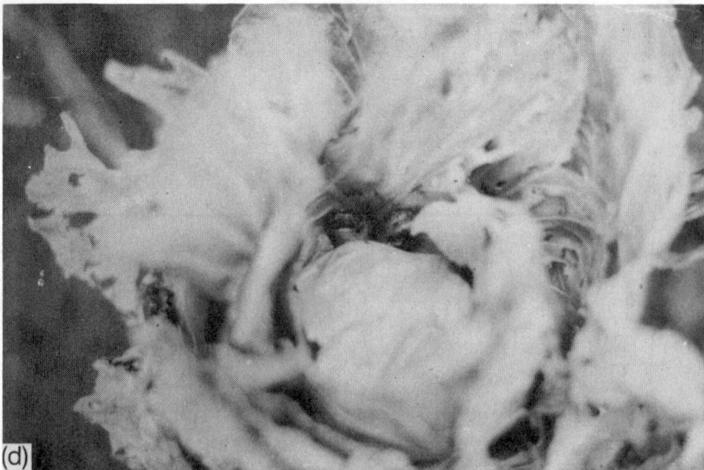

severe cases. Some may present with history of convulsion or psychosis. Mild constitutional symptoms such as malaise, anorexia, and general aching are usual.

Paraesthesia of the trunk and extremities indicating peripheral-nerve injury may be observed. Generalized motor weakness and paraplegia due to spinal-cord involvement may be noted in some severe cases. Cough, audible rales, and radiographic features of pneumonitis have been recognized in very severe cases; *A. cantonensis* has been found in the lungs at autopsy. Cranial nerves are sometimes involved, particularly the optic, facial, and abducens nerves (Fig. 5). Bilateral or unilateral amblyopia of varying degree, associated with abnormal fundi, is not uncommon. Diplopia, abnormal visual fields, optic atrophy, and periorbital oedema are seldom seen. *A. cantonensis* larvae have been recovered from the eye chambers in many cases (Fig. 6). Retinal haemorrhage and detachment are important ocular complications.

Specific inquiries about consumption of raw or rare food within 2 to 4 weeks of the onset of headache usually yields a positive response. Some may give a history of nausea, vomiting, abdominal discomfort, and urticarial rash soon after ingestion of the suspected food.

LABORATORY FINDINGS

The peripheral blood usually shows slight leucocytosis with 10 to 50 per cent eosinophilia persisting for about 3 months.

Lumbar puncture, the single most useful diagnostic test, must be done in all suspected cases. The opening pressure is usually high, in some cases over 500 mm of cerebrospinal fluid. The fluid may be clear or turbid, colourless or slightly xanthochromic but not purulent. The pleocytosis is usually in the range of 500 to 2000/mm^3. Red blood cells may be seen occasionally. Eosinophilic pleocytosis varies from 10 per cent to over 90 per cent. The predominant cells may, however, be lymphocytes, and some neutrophils may also be found. Eosinophilic pleocytosis reaches a peak around the second week after the first symptom and gradually disappears over 3 months. In a few cases, the pleocytosis may recur during the second month with return of some symptoms. The protein concentration is high but the sugar concentration is normal. Spinal

Fig. 3 Note the immense cellular reaction around the dead worm (a) compared to that around the live one (b).

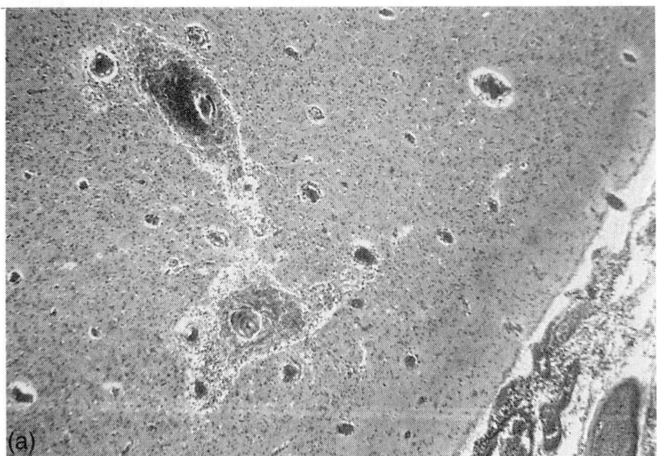

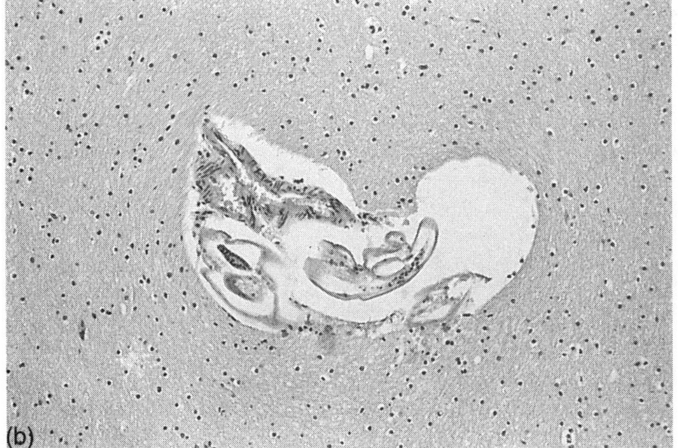

Fig. 4 Haemorrhages of the brain in cerebral angiostrongyliasis (a) compared to the massive haemorrhage in cerebral gnathostomiasis (b).

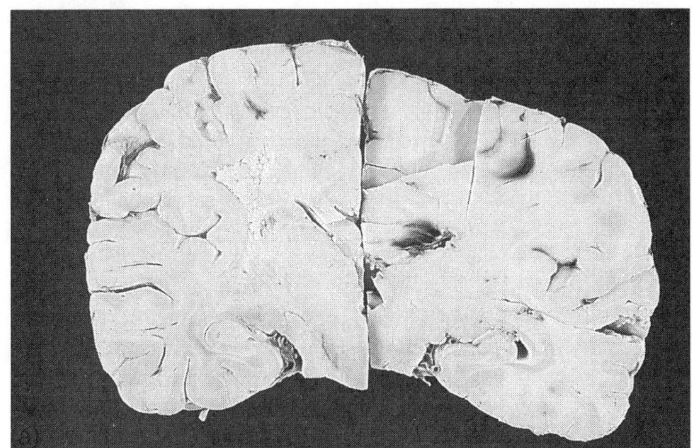

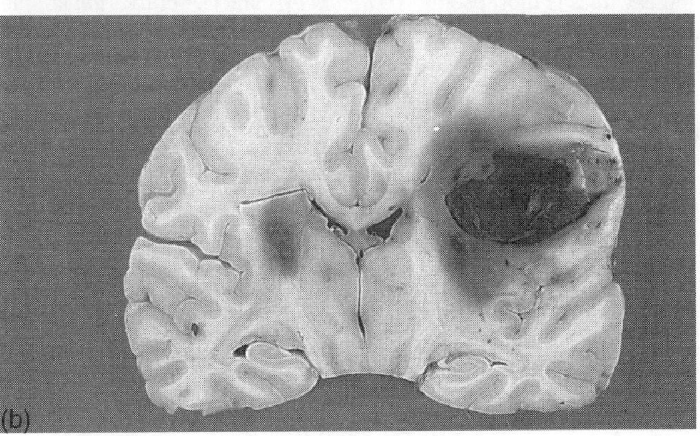

Fig. 5 Patient in semicomatose stage with abducens nerve paralysis.

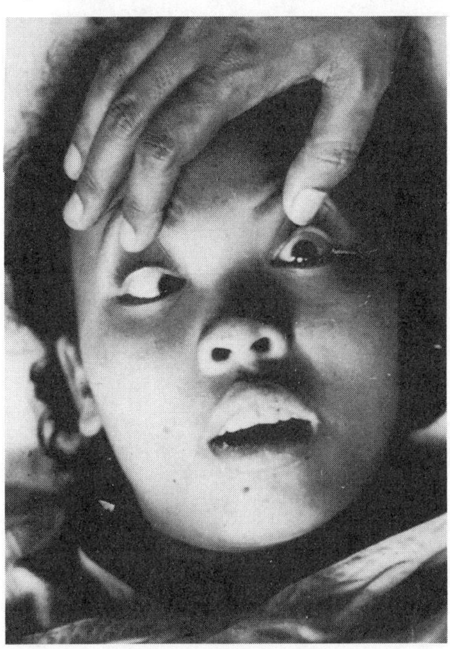

fluid should be examined closely under a bright light with the help of a hand lens to detect tiny moving larvae (Fig. 7). In Taiwan the recovery rate of worms in the spinal fluid is much higher than elsewhere, ranging from 6.4 to 30 per cent.

Other investigations, including biochemical tests, electroencephalogram, brain scan, and cerebral angiography, are of no diagnostic value. Some abnormalities have been observed in computerized axial tomographs of the brain.

DIAGNOSIS

Cerebral angiostrongyliasis should always be suspected if a patient who resides in or recently visited the known endemic area presents with a history of typical symptoms and eosinophilic pleocytosis within 1 month of eating snails, shrimps, etc. A definite diagnosis can only be made by recovering *A. cantonensis* larvae from the spinal fluid or ocular chambers, or at autopsy. Enzyme-linked immunosorbent assay, with antigen prepared from fourth-stage larvae, may be used as supportive evidence.

DIFFERENTIAL DIAGNOSIS

In spite of the fact that eosinophilic pleocytosis has been observed rarely in tuberculous meningitis, neurosyphilis, and multiple sclerosis, for practical purposes it indicates a parasitic infection of the central nervous system: *A. cantonensis*, *Gnathostoma spinigerum*, *Paragonimus westermani*, and schistosoma. Epidemiological information in different geographical areas is most useful. *A. cantonensis* and *G. spinigerum* are the most frequently encountered. *G. spinigerum* should be suspected if the patient develops paralysis of the extremities following severe radicular pain or impairment of the sensorium with bloody or xanthochromic spinal fluid and eosinophilic pleocytosis (Table 1).

Table 1 *Major clinical features of eosinophilic meningitis due to* A. cantonensis *(484 cases) and* G. spinigerum *(162 cases)*

	A. cantonensis %	*G. spinigerum* %
Severe headache	98.0	71.0
Neck pain	64.0	51.0
Vomiting	38.0	36.0
Visual impairment	40.0	42.0
Paraesthesia	37.0	6.0
Fever	33.0	26.0
Severe radiculitis	0.0	37.0*
Sensorium impairment	6.0	27.0*
Neck stiffness	14.8	20.5
Kernig positive	5.6	7.5
Facial paralysis	4.0	3.7
Abducens paralysis	3.3	3.1
Visual acuity impairment	16.1	21.1
Abnormal fundi	12.4	13.7
Eyelid oedema	1.0	9.0
Paraparesis, paraplegia	0.8	67.7*
Bloody or xanthochromic cerebrospinal fluid	1.0	64.0*

*Significant points for differential diagnosis.

Fig. 6 A living *A. cantonensis* larva in the posterior chamber of a patient's eye.

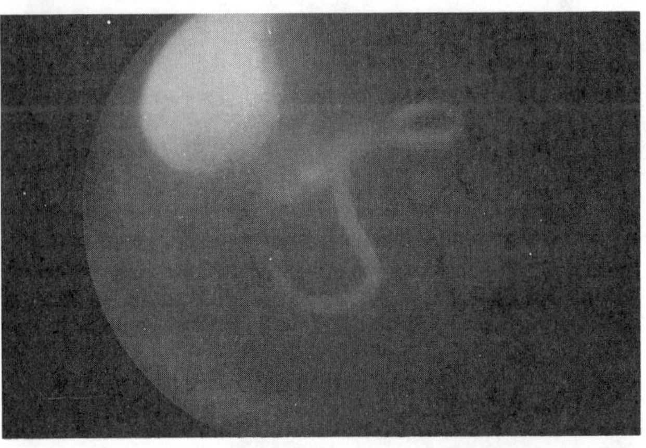

Fig. 7 *A. cantonensis* larvae recovered from the cerebrospinal fluid.

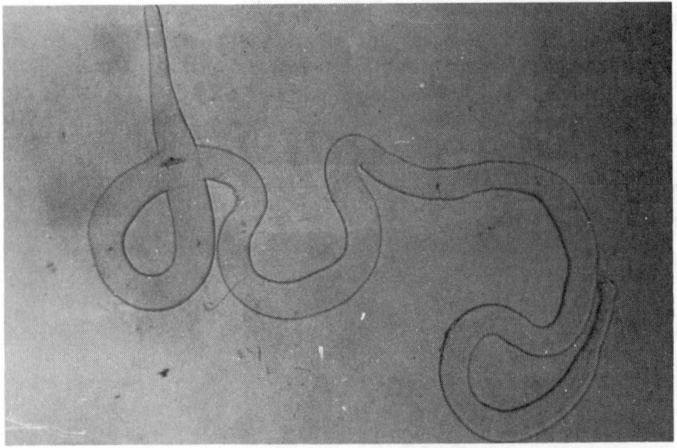

TREATMENT AND CLINICAL COURSE

Because this is a self-limiting disease in most cases, an effective anthelminthic, even if available, should not be given because the reaction to the dead worms in the brain can be disastrous, leading to clinical deterioration or even death. Headache usually subsides dramatically, but temporarily, after each lumbar puncture. The tap should therefore be repeated at intervals of 3 to 7 days until there is a definite clinical as well as laboratory improvement. Analgesics and sedatives are helpful. Based on the immunopathological concept, corticosteroids, such as prednisolone, in a dose of 30 to 60 mg daily, have been advocated in critical cases with cerebral depression, or in those with cranial-nerve involvement, but no benefit has been confirmed in milder cases.

Fig. 8 Section of a human caecum showing three ova of *A. costaricensis* with cellular infiltration mostly of eosinophils (by courtesy of Dr Pedro Morera, University of Costa Rica).

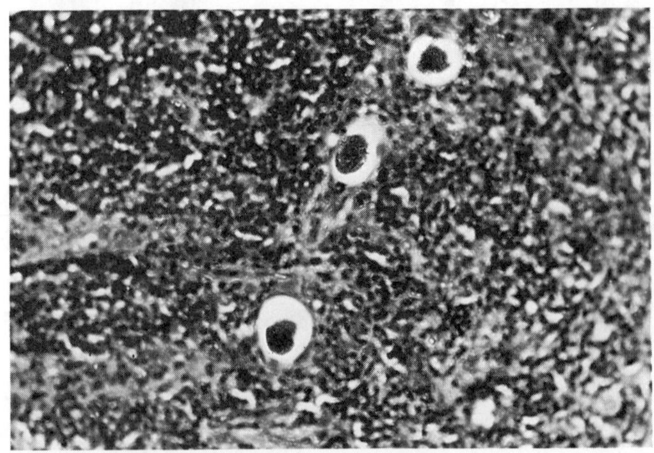

Although clinical symptoms persist for only 2 to 4 weeks, the neurological deficit may last longer. In some patients, relapse of acute symptoms may occur after 2 months of illness, probably representing a reaction to some dead worms in the brain.

Angiostrongylus in the eye should be removed surgically, but complications are inevitable if the posterior chamber is involved.

The overall mortality rate is low: 3.7 per cent in Taiwan, 0.5 per cent in Thailand, and none in Tahiti. However, the fatality among specific groups of patients may be as high as 25 per cent. Patients usually die in coma 2 to 4 weeks after the onset. Energetic neurological and cardiopulmonary intensive care during the acute stage can be life saving. As there is no specific treatment, preventive measures through public education are necessary.

Angiostrongyliasis costaricensis

Eosinophilic gastroenteritis is a clinical syndrome of unknown aetiology. Parasites, such as *Eustoma rotundatum*, *Anisakis*, *G. spinigerum*, and *A. costaricensis* are, however, capable of producing eosinophilic gastroenteritis or granuloma.

PATHOGENESIS

A. costaricensis lives in the mesenteric arteries of cotton rats (*Sigmodon hispidus*), *Rattus rattus*, and some other rodents. First-stage larvae hatch from eggs in the intestinal capillaries and enter the intestine. Slugs (*Vaginulus plebelus*), which ingest the larvae in rat faeces, serve as intermediate hosts in which second- and third-stage larvae develop. Human beings accidentally ingests vegetable leaves smeared with mucous secretion of slugs containing infective larvae. Man is not a definitive host, yet the female worms are capable of producing fertile but unhatched eggs. The lesions are confined to the ileocaecal region (Fig. 8). Oedema and thickening of the intestinal wall with miliary, yellowish, granulomatous inflammation of the appendix, terminal ileum, caecum, or ascending colon are observed. Regional lymph nodes, liver, omentum, and testicles are occasionally involved. Arteritis or thrombosis of arteries by the 2–4 cm long, filiform, adult worms may be noted. Microscopy of the lesions shows eosinophilic infiltration and characteristic thin-walled eggs or larvae of *A. costaricensis*.

CLINICAL FEATURES

The disease mainly attacks children. The incubation period is unknow. Patients experience high fever for 2 to 4 weeks, anorexia, vomiting, and right-sided, particularly right iliac fossa, abdominal pain resembling that of acute appendicitis. Some present features of partial or complete intestinal obstruction. Ectopic migration of the worms to the liver causing hypereosinophilia with hepatomegaly has been recognized. Physical examination reveals tenderness or a tender mass in the right inferior quadrant and tenderness on rectal examination. Leucocytosis of 10 to 50×10^9/l with 11 to 82 per cent eosinophilia is a constant finding. Radiographs may show spasticity, filling defects, and irritability at the caecum and ascending colon. Serodiagnosis may be helpful in chronic as well as acute cases.

DIAGNOSIS AND TREATMENT

The diagnosis should be considered in children with features of appendicitis, inflammatory bowel disease, or ileocaecal mass associated with blood eosinophilia. Definitive diagnosis and treatment are best achieved by surgical exploration and resection of affected bowel. Medical treatment with thiabendazole has achieved inconclusive results. In the majority of cases, appendectomy, ileocolonic resection, right hemicolectomy, or colostomy were done. Two patients died out of 114 who received both surgical and medical treatment.

REFERENCES

Kliks, M.M., Kroenke, K., and Hardman, J.M. (1982). Eosinophilic radiculomyeloencephalitis: an angiostrongyliasis outbreak in American Samoa related to ingestion of *Achatina fulica* snails. *American Journal of Tropical Medicine and Hygiene*, **31**, 1122–44.

Loria-Cortes, R. and Lobo Sanahuja, J.F. (1980). Clinical abdominal angiostrongylosis. A study of 116 children with intestinal eosinophilic granuloma caused by *Angiostrongylus costaricensis*. *American Journal of Tropical Medicine and Hygiene*, **29**, 538–44.

Morera, P. (1973). Life history and redescription of *Angiostrongylus costaricensis* Morera and Cespedes, 1971. *American Journal of Tropical Medicine and Hygiene*, **22**, 613–21.

Morera, P., Perez, F., Mora, F., and Castro, L. (1982). Visceral larvae migrans like syndrome caused by *Angiostrongylus costaricensis*. *American Journal of Tropical Medicine and Hygiene*, **31**, 67–70.

Punyagupta, S., Juttijudata, P., and Bunnag, T. (1975). Eosinophilic meningitis in Thailand. Clinical studies of 484 typical cases probably caused by *Angiostrongylus cantonensis*. *American Journal of Tropical Medicine and Hygiene*, **24**, 921–31.

Punyagupta, S., Bunnag, T., and Juttijudata, P. (1990). Eosinophilic meningitis in Thailand. Clinical and epidemiological characteristics of 162 patients with myeloencephalitis probably caused by *Gnathostoma spinigerum*. *Journal of Neurological Sciences*, **96**, 241–56.

Yii, C.Y. (1976). Clinical observations on eosinophilic meningitis and meningoencephalitis caused by *Angiostrongylus cantonensis* in Taiwan. *American Journal of Tropical Medicine and Hygiene*, **25**, 233–49.

7.14.9 Gnathostomiasis

PRAVAN SUNTHARASAMAI

Gnathostomiasis in man is an extraintestinal infection with, in most cases, larval or immature *Gnathostoma spinigerum*, a nematode parasite (order Spirurida) that lives in the stomachs of cats and dogs. The disease is characterized by intermittent and migratory space-occupying lesions in the skin and less commonly in the internal organs, resulting from inflammation or haemorrhage. Occasional deaths are due to the invasion of the central nervous system. It is known by the following local names: *tuachid* (Thailand), *chokofushi* (Japan), and Shanghai rheumatism or Nanching Consular disease (China).

Aetiology

At present, four species of gnathostomes are known to infect man (Table 1). In general, the adults of the gnathostomes live in the upper gastrointestinal tract of the definitive hosts, which for *G. spinigerum*, the most thoroughly studied species, include dog, cat, tiger, leopard, golden cat, leopard cat, jungle cat, ocelot, lynx, lion, otter, opossum, mink, and racoon. Cyclops, the first intermediate host, ingests the sheathed, first-stage larvae, which hatch in water from ova shed with the host's faeces. The third-stage larvae (Fig. 1) are found in the walls of viscera and in muscles of second intermediate hosts, such as fish, frog, snake, lizard, chicken, duck, rat, pig, and mongoose, which have ingested the infected cyclops or the infected flesh of another second intermediate host. Only the consumption of the third-stage larvae by a definitive host can lead to the development of mature male and female worms in the stomach; otherwise those fishes, amphibians, reptiles, birds, and other mammals become only infectious, paratenic hosts.

Consumption of the raw or undercooked flesh of second intermediate and paratenic hosts is the most common mode of transmission. Skin penetration by worms after contamination of the skin of food preparers by infected meat, or the use of such flesh as a poultice, are less important. Ingestion of infected cyclops can induce infection in mice, and is another, but not yet proven, mode of transmission in man.

Table 1 *Gnathostoma spp. infecting man*

Species	Definitive hosts	Second intermediate and paratenic hosts	Geographical distribution
G. spinigerum	Felines and canines	Fish, amphibians, reptiles, and mammals	Asia, Oceania, Central and South America
G. hispidum	Pig	Loaches, amphibians, birds, and mammals	Asia, Europe
G. doloresi	Swine and wild boar	Amphibians and reptiles	Asia, Oceania
G. nipponicum	Weasel	Loaches and snakes	Japan

Prenatal transmission can occur, as *G. spinigerum* larvae have been recovered in neonates as young as 3 days old. Venereal transmission is unlikely, even though larvae have been found in both male and female genitalia.

The *G. spinigerum* parasites recovered from man are third-stage larvae (0.34–0.63 mm wide, 2.2–3.5 mm long), immature males (0.60–1.05 mm wide, 4.63–9.35 mm long), immature females (0.83–1.0 mm wide, 3.83–16.25 mm long), or mature males (1.0–1.25 mm wide, 9.9–12.5 mm long). Their stage of development does not correlate with the duration of the clinical illness. Infection with more than one larva is rare.

Geographical distribution

Human infections with *G. spinigerum* have been reported frequently in Thailand and Japan, and sporadically in Australia, Bangladesh, Burma, China, Ecuador, India, Indonesia, Laos, Malaysia, Mexico, the Philippines, Sri Lanka, and Vietnam. Animal infections also occur in Palestine, the United States, the former USSR, and Zimbabwe. Prevalence in Bangkok, Thailand, has been estimated to be 4/1000 people. Infections in man have been recorded in places far away from areas of natural occurrence of the gnathostomes due to migration of, particularly, the paratenic human hosts, who carry this long-lived parasite with them.

Human infections with the other three species have been reported from Japan. However, it appears that the Japanese acquire *G. hispidum* from infected loaches imported from China; *G. doloresi* and *G. nipponicum* occur naturally in Japan.

There have been recent claims from Mexico of a new species of Gnathostoma that can infect man, but the evidence that this is a distinct species, rather than a subspecies of *G. spinigerum* is inconclusive.

Pathology and pathogenesis

After being ingested, the larva penetrates the gut wall and migrates to the liver before wandering, perhaps randomly, through almost any tissue except bone. The migration appears to be facilitated by production of enzymes and the organism's cuticular architecture and musculature. As the worm migrates the tissue is destroyed, producing track-like spaces together with varying degrees of haemorrhage and eosinophil-associated acute inflammation that may be the result of an immunological reaction and toxic products of the parasites (Figs 2 to 4). Oedema is prominent in some skin lesions, while multiple and sometimes large areas of haematoma are typical of spinal cord and brain involvement. In a more stationary lesion the eosinophil-associated zone will be surrounded by granulomatous changes, occasional multinucleate cells, and histiocytes filled with Charcot–Leyden crystals. Onion-like, perivascular fibrous thickening of small arteries and eosinophilic endarteritis with thrombosis are also observed. The draining lymph nodes show follicular hyperplasia with marked eosinophilic infiltration within medullary cords and sinusoids.

Fig. 1 Scanning electron micrograph of the head bulb of a third-stage larva of the gnathostome (by courtesy of Mr Win Chaeychomsri).

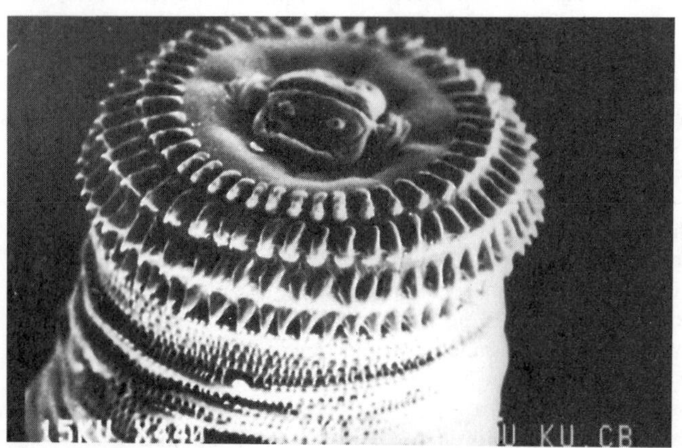

Fig. 2 Sections of brain and spinal cord showing haemorrhagic tracts due to the migration of a gnathostome larva (by courtesy of Professor Rangsan Panyadhanya).

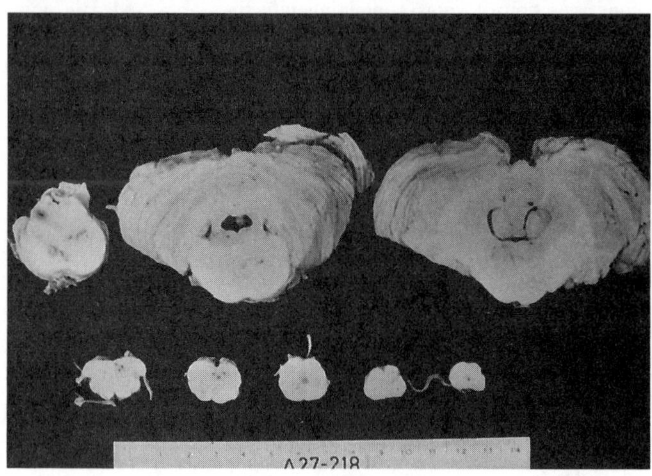

Fig. 3 A cross-section of a gnathostome larva and tracts of inflammation and haemorrhage (by courtesy of Dr Prakit Rodprasert).

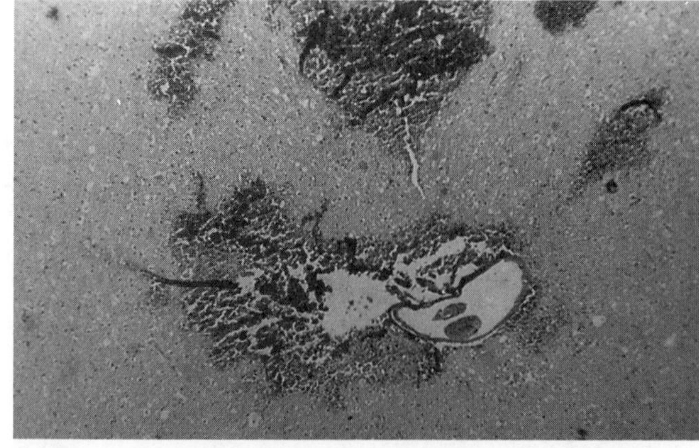

Symptoms and signs result from space-occupying effects of the inflammatory lesion or haemorrhage, mechanical destruction of tissues and blood vessels or disruption of blood supply, and vary according to the sites and sizes of the lesions induced intermittently along the migratory route.

Clinical features

After consumption of infected flesh, nausea, vomiting, and abdominal pain may occasionally be noted within 1 to 2 days, and a syndrome consisting of fever, pain in the right upper quadrant of the abdomen, chest pain, dry cough, and hypereosinophilia may develop within 1 to 2 weeks. The patients usually present with only one of the following forms of the infection.

CUTANEOUS FORMS

Gnathostomal creeping eruption

This is extremely rare. The serpigenous track (Fig. 5) is similar to, but bigger and more variable in depth than those caused by dog or cat hookworm larvae. A trail of subcutaneous haemorrhage is sometimes observed.

Cutaneous migratory swelling

This is the most common manifestation of human gnathostomiasis (Fig. 6). The first swelling may develop 3 to 4 weeks after ingestion. However, incubation periods in most cases are unknown. Swelling can occur anywhere and may recur close to the original site (Fig. 7) or at a distance. When the parasite moves into the forearm or lower leg and ankle, further swelling is usually distal to the elbow or the knee. Swelling develops rapidly and usually lasts for about 1 to 2 weeks. Frequently it is extensive, involving the whole wrist or hand. Swelling of the digits or plantar surfaces can be very painful and incapacitating. The degree of pain in most places is unrelated to the size of the swelling. Itching is the main associated symptom. The overlying skin is normal in colour or occasionally erythematous. The oedema is non-pitting. Regional lymphadenitis and fever are usually absent. When swelling involves the eyelid,

Fig. 4 (a) Section showing a gnathostome larva under the skin; the higher magnified figure (b) shows four rows of cuticular spines of the head bulb (by courtesy of Dr Mario Riganti).

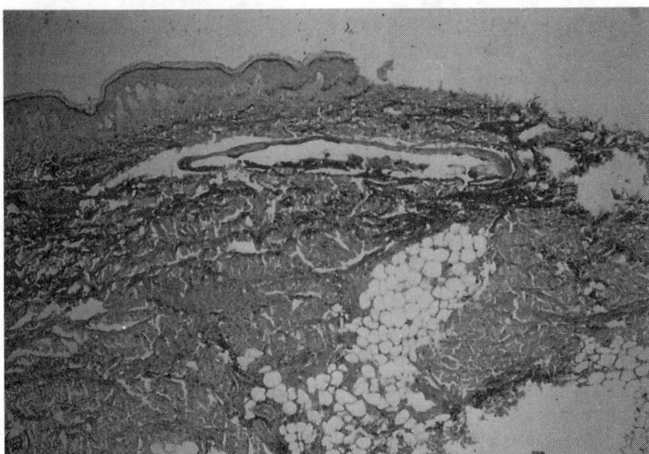

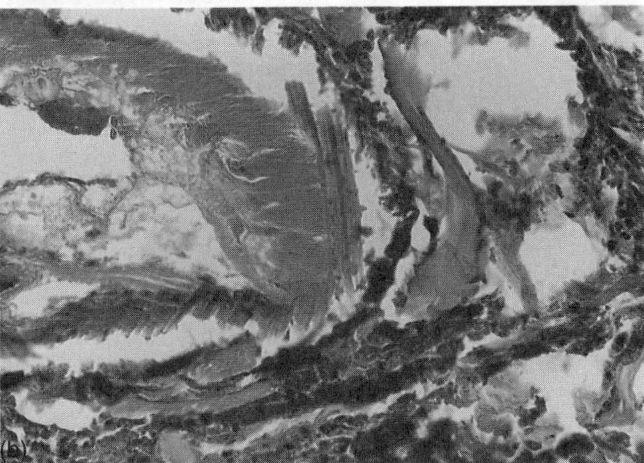

Fig. 5 Creeping eruption around the left thigh. (Reproduced from Bhaibulaya and Charoenlarp (1983), by permission.)

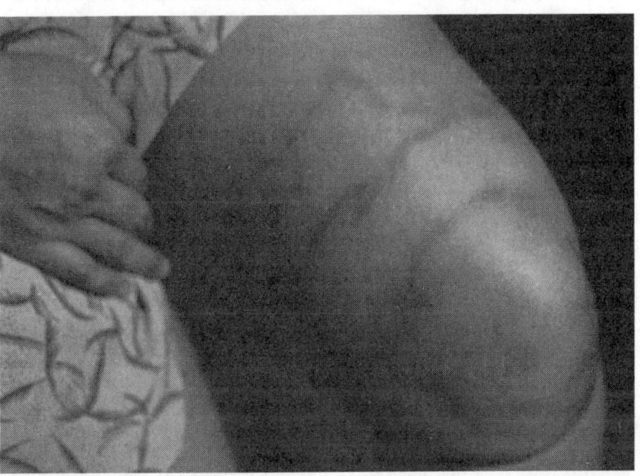

Fig. 6 Gnathostoma cutaneous swelling of (a) the back (b) and the hand in two patients.

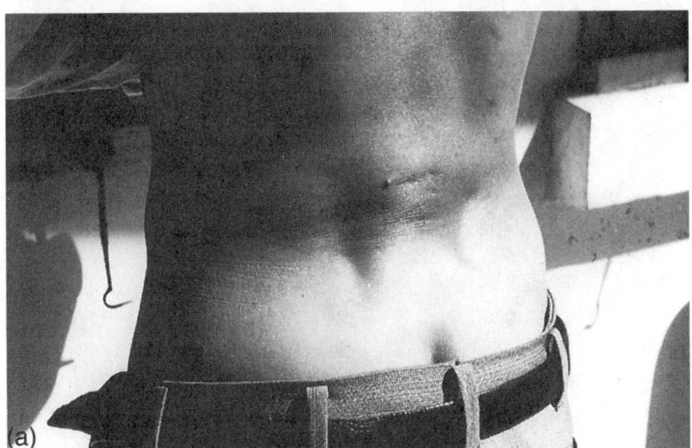

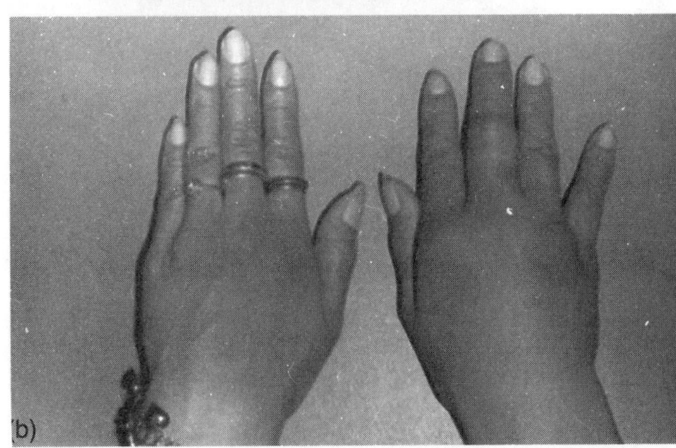

chemosis (Fig. 8) and conjunctival haemorrhage may be observed. The worms can escape spontaneously through the skin (Figs. 7 and 8), the gingiva, or the conjunctiva. The interval between episodes of swelling varies from a few days to a few months and rarely 1 to 2 years. The illness may recur for 20 years. In cases where reinfection could be excluded, persistence of infection for 3.5 years has been observed.

VISCERAL FORMS

Spinocerebral gnathostomiasis

Involvement of the central nervous system (Figs. 9 and 10) commonly starts with intermittent, agonizing, shooting pains with paraesthesia of a limb or a segment of trunk, followed by paraplegia with urinary retention and, rarely, quadriplegia. Sensation is correspondingly impaired and the Brown–Séquard syndrome is sometimes seen. A few patients present with severe headache and vomiting, followed very quickly by coma, cranial-nerve palsies, and hemiplegia, resembling a cerebrovascular accident. Physical findings, other than the usual signs of meningeal irritation, depend on the size of the lesions, but a rapidly advancing or changing pattern of neurological deficit is characteristic of the infection. Cutaneous migratory swelling precedes or follows the episode in only a few of these patients. Eosinophilic meningitis without focal neurological deficit occurs occasionally.

Ocular gnathostomiasis

The gnathostome can be found in the anterior chamber (Fig. 11), the vitreous humour, and the retina. Inflammation and destruction markedly impair vision. The parasite usually migrates through the sclera or the cornea, but may die in the vitreous humour.

Intra-abdominal and oral gnathostomiasis

These can induce intestinal obstruction, or cause a painful intra-abdominal mass. It is very likely that in some cases the infection may terminate spontaneously when the worm escapes unnoticed into the lumen of the gastrointestinal tract and is expelled with the faeces, as spontaneous escape through the mucosa of the mouth has been observed.

Pulmonary and respiratory gnathostomiasis

The parasites have been found in the sputum of patients with eosinophilic pneumonitis, or following symptoms indicating irritation of the upper respiratory tract.

Genitourinary gnathostomiasis

The parasites have been found in bloodstained urethral discharge, accompanying haematuria, in the glans penis, or in the uterine cervical mucosa.

Fig. 7 Migratory swelling in a 23-year-old male: (a) at the eyelids for 5 days when seen on 5 June 1986; (b) at the left side of the upper lip on 7 June 1986; (c) at the right side of the upper lip on 9 June 1986 when the larva was picked out by needle puncture and squeezing; (d) subsided condition on 10 June, 24 h after removal of the gnathostome.

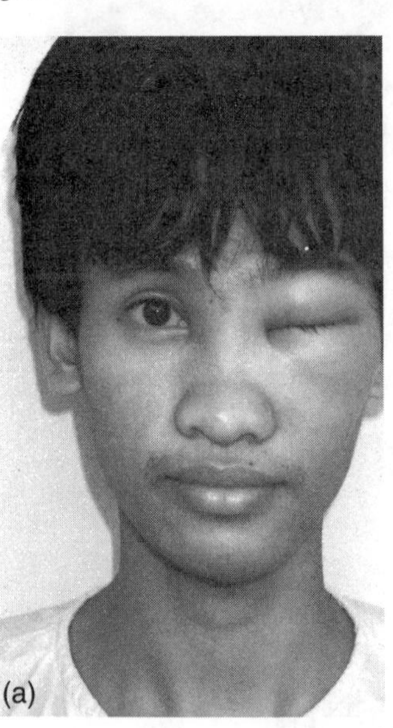

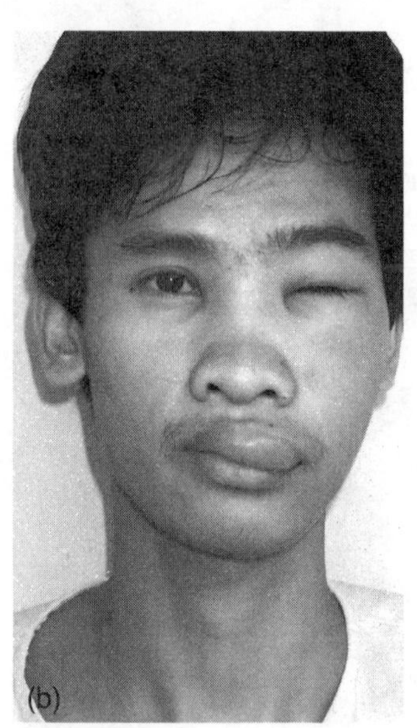

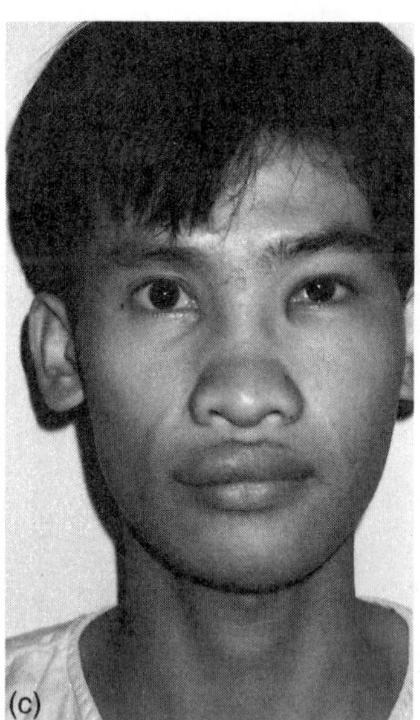

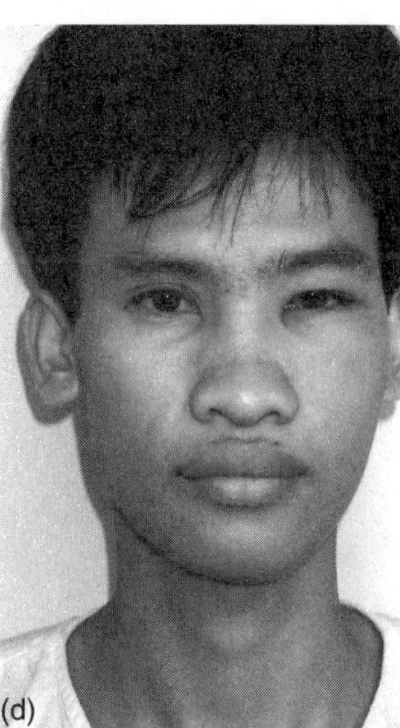

Fig. 8 (a) Chemosis of the right conjunctiva; (b) the gnathostome emigrated through the upper eyelid; (c) a small papule was still visible 1 week afterward but (d) there was no scar 1 month later.

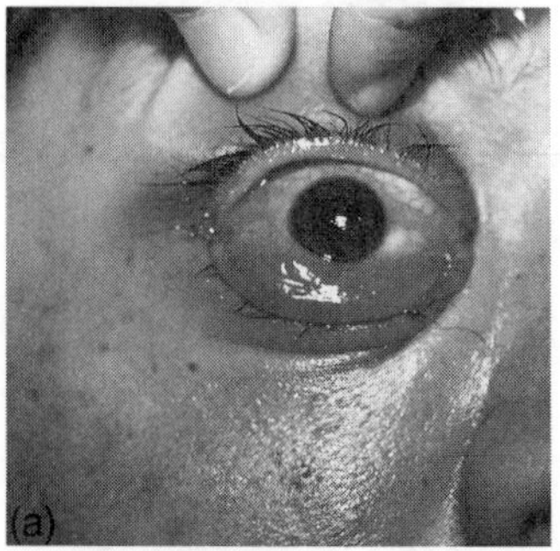

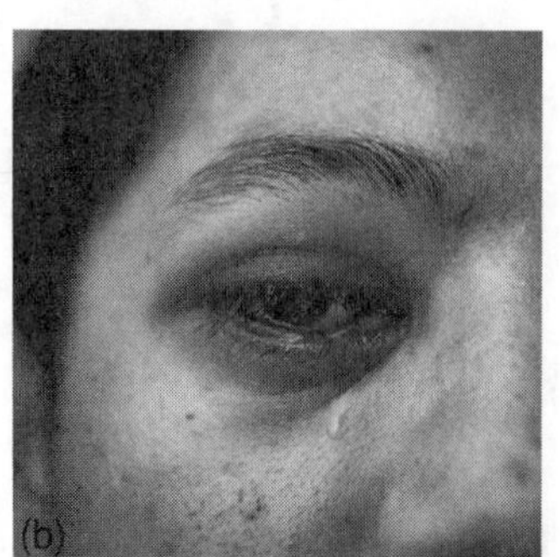

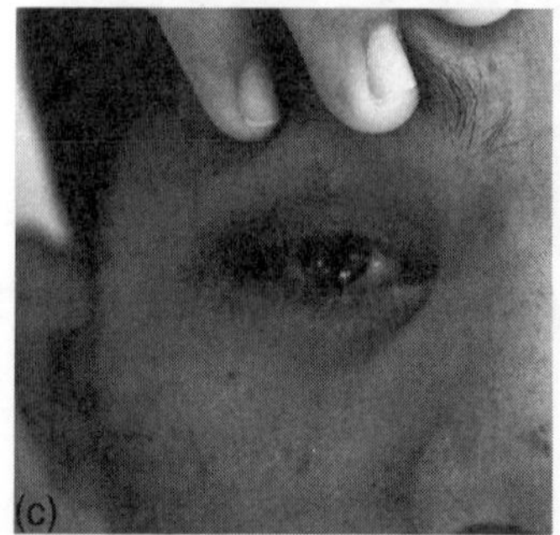

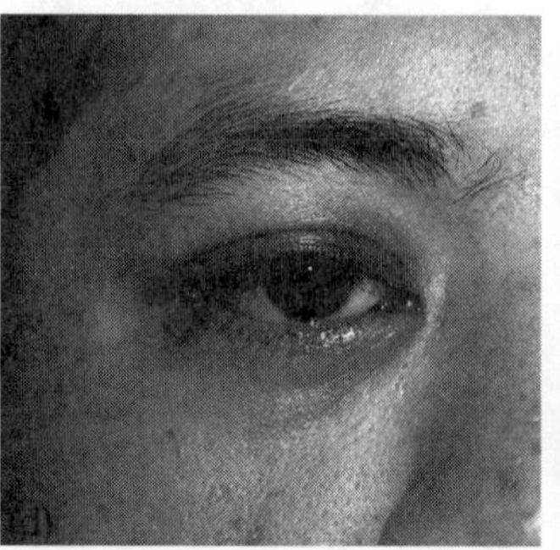

Auditory gnathostomiasis

The worms have been found in the external auditory canal in a patient with sensorineural hearing loss with tinnitus, and in another while penetrating the tympanic membrane.

These visceral manifestations are pertaining to the *G. spinigerum* infection and have not yet been reported in infections with other species of Gnathostoma.

Diagnosis

GENERAL

The diagnosis is suggested by clinical characteristics, and the geographical and dietary history. It is supported by finding eosinophilia and excluding other causes, and is definitive if the worm is obtained and identified.

IMMUNODIAGNOSIS

Immunodiagnosis is of limited use and availability. Immediate skin hypersensitivity using crude extracts of adults and larvae appears to be non-specific. An immunoenzyme test for IgG antibody against antigen from an aqueous extract of the third-stage larvae has been developed. A titre of 1:400 or above is indicative of this infection. As its specificity is 84 per cent, the test may be used as a screening test before using a more specific Western blot analysis for antibody reacting with 24 000-kDa glycoprotein.

Fig. 9 Computerized tomographic brain scan showing intracerebral haemorrhage in a 25-year-old woman who presented with transverse myelitis that progressed to quadriplegia and then respiratory arrest (by courtesy of Dr Prakit Rodprasert).

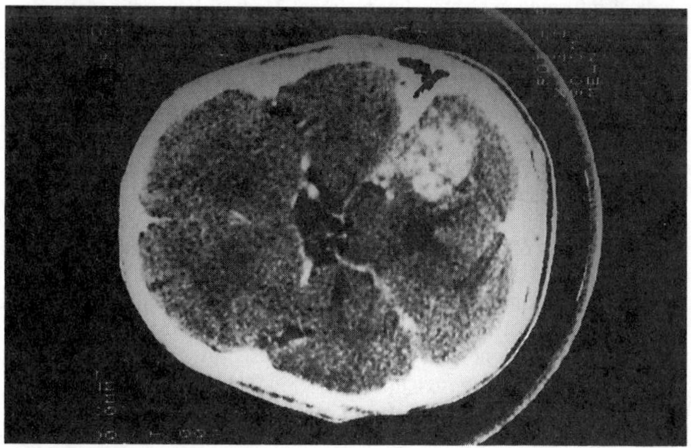

Fig. 10 Magnetic resonance image showing intraventricular haemorrhage in a patient presenting with sudden loss of consciousness and bloodstained eosinophil pleocytosis (by courtesy of Professor Thirawat Hemachudha).

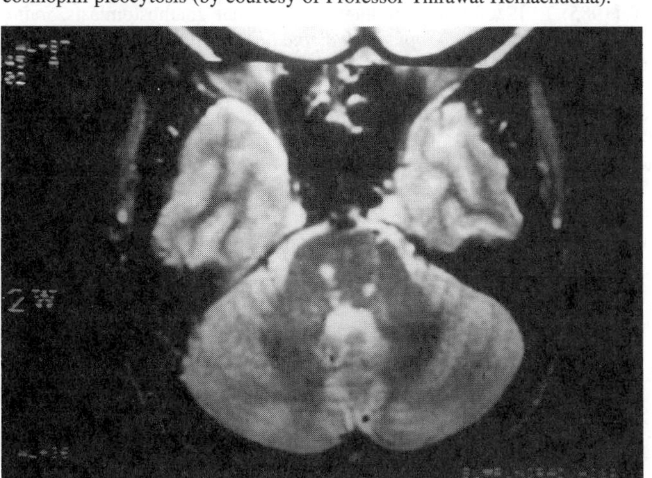

LABORATORY FEATURES

Blood eosinophilia occurs irregularly in about 60 per cent of cases of gnathostomiasis and, therefore, is not necessary in making presumptive diagnosis. The degree of eosinophilia also does not correlete with the clinical severity. With spinocerebral involvement the cerebrospinal fluid can be bloody, xanthochromic, or slightly turbid with a minor increase in protein content. The proportion of eosinophils is higher than expected from haemorrhage *per se*. Neutrophil pleocytosis is sometimes noted, but eosinophil pleocytosis is almost always found in the spinocerebral form of the infection.

Differential diagnosis

The familiar migratory cutaneous swelling should be differentiated from contact dermatitis and urticaria. Calabar swellings (caused by *Loa loa*) occur only in the Central African forest belt and are associated with microfilariae in the blood. With the first episode of swelling, the relatively mild symptoms and absence of signs of acute inflammation, the presence of eosinophilia, and the absence of regional lymphadenitis and fever suggest gnathostomiasis in patients in or from the endemic area. Stationary swelling must be differentiated from other infections such as fascioliasis, paragonimiasis, sparganosis, and dirofilariasis, and from non-infectious causes.

Paragonimus heterotremus infection was found in one patient with cutaneous migratory swelling after pneumonitis and empyema, but this infection is confined to a small area about 100 km north-east of Bangkok. Diseases most likely to be confused with gnathostomal creeping eruption are those caused by dog or cat hookworms, in which the track is smaller and the affected area has been exposed to contaminated materials (Chapter 7.14.4).

Gnathostomal aetiology is highly likely if rapidly advancing myelitis follows radiculitic pain, or if features of cerebral or subarachnoid haemorrhage occur in a person who is otherwise healthy but for a history of cutaneous migratory swelling and blood eosinophilia. Eosinophil pleocytosis is essential for the diagnosis, as is exclusion of non-helminthic encephalomyelitis and Guillain–Barré syndrome. Eosinophilic meningoencephalitis caused by *Angiostrongylus cantonensis* can produce severe headache, meningeal irritation, cranial-nerve palsies, and impaired consciousness, but the development is less dramatic. Development of meningoencephalitis after eating poorly cooked, freshwater

Fig. 11 Gnathostome larva in the anterior chamber (by courtesy of Dr Nisit Leelawong).

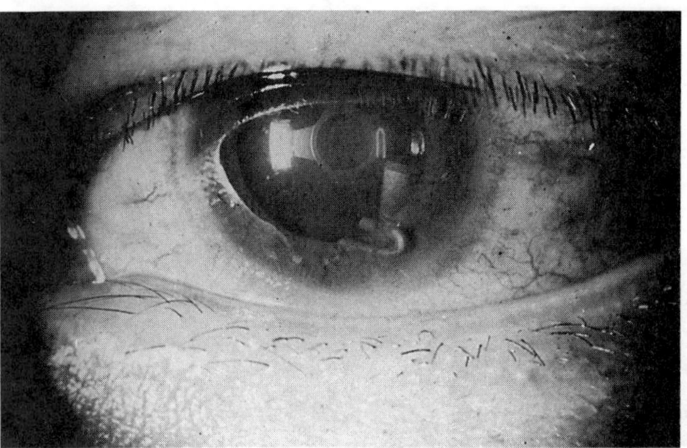

snails favours the diagnosis of *A. cantonensis* infection. Rarely, Angiostrongylus larvae can be identified in the cerebrospinal fluid. In the case of intraocular infection, the larvae of *A. cantonensis* can be distinguished by being thinner, longer, and folding. They appear in the eyeball 2 to 3 weeks after the manifestation of eosinophilic meningoencephalitis. The much smaller microfilariae of *Onchocerca volvulus*, found only in Africa, Latin America, and North Yemen, can be seen in the anterior chamber by slit-lamp examination.

The diagnosis of visceral gnathostomiasis depends mainly on the identification of the worm in surgical specimens and secretions such as sputum, urine or vaginal discharge. The presence of eosinophils in tissue sections and the migratory phenomenon strongly suggest this diagnosis.

Treatment

Surgical removal of the parasite is curative, but rarely possible. Various antiparasitic agents such as quinine, thiabendazole, and diethylcarbamazine have been tried without convincing effect. Metronidazole in a dose of 400 mg thrice daily for 21 days significantly reduces the recurrence rate, the duration of swelling, and the eosinophil count in the blood, but is not curative.

Recently, albendazole has been shown to have a unique effect on the worm movement: the gnathostome tends to migrate outward to the skin as a result of the treatment (in adult) with this drug at a dosage of 400 mg twice daily for 2 weeks (Fig. 12). The worms have been frequently recovered between day 2 and 14 by picking with a needle, excisional biopsy (see Fig. 4), or even by pinching with the patient's nails. However, the success rate was 6.2 to 7.3 per cent only. The recurrence rate of swelling was marked diminished in another study giving the drug for 3 weeks.

Efficacy of ultrasonic application for an apparently superficial infection needs appropriate evaluation. Supportive, symptomatic, and anti-inflammatory treatments are preferable to surgical attempts.

Prognosis

Cerebral gnathostomiasis can be fatal and blindness is usual in intraocular gnathostomiasis. The probability of central nervous or intraocular involvement is less than 1 per cent in patients with cutaneous migratory swelling. Intestinal obstruction may prove fatal if it is complete and prolonged, but more frequently the patient will lose a segment of gut because of a perhaps unnecessary operation.

Prevention

The infective larvae in the flesh of the second intermediate host can be killed by adequate heat or by chemicals. In the endemic area all dishes that contain raw or poorly cooked flesh of animals, particularly those of freshwater fish or chicken, must be avoided. Food preparers who have had prolonged exposure to potentially infected flesh should use gloves.

Fig. 12 Gnathostome larva obtaining from a patient treated with albendazole

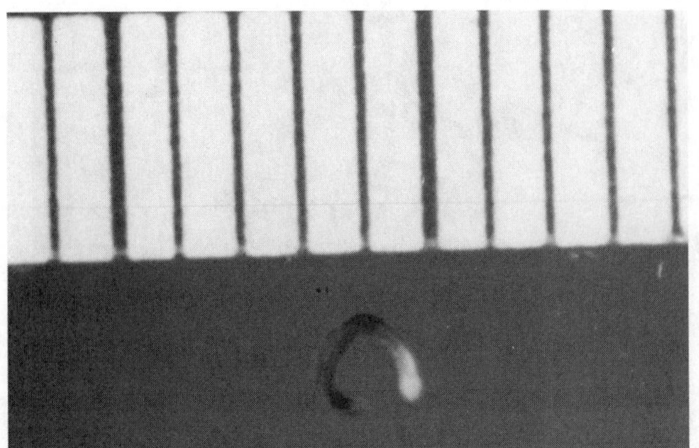

Other spirurida pathogenic in man

The order Spirurida includes the human pathogens Dracunculus (Guinea worm; Chapter 7.14.3), *Physaloptera caucasia* (a rare parasite of the upper gastrointestinal tract), *Thelazia callipaeda* (the cause of Oriental eye worm), *Gongylonema pulchrum* (the scutate threadworm, a parasite of the oesophagus and mouth), Rictularia, Cheilospirura and Spirocerca (very rare parasites of the eye or gut), and the filariae (see Chapter 7.14.2).

REFERENCES

Beaver, P.C., Jung, R.C., and Cupp, E.W. (1984). *Clinical parasitology*, pp. 335–349. Lea and Febiger, Philadelphia.

Bhaibulya, M. and Charoenlarp, P. (1983). Creeping eruption caused by *Gnathostoma spinigerum. Southeast Asian Journal of Tropical Medicine and Public Health*, **14,** 226–8.

Boongird, P., Phuapradit, P., Siridej, N., Chirachariyavej, T., Chuahirum, S., and Vejjaviva, A. (1977). Neurological manifestation of gnathostomiasis. *Journal of Neurological Science*, **31,** 279–91.

Daengsvang, S. (1968). Further observations on the experimental transmission of *Gnathostoma spinigerum. Annals of Tropical Medicine and Parasitology*, **62,** 88–94.

Daengsvang, S. (1980). *Monograph on the genus* Gnathostoma *and gnathostomiasis in Thailand*, SEAMIC Publication No. 21. Southeast Asian Medical Information Centre, International Medical Foundation of Japan, Tokyo.

Kraivicheina, P., Kulkumthorn, M., Yingyourd, P., Akarabovorn, P., and Paireepai, C. (1992). Albendazole for the treatment of human gnathostomiasis. *Transactions of the Royal Society of Tropical Medicine and Hygiene*, **86,** 418–21.

Miyazaki, I. (1960). On the genus Gnathostoma and gnathostomiasis, with special reference to Japan. *Experimental Parasitology*, **9,** 338–70.

Miyazaki, I. (1991). *An illustrated book of helminthic zoonoses*, SEAMIC Publication No. 62, pp. 368–409. Southeast Asian Medical Information Centre, International Medical Foundation of Japan, Tokyo.

Punyagupta, S., Bunnag, T., and Juttijudata, P. (1990). Eosinophilic meningitis in Thailand; clinical and epidemiological characteristics of 162 patients with myeloencephalitis probably caused by *Gnathostoma spinigerum. Journal of Neurological Science*, **96,** 241–56.

Rusnak, J.M. and Lucey, D.R. (1993). Clinical gnathostomiasis: case report and review of the English-language literature. *Clinics in Infectious Diseases*, **16,** 33–50.

Sirikulchayanonta, V. and Chongchitnant, N. (1979). Gnathostomiasis, a possible aetiologic agent of eosinophilic granuloma of the gastrointestinal tract. *American Journal of Tropical Medicine and Hygiene*, **28,** 42–4.

Suntharasamai, P., Desakorn, V., Migasena, S., Bunnag, D., and Harinasuta, T. (1985). ELISA for immunodiagnosis of human gnathostomiasis. *Southeast Asian Journal of Tropical Medicine and Public Health*, **16,** 274–9.

Suntharasamai, P., Riganti, M., Chittamas, S., and Desakorn, V. (1992). Albendazole stimulates outward migration of *Gnathostoma spinigerum* to the dermis in man. *Southeast Asian Journal of Tropical Medicine and Public Health*, **23,** 716–22.

Swanson, V.L. (1971). Gnathostomiasis. In *Pathology of protozoal and helminthic diseases with clinical correlation*, (ed. R.A. Marcial-Rojas), pp. 871–9. Williams and Wilkins, Baltimore.

Tapchaisri, P., Nopparatana, C., Chaicumpa, W., and Setasuban. P. (1991). Specific antigen of *Gnathostoma spinigerum* for immunodiagnosis of human gnathostomiasis. *International Journal of Parasitology*, **21,** 315–19.

7.15 Cestodes (tapeworms)

7.15.1 Hydatid disease

A. J. Radford

Echinococcosis, hydatidosis, and hydatid disease are synonyms for infection with the dog tapeworm, *Echinococcus granulosus*. *E.granulosus* infection is a cyclozoonosis, that is, a parasitic disease that man shares with other vertebrates but which requires at least one other vertebrate (but no invertebrate) host for completion of its lifecycle. Less common species infecting man include *E.multilocularis* and *E.vogeli*.

'Hydatidosis is not a tropical disease and it is unwise to dismiss (it) as a curiosity' (*Lancet*). Nor has it been recognized only recently. Hippocrates noted that 'when the liver is filled with water and bursts . . . the belly is filled with water and the patient dies'. In 1773, John Hunter made an accurate description of hydatid disease, noting that large and small hydatids were 'uniformly round and filled with clear water . . . in a transparent bag . . . of two coats . . . the inner surface covered with small hydatids . . . not so large as the heads of pins'. Hence the name, another medical bastardization of Latin and Greek, derives from *echinos* (Greek: hedgehog), *kokkos* (Greek: berry), *granulum* (Latin: small grain), and *hydatis* (Greek: drop of water).

Epidemiology

Although decreasing in prevalence in many countries, the worm is 'alive and well and living in many parts of the world'. It is widespread throughout the whole Euro-Asian land mass in northern and eastern Africa as well as southern and western South America, much of Canada, and in Australasia (Fig. 1). Overall there is an increasing pandemic. *E.multilocularis* is found in North America, the former USSR, Japan, parts of Central Europe, and Turkey. It causes alveolar hydatid disease.

Human beings today are intruders ('accidental hosts') in the lifecycle of *E.granulosus* and represent a 'dead end' for the parasite, whose most usual cycle is between sheep and dogs. Formerly, man would have taken his place in the lifecycle as a victim of predation and scavenging. Other animals, including camels, swine, buffaloes, kangaroos, deer, pigs, goats, and rodents, may also be intermediate hosts. Hydatids occur both in domestic and sylvatic (wild) forms but the disease is principally an enzootic of dogs. Other definitive hosts include foxes, wolves, and jackals. Recently, different strains of *E.granulosus* have been identified and these probably have different levels of pathogenicity in man. The lifecycle is shown in Fig. 2. Some equine strains of *E.granulosus* are probably unable to establish themselves in man.

Prevalence rates in excess of 50 per cent have been reported in horses in England, 50 to 90 per cent in cattle in Italy (and similar rates in Queensland, Australia), over 20 per cent of some Eskimo dog packs, and up to 100 per cent of dingoes in parts of Australia. A major factor in the appearance of hydatidosis in countries previously free from it is the importation of infected livestock in which diagnosis is difficult clinically and in which serological cross-reactions occur with closely related tapeworms such as *Taenia ovis* and *T. saginata*.

In Australia, rural rates are almost always higher and in certain areas specific cultural patterns result in higher prevalence, as in the Maoris of New Zealand (up to six times that of Europeans), and in the seasonally

Fig. 1 Distribution of hydatid disease. (Reproduced from Matossian *et al.* (1977). *Bulletin of the World Health Organization* **55,** 449, by permission.)

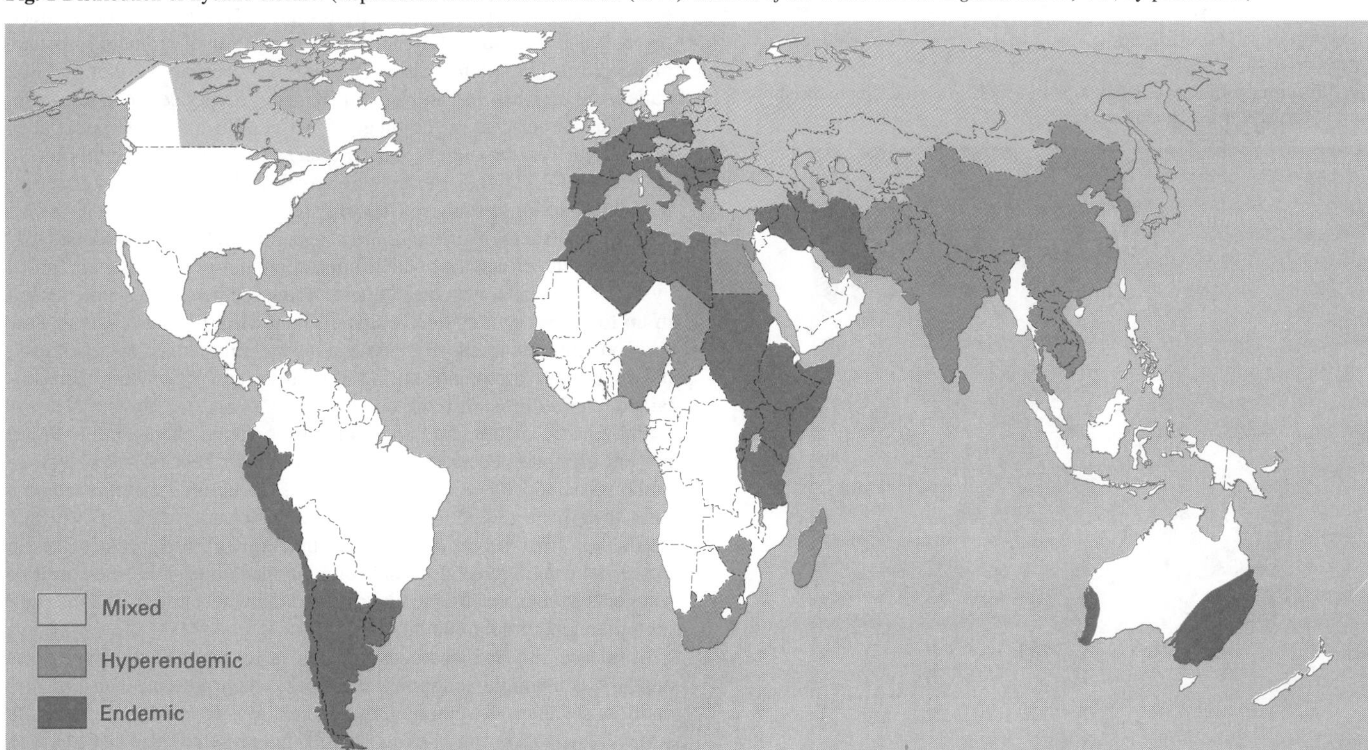

mobile sheep ranchers in the western United States. Wales has an annual incidence of 1.5 per million of the population, almost 10 times that of England. Rural Tasmania, before its campaign in 1960, had an annual hospital incidence of 274 per million per year. A prevalence of 1.6 per cent has been reported from northern Israel and 3.5 per cent in central Tunisia. Higher number of dogs per person, an easy familiarity with dogs, and ignorance of, or indifference to, the significance and prevalence of the disease are important factors in maintaining infection rates in humans. In microendemic areas, rates in excess of 10 per cent have been found using socio-epidemiological methods.

Lifecycle

The adult cestode worm is 3 to 9 mm long with three or four segments (proglottids). There may be several thousand adults in the jejunum of an infected animal. The terminal segment is the longest and broadest, giving the adult worm a tapered bottle shape (Fig. 3). This segment is gravid and shed every 2 weeks; on rupture it releases 500 to 800 eggs into the intestine. These are passed in faeces on to the ground, where herbivores incidentally ingest them while grazing. They are viable in dry conditions for up to a year but are sensitive to heat. Human beings most commonly ingest them after handling dogs with contaminated hair, or by consuming contaminated vegetables or water. Carnivores acquire the parasite by consuming the infected viscera of intermediate hosts. For *E.granulosus*, this most commonly occurs when dogs devour sheep livers and lungs, and for *E.multilocularis* when foxes or cats consume infected rodents.

Fig. 2 Lifecycle of *E. granulosus*.

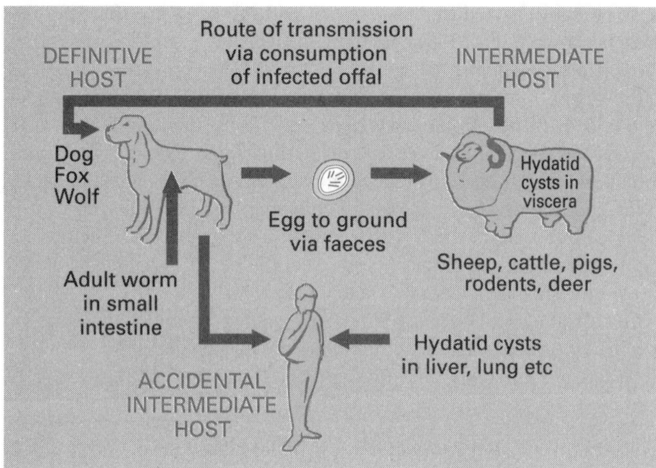

Fig. 3 Electron microscope photograph of a hydatid worm. (Reproduced by courtesy of Dr R.C.A. Thompson, Perth.)

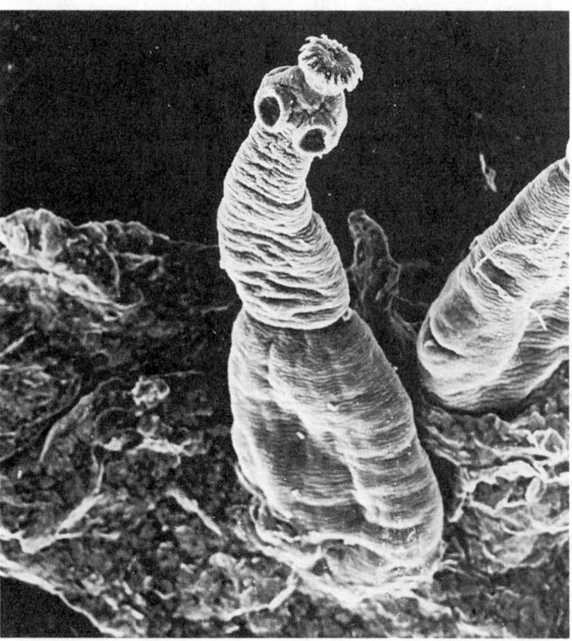

In the intermediate host, eggs hatch in the alkaline duodenum and the emergent hexacanth embryo (with its three pairs of cephalic hooks) passes through the intestinal wall into the portal and lymphatic systems and thence most commonly to the liver or lungs, but may pass on from the lungs to any other organ of the body. When it settles, the embryo develops into a simple cyst with an outer, elastic, laminated layer and a more fragile, inner, germinal layer of epithelial cells from which bud brood capsules. Both capsules and protoscoleces may break off forming 'hydatid sand' on the floor of the cyst. Growth is slow, taking 3 months to reach 4 to 5 mm in size, and 5 to 6 months to become 20 mm in size and infective. In the case of *E.granulosus* the cyst is single and filled with clear fluid, but for *E.multilocularis* the cyst is an 'alveolar' or honey-combed structure. In *E.granulosus* the simple cyst sometimes forms daughter cysts.

Clinical features

There are no specific local or general symptoms and signs of hydatid disease. The diagnosis is usually made in young adults and in most series there is a predominance of males, which can be attributed to their closer relationship to infected dogs. Most infestations are diagnosed as incidental findings at radiographic examination for non-related complaints. The most common symptoms and signs are secondary to the progressive expansion of cysts and are either those of a space-occupying lesion, or obstructive features secondary to direct pressure, or those due to embolization.

The distribution and manifestations of hydatidosis are both ubiquitous and protean, but liver and lung involvement is most common, and in only about 10 per cent of patients is neither organ involved. Almost every organ has been involved, from brain, heart, spleen, biliary tract, thyroid, and parotid to tongue, tooth, bone, broad ligament, prostate, bladder, tonsil, pulmonary artery, and inferior vena cava. Amongst 1802 patients in an Australasian Hydatid Register, 63 per cent had lesions in the liver, 25 per cent in the lung, 25 per cent in muscle, 3 per cent in bone, 2 per cent in kidney, and 1 per cent each in spleen and brain. In 20 per cent of patients, multiple organs were involved. In other series, pulmonary lesions are more frequent.

With the exception of *E.multilocularis*, human beings are remarkably tolerant of the effects of hydatid infestation and wall off the laminated cyst of the parasite, which calcifies in about 3.5 per cent of patients and in up to 25 per cent of liver lesions. The growth of most cysts is slow and sometimes is arrested. Many lesions are only picked up at autopsy, having been asymptomatic during life. The largest lesion described contained over 50 litres of fluid.

Pulmonary lesions are most commonly found incidentally. When present, symptoms consist of a cough in 60 per cent of cases, with or without haemoptysis. Coughing up pieces of ruptured membrane and a salty taste from cyst fluid occurs in 20 per cent of patients. Multiple lesions occur in 40 per cent and are bilateral in 20 per cent of cases. Lower-lobe involvement is more common than upper-lobe, the posterior segments being more frequently involved than the anterior, and the right lobe more commonly than the left.

Similarly, in liver disease most lesions are silent and are found accidentally as a simple abdominal mass but, when present, pain and discomfort are the most common symptoms. Where lesions are near the surface, fluctuation and a 'hydatid thrill' may be elicited. The right lobe is involved in 75 per cent of cases and about one-third of cysts are solitary. In endemic regions up to 2 to 3 per cent of all intracerebral lesions are hydatid cysts. Presentation of such lesions relates to a rise in intracranial pressure, with signs and symptoms progressing over 2 to 6 months according to the site of localization.

Complications are the most common form of presentation of hydatid disease. At the time of diagnosis, 36 to 40 per cent of hepatic cysts and 27 to 67 per cent of pulmonary ones have ruptured or become secondarily infected.

E.multilocularis infections are more invasive, akin to a locally invasive malignancy. Anaphylaxis, which may be fatal, can follow rupture but bronchopulmonary or hepatobiliary obstruction, and fistulae, are more common complications. Long-bone lesions may result in spontaneous fracture. Bladder involvement with hydatiduria may also occur. Fifty years ago over 30 per cent of these complications were fatal.

Diagnosis

'Where were you born and where have you been living over the past several decades?' are important components of the clinical history. The absence of an appropriate geographical history and no contact with dogs makes the diagnosis unlikely.

Over 90 per cent of pulmonary diagnoses can be made by radiography, which indicates well-defined, solitary or multiple lesions. Lesions are usually round and uniform unless surrounding pneumonitis or atelectasis occurs, but occasionally they calcify if the parasite dies. Multicystic lesions of *E.multilocularis* infections show notching and budding of cyst walls, which vary from 1 to 20 cm in diameter. Various, almost pathognomonic, radiological appearances may occur. These give rise to 'crescent', 'double arch', or 'water-lily' signs as a result of bronchopulmonary fistulous formation and collapse of the cyst wall. A fluid level may be present after rupture (Fig. 4). Thin- or thick-walled cavitation may occur, requiring a differential diagnosis from pulmonary abscess. A pleural reaction occurs in about one-third of cases. Sputum microscopy may reveal invaginated or evaginated protoscolices, even when immunodiagnostic tests are negative. A plain radiograph of the abdomen reveals about a third of cases of hepatic disease, and may reveal 'white line' images for almost the full circumference of the walled cyst. Intralesional gas bubbles may be present if hepatobronchial fistulae have formed. The right hemidiaphragm is deformed and elevated in almost half of liver lesions. Skull radiographs may show signs of increased intracranial pressure with asymmetrical growth or thinning of the underlying bone.

Next to plain radiographs, computerized tomography and/or magnetic resonance imaging, where available, is the best aid to visualization of the lesion, especially in the skull. Ultrasonography, and to a lesser extent radionuclide scintigraphy with technetium-99 are of value, especially in abdominal imaging (the former being cheaper and non-invasive). The appearances are usually pathognomonic (Figs. 5 and 6). By accurate localization and identification of the number, size, and the most external sites, these techniques minimize the chance of accidental tapping or tearing of cysts at surgery. In the case of liver lesions they usually differentiate hydatid cysts from malignant metastases, hepatomata, angiomata, and abscesses (Figs. 7 and 8). The appearances of intracranial lesions are cystic, spherical with a sharp border, a central absorptive value similar to cerebrospinal fluid, and usually with significant ventricular distortion and a shift of midline structures. There is a lack of enhancement and of the perifocal oedema seen in cerebral abscesses, or of solid portions and perifocal oedema seen in cystic tumours (Figs. 5 and 6).

Fig. 4 Large hydatid cyst of the right lung showing evidence of bronchopleural fistula. (Reproduced by courtesy of Professor M.R. Sage, Adelaide.)

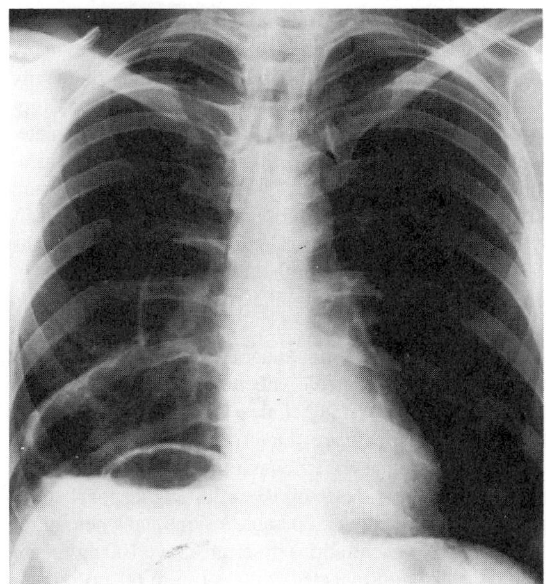

Fig. 5 Ultrasound showing large cyst of the liver with daughter cysts. (Reproduced by courtesy of *Medical Journal of Australia*, Professor G.A. Kune, Melbourne.)

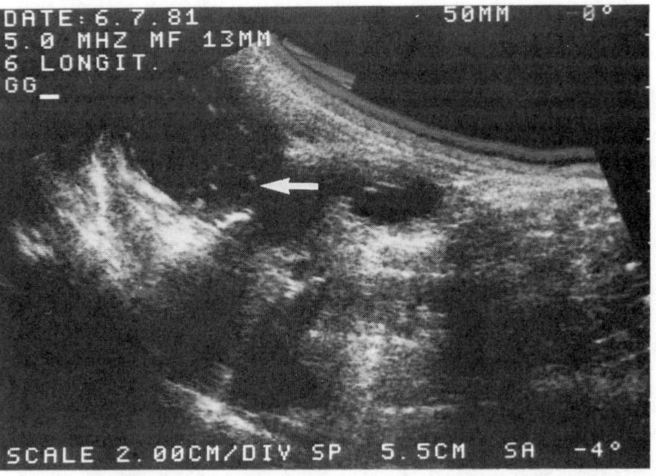

Fig. 6 Radionuclide delineation of large univesicular cyst. (Reproduced by courtesy of *Medical Journal of Australia*, Professor G.A. Kune, Melbourne.)

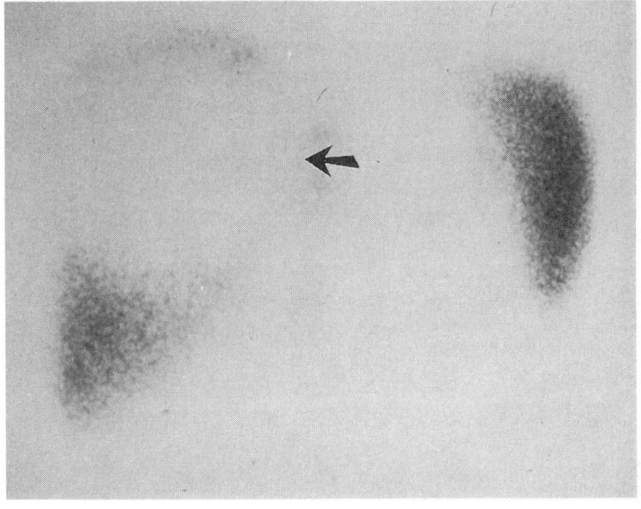

IMMUNODIAGNOSIS

Since the first complement fixation test for hydatid disease in 1906 an immense array of immunodiagnostic techniques has been developed to assist in individual diagnosis and in seroepidemiological surveys. With every method the single intact pulmonary cyst gives the fewest positive results, apparently because the concentration of antibodies is close to zero until the cyst leaks or ruptures. Eosinophilia occurs in only 20 per cent of patients.

The intradermal Casoni test developed in 1911 is the best known. It has a wide range of positivity, reported variously from less than 40 to over 90 per cent. Up to 15 per cent false positives are reported, especially in the presence of taeniasis, leishmaniasis, carcinomatosis, cirrhosis, and collagen disease. Diluted antigen decreases sensitivity but increases specificity, while the use of low nitrogen concentration increases sensitivity. The 'intermediate' reaction is read as positive if induration is over 25 mm in diameter at 20 to 30 min, and is more reliable than the 'delayed' reaction.

At present the immunoelectrophoresis test is the most specific and the most sophisticated in general use. Its sensitivity is lower than that of some other tests but is improved by concentration of serum. False-negative reports of up to 20 per cent occur, mainly in patients with intact cysts and for the reasons stated above. Although precipitin bands at points 3 and 4 occur, it is the Arc 5 band which is used as the marker.

Fig. 7 CT scan of the liver showing multiple cysts just under the capsule and around the porta hepatis. (Reproduced by courtesy of Professor M.R. Sage, Adelaide.)

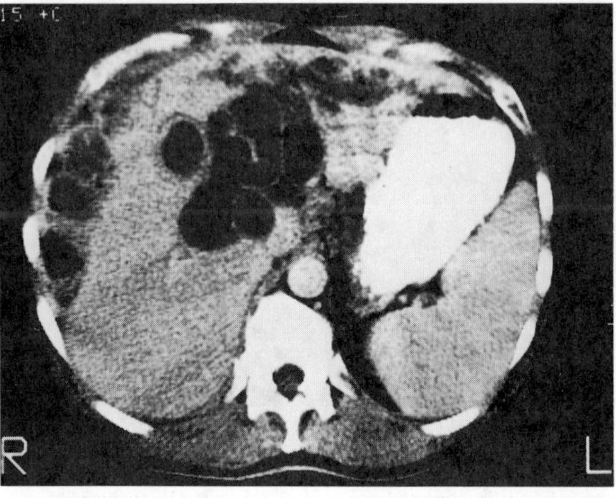

Fig. 8 CT scan of the abdomen showing several daughter cysts within the peritoneal cavity. (Reproduced by courtesy of Professor M.R. Sage, Adelaide.)

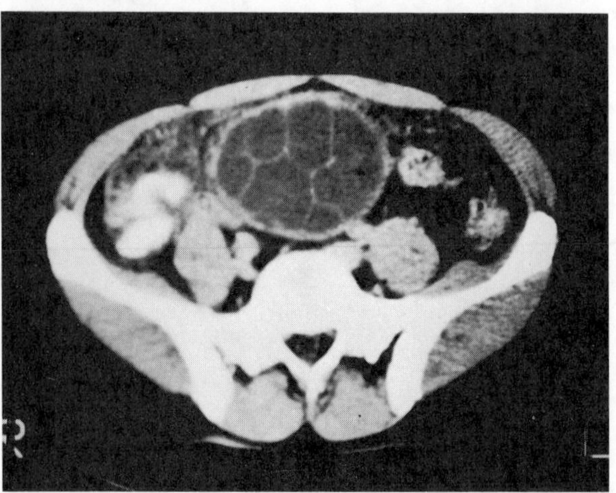

Whole sheep hydatid cyst fluid is the best source of antigen. Reactions also occur with *E.vogeli* and *E.multilocularis*. Positives occur only if active disease is present or within 12 months after surgery; a few remain positive even longer. The complement fixation test is positive in up to 80 per cent of patients and also usually returns to normal within a year of surgery whereas the indirect haemaglutination test may continue to remain positive even after 2 years. The latex agglutination test is a good screening test with high specificity and few false positives. Improved techniques produce up to 90 per cent sensitivity for all tests.

Radioimmunoassay, the radio-allergosorbent test, and enzyme immunoassay give up to 95 per cent positive results in confirmed cases. Latex agglutination or indirect haemaglutination as a screen, and immunoelectrophoresis (or complement fixation or indirect fluorescent antibody) as a confirmation test appear the best tools for specific diagnosis.

Management

Surgery, often using laser techniques, is the main line of treatment and may be technically very demanding. It carries a mortality rate of 1 to 3 per cent and a recurrence rate of 10 or more per cent when rupture occurs or has occurred. Rupture on cyst enucleation is reported in up to half of the cases, after which anaphylactic shock may occur immediately, as may infection in the days or weeks that follow. Several techniques are used to sterilize the contents of the cysts before enucleation is attempted by a small aspiration followed by the injection of a scolicide. Alcohol and 20 per cent hypertonic saline have both been used but less absorbable and less toxic are 1 per cent aqueous or polyvinylpyrrolidone iodine, aqueous cetrimide (1/1000), or 0.5 per cent silver nitrate solution. Low viscosity of the iodine solution gives rapid diffusion and complete sterilization within a few minutes. A technique to minimize rupture and allow controlled evacuation of all parasitic material has been developed by strengthening the friable outer layer through freezing it with CO_2 gas in a steel cone over the incision site. In pulmonary disease, simple enucleation, cystectomy, wedge or segmental resection, lobectomy or pneumonectomy may be required. Cystectomy, with or without resection, may be done for liver disease and the common bile duct should always be explored in these cases. Omentoplasty has been reported to reduce morbidity to 2.5 per cent.

The following technique was found to be effective in a large series of Tibetan patients with predominantly hepatic hydatid cysts. Most operations were done under local anaesthetic. The liver surface was sutured to the parietal peritoneum to prevent spillage into the peritoneal cavity, then the cyst was punctured and sucked out. The opening was enlarged and the cyst and any daughter cysts painted with formalin solution, after which the rubbery cyst wall was extracted with sponge forceps and the remaining liver cavity painted with formalin solution. The wound was then firmly closed with sutures. Marsupialization or drainage inevitably resulted in sepsis. Occasionally it was necessary to aspirate the cavity percutaneously once or twice. Some of the larger cysts had already ruptured into the biliary tract and were filled with bile-stained, mushy material. After this material had been removed it was found best to anastomose the cavity to the gut by a 'roux-en-Y' opening into the jejunum (Dr R.M. Clarke, personal communication). Even simple puncture aspiration of cysts followed by a scolicide injection has had good results where extensive surgery has not been suitable.

In intracerebral lesions, limited but significant expansion of the brain occurs postoperatively.

There may be a place for medical treatment at some future date. The benzimidazole derivatives mebendazole, albendazole, fluoromebendazole, and combendazole are undergoing clinical trials. None has consistently demonstrated either its efficiency in man or its safety at prolonged high dosage, although occasional reductions in the size of lesions with mebendazole are reported using doses of 10 to 200 mg/kg for 4 to 13 months. It is probably worth using in inoperable lesions and where intraperitoneal spillage occurs. Concentrations in serum above 100 ng/ml are recommended. Some trials with repeated courses (up to 60!) of albendazole in doses varying from 10 to 20 mg/kg a day for 30 days are showing promising results and some 'cures' have been reported.

Control

Hydatid programmes have been some of the world's most successful public health measures against any communicable disease. It may be significant that the most effective campaigns have been on islands with relatively small populations, especially Iceland, New Zealand, Tasmania, and Cyprus. During the nineteenth century, Iceland had the world's highest prevalence of hydatidosis, with up to a third of all autopsies showing evidence of disease. It is now hydatid free. Tasmania reduced the annual incidence from about 15 cases per 100 000 before 1965 to 1/100 000 in 1983, the annual prevalence in dogs from 12.7 to 0.04 per cent, and that of 'full mouth' sheep from 52 to 0.8 per cent over the same period. The transmission of the disease to man appears to have stopped in 1972 as no new surgical case has been reported in a person under 10 years of age since then.

This campaign had one principal objective—'to prevent dogs from getting offal'—thereby interrupting the lifecycle of the parasite (see Fig. 2). It started with an intensive education campaign based on geographically defined areas with maximum community involvement. In due course the Department of Primary Industry was able to use the power available under the stock diseases legislation in what was correctly seen as a response to public opinion. Used late in the campaign to mop up resistant pockets of 'delinquent human behaviour', these measures were highly effective and popular.

Effective control measures include:

1. The prevention of infection of dogs by their exclusion from slaughtering areas and the installation of deep offal pits or incineration systems.
2. Raising the level of public and, especially, farmers' awareness and participation in the project with literature, media, and school programmes.
3. On-site farm visits with individual contacts and the demonstration of dogs' infection by purgation with arecoline hydrobromide (15–30 mg). Such purgation does not constitute treatment (which may be effected by praziquantel, or epsiprantal, mebendazole, nitroscanate, or bunamidine).
4. Control of stray dogs is also important in some areas.
5. Legislation, which may be preceded or accompanied by incentives but, is probably always necessary to effect control or eradication.
6. Dog immunization is a real possibility for the future.

Control or eradication of sylvatic disease is much more difficult.

Other hydatidiform cysts

Other important taeniid larval infections of man that may cause the development of bladder-like structures in tissues include *Cysticercus cellulosae*, the larvae of *T.solium* (see Chapter 7.15.3), *C.bovis*, the larva of *T. saginata* and *Coenurus cerebralis*, the larval form of *T. (Multiceps) multiceps* in sheep, which appears to be morphologically indistinguishable from the larvae of *M. serialis* of rabbits and rodents, and *T. brauni*, one of the tape-worms of African dogs. An enzyme immunoassay has been developed for *T.solium cysticerci.*

Coenurus, the 'gill' worm, is a common parasite of dogs that causes blind staggers in its intermediate host, sheep. Dogs become infected by eating infected sheep's brain. Most human reports are from Africa, but occasionally it is seen in the United Kingdom, the United States, and France. It is more common in children. There are some variations in clinical presentation. The cerebral forms produce effects due to raised intracranial pressure or focal signs, and may involve the spinal cord. They are usually unilocular but occasionally huge cysts develop that look like a bunch of grapes, most of which are sterile. On rupture, cysts may produce signs of a toxic psychosis. Many African patients present with solitary and asymptomatic subcutaneous lumps, usually on the chest wall, which are possibly caused by a different species. They are slow growing, may be present for months, and require differentiation from sebaceous or epidermal cysts and from lipomata. On section, cysts show a narrow zone of fibrous tissue with infiltration by lymphocytes and eosinophils. Lesions may also occur in the eye, and especially with *M. serialis*, whose cysts bud both externally and internally.

REFERENCES

Abbassioun, K. Rahmat, H., Ameli, N.O., and Tafazouli, M. (1978). Computerized tomography in hydatid cyst of the brain. *Journal of Neurosurgery*, **49**, 408–11.

Beard, T.C. (1969). Hydatid control. A problem in health education. *Medical Journal of Australia*, **2**, 456–9.

Beggs, I. (1983). The radiological appearances of hydatid disease of the liver. *Clinical Radiology*, **34**, 555–63.

Editorial (1976). The invisible worm. *Lancet*, **ii**, 552–3.

McConnell, J.D. and Green, R.J. (1979). The control of hydatid disease in Tasmania. *Australian Veterinary Journal*, **55**, 140–5.

Matossian, R.M. (1977). The immunological diagnosis of human hydatid disease. *Transactions of the Royal Society of Tropical Medicine and Hygiene*, **71**, 101–3.

Matossian, R.M., Rickard, M.D., and Smith, J.D. (1977). Hydatidosis: a global problem of increasing importance. *Bulletin of the World Health Organization*, **55**, 499–507.

Morris, D.L. and Richards, K.S. (1992) *Hydatid disease: current medical and surgical treatment.* Butterworth-Heinemann, Oxford.

Templeton, A.C. (1968). Human *Coenurus* infection. A report of 14 cases from Uganda. *Transactions of the Royal Society of Tropical Medicine and Hygiene*, **62**, 251–5.

Thompson, R.C.A. (ed.) (1986). The biology of Echinococcus and hydatid disease. George Allen and Unwin, London.

Wainwright, J. (1957). *Coenurus cerebralis* and racemose cysts of the brain. *Journal of Pathology and Bacteriology*, **73**, 347–54.

7.15.2 Gut cestodes

R. KNIGHT

The cyclophyllidean tapeworms maintain anchorage to the host small-gut mucosa by means of a holdfast structure called the scolex, which bears a circlet of four adhesive suckers, and usually an evertible rostellum that lies centrally between them (Fig 1a,b). The rostellum may have one or more circlets of hooks. The rest of the body forms the strobila and consists of a chain of flattened proglottids, which bud behind the scolex. The worms change their site of attachment regularly, and are surprisingly motile. Gravid proglottids are lost from the end of the strobila and are replaced by others that have matured as they pass down the strobila. Each proglottid possesses a complete set of hermaphroditic sex organs; the genital openings are marginal. Eggs accumulate in the uterus of gravid proglottids and only enter the faecal stream when the proglottids are disrupted. In many species the eggs enter the environment within intact proglottids. In either case the eggs are embryonated and contain a hexacanth embryo (onchosphere) that bears three pairs of hooks. The eggshells have two membranes; but in Taenia the outer is lost early and the inner forms the thick embryophore. After ingestion by the intermediate host, eggs hatch and the released hexacanth embryo bores its way into the mucosa. The larval stages of the parasite are generally cystic; the embryonic scolex, the protoscolex, is visible within, usually in an invaginated mode. The cycle is completed when the larval stage, within the intermediate host or its tissues, is eaten by the definitive host; the protoscolex evaginates and attaches to the gut mucosa.

In three species, human beings are a regular part of the lifecycle

(Table 1; Figs. 2, 3 and 4); in the rest they are an accidental host (see Table 2 below). The two *Taenia* spp. are unique among all human infections in that they are zoonoses, that is infections derived from vertebrates, but man is an obligatory host. For this reason they are described as anthropozoonoses. Symptoms result from local hypersensitivity reactions to the worm and its scolex, and altered gut motility due to the physical mass of the worm. Patients often become aware of proglottids in their faeces. Some patients report poorly defined systemic symptoms, which may have an immunological basis. A blood eosinophilia up to 10 per cent can occur with any gut cestode.

Taenia saginata

GEOGRAPHIC DISTRIBUTION

The beef tapeworm is prevalent where cattle have access to human faeces and where man eats undercooked beef. The highest prevalence is in Africa, particularly in eastern and north-eastern parts; it is also common in many countries in the Middle East, South America, and South-East Asia. Prevalence is now very low in the United States, Canada, and Australia. It still persists endemically in Western Europe; but eastwards prevalence increases progressively across Europe and into the former USSR.

Fig. 1 (a) *Taenia solium* showing scolex with four suckers and a double row of hooks (× 250). (b) *Taenia saginata* showing scolex with four suckers and no hooks (× 250). (By courtesy of Professor V. Zaman.)

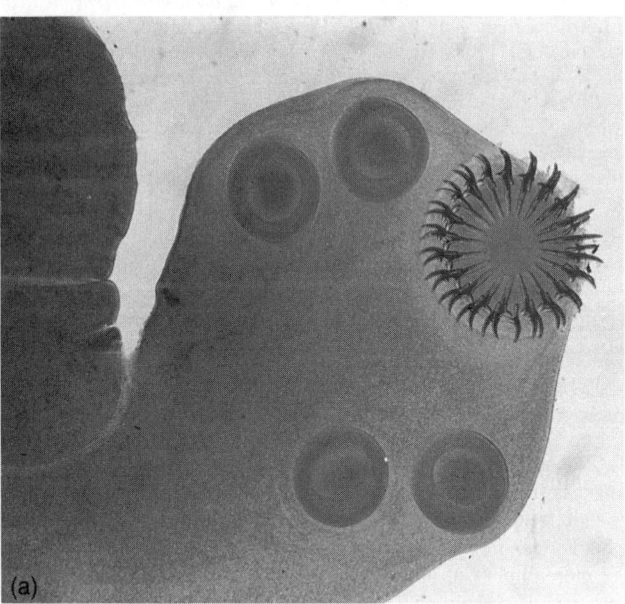

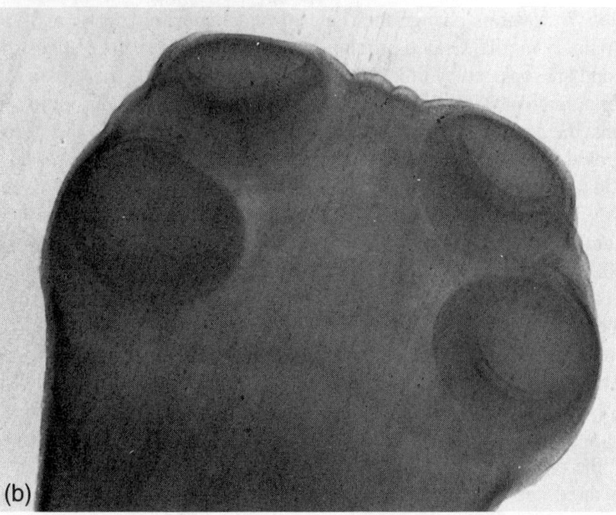

EPIDEMIOLOGY

Gravid proglottids are passed at defaecation, often in short chains; free eggs also occur in faeces. The whitish proglottids, approximately 2 to 3 cm long, are actively motile, elongating and contracting. Eggs persist on pasture for many months and can survive most forms of sewage treatment. Cattle have access to human faeces on farms, at camp sites and recreation areas, and on railway lines. Infected herdsmen can initiate epizootics. Eggs may be dispersed by flies and dung beetles, and seabirds can ingest proglottids in estuarine waters and deposit them in their faeces on inland pastures.

In cattle, cysticerci occur in striated muscle; they are whitish, ovoid, and measure 8 by 5 mm; they contain an invaginated protoscolex with no hooks. They become infective within 12 weeks and remain viable in the living host for 2 years; they are viable in stored, chilled meat for several weeks but are killed at −20°C within 1 week. The prepatent period in man is 3 months and worms may live 30 years. Cattle develop protective immunity to new infection. Prevalence in cattle is best estimated by carcass inspection.

Among Taiwan aboriginals a strain of this species is transmitted by eating raw pig or wild boar liver; the protoscolex of the cysticercus bears hooks.

CLINICAL FEATURES

Most worms are solitary; multiple worms are more common in high-transmission areas and probably arise by simultaneous infection. Most patients are first aware of the worm by seeing proglottids on faeces. Sooner, or later, they will experience active worm migration through the anus, and this may induce an anxiety response. Many have no other symptoms, but others complain of nausea and upper abdominal pains, often relieved by food. A few patients eat to relieve symptoms. In children, impaired appetite can have nutritional consequences. Some patients have symptoms suggestive of hypoglycaemia, namely dizziness and sweating. Pruritus ani is common. The worm may be visible on small-bowel barium studies.

Proglottids are found in a variety of surgical specimens but a pathogenic role is often difficult to establish. Thus they are found in resected appendices, and occasionally obstruct the small intestine, pancreatic duct, or bile duct. After gut perforation they can occur in the peritoneum. Proglottids are recorded in the gallbladder, and eggs have been found in gallstones.

DIAGNOSIS

The typical eggs may be found in faeces, but this is an insensitive method; perianal swabs are also useful. Eggs are indistinguishable from those of *T. solium*; patients should be asked to bring worm specimens. Unless the proglottid is fully gravid the number of uterine branches is an unreliable diagnostic character. Another morphological feature is the presence of a vaginal sphincter; this is absent in *T. solium*. In human surveys in endemic areas a 24-h faecal collection after an anthelminthic will give the most reliable prevalence.

TREATMENT

Niclosamide, 2 g, is given to adults and older children as a single morning dose on an empty stomach; the tablets should be chewed. Children of 2 to 6 years should receive 1 g, and those below 2500 mg. The alternative is praziquantel, 5 to 10 mg/kg as a single dose after a light breakfast. After either drug the proximal part of the worm disintegrates in the gut and the scolex cannot be found. Failure of proglottids to reappear within 3 to 4 months indicates cure.

Table 1 *Major gut cestodes infecting man*

	Taenia saginata (beef tapeworm)	*Taenia solium* (pork tapeworm)	*Hymenolepis nana* (dwarf tapeworm)
Intermediate hosts	Cattle, water buffalo, other bovids, reindeer	Pig, wild boar Accidentally in man	None; but see Table 2 for murine subspecies
Length	4–12 m	3–5 m	25–40 mm
Number of proglottids	2000 (mean)	700–1000	200 (mean)
Gravid proglottid	Longer than wide 20–30 × 5–7 mm	Longer than wide 18–25 × 5–7 mm	Transverse 0.8 × 0.2 mm
Scolex	No rostellum No hooks	Rostellum with double circlet of 22–32 large and small hooks	Rostellum with single circlet of 20–30 minute hooks
Gravid uterus	15–20 lateral branches	7–13 lateral branches	Bilobed
Testes	800–1200	394–534	3
Ovary	2-lobed	3-lobed	2-lobed
Egg (contains hexacanth embryo)	Embryophore shell is radially striated and 31–40 μm in diameter	Embryophore shell is radially striated and 31–40 μm in diameter	Oval, 30–47 μm long; two membranes; 4–8 filaments arise from each pole of inner membrane

CONTROL

This can be very successful. It employs health education concerning raw beef, meat inspection, sanitation and hygiene on cattle farms, and proper sewage treatment and disposal. Mass treatment of herd contacts, or whole adult populations, are the most effective short-term measures when endemicity is high. *T. saginata* causes great economic loss to the beef industry in some developing countries.

Taenia solium

The pork tapeworm is generally much less common than the beef tapeworm. Its clinical importance relates to cysticercosis (see Chapter 7.15.3), the occurrence of larval forms in human tissue. This arises when eggs hatch in the upper gut and man becomes an accidental intermediate host. *T. solium* is now very rare in North America and Western Europe, but it remains common in much of subSaharan Africa, and in China, India, and other parts of Asia. High prevalences occur in Mexico and several South American countries.

EPIDEMIOLOGY

Unlike *T. saginata*, the proglottids do not migrate actively *per anum*. The eggs have the same resistant qualities. In the pig, muscle cysticerci produce 'measly pork'; the cysts are most numerous in the tongue, masseter, heart, and diaphragm, but also occur in the brain. When eaten by man in undercooked pork the worms mature in 5 to 12 weeks.

The distribution of human cysticercosis is much more limited than that of *T. solium*; this implies that internal autoinfection from disrupted proglottids is rare. Conditions favouring the cysticercosis include poor personal hygiene, which facilitates external autoinfection and contaminated fingers among food handlers. Faecal pollution of the peridomestic environment, irrigation water or cultivated vegetables are also important. In parts of Africa, tapeworm proglottids are used in traditional medicine. In the absence of these factors, *T. solium* can be endemic with only very sporadic cases of cysticercosis. Cysticercosis is a major health problem in Mexico, some South American countries, and to a lesser

Fig. 2 Lifecycle of *Taenia solium*. (Adapted by Professor V. Zaman from Center for Disease Control, Atlanta, Georgia, USA.)

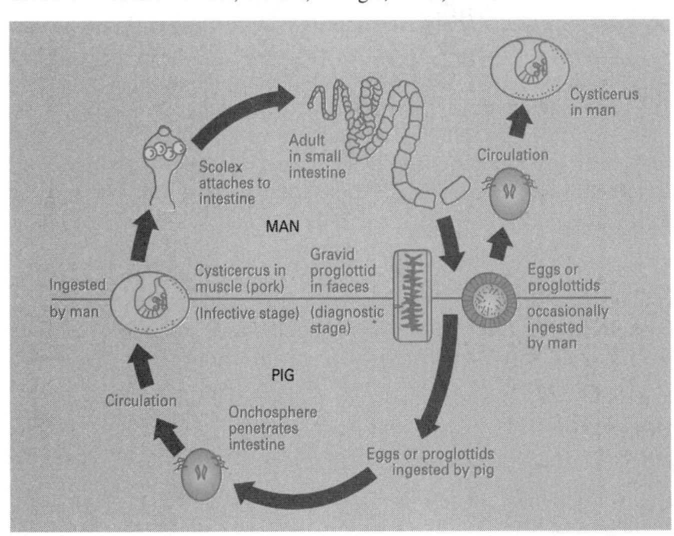

Fig. 3 Lifecycle of *Taenia saginata*. (Adapted by Professor V. Zaman from Center for Disease Control, Atlanta, Georgia, USA.)

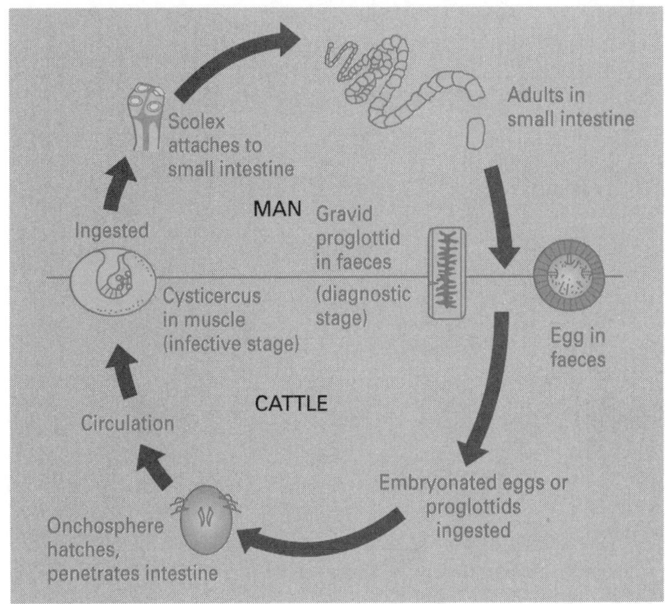

Table 2 *Accidental gut cestodes that infect man*

Species	Geographic distribution	Definitive hosts	Intermediate hosts	Length and width (max)	Shape of gravid proglottid	Other features
Hymenolepis nana fraterna	Worldwide	Mouse, rat	Fleas, beetles	2.5–9 cm 0.5–1 mm	Very transverse	Murine form of *H.nana*; the egg is identical
H. diminuta (rat tapeworm)	Worldwide	Rat	Fleas, beetles, cockroaches	20–60 cm 3–4 mm	Very transverse	Egg like *H. nana* but yellow outer membrane and no filaments; 60–85 μm
Dipylidium caninum	Worldwide	Dog, cat	Fleas and dog louse	10–70 cm 2.5–3 mm	Elongate, wider in middle	Double set of sex organs. Egg capsules with 8–15 eggs
Bertiella studeri	S. and S.E. Asia, Africa, Cuba	Primates	Oribatid mites	27–30 cm 6–10 mm	Much wider than long	Inner eggshell bears bicornuate knob
B. mucronata	S. and C. America	Primates	Oribatid mites	15–45 cm	Transverse	As above
Mathevotaenia symmetrica	Thailand	Rats	Beetles	13 cm 1–2 mm	Elongate	Capsule surrounds individual egg
Inermicapsifer madagascariensis	Malagasy, Africa, C. America, Cuba	Rats	'Arthropod'	26–42 cm 2.6 mm	Slightly elongate, white and opaque	Egg capsules with 6–11 eggs
Raillietina celebensis	East Asia, Australia	Rats	Ant	16–60 cm 3mm	As above	Egg capsules with 1–4 eggs
R. demerariensis	Guyana, Cuba Ecuador	Rats	'Insect'	Up to 60 cm 2–3 mm	As above	Egg capsule with 8–10 eggs
R. siriraji	Thailand	Rats	Cockroach	As above	As above	As above
Mesocestoides variabilis	Rwanda, Japan, Greenland, USA, Korea	Carnivores (fox, skunk, etc.); birds of prey	Mites (1st host) Amphibia, reptiles, birds and mammals (2nd hosts)	40 cm 2 mm	Longer than broad	Median genital pore Larval worms can occur in man, in muscle and subcutaneous tissue

Fig. 4 Lifecycle of *Hymenolepis nana*. (Adapted by Professor V. Zaman from Center for Disease Control, Atlanta, Georgia, USA.)

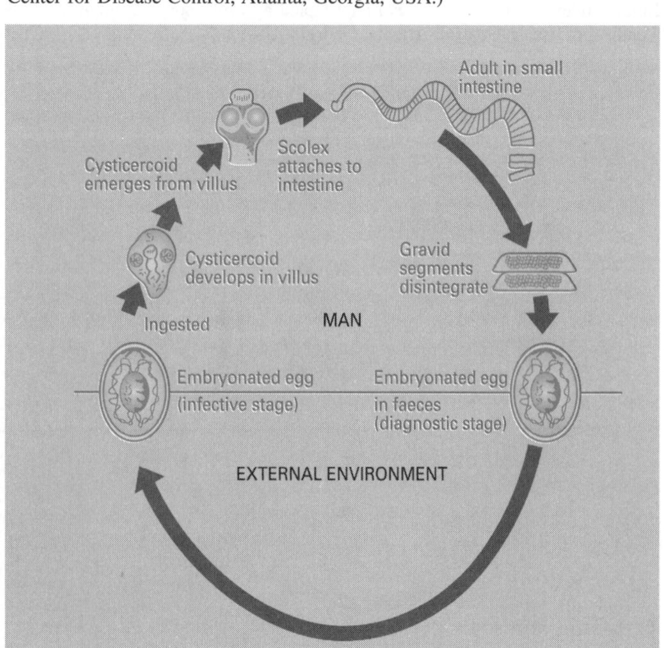

extent in Africa and Asia. In 1969, *T. solium* was introduced from Bali into the highlands of Indonesian New Guinea, where the disease is now one of great importance.

PATHOLOGY OF CYSTICERCOSIS

Cysts occur especially in striated muscle, subcutaneous tissue, the nervous system, and the eye. Many remain clinically silent until the parasite dies after 3 to 5 years, when vigorous inflammatory and hypersensitivity reactions may occur; later lesions may calcify. In the brain, particularly in the subarachnoid and the ventricular system, atypical racemose cysts may occur. They appear as irregular or grape-like clusters of cysts that have no protoscolex; they can be mistaken pathologically for non-parasitic cysts.

CLINICAL FEATURES

Symptoms due to the adult worms are similar to those of *T. saginata* but are often milder and not associated with pruritus ani.

DIAGNOSIS

Adult worm infection is detected as for *T. saginata*. Methods for detecting faecal antigen are available and have great potential use in epidemiological studies.

TREATMENT AND CONTROL

Adult worms are treated as for *T. saginata*. Drugs causing vomiting must be avoided; it should be remembered that the faeces will be potentially highly infective for several days, both for the patient and attendants. For the treatment of cysticercosis, see Chapter 7.15.3. Control measures are similar to those of *T. saginata* but local risk factors for human cysticercosis must receive special attention.

Hymenolepis nana

The dwarf tapeworm is the most common cestode in man; it is also the smallest. When worm loads are high it causes more gut pathology than any other species. It is common in most developing and tropical countries. The lifecycle normally involves only man (Fig. 4). Fully embryonated infective eggs are passed in the faeces; gravid proglottids normally disintegrate completely in the gut. Infection is commonly direct, but also by the other faecal–oral routes. Eggs hatch in the jejunum and the hexacanth embryo bores into a villus where it transforms into a cysticercoid larva. After 4 to 6 days it re-enters the gut, everts the scolex, and attaches to the mucosa; eggs appear in the faeces within 12 days. The life-span is 3 months. The eggs are delicate and survive less than 10 days in the environment. Prevalence is usually much higher in children than adults; outbreaks can occur in families and institutions. External autoinfection is common in high-risk groups and enables high worm loads to build up. In addition, internal autoinfection occurs when there is gut stasis or retroperistalsis. Because of the importance of direct transmission, this infection may be common in arid environments such as Western Australia.

CLINICAL FEATURES

In heavily infected people, especially children, up to 1000 or more worms may be present. Mucosal damage caused by both larval and adult worms leads to protein loss and sometimes malabsorption. Abdominal pains and anorexia are common. An association with phlyctenular conjunctivitis is reported in Egypt.

Immunosuppressant or steroid therapy, particularly in lymphoma patients, can lead to the development of bizarre cystic larval forms in the gut wall, mesenteric nodes, liver, and lungs. A similar condition can be produced in immunosuppressed mice.

DIAGNOSIS AND TREATMENT

Eggs can be detected in faeces using concentration methods. Proglottids are rarely found in faeces, except after treatment.

Praziquantel in a single dose of 25 mg/kg is the most effective drug. If niclosamide is used, a 7-day course is needed to ensure that larval stages are killed when they re-enter the gut lumen. The dose on the first day is as for *T. saginata*; on the remaining days one half of this dose is given. Relapses often result from persistence of eggs in the patient's environment.

Accidental gut cestodes

A number of species are detailed in Table 2. All have arthropods as intermediate hosts, the larval cysticercoid stage being in the haemocele; the lifecycles of some species are unknown. The normal definitive host becomes infected by eating the arthropod intentionally, or accidentally. The means by which man becomes infected is sometimes not clear, but fleas, small beetles, and mites are easily overlooked in food. *Dipylidium caninum* infection occurs in children who have groomed their pet (Fig. 5). Infections with Bertiella are mostly in owners of pet monkeys, but oribatid mites are common in fallen fruit especially mangoes. Children may eat insects deliberately, and this appears to be the mode of infection by *R. siriraji* in Bangkok. Beetles are used for medicinal purposes in parts of Thailand and Malaysia, and this is the most likely route by which Mathevotaenia is acquired.

H. n. fraterna is the murine strain of the human parasite *H. nana*, and *H. diminuta* (Fig. 6) also infects rodents. They are rare in human beings; both human and murine subspecies of *H. nana* will infect Tribolium beetles. In many of these species the eggs are in capsules that are released when the proglottid disintegrates in the gut, or more commonly, in the faecal mass. Mesocestoides is unique among these parasites in three respects: two intermediate hosts are required; the genital opening is medioventral rather than at the margin of the proglottid as in all other

Fig. 5 Lifecycle of *Dipylidium caninum*. (Adapted by Professor V. Zaman from Center for Disease Control, Atlanta, Georgia, USA.)

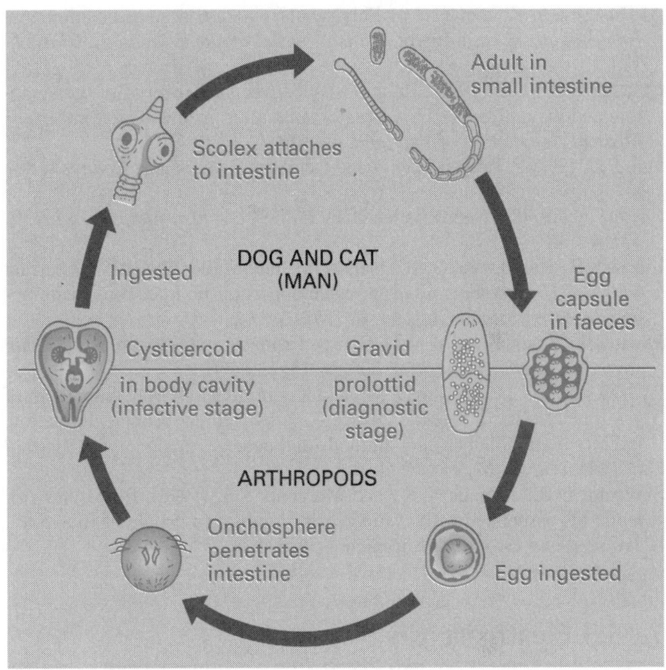

Fig. 6 Lifecycle of *Hymenolepis diminuta*. (Adapted by Professor V. Zaman from Center for Disease Control, Atlanta, Georgia, USA.)

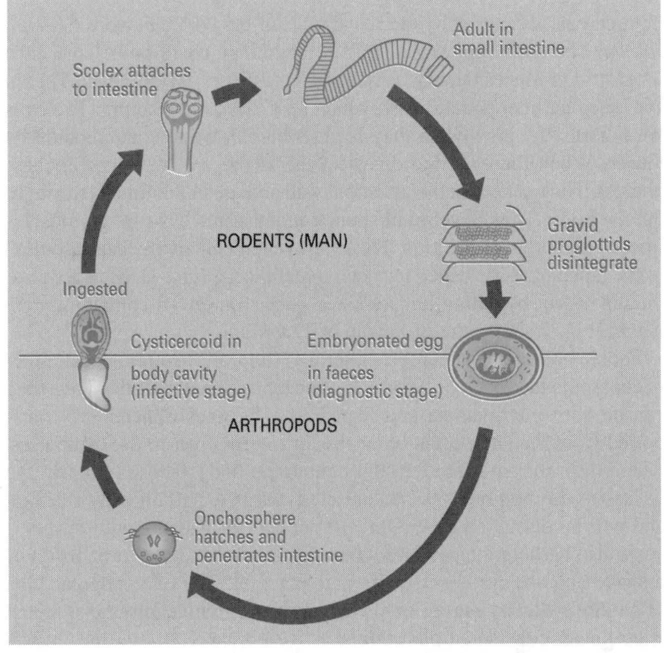

cyclophyllidean tapeworms; larval worms can occur in man when mites are ingested.

Many patients will present because they have passed proglottids; *D. caninum* actively migrates out of the anus, like *T. saginata*. Faecal examinations of persons with abdominal complaints may reveal unusual eggs or egg capsules. Poorly defined systemic and allergic complaints are common. Treatment is as for *T. saginata*.

Recognition of these parasites is of epidemiological interest and may indicate potential transmission of other zoonotic pathogens. It is certain that all these parasites are under-reported. Unusual proglottids or eggs should be preserved in formol saline and sent to a parasitologist.

REFERENCES

Al-Hussaini, M.K. *et al.* (1979). Phlyctenular eye disease in association with *Hymenolepis nana* in Egypt. *British Journal of Ophthalmology*, **63,** 627–31.

Chitchang, S. *et al.* (1985). Relationship between the severity of the symptom and the number of *Hymenolepis nana* after treatment. *Journal of the Medical Association of Thailand*, **68,** 424–6.

Fan, P.C. (1988). Taiwan *Taenia* and taeniasis. *Parasitology Today*, **4,** 86–8.

Flisser, A. (1988). Neurocysticercosis in Mexico. *Parasitology Today*, **4,** 131–7.

Lucas, S.B., Hassounah, O.A., Doenoff, M., and Muller, R. (1979). Aberrant forms of *Hymenolepis nana*: possible opportunistic infections in immunosuppressed patients. *Lancet*, **ii,** 1372–3.

Pawlowski, Z. and Schultz, M.G. (1972). Taeniasis and cysticercosis (*Taenia saginata*). *Advances in Parasitology*, **10,** 269–343.

Rydzewski, A.K., Chisholm, E.M., and Kagan, I.G. (1975). Comparison of serological tests for human cysticercosis by indirect haemagglutination, indirect immunofluorescent antibody and agar gel precipitation. *Journal of Parasitology*, **61,** 154–5.

Subianto, D.B., Tumada, L.R., and Morgono, S.S. (1978). Burns and epileptic fits associated with cysticercosis in mountain people of Irian Jaya. *Tropical and Geographic Medicine*, **30,** 275–8.

7.15.3 Cysticercosis

D. Overbosch

Introduction and life-cycle

Cysticercosis is caused by the larval stage of the pork tapeworm, *Taenia solium*. The adult tapeworm lives in the human small bowel and each proglottid produces thousands of eggs. For further development, *Taenia* spp. need an intermediate host, which for *T. solium* is the pig. The eggs are ingested by pigs when they feed on human waste contaminated by faeces. When the eggs are digested, the larvae are liberated (onchospheres). They penetrate the intestinal wall and are disseminated throughout the body. They develop in about 2 months into cysts in the muscles (meat!) and brain of the pigs. The cysts, which contain the head (scolex) of the tapeworm, are called cysticercus cellulosae (Fig. 1). Man acquires the tapeworm by eating undercooked pork (Bar-B-Q!) containing cysticerci. Fig. 2 shows the life-cycle of *T. solium*.

People contract cysticercosis after ingestion of *T. solium* eggs, either in contaminated food or by autoinfection (anus–hand–mouth). Thus they can be both intermediate and final host. The onchospheres are transported from the gut via the bloodstream and the liver to the capillaries, where they encyst at random throughout the body. Those found in the tissues of the nervous system, muscles, and eye are clinically relevant and will be discussed here. Only 10 per cent of patients with cysticercosis also harbour a tapeworm; consequently only a small proportion of patients acquire cysticercosis by autoinfection. The once popular idea of autoinfection by regurgitation of gravid proglottids into the stomach is no longer considered plausible.

In contrast to Echinococcus, one cysticercus contains only one larval scolex so that a single egg of *T. solium* cannot lead to more than one parasitic lesion in the human body. The incubation period for cysticercosis varies from several months to up to 30 years, the average being 5 years. Cysticerci may survive for up to 10 years in the body. The World Health Organization estimates that over 2.5 million people in the world are infested with the pork tapeworm but a far higher number have cysticercosis. *T. solium* cysticercosis occurs especially in countries with poor hygienic conditions and a lack of meat inspection. Central America (Mexico), South America, parts of Africa, India, and South-East Asia are endemic areas. Cysticercosis does not occur in Islamic countries via the intermediate host, as pork is not eaten there. An increasing number of cases of cysticercosis are found in industrialized countries (e.g. the United States, Australia, and Europe) due to increased travel into and immigration from the Third World. Many travellers are not properly instructed in ways of avoiding infectious and parasitic diseases in Third World countries, rendering them especially vulnerable.

History

The first author to describe cysticercosis in pigs was probably Hippocrates, followed by Aristophanes and Aristotle. Paranoli, Gessner, and Rummler described cysts in the brain in the sixteenth century; Malpighi identified them as parasites in 1686. The seventeenth-century Dutch

Fig. 1 Excised cysticercus (top), diameter 1.5 cm, and magnified head of the scolex (bottom), clearly showing the suckers and hooks.

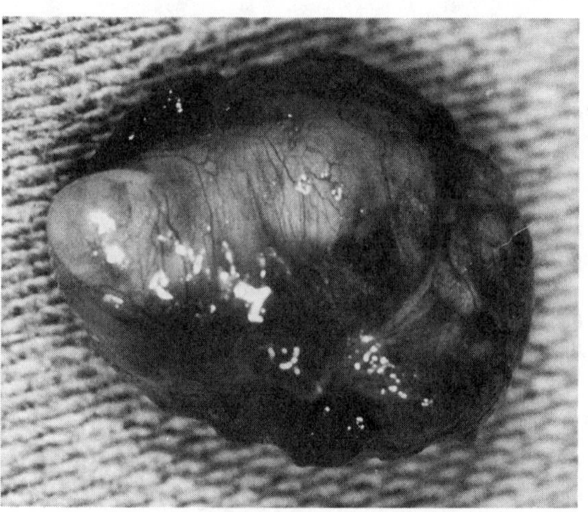

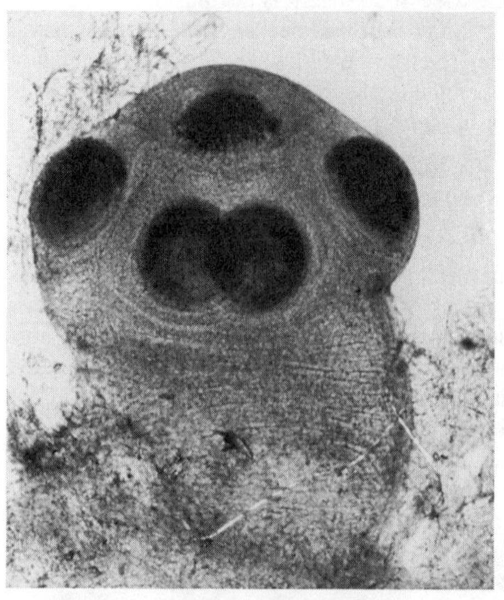

physicians Van Beverwijck and Blanckaert made the association between the excretion of worms and the occurrence of epileptic fits, while Virchow described the racemose form of cysticercosis. Weinberg developed the first serological test, a complement fixation test, in 1909. McArthur, Dixon, and Hargreaves described in detail the clinical patterns and sequelae of cysticercosis among British soldiers in the Indian Army. No medical treatment existed until 1980 when the first patients were given praziquantel by Rim in Korea and Robles and Chavarra in Mexico. Since 1983, albendazole has also been used for the treatment of cysticercosis.

Pathogenesis and clinical pattern

Cysticercosis is characterized by a large variety of clinical manifestations, but the three most clinically relevant are cysticercosis of the central nervous system (neurocysticercosis), muscular and subcutaneous cysticercosis, and ocular cysticercosis. These forms can be either symptomatic or asymptomatic and combinations of them frequently occur.

NEUROCYSTICERCOSIS

The clinical manifestations of neurocysticercosis depend on the number and localization of the cysticerci in the central nervous system as well as the inflammatory reaction around them. The clinical picture is therefore highly diverse, ranging from asymptomatic to severe neurological disease. The cysticerci lodge in various parts of the brain, such as the cortex, the ventricles, and/or the basal cisterns. This determines the clinical pattern of the neurocysticercosis (Fig. 3).

Neurocysticercosis can be divided into active and inactive forms (Table 1). The active form occurs in association with living and degenerating parasites; inactive disease arises from the effects of the resulting granulomas, calcifications or fibrosis.

Neurocysticercosis becomes manifest predominantly as epilepsy, especially in the case of cortical cysts. Elevated intracranial pressure occurs when arachnoiditis blocks the basal cisterns; hydrocephalus develops when cysts block the intraventricular foramina. The latter is encountered especially in the so-called racemose form in which clusters of cysts, resembling bunches of grapes, are located in the ventricles. As this form is often found in the basal cisterns, it may also lead to basal meningitis and cranial-nerve dysfunction.

Table 1 *Classification of neurocysticercosis*

Active	Inactive
Arachnoiditis	Parenchymal calcifications
Meningeal inflammation	Meningeal fibrosis
Parenchymal cysts	
Vasculitis	
Mass effect	
Intraventricular cysts	
Spinal cysts	

According to Sotelo *et al.* (1985).

Multiple frontal cysts cause dementia, especially in children. In India, cerebral lesions can be so numerous as to give a 'starry sky' appearance on computerized tomographic (**CT**) or magnetic resonance imaging (**MRI**). Fairly large brain infarcts are attributable to vasculitis. Epilepsy and focal neurological deficits occur in both active and inactive disease, depending upon the inflammatory reaction induced within the host or the presence of scar formation or calcification, respectively. Frequently there is a combination of the various manifestations of active neurocysticercosis. In inactive neurocysticercosis, calcified cysts often cause epilepsy. Subarachnoidal fibrosis is a sequel of arachnoiditis and may result in hydrocephalus and permanent cranial-nerve dysfunction. In about half of patients, active and inactive disease combine. Spinal cysticercosis can cause compression resulting in paresis, radicular symptoms, or cauda equina syndrome.

Fig. 2 Lifecycle of *Taenia solium*. The recumbent human figure on the right was reproduced from 'The good Samaritan', drawing, Dutch School, eighteenth century (author's collection) (reproduced from Overbosch (1992), with permission).

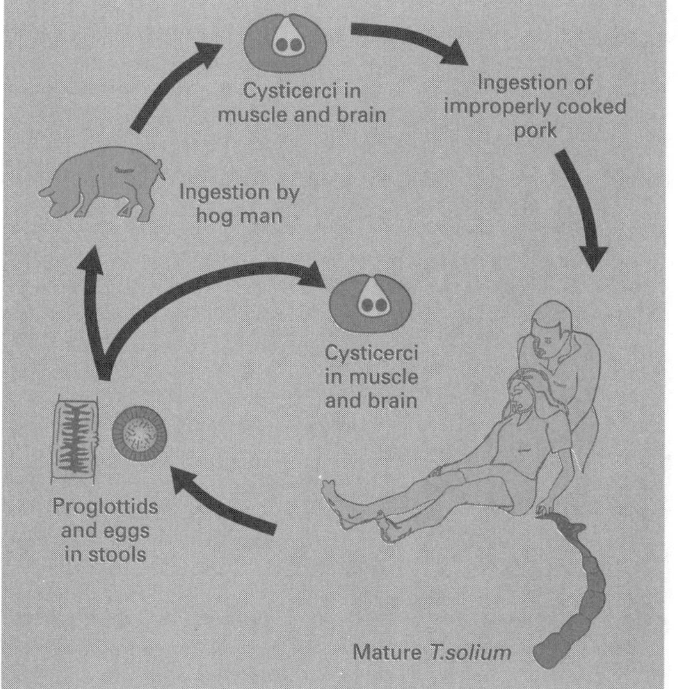

Fig. 3 Sections of the brain of a patient with parenchymal neurocysticercosis (by courtesy of Professor Dr E. Jung, E. Merck, Darmstadt, Germany).

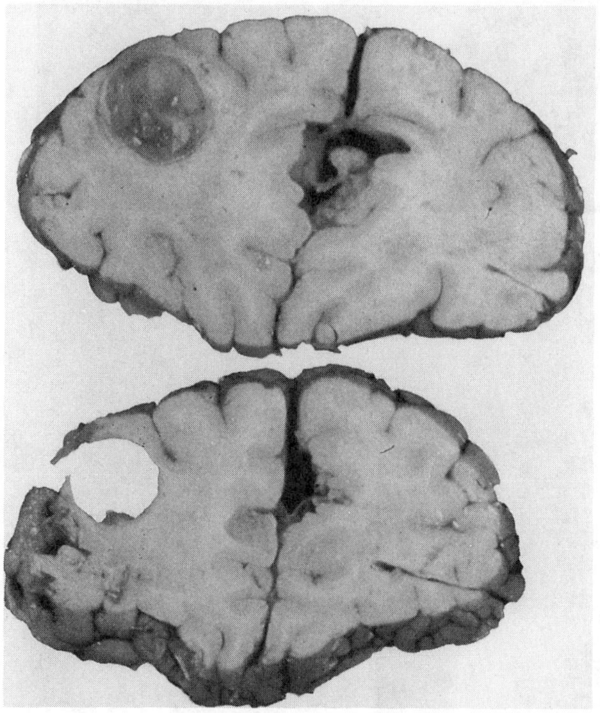

MUSCULAR AND SUBCUTANEOUS CYSTICERCOSIS

These frequently go unrecognized, unless the localization causes discomfort or nerve dysfunction. The diagnosis is suggested upon palpation of the typical firm, round, painless, bean-sized subcutaneous nodules. Radiographs may by chance reveal multiple calcifications in the muscles. They can disappear within several days or appear suddenly, thus seeming to migrate. In India, massive infection results in a syndrome of pseudohypertrophy of the calves and cardiac involvement, together with features of neurocysticercosis including intractable epilepsy, spinal-cord lesions, and unilateral blindness.

OCULAR CYSTICERCOSIS

Ocular cysticercosis occurs in about 25 per cent of all patients with cysticercosis. The parasite probably enters the eye via the posterior ciliary artery and lodges in the macular part of the subretinal space (Fig. 4). It may reach the vitreous cavity after perforation of the retina. Ocular cysticercosis may lead to severe impairment of vision, blindness or atrophy of the eye. Of 520 cases described by Kruger-Leite *et al.*, 35 per cent were subretinal, 22 per cent vitreal cavity, 72 per cent retinal and vitreal, and 22 per cent subconjunctival. In only 5 per cent of cases were parasites seen in the anterior chamber (Fig. 5).

The patient may experience blurring of vision and note slow movements of the parasite, often induced by light, for example the light of the examining ophthalmoscope.

Fig. 4 Subretinal cysticercus as seen by indirect ophthalmoscopy (above) and section through excised cysticercus (below) (by courtesy of Professor Stilma, State University Hospital Utrecht, The Netherlands).

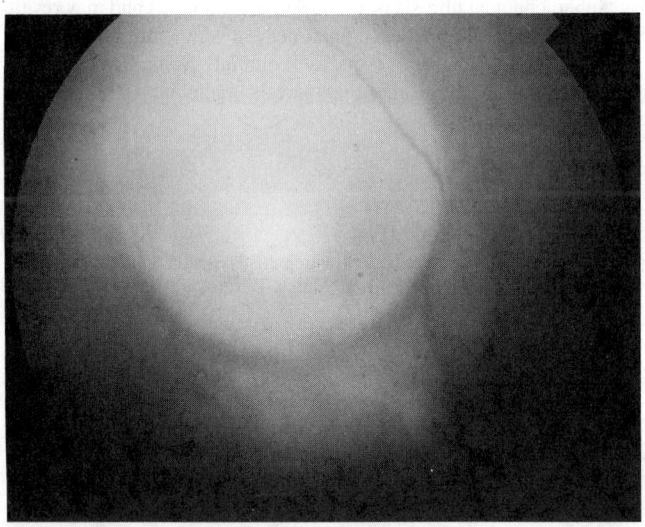

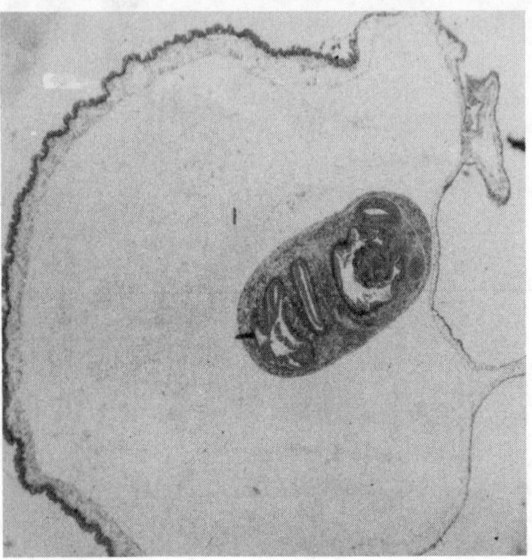

Diagnosis

The ultimate proof of parasitic infection lies in demonstration of the parasite. In the past the diagnosis of neurocysticercosis was only suspected if patients with epilepsy from endemic areas had subcutaneous nodules that, on excision, contained the characteristic parasite. However, only 25 per cent of the patients with neurocysticercosis have such subcutaneous nodules. Plain radiographs of the extremities or CT scanning may also reveal calcified subcutaneous or muscular nodules (Fig. 6). However, calcifications usually occur in a later stage of the disease. In Western countries, patients usually seek medical attention sooner after the onset of the disease.

Two major developments have made the diagnostic work-up for neuro-

Fig. 5 Cysticercus in the anterior chamber of the eye.

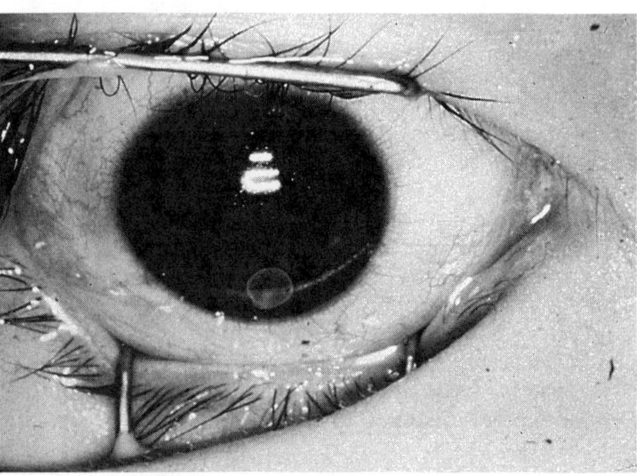

Fig. 6 Calcified cysticercus as seen on a plain radiograph of the thigh.

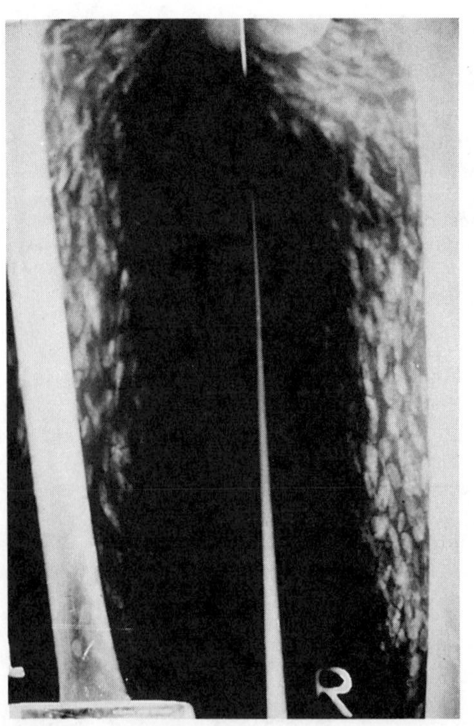

cysticercosis considerably easier: first, the introduction of CT and MRI, and second, the development of specific serological reactions against *T. solium* cysticercosis. CT is especially helpful in detecting cysticerci, which show up as hypodense areas in which the head of the scolex can often be discerned (Fig. 7). Degenerating lesions produce ring-enhancing images. Old, inactive lesions are seen as calcified, hyperdense spots (Fig. 7). CT scans also show enlarged ventricles (Fig. 8).

MRI is applied mainly to acquire images of active neurocysticerci, the best results being obtained with gadolinium as contrast and T_1-weighted image (Fig. 9). Calcified lesions are not visualized by MRI. The two methods of imaging are considered complementary for the demonstration of neurocysticercosis.

Fig. 7 Computerized tomographic scan of the brain, showing active and calcified lesions simultaneously (by courtesy of Dr T.E. Nash, National Institutes of Health, Bethesda, MD, USA).

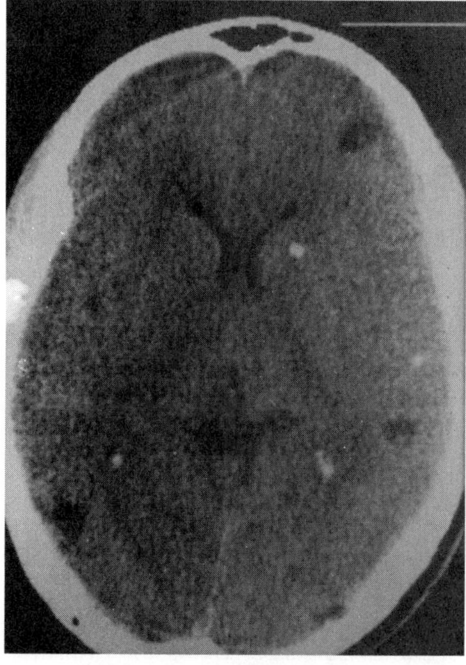

Fig. 8 Computerized tomographic scan of the brain, showing widened ventricles due to blocking of the intraventricular foramina (by courtesy of Dr T.E. Nash, National Institutes of Health, Bethesda, MD, USA).

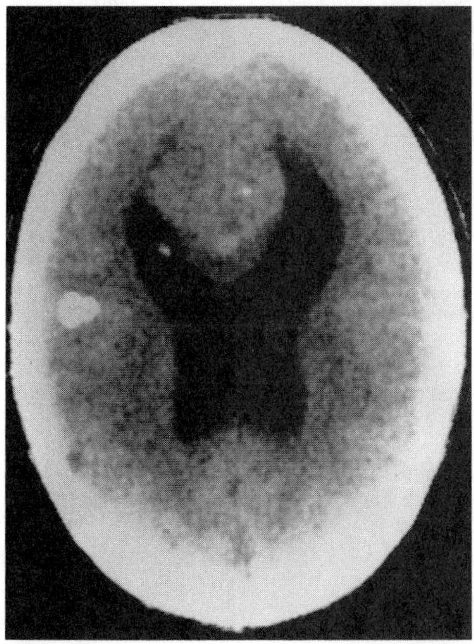

Serological tests may be essential for establishing the diagnosis. The complement fixation and immunofluorescence antibody tests had rather low sensitivity and cross-reactivity with other parasitic diseases. They have now been replaced by an enzyme immunoassay using *T. solium* extracts as antigen. More recently, an enzyme-linked immunoelectrotransfer blot assay has been developed; it is claimed that this has an almost 100 per cent specificity and sensitivity for cysticercosis. It is, however, not yet widely available.

For immunodiagnosis, serum is considered superior to cerebrospinal fluid, which may reveal lymphocytic pleocytosis, sometimes with eosinophilia. An elevated pressure at the opening tap, a high protein and low glucose concentration are other non-specific findings for neurocysticercosis in cerebrospinal fluid. In parenchymal neurocysticercosis there may be no abnormalities of cerebrospinal fluid at all, while in inactive disease, the fluid is completely normal in about 40 per cent of cases.

The diagnosis of neurocysticercosis can thus be difficult, especially when the serological reactions are negative and the intracerebral lesions are scarce and non-specific. Spinal cysticercosis can be demonstrated by myelography, CT, and MRI. Ocular cysticercosis can be seen at indirect ophthalmoscopy; however, if the vitreous or anterior chamber is opaque, ultrasound offers an adequate imaging alternative.

Differential diagnosis

The differential diagnosis of neurocysticercosis includes cerebral tumour or metastasis, benign intracranial hypertension, cerebral toxoplasmosis (especially in patients with AIDS) and, if a calcification is seen, a tuberculoma. Arteriovenous malformations, echinococcosis, syphilitic gumma, bacterial or amoebic cerebral abscesses, paragonimiasis, and cerebral localizations of schistosomiasis (especially *S. japonicum*) may also be considered. Epilepsy occurs in about 30 per cent of cases of astrocytoma and also in cerebral metastases, toxoplasmosis, and cerebral schistosomiasis.

CT scanning cannot easily differentiate between these and neurocysticercosis. Calcifications are frequently seen on CT scans of oligodendroglioma, toxoplasmosis, paragonimiasis, and tuberculomas. Multiple intracerebral lesions may occur in cerebral metastases, tuberculosis, sarcoidosis, and toxoplasmosis.

Fig. 9 Magnetic resonance image of the brain, showing active lesions of neurocysticercosis.

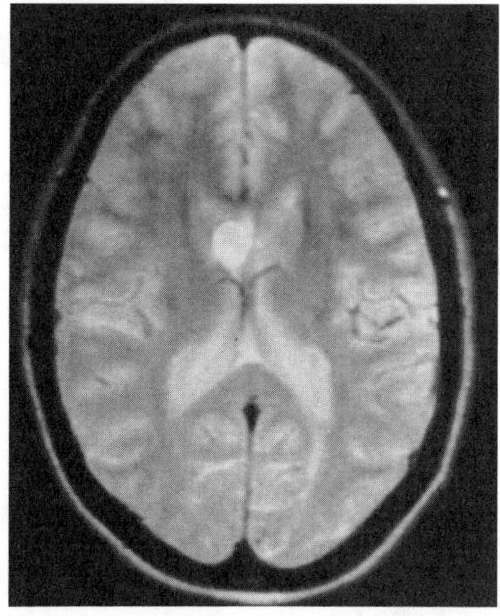

It is sometimes almost impossible to differentiate between a cerebral tumour or metastasis and neurocysticercosis. For patients from endemic areas with intracerebral lesions and positive serological tests, the reactions may well be associated with earlier or extracerebral cysticercosis and surgery must be undertaken even when neurocysticercosis is seriously considered. In non-endemic areas, cysticercosis can be mistaken for a malignant disorder when the serology is negative or inconclusive with very low titres. Sometimes it is then necessary to give a trial course of antiparasitic drugs before neurosurgery. Obviously a search for a primary tumour is warranted in such cases.

Muscular calcifications also occur in trichinosis. Cystic lesions of the eye, other than cysticercosis, may be due to echinococcosis or coenuriasis, which is caused by the larva of *T. multiceps*.

Treatment

Until the early 1980s, neurocysticercosis could only be treated symptomatically with antiepileptics or glucocorticosteroids to diminish the inflammatory reaction around degenerating cysts. Neurosurgical removal of intraventricular cysts that cause obstruction or the introduction of ventriculoatrial or ventriculoperitoneal shunts in case of (imminent) hydrocephalus is still a common procedure. Spinal-cord decompression or laminectomy may relieve paresis or radicular symptoms.

DRUG THERAPY

Praziquantel is a potent drug against cysticercosis. The generally recommended dose is 50 to 75 mg/kg a day orally for 2 to 3 weeks. The effectiveness of praziquantel against parenchymal neurocysticercosis is 60 to 85 per cent. It has remarkably few side-effects. However, in patients with massive infections the induction of treatment may cause a severe inflammatory reaction around degenerating cysticerci. This can aggravate symptoms and lead to cerebral oedema and even death. Therefore glucocorticosteroids are generally recommended as prophylaxis against the inflammatory response.

Praziquantel is metabolized rapidly and most probably eliminated by the P450 metabolic pathway in the liver (first-pass effect). Consequently, its bioavailability is low. When only a small proportion of the active drug reaches the circulation, small variations in metabolism will have a marked effect on the bioavailability and consequently on the results of treatment. There is, however, no clear relation between plasma concentrations and therapeutic efficacy.

It has been suggested that dexamethasone decreases the bioavailability of praziquantel, but this has not been confirmed. The bioavailability of praziquantel is further reduced by antiepileptic drugs, which are known to induce its metabolism in the liver, whereas praziquantel is even capable of inducing its own metabolism. A possible means of effectively blocking the metabolism of praziquantel is the coadministration of a drug that inhibits the P450 cytochrome metabolic pathway in the liver, for example cimetidine. In this manner much higher concentrations of praziquantel can be achieved.

Albendazole is a new benzimidazole derivative that is equally effective against parenchymal, neurocysticercosis and may even prove to be superior to praziquantel for arachnoidal cysticercosis. However, it has more side-effects than praziquantel, for example on bone marrow and liver; it also has mutagenic and teratogenic properties. The generally accepted dose for albendazole is 15 mg/kg orally for 30 days. Higher doses are probably not safe. The effectiveness of albendazole against intraparenchymal neurocysticercosis is 80 to 90 per cent. Shorter courses have been reported to be as effective as the 30-day course.

Both praziquantel and albendazole are equally ineffective against intraventricular or meningeal cysticerci. Praziquantel enters the cerebrospinal fluid rapidly and completely. In the destruction of parasites, immunological mechanisms play a part in addition to the direct toxic effect of the drug. Most probably the intraventricular space is an 'immunologically privileged site', where host immunological activity is ineffective against the parasite even when antiparasitic chemotherapy is given. Muscular and subcutaneous cysticercosis can be treated quite successfully with either drug.

Ocular cysticercosis

This is usually treated surgically. Glucocorticosteroids have to be given both locally and systemically to prevent an intense inflammatory reaction. Scarce and conflicting reports on successful treatment of ocular cysticercosis with praziquantel need to be confirmed in the future and, as yet, do not justify medical treatment in this condition. Diathermy, photocoagulation, or cryotherapy have not been studied extensively enough to be generally recommended.

Course and prognosis

The long-term follow-up of a disease that is endemic to the Third World and that is so polymorphic is very difficult. Before chemotherapy, mortality in the first 10 years after the onset of symptoms was 30 to 50 per cent. Chemotherapy has now greatly reduced mortality and the frequency of seizures has fallen significantly. Parenchymal neurocysticercosis and subcutaneous cysticercosis can be cured medically.

Untreated ocular cysticercosis carries has a bad prognosis. The success of surgical removal of the cyst depends on its site; a subretinal cyst has a better prognosis with regard to vision than an intravitreal or intraciliary cyst.

REFERENCES

Couldwell, W.T., Zee, C.S., and Apuzzo, M.L. (1991). Definition of the role of contemporary surgical management in cisternal and parenchymatous cysticercosis cerebri. *Neurosurgery*, **28,** 231–7.

Del Brutto, O.H., Sotelo, J., and Roman, G.C. (1993). Therapy for neurocysticercosis: a reappraisal. *Clinical Infectious Diseases*, **17,** 730–5.

Flisser, A. (1988). Neurocysticercosis in Mexico. *Parasitology Today*, **4,** 131–7.

Frohberg, H. (1989). The toxicological profile of praziquantel in comparison to other anthelminthic drugs. *Acta Leidensia*, **57,** 201–15.

Garcia, H.H. *et al.* (1991). Diagnosis of cysticercosis in endemic regions. *Lancet*, **338,** 549–51.

Kruger-Leite, E., Jalkh, A.E., Quiroz, H., and Schepens, C.L. (1985). Intraocular cysticercosis. *American Journal of Ophthalmology*, **99,** 252–7.

Lotz, J., Hewlett, R., Alheit, B., and Bowen, R. (1988). Neurocysticercosis: correlative pathomorphology and MR imaging. *Neuroradiology*, **30,** 35–41.

Overbosch, D. (1992). Neurocysticercosis. An introduction with special emphasis on new developments in pharmacotherapy. *Schweizerische Medizinische Wochenschrift*, **122,** 893–8.

Sotelo, J., Escobedo, F., Rodriguez-Carbajal, J., Torres, B., and Rubio-Donnadieu, F. (1984). Therapy of parenchymal brain cysticercosis with praziquantel. *New England Journal of Medicine*, **310,** 1001–7.

Sotelo, J., Guerrero, V., and Rubio-Donnadieu, F. (1985). Neurocysticercosis: a new classification based on active and inactive forms. *Archives of Internal Medicine*, **145,** 442–5.

Sotelo, J., Escobedo, F., and Penagos, P. (1988). Albendazole vs praziquantel for therapy for neurocysticercosis: a controlled trial. *Archives of Neurology*, **45,** 532–4.

Takayanagui, O.M. and Jardim, E. (1992). Therapy for neurocysticercosis: comparison between albendazole and praziquantel. *Archives of Neurology*, **49,** 290–4.

Teitelbaum, G.P. *et al.* (1989). MR imaging of neurocysticercosis. *American Journal of Radiology*, **153,** 857–66.

Vazquez, V. and Sotelo, J. (1992). The course of seizures after treatment for cerebral cysticercosis. *New England Journal of Medicine*, **327,** 696–701.

Wilson, M. *et al.* (1991). Clinical evaluation of the cysticercosis enzyme-linked immunoelectrotransfer blot in patients with neurocysticercosis. *Journal of Infectious Diseases*, **164,** 1007–9.

7.15.4 Diphyllobothriasis and sparganosis

SEUNG-YULL CHO

Diphyllobothriasis

Diphyllobothriasis is an intestinal infection with tapeworms belonging to the genus Diphyllobothrium. The most important species is *D. latum*, which is commonly called, fish tapeworm or broad tapeworm.

BIOLOGY AND EPIDEMIOLOGY

Human diphyllobothriasis is contracted by consuming raw fish, such as pike, turbot, perch, and salmonids, that have plerocercoid larvae. In the human intestine the plerocercoid develops into an adult (usually one per person) that is 5 to 6 m long and 0.8 to 1.5 cm wide. An adult produces a million eggs each day. Eggs are 65×45 μm. In fresh water, eggs embryonate to a coracidium. The swimming coracidium is taken up by zooplankters such as *Cyclops strenuus* and *Eudiaptomus gracilis*, and develops into a procercoid larva. This larva is then infects freshwater fish, which in turn are eaten by larger salmonid fish, in which the plerocercoid develops. The plerocercoid larva, which is infective to man, is 1 to 1.5 cm long and 1 mm wide, and is found in the muscle and peritoneal cavity of fish.

The highest incidence of human cases is in the Baltic region, especially in Finland, and throughout Siberia. Villages used to exist where 80 per cent of the population were infected. In Switzerland, northern Italy, lake regions of North America, north-east China, Korea, and Japan, cases are not uncommon. People may be infected by other *Diphyllobothrium* species of bears, whales, seals, or birds. These tapeworms are also acquired by eating marine fish. For example, *D. yonagoense*, *D. nihonkaiense* etc. in Japan and *D. pacificum* in Chile and Peru are intestinal parasites of seals. In Alaska, human infections with *D. ursi*, *D. dendriticum*, *D. lanceolatum*, *D. dalliae* etc. of birds or bears may be acquired by eating infected marine fish.

The habit of eating sliced raw fish creates the opportunity for infection. The Russian custom of eating raw pike roe and Jewish *gefuellte fisch* also leads to infection. Prevention is achieved by freezing fish at −18°C or lower for 1 day.

CLINICAL MANIFESTATIONS

Infection usually causes few symptoms. Abdominal discomfort, fatigue, diarrhoea alternating with constipation, dizziness, and urticaria may be the vague presenting symptoms. Vomiting up a tapeworm and intestinal obstruction due to a mass of worms occurs very rarely. Strips of gravid segments, 10 to 80 cm long, may be passed with the stools and noticed by the patient.

Tapeworm pernicious anaemia is associated with *D. latum* infection. In these patients, elimination of the tapeworm results in progressive improvement of the anaemia itself. Clinical manifestations, including haematological and neurological disorders, are essentially the same as in classical pernicious anaemia. Most of these patients are Finnish. For more details of tapeworm anaemia the monograph of von Bornsdorff (1977) should be consulted.

DIAGNOSIS AND TREATMENT

Clinical symptoms are rarely responsible for raising the suspicion of diphyllobothriasis. Racial and geographical origin and predilection for raw fish provide the clue to a diagnosis that can be confirmed by identifying the characteristic eggs in stool by microscopy. Discharged, long chains of worm segments are the best material for morphological identification. In endemic areas, all patients with pernicious anaemia should have their stools examined.

Treatment is simple and effective. Niclosamide, in a single adult dose of 2 g, or praziquantel in a single dose of 10 mg/kg body weight are the drugs of choice. Identification of an expelled scolex confirms a complete cure.

Sparganosis

Sparganosis is a zoonotic infection caused by the larval tapeworms of *Spirometra mansoni* or *S. mansonoides*. These tapeworm larvae invade a variety of tissues and organs.

BIOLOGY

The white, slender, tapeworm larva without round suckers is called a sparganum (= plerocercoid) when it is found in tissues or body cavities of terrestrial vertebrates. The length varies from one to scores of centimetres. When larva-infected hosts are eaten by carnivorous mammals, the sparganum matures to an adult in their small intestine. Within 5 to 6 days the adult worm produces operculated eggs. Germ cells in the egg become a coracidium. When the swimming coracidium is taken up by freshwater zooplankters such as *Cyclops leuckarti*, it develops into a procercoid larva. When the procercoid is ingested by terrestrial vertebrates including man, it becomes a sparganum (Fig. 1).

EPIDEMIOLOGY

Human sparganosis has a low prevalence throughout the world, but improved medical services have increased its recognition. The infection is contracted by eating either the procercoid or the sparganum. The procercoid larva in the infected cyclops may be swallowed accidentally when people drink unfiltered water.

The most endemic areas for sparganosis are in Asia such as Japan, Korea, China, Vietnam and South-East Asia, where traditional habits contributed to the higher incidence. Poultry, frogs, and snakes are important sources. Some people believe that eating these animals raw is beneficial for physically feeble children and for tuberculosis or arthritis. Others believe that live vipers are a tonic. Raw pork may be a source of infection. The practice of applying poultices of frog or snake skin to an inflamed eye or abscess was common in the pre-antibiotic era in southern China and Vietnam. In these instances a sparganum in the herpetile skin could invade directly through conjunctiva or friable abscess wall. Sparganosis is, therefore, a disease of rural people or of those who seek the rural life.

Fig. 1 A sparganum surgically removed from a subcutaneous mass.

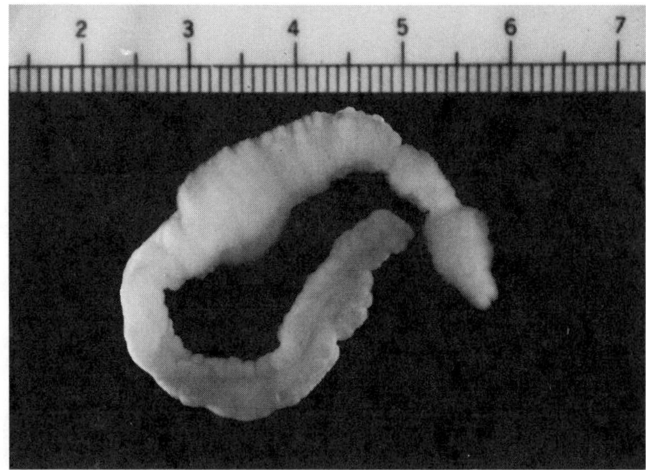

PATHOLOGY AND CLINICAL MANIFESTATIONS

The ingested procercoid larva or sparganum actively penetrates the host's intestinal wall to reach the peritoneal cavity, whence it begins to migrate systemically. The worm usually lodges in subcutaneous tissue or muscle in the chest or abdominal walls, limbs, or scrotum. Orbital sparganosis is also common. Urinary tract, pleural cavity, pericardial sac, and abdominal viscera are other reported sites where symptoms of inflammation are produced. The worm may slowly migrate in the body. A lump appears then spontaneously disappears, only to reappear some weeks or months later at a site remote from the first. There is redness and itching of overlying skin; local bleeding and acute suppurative necrosis may occur. Since imaging diagnosis by computerized tomography and magnetic resonance became available, granulomatous lesions due to sparganum have been increasingly recognized in brain and spinal canal.

Histologically the lesion is a granuloma formed along the tortuous track of focal necrosis caused by the migration. The larva and its tracks are surrounded by zones of necrotic debris and lymphohistiocytic reaction. Heavy eosinophilic infiltration with Charcot–Leyden crystals is usually found. The inflammatory reaction often extends into surrounding muscle or fat tissue. Part of a dead worm may be found in the tissues, leaving its calcareous corpuscles, which are engulfed by histiocytes. The sparganum may survive more than 5 years in an infected individual. In general only a few worms infect each patient.

Fig. 2 Sparganum proliferum in the subcutaneous tissue of the thigh of a 24-year-old Japanese woman. She had elephantoid swellings of abdomen and thigh and eventually died. The figure shows multiple transverse and tangential sections of a proliferating sparganum (*arrows*). Although in section the worm appears as multiple spargana, each cross section probably represents a continuous branching worm. The pair in the lower right appear to be close to a bifurcation. Each section of sparganum is surrounded by a band of fibrous tissue. Movat, X14.5. (Armed Forces Institute of Pathology Photograph, Negative No. 76-6318.)

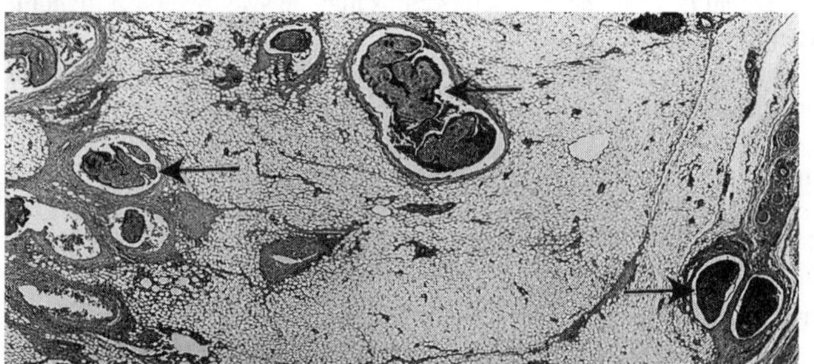

Sparganum proliferum is an acephalic, branched, proliferating larva that is histologically similar to a non-proliferating sparganum. In very rare human infections, the larvae are found in thousands in subcutaneous tissue and internal organs (Fig. 2). This infection has been reported in Japan, and North and Latin American countries. The biology of this larva is still unknown.

DIAGNOSIS AND TREATMENT

Diagnosis of sparganosis is rarely made preoperatively. In most cases, definitive diagnosis is made incidentally by recovering the worm at surgery. The sparganum is a white, ribbon-shaped, moving worm with transverse wrinklings and peristaltic waves. Preoperative diagnosis of cerebral sparganosis is made with high confidence when computerized tomography of the brain shows an enhancing nodule with changing shape or position, calcifications, and degeneration of white matter, together with positive specific antibody in serum and cerebrospinal fluid. The tomographic findings are similar to those of a brain tumour or cerebral infarction.

The excision of a mass or removal of the worm from the lesion is therapeutic in itself. Repeated surgery is needed when the patient has multiple lesions. No drugs are known to be effective for sparganosis.

The prognosis is excellent in almost all cases when surgically treated. Cerebral sparganosis is complicated by epilepsy and hemiparesis. All *S. proliferum* infections have proved fatal (Fig. 2).

REFERENCES

Chang, K.H., Chi, J.G., Cho, S.Y., Han, M.H., Han, D.H., and Han, M.C. (1992). Cerebral sparganosis: analysis of 34 cases with emphasis on CT features. *Neuroradiology*, **34,** 1–8.

Moulinier, R., Martinez, E., Torres, J., Noya, O., de Noya, B.A., and Reyes, O. (1982). Human proliferative sparganosis in Venezuela. *American Journal of Tropical Medicine and Hygiene*, **31,** 358–63.

von Bonsdorff, B. (1977). *Diphyllobothriasis in man.* Academic Press, London.

7.16 Trematodes (flukes)

7.16.1 Schistosomiasis

A. E. Butterworth and J. E. P. Thomas

Introduction

Schistosomiasis is the generic term given to disease caused by parasitic blood flukes of the genus Schistosoma (class Trematoda of the phylum Platyhelminthes or flatworms). An older, non-scientific name, still commonly encountered in the literature and in many developing countries in Africa and elsewhere, is bilharzia. Farley provides an excellent and detailed history of bilharzia, including developments in research and control up to the 1970s; up-to-date information is provided in a new edition of the definitive textbook by Jordan *et al.* (1993).

Three major species (*Schistosoma mansoni, S. haematobium*, and *S. japonicum*) and two minor species (*S. mekongi* and *S. intercalatum*) are estimated to affect about 200 million people in over 70 different countries, mainly in Africa, the Middle East, South America and the Caribbean, China, the Philippines, and parts of South-East Asia. There are also important schistosomes of domestic animals. The disease is usually characterized by chronic infection, with adult worms slowly accumulating over a period of 10 to 20 years from early childhood onwards, and with a progressive deposition of eggs in the tissues leading to granulomatous reactions and subsequent fibrosis in the intestines and liver (*S. mansoni* and *S. japonicum*) or in the bladder and urinary tract (*S. haematobium*). Depending on the species, this in turn leads to long-term sequelae of chronic bloody diarrhoea, portal hypertension with hepatosplenomegaly, oesophageal varices and haematemesis, or obstructive uropathy associated with renal damage. Less commonly observed manifestations include a cercarial dermatitis that develops within minutes or hours after exposure, a syndrome of acute schistosomiasis ('Katayama fever') that develops within a few weeks of an initial infection, and a variety of other long-term sequelae that follow the deposition of eggs in the lungs (cor pulmonale) or central nervous system (focal epilepsy, generalized encephalitis, or transverse myelitis). *S. mekongi* and *S. intercalatum* are uncommon species that cause disease resembling that induced by *S. japonicum* and *S. mansoni*, respectively; they are not discussed in detail.

Lifecycle

The lifecycle of all schistosomes is characterized by a requirement for two hosts: a 'definitive' vertebrate host, in which sexual maturation and mating of the adult worms occurs, and an 'intermediate' invertebrate host, in which asexual replication occurs. The schistosomes that affect man may also affect other mammals, which act as reservoir hosts. This is important in the case of *S. japonicum*, in which cattle, water buffalo, pigs, dogs, and rodents serve as major reservoirs; possible but less important in the case of *S. mansoni*, in which non-human primates and some rodents can sometimes act as reservoirs; and unimportant in the case of *S. haematobium*. The invertebrate host is invariably an aquatic or amphibious snail of certain restricted genera, depending on the species of parasite. Transmission between the two hosts is achieved by free-living stages of the parasite: cercariae released from infected snails into the water penetrate directly through the skin of potential vertebrate hosts, while eggs passed out in the excreta of infected vertebrates hatch upon contact with water to release the larval miracidia, which directly invade new snails. Thus, schistosomiasis is essentially a disease associated with fresh water in habitats that are suitable for the propagation of the snail intermediate host.

The basic lifecycle is similar for the three main species that affect man. The infective cercariae released from the snail are small, multicellular organisms, about 200 μm long and just visible to the naked eye in heavily contaminated water (Fig. 1). The cercaria, which is surrounded by a water-resistant glycocalyx, is composed of two parts: the head, which bears anterior and ventral suckers and which will eventually go on to form the adult worm, and a forked muscular tail that allows active movement in the water. Cercariae of *S. mansoni* and *S. haematobium* are released from the snails during periods of daylight, and move vertically in water, alternating between active movement towards the surface and slow sinking. Those of *S. japonicum* are released later in the afternoon or evening and tend to move to and remain at the surface of the water. Cercariae can remain infective for up to 24 h, although under field conditions their viability is usually less. If, during this time, they come into contact with an appropriate host, they attach to the skin through their suckers, shed their tails, discharge the proteolytic contents of their preacetabular glands, and penetrate the epidermis within minutes. During this time the skin must remain immersed in water, or at least moist; rapid drying kills the organism. Immediately after skin penetration, the cercarial glycocalyx is shed and the young larva, now referred to as a schistosomulum (Fig. 2), produces an extra layer to the outer membrane that covers its syncytial tegument. The new double lipid bilayer is unique to the blood flukes, and may represent an adaptation to survival in potentially immune hosts.

Fig. 1 The free-living, infective stage (cercaria) of *Schistosoma mansoni*; note the forked, muscular tail.

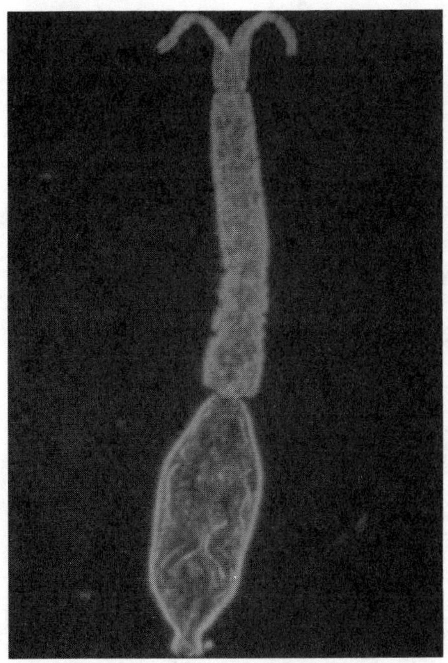

Following skin penetration, the schistosomula remain at the dermal–epidermal junction for 48 h, where many (up to 60 per cent in experimental animals) die, even in non-immune hosts. The remainder migrate via the bloodstream to the lungs, whence they can be recovered in experimental animals between 4 and 7 days after infection, and then again via the bloodstream to the liver, where, in the case of *S. mansoni*, they begin to arrive at about 10 to 12 days (shorter for *S. japonicum* and longer for *S. haematobium*). Experiments in mice indicate that schistosomula can cross the pulmonary and systemic circulation two or three times, with a proportion being retained in the hepatic portal system on each passage. Once within the hepatic portal system, the schistosomula mature and differentiate into adult worms, form pairs, and migrate against the portal blood flow to take up their final position in small venules draining the large and, to a lesser extent, the small intestine (*S. mansoni* and *S. japonicum*) or the bladder and ureters (*S. haematobium*).

The male and female worms, 1 to 2 cm long, are morphologically distinct (Fig. 3). The shorter and flatter male envelopes the female in its gynaecophoric canal or schist, and the pairs remain permanently coupled, with the male attaching itself to the venule wall by means of a ventral sucker. Both sexes absorb nutrients through the tegument and also ingest blood cells, but the female, because of its high metabolic requirement for egg laying, feeds more actively than the male. In both sexes the intestine is close-ended, and the intestinal contents, including the characteristic, insoluble haematin-like pigment derived from ingested red cells, are regurgitated. Adult worms live for 3 to 7 years on average (although active infection has been reported in individuals who have left an endemic area up to 30 years previously), during which time the female worm produces eggs at the rate of 300 a day (*S. mansoni*) to 3000 a day (*S. japonicum*).

The mature female starts to lay eggs after about 5 to 7 weeks (*S. japonicum* and *S. mansoni*) or 10 to 12 weeks (*S. haematobium*). The eggs are characteristic of each species, and identification of eggs in the

Fig. 2 The young larva (schistosomulum) of *S. mansoni*, immediately after cercarial penetration of the skin.

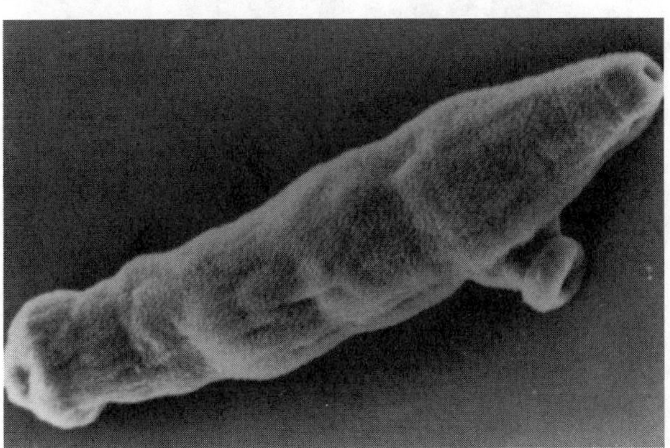

excreta is a key element in diagnosis. All contain a larval stage, the miracidium, surrounded by a thick, rigid shell containing cross-linked tyrosine residues. The shells of *S. mansoni* and *S. haematobium* are ellipsoid, measuring 60 to 70 × 140 to 160 μm: those of *S. haematobium* have a sharp terminal spine, while those of *S. mansoni* have a distinctive lateral spine (Fig. 4). The eggs of *S. japonicum* are more nearly spherical, measuring about 70 × 90 μm, with a small knob. Once deposited by the female, the eggs can lodge in the tissues (intestines and liver, or bladder and ureter, depending on the species), where they elicit the development of a cellular, granulomatous reaction, which, with its ensuing fibrosis, is responsible for most of the chronic tissue damage and disease that is described below.

Of particular interest is the tissue damage caused by the eggs of *S. mansoni* and *S. japonicum* as they are swept back to the liver by the portal system causing vascular and granulomatous changes. The granulomatous pylephlebitis and peripylephlebitis is responsible for the portal hypertension, while granulomata with subsequent fibrosis develop in the liver causing periportal fibrosis. With many collaterals developing, the eggs may not be caught up in the portal circulation but may be diverted to the pulmonary circulation. Here the same combination of vascular and granulomatous changes is responsible for the rarer pulmonary hypertension and pulmonary fibrosis. Occasionally, schistosomes, and hence their eggs, may enter the valveless visceral pelvic veins or haemorrhoidal veins and so reach the vertebral plexus. The ova reaching the spinal cord will again cause vascular and granulomatous changes in the lower spinal cord, cauda equina and conus medullaris, with resultant paraparesis as described in the clinical picture below.

Alternatively, the eggs can pass out through the intestinal or bladder wall into the lumen, from where they are released in the excreta into the environment. Passage through the tissues is aided by the release from eggs of proteolytic and other substances through micropores in the eggshell; these substances are also strongly antigenic, and the immune response, as well as causing host tissue damage, may also contribute to egg excretion.

Eggs that are carried to or deposited in fresh water rapidly hatch, releasing a free-living form, the miracidium. This is a ciliated and actively motile organism that lives for about 6 h and that moves randomly in the water. When it encounters a suitable snail host, the mira-

Fig. 3 Adult worms of *S. mansoni*: the short, flat male encloses the long, pigmented female in its gynaecophoric canal.

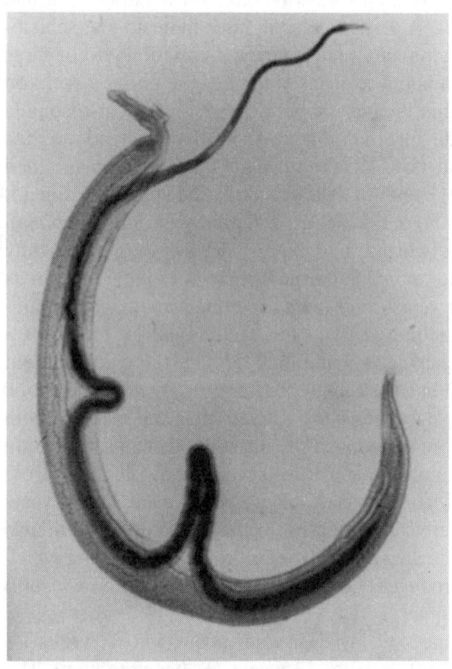

Fig. 4 Egg of *S. mansoni*; note the distinctive lateral spine.

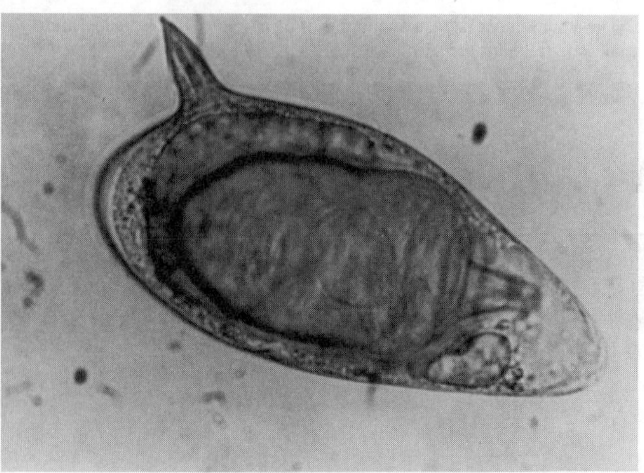

Fig. 5 *Biomphalaria glabrata*, an intermediate host of *S. mansoni* from South America.

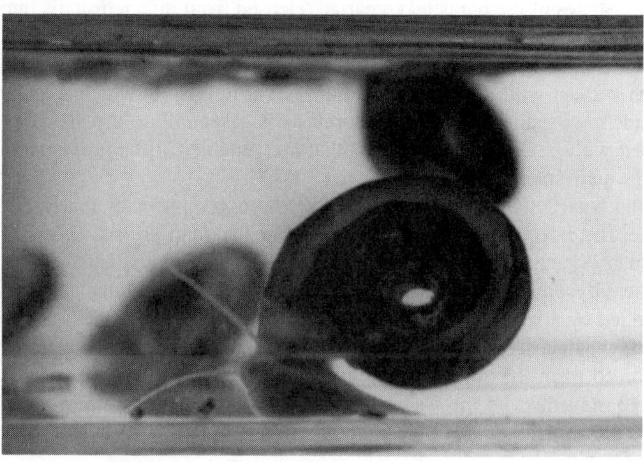

Fig. 6 Collecting snails from a schistosome-infested pool in Kenya.

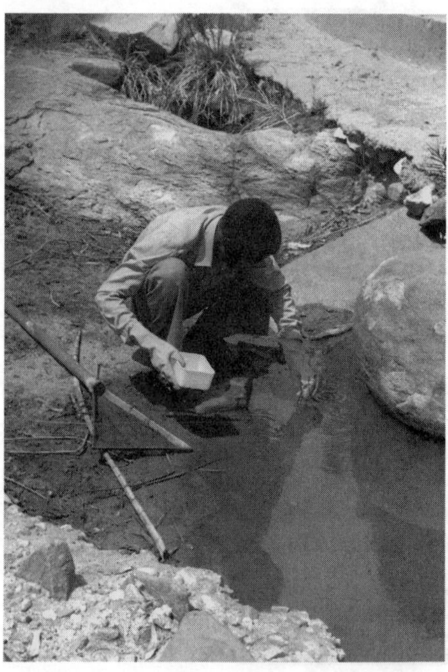

cidium actively penetrates into the body of the snail, aided by the release of enzymatic secretions, and transforms into a primary sporocyst. Within the primary sporocyst, secondary sporocysts are formed by budding, are released and migrate to the snail's hepatopancreas. Here, a further asexual replication occurs, leading eventually (4 to 6 weeks after infection of the snail) to the release of large numbers of the infective larvae, the cercariae. Infected snails can live for several months, releasing up to 1000 cercariae a day.

There is a considerable restriction on the type of snails that can act as intermediate hosts, and the distribution of such snails is a major factor that limits the distribution of schistosomiasis. In the case of *S. mansoni*, they are confined to aquatic snails of the genus Biomphalaria, especially *B. pfeifferi* in subSaharan Africa and *B. glabrata* (Fig. 5) in South America. These snails mainly inhabit small pools (Fig. 6) and weedy, slowly flowing or static streams or irrigation canals, but any body of fresh water should be regarded as a possible habitat, and therefore potentially a source of schistosome infection. *S. haematobium* is also carried by aquatic snails, in this case of the genus Bulinus. Both *Biomphalaria* and *Bulinus* spp. can withstand prolonged and severe desiccation by aestivating, a process in which they bury themselves in muddy substrates, retract into their shells, and seal the apertures with a layer of mucus. In this way, snail populations and transmission can be maintained even in prolonged drought. Snail populations are usually washed out of streams or small rivers during intense or prolonged rainy seasons, but are repopulated from egg masses deposited on vegetation. In contrast, *S. japonicum* is carried by amphibious snails of the genus Oncomelania. These are found in a wide variety of habitats, including not only small streams, pools, and irrigation canals, but also cultivated or fallow wet land, especially rice paddy-fields.

Distribution

Human schistosomiasis is widely, albeit focally, distributed in 74 countries, especially in Africa. *S. mansoni* is found in most countries south of the Sahara, as well as Madagascar, the Nile delta and part of the Nile valley in Egypt, Saudi Arabia, Yemen, Oman, and Libya. In South America, it is found primarily in northern and eastern Brazil, as well as Venezuela and Surinam, while in the Caribbean Puerto Rico and several of the smaller islands (Saint Lucia, Antigua, Montserrat, Martinique, Guadeloupe, Dominican Republic) are infested. *S. haematobium* is not found in the New World, but is again widely distributed throughout much of subSaharan Africa and Madagascar. It is also more widely distributed than *S. mansoni* in North Africa and the Middle East, being found throughout much of the Nile valley and delta, Morocco, Algeria, Tunisia, and Libya, as well as Saudi Arabia, Yemen, Syria, Lebanon, Turkey, Iraq, and Iran. *S. japonicum* is confined to the Far East: it is no longer found in Japan, but remains widespread in China and the Philippines, together with a few small foci in Indonesia. The two minor species, *S. intercalatum* and *S. mekongi*, are much more restricted in their distribution, the former being found in some countries in West and Central Africa, the latter in the Mekong valley in Laos and Cambodia. Recent estimates from the World Health Organization are that 200 million people are infected with one or other of the various species of schistosome, and that 500 to 600 million people, living in poor conditions in endemic areas, are at risk of infection. The reviews by Chen and Mott (1989) and World Health Organization (1988) give detailed information on how much morbidity and resulting mortality can be expected with *S. haematobium* and *S. mansoni*.

Aspects of transmission

Some general features of transmission and infection are common to all three of the major species of schistosome that infect man. The first and possibly most important point is that, as with other parasitic helminths in their definitive hosts but in contrast to most other infectious agents, the adult worms do not replicate. Each cercaria has the opportunity to become a single worm; infection is acquired cumulatively over a period of years; and each female worm has the capacity to deposit several hundred eggs a day for a period of several years. Because most of the manifestations of disease are attributable to the retention of eggs in the tissues, with ensuing fibrosis, it should follow that the severity of disease is related to the intensity of infection (that is, the numbers of adult worms present), as well as to its duration: and such a relation has now been demonstrated in many studies in endemic communities.

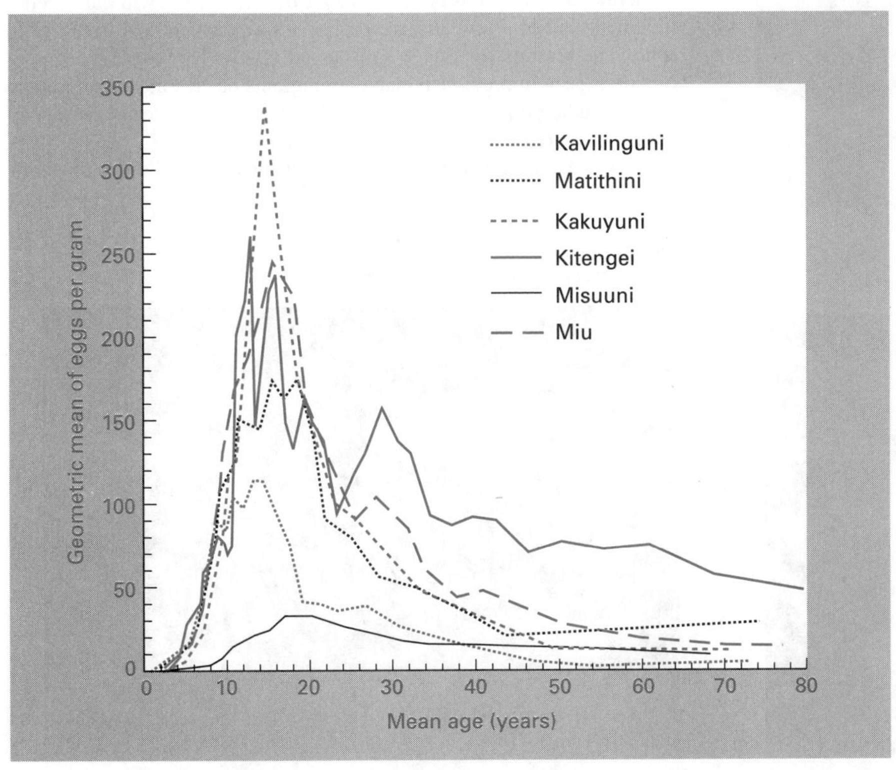

Fig. 7 Typical age-intensity profiles of *S. mansoni* infection from six communities in Machakos District, Kenya (reproduced from Fulford *et al.* (1992) with permission).

A second important feature, as with other helminths, is that the distribution of adult worms in a host population, as reflected by egg output in the faeces, is highly overdispersed or aggregated. Even in a community in which the overall prevalence of infection is high, most individuals have only light infections, which cause little morbidity, while a few individuals have very heavy infections that may lead to severe disease. The reasons for such aggregation are unclear but potentially diverse, and may include a genetic predisposition to heavy or light infections, a heterogeneity in the acquisition of protective immunity, or a heterogeneity, which may be both geographical and behavioural, in exposure to infection. In this context, it should be noted that, even within a small, highly endemic area, transmission is often very focal, reflecting the heterogeneous distribution of infected snails; and such foci can vary markedly from year to year, as local changes in climate and habitat affect snail populations.

Thirdly, the shape of the distribution of infection by age in communities living in endemic areas is characteristically convex. This is seen both for prevalence of infection (that is, the proportion of individuals in each age group who have detectable infection) and for mean intensity of infection (that is, the mean worm burden for each age group, measured indirectly as described below by counting the number of eggs excreted in the faeces or urine) (Fig. 7). A typical picture is that young children start to become infected from about the age of 3 to 4 years, when they start to have regular contact with infected water (Figs. 8 and 9). Both prevalence and mean intensity then rise sharply, reaching a peak during or towards the end of the second decade of life. Thereafter, both prevalence and, more markedly, intensity of infection decline in the older age groups. There appear to be several reasons for this decline. First, the adult worms from infections acquired early in life, having a limited mean life-span of about 3 to 7 years, progressively die. Secondly, in most cultures, adults have less contact with infected water than children and young teenagers, and therefore less exposure to new infections. Water contact patterns vary markedly between communities, and to a certain extent within communities, depending on annual or seasonal climatic patterns. As a broad generalization, children have frequent, prolonged, and extensive body contact through swimming, bathing or playing, as well as some household chores such as drawing water or tending animals. In adults, water contact is more generally associated with bathing or with washing clothes or utensils: but a variety of particular occupations also involve extensive contact with infective water, including fishing, cleaning irrigation canals, drawing water for small-scale irrigation, and working in rice paddies.

Fig. 8 Children crossing a stream infested with *S. mansoni* in Kenya. (The man on the rock is observing water-contact behaviour.)

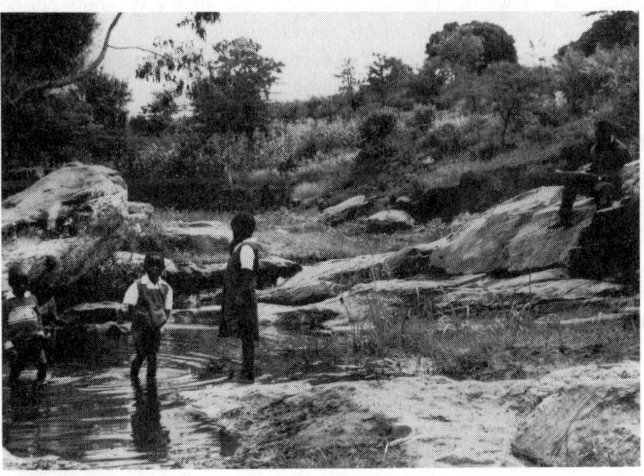

Fig. 9 Children in a paddy-field infested with *S. japonicum* in Leyte, Philippines.

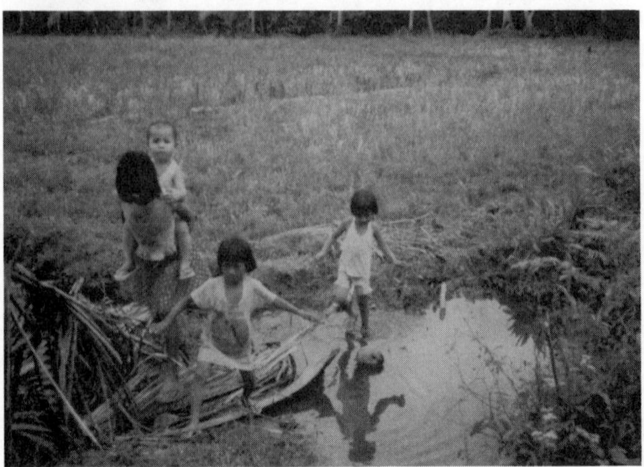

There is also a substantial body of evidence, largely from studies of reinfection after treatment under conditions of observed exposure, that older children and adults slowly develop an immunity to reinfection. This may be mediated by IgE antibodies with specificity for adult worm antigens. The mechanism of this protective immunity remains unproven, although a variety of antibody-dependent, cell-mediated cytotoxicity reactions, mediated by eosinophils and other effector cell types, can be shown to be active *in vitro* against the young, migrating schistosomulum that is probably the main target for immune attack (Fig. 10). In contrast to adults, young children remain susceptible to reinfection: even though they show a range of immune responses to schistosome antigens, such responses fail to mediate protection and may actually block the effect of potentially protective responses.

One consequence of the relative lack of infection among adults is that, in communities living in endemic areas, schistosomiasis is usually perceived as a disease of children of primary school age. The late sequelae of infection, resulting from fibrosis of egg granulomata, may affect and even kill older children and adults, but these are rare events in comparison with the extensive, although milder, morbidity that is seen in the younger age groups. A typical picture in an area of high transmission is that a majority of young children are infected and have detectable signs or symptoms; in most of these children there is a spontaneous reduction in clinical morbidity as they grow older, even without specific treatment, but in a few, disease progresses to a severe and irreversible state. The reasons for this are discussed below. However, a different picture is seen in previously naive immigrants or visitors to an endemic area (including foreign tourists or workers), in whom severe disease may develop as a result of new infection at any age.

A second consequence of the high intensities of infection among chil-

Fig. 10 Human eosinophils adhering to an antibody-coated schistosomulum: one of several possible effector mechanisms of immunity.

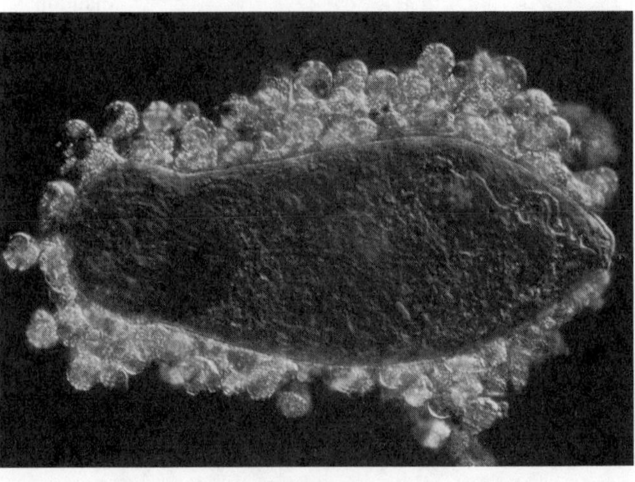

dren is that it is they who contribute most to contamination of the environment with excreted eggs, and hence to continued transmission. In the case of *S. haematobium*, contamination occurs when urine is voided (by both sexes and all ages) directly into water, especially during bathing. In the case of *S. mansoni* and *S. japonicum*, in contrast, defaecation directly into water is relatively uncommon. Instead, faeces are deposited, for example, among bushes on the banks of streams. Eggs survive in drying faeces only for a few days. They may be flushed by rain into the water bodies, but this occurs largely during rainy seasons when snail populations may be low. Instead, during the dry seasons, faeces containing eggs may reach water by a variety of means: by washing of soiled clothes, by washing the anal region after defaecation, on cattle hooves or chicken claws, or even by dogs that drink water after eating faeces. None of these methods is particularly efficient, but the reproductive capacity of the organism is such that transmission is very adequately maintained even if only a small number of eggs hatch and go on to infect snails.

In many circumstances, and in particular in communities that have been settled for some generations in endemic areas, the parasite and its human host have reached a state of relative equilibrium; transmission continues, but at fairly low levels, and severe disease may be uncommon. This has led to the view, recently expressed, that schistosomiasis is a disease of minor public-health importance. However, this is an over-optimistic attitude. The increasing pressure on land usage, resulting from overpopulation, that is occurring throughout much of the tropics leads continuously to attempts to develop new land for agricultural purposes. Such attempts frequently involve water development projects, including the construction of dams and other large or small irrigation schemes. Such projects, in turn, frequently lead to the creation of conditions that are ideal for transmission of schistosomiasis; and, as immigrants to such schemes, or migrant workers employed on a temporary basis, may come from non-endemic areas, they rapidly acquire heavy and clinically severe infections. Historically, the most serious example of this was the increase in schistosomiasis in Egypt that followed the changes in irrigation practices associated with the expansion of the cotton industry and with the construction of the low and high dams at Aswan in the 1930s and 1960s, respectively. However, there have been many more recent examples. These include the high prevalence of severe schistosomiasis seen in large-scale irrigation schemes, such as the Gezira in the Sudan; other smaller but equally severe situations, such as the epidemic of schistosomiasis recently observed in the town of Richard Toll in Senegal, following the construction in 1986 of a barrage across the Senegal River; and the very common situation that is seen following settlement by individual families of new, semiarid areas. In Africa in particular, schistosomiasis remains a disease of considerable public-health, as well as individual, importance.

Pathogenesis and clinical features

Although there are individual differences, especially in the anatomical location and hence the clinical consequences of the lesions, the underlying pathology is similar for all species of schistosome. Four main phases can be identified, which are associated respectively with: (i) invasion of the skin by cercariae, and the subsequent migration of schistosomula through the lungs; (ii) maturation of the adult worms, and early egg laying; (iii) established infection, with disease mainly attributable to the granulomatous reactions around the deposited eggs; and (iv) late infection, with irreversible lesions caused by extensive fibrosis of the granulomata and the surrounding tissues.

STAGE OF INVASION: CERCARIAL DERMATITIS

Penetration of the skin by cercariae, both of species that cause human disease and of avian or other 'non-human' schistosomes, can be associated with a dermatitis (cercarial dermatitis or 'swimmer's itch'). In the case of the non-human schistosomes, cercarial dermatitis can occur after primary exposure as well as after re-exposure, and is associated with the death of cercariae in the skin; it may be observed both in areas endemic for human schistosomiasis and in non-endemic regions, such as Western Australia and the Great Lakes of Canada. In the case of the human schistosomes, mainly *S. mansoni* and *S. japonicum*, dermatitis follows re-exposure in older and putatively immune individuals. A transient immediate hypersensitivity reaction that occurs 10 to 15 min after exposure is followed by a more prolonged, delayed reaction, which develops after 12 to 24 h and may persist for up to 15 days. The lesion is characterized by a small, red, pruritic, macular rash, which progresses to papules, possibly accompanied by vesicle formation and oedema. Pustules may form if secondary infection occurs, and residual pigmentation may persist for months. The differential diagnosis is from conditions such as contact dermatitis, exposure to poison ivy, scabies, impetigo, and insect bites. The distinguishing features are a history of exposure to potentially infective water, followed by the development within 24 h of an intensely pruritic rash whose distribution corresponds to those parts of the body that were immersed. Treatment of the dermatitis itself is usually unnecessary, although topical corticosteroid creams or oral or parenteral antihistamines can be used.

The subsequent migration of schistosomula through the lungs to the liver, a few days after exposure, can be associated with transient fever, cough and pulmonary infiltrates, as well as myalgia and abdominal pain. This stage is difficult to identify, although there is commonly an eosinophilia.

STAGE OF MATURATION: ACUTE SCHISTOSOMIASIS

The development of adult worms during the first 5 weeks after infection, and thereafter the early stages of egg deposition, can be associated with a severe, systemic reaction resembling serum sickness. This syndrome of 'acute schistosomiasis', which can be fatal, is most commonly seen with *S. japonicum* infection, in which it is referred to as Katayama fever, and in which it can occur in both newly exposed and re-exposed individuals. Acute disease in schistosomiasis japonica can reach epidemic proportions: in 1950, for example, in one village of 7000 people in Jiangsu province in China, 1335 individuals died of acute infection. It is also seen, although less commonly, in *S. mansoni* infection, especially in individuals who are newly exposed to infection for the first time as adults. It is uncommon in *S. haematobium* infection.

The presenting symptoms of acute schistosomiasis include fever, rigors, sweating, headache, malaise, muscular aches, profound weakness, an unproductive, irritating cough, abdominal pain or swelling, nausea, vomiting, diarrhoea, and loss of weight. Physical signs include pyrexia (intermittent or remittent with evening peaks), oedema, a generalized soft lymphadenopathy, a tender enlarged liver, possibly with jaundice, a slightly enlarged and soft spleen, and some chest signs. Patients may also become confused or stuporose, or show visual impairment or papilloedema. Severe central-nervous manifestations can also occur and are discussed separately below.

The differential diagnosis includes other infections, such as typhoid, brucellosis, infectious mononucleosis, miliary tuberculosis, invasive ankylostomiasis, strongyloidiasis, visceral larva migrans and trichinosis, and non-infectious conditions such as sarcoidosis and the connective tissue disorders. A leucocytosis with an eosinophilia of 10 to 75 per cent alerts one to the possibility of a helminth infection, while total IgE, IgM, and IgG levels and antischistosome antibodies are elevated at an early stage. Eggs become detectable in the faeces about 6 weeks after exposure.

The aetiology of acute schistosomiasis remains somewhat obscure. It usually develops at about the time that egg laying starts, and is associated with massive and florid granulomatous reactions around eggs deposited in the tissues. However, the syndrome may also precede egg laying, developing as early as 9 to 13 days after exposure; in this case, it may be associated with reactions to maturing worms as they die, and with the formation and systemic deposition of immune complexes.

STAGE OF ESTABLISHED INFECTION

This is the stage that is commonly observed in children living in endemic areas. The main pathogenic event, which has been extensively studied in animal models of schistosome infection, is a cellular, granulomatous reaction around eggs deposited in the tissues (Fig. 11). In *S. mansoni* and *S. haematobium* infections, the egg granuloma is a T lymphocyte-mediated process of a delayed hypersensitivity type, and is composed of lymphocytes and macrophages, with also a high percentage of eosinophils. Recent evidence suggests a major role for tumour necrosis factor-α in the induction of the granuloma. As is the case in other conditions, such as leprosy, the granuloma, as well as causing host tissue damage and disease, may also serve to protect the host against the more deleterious effects of toxic egg products, which, in animals that are deprived of T cells and that fail to mount a granulomatous reaction to *S. mansoni* eggs, cause extensive necrosis of hepatic parenchymal cells and more severe disease. In *S. japonicum* infection the local formation of immune complexes at the site of egg deposition is also an important pathogenic event.

The clinical manifestations of granuloma formation depend on the anatomical location of the lesions, and hence on the species of parasite. In *S. haematobium* infection, eggs are deposited mainly in the bladder and the lower end of the urinary tract (although the few that are deposited in the rectum can aid in diagnosis through rectal biopsy). Schistosomal cystitis is associated with varying degrees of hypogastric discomfort, suprapubic pain, frequency, dysuria, haematuria, proteinuria, and pyuria. The pyuria is typically abacterial, and becomes bacterial only after invasive investigations such as cystoscopy or after obstructive uropathy has developed. The haematuria is characteristically terminal, due to involvement of the trigone of the bladder. The prevalence and severity of the haematuria are related to the intensity of egg output, and in communities in which *S. haematobium* infection is heavily endemic, haematuria among boys is still considered to be part of the normal process of maturation. In addition, ureteric obstruction may occur as a consequence of granulomatous reactions to eggs in either the ureters or the bladder; in contrast to the later, chronic lesions associated with fibrosis, these acute lesions usually reverse spontaneously after antischistosomal chemotherapy, leaving little residual damage.

In *S. mansoni* and *S. japonicum* infections, eggs are deposited and granulomata form in the intestines, mainly the large intestine, and the liver. This stage is very frequently asymptomatic: this is a potential danger, as the condition can pass unnoticed until the stage of irreversible complications. Classical symptoms develop in a minority of individuals with heavy infections, and include hypogastric pain, diarrhoea, and the passage of blood or mucus in the stool. The liver, especially the left lobe, may be enlarged and tender; the spleen may also be enlarged, but is usually soft. At this stage, before fibrosis has developed, the condition is entirely reversible by specific antischistosome treatment.

Fig. 11 Granulomatous reaction around an egg of *S. mansoni* in the liver.

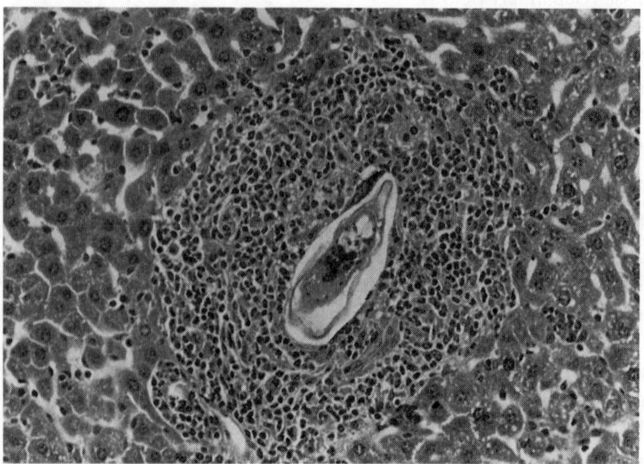

STAGE OF LATE INFECTION AND SEQUELAE

Two opposing processes govern the subsequent progression of disease in untreated individuals. On the one hand, egg deposition is diminished, as the worm burden declines in older individuals; it has also been suggested that there is a suppression of egg output by female worms in older individuals, although the evidence that this occurs in man is still uncertain. In addition, those eggs that are newly deposited elicit smaller granulomata and less severe tissue reactions than those that are deposited early in infection. This phenomenon, which has been referred to as 'modulation', has been variously attributed to the action of suppressor T cells, of non-specific macrophage-derived factors, and of either T cells or antibodies with anti-idiotypic specificity. On the other hand, although some granulomata from the early stages of infection may resolve entirely as the egg dies, others may progress to fibrosis. It is this fibrosis, which is also a T cell-dependent event attributable to the release of soluble mediators, that is responsible for the severe late sequelae of infection. It is for this reason that it is important to treat established infections in young children, even if they are asymptomatic.

Individuals vary considerably in their propensity to develop late sequelae, for reasons that are still poorly understood. Intensity and duration of infection are major determinants, but other factors are also involved. These include particularly the genetic background of the host. In studies in Brazil and St Lucia it has been found that people of black African origin are less likely to develop severe hepatosplenic disease from *S. mansoni* infection than are Caucasians or people of Asian origin; this may account in part for the low prevalence of severe schistosomiasis mansoni in endemic communities in Africa south of the Sahara, and for the high incidence of severe disease among Caucasian visitors to an endemic area. The nature of the genetic factors involved remains unclear, although some studies suggest an HLA association: in Egypt, HLA-A1 and -B5 have been associated with severe hepatosplenic schistosomiasis mansoni, while in the case of *S. japonicum* infection, HLA-DR and -DQ have been implicated in the differential regulation of immune responses to egg antigens. In addition, apart from host genetic constitution, other factors that may contribute to the presence or absence

Fig. 12 Intravenous pyelogram in a patient with obstructive uropathy due to chronic *S. haematobium* infection (photograph by courtesy of Dr D. Ndlovu, Harare, Zimbabwe).

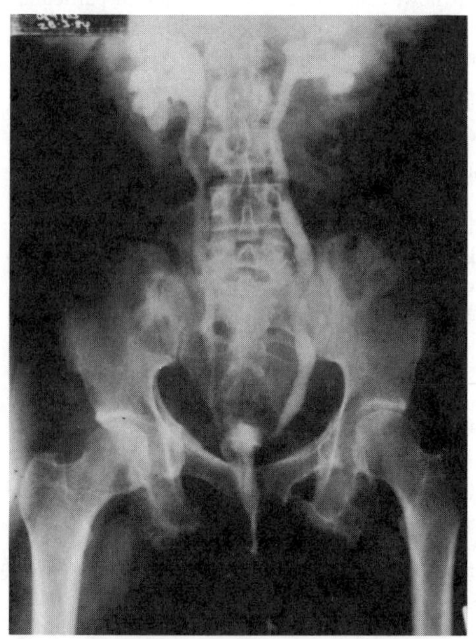

of severe disease may include parasite strain differences; maternal infection status, in that offspring of infected mothers may be primed to mount a 'modulated' type of response at first infection; nutritional status; and interactions with other infections, including particularly malaria, hepatitis, and other intestinal helminths.

In urinary schistosomiasis, the common late complication, and the reason why the infection is of clinical and public-health importance, is an irreversible obstructive uropathy (Fig. 12), which can progress to uraemia. Calculus formation is common, as is secondary infection, usually due to *Escherichia coli*, or *Pseudomonas, Klebsiella, Enterobacter*, or *Salmonella* spp. Various changes occur in the bladder, including calcification, ulceration, and papillomas, while at cystoscopy 'sandy patches', composed of large numbers of eggs surrounded by dense fibrous tissue with an atrophic mucosal surface, are characteristically seen in the bladder walls. As the bladder lesions develop, there may be symptoms of nocturia, precipitancy, retention of urine, dribbling, and severe pain. The ureters are less heavily and less frequently affected than the bladder, but their involvement is an important cause of chronic morbidity; bilateral ureteric involvement is common, although lesions may predominate more on one side. The ureteric pathology is usually asymptomatic, but may lead to ureteric colic. An association has also been described between *S. haematobium* infection and the development of squamous cell carcinoma of the bladder. In Africa and the Middle East, in contrast to Europe and North America, carcinoma of the bladder is one of the more common malignant tumours, accounting (in one study) for 27 per cent of all tumours in Egypt, and affecting young and middle-aged adults. Causality is not proven, but is suggested by the finding that the prevalence of carcinoma of the bladder is correlated with the intensity of *S. haematobium* infection.

In *S. mansoni* and *S. japonicum* infections, the later stages present as either intestinal or hepatosplenic disease. Intestinal schistosomiasis is associated with granuloma formation, inflammation, fibrosis, and sometimes polyposis, primarily in the large intestine. The differential diagnosis includes irritable bowel syndrome, amoebiasis, giardiasis, other intestinal helminths, ulcerative colitis, Crohn's disease, and tuberculosis, as well as malignancies. In schistosomiasis mansoni, there is intermittent diarrhoea, with or without the passage of blood or mucus; the colon may be tender. In between the episodes of diarrhoea, the stools are normal. Polyposis coli occurs mainly in Egypt, and is a more severe syndrome with bloody diarrhoea, severe anaemia, a protein-losing enteropathy, and ascites. In schistosomiasis japonica, the stomach may also be involved, with gastric bleeding and pyloric obstruction. In both infections, involvement of the small intestine is rare.

Fig. 13 Kenyan child with severe hepatosplenic schistosomiasis mansoni.

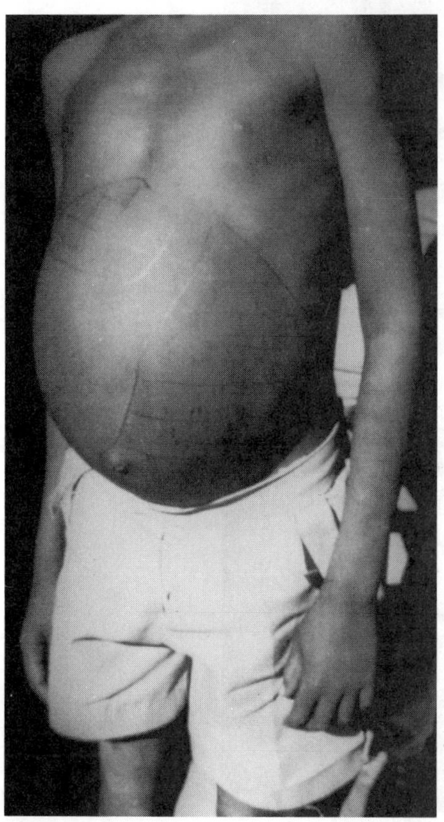

Hepatosplenic disease is the most severe chronic manifestation of both *S. mansoni* and *S. japonicum* infection (Fig. 13). The characteristic lesion in the liver is a presinusoidal periportal fibrosis referred to as Symmers' or 'clay pipe stem' fibrosis (so called because it resembles an old-fashioned clay pipe in cross-section, with a thick white wall and a narrow lumen). Typically, there is no bridging between the fibrous tracts and no nodule formation or hepatic parenchymal cell damage; in fact, hepatic function usually remains normal. The liver is usually enlarged, but may be of normal size or even shrunken. The presinusoidal fibrosis leads to portal hypertension, and the spleen is enlarged due to chronic passive congestion and reticuloendothelial hyperplasia. The condition develops insidiously, and usually presents during the second or third decades of life. The patients may be asymptomatic, or may complain of a left hypochondrial mass with discomfort, fullness, and anorexia. During the early stages, the liver is enlarged, especially the left lobe, smooth, firm and sometimes tender; later, it becomes hard and nodular, and may decrease in size. The spleen is enlarged, often massively, and is firm, smooth, and non-tender. There may be evidence of anaemia, and ascites also occurs, especially in *S. japonicum* infection: this is attributable both to the portal hypertension and to hypoalbuminaemia, resulting from either intestinal loss, or renal loss in the nephrotic syndrome, or reduced synthesis. There may be reduced growth, infantilism, amenorrhoea, or loss of libido, depending on age and sex. Evidence of hepatic dysfunction is not common, except where there is associated hepatitis B infection or after repeated gastrointestinal bleeding ('decompensated' hepatosplenic disease). Most important, 80 per cent of individuals with hepatosplenic schistosomiasis have oesophageal varices detectable by endoscopy; there may also be periumbilical or 'Medusa head' collaterals.

The most severe, and potentially fatal, complication of hepatosplenic schistosomiasis is bleeding from oesophageal varices leading to haematemesis, melaena, or both. Blood loss is frequently massive, and exsanguination is the usual cause of death rather than hepatic coma. Repeated episodes of gastrointestinal bleeding, preceding a terminal event, are characteristic.

The differential diagnosis of hepatosplenic schistosomiasis includes kala-azar (visceral leishmaniasis) and the tropical splenomegaly syndrome associated with recurrent malaria, as well as leukaemia, lymphoma, and alcoholic or viral cirrhosis.

OTHER MANIFESTATIONS

Central nervous system

This is a serious complication that may be more common than was previously thought, especially in acute infection with *S. mansoni* or *S. haematobium*. For example, in one study in Kenya, 15 out of 18 expatriate students who acquired schistosomiasis mansoni while swimming developed acute central-nervous disease, of whom two developed paraplegia. In a further study from Brazil, five cases of paraplegia were described among 26 members of (separate) swimming parties who developed acute schistosomiasis. In *S. mansoni* and *S. haematobium* infections, lesions are most frequently observed in the spinal cord following acute infection; a myelopathy results from the inflammatory reaction that accompanies the deposition of eggs in venules in and around the spinal cord. An eosinophilic pleocytosis may be detected in the cerebrospinal fluid, and myelography and computerized tomographic or magnetic resonance scans are of value, in addition to a history of exposure and the detection of faecal eggs. In contrast, although cerebral lesions can also occur with chronic *S. mansoni* infection, they are usually more common in chronic *S. japonicum* infections, in which they often present as focal epilepsy.

Although a paraparesis is seen most commonly during acute schistosomiasis due to *S. mansoni* (and rarely *S. haematobium*), it may also be a late complication of *S. mansoni* in endemic areas with heavy worm loads. Like most schistosomal lesions there are vascular and granulomatous changes. In the acute cases these are seen on MRI scans as diffuse swelling of the lumbar cord with central softening or cyst formation. In the late chronic cases the presentation is more that of a slowly developing space-occupying lesion, usually in the region of the cauda equina.

Pulmonary

Deposition of eggs can also occur in the lungs. This is particularly seen as a complication of hepatosplenic schistosomiasis, in which the opening of portosystemic collaterals allows the passage of large numbers of eggs from the portal vein directly to the lungs, bypassing the liver. Granulomatous reactions and fibrosis develop in the pulmonary vasculature, together with arteritis, medial hypertrophy, and diffuse intimal arteriolar proliferation, leading to pulmonary hypertension and/or cor pulmonale. Symptoms include fatigue, palpitations, dyspnoea on exertion, cough and occasional haemoptysis, with electrocardiographic and echographic abnormalities. Patients may progress to decompensation with congestive cardiac failure, or sudden death may follow cardiovascular collapse.

Renal

Renal lesions commonly occur in chronic *S. mansoni* infection in Brazil, especially in those with hepatosplenic disease, and consist of a chronic glomerulonephritis with deposition in the mesangial area of immunoglobulins, complement components, and schistosome antigens. The condition may present as the nephrotic syndrome, as hypertension, or as simple proteinuria, and appears to develop only slowly, perhaps 10 or more years after the onset of hepatosplenic disease. A similar condition has been reported from Egypt, especially when *S. mansoni* infection is associated with chronic persistent salmonella bacteraemia. It has been suggested that, in this association, the adult schistosomes serve as a reservoir of salmonella; although antibiotic therapy is effective, the bacteraemia frequently recurs unless the underlying schistosome infection is also treated.

Miscellaneous

Various other complications of infection with one or other schistosome species have also been described or suggested, including an endocrine presentation resembling hypopituitarism, due to diminished levels of somatomedins; chronic dermatitis, due to ectopic eggs; musculoskeletal involvement, including an inflammatory polyarthritis, in schistosomiasis mansoni; osteomalacia in schistosomiasis haematobium, resulting from tubular lesions in association with obstructive uropathy; and lesions of the uterine cervix resembling carcinoma of the cervix.

S. intercalatum infection usually presents with diarrhoea. *S. mekongi* infection is usually asymptomatic but may produce a clinical picture similar to that of *S. japonicum*.

Diagnosis and investigations

The key features in the individual diagnosis of infection are a history of exposure to potentially contaminated water (especially in travellers recently returned to temperate countries from an endemic area) and the qualitative demonstration of viable eggs in the excreta. In addition, in epidemiological studies, it is usually necessary to obtain a quantitative estimate of egg output. In the case of *S. haematobium*, this can be achieved by collecting urine at a fixed time of day, usually midday (because egg excretion shows a diurnal variation), and passing a known volume (usually 10 ml) through polycarbonate (Nuclepore®) or polyamide (Nytrel®) membranes held in an appropriate filter support, followed by microscopical examination of the membrane and counting of eggs. In *S. mansoni* and *S. japonicum* infections the method usually adopted now is the Kato thick-smear technique. A stool sample is collected and passed through a wire-mesh sieve to remove large, particulate material. Portions of 50 mg of the sieved material are dispensed, with the aid of a metal template, on to microscope slides, and pressed out under coverslips of cellophane previously soaked in a glycerol solution. After leaving for 6 to 24 h to allow the preparation to clear, all the eggs on the slide are counted. The main problem in obtaining quantitative estimates of schistosome infection is the degree of variation between different samples. This problem, which is particular severe in *S. haematobium* and *S. japonicum* infections (in which eggs are deposited and excreted in clumps), may be partially overcome by collecting repeated samples on three to five occasions. Intensity of infection is expressed either as an absolute figure (eggs per 10 ml of urine or per gram of faeces) or as a series of strata (for example, < 1, 1–100, 101–400, and > 400 eggs/10 ml).

In previously unexposed visitors to endemic areas, even light infections can cause significant morbidity and may be difficult to detect by examination of excreta. In this case, examination of a rectal biopsy for

Fig. 14 (a) Liver in a patient with hepatosplenic schistosomiasis mansoni, seen at laparoscopy; note the fibrous bands across an otherwise normal liver, and the dilated veins on the inner surface of the peritoneum. (b) Enlarged spleen in a patient with hepatosplenic schistosomiasis mansoni, seen at laparoscopy; note the dilated veins on the inner surface of the peritoneum. (Photographs by courtesy of Dr A. Wiles, Harare, Zimbabwe.)

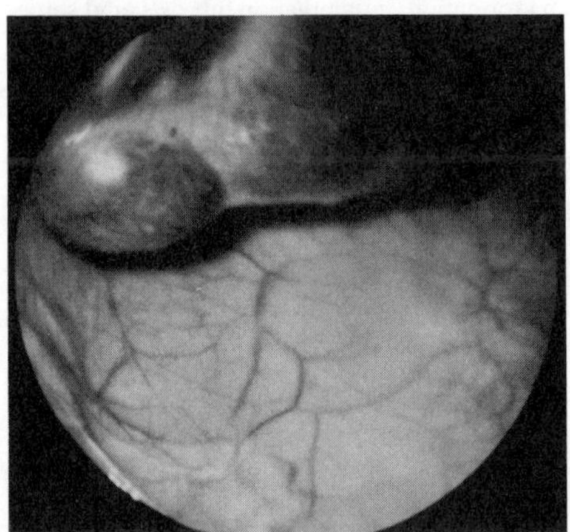

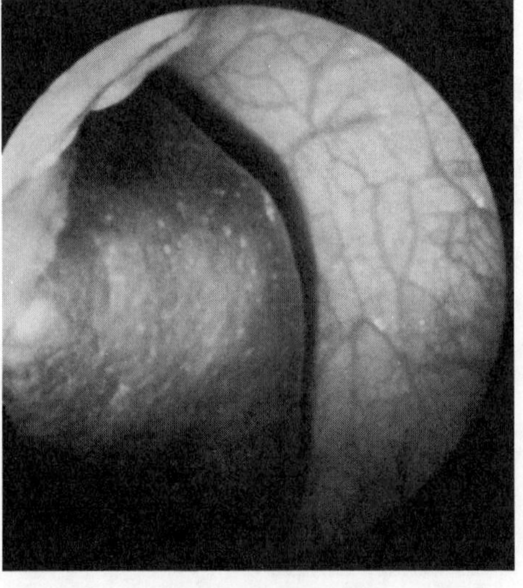

intact eggs may prove more sensitive; it can be positive in both intestinal and urinary schistosomiasis.

Immunological tests for schistosomiasis can be useful, but have not replaced the identification of viable eggs as the 'gold standard'. A wide variety of assays for the detection of antischistosome antibodies has been developed, often based on enzyme immunoassay or immunofluorescence. The sensitivity and specificity of such tests are variable, and depend on the nature of the antigen employed: at present, a crude egg-antigen extract (SEA) or a purified component of this extract (CEF6) give the best results, although various recombinant antigens are becoming available. These tests can be particularly useful in, for example, the screening of expatriates who have recently returned home from an endemic region. However, a major problem with such tests, when used in endemic areas, is that they do not distinguish between current active infection and previous infection that has either resolved spontaneously (following death of adult worms) or been removed by chemotherapy. Instead, therefore, considerable attention is being paid at present to the development of tests based on the detection of circulating antigens, in particular a circulating anodic antigen (CAA) that is released from the gut of the adult worm. These tests have two advantages. First, they depend on the presence of active, current infection, and can therefore be used, for example, to monitor the effect of chemotherapy in either the individual or the community. Secondly, they provide a direct measure of the adult worm burden, thereby overcoming the potential problems that egg output by female worms may be temporarily or permanently suppressed, or that eggs are being retained in the tissues rather than excreted. Such tests are not available for general use at the time of writing, but are likely to become widely available during the next few years.

Additional diagnostic tools are useful in epidemiological studies and in large-scale control programmes. These include, for *S. haematobium*, the use of reagent strips to detect haematuria and proteinuria as criteria for treatment, thereby obviating the need for microscopy; and, in all the species, the use of portable ultrasonographic equipment to make field investigations of the levels of disease in a community. This very valuable technique has been used for several years in urinary schistosomiasis; it has only recently been introduced in intestinal schistosomiasis, in particular for the detection of hepatic fibrosis, in which it is offering a much needed objectivity to the assessment of morbidity and its reversibility by chemotherapy.

In the individual a variety of additional procedures may be required, depending on the type of disease observed. In the investigation of chronic urinary schistosomiasis, for example, these may include intravenous pyelography and computerized tomography, as well as ultrasonography. In the central-nervous manifestations of acute schistosomiasis, the intensity of infection may be too low for eggs to be detected in the excreta; in this case, the simultaneous demonstration of antibodies in the serum and cerebrospinal fluid is of value. In chronic intestinal schistosomiasis, sigmoidoscopy and barium enema may help in determining the severity of disease. In hepatosplenic disease, apart from ultrasonography and fibreoptic endoscopy, investigations may include laparoscopy (Fig. 14) and splenoportography. Percutaneous liver biopsies do not yield enough material to allow the diagnosis of Symmers' fibrosis in most patients and, if it is important to exclude other causes of hepatic fibrosis, surgical biopsies are more reliable.

Treatment and prognosis

During the last 15 years, the treatment of schistosomiasis has been radically altered by the introduction of new drugs that are both effective and safe. Originally, trivalent antimony compounds, such as antimony sodium tartrate, were the only effective medication against all species of schistosome, but they had to be given by injection over long periods, and they caused much toxicity, numerous side-effects, and sometimes death. Subsequently, lucanthone was introduced as the first oral preparation active against *S. haematobium* but, like the purified derivative hycanthone, which was given by intramuscular injection, it had severe side-effects. Niridazole, an oral preparation related to metronidazole, was active against all species of parasite but caused severe mental disorders, especially in those with advanced liver involvement.

The use of all these drugs has been discontinued, although references to them may be found even in quite recent literature. Subsequently, two drugs were introduced that are still sometimes used. Metrifonate is an inexpensive organophosphorus compound that is active only against *S. haematobium* and that can be given orally. It has few side-effects, including rare cholinergic symptoms, and its main disadvantage is that it has to be given in widely spaced doses (usually 7.5 mg/kg body weight, once every 2 weeks on up to three occasions each year). This can be a large problem, in particular in national control programmes. In some circumstances, however, the low cost of the drug may outweigh this disadvantage. Oxamniquine (Vansil) is active only against *S. mansoni*; it is presented either as a capsule or as a paediatric syrup, and again has to be given in divided doses at intervals of 12 to 24 h, the total dose varying according to the geographical location and ranging from 15 mg/kg (West Africa and South America) to 60 mg/kg (southern Africa, Egypt, and Sudan). It is not recommended for use in early pregnancy. Its main disadvantage is that it can cause severe dizziness, as well as epileptiform convulsions, in a small minority of individuals. It was extensively used in a national control programme in Brazil in the late 1970s, where there was evidence for the emergence of drug resistance.

More recently, both of these drugs have tended to be replaced by praziquantel (e.g. Biltricide). This is a bitter-tasting, pyrazino-isoquinolinone compound, presented as a tablet, that is highly effective against all schistosome species when given orally, as well as against other trematodes and adult cestodes. Complete cure is achieved in up to 85 per cent of treated individuals; in those who are not cured, egg counts are reduced by 95 per cent or more. In endemic areas, this level of efficacy is acceptable, as very light residual infections do not lead to severe morbidity, and as the development of immunity to new infections may in fact be assisted by the continued presence of a few adult worms. A single dose of 40 mg/kg is usually sufficient for *S. mansoni* and *S. haematobium* infections; for *S. japonicum*, especially heavy infections, a total of 60 mg/kg, given in three doses at intervals of 4 h or two doses at intervals of 6 to 48 h, is preferable. In patients who are not cured by the initial treatment the same dose can be repeated at weekly intervals for 2 weeks, or on two successive days. Although not teratogenic, it is not recommended for use in the first trimester of pregnancy. Otherwise there are no contraindications. A minute proportion of the total maternal dose (less than 0.003 per cent) is excreted in milk and so breast feeding may be regarded as safe. The drug is well tolerated, and can be given without supervision. Side-effects include abdominal pain, which occurs in about 10 per cent of treated individuals, is related to intensity of infection, probably reflects the death of adult worms, and resolves spontaneously over some hours; treatment is rarely required. Urticarial skin reactions and periorbital oedema may occur in about 2 per cent of treated individuals; again, this disappears spontaneously over a matter of days. General side-effects including headache, dizziness, fever, and fatigue also occur. There have been no definitive reports of the development of drug resistance. In experimental animal models, praziquantel acts synergistically with the immune system in killing the parasite (by exposing antigenic determinants that subsequently form a target for antibody-mediated attack), but there is no good evidence yet that this occurs in man. The only serious disadvantage of praziquantel is its relatively high cost, which may cause difficulties in large-scale national control programmes that have access to only limited hard currency.

Apart from the specific treatment of the schistosome infection, additional measures are required for the management of particular conditions. In acute schistosomiasis, the addition of corticosteroid treatment to specific antischistosomal therapy with oxamniquine or praziquantel has been found to be beneficial. This needs to be initiated early, especially if there is evidence of transverse myelitis. The use of praziquantel in the treatment of cerebral schistosomiasis in *S. japonicum* infections is safe and effective, leading to rapid dissipation of cerebral oedema and resolution of cerebral masses.

The management of schistosomal portal hypertension, and the management or prevention of bleeding from oesophageal varices, is controversial and beyond the scope of this chapter; the reader is referred to reviews by Lambertucci and by Davis in Jordan *et al.* (1993). In brief, available options include: (i) endoscopic sclerotherapy; (ii) portasystemic shunts, among which distal splenorenal shunts are preferred; (iii) surgical devascularization; and (iv) β-adrenergic blockade with drugs such as propranolol or nadolol. Patients with schistosomal oesophageal varices who have not previously bled have an estimated 30 per cent lifetime chance of bleeding, which varies according to the size of the varices and the functional state of the liver. Depending on these factors, endoscopic sclerotherapy may be considered; and, in a meta-analysis of earlier studies, a significant reduction has been demonstrated in initial bleeding in patients receiving β-blockers. However, a problem with β-blockers is that their long-term administration under field conditions may be difficult or impossible. Patients who have already bled have an estimated 70 per cent chance of rebleeding. Endoscopic sclerotherapy should be considered as the initial measure; if this fails, due to ulceration or rebleeding, then either a shunting procedure or surgical devascularization may be undertaken. β-Blockade has not been shown to have a significant effect in preventing rebleeding, but does reduce mortality in patients who also have cirrhosis.

The prognosis of schistosomiasis depends on the species, the intensity of infection, and the stage at which the infection is detected and treated. In a majority of infected individuals, infection remains asymptomatic or mild, even in the absence of treatment. However, the minority of individuals who do develop morbidity is sufficiently great, at the level of the community and of the national health structure, that both treatment of infected individuals and attempts at control are usually warranted (see below). Acute schistosomiasis can be fatal, or can leave to severe residual damage to the central nervous system, but responds well to antischistosomal therapy with steroids if started sufficiently early. Early infections respond extremely well to antischistosomal therapy, leaving little or no residual damage, the main problem being that, if treatment (especially of young children) is carried out only at the individual level, the patient will rapidly become re-exposed and reinfected unless control measures are undertaken at the community level. Late infections with fibrosis respond less well to specific antischistosomal therapy (although, for example, some regression of hepatosplenic disease after treatment has been claimed); the main purpose of treatment at this stage is to prevent the further progression of disease, while the consequences of fibrosis are managed in other ways.

Prevention and control

Individual protection against infection is achieved by avoiding contact with all potentially contaminated fresh water in endemic areas; for example, by wearing boots and other waterproof clothing. Such water should be boiled before drinking, or left to stand for at least 2 days before use for other purposes such as washing. Should contact with water occur, the skin should be immediately rubbed vigorously with a towel; the water should not be allowed to evaporate, as this aids cercarial penetration. Soap and alcohol also kill cercariae, and cercaricidal barrier creams can be used.

Thus, prevention of infection in occasional visitors to an endemic area is relatively straightforward, provided that contact with water is not a necessary part of their work (e.g., members of armed forces) or recreation (e.g., fishing, swimming or sailing). However, in most endemic regions, the local residents do not have the luxury of being able to avoid contact with water; it is a necessary part of their daily activities. In such regions, the control of schistosomiasis is extremely difficult, and requires a many-pronged and integrated attack at the community level. This sort of integrated approach has a long history of success, since its early application in Venezuela in the 1940s, and subsequently in Japan (where transmission of *S. japonicum* no longer occurs) and China. The methods used may be either specific for schistosomiasis (such as chemotherapy and snail control) or non-specific, affecting a variety of water-borne diseases (such as sanitation, clean water supplies, and health education). They may be delivered through centrally organized, 'vertical', national control programmes with a highly hierarchical structure, but the preference nowadays is for 'horizontal' programmes, organized through primary health-care services at the community level. It is also worth noting that emphasis is now given to control, rather than to eradication, of infection. Because morbidity develops primarily in the most heavily infected individuals, the aim is to reduce the mean intensity of infection in a community to levels at which significant morbidity does not occur.

Since the introduction of modern drugs, especially praziquantel, the main tool for control has been community-based chemotherapy, which can be delivered in a variety of ways. Mass chemotherapy involves the treatment of all individuals in those communities in which prevalence reaches a given level, without diagnosis of individual infections. This approach, which has been extensively used in a national control programme in Brazil, has the advantage eliminating the labour and costs involved in diagnosis. However, this may be outweighed by the high cost, often in foreign hard currency, of drugs. An alternative approach is selective chemotherapy of individuals with previously diagnosed infection. This may involve treatment of either all infected individuals in a community or, in a further attempt to reduce drug costs, particular groups in the community. For example, treatment may be given to those with heavy infections, as they are the ones who may go on to develop severe illness. An alternative approach, which has proved valuable, is to concentrate on children, by conducting both diagnosis and treatment in the primary schools rather than in the wider community; this group of primary schoolchildren usually includes the most heavily infected members of the community, as well as those who contribute most to transmission.

An advantage of chemotherapy as a control measure is that, in addition to reducing transmission, it has an immediate impact on infection and illness in individual patients. However, other methods of reducing transmission are also valuable. In particular, snail control through the use of molluscicides such as niclosamide has a long history and, although it has recently been somewhat disparaged, has a useful role in certain circumstances; in particular, in large irrigation schemes in which molluscicides can be applied at a limited number of sites, and in rural areas in which molluscicides can be applied focally, and therefore cheaply, only at the appropriate times of year to those limited sites that actually contain infected snails. In addition, although biological control of snail populations by competitors and predators has had little practical application, environmental control of snail populations (for example, by periodic desiccation) is widely used. The provision of clean water supplies and sanitation is a desirable ideal, and inexpensive approaches (such as the use of boreholes and standpipes, and the provision of washing and laundry units) can be effective. Finally, a key element in any control programme is the close involvement of the community, with extensive health education, especially of children.

These measures, especially when appropriately applied in an integrated programme, can be very effective and have contributed to a successful reduction in schistosome morbidity in many endemic areas. However, a complete solution to the problem has not yet been reached. In particular, transmission may be reduced, but is rarely completely interrupted; reinfection after chemotherapy therefore occurs, especially in the younger, non-immune children. Control programmes therefore have to be continued indefinitely, with surveillance and retreatment being required at frequent intervals, perhaps every 1 to 4 years, and this may place excessive strain on national health budgets. New control measures are therefore still being sought, among which there are reasonable prospects for vaccination in the foreseeable future. Recombinant vaccine antigens have been prepared and tested in experimental animal models, and are awaiting development for clinical trials.

REFERENCES

Amiri, P. *et al.* (1992). Tumour necrosis factor alpha restores granulomas and induces parasite egg-laying in schistosome-infected SCID mice. *Nature*, **356,** 604–7.

Anderson, R.M. and May, R.M. (1985). Helminth infections of humans: mathematical models, population dynamics and control. *Advances in Parasitology*, **24,** 1–101.

Boros, D.L. (1986). Immunoregulation of granuloma formation in murine schistosomiasis. *Annals of the New York Academy of Sciences*, **465,** 313–23.

Boros, D.L., Pelley, R.P., and Warren, K.S. (1975). Spontaneous modulation of granulomatous hypersensitivity in schistosomiasis mansoni. *Journal of Immunology*, **114,** 1437–41.

Capron, M., and Capron, A. (1994). Immunoglobulin E and effector cells in schistosomiasis. *Science*, **264,** 1876–7.

Chen, M.G. and Mott, K.E. (1989). Progress in assessment of morbidity due to *Schistosoma haematobium* infection. A review of the recent literature. *Tropical Diseases Bulletin*, **86,** R1–36.

Colley, D.G. *et al.* (1986). Immune responses during human schistosomiasis. XII. Differential responsiveness in patients with hepatosplenic disease. *American Journal of Tropical Medicine and Hygiene*, **35,** 793–802.

de Jonge, N., Boerman, O.C., and Deelder, A.M. (1989). Time-resolved immunofluorometric assay (TR-IFMA) for the detection of the schistosome circulating anodic antigen. *Transactions of the Royal Society of Tropical Medicine and Hygiene*, **83,** 659–63.

Demeure, C.E. *et al.* (1993). Resistance to *Schistosoma mansoni* in humans: influence of the IgE/IgE4 balance and IgG2 in immunity to reinfection after chemotherapy. *Journal of Infectious Diseases*, **168,** 1000–8.

Dunne, D.W. *et al.* (1992). Immunity after treatment of human schistosomiasis mansoni: association between IgE antibodies to adult worm antigens and resistance to reinfection. *European Journal of Immunology*, **22,** 1483–94.

Farley, J. (1991). *Bilharzia: a history of imperial tropical medicine*. Cambridge University Press.

Fulford, A.J.C., Butterworth, A.E., Sturrock, R.F., and Ouma, J.H. (1992). On the use of age-intensity data to detect immunity to parasitic infections, with special reference to *Schistosoma mansoni* in Kenya. *Parasitology*, **105,** 219–27.

Hagan, P., Blumenthal, U.J., Dunn, D., Simpson, A.J., and Wilkins, H.A. (1991). Human IgE, IgG4 and resistance to reinfection with *Schistosoma haematobium*. *Nature*, **349,** 243–5.

Homeida, M. *et al.* (1988). Diagnosis of pathologically-confirmed Symmers' periportal fibrosis by ultrasonography: a prospective blinded study. *American Journal of Tropical Medicine and Hygiene*, **38,** 86–91.

Jordan, P., Webbe, G., and Sturrock, R.F. (ed.) (1993). *Human schistosomiasis*. CAB International, Wallingford.

Lambertucci, J.R. (1989). A new approach to the treatment of acute schistosomiasis. *Memorias do Instituto Oswaldo Cruz*, **84,** 23–30.

Neves, J., Marinho, R.P., De Aranjo, P.K., and Raso, P. (1973). Spinal cord complications of acute schistosomiasis mansoni. *Transactions of the Royal Society of Tropical Medicine and Hygiene*, **67,** 782–92.

Parra, J.C. *et al.* (1991). Granulomatous hypersensitivity to *Schistosoma mansoni* egg antigens in human schistosomiasis. II. *In vitro* granuloma modulation induced by polyclonal antiidiotypic antibodies. *Journal of Immunology*, **147,** 3949–54.

Scrimgeour, E.M.T. (1991). Involvement of the central nervous system in *Schistosoma mansoni* and *Schistosoma haematobium* infection. *Brain*, **108,** 1023–38.

Siongok, T.K.A. *et al.* (1976). Morbidity in schistosomiasis mansoni in relation to intensity of infection: study of a community in Machakos, Kenya. *American Journal of Tropical Medicine and Hygiene*, **25,** 273–84.

Thomas, J.E., Bassett, M.T., Sigola, L.B., and Taylor, P. (1990). Relationship between bladder cancer incidence, *Schistosoma haematobium* infection, and geographical region of Zimbabwe. *Transactions of the Royal Society of Tropical Medicine and Hygiene*, **84,** 551–3.

World Health Organization (1985). *Report of a WHO expert committee: the control of schistosomiasis*, Technical Report Series No. 728. WHO, Geneva.

World Health Organization (1988). *Progress in assessment of morbidity due to* Schistosoma mansoni *infection: a review of recent literature*, WHO/Schisto/88-97, pp. 1–66 (distribution limited).

Wyler, D.J. (1992). Why does liver fibrosis occur in schistosomiasis? *Parasitology Today*, **8,** 277–9.

7.16.2 Liver fluke diseases of man

SWANGJAI PUNGPAK and DANAI BUNNAG

Flukes of the genera Opisthorchis, Clonorchis, Fasciola, and, rarely, Dicrocoelium infect the liver, or, more correctly, the biliary tract of man. *Opisthorchis viverrini, O. felineus*, and *Clonorchis sinensis*, the most important species, infect millions of people in Eastern Europe and the Far East, but most have no symptoms. Infection is usually recognized when ova are found in the stools during routine examination.

Table 1 lists species of liver fluke infecting human beings.

Opisthorchiasis

The causative agents, *O.viverrini* (Fig. 1(f)) and *O.felineus*, are similar in shape and arrangement of their internal organs.

The egg is yellowish brown and oval with an operculum resting on shoulders with, or without, a tubercle-like knob at the abopercular end (Fig. 2(b)). It contains a miracidium when laid. The ratio of length to breadth of *O.felineus* is about 3:1 (about 30 × 11 μm) and of *O.viverrini* approximately 2:1 (about 28 × 15 μm).

LIFECYCLE (FIG. 3)

The adult worms live in the distal bile ducts and gallbladder. Fully developed eggs are carried in the bile and passed out in faeces. On reaching water the eggs are eaten by snails, the first intermediate hosts, in which they hatch. In the snail the miracidia develop further through the stages of sporocyst, redia, and cercaria. The mature cercariae are released from the snail into the water after 6 to 8 weeks, and then penetrate the muscle of susceptible freshwater fish to develop into metacercariae. The metacercariae mature and reach an infective stage in 6 weeks. Consumption of infected fish results in infection of the definitive host. When the metacercariae are liberated by digestion, they enter the duodenum then migrate to the bile ducts, where they mature within 4 weeks and begin to produce eggs. The lifespan of these flukes is over 10 years.

The snail intermediate host for *O.felineus* is *Bithynia leachii* and for *O.viverrini, B.siamensis goniomphalus, B.funiculata*, and *B.siamensis siamensis (= B.leavis)*. Many species of cyprinoid fish or carp serve as second intermediate hosts in Central, East, and South Europe, Siberia, and South-East Asia. *Cyclocheilicthys siaja* is the most important in Thailand. Cats, dogs, and many fish-eating mammals are definitive hosts. Golden hamsters, mice, and guinea-pigs make good laboratory models.

EPIDEMIOLOGY

O.viverrini is endemic in northern and north-eastern Thailand, Laos, and Cambodia, while *O.felineus* has been reported from Central, East and South Europe, Siberia, and some areas of the Far East.

The prevalence of *O.viverrini* in Thailand has risen each year, and in 1991 it was estimated that about 8.7 million Thais harboured the fluke. This is explained by the rapid growth of the human population and increased number of snail and fish intermediate hosts. Development of water reservoirs and irrigation systems, lack of proper sanitation facilities, and the popular practice of consuming raw fish continue to provide suitable conditions for propagation of the infection. The prevalence in some villages is over 90 per cent. Even infants are infected, for mothers

Table 1 *Human liver flukes*

Species	Geographical distribution	Definitive hosts other than man	Source of infection	Size of adults (mm)	Size of ova (μm)
Clonorchis sinensis	Far East	Dog, cat, rat, rabbit	Freshwater fish	10–25 × 3–5	27–35 × 12–19.5
Dicrocoelium dendriticum	Sheep- and cattle-raising areas	Sheep, goat, deer, other herbivorous and omnivorous mammals	Ants (accidentally ingested with food)	6.0–10.0 × 1.5–2.5	36–45 × 22–30
Eurytrema pancreaticum	Japan	Sheep, hare, rabbit	Grasshopper	8–16 × 5.5–8	40–50 × 23–34
Fasciola gigantica	Sheep- and cattle-raising areas	Cattle, water buffalo, herbivorous mammals	Vegetations such as watercress	29–36 × 8	125–157 × 60–100
F. hepatica	Sheep- and cattle-raising areas	Sheep, cattle, herbivorous and omnivorous mammals	Vegetations such as watercress	20–30 × 8–12	130–145 × 70–90
Opisthorchis felineus	Eastern Europe, Vietnam	Dog, cat, rat, pig, beaver, seal, rabbit, and night heron	Freshwater fish	10–18 × 1.25–2.5	26–30 × 10–15
O. viverrini	Thailand, Laos	Dog, cat, piscivorous mammals	Freshwater fish	6.0 × 2.0	26 × 13

start to supplement their babies' diets when they are only a few weeks old. The most famous dish (*Koi Pla*'), which is prepared from chopped raw cyprinoid fish, is consumed regularly by almost everyone in the village, from infants to the elders. The largest numbers of flukes are generally found in patients over the age of 40 years, because of accumulation of flukes from repeated infections, lack of protective immunity, and the flukes' long life-span.

There are about 2.5 million cases of *O.felineus* infection, with a prevalence rate as high as 8.5 per cent, in some areas of the Commonwealth of Independent States. In western Siberia, people are fond of consuming raw freshwater fish and 1-day-old salted fish. Newly arrived immigrants acquire infections during their first year of residence. Cats and dogs may play a part in transmission.

PATHOLOGY AND PATHOGENESIS

The pathological changes are more or less related to the intensity and the duration of the infection, and are most commonly seen in older patients with large numbers of flukes. They result from mechanical irritation, toxic substances, the immunological response of the host, and secondary bacterial infection. The flukes live in the biliary tree, cystic duct, gallbladder, and rarely in the pancreatic duct; lesions are mainly confined to the biliary system. Histological examination shows varying stages of epithelial-cell hyperplasia, proliferation, and desquamation (Fig. 4). In heavy and severe infections, there is obstruction of the biliary tract, bile retention, hyperplasia of the biliary system with glandular proliferation of papillomatous and adenomatous cholangitis, periductal infiltration with eosinophils and round cells, and fibrosis with necrosis and atrophy of hepatic cells (Fig. 4). There is uniform dilatation of intrahepatic bile ducts with distal clubbing or cyst formation. In late cases, large cysts may develop. The gallbladder may be enlarged to 10 to 20 cm in length and contains white bile (Fig. 5). The epithelial lining is grossly hypertrophic and glandular. Lithiasis of the bile duct or the gallbladder is associated with opisthorchis infection. Eggs and debris of dead parasites are found in the centre of stones (Fig. 6).

At autopsy, severe opisthorchiasis has been associated with cholangitis, cholecystitis, pancreatitis, and cholangiocarcinoma. Frank cirrhosis is unusual. At autopsy, as many as 20 000 worms have been found in one patient.

CLINICAL MANIFESTATIONS

Most patients are asymptomatic or have a benign clinical course and are diagnosed on routine stool examination. The clinical manifestations depend on the patient's age or the duration of infection, number of flukes, and the patient's general health. In endemic areas where infection begins early in life there are practically no characteristic symptoms or signs that can be attributed to the flukes. This may be because the infections are light. Repeated infections result in accumulation of flukes, reaching a maximum around the fifth decade when symptoms appear. There is dull pain and discomfort in the right hypochondrium that sometimes spreads to the epigastrium and the left hypochondrium and often lasts 1 to 2 h in the late afternoon. These pains occur over a period of a few days to a few weeks and recur for months or years. As the disease progresses, pain becomes persistent over weeks and months, by which time the patient is unable to cope with work. A peculiar, hot, cutaneous sensation is commonly felt over the abdomen or the back. Other symptoms are lassitude, loss of taste, anorexia, flatulence, diarrhoea, prolonged low-grade fever, and hepatomegaly. Weight loss and slight pedal oedema, due to associated malnutrition, are not uncommon. The gallbladder is enlarged and functions poorly (Figs. 7 and 8). The liver is usually enlarged and has a firm consistency. In mild cases the liver function profile is generally normal.

Severe manifestations are rare. Relapsing pyogenic cholangitis and cholangiocarcinoma are fatal.

Acute symptoms on exposure have only been reported in opisthorchiasis felineus, they include a 2- to 3-week prepatent period, irregular high fever, occasional facial oedema, lymph-node enlargement, myalgia, arthralgia, rash, and eosinophilia. Allergic hepatitis has been observed in severe cases.

DIAGNOSIS

In patients who have entered an endemic area (e.g. Eastern Europe, the Commonwealth of Independent States, Laos, and Thailand) who have consumed raw or inadequately cooked fish and are suffering from vague gastrointestinal symptoms, cholangitis, or gallbladder enlargement, the diagnosis of opisthorchiasis should be suspected. Definite diagnosis is made by finding opisthorchis eggs in faeces or bile. However, it is very

Fig. 1 Adult liver flukes of humans. (a) *Fasciola gigantica* (3.6 cm). (b) *Fasciola hepatica* (3 cm). (c) *Eurytrema pancreaticum* (9 mm). (d) *Dicrocoelium dendriticum* (10 mm). (e) *Clonorchis sinensis* (11 mm). (f) *Opisthorchis viverrini* (7 mm). (By courtesy of Prayong Radomyos, Faculty of Tropical Medicine, Mahidol University, Bangkok.)

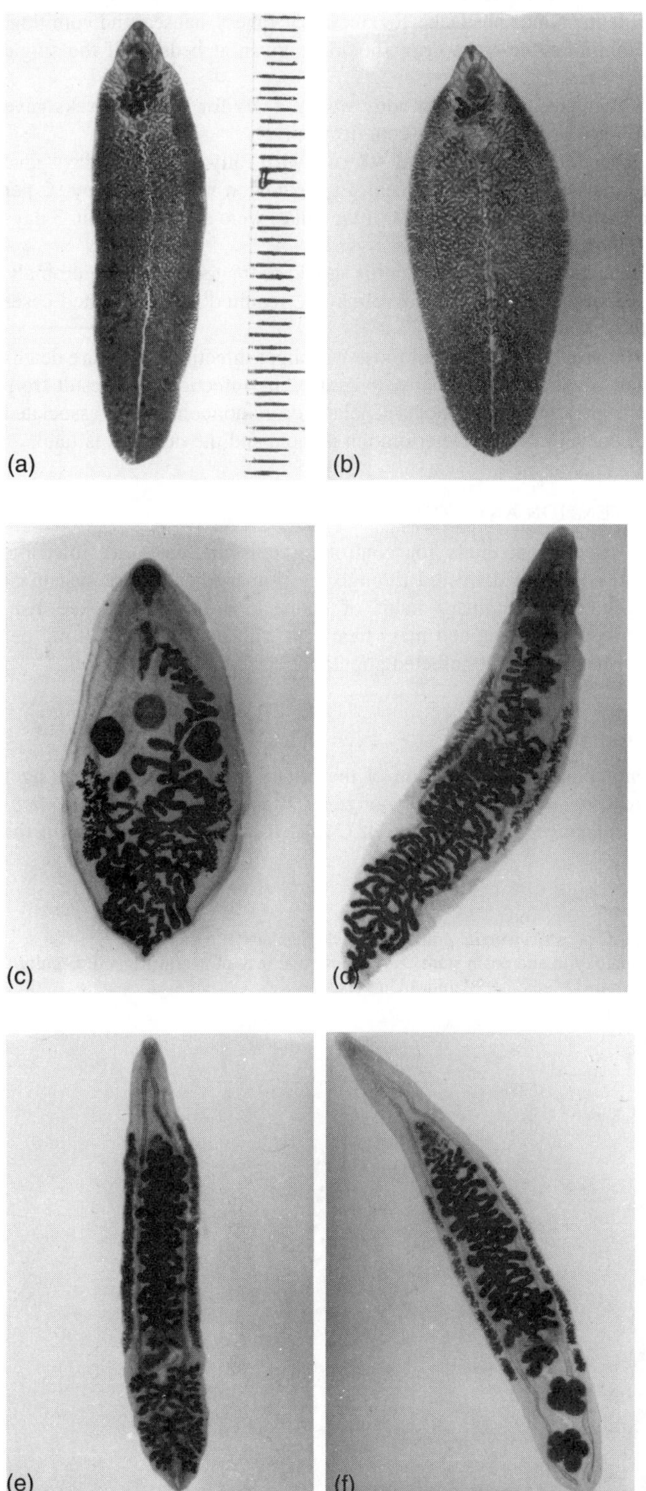

Fig. 2 Ova of human liver flukes. (a) *Clonorchis sinensis*. (b) *Opisthorchis viverrini*. (By courtesy of Prayong Radomyos, Faculty of Tropical Medicine, Mahidol University, Bangkok.)

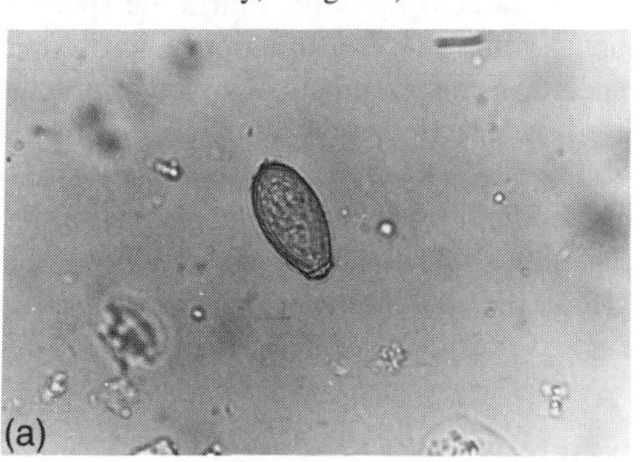

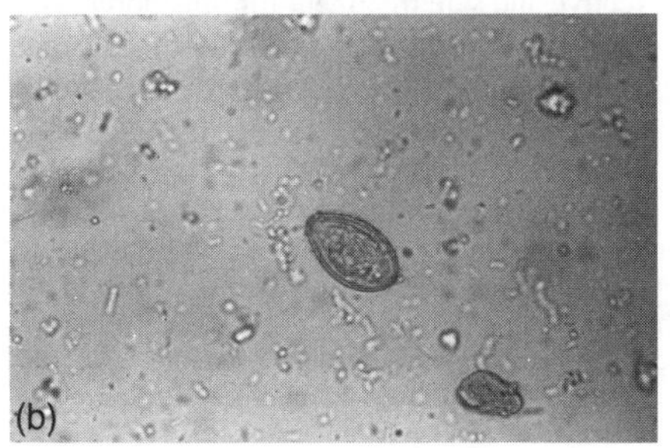

Fig. 3 Lifecycle of *Opisthorchis viverrini*.

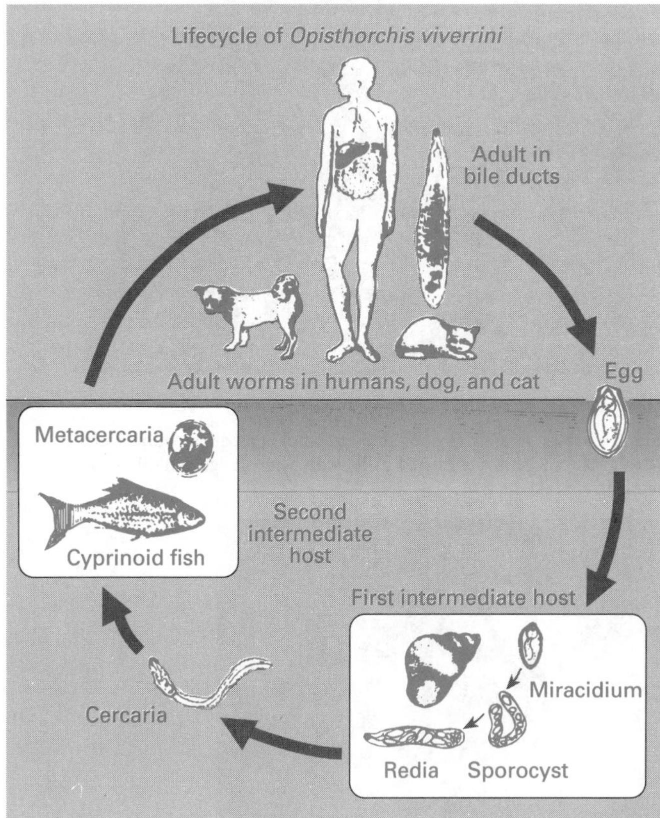

difficult to differentiate the ova of opisthorchis from those of the tiny intestinal flukes. Only the identification of the adult worms after anthelminthic treatment, at operation or at autopsy will confirm the species. In light infections or in patients with biliary obstruction, microscopic examination of the clinical specimens may not be diagnostic. Immunodiagnosis is useful in these situations. Detection of parasite antigens using specific monoclonal antibodies and enzyme immunoassay and DNA hybridization is highly specific. To exclude cholangiocarcinoma, ultrasonography and liver scanning or other non-invasive radiological techniques are of value. However, definite histological diagnosis requires tissue biopsy.

TREATMENT AND PROGNOSIS

Praziquantel is a highly effective and safe treatment for opisthorchiasis. A 1-day regimen of 25 mg/kg body weight three times after meals, and a single dose of 40 mg/kg body weight yielded 100 and 91 per cent cure rates, respectively. In heavy infections a single dose of 50 mg/kg body weight gave a cure rate of 97 per cent. Most flukes are expelled dead and damaged with peeling integument (Fig. 9); those still viable are elongated. Eggs disappear from the stool in 1 week while the clinical symptoms and the enlarged, dysfunctioning gallbladder take a few months to return to normal. Side-effects, which are usually mild and transient, include headache, dizziness, sleepiness, nausea, and vomiting. To minimize these the drug should be given at bedtime if the single dose regimen is used.

Mebendazole, 30 mg/kg body weight a day for 3 and 4 weeks gave cure rates of 89 and 94 per cent, respectively.

Albendazole at a dosage of 400 mg twice daily for 3 and 7 days gave cure rates of 40 and 63 per cent. Egg excretion was reduced by 92 per cent after each regimen. Most of the flukes were expelled within 3 days of treatment.

Relapsing pyogenic cholangitis should be treated with antimicrobials. A palliative surgical procedure may be required in complicated cases with obstructive jaundice.

The prognosis is good in those with light infections. The rare deaths occur in patients with heavy, long-standing infections and result from cholangitis and septic shock. Cholangiocarcinoma has been associated with opisthorchiasis. Deterioration is rapid and the outcome is fatal.

Fig. 4 Liver fluke. The liver shows marked dilation, distortion, and glandular proliferation of the bile ducts, one of which demonstrates a cross-section of a liver fluke, in the lumen. The bile ducts are surrounded by thickened fibrous connective tissue. A chronic inflammatory infiltration composed of lymphocytes, mononuclear cells, and eosinophils is discernible. (By courtesy of M. Riganti, Faculty of Tropical Medicine, Mahidol University, Bangkok, Thailand.)

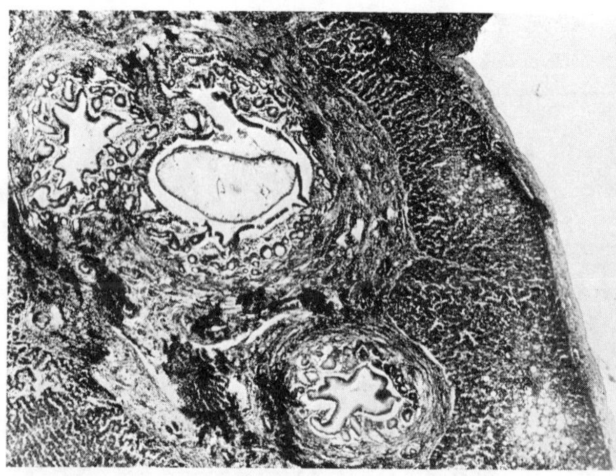

Fig. 5 Ultrasonography (by portable machine) in a patient with severe opisthorchiasis, showing dilated gallbladder with sludge and dilatation of intrahepatic bile ducts.

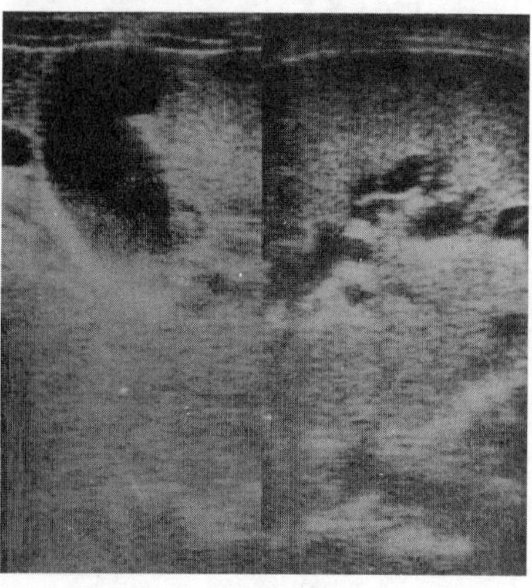

PREVENTION AND CONTROL

The effective methods for controlling opisthorchiasis are intensive health education delivered through the primary health-care system to discourage the culinary habit of eating raw or undercooked fish, improved sanitation, and mass treatment with praziquantel, 40 mg per kg, at bedtime to the infected population to reduce transmission.

Clonorchiasis

Clonorchiasis is an infection of the biliary tract by the Chinese liver fluke *Clonorchis sinensis* (synonyms: *Distoma sinensis, Distoma hepatis innocuum, O.sinensis*, etc.). *C.sinensis* should be included in the

Fig. 6 Ova of *O.viverrini* embedded in the nucleus of a gallstone. Haematoxylin and eosin stain, × 400. (By courtesy of Mario Riganti, Faculty of Tropical Medicine, Mahidol University.)

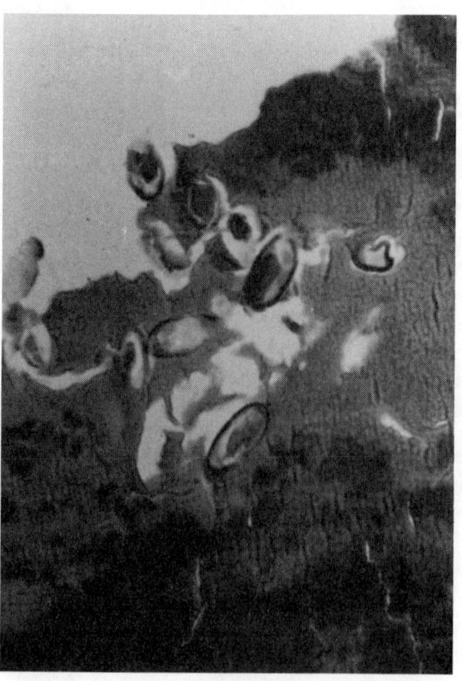

genus Opisthorchis, but the genus Clonorchis is so well established that most parasitologists prefer to retain this generic name.

AETIOLOGY

C.sinensis is larger than *O.felineus* and *O.viverrini* (see Fig. 1(e)) being 10 to 25 mm long and 3 to 5 mm wide. The egg is small (20–30 μm long and 15 to 17 μm wide) (see Fig. 2(a)), resembles the egg of *O.viverrini* but is broader than that of *O.felineus.*

The lifecycle of *Clonorchis* is similar to that of Opisthorchis (see Fig. 3). The first hosts for *C.sinensis* are hydrobid snails: *Parafossarulus manchouricus* in most endemic areas; *Bulinus fuschianus* and *Alocinma longicornis* in other areas. Many cyprinoid fish or carp serve as second intermediate hosts; at least 49 species in China, 29 in Korea, 27 in Japan, and 15 in Taiwan have been found to be infected with *C.sinensis* metacercariae. Reservoir (definitive) hosts include dogs, cats, mink, rats, and other fish-eating mammals.

EPIDEMIOLOGY

Human clonorchiasis is endemic in Japan, Korea, China, Taiwan, and Vietnam, where the first and second intermediate hosts are found and where the population is accustomed to consume raw fish. Although many cases have been reported from Hong Kong, neither the snail nor fish intermediate host are indigenous to that area. Infected fish comes from China and is shipped in daily to provide the Hong Kong population with *Yu Shun Chuk* (raw fish congee). Clonorchiasis has been reported in the United States, Canada, France, Australia, and other countries, because of increased travel and the resettlement of refugees.

Throughout most of the endemic area, fish are kept in ponds fertilized with human and animal faeces. It has been estimated that over 20 million

Fig. 8 The same patient as in Fig. 7. Intravenous cholecystogram. The common bile duct (CBD) was moderately distended (1.5 cm) on day 0. On day 60 and day 180 there was little change. It became normal at 16 months. GB, gallbladder. (By courtesy of Tula Dhiensiri, Khon Kaen Hospital, Thailand.)

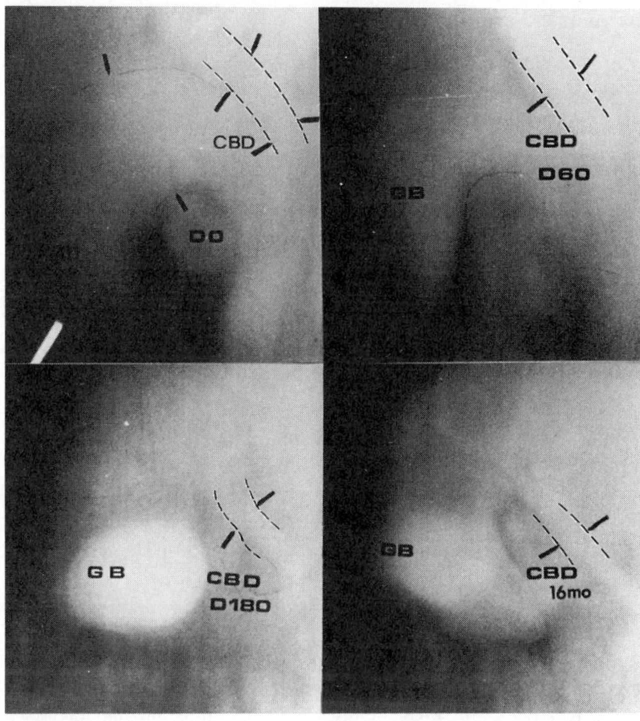

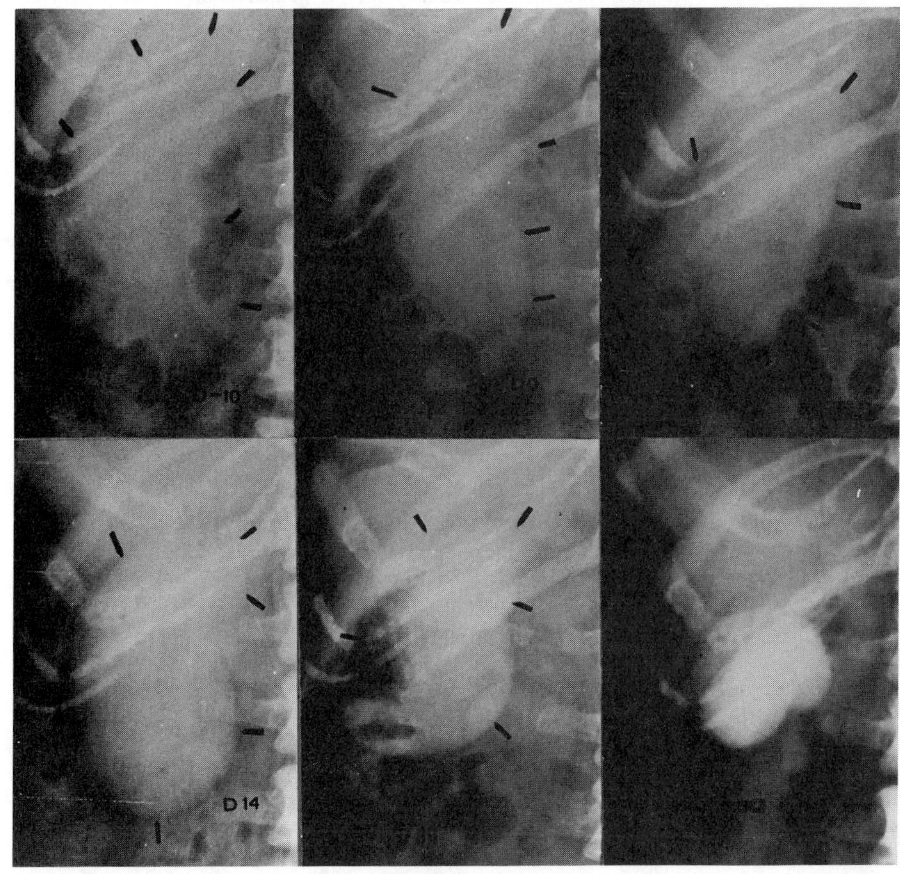

Fig. 7 Oral cholecystography. The gallbladder on days 10 and 0 was extra large (81 cm^2) and showed moderate/poor opacification. After treatment, the function gradually improved and the size decreased becoming normal on day 180.

people in China and over 0.5 million in Korea are infected. There has been some recent reduction in prevalence due to effective national control programmes and other factors responsible for a decrease in the snail population—for instance, industrialization, insecticide pollution of water, and land reclamation.

PATHOLOGY, PATHOGENESIS, AND CLINICAL MANIFESTATIONS

These are similar to those of opisthorchiasis. Acute symptoms occur rarely; anorexia, epigastric pain, diarrhoea, and leucocytosis with eosinophilia were reported in two patients 10 to 26 days after they consumed inadequately cooked fish that were massively infected. Cholangitis, cholelithiasis, pancreatitis, and cholangiocarcinoma are common complications of chronic infection and can be fatal.

DIAGNOSIS

Clonorchis eggs resemble those of heterophyids, but have prominent opercular shoulders and often a small spine-like process at the abopercular end (see Fig. 2(a)). The eggs must be differentiated from those of other opisthorchis flukes; clonorchis eggs look more like electric light bulbs, but differentiation can be difficult, even for experts. Identification of adult flukes provides the best means of making a species diagnosis.

TREATMENT

The drug of choice is praziquantel, 25 mg/kg body weight after meals three times daily for 1 or 2 days. These regimens yielded cure rates of 85 and 100 per cent, respectively. In China, albendazole has been claimed to yield 90 to 100 per cent cure in dosages of 5 and 10 mg/kg for 7 days.

PROGNOSIS, PREVENTION, AND CONTROL

These are essentially the same as for opisthorchiasis.

Fascioliasis

Fascioliasis is an infection caused by the sheep liver fluke *Fasciola hepatica* (synonyms: *Distoma hepaticum, F.californica, F.halli*, etc.) or *F.gigantica*.

Fig. 9 Scanning electron micrography of damaged opisthorchis eggs after praziquantel treatment. × 1800. (By courtesy of Emsri Pongponratn, Faculty of Tropical Medicine, Mahidol University, Bangkok.)

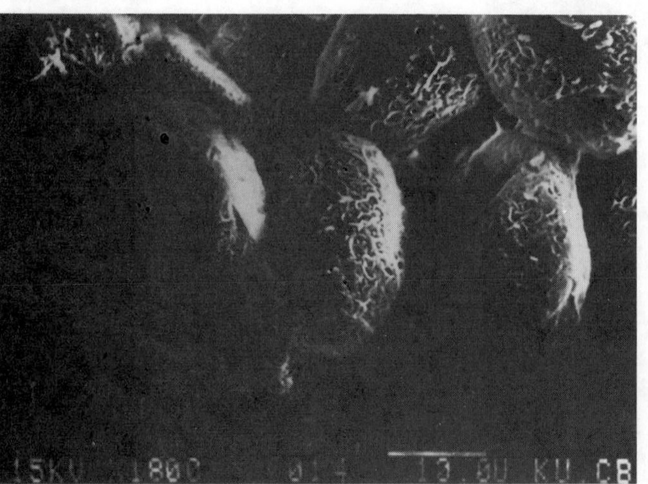

AETIOLOGY

F. hepatica is a brownish, large, flat, broad, leaf-shaped trematode (20–30 × 8–13 mm) (see Fig. 1(b)). The integument of the anterior portion is covered with scale-like spines. A distinct cephalic cone gives a characteristic shouldered appearance. The egg is large, ovoid, with an inconspicuous operculum (130–150 μm in length and 60–90 μm in width).

Adult *F.hepatica* live in the large biliary ducts. Eggs, passed in the host's faeces, require a period of 9 to 15 days for the miracidium to develop and hatch in water of 22 to 25°C; they may remain viable, if kept moist, for up to 9 months at lower temperatures. The miracidium penetrates various lymnaeid snails, the first intermediate hosts. Within the snail's tissue, the development of rediae, daughter rediae, and cercariae requires 4 to 5 weeks. The cercariae emerge from the snail, encyst on various kinds of aquatic vegetation, and even swim freely in the water and develop into metacercariae.

Infection may develop in a wide range of susceptible mammals, the definitive hosts, when they consume infected vegetation or ingest the encysted metacercariae in water. Most human infection is by eating fresh watercress or drinking water contaminated with metacercariae. Metacercariae excyst in the duodenum and penetrate the intestinal wall to enter the peritoneal cavity. Then they invade the liver capsule and migrate through the parenchyma to the bile ducts. They mature in about 3 to 4 months. The lifespan of these flukes is 3 years in rabbits and at least 5 years in sheep.

Numerous species of snail, both amphibious and aquatic, serve as intermediate hosts. The most important definitive hosts are sheep but other herbivores including goats, cattle, horses, camels, vicuña, hogs, rabbits, and deer are commonly infected; even dogs may harbour the flukes.

F.gigantica (or *F.aegyptica*) may attain a length of 7.5 cm. It is more lanceolate and has a less distinct cephalic cone than *F.hepatica* (see Fig. 1(a)). The eggs are larger (160–190 × 70–90 μm). The lifecycle is similar but the snail intermediate host is *Lymnaea natalensis* in Africa, and *L. auricularia* and *L. acuminata* in Asia.

EPIDEMIOLOGY

Fascioliasis is an important veterinary problem in sheep-raising areas. Because of the wide range of definitive and intermediate hosts the disease is geographically widespread. Human infection is most common where watercress is eaten. Sporadic human fascioliasis hepatica has been reported from many parts of the world including mainland United States and Hawaii, Europe including Britain, the Middle East, Asia, and Africa, with extensive outbreaks in France and Cuba. Human fascioliasis gigantica has been reported occasionally from Africa, Asia, and Hawaii.

PATHOLOGY AND PATHOGENESIS

In experimental animals the excysted metacercariae produce some necrosis of the hepatic parenchyma with fibrosis, cellular infiltration, and abscess formation. Sheep heavily infected with *F.hepatica* develop 'liver rot'. Adult flukes may cause hyperplasia, desquamation, thickening, and dilation of the bile ducts. The amount of damage is correlated with worm load: 600 flukes will kill a sheep.

Human fascioliasis is usually mild, but in rare cases of heavy infection there is hyperplasia, necrosis, cystic dilation, and leucocytic infiltration of the bile ducts, and subcapsular haematoma. The liver is enlarged, with multiple nodules that are found to be eosinophilic abscesses. Rarely, a fluke may block the common bile duct. Wandering of flukes in liver parenchyma may result in internal haemorrhage. Migratory tracks can be found in the liver and other organs. They are filled with necrotic cellular debris, with considerable numbers of eosinophils infiltrating around the tracks. Ectopic facioliasis is also common. The flukes in ectopic lesions never achieve maturity. They may be calcified or lead to granuloma formation.

The fluke feeds on blood and may consume 0.2 ml of blood per day.

Urticaria, granuloma, eosinophilia, and eosinophilic hyperplasia of the bone marrow may be provoked by the fluke's antigens. Various types of antibodies, precipitins, and haemagglutinins can be detected in the serum. Serum transpeptidases, alkaline phosphatase, bilirubin, thymol turbidity, cephalin flocculation, and gammaglobulin concentrations and the erythrocyte sedimentation rate may be abnormal.

CLINICAL MANIFESTATIONS

Human fascioliasis is usually mild and related to the phase of the infection. There are three phases: migratory or acute, latent, and obstructive or chronic.

Migratory or acute phase

During the migratory period, in which the immature flukes travel from the gut lumen to bile ducts, patients may develop acute dyspepsia, anorexia, nausea, vomiting, abdominal pain (especially in the epigastrium or right upper quadrant), fever, headache, liver enlargement and tenderness, and urticaria with marked eosinophilia. Severe illness, with prostration, wasting, and jaundice, is unusual. A variety of allergic symptoms may also occur. Acute symptoms may persist for several months.

Latent phase

When the flukes become mature, they lodge in the biliary passage and initiate oviposition, but there are usually no symptoms. Diagnosis is by finding eggs in the duodenal fluid or stool. This phase can last for months or years.

Obstructive or chronic phase

Adult flukes in the bile ducts cause inflammation and obstruction. Some patients have pain in the right hypochondrium and epigastrium, dyspepsia, diarrhoea, nausea, vomiting, hepatomegaly, and jaundice. Eosinophilia, dysproteinaemia, and altered liver function tests are frequent. If the extrahepatic bile ducts are occluded the symptoms will be those of cholangitis or cholecystitis. There may be bleeding into the bile ducts due to mechanical injury by the flukes. Massive haemorrhage can lead to death. Sclerosing cholangitis and biliary cirrhosis following prolonged heavy infection may occur.

Flukes occasionally migrate to ectopic sites such as the intestinal wall, lungs, heart, brain, and skin, where they may cause pluritic pain, nodules, or abscesses.

The acute nasopharyngitis known as *halzoun* in Lebanon or *marrara* in Sudan may be an allergic response to larval flukes eaten in raw sheep or goat liver. Other causes of this syndrome are the pentastome *Linguatula serrata*, the catfish fluke *Isoparorchis hypselobagri*, and aquatic leeches such as *Limanatis nilotica* and *Dinobdella ferox*.

DIAGNOSIS

In enzootic areas, fascioliasis is suspected in patients suffering from fever, hepatomegaly, and eosinophilia who give a history of consuming freshwater plants. Serological tests are particularly useful early in the acute phase of illness while the flukes are still immature, before ova appear in the faeces, and also in the ectopic type. Using purified somatic or excretory–secretory antigen, immunofluorescence and enzyme immunoassay are highly sensitive and specific. Liver biopsy may be helpful in some cases.

Chronic fascioliasis is diagnosed by finding the characteristic eggs in stools or material obtained by duodenal or biliary drainage. Typical radiolucent shadows of flukes may be shown by cholangiography. Ultrasonography and computerized tomography are useful in the demonstration of pathological lesions in the liver and biliary tracts. Spurious infections should be ruled out by placing the patients on a liver-free diet for a few days and repeating the examination. Fascioliasis can be excluded on geographical grounds. The eggs of *F.hepatica* and *F. buski* are difficult to distinguish. Recovery of adult flukes by surgical exploration, after anthelminthics, or at autopsy will confirm the diagnosis.

TREATMENT AND PROGNOSIS

Bithionol, emetine hydrochloride (adults, 30 mg by intramuscular injection daily for 18 days), and chloroquine (children, 5 mg/kg a day by mouth for 3 weeks) have been shown to be effective. The efficacy of praziquantel in human fascioliasis is doubtful. Many studies have shown that praziquantel failed to cure fasciola infection. Recently, patients with fascioliasis have been successfully treated with triclabendazole in a single dose of 10 mg/kg.

The prognosis of human fascioliasis is good. Most patients recover spontaneously after the evacuation of flukes through the intestinal tract.

PREVENTION AND CONTROL

Human fascioliasis is prevented by not eating fresh aquatic plants especially watercress, by boiling drinking water, and thoroughly cooking sheep and goat liver. Long-range control measures are elimination of snail intermediate hosts by draining sheep pastures and treating with molluscicides (e.g., copper sulphate or Frescon), and eradication of the infection from definitive, herbivorous animals.

Dicrocoeliasis

Dicrocoeliasis is caused by *Dicrocoelium dendriticum* (synonyms: *Fasciola lanceolata, Fasciola dendritica, Distomum lanceolatum*, etc.) or *Dicrocoelium hospes*.

D. dendriticum is transparent, flat, and lanceolate measuring 5 to 15 × 1.5 to 2.5 mm (see Fig. 1(d)).

The eggs are dark brown (38–45 × 22–30 μm), slightly flattened on one side, thick-shelled with a large operculum, and contain a fully developed miracidium when laid. *D.hospes* is shorter and more slender.

The adult flukes live in the biliary passages of sheep and cattle. The eggs are passed out in the faeces. If ingested by land snails, the first intermediate host, the eggs undergo a developmental cycle and cercariae are finally released in slime balls shed by the snail on vegetation as it crawls along. The cercariae develop into infective metacercariae only if ingested by ants, the second intermediate hosts. Infected ants are ingested inadvertently by grazing herbivores. The metacercariae excyst and migrate to the biliary tract. People also become infected by eating infected ants.

The land snails' first intermediate hosts are those of the genus Helicella whereas ant second intermediate hosts include *Formica fusca* and *F.rufibarbis*.

EPIDEMIOLOGY

Dicrocoeliasis is enzootic in sheep, goats, deer, and other herbivores. It is commonly seen in Europe, Turkey, North Africa, parts of Asia, and sometimes in America. Spurious human infections are common and result from the consumption of raw infected liver. True human infections are rare but have been reported from Europe, Egypt, Iran, Nigeria, Ivory Coast, and China.

PATHOLOGY, PATHOGENESIS, AND CLINICAL MANIFESTATIONS

The flukes usually move from the biliary capillaries to the main ducts and to the gallbladder, where they mature. Symptoms of human dicrocoeliasis are mild. In heavy infections, vague biliary and gastrointestinal disturbances including abdominal distress, flatulence, biliary colic, vomiting, diarrhoea, or constipation have been reported. The liver may be enlarged.

DIAGNOSIS

Diagnosis is usually made by finding the characteristic ova in faeces, bile, or duodenal fluid. Spurious infections must be ruled out by repeated stool examinations. Recovery of adult flukes after anthelminthics, at surgery, or at autopsy may be necessary for specific diagnosis.

TREATMENT

Praziquantel in the same dose as for opisthorchiasis is recommended.

PREVENTION AND CONTROL

As human infection is generally accidental, no preventive measures can be expected to be effective; however, raw vegetables should not be eaten in the endemic area.

REFERENCES

Bunnag, D. and Harinasuta, T. (1981). Studies on the chemotherapy of human opisthorchiasis. III. Minimum effective dose of praziquantel. *Southeast Asian Journal of Tropical Medicine and Public Health*, **12,** 413–17.

el-Shiek Mohamad, A.R. and Mummery, V. (1990). Human dicrocoeliasis. Report on 208 cases from Saudi Arabia. *Tropical Geographic Medicine*, **42,** 1–7.

Hardman, E.W., Jones, R.L.H., and Davies, A.H. (1970). Fascioliasis a large outbreak. *British Medical Journal*, **iii,** 502–5.

Laird, P.P. and Boray, J.C. (1992). Human fascioliasis successfully treated with triclabendazole. *Australia and New Zealand Journal of Medicine*, **22,** 45–7.

Liu, Y.H. *et al.* (1991). Experimental and clinical trial of albendazole in the treatment of clonorchiasis sinensis. *Chinese Medical Journal*, **104,** 27–31.

Rim, H.J., Lyy, K.S., Lee, J.S., and Joo, K.H. (1980). Clinical efficacy of Praziquantel (EMBAY 8440) against *Clonorchis sinensis* infection in man. *Annals of Tropical Medicine and Parasitology*, **75,** 27.

Sadun, E.H. (1955). Studies on *Opisthorchis viverrini* in Thailand. *American Journal of Hygiene*, **62,** 31–115.

Schwartz, D.A. (1980). Helminths in the induction of cancer. *Opisthorchis viverrini, Clonorchis sinensis* and cholangiocarcinoma. *Tropical Geographic Medicine*, **32,** 95–100.

Strauss, W.G. (1962). Clinical manifestations of clonorchiasis. A controlled study of 105 cases. *American Journal of Tropical Medicine and Hygiene*, **11,** 625–30.

Yu, S., Zhong, H., and Cao, W. (1970). Acute chlonorchiasis: report of 2 cases. *Chinese Medical Journal*, **92,** 423.

7.16.3 Lung flukes (paragonimiasis)

SIRIVAN VANIJANONTA

Many species of *Paragonimus* have been described, of which at least 15 cause disease in man (Table 1). *Paragonimus westermani* is the most common and widespread but *P. africanus*, *P. uterobilateralis* (West Africa), *P. ilokstuenensis* (China), and *P. peruvianus* (South America) also infect man. *P. heterotremus* (Thailand, Laos), *P. szechuanensis*, and *P. hueitungensis* can cause cutaneous paragonimiasis.

The adult flukes are reddish-brown and pea-shaped (Fig. 1). They are 0.8 to 1.6 cm in length, 0.4 to 0.8 cm in width, and 0.3 to 0.5 cm thick, with cuticular spines on the integument. Typically they are encapsulated in cysts adjacent to the bronchi. The eggs are golden brown and ovoid in shape (80–120 × 50–60 μm) (Fig. 2).

Lifecycle (Fig. 3)

Adult flukes encyst in the lung. Ova are expelled through the bronchi and expectorated with sputum or swallowed and passed with faeces. They hatch in fresh water after a few weeks. The resulting miracidia then infect various species of freshwater snail in which they form sporocysts, rediae, and daughter rediae. Metacercariae develop in susceptible freshwater crabs and crayfish (Fig. 4). Infection results from ingestion of viable metacercariae in raw or insufficiently cooked crabs and crayfish. Metacercariae excyst in the peritoneal cavity, where they grow and become young flukes. Most of these will then reach the lung by passing through the peritoneal cavity, diaphragm, and pleural cavity, and finally encyst in the lung parenchyma. Tunnels may be formed during their migration. Encysted flukes mature over a period of 6 to 8 weeks and eggs are produced in 10 to 12 weeks. The circuitous routes of migration allow young flukes to lodge and mature in ectopic locations. The reservoir hosts are wild and domestic felines that feed on crabs and crayfish. Freshwater snails that serve as the first intermediate hosts are Thiaridae, Hydrobilidae, and Pleuroceridae. The second intermediate hosts are the freshwater and brackish-water crabs *Eriocheir japonicus* (Fig. 5), *Tiwaripotamon beusekomae* (Fig. 6) and *Potamon smithiasis*, or crayfish of the genus Cambaroides, such as *C. japonicus* in Japan, and *C. similis*, *C. dauricus*, *C. sckrenki* in China and Korea.

Epidemiology

Paragonimiasis is an important zoonosis. Human beings enter the lifecycle accidentally. However, in some areas human paragonimiasis may be common enough for person-to-person transmission to occur. Human infection is limited in its distribution to places where there are contributory factors that facilitate the lifecycle: reservoir hosts, suitable environment, first and second intermediate hosts, and dietary habits. The three major foci of this disease are in Asia, Africa, and Central and South America. In Asia, endemic areas are in China, Japan, Taiwan, Korea, the Philippines, Thailand, Laos, Vietnam, and Myanmar. The principal parasites are *P. westermani*, *P. skjabini*, and *P. heterotremus*. In Africa, the disease is endemic in eastern Nigeria, the Cameroons, the Congo valley, and Zaire. In Nigeria the dominant parasite is *P. uterobilateralis*, while in the Cameroons and Zaire, *P. africanus* predominates. *P. mexicanus*, *P. peruvianus*, and *P. caliensis* are causative agents in Mexico, Guatemala, Honduras, Costa Rica, Ecuador, Colombia, Peru, and Paraguay.

Transmission of *Paragonimus* spp. to man occurs mostly through ingestion of metacercariae in the second intermediate host. Paratenic hosts infected with immature worms also contribute to animal and human disease.

Pathology and pathogenesis

The pathogenesis of human paragonimiasis is unknown. In experimental animals the larval flukes penetrate the intestinal wall and reach the peritoneal cavity, then pass through the diaphragm and pleura to the lung. They cause irritation, acute inflammatory reactions, traumatic tracts, pressure effects, haemorrhage, and necrosis in affected tissues. Pathological findings in the pleural cavity include turbid and haemorrhagic fluid containing numerous pus cells and eosinophils. Acute, diffuse, fibrinoexudative peritonitis may also occur. Abscess cavities containing young flukes are then formed and become enclosed in a fibrous capsule. Mature cysts adjacent to the bronchial system may rupture into it and the cystic contents are expectorated with sputum or swallowed and passed with faeces. Single or multiple cysts may occur, usually in the lower lobes of the lungs.

Extrapulmonary pathological changes may be caused by aberrant migratory flukes. Cysts, abscesses, and granulomas may be found in the

Table 1 *Human lung flukes (and other tissue trematodes)*

Species	Geographical distribution	Definite hosts other than man	Source of infection	Size of adults (mm)	Size of ova (μm)
Paragonimus africanus	Cameroons	Mongoose, civet cat, dog	Freshwater crabs (*Sudanautes africanus, S. pelii*)	16–17 × 10	65.1–113 × 36.8–62.3
P. caliensis	Peru, Ecuador, Colombia, Mexico, Honduras, El Salvador	*Didelphys marsupialis* *Philander opossum*	Freshwater crabs	7.6–13.3 × 4.2–6.4	70–92 × 38–54
P. compactus	India	*Herpestes myula* *Mungos mungo*	—	4.7–9 × 3.5–5.6	
P. heterotremus (P. tuanshanensis)	Thailand, Laos, China	Cat, dog, leopard, rat	Freshwater crabs	11–14.2 × 5.5–7.1	77–80.1 × 40.4–55.5
P. hueitungensis	China	Cat, dog	Freshwater crabs, crayfish, shrimps	—	—
P. kellicotti	Peru, Ecuador, other Latin American countries	Mink, crayfish-eating mammals, cat, dog, pig	Freshwater crabs *Cambarus* spp.	3–20 × 2.0–7.7	77.5–87.5 × 52.5–65
P. mexicanus	Mexico, Guatemala, Panama, Ecuador, Peru, Costa Rica	Opossum	Freshwater crabs	13.5–14.8 × 6.6–7.9	59.5–78.5 × 38.5–49
P. miyazakii	Japan	Cat, dog, rat, boar	Freshwater crabs	9.2–12.5 × 5.0–6.0	62–81 × 39–52
P. ohirai	Japan	Pig, dog, rat	Freshwater crab	7.2–10.11 × 4.1–50	64–87 × 42–54
P. peruvianus	Peru	Cat	Freshwater crabs	11.6–13.3 × 5.8–7.6	75–86 × 44–53
P. philippinensis (P. filipinus)	Philippines	Cat, dog	Freshwater crabs	—	—
P. pulmonalis	Japan, Korea, Taiwan	Cat, dog	Freshwater crabs, crayfish, shrimps		
P. rudis	Brazil Guatemala	*Lutra braziliensis* *Mustela vison* *Mephitis macroura*	Freshwater crab	12.72 × 6.936	67–71 × 46
P. skrjabini (P. szechuanensis)	China	*Paguma larvata*, cat, dog	Freshwater crabs, crayfish, shrimps	13.13 × 5.43	71 × 48
P. uterobilateralis	Cameroons, Liberia, Nigeria	Cat, dog	Freshwater crabs	5–7 × 4–5	62.3–73.6 × 34–50.9
P. westermani	Worldwide	Tiger, cattle, crayfish-eating mammals	Freshwater crabs, crayfish, shrimps	7.5–16 × 4–6	80–100 × 48–60
P. westermani ichunensis	China	Cat, dog, tiger, leopard, wolf, carnivorous animals of Felidae and Canidae families	Freshwater crabs, crayfish, shrimps	—	—
Other tissue trematodes:					
Achillurbania nouveli	China	*Felis pardus*	—	9.5–11 × 4.5–6.0	55–64 × 32–36
Poikilorchis congolensis	Zaire, Sarawak	Leopard, giant rat	Freshwater crab?	7.6 × 3.9	56–68 × 33–41

abdominal viscera, subcutaneous tissue, muscles, genital organs, and the brain. *P. heterotremus* and *P. skjabini* also create migratory subcutaneous swellings.

Clinical manifestations

The clinical manifestations are divided into acute and chronic phases. The acute phase occurs after the consumption of an improperly cooked, infected crab or crayfish. The incubation period varies from a few days to weeks. The severity of symptoms usually correlates with worm load. Invasion and migration by young flukes causes inflammatory and allergic responses such as fever, rashes, urticaria, abdominal pain, and discomfort and a feeling of tightness in the chest. Acute symptoms are rarely serious and patients progress the chronic stage.

Chronic manifestations are classified as pulmonary and extrapulmonary.

PULMONARY PARAGONIMIASIS

The most remarkable clinical feature is a chronic, productive cough with jam-like, browish-red sputum. Other symptoms include breathlessness, chest pain, unilateral or bilateral pleural effusions, and empyema. Occasional patients may have haemoptysis following heavy work or exertion, while pneumothorax rarely occurs.

Pulmonary paragonimiasis is an insidious and persistent lung disease. Patients have surprisingly good general health and usually show few abnormalities on physical examination. A minority of symptomatic patients have normal chest radiographs. Abnormal findings include linear infiltrations, exudative pneumonia, localized pleural effusion, and nodular or cystic lesions (see Fig. 7). These lesions are predominantly found in the basilar and peripheral regions of both lower lung fields. Cysts may be single or multiple; the most characteristic radiographic feature is a ring shadow with a crescentic opacity along one side of the border resembling the corona phase of a solar eclipse. Other findings are pleural effusion and thickening, and calcification. Long-standing, extensive lesions with fibroatelectasis resemble the lesions of chronic pulmonary tuberculosis.

EXTRAPULMONARY PARAGONIMIASIS

Extrapulmonary paragonimiasis is caused by the aberrant migration of larval and young adult flukes to any organ. Migratory swelling of subcutaneous tissues may also occur.

Fig. 1 Adult lung flukes: (a) *Paragonimus heterometrus* (1.5 cm); (b) *P. westermani* (1.5 cm). (By courtesy of Prayong Radomyos, Bangkok.)

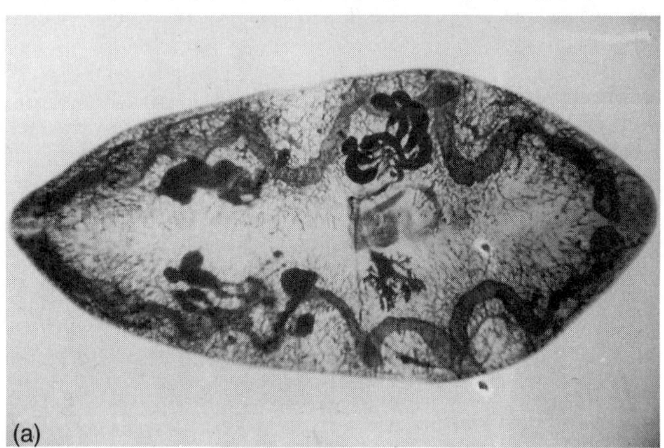

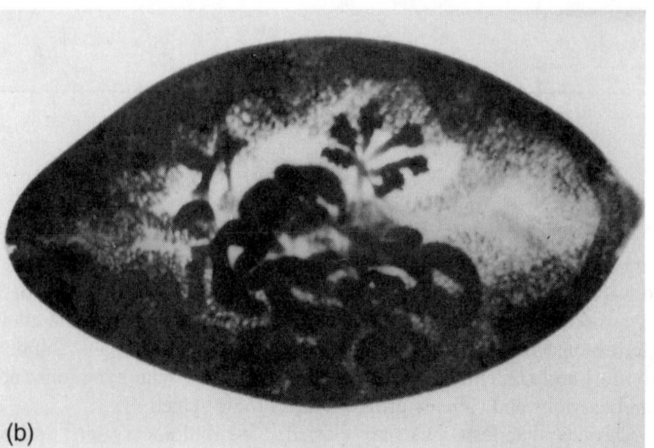

Fig. 2 Ova of lung flukes: (a) *Paragonimus heterometrus*; (b) *P. westermani*. (By courtesy of Prayong Radomyos, Bangkok.)

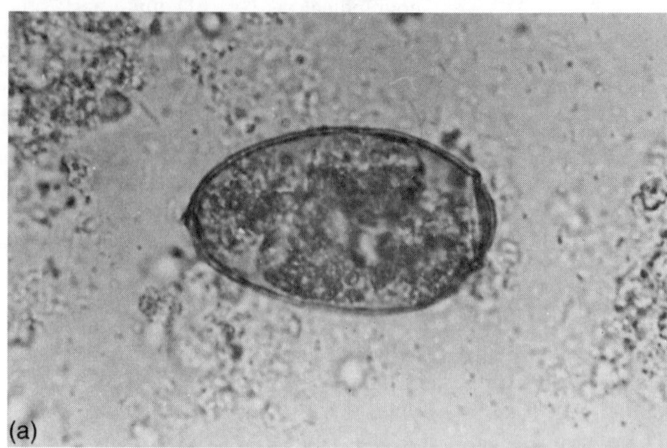

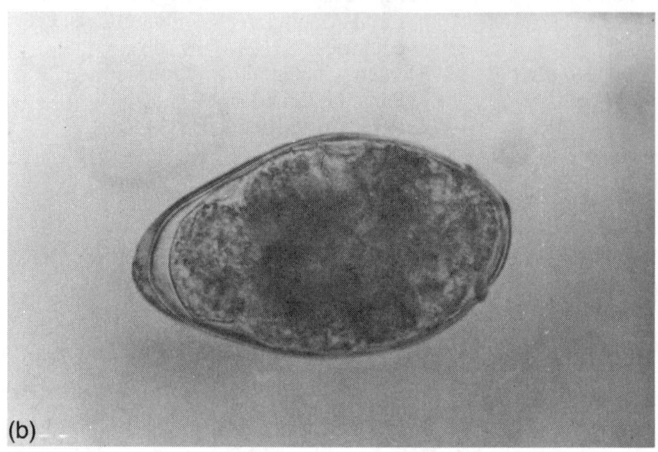

Fig. 3 Lifecycle of *Paragonimus westermani*.

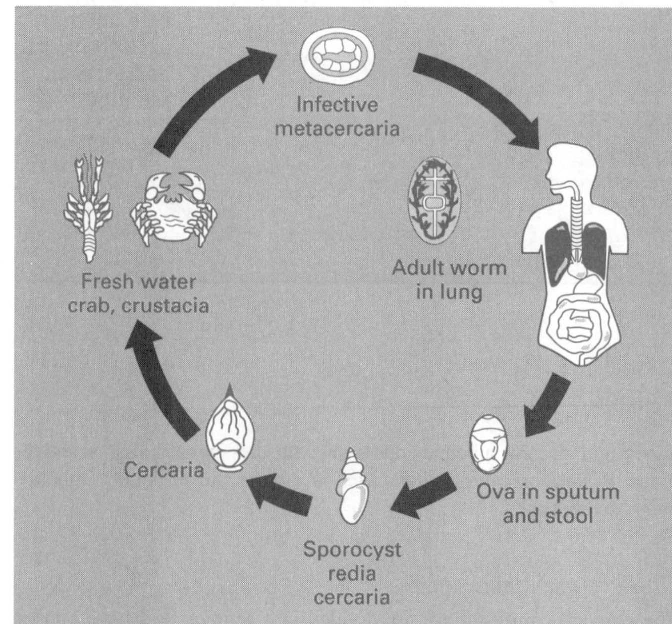

CEREBRAL PARAGONIMIASIS

The clinical symptoms are similar to those of a cerebral space-occupying lesion, and are related to the site of the lesion. However, one or more syndromes may be present. Epiletic seizures are common, or patients may develop mental disturbances of the schizoid and paranoid type. Increased intracranial pressure induces persistent intense headache, nausea, vomiting, papilloedema, diplopia, and loss of visual acuity. Patients with paragonimus cysts in the basal meninges will present with meningeal symptoms that include increased intracranial pressure, obstructive hydrocephalus, arterial thrombosis, and stroke. On rare occasions, patients may suffer from cerebellopontine-angle syndrome with tinnitus, progressive deafness, nystagmus, dysphagia, and hiccups.

SPINAL-CORD PARAGONIMIASIS

Spinal involvement produces progressive weakness, sensory impairment of the lower extremities, paralysis, and back pain.

INTRA-ABDOMINAL PARAGONIMIASIS

Paragonimus spp. may create migratory tracts or pressure effects leading to necrosis of the spleen, liver, small- and large-intestinal wall, and cause non-specific abdominal signs and symptoms.

SUBCUTANEOUS PARAGONIMIASIS

P. skjabini, *P. westermani*, and *P. heterotremus* cause migratory subcutaneous nodules.

Diagnosis

Pulmonary paragonimiasis should be excluded in any subject from an endemic area who presents with a chronic productive cough and jam-like, browish-red or 'rusty' sputum. Definitive diagnosis is made by observing the characteristic ova in sputum, pleural effusion, or stool, or flukes in biopsy specimens. Expectoration of intact flukes has been reported. Other supportive evidence is obtained by chest radiographs, which show the characteristic shadows of single or multiple cysts in the lungs (Fig. 7). Computerized tomography of the chest is also helpful (Fig. 8)

Serology is essential in the diagnosis of extrapulmonary paragonimiasis. Enzyme immunoassay and dot enzyme immunoassay are both highly sensitive and specific, as is counter-immunoelectrophoresis using adult or free metacercariae as a source of antigen. Other less sensitive but more specific tests include complement fixation and indirect haemagglutination. Intradermal skin tests have been used for epidemiological surveys.

Differential diagnosis

Pulmonary paragonimiasis should be differentiated from pulmonary tuberculosis, melioidosis, lung abscess, and lung tumours.

Extrapulmonary paragonimiasis should be differentiated from other diseases that produce similar clinical manifestations in affected organs. For example, cerebral paragonimiasis should be differentiated from cerebral cysticercosis, meningoencephalitis, brain abscess, and tumours.

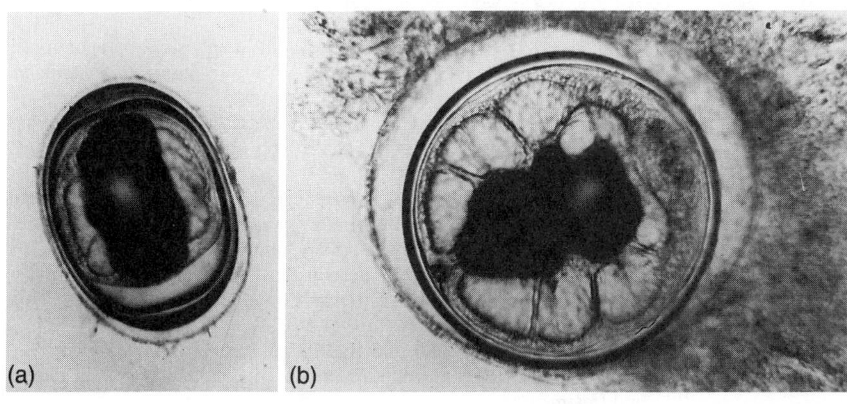

Fig. 4 Metacercariae of lung flukes in crabs, the second intermediate hosts: (a) *Paragonimus heterometrus*; (b) *P. westermani*. (By courtesy of Prayong Radomyos, Bangkok.)

Fig. 5 Freshwater crab *Eriocheir japonicus*, the second intermediate host of Paragonimus.

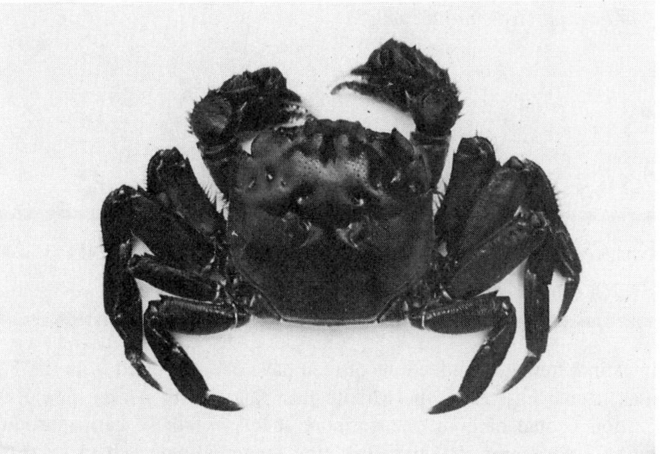

Fig. 6 Freshwater crab *Tiwaripotamon beusekomae*, the second intermediate host of *P. heterometrus*.

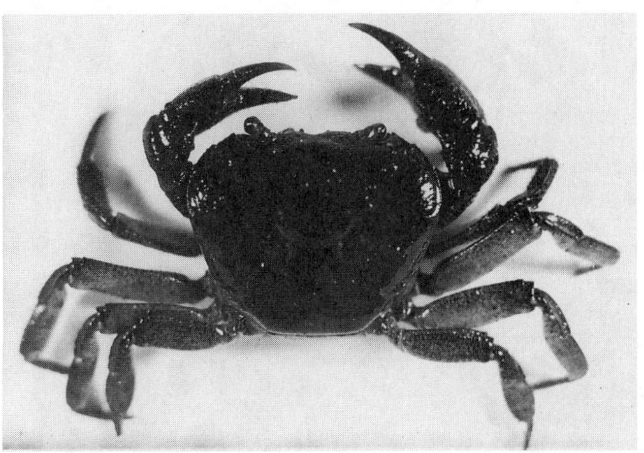

Subcutaneous paragonimiasis may resemble gnathostomiasis, sparganosis, loiasis, or onchocerciasis.

Treatment

SPECIFIC

The drug of choice is praziquantel at a dosage of 75 mg/kg per day in three divided doses for 2 to 3 days. The cure rate is nearly 100 per cent in multicentre studies. The symptoms rapidly improve in a few days. Eggs disappear from the sputum in few weeks. Radiological improvement takes months, depending on the extent and chronicity of the disease. During treatment of cerebral paragonimiasis, convulsions, seizures, coma, and behaviour changes may develop. As a result of parasite death brain oedema and host–parasite interaction may cause intracranial pressure. Therefore, treatment should proceed with caution, and the dose adjusted if necessary. Dexamethasone cover has been suggested.

Fig. 7 Pulmonary paragonimiasis: posteroanterior radiograph showing thick-walled cystic lesion in the right upper lobe with pericystic fibrosis. (Copyright Dr S. Vanijanonta.)

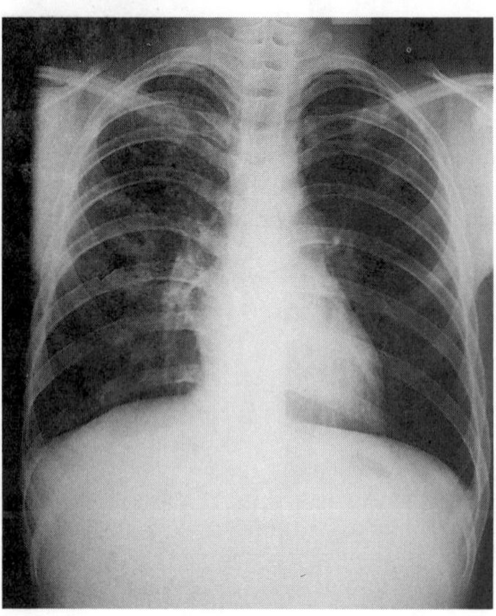

Fig. 8 Pulmonary paragonimiasis: CT scan showing thick-walled cystic lesion in the left upper lobe with pericystic fibrosis and a fibrocalcific lesion in the right upper lobe. (Copyright Dr S. Vanijanonta.)

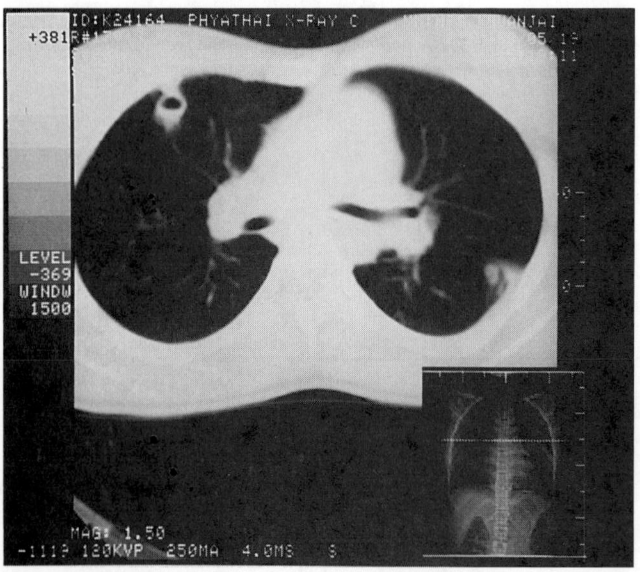

SYMPTOMATIC AND SUPPORTIVE

These treatments, including blood transfusion, bronchodilators, anticonvulsants, and analgesics, are also important.

Prognosis

Pulmonary paragonimiasis is rarely fatal and the lesions may calcify or completely resolve in a few years. Cerebral paragonimiasis may cause chronic morbidity such as epilepsy, mental changes, and neurological sequelae.

Prevention and control

Effective control measures are directed towards interruption of the lifecycle. However, control and eradication of intermediate hosts is impracticable; therefore, health education, changing the social and dietary customs, and mass treatment of infected people in an endemic area are more effective for prevention and control.

REFERENCES

Chen, G.U., Guo, Y.F., Sha, R.J., Chen, H., and Lin, L.B. (1986). Counterimmunoelectrophoresis in detecting antibodies in experimental paragonimiasis. *Chinese Journal of Zoonoses*, **2,** 58.

Chung, H.L., Ho, L.Y., Hsu, C.P., and Ts'ao, W.J. (1981). Recent progresses in studies of paragonimus and paragonimiasis control in China. *Chinese Medical Journal*, **94,** 483–94.

Jun-ichi, I. (1987). Evaluation of ELISA for the diagnosis of paragonimiasis westermani. *Transactions of the Royal Society of Tropical Medicine and Hygiene*, **81,** 3–6.

Miyazaki, I. (1982). Paragonimiasis. In *CRC Handbook Series in Zoonoses*, Section C, *Parasitic zoonoses*, Vol.III, pp. 143–64. Lea and Febiger, Philadelphia.

Miyazaki, I. and Harinasuta, T. (1966). The first case of human paragonimiasis caused by *Paragonimus heterotremus* (Chen *et* Hsia 1964). *Annals of Tropical Medicine and Parasitology*, **60,** 509.

Pariyanonda, S. *et al.*, (1990). Serodiagnosis of human paragonimiasis caused by *Paragonimus heterotremus*. *Southeast Asian Journal of Tropical Medicine and Public Health*, **21,** 103–7.

Vanijanonta, S., Bunnag, D., and Harinasuta, T. (1984). *Paragonimus heterotremus* and other paragonimus spp. in Thailand: pathogenesis, clinical and treatment. *Drug Research*, **34,** 1186–8.

Vanijanonta, S., Bunnag, D., and Harinasuta, T. (1984). Radiological findings in pulmonary paragonimiasis heterotremus. *Southeast Asian Journal of Tropical Medicine and Public Health*, **15,** 122–8.

Zhang, Y.Q., Hou, L.P., Gui, S.H., Wen, Y., and Zu, Z.B. (1986). The significance of dot-ELISA in diagnosis of paragonimiasis. *Chinese Journal of Internal Medicine*, **25,** 679–81.

7.16.4 Intestinal trematodiasis

KHANYING TRANAKCHIT HARINASUTA AND PRAYONG RADOMYOS

Intestinal trematode infections of man have been reported from the Far East, South-East Asia, the Middle East, and North Africa. Some 50 million people harbour one or more species of these hermaphrodite flukes. Information on their distribution, epidemiological characteristics, and pathological effects is very limited. Thus, it is not possible to comment on the public health importance of these infections. More research is needed to reveal the real extent of morbidity. More than 50 species have been reported in man (see Table 1; Figs. 1 and 2) but only a few are known to cause morbidity. These include *Fasciolopsis buski, Heterophyes heterophyes, Metagonimus yokogawai*, and *Gastrodiscoides hominis. Fasciolopsis buski* is the most important.

Fasciolopsiasis

Fasciolopsiasis is caused by the giant intestinal fluke *Fasciolopsis buski* (synonyms: *Distomum crassum, D. rathouisi, F. rathouisi, F. fülleborni, F. goddardi* etc.).

F. buski is the largest intestinal fluke (50–75 mm × 8–20 mm, 0.5–3 mm thick). It is fleshy, reddish beef coloured, elongate, and ovoid in shape (Fig. 1(e)). There is no cephalic cone.

The large hen's egg-shaped ovum is yellowish-brown, with a clear, thin shell and small operculum at one end (130–140 μm × 80–85 μ) (Fig. 2(e)). It is undeveloped when laid.

The adult flukes are found in the small intestine of pigs and man. The eggs are passed with faeces. On reaching the water, miracidia develop in 4 to 8 weeks, enter snails, the first intermediate host, forming sporocysts, rediae, and cercariae. The cercariae then swim out and encyst on water plants and develop into metacercariae in approximately 4 weeks. When pigs or humans ingest freshwater plants, the metacercariae excyst in the duodenum. They attach themselves to the mucosa and in about 90 days develop into mature worms. The life-span of the fluke is only 1 year.

The snail hosts include *Segmentina, Hippeutis*, and *Gyraulus* spp.

The edible water plants are water caltrop (*Trapa bicornis* (Fig. 3) *T. natans*) water morning glory (*Ipomoea aquatica*), water chestnut (*Eliocharis tuberosa*), water bamboo (*Zizania aquatica*), and watercress (*Neptunia oleracea*).

EPIDEMIOLOGY

In 1947 it was estimated that over 10 million people in the Far East were infected with *F. buski*. Most of the infections were from mainland China. Fasciolopsiasis is endemic in Taiwan, Thailand, Laos, Bangladesh, and India, but the distribution is limited and the prevalence rates are low. The present prevalence of the disease is unknown. Human infections have been reported from Japan, the Philippines, Malaysia, and a number of Western countries, but it is probable these were from people who had migrated from endemic areas, or the eggs were misidentified.

Fasciolopsiasis seems to be restricted to areas where people raise water plants and pigs, and to populations that commonly eat freshwater plants. In many farms, pigs are kept near the ponds where water plants are grown. Pig excreta are washed into the ponds where there are plenty of snail intermediate hosts. Water plants are fed to pigs and the cycle of *F. buski* is continued.

Humans are infected by consuming raw stems, leaves, and pods of water plants. Another means of acquiring the infection is by peeling with the teeth the outer layers of the plant where metacercariae are encysted. In central Thailand, where water caltrops are cultivated in canals along the side of the road, schoolchildren on their way to and from school enjoy picking them and eating them fresh. This explains the high prevalence of fasciolopsiasis among children in these areas.

PATHOLOGY

The flukes attach themselves to the duodenal and jejunal mucosa. The effects are traumatic, obstructive, and toxic. Localized inflammation is usually followed by ulceration at the site of attachment and there may be bleeding from deep erosions. The flukes disturb the secretion of intestinal juice and provoke mucous discharge. In severe cases there is profound intoxication and sensitization from absorption of the fluke metabolites. Eosinophilic leucocytosis is a common blood picture.

CLINICAL FEATURES

Most of the infections are light and asymptomatic. In heavy infections, the first symptoms are diarrhoea with hunger pains, simulating peptic ulcer. At first, diarrhoea and constipation alternate, but later diarrhoea becomes persistent. The stool is greenish-yellow and foul smelling, and contains undigested food. The appetite is usually normal or even excessive, but some patients are anorexic, nauseated, and are vomiting. In severe cases, oedema of face, trunk, and limbs, and ascites develop; the skin becomes dry and rough, and there is marked prostration. Protein-losing enteropathy is a possible mechanism. Heavy worm load may cause intestinal obstruction. Death is rare.

DIAGNOSIS

Flukes and ova are passed in the stool or may be vomited up. They must be distinguished from those of other large species such as *Echinostoma* sp., *Fasciola hepatica*, and *F. gigantica*.

DIFFERENTIAL DIAGNOSIS

The symptoms associated with heavy infections may be confused with those of giardiasis, massive gut nematode infection, peptic ulcer, and other causes of bowel obstruction. Generalized oedema may suggest nephrotic syndrome and other causes of hypoproteinaemia.

TREATMENT

The drug of choice is praziquantel in a single dose of 15 mg after supper, before retiring to bed. It is very effective: the fluke will be expelled on the following day. A single dose of niclosamide, 150 mg/kg daily for 1 or 2 days, a single dose of tetrachloroethylene, 0.1 mg/kg, or albendazole, 200 mg for 2 days, are less effective.

PROGNOSIS

Light infections carry a good prognosis. In most cases spontaneous cure usually occurs after 1 year, but in untreated heavy infections the prognosis can be grave.

PREVENTION

Water plants should be cooked or grown in ponds that are not contaminated with human or pig faeces. Molluscicides can be used to eradicate the snail vectors.

Echinostomiasis

There are more than 30 genera of the family Echinostomatidae and about 12 species have been reported in man. The common species are *Echinostoma ilocanum* (Fig. 1(a)), and *E. lindoense*. The other species are *E. malayanum* (Fig. 1(b)), *E. revolutum* (Fig. 1(c)), *E. recurvatum, E. melis* (*E. jassyense*), *E. macrochis, E. cinetorchis, Hypoderaeum conoideum* (Fig. 1(l)), *Echinochasmus perfoliatus, Paryphostomum sufrartyfex*, and *Himasthla muehlensi*.

The echninostome flukes have a characteristic horseshoe-shaped collar of one or two rows of straight spines surrounding the dorsal and lateral sides of the oral sucker. The flukes are elongated and of moderate size (5–15 mm × 1–2 mm) with slightly tapering, rounded ends. The cuticle of the anterior portion of the body is covered by minute scale-like spines. The species differ in the extent and distribution of these spines.

Table 1 *Human intestinal flukes*

Species	Geographical distribution	Definitive hosts other than man	Source of infection	Size of adult (mm)	Size of ova (μm)
Alaria americana	USA, Canada	Wild carnivores	Frog	4–5 × —	106–134 × 64–80
Apophallus donicus	USA	Dog, cat, rat, fox, rabbit	Freshwater fish	1.12–1.3 × 0.58–0.72	35 × 25
Artyfechinostomum mehrai	India	Rat, pig	Snail	4.84–8.36 × —	96 × 64
Centrocestus armatus	Japan	Cat, dog, rat, mouse, rabbit, heron	Fish	0.35–0.63 × 0.182–0.294	28.6–32.8 × 15.9–17
C. canimus	Taiwan	Dog, cat, rat	Fish	0.4–0.45 × 0.21–0.247	32.5–35 × 17.5–20
C. cuspidatus	Egypt, Formosa	*Milvus parasiticus*, chicks, rats	Fish	0.5–0.8 × 0.25–0.35	30–35 × 15–20
C. formosanus	Taiwan, South China, Philippines	Rat, cat, dog, chicken, duck	Fish, frog		
C. kurokawai	Japan		Fish	0.35–0.515 × 0.175–0.225	33–40 × 17–21
C. longus	Formosa	—			
Cryptocotyle lingua	Greenland	Cat, dog, rat		1.2–2.0 × 0.4–0.9	42–48 × 20–22
Diorchitrema formosanus	Taiwan	Cat, rat	Fish	0.324–0.558 × 0.126–0.21	18–24 × 12–15
D. pseudocirratum	Hawaii, Philippines	Dog, cat	Fish	0.3–0.6 × 0.2–0.3	18–21 × 9–12
Echinochasmus japonicus	China, Korea	Cat, dog, rat, mouse, chick	Fish	0.6–0.9 × 0.16–0.18	77–90 × 51–57
E. perfoliatus	Japan, Italy Romania, Russia, Northern Asia, Egypt, Taiwan	Cat, dog, hog Fox, rat, wild boar	Fish Fish	3–4 × 0.6–1.0	90–135 × 55–95
Echinoparyphium paraulum	USSR (former)	Duck, geese, swans, dove			
E. recurvatum	Taiwan, Indonesia, Egypt	Birds, mammals, wild rat	Tadpole, frog, snail	1.9–7.3 × 0.4 × 0.85	88–111 × 54–75
Echinostoma cinetorchis	Japan, Taiwan	Rat	Tadpole, frog	5.57–21.23 × 1.28–3.7	96–100 × 61–70
E. hortense	Japan	Dog, rat	Loaches, frogs	8.2–14 × 0.93–1.6	110–126 × 61–70
E. ilocanum	Indonesia, Philippines, China, Thailand, Malaysia	Dogs, rats, mice	Freshwater mollusc	4–8 × 0.55–1.0	86–116 × 52–70
E. jassyense	Romania, China	Unknown	Tadpole	5.5–7.5 × 1.2	132–154 × 75–85
E. lindoense	Celebes, Brazil	Rat, bird	Snail	13–22 × 2.5–3.0	92–124 × 65–76
E. macrochis	Japan	Rat	Snails	3.3–4.2 × 0.68–0.86	81–89 × 54–58
E. malayanum	Indonesia, China, Thailand, Malaysia	Field rat	Snail, tadpole, fish	5–10 × 2.5	137 × 75.5
E. revolutum	Indonesia, China, Thailand, Taiwan, Malaysia	Duck, goose, chicken, rat	Clam, tadpole, snail	21–26 × 2.0–3.5	104–112 × 64–72
Episthmium caninum	Thailand	Dog	Fish	1.0–1.5 × 0.4–0.75	84 × 50–60
Fasciolopsis buski	China, Taiwan, Laos, Bangladesh, India, Thailand	Pig, dog	Water plants (water caltrops, water morning glory, water bamboo, watercress)	20–75 × 8–20	130–140 × 80–85
Gastrodiscoides hominis	India, Burma, Malaysia, Vietnam, British Guiana, Kazakhstan, Thailand	Pig, field rats, monkey, Nepu mouse deer	?	4–8 × 3–4	150 × 72
Haplorchis microrchis	Japan	Dog, cat	Fish	0.396–0.756 × 0.17–0.288	27.2–30 × 14.4–16

Species	Geographical distribution	Definitive hosts other than man	Source of infection	Size of adult (mm)	Size of ova (μm)
H. pleurolophocerca	Egypt	Cat	*Gambusia affinis*		
H. pumilio	Taiwan, Philippines, Thailand, Egypt	Dog, cat, night heron	Fish	0.32–0.42 × 0.135–0.17	29–32 × 15.5–17.5
H. taichui	Taiwan, Philippines, Thailand, Pakistan	Dog, cat	Fish	0.45–0.89 × 0.21–0.4	24–28 × 12–15
H. vanissimus	Philippines	?	Fish	0.375–0.512 × 0.25–0.312	25–30 × 18–21
H. yokogawai	Taiwan, Indonesia, Philippines, Thailand, South China	Dog, cat	Fish	0.468–0.64 × 0.184–0.218	20.4–33 × 10.5–16.5
Heterophyes heterophyes	Egypt, Korea, China, Taiwan, Philippines	Cat, dog, rat, fox, wolf, birds, weasel, mammals	Freshwater or brackish-water fish	1–1.7 × 0.3–0.4	28–30 × 15–17
H. katsuradai	Japan	Dog	Fish	0.61–0.89 × 0.40–0.47	25.3–25.9 × 14.3–15
H. nocens	Japan	Dog, cat, rat	Fish	0.9–1.1 × 0.4–0.53	28 × 15.5
Heterophyopsis continua	Japan	Dog	Fish	1.97–2.05 × 0.24–0.28	25–26 × 14–16
Himasthla muehlensi	Germany	Gulls, bird	Clam, mollusc	11–18 × 0.41–0.67	114–149 × 62–85
Hypoderaeum conoideum	Thailand	Duck, fowl	Snail, tadpole	6–12 × 1.3–2.0	95.2–108 × 61.2–68
Metagonimus minutus	Taiwan	Cat, mouse (exper.)	Fish	0.432–0.504 × 0.252–0.396	21–24 × 12–15
M. yokogawai	China, Japan, Taiwan, Korea, Philippines, The Balkans, Russia, Spain, Rumania, East Indies	Dog, cat, hog, pelican	Fish	1–2.5 × 0.4–0.75	26–28 × 15–17
Paryphostomum sufrartyfex	India	Hog, dog, rat	*Digoniostoma pulchella*	9.0 × 2.5	90–125 × 60–75
Phaneropsolus bonnei	Thailand, Indonesia	Bat, monkey	Dragonfly naiad	0.48–0.78 × 0.22–0.35	27–29 × 10–12
P. spinicirus	Thailand	?	?	0.55–0.76 × 0.43–0.63	27–33 × 13–16
Plagiorchis harinasutai	Thailand	?	?	1.75–1.87 × 0.60–0.65	32.63–33.75 × 16.88–18.0
P. javensis	Indonesia	Bird, bat	Larval insect	1.82 × 0.68	36 × 22–24
P. muris	Japan	Bird, dog, rat	Snail, aquatic insects	0.8–2.0 × 0.24–0.84	36 × —
P. philippinensis	Philippines	Bird, rat	Larval insect?	1.5–2.0 × 0.385–0.435	28–30 × 19–21
Procerovum calderoni	Philippines	Cat, dog	Fish	0.47–0.55 × 0.25–0.26	21–25 × 11–15
P. varium	Japan	Cat, bird	Fish	0.256–0.378 × 0.125–0.157	25–29 × 12–18
Prosthodendrium molenkampi	Thailand, Indonesia	Bat, monkey, rat	Dragonfly naiad, crab	0.55–0.92 × 0.41–0.77	20–28 × 9–14
Pygidiopsis summa	Korea	Bird, cat, dog, rat	Fish	0.49–0.76 × 0.25–0.44	21–23 × 11–14
Spelotrema brevicaeca	Philippines	Bird	Crab	0.5–0.7 × 0.3–0.4	15–16 × 9.4–10
Stellantchasmus amplicaecalis	Taiwan	Dog, cat, rat	Fish	0.45–0.648 × 0.198–0.324	22–24 × 8–14.4
S. falcatus	Japan, Hawaii, Philippines, Thailand	Dog, cat	Fish	0.428–0.585 × 0.187–0.335	21.5–23.1 × 12–13.2
Stictodora fuscata	Japan	Cat, bird	Fish	0.59 × 0.23	36–38 × 22–23
Watsonius watsoni	South-West Africa	Baboon monkey	Water plants?	8–10 × 4–5	122–130 × 75–80

Fig. 1 Adult intestinal flukes of man: (a) *Echinostoma ilocanum* (8 mm); (b) *E. malayanum* (12 mm); (c) *E. revolutum* (12 mm); (d) *Episthmium caninum* (1 mm); (e) *Fasciolopsis buski* (5.3 cm); (f) *Gastrodiscoides hominis* (9 mm); (g) *Haplorchis pumilio* (0.7 mm); (h) *H. taichui* (0.76 mm); (i) *H. yokogawai* (0.47 mm); (j) *Heterophyes heterophyes* (1.7 mm); (k) *H. h. nocens* (1.2 mm); (l) *Hypoderaeum canoideum* (10 mm); (m) *Metagonimus yokogawai* (1.3 mm); (n) *Plagiorchis harinasutai* (1.87 mm); (o) *Phaneropsolus bonnei* (0.65 mm); (p) *Prosthodendrium molenkampi* (0.8 mm); (q) *Stellantchasmus falcatus* (0.43 mm). (Copyright P. Radomyos.)

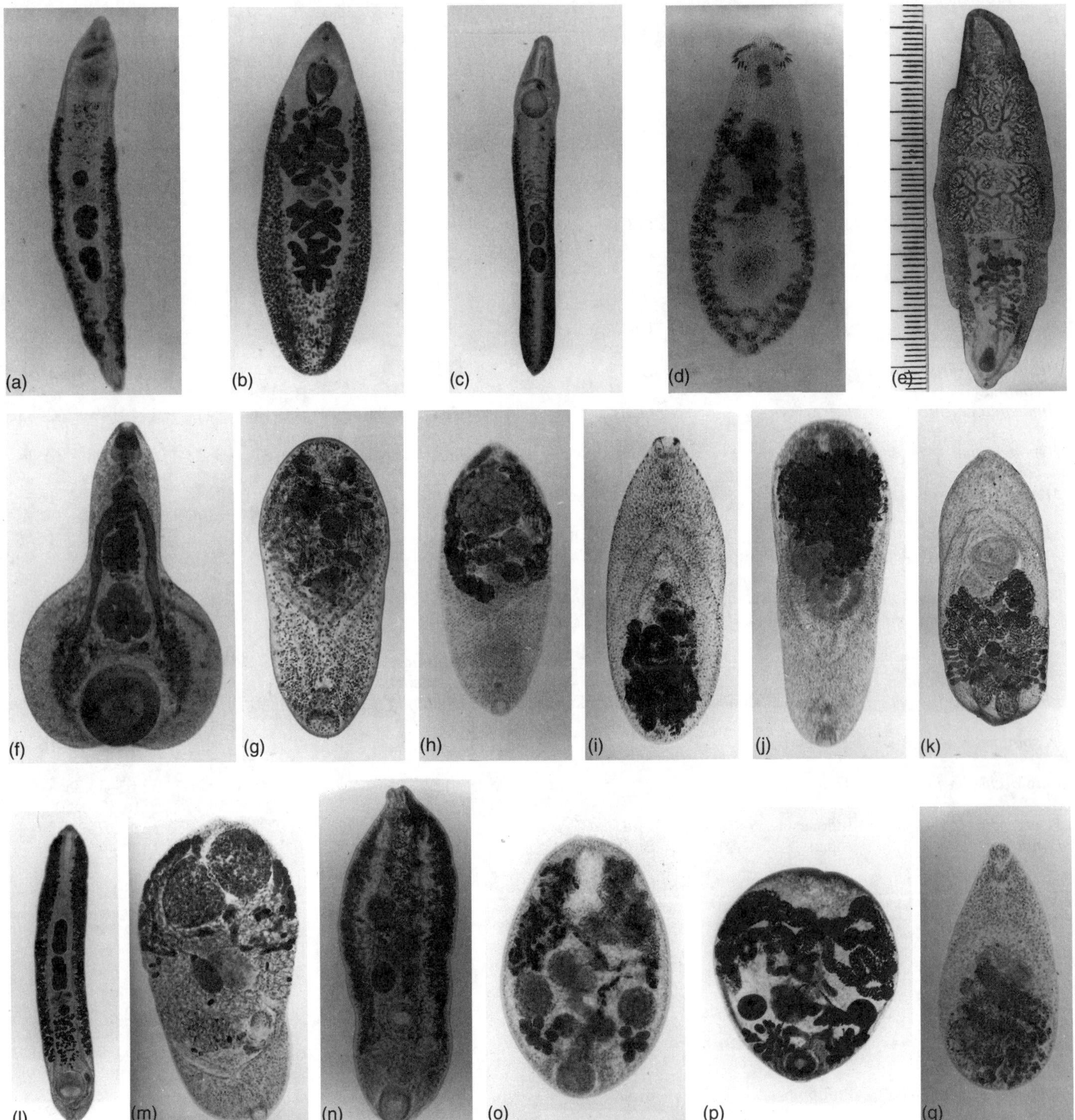

The eggs are large (83–154 μm × 53–95 μm), yellow to yellowish-brown in colour, thin-shelled, operculated, and ellipsoid. They are immature when passed in faeces (Fig. 2(a–d)).

LIFECYCLE

The flukes live in the small intestine and the eggs are passed in faeces. On reaching water, the miracidium develops, hatches, and enters a snail, the first intermediate host. It then develops into sporocyst, mother rediae, daughter rediae, and cercariae. The cercariae escape to infect the second intermediate host, Pila snails, fish, and tadpoles, or they encyst on vegetation. When humans and definitive hosts ingest the second intermediate host in an inadequately cooked form they become infected.

EPIDEMIOLOGY

Echinostoma is an intestinal fluke of birds and mammals; on occasions, human beings become infected. It is common in Indonesia and the Philippines, in places where there is an abundance of the intermediate hosts and lack of sanitary facilities that play an important role in the prevalence of human echinostomiasis. In some villages in north-eastern Thailand, the prevalence rate is around 50 per cent. *E. malayanum, Hypod-*

Fig. 2 Ova of human intestinal flukes: (a) *Echinostoma ilocanum*; (b) *E. malayanum*; (c) *E. revolutum*; (d) *Episthmium caninum*; (e) *Fasciolopsis buski*; (f) *Gastrodiscoides hominis*; (g) *Haplorchis pumilio*; (h) *H. taichui*; (i) *H. yokogawai*; (j) *Hypoderaeum canoideum*; (k) *Metagonimus yokogawai*; (l) *Phaneropsolus bonnei*; (m) *Prosthodendrium molencampi*; (n) *Stellantchasmus falcatus*. (Copyright P. Radomyos.)

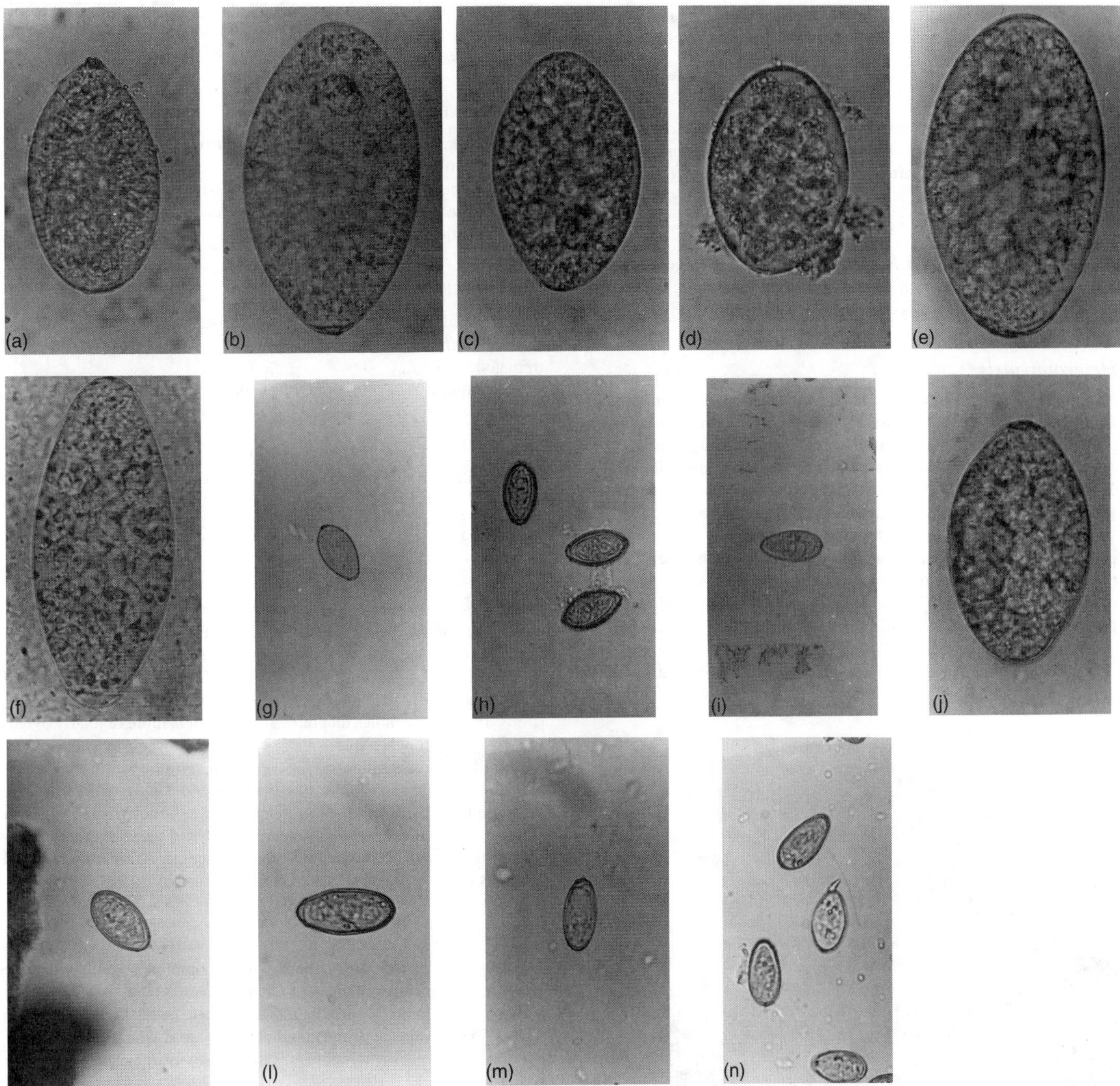

eraeum conoideum, E. revolutum, and *E. ilocanum* have been reported. A few decades ago, *E. lindoensis* was very common in Lindu Lake, Sulawesi (Celebes), and Indonesia, but it has now disappeared; this may be due to the introduction of *Tilapia mossambica* fish in 1951. The snail hosts have dwindled in numbers as there was competition for food with the fish.

PATHOLOGY

The flukes attach by an oral circlet of spines to the mucosa of the small intestine, especially the jejunum, causing little damage to the tissues. Heavy infections may produce catarrhal inflammation of the intestinal mucosa.

CLINICAL FINDINGS

Heavy worm loads may cause vague abdominal complaints of flatulence and loose motions. In children, diarrhoea, abdominal pain, anaemia, and oedema, reminiscent of fasciolopsiasis buski, have been reported.

DIAGNOSIS

The diagnosis is made by recovering eggs from faeces. However, it is impossible to differentiate between species except by examining adult worms recovered in faeces after anthelminthics or recovered at autopsy.

TREATMENT

All drugs recommended for *F. buski* infection are effective. The prognosis is good. The infection can be prevented by thoroughly cooking and avoiding raw Pila snails and other second intermediate hosts.

Heterophyiasis

More than 10 species of minute heterophyid flukes have been found in man (Table 1); *Heterophyes heterophyes* (synonyms: *Distoma heterophyes, H. aegyptiaca, H. nocens* etc.) is the most common.

Heterophyes heterophyes is a pyriform, grey, very small fluke (1.0–1.76 × 0.3–0.7 mm). The cuticle is covered with scales that are closely set and most numerous in the anterior portion of the body.

The egg is the same size as that of *Clonorchis sinensis* (20–30 µm × 15–17 µm). It contains a ciliated miracidium when deposited. It hatches after being ingested by freshwater or brackish-water snails, the first intermediate hosts. The cercariae emerge from the snail and enter freshwater or brackish-water fish.

The proven snail hosts are *Pirenella conica* in the Middle East, and *Cerithidea cingulata* and *Tympanotonus micropterus* in the Far East.

Fig. 3 Water caltrop (*Trapa bicornis*). (Copyright P. Radomyos.)

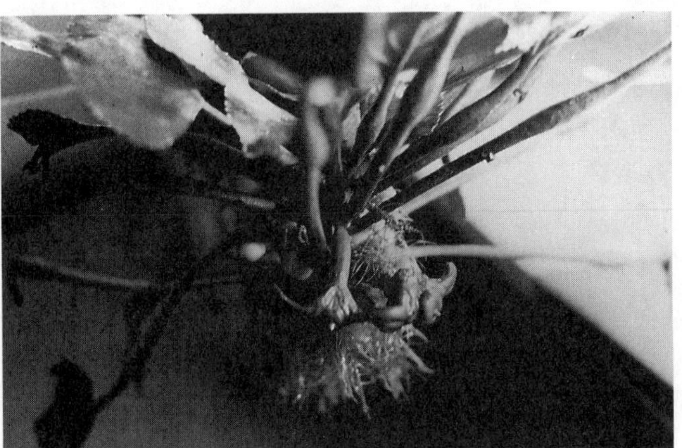

The fish second intermediate hosts are the mullet (*Mugil cephalus*), minnow (*Gambusia affinis*), and *Acanthogobius* in Japan.

EPIDEMIOLOGY

Human infection is common in Egypt, Iran, the Far East, Japan (*H. katsuradai*), South Korea, Taiwan, China, and the Philippines (*H. brevicaeca*). The fluke inhabits the small intestine of man, cat, dog, fox, bird, and other fish-eating mammals. People are infected by eating infected raw fish.

PATHOLOGY

Flukes attach to small-bowel mucosa producing shallow ulcers and a mild inflammatory response. Ova deposited in the bowel wall may enter blood vessels and embolize to the heart and central nervous system. In the Philippines, severe cardiac damage was described in former times. The heart is dilated, there are subepicardial haemorrhages and myocardial damage caused by occlusion of vessels by the ova. Ova stick to the mitral valve, which becomes thickened and calcified.

CLINICAL FEATURES

Dyspepsia and gastroenterocolitis with mucous diarrhoea are common. Cardiac involvement may produce chronic congestive cardiac failure or there may be sudden death caused by massive coronary embolization. This disease was said to be responsible for more than 14 per cent of cardiac deaths in the Philippines.

DIAGNOSIS

This is based on the recovery of characteristic eggs in the faeces, but it is very difficult to differentiate from eggs of other heterophyid trematodes.

Prevention is by avoiding raw or undercooked fish.

TREATMENT

Praziquantel at a single dose of 15 to 25 mg/kg may be effective. Hexylresorcinol, tetrachloroethylene, and bephenium are also effective. The prognosis is good except when the brain and heart are involved.

Metagonimiasis

Metagonimus yokogawai (synonyms: *Heterophyes yokogawai, Loxotrema ovatum, M. ovatus, Yokogawa yokogawai, Loossia romanica, L. parva, L. dobrogiensis, M. romanicus* etc.) is the smallest human fluke (1–2.5 mm × 0.4–0.7 mm) and resembles *H. heterophyes* in size and shape (Fig. 1(m)). The cuticle is covered with small spines. The egg (27 µm × 16 µm) resembles that of *C. sinensis* but is more regularly ovoid. It is fully mature when laid.

The lifecycle is similar to *Heterophyes heterophyes*. The first intermediate hosts are *Semisulcospira libertina* and *Thiara granifera*. The second intermediate hosts are salmonoid and cyprinoid fish. Sweet fish (*Plecoglossus altivelis*) and silver carp (*Carassius carassius*) are important hosts in Japan, Taiwan, and Korea. Metacercariae are usually found in scales (Fig. 4), fins, and subcutaneous tissues of the fish.

EPIDEMIOLOGY

M. yokogawai is believed to be the most common heterophyid fluke infection in the endemic areas of China, Japan, Korea, and Taiwan. It has also been reported from Siberia, Manchuria, Israel, the Balkans, and Spain. The prevalence of metagonimiasis in areas where there are clonorchiasis and other heterophyids is difficult to estimate as the eggs are similar.

People are infected by eating raw or undercooked fish.

PATHOLOGY

The flukes invade the mucosa of the small intestine, the duodenum or the jejunum causing inflammation, granulomatous infiltration, and ulceration. They ultimately become encapsulated. On rare occasions, eggs deposited in the tissues are carried by the bloodstream and deposited in other organs.

CLINICAL FINDINGS

The infection causes either mild diarrhoea or no symptoms. When eggs are carried by the bloodstream and lodge in other tissues, serious manifestations may result.

DIAGNOSIS

The diagnosis is based on the recovery of eggs in stools. The eggs resemble those of *C. sinensis* but the shell is thicker around the operculum of *C. sinensis*. The eggs of *M. yokogawai* are indistinguishable from those of *H. heterophyes*.

Gastrodisciasis

Gastrodiscoides hominis (synonym: *Gastrodiscus hominis*) is an aspinous fluke. When alive it is bright pinkish, very expansile (8–14 mm × 5–8 mm) and pyriform in outline, with a conical anterior and a discoidal posterior portion (Fig. 1(f)). A huge acetabulum occupying the ventral posterior portion of the fluke bears a characteristic notch at its posterior extremity. The eggs are greenish brown and immature when laid (152 μm × 60 μm (Fig. 2(f)). The lifecycle is not known but it is probably similar to those of amphistomes. The cercariae probably encyst on vegetation.

EPIDEMIOLOGY

G. hominis is a common parasite in Assam, Bengal, Bihar, and Orissa in India. Human infections have also been reported from Burma, Malaysia, Vietnam, British Guyana, Kazakhstan in the former USSR, and Thailand.

Reservoir hosts include pigs in India and deer in Malaysia.

PATHOLOGY

G. hominis attaches to the mucosa of the caecum and ascending colon. The pathology in man and pig may be similar. At the site of attachment the mucosa is dragged out by the acetabulum, forming a minute papilla in the sharply defined circular imprint made by the discoidal region of the fluke. There is surface desquamation of the mucosa. Both the mucosa and submucosa show infiltration with eosinophils, lymphocytes, and plasma cells.

Fig. 4 Metacercariae of *Metagonimus yokogawai* in scale of the fish, which is the second intermediate host. (Copyright P. Radomyos.)

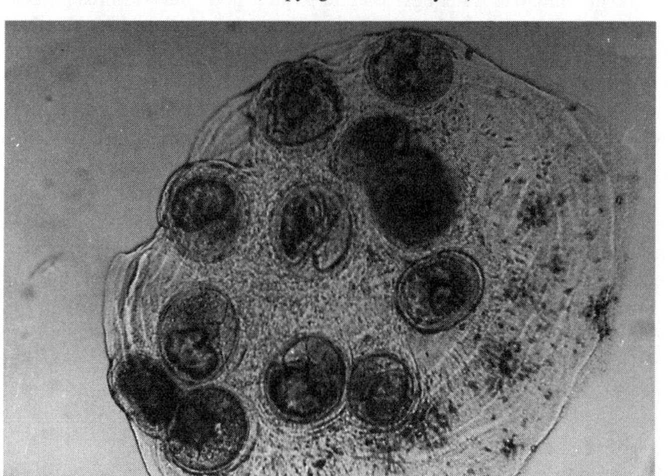

CLINICAL FINDINGS

The flukes live in the caecum in large numbers, usually producing no symptoms. Mucous diarrhoea associated with gastrodisciasis has been recorded.

DIAGNOSIS

The diagnosis is based on the finding of characteristic ova or adult flukes after anthelminthic. The ova resemble those of *Fasciolopsis buski* but are narrower and have a greenish-brown colour. The adult fluke may be identified readily by its pyriform shape, bright pinkish colour, and huge notched acetabulum.

TREATMENT

Praziquantel at the same dosage used in fasciolopsiasis may be effective.

Alariasis

In North America, various species of Alaria are parasites, in their adult fluke stage, in the gut of wild carnivores such as wolves, foxes, bobcats, martens, and skunks. Ova passed in faeces hatch in water, invade snails (genus Helisoma) from which cercariae eventually emerge and infect frog tadpoles. One fatal human infection with *Alaria americana* was assumed to have resulted from eating raw frogs' legs, and another eye infection to direct penetration by the infective mesocercarial stage while frogs were being prepared for the table. Treatment has never been attempted, but praziquantel, bithionol or niridazole might be effective.

Other minor genera of intestinal flukes, occasionally reported as human infections include *Eurytrema*, *Haplorchis* (Fig. 1(g–i) Fig. 2(g–i)), *Plagiorchis* (Fig. 1(n)), *Episthmium* (Fig. 1(d)), *Prosthodendrium* (Fig. 1(p), Fig. 2(m)), and *Phaneropsolus* (Fig. 1(o), Fig. 2(l)).

REFERENCES

Africa, C.M., De Leon, W., and Garcia, E.Y. (1935). Heterophyidiasis: II Presence of ova in sclerosed mitral valves with other chronic lesions in the myocardium. *Journal of the Philippines Medical Association*, **15,** 583–592.

Bunnag, D., Harinasuta, T., and Radomyos, P. (1983). Clinical trial of praziquantel on fasiolopsiasis buski. *South-East Asian Journal* of *Tropical Medicine and Public Health*, **14,** 216–219.

Carney, W.P., Sudomo, M., and Purnomo (1980). Echinostomiasis: a disease that disappeared. *Tropical and Geographic Medicine*, **32,** 101–106.

Cross, J.H. (1969). Fasciolopsiasis in Southeast Asia and the Far East. In *Schistosomiasis and other snail-transmitted helminthiasis, Proceedings of the 4th South-East Asian seminar on parasitology and tropical medicine*, (ed. C. Harinasuta), pp. 177–199. Manila, Philippines.

Manning, G.S. and Lertprasert, P. (1973). Studies on the life cycle of *Phaneropsolus bonnei* and *Prosthodendrium molenkampi* in Thailand *Annals of Tropical Medicine and Parasitology*, **67,** 361–365.

Radomyos, P., Bunnag, D., and Harinasuta, T. (1984). Worms recovered in stools following praziquantel treatment. *Arzneimittelforschung/Drug Research, 34(II)*, **9b,** 1186–1188.

Radomyos, P., Radomyos, B., and Tungtrongchitr, A. (1994). Multi-infection with helminths in adults from northeast Thailand as determined by post-treatment fecal examination of adult worms. *Tropical Medicine and Parasitology*, **45,** 133–5.

Suntharasamai, P. *et al.* (1974). Comparative clinical trial of niclosamide and tetrachlorethylene in the treatment of *Fasciolopsis buski* infection. *South-East Asian Journal* of *Tropical Medicine and Public Health*, **5,** 556.

7.17 Non-venomous arthropods

A. J. Radford and J. Paul

There are more than a million species in the phylum Arthropoda, a few hundred of which are of great medical importance. Nearly all the significant taxa belong to the classes Insecta (flies, fleas, lice, cockroaches, eye-frequenting moths, pharoah's ants) and Arachnida (mites and ticks). Non-venomous arthropods may be medically important by causing mechanical injury, as specific and passive vectors of infection, as allergens, and as a source of phobias. The most important organisms are those that gain nourishment by feeding on human tissues, blood, secretions or wounds; as such they may be directly destructive, painful or irritating, or specific or passive vectors of infection. Many blood-sucking arthropods are predatory, making transient visits to humans for a blood meal, while the human louse, *Pediculus humanus* (L.), the pubic louse, *Pthirus pubis* (L.), and the human flea, *Pulex irritans* (L.), are long-term human residents. The scabies mite, *Sarcoptes scabiei* (L.) is a skin parasite, and the follicle mite, *Demodex follicularum* (Simon), is well-adapted to the human host and rarely troublesome. Besides feeding on man, arthropods may inflict bites when threatened. Some may accidentally enter various orifices of the body. The larvae of several species of fly and a few types of beetle are facultative parasites of wounds or may temporarily dwell in the intestine when accidentally swallowed. Some Diptera are obligate parasites, causing dermal, wound, and nasopharyngeal myiasis. Without having direct contact with man, several arthropod species, including some of the Crustacea, are hosts of certain stages of human parasites. Arthropods that feed on human food, wounds, and faeces, notably cockroaches and flies, are potential passive vectors of bacterial and viral infections. A number of moths and some flies specialize in feeding on eye secretions and are potential vectors of eye infections. Arthropods that feed on man often cause local allergy, whilst arthropod antigens may serve as inhalent allergens. There are phobias directed at various arthropods.

General management principles include identification of the arthropod, recognition of associated risks, and removal, destruction or avoidance of the organism. Arthropods for identification by a specialist may be sent as dry specimens, wrapped in tissue in a plastic box, while the softer larvae, mites, and ticks may be preserved in 70 per cent ethanol, or 10 per cent formalin. All arthropods can be controlled with insecticides. Vectors may be avoided by use of repellents, bed nets impregnated with pyrethrum insecticide, and appropriate clothing. Parasites may be removed mechanically or treated with insecticides.

Parasites

Order: Diptera

Myiasis

Myiasis is the infestation of living animals by the larvae of flies (Diptera). It may be classified according to the anatomical site; so there are dermal, subdermal, wound, nasopharyngeal, orbital, ophthalmic, aural, urogenital, and intestinal myiases. Many species of fly can cause myiasis, but the majority are opportunists whose saprophagous larvae normally dwell in and feed on decaying organic matter such as carrion. They are thus equipped to flourish in necrotic wounds. Such maggots usually confine themselves to dead tissue and may even benefit the healing process. For centuries, maggots have been used to debride necrotic wounds. There is no dipterous obligate intestinal parasite of man. Intestinal myiasis may be caused by coprophagous larvae that invade the rectum of a debilitated host or by resilient maggots, such as those of the false stable fly, *Muscina stabulans* (Fallén), and the cheese skipper, *Piophila casei* (L.), that survive in the intestine when swallowed in infested food and may cause intestinal disturbance and scarring. Intestinal myiasis may also be spurious, being suspected on the grounds of finding rapidly hatching larvae on freshly passed faeces. No species is dependent on completing its lifecycle within the urinary system, but several genera of saprophagous flies may cause urogenital myiasis, notably *Fannia* spp., which may invade the urinary tract as well as wounds. Besides flies with a saprophagous background, there are myiasis flies whose larvae are specialist piercers, blood suckers, and burrowers. A limited number of flies are obligate parasites of living animal tissues and a few species are closely associated but not specific to man. These include predatory blood-sucking species, the most important being the Congo floor maggot, *Auchmeromyia luteola* (Fab.), as well as more permanent residents, which show various degrees of adaptation to the human host. In particular, the Tumbu fly, *Cordylobia anthropophaga* (Blanchard), in the Afrotropical region, and the human bot fly, *Dermatobia hominis* (L.), in the neotropical region, are locally common causes of dermal myiasis. The New World screw-worm, *Cochliomyia hominivorax* (Coquerel), is a cause of nasopharyngeal, genital, and wound myiasis in the Americas, where as well as being detrimental to livestock it may cause mutilating and fatal injuries to man. The Old World screw-worm, *Chrysomya bezziana* (Villeneuve), and Wohlfahrt's wound myiasis fly, *Wohlfahrtia magnifica* (Schiner), which are obligatory wound myiasis species, probably arose from saprophagous ancestors, as both species have congeners that are carrion feeders, but may sometimes cause wound myiasis. For the taxonomist, there are large catalogues of myiasis-causing species. Identifying specimens is the job of an entomologist. Many cases of myiasis are self-limiting and relatively harmless, but aural, nasopharyngeal, and malign wound myiasis are potentially lethal entities that may require removal of the larvae and possibly reconstructive surgery.

Dermal myiasis

In the lowland forests of the American tropics, the human bot fly, *D. hominis*, is a common cause of dermal myiasis. The adult fly is seldom seen. The female lays her eggs on biting arthropods, such as mosquitoes, and the eggs hatch when in contact with a warm-blooded mammal or bird and pierce the skin. The larval stage (Fig. 1) lasts about 10 weeks, a boil with a small aperture forming as the larva grows. Such boils are not infrequently seen in Europeans returning from the neotropics. The lesion may not be noticed until quite large, the full-grown larva reaching over a centimetre in length. If in an inconspicuous site, such as the back or scalp, the first thing that the patient may notice is sporadic pain caused by the moving, spiny larva. Unless in an unusual site, such as close to the eye, infestation is generally harmless; if left alone, the insect will reach maturity and leave of its own accord. Secondary infection of the wound is the most common complication. In areas where the insect is well known there are numerous, but not always successful, remedies for removing larvae, including the application of raw meat or glue to the lesion. Larvae may be removed by means of a simple incision. Partial removal of the larva may result in a local granulomatous reaction, a hazard of squeezing out the larva.

The Tumbu fly, *C. anthropophaga*, is widespread in the Afrotropical region. The female oviposits on sand and also on clothes left out to dry.

Babies' nappies are a common site of oviposition. Ironing destroys the eggs. Contact with viable ova on clothing leads to infestation. The larvae pierce the skin and grow rapidly but may not be noticed for several days until an obvious and uncomfortable boil has formed, which oozes serosanguinous fluid. Infestation can be associated with fever and lymph node enlargement. Larvae reach maturity in about 10 days. They may be removed by forceps through a simple incision. Alternatively, paraffin or petroleum jelly may be applied to the boil aperture. This excites the larva, which may be expressed from the lesion.

Horse bot flies, *Gasterophilus* spp., lay their eggs on the hairs of animals, mainly equines, whence the larvae make their way to the stomach where they mature. Young larvae can pierce human skin, where they wander around for a week or so, causing intense itching. The infestation is self-limiting in man. The larvae of warble flies, *Hypoderma* spp., occasionally cause dermal myiasis in man.

Predatory sanguivorous myiasis

The Congo floor maggot, *A. luteola*, from tropical Africa, is a predatory blood-sucking species whose visits to man are limited to the 10 to 20 min needed to puncture the skin and obtain a blood meal. Each maggot feeds once nightly and otherwise conceals itself on hut floors. The maggots are a nuisance and can cause pain at the time of feeding and irritation afterwards. Maggots can be avoided by sleeping on a raised bed.

Fig. 1 (a) Two, third larval instars of the human bot fly (*Dermatobia hominis*) (approx. 13 mm long) extracted from a facial 'boil' in a European who had been visiting Guyana. (b) Larva of *Dermatobium hominis*, initially infesting the scalp of a young child in Panama. The larva made a 4-mm diameter hole in the anterior fontanelle and entered the frontal lobe of the brain. The child died of malaria. (Armed Forces Institute of Pathology photograph, neg. no 50807.)

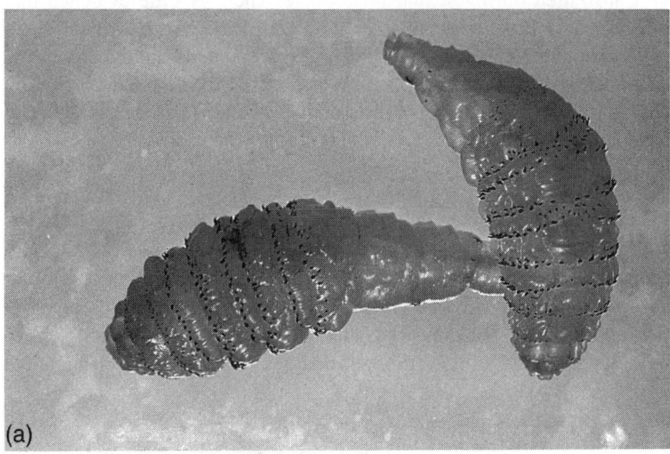

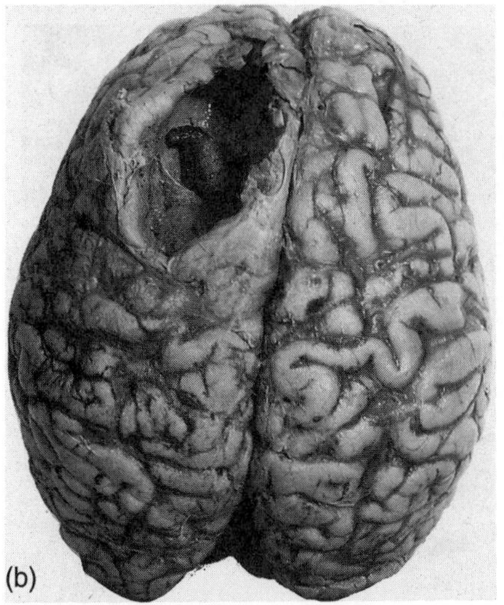

Wound myiasis

Many dipterous species are known to cause wound myiasis, but most of them are facultative feeders on necrotic tissue and are rarely very destructive to the host, although the presence of maggots in a wound may cause distress. Debridement and wound cleaning are all that are needed to control such infestation. Wounds may become a source of secondary bacterial infection and tetanus.

The Old World screw-worm, *C. bezziana*, of Africa and southern Asia, Wohlfaht's wound myiasis fly or spotted flesh fly, *W. magnifica*, of North Africa, and the New World screw-worm, *C. hominivorax*, of the Americas, are the principal causes of malign myiasis in man. Their larvae are obligate parasites of living tissue. Batches of eggs are laid on wounds, in ears, and on mucous membranes. The larvae (Fig. 2) burrow in groups into healthy tissue, causing widespread destruction that may be mutilating or fatal (Fig. 3). Secondary bacterial infection or secondary wound myiasis may ensue. All species may cause nasopharyngeal, aural, orbital, genital, and malign wound myiasis. Infestation is best avoided by cleaning and dressing wounds as they occur. Treatment involves surgical removal of the larvae, debridement of affected tissue, wound cleaning, and treatment of secondary infection.

Ophthalmic myiasis

Nasal bot flies, *Oestrus* spp., naturally parasitize various herbivorous mammals. They are larviparous and drop their larvae into the nostrils of the host. Dropped into human eyes they cause a self-limiting conjunctivitis. Larvae of warble flies, *Hypoderma* spp., are more dangerous: they may burrow into the eye, resulting in pain, nausea, and blindness, and must be surgically removed.

Canthariasis

Infestation of the body by beetles or their larvae is called canthariasis. It may be confused with, and is much rarer than, myiasis. Larvae swallowed in infested food may temporarily dwell in the intestines, causing discomfort and may be detected in excreta. Adult scarabid dung beetles have been reported to invade the rectum of patients in Sri Lanka.

Fig. 2 Larvae of the New World screw-worm (*Cochliomyia hominivorax*) (approx. 8 mm long) extracted from the wound illustrated in Fig. 3. These were sent to the Natural History Museum, London, where they were identified. Larvae of the secondary myiasis species, *C. macellaria*, were also found in the sample and were probably collected from the edges of the wound. (By courtesy of Dr Martin J.R. Hall, Medical and Veterinary Division, The Natural History Museum, London.)

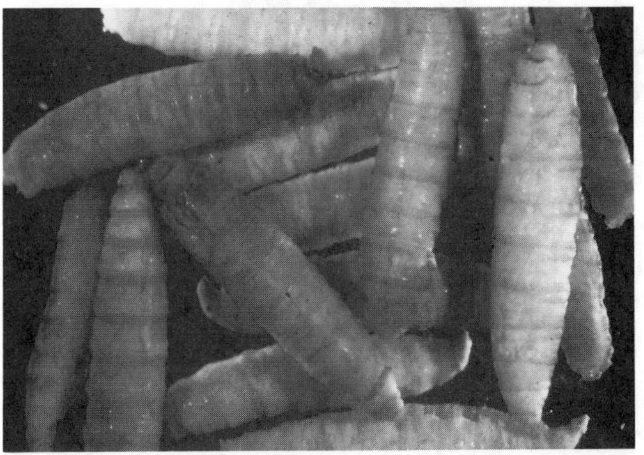

Lice

Order: Pthiraptera
Family: Pediculidae

To a louse, on seeing on a lady's bonnet at church:

Ye ugly creepin', blastit wonner;
Detested, shunn'd, by saunt and sinner
How dare ye set your fit upon her.
Sae fine a lady
Gae somewhere else, and seek your dinner
On some poor body.
(Robert Burns)

Lice have had a long association with man and have even been found on ancient mummies in Egypt. Once known as 'pearls of poverty', they were regarded as a sign of sainthood—Thomas à Becket's clothes were noted to crawl with them after his death.

The two varieties (head and body) of human pediculus (Latin: louse) are morphologically quite distinct. Although they may coexist, there is no correlation between their prevalence densities, that is, they are 'spatially and ecologically isolated'. Where double infestation occurs, the areas of overlap are less than 1 per cent, indicating that the habitat of one is unsuitable for the other. *Pthirus* is the correct name for the pubic louse, the original description containing a printing error of *Phthirus* (Greek: louse).

*Head louse infestation (*Pediculus humanus capitis*)*

An increasing prevalence was reported throughout Europe during the 1960s, 1970s and 1980s. It is lower before preschool age but is by no means uncommon in adults. There is a wide variation in cultural response to infestation. In some communities it is not only regarded as normal, it has positive social significance (Fig. 4), while in upper strata of more industrialized societies, infestation is usually viewed with shock and abhorrence, and, if contracted, may become a cause of shame and embarrassment. Widely varying prevalence rates have been reported in parts of Britain, from a high 30 per cent in the early 1940s, and 23 per cent in the lower socioeconomic groups of Teeside in the 1970s, 4 to 10 per cent in Glasgow, and slightly less in Northern Ireland, to current estimates of 2 to 3 per cent for the United Kingdom as a whole. Rates in females usually outnumber those in males by approximately 3:1. In the New World, rates of 22.5 per cent in females and 17 per cent in males in Chile, and an average for whites of 7 per cent in males and 10 per cent in females in the United States, with a lower rate in blacks, have been noted. It has been estimated that 6 to 12 million cases occur annually in the United States at a cost of $363 million a year. In Malaysia, one study reported rates of over 30 per cent in some states, with a racial variation between Indians (28.3 per cent), Malays (18.9 per cent), and Chinese (4.6 per cent). In Taiwan, 40 per cent of girls in three girls' schools were infected, with up to 66.7 per cent in one primary class. Similarly high rates are also reported from East and West Africa.

Head lice, like scabies, have no respect for class. The rise in prevalence in Europe may reflect increasing resistance to DDT or increased social mixing between groups in society. An increased incidence has been reported in warmer months.

Lice are blood, not debris, feeders. Studies show that hygiene, or rather lack of it, is not a principal factor in their epidemiology. Hair length has been shown to correlate with prevalence in some studies but not in others. A persistence of these beliefs is a barrier to control. Other possible factors, largely unproven, include apathy by health authorities, ignorance, increased tourism, migrant labour, and communal living. While most transmission is among younger age groups, and is usually effected by direct contact or by shared combs and brushes, lice can also be transmitted during sexual intercourse. There is little evidence that lice are significant reservoirs for infections other than pyogenic skin bacteria, though they can be experimentally infected with the organisms which cause typhus and relapsing fever. Extensive community education and ready access to treatment is essential as control can be expensive in terms of personnel.

BIOLOGY

Adult lice are 3 to 4 mm long with colour variations from dirty white to grey-black (Fig. 5). They are scalp rather than hair dwellers, living very close to the skin where food, moisture, warmth, and ovipositing sites are readily available. They attach to the hair base by strong, crab-like claws and suck blood through a stylet. An anticoagulant in saliva

Fig. 3 Fatal myiasis (New World screw-worm): historical illustration of a 50-year-old Honduran woman who complained of a small chronic ulcer on the right cheek; on admission to hospital she was found to have a huge ulcer exposing the bones of the face and forehead and destroying the tissues of the cheek and face, right eye, and orbit; more than 300 larvae were removed (see Fig. 2). (Harrison, J.H.H. (1908). A case of myiasis. *Journal of Tropical Medicine and Hygiene*, XI, 20.)

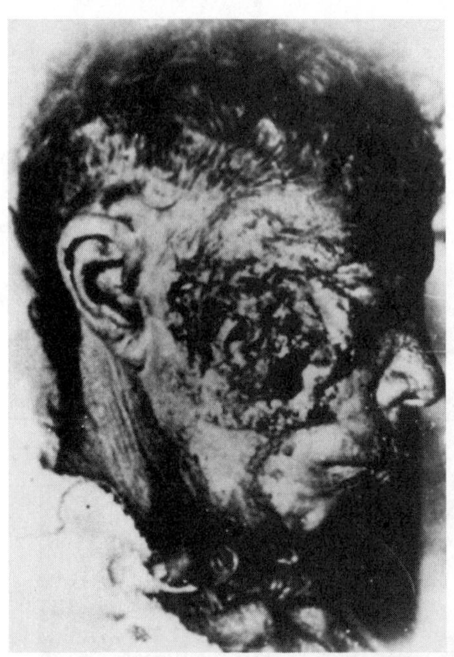

Fig. 4 Delousing: a family affair in Papua New Guinea.

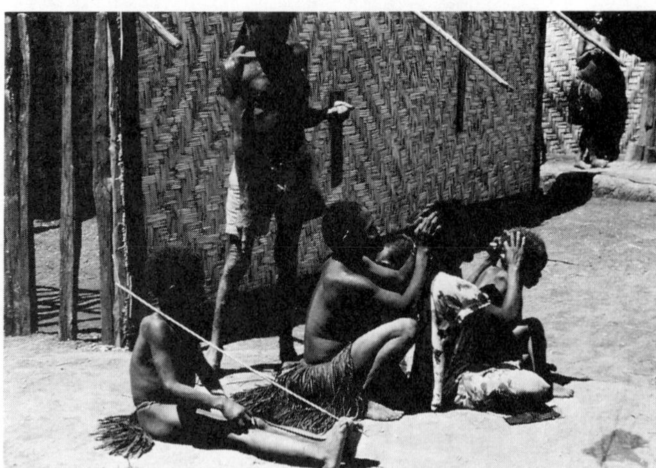

provides increased flow and may, together with the sensation caused by the movement of the arthropods, be the cause of irritation. Adults are very difficult to dislodge but once damaged tend to die quickly. They readily resist washing by closing over their breathing apparatus. An average infestation is 5 to 10 lice per head. Eggs are produced at a rate of six to eight per day and are well dispersed over the scalp. Immature forms (nymphs) pass through three moults (instars) over 7 to 16 days; the warmer the environment the shorter the incubation period. During a lifetime of 30 to 40 days, up to 300 eggs are laid. These are placed within 1 cm of the scalp and are strongly cemented to the base of the hair, growing out at a rate of 1 cm a month. Thus, the duration of infection can be measured by the distance of the ovoid egg containers, 'nits', from the scalp (Fig. 6).

Fig. 5 Adult specimen of *Pediculus humanus*. (Reproduced by courtesy of R.V. Southcott, Adelaide, South Australia.)

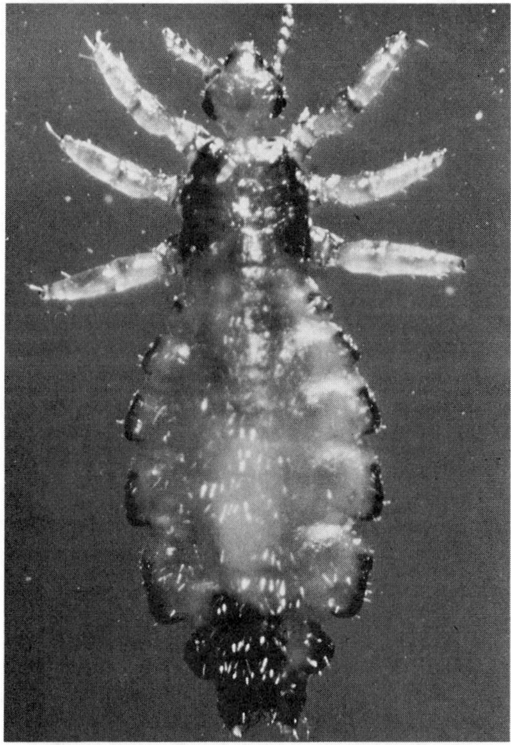

Fig. 6 Nits attached to hair. (Reproduced by courtesy of D. Hill, Adelaide.) Photograph showing several hair fibres with numerous egg cases attached from a patient with pediculosis.

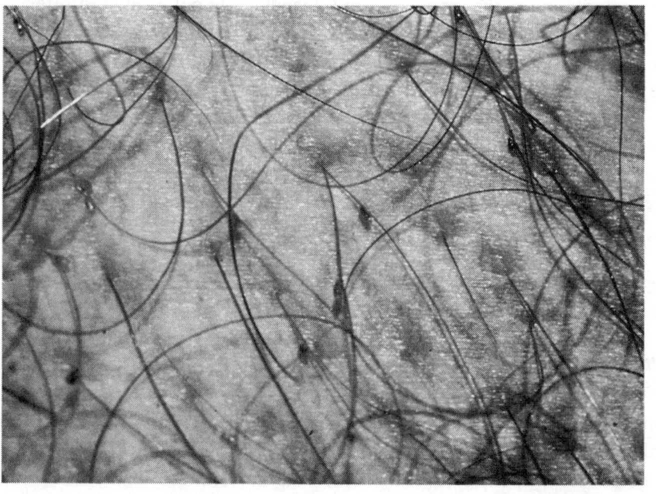

CLINICAL FEATURES

Variable but often intense itching is the predominant symptom. Therefore, inattention or observation of persistent scratching of the scalp by teacher or parent may alert one to the diagnosis. Secondary infection may cause impetigo or furunculosis and consequent cervical adenitis, leading to the diagnosis. Occasionally a 'cap' of debris may form over the scalp with the lice attached to the base of hairs underneath.

Diagnosis is most commonly confirmed through finding the white, empty nits firmly adherent to hairs, and a more careful inspection will reveal the lice attached to hairs near the scalp. Differential diagnosis includes seborrhoeic scales ('dandruff'), hair-spray, soap flakes, and hair casts, all of which readily brush off.

*Body louse infestation (*Pediculus humanus humanus*)*

Unlike their loftier, smaller relative, body lice may be associated with the transmission of serious infections. These include the often fatal, louse-borne or epidemic typhus (*Rickettsia prowazekii*) (see Chapter 7.11.37), the less serious trench fever (*Bartonella quintana*) (see Chapter 7.11.40), and epidemic relapsing fever (*Borrelia recurrentis*) (see Chapter 7.11.30, 7.11.31). Body lice may also play a part in the spread of salmonella infections and some of the taenias, such as the dog tapeworm, *Dipylidium caninum* (Section 7.15). Rickettsiae, spirochaetes, and tubercule bacilli have been shown experimentally to be capable of multiplication in lice. Evidence is less convincing for *Bartonella bacilliformis* and *Toxoplasma gondii* transmission. People are infected through inoculation by contaminated faeces being scratched into the skin, or through mucous membranes or conjunctivae. Less commonly, inoculation occurs through crushing of lice into the skin. With rickettsial infections, the epithelial cells of the louse midgut are involved, and once so the louse remains infected for life. On rupture of these cells into the digestive tract, large numbers of pathogens are released.

Body lice are a clothing rather than a body infestation and are found especially on the mentally defective and on the socially deprived, giving rise to the synonym 'vagabond's disease'.

Although eggs are most commonly found on the seams of clothing, where there is greatest access to body contact thus facilitating the feeding of young, they may also be found on body hair. The incubation period is from 6 to 15 days. Adults are 10 to 20 per cent larger than adult head lice. Gregarious by nature, they are said to be attracted to each other by smell. Feeding points produce pinpoint macules, which may provide portals of entry for pyogenic bacteria by excoriation and resolve leaving pigmented scars.

*Pubic or crab louse (*Pthirus pubis*)*

Sexual intercourse is the most common form of transmission of pthirus, giving rise to the synonym 'butterfly of love', which name also indicates its triangular shape (Fig. 7). Fomite transmission is very uncommon as adults rarely leave the body unless damaged or dying. Transmission from toilet seats, whilst possible, is therefore most unlikely. In contrast to pediculosis, incidence has been noted to increase in cooler months. Children may be affected by direct contact with infested adults or other children, and about 1 per cent of head lice in their age group are *Pthirus* spp.

Adult crab lice live about 1 month. They are broader in the upper abdomen than other lice, and their second and third pairs of legs are stouter. They vary in colour from dirty white through yellow to grey. Pthirus is a voracious feeder, taking up to 12 meals a day, largely of tissue fluid.

CLINICAL FEATURES

Itching and irritation are the major presenting symptoms, especially in the inguinal, pubic, lower abdominal, and perineal hair areas. Axillary, arm, and thigh hair infestation also occurs but is less common. Skin lesions may appear as blue-grey macules or, if excoriated, as reddish pustules. Involvement of eyebrows and eyelashes has given rise to the term 'phthirus palpebrarum'; this is more common in childhood infestations and gives rise to a typical blepharoconjunctivitis, sometimes with a bloodstained discharge at the eyelid margins (see Fig. 8). Careful observation with a loop reveals adult lice towards the roots of affected lashes.

MANAGEMENT

For head lice

In many parts of Europe, increasing resistance of head lice to the chlorinated hydrocarbons (DDT) has made organophosphorous insecticides the drugs of choice. An additional advantage of malathion as an 0.5 per cent alcohol lotion or shampoo, with or without dicophane, and of 10 per cent crotamiton lotion or carbaryl (0.5 per cent liquid), is that they are ovicidal as well as pediculicidal. More recently, less toxic phenothrins such as permethrin (0.5–1 per cent) shampoo have been shown to be equally effective and without the rare central nervous side-effects of some other treatments. Their chemical binding properties with hair ensure that there is a persistence of action for 4 weeks.

Head shaving is not necessary. With lotions, sprinkle the solution into the palm of the hand and, avoiding the eyes, work well into the scalp. Repeat until the whole head is moist and allow to dry naturally. Although single, thorough applications achieve cure rates of approximately 100 per cent, some authorities recommend a second application a few days later as no pediculicide is 100 per cent ovicidal. Malathion, which also has a musty smell, should be avoided in pregnancy. Artificial heat should be avoided as it will denature malathion, which is also inflammable. With shampoos, wet the hair, lather and work well into the scalp, leave for 5 min and repeat. Wash the head in 12 h and use a tight comb while the hair is wet to assist in nit removal. Vinegar solution also assists in removal of nits. In areas of non-resistance, DDT, 2 to 5 per cent emulsion or 10 per cent powder, and 1 per cent γ-benzene hexachloride (**BHC**) shampoo (5–10 ml) can be used but require a repeat application 1 to 2 weeks later to kill recently hatched, immature forms.

Where secondary infection follows, topical antimicrobials such as chlorhexidine and, where substantial adenitis has occurred, oral antibiotics or co-trimoxazole are required. Treatment failure is often due to reinfestation from within the family, up to a third of whom may be infested. Therefore a thorough inspection of family and close contacts is necessary.

Fig. 7 Adult specimen of *Pthirus pubis*. (Reproduced by courtesy of R.V. Southcott, Adelaide, South Australia.)

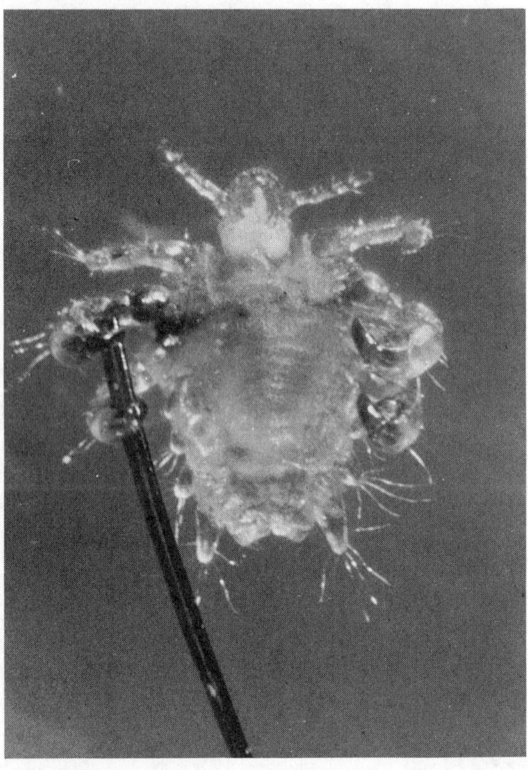

Fig. 8 Phthirus palpebrarum. (Reproduced by courtesy of D. Hill, Adelaide.)

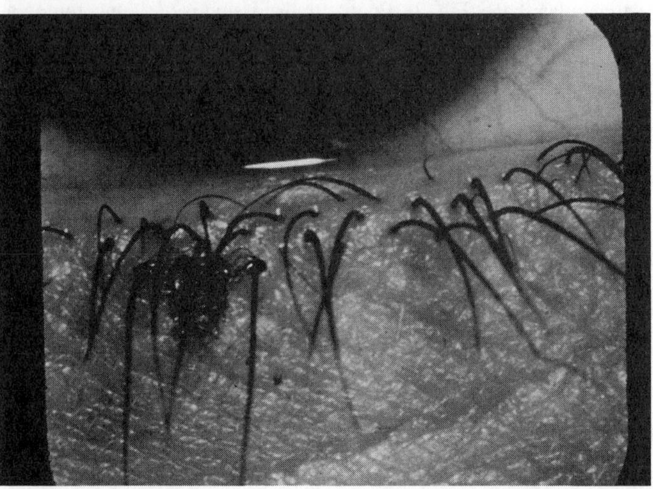

For body lice

Malathion, DDT, or BHC as for head lice are effective. Clothes are readily disinfected by boiling or hot-water machine laundering and ironing.

Pubic lice

As for head and body lice, shaving affected areas is not necessary. Mechanical removal of adults by forceps may be done but is often difficult because of their strong attachment to hair by claws. Yellow oxide of mercury ointment (1 per cent) twice daily for a week or a single application of one or two drops of 20 per cent fluorescein may be used for eyebrow/lash involvement. The usual method of spread of pubic lice should alert the physician to exclude other concomitant venereal diseases, especially asymptomatic gonorrhoea. All sexual partners and, for children, adult family contacts require inspection and treatment as necessary.

There is no reason for a child to be excluded from school immediately after treatment for lice.

Parasitophobia

Parasitophobia is the erroneous and unshakeable belief in skin infestation with a parasite. Rarely, severe forms may present as toxic psychosis, dementia praecox, involutional melancholia or paranoia, and require psychiatric management. Much more common is the stigma attached (especially by parents and teachers) to the false belief of a relation between infestation and poor hygiene. Sympathetic explanation of the ubiquity of lice, their method of spread, and the effectiveness of simple treatment may be required; indeed it should be an integral part of management as the worry is often unvoiced.

Fleas

Order: Siphonaptera.
Family: Pulicidae

There are 2000 species of these temporary obligate, blood-sucking parasites of many animals that include rats, cats, dogs, poultry, horses, and pigs as well as people (Fig. 9). Over 20 species attack man.

The adult spends little time on the host. Ovipositing usually occurs among the hairs of the host (or in its nest). The incubation period varies from 1 to 3 weeks. *Pulex irritans* is the most common offender, together with *Ctenocephalides felis* and *C. canis*. The most common manifestation of flea infestation is their bite. However, they can also be vectors to man of the plague (Chapter 7.11.16), especially by *Xenopsylla* spp., the milder murine typhus (*R. typhi*), Q fever, *Coxiella burneti* (Chapter 7.11.39), listeriosis, salmonellosis, the dog tapeworm, *Dipylidium caninum* (Section 7.15), *Borrelia burgdorferi* (Lyme disease), and haemorrhagic fever.

The usual presentation is a small series of linear, erythematous papules, especially along pressure areas such as belt and bra lines, accompanied by varying degrees of itchiness. There is wide variation in the degree of erythematous reaction and the degree of itching, which is often delayed several hours and may persist for several days. A central bite point may be visible in lesions (Fig. 10). Pathogens are most commonly transmitted by scratching organisms from the flea faeces into excoriated skin lesions or into mucous membranes.

Fig. 9 An adult flea. (Reproduced by courtesy of D. Hill, Adelaide.)

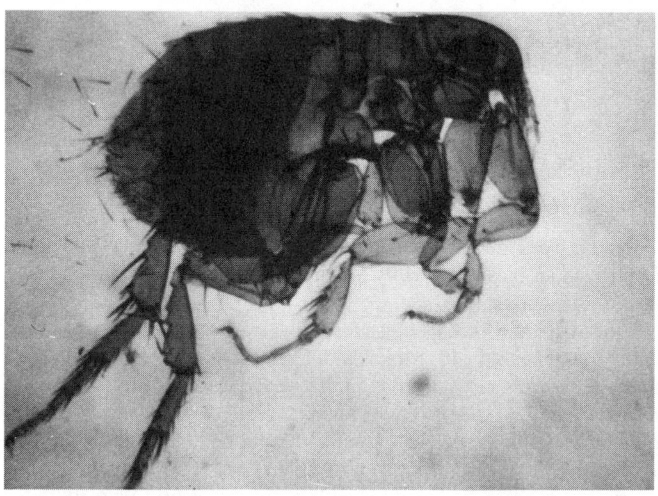

Fig. 10 Fleabites. Erythematous maculopapule with central bite point visible. (Reproduced by courtesy of D. Hill, Adelaide.)

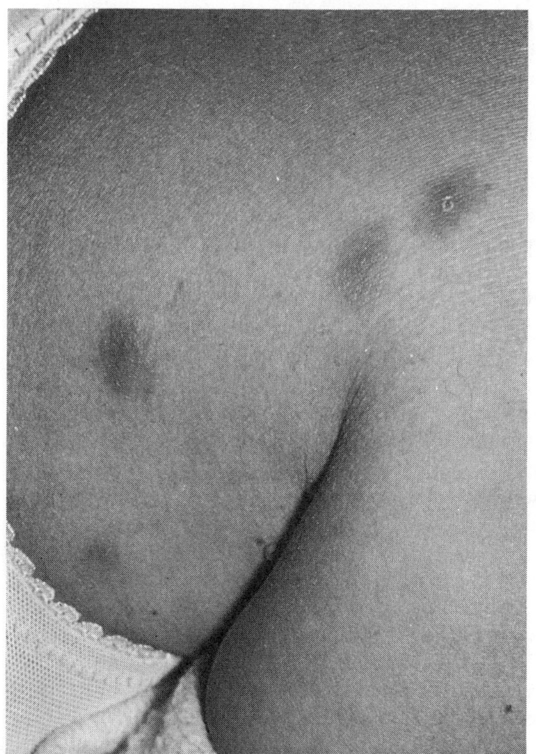

Management consists of local calamine lotion or systemic antihistamine if irritation is severe. More important is the use of a long-acting insecticide such as methoprene (inside the house, alongside base boards, in floor and wall cracks, and under furniture) and of 5 to 10 per cent carbaryl (outside), together with deflea-ing all cats and dogs in the house.

Family: Tungidae

The most troublesome flea to man is *Tunga penetrans*, the 'chigoe', 'jigger', 'chigger' (but see scrub mites, also known as 'jiggers' or 'chiggers', below) or 'sand flea' found in Africa and the tropical Americas but not in Asia. Normally only 1 mm in length, the reddish-brown gravid female may swell to almost 1 cm across, after burrowing into the skin (Fig. 11). Irritation may be extreme. Under the toe nails (very painful), between the toes, and the soles of the feet are the sites of predilection. Secondary infection and ulceration may occur, and tetanus or gangrene are occasional complications. The female may become completely embedded except for a minute aperture. Surgical enucleation is required.

Bed bugs

Order: Hemiptera
Family: Cimidae

The common bed bug, *Cimex lenticularis* (Fig. 12), has been an annoying companion of man for a long time. Both *C. lenticularis* and its virtually identical tropical relation *C. hemipterus* occur in both hemispheres. A second genus, *Leptocimex boneti*, is found in tropical Africa. Other *Cimex* spp. may also attack man. Bed bugs can facilitate the transmission of relapsing fever (*Borrelia recurrentis*) and possibly hepatitis, with which they have been infected experimentally and have transmitted hepatitis B virus to non-human primates.

They are nocturnal bugs that hide in the crevices of beds by day and sally forth at night, often in great numbers. Transmission can also occur from clothing contact, for example, when sitting next to someone in public transport. The young are white-yellow and the adults red-brown in colour. Through a long stiletto mouthpiece they can complete a meal in less than 10 min.

As with fleas there is a great variation in the effect of bites, from minimal to marked irritation and swellings of purplish hue, caused by sensitization to saliva (Fig. 13). The bumps may persist for several days. No specific therapy is necessary, other than calamine lotion and a short course of antihistamines or local steroid when local reaction is marked.

Fig. 11 Histological section of female chigger flea (*Tunga penetrans*) in a foot lesion excised from a European visitor to Venezuela. (Reproduced by courtesy of N. Riley, Guildford, UK.)

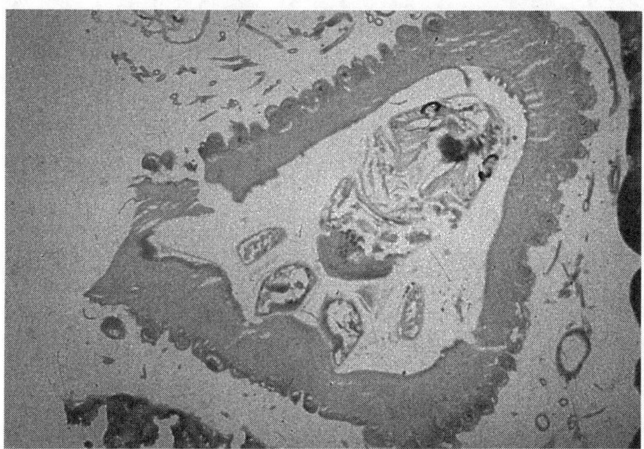

As with fleas, eradication of the parasite with a long-acting pesticide is required for other than casual bites.

Family: Reduviidae

The subfamily of triatomine bugs are the most important medically for their role in the transmission of South American trypanosomiasis (Chagas' disease). They are known by a variety of local names but most commonly as 'kissing' bugs for the lesions they produce around the eyes and mouth, 'cone-nose' bugs from the shape of their probosis, and, inappropriately, 'assassin' bugs because of the lethal effect of other subfamilies on some insects. The most important genera are Rhodnius, Panstrongylus, and Triatoma. There are five tribes of triatome bugs distributed especially across Central Africa and the tropics, but they also occur in parts of Asia, Australasia, and the Pacific.

There are more rural than domestic triatome species. Both are haematophagous. The former live on wild animals and the latter in the cracks and crevices of mud houses, sallying forth at night to forage for a blood meal.

The pain of their bites is very variable, from unnoticed to quite marked. They vary in length from a few millimetres to almost 3 cm in the case of some females.

Control of the bugs is achieved through improved housing, elevation of bedding, and spraying regularly with organochlorine preparations such as BHC or dieldrin, or one of the organophosphates, carbamates or pyrethroids, which require less frequent application but are more expensive.

Fig. 12 Adult specimen of *Cimex lenticularis*. (Reproduced by courtesy of R.V. Southcott, Adelaide, South Australia.)

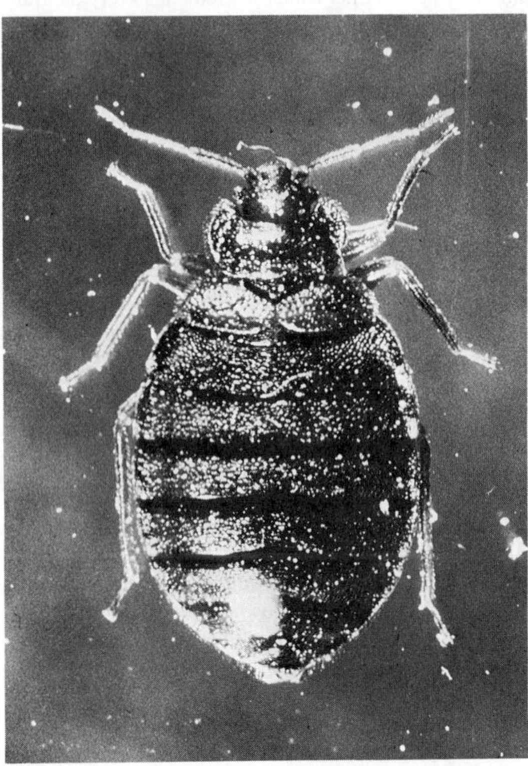

Fig. 13 Erythematous macules of bed bugs. (Reproduced by courtesy of D. Hill, Adelaide.)

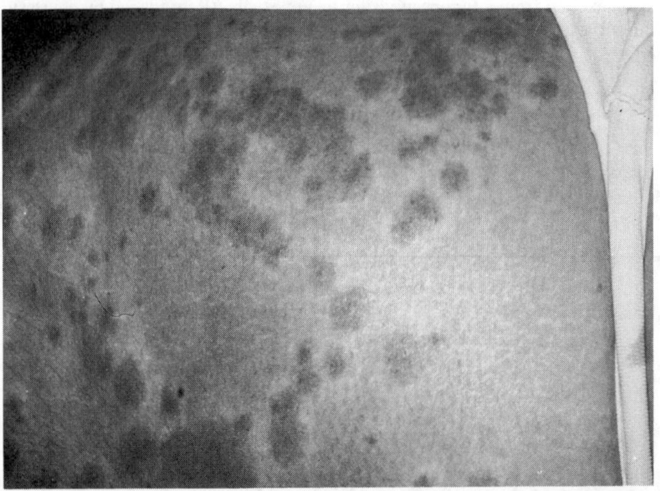

Arachnids

Order: Acarina
Family: Sarcoptidae

*Scabies (*Sarcoptes scabei *var.* hominis*): the itch mite*

EPIDEMIOLOGY

Benomo in 1687 first drew attention to the causal relation between mite and itch, so scabies is probably the first infection for which the known cause was found.

Two pandemics, each lasting about 15 years, occurred in the twentieth century, with peaks in 1918 and 1945. Each had a 30-year cycle. A third pandemic is current in the 1980s and 1990s. Explanations for this pattern are not clear. Changes in herd immunity levels are not the answer as epidemics would take about 45 years to build up a non-sensitized population and this would produce 60-year and not 30-year cycles. While the greatest peaks occurred at the ends of the two World Wars, both the epidemics started in Europe beforehand, and also occurred in countries not significantly involved. The increase during the last decade is worldwide.

Scabies is a disease both of the clean and the dirty. Denmark, where scabies is a notifiable disease, has reported a million cases since 1900. The prevalence there is identical to that at the turn of the century—about 2 per 1000—despite a marked improvement in the standards of living, so a poor standard of living has little basis as a significant aetiological factor. Armed forces' personnel have very high standards of hygiene and diet but in a United States naval study, rates increased eightfold in less than a decade without any concomitant change in the prevalence of gonorrhoea, syphilis, or body lice. Thus, while scabies can be transmitted during intercourse, promiscuity is unlikely to be the major factor in the current epidemic. Prevalence in the West is usually under 5 per cent but may reach 100 per cent in selected groups in less developed countries. The prevalence in the United Kingdom today is between 2 and 4 per cent, and the incidence in dermatological practice in the United States is similar.

Transmission is greater where there is a higher density of infestation. Winter levels exceed those of summer in northern Europe but the provinces in Denmark show no greater prevalence than the capital. Higher rates occur in the tropics where the disease is usually endemic. Increased prevalence has been found in Africa during colder, drier months. While poorer living conditions, greater illiteracy, and lower resistance may exist in such settings, there is also much greater skin-to-skin contact, especially between siblings. Fomites appear to play little part, as repeated experiments with volunteers have failed to facilitate transmission, especially where clothes are washed and ironed regularly. However, studies have indicated prolonged survival of mites in clothes, especially when conditions were cool and humid. Nosocomial infections occur in nursing homes and mental hospitals, where it often presents as a non-specific pruritic eruption and where staff are unfamiliar with the less known but more infectious Norwegian form of the disease (see Fig. 17).

Scabies is most commonly a 'family affair' with a secondary attack rate within families as high as 38 per cent. There is a fairly uniform age distribution until about the age of 45 years after which there is a marked fall in prevalence (Fig. 14). Friends are the most common point source and the greater tendency of girls to hold hands may be the significant factor in the greater prevalence in females, which, in industrial countries, outnumbers that in males by 3:2.

Zoonotic scabies has a shorter incubation period and is usually self-limiting over a few months because these mites do not propagate on human skin. Direct transmission from dogs, pigs, horses, and cats is not uncommon, and occurs especially from external ear, periorbital, back, and abdominal lesions to points of contact. *Sarcoptes scabei* var. *hominis* is distinguishable morphologically from var. *canis*, var. *equi.*, and var. *suis*. *Otoedres cati* is smaller, rounder, and rarely affects man. Animal sources can initiate mini-epidemics within families. In Asia, infestations from buffaloes may occur.

LIFECYCLE

The female mite averages 0.4 × 0.3 cm in size and is about twice the size of the male. It is virtually headless apart from its 'jaws' (Fig. 15). There are four pairs of legs, the front two end in suckers. In the female the third and fourth pair are 'trailers' but in the male the fourth pair also has suckers. Adults can move at the rate of 2.5 cm/min.

Only the adult female of the human variety burrows. She does this under the cornified layer at its junction with the stratum granulosum, continually extending her burrow about 2 mm a day, leaving eggs (two to three per day) and faecal pellets in her wake. The eggs hatch in 3 to 4 days producing six-legged larvae that evolve into eight-legged nymphs 3 days later. These moult once or twice before reaching adulthood; the whole process taking 10 to 14 days. Fewer than 10 per cent of eggs mature into adults, which survive about 30 days.

Almost all initial infections 'take' but there are generally no symptoms and few signs for the first 4 to 6 weeks during which period sensitization occurs. Over ensuing weeks and months a measure of immunity builds up as only 60 per cent of reinfestations, establish themselves and then with lower density loads. With reinfestation, irritation is almost instantaneous. The sensitization is due to mite saliva, faecal material, or both. Infestations in temperate countries are relatively light, with 50 per cent having fewer than six adults and only 4 per cent having greater than 50 in United Kingdom reports.

Fig. 14 Age pattern of scabies 1963–9 and 1970–75, Denmark. (Reproduced from Christophersen (1978). *Archives of Dermatology*, **114**, 749, by permission.)

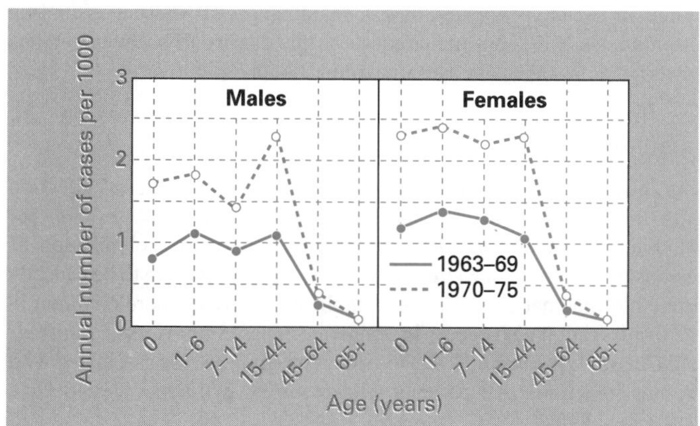

CLINICAL FEATURES

Itching is the hallmark of scabies infestation. It is often worse at night or after a hot shower, possibly due to activation of the mite. The itch can be excruciating and lead to excoriation with soiling of bed linen and haemorrhagic crusting of lesions. Scabies is a very polymorphic disease. Lesions of papular urticaria, eczema, and pyoderma tend to be symmetrical, while papulovesicular lesions with or without eczematous dermatitis are the most common form (Fig. 16). The vesicles are 2 to 3 mm in diameter. Macules, pustules, and scaly plaques also occur. In two-thirds of cases, lesions are confined to the dorsal surface of the interdigital spaces and to the flexor surface of wrists, with at least one lesion being found here in 85 per cent of patients. Occasionally it can be very widespread over much of the body. The palms and soles are less com-

Fig. 15 Adult specimen of *Sarcoptes scabei*. (Reproduced by courtesy of R.V. Southcott, Adelaide, South Australia.)

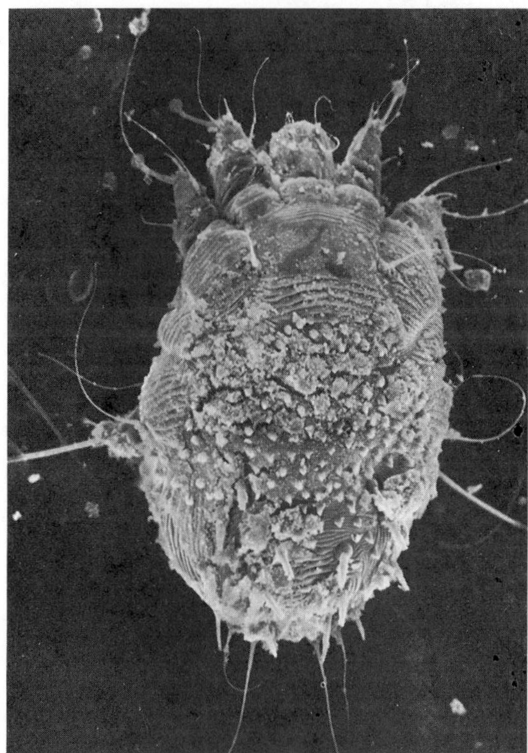

Fig. 16 Papulovesicular lesions of scabies.

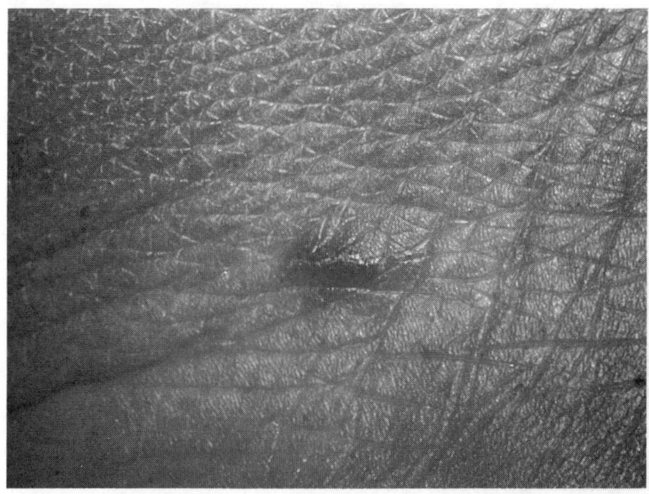

monly affected in adults. Lesions may also occur around the elbows, anterior axillary folds, the breasts, periumbilicus, belt line, lower buttocks, thighs, penis (including glans), the scrotum, below the ankles, and even subungually. The face and scalp are usually involved only in infants, in whom lesions may also be bulbous. In long-standing cases, lichenification is not uncommon (see Fig. 17).

The characteristic burrows are from 3 to 15 mm long and irregular in direction (Fig. 16). They may be difficult to identify and are said to be less common in the current epidemic in industrial countries. Burrows may be more easily felt than seen. (In scabies transmitted from animals they are absent or less common and areas involved tend to be more localized. Interdigital webs and genitalia are usually spared in canine scabies.) There are usually many more lesions than burrows as larval mites do not burrow, only imbed. Periumbilical lesions tend to be eczematous and spoke-like in distribution. Scrotal and penile lesions are reddish and nodular but never discharge unless secondarily infected (Fig. 18). In adults, especially where there has been recent contact with an unstable partner and where perineal lesions are present, other venereal diseases should be excluded; up to 15 per cent of infected adult females have been shown to have asymptomatic gonorrhoea. A less common syndrome of recurrent vesicles and pustules, which persists for many months despite repeated treatments, has recently been described in some Asian refugees in the United States.

The nodular variety may persist for months or years and the Norwegian form especially so. It is so named because it was first described in Norwegian leprosy patients. This variant is more commonly found in the elderly, the incapacitated, and the mentally retarded (especially in patients with Down's syndrome), and at any age in the tropics. In all these groups, presentation for treatment is often delayed. Thick, white or yellowish scales or plaques may be widespread and may involve the palms and the soles. Nail dystrophy is common. The diagnosis is occasionally masked in the immunosuppressed, including patients with AIDS in whom the Norwegian form is now a recognized complication.

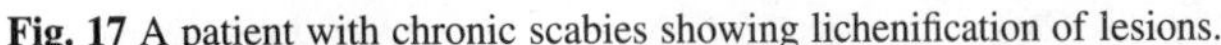

Fig. 17 A patient with chronic scabies showing lichenification of lesions.

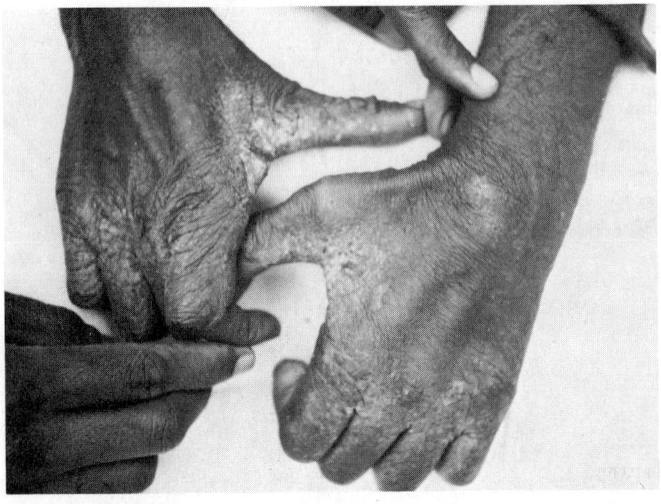

Fig. 18 Penile scabies with erythematous nodular lesions of the dorsum and glans. (Reproduced by courtesy of D. Hill, Adelaide.)

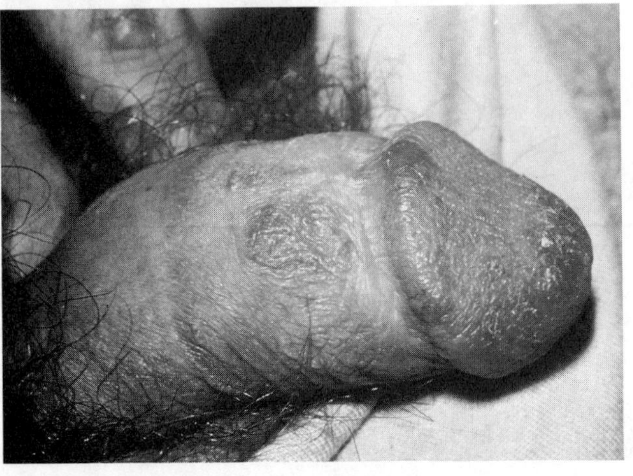

DIAGNOSIS

The characteristic appearance is often sufficient, especially in an epidemic. A hand lens may assist in teasing a female adult out of her burrow with a needle. The burrow is intradermal and therefore not deep. Alternatively, a drop of oil placed on the lesion, half-a-dozen brisk scrapes with a scalpel blade, and application of the material to a slide will reveal some combination of faecal pellets, eggs, and females on microscopy (× 10). Scrapings are often negative in zoonotic forms because adults do not burrow. A punch biopsy is rarely necessary but reveals characteristic histopathological appearances of egg or mite debris, with or without the female mite, in a non-specific dermatitis or granuloma. In epidemics or institutional outbreaks at least one mite should be identified to confirm the diagnosis.

HISTOPATHOLOGY

There is a perivascular cellular infiltrate in both the superficial and deep layers of the epidermis. Histiocytes, lymphocytes (predominantly T cells), and eosinophils are found in varying proportions. Polymorphonuclear leucocytes are also present when excoriation and secondary infection occur. Spongiotic vesiculation occurs in the papulovesicular type, a dense cellular reaction in the nodular variety, and, in the Norwegian form of the disease, a hyperkeratotic psoriaform dermatitis characterized by ortho- and parakeratosis with intraepidermal pustules related to mites and eggs is seen. Eggs, larvae, and adults are abundant in this variety, episodic in papulovesicular biopsies, and rare in the nodular form. IgE is sometimes found in the walls of upper dermal blood vessels by direct, but not indirect, immunofluorescence, and some humoral immune responses have been described.

DIFFERENTIAL DIAGNOSIS

Scabies, like syphilis, has been called 'a great imitator'. Any of the pruritic dermatoses needs to be considered but the complete sparing of the head is unusual in other dermatoses. Papular urticaria, especially if asymmetrical with sparing of hands and feet in children, is sometimes caused the bites of fleas or mosquitoes. Another diagnosis to be excluded is dermatitis herpetiformis (elbows, knees, scalp, shoulders, and buttock lesions occur). Other causes of pruritis or eczema are discussed in Section 23. Norwegian scabies may imitate psoriasis and erythroderma. When in doubt, histopathological examination of unusual lesions is essential, since it is not uncommon for this disease to occur in persons suffering from other diseases, including lymphoma.

COMPLICATIONS

The most common complication is local secondary bacterial infection with or without secondary adenitis (Fig. 19). The most serious, but uncommon, outcome is glomerulonephritis following colonization of lesions by nephritogenic streptococci, but it does not seem to be causally related to rheumatic fever. This complication may be more common in the tropics, but it also occurs in temperate zones. *Staphylococcus aureus* and *Corynebacterium diphtheriae* infections may also be associated with scabies infections. All patients with recurrent pyoderma should have scabies excluded.

TREATMENT

All members of a household or community must be treated simultaneously. After soaking (in a hot bath) to soften vesicles, scrub the lesions, fingers, and nails with a firm brush. Where secondary infection is present, scrubbing is unnecessary (and painful) due to epidermal maceration. It is not essential in an institute for the mentally handicapped or senile dementia, where bathing may be resented. To decrease percutaneous absorption, dry and cool the skin before applying benzyl benzoate, 25 per cent, as an emulsion or as an alcoholic lotion. Pyrethrum has been a well-known treatment since ancient times in India and its derivative permethrin has been shown to be effective as a 2.5 to 5 per cent cream, as has the very cheap 10 per cent sulphur in cold cream or pork fat. Apply thinly all over from the neck to the soles of the feet but rub well into burrows; the whole skin surface should be treated and not just the itchy areas; wash off after 6 to 24 h. Because of some percutaneous absorption, BHC is best avoided in pregnant women and infants. BHC is probably the best treatment in Caucasians because they have increased sensitivity and greater reactions with benzyl benzoate than those with darker skin. Repeat in 1 week. About 30 g is required for an adult. Other effective medicaments include crotamiton (10 per cent) cream or lotion and monosulfiram (25 per cent) diluted with two to three parts of water. Repeat with a second application 2 or 3 days later. Crotamiton is occasionally irritating and, with monosulfiram, alcohol consumption needs to be avoided as it is similar in effect to disulfiram (Antabuse).

The itchiness can be troublesome and may require an oily calamine solution or even a systemic antihistamine preparation. Itching may persist for some time (weeks or months) after basic therapy. Very rarely a short course of corticosteroids, such as prednisolone, 40 mg daily for 3 to 7 days, may be required. Menthol or phenol (0.25–0.5 per cent) may also help. Family and sexual contacts need to be checked and treated if complete clearance is to be achieved. Recurrence is common unless all family members (and sexual partners) are treated simultaneously. Where secondary bacterial infection occurs, local antimicrobials are also necessary. Where such lesions are confluent or where adenitis occurs, a course of systemic antibiotics is advised.

For the crusted Norwegian form a strong keratolytic agent such as salicylic acid may be required several times before using a scabicide. When nodules persist a nightly application of targel may help. As the mite cannot survive dry heat, exposure of the whole body and clothing to the midday sun is effective and useful under drought conditions. Energetic mass treatment by mobile teams has benefited affected tribes in India and South America.

Fig. 19 Secondarily infected scabies in mother and child. (Reproduced with permission from Reeves and Maibach (1984). *Clinical dermatology illustrated: a regional approach.* ADIS Health Science Press, Australia.)

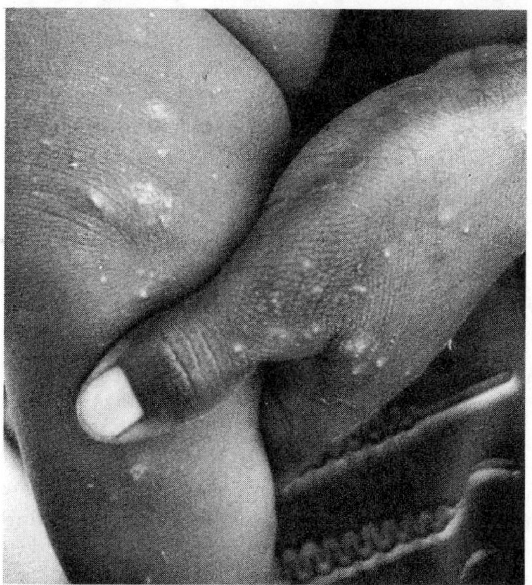

Acarinophobia

Acarinophobia (phobia about mites) will affect some patients, who will require reassurance that scabies is a not a respecter of persons and that treatment is easy and effective. Tetmasol soap may be issued to casual contacts such as cleaners, cooks, and others staffing homes for elderly people or other institutions. Hot-water washing machines, dry cleaning, and ironing will kill any mites.

Follicle mite

Family: Demodicidae

Demodex folliculorum and *D. brevis* are found in man, but the role of these obligatory parasites as the cause of any definitive pathology is still disputed. The former aggregate around hair follicles and in the orifices whilst *D. brevis* usually appears solitarily in sebaceous glands. They are very small (0.1–0.45 mm long) and are most commonly found on the nose, in the nasolabial folds, and on the eyebrows. Infestation rates vary from 10 to 100 per cent and increase with age.

Blepharitis, with or without the loss of eye lashes, a seborrhoeic dermatitis, perioral rosacea, and granulomatous acne may occur (Fig. 20). Histopathological features include follicular dilation, perifollicular inflammation, and a homogeneous eosinophilic aggregate around the mites. In summary, both (species) seem minor pathogens, merely harvesting the cells of their respective habitats.

Other mites

The tropical rat mite (*Ornithonyssus bacoti*), though not confined to the tropics, can give a painful bite and a generalized papular dermatitis, especially on the limbs. The itching can be intense and last for several weeks. It is most common in laboratory workers.

Fig. 20 Dermodex 'seborrhoea' (copyright A.J. Radford).

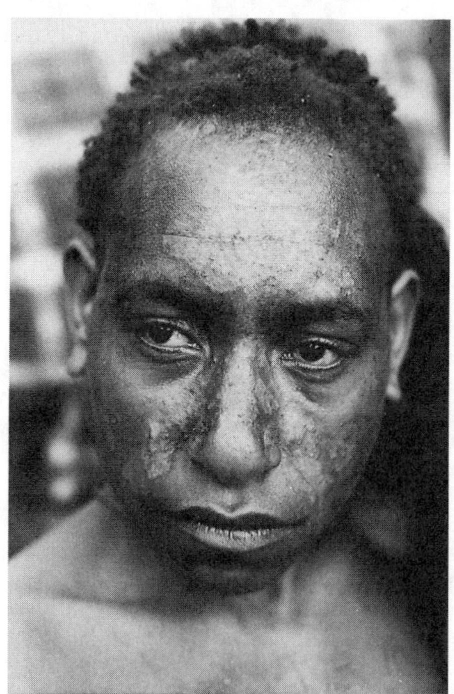

Table 1 *Taxonomic arrangement of medically important Diptera*

Family	Subfamily	Genus (and species)	Medical importance
Suborder Nematocera			
Culicidae (mosquitoes)	Anophelinae	*Anopheles*	BS, V—malaria, filariasis, viruses
	Culicinae	*Aedeomyia*	BS, V—filariasis, viruses
		Aedes	BS, V—filariasis, viruses
		Culex	BS, V—filariasis, viruses
		Culiseta	BS, V—filariasis, viruses
		Deinocerites	BS, V—viruses
		Haemagogus	BS, V—viruses
		Mansonia	BS, V—viruses
		Psorophora	BS, V—viruses
		Sabethes	BS, V—viruses
		Wyeomyia	BS, V—viruses
Phlebotomidae (sand flies)		*Phlebotomus*	BS, V—*Leishmania* spp.
		Lutzomyia	BS, V—*Leishmania* spp., *Bartonella bacilliformis*
Simuliidae (black flies)		*Simulium*	BS, V—*Onchocerca volvulus*, haemorrhagic syndrome of Altimira
Ceratopogonidae (biting midges)		*Culicoides*	BS, V—*Dipetalonema perstans, Mansonella ozzardi*
Suborder Brachycera			
Tabanidae (horse flies)		*Haematopota*	BS
		Tabanus	BS
		Pangonia	BS
		Chrysops	BS, V—*Loa loa*
Suborder Cyclorrhaphia			
Glossinidae (tsetse flies)		*Glossina*	BS, V—African trypanosomiasis
Muscidae		*Fannia*	Myiasis
		Musca	Myiasis, V
		Stomoxys	Myiasis
Calliphoridae		*Auchmeromyia luteola*	BS/myiasis
		Calliphora	Myiasis
		Cochliomyia hominivorax	Myiasis
		C.macelleria	Myiasis
		Cordylobia anthropophaga	Myiasis
		Wohlfahrtia magnifica	Myiasis
Piophilidae		*Piophila casei*	Myiasis
Oestridae		*Hypoderma*	Myiasis
		Dermatobia hominis	Myiasis
Gasterophilidae		*Gasterophilus*	Myiasis
Hippoboscidae		*Melophagus*	BS

BS, blood sucker; V, vector.

Cheyletiella, a non-burrowing mite of rabbits, dogs and man, may produce recurrent, intensely pruritic, grouped red papules on the trunk and thighs.

The straw or grain mite (*Pyemotes* spp.) causes papular or varicelliform eruptions, especially on the arms and legs. The condition is self-limiting. Quite large epidemics of seasonal dermatitis may occur.

The scrub mites (also called 'jiggers' or 'chiggers'), Trombiculidae, whose normal hosts are rodents, are particularly likely to infest military personnel on manoeuvres. They transmit scrub typhus (see Chapter 7.11.38). Uniforms treated with permethrin (0.125 cm^2) afford reasonable protection. Gamasidea mites have been experimentally infected with haemorrhagic fever virus, and *Borrelia burgdorfei* (Lyme disease) has been isolated from several species of ticks.

The role of house mites (*Dermatophagoides* spp. and *Dermanyussus* spp.) in asthma is discussed elsewhere (see Section 17). They may also cause cutaneous papular or generalized eczematous eruption.

Eye-frequenting Lepidoptera

Some nocturnal moths of the families Pyralidae, Noctuidae, and Geometridae in Africa and South-East Asia habitually feed on the lachrymal secretions of wild and domesticated herbivorous mammals. They may also visit human eyes, causing a certain amount of discomfort and may transmit eye infections, including trachoma and viral conjunctivitis. They may also cause mechanical damage to the cornea. The moths stimulate the flow of secretions by vibrating and probing with their probosces. Implicated species include *Lobocraspis griseifulva* (Hpsn.), *Arcy-*

ophora spp. and *Filodes fulvidorsalis* (Hbn.). *Calyptra eustrigata* (Hmps.) is a skin-piercing, blood-sucking noctuid from Malaysia. Such Lepidoptera may be avoided by sleeping under a net.

Blood-sucking flies (Table 1)

Numerous species of fly are specialized sanguivores. Most of them belong to the suborder Nematocera (mosquitoes, sand flies, black flies, biting midges) and family Tabanidae of the suborder Brachycera (horse flies, clegs). The tsetse flies, *Glossina* spp., are in the suborder Cyclorrhapha. All of these flies are at least a nuisance: the bites are often painful and associated with allergy. More importantly, biting flies transmit some of the most important human diseases and a large number of zoonotic infections. Important biting flies and their medical associations are listed in Table 1. Biting flies can be largely avoided by avoiding their favoured habitats, staying indoors when they are active, and by using bed nets, appropriate clothing, and insect repellents. Systemic antihistamines are often useful in treating allergic reactions to bites.

Mosquitoes

The true mosquitoes constitute the family Culicidae, whose early stages are dependent on stagnant water. Mosquitoes fly at various times of the day, depending on the species. The females of medically important mosquitoes suck blood from warm-blooded vertebrates. Malaria is transmitted exclusively by *Anopheles* spp., many of which are suitable vectors, including the *A. gambiae* (Giles) complex and *A. funestus* (Giles) in Africa, *A. albimanus* (Wiedemann) and *A. albitarsis* (Lynch Arribálzaga) in the Americas, and *A. stephensi* (Liston), *A. fluviatilis* (James), and *A. culcifacies* (Giles) in Asia. Anophelines are also important vectors of Bancroftian and Malayan filariasis. Numerous mosquito genera are vectors of viral disease.

Other biting flies

Black flies, *Simulium* spp., depend on well-oxygenated water for their early stages. Adults transmit onchocerciasis. Black flies are also associated with the haemorrhagic syndrome of Altimira in Brazil, but no infectious micro-organism or parasite has been implicated. Black flies generally bite during the day. Loaiasis is transmitted by several *Chrysops* spp. that frequent forests in West Africa and bite during the day. Sand flies bite at night and occur in a variety of habitats. They transmit leishmaniasis and, in South America, bartonellosis. Tsetse flies occur in moister areas of tropical Africa. They are conspicuous and diurnal.

Insects and hygiene

Flies

Many species of fly, mostly of the suborder Cyclorrhapha, frequent human and animal food, wounds, eyes, and faeces. Such flies vomit and defaecate wherever they feed. Numerous pathogenic bacteria and viruses have been isolated from flies, which may therefore serve as passive vectors of bacterial and viral diseases. Flies of the genus Musca are considered to be major vectors of trachoma.

Pharaoh's ants

Pharaoh's ants, *Monomorium pharaonis* (L.), commonly infest hospitals, where they invade sterile packs and wound dressings. They are potential passive vectors, as bacteria, including *Salmonella* spp. and *Staphylococcus* spp., have been isolated from these ants, which should, therefore, be controlled with insecticides.

Cockroaches

> Depuis très longtemps, on soupçonne les Blattes d'être les vecteurs de maladies transmissible diverses, . . . (Graffar and Mertens, 1950)

Cockroaches are omnivorous scavengers and of the 3500 species, a few have become cosmopolitan synanthropes, which share the ability to be a nuisance to man for several reasons: their affinity for human food, wounds, and faeces, and their considerable motility implicate them as being passive vectors of disease; they are a source of allergens; their appearance and general demeanour, their characteristic smell and occurrence, often in large numbers cause distress and loathing; they occasionally bite. The important worldwide species are the common cockroach, *Blatta orientalis* (L.), the American cockroach, *Periplaneta americana* (L.), the German cockroach, *Blattella germanica* (L.), and the banded cockroach, *Supella longipalpa* (Fab.). Other species are important locally. The medically important species are mostly of tropical origin and require temperatures of 25 to 33 °C, except for *B. orientalis*, which will tolerate 20°C. In cooler climates they are therefore restricted to permanently heated areas and can occur in large numbers in hospitals and in sewers. Many pathogenic viruses, including poliomyelitis virus and coxsackie virus A, and bacteria, including *Shigella* spp., have been isolated from cockroaches. There is evidence that cockroaches acted as passive vectors of hepatitis A during an outbreak in California and of *Salmonella typhimurium* in a paediatric ward in Belgium. Cockroaches are potential allergens, 7.5 per cent of healthy persons being skin-test positive in one study. Cockroaches wander over sleepers and are attracted to nasal and oral secretions. Herpes blattae is a dermatitis described from Reunion and attributed to cockroach allergy. Cockroaches sometimes wander into ears and nostrils, where they become trapped or reluctant to leave. Lignocaine spray is reported to hasten the exit of such visitors. Cockroaches are especially hazardous in hospitals, where their presence should be monitored and controlled.

REFERENCES

Myiasis

Alexander, J.O'D. (1984). *Arthropods and human skin.* Springer-Verlag, Berlin.

Smith, K.G.V. (ed.) (1973). *Insects and arthropods of Medical importance.* British Museum (Natural History), London.

Zumpt, F. (1965). *Myiasis in man and animals in the old world.* Butterworth, London.

Lice

Busvine, J.R. (1978). Evidence from double infestations of the specific status of human head lice and body lice. *Systematic Entomology*, **3,** 1–8.

Donaldson, R.J. (1976). The head louse in England. *Royal Society of Health Journal*, **96,** 55–7.

Editorial (1979). Head lice in the seventies. *Lancet*, **ii,** 130–1.

Maunder, J.W. (1977). Parasites and man. Human lice—biology and control. *Royal Society of Health Journal*, **97,** 29–32.

Morley, W.N. (1977). Body infestations. *Scottish Medical Journal*, **22,** 211–16.

Arachnids

Arlian, L.G., Runyon, R.A., Sorlie, L.B., and Ester, S.A. (1984). Survival and infectivity of *Sarcoptes scabei* vars *canis* and vars *hominis*. *Journal of the American Academy of Dermatology*, **15,** 594–8.

Christopherson, J. (1978). The epidemiology of scabies in Denmark, 1900 to 1975. *Archives of Dermatology*, **114,** 747–50.

Harwood, R.F. and James, M.T. (1979). *Entomology in human and animal health.* Macmillan, New York.

Medleau, L. and Miller, W.H. (1983). Flea infestation and its control. *International Journal of Dermatology*, **22,** 378–9.

Mellanby, K. (1972). *Scabies*, (2nd edn). Classey, Hampton, Middlesex.

Nutting, W.B. and Green, A.C. (1976). Pathogenesis associated with hair follicle mites (*Demodex* spp.) in Australian aborigines. *British Journal of Dermatology*, **94,** 307–12.

Taplin, D. (1984). Scabies in the tropics. Proceedings: Fifth World Congress of Tropical Dermatology, Mexico.

Witkowski, J.A. and Parish, L.C. (1984). Scabies. Subungualaneas harbor mites. *Journal of the American Medical Association*, **252**, 1318–19.

Eye-frequenting Lepidoptera

Bänziger, H. and Büttiker, W. (1969). Records of eye-frequenting Lepidoptera from man. *Journal of medical Entomology*, **6**, 53–8.

Büttiker, W. and Bezuidenhout, J.D. (1974). First records of eye-frequenting Lepidoptera from South West Africa. *Journal of the Entomological Society of South Africa*, **37**, 73–8.

Blood-sucking flies

Pinheiro, F.P., Bensabath, G., Costa, D., Jr., Maroja, O.M., Lins, Z.C., and Andrade, A.H.P. (1974). Haemorrhagic syndrome of Altamira. *Lancet*, **i**, 639–42.

Smith, K.G.V. (ed.) (1973). *Insects and arthropods of medical importance*. British Museum (Natural History), London.

Insects and hygiene

Baker, L.F. (1981). Pests in hospitals. *Journal of Hospital Infection*, **2**, 5–9.

Beatson, S.H. (1972). Pharoah's ants as pathogen vectors in hospitals. *Lancet*, **i**, 425–7.

Cornwell, P.B. (1968). *The cockroach*, Vol. 1. Rentokil, London.

Graffar, M. and Mertens, S. (1950). Le role des blattes dans la transmission des salmonelloses. *Annales de l'Institut Pasteur*, **79**, 654–60.

O'Toole, K., Paris, P.M., and Stewart, R.D. (1985). Removing cockroaches from the auditory canal: controlled trial. *New England Journal of Medicine*, **312**, 1197.

Richman, P.G., Khan, H.A., Turkeltaub, P.C., Malveaux, F.J., and Baer, H. (1984). The important sources of German cockroach allergens as determined by RAST analysis. *Journal of Allergy and Clinical Immunology*, **73**, 590–5.

Roth, L.M. and Willis, E.R. (1957). The medical and veterinary importance of cockroaches. *Smithsonian Miscellaneous Collection*, **134**, 1–147.

Sheard, A. (1922). Cockroach in the nasal passages. *British Medical Journal*, **i**, 982.

Tarshis, I.B. (1962). The cockroach—new suspect in the spread of infectious hepatitis. *American Journal of Tropical Medicine and Hygiene*, **2**, 705–11.

7.18 Pentastomiasis (porocephalosis)

D. A. Warrell

The pentastomida, pentastomes or 'tongue worms' inhabit the respiratory tracts of vertebrates, where they feed on blood and other tissues. There are more than 100 species, classified into two orders, Cephalobaenida (e.g. genus Raillietiella) and Porocephalida (e.g. genera Linguatula, Armillifer, Leiperia, and Sebekia). About 10 species are known to be capable of causing zoonotic infections in man. Pentastomida should probably be classified as arthropods but they have also been grouped with the Branchiuran crustacea, with annelids, and in a separate phylum. The name pentastome derives from their having two pairs of anterior hooks and a mouth, giving the impression of five stomata (Fig. 1). In man, visceral pentastomiasis is most often caused by *Linguatula serrata* or *Armillifer armillatus* and nasopharyngeal pentastomiasis (halzoun or Marrara syndrome) is usually caused by *L. serrata*, although other helminthic parasites have been implicated.

Linguatula

L. serrata has been reported from Europe, the Middle East, Africa and North, Central, and South America, but not from Asia. The names *Linguatula* and tongue worm describe the flattened shape particularly of the adult female. Their surface bears numerous annular grooves. Dogs, foxes, and wolves, the definitive hosts, harbour adults and nymphs in their upper respiratory tract and shed them in their nasal secretions and hence saliva and faeces. The intermediate hosts, herbivorous animals, ingest the ova, which hatch in the lumen of the gut releasing larvae that burrow into the tissues and encyst. When the intermediate host is eaten by the definitive host, nymphs hatch from the cysts and migrate to the lungs and nasopharynx, where they mature.

CLINICAL FEATURES

If humans ingest Linguatula ova, the resulting cysts, which usually develop in the liver, do not cause symptoms unless they obstruct or compress, for example, the filtration angle of the anterior chamber of the eye, biliary or respiratory tracts, meninges or brain. However, ingestion of cysts containing third-stage larvae in raw liver and lymph nodes of sheep, goats, cattle, and lagomorphs can result in acute nasopharyngitis, known as halzoun, Marrara syndrome, or nasopharyngeal pentostomiasis. This has been reported from the Middle East, especially Lebanon, Greece, and the Sudan. In the human stomach, larvae escape from the cysts and migrate up the oesophagus to the mucosae of the nasopharynx. Within a few hours of eating the infected viscera there is intense irritation of the upper respiratory and gastrointestinal tracts associated with coughing, sneezing, rhinorrhoea, retching, vomiting, lacrimation, haemoptysis, epistaxis, cervical lymphadenopathy, transient deafness, difficulty in speaking, dysphagia, wheezing, and dyspnoea. Larvae can be found in sputum and vomitus. Patients usually recover in 1 or 2 weeks but deaths have resulted from acute upper-airway obstruction. These features suggest a hypersensitivity reaction. Halzoun has also been attributed to flukes (*Fasciola hepatica*) and nematodes (*Mammomonogamus laryngeus*) ingested in raw sheep and goat liver and to leeches (*Limnatis nilotica* and *Dinobdella ferox*). Very rarely, larvae may develop to adults in the human nasal cavity.

Fig. 1 Adult pentastomid showing mouth (arrowed) and lateral hooks giving the appearance of five stomata. Scanning electron micrograph, × 400 (by courtesy Professor Viqar Zaman).

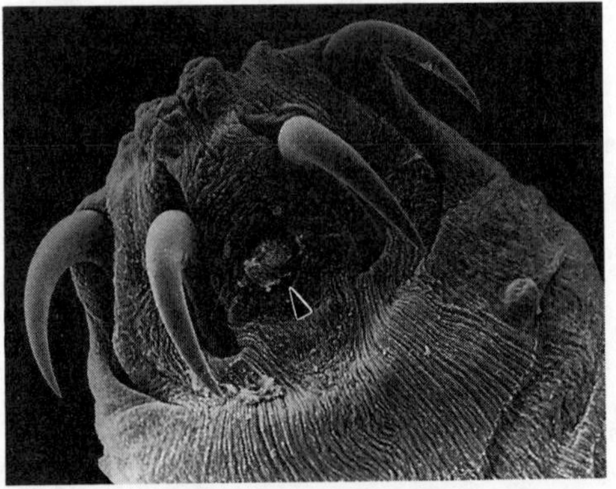

Armillifer (Porocephalus) *spp.*

These are also annulated, non-segmented parasites (Fig. 2). The adults, up to 20 cm long, inhabit the respiratory and digestive tracts of snakes, especially those of the genera Python, Boaedon and Bitis, and other vertebrates. Ova are shed in the snake's nasal secretions and are picked up by herbivorous mammals. Larvae encyst in the tissues of these intermediate hosts and will develop further to the stage of nymphs if ingested by another animal, but develop to adults only in snakes. Humans may ingest ova by drinking water contaminated by snakes, or they may ingest living encysted larvae in raw snake meat eaten as part of ju-ju rituals (West Africa), or inadequately cooked snake (Temuan tribe of Malaysian aborigines and in Benin and other West African countries). Ingested eggs hatch in the gut, releasing larvae that burrow into the tissues, where they develop into nymphs. Wriggling nymphs have been discovered beneath the visceral peritoneum at laparotomy.

Human infections with the larvae or nymphs of the following species of Armillifer have been reported: *A. armillatus* (18–22 annular rings)—Africa (Egypt, Senegal, The Gambia, Ghana, Benin, Nigeria, Cameroon, Zaire, and Zimbabwe); *A. grandis*—Zaire; *A. moniliformis* (30 annular rings)—Malaysia, Philippines, Indonesia, Tibet and Australia; *A. najae*—India.

CLINICAL FEATURES

The most common evidence of Armillifer infection is the discovery of calcified nymphs (Fig. 2) on radiographs of the abdomen and chest (Fig. 3). These appear as discrete, crescent-shaped, soft-tissue calcifications, 4 × 4 mm in size. In West Africa they are seen particularly in the right upper quadrant and are situated beneath the peritoneum covering the liver. In Ibadan, Nigeria, these shadows were seen in 2 per cent of adult men and 4 per cent of adult women. Hundres of calcified encysted nymphs have been found in the peritoneum at laparotomy or at autopsy in the liver (Fig. 4), spleen, gut wall and lumen, lungs, cirrhosal cavities,

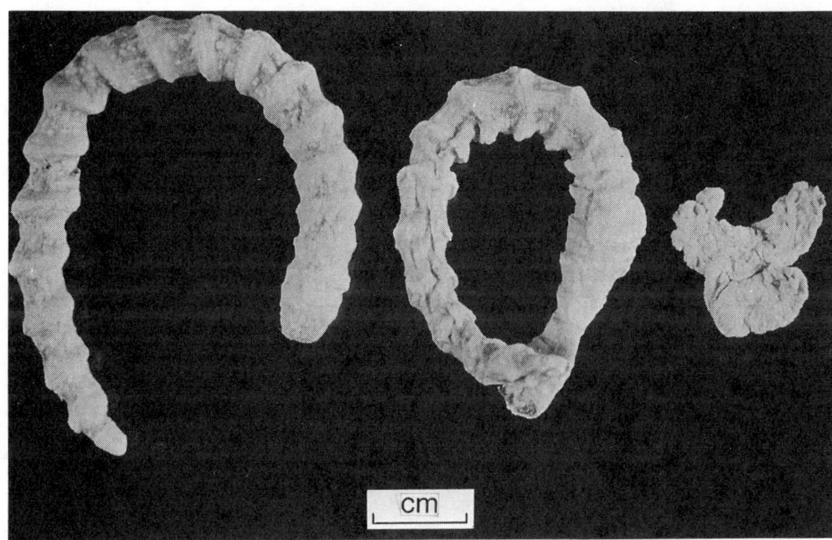

Fig. 2 *Armillifer armillatus*. Left: two adults found in the lungs of a Gaboon viper (*Bitis gabonica*). Right: calcified nymph from the mesentery of a Ghanaian patient. (By courtesy of Dr G. M. Ardran.)

Fig. 3 Typical radiographic appearance of calcified nymphs of *Armillifer armillatus* in the abdominal cavity of a Ghanaian patient. (By courtesy of Dr G. M. Ardran.)

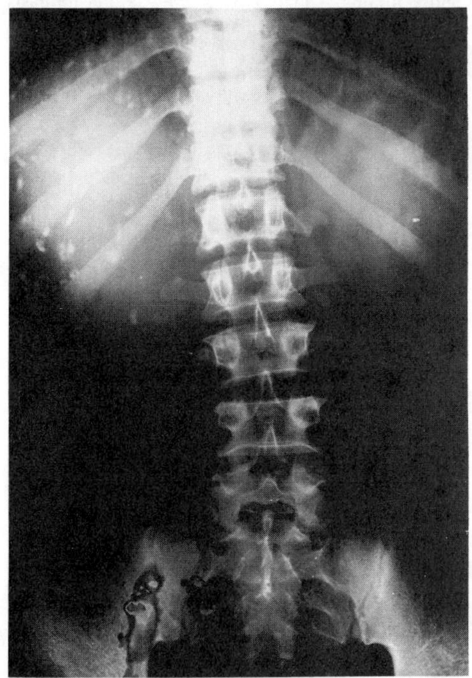

Fig. 4 Encysted nymph/larva of *Armillifer armillatus* in human liver. The outer layer of the parasite (arrowed) lines the cyst wall. Acidophilic glands (ag), intestine (in). × 21. (Armed Forces Institute of Pathology photograph, negative number 75-2703.)

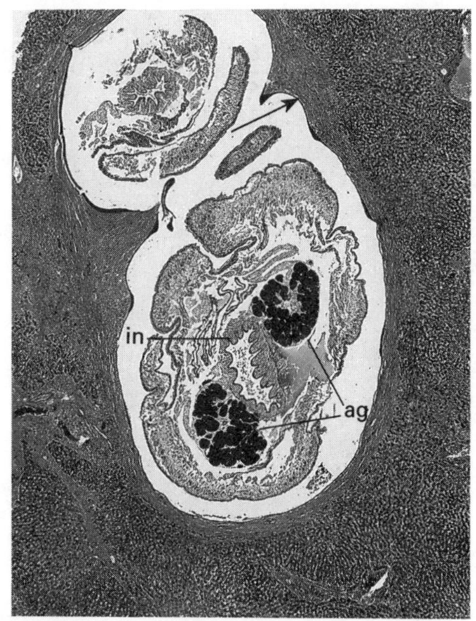

central nervous system, eye, and elsewhere in 27 per cent of cases in The Congo (*A. armillatus* and *A. grandis*), in 6 to 13 per cent in Cameroon (*A. armillatus*), and in 45 per cent in Malaysian Orang Asli (*A. moniliformis*).

Armillifer infection is usually symptomless or causes vague abdominal pain. Serious inflammatory and obstructive effects have been described in the gut, lungs, biliary tract, pericardium, central nervous system, and anterior chamber of the eye. Severe acute reactions may be related to hypersensitivity or perhaps to massive infection such as might follow ingestion of a gravid female. Migration of large numbers of larvae from the gut into the tissue might produce abdominal pain and obstructive jaundice. A few fatal cases have been reported, including one patient who died from intestinal obstruction caused by nymphs of *A. armillatus*. There has been some suggestion from Nigeria and Zaire that Armillifer infection might be associated with malignancy of the colon and elsewhere.

Other pentastomid infections

Human infections with *Leiperia cincinnalis* have been described in Africa, and subcutaneous infections by *Railliettiella gehyrae* and *R. hemidactyli* in Vietnam and by *Sebekia* spp. in Costa Rica. In Vietnam, infection with Railliettiella follows the swallowing of small live lizards for medicinal purposes.

Diagnosis

The radiographical appearances of calcified pentastomid nymphs are distinctive (Fig. 3). Pentastomes may be discovered at surgery or autopsy. In the liver (Fig. 4), intestinal wall, mesentery, mesenteric lymph nodes, peritoneum or lung, viable encysted larvae or granulomas containing necrotic pentastomes or their moulted cuticles may be identified. Initially, encysted larvae excite little or no tissue reaction, but the granulomata are surrounded by hyalinized or calcified fibrous tissue. In tissue sections, pentastomes can be distinguished from helminths. In infected patients, antibodies to Armillifer have been detected by fluorescence.

Treatment

There is no specific treatment for pentastomiasis. Obstruction and compression should be relieved surgically. Hypersensitivity phenomena should be treated with adrenaline, antihistamines, and corticosteroids. Infections can be prevented if all meat is thoroughly cooked.

Other zoonoses transmitted from reptiles to man

The most important of these is salmonellosis transmitted from chelonians (tortoises, turtles, terrapins) and from snakes and lizards. In Britain, 38 per cent of imported tortoises (*Testudo* spp.) contain salmonellae; in the United States, 14 per cent of reported salmonellosis cases were attributable to pet terrapins as were up to 17 per cent of cases of infant salmonellosis in Puerto Rico. The species include *S. typhimurium*, *S. muenchen*, *S. ealing*, *S. volta*, *S. alachua*, and *S. java*. *S. marina* is associated with iguanas.

Other infections transmissible from reptiles to man include *Arizona hinshawii* (in snake powder, Pulvo de Vibora, made from rattlesnakes), *Plesiomonas shigelloides*, *Edwardsiella tarda*, leptospirosis, Q fever, sparganosis, capillariasis, strongyloidiasis, mesocestoidiasis, and infestation with the mite *Ophionyssus natricis*. Potential zoonoses include *Mycobacteria*, *Pseudomonas*, other *Aeromonas* spp., Proteus, and some togaviruses (such as Western equine encephalitis in garter snakes in western North America) and herpesviruses.

REFERENCES

Adran, G.M. (1948). Armillifer armillatus. A note of three cases of calcification in man. *British Journal of Radiology*, **21,** 342–5.

Dollfus, R.P. and Canet, J. (1954). Sur en Pentostomatidae *Raillietiella hemidactyli* suppose susceptible de parasiter l'homme consecutivement a l'ingestion des lezards vivants. *Bulletin de la Société de Pathologie Exotique*, **47,** 401–7.

Editorial (1981). Reptilian salmonellosis. *Lancet*, **ii,** 130–1.

Fain, A. (1975). The Pentastomida parasitic in man. *Annales de la Société Belgique de Medecine Tropicale*, **55,** 59–64.

Frank, W. (1981). Endoparasites. In *Diseases of reptiles*, Vol. 1, (ed. J.E. Cooper and O.F. Jackson), pp. 291–358. Academic Press, London.

Haugerud, R.E. (1989). Evolution in the Pentastomids. *Parasitology Today*, **5,** 126–32.

Prathap, K. (1981). Pentastomiasis. *Annals of the Academy of Medicine Singapore*, **10,** 132–5.

Prathap, K., Lau, K.S., and Bolton, J.M. (1969). Pentastomiasis: a common finding at autopsy in Malaysian aborigines. *American Journal of Tropical Medicine and Hygiene*, **18,** 20–7.

Riley, J. (1986). The biology of pentastomids. *Advances in Parasitology*, **25,** 45–128.

Schacher, J.F., Saab, S., Germanos, R., and Boustany, N. (1969). The aetiology of halzoun in Lebanon: recovery of *Linguatula serrata* nymphs from two patients. *Transactions of the Royal Society of Tropical Medicine and Hygiene*, **63,** 854–8.

Self, J.T., Hopps, H.C., and Williams, A.O. (1975). Review. Pentastomiasis in Africans. *Tropical and Geographic Medicine*, **27,** 1–13.

7.19 Infectious disease syndromes

7.19.1 Fever of unknown origin

D. T. DURACK

Fever is a common factor in most fields of medical practice. The special problem of prolonged fevers has occupied a prominent position in clinical science since the introduction of routine thermometry by Wunderlich 125 years ago. In 1955, at the beginning of the antibiotic era, Keefer and Leard wrote that fever of unknown origin '. . . perplexes both the physician and the patient, and has not become less important with the introduction of new agents for the combating of acute infections'. Today, patients with fever of unknown origin still can be perplexing, but different clinical issues have evolved with the advent of new diseases, therapies, and diagnostic tests, especially advanced imaging techniques.

Definitions and terminology

Normal body temperature is 37.0°C or 98.6°F. The normal range is quite wide, and for several reasons it is difficult to define precisely. Body temperature is most often estimated by measurements taken in the mouth for reasons of convenience, but oral temperatures can be affected by mouth breathing, by the respiratory rate, and by recent drinking of hot or cold liquids. The core body temperature is more closely reflected by rectal measurements, which are usually 0.3 to 0.6°C higher than oral measurements. Heavy exercise can raise the core temperature of healthy people by 2°C or more. Another factor is normal circadian variation, which cycles through a range of ± 0.5°C (0.9°F) daily, with lowest temperatures occurring between 4.00 and 6.00 a.m. and highest between 4.00 and 8.00 p.m. The normal circadian rhythm varies between individuals and is likely to be affected by jet travel between time zones, by work and sleep patterns, and by illnesses. The menstrual cycle affects the baseline temperature of normal women by 0.3 to 0.5°C, with a small spike at ovulation and higher temperatures from about the 15th to the 25th days of a 28-day cycle. In addition to these factors, there is considerable variation in normal temperature patterns between individuals. Some normal young people, especially women, persistently exhibit slightly 'high' temperatures that are of no significance unless the subject perceives them as fever needing medical attention. This common condition may be termed 'habitual hyperthermia', a comforting term of art that may help physicians to resist pressures to investigate such patients excessively for possible causes of fever.

Fever and hypothermia may be defined as core body temperatures above or below the normal range, allowing for all the factors listed above. For practical clinical purposes, the author's rule of thumb is to consider oral or rectal temperatures falling outside the range 35.5 to 38.0°C (95.9–100.4°F) as abnormal. Specific circumstances should be considered: for example, an oral temperature of 37.3°C taken in the morning could represent significant fever in an individual patient.

The terms 'fever of unknown origin' (FUO) and 'pyrexia of unknown origin' (PUO) are interchangeable; fever of unknown origin will be used in this discussion. Use of clear definitions for fever of unknown origin promotes a rational diagnostic approach. Fever of unknown origin was previously defined as an illness of more than 3 weeks' duration, with fever higher than 101°F documented on several occasions, without a diagnosis after 1 week of evaluation in hospital. This definition has been useful for 30 years, but today should be revised and extended to describe undiagnosed fevers in patients with AIDS, patients with severe neutropenia, and patients who develop complications during a period in hospital. Table 1 lists definitions for four distinct groups of prolonged fevers: classical, nosocomial, neutropenic, and human immunodeficiency virus (**HIV**)-associated fever of unknown origin.

Symptoms and signs of fever of unknown origin

The symptoms and signs are highly variable in patients with fever of unknown origin. Some have trivial symptoms, others may be incapacitated by debilitating chills, rigors, and sweats. The clinical findings may be limited to manifestations of the fever itself, or may reflect the underlying disease. The physician should evaluate every symptom or sign, especially new ones, as potential clues to the primary diagnosis.

Certain diseases can produce characteristic patterns of fever, notably malaria, brucellosis, typhoid fever, and some lymphomas. Despite these classical associations, in practice the shape of the fever curve is seldom of major practical value in diagnosis of fever of unknown origin. Individual variation and the common use of analgesics with antipyrexial effects confuse the picture. The clinical characteristics of drug-induced fevers are highly variable, despite the common misconception that they are usually low-grade fevers with relatively little variation from peak to trough, and relatively low pulse rate.

Classical fever of unknown origin

The causes of classical fever of unknown origin are legion. Most can be included under five simple categories: infections, malignancies, connective tissue diseases, miscellaneous conditions including factitious fever and habitual hyperthermia, and undiagnosed cases (Fig. 1). Within the first three categories, certain diagnoses predominate (Tables 2 and 3). The leading infectious aetiologies for classical fever of unknown origin are intra-abdominal infections, tuberculosis, complicated urinary-tract infections, and endocarditis. The leading malignancies are lymphomas (especially Hodgkin's disease), leukaemias, and some solid tumours including adenocarcinomas and hypernephromas. Vasculitides including the temporal arteritis–polymyalgia syndromes, Still's disease, systemic lupus erythematosus, and rheumatic fever are important among the connective tissue diseases. Among the miscellaneous conditions that can cause fever of unknown origin, alcoholic hepatitis and granulomatous conditions such as sarcoidosis or granulomatous hepatitis are important. Self-induced or factitious fever is surprisingly common. Some of the many other miscellaneous, uncommon, or rare diseases that can cause fever of unknown origin are listed in Table 4. In all published series, a sizeable subgroup of patients with fever of unknown origin remains undiagnosed (Fig. 1).

FEVER OF UNKNOWN ORIGIN IN CHILDREN: SPECIAL FEATURES

The proportion of cases of fever of unknown origin due to infections is higher in children, and the proportion due to malignancy is correspondingly lower. Infections that are particularly common in children are viral syndromes and urinary-tract infections. Still's disease and rheumatic fever are more likely to cause fever of unknown origin in children than in adults, and children are less likely to have factitious fever. The overall mortality of fever of unknown origin in children is lower than in adults.

Table 1 *Summary of definitions and major features of four types of fever of unknown origin (FUO)*

	Classical FUO	Nosocomial FUO	Neutropenic FUO	HIV-related FUO
Definition	> 38.0°C, > 3 weeks, > 2 visits or 3 days in hospital	> 38.0°C, > 72 h, not present or incubating on admission	> 38.0°C, > 72 h, < 1000 PMNs/mm³, negative cultures after 48 h	> 38.0°C, > 4 weeks for outpatients, > 3 days for inpatients, HIV infection confirmed
Patient location	Community, clinic or hospital	Acute-care hospital	Hospital or clinic	Community, clinic or hospital
Leading causes	Malignancy, infections, inflammatory conditions, undiagnosed, habitual hyperthermia	Nosocomial infections, postoperative complications, drug fevers	Majority due to infections, but aetiology documented in only 40–60%	HIV, typical and atypical mycobacteria, CMV, lymphomas, toxoplasmosis
History emphasis	Travel, contacts, animal and insect exposure, immunizations, family history	Operations and procedures, devices, anatomical considerations, drug treatment	Stage of chemotherapy, drugs administered	Drugs, exposures, risk factors, travel, contacts, staging of HIV infection
Examination emphasis	Abdomen, lymph nodes, spleen, joints, muscles, arteries	Wounds, drains, devices, sinuses, urine	Skin folds, i.v. sites, lungs, perianal area	Mouth, skin, lymph nodes, eyes, lungs, perianal area
Investigation emphasis	Imaging, biopsies, sedimentation rate, PPD	Imaging, bacterial cultures	Chest radiograph, bacterial cultures	Blood and lymphocyte count; serologies; chest radiograph; stool examination; biopsies of lung, bone marrow, liver; cultures and cytology; brain imaging
Management	Observation, outpatient temperature chart, investigations, avoid empirical drug treatments	Depends on situation	Antimicrobial treatment protocols	AZT, antimicrobial treatment protocols, revision of treatment regimens, nutrition
Time course of disease	Months	Weeks	Days	Weeks to months
Tempo of investigation	Weeks	Days	Hours	Days to weeks
Mortality (attributable to the cause of FUO)	Moderate	Moderate	Low	High

AZT, azidothymidine; CMV, cytomegalovirus; HIV, human immunodeficiency virus; PMN, polymorphonuclear leucocyte; PPD, purified protein derivative.

Adapted from Durack, D.T. and Street, A.C. (1991). Fever of unknown origin-reexamined and redefined. In *Current clinical topics in infectious diseases*, Vol. 11, (ed. J.S. Remington and M.N. Swartz), pp. 35–51. Blackwell Scientific, Boston.

FEVER OF UNKNOWN ORIGIN IN THE ELDERLY: SPECIAL FEATURES

In patients over 65 years old, intra-abdominal abscesses (including hepatic abscesses), malignancies, and vasculitides form a high proportion of cases of fever of unknown origin. The proportion of fevers of unknown origin that remain undiagnosed in elderly people is only about half that in children and younger adults. The higher rate of underlying malignancies in any series of elderly patients with fever of unknown origin means that the long-term prognosis is less favourable than in a younger group. The temporal arteritis–polymyalgia rheumatica syndromes are particularly important because they are common in elderly people and their many non-specific symptoms may be missed or misdiagnosed. The diagnosis is easily suspected if the erythrocyte sedimentation rate is over 100 mm/h, but easily overlooked if this test is not made. Other connective tissue diseases are less common than in younger patients. Bacterial prostatitis and related urinary-tract infections are more common, owing to prostatic hypertrophy in elderly men. In developed countries, endocarditis has become more common in older patients. Occult pulmonary emboli always should be considered in the differential diagnosis. Factitious fever is rare in elderly people.

Nosocomial fever of unknown origin

Fever that develops and remains undiagnosed in an inpatient in an acute-care hospital is termed nosocomial fever of unknown origin. Usually these patients are being treated for one or more major pre-existing conditions, and have many possible reasons for developing fever. Several of these may be contributing simultaneously to the development of fever. After common bacterial infections such as pneumonia, urinary-tract infection, and bacteraemia have been excluded, many other infections remain in the differential diagnosis. Important examples are local or disseminated candidiasis, *Clostridium difficile* diarrhoea or colitis, cytomegalovirus infection, hepatitis, sinusitis (especially if the patient is intubated), and intravascular line-related infections or endocarditis. The possibility that a non-infectious inflammatory condition such as

Table 2 *Listing of infections causing fever of unknown origin, from selected studies in the USA or overseas*

Location	Connecticut	Washington	Rhode Island	Spain	Belgium	India	Total
Years	1952–1957	1970–1980	1984–1990	1968–1981	1980–1989	1974–1989	1952–1990
Number of patients	100	105	86	133	199	150	773
Abscess:							
Any site	11[a]	10	13	3	4	3	7
Abdominal	11	10	10	N/A	2	2	7
Mycobacterial infection	11	5	5	11	5	25	10
Endocarditis	5	0	5	2	2	3	3
Urinary-tract infection	3	3	0	1	1	0	1
Viral:	0	4	5	0	5	0	2
CMV	0	4	2	0	4	0	2
EBV	0	0	1	0	0	0	<1
HIV	0	0	1	0	1	0	<1
Amoebic abscess	0	1	2	0	0	3	1
Kala-azar	0	0	0	0	0	5	1
Leishmaniasis	0	0	0	2	0	1	<1
Brucellosis	1	0	0	3	0	0	<1

[a]All figures are percentages. CMV, cytomegalovirus; EBV, Epstein–Barr virus; HIV, human immunodeficiency virus; N/A = not applicable.

Adapted from Miller, W.C. and Durack, D.T. (1994). Fever of unknown origin in the 1990s: a rational diagnostic approach. *Hospital Medicine*, **30** (in press).

Table 3 *Percentage of patients with malignancies or connective tissue diseases from selected studies of fever of unknown origin in the USA or overseas*

Location	Connecticut	Washington	Rhode Island	Spain	Belgium	India	Percentage of this category	Percentage total
Years	1952–1957	1970–1980	1984–1990	1968–1981	1980–1989	1974–1989		
Number of patients	100	105	86	133	199	150		
Malignancies								
Lymphomas:	6[a]	11	16	12	1	7	41	9
Non-Hodgkin's	4	7	8	4	0	N/A	19	5
Hodgkin's	2	4	6	8	1	N/A	21	4
Leukaemia	2	5	0	0	2	5	11	2
Other hematological malignancies	0	6	2	0	1	2	7	2
Solid tumours	9	11	8	6	4	9	34	8
Connective tissue diseases								
Still's disease	2	4	6	1	3	0	19	3
Polyarteritis nodosa	0	2	1	8	2	0	15	2
Systemic lupus erythematosus	5	0	2	1	1	7	24	3
Temporal arteritis	2	1	1	3	8	0	15	3
Polymyalgia rheumatica	0	0	0	0	1	0	<1	<1
Rheumatic fever	6	1	1	0	0	0	10	1

[a]All figures are percentages. N/A = not applicable.

Adapted from Miller, W.C. and Durack, D.T. (1994). Fever of unknown origin in the 1990s: a rational diagnostic approach. *Hospital Medicine*, **30** (in press).

acalculous cholecystitis, gout or pseudogout has flared during the admission to hospital for another condition should be considered. Occult pulmonary emboli are an important cause of nosocomial fever of unknown origin. Drug fever is especially common in this patient group.

Neutropenic fever of unknown origin

The number of patients with neutropenia caused by cytotoxic chemotherapy for various diseases is increasing, although the duration of neutropenia is now being curtailed by administration of colony-stimulating factors. Fevers in neutropenic patients are very different from the classical fever of unknown origin defined above. The leading causes of neutropenic fever of unknown origin are bacteraemias, pneumonias, and skin/soft tissue infections. Urinary-tract infections are less common than in nosocomial fevers of unknown origin. Focal bacterial infections of intravascular lines and puncture wounds, skin folds, and the perianal area all are common, often associated with bacteraemia. In the early stages of neutropenia, fevers are usually caused by bacteria but if neu-

Table 4 *Some miscellaneous, uncommon, or rare causes of fever of unknown origin (in alphabetical order)*

Alcoholic hepatitis
Atrial myxoma
Behçet's syndrome
Chronic meningitis
Carcinomatous meningitis
Cyclic neutropenia
Drug fever and other hypersensitivities
Erythema multiforme
Fabry's disease
Granulomatous hepatitis
Granulomatous peritonitis
Haemoglobinopathies
Haemolytic anaemias
Histiocytosis X
Inflammatory bowel disease
Lymphomatoid granulomatosis
Myeloproliferative syndromes
Pancreatitis
Paroxysmal haemoglobinurias
Pericarditis
Periodic fever
Phaeochromocytoma
Pulmonary emboli
Postpericardiotomy syndrome
Retroperitoneal fibrosis
Sarcoidosis
Serum sickness
Thrombotic thrombocytopenic purpura
Thrombophlebitis
Thyroiditis and thyrotoxicosis
Wegener's granulomatosis
Whipple's disease

tropenia persists, fungal, viral, and other conditions become relatively more common. However, this well-known sequence loses diagnostic value when the patient has received multiple cycles of chemotherapy and antimicrobial drugs.

The natural history of neutropenic fever of unknown origin tends to be much shorter than that of the classical FUO. Onset of fever often occurs within days of onset of neutropenia; immediate empirical treatment is usually given, and improvement often is rapid. The aetiology of these fevers often remains unconfirmed. In the majority of neutropenic fever of unknown origin the fever is likely due to infection, but the causative organism(s) will be identified in only 40 to 60 per cent. Recurrent episodes are likely as long as the patient remains neutropenic.

HIV-associated fever of unknown origin

A self-limiting period of fever often occurs during primary HIV infection. After a long asymptomatic interval, fevers of known and unknown origin are extremely common during the later stages of HIV infection. This justifies the introduction of the term 'HIV-associated fever of unknown origin' in the definitions listed above. The single most common cause of fever of unknown origin in this situation is atypical mycobacterial infection, which eventually affects up to 40 per cent of AIDS patients in developed countries before death. In developing countries, typical tuberculosis is more common. Many other diagnoses must be considered, especially disseminated cryptococcosis, toxoplasmosis of the central nervous system, lymphomas, and infection with other unusual pathogens. Recently, *Rochalimaea* spp., which cause bacillary angiomatosis and peliosis hepatitis, have also been found to cause febrile bacteraemic syndromes and endocarditis in AIDS patients. In the appropriate geographical regions, disseminated histoplasmosis and coccidioidomycosis must be considered.

Approach to investigation of fever of unknown origin

Efficient and economical investigation of an fever of unknown origin is an art based upon knowledge and sound judgement. First, a meticulous history should be taken, and a complete physical examination made. The results of chest radiography, routine blood count, differential cell count, erythrocyte sedimentation rate, and serum biochemistry should be immediately available. A raised serum uric acid could signal rapid cell turnover in lymphoma, and alkaline phosphatase can indicate liver involvement. The peripheral blood smear should be examined carefully for abnormalities such as thrombocytosis, leukaemoid reactions, presence of nucleated red blood cells, and other clues that the marrow is reacting to a pathological stimulus. These initial clinical and laboratory findings should be pondered in relation to the tempo of disease progression before deciding upon the next round of investigations. What major tests have already been done elsewhere? Repetition of costly radiographs and scans may be unnecessary. Can further testing be safely postponed? Sometimes more will be learned by waiting, or the fever of unknown origin may resolve spontaneously.

The next level of investigation will usually involve blood cultures, skin testing for delayed hypersensitivity, and selected serological tests. In older patients, tests for prostate-specific antigen and carcinoembryonic antigen should be obtained. If infective endocarditis seems likely, echocardiography should be used.

The order in which further major investigations are performed requires careful consideration of the likely yield, risks, and costs of each. Because many fevers of unknown origin are associated with intra-abdominal conditions, computerized tomography (**CT**) of the abdomen is often valuable. Sinus radiographs and pulmonary CT can reveal the lesions of Wegener's granulomatosis. Radiographs of the bowel with contrast can reveal an abnormality for further investigation. Gastrointestinal endoscopy with biopsy is often appropriate if symptoms or imaging studies suggest enteric conditions such as inflammatory bowel disease or cancer. Adjunctive imaging with magnetic resonance scan,

Fig. 1 The five main aetiological categories of fever of unknown origin, comparing their frequency in three geographical areas. Adapted from Miller, W.C. and Durack, D.T. (1994). Fever of unknown origin in the 1990s: a rational diagnostic approach. *Hospital Medicine*, **30** (in press).

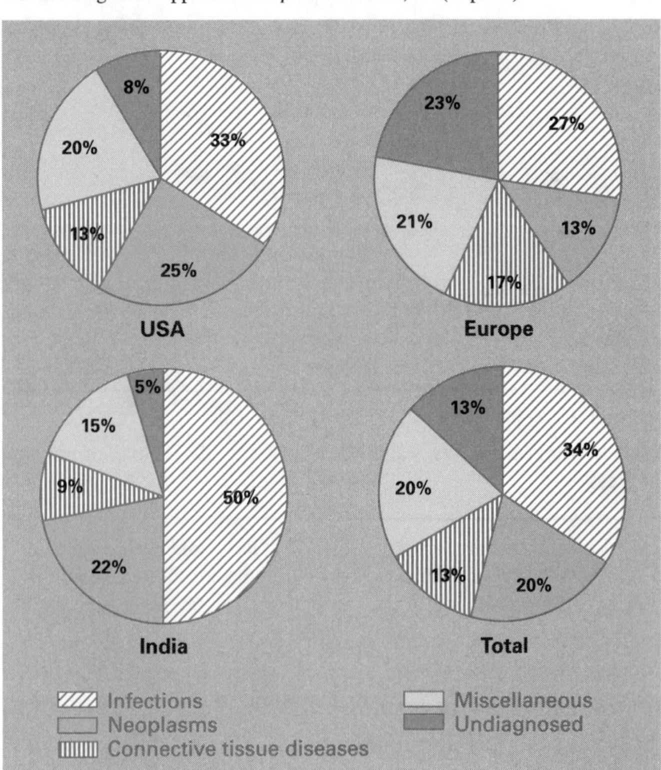

^{67}Ga-or ^{111}In-labelled leucocytes can be helpful, but these tests should be used selectively because they are costly, and of limited sensitivity; the chance that one of these will reveal a diagnosis is quite low if radiographs and CT scans are negative. If the echocardiogram is indeterminate but endocarditis still seems likely, transoesophageal echocardiography should be used.

Biopsies of bone marrow, lymph nodes, lung tissue, liver, skin, and temporal arteries or other vessels are essential for diagnosis of many fevers of unknown origin. Exploratory laparotomy, previously often done for diagnosis of fever of unknown origin, is now rarely necessary because of improved imaging techniques.

Treatment

Treatment of the fever itself is indicated if it distresses the patient, if it exacerbates heart failure, or if it is high enough to cause a catabolic state, interfering with maintenance of nutrition. Otherwise, the temperature curve can be observed in the absence of treatment, often yielding useful new information while investigations continue. If the fever must be treated, aspirin, paracetamol, or a non-steroidal anti-inflammatory drug in standard doses will usually suffice. A regular schedule rather than occasional or 'when required' dosing is recommended, to avoid the discomfort and sweating that may accompany wide temperature swings.

If an aetiological diagnosis cannot be made at first in a patient with classical fever of unknown origin, it is usually best to withhold treatment while observing the patient's progress at regular intervals. If he or she is too ill to permit prolonged observation, empirical treatment for fever of unknown origin may be considered. The most common choice for a therapeutic trial is corticosteroid. The recommended dose for an adult is prednisone, 30 mg twice daily, or the equivalent dose of another corticosteroid.

For neutropenic fever of unknown origin, the approach to treatment is quite different. After promptly making a focused physical examination, obtaining a chest radiograph, and sending blood and urine for culture, empirical broad-spectrum antibacterial therapy should be started immediately, before results of laboratory tests are available. Later, antifungal or antiviral therapy may be added according to the patient's progress and the results of investigations.

For HIV-associated fever of unknown origin, the physical examination should include retinoscopy to look for possible cytomegalovirus retinitis. If the chest radiograph is abnormal or the patient is hypoxic, bronchial washings or biopsy may reveal a pathogen such as Pneumocystis, Cryptococcus, cytomegalovirus, or mycobacteria. Direct staining of stool may reveal mycobacteria. The results of blood cultures for mycobacteria and unusual bacteria such as Rhodococcus or Rochalimaea should be awaited before further invasive tests are done. If the fever remains undiagnosed at this stage, bone marrow and liver biopsies are most likely to be informative. Once the cause of HIV-associated fever of unknown origin has been diagnosed, specific treatment regimens described in Chapter 7.10.29 can be prescribed.

Prognosis

Classical fever of unknown origin is a serious condition. Although most of the causes of this type of fever of unknown origin can be treated, the 1-year mortality is 20 to 30 per cent. Obviously, this varies depending upon the underlying disease and the age of the patient. If a patient has an fever of unknown origin lasting more than 6 to 12 months, the likelihood that a specific diagnosis will be made decreases, and the prognosis improves.

The prognosis for nosocomial fever of unknown origin varies according to the underlying diagnoses. The short-term prognosis for neutropenic fever of unknown origin is excellent, with over 90 per cent response to empirical antimicrobial therapy with appropriate modifications as time passes. The long-term prognosis is determined by the underlying diagnosis. Most of the causes of HIV-associated fever of unknown origin can be treated, but these patients have a poor prognosis, with death likely within 1 year. This may be due to HIV disease itself, which is usually advanced by the time the patient has fever of unknown origin. Atypical mycobacteria (which are the most common cause of HIV-associated fever of unknown origin) can be suppressed but not cured, and are likely to develop resistance to therapy. Finally, the patient remains at continual risk for development of other complications of AIDS.

REFERENCES

Barbado, F.J. *et al.* (1984). Fever of unknown origin: a survey on 133 patients. *Journal of Medicine*, **15**, 185–92.

Durack, D.T. and Street, A.C. (1991). Fever of unknown origin—reexamined and redefined. *Current Clinical Topics in Infectious Diseases*, **11**, 35–51.

Esposito, A.L. and Gleckman, R.A. (1978). Fever of unknown origin in the elderly. *Journal of the American Geriatrics Society*, **26**, 498–505.

Ghose, M.K., Shensa, S., and Lerner, P.I. (1976). Arteritis of the aged (giant cell arteritis) and fever of unexplained origin. *American Journal of Medicine*, **60**, 429–36.

Gleckman, R.A. and Esposito, A.L. (1986). Fever of unknown origin in the elderly: diagnosis and treatment. *Geriatrics*, **41**, 45–52.

Gleckman, R., Crowley, M., and Esposito, A. (1977). Fever of unknown origin: a view from the community hospital. *American Journal of Medical Sciences*, **274**, 21–5.

Greenberg, S.B. and Taber, L. (1991). Fever of unknown origin. In *Fever: basic mechanisms and management*, (ed. P. Mackowiak), pp. 183–95. Raven Press, New York.

Jackson, R.D. and Mysiw, W.J. (1991). Fever of unknown origin following traumatic brain injury. *Brain Injury*, **5**, 93–100.

Kazanjian, P.H. (1992). Fever of unknown origin: review of 86 patients treated in community hospitals. *Clinical Infectious Diseases*, **15**, 968–73.

Keefer, C.S. and Leard, S.E. (1955). *Prolonged and perplexing fevers*, Little, Brown, Boston.

Kluger, M.J. (1979). *Fever: its biology, evolution, and function*. Princeton University Press.

Knockaert, D.C. (1992). Diagnostic strategy for fever of unknown origin in the ultrasonography and computed tomography era. *Acta Clinica Belgica*, **47.2**, 100–16.

Knockaert, D.C., Vanneste, L.J., Vanneste, S.B., and Bobbaers, H.J. (1992). Fever of unknown origin in the 1980s. An update of the diagnostic spectrum. *Archives of Internal Medicine*, **152**, 51–5.

Larson, E.B., Featherstone, H.J., and Petersdorf, R.G. (1982). Fever of undetermined origin: diagnosis and follow-up of 105 cases, 1970–1980. *Medicine*, **61**, 269–92.

Leibovici, L., Cohen, O., and Wysenbeek, A.J. (1990). Occult bacterial infection in adults with unexplained fever. Validation of a diagnostic index. *Archives of Internal Medicine*, **150**, 1270–2.

Mackowiak, P.A. (ed.) (1991). *Fever: basic mechanisms and management*. Raven Press, New York.

Mackowiak, P.A., Wasserman, S.S., and Levine, M.M. (1993). A critical appraisal of 98.6°F, the upper limit of the normal body temperature, and other legacies of Carl Reinhold August Wunderlich. *Journal of the American Medical Association*, **268**, 1578–80.

MacSweeney, J.E., Peters, A.M., and Lavender, J.P. (1990). Indium labelled leucocyte scanning in pyrexia of unknown origin. *Clinical Radiology*, **42**, 414–17.

Petersdorf, R.G. and Beeson, P.B. (1961). Fever of unexplained origin: report on 100 cases. *Medicine*, **40**, 1–30.

Prego, V., Glatt, A.E., Roy, V., Thelmo, W., Dinesoy, H., and Raufman, J.P. (1990). Comparative yield of blood culture for fungi and mycobacteria, liver biopsy, and bone marrow biopsy in the diagnosis of fever of undetermined origin in human immunodeficiency virus-infected patients. *Archives of Internal Medicine*, **150**, 333–6.

Sharma, B.K., Kumari, S., Varma, S.C., Sagar, S., and Singh, S. (1992). Prolonged undiagnosed fever in Northern India. *Tropical and Geographical Medicine*, **44**, 32–6.

Steele, R.W., Jones, S.M., Lowe, B.A., and Glasier, C.M. (1991). Usefulness of scanning procedures for diagnosis of fever of unknown origin in children. *Journal of Pediatrics*, **119**, 526–30.

Suga, K. *et al.* (1991). The role of gallium-67 imaging in the detection of foci in recent cases of fever of unknown origin. *Annals of Nuclear Medicine*, **5**, 35–40.

Syrjala, M.T., Valtonen, V., Liewendahl, K., and Myllyla, G. (1987). Diagnostic significance of indium-111 granulocyte scintigraphy in febrile patients. *Journal of Nuclear Medicine*, **28,** 155–60.

Zoutman, D.E., Ralph, E.D., and Frei, J.V. (1991). Granulomatous hepatitis and fever of unknown origin. An 11-year experience of 23 cases with three years' follow-up. *Journal of Clinical Gastroenterology*, **13,** 69–75.

7.19.2 Septicaemia

P. A. MURPHY

Septicaemia is a term used to denote those clinical states in which bacteria are present in the bloodstream and cause systemic symptoms such as fever and hypotension. It is the most common cause of the systemic inflammatory response syndrome. However, the manifestations of septicaemia can also be induced by non-bacterial infectious agents, by non-living bacterial or fungal products, or by a variety of non-infectious conditions such as major trauma, burns, or pancreatitis. Septicaemia is an acute condition; most cases of infective endocarditis or miliary tuberculosis would not be included, even though many of the symptoms and signs are the same. Lastly, septicaemia has a connotation of urgency; unless the right things are done quickly, the patient is likely to die.

The aetiology of septicaemia

Almost any bacterium known to man may cause septicaemia on occasion. However, some organisms do so regularly in healthy people, while others need considerable assistance even to cause disease in sick people. Anything is possible, but not everything is equally frequent, and useful clinical information can be gained from a consideration of the circumstances under which the septicaemia arose. This matters because the initial therapy must usually be undertaken in the absence of bacteriological information, and it is important to guess right.

All septicaemias start from some kind of infected focus. If that focus is obvious clinically, one regards the septicaemia as 'secondary'. Finding a focus is important for several reasons. If Gram stains of pus, sputum, urine, and so forth are positive, that provides early information about the species probably responsible for sepsis. Even if stained smears are not helpful, the site of primary infection enables one to make a better guess at the cause of the sepsis. Removal or drainage of the focus will go a long way towards curing the septicaemia. In fact, if an undrained focus of infection is allowed to persist, the patient will probably remain septicaemic even though the organisms in the abscess and the bloodstream are completely susceptible to the antibiotics being used. Such patients generally die. Lastly, if a focus really cannot be found, that influences both the intensity and duration of therapy. With Gram-negative rods, one would be reassured, and treat for 5 to 7 days. With *Staphylococcus aureus*, one would assume that the patient probably had endocarditis, and would treat for at least 4 weeks. This may sound curious, but is based on the fact that Gram-negative endocarditis is rare, and need not be considered in the absence of compelling clinical evidence. On the other hand, about half of patients with staphylococcal sepsis and no evident focus prove eventually to have endocarditis.

Almost any organism may cause a secondary septicaemia. Some are high-grade pathogens such as the pneumococcus, following its usual path of nasopharyngeal colonization to pneumonia to sepsis. At the other end of the spectrum are organisms such as *Pseudomonas thomasii*, which causes disease only if it is allowed to grow in intravenous fluids and then is infused into the patient. The essence of secondary septicaemia is that some circumstance allows the generation of a large local population of organisms, which may be virulent, but do not have to be. From the local lesion, organisms are fed into the bloodstream.

'Primary' septicaemias are those without a clinically obvious focus of infection. Of course, there always is a portal of entry, but it may be subtle. Meningococcal nasopharyngitis, trivial staphylococcal folliculitis, or the intestinal ulcers that develop in people on chemotherapy are examples. Because there is no large local population, the organisms have to be capable of maintaining themselves in the bloodstream. In one kind of primary septicaemia, high-grade capsulated extracellular pathogens infect reasonably normal people. In the other kind, organisms of low virulence invade persons whose defences have been abrogated by disease or its treatment.

PRIMARY SEPTICAEMIA ACQUIRED IN THE COMMUNITY

Most patients in this class are not in the best of health. They are old, alcoholic, malnourished, or suffer from various debilitating diseases such as cirrhosis or diabetes. None the less they have some defences, and a relatively few organisms cause most of the septicaemias (Table 1). This table refers to adults: a list for children would be headed by the pneumococcus and *Haemophilus influenzae*, and a neonatal one by Gram-negative rods and Group B streptococci. The list is in approximate order of frequency for times when salmonellae and meningococci are not epidemic. The pneumococcus is third on the list only because the pneumonia is generally apparent in adults with pneumococcal sepsis. Noteworthy is the position of the Gram-negative rods so common in hospitals: if there is no urinary-tract infection or other local pathology, these are rare causes of sepsis acquired outside hospital. Occasionally, however, one sees Gram-negative sepsis in fishermen or other people who sustain cutaneous injuries that allow water organisms such as *Vibrio vulnificus* access to the tissues. Primary fungal septicaemia in patients outside hospital is virtually unheard of.

Gonococcal septicaemia is common in young people, but is usually mild and subacute. Septicaemia with shock acquired in the community by a healthy person is a great rarity. One should think of infection with unusual, very virulent organisms such as those of plague, anthrax, and tularaemia. If these can be ruled out, then the most likely culprits are *Staph. aureus* and the meningococcus. Persons who inject themselves with illegal drugs frequently develop acute infective endocarditis, which may be right-sided and difficult to diagnose. The most common cause is *Staph. aureus*, followed by yeasts, Pseudomonas and Serratia.

COMMUNITY-ACQUIRED SEPTICAEMIA WITH A LOCAL FOCUS

Common foci for the origin of sepsis are listed in Table 2, along with the classes of organisms most likely to be responsible. Although it is true that septicaemia from a local focus can occur in healthy people, this is rare. Most of the people who develop generalized sepsis from a pneumonia or a urinary-tract infection are old, malnourished, or suffer from debilitating diseases such as diabetes mellitus.

Well over half of urinary-tract infections are caused by *Escherichia coli*, and most of the rest by other Gram-negative rods. A Gram stain of the spun urinary sediment is a reliable guide to those few cases where enterococci or staphylococci are responsible.

Skin ulcers and areas of cellulitis generally have a Gram-positive flora of streptococci or staphylococci. Lesions around the perineum may be contaminated by aerobic Gram-negative rods. However, if there is frank cellulitis of the perineum, or a decubitus ulcer, anaerobes such as *Bacteroides fragilis* are the only organisms present in the bloodstream in half the cases, and are one component of the mixture in others. One should never forget that *Clostridium perfringens* is normal in human faecal flora and may also cause buttock cellulitis. The skin often shows haemorrhagic blebs, and Gram stains of exudate show large Gram-positive rods. The ischaemic or diabetic foot is usually infected with a mixed flora dominated by anaerobes.

When pneumonia is the obvious focus, and the patient has not been treated with antibiotics, the pneumococcus is first and the rest nowhere.

Table 1 *The common causes of community-acquired 'primary' septicaemia in adults*

Neisseria gonorrhoeae
Staphylococcus aureus
Streptococcus pneumoniae
Strep. pyogenes, groups A–T
Non-typhoidal salmonellae
Strep. faecalis
Neisseria meningitidis
Listeria monocytogenes
Escherichia coli, Pseudomonas, etc.

Table 2 *Common sites from which septicaemia arises in relatively normal patients*

Site	Likely bacterial causes of sepsis
Urine	Aerobic Gram-negative rods (90%)
	Aerobic Gram-positive cocci (10%)
Skin	Gram-positive cocci
Respiratory	*Streptococcus pneumoniae*
Abdominal:	
Gallbladder	Aerobic Gram-negative rods, *Strep. faecalis*
Bowel perforations	Aerobic Gram-negative rods
Pelvic inflammatory disease	*Neisseria gonorrhoeae*
	Mixed anaerobes

Klebsiella pneumonia may occur primarily in alcoholics; most other Gram-negative rod pneumonias occur in patients with bronchitis who have received tetracycline or other antibiotics. Staphylococcal pneumonia is most common as a complication of influenza. Both staphylococcal and Gram-negative rod pneumonias are easily diagnosed on Gram stain, and neither commonly causes a lobar infiltrate. Occasionally, *H. influenzae* causes pneumonia and septicaemia in an adult, and another organism seen from time to time is Acinetobacter. In both cases, sputum Gram stains show Gram-negative coccobacilli.

If the respiratory focus is a nasal sinus or the middle ear, more organisms need to be considered. Acute otitis media is a rare disease in adults; the most usual causes are the pneumococcus, and other streptococci, and spread to the bloodstream is exceptional. Acute sinusitis is very common in adults; again the pneumococcus is the most usual cause and again septicaemia is rare. Much more likely as a cause of sepsis are chronic otitis media and chronic sinusitis. Complications such as cholesteatomas and infective necrosis of bone are usually present, and the sepsis is precipitated by invasion and thrombosis of one of the cerebral veins. The bacterial flora is usually of mixed anaerobes, and the most likely aerobes are staphylococci and Gram-negative rods.

Abdominal catastrophes usually present as such. However, cholecystitis can be completely silent, especially in an old person, and may give rise to septicaemia with Gram-negative rods or enterococci. Similarly, diverticulitis or appendicitis in an old person may cause few local symptoms. Despite the very large numbers of anaerobes in colonic contents, the organisms in the bloodstream are usually Gram-negative aerobic rods. However, if the patient has an abscess, Bacteroides or other anaerobes may cause septicaemia.

Young women may acquire septicaemia because of pelvic inflammatory disease. Gonorrhoea is probably the most frequent single cause. Infected abortions are now uncommon, but infections of intrauterine devices are quite frequent. Postpartum infections due to retained products of conception are also seen. Most pelvic infections cause septicaemia with *E. coli*, group B streptococci, or anaerobic cocci. Often several organisms infect the bloodstream simultaneously.

SEPTICAEMIA IN HOSPITAL

Septicaemia in patients in the hospital is no different in principle from sepsis in the community. However, it is vastly more frequent, for a number of reasons. The most important reasons from the diagnostic point of view are the portals of entry for organisms that are provided by surgical wounds, urinary and vascular catheters, and the other impedimenta of modern medicine. General factors such as old age, steroid treatment, and diabetes make it more likely that patients will get septicaemia but do not greatly influence the route. However, patients with severe neutropenia are so susceptible to infection that bacteria may invade from trivial local lesions, or from no visible lesion at all.

The most common focus of infection is the urinary tract; it is estimated that 10 per cent of all patients in hospital have an indwelling urinary catheter, and that even with the best care, 25 per cent of those will be infected by the fourteenth day. The most common organism is still *E. coli*, but because of the strong selective pressure of antibiotics, it now causes only one-third of cases. Other Gram-negative rods such as Klebsiella, Proteus, Serratia, and Pseudomonas account for most of the remaining cases, and the enterococcus is the most common Gram-positive species. In forming an opinion of the likely cause in any particular patient, there are two main considerations. First, if the patient's urine is known to be infected with, say, *Enterobacter cloacae*, then that organism is the most likely cause of the sepsis. Second, in most hospitals particular organisms are troublesome on particular wards at particular times. If it is known that three patients on a particular urology ward developed septicaemia with *Serratia marcescens* in the last 10 days, then when a fourth patient on that ward develops sepsis, the serratia is probably the culprit.

The next most common source of sepsis is probably the surgical wound. Included in this category are deep-seated processes such as mediastinitis, leaking intestinal anastomoses, vaginal-cuff infections, and infections of the renal transplant bed. In any of these there may be no evidence of infection in the surface incision. If the patient has recently had an operation, one should be very loathe to consider any other source of sepsis. The bacteria likely to be responsible vary with the site of incision; one expects *Staph. aureus* or *epidermidis* after cranial surgery, *E. coli* or mixed anaerobes after a gynaecological operation.

Intravenous-line sepsis is rare if the device has been in place less than 24 h, and is uncommon before 48 h. Lines maintained for long periods, such as hyperalimentation lines, inevitably become infected unless cared for by special teams. The most troublesome area for line sepsis in most hospitals is the intensive care unit. It is not uncommon for a patient to have a peripheral line, a central line, a Swan–Ganz catheter, and an arterial line, all inserted in haste under conditions of dubious sterility, and all maintained for several days.

There are several distinct types of line sepsis. Sometimes the infusion fluid is contaminated, especially if additives have been necessary. In bottles containing glucose as the only nutrient, the organism is almost always Klebsiella, Enterobacter, or Serratia, as these organisms can grow fairly well in such solutions. Hyperalimentation solutions support the growth of yeasts such as *Candida albicans*.

In other types, the fluid is sterile, but there is cellulitis of the puncture wound, infection of the plastic catheter, or septic thrombophlebitis. The risk of septicaemia from a peripheral line is highest for cut-downs, and least for steel needles (Table 3). *Staph. aureus* accounts for about a third of cases with a demonstrated cause; most of the remaining cases are due to *Staph. epidermidis*, Klebsiella, Pseudomonas, and *C. albicans* in roughly equal proportions.

A very common source of sepsis in patients in hospital is the chest. Some cases have straightforward illnesses such as post-influenzal pneu-

Table 3 *Incidence of intravenous-line sepsis with various devices*

Device	Incidence of sepsis (%)
Hyperalimentation lines	12.0
Cut-downs	6.5
Subclavian plastic cannulae	3.8
Peripheral plastic cannulae	0.5
Steel needles	0.2

Modified from Rhame *et al.* (1979).

mococcal pneumonia, which are entirely analogous to the same diseases developing in the community. Most cases, however, develop in patients who aspirate pharyngeal contents for one reason or another. Many are weak or obtunded; others have had abdominal operations and are recumbent with nasogastric tubes in place. Nosocomial pneumonia is particularly frequent in patients on respirators. Most such patients have been treated with antibiotics, and pneumonia with septicaemia is almost always caused by aerobic Gram-negative rods.

On obstetric and gynaecological wards, sepsis is usually associated with infection of the pregnant or recently pregnant uterine cavity. Attempts to induce abortion by intra-amniotic injections of urea or saline, prolonged labour with ruptured membranes, or the retention of products of conception are the usual predisposing factors. The most dangerous organism is the group A *Streptococcus pyogenes*, but this has become rare. Most cases now are caused by other streptococci, including Group B, viridans, and enterococcal strains; anaerobic cocci; and aerobic Gram-negative rods such as *E. coli*, Klebsiella, and Proteus. Serratia and Pseudomonas are very uncommon; *Bacteroides fragilis* is a major pathogen occasionally.

Burned patients are very susceptible to septicaemia because the dead skin rapidly becomes colonized with bacteria, often in concentrations of 10^8 organisms/g. The organism causing septicaemia is almost always that most prominent in the burn at the time, and on good burn units this information is available. There is a predictable progression in the species of organisms that colonize the burn. In the first week after injury, sepsis is usually caused by Gram-positive cocci. Later, Gram-negative rods such as Pseudomonas or *Providencia stuartii* cause most cases. If the burn remains unhealed for weeks, *C. albicans*, and other yeasts may take over.

A very important patient population is those who do not have normal defences against infection. By far the most important defect is the lack of mature neutrophils; septicaemia becomes progressively more common as the absolute neutrophil count falls below 500/mm^3. Such patients are susceptible to all the usual hospital-acquired infections, but in addition are constantly in danger of being overwhelmed by their own flora. They often have several episodes of septicaemia. The initial ones are generally caused by organisms such as *E. coli* and Klebsiella, which are from the normal enteric flora. Antibiotics select out resistant organisms, and subsequent episodes are due to organisms such as Enterobacter or Pseudomonas, which are rarely found in the faeces of normal people. Fungaemias due to *Candida* spp. or to *Torulopsis glabrata* also become common. At all stages of the illness, 10 to 20 per cent of septicaemias are caused by Gram-positive species such as *Staph. aureus*.

The prevention of septicaemia

Septicaemia is a dangerous illness, with an appreciable mortality even in fundamentally healthy people. We have no control over cases arising in the community, but most of the cases arising in hospital are preventable. Infection control is humdrum, devoid of excitement, and essential. It is best not left to physicians, as few of them are temperamentally suited to carry it out. However, physicians should be made to follow the rules. They must not take down septic wound dressings with bare hands and move to the next patient without washing. They must not irrigate urinary catheters in half a minute between other commitments. They must not be allowed to flout the rules about isolation of infected patients. Every study ever done has shown that physicians ignore protocol far more often than nurses or other personnel. Physicians can make a large contribution to infection control by reducing the number of invasive procedures used, and especially by restricting their duration. Surgeons can contribute by following the fundamental principles of surgery in clean procedures, and by the proper use of drains and antibiotics when infection is probable. If it is known that a patient will be aplastic for some time, the incidence of septicaemia can be reduced by selective decontamination of the gut. The aim is to kill the aerobic Gram-negative rods that are the most common causes of septicaemia while leaving the anaerobic population intact. The antibiotic most often used is norfloxacin.

Clinical features

Septicaemia is one of the very few clinical situations in which the patient can give little useful information. He or she may complain of fever, rigors or headache, may simply feel awful, or may be too obtunded to complain of anything. Frequently, septicaemia develops in a patient already gravely ill from some other process, and incapable of communicating with attendants. The responsibility therefore rests squarely on the doctor.

Septicaemia should be suspected whenever there is an acute change in the patient's condition. Almost all patients develop some fever, and those in reasonably good condition usually exceed 39°C. Failure to develop a temperature greater than 37.6°C is a bad prognostic sign, and patients whose body temperature stays subnormal virtually all die. Chills and rigors simply mean that the temperature is rising rapidly, they have no independent significance, and the number of rigors gives no clue to the organism.

If the patient is closely observed, certain signs may be seen even before fever. Unexplained apprehension, lethargy, and clouding of consciousness are commonly noticed by alert relatives or nurses. Tachypnoea and respiratory alkalosis is another early sign. Occasionally, someone will notice that the patient's hands are unusually warm.

Hypotension usually follows fever, but if a large number of organisms has been suddenly introduced into the circulation, it may be the initial sign. Hypotension is due to peripheral vasodilation and the cardiac output is high or comparatively high. Cardiac outputs of 20 l/min may be seen in healthy young men; more modest outputs of 7 to 8 l/min may represent the maximum in a frail, elderly patient. By the time most patients come under observation, much fluid has been lost from the circulation through leaky capillaries into the tissues. Cardiac output falls, and the patient appears pale, cold, and clammy.

The pulmonary vascular resistance is persistently elevated, and very early on the arterial oxygen tension becomes subnormal. At least some of this pulmonary dysfunction is due to obstruction of pulmonary arterioles with microthrombi: much of the rest appears to be due to leaky pulmonary capillaries. Severe forms of pulmonary dysfunction are associated with gross hypoxaemia, visible infiltrates on chest radiographs, and other features of the adult respiratory-distress syndrome. There is also disorder of the microcirculation in non-pulmonary tissues; the oxygen consumption is subnormal from the outset, and becomes grossly so terminally. However, the mixed venous $P\text{O}_2$ is generally normal because much arterial blood is shunted past the tissues.

If the patient is already severely ill, septicaemia may present as unexplained deterioration. Bleeding, thrombocytopenia or leucocytosis may be noticed. Leucopenia may also occur if the patient's marrow reserves of neutrophils become exhausted. Oliguria or anuria, jaundice, or cardiac failure may follow inadequate perfusion of those organs. Organic psychoses of many varieties may occur for the same reason. Some cases present with ecthyma gangrenosum or other skin lesions.

Management

The management of septicaemia can be discussed in terms of what we do now, and what we will probably do in the future. At present, the essentials in the management of septicaemia are to cut off the inflow of organisms to the bloodstream, to kill or inhibit those already there, and to restore the perfusion of vital organs. All other considerations are secondary, and time should not be wasted on them initially. Bleeding, delirium, and pulmonary and renal failure will generally take care of themselves if the essentials have been achieved. Operationally, the initial steps are the removal or drainage of the source of sepsis if that is possible, the selection of a suitable antibiotic or antibiotics, and the infusion of large quantities of fluid intravenously. Steps in resuscitation in severe sepsis are outlined in Table 4.

Table 4 *Resuscitation in severe sepsis*

The values to aim at are:
Cardiac index 4.5 l/min per m²
Oxygen delivery (through aortic valve) 800 ml/min per m²
Oxygen consumption 170 ml/min per m²
If left atrial pressure is < 18 mmHg, give:
2 u packed red cells if the haemotocrit is < 33
500 ml hydroxyethyl starch if haematocrit > 33
Repeat until left atrial pressure is 15–18 mmHg
If left atrial pressure is 15–18 mmHg and values are still low:
Give dobutamine starting at 2 μg/kg per min
If dobutamine benefit has maximized:
Try dopamine starting at 2 μg/kg per min

Modified from Tuchschmidt *et al.* (1991).

CLINICAL ASSESSMENT

The experienced clinician makes a *gestalt* assessment of the severity of the patient's state, taking many factors into consideration, often unconsciously. The bedside chart shows the height of the fever and the speed of its rise. The pulse rate and blood pressure are measured if not charted. A look at the patient from the foot of the bed may show apathy, clouding of consciousness, or tachypnoea. Other associated findings may include skin rashes or jaundice. A rapid search for the source of the infection follows. In a patient from outside the hospital, one looks for signs of cutaneous ulcers, pneumonia, local or generalized peritonitis, pyelonephritis, and pelvic inflammatory disease. In a patient already in the hospital, one thinks first of intravascular catheters and monitoring devices, urinary catheters, surgical wounds and deep infections of recent operation sites, pneumonia, and decubitus ulcers. Parenthetically, one should not forget common non-infectious problems such as drug reactions and pulmonary emboli. This rapid assessment should take no more than 30 min. A tentative diagnosis is made, together with a guess at the responsible organism. The most useful diagnostic specimens are taken for culture; these will always include two blood cultures, together with urine, pus, sputum, and cerebrospinal fluid as appropriate. Treatment must be got under way immediately. Radiographs, sonograms, computerized tomographic scans, and other time-wasting investigations should be deferred until the patient's condition stabilizes.

DIFFERENTIAL DIAGNOSIS

There is a very large number of causes of fever, and if there is no evidence of shock it may be reasonable to consider drug reactions, viral infections, and various other non-urgent diagnoses, even to the point of deferring treatment. But the more acute the onset of fever, the higher the value it reaches, and the sicker the appearance of the patient, the more likely it is that bacteria are in the bloodstream. Treatment should not be delayed, unless bacterial sepsis is thought to be an improbable explanation of the patient's state. Even then, the patient should be closely observed for evidence of deterioration until the situation clarifies. If the patient is neutropenic, there is no case for delay. It is true that only about half of the febrile episodes occurring in neutropenic patients can be shown to be due to bacterial infection. But untreated sepsis in such patients is generally fatal within 24 h.

If patients suddenly develop both fever and shock, they should be treated for septicaemia unless there is cast-iron evidence of some other cause. One can imagine circumstances where pulmonary embolism or myocardial infarction might present in this way. Intraperitoneal or retroperitoneal bleeding, or even bleeding into the gastrointestinal tract, might cause confusion. But the shock must be treated in any event, and 2 days of antimicrobial therapy is unlikely to be harmful. If one attempts to be always correct in urgent situations, the likely result is that patients will deteriorate irreversibly while time is frittered away.

TREATMENT

Antimicrobial selection

It is important not to waste too much time on this. Most organisms are somewhat sensitive to most antimicrobials. Even in leukaemic patients, antimicrobial regimens that are theoretically unsuitable for the organism which eventually grows out of the bloodstream often lead to clinical improvement. There is evidence that the sensitivity or resistance of the organisms in the bloodstream to the antibiotics prescribed during the first 24 h of the patient's stay in the hospital makes little difference to mortality (although the continued use of inappropriate antimicrobials on day 2 and subsequently does lead to increased mortality). The use of antimicrobials such as cefotaxime and piperacillin, which have greatly increased antibacterial activity and a broader spectrum, has conspicuously not led to improved mortality rates for septic people. The mortality of sepsis has remained stable at about 30 per cent for 25 years. There is no published evidence that any antimicrobial is more effective for septicaemia than another, provided that the organisms are sensitive to both agents. All this suggests that much of the agonizing about just which antimicrobial should be used for a particular patient is inappropriate. It is better to do anything than to do nothing.

The antimicrobials usually selected for treatment of presumed septicaemia are the third-generation cephalosporins such as ceftriaxone or an extended-spectrum penicillin such as ticarcillin in combination with a β-L lactamase inhibitor. Reasonable people differ over whether or not to add an aminoglycoside; personally I only use gentamicin and its relatives if there is a probability of Pseudomonas, if the septicaemia is overwhelming, or if the patient is neutropenic.

A few treatable organisms are completely resistant to cephalosporins and aminoglycosides. Rickettsiae can cause septic shock, and both typhus and Rocky Mountain spotted fever should be thought of in appropriate parts of the world. Occasionally, psittacosis presents with very high fever and few or no pulmonary signs. Some young women have salpingitis caused by chlamydiae. Chlamydial and rickettsial infections respond to tetracycline. Malaria should be specifically excluded by the examination of blood smears if it is conceivable that the patient might have acquired it by any route including transfusions. *C. albicans* can cause intravenous-line sepsis in normal patients or septicaemia in debilitated ones. Fungal sepsis is seldom immediately lethal, and most oncology units do not treat for it in the first instance, particularly as amphotericin B is so toxic. Some of the viral haemorrhagic fevers are susceptible to chemotherapy (see Chapter 7.10.20). However, if the patient has been to Africa, or works with monkeys, they are worth remembering because several of them pose an infection hazard to the attendants.

There is experimental evidence that β-lactams whose principal target is penicillin-binding protein (**PBP**) 3 cause lysis of bacteria with release of large amounts of soluble endotoxin. β-Lactams whose main target is PBP2 kill with little or no endotoxin release. This has not yet been shown to make any difference to mortality from sepsis in animals or man, but if such differences were shown, one would obviously prefer to use a PBP2-specific agent. Following the same idea, an antimicrobial that kills without lysis (a quinolone) may prove preferable to any β-lactam, and a clinical trial on this point is in progress.

Whatever antimicrobial regimen is chosen, it should be given intravenously in large doses. When the blood cultures are reported, the sensitivities as measured in the laboratory should be checked against the antimicrobial regimen that is being given. If the regimen appears to be inadequate, one should strongly consider changing it, even if the patient appears to be improving. There is no place for half measures in the treatment of septicaemia: an initial mistake in antimicrobial selection is not usually disastrous, but persistence in error commonly is.

INTRAVENOUS FLUID THERAPY

A large bore intravenous line should be inserted as soon as possible. Through it one gives fluid until the haemodynamic measures normalize, or until there is evidence of fluid overload. There is no evidence that any particular formula of intravenous fluid is better than normal saline. Usually, saline containing some potassium, glucose, and a substrate metabolizable into bicarbonate is given, on the assumption that those additions are harmless and may be useful. Solutions containing albumin or other colloids such as hydroxyethyl starch can be used if available because they may better retain fluid in the bloodstream. If the patients hematocrit is below 33 per cent, then enough whole blood or packed red cells should be given to get the haematocrit above that percentage.

Under most circumstances, when the patient is not desperately ill, this process can be monitored by ordinary clinical methods. The pulse rate, blood pressure, and respiratory rate should be measured and recorded at regular intervals. In most patients it is best to catheterize the urinary bladder to provide accurate information about urine flow. One watches the jugular veins and regularly listens for crepitations at the lung bases.

A good starting dose of fluid would be 1 litre of Ringers' lactate in the first hour. If marked hypotension is present, it could be given faster and rapidly followed by a second litre. One would then reassess the patient. If the blood pressure has risen to normal, the pulse has slowed somewhat, respiration is no faster, the patient is alert and orientated, and urine flow exceeds 75 ml/h, well and good. One would slow the rate of fluid administration to perhaps 1 litre every 6 h and await events.

If the patient remains hypotensive and there is no evidence of fluid overload, one should continue to give fluid, but also look for other correctable problems. The arterial oxygen saturation or Po_2 should be checked; if these are not over 90 per cent or 65 mmHg, respectively, the patient should be given oxygen, and intubated if necessary. Obvious electrolyte abnormalities should be corrected. Patients commonly have normal or near normal serum sodium and potassium, but very low levels of phosphate or magnesium. Severe hypoglycaemia should also be corrected.

The correction of acidosis is controversial. Certainly if the arterial pH is below 7.2, most physicians would cautiously give bicarbonate. However there is no evidence, in people or in animals, that this is beneficial, and total correction of pH into the normal range is positively harmful. It seems to be true that if the patient's circulatory state can be improved, the acidosis will take care of itself, and that if that cannot be done, bicarbonate will not change the outcome.

If the patient fails to respond to simple management, or is desperately ill to start with, the full resources of an intensive care unit should be used if available. One can install a central venous catheter, a Swan–Ganz catheter, and a radial-artery catheter. The arterial, central venous, and pulmonary capillary-wedge pressures should be monitored, and regular samples of arterial blood for pH, oxygen, and carbon dioxide, and venous blood for electrolytes should be taken. The cardiac output should be measured from time to time, usually by thermodilution. If the patient's respiratory function is unsatisfactory, intubate the trachea and supply room air enriched with oxygen, varying the Fio_2, the tidal volume, the end-expiratory pressure, and the respiratory rate, as appropriate. A urinary catheter is installed to measure hourly urine flow.

With all this equipment, fluid therapy can be much more aggressive. One gives fluid until the cardiac output reaches a plateau or the pulmonary capillary-wedge pressure reaches 18 mmHg. If pulmonary oedema develops, the end-expiratory airway pressure is increased cautiously until the oedema goes away.

VASOCONSTRICTORS AND INOTROPES

If the patient has failed to respond to maximal fluid repletion, and remains hypotensive with a now raised left-atrial pressure, one is in deep trouble. The use of inotropes and vasoconstrictors has in the past been controlled by using them to achieve some predetermined mean arterial pressure that was thought to be adequate. The raised blood pressure was often achieved by inducing peripheral vasoconstriction and, even worse, tissue ischaemia. Death rates for such patients were well over 80 per cent.

A more modern concept starts from the premise that the principal function of the circulation is to transport oxygen to the tissues. Inotropes and vasoconstrictors are useful if they improve oxygen delivery, and harmful if they reduce it. The level of the blood pressure *per se* is unimportant.

There is evidence that the oxygen consumption of septic patients is limited by oxygen delivery. If more oxygen is supplied, they use it. To be precise, the 'normal' oxygen consumption of a septic patient should be 3.5 ml/kg per min, and in order to achieve that, 15 ml oxygen/kg per min need to be delivered through the aortic valve. Virtually all patients still in shock after fluid repletion have oxygen consumptions below 3.5 ml/kg per min. It should be noted that a normal person at rest also consumes 3.5 ml oxygen/kg per min. However, this is achieved by delivering 12 to 14 ml of oxygen/kg per min through the aortic valve. If this figure is reduced to 8 to 10 ml/kg per min, a normal person can maintain oxygen consumption by increasing the amount of oxygen extracted from each millilitre of blood. In sepsis, the peripheral circulation is disordered, stagnant, and largely bypassed. It is so inefficient that increasing oxygen extracted per ml of blood is not possible and oxygen consumption is limited by the amount supplied.

If the cardiac output, haemoglobin concentration and arterial oxygen tension or saturation are all known, then oxygen delivery through the aortic valve can be determined. If it is subnormal, then therapeutic changes should be made to try and raise it. The haemoglobin and arterial oxygen saturation should be raised above 33 and 90 per cent, respectively, if that has not already been done. The best stimulus for improved oxygen delivery turns out to be dobutamine, which improves left-ventricular stroke volume, but has little effect on blood pressure. The initial dose should be 2 μg/kg per min, with increments every 10 min until cardiac output and oxygen delivery stop increasing. Fluid repletion can be precisely controlled by raising the left atrial pressure until oxygen delivery reaches a plateau. In many patients, that occurs at 15 mmHg, and left atrial pressures of 18 mm and above are deleterious. Selective vasoconstrictors such as dopamine may slightly improve oxygen delivery above that obtainable from the use of dobutamine. General vasoconstrictors such as noradrenaline usually do not improve tissue oxygenation, and may reduce it.

There are no controlled trials of this mode of using inotropes and vasoconstrictors. However, in one published series, mortality was only 4 per cent in patients whose measures for oxygen delivery could be normalized in this way.

REMOVAL OF SEPTIC FOCI

If a patient in hospital develops septicaemia and no other source is evident, it is advisable to remove all intravascular devices. If they must be replaced, completely new systems should be inserted in vessels far removed from the old sites. If vascular access is limited and a line is precious, one can compromise by changing the device over a wire, and making a quantitative culture of the old line. If that culture is negative, the new line can be left in place. However, if culture of the old line is positive, then the new line must be removed and a new site selected. If there is evidence of suppurative thrombophlebitis, the affected segment of vein must be removed surgically or the septicaemia will probably continue.

Localized collections of pus such as empyema or subphrenic abscess should be drained. This is best done by radiologists, using computerized tomographic or ultrasonic guidance. Foci that are acutely infected but where there is no frank abscess formation are usually left alone in the first instance. Cholecystitis, pneumonia, sinusitis, and pelvic inflammatory disease will all generally respond to antibiotic therapy. If an operation is thought necessary, it can be done later when the patient's condition is stable and the local inflammation has subsided. If the patient has extensive phlegmonous inflammation, but no localized collection, amputation or massive debridement may be life saving.

ANTICOAGULATION

Disseminated intravascular coagulation is common in Gram-negative sepsis, and also occurs in Gram-positive infections, but there is no evidence that preventing it by the use of heparin makes any difference to the outcome of sepsis. However, heparin therapy is life saving for septic pelvic thrombophlebitis in women, and sometimes for suppurative thrombophlebitis of central veins that cannot be surgically excised. Antimicrobial therapy alone does not cure these patients; they continue to have septic pulmonary emboli, abscesses, and empyemas. The addition of heparin generally leads to cure.

OTHER SUPPORTIVE MEASURES

Septicaemic patients are usually already gravely ill with some other process. They will need all the usual measures for their underlying condition. They may also develop organ failure because of sepsis. It may be necessary to manage postoperative ileus, epileptic fits, and hepatic, renal, or pulmonary failure.

Prognosis

It is important not to be unreasonably optimistic, particularly when talking to relatives. In all infections, there is a 'point of no return' after which antimicrobial therapy ceases to influence the outcome. Even with the best care, many patients die.

The most important single factor is the patient's general condition; this was first shown by McCabe and Jackson, and every study since has confirmed it. The mortality also rises with age; most of the excess deaths are attributable to cardiac and pulmonary problems, and to tumours. The species of organism is of some consequence; *Ps. aeruginosa* consistently causes high mortality, probably because of its exotoxin. Other Gram-negative rods, including Bacteroides, cause mortalities in the range of 25 to 40 per cent in most series, and there is little difference between species. Gram-positive sepsis may be overwhelming, but overall the mortality is lower, perhaps 10 to 20 per cent.

When death is attributable mainly or entirely to infection, it is often due not so much to the septicaemia as to the consequences of infection in the primary site. Extensive pneumonia, meningitis, or widespread intraperitoneal infection may be impossible to deal with, or may lead to such debilitation that the patient expires of the diseases of the bedridden—bedsores, pulmonary emboli, and bronchopneumonia.

The presence of shock suggests a large dose of organisms, and, not surprisingly, mortality in shocked patients is two or three times that of comparable patients with normal blood pressure. This applies whatever the species of organism. The excess mortality almost all occurs in the first 48 h, and is directly attributable to septicaemia. A normal or subnormal temperature in the presence of septicaemia is also a very bad prognostic sign.

The effect of antibiotic therapy on prognosis is discernible, but not as great as might be expected. Patients treated with antimicrobials to which the organisms are sensitive do survive better than those in whom the treatment was not appropriate. However, the general condition, and the presence or absence of shock, are powerful independent variables.

Septicaemia persisting in the face of therapy

If the patient remains febrile and sick after 48 h of therapy, a total reassessment should be made. The most important is a complete physical examination looking for infectious foci that might have become apparent since admission. Examination should be detailed, including the fundi, the entire skin surface, and rectal and vaginal examinations. New blood cultures, and cultures of anything else that might be helpful, should be obtained.

If the original blood cultures were positive, and the antimicrobial therapy was inappropriate, it should be changed if not already done. If the original blood cultures were positive and the organisms were sensitive to the antimicrobials employed, then it is probable that the patient has undrained pus somewhere, and search for that should be made by radiographs, sonograms, computed tomography or indium-111 scans, as seem appropriate.

The antimicrobial regimen should be reviewed to make certain that the route, frequency, and dosage are adequate; subtherapeutic doses are particularly common with aminoglycosides. It is often useful to measure antimicrobial levels in blood. Neutropenic patients, and those with large foci of infected tissue, respond very slowly, even when the antimicrobial regimen is adequate. In such patients, it may be right to persist with the same therapy, provided that one is reasonably certain there are no other adverse factors.

If the original blood cultures are negative, and the patient remains febrile, the antimicrobials should be discontinued, and two new ones substituted. The only exception to this rule is if some acceptable non-infectious cause of the symptoms has declared itself. A search for deep infected foci should be made as outlined above. In neutropenic patients, one should probably add amphotericin B at this stage, as Candida and other yeasts may take some days to grow out of the original blood cultures.

Failure to respond to two different antimicrobial regimens, with no evidence of local sepsis and no response to antifungal drugs, suggests that the diagnosis of septicaemia was wrong. Many fevers in patients in hospital are caused by drug reactions, tumours, or viral infections of diverse types. High, spiking fever may persist for months in alcoholic hepatitis. The best way of managing such situations is to withdraw antibiotics while carefully observing the patient and reculturing as indicated.

Experimental treatment

There is tremendous interest in improving the outcome in sepsis by interfering with one or more of the pathogenetic steps that are thought to be important. It must be admitted at the outset that most published studies to this point have been failures. We have been naïve in assuming that reagents which protect healthy animals when given soon after bacterial challenge will necessarily help patients whose sepsis has been going on for hours or days. But we have learned from the failures: if we are to help our patients we must find a late reaction that is critically important rather than an early one.

The use of antimicrobials that do not cause bacterial lysis, and that minimize the release of endotoxin and peptidoglycan, was referred to above, and may prove to be important.

Monoclonal anti-endotoxin antibody was tried in man in two large controlled trials. There was an improved outcome in patients who had

Gram-negative sepsis with shock. However, for unclear reasons, the mortality in patients who did not have Gram-negative bacteraemia was actually slightly increased and, as such patients were the majority, the overall mortality was not significantly different. Furthermore, the methodology of the trial was seriously criticized, and it may well be that the treated and placebo group were not truly comparable. Finally, the antibody was inordinately expensive: if it had been used in my hospital it would have consumed more than half the budget available for all drugs. For all these reasons, the United States Food and Drug Administration did not approve the antibody for clinical use.

Steroids are another mode of treatment that have an excellent experimental foundation but proved to be useless in the treatment of septic patients. The probable reason for the failure is that steroids prevent transcription of the genes for interleukin (**IL**) 1 and tumour necrosis factor (**TNF**) into mRNA. However, 30 min after a macrophage has been exposed to endotoxin the transcripts have been made, and steroids do not affect synthesis and secretion of IL-1 and TNF proteins. We do not see our septic patients soon enough for steroids to be effective. It was shown in two large trials that steroids were ineffective overall, and were actually deleterious in some subgroups. Therefore, steroids are not currently recommended for the treatment of any form of sepsis.

A clinical trial of the opiate antagonist naloxone in human patients did not affect mortality.

Clinical trials of antibody to TNF-α and of the IL-1-receptor antagonist protein are in progress. Preliminary results for antiTNF-α were not very encouraging. According to the *Wall Street Journal*, which is generally reliable, the same is true for the IL-1-receptor antagonist. Even if these products do prove to have some protective activity, they are proteins and will be very expensive. No purpose is served by developing a reagent that no one can afford to use.

The greatest clinical activity currently concerns antagonists of platelet-activating factor (**PAF**). PAF binds to a high-affinity receptor on neutrophils, and there are analogues that bind to the receptor, block PAF access, but have no agonist activity of their own. These agents are drugs, simple organic chemicals that can be synthesized by the kilogram for not much money. One of them has a serum half-life of 48 h, they do not appear to be toxic, and the results of animal experiments are very encouraging. Clinical trials in septic patients are in progress, but not even preliminary results are available.

Other endstage reactions of sepsis that might be usefully inhibited may be rapidly reviewed. Many intracellular signalling mechanisms depend upon calcium entry from the exterior of the cell. Calcium-channel blockers might antagonize release of arachidonate derivatives, PAF, polymorph granules, or endothelial-cell expression of selectins. Antagonists of proteolytic enzymes might reduce the damage caused by highly activated polymorphs and macrophages, and scavengers of the hydroxyl radical might reduce damage to endothelial-cell membranes. Free-radical scavengers are simple molecules such as histidine and mannitol, which could be produced inexpensively.

Obviously, many of these experimental approaches are going to founder for one reason or another. However, in sepsis as in other areas of infectious disease, the next great advance is going to come from the control of the inflammatory response.

REFERENCES

Altemeier, W.A., Burke, J.F., Pruitt, B.A., and Sandusky, W.R. (ed.) (1976). *Manual on control of infections in surgical patients*. Lippincott, Philadelphia.

Beal, A.L., and Cerra, F.B. (1994). Multiple organ failure syndrome in the 1990's. *Journal of the American Medical Association*, **271**, 226–33.

Bodey, G.P., Buckley, M., and Sathe, Y.S. (1966). Quantitative relationships between circulating leukocytes and infection in patients with acute leukemia. *Annals of Internal Medicine*, **64**, 328–40.

Bodey, G.P. (1986). Infection in cancer patients. A continuing association. *American Journal of Medicine*, **87**, (Suppl. 1A), 11–26.

Bone, R.C. *et al.* (1987). A controlled clinical trial of high dose methyl prednisolone in the treatment of severe sepsis and septic shock. *New England Journal of Medicine*, **317**, 653–8.

Bryan, C.S., Reynolds, K.L., and Branner, E.R. (1983). Analysis of 1186 episodes of Gram-negative bacteremia in non-university hospitals: the effects of antimicrobial therapy. *Reviews of Infectious Diseases*, **5**, 639–38.

Corrigna, J.C. and Kiernat, J.F. (1975). Effect of heparin in experimental Gram-negative septicaemia. *Journal of Infectious Diseases*, **131**, 138–43.

Exley, A.R. *et al.* (1990). Monoclonal antibody to TNF in severe septic shock. *Lancet*, **335**, 1275–7.

Fisher, C.J. *et al.* (1993). Influence of an anti-TNF monoclonal antibody on cytokine levels in patients with sepsis. *Critical Care Medicine*, **21**, 318–27.

Fisher, C.J., *et al.* (1994). Recombinant human interleukin 1 receptor antagonist in the treatment of patients with sepsis syndrome: results from a randomized, double-blind, placebo controlled trial. *Journal of the American Medical Association,* **271**, 1836–43.

Galpin, J.E., Chow, A.W., Bayer, A.S., and Guze, L.B. (1976). Sepsis associated with decubitus ulcers. *American Journal of Medicine*, **61**, 346–50.

Hayes, M.A., Timmins, A.C., Yau, E.H.S., Palazzo, M., Hinds, C.J., and Watson, D. (1994). Elevation of systemic oxygen delivery in the treatment of critically ill patients. *New England Journal of Medicine,* **330**, 1717–22.

Hinshaw, L. *et al.* (1987). Effect of high dose glucocorticoid therapy on mortality in patients with clinical signs of systemic sepsis. *New England Journal of Medicine*, **317**, 659–65.

Jackson, J.J. and Kropp, H. (1992). Betalactam induced release of free endotoxin: *in vitro* comparison of penicillin binding protein (PBP)2 specific imipenem and PBP3 specific ceftazidime. *Journal of Infectious Diseases*, **165**, 1033–41.

Kreger, B.E., Craven, D.E., and McCabe, W.R. (1980). Gram-negative bacteremia. Re-evaluation of clinical features and treatment in 612 patients. *American Journal of Medicine*, **68**, 344–55.

Ledger, W.J. and Peterson, E.P. (1970). The use of heparin in the management of pelvic thrombophlebitis. *Surgery, Gynecology and Obstetrics*, **131**, 1115–21.

Louie, T.J., Bartlett, J.G., Tally, F.P., and Gorbach, S.L. (1976). Aerobic and anaerobic bacteria in diabetic foot ulcers. *Annals of Internal Medicine*, **85**, 461–3.

McCabe, W.R., and Jackson, G.G. (1962). Gram-negative bacteremia. Clinical, laboratory and therapeutic observations. *Archives of Internal Medicine*, **110**, 856–64.

Maki, D.G. (1987). Nosocomial bacteremia: an epidemiologic overview. *American Journal of Medicine*, **70**, 719–32.

Martin, D.T. *et al.* (1984). Crystalloid versus colloid resuscitation in experimental haemorrhagic pancreatitis. *Surgery, Gynecology and Obstetrics*, **159**, 445–9.

Miller, P.J., and Wenzel, R.P. (1987). Etiologic organisms as independent predictors of death and morbidity associated with bloodstream infections. *Journal of Infectious Diseases*, **156**, 471–7.

Monif, G.R.G., and Baer, H. (1976). Polymicrobial bacteremia in obstetric patients. *Obstetrics and Gynecology*, **48**, 167–9.

Ognibene, F.P. *et al.* (1988). Depressed left ventricular performance: response to volume infusion in patients with sepsis and septic shock. *Chest*, **93**, 903–10.

Parker, M.M., and Parillo, J.E. (1983). Septic shock: hemodynamics and pathogenesis. *Journal of the American Medical Association*, **250**, 3324–7.

Platt, R. *et al.* (1982). Mortality associated with nosocomial urinary tract infection. *New England Journal of Medicine*, **307**, 637–42.

Rhame, F.S., Maki, D.G., and Bennett, J.V. (1979). Intravenous cannula-associated infections. In *Hospital infections* (ed. J.V. Bennett and P.S. Brachman) Ch. 25. Little Brown, Boston.

Safani, M. *et al.* (1989). Prospective, controlled, randomized trial of naloxone infusion in early hyperdynamic septic shock. *Critical Care Medicine*, **17**, 1004–9.

Singer, C., Kaplan, M.H., and Armstrong, D. (1977). Bacteremia and fungemia complicating neoplastic disease: a study of 364 cases. *American Journal of Medicine*, **62**, 731–42.

Stein, J.M. and Pruitt, B.A. (1970). Suppurative thrombophlebitis. A lethal iatrogenic disease. *New England Journal of Medicine*, **282**, 1452–5.

Tuchschmidt, J., Oblitas, D., and Fried, J.C. (1991). Oxygen consumption in sepsis and septic shock. *Critical Care Medicine*, **19**, 664–71.

Warren, H.S., Danner, R.L., and Munford, R.S. (1992). Anti-endotoxin monoclonal antibodies. (Editorial.) *New England Journal of Medicine*, **326,** 1153–7.

Ziegler, E.J. *et al.* (1991). Treatment of Gram-negative bacteremia and septic shock with HA-1A human monoclonal antibody against endotoxin: a randomized double blind placebo controlled trial. *New England Journal of Medicine*, **324,** 429–36.

7.19.3 Infection in the immunocompromised host

J. COHEN

One of the most distressing experiences in medicine is to see a patient cured of a serious underlying disease, only to die as a result of a complication of the treatment. While the benefits of immunosuppression have been enormous, there is no doubt that unwanted effects, and in particular serious infection, have proved to be a major drawback.

Classification

The term 'immunocompromised host' has no formal definition, but embraces a group of overlapping conditions in which the ability to respond normally to an infective challenge is in some way impaired. Nevertheless, it is helpful to think of such patients falling into one of three broad groups (Fig. 1).

Primary immunodeficiency syndromes

These are patients with congenital defects in immunity that render them more susceptible to infection. At the most extreme, children with severe combined immunodeficiency have virtually no functioning cellular or humoral immunity, and if unprotected they will die from infection within a few months of birth. In contrast, some patients with chronic granulomatous disease, an inherited defect in neutrophil function, remain undiagnosed until early adult life. A complete description of the diagnosis and management of this group of disorders is given in Chapter 5.3.

Secondary immunodeficiency syndromes

AIDS

AIDS (acquired immune deficiency syndrome) is a model for an acquired defect of immunity leading to an increased risk of infection.

Fig. 1 A classification of the immunocompromised host.

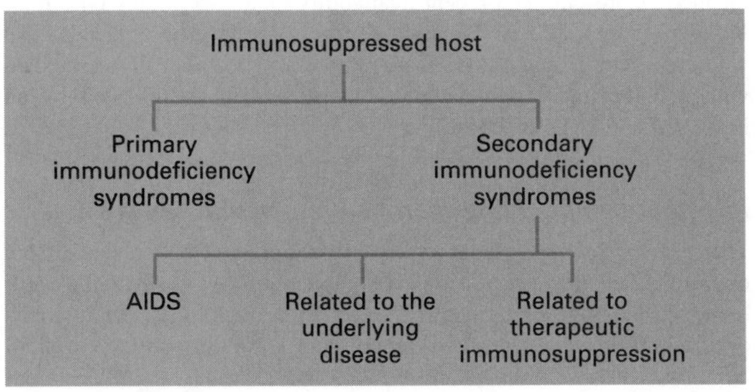

Although there are inevitably parallels with other groups of immunocompromised patients, it has become apparent that there are particular issues both in the diagnosis and management of infection in AIDS that warrant separate discussion (see Section 5).

Infection related to the underlying condition

The notion of opportunistic infection in the immunocompromised host is most familiar in patients with haematological malignancy or organ transplantation, discussed in detail below. Less obvious, but probably more numerous, are the many physiological conditions and other diseases associated with an increased incidence of infection. Neonates for example, whose immune system is still not fully mature, are especially susceptible to strains of *Escherichia coli* bearing the K1 antigen, and to infections caused by group B haemolytic streptococci and *Listeria monocytogenes.* The transient immunosuppression that accompanies pregnancy results in unusually severe infections with poliomyelitis, influenza, tuberculosis, pneumococcal meningitis, and falciparum malaria; herpes zoster, normally limited to a dermatome, may disseminate. In elderly people, many of the 'first line' mucosal defences are diminished and there is a functional decline in cell-mediated immunity, leading to more frequent and more severe infections. Repeated admissions to hospital and the use of indwelling, right-atrial catheters and other devices all contribute to increased exposure to nosocomial pathogens.

Infection is a prominent feature of many diseases in which host defences are impaired, often in a rather complex way (Table 1). These defects are usually mixed, and frequently poorly characterized, but the clinical problem is real. In malnutrition for example, infection due to mycobacteria and salmonellae is more common. *Pneumocystis carinii* pneumonia was first described in children with protein-calorie malnutrition. Patients with severe burns are at risk in different ways; the damage to the skin provides a ready portal of entry for micro-organisms, but in addition there are subtle defects in leucocyte chemotaxis. There is an extensive literature describing the multiple defects of host defence associated with alcohol abuse; clinically, this is reflected in an excess of lower respiratory-tract infections with *Streptococcus pneumoniae*, *Mycobacterium tuberculosis*, and *Klebsiella pneumoniae*.

Further examples are provided by the metabolic disorders such as uraemia or Cushing's disease, in which the excess endogenous steroid production can result in a pattern of opportunistic infections which mirrors that seen in patients receiving steroid therapy (see below). Diabetes mellitus is good example of a disease which is frequently complicated by infection, typically staphylococcal skin abscesses. Many investigations have been done to try and explain this; several groups have demonstrated abnormalities in neutrophil chemotaxis and phagocytosis, although whether these are causally related to the frequent infections is disputed. The association of an unusual fungal infection, invasive mucormycosis, with diabetic ketoacidosis provides a fascinating insight into both the subtleties and the complexities of host defences. Mucor is a mould that causes a destructive infection of the paranasal sinuses and sometimes spreads to the brain (see below and Section 24). Studies in diabetic mice showed that an uncharacterized serum component was present that hindered macrophages' attaching to fungal hyphae and also stimulated fungal sporulation. Similarly, normal human serum is inhibitory for these fungal spores, but serum obtained from patients with diabetic ketoacidosis has lost this property, and may even enhance growth. Curiously mucormycosis has recently been described as a complication in a quite unrelated clinical setting, that of iron overload associated with haemodialysis. Although iron plays an important part in the physiology of many micro-organisms, notably plasmodia, the reason for this particular association is unknown.

Splenectomy

Patients who have had their spleen removed, or who have functional (or more rarely congenital) asplenia, are at increased risk of certain infec-

Table 1 *Examples of conditions associated with impaired immune responses and an increased risk/severity of infection*

Extremes of life
Pregnancy
Malnutrition
Trauma/surgery
Haemodialysis
Cushing's disease
Intravenous drug abuse
Down's syndrome
'Vasculitic' diseases:
(Felty's syndrome, rheumatoid arthritis, etc.)
Splenectomy
Alcohol abuse
Spinal cord injury
Burns
Uraemia
Diabetes mellitus
Haemochromatosis
Severe liver disease

Table 2 *Organisms associated with severe infection as a complication of splenectomy*

Streptococcus pneumoniae
Other haemolytic streptococci
Haemophilus influenzae
Neisseria meningitidis
Capnocytophaga canimorsus
Babesia microti
Salmonella spp.
Plasmodium spp.
Escherichia coli

tions. The degree of risk is related to the underlying cause; overall, 4 to 12 per cent will suffer a serious infection, but this varies from 1.5 per cent following traumatic splenectomy to as high as 25 per cent in patients with thalassaemia. The relative risk of fatal infection is very much higher than in the general population; in the post-traumatic group for instance, the risk is up to 200 times higher. Serious infections are most common during the first 5 years following splenectomy, and particularly during the first year; recurrent infections occur in about 20 per cent of those affected. Approximately 50 per cent of infections are meningitis or bacteraemias, and most of the remainder are pneumonias. The organisms implicated are listed in Table 2. The encapsulated bacteria (*Strep. pneumoniae, Haemophilus influenzae, Neisseria meningitidis*) account for about 75 per cent of all infections. *Capnocytophaga canimorsus* (previously known as the DF2 bacillus, and associated with dog bites), and *Babesia* spp. (protozoal parasites of erythrocytes) are rare but well-described causes of overwhelming sepsis in these patients. (The role of the spleen in malaria is discussed in Chapter 7.13.2.) Infections caused by salmonellae (in particular osteomyelitis) are particularly linked to the functional hyposplenism seen in sickle-cell disease, and do not seem to occur with increased frequency in other groups of splenectomized patients.

The nature of the immunodeficiency that may follow splenectomy provides some explanation for this pattern of infection. Perhaps the two most important factors are the role of the spleen in generating an antibody response to polysaccharide antigens (hence the bacterial infections), and its ability to act as a phagocytic filter, especially for the removal of damaged or senescent erythrocytes (probably explaining the association with babesia and severe malaria). Other factors, too, may play a part; there is evidence of complement dysfunction, and of defective production of tuftsin, a small peptide that has some opsonic properties for bacteria.

Characteristically, these patients suffer a short prodrome followed by a fulminant illness with high fever and few specific clinical signs. Initially, the focus of infection may be obscure. Laboratory findings consistent with disseminated intravascular coagulation are common. Treatment is with high-dose intravenous antimicrobials and supportive care; a reasonable empirical regimen is ampicillin plus gentamicin.

All splenectomized patients and those with a non-functioning spleen should be given pneumococcal vaccine. The 14-valent vaccine, which had been available for some years, was replaced recently by a new 23-valent formulation. Patients who received the older vaccine should be revaccinated with the new. Revaccination should be considered every 6 years. In patients who are to undergo elective splenectomy the vaccine should be given at least 2 weeks preoperatively, but when this is not possible (e.g. following trauma), vaccination is still worthwhile. Vaccination will not remove the risk of infection completely, and for those at particularly high risk (e.g. children with sickle-cell disease) antimicrobial prophylaxis (penicillin or erythromycin) should be given as well. Many recommend lifelong penicillin prophylaxis, but its benefits have not been formally shown. Patient education is also important; they should be advised to wear a warning bracelet, and it may be worthwhile giving them a supply of amoxycillin and advising them to start treatment at the earliest signs of infection. It would be logical to give these patients the new *H. influenzae* b (Hib) vaccine as well, although clinical trials of efficacy in this group have not yet been done.

Other haematological conditions associated with an increased risk of infection, such as sickle-cell disease, spherocytosis, and thalassaemia are discussed in more detail elsewhere (see Section 22.4).

The final group of diseases considered here form a kind of no man's land between those in which infection is due to disordered underlying immunity, and those receiving therapeutic immunosuppression. Patients with conditions such as Hodgkin's disease, multiple myeloma, chronic lymphocytic leukaemia, and the large group of vasculitides (e.g. rheumatoid arthritis, systemic lupus erythematosus, polyarteritis nodosa, and others), all have impaired immunity as a consequence of their underlying disease, but because they also commonly receive treatment with immunosuppressive drugs it can be very difficult to attribute cause and effect.

In myeloma and chronic lymphocytic leukaemia the primary defect is hypogammaglobulinaemia, which is manifested clinically by an excess of bacterial infections, typically those caused by encapsulated organisms such as *Strep. pneumoniae* and *H. influenzae*. Reducing the frequency of these infections by active or passive immunization is one option that has been explored; pneumococcal vaccination is worthwhile but of limited benefit. Patients with myeloma often have only a modest rise in titres, and the increased catabolic rate of immunoglobulins results in a rapid loss of protection. In patients with particularly severe problems in whom antibody titres to pneumococcal capsular antigens have been shown to be low, revaccination should be considered. In one placebo-controlled trial, prophylaxis with intravenous immunoglobulin in chronic lymphocytic leukaemia was shown to confer a modest benefit; it has not been formally evaluated in myeloma and cannot be recommended at present. The recent availability of a vaccine for type b *H. influenzae* might also be beneficial for these patients, but no trials have yet been done. Hodgkin's disease, in contrast, is classically associated with a defect in cell-mediated immunity and is complicated by an increased incidence of infections such as varicella-zoster.

Infection complicating therapeutic immunosuppression

There is a growing number of immunosuppressed patients in whom opportunistic infection is a major complication. As well as the well-recognized risk groups, such as those with haematological malignancy or allograft recipients, immunosuppression is now a common component of the management of conditions as diverse as asthma, inflammatory bowel disease, and rheumatoid arthritis.

It has frequently been taught that the specific defect in host defences caused by the various different types of immunosuppression is mirrored in the types of infection that ensue. This is partly true. Neutropenic patients are likely to have bacterial sepsis, while a patient with sarcoidosis receiving high-dose steroids is more susceptible to cryptococcal meningitis, an infection normally contained by cellular mechanisms. However, many immunosuppressed patients have multiple risk factors; a bone-marrow transplant recipient may have been treated with corticosteroids and cyclosporin A for management of graft-versus-host disease, may be neutropenic, and may have an indwelling right-atrial catheter for feeding purposes. Each of these represents a substantial, and very different type of risk factor for infection, and it is important to remember that, in such patients, multiple pathogens can cause disease simultaneously. The following sections describe the management of some of the common clinical syndromes presenting as infection in immunosuppressed patients.

Common clinical syndromes

A general approach to management

Infections in immunosuppressed patients can progress with frightening rapidity; the early physical signs are often muted and the microbiological findings can be confusing. Patients need to be reviewed frequently and will often need empirical therapy, but this need not be totally 'blind'; a structured and informed assessment will generally allow a logical response to what are the most likely pathogens.

The history

This may reveal exposure to community-acquired infections such as varicella-zoster or tuberculosis, which can be particularly severe in immunocompromised patients. Past infections, should be noted; bronchiectasis, for instance, can be very troublesome in transplant recipients. A detailed travel history is important: patients who have visited certain parts of the United States may have been exposed to systemic mycoses such as histoplasmosis or coccidioidomycosis, which are not endemic here and are unfamiliar to many clinicians. Visitors to Central America or the Far East, even many years ago, may have acquired an asymptomatic infection with the nematode helminth *Strongyloides stercoralis*; immunosuppression can lead to overt disease (the hyperinfection syndrome), with a high mortality (see below).

Physical examination

This may be disappointing; immunosuppressed patients often do not mount a good inflammatory response. Thus there may only be a low-grade fever, a thin serous exudate may suffice for pus, and mild abdominal tenderness may be the only sign of peritonitis. Nevertheless, careful, and if necessary repeated, clinical examination is worthwhile, as signs of inflammation may become apparent only when immune function returns. Particular attention should be paid to the presence of new skin lesions. In neutropenic patients bacteraemias may be accompanied by striking embolic lesions (Fig. 2); Pseudomonas infections (and less commonly Klebsiella and Aeromonas) can cause a focal necrotic cellulitis referred to as ecthyma gangrenosum. Fungal infections present as indolent, locally invasive lesions; Aspergillus infections often have a black eschar (Fig. 3). Dermatophyte infections can become very extensive, but rarely invade systemically. The perianal area and the insertion sites of indwelling right-atrial catheters should be examined carefully. In non-neutropenic patients (typically those on high-dose corticosteroids or renal transplant recipients), *M. chelonei* causes crops of large, palpable nodules but rarely leads to deep-seated infection. Antimicrobial therapy should be guided by *in vitro* sensitivity testing, but despite this the infection may pursue a relapsing and remitting course. Aspiration and/or biopsy of any new skin lesion in immunosuppressed patient is well worthwhile, as it may quickly point to an otherwise unsuspected diagnosis.

Underlying disease

This can provide valuable clues. Neutropenia is a major risk factor for infection, and renders the patient susceptible to bacteraemias, particularly with Gram-negative organisms such as Escherichia and Pseudomonas. A patient with an obstructing bronchial neoplasm may develop a lung abscess due to inadequate drainage. Immunosuppressive drugs have a complex effect on many aspects of immune function, and the pattern of infections is often related to the underlying disease for which they are given. Corticosteroids are used widely; when given in doses exceeding 15 to 20 mg daily for long periods they increase susceptibility to infections with viruses, fungi, parasites, and bacteria such as *M. tuberculosis*, all organisms normally associated with cellular immune defences.

Duration of immunosuppression

This often has a profound effect on the type of infection that occurs, and this effect is well illustrated by comparing the 'timetables' of infections in renal transplant recipients with patients receiving bone marrow transplants (Fig. 4). In renal transplants there are three rather well-

Fig. 2 Embolic skin lesions in a neutropenic patient with *E.coli* septicaemia.

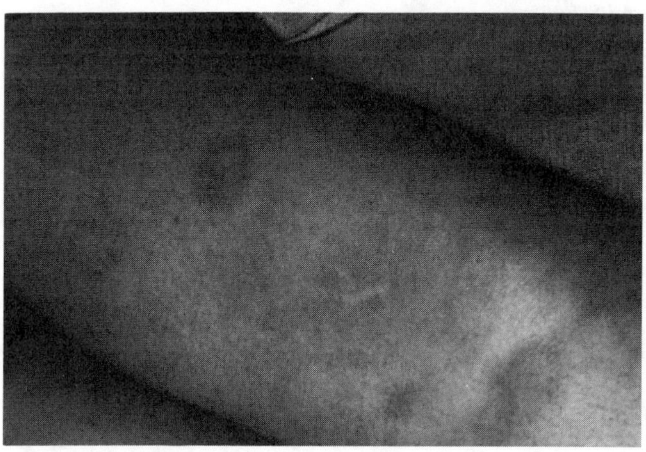

Fig. 3 Cutaneous aspergillosis: (left) scalp lesion in a bone-marrow transplant recipient; (right) palatal lesion in a patient with acute leukaemia.

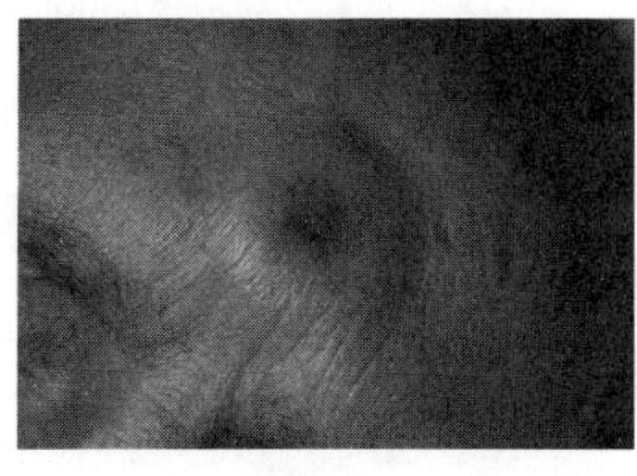

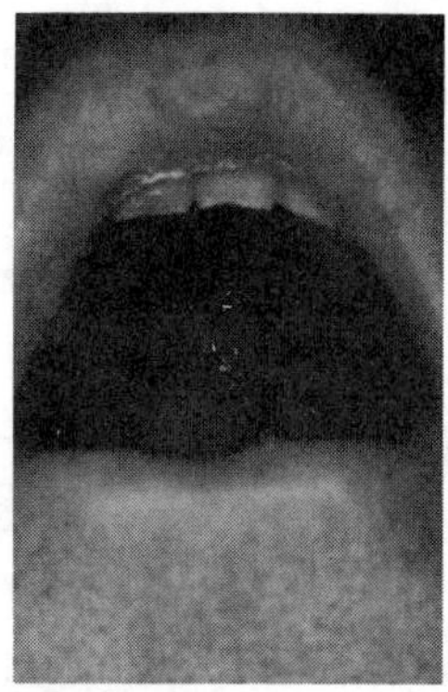

defined periods following the transplant during which the pattern of infection varies. In the first 6 weeks, bacterial infections predominate, typically surgical complications of the procedure or urinary infections. Between 6 weeks and 6 months post-transplant the patient is most at risk from the 'classical' opportunistic infections: Cryptococcus, Listeria, Mycobacteria, or Pneumocystis. As time continues and the intensity of immunosuppression declines, typical community-acquired infections become more common: influenza or respiratory syncytial virus, for instance. In bone marrow transplantation, the initial period of neutropenia is characterized by bacterial infections; later, when many patients receive high-dose corticosteroids for graft-versus-host-disease, cytomegalovirus and fungal infections (Candida and Aspergillus) develop. Varicella-zoster is a well-described late (in excess of 1 year) complication of bone marrow transplantation.

Speed of progression

An assessment of this is helpful in differential diagnosis and in deciding on empirical therapy. In neutropenic patients, the onset of fever is usually an indication for immediate empirical antimicrobial therapy (see below). In contrast, the response to a fever and new pulmonary infiltrates in a patient who is 8 months post-renal transplant will depend on the pace of the illness. Rapid deterioration over the space of a few hours will suggest a bacterial infection or a non-infectious cause, and will need urgent therapy; a more indolent presentation would point to a fungal or mycobacterial aetiology, and treatment can be delayed for a short period to try and establish the diagnosis.

Investigations

Specific investigations will depend on the clinical presentation. These are discussed below. It is important that diagnostic laboratories be made aware of the clinical problem because handling of specimens from immunosuppressed patients—and interpretation of the results—will often differ substantially from routine procedures. In addition, routine screening of transplant recipients and donors should include serological tests for cytomegalovirus, hepatitis B, and human immunodeficiency virus.

Pyrexia of unknown origin (PUO)

In neutropenic patients, fever is often the first and only sign of bacteraemia, and prompt action is necessary. In these cases, a PUO is defined as a fever of over 38°C sustained for 2 h, and not obviously due to an identifiable cause such as concomitant blood transfusion.

The risk of bacteraemia is directly related to the depth of the neutropenia; the incidence is greatest at white counts below 1×10^9/l, and particularly when the count falls to less than 0.1×10^9/l (Fig. 5). Some years ago, the most common isolates were Gram-negative bacteria such as *E. coli* and klebsiellae, generally derived from the patient's gut flora, and *Pseudomonas aeruginosa*, a common environmental pathogen. Gram-negative bacteraemia in neutropenic patients carried a very high mortality, and led to the introduction of a number of preventative strategies such as gut decontamination and the use of prophylactic antimicrobials. Although these approaches have not been entirely successful, the incidence of Gram-negative bacteraemias has declined substantially, and in many units Gram-positive organisms, notably coagulase-negative staphylococci (*Staph. epidermidis*) and viridans streptococci are now the most common isolates. Certain organisms are notable for their absence; *H. influenzae* and anaerobes, for instance, almost never cause bacteraemia in this population, an important consideration when contemplating empirical chemotherapy.

The clinical features are entirely non-specific. Occasionally a focus is suggested by erythema around the point of entry of an indwelling catheter, a finding often associated with staphylococcal infection. Septic shock is infrequent, although it can be associated with viridans streptococci; endocarditis is surprisingly rare.

Blood cultures should be drawn before starting antimicrobial treatment. Ideally two sets should be obtained, at least one of which should be from a peripheral vein (rather than an indwelling catheter), although this is not always possible. Culturing larger volumes of blood (e.g. 30 ml compared to the more conventional 10 ml) will increase the yield, and a policy should be agreed with the microbiology department. Appropriate samples must also be taken from other potential foci of infection. Nevertheless, it has been one of the enduring frustrations of this subject

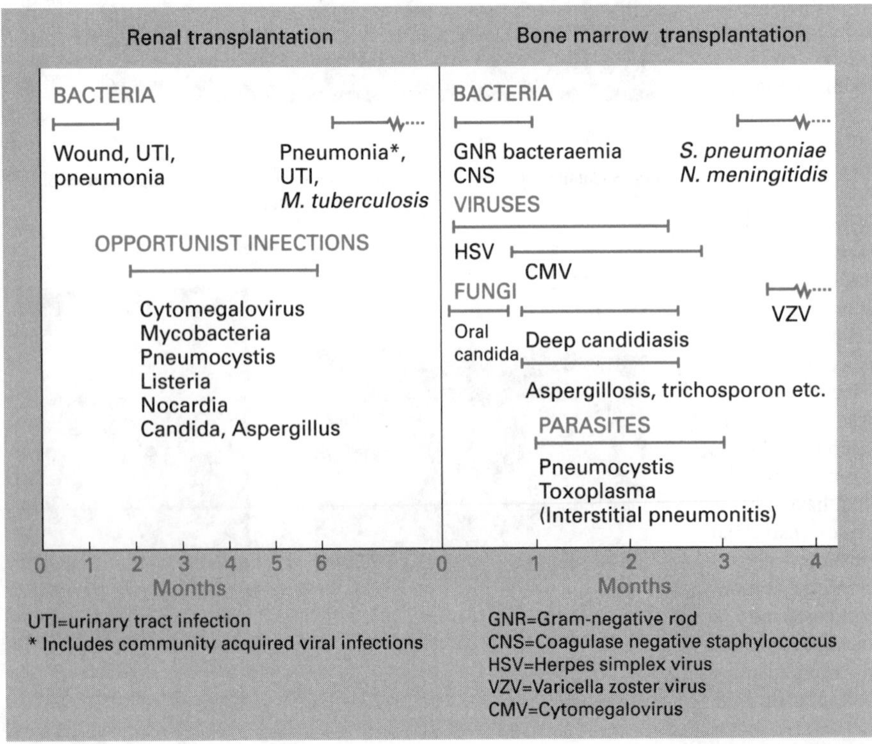

Fig. 4 A scheme representing a timetable for the development of infective complications in renal and bone-marrow transplant recipients.

that even the most rigorous of microbiological investigations in the febrile neutropenic patient will yield only some 40 to 50 per cent of positive cultures. This has not been explained; some studies have suggested that it is due to endotoxaemia in the absence of bacteraemia, but the data are inconclusive. However, it is clear that treatment must begin before the results of the cultures are available; delay will lead to unacceptable fatalities.

The choice of the initial empirical antimicrobial regimen for the febrile neutropenic patient has been the subject of intense investigation. The ideal regimen should be safe and have good bactericidal activity against all the common pathogens. No single regimen is perfect; much will depend on the availability (and cost) of antimicrobials in a given institution, and on local patterns of antimicrobial susceptibility. The two well-validated regimens are, first, the combination of an antipseudomonal penicillin and an aminoglycoside (for example, piperacillin plus gentamicin), or the use of a single, extended-spectrum cephalosporin, such as ceftazidime. Both regimens are very active against all the common Gram-negative organisms, but are relatively ineffective at treating Gram-positive bacteria such as coagulase-negative staphylococci, nowadays a common problem. Unfortunately, the only drugs that are reliably active against these organisms are glycopeptides such as vancomycin. Some clinicians have advocated adding vancomycin to the initial empirical regimen. The disadvantage of this approach is the toxicity (and cost) of vancomycin, which may not be justified because, unlike the Gram-negative infections, coagulase-negative staphylococci rarely cause death. Several prospective clinical trials which have evaluated this strategy have suggested that vancomycin can usually be withheld until the results of blood cultures are known.

In patients who respond to the initial regimen the treatment should be continued for at least 7 days, and ideally until the neutrophil account has returned to above 0.5×10^9/l. Sometimes this is not possible; the patient may have a persistent or unresponsive neutropenia (e.g. aplastic anaemia, or following bone marrow transplantation). In these cases, treatment is usually cautiously stopped after an arbitrary period such as 14 days; rebound bacteraemias can occur and will need further treatment.

A much more difficult problem is the patient who remains febrile.

Fig. 5 The relation between neutrophil count and the risk of invasive, Gram-negative infection. (Reproduced from Bodey *et al.* (1966). *Annals of Internal Medicine*, **64**, 328–40, with permission.)

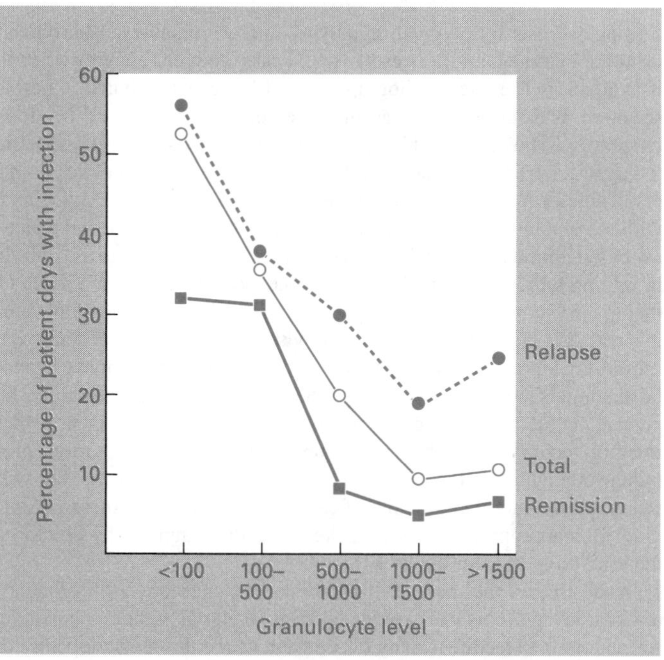

Table 3 *Conditions that commonly present as fever of unknown origin in non-neutropenic, immunosuppressed patients*

Infections
Tuberculosis
Cytomegalovirus
Toxoplasmosis
Non-infective causes
Drug reactions
Malignancy (particularly lymphoma)
Recrudescence of the underlying disease

Where the blood cultures are positive the antimicrobial may be modified as necessary, for example by the addition of vancomycin. If an indwelling right-atrial catheter is incriminated as the possible source (the blood cultures will not necessarily be positive), most clinicians will try to treat the infection without removing the line; however, this is rarely successful in the case of line-associated infections caused by Gram-negative bacteria or yeast. A common problem is the patient who continues to have high, swinging fevers in the absence of any obvious focus or positive microbiological findings. Sometimes repeated clinical examination or investigations will provide a clue: a new infiltrate on chest radiograph, for instance. In this situation, deep fungal infection becomes more likely. The few clinical trials that have addressed this problem conclude that persistent fever for 72 h should be treated by the addition of amphotericin B. At least 0.3 mg/kg should be given in the first 24 h, and this should be increased to 0.5–0.75 mg/kg a day thereafter.

Fever of unknown origin in the non-neutropenic immunosuppressed patient is a completely different problem. It is rarely an immediate threat to life, and the wide differential diagnosis means that it is generally better to pursue the cause rather than embark on empirical therapy. Frequently, clinical examination and simple investigations will point to a likely source, but some conditions may present with fever alone (Table 3), and investigations should be designed with these in mind.

Fever and new pulmonary infiltrates

The development of fever and new pulmonary infiltrates is one of the most challenging clinical problems in this group of patients. Pneumonia is the most common infective cause of death in immunocompromised patients. In the presence of diffuse airspace disease the mortality approaches 50 per cent, irrespective of the underlying defect in host defence, although the epidemiological background varies both between different patient groups and at different times, reflecting the intensity of the immunosuppression (Table 4).

The condition can progress extremely quickly, and conventional diagnostic procedures may be unhelpful. The list of possible causes is so daunting (Table 5) that clinicians might be tempted to use multiple antimicrobial agents empirically, sometimes to the patient's detriment. It is often impossible to 'guess' with any certainty the precise cause of the problem (indeed, it can be dangerous to do so, as it is not uncommon for multiple causes to be present simultaneously), but by considering the available information one can construct a 'short list', which will guide further investigation and treatment.

The initial evaluation should follow the approach outlined above, in particular making an assessment of the intensity of the immunosuppression and the speed of progression of the pulmonary disease. The main purpose is to determine the need for empirical therapy, either because the clinical picture is suggestive of a 'simple' bacterial pneumonia, or because of a potentially more serious, progressive course of uncertain aetiology. Factors that would favour a bacterial cause include the presence of neutropenia, a rapid clinical evolution (e.g. deterioration over a period of 12 h), progressive hypoxia, a sputum Gram stain showing a marked predominance of a single bacterial morphology (even in

Table 4 *The aetiology of the 'febrile pneumonitis' syndrome in different patient groups*

	Renal transplant	Bone marrow transplant
< 1 month	Aspiration Nosocomial LRTI	Aspiration Nosocomial LRTI Aspergillus
1–3 months*	Cytomegalovirus Pneumocystis Aspergillus Nocardia Mycobacteria Mucor	Cytomegalovirus Pneumocystis Aspergillus Respiratory syncytial virus Mycobacteria Mucor Non-infective causes
> 3 months*	Influenza Legionella Common respiratory bacteria	Varicella-zoster GVHD Common respiratory bacteria and viruses

LRTI, lower respiratory-tract infection; GVHD, graft-versus-host disease.

*6 months in renal transplants. Includes idiopathic interstitial pneumonitis in bone-marrow transplant recipients.

Modified from Wilson *et al.* (1985).

Table 5 *Causes of fever and new pulmonary infiltrates in the immunocompromised host*

INFECTIONS

Bacterial

Conventional respiratory pathogens:
  S.pneumoniae; *H.influenzae*; Klebsiella
Nosocomial pathogens:
  E.coli; *Pseudomonas* spp.; *Legionella* spp.
'Atypical' organisms:
  Chlamydia psittaci, C.pneumoniae; mycoplasmas
Mycobacteria and related organisms:
  Mycobacterium tuberculosis; atypical mycobacteria; Nocardia
Other unusual organisms:
  Listeria, Bacillus spp.

Viral

Herpes viruses:
  Cytomegalovirus; herpes simplex; Varicella-zoster
Respiratory viruses:
  Respiratory syncytial virus; (para)influenza; adenovirus; measles

Fungi

Systemic mycoses:
  Blastomycosis; histoplasmosis; coccidioidomycosis
Opportunistic mycoses:
  Candida; Aspergillus; Mucor; Cryptococcus
Other rare fungi:
  Trichosporon; Pseudallescheria

Parasites

  Pneumocystis; Strongyloides; Toxoplasma

NON-INFECTIVE CAUSES

Pulmonary pathology

  Pulmonary oedema; pulmonary infarction/emboli; pulmonary haemorrhage
  Primary or secondary malignancy

Other causes

  Drugs (e.g. busulphan)
  Activity of the underlying disease (e.g. systemic lupus)
  Radiation pneumonitis

the absence of neutrophils), or a chest radiographic appearance that has worsened significantly over a short period. High fever is not necessarily a part of this syndrome; indeed, it is important to emphasize that this rapidly evolving clinical picture is not inevitably due to infection. Non-infective causes such as acute lung haemorrhage or pulmonary oedema can present in an identical fashion, and the most appropriate therapy may be diuretics rather than antimicrobials. However, antimicrobials will often need to be given as well because of what has been termed 'infection-provoked relapse'. In immunologically mediated diseases such as systemic lupus erythematosus or antiglomerular basement-membrane (**GBM**) disease (Goodpasture's syndrome), infection can precipitate a relapse of the underlying disease. Thus the development of fever and new pulmonary shadows in a patient with anti-GBM disease may be primarily due to lung haemorrhage associated with a rise in anti-GBM antibodies, but this can be precipitated in turn by an infection that need not necessarily be in the lung. Treatment must be directed both towards improving oxygenation and the underlying infection.

Certain baseline investigations should be done even if urgent treatment is needed. Blood cultures should always be obtained, and sputum if it is available. A chest radiograph and arterial blood-gas analysis are essential. The initial treatment will be dictated by the clinical circumstances, but the temptation to use a complex regimen to provide very broad-spectrum cover is best avoided. Rapid clinical deterioration is most often caused by bacterial infections; if community acquired, a combination of an extended-spectrum cephalosporin plus erythromycin will be appropriate. For hospital-acquired infections, a cephalosporin (combined with an aminoglycoside if there is strong evidence of Pseudomonas infection) is reasonable. Where staphylococcal infection is suspected, flucloxacillin plus an aminoglycoside should be used. Unusual ('opportunistic') organisms such as mycobacteria, nocardiae, or cytomegalovirus rarely cause such a rapid clinical deterioration and it is extremely difficult to distinguish them on clinical grounds alone. For these reasons, the addition of further empirical agents is usually not warranted. A possible exception is Pneumocystis pneumonia (see below).

In patients in whom immediate empirical therapy is not necessary, additional diagnostic procedures can be done. These should include serological tests for atypical organisms, and examination of blood and urine for cytomegalovirus (tests for viral early antigens are very helpful, if available). The chest radiograph should be repeated, but it is not as sensitive as arterial blood-gas measurements, which should be done twice daily. The radiographic appearances are rarely sufficiently specific to suggest a precise diagnosis, although they can provide helpful pointers (Table 6). Thus a bilateral, interstitial, midzone infiltrate associated with marked hypoxia is typical of Pneumocystis pneumonia, and a pleural-based infarct is suggestive of Aspergillus. However, there are pitfalls in relying on the radiographic appearance alone to guide the choice of therapy. First, no radiographic appearance is pathognomonic of any single pathological process; cytomegalovirus or pulmonary oedema can mimic Pneumocystis, for example, and Legionella pneumonia cannot be distinguished from Aspergillus. Secondly, multiple agents can be present simultaneously, and each may require separate treatment. Other imaging techniques, such as computerized tomography, can often provide useful additional information on the extent of the process, but will rarely allow a more precise identification of the cause. For these reasons it is often appropriate to try to make a specific diagnosis by obtaining material directly from the bronchial tree.

In most cases the method of choice is bronchoscopy with bronchoalveolar lavage. This can provide adequate material without incurring a serious risk of bleeding (many of the patients are thrombocytopenic) or

Table 6 *Clinical and radiological syndromes associated with pneumonia in the compromised host*

	Acute	Subacute
Consolidation	Common LRTI bacteria Legionella Pulmonary embolism	Nocardia Fungi (Aspergillus and Mucor) Mycobacteria Tumour
Nodular infiltrate:		
Single		Tumour Mycobacteria
Multifocal		Nocardia *Staph.aureus*
Diffuse interstitial infiltrates	Pulmonary oedema Pulmonary haemorrhage Acute RSV infection	PCP Cytomegalovirus Radiation Drugs

'Acute' refers to changes developing over approx. 24 h.

LRTI, lower respiratory-tract infection (i.e. *Strep.pneumoniae, H. influenzae*); RSV, respiratory syncytial virus; PCP, *Pneumocystis carinii* pneumonia.

Modified from Rubin and Young (1988).

pneumothorax. In most series, bronchial brush or transbronchial biopsy specimens produce only a marginal increase in the diagnostic yield, and are usually not done unless the clinical picture is suggestive of a non-infective process such as an infiltrating tumour. Percutaneous needle biopsies or drill biopsies offer no significant advantage. The highest yield is from an open lung biopsy, but this should not usually be done as a first-line procedure.

Whichever method is used, it is essential that the diagnostic laboratories are informed to ensure that the specimen is handled appropriately. Even under optimum conditions, however, the diagnostic rate rarely exceeds 70 per cent, although the reasons for this are not clear. Newer procedures such as the use of immunofluorescence microscopy for Pneumocystis may help to improve this. In bone-marrow transplant recipients the syndrome of idiopathic interstitial pneumonitis is well recognized. It develops during the first 3 months after the transplant and presents as diffuse interstitial alveolitis associated with fever, cough, and progressive hypoxia. It is clinically indistinguishable from pneumonitis due to Pneumocystis or cytomegalovirus, yet extensive investigations have failed to reveal a microbial cause; it is most likely a combined effect of the conditioning regimen and pulmonary graft-versus-host disease. There is no specific treatment and the mortality is 70 per cent or more.

A difficult problem is the management of a patient with a non-diagnostic bronchoscopy who continues to deteriorate and in whom the suspicion of occult infection remains. Empirical therapy can never be totally comprehensive, and a judgement must be made of the most probable causes. An extended-spectrum cephalosporin plus erythromycin will provide cover against likely bacterial pathogens, and flucloxacillin should be added if *Staph.aureus* is suspected. If tuberculosis is likely, three agents should be used (such as rifampicin, isoniazid, and pyrazinamide). Pneumocystis and cytomegalovirus are difficult to tell apart on clinical grounds alone and often occur together; high-dose co-trimoxazole and ganciclovir are the drugs of first choice.

Acute neurological syndromes

A large number of conventional and opportunistic pathogens can lead to neurological infection in immunocompromised patients. Although there is some degree of overlap, the underlying defect in host defence is a often a good indicator of the likely cause (Table 7).

The clinical features may help suggest the diagnosis. Meningitic syndromes are more likely to be associated with conventional bacterial infections, listeriosis and tuberculosis, as well as fungi such as Cryptococcus and Candida. In contrast, infections with Toxoplasma, Aspergillus or Nocardia more commonly present as space-occupying lesions. Pure encephalitic syndromes are less common, but can occur with herpes simplex virus (although curiously, herpes simplex encephalitis is remarkably uncommon in immunocompromised patients, despite the frequency of reactivation of cutaneous infection). One characteristic presentation that occurs in immunocompromised patients is rhinocerebral mucormycosis. It is a progressive, destructive infection caused by Mucor and related moulds, which usually begins in the paranasal sinuses and spreads caudally to involve the orbits or the frontal lobes of the brain. It is seen particularly in patients with uncontrolled diabetes mellitus or as a complication of neutropenia.

The speed of progression can also be helpful: bacterial infections generally proceed rapidly, while fungi and parasites pursue a more indolent course. While these generalizations are often helpful, it must be emphasized that they are not absolute; exceptions are common, and there is no substitute for obtaining a precise diagnosis. Examination of the skin (see below) and fundoscopy may be valuable. Retinitis is not usually a feature of systemic infection with toxoplasma or cytomegalovirus in immunocompromised patients but in contrast, candidal endophthalmitis may be the only manifestation of deep-seated infection.

Examination of the cerebrospinal fluid is mandatory. A high index of suspicion is necessary, as the clinical features of meningitis are often muted in these patients. An unexplained low-grade fever and mild headache may be the only clues; frank meningism, photophobia or focal neurological signs are late and often ominous developments. It is preferable to obtain a CT scan before proceeding, but if this is not possible lumbar puncture should not be delayed, unless there are clear signs of raised intracerebral pressure or lateralizing neurological signs. Examination of the cerebrospinal fluid should include direct microscopy for (myco)bacteria and fungi, and culture. The cryptococcal latex agglutination test is sensitive and specific; it is better than the India ink test, and should be done on all samples of cerebrospinal fluid from immunosuppressed patients. Other procedures that can be done (in consultation with the laboratory) include antigen tests for the pneumococcus, serological tests for fungi using cerebrospinal fluid and serum, and the demonstration of specific antibody production or DNA sequences by the polymerase chain reaction (e.g. for herpes simplex and papovaviruses).

The cerebrospinal fluid may reveal only non-specific abnormalities. Certain organisms are notable for their absence on direct microscopy: mycobacteria are seen in less than 10 per cent of cases, Nocardia and Aspergillus only very rarely. A predominance of lymphocytes suggests partially treated bacterial infection, tuberculosis or a viral aetiology but not infection with Listeria, despite its specific name. A low concentration of glucose in cerebrospinal fluid points to tuberculosis but is not specific. Sometimes the only abnormality is a modest elevation of the cerebrospinal fluid protein; this should never be ignored, even in the apparent absence of other features of neurological infection. Where appropriate, cytological examination of the cerebrospinal fluid should be done to exclude carcinomatous, lymphomatous, or leukaemic meningitis, which can mimic an acute infective presentation.

A chest radiograph can be surprisingly helpful. Certain neurological infections are often associated with pulmonary disease; these include Legionella, tuberculosis, Aspergillus, Mucor, and Nocardia. A CT brain scan, which should be contrast enhanced, is valuable. Focal, usually enhancing lesions are particularly associated with pyogenic abscesses and toxoplasmosis. Tuberculomas (and even less often, cryptococcomas) can appear as single lesions. The appearances may suggest herpes simplex encephalitis or progressive multifocal leucoencephalitis (see Section 24). The place of magnetic resonance imaging has not yet been defined. It appears to be better than CT scanning for abnormalities of

Table 7 *Organisms causing neurological infections in different patient groups*

	Bacteria	Fungi	Parasites	Virus
Neutropenia	Enterics	Candida Aspergillus Mucor		
T-cell/monocyte defect	Listeria Legionella Nocardia Mycobacteria	Cryptococcus Aspergillus Mucor Coccidioides	Toxoplasma Strongyloides	Varicella-zoster Herpes simplex Papovavirus
Splenectomy	*Strep. pneumoniae* *Haemophilus influenzae* Neisseria			

the brain-stem (e.g. the basal meningitis associated with cryptococcal infection), and occasionally reveals lesions in toxoplasmosis that are not seen on CT scans. It may be particularly helpful in avoiding a brain biopsy when a diagnosis of progressive multifocal leucoencephalitis is considered.

Other investigations are sometimes helpful. Any new skin lesions should be biopsied; a nasal biopsy may reveal Mucor. An electroencephalogram is not helpful, unless herpes encephalitis is suspected. Brain biopsy is done rarely; it was sometimes indicated to make a specific diagnosis of toxoplasmosis or progressive multifocal leucoencephalitis but it is rapidly being superseded by newer techniques such as the use of the polymerase chain reaction with cerebrospinal fluid, and it should not be considered unless empirical therapy has failed and there is a real prospect of therapeutic benefit to the patient.

When the initial examination and investigations reveal the probable diagnosis, treatment is straightforward. If the cerebrospinal fluid is not diagnostic but bacterial infection cannot be excluded, empirical antimicrobials should be given immediately. An extended-spectrum cephalosporin such as cefotaxime is suitable. Empirical antituberculosis therapy should be with three drugs (see above). A common dilemma is the patient with clinical and radiological features of toxoplasmosis; serological tests for toxoplasmosis are not specific in this setting, and although other infections cannot be excluded with certainty it is better to start empirical therapy with pyrimethamine and sulphadimidine. Cerebral aspergillosis and mucormycosis have a very poor prognosis; treatment should be begun with high-dose amphotericin B, and surgical debridement considered if possible. There is no effective treatment for progressive multifocal leucoencephalitis.

Acute gastrointestinal syndromes

The organisms associated with specific gastrointestinal syndromes in these patients are shown in Table 8.

Severe stomatitis is a common complaint in immunosuppressed patients. Its assessment is hampered by the fact that the three most common causes, Candida, Herpes simplex, and chemotherapy-induced mucositis, are clinically indistinguishable and can coexist and cause disease together. For these reasons, the diagnosis should always be confirmed by microscopy and culture. Herpetic stomatitis in particular can be atypical in these patients; the classical appearance of groups of small vesicles is unusual, and a more common presentation is ulceration, which can be extensive (Fig. 6). In profoundly immunosuppressed patients, such as bone-marrow transplant recipients, oral candidiasis is very common, and in patients who are seropositive before transplant, reactivation of herpes simplex almost universal. For these reasons, prophylaxis is usually given. Acyclovir is extremely effective for herpes simplex virus; prevention of mucosal candidiasis is less successful, although the new triazole agents, such as fluconazole, seem promising.

Both herpes simplex virus and Candida can cause oesophagitis, generally (but not exclusively) as an extension of oral disease. Oesophagoscopy with brush cytology and/or biopsy is the investigation of choice. Proven oesophageal candidiasis should be regarded as 'invasive' disease and treated with systemic antifungals (amphotericin B or fluconazole).

A large number of organisms can cause acute diarrhoea. Non-infective conditions such as radiation enteritis, drugs, and graft-versus-host disease must be included in the differential diagnosis. There are no distinguishing clinical features, and diagnosis depends on microbiological examination of the faeces. The request should be discussed with the laboratory to ensure that the specimen is processed appropriately.

The diarrhoea caused by *Clostridium difficile* is usually due to a pseudomembranous colitis, but neutropenic patients may develop a fulminating, invasive colitis associated with clostridial bacteraemia and a high mortality. The nematode *Strongyloides stercoralis* can be carried asymptomatically for many years after exposure. Strongyloidiasis has recently been recognized as a complication of infection with human T-cell leukaemia virus type 1, and also occurs secondarily to immunosuppression (typically with high dose corticosteroids and in solid-organ transplant recipients). A rise in the worm burden results in the hyperinfection syndrome, which may present as pneumonitis or intermittent intestinal obstruction. The worms can carry enteric bacteria through the gut wall, resulting in polymicrobial bacteraemias, and in the same way, Gram-negative meningitis when the worms penetrate the cerebrospinal fluid. Treatment is with extended courses of thiabendazole or mebendazole.

Giardiasis is particularly associated with hypogammaglobulinaemia, and, curiously, is rarely seen in other groups. Cryptosporidium, Microsporidia, and Isospora are now well-recognized causes of severe and sometimes chronic diarrhoea in AIDS patients, but may also occur in other, less severely immunocompromised patients. Among the viruses, the most difficult problem is cytomegalovirus. There is no doubt that it can cause a severe colitis, and in these cases ganciclovir is beneficial. The diagnosis should be confirmed by biopsy, but ultimately may depend on the result of a therapeutic trial because demonstration of the organism does not necessarily indicate that it is causing disease.

Mild abnormalities of 'liver function tests' are a common accompaniment of many systemic infections, but hepatitis is a particular feature of both toxoplasmosis and cytomegalovirus infection. Immunosuppressed patients frequently need blood transfusions, and for this reason blood-borne hepatitis viruses have been a particular problem. Historically, interest has been focused on hepatitis B, but, since the advent of effective screening, hepatitis C (and latterly, hepatitis D and E) have assumed greater importance. Immunosuppressed patients are more often exposed to these infections, and the severity of the acute illness and the long-term consequences can differ markedly from the course in the non-compromised host.

An increased prevalence of hepatitis B has been found in patients on chronic haemodialysis (10 per cent), and those with Hodgkin's disease

Table 8 *Gastrointestinal syndromes in the immunocompromised host*

	Bacteria	Fungi	Parasites	Virus
Oral infection		Candida		Herpes simplex
Diarrhoeal syndromes	*C. difficile*	Candida	Giardia	Enterovirus
	Mycobacteria		Isospora	Adenovirus
	Salmonellae		Cryptosporidia	Cytomegalovirus
	Shigellae		Microsporidia	Rotavirus
			Strongyloides	
Hepatic syndromes		Candida	Toxoplasma	Cytomegalovirus
				Hepatitis B
				Hepatitis C, D, E
				Herpes simplex
				Varicella-zoster

(8 per cent) and lepromatous leprosy (20 per cent). The acute hepatitic episode is generally mild, often anicteric, and may pass unnoticed. However, persistent viral replication (hepatitis e antigenaemia) and the development of complications associated with chronic infection are more likely. In countries where transfusion-associated hepatitis B is now rare, this problem has largely disappeared. Nevertheless, the possibility of acquiring infection from a clinically inapparent source is real, and emphasizes the need to immunize staff. Hepatitis B vaccine is safe to give to immunosuppressed patients, although they should receive a double-dose regimen as the seroconversion rate is not as high as in healthy individuals.

Although it is likely that infection with the other hepatitis viruses occurs in immunosuppressed patients, the problem has not yet been defined clinically or epidemiologically.

A particular form of systemic candidiasis has been called chronic hepatosplenic candidiasis (although other organs can be involved, and the syndrome is better referred to as chronic systemic candidiasis). The patient presents with unremitting fever and occasionally abdominal pain; palpable hepatomegaly is unusual. Typically the neutrophil count has returned to normal after a recent course of chemotherapy for acute leukaemia; alkaline phosphatase is markedly raised and there may be hyperbilirubinaemia, but microbiological investigations (including blood cultures) are negative. The diagnosis is made by ultrasonography or CT scan of the abdomen, which reveals multiple intrahepatic (or less commonly, splenic) abscesses. Unfortunately, culture or histological evidence of this organism can be found in only about a third of cases. Treatment has been difficult; conventional therapy with amphotericin B (even with the addition of flucytosine) has often failed, but the use of a liposomal formulation of amphotericin B and fluconazole has produced encouraging results.

Fig. 6 An extensive herpetic lesion in a patient with lymphoma.

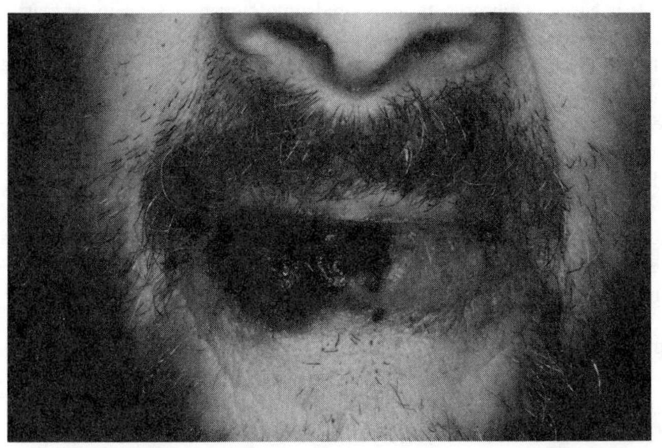

REFERENCES

EORTC International Antimicrobial Therapy Cooperative Group. (1990). Gram-positive bacteraemia in granulocytopenic cancer patients. *European Journal of Cancer*, **26**, 569–74.

Hooper, D.C., Pruitt, A.A., and Rubin, R.H. (1982). Central nervous system infection in the chronically immunosuppressed. *Medicine (Baltimore)*, **61**, 166–88.

Orr, K.E. and Gould, F.K. (1992). Infection problems in patients receiving solid organ transplants. *Reviews in Medical Microbiology*, **3**, 96–103.

Pizzo, P.A. (ed). (1993). Infectious complications in the immunocompromised host II. *Hematology/Oncology Clinics of North America*, **7**, 919–1099.

Rubin, R.H. and Johnson, P.L. (eds). (1990) Pulmonary infection in solid organ transplant recipients. *Seminars in Respiratory Infections*, **5**, 1–89.

Rubin, R.H. and Young, L.S. (1994). *Clinical approach to infection in the compromised host*, (3rd edn). Plenum, New York.

Sable, C.A., and Donowitz, G.R. (1994). Infections in bone marrow transplant recipients. *Clinical Infectious Diseases*, **18**, 273–84.

Warnock, D.W. and Richardson, M.D. (1991). *Fungal infection in the compromised patient*, (2nd edn). Wiley, Chichester.

7.19.4 Chronic fatigue syndrome (postviral fatigue syndrome and myalgic encephalomyelitis)

M. Sharpe

DEFINITION

The terms chronic fatigue syndrome, postviral fatigue syndrome, neurasthenia, and myalgic encephalomyelitis have been used to describe an idiopathic syndrome of chronic fatigue and disability, often associated with a history of preceding infection. The nature, pathology, and aetiology of this syndrome remain controversial and the purely descriptive term chronic fatigue syndrome is generally preferred. Working definitions of the syndrome for the purpose of research have been published in the United States, the United Kingdom, and in Australia. All these definitions require that the patient's main complaint is of excessive and disabling fatigue, although other symptoms such as muscle pain and poor concentration are typically present. The illness must be of at least 6 months' duration, and other causes of fatigue excluded (Table 1). The component parts of this definition merit further examination.

What is fatigue?

The word fatigue can have many meanings. An objective definition is provided by physiology as failure to sustain force or power output. The subjective experience of fatigue is much less precisely defined, however,

Table 1 *Definition of chronic fatigue syndrome*

1. Principal complaint of fatigue
2. Other symptoms commonly present
3. Impairment of functioning
4. Duration at least 6 months
5. Other conditions excluded

and does not bear any close relation to objective fatigue. Furthermore, patients use words like tiredness and fatigue to describe a variety of subjective experiences. These can be divided broadly into physical fatigue and mental fatigue. Physical fatigue may refer to the experience of lack of energy, lack of endurance, and muscular weakness. Mental fatigue can be subdivided into poor concentration and memory, lack of interest in activities, and daytime sleepiness. Time spent elucidating the precise nature of the patient's complaint will help in the differential diagnosis (see below).

When is fatigue abnormal?

Fatigue occurring after physical or mental exertion, which resolves with rest, is a normal phenomenon. It is necessary, therefore, to set a threshold beyond which fatigue is judged abnormal. When making this judgement the physician should consider whether the fatigue is disproportionate to the level of exertion and whether it is relieved by a reasonable period of rest. There is no objective measure of the feeling of fatigue and the clinician must rely on the patient's report. Definitions of chronic fatigue syndrome do not specify the severity of fatigue that is to be considered abnormal, but rather require that the there is an associated and significant impairment of functioning.

Which other symptoms?

Patients with chronic fatigue syndrome commonly complain of symptoms other than fatigue and these are described under clinical features below. Some definitions of chronic fatigue syndrome require that the patient has a specified number of such associated symptoms, others do not. The precise number of symptoms is probably of little importance.

Why 6 months?

An illness duration of 6 months is used to define chronicity for purposes of research. It has the benefit of excluding short-lived states of fatigue that can follow any illness.

What conditions must be excluded?

Fatigue is a symptom of many, if not most, medical and psychiatric conditions. The term chronic fatigue syndrome is, however, usually reserved for patients in whom the fatigue remains medically unexplained or 'idiopathic', even after careful clinical assessment. It is generally agreed that patients with definite organic disease should be excluded. There is, however, less agreement about patients who meet criteria for psychiatric diagnoses. Some investigators consider that patients with anxiety and depression have an adequate explanation for the fatigue and should be excluded but others do not. Although an important issue for researchers, the clinician should be pragmatic.

Speculative diagnoses and chronic fatigue syndrome

For cases where the fatigue remains unexplained by identifiable pathological processes, a number of hypothetical disease entities have been proposed. These include, among others, myalgic encephalomyelitis, postviral fatigue syndrome, chronic active Epstein–Barr virus infection, hypoglycaemia, and candidiasis. All these conditions purport to identify a pathological basis for the patient's symptoms.

Myalgic encephalomyelitis (ME) was a term coined after an epidemic of unexplained symptoms and signs in the medical and nursing staff of the Royal Free hospital in 1955. This term continues to be used by patients, and by some doctors. So far there is no convincing evidence that it is a specific condition, however, and no support for the presence of the inflammation of the central nervous system it implies. Postviral fatigue syndrome refers to a chronic fatigue syndrome in which a viral infection is presumed to have been a causal factor. A fatigue state does undoubtedly occur following many illnesses, and may be particularly prolonged after acute infection with Epstein–Barr virus. The role of infection in chronic fatigue states is less clear. Hypoglycaemia can undoubtedly cause fatigue and other symptoms, but it is rarely, if ever, demonstrated in non-diabetic patients with chronic fatigue syndrome. Candidiasis, a condition due to an alleged overgrowth of *Candida albicans* in the gut, is also supposed to occur in patients with chronic fatigue syndrome, but there is no scientific evidence to support this claim.

The use of these unvalidated diagnoses is generally unhelpful. On the one hand they may prevent the doctor from making an adequate search for treatable illness, and on the other serve to reinforce the patient's belief in illness and fear of a non-existent sinister pathology. It is therefore preferable to avoid their use and to consider chronic fatigue syndrome as a syndrome rather than as a specific disease.

EPIDEMIOLOGY

Fatigue

Surveys in the United Kingdom and United States indicate that the symptom of persistent fatigue is experienced by as many as one-quarter of the general population at any one time. Fatigue is associated with anxiety, depression, and inactivity, is more common in females, and may also be associated with low blood pressure. Fatigue appears to be a common symptom in all parts of the world, although there are few systematic epidemiological data.

Fatigue is also a common complaint among patients attending primary-care and hospital outpatient clinics. In primary care the condition has been referred to as 'tired all the time' (TAT). In the majority of such cases the symptom is transient and not associated with functional impairment. Consequently, the prevalence of chronic fatigue syndrome as defined above is much lower than that of the symptom of fatigue. A recent population study in the United Kingdom found that 20 per cent of the sample complained of excessive fatigue, but less than 1 per cent could be regarded as having chronic fatigue syndrome.

Chronic fatigue syndrome

Chronic, medically unexplained fatigue is not a new phenomenon. Patients with similar symptoms presenting at the turn of the century were given a diagnosis of neurasthenia, a category recently reintroduced into the *International Classification of Diseases* (10th edn). Diagnostic fashion has varied over the ensuing decades and patients with similar symptoms have been given a variety of tentative diagnoses including chronic brucellosis, chronic active Epstein–Barr virus infection, and chronic nervous exhaustion. It is unclear whether renewed interest in the condition reflects a real change in prevalence, or merely increased medical recognition.

Most cases of chronic fatigue syndrome currently seen in primary-care and hospital practice have arisen sporadically and present individually, although apparent epidemics have also been described. Patients may be referred to any of a variety of medical specialities depending on the interest of local consultants. Because there is often a history of infection at onset, referrals are commonly made to infectious disease clinics. Others specialities receiving referrals include general medicine, neurology, and occasionally psychiatry. Case series from both primary-care and hospital outpatient clinics indicate that patients are most commonly aged between 20 and 40 years, with a predominance of females. The syndrome is also seen in children and adolescents.

Epidemics

Epidemics of a similar syndrome have been described from various parts of the globe. The occurrence of epidemics would appear to favour an infective causation, and a variety of agents has been considered responsible. The nature of these epidemics remains controversial, however. Questions have been raised about whether these were true epidemics or the consequence of an artificial linking of cases by doctors, and also whether the clinical picture reported in such apparent epidemics is really similar to that of patients presenting sporadically. Where large clusters of cases have occurred, alternative explanations have been put forward, including that of 'mass hysteria'. A lack of comprehensive data about such possible epidemics means that these questions remain unanswered.

AETIOLOGY

The cause of chronic fatigue syndrome remains controversial and indeed it is most unlikely that a single cause for the syndrome will be identified. Possible causes may be divided into three main categories:

(1) unidentified organic disease;
(2) depressive and anxiety disorders;
(3) poorly understood or hypothetical causes.

Unidentified organic disease

A variety of organic diseases may present with the symptom of fatigue (see Management below). If the disease is easily diagnosed, little is added by giving the patient an additional diagnosis of chronic fatigue syndrome. In a minority of cases an organic disease will be the cause of the fatigue but is not apparent on initial assessment.

Depressive and anxiety disorders

The presence of depression and anxiety may not be obvious in patients presenting with chronic fatigue syndrome, especially if they minimize expressions of emotional distress and emphasize the associated somatic symptoms. This type of presentation of emotional disorders has been referred to as somatization. When patients with chronic fatigue are systematically assessed, it is found that many can be given diagnoses of depressive and anxiety disorders. As many as half of the patients seen in hospital clinics may be significantly depressed and a further quarter suffering from severe anxiety. It has consequently been suggested that these patients might be better regarded as suffering from depression or anxiety than from chronic fatigue syndrome. However, the diagnosis of depression is also based solely on symptoms, and does not itself identify a specific disease process. There are therefore several possible ways in which depression and chronic fatigue syndrome could be associated:

(1) depression could occur as a consequence of having an unpleasant and disabling condition such as chronic fatigue syndrome;
(2) depressive disorder could explain the symptoms of chronic fatigue syndrome;
(3) depression could co-occur with chronic fatigue syndrome as a result of a common cause (such as infection, or personality).

On balance the evidence suggests that depression and anxiety, in conjunction with the psychological, social, and behavioural factors described below, are sufficient to explain the symptoms in a significant proportion of patients. The evidence supporting this conclusion is that first, the somatic symptoms of depression and anxiety are remarkably similar to those of chronic fatigue syndrome; second, the prevalence of depressive disorder in patients with chronic fatigue syndrome has been found to be much higher than in patients with disabling organic diseases; third, patients with chronic fatigue syndrome have commonly suffered previous episodes of severe depression. Furthermore, careful enquiry frequently reveals a history of severe losses and other stresses preceding the onset of chronic fatigue syndrome. Why then do such patients present to physicians with fatigue, and not to psychiatrists with depression? The answer to this question is likely to be found in a mixture of ignorance amongst both patients and doctors about the somatic manifestations of emotional disorders, and in the stigma associated with a psychiatric diagnosis.

Other aetiological factors

Not all cases are adequately explained by either occult organic disease or by emotional disorder. The cause of fatigue in such cases is the subject of considerable controversy. A number of explanations have been proposed. It is helpful when considering such causes to distinguish between predisposing, precipitating, and perpetuating causes. The factors that perpetuate symptoms and disability may differ from those that precipitate it, and from those that predisposed the individual in the first place. Hence, certain individuals may be predisposed to develop chronic fatigue syndrome by virtue of personality or other vulnerability. The condition may be precipitated in those individuals by infection or by psychological stress. However, in established cases the most important factors to consider are those that act to perpetuate the condition and thereby to prevent recovery. These perpetuating factors may be multiple, and may differ between patients. It is necessary to assess each patient individually in order to determine the relative contribution of the possible perpetuating factors in that person's illness. The causes to be considered are listed below.

Chronic infection

Although patients frequently give a history of acute infection at onset, the role of chronic infection in perpetuating the condition is doubtful. Virus particles and antibodies to various micro-organisms can be detected in a proportion of patients, but both their specificity to chronic fatigue syndrome, and their role in causing symptoms is uncertain.

Immune dysfunction

Dysfunction of the immune system has been suggested as a cause of chronic fatigue syndrome because it may predispose to persistent or recurrent infection, or may itself cause symptoms as a result of abnormal levels of interferon or interleukins. There is evidence of relatively minor immune abnormalities in a proportion of patients, but no consistent abnormality has been established. The possibility that the abnormalities observed are the consequence of other processes such as depressive disorder, distress, or inactivity has not been effectively excluded.

Muscle dysfunction

The symptoms of weakness and muscular pain have led investigators to examine muscle tissue and to test muscular function. Examination of muscle tissue has yielded evidence suggestive of persistent virus in a minority of cases but muscle function has been found to be normal. Exercise capacity is reduced and subjective effort is greatly increased, however.

Inactivity

Clinical experience indicates that many (but not all) patients with chronic fatigue syndrome are profoundly inactive, some resorting to prolonged periods of complete bedrest. The effects of inactivity have been well researched. Even brief periods of inactivity in healthy young males result in muscle wasting, changes in the cardiovascular response to exertion, and consequent intolerance of activity.

Dysfunction of the central nervous system

Much recent investigation has focused on possible abnormalities in central nervous function. Abnormalities have been found in cognitive function, neuroendocrine function, and neuroimaging. Such abnormalities also occur in depression and anxiety and their specificity to chronic fatigue syndrome remains to be established.

Sleep disorder

Most patients with chronic fatigue syndrome complain of abnormal sleep, and particularly of feeling unrefreshed on waking. Many have developed a pattern of sleeping during the day. Chaotic patterns of sleeping, sleep deprivation, and excess sleep may all contribute to daytime fatigue.

Psychological factors

Patients' responses to illness are varied, and premorbid personality factors may influence their rate of recovery. Furthermore, certain specific ways of coping with chronic fatigue may tend to perpetuate it. These include prolonged bedrest, excessive avoidance of activities, repeated seeking of ineffective medical care, and avoidance of ongoing psychological and social problems. In some cases being ill may appear to have resolved major conflicts in the patient's personal life.

Social factors

Illnesses occurring in the absence of demonstrated physical disease are frequently regarded as 'not real', 'all in the mind', as revealing personal weakness, and as not being reason for exemption from daily demands. Proven organic disease on the other hand, particularly if validated by a doctor, is rarely considered to be the responsibility of the afflicted, merits sympathy, and excuses the sufferer from the demands of others. Patients without a 'physical' label for their illness may therefore experience difficulty in explaining their disability to friends, family, and employers and request a 'physical' disease label from their doctor. It is important that the doctor is aware of the strength of feeling that may be associated with this issue; if it is mishandled a breakdown in the doctor–patient relationship may result.

Information about chronic fatigue syndrome or myalgic encephalomyelitis, whether from doctors, patient groups, or the media, which leads patients to see their illness as mysterious, with a poor prognosis, and untreatable other than by rest is unhelpful and may even tend to perpetuate illness in some individuals.

CLINICAL FEATURES

The common symptoms of chronic fatigue syndrome are chronic mental and physical fatigue, exacerbated by activity and often associated with muscular pain. Patients often report being able to perform for brief periods, but subsequently experiencing severe fatigue for hours or days thereafter. Other symptoms commonly reported include unrefreshing sleep, dizziness and breathlessness, headache, tender lymph glands, and symptoms of irritable bowel syndrome. The patient often describes day-to-day fluctuations in their symptoms, irrespective of activity. Periods of almost complete recovery may be followed by relapse, often sufficiently severe to make normal daily activity impossible. Depression and anxiety are also common, and a proportion of patients suffer panic attacks. Patients and their relatives may hold strong beliefs about the nature and aetiology of their illness (see Aetiology), and these may be of importance when planning management.

Physical examination is typically unremarkable. Complaints of fever and lymphadenopathy are usually found to be within normal variation when assessed. The presence of definite physical signs should not be ascribed to the syndrome and requires an alternative explanation.

MANAGEMENT

Assessment

It is important carefully to assess the patient for treatable organic and psychiatric illness. Although identifiable organic disease is relatively uncommon in patients presenting with chronic fatigue, reasonable measures to exclude it should be taken. This is particularly the case if the patient presents with a self-diagnosis. A careful history and physical examination should be made in all cases.

The history should include enquiry into the taking of prescribed and non-prescribed drugs. Sedatives, β-blocking drugs, chronic alcohol and drug abuse can all cause fatigue. It is also important to enquire about stresses in the patient's life and work. The patient and his or her spouse should be asked about their own understanding of, and beliefs about, the illness, and how they currently cope with it. Such enquiry may reveal inaccurate beliefs and unhelpful coping behaviours such as prolonged bedrest, or determined but ineffective efforts to perform.

Table 2 *Conditions to be considered in the differential diagnosis of chronic fatigue syndrome*

General
Occult malignancy
Autoimmune disease
Endocrine disease
Cardiac, respiratory, or renal failure
Neurological
Disseminated sclerosis
Myasthenia gravis
Parkinson's disease
Infectious disease
Chronic active hepatitis (B or C)
Lyme disease
Human immunodeficiency virus
Tuberculosis
Respiratory disease
Nocturnal asthma
Obstructive sleep apnoea
Chronic toxicity
Alcohol
Solvents
Heavy metals
Irradiation
Psychiatric
Major depressive disorder
Dysthymia
Anxiety and panic disorder

Almost any organic disease may present with unexplained fatigue and the differential diagnosis of idiopathic chronic fatigue syndrome is large (Table 2). The nature of the fatigue may offer useful clues. Muscular disease should be considered if the patient has no psychological symptoms, and especially if they have a family history. If the patients complaint of fatigue includes prominent sleepiness, a specific sleep disorder should be considered. In particular, prominent night-time snoring and morning headaches in the obese patient raise the possibility of obstructive sleep apnoea.

It is particularly important to carry out a careful assessment of the mental state. Depression is suggested by fatigue that is worse in the morning and accompanied by loss of motivation, interest, and pleasure. Other symptoms of depression should be sought, including sadness, loss of appetite and weight, and feelings of pessimism and failure. If there is evidence of depression, it is essential to ask about suicide plans. Chronic anxiety is associated both with fatigue and with many of the symptoms of chronic fatigue syndrome such as muscle pain, impaired concentration, and poor sleep. Psychiatric self-rating scales such as the Hospital Anxiety and Depression (HAD) scale may be a useful adjuvant to the clinical interview.

It is important to note that the patient may not reveal the extent of his or her distress. In particular they may be reluctant to say they have been depressed if they think this will result in their physical complaints being dismissed. The physician should let the patient know that s/he takes their complaints seriously and that depression is understandable in their circumstances. Patients should be asked about specific disease fears (cancer, leukaemia, HIV for example) as these may be the reason for their seeking medical advice.

Extensive laboratory investigation is likely to be unrewarding. In particular, virological investigations, even if positive, are usually unhelpful in planning management when fatigue is chronic. It is recommended, however, that all patients should have a full blood count, erythrocyte sedimentation rate or C-reactive protein, basic biochemical screen, urinalysis, and possibly thyroid function and antinuclear antibody tests. Any further investigation must be determined by the clinical findings and differential diagnosis under consideration. The assessing physician should retain an open mind. If organic disease is suspected but not apparent, a period of outpatient observation is often the best course of action.

Treatment

In all cases the doctor should take the opportunity to educate the patient about his or her condition, and should correct misconceptions about its cause and appropriate treatment. In particular, it is useful to tell the patient that there is no evidence that their particular illness is due to a chronic viral infection. In many cases it is possible to offer a more positive and less sinister explanation. Such an explanation would distinguish between viral infection as a precipitating cause, and factors such as depression and anxiety and the physiological effects of inactivity as factors perpetuating the illness.

The adverse effects of prolonged bedrest should be explained and this behaviour strongly discouraged. The patient should be encouraged to adopt a consistent but gradually increasing level of activity, avoiding extremes of both inactivity and exertion. Patients should, however, be warned that even gradual increases in activity may produce an increase in symptoms, but that this will be temporary.

It is worth considering the prescription of an antidepressant drug. It is advisable to choose a non-sedating type and to start with as low a dose as possible, as patients with chronic fatigue syndrome may be particularly sensitive to side-effects. Low doses of antidepressant drugs may reduce anxiety, improve the quality of sleep, and reduce pain. If there is evidence that the patient has a depressive disorder, whatever the cause, it is important to give the antidepressants in an adequate dose for an adequate period. Referral to a psychiatrist should be considered in such cases.

There is no specific treatment for chronic fatigue syndrome that remains idiopathic after full medical and psychiatric assessment. The best management is pragmatic, aimed at helping the patient to regain physical, occupational, and social functioning. Many patients will have severe ongoing difficulties in their work or relationships. These may need to be removed or the patient's ability to cope with them improved before recovery is possible. For some patients, long-term follow-up may be helpful in encouraging them to persevere with such an approach and in reducing the risk of possible iatrogenic harm from repeated medical investigation and failed therapy.

Although many treatments have been proposed for idiopathic chronic fatigue syndrome, few of these have been adequately evaluated. Ineffective treatments include the antiviral drug acyclovir and anticandidal treatments. Several other therapies have gained preliminary support in clinical trials, including magnesium injections, immunoglobulin infusions, and fish oil, but none of these agents has been convincingly demonstrated to be efficacious. Such treatments may be expensive and even harmful, and distract both patient and doctor from efforts at rehabilitation, which are more likely to effective in the longer term. Patients should be discouraged from pursuing unproven treatments unless they are part of a carefully conducted clinical trial.

There is evidence that patients with severe and chronic chronic fatigue syndrome may benefit from referral to a psychiatric or psychological treatment service for specific psychological therapy. If available a specialist liaison psychiatry service may be best placed to offer effective treatment in a setting acceptable to the patient. Referrals for psychological therapy should be explained to the patient in a positive way. There may also be a role for physiotherapy as part of the patient's rehabilitation programme.

PROGNOSIS

The prognosis for full recovery from chronic fatigue is good in patients seen in general practice, but poor in those severe enough to be referred to hospital clinics. The proportion of patients returning to normal functioning improves with time, however, and by 2 years after assessment only a minority remain functionally impaired. The prognosis for patients who receive more vigorous rehabilitative treatment is not yet known, but appears to be considerably better. There is no mortality associated with chronic fatigue syndrome. There is, however, a risk of death by suicide in patients whose fatigue is associated with depression.

REFERENCES

Kroenke, K. (1989). Chronic fatigue: frequency, causes, evaluation, and management. *Comprehensive Therapy*, **15,** 3–7.

Shafran, S.D. (1991) The chronic fatigue syndrome. *American Journal of Medicine*, **90,** 730–9.

Sharpe, M.C., *et al.* Chronic Fatigue Syndrome: guidelines for research. *Journal of the Royal Society of Medicine*, **84,** 118–121.

Sharpe, M.C. (1991) Psychiatric management of PVFS. *British Medical Bulletin*, **47,** 989–1006.

Chronic fatigue syndrome, CIBA Foundation Symposium No. 173. (1993). Wiley, Chichester.

Wessely, S. (1990) Old wine in new bottles: neurasthenia and 'ME'. *Psychological Medicine*, **20,** 35–53.

Section 8 *Chemical and physical injuries and environmental and occupational diseases*

8.1 Poisoning

8.1.1 Introduction and epidemiology

T. J. MEREDITH, J. A. VALE, AND A. T. PROUDFOOT

In the minds of most people, not least those of doctors, the term poisoning suggests an acute event demanding immediate care and attention. This may be so, but poisoning may take other forms. The consequence is not always immediate after a single dose—so-called acute poisoning. Prolonged uptake may result in cumulation, as with many heavy metals, and the damage may arise only after prolonged exposure—that is, chronic poisoning.

The intrinsic toxicity of the noxious agent involved cannot be judged solely by the LD_{50} in animal studies, for species differences may be great, and extrapolation from animal data is therefore extremely difficult.

Exposure, by oral, inhalational, cutaneous, or other routes, should not itself be equated with poisoning. Uptake is necessary for there to be a toxic effect, and even if this occurs, poisoning does not necessarily result: for example, the dose may be too small or the individual may not be susceptible.

If true poisoning does occur, the ensuing clinical syndrome may be distinctive: for example, fixed dilated pupils, exaggerated tendon reflexes, extensor plantars, depressed respiration, and cardiac tachyarrhythmias suggest tricyclic antidepressant poisoning; and anaemia, constipation, colic, and motor nerve palsies are indicative of lead poisoning. Otherwise, with a whole range of psychotropic medications there may be only non-specific central nervous depression, respiratory embarrassment, and hypotension. In some instances, distinctive sequelae may not appear until many years have elapsed as, for example, with carcinoma of the oesophagus following ingestion of corrosives or hepatic haemangiosarcoma from vinyl chloride exposure.

Poisoning may be accidental or deliberate. It is usually accidental in small children, and in adults it is usually deliberate with parasuicidal, suicidal, or, rarely, homicidal intent.

Thus, the medical approach to poisoning should never be confined to cause and effect. The whole aetiology must be taken into account, especially in cases where litigation may follow, for example in the event of an occupational mishap with a chemical. It is therefore important that the doctor concerned, having instituted any necessary life-saving measures, should take a careful history, retain all pertinent evidence such as suicide notes, biological specimens, and the like, and make a meticulous record of symptoms, signs, progress and outcome.

Epidemiology

Few health care professionals would deny that poisoning, accidental or deliberate, is a common problem in most countries throughout the world. Yet it is remarkably difficult to obtain reliable statistics on the absolute morbidity or mortality resulting from poisoning, even in those countries with comparatively advanced systems for collection of population health data. The following observations are based primarily on data from the United Kingdom and the United States but, wherever appropriate, observed variations in patterns of poisoning in other countries are noted.

Hospital admissions due to poisoning

Poisoning from accidental or deliberate ingestion or inhalation of drugs or chemicals is a common acute medical emergency requiring hospital admission. In the period 1957–1976, the annual number of hospital admissions due to acute poisoning in England and Wales rose steadily from less than 20 000 to more than 125 000. Since then, there has been a decline in the incidence of self-poisoning in England to approximately 100 000 each year.

Despite this decline self-poisoning still accounts for more than 10 per cent of acute adult medical admissions. However, the true incidence of acute poisoning may be as much as three times that of the hospital admission rate.

In the United Kingdom, with the exception of young children, females predominate in all age groups in those admitted to hospital because of acute poisoning, and there is a marked preponderance in those aged 15 to 44 years. Many paediatric episodes are poisoning scares, rather than true poisonings, while the majority of adult patients who poison themselves are not suicidal.

In Western Europe and North America, drugs have always been the most common agents taken by adults and rank second only to household products as the substances most often ingested by children. In the United Kingdom, alcohol is taken in addition to the drug overdose in 60 per cent of males and 40 per cent of females, and at least one-third of self-poisoning episodes involve one or more drugs. Approximately two-thirds of adults ingest drugs that have been prescribed for themselves or a close relative, and so the pattern of self-poisoning in the community reflects prescribing habits. In part this accounts for the changing pattern observed in the drugs used for self-poisoning: barbiturates and non barbiturate hypnotics have become less common causes of poisoning, while use of other psychotropic agents such as the benzodiazepines and tricyclic antidepressants in overdose is now more frequent; analgesic poisoning also occurs more commonly than previously. There has been a similar pattern of change in Norway and central Europe.

Within Europe there are variations from country to country. In Finland, for example, alcohol, cardiovascular drugs, and psychotropics are the most common causes of poisoning. Outside Europe, and in developing countries in particular, the situation is often very different. In Sri Lanka, for example, agrochemicals account for nearly 60 per cent of all poisonings; such agents account for less than 1 per cent of hospital admissions for poisoning in England and Wales. In South Africa, the pattern of poisoning in the white population mirrors that in North America and Western Europe, whereas that observed in black South Africans is very different, with kerosene (paraffin) and traditional medicines accounting for the majority of hospital admissions (and deaths) attributable to poisoning. In countries where malaria is prevalent, poisoning by antimalarials is an additional cause of morbidity and mortality.

Deaths from poisoning

In contrast to the rise and more recent fall in the hospital admission rate for poisoning in England and Wales, deaths from acute poisoning have decreased over the last 25 years and, since 1972, they have remained virtually constant at 4000 per annum. The lack of change in the mortality rate over the last 20 years is particularly striking, because this period follows the substitution of 'natural gas' for 'town gas', which led directly to a fall in carbon monoxide deaths from nearly 4000 in 1963 to just over 1000 per annum 10 years later.

Despite relatively little change in the overall mortality statistics for acute poisoning in England and Wales, there have been very substantial changes in the agents responsible. Deaths from barbiturates and non-barbiturate hypnotics have fallen, while those due to analgesics and psychotropic agents have risen. Deaths from carbon monoxide have shown a slow but steady increase since 1975, reaching just over 1500 in 1991. Increasing numbers of young men (14–24 years) in the United Kingdom are committing suicide. Self-poisoning with car exhaust fumes (containing carbon monoxide) is currently the most common means of doing so.

In England and Wales, most patients who die as a result of poisoning do so at home, the inpatient mortality being less than 1 per cent of all cases admitted to hospital. The age and sex distribution of deaths attributed to acute poisoning is very different from that for admissions—there are fewer patients in the age range 15 to 44 years (where males predominate over females) and more in the older age categories.

A similar pattern of causes of death has been observed elsewhere in Western Europe and in North America, but in many developing agricultural countries, agrochemicals (cholinesterase inhibitors, organochlorines, and other pesticides) more commonly predominate. It has been estimated that, globally, pesticides account for 1 million serious unintentional poisonings and 2 million hospitalized suicide attempts annually, predominantly in developing countries. The mortality rate from poisoning is to some extent determined by the lethality of the agents involved, which in turn results in regional differences in mortality rates which are often much higher in developing countries.

Childhood poisoning

In the period April 1989 to March 1990, the latest year for which figures are available for England, nearly 18 000 children aged 0–14 years were admitted to hospital ostensibly because of ingestion of a poison; 70 per cent were aged 4 years or less. Although hospital admission rates for children may be declining, it is estimated that as many as 41 000 poisoning incidents occur in children aged 4 years or less in the United Kingdom each year. In the United States, the figures of the American Association of Poison Control Centers National Data Collection System for 1992 record more than 1 million so called 'poison exposures' in children less than 6 years of age.

Children aged less than 5 years are particularly active and exploratory and have a strong impulse to put things into their mouths. These characteristics predispose to accidental poisoning, which in Western Europe is particularly likely to occur when parents are inattentive or neglectful, as at times of family crises. The vast majority (80–85 per cent) of cases occur in the child's own home, and in many instances the substances involved are out of their usual storage place or have been put into some other container; grandparents, for example, may find it convenient to remove drugs from child-resistant closures because they themselves have difficulty opening this type of packaging.

A child may also be poisoned by an adult who administers a toxic substance by mistake, and rarely a parent may poison a child as a form of abuse, sometimes with fatal consequences. In addition, older (typically 10–16 years) emotionally disturbed children may deliberately poison themselves.

Although in North America and Western Europe, young children (aged 4 years or less) more commonly ingest household products than drugs, this is not the case when children of all ages are considered. In England and Wales, analgesics account for 20 per cent of cases; a further 40 per cent ingest other pharmaceutical preparations. Iron, tricyclic antidepressants, benzodiazepines, paracetamol, and contraceptive pills are the agents most commonly involved; the remainder are poisoned by a variety of household products (bleaches, detergents and disinfectants, and petroleum distillates such as turpentine substitute), alcohol, garden plants, and seeds. In recent years, abuse of volatile substances has become an increasing problem in adolescents, a subject that is dealt with in detail in Chapter 8.3.3. In developing countries the pattern is rather different, with accidental poisoning due to hydrocarbons (especially paraffin) and traditional medicines, snake bites, and arthropod stings being more common.

As far as childhood deaths are concerned, poisoning accounts for a very small proportion indeed when measured against the total mortality of children under 10 years of age. In England and Wales, carbon monoxide remains the most common cause of childhood death due to poisoning (Table 1), and tricyclic antidepressant ingestion carries a relatively high mortality when the infrequency with which children ingest these drugs in overdose is considered. Non-medicinal products account for few deaths in the United Kingdom, but in the United States petroleum distillates, pesticides, and cleaning and polishing agents are still significant contributory causes.

Table 1 *Deaths from poisoning in children aged less than 10 years (England and Wales, 1968–1991,* n *= 2423)*

	Number of deaths	
Poison (ICD code)	1968–1973[a]	1974–1991[b]
Carbon monoxide (986)	631	926
Other gases, fumes or vapours (987)	5	461[c]
Antidepressants (969.0)	—	45
Opiates and related compounds (965.0)	—	19
Barbiturates (967.0)	—	17
Salicylates (965.1)	—	13
Lead (984)	9	9
Other drugs/medicines (960–979)	134	99
Other (non-medicinal) poisons (980–989)	26	29
Total (960–989)	805	1618

[a]Source: Registrar-General (1968–1973).

[b]Source: Office of Population Censuses and Surveys (1974–1991b).

[c]Coding change from 1979.

REFERENCES

Casey, P. and Vale, J.A. (1994). Deaths from pesticide poisoning in England and Wales: 1945–1989. *Human and Experimental Toxicology,* **13,** 95–101.

Kasilo, O.M.J. and Nhachi, C.F.B. (1992). A pattern of acute poisoning in children in urban Zimbabwe: ten years experience. *Human and Experimental Toxicology,* **11,** 335–40.

Litovitz, T.L., Holm, K.C., Clancy, C., Schmitz, B.F., Clark, L.R., and Oderda, G.M. (1993). 1992 Annual report of the American Association of Poison Control Centers Toxic Exposure Surveillance System. *American Journal of Emergency Medicine,* **11,** 494–555.

Meredith, T.J. and Vale, J.A. (1984). Epidemiology of analgesic overdose in England and Wales. *Human Toxicology,* **3,** 61S–74S.

Wiseman, H.M., Guest, K., Murray, V.S.G., and Volans, G.N. (1987). Accidental poisoning in childhood: a multicentre survey. 1. General epidemiology. *Human Toxicology,* **6,** 293–301.

Woolf, A.D. and Lovejoy, F.H (1993). Epidemiology of drug overdose in children. *Drug Safety,* **9,** 291–308.

8.1.2 Clinical and metabolic features and general principles of management

A. T. PROUDFOOT, J. A. VALE, AND T. J. MEREDITH

Diagnosis

Ideally, diagnosis of acute poisoning requires that the doctor not only establish that exposure to a poison (whether by ingestion, injection, inhalation, or skin contamination) has occurred, but also its chemical

Table 1 *Common feature clusters*

Feature cluster	Likely poisons
Coma, hypertonia, hyperreflexia, extensor plantar responses, myoclonus, strabismus, mydriasis, sinus tachycardia	Tricyclic antidepressants—less commonly orphenadrine, thioridazine
Coma, hypotonia, hyporeflexia, plantar responses, flexor, or non-elicitable, hypotension	Barbiturates, benzodiazepines and alcohol combinations, severe tricyclic antidepressant poisoning
Coma, miosis, reduced respiratory rate	Opioid analgesics
Nausea, vomiting, tinnitus, deafness, sweating, hyperventilation, vasodilation, tachycardia	Salicylates
Restlessness, agitation, mydriasis, anxiety, tremor, tachycardia, convulsions, arrhythmias	Sympathomimetics

composition and magnitude so that the features likely to develop can be anticipated and risk assessed. As in any other branch of medicine, diagnosis of acute poisoning is based on the patient's history and on a combination of circumstantial evidence, the findings on physical examination, and appropriate investigations when a history is not available. However, in acute poisoning, there are many obstacles to establishing the information required. Young children may not be able to give a history and adults are often unreliable while physical signs are rarely diagnostic. Similarly, circumstantial evidence may not be available, be only tentative or misleading, and laboratory diagnosis can never be fully comprehensive.

History

Since accidental poisoning in childhood is most common between the ages of 9 months and 5 years, an unequivocal history is unlikely to be forthcoming from the victim but may be obtainable from older witnesses. Clearly, however, statements about amounts must be interpreted with caution since knowledge of the quantities in original containers is frequently inaccurate or unknown.

In contrast, about 90 per cent or more of adults presenting with acute poisoning are conscious or only slightly drowsy and there would seem little reason why diagnosis of self-poisoning on the basis of the history should be difficult. Indeed, although a small number of patients adamantly deny having taken poisons, the majority usually admit to it without hesitation although problems arise in trying to establish precisely the nature and quantity of what has been taken. Comparison of patients' statements with poisons detected by laboratory analysis of blood or urine consistently reveals major differences in about half the cases. In consequence, patients are often thought to be deliberately untruthful. However, surprise at these findings may merely reveal a lack of medical insight into the circumstances under which self-poisoning occurs. It is commonly an impulsive act with the patient ingesting the contents of the first bottle that comes to hand, often when considerably under the influence of alcohol. Moreover, although about 60 per cent of episodes involve drugs prescribed for the victims or their relatives, like many other patients, they are often ignorant of their names.

If these considerations make it difficult to establish the nature of the poison, it is hardly surprising that they should make the amounts involved even more suspect. Few patients count the number of tablets they consume and it is impossible for patient or doctor to know what constitutes a 'handful', 'bottleful', or similar arbitrary quantity.

Circumstantial evidence

Circumstantial evidence becomes important in the diagnosis of acute poisoning when patients are either unable to give a history (as is likely to occur with young children, adults who are educationally subnormal or demented and those who are unconscious) or are unwilling to do so. However, although circumstantial evidence may strongly suggest poisoning, it is seldom incontrovertible. It takes several forms.

Circumstances under which found

Accidental poisoning in infants is frequently suspected from the circumstances under which they are found. The mother may return to the kitchen or bathroom to find her child with some substance all over his hands, face, and clothing, or surrounded by pills, one of which he is eating. The assumption that more has been ingested may or may not be correct and the amount swallowed is a matter of speculation. Similarly, adults may be found unconscious with tablet particles around the mouth or on clothing as the only clue to diagnosis. More often, the presence of empty drug containers with occasional tablets or capsules in close proximity to the patient suggests the diagnosis. Less commonly, they are found unconscious or dead in some remote location. The lack of personal effects to indicate who they are or where they live may suggest a desire not to be identified and should arouse suspicion of drug overdosage. Self-poisoning is a common cause of coma in previously healthy young adults. Protestations by relatives that patients would never take overdoses are usually wrong.

Suicide notes

Suicide notes are reliable indicators of drug overdosage in the absence of physical violence as a cause of coma. The note may specify what has been taken in addition to expressing despair, futility, worthlessness, and remorse.

Features

There are few symptoms or physical signs which cannot be attributed to one poison or another. However, a clinical feature rarely arises in isolation and clusters of features are of much greater diagnostic value. Those most commonly encountered in present-day practice are given in Table 1.

Conscious patients with abnormal behaviour, perhaps in combination with auditory and visual hallucinations, may have ingested amphetamines, phenycyclidine, LSD, 'magic' (psilocybin-containing) mushrooms, and drugs such as the older antihistamines and tricyclic antidepressants which have marked anticholinergic actions. Occasionally a patient with severe salicylate intoxication who cannot give a history despite being conscious, shows hyperventilation, sweating, flushing, and tachycardia suggesting a diagnosis which can then be confirmed by the laboratory.

Drowsiness, ataxia, dysarthria, and nystagmus are common after ingestion of benzodiazepines. Coma with hypotonia and hyporeflexia may follow, particularly if alcohol has also been taken. Hypotension, hypothermia, and respiratory depression are rare. All of these features, however, may occur after overdosage with outmoded drugs such as barbiturates, methaqualone, meprobamate, and ethchlorvynol which are still occasionally prescribed. In present-day clinical practice, tricyclic antidepressants remain among the most common CNS depressants encountered in overdosage and cause hypertonia, hyperreflexia, extensor plantar responses, and dilated pupils. Sinus tachycardia and prolongation of the QRS interval on the electrocardiogram support a diagnosis of intoxication with these drugs. Hypotension and hypothermia are uncommon. Tricyclic antidepressants and non-steroidal anti-inflammatory agents, particularly mefenamic acid, are the most common causes of seizures after drug overdosage. Coma with pinpoint pupils and a reduced respiratory rate is virtually diagnostic of overdosage with opioid analgesics and is an indication for a therapeutic trial of naloxone. Many patients with opioid poisoning will be habitual drug abusers and have venepuncture marks and evidence of venous tracking in the antecubital fossae. Alcohol may be smelt on the breath as may solvents such as toluene, acetone, or xylene as the result of 'sniffing' glues, cleaning agents, or other preparations. Skin blisters occur in poisoning by many drugs (see below) but rarely in coma due to other causes. Burns around the lips or in the buccal cavity or pharynx indicate ingestion of corrosives (see Chapter 8.3.5) including paraquat.

Lateralizing neurological signs

Since most serious poisonings are associated with impairment of consciousness, neurological signs are particularly important. Lateralizing signs (unless they are attributable to a known neurological disease) virtually exclude a diagnosis of acute poisoning. Such findings have been recorded with barbiturate and phenytoin overdosage but so rarely that the general rule is not significantly compromised. A possible exception is transient inequality of pupil size. This has been reported only rarely in acute poisoning but is not an uncommon finding in normal individuals (e.g. due to Holmes–Adie pupils) but clinical experience suggests that it occurs more frequently in poisoning than seems apparent from the literature.

Decerebrate and decorticate movements

Unconscious poisoned patients may respond to painful stimuli with flexor and extensor limb movements of the type seen in decorticate and decerebrate states. However, in poisoning, these signs do not indicate irreversible brain damage and patients showing them can be expected to recovery fully. Hypoglycaemia must be excluded in these cases.

Strabismus, and internuclear and external ophthalmoplegia

Several recent reports have drawn attention to the occurrence of a variety of ocular signs including strabismus, internuclear ophthalmoplegia, and total external opthalmoplegia, not previously described in acute poisoning by psychtropic drugs.

Strabismus has now been described in poisoning with phenytoin, carbamazepine, and tricyclic antidepressants. Usually the optic axes diverge in the horizontal plane but in some patients there is additional vertical deviation. It is present transiently and only in patients who are unconscious. Dysconjugate, roving eye movements may also be seen if both eyes are observed for a period of time. It is important to know that such abnormalities occur so that they are not misattributed to intracranial vascular lesions or some other pathology requiring surgical intervention.

Dysconjugate eye movements may become apparent only when oculovestibular reflexes are examined by caloric stimuli. Installation of ice-cold water into the external auditory meatus should make both eyes turn to the side irrigated and failure of one eye to deviate is evidence of internuclear ophthalmoplegia and a lesion of the medial longitudinal fasciculus. This has been reported in poisoning with a variety of drugs including tricyclic antidepressants, phenothiazines, benzodiazepines, barbiturates, and ethanol and can be detected in 10 per cent of cases if caloric tests are carried out. Both sides are usually affected but internuclear ophthalmoplegia on testing one side only also occurs in acute poisoning.

Table 2 *Coma grading scheme*

Grade of coma	Description
I	Drowsy but responds to vocal command
II	Unconscious but responds to minimal stimuli
III	Unconscious and responds only to maximal painful stimuli
IV	Unconscious and no response to pain

In some cases, cold-induced lateral eye movements are followed after an interval of 5 to 15 s by forced downward gaze lasting several minutes but the suggestion that the latter may be diagnostic of drug-induced coma requires further study before acceptance.

It is widely accepted that absence of oculocervical and oculovestibular responses indicates severe brain-stem damage and the likelihood that the patient will not survive. However, this is not the case in acute poisoning where these reflexes may be abolished in patients who subsequently make a full recovery.

Management

Antidotes and methods to enhance elimination are available for only a very small number of poisons and the management of the great majority of poisoned patients is based on what has been called 'an orderly if unspectacular regimen of supportive therapy'.

Emergency treatment

A small but significant number of poisoned patients arrive at hospital with respiratory obstruction, ventilatory failure, or in cardiorespiratory arrest. In these cases, conventional resuscitation takes precedence over detailed assessment of the patient and attempts to obtain a history. The opioid antagonist, naloxone, can be of inestimable value in emergency treatment. It is safe and should be used whenever there is the slightest suspicion that an opioid may be involved. Its use may transform a desperate situation for the better within seconds and even if it is given inappropriately, it is highly unlikely to have adverse effects.

Supportive care

Unconscious patients need scrupulous attention to respiration, hypotension, hypothermia, and other complications if they are to survive. Expert nursing is as important as medical measures.

AIRWAY

Establishment and maintenance of an adequate airway is of paramount importance in the management of unconscious poisoned patients. The airway may be obstructed by the tongue falling back, dental plates being dislodged, other foreign bodies, buccal secretions, vomitus, and flexion of the neck. In the first instance, the neck should be extended and the tongue and jaw held forward. Secretions in the oropharynx must be removed and an oropharyngeal airway should be inserted before turning the patient into a semiprone position. If the cough reflex is absent, an endotracheal tube should be inserted to prevent aspiration into the lungs and allow regular aspiration of bronchial secretions. It is then important to ensure that the inspired air is adequately warmed and humidified.

VENTILATION

Once a clear airway has been established the adequacy of spontaneous ventilation should be assessed from the results of arterial blood gas and pH measurements. These should be carried out in all patients in grade III or IV coma (Table 2) irrespective of the presence or absence of features suggesting inadequate gas exchange. Unconscious poisoned patients often have a mild, mixed respiratory and metabolic acidosis with carbon dioxide tensions at the upper limit of normal and oxygen tensions which fall with increasing depth of coma. Increasing the oxygen content of the inspired air is often sufficient to correct hypoxia. Patients with respiratory failure ('carbon dioxide retention') should have an endotracheal tube inserted to reduce the respiratory dead space and thereby increase alveolar ventilation. If this does not reduce carbon dioxide tensions, assisted ventilation is indicated. High inspired oxygen concentrations are imperative in patients with carbon monoxide and cyanide poisoning and in pulmonary oedema resulting from inhalation of irritant gases.

HYPOTENSION

Hypotension in acute poisoning can be due to a variety of factors including a relative reduction in the intravascular volume secondary to expansion of the venous capacitance bed, metabolic acidosis, arrhythmias, the cardiodepressant effects of some drugs, and blood or fluid loss into the gut. Correct management of individual cases obviously depends on accurate identification of the causes. Young patients are generally not at risk of cerebral or renal damage unless the systolic blood pressure falls below 80 mmHg but in those over the age of 40 years it is preferable to keep the systolic blood pressure above 90 mmHg. Hypotension often responds to elevation of the foot of the bed by 15 cm and if this is unsuccessful a central venous line should be inserted and the intravascular volume expanded as necessary. Dopamine (2.5–20 μg/kg.min) and dobutamine (5–40 μg/kg.min) are indicated if hypotension is resistant to these measures. The possibility of using techniques to enhance elimination of the poison from the body should then be considered.

ARRHYTHMIAS

Although many poisons are potentially cardiotoxic, the incidence of serious cardiac arrhythmias in acute poisoning is very low. Tricyclic antidepressants, β-adrenoceptor blocking drugs, chloral hydrate, cardiac glycosides, amphetamines, and bronchodilators (particularly theophylline and its derivatives and antimalarial drugs) are the most likely causes. Cardiotoxicity usually occurs together with other features of severe poisoning including metabolic acidosis, hypoxia, convulsions, respiratory depression, and abnormalities of electrolyte balance which should be corrected before considering the use of antiarrhythmic drugs. The latter have narrow therapeutic ratios and their use may further impair myocardial function. In general, drug therapy should only be given for persistent, life-threatening arrhythmias associated with peripheral circulatory failure. The drug used must be selected from a knowledge of the pharmacology and toxicology of the poison involved and in such a way that it will not further compromise cardiac function. Lignocaine is probably the drug of choice for serious ventricular tachydysrhythmias since its half-life is short and the dose can be adjusted more readily.

CONVULSIONS

Convulsions are potentially life-threatening because they cause hypoxia and metabolic acidosis and may precipitate cardiac arrhythmias and arrest. Short isolated convulsions do not require treatment but those which are recurrent or protracted should be suppressed with intravenous diazepam. This drug is highly effective in adequate doses and alternatives are seldom needed. However, it is important to remember that giving benzodiazepines in this way may potentate the respiratory depressant effects of other poisons and further complicate management. The combination of convulsions, coma and vomiting, which may occur with overdosage of theophylline derivatives, is particularly dangerous and in these circumstances it may be preferable to paralyse the patient, insert an endotracheal tube, and start assisted ventilation. However, although this ensures control of the airway and oxygenation, thus avoiding the risk of inhalation of gastric contents, it does not suppress seizure activity; cerebral function must therefore be monitored and parenteral anticonvulsants given as required.

HYPOTHERMIA

Any poison which depresses the central nervous system may impair temperature regulation and cause hypothermia, especially when discovery of the patient is delayed and environmental temperatures are low. This important complication may be missed unless temperature is recorded rectally using a low reading thermometer. In severe cases, peripheral and core temperatures should be monitored. Treatment includes nursing the patient in a warm room (27–29 °C) and a heat conserving 'space blanket'. Cold intravenous fluids should be avoided and bottles for use should be stored in the room or the lines should pass through a heating device.

HYPERTHERMIA

Rarely, body temperature may increase to potentially fatal levels after overdosage with central nervous system stimulants such as cocaine, amphetamines, phencyclidine, monoamine oxidase inhibitors, and theophylline and its derivatives. In such cases, muscle tone is often grossly increased and convulsions and rhabdomyolysis are common. Cooling measures including administration of chlorpromazine are indicated and dantrolene should be given to reduce muscle tone.

ACID–BASE ABNORMALITIES

Acid–base disturbances commonly accompany coma due to drugs. Acute respiratory acidosis is less common than might be expected but some elevation of arterial carbon dioxide tensions towards the upper limit of normal is usual. This, in combination with mild hypoxia in the deeper grades of coma, produces overall acidaemia. In general, acidosis should be prevented and managed by ensuring adequate ventilation, oxygenation and tissue perfusion, and control of convulsions rather than by giving bicarbonate. However, a number of poisons, particularly methanol and ethylene glycol, cause life-threatening metabolic acidosis which should be corrected by infusion of sodium bicarbonate.

Acute respiratory alkalosis, often in combination with a minor metabolic acidosis, is commonly found in acute salicylate overdosage. The metabolic component may require treatment if it is the dominant feature and is causing overall acidaemia. Respiratory alkalosis should not be treated.

ELECTROLYTE ABNORMALITIES

Electrolyte abnormalities may result from acid–base disturbances or the direct effects of poisons. Massive tissue damage, usually rhabdomyolysis, may allow potassium to leak from cells leading to potentially lethal hyperkalaemia. Cardiac glycosides cause hyperkalaemia secondary to loss from cells due to inhibition of the membrane sodium–potassium pump while the reverse occurs with sympathomimetic drugs. Oxalic acid and ethylene glycol (which is metabolized to oxalic acid) may cause hypocalcaemia by leading to the formation of insoluble calcium oxalate which is deposited in tissues. Similarly, ingestion of fluorides is also a possible cause of hypocalcaemia but the amounts children tend to ingest in the form of tablets to prevent dental caries seldom cause serious problems. Ingestion of potassium salts, even in sustained release formulations, may lead to hyperkalaemia and fatal arrhythmias.

BLADDER CARE

Urinary retention is a common complication of acute poisoning, particularly with tricyclic antidepressants and other drugs which have marked anticholinergic actions. However, bladder catheterization is all too often an unthinking measure in unconscious poisoned patients. Coma *per se* is not an indication for bladder catheters in poisoned patients, the great majority of whom regain consciousness within 12 h. The bladder can usually be induced to empty reflexly (provided it is not allowed to become grossly over-distended) by applying gentle suprapubic pressure. Catheterization should be reserved for those patients in whom suprapubic pressure is insufficient to empty the bladder, and in those thought to be developing renal failure.

SKIN, MUSCLE, AND NERVE LESIONS

Skin blisters may be found after poisoning with a wide variety of drugs including barbiturates, tricyclic antidepressants and benzodiazepines, and non-drug toxins. They often occur over bony prominences which have been subjected to pressure and less frequently at sites where two skin areas have been in contact, e.g., the inner aspects of the knees. They should be managed as partial thickness burns. Rhabdomyolysis is a further possible result of immobility and may occur in combination with skin lesions or independently. Drug overdosage is the most common non-traumatic cause of this condition and it may lead to acute renal failure and, rarely, to ischaemic muscle contractures and long-term disability. Similarly, peripheral nerves such as the radial, ulnar, and common peroneal may be damaged by direct pressure while the patient is unconscious or by being entrapped in fibrosing muscle after rhabdomyolysis.

Antidotes

Naloxone for opioid analgesics, oxygen for carbon monoxide, and, possibly, flumazenil for benzodiazepines are the only antidotes commonly needed in the management of unconscious poisoned patients. Methionine and *N*-acetylcysteine are used frequently for paracetamol overdosage. Other antidotes of proven value are listed in Table 3 together with brief details of dosage. They are seldom required and although their use in correct circumstances may be life-saving, some are toxic in their own right and the reader is recommended to seek further advice from a poisons information service. Antivenoms for bites and stings by venomous animals are discussed in Section 8.4.

Prevention of absorption of the poison

Prevention of absorption of poisons through the lungs obviously requires removal from the toxic atmosphere and occasionally removal of soiled clothing. The latter is also necessary when absorption is thought to have been percutaneous and, in addition, the contaminated skin should be thoroughly washed with soap and water. Measures to limit further absorption of ingested poisons include emptying the stomach, either by inducing emesis or by gastric aspiration and lavage, the administration of oral adsorbents, particularly activated charcoal, and the use of whole bowel irrigation.

EMPTYING THE STOMACH

The stomach is emptied in the hope of retrieving potentially toxic amounts of poison from the stomach, thereby preventing its absorption and reducing morbidity and mortality.

TECHNIQUES

Gastric lavage and induced emesis are the methods available. The technique of gastric lavage is given in Table 4. Emesis may be induced by mechanical and chemical means. Provoking gagging by stimulating the pharynx with the fingers is simple, widely practised (particularly in the treatment of children), and does not appear to carry any particular risks. However, it is frequently ineffective. Syrup of ipecacuanha is the emetic of choice; it should be given in doses of 10 to 30 ml followed by a glass of water or fruit juice and may be repeated once if vomiting does not occur within 20 min. Ipecacuanha is an extract of the dried root of *Cephaelis ipecacuanha* or *C. acuminanata*, both of which grow in South America and contain several alkaloids including cephaeline and emetine which are the active ingredients. These irritate the gastrointestinal tract and stimulate the medullary vomiting centre; small doses induce vomiting in about 95 per cent of patients, whether children or adults, within 30 to 45 min. Deaths have occurred from the use of salt and copper sulphate solutions and their use is deplored.

Table 3 *Antidotes of proven value in poisoning due to drugs and chemicals*

Poison	Antidote
Anticoagulants (oral)	Vitamin K
Arsenic	Dimercaprol DMAS, DMPS
Benzodiazepines	Flumazenil
β-Adrenoceptor blockers	Atropine Glucagon
Carbon monoxide	Oxygen
Cyanide	Amyl nitrite Sodium nitrite Sodium thiosulphate Dicobalt edetate
Digoxin	Digoxin-specific Fab antibodies
Ethylene glycol	Ethanol
Iron salts	Desferrioxamine
Lead (inorganic)	Sodium calcium edetate DMSA DMPS
Methaemoglobinaemia	Methylene blue
Methanol	Ethanol
Mercury (inorganic)	Dimercaprol Penicillamine DMSA, DMPS
Opioids	Naloxone
Organophosphate insecticides	Atropine Pralidoxime
Paracetamol	Methionine *N*-acetylcysteine

Table 4 *Gastric aspiration and lavage procedure*

1. Ensure the availability of functioning powerful suction before starting
2. If the patient is very drowsy or unconscious confirm that a vigorous cough reflex is present—if not, do not attempt lavage unless an endotracheal tube is inserted
3. Place the patient in the left lateral position
4. Elevate the foot of the bed so that the mouth and throat are at a level lower than the larynx and trachea
5. Pass a lubricated lavage tube. In the adult, 50 cm will reach the stomach
6. Confirm that the end of the tube is in the stomach by either aspirating gastric contents or by blowing some air down the tube while auscultating over the left hypochondrium
7. Aspirate gastric contents and save 50 ml in case a sample is needed for laboratory analysis
8. Carry out lavage by pouring aliquots of 300–400 ml tepid water down the tube siphoning off between each. Repeat this process until the returning fluid is clear of drug particles
9. Occlude the proximal end of the tube before withdrawing it from the oesophagus into the pharynx to avoid aspiration of fluid in the tube

EFFICACY

While in theory, gastric emptying seems an eminently sensible measure after ingestion of a poison, in practice its value is much more controversial. It is now apparent that gastric lavage (a) retrieves toxicologically significant quantities of drugs in only a small proportion of cases, particularly if carried out later than 1 h after ingestion, (b) usually yields amounts of drug which could be inactivated as effectively by giving adsorbents, (c) does not appear to alter the course of minor and moderate poisoning, (d) does not empty the stomach completely in many cases, and (e) may increase the severity of poisoning by flushing drug from the stomach into the small bowel, thus facilitating rapid absorption.

Induced emesis may not be any more effective. Much of the evidence supporting its use is derived from experiments in volunteers given relatively small doses of drugs in the fasting state rather than from acutely poisoned patients. However, efficient induction of emesis does not necessarily mean that important amounts of poison are being ejected. Moreover, no clinical trial has demonstrated efficacy.

It is self-evident that lavage is the only practicable method of gastric emptying in unconscious patients and that the passage of stomach tubes of sufficiently wide bore is impossible in small children.

The use of lavage and syrup of ipecacuanha outside hospital, other than by fully trained personnel, could be dangerous. Even with syrup of ipecac, there is increasing evidence of excessive and unacceptable adverse effects (see below). In general, therefore, we do not recommend that ipecacuanha should be available in the home or first-aid units. Exceptions might be made when patients are a considerable distance from doctors and for full-time units in industrial settings where there is considered to be a high risk of ingestion of poisons and the staff have been appropriately trained.

HAZARDS OF GASTRIC EMPTYING

Gastric lavage carries a number of potentially serious hazards. Stomach contents may be aspirated into the lungs unless the patient has a vigorous cough reflex or the airway is protected with an endotracheal tube. Perforation of the oesophagus is fortunately a rare complication. Significant hypoxia may develop and possibly predispose to the onset of cardiac arrhythmias. Similarly, the use of syrup of ipecacuanha is not without adverse effects. Serious morbidity is rare but protracted vomiting beyond the time when toxin might be ejected is not uncommon and diarrhoea, abdominal pain, drowsiness, and irritability occur in 10 to 15 per cent of cases. Aspiration pneumonia occurs in 5 per cent of conscious patients. Large doses cause CNS depression and are cardiotoxic.

INDICATIONS FOR GASTRIC EMPTYING

It has always been, and probably will remain, difficult to identify the patient who will benefit from gastric emptying. As indicated above, gastric emptying is only indicated when it is considered that a potentially toxic amount of poison has been ingested, that it is likely that significant amounts remain in the stomach and that the risk of complications from the method used is justified. Ideally, therefore, a decision should be based on knowledge of the toxicity of the substance or product, the amount involved, its effect on gastric emptying and the time since ingestion. The first of these is probably the most important consideration and, if not already known, can be rapidly obtained from the poisons information services; the amounts ingested and the time that has elapsed are frequently little more than speculative. Many of the drugs currently and commonly encountered in poisoning episodes are less toxic than those of a few decades ago and the need for gastric emptying should be less now than previously. Experience suggests, however, that both methods are considerably over-used, partly because of uncertainty about the amount taken and the time of ingestion and perhaps partly from fear of retribution should the stomach not be emptied and the outcome of the poisoning be other than full recovery. Acting 'safe' is therefore common. In other instances, however, gastric emptying may be an unthinking routine or, in the case of gastric lavage, done in the belief (for which there is no evidence) that the procedure will deter the recipient from further episodes of self-poisoning.

There is no dispute that clinically severe poisoning remains an indication for gastric emptying. Commonly, this will mean that the patient is unconscious and that gastric lavage (subject to the contraindications below) is the only available method. In these patients the time since ingestion may be less relevant since it is obvious that a toxic dose has been ingested and the gastrointestinal stasis which often accompanies deep coma can delay gastric emptying. The drugs most likely to be the cause include the tricyclic antidepressants which, like other drugs with anticholinergic effects and opioid analgesics may delay gastric emptying. In addition, large amounts of salicylate may adhere in the stomach. However, there is no evidence from controlled clinical studies that performing lavage later than 1 h after overdose is effective and no study has demonstrated reduced inability and mortality following the use of gastric lavage.

In less severe poisoning, decisions about gastric emptying are even more difficult. While the toxicity of the substance or product remains important, the time since ingestion increasingly becomes the dominant consideration. Gastric emptying can reasonably be omitted from management if the patient presents later than 1 h after overdose. It has been suggested that exceptions to this generalization are patients with anatomical reasons for delayed gastric emptying, ingestion of drugs specifically formulated to release their active ingredient slowly (notably theophylline preparations), substances which require metabolic activation before becoming toxic (e.g. paracetamol, methanol, ethylene glycol, and some organophosphate insecticides), and those to which tissues appear to react only slowly (e.g. lithium salts and monoamine oxidase inhibitors). However, clinical studies have not demonstrated that the routine use of gastric lavage in these circumstances has been beneficial.

CONTRAINDICATIONS TO GASTRIC EMPTYING

Gastric lavage must not be carried out and emetics must not be given unless the patient has a vigorous cough reflex or an endotracheal tube has been inserted since lavage fluid or gastric contents may be aspirated into the lungs. For the same reason, and because of their propensity to spread rapidly within the lungs and cause severe pneumonitis, ingestion of petroleum distillates is a contraindication to the use of either of these methods. Ingestion of corrosive poisons greatly increases the risk of perforating the oesophagus or stomach during lavage and, in general, the procedure is best avoided (see Chapter 8.3.5).

ORAL ADSORBENTS

The use of orally administered adsorbents to reduce absorption should be considered as an alternative or adjunct to gastric lavage. Of the numerous adsorbents which have been recommended over the years, activated charcoal is rightly the most widely used. In all comparative studies it is proved the best. Cholestyramine has been advocated for poisoning with warfarin and the super-warfarins.

Activated charcoal

The description 'activated' applied to charcoal relates to the process whereby the number of pores and channels throughout individual particles is greatly increased, correspondingly enlarging the surface area to which poisons may be adsorbed. *In-vitro* studies confirm that charcoal is an effective adsorbent of a wide range of drugs and chemicals and experiments using therapeutic doses of drugs in human volunteers have shown that when given within 1 h of ingestion it can reduce absorption of most drugs commonly taken in overdosage. If given later than 1 h, the efficacy of charcoal is severely reduced. Unfortunately, it is much more difficult to demonstrate its value in clinical poisoning although there is evidence that it is more effective than syrup of ipecacuanha and gastric lavage in preventing absorption after paracetamol overdosage.

Adverse effects

Oral activated charcoal is usually free from serious toxicity but is unpalatable and compliance with treatment may be poor. Vomiting is common and in unconscious patients inhalation into the lungs is a possibility if the airway is not adequately protected. Depending on the preparation used, diarrhoea or constipation may result, the latter occasionally being so severe that intestinal obstruction requiring surgery develops. Rarely, charcoal bezoar formation in the stomach has been reported. Oral antidotes (e.g. methionine) may be strongly adsorbed on to charcoal which should not be administered along with these drugs.

Dosage

Activated charcoal is most easily administered as a finely divided powder in water and is best tolerated if given via a nasogastric tube. The effective ratio of charcoal to estimated amount of poison to be adsorbed is of the order of 10:1. It is therefore most likely to be useful when small quantities of poison produce major effects (e.g. tricyclic antidepressants and theophylline derivatives). In contrast, it is unlikely to be of value when large amounts of poison are required before there is any risk of serious toxicity; for example, 150 g of charcoal would be required to adsorb 15 g of aspirin or paracetamol and few, if any, patients would tolerate this dose. In general, 50 to 100 g should be given to adults who have taken a substantial overdose of a toxic substance within the previous 1 h. If sustained release formulations (e.g. theophylline derivatives) or drugs which delay gastric emptying have been taken (e.g. tricyclic antidepressants and opioid analgesics) the time interval for administration of charcoal can be extended and repeated doses may be indicated (see below).

Methods of elimination

Once a poison has been absorbed and providing there is no antidote, it is reasonable to consider the use of treatments that might speed its elimination from the body. Formerly, forced diuresis, peritoneal and haemodialysis, charcoal haemoperfusion and, less commonly, plasmapheresis were the techniques of choice. In recent years, however, it has been shown that repeated oral doses of activated charcoal given over many hours significantly shorten the plasma half-life of many drugs. Being non-invasive, it is the obvious first measure to be taken to enhance their elimination.

REPEATED DOSES OF ORAL ACTIVATED CHARCOAL

Repeated doses of activated charcoal aid the elimination of some drugs from the circulation by interrupting their enterohepatic circulation and adsorbing that which diffuses into the intestinal juices. The rate of transfer of the latter is dependent upon the blood supply to the gut, the area of mucosa available for transfer, and the concentration gradient of the drug across the mucosa. The adsorptive capacity of charcoal is such that zero concentrations are present in luminal fluid and that the diffusion gradient remains as high as possible. The process has been termed 'gut dialysis' since, in effect, the intestinal mucosa is being used as a semi-permeable membrane. Studies in poisoned patients have shown that giving repeated doses of oral activated charcoal is an effective way of shortening the plasma half-life of carbamazepine, dapsone, phenobarbitone, quinine, salicylate, and theophylline and, in some cases, is as effective as charcoal haemoperfusion. Recommended adult doses of charcoal for this purpose are 50 to 100 g initially, followed by 50 g four-hourly until charcoal appears in the faeces or recovery occurs.

INVASIVE METHODS OF ENHANCING ELIMINATION OF POISONS

Methods such as forced diuresis, peritoneal dialysis, haemodialysis, charcoal haemoperfusion, and plasmapheresis can be used to enhance the elimination of absorbed toxins. However, their use is invasive, either physically or biochemically.

Indications for use

Supportive therapy is all that the vast majority of poisoned patients require. The use of invasive procedures to remove poisons from the circulation is seldom indicated. They should be employed only when (a) clinically significant quantities of the poison can be removed by the technique, (b) the clinical condition of the patient is serious, and (c) the poison is present in the blood in sufficiently high concentrations for significant amounts to be available for removal. In practice there will sometimes be a delay in obtaining the plasma concentration of the poison and a decision to start treatment on clinical grounds alone can be justified if the clinical risks appear to be extreme and the use of the procedure can be reviewed within a few hours. However, it is not valid to use these techniques in hope alone; their use should be confined to ill patients, guided by knowledge of the pharmacokinetic properties of the poison and carefully monitored with appropriate measurements of the concentration of toxin in body fluids as well as clinically.

FORCED DIURESIS

In the past, forced diuresis enjoyed extensive use in the treatment of acute poisoning if only because it did not require special equipment and could be instituted rapidly and in any hospital. However, there was considerable ignorance of its rationale and its use for some toxins was not always justified.

Pharmacokinetic principles

The efficacy of forced diuresis depends on two factors. First, only if the poison is excreted unchanged by the kidney or as active metabolites can one expect its elimination to be enhanced by increasing urine flow. Secondly, since most drugs are partly reabsorbed from the urine as it flows through the renal tubules and, as elsewhere in the body, reabsorption is confined to unionized, lipid-soluble molecules. Increasing the concentration of ionized drug in the urine should reduce reabsorption and further enhance elimination. This is achieved by manipulating urine pH. Thus, elimination of weakly acidic compounds such as salicylates, phenobarbitone, and phenoxyacetate herbicides is enhanced by rendering the urine alkaline and that of amphetamines and phencyclidine by making the urine acid. Most drugs, however, are either degraded by the liver to non-toxic metabolites or have such large volumes of distribution that there is insufficient active drug elimination in urine for forced diuresis to be of any value. Although a small amount of active drug is eliminated in this way and its elimination can be dramatically increased by alkaline diuresis, the amount removed is insignificant compared to that removed by hepatic metabolism. Equally important, it is now generally accepted that alteration of urine pH is more important than urine flow and in recent years there has been a trend away from forcing a diuresis (i.e. infusing large volumes of fluid) to attempting to alter urine pH alone.

FORCED ALKALINE DIURESIS

In practice, inducing an alkaline diuresis is only commonly used in poisoning by salicylates and phenoxyacetate herbicides (Chapter 8.3.8). Even with these toxins, however, its role is diminishing with the advent of repeated oral activated charcoal. The use of alkaline diuresis in salicylate intoxication is discussed in Chapter 8.2.1. If indicated, a suitable regime for adults is to infuse 0.5 litres of 0.9 per cent saline, 0.5 lities of 5 per cent dextrose, and 0.5 litres of 1.26 per cent sodium bicarbonate in rotation at a rate of 0.5 l/h. Urinary pH should be monitored using narrow-range indicator paper and the infusion fluids adjusted to maintain it between 7.5 and 8.5 by substituting bicarbonate for saline or vice versa. A fall in plasma potassium concentration is likely; plasma electrolytes should therefore be monitored and supplements given as necessary.

FORCED ACID DIURESIS

Although, theoretically, induction of an acid diuresis should increase the elimination of basic drugs such as amphetamines, there is seldom any need to use it and no evidence that it is of value in cases of poisoning.

DIALYSIS

Dialysis in acute poisoning is most commonly indicated for the treatment of acute renal failure and only infrequently to increase elimination of poisons. It is an inefficient way of trying to remove most poisons. The rate of elimination across the dialysis membrane depends upon a number of variables including the molecular weight of the toxin, the extent to which it is protein bound, the concentration gradient, and pH of blood and dialysate. Haemodialysis is more efficient than peritoneal dialysis and of value in severe poisoning with salicylates, phenobarbitone, methanol, ethanol ethylene glycol, lithium, and chlorates. Peritoneal dialysis is useful for the removal of the same toxins when haemodialysis is not available or when renal failure complicates poisoning due to phenobarbitone or salicylates.

HAEMOPERFUSION

Although haemoperfusion was a major advance in the treatment of some of the most serious forms of poisoning of 20 years ago, its present day application is extremely limited as a result of the greatly reduced incidence of overdosage with barbiturates, meprobamate, glutethimide, and methaqualone. Unfortunately, it does not remove tricyclic antidepressants. Repeated doses of activated charcoal have been shown to produce similar drug clearances in many cases.

Poisons information services

The general principles of management of acute poisoning outlined in this chapter and in those which follow should provide adequate guidelines for the treatment of most poisoned patients. It will be clear, however, that in many cases there will be additional problems which are not immediately answered. For this reason most countries have established information centres to provide information on the ingredients, toxicity, and treatment of poisoning with a vast range of products and also provide an opportunity to discuss complex and difficult clinical problems with clinicians experienced in the management of cases of poisoning.

8.2 Poisoning by drugs

8.2.1 Poisoning caused by analgesic drugs

T. J. MEREDITH, J. A. VALE, and A. T. PROUDFOOT

Paracetamol (acetaminophen)

Paracetamol has a justified reputation as an effective analgesic which, in therapeutic doses, is thought to be safer than aspirin. Although it was first synthesized at the end of the 19th century, it is only since 1956 that paracetamol has been actively marketed in the United Kingdom; in the United States it has been available since 1952 as acetaminophen. Unlike the case of aspirin, paracetamol overdosage is likely to cause hepatic and renal damage and, in some cases, death from fulminant hepatic failure.

MECHANISM OF TOXICITY

The toxicity of paracetamol is related to its metabolism. In therapeutic doses, 60 to 90 per cent is metabolized by conjugation to form paracetamol glucuronide and sulphate. A much smaller amount (5–10 per cent) is oxidized by mixed function oxidase enzymes to form a highly reactive compound (*N*-acetyl-*p*-benzoquinoneimine, NAPQI) which is then immediately conjugated with glutathione and subsequently excreted as cysteine and mercapturate conjugates. Only 1 to 4 per cent of a therapeutic dose of the drug is excreted unchanged in the urine.

In overdose, larger amounts of paracetamol are metabolized by oxidation because of saturation of the sulphate conjugation pathway. As a result, liver glutathione stores become depleted so that the liver is unable to 'deactivate' the toxic metabolite. The reactive metabolite has a high affinity for cell protein and binds to liver cell macromolecules. However, covalent binding of NAPQI to cell structure nucleophiles is not thought to be directly responsible for paracetamol-induced hepatic necrosis. NAPQI is believed to have two separate but complementary effects. Firstly, it reacts with glutathione, thereby depleting the cell of its normal defence against oxidizing damage. Secondly, it is a potent oxidizing as well as arylating agent; it inactivates key sulphydryl groups in certain enzymes, particularly those controlling calcium homeostasis. Inhibition of membrane calcium translocase activity and impairment of microsomal calcium uptake leads to a marked increase in cytosolic calcium concentration, which causes depolymerization of microtubules and contraction of microfilaments, with consequent disruption of cellular architecture and function. The activity of the mixed function oxidase enzyme system and the size of liver glutathione stores may be modified by pharmacological means.

Paracetamol-induced renal damage probably results from a mechanism similar to that which is responsible for hepatotoxicity, that is, by formation of NAPQI, although in the kidney this is generated by prostaglandin endoperoxide synthetase rather than by cytochrome P450-dependent mixed function oxidases.

CLINICAL FEATURES (TABLE 1)

As would be expected from the mechanism of toxicity, the severity of paracetamol poisoning is dose-related. An absorbed dose of 15 g (200 mg/kg) or more is potentially serious in most patients. There is, however, some variation in individual susceptibility to paracetamol-induced hepatotoxicity and patients with pre-existing liver disease, those with a high alcohol intake, and those receiving enzyme-inducing drugs should be considered to be at greater risk. Individuals with HIV-related disease also appear to be susceptible to paracetamol-induced hepatic damage. It is uncommon for young children to develop paracetamol-induced liver or renal damage, probably because they ingest relatively small amounts in overdose.

Following the ingestion of an overdose of paracetamol, patients usually remain asymptomatic for the first 24 h or, at the most, develop anorexia, nausea, and vomiting. Liver damage is not usually detectable by routine liver function tests until at least 18 h after ingestion of the drug, and hepatic tenderness and abdominal pain are seldom exhibited before the second day. Maximum liver damage, as assessed by plasma

Table 1 *Clinical, biochemical, and haematological features of paracetamol poisoning* (> 200 mg/kg)

Day 1
Asymptomatic
Nausea, vomiting, abdominal pain, anorexia
Day 2
May become asymptomatic
Vomiting
Hepatic tenderness ± generalized abdominal pain
Occasionally, mild jaundice
Day 3 (in severe untreated poisoning)
Jaundice → liver failure → hepatic encephalopathy
Back pain + renal angle tenderness → renal failure
Disseminated intravascular coagulation
Cardiac arrhythmias → cardiac arrest
Pancreatitis
Biochemical and haematological abnormalities
Biochemical
AST/ALT ↑ ↑
Bilirubin ↑
Blood sugar ↓
Creatinine ↑
Lactate ↑
Phosphate ↓
Amylase ↑
Haematological
PT ↑
Platelets ↓
Clotting factors II ↓ V ↓ VII ↓

alanine or aspartate aminotransferase (ALT, AST) activity or prothrombin time, occurs 72 to 96 h after ingestion. Hepatic failure, manifested by jaundice and encephalopathy, may then develop between the third and fifth day (Table 2) with the rate of clinical deterioration reflecting the severity of the overdose. More usually there is prolongation of the prothrombin time and a marked rise in aminotransferase activity without the development of fulminant hepatic failure. Renal failure due to acute tubular necrosis develops in about 25 per cent of patients with severe hepatic damage and in a few without evidence of serious disturbance of liver function. Other features, including hypoglycaemia and hyperglycaemia, cardiac arrhythmias, pancreatitis, gastrointestinal haemorrhage, and cerebral oedema may all occur with hepatic failure due to any cause and are not direct consequences of paracetamol toxicity.

There are two additional metabolic complications of paracetamol overdosage: hyperlactataemia and metabolic acidosis, and hypophosphataemia. Paracetamol can cause metabolic acidosis at two distinct periods after overdosage. Transient hyperlactataemia is frequently found within the first 15 h of ingestion of paracetamol in all but minor overdoses. This appears to be due to inhibition of mitochondrial respiration at the level of ubiquinone and increased lactate production, and may be associated with a metabolic acidosis; it is rarely of clinical consequence, although in very severe paracetamol poisoning (plasma paracetamol concentration > 500 mg/l at 4 h after ingestion) the acidosis may be associated with coma. The second phase of hyperlactataemia and acidosis occurs in those patients who present late and go on to develop hepatic damage; in this instance decreased hepatic lactate clearance appears to be the major cause, compounded by poor peripheral perfusion and increased lactate production. The development of lactic acidosis consequent upon paracetamol-induced liver damage is associated with a poor prognosis.

Hypophosphataemia is a recognized complication of acute liver failure, including that due to paracetamol, and may contribute to morbidity and mortality by inducing mental confusion, irritability, coma, and abnormalities of platelet, white cell and erythrocyte function. Phosphaturia appears to be the principal cause of hypophosphataemia in paracetamol poisoning; it may occur in the absence of fulminant hepatic failure and indicates paracetamol-induced renal tubular damage.

Table 2 *Clinical course of severe (untreated) paracetamol poisoning*

Clinical features	Hours after ingestion
Sudden coma due to hypoglycaemia	24–72
Grade 3 hepatic encephalopathy*	> 72
Grade 4 hepatic encephalopathy*	96–120
Brain-stem coning	> 96

Prediction of liver damage

In the early stages following ingestion of a paracetamol overdose, most patients have few symptoms and no physical signs. There is thus a need for some form of assessment which estimates the risk of liver damage at a time when the liver function tests are still normal. Details of the dose ingested may be used but, in many cases, the history is unreliable and, even when the dose is known for certain, it does not take account of early vomiting and individual variation in response to the drug. However, a single measurement of the plasma paracetamol concentration is an accurate predictor of liver damage provided that it is taken not earlier than 4 h after ingestion of the overdose. Information gained from several large studies has enabled the production of a graph which may be used for prediction of liver damage and which serves as a guide to the need for specific treatment with either oral methionine or intravenous or oral *N*-acetylcysteine (Fig. 1). Sixty per cent of patients whose plasma paracetamol concentration falls above a line drawn between 200 mg/l (1.32 mmol/l) at 4 h and 50 mg/l (0.33 mmol/l) at 12 h after the ingestion of the overdose are likely to sustain liver damage (ALT or AST > 1000 i.u./l) unless specific protective treatment is given. When more than 12 h have elapsed after ingestion, the plasma paracetamol level is still of value and should be considered in conjunction with changes in the prothrombin time (see below) when assessing the prognosis of an individual patient. Patients with pre-existing liver disease, alcohol abusers, and those receiving enzyme-inducing drugs are at greater risk of paracetamol-induced liver damage and treatment should be indicated therefore at lower plasma paracetamol concentrations.

Fig. 1 Graph for use in prediction of liver damage caused by paracetamol and the need for administration of specific protective treatment (see text for further details).

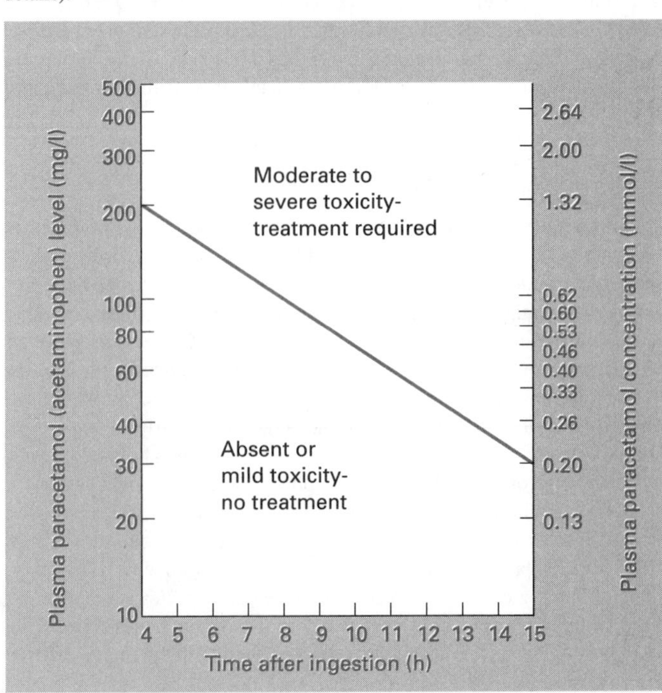

Prognostic factors

The overall mortality of paracetamol poisoning in untreated patients is only of the order of 5 per cent. The prothrombin time is usually the first liver function test to become abnormal and, for this reason, it is of particular value in assessing the prognosis of an individual patient. The more rapid the increase in prothrombin time, the worse the prognosis of the patient. A prothrombin time of more than 20 s at 24 h after ingestion indicates that significant hepatic damage has been sustained, and a peak prothrombin time of more than 180 s is associated with a chance of survival of less than 8 per cent.

Acid–base disturbances are also a good guide to prognosis. Systemic acidosis developing more than 24 h after overdose indicates a poor prognosis; patients with a blood pH below 7.30 at this time have only a 15 per cent chance of survival. In addition, a rise in serum creatinine concentration is associated with poor survival; patients with a serum creatinine concentration above 300 μmol/l have only a 23 per cent chance of survival.

A recent study of prognostic indicators in established paracetamol-induced fulminant hepatic failure treated conventionally compared the sensitivity (percentage of patients who died with a positive test), predictive accuracy (percentage of patients whose outcome was predicted accurately), positive predictive value (percentage of patients with a positive test who died), and specificity (percentage of survivors with a negative test) of measurement of Factors V and VIII with conventional tests. (Factor V is vitamin K-dependent and levels fall in liver failure; levels of Factor VIII rise in patients with liver failure.) An admission pH below 7.30 with a serum creatinine concentration above 300 μmol/l and a prothrombin time above 100 s in Grade III–IV encephalopathy has a sensitivity, predictive accuracy, positive predictive value and specificity of 91, 86, 83, and 91, respectively. However, a Factor VIII/V ratio above 30 had comparable values of 91, 95, 100, and 100.

MANAGEMENT

Gastric lavage may be of value if performed within 1 h of overdose, though one clinical study suggests that activated charcoal is superior, but its use then precludes the administration of oral antidotes because of their adsorption by charcoal. Parenteral fluid replacement should be given for the first 1 to 2 days after overdose if nausea persists or vomiting occurs.

From knowledge of the mechanism of toxicity, it may be predicted that replenishment of glutathione stores would be of value. Two substances, methionine and *N*-acetylcysteine have emerged as effective protective agents, provided that they are administered within 8 to 10 h of ingestion of the overdose (Table 3). Both substances act by replenishing cellular glutathione stores, though *N*-acetylcysteine may also repair oxidative damage caused by NAPQI either directly or, more probably, through the generation of cysteine and/or glutathione. It may also act as a source of sulphate and so 'unsaturate' sulphate conjugation. Methionine appears more effective when given orally than when administered intravenously, whereas oral *N*-acetylcysteine induces vomiting in most patients, the intravenous route therefore being preferred. Both substances must be given within 8 to 10 h of ingestion of the paracetamol overdose to prevent the development of hepatic damage completely; thereafter, the protective effects decline rapidly. Up to 10 per cent of patients treated with intravenous *N*-acetylcysteine develop rash, angioedema, hypotension, and bronchospasm. These reactions which follow the bolus dose of *N*-acetylcysteine are seldom serious and no fatalities have so far been reported in those receiving the regimen outlined in Table 3. If such reactions do occur, the infusions should be discontinued for 1 to 2 h and an antihistamine such as chlorpheniramine or terfenadine should be given.

Enhanced elimination by forced diuresis or dialysis has no role to play in the management of paracetamol poisoning. Haemoperfusion has been advocated for the treatment of patients who present too late for the effective administration of protective agents but before the onset of liver failure. There is no substantive evidence at present that the use of this technique confers any benefit.

Table 3 *Treatment of paracetamol poisoning*

Methionine (orally) 2.5 g initially, then 2.5 g 4-hourly for a further three doses. Total dose 10 g methionine over 12 h
N-acetylcysteine (intravenously) 150 mg/kg over 15 min, then 50 mg/kg in 500 ml of 5% dextrose in the next 4 h and 100 mg/kg in 1000 ml of 5% dextrose over the ensuing 16 h. Total dose 300 mg/kg over 20 h
N-acetylcysteine (orally) 140 mg/kg initially, then 70 mg/kg every 4 h for 17 additional doses. Total dose 1330 mg/kg over 72 h

Note: In patients with liver failure *N*-acetycysteine may be continued intravenously (100 mg/kg in 1000 ml of 5% dextrose over 16 h) until recovery occurs.

Fortunately, only a minority of patients present more than 10 to 24 h after an overdose of paracetamol but, in these cases, the morbidity and mortality is greater and the correct treatment is that intended to prevent or support hepatic failure, though the use of *N*-acetylcysteine has been advocated. Ten per cent glucose solution should be administered to prevent the onset of hypoglycaemia. Correction of severe coagulation abnormalities (prothrombin time > 100 s) may be attempted using fresh frozen plasma. Although there is no evidence that this prevents gastrointestinal haemorrhage, bleeding can be catastrophic if it does occur. Fresh frozen plasma will also be required to cover the insertion of intracranial pressure monitoring apparatus. An H_2-receptor antagonist will reduce the risk of gastrointestinal bleeding from 'stress' ulceration/erosions. If acute renal failure supervenes, then this should be managed conventionally.

Current evidence suggests that if fulminant hepatic failure does supervene, the use of continued intravenous *N*-acetylcysteine (see Table 3 for regimen) is likely to reduce morbidity and mortality. This beneficial effect is observed even after the onset of encephalopathy and other signs of severe liver damage and has been shown to be associated with an increase in oxygen tissue delivery and consumption. It has been suggested that this effect is due to improved microcirculatory blood flow as a result of restoration of full activity of endothelium-derived relaxing factor by replenishment of sulphydryl groups. In one study the survival rate in 25 patients with paracetamol-induced fulminant hepatic failure was 20 per cent, with an incidence of cerebral oedema and of hypotension requiring inotropic support of 68 and 80 per cent, respectively. With *N*-acetylcysteine, the comparable figures in 25 matched patients were 48 per cent (survival rate), 40 per cent (cerebral oedema), and 48 per cent (hypotension) respectively.

Liver transplantation has been performed successfully in patients with paracetamol-induced fulminant hepatic failure, using criteria outlined above (see under Prognostic factors) to identify those individuals who would otherwise be likely to die. However, there has been no formal study to compare the value of transplantation with *N*-acetylcysteine in fulminant hepatic failure.

FURTHER READING

Keays, P., *et al.* (1991). Intravenous acetylcysteine in paracetamol induced fulminant hepatic failure: a prospective controlled trial. *British Medical Journal*, **303,** 1026–9.

Meredith, T.J. and Vale, J.A. (1992). Poisoning due to paracetamol, salicylates, and diflunisal. In *Therapeutic applications of NSAIDs: subpopulations and new formulations.* (ed. J.P. Famaey and H.E. Paulus), pp. 67–96. Marcel Dekker, New York.

O'Grady, J.G., *et al.* (1991). Liver transplantation after paracetamol overdose. *British Medical Journal*, **303,** 221–3.

Pereira, L.M.M.B., Langley, P.G., Hayllar, K.M., and Williams, R. (1989). Coagulation factor V and VIII/V ratio as predictors of outcome in paracetamol induced fulminant hepatic failure: relation to other prognostic indicators. *Gut*, **33,** 98–102.

Prescott, L.F., Illingworth, R.N., Critchley, J.A.J.H., Stewart, M.J., Adam, R.D., and Proudfoot, A.T. (1979). Intravenous *N*-acetylcysteine: the treatment of choice for paracetamol poisoning. *British Medical Journal*, **2,** 1097–100.

Rumack, B.H. Peterson, R.C., Koch, G.G., and Amara I.A. (1981). Acetaminophen overdose. *Archives of Internal Medicine*, **141,** 380–5.

Vale, J.A., Meredith, T.J., and Goulding, R. (1981). Treatment of acetaminophen poisoning: the use of oral methionine. *Archives of Internal Medicine*, **141,** 394–6.

Salicylates

Despite the introduction of alternative 'mild' analgesic agents in recent years, aspirin (acetylsalicylic acid) is still used commonly and is found in most household medicine cabinets. It is not surprising, therefore, that aspirin poisoning is a common cause for admission to hospital. Although accidental consumption of aspirin by young children has been reduced in both the United Kingdom and the United States as the result of new legal requirements for child-resistant packaging, iatrogenic overdose in children is not uncommon. Moreover, aspirin remains the drug of choice for many adults who choose deliberately to poison themselves. Although ingestion of aspirin tablets represents the most frequent cause of salicylate poisoning, percutaneous absorption of salicylic acid (used in keratolytic agents), and ingestion of methyl salicylate ('oil of wintergreen') are occasionally responsible. Methyl salicylate is particularly toxic because of rapid absorption, and one teaspoonful (5 ml) contains the equivalent of 6.9 g of aspirin. In neonates, infants, and children, salicylate intoxication may occur inadvertently through placental transfer, breast milk, or by the application of teething gels to the gums.

Studies in the United States have suggested an association between Reye's syndrome and the use of salicylates. Salicylates should not be used therefore in children under the age of 12 years unless specifically indicated for a childhood rheumatic condition.

PHARMACOKINETICS AND TOXICITY

In therapeutic doses, aspirin is absorbed rapidly from the stomach and small intestine, but in overdose, absorption may occur more slowly and the plasma salicylate concentration may continue to rise for up to 24 h.

The pharmacokinetics of elimination of aspirin are an important determinant in the development of salicylate toxicity. The biotransformation pathways concerned with the formation of salicyluric acid and salicylphenolic glucuronide (Fig. 2) are saturable, a fact which has the following clinical consequences: (i) the time needed to eliminate a given fraction of a dose increases with increasing dose; (ii) the steady-state plasma concentration of salicylate, particularly that of the pharmacologically active non-protein-bound fraction, increases more than proportionately with increasing dose; and (iii) as the metabolic pathways of elimination become saturated, renal excretion of salicylic acid becomes increasingly important, a pathway which is extremely sensitive to changes in urinary pH.

Fig. 2 The principal biotransformation pathways of aspirin.

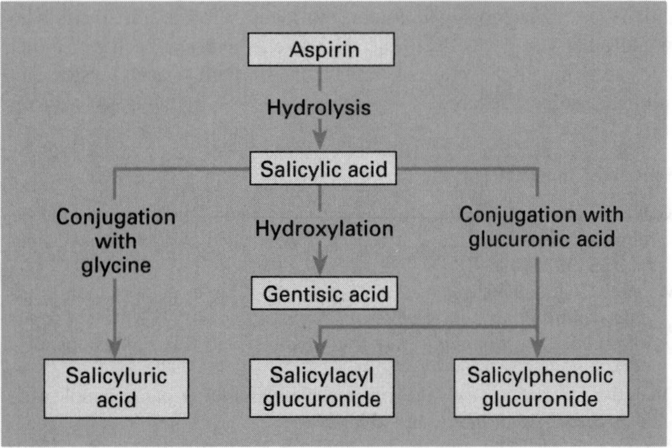

METABOLIC EFFECTS

When ingested in overdose, salicylates directly stimulate the respiratory centre to produce both increased depth and rate of respiration, thereby causing a respiratory alkalosis (Fig. 3). At least part of this effect on the respiratory centre has been shown to be due to local uncoupling of oxidative phosphorylation within the brain-stem. In an attempt by the body to compensate, bicarbonate, accompanied by sodium, potassium, and water, is excreted in the urine. Dehydration and hypokalaemia result, but more importantly, the loss of bicarbonate diminishes the buffering capacity of the body and allows an acidosis to develop more easily. Very high concentrations of salicylates in the brain depress the respiratory centre and may further contribute to the development of acidaemia.

Simultaneously, a variable degree of metabolic acidosis develops, not only because of the presence of salicylic acid itself, but also because of interference with carbohydrate, lipid, protein, and amino acid metabolism by salicylate ions (Fig. 3). Inhibition of citric acid cycle enzymes causes an increase in circulating lactic and pyruvic acids. Salicylates stimulate fat metabolism and cause increased production of the ketone bodies, β-hydroxybutyric acid, acetoacetic acid, and acetone. Dehydration and lack of food intake because of vomiting further contribute to the development of ketosis. Protein catabolism is accelerated, protein synthesis diminished, and aminotransferases (responsible for the interconversion of amino acids) inhibited. Increased circulating blood levels of amino acids result, together with aminoaciduria; this latter feature is further enhanced by inhibition of active tubular reabsorption of amino acids. The aminoaciduria increases the solute load on the kidneys and, thereby, increases water loss from the body.

A primary toxic effect of salicylates in overdose is uncoupling of oxidative phosphorylation (Fig. 3). ATP-dependent reactions are inhibited and oxygen utilization and carbon dioxide production increased. Energy normally used for the conversion of inorganic phosphate to ATP is dissipated as heat. Hyperpyrexia and sweating result causing further dehydration. Fluid loss is enhanced because salicylates stimulate the chemoreceptor trigger zone and induce nausea and vomiting and, thereby, diminish oral fluid intake. If dehydration is sufficiently marked, low cardiac output and oliguria will aggravate the metabolic acidosis already present which, if severe, can itself diminish cardiac output.

Glucose metabolism also suffers as a result of uncoupled oxidative phosphorylation because of increased tissue glycolysis and peripheral demand for glucose (Fig. 3). This is seen principally in skeletal muscle and may cause hypoglycaemia. The brain appears to be particularly sensitive to this effect and neuroglycopenia can occur in the presence of a normal blood sugar level when the rate of utilization exceeds the rate at which glucose can be supplied from the blood. Increased metabolism and peripheral demand for glucose activates hypothalamic centres resulting in increased adrenocortical stimulation and release of adrenaline. Increased glucose 6-phosphatase activity and hepatic glycogenolysis contribute to the hyperglycaemia which is sometimes seen following the ingestion of large amounts of salicylate. Increased circulating adrenocorticosteroids exacerbate fluid and electrolyte imbalance.

Although rarely a practical problem, salicylate intoxication may be accompanied by hypoprothrombinaemia due to a warfarin-like action of salicylates on the physiologically important vitamin K_1 epoxide cycle. Vitamin K_1 is necessary for the post-translational γ-carboxylation of specific glutamyl residues on clotting factors II, VII, IX, and X. Vitamin K is converted to vitamin K 2,3-epoxide and then reconverted to vitamin

K_1 by a reductase enzyme competitively inhibited by warfarin and salicylates.

CLINICAL FEATURES AND ASSESSMENT OF SEVERITY OF SALICYLATE INTOXICATION

The dose of salicylate ingested and the age of the patient (see below) are the principal determinants of the severity of an overdose, but prior therapeutic administration of aspirin will increase the toxicity of an acutely ingested overdose. The plasma salicylate concentration should be determined on admission, but it is important to repeat it 2 h later to make sure that the concentration is not continuing to rise because of slow absorption. If the concentration has risen, the level should be repeated after a further 2 h. Generally speaking, plasma salicylate levels that lie between 300 and 500 mg/l 6 h after ingestion of an overdose are associated with only mild toxicity, levels between 500 and 700 mg/l are associated with moderate toxicity, and levels in excess of 700 mg/l confirm severe poisoning.

Salicylate poisoning of any severity is associated with sweating, vomiting, epigastric pain, tinnitus, and deafness (Table 4). The latter features are due to increased labyrinthine pressure and/or an effect on the hair cells of the cochlea. Early loss of consciousness does not occur following the ingestion of a salicylate overdose, unless an hypnotic or sedative drug has been taken as well.

Young children quickly develop a metabolic acidosis following the ingestion of aspirin in overdose but, by the age of 12 years, the usual adult picture of a combined dominant respiratory alkalosis and mild metabolic acidosis is seen. Dehydration and electrolyte imbalance occur quickly due to the combination of the above factors. To some extent, the presence of an alkalaemia protects against serious salicylate toxicity because salicylate remains ionized and unable to penetrate cell membranes easily. Development of acidaemia allows salicylates to penetrate tissues more readily and leads, in particular, to CNS toxicity characterized by excitement, tremor, delirium, convulsions, and stupor and coma. Very high plasma salicylate concentrations cause paralysis of the respiratory centre and cardiovascular collapse due to vasomotor depression.

Table 4 *Clinical features of salicylate poisoning*

Nausea, vomiting, and epigastric discomfort
Irritability, tremor, tinnitus, deafness, blurring of vision
Hyperpyrexia, sweating, dehydration
Tachypnoea and hyperpnoea
Non-cardiogenic pulmonary oedema
Acute renal failure
Mixed respiratory alkalosis and metabolic acidosis (except in children who usually develop metabolic acidosis alone)
Hypokalaemia, hypernatraemia, or hyponatraemia
Hyperglycaemia or hypoglycaemia
Hypoprothrombinaemia (rare)
Confusion, delirium, stupor, and coma (in severe cases)

Pulmonary oedema is seen occasionally in salicylate poisoning, and although this is often due to fluid overload as a result of treatment, it may be non-cardiac and occur in the presence of hypovolaemia. In these circumstances, the pulmonary oedema fluid has the same protein and electrolyte composition as plasma, suggesting increased pulmonary vascular permeability. It is possible that an effect of aspirin on prostaglandin or leukotriene synthesis and platelet function is responsible for the increased microvascular leak of proteins and fluid.

Although aspirin overdose may be complicated by inhibition of platelet aggregation and hypoprothrombinaemia, gastric erosions and gastrointestinal bleeding are rare following salicylate overdose. Oliguria is sometimes seen in patients following the ingestion of salicylates in overdose. The most common cause is dehydration but, rarely, acute renal failure or inappropriate secretion of antidiuretic hormone may occur.

Whilst the urinary pH may be alkaline in the early stages of salicylate overdose, it soon becomes acid. Measurement of arterial blood gases, pH, and standard bicarbonate may show a respiratory alkalosis in the early stages of salicylate intoxication accompanied by the development of a metabolic acidosis. The plasma potassium concentration is often low; rarely, the blood sugar may be high.

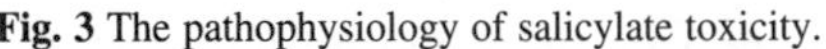
Fig. 3 The pathophysiology of salicylate toxicity.

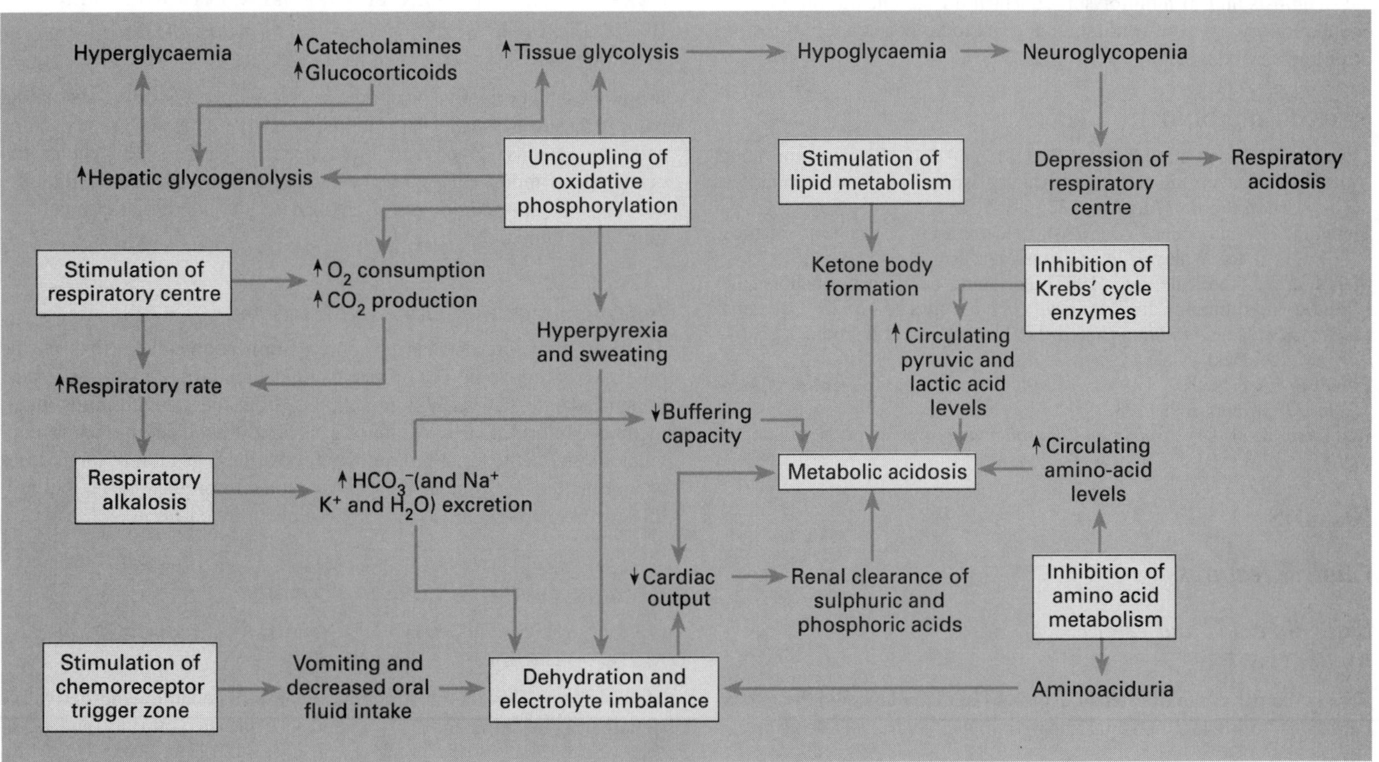

MANAGEMENT (TABLE 5)

Gastric lavage may be of value if performed within 1 h of overdose. Exceptionally, significant amounts of salicylate may be retrieved if lavage is performed later than 1 h, as tablets of aspirin may adhere to each other to form a large mass in the stomach resulting in slow absorption. Activated charcoal not only effectively adsorbs salicylate and reduces absorption but also increase salicylate elimination.

Fluid and electrolyte replacement is particularly important and special attention should be paid to potassium supplementation. Severe metabolic acidosis requires at least partial correction with bicarbonate. Sedatives and respiratory depressant drugs should be avoided because they may hasten the development of acidaemia and CNS toxicity. Mild cases of salicylate poisoning may be managed with either oral or parenteral fluid and electrolyte replacement only. Patients who exhibit symptoms or signs of salicylism and whose blood salicylate levels are in excess of 500 mg/l (or lower if acidaemia is present) should receive specific elimination therapy. An alkaline diuresis is most often used for this purpose. The pH of the urine during this procedure is of far greater importance than the volume of urine excreted. The urinary pH should be in excess of 7.5 and should ideally lie between 8.0 and 8.5. If it proves difficult to achieve this degree of urinary alkalinization without causing the blood pH to rise above 7.6, then any potassium deficit should be fully corrected.

As an alternative, and if the patient is not vomiting, repeat dose activated charcoal (50 g 4-hourly) may be employed orally; good salicylate clearance rates may be achieved. Rarely, patients prove refractory to alkaline diuresis and/or charcoal therapy, or these therapies may be contraindicated. Haemodialysis may then prove necessary to remove salicylate from the body. Haemodialysis is the treatment of choice for severely poisoned patients, particularly those with features of central nervous system toxicity and metabolic acidosis and has the advantage that it enables simultaneous correction of acid–base and fluid and electrolyte imbalances.

Pulmonary oedema occasionally complicates salicylate toxicity. Fluid overload should be excluded so far as possible but, if increased pulmonary vascular permeability is suspected, measurement of the pulmonary artery wedge pressure may be needed both for confirmation of the diagnosis and to monitor subsequent fluid administration. Positive end expiratory pressure ventilation appears to be beneficial in this form of pulmonary oedema.

FURTHER READING

Chapman, B.J. and Proudfoot, A.T. (1989). Adult salicylate poisoning: deaths and outcome in patients with high plasma salicylate concentrations. *Quarterly Journal of Medicine*, **72,** 699–707.

Meredith, T.J. and Vale, J.A. (1984). Epidemiology of analgesic overdose in England and Wales. *Human Toxicology*, **3,** 61S–74S.

Meredith, T.J. and Vale, J.A. (1992). Poisoning due to paracetamol, salicylates, and diflunisal. In *Therapeutic applications of NSAIDs: subpopulations and new formulations*. (ed. J.P. Famaey and H.E. Paulus), pp. 67–96. Marcel Dekker, New York.

Proudfoot, A.T. (1983). Toxicity of salicylates. *American Journal of Medicine*, **75,** (Suppl.), 99–103.

Rainsford, K. (1984). *Aspirin and the salicylates*. Butterworths, London.

NSAIDS

Clinical features

Salicylic acids and esters

BENORYLATE

This is the paracetamol ester of aspirin (4-acetamidophenyl 2-acetoxybenzoate); following intestinal absorption, it is hydrolysed to paracetamol and salicylic acid. The clinical features of poisoning are therefore due to these last compounds; the effects of salicylate tend to predominate.

Table 5 *Treatment of salicylate poisoning*

Gastric aspiration and lavage up to 1 h after ingestion
Correction of dehydration either orally or parenterally
Correction of hypokalaemia
Correction of hypoglycaemia
Correction of severe metabolic acidosis with intravenous bicarbonate
Tepid sponging for hyperpyrexia
Alkaline diuresis if blood salicylate level > 500 mg/l, (particularly if metabolic acidosis is present)
Consider haemodialysis if neurological features are present and blood salicylate concentration > 700 mg/l or if severe acidosis supervenes)

DIFLUNISAL (5-(2,4-DIFLUOROPHENYL) SALICYLIC ACID)

Diflunisal is a potent analgesic and antipyretic drug. Ingestion in overdose may cause nausea, vomiting, and diarrhoea; in more serious cases, tinnitus, hyperventilation, drowsiness, sweating, tachycardia, and hypotension can also develop. Coma, cardiorespiratory arrest and death have been described.

Phenylacetic (arylacetic) acid derivatives

ALCLOFENAC, DICLOFENAC, FENTIAZAC

Phenylacetic acid derivative poisoning is less serious and headache, dizziness, nausea, and abdominal discomfort are the most common clinical features. It is possible that gastrointestinal bleeding, confusion, hypotonia, tinnitus and auditory hallucinations may also occur.

Phenylpropionic (arylpropionic) acid derivatives

CARPROFEN, FENBUFEN, FENOPROFEN, FLURBIPROFEN, IBUPROFEN, KETOPROFEN, NAPROXEN, PIRPROFEN, TIAPROFENIC ACID

Propionic acid derivative poisoning causes nausea, vomiting, abdominal pain, drowsiness, headache, tinnitus, ataxia, stupor, and, rarely, coma and convulsions. Hypoventilation, bronchospasm, and hypotension occur; more importantly, gastrointestinal haemorrhage and renal failure are rare but reported complications. These and additional clinical features are summarized in Table 6.

Indomethacin, sulindac, and tolmetin

There are far more data on poisoning from indomethacin than on the other two compounds. The principal clinical features of overdose appear to be headache, nausea, abdominal pain, drowsiness, and tinnitus. Indomethacin and sulindac may induce gastrointestinal bleeding; coma, convulsions and acute renal failure may follow the ingestion of large doses of indomethacin. Sulindac has been reported to produce acute, but rapidly reversible, agranulocytosis following an overdose.

Fenamic (anthranilic) acid derivatives

FLUFENAMIC ACID, MECLOFENAMIC ACID, MEFENAMIC ACID, TOLFENAMIC ACID

Mefenamic acid is the most common cause of fenamic acid derivative (fenamate) poisoning and is associated with nausea, vomiting, and, occa-

Table 6 *Clinical features of poisoning from phenylpropionic acid derivatives*

Nausea, vomiting, abdominal pain and tenderness, haematemesis
Headache, tinnitus, hyperventilation, sinus tachycardia
Haematuria, proteinuria, renal angle tenderness, acute renal failure
Hypotension, hypothermia, hypoprothrombinaemia
Drowsiness, coma, respiratory depression
Nystagmus, diplopia

Table 7 *Clinical features of poisoning from phenylbutazone and oxyphenbutazone*

Nausea, vomiting, abdominal pain, gastrointestinal haemorrhage, diarrhoea
Restlessness, agitation, disorientation, hyperthermia, tinnitus, deafness
Respiratory alkalosis (due to hyperventilation), metabolic acidosis, hyperglycaemia, sodium and water retention
Hypotension, sinus tachycardia, cardiorespiratory collapse, sometimes followed by cardiac arrest
Coma, convulsions, nystagmus, hypertonia, hyper-reflexia, extensor plantar responses
Hepatic dysfunction, cholestatic jaundice
Acute renal failure
Hypoprothrombinaemia, thrombocytopenia, leucopenia, leucocytosis, haematuria, red discoloration of urine (due to metabolite)

sionally, bloody diarrhoea. Drowsiness, dizziness, and headaches are common and hyper-reflexia, muscle twitching, convulsions, cardiorespiratory arrest, hypoprothrombinaemia, and acute renal failure have been reported. In a study of 29 cases of mefenamic acid poisoning, convulsions were noted in 38 per cent of patients, although only rarely were they persistent.

Benzotriazine derivatives

AZAPROPAZONE

Although azapropazone is a derivative of pyrazolinedione in much the same way as phenylbutazone, it has been argued that it should be classified separately because of structural, spectroscopic and chemical differences. Certainly, the clinical features of toxicity following overdosage appear very different to those of phenylbutazone; in particular, bone marrow suppression does not occur. Clinical features of azapropazone poisoning include nausea, vomiting, epigastric pain and haematemesis; giddiness, abnormal limb movements, hyperventilation, coma, and acute renal failure have also been reported.

Pyrazolones and pyrazolidines

FEPRAZONE, OXYPHENBUTAZONE, PHENYLBUTAZONE

Poisoning due to pyrazolones may be serious, and it is usually due to phenylbutazone. This may become less common now that use of oxyphenbutazone and phenylbutazone has been restricted in some countries. Minor overdoses cause nausea, vomiting, abdominal pain, and drowsiness. More seriously poisoned patients may develop life-threatening complications (Table 7).

Table 8 *Clinical features of piroxicam poisoning*

Nausea, vomiting, diarrhoea, abdominal (often epigastric) pain
Gastrointestinal bleeding (due to peptic erosions)
Dizziness, blurred vision, excitability, hyperventilation
Hyper-reflexia, coma, convulsions
Haematuria, proteinuria, acute renal failure
Hepatic dysfunction, hypoprothrombinaemia

Aminophenazone, antipyrine, metamizole, and propyphenazone

Aminophenazone (aminopyrine, amidopyrine), antipyrine (phenazone), metamizole (dipyrine), and propyphenazone remain available in some countries, often as 'over-the-counter' remedies. Following ingestion of these compounds there is progressive impairment of consciousness, convulsions occurring with aminopyrine and propyphenazone. Sudden respiratory arrest can ensue and may be followed by cardiac arrest which is induced both by hypoxia and a direct toxic effect on the myocardium and conduction system. Less commonly, hepatorenal damage is observed.

Floctafenine and glafenine

Glafenine is a 4-amino-7-chloro derivative of quinolone and has been widely used in Europe for many years as a non-steroidal analgesic agent. Floctafenine is a derivative of glafenine with some anti-inflammatory activity as well as analgesic properties. Glafenine has a particular propensity to cause renal failure when taken in overdose, and in one large series it occurred in 30 per cent of cases. Renal failure tends to be accompanied by oliguria or anuria together with lumbar pain; renal biopsy may be normal or may show evidence of interstitial or tubular necrosis. Recovery is the rule although a period of haemodialysis may be required. A direct nephrotoxic effect appears to be responsible in the majority of cases, although in some cases renal failure appears to have been precipitated by hypotension (due to anaphylaxis) or haemolysis. Floctafenine toxicity appears to be similar to that of glafenine.

Oxicams

PIROXICAM

Piroxicam is structurally distinct from other NSAIDs. The clinical features of piroxicam overdose are summarized in Table 8.

Indole acetic acid derivatives

ETODOLAC

Clinical features of toxicity include hypoprothrombinaemia and neutropenia; a false positive test for urinary bilirubin may be found, due to phenolic metabolites of etodolac.

Management

Activated charcoal adsorbs propionic acid derivatives, fenamates, and phenylbutazone, and 50 to 100 g may reasonably be left in the stomach after gastric lavage in poisoning by these and other NSAIDs if the patient presents less than 1 h after overdose. Diazepam, (5–10 mg intravenously) should be given for convulsions. H_2-receptor antagonists are often administered prophylactically, though there is no definite evidence that their use prevents the development of gastrointestinal bleeding. As most NSAIDs are highly protein-bound and extensively metabolized, forced diuresis, dialysis, and haemoperfusion are unlikely to enhance elimination significantly, though this approach has been advocated in the case of phenylbutazone poisoning. Repeated doses of oral activated charcoal (50 g 4- hourly) are likely to increase the non-renal elimination of propionic acid derivatives, fenamates, and phenylbutazone.

FURTHER READING

Meredith, T.J. and Vale, J.A. (1992). Poisoning due to NSAIDs. In *Therapeutic applications of NSAIDs. Subpopulations and new formulations*. (ed. J.P. Famaey and H.E. Paulus), pp. 67–96. Marcel Dekker, New York.

Opiates

Acute opioid overdose occurs commonly in 'addicts', in whom the presence of venepuncture marks and thrombosed veins in the arms and legs should prompt the diagnosis. The opioid group of drugs includes buprenorphine, codeine, dihydrocodeine, dextromoramide, dextropropoxyphene, diamorphine (heroin), dipipanone, diphenoxylate, etorphine, loperamide, methadone, morphine, pentazocine, and pethidine.

CLINICAL FEATURES

The cardinal signs of opioid overdose are pinpoint pupils, reduced respiratory rate (often accompanied by cyanosis), and coma. The depressant effects of opioids are exacerbated by the concomitant ingestion of alcohol; for example, the ingestion of dextropropoxyphene in excess together with alcohol may be followed by sudden, severe respiratory depression. These effects are most marked when 'non-addicts' ingest dextropropoxyphene or dihydrocodeine in overdose. Hypotension, due to peripheral vasodilation, occurs in less than 10 per cent of cases. Paradoxically, hypertension may accompany pentazocine overdose. Hypothermia and hypoglycaemia may also complicate the clinical picture of opioid poisoning.

Heroin (diamorphine) is the opioid most frequently abused. It is self-administered by intravenous injection ('main-lining'), inhalation (smoking), or via the nose ('snorting'). As many as 50 per cent of heroin overdose victims develop non-cardiogenic pulmonary oedema, the majority of whom, in turn, develop bacterial pneumonia. The prognosis is particularly poor in this group of patients. It should be noted, though, that any opioid may cause non-cardiogenic pulmonary oedema.

Although skeletal muscles are usually flaccid in opiate overdose, codeine, dextropropoxyphene, and pethidine cause increased muscle tone, twitching, and convulsions. Rhabdomyolysis has been reported in association with poisoning due to diamorphine, dihydrocodeine, dipipanone, methadone, and morphine. Hyperkalaemia, hyperuricaemia, acute tubular necrosis, and renal failure may then supervene.

Diphenoxylate is used as an antidiarrhoeal agent in conjunction with atropine, and paediatric poisoning due to the ingestion of this antidiarrhoeal preparation is not uncommon.

MANAGEMENT

The treatment of choice in opioid overdose is naloxone, a pure narcotic antagonist with no intrinsic agonist activity. Naloxone is used to reverse severe respiratory depression and coma due to opioid poisoning. The adult dose is 0.4 to 1.2 mg, given either intravenously or, less satisfactorily, intramuscularly; the dose in children is 5 to 10 μg/kg body weight. If the diagnosis of opioid poisoning is correct, the patient should improve within 1 min with an increase in respiratory rate, an improvement in the level of consciousness and dilation of the pupils. In severe opioid poisoning, larger initial doses of naloxone (e.g. 2.4 mg) may be required to obtain the desired response. The duration of action of naloxone is often less than that of the drug taken in overdose and, for this reason, careful observation of the patient is necessary. Repeated doses of naloxone should be given as required.

In opioid-dependent subjects, naloxone may rarely precipitate a withdrawal syndrome similar to that seen after the abrupt withdrawal of opioids (except that it occurs within minutes of administration of the naloxone). The severity and duration of the syndrome are related to the dose of the antagonist and the degree of dependence but it usually subsides within 2 h. Ventricular tachyarrhythmias have been observed during acute withdrawal from opioids induced by naloxone.

Buprenorphine, an opioid agonist–antagonist analgesic similar to pentazocine, is unusual in that the analgesic and respiratory depressant effects of the drug are only partially reversed by naloxone. Although doxapram may be used to stimulate respiration, assisted ventilation may be required in cases of severe buprenorphine poisoning.

Gastric aspiration and lavage and the administration of activated charcoal may be of value if an opioid has been ingested in overdose and presentation is early.

The development of non-cardiogenic pulmonary oedema may necessitate the use of assisted ventilation with positive end-expiratory pressure (PEEP); antibiotics will be required to treat secondary bacterial infection. Hyperkalaemia and renal failure, as a result of rhabdomyolysis, should be treated conventionally.

8.2.2 Poisoning from antidepressants, hypnotics, antihistamines, anticonvulsants, and antiparkinsonian drugs

A. T. PROUDFOOT, J. A. VALE, AND T. J. MEREDITH

Tricyclic antidepressants and benzodiazepines, the ubiquitous hypnotics and sedatives, are the major causes of clinical problems with drugs which depress the central nervous system. In many countries, barbiturates have now all but disappeared and should seldom be encountered in overdosage. Others such as glutethimide, methaqualone, and ethchlorvynol are no longer available. However, meprobamate and chloral hydrate and its related compounds retain limited popularity.

Poisoning from antidepressants

At present, on average, one person dies from overdosage with tricyclic antidepressants, alone or in combination with other agents, each day in England and Wales. There are two main reasons for this. First, these drugs are still the most widely used for the treatment of depression and secondly, they are given to patients who are depressed and, therefore, intrinsically more likely to poison themselves.

Tricyclic antidepressants

Tricyclic antidepressants have complex actions which account for the diverse nature of the features seen after overdosage. They block the reuptake of noradrenaline into peripheral and intracerebral neurones thereby increasing the concentration of monoamines in these areas. They also have anticholinergic actions and class 1 antiarrhythmic (quinidine-like) activity.

CLINICAL FEATURES

Features of poisoning typically appear within 30 to 60 min after ingestion of an overdose and usually reach maximum intensity in 4 to 12 h.

Drowsiness, sinus tachycardia, dry mouth, dilated pupils, urinary retention, increased reflexes, and extensor plantar responses are the most common features of mild poisoning. Severe intoxication leads to coma, often with divergent strabismus secondary to internuclear ophthalmoplegia, and to convulsions in about 6 per cent of cases. In deep coma the plantar, oculocephalic, and oculovestibular reflexes may be temporarily abolished. Skin blisters and rhabdomyolysis may be present.

Sinus tachycardia, secondary to loss of vagal tone, is very common and the dose-related quinidine-like action decreases myocardial contractility and delays conduction particularly in the bundle of His and the more peripheral ventricular conduction system. As a result the ECG is often bizarre. The PR and QRS intervals increase and the P waves diminish in amplitude and may be completely obscured by the preceding T wave. These changes, in conjunction with the increased heart rate, not infrequently make differentiation between ventricular tachycardia and supraventricular tachycardia with aberrant conduction difficult, if not impossible. Serious arrhythmias, particularly ventricular tachycardia, sometimes of the *torsade-de-pointes* variety, occur in only about 4 per cent of cases. The blood pressure and cardiac output fall due to a combination of arrhythmias, negative inotropic effects, and the relative hypovolaemia which is seen in many types of poisoning. The combined effect is to produce metabolic acidosis and cardiorespiratory depression which are the major causes of death.

TREATMENT

The great majority of patients poisoned with tricyclic antidepressants recover with no more sophisticated measures than those indicated under supportive therapy. Potentially lethal complications such as convulsions and arrhythmias are most common within 6 h of overdosage. It is uncommon for coma to last for more than 24 h and most severely poisoned patients recover consciousness within 48 h.

Subject to the conditions outlined above, gastric lavage should be considered in adults when more than 250 mg of the drug has been taken, though the results from clinical studies are disappointing overall. Absorption of drug from the gut may also be reduced by the oral administration of activated charcoal given as a drink or left in the stomach after gastric lavage. A dose of 50 to 100 g should be sufficient in most adults, though after massive overdoses up to 200 g has been given with encouraging results, possibly because drug elimination may also be increased.

Management of tricyclic antidepressant-induced cardiotoxicity poses serious difficulties. In general, the natural inclination to use antiarrhythmic drugs to treat tachycardia and arrhythmias should be resisted. Tricyclic antidepressants have intrinsic class 1 activity and giving disopyramide, lignocaine and β-adrenoceptor blocking drugs may only make matters worse. In cases where an acceptable cardiac output is maintained, antiarrhythmic drugs are not only unnecessary, but are positively contraindicated. Attention to supportive measures, particularly adequate oxygenation, control of convulsions and correction of acidosis will generally be more rewarding. Sodium bicarbonate (50 mmol intravenously over 20 min) should be given even if there is no acidosis. Lignocaine (50–100 mg intravenously) may be tried cautiously if ventricular tachycardia is compromising cardiac output.

Physostigmine salicylate, a cholinesterase inhibitor, has no role in the treatment of tricyclic antidepressant poisoning. When benzodiazepines have been taken in overdosage together with tricyclic antidepressants flumazenil may unmask the tricylic antidepressant induced seizure potential and should therefore be used with caution.

Only a very small proportion of the body load of tricyclic antidepressants circulates in the vascular compartment and forced diuresis and haemodialysis are therefore of no value. Nor is there convincing evidence that charcoal haemoperfusion is effective. High plasma clearances can be obtained but only small amounts of drug are removed by this technique as would be expected from the large volume of distribution.

Delirium with auditory and visual hallucinations is a frequent and troublesome complication during the recovery phase. Sedation with oral or intravenous diazepam may be required.

REFERENCES

Caravati, E.M. and Bossart, P.J. (1991). Demographic and electrocardiographic factors associated with severe tricyclic antidepressant toxicity. *Clinical Toxicology*, **29,** 31–43.

Dziukas, L.J. and Vohra, J. (1991). Tricyclic antidepressant poisoning. *Medical Journal of Australia*, **154,** 344–50.

Amoxapine

Amoxapine is closely related to the tricyclic antidepressants and has the same effects in overdosage. However, it is associated with a greater frequency of seizures, rhabdomyolysis and acute renal failure.

Treatment is the same as for tricyclic antidepressants with particular attention to early detection of possible muscle damage and renal impairment.

Maprotiline

Although maprotiline is chemically related to the tricyclic antidepressants, the presence of a bridge across the central ring converts it into a three-dimensional tetracyclic structure. It therefore shows most of the pharmacological and toxicological properties of tricyclic antidepressants and treatment should be according to the principles outlined above.

Mianserin

Mianserin has a four-ringed structure and is believed to act in depression by increasing noradrenaline turnover. Drowsiness is a common side-effect of overdose but deep coma, convulsions, cardiotoxicity, and respiratory depression have not been reported, except when other drugs have been taken in addition. Treatment is symptomatic. Gastric lavage should be performed if a substantial overdose has been ingested and the patient presents within 1 h.

Monoamine-oxidase inhibitors

These drugs are now used less frequently in the treatment of depression and poisoning with them is correspondingly uncommon. The onset of features may be delayed for 12 to 24 h after acute overdosage and are due principally to increased sympathetic activity. They include excitement, restlessness (which may be extreme), hyperpyrexia, hyperreflexia, convulsions, opisthotonos, rhabdomyolysis, and coma. Cardiovascular effects include sinus tachycardia, and either hypotension or hypertension.

Treatment of overdosage is essentially supportive. Control of convulsions and marked excitement with drugs such as diazepam or chlormethiazole may be necessary to reduce blood pressure and minimize the risk of hyperpyrexia and rhabdomyolysis. Dantrolene may also be indicated for the latter purpose. Hypotension should, in the first instance, be treated by fluid replacement to restore a normal circulating blood volume. The use of sympathomimetic drugs should clearly be avoided. Hypertension should be treated by the administration of an α-adrenoceptor blocker, such as chlorpromazine, phentolamine, or phenoxybenzamine.

Fluoxetine and fluvoxamine

Fluoxetine and fluvoxamine are new antidepressants which are effective by virtue of their ability to inhibit serotonin reuptake. Experience of overdosage with them is limited but doses of up to 3.6 mg/kg body weight do not appear to cause toxicity. Larger amounts are relatively safe unless potentiated by ethanol. They lack the anticholinergic actions of the tricyclic antidepressants. Most patients will show no signs of toxicity but drowsiness, nausea, diarrhoea, and sinus tachycardia have been reported. Rarely, junctional bradycardia, seizures, and hypertension have been encountered and influenza-like symptoms may develop after a day or two.

Supportive measures are all that are required. Activated charcoal will reduce absorption.

REFERENCE

Borys, D.J., *et al.* (1990). The effects of fluoxetine in the overdose patient. *Clinical Toxicology*, **28,** 331–40.

Viloxazine

This antidepressant is not widely used. Information on overdosage is scanty. It does not have the anticholinergic actions of tricyclic antidepressants. Drowsiness, coma, tachycardia, and hypotension are the most likely features. Supportive measures are all that are required. Activated charcoal may reduce absorption.

Poisoning with hypnotics and tranquillizers

Benzodiazepines

The benzodiazepines comprise one of the most important groups of psychotropic drugs in present-day medical practice. They are widely used as tranquillizers, hypnotics, and sedatives. Chlordiazepoxide and diazepam are still commonly prescribed but other early members of the group (particularly nitrazepam and flurazepam) have largely been displaced by newer, shorter-acting compounds such as temazepam, lorazepam, and triazolam. However, there is no reason to believe that the toxicity of the latter group in overdosage will be any different. Bromazepam, clonazepam, desmethyldiazepam, flunitrazepam, medazepam, and prazepam are among the most recent additions to this extensive family of drugs.

CLINICAL FEATURES

Although many benzodiazepines have active metabolites which account for their sometimes prolonged sedative effects, they all share a remarkable safety when taken alone in overdosage. As many as 70 or 80 tablets of any of them are unlikely to produce anything more than mild effects in most adults. However, this is not always the case and it cannot now be said that overdosage with these drugs is never without harm. There is some degree of individual variation in response to them and some otherwise healthy elderly people, in particular, respond to an overdose with prolonged toxicity but it is seldom life-threatening. More important, benzodiazepines potentiate the effects of other CNS depressants, particularly alcohol, tricyclic antidepressants, and barbiturates. Dizziness, drowsiness, ataxia, and slurred speech are the usual features while coma, respiratory depression, and hypotension are uncommon and usually mild. Of all the benzodiazepines, flurazepam is most likely to cause significant CNS depression.

TREATMENT

Supportive measures are the only treatment usually required. Gastric aspiration and lavage is of doubtful benefit when these drugs have been taken and is unnecessary unless the overdose exceeds 30 therapeutic doses in an adult and the patient presents within 1 h. In rare cases of severe poisoning, the use of the specific benzodiazepine antagonist, flumazenil, may be indicated. The dose is 0.5 mg intravenously over 30 s and, if necessary, a further 0.5 mg over 30 s. Most patients will respond to a total dose of between 1 and 3 mg.

REFERENCES

Hojer, J., Baehrendtz, S., and Gustafsson, L. (1989). Benzodiazepine poisoning: experience of 702 admissions to an intensive care unit during a 14-year period. *Journal of Internal Medicine*, **226,** 117–22.

Kulka, P.J. and Lauven, P.M. (1992). Benzodiazepine antagonists. An update of their role in the emergency care of overdose patients. *Drug Safety*, **7,** 381–6.

Chlormethiazole

Coma, respiratory depression, reduced muscle tone, hypotension, and hypothermia may result from chlormethiazole overdose. Excessive salivation is sometimes a prominent feature and the characteristic odour of chlormethiazole is often detected on the breath and in gastric lavage fluid. Treatment is supportive.

Barbiturates

The barbiturates include amylobarbitone, butobarbitone, cyclobarbitone, heptabarbitone, hexabarbitone, pentobarbitone, and quinalbarbitone, which are conventionally regarded as being short- or medium-acting, and phenobarbitone and barbitone which are long-acting. However, this classification has little toxicological merit except that the more lipid soluble, shorter-acting preparations are commonly associated with more serious poisoning than phenobarbitone and barbitone which are much more water soluble.

CLINICAL FEATURES

Impairment of consciousness, respiratory depression, hypotension, and hypothermia are typical of barbiturate poisoning and, in common with all forms of hypnotic overdose, are potentiated by alcohol and benzodiazepines. There are no specific neurological signs.

Hypotonia and hyporeflexia are the rule and the plantar responses are either flexor or absent. Hypotension is due not only to depression of medullary centres but also to peripheral venous pooling and myocardial depression. Skin blisters occur in approximately 6 per cent of cases and rhabdomyolysis may develop. During recovery from coma with or without hypothermia, it is common to observe a peak of temperature which cannot be explained by infection. Most deaths result from respiratory complications, in particular, adult respiratory distress syndrome ('shock lung').

TREATMENT

Gastric aspiration and lavage and intensive supportive measures should be used as appropriate. Induction of an alkaline diuresis (Chapter 8.1.2) is effective only in barbitone and phenobarbitone poisoning and has no place in the treatment of other forms of barbiturate intoxication. Although charcoal haemoperfusion is the technique of choice for severely poisoned patients, both phenobarbitone and barbitone can be removed efficiently by repeated doses of oral and activated charcoal.

Meprobamate

Meprobamate is still used as a sedative and tranquillizing agent. Coma, respiratory depression, and hypotension are the usual features of overdosage. Hypotension may be marked and pulmonary oedema has been reported in some patients. Gastric aspiration and lavage should be performed where appropriate. Treatment is supportive. Haemoperfusion may be necessary in very severely poisoned patients.

Chloral hydrate, dichloralphenazone, and triclofos

These drugs are metabolized in the liver by alcohol dehydrogenase to trichlorethanol, the active compound. This, in turn, is further metabolized to trichloroacetic acid and trichloroethanol glucuronide which are inactive.

The clinical features of acute overdosage with chloral hydrate and its derivatives are similar to those of barbiturate poisoning, although a retrosternal burning sensation accompanied by vomiting may be prominent in the early stages. Cardiac arrhythmias, particularly supraventricular tachycardias and ventricular premature beats, have been described in chloral hydrate poisoning and are often abolished by β-adrenoceptor blocking drugs, provided respiratory depression and hypoxia have been corrected.

Treatment consists of gastric aspiration and lavage, where appropriate, and intensive supportive therapy. Repeated doses of oral charcoal and haemoperfusion should be considered in severely poisoned patients.

Phenothiazines

The phenothiazines are used principally as antiemetics and antipsychotic drugs and may be given orally, alone or in combination with depot phenothiazines such as flupenthixol and fluphenazine. They block peripheral cholinergic and α-adrenergic receptors, reuptake of amines, and the effects of histamine and 5 hydroxytryptamine.

CLINICAL FEATURES

The features of overdosage include impairment of consciousness and hypotension but respiratory depression is seen only in severe poisoning. Hypothermia may be present, particularly after overdosage with chlorpromazine, perphenazine, and promazine. These drugs also seem more prone to cause hypotension, while anticholinergic effects with tachycardia, ECG changes (prolongation of Q-T interval and T wave abnormalities) and arrhythmias are most common with overdosage of thioridazine and mesoridazine and acute spasmodic torticollis, oculogyric crises, and orolingual dyskinesias with trifluperazine and prochlorperazine. Other extrapyramidal features, such as rigidity, tremor, restlessness, and tardive dyskinesia are more likely to be the result of long-term therapeutic doses.

TREATMENT

Treatment is supportive and gastric aspiration and lavage should be performed where appropriate. Acute dystonic reactions may be abolished by a variety of drugs; benztropine 1–2 mg or procyclidine 5–10 mg intravenously is appropriate for an adult and diphenhydramine 2 mg/kg body weight (to a maximum of 50 mg) should suffice for a child.

REFERENCES

Baker, P.B., *et al.* (1988). Hyperthermia, hypertension, hypertonia, and coma in a massive thioridazine overdose. *American Journal of Emergency Medicine*, **6,** 346–9.

Li, C. and Gefter, W.B. (1992). Acute pulmonary edema induced by overdosage of phenothiazines. *Chest*, **101,** 102–4.

Marrs-Simon, P.A. *et al.* (1988). Cardiotoxic manifestations of mesoridazine overdose. *Annals of Emergency Medicine*, **17,** 1074–8.

Butyrophenones

The butyrophenones (benperidol, haloperidol, and triperidol) are also used as antipsychotic and neuroleptic agents. Overdosage may result in drowsiness and hypotension, but extrapyramidal effects, particularly acute dystonic reactions, are among the most dramatic consequences. Treatment is supportive. Acute extrapyramidal features should be treated as above (see phenothiazines).

Lithium carbonate

The therapeutic index of lithium is low and toxicity is usually the result of therapeutic overdosage rather than deliberate self-poisoning.

CLINICAL FEATURES

Features of intoxication include thirst, polyuria, diarrhoea, and vomiting, and, in more serious cases, impairment of consciousness, hypertonia, and convulsions. Measurement of the serum lithium concentration confirms the diagnosis, toxicity usually being associated with concentrations above 1.5 mmol/l. However, acute massive overdosage may produce much higher concentrations without causing toxic features, at least initially.

TREATMENT

Treatment is supportive together with measures to enhance the rate of elimination of lithium. The decision to use the latter is based on the severity of features and a serum lithium concentration greater than 3 mmol/l. Forced diuresis is effective but there is doubt about the need for alkalinization and its use is commonly complicated by hypernatraemia and increased plasma osmolality; the infusion of low dose dopamine (2.5 μg/kg/min) may be an effective alternative. Peritoneal dialysis or haemodialysis may be needed if renal function is impaired and in severe poisoning; peritoneal dialysis is much less effective than haemodialysis. However, the efficacy of all of these techniques is limited by the relatively slow rate of movement of lithium ions across cell membranes. It is easy to reduce serum lithium concentrations but they frequently rebound when treatment is stopped and clinical improvement is much slower.

REFERENCES

Groleau, G., *et al.* (1987). Lithium intoxication. Manifestations and management. *American Journal of Emergency Medicine*, **5,** 527–32.

Szerlip, H.M., Heeger, P., and Feldman, G.M. (1992). Comparison between acetate and bicarbonate dialysis for the treatment of lithium intoxication. *American Journal of Nephrology*, **12,** 116–20.

Poisoning with anticonvulsants

Carbamazepine

Carbamazepine is structurally related to the tricyclic antidepressants and has similar anticholinergic actions. Overdosage may therefore result in a dry mouth, drowsiness, coma, and convulsions. Cardiotoxicity similar to that seen in tricyclic antidepressant poisoning also occurs but is uncommon. Relapse into coma has been described during the course of recovery. Treatment should include gastric lavage, if appropriate, and supportive therapy. Diazepam may be required to treat convulsions. Recovery is slow and may be hastened by giving regular activated charcoal (section 8.1.2) in a dose of 50 g orally every 4 h.

REFERENCES

Boldy, D.A.R., Heath, A., Ruddock, S., Vale, J.A., and Prescott, L.F. (1987). Activated charcoal for carbamazepine poisoning. *Lancet,* **1,** 1027.

Durelli, L., Massazza, U., and Cavallo, R. (1989). Carbamazepine toxicity and poisoning. *Medical Toxicology and Adverse Drug Experience*, **4,** 95–107.

Phenytoin

Acute overdosage of phenytoin results in nausea, vomiting, headache, tremor, cerebellar ataxia, nystagmus, and, rarely, loss of consciousness. Treatment should include gastric aspiration and lavage, where appropriate, together with supportive therapy. Oral activated charcoal (as indicated under carbamazepine) may be useful.

REFERENCES

Masur, H., *et al.* (1990). Cerebellar atrophy following acute intoxication with phenytoin. *Neurology*, **40,** 1800.

Murphy, J.M., Motiwala, R., and Devinski, O. (1991). Phenytoin intoxication. *Southern Medical Journal*, **84,** 1199–204.

Sodium valproate

Sodium valproate in overdose causes impairment of consciousness and respiration. Gastric lavage is of limited value because of the rapid absorption of the drug. Treatment is symptomatic and supportive.

Primidone

Primidone is converted to the two active metabolites, phenobarbitone and phenylethyl malonamide. The clinical features and management of primidone poisoning are as for barbiturate poisoning. Again, regular oral charcoal may be beneficial.

REFERENCE

Lehmann, D.F. (1987). Primidone crystalluria following overdose. *Medical Toxicology*, **2,** 383–7.

Ethosuximide and methsuxemide

The ingestion of either agent may cause anorexia, nausea, vomiting, dizziness, ataxia, drowsiness, and coma. Treatment is supportive and gastric lavage should be performed if appropriate.

Sulthiame

Sulthiame is a sulphonamide derivative and a weak inhibitor of carbonic anhydrase. Overdose results in headache, vomiting, ataxia, vertigo, and hyperventilation. Hyperreflexia, clouding of consciousness and catatonia may also develop, and renal tubular obstruction due to crystalluria (in acid urine) has been reported. Treatment is supportive. The urine should be kept alkaline to avoid renal impairment.

Poisoning with antihistamines

Two generations of antihistamines are now available; the early ones, include brompheniramine, chlorpheniramine, cyclizine, diphenhydramine, mepyramine, methapyrilene, promethazine, trimeprazine, and tripelennamine while the newer agents include astemizole and terfenadine. The toxicity of the two groups varies.

The older antihistamines have anticholinergic actions and their effects are therefore similar to the tricyclic antidepressants although the more serious features such as convulsions, coma, respiratory depression, and arrhythmias (other than sinus tachycardia) are very uncommon and death from these drugs alone is rare. Treatment is largely supportive as described under tricyclic antidepressants.

Information on the effects of overdosage with astemizole and terfenadine is limited but they appear to lack the anticholinergic actions of the older antihistamines. The main toxic effects have been cardiac with prolongation of the QT_c interval and ventricular tachycardia, including the *torsade-de-pointes* type, in children and adults. Associated giant U waves have been described. Convulsions have been caused by terfenadine in overdosage.

Supportive care is probably all that will be required by the majority of patients who ingest overdoses of these drugs. Oral activated charcoal may be given but it did not prevent cardiotoxicity in some children. The patients should be observed for about 12 h with cardiac monitoring if the QT interval is prolonged. Intravenous magnesium sulphate may abolish serious ventricular arrhythmias.

REFERENCES

Farrell, M., Heinrichs, M., and Tilbelli, J.A. (1991). Response of life threatening dimenhydrinate intoxication to sodium bicarbonate administration. *Clinical Toxicology*, **29,** 527–35.

Hildago, H.A., and Mowers, R.M. (1990). Anticholinergic drug abuse. *Drug Intelligence and Clinical Pharmacy*, **24,** 40–1.

Hoppu, K., *et al.* (1991). Accidental astemizole overdose in young children. *Lancet*, **338,** 538–40.

Leor, J., *et al.* (1991). Giant U waves and associated ventricular tachycardia complicating astemizole overdose: successful therapy with intravenous magnesium. *American Journal of Medicine*, **91,** 94–7.

Rinder, C.S., *et al.* (1988). Survival in complicated diphenhydramine overdose. *Critical Care Medicine*, **16,** 1161–2.

Spiller, H.A., Picciotti, M., and Perez, E. (1989). Accidental terfenadine ingestion in children. *Veterinary and Human Toxicology*, **31,** 154–56.

Poisoning with antiparkinsonian drugs

Like the tricyclic antidepressants and older antihistamines, drugs such as amantidine, benzhexol, and orphenadrine, which are used in the treatment of Parkinson's disease, also have anticholinergic effects in overdosage. Orphenadrine is probably the most toxic and has caused deaths. The features of poisoning are similar to those of the tricyclic antidepressants and should be managed in the same way.

REFERENCES

Danze, L.K. and Langdorf, M.I. (1991). Reversal of orphenadrine-induced ventricular tachycardia with physostigmine. *Journal of Emergency Medicine*, **9,** 453–7.

Fahy, A., *et al.* (1989). Serial serum drug concentrations and prolonged anticholinergic toxicity after benztropine (Cogentin) overdose. *American Journal of Emergency Medicine*, **7,** 199–202.

Snoey, E.R. and Bessen, H.A. (1990). Acute psychosis after amantidine overdose. *Annals of Emergency Medicine*, **19,** 668–70.

8.2.3 Poisoning from cardiovascular drugs

J. A. VALE, A. T. PROUDFOOT, AND T. J. MEREDITH

Angiotensin converting enzyme inhibitors

Angiotensin converting enzyme (ACE) inhibitors (captopril, cilazapril, enalapril, fosinopril, lisinopril, perindropril, quinapril, ramipril) block the conversion of angiotensin I to angiotensin II.

CLINICAL FEATURES

Anorexia, nausea, abdominal discomfort, headache, and paraesthesiae have been reported. In addition, hypotension (which may be mediated by the endogenous opioid system), sinus tachycardia, bronchospasm, and hyperkalaemia may develop. Fatalities have been reported.

TREATMENT

If the patient presents within 1 h of a substantial overdose, gastric lavage should be undertaken or activated charcoal administered. Supportive therapy should then be employed, including volume expansion with plasma expanders for hypotension. There is increasing evidence that naloxone can reverse ACE inhibitor-induced hypotension and a dose of 0.8 to 1.2 mg should be administered in these circumstances. Marked hyperkalaemia may require an intravenous infusion of glucose (50 g) and soluble insulin (15 units).

REFERENCES

Augenstein, W.L., Kulig, K.W., and Rumack, B.H. (1988). Captopril overdose resulting in hypotension. *Journal of the American Medical Association*, **259,** 3302–5.

Varon, J. and Duncan, S.R. (1991). Naloxone reversal of hypotension due to captopril overdose. *Annals of Emergency Medicine*, **20,** 1125–7.

α-Adrenoceptor blocking drugs

The α-adrenoceptor blocking drugs (doxazosin, indoramin, phenoxybenzamine, phentolamine, prazosin, terazosin, thymoxamine, and tolazoline) act peripherally to cause vasodilatation.

Phenoxybenzamine has a prolonged duration of action due to stable covalent binding at α-receptors in contrast to the other drugs which all act as competitive, rather than non-competitive, inhibitors.

CLINICAL FEATURES

The main features of overdose are severe hypotension and reflex sinus tachycardia. Nausea, vomiting, diarrhoea, and epigastric pain may also occur, together with nasal congestion, dry mouth, flushing, miosis, drowsiness, and coma. Hypothermia, respiratory depression, and convulsions may be observed in severely poisoned patients.

TREATMENT

Gastric lavage should be undertaken or activated charcoal (50–100 g) administered if the patient presents within 1 h of a substantial overdose. Severe hypotension should be treated with plasma expanders to achieve an adequate circulating blood volume, followed by the use of either dopamine (5–20 μg/kg.min), or dobutamine (5–40 μg/kg.min) by intravenous infusion. If hypotension proves refractory to these measures, noradrenaline (2.5–10 μg/min by intravenous infusion) may be used cautiously. Diazepam (5–10 mg intravenously) should be given for convulsions.

Antiarrhythmic drugs

Class 1A (disopyramide, procainamide, quinidine)

Disopyramide

Disopyramide possesses membrane stabilizing activity and prolongs the action potential of normal cardiac cells. Anticholinergic effects are common even at therapeutic dosage.

CLINICAL FEATURES

Disopyramide overdose causes a steady decline in cardiac output, though the blood pressure is usually well maintained until, in a few patients, peripheral circulatory failure supervenes suddenly and unpredictably. This may be associated with respiratory depression, pulmonary oedema, and serious cardiac arrhythmias with prolonged intraventricular conduction times. The mortality is high in severely poisoned patients.

TREATMENT

Gastric lavage should be undertaken or activated charcoal (50–100 g) administered if a substantial overdose has been ingested less than 1 h previously. Supportive measures, including the correction of acidosis and hypokalaemia, should be employed in all cases. An indwelling arterial cannula with constant blood pressure monitoring will provide immediate warning of cardiovascular collapse. An isoprenaline infusion (5–50 μg/min) is the treatment of choice for hypotension. Cardiodepressant drugs, such as quinidine and procainamide, should be avoided in the treatment of arrhythmias as they may increase mortality. If asystole occurs, transvenous pacing should be tried but the ventricular response is often poor. Haemoperfusion may be of value in those who are severely poisoned.

REFERENCE

Hayler, A.M., Holt, D.W., and Volans, G.N. (1978). Fatal overdosage with disopyramide. *Lancet*, **i,** 968–9.

Procainamide

Procainamide is metabolized to an active metabolite, *N*-acetylprocainamide, which may itself produce toxicity either following overdose or in the presence of renal failure.

CLINICAL FEATURES

Overdose may lead to anorexia, nausea, vomiting, and diarrhoea. Cardiac arrhythmias, including *torsade de pointes*, may also develop and rapid intravenous injection of procainamide has led to collapse, convulsions, hypotension, and death. Severe procainamide intoxication has also been complicated by respiratory failure.

TREATMENT

If the drug has been ingested, gastric lavage should be undertaken if the patient presents within 1 h of taking a substantial overdose or, alternatively, activated charcoal (50–100 g) may be administered. Treatment is symptomatic and supportive. Haemodialysis appears to be more effective in increasing elimination than haemoperfusion.

REFERENCE

Domoto, D.T., Brown, W.W., and Bruggensmith, P. (1987). Removal of toxic levels of *N*-acetylprocainamide with continuous hemofiltration or continuous arteriovenous hemodiafiltration. *Annals of Internal Medicine*, **106,** 550–2.

Quinidine

Quinidine, unlike lignocaine, has an effect on repolarization thereby prolonging total action potential duration. Quinidine and quinine (Chapter 8.2.9) are optical isomers and share many pharmacological properties, although quinine is more oculotoxic and quinidine is more cardiotoxic in overdose.

CLINICAL FEATURES

Nausea, vomiting, abdominal pain, diarrhoea, and sinus tachycardia may occur, but in more serious poisoning, collapse with impairment of consciousness (due to ventricular arrhythmias), convulsions, rapid shallow breathing, hypotension, pulmonary oedema, and cardiorespiratory arrest are observed. Hypotension is due to depressed myocardial contractility and peripheral vasodilation. Cardiac arrhythmias may include ventricular tachycardia (*torsade de pointes*) and ventricular fibrillation; depression of automaticity and intracardiac conduction leads to QRS and QTc interval prolongation, bundle-branch block, sinus bradycardia, sinoatrial block, sinus pauses and sinus arrest, atrioventricular block, junctional or ventricular bradycardia, and asystole. Pulmonary oedema and acute renal failure have been described and hypokalaemia, hypocalcaemia, hypoglycaemia, hypophosphataemia, hypomagnesaemia, and metabolic acidosis have been reported in severe cases.

TREATMENT

Gastric lavage should be employed if the patient presents within 1 h of ingestion or, alternatively, activated charcoal (50–100 g) may be administered. Symptomatic and supportive measures should be given and electrolyte and acid–base disturbance should be corrected as necessary. Clinically significant brady- and tachyarrhythmias may respond to isoprenaline; overdrive pacing may be required if *torsade de pointes* occurs. Plasma expanders should be given for hypotension but if the response is poor, an inotrope should be administered.

REFERENCE

Kim, S.Y. and Benowitz, N.L. (1990). Poisoning due to Class 1A antiarrhythmic drugs: quinidine, procainamide and disopyramide. *Drug Safety*, **5,** 393–420.

Class 1B (lignocaine, mexiletine, tocainide)

Lignocaine, mexiletine, and tocainide depress the fast inward sodium current in cardiac muscle, lengthen the effective refractory period, and delay the return of excitability; the resting membrane potential is unaffected. Intoxication with these agents, particularly lignocaine, occurs most often as a result of therapeutic overdosage, for example, in coronary and intensive care areas. Exceptionally, topical absorption of lignocaine may result in systemic toxicity, particularly in children.

CLINICAL FEATURES

Poisoning with these agents induces nausea, vomiting, paraesthesiae, tremor, drowsiness, dizziness, dysarthria, diplopia, nystagmus, ataxia, confusion, convulsions, and coma. Sinus bradycardia, heart block, and hypotension may develop in severe poisoning and cardiac arrest may ensue; mexiletine may also cause atrial fibrillation.

TREATMENT

Gastric lavage should be considered if an overdose has been ingested less than 1 h before presentation or activated charcoal (50–100 g) should be administered. Diazepam (5–10 mg intravenously) should be given for convulsions, if they are not short-lived, and atropine (1–2 mg intravenously) should be administered for sinus bradycardia. Inotropic support such as dobutamine (5–40 μg/kg.min) or isoprenaline (5–50 μg/min) by intravenous infusion may become necessary if heart block or severe hypotension supervene. Pacing may be attempted but the ventricular response is usually poor. Tocainide elimination is increased significantly with haemodialysis.

REFERENCE

Denaro, C.P. and Benowitz, N.L. (1989). Poisoning due to class 1B antiarrhythmic drugs: lignocaine, mexilitine and tocainide. *Medical Toxicology*, **4,** 412–28.

Class 1C (flecainide)

Even when administered therapeutically, flecainide may cause dizziness, visual disturbances, headache, heart failure, conduction system disorders, and ventricular arrhythmias. Ataxia, dyspnoea, and convulsions have been reported in animal studies.

CLINICAL FEATURES

The features of overdose are predictable from the drug's known side-effects and include hypotension, bradycardia, intraventricular conduction abnormalities, atrioventricular block, and ventricular tachycardia. In severe cases convulsions and cardiorespiratory failure occur and fatalities have been reported.

TREATMENT

If the patient presents within 1 h of ingesting a substantial overdose, gastric lavage should be considered or, alternatively, activated charcoal (50–100 g) may be administered. Supportive measures should then be employed as no specific antidote is available, though lignocaine has been found to be of value in controlling ventricular tachycardia after overdose. There is evidence from volunteer studies that acidification of the urine will increase flecainide elimination; haemodialysis and haemofiltration are of no benefit.

REFERENCE

Winkelmann, B.R. and Leinberger, H. (1987). Life-threatening flecainide toxicity: a pharmacodynamic approach. *Annals of Internal Medicine*, **106,** 807–14.

Class III (amiodarone)

CLINICAL FEATURES

Acute overdose with amiodarone is uncommon and severe features are unusual. Nausea, vomiting, headaches, flushing, paraesthesiae, ataxia, tremor and vertigo, marked bradycardia, and hypotension can occur. Prolongation of the QT interval, T wave inversion, and ventricular tachycardia may be seen on the electrocardiogram.

TREATMENT

Gastric lavage should be undertaken or activated charcoal administered if the patient presents within 1 h of a substantial overdose. Inotropic support should be given for severe hypotension: dopamine (5–20 μg/kg.min) or dobutamine (5–40 μg/kg.min) by intravenous infusion may be given once an adequate circulating blood volume has been established. Cholestyramine (4 g four hourly) may increase amiodarone elimination; in animal studies charcoal does not appear to confer this benefit.

REFERENCE

Goddard, C.J.R. and Whorwell, P.J. (1989). Amiodarone overdose and its management. *British Journal of Clinical Practice*, **43,** 184–6.

β-Adrenoceptor blocking drugs

β-Adrenoceptor blocking drugs (acebutolol, atenolol, betaxolol, bioprolol, carteolol, celiprolol, esmolol, metoprolol, nadolol, oxprenolol, penbutolol, pindolol, propranolol, sotalol, timolol) antagonize the effects of endogenous catecholamines on the heart and other tissues by competitive inhibition at β-adrenoceptors. In overdose these drugs exhibit a marked negative inotropic action.

CLINICAL FEATURES

Sinus bradycardia may be the only feature following a small overdose, but if a substantial amount has been ingested, coma, convulsions (particularly with propanolol), profound bradycardia, and hypotension may occur. Other cardiovascular and neurological effects include drowsiness, delirium, hallucinations, low-output cardiac failure, and cardiorespiratory arrest (asystole or ventricular fibrillation). Bronchospasm and hypoglycaemia occur rarely.

First degree heart block, intraventricular conduction defects, right and left bundle branch block, ST segment elevation, ventricular extrasystoles, and disappearance of the P wave may be noted on the electrocardiogram. Sotalol has been reported to cause QT interval prolongation and ventricular arrhythmias and asystole may follow severe overdose from any β-adrenoceptor blocking drug.

TREATMENT

A delay in treatment may be fatal in patients who are severely poisoned with a β-adrenoceptor blocking drug. If an overdose is suspected, the blood pressure and cardiac rhythm of the patient should be monitored immediately in an intensive care area and supportive measures implemented. Gastric lavage should be considered in adults who have ingested more than 10 therapeutic doses less than 1 h previously; atropine (0.6–1.2 mg intravenously) may prevent vagal-induced cardiovascular collapse during this procedure.

Glucagon is the drug of choice for severe hypotension and should be given in a bolus dose of 50 to 150 μg/kg (typically, 10 mg in an adult) over 1 min, followed by an infusion of 1 to 5 mg/h according to response. Glucagon acts by bypassing the blocked β-receptor, thus activating adenyl cyclase and promoting formation of cyclic AMP from ATP; cyclic AMP in turn exerts a direct β-stimulant effect on the heart.

Insertion of a temporary transvenous pacemaker wire and the use of intravenous atropine (0.6–3.0 mg; 50 μg/kg in a child) and isoprenaline (5–50 μg/min intravenously) or other inotropic agents, have been recommended but are probably less effective than glucagon, even when used in high doses. Occasionally, convulsions associated with β-blocker poisonings are sustained and diazepam (5–10 mg intravenously) may be needed. If bronchospasm supervenes, salbutamol (albuterol) by nebulizer, or aminophylline by intravenous infusion, should be employed. Hypoglycaemia should be corrected with intravenous glucose.

REFERENCE

Critchley, J.A.J.H. and Ungar, A. (1989). The management of acute poisoning due to β-adrenoceptor antagonists. *Medical Toxicology*, **4**, 32–45.

Calcium-channel blockers

Calcium-channel blockers (amlodipine, diltiazem, felodipine, isradipine, nicardipine, nifedipine, nimodipine, verapamil) interfere with the inward transmembrane passage of calcium ions in myocardial cells, the cells within the specialized conducting system of the heart, and the cells of vascular smooth muscle. Hence, myocardial contractility may be reduced, the formation and propagation of electrical impulses within the heart may be depressed, and coronary or systemic vascular tone may be diminished. Calcium-channel blockers differ in their predilection for the various possible sites of action, so that the features of overdose may differ in severity depending on the agent ingested.

CLINICAL FEATURES

In overdose, calcium-channel blockers cause nausea, vomiting, dizziness, slurred speech, confusion, sinus bradycardia and tachycardia, prolonged atrioventricular conduction, atrioventricular dissociation, hypotension, pulmonary oedema, respiratory arrest, convulsions, coma, hyperglycaemia, and metabolic acidosis. The ingestion of a large overdose is associated with a poor prognosis, particularly in patients with ischaemic heart disease and in those taking β-adrenergic blocking agents therapeutically.

TREATMENT

Gastric lavage should be considered in all patients who present within 1 h of a substantial overdose or, alternatively, 50 to 100 g of activated charcoal may be administered. Symptomatic and supportive measures should be instituted and calcium gluconate (10–20 ml of 10 per cent solution intravenously) may reverse prolonged intracardiac conduction times but inotropic support with dobutamine (5–40 μg/kg.min) or isoprenaline (5–50 μg/min) by intravenous infusion, will also be needed to maintain cardiac output in severe cases.

REFERENCE

Pearigan, P.D. and Benowitz, N.L. (1991). Poisoning due to calcium antagonists. *Drug Safety*, **6**, 408–30.

Clonidine

Clonidine exerts its hypotensive action by reduction of sympathetic tone mediated by a central effect on postsynaptic α_2-adrenoceptors in the medulla. Clonidine decreases heart rate, cardiac output, and total peripheral resistance. In the presence of high plasma clonidine concentrations, peripheral α_2-agonist activity predominates and accounts for those instances of vasoconstriction and hypertension reported following clonidine overdose.

CLINICAL FEATURES

A review of 170 cases indicates that poisoning with this drug may be severe and life-threatening, particularly in children, though no deaths occurred in this particular series. In contrast to other reports, peripherally mediated α-sympathomimetic effects (such as hypertension and severe vasoconstriction) were unusual while bradycardia, hypotension, coma, and respiratory depression (due to the central effects of the drug) were common. The duration of toxic effects is normally about 16 h, but it may extend to several days in severe overdose.

TREATMENT

Gastric lavage should be considered or activated charcoal (50–100 g) administered if a patient presents within 1 h following a substantial overdose. Bradycardia is usually reversed by atropine (0.6–2.4 mg intravenously). The use of α-adrenergic blocking drugs (tolazoline or phentolamine) has been advocated in severely poisoned patients in order to block both the peripheral and central actions of clonidine but experience with these agents is limited and the complicated pharmacology of clonidine suggests that their action may be unpredictable. Severe hypotension should first be treated with a plasma expander and then, if necessary, an inotropic agent such as dobutamine (5–40 μg/kg.min)may be given by intravenous infusion. The use of naloxone has been advocated but its benefit is inconsistent and it may produce hypertension. Sodium nitroprusside (50–400 μg/min)by intravenous infusion is the most effective agent for management of severe hypertension and peripheral vasoconstriction.

Although forced diuresis has been employed in the treatment of clonidine poisoning, renal elimination is not increased.

REFERENCES

Stein, B. and Volans, G.N. (1978). Dixarit overdose: the problem of attractive tablets. *British Medical Journal*, **2**, 667–8.

Wiley, J.F., Wiley, C.C., Torrey, S.B., and Henretig, F.M. (1990). Clonidine poisoning in young children. *Journal of Pediatrics*, **116**, 654–8.

Digoxin and digitoxin

Toxicity occurring during chronic administration of these cardiac glycosides is common, while acute poisoning from digoxin and digitoxin is infrequent, though the mortality may be as high as 20 per cent after a substantial overdose, particularly if digoxin-specific antibody fragments are not employed.

CLINICAL FEATURES

Nausea, vomiting, dizziness, anorexia, and drowsiness are common. Confusion, diarrhoea, visual disturbances, and hallucinations may also occur. Sinus bradycardia, often marked, is the earliest cardiotoxic effect and may be followed by supraventricular arrhythmias with or without heart block, ventricular premature beats, and ventricular tachycardia. Hyperkalaemia occurs due to inhibition of the Na^+-K^+ activated ATPase pump. The diagnosis may be confirmed by measurement of the serum digoxin concentration.

TREATMENT

Gastric lavage should be employed in all patients with a history of a substantial overdose less than 1 h previously. Alternatively, activated charcoal (50–100 g) may be administered to reduce absorption and repeated doses will also enhance elimination. Potassium supplements should not be given until the serum potassium concentration is known as severe poisoning is commonly associated with hyperkalaemia. This may be treated with a glucose and insulin infusion or, if very severe, by the use of sodium resonium ion-exchange resins, or dialysis.

Sinus bradycardia, ventricular ectopics, atrioventricular block, and sinoatrial standstill or block are often reduced or abolished by atropine (1.2–2.4 mg). Ventricular ectopics alone should not be treated unless cardiac output is impaired. Ventricular tachydysrhythmias may be treated with intravenous lignocaine, atenolol, phenytoin, or amiodarone; if clinically significant and persistent, digoxin-specific antibody fragments should be considered. Failure to achieve a satisfactory cardiac output by drug therapy in patients with bradycardia, atrioventricular block or sinus arrest is an indication for insertion of a right ventricular pacing wire or, if available, the administration of digoxin-specific antibody fragments (which will also benefit digitoxin poisoning) (6–8mg/kg body weight). Unlike whole antibodies, Fab antibody fragments lack complement-fixing activity, they are not susceptible to immune degradation, and neither are they immunogenic. Their low molecular weight (50-kDa) permits high renal clearance of the Fab fragment–digoxin complex by glomerular filtration. Fab antibody fragments are now generally available but are expensive, though an improvement in the patient's condition should occur within 20 to 40 min.

Forced diuresis does not increase the renal clearance of digoxin once it has become tissue-bound, and peritoneal dialysis, haemodialysis, and haemoperfusion do not significantly increase the elimination of the drug because of its large volume of distribution (7 l/kg).

Haemoperfusion may be more effective in the treatment of digitoxin poisoning because of its small volume of distribution (0.5 l/kg). However, if available, digoxin-specific antibody fragments are to be preferred to haemoperfusion.

REFERENCES

Kelly, R.A. and Smith, T.W. (1992). Recognition and management of digitalis toxicity. *American Journal of Cardiology*, **69,** 108G–119G.

Smith, T.W. (1991). Review of clinical experience with digoxin immune Fab (Ovine). *American Journal of Emergency Medicine*, **9,** 1–6 (suppl. 1).

Woolf, A.D., Wenger, T., Smith, T.W., and Lovejoy, F.H. (1992). The use of digoxin-specific Fab fragments for severe digitalis intoxication in children. *New England Journal of Medicine*, **326,** 1739–44.

Diuretics

Most overdoses involving diuretics are minor, although inevitably some disturbance of fluid and electrolyte balance will result. When combined diuretic and potassium formulations are ingested, the potassium content is likely to pose the greater risk. More serious consequences are likely if a potassium-sparing diuretic has been ingested.

CLINICAL FEATURES

Symptoms and signs of toxicity include anorexia, nausea, vomiting, diarrhoea, profound diuresis, dehydration, and hypotension. In addition, dizziness, weakness, muscle cramps, tetany, and occasionally gastrointestinal bleeding may be seen. The electrolytic and metabolic disturbances that may be observed include hyponatraemia, hypoglycaemia or hyperglycaemia, hyperuricaemia, hypokalaemia, and metabolic alkalosis. Hyperkalaemia may develop following the ingestion of combined diuretic and potassium preparations and potassium-sparing diuretics, such as amiloride, spironolactone, or triamterene, and small-bowel ulceration and stricture formation has followed poisoning due to diuretics with an enteric-coated core of potassium chloride. In addition, to these features, prolonged use of diuretics may lead to severe potassium depletion with cardiac arrhythmias and impaired urinary concentrating ability due either to hypokalaemic nephropathy or nephrogenic diabetes insipidus.

TREATMENT

Symptomatic and supportive therapy should be employed with correction of fluid and electrolyte imbalance. Patients with hyperkalaemia due to the ingestion of potassium-sparing diuretics may need a glucose and insulin infusion followed by oral or rectal administration of an ion-exchange resin.

Hydralazine

Hydralazine acts directly on smooth muscle to cause arteriolar vasodilation.

CLINICAL FEATURES

Overdose causes anorexia, nausea, vomiting, diarrhoea, headache, flushing, hypotension, sinus tachycardia, and cardiac arrhythmias. Marked ST segment depression on ECG has been observed.

TREATMENT

If the patient presents within 1 h, gastric lavage should be undertaken or activated charcoal (50–100 g) administered. In common with most cases of poisoning due to vasodilator agents, simple measures such as keeping the patient flat in bed or elevation of the lower limbs are all that are usually required. Mobilization requires supervision as syncope may result from postural hypotension. Severe hypotension should be treated with plasma expanders and either dopamine (5–20 μg/kg.min) or dobutamine (5–40 μg/kg.min) by intravenous infusion. If these inotropic agents are ineffective, then noradrenaline (2.5–10 μg/min) by infusion may be tried cautiously.

REFERENCE

Smith, B.A. and Ferguson, D.B. (1992). Acute hydralazine overdose: marked ECG abnormalities in a young adult. *Annals of Emergency Medicine*, **21,** 326–30.

Methyldopa

In central noradrenergic neurones, methyldopa is metabolized to α-methylnoradrenaline, which is a specific agonist for α_2-receptors.

CLINICAL FEATURES

There are few well-documented cases of serious methyldopa poisoning, but dizziness, drowsiness, hypotension, and bradycardia or tachycardia may be seen. Extrapyramidal signs, hypothermia, and coma also occur.

TREATMENT

Gastric lavage should be performed in patients who present within 1 h of ingestion of a substantial overdose. Simple measures to prevent postural hypotension should be instituted but, in more serious cases, a plasma expander and inotropic agent such as dobutamine (5–40 μg/kg.min) by intravenous infusion may be necessary. Benztropine (1–2 mg intravenously) should be given if extrapyramidal signs are troublesome. Haemodialysis has been reported to remove 60 per cent of a therapeutic dose of methyldopa in patients. However, in view of the relative lack of toxicity of this drug in overdose, this procedure is not recommended as routine management.

REFERENCE

Shnaps, Y., Almog, S., Halkin, H., and Tirosh, M. (1982). Methyldopa poisoning. *Clinical Toxicology*, **19**, 501–3.

Nitrates

Organic nitrates (glyceryl trinitrate, isosorbide mononitrate and dinitrate, pentaerythritol tetranitrate) are used as vasodilating agents in the treatment of patients with ischaemic heart disease. They are believed to act within smooth muscle cells by release or formation of nitric oxide that then reacts with sulphydryl groups to form *S*-nitrosothiols. These in turn activate guanylate cyclase, increase guanine monophosphate levels, and cause relaxation of vascular smooth muscle.

CLINICAL FEATURES

The symptoms and signs caused by nitrates in overdose are due primarily to excessive arteriolar and venous dilation. Headache and vomiting are common, accompanied by flushing of the skin and dizziness. Sinus tachycardia, severe orthostatic hypotension, and syncope may develop. Convulsions and coma may be seen in severely poisoned patients. In contrast to poisoning by inorganic nitrates, methaemoglobinaemia is seen very rarely.

TREATMENT

Give activated charcoal (50–100 g) if a substantial overdose has been ingested less than 1 h previously. Mild hypotension may be treated by placing the patient in a head-down position but more severe hypotension will require plasma expanders. If hypotension proves refractory to these measures, then a vasopressor agent, such as noradrenaline (2.5–10 μg/min by intravenous infusion), or methoxamine (5–10 mg intravenously) should be tried cautiously. As organic nitrates undergo extensive 'first pass' metabolism in the liver, there is little point in attempting to accelerate excretion of these compounds from the body.

Sodium nitroprusside

Sodium nitroprusside is a potent, rapidly acting, and short-lasting intravenous vasodilator which is converted *in vivo* to nitric oxide and cyanide. Nitric oxide induces vasodilation and hypotension and is responsible not only for the therapeutic benefit of sodium nitroprusside but also for some of its toxicity. Accumulation of cyanide occurs if the normal endogenous detoxification processes are overwhelmed by too high an infusion rate of nitroprusside (> 2 μg/kg.min for several hours or > 8 μg/kg.min for 10 min). The risk of thiocyanate toxicity increases when sodium nitroprusside is infused continuously for more than 24 to 48 h, especially if renal function is impaired.

CLINICAL FEATURES

Hypotension is the major side-effect of treatment and may be corrected by a change in infusion rate. The development of metabolic (lactic) acidosis is usually the first indication of cyanide toxicity (see Section 8.3 for other features). Thiocyanate accumulation may lead to anorexia, nausea, lethargy, fatigue, and psychosis.

TREATMENT

During prolonged infusions the blood cyanide and thiocyanate concentrations should be measured and should not exceed 1 mg/l and 100 mg/l, respectively. The risk of toxicity can be reduced (or even abolished) by not exceeding the recommended infusion rates and/or by giving sodium thiosulphate or hydroxocobalamin intravenously. Cyanide toxicity should be treated conventionally (see Section 8.3).

REFERENCE

Vesey, C.J., Cole, P.V., and Simpson, P.J. (1976). Cyanide and thiocyanate concentrations following sodium nitroprusside infusion in man. *British Journal of Anaesthesia*, **48**, 651–60.

8.2.4 Poisoning caused by respiratory drugs

A. T. Proudfoot, J. A. Vale, and T. J. Meredith

β_2-Agonists

Poisoning with β_2-agonists, including fenoterol, pirbuterol, reproburerol, rimiterol, salbutamol, and terbutaline, has followed deliberate and accidental ingestion of these drugs and may also result from confusion over the difference between oral and parenteral doses.

CLINICAL FEATURES AND MECHANISMS OF TOXICITY

These include a feeling of excitement, hallucinations, and agitation, accompanied by palpitation, tachycardia, tremor, and peripheral vasodilatation. More serious complications such as hypokalaemia, ventricular tachyarrhythmias, ECG changes of myocardial ischaemia, pulmonary oedema, convulsions, hyperglycaemia, and lactic acidosis are uncommon. The hypokalaemia is the result of movement of potassium from the extracellular pool into cells and is secondary to increased cell membrane Na^+/K^+ ATPase activity, stimulated by catecholamines and β_2-agonists and mediated via increased intracellular 3,5-cyclic AMP concentrations. Hyperglycaemia and hyperinsulinism may potentiate the intracellular potassium shift. β_2-Agonists also increase ventilation and the resulting respiratory alkalosis will exacerbate the hypokalaemia observed in poisoning with these agents.

TREATMENT

The stomach should be emptied if the patient presents within 1 h and if a substantial dose has been ingested. In addition, symptomatic and supportive measures should be employed. Hypokalaemia should be corrected as soon as possible by the administration of an infusion of potassium at a rate of 40 to 60 mmol/h diluted in 5 per cent dextrose. A non-selective β-blocker, such as propranolol (1–5 mg by slow intravenous injection) will also reverse β_2-agonist-induced hypokalaemia and may be needed if myocardial ischaemia occurs as a result of the tachyarrhythmia. However, its use may exacerbate pre-existing chronic air flow obstruction. Methods to increase elimination have no role.

REFERENCE

Jarvie, D.R., Thompson, A.M., and Dyson, E.H. (1987). Laboratory and clinical features of self-poisoning with salbutamol and terbutaline. *Clinica Chimica Acta*, **168,** 313–22.

Theophylline

Poisoning may complicate therapeutic use as well as being the result of deliberate self-poisoning. It is important to establish at an early stage the precise theophylline product involved in a poisoning incident since many of them are sustained-release formulations. As a consequence, peak plasma concentrations of the drug are frequently not attained until 6 to 12 h after overdosage and the onset of toxic features is correspondingly delayed.

CLINICAL FEATURES

The clinical features of theophylline poisoning correlate with plasma theophylline concentrations to only a limited extent. Most symptomatic patients have concentrations in excess of 25 mg/l and although convulsions have been reported with such concentrations, they are seen more commonly when concentrations are greater than 50 mg/l. Some patients have been reported free from serious neurological or cardiological effects despite very high plasma theophylline concentrations. It is therefore important that each patient be assessed and managed individually according to the clinical features as well as plasma drug concentrations.

The features of theophylline toxicity are complex. They include nausea, vomiting, and hyperventilation secondary to stimulation of medullary centres; haematemesis, abdominal pain, and diarrhoea due to local effects on the gastrointestinal tract; sinus tachycardia and supraventricular and ventricular arrhythmias due to myocardial stimulation and catecholamine release; hypotension due to decrease in peripheral resistance; and restlessness, irritability, headache, hyperreflexia, tremors, and convulsions due to CNS stimulation. Hypokalaemia results from the mechanisms described in the section on β_2-agonists while hyperventilation results in respiratory alkalosis and convulsions and hypotension in metabolic acidosis.

ASSESSMENT OF THE SEVERITY OF POISONING

The severity of theophylline intoxication is important in deciding management. Plasma potassium concentrations of less than 2.6 mmol/l, acidaemia, hypotension, seizures, and arrhythmias are indications for urgent measurement of the plasma theophylline concentration. Patients require close observation to detect the onset of delayed toxicity and it may be necessary to repeat the measurement of the plasma theophylline concentration a few hours after admission.

TREATMENT

Patients who have taken a significant overdose of theophylline and who present within 1 h of ingestion should have gastric lavage. Administration of activated charcoal (by nasogastric tube, if necessary) is particularly important; 50 to 100 g initially followed by 50 g four-hourly may reduce theophylline absorption and will enhance its systemic elimination. Intractable vomiting is rarely alleviated by even substantial doses of older antiemetics but may be helped by ondansetron, 8 mg intravenously in an adult. Gastrointestinal haemorrhage may require blood transfusion and ranitidine is the H_2-receptor blocker of choice since cimetidine slows the metabolism of theophylline. Tachyarrhythmias may be induced by the rapid flux of potassium across cell membranes and early correction of hypokalaemia may prevent their development. The plasma potassium concentration should therefore be measured on admission and at hourly intervals thereafter while the patient is symptomatic. Potassium supplements will be needed in almost all cases and doses of up to 60 mmol/h may be required at the outset. Non-selective β-adrenoceptor blocking drugs, such as propranolol, may also be useful in the treatment of tachyarrhythmias secondary to hypokalaemia. Convulsions should be managed as described in Chapter 8.1.2.

Although charcoal haemoperfusion increases theophylline clearance at 2 to 6 times the endogenous rate and reduces circulating theophylline concentrations, its use should seldom be necessary. Repeat dose oral charcoal should suffice in most cases, even in severe poisoning. Haemoperfusion should be reserved for those in whom intractable vomiting or recurrent seizures make oral charcoal impracticable or hazardous.

REFERENCES

Janss, G.J. (1990). Acute theophylline overdose treated with whole bowel irrigation. *South Dakota Journal of Medicine*, **43,** 7–8.

Sessler, C.N. (1990). Theophylline toxicity: clinical features of 116 consecutive cases. *American Journal of Medicine*, **88,** 567–76.

Isoniazid

Poisoning with isoniazid is potentially very serious, but uncommon except in certain ethnic groups (for example, North American Indians) in whom the incidence of tuberculosis, and hence availability of antituberculosis drugs, is high.

MECHANISMS OF TOXICITY

Isoniazid prevents the activation of pyridoxine, depresses tissue concentrations of its coenzyme form, pyridoxal 5-phosphate, and brain concentrations of γ-aminobutyric acid (GABA), thus leading to seizures. The associated metabolic (predominantly lactic) acidosis may be the consequence of seizures but accumulation of 3-hydroxybutyrate may also contribute. Pyridoxine is thought to act specifically in isoniazid poisoning by maintaining concentrations of GABA, thus preventing the development of convulsions and acidosis.

CLINICAL FEATURES

The ingestion of 80 to 150 mg isoniazid/kg body weight is likely to cause severe poisoning. Within 30 to 120 min of ingestion, nausea, vomiting, slurred speech, dizziness, and visual hallucinations may develop. Stupor, coma, and convulsions follow rapidly and may be associated with hyperthermia, hyperreflexia, extensor plantar responses, and, later, rhabdomyolysis. In addition, dilated pupils, sinus tachycardia, and urinary retention may be observed. In severe cases, hypotension may cause acute renal failure if uncorrected and respiratory failure may ensue. Marked metabolic (lactic) acidosis is common. Less commonly, hyperglycaemia, ketoacidosis, glycosuria, and ketonuria are found.

TREATMENT

Supportive measures, including the correction of metabolic acidosis, should be instituted immediately if the patient is unconscious. If the airway can be protected, and the patient presents within 1 h, gastric lavage should be carried out and 50 g of activated charcoal instilled into the stomach. Convulsions must be controlled but conventional treatments are commonly ineffectual. Pyridoxine intravenously in a dose 1 g for 1 g of isoniazid ingested should be given. When the ingested dose of isoniazid is unknown, an initial intravenous dose of 5 g pyridoxine should be given. The use of diazepam and pyridoxine is synergistic and both should be given to those with convulsions. The 5-g dose of pyridoxine may be repeated if convulsions persist (in one case 52 g pyridoxine were given intravenously without ill effects).

Charcoal haemoperfusion is the most effective technique for enhancing the elimination of isoniazid from the circulation but its use should rarely be necessary provided appropriate supportive measures and adequate and repeated doses of pyridoxine and diazepam are given.

REFERENCE

Gurnani, A., Chawla, R., Kundra, P., and Bhattacharya, A. (1992). Acute isoniazid poisoning. *Anaesthesia*, **47**, 781–3.

Rifampicin (rifampin)

Although rifampicin is used as first-line treatment for tuberculosis in most developed countries, poisoning with the drug is far less common than with isoniazid.

CLINICAL FEATURES

Poisoning with rifampicin results in the so-called 'red man syndrome' which can be fatal. The skin, and subsequently the sclerae, become yellow-orange in colour (the colour of a boiled lobster) and the skin discoloration may be removed by washing. These appearances are due to the intense colour of rifampicin and its metabolites which are distributed throughout the body. In addition, nausea, vomiting, abdominal pain, pruritus, a sensation of the skin burning, and convulsions, have been observed. Less commonly, marked oedema of the forehead, cheeks, chin, and lips, with associated eosinophilia, has occurred. Elevation in serum activities of hepatic enzymes and bilirubin have been noted. Sudden death has also been recorded in two patients, due probably to cardiorespiratory arrest.

TREATMENT

Treatment is supportive and symptomatic. Gastric lavage should be carried out when a substantial overdose has been ingested and the patient presents within 1 h of overdose.

REFERENCE

Holdiness, M.R. (1989). A review of the red man syndrome and rifampicin overdosage. *Medical Toxicology and Adverse Drug Experience*, **4**, 444–51.

8.2.5 Poisoning caused by drugs acting on the gastrointestinal system

J. A. Vale, A. T. Proudfoot, and T. J. Meredith

Bismuth chelate

Bismuth chelate (tripotassium dicitratobismuthate) is effective in healing peptic ulcer and it appears to have a particular beneficial effect on *Helicobacter pylori*-associated gastritis. A wide variety of toxic effects have been reported from the administration of different bismuth compounds but the clinical features reported below relate particularly to the ingestion of bismuth chelate.

MECHANISM OF TOXICITY

Although bismuth absorption from bismuth chelate is low after a therapeutic dose, a significant quantity of bismuth may be absorbed after overdose. Renal toxicity is dose-dependent in animals and is directed primarily towards the tubular epithelial cells.

CLINICAL FEATURES

Self poisoning with large doses of bismuth chelate has caused (reversible) renal failure, usually between 2 and 10 days after overdose and at least one death. During prolonged (and sometimes high dose) therapy, bismuth-induced encephalopathy has been reported.

TREATMENT

If a patient presents within 1 h of a substantial overdose of bismuth chelate, gastric lavage should be considered. Dimercaprol can lower brain bismuth concentrations in animals though there is no evidence that it can prevent nephrotoxicity. DMSA and DMPS may be effective oral alternatives to dimercaprol.

REFERENCES

Playford, R.J. *et al.* (1990). Bismuth induced encephalopathy caused by tripotassium dicitrato bismuthate in a patient with chronic renal failure. *Gut*, **31**, 359–60.

Taylor, E.G. and Klenerman, P. (1990). Acute renal failure after colloidal bismuth subnitrate overdose. *Lancet*, **335**, 670–1.

Co-phenotrope

Co-phenotrope is a mixture of diphenoxylate hydrochloride (2.5 mg) and atropine (0.25 mg) and is used in the treatment of diarrhoea.

MECHANISM OF TOXICITY

The active metabolite of diphenoxylate, diphenoxylic acid, is a more potent and long-acting opioid than diphenoxylate. The combination of diphenoxylate and atropine reduces gastric emptying and intestinal motility and, for this reason, the onset of toxicity following an overdose may be delayed for up to 12 h.

CLINICAL FEATURES

Respiratory depression is the major complication of diphenoxylate poisoning and, typically, a gradual reduction in the respiratory rate is followed by apnoea. Vomiting, abdominal pain, drowsiness, and coma also occur. Even though co-phenotrope tablets incorporate only a small amount of atropine this is often toxic to children under 5 years and several deaths have been reported. Tachycardia, anxiety, restlessness, and flushing may be observed but the pupils are more often constricted (due to diphenoxylate) than dilated. Hypotension, loss of tendon reflexes, and convulsions occur in severe cases and relapse is not uncommon during the course of recovery.

TREATMENT

Repeated doses of naloxone (or an infusion) may be necessary to reverse respiratory depression because of the long duration of action of diphenoxylate and the prolonged absorption of the drug due to intestinal stasis. Emesis is inappropriate because of the risk of aspiration but lavage may be appropriate in an adult presenting within 1 h of a substantial overdose before toxicity develops; activated charcoal (50–100 g) may also reduce absorption significantly.

REFERENCE

McCarron, M.M., Challoner, K.R., and Thompson, G.A. (1991). Diphenoxylate–atropine (Lomotil) overdose in children: an update (report of eight cases and review of the literature). *Pediatrics*, **87,** 694–700.

H_2-receptor antagonists (cimetidine, famotidine, nizatidine, ranitidine)

Although H_2-receptor antagonists are very widely prescribed, and therefore available, surprisingly few cases of overdose have been reported and many of these have involved the ingestion of other drugs.

CLINICAL FEATURES

Most patients remain asymptomatic. In a few, drowsiness, dryness of the mouth, slurred speech, dizziness, confusion, vomiting, and abdominal discomfort have been reported. Rarely, bradycardia, respiratory depression, and coma may result.

TREATMENT

Gut decontamination is unnecessary and supportive and symptomatic measures should be employed as necessary. Although forced diuresis has been employed in one case, no supporting evidence of efficacy was given.

REFERENCE

Krenzelok, E.P., Litovitz, T., Lippold, K.P., and McNally, C.F. (1987). Cimetidine toxicity: an assessment of 881 cases. *Annals of Emergency Medicine*, **16,** 1217–22.

Metoclopramide

Metoclopramide, a chlorbenzamide derivative, is used as an antiemetic.

CLINICAL FEATURES

Extrapyramidal signs, including torticollis, hypertonia, oculogyric crises, facial grimacing, diplopia, trismus, nystagmus, rhythmic protrusion of the tongue, and opisthotonos have been reported, accompanied by agitation and anxiety and, rarely, by oedema of the tongue, periorbital oedema, and convulsions. To prevent persistent and disabling movement disorders, long-term use of metoclopramide should be avoided.

TREATMENT

In addition to measures to reduce absorption, if these are appropriate, benztropine (1–2 mg in an adult), should be given intravenously if extrapyramidal features are present. Alternatively, diazepam (5–10 mg intravenously) is effective and has the additional advantage of alleviating anxiety and agitation.

REFERENCES

Low, L.C.K. and Goel, K.M. (1980). Metoclopramide poisoning in children. *Archives of Disease in Childhood*, **55,** 310–12.

Miller, L.G. and Jankovic, J. (1989). Metoclopramide-induced movement disorders. *Archives of Internal Medicine*, **149,** 2486–92.

8.2.6 Poisoning by haematinics and vitamins

A. T. Proudfoot, J. A. Vale, and T. J. Meredith

Iron preparations

Most medicinal iron preparations are ferrous salts which must be oxidized to the ferric state before being absorbed and stored in the liver and reticuloendothelial system. Iron overdosage is much more common in preschool children than in adults, and the attractive colours of the tablets and their resemblance to sweets have long been held responsible for accidental poisoning in this age group. Toxic features are unlikely unless more than 60 mg of elemental iron/kg body weight has been ingested. Poisoning is therefore seldom severe and deaths are rare.

MODE OF TOXICITY

Iron salts have complex actions, including direct corrosive effects on the upper gastrointestinal tract and potentially serious effects on the circulation; at a cellular level they tend to concentrate around mitochondrial cristae where they may act as an electron 'sink', thereby interfering with intermediary metabolism.

FEATURES OF POISONING

The course of iron poisoning is conventionally divided into four phases.

Phase 1

The first phase starts immediately after ingestion and lasts about 6 h. It is characterized by nausea, vomiting, abdominal pain, and diarrhoea, all of which result from direct irritation of the gut. The gastric and upper small bowel mucosae may be stained and impregnated with iron and become ulcerated, the severity of these changes decreasing with distance from the stomach. The disintegrating tablets may make the vomitus and stools grey or black in colour. Polymorph leucocytosis and hyperglycaemia are common. Iron tablets in the upper gut may be visible in a straight abdominal radiograph, particularly if it is taken within 2 h of alleged ingestion and is helpful in confirming overdosage in doubtful cases.

A small number of patients develop more serious features such as haematemesis, hypotension, coma, and shock which may be fatal.

Phase 2

This phase lasts from about 6 to 24 h after ingestion and is a period during which patients improve symptomatically. Indeed, most do not progress further.

Phase 3

During this phase, 12 to 48 h after ingestion, a small minority of patients deteriorate, often with profound shock, metabolic acidosis, and features which are due to acute renal tubular and hepatocellular necrosis. Liver failure and its complications develop and may be fatal. The extent of liver damage is varied from almost complete necrosis in some areas to only the periportal areas in others.

Phase 4

This is the period 2 to 6 weeks after ingestion. The features at this stage are those of high intestinal obstruction by a stricture formed at the site of corrosive damage to the mucosa, usually the pyloric antrum. Children are most likely to be affected.

ASSESSMENT OF THE SEVERITY OF POISONING

The estimated lethal dose of elemental iron is 180 to 300 mg/kg body weight, but the amount ingested is not a reliable method of assessing the severity of poisoning. Shock and coma indicate severe poisoning. Other clinical features are less useful, but a white cell count above 15 000 mm^3 and blood glucose level above 8.3 mmol/l (> 150 mg/dl) in the 6 h after ingestion and the presence of tablets on the abdominal radiograph correlate with serum iron concentrations above 54 μmol/l. However, these indicators are no substitute for emergency estimation of the serum iron concentration. If these concentrations exceed predicted normal iron binding capacity (usually > 90 μmol/l) free iron is circulating and treatment is needed. However, measurement of the total iron binding capacity in acute iron overdosage may give misleading results and is not recommended.

TREATMENT

Reducing absorption

The stomach should be emptied if more than 20 mg of elemental iron/kg body weight has been taken in the previous 4 h. Addition of bicarbonate, phosphates and desferrioxamine to lavage fluids, recommended in the past, does not reduce absorption further. Indeed, the use of desferrioxamine in this manner may actually increase iron absorption. Whole bowel irrigation may have a role if a large amount (particularly of a slow release formulation) has been ingested and has already passed through the pylorus.

Severe poisoning with coma or shock

The specific iron chelating agent, desferrioxamine, should be given without delay and, if necessary, before the result of the serum iron concentration is available. The dose is 15 mg/kg body weight/h intravenously and the total amount infused should not exceed 80 mg/kg in 24 h. Clinical improvement can be expected within an hour or two, after which the rate of infusion may be reduced. There is no simple or readily available method of deciding when to stop desferrioxamine administration; the clinical state of the patient is probably the most appropriate guide. Desferrioxamine may also be given intramuscularly in a dose of 2 g for an adult and 1 g for a child.

Hypotension due to desferrioxamine-induced histamine release may develop if the recommended rate of administration is exceeded. Other adverse effects include hypersensitivity reactions and, rarely, anaphylaxis. Pulmonary oedema and adult respiratory distress syndrome attributed to desferrioxamine have been reported in patients given 15 mg/kg for 65 h and longer. Optic neuropathy, hearing loss, and cataracts have developed after long-term use in iron overload states.

Poisoning without coma or shock

Unfortunately, indiscriminate administration of desferrioxamine cannot be recommended. Patients who are not severely poisoned clinically but who have sufficient circulating free iron to justify use of the antidote must therefore be identified in the manner described above.

Overdosage without features

Patients who have taken overdoses of iron preparations and have not developed features of poisoning within 6 h have probably not ingested toxic amounts. They do not require treatment or observation. Those who present earlier than 6 h should be assessed as described above and treated accordingly.

Supportive measures

Only a small minority of patients will require supportive measures in addition to those described above. Attention to the airway and ventilation is obviously important if consciousness is impaired and fluid and electrolytes should be replaced as necessary. Blood transfusion may be required if there has been significant haemorrhage. Liver and renal function should be monitored and failure managed conventionally.

OVERDOSAGE IN PREGNANCY

Overdosage with iron salts during pregnancy should be treated as under other circumstances. Limited evidence indicated that desferrioxamine is not fetotoxic or teratogenic and to withhold it when it is indicated may be fatal.

REFERENCES

Klein-Schwartz, W., *et al.* (1990). Assessment of management guidelines. Acute iron ingestion. *Clinical Pediatrics*, **29**, 316–21.

Schauben, J.L., Augenstein, W.L., Cox, J., and Sato, R. (1990). Iron poisoning: report of three cases and a review of therapeutic intervention. *Journal of Emergency Medicine*, **8**, 309–19.

Folic acid

Overdosage with this vitamin does not cause toxic features. No treatment is necessary.

Pyridoxine

The daily adult requirement of pyridoxine (vitamin B_6) is 2 to 4 mg but high doses (> 2–3 g/day) have been used for the treatment of a variety of conditions including the premenstrual syndrome, carpal-tunnel syndrome, schizophrenia, and hyperactivity in childhood. Prolonged daily intake of doses of 50 to 300 mg in women has been reported to cause headaches, irritability, tiredness, shooting pains, circumoral and limb paraesthesiae, numb extremities, clumsiness, and ataxia, indicating a sensory neuropathy. Vibration sense is usually most severely affected.

Diagnosis requires a high index of suspicion. Considerable symptomatic improvement occurs within 2 months of stopping the drug but objective evidence of sensory impairment may persist much longer. There is no specific treatment.

8.2.7 Poisoning by endocrine drugs

A. T. PROUDFOOT, J. A. VALE, AND T. J. MEREDITH

Hypoglycaemic agents

Intentional overdose with insulin and oral hypoglycaemic agents is uncommon and is often difficult to recognize. Despite the massive doses of insulin frequently injected on such occasions, the degree of hypoglycaemia is sometimes surprisingly mild, though it may persist for several days. However, deaths from insulin and sulphonylurea overdosage have been reported. Chlorpropamide and glyburide (available only in the United States) are the oral agents most commonly ingested. Chlorpropamide, because of its long half-life, may, in overdose, induce hypoglycaemia for a considerable period of time. In all cases of poisoning with hypoglycaemic agents prompt diagnosis and treatment is essential if death or cerebral damage from neuroglycopenia is to be prevented.

CLINICAL FEATURES

Features of overdosage include drowsiness, coma, twitching, convulsions, depressed limb reflexes, extensor plantar responses, hyperpnoea, pulmonary oedema, tachycardia, and circulatory failure. Hypoglycaemia is to be expected and hypokalaemia, cerebral oedema, and metabolic acidosis might occur. Neurogenic diabetes insipidus and persistent vegetative states are possible long-term complications. Cholestatic jaundice has been described as a late complication of chlorpropamide poisoning.

TREATMENT

The blood or plasma glucose concentration should be measured urgently and intravenous glucose (50 ml of 50 per cent solution) given. Glucagon (1–2 mg intravenously) may also be tried but may be ineffective. Thereafter, gastric lavage should be performed if the patient has presented early after the ingestion of an oral preparation.

Recurring hypoglycaemia is highly likely. A continuous infusion of glucose together with carbohydrate-rich meals are required in cases of severe insulin overdosage, though there may be difficulty in maintaining normoglycaemia. In the case of sulphonylurea overdosage, however, further glucose (although its administration may be unavoidable) only serves to increase already high circulating insulin concentrations. Diazoxide has therefore been recommended since it increases blood glucose concentrations and raises circulating catecholamine concentrations while blocking insulin release. The dose is 1.25 mg/kg body weight intravenously over 1 h, repeated at six-hourly intervals if necessary.

REFERENCES

Erickson, T., *et al.* (1991). Acute oral hypoglycemic ingestions. *Veterinary and Human Toxicology*, **33,** 256–8.

Kaminer, Y. and Robbins, D.R. (1988). Attempted suicide by insulin overdose in insulin-dependent diabetic adolescents. *Pediatrics*, **81,** 526–8.

Palatnick, W., Meatherall, R.C., and Tenenbein, M. (1991). Clinical spectrum of sulfonylurea overdose and experience with diazoxide therapy. *Archives of Internal Medicine*, **151,** 1859–62.

Samuels, M.H. and Eckel, R.H. (1989). Massive insulin overdose: detailed studies of free insulin levels and glucose requirements. *Journal of Toxicology–Clinical Toxicology*, **27,** 157–68.

Thyroxine and tri-iodothyronine

Acute overdosage with thyroid hormones is uncommon. Not surprisingly, thyroxine is the agent most commonly involved.

CLINICAL FEATURES

Probably only a small percentage of patients who ingest large amounts of thyroid hormones develop features of toxicity. Symptoms develop within a few hours with tri-iodothyronine (T_3) and after 3 to 6 days with thyroxine (T_4). They tend to resolve in about the same time as they take to develop. Mental confusion, agitation, irritability and hyperactivity with sinus tachycardia, tachypnoea, pyrexia, and dilated pupils are common while atrial fibrillation, sweating, loose stools, and the ocular features of hyperthyroidism are rare. Convulsions developed in one child.

Serum T_4 and T_3 concentrations which are many times normal values may be attained while those of TSH fall.

TREATMENT

Empty the stomach if more than 2 mg of thyroxine has been ingested within the preceding 1 h. Activated charcoal may be valuable. Serum T_4 and T_3 concentrations should be measured in blood taken 6 to 12 h after ingestion since a normal result precludes the possibility of delayed toxicity and allows the patient to be discharged. Those with high T_4 concentrations should be reviewed for evidence of toxicity on the fourth or fifth day after ingestion. Patients who develop toxicity should be given propranolol for 5 days.

REFERENCES

Berkner, P.D., Starkman, H., and Person, N. (1991). Acute L-thyroxine overdose; therapy with sodium ipodate: evaluation of clinical and physiologic parameters. *Journal of Emergency Medicine*, **9,** 129–31.

Lin, T.-H., Kirkland, R.T., and Kirkland, J.L. (1988). Clinical features and management of overdosage with thyroid drugs. *Medical Toxicology*, **3,** 264–72.

8.2.8 Poisoning from antimicrobials

A. T. PROUDFOOT, J. A. VALE, AND T. J. MEREDITH

It is uncommon for antimicrobials to be taken in gross overdosage and when they are, they seldom seem to cause toxic effects. The majority of patients will have no symptoms and require no treatment. Transient nausea, vomiting and diarrhoea may occur and, in rare cases, may require symptomatic measures. Renal failure has been recorded after overdosage with co-trimoxazole, pancreatitis with erythromycin, and haemorrhagic cystitis with amoxicillin but only in single case reports.

REFERENCES

Berger, T.M. *et al.* (1992). Acute pancreatitis in a 12 year old girl after an erythomycin overdose. *Pediatrics,* **90,** 624–6.

Bright, D.A., *et al.* (1989). Amoxicillin overdose with gross hematuria. *Western Journal of Medicine*, **150,** 698–9.

Goff, D. (1989). Renal failure induced by co-trimoxazole. *Hospital Therapy*, **14,** 61–7.

Gumaste, V.V. (1989). Erythromycin-induced pancreatitis. *American Journal of Medicine*, **86,** 725.

8.2.9 Poisoning from cinchona alkaloids and other antimalarials

P. A. WINSTANLEY

Chloroquine

Chloroquine overdose is probably the most common form of self-poisoning with drugs in Africa, the Far East, and West Pacific and is a growing problem in Europe.

Clinical features

Toxicity can result from doses greater than 1 g (about six tablets) in adults. Cardiovascular effects are severe and develop rapidly. In some cases cardiorespiratory arrest is the first clinical manifestation of poisoning, but hypotension, resulting mainly from negative inotropic effects, usually precedes it and may progress to cardiogenic shock and pulmonary oedema. Electrocardiographic abnormalities, bradyarrhythmias, and tachyarrhythmias are common and are similar to those of quinine (see below). Visual disturbance, agitation, drowsiness, acute psychosis, dystonic reactions, seizures, and coma may ensue. Hypokalaemia is common and may be due to potassium channel blockade.

Treatment

Gastric lavage should be considered if the patient presents within 1 h or, alternatively, activated charcoal (50–100 g) should be administered. Supportive measures should be employed and hypokalaemia corrected as there is no specific antidote and there are no means of increasing drug clearance. There is evidence that mechanical ventilation, the administration of adrenaline (0.25 μg/kg.min) and the use of high-doses of diazepam (1 mg/kg as a loading dose and 0.25–0.4 mg/kg.h maintenance) may reduce the mortality to 10 per cent even in severe poisoning. Diazepam may be of benefit because it competes for cardiac chloroquine receptors.

Dapsone

Dapsone is available formulated alone or in combination with pyrimethamine (as Maloprim).

Clinical features

Dapsone poisoning can be severe and results not only in methaemoglobinaemia but also in haemolysis, hepatitis, drowsiness, coma, seizures, and metabolic acidosis.

Treatment

If presentation after overdose is within 1 h, gastric lavage should be considered or, alternatively, activated charcoal (50–100 g) may be administered. Administration of repeat doses of activated charcoal seems to have comparable efficacy to haemodialysis in increasing dapsone elimination. Methylene blue (1–2 mg/kg) should be given intravenously over 5 min for severe methaemoglobinaemia.

Mefloquine

Clinical features

Poisoning may result in vertigo, visual disturbance, hypotension, and tachycardia.

Treatment

Treatment is supportive as there are no means of enhancing mefloquine elimination.

Primaquine

Clinical features

Primaquine poisoning is rare, though toxicity is frequent if more than 60 mg is ingested in one day. Headache, nausea, abdominal pain, and methaemoglobinaemia may occur and haemolytic anaemia and leucopenia have been observed, especially in patients with glucose 6-phosphate dehydrogenase deficiency.

Treatment

Gut decontamination should be considered if presentation is within 1 h. If methaemoglobinaemia exceeds 40 per cent, methylene blue (1–2 mg/kg) should be administered intravenously over 5 min.

Proguanil

Clinical features

Proguanil is less dangerous in overdose than any other antimalarial. Overdoses as high as 14.5 g have been survived without sequelae. Gastrointestinal upset and abdominal pain occur and temporary bone marrow depression and hair loss may be seen.

Treatment

Management is supportive and symptomatic

Pyrimethamine

Pyrimethamine is formulated alone (Daraprim) and in combination with sulphadoxine (Fansidar) or dapsone (Maloprim).

Clinical features

In children, toxicity is seen readily with doses greater than 25 mg. Coma, seizures, apnoea, pyrexia, visual impairment, and deafness may occur.

Treatment

Gut decontamination should be considered if the patient presents early. Supportive measures should then be employed as there are no proven means of enhancing drug elimination.

Quinine

Quinine poisoning is uncommon. Most cases involve young adults who ingest the drug deliberately; a minority are iatrogenic or result from attempted abortion or adulterated heroin.

Clinical features

Toxicity can be seen with doses as low as 2 g in adults. About 40 per cent of patients develop ocular features, which may be unilateral, including blindness, contracted fields, scotoma, dilated pupils, blurred disc margins, macular oedema, arteriolar spasm, and late optic atrophy. Oculotoxicity is related to plasma concentration, becoming likely when concentrations exceed 10 mg/l. Visual loss is permanent in about 50 per cent of cases. Prolongation of the QT interval, widening of QRS complexes, non-specific T wave changes, sinus arrest, sinus bradycardia, heart block, ventricular tachycardia, and ventricular fibrillation may be observed on ECG. Hypotension can occur but is less of a problem than with chloroquine. Cinchonism, which comprises tinnitus, deafness, vertigo, nausea, headache, and diarrhoea, is common at plasma concentrations greater than 5 mg/l. Coma and seizures can occur at high plasma quinine concentrations. Hypoglycaemia may occur due to drug-induced insulin secretion and hypokalaemia has also been reported, and is probably due to potassium channel blockade. In malaria, high quinine concentrations are tolerated without serious toxicity: this may be due to increased binding of the drug to acute phase reactants.

Treatment

If the patient presents within 1 h of overdose, the stomach should be emptied or, alternatively, activated charcoal (50–100 g) should be administered. Repeated doses of activated charcoal have been shown to increase quinine clearance even after parenteral overdose. Forced acid diuresis, charcoal haemoperfusion, and haemodialysis do not increase quinine elimination and no consistent benefit has been found from stellate ganglion block or the use of calcium-channel blockers.

Sulphadoxine

This is available in combination with pyrimethamine (Fansidar).

Clinical features

In overdose sulphadoxine can cause methaemoglobinaemia, but otherwise only produces mild effects.

Treatment

Supportive care should be given and methylene blue (1–2 mg/kg) should be administered over 5 min for cases of severe methaemoglobinaemia.

REFERENCES

Dyson, E.H., Proudfoot, A.T., Prescott, L.F., and Heyworth, R. (1985). Death and blindness due to overdose of quinine. *British Medical Journal*, **291,** 31–3.

Jaeger, A., Sauder, P., Kopferschmitt, J., and Flesch, F. (1987). Clinical features and management of poisoning due to antimalarial drugs. *Medical Toxicology*, **2,** 242–73.

Looareesuwan, S., *et al.* (1986). Cardiovascular toxicity and distribution kinetics of intravenous chloroquine. *British Journal of Clinical Pharmacology*, **22,** 31–6.

Riou, B., Barriot, P., Rimailho, A., and Baud, F. (1988). Treatment of severe chloroquine poisoning. *New England Journal of Medicine*, **318,** 1–6.

8.2.10 Poisoning from drugs of abuse

A. T. Proudfoot, J. A. Vale, and T. J. Meredith

Classification

The drugs or substances of abuse can be classified into three main groups; those which alter perception, those which stimulate the brain and those which depress it. Inevitably these groups overlap to some extent. Substances which predominantly depress the CNS often arouse and disinhibit behaviour before exerting their main action (e.g. ethanol and barbiturates) while, conversely, drugs which initially stimulate the brain can impair consciousness if taken in sufficient quantity. There are similar parallels in clinical toxicology; anticonvulsants in overdosage can cause seizures and antiarrhythmic drugs arrhythmias.

Methods of abuse

Virtually every possible route of drug absorption has been used for substances which are abused. The method of choice depends to a large extent on the nature of the substance in question and the desired intensity of effect on the brain of the user. Ingestion is clearly convenient and may be the only route possible with some substances because of their physical characteristics, especially the extent to which they are water soluble. However, absorption from the gut is relatively slow and the impact of the drug on the brain correspondingly muted unless large quantities are taken. Drugs such as ethanol, the benzodiazepines, chlormethiazole, some opioid analgesics (particularly, codeine, dihydrocodeine, and pentazocine), sympathomimetics, anticholinergic drugs, and plant preparations are taken in this way. The speed of absorption can be increased by inhaling the substance but this is possible with only a small range of materials. Nicotine from tobacco is the most common example but volatile substances, particularly organic solvents, cannabis, narcotic analgesics, phencyclidine, cocaine, and organic nitrites can also be taken by this route. Absorption through the skin or mucous membranes is not a popular route except in the case of cocaine. Cocaine is commonly dissolved and the solution sniffed up into the nostrils where part is absorbed, a technique commonly referred to as snorting. Some is no doubt swallowed in the process. Injection is the fastest method of getting drugs to the brain in high concentration. Subcutaneous injection is known as 'skin popping' and that into veins as 'mainlining'. The latter is the preferred route for the most potent opioid analgesics.

The hazards of drug abuse

ACCIDENTAL OVERDOSAGE

Drug abusers seek intoxication with the substance of their choice but the amount they take is usually arbitrary and the potency may vary considerably from one time to another and from one source to another. Accidental overdosage is a constant risk, less with some routes of administration than others. Effects of smoking and other methods of inhalation require top-up at regular, brief intervals for their continuation and this process is inhibited by intoxication, thereby preventing serious toxicity. This is not the case however, when intoxication is from the atmosphere (e.g. an enclosed small room or a plastic bag placed over the head). Not surprisingly, intravenous injection carries the greatest risk of accidental overdosage and once done, the drug cannot be retrieved. This problem is probably due to the inexperience of the user or to unexpected increases in the potency of street drug. Drug pushers are likely to 'cut' (i.e. dilute) what is sold on the streets when supplies of high quality drug fall and during this period users may increase the amounts they inject so that they can continue to experience a 'rush'. If they continue with these amounts when, unknown to them, the potency of the street drug has increased, there is obviously a serious risk of accidental overdosage.

DELAYED PRESENTATION

Since abuse is often illegal and intoxication is the objective, drug users are usually anxious not to attract attention to themselves. Mild to moderate poisoning is therefore unlikely to come to medical notice and on occasions even individuals who become unconscious or seriously ill in other ways may not be referred for medical help immediately. They are often simply observed or given rudimentary 'care' by their less intoxicated fellow users until they improve or their colleagues are finally forced to accept that something serious is amiss. Unfortunately, the reluctance to accept what, even to the uninitiated, must often be obvious means that there may occasionally be delays of several hours during which hypotension and hypoxia can cause irreversible brain damage.

CONTAMINANTS

Some of the apparent complications of drug misuse may not be due to the primary drug but to the substances such as talc which are often used to cut it before it is sold to the user. In other cases, contaminants are the result of the way in which the drug is prepared for injection e.g. passage through cigarette filters or cotton wool. These are the cause of the long-term, progressive, granulomatous pulmonary lesions while others, particularly quinine, may be responsible for some of the more acute toxic phenomena and possibly even deaths.

NON-DRUG HAZARDS

The non-drug related hazards of drug abuse are well-known. They include infections with hepatitis B, etc., and HIV, bacterial infections causing skin abscesses, thrombophlebitis and endocarditis, moniliasis and inadvertent intra-arterial injection leading to digital gangrene. These lesions will not be discussed here.

Body packing

A potential source of poisoning and death unique to illicit drugs is the phenomenon of body packing. This is the term given to the practice of smuggling these drugs by making them up into small packets which are then swallowed for later retrieval from vomitus or faeces (the practitioners being called 'swallowers') or inserted into the vagina or rectum (the 'stuffers'). The number of quite large packets that can be concealed in this way is surprising; 103, each the size of a small egg, and with a combined weight of over 580 g were reported in one case. The obvious discomfort and hazards of this technique are such that it is reserved for the financially most lucrative preparations such as high quality cannabis, cocaine, heroin, and morphine. The corollary is that they are also potentially the most toxic. The purity of heroin in some Australian cases varied from 29 to 85 per cent and there is clearly a grave risk of overdosage should one or more packets burst allowing absorption through the intestinal, rectal, or vaginal mucosae. The choice of wrapping is therefore of considerable medical importance since it not only determines the ease with which they can be removed but also the risk of disintegration and that of drug leaching out while traversing the gut. Condoms, foil, cellophane, and other wrappings are used. In addition to these toxic hazards, the body packer is at risk of acute intestinal obstruction.

MANAGEMENT OF BODY PACKERS

The vagina can be cleared of packets relatively easily and safely but attempts at manual evacuation of the rectum may lead to rupture of packets and systemic toxicity from rectal absorption. Packets in the stomach may be retrieved by inducing emesis but the management of packets which have passed through the pylorus is controversial. The current trend is towards as conservative an approach as possible, resorting to surgery only when obstructive features develop or intra-abdominal packets rupture and cause systemic toxicity. The majority of cases should simply be observed while given laxatives or other measures to speed transit through the gut. Two recent series have shown that 'swallowers' can be satisfactorily managed medically using bulk laxatives with or without bowel stimulants such as bisacodyl.

Abdominal radiography may yield information about the physical characteristics of the wrappings which, together with the nature of the drug they contain, is crucial in deciding whether a conservative or a surgical approach should be adopted. Emergency surgery should not be the automatic response to identification of drug packages in the gut, particularly if the drug involved is cannabis or an opioid analgesic since the toxicity of the former is unlikely to be serious and the effects of the latter can be reversed by naloxone. On the other hand there may a stronger case for early surgical intervention for packets containing amphetamines or cocaine since massive overdosage with these substances carries a significant morbidity and mortality and is less readily treated.

Cannabis

Cannabis is obtained from the plant *Cannabis sativa* which grows extensively in various parts of the world, particularly South America. Preparations of different parts of the plant have common names. Resin and oil are obtained from the flowering tops while the considerably less potent 'grass' is derived from the leaves and stems. Marihuana is obtained from any part. The plant contains many active substances of which the most important are the tetrahydrocannabinols which are responsible for the mental effects.

Smoking is the common route of use of cannabis. It is occasionally ingested and, rarely, made into a 'tea' and injected intravenously. Cannabis use is usually a group activity.

CLINICAL FEATURES

Euphoria with drowsiness and distorted and heightened images, colours, and sounds are the usual effects of this compound. Tactile sensations may also be altered. A tachycardia is often present and heavy use may lead to conjunctival suffusion, tachycardia, hypotension, and ataxia. Higher doses induce visual and auditory hallucinations, confusion, depersonalization, and panic. Cannabis is clearly used because some people find the distortion of perception pleasurable but novice users may react with panic attacks which prompt them or their friends to seek medical help. However, accident and emergency presentations for this reason are very uncommon despite the probable widespread use of the drug and it must be deduced that most cannabis users cope without difficulty with the sensations it induces.

Intravenous injection of cannabis infusions leads to an altogether more serious illness. Within a few minutes, there is nausea, vomiting, and chills followed after an interval of an hour or so by profuse watery diarrhoea, tachycardia, hypotension, and arthralgia. A marked neutrophil leucocytosis is often present and hypoglycaemia has been reported in some cases. There may also be transient renal failure. Whether long-term use leads to psychosis is a matter of controversy.

TREATMENT

Most patients will settle with reassurance and comforting. Sedation with intravenous diazepam may be required for a small minority whose behaviour is disruptive or who are clearly very distressed. Those who have injected cannabis infusions should be treated supportively with particular attention to intravascular volume expansion and correction of hypoglycaemia. This will usually be sufficient to restore normal blood pressure and considerable general improvement can be expected within 24 h. Cannabis body packers should be managed as described above.

Lysergic acid diethylamide

As with cannabis, individuals intoxicated with lysergic acid diethylamide (LSD) rarely present to the medical services.

CLINICAL FEATURES

The ability of LSD to distort reality is well known. Visual hallucinations, distortion of images, agitation, excitement, dilated pupils, tachycardia, hypertension, hyperreflexia, tremor, and hyperthermia are common. Auditory hallucinations are said to be rare but colours may be heard and sounds seen. Time seems to pass very slowly and behaviour may become disturbed with paranoid delusions necessitating sedation or physical restraint. The latter has led to rhabdomyolysis and acute renal failure. Coma, respiratory arrest, and coagulation disturbances have been described in eight individuals who snorted large amounts of pure LSD. Flashbacks in which the effects of LSD may be re-experienced without further exposure to the drug occur in about 15 per cent of users for several years and are not explained.

TREATMENT

Most individuals will require little more than reassurance and sedation. Supportive measures are all that can be offered those who are seriously ill.

Phencyclidine

Phencyclidine (PCP) was developed for use as an anaesthetic in the late 1970s but quickly abandoned mainly because of an unacceptably high incidence of postoperative psychotic reactions and to some extent because it was superseded by the related compound ketamine. Phencyclidine is easily synthesized and several variants probably circulate. It has a number of pseudonyms including PCP, Pea Ce Pill, hog, goon, crystal, and angel dust. PCP is usually smoked in combination with tobacco and less frequently with marijuanha but it may also be ingested or injected. Its mode of action is not clear. Cerebrospinal fluid concentrations may be three or four times higher than those in serum and take much longer to clear.

CLINICAL FEATURES

Poisoning with PCP has been reported throughout a wide age range. In young children it is often the result of accidental ingestion but it is possible that it can be caused by inhalation as intoxication has occurred in children in the same room as adults smoking the drug.

The pleasurable effects of phencyclidine include initial euphoria, a feeling of dissociation, numbness, perceptual distortion, and hallucinations which are usually visual in type. Nystagmus, hypertension, and tachycardia are common but there is lack of agreement about whether hypothermia occurs more frequently than hyperthermia. As with other substances which distort perception, some users find these effects intolerable and present to medical services. More severe intoxication may be complicated by hypersalivation, profuse sweating, generalized seizures, prolonged psychotic reactions, dystonias, and hypoglycaemia. Rhabdomyolysis and acute renal failure are common.

Behavioural disturbances are common. Some individuals become disorientated and confused with inappropriate affect while others develop a catatonic syndrome with stupor, posturing, catalepsy, mutism, and staring. The greatest clinical and social problems, however, are caused by the substantial minority whose behaviour becomes bizarre with excitement, agitation, and a tendency to violence. Rarely, intracranial haemorrhage and malignant hyperthermia with subtotal necrosis of the liver have been reported.

TREATMENT

Supportive measures are all that will be required in the majority of individuals with mild intoxication. If behaviour is disturbed or if coma, convulsions, or sweating are present it is important to measure the plasma glucose concentration and treat hypoglycaemia if it is found. Following that sedation may be necessary and the drug chosen will to a large extent be dictated by the ease with which the patient can be handled. Oral diazepam may suffice but chlorpromazine may be the drug of choice particularly if hypertension is a problem and convulsions have not occurred. Unconscious patients will require appropriate care.

The plasma activity of muscle enzymes and renal function should be monitored to detect rhabdomyolysis as early as possible and to initiate measures to minimize the risk of renal tubular necrosis. Diphenhydramine by intramuscular injection has been reported rapidly to abolish acute dystonic reactions induced by PCP.

Measures intended to increase the elimination of absorbed PCP have been recommended. Acidification of the urine enhances renal elimination and continuous gastric suction may be of some value in unconscious patients by removing PCP secreted in gastric juice, thereby preventing reabsorption further down the gut.

REFERENCE

Patel, R. and Connor, G. (1985–86). A review of thirty cases of rhabdomyolysis-associated acute renal failure among phencyclidine users. *Clinical Toxicology*, **23**, 547–56.

Anticholinergic substances

It would be a mistake to believe that drug abuse is confined to the potent narcotic analgesics, cocaine and cannabis, which tend to attract the attention of the media. A large number of other substances are widely misused in the search for a 'buzz' or in desperation resulting from lack of the drugs of first choice. Anticholinergic substances feature high on the list of occasional alternatives. Plants have been used for many years, particularly the *Datura* species which grow in many countries throughout the world and which contain atropine, hyoscine, and hyoscyamine among other alkaloids. In England *Datura stramonium* has long been known as the mad apple because of its ability to induce hallucinations and has been abused. However, its anticholinergic actions found a therapeutic role in the treatment of asthma by making dried leaves into cigarettes. These, in turn, have been eaten rather than smoked in the search for kicks. Not only are the leaves eaten or made into a tea but the long flowers known as angels' trumpets have been used similarly. In the United States, *D.stramonium* is known as the Jimsonweed and has been widely abused.

Anticholinergic substance abuse is not confined to plants. A large number of drugs currently used in medicine have these properties among others and have been misused. The problem of adolescents ingesting antihistamines, particularly cyclizine which can be bought over-the-counter in many countries, was first reported in 1968 and continues today, albeit not on a large scale. Similarly, concern has been expressed that addicts abuse antiparkinsonian drugs such as benzhexol, benztropine, orphenadrine, and biperiden. Even tricyclic antidepressants are thought to have been abused.

The features and management of intoxication with these substances is considered elsewhere (Chapter 8.2.2).

Amphetamines

Amphetamine, dexamphetamine, methamphetamine, and 'ecstasy' (3,4-methylenedioxymethamphetamine, MDMA) stimulate the central nervous system causing increased alertness and self-confidence, initial euphoria, more extrovert behaviour, increased talkativeness with rapid speech, lack of desire to eat or sleep, tremor, dilated pupils, tachycardia, and hypertension. More severe intoxication is associated with excitability, agitation, paranoid delusions, hallucinations with violent behaviour, hypertonia, and hyperreflexia. Convulsions, rhabdomyolysis, hyperthermia, and cardiac arrhythmias may develop in the worst cases. Hyperthyroxinaemia may be found in chronic users. Rarely, intracerebral and subarachnoid haemorrhage, acute cardiomyopathy, and cardiac arrhythmias occur and may be fatal.

TREATMENT

The stomach should be emptied if more than 10 tablets have been ingested by an adult in the preceding 1 h. Supportive measures should be instituted as indicated. Sedation may well be required and chlorpromazine has been recommended although droperidol and diazepam have their advocates. The peripheral sympathomimetic actions of amphetamines may be antagonized by β-adrenergic blocking drugs. Acidification of the urine has been reported to increase the renal elimination of methamphetamine five-fold.

REFERENCES

Derlet, R.W., Rice, P., Horowitz, B.Z., and Lord, R.V. (1989). Amphetamine toxicity: experience with 127 cases. *Journal of Emergency Medicine*, **7**, 157–61.

Henry, J.A., Jeffreys, K.J., and Dawling, S. (1992). Toxicity and deaths from 3,4-methylenedioxymethamphetamine (''ecstasy''). *Lancet*, **340**, 384–7.

Cocaine

In recent years there has been a considerable increase in the illicit use of cocaine. Cocaine is a powerful local anaesthetic and vasoconstrictor and may be abused by smoking, ingestion, injection, or by 'snorting' it intranasally. Not surprisingly, overdosage has occurred. Not only are users at risk, but also body packers. In the United States, 'street' cocaine is sometimes purified by dissolving it in an aqueous alkaline solution and extracting the cocaine into ether which is then evaporated to leave crystals of relatively pure or 'freebase' cocaine. 'Crack' (cocaine without the hydrochloride moiety) is also used widely. Other drugs such as ethanol, cannabis, and conventional hypnotics and sedatives are frequently taken with cocaine to reduce the intensity of its less pleasant effects.

CLINICAL FEATURES

The features of cocaine overdosage are similar to those of amphetamine. In addition to euphoria, it also has sympathomimetic effects including agitation, tachycardia, hypertension, sweating, and hallucinations. Prolonged convulsions with metabolic acidosis, hyperthermia, rhabdomyolysis, ventricular arrhythmias, and cardiorespiratory arrest may follow in the most severe cases. Less common features include dissection of the aorta, myocarditis, myocardial infarction, dilated cardiomyopathy, subarachnoid haemorrhage, cerebral haemorrhage, and cerebral vasculitis.

A number of rare complications of the method of use of cocaine have also been reported. These include pulmonary oedema after intravenous injection of freebase cocaine and pneumomediastinum and pneumothorax after sniffing it. In addition, chronic 'snorting' has caused perforation of the nasal septum and CSF rhinorrhoea due to thinning of the cribriform plate and pulmonary granulomatosis.

TREATMENT

Users who are intoxicated may require sedation with diazepam to control agitation or convulsions. Measures to prevent further absorption are usually irrelevant. Hypertension and severe tachycardia may be controlled with a β-adrenergic blocking drug but, in one case at least, the use of propranolol caused paradoxical hypertension. Accelerated idioventricular rhythm should not normally require treatment but ventricular fibrillation and asystole should be managed in the usual way.

REFERENCES

Brown, E., Prager, J., Lee, H.-Y., and Ramsey, R.G. (1992). CNS complications of cocaine abuse: prevalence, pathophysiology, and neuroradiology. *American Journal of Roentgenology*, **159,** 137–47.

Kloner, R.A., Hale, S., Alker, K., and Rezkalla, S. (1992). The effects of acute and chronic cocaine use on the heart. *Circulation*, **85,** 407–19.

Lange, R.A., *et al.* (1990). Potentiation of cocaine-induced vasoconstriction by beta-adrenergic blockade. *Annals of Internal Medicine*, **112,** 897–903.

Rubin, R.B. and Neugarten, J. (1992). Medical complications of cocaine: changes in pattern of use and spectrum of complications. *Clinical Toxicology*, **30,** 1–12.

Silva, M.O., *et al.* (1991). Hepatic dysfunction accompanying acute cocaine intoxication. *Journal of Hepatology*, **12,** 312–15.

Other CNS stimulants

A number of other substances which stimulate the central nervous system lend themselves to abuse, largely through being available without prescription. They therefore appeal to adolescents and young adults. They include phenylpropanolamine, caffeine, ephedrine, pseudoephedrine, and propylhexedrine.

Their effects are similar to those of amphetamines and treatment of overdosage is mainly supportive with sedation and perhaps β-adrenergic blocking drugs.

REFERENCE

Price, K.R. and Fligner, D.J. (1990). Treatment of caffeine toxicity with esmolol. *Annals of Emergency Medicine*, **19,** 44–6.

Opioid analgesics

These are discussed in Chapter 8.2.1.

8.2.11 Poisoning due to miscellaneous drugs

J. A. VALE, A. T. PROUDFOOT, AND T. J. MEREDITH

Anticoagulants (oral)

Warfarin is the most commonly used oral anticoagulant; nicoumalone and phenindione are seldom used. Anticoagulants are also used as rodenticides and the majority of these agents are more potent antagonists of vitamin K_1 than warfarin.

MECHANISM OF TOXICITY

Anticoagulants interfere with synthesis of clotting factors II, VII, IX, and X by inhibiting the regeneration of vitamin K_1 from its biologically inactive metabolite vitamin K_1 2,3-epoxide. Vitamin K is an obligatory cofactor for the enzyme that carboxylates specific glutamate residues in blood coagulation proteins (factors II, VII, IX, and X, and proteins C, S, Z, and M). Vitamin K is first reduced to a biologically active hydroquinone form (vitamin KH_2) by an NAD(P)H-dependent reductase. This reductase and the one responsible for cycling vitamin K epoxide (formed as a consequence of the carboxylation reaction) back to vitamin K is irreversibly inhibited by warfarin and other anticoagulants. Vitamin K is an effective antidote in anticoagulant overdose because it stimulates formation of vitamin KH_2 through an alternative warfarin-resistant enzyme pathway.

CLINICAL FEATURES

Gastrointestinal bleeding, haematuria, and bruising are the commonest features, though the most common site of fatal haemorrhage is intracranial. The risk of haemorrhage depends on the dose of anticoagulant ingested acutely, the pre-existing coagulation state, and the appropriateness of medical care.

TREATMENT

If the INR is less than 5 and the patient is not bleeding and continuing anticoagulation is required, no immediate treatment beyond temporarily discontinuing the anticoagulant is usually required. If continuing anticoagulation is not intended, the INR is greater than 5 and severe bleeding has occurred, vitamin K_1 (phytomenadione) 5 mg should be given slowly intravenously. In less severe cases of bleeding give phytomenadione 1 mg slowly intravenously. The INR will shorten within 10 h but, if haemorrhage is major, fresh-frozen plasma should be given in addition.

REFERENCES

Dowd, D., Ham, S.W., and Geib, S.J. (1991). Mechanism of action of vitamin K. *Journal of the American Chemical Society,* **113,** 7734–43.

Wallin, R. and Martin L.F. (1987). Warfarin poisoning and vitamin K antagonism in rat and human liver. *Biochemical Journal,* **241,** 389–96.

Disulfiram

Disulfiram is used as an adjunct in the treatment of chronic alcohol abuse and it has also been employed in the management of nickel dermatitis.

MECHANISM OF TOXICITY

Disulfiram inhibits the activity of a wide range of enzymes including aldehyde dehydrogenase, fructose 1,6-diphosphate and succinic dehydrogenase (so that glycolysis, the pentose phosphate pathway, and the tricarboxylic acid cycle are affected), hepatic microsomal drug-metabolizing enzymes, xanthine oxidase, and dopamine β-hydroxylase (with consequent reduction of noradrenaline synthesis). The main metabolite, diethyldithiocarbamate, is a potent metal chelator and also inhibits aldehyde dehydrogenase and dopamine β-hydroxylase. Carbon disulphide, a further metabolite, may account for some of the side-effects observed during disulfiram therapy.

CLINICAL FEATURES

Acute poisoning

Adult cases are invariably alcoholics and are thus likely to have been taking disulfiram prior to the overdose and to be malnourished. These two factors may well explain the frequency of neuropsychiatric features. One patient presented with aggressive and confused behaviour, pyrexia, and mild ketosis; all symptoms resolved within 7 days of admission. Other chronic alcohol abusers have developed a sensorimotor neuropathy, flaccid tetraparesis, and encephalopathy after overdose though these features may have been exacerbated by pre-existing malnourishment. Vomiting for several days, abdominal pain, and diarrhoea were reported in a patient who ingested 18 g of disulfiram.

Several cases of paediatric poisoning have been reported. Drowsiness, pyrexia, hypotonia, ataxia, uncontrollable and inappropriate arm movements, irritability and speech difficulties, hallucinations, coma, and hyper-reflexia were the major features.

Disulfiram–ethanol reaction

When taken together (even small amounts of alcohol may produce a reaction) a variety of unpleasant effects may occur including nausea, vertigo, anxiety, blurred vision, hypotension, chest pain, palpitations, tachycardia, facial flushing, and throbbing headache. Symptoms usually last for 3 to 4 days but may persist for a week. Occasionally the reaction is very severe with respiratory depression, cardiovascular collapse, cardiac arrhythmias, coma, cerebral oedema, hemiplegia, and convulsions: fatalities have been reported.

REFERENCES

Kirubakaran, V., Liskow, B., Mayfield, D., and Faiman, M.D. (1983). Case report of acute disulfiram overdose. *American Journal of Psychiatry*, **140,** 1513–14.

Manoguerra, A.S. and Kearney, T.E. (1982). Acute disulfiram toxicity. *Veterinary and Human Toxicology*, **24,** 282.

Sodium chloride

Poisoning with sodium chloride is uncommon but has occurred accidentally (e.g. addition of salt instead of sugar to infant feeds), as a result of deliberate intent (e.g. as a form of child abuse), or iatrogenically (e.g. use of hypertonic saline in gastric lavage or too rapid administration of saline during treatment of hyponatraemia).

MECHANISM OF TOXICITY

An increase in plasma sodium will increase plasma osmolality causing a shift of water from the intracellular to the extracellular space. CNS cell dehydration results in distended cerebral vessels and subarachnoid, subdural, and intravascular haemorrhages may follow; these changes may be compounded by overzealous rehydration.

CLINICAL FEATURES

Poisoning with sodium chloride can induce vomiting, increased thirst, anorexia, fever, hypotonia, lethargy, dehydration, 'shut-down' extremities, irritability, muscular rigidity, convulsions, and coma. Hypernatraemia, increased plasma and urine osmolality, hyperglycaemia, metabolic acidosis, and hypocalcaemia may ensue. In severe cases pulmonary oedema and congestive heart failure may develop.

TREATMENT

The aim is to lower the serum sodium concentration slowly so that cerebral oedema, pulmonary oedema, convulsions, and coma do not occur. Five per cent dextrose, then hypotonic saline solutions, should be given intravenously, but in severe cases complicated by renal insufficiency, haemodialysis (peritoneal dialysis is less efficient) should be considered. Hyperglycaemia should not be corrected by insulin as this may induce cerebral oedema.

REFERENCES

Addleman, M., Pollard, A., and Grossman, R.F. (1985). Survival after severe hypernatremia due to salt ingestion by an adult. *American Journal of Medicine*, **78,** 176–8.

Finberg, L. (1973). Hypernatremic (hypertonic) dehydration in infants. *New England Journal of Medicine*, **289,** 196–8.

8.3 Poisoning by chemicals

8.3.1 Poisoning from household products

T. J. MEREDITH, J. A. VALE, AND A. T. PROUDFOOT

There is a commonly held belief that household products contain a wide range of highly toxic chemicals, and so the ingestion of these substances by children is a frequent cause for alarm in parents and doctors alike. So-called poisoning from household products is more often the result of accidental than deliberate ingestion, mostly involves young children and is not usually serious. Even when the toxicity of a household product is high, the risk it poses is usually low, certainly following accidental poisoning. However, adults intent on suicide may, by deliberately swallowing massive quantities, succeed in killing themselves.

The enormous variety of domestic products prevents generalization about their chemical composition, but some comments can be offered about the toxicological properties of the principal groups.

Antiseptics and disinfectants

Once these solutions commonly contained phenol but this is now usually replaced by small quantities of either chlorophenol or chloroxylenol, which although less toxic than phenol can be hazardous if ingested in large quantities. More dangerous is isopropyl alcohol, which possesses approximately double the potency and toxicity of ethyl alcohol and may form 40 per cent of some disinfectant solutions.

Ingestion of a significant quantity of either an antiseptic or disinfectant results in a sensation of burning in the mouth and throat, followed by drowsiness, stupor, depression of respiration, and coma. Up to 15 per cent of the isopropyl alcohol ingested is converted to acetone, and ketonuria may therefore be detected.

The fatal dose of isopropyl alcohol can be as little as 100 ml in an adult, and so gastric aspiration and lavage is indicated if more than the equivalent of a mouthful has been swallowed. Otherwise symptomatic and supportive care should be given; in severely poisoned patients, haemodialysis may be indicated to remove the isopropyl alcohol.

Dishwashing liquids, fabric conditioners, and general household detergents

Most of these products, including carpet shampoo, dishwashing rinse aid for dishwashing machines, fabric washing powder and flakes, and scouring liquids, creams, and powders, contain, as their principal active ingredient, surfactants, which are chemicals that contain both hydrophilic and lipophilic groups to allow fat-soluble substances to be dispersed in aqueous media.

There are three types of surfactant, of differing toxicity: anionic surfactants, which have a negative electrical charge on the lipophilic groups; cationic surfactants, which have positive charges; and non-ionic surfactants which have no charge at all on the lipophilic groups.

Anionic detergents irritate the skin by removing natural oils and cause redness, soreness, and even a papular dermatitis. Ingestion may cause mild gastrointestinal irritation, nausea, vomiting, and diarrhoea. Non-ionic surfactants irritate the skin only slightly and appear to be completely harmless when ingested. Cationic surfactants are much more toxic than the others but are rarely found in household cleaning materials.

After ingestion of products containing either a non-ionic or anionic surfactant, liberal amounts of water or milk should be administered. If a cationic surfactant is involved, advice should be sought from a poisons information centre.

Bleaches and lavatory cleaners

Household bleach is normally a 3 to 6 per cent solution of sodium hypochlorite. Ingestion may cause a burning sensation in the mouth, throat, and oesophagus, accompanied by a sensation of thirst, vomiting, and abdominal discomfort. It is rare for household, as opposed to industrial, bleach preparations to cause harm, though pharyngeal and laryngeal oedema may occasionally be encountered. The properties of industrial bleaches are reviewed in Chapter 8.3.5.

When small quantities of bleach have been ingested, liberal fluids by mouth are all that is required. Gastric aspiration and lavage should only be considered if concentrated bleach has been swallowed less than 1 h primarily.

Household bleach may give rise to toxic gases. This occurs when several cleaning agents are mixed together in the lavatory bowl. Hypochlorite bleach mixed with ammonia produces chloramine gas which causes nausea and respiratory irritation. More dangerous is the mixture of bleach and powder lavatory cleaners containing bisulphites which themselves normally evolve chlorine. This results in the formation of oxides of sulphur. Inhalation of these gases may result in severe respiratory irritation and even pulmonary oedema. Supplemental humidified oxygen and a β_2-agonist such as salbutamol (albuterol) by nebulizer may be needed. If the response is poor, corticosteroids should be considered.

Lavatory sanitizers and deodorants

Solid lavatory sanitizer or deodorant blocks normally contain paradichlorobenzene. Ingestion may cause nausea, vomiting, diarrhoea, and abdominal pain. Symptomatic and supportive treatment is all that is required unless many grams have been ingested in which case gastric lavage should be undertaken if the patient presents soon after ingestion.

REFERENCES

Gosselin, R.E., Smith, R.P., and Hodge, H.C. (1984). *Clinical toxicology of commercial products*. 5th edn. Williams & Wilkins, Baltimore.

Meredith, T.J. and Vale, J.A. (1981). Poisoning due to household products. In *Poisoning: diagnosis and treatment* (eds J.A. Vale and T.J. Meredith), pp. 160–7. MTP/Update, London.

8.3.2 Poisoning by alcohols and glycols

J. A. Vale, A. T. Proudfoot, and T. J. Meredith

General mechanisms of toxicity

Benzyl alcohol, ethanol, isopropanol, methanol, ethylene glycol, diethylene glycol, and propylene glycol are CNS depressants which are rapidly absorbed from the upper gut and oxidized initially and principally by hepatic (and in the case of ethanol, gastric) alcohol dehydrogenase and then (with the exception of isopropanol) by aldehyde dehydrogenase to acids. Systemic complications arise as a result of the disruption of normal control of the hepatic NAD^+:NADH ratio (which inhibits gluconeogenesis and lactate conversion) and from the accumulation of metabolic products which are toxic and cause acidosis. The diagnosis of ethanol, methanol, ethylene glycol, diethylene glycol, and propylene glycol poisoning must therefore be considered in any patient who presents with metabolic acidosis of unknown origin. It should be remembered that many antifreeze solutions now contain significant quantities of methanol as well as ethylene glycol.

Alcohols

Benzyl alcohol

Benzyl alcohol has been used as a preservative in intravascular flush solutions and in drug formulations.

MECHANISM OF TOXICITY

Benzyl alcohol is metabolized to benzoic acid which is then conjugated with glycine in the liver and excreted as hippuric acid. The immature liver's capacity to metabolize benzoic acid is limited and when exceeded leads to accumulation of this metabolite and the development of metabolic acidosis.

CLINICAL FEATURES

In 1982, a syndrome consisting of metabolic acidosis, convulsions, neurological deterioration (due to intraventricular haemorrhage), gasping respirations, hepatic and renal abnormalities, cardiovascular collapse, and death was described in small premature infants between 2 and 14 days of age. The removal of benzyl alcohol solutions from neonatal units led to a considerable reduction both in morbidity and mortality and in particular there was a reduction in cases of kernicterus and intraventricular haemorrhage.

REFERENCE

Jardine, D.S. and Rogers, K. (1989). Relationship of benzyl alcohol to kernicterus, intraventricular hemorrhage, and mortality in preterm infants. *Pediatrics*, **83**, 153–60.

Ethanol (ethyl alcohol)

Ethanol is commonly ingested in beverages before, or with, the deliberate ingestion of other substances in overdose. Ethanol is also used as a solvent and is found in many cosmetic and antiseptic preparations. It is rapidly absorbed through the gastric and intestinal mucosae and approximately 95 per cent is oxidized to acetaldehyde and then to acetate; the remainder is excreted unchanged in the urine and to a lesser extent in the breath and through the skin.

Ethanol acts as a central nervous depressant which in small doses interferes with cortical function but which in large doses may depress medullary processes. The effects of alcohol exacerbate those of other central nervous system depressants, in particular, hypnotic agents. The fatal dose of ethanol alone is between 300 and 500 ml absolute alcohol, if this is ingested in less than 1 h (strong spirits, such as whisky and gin, contain 40–55 per cent ethanol).

CLINICAL FEATURES

The clinical features of ethanol intoxication are well known and are generally related to blood concentrations.

Mild intoxication (500–1500 mg/l) Emotional lability, and slight impairment of visual acuity, muscular co-ordination, and reaction time.

Moderate intoxication (1500–3000 mg/l) Visual impairment, sensory loss, muscular inco-ordination, slowed reaction time, slurred speech.

Severe intoxication (3000–5000 mg/l) Marked muscular inco-ordination, blurred or double vision, sometimes stupor and hypothermia, and occasionally hypoglycaemia and convulsions.

Coma (> 5000 mg/l) depressed reflexes, respiratory depression, hypotension, and hypothermia. Death may occur from respiratory or circulatory failure or as the result of aspiration of stomach contents in the absence of a gag reflex.

Severe hypoglycaemia may accompany alcohol intoxication due to inhibition of gluconeogenesis. This occurs more commonly in children than in adults. Typically, alcohol-induced hypoglycaemia occurs within 6 to 36 h of ingestion of a moderate to large amount of alcohol by either a previously malnourished individual or one who has fasted for the previous 24 h. The patient is often in coma and hypothermic: the usual features of hypoglycaemia such as flushing, sweating, and tachycardia are frequently absent. Rarely lactic acidosis may also complicate acute ethanol intoxication in patients with severe liver disease, pancreatitis, sepsis, or those receiving biguanides. Furthermore, hypovolaemia, a frequent accompaniment of severe intoxication predisposes to lactic acidosis. Ketoacidosis, due to a combination of dehydration, glycopenia, increased lipolysis, and ketogenesis may develop in alcoholics who have recently indulged in very heavy drinking. Acute renal failure has also been described.

TREATMENT

Gastric lavage has not been shown to be of benefit in ethanol poisoning. Supportive measures are all that are required for the great majority of patients. Fructose should not be given as it may cause both acidosis and hyperuricaemia as well as retrosternal and epigastric discomfort; furthermore, the clinical benefit obtained by accelerating ethanol oxidation is negligible. Hypoglycaemia is usually unresponsive to glucagon and therefore intravenous glucose (50 ml of 50 per cent solution) should be given. The management of lactic acidosis will require not only the correction of hyperglycaemia, hypovolaemia, and circulatory insufficiency, if present, but also the judicious intravenous infusion of sodium bicarbonate. Alcoholic ketoacidosis may usually be corrected by the infusion of 5 per cent dextrose alone; insulin is not necessary except in diabetics. The use of haemodialysis should be considered if the blood ethanol concentration exceeds 5000 mg/l and/or if metabolic acidosis is present.

REFERENCES

O'Neill, S., Tipton, K.F., Prichard, J.S., and Quinlan, A. (1984). Survival after high blood alcohol levels. *Archives of Internal Medicine*, **144**, 641–2.

Ragan, F.A., Samuels, M.S., and Hite, S.A. (1979). Ethanol ingestion in children. *Journal of the American Medical Association*, **242**, 2787–8.

Isopropanol (isopropyl alcohol; 2-propanol)

Isopropanol is used as a sterilizing agent and as rubbing alcohol. It is also found in aftershave lotions, disinfectants and window-cleaning solutions.

CLINICAL FEATURES

Intoxication can result both from ingestion and skin absorption. Isopropanol is oxidized in the liver to acetone. The effects of isopropanol on the CNS are qualitatively similar to those of ethanol but they are both more severe and persistent. In addition to coma and respiratory depression, and the odour of acetone on the breath, gastritis, haematemesis, hypotension, hypothermia, renal tubular necrosis, acute myopathy, and haemolytic anaemia have been described; cardiac arrest has occurred. The development of hypotension is a poor prognostic feature.

TREATMENT

Gastric lavage should be employed if the patient presents no more than 1 h after ingestion. In addition to supportive measures, haemodialysis should be employed in severely poisoned patients as it not only removes isopropanol but it also shortens the duration of coma. Peritoneal dialysis is less effective. No advantage is to be gained by infusing ethanol to block alcohol dehydrogenase as the toxicity of isopropanol is due principally to the parent compound.

REFERENCES

IPCS. (1990). *Environmental Health Criteria 103. 2-Propanol.* WHO, Geneva.

Lacouture, P.G., Wason, S., Abrams, A., and Lovejoy, F.H. (1983). Acute isopropyl alcohol intoxication: diagnosis and management. *American Journal of Medicine*, **75**, 680–6.

Pappas, A.A., Ackeman, B.H., Olsen, K.M., and Taylor, E.H. (1991). Isopropanol ingestion; a report of six episodes with isopropanol and acetone serum concentration time data. *Clinical Toxicology*, **29**, 11–21.

Methanol (methyl alcohol)

Methanol is used widely as a solvent and to denature ethanol. It is also found in antifreeze solutions, paints, duplicating fluids, paint removers, varnishes, and shoe polishes. The ingestion of as little as 10 ml of pure methanol has caused permanent blindness and 30 ml is potentially fatal although individual susceptibility varies widely. Toxicity may also occur as a result of inhalation or percutaneous absorption. Methylated spirits consists of 5 per cent methanol and 95 per cent ethanol and contrary to popular opinion, toxicity is due mainly to the presence of the latter component.

MECHANISMS OF TOXICITY

In humans, methanol is metabolized by alcohol dehydrogenase and catalase enzyme systems to formaldehyde and formic acid. The concentration of formate increases greatly and is accompanied by accumulation of hydrogen ions causing metabolic acidosis, due in part to formate induced inhibition of mitochondrial respiration. Depression of the hepatic NAD^+:NADH ratio inhibits gluconeogenesis from lactate and further increases the tendency to acidosis. It is not certain whether the visual toxicity of methanol is due to the local formation of formaldehyde in the retina by alcohol dehydrogenase (required for the utilization of vitamin A) or to interruption of axoplasmic flow in the optic nerve as a result of inhibition of cytochrome oxidase activity by formate ions.

CLINICAL FEATURES

Methanol causes mild and transient inebriation and drowsiness when ingested alone. After a latent period of 8 to 36 h, nausea, vomiting, abdominal pain, headaches, dizziness, and coma supervene. Blurred vision and diminished visual acuity may occur and the presence of dilated pupils, unreactive to light, suggests that permanent blindness is likely to ensue. A severe metabolic acidosis develops in serious cases and this may be accompanied by hyperglycaemia and a raised serum amylase activity. Blood methanol concentrations greater than 500 mg/l confirm serious poisoning. Mortality increases with the severity and duration of the metabolic acidosis. Survivors may show permanent neurological sequelae including blindness, rigidity, hypokinesis, and other parkinsonian-like signs; these features follow the development of optic neuropathy and putaminal necrosis.

TREATMENT

Gastric lavage should be considered in patients who present less than 1 h after ingestion. Thereafter, the treatment of methanol poisoning is directed towards, first, the correction of metabolic acidosis; secondly, the inhibition of methanol oxidation; and thirdly, the removal of circulating methanol and its toxic metabolites. Substantial quantities of buffer base (often as much as 2 mol) usually bicarbonate, may be required and, since this must be accompanied by sodium, hypernatraemia and hypervolaemia result.

There is good evidence that ethanol inhibits methanol oxidation when taken together or given early in poisoning. However, if admission plasma concentrations show that most of the methanol has already been metabolized, ethanol administration may not be of benefit and might exacerbate the acidosis. A loading dose of 50 g ethanol orally (conveniently given as approximately 125 ml of gin, whisky, or vodka) should be given followed by an intravenous infusion of 10 to 12 g ethanol/h to produce blood concentrations of approximately 1 g/l. The infusion should be continued until methanol is undetectable in the blood. Plasma ethanol and methanol concentrations should be measured frequently for ideal management.

To maintain these high ethanol concentrations the rate of administration of intravenous ethanol may have to be increased in some cases. Patients with induced liver enzymes (e.g. those with a history of alcohol or drug abuse) may require 12 to 15 g/h and those undergoing haemodialysis (see below), 17 to 22 g/h, since ethanol is readily dialysable. When peritoneal dialysis is being employed, ethanol may be added to the dialysate fluid (1–2 g/l of dialysate) once the required blood ethanol concentration has been achieved. 4-Methylpyrazole, a competitive inhibitor of alcohol dehydrogenase is under investigation in humans, but it can cause hepatotoxicity.

Dialysis is indicated when a patient has ingested more than 30 g of methanol, or develops metabolic acidosis, mental, visual, or fundoscopic abnormalities attributable to methanol, or a blood methanol concentration in excess of 500 mg/l. Haemodialysis is two to three times more efficient than peritoneal dialysis. Folinic acid (30 mg IV six hourly) may protect against ocular toxicity by accelerating formate metabolism.

REFERENCES

Anon. (1983). Methanol poisoning. *Lancet*, **i**, 910–12.

Jacobsen, D., Jansen, H., Wiik-Larsen, E., Bredesen, J.E., and Halvorsen, S. (1982). Studies on methanol poisoning. *Acta Medica Scandinavica*, **212**, 5–10.

McCoy, H.G., Cipolle, R.J., Ehlers, S.M., Sawchuk, R.J., and Zaske, D.E. (1979). Severe methanol poisoning. Application of a pharmacokinetic model for ethanol therapy and hemodialysis. *American Journal of Medicine*, **67**, 804–7.

Swartz, R.D., *et al.* (1981). Epidemic methanol poisoning: clinical and biochemical analysis of a recent episode. *Medicine*, **60**, 373–82

Glycols

Diethylene glycol

Diethylene glycol is used mainly in polyester resins and polyols, as a humectant in the tobacco industry and as a solvent. It achieved notoriety in 1985 when it was discovered that for some years it had been added to wines produced in Austria, Germany and Italy to improve their ''body'' and sweetness.

MECHANISM OF TOXICITY

Animal studies suggest that diethylene glycol is first oxidized by alcohol dehydrogenase to 2-hydroxyethoxyacetaldehyde which is rapidly oxidized by aldehyde dehydrogenase to 2-hydroxyethoxyacetic acid (HEAA). Inhibition of alcohol dehydrogenase by the administration of pyrazole decreased the formation of HEAA.

CLINICAL FEATURES

In 1937, as a result of a pharmaceutical accident, at least 76 deaths followed the use of elixir of sulphanilamide–Massenfill containing 72 per cent diethylene glycol. Nausea, vomiting, and abdominal pain occurred frequently and were followed by the development of jaundice, pulmonary oedema, coma, and renal failure in most cases. More recently, the clinical course of seven children accidentally poisoned with diethylene glycol has been described. After a prodromal febrile illness the children presented at hospital with vomiting, impaired consciousness, dehydration, oliguria, hepatomegaly, and metabolic acidosis. Despite supportive treatment and, in two cases, the use of dialysis and mechanical ventilation, all seven children died within 9 days of admission. More recently, five adults died after the application of a burn cream containing diethylene glycol. In addition, there is a report of a 65-year-old man who became comatose after ingesting 150 ml of diethylene glycol. He also developed metabolic acidosis, renal failure, and oxaluria. In addition to the correction of the acidosis he required mechanical ventilation and dialysis but made a full recovery.

TREATMENT

Supportive measures to treat dehydration and to correct metabolic acidosis should be instituted promptly. Ethanol should be administered intravenously to block diethylene glycol metabolism (for dosage see methanol poisoning) and dialysis/filtration should be employed if renal failure supervenes.

REFERENCES

Bowie, M.D., and McKenzie, D. (1972). Diethylene glycol poisoning in children. *South African Medical Journal*, **46**, 931–4.

Cantarell, M.C., Fort, J., Camps, J., Sans, M., Piera, L., and Rodamilans, M. (1987). Acute intoxication due to topical application of diethylene glycol. *Annals of Internal Medicine*, **106**, 478–9.

Geiling, E.M.K., and Cannon, P.R. (1938). Pathologic effects of elixir of sulfanilamide (diethylene glycol) poisoning. A clinical and experimental correlation: final report. *Journal of the American Medical Association*, **111**, 919–26.

Ethylene glycol (1,2-ethanediol)

Ethylene glycol has a variety of commercial applications and it is commonly used as an antifreeze fluid in car radiators. Its sweet taste and ready availability have contributed to its popularity as a suicide agent and as a poor man's substitute for alcohol.

It is thought that the minimum lethal dose of ethylene glycol is about 100 ml for an adult, although recovery after treatment has been reported following the ingestion of up to 1 litre.

MECHANISM OF TOXICITY

Ethylene glycol itself appears to be non-toxic. Until metabolized it has no effect on respiration, the citric acid cycle, or other biochemical pathways. Metabolism takes place in the liver and kidneys and may be explained on the basis of accumulation of the following four metabolic products.

1. Aldehydes, which inhibit oxidative phosphorylation, cellular respiration, and glucose metabolism, protein synthesis, DNA replication and ribosomal RNA synthesis, central nervous system respiration, and serotonin metabolism. Aldehydes also alter central nervous system amine levels. (Cerebral symptoms occur 6 to 12 h after the ingestion of ethylene glycol and coincide with the maximum production of aldehydes.)
2. Glycolate which has been shown to be largely responsible for the development of the marked acidosis in overdose.
3. Oxalate, which causes renal damage and acidosis. It is thought, however, that less than 5 per cent of an ingested dose of ethylene glycol is converted to this substance. The production of oxalate is also important in that it chelates calcium ions to form insoluble calcium oxalate crystals: hypocalcaemia may result. As well as renal intratubular obstruction, impairment of cerebral function follows deposition of calcium oxalate in the brain.
4. Lactic acid is produced as the result of the formation of large amounts of reduced nicotinamide adenine dinucleotide (NADH) during breakdown of ethylene glycol, preventing flow of carbon through the citric acid cycle.

CLINICAL FEATURES

The clinical features of ethylene glycol poisoning may be divided into three stages depending on the time after ingestion (Table 1). The severity of each stage and the progression from one stage to the next depends on the amount of ethylene glycol ingested. Death may occur during any of the three stages. An ethylene glycol concentration in excess of 500 mg/l indicates severe poisoning.

Table 1 *Clinical features of ethylene glycol poisoning*

Stage 1 (30 min–12 h): gastrointestinal and nervous system involvement
Patient appears intoxicated with alcohol (but no ethanol on breath)
Nausea, vomiting, haematemesis
Coma and convulsions (often focal)
Nystagmus, ophthalmoplegias, papilloedema, depressed reflexes, myoclonic jerks, tetanic contractions, V, VII, VIII nerve palsies
Stage 2 (12–24 h): cardiorespiratory system involvement
Tachypnoea
Tachycardia
Mild hypertension
Pulmonary oedema
Congestic cardiac failure
Stage 3 (24–72 h): renal involvement
Flank pain
Renal angle tenderness
Acute tubular necrosis

TREATMENT

Early diagnosis and appropriate therapy significantly reduce the mortality from ethylene glycol posioning. In addition to gastric lavage to prevent further absorption and to confirm the diagnosis, supportive measures to combat shock, respiratory distress, hypocalcaemia, and metabolic acidosis should be instituted. Thereafter, treatment has two main aims. Firstly, the use of ethanol as a competitive inhibitor of ethylene glycol metabolism (see methanol above for regimen) and secondly, the use of dialysis to increase elimination of the substance from the body.

The half-life of ethylene glycol is about 3 h in humans and for this reason an ethanol infusion should be started as soon as possible, and continued until ethylene glycol can no longer be detected in blood (see methanol poisoning). 4-Methylpyrazole, a competitive inhibitor of alcohol dehydrogenase, has also been employed with encouraging results, but it may be hepatotoxic.

Ethylene glycol, its aldehyde metabolites and glycolate may be removed by either peritoneal or haemodialysis though the latter is two to three times more efficient. Oxalate, however, is poorly dialysable. In addition, it may be necessary to treat the uraemic complications of ethylene glycol poisoning with dialysis and to use haemodialysis/ultrafiltration to correct the sodium overload that can result from the necessary, but sometimes overjudicious, correction of the metabolic acidosis with sodium bicarbonate. Dialysis should be continued until ethylene glycol is no longer detectable in the blood.

REFERENCES

Jacobsen, D., Ovrebo, S., Ostborg, J., and Sejersted, O.M. (1984). Glycolate causes the acidosis in ethylene glycol poisoning and is effectively removed by hemodialysis. *Acta Medica Scandinavica*, **216,** 409–16.

Jacobsen, D., Hewlett, T.P., Webb, R., Brown, S.T., Ordinario, A.T., and MacMartin, K.E. (1988). Ethylene glycol intoxication; evaluation of kinetics and crystalluria. *American Journal of Medicine*, **84,** 145–52.

Propylene glycol (1,2-propanediol)

Propylene glycol is used widely as a preservative and as a vehicle for both oral and intravenous medications; some formulations contain up to 50 per cent propylene glycol. In addition, propylene glycol contained in preparations used for treating burns may be absorbed percutaneously in significant amounts to cause toxicity. Low birth weight infants are particularly at risk.

MECHANISM OF TOXICITY

Propylene glycol is oxidized to lactic acid and pyruvate and may produce a clinically significant metabolic (lactic) acidosis.

CLINICAL FEATURES

The ingestion of substantial quantities of propylene glycol or its administration to neonates or those in renal failure may produce significant toxicity including the development of convulsions, coma, cardiac arrhythmias, hepatorenal damage, intravascular haemolysis, metabolic acidosis, and increased serum osmolality.

TREATMENT

Gastric lavage should be considered if the patient presents soon after ingestion. Metabolic acidosis should be corrected by the administration of sodium bicarbonate. Renal failure and respiratory depression should be treated conventionally. Haemodialysis can remove propylene glycol efficiently.

REFERENCE

MacDonald, M.G., Getson, P.R., Glasgow, A.M., Miller, M.K., Boeckx, R.L., and Johnson, E.L. (1987). Propylene glycol: increased incidence of seizures in low birth weight infants. *Pediatrics*, **79,** 622–5.

8.3.3 Poisoning from hydrocarbons and chlorofluorocarbons and volatile substance abuse

J. A. VALE, A. T. PROUDFOOT, AND T. J. MEREDITH

Alkanes

Methane, ethane, propane, butane

Natural gas contains methane and ethane, and LPG (liquefied petroleum gas, 'bottled gas') contains propane and butane (and sometimes propylene and butylene). Methane and ethane are pharmacologically inert and can be tolerated in high concentrations without the production of any toxic effects. Both gases, however, if present in very high concentration (> 80 per cent), may produce asphyxia in poorly ventilated areas, as a result of oxygen deprivation. Propane and butane may cause vertigo and drowsiness and, at high concentrations, propane may act as an asphyxiant.

n-Hexane

n-Hexane is probably the most highly toxic alkane. When ingested it causes nausea, dizziness, CNS excitation and then depression, and presents an acute aspiration hazard. Following inhalation, either inadvertently or deliberately, similar symptoms occur with, additionally, the development of a progressive sensorimotor neuropathy in cases of chronic exposure.

REFERENCE

Low, L.K., Meeks, J.R., and Mackerer, C.R. (1987). The aliphatic hydrocarbons. In *Ethel Browning's Toxicity and Metabolism of Industrial Solvents* (ed. R. Snyder), 2nd edn, pp. 253–335. Elsevier, Amsterdam.

Paraffin oil (kerosene)

Paraffin oil (kerosene) has three physical properties accounting for its toxicity. Its low viscosity and surface tension allow it to spread rapidly throughout the lungs when aspirated after ingestion. Its low vapour pressure makes it unlikely to cause poisoning by inhalation.

CLINICAL FEATURES

Repeated local application to the skin results in dryness, dermatitis, and, rarely, genital ulceration and epidermal necrolysis. Pulmonary toxicity may occur within 1 h of ingestion and is characterized by pyrexia, cough, tachypnoea, tachycardia, basal crepitations, and cyanosis. Nonsegmental consolidation or collapse is seen radiologically, involving the middle and lower zones predominantly and often bilaterally. Later and rarely, pneumatocele formation, pneumothorax, pleural effusion, or pulmonary oedema may occur.

There is now good evidence, based on observations in both animals and man, that the pulmonary features are due to aspiration rather than a direct toxic effect following absorption from the gut, although this may occur if a very high dose is ingested.

Paraffin ingestion causes respiratory symptoms, skin bullae, a burning sensation in the mouth and throat, vomiting, diarrhoea, abdominal pain, and mild hepatomegaly with hepatic dysfunction and in severe cases atrial fibrillation/flutter and ventricular fibrillation (due to myocardial sensitization to circulating endogenous catecholamines).

It is possible for a patient to have pulmonary symptoms without radiological abnormalities and conversely to have radiological abnormalities but no symptoms. Radiological features occur more commonly than symptoms and almost all patients who develop either pulmonary symptoms or abnormal radiological findings do so within 8 h of ingestion of paraffin oil. The radiological abnormalities are usually maximal within 72 h.

TREATMENT

Gastric lavage and emesis should be avoided because of the increased risk of chemical pneumonitis, but lavage may be considered in those adults who ingest very large quantities of paraffin oil, if the airway can be protected and the procedure can be carried out within the first hour. There is no evidence that corticosteroids and antibiotics reduce morbidity or mortality; mechanical ventilation with positive and expiratory pressure may be necessary in severe cases of aspiration.

REFERENCES

Anas, N., Namasonthi, V., and Ginsburg, C. (1981). Criteria for hospitalizing children who have ingested products containing hydrocarbons. *Journal of the American Medical Association*, **246,** 840–3.

Baldachin, B.J., and Melmed, R.N. (1964). Clinical and therapeutic aspects of kerosene poisoning: a series of 200 cases. *British Medical Journal*, **2,** 28–30.

Beamon, R.F., Siegel, C.J., Landers, G., and Green, V. (1976). Hydrocarbon ingestion in children: a six-year retrospective study. *Journal of the American College of Emergency Physicians*, **5,** 771–5.

Cachia, E.A., and Fenech, F.F. (1964). Kerosene poisoning in children. *Archives of Diseases of Childhood*, **39,** 502–4.

Petrol (gasoline)

Petrol is a complex mixture of hydrocarbons containing a small proportion of non-hydrocarbon additives such as 'antiknock' agents, antioxidants, rust inhibitors, and dyes.

CLINICAL FEATURES

Acute exposure

Following the inhalation of petrol, dizziness and irritation of the eyes, nose and throat may occur within 5 min followed by euphoria, headache, and blurred vision. If inhalation continues, or if significant quantities of petrol are ingested, then excitement and depression of the nervous system occurs; inco-ordination, restlessness, excitement, confusion, disorientation, hallucinations, ataxia, nystagmus, tremor, delirium, coma, and convulsions may be seen. The inhalation of high concentrations of petrol, such as those encountered by workmen cleaning storage tanks or those sniffing petrol, may cause immediate death. In these circumstances, it is probable that the myocardium is sensitized to circulating catecholamines with precipitation of ventricular fibrillation. High concentrations of petrol vapour can also cause death from acute respiratory failure. Chemical pneumonitis may occur as in paraffin oil ingestion (see above) and the clinical features and management are then identical. In addition, intravascular haemolysis, hypofibrinogenaemia and cardiorespiratory arrest have been reported together with, in one patient, epiglottitis so severe that near total airway obstruction resulted.

Chronic exposure

Chronic exposure to petrol (gasoline) vapour, such as occurs in men engaged in cleaning storage tanks or in children who habitually sniff gasoline, may lead to both chronic hydrocarbon and organic lead poisoning. Tetraethyl lead (the 'antiknock' additive) is non-toxic, but this substance is converted in the liver to the toxic metabolite triethyl lead. Triethyl lead may further be degraded to inorganic lead.

Chronic exposure to the hydrocarbon content of petrol leads to gastrointestinal disease (anorexia, nausea, vomiting, and diarrhoea), cardiovascular disease (relative bradycardia and hypotension), neurological disease (muscle weakness, brisk reflexes, extensor plantar responses, tremor, chorea, and convulsions) and neuropsychological disease (insomnia, irritability, restlessness, anxiety, loss of short-term memory, mania, and suicidal tendencies). Acute myopathy and myoglobinuria have been reported in one case and hepatorenal damage has been described occasionally. The lead content of petrol may give rise to anaemia, cerebellar dysfunction, myoclonus, and encephalopathy.

TREATMENT

Following removal from exposure, supportive measures provide the basis of treatment. Gastric lavage and emesis will increase the risk of aspiration and chemical pneumonitis, though lavage could be considered, with protection of the airway, if a large amount of petrol was ingested by an adult and the procedure could be performed within 1 h.

In the case of occupational exposure to petrol, scrupulous attention to hygiene, the provision of protective clothing and facilities for these to be laundered and adequate washing and showering facilities are all essential. The treatment of lead poisoning is described in Chapter 8.3.6. Petrol 'sniffers' will also require intensive psychosocial support.

REFERENCES

Coulehan, J.L., *et al.* (1983). Gasoline sniffing and lead toxicity in Navajo adolescents. *Pediatrics*, **71,** 113–17.

Fortenberry, J.D. (1985). Gasoline sniffing. *American Journal of Medicine*, **79,** 740–4.

Hansen, K.S. and Sharp, F.R. (1978). Gasoline sniffing, lead poisoning and myoclonus. *Journal of the American Medical Association*, **240,** 1375–6.

Kovanen, J., Somer, H., and Schroeder, P. (1983). Acute myopathy associated with gasoline sniffing. *Neurology*, **33,** 629–31.

Robinson, R.O. (1978). Tetraethyl lead poisoning from gasoline sniffing. *Journal of the American Medical Association*, **240,** 1373–4.

Benzene poisoning

Benzene is a colourless, volatile liquid with a pleasant odour. It is an ingredient in many paints and varnish removers and some petrols. It is also the primary raw material for styrene, phenol, nylon intermediates, and for synthetic detergents of the alkylaryl sulphonate type.

MECHANISMS OF TOXICITY

Following exposure, about 10 per cent of inhaled benzene is excreted unchanged in the breath. The remainder is metabolized by hepatic mixed function oxidase enzymes found predominantly in the liver, but also in the bone marrow, which is the target organ of benzene toxicity. The oxidizing moieties produced by these enzymes probably involve a cascade of reactive oxygen species, including free radicals, which may contribute to cell damage. The hydroxylated benzenes can undergo conjugation reactions to form glucuronides and sulphate esters, or can be further oxidized to benzoquinones, which can bind covalently to macromolecules. Small amounts of absorbed benzene are oxidized completely to carbon dioxide and excreted subsequently in the breath.

Benzene induces pancytopenia by disrupting cell production from the pluripotent stem-cell stage to the functional stage. There is also good evidence that benzene is carcinogenic.

CLINICAL FEATURES

Acute exposure

Acute poisoning results when benzene is ingested or inhaled occupationally, accidentally, or with suicidal or parasuicidal intent. Euphoria, dizziness, weakness, headache, blurring of vision, mucous membrane irritation, tremor, ataxia, chest tightness, respiratory depression, cardiac arrhythmias, coma, and convulsions have been reported. Direct skin contact with liquid benzene may produce signs of marked irritation due to the defatting action of the solvent.

Chronic exposure

The toxic effects of chronic poisoning may not become apparent for months or years after initial contact and indeed they may develop after all exposure has ceased.

Anorexia, headache, drowsiness, nervousness, and irritability are well described. Anaemia (including aplastic anaemia), leucopenia, thrombocytopenia, pancytopenia, leukaemia (particularly of the myelomonocytic type), lymphomas, chromosomal abnormalities, and cerebral atrophy have been reported. In chronic poisoning a steady decrease in the cellular elements of the blood or bone marrow indicate a poor outcome. However, patients have recovered after as long as a year of almost complete absence of formation of new blood cells. A dry, scaly dermatitis may develop on prolonged or repeated skin exposure to liquid benzene.

TREATMENT

Following removal from the contaminated atmosphere, treatment should be directed towards symptomatic and supportive measures. Even if the patient presents soon after ingestion, gastric lavage is still hazardous as aspiration is likely to occur.

REFERENCES

Cavender, F. (1994). Benzene. In *Patty's Industrial Hygiene and Toxicology*. (ed. G.D. Clayton and F.E. Clayton), Vol IIB, 4th edn., pp. 1306–26. John Wiley & Sons, Inc, New York.

Fielder, R.J. (1982). *Toxicity Review. Benzene*. HMSO, London.

Snyder, C.A. (1987). Benzene. In *Ethel Browning's Toxicity and Metabolism of Industrial Solvents* (ed. R. Snyder), 2nd edn., pp. 3–37. Elsevier, Amsterdam.

Carbon tetrachloride (tetrachloromethane)

Carbon tetrachloride was once widely used as a dry-cleaning chemical, degreasing agent, and fire extinguisher. International regulations have now restricted carbon tetrachloride to laboratory and industrial usage and a complete ban is anticipated by the year 2000. Most carbon tetrachloride produced currently goes into the synthesis of chlorofluoromethane refrigerants (which are also to be banned), other solvents, and aerosol propellants.

MECHANISMS OF TOXICITY

Before toxicity occurs, carbon tetrachloride must be activated by the cytochrome P450-dependent reductase system with NADPH supplying electrons via cytochrome C reductase. The trichloromethyl free radical formed binds covalently to proteins and lipids and initiates peroxidation of polyenoic fatty acids with the release of chloroform. Small amounts of hexachloroethane are also formed as a result of condensation of two trichloromethyl free radicals. The trichloromethyl free radical is able to bind covalently to microsomal lipid and protein and oxygenation leads to the formation of trichloromethyl free radical, which itself is able to initiate lipid peroxidation of the endoplasmic reticulum. Conversion to trichloromethylhydroperoxide and trichloromethanol with subsequent dehydrohalogenation generates phosgene, which may be responsible for the majority of covalent binding and tissue necrosis that occurs. Phosgene reacts with tissue water to form chloride ion and carbon dioxide (a major metabolic product of carbon tetrachloride) and with gluthathione to form diglutathionyl dithiocarbonate. *In vitro*, cysteine traps phosgene to prevent covalent binding by generating the substance 2-oxothiazolidine-4-carboxylic acid. Cysteine also acts as a precursor of glutathione which in turn also reacts with phosgene to form the inactive metabolite, diglutathionyl dithiocarbonate. Early administration of *N*-acetylcysteine may, therefore, prevent hepatorenal damage.

Exposure to even low concentrations of carbon tetrachloride causes fatty degeneration of the liver, while high concentrations cause centrilobular necrosis of the liver, fatty degeneration, and necrosis of renal tubules. The hepatic accumulation of lipid is related to injury of the endoplasmic reticulum and disruption of the mechanism for moving lipid out of the hepatocyte through coupling of triglycerides to a lipoprotein carrier. Hepatic necrosis is due to a different mechanism associated with intracellular release of lysosomal enzymes, injury to mitochondria, and loss of cytoplasmic enzymes and coenzymes.

CLINICAL FEATURES

Acute exposure

The immediate effects of acute exposure to carbon tetrachloride include nausea, vomiting, abdominal pain, and diarrhoea. High concentrations cause dizziness, confusion, coma, respiratory depression, hypotension, and occasionally convulsions. If exposure is not terminated immediately, death may follow from respiratory failure. Sudden death sometimes results because of ventricular fibrillation due to cardiac sensitization to circulating catecholamines. If the patient recovers consciousness, anorexia and nausea may occur and persist or, alternatively, the patient may remain asymptomatic until hepatorenal damage supervenes which may be delayed, unusually up to 2 weeks. Hepatic enzyme activities become elevated before jaundice supervenes and a tender swollen liver develops. Serum aspartate aminotransferase activities in excess of 25 000 i.u./l have been reported following acute nonfatal carbon tetrachloride poisoning. Maximal liver damage probably occurs within 48 h of an acute exposure and may progress to fulminant hepatic failure accompanied by hepatic encephalopathy. Renal impairment due to acute tubular necrosis is common and may develop in the absence of hepatic dysfunction. Costovertebral angle pain, proteinuria, oliguria and, anuria occur from 1 to 7 days after exposure. Rarely, cerebellar dysfunction, cerebral haemorrhage, optic atrophy, and parkinsonism may occur.

A plain film of the abdomen may confirm that ingestion has occurred (Fig. 1).

There is marked variation in individual susceptibility to carbon tetrachloride toxicity and some individuals are unaffected by exposures that seriously poison other workers. Alcohol and previous liver and kidney damage render the individual more susceptible (probably because of glutathione depletion in the case of ethanol) and trichloroethylene and isopropyl alcohol may potentiate hepatotoxicity.

Chronic exposure

Repeated daily exposures to low concentrations of carbon tetrachloride may also cause hepatic and renal damage. In addition, cirrhosis of the liver and late development of hepatoma have been reported. Prolonged exposure to carbon tetrachloride has also been associated with polyneuritis, various visual disturbances (blind spots, spots before the eyes, a visual 'haze', and restriction of visual fields), anaemia, and occasionally mild jaundice. Fatal aplastic anaemia has also been described.

TREATMENT

After removal from exposure, conventional symptomatic and supportive measures should be instituted with special attention being paid to hepatic and renal function. Peritoneal or haemodialysis may be required for renal failure. For the reasons given above, if the patient presents within 12 h of exposure *N*-acetylcysteine should be given to prevent or, at least, ameliorate hepatorenal damage and the following regimen has been proposed: *N*-acetylcysteine (150 mg/kg) in 250 ml of 5 per cent dextrose intravenously over 15 min, followed by an infusion of 50 mg/kg in 500 ml of 5 per cent dextrose in 4 h and 100 mg/kg in a litre of 5 per cent dextrose over the next 16 h (total 300 mg/kg in 20 h).

REFERENCES

Brattin, W.J., Glende, E.A., and Recknagel, R.O. (1985). Pathological mechanisms in carbon tetrachloride hepatotoxicity. *Journal of Free Radicals in Biology and Medicine*, **1**, 27–38.

Louria, D.B. and Bodgen, J.R. (1980). The dangers from limited exposure to carbon tetrachloride. *CRC Critical Reviews in Toxicology*, **7**, 177–88.

Ruprah, M., Mant, T.G.K., and Flanagan, R.J. (1985). Acute carbon tetrachloride poisoning in 19 patients: implications for diagnosis and treatment. *Lancet*, **i**, 1027–9.

Chloroform (trichloromethane)

Chloroform is a colourless, volatile liquid with a characteristic odour and sweet taste. It was once used extensively as an anaesthetic agent but because of liver injury, often delayed, and to a lesser extent cardiac sensitization, it is no longer employed for this purpose. Chloroform is now used in industry and in the laboratory as a chemical intermediate and solvent. It is sometimes incorporated into pharmaceutical preparations for its solvent and local anaesthetic properties. In laboratory animals, chloroform is an established carcinogen and for this reason the FDA has prohibited its use in drugs, cosmetics, cough medicines, and toothpaste.

MECHANISMS OF TOXICITY

Chloroform acts primarily as a narcotic and anaesthetic agent and the inhalation of as little as 10 ml may result in fatal central nervous system

Fig. 1 Plain abdominal radiograph in a patient who ingested carbon tetrachloride.

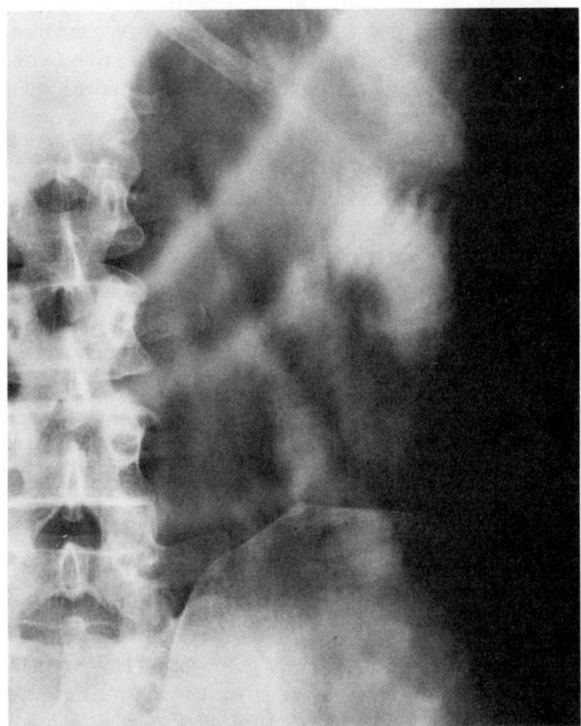

depression. High concentrations of chloroform and chronic or repeated exposure lead to liver and kidney damage. Chloroform is highly lipid soluble and rapidly penetrates into cells where it is metabolized by the microsomal cytochrome P450-dependent mono-oxygenases to trichloromethanol, which spontaneously decomposes to form hydrochloric acid and phosgene. Phosgene reacts with water to produce chloride ion and carbon dioxide and with glutathione to form diglutathionyl dithiocarbonate. *In vitro*, cysteine traps phosgene to prevent covalent binding by forming 2-oxothiazolidine-4-carboxylic acid. Cysteine also acts as a precursor of glutathione to increase formation of diglutathionyl dithiocarbonate. It is, therefore, possible that early administration of *N*-acetylcysteine will protect against hepatorenal damage following chloroform exposure.

Clinical features

The effects of single or short-term exposure to chloroform depend on the concentration to which the patient has been exposed. A level of 200 to 300 p.p.m. is the lowest that can be detected by smell, and up to 400 p.p.m. can be tolerated for 30 min without effect. Single exposures to 1000 p.p.m. cause nausea, vomiting, and dizziness with after-effects of headache and fatigue; concentrations of 1000 to 4000 p.p.m. cause serious disorientation; 14 000 to 16 000 p.p.m. cause rapid loss of consciousness.

Exposure to high concentrations of chloroform is accompanied by conjunctival irritation and blepharospasm, irritation of the mucous membranes and skin, and dilation of the pupils with a diminished light-reflex. Narcosis is usually preceded by a phase of excitement, followed by loss of tendon reflexes, sensation, and then consciousness. Respiratory depression and hypotension may be observed and convulsions may occur either as a result of hypoxia or carbon dioxide retention. High concentrations of chloroform sensitize the heart to circulating catecholamines with resultant ventricular tachyarrhythmias.

A plain film of the abdomen may confirm that ingestion has occurred.

TREATMENT

After removal from exposure conventional symptomatic and supportive treatment should be instituted, including, as necessary, assisted ventilation for respiratory depression and plasma expanders and inotropes for hypotension. Hypercapnia and hypokalaemia should be corrected. Hepatorenal function should be monitored. For the reasons given above, if the patient presents within 12 h of exposure, *N*-acetylcysteine should be given, using the following dosage regimen, to prevent or, at least, ameliorate hepatorenal damage: *N*-acetylcysteine (150 mg/kg intravenously) over 15 min in 250 ml of 5 per cent dextrose, followed by an infusion of 50 mg/kg in 500 ml of 5 per cent dextrose in 4 h and 100 mg/kg in a litre of 5 per cent dextrose over the next 16 h (total 300 mg/kg in 20 h).

REFERENCES

Challen, P.J.R., Hickish, D.E., and Bedford, J. (1958). Chronic chloroform intoxication. *British Journal of Industrial Medicine*, **15**, 243–9.

Pohl, L.R. (1979). Biochemical toxicology of chloroform. In *Reviews in Biochemical Toxicology* (ed. E. Hodgson, J.R. Bend, and R.M. Philpot), pp. 79–107. Elsevier/North-Holland, New York.

Methyl bromide (bromomethane)

Methyl bromide is a colourless, odourless gas at ordinary temperatures and, therefore, dangerous concentrations may accumulate without warning. In the past it was used in fire extinguishers, as a refrigerant and as a delousing agent, but these uses have been abandoned following fatalities. Methyl bromide has high penetrating power and is non-flammable and explosive; these features explain its increasing use as a disinfectant to fumigate soil, a wide range of commodities, grain, warehouses, and mills. Its high density causes it to settle at floor level.

MECHANISM OF TOXICITY

Methyl bromide is absorbed readily through the lungs and is excreted largely unchanged by the same route. The remainder is metabolized and inorganic bromide is excreted in the urine. The mechanism of toxicity is uncertain but methyl bromide appears to have an affinity for intracellular proteins, particularly those with sulphydryl groups. Although determination of bromide in the blood is useful in establishing whether exposure to methyl bromide has occurred, bromide ion concentrations correlate poorly with severity of poisoning. Thus, in cases of methyl bromide poisoning, toxicity may be observed with bromide concentrations as low as 30 mg/l and death may occur at concentrations of 80 to 100 mg/l. In contrast, bromide poisoning caused by inorganic bromides is usually not clinically manifest until concentrations as high as 500 to 1000 mg/l are reached.

CLINICAL FEATURES

Acute exposure

There may be a latent period of up to 12 h before toxic symptoms occur. Symptoms include dizziness, headache, nausea, vomiting, abdominal pain, malaise, transient blurring of vision, diplopia, and breathlessness. In severe cases, coma, status epilepticus, tremor, ataxia, hyporeflexia, paraesthesiae, hallucinations, acute psychosis, and polyneuropathy may be found. Proteinuria, oliguria (due to renal tubular and cortical necrosis), and jaundice have been described. An illness resembling Reye's syndrome occurred in a child poisoned with methyl bromide. Death in the early stages is most likely to be due to pulmonary oedema, and, if late, to circulatory failure. The prognosis is likely to be good if the patient survives for 2 days after the onset of symptoms.

Chronic exposure

Long-term exposure to methyl bromide may lead to a chronic polyneuropathy, lethargy, personality changes, an intolerance to alcohol, dysarthria, and epilepsy.

TREATMENT

The casualty should be removed promptly from the contaminated atmosphere and undressed, as methyl bromide can penetrate clothing and rubber gloves. Contaminated skin should be washed with water. Blistered areas should be covered with a sterile dressing. Convulsions may be treated with diazepam (5–10 mg intravenously) repeated as necessary. Pulmonary oedema should respond to supplemental oxygen, bronchodilators, and diuretics. Mechanical ventilation with positive end expiratory pressure may be necessary in the seriously poisoned patient.

REFERENCES

Shield, L.K., Coleman, T.L., and Markesbery, W.R. (1977). Methyl bromide intoxication: neurologic features, including simulation of Reye syndrome. *Neurology*, **27**, 959–62.

Zatuchni, J. and Hong, K. (1981). Methyl bromide poisoning seen initially as psychosis. *Archives of Neurology*, **38**, 529–30.

Zwaveling, J.H., de Kort, W.L.A.M., Meulenbelt, J., Hezemans-Boer, M., Van Vloten, W.A., and Sangster, B. (1987). Exposure of the skin to methyl bromide: a study of six cases occupationally exposed to high concentrations during fumigation. *Human Toxicology*, **6**, 491–45.

Methyl chloride (chloromethane)

Methyl chloride is a colourless gas used as a chemical intermediate, particularly in methylating reactions in the production of butyl rubber, tetramethyl lead, and other products, as well as a blowing agent for some polystyrene foams. Absorption may occur through the skin although the principal route is by inhalation.

MECHANISMS OF TOXICITY

In rats, methyl chloride is metabolized to formate, which is then further metabolized primarily by folic acid-dependent pathways. It is ultimately incorporated into tissue macromolecules or oxidized to carbon dioxide.

The lack of accumulation of formate suggests that the toxicity of methyl chloride is not due to formate poisoning. It has now been shown that methyl chloride can cause marked glutathione depletion suggesting an alternative route of metabolism which may explain its hepatorenal toxicity.

CLINICAL FEATURES

Acute exposure

The appearance of symptoms may be delayed and can persist for several hours or days once exposure has ceased. Methyl chloride is a potent CNS depressant and may also cause hepatic, renal, and haematological damage. Following acute poisoning, many patients develop gastrointestinal disturbances (nausea, vomiting, abdominal pain, and diarrhoea), headache, drowsiness, giddiness, ataxia, convulsions, and coma.

Chronic exposure

Chronic exposure may lead to confusion, blurring of vision, slurred speech, staggering gait, and convulsions.

TREATMENT

After evacuation from exposure and removal of contaminated clothing, treatment is symptomatic and supportive. It is possible that glutathione repletion with the aid of *N*-acetylcysteine may be of value though to date there is no experimental or clinical evidence to support its use.

REFERENCES

Hansen, H., Weaver, N.K., and Venable, F.S. (1958). Methyl chloride intoxication: report of fifteen cases. *Archives of Industrial Hygiene and Occupational Medicine*, **8,** 328–34.

Repko, J.D. (1981). Neurotoxicity of methyl chloride. *Neurobehavioural Toxicology and Teratology*, **3,** 425–9.

Scharnweber, H.C., Spears, G.N., and Cowles, S.R. (1974). Chronic methyl chloride intoxication in six industrial workers. *Journal of Occupational Medicine*, **16,** 112–13.

Methyl iodide (iodomethane)

Methyl iodide is a colourless liquid used as a chemical intermediate. Consequently, poisoning is unusual and fewer than 10 cases have been reported in the literature. Between 50 and 90 per cent of an inhaled dose is retained in the body. Skin absorption also occurs.

CLINICAL FEATURES

Methyl iodide acts primarily as a central nervous system depressant but lung irritation and renal damage may occur. Initial symptoms, which may be delayed, include lethargy, somnolence, slurred speech, ataxia, and visual disturbances. Clothing contaminated with methyl iodide may cause skin irritation and local burns as well as systemic effects following absorption.

TREATMENT

Contaminated clothing should be removed and the casualty placed in a non-contaminated environment. Thereafter, treatment is symptomatic and supportive.

REFERENCES

Appel, G.B., Galen, R., O'Brien, J., and Schoenfeldt, R. (1975). Methyl iodide intoxication. A case report. *Annals of Internal Medicine*, **82,** 534–6.

Methylene chloride (dichloromethane)

Methylene chloride is a common ingredient in paint removers and is used as a solvent for plastic films and cements and also as a degreaser and aerosol propellant.

MECHANISM OF TOXICITY

Owing to its volatility, high atmospheric concentrations of methylene chloride may develop rapidly within poorly ventilated areas. Following inhalation or ingestion methylene chloride is metabolized by mixed function oxidases to carbon dioxide and carbon monoxide. Carboxyhaemoglobin concentrations of 3 to 10 per cent are commonly attained, although higher concentrations have been reported (e.g. a carboxyhaemoglobin concentration of 40 per cent in one subject more than 12 h after cessation of exposure).

The addition of methanol to paint removers extends the biological half-life of carboxyhaemoglobin derived from methylene chloride. Furthermore, it has been shown that smokers or physically active workers exposed to methylene chloride have higher blood carboxyhaemoglobin concentrations than do non-smokers or those with sedentary occupations. Patients with ischaemic heart disease are at particular risk from carboxyhaemoglobin concentrations of more than 5 per cent and the mortality may be higher in these subjects exposed to methylene chloride.

CLINICAL FEATURES

Acute exposure

Skin contact with liquid methylene chloride can be painful. Following inhalation, dizziness, tingling and numbness of the extremities, throbbing headache, nausea, irritability, fatigue, and stupor have been reported. Severe and prolonged exposure may lead to irritative conjunctivitis, lacrimination, respiratory depression, and death. Hepatorenal dysfunction and pulmonary oedema have also been described. In addition, if high concentrations of carboxyhaemoglobin are present, the features of acute carbon monoxide poisoning may occur, although these tend to be mild even in the presence of very high carboxyhaemoglobin concentrations.

Chronic exposure

The possibility that chronic exposure to methylene chloride might result in chronic carbon monoxide poisoning has been suggested. However, an epidemiological analysis of a male population exposed to methylene chloride for up to 30 years found no significant excess mortality compared with matched controls.

TREATMENT

Prompt removal from exposure prior to death usually results in complete recovery. Thereafter, treatment is supportive and should include the use of supplemental oxygen.

REFERENCES

Illing, H.P.A. and Shillaker, R.O. (1985). *Toxicity Review. Dichloromethane (Methylene Chloride)*. HMSO, London.

Stewart, R.D., Fisher, T.H., Hosko, M.J., Peterson, J.E., Baretta, E.D., and Dodd, H.C. (1972). Experimental human exposure to methylene chloride. *Archives of Environmental Health*, **25**, 342–8.

Stewart, R.D. and Hake, C.L. (1976). Paint-remover hazard. *Journal of the American Medical Association*, **235**, 398–401.

Styrene (vinyl benzene)

Styrene is a colourless to yellow liquid with a pleasant, sweet odour at low concentrations. Styrene monomer is an important industrial chemical agent used for the production of plastic, as a modifying additive for resins, as a dental filling component, as a chemical reaction intermediate, as a component in agricultural products, and as a stabilizing agent in a variety of products. Polystyrene is prepared from the polymerization of styrene monomer under the influence of organic peroxides such as benzoyl peroxide and lauroyl peroxide. Styrene is highly reactive and may polymerize prematurely in storage containers unless inhibitors, usually phenols, are added.

MECHANISM OF TOXICITY

Styrene is oxidized to styrene oxide and then hydrated to styrene glycol; styrene oxide can bind covalently to cellular macromolecules probably due to depletion of glutathione. Styrene is excreted mainly as mandelic acid and phenylglyoxylic acid with approximately 2 per cent of an inhaled dose being exhaled in unchanged form; hippuric acid is also a minor metabolite. Non-excreted styrene may accumulate in subcutaneous adipose tissue, which is thought to be the basis of the observed lag phase in styrene excretion; a weekend has been shown to be insufficient time to excrete all the metabolites of an high inhaled dose of styrene.

CLINICAL FEATURES

Acute exposure

Although inhalation is the most common route of exposure, absorption of styrene may also occur through the skin and gut. Styrene is irritant to the eyes, skin, mucous membranes, and respiratory system. At a concentration of 800 p.p.m., immediate eye and throat irritation occurs, accompanied by increased nasal mucous secretion, a metallic taste in the mouth, drowsiness, and vertigo. Higher concentrations of styrene may cause CNS depression.

Chronic exposure

Although there have been a number of studies of industrial exposure to styrene, many of the observations made have been non-specific, and few studies have included satisfactory air concentration figures to substantiate their findings. An average chronic exposure of 150 p.p.m. or higher has resulted in a prolonged simple reaction time. A clinical study of production workers revealed lower respiratory and prenarcotic symptoms, but no abnormalities of liver function, even at high exposure levels. In contrast, some Russian reports have indicated more serious problems. One study of petroleum workers producing synthetic rubber suggested that half the work force suffered abnormalities of gastric acid secretion and liver and pancreatic function. Anaemia, leucopenia, reticulocytosis, reduced coagulability, and a rise in capillary permeability were also reported, and changes in blood protein composition and cholinesterase activity were described. Another group of workers, in whom occupational exposure to styrene was monitored using mandelic acid excretion, showed changes in psychological function, abnormal EEGs, and occasional peripheral nerve lesions.

In a more rigorous study, men exposed to styrene in the building of glass-fibre boats showed no convincing changes in most objective tests of performance when compared to a control group. However, those workers with high blood styrene levels reported greater subjective feelings of physical and mental tiredness at the end of the day and had consistently slower reaction times in both the morning and the afternoon. In all three groups, scores in the tests worsened through the day, but deterioration was greatest in the high styrene exposure group. Even so, it may be the effects of the exercise itself which were responsible for the findings.

TREATMENT

If acute exposure has occurred, the subject should be removed from further exposure, the skin washed, and the eyes irrigated. Central nervous system effects should be treated symptomatically and supportively. Urinary mandelic acid concentrations may be of value in estimating the level of occupational exposure. Potentially, *N*-acetylcysteine could be of value in preventing hepatic damage.

REFERENCE

Vainio, H. and Hietanen, E. (1987). Styrene. In *Ethel Browning's Toxicity and Metabolism of Industrial Solvents*, (ed. R. Snyder), 2nd edn., pp. 199–208. Elsevier, Amsterdam.

Tetrachloroethylene (perchloroethylene)

Tetrachloroethylene is a colourless, non-flammable liquid with a chloroform-like odour. It is used widely as an industrial solvent particularly for dry-cleaning and degreasing. Poisoning may occur by inhalation or ingestion.

MECHANISMS OF TOXICITY

A considerable proportion of an inspired dose is exhaled unchanged, and that retained is excreted only slowly (half-life approximately 144 h). Tetrachloroethylene first undergoes epoxidation followed by intramolecular rearrangement to give rise to trichloracetyl acid chloride, which is hydrolysed to trichloroacetic acid, the major urinary metabolite. The capacity of man to metabolize tetrachloroethylene is limited when inhaled concentrations are high.

CLINICAL FEATURES

Following inhalation or ingestion, there is depression of the central nervous system; nausea and vomiting may occur and persist for several hours. Irritation of the eyes, nose, and throat may occur. Hepatic and renal dysfunction may also develop and ventricular arrhythmias and non-cardiogenic pulmonary oedema have been reported. It has now been shown in animals that tetrachloroethylene sensitizes the myocardium, albeit weakly, to catecholamine-induced cardiac arrhythmias.

A plain film of the abdomen may confirm that ingestion of tetrachloroethylene has occurred.

TREATMENT

After removal from exposure, treatment is supportive and symptomatic.

REFERENCES

Illing, H.P.A., Mariscotti, S.P., and Smith, A.M. (1987). *Toxicity Review. Tetrachloroethylene. (Tetrachloroethene, Perchloroethylene)*. HMSO, London.

IPCS. (1984). *Environmental Health Criteria 31. Tetrachloroethylene.* WHO, Geneva.

Mutti, A., *et al.* (1992) Nephropathies and exposure to perchloroethylene in dry-cleaners. *Lancet*, **340,** 189–93.

Toluene poisoning

Toluene has much lower volatility and toxicity than benzene. It is used extensively as a solvent in the chemical, rubber, paint, glue, and pharmaceutical industries and as a thinner for inks, perfumes, and dyes. Certain industrial solvent mixtures, containing predominantly toluene have been reported to cause bone-marrow failure. It is now thought that these mixtures were contaminated with benzene, since animal studies have failed to demonstrate any convincing myelotoxic effect of toluene.

METABOLISM

Following inhalation or ingestion, toluene is oxidized to benzoic acid and in turn conjugated with glycine to form hippuric acid or with glucuronic acid to yield benzoylglucuronates. Hippuric acid and benzoylgluconic acid are excreted in the urine and the former metabolite has been used as a marker of occupational exposure, though this is unreliable particularly at low levels of toluene exposure.

CLINICAL FEATURES

Acute poisoning results in euphoria, excitement, dizziness, confusion, increased lacrimation, headache, nervousness, nausea, tinnitus, ataxia, tremor, and coma. Chronic poisoning may give rise to muscle weakness, abdominal pain and haematemesis, cerebellar abnormalities (which may be persistent), optic neuropathy, peripheral neuropathy, altered mental state, dementia, hearing loss, hypokalaemia (including hypokalaemic periodic paralysis), hypophosphataemia, hyperchloraemia, metabolic acidosis, and hepatorenal disease, including distal renal tubular acidosis and urinary calculi. Recently, hypothalamic dysfunction and central sleep apnoea have been described in association with chronic toluene exposure.

TREATMENT

If poisoning results from inhalation, whether accidental or intentional as in volatile substance abuse (see below), the patient should be removed from the contaminated environment. Thereafter, treatment consists of symptomatic and supportive measures.

REFERENCES

Antti-Poika, M., Kalliokoski, P., and Hanninen, O. (1987). Toluene. In *Ethel Browning's Toxicity and Metabolism of Industrial Solvents.* (ed. R. Snyder), 2nd edn., pp. 38–63, Elsevier, Amsterdam.

Bell, G.M., Battershill, J.M., and Shillaker, R.O. (1989). *Toxicity Review. Toluene.* HMSO, London.

Cavender, F. (1994). Toluene. In *Patty's Industrial Hygiene and Toxicology.* (ed. G.D. Clayton and F.E. Clayton), Vol IIB, 4th edn., pp. 1326–32. John Wiley & Sons, Inc, New York.

IPCS. (1985) *Environmental Health Criteria 52. Toluene.* WHO, Geneva.

Streicher, H.Z., Gabow, P.A., Moss, A.H., Kono, D., and Kaehny, W.D. (1981). Syndromes of toluene sniffing in adults. *Annals of Internal Medicine*, **94,** 758–62.

1,1,1-Trichloroethane (methyl chloroform)

1,1,1-Trichloroethane is a colourless, non-flammable liquid with high volatility widely used as a solvent in industry, in the office (e.g. typewriter correction fluid) and at home (e.g. water-proofing aerosol products).

MECHANISM OF TOXICITY

1,1,1-Trichloroethane has low systemic toxicity because only small amounts of trichloroacetic acid and trichloroethanol are formed. Most of an inhaled dose is expired unchanged. Concomitant ingestion of ethanol is known to enhance toxicity.

CLINICAL FEATURES

Acute exposure

Following inhalation of a sufficiently large dose, CNS depression occurs in proportion to the amount inhaled; hepatic and renal dysfunction may also result. Deaths have followed exposure to very high concentrations in unventilated tanks. In such cases death may either be due to CNS depression, culminating in respiratory arrest, or to fatal arrhythmias as a result of myocardial sensitization to circulating catecholoamines in the presence of hypoxia. Inhalation of a weather-proofing aerosol containing 96.6 per cent 1,1,1-trichloroethane has been reported to give rise to transient shortness of breath, constricting chest pain, cough, and myalgia. Animal data suggest that ingestion may result not only in the above features but also pulmonary aspiration and haemorrhage.

Chronic exposure

Chronic exposure is not thought to produce hepatic, renal, or cardiovascular damage, although cirrhosis has been reported following repeated exposure to a combination of this agent and trichloroethylene.

TREATMENT

The casualty should be removed from the contaminated environment. Thereafter treatment is symptomatic and supportive.

REFERENCES

Fielder, R.J. and Williams, S.D. (1984). *Toxicity Review. 1,1,1-Trichloroethane.* HMSO, London.

Hodgson, M.J., Heyl, A.E., and Van Thiel, D.H. (1989). Liver disease associated with exposure to 1,1,1-trichloroethane. *Archives of Internal Medicine*, **149,** 1793–979.

IPCS. (1992) *Environmental Health Criteria 136. 1,1,1-Trichloroethane.* WHO, Geneva.

Trichloroethylene

Trichloroethylene is a colourless, volatile liquid used widely as an industrial solvent, particularly in metal degreasing and extraction processes.

MECHANISMS OF TOXICITY

Trichloroethylene is absorbed readily from the gut and through the skin and lungs. Following inhalation, 16 to 28 per cent of absorbed trichloroethylene is excreted unchanged in the breath. It is metabolized by the enzymes of the mixed function oxidase system to the transient metabolite trichloroethylene epoxide. The epoxide may undergo intramolecular rearrangement to trichloroacetaldehyde which is then hydrolysed to chloral hydrate. Trichloroethylene epoxide may be the reactive metabolite that binds irreversibly to protein and nucleic acids to cause cell toxicity.

Subsequent metabolism of chloral hydrate by alcohol dehydrogenase and chloral hydrate dehydrogenase yields trichloroethanol and trichloroacetic acid, which are excreted in the urine, the former mainly as the glucuronide and the latter as the free acid. Carbon dioxide, which arises from the metabolism of chloral hydrate and trichloroacetic acid, is excreted in the breath. The principal metabolite, trichloroacetic acid, may be found in the urine several weeks after exposure.

It has been demonstrated in rabbits poisoned with trichloroethylene that ethanol increases the likelihood of catecholamine-induced arrhythmias and that the occurrence of arrhythmias is related to trichloroethylene rather than its metabolites. Furthermore, it has been shown that the concomitant administration of ethanol and trichloroethylene results in higher concentrations of trichloroethylene and lower concentrations of trichloroacetic acid in animals treated with ethanol. This may be explained by the fact that ethanol competitively inhibits the conversion of chloral hydrate by alcohol dehydrogenase to trichloroethanol and trichloroacetic acid. In the presence of heat, light, or an alkaline solution (e.g. concrete or tile-filling materials), non-stabilized trichloroethylene decomposes to more toxic products (dichloroacetylene, phosgene, carbon monoxide); dichloroacetylene may be responsible for cranial nerve palsies seen in some patients poisoned by trichloroethylene.

CLINICAL FEATURES

Acute exposure

Following inhalation, ingestion or dermal absorption, central nervous system depression occurs and there may be associated and prolonged nausea and vomiting. One study showed that exposure to trichloroethylene concentrations of between 90 and 130 p.p.m. reduced significantly the efficiency with which various psychophysiological tests were performed. Hepatic and renal dysfunction can follow, and death has been reported, probably caused by catecholamine-induced ventricular arrhythmias. 'Degreaser's flush' (in which the skin on the face and arms becomes markedly reddened) may occur if ethanol is consumed shortly before or after exposure to trichloroethylene. Cranial nerve damage, (particularly trigeminal neuropathy), cerebellar dysfunction, and convulsions have been described.

A plain abdominal film of the abdomen may demonstrate the presence of this chlorinated hydrocarbon in the gut.

Chronic exposure

Following chronic exposure (as in paint-solvent abusers), weight loss, nausea and anorexia, fatigue, visual impairment, dermatitis, and, rarely, jaundice have been described. Cirrhosis and portal hypertension have followed repeated bouts of acute hepatotoxicity caused by trichloroethylene.

TREATMENT

Removal from exposure will reduce CNS depression, and thereafter, whether trichloroethylene has been inhaled, ingested, or absorbed through the skin, treatment is supportive and symptomatic.

REFERENCES

Fielder, R.J., Lowing, R.K., and Shillaker, R.O. (1982). *Toxicity Review. Trichloroethylene.* HMSO, London

IPCS. (1985). *Environmental Health Criteria 50. Trichloroethylene.* WHO, Geneva.

Vinyl chloride (monochloroethylene, chloroethene)

Vinyl chloride is a colourless, highly flammable, and explosive gas. It is usually handled as a liquid under pressure, and in this form it polymerizes readily, at temperatures in the range of 40 to 70 °C, by exothermic reaction to form polyvinyl chloride (PVC). In addition, to its use as an intermediate in the manufacture of plastic, vinyl chloride is also used in the production of 1,1,1-trichloroethane and as a component of aerosol propellant mixtures. Vinyl chloride was recognized as having a narcotic action as early as 1933, when it was considered for use as an anaesthetic agent but was abandoned because it was found to induce cardiac arrhythmias at the 10 to 20 per cent concentration necessary to produce surgical anaesthesia. In 1949, hepatitis-like changes were reported in the livers of exposed Russian workers, and in 1966 acro-osteolysis was described in vinyl chloride autoclave cleaners in Belgium. Subsequently, as the result of an epidemiological study of men who had previously worked as autoclave cleaners in a PVC polymerization plant, it was recognized that vinyl chloride was also a cause of angiosarcoma of the liver. Since then, vinyl chloride has been shown to have other carcinogenic effects.

MECHANISMS OF TOXICITY

The main route of absorption of vinyl chloride is through the lungs, although some skin penetration does occur. Experiments with volunteers have shown that 42 per cent of an inhaled dose is retained in the lungs regardless of the atmospheric concentration. Metabolism of vinyl chloride to a reactive metabolite appears to be necessary before toxic effects are seen. Two toxic metabolites, chloroethylene oxide and chloroacetaldehyde, are formed as the result of biotransformation of vinyl chloride by hepatic microsomal mixed-function oxidase enzymes. The epoxide derivative has been shown to bind covalently to DNA, RNA, and protein, while chloroacetaldehyde is a known mutagen. Detoxification of these metabolites occurs mainly by conjugation with glutathione, catalysed by hepatic glutathione transferases; the conjugates are excreted in the urine as substituted cysteine derivatives. Dose-dependent depletion of the hepatic pool of cysteine and glutathione has been shown to accompany biotransformation of vinyl chloride. In rats, the prior administration of either cysteine or methionine protects against vinyl chloride-induced hepatotoxicity. It seems probable that once hepatic glutathione stores are depleted beyond a certain critical point, the liver is no longer protected against hepatotoxic vinyl chloride metabolites. A further metabolic pathway also has been described via alcohol dehydrogenase involving sequential oxidation to 2-chloroethanol, chloroacetaldehyde, and monochloracetic acid. This pathway is also saturable at high exposure levels.

It has also been postulated that the various features of vinyl chloride disease may have an immunological basis.

CLINICAL FEATURES

Acute exposure

Acute exposure to vinyl chloride results in CNS depression, but concentrations need to be in excess of 10 000 p.p.m. before this effect becomes noticeable. Exposure of volunteers to 20 000 p.p.m. for 5 min caused dizziness, light-headedness, nausea, and dulling of vision.

Chronic exposure

Acro-osteolysis has been described in workers engaged in the hand-cleaning of autoclaves. The syndrome has three main components: (1) Raynaud's phenomenon, which affects the fingers and sometimes the toes, (2) skin changes resembling scleroderma on the back of the hands or distal third of the flexor aspect of the forearm, and (3) bony changes of the terminal phalanges of the fingers and sometimes the toes, radial and ulnar styloid processes, sacroiliac joints, and lower poles of the patellas. The radiological appearances in the phalanges are those of band-like translucencies due to bony absorption. If the condition is advanced, complete destruction of the tuft of the phalanx and partial or complete occlusion of the digital arteries may occur. Epidemiological surveys of autoclave cleaners have suggested an incidence of about 3 per cent, although the condition is virtually unknown in workers with less than 12 months' exposure.

Angiosarcoma of the liver is a rare tumour, but worldwide since 1974 more than 130 cases have been described in vinyl chloride autoclave cleaners. The median latency period before development of the tumour is approximately 20 years, although it may range from 10 to 40 years. The duration of exposure in each case ranges from about 4 to 30 years, with a median of just under 20 years. Hepatic fibrosis, often associated with splenomegaly and portal hypertension also has been reported in vinyl chloride workers. Hepatic fibrosis, which can be demonstrated in livers both with and without angiosarcoma, is of the periportal type and is accompanied frequently by capsular thickening. In addition, vinyl chloride particles have been demonstrated in the livers of haemodialysis patients and are thought to be due to fragmentation of dialysis tubing within the blood pumps necessary for haemodialysis.

Exposure to vinyl chloride may also be associated with the development of cancer of the liver, biliary tract and brain, though the latter association has not been confirmed in some studies. Chromosomal abnormalities, mainly breakages, in exposed vinyl chloride workers have been reported.

TREATMENT

Preventive measures, adopted worldwide, and designed to protect against angiosarcoma of the liver, should also prevent other adverse effects. Symptoms due to osteo-acrolysis do not improve significantly after removal from exposure, but radiographic improvement of the phalangeal lesions, with recalcification, has been demonstrated.

REFERENCES

Simonato, L., *et al.* (1991). A collaborative study of cancer incidence and mortality among vinyl chloride workers. *Scandinavian Journal of Work and Environmental Health*, **17,** 159–69.

Uzych, L. (1988). Human male exposure to vinyl chloride and possible teratogenic and mutagenic risks: a review. *Human Toxicology*, **7,** 517–27.

Ward, A.M., Udnoon, S., Watkins, J., Walker, A.E., Darke, C.S. (1976). Immunological mechanisms in the pathogenesis of vinyl chloride disease. *British Medical Journal*, **1,** 936–938.

Wong, O., Whorton, M.D., Foliart, D.E., Ragland, D. (1991). An industry-wide epidemiologic study of vinyl chloride workers, 1942–1982. *American Journal of Industrial Medicine,* **20,** 317–34.

Xylenes

The three isomers of xylene, which possess similar properties, are used widely as solvents in paints, lacquers, pesticides, gums, resins, adhesives, and the paper coating industry. Commercial xylene usually consists of 75 to 85 per cent of the *m*-isomer and only about 5 per cent of the *p*-isomer.

METABOLISM

Following inhalation or skin exposure, xylene is metabolized predominantly by oxidation of a methyl group to the corresponding *o*-,*m*-, or *p*-toluic acids and excreted in the urine either free or conjugated with glycine as methylhippuric acid which may be used as an index of exposure, though the concentration will be artefacturally reduced if aspirin is taken regularly. Coadministration of ethanol inhibits xylene metabolism so that blood xylene concentrations increase two-fold approximately.

CLINICAL FEATURES

Acute exposure

Following inhalation, dizziness, excitement, flushing of the face, eye irritation, drowsiness, inco-ordination, ataxia, tremor, confusion, coma, respiratory depression, and catecholomine-induced ventricular arrhythmias may occur. Hepatorenal damage also has been described. Immersion of the hand in liquid xylene may result in erythema and a burning feeling, with some scaling of the skin.

Chronic exposure

Repeated skin contact results in defatting and local irritation. Chronic exposure to xylene may cause subtle neurological damage but this has yet to be confirmed.

TREATMENT

Treatment is supportive.

REFERENCE

Riihimaki, V. and Hanninen, O. (1987). Xylenes. In *Ethel Browning's Toxicity and Metabolism of Industrial Solvents.* (ed. R. Snyder). 2nd edn., pp. 64–84. Elsevier, Amsterdam.

Chlorofluorocarbons (CFCs)

CFCs are derived by the partial or complete substitution of the hydrogen atoms in methane and ethane with both chlorine and fluorine atoms (see Table 1). CFCs were developed as refrigerants some 60 years ago but have been used as propellants in aerosols, as blowing agents in foam insulation products, and as intermediates for plastics. The aerosol propellant market which previously consumed half of the total production is currently a minor application due to international restrictions. This global concern arises because high energy radiation splits chlorine off from CFCs in the stratosphere; chlorine radicals destroy ozone, allowing UV-B radiation to penetrate to the earth's surface.

Table 1 *Chlorofluorocarbons*

Chemical name	Common name
Trichlorofluoromethane	CFC-11, Freon 11
Dichlorofluroethane	HCFC 141b
Dichlorodifluoromethane	CFC-12, Freon 12
Dichlorotrifluorethane	HCFC 123
Chlorotrifluoromethane	CFC-13
Chlorodifluoromethane	Freon 22, HCFC 22
1,2-difluoro-1,1,2,2-tetrachloroethane	CFC-112
1,1-difluoro-1,2,2,2-tetrachloroethane	CFC-112a
1,1,2-trichloro-1,2,2-trifluorethane	CFC-113, Freon 113
1,1,1-trichloro-2,2,2-trifluoroethane	CFC-113a
1,2-dichloro-1,1,2,2-tetrafluoroethane	CFC-114
1,1-dichloro-1,2,2,2-tetrafluoroethane	CFC-114a
1-chloro-1,1,2,2,2-pentafluoroethane	CFC-115, Freon 115

CLINICAL FEATURES

Acute exposure

Inhalation of CFCs may result in a tingling sensation, humming in the ears, apprehension, slurred speech, and decreased performance in psychological tests. Exposure to high CFC concentrations may result in clinically significant arrhythmias, coma, and respiratory depression; fatalities have occurred particularly after CFC abuse (see below under Volatile Substance Abuse).

Chronic exposure

A sensorimotor neuropathy developed in a laundry worker exposed for several years both to CFC 113 and tetrachloroethylene and in a refrigerator repair worker. However, epidemiological studies in exposed workers have not confirmed these findings.

REFERENCES

IPCS. (1990). *Environmental Health Criteria 113. Fully Halogenated Chlorofluorocarbons.* WHO, Geneva.

IPCS. (1991). *Environmental Health Criteria 126. Partially halogenated chlorofluorocarbons (Methane derivatives).* WHO, Geneva.

IPCS. (1992). *Environmental Health Criteria 139. Partially halogenated chlorofluorocarbons (Ethane derivatives).* WHO, Geneva.

Volatile substance abuse

Solvent abuse may be defined as the intentional inhalation of volatile organic chemicals other than conventional anaesthetic gases. This definition includes the inhalation of organic solvents and vapours (whether pure or in combination with other non-volatile ingredients), hydrocarbon mixtures such as petrol (gasoline), and aerosol propellants.

Volatile substances are either 'bagged' (sprayed into a plastic bag and then inhaled until the subject passes out) or 'huffed' (sprayed on to a cloth held to the mouth). Glue is most often sniffed from a potato crisp bag and repeated abuse in this manner leads to the development of erythmatous spots around the mouth and nose ('glue-sniffer's rash'). The composition of products commonly abused is shown in Table 2. Most solvent abusers are male and adolescent and indulge in the habit as a group activity. Boys may take up glue sniffing as a relief from boredom, in response to peer group pressure, out of curiosity, or in an attempt to gain status. Most youngsters sniff solvents for a short time and on few occasions; only a few become dependent chronic users, and many of these 'mature out' of the solvent habit. Solvent misuse may, however, also occur in adults. Some studies have found a higher incidence of solvent abuse in children from single-parent families and families with paternal unemployment.

Table 2 *Solvent composition of products commonly abused*

Products inhaled	Chemical constituents
Glues/adhesives	Toluene, benzene, xylene, acetone, *n*-hexane
Cleaning fluids	Trichloroethylene, tetrachloroethylene, 1,1,1-trichloroethane, carbon tetrachloride, toluene
Fire extinguishers	Bromochlorodifluoromethane
Petrol (gasoline)	Hydrocarbons, tetraethyl lead
Aerosols	Fluorocarbons
Lighter refills	Butane
Acrylic paint	Toluene
Paints, varnishes, lacquers	Trichloroethylene, methylene chloride, toluene
Polystyrene cements	Acetone, toluene, trichloroethylene
Dyes	Acetone, methylene chloride
Nail-polish remover	Acetone, amyl acetate

Clinical features

The clinical features of intoxication with volatile substances are similar to those of alcohol intoxication with initial CNS stimulation followed by depression. Other symptoms may include euphoria, blurring of vision, tinnitus, slurring of speech, ataxia, feelings of omnipotence, headache, abdominal pain, anorexia, nausea, vomiting, jaundice, chest pain, bronchospasm, impaired judgement, irritability, and excitement. Less often a delerious state is seen, with clouding of consciousness and hallucinations. Many chronic users report transient psychotic symptoms which often have an affective component. Convulsions, status epilepticus, and coma may occur. Self-destructive and antisocial acts may be carried out by people under the influence of volatile substances. Psychological dependence and tolerance may develop, but physical dependence is rare. Volatile substance abuse may be associated with the abuse of alcohol and multiple illicit drugs.

Volatile substance abuse should be suspected if groups of adolescents or individuals behave is if they are drunk. The hair, breath, or clothing may smell of solvent and the clothing is often stained. Unexplained listlessness, anorexia, and marked moodiness are suggestive of chronic abuse. Poor school adjustment and scholastic performance have been noted in chronic glue sniffers apparently due to lack of motivation.

'Glue sniffing'

Glues are volatile, semiliquid preparations which usually contain an aromatic hydrocarbon as the vehicle. Fortunately, benzene itself has now been replaced by toluene and other aromatic hydrocarbons in most commercially available products. For this reason, glue sniffing is now attended by fewer short- and long-term complications than was previously the case. The inhalation of glues, however, remains hazardous and can be fatal.

The physical sequelae of prolonged glue sniffing include aplastic anaemia and acute hepatic and renal damage. Features of renal toxicity include proteinuria, haematuria, distal renal tubular acidosis, and recurrent urinary calculi. Irreversible neurological sequelae such as optic atrophy, encephalopathy, cerebellar degeneration, and equilibrium disorders have been reported in adults who are chronic abusers. Toluene inhalation may cause encephalopathy in children. Neurological damage may occur after 'sniffing' of less than 1 year's duration and symptoms may progress for up to 3 months after the habit has been abandoned. Glues containing *n*-hexane and toluene have been associated with the development of muscle weakness and atrophy and sensory impairment of either the 'glove and stocking' or sensorimotor type, with or without muscle atrophy. It is not certain whether the polyneuropathy is due to *n*-hexane alone or to the combination of *n*-hexane and toluene.

A review of adults who had sniffed toluene indicated three major patterns of presentation: (1) muscle weakness, (2) gastrointestinal complaints (abdominal pain, haematemesis), and (3) neuropsychiatric disorders (altered mental status, cerebellar abnormalities, peripheral neuropathy). In addition, hypokalaemia, hypophosphataemia, and hyperchloraemia were common. Rhabdomyolysis occurred in 40 per cent of cases. Cardiac and haematological toxicity due to toluene appears to be uncommon.

Petrol (gasoline) sniffing

Petrol is a complex mixture of hydrocarbons containing a small proportion of non-hydrocarbon additives such as 'antiknock' agents, antitoxidants, rust inhibitors and dyes.

Abusers of petrol have reported that 15 to 20 breaths of the vapours are sufficient to produce intoxication for 3 to 6 h. The lipid solubility of the components of petrol ensures rapid absorption from lungs and symptoms start within 3 to 5 min.

The euphoria of mild intoxication may be accompanied by nausea and vomiting. After prolonged inhalation, or rapid inhalation of highly concentrated vapour, the 'sniffer' may experience a phase of violent excitement followed by loss of consciousness and coma. While unconscious, the subject may suffer convulsions and the pupils may become fixed and dilated or unequal. Nystagmus and conjugate deviation of the eyes may be observed.

Death from inhalation of petrol vapour is rare, but may occur due either to respiratory depression or to ventricular fibrillation from cardiac sensitization by the aromatic fractions of petrol. Cerebral and pulmonary oedema and renal and hepatic damage have been noted at autopsy. The greater danger from petrol 'sniffing' is related to the long-term effects of chronic exposure which include loss of appetite and loss of weight, neurasthenia, muscle weakness, and cramps. Abnormal EEGs have been reported and permanent neuropsychological damage may develop. Encephalopathy in petrol sniffers may also be due to tetraethyl lead added to petrol as an 'antiknock' agent.

The deliberate abuse of hydrocarbon mixtures other than petrol is unusual, although a 'huffer's' neuropathy, similar to the Guillain-Barré syndrome has been described following inhalation of a lacquer thinner.

Chlorinated hydrocarbon abuse

Inhalation of chlorinated hydrocarbons causes a sense of euphoria, and sometimes excitement, associated with headache, dizziness, nausea,

Table 3 *Urinary metabolites used to monitor solvent exposure*

Solvent	Metabolite
Benzene	Phenol
Styrene	Mandelic acid and phenylglyoxylic acid
1,1,1-Trichloroethane	Trichloroacetic acid and trichloroethanol
Trichloroethylene	Trichloracetic acid and trichloroethanol
Toluene	Hippuric acid
Xylene	Methylhippuric acid (toluic acid)

vomiting, stupor, coma, and convulsions. Abuse of carbon tetrachloride may lead to acute renal failure and centrilobular hepatic necrosis. Trichloroethylene abuse has, on rare occasions, led to similar effects and it has also been associated with cranial nerve damage, particularly affecting the optic and trigeminal nerves. Both carbon tetrachloride and trichloroethylene sensitize the myocardium to circulating catecholamines, and fatal ventricular arrhythmias may result. Abuse of a proprietary stain-removing product containing 1,2-dichloropropane has been reported to cause the haemolytic-uraemic syndrome.

Toxicity due to aerosol inhalation

The most commonly abused aerosol propellants are the chlorofluorocarbons (CFCs) (see above) of which those most widely employed are trichloromonofluoromethane (Freon 11), dichlorodifluoromethane (Freon 12), and dichlorotetrafluoroethane (CFC 114).

Sudden death following inhalation of CFC aerosol propellants was first described in 1968. Since then, several hundred deaths in teenagers have occurred from this cause and death has often been preceded by some form of excessive exercise or stress. No anatomical abnormalities to account for the deaths were found at autopsy and it is likely that the fatalities were due to cardiac arrhythmias. Animal experiments have shown that CFCs readily sensitize the heart to asphyxia-induced sinus bradycardia and asystole, an effect which persists after exposure to the CFC ceases. At the same time, CFCs sensitize the heart to circulating catecholamines and ventricular tachycardia and fibrillation may occur as a consequence.

One death from exposure to a CFC propellant was that of a Canadian youth who continually inhaled a lipid aerosol containing soyabean extract, used to prevent food sticking to cooking pans. He died from acute adult respiratory distress syndrome rather than cardiac causes. Laboratory experiments suggested that Freons 11 and 12 had interfered with surfactant function.

Diagnosis and management of volatile substance abuse

The clinical features described above and the circumstances in which patients are found usually point to the diagnosis, but confirmation may be obtained by detection of solvents in blood or, in some cases of volatile substance abuse, metabolites may be detected in the urine (Table 3).

Prevention is by far the most important aspect of management of volatile substance abuse and every opportunity should be taken to educate adolescents about the serious short- and long-term hazards of 'sniffing'. Minimal, non-dramatic intervention at an early stage with the participation of parents is often effective. Particular attention should be paid to the lonely, dependent chronic abuser with emotional problems who may also be using more dangerous substances. Health education, improved recreational facilities, and help for single parents and those with alcohol, physical, marital, and psychiatric problems have proved to be useful.

Acute intoxication from volatile substance abuse is usually brief and self-limiting. If respiratory depression and cardiac arrhythmias supervene they should be treated conventionally. Renal and hepatic failure may require further supportive measures and dialysis.

REFERENCES

Anon. (1988). Complications of chronic volatile substance abuse. *Lancet*, **ii,** 431–2.

Streicher, H.A., Gabow, P.A., Moss, A.H., Kono, D., and Kaehny, W.D. (1981). Syndromes of toluene sniffing in adults. *Annals of Internal Medicine*, **94,** 758–62.

8.3.4 Poisoning by inhalational agents

J. A. Vale, A. T. Proudfoot, and T. J. Meredith

Acetone

Acetone is a clear liquid with a characteristic pungent odour and sweet taste. It is used widely in industrial and household products, in glues and as a chemical intermediate.

METABOLISM

Isopropanol is metabolized to acetone *in vivo*. Once absorbed either through the lungs or gut, acetone is exhaled unchanged or metabolized to carbon dioxide; only about 1 per cent of the uptake is excreted unchanged in the urine. If exposure is high accumulation of acetone may occur.

CLINICAL FEATURES

Acetone is highly volatile and its vapour has an irritating effect on the mucous membranes of the eyes, nose, and throat. Intoxication results in headache, excitement, restlessness, chest tightness, incoherent speech, nausea and vomiting (occasionally gastrointestinal bleeding has been reported), coma, and convulsions. Hyperglycaemia has been observed.

TREATMENT

If toxicity has followed inhalation, remove from exposure. Thereafter, supportive measures should be given with correction of hyperglycaemia, as necessary. There is no evidence that gut decontamination is of value after ingestion.

REFERENCE

Ross, D.S. (1973). Acute acetone intoxication involving eight male workers. *Annals of Occupational Hygiene*, **16,** 73–5.

Ammonia

Ammonia, a colourless gas with a strong irritating odour, is available in aqueous form for industrial and household applications and is used in the manufacture of chemicals such as plastics, pesticides, and detergents, and as a commercial refrigerant gas. Most of the ammonia produced by industry is used for fertilizer.

CLINICAL FEATURES

Ammonia may be absorbed by inhalation, ingestion, or percutaneously if the concentration of liquid ammonia is high enough to cause skin injury. Once absorbed, it is converted to ammonium hydroxide and other salts, including ammonium carbonate, and then to urea. When in contact with moist mucosal membranes, ammonia reacts with water to form ammonium hydroxide, which causes irritation to the eyes, upper respiratory tract, and pharynx. Exposed surfaces may develop chemical burns, blisters, thrombosis of surface vessels, and severe local oedema which may lead to respiratory obstruction and death, if the larynx and glottis are also involved. High inhaled concentrations may cause dyspnoea and pulmonary oedema and may result in airways damage and reduced gas transfer for up to 3 years.

TREATMENT

The casualty should be removed from the contaminated area. The eyes should be irrigated with water or saline (0.9 per cent) for 15 to 30 min and an ophthalmic opinion sought as permanent blindness may result. Pulmonary complications should be treated with humidified supplemental oxygen, bronchodilators, and, if necessary, assisted ventilation with positive end-expiratory pressure. Although widely employed, there is no conclusive evidence that diuretics and corticosteroids alter the prognosis. Patients who survive for 24 h are likely to recover fully.

REFERENCES

Caplin, M. (1941). Ammonia-gas poisoning. Forty-seven cases in a London shelter. *Lancet*, **ii,** 95–6.

Flury, K.E., Dines, D.E., Rodarte, J.R., and Rodgers, R. (1983). Airway obstruction due to inhalation of ammonia. *Mayo Clinic Proceedings*, **58,** 389–93.

Levy, D.M., Divertie, M.B., Litzow, T.J., and Henderson, J.W. (1964). Ammonia burns of the face and respiratory tract. *Journal of the American Medical Association*, **190,** 95–8.

Taplin, G.V., Chopra, S., Yanda, R.L., and Elam, D. (1976). Radionuclidic lung-imaging procedures in the assessment of injury due to ammonia inhalation. *Chest*, **69,** 582–6.

Walton, M. (1973). Industrial ammonia gassing. *British Journal of Industrial Medicine*, **30,** 78–86.

Arsine

Arsine is a colourless, non-irritating gas that is produced as a result of nascent hydrogen in the presence of arsenic or by the action of water on a metallic arsenide.

MECHANISM OF TOXICITY

Arsine binds with oxidized haemoglobin causing marked haemolysis of sudden onset by a mechanism not yet elucidated. Acute tubular necrosis then develops.

CLINICAL FEATURES

Acute exposure

There is usually a delay of some 2 to 24 h after exposure before the onset of headache, malaise, weakness, dizziness, breathlessness, migratory abdominal pain, fever, tachycardia, tachypnoea, nausea, and vomiting. A bronze skin colour is noted in some patients but most have the typical appearance of a jaundiced patient. Acute renal failure is observed by the third day after substantial exposure and the urine is dark red then brown before anuria ensues. Investigations will show leucocytosis, reticulocytosis, elevated plasma haemoglobin, and haemoglobinuria. Historically, the mortality has been as high as 25 per cent.

Chronic exposure

Severe anaemia has been reported in workers engaged in the extraction of gold.

TREATMENT

The treatment of choice if haemolysis is severe is exchange transfusion and, if renal failure ensues, haemodialysis/filtration. Dimercaprol is of no value. The role of alkaline diuresis is controversial.

REFERENCES

Fowler, B.A. and Weissburg, J.B. (1974). Arsine poisoning. *New England Journal of Medicine*, **291,** 1171–4.

Wilkinson, S.P., *et al.* (1975). Arsine toxicity aboard the Asia freighter. *British Medical Journal*, **3,** 559–63.

Carbon dioxide

Carbon dioxide is a colourless gas that is also available commercially as a solid for refrigeration purposes ('dry ice'). It is a normal constituent of the atmosphere, but high concentrations may accumulate in wells, silos, manholes, and mines. It is a byproduct of ammonia production, lime kiln operations, and fermentation. It is thought that carbon dioxide was the main cause of the Lake Nyos disaster in 1986 when more than 1700 inhabitants of the Northwest Province of Cameroon died.

MECHANISMS OF TOXICITY

Carbon dioxide has been evaluated as a possible anaesthetic agent but although a mixture of 30 per cent (300 000 p.p.m.) carbon dioxide in air induces anaesthesia, adverse effects have precluded its use. Animal studies have confirmed that the prime cause of death is not hypoxia but high carbon dioxide concentrations. Concentrations greater than 35 per cent produce CNS, cardiac, and respiratory depression, whereas lower concentrations stimulate the respiratory centre.

CLINICAL FEATURES

Dyspnoea, headache, dizziness, sweating, restlessness, paraesthesiae, and sinus tachycardia are features after modest carbon dioxide exposure (up to 100 000 p.p.m.). Higher concentrations produce psychomotor agitation, myoclonic twitches, eye flickering, coma, and convulsions. Death occurs from acute cardiorespiratory depression. In the Lake Nyos disaster, survivors complained most commonly of cough, skin lesions resembling burns (possibly secondary to coma), limb swelling, headache, lethargy, and fever.

Skin contact with 'dry ice' may result in frostbite and local blistering.

TREATMENT

The casualty should be removed from the contaminated environment without the rescuer being put at risk. Thereafter, supportive care should be employed.

REFERENCES

Baxter, P.J., Kapila, M., and Mfonfu, D. (1989). Lake Nyos disaster, Cameroon, 1986: the medical effects of large scale emission of carbon dioxide? *British Medical Journal*, **298,** 1437–41.

Williams, H.I. (1958). Carbon dioxide poisoning—report of eight cases, with two deaths. *British Medical Journal*, **2,** 1012–14.

Carbon disulphide

Carbon disulphide is used as a fumigant for grain and as a solvent, particularly in the rayon industry. It is a clear, colourless, volatile liquid, with an odour like that of decaying cabbage. However, the foul odour is insufficient to give adequate warning of hazardous concentrations. Inhaled carbon disulphide reacts with free amino groups of proteins and amino acids to form dithiocarbamates, which in turn inhibit protein synthesis and which have been implicated in disturbances of trace metal balance. In animals, carbon disulphide is metabolized by cytochrome P450-dependent enzymes to carbonyl sulphide and carbon dioxide, which are predominantly excreted in expired air. Less than 1 per cent of free carbon disulphide is eliminated in the urine and about 5 per cent is eliminated unchanged through the lungs. The metabolite, 2-thiothiazolidine-4-carboxylic acid, appears to be a reliable marker of exposure.

CLINICAL FEATURES

Acute exposure

Although acute poisoning is rare, chronic industrial exposure is common. Absorption occurs through the skin as well as by inhalation. Carbon disulphide, due to its potent defatting activity, causes reddening, cracking, and peeling of the skin and a burn may occur if contact continues for several minutes. Splashes of carbon disulphide in the eye cause immediate and severe irritation. Acute inhalation may result in irritation of the mucous membranes, blurred vision, nausea and vomiting, headache, delirium, hallucinations, coma, tremor, convulsions, and cardiac and respiratory arrest.

Chronic exposure

There is considerable epidemiological evidence to suggest that chronic industrial exposure to carbon disulphide may lead to the development of atherosclerosis and coronary heart disease. In addition, sleep disturbances, fatigue, anorexia, and weight loss are common complaints among workers in the industry. Intellectual decline, depression, stereotyped behaviour, and ocular changes (central scotoma, discrete pigmentary changes in the posterior pole, and choroidal microvascular lesions) have been described, as well as cerebellar and extrapyramidal signs, hepatic damage, and permanent impairment of reproductive performance; evidence for renal toxicity is not strong.

Numerous cohort studies undertaken since the 1930s have demonstrated an increased incidence of cardiovascular disease among workers exposed to carbon disulphide. Despite improvements in ventilation since then, subsequent studies continue to show an increased mortality among this group of workers despite much lower levels of carbon disulphide in the workplace.

TREATMENT

Treatment involves removal from exposure, washing contaminated skin, irrigation of the eyes with water, and supportive measures. In the majority of cases, however, preventive measures to keep carbon disulphide concentrations in the workplace as low as possible are more important and should be applied vigorously.

REFERENCES

Fielder, R.J. and Shillaker, R.O. (1981). *Toxicity Review. Carbon disulphide*. HMSO, London.

IPCS (1979) *Environmental Health Criteria 10. Carbon disulphide*. WHO, Geneva.

Spyker, D.A., Gallanosa, A.G., and Suratt, P.M. (1982). Health effects of acute carbon disulfide exposure. *Clinical Toxicology*, **19,** 87–93.

Carbon monoxide

Carbon monoxide is a tasteless, odourless, colourless, and non-irritating gas produced by incomplete combustion of organic materials. It is produced endogenously in humans from the α-methyl carbon atom of the protoporphyrin ring during the catabolism of haemoglobin. Normal endogenous production of carbon monoxide is sufficient to maintain a resting carboxyhaemoglobin level of 1 to 3 per cent in urban non-smokers and 5 to 6 per cent in smokers (cigarette smoke contains about 4 per cent carbon monoxide).

Although the mortality due to carbon monoxide poisoning has fallen in the United Kingdom since the introduction of natural gas to domestic households, approximately 1500 deaths still occur annually in England and Wales from this cause and carbon monoxide remains the main toxicological cause of death in children in the United Kingdom Worldwide, common sources of carbon monoxide are car exhaust fumes, improperly maintained and ventilated heating systems, smoke from all types of fire, and household gas (if supplies have not been converted to natural gas). Carbon monoxide derived from domestic heating systems is a major cause of accidental death in the developing world. Inhalation of methylene chloride (found in paint strippers) may also lead to carbon monoxide poisoning as a result of hepatic metabolism (see Chapter 8.3.3).

MECHANISMS OF TOXICITY

Symptoms and signs that follow inhalation of carbon monoxide are the result of tissue hypoxia. The affinity of haemoglobin for carbon monoxide is approximately 240 times greater than that for oxygen. Carbon monoxide combines with haemoglobin to form carboxyhaemoglobin, reducing the total oxygen-carrying capacity of the blood and shifting the oxygen dissociation curve to the left. However, the binding of one or more carbon monoxide molecules to haemoglobin also induces an allosteric modification in the remaining oxygen-binding sites. As a result, the affinity of the remaining haem groups for oxygen is increased, and the oxygen dissociation curve is distorted as well as being shifted to the left. The resulting tissue hypoxia is thus far greater than that which would result from simple loss of oxygen-carrying capacity. Recent evidence suggests that carbon monoxide toxicity may also be due to direct inhibition of cellular respiration as a result of reversible binding to other haem proteins, particularly cytochrome oxidase a,a_3, where it acts in the same way as cyanide. Although inhibition of cellular respiration had only been thought to occur in conditions of established tissue hypoxia (because the affinity of cytochrome oxidase for oxygen is much greater than that for carbon monoxide), this view is now challenged. Carbon monoxide mediated brain lipid peroxidation may play a role in the development of delayed neuropsychiatric sequelae.

CLINICAL FEATURES

The clinical features of carbon monoxide poisoning are summarized in Table 1. The symptoms of moderate exposure to carbon monoxide are mild and may even be mistaken for a viral illness and for this reason it is important that the diagnosis is always borne in mind. The severity of poisoning following exposure to carbon monoxide depends on the concentration of carbon monoxide in the inspired air, the length of exposure, and the general health of the exposed individual. Elderly patients and those with pre-existing cardiorespiratory disease are at greater risk. The symptoms and signs of toxicity can be correlated with the maximum blood carboxyhaemoglobin concentration achieved under experimental conditions before treatment is instituted. Unfortunately, in clinical practice, the maximum carboxyhaemoglobin concentration is rarely known with certainty. A carboxyhaemoglobin level of less than 10 per cent is not normally associated with symptoms and 10 to 30 per cent carboxyhaemoglobin may cause only headache and mild exertional dyspnoea. It is known that even low concentrations of carbon monoxide produce significant effects on cardiac function during exercise in subjects with coronary artery disease. Transmural myocardial infarction has been reported in a 38-year-old worker whose carboxyhaemoglobin level did not exceed 25 per cent. Coma, convulsions, and cardiorespiratory arrest may be expected to occur with carboxyhaemoglobin concentrations in

Table 1 *Immediate and late clinical features of carbon monoxide poisoning*

Agitation, mental confusion, headache (usually frontal and band-like, sometimes occipital)
Nausea and vomiting, incontinence (occasionally), haematemesis, melaena
Hyperventilation, pulmonary oedema, respiratory failure, Cheyne-Stokes respiration
Metabolic acidosis
Bullous lesions
Hyperpyrexia
Loss of consciousness, hypertonia, hyper-reflexia
Extensor plantar responses, papilloedema, convulsions
Monoplegia or hemiplegia, peripheral neuropathies
Cerebral, cerebellar, and midbrain damage (parkinsonism, akinetic mutism)
Myocardial ischaemia and infarction
Arrhythmias and ECG changes: atrial fibrillation, prolonged PR interval, AV block, bundle-branch block, ventricular extrasystoles, prolonged QT interval, ST depression
Decrease in light sensitivity and dark adaptation, retinal haemorrhages
Hearing loss (central type due to ischaemia of cochlea and brain-stem nuclei)
Acute renal failure
Muscle necrosis
Thrombotic thrombocytopenic purpura
Late neuropsychiatric sequelae

excess of 60 per cent. Coma may ensue before other symptoms if the rise in carboxyhaemoglobin has been unusually rapid. Similarly, the development of neuropsychiatric problems after recovery from carbon monoxide intoxication may develop insiduously over a number of weeks. These neuropsychiatric changes may include intellectual deterioration, memory impairment, cerebral, cerebellar, and midbrain damage (e.g. parkinsonism, akinetic mutism) and change in personality typified by increased irritability, verbal aggressiveness, violence, impulsiveness, and moodiness.

TREATMENT

The patient should be removed from exposure and 100 per cent oxygen administered using a tightly-fitting face mask. Endotracheal intubation and mechanical ventilation may be required in those who are unconscious. The administration of oxygen should be continued until the carboxyhaemoglobin level is less than 10 per cent.

The use of hyperbaric oxygen therapy has been advocated as a means of preventing, diminishing the severity of, or treating delayed neuropsychiatric sequelae following carbon monoxide exposure. Unfortunately it is not possible to identify with certainty those patients at particular risk of developing such sequelae, though criteria employed currently include a measured carboxyhaemoglobin level of 40 per cent or greater, a history of loss of consciousness, or persistent neurological or cardiac abnormalities. There remains controversy over the value of hyperbaric oxygen therapy in this context and it is possible that 100 per cent normobaric oxygen with elective ventilation would confer the same benefit. Moreover, to transfer a patient to a hyperbaric oxygen chamber and then to achieve full working pressure may take too long to make hyperbaric oxygen practicable even in cases of severe carbon monoxide poisoning.

In addition to the specific therapy outlined above, general symptomatic and supportive measures will be required. Diazepam, (5–10 mg intravenously) repeated as necessary, is the agent of choice for the management of convulsions. Although corticosteroids have been advocated for the treatment of cerebral oedema, there is no definite evidence as to their efficacy; mannitol may be of value.

REFERENCES

Burney, R.E., Wu, S-C., and Nemiroff, M.J. (1982). Mass carbon monoxide poisoning: clinical effects and results of treatment in 184 victims. *Annals of Emergency Medicine*, **11,** 394–9.

Choi, I.S. (1983). Delayed neurologic sequelae in carbon monoxide intoxication. *Archives of Neurology,* **40,** 433–35.

IPCS (1979).*Environmental Health Criteria 13. Carbon monoxide*. WHO, Geneva.

Meredith, T., and Vale, A. (1988). Carbon monoxide poisoning. *British Medical Journal,* **296,** 77–9.

Myers, R.A.M., Snyder, S.K., and Emhoff, T.A. (1985). Subacute sequelae of carbon monoxide poisoning. *Annals of Emergency Medicine,* **14,** 1163–7.

Piantidosi, C.A. (1987). Carbon monoxide, oxygen transport, and oxygen metabolism. *Journal of Hyperbaric Medicine,* **2,** 27–44.

Raphael, J-C., *et al.* (1989). Trial of normobaric and hyperbaric oxygen for acute carbon monoxide intoxication. *Lancet*, **ii,** 414–19.

Sokal, J.A. and Kralkowska, E. (1985). The relationship between exposure duration, carboxyhemoglobin, blood glucose, pyruvate and lactate and the severity of intoxication in 39 cases of acute carbon monoxide poisoning in man. *Archives of Toxicology*, **57,** 196–9.

Symposium (1985). Carbon monoxide poisoning. *Clinical Toxicology*, **23,** 247–326.

Chlorine

Chlorine is a greenish-yellow gas at room temperature and atmospheric pressure, although it is normally transported as a pressurized liquid. Exposure after spillage may be prolonged because the density of chlorine gas is greater than that of air, causing it to remain near ground level. Chlorine has a pungent odour that can usually be detected by smell at concentrations of less than 0.5 p.p.m., though some workers chronically exposed to the gas become anosmic.

Although millions of tons of chlorine are used annually in the manufacture of chemical, plastics, and paper, and in the purification of water and sewage, surprisingly few industrial deaths are recorded. Poisoning has followed transportation mishaps, industrial accidents affecting both the workforce and the surrounding population, school chemistry experiments, the mixing of acidic lavatory-cleaning agents with bleaches containing sodium hypochlorite, and accidental release of chlorine in the plant room of swimming-pools. Voluntary chlorine inhalation for pleasure has also been reported.

MECHANISMS OF TOXICITY

The severity of injury due to chlorine is directly related to the concentration of the gas, the duration of exposure, and the water content of tissues exposed. While the mechanism of toxicity is not understood in detail, molecular chlorine, a strong oxidizing agent, is known to react with many functional groups in cell components and it can form chloramines and oxidize thiol radicals. In addition, chlorine reacts with tissue water to form hypochlorite and hydrochloric acid, and it may generate oxygen free radicals. It is noteworthy that chlorine gas is some 30 times more irritant to the respiratory tract than hydrogen chloride.

CLINICAL FEATURES

Symptoms of exposure to chlorine begin within minutes and include irritation of the mucous membranes of the eyes, nose, and throat, followed by cough, breathlessness, expectoration of white sputum (which may be bloodstained) chest pain and tightness, abdominal pain, nausea, headache, dizziness, and palpitations due to ventricular ectopic beats.

Laryngeal oedema may cause hoarseness of the voice and stridor, and cardiac arrest may occur secondary to hypoxia.

Workers habituated to low levels of chlorine gas are more tolerant than the general population, suggesting that hyperventilation and bronchospasm are at least partly due to afferent nerve irritation, though bronchial mucosal oedema may contribute to airways obstruction. Restrictive as well as obstructive defects arise in those who have inhaled sublethal amounts, presumably because of interstitial oedema. In addition, gas diffusion is impaired, leading to arterial hypoxaemia. In very severe cases, non-cardiogenic pulmonary oedema may supervene with rapid onset of respiratory failure. Arterial blood-gas analysis reflects the extent of pulmonary involvement, ranging from mild respiratory alkalosis to metabolic acidosis with profound hypoxaemia. Survival is usually followed by complete resolution of the pulmonary defects.

TREATMENT

The first priority is to remove the casualty from exposure. Rescuers may minimize their exposure by using either breathing apparatus or a makeshift gas mask consisting of a water-soaked cloth held to the face. Casualties who have been exposed only slightly and who are symptomless should be advised to rest for 12 h and to report to their medical practitioner if symptoms develop (which is unlikely). Conjunctival irritation should be treated by copious irrigation with water or saline and the eyes examined with fluorescein for corneal defects. Skin burns due, for example, to direct trauma from a jet of escaping chlorine, should also be extensively irrigated and treated coventionally.

The respiratory effects of chlorine are potentially lethal and patients with respiratory symptoms persisting beyond the period of exposure should be admitted to hospital in case they require bronchodilators and humidified oxygen. Although inhaled nebulized sodium bicarbonate has been advocated to counteract the potential damage caused by hydrogen chloride, no clinical trial has demonstrated efficacy. Some will also require mechanical ventilation with positive end-expiratory pressure, particularly if non-cardiogenic pulmonary oedema develops. Frusemide has been reported to be of value in these circumstances. Corticosteroids have been employed (particularly in the hope of preventing broncholitis obliterans) but their role is not established and prophylactic antibiotics have not been shown to be effective in preventing infection. Correction of serious metabolic acidosis with intravenous sodium bicarbonate may be necessary. The rarity of severe poisoning and the negligible mortality reflects not so much the efficacy of supportive treatment as the care with which this agent is now usually handled.

REFERENCES

Anon. (1984). Chlorine poisoning. *Lancet*, **i**, 321–2.

IPCS. (1982). *Environmental Health Criteria 21. Chlorine and hydrogen chloride*. WHO, Geneva.

Kaufman, J. and Burkons, D. (1971). Clinical, roentgenologic, and physiologic effects of acute chlorine exposure. *Archives of Environmental Health*, **23**, 29–34.

Weill, H., George, R., Schwarz, M., and Ziskind, M. (1969). Late evaluation of pulmonary function after acute exposure to chlorine gas. *American Review of Respiratory Diseases*, **99**, 374–9.

Cyanide

Hydrogen cyanide and its derivatives (acetonitrile, acrylonitrile, cyanamide, cyanides, nitroprusside, and thiocyanates) are used widely in industry. It is estimated that worldwide some 3.5 million tons of cyanide are manufactured each year. Hydrogen cyanide is found in the workplace both as a gas and as a liquid. Cyanides are found in electroplating solutions, fertilizers, fumigant mixtures, metal polishes, and rodenticides and acrylonitrile is used in the production of synthetic rubber. Sodium nitroprusside is used to treat severe hypertension, to induce hypotension during surgical procedures, and to reduce myocardial afterload following infarction or in cases of refractory congestive cardiac failure. Prolonged or excessive use of nitroprusside may lead to cyanide toxicity and metabolic acidosis.

Hydrogen cyanide and other organic cyanides are released during the thermal decomposition of polyurethane foams used in the manufacture of furniture and they contribute to mortality in smoke-inhalation victims. Cyanide poisoning may also result from the ingestion of the cyanogenic glycoside, amygdalin (vitamin B_{17}) which is found in the kernels of almonds, apples, apricots, cherries, peaches, plums, and other fruits. Other sources of amygdalin include cassava beans, choke-cherries, jet beans, and the non-approved anticancer agent, Laetrile.

Over the last 20 years, more than 400 deaths have been recorded in England and Wales as being due to cyanide poisoning. Some have arisen as the result of accidental exposure in industry, but most were due to suicide or homicide. In the United States, seven deaths occurred in Chicago in September 1982 when over-the-counter extra-strength Tylenol capsules were criminally adulterated with cyanide and similar adulteration has been attempted subsequently.

MECHANISMS OF TOXICITY

Cyanide reversibly inhibits cellular enzymes which contain ferric iron, notably cytochrome oxidase a,a_3. This enzyme is the terminal member of the mitochondrial electron transport chain which traps electrons liberated in the tricarboxylic acid cycle and then transfers them to mediate the formation of water from oxygen and hydrogen. In the presence of cyanide, electron transfer is blocked, the tricarboxylic acid cycle is paralysed, and cellular respiration ceases.

CLINICAL FEATURES

Acute exposure

The ingestion by an adult of 50 ml of (liquid) hydrogen cyanide or 200 to 300 mg of one of its salts is likely to prove fatal. The onset of poisoning is hastened by the presence of an empty stomach and high gastric acidity but symptoms may be delayed for up to 4 h if a cyanide salt is taken on a full stomach. Delayed absorption may also result from skin splashes when either soaked clothing or the stratum corneum may act as a reservoir. Inhalation of hydrogen cyanide gas may produce symptoms within seconds and death within minutes.

Acute poisoning is characterized by dizziness, headache, palpitations, anxiety, a feeling of constriction in the chest, dyspnoea, pulmonary oedema, confusion, vertigo, ataxia, coma, and paralysis. Cardiovascular collapse, respiratory arrest, convulsions, and metabolic acidosis are seen in severe cases. Cyanosis may occur, and the classical 'brick-red' colour of the skin is noted occasionally. There is sometimes an odour of bitter almonds on the breath, but the ability to detect it is genetically determined and some 40 per cent of the population are unable to do so.

Chronic Exposure

Chronic exposure results predominantly in neurological damage which can include ataxia, peripheral neuropathies, optic atrophy, and nerve deafness. Toxic amblyopia associated with heavy cigarette smoking has been attributed to the cyanide content of tobacco and epidemiological studies in Southern Nigeria strongly suggest that tropical ataxic neuropathy is related to the chronic ingestion of cassava root, which contains an amygdalin derivative. Abnormalities of cyanide metabolism have been described in juvenile optic atrophy and in Leber's disease.

TREATMENT

Cyanide poisoning is a medical emergency, although specific antidotal treatment may not always be necessary. Where appropriate, the patient should be removed from the source of exposure, contaminated clothing discarded, and the skin washed with soap and water. Gastric aspiration and lavage should be undertaken if cyanide has been ingested but this procedure must not delay treatment if symptoms or signs of toxicity are present. It may be difficult to differentiate between the genuine fear and anxiety of a patient and the early symptoms of cyanide poisoning (anxiety, excitement, sweating, faintness). However, a patient who has been exposed to hydrogen cyanide gas and who remains conscious on arrival at hospital 30 min later is unlikely to require antidotal therapy.

Dicobalt edetate

Cobalt compounds form stable inert complexes with cyanide (cobaltocyanides and cobalticyanides). Dicobalt edetate (Kelocyanor), if available, is the treatment of choice for confirmed cyanide poisoning and should be given intravenously in a dose of 300 to 600 mg over 1 min, with a further 300 mg if recovery does not occur within 1 min. It should be administered only if the diagnosis is certain because, in the absence of cyanide, this drug may cause serious side-effects including vomiting, tachycardia, hypertension, chest pain, and facial and palpebral oedema. These reactions are usually self-limiting and are thought to be due to the presence of free cobalt in the formulation, which also enhances the efficacy of dicobalt edetate. Glucose is advocated following dicobalt edetate because early animal experiments suggested that this reduced the toxic effects of the antidote; such an infusion will not be necessary if the antidote has been used appropriately as all cobalt will be bound to cyanide.

Oxygen

The administration of oxygen, which acts synergistically with other cyanide antidotes, is of paramount importance in the treatment of cyanide poisoning. Oxygen is believed to prevent inhibition of cytochrome oxidase, a,a_3 and to accelerate its reactivation. Oxygen should always be given to patients with cyanide poisoning and a number of cases have now been described where serious cyanide toxicity has been treated successfully with vigorous supportive (including oxygen), but non-specific, therapy alone.

Sodium nitrite, sodium thiosulphate, 4-dimethylaminophenol

The principal route of detoxification of cyanide in the body is the conversion of cyanide to thiocyanate which is catalysed by the enzyme, rhodanase, present in liver and muscle. Thiosulphate is required for this reaction as a source of sulphane sulphur. Thiosulphate penetrates cell membranes slowly, and for this reason there has been doubt in the past about its value as a cyanide antidote. However, recent evidence suggests that thiosulphate replenishes a pool of sulphane sulphur bound to serum albumin, and there is evidence from animal experiments that thiosulphate acts quickly as a cyanide antidote. Another means of inactivating cyanide is to convert a portion of the body's haemoglobin to methaemoglobin which contains ferric iron that binds cyanide. Methaemoglobinaemia may be induced by the administration of either a nitrite or 4-dimethylaminophenol (4-DMAP). Almost 40 per cent of the haemoglobin in the body may be converted to methaemoglobin without untoward effect, though loss of oxygen-carrying capacity does result. Although the affinity of cyanide for methaemoglobin for cyanide is less than that of cytochrome oxidase, the presence of a large circulating methaemoglobin pool diminishes cyanide toxicity by binding cyanide ion before tissue penetration occurs. Nitrites may also mitigate cyanide toxicity by virtue of their vasodilatory actions and improvement of tissue perfusion. 4-DMAP (4-dimethylaminophenol) is another means of inducing methaemoglobinaemia, though the amount produced may be unexpectedly high. High doses may cause acute tubular necrosis and Heinz-body anaemia; mutagenesis and teratogenesis have been reported in cell cultures.

Inhalation of amyl nitrite was recommended in the past in order to produce rapid methaemoglobinaemia, but only low circulating concentrations of methaemoglobin were achieved and its use was discontinued. However, it is now believed that amyl nitrite has a role in combating cyanide-induced shock by improving coronary perfusion. For this reason, the administration of 1–2 ampoules amyl nitrite using an Ambu bag is recommended as first aid treatment.

If dicobalt edetate is not available, the treatment of choice for cyanide poisoning is a combination of sodium nitrite (10 ml of a 3 per cent solution (300 mg) IV over 5–20 min) and sodium thiosulphate (50 ml of a 25 per cent solution (12.5 g) IV over 10 min).

Hydroxocobalamin

Hydroxocobalamin may be used in the treatment of cyanide poisoning since a minor route of cyanide metabolism involves the formation of cyanocobalamin (vitamin B_{12}) from hydroxocobalamin. One mole of hydroxocobalamin inactives one mole of cyanide but on a weight-for-weight basis, 50 times more hydroxocobalamin is needed than cyanide because hydroxocobalamin is a far larger molecule. Although used with sodium thiosulphate as standard treatment in France (in a dose of 10 ml of a 40 per cent solution IV over 20 min), concentrated formulations of hydroxocobalamin are not yet freely available in most other countries.

REFERENCES

Anderson, R.A. and Harland, W.A. (1982). Five deaths in the Glasgow area: III The role of hydrogen cyanide. *Medicine, Science and the Law*, **22,** 35–40.

Ballantyne, B. and Marrs, T.C. (1987). *Clinical and Experimental Toxicology of Cyanides*. Wright, Bristol.

Blanc, P., Hogan, M., Mallin, K., Hryhorczuk, D., Hessel, S., and Bernard, B. (1985). Cyanide intoxication among silver-reclaiming workers. *Journal of the American Medical Association*, **253,** 367–71.

Meredith, T.J., Jacobsen, D., Haines, J.A., Berger, J-C., and van Heisjt, A.N.P. (1993). *IPCS/CEC evaluation of antidotes series. Antidotes for poisoning by cyanide.* Cambridge University Press, Cambridge, UK.

Way, J.L. (1984). Cyanide intoxication and its mechanism of antagonism. *Annual Reviews of Pharmacology and Toxicology*, **24,** 451–81.

Formaldehyde

Formaldehyde is a flammable, colourless gas with a pungent odour. It is most commonly available commercially as a 30 to 50 per cent w/w aqueous solution (with added stabilizers, e.g. methanol, to prevent polymerization). Formaldehyde is an important raw material in the synthesis of organic compounds and is used as a preservative in cosmetics and other consumer goods. Approximately 80 per cent of production is used for plastic and resin manufacture (urea-formaldehyde resins, phenolic resins, polyacetyl resins and formaldehyde-melamine resins, melamine-urea-formaldehyde resins) and the production of chemical intermediates.

METABOLISM

Formaldehyde is oxidized rapidly to formic acid and then converted more slowly to carbon dioxide and water; some formic acid is excreted in the urine.

CLINICAL FEATURES

Acute exposure

Severe irritation of the mucous membranes of the eyes, nose, and upper airways occurs after minimal exposure to low concentrations of formaldehyde, which tends to prevent higher exposure (> 5 p.p.m.) in even the most tolerant subjects. Substantial exposure may result in severe bronchospasm, pulmonary oedema and death.

Formaldehyde solutions splashed into the eye have caused corneal damage and skin contamination has resulted in dermatitis. Spillage of phenol–formaldehyde resin on to the skin has produced extensive necrotic skin lesions, fever, hypertension, adult respiratory distress syndrome, proteinuria, and renal impairment. Ingestion of formaldehyde solution has resulted in severe corrosive damage to the buccal cavity and tonsils, oesophagus, and stomach with ulceration, necrosis, (and subsequent fibrosis, and contracture), and accompanying circulatory shock, metabolic acidosis (due in part to high formate concentrations), respiratory insufficiency, and renal impairment. Death may follow ingestion of less than 100 ml in an adult.

Chronic exposure

Skin irritation and dermatitis have been observed frequently and allergic sensitization to formaldehyde solutions or resins has been reported. No long-term lung damage appears to occur. There is some evidence that formaldehyde is a human carcinogen.

TREATMENT

Supportive measures, including the correction of acid–base disturbance, should be given. Haemodialysis is only moderately effective in increasing formate elimination.

REFERENCES

Fielder, R.J. (1981). *Toxicity Review. Formaldehyde.* HMSO, London.

IPCS. (1989). *Environmental Health Criteria 89. Formaldehyde.* WHO, Geneva.

Hydrogen fluoride (hydrofluoric acid)

Hydrogen fluoride is a corrosive, fuming, nearly colourless liquid (hydrofluoric acid) at ordinary pressures below 19 °C; above 19 °C it is gaseous. Hydrogen fluoride is very soluble in cold water and for this reason it fumes strongly in moist air. Its aqueous solutions dissolve glass, reacting to form gaseous silicon fluoride. Hydrogen fluoride is used extensively in industry and storage of hydrofluoric acid for this purpose leads to danger from spills.

MECHANISMS OF TOXICITY

Hydrogen fluoride produces liquefactive necrosis of tissues as a result of the formation of a soluble salt. Absorbed fluoride ion chelates calcium and lowers the serum ionized calcium concentration. Calcium binding is also thought to be responsible for disturbances of coagulation. Fluoride directly inhibits many enzyme systems, including glycolytic enzymes, cholinesterases, and enzymes in which magnesium and manganese are present. In addition, there appears to be a direct toxic effect of fluoride on nerve tissue and muscle and depression of vasomotor and smooth-muscle tone may also occur.

CLINICAL FEATURES

Inhalation of hydrogen fluoride causes a choking sensation, cough, dyspnoea, cyanosis, and laryngeal and pulmonary oedema. Ingestion of hydrofluoric acid leads within minutes to nausea, vomiting, abdominal pain, diarrhoea, and to severe corrosive damage to the upper gastrointestinal tract. Significant systemic absorption may also occur by the dermal route. Following absorption by whatever route, hypocalcaemia results and causes weakness, paraesthesiae, tetany, and convulsions. Hypotension and cardiac arrhythmias, including ventricular fibrillation, may be observed. Central effects of fluoride cause confusion, clouding of consciousness, and coma. Hepatic and renal failure may develop and petechial skin haemorrhages may be seen before death.

Skin contact with anhydrous hydrogen fluoride produces severe burns that are felt immediately. Concentrated aqueous solutions also cause an early sensation of pain but more dilute solutions may give no warning of injury. If the solution is not removed promptly, penetration of the skin by fluoride ion may occur, leading to painful ulcers which heal only slowly.

TREATMENT

Following inhalation of hydrogen fluoride, the casualty should be removed immediately from the contaminated atmosphere. Exposed skin areas should be bathed with copious quantities of water. Further treatment is symptomatic and supportive. Mechanical ventilation with positive end-expiratory pressure may be needed to treat pulmonary oedema.

If hydrofluoric acid has been ingested, gastric aspiration and lavage or emesis should be withheld, and copious fluids and demulcents (e.g. milk) administered by mouth. If the patient is able to swallow, soluble calcium tablets (10–20 g), should be given by mouth, followed by an intravenous injection of 10 ml of 10 per cent calcium gluconate solution. Symptomatic and supportive measures should be employed thereafter.

Skin contact requires thorough washing of the affected area with copious quantities of water for 20 min, even if there is no apparent burn or pain. Skin burns should be coated repeatedly with 2.5 per cent calcium gluconate gel, but if the gel is unavailable, immersion of the skin in iced water until the pain subsides is often helpful. If the pain does not subside, 10 per cent calcium gluconate solution (up to 0.5 ml/cm^2) should be injected under the burn area. Alternatively, calcium gluconate may be given intra-arterially and this approach is more effective therapeutically than the subcutaneous route.

REFERENCES

Braun, J., Stob, H., and Zober, A. (1984). Intoxication following the inhalation of hydrogen fluoride. *Archives of Toxicology*, **56,** 50–4.

Henry, J.A. and Hla, K.K. (1992). Intravenous regional calcium gluconate perfusion for hydrofluoric acid burns. *Clinical Toxicology,* **30,** 203–7.

McCulley, J..P, Whiting, D.W,, Petitt, M.G., and Lauber, S.E. (1983). Hydrofluoric acid burns of the eye. *Journal of Occupational Medicine*, **25,** 447–50.

Vance, M.V., Curry, S.C., Kunkel, D.B., Ryan, P.J., and Ruggeri, S.B. (1986). Digital hydrofluoric acid burns: treatment with intraarterial calcium infusion. *Annals of Emergency Medicine*, **15,** 890–6.

Hydrogen sulphide

Hydrogen sulphide is a colourless gas which smells of rotten eggs, although high concentrations cause olfactory nerve paralysis. Workers in the petrochemical industry, gas industry and in tanning are particularly at risk from exposure to hydrogen sulphide. The gas is also found in mines and sewers and is liberated from decomposing fish (a hazard in fishing boats if the hold is filled with 'trash' fish used for making fish meal) and liquid manure systems.

MECHANISMS OF TOXICITY

It is now thought that the serious sequelae following exposure to high concentrations of hydrogen sulphide are due principally to inhibition of cytochrome oxidase, and there is evidence that this agent is an even more potent inhibitor of cytochrome oxidase than cyanide.

CLINICAL FEATURES

Exposure to low concentrations leads to blepharospasm, pain and redness in the eyes, blurred vision, and coloured haloes round lights. Headache, nausea, dizziness, drowsiness, sore throat, and cough may also occur. With exposure to higher concentrations, cyanosis, confusion, pulmonary oedema, coma, and convulsions are common. Mortality is approximately 6 per cent in this latter group, largely as a result of respiratory arrest, though the morbidity from traumatic injuries also contributes.

TREATMENT

The casualty should be moved to fresh air from the contaminated atmosphere, but because of the risk of sudden respiratory arrest it is essential that the rescuer dons breathing apparatus beforehand.

The excretion of sulphide can be accelerated by the formation of sulphmethaemoglobin and it has been shown in mice that the efficacy of sodium nitrite (which converts haemoglobin to methaemoglobin) is superior to that of oxygen alone in the treatment of acute hydrogen sulphide poisoning. Hence, it would seem reasonable to administer 10 ml of a 3 per cent sodium nitrite solution intravenously over 2 to 3 min, though the value of this treatment in humans has not been established.

REFERENCES

Beauchamp, R.O., Bus, J.S., Popp, J.A., Boreiko, C.J., and Andjelkovich, D.A. (1984). A critical review of the literature on hydrogen sulfide toxicity. *CRC Critical Reviews in Toxicology*, **13,** 25–97.

Burnett, W.W., King, E.G., Grace, M., and Hall, W.F. (1977). Hydrogen sulfide poisoning: review of 5 years' experience. *Canadian Medical Association Journal*, **117,** 1277–80.

IPCS. (1981). *Environmental Health Criteria 19. Hydrogen sulfide*. WHO, Geneva.

Prior, M.G., Roth, S.H., Green, F.H.Y., Hulbert, W.C., and Reiffenstein, R. (1989). *Proceedings of an International Conference on Hydrogen Sulphide Toxicity*. University of Alberta, Edmonton.

Isocyanates

Diisocyanates are used commercially to produce polyurethanes (polymers of diisocyanates and polyglycols), and toluene diisocyanate, diphenylmethane diisocyanate, and hexamethylene diisocyanate are recognized causes of asthma in sensitized subjects. Approximately 90 per cent of diisocyanate production is used in the manufacture of foam products (cushions, mattresses, packaging material, and thermal and noise insulation), most of the remainder contributing to polyurethane protective coating materials such as paints and varnishes. The majority of people affected by diisocyanate asthma are employed in its manufacture, transport, or subsequent use in the production or application of polyurethane.

Methyl isocyanate

Leakage of methyl isocyanate vapour from a chemical plant in Bhopal, India in 1984 led to the death of more than 2000 people within 12 to 72 h and 90 000 casualties required medical treatment. Methyl isocyanate is known to be intensely irritating to the eyes, nose, and throat. Lacrimation, sore throat, a choking sensation, coughing, and vomiting develop quickly after exposure. Subsequent corneal ulceration and opacities (some 50 000 people were blinded at Bhopal, many of them permanently) and pulmonary oedema, accompanied by secondary infection, were the most common complications responsible for the high morbidity and mortality. Exposure to methyl isocyanate may also have resulted in a significantly higher loss of pregnancies and neonatal mortality. Animal studies have demonstrated that methyl isocyanate produces hyperglycaemia, lactic acidosis, uraemia, hypotension, and hypothermia, as well as long-term pulmonary impairment after a single exposure.

TREATMENT

The patient should be removed immediately from the contaminated environment. Subsequent treatment is symptomatic and supportive since no specific therapy is known. The eyes should be irrigated with water or saline (0.9 per cent) for 15 to 30 min and an ophthalmic opinion sought, as permanent blindness may ensue. The pulmonary complications should be treated with humidified supplemental oxygen and bronchodilators. The use of mechanical ventilation with positive end expiratory pressure may be life-saving in severe cases. Antibiotics will be required if pneumonia supervenes.

REFERENCES

Anon. (1984). Calamity at Bhopal. *Lancet*, **ii,** 1378–9.

IPCS. (1987). *Environmental Health Criteria 75. Toluene diisocyanate*. WHO, Geneva.

Jeevaratnam, K., Vijayaraghavan, R., Kaushik, M.P., and Vaidyanathan, C.S. (1990). Acute toxicity of methyl isocyanate in mammals. II. Induction of hyperglycemia, lactic acidosis, uraemia and hypothermia in rats. *Archives of Environmental Contamination and Toxicology*, **19,** 314–18.

Nitrogen dioxide

Nitrogen dioxide is a largely insoluble, brown, mildly irritating gas that is usually found in association with its dimer, nitrogen tetroxide. Nitrogen dioxide occurs naturally as a result of bacterial action on nitrogenous compounds. However, the main source of atmospheric nitrogen dioxide is the combustion of fossil fuels as in open fires, domestic or industrial boilers, or motor vehicles. Combustion yields nitric oxide and nitrogen dioxide. In the air, more nitrogen dioxide is formed by gradual oxidation of nitrogen by photochemical reactions that require the presence of volatile hydrocarbons. Fermentation of silage produces high concentrations of this gas within 2 days of filling the silo. Farm workers who enter silos have experienced an acute respiratory illness and fatalities have occurred. Nitrogen dioxide is also a byproduct of many industrial processes and leaks have produced illness in firemen. Occupational exposure has led to respiratory symptoms in other circumstances. Three American astronauts who were exposed to about 250 p.p.m. of nitrogen dioxide for 4 to 5 min, owing to the inadvertent firing of the reaction control system in the Apollo–Soyuz spacecraft, had radiological evidence of pulmonary oedema the day after splashdown.

CLINICAL FEATURES

The clinical features following acute exposure to high concentrations of nitrogen dioxide depend on the concentration and duration of exposure to the gas. Since nitrogen dioxide is only a mild upper respiratory tract irritant, modest acute exposure (< 50 p.p.m.) for a short time often produces no immediate symptoms, although throat irritation, cough, transient choking, tightness in the chest, and sweating have been observed. By contrast, exposure to a massive concentration of nitrogen dioxide such as that found in a silo, can produce severe and immediate hypoxaemia, which may be fatal. Methaemoglobinaemia may also be induced in these circumstances and compound the pre-existing hypoxaemia. In less severe cases, the onset of symptoms may be delayed for a few hours (typically 3–36 h) and the patient then develops dyspnoea, chest pain (which may be pleuritic), haemoptysis, tachycardia, headache, conjunctivitis, generalized weakness, and dizziness (which may be due to hypotension). Bronchiolitis obliterans is a late complication.

TREATMENT

Most patients will make an uneventful recovery with bronchodilator and corticosteroid therapy but a few will become acutely ill with cough, wheeze, frothy bloodstained sputum, increasing dyspnoea, restlessness, and fever. Pulmonary oedema may also occur in those who were previously symptom free. The oedema responds poorly to diuretics; corticosteroids and mechanical ventilation with positive end-expiratory pressure offer the best hope of reducing the mortality, which may be as high as 40 per cent in severe cases. Patients may relapse after recovery, and this is more likely if corticosteroids are discontinued prematurely. Not only may a second episode of pulmonary oedema occur but also bronchiolitis obliterans may develop within 2 to 6 weeks. When extensive and untreated, this complication may be fatal, but corticosteroids are highly effective if continued for at least 2 months.

REFERENCE

Berglund, M., Boström, C.-E., Bylin, G., *et al.* (1993). Health risk evaluation of nitrogen oxides. *Scandinavian Journal of Work, Environment and Health,* **19 (Suppl.2),** 1–72.

Phosgene

Phosgene is a colourless gas, responsible for more than 80 per cent of deaths caused by gas during the First World War. Phosgene is now used for the synthesis of isocyanates, polyurethane and polycarbonate resins, dyes, and pharmaceutical intermediary products. In addition, many paint removers and dry cleaning fluids contain chlorinated hydrocarbons that may decompose to phosgene in the presence of fire or heat.

MECHANISM OF TOXICITY

Following inhalation, phosgene reacts with water to produce chloride ion and carbon dioxide, and with glutathione to form diglutathionyl dithiocarbonate. It is only when hepatic and renal stores of glutathione become depleted beyond a critical level that covalent binding occurs between phosgene and cell macromolecules, with resultant hepatic and renal necrosis.

CLINICAL FEATURES

Exposure to phosgene causes irritation of the eyes, dryness or burning sensation in the throat, cough, pain in the chest, and nausea and vomiting. The severity of these initial symptoms is no guide to prognosis since casualties with severe symptoms may fail to develop any serious lung damage, whereas others with little initial irritation may later develop fatal pulmonary oedema. Following these initial symptoms, there is usually a latent period during which the casualty suffers little discomfort and has no abnormal chest signs. This period may last between 30 min and 24 h (rarely, 72 h). The latent period is followed by the development of pulmonary oedema due to increased capillary permeability; circulatory collapse may follow. Of the fatal cases, some 80 per cent die within 48 h of exposure. The subsequent development of bronchopneumonia accounts for a number of deaths after this period.

TREATMENT

There is as yet no proven specific therapy for phosgene-induced pulmonary injury, though claims for the efficacy of hexamethylenetetramine (methenamine) have been made and, in turn, strongly refuted. Cysteine has been shown *in vitro* to trap phosgene to form the metabolite, 2-oxothiazolidine-4-carboxylic acid. It is possible, therefore, that the administration of *N*-acetylcysteine may confer some protection against the toxic effects of phosgene. Supplemental oxygen should be administered and bronchodilators may be helpful. The place of steroids has not yet been established. The use of mechanical ventilation with positive end-expiratory pressure may be life-saving in severe cases. Antibiotics will be required if pneumonia supervenes.

REFERENCE

Diller, W.F. and Zante, R. (1985). A literature review: therapy for phosgene poisoning. *Toxicology and Industrial Health,* **1,** 117–28.

Phosphine

Phosphine is a colourless gas with a fish-like odour and is used as a fumigant against insects and rodents in stored grain, particularly in grain elevators and, increasingly, aboard ships. It is also used to treat silicon crystals in the semiconductor industry.

CLINICAL FEATURES

Fatigue, nausea, vomiting, diarrhoea, chest tightness, breathlessness, productive cough, dizziness, and headache are common features of acute exposure to phosphine. Acute pulmonary oedema, hypertension, cardiac arrhythmias, and convulsions have been described in severe cases of poisoning. Jaundice, ataxia, intention tremor, and diplopia may be found on examination. Focal myocardial infiltration with necrosis, pulmonary oedema, and widespread small-vessel injury were found at postmortem examination in a child who died.

TREATMENT

The casualty should be removed from exposure as soon as possible. Thereafter, treatment is supportive and symptomatic. The value of steroids in preventing pulmonary damage (which may be delayed) has not been established.

REFERENCES

Wilson, R., Lovejoy, F.H., Jaeger, R.J., and Landigan, P.L. (1980). Acute phosphine poisoning aboard a grain freighter: epidemiologic, clinical and pathological findings. *Journal of the American Medical Association,* **244,** 148–50.

IPCS. (1988). *Environmental Health Criteria 73. Phosphine and selected metal phosphides.* WHO, Geneva.

Smoke

Smoke consists of a suspension of small particles in hot air and gases. It has a particulate phase and a gaseous phase. The particles consist of carbon and they are coated with combustion products such as organic acids and aldehydes. The majority of particles measuring less than 1 to 3 μm are filtered out by the nasal, oral and pharyngeal mucosae, but the acids and aldehydes coating these particles cause symptoms of local irritation, e.g. lacrimation, burning of the throat, and nausea and vomiting when swallowed. Inhalation of some of the small particles into the airways contributes to the bronchospasm that can occur following inhalation of smoke.

The gaseous phase of smoke has an extremely variable composition, but carbon dioxide and carbon monoxide are always present and constitute the bulk of this fraction. The gaseous phase of smoke may contain other toxic gases, including pulmonary irritants such as acrolein, ammonia, chlorine, hydrogen chloride, nitrogen dioxide, phosgene, and sulphur dioxide.

The adverse effects of smoke not only result from its chemical composition but also from the fact that the particulate and gaseous fractions are space-occupying and they can rapidly fill an enclosed space at the expense of air. The duration of exposure and the occurrence of that exposure in a confined space are two factors that determine the severity of the pulmonary consequences of smoke inhalation. Thermal injury to the lungs is not thought to play a significant role, since under usual circumstances heat does not enter the trachea because of the rapid cooling that occurs in the larynx.

The increased use of synthetic plastic materials in the construction of buildings in recent years has presented special problems. Thermal decomposition of polyurethane foams and synthetic polymers containing acrylonitrile produces substantial quantities of free hydrogen cyanide gas and other organic cyanides. Characteristics of fires involving plastics are extremely high temperatures (plastic possesses a heat of combustion 2.5 times that of other combustible materials), very high burning rates, and high-density smoke. Polyvinyl chloride (PVC) has been reported to produce smoke 4 to 14 times more dense than that from fires involving constructional timber under similar conditions. PVC is very widely used within domestic and office environments and there are 75 known products of combustion, some of which are generated at relatively low temperatures (200 to 300 °C). Upon complete combustion each kilogram of PVC can produce about 0.4 kg of hydrogen chloride gas. Other important products of PVC combustion include carbon monoxide, chlorine, and phosgene, together with benzene, naphthalene, toluene, vinyl chloride, and xylenes.

CLINICAL FEATURES

Adverse respiratory effects resulting from smoke inhalation range from mild irritation of the upper airways to severe tracheobronchitis, bronchospasm, pulmonary oedema, and bronchopneumonia, often resulting in pulmonary insufficiency and death. Laryngitis and laryngeal oedema can also occur and they may progress to complete laryngeal obstruction over a period of several hours. Acute upper airways obstruction can occur at any time from retained secretions when glottal oedema is present. Inhalation of pulmonary irritants may lead to transient but often marked hypoxaemia and small airways obstruction in the absence of any notable respiratory symptoms. These latter features appear to be more common in smokers than in non-smokers, but there is no evidence that acute smoke inhalation *per se* leads to the onset of chronic respiratory symptoms or chronic functional respiratory impairment. Acute hypoxaemia may be associated with the occurrence of frequent ventricular premature beats and tissue hypoxia due to elevated carboxyhaemoglobin levels may lead to chest pain and cardiac arrhythmias in subjects with pre-existing ischaemic heart disease. Additional clinical features due to specific pulmonary irritants and toxins should be sought under the appropriate headings above.

TREATMENT

After removal of the casualty from further exposure to smoke, supplemental humidified oxygen should be administered, together with a nebulized bronchodilator as necessary. Arterial blood gases should be measured and a serum carboxyhaemoglobin concentration obtained. If there is any likelihood of exposure to burning plastics or pulmonary irritants, then serial blood gas analyses may need to be undertaken for at least 48 h after admission to hospital. Early fibreoptic laryngoscopy or bronchoscopy may assist the diagnosis and enable the severity of any subglottal injury to be determined. It has also been suggested that the early administration of high-dose corticosteroids protects against pulmonary injury but, as yet, there is no incontrovertible evidence that this is true in humans.

REFERENCES

Charnock, E.L. and Meehan, J.J. (1980). Postburn respiratory injuries in children. *Pediatric Clinics of North America*, **27**, 661–76.

Clark, C.J., Reid, W.H., Gilmour, W.H., and Campbell, D. (1986). Mortality probability in victims of fire trauma: revised equation to include inhalation injury. *British Medical Journal*, **292**, 1303–5.

Dyer, R.F. and Esch, V.H. (1976). Polyvinyl chloride toxicity in fires: hydrogen chloride toxicity in fire fighters. *Journal of the American Medical Association*, **235**, 393–7.

Genovesi, M.G., Tashkin, D.P., Chopra, S., Morgan, M., and McElroy, C. (1977). Transient hypoxaemia in firemen following inhalation of smoke. *Chest*, **71**, 441–4.

Head, J.M. (1980). Inhalation injury in burns. *American Journal of Surgery*, **139**, 508–12.

Loke, J., Farmer, W., Matthay, R.A., Putman, C.E., and Walker-Smith, G.J. (1980). Acute and chronic effects of fire fighting on pulmonary function. *Chest*, **77**, 369–73.

Symington, I.S., Anderson, R.A., Thomson, I., Oliver, J.S., Harland, W.A., and Kerr, J.W. (1978). Cyanide exposure in fires. *Lancet*, **ii**, 91–2.

Sulphur dioxide

Sulphur dioxide is a colourless gas which has a pungent irritating odour. The combustion of fuels for heating and power generation results in environmental pollution from this cause. Sulphur dioxide is also employed in the manufacture of sulphuric acid and is a potential occupational problem in paper mills, steel works and oil refineries.

MECHANISM OF TOXICITY

The irritant effects of sulphur dioxide are though to be caused by the rapidity with which it forms sulphurous acid on contact with moist membranes.

CLINICAL FEATURES

Following exposure to sulphur dioxide, lacrimation, rhinorrhoea, cough, increased bronchial secretions, bronchoconstriction, and, in severe cases, pulmonary oedema and respiratory arrest occur. Corneal burns can follow eye exposure and liquefied sulphur dioxide can cause skin burns. Survivors of massive sulphur dioxide exposure have shown a chronic obstructive defect in serial pulmonary studies along with bronchial hyperactivity.

TREATMENT

After removal from exposure, admission to hospital for observation is mandatory in severe cases to ensure that delayed pulmonary oedema is treated effectively. Symptomatic and supportive measures should be given and, if necessary, mechanical ventilation with positive end-expiratory pressure should be undertaken if diuretics alone do not control pulmonary oedema; the role of corticosteroids is uncertain. The eyes and skin should be irrigated with water, if exposure has occurred.

REFERENCE

IPCS. (1979). *Environmental Health Criteria 8. Sulfur oxides and suspended particulate matter*. WHO, Geneva.

8.3.5 Poisoning due to corrosive substances

T. J. MEREDITH, J. A. VALE, AND A. T. PROUDFOOT

Of the many chemicals used in the world today, a large proportion possess irritant or corrosive properties but epidemiological studies suggest that the incidence of poisoning from such agents is, in most countries, fairly low. Occupationally, an increasing awareness of the related dangers has led to precautions which mitigate the harm to workers. Yet it is still possible for adults to procure strong corrosives for suicidal acts, though the tendency nowadays is for those intent upon self-destruction to choose less aversive products, chiefly drugs. In addition to deliberate acts, accidents with excoriating chemicals can still beset adults, and substances of this kind are still left within the reach of small children who may ingest them.

Mode of action and clinical features of toxicity

Although acids and alkalis have rather different pathological effects, the clinical consequences of exposure may be grouped into those that result from contact with skin or mucous membranes and those that result from ingestion.

On the skin, according to the nature of the chemical and its concentration, there may be reddening, inflammation, blistering, ulceration, and penetrating necrosis, with pain at the site. The trauma may, however, remain localized. Similarly, in the eye, there may be conjunctival and/or corneal irritation and ulceration, with or without penetration and more profound tissue disorganization. In other instances, for example as with hydrofluoric acid, the chemical may give rise not only to circumscribed physicochemical changes, but may be absorbed to cause systemic toxicity.

The primary impact of corrosives and irritants by mouth is on the lips, tongue, mouth, pharynx, oesophagus, and stomach. Depending on the degree to which this advances there may be reactionary oedema, for which the larynx is a prime target, serous exudation, and even perforation. Eventually healing may be achieved by cicatrization and stenosis. Again, superimposed upon these primary anatomical lesions, the chemical may be absorbed to demonstrate its toxicity upon other organs and tissues.

ACIDS

Inorganic acids encountered in cases of poisoning include hydrochloric, hydrofluoric, nitric, phosphoric, and sulphuric acids; organic acids encountered include acetic, formic, lactic, and trichloroacetic acids. Hydrochloric acid is used in many industrial processes, particularly those involving brick, pottery, glass, and ceramics. Car battery acid typically contains 28 per cent sulphuric acid, and proprietary cleaning agents and antirust compounds are often comprised of a mixture of hydrochloric and phosphoric acids.

On the skin these behave characteristically as corrosives. When ingested, acids flow rapidly along the lesser curvature of the stomach to the prepyloric region where they pool because of spasm of the pylorus and antrum to cause almost instantaneous coagulative necrosis of one or more layers of the stomach. Typically, acids spare the oesophagus (except in 20 per cent of cases) because of rapid transit and resistant squamous epithelium.

Corrosive acid ingestion is characterized by immediate pain in the mouth, pharynx, and abdomen, intense thirst, vomiting, haematemesis, and diarrhoea. The combination of pain and almost immediate mucosal oedema results in difficulty in swallowing and drooling of saliva. Gastric and oesophageal perforation may occur, with resultant chemical peritonitis. Non-gastrointestinal features of corrosive acid ingestion include hoarseness, stridor, respiratory distress, and laryngeal and epiglottic oedema. Circulatory shock, metabolic acidosis, leucocytosis, acute tubular necrosis, renal failure, hypoxaemia, respiratory failure, intravascular coagulation, and haemolysis may also occur.

Formic acid ingestion in particular is associated with the development of systemic acidosis, haematuria, and renal damage. Hydrofluoric acid ingestion causes chelation of calcium, with resultant weakness, paraesthesiae, tetany, convulsions, and disturbed coagulation.

Late clinical features of corrosive acid ingestion include antral or pyloric stenosis (in nearly 80 per cent of cases), jejunal stricture formation, achlorhydria, protein-losing gastroenteropathy, and gastric carcinoma.

ALKALIS

Alkaline substances commonly encountered in cases of poisoning include drain, lavatory, and pipe cleaners (sodium hydroxide), dishwashing detergents (sodium carbonate, sodium silicate, sodium tripolyphosphate), denture cleaning tablets (sodium perborate, sodium phosphate, sodium carbonate), urinary glucose testing tablets (sodium hydroxide), water sterilizing tablets (sodium dichloroisocyanurate), and alkaline disc batteries.

Another alkaline substance commonly encountered is sodium hypochlorite, which in solution (pH 11–12) is widely sold as a bleaching agent. In the stomach it gives rise to hypochlorous acid. Such is its concentration in most domestic brands, however, that symptoms are usually minor, or negligible, unless huge quantities of the undiluted formulation are deliberately swallowed, in which case the line of treatment should follow that for other alkalis as set out below.

The pathological consequence of exposure to alkalis in general is different from that following acid exposure—alkalis cause liquefactive necrosis within seconds, with saponification of tissue fat and formation of soluble proteinates. When ingested, alkalis typically damage the oesophagus and, in 80 per cent of cases, spare the stomach because of the protective effect of gastric acid. There is little immediate oral discomfort but subsequently a burning sensation develops in the mouth and pharynx, together with epigastric pain, vomiting, and diarrhoea. Oesophageal ulceration with or without perforation may occur; in the former instance, mediastinitis, pneumonitis, cardiac injury, and tracheo-oesophageal and aortoenteric fistulae may develop. In 20 per cent of cases, gastric injury (bleeding, perforation) also occurs. Non-respiratory features include hoarseness, stridor, respiratory distress, and laryngeal and epiglottic oedema. Late sequelae include oesophageal stricture formation, at anatomically narrow sites (cricopharyngeus, aortic arch, carina, diaphragmatic hiatus) and carcinoma of the oesophagus.

Management

Treatment of acid or alkali burns to the skin consists of liberal irrigation with water, or saline, and the application of dressings as for a thermal burn. Where the affected area is extensive, skin grafting may be necessary later. Similarly, an eye into which an acid or alkali has found its way should be irrigated at once, preferably with saline or else with water, the instillation of a local anaesthetic sometimes being indicated to relieve pain locally and to overcome blepharospasm. Thereafter, specialist ophthalmic advice should be sought.

Lime, or quicklime, is an alkaline substance that can prove very troublesome if particles get into the eye. The local reaction in the conjunctiva and cornea is that to be expected from any alkali. Irrigation alone, however, may not be sufficient, for any particulate lime adherent to the surface of the eye must be physically removed, preferably under local anaesthetic cover.

Corrosive substance ingestion

Attention should first be given to the airway, to establish that it is clear; endotracheal intubation, cricothyroidectomy or tracheostomy may be required for life-threatening pharyngeal or laryngeal oedema. Opioids or opiates may be required for analgesia.

ALKALIS

Induced emesis and gastric aspiration and lavage are contraindicated, as is dilution or neutralization of the alkali. Factors influencing the extent and severity of tissue damage, and the need for and nature of treatment, include:

quantity ingested;

physical form (liquid rather than solid preparations are far more likely to result in stricture formation);

concentration;

pH (a pH of < 11.4 tends to be associated with superficial muco-

sal ulceration only, whereas one of > 12.5 is associated with oesophageal necrosis and stricture formation);
viscosity;
duration of contact;
transit time;
presence or absence of food;
presence or absence of oesophageal reflux;
premorbid gastrointestinal tract condition;
titratable acid/alkaline reserve (a measure of alkalinity that correlates more closely than pH with resultant tissue damage).

In children, the presence of two or more of the signs, drooling, vomiting, or stridor, is associated with moderate or severe oesophageal lesions. However, as a general rule, the presence or absence of symptoms and/or oropharyngeal burns correlates poorly with the presence or absence of oesophageal damage at endoscopy, and should not, therefore, be used to determine whether or not to undertake this procedure.

Diagnostic panendoscopy (to beyond the site of the first observable oesophageal/gastric lesion, even if deep penetrating and/or circumferential oesophageal burns are present) should be performed within 12 to 24 h of alkali ingestion. If perforation of the gastrointestinal tract is suspected or if severe hypopharyngeal burns are present then as an alternative radiographic studies using water-soluble contrast media may be performed, though with caution because of the risk of aspiration.

Patients with first-degree oesophageal burns (erythema and oedema) may be discharged home if they are able to take fluids orally. Patients with second-degree burns (erythema, blistering, superficial ulceration, fibrinous exudate) should be admitted and given total parenteral nutrition during the initial catabolic phase. Oral fluids can normally be given by day 7, and solids as tolerated thereafter. Patients with third-degree burns (erythema, deep ulceration, friability, eschar formation, perforation) should be managed in an intensive care unit. Total parenteral nutrition (or a feeding jejunostomy) will be required until the gastrointestinal lesions have healed. If at endoscopy there are observable second- or third-degree oesophageal burns or evidence of gastric necrosis, or if there is a history of alkali ingestion and a persistently alkaline gastric pH, then laparotomy should be performed and necrotic tissue resected.

The role of corticosteroids in the prevention of oesophageal stricture following alkali ingestion remains controversial. The evaluation of published studies is hampered by a number of factors, including: (i) a lack of, or variability in, burn classifications (for allocation to treatment groups); (ii) difficulty in differentiating second-degree from third-degree burns at endoscopy; and (iii) use of varying corticosteroid treatment regimens with and without antibiotics and with or without oesophageal dilation. However, it appears that use of corticosteroids does not alter the incidence of stricture formation, which seems to correlate better with the severity of the burn at presentation. However, use of corticosteroids may decrease the need for surgical repair of strictures arising from second- or third-degree burns if they are used in conjunction with either anterograde or retrograde oesophageal dilation. Steroid employed are methylprednisolone (40 mg IV eight-hourly in adults) or prednisolone (2 mg/kg.day IV, until oral intake is resumed, when an equivalent dosage of prednisolone can be given orally and tapered off over a period of 3 to 6 weeks). A broad-spectrum antibiotic (such as ampicillin, tetracycline, erythromycin, or clindamycin) should be given at the same time as the corticosteroid.

Alternative strategies employed to prevent the development of oesophageal strictures include the use of a nasogastric tube alone or, experimentally, lathyrogens (β-aminoproprionitrile), penicillamine, *N*-acetylcysteine, and sodium polyacrylate.

ACIDS

Careful gastric aspiration is indicated though, as with alkalis, dilution and/or neutralization is contraindicated. Panendoscopy should be undertaken as a matter of urgency. Patients with Grade 1 (oedema or hyperaemia of mucosa) or Grade 2a (superficial, localized ulcerations, friability, blisters) oesophageal or gastric burns may be admitted to a general medical ward. Patients with Grade 2b (Grade 2a findings plus circumferential ulceration) or Grade 3 (multiple, deep ulceration, areas of necrosis) burns should be admitted to an intensive care unit. Total parenteral nutrition may be required. Corticosteroids confer no benefit and may mask abdominal signs of perforation; antibiotics should be given for established infection only.

In view of the high morbidity rate associated with acid-induced upper gastrointestinal perforation and the high incidence of late complications requiring surgery, laparotomy with resection of necrotic tissue and surgical repair is recommended: (i) when endoscopy reveals evidence of Grade 3 burns with full-thickness necrosis (blackened, ulcerated mucosa) of the stomach or oesophagus; or (ii) if symptoms or signs of gastrointestinal perforation are evident at the time of initial presentation.

LONGER-TERM MANAGEMENT OF CORROSIVE SUBSTANCE INGESTION

Both alkali and acid injuries may result in stricture formation requiring either long-term dilation therapy or surgical repair. An associated risk of malignancy dictates the need for life-long monitoring. The mean latent period for development of carcinoma of the oesophagus following alkali ingestion is more than 40 years.

Phenol

Phenol, or as it was once more commonly named 'carbolic acid', is another intense corrosive which does not feature in suicide at the present time as commonly as it did in the past. Its presence is nearly always recognizable by its odour and, distinctively, the pain to which it gives rise is much less than might be expected. This is due to its damage to the afferent nerve endings.

If phenol is spilled on the skin, pain is followed promptly by numbness. The skin becomes blanched, and a dry opaque eschar forms over the burn. When the eschar sloughs off, a brown stain remains. Phenol penetrates intact skin rapidly and systemic toxicity is common, though the severity of poisoning is determined by the concentration of phenol in solution and the surface area of skin exposed. Phenol vapour is well absorbed through the lungs. By mouth, there is a clinical picture of corrosive poisoning with vomiting, abdominal pain, and gastrointestinal haemorrhage, an identifying odour of carbolic acid, eschars, and, again, systemic phenol toxicity.

Systemic phenol poisoning is indicated by central nervous system depression, with coma, loss of vasoconstrictor tone, and hypothermia, together with cardiac and respiratory depression. An initial phase of central nervous system stimulation, and rarely convulsions, has sometimes been observed in children. Phenol poisoning is associated with markedly pigmented urine and though this is due in part to metabolites of phenol, Heinz body haemolytic anaemia as well as methaemoglobinaemia and hyperbilirubinaemia are recognized clinical features of phenol toxicity. Renal complications are seen frequently, due to: (i) excretion of unconjugated phenol, which is directly toxic to renal glomeruli and tubules; (ii) renal ischaemia due to hypotension; and (iii) formation of obstructive casts due to precipitation of haemoglobin.

MANAGEMENT

Emesis should not be induced but gastric aspiration and lavage may be undertaken provided that this is not contraindicated by the presence of severe oropharyngeal burns. Contaminated eyes and skin should be irrigated thoroughly with copious amounts of water as soon as contaminated clothing has been removed, with attending personnel taking care not to contaminate themselves. Otherwise, symptomatic and supportive care is indicated, including as necessary the use of methylene blue (1–2 mg/kg IV slowly) for methaemoglobinaemia, and peritoneal or haemodialysis for renal failure. The possibility of oesophageal stricture formation following phenol ingestion, though rare, should be borne in mind on follow-up.

REFERENCES

Anderson, K.D., Rouse, T.M., and Randolph, J.G. (1990). A controlled trial of corticosteroids in children with corrosive injury of the esophagus. *New England Journal of Medicine*, **323,** 637–40.

Ferguson, M.K., Migliore, M., Staszak, V.M., and Little, A.G. (1989). Early evaluation and therapy for caustic esophageal injury. *American Journal of Surgery*, **157,** 116–20.

Gaudreault, P., *et al.* (1983). Predictability of esophageal injury from signs and symptoms: a study of caustic ingestion in 378 children. *Pediatrics*, **71,** 767–70.

Gosselin, R.E., Smith, R.P., and Hodge, H.C. (1984). Phenol. In *Clinical Toxicology of Commercial Products*. 5th edn. pp. III–344–348, Williams & Wilkins, Baltimore.

Sugawa, C. and Lucas, C.E. (1989). Caustic injury of the upper gastrointestinal tract in adults: a clinical and endoscopic study. *Surgery*, **106,** 802–7.

8.3.6 Poisoning from metals

T. C. AW AND J. A. VALE

Metals are elements that are generally shiny, solid (except mercury), tough, malleable, ductile, and are good conductors. Eighty of the 105 elements in the periodic table are classed as metals, although less than half of these have caused toxic effects in man. Metals and their organic or inorganic salts are widely used in industry. Some metals such as zinc, magnesium, and chromium are essential dietary nutrients although excessive amounts can be harmful. Exposure to metals and their salts, either from inhalation of dust or ingestion of particles, has led to acute and chronic metal poisoning. Exposure may be occupational, domestic, or environmental, and can be acute or chronic, accidental or intentional.

Aluminium (aluminum)

Aluminium is the most abundant metal on earth, occurring in natural rocks as mica, feldspar, and bauxite. It is a light metal which resists corrosion and is a good conductor of both heat and electricity. It is used in packaging materials, kitchen utensils, car and aeroplane construction, paints, insulating materials, cosmetics, and foods. Aluminium hydroxide is used as an antacid and as a phosphate binder in the management of chronic renal failure. Aluminium sulphate is employed for water purification and in paper manufacture.

Aluminium may be absorbed orally and by inhalation. More than 90 per cent of absorbed aluminium is bound to transferrin which does not cross the blood-brain barrier readily. The remaining 10 per cent is associated with low molecular weight complexes, such as citrate, which can accumulate in brain tissue. Most body aluminium is stored in bone and the liver. Aluminium is excreted mainly via the kidneys.

CLINICAL FEATURES

Acute poisoning

Ingestion of soluble aluminium salts such as aluminium sulphate gives rise to burning in the mouth and throat, nausea, vomiting, diarrhoea, abdominal pain, hypotension, seizures, haemolysis, haematuria, and, rarely, hepatorenal failure. Topical aluminium sulphate may be irritant to the skin and eyes. By contrast, insoluble aluminium salts, such as aluminium oxide, do not produce an acute toxic response.

In 1988, 20 tonnes of concentrated aluminium sulphate were accidentally discharged into a water reservoir in North Cornwall, England and this was distributed via the community water supply. A variety of acute symptoms were reported among local residents and holidaymakers. These included gastrointestinal disturbance, rashes, and mouth ulcers. Some 400 people continued to experience longer-term symptoms such as joint and muscle pains, malaise, fatigue, and memory problems. An advisory group reviewed the incident and concluded that there was no convincing evidence of harmful accumulation of aluminium, nor greater prevalence of ill-health due to the distribution of contaminated water.

Chronic poisoning

Inhalation of 'stamped aluminium powder', which is produced by grinding hard unmelted aluminium, can cause a persistent cough and breathlessness due to lung fibrosis; pneumothorax is a recognized complication. Occupational asthma has also been described. Workers involved in aluminium production may be at increased risk of developing lung cancer but concomitant exposure to other agents has prevented a firm conclusion about its carcinogenic potential.

There is substantial evidence that aluminium is a neurotoxin. 'Dialysis dementia' involves the accumulation of aluminium, mainly in the brain, in patients on haemodialysis where the dialysis water contains significant amounts of aluminium, usually as aluminium sulphate. Aluminium poisoning in these circumstances may be enhanced by the administration of oral aluminium hydroxide as a phosphate binder. Typical features include speech and memory disturbances, altered personality, dementia, apraxia, myoclonic jerks, and seizures. The disease is progressive and usually fatal. Renal failure without dialysis may also lead to the accumulation of aluminium due to decreased clearance.

The role of aluminium is the aetiology of Alzheimer's disease remains unclear. There are reports of a geographical association between the incidence of Alzheimer's disease and high concentrations of aluminium sulphate in drinking water. Some patients with Alzheimer's disease have elevated brain aluminium concentrations, particularly in the neurofibrillary tangles which are characteristic of this form of dementia. Mortality studies in aluminium plant workers, however, have not shown excess mortality from dementia although neuropsychiatric symptoms have been reported more frequently in those who are exposed occupationally to aluminium than in controls.

There is experimental evidence that aluminium inhibits bone mineralization and aluminium toxicity may contribute, therefore, to osteomalacia in renal osteodystrophy. There are also reports of contact allergy to aluminium but this is extremely rare.

MEDICAL SURVEILLANCE

Aluminium toxicity should be considered in those who are exposed occupationally to aluminium dust and who develop respiratory or neuropsychiatric symptoms, and in patients with renal failure who may be at risk of aluminium retention. Useful indicators of exposure include the 24-h urine aluminium excretion (normal range < 15 μg/24 h) and the blood aluminium concentration (normal range < 10 μg/l).

TREATMENT

Desferrioxamine increases aluminium excretion in humans and in experimental animals and there are reports of neurocognitive improvement following desferrioxamine therapy in aluminium-toxic dialysis patients and in patients with Alzheimer's disease. However, there is concern about the long-term use of desferrioxamine because of reports of hypotension, gastrointestinal upset, porphyria cutanea tarda-like lesions, and transient visual disturbances. It has been proposed, therefore, that desferrioxamine should be employed in dialysis patients only when symptoms demand treatment and when patients can be monitored regularly for toxicity.

REFERENCES

Elinder, C-G. and Sjogren, B. (1986). Aluminum. In *Handbook on the Toxicology of Metals*. (ed. L. Friberg, G.F. Nordberg, and V.B. Vouk.) 2nd edn. Volume II. pp. 1–25. Elsevier, Amsterdam.

McCarthy, J.T., Milliner, D.S. and Johnson, W.J. (1990). Clinical experience with desferrioxamine in dialysis patients with aluminium toxicity. *Quarterly Journal of Medicine*, **74,** 257–76.

Arsenic

Arsenic is termed a metalloid as it has properties of both metals and non-metals. It forms both trivalent (e.g. arsenic trioxide, arsenious acid, and arsenites) and pentavalent (e.g. arsenic pentoxide, arsenic acid, and arsenates) derivatives. Inorganic arsenical compounds may generate arsine gas (see Chapter 8.3.5) when in contact with acids and reducing metals (e.g. iron and zinc) or with sodium hydroxide and aluminium. Arsenic is used in the electronics industry, in the production of special types of crystal and optical glass, in hardening lead and copper alloys, in the manufacture of fireworks, and as a wood preservative and pesticide. It is a byproduct of copper smelting. Some 90 per cent of an ingested dose of most inorganic trivalent and pentavalent arsenicals is absorbed, the exception being some insoluble compounds such as arsenic selenide. Soluble arsenical compounds can be absorbed by inhalation but skin absorption is generally poor. In exposed individuals high concentrations of arsenic are present in bone, hair, and nails. The half-life is in the range of 1 to 3 days. Excretion is predominantly in the urine as mono- and dimethyl-derivatives.

CLINICAL FEATURES

Acute poisoning

This can follow accidental, suicidal, or deliberate ingestion, the toxicity being largely dependent on the water solubility of the ingested compound. Within 2 h of substantial ingestion of a soluble arsenical compound, severe haemorrhagic gastritis or gastroenteritis may ensue with collapse and death usually within 4 days. A metallic taste, salivation, muscular cramps, facial oedema, difficulty in swallowing, hepatorenal dysfunction, convulsions, and encephalopthy are reported. A peripheral neuropathy (predominantly sensory), striate leukonychia (Mees' lines) and hyperkeratotic, hyperpigmentated skin lesions are common in those surviving a near fatal ingestion. In moderate or severe arsenic poisoning investigations may show anaemia, leucopenia, thrombocytopenia, and disseminated intravascular coagulation. ECG abnormalities have been reported and include QT prolongation and ventricular arrhythmias.

Exposure to arsenic trioxide and trichloride dust causes irritation of the eyes, nose, throat, and lower respiratory tract. Corrosive skin damage may follow skin contact with arsenical compounds such as arsenious acid and arsenic trichloride.

Chronic poisoning

The ingestion of arsenic in contaminated drinking water or in 'tonics' containing inorganic trivalent arsenical compounds has led to progressive weakness, anorexia, nausea, vomiting, stomatitis, colitis, increased salivation, epistaxis, bleeding gums, conjunctivitis, weight loss, and low grade fever. Characteristically there is hyperkeratosis of the palms and soles of the feet, 'raindrop' pigmentation of the skin, and 'Mees' lines' on the nails. There is an increased risk of skin cancer (usually squamous cell epithelioma) in affected individuals. A symmetrical peripheral neuropathy is typical. Sensory symptoms predominate but motor involvement is recognized and may cause confusion with the Guillain-Barré syndrome. Central nervous system effects such as hearing loss, psychological impairment and EEG changes have been reported. Other chronic effects include disturbances of liver function and ulceration and perforation of the nasal septum. Chronic exposure to trivalent and pentavalent forms of arsenic has been linked to excess lung cancer and lung cancer occurring in lead, tin, and copper smelter workers has been attributed to arsenic.

MEDICAL SURVEILLANCE

Blood arsenic concentrations correlate poorly with exposure. Arsenic concentrations in hair and nails have been used to indicate chronic systemic absorption, although its use as a biological monitoring tool for occupational exposure to airborne arsenic is limited. Urinary arsenic concentrations correlate closely with airborne arsenic concentrations in arsenic-exposed workers. Because certain marine organisms (especially mussels) may accumulate large amounts of organoarsenicals, it is advisable that workers refrain from eating seafood for at least 48 h before urine collection. A 24-h urine collection is the most reliable sample for these measurements. Regular examination of the skin should be included in an occupational health screening programme and workers with evidence of excessive arsenic exposure should be monitored long term to detect the development of occupationally-related malignancy.

TREATMENT

Traditionally, dimercaprol (British Anti-Lewisite, BAL) has been the recommended chelator in the treatment of arsenic poisoning. There is now increasing evidence, however, that DMSA (succimer) and DMPS (unithiol) may be preferable. They are more effective in reducing the arsenic content of tissues and, unlike dimercaprol they do not cause accumulation of arsenic in the brain. DMSA and DMPS may be given orally (in a dose of 30 mg/kg body weight daily), whereas dimercaprol must be given by deep intramuscular injection (2.5–5 mg/kg four hourly for 2 days followed by 2.5 mg/kg intramuscularly twice daily for 1 to 2 weeks).

REFERENCES

Fielder, R.J., Dale, E.A., and Williams, S.D. (1986). *Toxicity Review 16. Inorganic arsenic compounds*. HMSO, London.

IPCS. (1981). *Environmental Health Criteria 18. Arsenic*. WHO, Geneva.

Cadmium

Cadmium is used in plating, in nickel–cadmium batteries, as a component of various alloys and solders, as a PVC stabilizer, and is contained in some pigments, paints, and pottery. Exposure also occurs in areas around non-ferrous mines and smelters. Tobacco is an important source of cadmium uptake in smokers (up to several hundred μg/day) whereas in non-smokers the major route of exposure is via food.

Cadmium compounds are poorly absorbed orally but are well absorbed through the lungs. Cadmium is then deposited in the liver and kidneys as a complex with metallothionein. Cadmium is excreted primarily in the urine but only very slowly so that the half-life of cadmium is some 10 to 30 years.

CLINICAL FEATURES

Acute poisoning

Inhalation of cadmium oxide fumes produced in welding or cutting has led to the development of severe lung damage and death. Often there are no initial symptoms but after some 4 to 10 h there is increasing respiratory distress. Dyspnoea, cough and chest pain are accompanied frequently by chills and fever. Severe pulmonary oedema may develop, or chemical pneumonitis in less severe cases. Recovery may be complicated by progressive pulmonary fibrosis.

The ingestion of cadmium salts (> 3 mg/kg body weight) may lead to gastrointestinal disturbance which, in severe cases, may progress to circulatory collapse, acute renal failure, pulmonary oedema, and death.

Chronic poisoning

Repeated exposure to cadmium leads to renal tubular dysfunction, and, at a later stage, emphysema. Tubular dysfunction may be detected by the measurement of low molecular weight proteins such as β_2-microglobulin, retinol binding protein, α-microglobulin and *N*-acetyl-β-glucosaminidase in the urine. Though the amount of tubular proteinuria is a reasonable measure of cadmium exposure, it is clinically unimportant unless there is glomerular dysfunction. There are a few reports of cadmium-induced albuminuria but an association between chronic cadmium exposure and glomerular damage has not been confirmed. Glycosuria, aminoaciduria, hypercalciuria, an increased incidence of renal stones, and osteomalacia may result from severe tubular damage. Itai-Itai disease refers to the outbreak of osteomalacia reported in post-menopausal Japanese women living in areas where the water used for crop irrigation was contaminated with cadmium. Cadmium-induced osteomalacia is due probably to a combination of tubular calcium and phosphate loss and impaired renal calcitriol synthesis. Less common features of chronic cadmium exposure include anosmia, anaemia, teeth discoloration, and neuropsychological impairment.

Deaths from emphysema more usually follow repeated exposure to cadmium fumes, rather than to cadmium dust and the risk of developing emphysema is increased in individuals with an α-antitrypsin deficiency. No relationship has been confirmed between cadmium exposure and hypertension. Workers repeatedly exposed to high concentrations of cadmium have developed carcinoma of the prostate or lung and it is likely that a causal association exists.

MEDICAL SURVEILLANCE

Medical surveillance of exposed workers includes periodic assessment of blood and urine cadmium concentrations and the quantification of small molecular weight urinary proteins. It is now thought that measurement of the urinary excretion of both retinol binding protein and *N*-acetyl-β-glucosaminidase are the best screening tests. Lung function tests do not show a dose–response relationship with cadmium exposure and cannot be used as a screening test in workers exposed to cadmium fumes, although lung function should be monitored in those with high blood or urine cadmium concentrations.

TREATMENT

Animal studies suggest that oral DMSA (succimer) is an effective antidote for acute oral cadmium intoxication but that DPTA (as the salt calcium trisodium pentetate) is more effective parenterally; *N*-acetylcysteine and dimercaprol are of no benefit. There is, however, no clinical evidence that a substantial body burden of cadmium may be chelated by any currently available antidote.

REFERENCES

Fielder, R.J. and Dale, E.A (1983). *Toxicity Review 7. Cadmium and its compounds*. HMSO, London.

IPCS. (1992). *Environmental Health Criteria 134. Cadmium*. WHO, Geneva.

IPCS. (1992). *Environmental Health Criteria 135. Cadmium—environmental aspects*. WHO, Geneva.

Chromium

Chromium is mined from chromium ore and exists in several oxidation states which vary in their water solubility, industrial application, and toxicity; all exist in solid form except chromyl chloride which is a liquid. Virtually all natural sources of chromium are in the trivalent form. All forms of hexavalent chromium are produced via various manufacturing processes. Chromium compounds are used for metal plating, production of pigments, in steel and alloy manufacture, as a component of anticorrosion paints and wood preservatives, and in leather tanning. Chromium(III) is an essential dietary trace element which serves to potentiate the effects of insulin.

There is no good evidence that chromium(II), chromium(III), and chromium(IV) compounds are dangerous but chromium(III) compounds have produced skin sensitization. Chromium(VI) is the most important toxicologically because it can cross cell membranes readily. In contrast, chromium(III) compounds are confined to the extracellular space.

Chromium is absorbed mainly by inhalation and, to a lesser extent via the skin or gastrointestinal tract. Hexavalent chromium compounds are generally better absorbed than trivalent chromium compounds and, understandably, soluble chromium compounds such as sodium(VI) chromate are absorbed more readily than insoluble compounds such as chromium(III) oxide. Chromium is excreted via the kidney.

CLINICAL FEATURES

Acute poisoning

Inhaled soluble chromium(VI) compounds, such as sodium and potassium chromate and dichromate, are highly irritant to mucous membranes and may lead to inflammation of the nasal mucosa that persists for several days. Inhalation of chromium(VI) trioxide (chromic acid) causes cough, headache, chest pain, dyspnoea, and cyanosis.

Accidental or deliberate ingestion of highly water soluble chromium(VI) compounds leads within minutes to nausea, vomiting, abdominal pain, diarrhoea, and a burning sensation in the mouth, throat, and stomach; gastrointestinal haemorrhage is a frequent complication. Methaemoglobinaemia, haemolysis, and disseminated intravascular coagulation have been reported. Death may ensue within hours but those surviving the acute phase may go on to develop renal and hepatic failure.

Concentrated solutions of chromic acid used in the electroplating industry have a very low pH; accidental splashes produce severe burns. Percutaneous absorption may lead to systemic features. There are reports of kidney and liver failure developing in workers who have fallen into chromic acid solutions or been splashed with 50 per cent solutions of hot potassium dichromate or sodium chromate and dichromate; fatalities have occurred. Eye contact with concentrated chromic acid results in severe conjunctival congestion and necrosis with corneal oedema and opacification. Similar effects have been reported following splashing with hot solutions of sodium chromate and dichromate.

Chronic poisoning

'Chrome ulcers' may develop after repeated topical exposure to chromium(VI) compounds. They have a well-defined circular margin with raised edges and a central cavity filled with exudate or a tenacious crust which may penetrate to bone. The ulcers usually develop at a site of previous skin damage, which may be trivial. The severity of the lesion depends on the frequency and duration of skin contamination. Chromium(VI) compounds are also skin sensitizers and contribute to the development of cement dermatitis and contact dermatitis from paint primer, tanned leather, tattoo pigments, and matches.

Inhalation of chromium(VI) compounds has led to atrophy, ulceration, and perforation of the nasal septum. Pharyngeal and laryngeal ulcers may also occur. Asthma may be precipitated by exposure to fumes during stainless steel welding or to mists of chromium compounds (e.g. zinc chromate spray). Lung fibrosis, bronchitis and emphysema result from occupational exposure to chromium. Proximal tubular damage with increased urinary excretion of retinol binding protein and β_2-microglobulin may also ensue.

There is good evidence that workers exposed to chromium(VI) have an increased mortality from lung cancer. Lung cancer is a prescribed disease in occupations which involve exposure to strontium chromate, zinc chromate, or calcium chromate.

MEDICAL SURVEILLANCE

The skin of the hands and arms should be inspected periodically in those working with chromic acid or solutions of chromium(VI) compounds. Simple preventive measures such as wearing gloves and frequent hand washing will reduce occupational chromium exposure. Respiratory symptoms should be investigated in those exposed to chromates. Pre- and post-shift urinary chromium concentrations at the end of a working week can be measured, but chrome contamination of urine samples must be avoided.

TREATMENT

Ascorbic acid has been proposed as a topical and systemic antidote for chromium(VI) compounds, as it reduces these to the less toxic chromium(III) compounds. Topical 10 per cent ascorbic acid, as an ointment or in solution, has led to dramatic resolution of occupational chromium dermatitis but there is no clinical evidence that the systemic administration of ascorbic acid, or any other reducing agent, lessens morbidity or mortality in severe chromium poisoning. Topical preparations containing sodium calcium edetate may also afford some protection to the skin but there is no undisputed evidence that systemic chelation treatment is beneficial in chromium poisoning. Haemodialysis effectively removes chromium from the blood but the high tissue uptake limits the value of this treatment when used alone. The dialysis clearance of chromium is no better than the renal clearance, provided an adequate diuresis is maintained. It is important, therefore, that adequate fluid resuscitation is given promptly to patients with severe chromium poisoning.

REFERENCES

Fairhurst, S. and Minty, C.A. (1989). *Toxicity Review 21. The toxicity of chromium and inorganic chromium compounds.* HMSO, London.

IPCS. (1988). *Environmental Health Criteria 61. Chromium.* WHO, Geneva.

Cobalt

Cobalt is a relatively rare element that usually exists in association with nickel, silver, lead, copper, and iron ores. It is used in steel alloys, in the manufacture of magnets, and in the hard metal industry as a binder for tungsten carbide. It is an essential dietary trace element available as a component of vitamin B_{12} (cyanocobalamin).

Cobalt can be absorbed orally and by inhalation. After ingestion, approximately 80 per cent is excreted in the urine and small amounts appear in the faeces and sweat. Most of the absorbed cobalt is excreted within days but a small proportion of the retained metal has a biological half-life of approximately 2 years. The normal body burden of cobalt is about 1.1 mg. Approximately 43 per cent is in muscle; high concentrations of cobalt are also found in the liver, kidneys, heart, hair and nails.

CLINICAL FEATURES

Acute poisoning

Cobalt salts are relatively non-toxic but their ingestion may lead to gastrointestinal disturbance. A 6-year-old boy developed nausea, vomiting, and a transient neutropenia after swallowing a drink to which he had added about 2.5 g of cobalt chloride from a crystal-growing set.

Chronic poisoning

Occupational exposure to cobalt dust occurs mainly in the tungsten carbide industry and causes 'hard metal' pneumoconiosis with interstitial fibrosis. This usually develops after several years of exposure to high concentrations of cobalt and may prove fatal. There is also a higher incidence of bronchitis and emphysema among cobalt workers. Occupational asthma has been reported.

Chronic occupational exposure also leads to anosmia, auditory nerve damage, visual disturbance, irritability, headache, memory deficit, weakness, peripheral neuropathy, gastrointestinal disturbance, and weight loss. There is no firm evidence that cobalt is carcinogenic and assessment of cancer risk is often confounded by a simultaneous exposure to nickel and arsenic.

Chronic ingestion of cobalt causes polycythaemia, which, in the past led to its use in the treatment of anaemia. Cobalt inhibits the iodination of tyrosine and therefore can cause goitre. A 13-month-old baby developed clinical and biochemical hypothyroidism after 1 year's treatment of iron deficiency with a commercial iron-cobalt preparation. The child also showed persistent anaemia with polycythaemia, cardiomegaly, and hypertrichosis. The haematological abnormalities, hypothyroidism, and cardiomegaly resolved when the treatment was stopped.

Congestive cardiomyopathy has been reported in people who drank large quantities of beer to which cobalt had been added as a foam stabilizer; pericardial effusion and polycythaemia were also present in the majority. It is believed that alcohol also contributed to the cardiotoxicity observed in these cases, as the absolute quantities of cobalt involved were small. Fatal cardiomyopathy has occurred following occupational exposure.

Simultaneous allergies to nickel and to cobalt are frequent and there is some evidence of a mutual enhancing effect of contact sensitization to one metal in the presence of the other.

TREATMENT

If the patient presents early after oral ingestion of a cobalt salt, gastric lavage should be considered. In two studies DMSA (succimer) significantly reduced mortality in mice poisoned with cobalt chloride but in another study, DTPA (as the salt calcium trisodium pentetate) was more effective than DMSA. No satisfactory human studies have yet been performed.

REFERENCES

Domingo, J.L. (1989). Cobalt in the environment and its toxicological implications. *Reviews of Environmental Contamination and Toxicology*, **108,** 105–32.

Elinder, C-G. and Friberg, L. (1986) Cobalt. In *Handbook on the Toxicology of Metals.* (ed. L. Friberg, G.F. Nordberg, and V.B. Vouk) 2nd edn. Volume II. pp. 211–32. Elsevier, Amsterdam.

Mucklow, E.S., Griffin, S.J., Trevor Delves, H., and Suchak, B. (1990). Cobalt poisoning in a 6-year-old. *Lancet*, **335,** 981.

Copper

Copper is used for pipes and roofing material, in alloys and as a pigment. It is a component of several enzymes, including tyrosinase and cytochrome oxidase, and is essential for the utilization of iron. Copper sulphate is used as a fungicide, an algicide, and in some fertilizers.

Approximately one-third of an ingested copper salt is absorbed and in the blood 80 per cent is bound to caeruloplasmin. Most absorbed copper is deposited in the liver bound to copper-chelating proteins such as metallothionein. Copper is eliminated mainly via bile with only 4 per cent of the absorbed dose excreted in the urine. Copper can cross the placenta.

CLINICAL FEATURES

Acute poisoning

Acute copper poisoning usually results from the ingestion of contaminated foods or from accidental or deliberate ingestion of copper salts. Following a substantial ingestion of a copper salt there is profuse vomiting with abdominal pain, diarrhoea, headache, dizziness, and a metallic taste. Gastrointestinal haemorrhage, haemolysis, and hepatorenal failure may ensue and fatalities have occurred. Body secretions may have a green or blue discoloration. Copper sulphate solutions used as an antiseptic on open wounds may also be absorbed and give rise to systemic effects. Three patients undergoing haemodialysis using a unit with a copper heating coil developed acute copper poisoning with gastrointestinal upset, pancreatitis, and myoglobinuria. Accidental ingestion of melted copper has caused oesophageal stricture.

Occupational exposure to copper fumes (during refining or welding) or to copper-containing dust causes 'metal-fume fever' with upper respiratory tract symptoms, headache, fever, and myalgia.

Chronic poisoning

Chronic occupational copper poisoning causes general malaise, anorexia, nausea, vomiting, and hepatomegaly. Contact dermatitis, pulmonary granulomata, and pulmonary fibrosis have also been described. There is no convincing evidence that copper is carcinogenic in humans.

Wilson's disease is an inborn error of metabolism characterized by excessive accumulation of copper in the liver, brain, kidneys, and cornea. The clinical features and management are described in Chapter 11.7.

MEDICAL SURVEILLANCE

Prior to employment involving exposure to copper, employees should be examined for abnormalities of respiratory and liver function and screened for Wilson's disease. Urine copper concentrations are useful in screening copper-exposed workers.

TREATMENT

Although vomiting occurs invariably following the ingestion of many copper salts, gastric lavage may be of value in reducing copper absorption if presentation is early. Blood copper levels correlate well with the severity of intoxication: a blood copper concentration less than 3 mg/l indicates mild to moderate poisoning, whereas a concentration in excess of 8 mg/l confirms severe intoxication. D-Penicillamine enhances copper chelation in Wilson's disease and has been used in both acute and chronic copper poisoning at a dose of 25 mg/kg body weight daily until recovery. There is now animal evidence to suggest that *N*-acetylcysteine and DMPS (unithiol) are of similar efficacy.

REFERENCE

Aaseth, J. and Norseth, T. (1986). Copper. In *Handbook of the Toxicology of Metals*. (ed. L. Friberg, G.F. Nordberg, and V.B. Vouk). 2nd edn. Volume II. pp. 233–54. Elsevier, Amsterdam.

Beliles, R.P. (1994). Copper. In *Patty's Industrial Hygiene and Toxicology*. (ed G.D. Clayton and F.E. Clayton) 4th edn. Volume II, Part C. pp 1999–2006. John Wiley and Sons Inc., New York.

Lead

Lead is a naturally occurring element that has been used since the beginning of civilization. Many industrial activities, and particularly its use in petrol (gasoline), have led to its wide distribution so that all humans have lead in their bodies. Lead poisoning is a wholly preventable disease.

Exposure to lead occurs in the reclamation of lead from scrap metal, in the demolition and flame-cutting of old railway bridges previously painted with lead paint, and in the manufacture of storage batteries and ceramics. Children with pica who chew on lead-painted railings in homes, or who eat contaminated soil, have developed lead poisoning. As a consequence of lead leaching out of the glazing material, poisoning has also been described in individuals who have consumed drinks from lead-glazed mugs. Ingestion of lead-based powders in paints and imported baby tonics has also caused lead poisoning. Use of lead-containing cosmetics such as 'surma' applied to the face in Asian communities has resulted in lead intoxication. Rarely, lead acetate has been injected intravenously with suicidal intent. Tetraethyl lead, which is used as an antiknock agent in leaded petrol, can be absorbed systemically by inhalation, ingestion, and through the skin. Transplacental transfer of lead from mother to fetus results in reduced viability of the fetus, reduced birth weight, and premature birth.

Recently the Centers for Disease Control in Atlanta have revised the concentration of lead at which intervention is indicated from 250 μg/l down to 100 μg/l, as some adverse health effects have been observed in young children at the lower concentration. It has been estimated that in the United States 4 million children are at risk of lead poisoning and that 1 million workers are exposed to lead.

Once lead is absorbed into the body either via ingestion (approximately 10–15 per cent is absorbed) or inhalation (almost 100 per cent is absorbed) it is mainly (95 per cent) deposited in the bones and teeth. Of the lead in the blood, 99 per cent is associated with erythrocytes. As the body accumulates lead over many years and releases it into the urine only slowly, even small doses can in time lead to intoxication. The total body burden of lead correlates better with the risk of toxicity than the blood concentration alone.

CLINICAL FEATURES

Because of differences in individual susceptibility, symptoms of lead poisoning and their onset may vary. Mild intoxication may result in no more than lethargy and occasional abdominal discomfort, whereas abdominal pain (which is usually diffuse but may be colicky), vomiting, lethargy, constipation, and encephalopathy develop in more severe cases. Lead colic was first described by Hippocrates and, on occasions, has been incorrectly managed surgically as a case of an acute abdomen. Encephalopathy (seizures, mania, delirium, coma) is more common in children than in adults. Classically, lead poisoning results in foot drop attributable to primary motor peripheral neuropathy; wrist drop occurs only as a late sign of lead intoxication.

Renal effects include reversible renal tubular dysfunction causing glycosuria, aminoaciduria, and phosphaturia, and irreversible interstitial fibrosis with progressive renal insufficiency leading to hypertension.

Although a bluish discoloration of the gum margins is well described it is now uncommon. Perhaps poor dental hygiene as well as deposition of lead sulphide is required for this sign.

Lead depresses the enzymes responsible for haem synthesis and shortens erythrocyte life-span leading to a microcytic or normocytic hypochromic anaemia. In severe cases of intoxication a haemolytic anaemia may occur. Basophilic stippling of erythrocytes is due to nuclear remnants. Lead blocks the conversion of δ-aminolaevulinic acid to porphobilinogen by blocking the enzyme aminolaevulinic acid dehydrase. This leads to an increase in δ-aminolaevulinic acid in blood and urine. Lead also inhibits ferrochelatase which results in elevated free erythrocyte protoporphyrin (FEP) levels. There is a concomitant increase in urinary coproporphyrins and FEP, commonly assayed as zinc protoporphyrin.

An elevated zinc protoporphyrin concentration (> 350 μg/l) reaches a steady state in the blood only after the entire population of circulating erythrocytes has turned over (approximately 120 days). Consequently, it lags behind blood lead concentrations and is an indirect measure of long-term lead exposure. Moreover, zinc protoporphyrin is not a good screening test as it is not sensitive at the lower levels of lead poisoning.

MEDICAL SURVEILLANCE

The current practice in the United Kingdom and other European countries is to recommend stopping work with lead where a worker's blood lead concentration is shown to be above 700 μg/l. In workers exposed to organic lead compounds, the urinary lead concentration (> 150 μg/l) is a good indicator of exposure.

TREATMENT

Primary prevention (the elimination of lead hazards for children and exposed workers), must receive due public health attention. The social dimension of the problem must also be recognized: simply giving children chelators and then returning them to a contaminated home environment is of no value. Similarly, if an occupational source of lead exposure is implicated, a thorough evaluation of the workplace, other exposed workers, and the systems for handling lead at work is appropriate.

The decision to use chelation therapy is based not only on the blood lead concentration but also on the symptoms present and, if available, an estimate of the total body burden of lead using X-ray fluorescence. In molar equivalent doses sodium calcium edetate is approximately four times more efficient than DMSA (succimer) in increasing lead excretion but it must be given intravenously rather than orally which requires admission to hospital. In severe acute lead poisoning, particularly of an occupational kind, sodium calcium edetate (75 mg/kg body weight/day for 5 days) provides rapid relief of symptoms with minimal risk of adverse effect; a second course may be given a week after the first. Although zinc excretion is increased with sodium calcium edetate more than with DMSA, this is not clinically relevant if only a few courses of chelation are required. If hydration is maintained during chelation proximal tubular damage is not usually observed. DMSA (30 mg/kg body weight) is an effective oral chelator and may be given to outpatients. Though adverse effects have been reported these do not appear to be life-threatening but more data are required. Data on the therapeutic efficacy of DMPS (unithiol) are insufficient, at present, to make a judgement, though the frequency of adverse effects reported to date suggests that DMSA may be the oral chelator of choice. Penicillamine (0.5–1.5 g daily in an adult (20 mg/kg body weight daily in a child)) is an alternative oral chelating agent in those countries where DMSA is not available.

Chelation therapy has no prophylactic role and the practice of providing daily milk to lead-exposed workers to reduce lead absorption is of no proven value. Chelation therapy in organic lead poisoning is ineffective.

REFERENCES

CDC. (1991). *Preventing lead poisoning in young children.* US Department of Health and Human Services, Washington.

Tsuchiya, K. (1986). Lead. In *Handbook on the Toxicity of Metals*, (ed. L. Friberg., G.F. Nordberg, and V.B. Vouk), 2nd edn. Volume II. pp. 298–353. Elsevier, Amsterdam.

Manganese

Manganese is an essential dietary trace element which serves as an enzyme cofactor in phosphorylation reactions and in cholesterol and fatty acid synthesis. In industry it is used as a deoxidizing agent in steel manufacture and as a constituent of alloys. Other uses include the manufacture of dry cell batteries, as an oxidizing agent for coating electrodes, in textile bleaching, in glass manufacture, and as a constituent of fertilizers. Organomanganese compounds are used as additives in unleaded petrol and as pesticides.

Manganese can be absorbed by inhalation and ingestion. Less than 5 per cent of an ingested dose is absorbed but this is higher in iron-deficient subjects, probably due to a shared transport system. In the blood, manganese is mainly bound to transferrin and accumulates preferentially in tissues rich in mitochondria, such as the liver, pancreas, kidneys, and gastrointestinal tract. Excretion is principally via the faeces; less than 1 per cent appears in the urine. The biological half-life of manganese is 37 days, although clearance from the brain occurs more slowly. Manganese crosses the placenta and also appears in human milk.

CLINICAL FEATURES

Acute poisoning

Inhalation of manganese dioxide may cause an acute pneumonitis with marked dyspnoea which resolves without complication in those removed from exposure. Until the installation of a dust collector, children living in the vicinity of a ferromanganese plant were reported to have a higher incidence of upper respiratory tract symptoms than controls. Acute pancreatitis has also been reported in a patient treated with a haemodialysis solution contaminated with manganese.

Chronic poisoning

Chronic manganese poisoning occurs most commonly after prolonged exposure to manganese dust in an inadequately ventilated environment. In addition, occupational exposure to pesticides containing manganese may result in manganese intoxication. Chronic manganese poisoning has also been reported in a man treated for 31 months with total parenteral nutrition to which manganese supplements had been added.

Characteristically chronic manganese poisoning affects the extrapyramidal system. Symptoms may appear after only a few months exposure but more usually do so after 1 to 2 years. Initial features are largely subjective with complaints of apathy and asthenia, anorexia, and headache. These are followed by speech disturbances, sometimes with muteness, a mask-like facies, decreased ability to perform skilled movements, emotional lability, and exaggerated tendon reflexes. In established cases rigidity, bradykinesia and tremor are the main features, though the tremor is usually of an intention type rather than the resting tremor typical of Parkinson's disease. Micrognathia is also a feature and irritability, restlessness, and hallucinations, together with autonomic disturbances such as increased salivation and sweating have been reported.

An increased morbidity and mortality rate from pneumonia and bronchitis have been found among workers exposed to manganese dust. There are reports of manganese associated neutropenia, polycythaemia, hypercalcaemia, and impotence. Manganese is not carcinogenic in humans.

Chronic manganese poisoning is irreversible. At autopsy manganese is frequently concentrated in the basal ganglia, a finding consistent with the observed extrapyramidal features.

MEDICAL SURVEILLANCE

The laboratory diagnosis of chronic manganese poisoning is non-specific. Concentrations in body fluids are often not helpful as there is no direct correlation between blood and urine manganese concentrations and the occurrence or severity of poisoning. The diagnosis is therefore made clinically and from the history of occupational exposure.

TREATMENT

Chelation therapy with sodium calcium edetate may be of value in the early stages but no improvement can be expected once there is neurological damage. Therapeutic trials with levodopa and serotonin have been undertaken but there is no convincing evidence of long-term benefit. Intravenous sodium *p*-aminosalicylic acid has been reported to be of value in two cases of chronic manganese poisoning but the mechanism is unclear.

REFERENCES

IPCS.(1981). *Environmental Health Criteria 17. Manganese.* WHO, Geneva.

Saric, M. (1986). Manganese. In *Handbook on the Toxicology of Metals.* (ed. L. Friberg, G.F. Nordberg, and V.B. Vouk) 2nd edn. Volume II. pp. 354–86. Elsevier, Amsterdam.

Shuqin, K., Haishang, D., Peiyi, X., and Wanda, H. (1992). A report of two cases of chronic serious manganese poisoning treated with sodium para-aminosalicylic acid. *British Journal of Industrial Medicine,* **49,** 66–9.

Mercury

Mercury is the only metal which is liquid at room temperature. It exists in three forms, metallic (Hg^0), mercurous (Hg_2^{2+}) and mercuric (Hg^{2+}). Metallic mercury is very volatile and when spilt has a large surface area so that high atmospheric concentrations are produced in an enclosed space when environmental temperature is high. In addition to simple salts, such as chloride, nitrate, and sulphate, mercuric mercury forms organometallic compounds, where mercury is covalently bound to carbon, such as methyl-, ethyl-, phenyl-, and methoxyethyl mercury.

Metallic mercury is used in batteries, dental amalgam, and in scientific and medical instruments such as thermometers, barometers, and sphygmomanometers. Metallic mercury is also used as the cathode in the Castner–Kellner process for the electrolysis of brine to produce chlorine gas. Methyl mercury has been used as a fungicide.

Occupational exposure to inorganic mercury has occurred in mercury mines, chloroalkali plants, thermometer factories and in health service maintenance workers responsible for repairing broken sphygmomanometers. Accidents in dental surgeries have led to mercury vapour poisoning in dentists and dental nurses.

Non-occupational exposure to mercury occurs principally from dietary intake and to a minor extent from dental amalgam. Many foodstuffs contain small amounts of inorganic mercury but organic mercury compounds bioaccumulate in the aquatic food chain so that certain fish (e.g. trout, pike, bass, and tuna) contain significant amounts of methylmercury. The Minamata Bay disaster in 1956 resulted from methylmercury poisoning when mercury in a factory effluent was discharged into the bay. The mercury was concentrated up the food chain and affected members of the community living around the bay. The use of methylmercury as a fungicide led to an outbreak of mercury poisoning in Iraq in the early 1970s, when bread was made with contaminated grain. Creams and soaps containing inorganic mercury have been marketed as skin toners to lighten the complexion; these products are now banned in the EC and North America.

The absorption of mercury depends on its chemical form. Inhaled mercury vapour is absorbed rapidly and oxidized to Hg^{2+} in erythrocytes and other tissues. Prior to oxidation, absorbed mercury vapour can cross the blood–brain barrier but the divalent ion oxidation product serves to trap mercury in the brain. Mercury vapour is also absorbed via the skin, at an average rate of 0.24 ng/cm^2/min. Less than 1 per cent of an ingested dose of metallic mercury reaches the systemic circulation. Organic mercuric salts are better absorbed following ingestion than are inorganic mercuric salts. Organic mercury compounds cross the blood–brain barrier readily to accumulate in the brain. In contrast the kidney is the main storage organ for inorganic mercury compounds. *In vivo,* mercury is bound to metallothionein which serves a protective role since renal damage is caused only by the unbound metal. Mercury is excreted mainly in urine and faeces although a small amount of absorbed inorganic mercury is exhaled as mercury vapour. The half-life of most body mercury is 1 to 2 months but a small fraction has a half-life of several years.

CLINICAL FEATURES

Acute poisoning

Acute inhalation of mercury vapour causes headache, nausea, cough, chest pain, bronchitis, and pneumonia. In a few individuals renal damage from such acute exposure may produce gross proteinuria or nephrotic syndrome. In addition, a fine tremor and neurobehavioural impairment occurs and peripheral nerve involvement has also been observed. Kawasaki disease has been reported in exposed children.

Ingestion of metallic mercury is usually without severe systemic effects as metallic mercury is poorly absorbed from the gastrointestinal tract. However, mercuric chloride or other inorganic mercuric salts cause an irritant gastroenteritis with corrosive ulceration, bloody diarrhoea, and abdominal cramps, and may lead to circulatory collapse and shock. The ingestion of disc batteries containing mercuric oxide usually results in uneventful spontaneous passage through the gastrointestinal tract but potentially toxic mercury levels may result if the battery opens in transit. Mercurous compounds are less soluble, less corrosive, and less toxic than mercuric salts. Ingestion of mercurous chloride in teething powder has led to 'pink disease' or acrodynia in infants. This condition presents as fever with a pink-coloured rash, irritability, photophobia, painful and swollen extremities, hyperkeratosis, and hypersecretion of sweat glands. It is believed to be a hypersensitivity response to the mercurous chloride. There are reports of deliberate intravenous or subcutaneous metallic mercury injection. Accidental injection also has occurred after injury from broken thermometers and, in the past, following gas analysis procedures using mercury as a syringe sealant. Intravascular mercury may result in pulmonary venous or peripheral arterial embolism. Subcutaneous mercury initiates a soft-tissue inflammatory reaction with granuloma formation. Signs of systemic mercury toxicity are rare following metallic mercury injection.

Chronic poisoning

Chronic poisoning from inorganic mercury compounds or mercury vapour is characterized by non-specific early symptoms such as anorexia, insomnia, abnormal sweating, headache, and lassitude. The classical features of chronic mercury poisoning are increased excitability, tremor, gingivitis, and hypersalivation. Other central nervous system effects are extreme shyness, personality changes, and memory and intellectual deterioration. Emotional lability ('mercurial erethism') is thought to be responsible for the phrase 'mad as a hatter' which refers to felt hat makers who were exposed to hot mercuric nitrate used for treating the felt. The fine tremor causes the characteristic changes in handwriting seen in affected individuals and the term 'hatter's shakes' is a reference to this effect in mercury-exposed hatters. Severe cases develop frank psychosis with suicidal tendency and hallucinations. Systemically absorbed mercury may also be deposited on the lens of the eye giving rise to a permanent discoloration of the anterior capsule of the lens which does not affect visual acuity (mercurialentis). Both glomerular and tubular damage may follow chronic exposure to mercury and renal tubular acidosis has been described in children.

Exposure to organic mercury compounds usually involves aromatic derivatives such as phenyl mercuric acetate and phenyl mercuric benzoate, or aliphatic compounds such as methylmercury and ethylmercury chloride. The Minamata Bay incident was due to methylmercury poisoning. In the early 1970s another outbreak occurred in Iraq following consumption of bread made from flour from seeds treated with methylmercury. The main features of organic mercury poisoning are paraesthesiae of the lips, hands and feet, ataxia, tremor, dysarthria, constriction of visual fields, deafness, and emotional and intellectual changes. There is often a latent period of several weeks between the last exposure and the development of symptoms.

MEDICAL SURVEILLANCE

Surveillance of workers exposed to mercury and its salts should include measurement of urinary mercury concentrations and tubular protein excretion. Urinary mercury concentrations give an indication of long-term exposure and absorption, whereas blood mercury concentrations are a better measure of recent acute exposure. Clinical effects are unlikely in those with urinary mercury concentrations less than 250 μg/l; a concentration of 30 μg/l in the urine has been suggested as an upper limit for exposure to organic mercury.

TREATMENT

Even prompt removal from exposure to mercury vapour may not prevent the development of serious sequelae. In those who do develop symptoms no antidote has been shown to be effective. Early intensive supportive measures are of paramount importance in the management of the severe gastrointestinal complications caused by the ingestion of mercuric salts, such as mercuric chloride. In these circumstances gastric lavage is best avoided as significant oesophageal erosions may be present. Traditionally, dimercaprol (British Anti-Lewisite, BAL) has been used in the treatment of inorganic mercury poisoning. Oral DMSA (succimer) and DMPS (unithiol) (30 mg/kg body weight) have been shown significantly to enhance mercury elimination, protect against renal damage and increase survival. In some animal studies DMPS appears to be significantly better than DMSA in reducing the total body mercury burden, renal deposition of mercury, and mortality.

Both DMSA and DMPS appear to be of value in the treatment of methylmercury poisoning though some studies in animals suggest that DMSA is superior to DMPS whereas preliminary clinical studies suggest the reverse. There is no effective treatment for chronic mercury poisoning as neither DMSA nor DMPS can mobilize mercury deposited in the brain.

REFERENCES

Berlin, M. (1986). Mercury. In *Handbook on the Toxicology of Metals*. (ed. L. Friberg, G.F. Nordberg and V.B. Vouk) 2nd edn. Volume II. pp. 387–445. Elsevier, Amsterdam.

IPCS. (1990). *Environmental Health Criteria 101. Methylmercury.* WHO, Geneva.

IPCS. (1991). *Environmental Health Criteria 118. Inorganic mercury.* WHO, Geneva.

Nickel

Nickel is an ubiquitous trace metal that is mined in the form of sulphide ore. It is used primarily for producing stainless steel and other alloys. In the Mond process nickel is reacted with carbon monoxide to produce nickel carbonyl, an intermediate compound in nickel purification, that is used as a catalyst in the petroleum, plastic, and rubber industries. Nickel compounds have been divided into nickel carbonyl, soluble nickel salts (e.g. acetate, bromide, chloride, chloride hexahydrate, nitrate, subsulphide, sulphate), insoluble nickel compounds (e.g. arsenate, carbonate, hydroxide, oxide, phosphate), and metallic nickel. Nickel sulphate is used for electroplating and nickel hydroxide is a component of nickel–cadmium batteries.

Nickel can be absorbed both orally and by inhalation. Vaporized nickel carbonyl is the most readily absorbed form of inhaled nickel, followed by its soluble salts. Approximately 75 per cent of inspired particulate nickel is retained and two-thirds of this is swallowed via mucociliary clearance of inhaled particles. Gastrointestinal absorption of nickel depends on the solubility of the nickel salt and whether other substances are co-ingested. In the blood nickel is transported bound principally to albumin. Nickel is concentrated in the kidneys, liver, and lungs and is excreted primarily in the urine. Nickel crosses the placenta; it is present in the fetus and is also passed to the child in maternal milk.

CLINICAL FEATURES

Acute poisoning

Nickel carbonyl is a colourless, volatile liquid which, when inhaled, leads, within a few minutes, to dizziness, headache, vertigo, nausea, vomiting, cough, and dyspnoea. In many cases these symptoms disappear and there follows a symptom-free period lasting several days before the start of tachypnoea, dyspnoea, haemoptysis, cyanosis, chest pain, vomiting, tachycardia, weakness, and muscle fatigue. Paraesthesiae, diarrhoea, abdominal distension, delirium, and convulsions have also been reported. Death may occur 4 to 11 days after exposure from cardiorespiratory failure. Postmortem findings include epithelial and endothelial cell damage leading to pulmonary oedema and haemorrhage and interstitial pneumonitis; cerebral haemorrhage has also been observed.

There is relatively little information on the acute toxicity of soluble nickel salts in humans, though at high concentrations they are primary skin and eye irritants. Workers at an electroplating plant who drank water accidentally contaminated with nickel sulphate experienced nausea, vomiting, diarrhoea, abdominal pain, headache, cough, and breathlessness which persisted for up to 2 days. A 2-year-old child died 4 h after ingesting 15 g of nickel sulphate crystals. A group of dialysis patients accidentally infused with a nickel-containing dialysate all suffered nausea and most reported vomiting, weakness, and headache. There is some evidence in animals that high plasma nickel concentrations may induce coronary artery vasoconstriction.

Chronic poisoning

Chronic exposure to aerosols of nickel salts may lead to chronic rhinitis and nasal sinusitis and in rare cases to anosmia and perforation of the nasal septum. Inhaled nickel can produce an allergic (Type I hypersensitivity) respiratory reaction manifest as bronchial asthma with circulating IgE antibodies to nickel. Pulmonary eosinophilia (Loeffler's syndrome) due to a type III hypersensitivity reaction to nickel has also been described.

A significant increase in deaths from non-malignant respiratory disease or pneumoconiosis has also been observed in nickel refinery workers. There is evidence that occupational exposure to nickel may cause cancer of the lung and nasal sinuses. Roasting sulphide ores at high temperature in dusty conditions produces the highest risk.

The exact aetiological agent is unknown, although nickel sulphate, nickel oxide, and nickel subsulphide have been suspected. There have also been reports of an increased incidence of laryngeal cancer, though this has not yet been confirmed.

Metallic nickel and nickel salts cause allergic contact dermatitis. This is often described as 'nickel-itch' and can occur occupationally and from contact with nickel in jewellery, coins, and other nickel-plated objects. The prevalence of nickel dermatitis may be as high as 10 per cent in females and 1 per cent in males and is due to a Type IV delayed hypersensitivity response, although nickel-induced urticaria, probably the result of a Type I immediate hypersensitivity reaction, has also been described.

MEDICAL SURVEILLANCE

Nickel concentrations in finger nails can indicate occupational nickel exposure but surface contamination of nail samples make this an unsuitable method for routine surveillance. The nickel concentration in a spot urine sample is useful for screening although a 24-h collection provides a more accurate indication of nickel exposure. A urine nickel concentration greater than 500 μg/l indicates severe poisoning.

TREATMENT

Blood nickel concentrations immediately following exposure to nickel carbonyl provide a guide as to severity of exposure and the need for chelation therapy. DMPS (unithiol) enhances the urinary excretion of nickel in nickel-intoxicated animals and diethyldithiocarbamate and disulfiram (which is metabolized to diethyldithiocarbamate) are effective agents in the treatment of nickel dermatitis, but their role in the treatment of acute severe nickel carbonyl poisoning has not been confirmed in a controlled clinical study.

REFERENCES

Fairhurst, S., and Illing, H.P.A. (1987). *Toxicity Review 19. The toxicity of nickel and its inorganic compounds.* HMSO, London.

IPCS. (1991). *Environmental Health Criteria 108. Nickel.* WHO, Geneva.

Kaaber, K., Menne, T., Veien, N., and Hougaard, P. (1983). Treatment of nickel dermatitis with Antabuse; a double blind study. *Contact Dermatitis*, **9**, 297–9.

Thallium

Thallium has been used as a rodenticide, in the manufacture of optical and electrical equipment, as a catalyst in organic synthesis, and in isotopic form for medical imaging of the myocardium. Poisoning is rarely from occupational exposure; most cases of intoxication have occurred as a result of accidental (e.g. cocaine contaminated with thallium) or suicidal ingestion or the criminal administration of thallous salts. Atmospheric pollution may occur as a result of coal-burning power plants and from smelting copper, lead, or zinc.

Absorption of thallous salts (particularly the more soluble salts such as sulphate, acetate, or carbonate) is rapid following ingestion, inhalation, and even skin contact. Following absorption, high thallium concentrations are found in the kidneys, brain, and heart, and excretion occurs both in the urine and faeces. Thallium can also cross the placenta. Observation in a single human case of poisoning suggests a half-life of some 30 days. Blood thallium and urine thallium concentrations above 100 μg/l and 200 μg/l respectively are toxic.

The exact mechanism of toxicity is unknown but may involve disruption of sulphydryl groups on the mitochondrial membrane and interference with the function of sodium-potassium ATPase for which thallium has an affinity 10 times higher than that of potassium. In addition, thallium may interfere with riboflavin homeostasis leading to dermatitis, alopecia, and neuropathy.

CLINICAL FEATURES

Acute poisoning

Within a few hours of ingestion, nausea, vomiting, and abdominal pain develop and, less commonly, gastrointestinal bleeding occurs which may be severe. Paralytic ileus and parotid (sialadenosis) and pancreatic damage have also been documented. After a few days, paraesthesiae, painful and tender extremities, and weakness supervene and may be accompanied by confusion, delirium, convulsions, cardiorespiratory depression, and death. If death does not occur within the first week, ataxia, tremor, and muscular atrophy predominate with ptosis, ophthalmoplegia, retrobulbar neuritis, facial paralysis, optic atrophy, and defective colour vision developing. Characteristically, alopecia develops within 1 to 3 weeks and it is often this sign which leads to the diagnosis being made.

Tachycardia and hypertension may occur possibly due either to vagal denervation or increased secretion of catecholamines secondary to the effect of thallium on chromaffin cellular ATP. Bradycardia and hypotension have also been reported in severe cases and may result from a direct action of thallium on the sinus node and on myocardial contractility. Hepatic and renal necrosis may develop. In the first week, there is often a sudden onset of acne which may be severe and complicated by necrotic lesions. Sweat glands and sebaceous glands are destroyed and the skin becomes dry and slightly scaly. Nail growth is impaired with the development of ridges (Mees' lines). Anaemia, leucocytosis, eosinophilia, and lymphopenia have been reported.

Chronic poisoning

Following repeated small exposures, the patient insidiously develops a distal neuropathy initially with sensory and then motor loss, which spreads proximally. Cranial nerves may become involved and respiratory paralysis is recognized. Ataxia, tremor, and marked tenderness of the soles, together with personality changes and severe loss of intellectual function may result.

TREATMENT

If a patient presents soon after the ingestion of a thallium salt, the use of gastric lavage should be considered. However, most patients present, or at least the diagnosis is only made, days, weeks, or even months after exposure so that chelation therapy is likely to be more productive therapeutically than measures to reduce absorption. Thallium ions are excreted, like those of potassium, through the kidneys and into the gastrointestinal tract via the saliva, the bile, and through the intestinal mucosa. It is possible to sequester thallium ions in the gut and prevent reabsorption by the oral administration of colloidally soluble Prussian (Berlin) blue (potassium ferrihexacyanoferrate(II)) (250–300 mg/kg.day (approximately 10 g twice daily for an adult)). Thallium ions are exchanged for potassium ions in the lattice of the Prussian blue molecule and are subsequently excreted in faeces. During treatment with Prussian blue, plasma levels of thallium fall and urine excretion declines exponentionally. In contrast, faecal excretion of thallium is detectable even when urine excretion of the metal has ceased and, therefore, administration of Prussian blue should be continued until thallium can no longer be detected in the faeces.

Prussian blue reduced the half-life of thallium from 4 to 2 days in rats. Human experience has confirmed the value of Prussian blue in thallium intoxication, though neurological damage may be permanent even if chelation therapy has been employed. It is possible that the administration of intravenous potassium might further enhance the excretion of thallium into the gut. In contrast, oral potassium supplements should theoretically be avoided because they are likely to interfere with the exchange between potassium and thallium ions in the gut and so increase the signs of poisoning, though this has not always been observed.

Other agents such as dithizone and sodium diethyldithiocarbamate (dithiocarb), while enhancing thallium elimination, also cause thallium redistribution, are inherently toxic, and should not be employed. In a single animal study, activated charcoal was shown to enhance thallium elimination. Although it has been proposed that large doses of activated charcoal should be administered together with Prussian blue, the efficacy of chelation may be lessened due to the development of severe constipation which may further exacerbate thallium-induced paralytic ileus. Peritoneal dialysis, haemodialysis, and haemoperfusion have not been shown to be of clinical benefit in thallium intoxication, though clearance is increased. Although forced diuresis is of value, the presence of thallium-induced renal impairment may preclude its use.

Physiotherapy is valuable in ensuring successful rehabilitation and attention to mouth hygiene is important as stomatitis is often present.

REFERENCES

Cavanagh, J.B., Fuller, N.H., Johnson, H.R.M., and Rudge, P. (1974). The effect of thallium salts, with particular reference to the nervous system changes. *Quarterly Journal of Medicine*, **43,** 293–319.

Gastel, B. (1978). Thallium poisoning. *John Hopkins Medical Journal*, **142,** 27–31.

Grand Rounds—Guy's Hospital. (1993). Thallium poisoning. *British Medical Journal*, **306,** 1527–9.

Wainwright, A.P., Kox, W.J., House, I.M., Henry, J.A., Heaton, R., and Seed, W.A. (1988). Clinical features and therapy of acute thallium poisoning. *Quarterly Journal of Medicine*, **69,** 939–44.

Vanadium

Most commercially available vanadium is in the form of vanadium pentoxide (V_2O_5) which is used as a catalyst in chemical processes including the production of sulphuric acid and in catalytic converters. Vanadium (as ferrovanadium) is used to increase the hardness of steel alloys. Vanadium is found in some sources of crude oil (e.g. Venezuelan crude) and is a byproduct in oil-fired boilers and furnaces. Exposure to vanadium also occurs in glazing. Most cases of poisoning have occurred during the cleaning of oil-fired burners or gas turbines.

Absorption of vanadium from the gut is poor (1–2 per cent) whereas approximately 25 per cent of an inhaled dose of a soluble vanadium compound is absorbed; the skin is a minor route of absorption in man. Vanadium is bound to transferrin and accumulates in bone and kidney. The half-life in man has been estimated to be 42 days. Excretion is almost entirely in the urine.

CLINICAL FEATURES

Acute poisoning

Inhalation of vanadium causes irritation of mucous membranes, with rhinitis, conjunctivitis, tracheobronchitis, and epistaxis. Pneumonitis may occur after substantial inhalation but is often delayed for 1 to 6 days. In such cases there may also be gastrointestinal upset with diarrhoea and vomiting and neurological features including headache, weakness, tremor, and neurosis have been observed.

Chronic poisoning

Chronic bronchitis and asthma have been described after repeated vanadium exposure, although obstructive lung defects are usually transient and resolve when exposure ceases. Chronic vanadium poisoning may produce greenish-black discoloration of the tongue though this disappears within a few days of the end of exposure. There is conflicting evidence as to whether chronic vanadium poisoning causes depressive illness. There is no evidence that vanadium is carcinogenic in man.

Medical surveillance

Spot-urine vanadium concentrations are useful for screening although measurement of the 24-h urine vanadium excretion, together with the blood vanadium concentration, more accurately reflect toxic exposure. The reference range for urine vanadium is less than 10 μg/l and removal from exposure is suggested if the urine vanadium concentration exceeds 50 μg/l.

TREATMENT

Ascorbic acid, sodium calcium edetate, and desferrioxamine were found to be effective in enhancing vanadium elimination in animals and dimercaprol has been used to increase elimination in two occupational cases. Fortunately, in the majority of cases, symptoms are mild and no more than symptomatic and supportive treatment is required.

REFERENCES

IPCS. (1988). *Environmental Health Criteria 81. Vanadium.* WHO, Geneva.

Lagerkvist, B., Nordberg, G.F., and Vouk, V. (1986). Vanadium. In *Handbook on the Toxicity of Metals*, (ed. L. Friberg., G.F. Nordberg, and V.B. Vouk), 2nd edn. Volume II. pp. 638–663. Elsevier, Amsterdam.

Zinc

Zinc is an essential trace element. Over 70 metalloenzymes are known to require zinc for their function. It is used in the manufacture of alloys, as a component of brass, as a case for batteries, in dyes and paints, for electroplating, and in soldering fluxes. In human toxicology the most important zinc salts are zinc chloride and zinc oxide. Zinc oxide fumes are emitted in any process involving molten zinc and are the most common case of metal fume fever. Exposure to zinc chloride occurs in soldering, in the manufacture of dyes, paper, and deodorants, and on military exercises when it is used as a smoke screen.

Poisoning has followed the accidental or deliberate ingestion of elemental zinc and zinc chloride and fatal intoxication has followed inadvertent intravenous administration. Inhalation of zinc chloride and oxide may lead to acute nasopharyngeal and respiratory damage.

Gastrointestinal zinc absorption is dependent on mucosal metallothionein which sequesters zinc within erythrocytes. Intravascular zinc is bound to transferrin and is transported to the liver and muscle to be stored as a metallothionein complex. Zinc may be absorbed through broken skin when zinc oxide paste is used to treat wounds and burns. Approximately 75 per cent of ingested zinc is eliminated in faeces with small amounts in urine and sweat. The half-life exceeds 300 days.

CLINICAL FEATURES

Acute poisoning

Following the ingestion of zinc or one of its salts, vomiting, diarrhoea, fever, lethargy, muscle pain, and stiffness may occur and profound anaemia has been reported. Ingestion of zinc chloride has led to erosive pharyngitis, oesophagitis, and haematemesis. Acute renal failure and pancreatitis have also been recorded after ingestion. Topical exposure to zinc chloride causes ulceration and dermatitis of the exposed skin. Zinc chloride is highly irritant to the eye.

Metal fume fever was described as early as 1669 in brass foundry workers as 'brass foundryman's ague'. Symptoms of metal fume fever occur up to 24 h after exposure to zinc oxide fumes. It presents as an influenza-like illness with headache, fever, sweating, chest tightness and discomfort, and joint pains. Typically symptoms appear after the weekend, thereby giving rise to the term 'Monday morning fever'. The illness usually has an excellent prognosis and the symptoms often improve towards the end of the working week as some short-term immunity from further symptoms develops. Metal fume fever is unlikely to occur if exposure is kept below 5 mg/m^3. It has been shown that inhalation of zinc oxide fumes is associated with a dose-dependent marked inflammatory response in the lung even if clinical symptoms do not occur. There is an increase in the polymorphonuclear leucocyte count in bronchoalveolar lavage fluid and it has been proposed that cytokines may play a part both in the recruitment to the lung of inflammatory cells and in the systemic manifestations of metal fume fever.

In contrast to the relatively mild clinical course after zinc oxide inhalation, exposure to zinc chloride ammunition bombs (hexite) has led to the development of fatal adult respiratory distress syndrome.

Chronic poisoning

Repeated exposure to zinc oxide may cause liver dysfunction and papular folliculitis. Chronic excessive ingestion of zinc supplements (zinc sulphate) may induce reversible anaemia and leucopenia secondary to a relative copper deficiency. Zinc chromate is a suspected human lung carcinogen.

TREATMENT

Symptomatic and supportive measures should be employed following the ingestion of elemental zinc or one of its salts. If the eyes are affected they should be promptly irrigated with copious volumes of water. Careful endoscopic examination is required following zinc chloride ingestion. The possible late development of the adult respiratory distress syndrome (ARDS) must be considered if zinc chloride or zinc phosphide has been inhaled. Animal studies suggest that DTPA (as the salt calcium trisodium pentetate) and sodium calcium edetate are the most effective chelating agents, but no formal clinical trials have been undertaken in humans.

REFERENCES

Elinder, C.-G. (1986). Zinc. In *Handbook on the Toxicity of Metals*, (ed. L. Friberg., G.F. Nordberg, and V.B. Vouk), 2nd edn. Volume II. pp. 664–79. Elsevier, Amsterdam.

Hjortso, E., *et al.* (1988). ARDS after accidental inhalation of zinc chloride smoke. *Intensive Care Medicine*, **14,** 17–24.

Potter, J.L. (1981). Acute zinc chloride ingestion in a young child. *Annals of Emergency Medicine*, **10,** 267–9.

8.3.7 Poisoning in conflict

R. L. Maynard and T. C. Marrs

From ancient times, the military advantages of using noxious chemicals have been recognized. The enemy may be killed or disabled and denied material or ground. To use, or merely threaten to use, chemical warfare agents has a powerful psychological effect. The First World War exploited chemicals to the full, among them mustard gas (*bis*-2-chloroethylsulphide), which is alleged to have been used in military operations as late as 1986. Since 1918, a number of pharmacologically potent chemicals have been discovered which might be used in warfare. The most important are the organophosphorus cholinesterase inhibitors commonly known as the nerve agents, with a lethal dose of about 1 mg. However, the range of possible agents is very wide if it is accepted that any readily available material as toxic as, or more toxic than, hydrogen cyanide may be used. Some examples of relative toxicities are given in Table 1. Dissemination of any of these chemicals as gases, vapours, aerosols (smoke), or as coarse droplets is technically feasible and intoxication may be via the lungs or/and skin. Many of the chemicals used during the First World War were mainly irritant to the eyes and upper respiratory tract. The temporary incapacitation which they produced had little value in warfare but chemical irritants have been used in the testing of military respirators, military training for chemical defence and by the police in riots and when hostages have been taken (riot control agents).

There are a number of important differences between intoxications produced by the military use of chemical weapons and those resulting from the accidental or deliberate use of poisons elsewhere. In war, the toxic material is used to produce casualties, put the individuals under attack at a disadvantage by forcing them to wear protective clothing, to deny them access to contaminated terrain, equipment or stores, including food, and to lower morale. Because of vagaries of wind and weather which determine the pattern of dispersion of the agent it is unlikely that all those attacked will become casualties, but many will be affected. The doctor's task includes triage, decontamination of casualties, and first-aid measures as well as conventional treatment. Non-casualties must be instructed about the safe disposal or decontamination of residual agent which may otherwise produce late casualties, possibly in the medical team itself. The difficulties which occur at every stage of this process are exemplified by the disaster at Bhopal, India in December 1984 where, within the space of a few hours, the release of a gas cloud of methyl isocyanate produced in excess of 50 000 casualties, most of whom had some degree of pulmonary oedema and eye injuries, and more than 2000 died (see Chapter 8.3.4).

Decontamination of casualties

War 'gases' have been categorized as persistent and non-persistent; persistent agents such as mustard gas call for careful decontamination, which should be done as soon as possible, preferably within minutes, if the skin or eyes are affected. Contaminated clothing and other objects should also be dealt with quickly for they will be a source of danger either from the low concentration of vapour they produce or from secondary skin contamination caused by handling.

Contaminated materials can be handled safely if rubber gloves and a respirator are worn but many agents will slowly penetrate most types of rubber, and gloves should be discarded promptly after the task is completed. The agents may be destroyed by solvents, adsorbents, or by weathering. A simple method is to use a slurry of bleaching powder in water applied liberally with a brush. Burning carries the risk of producing a vapour. For the casualties themselves, suspected areas of contamination should be dusted liberally with fullers' earth, or washed with copious quantities of hot soapy water, but agents removed in this way are still potentially dangerous.

Further discussion of decontamination can be found in *Medical manual of defence against chemical agents.* (1986). 6th edn. HMSO, London.

Sulphur mustard

Sulphur mustard (mustard gas or H), nitrogen mustard, and sesqui mustard are vesicant compounds. Only sulphur mustard has been used much in chemical warfare. It was used first by the Germans on 12 July 1917 at Ypres producing 14 276 British casualties during the first 3 months and some 168 000 casualties by the end of the war with a case fatality of 2 to 3 per cent. Mustard was the most effective chemical weapon introduced during the First World War.

Italian forces used sulphur mustard extensively during the invasion of Ethiopia in 1936, and in 1984 Iran accused Iraq of using it.

The name mustard was used by soldiers during the First World War because of the smell. It is an oily liquid at room temperature. The vapour passes through clothing and penetrates and is absorbed through the skin producing local and systemic effects. It may be delivered by artillery shell, rocket, bomb, or aircraft spray. It is persistent and ground may remain contaminated for long periods in cold weather. Protected troops can withstand an attack but unprotected, inexperienced troops suffer badly. Exposed drinking water may be contaminated by dangerous oily surface film of mustard.

Sulphur mustard is an alkylating agent. The therapeutically more useful compound nitrogen mustard has been investigated in detail: it is converted in the body to an active ethylenimonium intermediate which binds to a range of molecules including proteins, enzymes, and nucleic acids. Sulphur mustard is converted in part to a similar sulphonium ion. The binding of these compounds to guanine residues causes severe disruption of DNA structure and function. Repair of the DNA damage occurs in some cells but the process of repair can itself lead to further impairment of cellular function. Damage to DNA will have profound

Table 1 *Relative toxicities of some synthetic and naturally occurring poisons compared with the nerve agent sarin*

			10^3 = sarin (GB) = 10^3 nerve agent			
			Decreasing toxicity ↓	Increasing toxicity ↓		
Tabun (GA)	10^3–10^4	Aconitine			10^3–10^2	Russell viper venom
		Physostigmine				Amanitine
Methylfluoroacetate		Strychnine				D-Tubocurarine
Hydrogen cyanide	10^4–10^5					Ricin saxitoxin
Mustard gas						Curare abrin
Parathion					10^2–1	Batrachotoxin
Phosgene					1–10^1	Palytoxin
					10^{-1}–10^{-2}	Palytoxin
					10^{-2}–10^{-3}	Tetanus toxin
Arsine					10^{-3}–10^{-4}	Botulinus toxin
Chlorine	10^5–10^6					
White arsenic						

Reproduced from Beswick (1983), with permission.

effects upon rapidly dividing tissues, and bone marrow depression, hair loss, and gut effects are well recognized. The lethal toxicity of sulphur mustard for various species is given in Table 2. Nitrogen mustard and to a lesser extent sulphur mustard has direct effects on the central nervous system: nausea and vomiting, convulsions, and progressive muscular paralysis.

Clinical features

Typically, there is a latent period of up to 2 to 4 h after exposure to vapour before symptoms and signs appear (Table 3). Hypersensitivity to low concentrations has been reported. The symptoms and signs depend upon the mode of exposure. Liquid will produce similar effects but local vesication will be more marked. Fatalities may result from bronchopneumonia complicated by severe damage to the bone marrow. Deaths usually occur 2 days and 4 weeks after exposure and rarely occur within 24 h.

Treatment

First aid measures

These are of the greatest importance since there is no specific therapy. A respirator and adequate protective clothing must be worn when dealing with contaminated individuals.

1. Patients should be removed from the source of the sulphur mustard vapour.
2. Those severely affected should not be allowed to walk (this was recommended during the First World War but is not likely to be as important in cases of sulphur mustard poisoning as in cases of phosgene poisoning (Chapter 8.3.4).
3. Clothing should be removed and affected areas washed with soap and water.
4. Liquid contamination of eyes should be rinsed out immediately using 0.9 per cent saline solution, if available, or water.

Therapeutic measures

There is no specific therapy. A number of palliative approaches have been suggested. Cysteine can reduce the antitumour effects of alkylating agents presumably by providing alternative binding sites to those of DNA; its use has been suggested but its efficacy is unproven.

1. Skin. For areas of erythema and minor blistering bland calamine lotions are suggested. Recently, beclomethasone-dipropionate cream has been used, but it is unlikely to enhance healing. Areas of deeper burning are difficult to manage. Standard thermal burn therapy, e.g. silver sulphadiazine cream may play a useful role in preventing secondary infection. Full thickness burns will not heal without grafting.
2. Eyes. Early decontamination is critical. Attempts to decontaminate the eye when more than 5 min have passed since liquid contamination are likely to be valueless. Topical prednisolone drops (1 per cent), ascorbate (potassium ascorbate 10 per cent), and citrate (sodium citrate 10 per cent) drops (each once per

Table 2 *Toxicity of sulphur mustard*

Species	LD_{50} skin (mg/kg)	LD_{50} intravenous (μg/kg)	LD_{LC} (mg/kg)
Rat	9	700	
Mouse	92	8600	
Dog	20		
Rabbit	100	1100	
Humans			64

LD_{LC} is the lowest recorded lethal dose.

Table 3 *Signs and symptoms of sulphur mustard poisoning*

Time after exposure	Symptoms and signs
20–60 min	Nausea, retching, vomiting, and eye smarting have occasionally been observed
2–6 h	Nausea, vomiting, fatigue, headache
	Inflammation of the eyes, lacrimation, blepharospasm, photophobia, rhinorrhoea
	Reddening of face and neck
	Soreness of throat
	Increase in pulse and respiratory rate
24 h	General increase in severity of above effects
	Inflammation of inner thighs, axillae, genitalia, buttocks, followed by onset of blister formation
	Blisters are large, filled with yellow fluid and may be pendulous
48 h	Condition generally worsened
	Blistering more marked, swelling of genitalia
	Bronchitis established with expectoration of mucopus and necrotic slough
	Temperature, pulse, and respiratory rate increased

hour, i.e. half-hourly drops, for all the working day, until a stable epithelium has reformed) are recommended. Local anaesthetics such as amethocaine hydrochloride (0.5 per cent) but not cocaine, which may produce corneal sloughing and mydriatics, e.g. 0.5 per cent hyoscine, are suggested. Topical antibiotics e.g. chloramphenicol, should be used to prevent secondary infection.

3. Respiratory system. Codeine linctus may ease severe coughing. An antimicrobial, but not one liable to induce further bone marrow depression, is recommended. Adult respiratory distress syndrome may occur in severe cases. This should be managed as described elsewhere.
4. Bone marrow depression resulting from sulphur mustard poisoning has been considered irreversible but colony stimulating factor may be worth a therapeutic trial. If there is severe aplastic anaemia, platelet and granulocyte transfusions and bone marrow transplantation should be considered.
5. Haemodialysis and haemoperfusion have both been suggested as general measures but their efficacy is uncertain. Vomiting may be controlled by phenothiazine-like drugs.

Long-term effects

Long-term ophthalmic problems including corneal ulceration and blindness occur in a small minority of cases. Sulphur mustard is a known carcinogen and studies of American soldiers exposed during the First World War and Japanese factory workers revealed an increased incidence of lung cancer (and chronic bronchitis).

Lewisite

Lewisite (2-chlorovinyl-dichlorarsine), one of a group of 'arsenical vesicants', was suggested as a chemical weapon at the end of the First World War but was never manufactured in large quantities and has not been used in war. Soon after its discovery it was nicknamed the 'Dew of Death' on account of its very dangerous properties.

Ethyldichlorarsine and phenyldichlorarsine ('The Dicks') were used to a limited extent during the First World War. Phenyldichlorarsine produces nasal irritation in a concentration of one part in 50×10^6, is intolerable at one part in 1×10^6, and was referred to as 'sneeze-gas'.

Impure lewisite has an odour of geraniums but in the pure state it has only a faint odour. It is absorbed rapidly through the skin and mucous membranes. Its distribution in the body is assumed to follow that of other arsenical compounds and heavy deposits in the liver, kidney, wall of the gut, spleen, and lung would be expected. Lewisite is a liquid and may be disseminated by shells, bombs, rockets, and aircraft spray. Contamination may occur by contact with liquid or by inhalation of evolved vapour. Its use as a chemical weapon is limited because of rapid hydrolysis and difficulties in maintaining effective vapour concentrations. In dry climates it might be expected to be very effective.

Toxicity figures for lewisite in humans are not known. The effect of lewisite is thought to be due to the combining of the arsenical part with lipoic acid to form a cyclic compound: lipoic acid is an essential part of the pyruvate dehydrogenase system acting as a coenzyme in the formation of acetyl CoA from pyruvate.

Clinical features

In animals, exposure causes immediate eye irritation. Coughing, sneezing, profuse nasal mucus discharge, salivation, and lacrimation follow rapidly. Liquid contamination of the skin causes erythema immediately and vesication within a few hours. Lewisite is a more powerful vesicant than sulphur mustard but healing probably occurs earlier. The eye and skin effects are likely to be maximal between 4 and 8 h after exposure. Victims are rapidly incapacitated, unable to see, and hardly able to breathe. Severe lung injury produces pulmonary oedema and death from respiratory failure. Heavy skin contamination (e.g. 1.4 ml of lewisite) can lead to absorption of fatal amounts of arsenic.

Blindness follows contamination of the eye with liquid lewisite unless there is very prompt decontamination.

Treatment

1. First aid (as for mustard gas).
2. Therapy. Dimercaprol (British Anti-Lewisite, BAL) developed during the Second World War was shown, in animal experiments, to protect against the effects of lewisite and to reverse the enzyme inhibition it produced. It is applied as drops (5–10 per cent in vegetable oil) into the conjunctival sacs of affected eyes as an urgent measure. Skin lesions should be treated with dimercaprol ointment. Application of the ointment to damaged areas may produce an intense burning sensation which disappears in about 30 min to be replaced by an alleviation of the pretreatment irritation. The ointment is applied daily. Dimercaprol can also be given intramuscularly to antagonize the systemic effects of the absorbed arsenical. Dimercaprol is specific in opposing the effects of lewisite, but the risk of bronchopneumonia in patients who have inhaled lewisite vapour probably justifies the use of prophylactic antimicrobials. DMSA (succimer), DMPS (unithiol), and DMPA have been developed more recently and should be considered as possible alternatives to BAL.

The nerve agents

The nerve agents, a group of the most toxic chemical warfare agents, are powerful organophosphorus inhibitors of acetylcholinesterase. Similar compounds are widely used as insecticides.

These compounds have been known since 1854, and their toxicity recognized in the 1930s. In the Second World War a great many such compounds were synthesized in Germany. With the exception of the highly toxic V agents no significant additions have been made to the short list of tabun (GA), sarin (GB) (Fig. 1), and soman (GD) known since the Second World War.

Clinical features

The pattern of symptoms and signs following exposure to nerve agents is partly dependent upon the route of exposure. Miosis, a characteristic

Fig. 1 Structural formulae of nerve agents.

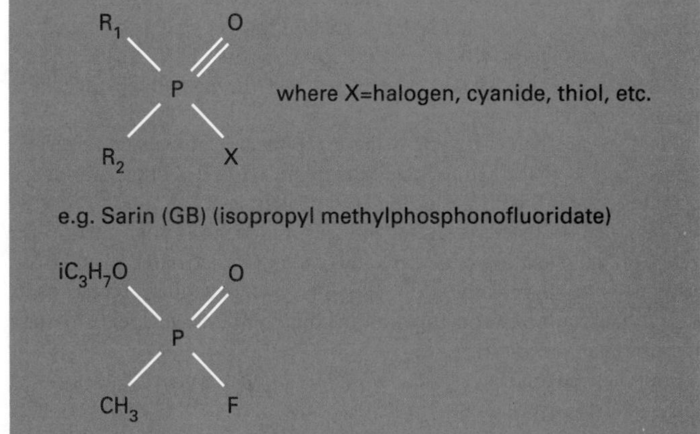

Table 4 *Symptoms and signs following exposure to sarin (GB) vapour*

Frontal headache
Eye pain
Tightness in chest
Rhinorrhoea
Conjunctival injection
Miosis
Increased sweating
Increased salivation
Abdominal cramps
Nausea and vomiting
Involuntary micturition and defecation
Muscular weakness
Fasciculation
Tremor
Restlessness
Ataxia
Convulsions
Respiratory paralysis

sign of vapour exposure is mainly due to local absorption of the nerve agent. Likewise, local fasciculation following liquid contamination of skin is not necessarily a sign of systemic poisoning. Nerve agents are likely to be encountered either as gases (GA or GB) or as liquids (VX and GD), delivered as sprays, or in bombs and shells. GD is a volatile liquid and so also produces a vapour. A synopsis of the effects of acute exposure to GB is given in Table 4.

The rate of development of symptoms and signs varies with the route of exposure and dose. Potentially lethal exposure to GB produces noticeable effects within a few minutes; death, resulting from respiratory failure, may follow within 5 to 15 min.

Treatment

Post-exposure therapy

The cornerstone of therapy is atropine, which competitively blocks acetylcholine at muscarinic receptors, ameliorating the parasympathomimetic effects of anticholinesterase compounds. Atropine has mild or negligible effects on the neuromuscular junction (nicotinic receptors), the autonomic ganglia (nicotinic receptors), and CNS synapses protected by the blood–brain barrier. Atropine should be given as soon as possible after exposure. Large doses may be required, 2 mg of atropine sulphate intravenously, or if necessary intramuscularly, should be given every 5 min until the parasympathomimetic effects (e.g. bradycardia, salivation) are reversed. Automatic injection devices are widely used by military personnel for self-administration after nerve agent poisoning. These always contain atropine with a variety of other drugs. Overdoses of atropine may be given and so close monitoring is needed. As much as 30 mg of atropine may be required during the first 24 h. At the end of that period atropine should be stopped and the patient observed for return of cholinergic signs.

The second line of therapy is the use of acetylcholinesterase reactivators such as pralidoxime, obidoxime, and HI-6. This reactivation of enzyme reduces the effects of the accumulated acetylcholine so reversing the effects of the nerve agent. Unlike atropine this is not a muscarinic receptor-dependent effect and is effective at a wider range of pharmacological sites, especially at the neuromuscular junction. Oximes such as pralidoxime have little effect on the binding of nerve agents to cholinesterase at sites in the CNS.

Early administration is essential. Pralidoxime mesylate (2 g) is given intravenously over about 4 min (not more than 500 mg/min) and repeated 4 to 6 hourly. Too rapid administration may cause weakness, blurred vision, dizziness, headache, nausea, and tachycardia.

Treatment of GD poisoning presents particular problems because the dialkylphosphoryl-enzyme complex loses an alkyl group ('ageing') to form a monoalkylphosphoryl–enzyme complex. This 'aged' complex is refractory both to spontaneous reactivation and to oxime-induced reactivation. 'Ageing' occurs to some extent with most anticholinesterase organophosphates but it is so rapid with GD (a matter of minutes) that spontaneous reactivation does not occur and oximes are ineffective, with the possible exception of HI-6.

The third drug which has proved useful in the treatment of nerve agent poisoning in animals is diazepam. This is thought to act by its central anticonvulsive properties and is effective against muscle fasciculation. It is recommended in doses of 5 mg intravenously every 10 min to a maximum dose of 15 mg. Respiratory depression may occur.

General supporting therapy is essential. Mechanical ventilation with oxygen enriched air via an endotracheal tube is recommended. Removal of bronchial secretions is also necessary, but the drying of such secretions by atropine makes this difficult.

Pretreatment with carbamate anticholinesterase compounds

Reversible binding of a proportion of cholinesterase to a carbamate, such as pyridostigmine protects it from inactivation by a nerve agent. This is likely to be particularly valuable where GD gives rise to an aged nerve agent–enzyme complex. Pyridostigmine bromide (30 mg, 8 hourly) should be given by mouth prior to exposure to nerve agent.

Riot control agents

Noxious smokes produced by burning sulphur and pitch have long been used to drive people away from occupied ground or fortifications. The deliberate selection of chemicals which cause lacrimation and severe upper respiratory tract irritation for this purpose dates only from the beginning of this century. In 1912, the Paris police used ethyl bromoacetate to overcome armed criminals and in 1914, the French army used the same material loaded into artillery shells to harass the enemy on the Western front. More than 30 chemicals have been used to produce irritant effects. Of these only the arsenicals (see lewisite above), 2-chloroacetophenone (CN), dibenzoxazepine (CR), and orthochlorobenzylidene malononitrile (CS) deserve specific mention. CN, CR, and CS might well be used in this way because their effects, confined to the eyes and the upper respiratory tract, are brief (perhaps 15 min at the most) and completely reversible. They are crystalline solids; CN colourless, CR yellow and CS white. CR is stable and persistent, but CS hydrolyses comparatively quickly (half-life about 15 min) to non-irritant products.

All three compounds can be dispersed as liquids in organic solvents, powders, and as smokes. Private possession of these devices is illegal in the United Kingdom, but elsewhere self-protection devices such as 'Mace' and 'The Federal Streamer' (CN) and 'The Paralyser' (CS) may be available.

Liquid dispersal

CN has been marketed for personal protection as the tear gas gun. These are available to the public in a few countries. They operate by the explosive discharge of CN powder at short range with the eyes as a prime target. The risk of eye injury is greater with these devices than with liquids because of blast and heat hazards and the possibility that crystalline CN may be driven into the conjunctiva.

CS powder has been dispersed without explosives, for example, by air blowers in the Vietnam War. Ninety per cent of micropulverized CS (particle diameter average 5 μm, maximum 10 μm) is formulated with 10 per cent of similarly-sized silica particles. These particles will mainly affect the eyes, nose, and mouth unlike smokes which involve the upper respiratory tract more. Avoiding an explosive dispersion eliminates blast and heat which add to the danger of tear gas guns. The effects and their duration resemble those of CS smoke.

Smoke dispersal

CN, CS, and CR are readily dispersed as smokes by heating them with potassium chlorate, lactose, and kaolin. The vaporized irritant condenses in the air to form droplets of about 1 μm diameter.

Riot control smoke clouds are easily seen. Their main effect, persistent but non-disabling eye irritations, may occur at concentrations as low as 0.3 mg/m^3 (CN), 0.004 mg/m^3 (CS), and 0.002 mg/m^3 (CR). Above concentrations of 35 mg/m^3 (CN), 5 mg/m^3 (CS), and 1 mg/m^3 (CR) full effects develop. The eyes become painful almost immediately and there is a tight uncontrollable blepharospasm, with lacrimation. There is a burning sensation in the nose and mouth with rhinorrhoea and salivation. Breathing becomes irregular, there is tightness of the chest, substernal pain, and coughing. Minutes later, the skin becomes sore. In men the shaving area is particularly affected. In more severe cases swallowing of contaminated saliva causes epigastric discomfort, retching or vomiting. Most affected individuals will quickly seek fresh air where recovery is substantially complete within 15 min. However, at least five human deaths have been reported caused by explosion of CN grenades in enclosed spaces.

Possible complications and treatment

Treatment is seldom required. All the compounds are highly potent stimulators of sensory nerve endings but appear to have few other pharmacological properties. First, patients and their clothing should be decontaminated.

Eyes

Eye pain is usually accompanied by an increase in intraocular pressure. The risk of glaucoma should be considered in those over 40 years old. Gross contamination of the eye causing structural damage is a very rare possibility, but high concentrations of CN may cause keratitis and chemosis.

Skin

Reversible erythema is usual. Contamination of wounds should not influence their healing in anyway. Gross persistent contamination with solid material, especially CN, may cause blistering.

Cardiovascular system

Tachycardia and hypertension reflect the degree of exposure and are associated with pain and fright. They peak within several minutes and, as the discomfort diminishes, return to normal. Hypertensive individuals may need to be observed.

Respiratory system

Bronchospasm has not been observed but laryngeal spasm associated with cold or resulting from a coughing spasm might occur. Sufferers from chronic bronchitis are not particularly vulnerable but asthmatics who have reactive airways should be monitored carefully.

Central nervous system

Riot control agents are used in circumstances of emotional stress and produce effects which themselves are stressful. All but the most hardened of individuals can be expected to show signs of acute anxiety at least. Reassurance is the main feature of treatment.

REFERENCES

Almqvist, X., and Wiksell, X. (1971). *The problems of chemical and biological warfare*. Vols. I to IV. Stockholm International Peace Research Institute, Stockholm.

Aposhian, H.V. (1984). DMSA, DMPS and DMPA—as arsenic antidotes. *Fundamental and Applied Toxicology*, **4**, S58–S70.

Ballantyne, B. (1971). Riot control agents—biomedical and health aspects of the use of chemicals in civil disturbances. *Medical Annual*, pp. 7–41, John Wright, Bristol.

Beebe, G.W. (1960). Lung cancer in World War I veterans: possible relation to mustard gas injury and the 1918 influenza epidemic. *Journal of the National Cancer Institute*, **25**, 1231–52.

Beswick, F.W. (1983). Chemical agents used in riot control and warfare. *Human Toxicology*, **2**, 247–56.

British Medical Journal (1940). Gas injuries to the eye. *British Medical Journal*, 1986.

Foster, J. (1939). Ophthalmic injuries from mustard gas (DES). *British Medical Journal*, 1181–3.

Fox, M. (1980). The genetic toxicology of nitrogen and sulphur mustard. *Mutation Research*, **75**, 131–68.

Graziano, J.H. (1978). The pharmacology of 2,3-dimercaptosuccinic acid and its potential use in arsenic poisoning. *Journal of Pharmacology and Experimental Therapeutics*, **207**, 1051–8.

Grob, D. (1953). The effects and treatment of nerve agent poisoning. *American Journal of Medicine*, **14**, 52–63.

Haldane, J.B.S. (1925). *Callinicus, a defence of chemical warfare*. Kegan Paul, Trench, Trubner and Co. Ltd., London.

HMSO (1986). *Medical manual of defence against chemical agents*. 6th edn, JSP 312. HMSO, London.

Holmstedt, B. (1959). Pharmacology of organophosphorus cholinesterase inhibitors. *Pharmacological Reviews*, **11**, 567–688.

Ireland, M.W. (1926). Medical aspects of gas warfare. *The Medical Department of the United States Army in World War I*. Vol. XIV. Government Printing Office, Washington.

Inns, R.H. and Marrs, T.C. (1992) Prophylaxis against anticholinesterase poisoning. In *Clinical and Experimental Toxicology of Organophosphates and Carbamates*. (ed. B. Ballantyne and T.C. Marrs), pp. 633–7. Butterworth-Heinemann, Oxford.

Koelle, G.B. (ed). (1963). Cholinesterase and anticholinesterase agents. *Handbuch der experimentellen Pharmakologie*. Vol 15, Springer-Verlag, Berlin.

Lentz, K. (1981). 2,3-Dimercaptosuccinic acid in human arsenic poisoning. *Archives of Toxicology*, **47**, 241–3.

Marrs, T.C. (1991). Toxicology of oximes used in organophosphorus poisoning. *Adverse Drug Reactions Reviews*, **10**, 61–73.

Maynard, R.L. and Beswick, F.W. (1992). Organophosphorus compounds as chemical warfare agents. In *Clinical and Experimental Toxicology of Organophosphates and Carbamates* (ed. B. Ballantyne, and T.C. Marrs), pp. 373–85, Butterworth-Heinemann, Oxford.

Ministry of Home Security Air Raid Precautions Department. (1940). *The detection and identification of war gases*. Chemical Publishing Company Inc., New York.

Peters, R. (1945). British anti-Lewisite (BAL). *Nature*, **156**, 616–19.

Peters, R. (1948). Development and theoretical significance of British anti-Lewisite (BAL). *British Medical Bulletin*, **5**, 313–18.

Renshaw, B. (1946). Mechanisms in production of cutaneous injuries by sulfur and nitrogen mustards. In *Chemical warfare agents and related chemical problems*, Vol I, pp. 479–518. US Office of Science Research and Development, National Defence Research Committee, Washington DC.

Taylor, P. (1980). Anticholinesterase agents. In *The pharmacological basis of therapeutics* (ed. L.S. Goodman and A. Gilman). 6th edn. Macmillan, Basingstoke.

Willems, J.L. (1989). Clinical management of mustard gas casualties. *Annales Medicina Militaris Belgica*, **3,** 51–61.

Yamada, A. (1986). On the late injuries following occupational inhalation of mustard gas with special reference to carcinoma of the respiratory tract. *Acta Pathologica Japonica*, **13,** 131–55.

8.3.8 Pesticides

A. T. PROUDFOOT AND J. A. VALE

Pesticides are a diverse group of chemicals which share only one property—they are toxic to one or more species of organism. The main groups of pesticides are herbicides, insecticides, molluscicides, fungicides, and rodenticides with herbicides accounting for about 75 per cent of the total tonnage of active ingredients produced annually. In developed countries the amounts of pesticides which can be applied, the target species, and the conditions under which they should be used (including the time of the year, method of application, and protective equipment for operators) are specified by regulatory authorities after detailed consideration of their efficacy, toxicology, and environmental impact. Like drugs, pesticide formulations often contain substances other than the active ingredient(s) including emulsifiers, surfactants, and solvents, and the last, in particular, may contribute to the toxicity of the product.

Theoretically, acute poisoning with pesticides could occur at various stages from their manufacture through to exposure to treated produce. Clearly, however, the hazards are greater at some stages than others. For example, major disasters excepted, poisoning during manufacture is extremely unlikely because of the engineering controls and other safety measures built into manufacturing processes. In contrast, the dilution of pesticides at the site of use, correct application, and observance of operator safety recommendations are virtually impossible to control, particularly when the climatic factors under which they are used and the extent to which workers are educated in their use vary enormously. It would be wrong, however, to think that all acute pesticide poisoning is the result of recommended use. Some, particularly paraquat, are deliberately ingested or injected in attempts to commit suicide and the outbreaks of carbamate and organophosphate poisoning which have been reported after consumption of hydroponically grown melons and cucumbers were almost certainly due to inappropriate application of these pesticides.

In addition to acute poisoning, there is concern in some sections of society over the longer-term intake of pesticide residues and their breakdown products which are present, usually in minute amounts, in water and the food of humans and other animals. The extensive use of pesticides in present-day agriculture and horticulture makes it virtually impossible to avoid such exposure and ingestion is sometimes blamed for a variety of ailments including allergies, infertility, some forms of malignant disease, and neurological disorders.

REFERENCES

British Medical Association (1992). *Pesticides, Chemicals and Health.* Edward Arnold, London.

Lamminpaa, A., and Riihimaki, V. (1992). Pesticide-related incidents treated in Finnish hospitals—a review of cases registered over a 5-year period. *Human and Experimental Toxicology*, **11,** 473–9.

Proudfoot, A.T. and Dougall, H. (1988). Poisoning treatment centre admissions following acute incidents involving pesticides. *Human Toxicology*, **7,** 255–8.

Herbicides

Bipyridilium herbicides

The bipyridilium herbicides include diquat, morfamquat, and paraquat, the last being the one most commonly encountered in clinical toxicology since it is used for committing suicide.

CLINICAL FEATURES

Occupationally, carelessness in handling paraquat has led to reversible changes in the finger nails and inhalation of spray may cause pain in the throat and epistaxis. Skin splashes which are promptly and thoroughly washed should not cause problems but prolonged dermal exposure may cause burns and, very rarely, may enable enough paraquat to be absorbed to cause serious and fatal systemic poisoning. Splashes in the eyes cause blepharospasm, lacrimation, and corneal ulceration.

Potentially lethal poisoning is most common after ingestion of paraquat. Probably no more than 5 per cent of the ingested amount is absorbed but absorption is rapid, the volume of distribution is high, and there is energy-dependent accumulation in some organs (particularly the lungs). Elimination is mainly through the kidneys.

The features of toxicity are largely dependent on the amount of paraquat swallowed. Ingestion of 6 g or more of paraquat ion is likely to be fatal within 24 to 48 h while 3 to 6 g is likely to lead to a more protracted, but still fatal, course. Nausea, vomiting, abdominal pain, and diarrhoea, rapidly followed by peripheral circulatory failure, metabolic acidosis, impaired consciousness, convulsions, and increasing breathlessness and cyanosis secondary to acute pneumonitis, are the features of ingestion of large amounts of paraquat. With smaller amounts, the cardiovascular and CNS complications are not seen and the course of poisoning is dominated by alimentary features, particularly painful ulceration of the mouth, tongue, and throat, which makes it very difficult to swallow, speak, and cough. Perforation of the oesophagus with subsequent mediastinitis has been reported. Mild jaundice may be seen and renal failure is usually severe and may require treatment by haemodialysis. Breathlessness, tachypnoea, widespread crepitations, and central cyanosis may be present by 5 to 7 days after ingestion and progress relentlessly until the patient dies from hypoxia a few days later.

Ingestion of 1.5 to 2.0 g of paraquat causes nausea, vomiting and diarrhoea, and mild renal tubular necrosis while liver damage is uncommon. Pain in the throat is common but ulceration is unusual. Respiratory involvement may not be apparent till 10 to 21 days after ingestion. Breathlessness, basal crepitations, and bilateral chest radiographic opacities develop and progress till the patient dies of respiratory failure as late as 5 or 6 weeks after taking the paraquat. At autopsy the lungs are found to be heavy and rubbery due to extensive intra- and interalveolar fibrosis.

DIAGNOSIS

The diagnosis of poisoning is usually made on the basis of the history and can be readily confirmed by a simple qualitative test on urine. This test is of particular value in accidental inhalation or ingestion of very small quantities and if performed on urine passed within 4 h of alleged ingestion; a negative test indicates that not enough has been taken to cause problems.

TREATMENT

There is no evidence that the outcome of paraquat poisoning can be altered by any form of intervention. It is traditional to empty the stomach despite the corrosive effects of the toxin but administration of activated charcoal is probably more effective in reducing absorption.

Symptomatic measures including antiemetics, mouth washes, and analgesics are indicated and intravenous fluids may be necessary to

Table 1 *Chlorophenoxyacetate herbicides*

Chemical name	Other names
2,4-Dichlorophenoxy acetic acid	2,4-D
4-(2,4-Dichlorophenoxy) butyric acid	2,4-DB
2-(2,4-Dichlorophenoxy) propionic acid Dichlorprop	2,4-DP, DCPP,
2,4,5-Trichlorophenoxy acetic acid	2,4,5-T
2-(2,4,5-Trichlorophenoxy) propionic acid	2,4,5-TP, fenoprop
4-Chloro-2-methylphenoxyacetic acid	MCPA
4-(4-Chloro-2-methylphenoxy) butyric acid	MCPB
2-(4-Chloro-2-methylphenoxy) propionic acid	MCPA, mecoprop

replace gastrointestinal losses. Skin ulcers should be treated as burns. Unfortunately, currently available techniques for enhancing the elimination of poisons appear incapable of rapidly removing toxicologically significant quantities of paraquat. Equally, there is no evidence that corticosteroids, drugs to prevent free radical formation, free radical scavengers, immunosuppressive agents, radiotherapy to the lungs, or lung transplantation reduce mortality. The prognosis in individual cases can be predicted from the plasma paraquat concentration related to the time from ingestion. Patients whose levels do not exceed 2.0, 0.6, 0.3, 0.16 mg/l at 4, 6, 10, and 16 h after ingestion will almost certainly survive without treatment while those with higher concentrations are very likely to die regardless of treatment. Any patient whose plasma paraquat concentration exceeds 0.1 mg/l after 25 h is also unlikely to survive and should therefore be kept as comfortable as possible. Poisons information services will advise on the interpretation of plasma paraquat concentrations.

REFERENCES

Pond, S.M. (1990). Manifestations and management of paraquat poisoning. *Medical Journal of Australia*, **152,** 256–9.

Second European Symposium on Paraquat Poisoning. (1987). *Human Toxicology* **6,** 3–98.

Chlorates

Sodium chlorate and potassium chlorate are powerful oxidizing agents and are highly toxic if ingested. The early features include nausea, vomiting, diarrhoea, abdominal pain, and cyanosis secondary to methaemoglobinaemia. Intravascular haemolysis occurs causing hyperkalaemia, jaundice, and oliguric renal failure.

Management includes emptying the stomach if the patient presents within 1 h of ingestion. Methaemoglobinaemia can be corrected by slow intravenous injection of methylene blue (1–2 mg/kg body weight) which may have to be repeated. Blood transfusion may be required. Plasma potassium concentrations should be monitored and reduced if necessary. Haemodialysis will remove chlorate in addition to possible being necessary for the management of renal failure and hyperkalaemia. Plasmapheresis may also have a role since it will remove chlorate, circulating free haemoglobin, and red cell stroma and thus help prevent the development of renal failure.

Chlorophenoxyacetate herbicides

The chlorophenoxyacetate herbicides (Table 1) include the substances popularly referred to as 'hormone' weedkillers and are used widely in agriculture and by the public. Most instances of serious poisoning have been due to deliberate ingestion but few cases have been reported. These herbicides are often co-formulated with dicamba which is of low toxicity and ioxynil and bromoxynil which uncouple oxidative phosphorylation.

Ingestion causes burning in the mouth and throat, nausea, vomiting, and abdominal pain. The face may be flushed and there is often profuse sweating and fever. CNS depression leading to deep, prolonged coma, hyperventilation, carpopedal spasm, hypotension, hypoglycaemia, hypocalcaemia, metabolic acidosis, and pulmonary oedema may develop. ECG abnormalities and skeletal muscle damage leading to proximal myopathy have been reported.

Management includes emptying the stomach and supportive measures as indicated by the patient's clinical state. Alkalinization of the urine (see Chapter 8.1.2) is indicated for severe poisoning since it considerably enhances elimination of 2,4-dichlorophenoxy acetic acid (2,4-D) and dichlorprop and, to a lesser extent, mecoprop which are moderately strong acids. Alkalinization of the urine probably does not have a beneficial effect on the elimination of other phenoxyacetates and does not affect that of ioxynil. Haemodialysis would be expected to enhance the elimination of these compounds and may have a role in severe intoxication.

REFERENCES

Durakovic, Z., *et al.* (1992). Poisoning with 2,4-dichlorophenoxyacetic acid treated by hemodialysis. *Archives of Toxicology*, **66,** 518–21.

Flanagan, R.J., *et al.* (1990). Alkaline diuresis for acute poisoning with chlorophenoxy herbicides and ioxynil. *Lancet*, **335,** 454–8.

Glyphosate-containing herbicides

Glyphosate-containing herbicides are amongst the most recent to have become available. They usually contain the isopropylamine salt together with a surfactant which has recently been changed. The original surfactant was probably the main cause of toxicity.

The most prominent effects are on the alimentary tract with burning in the mouth and throat, nausea, vomiting, dysphagia, and diarrhoea being the main features. Upper gastrointestinal haemorrhage is a much less common complication. A polymorph leucocytosis is usual. Hypotension, tachycardia, bradycardia, acute chemical pneumonitis, oliguria, haematuria, and metabolic acidosis may be seen in severe poisoning.

Management is largely symptomatic and supportive. Intravenous fluids or blood may be required. Respiratory and renal failure should be managed conventionally. The toxicokinetics of glyphosate in man are not known and rational use of elimination procedures is therefore not possible.

REFERENCES

Menkes, D.B., Temple, W.A., and Edwards, I.R. (1991). Intentional self-poisoning with glyphosate-containing herbicides. *Human and Experimental Toxicology*, **10,** 103–7.

Talbot, A.R., *et al.* (1991). Acute poisoning with a glyphosate-surfactant herbicide (''Round-up''): a review of 93 cases. *Human and Experimental Toxicology*, **10,** 1–8.

Tominack, R.L., *et al.* (1991). Taiwan National Poison Center survey of glyphosate-surfactant herbicide ingestions. *Clinical Toxicology*, **29,** 91–109.

Triazine herbicides

This class of herbicides includes atrazine and simazine which are currently of concern because their concentrations in drinking water exceed internationally agreed levels rather than because they are toxic. Indeed, there is no evidence that even large amounts cause serious effects in humans. However, it has recently been alleged that inhalation of amitrole caused partially reversible pulmonary alveolar damage.

Insecticides

Organophosphorus compounds

Organophosphorus insecticides are among the most widely used pesticides throughout the world. They vary widely in their toxicity and while some are directly toxic, others such as malathion, have to be metabolized before being effective.

MODE OF ACTION

Organophosphate insecticides inhibit cholinesterases, causing accumulation of acetylcholine at central and peripheral cholinergic nerve endings, including neuromuscular junctions. The speed of onset and severity of poisoning depend on a combination of factors including the rate at which the insecticide phosphorylates (inactivates) the enzyme, the rate of spontaneous hydrolysis of the phosphorylated enzyme to release active enzyme, and the rate at which the phosphorylated enzyme changes chemically ('ages') into a form that is incapable of being reactivated to yield functional cholinesterase. Once the last has happened, recovery of acetylcholinesterase activity depends on synthesis of new enzyme by the liver which will take weeks in severe cases.

CLINICAL FEATURES

The features of organophosphate insecticide poisoning are dose related. Minor exposure may produce subclinical poisoning in which there is reduction of cholinesterase activity but no symptoms or signs. Poisoning is characterized by anxiety, restlessness, insomnia, nightmares, tiredness, dizziness, headache, and muscarinic features such as nausea, vomiting, abdominal colic, diarrhoea, tenesmus, sweating, hypersalivation, and chest tightness. Miosis may be present. Nicotinic effects follow with fasciculation and flaccid paresis of limb muscles, respiratory muscles, and, occasionally, various combinations of extraocular muscles. Respiratory failure ensues and is exacerbated by the development of pulmonary oedema and by the retention in the bronchi of large amounts of respiratory secretions. Consciousness is impaired in severe poisoning and convulsions may occur. Hyperglycaemia and glycosuria have been reported though ketonuria is absent. Rarely, complete heart block and arrhythmias occur.

DIAGNOSIS

Diagnosis of organophosphate pesticide poisoning is difficult in the absence of a history of exposure and requires a high index of suspicion. Gastroenteritis is a common erroneous diagnosis and the finding of glycosuria and hyperglycaemia may prompt consideration of diabetes mellitus and its complications. Miosis is an important diagnostic sign but is not invariable. Once raised, the diagnosis can be confirmed by demonstrating reduced plasma, but preferably erythrocyte, cholinesterase activity. However, the extent of reduction correlates only crudely with the severity of poisoning. In subclinical poisoning cholinesterase activity may be reduced by up to 50 per cent while mild, moderate, and severe acute poisoning are associated with reduction of cholinesterase activity to approximately 20 to 50 per cent, 10 to 20 per cent, and less than 10 per cent of normal respectively.

TREATMENT

Subclinical poisoning does not require treatment other than appropriate measures to prevent further absorption of the poison. The patient should be kept under observation for about 24 h to ensure that delayed toxicity does not develop. The management of symptomatic organophosphate poisoning involves supportive measures and judicious administration of antidotes. Soiled clothing should be removed and contaminated skin washed with soap and water prevents further absorption. The stomach should be emptied if the poison has been ingested less than 1 h previously. Activated charcoal may be given. A clear airway, effective removal of respiratory secretions, and correction of hypoxia are essential using endotracheal intubation and assisted ventilation if necessary. The early use of diazepam may reduce morbidity and mortality; 5 to 10 mg intravenously for an adult reduces anxiety and restlessness but larger doses may be required to control convulsions.

Atropine (2 mg intravenously every 10–30 min for an adult depending on the severity of poisoning) should be given to reduce bronchorrhoea and bronchospasm or until signs of atropinization (flushed dry skin, tachycardia, dilated pupils, and dry mouth) develop. As much as 30 mg and occasionally much more may be required in the first 24 h. Children should be given 0.02 mg/kg body weight but may require up to 0.05 mg/kg.

Oximes such as pralidoxime mesylate (P2S), pralidoxime chloride (2-PAM chloride, 2-PAMCl) or obidoxime (Toxogonin) reactivate phosphorylated cholinesterases. Pralidoxime is preferred because it is less likely to cause hepatic damage and should be given together with atropine to every symptomatic patient. The dose is 30 mg/kg body weight by slow intravenous injection or 7.5 mg/kg body weight/h by continuous infusion after two initial bolus doses 4 h apart.

Improvement in the patient's condition (particularly cessation of convulsions and fasciculation, improvement in muscle power, and recovery of consciousness) will usually be apparent within 30 min. Further bolus doses of the mesylate may be given four-hourly and the chloride six-hourly and may have to be given for several days in severe cases. Alternatively, an infusion of pralidoxime 7.5 mg/kg body weight/h may be administered. Monitoring of cholinesterase activity may be used together with clinical signs to guide the duration of therapy. Giving pralidoxime usually necessitates reducing the dose of atropine and may unmask atropine toxicity.

COMPLICATIONS

A small number of patients develop what has been called the intermediate syndrome which comprises cranial nerve and brain-stem lesions and a proximal neuropathy starting 1 to 4 days after acute intoxication and persisting for 2 to 3 weeks. Respiratory failure secondary to muscle weakness is a potential complication. The aetiology of this syndrome is uncertain but is probably due to inadequate oxime therapy.

A variety of longer-term complications may develop including tiredness, insomnia, inability to concentrate, depression, and irritability. A peripheral neuropathy starting 2 weeks after exposure and mainly affecting the lower limbs is also well recognized. Axonal degeneration of large myelinated motor and sensory fibres has been demonstrated and is thought to be caused by inhibition of neuropathy target esterase.

REFERENCES

Ballantyne, B. and Marrs T.C. *Organophosphates and Carbamates*. Butterworth-Heinemann, Oxford, 1992.

Benson, B.(J.), Tolo, D, McIntyre, M. (1992). Is the intermediate syndrome in organophosphate poisoning the result of insufficient oxime therapy? *Clinical Toxicology*, **30**, 347–9.

De Bleeker, J., *et al.* (1992). Prolonged toxicity with intermediate syndrome after combined parathion and methyl parathion poisoning. *Clinical Toxicology*, **30**, 333–45.

Karalliedde, L. and Henry, J.A. (1993). Effects of organophosphates on skeletal muscle. *Human and Experimental Toxicology*, **12,** 289–96.
Senanayake, N., de Silva, H.J., and Karalliedde, L. (1993). A scale to assess severity in organophosphorus intoxication: POP scale. *Human and Experimental Toxicology*, **12,** 297–9.

Carbamate insecticides

Like organophosphorus compounds, carbamate insecticides combine with cholinesterases and inhibit their function. However, the duration of this effect is comparatively short-lived since the carbamate–enzyme complex tends to dissociate spontaneously. The features of intoxication are similar to those of organophosphate poisoning but seldom so severe. Symptomatic cases require atropine, but the use of oximes is contraindicated and so long as the exposure is not overwhelming, fairly rapid recovery is the rule.

Gamma-hexachlorocyclohexane

Gamma-hexachlorocyclohexane (lindane, gamma-benzene hexachloride) is used widely in agriculture and for the treatment of scabies and pediculosis. Its main toxic effects are on the central nervous system with rapid loss of consciousness and the development of myoclonus, hypertonia, hyperreflexia, convulsions, and rhabdomyolysis. Metabolic acidosis, disseminated intravascular coagulation, renal tubular and hepatocellular necrosis, pancreatitis, and proximal myopathy have been reported.

Treatment is symptomatic and supportive. The stomach should be emptied if the poison has been taken within 1 h and any acid–base abnormality corrected once convulsions have been controlled. Recovery can be expected within 24 to 48 h.

REFERENCE

IPCS (1991). *Environmental Health Criteria 124. Lindane*. WHO, Geneva.

Aluminium phosphide

Aluminium phosphide reacts with moisture in the air to produce phosphine (see Chapter 8.3.7), a gas with a garlic-like odour. Exposure to phosphine causes lacrimation, rhinorrhoea, cough, breathlessness, chest tightness, dizziness, nausea, and drowsiness. Pulmonary oedema and jaundice may develop later. Ingestion of aluminium phosphide causes vomiting, epigastric pain, peripheral circulatory failure, severe metabolic acidosis, and renal failure in addition to many of the features induced by inhalation of phosphine. Treatment is symptomatic and supportive. The stomach should be emptied if the poison has been ingested within 1 h.

REFERENCES

Misra, U.K., Tripathi, A.K., Pandey, R., and Bhargwa, B. (1988). Acute phosphine poisoning following ingestion of aluminium phosphide. *Human Toxicology*, **7,** 343–5.
Sharma, A. and Gathwala, G. (1992). Oral aluminium phosphide poisoning in Indian children. *Journal of Tropical Medicine and Hygiene*, **95,** 221–2.

Pyrethrum and synthetic pyrethroids

Acute poisoning with this group of insecticides is rare. In the most severe cases, coma, convulsions, and pulmonary oedema are the major problems and symptomatic and supportive care is all that can be offered. These insecticides are best known for their ability to cause facial dysaesthesiae as a complication of occupational exposure. These symptoms last only a few hours at most and do not require treatment other than reassurance of the patient that long-term consequences do not occur.

Rodenticides

Warfarin and anticoagulant varieties

Anticoagulant-containing rodenticides are widely used. Initially warfarin was the agent used but concern about resistance of rodents to it has led to the introduction of substances such as brodifacoum, bromodiolone, coumatetralyl, difenacoum, chlorophacinone, and flocoumafen which are commonly referred to as 'superwarfarins'. They are characterized by durations of action which are measured in weeks and months.

Warfarin-containing rodenticides are commonly marketed as prepared baits in which small amounts of the active agent are mixed with cereal. Children are most likely to ingest them but, fortunately, they seldom seem to eat the large amounts necessary to cause serious effects. Deliberate self-poisoning is a more likely cause of morbidity after ingestion of these compounds and, occasionally, is not disclosed causing diagnostic difficulty.

Only a small minority of patients who ingest anticoagulant rodenticides will develop symptoms. Spontaneous bleeding is the usual consequence in those who do, and is generally from the nose, gums, and gastrointestinal and urinary tracts. Less commonly there may be haemorrhage into the skin and brain. Inevitably, there are delays before the maximum anticoagulant effect is reached and with the superwarfarins, some degree of anticoagulation may be induced for weeks or months despite treatment.

Treatment has to be tailored to individual circumstances. It is doubtful if gastric emptying will be of value unless a very large amount has been consumed within the preceding 1 h. Repeated oral administration of adsorbents such as cholestyramine not only prevent absorption but also shorten the plasma half-life of anticoagulant already absorbed. If it is thought that only a small amount has been ingested, no action is required other than to measure the prothrombin time at about 36 to 48 h. Alternatively, vitamin K_1 (5-10 mg intravenously for an adult) could be given intravenously as a prophylactic measure. The latter is also indicated if significant, asymptomatic prothrombin time prolongation has occurred, and if bleeding is already evident, fresh frozen plasma will be necessary for immediate control since vitamin K_1 will not be effective for about 24 h. Repeated doses of vitamin K may be required depending on the amount and specific nature of the compound involved. Monitoring of the prothrombin time will be necessary to determine the need for further treatment.

REFERENCES

Routh, C.R., *et al.* (1991). Superwarfarin ingestion and detection. *American Journal of Hematology*, **36,** 50–4.
Travis, S.F., *et al.* (1993). Spontaneous hemorrhage associated with accidental brodifacoum poisoning in a child. *Journal of Pediatrics*, **122,** 982–4.
Weitzel, J.N., *et al.* (1990). Surreptitious ingestion of a long-acting vitamin K antagonist/rodenticide, brodifacoum: clinical and metabolic studies of three cases. *Blood*, **76,** 2555–9.

Alpha-chloralose

Alpha-chloralose, when used as a rodenticide, is also marketed as cereal baits containing 4 per cent while technical alpha-chloralose (about 90 per cent pure) is used against moles and is occasionally encountered in self-poisoning episodes. The toxic amount for an adult is said to be 1 g and for an infant, 20 mg/kg body weight.

Toxic amounts of alpha-chloralose cause severe CNS excitation with hypersalivation, increased muscle tone, hyper-reflexia, opisthotonus, and convulsions. Rhabdomyolysis is a potential complication. Coma, generalized flaccidity, and respiratory depression may follow.

No treatment is required for most children who ingest alpha-chloralose baits. Supportive measures are necessary when very large amounts of bait or the technical compound is involved. Gastric emptying should not be carried out since the stimulation may provoke seizures. Repeated doses of oral activated charcoal may have a role if a clear airway can be maintained.

REFERENCE

Thomas, H.M., Simpson, D., and Prescott, L.F. (1988). The toxic effects of alpha-chloralose. *Human Toxicology*, **7**, 285–7.

Molluscicides

Metaldehyde

Metaldehyde in the form of pellets is widely used for killing slugs and in some countries as a solid fuel. Small children and animals are most likely to ingest metaldehyde but the consequences are rarely serious. Nausea, vomiting, abdominal pain, and diarrhoea often occur 1 to 3 h after ingestion of any amount while more than 100 mg/kg body weight may cause hypertonia, convulsions, impairment of consciousness, and metabolic acidosis. Hepatic and renal tubular necrosis may become apparent after 2 to 3 days.

The stomach should be emptied if more than 50 mg/kg has been ingested within 1 h. Treatment thereafter is supportive.

REFERENCE

Longstreth, W.T. and Pierson, D.J. (1982). Metaldehyde poisoning from slug bait ingestion. *Western Journal of Medicine*, **137**, 134–7.

8.4 Venoms, toxins, and poisons of animals and plants

8.4.1 Injuries, envenoming, poisoning, and allergic reactions caused by animals

D. A. WARRELL

Mechanical injuries caused by animals

Wild mammals that have killed or severely mauled humans include lion (Fig. 1), tiger, leopard, jaguar, hyena (Fig. 2), wolf, bear, elephant, hippopotamus, buffalo, musk ox, moose, and wild pig. Serious injuries by birds are extremely rare but ostriches have caused fatal injuries. There are about 100 shark attacks reported each year, 50 of them fatal. Most occur between latitudes 30 °N and 30 °S. Other fish capable of causing severe mechanical trauma are barracuda, moray and conger eels, garfish, groupers, and stingrays (see below). Tiny Amazonian catfish (*Vandelia wieneri* and *V.cirrhosa*, Spanish—'canero', Portuguese—'candirú') are the only vertebrate parasites of humans (Plate 1). Attracted by urine, these 5-cm long fish may enter the urethra, vulva, or anus of swimmers causing pain, bleeding, and obstruction. Their spines make them difficult to remove. The 'electric eel' (*Electrophorus electricus*) of South American rivers can discharge up to 650 V, 1 A, 400 times per second, a shock capable of killing an adult. The electric catfish (*Malopterurus electricus*) of African rivers, discharges 90 V at 0.1 A and is not dangerous. The marine torpedo rays can produce a dangerous shock in salt water of 80 V at high amperage. Crocodiles kill about 1000 people each year in Africa (*Crocodilus niloticus*). In Asia, the most important species

Fig. 1 Dr David Livingstone's left humerus with malunited fracture resulting from an attack by a wounded lion at Mabotsa, 220 miles north of Kuruman (South Africa) in 1843. (By courtesy of Professor P.D. Marsden, Brasilia.)

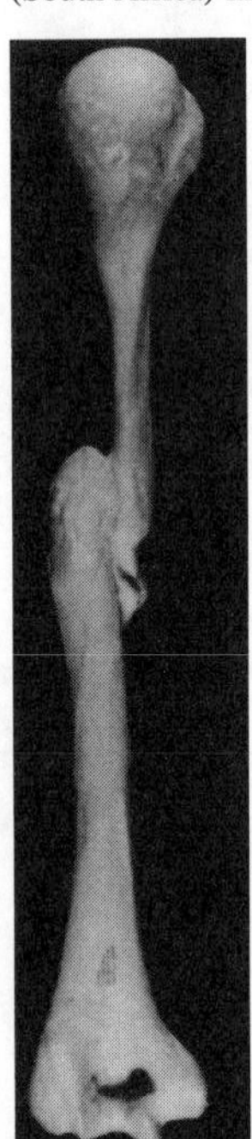

Fig. 2 Severe facial injuries in an Ethiopian boy who was seized by the face by a hyena. (Copyright D.A. Warrell.)

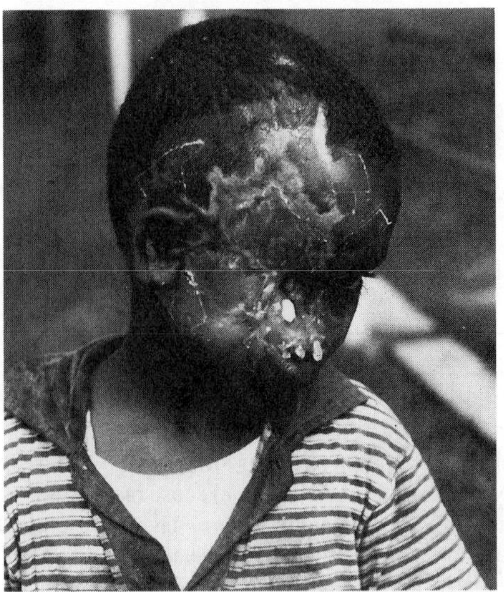

is the salt water or estuarine crocodile (*C.porosus*). In northern Australia seven people have been taken by this species since 1974 and there have been 12 other suspected cases in recent years. Giant pythons have attacked, killed, and even swallowed people in Indonesia (*Python reticulatus*), Africa (*P.sebae*), and South America (*Eunectes murinus*). Collisions between vehicles and deer cause more than one hundred injuries each year in Kentucky and are also common in other areas. In the United States, injuries to horse riders result in more than 46 000 visits to casualty departments each year and at least 20 deaths.

Dog bites

Bites by domestic dogs are common in most parts of the world. An estimated six million dogs live in England and Wales: 209 000 patients bitten by dogs attend hospitals each year (4.2 per 1000 population) and 31 000 of them develop *Pasteurella multocida* wound infections. In Los Angeles, the incidence of animal bites was 664 per 100 000 population in 1956. Approximately 600 000 people are bitten by dogs each year in the United States. In Israel, the incidence of bites is 447 per 100 000 population per year. In Canberra, Australia, 184 children per 100 000 population attended hospital after dog bites in 1977–78. In Britain, there were 701 injuries and 10 deaths attributed to animals in 1975. Reports of 11 deaths from dog bites were collected in a 2-year period in the United States.

Other domestic animals which have caused severe injuries or deaths include camels, cattle, water buffalo, sheep, pigs, cats, and even ferrets.

Clinical features

Teeth, tusks, claws, horns, and spines produce lacerating, penetrating, and crushing injuries. Severe facial and eye injuries are common, for example, among nomadic cattle herders such as the Fulani of Sahel. Pneumothorax, haemothorax, and perforation of the peritoneal cavity and bowel have been reported. Even dog bites may cause compound fractures and kicks by horses or camels are capable of producing fractures or more severe injuries. Among nine cases of camel injury at a durbar in north-western Nigeria, there were two compound and two simple fractures, a dislocation, crush injury, and two lacerations caused by bites and kicks. There is a high risk of infection in wounds inflicted by animals. In England, 30 per cent of dog bite wounds became infected, in half the cases by *Pasteurella multocida*. A wide range of micro-organisms have been implicated, including anaerobic bacteria, as teeth and claws may be contaminated with rotting meat. Large bovines may trample and kneel on the victim producing severe crush injuries.

Treatment

All wounds inflicted by animals should be thoroughly cleaned with soap and water as soon as possible; suitable antiseptics include iodine and alcohol solutions. The use of prophylactic antimicrobials such as co-trimoxazole has not proved effective in dog bite wounds, but is probably justified in the case of multiple or severe wounds and in those at the sites associated with a high risk of infection such as the face and hands. Severe trauma must be assessed in hospital. Emergency surgery may be required with replacement of blood loss; attention to local mechanical complications such as fractures, tension pneumothorax, damage to large blood vessels, perforation of the bowel, and lacerations of other abdominal viscera; and thorough débridement of dead tissue with removal of foreign material, teeth, etc; irrigation, drainage, and delayed closure. In these cases infection must be prevented by using a combination of penicillin, aminoglycoside (such as gentamicin), and metronidazole.

REFERENCES

Barss, P.G. (1982). Injuries caused by garfish in Papua New Guinea. *British Medical Journal*, **284,** 77–9.

Barss, P. and Ennis, S. (1988). Injuries caused by pigs in Papua New Guinea. *Medical Journal of Australia*, **149,** 649–56.

Baxter, D.N. *et al.* (1984). The deleterious effects of dogs on human health. *Community Medicine*, **6,** 29–36, 185–97, 198–203.

Campbell, G.D. and Smith, E.D. (1993). The 'problem' of shark attacks upon humans. *Journal of Wilderness Medicine*, **4,** 5–10.

Caras, R.A. (1975). *Dangerous to man*. Holt, Rinehart and Winston, New York.

Clarke, J. (1969). *Man is the prey*. Andre Deutsch, London.

Coppleson, V.M. (1958). *Shark attack*. Angus and Robertson, Sydney.

Langley, R.L. (1994). Fatal animal attacks in North Carolina over an 18-year period. *American Journal of Forensic Medicine and Pathology* **15,** 160–7.

Middaugh, J.P. (1987). Human injury from bear attacks in Alaska, 1900–1985. *Alaska Medicine*, **29,** 121–6.

Wallet, T. (1978). *Shark attack and treatment of victims in South African waters*. Purnell, Cape Town.

Venomous animals

For predation or defence, some animals secrete venoms which are injected into the prey or enemy through fangs, chelicerae, stings, spines, hairs, nematocysts, or other specialized venom organs, or are squirted on to absorbent mucous membranes by 'spitting' snakes, scorpions, and millipedes. Poisoning may result from ingestion of aquatic animals (see below). Allergic reactions to injected venoms (for example, of Hymenoptera) and ingested poisons (for example, ciguatera) create a more common medical problem than do their direct toxic effects.

REFERENCES

Junghanss, T. and Bodio, M. (1995). *Notfal-Handbuch Gifttiere. Diagnose–Therapie–Biologie*. Georg Thieme Verlag, Stuttgart.

Meier, J. and White, J. (1995). *Clinical toxicology of animal venoms*. CRC Press, Boca Raton.

Venomous mammals

Male duck-billed platypuses (*Ornithorhynchus anatinus*) have venomous spurs on their hind limbs. These aquatic, egg-laying mammals of eastern Australia inflict at least one sting a year on humans in Victoria, but fewer than 20 cases have been reported. There is agonizing local pain, persistent local swelling with a risk of compartmental syndromes, inflammation and regional lymphadenopathy. These effects are not life-threatening and there is no specific treatment. Several species of Insectivora produce venomous saliva conducted into bite wounds by curved and sometimes grooved lower incisors. Venomous species include Haitian and Cuban solenodons (*Solenodon paradoxus*, *Atopogale cubanus*), European water shrew (*Neomys fodiens*), Mediterranean shrew (*N.anomalus*) and the North American short-tailed shrew (*Blarina brevicauda*). Their bites can produce fatal envenoming in rodents and lagomorphs but in humans bites occasionally result in local pain, swelling, and inflammation. Anaphylactic shock and coma have followed bites by the slow loris (*Nycticebus coucang*) of southern Asia. Saliva of vampire bats (Desmodontinae) contains various toxins which promote the flow of blood from the animal on which they are feeding.

REFERENCES

Bucherl, Buckley, E.E., and Deulofeu, V. (eds) (1968). *Venomous Animals and their Venoms*. Vol.1. pp. 15–50. Academic Press, New York.

Dufton, M.J. (1992). Venomous animals. *Pharmacology and Therapeutics*, **53,** 199–215.

Hawkey, C.M. (1988). Salivary antihemostatic factors. In *Natural History of Vampire bats*. (ed. A.M. Greenhall and U. Schmidt), pp. 133–41. CRC Press, Boca Raton.

Venomous snakes

Among the 500 species of venomous snake (families Atractaspididae, Viperidae, Elapidae, and Hydrophiidae) fewer than 200 have been responsible for severe envenoming of humans ending in death or permanent disability. Colubridae, the largest family of snakes, have been regarded as harmless, but an increasing number of species, currently more than 40, are being recognized as capable of envenoming humans, in some cases fatally. Since the distinction between venomous and non-venomous species is uncertain, bites by any snake should be avoided and patients bitten by any species should be assessed carefully.

Fig. 3 Back fangs of the South American colubrid snake *Philodryas olfersii*. A case of fatal envenoming by this species has been reported from Brazil. (Copyright D.A. Warrell.)

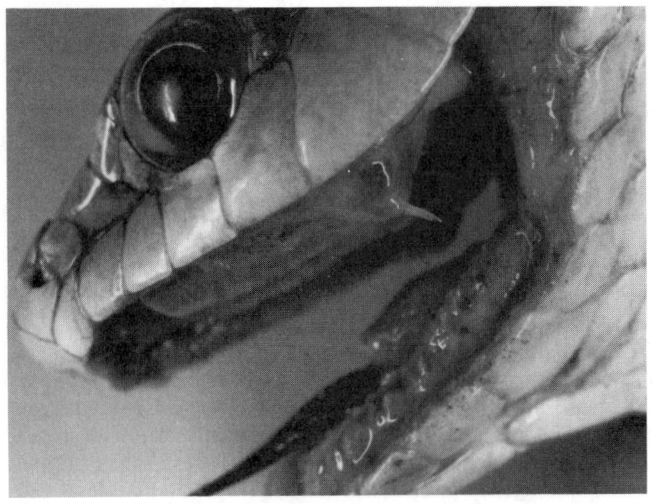

Fig. 4 Burrowing asp (*Atractaspis engaddensis*) showing side-stabbing action with one of the long fangs (arrow) (in this case through a membrane). (Photograph by courtesy of Dr I. Golani and Professor E. Kochva, Tel Aviv.)

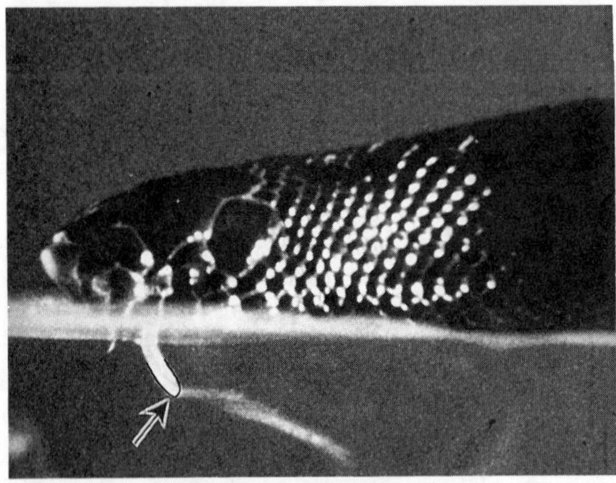

Distribution of venomous snakes

Regions free of venomous snakes include the Antarctic, most of the islands of the western Mediterranean, Atlantic, and Caribbean, Madagascar, New Caledonia, New Zealand, Hawaii and most of the other Pacific islands, Ireland, Iceland, and Chile. Elsewhere, venomous snakes are widely distributed up to altitudes of more than 5300 m (*Agkistrodon himalayanus*), within the Arctic Circle (*Vipera berus*), in the Indian and Pacific Oceans as far north as Siberia (*Pelamis platurus*), and in some freshwater lakes (*Hydrophis semperi*).

CLASSIFICATION

All medically important species possess one or more pairs of enlarged teeth or fangs in the upper jaw. These penetrate the skin of their victim and conduct venom through a groove or closed channel into the tissues.

Colubridae

The short, immobile fangs are at the back of the mouth (Fig. 3). Most of the common and familiar non-venomous species belong to this large family, for example, the British grass snake and smooth snake. Three African species, the boomslang (*Dispholidus typus*) and the vine, twig, or bird snake (*Thelotornis kirtlandii* and *T.capensis*), the Japanese yamakagashi (*Rhabdophis tigrinus*), the southeast Asian red-necked keelback (*R. subminiatus*), the Australasian brown tree snake (*Boiga irregularis*), and the South American *Philodryas olfersii* (Fig. 3) have caused severe envenoming or death.

Atractaspididae

The African and middle eastern burrowing asps or stiletto snakes, also known as burrowing or mole vipers or adders, strike sideways, impaling their victims on a long front fang protruding through the partially closed mouth (Fig. 4). Members of other genera, such as the Natal black snake (*Macrelaps microlepidota*) have fangs at the posterior end of the maxilla.

Three species have caused fatal envenoming: *Atractaspis microlepidota*, *A.engaddensis*, and *A.irregularis*.

Elapidae

This family includes cobras (Fig. 5), kraits, mambas, shield-nose snakes, coral snakes, garter snakes, and Australasian venomous snakes (Fig. 6).

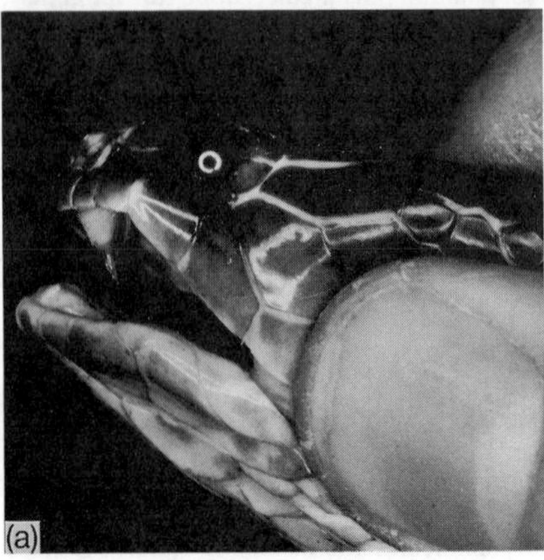

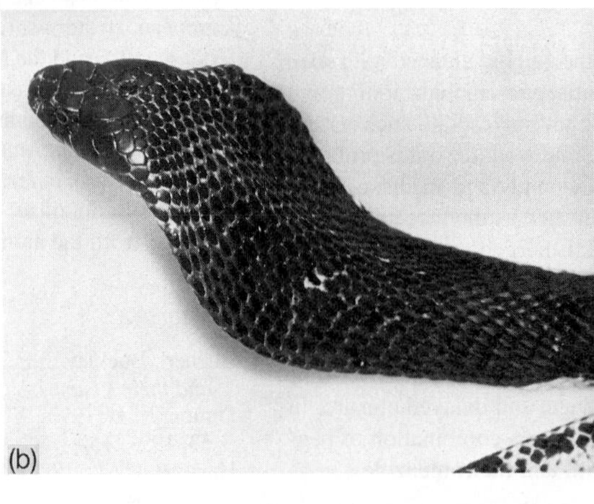

Fig. 5 Cobras. (a) Short front fang of the Sri Lankan cobra (*Naja naja*) a typical elapid snake. (b) Hood of Thai spitting cobra (*Naja siamensis*). (Copyright D.A. Warrell.)

The short, front fangs are immobile (Fig. 5). Several African and Asian species (rinkhals and spitting cobras) can eject their venom from the tips of the fangs as a fine spray for a distance of a few metres into the eyes of an enemy.

Hydrophiidae

The medically important sea snakes have short, fixed front fangs (Fig. 7).

Viperidae

The front fangs are long, curved and capable of a wide range of movement (Fig. 8). The subfamily Crotalinae comprises the American rattlesnakes (Fig. 9), moccasins, lance-headed vipers, and Asian pit vipers which possess a heat-sensitive pit organ behind the nostril (Fig. 10). The vipers and adders of Europe, Africa and Asia (subfamily Viperinae) have no pit organ.

Incidence and importance of snake bites

Snake bite is an important problem of the rural tropics; its incidence is usually underestimated because of the lack of reliable data. In Africa, the saw-scaled or carpet viper (*Echis* sp.), puff adder (*Bitis arietans*), and spitting cobra (*Naja nigricollis, N. mossambica*, etc.) are the most important species. In the Benue Valley of northeastern Nigeria, *E. ocellatus* (Fig. 11) causes some 500 bites per 100 000 population per year with a mortality of 12 per cent and in northern Ghana the same species is responsible for 86 bites per 100 000 population with a mortality of 28 per cent. *Echis* sp., whose geographical range extends through the northern half of Africa and the Middle East to India, probably bite and kill more people than any other species of snake. In the Indian subcontinent, the most important species are cobra (*Naja naja*) (Fig. 5), common krait (*Bungarus caeruleus*), Russell's viper (*Daboia russelii*) (Fig. 8), and *E. carinatus*. Each year more than 1000 people die of snake bite in Maharashtra State alone, and in Sri Lanka there are 60 000 bites and 900 deaths (6 per 100 000 population) per year. In southeast Asia the Malayan pit viper (*Calloselasma rhodostoma*), *D. russelii*, green pit vipers (e.g. *Trimeresurus albolabris*), and the monocellate cobra (*N. kaouthia*) cause most bites and deaths. In Burma, Russell's viper bite has been as high as fifth among causes of death, with an annual mortality of 2000 or more (15 per 100 000 population). In Central and South America, medically important species include rattlesnakes (e.g. *C. durissus terrificus*) (Fig. 9), *Bothrops atrox* ('fer de lance'), *B. asper*, and *B. jararaca*. Earlier this century there were at least 200 snake bite deaths each year in Brazil and in the 1950s and 1960s there were more than 100 deaths each year in Venezuela. In the United States of America there are approximately 45 000 bites per year, 7000 of which are caused by venomous species, with 9 to 14 deaths per year. Most deaths are caused by the eastern and western diamond-back rattlesnakes (*C. adamanteus* and *C. atrox*). In the Amami and Okinawa islands of Japan, the habu (*T. flavoviridis*) (Fig. 10) inflicted an average of 610 bites with 5.6 deaths per year during the 1960s. In Britain, the adder or viper (*Vipera berus*) is the only venomous species (Fig. 12). More than 200

Fig. 6 Papua New Guinean taipan (*Oxyuranus scutellatus canni*), an Australasian elapid snake. (Copyright D.A. Warrell.)

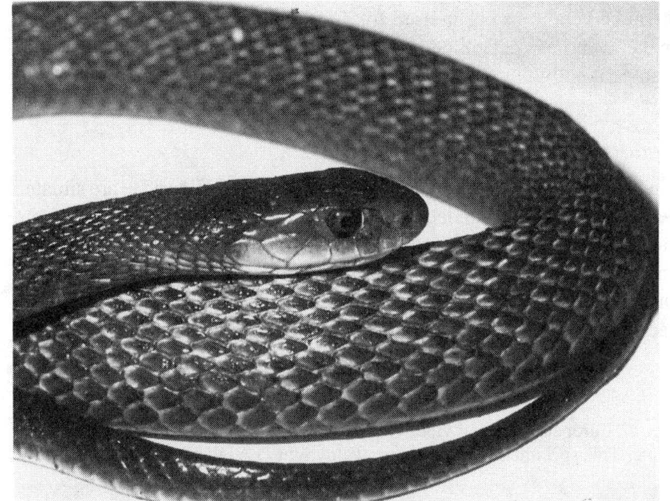

Fig. 7 Short front fangs of the laticaudine sea snake (sea krait) *Laticauda colubrina*. (Copyright D.A. Warrell.)

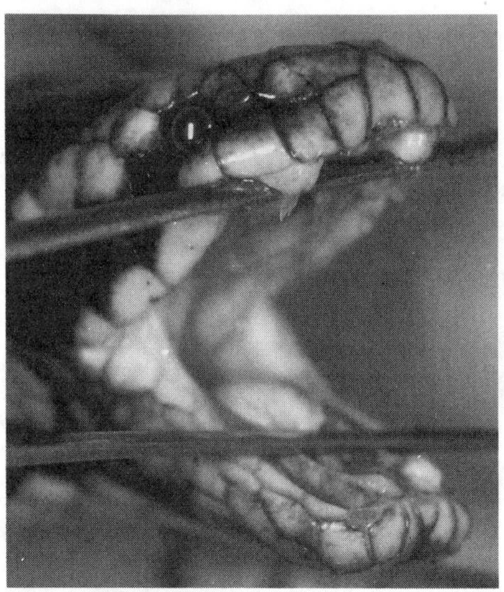

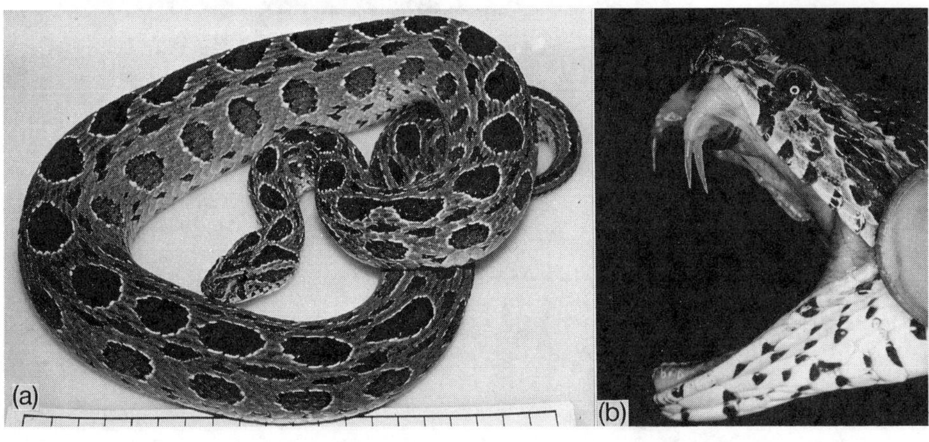

Fig. 8 Russell's vipers (a) Thai Russell's viper (*Daboia russelii siamensis*), a typical viperine snake (scale in cm) (b) Long hinged front fangs (reserve fang on the left side) in dental sheath. (Copyright D.A. Warrell.)

people are bitten each year but only 14 deaths have been reported since 1876. In Sweden, this species causes 150 to 200 hospital admissions each year and 44 deaths between 1911 and 1978, and in Finland, 21 deaths in 25 years with an annual incidence of almost 200 bites. *Vipera aspis* causes most bites in France, while *V. ammodytes* is important in eastern Europe.

In Australia there was an average annual death rate of 11.4 before antivenoms were introduced in the 1930s, more than 200 bites per year with an average of 4.5 deaths per year during the 30 years up to 1977, and 18 deaths during the 10-year period 1981–1991. The principal causes of death are eastern brown snake (*Pseudonaja textilis*), tiger snake (*Notechis scutatus*), taipan (*Oxyuranus scutellatus*) (Fig. 6), and death adder (*Acanthophis* sp.). The highest snake bite mortalities, up to 24 per cent of all adult deaths, are suffered by hunter-gatherer tribes of Brazil, Venezuela, Ecuador, Tanzania, and Papua New Guinea.

Fig. 9 South American tropical rattlesnake or cascabel (*Crotalus durissus cascavella*).

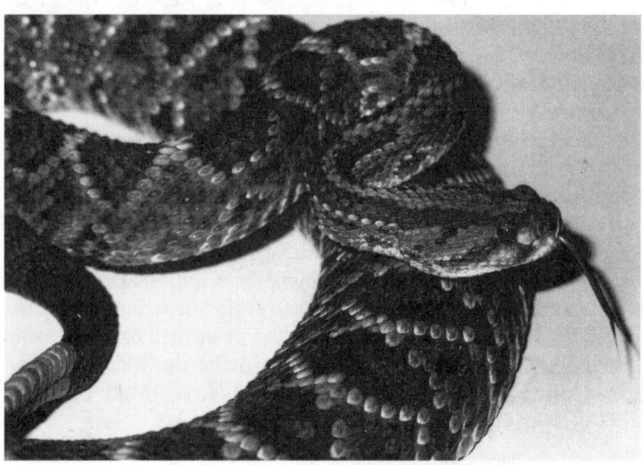

Fig. 10 Heat sensitive pit organ (between eye and nostril) in a Japanese habu (*Trimeresurus flavoviridis*). (Copyright D.A. Warrell.)

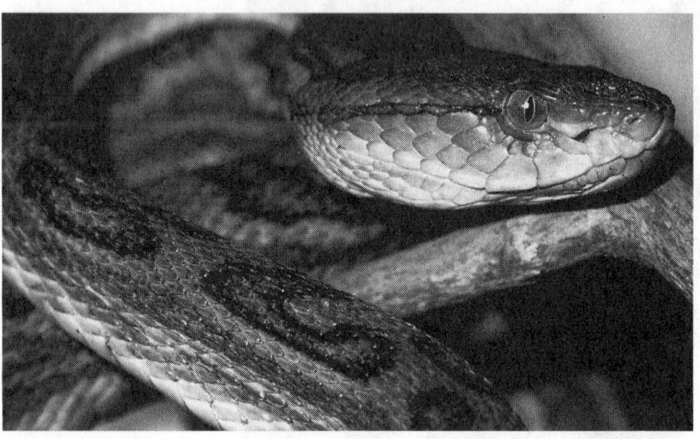

Fig. 11 Saw-scaled or carpet viper from West Africa (*Echis ocellatus*). (Copyright D.A. Warrell.)

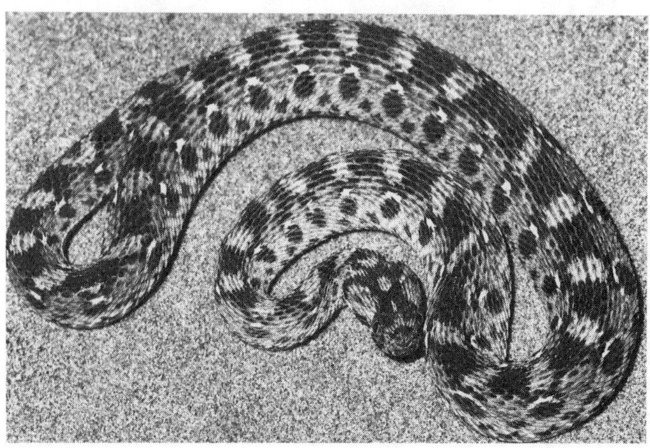

Epidemiology

Most snake bites are inflicted on the lower limbs of farmers, plantation workers, herdsmen, and hunters in the rural tropics. Usually the snake is trodden on at night or in undergrowth. Some species such as the Asiatic kraits (*Bungarus sp.*) and African spitting cobras (*N. nigricollis*) enter dwellings at night and bite people who are asleep. Snakes do not bite without provocation, but this may be an inadvertent tread or touch. In Europe and North America snakes are increasingly popular 'macho' pets: in these countries many bites are inflicted on the hands of people who are picking up the snake and in the United States, 25 per cent of bites result from snakes being attacked or handled. Serious bites by back-fanged (colubrid) snakes usually occur only under these conditions. Seasonal peaks in the incidence of snake bite are associated with agricultural activities, such as ploughing before the annual rains in the West African Sahel and the rice harvest in southeast Asia, or to fluctuations in the activity or population of venomous snakes. Severe flooding, by concentrating the human and snake populations, has given rise to epidemics of snake bite in Colombia, Pakistan, India, Bangladesh, and Vietnam. Penetration of jungle areas during construction of new highways and irrigation and hydroelectric schemes has led to an increased incidence of snake bite in Brazil and Sri Lanka. Snake bite or injection of snake venom has been used for murder and suicide, and some crude snake venoms or refined venom procoagulants have been used therapeutically.

Venom apparatus

The venom glands of Elapidae, Hydrophiidae, and Viperidae are situated behind the eye, surrounded by compressor muscles (Fig. 13). A venom duct opens within the sheath at the base of the fang and venom is conducted to its tip through a canal. In Colubridae, venom secreted by Duvernoy's gland tracks down grooves in the anterior surfaces of the back fangs (Fig. 3). The average quantity of venom injected at a strike

Fig. 12 European adder or viper (*Vipera berus*), Britain's only venomous snake. This specimen is 50 cm long. (Copyright D.A. Warrell.)

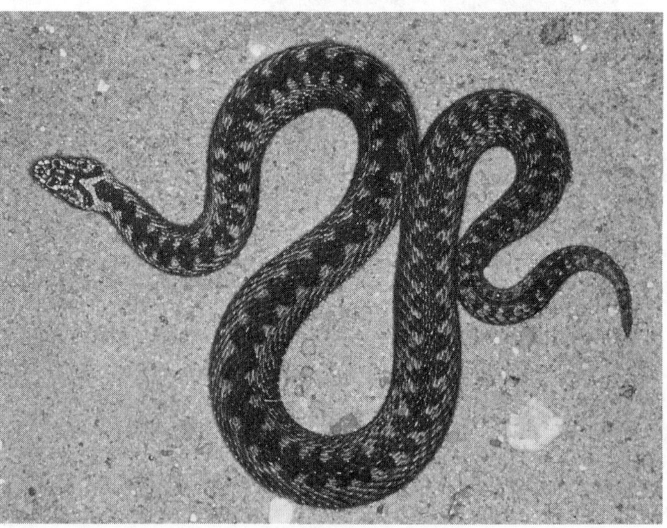

is approximately 60 mg in *N. naja*, 13 mg in *E. carinatus*, 63 mg in *D. russelii*, and 32 mg in *V. palaestinae* (dry weights). The amount injected into human patients is very variable so that a proportion of them suffer only negligible envenoming. More than half of those bitten by the Malayan pit viper (*C. rhodostoma*) and Russell's viper show only trivial effects. *Vipera palaestinae* uses only about one-tenth of the content of its venom gland at each strike, whereas *D. russelii* exhausts more than three-quarters of the supply at the first strike. There is no support for the popular belief that snakes are less dangerous after they have eaten.

Venom properties

Snake venoms may contain 20 or more components. More than 90 per cent of the dry weight is protein, in the form of enzymes, non-enzymatic polypeptide toxins, and non-toxic proteins. The role of enzymes in envenoming is most clearly seen in the case of venom procoagulants. For example, *D. russelii* venom contains a serine protease which activates factor X and an arginine ester hydrolase which activates factor V. The zinc metalloproteinase, ecarin (*E. carinatus*) and the serine proteases oscutarin (*O. scutellatus*) and notecarin (*N. scutatus*) activate prothrombin. Many crotaline venoms contain thrombin-like proteases which cleave the fibrinogen molecule, for example, ancrod (*C. rhodostoma*), batroxobin (*B.atrox*), and crotalase (*C. adamanteus*). Phospholipase A_2 (lecithinase) is the most widespread venom enzyme. It may contribute to myotoxicity, neurotoxicity, cardiotoxicity, haemolysis, and increased vascular permeability. Hyaluronidase promotes spread of venom. L-Amino acid oxidase is responsible for the bright yellow colour of some viper venoms.

Fig. 13 Venom apparatus of viperine and crotaline snakes. (a) Venom gland of Palestine viper (*Vipera palaestinae*); (b) Venom gland of Western rattlesnake (*Crotalus viridis*). C = compressor glandulae muscle; VG = venom gland; AG = accessory gland; F = fang. (Dissection by Professor E. Kochva, reproduced from Gans, C. and Gans, K.A. (eds.), 1978, *Biology of the reptilia*, vol 8. Academic Press, London, by permission.)

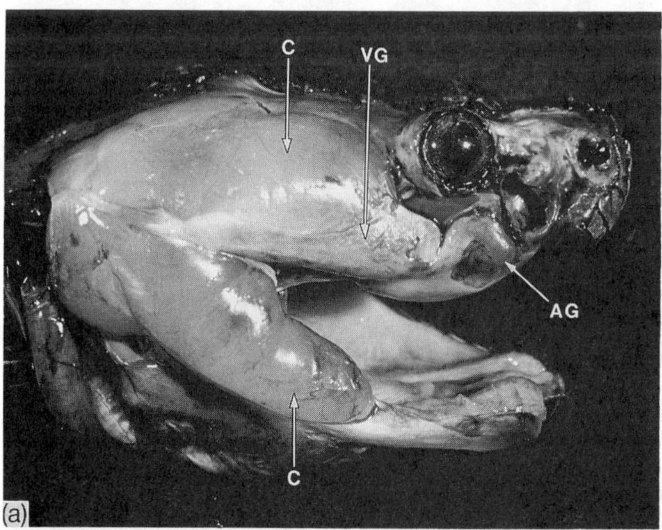

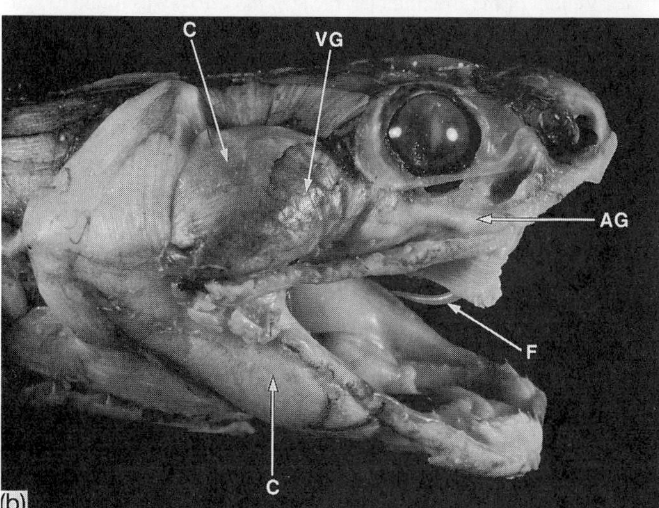

POLYPEPTIDE TOXINS (NEUROTOXINS)

Postsynaptic (α-) neurotoxins such as α-bungarotoxin and cobrotoxin, contain about 60 to 62 (short chain) or 66 to 74 (long chain) amino acid residues and bind to acetylcholine receptors at the motor end-plate. Toxic phospholipases A_2 can block neuromuscular transmission by acting pre- or postsynaptically and can damage skeletal muscle. They include the presynaptic (β-) neurotoxins, β-bungarotoxin, crotoxin and taipoxin. Presynaptic neurotoxins block the release of acetylcholine at the neuromuscular junction.

PHARMACOLOGY

The neurotoxins of Elapidae and Hydrophiidae are rapidly absorbed into the bloodstream, whereas the much larger molecules of Viperidae venoms are taken up more slowly through lymphatics. Venoms of the spitting cobras and rinkhals can be absorbed through the intact cornea, causing systemic envenoming and even death in animals. Envenoming after ingestion of snake venom has not been reported in humans. Most venoms are concentrated and bound in the kidney and some components are eliminated in the urine. Crotaline venoms are selectively bound in the lungs, concentrated in the liver and excreted in bile, while neurotoxins such as α-bungarotoxin, are tightly bound at neuromuscular junctions. Most venom components do not cross the blood–brain barrier.

Pathophysiology

Swelling and bruising of the bitten limb result from increased vascular permeability induced by proteases, phospholipases, membrane-damaging polypeptide toxins, and endogenous autacoids released by the venom, such as histamine, 5-hydroxytryptamine, and kinins. Venoms of some of the North American rattlesnakes and viperine species cause a generalized increase in vascular permeability resulting in hypovolaemia, haemoconcentration, hypoalbuminaemia, albuminburia, serous effusions, pulmonary oedema, and, in the case of Burmese *D. russelii*, conjunctival and facial oedema (Fig. 14). Tissue necrosis near to the site of

Fig. 14 Gross bilateral conjunctival oedema (chemosis) in a Burmese rice farmer 48 h after being bitten by a Russell's viper (*Daboia russelii siamensis*). (Copyright D.A. Warrell.)

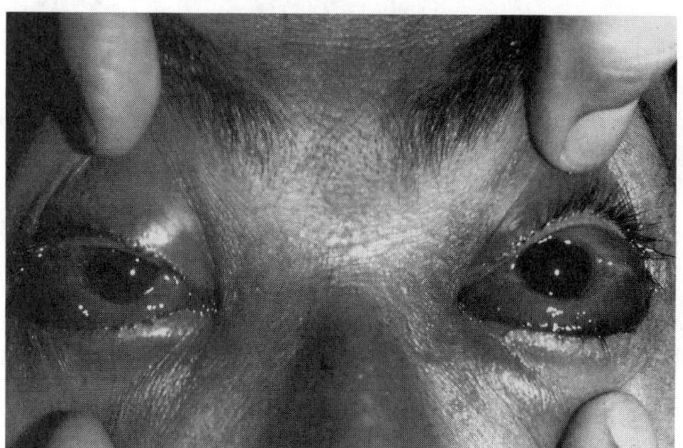

Fig. 15 Amino-acid sequences of endothelins and sarafotoxins (from the venom of *Atractaspis engaddensis*) (redrawn from Sokolovsky, M. (1992) *Journal of Neurochemistry*, **59,** 809–821).

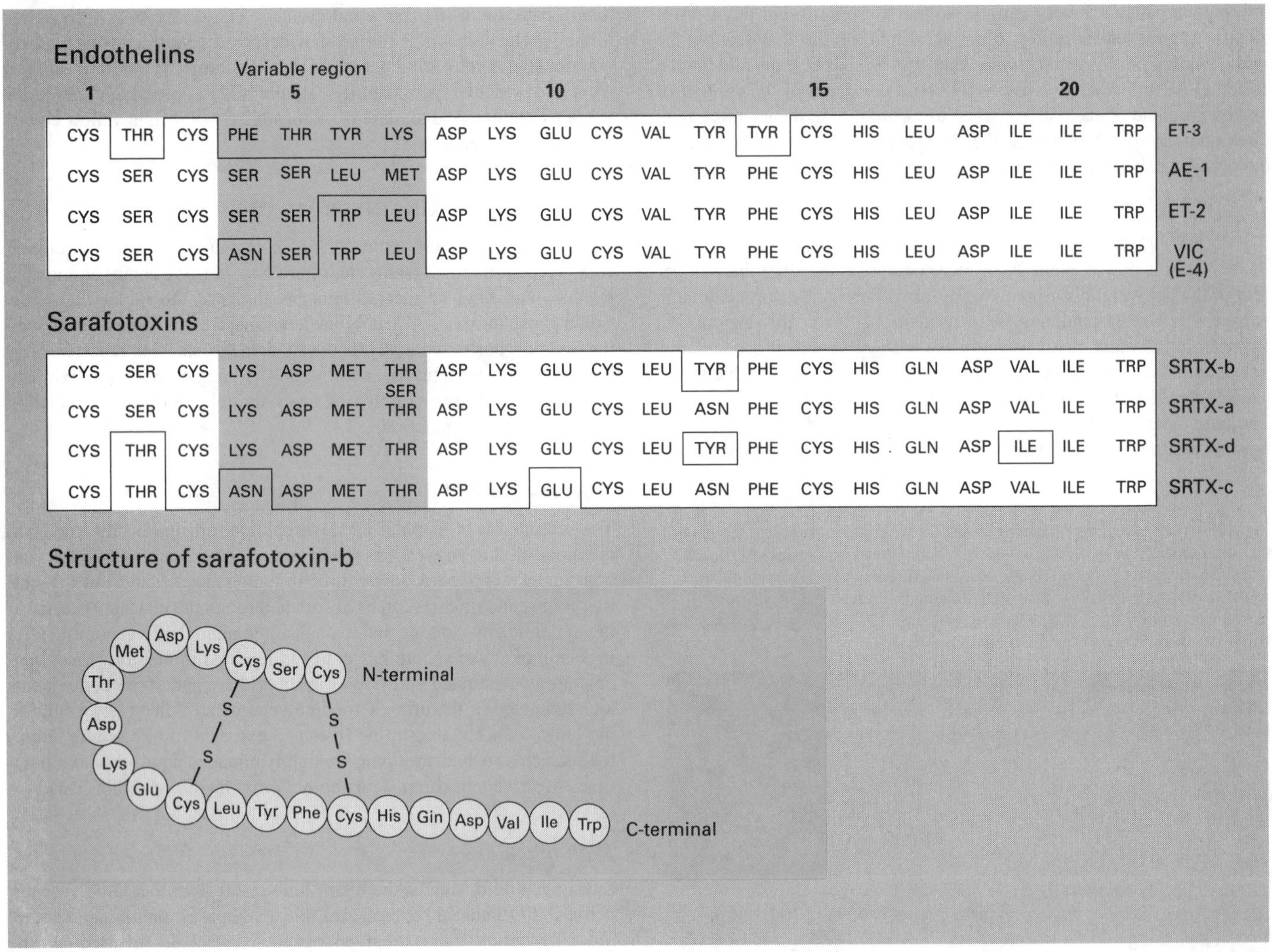

Endothelins

Variable region

1				5					10					15					20		
CYS	THR	CYS	PHE	THR	TYR	LYS	ASP	LYS	GLU	CYS	VAL	TYR	TYR	CYS	HIS	LEU	ASP	ILE	ILE	TRP	ET-3
CYS	SER	CYS	SER	SER	LEU	MET	ASP	LYS	GLU	CYS	VAL	TYR	PHE	CYS	HIS	LEU	ASP	ILE	ILE	TRP	AE-1
CYS	SER	CYS	SER	SER	TRP	LEU	ASP	LYS	GLU	CYS	VAL	TYR	PHE	CYS	HIS	LEU	ASP	ILE	ILE	TRP	ET-2
CYS	SER	CYS	ASN	SER	TRP	LEU	ASP	LYS	GLU	CYS	VAL	TYR	PHE	CYS	HIS	LEU	ASP	ILE	ILE	TRP	VIC (E-4)

Sarafotoxins

CYS	SER	CYS	LYS	ASP	MET	THR	ASP	LYS	GLU	CYS	LEU	TYR	PHE	CYS	HIS	GLN	ASP	VAL	ILE	TRP	SRTX-b
CYS	SER	CYS	LYS	ASP	MET	SER THR	ASP	LYS	GLU	CYS	LEU	ASN	PHE	CYS	HIS	GLN	ASP	VAL	ILE	TRP	SRTX-a
CYS	THR	CYS	LYS	ASP	MET	THR	ASP	LYS	GLU	CYS	LEU	TYR	PHE	CYS	HIS	GLN	ASP	ILE	ILE	TRP	SRTX-d
CYS	THR	CYS	ASN	ASP	MET	THR	ASP	LYS	GLU	CYS	LEU	ASN	PHE	CYS	HIS	GLN	ASP	VAL	ILE	TRP	SRTX-c

Structure of sarafotoxin-b

Asp Met Lys Cys Ser Cys N-terminal
Thr Asp Lys Glu S S S S
Cys Leu Tyr Phe Cys His Gin Asp Val Ile Trp C-terminal

Fig. 16 Haemorrhagin activity. An erythrocyte (E) spurting through an open endothelial junction (J) between endothelial cells (En) from the lumen (L) of rat mesenteric blood vessel, 5 min after exposure to habu (*Trimeresurus flavoviridis*) venom. Note extensive destruction of the basement membrane (Bm), and failure of the platelet (P) to undergo viscous metamorphosis. (By courtesy of Dr A. Ohsaka and Academic Press, from Ohsaka, A., Suzuki, K., and Ohashi, M. (1975). *Microvascular Research*, **10,** 208.)

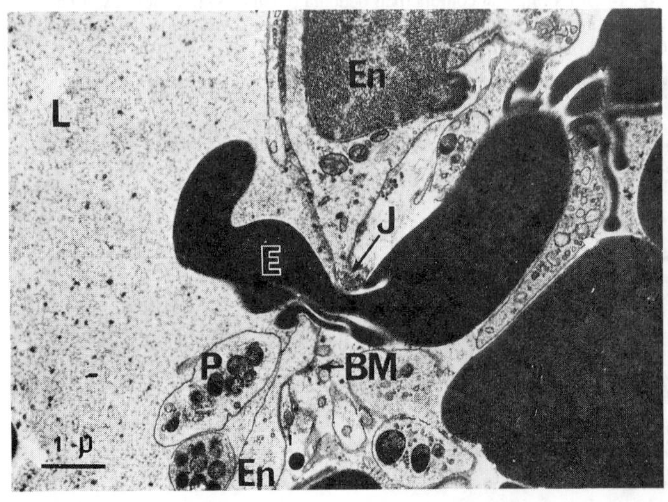

the bite is caused by myotoxic and cytolytic factors: in some cases, ischaemia resulting from thrombosis, intracompartmental syndrome, or a tight tourniquet may contribute. Causes of hypotension and shock include hypovolaemia, vasodilatation, and myocardial dysfunction. Some venoms release vasodilating autacoids such as histamine and kinins. Venom of the Brazilian jararaca (*B. jararaca*) was found to activate bradykinin and, through a bradykinin-potentiating peptide, to prolong its hypotensive effect by inactivating the peptidyl dipeptidase responsible both for destroying bradykinin and converting angiotensin I to angiotensin II. This led to the synthesis of ACE inhibitors. Bradykinin-potentiating and ACE-inhibiting peptides have subsequently been found in a number of other crotaline venoms (genera Bothrops and Agkistrodon). Four sarafotoxins have been isolated from the venom of the Israeli burrowing asp (*Atractaspis engaddensis*) (Fig. 4). They show about 60 per cent sequence homology with endothelins, also 21 amino acid polypeptides, with which they share potent vasoconstrictor/vasodilator properties (Fig. 15). Snake venoms can cause haemostatic defects in a number of different ways: venom procoagulants can activate the blood clotting cascade at various sites. Some Viperidae venoms contain fibrinogenases which degrade fibrinogen directly, others activate endogenous plasminogen. Venoms may induce or inhibit platelet aggregation. Spontaneous systemic bleeding is caused by haemorrhagins which damage vascular endothelium (Fig. 16). The combination of defibrination, thrombocytopenia, and vessel wall damage can result in massive and incontinent bleeding, a common cause of death after bites by Viperidae. Many venoms are haemolytic *in vitro*, but clinically significant intravascular haemolysis, apart from mild microangiopathic haemolysis associated with disseminated intravascular coagulation, is seen only after bites by *D. russelii* (Sri Lanka and India), some Bothrops, Australasian elapid, and colubrid species. Acute renal tubular necrosis may be caused by severe hypotension, disseminated intravascular coagulation (*D. russelii*), a direct nephrotoxic effect of the venom (*D. russelii*) and myoglobinuria secondary to generalized rhabdomyolysis (Hydrophiidae, Australasian elapids, *D. russelii* in Sri Lanka and India and *C. d. terrificus*). Neurotoxic polypeptides and phospholipases block neuromuscular transmission causing death by bulbar or respiratory paralysis.

Clinical features

Fear and effects of treatment as well as the venom contribute to the symptoms and signs in those bitten by snakes. Even patients who are not envenomed may feel flushed, dizzy, and breathless and may notice constriction of the chest, palpitations, sweating, and acroparaesthesiae. Tight tourniquets may produce congested and ischaemic limbs; local incisions at the site of the bite may cause bleeding and sensory loss and herbal medicines often induce vomiting. The earliest symptoms directly attributable to the bite are local pain and bleeding from the fang punctures, followed by pain, tenderness, swelling and bruising extending up the limb, lymphangitis, and tender enlargement of regional lymph nodes. Early syncope, vomiting, colic, diarrhoea, angio-oedema, and wheezing may follow bites by some snakes (e.g. European Vipera, *D. russelii*, *Bothrops* sp., Australian elapids, and *Atractaspis engaddensis*). Nausea and vomiting are common symptoms of severe envenoming.

BITES BY COLUBRIDAE (BACK-FANGED SNAKES)

Patients with severe or fatal envenoming experience repeated vomiting, colicky abdominal pain and headache, widespread systemic bleeding including extensive ecchymoses (Fig. 17), incoagulable blood, intravascular haemolysis, and renal failure. In some cases (Fig. 18) local swelling and bruising may be the only results of envenoming. Envenoming may develop slowly over several days.

Fig. 17 Brazilian patient who was bitten by the back-fanged snake *Philodryas olfersii* (see Fig. 3), showing swelling of the bitten arm and extensive ecchymoses. (By courtesy of Dr João Luiz Costa Cardoso, São Paulo, Brazil.)

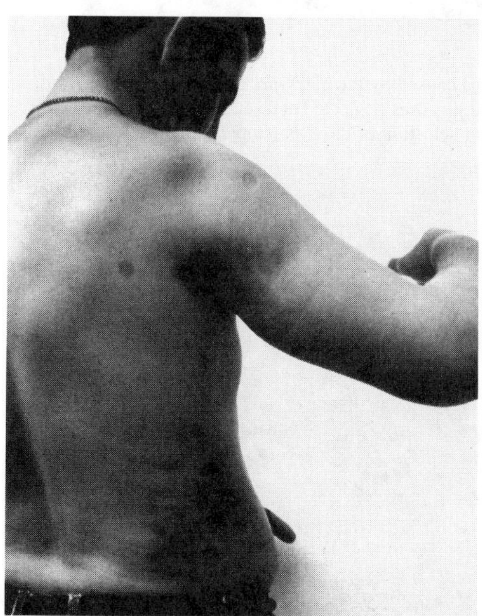

BITES BY ATRACTASPIDIDAE (BURROWING ASPS OR STILETTO SNAKES; NATAL BLACK SNAKE)

Local effects include pain, swelling, blistering, necrosis, and tender enlargement of local lymph nodes. Violent gastrointestinal symptoms (nausea, vomiting, and diarrhoea), anaphylaxis (dyspnoea, respiratory failure), and ECG changes (A-V block, ST, T wave changes) have been described in patients envenomed by *A. engaddensis*.

BITES BY ELAPIDAE (COBRAS, KRAITS, MAMBAS, CORAL SNAKES, AND AUSTRALASIAN SNAKES)

Bites by kraits, mambas, coral snakes, and some cobras (e.g. *N. haje* and *N. nivea*) produce minimal local effects, but the venoms of African spitting cobras (*N. nigricollis*, *N. mossambica*, etc.) and Asian cobras *N. naja*, *N. kaouthia*, *N. sumatrana*, etc.) cause tender local swelling, blistering, and superficial necrosis which may be extensive (Fig. 19). However, elapid venoms are best known for their neurotoxic effects. Early symptoms, before there are objective neurological signs, include

Fig. 18 Swelling of the left hand in a zoo-keeper who was bitten by the South American false cobra (*Hydrodynastes* or *Cyclagras gigas*). (By courtesy of Mr Dave Ball, London.)

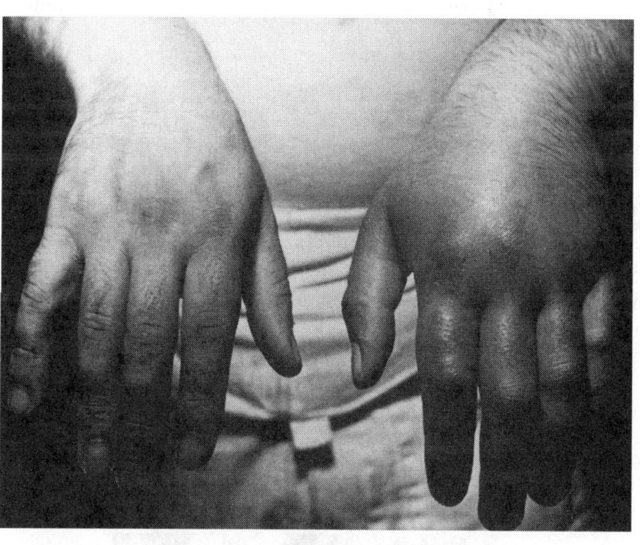

Fig. 19 Extensive necrosis of skin and subcutaneous tissues in a Nigerian girl bitten 9 days previously on the elbow by a black-necked or spitting cobra (*Naja nigricollis*). (Copyright D.A. Warrell.)

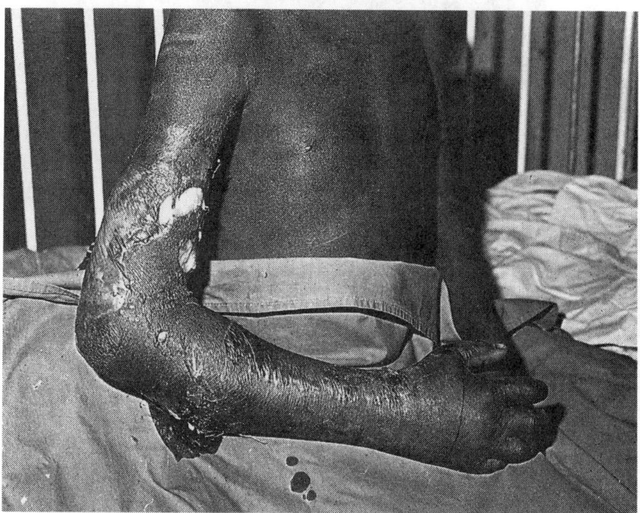

vomiting, 'heaviness' of the eyelids, blurred vision, paraesthesiae around the mouth, hyperacusis, headache, dizziness, vertigo, hypersalivation, congested conjunctivae, and 'gooseflesh'. Paralysis is first detectable as ptosis and external ophthalmoplegia appearing as early as 15 min after the bite, but sometimes delayed for 10 h or more. Later the face, palate, jaws, tongue, vocal cords, neck muscles, and muscles of deglutition may become paralysed (Fig. 20). Respiratory failure may be precipitated by airway obstruction at this stage, or later after paralysis of intercostal muscles and diaphragm. Neurotoxic effects are completely reversible either acutely in response to antivenom or anticholinesterases (e.g. following bites by Asian cobras, some Latin American coral snakes—Micrurus, and Australasian death adders—Acanthophis) or they may wear off spontaneously in 1 to 7 days.

Envenoming by terrestrial Australasian snakes produces three main groups of symptoms: neurotoxicity (Fig. 21), haemostatic disturbances and, rarely, generalized rhabdomyolysis and renal failure. Painful regional lymph nodes are a useful sign of impending systemic envenoming, but local signs are usually mild. Early symptoms include vomiting, headache, and syncopal attacks.

Patients 'spat' at by spitting elapids may develop venom ophthalmia. There is intense pain in the eye, blepharospasm, palpebral oedema, and leucorrhoea (Fig. 22). Corneal erosions can be seen by slit lamp or fluorescein examination in more than half the patients spat at by *N. nigricollis*. Rarely, venom is absorbed into the anterior chamber causing hypopyon and anterior uveitis. Secondary infection of corneal abrasions may lead to permanent blinding opacities or panophthalmitis (Fig. 22).

BITES BY HYDROPHIIDAE (SEA SNAKES AND SEA KRAITS)

Patients envenomed by sea snakes notice headache, a thick feeling of the tongue, thirst, sweating, and vomiting. Some 30 min to 3.5 h after the bite there is generalized aching, stiffness, and tenderness of the muscles (Fig. 23). Trismus is common. Later there is generalized flaccid paralysis as in elapid neurotoxicity (Fig. 24). Myoglobinuria appears 3 to 8 h after the bite. Myoglobin and potassium released from damaged skeletal muscles can cause renal failure, while hyperkalaemia may precipitate cardiac arrest.

Fig. 20 Neurotoxic envenoming. Ptosis, ophthalmoplegia and inability to open the mouth and protrude the tongue in a Sri Lankan patient envenomed by the common krait (*Bungarus caeruleus*). (Copyright D.A. Warrell.)

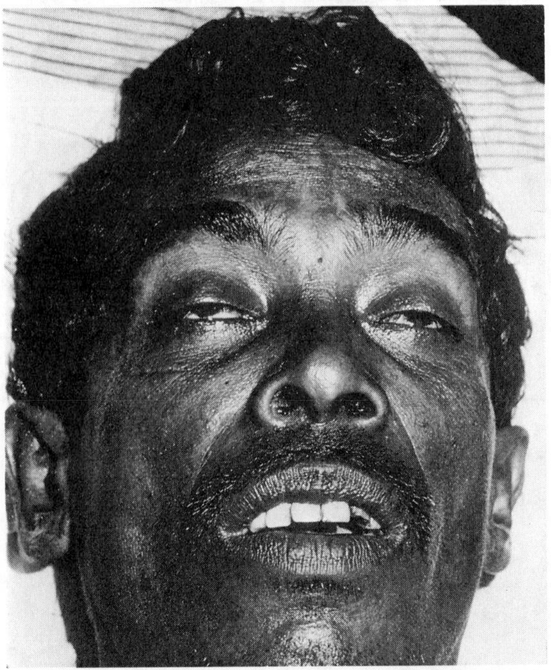

BITES BY VIPERIDAE (VIPERS, ADDERS, RATTLESNAKES, LANCE-HEADED VIPERS, MOCCASINS, AND PIT VIPERS)

Venoms of Viperidae usually produce more severe local effects than other snake venoms. Swelling may become detectable within 15 min but is sometimes delayed for several hours. It spreads rapidly and may involve the whole limb and adjacent trunk. There is associated pain and tenderness in regional lymph nodes. Bruising, blistering, and necrosis may appear during the next few days (Fig. 25). Necrosis is particularly frequent and severe following bites by some rattlesnakes, lance-headed vipers (genus Bothrops), Asian pit vipers, and African giant vipers (genus Bitis). When the envenomed tissue is contained in a tight fascial compartment such as the pulp space of digits or anterior tibial compartment ischaemia may result (Fig. 26). If there is no swelling 2 h after

Fig. 21 Generalized paralysis, including ptosis, external ophthalmoplegia, inability to open the mouth, protrude the tongue, swallow, or speak, and respiratory paralysis requiring mechanical ventilation in a Papua New Guinean man bitten 24 h previously by a taipan (*Oxyuranus scutellatus canni*). (Copyright D.A. Warrell.)

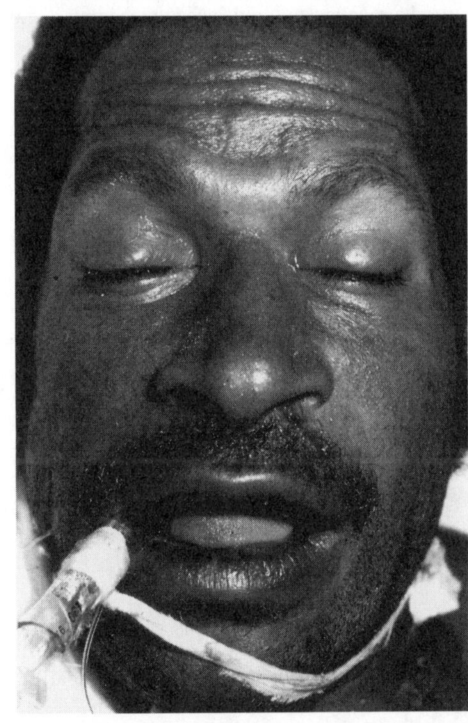

Fig. 22 Venom ophthalmia caused by the black-necked spitting cobra (*Naja nigricollis*). The corneal injury was neglected and secondary infection developed, necessitating enucleation of the eye. (Copyright D.A. Warrell.)

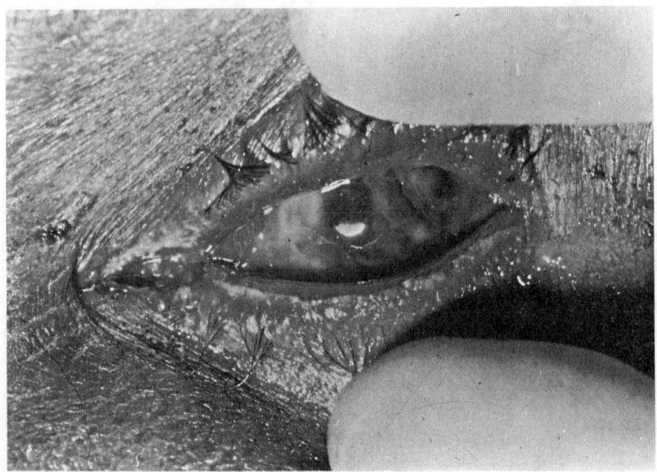

a viper bite it is usually safe to assume that there has been no envenoming. However, fatal envenoming by a few species can occur in the absence of local signs (e.g. *C.d. terrificus*, *C. scutulatus*, and Burmese Russell's viper). Haemostatic abnormalities are characteristic of envenoming by Viperidae. Persistent bleeding from fang puncture wounds, venepuncture or injection sites, other new and partially healed wounds, and postpartum suggests that the blood is incoagulable. Spontaneous systemic haemorrhage is most often detected in the gingival sulci (Fig. 27). Epistaxis, haematemesis, cutaneous ecchymoses, haemoptysis, subconjunctival, retroperitoneal, and intracranial haemorrhages (Fig. 28) are also reported. Patients envenomed by the Burmese Russell's viper may bleed into the anterior pituitary (Sheehan's syndrome) (Fig. 29). Hypotension and shock are common in patients bitten by some of the North American rattlesnakes (e.g. *C. adamanteus*, *C. atrox*, and *C. scutulatus*), *Bothrops*, *Daboia*, and *Vipera* species (e.g. *V. palaestinae* and *V. berus*). The central venous pressure is usually low and the pulse rate rapid suggesting hypovolaemia for which the usual cause is extravasation of fluid into the bitten limb. Patients envenomed by Burmese Russell's vipers show evidence of generally increased vascular permeability (Fig. 14). Direct myocardial involvement is suggested by an abnormal ECG or cardiac arrhythmia. Patients envenomed by some species of the genera Vipera and Bothrops may experience transient recurrent syncopal attacks associated with features of an autopharmacological or anaphylactic reaction such as vomiting, sweating, colic, diarrhoea, shock, and angio-oedema. These symptoms may appear as early as 5 min or as late

Fig. 23 Trismus, generalized myalgia, and muscle stiffness (resistance to passive movement) in a Malaysian patient envenomed by a sea snake, probably *Enhydrina schistosa*. (By courtesy of the late Dr H.A. Reid.)

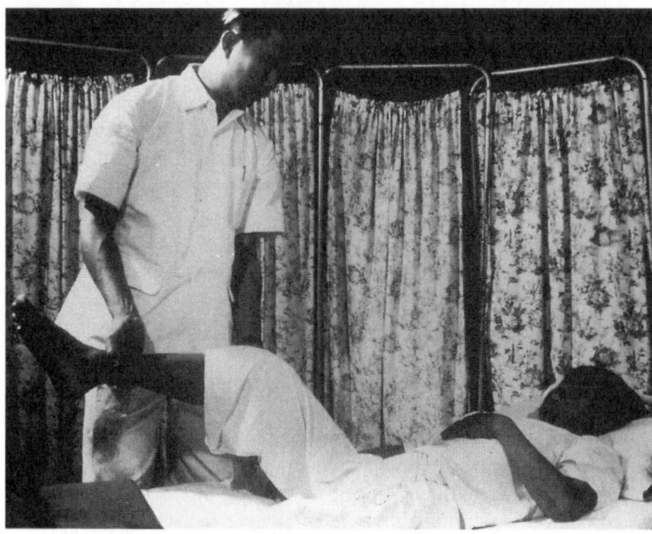

Fig. 24 Ptosis and external ophthalmoplegia in a Malaysian fisherman bitten by a sea snake (probably *Enhydrina schistosa*). (By courtesy of the late Dr H.A. Reid.)

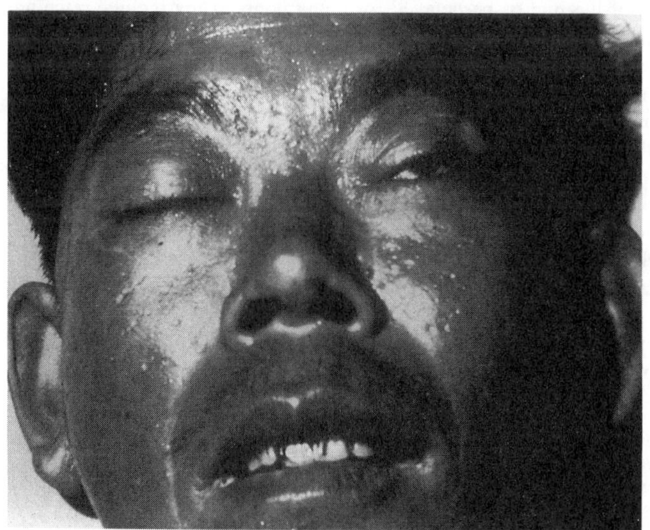

Fig. 25 Severe blistering in a Thai boy bitten on the leg by a Malayan pit viper (*Calloselasma rhodostoma*). (Copyright D.A. Warrell.)

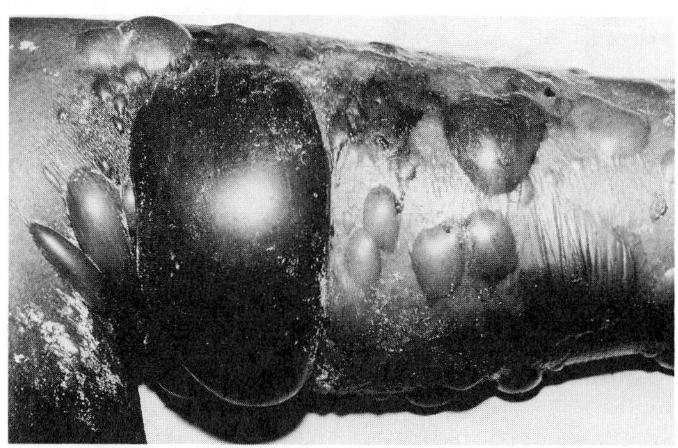

Fig. 26 Extensive necrosis of skin and muscle including the contents of the anterior tibial compartment. The periosteum has been drilled to encourage granulation (same patient as in Fig. 25). (Copyright D.A. Warrell.)

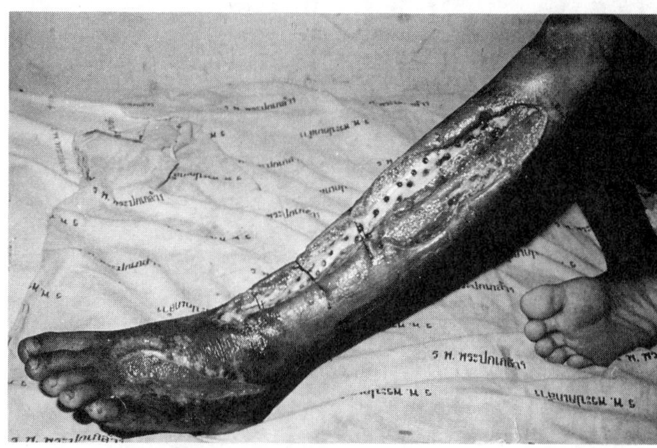

Fig. 27 Bleeding from gingival sulci in a Nigerian patient bitten by *Echis ocellatus*. (Copyright D.A. Warrell.)

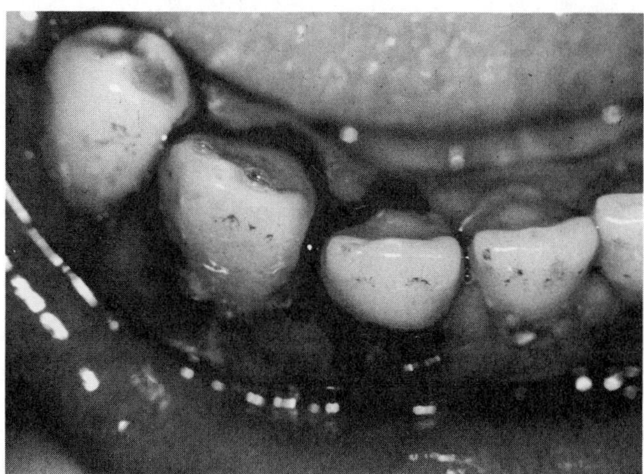

as many hours after the bite. Renal failure is the major cause of death in patients envenomed by some species of Viperidae. Victims of Russell's viper may become oliguric within a few hours of the bite and have loin pain suggesting renal ischaemia. Neurotoxicity, resembling that seen in patients bitten by Elapidae, is a feature of envenoming by a few species of Viperidae (e.g. *C. d. terrificus*, Far Eastern *Agkistrodon* sp., *Bitis atropos*, and Sri Lankan *D. russelii pulchella*). There is evidence of generalized rhabdomyolysis (Fig. 30). Progression to respiratory or generalized paralysis is unusual.

Fig. 28 Cerebral haemorrhage in a Burmese victim of Russell's viper (*Daboia russelii siamensis*). (By courtesy of Dr U Hla Mon, Yangon, Myanmar.)

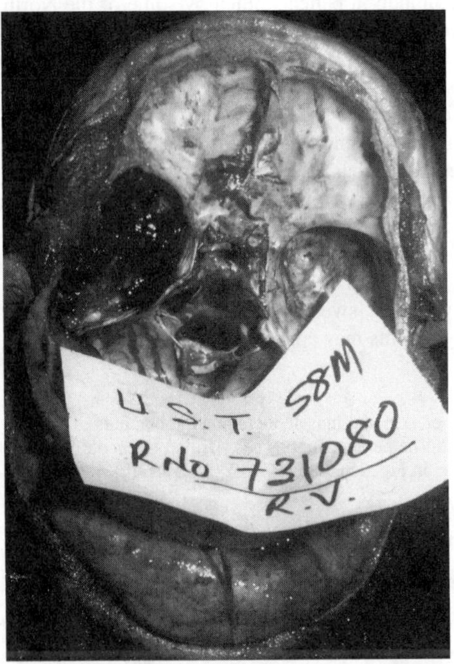

Fig. 29 Haemorrhage of anterior pituitary in a Burmese patient who died after being bitten by a Russell's viper (*Daboia russelii siamensis*). (By courtesy of Dr U Hla Mon, Yangon, Myanmar.)

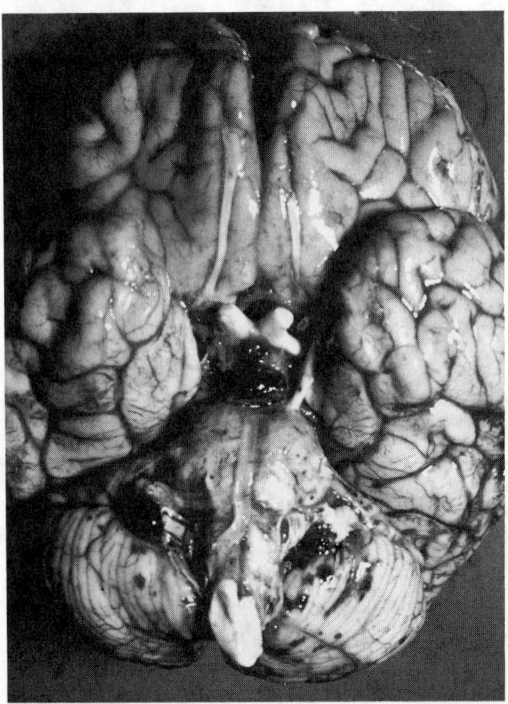

ENVENOMING BY EUROPEAN VIPERS

The common viper, or adder (*V. berus*) (Fig. 12) is the only venomous snake found in Britain. This species occurs in England, Wales, and Scotland and extends across northern Europe into the Arctic Circle and through Asia as far east as Sakhalin Island and south to northern Korea. Four other vipers are widely distributed in mainland Europe: the nose-horned or sand viper (*V. ammodytes*) in the Balkans, Italy, Austria, and Romania; the asp viper (*V. aspis*) in France, Spain, Germany, Switzerland, and Italy; Lataste's viper (*V. latasti*) in Spain and Portugal, and Orsini's viper (*V. ursinii*). The Montpellier snake (*Malpolon monspessulanus*) is a large back-fanged colubrid snake whose bite can cause transient mild systemic symptoms.

CLINICAL FEATURES OF EUROPEAN VIPER BITE

Symptoms are similar but in roughly decreasing order of severity as follows: *V. ammodytes, V. aspis, V. berus, V. latasti, V. ursinii.*

Early pain at the site of the bite is common but may be absent. Local swelling usually appears within a few minutes but is sometimes delayed for 30 min or longer. Local blisters containing blood are uncommon. Swelling and bruising may advance to involve the whole limb within 24 h and extend on to the trunk. A few cases of intra-compartmental syndromes and necrosis have been described. Pain, tenderness, and enlargement of local lymph nodes is sometimes noticeable within hours. Marked lymphangitis and bruising of the affected limb appears within a day or two. Dramatic early systemic symptoms may appear within 5 min of the bite or be delayed for many hours. They include retching, vomiting, abdominal colic, diarrhoea, incontinence of urine and faeces, sweating, shock, vasoconstriction, tachycardia, and angio-oedema of the face, lips, gums, tongue, throat and epiglottis, urticaria, and bronchospasm. These symptoms may persist for as long as 48 h. Hypotension is the most important sign. It usually develops within 2 h, may be transient, resolving spontaneously within 2 h, or persistent, recurrent, or progressive and fatal. ECG changes include flattening or inversion of T waves, ST elevation, second degree heart block and cardiac brady- and tachy-arrhythmias, atrial fibrillation, and myocardial infarction. Defibrinogenation (incoagulable blood) or milder degrees of coagulopathy and spontaneous bleeding into the gastrointestinal tract, lungs (Fig. 31), or urinary tract are uncommon. Other clinical features include fever, drowsiness and rarely, coma and seizures secondary to hypotension or

Fig. 30 Brazilian girl bitten 24 h previously by a tropical rattlesnake (*Crotalus durissus terrificus*). She has bilateral ptosis, paralysis of the facial muscles, and gross myoglobinuria resulting from generalized rhabdomyolysis. (Copyright D.A. Warrell.)

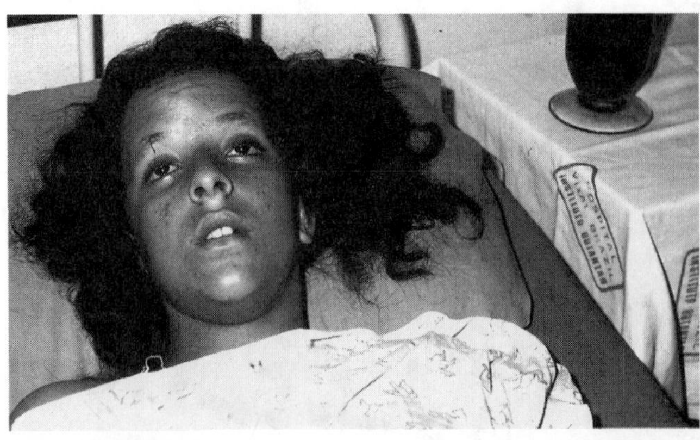

cerebral oedema, respiratory distress, pulmonary oedema, cerebral oedema, acute renal failure, cardiac arrest, intrauterine death, acute gastric dilatation, and paralytic ileus. Laboratory findings include neutrophil leucocytosis (more than 20 000/μl in severe cases), thrombocytopenia, initial haemoconcentration, and later anaemia resulting from extravasation into the bitten limb and rarely haemolysis, elevation of serum creatine phosphokinase, and metabolic acidosis. Deaths have occurred from 6 to 60 (average 34) h after the bite. Most adder bites cause only trivial symptoms, but patients must be assessed individually. Children may be severely envenomed: in a recent French series there were three deaths in a group of seven children aged between 30 months and 10 years. The dangers of adder bite should not be underestimated. Antivenom treatment of adder bite is discussed below.

Laboratory investigations

The peripheral neutrophil count is raised to 20 000 cells per μl or more in severely envenomed patients. Initial haemoconcentration, resulting from extravasation of plasma (*Crotalus* species and Burmese *D. russelii*), is followed by anaemia caused by bleeding or, more rarely, haemolysis. Thrombocytopenia is common following bites by pit vipers (e.g. *C. rhodostoma*, *Crotalus viridis helleri*) and some Viperidae (e.g. *Bitis arietans* and *D. russelii*), but is unusual after bites by *Echis* species. A useful test for venom induced defibrinogenation is the simple 20 min whole blood clotting test (20 WBCT). A sample of a few ml of venous blood is placed in a new clean, dry, glass test tube, left undisturbed for 20 min, and then tipped to see if it has clotted or not. Incoagulable blood indicates systemic envenoming and may be diagnostic of a particular species (for example *Echis* species in Africa). More sensitive tests which are simple to perform are whole blood or plasma prothrombin times, or detection of elevated FDP by agglutination of sensitized latex particles (Thrombo Wellco Test). Patients with generalized rhabdomyolysis show a steep rise in serum creatine phosphokinase, myoglobin, and potassium. Black or brown urine suggests generalized rhabdomyolysis or intravascular haemolysis. Concentrations of serum enzymes such as creatine phosphokinase and aspartate aminotransferase are moderately raised in patients with severe local envenoming, probably because of local muscle damage at the site of the bite. High concentrations suggest generalized rhabdomyolysis. Urine should be examined for blood/haemoglobin, myoglobin and protein, and for microscopic haematuria and red cell casts. Electrocardiographic abnormalities such as sinus bradycardia, ST-T changes, various degrees of atrioventricular block, and hyperkalaemic changes may be seen.

Fig. 31 Chest radiograph of a 9-year-old girl, 3 days after being bitten by *Vipera berus*, showing interstitial pulmonary bleeding. (By courtesy of Dr R. Pugh, Hull and *The Practitioner*.)

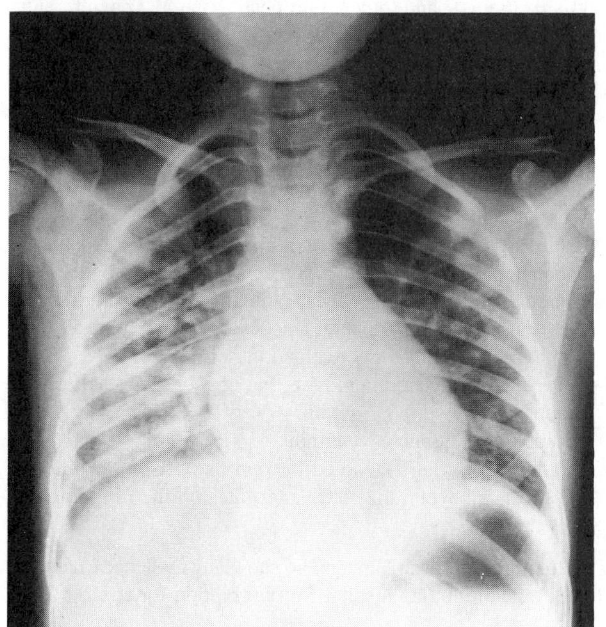

IMMUNODIAGNOSIS

Specific snake venom antigens have been detected in wound swabs, aspirates or biopsies, serum, urine, CSF and other body fluids. Of the various techniques for their detection, radioimmunoassay is probably the most sensitive and specific, but enzyme immunoassay (EIA) has been the most widely used. Under ideal conditions, relatively high venom antigen concentrations (wound swabs or aspirates) may be detected quickly enough (<10 min) to allow the selection of the appropriate monospecific antivenom. A commercial test kit for Australian elapids is produced by CSL, Melbourne. For retrospective diagnosis, including forensic cases, tissue around the fang punctures, wound and blister aspirate, serum, and urine should be stored for EIA immunodiagnosis.

Management of snake bite

FIRST AID

The patient should be reassured and moved to the nearest hospital or dispensary as quickly, comfortably, and passively as possible. The bitten limb should be immobilized, as far as is practicable, with a splint or sling.

Most traditional first aid methods are potentially harmful and should not be used. Local incisions and suction are more likely to introduce infection, damage tissues, and give rise to persistent bleeding than to remove significant amounts of venom from the wound. Potassium permanganate and ice packs may potentiate local necrosis. Electric shocks may relieve local pain but are potentially dangerous and have not been proved to affect the course of envenoming. Tourniquets and compression bands are potentially dangerous as they can cause gangrene (Fig. 32), increased fibrinolysis and bleeding in the occluded limb, peripheral nerve palsies, and intensification of local signs of envenoming. The use of such methods is justified only in the case of bites by dangerously neurotoxic elapids, sea snakes, and Australasian snakes when the delay in reaching medical care is likely to be more than 30 min but less than 2 or 3 h. In these particular circumstances, the development of respiratory paralysis may be delayed until the patient has reached a place where they can be resuscitated.

The pressure immobilization method developed by Sutherland and his colleagues in Australia involves firm but not tight bandaging of the entire bitten limb with a long crepe bandage, starting over the site of the bite and incorporating a splint. Experimentally, in animals, this method exerted a pressure of about 55 mmHg and was effective in pre-

Fig. 32 Gangrene of forearm in a Thai patient who applied a tight tourniquet above the elbow for several hours after being bitten by a Malayan pit viper (*Calloselasma rhodostoma*). (Copyright D.A. Warrell.)

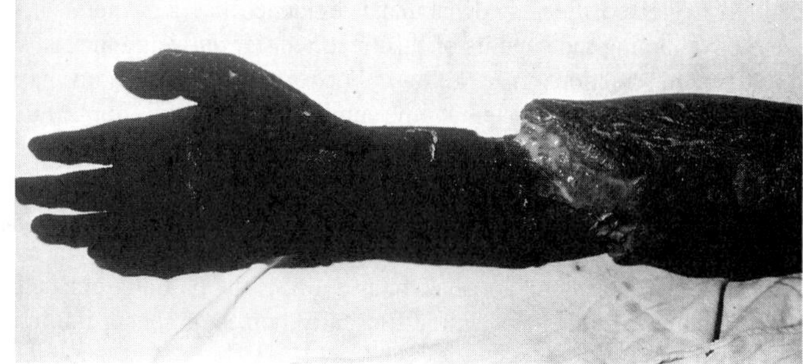

venting systemic uptake of Australian elapid and other venoms. Advocates of the method suggest that the venom may be inactivated by the tissues, but it seems possible that the devastating local effects of many snake venoms might be increased. Clinical studies are needed to assess the risks and benefits of this interesting technique.

Pursuing and killing the snake is not recommended, but if the snake has been killed it should be taken with the patient to hospital but must not be handled as even a severed head can inject venom.

Patients being transported to hospital should lie on their side to prevent aspiration of vomit. Persistent vomiting can be treated with chlorpromazine by intravenous injection (25–50 mg for adults, 1 mg/kg for children). Syncope, shock, angio-oedema, and other autonomic symptoms can be treated with 0.1 per cent adrenaline by subcutaneous injection (0.5 ml for adults, 0.01 ml/kg for children) and an antihistamine such as chlorpheniramine maleate by intravenous injection (10 mg for adults, 0.2 mg/kg for children). Patients with incoagulable blood will develop haematomas after intramuscular and subcutaneous injections, and so the intravenous route should be used whenever possible. Respiratory distress and cyanosis should be treated by clearing the airway, giving oxygen, and, if necessary, assisted ventilation. If the patient is unconscious and no femoral or carotid pulses can be detected, cardiorespiratory resuscitation should be started immediately.

HOSPITAL TREATMENT

Clinical assessment

In most cases of snake bite there are uncertainties about the species, quantity, and composition of venom injected that can be resolved only by admitting the patient for at least 24 h of observation. Local swelling is usually detectable within 15 min of significant pit viper envenoming and within 2 h of envenoming by most other vipers, but does not develop in patients bitten by some neurotoxic species such as kraits, coral snakes, and sea snakes. Fang marks may be invisible. Tender enlargement of regional lymph nodes draining the bitten area is an early sign of envenoming by Viperidae, some Elapidae, and Australasian elapids. All the tooth sockets should be examined meticulously as this is usually the first site of spontaneous bleeding: other common sites are nose, conjunctivae, skin, and gastrointestinal tract. Bleeding from venepuncture sites and other wounds implies incoagulable blood. Hypotension and shock are important signs of hypovolaemia or cardiotoxicity, seen particularly in patients bitten by North American rattlesnakes and some Viperinae (eg *V. berus, D. russelii, V. palaestinae*). Ptosis is the earliest sign of neurotoxic envenoming. Respiratory muscle power should be assessed objectively, for example, by measuring vital capacity. Trismus and generalized muscle tenderness suggest rhabdomyolysis (Hydrophiidae). If a procoagulant venom is suspected, coagulability of whole blood should be checked at the bedside using the simple 20 min whole blood clotting test.

ANTIVENOM TREATMENT

The most important decision in the management of a patient bitten by a snake is whether or not to give antivenom, the only specific treatment for envenoming. Although the clinical testing of antivenoms has been relatively neglected, there is now abundant evidence that in patients with severe envenoming the benefits of this treatment far outweigh the risks of antivenom reactions (see below). For example, antivenom has reduced the mortality of systemic envenoming by *Echis* sp. from 20 to 3 per cent and by *C. d. terrificus* from 74 to 12 per cent. Antivenoms have also proved effective in reversing hypotension caused by *V. berus* envenoming and coagulopathies caused by *D. russelii, C. rhodostoma, T. albolabris*, and *Oxyuranus scutellatus*. Antivenom, also known as antivenin, antivenene, and antisnakebite serum, is the partially purified immunoglobulin ($F(ab')_2$) of animals, usually horses or sheep, immunized with venom. The new generation of antivenoms will be affinity purified specific Fab fragments raised in sheep.

General indications for antivenom

Antivenom is indicated if there are signs of systemic envenoming such as:

1. Haemostatic abnormalities such as spontaneous systemic bleeding, incoagulable blood, or thrombocytopenia
2. Neurotoxicity
3. Hypotension and shock, abnormal ECG, or other evidence of cardiovascular dysfunction
4. Impaired consciousness of any cause
5. Generalized rhabdomyolysis.

Supporting evidence of severe envenoming is a neutrophil leucocytosis, elevated serum enzymes such as creatine phosphokinase and aminotransferases, haemoconcentration, severe anaemia, myoglobinuria, haemoglobinuria, methaemoglobinuria, hypoxaemia, and acidosis.

In the absence of systemic envenoming, local swelling involving more than half the bitten limb, extensive blistering or bruising, bites on digits, and rapid progression of swelling are indications for antivenom, especially in patients bitten by species whose venoms are known to cause local necrosis (e.g. Viperidae, Asian cobras, and African spitting cobras).

Special indications for antivenom

Some developed countries can afford a wider range of indications.

United States and Canada

After bites by the most dangerous rattlesnakes (*C. atrox, C. adamanteus, C. viridis, C. horridus*, and *C. scutulatus*) antivenom therapy should be given early, before systemic envenoming has become obvious. Rapid spread of local swelling is considered to be an indication for antivenom as is immediate pain or any other symptom or sign of envenoming after bites by coral snakes (*Micruroides euryxanthus* and *Micrurus fulvius*).

Australia

Antivenom should be given to any patient with proved or suspected snake bite if there are tender regional lymph nodes or any other evidence of systemic spread of venom and in anyone effectively bitten by an identified highly venomous species.

Europe

(Adder—*Vipera berus*—and other European Vipera). Zagreb antivenom, or the new Therapeutic Antibodies Inc Fab antivenom (Table 1) is indicated to prevent morbidity and reduce the length of convalescence in patients with moderately severe envenoming as well as to save the lives of severely envenomed patients. Indications are:

1. Fall in blood pressure (systolic to < 80 mmHg or by more than 50 mmHg from the normal or admission value) with or without signs of shock;
2. Other signs of systemic envenoming (see above) including spontaneous bleeding, coagulopathy, pulmonary oedema or haemorrhage (shown by chest radiograph), ECG abnormalities, and a definite peripheral leucocytosis (more than 15 000/μl) and elevated serum creatine kinase;
3. Severe local envenoming—swelling of more than half of the bitten limb developing within 48 h of the bite—even in the absence of systemic envenoming;
4. In adults, swelling extending beyond the wrist after bites on the hand or beyond the ankle after bites on the foot within 4 h of the bite.

Patients bitten by European Vipera who show any evidence of envenoming should be admitted to hospital for observation for at least 24 h.

Table 1 *Guide to initial dosage of some important antivenoms*

Species: Latin name	Species: English name	Manufacturer, antivenom	Approximate initial dose
Acanthophis sp.	Death adder	CSL,* monospecific	3000–6000 units
Bitis arietans	Puff adder	Behringwerke North/Central Africa; SAIMR[d] polyspecific	80 ml
Bothrops jararaca	Jararaca	Brazilian manufacturers Bothrops polyspecific	20 ml
Bungarus caeruleus	Common krait	Haffkine polyspecific	100 ml
Calloselasma (Agkistrodon) rhodostoma	Malayan pit viper	Thai Red Cross (Saovabha), Bangkok, monospecific	100 ml
		Thai Government Pharmaceutical Organization, monospecific	50 ml
Crotalus adamanteus	Eastern diamondback rattlesnakes	Wyeth (Crotalidae) polyspecific	30–100 ml
C. atrox	Western diamondback rattlesnakes		
C. viridis subspecies	Western rattlesnakes		
Daboia (Vipera) russelii	Russell's vipers	Burma Pharmaceutical Industry, monospecific	40 ml
		Haffkine polyspecific	100 ml
		Thai manufacturers, monospecific	50 ml
Echis sp.	Saw-scaled or carpet vipers	SAIMR,[d] Echis, monospecific	20 ml
		Behringwerke, North Africa/Near and Middle East, polyspecific	100 ml
Hydrophiidae	Sea snakes	CSL,* sea snake/tiger snake	1000 units
Naja kaouthia	Monocellate Thai cobra	Thai Red Cross, monospecific	100 ml
N. naja	Indian cobra	Haffkine; Central Research Institute, Kasauli; Serum Institute of India, polyspecific	100 ml
Notechis scutatus	Tiger snake	CSL,* monospecific	3000–6000 units
Pseudechis textilis	Eastern brown snake		
Oxyuranus scutellatus	Taipan	CSL,* monospecific	12 000 units
Trimeresurus albolabris	Green pit viper	Thai Red Cross, monospecific	100 ml
Vipera berus	European adder	Immunoloski Zavod-Zagreb Vipera polyspecific	10 ml
		Therapeutic Antibodies (Inc.), Fab monospecific 'Beritab'	100–200 mg
V. palaestinae	Palestine viper	Rogoff Medical Research Institute, Tel Aviv, Palestine viper monospecific	50–80 ml

* Commonwealth Serum Laboratories, Australia.

[d] South African Institute for Medical Research.

Antivenom should be given whenever there is evidence of systemic envenoming [(1) or (2) above] even if its appearance is delayed for several days after the bite.

Prediction of antivenom reactions

Skin and conjunctival tests do not predict early (anaphylactic) or late (serum sickness type) antivenom reactions and should not be used.

Contraindications to antivenom

Atopic patients and those who have reacted previously to equine antiserum are at increased risk of developing severe antivenom reactions. In such cases, antivenom should be given only if there are definite signs of severe systemic envenoming. Reactions may be prevented or ameliorated by pretreatment with subcutaneous adrenaline, antihistamine, and hydrocortisone or continuous intravenous infusion of adrenaline while antivenom is being given. Rapid desensitization is not recommended.

Selection and administration of antivenom

Antivenom should be given only if its stated range of specificity includes the species responsible for the bite. Opaque solutions should be discarded as precipitation of protein indicates loss of activity and increased risk of reactions. Expiry dates quoted on ampoules are often very conservative, for commercial reasons. Liquid and lyophilized antivenoms stored below 8 °C usually retain most of their activity for 5 years or more. Monospecific (monovalent) antivenom is ideal if the biting species is known. Polyspecific (polyvalent) antivenoms are used in many countries because of the difficulty in identifying the species responsible for bites. Polyspecific antivenoms may be just as effective as monospecific ones but contain less specific activity per unit of immunoglobulin. Apart from the venoms used for immunization in the production of antivenoms, there may be a range of paraspecific activity. For example, Commonwealth Serum Laboratories' 'tiger-sea snake antivenom' neutralizes many hydrophiid and even elapid venoms, and South African Institute for Medical Research's 'polyvalent antivenom', which is raised against the venoms of 10 species, has paraspecific activity against a further five.

It is almost never too late to give antivenom while signs of systemic envenoming persist, but, ideally, it should be given as soon as it is indicated. Antivenom has proved effective up to 2 days after hydrophiid bites and in patients still defibrinated weeks after bites by Viperidae. In contrast, local envenoming is probably not reversible unless antivenom is given within a few hours of the bite. The intravenous route is the most effective. Infusion of antivenom diluted in approximately 5 ml of isotonic fluid/kg body weight is easier to control than intravenous 'push' injection of undiluted antivenom given at the rate of about 4 ml/min, but there is no difference in the incidence or severity of antivenom reactions in patients treated by these two methods.

Dose of antivenom

Manufacturers' recommendations are based on mouse protection tests and may be very misleading. Few clinical trials have been performed to establish appropriate starting doses, and in most countries antivenom is used empirically. Many hospitals in the rural tropics give a standard dose of 1 to 2 ampoules to every patient who claims to have been bitten, irrespective of clinical severity. This practice squanders scarce, expensive antivenom and exposes non-envenomed patients to the risk of reactions. Some suggested initial doses are given in Table 1. Children should be given the same dose as adults.

Response to antivenom

Often, there is marked symptomatic improvement soon after antivenom has been injected. In shocked patients, the blood pressure may rise and consciousness return (*C. rhodostoma, V. berus, Bitis arietans*). Neurotoxic signs may improve within 30 min (*Acanthophis* sp.,*N. kaouthia*), but usually take several hours. Spontaneous systemic bleeding usually stops within 15 to 30 min and blood coagulability is restored within 6 h of antivenom, provided a neutralizing dose has been given. More antivenom should be given if severe signs of envenoming persist after 1 to 2 h, or if blood coagulability is not restored within about 6 h. Systemic envenoming may recur hours or days after initially good response to antivenom. This is explained by continuing absorption of venom from the injection site and the clearance of antivenom from the bloodstream. The apparent serum elimination half-lives of antivenoms in envenomed patients range from 26 to 95 h. Envenomed patients should therefore be assessed daily for at least 3 or 4 days.

Antivenom reactions

Early (anaphylactic) reactions develop within 10 to 180 min of starting antivenom in 3 to more than 80 per cent of patients. The incidence increases with dose and decreases when more highly refined antivenom is used and administration is by intramuscular rather than intravenous injection. The symptoms are itching, urticaria, cough, nausea, vomiting, other autonomic manifestations, fever, and tachycardia. Up to 40 per cent of patients with early reactions develop systemic anaphylaxis: hypotension, bronchospasm, and angio-oedema. Deaths are rare but individual cases, such as the asthmatic boy who died from anaphylactic shock after Pasteur antivenom in England in 1957, have been widely publicized and have led to an unreasonable rejection of antivenom treatment. Early antivenom reactions are unlikely to be type I IgE-mediated hypersensitivity reactions to equine serum protein. They are probably the result of complement activation by immune complexes or aggregates of IgG.

Pyrogenic reactions result from contamination of the antivenom with endotoxin-like compounds. Fever, rigors, vasodilatation, and a fall in blood pressure develop 1 to 2 h after treatment. In children, febrile convulsions may be precipitated. Late reactions of serum sickness type may develop 5 to 24 (mean 7) days after antivenom. The incidence of these reactions and the speed of their development increases with the dose of antivenom. Clinical features include fever, itching, urticaria, arthralgia (including the temporomandibular joint), lymphadenopathy, periarticular swellings, mononeuritis multiplex, albuminuria, and rarely encephalopathy. This is a classical immune complex disease.

Treatment of antivenom reactions

Adrenaline (epinephrine) is the effective treatment for early reactions; 0.5–1.0 ml of 0.1 per cent solution (1 in 1000, 1 mg/ml) is given by subcutaneous injection to adults (children 0.01 ml/kg) at the first signs of a reaction. The dose may be repeated if the reaction is not controlled. Patients with profound hypotension, severe bronchospasm or laryngeal oedema may be given adrenaline by slow intravenous injection (0.5 mg diluted in 20 ml of iosotonic saline in 10–15 min). An antihistamine, such as chlorpheniramine maleate (10 mg for adults, 0.2 mg/kg for children) should be given by intravenous injection to combat the effects of histamine release during the reaction. Pyrogenic reactions are treated by cooling the patient and giving antipyretics. Late reactions respond to an oral anthistamine such as chlorpheniramine (2 mg six hourly for adults, 0.25 mg/kg.day in divided doses for children) or to oral prednisolone (5 mg six hourly for 5 to 7 days for adults, 0.7 mg/kg.day in divided doses for children).

SUPPORTIVE TREATMENT

Neurotoxic envenoming

Bulbar and respiratory paralysis may lead to death from aspiration, airway obstruction, or respiratory failure. A clear airway must be maintained and, once there is pooling of secretions and if respiratory distress develops, a cuffed endotracheal tube should be inserted or tracheostomy performed. Provided they are adequately ventilated, patients with neurotoxic envenoming remain fully conscious with intact sensation. Patients have been effectively ventilated manually (by Ambu bag or anaesthetic bag), as in the 1952 poliomyelitis epidemic in Copenhagen, for 30 days and have recovered after 10 weeks of mechanical ventilation. Although artificial ventilation was first suggested for neurotoxic envenoming more than 100 years ago, patients continue to die because they are denied this simple procedure. Anticholinesterases have a variable but potentially useful effect in patients with neurotoxic envenoming especially when postsynaptic neurotoxins are involved. The 'Tensilon test' should be done in all cases of severe neurotoxic envenoming as with suspected myasthenia gravis. Atropine sulphate (0.6 mg for adults, 50 μg/kg for children) is given by intravenous injection followed by an intravenous injection of edrophonium chloride (10 mg for adults, 0.25 mg/kg for children). Patients who respond convincingly can be maintained on neostigmine methyl sulphate (50–100 μg/kg) and atropine (four hourly for by continuous infusion).

Hypotension and shock

If the central venous pressure is low or there is other clinical evidence of hypovolaemia, a plasma expander, preferably fresh whole blood or fresh frozen plasma, should be infused. If there is evidence of increased capillary permeability (e.g. facial and conjunctival oedema, serous effusions, haemoconcentration, hypoalbuminaemia, etc.) it may be safer in the long term to rely on a selective vasoconstrictor such as dopamine (starting dose 2.5–5 μg/kg.min by intravenous infusion). Delayed hypotension developing about 1 week after bites by Burmese *D. russelii* may respond to intravenous hydrocortisone.

Oliguria and renal failure

Urine output, serum creatinine, urea, and electrolytes should be measured each day in patients with severe envenoming and in those bitten by species known to cause renal failure (e.g. *D. russelii, C d terrificus, Bothrops* species, sea snakes). If urine output drops below 400 ml in 24 h, urethral and central venous catheters should be inserted. If urine flow fails to increase after cautious rehydration and diuretics (e.g. frusemide up to 1000 mg IV), dopamine (2.5 μg/kg.min by intravenous infusion) should be tried and the patient placed on strict fluid balance. If these measures are ineffective, haemofiltration or peritoneal or haemodialysis is usually required. In Rangoon, the mortality of established renal failure following *D. russelii* envenoming has been reduced to less than 30 per cent by using peritoneal dialysis, usually for only 72 h.

Local infection at the site of the bite

Bites by some species (e.g. *Bothrops* sp., *C. rhodostoma*) are likely to be complicated by local infections caused by bacteria in the snake's venom or on its fangs. This should be prevented with penicillin, chloramphenicol, or erythromycin and a booster dose of tetanus toxoid, especially if the wound has been incised or tampered with in any way. An aminoglycoside such as gentamicin should be added if there is evidence of local necrosis.

Management of local envenoming

Bullae are best left intact. The bitten limb should be nursed in the most comfortable position. Once definite signs of necrosis have appeared (blackened anaesthetic area with putrid odour or signs of sloughing) surgical débridement, immediate split skin grafting, and broad-spectrum antimicrobial cover are indicated. Increased pressure within tight fascial compartments such as the digital pulp spaces and anterior tibial compartment may cause ischaemic damage. This complication is most likely after bites by North American rattlesnakes such as *C. adamanteus*, and bites by *Calloselasma rhodostoma, Trimeresurus flavoviridis, Bothrops* sp., and *Bitis arietans*). The signs are excessive pain, weakness of the compartmental muscles and pain when they are passively stretched, hypoaesthesia of areas of skin supplied by nerves running through the compartment, and obvious tenseness of the compartment. Detection of arterial pulses does not exclude intracompartmental ischaemia. The opening pressure required for very slow infusion of isotonic saline by pump through a cannula inserted into the anterior tibial compartment is a measure of intracompartmental pressure. Pressures exceeding 45 mmHg are associated with a high risk of ischaemic necrosis. In these circumstances, fasciotomy may be justified but this should not be contemplated until blood coagulability and a platelet count of more than 50 000/μl have been restored. Animal studies have suggested that muscles sufficiently envenomed and swollen to cause intracompartmental syndromes are already irreversibly damaged. Early adequate antivenom treatment will prevent the development of intracompartmental syndromes in most cases.

Haemostatic disturbances

Once specific antivenom has been given to neutralize venom procoagulants, restoration of coagulability and platelet function may be accelerated by giving fresh whole blood, fresh frozen plasma, cryoprecipitates (containing fibrinogen, Factor VIII, fibronectin, and some factors V and XIII) or platelet concentrates. Heparin has been recommended for a variety of snake bites and has been used, sometimes with disastrous results. The strongest theoretical case for the use of heparin is in patients bitten by *D. russelii* who show definite evidence of disseminated intravascular coagulation (e.g. prolonged whole blood prothrombin time and elevated serum fibrin degradation products) but whose blood is still coagulable. Heparin did not prove beneficial in patients envenomed by *Echis ocellatus* whose venom activates prothrombin, producing a thrombin which is not neutralized by heparin.

Other drugs

Corticosteroids, antifibrinolytic agents such as trasylol and ϵ-aminocaproic acid, antihistamines, trypsin, and a variety of traditional herbal remedies, have been used but none has proved clinically effective and most are potentially harmful.

TREATMENT OF SNAKE VENOM OPHTHALMIA

When cobra venom is 'spat' into the eyes, first aid consists of irrigation with generous volumes of water or any other bland liquid which is available. Unless a corneal abrasion can be excluded by fluorescein staining or slit lamp examination, treatment should be the same as for any corneal injury: a topical antimicrobial such as tetracycline or chloramphenicol should be applied. Instillation of diluted antivenom seems logical, but it may prove irritant, is of uncertain benefit, and is not currently recommended. Instillation of 0.5 per cent adrenaline drops is said to relieve pain and inflammation.

Interval between bite and death and prognosis

Exceptionally, patients may die 'a few minutes' (reputedly after a bite by the king cobra, *Ophiophagus hannah*) or as long as 41 days (*E. carinatus*) after snake bite. However, most deaths occur about 8 h after cobra bites (*N. naja*), 18 h after krait bites (*Bungarus caeruleus*), 16 h after North American rattlesnake bites (*Crotalus* sp.), 3 days after *D. russelii* bites, and 5 days after Echis bites. Even when the fangs of a highly venomous snake have pierced the skin, envenoming is not certain. About 20 to 50 per cent of patients bitten by American crotalines, *C. rhodostoma* and *D. russelii*, show absolutely no evidence of envenoming and as many as 80 per cent of those bitten by sea snakes and 50 per cent by *C. rhodostoma* and *D. russelii* develop trivial or no envenoming. Antivenom has reduced dramatically the mortality from snake bite. Prognosis is worst in infants and the elderly but children often do well despite the larger dose of venom injected relative to their body weight.

Prevention of snake bites

To reduce the risk of bites, snakes should never be disturbed, attacked, cornered, or handled even if they are thought to be a harmless species or appear to be dead. Venomous species should never be kept as pets or as performing animals. In snake infested areas, boots, socks, and long trousers should be worn for walks in undergrowth or deep sand and a light should always be carried at night. Collecting firewood, dislodging logs and boulders with bare hands, pushing sticks or digits into burrows, holes, and crevices, climbing rocks and trees covered with dense foliage, and swimming in overgrown lakes and rivers are particularly hazardous activities. Unlit paths and gutters are especially dangerous after heavy rains. To prevent sea snake bites fishermen should not touch these animals when they are caught in nets or on lines, and swimmers and divers should not aggravate them and should avoid wading in the sea, especially in sand or near coral reefs. It is futile and ecologically undesirable to attempt to exterminate venomous snakes. Various substances toxic to snakes, such as insecticides and methyl bromide, have been used to keep human dwellings free of these animals. However, no effective but harmless snake repellent is yet available.

IMMUNIZATION AGAINST ENVENOMING

The idea of inducing protective levels of antibodies against lethal venom components by pre-exposure immunization in high risk populations is an attractive one. This has been tried with inconclusive results against *T.flavoviridis* in the Ryukyu and Amami Islands of Japan and has been contemplated to protect rice farmers against *D.russelii* in Burma. For protection, a high titre of circulating antibody would have to be present at the time of the bite. An accelerated secondary response stimulated by the venom antigen injected at the time of the bite would be too late to be useful.

REFERENCES

Bücherl, W., Buckley, E.E. and Deulofue, V. (eds) (1968, 1971). *Venomous animals and their venoms*. Vols. 1 and 2. Academic Press, New York.

Cardoso, J.L.C., *et al.* (1993). Randomized comparative trial of three antivenoms in the treatment of envenoming by lance-headed vipers (*Bothrops jararaca*) in São Paulo, Brazil. *Quarterly Journal of Medicine*.

Douglas, W.W. (1985). Polypeptides—angiotensin, plasma kinins and others. In: *The Pharmacological Basis of Therapeutics* (eds. Goodman and Gilman). Macmillan, New York.

Gans, C. and Gans, K.A. (eds) (1978). *Biology of the reptilia*. Vol 8. Academic Press, London.

Gopalakrishnakone, P. (ed). (1994) *Sea snake toxinology*. National University of Singapore Press.

Gopalakrishnakone, P. and Chou, L.M. (eds). (1990). *Snakes of medical importance (Asia-Pacific Region)*. National University of Singapore Press.

Harvey, A.L. (ed) (1991). *Snake toxins. International encyclopedia of pharmacology and therapeutics*. Section 134. Pergamon, New York.

Lee, C-Y. (ed), (1979). Snake venoms. *Handbook of experimental pharmacology* Vol 52. Springer-Verlag, Berlin.

Malasit, P., *et al.* (1986). Prediction, prevention and mechanism of early (anaphylactic) antivenom reactions in victims of snake bites. *British Medical Journal*, **292,** 17–20.

Myint-Lwin, *et al.* (1985). Bites by Russell's viper (*Vipera russelli siamensis*) in Burma: haemostatic, vascular and renal disturbances and response to treatment. *Lancet*, **ii,** 1259–64.

Reid, H.A. (1976). Adder bites in Britain. *British Medical Journal*, **2,** 153–6.

Reid, H.A., Thean, P.C., Chan, K.E., and Baharom, A.R. (1963). Clinical effects of bites by Malayan viper (*Ancistrodon rhodostoma*). *Lancet*, **i,** 617–21.

Russell, F.E. (1980). *Snake venom poisoning*. Lippincott, Philadelphia.

Sokolovsky, M. (1992). Short review. Structure–function relationships of endothelins, sarafotoxins and their receptor subtypes. *Journal of Neurochemistry*, **59,** 809–21.

Sutherland, S.K. (1983). *Australian animal toxins. The creatures, their toxins and care of the poisoned patient.* Oxford University Press, Melbourne.

Theakston, R.D.G. and Warrell, D.A. (1991). Antivenoms: a list of hyperimmune sera currently available for the treatment of envenoming by bites and stings. *Toxicon*, **29,** 1419–70.

Tu, A.T. (ed). (1991). *Handbook of natural toxins*. Vol. 5. Reptile venoms and toxins. Marcel Dekker Inc., New York.

Warrell, D.A. (1990). Treatment of snake bite in the Asia–Pacific region: a personal view. In: *Snakes of medical importance (Asia–Pacific region)*. (ed. P. Gopalakrishnakone and L.M. Chou. Singapore University Press.

Warrell, D.A., *et al.* (1977). Poisoning by bites of the saw-scaled or carpet viper (*Echis carinatus*) in Nigeria. *Quarterly Journal of Medicine*, **46,** 33–62.

Warrell, D.A., *et al.* (1976). Necrosis, haemorrhage and complement depletion following bites by the spitting cobra (*Naja nigricollis*) *Quarterly Journal of Medicine*, **45,** 1–22.

Venomous lizards

Only two species, the gila monster (*Heloderma suspectum*) and Mexican beaded lizard (*H.horridum*), are venomous (Plate 2). They occur in the southwestern United States, western Mexico, and Central America and reach about 60 to 80 cm in length. Venom is secreted by glands in the lower jaw and is conducted along the grooved mandibular teeth. Humans are rarely bitten. The lizard clings on with a bulldog-like grip. There is immediate severe local pain and tender swelling of regional lymph nodes. Systemic symptoms include weakness, dizziness, hypotension, syncope, sweating, rigors, tinnitus, nausea, vomiting, leucocytosis, and ECG changes. The venom contains toxins, enzymes and 5-hydroxytryptamine. There are no reliable reports of fatalities but in one patient envenomed by *H.suspectum* there was severe refractory hypotension resulting in myocardial infarction and renal failure and coagulopathy. Specific antivenom is not available. Strong analgesia may be required. Hypotension should be treated with plasma expanders and, if persistent, with a selective vasoconstrictor such as dopamine.

REFERENCES

Bogert, C.M. and Martin del Campo, R. (1956). The Gila monster and its allies. *Bulletin of the American Museum of Natural History*, **109,** 1–238.

Hooker, K.R. and Caravati, E.M. (1994). Gila monster envenomation. *Annals of Emergency Medicine,* **24,** 731–5.

Russell, F.E. and Bogert, C.M. (1981). Gila monster, venom and bite—a review. *Toxicon*, **19,** 341–59.

Tu, A.T. (1991). A lizard venom: Gila monster (genus Heloderma). In: Handbook of natural toxins (ed). A.T. Tu. Vol. 5, pp. 755–730. Marcel Dekker Inc., New York.

Poisonous amphibians

The moist skin of amphibians such as frogs, toads, newts, and salamanders is an accessory respiratory organ which is protected from microorganisms by highly toxic secretions. The bitter flavour and lethal effects of these secretions and the vivid warning coloration of many species is a defence against predators. The skin of the 'poison dart frogs' (Dendrobatidae) (Plate 3) of Central and South America contain alkaloids such as batrachotoxins (*Phyllobates* species) which block sodium channels, have a mouse subcutaneous LD_{50} of only 2 μg/kg and are used by some Colombian Indians to coat the tips of their darts. The skin of the Ecuadorean poison frog (*Epipedobates tricolor*, Dendrobatidae) contains a number of alkaloids including pumiliotoxin 251D and epibatidine, a potent non-opioid analgesic. Some toads can squirt venom from their parotid glands and when licked or put in the mouth by dogs or children or when ingested as part of a Chinese traditional medicine, severe or even fatal poisoning may result. Symptoms include hypersalivation, cyanosis, cardiac arrhythmias, and generalized convulsions (for example Colorado River toad, *Bufo alvarius*). The digoxin-like toxin, bufotalin may cause atrial fibrillation with a slow ventricular rate and periods of ventricular asystole.

The skin of three species of newts, genus Taricha, from the western United States, contains tarichatoxins identical to tetrodotoxin also found in some frogs, fish, crustaceans, and octopuses (see below). Tetrodotoxin can be absorbed through the gastric mucosa, explaining the death of a man who swallowed a 20-cm long Oregon rough-skinned newt (*Taricha granulosa*). The patient developed paraesthesia of the lips, progressing to more generalized numbness and weakness and had a cardiopulmonary arrest about 2 h after swallowing the newt.

REFERENCES

Bradley, S.C. and Klika, L.J. (1981). A fatal poisoning from the Oregon rough skinned newt (*Taricha granulosa*) *Journal of the American Medical Association*, **246,** 247.

Hitt, M. and Ettinger, D.D. (1986). Toad toxicity. *New England Journal of Medicine*, **314,** 1517–8.

Kwan, T., Dino Paiusco, A. and Kohl, L. (1992). *Digitalis toxicity caused by toad venom. Chest*, **102,** 949–50.

Myers, C.W., Daly, J.W., and Malkin, B. (1978). A dangerously toxic new frog (Phyllobates) used by the Emberá Indians of Western Colombia with discussion of blowgun fabrication and dart poisons. *Bulletin of the American Museum of Natural History*, **161,** Art. 2, pp 307–66.

Spande, T.F., *et al.* (1992). Epibatidine: a novel (chloropyridyl) azabicycloheptane with potent analgesic activity from an Ecuadorean poison frog. *Journal of the American Chemical Society*, **114,** 3475–8.

Thomas, M., David, J.M., and Jouglard, J. (1989). Le crapaud animal vénimeux. Expérience du centre anti-poisons de Marseille. *Journal de Toxicologie Clinique et Experimentale*, **9,** 368–70.

Poisonous birds

The feathers and skin and breast muscles of three species of pitohui or thickhead (Plate 3(a)) passerine birds from New Guinea (genus Pitohui, Pachycephalidae) were found to contain homobatrachotoxin, a potent steroidal alkaloid which activates sodium channels and was originally isolated from the skin of South American poison dart frogs (Phyllobates, Dendrobatidae—see above). Poisonous pitohuis have an unpleasant peppery odour and their skin has a bitter flavour. Contact with feathers causes numbness and burning of the tongue, lips, or skin wounds and sneezing. This may be a protective mechanism, and the striking 'warning' coloration of the hooded pitohui (*P.dichrous*) (Plate 4) may be the subject of müllerian mimicry by less poisonous species. Judging by their reputation in Papua New Guinea, other species, including birds of paradise and the blue-capped Ifrita (*Ifrita kowaldi*) may also prove to have poisonous tissues.

REFERENCE

Dumbacher, J.P., *et al.* (1992). Homobatrachotoxin in the genus Pitohui: chemical defense in birds? *Science*, **258,** 799–800.

Venomous fish

More than 100 species of fish can inflict dangerous stings on humans. Venom is injected through spines in front of the fins and tail and in the gill covers. The Indo-Pacific region and other tropical waters have the richest venomous fish fauna, but dangerous species such as sharks, chimaeras, and weevers also occur in temperate northern waters and a number of large rivers in South American, West Africa, and southeast Asia are inhabited by freshwater stingrays (Potamotrygon). The following groups are capable of fatal envenoming: Squaliformes (sharks and dogfish), Rajiformes (stingrays and mantas), Siluroidei (catfish), Trachinidae (weevers), Scorpaenidae (scorpionfish and stonefish), and Uranoscopidae (stargazers and stonelifters). Venom glands are embedded in grooves in the spines or, in the case of stingrays, lie beneath a membrane covering the long barbed precaudal spine.

Incidence and epidemiology

Weeverfish are common around the British coast especially in Cornwall. Hundreds of stings occur each year with a peak incidence in August and September. Fifty-eight cases were seen at one hospital at Pula on the Adriatic coast over 13 years. It has been estimated that there are 1500 stings by rays and 300 stings by scorpionfish in the United States each year. Stings by venomous freshwater rays (*Potamotrygon hystrix, P.motoro*) are common in the Amazon region of Brazil and especially in Acré. In four years, 81 cases of stonefish (Synaceja) sting were seen in Pulau Bukom Hospital near Singapore. Ornate, but aggressive and venomous members of the genera Pterois and Dendrochirus (lion, zebra, tiger, turkey or red fire fish) (Plate 5), which are popular aquarium pets, may sting their owners on the fingers. Most fish stings are inflicted on the soles of the feet of people wading near the shore or in the vicinity of coral reefs. Venomous fish are effectively camouflaged (Synanceja) or lie partly covered by sand. Stingrays lash their tails at the intruding limb and usually impale the ankle (Plate 5). Fatal fish stings are very rarely reported.

Venom composition

The instability of most fish venoms at normal ambient temperatures has made them difficult to study. Stingray and weeverfish venoms contain peptides, enzymes, and a variety of vasoactive compounds such as kinins, 5-hydroxytryptamine, histamine, and catecholamines. Pharmacological effects include increased vascular permeability, local necrosis, direct actions on cardiac skeletal and smooth muscle resulting in ECG changes, hypotension, paralysis, and central nervous system depression.

Clinical features

Immediate sharp, agonizing pain is the dominating symptom. Hot, erythematous swelling extends up the stung limb and may persist with pain for several days and be complicated by necrosis and secondary infection, particularly if the spine remains embedded in the wound. (Plate 6). Stingray spines, which are up to 30 cm long, can cause severe lacerating injuries especially to the lower legs, but if the victim inadvertently lies on the ray or falls on to it, the spine may penetrate the thoracic or abdominal cavities with fatal results.

Systemic effects are uncommon after weever stings (Trachinidae) but patients stung by rays or Scorpaenidae (scorpion- and stonefish) may develop nausea, vomiting, signs of autonomic nervous system stimulation, such as diarrhoea, sweating and hypersalivation, cardiac arrhythmias, hypotension, respiratory distress, acute pulmonary oedema, neurological signs, and generalized convulsions. Patients have died within an hour of being stung by *Synanceja verrucosa.*

Treatment

Pain is alleviated by immersing the stung limb in water which is uncomfortably hot (less than 45 °C) but not scalding. Temperature can be assessed with the unstung limb. Addition of magnesium sulphate is not necessary. Injection of local anaesthetic is less effective even when applied as a ring block in the case of stung digits but local nerve block with 0.5 per cent plain bupivacaine does seem to work. The venomous spine, which may be barbed, fragments of membrane, and other foreign material, should be removed as soon as possible. Systemic effects must be treated symptomatically. An adequate airway should be established and cardiorespiratory resuscitation may be needed. Severe hypotension may respond to adrenaline and bradycardia to atropine. The Commonwealth Serum Laboratories in Australia manufacture an antivenom specific for *Synaceja trachynis, S.verrucosa* and *S.horridus*. This has paraspecific activity against the venoms of the North American scorpionfish (*Scorpaena guttata*) and some other members of the Scorpaenidae. One ampoule (2 ml or 2000 units) is given intravenously for each two puncture marks found at the site of the sting. The dose is increased for patients with severe symptoms.

Prevention

Fish stings can be prevented by employing a shuffling gait when wading, by avoiding handling living or dead fish, and by keeping clear of fish in the water especially in the vicinity of tropical reefs. Footwear is protective against most species except stingrays.

REFERENCES

Castex, M.N. (1967). Fresh water venomous rays. In: *Animal toxins* (ed. F.E. Russell and P.R. Saunders. pp. 167–76. Pergamon, Oxford.

Edmunds, C. (1989). *Dangerous marine creatures.* Reed, Frenchs Forest, New South Wales.

Halstead, B.W. (1988). *Poisonous and venomous marine animals of the world* (second revised edition). Darwin Press, Princeton.

Halstead, B.W., Auerbach, P.S., and Campbell, D.R. (1990). *A colour atlas of dangerous marine animals.* Wolfe, London.

Lehmann, D.F. and Hardy, J.C. (1993). Stonefish envenomation. *New England Journal of Medicine*, **329,** 510–1.

Maretić, Z. (1973). Some epidemiological, clinical and therapeutic aspects of envenomation by weever fish sting. In: *Toxins of animal and plant origin* (ed. A. De Vries and E. Kochva). pp. 1055–65. Gordon and Breach, New York.

Sutherland, S.K. (1983). *Australian animal toxins. The creatures, their toxins and care of the poisoned patient.* Oxford University Press, Melbourne.

Williamson, J. and Exton, D. (1985). *The marine stinger book.* 3rd edn. Queensland Centre Surf Life-Saving Association of Australia, Brisbane.

Poisoning by ingestion of aquatic animals

Acute gastrointestinal symptoms ('food poisoning') after eating seafood are usually caused by bacterial or viral infections such as *Vibrio para-*

haemolyticus (crustaceans, especially shrimps), *V. cholerae* (crabs and molluscs), non-O group 1 *V. cholerae* (oysters), *V. vulnificus* (oysters), *Aeromonas hydrophila* (frozen oysters), *Plesiomonas shigelloides* (oysters, mussels, mackerel, cuttlefish), *Shigella* sp, (molluscs), *Campylobacter jejuni* (clams), *Salmonella typhi* (molluscs), hepatitis A virus (molluscs, especially clams, and oysters), Norwalk virus (clams and oysters), and astro- and calici viruses (cockles). Botulism has been caused by eating smoked fish and canned salmon, and in Japan and elsewhere, fish and molluscs became contaminated with methyl mercury from industrial waste, causing severe neurological damage and fetal abnormalities ('Minamata disease').

Toxins in seafood may also give rise to gastrointestinal neurotoxic and histamine-like symptoms. Two main syndromes are described.

Gastrointestinal and neurotoxic syndromes

Symptoms include the following: acute nausea, vomiting, abdominal colic, tenesmus, and watery diarrhoea associated with paraesthesia of the lips, buccal cavity, and extremities; distorted temperature perception so that cold objects impart a burning sensation like dry ice; myalgia, progressive flaccid paralysis, ataxia, cardiovascular disturbances, bradycardia, and rashes. Important causes of this syndrome are discussed below.

1. Ciguatera fish poisonings

Symptoms develop 1 to 6 h (extreme range, minutes to 30 hours) after eating fish such as groupers, snappers, parrot fish, mackerel, moray eels, barracudas, and jacks. These are warm water shore or reef fish. The global incidence is thought to be 50 000 cases per year. In the Pacific region, e.g. in New Caledonia, where 3009 cases with 0.1 per cent mortality were reported during a 14-year period, the toxins responsible, including ciguatoxin, maitotoxin, and scaritoxin, are ultimately derived along the food chain from benthic dinoflagellates such as *Gambierdiscus toxicus* and are concentrated in the liver, viscera, and gonads, especially of large fish. Increasing importation of exotic fish from the Caribbean and elsewhere has led to cases of ciguatera in Britain. A rapid and sensitive test has been developed for detecting toxin in fish using a monoclonal antibody and EIA. Gastrointestinal symptoms resolve within a few hours, but paraesthesiae may persist for a week or even months. Similar symptoms may follow ingestion of marine turtles in the Indo-Pacific area. The mortality of ciguatera fish poisoning is less than 10 per cent.

2. Tetrodotoxin poisoning

Scaleless porcupine, sun, puffer, and toad fish (order Tetraodonitiformes) may become highly poisonous at certain seasons, such as May to June, the spawning season in Japan. Tetrodotoxin, an aminoperhydroquinazoline, is one of the most potent non-protein toxins known. It produces neurotoxic and cardiotoxic effects by blocking the sodium ion flux through excitable membranes and prolonging nerve conduction. It is concentrated in the ovaries, viscera, and skin of tetraodontiform fish and it is also found in the skin of newts (genus Taricha), frogs (genus Atelopus) and salamanders, the saliva of octopuses, from the digestive glands of several species of gastropod mollusc and a starfish, flat worm (Planorbis), and Nemertine worms in Japan, and is produced by some bacteria.

Puffer fish ('fugu') is particularly popular in Japan where, despite stringent regulations, there are 250 cases of tetrodotoxin poisoning each year with a 60 per cent mortality. Neurotoxic symptoms develop within 10 to 45 min and death from respiratory paralysis usually occurs between 2 and 6 h after eating the fish. There may be no gastrointestinal symptoms. Erythema, petechiae, blistering, and desquamation may appear.

An unusually severe case became apnoeic and deeply comatose with brain-stem areflexia and developed cerebral diabetes insipidus attributed to central action of tetrodotoxin on the neurohypophysis. He recovered consciousness after 36 h.

3. Paralytic shellfish poisoning

Bivalve molluscs, such as mussels, clams, oysters, cockles, and scallops, as well as xanthid, coconut, and horseshoe crabs may acquire tetrahydropurine neurotoxins such as saxitoxin from dinoflagellates such as *Gonyaulax* species. These dinoflagellates may be sufficiently abundant during the warmer months of May to October to produce a 'red tide'. The dangerous season is signalled by the deaths of large numbers of fish and sea birds. Symptoms develop within 30 min of ingestion and may progress to fatal respiratory paralysis within 12 h in 8 per cent of cases. Milder symptoms without paralysis can follow the ingestion of molluscs contaminated by neurotoxins from *Ptychodiscus brevis* which also causes a 'red tide'. As mentioned above, several Japanese species of gastropod mollusc have been found to contain tetrodotoxin and there has been one case of serious poisoning. In the United Kingdom there have been several outbreaks of neurotoxic red whelk (*Neptunea antiqua*) poisoning attributable to tetramine.

Histamine-like syndrome (scombrotoxic poisoning)

The red flesh of scombroid fish (tuna, mackerel, bonito, and skipjack) and of canned non-scombroid fish, such as sardines and pilchards, may be decomposed by the action of bacteria such as *Proteus morgani* and *Klebsiella pneumoniae*, which convert muscle histidine into saurine, histamine, and unidentified toxins; 100 g of spoiled fish may contain almost 1 g of histamine. Histamine absorbed from the gut is normally broken down by *N*-methyl-transferase and diamine oxidase (histaminase), but if the histamine concentration is very high, or the patient is taking a diamine oxidase inhibitor such as isoniazid (as antituberculosis chemotherapy) scombrotoxic poisoning may result. Toxic fish may produce a tingling or smarting sensation in the mouth when eaten. Within minutes or up to a few hours after ingestion, flushing, burning, sweating, urticaria, and pruritus may develop with headache, abdominal colic, nausea, vomiting, diarrhoea, bronchial asthma, giddiness, and hypotension.

Diagnosis and treatment

The differential diagnosis includes bacterial and viral food poisoning and allergic reactions. No specific treatments or antidotes are available but gastrointestinal contents should speedily be eliminated by emetics and purges. Activated charcoal adsorbs saxitoxin and other shellfish toxins. Mannitol has been advocated for ciguatera poisoning. Atropine is said to improve gastrointestinal symptoms and sinus bradycardia in patients with gastrointestinal and neurotoxic poisoning. Calcium gluconate may relieve mild neuromuscular symptoms. Oximes and anticholinesterases appear ineffective in ciguatera and tetrodotoxin poisoning, respectively. Patients who develop respiratory paralysis should be intubated and ventilated even if the neurological signs suggest extensive brain damage. The symptoms of scombrotoxic poisoning can be alleviated with antihistamines and bronchodilators.

Prevention

Ciguatera toxin, tetrodotoxin, and many other marine toxins are heat stable so cooking does not prevent poisoning. Some toxins are fairly water soluble and may be leached out by soaking, so water in which fish are cooked should not be drunk. In tropical areas, the flesh of fish should be separated as soon as possible from the head, skin, intestines, gonads, and other viscera which may contain high concentrations of toxin. All scaleless fish should be regarded as potentially tetrodotoxic and very large fish carry an increased risk of being ciguatera-toxic. Moray eels should never be eaten because of the high risk of unusually rapid and severe ciguatera fish poisoning. Scombroid poisoning can be prevented by eating fresh fish or by freezing them as soon as possible after they are caught. Shellfish should not be eaten during the dangerous seasons and when there are red tides.

REFERENCES

Bagnis, R.A., *et al.* (1979). Clinical observations on 3009 cases of Ciguatera (fish poisoning) in the Southern Pacific. *American Journal of Tropical Medicine and Hygiene*, **28,** 1067–73.

Eastaugh, J. and Shepherd, S. (1989). Infections and toxic syndromes from fish and shellfish consumption. A review. *Archives of Internal Medicine*, **149,** 1735–40.

Halstead, B.W. (1988). *Poisonous and venomous marine animals of the world.* 2nd revised edition. Darwin Press, Princeton.

Hughes, J.M. and Merson, M.H. (1976). Fish and shellfish poisoning. *New England Journal of Medicine*, **296,** 1117–20.

Scheuer, P.J. (1987). Recent developments in ciguatera research. In: *Natural toxins: animal, plant and microbial* (ed. J.B. Harris). Oxford University Press, Oxford.

Scoging, A.C. (1991). Illness associated with seafood. *Communicable Disease Reports*, **1,** R117–122.

Tambyah, P.A., *et al.* (1994). Central-nervous-system effects of tetrodotoxin poisoning. *Lancet*, **343,** 538–9.

Trishnananda, M., *et al.* (1966). Poisoning following the ingestion of the horseshoe crab (*Carcinoscorpius rotundicauda*): report of four cases in Thailand. *Journal of Tropical Medicine and Hygiene*, **69,** 194–6.

Uragoda, C.G. and Kottegoda, S.R. (1977). Adverse reactions to isoniazid on ingestion of fish with a high histamine content. *Tubercle*, **58,** 83–9.

World Health Organization (1984). *Aquatic (marine and fresh water) biotoxins.* Environmental Health Criteria, 37, WHO, Geneva.

Poisoning by ingestion of carp's gallbladder

In parts of the Far East, the raw bile and gallbladder of various species of freshwater carp (e.g. the grass carp *Ctenopharyngodon idellus*, 'plaa yeesok' *Probarbus jullienii*) are believed to have medicinal properties. Patients in China, Taiwan, Hong Kong, Thailand, and elsewhere have developed acute abdominal pain, vomiting, and watery diarrhoea 2 to 18 h after drinking the raw bile or eating raw gallbladder of these fish. One patient developed flushing and dizziness. Hepatic and renal damage may develop, progressing to oliguric or non-oliguric acute renal failure (acute tubular necrosis). The hepatonephrotoxin has not been identified, but is heat stable and may be derived from the carps' diet.

REFERENCES

Chan, D.W.S., Yeung, C.K., and Chan M.K. (1985). Acute renal failure after eating raw fish gall bladder. *British Medical Journal*, **290,** 897.

Yip, L.L. (1981). Toxic material from the gall-bladder of the grass carp (*Ctenopharyngodon idellus*). *Toxicon*, **19,** 567–9.

Venomous marine invertebrates

Coelenterates (jellyfish, cubomedusoids, sea wasps, Portuguese-men-o'-war or bluebottles, hydroids, sea anemones, etc.)

The tentacles of cnidarian coelenterates are armed with nematocysts (stinging capsules) which produce lines of painful irritant weals on the skin of swimmers unlucky enough to make contact with them. Coelenterate venoms contain or release vasoactive substances such as histamine and kinins which cause immediate excruciating pain, inflammation, and urticaria.

EPIDEMIOLOGY

The most dangerous species, the box jellyfish, cubomedusoid, sea wasp, or indringa (*Chironex fleckeri*) of northern Australia, has caused more than 70 deaths this century. Most stings occur in December and January. Fatal jellyfish stings in the Indo-Pacific region from India, north to the Philippines and east to Bougainville Island, are attributable to *Chiropsalmus quadrumanus* and *C. quadrigatus* (Plate 7). Fatal stings have also been inflicted by the Atlantic Portuguese man-o'-war (Physalia) and the Chinese jellyfish *Stomolophus nomurai*. Many stings in northern Queensland are caused by *Carukia barnesi* (Irukandji stings). Hundreds of thousands of swimmers off the northern Adriatic coast were stung by a plague of *Pelagia noctiluca* during the summers of 1977 to 1979. Stings by the sea anemone, *Anemonia sulcata*, are also reported from the Adriatic coast.

CLINICAL FEATURES

Nematocyst stings may leave a diagnostic pattern on the skin: *C. fleckeri* produces wide striated brownish purple weals (Plate 8), whereas *C. barnesi* causes a transient erythematous macule and the Portuguese man-o'-war (Physalia) produces chains of oval weals surrounded by erythema. Immediate severe pain is the most common symptom. Chirodropids (genera Chironex and Chiropsalmus) cause the most severe systemic symptoms such as respiratory arrest, generalized convulsions, pulmonary oedema, and cardiac arrest within minutes of the accident. Other systemic effects include cough, nausea, vomiting, abdominal colic, diarrhoea, rigors, severe musculoskeletal pains, and profuse sweating. 'Irukandji' syndrome consists of severe musculoskeletal pain, anxiety, trembling, headache, piloerection, sweating, tachycardia, hypertension, and pulmonary oedema starting about 30 min after a sting by *C. barnesi* and persisting for hours. *Physalia* species can also cause severe systemic envenoming including respiratory distress, muscle pains, spasms, and coma, intravascular haemolysis, and renal failure.

TREATMENT

Patients stung by jellyfish must get out of the water as soon as possible. The aim is to prevent further discharge of nematocysts on fragments of tentacles stuck to the skin. Alcoholic solutions such as methylated spirits or suntan lotion, the traditional remedy, have now been shown to cause massive discharge of nematocysts! Commercial vinegar or 3 to 10 per cent aqueous acetic acid are, however, effective for Chironex, Chiropsalmus, Carukia, and Physalia, and baking soda and water (50 per cent w/v) is effective for the widely distributed Atlantic genus, Chrysaora. Ice packs can be applied. In patients with extensive stings, firm crepe bandaging of the whole stung limb (after inactivation of nematocysts), or the application of tourniquets proximal to the stung areas may produce a useful delay in the absorption of venom. Cardiorespiratory resuscitation has proved life-saving in several Australian patients who became cyanosed, comatose, and pulseless. A specific 'sea wasp' antivenom for *C. fleckeri* is manufactured in Australia and can be given by intramuscular injection into the anterior thigh by first aiders in patients with extensive stings from chirodropids.

PREVENTION

Bathers, especially children, should keep out of the sea at times of the year when dangerous coelenterates are prevalent, especially when warning notices have been put up, or bathe in 'stinger-resistant' enclosures. Wet or 'Lycra' suits and other clothing will protect against nematocyst stings. Divers should avoid surfacing underneath coelenterates by looking upwards during the ascent.

Echinodermata (starfish and sea urchins)

These animals are protected by hard exoskeletons with numerous long, sharp projecting spines and grapples (globiferous pedicellariae) (Plate 9) which can release venom when embedded in the skin. Severe pain and local swelling may result and sometimes systemic effects such as syncope, numbness, generalized paralysis, aphonia, respiratory distress, cardiac arrhythmias, and even death. Embedded fragments of spines may lead to secondary infection and chronic granulomas or damage to bones and joints (Fig. 33).

TREATMENT

Skin penetrated by the spines, usually the soles of the feet, should be softened with 2 per cent salicylic acid ointment or acetone. The spines can then be squeezed out or removed surgically. No antivenoms are available.

Mollusca (cone shells and octopuses)

The 500 species of cone shells (genus Conus) are carnivorous marine snails which harpoon their prey (fish, polychaete worms, and other molluscs), implanting a radular tooth charged with venom containing a mixture of small (10–30 amino acid) peptide toxins. These include conotoxins which block acetylcholine receptors and voltage-sensitive Ca^{2+} and Na^{+} channels, conantokins, and conopressins. Cone shells are attractive and valuable collector's items. People who pick them up may be stung. Symptoms of envenoming are local paraesthesia, numbness, and paralysis which proved fatal in eight of 30 reported cases (Plate 10).

Two species of small octopus found in the Australian and West Pacific region (blue ringed octopus—*Octopus maculosus* and *O. lunulatus*—Plate 11) can inject salivary tetrodotoxin when they bite swimmers using their powerful beaks. These bites are painful and cause local bleeding, swelling, and inflammation. Severe neurotoxic symptoms, and even fatal generalized paralysis, may develop within 15 min of the bite.

TREATMENT

No antivenoms are available. Cardiorespiratory resuscitation and mechanical ventilation may be required.

REFERENCES

Beadnell, C.E., *et al.* (1992). Management of a major box jellyfish (*Chironex fleckeri*) sting. *Medical Journal of Australia*, **156,** 655–8.

Fig. 33 Results of repeated injuries by black sea urchins (*Stomopneustes variolaris*) at Wellawatte, Sri Lanka. (By courtesy of Dr Malik Fernando, Colombo, Sri Lanka.)

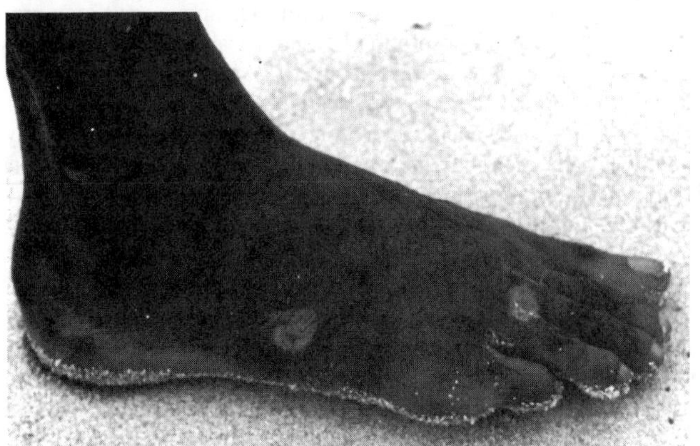

Burnett, J.W., *et al.* (1994). Serious *Physalia* (Portuguese man o'war) stings: implications for scuba divers. *Journal of Wilderness Medicine*, **5,** 71–6.

Fenner, P.J., *et al.* (1993). First aid treatment of jelly fish stings in Australia. *Medical Journal of Australia*, **158,** 498–501.

Halstead, B.W. (1988). *Poisonous and venomous marine animals of the world* (2nd revised edition). Darwin Press, Princeton.

Martin, J.C. and Audley I. (1990). Cardiac failure following Irukandji envenomation. *Medical Journal of Australia*, **153,** 164–6.

Olivera, B.M., *et al.* (1991). Conotoxins. *Journal of Biological Chemistry*, **266,** 22067–70.

Sutherland, S.K. (1983). *Australian animal toxins. The creatures, their toxins and care of the poisoned patient.* Oxford University Press, Melbourne.

Williamson, J. and Exton, D. (1985). *The marine stinger book.* 3rd edn. Surf Life Saving Association of Australia, Queensland State Centre Inc., Brisbane.

Venomous arthropods

Hymenoptera (bees, wasps, yellowjackets, hornets, and ants)

The commonest and most severe Hymenoptera stings are caused by members of the families Apidae (e.g. the honey bee, *Apis mellifera*, bumble bees, etc), Vespidae (e.g. wasps, genera Polistes and Paravespula; American yellowjackets and 'hornets', genera Vespula and Dolichovespula; and European and Asian true hornets, genus Vespa), and Formicidae (e.g. fire ants, genus Solenopsis). Allergic reactions to single Hymenoptera stings are common, whereas toxic reactions resulting from many stings are rare, except in Middle and South America. Venom allergens include phospholipases A, hyaluronidase, acid phosphomonoesterases, and melittin (*A. mellifera*). Non-allergenic compounds include vasoactive amines such as histamine, 5-hydroxytryptamine, catecholamines and kinins, cholinesterase (in the venom of the common European wasp (*Paravespula germanica*), pheromones, and 2-methylpiperidine alkaloids in Solenopsis (fire ant) venoms.

Epidemiology

Sixty-one people died from insect stings in England and Wales between 1959 and 1972 and in the United States there are between 40 and 50 deaths a year. These figures are probably underestimates, as deaths caused by anaphylaxis following insect stings may be attributed to secondary phenomena, such as myocardial infarction and cerebrovascular accident. The incidence of systemic reactions to Hymenoptera stings has been reported as 0.4 to 0.8 per cent in children. In an adult population in the United States, the prevalence of systemic allergic sting reactions was 4 per cent; 20 per cent of this population showed evidence of venom hypersensitivity (skin tests or radioallergosorbent test, RAST). In Britain, most patients allergic to bee venom are beekeepers or their relatives. Since the escape of swarms of African honey bees (*A. m. scutellata*) in Rio Claro, Brazil, in 1957, this aggressive strain has spread throughout Latin America and north to the southern states of the United States. About 30 deaths from mass attacks by these bees have been reported each year. Two species of fire ants, *Solenopsis richteri* and *S. invicta*, were imported into the United State from South America in 1918 and have now spread to 13 southern states where an estimated 2.5 million individuals are stung each month. The incidence of systemic allergic reactions is about 4 per 100 000 population per year, and there have been fatal reactions.

Clinical features

TOXIC EFFECTS

In non-sensitized individuals, a sting, which, in the case of Vespidae and Apidae, introduces about 50 μg of venom, will rapidly produce a hot, red, painful swelling and weal a few centimetres in diameter, which persists for a few hours. These effects are dangerous only if the airway is obstructed, for example, after stings on the tongue. As few as 30 stings can cause fatal systemic envenoming in children, but children and adults have survived more than 1000 stings by *A. mellifera*. In some patients, symptoms suggested histamine toxicity (vasodilatation, hypotension, vomiting, diarrhoea, throbbing headache, coma, and bronchoconstriction). In Latin America, victims of attacks by *A. m. scutellata* have shown evidence of generalized rhabdomyolysis (grossly elevated serum creatine phosphokinase, aminopeptidases, and myoglobin), intravascular haemolysis, hypercatecholaminaemia (hypertension, pulmonary oedema, myocardial damage), bleeding, hepatic dysfunction, and acute renal failure (Plate 12). In nonsensitized people Solenopsis sting produces pain, itching, swelling, and erythema around a central weal which last a few hours and later vesicles or pustules (Plate 13). In an unsensitized patient an estimated 10 000 *S. invicta* stings caused no systemic envenoming.

ALLERGIC EFFECTS

Clinical suspicion of venom hypersensitivity arises when there are progressively severe local reactions to successive stings or when systemic symptoms follow a sting. Patients may die within minutes of the sting. Systemic symptoms include tingling scalp, itching of the palms, soles, axillae, and perineum (becoming generalized), flushing, dizziness, syncope, wheezing, abdominal colic, uterine contraction, diarrhoea, incontinence of urine and faeces, tachycardia, and visual disturbances, all developing within a few minutes of the sting. Over the next 15 to 20 min, urticaria, angio-oedema, oedema of the glottis, profound hypotension, and coma may develop. Guillain-Barré syndrome, neuralgic amyotrophy, optic neuritis, multiple sclerosis, other allergic demyelinating disorders, and encephalopathy have been described. A few patients develop serum sickness a week or more after the sting. Many patients with sting allergy have other evidence of an atopic disposition. Reactions are greatly enhanced by β- blockers and non-steroidal anti-inflammatory agents.

Diagnosis of venom hypersensitivity

Type I hypersensitivity is confirmed by detecting venom specific IgE in the serum using RAST. Intradermal skin tests using dialysed freeze dried pure specific venoms are also diagnostic. In patients who have suffered a systemic reaction, there is a 50 to 60 per cent risk of a similar or more severe reaction to the next sting. Those who have had a marked local but no systemic reaction have a 5 to 10 per cent chance of a systemic reaction when stung again. Children who have generalized urticaria after a sting have only a 10 per cent chance of a systemic reaction when restung. Hypersensitivity to venom may be lost spontaneously especially by children and young adults. The RAST test has been used for postmortem diagnosis of Hymenoptera sting anaphylaxis.

Treatment

The barbed stings of Apidae remain embedded at the site of the sting and continue to inject venom, so they should be removed immediately by scraping with a blade or fingernail. Wasp stings may become infected (Plate 14). Domestic meat tenderizer (papain) diluted roughly 1:5 with tap water is said to produce immediate relief of pain. Ice packs and aspirin are also effective. Systemic but not topical antihistamines can be used for more severe local reactions. Vespids can withdraw their stings and sting repeatedly. Massive local reactions can be treated with a short course of corticosteroid. Systemic anaphylaxis must be treated with 0.1 per cent (1:1000) adrenaline (0.5–1 ml for adults, 0.01 mg/kg for children) given by subcutaneous or intramuscular injection, or, if the patient is unconscious or pulseless, by intravenous injection. In rare cases, blood pressure fails to respond even to large doses of adrenaline and plasma expanders. These patients should be given cardio-respiratory resuscitation, selective bronchodilators such as salbutamol, selective vasoconstrictors such as dopamine, and intravenous antihistamines such as chlorpheniramine maleate (10 mg for adults, 0.2 mg/kg for children). Corticosteroids are not useful in the treatment of severe systemic anaphylaxis. Patients who know they are hypersensitive to venom should wear an identifying tag (such as provided by Medic-Alert in Britain) as they may be discovered unconscious after being stung. They should be trained to give themselves adrenaline subcutaneously and should always carry a preloaded syringe of adrenaline for this purpose. Adrenaline delivered by a pressurized inhaler ('Medihaler-Epi') will relieve bronchospasm, but the amount of drug absorbed is insufficient to combat other effects of anaphylaxis unless at least 20 puffs are taken (10–15 for children) and the effect is more transient than with injected adrenaline. Respiratory tract obstruction and shock are the main causes of death.

Severe envenoming from multiple Hymenoptera stings should be treated with adrenaline, intravenous antihistamines (doses as above), and corticosteroids. Intensive care is essential. Intravenous mannitol and bicarbonate may reduce the risk of 'pigment nephropathy' as in patients with crush syndrome. Since no antivenom is available, exchange transfusion or plasmapheresis might be considered to remove venom in severe cases. Renal dialysis is often needed.

Prevention

Patients over the age of 25 years who have a history of systemic anaphylaxis following a sting and who have evidence of hypersensitivity (venom specific IgE detectable in the serum or a positive skin test) should be considered for desensitization with pure specific venoms. This treatment has proved to be significantly more effective than placebo or the previously used whole body extracts of Hymenoptera in preventing anaphylactic reactions to sting challenge. In the United Kingdom, the Committee on Safety of Medicines ruled, in October 1968, that desensitization could be carried out only where there were facilities for full cardiorespiratory resuscitation. Patients should be kept under observation for at least 2 h after treatment. Desensitization usually involves weekly visits to the hospital for at least 8 weeks while gradually increasing doses of venom are given. When protection has been demonstrated by the patient's ability to tolerate 100 μg of venom (equivalent to two stings) they are ready for maintenance therapy, usually 100 μg of venom every 4 to 8 weeks. With this regimen, serum venom specific IgE may decline and specific IgG may increase. After 2 years of maintenance desensitization up to 90 per cent of subjects will remain protected against systemic reactions if they stop treatment. Desensitization is complicated by systemic reactions in 5 to 15 per cent of patients and by large local reactions in 50 per cent. Currently, only whole body extracts of fire ants are available for desensitizing hypersensitive subjects.

Most people are stung by apids or vespids when they inadvertently crush the insects or interfere with their nests (i.e. bee keepers). Wasps congregate where sweet things are manufactured or consumed, in orchards, vineyards, and, since they are carnivorous, where meat is being served. Vespidae are attracted by brightly coloured floral patterns and perfumes. Some hornets are so aggressive that their nests must be eradicated before their territory can be used for agricultural purposes.

REFERENCES

Anon. (1994). Adrenaline for anaphylaxis. *Drug and Therapeutics Bulletin*, **32,** 19–21.

British Society for Allergy and Clinical Immunology. (1993). Position paper on allergen immunotherapy. Report of a BSACI working party. *Clinical and Experimental Allergy*, **23,** Suppl. 3, 1–44.

de Shazo, R.D., Butcher, B.T., and Banks, W.A. (1990). Reactions to the stings of the imported fire ant. *New England Journal of Medicine*, **323,** 462–6.

Diaz, J.D., *et al.* (1988). Multiple stings by imported fire ants (*Solenopsis invicta*), without systemic effects. *Southern Medical Journal,* **82,** 775–7.

França, F.O.S., *et al.* (1994). Severe and fatal mass attacks by "killer" bees (Africanized honey bees-*Apis mellifera scutellata*) in Brazil: clinic pathological studies with measurement of serum venom concentrations and a review of the literature. *Quarterly Journal of Medicine*, **87,** 269–82.

Frankland, A.W. and Lessof, M.H. (1980). Allergy to bee stings: a review. *Journal of the Royal Society of Medicine*, **73,** 807–10.

Hunt, J.Jr, Valentine, M.D., Sobotka, A.K., Benun, A.W., Amodie, F.J., and Lichtenstein, L.M. (1978). A controlled trial of immunotherapy in insect hypersensitivity. *New England Journal of Medicine*, **299I,** 157–61.

Mueller, U.R. (1990). *Insect sting allergy. Clinical picture, diagnosis and treatment.* Gustav Fischer, Stuttgart.

Piek, T. (1986). *Venoms of the Hymenoptera. Biochemical, Pharmacological and Behavioural Aspects.* Academic Press, London.

Smith, P.L., *et al.* (1980). Physiologic manifestations of human anaphylaxis. *Journal of Clinical Investigation*, **66,** 107.

Winston, M.L. (1992). Killer bees. *The Africanized honey bee in the Americas.* Harvard University Press, Cambridge, MA.

Venomous lepidoptera

Contact with the stinging hairs of many species of adult moths or their larvae (caterpillars) can cause contact dermatitis, urticating lesions or, in some cases, systemic envenoming. 'Lepidopterism' describes effects of contact with imago or caterpillar, and 'erucism' contact with caterpillars. Venomous lepidoptera are found in all parts of the world but most cases of lepidopterism are reported from Middle and Southern America. Examples of severe cutaneous urticating eruptions are those caused by caterpillars of the genus Megalopyge (called 'pussmoths' in the southern United States) (Plate 15) and by adult female moths of the genus Hylesia which have on their abdomens barbed setae ('flechettes') (Plate 16). Epidemics of stings by these moths have been described especially from coastal areas of Brazil, Peru, Venezuela, and Mexico. Caterpillars of the genus Lanomia can inject a fibrinolytic haemolymph resulting in defibrinogenation, spontaneous bleeding into the skin, urinary tract, and even fatal intracranial haemorrhage (Plate 17). Contact with caterpillars of *Lonomia achelous* produces a bleeding diathesis characterized by decreased plasma fibrinogen factor V, factor XIII, and plasminogen concentrations, increased fibrin degradation products and fibrinolytic activity, but a normal platelet count.

In Pará State, Brazil, rubber tappers are frequently in contact with caterpillars of *Premolis semirufa* whose stinging hairs can cause a disabling arthritis of the hands ('pararama').

Venomous coleoptera (beetles)

Two families of beetles can exude vesicating liquids. The most famous is 'Spanish fly'—*Lytta vesicatoria* (Meloidae—blister beetles) which contains cantharidin which causes blistering when applied to the skin and priapism (hence its reputation as an aphrodisiac) and renal failure when given systemically or absorbed after ingestion of the legs of frogs which have fed on meloid beetles.

'Nairobi eye' and similar blistering conditions in Australia and southeast Asia are caused by species of the genus Paederus (Staphylinidae) (Plate 18). A typical skin lesion (dermatitis linearis) consists of erythema, itching, and blistering caused by inadvertently crushing and smearing the beetle (Plate 19). Systemic symptoms such as fever, arthralgia, and vomiting may arise in severe cases. The active principle pedrin is the most complex non-proteinaceous insect toxin known. Treatment is palliative. The toxin is easily spread to other sites such as the eye by fingers.

REFERENCES

Arocha-Piñango, C.L., *et al.* (1988). Fibrinolytic and procoagulant agents from a saturnidae moth caterpillar. In: *Hemostasis and Animal Venoms*, (ed. H. Pirkle and F.S. Markland. pp. 223–40. Marcel Dekker, New York.

Eisner, T., *et al.* (1990). Systemic retention of ingested cantharidin by frogs. *Chemoecology*, **1,** 57–62.

Frank, J.H. and Kanamitsu, K. (1987). Paederus, sensulato (Coleoptera: Staphylinidae): natural history and medical importance. *Journal of Medical Entomology*, **24,** 1555–91.

Roberts, J.I. and Tonking, H.D. (1935). Notes on an East African vesicant beetle, *Pederus crebripunctatus* Epp. *Annals of Tropical Medicine and Parasitology*, **29,** 415–20.

Southcott, R.V. (1989). Injuries from Coleoptera. *Medical Journal of Australia,* **151,** 654–9.

Scorpions (Scorpiones: Buthidae, Scorpionidae)

Species capable of inflicting fatal stings occur in North Africa and the Middle East (genus Androctonus, Buthus, and Leiurus); South Africa (Parabuthus); India (*Mesobuthus tamulus*); North, Central, and Southern America, and Trinidad (Tityus (Plate 20) and Centruroides).

Epidemiology

In southern Libya there were 900 stings with 7 deaths per 100 000 population in 1979. There have been no deaths from scorpion sting in the United States since 1968, but in Mexico there are between 1000 and 2000 deaths each year with an incidence of 84 deaths per 100 000 population per year in Colima state. Mortality is about 50 per cent in children less than 4 years old. In Trinidad, where stings by *Tityus trinitatis* are an occupational hazard of sugar cane and cocoa planters, there were 33 deaths in a group of 698 cases. Mortality was 25 per cent among children under 5 years compared to 0.25 per cent in adults. In Brazil, mortality was about 1 per cent in adults and 15 to 25 per cent in children less than 6 years old. In Algeria there were an average of 1260 stings and 24 deaths per year. In India there are many cases of scorpion stings with fatalities in adults and children.

Clinical features

Local intense pain is the most common symptom. There may be slight local oedema and tender enlargement of regional lymph nodes. Systemic symptoms may develop within minutes or be delayed for as much as 24 h. There is some variation in symptoms depending on the species and geographical area. Scorpion venoms stimulate the sustained release of acetylcholine and catecholamines, usually resulting in initial cholinergic and later adrenergic symptoms. Early symptoms include vomiting, profuse sweating, piloerection, alternating brady- and tachycardia, abdominal colic, diarrhoea, loss of sphincter control, and priapism. Later, severe life-threatening cardiorespiratory effects may appear: hypertension, shock, tachy- and bradyarrhythmias, ECG changes (Fig. 34) and pulmonary oedema (Fig. 35) with or without evidence of myocardial dysfunction. Severe cardiovascular complications are particularly associated with stings by *Leiurus quinquestriatus*, *Mesobuthus tamulus*, and *Tityus* species. Stings by North American *Centruroides sculpturatus* produce neurotoxic effects such as fascicultion, spasms, respiratory paralysis, and convulsions. Victims of the Trinidad black scorpion (*Tityus trinitatis*) develop severe abdominal pain with nausea, vomiting and haematemesis, hyperglycaemia, and biochemical evidence of acute pancreatitis. Victims of *Hemiscorpius lepturus* (Iran and Iraq) develop a macular lesion at the site of the sting which may blister and become necrotic resulting in sloughing of a large area of skin (Plate 21).

Treatment

Pain responds temporarily to local infiltration or ring block with local anaesthetic. Local injection of emetine or dehydroemetine is said to relieve the pain but may cause necrosis. Parenteral opiate analgesics, such as pethidine or morphine, may be required, but are alleged to be dangerous in victims of *C. sculpturatus*.

Antivenom is manufactured in a number of countries. Its use is strongly advocated in Africa and the Americas, but ancillary pharmacological treatment is regarded as being much more important in the Middle East and India. However, if specific antivenom is available it should be administered intravenously as soon as possible in patients with systemic envenoming and in young children stung by dangerous species, even before the development of these symptoms. Patients with cardiovascular symptoms benefit from vasodilator treatment with α-blockers (e.g. prazosin), calcium-channel blockers (e.g. nifedipine), or ACE inhibitors (e.g. captopril). Atropine should not be used except in cases of life-threatening sinus bradycardia. The use of cardiac glycosides and β-blockers is controversial. Anticonvulsants such as phenobarbitone are recommended for neurotoxic symptoms.

Prevention

Scorpions can be kept out of houses by including a row of ceramic tiles in the outside wall, making the doorsteps at least 20 cm high and using residual insecticides, such as 1 per cent lindane or dieldrin powders.

REFERENCES

Amaral, C.F.S., *et al.* (1991). Electrocardiographic, enzymatic and echocardiographic evidence of myocardial damage after *Tityus serrulatus* scorpion poisoning. *American Journal of Cardiology*, **67**, 655–7.

Amaral, C.F.S., De Rezende, N.A., and Freire-Maia, L. (1993). Acute pulmonary edema after *Tityus serrulatus* scorpion sting in children. *American Journal of Cardiology*, **71**, 242–5.

Bawaskar, H.S. and Bawaskar, P.H. (1992). Management of the cardiovascular manifestations of poisoning by the Indian red scorpion (*Mesobuthus tamulus*). *British Heart Journal*, **68**, 478–80.

Bettini, S. (ed.) (1978). *Athropod venoms. Handbook of experimental pharmacology*. Vol. 48, p. 279. Springer-Verlag, Berlin.

Bücherl, W. and Buckley, F.E. (eds.) (1971). *Venomous animals and their venoms*. Vol. 3, p. 311. Academic Press, New York.

Dehesa-Dávila, M. (1989). Epidemiological characteristics of scorpion stings in Léon, Guanajuato, México. *Toxicon*, **27**, 281–6.

Gueron, M., Ilia, R., and Sofer, S. (1992). The cardiovascular system after scorpion envenomation. A review. *Clinical Toxicology*, **30**, 245–8.

Keegan, H.L. (1980). *Scorpions of medical importance*. University Press of Mississippi, Jackson.

Mazzotti, L. and Bravo-Becherelle, M.A. (1963). Scorpionism in the Mexican Republic. In *Venomous and poisonous animals and noxious plants of the Pacific region*. (ed. H.L. Keegan and W.V. MacFarland), pp. 119–131. Pergamon Press, Oxford.

Polis, G.A. (ed.) (1990). *The Biology of Scorpions*. Stanford University Press, Stanford.

Radmanesh M. (1990). Clinical study of *Hemiscorpion lepturus* in Iran. *Journal of Tropical Medicine and Hygiene*, **93**, 327–32.

Waterman, J.A. (1938). Some notes on scorpion poisoning in Trinidad. *Transactions of the Society of Tropical Medicine and Hygiene*, **31**, 607–24.

Spiders (Araneae)

All but one family of this enormous order are venomous, but few species have proved dangerous to humans. Spiders bite with a pair of small

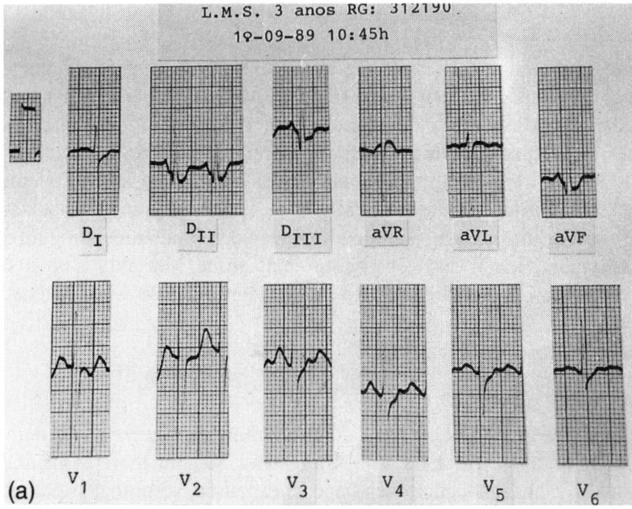

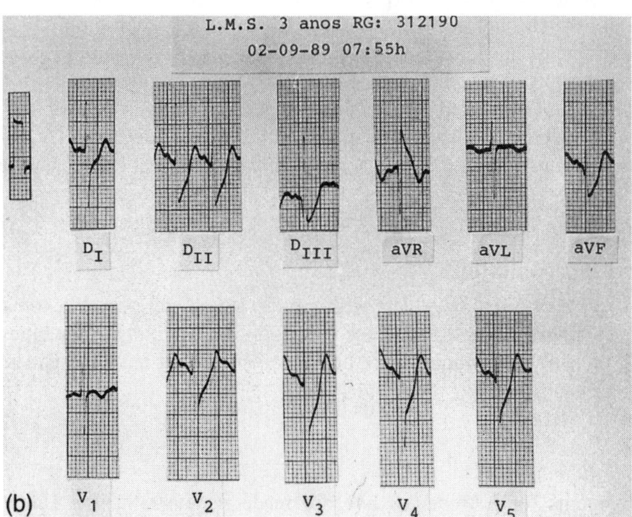

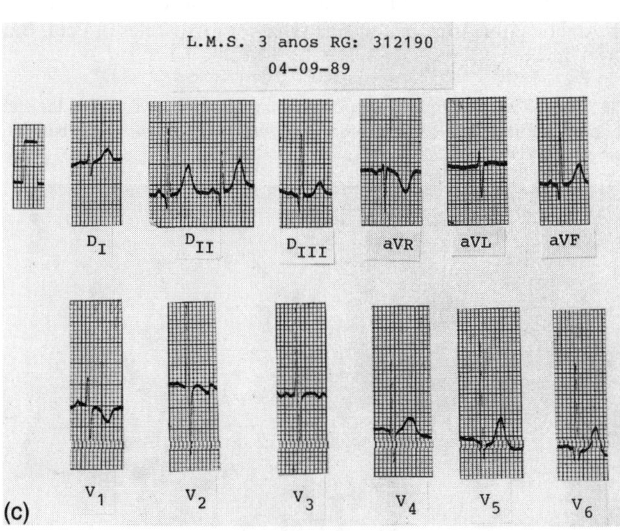

Fig. 34 Electrocardiographic changes caused by envenoming by the Brazilian scorpion (*Tityus serrulatus*). (By courtesy of Dr Carlos Amaral, Belo Horizonte, Brazil.) (a) ECG of 3-year-old girl 2 h after the sting, showing sinus tachycardia and mild T wave and ST segment changes in inferior and anterior leads. (b) Same patient 24 h after the sting showing sinus tachycardia with marked ST down sloping and ST displacement in inferior and anterolateral leads. (c) ECG of the same patient 3 days after the sting showing return to normal sinus rhythm and ST pattern.

fangs, the chelicerae, to which the venom glands are connected (Plate 22). There are four medically important genera of venomous spiders: Loxosceles cause necrotic araneism and Latrodectus, Phoneutria, and Atrax cause neurotoxic araneism.

Epidemiology

Loxosceles laeta is widely distributed and causes many bites in central and Southern America, especially in Chile, where the mortality ranges from 1 to 17 per cent. *Loxosceles reclusa*, the brown recluse spider, has caused at least 200 bites and six deaths in the United States this century. More than 60 cases were reported from Texas between 1959 and 1962. Bites by *L. rufescens* have been reported from the Mediterranean region, North Africa, and Israel. Most Loxosceles bites occur in bedrooms while people are asleep or dressing and in the United States a number of men were bitten on the genitalia while they sat on outdoor lavatories in which the spiders had spun their webs. *Latrodectus tredecemguttatus* (sometimes referred to, loosely, as 'tarantula') lives in fields in Mediterranean countries and has been responsible for a series of epidemics of bites. In Italy, 946 cases were reported between 1946 and 1951. *Latrodectus hasselti*, the Australian redback spider, causes up to 340 bites each year in Australia and 20 deaths have been reported. The black widow spider (*L. mactans*) was responsible for 63 deaths in the United States between 1950 and 1959. Other species of Latrodectus are found in Latin America (Plate 23). *Phoneutria nigriventer* (Plate 24), the banana spider, causes bites and deaths in South American countries. These spiders have been imported to temperate countries on bunches of bananas and have been responsible for a few bites and deaths. The funnel web spiders (genus Atrax) are restricted to south-eastern Australia and Tasmania. The Sydney funnel web spider (A. robustus) occurs only within a 160-mile (256 km) radius of Sydney. The aggressive males of this species caused at least 13 deaths between 1927 and 1980. In England, mild neurotoxic araneism has been described after bites by *Steatoda nobilis* (Theridiidae) and the woodlouse spider (*Dysdera crocota*).

Fig. 35 Pulmonary oedema caused by *Tityus serrulatus* envenoming. (By courtesy of Dr Carlos Amaral, Belo Horizonte, Brazil.) (a) Chest radiograph of 9-year-old girl 24 h after the sting showing alveolar infiltrates over both lungs with air bronchograms. The heart size is increased. (b) Chest radiograph of 7-year-old girl 10 h after the sting showing bilateral pulmonary oedema with enlarged heart.

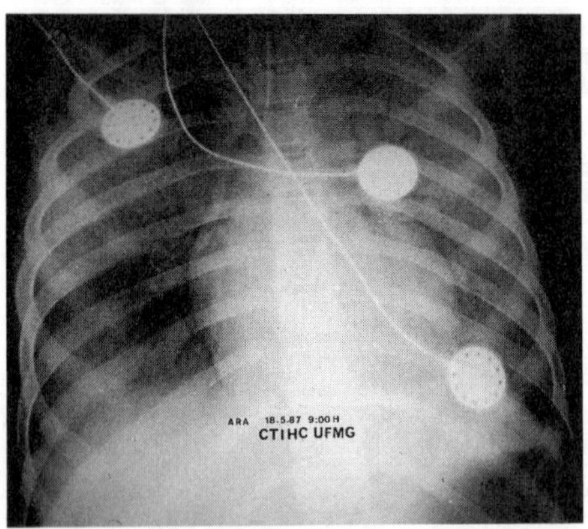

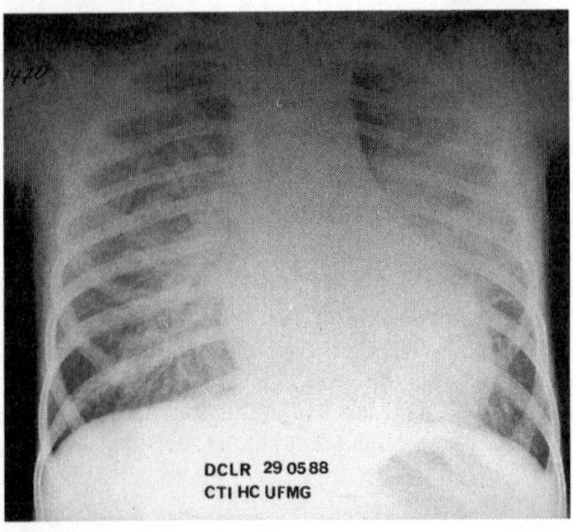

Necrotic araneism

There is burning at the site of the bite with swelling and development of a characteristic macular lesion (Plate 25) which becomes violaceous and then turns into a blackened eschar (Plate 26) that sloughs in a few weeks, sometimes leaving a necrotic ulcer. The necrotic area may, rarely, cover an entire limb. Facial lesions may cause much oedema (Plate 27). Thirteen per cent of cases have systemic symptoms such as fever, scarlatiniform rash, jaundice, and haemoglobinuria resulting from intravascular haemolysis. Renal failure may ensue. Mortality is about 6 per cent of all reported cases and 30 per cent of those with systemic envenoming.

Neurotoxic araneism

The bite is very painful but local signs are minimal (*Lactrodectus mactans*) or moderate (L. hasselti). After about 30 min there is painful regional lymphadenopathy, then headache, nausea, vomiting, sweating, 'gooseflesh' (horripilation) (Fig. 36), and painful muscle spasms and tremors which may be severe enough to embarrass respiration. Other features include tachycardia, hypertension, restlessness, irritability, psychosis, priapism, and rhabdomyolysis. The 'facies latrodectismica' is a painful grimace caused by facial spasm and trismus associated with swollen eyelids, congested conjunctivae, flushing and sweating (*L. tredecemguttatus*). Similar effects are seen in patients bitten by Phoneutria and Atrax.

First aid treatment

In the case of bites by spiders with rapidly acting and potent venoms, such as *Atrax robustus*, firm crepe bandaging and splinting of the bitten limb or a tight tourniquet may delay venom spread until the patient reaches hospital.

Specific treatment

Antivenoms for Latrodectus bite are made in Australia, the United States, the Russian Federation, Italy, Yugoslavia, South Africa, and South America; for Atrax bite in Australia; for Loxosceles in Peru, Bra-

Fig. 36 'Gooseflesh' (horripilation), piloerection, and local sweating at the site of a bite by the Brazilian 'banana spider' (*Phoneutria nigriventer*) 1 h before. (Copyright D.A. Warrell.)

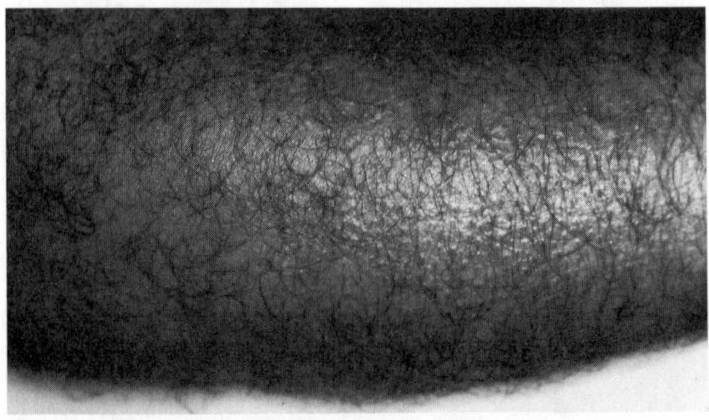

zil, and Argentina; and for Phoneutria in Brazil. Neurotoxic araneism seems more responsive to antivenom than does the necrotic type.

Supportive treatment

Oral dapsone (100 mg twice daily) is said to reduce the extent of necrotic lesions. Calcium gluconate (10 ml of a 10 per cent solution, given by slow intravenous injection) relieves the pain of muscle spasms caused by Latrodectus venom rapidly and more effectively than muscle relaxants such as diazepam or methocarbamol. Antihistamines, corticosteroids, β-blockers, and atropine have also been advocated.

REFERENCES

Bettini, S. (ed.) (1978). Arthropod venoms. *Handbook of experimental pharmacology*. Vol 48, p.121. Springer-Verlag, Berlin.

Clark, R.F., *et al.* (1992). Clinical presentation and treatment of black widow spider envenomation: a review of 163 cases. *Annals of Emergency Medicine*, **21,** 782–7.

Maretić, Z. and Lebez, D. (1979). *Araneism with special reference to Europe*. Novit, Pula-Ljubjan, Yugoslavia.

Southcott, R.V. (1976). Arachnidism and allied syndromes in the Australian region. *Records of Adelaide Childrens Hospital*, **1,** 97–186.

Sutherland, S.K. (1983). *Australian animal toxins. The creatures, their toxins and care of the poisoned patient*. Oxford University Press, Melbourne.

Warrell, D.A., *et al.* (1991). Neurotoxic envenoming by an immigrant spider (*Steatoda nobilis*) in southern England. *Toxicon*, **29,** 1263–5.

Ticks (Acari)

Taxonomy and epidemiology

Ticks, with mites, form the order Acari of the class Arachnida. Adult females of about 34 species of hard tick (family Ixodidae) and immature specimens of nine species of soft ticks (family Argasidae) have been implicated in human tick paralysis. The tick's saliva contains a neurotoxin which causes presynaptic neuromuscular block and decreased nerve conduction velocity. The tick embeds itself in the skin with its barbed hypostome introducing the salivary toxin while it engorges with blood.

Although tick paralysis has been reported from all continents, most cases occur in western North America (*Dermacentor andersoni*), eastern United States (*D. variabilis*) and eastern Australia from north Queensland to Victoria (*Ixodes holocyclus* known as the bush, scrub, paralysis, or dog tick). In British Columbia there were 305 cases with 10 per cent mortality between 1900 and 1968. About 120 cases have been reported in the United States and in New South Wales there were at least 20 deaths between 1900 and 1945.

Clinical features

Ticks are picked up in the countryside or from domestic animals, particularly dogs, in the home. A majority of patients and almost all fatal cases are children. After the tick has been attached for about 5 or 6 days a progressive ascending, lower motor neurone paralysis develops with paraesthesiae. Often a child, who may have been irritable for the previous 24 h, falls on getting out of bed first thing in the morning and is found to be weak or ataxic. Paralysis increases over the next few days: death results from bulbar and respiratory paralysis and aspiration of stomach contents. Vomiting is a feature of the more acute course of *Ixodes holocyclus* envenoming.

This clinical picture is often misinterpreted as poliomyelitis, although in North America the peak incidence of tick paralysis is earlier in the year than the epidemic season for poliomyelitis. Other neurological conditions including Guillain-Barré syndrome, paralytic rabies, Eaton–Lambert syndrome, myasthenia gravis, or botulism may also be suspected. Diagnosis depends on finding the tick, which is likely to be concealed in a crevice, orifice, or hairy area of the body. The scalp is the most common place. Fatal tick paralysis has been caused by a tick attached to the tympanic membrane.

Treatment

The tick must be detached without being squeezed. It can be painted with ether, chloroform, paraffin, petrol, or turpentine, or prised out between the partially separated tips of a pair of small curved forceps. Following removal of the tick there is usually rapid and complete recovery; but in Australia, patients have died after the tick has been detached. An antivenom, raised in dogs, is available in Australia and, recently, rabbits have been used to produce an antitoxin against *I. holocyclus* saliva. This is recommended for severely affected or very young patients; 20 to 30 ml is given intravenously.

REFERENCES

Gothe, R., Kunze, K., and Hoogstraal, H. (1979). The mechanism of pathogenicity in the tick paralyses. *Journal of Medical Entomology*, **16,** 357–369.

Murnaghan, M.F. and O'Rourke, F.J. (1978). Tick paralysis. In *Arthropod Venoms. Handbook of experimental pharmacology*. Vol. 48 (ed. S. Bettini), p. 419. Springer-Verlag, Berlin.

Pearn, J. (1977). The clinical features of tick bite. *Medical Journal of Australia*, **2,** 313.

Stone, B.F. (1987). Toxicoses induced by ticks and reptiles in domestic animals. In *Natural toxins: Animal, plant and microbial* (ed. J.B. Harris). Oxford University Press, Oxford.

Centipedes (Chilopoda)

Many species of centipede can inflict painful bites (Fig. 37) producing swelling, inflammation, and lymphangitis. Systemic effects such as vomiting, headache, cardiac arrhythmias, and convulsions are extremely rare and the risk of mortality was probably greatly exaggerated in the older literature. The most important genus is Scolopendra which is distributed throughout tropical countries. Local treatment is the same as for scorpion stings. No antivenom is available.

Millipedes (Diplopida)

Most species possess glands in each of their body segments which secrete, and in some cases squirt out, irritant liquids for defensive purposes. These contain hydrogen cyanide and a variety of aldehydes,

Fig. 37 Venom jaws of a Thai centipede (*Scolopendra* sp.). (Copyright D.A. Warrell.)

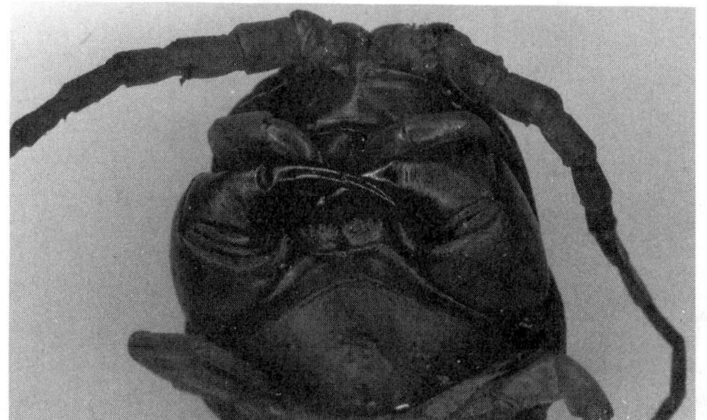

esters, phenols, and quinonoids. Members of at least eight genera of millipedes have proved injurious to humans. Important genera are Rhinocricus (Caribbean), Spirobolus (Tanzania), Spirostreptus and Iulus (Indonesia), and Polyceroconas (Papua New Guinea). Children are particularly at risk when they handle or try to eat these large arthropods. When venom is squirted into the eye, intense conjunctivitis results and there may be corneal ulceration and even blindness. Skin lesions are initially stained brown or purple, blister after a few days, and then peel. First aid is generous irrigation with water. Eye injuries should be treated as for snake venom ophthalmia (see above).

REFERENCES

Bettini, S. (ed.). *Arthropod venoms. Handbook of experimental pharmacology*, Vol. 48. Springer-Verlag, Berlin.

Radford, A.J. (1975). Millipede burns in man. *Tropical Geography*, **27**, 279–87.

Leeches (Phylum Annelida, Class Hirudinea)

Leeches are blood-sucking, hermaphroditic, egg-laying annelids which have elongated annulated bodies. They attach themselves to leaves, rocks, or the host by a posterior sucker. To feed, the leech applies its anterior sucker containing the mouth armed with three radially arranged jaws which make a Y-shaped incision. Blood is sucked out by the action of the muscular pharynx. To prevent blood clotting, the saliva contains a histamine-like vasodilator and anticoagulants, such as hirudin from the medicinal leech (*Hirudo medicinalis*) which inhibits thrombin and factor IXa, haementin from *Haementeria ghilianii* which is directly fibrinolytic, and haementerin from *H. depressa* (= *H. lutzi*) (Fig. 38), a plasminogen activator. Other enzymes include esterases, antitrypsin, antiplasmin, and antielastase. Recombinant hirudin is now produced as a therapeutic anticoagulant. The medicinal leech is still used by plastic surgeons to reduce haematomas under skin grafts; the wound may become infected with *Aeromonas hydrophila* which lives symbiotically in the leech's gut.

Two groups of leeches cause human morbidity and even mortality in tropical countries.

Land leeches

Species of the genera Haemadipsa and Phyrobdella are 1 to 8 cm long. They infest, often in enormous numbers, the damp, leafy floor and low vegetation of rain forests, choosing game trails and watering places. By standing on the posterior sucker and waving the anterior sucker, they can sense their prey with amazing efficiency. They drop on to the prey or pursue with a looping or lashing motion. These leeches usually attach themselves to the lower legs or ankles and are adept at penetrating clothing, even long trousers tucked into socks and lace-up boots. The bite is usually painless and the infested person may not realize what has happened until he hears a squelching sound, notices that his feet are warm and wet and sees blood welling over the tops of the boots. Land leeches ingest about 1 ml of blood in 1 h and then drop off, but the wound continues to bleed for some time and forms a fragile clot.

Fig. 38 Aquatic leech (*Haementeria depressa* = *H. lutzi*) from Brazil. Lateral (above) and dorsal (below) views, showing posterior foot process on the right and anterior sucker with mouthparts on the left. Scale in cm. (Copyright D.A. Warrell.)

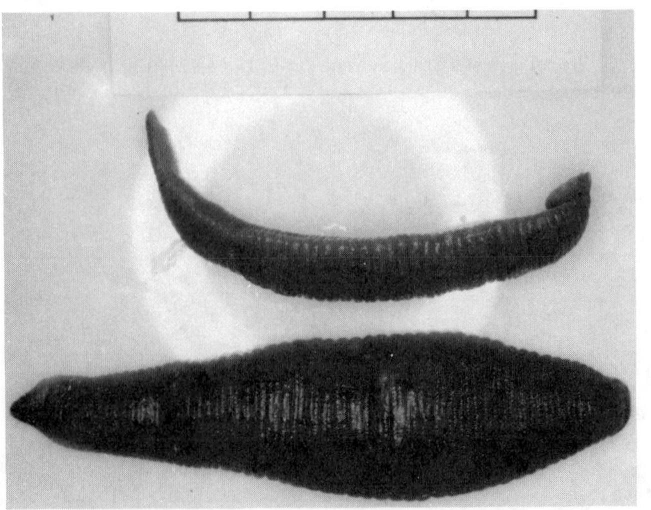

Aquatic leeches

These species may be swallowed by those who drink stagnant water or even mountain stream water or they may attack bathers, entering the mouth, nostrils, eyes, vulva, vagina, urethra, or anus. The enormous brightly coloured buffalo leech (*Hirudinaria manillensis*) of South-east Asia, is up to 16 cm long and can ingest 1 ml of blood in 10 min. *Limnatis nilotica* occurs around the Mediterranean, Middle East, and North Africa and *L. paluda* in the Middle East. *Myxobdella africana* occurs in East Africa. *Dinobdella ferox* (5 cm long) occurs in Asia. Some aquatic leeches are very slow feeders and may remain attached for days or even weeks.

Clinical features

The main effect is blood loss, but other symptoms include pain caused by the bite, secondary infection, a residual itching, and phobia. Ingested aquatic leeches usually attach to the nose or pharynx but may penetrate the trachea, bronchi, or oesophagus. *Hirudinaria manillensis* entering through the anus can reach the rectosigmoid junction of the bowel causing perforation and peritonitis. Patients with a leech in the pharynx often have a feeling of movement at the back of the throat with cough, hoarseness, stridor, breathlessness, epistaxis, haemoptysis, haematemesis and severe anaemia. Fatal upper airway obstruction may result. Bleeding may persist for up to a week after the leech has dropped off. In rural Thailand, vaginal bleeding in girls who have swum in ponds or canals is often attributable to infestation by aquatic leeches. Sexual abuse may be wrongly inferred if this diagnosis is not considered. Transmission of rinderpest and other viruses, leptospirosis, and *Trypanosoma cruzi* has been suggested but not proved. Secondary infection of medicinal leech bites by *Aeromonas hydrophila* has been described.

Treatment

Leeches will detach if a grain of salt, a lighted match, or a cigarette, alcohol, turpentine, or vinegar are applied. Local bleeding can be stopped by applying a styptic, such as silver nitrate or a firm dressing. Aquatic leeches which have penetrated the respiratory, upper gastrointestinal, or genitourinary tracts, or the rectum must be removed by endoscope. Spraying with 30 per cent cocaine, 10 per cent tartaric acid, or dilute (1:10 000) adrenaline makes the leech detach in the nasopharynx, larynx, trachea, or oesophagus, while irrigation with concentrated salt solution may be effective in the genitourinary tract and rectum. Leeches should not be pulled off so roughly that the mouth parts are left in the wound as this will lead to a chronic infection. Antimicrobial treatment of secondary bacterial infections (e.g. of *Aeromonas hydrophila* with cefuroxime or a quinolone) may be required.

Prevention

This can be achieved by impregnating clothing, especially the bottoms of trousers and socks, with repellants such as dibutyl phthalate and diethyl toluamide. They may also be applied to the skin and the inside and outside of footwear. If these compounds are not available, invasion of footwear during jungle walks can be prevented, rather messily, by rolling a rope of tobacco in the tops of the socks and keeping the feet well soaked with water. Children should be discouraged from bathing in leech-infested waters and all drinking water should be boiled or filtered.

REFERENCES

Adams, S.L. (1988). The medicinal leech. A page from the Annelids of Internal Medicine. *Annals of Internal Medicine*, **109,** 399–405.

Cameron, A. (1950). Haematemesis from leeches. *British Medical Journal*, **3,** 679–80.

Cundall, D.B. (1986). Severe anaemia and death due to the pharyngeal leech *Myxobdella africana*. *Transactions of the Royal Society of Tropical Medicine and Hygiene*, **80,** 940–4.

Editorial. (1992). Hirudins: return of the leech? *Lancet*, **340,** 579–80.

Harrison, J.L. (1953). Leeches. *Medical Journal of Malaya*, **8,** 180–5.

Keegan, H.L. (1963). Leeches as pests of man in the Pacific region. In *Venomous and poisonous animals and noxious plants of the Pacific region* (ed. H.L. Keegan and W.R. McFarlane), pp. 99–104. Pergamon Press, Oxford.

Kelen, E.N.A. and Rosenfeld, G. (1975). Fibrinogenolytic substance (hementerin) of Brazilian blood-sucking leeches (*Haementeria lutzi* Pinto 1920). *Haemostasis*, **4,** 51–64.

Sawyer, R.T. (1986). *Leech biology and behaviour*. Oxford University Press, Oxford.

Snower, D.P., Ruef, C., Kuritza, A.P., and Edberg, S.C. (1989). *Aeromonas hydrophila* infection associated with the use of medicinal leeches. *Journal of Clinical Microbiology*, **27,** 1421–2.

Stammers, F.M.G. (1950). Observations on the behaviour of land leeches (genus Haemadipsa). *Parasitology*, **40,** 237–46.

8.4.2 Poisonous plants and fungi

M. R. COOPER and A. W. JOHNSON

Although potentially poisonous plants are abundant in both urban and rural environments, poisoning by plants is not common. In general about 5 to 10 per cent of enquiries to poisons centres concern plants, and in the majority of these cases there are no symptoms or only mild to moderate gastrointestinal irritation. The most frequent enquiries about plants in temperate zones involve fruits and seeds. Of these, some including the cherry laurel (*Prunus laurocerasus*) and laburnum (*Laburnum anagyroides*) are toxic, while others are not or only mildly so: rowan (*Sorbus aucuparia*), *Mahonia* spp., *Cotoneaster* spp., honeysuckle (*Lonicera* spp.), firethorn (*Pyracantha* spp.), Christmas cherry (*Solanum pseudocapsicum*), sweet pea (*Lathyrus odorata*), and barberry (*Berberis* spp.). There are, however, a few plants and fungi that are dangerously toxic and can cause death. These include deadly nightshade (*Atropa belladonna*), yew (*Taxus baccata*), oleander (*Nerium oleander*), yellow oleander (*Thevetia* spp.), and the death cap fungus (*Amanita phalloides*). Castor beans (*Ricinus communis*) and jequirity beans (*Abrus precatorius*) contain lectins that are among the most poisonous substances known. Correct identification of the plant involved is thus of primary importance for determining whether it is harmless, potentially toxic, or dangerously so. Even when a potentially toxic plant has been identified it is not easy to predict its effects because of the variations in the toxicity of individual plants and different plant communities, the amount ingested and the susceptibility of the individual. As there are no specific antidotes to most plant poisons, treatment is mainly directed towards elimination of the poison and support of essential functions so that the body can respond to and deal with the toxins and the damage caused. The general principles of treating plant poisoning are the same as for poisoning from any other source (see Chapter 8.1.2); only guidelines are included in the text and tables of this chapter.

We should like to thank the following for permission to reproduce photographs from their collections: A.R.G. Mundell (ARGM), G.T. Cooper (GTC), S. Berrett (SB), and D.P. Dimmock (DPD).

The risk

The majority of plant ingestions are in young children and involve berries or house plants. Older children may eat berries or other small fruits and seeds found in their gardens or playgrounds, and as they investigate further afield the variety of plants available increases. In gathering wild plants for food or experimenting with hallucinogenic plants and mushrooms serious errors in identification are sometimes made. In adults, poisoning usually results from such mistakes, with most fatalities occurring from eating some highly toxic fungus. Poisoning by plants has also been reported in mentally disturbed patients or in suicide attempts.

Farm crops and grazing land are sometimes contaminated with poisonous weeds, so that parts of these and their toxins may find their way into foodstuffs or even into milk from cows feeding on plants, such as white snakeroot (*Eupatorium rugosum*) found in the United States. Occasionally, poisoning has arisen from eating honey produced by bees that have collected nectar from poisonous plants, e.g. rhododendron (*Rhododendron ponticum*).

Another source of human poisoning is self-medication with herbal preparations that may contain plant toxins. This type of poisoning is more common in cultures relying on traditional indigenous medicines, but cases have also occurred in more developed countries where interest in the use of herbal medicine is growing as people endeavour to use 'natural' remedies.

The toxins

Numerous chemical compounds are recognized as being responsible for the toxic effects produced by poisonous plants. Their names have usually been derived from the botanical names of the plants concerned, e.g. solanine from *Solanum* species and coniine from *Conium maculatum*. Traditionally the toxins have been classified as secondary plant metabolites, and include alkaloids, glycosides (cardiac, cyanogenic, goitrogenic, and saponic), oxalates, phenols, photosensitizing agents, tannins, volatile oils, proteins, peptides and amino acids. Classification of poisonous plants on the basis of these chemical groups is of little diagnostic or therapeutic significance, as substances within these groups produce different effects on the body, while some plants contain several toxic substances belonging to different chemical groups. Many of the toxic secondary plant metabolites increase in concentration in plant tissues in response to stresses, such as drought, or attack by pathogenic microorganisms or herbivorous arthropods; the toxins, therefore, may have a defensive role in the plant. This helps to explain the variations in toxicity of different plants, with toxin content increasing to meet the danger to the plant. Not all parts of a so-called poisonous plant are necessarily poisonous. For instance the seeds of yew (*Taxus baccata*) are highly toxic, and sudden death can occur if they are chewed, yet the surrounding red fleshy cup (aril) can be eaten without harmful effects. The red leaf stalks of rhubarb (*Rheum rhaponticum*) are edible when cooked and are commonly used as a dessert, but the green leaf blades have a high oxalate content and should never be eaten. The toxins are not necessarily distributed uniformly throughout a plant, but may be present in greater concentrations in certain parts. The concentration of these substances can also vary with the stage of growth and the growing conditions of the plant. Ingestion of plant materials containing chemical residues (from agricultural sprays or atmospheric pollution) can also lead to poisoning.

The effects

Once a plant has been identified the relevant textbooks and databases can be consulted to ascertain its likely toxic effects. Often, however, it is not known what plant or part of the plant has been eaten, or how much. A preliminary classification of plant poisoning can be based on the early signs and symptoms, with the plants being grouped according to those producing:

1. Irritation of the alimentary tract
   (a) mouth and throat
   (b) stomach and intestine
   (c) delayed gastroenteritis
2. Cardiovascular disturbances
3. Nicotine-like actions
4. Atropine-like actions
5. Central nervous effects, convulsions, hallucinations
6. Effects caused by hydrocyanic acid
7. Toxicity to the liver
8. Toxicity to the kidneys
9. Dermatitis

The range and severity of the toxic effects depend on the quantity of plant material eaten and the sensitivity of the individual. The above groups are not mutually exclusive; they are only a guide, with the effects of some plants falling into more than one group.

IRRITATION OF THE ALIMENTARY TRACT (TABLE 1 AND PLATES 1–6)

The mouth then the stomach and the rest of the digestive system are usually the first parts of the body to be affected when poisonous plants are eaten. Some plants that have very irritant sap, such as dumb cane (*Dieffenbachia* spp.), mezereon (*Daphne mezereum*), cuckoo pint (*Arum maculatum*), spurges (*Euphorbia* spp.), and black bryony (*Tamus communis*) give rise at once to soreness, reddening and even blistering of the lips and mouth. With most plants the first signs of poisoning are nausea, abdominal pain, and vomiting. In many cases the vomiting eliminates the poisonous substances and prevents the development of further toxic effects. Elimination of the poisonous substances is also promoted by diarrhoea, another very common reaction to eating poisonous plants.

Treatment

If vomiting has not occurred spontaneously, gastric emptying should be ensured by lavage or use of an emetic; fluid and electrolyte balance must be maintained.

CARDIOVASCULAR DISTURBANCES (TABLE 2 AND PLATES 7–13)

In addition to the well-known effects of foxglove (*Digitalis purpurea*) and its constituents, there are various other plants that contain cardiac glycosides producing the digitalis-like effects seen in digoxin overdosage (see Chapter 8.2.3).

Treatment

Ingested material should be removed, but not with ipecacuanha as this can also have effects on the heart. The Fab fragments of digoxin-specific antibody (Digibind) are not just specific for digoxin but can also be used to reverse the toxic effects of many of the other cardiac glycosides. Poisoning by the highly toxic alkaloids in aconite (*Aconitum* spp.) should always be treated as an emergency.

NICOTINE-LIKE ACTIONS (TABLE 3 AND PLATE 14)

Nicotine and other alkaloids with similar actions such as coniine from hemlock (*Conium maculatum*) first stimulate and then paralyse all autonomic ganglia. Centrally, small doses cause respiratory stimulation, while large doses produce convulsions and arrest of respiration.

Treatment

This should be symptomatic. Gastric lavage rather than ipecacuanha-induced emesis is recommended because of the rapid onset of the effects of nicotine.

ATROPINE-LIKE ACTIONS (TABLE 4 AND PLATE 15)

Atropine and hyoscine competitively inhibit the muscarinic effects of acetylcholine and block the parasympathetic nervous system. Their actions on the central nervous system differ qualitatively in that atropine first has stimulatory then depressive effects, whereas hyoscine generally has only a depressive effect. Both cause death by depression of the respiratory centre. The clinical signs of poisoning produced by plants in this group vary with the relative proportions they contain of atropine and hyoscine.

Treatment

Ipecacuanha can be used to induce emesis if given within 30 min of ingestion, otherwise gastric lavage should be performed. Physostigmine has been recommended for treatment of the central and peripheral effects, but it is not clear that this is superior to supportive management.

CENTRAL NERVOUS EFFECTS (TABLE 5 AND PLATE 16)

Although a number of plants contain convulsant substances, actual clinical cases have mainly involved Umbelliferae, whose leaf stalks have been mistaken for celery and roots for parsnips. Ingestion of unripe fruits of akee (*Blighia sapida*) causes Jamaican vomiting sickness, which is characterized by hypoglycaemia and convulsions. Plants that contain hallucinogenic compounds, e.g. cannabis (*Cannabis sativa*), are smoked, chewed, eaten, or infused in water to make teas.

Treatment

Convulsions must be controlled and respiration supported; it will then be possible to wash out the stomach safely. Patients who have taken hallucinogens require reassurance and supportive treatment.

HYDROCYANIC ACID TOXICITY

Although many plants contain cyanogenic glycosides in trace amounts, there are some which have relatively high concentrations that are potentially toxic. There is no obvious pattern in the family or genus where high concentrations are found, and even closely related species and individual plants of the same genus may differ greatly in their content of cyanogenic glycosides. In the potentially toxic species the highest concentrations are usually found in the leaves, but high concentrations also occur in seeds, roots, and other tissues. The most likely sources of human poisoning are the kernels of fruits of *Prunus* species (almonds, apricots, cherries, peaches, etc.) or of loquat (*Eriobotrya japonica*), a large number of apple pips (*Malus* spp.), the berries or leaves of the cherry laurel (*Prunus laurocerasus* (Plate 17), or inadequately prepared cassava (*Manihot esculenta*). The symptoms include vomiting, abdominal pain, weakness, coma, and tetanic convulsions.

Treatment

This is the same as for cyanide poisoning from any source (see Chapter 8.3.4). Mild cases may require only gastric lavage and supportive care.

LIVER DAMAGE

Various species of the Compositae (*Senecio* spp.), Leguminosae (*Crotalaria* spp.) and Boraginaceae (*Heliotropium* and *Symphytum* spp. (Plate 18)) as well as some other plant families contain pyrrolizidine alkaloids, which principally affect the liver. Human poisoning has occurred as a result of the contamination of cereal crops by these plants and their consequent incorporation into bread, and their use in herbal

Table 1 *Plants that irritate the alimentary tract*

	Plants	Toxic agents	Symptoms and signs	Treatment
Irritation of mouth and throat	Araceae: *Arum maculatum* (cuckoo pint) (Plate 1); *Dieffenbachia* spp. (dumb cane); *Philodendron* spp. (elephant's ear)	Calcium oxalate	Burning sensation; dysphagia; salivation; oedema	Intense pain in the mouth may need relief, e.g. with pethidine; fluids and soft food
	Tamus communis (black bryony) (Plate 2)	Probably calcium oxalate		
	Daphne spp. (mezereon, spurge laurel)	Diterpene esters		
	Euphorbia spp. (Plate 3)			
Irritation of stomach and intestines	*Aloe* spp.	Anthraquinones	Salivation, vomiting, abdominal pain, diarrhoea; effects on CNS, renal, and cardiovascular systems if absorbed	Gastric lavage; demulcents; correct fluid and electrolyte levels; prevent severe hypotension; possibly haemodialysis
	Frangula alnus (alder buckthorn)			
	Rhamnus cathartica (buckthorn)			
	Arum maculatum (cuckoo pint) (Plate 1)	Calcium oxalate		
	Laburnum anagyroides (laburnum) (Plate 4)	Cytisine		
	Jatropha spp.	Lectins		
	Amaryllidaceae: *Narcissus* spp. (daffodil etc.)	Lycorine		
	Anemone spp.	Protoanemonin		
	Clematis spp.			
	Helleborus spp. (hellebores, Christmas rose)			
	Ranunculus spp. (buttercups)			
	Aesculus hippocastanum (horse chestnut)	Saponins		
	Hedera helix (ivy)			
	Viscum album (mistletoe)	Viscotoxins		
	Actaea spp. (baneberry)	Unknown		
	Bryonia dioica (white bryony)			
	Ilex aquifolium (holly)			
	Lantana camara			
	Ligustrum vulgare (privet)			
	Phytolacca americana (pokeweed)			
	Symphoricarpos alba (snowberry)			
	Wisteria spp.			
Delayed gastroenteritis	*Colchicum autumnale* (autumn crocus)	Colchicine	No symptoms for 1 h to 2 days; severe vomiting and diarrhoea with blood; disturbance of CNS, renal, and cardiovascular functions	Cautious gastric lavage; demulcents; allow diarrhoea, but monitor fluid and electrolyte levels; control abdominal pain, e.g. with pethidine; assist respiration; consider haemodialysis
	Gloriosa superba (glory lily)			
	Abrus precatorius (jequirity bean)	Lectins		
	Ricinus communis (castor bean) (Plate 5)			
	Robinia pseudoacacia (false acacia)			
	Parthenocissus spp. (Virginia creeper)	Oxalic acid		
	Rumex spp. (dock, sorrel)			
	Solanum spp. (potato, bittersweet, black nightshade) (Plate 6)	Solanine		
	Euonymus europaeus (spindle)	Unknown		

Table 2 *Plants that cause cardiovascular disturbance*

Plants	Toxic agents	Symptoms and signs	Treatment
Aconitum napellus (monkshood) (Plate 7) *Delphinium* spp. (larkspur)	Aconitine	Tingling, burning, and numbness of mouth and lips; dysphagia, salivation, nausea and vomiting; tingling in fingers and face; headache; blurred vision; bradycardia; muscular weakness; dyspnoea; death in 1–6 h	**Emergency** Evacuate stomach immediately; atropine, antiarrhythmic agents, and possibly intravenous calcium and magnesium; assist respiration
Kalmia latifolia (mountain laurel) *Menziesia* spp. *Pieris* spp. *Rhododendron ponticum* (Plate 8)	Andromedotoxins	Burning in mouth; after several hours salivation, vomiting and diarrhoea; headache; muscular weakness; bradycardia; hypotension; sometimes convulsions and coma	Gastric lavage; maintain fluid and electrolyte levels; assist respiration; atropine
Convallaria majalis (lily of the valley) *Digitalis purpurea* (foxglove) (Plate 9) *Hyacinthoides non-scripta* (bluebell) *Nerium oleander* (oleander) (Plate 10) *Scilla* spp. (squill) *Thevetia* spp. (yellow oleander)	Cardiac glycosides	Irritation of mouth; vomiting, diarrhoea, abdominal pain; headache; cardiac arrhythmias	Gastric lavage; potassium if hypokalaemia occurs; monitor ECG and give antiarrhythmic agents if needed (see digoxin overdose, Chapter 8.2.3)
Veratrum spp. (false hellebores) (Plate 11)	Protoveratrines	Epigastric burning, salivation, and emesis; sweating, confusion, bradycardia, and hypotension	Gastric lavage; atropine; vasoconstrictive agents if hypotension severe; assist respiration
Taxus baccata (yew) (Plate 12)	Taxines	As for protoveratrines but also cardiac arrhythmias; cyanosis; dyspnoea; coma	**Emergency** As for protoveratrines; monitor ECG; consider temporary pacemaker
Zigadenus spp. (death camas) (Plate 13)	Veratrine	As for protoveratrines but vomiting may be delayed; drowsiness and coma	As for protoveratrines
Phoradendron flavescens (American mistletoe)	Unknown	Nausea, vomiting, diarrhoea; sweating; apathy; hypotension	Emetics or gastric lavage; atropine

medicines and bush teas. These alkaloids can produce acute damage to the liver (veno-occlusive disease), which has occurred, mainly in children, in Jamaica, India, and Afghanistan. Symptoms, including nausea, abdominal pain and distension, hepatomegaly, and sometimes fever and vomiting, first appear a few days after ingestion. A chronic cirrhosis of the liver can occur in people ingesting small quantities of pyrrolizidine alkaloids over a long period.

Treatment

This can only be supportive, as once absorbed there is no specific method of preventing the toxic effects of these alkaloids.

KIDNEY DAMAGE

Kidney failure occurs after ingestion of plants rich in oxalates e.g. the leaves of rhubarb (*Rheum rhaponticum*) and dock (*Rumex crispus*).

Treatment

An emetic should be given, followed by generous fluid replacement to promote renal excretion of the oxalates.

DERMATITIS

This usually results from the direct action of plants on the skin, e.g. the stinging hairs of the stinging nettle (*Urtica dioica*), the irritant diterpene-containing latex of *Euphorbia* spp., or the calcium oxalate crystals of *Dieffenbachia* spp. and other members of the Araceae family. There are also allergic forms of dermatitis that result from hypersensitivity to plant allergens. The most common form of direct contact allergic dermatitis in the United States is caused by poison ivy (*Toxicodendron radicans*) and western poison oak (*Toxicodendron diversilobum*), and in the United Kingdom by primula (*Primula obconica*), but such cutaneous hypersensitivity can occur to a very large number of vascular plants. Some plants contain phototoxic chemicals that increase the reactivity of the skin to ultraviolet light. Exposure to sunlight after eating fat hen (*Chenopodium album*), orache (*Atriplex purpurea*), or other members of the Chenopodiaceae has resulted in severe skin damage. Psoralens (furocoumarins) are present in various members of the Umbelliferae, including giant hogweed (*Heracleum mantegazzianum* (Plate 19)) and parsnips (*Pastinaca sativa*) and also celery (*Apium graveolens*) when infected with the pink rot fungus (*Sclerotinia sclerotiorum*). Other psoralen-containing plants are rue (*Ruta graveolens* (Plate 20)) and the gas plant (*Dictamnus albus*), both in the Rutaceae family. The lesions are similar to those of contact dermatitis with papules, vesicles, and enormous bullae localized to exposed areas of skin. Hyperpigmentation often occurs and can last for several months.

Treatment

The source should be identified and avoided, and relief given for itching and inflammation.

Table 3 *Plants with nicotine-like actions*

Plants	Toxic agents	Symptoms and signs	Treatment
Conium maculatum (hemlock) (Plate 14)	Coniine	Irritation of mouth; salivation, nausea and persistent vomiting; vertigo, headache; sweating; confusion, delirium, hallucinations, fasciculation, and convulsions; possibly paralysis and coma	Gastric lavage; assist respiration; manage convulsions; give antihypotensive drugs
Gelsemium sempervirens (yellow jessamine)	Gelsemine and other alkaloids		
Laburnum anagyroides (laburnum) (Plate 4)	Cytisine		
Lobelia spp.	Lobeline		
Nicotiana tabacum (tobacco)	Nicotine		

Table 4 *Plants with atropine-like actions*

Plants	Toxic agents	Symptoms and signs	Treatment
Atropa belladonna (deadly nightshade) (Plate 15)	Tropane alkaloids	Photophobia and visual disturbance due to mydriasis and loss of accommodation; dry mouth and intense thirst; hot, dry, flushed skin, sometimes erythematous rash; tachycardia; fever, headache, confusion, delirium, hallucinations; urinary retention; constipation; convulsions, stupor, coma, and respiratory failure	Prompt gastric lavage; slow intravenous infusion of physostigmine; sedate, and control convulsions; external cooling; pilocarpine eye drops
Brugmansia (angel's trumpet)			
Cestrum spp. (jessamine)			
Datura stramonium (thorn apple)			
Hyoscyamus niger (henbane)			

Fungi (Table 6 and Plates 21–23)

Of the many thousands of higher fungi (mushrooms, toadstools, and brackets) that have been identified, only a few are used regularly for food. Some that grow in the wild are very good to eat, but a few are dangerously poisonous. The toxicity of many is not known. Most cases of poisoning (mycetismus) result from mistaken identification. It is not without significance that in countries where it is common practice to collect and eat wild fungi, and also among those who choose to eat so-called 'natural' foods, there are more cases of fungal poisoning.

With fungi there is even greater variation than with vascular plants in the susceptibility of individuals, and even of the same individual on different occasions. The toxicity of fungi may vary with location, season and in different years, while even fungi considered to be edible, including the cultivated mushroom (*Agaricus bisporus*), can sometimes cause poisoning, especially if old, damaged, raw, or inadequately cooked.

An indication of what type of fungal toxin has been ingested can be gained, in the absence of specimens for identification, by ascertaining how quickly symptoms appeared and how quickly they abated. The latter is of particular importance as it may indicate the complete resolution of the toxic episode, or may signal the start of a latent period before further, more severe signs appear. Gastrointestinal disturbances are by far the most common symptoms; these usually appear within 2 h and eliminate most of the toxin so that most patients require no or only symptomatic treatment. Some hallucinogenic fungi (magic mushrooms) may also have no lasting effects. The life-threatening conditions (especially liver and kidney failure) follow apparent recovery from gastrointestinal symptoms that start 6 to 24 h after ingestion or occur after a latent, symptomless period of several days' duration.

Cases of fungal poisoning can be classified into those that develop signs of toxicity:

1. Within 2 h
   (a) mainly gastrointestinal
   (b) sweating, vertigo
   (c) delirium, deep sleep
   (d) hallucinations
   (e) associated with drinking alcohol
2. After 6 h or up to several days
   (a) severe vomiting and diarrhoea
   (b) oliguria, anuria
   (c) abdominal discomfort, severe headache.

SYMPTOMS THAT DEVELOP WITHIN 2 HOURS

Most cases of fungal poisoning fall into this category.

Gastroenteritis

Symptoms involving only the gastrointestinal tract account for the majority of these cases, and can result from eating any of a wide range of fungi. The symptoms vary from nausea, mild stomach-ache, or abdominal pain to severe emesis and profuse diarrhoea, which may persist for more than 24 h. In most cases symptomatic treatment, with fluid therapy as indicated, is all that is required, but it should always be borne in mind that initial gastrointestinal disturbances may precede some of the life-threatening fungal intoxications.

Sweating

This, associated with nausea, headache, visual disturbances, vertigo, hypotension, and some incoordination results from the parasympathomimetic effects of muscarine, which is present in many *Inocybe* and some *Clitocybe* species. There are only trace amounts of muscarine in *Amanita muscaria*, after which this toxin was named.

Mental confusion and sleep

Fungi that contain ibotenic acid and its derivative muscimol (*Amanita pantherina*, *A. muscaria*, and *A. strobiliformis*) affect psychomotor functions, and cause gastrointestinal disturbances. Dizziness, delirium and euphoria are common symptoms, sometimes associated with erratic, or even manic behaviour; deep sleep usually follows. These fungi can have very serious effects on children.

Table 5 *Plants that affect the central nervous system*

	Plants	Toxic agents	Symptoms and signs	Treatment
Convulsants	Umbelliferae: *Cicuta virosa* (cowbane)	Cicutoxin	Nausea, salivation, vomiting; tremors then severe intermittent seizures, exhaustion and respiratory failure	Control convulsions e.g. with barbiturates or diazepam; support respiration
	Oenanthe crocata (hemlock water dropwort) (Plate 16)	Oenanthetoxin		
	Blighia sapida (akee)	Hypoglycin A	Vomiting; convulsions; coma	Maintain fluid and electrolyte balance
	Coriaria myrtifolia	Coriariamyrtin	Convulsions	Maintain airway; support respiration; control convulsions
	Karwinskia humboldtiana	Anthracenones	Ascending paralytic neuropathy	Supportive
	Melia azedarach (chinaberry)	Tetranortriterpenes	Ataxia; mental confusion; stupor; sometimes vomiting and diarrhoea; convulsions	Symptomatic
	Menispermum canadense (moonseed)	Various alkaloids	Convulsions	Maintain airway; support respiration; control convulsions
	Podophyllum peltatum (May apple)	Podophylloresin	Vomiting; convulsions; coma	Symptomatic
	Strychnos nux-vomica (nux vomica)	Strychnine and brucine	Stiffness of face and neck muscles; reflex excitability; severe tetanic convulsions, and medullary paralysis	Gastric lavage when convulsions are controlled
Hallucinogens	*Cannabis sativa* (Indian hemp, hashish, pot etc.)	Tetrahydrocannabinols	Nausea; thirst; euphoria; tremor; drowsiness; hallucinations	Do not leave alone; reassurance and support to control panic
	Catha edulis (khat)	Alkaloids	Amphetamine-like effects	
	Ipomoea spp. (morning glory)	Lysergic acid and ethylamides	As cannabis above; also mydriasis and other sympathomimetic effects	
	Lophophora williamsii (peyote)	Mescaline	In 3–6 h vomiting and abdominal pain; lethargy; delirium; tachycardia; hypertension	
	Myristica fragrans (nutmeg)	Myristicin	Hallucinations; vomiting; sympathomimetic effects; tension; anxiety	
	Vinca spp. (periwinkle)	Vincristine and vinblastine	As cannabis above; also alopecia and paraesthesia	

Hallucinations

Psilocybin, a tryptamine derivative with hallucinogenic properties, is found in *Psilocybe* species and several other genera of (usually small) fungi, often called collectively 'magic mushrooms'. These fungi are eaten because of their psychoactive properties. They generally produce a feeling of relaxation, with visual effects, especially heightened perception of colour and shapes. The sensations may, however, be characterized by tension, agitation, and nausea; sometimes frightening flashbacks occur.

Alcohol-associated effects

When alcohol is taken at the same time as some fungi (notably *Coprinus atramentarius*, but also *Clitocybe clavipes*) or up to 5 days after they are eaten, a reaction similar to that induced by disulfiram (Antabuse) used for treating alcoholics (see Section 28) is produced. The skin becomes flushed and mydriasis, nausea, and hypotension can occur as a result of the accumulation of acetaldehyde because the toxin (named coprine in *C. atramentarius*) blocks the liver enzyme aldehyde dehydrogenase.

SYMPTOMS WITH DELAYED ONSET

Gastroenteritis

Digestive system disturbances that appear several hours or even days after ingestion are characteristic of the most severe types of fungal poisoning. By far the most common cause of death from plant ingestions is the death cap (*Amanita phalloides*). Specimens of this mushroom vary in size and cap colour (from almost white to yellowish green) and they are sometimes confused with edible species. The active toxins in this mushroom and some others are cyclopeptides, called amatoxins. Persistent emesis and profuse diarrhoea begin 6 to 24 h after ingestion (commonly about 12 h). A period of apparent recovery often follows, then

Table 6 *Poisonous fungi*

	Fungi	Toxic agents	Symptoms and signs	Treatment
Severe poisoning (symptoms with delayed onset)	*Amanita phalloides* (death cap) (Plate 21) *Amanita verna* (fool's mushroom) *Amanita virosa* (destroying angel) *Galerina* spp. *Lepiota cristata*	Amatoxins	Onset delayed 6–12 h. Vomiting, abdominal cramps, and severe diarrhoea (often with blood); thirst, albuminuria, haematuria, anuria; jaundice in 2–3 days; prostration, peripheral circulatory collapse, convulsions, hepatic coma, and death in 3–8 days	**Emergency** Gastric and colonic lavage; forced diuresis; immediate haemodialysis; possibly chemotherapy (infusion of very large doses of penicillins and silybin)
	Cortinarius orellanus *Cortinarius speciosissimus* *Cortinarius splendens*	Orellanin	Nausea, vomiting, and diarrhoea after 2–14 days; sweating; intense thirst; muscular and abdominal pain; signs of liver and kidney damage; drowsiness, convulsions, and death	**Emergency** Remove toxins from body by all possible means; consider kidney transplant
	Gyromitra esculenta (false morel)	Gyromitrin	Vomiting, diarrhoea and headache after 6–24 h; sometimes delirium, coma, and death	Gastric and colonic lavage; activated charcoal: maintain fluid and electrolyte balance; forced diuresis; pyridoxine hydrochloride to support liver function
Less severe poisoning (symptoms within 2 h)	*Clitocybe* spp. *Inocybe* spp.	Muscarine	Sweating; nausea; headache, vertigo and incoordination; hypotension	Gastric lavage if no emesis; intravenous or intramuscular atropine
	Amanita muscaria (fly agaric) (Plate 22) *Amanita pantherina* (panther cap) *Amanita strobiliformis*	Ibotenic acid/ muscimol	After 30 min—3 h symptoms similar to alcohol intoxication; sometimes euphoria and illusions, muscular cramps, deep sleep, or coma	Give emetics and purgatives. Do not give atropine, diazepam or barbiturates as these potentiate the action of muscimol
	Conocybe spp. *Gymnopilus* spp. *Panaeolina foenisecii* *Panaeolus* spp. *Pluteus* spp. *Psilocybe* spp. (magic mushrooms)	Psilocybin	Hallucinations; relaxation or tension; sometimes gastroenteritis	Usually not needed; possibly give sedatives; do not leave alone
	Stropharia spp.	Possibly psilocybin		
	Clitocybe clavipes	Possibly coprine	Only with alcohol. Flushed skin; mydriasis; nausea; tingling arms and legs, rapid pulse, palpitations	Symptomatic (usually not needed); possibly give sedatives
	Coprinus atramentarius (common ink cap)	Coprine		
	Agaricus placomyces *Agaricus xanthodermus* (yellow-staining mushroom) *Armillaria mellea* (honey fungus) *Boletus satanas* *Chlorophyllum molybdites* *Entoloma* spp. *Hebeloma* spp. *Hygrocybe* spp. *Hypholoma fasciculare* (sulphur tuft) (Plate 23) *Lactarius* spp. *Macrolepiota rhacodes* *Megacollybia platyphylla* *Omphalotus olearius* *Ramaria formosa* *Russula* spp. *Scleroderma* spp. *Tricholoma pardinum*	Mostly not known	With some, only if eaten raw. Gastrointestinal disturbances of varying severity	Usually not needed; possibly emetics, gastric lavage and purgatives
	Clitocybe gibba *Marasmius oreades*	Hydrocyanic acid	See cyanide poisoning (Chapter 8.3.4)	See cyanide poisoning (Chapter 8.3.4)

rapid deterioration. Despite emergency treatment to remove the toxins from the body and the maintenance of fluid and electrolyte levels, 10 to 15 per cent of ingestions of half a cap or more result in death from liver and kidney failure.

Liver and kidney damage

Poisoning characterized by oliguria and anuria after a latent period of 3 days to about 2 weeks (sometimes preceded by gastritis) is typical of the group of brownish-orange *Cortinarius* spp. that contain the bipyridyl toxins orelline and orellanin. Death can result from renal failure; kidney transplantation should be considered.

Vomiting and headache

Gastrointestinal symptoms associated with headache, cramps, delirium, and sometimes coma that appear 6 to 24 h after ingestion, or inhalation of cooking vapour are indicative of poisoning by the false morel (*Gyromitra esculenta*). Monomethylhydrazine is liberated from gyromitrin present in the fungus.

ALLERGIC REACTIONS

A few fungi, notably the roll-rim cap (*Paxillus involutus*), previously eaten with impunity or producing only very mild symptoms may suddenly give rise to an immunohaemolytic anaemia in which decreased haemoglobin levels result in shock and even renal insufficiency.

Allergic skin reactions, e.g. pruritus with the shiitake mushroom (*Lentinus elodes*), and respiratory allergies from inhaling spores of oyster mushrooms (*Pleurotus ostreatus*), and puffballs (*Lycoperdon* spp.) have been reported. The best-known example of respiratory allergy from spore inhalation is the condition called farmer's lung that results from inhaling spores of the mould *Faenia rectivirgula* that is sometimes present on grain or hay.

ERGOTISM (ST ANTHONY'S FIRE OR 'IGNIS SACER' (SEE ALSO CHAPTER 7.11.2))

The ascomycete *Claviceps purpurea* (Plate 24) is the cause of a disease of cereal crops in which hard purplish-black fruiting bodies (sclerotia) of the fungus develop in the seed head, replacing some or all of the grains. Rye is the most frequent host, but the disease occurs in other cereals and also in wild grasses that may be reservoirs of infection for grain crops. Ergot contains several alkaloids that have been studied extensively; among them are toxic and pharmacologically active substances.

Epidemics of human and animal disease occur when grain contaminated with ergot is used for food. The most usual form of the disease occurs after contaminated flour has been eaten in relatively small quantities over a long period. The alkaloids have a vasoconstrictive action resulting in tingling, pain, and occasional swelling of the extremities with characteristic burning sensations followed by numbness. The extremities may become gangrenous, with loss of parts of digits or ears. A less common, acute, convulsive form of ergot intoxication occurs when larger amounts of ergot are consumed over a short period. This form is characterized by vertigo, trembling, headache, muscular cramps, and convulsions; hallucinations may be experienced. Now that the possible effects of eating ergotized grain are better known, there are fewer cases of ergotism associated with food; most cases result from the deliberate ingestion of ergot preparations for hallucinogenic or abortifacient purposes (the alkaloids stimulate the action of uterine smooth muscle).

MYCOTOXINS

In recent years there has been a great deal of interest in the possible adverse effects of mycotoxins produced in certain foods by mould fungi. The moulds develop on growing crops, particularly if wet and harvested late, but occur mainly in cereal grains, rice or nuts stored under damp, inadequately ventilated conditions. The toxins may be present in the absence of visible signs of mould and are not necessarily associated with any alterations in taste. The main classes of mycotoxins are aflatoxins (from *Aspergillus* spp.), ochratoxins (from *Aspergillus* and *Penicillium* spp.), trichothecenes (from *Fusarium* spp.), and zearalenone (from *Fusarium* spp.); these and several others have been detected in food and animal feeds.

The role of mycotoxins in some animal diseases is now well understood; they can damage the liver, kidneys, skin, respiratory tract, and cardiac, nervous, and reproductive systems. Several mycotoxins are potent carcinogens and, largely because of this, sophisticated methods of detection at very low concentrations (a few parts per billion) have been developed. Their possible role in human disease is still being elucidated. There is fairly substantial evidence that the alimentary toxic aleukia (pancytopenia) associated with fatalities in Russia in the Second World War was caused by T-2 toxin, a trichothecene. *Penicillium* spp. that produce ochratoxins are often found in areas where the chronic kidney disease known as Balkan nephropathy is endemic. A condition called cardiac beri-beri in the Far East may be linked with the mycotoxin citreoviridin, found mainly in rice contaminated with *Penicillium citreonigrans*. Most work has been done on aflatoxins; these are suspected of causing hepatitis, hepatocarcinoma, alveolar cell carcinoma, and colonic cancer. Aflatoxin metabolites occur in the milk of animals that have consumed them, and the possibility of human exposure by this route has been studied; the actual risk is speculative.

Food plant toxicity

Many common food plants contain significant amounts of toxins. With experience over long periods of time, the plants containing major toxins have been recognized and eliminated from the diet or methods of detoxification found, but despite this accumulated knowledge, isolated cases or large outbreaks of poisoning from food plants still occur. When eaten as part of a mixed diet, it is unlikely that symptoms of poisoning will result, but when dangerously poisonous or inadequately processed or stored plant parts that contain toxins are eaten, serious poisoning can result. In times of food shortage, plant material not generally used is eaten (e.g. flower bulbs), or such food as is available is eaten as the major, or only constituent of the diet and poisoning can result. There is some evidence that enthusiasts who eat raw plants and also vegetarians are at a greater risk than those on more conventional diets because of the toxins present naturally in the type of food they eat. Errors or the deliberate substitution of foods of similar appearance, e.g. the neurotoxic seeds of a cultivated vetch (*Vicia sativa*) for red lentils (*Lens culinaris*), have led to poisoning. More subtle influences of food plants have been identified recently that are described as antinutritive, rather than directly toxic; various enzyme inhibitors and antivitamin factors belong to this group. The main toxins present in plants used regularly for food include lectins, cyanogens, alkaloids, oxalates, and polyphenols (mainly tannins).

Lectins

These phytohaemagglutinins are glycoproteins present in a number of plants; beans, belonging to the Leguminosae family, are the main food source, although they are also present in cereals and potatoes. The lectins in many beans are not readily digested by pepsin, and have a strong affinity for the intestinal mucosa. Here they prevent absorption of carbohydrates. Fortunately adequate cooking destroys these lectins, but eating raw or incompletely cooked beans can cause diarrhoea in the short term or in acute exposure, and long-term exposure can lead to retarded growth and may even be fatal.

Cyanogens

Cyanogenic glycosides are present in the staple foods of some populations. In this category are cassava, sweet potato, and yam, all of which can be made safe to eat by adequate soaking, drying, or fermentation.

Table 7 *Herbal preparations of known toxicity*

Preparation	Plants	Constituents	Toxic effects
Aristolochia	*Aristolochia* spp.	Phenanthrene derivatives	Nephrotoxicity; carcinogenicity
Herbal teas (bush teas, tisanes)	*Crotalaria* spp. *Heliotropium* spp. *Senecio* spp. *Symphytum* spp. (comfrey) (Plate 18)	Pyrrolizidine alkaloids	Hepatic veno-occlusion, cirrhosis and liver failure; resembles Reye's syndrome
	Piper methysticum (kava-kava)	Dihydromethysticin, kava pyrones	Nervous stimulation then relaxation; ataxia; somnolence; visual and hearing defects
	Datura stramonium (thorn apple)	Atropine and related alkaloids	Hallucinations, drowsiness
	Sassafras albidum	Safrole	Hepatotoxicity
Ginseng	*Panax* spp. *Eleutherococcus* spp.	Steroids and saponic glycosides	Excitation and arousal; tremors; hypertension; oestrogenic activity
Gossypol (alleged male contraceptive)	*Gossypium* spp.	Gossypol	Possible hypokalaemia and sterility
Liquorice	*Glycyrryhiza glabra*	Glycyrrhizin and glycyrrhizinic acid	Hypokalaemia; hypertension; oedema
Pennyroyal (abortifacient)	*Mentha pulegium* *Hedeoma pulegioides*	Pulegone	Liver necrosis
Laetrile (alleged anti-cancer agent)	*Prunus* spp.	Amygdalin and/or other cyanogenic glycosides	Cyanide poisoning

Other sources include legume pulses, e.g. lima beans, and the pips or kernels of some fruits, e.g. apples and bitter almonds.

Alkaloids

Dangerously high quantities of alkaloids may develop in some plant foods, e.g. potato tubers that have sprouted or been stored in the light and become green. The green colour is chlorophyll and is harmless, but under conditions where greening occurs the glycoalkaloid solanine and its derivatives will also have been produced. The alkaloid exhibits anticholinesterase activity, resulting in diarrhoea, listlessness, and even impaired respiration.

Oxalates

These accumulate in some food plants, e.g. rhubarb (*Rheum rhaponticum*), of which only the red leaf stalks should be eaten, and then only after cooking. Oxalates have also caused poisoning when wild *Rumex* species have been used as a major constituent of a meal, e.g. sorrel soup.

Polyphenols

It has been suggested that polyphenols are a possible cause of upper digestive tract cancers that develop after eating sorghum, or taking teas or alcoholic drinks containing high concentrations of tannins.

There are particular types of plant poisoning that are restricted to certain parts of the world or certain races. In Algeria and India a paralytic disease, lathyrism, results from eating a diet composed mainly of chick peas (*Lathyrus sativus*), which contain a neurotoxic amino acid. A genetic deficiency of the enzyme glucose 6-phosphate dehydrogenase among natives of parts of North Africa, the Middle East, and the Mediterranean islands results in the disease called favism when broad (fava) beans (*Vicia fava*) are eaten, as affected individuals are unable to digest the hydrolysis products of the glycosides vicine and convicine present in the beans. In Mozambique, the seeds of *Mucuna pruriens* are eaten and cause poisoning, and in the Pacific Islands, flour is ground from the cones of cycads (e.g. *Zamia* species) which contain the glycoside cycasin. Fruits of akee (*Blighia sapida*), especially when eaten unripe, produce the gastrointestinal syndrome known as Jamaican vomiting sickness. These fruits contain the antiriboflavin substance, hypoglycin A, which causes hypoglycaemia as a result of inhibition of gluconeogenesis. The vomiting is a central effect and may be associated with convulsions and coma. The possible human toxicity of bracken fern (*Pteridium aquilinum*) has been studied extensively because of its several known toxic effects in grazing animals. There is some evidence for an association between eating the young fronds of bracken and tumours of the digestive system, mainly in Japan. Claims of possible carcinogenicity have also been made following the inhalation of bracken spores, but evidence accumulated to date is not conclusive.

Herbal medicines (Table 7)

Although many pharmaceutical preparations in current use were derived originally from plants, the stringent testing and clinical trials that are compulsory before they can be marketed make them potentially much safer to use than plant extracts or the plants themselves, which contain complex mixtures of non-standardized substances in unknown proportions. Some herbal preparations are undoubtedly efficacious in treating the condition for which they are used, but may also have underlying harmful effects that are not immediately obvious, e.g. carcinogenicity, hepatotoxicity, or teratogenicity.

Poisoning has occurred from using herbal preparations that contain other more poisonous plants inadvertently gathered with those intended for use, or through the inclusion of heavy metal compounds that are often added, particularly to Chinese medicines.

The labelling of herbal preparations is undergoing investigations in some countries, as ingredients not listed on the contents label are sometimes included to enhance their action. Ginseng preparations, for example, have been found adulterated by cheaper ingredients, and some so-called herbal medicines also contain orthodox drugs. Further complications can arise if orthodox and herbal medicines are taken simultaneously, as there may be synergic or potentiating effects.

Sources of further information

In this brief review it has been possible to mention by name only a few of the plants that can cause poisoning. The potentially toxic species present in the different regions and countries of the world obviously vary greatly, as do their whole floras. There are now, however, about 250 poison information centres worldwide that are well aware of their local toxic plants. A list of these centres has been prepared and is kept up to date for the World Federation of the Association of Clinical Toxicology Centres by Jacques Descôtes, of the Centre Anti-Poison, Lyon, France.

A problem frequently encountered by the poison centres is the inability of their callers to identify accurately the plant that is thought to have caused poisoning. An attempt to remedy this is being made in the United Kingdom, where a computerized image-based system for plant identification (e.g. by leaf shape, flower, and fruit type) is being developed jointly by Dr Virginia Murray and Christine Leon of the National Poisons Unit, Guy's and St Thomas' NHS Hospital Trust, London, and the Royal Botanic Gardens, Kew. The system, called PLATO (PLAnt TOxins), includes a selection of poisonous plants, their clinical effects, non-toxic plants that are frequently the subject of enquiries, and also some 'look-alike' plants; it is currently being evaluated in hospital accident and emergency departments in the United Kingdom. The application of PLATO to meet the needs of other countries is also being investigated.

FURTHER READING

Albert, A. (1987). *Xenobiosis. Foods, drugs and poisons in the human body.* Chapman and Hall, London.

Bresinsky, A., and Besl, H. (1990). *A colour atlas of poisonous fungi.* Wolfe Publishing Ltd, London.

Connor, H.E. (1977). *The poisonous plants in New Zealand.* E.C. Keating, Government Printers, Wellington, New Zealand.

Cooper, M.R., and Johnson, A.W. (1984). *Poisonous plants in Britain and their effects on animals and man.* Her Majesty's Stationery Office, London.

Cooper, M.R., and Johnson, A.W. (1988). *Poisonous plants and fungi. An illustrated guide.* Her Majesty's Stationery Office, London.

Ellenhorn, M.J., and Barceloux, D.G. (1988). *Medical toxicology. Diagnosis and treatment of human poisoning.* Elsevier, New York. Ch. 41. Plants—mycotoxins—mushrooms.

Everist, S.L. (1981). *Poisonous plants of Australia.* 2nd edn. Angus and Robertson Publishers, Sydney.

Frohne, D., and Pfänder, H.J. (1984). *A colour atlas of poisonous plants.* Wolfe Publishing Ltd, London.

Lampe, K.F., and McCann, M.A. (1985). *AMA handbook of poisonous and injurious plants.* American Medical Association, Chicago.

Lang, D. C. (1987). *The complete book of British berries.* Threshold Books Ltd, London.

Lovell, C.R. (1993). *Plants and the skin.* Blackwell Scientific Publications, Oxford.

Murray, V., Leon, C., and Knott, C. (1992). Identifying poisonous plants and fungi: the design and development of an image-based computer system. *Toxicon,* **30,** 538.

Penn, R.G. (1985). Adverse reactions to herbals and other unorthodox medicines. In *Iatrogenic diseases* (ed. P.F. D'Arcy and J.P. Griffin), 3rd edn, pp. 898–918. University Press, Oxford.

Pain, S. (1994). PLATO solves doctors' poison dilemmas *New Scientist,* **143,** No. 1938, 18.

Reddy, C.S., and Hayes, A.W. (1989). Food-borne toxicants. In *Principles and methods of toxicology.* 2nd edn, (ed. A.W. Hayes), pp. 67–110. Raven Press, New York.

Roth, L., Daunderer, M., and Kormann, K. (1987). *Giftpflanzen Pflanzengifte.* 3rd edn. Ecomed Verlagsgesellschaft, Landsberg, Munich.

Verdcourt, B., and Trump, E.C. (1969). *Common poisonous plants of East Africa.* Collins, London.

Watt, J.M. and Breyer-Brandwijk, M.G. (1962). *The medicinal and poisonous plants of southern and eastern Africa.* 2nd edn. E. & S. Livingstone Ltd, Edinburgh.

8.5 Occupational and environmental health and safety

8.5.1 General introduction

E. S. HODGSON AND J. M. HARRINGTON

Definition and scope

Occupational health is a multidisciplinary subject concerned with the effect of work upon employees' health and personal health upon ability to work. It is particularly concerned with prevention, but has been and will continue to be involved with the identification, investigation, and (perhaps) treatment of work-related ill health.

Successful occupational health practice requires informed and willing cooperation from management and workers. Inevitably, the health of individuals at work is affected by the general environment, and it is increasingly recognized that occupational and environmental health are closely allied disciplines requiring joint investigation of circumstances which lead to health deficits. For instance, the effect of poor external air quality (due perhaps to a mixture in the atmosphere of industrial chemicals and internal combustion engine exhaust) may complicate any health effects of airborne industrial by-products at work (Chapter 8.5.5(f)). Further variables will include pre-existent latent or overt disease, genetic factors, diet, and personal habits. The environmental scientist or physician is increasingly involved with occupational health specialists in investigating work factors, such as noise, radiation, and particulate emissions which inevitably spill over into the general environment.

The related discipline of safety engineering is concerned with the prevention and investigation of accidents at work which may be caused by workplace or job design, inadequate training and supervision, and failure to recognize the inherent hazards and consequent physical risks resulting of work procedures (Chapter 8.5.4).

Occupational and environmental health and safety are inextricably entwined in investigating and delivering the International Labour Office/World Health Organization requirements of 'the prevention amongst workers of departures from health caused by their working conditions' and 'the protection of workers . . . from risks from factors adverse to health'.

Those involved must aim to create fundamental awareness amongst workers and management that healthy and safe working practices are crucial to the maintenance of good general health. This will require the skills of occupational physicians and nurses, toxicologists, epidemiologists, occupational hygienists, ergonomists, safety engineers, and ultimately (when all else fails!) lawyers. Many of these skills overlap and there is much blurring of the division between clinical and non-clinical professionals. For instance, occupational physicians, safety and ventilation engineers, and hygienists may advise jointly on methods to control occupational lung disease using a combination of ventilation, respiratory protection, and health surveillance. The role of the occupational hygienist who is responsible for measuring, monitoring and modifying the working environment is discussed in more detail in Chapter 8.5.2.

History of occupational disease

Stone Age flint knappers were almost certainly exposed to aerosols of silica dust in the course of their work. However, life expectancy then was probably shorter than the pathogenesis of silicosis. Some industries like mining have always been a hazardous business. The ancient Egyptians recognized this by restricting such work to slaves and criminals. Workers in skilled trades in ancient times were almost certainly exposed to high levels of contamination (Plate 1). By the Middle Ages, the plight of the free miner had been recognized by Agricola (1494–1535) and Paracelsus (1493–1541). Agricola not only described the 'galloping consumption' of Carpathian miners but also proposed ways of reducing the dust in mines by improved ventilation.

Nevertheless the first authoritative treatise on occupational disease was written by Ramazzini (1633–1764). His book *De Morbis Artificium* is still unparalleled for its classic descriptions of many occupational diseases ranging from mercurialism in mirror workers to an account of repetitive strain injury in clerical workers. The Industrial Revolution in Britain brought occupational diseases to the attention of Parliament largely through the work of philanthropists like Robert Owen, Robert Peel, and Lord Shaftesbury. Early legislation to control the worst vicissitudes of factory labour was emasculated by Parliament but the process had begun. The First Act of 1802 was followed by others leading to the 1833 Act which saw the start of the Factory Inspectorate.

By the early 20th century the toxic effects of arsenic, mercury, phosphorus, and lead were so common that notification of these diseases became law and compensation for ill health was granted. Clearly, working conditions in the Western world have improved greatly since then but the recent revelations about factory life in Eastern Europe as well as the working conditions for many in Third World countries demonstrates an important tenet of occupational health practice. That is, while occupational disease may be preventable, the continued—often necessary—use of hazardous materials and processes ensures that many such diseases cannot be eliminated—only controlled.

Occupational health services

The notion that employers should provide health care for workers is hardly new. During the 14th century the Pope decreed that prostitutes should be examined regularly for evidence of sexually transmitted disease. Whether the results were significant epidemiologically is not recorded. The first recognizable occupational health service in England began in the mid-18th century when the London (Quaker) Lead Company recognized the adverse effect of mining on workers and provided health and welfare services in north-west England. Since then occupational health provision has expanded along different lines dependent upon the country.

The International Labour Organization (Convention 161; 1985) urged members 'to develop progressively occupational health services for all workers. . . . The provision made should be adequate and appropriate to the specific needs of the undertaking.'. Services are not universally available and interpretation of the requirements varies greatly between countries and employment sectors. Initially, most services arose from a mixture, part philanthropy, part self interest, the theory being that the healthy worker was likely to be more productive. Contemporary services range from total health care including primary care and hospital medicine (the states of Eastern Europe), to industry-specific systems concerned almost solely with the adverse health effects of a single industrial environment (the extractive, off-shore, and chemical industries). Services in the United States and much of Europe may include general health promotion and education.

Recent provision of occupational health services has increasingly followed the enactment of effective health and safety legislation. The Health and Safety at Work Act (1974) in the United Kingdom is an example. Some countries, such as the Commonwealth of Independent States, much of East and West Europe, and Scandinavia, require the provision of occupational health services by law. Statutory provision of such services in the United Kingdom and the United States is limited to particular industry sectors and specific occupational exposures such as ionizing radiation, heavy metals, fibrogenic materials, and carcinogens. In general, major Health and Safety Acts will 'enable' a variety of Government departments to create legislation in the form of 'Regulations' requiring action from employers in particular occupational and environmental circumstances.

The European Union adds an extra dimension to the process through 'Directives' requiring member states to modify or create legislation in response. Early 1993 saw new legislation in member states requiring improvements in general safety and health in the workplace environment, use of work and protective equipment, manual handling, and display screen working. This fundamental legislation augurs a major shift in employer and employee thinking and will require occupational physicians to reassess delivery of their services as 'competent'. Assessment of workplace hazard and risk will be mandatory. Whether such legislation will have a profound effect on occupational ill health is arguable.

An ideal 'menu' of such services depends on many variables including the industry sector, existing legislation, management/employee collaboration, the perception of hazard and risk, the availability of employment, and compensation for damage. However, basic services may provide:

1. Pre-placement assessment to ensure that the person/job fit in terms of physical ability, job requirements, and health profile is satisfactory.
2. Periodic health surveillance—dependent upon occupational and environmental exposure or work requirements.
3. Workplace inspection to advise on improvement in hazard control and job design.
4. Rehabilitation following illness/injury.
5. Adequate first aid to the required legal standard.
6. Advice to management and employees on developments in occupational health.

To deliver even such a basic service will require multidisciplinary teams including trained physicians, hygienists, and nurses.

Developments will be tempered primarily by the economic climate, perceptions of what constitutes occupationally mediated disease, and political will. However, an exponential rise in legal action, insurance costs, and compensation will play a significant part in persuading management that competent occupational health services are an absolute requirement of profitable organizations.

Prevention

The prevention of occupational disease depends upon recognition of the condition as occupational, assessment of the effect of exposure, control of the problem at source, monitoring of control systems, and perhaps health surveillance of those exposed using suitable techniques. A potent prevention technique is total substitution by less hazardous material for the substance in question. When substitution is impracticable, reduction of exposure is crucial, allied to training of workers using carefully designed procedures to reduce exposure (Chapter 8.5.2). Work schedules and hours may be also altered to reduce exposure time.

Recognition of disease as occupational is not straightforward and conditions which are considered so in the United Kingdom may not be considered thus elsewhere. The European Union is currently proposing a harmonization of national lists of occupational disease (Chapter 8.5.5).

Health surveillance, that is the assessment of effect of exposure on individuals, may be required by statute or form part of good occupational health practice. Methods should identify early change which whilst significant does not indicate permanent pathological effect. Control of further exposure will often see a return to the same biological state as before. Such surveillance must be sensitive and specific for the condition being sought. It is rarely appropriate to use the classical medical examination as a surveillance technique. An example of appropriate health surveillance is the use of respiratory history, and peak flow measurement in the prevention of occupational asthma in animal handlers where the history indicates relevant symptomatology (rhinitis, mucus membrane irritation, cough, or wheeze). Steps should be taken to reduce further exposure in such circumstances. Where occupationally related asthma is established, increased personal protection may be required, and occasionally a job change although this is an admission of failure.

Many health and safety jurisdictions require specific types of health surveillance for particular exposures often based on an imperfect understanding of the sensitivity and specificity of particular examination techniques. Chest radiography, for example, has little to offer health surveillance apart from its accepted place in pneumoconiosis.

Compensation of occupational diseases

In the early years of Western industrialized society, if a worker acquired an occupationally related disease or injury, the chances of compensation were slim, resting as they did on a successful common law suit against the employer for negligence. Such cases are still notoriously difficult to win. However, by the turn of the century, many countries in Europe as well as in the United States had passed Workman's Compensation Laws of one sort or another. Such schemes were usually restricted to specified diseases or occupations. For example, the 1897 Act in Britain was for accidents only, with six diseases added in the 1906 Act. Today the Industrial Injuries Scheme extends to over 65 diseases.

The principles underlying such schemes are that there should be 'no fault' that the disease should be, with reasonable certainty, caused by work and that the benefit claimed should offset job loss, wage earning deficit, disability, or provide death benefit to the next of kin. Whilst the scheme in Britain has suffered considerable erosion over the last 10 years, similar schemes exist in one form or another in all member countries of the European Union, excepting The Netherlands where ill-health compensation is of a more general nature. Advice on proposed additions to the list of compensatable diseases is made in 11 Member States by government appointed advisory groups. In Britain, this group is the Industrial Injuries Advisory Council which reports to the Secretary of State for Social Security.

New European Union recommendations propose a harmonization of national schemes. At present, the Commission is finalizing its list of compensatable diseases along with their diagnostic and workplace exposure criteria. It is likely to propose adoption of the list in all member states in 1993. In addition the European Commission wishes to see the introduction of a concept to aid those who can prove they have an occupationally related disease which is not on the standard list—the so-called 'individual proof' system. In Britain such a dual system of specified agents and individual claim opportunity only exists for asthma. No specific agents are listed for dermatitis.

It is important that the clinician is aware of such schemes. If the disease and work exposure seem related, and are listed, the patient should be advised to claim for compensation.

FURTHER READING

Adams, R.M. (1990). *Occupational Skin Disease.* 2nd edn. W.B. Saunders, Philadelphia.

Cox, R.A.F. (ed.) (1995). *Fitness to Work. The Medical Aspects*, 3rd edn. A joint report of the Royal College of Physicians of London and the Faculty of Occupational Medicine. Oxford Medical Publications, Oxford.

Harrington, J.M. and Gill, F.S. (1992). *Occupational Health*, 3rd edn. Blackwell Scientific Publications, Oxford.

International Labour Office (1988). *Encyclopaedia of Occupational Health and Safety*. 3rd edn. International Labour Office, Geneva.

Levy, B.S. and Wegman, D.H. (1988). *Occupational Health*, 2nd edn. Little Brown and Company, Boston.

Parkes, W.R. (ed). (1994). *Occupational Lung Disorders.* 4th edn. Butterworth & Co, London.

Raffle, P.A.B., Adams, P., Baxter, P.S., and Lee, W.R.(eds,). (1995). *Hunter's Disease of Occupation.* 9th edn. Hodder & Stoughton, London.

Waldron, H.A. (ed.). (1992). *Occupational Health Practice*, 3rd edn. Butterworth & Co, London.

8.5.2 The investigation of occupational disease

J. M. Harrington and E.S. Hodgson

The clinical approach and biological monitoring

The investigation of occupational disease requires all the traditional skills of the physician, including a careful and detailed history, appropriate physical examination, intimate knowledge of the workplace (including an understanding of the technology, substances used, and exposures) and subsequent laboratory investigation which itself increasingly calls for the use of sensitive and specific biological monitoring. Such investigation should establish whether an adverse health effect is due to the working environment. Knowledge of the literature with particular reference to studies related to the exposure in question is essential. A high 'index of suspicion' triggered by knowledge of the working environment should point the occupational clinician in the appropriate direction. Traditionally, occupational health has tended to react to situations rather than anticipate or 'pro-act', but the situation is changing.

Reactive investigations have involved the occupational physician in the clinical investigation of workers (with, for example, an eczematous eruption) subsequently shown by history of exposure and patch testing to be due to a substance at work. More recently occupational physicians have looked with increasing care at substances used at work and, where it is clear that they resemble those which may already have caused problems, they have created a prospective system of health surveillance using standard epidemiological techniques to identify early biological change in the hope of preventing adverse effects. This prospective approach is increasingly required by legislation which may on occasion define the forms of health surveillance to be undertaken.

Fundamental to the appropriate investigation of potentially occupationally related disease is a detailed occupational history which will look chronologically at the workers' jobs, the period of employment, substance exposure, and special environment during work. Along with a symptom review it is probable that the history will be of more use than physical examination, particularly where physical signs have disappeared perhaps due to changed job environments or better workplace control.

Biological monitoring, which is the estimation of the substance (or metabolite) in a biological fluid such as blood, urine, exhaled air, or sweat, is a technique increasingly used to assess individual exposure and therefore risk. Direct readings of cadmium, lead, and mercury in blood and/or urine may be appropriate for relevant exposure and for lead are required by statute in most countries. Measurement of carboxyhaemoglobin in blood or exhaled air is a sensitive measure of exposure to carbon monoxide from the products of combustion whilst urinary trichloroacetic acid may be of use in assessing exposure to 1,1,1-trichloroethane. Such monitoring has its difficulties.

1. Rapidly acting substances are usually unsuitable for such testing as the effect is likely to be experienced long before the results of testing become available.
2. Only a small number of substances and metabolites can be accurately assessed in biological fluids using present techniques.

There must be valid and repeatable analytical methods for measurement. Careful inter- and intra-laboratory audit is required to ensure that results are repeatable, accurate, and interpretable in terms of health effect and risk. The timing of biological sampling is crucial. Agents with a half-life of less than 5 h can normally be sampled at any time during exposure, for example:

1. n-Hexane—exhaled air estimation
2. Toluene—urinary hippuric acid

Agents with a half-life of over 10 h should be sampled at the end of the working week. These include trichloroethylene (measured by urinary concentrations of trichloroacetic acid) and ethyl chloroform (end-exhaled air methyl chloroform). It must be remembered that the measurement of many biological agents, particularly metabolites, is non-specific and some are seen after exposure to different chemicals which are often contained in complex mixtures within the working environment.

The American Conference of Government Industrial Hygienists (ACGIH) has defined the biological exposure index (BEI). This compares the levels found in individuals exposed to the index chemical with workers inhaling the chemical at a level in air at the 'threshold limit value' or TLV. In the United States this is the level below which employers are required to keep exposures by all practicable means. An updated list is published annually giving threshold limit values of over 500 chemicals. The Health and Safety Executive in the United Kingdom publishes a similar list of threshold limit value equivalents. Different nomenclatures include occupational exposure limits (OEL), maximum allowable concentrations (MAC), and occupational exposure standards (OES). Strict inter-country comparison should not be attempted and caution must be exercised in interpreting levels when investigating occupational disease.

The use of environmental monitoring of substance concentration in air, radiation type (ionizing and non-ionizing), and pressure (noise and vibration) is a powerful tool in the occupational physician's armamentarium for investigating occupational disease. Comparison of workplace exposures in various working environments may give a clue to the likelihood of occupational disease being present. Biological and environmental monitoring requires the co-operation of management and workers; the expertise of laboratory services and occupational hygienists, are also an essential part of the investigative process.

Crucial to the investigation of occupational disease is an intimate knowledge of the workplace. It cannot be stressed too highly that occupational physicians must be totally familiar with the technology, exposures, and environments they are investigating. Occupational physicians may wish to use the 'walk through' visit of a working environment to familiarize themselves with new situations and working practices. Expert advice will be required from line management and local safety practitioners who are completely familiar on a day-to-day basis with the workplace. A detailed understanding of the job descriptions of the individuals being investigated is also important. Many jargon or local dialect words are used to describe jobs and processes and these must be thoroughly understood. It may be necessary for the physician to observe individuals at work for an extended period of time, perhaps using photography or video to record events. It is also useful to ask employees to indicate where they feel the difficulties lie with particular reference to pockets of high exposure and adverse environmental conditions that may occur only once or twice during the working day. It is surprising how often the recorded opinions of management and employees differ markedly and it is not unusual to be convinced that the two groups are talking about entirely different employment circumstances. The independent observations of the trained occupational physician may indicate the hidden points of contact which will throw light on the disease process being investigated.

Workplace exposure and control

The investigation of work-related ill health cannot be restricted to clinical recognition. For the purposes of prevention especially, it is essential to study workplace exposure and to institute appropriate environmental control. Occupational hygiene is the environmental science of identifying and evaluating the physical, chemical, or biological hazards in the workplace and then devising ways to control or eliminate those hazards. The practitioners are usually science or engineering graduates who attempt to collate toxicological information on the noxious agent with its behaviour in air or in combination with other agents, measure its concentrations near the worker, and then design control procedures. For example, these could be ventilation systems, noise abatement measures, or radiation protection programmes. It is important to emphasize that the occupational hygienist and the occupational physician undertake complementary and overlapping roles. Rarely is either sufficient to cover all aspects of the disease–exposure relationship on their own. Indeed, one could justifiably contend that the safety engineer is the third essential player in this team approach. Whilst most organizations of any size have a designated safety officer, only the largest companies employ a trained hygienist. Smaller companies either use untrained personnel, hire academics or consultants on an *ad-hoc* basis, or do without. Yet for the effective evaluation of workplace exposure and particularly for their efficient control, trained expertise is essential.

EXPOSURE ASSESSMENT

In the past, the need for a formal exposure assessment has usually followed the discovery of a workplace health effect. The advent of more broadly based workplace regulations—such as the Control of Substances Hazardous to Health Regulations, UK (1988)—has seen the required growth in workplace assessments without overt evidence of a health problem in that particular environment.

Such a survey requires the hygienist to undertake several steps.

Collect background information on processes and hazards;
Visit the workplace to review actual procedures and potential risks;
Evaluate these procedures and decide on a sampling strategy for monitoring workforce exposures;
In the light of these measurements, institute control measures to eliminate or minimize exposure to below published occupational exposure limits;
Continue monitoring to audit the efficiency of control measures.

Whilst the range of possible exposures and agents is legion, some general principles are relevant here for the more common problems of modern industry. Most hazardous materials gain entry to the body by inhalation or skin absorption. Air sampling procedures should involve, where feasible, both area sampling and personal dosimetry. The choice of sampler depends upon the agent(s) to be sampled, ranging from direct reading instruments such as detector tubes or noise or radiation dosimeters to sample collectors for dusts and gases or vapours. Such collectors may filter the air drawn through the instrument by a pump, dissolve the relevant agent in a bubbler, or adsorb it on charcoal in a tube. Personal sampling must take into account the work cycle and the specific operator characteristics of the job. Where skin absorption is a problem, measurement techniques are much less accurate, involving, for example, skin wipes or cloth patches, but close observation of the mode of exposure may suffice. The other aspect of worker sampling (biological monitoring) is discussed above.

EXPOSURE CONTROL

Having established the worker exposure characteristics, it is vital to ensure that effective control measures to minimize exposure are in place. Three principles underlie control measures.

Substitution of the hazardous agent;
Limitation of release from the source;
Limitation of contact with the worker.

Clearly substitution is the safest option but frequently not feasible. Therefore, the degree of control is dependent on the degree of hazard and on the effects which failure to control would have on the workforce. Cost is a factor which cannot be ignored. For example, although personal protective equipment (PPE) may be a cheaper option than engineering controls, it is rarely justified as a front line control measure unless the exposure is limited to short, scheduled activities.

Limitation of airborne release can range from total enclosure of the process to some form of local exhaust ventilation. Exhaust ventilation usually involves a hood close to the emission source with the offending agent being ducted away from the site to a filter system or a collection chamber usually by means of a fan-assisted draught. For noise, a system of enclosure with or without baffles is necessary, though the simplest (but often most expensive) workplace option is to buy quieter machinery. For ionizing radiation, shielding and interlocks are required commensurate with the type of radiation. For all these exposures, distance from the worker is another valuable protection factor. Thus, a process which operates automatically or semi-automatically may require little operator involvement. Such a separation of process and worker may allow personal protection equipment to be used, thus obviating expensive engineering control.

Personal protective equipment may range from gloves and overalls to total enclosure in an air-fed suit, or, for noise, from ear plugs to ear muffs. It is important to remember that failure to wear the appropriate equipment for the whole of the time in the area can be almost as inappropriate as not wearing it at all. Furthermore the equipment must be regularly and efficiently maintained, be appropriate for the task (i.e. the filter in the mask must be the correct one for the exposure and the agent), and fit the individual correctly. Even such apparently unimportant factors as the presence of a beard may vitiate an otherwise correct mask and filter. The wrong glove material may actually aid skin absorption although the operator is lulled into a false sense of security because he or she is wearing something which appears protective.

In short, the process of monitoring workplace exposure and instituting control measures is a skilled business which should only be undertaken by trained specialists. Anything less could be a recipe for disaster.

8.5.3 The main occupational diseases

8.5.3(a) Occupational dermatology

I. FOULDS

An occupational dermatosis is a pathological condition of the skin for which occupational exposure can be shown to be a major contributory factor. However, most dermatologists prefer to limit their concept of occupational dermatoses to cutaneous abnormalities primarily caused by components of the work environment, or a skin disease which would not have occurred if the patient had not been doing the work of that occupation.

Legal definitions of occupational dermatoses vary considerably between countries. In the United Kingdom the majority are defined by Prescribed Disease D5 of the Department of Health and Social Security as 'non-infective dermatitis of external origin (including chrome ulceration of the skin but excluding dermatitis due to ionising particles or electromagnetic radiation other than radiant heat)'. However, this definition may exclude newly described dermatoses, and in the case of occupationally acquired hypomelanosis a new category (Prescribed Disease C25) was necessary.

Incidence

The true incidence of occupational dermatoses is difficult to obtain as in some countries occupational accidents and illnesses are not differentiated, and others fail to separate dermatitis from other skin diseases. Dermatoses comprise from 20 to 70 per cent of all occupationally acquired disease. In many countries, between 20 to 90 per cent are dermatitis, determined by the industrial spectrum of the country and to a large extent by the awareness of an interested dermatologist. In the United Kingdom a million days a year may be lost due to dermatitis. The diagnosis and management is discussed elsewhere (Section 23).

There is a belief amongst some managers and even some doctors that individuals with dermatitis set out to obtain whatever they can in the way of compensation but in reality this is far from the truth. With high unemployment, many individuals are reluctant to seek help in case they are labelled as suffering from industrial dermatitis and are then transferred to less skilled work with loss of bonuses or even their jobs. Once labelled as suffering from dermatitis, the chances of finding alternative employment may be remote.

Many employers believe that they do not have a problem with dermatitis but careful inspection of employees' shows that dermatitis may be present in up to a third of the workforce. Therefore, not only is there considerable lost time due to dermatitis but suffering due to discomfort, depression, and social ostracism is impossible to quantify.

The attitude of employees and employers to dermatitis

Like many skin diseases there are many myths attached to dermatitis. Unfortunately, there still exists the 'leper approach' to people with dermatitis. Many people believe that dermatitis is infectious and can be passed on by towels and touching; this results in the affected individual becoming socially isolated. Under no circumstances should dermatitis be regarded as infectious. It can only be acquired by wear and tear occurring to the skin or by the development of an allergy to a substance that has been in contact with the skin. Affected individuals, therefore, should not have unnecessary restrictions placed on them.

When a person develops severe occupational dermatitis it is often apparent to their colleagues; after discussion others may think that their own skin problems are also occupationally related. However, since skin diseases are common and more than 3000 are known, individual problems may well be falsely attributed to a work related cause. With outbreaks of apparent dermatitis great care is needed in handling the situation to identify the causes and identify those with occupationally related problems from those with other skin diseases. It may be necessary to ask for the help of a dermatologist with a special knowledge of industrial dermatitis if the confidence of the workforce is to be maintained.

Barrier creams

It should be recognized that there is no cream which actually provides a barrier preventing penetration of substances into the skin. In fact, in some situations they may actually enhance penetration. Although numerous formulations are available, in practice they divide into those suitable for dry or for wet work. The main benefit they offer is obtained from their bases, such as lanolin, which may help to improve the hydration (suppleness) of the skin, with the result that, when cleansers are used, less degreasing of the skin occurs. In theory this may help to reduce irritant contact dermatitis from repeated hand washing. There is no evidence that barrier creams protect against sensitizers and occasionally sensitization may occur to some of the constituents of the cream. In addition, the use of a barrier cream may give an employee a false sense of security and lead to increased skin abuse.

Skin cleansing

When substances remain on the skin after the working day, the risk of irritation or sensitization is increased. The most efficient skin cleansers, however, are often the most irritant of substances due to their solvent or detergent content. If cleansers are too mild for the task, workers will often use degreasing agents in the manufacturing process, for example solvents or paraffins to obtain adequate cleansing. Although these substances will cleanse they are potentially very irritant with repeated use. It is often not appropriate to provide one type of cleanser for different jobs. Cleansers should be chosen to provide adequate cleansing in a short period of time without having too strong a degreasing effect.

After-work creams

There are many such creams which are in essence moisturizers and which have the benefit of increasing the hydration of the skin following cleansing at the end of the day. They are of particular benefit in occupations where excessive drying of the skin may occur. Their use should be encouraged where hot air driers are used as these tend to dry the skin unduly.

Skin protection

In industrial situations the hands and forearms are most at risk. The use of proper gloves, coupled with a high standard of hygiene, can minimize contact and provide adequate protection. In many industrial situations where moving machinery is present, wearing gloves may pose a potential danger. Even when gloves are used, they may be taken off to undertake tasks requiring manual dexterity, resulting in contaminated hands being placed back inside the gloves.

When powders are being handled, the operator may not be aware of possible entry through the cuff. This can be prevented by the wearing of gauntlets or arm-bands, or by tucking sleeves underneath the cuff. Regular washing or changing of gloves will help to reduce contamination from the surface. Irritants or allergens may also enter through tears in the gloves or by direct penetration.

A wide range of materials have been used to manufacture protective clothes, including cotton, leather, nylon, glass fibre, acrylonitrile, rubber, neoprene, butyl rubber, viton, polyurethane, PVC, PVA, and Teflon. Several systems for the direct determination of permeability have been devised, based on the measurement time for the chemical to be detected on the inside of the material when the outside surface is placed in contact with the liquid. They vary in the way the sample of the material is held, and the size and the shape of the material tested. Measurements of permeability may thus be misleading if different protective clothing is being compared.

The ratings found in glove manufacturers catalogues, such as 'good', 'excellent', or 'superior', usually relate to physical properties such as abrasion resistance, elongation, and tear resistance, but do not give information on breakthrough times or permeation rates, which are important in determining the degree of chemical protection. When deciding whether or not a particular material will give adequate protection in a specific application, a number of factors must be taken into account. The toxic properties of the chemical involved must be known so that, should over-exposure occur, it can be clearly identified. The period, frequency, severity, and type of exposure are important in defining the insult the protective material must resist. The type of work, and the degree of manual dexterity required in the case of gloves, gives a guide to the needs for flexibility and strength.

Non-dermatitic occupational dermatoses

These form a significant minority of occupational dermatoses and awareness of their existence is important for those involved in managing skin patients. The more important are briefly mentioned below.

1. Psoriasis (see Section 23) may erupt at sites of injury or as a response to friction in manual workers. When this occurs on the hands, it may be confused with dermatitis although vesicles (blisters) are not found in psoriatic skin.
2. Infections, such as anthrax due to exposure to contaminated bones or wool, is well recognized, albeit rare in the United Kingdom. Warts caused by the human papilloma virus occur more commonly in some occupational groups such as butchers and poultry processing workers. Fungal infections are common and may be occupationally acquired. Perhaps the most common example is tinea pedis (athlete's foot) in miners using communal changing facilities. Cattle ringworm (trichophyton mentagrophytes) occurs in farm workers and may extend into the deeper subcutaneous tissues requiring systemic therapy. Orf, (Plate 1) a pox virus, occurs in sheep handlers (see Chapter 7.10.9). Other occupationally acquired infections which may have a cutaneous component include brucellosis, glanders, ankylostomiasis, and leptospirosis.
3. Chronic paronychia due to Candida occurs in those exposed to wet work, e.g. in nursing, in catering, and in housewives. Separation of the nail plate from the nail bed (onycholysis) may occur in those exposed to solvents and koilonychia may occur as a response to trauma of the finger pulps.
4. Acne may be caused by a variety of chemicals including oils, coal tar, and petroleum products. Chloracne (Plate 2) is a particularly refractory form of acne caused by halogenated aromatic chemicals, which may also cause systemic toxicity. Mild cases may be difficult to differentiate from conventional acne but multiple comedones (blackheads) are found over the malar regions. Chlorphenols used as insecticides, fungicides, and herbicides and polychlorinated biphenyls used as insulators or as a contaminant of cooking oil can cause chloracne. For example, exposure to 2,3,6,7-tetrachlorodibenzodioxin caused severe systemic and cutaneous symptoms in the population over a wide area around Ceveso in Italy.
5. Vitiligo may be occupationally acquired. Several substituted phenols including *p*-tert-butyl phenol and monobenzyl ether of hydroquinone may cause hypomelanosis indistinguishable from vitiligo.
6. Scleroderma may be caused by exposure to vinyl chloride, and has been caused by trichlorethylene and organic solvents. Scleroderma-like lesions have also been reported in people exposed to epoxy resin fumes and silicosis associated with scleroderma has been reported in miners.
7. A variety of chemicals may cause alteration of skin pigment, including mercury, and silver (which causes argyria).

8.5.3(b) Occupational cancer

J. M. Harrington

Background

Although many accounts of occupational cancer start with Percival Pott's description in 1775 of chimney sweep's scrotal cancer, there is good reason to go back further—even though the earliest accounts do not propose the link between occupation and cancer.

Agricola's account of the illnesses of Carpathian silver miners includes evidence of a rapidly progressive and fatal lung disorder. The fact that these mines contain uranium ore suggests that radon gas exposures may well have been high enough to cause lung cancer in the miners. Nevertheless, it is Pott's description of an excess risk of scrotal cancer in postpubertal chimney sweeps which first raised the possibility that chemicals—particularly polynuclear aromatic hydrocarbons—cause cancer. Confirmatory evidence from animal experiments did not arrive until 1915 and the first carcinogenic hydrocarbon was identified by Kennaway in 1924 as 1:2:5:6 dibenzanthracene (dibenz[*a*,*h*]anthracene).

Whilst the polynuclear aromatic hydrocarbons were generating interest as skin carcinogens, clinical observations of dyestuff workers were suggesting a link between bladder cancer and aromatic amines. In 1895, Rehn described three cases in a group of 45 workers in Germany involved in the preparation of fuchsin. Further reports followed from other countries and the classic studies of Case and his coworkers in the 1950s showed that 2-naphthylamine and benzidine were human carcinogens in the manufacturing industry and in the user industry (2-naphthylamine was a contaminant of the antioxidant used in tyre manufacture). Rehn's discovery added a new element to the knowledge of carcinogenesis, that is, that an organ distant from the point of first contact could bear the main force of the carcinogenic effect. In other words, the carcinogenic influence is greatest where the concentration is most prolonged and most intense.

In the same year that Rehn made his discovery, Roentgen discovered X-rays and 3 years later, the Curies isolated radium. Unfortunately, knowledge of the carcinogenic properties of ionizing radiation came from the skin and bone marrow cancers suffered by these early pioneers with confirmatory animal data following soon after. The bone sarcomata noted in laboratory animals was followed by human evidence in the 1930s among the luminous dial painters who used radium-235 and mesothorium. The inventor of the luminous paint, Dr von Sochocky, died of aplastic anaemia in 1928. Again in the 1930s, case reports were appearing of lung cancer (an unusual tumour in those days) in workers exposed to asbestos fibre. In asbestosis cases the incidence was reported as 18 per cent and reports of pleural mesothelioma followed a decade or so later.

Thus, within a century of Rehn's discovery, chemical carcinogenesis had become a well-recognized phenomenon with much of the evidence coming from occupational studies.

Diagnosis

Clinical acumen remains of paramount importance. It is the clinician who has played the major role in discovering new causes of cancer with confirmatory evidence coming from laboratory studies and epidemiological investigations. Establishing that a particular exposure causes human cancer involves all these elements and others. A schematic representation of the links between sources of evidence is shown in Fig. 1. To be reasonably certain that a workplace exposure causes a particular cancer, good quality epidemiological studies are essential. Further evidence from animal experiments, genotoxicity studies, and case reports add weight to the assertion but are insufficient in themselves.

Fig. 1 The scientific basis for establishing occupational causality.

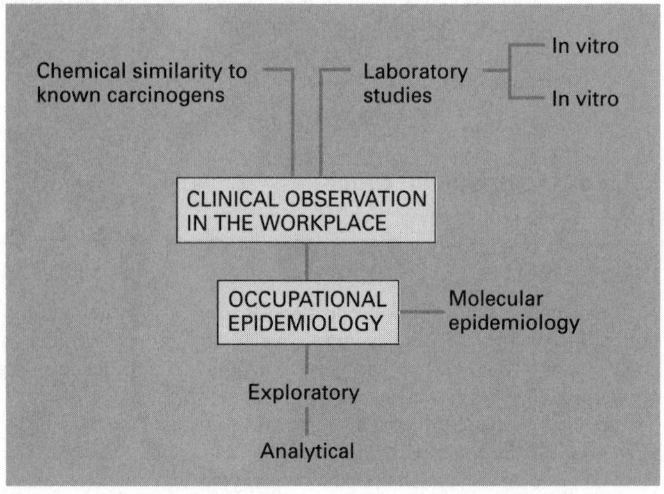

Such information is collated and interpreted by various national and international agencies. The most reliable source is the Monograph Series of the International Agency for Research on Cancer (IARC) based in Lyon. To date they have published over 50 such monographs with several updating supplements. When a patient is diagnosed as having cancer, it is important that the clinician should review the occupational history to consider an occupational cause. If such a cause seems probable, enquires should be made to see if state compensation is available for that cancer and that workplace exposure.

Attribution of cancer to occupational causes

The most widely accepted estimates of the proportion of all cancers attributable to occupational exposures is 4 per cent with a range of 2 to 8 per cent for a typically industrially developed country like the United States. For that proportion of the population (20 per cent or so) in which occupationally related cancers are almost exclusively concentrated (manual workers aged 20 or over, in mining, agriculture, and industry broadly defined), perhaps as much as one cancer in every five may be attributed to workplace exposure.

In addition, it is necessary to consider other exposures which may interact with workplace exposures. These are particularly relevant when considering the relative effectiveness of removing or reducing exposure to one or more agents acting jointly. Few good studies have been completed on interaction but there is good evidence for the multiplicative effects of cigarette smoking and asbestos exposure in the genesis of lung cancer. Besides asbestos, interactions have been demonstrated to be at least additive for tobacco consumption and exposure to arsenic, nickel, and ionizing radiation. By analogy it is possible to envisage interaction between these workplace agents—as might occur in the mining industry.

Important examples of occupational exposures causing cancer

There is insufficient space in a text of this kind to describe the tens of agents or processes which have been causally linked to human cancer let alone to the hundreds of such exposures for which the evidence is somewhat more tentative. More detailed accounts may be found in the IARC Monographs or the standard texts in occupational medicine. Some important exposures are highlighted here with a summary of the causally linked processes (Table 1) and agents (Table 2). Ionizing radiation is dealt in Chapter 8.5.5(i).

Polynuclear aromatic hydrocarbons

Polynuclear aromatic hydrocarbons are members of a large and complex group of compounds mainly generated during the incomplete combustion of carbonaceous products of which the combustion of coal and oil comprise the most important occupational exposures. Cigarette smoke, of course, contains a number of these compounds and it is thus often difficult to distinguish lifestyle from occupational factors in populations employed in these occupations. The site of action of these compounds is mainly the lung, skin, and bladder. The industries most prominently linked to such exposures are coke ovens, gas production, steel industries, aluminium refineries, and iron and steel foundries; workers exposed to soot, pitch, tar, and petroleum product exhaust fumes are also at risk.

Table 1 *Industrial processes causally associated with human cancer*

Exposure	Human target organ
Aluminium production	Lung, bladder (lymphoma, oesophagus, stomach)
Auramine, manufacture of	Bladder
Boot and shoe manufacture and repair	Leukaemia, nasal sinus (bladder, digestive tract)
Coal gasification	Skin, lung, bladder
Coke production	Skin, lung, kidney
Furniture and cabinet making	Nasal sinus
Haematite mining, underground, with exposure to radon	Lung
Iron and steel founding	Lung (digestive tract, genitourinary tract, leukaemia)
Isopropyl alcohol manufacture, strong-acid process	Nasal sinus (larynx)
Magenta, manufacture of	Bladder
Painters (occupational exposure as)	Lung (oesophagus, stomach, bladder)
Rubber industry	Bladder, leukaemia (lymphoma, lung, renal tract, digestive tract, skin, liver, larynx, brain, stomach)

(Suspected target organs in parentheses.)

Source (Tables 1 and 2): IARC Monographs Vol. 1–54 (Harrington and Saracci 1993 in *Hunter's Disease of Occupation* 8th edn.).

Table 2 *Chemicals and groups of chemicals causally associated with human cancer for which exposure has been mostly occupational*

Exposure	Human target organ
4-Aminobiphenyl	Bladder
Arsenic and arsenic compounds*	Skin, lung (liver, haematopoietic system, gastrointestinal tract, kidney)
Asbestos	Lung, pleura, peritoneum, gastrointestinal tract, larynx
Benzene	Leukaemia
Benzidine	Bladder
Bis(chloromethyl) ether and chloromethyl methyl ether (technical grade)	Lung
Chromium compounds, hexavalent*	Lung (gastrointestinal tract)
Coal-tars	Skin, lung (bladder)
Coal-tar pitches	Skin, lung, bladder (gastrointestinal tract, leukaemia)
Inorganic acid mists (strong) containing sulphuric acid	Larynx
Ionizing radiation	Leukaemia, bone, skin, and other organs depending on exposure and type of radiation
Mineral oils, untreated and mildly treated	Skin (respiratory tract, bladder, gastrointestinal tract)
Mustard gas (sulphur mustard)	Lung, larynx, pharynx
2-Naphthylamine	Bladder (liver)
Nickel and nickel compounds*	Nasal sinus, lung (larynx)
Radon	Lung
Shale-oils	Skin (colon)
Soots	Skin, lung
Talc containing asbestiform fibre	Lung (pleura)
Vinyl chloride	Liver, lung, brain, lymphatic and haematopoietic system (gastrointestinal tract)

* The evaluation of carcinogenicity to humans applies to the group of chemicals as a whole and not necessarily all individual chemicals within the group.

(Suspected target organs in parentheses.)

Aromatic amines

Aromatic amines are a group of chemically similar compounds which have particular importance as dyestuffs or antioxidants or as intermediates in dye production. Some are known human bladder carcinogens, and a larger number are known animal carcinogens for which human data are limited or lacking. The more potent carcinogens are now banned and previous excess risks of bladder cancer in, for example, the dyestuffs and rubber industries have largely disappeared. Bladder cancer remains, however, a numerically important tumour and further work to delineate other potential occupational carcinogens is still required.

Metals and metalloids

The most important carcinogenic elements of this group are arsenic, chromium, and nickel. Arsenic and its compounds cause lung and skin cancer and these risks occur in the extraction of metalliferous ores (which are frequently contaminated by arsenic compounds) and in the now limited use of arsenic in pesticides and other industrial usages. Hexavalent chromium compounds, used in the pigment and plating industries, have been shown to cause lung cancer. Lung and nasal cancer is associated with the refining of nickel and the most likely causative agents are the oxidic and sulphidic nickel compounds. Other metals for which there is less clear-cut evidence of carcinogenicity include beryllium and cadmium.

Other organic compounds

Benzene is widely used both as the base compound and as an important building block in the organic chemical industry. It causes leukaemia and aplastic anaemia. Vinyl chloride monomer, which is the starting point for polyvinyl chloride, causes angiosarcoma of the liver. The most potent lung carcinogens are apparently the chloromethyl ethers which are used in ion exchange resins. Other suspect organic compounds include acrylonitrile, diethyl sulphate, epichlorhydrin, ethylene oxide, formaldehyde, and tetrachloroethylene.

Industrial processes

Some processes listed in Table 1 are linked to specific exposures, such as polycyclic aromatic hydrocarbons in aluminium production and radon in underground mining. For others such as boot and shoe manufacture, furniture making, and painting, the specific relevant exposures have not been identified. For painting, the exposure characteristics such as construction sites may be as important as paint constituents. In the past asbestos and chromates were used in some paints but these have been removed or are being phased out. The paint manufacturing industry has not been shown to carry an excess risk of cancer.

8.5.3(c) Musculoskeletal disorders

R. W. JUBB

Musculoskeletal disorders are common in the general population and their suspected relationship to specific occupations or activities can often be difficult to confirm. The epidemic of repetitive strain injury in Australia during the 1980s highlighted the complex interaction of symptoms, group perceptions, and employment.

An incidence of about 2 per cent has been quoted for certain repetitive strain disorders but it is not clear why the remaining 98 per cent of the workforce are spared. Because the rheumatic diseases are common, it is likely that some employees will have a recognized medical disease to account for their symptoms.

In any patient presenting with musculoskeletal symptoms, it is important to consider their leisure interests as well as their occupation. Increased leisure time has resulted in an epidemic of sports-related symptoms that have parallels with certain occupational diseases. The diagnosis and clinical management are usually similar, although the interplay of psychological factors is often different.

Pain and disability arising in a discrete anatomical region (regional pain syndromes) are a common presentation of occupationally related conditions. However, this classification is not particularly useful and a more precise diagnosis should be attempted; this grouping gives no guidance as to diagnosis, management, or prognosis.

Rheumatic diseases affecting occupation

Sometimes the patient will already have a known rheumatic disease, such as rheumatoid arthritis, and the effect that this has on his or her performance at work will have to be assessed. The fluctuating nature of most forms of arthritis makes precise predictions difficult. Physical disability often improves despite persistence of the disease. This is due both to the beneficial effects of treatment and to the patient's adaptation to the consequences of the disease.

Often the presenting 'occupational' complaint will be the first indication of a chronic rheumatic disease. An example is the insidious back pain of ankylosing spondylitis. This diagnosis should always be considered in young men presenting with back pain at work, especially if there is prolonged morning stiffness affecting the back. Radiological confirmation may take several years.

Isolated carpal tunnel syndrome can be a presenting feature of rheumatoid arthritis, hypothyroidism, and systemic lupus erythematosus (SLE), as well as being of occupational or idiopathic origin. Synovitis in rheumatoid arthritis and SLE affects both the lining of the joint and the tendon sheath. The development of tenosynovitis as a presenting problem may be mistaken for an occupational disease. Nerve root entrapment neuropathies are very common in cervical and lumbar spondylosis, and are often attributed to occupational activity.

Occupation causing a rheumatic disease

All the tissues of the musculoskeletal system can be affected by occupationally related disorders. Involvement of the joint may lead to arthritis with traumatic synovitis and eventually degenerative changes. Inflammation of the periarticular tissues causes a range of conditions including tenosynovitis, bursitis, fasciitis, and tendinitis. The muscles can suffer from cramp, fatigue, and inflammation. The nervous system is affected with entrapment neuropathies and reflex dystrophies. The bones are subject to stress fractures, impact fractures, and remodelling defects.

Research in this field has been hampered by the problem of collecting appropriate control information. The frequency of musculoskeletal problems in the general population emphasizes the importance of adequate control data; not only age and sex but also family history, past history, and leisure activities should be considered. In addition, the definition of the various occupational conditions is often imprecise or ambiguous. The majority of clinical features are subjective and there are few suitable objective measures. Add to this the inevitable medicolegal implications and it is clear why this is a difficult area in which to perform clinical research.

The effect of occupation on the musculoskeletal system can usefully be considered in four categories; sometimes there will be a combination of contributing factors in a particular disorder.

1. Repeated heavy impact loading

Some jobs inevitably put considerable physical stress on the bones and joints. Examples are coal-face workers, farmers, and less obviously professional dancers. In these and similar occupations the joints are subjected to frequent heavy impact loading. A high incidence of degenerative changes are found in certain joints after prolonged exposure to this physical insult. The rheumatological consequence is the development of osteoarthritis. Even though there is a clear association between the arthritis and the occupation, genetic factors could be involved in groups such as farmers and miners.

Similar impact loading on the bursae can lead to bursitis with subsequent infection and cellulitis. The most common site is the knee which can be affected in any occupation that involves prolonged kneeling—for example, beat knee in miners.

2. Repetitive low impact trauma

Repeated low impact trauma is thought to lead to the development of repetitive strain injury. This problem has become increasingly common over the past decade. A variety of terms have been used including overuse syndrome, chronic occupational pain and cumulative trauma disorder, and work related upper limb disorders.

Commonly affected groups of workers are assembly-line workers, keyboard operators, musicians, cleaners, hairdressers, butchers, and machine operators. The wrist and forearm are the anatomical regions most frequently affected, although symptoms are often very diffuse with involvement of the shoulder and neck as well. Tendinitis, fasciitis, and myositis are diagnostic labels used for the complaints in which pain, fatigue, cramp, swelling, and tenderness are all symptoms.

A suggested definition for overuse syndrome in musicians is 'pain and demonstrable tenderness in the muscle group and joint ligaments which have been taken beyond their biological tolerance'. Although this seems a reasonable statement of the clinical problem it is clear that it is too ambiguous for any reproducible research studies.

Treatment includes rest, splinting (but not of the shoulder), analgesics, and non-steroidal anti-inflammatory drugs. Localized areas of inflammation will respond to local injections of corticosteroids. Physical therapy procedures can be tried and occasionally surgery.

3. Ergonomic problems

The design of an individual's workplace can have a direct effect on the development of musculoskeletal symptoms. The differences in size and shape of the worker can result in many problems. For example, tall people in small cars or short people working on assembly lines built for the average height and reach may develop pain and stiffness in the neck and back that is more related to their own shape than an inherent problem with the occupational activity. In these situations attention to the work equipment needs of the individual will usually correct the problem.

Sometimes the design of a work station is poor resulting in a high incidence of musculoskeletal problems, whatever the size and shape of the worker. Industrial design is increasingly taking account of this type of issue but often the problem will only become apparent if there is an aware and vigilant management.

4. High risk occupations

Many occupations are inherently hazardous with a high risk of sustaining an occupationally related problem, for example, acute trauma causing fractures and joint damage in construction workers, miners, and deep sea fishermen. Other specific hazards include avascular necrosis from decompression sickness in tunnellers and divers, acro-osteolysis in certain chemical industries, and septic bone and joint lesions from brucellosis in meat process workers. Employees in these occupations are often aware of the relevant diseases.

History, examination, and investigations

Musculoskeletal symptoms associated with specific occupations require detailed examination and documentation. It should be assumed that there will be medicolegal implications at some time in the future and an accurate description of the abnormal clinical features at the time of presentation is invaluable; a note of 'tenosynovitis' or 'frozen shoulder' is inadequate (although possibly correct).

The common symptoms include pain (localized or referred), stiffness, fatigue, swelling, cramp, numbness and paraesthesia, and loss of function. The timing and nature of these symptoms are important. Associated signs include tenderness, heat changes, colour changes, deformity, swelling, crepitus, effusions, neurological deficit, and abnormalities of muscle function.

Many of the investigations are to exclude an underlying medical condition. ESR and C-reactive protein are simple markers of the acute phase response associated with an inflammatory systemic illness. Measurement of rheumatoid factor, antinuclear factor, thyroid stimulating hormone, urate, and creatine phosphokinase are all helpful in appropriate cases. Radiographs of hands and feet can demonstrate erosive inflammatory arthritis in the absence of any symptoms in the eroded joint. Nerve conduction studies are particularly useful in suspected cases of carpal tunnel syndrome and ulnar neuropathy, and electromyography can help delineate muscle pathology.

Magnetic resonance imaging has tremendous diagnostic potential for many 'soft tissue' injuries and occupationally related disorders. As this facility becomes more accessible, it is, hopefully, going to be the technical breakthrough that this field of research has been awaiting.

8.5.3(d) Neurological disorders

E. L. BAKER

Neurological disorders caused by chemical exposures

Central nervous system effects

Chemical exposures, primarily encountered by workers in manufacturing, construction, and agricultural jobs, can cause transient and persistent central nervous system (CNS) effects (Table 1). Transient CNS dysfunction is most commonly caused by exposure to volatile organic solvents, to organophosphate insecticides, or to carbon monoxide. In each instance, these substances, acting through different mechanisms, may cause CNS dysfunction ranging from acute intoxication manifested by light-headedness and dizziness to loss of consciousness and even death. Persistent CNS sequelae may occur following one exposure episode if exposure levels are high and time of exposure is prolonged.

Persistent CNS dysfunction, manifesting as neurobehavioural performance deficits, has been reported following chronic exposure to moderate concentrations of various agents encountered in the workplace and occasionally in the environment. This syndrome, chronic toxic encephalopathy, consisting primarily of memory impairment, impaired psychomotor function, and mood disorders, has been seen following chronic exposure to lead, styrene, and certain organic solvents. In more severe cases, the deficits persist, but do not progress, following cessation of exposure. If behavioural symptoms are present without evidence of abnormal neurobehavioural tests (i.e. organic affective syndrome) reversal of these manifestations usually occurs following exposure cessation.

Peripheral nervous system effects

Exposure to certain agents (Table 2) may cause either motor or sensorimotor polyneuropathy. Rarely, lead exposure, at high levels for long periods, may cause upper extremity motor neuropathy, consisting of wrist extension weakness or wrist drop. Certain substances (e.g. acrylamide, hexacarbon solvents, and certain organophosphorus compounds) may act as axonal toxins causing a mixed sensorimotor polyneuropathy manifesting as symmetrical, distal sensory loss. Upon removal from exposure, the symptoms usually recede over a period of months with modest or no residual damage.

Other nervous system effects

A variety of other neurological effects have been reported following exposure to toxic agents in the environment (Table 3). In most cases, symptoms recede following exposure cessation.

Neurological disorders caused by physical factors

Repetitive trauma disorders (see also Chapter 8.5.3(c))

A dramatic increase in the occurrence of carpal tunnel syndrome, and other repetitive trauma disorders, has been noted in recent years. Although a portion of the increase may be attributable to increased awareness by clinicians, most of the change is related to changing job demands. Jobs which require repetitive flexion and extension of the wrist, along with application of significant force, are associated with high rates of carpal tunnel syndrome. Management of the disorder is best accomplished by consideration of the ergonomic characteristics of the work tasks and by job redesign based on ergonomic principles. Hand surgery and other forms of medical and surgical treatment should not be substituted for proper job redesign; if this is done, the disorder will often recur and the patient may well become permanently disabled.

Entrapment neuropathies

In certain occupations, sustained postures (such as working overhead) may cause muscular hypertrophy or other changes resulting in entrapment of nerve roots or individual nerves. Such conditions are diagnosed by obtaining a careful work history and managed by modification of the work environment.

Vibration-induced neuropathy (see also Chapter 8.5.5(e))

Certain jobs, involving the use of vibrating hand tools or pneumatic drills, may be responsible for the occurrence of peripheral neuropathy. These disorders may originate from a combination of physical trauma to the nerve itself as well as damage to blood vessels which supply the nerves.

8.5.3(e) Cardiovascular system

J. M. HARRINGTON

Cardiovascular disease is the major cause of mortality and morbidity in industrialized countries. The subject is extensively covered elsewhere in this book (Section 15). While the association between personal

Table 1 *Central nervous system syndromes caused by workplace toxins*

Disorders	Manifestations	Causal agents
Acute intoxication	Light-headedness Loss of consciousness Death (rare)	Carbon monoxide Organic solvents Organophosphate insecticides
Organic effective syndrome	Fatigue Irritability Depression	Organic solvents Lead Mercury Styrene
Chronic toxic encephalopathy	Symptoms (as noted above) Impaired neurobehavioural test performance	Organic solvents Lead Carbon monoxide (rare)
Psychosis	Marked emotional instability	Carbon disulphide Manganese (rare) Toluene (rare)

Table 2 *Peripheral nervous system syndromes caused by workplace toxins*

Disorders	Manifestation	Agent
Motor neuropathy	Wrist weakness	Lead
Mixed sensorimotor neuropathy	Symmetrical distal sensory loss; mild motor dysfunction	Acrylamide Arsenic Carbon disulphide Carbon monoxide (rare) DDT (rare) n-Hexane Methyl n-butyl ketone Mercury Organophosphorus compounds (selected agents)

Table 3 *Other neurological manifestations*

Manifestation	Agent
Ataxic gait	Acrylamide Chlordane Chlordecone (Kepone) DDT Manganese Methyl mercury
Bladder neuropathy	Dimethylaminopropionitrile
Constricted visual fields	Organic mercury
Cranial neuropathy	Carbon disulphide Trichlorethylene
Headache	Lead Nickel
Impaired visual activity	n-Hexane Methanol Organic mercury
Increased intracranial pressure	Organotin compounds
Opsoclonus	Chlordecone (Kepone)
Paraplegia	Organotin compounds
Parkinsonism	Carbon disulphide Carbon monoxide Manganese
Seizures	Lead Organic mercury Organochlorine insecticides Organotin compounds
Tremor	Carbon disulphide Chlordecone (Kepone) DDT Manganese Mercury

risk factors and cardiovascular disease is well known, less attention has been paid to occupational and environmental influences in the pathogenesis of these diseases.

First to consider are the occupational influences associated with lifestyle. There is good evidence from the classic studies on London bus drivers and conductors that sedentary workers have a higher risk of ischaemic heart disease than workers with a more active job. Much attention has focused recently on job stress and heart disease. The scientific evidence to support this is by no means incontrovertible. It is clear that the so-called ‘Type A’ personalities express more anger and hostility than ‘Type B’ and that such traits may encourage certain individuals to self select for certain jobs. What is clear is that the professional and managerial groups seem to experience less heart disease than manual workers despite the work environment of job pressure and decision making of the former group. Perhaps the physical and chemical stresses of the shop floor environment are more important influences these days or perhaps the professional groups have taken greater heed of the advice to reduce their personal lifestyle risk factors.

There is good evidence linking some chemical exposures to cardiovascular disease. Carbon disulphide, which is used in the viscose rayon industry, had been clearly associated with heart disease, possibly due to hypercholesterolaemia. However, recent research suggests that part (at least) of this cardiovascular effect may be due to an acute myotoxic effect leading to fatal arrhythmias. Such arrhythmias can also be caused by exposure to chlorinated organic solvents such as trichloroethylene. Other chemicals such as nitroglycerine are potent vasodilators and the effect is greatest after a period away from exposure—thus, the so called ‘Monday morning death’ syndrome in the makers and users of explosives. Vinyl chloride monomer has a peripheral vascular effect leading to Raynaud’s phenomenon.

The cardiovascular effects of exposure to metals are largely secondary. Lead, cadmium, and mercury can cause cardiovascular disease subsequent to their nephrotoxic effects. However, cobalt has been shown to cause cardiomyopathy by a direct effect on cardiac muscle.

The toxic industrial gases produce their effect secondary to anoxia. The most ubiquitous is carbon monoxide. Whilst these effects are well described at high exposure concentration, the effects of chronic low dose exposure to carbon monoxide are disputed although there is supporting evidence in animals so exposed but also fed on a diet rich in saturated fats. It is important to note that the paint-stripper methylene chloride is metabolized to carbon monoxide.

Of exposure to physical agents, it is known that vibration transmitted to the hands causes peripheral vascular disease probably due to damage to the neurovascular bundle. Cold can, of course, cause frostbite but the influence of noise is less clear cut. Acute high exposure to noise is known to raise blood pressure but although prolonged exposure to such noise can cause deafness, no cardiovascular effects have been clearly substantiated.

Finally, recent research has added considerable weight to the long-held assertion that workers on rotating shifts have an increased risk of ischaemic heart disease.

8.5.3(f) Genitourinary system

J. M. Harrington

The kidney plays a crucial role in the excretory and detoxification mechanisms of the body. Perhaps the most effective detoxification manoeuvre of the liver is to increase the polarity or acidity of the absorbed substance. This, in turn, increases the water solubility of the compound and hence its renal excretion. The kidney, therefore, bears the brunt of many toxic chemical exposures. Some toxic substances do reach the kidney unchanged but most are metabolized to some extent or other. Some, such as cadmium, become sequestered in the renal cortex whilst others, such as the aromatic amines stay in the bladder long enough and at high enough concentration to induce malignant change in the transitional cell epithelium.

Sudden, severe exposures to some chemicals can cause acute nephropathy. Such compounds may directly damage the kidney due to their intrinsic nephrotoxicity or may induce secondary damage due to prerenal effects such as the haemolysis following arsenic exposure. Hypovolaemic shock can also follow acute fluid loss or extreme heat whilst post-traumatic renal failure can follow crush injuries or high voltage electric shock both of which cause muscle necrosis. Chronic lower dose exposure leading to nephropathy are more commonly associated with metals or organic solvents.

The metals most commonly implicated in renal disease are mercury, cadmium, lead, and, perhaps, uranium. Exposure to mercury resulting in acute tubular necrosis or the nephrotic syndrome is most unusual these days. Under present day conditions workplace exposures to inhaled mercury vapour or absorbed mercury salts are more likely to cause mild proteinuria and limited tubular dysfunction. Biological monitoring of mercury-exposed workers has thus, of necessity, become more sophisticated. Sensitive tests of urinary enzymes, such as n-acetyl-β-D-glucosamidase, are necessary to detect those subtle effects. Similarly, modern industrial exposures to cadmium rarely result in the proximal or distal tubular dysfunction or renal cortical damage that was more prevalent in the past. However, cadmium is only slowly leached from the renal cortex and it is thus, even now, a potentially serious long-term cumulative poison. The environmental cadmium contamination which caused widespread tubular dysfunction with hypercalcuria and osteomalacia in multiparous postmenopausal Japanese women (Itai-Itai disease) has not been described in Western workers. Lead nephropathy is also a rarity nowadays. Lead is capable of causing damage to all parts of the nephron and lead nephritis was not uncommon in the early part of this century. Again, more subtle tests of renal enzymes are needed to assess modern lead exposure effects on the kidney. Soluble uranium compounds such as the hexafluoride have been shown, following acute accidental exposure, to be potent nephrotoxins, but such renal damage is largely unknown in a well controlled modern facility.

Chlorinated aliphatic solvents such as carbon tetrachloride and chloroform can cause the hepatorenal syndrome. The renal damage is largely an effect on the proximal tubular epithelium which can lead to tubular necrosis and acute oliguric renal failure. Whilst there are a number of case reports of glomerulonephritis following exposure to organic solvents (not necessarily the halogenated aliphatics) a causative role has not been established. The weight of evidence from case control studies of workers exposed to solvents also suggests an excess risk of glomerulonephritis. The mechanism is unclear but a link with Goodpasture's syndrome suggests possible autoimmune damage to the glomerular basement membrane.

Although the prostate possesses the curious ability to concentrate (and excrete) heavy metals, little evidence exists of occupationally caused prostatic disease. Earlier reports of a link between cadmium exposure and prostatic cancer have not been corroborated by more recent careful studies. Cancers of the urinary tract associated with occupational exposure to aromatic amines and polynuclear aromatic hydrocarbons are described in Chapter 8.5.3(c).

8.5.3(g) Gastrointestinal tract

E. S. Hodgson

In toxicological terms the gastrointestinal tract is a semipermeable membrane second only to the lung. Many elements and chemicals are efficiently transported across the gastrointestinal mucous membrane to their ultimate target organs—the most common being the liver.

However, relatively few chemicals cause direct damage to the alimentary tract. Acute gastroenteritis may be caused by the ingestion of the soluble salts of several metals, in particular arsenic, antimony, cadmium, mercury, thallium, and zinc. This is usually acute and reversible. Inorganic lead ingestion may cause acute intestinal colic but this is not always seen in chronic intoxication. Acute poisoning with organophosphorus insecticides (e.g. Dichlorvos, Parathion) may initially present with vomiting, diarrhoea, and severe abdominal pain probably initiated by the rapid effects such substances have on blood cholinesterase activity. Ingestion of many aromatic and aliphatic hydrocarbons will cause nausea and vomiting and perhaps gastritis from direct irritant effects. Corrosive liquids such as phenol and its derivatives, and mineral acids and alkalis, as well as the reactive metal salts are likely to cause severe mucosal burns with possible oesophageal perforation. Permanent damage is the rule with stenosis and is accompanied by extensive scarring of the oral cavity. Such effects are occasionally seen in work situations, usually due to lack of proper facial or personal protective equipment, but poisoning by ingestion is more commonly associated with accidents to children or suicide attempts in adults.

Peptic ulceration has traditionally been thought to be associated with shift work, perhaps due to disordered diet and stress related factors.

The liver is frequently at risk from occupational exposures. A wide variety of substances cause different types of hepatocellular injury which may eventually lead to cirrhosis and liver failure (Table 1).

Hepatitis viruses and infection with leptospirosis species may cause hepatic cell damage with jaundice (see Chapter 8.5.3(i)). Consumption of alcohol will inevitably enhance the effects of toxic substances on the liver and cases of rapidly advancing liver disease have been recorded in workers exposed to 1,1,1-trichlorethane or (formerly) trichloroethylene who are in the habit of drinking during their shift. Organic solvents, in particular the chlorinated hydrocarbons, nitrobenzenes, and chlorinated naphthalenes have been reported as causes of hepatocellular necrosis often leading to chronic liver dysfunction. Chronic arsenic poisoning in those using pesticide sprays in vineyards may include liver damage and

Table 1 *Effects of occupationally related hepatotoxins*

	Substance	
Effect	Organic	Inorganic
Centrilobular necrosis	Acrylonitrile	Antimony
	Carbon tetrachloride	Arsenic
	Chlorinated hydrocarbon insecticides	Boranes
	Chlorinated naphthalenes	Phosphorus (Yellow)
	Dimethyl hydrazine	Selenium
	Dimethyl nitrosamine	Thallium
	Dinitrophenol	
	Ethyl alcohol	
	Halothane	
	Methyl chloride	
	Nitrobenzene	
	Phenol	
	Polychlorinated diphenyls	
	Tetrachloroethylene	
	1,1,1-Trichloroethane	
	Trichloroethylene	
	Trinitrotoluene	
	Toluene	
	Vinyl chloride	
Hepatic effect	Halothane	
	Viral hepatitis	
	Leptospirosis	
Cholestatic cholangiolytic	Methylene dianiline	
	Organic arsenicals	
	Toluene diamine	
	4,4′-Diaminodiphenyl methane	

From Harrington and Gill (1991).

frank cirrhosis in cases of prolonged heavy exposure, which may be superimposed on high alcohol consumption.

Vinyl chloride monomer, the precursor of polyvinyl chloride (PVC) is a carcinogen particularly noted for its effect on the liver giving rise to angiosarcoma which may be preceded by a non-cirrhotic portal fibrosis.

The control of occupationally induced gastrointestinal disease relies especially upon good process design to reduce exposure of the workforce as far as is practicable. It may be necessary to exclude those with alcohol problems or frank alcoholic liver damage from such exposure.

8.5.3(h) The haemopoietic system

E. S. Hodgson

The haemopoietic system is particularly sensitive to the effect of a range of workplace substances. Micro-organisms may also affect the blood and this is discussed elsewhere (Section 7 and Chapter 8.5.3.(i)).

Ionizing radiation particularly affects rapidly dividing cells and thus the bone marrow is at especial risk. Doses between 1 and 10 Gy lead to an early decrease in peripheral lymphocyte count followed by reduction in all white cell elements within 3 weeks giving increased risk of infection with bleeding and petechial haemorrhages. Recovery may be possible and is discussed elsewhere (Chapter 5.3). The possibility of leukaemia from low dose radiation remains controversial.

The element most frequently associated with bone marrow damage is inorganic lead which produces anaemia by direct action upon the enzymes involved in haem synthesis and also by haemolysis of red cells. The early and specific effects on haem enzymes allow sensitive testing of low level lead absorption and this is a fundamental tool in accurate health surveillance of exposed workers. Haemolysis is also caused by arsine which may be liberated in the smelting and refining of metal, galvanizing processes, and certain soldering techniques.

Benzene has a profound influence on the haemopoietic system causing complex effects including early deficiency of platelets, and perhaps mild haemolysis and pancytopenia. Aplastic anaemia was the major effect reported historically although lymphoid and myeloid leukaemias have been described in some cases. Exposure to benzene is carefully controlled under most health and safety jurisdictions. Styrene has been implicated in an excess of leukaemia in those exposed but most short chain alkyl benzenes do not exhibit the haemotoxic effects of the parent benzene. Methaemoglobinaemia traditionally associated with the aniline dye industry is more likely nowadays to be associated with the nitrated aromatic compounds, in particular nitrobenzenes and toluenes. Individual response to these compounds is highly idiosyncratic and monitoring procedures must be supplemented by careful clinical appraisal to detect the early adverse signs of relative tissue hypoxia. Carbon monoxide inhalation giving rise to carboxyhaemoglobinaemia may occur in a variety of occupations. Fire fighters are known to be exposed to high levels during fire fighting but should be protected by breathing apparatus although this is not always worn. A variety of industrial processes involving combustion as well as the use of methylene chloride as a paint stripper have given rise to carbon monoxide poisoning. Commercial garages may produce high levels of carbon monoxide in the absence of appropriate scavenging systems and workers in traditional communities using open fires to heat enclosed work places may suffer the consequences of inadequate combustion and ventilation. Low level tissue hypoxia whilst not life threatening may cause a prolonged decrement in job performance.

The possibility that many chemicals, in particular the organic solvents, may produce a biological effect on the haemopoietic systems, cannot be discounted. It is likely that with the development of more sophisticated biological monitoring systems these possibilities will be elucidated.

8.5.3(i) Infections

E. S. Hodgson

Hookworm is perhaps the most common occupational disease worldwide, infecting many barefoot agricultural workers in developing tropical economies. Indeed, the zoonoses as a group contribute significantly to economic deficit in most traditional economies, causing significant morbidity and mortality in the working population.

Micro-organisms and invertebrates of many groups can be acquired by workers across the job spectrum. Brucellosis, leptospirosis, Q fever, and a variety of gastrointestinal infections are recorded in farm workers in Europe. Any workers exposed to environments contaminated by animal excreta, body fluids, or carcasses are at risk from indigenous micro-organisms. Thus, tularaemia has been seen in hunters, veterinary surgeons, and butchers in most of the Northern hemisphere, but not in the United Kingdom. Engineers, scientists, and field researchers working in remote areas may acquire a range of zoonoses including rabies, ornithosis, haemorrhagic fevers, and tick-borne conditions of varying severity. More recently, workers in the expanding occupation of 'leisure' worker, (perhaps teaching water-based, or country pursuits), have exhibited a range of zoonoses and geographically acquired infections. Deaths from leptospirosis in speleologists and canoeists have been recorded worldwide.

Business travellers are especially vulnerable to local infections particularly when travelling from temperate areas to the tropics. Gastrointestinal conditions are universal in such travellers, often associated with unfamiliar diets or rural trips, and can seriously disrupt delicate commercial negotiations. Sexually transmitted disease, including HIV, constitutes a major risk for the lonely and unwise traveller, with devastating effects on partners and family on return. Expatriate personnel are prey to the full range of local infections common to the area, and such conditions may be considered as occupationally related. International aid workers are heavily exposed to risk from poliomyelitis, tuberculosis, hepatitis A infection, and salmonellosis, especially during refugee crises. Malaria, increasingly drug resistant, continues to levy its toll on altruistic and commercially active expatriates.

Infectious hazards to health care and laboratory personnel are well documented and of increasing concern. The hepatitis viruses, particularly hepatitis B, pose a special risk, (via percutaneous inoculation and mucous membrane contact), in areas of high endemicity, and where care is provided to likely carriers. Legislation requiring assessment of such risks, control, and prevention is increasing rapidly in many jurisdictions, partly driven by increased employee perception, but mainly by adverse legal activity. Other hepatitis viruses, including hepatitis C and D (delta agent), are a potential hazard to clinical workers, but the actual 'risk' is unknown.

The hazard to such employees from HIV is low but transmission has occurred in dentists, surgeons, and nurses usually following percutaneous inoculation of considerable quantities of infected material. The risk is several orders of magnitude less than that from hepatitis B virus. Prion disease, such as Creutzfeldt-Jacob disease has been observed in mortuary and neurosurgical workers, but the epidemiology is obscure. Most micro-organism transmitted diseases have been seen in laboratory workers, although tuberculosis, viral hepatitis, and salmonellosis occur most frequently. Infections normally seen in childhood, such as chickenpox, mumps, and measles are seen in health care personnel, usually acquired in paediatric or primary care practice.

Prevention requires careful assessment of hazard and risk, detailed knowledge of the environment, scrupulously designed work systems, and rigorously applied training with frequent updating. Immunization plays a crucial part in the health surveillance of exposed workers. Managers must increasingly satisfy the demands of stricter legislation designed to protect workers exposed to infectious hazards. Health surveillance is now an established component of management systems.

8.5.3(j) Reproductive system

E. C. McCloy

Reproductive hazards may affect both the female and male reproductive cycles. They include agents producing developmental abnormalities in offspring. Their classification includes metals, organic chemicals, physical agents such as ionizing radiation, and microbiological organisms. All stages of the reproductive cycle may be vulnerable, from gametogenesis, through fertilization, implantation, embryo- and fetogenesis, to the newborn and maturing infant. Adverse pregnancy outcomes are fetal death, manifest as spontaneous miscarriage or stillbirth, prematurity, and low birth weight. Adverse outcomes affecting the offspring include congenital abnormality, development delay, and, perhaps, childhood malignancy.

For some individual reproductive toxins sufficient clinical and scientific evidence has accumulated following high exposure, either accidentally or as a result of previous adverse working environments, to allow definite conclusions to be drawn regarding their reproductive toxicity. For other substances associations have been made through hypotheses generated by epidemiological studies on adverse reproductive outcomes in occupations in which the particular substance is the major environmental toxin. However, abnormal outcomes associated with occupational exposures have to be set against the natural outcomes of an event and difficulties in relating exposure, both in terms of dose and time, to the observed effect. From these sources it can be said that there may be increased risk of the following outcomes through exposure to either the particular substance or employment in the broad occupational category.

Gametogenesis

Impaired male fertility with exposure to lead; the nematocide 1,2-dibromo-3-chloropropane (DBPC); ethylene dibromide, an active ingredient of several pesticides; employment in mild steel welding.

Spontaneous miscarriages

Employment in agriculture, horticulture, food and beverage industries, and in some health care occupations; employment in manufacturing industries and microelectronic assembly, which have, in common, exposure to solvents.

Stillbirth

Employment in agriculture, horticulture, and the leather industries.

Prematurity and low birth weight

The presence of ergonomic stressors such as lifting heavy weights and shift work, has been shown to retard fetal growth and increase the risk of preterm birth.

Congenital abnormality

Specific association has been shown between exposure to methyl mercury in pregnancy and characteristic facial abnormalities, as well as exposure to solvents and the occurrence of cleft palate.

Developmental

Neurobehavioural defects in children are associated with fetal lead levels above 20 μg/dl although pregnant women are permitted to continue working whilst their blood lead is below 40 μg/dl. Developmental delay is associated with maternal exposure to polychlorinated biphenyls which are secreted in breast milk, and cerebral palsy with maternal exposure to methyl mercury.

Childhood cancer

Associations have been published between leukaemia and paternal exposure to radiation; brain cancer and paternal employment in agriculture, the construction industry, machine repair and installation, and electrical assembly; non-specific malignancy and parental exposure to chemicals including paints, petroleum products, pesticides, and metals.

Summary

Improved control of environmental levels of xenobiotics has removed, for many employees, the harmful effects that some substances had on the reproductive cycle. Evidence for reproductive effects from occupations must be sought from prospective epidemiological studies with early identification of fertilization and concomitant measure of exposure levels with each stage of the reproductive cycle.

8.5.3(k) Neuropsychological disorders

A. Spurgeon

Psychiatric disorders and cognitive impairment have been associated with exposure to a number of industrial agents, notably organic solvents, organophosphorus pesticides, and some metals.

Organic solvents

Inhalation of a number of volatile aromatic and aliphatic organic compounds used as industrial solvents (e.g. toluene, styrene, trichlorethylene) may result in acute narcotic effects. Typical industrial exposures involve more than one solvent and effects are usually assumed to be additive although occasionally synergistic effects may occur. Acute effects are usually rapidly reversed on removal from exposure. Long-term low level exposure may result in chronic toxic encephalopathy characterized by depressive symptoms and disturbances of mood and by cognitive impairment involving learning, memory, control of attention, and visual motor skills. Effects on cognitive functioning may be subtle and occur in the absence of psychiatric or other symptoms. The level and duration of exposure required to produce these effects is controversial. Severe toxic encephalopathy characterized by progressive and global intellectual deterioration and personality disturbance has been observed in some workers with very high or very long exposure but this is now rarely seen clinically. Since most exposures are to solvent mixtures information on the specific effects of particular compounds is limited. However, carbon disulphide is known to have particularly severe effects on emotional and cognitive functioning at relatively low concentrations.

Organophosphorus pesticides

Exposure to organophosphorus compounds typically occurs in agricultural workers involved in crop spraying or sheep dipping and may result from inhalation or absorption through intact skin. The principal action of organophosphates is the inhibition of acetylcholinesterase producing initial symptoms of fatigue followed by restlessness and irritability. A variety of symptoms of emotional disturbance including depression and anxiety may occur shortly after exposure and persist for many months. This may be accompanied by generalized impairment of cognitive functioning, including effects on learning and memory processes, control of attention, psychomotor speed, and expressive language.

Metals

Neuropsychological effects have most commonly been observed in relation to lead, mercury, and manganese exposure.

Lead

Acute encephalopathy resulting from poisoning is now uncommon in industrial settings. However, subtle effects on cognitive functioning relating particularly to visual motor skills and memory processes, have been observed in lead workers. Emotional disturbances, characterized by depression and confusion, have also been reported in those with long-term exposure.

Mercury

Inhalation of mercury vapour commonly results in the condition termed 'erethism' characterized by irritable behaviour, depression, and fatigue. Intellectual impairment involving visual motor skills, memory, and attentional control may also occur. Disturbances of behaviour and cognitive functioning often precede the development of motor system abnormalities typical of chronic mercury poisoning. In severe cases a parkinsonian syndrome may develop.

Manganese

Intoxication resulting from manganese exposure initially produces symptoms of drowsiness, poor co-ordination, and impaired speech which may be accompanied by psychiatric disturbances including insomnia, hallucinations, and aggressive behaviour. Subsequently parkinsonian-like symptoms of increasing severity may develop, often accompanied by psychotic behaviour.

Other neurotoxic metals commonly encountered in the workplace are aluminium, arsenic, and organic tin compounds. However, neuropsychological abnormalities associated with occupational exposure have occurred only in isolated cases in modern industrialized countries.

8.5.4 Occupational safety

R. T. Booth

Introduction

Accidents at work occur in diverse circumstances and settings. Although a small number of serious accidents result from component, structural, or process failures, the vast majority of accidents are associated with dangers that form an everyday part of working life, for example, contact with moving machinery, falls, cuts from material being handled, slipping on or striking against objects, and injuries from hand tools. Notwithstanding the diversity of accident experience, there is now broad agreement that the principles of safety management apply equally to the control of all these situations, and indeed to the control of health hazards at work.

In Great Britain, approximately 600 people receive fatal injuries as a result of work accidents every year, and about 1.4 million suffer injuries. But the problem is not adequately described merely by listing the historical evidence of harm. Preventive effort must also be devoted to risk assessment and control of hazards with serious potential before the first accident leading to casualties occur. In the last decade of the 20th century the United Kingdom is experiencing the most fundamental changes in health and safety regulation than perhaps at any time since the introduction of the first safety legislation in the mid-19th century. The changes in law result from the introduction in the United Kingdom of European Union health and safety directives associated with the introduction of the Single Market in January 1993. The new regulations build on the skeleton framework for safety management contained in the Health and Safety at Work Act 1974. The regulations specify in detail the steps that employers must take to plan for safety, identify hazards,

Table 1 *Kinds of accident: fatal and non-fatal major[1] injuries to employees for Great Britain. Numbers averaged for the 4 years 1987/88–1990/91*

	Fatal injuries		Non-fatal major injuries	
Kind of accident	No.	%	No.	%
Contact with moving machinery	26	6.4	1962	9.8
Struck by moving/falling object	53	13.2	2616	13.0
Struck by moving vehicle	57	14.2	754	3.8
Struck against something fixed or stationary	2	0.6	785	3.9
Injured while handling lifting or carrying	1	0.2	1350	6.7
Slip, trip or fall on same level	5	1.2	5816	29.0
Falls from heights	91	22.5	4350	21.7
Trapped by something collapsing or overturning	31	7.6	229	1.1
Drowning or asphyxiation	14	3.5	25	0.1
Exposure to or contact with a harmful substance	11	2.6	771	3.8
Exposure to fire	7	1.7	111	0.6
Exposure to explosion	8	1.9	81	0.4
Contact with electricity or electrical discharge	22	5.4	303	1.5
Injured by an animal	2	0.4	76	0.4
Other kind of accident	24	6.0	735	3.7
Injuries not classified by kind[2]	51	12.7	112	0.6
Totals	402	100.0	20 073	100.0

[1] Major injuries are defined under RIDDOR, and include fractures, amputations, losses of consciousness due to lack of oxygen, and any injury that results in the person injured being admitted immediately into hospital for more than 24 h.

[2] This figure includes the 167 fatalities in the Piper Alpha disaster in 1988. The average for the other 3 years was 10 fatalities not classified by kind.

Derived from Table 9 of Department of Employment (1992).

assess risks, and select appropriate controls; controls that should be appropriate and effective in the context of each employer's operations.

In parallel with these legal developments, substantial progress has been made in identifying and classifying the crucial ingredients of effective safety management, and the approach companies should adopt to improve their safety performance. It is now clear that safety management and corporate management generally should share a common approach. The influence of safety culture, a subset of the overall organizational culture, is now understood to be a key predictor of safety performance. Indeed, aspects of the overall culture (for example, the effectiveness of communications generally in an organization) may have more influence on accident rates than many elements of mainstream safety programmes.

A series of major accidents in transportation and in offshore oil exploration in the late 1980s have demonstrated the disastrous consequences of weaknesses in safety organization and culture. A significant finding of the inquiry reports was that managers in the organizations concerned shared a fallacious belief that they were working in organizations with total commitment to safety and with effective safety systems. The inquiry reports emphasized the priority that enterprises must attach to objective prediction and measurement of safety performance.

The aims of this chapter are to describe:

- The size of the occupational accident problem;
- The development of theories which have sought to explain the process of accident causation;
- The evolution of the principles of safety management, and the concept of safety culture;
- The way statutory requirements now underpin contemporary perceptions of the most effective methods for accident prevention;
- The key elements of safety management: risk assessment, and safety performance measurement.

The chapter draws heavily on the introductory sections of the report *Organising for Safety* (Health and Safety Commission 1993), and adopts a similar approach to that of the report *Successful Health and Safety Management* (Health and Safety Executive 1991).

The size of the problem

In 1990/91, a typical year, 346 employees were killed at work in Great Britain. In addition 87 self-employed persons and 139 members of the public received fatal injuries as a result of work activities. The statistical evidence of non-fatal accidents is more difficult to state with precision. Accidents caused by work activities in Great Britain should be reported to the relevant enforcing authority under the terms of the Reporting of Injuries, Diseases and Dangerous Occurrences Regulations 1985 (RIDDOR). However the findings of the recent Labour Force Survey suggest that only about 30 per cent of all reportable accidents to employees are in fact reported. Moreover, the reporting levels vary sharply in different employment sectors, varying from 80 per cent in the energy sector to 17 per cent in agriculture. It appears that only about 5 per cent of reportable accidents to the self-employed are reported. In 1991, The Health and Safety Executive have published evidence based on reported accidents that suggest that accident performance in Great Britain compares very favourably with other industrialized countries. The findings of the Labour Force Survey would suggest that part, and perhaps a substantial part, of the explanation for the difference is explained by under-reporting, and also by differences in reporting criteria.

Table 1 shows the pattern of accident causation in terms of kinds of accident. The table reveals that the kinds of accident that lead to fatal injuries are in some cases markedly different from the kinds that lead to major injuries. Falls on one level are the greatest cause of major injuries but, not surprisingly, only involve a small number of fatalities. Falls from heights and being struck by moving/falling objects contribute substantially to both severity categories.

Table 2 shows the nature of fatal and major injury accidents. The data

Table 2 *Nature of injury: fatal and non-fatal major[1] injuries to employees for Great Britain. Numbers averaged for the 4 years 1987/88–1990/91*

	Fatal injuries		Non-fatal major injuries	
Kind of accident	No.	%	No.	%
Amputation	1	0.4	1692	9.0
Loss of sight of eye	0	0.0	20	0.1
Fracture	56	17.8	13 658	72.3
Dislocation	0	0.0	36	0.2
Concussion and internal injuries	20	6.2	151	0.8
Lacerations and open wounds	6	1.8	645	3.4
Contusions	41	13.1	382	2.0
Burns	14	4.4	863	4.6
Poisonings and gassings	23	7.2	229	1.2
Sprains and strains	1	0.2	155	0.8
Superficial injuries	1	0.4	292	1.5
Natural causes	1	0.2	5	0.0
Other injuries caused by contact with electricity	16	5.2	78	0.4
Injuries of more than one of the other natures	46	14.8	254	1.3
Injuries not elsewhere specified	17	5.5	71	0.4
Injury not known	72	23.0	365	1.9
Totals	314	100.0	18 895	100.0

[1] See footnote 2 of Table 1.

Derived from Table 15 of Departmnt of Employment (1992).

reveal that fractures, contusions, and multiple injuries together account for approximately 46 per cent of fatal injuries. Nearly three-quarters of all major injuries are attributable to fractures. Perhaps the most curious feature of the fatal accident data is that the nature of injury was unknown in no less than 23 per cent of cases.

The evolution of safety management and law

Accident prevention requires the creation, and maintenance, of a safe working environment, and the promotion of safe behaviour—the avoidance of error—by people working with hazards. However, safety management effort has traditionally been directed at the prevention of repetitions of accidents that have already occurred, largely on the basis of information derived from detailed accident investigations. Accidents meriting investigation usually involve a casualty, and it is not surprising that the behaviour of those who are injured may dominate the minds of the investigators. The main reason why safety management has concentrated on reactive prevention is simply that it is a good deal easier than proactive prevention. Assessing risks and devising preventive plans without the help of accident data is difficult: it involves weighing the probabilities of a wide range of unwanted outcomes, and preparing an integrated control plan to cope with all the hazards detected. In contrast, preventing the recurrence of a particular accident is a self-contained problem with an apparently self-evident solution.

Key features of the traditional approach, based on early models of accident causation were the search for a primary accident cause; and the debate as to whether the primary cause was an unsafe act or an unsafe condition.

Most practical accident prevention involved the preparation of a safety rule designed to prevent a recurrence of the unsafe act, or a physical safeguard to remedy the unsafe condition, most proximate to the accident. Much of the corpus of traditional United Kingdom health and safety legislation contains rules and physical standards derived as has been described. A satisfactory feature of the introduction of the new European Union led law referred to above is the phased repeal of much archaic safety law.

The causation debate, clouded by sterile political overtones and a desire to apportion blame, has often missed three crucial, and interrelated, issues.

The concept of a single primary accident cause is a bizarre simplification of a complex multicausal process. Moreover, the term 'unsafe act' embraces a wide range of human errors, including both unintentional errors and intentionally risky behaviour (violations).

The distinction between the contribution of unsafe conditions and unsafe acts in causation has masked the more important distinction between the relative contribution of conditions and behaviour in prevention and the need for prevention plans to promote both safe conditions and safe behaviour.

The argument has focused almost exclusively on the errors made by the people who have had the accidents, not the managers and engineers whose errors (remote in time and place from the location of an accident) may have created a climate and a physical environment where errors by people at risk are made more likely or more serious. Unsafe acts create conditions where unsafe acts may lead to accidents. Reason (1990) calls the remote errors by managers latent or decision failures, and the errors by people directly at risk active failures.

Whatever the merits—and achievements—of the safety management approach just described, it was clearly inadequate to cope with major hazards in rapidly developing technologies. Here preventive measures may be rendered obsolete by each technical advance, and the occurrence of the first accident may itself be intolerable. But the weakness of the method is not confined to high-risk and rapidly-advancing technologies. The essential point is that rules and safeguards devised in the aftermath of disagreeable accidents may be over zealous (as perceived some years after the accident), and conflict with the needs of both employers and employees to get the job done. Both parties may tacitly conspire to evade the safety rules or to defeat the physical safeguards. Moreover the measures taken to prevent one specific accident may conflict with the measures adopted to prevent a different accident, and with production-oriented rules. Rule books (and indeed legislation) drawn up in this way are likely to become in time both incomprehensible and contradictory. At least two company rules may exist for any situation: the rule to get the job done in time, and a more demanding rule that may be invoked when things go wrong.

The Robens Committee report

The Robens Committee (Committee on Safety and Health at Work, 1972), whose report created the framework and philosophy of the Health and Safety at Work Act 1974, described in detail the shortcomings of safety management as it had evolved in industry in the United Kingdom. The report stated 'the most important single reason for accidents at work is apathy', and continued:

> 'The primary responsibility . . . lies with those who create the risks and those who work with them . . . Our present system encourages too much reliance on state regulation and rather too little on responsibility and voluntary self generating effort. . .'
>
> 'It is not to underrate the importance of physical safeguards to say that the preoccupation with the physical environment has tended to dominate this field, to the neglect of the equally important human and organisational factors such as the role of training . . . the arrangements for monitoring safety performance, or the influence of work systems on management and behaviour.' . . .
>
> 'There are two essential ingredients for better management performance in this field—explicit policy objectives, and effective organisation in which individual responsibilities are clearly defined.'

Robens, having noted that companies with excellent safety records in the United Kingdom and overseas prepared policy statements setting out their safety objectives, recommended that the preparation of a safety policy should become a statutory duty upon all but the smallest companies.

Robens advocated self-regulation: the doctrine that competent and committed employers, in consultation with their workforce, would identify hazards, assess risks, and implement preventive measures, within a framework of law and standards developed nationally with the participation of all parties. Traditional prescriptive law promoted at best grudging, unthinking compliance. The idea of the new law was to promote proactive safety management, and enthusiastic compliance by everyone involved. Robens said:

> 'We need a more effectively self-regulating system. This calls for the acceptance and exercise of appropriate responsibilities at all levels within industry and commerce—it calls for better systems of safety organisation, for more management initiatives and for more involvement of work people themselves . . .'

Robens used the phrase self-regulation to describe elements of what would now be termed safety culture. Crucially Robens argued that the character and scope of the law as it had evolved was a hindrance to the promotion of self-regulation, and hence to the promotion of a good safety culture.

Self regulation after Robens

The Robens diagnosis was accepted by government, but the cure proposed—or more accurately the cure adopted—was not sufficiently radical or targeted. The proposals did not take account of the diversity of employers, or the very real difficulties that employers would have in understanding what they had to do in practice. They underestimated the extent to which the dead hand of traditional law and beliefs would continue to militate against the development of self-regulation. One commentator in 1987 suggested that self-regulation 'works' only within a very narrow range of employers with clear, self-interested, reasons for compliance. Most employers were described as amoral calculators whose unwritten safety policy was to do as little with which they could get away. Such employers would implement safety improvements only when set out in detail and enforced by an inspector. It was perhaps naive to believe that the imposition of a duty to write a safety policy would transform amoral calculators into willing self-regulators.

The introduction in January 1993 of European Union-driven safety regulations, and particularly the Management of Health and Safety at Work Regulations 1992, taken together with the phased repeal of archaic safety law, offers a new chance to employers to develop self-regulation as envisaged by Robens. The distinctive feature of traditional safety law was that it was prescriptive in outcome—the law specified the hazards and preventive measures (typically guards to machinery). In contrast the new regulations are mainly prescriptive in process—the law specified the steps which an employer should take to identify hazards, assess risks, and select, implement, and monitor preventive measures.

Proactive safety management

Accident investigations and prevention programmes must address the following distinctive elements of the accident causation process.

1. Multicausality

Very few accidents, particularly in large organizations and complex technologies, are associated with a single cause. Rather, accidents happen as a result of a chance concatenation of many distinct causative factors, each one necessary but not sufficient to cause a final breakdown. It follows that the coverage of prevention plans should seek to permeate all aspects of the organization's activities. Moreover, accident investigators should continue to seek out further causative factors even when a familiar, abnormal event is found which is therefore accepted as explanation, and a cure is known.

2. Active and latent failures

Active failures are errors which have an immediate adverse effect. They are equivalent to the unsafe acts discussed earlier. In contrast, latent failures lie dormant in an organization for some time, only becoming evident when they combine with local triggers. The triggers are the active failures—unsafe acts, and unsafe conditions (for example, a mechanical failure). The recognition of the importance of latent failures is useful because it emphasizes the role of senior managers in causation, and draws attention to the scope for detecting latent failures in the system well before they are revealed by active failures.

3. Skill-, rule-, and knowledge-based errors, and violations

The standard framework for classifying error is the skill–rule–knowledge based model proposed by Rasmussen in 1987.

Skill-based errors involve 'slips' or 'lapses' in highly practised and routine tasks. At a rather more complex level a person has to look at a situation and classify it into a familiar category as the basis for action; if it is mis-classified, this may be called a rule-based error, or mistake. Knowledge-based errors describe the most complex cases where people fail to create an adequate new rule to cope with a situation. Violations, sometimes referred to as risk taking, comprise a further category of error.

Here a person deliberately carries out an action that is contrary to a rule, such as an approved operating procedure.

The success of training programmes depends on an adequate diagnosis of the nature of the errors likely to be made. For example, task analysis and training which fails to consider violations may prove wholly ineffective.

4. Hazard identification, risk assessment, and preventive action

The need to identify hazards, assess risks, and select, implement, and monitor preventive actions is an essential foundation of safety management—the avoidance of latent failures. It is also the foundation for safe personal behaviour in the face of danger—the avoidance of active failures.

To create and maintain a safe working environment, and to work safely in a dangerous environment people must have the appropriate knowledge and skills, and must know the rules, and be motivated, to:

(a) Identify hazards;
(b) Assess accurately the priority and importance of the hazards (risk assessment);
(c) Recognize and accept personal responsibility for dealing with the hazards in an appropriate way;
(d) Have appropriate knowledge about what should be done (including specified rules);
(e) Have the skills to carry out the appropriate necessary sequence of preventive actions, including monitoring the adequacy of the actions, and taking further corrective action.

The organization should be aware of circumstances where managers, supervisors, and other personnel may underestimate the magnitude of risks, overestimate their ability to assess and control risks, and have an impaired ability to cope with risks.

The aims of safety management

The primary aim of safety management is to intervene in the accident causation process and to break the causation chain. This involves preventing or detecting latent and active failures in the continuing process of hazard identification, risk assessment, control, and monitoring. However, the aim of safety management is not limited simply to hazard identification, control, and monitoring. Employers must plan for safety. Decisions have to be made, for example, about priorities for resource allocation, about training needs, about the appropriate risk assessment methodologies to be adopted, about the need for human reliability assessment, and about the choice of tolerable risk criteria. Safety criteria should underpin every decision made by the enterprise. Safety must be considered as an integral part of day-to-day decision-making. Moreover, an employer must establish organization and communications systems which facilitate the process of integrating safety within the management process, and which ensure that everyone in the organization is at least fully informed of safety issues, and ideally has had an opportunity to contribute to the debate.

Key functions of safety management

From the foregoing, the four key functions of the management of safety may be summarized as follows.

1. *Policy and planning*: determining safety goals, quantified objectives, and priorities, and a programme of work designed to achieve the objectives, which is then subject to measurement and review.
2. *Organization and communication*: establishing clear lines of responsibility and two-way communications at all levels.
3. *Hazard management*: ensuring that hazards are identified, risks assessed, and control measures determined, implemented, and subject to measurement and review.
4. *Monitoring and review*: establishing whether steps (i), (ii), and (iii) above are in place, in use, and work in practice.

The four key elements of safety management are underpinned by the requirements of the Management of Health and Safety at Work Regulations 1992.

Safety management and safety culture

The procedures and systems described above are necessary elements of an effective safety programme. But they are not the whole story. There is the danger that an organization's safety policies, plans, and monitoring arrangements which appear, on paper, to be well-considered and comprehensive may create an aura of respectability which disguises sullen scepticism or false perceptions among opinion formers at management and shop floor levels. The critical point is not so much the adequacy of the safety plans as the perceptions and beliefs that people hold about them. The next sections focus on the issues that determine whether the safety procedures just described are implemented with the full and enthusiastic support of the whole workforce, or whether the procedures are, at best, put into practice grudgingly and without thought, or at worst are honoured in the breach.

The concept of safety culture origins and definition of safety culture

The concept of safety culture was introduced in a seminal paper by Zohar in 1980, and reappeared in the nuclear safety debate by the International Nuclear Safety Advisory Group (INSAG) in their analysis of the accident at Chernobyl. The Agency has subsequently published an authoritative report in 1991 which elaborates the concept in detail and has defined safety culture as:

> '. . . that assembly of characteristics and attitudes in organisations and individuals which establishes that, as an overriding priority, nuclear plant safety issues receive the attention warranted by their significance'.

In 1991, the Confederation of British Industries described the culture of an organization as 'the mix of shared values, attitudes and patterns of behaviour that give the organisation its particular character. Put simply it is "the way we do things round here" '. They suggest that the 'safety culture of an organisation could be described as the ideas and beliefs that all members of the organisation share about risk, accidents and ill health'.

A possible shortcoming of the INSAG definition is that they use the term to describe only an ideal safety culture. The reference to shared ideas and beliefs by the Confederation of British Industries does not make explicit the need for shared action. Neither definition quite captures the necessary elements of competency and proficiency. The Health and Safety Commission (1993) suggests the following as a working definition.

SAFETY CULTURE

The safety culture of an organization is the product of individual and group values, attitudes, competencies, and patterns of behaviour that determine the commitment to, and the style and proficiency of, an organization's health and safety programmes.

Organizations with a positive safety culture are characterized by communications founded on mutual trust, by shared perceptions of the importance of safety, and by confidence in the efficacy of preventive measures.

Characteristics of organizations with a positive safety culture

A positive safety culture implies that the whole is more than the sum of the parts. The many separate practices interact to give added effect and, in particular, to allow all the people involved to share similar perceptions and adopt the same positive attitudes to safety: a collective commitment.

The synergy of a positive safety culture is mirrored by the negative synergy of organizations with a poor safety culture. Here the commitment to safety of some individuals is strangled by the cynicism of others, and the whole is less than the sum of the parts. This is evident in organizations where a strong commitment to safety resides only in the safety department.

The Confederation of British Industries has reported the results of a survey of 'how companies manage health and safety'. The idea of the culture of an organization was incorporated in the report's title *Developing a Safety Culture*. The dominant themes to emerge were:

1. The crucial importance of leadership and the commitment of the chief executive;
2. The executive safety role of line management;
3. Involvement of all employees;
4. Openness of communication;
5. Demonstration of care and concern for all those affected by the business.

The objective of these and related organizational features is to cultivate a coherent set of perceptions and attitudes that accurately reflect the risks involved and give high priority to safety as an integral part of workshop floor and managerial performance. What is critical is not so much the apparent quality and comprehensiveness of health and safety policy and procedures, but the perception of their necessity and their effectiveness by staff at all levels.

A constant theme in the discussion of safety culture is that it is a subset of, or at least profoundly influenced by, the overall culture of an organization. It follows that the safety performance of organizations is greatly influenced by aspects of management that have traditionally not been 'part of safety'. This view has been supported by an extensive research programme carried out by the United States Nuclear Regulatory Commission (NUREG). The expert judgement of the researchers who conducted the work is that the key predictive indicators of safety performance in the nuclear industry of the United States are, in rank order:

(i) Effective communication, leading to commonly understood goals, and means to achieve the goals, at all levels in the organization;
(ii) Good organizational learning, where organizations are tuned to identify, and respond to incremental change;
(iii) Organizational focus; simply the attention devoted by the organization to workplace safety and health;
(iv) External factors, including the financial health of the parent organization, or simply the economic climate within which the company is working, and the impact of regulatory bodies.

The point about these factors is that both (i) and (ii) above do not concern safety directly; they relate to all aspects of a company's culture. It follows that to make managers manage safety better it is necessary to make them better managers.

The conclusion drawn from this work and other studies, putting to one side the impact of external pressures and constraints, is that safety depends as much on organizational culture generally as on visible safety management activity. Crucially the best health and safety standards can arguably only be achieved by a programme which has a scope well beyond the traditional pattern of safety management functions.

The Health and Safety at Work Act requires all companies employing five or more people to prepare a health and safety policy. A written corporate statement on the safety policy and organization should be a crucial element in the promotion and maintenance of a positive safety culture within the organization and of high standards of safety awareness in the minds of both management and workforce.

The policy should provide the basis for a positive approach to the management of safety. For such a policy to be meaningful it must be more than a one-off event written to fulfil the letter of the Act; its objective should be to establish the corporate attitude to safety and the organizational framework through which the safety objectives can be assured. The importance of the written safety policy in creating an organizational climate and structure for safety assurance cannot be underestimated; neither can the need to keep the policy under regular, systematic review.

The written safety policy represents the formal, public corporate statement on safety as the foundation in the process of building a positive safety culture within an organization.

Monitoring safety performance

The conventional method many companies adopt to measure safety performance is simply to count the number of accidents. In fact accident data, on their own, provide a belated, and potentially misleading measure of safety performance. In many organizations there are not enough accidents to determine whether differences between sites or over time are due to real differences, or simply due to chance. Moreover, variations in the time individuals choose to take off for injuries deemed to be of similar severity influence company (and national) accident statistics.

The design of a health and safety monitoring system for an enterprise must address two crucial issues.

1. There is no single measure of safety performance that is unambiguous, and wholly resistant to abuse. Accident data should be used in conjunction with other performance measures;
2. Safety performance monitoring should not only be designed to check compliance; it should also be designed to promote compliance—the principle of 'what gets measured gets done'.

It follows that performance measures should be designed to permeate every activity and function within the organization, from top management decisions to shop floor behaviour. Moreover an organization needs a battery of distinctive tests incorporated in its safety programme, so that the limitations of one are balanced by the strengths of another. To a large extent, proprietary safety auditing techniques (described further below) aim to provide this all-embracing coverage. The measures should include checks to determine the adequacy of, and compliance with, hardware standards and systems of work. Moreover the arrangements for training, and training effectiveness should be monitored.

Safety auditing

Many employers have adopted and use a proprietary safety auditing system to measure their safety performance, and to identify aspects of their safety management where there is scope for improvement. A list of proprietary systems is given, for example, in the report from the Health and Safety Commission (1993) *Organising for Safety*. The audits typically comprise a checklist with about 500 questions, together with scoring system. The attraction of these audits is that companies can compare their safety management procedures against objective criteria. A disadvantage is that some companies might seek to improve their audit score in ways that do not, in fact, lead to real improvements in safety.

Safety training

Safety training provides the key to improved efforts in accident prevention. In the past too much training was of poor quality and of doubtful effectiveness. However, it is clear that safety training plays an essential part in the arrangements of companies with excellent safety records. In 1992, the Institution of Occupational Safety and Health published a safety training policy that emphasizes the need for:

1. Explicit training in organizations to promote and maintain a positive safety culture;
2. Training of senior managers to achieve competence in strategic safety management;
3. Training of managers and workpeople to achieve appropriate competence in hazard identification, risk assessment, and control;
4. Training of trainers for competence in safety training;
5. In-company evaluation of training effectiveness.

REFERENCES

Committee on Safety and Health at Work (Robens Committee). (1972). *Safety and Health at Work*. HMSO, London.

Department of Employment. (1992). *Health and Safety Statistics 1990–1991*. Employment Gazette Occasional Supplement No. 3, Vol. 100, No. 9. HMSO, London.

Hale, A.R. and Glendon, A.I. (1987). *Individual Behaviour in the Control of Danger*. Elsevier, Amsterdam.

Health and Safety Commission. (1993). *Third report: Organising for Safety. ACSNI Study Group on Human Factors*. HMSO, London 1993.

Health and Safety Executive. (1991). *Successful Health and Safety Management*. Health and Safety Series booklet HS(G) 65. HMSO, London.

Heinrich, H.W. (1969). *Industrial Accident Prevention*, 4th edn. McGraw Hill, New York.

International Nuclear Safety Advisory Group. (1991). *Safety Culture*. Safety Series No. 75-INSAG-4. International Atomic Energy Authority, Vienna.

Rasmussen, J., Duncan, K.D., and Leplat, J. (eds.) (1987). *New Technology and Human Error*. Wiley, New York.

Reason, J.T. (1990). *Human Error*. Cambridge University Press.

Zohar, D. (1980). Safety climate in industrial organisations: theoretical and applied implications. *Journal of Applied Psychology*, **65**, 96–102.

8.5.5 Environmental factors and disease

8.5.5(a) Heat

W. R. KEATINGE

Effects of heat on the body

In a hot environment thermal receptors in the skin initiate reflex vasodilatation and sweating through cholinergic sympathetic nerves. At a later stage, as the body temperature rises, deep receptors in the heat-loss centre in the preoptic region of the brain reinforce these responses. Vasodilatation is also directly produced by warming the blood vessels of the skin. Vasodilatation alone is able to dissipate resting metabolic heat production of the body as long as skin temperature is about 1°C or more below body core temperature. Conduction and convection in the air can keep skin temperature low enough to allow this in slowly moving air up to about 32°C, but in warmer air, or in cooler air during exercise, the heat produced can only be lost if sweat is formed and can evaporate to cool the skin. Sweat can be formed in larger amounts and with a lower salt content in heat-acclimatized than in unacclimatized people. If heat loss is insufficient, progressive rise in body temperature above 38°C leads to hyperventilation, to cerebral dysfunction involving irritability and confusion, and ultimately to cardiovascular collapse and cessation of sweating. As body temperature rises further, at about 41°C, heat denaturation of proteins causes damage to large cells of the cerebellum and cerebral cortex. Vascular endothelium, hepatic and renal cells, and striated muscle are then affected, and almost all cells of the body are killed if their temperature rises to 50°C for a few minutes. Surface burns represent heat necrosis of this kind from brief localized surface heating, but are not often associated with general overheating of the body core.

Heat stroke

Heat stroke describes the syndrome produced by over-heating of the body core. It can be produced in normal people by several hours of physical exercise in a hot, humid environment close to or above body temperature. Exercise in hot, dry air can cause heat stroke if sweating is limited, either by lack of acclimatization to heat, by the rare condition of congenital absence of sweat glands, by dehydration, or by a failure of sweating known as tropical anhydrosis which can follow prolonged exposure to hot climates. Tropical anhydrosis is usually preceded by the common tropical complaint of prickly heat, due to inflammation of sweat glands. After the inflammation subsides, the sweat glands may become functionless and form papules surmounted by vesicles. The face and axillae are not affected; sweating continues normally there. People with prickly heat recover rapidly, and people with tropical anhydrosis slowly, on return to cool surroundings but both conditions are liable to recur on subsequent prolonged exposure to heat.

In hot, humid air above body temperature heat stroke can develop even if sweating is normal, and in the absence of exercise. Many hours in a high temperature are normally required for a dangerous degree of over-heating, but in hyperbaric gas at high temperature uptake of heat by the body can be rapid, both at the body surface and from respiratory gas. Rapid deaths from heat stroke have accordingly occurred among divers in pressure chambers after the chamber temperature has risen as a result of difficulties with equipment.

Otherwise, heat stroke in sedentary people is usually associated with impairment of sweating and vasodilatation, either by drugs or disease. It is most commonly seen in psychiatric patients receiving drugs such as barbiturates or phenothiazines which depress reflex regulation of body temperature generally, or anticholinergic drugs which specifically suppress sweating and vasodilatation. General autonomic hypofunction due to diabetes is also a common cause of heat stroke in sedentary people. Old age without other obvious disability also seems to be associated with increased liability to heat stroke. A rare cause of a dangerous rise in body temperature is damage to the heat-loss centre in the preoptic region of the brain, usually by haemorrhage or encephalitis, or by a tumour or surgical interference with one. Shivering and vasoconstriction due to unrestrained action of the heat-gain centre in the hypothalamus can then cause a rapid and often fatal increase in body temperature even in temperate surroundings.

Diagnosis of heat stroke is generally easy, particularly in otherwise healthy people, from the history and the presence of irritability, confusion, headache, a hot, dry skin, and a deep body temperature (oral or rectal) close to or above 41°C. Blood pressure is normal in heat stroke until it falls in the terminal stage of cardiovascular collapse. There is initially respiratory alkalosis due to hyperventilation, often followed by metabolic acidosis due to accumulation of lactic acid as hepatic failure develops. Serum calcium may be low in severe cases due to calcium binding by proteins of damaged cells.

Treatment consists of immediate cooling. Mild cooling by sprinkling or sponging with tepid water which is allowed to evaporate on the skin, is often more effective than intense surface cooling by very cold water or refrigerated rubber blankets; mild cooling allows high blood flow in the skin to continue and to facilitate heat loss to the body surface. Rapidity of treatment is more important than the precise method used. In mild cases, recovery is generally rapid and complete, except in the ill or elderly when mortality is often due to other coexisting conditions. Patients with severe heat stroke may die suddenly, and if they recover may show lasting cerebellar or cerebral signs.

Postmortem examination may show little abnormality in cases of rapid death from heat stroke apart from degeneration of Purkinje cells and other large cells of the cerebellar and cerebral cortex. In less rapid deaths oedema and petechial haemorrhages, due to microvascular thrombosis occur in the brain, and sometimes in other tissues.

Water-depletion heat exhaustion

Severe cases result from deprivation of water in hot environments. They are often complicated by heat stroke. Unlike other forms of heat illness, water depletion can develop more rapidly in heat-acclimatized than in unacclimatized people because of their increased ability to sweat. The diagnosis is usually obvious from the history and from the presence of thirst, dehydration with sunken face and eyes, and elevated serum sodium and chloride. Haematocrit is normal since the water loss involves cell fluid and extracellular fluid proportionately. Death occurs when weight loss is 15 to 25 per cent of the body weight, and is due to excess concentration of salts in the body fluids. Contrary to some earlier views, present evidence indicates that shipwreck victims without fresh water cannot prolong survival by drinking seawater. Since seawater contains salts in higher concentration than can be excreted by the kidney, drinking of seawater accelerates death in victims of simple water depletion.

Treatment consists of giving up to 8 litres of water by mouth during the first 24 h, if the patient can swallow. In more severe cases, up to 5 litres of 5 per cent glucose should be given by intravenous drip.

Salt-depletion heat exhaustion

Salt depletion usually develops insidiously in people working in hot environments, particularly in unacclimatized people in whom loss of salt in sweat is relatively high. Sodium chloride intake of up to 20 g/day, in food and by salt tablets, may be needed to prevent it. The sodium chloride must be accompanied by an adequate intake of water and should not be given to people threatened by dehydration due to restricted supply of water.

Early cases show fatigue, weakness, headache, nausea, and sometimes vomiting. One characteristic symptom is the appearance of sudden, very painful muscle cramps (e.g. 'miner's cramp'), but these only develop if the salt depletion is associated with muscular exercise.

There are few physical signs in salt depletion apart from those of dehydration of the face and the skin generally, and often low blood pressure with marked postural hypotension. It is important to realize that serum sodium and chloride are normal in mild cases of salt deficiency since osmotic pressure is initially regulated at normal levels at the expense of falling blood volume. However, haematocrit is raised and so are plasma protein concentrations. Blood urea is often elevated. In severe cases, water is retained at the expense of osmotic pressure, and serum sodium and chloride fall. Treatment consists of giving 25 g sodium chloride in 5 litres of water by mouth, and then ensuring adequate daily salt intake. In severe cases, immediate intravenous infusion of 500 ml isotonic saline solution may be needed.

Gross examples of salt depletion are now rare, but it has been realized that minor degrees of it play an important role in heat exhaustion during exercise, and mortality among the elderly during hot weather (see Chapter 8.5.5(c)).

REFERENCES

Kew, M., Bersohn, I., Seftel, H. and Kent, G. (1970). Liver damage in heat stroke. *American Journal of Medicine*, **49**, 192–202.

Leithead, C.S. and Lind, A.R. (1964). *Heat stress and heat disorder*. Cassell, London.

McElroy, C. and Auerbach, P.S. (1983). Heat illness: current perspectives. In *Management of wilderness and environmental emergencies*, pp. 64–81. Macmillan, New York.

Oakley, E.H.N. (1987). Heat exhaustion. *Journal of World Accident, Emergency and Disaster Medicine*, **3**, 28–30.

Sprung, C.L., Portocarrero, C.J., Fernaine, A.V., and Weinberg, P.F. (1980). The metabolic and respiratory alterations of heat stroke. *Archives of Internal Medicine*, **140**, 665–9.

8.5.5(b) Drug-induced increases of body temperature

W. I. CRANSTON

Almost any drug can cause an otherwise unexplained pyrexia. There are several mechanisms which may explain this.

Some drugs can actually give rise to diseases, of which fever may be a presenting feature. Examples of this include antibiotic-induced colitis, drug-induced systemic lupus erythematosus, drug-related hepatitis, and infection consequent upon agranulocytosis which can be caused by numerous drugs.

Parenteral injection of drugs can sometimes cause fever by giving rise to local inflammatory changes. Intravenous injection of hypertonic solutions can do this, by causing local phlebitis. Fever commonly follows the injection of streptokinase. This particular reaction has been attributed to release of unspecified metabolites during thrombolysis; it is unlikely to result from contamination of the product by endotoxins as fever does not usually appear earlier than 12 h after such an injection, and the temperature response to intravenous endotoxin usually appears within 3 h.

Hypersensitivity has been quoted as the cause of many febrile reactions to drugs but frequently the evidence for this mechanism is not entirely convincing. However, this is probably the explanation for the fever seen in patients who have discontinued and then restarted rifampicin. Fever and eosinophilia have been observed following procainamide and methyldopa; in the latter case, abnormal liver function tests are not uncommon, and hepatitis may be the cause in many cases. Fever is often not due to the active agent itself but to other components of the product. The most common example of this is provided by vaccines, particularly those that contain antibiotics or egg protein to which the patient may be sensitive. Many vaccines contain endotoxin and cause fever because of inadvertent intravenous injection. They can also do so by production of a local inflammatory response.

Fever can follow antineoplastic treatment, particularly with bleomycin and asparaginase. These are derived from micro-organisms and endotoxin contamination may explain some of these instances. Injection of interferon commonly causes pyrexia, perhaps because the drug is obtained from leucocytes and the production of interferon may be accompanied by the release of leucocyte pyrogen.

There is a fairly convincing report of pyrexia following administration of misoprostol, in a patient with liver damage. As misoprostol has been reported to be beneficial in hepatorenal syndrome, this may become more common.

Although the nature of the neurotransmitters involved in the central nervous control of body temperatures remains uncertain, a number of drugs can cause fever in animals if introduced into the brain. These include monoamines, anticholinergics, arachidonic acid metabolites, and cimetidine. This kind of effect may explain the pyrexia produced in man by overdose of sympathomimetics, and monoamine oxidase inhibitors, with or without tricyclic antidepressants. Atropine overdosage also commonly causes pyrexia; this has been attributed to the prevention of sweating, but evidence for this is lacking.

In general, the management of drug-induced fever entails stopping the drug concerned, and usually the only treatment needed is mild skin cooling. Antipyretics are not required.

There are, however, two particularly dangerous forms of drug-induced fever, malignant hyperpyrexia and neuroleptic malignant syndrome.

Malignant hyperpyrexia

This is a dominantly inherited condition; though more than one gene may be involved in different families, it is probable that one resides on the long arm of chromosome 19, and may affect the ryanodine receptor. Skeletal muscle generates massive heat production in the presence of anaesthetic agents. Muscle contraction is caused by a postsynaptic effect, and muscle relaxants have no effect. The drugs most commonly incriminated are halothane and suxamethonium, although malignant hyperpyrexia has been reported with nitrous oxide and with epidural anaesthesia induced by lignocaine and bupivacaine. The condition still carries a high mortality and any suspicious family history should prompt further enquiry. An abnormal resting creatinine phosphokinase suggests the likelihood of this condition but a normal level does not exclude it. A similar condition can be provoked by poisoning with 'ecstasy', and it has also been reported after use of its analogue methylenedioxyamphetamine ('eve').

Usually, after induction of anaesthesia, muscle contraction develops and the skin becomes extremely hot; central temperature can rise by 1°C in a few minutes, and can rise to fatal levels. If it is suspected that the patient may be at risk, anaesthesia should be avoided if possible. If anaesthesia is essential, known inducing agents should be avoided. If time is available, premedication with oral dantrolene (5 mg/kg) should be given in the 24-h period before anaesthesia. This agent interferes with calcium efflux from the muscle cell and inhibits the contractile process. This drug has been shown to prevent anaesthetic-induced contraction of muscle biopsies from susceptible patients. Should unexpected malignant hyperpyrexia develop, the anaesthetic should be stopped, the patient ventilated and cooled, and intravenous dantrolene sodium given in a dose of 1 to 10 mg/kg. This drug is very alkaline and care must be taken not to allow it to extravasate. Metabolic acidosis is common and severe, and should be treated with sodium bicarbonate. Formal evidence of the effectiveness of sodium dantrolene in man is lacking for obvious ethical reasons.

Neuroleptic malignant syndrome

The other potentially lethal condition usually associated with hyperthermia is the neuroleptic malignant syndrome. The syndrome consists of hyperthermia, muscle rigidity, impaired consciousness, and tachycardia, and it appears to be an idiosyncratic reaction to therapeutic doses of phenothiazines, thioxanthine, and butyrophenones, all of which interfere with dopaminergic transmission in the central nervous system. The syndrome has been reported as beginning without fever, and it appears to affect 0.4 to 1.4 per cent of patients on neuroleptic drugs. Usually the syndrome develops early in a course of treatment or when the dose of drug is increased. Unlike malignant hyperpyrexia, it develops more insidiously over 1 to 3 days, and the recorded temperatures have not usually been as high as those in patients with malignant hyperpyrexia. There is a significant mortality of 15 to 25 per cent usually associated with respiratory failure or aspiration pneumonia. The increased muscle tone appears to be presynaptically excited: usually neuromuscular blocking agents will cause paralysis, and they can be used to treat neuroleptic malignant syndrome. Failure to realize this may have led to at least one fatality. During the illness, creatine phosphokinase levels are elevated and there is one report of elevated resting creatine phosphokinase in the asymptomatic children of a recovered patient.

The mechanism responsible for the condition is unknown but, if diagnosed, it should be treated in much the same way as malignant hyperpyrexia with attention to muscle relaxants, ventilation, and acidosis. Dantrolene has again been used in neuroleptic malignant syndrome. Generally, it has been reported as being of value, though there are cases where it was apparently ineffective. Because of the effect of these major tranquillizers on dopaminergic transmission, bromocriptine (a dopamine agonist) has been used to treat some patients but again the evidence of effectiveness is difficult to assess. Recovery generally takes several days until the tranquillizer responsible is cleared. Recovery is delayed further in patients who have received long-acting depot preparations such as fluphenazine. It is impossible to predict which patients are likely to develop this condition and prognosis depends upon its speedy identification. There are a number of anecdotal reports that, however improbably, ECT may be beneficial in neuroleptic malignant syndrome: it has even been employed with success in a woman with the syndrome who was 29 weeks pregnant.

REFERENCES

Granto, J.E., *et al.* (1983). Neuroleptic malignant syndrome: successful treatment with dantrolene and bromocriptine. *Annals of Neurology*, **14,** 89–90.

Kellam, A.M.P. (1987). The neuroleptic malignant syndrome, so-called. A survey of the world literature. *British Journal of Psychiatry*, **150,** 752–9.

Smego, R.A. and Durack, D.T. (1982). The neuroleptic malignant syndrome. *Archives of Internal Medicine*, **142,** 1183–5.

Velamoor, V.R., *et al.* (1994). Progression of symptoms in neuroleptic malignant syndrome. *Journal of Nervous and Mental Disease*, **182,** 168–73.

Verwiel, J.M., *et al.* (1994). Successful electroconvulsive therapy in a pregnant woman with neuroleptic malignant syndrome. *Nederlands Tijdschrift voor Geneeskunde*, **138,** 196–9.

8.5.5(c) Cold, drowning, and seasonal mortality

W. R. KEATINGE

Effects of cold on the body

Exposure to cold induces reflex vasoconstriction in the skin through noradrenergic sympathetic nerves, assisted by direct constrictor action of cold. This reduces body heat loss and also increases arterial pressure. If mean skin temperature falls below 33°C, reflex increases in muscle tone and shivering can increase heat production. The newborn infant does not shiver, but in a cold environment can increase heat production by metabolizing specialized brown fat, much of which is over the upper part of the back of the ribcage. This metabolism of brown fat is induced by noradrenergic sympathetic nerves which innervate the fat. Effects of acclimatization depend on the pattern of exposures to cold, but repeated brief exposures reduce vasoconstrictor and other responses to cold, leading to higher peripheral temperatures but greater loss of central body heat. These responses to cold enable most healthy and well-fed adults to maintain body temperature for many hours with skin temperatures as low as 12°C if the individual is fat, but only as low as 25 to 30°C if the individual is thin, and so has little internal insulation when vasoconstricted. Children are at a disadvantage because of a high surface area in relation to body mass. Most adults can maintain body temperature when lightly clothed in still air at about 5°C, but not in much colder air, or in less cold surroundings if external insulation is reduced by immersion in water or by wind and rain. Even fat people are liable to cool with skin temperatures below 12°C, since cold paralysis of the peripheral blood vessels then results in cold vasodilatation with rapid loss of heat, although exceptional individuals are resistant to this.

Hypothermia is usually defined by the presence of a deep body temperature, measured by reliable means, of less than 35°C. Reliable measurement of this may be made sublingually in air warmer than 24°C, in the external auditory meatus with servocontrolled external heating (zero gradient aural probe) in air warmer than 18°C, rectally in any environment if body temperature is reasonably stable, or oesophageally if the patient is not swallowing cold saliva. Rectal temperature is usually 0.2 to 0.5°C higher than the others, and lags behind them if deep body temperature is changing rapidly.

If the temperature of the heart and brain fall below 35°C, there is first listlessness and confusion, often with subsequent amnesia for events at the time of low body temperature. Consciousness is lost at a lower but variable temperature of 26 to 33°C. After an initial rise in cardiac output associated with shivering, cardiac output falls with slowed heart rate due to direct effects of cold on the cardiac muscle, and at a temperature of 17 to 26°C cardiac output becomes insufficient to supply even the reduced oxygen requirements of the cold tissues, so that death ultimately ensues unless the patient is rewarmed. Failure of haemoglobin to release normal amounts of oxygen, due to a shift of the dissociation curve to higher values of po_2, contributes to tissue anoxia. One consequence of impaired oxygenation of cardiac muscle is that atrial fibrillation may occur at temperatures of 28 to 35°C. Otherwise, slow cardiac activity can be maintained for a time by a normal or ectopic pacemaker at temperatures as low as 11°C. Respiration is depressed in hypothermia, but generally almost in proportion to metabolic needs, so that there is only slight respiratory acidosis. Accumulation of lactic acid from shivering in the early stages of cooling often produces some metabolic acidosis, but generally of mild degree unless very prolonged and severe hypothermia has resulted in anoxic liver damage. Glucose metabolism is depressed during hypothermia, and blood glucose and serum potassium rise as body temperature falls, and return to or below normal during recovery. Physiological cold diuresis at the start of exposure to cold ceases after a while, provided that deep body temperature remains near normal, but if hypothermia develops, inability of renal tubular cells to reabsorb sodium chloride and water at low temperature causes progressive loss of salt and water. Hypotension is therefore common when a victim of prolonged hypothermia is warmed and vasodilatation takes place. Gastric erosions and pancreatitis can occur in prolonged, severe hypothermia and may provide postmortem evidence of the cause of death.

Local cooling of the limbs can induce either non-freezing cold injury ('immersion injury' or 'trench foot'), or frostbite due to freezing of the tissues. Local cooling for many minutes below 12°C, without freezing, causes sensory and motor paralysis. This is due to block by low temperature of the sodium pump across cell membranes, with consequent net entry of sodium ions and ultimate inexcitability of nerve and muscle fibres. After short periods of cooling this recovers completely on warming, but after several hours at low temperatures nerve and muscle undergo lasting damage and subsequently degenerate when normal temperature and blood flow are restored.

Local cooling below − 0.54°C can freeze human tissues. This can happen in liquid sea-water, whose salt content depresses its freezing point to − 1.9°C. Unless the temperature is very low, only part of the tissue water freezes, leaving the remainder with an increased concentration of salts which denatures proteins. Endothelial cells of blood vessels are particularly vulnerable to such damage. When the tissue thaws the capillaries leak plasma and the red cells left behind may sludge, block the vessel, and then clot. Ischaemic necrosis produced in this way is responsible for most of the tissue damage in frostbite.

Prevention and management of hypothermia and cold injury

Immersion hypothermia

These cases usually result from shipwrecks. Most people of average fatness, without protection, develop a dangerous degree of hypothermia after several hours of immersion in water at 15 to 20°C. In colder water they may also suffer non-freezing immersion injury of the limbs and frostbite.

The most important measures are preventive. Body cooling during immersion and the risk of immersion injury can be reduced, and the risk of frostbite in the water virtually eliminated, by advising survivors who are abandoning ship to put on thick conventional clothing, including gloves and footwear. Body cooling in the water can also, surprisingly, be reduced by advising survivors to float still in lifejackets rather than exercising; exercise in cold water generally increases heat loss more than heat production. Wet suits of foam rubber, or waterproof suits, of course, provide excellent protection if they are available.

After an immersion victim is rescued, the immediate treatment is crucial, and some assessment must be made whether the patient is hypothermic, drowned, or both. This may be obvious from the circumstances or history, but in rough water mixed conditions are common. An immediate measure of body temperature is always useful. Rectal temperature by a low-reading thermometer is the most reliable method, though it must be remembered that it can lag 1 to 2°C behind cardiac temperature when body temperature is falling very rapidly.

People who have a body core temperature below about 31°C at the time of rescue, and who have not inhaled water, are liable to die suddenly during or shortly after rescue. The probable reason is ventricular fibrillation precipitated by catecholamine drive to the heart during exertion or postural hypotension. People should therefore if possible be rescued from cold water in the horizontal position, and with minimum exertion by the victim.

After rescue, the main principle of treatment in this and any other type of hypothermia is to prevent further heat loss by insulation until the patients can be moved into warm surroundings; to keep them recumbent; and to refrain from any other action such as unnecessary laryngeal intubation or external cardiac massage or intravenous adrenaline that can precipitate ventricular fibrillation. An immediate hot bath (not above 42°C) provides the quickest method of rewarming, but is seldom available within 30 min of rescue. After that time victims of immersion hypothermia who are still alive almost invariably recover if left recumbent in warm surroundings with mild heat input such as that from hot water bottles at 42°C. If ventricular fibrillation or cardiac arrest do occur, the patient should be taken straight to hospital where extracorporeal circulation, preferably by femoral bypass, gives the best chance of recovery.

After initial measures are taken, admission to hospital is always desirable if water is thought to have been inhaled, for chest radiograph and for possible intermittent positive pressure ventilation if late pulmonary oedema develops. Atrial fibrillation and ventricular ectopic beats, if present, usually cease as temperature rises and do not require treatment. Antifibrillatory agents should generally be avoided as they are liable to produce arrest or even induce fibrillation in deep hypothermia. Blood glucose, pH, and serum potassium may be measured, once a good flow of blood is restored to the limbs so that a venous sample can give meaningful information. However, attempts to correct apparent abnormalities of pH and potassium are rarely needed and should not be made unless the abnormalities are large and the patient is in poor general condition in spite of rising body temperature. They should never be made unless the validity of the blood sample itself, and of the assay and any temperature corrections made to it, are known without doubt to be dependable.

Immersion injury (non-freezing cold injury)

The limbs of people rescued from water below 12°C are initially often anaesthetic and paralysed. If the cooling lasts many hours they will, on warming, develop signs of immersion injury, becoming bright red, hot, oedematous, and painful. They should then be elevated to reduce oedema and analgesics given for the pain. During the next few weeks, muscle and nerve may degenerate, and physiotherapy is needed to prevent contractures. Partial denervation of blood vessels due to degeneration of their motor nerves often leads to vascular instability with excessive vasoconstriction in the cold and dilation in the heat. Some improvement in the disabilities is usual over the course of months as nerves regenerate, but disability may be permanent.

Table 1 *Hypoglycaemia and hypothermia induced by ethanol after exercise. All groups had taken 28 ml ethanol by mouth and then sat in air at 14 to 22°C for 80 min. Some had also taken approximately 60 g of glucose, and some had previously exercised for approximately 2 h, as indicated (means ± SE, seven experiments)*

	Exercise, no glucose	No exercise, no glucose	Exercise, glucose
Blood glucose (mmol/l)	1.77 ± 0.20	2.82 ± 0.17	4.96 ± 0.61
Rectal temperature (°C)	34.49 ± 0.34	36.82 ± 0.14	36.94 ± 0.14
Metabolic rate (kcal/m^2.h)	45.00 ± 2.90	76.10 ± 7.70	91.00 ± 10.40
Blood ethanol (mmol/l)	5.11 ± 0.29	5.12 ± 0.18	5.80 ± 0.74

Reproduced from Haight, J.S.J. and Keatinge, W.R. (1973). *Journal of Physiology*, **229,** 87–97, with permission.

Exposure without severe frostbite

Hillwalkers, climbers, and skiers who are inadequately clothed in air colder than 0°C are liable to both hypothermia and frostbite, and in air above 0°C to hypothermia alone. These conditions generally develop after people become lost, or immobilized by bad weather or injury, and have to spend one or more nights without shelter. However, hypothermia can develop during even mild exposure to cold if people take ethanol after exercise and without food, as inexperienced hillwalkers sometimes do. Two hours of exercise depletes the body's reserve of carbohydrate, and metabolism of ethanol leads to reduction of the pyruvate needed for gluconeogenesis, so that less than 30 ml of ethanol can then produce hypoglycaemia. This not only causes mental confusion but virtually eliminates the normal reflex vasoconstrictor and metabolic responses to cold, so that body temperature can fall to 33°C in as little as 80 min in slowly moving air at 20 to 22°C. Hypothermia due to ethanol hypoglycaemia should be considered when people who have taken insufficient ethanol to cause drunkenness are found confused, unconscious, or dead after relatively mild exposure to cold (Table 1).

Apathy and confusion on hillwalks can be produced by exhaustion as well as by hypothermia. A sublingual temperature measurement may exclude hypothermia if a low-reading thermometer is carried by the party, though false low readings can occur when the face is cold. If the reading is low, rectal temperature should therefore be measured. In cold air body temperature has usually fallen slowly and so is relatively stable at the time of rescue. Provided that there is no serious injury or frostbite, recovery is almost invariable if the victim is placed recumbent in a well-insulated sleeping bag until transport to warm surroundings. It is helpful in very cold air to control respiratory heat loss by a simple heat exchanger or heater. Since loss of plasma volume can be substantial during prolonged exposure, rapid rewarming can be dangerous. Even slow rewarming often lowers arterial pressure considerably. This can usually be controlled with recumbent posture and raising the legs, but 500 ml of saline or dextran intravenously is helpful. Depletion of body carbohydrate by prior exercise is common. Sugary drinks should be given, once body temperature is above 31°C and glucose can be metabolized.

Frostbite, if present, is obvious as hard, white areas of skin on the extremities. As long as it involves only parts of the fingers, toes, hands, or feet, it is best treated by sudden thawing in water no hotter than the observer can stand without discomfort. This allows optimal tissue recovery, probably because bloodflow returning is so rapid that it passes through damaged capillaries too rapidly to lose its plasma and block the vessels with sludged red cells. Subsequently, analgesics should be given for pain and the part elevated to reduce oedema. The skin may subsequently turn black, but then often sloughs off to leave almost normal tissue beneath. Surgery should be considered only after the necrotic region is fully delineated.

Exposure with massive frostbite

Exposure in very cold climates can result in massive freezing of most of the tissue of the limbs, together with general hypothermia. People in this condition sometimes survive slow rewarming in warm air without early medical help, but the best results seem to have been obtained by transporting them at once to hospital and rewarming them there at moderate speed under full biochemical control. Such people have extensive tissue damage from freezing, so that rapid thawing leads to massive release of potassium into the circulation, and to ventricular fibrillation. Haemodialysis, and extracorporeal circulation in cases of persistent ventricular fibrillation, may be needed for recovery.

Urban hypothermia

Causes

Urban hypothermia is a convenient term for hypothermia that develops in a patient's own home or elsewhere in built-up areas. In contrast to hypothermia at sea or on the hills, it is largely a condition of elderly people, and seldom due to cold stress alone. Despite popular perception that urban hypothermia kills tens of thousands of elderly people in Britain annually, death certificates show less than 200 deaths per year from hypothermia of all kinds, representing less than 1 per cent of total excess winter mortality. Surveys in east London showed first that this was not due to failure to diagnose hypothermia on admission to hospital, and secondly that when hypothermia was present it was almost always secondary to disease, alcohol, drugs, or injury. The most common cause was collapse, usually from cardiovascular or respiratory disease, while alone at home. Half of those who then became hypothermic, while lying helpless on the floor, were in heated rooms; 86 per cent of the rest had heating available but switched off, usually for the night. Alcohol was usually a factor in the smaller number of hypothermic patients found outdoors, many of whom had wandered away from a home, or lacked a fixed home. The relative importance of these factors varies, but reports of hypothermia from a wide range of countries show a high incidence of disease and alcohol, with alcohol the dominant factor in urban hypothermia in the United States.

Collapse and immobility due to these conditions can themselves produce hypothermia. In addition, hypoxia or ischaemic tissue, infection, hypoglycaemia due to alcohol or insulin, or malnutrition, can all impair metabolic and vasoconstrictor responses to cold. Hypothyroidism specifically reduces metabolic rate and α-adrenergic blocking drugs reduce vasoconstriction. Any central nervous depressant drug in high dosage can impair central thermoregulation, though they are not in practice a common cause of hypothermia. The fact that diseases causing collapse and hypothermia are much commoner in old age explains why elderly people are the main victims of urban hypothermia. Age itself may also impair thermoregulation though it is still controversial whether it does so significantly in the absence of malnutrition or disease.

Hypothermia in the absence of disease or alcohol, though rare, is important to recognize. People who die in this way can be mistaken for victims of violence, as confusion and loss of sensation of cold due to hypothermia sometimes cause the patients to shed clothing, damage furniture, and fall and injure themselves.

REFERENCES

Golden, F.St.C. and Rivers, J.F. (1975). Thoughts on immediate care: the immersion incident. *Anaesthesia*, **30,** 364–73.

Haight, J.S.J. and Keatinge, W.R. (1973). Failure of thermoregulation in the cold during hypoglycaemia induced by exercise and ethanol. *Journal of Physiology*, **229,** 87–97.

Maclean, D. and Emslie-Smith, D. (1977). *Accidental hypothermia*. Blackwell Scientific Publications, Oxford.

Seasonal mortality

In all except equatorial countries, mortality increases strikingly in winter. Heat waves can also increase mortality during the summer months in most countries, but overall cold-related mortality in winter greatly exceeds heat-related mortality in summer. This excess winter mortality is in fact generally greater in countries with mild winters such as Britain, Greece, and Italy than in countries such as Finland and Sweden where need for protection against cold in winter is more obvious.

Winter mortality

The number of cold-related excess deaths, taking minimum mortality in July as a baseline, is currently about 60 000 in England and Wales. Less than 1 per cent of these are due to hypothermia. About half of them are due to coronary and cerebral thrombosis, and about half of the rest to respiratory disease. The great majority occur in elderly people.

The deaths from coronary and cerebral thrombosis can be explained largely by haemoconcentration that occurs as part of the normal response to brief exposures to cold. Cold exposure just sufficient to cause shivering induces marked increases in red cell count, platelet count, plasma cholesterol, and blood viscosity before any important fall in body core temperature. Plasma fibrinogen also increases, without increase in the natural anticoagulant protein C whose low molecular size probably allows it to redistribute to the interstitial space. All of these changes increase the probability of arterial thrombosis in elderly people whose atheromatous arteries make them liable to thrombosis. Mortality statistics show that the peak in coronary deaths occurs about 1 day, and that in cerebral thrombosis deaths 3 days, after a cold day. The peak in respiratory deaths follows 2 to 3 weeks after a cold spell and may be due to reduced resistance to infection during persistent exposure to cold.

In accordance with this, in 20 years from 1964, in which central heating increased from 13 to 69 per cent of homes, excess deaths in winter from respiratory disease declined markedly, but deaths from coronary and cerebral thrombosis did not. The excess thrombotic deaths appear to be due largely to relatively brief outdoor excursions in the cold, including waits for public transport.

Deaths in heat waves

Only a small number of heat-related deaths are induced by immediate and direct effects of thermal stress, heat stroke, or dehydration. However, mortality statistics during heat waves show a large increase in deaths during heat waves. Unlike cold-related deaths, increased mortality in brief mild warm spells is often followed by compensating falls in mortality, suggesting that it occurs in people who are in any case close to death from other causes.

Heat waves associated with daily minima of environmental temperature above 17 to 20°C cause more important increases in mortality, particularly from coronary and cerebral thrombosis. These are not compensated by subsequent falls in mortality in the next few days. Experimental studies on volunteers suggest that haemoconcentration is again an important factor. In this case, haemoconcentration is caused by loss of salt in sweat. With water freely available, only enough water is drunk initially to restore normal osmotic pressure of the blood, so that the plasma volume declines. Consequently red cell and platelet counts, blood viscosity, and plasma cholesterol all increase and promote arterial thrombosis in elderly people with atheromatous arteries. Preventive measures are straightforward. In temperate countries such as Britain, light clothing, an open window, a fan, and if necessary sprinkling of water on clothing with the fan to provide air movement are almost always sufficient to prevent significant heat stress in vulnerable people. In hotter and humid climates air conditioning can give more sustained protection. Unacclimatized people are at particular risk, and elderly people from temperate regions should be advised not to go on holiday in hot countries if heat stress is likely to be unavoidable there.

REFERENCES

Bull, G.M. and Morton, J. (1978). Environment, temperature and death rates. *Age and Ageing*, **7,** 210–24.

Keatinge, W.R., Coleshaw, S.R.K., Easton, J.C., Cotter, F., Mattock, M.B., and Chelliah, R. (1986). Increased platelet and red cell counts, blood viscosity and plasma cholesterol during heat stress, and mortality from coronary and cerebral thrombosis. *American Journal of Medicine*, **81,** 795–800.

Keatinge, W.R., Coleshaw, S.R.K., Holmes, J., and Evans, S. (1989). Changes in seasonal mortality with improvement in home heating in England and Wales 1964–1984. *International Journal of Biometeorology*, **33,** 71–6.

Neild, P.J., Syndercombe-Court, D., Keatinge, W.R., Donaldson, G.C., Mattock, M., and Caunce, M. (1994). Cold-induced increases in erythrocyte count, plasma cholesterol and plasma fibrinogen of elderly people without comparable rise in protein C or factor X. *Clinical Science*, **86,** 43–8.

8.5.5(d) Diseases of high terrestrial altitudes

D. RENNIE

High altitude terrain and populations

Until the late 19th century, mountains were viewed by Europeans as dangerous, mysterious, hostile, and remote. Yet there is evidence that mountainous regions have, for many thousands of years, been the home of large and elaborate civilizations such as that of the Incas, which in the 15th century included Ecuador to the north and much of northern Chile and Argentina some 5000 km to the south, an empire of at least 12 million people. The Altiplano or high plateau of the Andes is still home to millions of descendants of these Incas, many of whom have never been below altitudes around 4000 m above sea level.

Temperature tends to determine the fauna and flora. Since, other things being equal, temperature falls with increasing altitude, the high altitude climate tends to be an arctic one. The snow line and tree line become lower with increasing distance from the equator and to live, work, hunt, and cultivate at altitudes above 3000 m is possible only within about 40° of the equator. This includes the Andes of Ecuador, Bolivia, Peru, and northern Chile, the Rocky Mountains in the United States, the high lands of east Africa, the Caucasus, the Pamirs, and the Himalayas, but does not include, for example, the European Alps.

The fall in temperature of some 1°C for every 150 m rise in altitude, irrespective of latitude, and the high winds increase the danger of cold injury. The low humidity contributes greatly to fluid loss and dehydration, as does the increased solar radiation which may be very much exaggerated by reflection from the snow. These factors are, however, common to most arctic environments and are discussed elsewhere.

The fact that so many people of diverse races have been born and have lived at such altitudes, and the fact that, excluding Antarctica, about 2.5 per cent of the land lies above 3000 m, gives high altitude physiology and medicine an economic, political, and cultural relevance. As modern transport brings the highest mountains within range of the meanest purse, tourists, hikers, mountaineers, and downhill and cross-country skiers, as well as mining engineers, geologists, and surveyors, are flocking up into the hills. Every day in July and August about 3600 people visit the summit of Pike's Peak in Colorado (4300 m) and there is now even a 42-km marathon race up and down that mountain. In 1950, three expert Western climbers first reached the base of the ice fall below Mount Everest's Western Cwm, at 5300 m. Twenty-five years later, in a mere 4 weeks, well over 500 inexpert tourists did so.

The vast majority of mankind lives below 1000 m altitude and, though there is this exponential rise in the numbers of lowlanders going to high altitude, they cannot assume that they can make the ascent with impunity.

Hypoxia

Though the proportion of oxygen in the air (20.93 per cent) is the same at every altitude, the atmospheric pressure, as was shown by Blaise Pascal on the Puy de Dome in his 'Great Experiment' of 1648, decreases with increasing altitude.

$$\text{Barometric pressure} = 760.e^{\frac{-\,\text{altitude}\,(m)}{7924}}.$$

The total atmospheric pressure at sea level (barometric pressure, P_B varies but is usually around 760 torr (mmHg) (101 kPa) and that due to oxygen (the partial pressure of oxygen) is 20.93 per cent of this, i.e. 159 torr (21.2 kPa). In the lung, the air is rapidly saturated with water vapour at body temperature. At any altitude this is 47 torr (6.25 kPa) at 37°C. The actual combined pressures of gas taken into the lungs is therefore $P_B - 47$) torr and the inspired oxygen tension (P_{IO_2}) is 20.93 per cent of this: $0.2093 \times (P_B - 47)$. At sea level this is $0.2093 \times (760 - 47) = 149$ torr (19.8 kPa). At about 5500 m the atmospheric pressure is about half that at sea level and at the summit of Everest (8848 m), allowing for the fact that the earth's atmosphere is an oblate spheroid—flattened at the poles—the atmospheric pressure is about 250 torr (33 kPa; one third that at sea level) and the partial pressure of oxygen is $0.2093 \times 250 = 52.3$ torr (7 kPa). The partial pressure of water, however, reduces the P_{IO_2} from 52.5 torr to $0.2093 \times (250 - 47) = 42.5$ torr (5.7 kPa). It is clear that the fraction of total inspired gas pressure due to water vapour, which at sea level is 6 per cent, increases with altitude. At the summit of Everest it will be nearly 19 per cent and at 19 200 m (63 000 feet), the total pressure of inspired gases would be a fatal 47 torr—fatal because all of it would be water vapour. Conversely, the proportion of inspired gas due to oxygen, which is 19.6 per cent at sea level, is reduced to 17 per cent at the summit of Everest and is, of course, zero at 19 200 m.

Following a plane's sudden decompression or a rapid balloon ascent, for example, a resting man, just up from sea level, would lose consciousness in a matter of minutes at altitudes between 6400 m and 7300 m (P_{AO_2} = 24–15 torr; 3.2–2 kPa) and in seconds above 7300 m (P_{AO_2} below 15 torr; 2 kPa), yet during 1 year (1978–9) a total of 14 men, on the three highest peaks in the world (Everest, K2, and Kanchenjunga) were not only fully conscious at rest more than 1000 m higher than this but were able to climb over difficult terrain in bad weather to their respective summits (8848 m, 8611 m, and 8598 m) all without the benefit of supplemental oxygen.

Acclimatization

These are obviously extreme examples, but anyone who has driven by car in a few hours from the coast up to mining towns of the Peruvian Andes at between 4000 and 4900 m, is immediately struck by the contrast between their own discomfort and helplessness and the energy with which the locals, after a hard shift in the mines, set about playing soccer. The difference consists of a myriad of physiological adjustments which collectively we call 'acclimatization'. As far as we can tell, it depends solely upon the length of exposure and the age when first exposed and has little if anything to do with genetic factors. It is not, therefore, an adaptation in the Darwinian sense and the physiologist has yet to demonstrate any discrete long-term adjustment that cannot be made by, say, Caucasians born at high altitude.

The processes of acclimatization, which affect every system in the body, proceed at different speeds but though changes may continue for many years thereafter, the time of greatest adjustment is in the hours and days after arrival at a higher altitude. During this early process, when the most marked changes are occurring, the newcomer to high altitude is not only comparatively weak and ineffectual but may suffer the signs and symptoms of acute mountain sickness, a disease which may itself be caused by the rapid physiological responses to the new and oxygen-deficient environment.

There are huge numbers of people who have ascended to high altitudes and, having had a measurable deficit in performance on arrival, but no signs or symptoms, have gradually acclimatized until their performance is identical with that of natives. The presence of acute mountain sickness, therefore, indicates that the early and most dramatic adjustments are not merely incomplete but distorted or deranged.

The changes that occur within the body, in response to hypoxia, affect every tissue and it is inappropriate to detail them here: there are excellent reviews of this subject at the end of this chapter. In general they may be briefly summarized as a series of adjustments which boost oxygen supply to the mitochondria by keeping the partial pressure of oxygen in the tissue capillaries as high as possible, by decreasing the distance oxygen has to diffuse in the tissues, and by increasing the concentrations of respiratory enzymes.

A few of the principal steps involved may be summarized thus:

Ventilation

When P_{AO_2} has fallen to 55 to 60 torr (7.3–7.9 kPa) at an altitude of about 2000 to 3000 m, the peripheral chemoreceptors are stimulated by hypoxia and ventilation is increased. This initial reaction is amplified over the next 3 or 4 days so that P_{AO_2} levels which are only very slightly lower than normal (as one would find, at, say, 1000 m altitude) now begin to stimulate ventilation. After a few weeks of sojourn, however, ventilation slowly decreases and this process continues for years, though ventilation is always higher in sojourners than in people who were born and have lived all their lives at altitude. With exercise, ventilation increases more at high altitude than at sea level and more in sojourners than in natives.

Driving respiration by hypoxia implies, from the point of view of carbon dioxide (CO_2), 'hyperventilation', since CO_2 is blown off, and a respiratory alkalosis develops. The P_{CO_2} falls in a linear manner with altitude, and the alkalosis is only partly compensated by a rise in urinary excretion of bicarbonate. The effect of this hypocarbia and alkalosis would normally be to inhibit respiration, as well as, for example, to diminish cerebral blood flow, but a heightened sensitivity of the respiratory centre to CO_2 tends to counteract this. The exact mechanisms by which changes in brain-stem extracellular [H^+] are produced during early and late exposure to high altitude and how they affect respiration are at present a matter of vigorous controversy.

The effect of the increased ventilation is rapidly to increase the alveolar oxygen pressure by reducing the oxygen gradient between ambient and alveolar air and by reducing P_{ACO_2}.

Pulmonary diffusion

Though no increase in pulmonary diffusing capacity occurs in sojourners at high altitude, natives have increased pulmonary diffusing capacity with a lowered alveolar–arterial oxygen gradient, associated with an increased capillary surface for diffusion. This is due to an opening up of pulmonary capillaries, and to polycythaemia which decreases the distance necessary for gaseous diffusion. There is no increase in pulmonary blood flow so the increase in lung capillary volume is equivalent to allowing the blood longer for gaseous equilibration.

In the newcomer to high altitude, exercise is accompanied by a marked fall in arterial oxygen saturation, in contrast to the unchanged values on exercise at sea level and this may be partly due to a limitation in diffusion. Pulmonary blood flow is unchanged and though ventilation increases in the newcomer at high altitude, there still seems to be an odd mismatch between ventilation and perfusion, possibly due to increased lung water or obstruction to some of the airways by oedema.

Circulation

Though there is an abrupt increase in cardiac output on ascent to high altitude, there follows a progressive decrease in stroke volume and maximal cardiac output is reduced at all levels of exercise including maximal exercise. There is no evidence for insufficient myocardial oxygenation and there is argument about whether or not the myocardium is actually depressed by the hypoxia. There is an immediate alteration in the distribution of blood flow. For example, coronary and cutaneous flow both fall, cerebral and retinal flow increase, renal flow temporarily decreases, and then, with acclimatization, returns to normal.

The oxygen-carrying ability of the blood is considerably increased by the massive increase in red cell production, in total red cell mass and, more importantly, in tissue capillarity. It is somewhat offset by the higher haematocrit which increases the blood viscosity and decreases the rate of flow. The shift in the oxy-haemoglobin dissociation curve to the right, which occurs on ascent and is due to an increase in red cell 2,3-diphosphoglycerate, favours unloading of oxygen to the tissues, but this particular adjustment is not now thought to be of much practical importance and is offset by the shift to the left caused by alkalosis.

Tissue adaptations

Apart from the very major role of increased tissue capillarity which reduces the average capillary-mitochondrial distance and so dramatically reduces the distance for diffusion, increased myoglobin facilitates oxygen diffusion and there is an increase both in mitochondrial density and in many enzymes of the respiratory pathway (e.g. in cytochrome oxidase).

Many alterations in the body that follow ascent are quite unexplained and it may be that these changes are not coping mechanisms at all but direct and deleterious results of the effect of hypoxia—or of other alterations such as alkalosis—upon the body. As a trivial example, one may quote the minimal increase in urine protein excretion of high altitudes, and, more importantly, the shifts of fluid from the extracellular to the intracellular compartments, or the failure of coronary artery blood flow to increase following ascent.

Oxygen uptake

Though the oxygen uptake at rest is not diminished even at very high altitudes, above an altitude of 1500 m the maximal oxygen uptake $\dot{V}O_2max$ falls about 10 per cent for each gain in altitude of 1000 m between 1500 and 6700 m and though it is improved by administration of pure oxygen, it does not return to normal until several days after descent. The cause of this drop in $\dot{V}O_2max$ has been debated. If, at any one altitude, the work load is increased, VO_2 may reach a maximum but ventilation, already increased at high altitude, is still able to increase further and so does not seem to be the factor limiting $\dot{V}O_2max$.

At altitude, as opposed to at sea level, arterial oxygen saturation falls with increasing exertion, but, at moderate altitudes, rises again near maximal exertion. There is probably no increase in alveolar–arterial oxygen gradient and because of the rise in haemoglobin, the amount of oxygen carried is kept up. Diffusion may be a little limited—this is controversial—but diffusion and the blood's oxygen carrying capacity are probably not factors limiting $\dot{V}O_2max$ either. After a few days at high altitude, however, maximal heart rate and particularly maximal cardiac stroke volume are reduced, the cause (a defect in myocardial contractility, for example) being unclear, and so the inability of the heart to go on increasing cardiac output seems to be the reason for the fact that $\dot{V}O_2max$ declines progressively with increases in altitude.

Extreme altitudes

Only serious climbers venture above altitudes of around 5800 m, where the atmospheric pressure is well below half that at sea level, but elaborate physiological measurements have been made at altitudes of 7500 m (P_B = 300 torr; 40 kPa).

At these extreme values, where every increment in height results in a precipitous fall in $\dot{V}O_2max$, the oxygen cost of the work of ventilation rises considerably and it assumes an even greater proportion of total oxygen cost when $\dot{V}O_2max$ is reduced to really low levels. Moreover, the maximal ventilation itself is reduced at such altitudes and in addition, there undoubtedly is a diffusion defect within the lungs which becomes very marked on exercise. This, together with the steady decline in maximal cardiac output causes maximal oxygen uptake to fall very precipitously when P_B is below 300 torr, reaching, at around 8000 m altitude, resting or basal levels of oxygen uptake, a figure of about 350 m/kg per min. The state of a climber at 8000 m who is comfortable resting in his tent but whose $\dot{V}O_2max$ is reached when he puts on his boots, for example, is interesting physiologically but is also, practically speaking, perilous.

Dr John West and his colleagues on the 1981 American Research Expedition to Everest, took alveolar gas samples from Dr Chris Pizzo on the summit (8848 m; barometric pressure 253 torr, 33.4 kPa). They report the following values: inspired PO_2 = 43 torr (5.68 kPa), and alveolar PO_2 = 35 torr (4.62 kPa). Estimated arterial gas values were: PO_2 = 28 torr (3.7 kPa); PCO_2 = 7.5 (0.99 kPa); pH = >7.7, oxygen saturation = 70 per cent. As West and others have noted, it is an extraordinary coincidence that the highest point on earth is the point where the best acclimatized and fittest athletes reach their physiological limit and find their $\dot{V}O_2max$ levels reduced to levels necessary to sustain life at rest. The atmospheric pressure in midsummer is about 11.5 torr (1.52 kPa) higher than in midwinter: a variation which could itself defeat a winter attempt without oxygen. A number of reports have suggested mild, possibly permanent defects in cognition in climbers who have ascended to extreme high altitudes.

Illness due to altitude

Acute mountain sickness

For centuries it has been known that when lowland dwellers climb mountains, some of them become ill. The illness, usually called acute mountain sickness, generally begins after a few hours, and is characterized by non-specific symptoms such as headache and vomiting. In the vast majority of people it is transient and trivial but in a few becomes progressive, severe, and may be fatal. It is to some extent relieved by breathing oxygen and it is cured by descent to sea level. Its cause is unknown.

Acute mountain sickness itself may be a miserable condition, but it is of concern to the physician practising in mountainous areas only because it may progress to one or both of two very serious conditions, high altitude pulmonary oedema and high altitude cerebral oedema, which are part of the syndrome of acute mountain sickness but which are often discussed separately from it. Reasons for classifying them together include the fact that pulmonary oedema never occurs without symptoms and signs of acute mountain sickness; that cerebral oedema seems clinically to be an exaggeration of acute mountain sickness; that they may coexist, and that all have the same predisposing and relieving factors: in particular, they only occur at high altitudes or in low pressure chambers, and they are relieved by descent.

SYMPTOMS AND SIGNS

Symptoms usually begin 24 to 48 h after ascent to a higher altitude, but sometimes begin in as little as 8 h or as many as 96 h. On arrival, the sufferer may have been aware of a curiously disordered breathing and some light headedness but frequently feels well and even euphoric. Within the passage of a few hours, an unaccustomed lethargy is experienced but sleep is fitful, disturbed by dreams, little bouts of breathlessness, and frequent arousals. On waking, the sufferer has a headache, often severe and occipital, which tends to diminish a little with activity but which may be unaffected by aspirin and codeine. He may vomit quite suddenly and nausea compounds his anorexia. Trying to keep up on his feet and active is made harder by dizziness and he may even lose his balance and fall. While the others organize the camp, he lies groaning in his sleeping bag, refusing food and dozing but the increasing periodicity of his respirations leads to frequent arousals and complaints of insomnia. After a day or two of rest, the symptoms disappear and are soon forgotten yet they may recur on further ascent to a greater altitude.

The signs are few: an irritable, depressed, but usually fit person, often, because he is starved, smelling of ketones and vomit, and holding his aching head. The most useful diagnostic sign is ataxia, best demonstrated by getting the patient to walk heel-toe (remembering that this may be awkward in boots and on snow) and then to turn around rapidly without staggering. Occasionally the patient, if he has been vomiting a great deal and especially if he has been taking diuretics, may be too dehydrated and hypotensive to stand up. At this stage crackles may be heard in more than a quarter of people examained.

In a few, the symptoms rapidly worsen with the onset of pulmonary oedema. Soon the breathlessness, even at rest, is extreme and may be accompanied by a dry cough. The patient, anxious and sometimes incoherent, becomes progressively more dyspnoeic and sometimes orthopnoeic. He is very cyanosed, though this is hard to judge in tents of differing colours. He may have a mild pyrexia (38.3°C). There is a pronounced tachycardia and sometimes mild hypotension. There are no signs of cardiac failure, but loud crackles can easily be heard all over the chest and frothy sputum, sometimes tinged with blood, wells out of the mouth and nose. At this point the patient, like anyone with severe acute pulmonary oedema, of whatever cause, is near death.

Pulmonary oedema, if very severe, tends to be accompanied by high altitude cerebral oedema but each syndrome may occur independently as features of acute mountain sickness. In cerebral oedema without pulmonary manifestations, the patient, having had progressively worsening symptoms of acute mountain sickness for 3 or 4 days (the range seems to vary from one day to as many as 21 days) becomes incoherent, hallucinated, and too ataxic and drowsy to stand up or look after himself. He may be unable to get out of his tent, or he may do so and then fall into a snow drift and lie there. Soon he is stuporose and snoring stertorously. His sleeping bag may be wet with urine and in a few hours he is in deepening coma. There are rarely any localizing signs—merely a generalized flaccid paralysis and pupillary reactions depending upon the depth of coma, though mild bilateral papilloedema is characteristic. In addition the bladder may be palpable.

PREDISPOSING FACTORS

Though males and females are equally likely to develop the acute mountain sickness syndrome, there are a number of factors which broadly predispose to acute mountain sickness (including pulmonary oedema and cerebral oedema), though it is important to remember the large differences in susceptibility between individuals.

1. Age. The incidence and severity of acute mountain sickness are inversely related to age and there is some evidence that young children are particularly susceptible to pulmonary oedema.
2. Previous acute mountain sickness. Most investigators have the strong impression that acute mountain sickness and in particular pulmonary oedema, are more common in those who have in the past suffered badly from these conditions.
3. Re-ascent. Workers in Colorado and Peru have both produced evidence that healthy high altitude dwellers are at unusually high risk from high altitude pulmonary oedema after brief descent to lower altitudes followed by re-ascent. Once again we lack the large epidemiological surveys necessary to test the truth of this assertion.
4. Speed of ascent. Whether on foot, or horseback, by train, or by air, the faster the ascent, the more likely and the worse the acute mountain sickness. In particular, the more nights spent on acclimatizing *en route*, the less the acute mountain sickness. There is good evidence for the wisdom of the climber's maxim: 'Climb high, sleep low.'
5. Altitude. The incidence and severity of acute mountain sickness following a 2000 m ascent to 5000 m from 3000 m are both much greater than from, say, 1000 m to 3000 m in the same amount of time.
6. Exertion. Independent of speed of ascent, severe exertion involved in the ascent (coping with snow; carrying loads) predisposes to acute mountain sickness.
7. Physiological functions measured at sea level. There is no good evidence that the incidence of acute mountain sickness relates to prior physical fitness as expressed by, say, maximal oxygen consumption, and much anecdotal evidence from many experienced observers that there is no such relationship. We know now, however, that statistically-speaking, the higher the vital capacity, the less the chance of acute mountain sickness and there is increasing evidence that susceptibility to acute mountain sickness is correlated with a poor ventilatory response to hypoxia, measured at sea level. Many other physiological functions have been measured at sea level but none usefully predict whether any one individual will develop acute mountain sickness.

There is no evidence that the presence of upper respiratory tract infection predisposes to acute mountain sickness, though pulmonary oedema must be distinguished from pneumonia. Nor is there evidence that the heat or cold at high altitudes influences acute mountain sickness, though once again such factors may complicate diagnosis. For example, the symptoms and signs of acute mountain sickness are identical with most of those found in hypothermia.

PATHOPHYSIOLOGY

The initiating cause of acute mountain sickness is hypoxia but it is probable that the disease is due to a combination of failed and exaggerated physiological adjustments to that hypoxia. We do not know why some people respond poorly to ascent. Reports of rare cases of patients with congenitally absent hypoxic ventilatory response who develop high altitude pulmonary oedema below 2000 m suggest that the respiratory centre might be primarily at fault. The individual's hypoxic ventilatory response at sea level is only a very rough predictor of acute mountain sickness, but people who have acute mountain sickness do, as a group, have lower arterial oxygen pressures and saturations at high altitudes than those who feel well. The extent of the lowering correlates well with the severity of acute mountain sickness, and this inadequate oxygenation is associated with high blood $P\text{CO}_2$ levels (and lower arterial pH), due to poorer ventilation. Whether as cause or result of the acute mountain sickness, they are therefore more hypoxic. Clearly, if they develop pulmonary oedema they will become yet more hypoxic and get into a vicious cycle of deepening hypoxia.

Perhaps as a result of the hypoxia (or relative hypercarbia), people with acute mountain sickness retain fluid and gain weight. Typically they have a pronounced antidiuresis on ascent which contrasts with the diuresis and the unchanged or even lowered weights of those who feel well. This antidiuresis is independent of the anorexia and vomiting of acute mountain sickness. On ascent, in people who feel well, as well as in those with acute mountain sickness, there is a movement of fluid into the cells from the plasma and interstitial fluid compartments. No one knows whether this movement is more pronounced in the brain, or in general greater in those people who will develop acute mountain sickness. At the same time there is a considerable hypoxic cerebral vasodilatation in people ascending to high altitude.

Milledge and his coworkers have noted that prolonged exercise at sea level causes sodium retention with a shift of fluid from the cells to the extra cellular space, due to increased renin and therefore aldosterone production. All studies have shown a reduction of aldosterone at altitude. When subjects at high altitude exercise there is a massive increase in renin production and a blunted aldosterone response due to diminished angiotensin converting enzyme (ACE) activity, itself due to hypoxia. These workers suggest that the reduction in ACE prevents fluid retention and hence reduces acute mountain sickness and that it is least marked in those most prone to acute mountain sickness.

A reasonable but not fully tested hypothesis to account for acute mountain sickness proposes that all the symptoms and signs and all the physiological abnormalities of the disease can be explained as being due to brain-stem and cerebral malfunction, itself due to minimal oedema of the respiratory and cardiovascular centres consequent upon the fluid shifts and the vasodilatation. In other words, in even mild acute mountain sickness, there is very mild (and transient) oedema within the brain and that, as the cerebral oedema increases, so do the symptoms, from headache and anorexia to coma. Hackett and his coworkers have shown oedema of the white matter on MRI examination of people with acute mountain sickness. This fits with the concept of a vasogenic oedema, perhaps due to a failure of vascular autoregulation and transmittal of increased pressures to the capillaries. Autopsies in people who have died from cerebral oedema have shown, besides oedema, numerous tiny haemorrhages from the capillaries. They have also shown arterial, capillary, and venous sludging and clotting. It is unlikely that these are primary events but more probably that the clotting system has been activated by the oedematous process which, by increasing intracranial pressure, has closed the cerebral capillaries.

The pathophysiology of high altitude pulmonary oedema is yet more obscure. Pulmonary oedema at sea level is known to follow numerous intracranial lesions including cerebral oedema, but the relationship at high altitude is unclear.

It is known that on ascent to high altitude, there is a shift in blood from the systemic 'capacitance vessels' (veins) to the pulmonary circuit. In addition, there is a brisk hypoxic pulmonary arterial vasoconstriction with a rise in pulmonary artery pressure. Neither of these processes causes the oedema but both contribute to it.

The oedema fluid of people suffering from high altitude pulmonary oedema at 4400 m on Mount McKinley has been shown to be very high in protein content, which is characteristic of a breakdown in vascular permeability, and not like that of 'high-pressure' cardiogenic pulmonary oedema. The oedema fluid also contains large numbers of cells, the vast majority of them macrophages as well as markers of chemotactic activity and inflammation. The fact that minor degrees of such breakdown occur early and frequently is suggested by the finding, in large studies at altitude, of a high incidence of pulmonary crackles in the asymptomatic newcomers, as well as by the finding in newcomers of an increased pulmonary liquid content.

The weight of evidence suggests that cardiac function is not really impaired. Pulmonary wedge pressures, reflecting average pulmonary venous pressures, are normal and so are atrial pressures when they have been measured. At autopsy, cuffs of oedema have been found around pulmonary arteries, as well as blebs of oedema within arteries and these may be associated with the thromboses that may be found at autopsy.

Four cases of high altitude pulmonary oedema have recently been described which are instructive. They all occurred after minimal exertion at modest altitudes and in each case the exceedingly rare anomaly of congenital absence of one pulmonary artery was revealed, suggesting that pulmonary hypertension and shearing forces due to a massively increased circulation (in these cases though one lung) might together contribute to high altitude pulmonary oedema. Experimentally, whether in dogs or sheep, this is very hard to reproduce, oedema occurring only when almost all but one upper lung lobe has been removed and the heart is assisted by pumps to force all the circulating blood through this tiny remnant of the pulmonary circulation. Nevertheless, most physiologists believe that in high altitude pulmonary oedema some lung capillary beds are closed off, whether by hypoxic vasoconstriction or by capillary wall oedema and thrombosis. There is, therefore, diversion of the whole circulation through the remaining widely patent capillaries which are damaged both by the increased pressure and the shear-stress of the large flow. As a consequence, they leak: pulmonary oedema.

INCIDENCE

Both the incidence and severity of acute mountain sickness depend upon the altitude and the terrain where they are assessed and upon the method of ascent used. Since there is wide individual variation in susceptibility, there is a wide variation in altitudes at which it has been reported. Also, as all the symptoms (which are found commonly in all sorts of maladies at sea level) and most of the signs are not specific to acute mountain sickness, and since there is variability in the criteria investigators use for diagnosing acute mountain sickness, it is impossible to give an exact value for the altitude at which it occurs. The difference in access and terrain has undoubtedly contributed to the belief, once held, that acute mountain sickness was a peculiarity of some mountain regions, particularly the Andes, and that it might be due to some local abnormality in the air. Eighty years ago the Andean mining towns could be reached in a few hours from the coast by railway, but to get the same altitudes of around 4500 m in the Himalayas required weeks of gradual trekking, riding, and travelling on foot. The Peruvians have had names for acute mountain sickness ('soroche', 'puna') for hundreds of years simply because one can go from coast to Altiplano in a very few days, even on foot, and very large numbers of people had to do so, going up to around 4000 m in the process. In contrast, the main trade route between Tibet and India, through central Nepal, passes through the Himalayas, squeezed between two mountains over 8000 m high but is itself at an altitude of only about 2400 m.

We now know that the atmosphere is less dense towards the poles so that the 250 mmHg isobar (which cuts through the summit of Everest (8848 m) at 27°59′N) is at a much lower altitude at the poles and much higher at the equator. Between altitudes of 2 and 16 km atmospheric pressure depends upon latitude since there is a large mass of cold air in the stratosphere above the equator. All this implies that acute mountain sickness might tend to occur at lower altitudes towards the poles, but this has yet to be tested, and other moderating factors such as mode of access and speed of ascent are likely to be far more important.

A fundamental problem in studying this problem is that though there are very many resorts and touring, climbing, and skiing areas at high altitudes, we do not have any really large-scale studies of acute mountain sickness and its complications which give us both the numbers affected (the numerator) and the population at risk (the denominator) so that true incidence may be calculated.

Suffice it to say that acute mountain sickness has been reported below 1550 m; that it is uncommon below 3000 m, and that the higher the altitude, the faster the ascent, and the greater the exertion (in load-carrying, dealing with difficult terrain, and so on), the higher the incidence and the worse the illness.

Because of difference in terrain, access, height, and criteria for diagnosis, and lack of both numerators and denominators, the incidence of acute mountain sickness has been reported variously as from fewer than 10 per cent to 60 per cent. Most large studies suggest that some symptoms, for example, a bad headache that is not relieved by 600 mg of aspirin, occur in over half of those lowlanders going to above 4000 m and that over 10 per cent of climbers have more than one severe symptom at that altitude. High altitude pulmonary oedema occurs in about 5 per cent of people at that altitude, but symptomless crackles in the lung in almost a quarter. Cerebral oedema is less common: occurring in perhaps 0.5 to 2 per cent. Since it usually takes several days to develop, it is unlikely to occur on mountains climbed in a day or two.

DIAGNOSIS

The differential diagnosis is small. For mild acute mountain sickness the non-specific symptoms mean that hypothermia, exhaustion, and dehydration should be considered. The effects of alcohol and marijuana may duplicate those of acute mountain sickness. The absence of diarrhoea speaks against, for example, dysentery or giardiasis. For pulmonary and cerebral oedema, only infectious diseases (pneumonia, or meningoencephalitis) are likely possibilities. It must be remembered that periodic breathing with apnoeic phases is normal at high altitude and not by itself a cause for alarm, though it may be very marked indeed and associated with very severe oxygen desaturation in cerebral oedema. In most high mountain settlements it is impossible to get chest radiographs or electrocardiographs or examine specimens of cerebrospinal fluid, even if such fluid could be obtained. Though high altitude pulmonary oedema may be accompanied by a slight fever, this is moderate, and the extreme tachycardia and tachypnoea and the absence of purulent sputum and of signs or symptoms of pleurisy are characteristic, as is gross cyanosis. Sometimes the pulmonary oedema is one-sided or there may have been an upper respiratory infection, both of which confuse the diagnosis. In cerebral oedema there is no meningism and little if any pyrexia, nor evidence of ear infection or of localizing signs. There is a striking absence of any signs of cardiac decompensation (cardiac enlargement; raised neck veins). Giving oxygen—which is expensive, often not available, and has to be given in 4 to 5 l/min amounts—frequently produces equivocal results as everyone at high altitude, with almost any illness or none at all, feels temporarily better on oxygen.

Whilst it is true that all illnesses, from laryngitis to haemorrhoids, which develop at high altitude, tend to improve much more rapidly at sea level, the very dramatic recovery in acute mountain sickness, and particularly in pulmonary and cerebral oedema on going down is so striking as to be diagnostic in itself. Numerous cases have been described of people unconscious and worsening at 4000 m who were fully conscious at 3000 m.

The physician who sees the patient on descent is, however, usually obliged to perform a battery of tests on the patient who, except in the case of very prolonged cerebral oedema, is recovering fast. The chest radiograph will show scattered fluffy patches of oedema; the electrocardiogram shows simple right ventricular hypertrophy and 'strain', and the cerebrospinal fluid will be normal.

PROPHYLAXIS

Acute mountain sickness and its complications are the consequence of ascent that for any one individual is too high or too fast and are therefore easily and completely preventable by going up slowly. It is essential for the physician to remember and stress the vast individual differences in susceptibility when advising people who are to take part in one of the many thousands of high altitude treks organized each year. These often have strict, cramped, and too optimistic schedules, and there is frequently great pressure on those who feel unwell to keep up with the rest of the party. It is essential that everyone should realize that acute mountain sickness, unless it is very mild, has ruined many an idyllic and expensive holiday and that it cannot be cured except by rest or temporary descent. They must be told very emphatically that high altitude pulmonary or cerebral oedema may be rapidly fatal, that they have a responsibility to keep an eye on their fellows, for the natural tendency is to leave people with headache and drowsiness to sleep it off, unwatched as they drift into coma. Everyone must know that to help a sick person down on his own feet is quick, easy, and safe, while a few hours later, when he is unconscious, 20 or 30 expert climbers may spend days in risking their lives trying to carry down that same patient. They should know that even in the 1990s, communications are frequently very faulty, planes and helicopters may not exist or may crash, or because of terrain and bad weather, may be unable to get near. They must know, therefore, that any rescue is chancy and dangerous to others.

Everyone, especially those who have flown to high altitude, has a personal duty to rest on arrival, to be sure to ascend at a pace that is personally comfortable (about 300 m per day above 3000 m with days of rest every 1000 m is usually a good pace), to spend nights as low down as possible and to climb less far each day as higher altitudes are reached. Time spent in acclimatizing to be able physically to work harder is also time spent in avoiding the miseries and dangers of acute mountain sickness. Since insensible water loss is increased due to the increased exertion, the extra ventilation and the dry air, every effort must be made to avoid dehydration, by drinking enough to urinate clear, dilute urine. The climber should also eat plenty, especially carbohydrates.

The drug acetazolamide, which is a carbonic anhydrase inhibitor, and was introduced in order, by its action in increasing urinary bicarbonate excretion, to counteract the respiratory alkalosis, reduces the incidence and severity of acute mountain sickness when taken before and during ascent. It probably works by decreasing cerebrospinal fluid formation and, more importantly, stimulating nocturnal respiration by causing an intracellular acidosis in the respiratory centre so that periodic episodes of apnoea, which are very common at altitude, are abolished and blood oxygen saturation is never allowed to fall. Its principal side effect is tingling in the hands, feet, and around the mouth. It is a matter of taste whether to recommend drugs such as acetazolamide except in the case of an emergency ascent, say for rescue, since slow ascent allowing time for acclimatization is so effective.

Dexamethasone, a glucocorticoid effective in the management of cerebral oedema, has been shown to prevent acute mountain sickness, while reducing the retinal arterial dilation that follows exposure to hypoxia. This is further evidence that acute mountain sickness is due to mild cerebral oedema, associated with the increased cerebral blood flow on ascent.

Energetic propaganda advising slow ascent and rest days and nights has been shown to lower the incidence of acute mountain sickness. There is evidence that sleeping tablets, which further lower the already lowered oxygen saturation during sleep should be avoided.

TREATMENT

First it is important to avoid sedatives and respiratory depressants. In mild acute mountain sickness, aspirin for the headache and rest are usually adequate. If not, the sufferer should descend 300 to 500 m and rest for a couple of nights. Occasionally an antiemetic should be given, and even intravenous fluids for dehydration. If there is ataxia or mild cerebral or pulmonary oedema, the patient should at once be assisted down 700 m to 1000 m, rested, and watched carefully. Controlled trials have now shown that acetazolamide increases oxygenation and relieves the symptoms of acute mountain sickness. If pulmonary oedema is severe or the patient is comatose, he must be immediately carried down at least 1000 m and further if recovery is not evident. While helicopters, etc., may be sent for at the same time and while oxygen, if available, should be administered (if the patient is comatose, tracheal intubation and sucking out of the airways must be performed, and the oxygen should be delivered at 5–6 l/min), it is essential to begin evacuation immediately because communications may be defective, helicopters are not always available or crash, oxygen may run out and is often ineffective, changes in weather can prevent evacuation, and people with pulmonary or cerebral oedema are in extreme danger of dying in a matter of hours, while a small decrease in altitude may improve them dramatically.

In pulmonary oedema, sit the patient up if this makes him comfortable. Give frusemide (20–40 mg orally) and morphine (15 mg intravenously). Both these drugs divert blood from the pulmonary to the systemic circuit. Frusemide causes a diuresis and morphine decreases anxiety and respiration rate.

The calcium blocker, nifedipine, has been shown to prevent high altitude pulmonary oedema in subjects who have had it before. Nifedipine reduces the excessive rise in pulmonary artery pressure that usually occurs in such people, and improves oxygenation, perhaps by improving the matching of perfusion to ventilation, by lessening the formation of oedema fluid, and by decreasing the inflammatory response. Its side-effects (hypotension and tachycardia) mean that its use should be limited to therapy of established oedema.

A portable, light-weight hyperbaric bag, made of impermeable nylon, has recently been developed. The victim lies inside while the air pressure is increased using a foot pump, by 104 torr. For example, at 4200 m, where ambient barometric pressure is 449 torr, the pressure in the bag, 553 torr, would be equivalent to an altitude of 2544 m. This is therefore equivalent to taking the patient down 1656 m. Controlled clinical trials now show the bag to be effective in acute mountain sickness and mild pulmonary oedema, and expeditions should consider taking such bags with them, though descent is still the best, quickest, and usually the safest therapy.

In cerebral oedema, intravenous dexamethasone in large doses (e.g. 16 mg) should be given to reduce the oedema. Intravenous infusion of hypertonic agents such as glycerol and mannitol have been used. They are logical and appropriate but are hard to set up in the mountains. A cuffed endotracheal tube should be passed, the lungs kept inflated and the bladder kept empty with a Foley catheter (all these devices should form part of the kit of a responsible physician travelling at high altitudes).

PROGNOSIS

This depends not merely on the altitude and terrain but on the speed with which early signs are noticed by the patient's colleagues and their determination and skill in evacuating him to lower altitudes immediately. There are numerous reports of deaths due to pulmonary oedema and to the rarer but more dangerous cerebral oedema. Once either of these has developed the patient probably has about a one-third chance of dying. If he recovers fully, it is probably that he will have no demonstrable physical after-effects and also likely that will be able to ascend to high altitudes again, but using great caution.

Retinal haemorrhage of high altitude

In 1969 it was noticed that some people flown to altitudes around 5600 m developed flame-shaped retinal haemorrhages. Retinal pathology occurring at between 4000 m and 8000 m altitude has now been confirmed by numerous studies.

On ascent, there is not merely a considerable increase in cerebral blood flow but in retinal blood flow also. Ophthalmoscopy around 5000 to 6000 m shows a 20 to 25 per cent increase in diameter of both arteries and veins, and striking increase in the tortuosity of these vessels (Fig. 1). The optic disc takes on a pink tinge and becomes suffused with blood due to capillary dilatation. This may delude the examiner into diagnosing papilloedema, a condition which may, as shown above, occur in

Fig. 1 The left optic fundus of a 26-year-old male climber photographed at 5900 m altitude. Both the veins and arteries are dilated and tortuous and there is hyperaemia of the optic disc as well as mild papilloedema. The climber had severe headache, nausea, and vomiting.

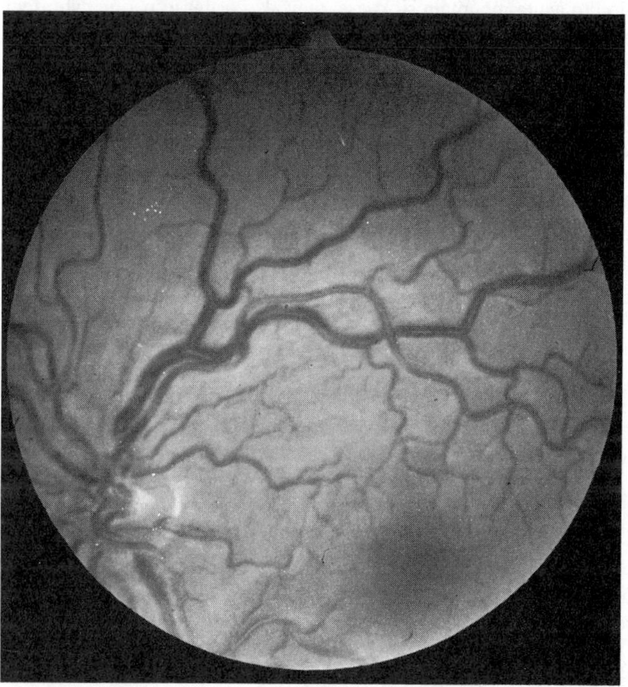

Fig. 2 The right optic fundus of a fit and symptomless 28-year-old male climber photographed at 5900 m altitude. The vessels are dilated, as in Fig. 1, but are less tortuous. There are numerous, scattered retinal haemorrhages.

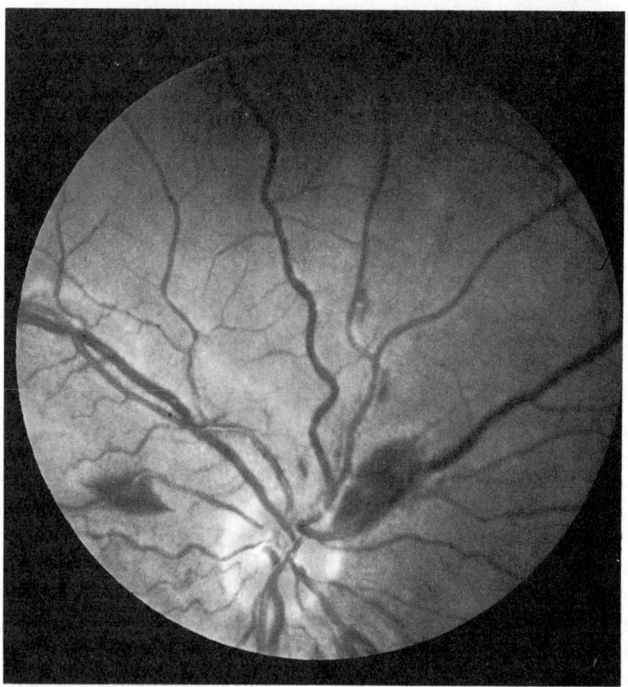

very ill subjects and be diagnostic of cerebral oedema. This vasodilatation is accompanied by a brisk increase in retinal blood flow.

At 5600 m studies have shown that one-third to one-half of people develop flame-shaped retinal haemorrhages (Fig. 2). Some further studies, carried out at 5900 m have confirmed this figure in fit, symptomless climbers descending from 7000 to 8000 m altitude. Clearly the exact figure depends upon whether pupillary dilators and retinal photography were used in the surveys. The haemorrhages are usually near the optic disc and may be of any size and number. Since they tend to occur adjacent to the disc and since the macula constitutes a tiny proportion of the area of the retina, it is not surprising that they are rarely noticed by those who develop them. Though their presence bears a statistical relation to acute mountain sickness, they also occur in people who feel very well.

It is not known whether the occurrence of haemorrhages relates to the unusual sheer stresses associated with an increased flow through dilated vessels. It may be that they are caused by transmittal of high thoracic pressures developed during straining or prolonged coughing, and transmitted through a vasculature dilated because of hypoxia. One study, at 5360 m, showed that fresh retinal haemorrhages developed in 7 of 34 people during maximal exercise. Their presence is reminiscent of the small haemorrhages found over the brain in high altitude cerebral oedema.

On descent, retinal blood flow, vascular diameter, and tortuosity all rapidly return to normal and the haemorrhages resolve, though when they impinge on the fovea, despite the fact that an observer can no longer see them, the victim may have a permanent blind spot. It is probable that the finding of retinal haemorrhages in someone at high altitude is not by itself a reason to counsel descent.

Peripheral oedema

Swelling of hands, face, and ankles may occur in climbers on ascent to high altitude and rarely there may be gross anasarca. The oedema is more common in women than in men though no association with menses has been found. It is associated with acute mountain sickness and pulmonary oedema but may occur by itself, and it is relieved by the diuresis that accompanies descent. Levels of antidiuretic hormone (ADH) are raised in severe acute mountain sickness but the relationship between ADH and peripheral oedema at high altitude is obscure. Treatment with a mild oral diuretic is easy. It should be noted that peripheral oedema may also follow long-continued daily hiking at sea level.

Other illnesses of high altitudes

Normal people frequently ask their physicians whether their hearts will be all right at high altitude. The physiological facts are that the normal heart is not limited by heights up to the top of Everest. Unhappily, the doctor has no tests that are sensitive or specific enough to give an accurate prediction, unless the patient has symptoms. Even then, among the millions of people who think they are well enough to ascend to high altitude, (35 million above 2439 m each year in the United States, of whom 2.9 million have hypertension and 456 000 have coronary disease) death rates seem very low. The doctor has to remind the prospective trekker that he or she is going on an adventure, and getting away from, among other things, good emergency medical treatment. The physician should be very hesitant to forbid any activity which may have great meaning to the patient, in the absence of actual, as opposed to theoretical, evidence that it is harmful.

On theoretical grounds (and occasionally this has been borne out by practical experience), people with diseases which limit ventilation (e.g. kyphoscoliosis, alveolar hypoventilation syndrome), diffusion (e.g. pulmonary fibrosis), circulation (e.g. general, as in heart failure or anaemia; specific as in vascular disease), and tissue adaptation, fare badly at high altitudes. Often, however, there is little evidence that any particular patient will succumb to the hypoxia. Doctors should remember that spas such as St Moritz, in Switzerland, have been receiving the sick for many centuries and that tuberculosis sanatoria at, say, Davos (1529 m) were places where people with lung disease were sent, and they should be cautious about the constraints they place on a patient's activities and frank about our ignorance.

On the other end of the spectrum, there are not enough people with abnormal haemoglobins shifting the oxyhaemoglobin dissociation curves to the left (e.g. Hb Andrew-Minneapolis) who can take on more oxygen and who do well at high altitude, for this sort of abnormality to make much difference to the average physician's practice.

In addition, some acclimatizing features may in themselves cause problems: the erythropoietic stimulus, to take an example, never shuts off above an altitude of about 5500 m: the consequent high viscosity of the blood makes it hard to pump and easy to clot and it is probably that, as in severe cyanotic congenital heart disease and chronic mountain sickness (see below), venesection is beneficial.

CHRONIC MOUNTAIN SICKNESS (MONGE'S DISEASE)

This is a clinical syndrome affecting a few very long-term residents at altitudes. It is to be distinguished from the persistent failure of a newcomer to adjust to the altitude which results in weeks or even months of acute mountain sickness. It usually occurs in men between the ages of 20 and 50, and the symptoms are of headache, dizziness, depression, irritability, and, most strikingly, drowsiness and even episodes of coma. The signs are those of severe polycythaemia and cyanosis with suffused, congested conjunctiva, ear lobes, cheeks, and lips, as well as clubbed finger nails. Signs of congestive heart failure may be present. The right heart may be enlarged on chest radiograph and there is evidence of right ventricular hypertrophy on ECG, itself a reflection of marked pulmonary hypertension.

These patients have a polycythaemia that is inappropriately high for the altitude, the haematocrit usually being in the high 70s. The total circulating red cell volume is increased, probably due to the arterial oxygen saturation which is very low, itself a reflection of inadequate ventilation as shown by the arterial $P\text{CO}_2$ which is high. All the symptoms, signs, and physiological abnormalities are cured by descent to sea level, and sufferers should move there permanently.

Where there is, for example, gross kyphoscoliosis, massive obesity, or a pneumoconiosis, it is possible to blame a specific defect for the excessive hypoxia and therefore the body's natural adjustments (for example, the great polycythaemia and pulmonary vasoconstriction) which themselves produce the syndrome. Where no such cause is found, it is probable that the cause lies in alveolar hypoventilation, similar to the alveolar hypoventilation syndrome that may occur at sea level, and due to a sluggish response to oxygen on the part of the peripheral chemoreceptors or to carbon dioxide on the part of the respiratory centre.

MYOCARDIAL INFARCTION

There is a low rate of coronary arterial disease in all indigenous populations studied at high altitudes, whether in the Andes, the Himalayas, or the Pamirs. Most workers find a reduction of cardiac output and of coronary arterial flow in such residents but how this relates to coronary disease is obscure.

It may be that as such indigenous populations tend to be more active physically, to eat differently and less (especially salt), when compared with people in the West, and to have lower serum lipids and less systemic hypertension, the reasons for the low prevalence of coronary disease and infarction has little to do with the altitude. However, it may have little to do with racial differences and to the factors listed above because most epidemiological evidence suggests that mortality from arteriosclerotic disease in the United States declines with increasing altitude of residence. Whether this is because mild arterial hypoxia 'trains' the myocardium to open more capillaries and thus makes it less vulnerable to occlusions is not known, nor is it clear whether the differences are due to migration down to lower altitudes of people liable to coronary disease.

The physician at sea level is often asked by people whether it is safe for them to go up to 3000 or 4000 m altitude to ski or to climb. Logic dictates that as the myocardium has no oxygen reserves, as myocardial oxygen extraction even at sea level leaves no room for improvement, and as coronary flow is decreased, people who have poor coronary circulation will be at great risk when they ascend from sea level and start hard exercise. There are, however, no credible studies to guide the physician. The few anecdotal reports suffer from the absence of a denominator, so we have no idea if such people are more or less likely to have suffered their infarct than when exercising at sea level. Moreover, age, state of training, cold, and a host of other variables confound the issue. A prudent physician might tell the patient not to go until they are fit to take exercise at sea level, but unless the patient has had a previous myocardial infarction, we have no evidence that an electrocardiogram, with or without exertion of breathing low oxygen mixtures simultaneously, has any predictive value at all, and the patients' previous history of fitness and of illness is likely to be far more useful. Since the predictive value of tests is critically dependent upon the prevalence of the condition, the usefulness of doing large numbers of such tests in the absence of symptoms is likely to be very low.

PULMONARY EMBOLI

Deep vein thrombosis tends to occur in climbers at very high altitudes partly because of the extreme polycythaemia and partly because of enforced inactivity due to storms. Pulmonary emboli, sometimes fatal, occur. Evacuation to lower altitudes and the administration of aspirin as an anticoagulant should be tried. More powerful anticoagulants require careful supervision of, say, prothrombin times, and this is impossible under the circumstances.

SICKLE-CELL ANAEMIA

Since cells containing HbS sickle, when hypoxic, become sticky and rigid, it is not surprising that homozygous cases of HbS (sickle-cell anaemia) are at great danger from high altitude. In Denver, at 1609 m, people who are heterozygotes (sickle-cell trait) apparently lead normal lives, but cases of splenic infarction in people with sickle-cell trait have been described in men at between 3500 and 4500 m. The effect of exercise is unclear. Clearly one should be cautious in advising anyone with sickle-cell trait to exercise at altitudes above about 2000 m.

REFERENCES

Hackett, P.H., and Roach, R.C. (1994). High altitude medicine and physiology. In *Management of Wilderness and Environmental Emergencies*, (ed. Paul S. Auerbach) 3rd edn. C.V. Mosby, St Louis.

Lenfant, C. and Sullivan, K. (1971). Adaptation to high altitude. *New England Journal of Medicine*, **284,** 1298–308.

Reeves, J.T. and Schoene, R.B. (1992). When lungs on mountains leak. *New England Journal of Medicine*, **325,** 1306–7.

Rennie, D. (1976). See Nuptse and die. *Lancet*, **ii,** 1177–9.

Rennie, D. (1986). The Great breathlessness mountains. *Journal of the American Medical Association*, **256,** 81–2.

Rennie, D. (1989). Will trekkers have heart attacks? *Journal of the American Medical Association*, **261,** 1045–6.

8.5.5(e) Aerospace medicine

J.A.C. HOPKIRK and D. M. DENISON

INTRODUCTION

Aerospace medicine concerns the welfare of man in flight.

PHYSICAL FEATURES OF THE ATMOSPHERE

The atmosphere is a uniformly mixed, oxygen-enriched gas that shields the ground below from thermal and other high-energy radiations above. Because it is held to the Earth by gravity and compresses under its own weight, it is denser close to the ground than further away. The long waves of infrared sunlight travel easily through the atmosphere, warming it very little but heating the ground below. The hot ground re-radiates some of this heat at other wavelengths, which are absorbed by carbon dioxide and water vapour, making the air close to the ground much warmer than that elsewhere. By contrast, the short waves of ultraviolet sunlight entering the upper atmosphere are absorbed by oxygen molecules early in their journey, creating a belt of warm ozone at high altitudes. Most of the other high-energy rays are also intercepted in the same region but generate secondary rays that extend lower down. Very few of these reach the ground. At sea level, air exerts a pressure of about 1 atm (760 mmHg; approx. 101 kPa), is variably moist, has a temperature that ranges from −60 °C to +60 °C, and moves at wind speeds from 0 to 160 km/h. With increasing altitude its temperature, pressure, and water content fall and wind speeds increase. Some of these features are summarized in Fig. 1. In general, on ascent, conditions become more severe and more uniform.

Atmospheric pressure

Although the Earth is almost perfectly spherical its atmosphere is not, being more extensive over the Equator than the Poles. On average the total gas pressure falls with altitude in a regular, almost exponential, way, halving every 18 000 ft. Thus it is easy to sketch a reasonable model of atmospheric pressure (i.e. half an atmosphere at 18 000 ft, a quarter at 36 000 ft, an eighth at 54 000 ft, a sixteenth at 72 000 ft, etc., as in Fig. 2). Because the oxygen content of the atmosphere (20.93 per cent) is constant to very high altitudes indeed, the same curve can be used to obtain the ambient oxygen pressure at any altitude, by rescaling the ordinate as shown in Fig. 2. The values obtained in this manner are slight overestimates because they make no allowance for the atmosphere's water-vapour content. Its water-vapour pressure is largely determined by temperature and introduces errors that are just significant at low altitudes where the air is warm. However, the oxygen pressure of physiological importance is that which exists in ambient air when it is warmed and wetted on entering the bronchial tree. This process necessarily raises water-vapour pressure to about 47 mmHg, regardless of the total gas pressure outside. Thus the oxygen pressure in moist inspired gas ($P\text{IO}_2$) fully saturated with water vapour at 37 °C is given by the relationship:

$$P\text{IO}_2 = F\text{IO}_2\,(\text{PB} - 47)$$

where $F\text{IO}_2$, the fractional concentration of oxygen in the inspirate, is 0.2093 when the air is inspired.

Atmospheric temperature

This drops more or less linearly with altitude, at about 2 °C/1000 ft, to the tropopause (40 000 ft), is stable at −56 °C up to about 80 000 ft and then rises to almost body temperature at about 150 000 ft, but by then air density is so low that its temperature is unimportant (cf. the dense cold air below).

Atmospheric ozone (O_3)

Ozone is formed by irradiation of diatomic oxygen molecules, which dissociate into atoms. At very high altitudes the ultraviolet irradiation is so intense that all oxygen exists in the monatomic form. Lower down those that are produced combine with oxygen molecules to form the triatomic gas O_3 (ozone) at concentrations from 1 to 10 parts/10^6. The ozonosphere normally exists between 40 000 and 140 000 ft, i.e from one-fifth to one-thirtieth of an atmosphere. Below 40 000 ft the irradiation is normally too weak for significant amounts of ozone to form. Concentrations of 1 part/10^6 at sea-level pressures cause lung irritation. Ten times that concentration can cause fatal lung oedema. Although the ozonosphere is at much lower pressure, aircraft ventilation systems can take it in and compress it to pressures at which pulmonary irritation is a real threat.

MECHANICAL ASPECTS

Propeller-driven aircraft need sufficient air to 'bite' on but not enough to slow them down. They fly best at altitudes below 30 000 ft. Jet aircraft are propelled by throwing a stream of hot gas behind them but they need atmospheric oxygen to ignite the fuel that does this. They fly best at altitudes below 65 000 ft. Rockets take an oxygen supply with them, and fly best in a vacuum.

Air permits vehicles to travel through it at very high speeds. Usually these are achieved and lost so gradually that the changes of pace pass unnoticed, but high-performance aircraft may make continuous high-speed turns that can be sustained for a minute or more. The radial accelerations that such turns produce are proportional to the square of the aircraft's speed and inversely proportional to the radius of its turning circle (as shown in Fig. 3). Because the aircraft turns by applying its broad wing surface to the air these accelerations are almost perpendicular to that surface and roughly parallel to the long axis of the people within. Usually aircraft make 'head to the middle' turns causing tissue fluids and loosely tethered organs like the liver and heart to fall footwards (positive 'g' or $+G_z$ accelerations). Occasionally the aircraft makes 'head-out' turns forcing these organs and fluids towards the head.

SUMMARY

In brief, the important features of the atmosphere are that its temperature and pressure fall and radiation intensities rise with altitude. In addition there is a poisonous belt of ozone at high altitude. The atmosphere also permits vehicles to travel at high speeds and make sustained severe accelerations.

The physiological problems posed by these stresses are extremely challenging but on the whole they only affect professional aircrew. One risk that is shared by all who fly, impinges on everyday life in many ways, and is a common feature of several diseases is hypoxia; it will be discussed first.

Hypoxia

Oxygen has a dual role in most animal cells, as it is life giving and extremely poisonous at the same time. In the form in which it exists in the air or dissolved in simple solution it is benign and only ionized with difficulty. However, once an electron is successfully attached to an oxygen molecule it becomes a highly corrosive superoxide ion, capable of pulling the (electron) linchpins from neighbouring molecules of all sorts and of forming a cascade of other highly destructive oxygen radicals. This is an essential feature of oxygen toxicity, which is discussed in Chapter 8.5.5(f). Superoxide dismutase and various peroxidases have evolved to protect most cells from the effects of spontaneous oxygen-radical formation, by quenching the ions as rapidly as they appear.

More recently in evolution, other enzymes have developed that can harness this property of oxygen molecules in a controlled way. There are three sorts. Firstly, there are the oxidases, which take oxygen and free electrons attracting hydrogen to make water. Quantitatively, cytochrome a_3 oxidase is the most important because, using oxygen as the ultimate electron sink, it allows many metabolic processes to proceed and at the same time unlocks and traps most of the energy the body needs (oxidative phosphorylation). However, there are several other oxidases that release the power but are unable to trap it. They are used to denature various unwanted products of metabolism.

Secondly, there are oxygenases, which take the oxygen molecule and introduce it into an organic molecule creating a new compound. Although these enzymes, of which there are many, only consume a small fraction of the body's total oxygen need, they are particularly important, because they are responsible for production and dismemberment of many critical compounds such as the amine transmitters of the brain.

Fig. 1 Some physical features of the Earth's atmosphere, showing the variations in barometric pressure, air temperature, and ozone concentration with altitude. (NB There is an international aviation safety convention that all altitudes are given in feet.) The shaded diagram on the left illustrates how the Earth's atmosphere is compressed under its own weight. The atmosphere absorbs much solar radiation.

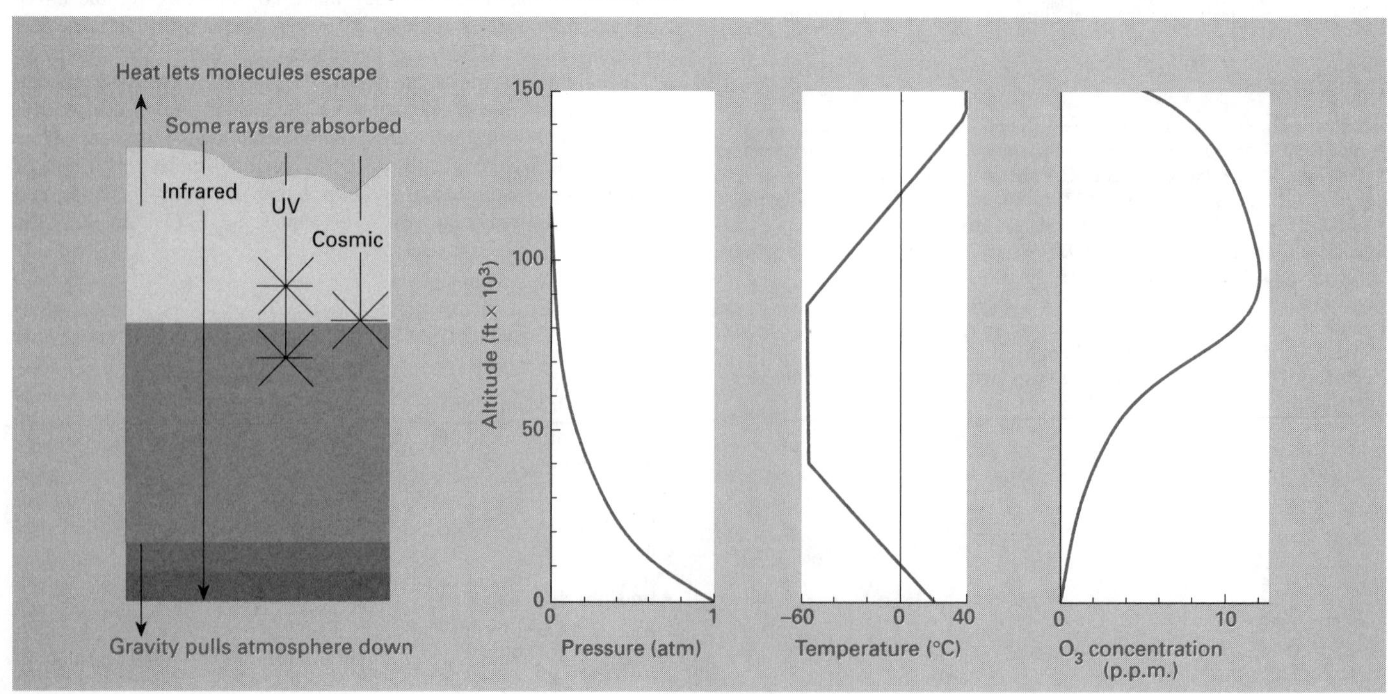

The third group of enzymes that handle oxygen has the attributes of both the other groups and so its members are called mixed function oxidases. They take one atom of an oxygen molecule and use it to make water as would an oxidase, but with another hand take the other atom of the oxygen molecule and put it into an organic moleculer as would an oxygenase. That atom takes hydrogen with it, so these enzymes are also known as hydroxylases. They too are responsible for many critical metabolic processes and for the denaturation of many drugs in the liver, kidney, and elsewhere.

These three groups of enzymes, which handle virtually all the oxygen uptake measured at the lips in man, differ from each other in a crucial respect, which is in their affinity for oxygen. That property can be described by a commonly used term in enzyme kinetics, the Michaelis constant (for oxygen). This constant (K_{mO_2}) is that partial pressure of oxygen which, when all other factors are equal, just allows an oxygen-consuming reaction to proceed at half its maximum velocity. The major oxidase (cytochrome a_3), which is the co-catalyst of oxidative phosphorylation, has a very high oxygen affinity and thus a very low K_{mO_2}, of 1 mmHg or less. That means this particular type of oxygen consumption, representing 80 to 90 per cent of the whole, can proceed full tilt down to very low levels of oxygen supply indeed. By contrast (Fig. 4), the other enzymes, which are quantitatively less important but qualitatively critical, have Michaelis constants for oxygen that vary from 5 to 250 mmHg. A fall in oxygen supply will influence these processes long before oxidative phosphorylation is affected and at times when overall oxygen consumption is diminished little if at all.

Although Fig. 2 describes how ambient oxygen pressure is related to altitude, it does not convey the measure of oxygen supply critical to man, namely the pressure of oxygen to be found in the lungs. That pressure is determined by two equations (Fig. 5). The alveolar ventilation equation states that alveolar CO_2 pressure ($P\text{ACO}_2$) depends only on CO_2 excretion ($M\text{CO}_2$) and alveolar ventilation ($V\text{A}$), so:

$$P\text{ACO}_2 = k(\dot{M}\text{CO}_2/\dot{V}\text{A}).$$

The alveolar air equation states that since at any one time there is a fixed trading ratio between oxygen uptake and CO_2 excretion ($R = \dot{M}\text{CO}_2/\dot{M}\text{O}_2$), alveolar oxygen pressure ($P\text{AO}_2$) can be calculated from the moist inspired oxygen pressure ($P\text{IO}_2$*) and alveolar $P\text{CO}_2$, so:

$$P\text{AO}_2 = P\text{IO}_2{}^* - (P\text{aCO}_2/\text{R})$$

Progressive hypoxia leads to a mild hyperventilation (i.e. rise in $\dot{V}\text{A}$ and fall in $P\text{ACO}_2$). Knowing this it is possible to sketch a graph of alveolar oxygen pressure against altitude as in Fig. 6(a).

When arterialized blood leaves a healthy lung it has an oxygen pressure some 10 mmHg less than that in the alveoli, due to uneven matching of ventilation to perfusion, some anatomical shunting, and an almost nominal obstacle to diffusion. In resting people, the alveolar–arterial oxygen gradient does not change much with altitude, although the relative importance of the factors contributing to it alter considerably; so,

Fig. 2 The variations of barometric pressure and ambient oxygen pressure with altitude.

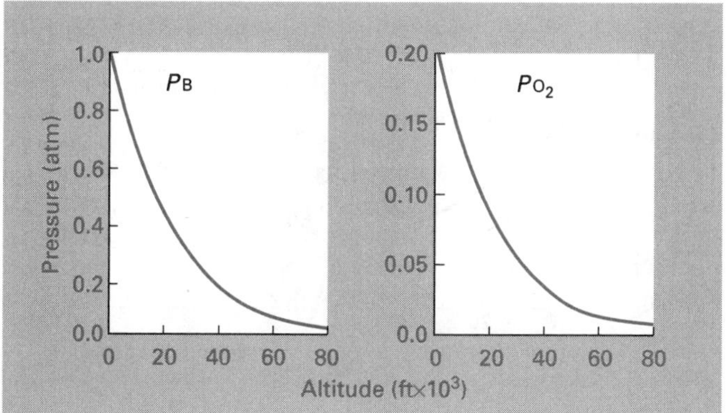

Fig. 4 Curves of oxygen uptake ($M\text{O}_2$) as a fraction of the theoretical maximum ($M\text{O}_2$max) against the partial pressure of oxygen ($P\text{O}_2$) for a family of oxygen-handling enzymes with Michaelis constants for oxygen ($K_m\text{O}_2$) from 1 to 250 mmHg.

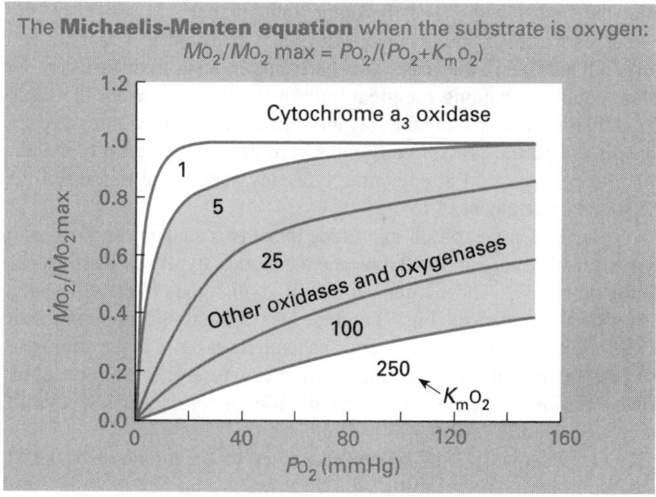

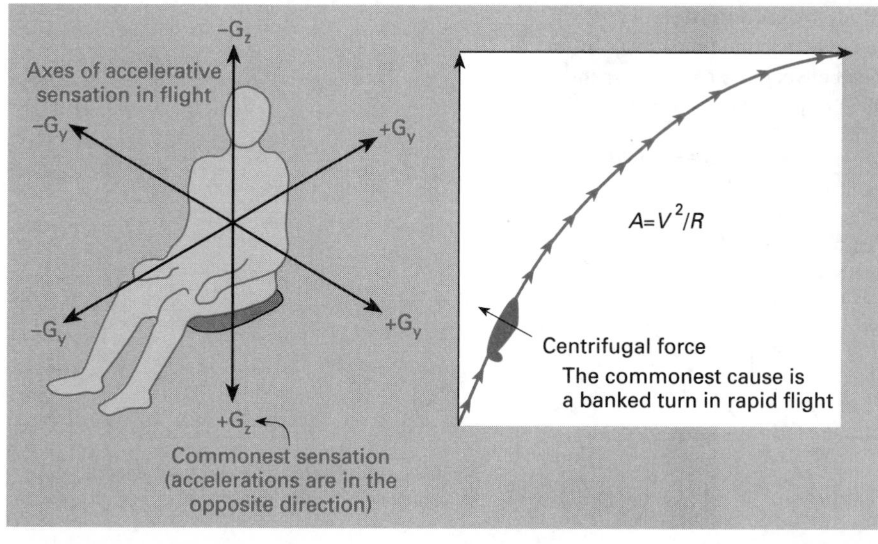

Fig. 3 The axes of acceleration in flight are labelled according to the sensations experienced by the aviator. Thus, when he is accelerated upwards (+G_z) he feels his body fluids and tissues sink towards his feet.

subtracting a further 10 to 15 mmHg describes the relation between arterial oxygen pressure and altitude (also shown in Fig. 6).

The most important change is the loss of the head of pressure driving oxygen from the alveoli to blood, as the fall in alveolar Po_2 is much greater than that in mixed venous Po_2 (because of the shape of the oxygen dissociation curve). As a result the alveolar–venous gradient for oxygen diffusion is smaller and equilibration slower than at ground level.

During the early part of the Second World War many reargunners who were quite alert breathing air while sitting in their turrets at 18 000 ft, lost consciousness when they attempted to crawl back into the body of the plane, at the same altitude. That occurred because exertion speeds up blood flow through individual capillaries in the lung, leaving even less time for oxygen equilibration. Because the obstacle to diffusion, which is nominal at ground level, is dominant at altitude, exertion leads to arterial desaturation not present at rest. The same phenomenon is seen at ground level in patients with fibrotic lung disease.

When systemic blood leaves the central arterial tree it loses a surprising amount of oxygen through the thin arteriolar walls. Some areas of the central nervous system, such as the part of the optic nerve around the central retinal artery and parts of the retina immediately adjacent to some of its branches, depend upon this diffusion for their supply of oxygen. The fall in this driving head (of arterial Po_2) may explain some of the visual impairment experienced on ascent to altitude. Most tissues do not get their oxygen in this way but receive it from the blood as it travels through the systemic capillaries. Until a few years ago it was supposed that there was a fairly even fall of Po_2 along the length of any capillary, with the oxygen diffusing radially, leaving a most deprived area (the 'lethal corner') at the outer limit of that part served by the venous end of the capillary. Nowadays it is believed that most of the oxygen floods out of the vessel very early in its course, to diffuse parallel to the capillary, holding the great bulk of the tissue at much the same Po_2 as in the blood leaving the servant venule. The arteriovenous oxygen content and partial-pressure differences are fixed by the ratio of metabolism to perfusion. In any respiratory steady state, local blood flow is the prime determinant of tissue Po_2.

People suddenly exposed to altitude make two adaptive responses to hypoxia, an increase in blood flow and the modest hyperventilation mentioned previously. These limit but do not abolish the effects of oxygen lack. The consequences (Fig. 7) include loss of night vision, impairment of the ability to learn complex and then simple tasks, a deterioration in the performance of already learnt skills, a progressive loss of muscular power (aerobic capacity), and eventually loss of consciousness, convulsions, and death.

As Fig. 7 shows, people suddenly exposed to an altitude of 10 000 ft and above are unreliable and physically weak. This altitude is taken as the ceiling above which it is mandatory to provide aviators with oxygen. To be safe, the ceiling that is actually used is almost always 8000 ft, at which barometric pressure is 565 mmHg, arterial oxygen pressure is around 55 mmHg (i.e. sitting just at the top of the sloping part of the oxyhaemoglobin dissociation curve, and venous oxygen pressures have only fallen by 1 to 2 mmHg. It is the maximum cabin altitude that is generally permitted in civilian passenger aircraft. There is some evidence that, even at this altitude, people tire more quickly and learn more slowly than at ground level. Some aircraft have a lower maximum to cabin altitude, but this requires a stronger and thus heavier cabin to contain the higher pressure, which makes the aircraft less economical to run and more difficult to get off the ground.

Two physiological features of altitude hypoxia are especially important in aviation. The first is a total lack of awareness that the mind is breaking down. This means that an affected individual cannot be relied on to take corrective action, however well trained. It follows that protective equipment has to be designed to sense the hypoxia and come into operation automatically. The second feature, known as the time of useful consciousness, describes how rapidly consciousness is lost and thus dictates how quickly this equipment must respond.

The time of useful consciousness is the interval after the onset of hypoxia during which an aviator can be relied on to act sensibly. This

Fig. 6 (a) Variations in moist-inspired, alveolar, and arterial oxygen pressure (Po_2) with altitude in normal men. (b) The conventional oxygen–haemoglobin dissociation curve of whole blood plotted to the same pressure scale as the left-hand graph, so that arterial O_2 content can be read directly (at the same horizontal level as the Po_2 curve. It also emphasizes that the arteriovenous oxygen content difference (a-v Δ) is proportional to the ratio of oxygen uptake (Mo_2) to local blood flow (Q).

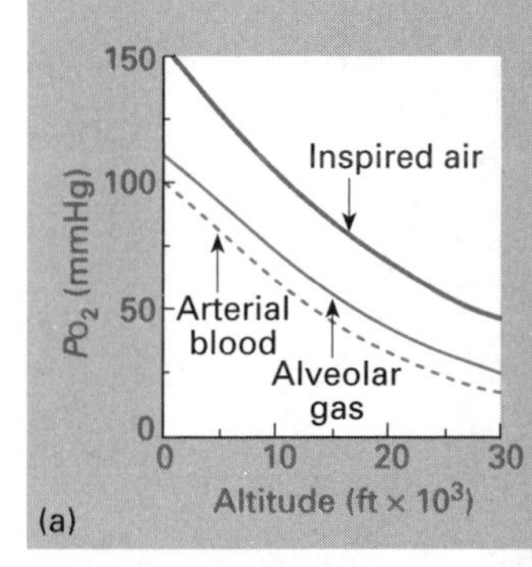

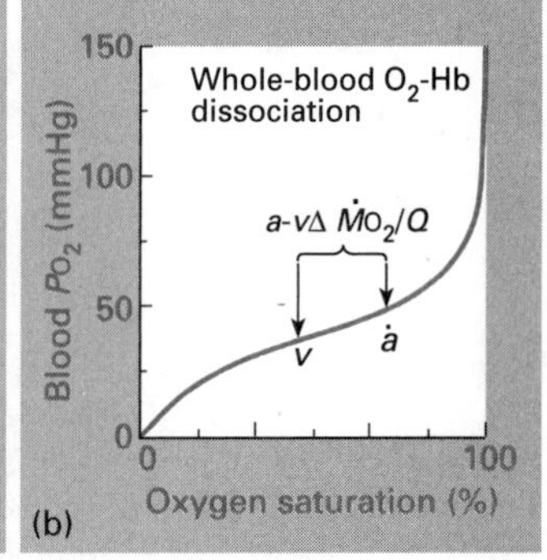

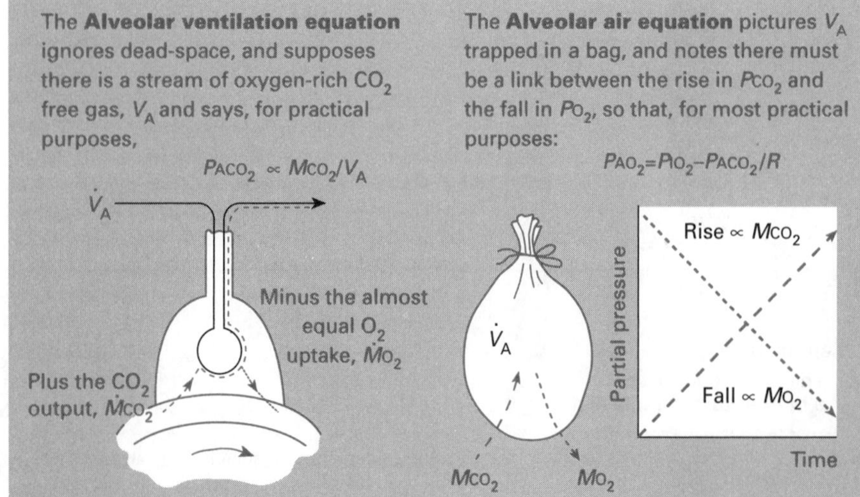

Fig. 5 Graphical representations of the alveolar ventilation and alveolar air equations.

is a difficult characteristic to test, as sophisticated abilities need to be sampled in an adequate and time-consuming way at moments when the level of consciousness may be changing rapidly.

Many studies have confirmed the general relation between this time interval and the altitude of sudden exposure, which is shown in Fig. 8(a). The time of useful consciousness diminishes from about 4 min at 25 000 ft to a minimum of roughly 15 s, which is reached at 35 000 to 40 000 ft. This asymptote represents the sum of the 7 s or so required for blood to travel from the lungs to the brain and the equal time needed for the brain to consume the oxygen that is already dissolved in its substance.

Some recent studies have defined the dose of hypoxia that can be suffered before useful consciousness is lost. In trained and healthy men breathing normally (i.e. with an alveolar $P\mathrm{CO}_2$ of 35–40 mmHg), it is equivalent on a curve of alveolar $P\mathrm{CO}_2$ against time, to an area of 150 'millimetre of mercury seconds', where $P\mathrm{CO}_2$ is less than 38 mmHg (Fig. 8(b)). However, this is sensitive to many other factors, of which the most important are the degree of hyperventilation and the acceleration that the person is exposed to at the time. Hyperventilation causes cerebral vasoconstriction, and 'positive g' opposes the upward flow of blood to the brain (see below). Sometimes deterioration in consciousness is quickened by vasovagal syncope, but more often the heart is beating quite rapidly as consciousness is lost. Exertion also quickens loss of consciousness, as mentioned previously, because it forces blood to rush through the lungs, leaving insufficient time for oxygen equilibration.

It is quite remarkable that resting, unadapted men suddenly exposed to the pressure that exists at the top of Mount Everest will lose consciousness in about 2 min, but after a few weeks of gradual exposure they are able to climb strenuously to the top without benefit of oxygen. All the available evidence suggests that exposure of at least 15 h a day is needed to produce sustained adaptation. No useful responses of this sort are ever seen in aviation. It is interesting that a very similar time per day is needed if chronic bronchitic and emphysematous patients are to benefit from long-term oxygen therapy.

The minimum cabin pressure of 565 mmHg (8000 ft), is sufficiently low to bring a normal person's arterial $P\mathrm{CO}_2$ along the plateau of the oxyhaemoglobin dissociation curve until it is sitting just at the top of the steep part (Fig. 6). Because their blood is still fully saturated with oxygen they will not be cyanosed at this altitude. At ground level, many people with chest diseases have arterial oxygen pressures that are as low as 55 to 60 mmHg (or even lower, in which case they become cyanosed). As they ascend to 8000 ft their arterial $P\mathrm{CO}_2$ will fall further. If their hypoxaemia at ground level is due to a mismatch of ventilation to perfusion, as is usually the case, the drop in arterial $P\mathrm{CO}_2$ will not be as extensive as in normal people (about 40 mmHg), but if it is due to diffusion defect associated with desaturation on exertion, as in some fibrotic conditions, it may be greater. However, in either event, it can be reversed completely by the administration of oxygen, because 30 per cent oxygen at 8000 ft is equivalent to breathing air at ground level. The medical services of all the major airlines can provide a personal oxygen supply for any passenger if they are given notice beforehand. (It is worth checking the altitudes of the patient's destination and of any stopping point en route at the same time.)

Fig. 7 A summary of the functional consequences of altitude hypoxia.

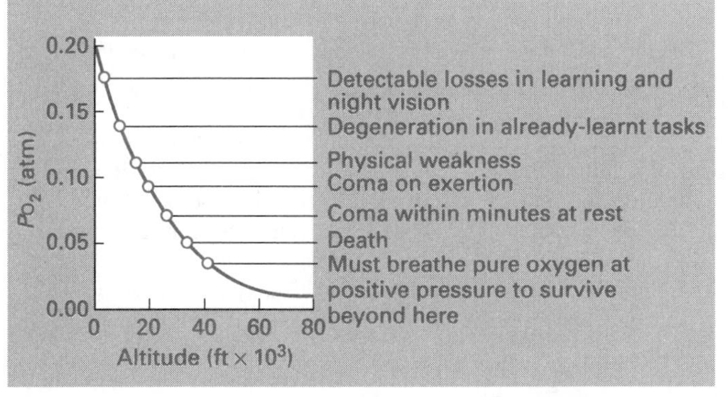

Oxygen equipment and pressure cabins

Aircraft that fly below 10 000 ft do not need any oxygen equipment at all. Most of those that fly higher have reinforced cabins capable of holding a higher pressure inside them than out. These are of two sorts, the high-differential type, seen in passenger and transport aircraft generally, and the low-differential variety found in military high-performance aircraft. The former, holding a high transmural pressure, usually prevent pressure falling below 565 mmHg (8000 ft). They provide an environment in which oxygen equipment is not needed routinely and the occupants breathe cabin air. However, it is always possible that the pressure-cabin system can fail, allowing the pressure within to fall to the level of that outside. This fall can be limited by descent to a lower altitude, but it is not always practical to put the aircraft into a very steep dive, for structural reasons. Similarly, it is not always practical to descend

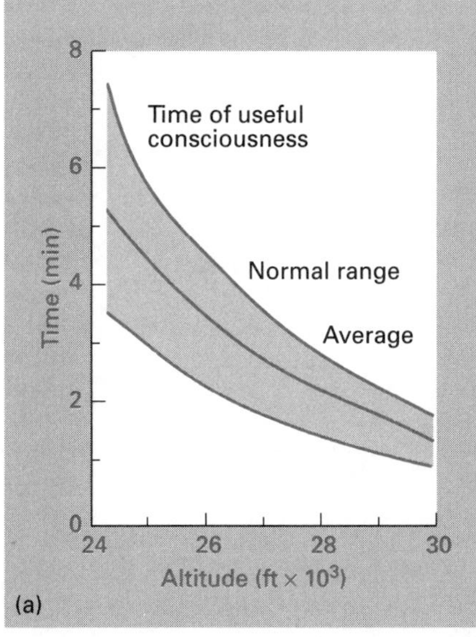

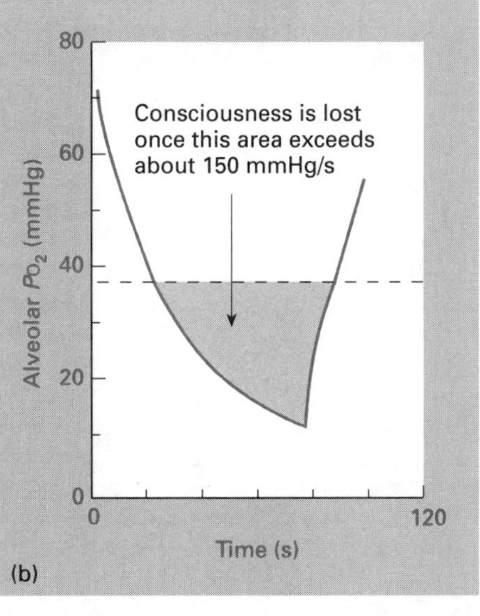

Fig. 8 (a) Variations in the time of useful consciousness with altitude. (b) One way of expressing the dose of hypoxia needed to bring about the loss of consciousness.

below 10 000 ft because, in mid-Atlantic for example, there may not be sufficient fuel for the vehicle to reach the nearest land through dense air. For these reasons, if there is a cabin-pressure failure, people can be exposed to a dangerously hypoxic environment for some time.

A high-differential cabin limits the vehicle's range and manoeuvrability. It also increases the risk of catastrophic damage if the fuselage is punctured. For these reasons, military high-performance aircraft are fitted with low-differential cabins. These usually prevent cabin pressure falling below 280 mmHg (equivalent to a pressure altitude of 25 000 ft). That is the level at which decompression sickness becomes a serious hazard (see below). In such aircraft, oxygen equipment is needed routinely.

The requirements such equipment must meet are demanding, and much ingenuity has gone into its design. In principle, it must

(1) conserve oxygen, which itself is heavy to carry;
(2) not allow the inspired oxygen pressure to rise above half an atmosphere (this avoids pulmonary oxygen toxicity and absorption atelectasis);
(3) not allow the inspired oxygen pressure to fall below about 100 mmHg, equivalent to breathing air at 8000 ft;
(4) therefore it must mix cabin air and stored oxygen in proportions that vary with cabin altitude and have to be regulated automatically.
(5) routinely, it must provide the air–oxygen mix at a slight positive pressure (safety pressure) to ensure that any leaks in the breathing system are outboard, because inward leaks of air cannot be detected but are dangerous;
(6) in the event of pressure-cabin failure at altitudes above 40 000 ft, it must deliver oxygen to the lung at pressures substantially greater than ambient air in such a way that the person can remain conscious and breath easily until the aircraft is brought below 40 000 ft, where pressure breathing is not required.

Devices the size of a matchbox can perform all these functions automatically, sensing the altitude, regulating the air-mix, providing the safety pressure and when necessary much greater overpressures, and at the same time constantly matching the volume demanded in response to respiratory pressure swings of at most a few mmHg. They usually deliver gas to an oronasal mask with a reflected edge seal; this is held on to the face by a harness capable of withstanding the greatest overpressure likely to be encountered.

Sometimes occupants have to escape from aircraft in flight. The faster the aircraft is travelling the more difficult this is to do. All modern fighters are equipped with ejector seats to launch them into the high-speed airstream and get them clear of the tail. Usually the person ejected free-falls in the seat until below 10 000 ft. This gets them through the cold hypoxic upper air as quickly as possible. A small seat- or suit-mounted emergency oxygen supply sees them safely through this stage.

Mechanical effects of pressure change

When any rigid gas-filled cavity (e.g. an aircraft cavity or a paranasal sinus) is exposed to an abrupt fall of external pressure, it tends to vent in an exponential manner, with a time-constant (i.e. time taken to follow 62 per cent of the external pressure change) that depends upon the volume of the cavity and the resistance of the pathway to the outside world (i.e. to the product RC in Fig. 9). If the external pressure change is gradual (i.e. if its time-constant is much longer than that of the cavity in question), the pressure in the cavity will almost exactly follow that outside, and the transmural pressure developed during the decompression will be slight. If the time-constant of the external pressure change is substantially shorter than that of the cavity, the transmural pressure will approach the magnitude of the decompression outside. This may be sufficient to rupture the cavity. If the wall of the cavity is pliable (as in the lung, gut, and middle ear), then part of the decompression is accommodated by expansion of the gas within, stretching the walls but limiting the maximum transmural pressures that can develop.

In civilian passenger and transport aircraft the climb from takeoff to cruise altitude takes about 30 min and involves a fall of about 200 mmHg in cabin pressure (to 8000 ft). The descent to ground, which involves an equivalent rise in cabin pressure, takes much the same time. Body fluids and tissues generally are virtually incompressible and do not alter shape to any important extent when these pressures are applied (cf. diving), but cavities such as the lungs, gut, middle ear, and facial sinuses, which do contain air, behave differently.

The thoracoabdominal wall is a floppy structure that can develop an internal pressure of 100 mmHg or so briefly but is normally flaccid and has a transmural pressure of a few millimetres of mercury. Thus, any gas inside the wall must be at a pressure very close to that outside, and must also follow Boyle's law. Ascent from ground level (760 mmHg) to 8000 ft (565 mmHg) will expand a given volume of gas in a completely pliable container by about 35 per cent, which is equivalent to a radial increase of 10 per cent if it were in a sphere or 18 per cent in a cylinder of fixed length. In the abdomen this may cause slightly uncomfortable gut distension in healthy people but it is not an important problem.

Expansion of gas in the chest is a different matter. The lungs can be thought of as a cluster of tubes and balloons of different sizes. A small balloon served by a wide-bore tube can empty freely and poses no threat,

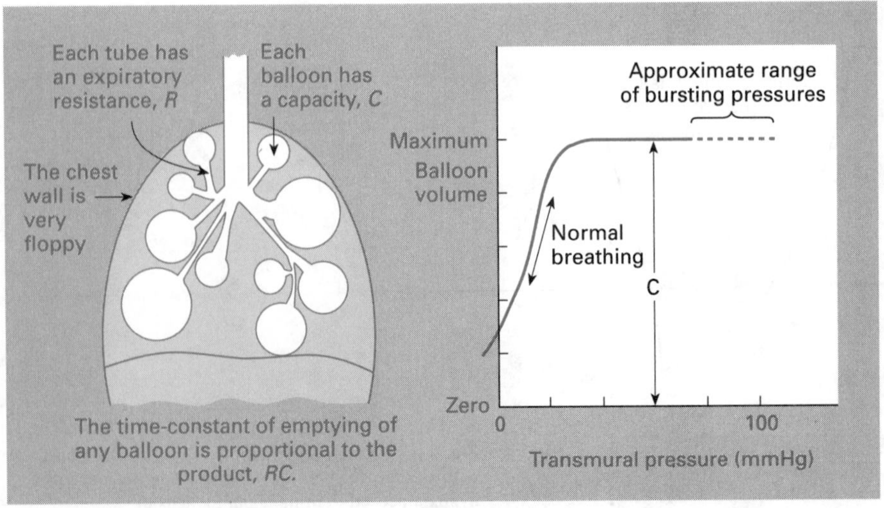

Fig. 9 A graphical summary of the factors determining lung rupture.

but the air in any space served by an inappropriately small airway will empty slowly and behave as 'trapped gas'. Because most spaces in the lung are only about half full during quiet breathing, they can accommodate the 35 per cent increase in volume that would accompany complete obstruction, without bursting. If there is a large obstructed space, a pneumothorax for example, this expansion can be functionally embarrassing. However, if any of the 'trapped gas' is already in a fairly tense container at ground level, there is a risk of lung rupture, because it has a bursting pressure of about 100 mmHg (cf. the 200 mmHg that are available on ascent to 8000 ft). The time-constant of emptying is about 1 s in the healthy lung (witness the normal forced expiratory volume in 1 s:forced vital capacity ratio) and even very diseased lungs can vent themselves over a minute or so. Most patients with obstructive chest disease are able to fly quite safely and should not be prevented from doing so, but those with very severe asthma, obviously tense cysts, or a pneumothorax should not fly. In this regard, flying in small helicopters and small private planes at low altitudes is perfectly acceptable.

The pressure cabins of civilian passenger aircraft are designed so that the failure of any single element (e.g. a window, an air intake, or a pressure-relief valve) will lead to a decompression that takes place over many seconds. In military aircraft, especially in high-performance fighters, decompressions are more likely and more rapid, perhaps taking a second or less, (as in 'through-canopy ejection'). To meet these circumstances, aircrew are trained to breath out throughout the decompression. Many experiments have shown that if they are correctly trained, healthy people can survive quite wide-range decompressions over such short times, but it is quite clear that anyone with obstructive lung disease would not. For this reason, aircrew medical examinations set stringent spirometric requirements (see below).

The cavity of the middle ear poses a separate problem since it vents easily but sometimes fails to fill because the lower part of the eustachian tube behaves as a non-return valve, especially when it is inflamed. As a result, the cavity equilibrates quite easily on ascent but does not refill on descent, and the ear-drum bows inwards, causing pain that can be severe. Patients with colds or a history of middle-ear infection should take a decongestant spray with them and use it before descent. In general, people who really cannot move their ear-drums outwards on performing a Valsalva manoeuvre are best advised to delay their flight.

The facial sinuses present a different hazard because their walls are rigid. If the sinus is obstructed before ascent, it will fail to vent and ultimately will hold a positive pressure of up to 200 mmHg. This is sufficient to obstruct the blood flow to the mucosa and may rupture the sinus. Occasionally, as with the thin roof of the ethmoid sinuses, this can force infected material through the floor of the skull, leading to cerebral abscess. If a sinus that was patent on ascent obstructed during descent, its cavity would contain a relative vacuum that could reach −200 mmHg. This is sufficient to cause gross mural oedema and to rupture some vessels, filling the cavity with blood. Occasionally, air-filled spaces in the teeth and jaw may behave in the same way (aerodontalgia).

DECOMPRESSION SICKNESS

One unexpected hazard that passengers in civil aircraft can experience is decompression sickness (see Chapter 8.5.5(f)). In principle, if the pressure around the person quickly falls to less than half its original value, the gas dissolved in blood and tissue fluids may come out of solution precipitously, forming bubbles and obstructing flow in small blood vessels. Although this cannot develop on simple ascents from ground level to 8000 ft, it may arise if the person has been scuba diving immediately before their flight. It is a particular hazard for holiday-makers on package tours, who often fly back home at night and have all day to swim beforehand. It is customary to advise people not to scuba dive to a depth greater than 30 feet in the 12 h before take-off. This condition should be kept in mind when looking at anyone who has developed neurological signs or symptoms during or soon after a flight. The correct treatment is immediate descent and ideally transfer to the nearest compression chamber, giving oxygen and other non-specific support meantime.

In aircraft with low-differential pressure cabins, the risk of developing decompression sickness is greater and people flying in them should not dive at all in the preceding 12 h. The time symptoms take to develop varies widely between individuals and shortens markedly as the altitude of exposure rises. A guide to these times and variability is given in Fig. 10.

Selection of aircrew and medical maintenance

INTRODUCTION

Because of the very high cost of training pilots, military forces and airlines demand the highest physical and mental standards on entry, to reduce the chance of a pilot's having to retire early on medical grounds. As far as airlines are concerned, aircrew need a current licence to fly, which is granted by the statutory licensing authority of the country concerned and in accordance with the recommendations of the International Civil Aviation Organization (ICAO). These recommendations are amended every 10 years or so. Most countries adhering to the United Nations adopt these recommended medical standards. In formulating medical standards, ICAO has to accept that some countries will lack the facilities for detailed biochemical and other assessments. For this reason the standards set by certain countries may in fact be higher than those expected by ICAO.

Risk

No aircraft flight is without risk. These risks include mechanical failure of the aircraft, adverse weather conditions, pilot error, and medical incapacitation of aircrew. Commercial flying, however, is very safe and with the best airlines and best aircraft the accident rate is approximately 1 in 2 million flying hours. Accidents in single-engine/single-pilot aircraft are more common. More common still are accidents in private pilot flying, where the fatal accident rate is about 1 in 50 000 h flown. About 80 per cent of all and 60 per cent of fatal accidents are due to some form of human failure. Medical conditions causing temporary or incomplete incapacitation are not uncommon in flight but are a rare cause of accidents. The most common cause of inflight incapacitation is acute gastroenteritis; acute vestibular problems and headache cause a few instances each. In dual-pilot commercial flying, however, accidents due to complete incapacitation are rare. With adequate incapacitation, training accidents should occur in less than 1 per cent of cases. The inter-

Fig. 10 The incidence of decompression sickness (percentage) at the end of 2 h of exposure to various altitudes in men at rest, or exerting themselves.

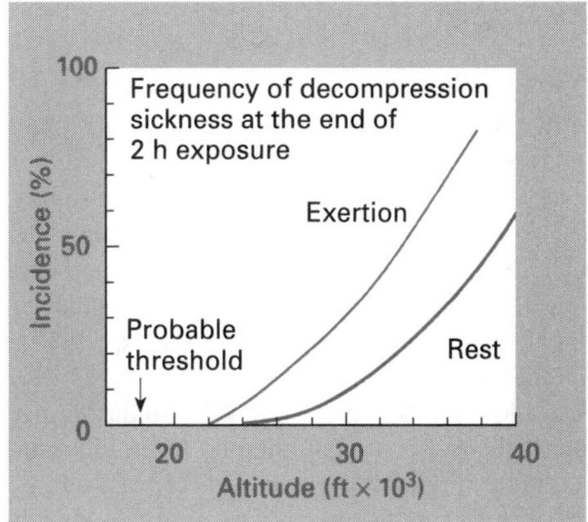

national target for flight safety is that an accident should occur in fewer than 1 in 10^7 aircraft flights and that failure of a single system, including the pilot, should occur in fewer than 1 in 10^8 flights. From this it can be calculated that in dual-pilot operations, with adequate incapacitation training, an acceptable risk of medical incapacitation is 1 per cent per year. Reductions below this will have little impact on flight safety and may actually increase accident rates by removing experienced aviators from flying. In areas where the intrinsic risk is greater, in crop spraying or military flying for example, risk assessment will be different.

Licensing structure

Civilian licensing authorities have the task of establishing the fitness to fly of an aircrew member. Physical standards are laid down in the United Kingdom by the Civil Aviation Authority. These standards differ according to the class of licence sought. There are three classes: Class 1—commercial pilot, airline transport pilot, and flight navigator and flight engineer; Class 2—private pilot, glider pilot, and balloon pilot; Class 3—air traffic controller. Fitness to fly is assessed for the duration of the appropriate licence. Restrictions may be imposed and the individual limited to a certain type of flying or, for example, only with a co-pilot. Military authorities differ in that they are the employing authorities as well as licensers for aircrew; they will take into account other factors such as long-term prognosis and the ability to operate in adverse physical conditions when considering their fitness to fly. Civilian employers, too, are concerned about the longer term and may be reluctant to employ aircrew with a history of illness that, although not disqualifying at the time, may lead to grounding in the future.

Because of the enormous financial investment involved in aircrew training the medical standards required for entry into pilot training are usually higher than those for trained pilots.

Medical considerations

Some medical conditions, hemiparesis, schizophrenia, convulsive disorders, and malignant disease for example, are obviously disqualifying because they render the crew member unable safely to perform the task. These will not be discussed further. Other conditions, for example most acute infections, are disqualifying when active but pose no threat when they have resolved. The conditions that cause most problems are those that are occult or have occult manifestations that may cause sudden incapacitation in the aviation environment. This last group includes most cardiovascular disease, the most common problem in clinical aviation medicine.

CARDIOVASCULAR DISEASE

Ischaemic heart disease

Over half the medical conditions leading to the loss of a licence in the United Kingdom are due to cardiovascular disease and most of these are due to coronary artery disease.

Asymptomatic coronary artery disease

This remains one of the major problems in clinical aviation medicine. There are many anecdotal reports of entirely asymtomatic aircrew dying suddenly of myocardial infarction. To attempt to screen for coronary disease, routine medical examinations of aircrew include standard electrocardiograms, which are scrutinized for signs of ischaemic heart disease. Unfortunately, particularly in young aircrew, minor changes in the ST segment may be entirely non-specific, but they do require elucidation. The standard procedure is to perform an exercise stress test. Unfortunately, this too has a low-positive predictive value in the young, asymptomatic population. If the test is normal, then no further investigation is required; if not, then gallium scintigraphy and coronary angiography may be needed to exclude significant coronary artery disease. It is usually accepted that a 50 per cent obstructive lesion on angiography constitutes significant disease and this would lead to the loss of licence.

Myocardial infarction

Myocardial infarction is disqualifying and in most instances aircrew will not regain flying status after an infarct. If studies after the event, including satisfactory left ventricular function and coronary angiography, meet laid-down criteria, limited certification may be considered after 1 year.

Coronary artery bypass grafting

Limited certification after coronary artery bypass grafting may also be considered, subject to repeated investigation to determine patency and absence of significant disease in the engrafted vessels. As long as ventricular function is good, individuals at low initial risk do well after bypass surgery and their mortality from coronary events is as low as in a matched control group. Follow-up studies on angioplasty are not as satisfactory and early restenosis is not uncommon; more stringent criteria for recertification should therefore apply.

Hypertension

As part of good medical practice, hypertension in aircrew should be investigated and treated. The following limits are recommended: age below 40 years, 145/90; age 40 to 49, 155/95, and age over 50, 160/100. If pressures above this level are sustained the aircrew member should be treated. Standard non-pharmacological methods are tried first and if these are unsuccessful drug therapy is initiated. Thiazide diuretics are recommended as first-line treatment and if this is unsatisfactory then a β-blocking agent added. A flight-simulator check is required before returning aircrew to flying taking β-blocking drugs. Angiotensin-converting enzyme inhibitors and calcium channel-blocking drugs may be considered if the standard regimen is unsatisfactory but initiation must be done with the subject off flying status and under close supervision. Again, a simulator flight is required before flying is resumed. If there are no other risk factors an aircrew member may be returned to flying status if the blood pressure can be kept within the above limits.

Arrhythmias

This is another area of great difficulty. Asymptomatic atrial and ventricular ectopic activity may be discovered on a routine electrocardiogram or on an exercise test made for some other reason. It is accepted that ventricular ectopic beats are probably not of any serious prognostic significance in the absence of underlying heart disease. If discovered, a full evaluation is required before returning to flying. Sustained ventricular tachyarrhythmias, paroxysmal atrial tachycardia, and paroxysmal atrial fibrillation are incompatible with flying. Well-controlled atrial fibrillation may allow limited flying, though the risk of systemic embolus must be taken into account. If a short-lived episode of atrial fibrillation has occurred as a result of an acute febrile episode, thyrotoxicosis, or excess caffeine or alcohol ingestion, then, after a full evaluation and appropriate treatment, return to flying may be allowed.

Thromboembolic disease

If acute pulmonary embolus develops after trauma or prolonged bedrest, then, following conventional anticoagulation, return to flying is usual. If no such preceding cause is present, clinical evaluation to exclude other causes such as an occult underlying malignancy must be undertaken. The risk of recurrence is that much greater and return to flying will be allowed only after a period of observation. Recurrent pulmonary embolus is permanently disqualifying.

Valvular disease and valve replacement

The risks of thromboembolism, arrhythmias, and heart failure in patients with significant aortic and mitral stenosis and mitral regurgitation are contraindications to flying. In those with mild aortic regurgitation who otherwise have a normal cardiac evaluation, flying may be allowed subject to regular review. The long-term problems with valve replacement include thromboembolism, valve failure, and endocarditis. Long-term anticoagulation will not allow flying. It is therefore likely that patients with valve replacement will be unfit to fly as aircrew.

Electrocardiographic abnormalities

First-degree heart block is often a manifestation of a high degree of physical conditioning and occurs together with sinus bradycardia in habitual exercisers. If it disappears on exercise or after atropine it may be ignored. Second-degree and complete heart block will usually be disqualifying. Isolated right bundle-branch block may develop over the years and as long as underlying heart disease is excluded is not a bar to flying. Left bundle-branch block is much more likely to be associated with organic heart disease and is usually incompatible with flying.

Pacemakers

A significant number of patients in whom pacemakers are implanted are below retiring age and some aircrew are therefore seen with this problem. In most instances the underlying cardiac condition will be disqualifying. A return to restricted flying would be considered in the rest only after a very full evaluation.

RESPIRATORY DISEASE

Asthma

People with asthma often have difficulty in assessing its true severity and aircrew with the condition may fly unaware of how severe it is. Exacerbations of asthma are often precipitated by upper respiratory infections. If such an exacerbation occurs when the aircrew member is overseas, there is considerable pressure on the individual to fly; alternatively, serious disruption of flight scheduling may result. An acute episode of asthma in flight is likely to interfere seriously with the flying task and has been reported to result in loss of control of the aircraft. Aircrew with very mild, intermittent asthma requiring only occasional treatment are fit to fly. Those with more continuous symptoms requiring regular suppressive medication, inhaled steroids, or cromoglycate are fit for restricted licensing provided their asthma is well controlled. Those whose symptoms persist in spite of medication or who have very reactive airways with unexpected attacks are unfit to fly.

Spontaneous pneumothorax

There is a high recurrence rate in simple spontaneous pneumothorax; 30 per cent after the first episode and 50 per cent after the second. Definitive treatment, usually pleurectomy, is recommended after a first pneumothorax before returning an individual to flying duty. Once this is accomplished, return to unrestricted flying is allowed.

Sarcoidosis

The chief anxiety about sarcoidosis in aircrew is the possible presence of occult myocardial involvement. This is associated with sudden incapacitation and death. All aircrew with sarcoidosis require a full cardiovascular evaluation, including rest, exercise, and 24 h electrocardiography and gallium scintigraphy. Those with evidence of cardiac involvement will be permanently grounded. In the absence of detectable cardiac involvement, with no evidence of disease activity and with normal pulmonary physiology, aircrew may return to restricted flying.

PSYCHIATRIC DISEASE

Alcohol use and abuse by aircrew

Aircrew are often placed in a high-risk environment for the use or abuse of alcohol. The flying task is often stressful and crew may use alcohol in an attempt to deal with this stress. They are often away from home, living in hotels abroad where alcohol is freely available and cheap. They are part of a team and the bar is the usual place to meet and socialize. There is the 'macho' culture, particularly of military pilots of fast jets, where 'a few beers' is a near essential part of the group behaviour. In general aviation accidents in the United States (this excludes commercial airline and military flying) the consumption of alcohol before flight is a significant contributory factor. In commercial and military flying, though the prevalence of heavy drinking is not different from that in general aviation, accidents due to alcohol are much less common. Alcohol is a depressant of central nervous functions and impairment of higher skills may be found at alcohol concentrations as low as 5.4 mmol/l. A standard drink of 15 g alcohol may result in a peak alcohol concentration of 4.3 to 8.7 mmol/l and even at these levels the complex task of flying an aircraft may be affected. Alcohol is metabolized by the body at an average rate of 8 g/h. It is evident that no pilot should fly while there is still a measurable amount of alcohol in his or her system. Measurable effects on vestibular function are, however, present for up to 34 h after moderate to heavy drinking, even when blood alcohol levels are at or near zero. In addition, hangover can significantly impair flying performance. In aircrew with a severe alcohol problem, withdrawal fits may occur during flight. The prevalence of heavy drinking in aircrew differs little from the general population and aircrew may underestimate the effect of a given amount of alcohol on their blood levels and the time required to metabolize this. Most airlines and military organizations insist on 8 h between 'bottle-to-throttle'. It is suggested that this is probably insufficient and that a 12-h rule for moderate drinking and 24 h for heavy drinking (five or more standard drinks) would be more appropriate.

The management of heavy drinking depends first on identifying the aircrew member affected. This may be difficult, as there is a tendency for other members to shield the person concerned. Once identified, specialist advice should be sought. If a significant alcohol problem is present, grounding is mandatory and no flying will be allowed until a substantial period of total abstinence is complete. Should drinking at any level recommence, grounding is permanent.

Psychotic and neurotic illness

Psychotic illness is a cause for permanent grounding. Anxiety or depressive states require grounding until remission occurs. Providing resolution is rapid and complete, return to flying may be allowed subject to regular review. Aircrew should not fly taking psychotropic medication.

Sleep disturbance

Sleep disturbance in aircrew is of great importance both in civilian and military flying. When pathological causes have been eliminated it usually has one of two causes, irregular flight schedules and jet lag. It is obviously inappropriate to have aircrew flying at times when their performance is suboptimal, and the organization of rosters and flight schedules should be undertaken with informed medical advice.

Passengers

INTRODUCTION

The stress of modern of travel should not be underestimated. Today, because of the necessity for a high degree of security, passengers on international flights are required to check in at least 2 h before departure. The modern airport, although sparing exposure to the elements, often has very long walkways and unless prior arrangements have been made it may be difficult to obtain help. Elderly travellers may find it difficult to cope, particularly if weighed down with hand baggage. With modern aircraft, individual stages are long, often over 12 h, adding considerably to the stress and exhaustion.

Passengers with no declared medical history may suffer an unexpected medical event in flight, such as a myocardial infarction. They may also be involved in cabin accidents. Passengers with a declared medical condition may, because of the various stresses involved with flight, have an exacerbation or complication of their declared condition. Airlines have a responsibility for providing medical and first-aid boxes, and adequate training of their flight attendants to deal with such emergencies. In addition, the major airlines have a medical department or have access to a suitably trained staff to provide passengers with pre-flight advice. All passengers requiring regular medication must remember to carry their drugs in their hand baggage.

IN-FLIGHT ACCIDENTS AND MEDICAL INCIDENTS

Accidents are rare and are usually due to sudden turbulence. If passengers are not restrained they may suffer trauma from being thrown around the cabin or they may be struck by objects that are improperly stowed. Modern passenger aircraft fly at altitudes where turbulence is less common and passengers are encouraged to wear seat belts at all times when seated. Regulations on stowage of cabin baggage have also been improved. In British Airways in 1979/80 there were 1063 accidents reported, of which eight were classed as major. It is noteworthy that half the accidents were to flight attendants. The risk of a passenger suffering a major accident in flight is $1{:}4.25 \times 10^6$. Over the same time there were 1328 medical incidents; in contrast to the accidents, very few of these involved aircrew. The risk for a passenger was 1:1300 per flight and if a medical condition had been declared the risk was 1:350 per flight. In-flight deaths are uncommon and between 1947 and 1967 there was a total of 90 in-flight deaths. As expected, the vast majority of these were cardiovascular, with myocardial infarction being the cause in 34 and heart failure in a further six; other causes included cancer (13) and cerebrovascular disease (7).

Aeromedical problems

Hypoxia

Most commercial airliners cabins are pressurized to 6000 to 8000 ft. At this altitude the partial pressure of oxygen in the alveoli will have fallen from about 13.5 to about 10 kPa. In the normal individual this will lead to a fall of about 3 per cent in the saturation of haemoglobin with oxygen. This is not of significance but, of course, in patients with cardio-respiratory disease it may be important.

Change in gas volume

With the decrease in ambient pressure there will be an increase in unrestrained gas volumes of 30 per cent. In the normal individual who is able to clear the ears and has no pockets of gas that cannot be voided, this may cause nothing more than slight discomfort in the ears and abdomen. If, however, the eustachian tube is blocked, otitic and sinus barotrauma may result. Passengers should not fly with sinusitis or otitis media, and those with upper respiratory infections should be treated with decongestants. For similar reasons, patients should not fly after recent ear surgery (particularly stapedectomy), eye surgery, laparotomy, thoracotomy or spontaneous pneumothorax unless a chest drain is in place. Plaster casts may expand if new and so should be split before travel.

SPECIFIC CONDITIONS

Respiratory

It is a common problem to be asked whether a patient with chronic respiratory disease is fit to fly. At 6000 ft the partial pressure of oxygen in the inspired air is 17 kPa. The approximate alveolar partial pressure at various cabin altitudes can be calculated from the alveolar gas equation and the arterial partial pressure estimated from this (Table 1).

Reduction in the partial pressure of inspired oxygen presents a potential hazard to patients with chronic airways obstruction. It is often recommended that supplemental oxygen should be provided if the arterial tension falls below 6.5 kPa. Equations to predict $P\text{AO}_2$ at altitude in normocapnoeic patients with chronic airways obstruction have been derived:

Table 1 *Calculation of alveolar partial pressure at various cabin altitudes*

Cabin altitude (ft × 10³)	Barometric pressure (kPa)	PO_2 approx. (kPa) Cabin	Alveolar	Arterial
0	100	21	13.5	12.8
2	93	19	12.3	11.8
6	80	16.7	10.1	8.4
8	74	15.5	9.0	7.9

$$Pa\text{O}_2\ \text{Alt} = 0.410(Pa_{\text{O}_2}\text{G}) + 17.650$$

$$Pa\text{O}_2\ \text{Alt} = 0.519(Pa_{\text{O}_2}\text{G}) + 11.855(\text{FEV}_1) - 1.760.$$

Where $Pa\text{O}_2$ Alt is the derived arterial oxygen tension in mmHg at a cabin altitude of 8000 ft, $Pa\text{O}_2$ G is the measured arterial oxygen tension at ground level in mmHg, and FEV_1 the forced expiratory volume in 1.

These provide an estimate of the 'worst case scenario'. If these provide a satisfactory result the patient can be considered fit to fly; those who have an unacceptably low result (< 6.5 kPa) should probably undergo hypoxic gas-inhalation testing or altitude-chamber testing. It must be emphasized that these equations apply only to chronic airways obstruction. For those with other forms of hypoxic chronic respiratory disease, further assessment will be necessary. In any form of respiratory disease, dyspnoea at rest is a contraindication to flying. If the predicted or measured altitude arterial oxygen tension is less than 6.5 kPa, then supplemental oxygen may be required in flight. The medical division of the airline should be contacted without delay for this to be arranged. Well-controlled asthma presents no problems in flight. Patients should be advised to take their medication as prescribed. Pressurized dose inhalers can be used quite safely at altitude.

Cardiovascular disease

The degree of hypoxia caused by an altitude of 6000 ft may cause deleterious effects in patients with unstable angina and they are therefore not fit to fly. Well-controlled angina with a good exercise tolerance at ground level is not a contraindication to flying. Patients who have recently had a myocardial infarction are at greater risk than the normal population. Although some airlines are willing to allow passengers to fly 2 weeks after an infarct, it is probably safer to advise waiting for 2 months. Uncontrolled cardiac failure is incompatible with flying. The stress of the airport procedures seems more of a problem than the flight itself and many of the problems occur on the ground. As a general rule, those with cardiac disease whose exercise tolerance at ground level is about 80 m and who can manage 12 stairs without symptoms should be able to fly safely. Those with even moderate exercise intolerance will require help at the departure and the arrival airport, and this must be arranged with the airline well before departure.

Neurological disease

Hypoxia adversely affects cerebrovascular disease and this together with the disorientating and tiring aspects of the journey may cause elderly people to become confused. Those who have had a history of nocturnal confusion should be accompanied by a friend or relative. Passengers should not fly within 3 weeks of a stroke. Tiredness, alcohol, and stress may increase the chance of a fit in epileptic passengers. Those whose fits have not been well controlled in the recent past should consider increasing their anticonvulsive medication before flight and continuing this until arrival. They should maintain the timing of their medication at their home time-zone and change this only in small increments when at their destination.

Psychiatric disease

Most psychiatric patients require only the care and courtesy afforded to other patients. They often do not regard themselves as ill and so may actively resent efforts to help them and they may also behave unpredictably. It is important, then, that they are accompanied by someone with whom they are familiar. Pre-flight briefing is also important so that they are not confronted with unexpected situations. All their medication should be continued and should be taken on a fixed time schedule to avoid the problems with changing times. Those on monoamine oxidase-inhibiting drugs should have tyramine-free diets arranged before they travel. It should be remembered that the anticholinergic effects of medication predispose to discomfort due to abdominal gas distension in flight and in heavily sedated patients this may be severe. Urinary retention is also a possibility. Heavy sedation also predisposes to deep venous thrombosis and barotrauma, and such patients are best managed supine on a stretcher. These can be arranged with the airline's medical department but it must be understood that a charge will be levied for the seat space occupied. If necessary, pre-flight sedation is best accomplished with chlorpromazine or benzodiazepines.

Haematological conditions

Severe anaemia will accentuate the problems of hypoxia and patients with a haemoglobin of less than 8 g probably should not fly without a full assessment, including hypoxic gas testing under controlled conditions. Pre-flight transfusion may be necessary. Sickle-cell crisis may be precipitated by the hypoxic conditions in people with sickle-cell haemoglobin C disease and sickle-cell β-thalassaemia. Such individuals should be encouraged not to fly. If, however, travel by air is essential, then additional inspired oxygen should be used throughout the flight. The risk of a sickle-cell crisis in straightforward sickle-cell disease is quite small and people with sickle-cell trait may fly safely in pressurized aircraft.

Ear, nose, and throat

The risks of otitic and sinus barotrauma in those with upper respiratory conditions has already been mentioned. Of greater importance is the risk of severe injury to the vestibulocochlear apparatus that may occur following middle-ear surgery. The replacement of the ossicles by a prosthesis allows transmission of pressure changes directly to the oval window from the tympanic membrane. In those in whom the maleus has been replaced, if there is obstruction of the eustachean tube, prosthesis displacement may occur with pressure changes, leading to severe damage. This is most likely to occur soon after surgery. When flying they should actively clear their ears at the onset of a descent and should continue to do so until on the ground. In those who have had more major surgery with an open tympanic cavity, such problems do not arise.

Endocrine

The most common endocrinological problem causing concern in passengers is insulin-dependent diabetes. The problems arise because of changing time-zones and the possibility of travel sickness. If possible, the best management is to stick to the departure time-zone as regards the injection of insulin and to cover this with food or snacks, which will be available from the cabin staff. On very long distance flights crossing numerous time-zones the airline's medical department should be notified to ensure that food is available at appropriate intervals. For those prone to travel sickness, prophylactic treatment is recommended.

Pregnancy

There is no excess risk of flying in pregnancy. To avoid confinement in the air, most airlines place a limit of 35 weeks. Of course this applies to the return journey as well and so passengers should plan their vacation to return before this.

Motion sickness

With modern high-flying aircraft this is rarely a problem. Those who are particularly susceptible should take an appropriate proprietary drug before the flight.

Gastrointestinal disease

Recent gastrointestinal haemorrhage is a contraindication to flying as distension has been associated with an increased risk of rebleeding. Patients with ileostomies and colostomies should be warned of the probability that they will produce an increased volume of gas at altitude and that they should therefore carry spare bags.

Deep venous thrombosis

There is a considerable body of anecdotal data that deep venous thrombosis may occur as a result of prolonged flight in seats which are often cramped and which restrict leg movements. There is now more direct evidence that this occurs and such thromboses have resulted in pulmonary embolus. This should therefore be taken into account when advising passengers who are at particular risk, for example those who have a previous history of venous thrombosis or pulmonary embolus, pregnant women, or those with clotting abnormalities. Such persons should be encouraged to perform leg exercises at fixed intervals through the flight and to walk the aisles if possible. If the medical department is contacted early, seats with good leg room or seats on the aisle can be prearranged. In those thought to be at very high risk the prescription of graduated compression stockings should be considered.

Jet lag

When flying east to west or vice versa (transmeridian flights) covering several time-zones there is often a disturbance of well-being that is known as jet lag. The symptoms include insomnia, tiredness, an inability to concentrate, loss of appetite, and irritability. This is of obvious importance in aircrew but is also of importance to business people who may make short transatlantic visits to conduct important affairs. Unless appropriate advice is taken they may schedule meetings at times when they are not best placed to make important decisions. Every human being experiences a regular alteration between sleep and wakefulness. This is innate but is also dependent on external cues such as light and darkness, and also social cues. Removal of these external influences, for example by sensory deprivation in caves, allows the innate diurnal variation to establish itself and this has a time constant in most individuals longer than 24 h (that is, most people are trying to extend their days and given no external clues would go to sleep an hour later each day). Travel from west to east results in delayed sleep. Initiation of sleep is often easy because the individual is going to bed so late, but sleep later in the night is disturbed as the time for rising at the home time-zone is reached. Adaptation occurs fairly rapidly. Important meetings should be scheduled after adaptation has been achieved. If this is not possible, then they should be arranged for a time at which full alertness would be expected at the home time-zone. The use of hypnotics that are rapidly eliminated and therefore free of hangover and accumulation is appropriate to sustain sleep for the first few nights when travelling west. Travelling east causes more of a disturbance because time-zone changes 'shorten' the traveller's day. This is against the normal tendency and adaptation is more prolonged. Initiation of sleep may be difficult because the traveller is going to bed in the afternoon of his or her home time-zone. A fast-acting hypnotic is required to initiate sleep. An appropriate hypnotic for both situations is temazepam, though if available brotizolam has been shown to be very effective.

REFERENCES

Aircraft Accident Digest No. 30 (1986). International Civil Aviation Organization, Montreal.

AMA Commission on Emergency Medical Services (1982). Medical aspects of transport aboard commercial aircraft. *Journal of the American Medical Association,* **247,** 1007–11.

Beighton, P.H. and Richards, P.R. (1968). Cardiovascular disease in air travellers. *British Heart Journal,* **30,** 367–72.
Bennett, G. (1988). Pilot incapacitation and aircraft accidents. *European Heart Journal,* **9**(suppl. G), 21–4.
Chaitman, B.R. *et al.* (1986). Should airline pilots be eleigible to resume active flight status after coronary bypass surgery? A CASS registry study. *Journal of the American College of Cardiology,* **8,** 1318–24.
Chamberlain, D. (1988). Ischaemic heart disease. *European Heart Journal,* **9**(suppl. G) 69–72.
Dillard, T.A., Berg, B.W., and Rajogopal, K.R. (1989). Hypoxaemia during air travel in patients with chronic obstructive pulmonary disease. *Annals of Internal Medicine,* **111,** 362–7.
Jones, D.R. (1980). Aeromedical transportation of psychiatric patients; historical review and present management. *Aviation and Space Environmental Medicine,* **51,** 709–16.
Ledermann, J.A. and Keshavarzian, A. (1983). Acute pulmonary embolism following air travel. *Postgraduate Medical Journal,* **59,** 104–5.
McIntyre, D., Moran, F., and Banham, S.W. (1982). Pulmonary embolism: a long-term follow up. *Postgraduate Medical Journal,* **58,** 222–5.
MacLaren, R.B. (1982). *Inflight medical care by flight attendants—an assessment of overall needs.* Preprints of the Aerospace Medical Association, pp. 305–6. Aerospace Medical Association, Washington DC.
Modell, J.G. and Mountz, J.M. (1990). Drinking and flying—the problem of alcohol use by pilots. *New England Journal of Medicine,* **323,** 455–61.
Moser, M. (1990). Fitness of civil aviation passengers to fly after ear surgery. *Aviation and Space Environmental Medicine,* **61,** 735–7.
Robertson, J.I.S. (1988). The management of hypertension in aircrew. *European Heart Journal,* **9**(suppl. G), 41–4.
Ross, S.M. and Ross, L.E. (1990). Pilots' knowledge of blood alcohol levels and the 0.04% blood alcohol concentration rule. *Aviation and Space Environmental Medicine,* **61,** 412–17.

8.5.5(f) Diving medicine

D.M. DENISON

We often think of humans as able creatures that have conquered the globe, but almost three-quarters of the Earth's surface is covered by sea, which they invade with very little success indeed. Other mammals, such as dolphins, explore it with much greater mastery because they have various features, such as a highly streamlined shape, a much thicker layer of subcutaneous fat, a more mobile chest wall, and bronchioles reinforced all the way to the alveoli, which men are unable to engineer or match for themselves except by very cumbersome means.

Because this is so, human divers are exposed to many hazards that marine mammals avoid. Frequently it is too late or too impractical to give divers specific help once they are in trouble, so diving medicine is largely concerned with prevention. It depends upon a thorough understanding of the job a diver must do and the risks he runs in completing it. In this sense, almost every diving accident is a failure of education or equipment design. However, many well-trained and well-equipped divers come to grief when they are driven or drive themselves beyond limits that are clearly understood but expensive to maintain.

This chapter begins with a description of the environment, which is usually dark, cold, and too deep to stay in without risk for much time. After discussing some features of the sea, and the basic but minor problems of vision, hearing, dexterity, and mobility, it concentrates on the major hazards of air embolism, inert gas narcosis, oxygen toxicity, decompression sickness, the high-pressure syndrome, and the difficulty of keeping warm. It finishes with notes on the selection and general medical care of divers, and some observations on long-term health effects of diving.

THE CONTOUR OF THE SEA BED

Most people have a hazy idea of the contour of the sea bed (Fig. 1). Leaving a typical shore, the sea bed falls away gently, with a slope of about 1:50 until it is 200 to 300 m deep. This shallow stretch is the Continental Shelf. It then angles more steeply (roughly 1:15), the Continental Slope, to descend to vast flat expanses of soft mud, known as the Abyssal Plains, which lie at depths of 3 to 6 km. These are interrupted by occasional mountain peaks and deep chasms. One of the mountains is slightly taller than Mount Everest. The deepest point is just over 11 km below the surface.

Various deep currents, arising from differences in water temperature and salinity, take regular courses across the Abyssal Plains, welling up the sides of the Continental Shelves as mineral-rich streams. These supply the vegetable life that exists in the sunlit upper zone. The animals that feed on these plants, or on each other, become concentrated in these waters so that 80 per cent of the biological wealth of the sea lies in the top 0.2 km, mainly close to the Continental Shelves. Put together, these sites form an area equal to that of Africa, infinitely more fertile, and, as yet unfarmed.

At the surface, regular tidal currents vary widely in velocity from point to point as they are accelerated or slowed down by features of the shore. They often exceed the speed at which humans can swim (Fig. 2(a), so that it may only be practical to dive in slack water, i.e. for an hour or two each day. Similarly, waves are often sufficiently tall to prevent a diver being launched into the sea or recovered with safety (Fig. 2(b)). These surface phenomena rarely penetrate below 100 m or so, but tidal currents can be tunnelled along marine canyons, and springs of fresh water, or falls of cold ocean water, can carry divers in unex-

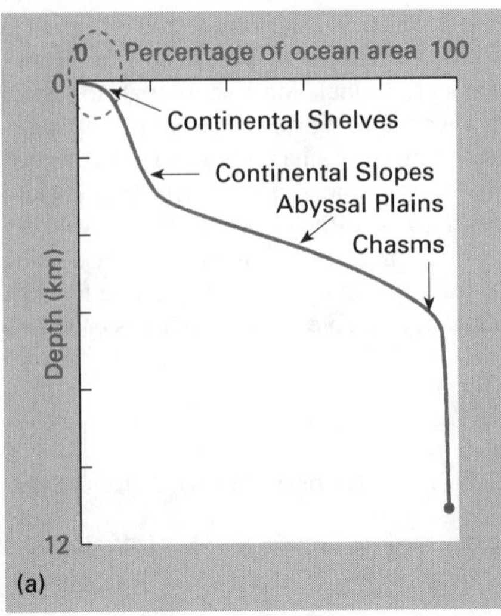

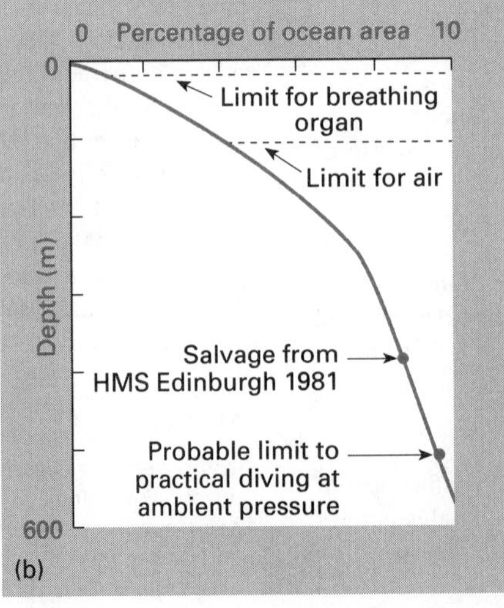

Fig. 1 (a) A cumulative depth versus area plot of the oceans. (b) A similar plot of the top 600 m, including the Continental Shelves.

pected directions without them necessarily being aware that they are moving at all.

VISION

Most recreational diving takes place in clear warm waters at placid times of the year, but many tasks in professional diving, e.g. harbour work, hull inspections and repairs, pipe-line surveys, oil-rig work, and wreck salvage, occur throughout the year, alongside or beneath large obstructions, in waters where simply finding the task, let alone completing it properly, may be very demanding indeed.

There are many reasons why this should be so. During the middle of the day about 5 per cent of the light falling on the surface of the sea is reflected back to the sky, but, whenever the sun is lower, much more is reflected, so dawn arrives late and dusk comes early to the sea. The light that does penetrate the surface is quickly altered by absorption and scattering. On average, intensity halves with every 1 or 2 m of descent. In consequence, even in very clear water, it is effectively 'night' below 80 m. However, even in shallow water, for example in harbours, near estuaries, close to wrecks, and after storms, sea-water can be very turbid, blurring the boundaries of objects to such an extent that the diver may have to be within 15 cm or so of the objects to see them at all. In these circumstances, artificial illumination is often ineffective because of back-scattering.

Normally, some 65 dioptres of refracting power are needed to focus parallel rays of light on the retina, and two-thirds of this refraction occurs at the air–cornea interface. Under water, this boundary is lost unless some form of gas-filled goggles or mask are worn. If they are worn, the additional glass–water boundary makes objects seem 30 per cent bigger and nearer than they actually are. This distortion is easily adjusted to but very often the margins of the goggles or mask restrict the visual fields severely giving the diver a blinkered, as well as blurred, view of his surroundings.

HEARING AND BLAST INJURY

Under water, localization of sound is poor because binaural cues disappear. They are lost because sounds are transmitted almost five times as fast and many times more efficiently through water than air. So there is very little alteration or delay as sound passes from ear to ear. Localization is also affected by echoes bouncing from the air–water interface above and the water–ground boundary below. The loss of air-conduction alone raises auditory thresholds by 30 to 60 dB. The neoprene-foam hoods that keep the head warm raise them by a further 30 dB or so.

The superior transmission of sound in water also increases susceptibility to blast injury. This is important, even in civilian fields, because plastic explosives are often used to free propellers from shafts or to ease buried objects from marine concretions, and the sort of detonation that would leave a human unharmed at 5 m range in air would be sufficient to kill at the same range under water. Damage is mainly due to abrupt decompression and recompression of the lungs, gut, and sinuses (see later). Gas-free tissues, such as the liver and spleen, are usually undamaged. The air-filled foam of some wet suits provides some protection.

DEXTERITY AND MOBILITY

Except for the surface waters of tropical seas, all of the oceans are too cold for individuals to stay long without insulation (Fig. 3). In air, they maintain body temperature at 37 °C with minimal effort when the air temperature is 18 to 24 °C, the zone of thermal neutrality. In water, this zone is higher and very narrow (35–35.5 °C). Loss of tactile discrimination and manual dexterity are major problems for divers working in cold water. In general, there is a steep loss of discrimination once finger-skin temperature drops below 8 °C, and there is a substantial loss of dexterity and grip-strength whenever the effective cold exposure of the

Fig. 3 Variations in sea temperature with site and depth. Note that water temperatures less than 20 °C are too cold for unclothed individuals to stay in for very long.

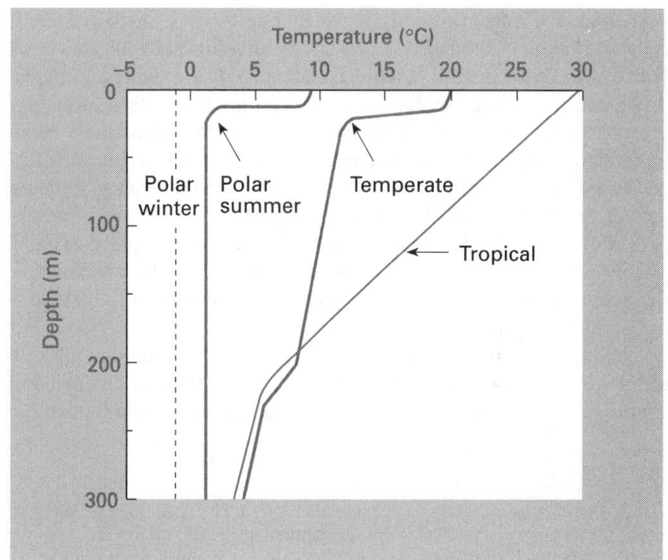

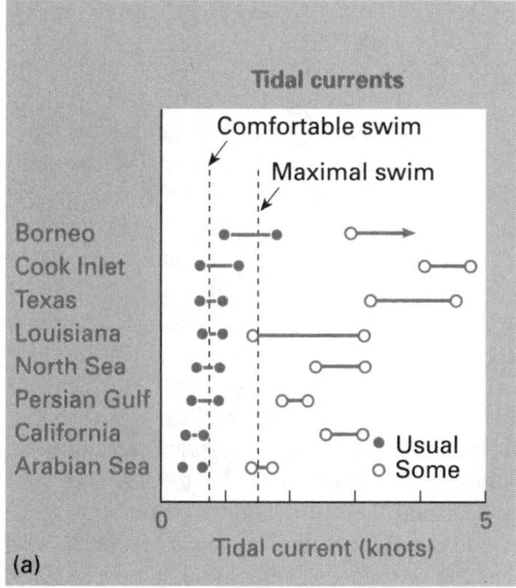

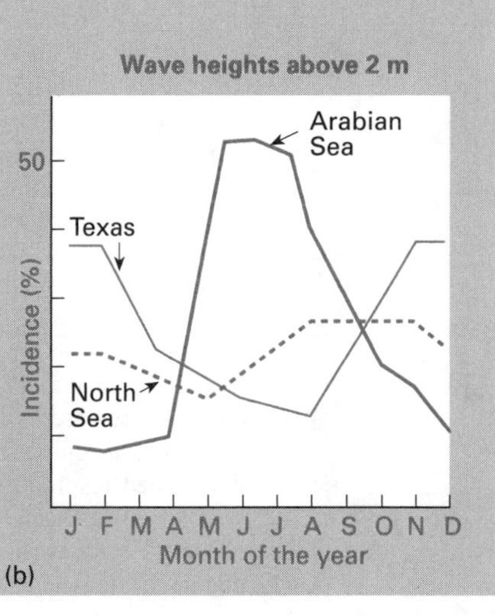

Fig. 2 (a) A plot of the usual and the not uncommonly seen tidal currents in eight diving sites around the world. (b) A plot of the percentage incidence of waves exceeding a height of 2 m at different times of the year in three of the diving sites.

forearm exceeds that of 20 °C water for 30 min. Re-examination of Fig. 3 indicates how easily such conditions are realized.

The most serious, and least tractable, problems of diving occur from working in a dense and viscous medium. Water is some 1300 times denser than air. Because it is virtually incompressible (the water at the deepest part of the ocean is 4 per cent denser than at the surface), ambient pressure rises linearly with depth. It does so, at very nearly 1 atm for every 10 m descent. Thus at 10 m depth, the surrounding pressure is 2 atm (one of water plus one of air), at 20 m it is 3 atm, and so on. Immersion in a fluid of this density makes the diver weightless and vertically unstable; it opposes any movement generating turbulent flow and exposes him to much higher pressures than on land. As water is also many times more viscous than air, it is useless as a ventilating fluid and opposes any body motion generating streamline flow.

When a diver enters water his body becomes 'weightless' because the density of sea-water, blood, tissue fluids, and the body as a whole are very nearly the same. As a result, his tissues are rehung on the skeleton, and blood and other fluids are displaced upwards, some 500 ml entering the chest, distending the large veins and the right atrium. Stretch receptors in the chest interpret this signal as an excess circulating volume and promote diuresis until the central distension is reduced to its normal value. When the man emerges from the water the normal hydrostatic gradient of body materials is unopposed and blood drops away from the chest, leaving the man hypovolaemic. Any negative pressure-breathing exaggerates this effect (see later).

Because the immersed body is weightless it can be displaced vertically with ease. Although this permits the diver to poise himself anywhere or examine the full height of a submerged rig at will, it is a great disadvantage, because he can no longer use his body weight to apply leverage or torque, or to stay in place when a current is running. More importantly, any vertical movement can quickly become uncontrolled because of the positive feedback between depth and buoyancy. Because the gas in the chest and abdomen is compressible, the deeper a breath-hold diver goes, the denser he becomes and the more rapidly he falls. The higher he rises, the less dense he becomes and the faster he ascends. Such changes should be seen in the context of the man's actual buoyancy and swimming power.

Although the rises of cardiac output and alveolar ventilation, with effort, are the same in air and water, much of the effort is dissipated in simply moving the limbs through the medium, making most tasks more tiring, and much less efficient below the surface than above (Fig. 4). The maximum sustained thrust that a swimmer can develop underwater is about 5 kg, which is just enough to propel him at about 1½ miles an hour. An opposing force of 5 kg, i.e. that weight on a string over a pully, would immobilize him. If a normally built man takes a full inspiration he is about 2.5 kg positively buoyant and so requires half of his maximum swim-power to descend. If he breathes out to residual volume he is about 2.5 kg negatively buoyant and needs half his maximum swim-power to ascend. The chest wall is a floppy structure that can only maintain a pressure difference equivalent to 1 or 2 m of sea-water, so the gas in the lungs is at virtually the same pressure as the water surrounding the chest. Thus a breath-hold diver leaving the surface with a full lung and diving 30 m (4 atm absolute) will compress his lung from total lung capacity to residual volume, forcing the man to use half his aerobic capacity to overcome positive buoyancy at the start of the dive and the same amount of effort to ascend. If he is wearing insulating clothing (e.g. a foam 'wet suit', normal buoyancy about 8 kg) the total changes in buoyancy are very close to maximum swimming capacity, leaving little margin for controlling unexpected ascent or descent.

Fig. 4 A comparison of oxygen consumption ($\dot{M}O_2$) when pedalling a cycle ergometer in air and underwater (a) at a constant speed (60 r.p.m.) and at a constant light load. Note the high cost of moving the limbs through water. Most people's aerobic capacity is about 2.5 litres O_2/min.

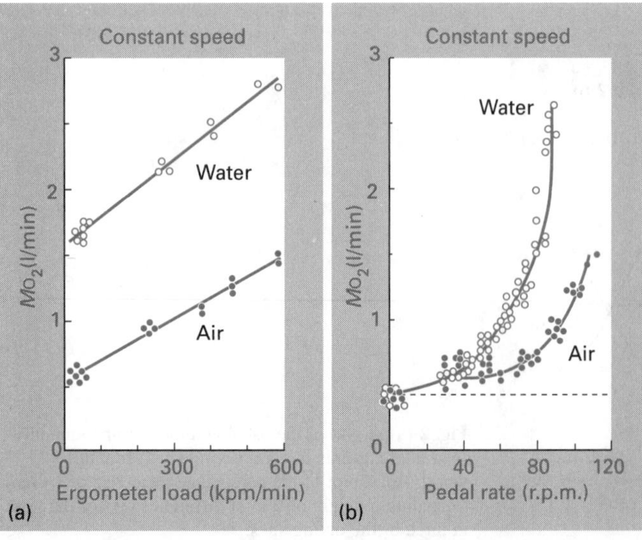

MECHANICAL EFFECTS OF COMPRESSION AND DECOMPRESSION

When a breath-hold diver descends the gas in his lungs is compressed by the surrounding water, according to Boyle's law, as just instanced. On return to the surface the gas will re-expand to its original volume, with no risk of lung rupture. However, if a diver has access to fresh gas at any time after leaving the surface, he can fill his lungs with enough gas to burst them on ascent, unless they are adequately vented. The principles that determine whether the lung will rupture have been mentioned in detail elsewhere (see Section 17): the lung can be considered as a cluster of tubes and balloons with bursting pressure of about 75 mmHg (1 m of sea-water) and time-constants of emptying that are normally close to 1 s. The latter may be grossly prolonged by injury, inhalation of water, or by disease. Divers are taught to exhale continuously whenever they ascend, and to ascend no faster than the bubbles they exhale. If people with healthy lungs ascend in this manner, the alveoli have time to empty sufficiently and the risk of lung rupture is very low. The mechanics of lung rupture are not clear. Contrary to common sense it does seem that people whose lungs are small for their body size but otherwise normal are at greater risk, perhaps because the chest wall can exert greater traction on the small lung. It appears also that people with entirely healthy lungs can rupture them simply by taking a vigorous deep breath, as in lung-function testing. Such episodes of spontaneous pneumomediastinum are usually asymptomatic. However, should they occur underwater the trapped gas will expand, causing serious injuries. For this reason, it presently seems wise to suggests that divers should never take extremely deep breaths underwater.

Lung rupture usually occurs in divers breath-holding while making emergency ascents after losing their gas supply. Central tears of lung tissue lead to mediastinal emphysema. Peripheral tears cause pneumothoraces. In both cases, but more commonly the former, gas may also enter the circulation as air emboli. Whether it is in the tissue, pleural space, or bloodstream, the escaped gas expands as the ascent continues, making matters worse. The victim usually notes dyspnoea, cough, or haemoptysis during the ascent, or no more than a few minutes later. If the tear is central he may also note dysphasia, voice change, or a sense of fullness in the throat or behind the sternum. On examination there may be surgical emphysema of the neck and upper chest, subcutaneous crepitus, increased cardiac dullness, or cardiac crepitus. If a pneumothorax has developed it is often accompanied by one-sided pleuritic pain, diminished respiratory movement, deviation of the trachea and apex beat, hyper-resonance, and distant breath sounds. If air embolism has occurred, there will be additional neurological signs. Patients with uncomplicated mediastinal and or superficial emphysema are treated by giving them pure oxygen to breathe, but they must never be positive-pressure ventilated. The oxygen accelerates bubble absorption by emptying the blood of inert gas so it is a more efficient sink for the gas in the bubble. After 2 or 3 days the emphysema will have subsided and the patient will be fit for release. Small pneumothoraces can be treated in the same way. If the pneumothorax is large it can be relieved in the ordinary way with a chest drain; however, if it is critically large at depth the patient should be recompressed immediately to reduce its size. This is rarely necessary for uncomplicated pneumothoraces. The chest drain must be clamped on compression and must be exposed to continuous suction at depth and during decompression.

If there is any evidence of air embolus, or any doubt about the diagnosis, the patient should immediately be laid semiprone, on his left side, with the head down and the buttocks up. He should be given oxygen, without positive-pressure ventilation, and be recompressed as soon as possible (details of recompression therapy are discussed below).

Lung rupture is the most worrying form of barotrauma (pressure damage) but others are more common. On descent, the diver may have difficulty in 'clearing his ears' because the mounting pressure on the outside of the drum is not balanced by an equal rise on the inner side, due to the valvular nature of the eustachian tube. This can be very painful, and may lead to drum rupture, but the strain on the drum usually resolves immediately on stopping the descent and ascending slightly. Sometimes the sinuses are affected on ascent or descent, in the same way. Pain on descent is always relieved by ascent. However, pain due to gas trapped in an obstructed space gets worse on ascent. Sometimes blood that has filled a sinus, and partly clotted during descent, is expelled in this manner as the diver returns to the surface. Occasionally, an ethmoid sinus may rupture into the cranial cavity. Usually, no specific treatment is needed for these injuries, but the diver is laid off diving until the cause has been established and he is fit to return. Pressure injuries also occur if the gas pressure inside the goggles, mask, or helmet does not keep pace with that outside. Sometimes, reversed-ear injury occurs because on descent the soft foam wet-suit helmet prevents a matching build-up of pressure in the external auditory canal, and the drum blows outwards.

INERT GAS NARCOSIS

Because the chest wall is a floppy structure, gas must be delivered to the diver at the same pressure as the water that surrounds him. This may be sent to him via an umbilical pipe from the surface, in which case it can flush through his helmet or face-mask continuously, which is wasteful of gas, but easily engineered, or it can supply a regulating valve that provides gas on demand only (surface-demand systems). Alternatively, the diver can take a self-contained underwater breathing apparatus (SCUBA) with him. This always feeds a demand regulator and rarely lasts for more than 1 h. Professional divers often use a combination of all three systems, i.e. a surface-demand supply for routine use, with a helmet-flushing capability for occasional comfort or emergency use, and a small, back-mounted gas supply ready in case the surface supply fails.

Nowadays, demand regulators and compensated outlet valves are well designed and there are few practical obstacles to providing the diver with gas at the right pressure. The composition of the gas to be breathed is a much more complex decision. Air can be breathed quite safely down to depths of 50 m, although tests of sophisticated cerebral function show there is already some impairment at 20 m. Below 50 m, mental deterioration becomes increasingly obvious, manifested by such actions as the diver offering his mouthpiece to neighbouring fish.

This condition is described as nitrogen narcosis or *'l'ivresse des profondeurs'*. It is a specific example of the more general condition of inert gas narcosis related to inhalation anaesthesia. An extension of the Meyer–Overton lipid solubility theory of anaesthesia supposes that the size or thickness of the nerve membrane, or some part of it, is dependent upon the size and number of gas molecules dissolved in it, and once the size or thickness of the membrane exceeds critical limits it cannot conduct an impulse. On descent breathing air, ambient and arterial nitrogen pressures rise, and more nitrogen dissolves in nerve membranes, making them thicker, until at a depth of about 50 m, interference in neural transmission becomes obvious functionally. Replacing the nitrogen molecules with smaller and less numerous helium molecules allows the membrane to shrink to an acceptable size and the impairment of function regresses (cf. replacing nitrogen molecules by bulkier xenon molecules, which is sufficient to cause anaesthesia at sea level). As would be expected, these changes in function develop within a few minutes and are rapidly reversible, because they depend purely on the process of passive chemical solution.

If men breathe an oxygen–helium mix, rather than air, they can descend to the lowermost parts of the Continental Shelves (730 m) without narcosis. Thus, nitrogen narcosis is a wholly preventable hazard in diving, which if it occurs by accident can be completely reversed within minutes, by ascent, and therefore needs no treatment. Unfortunately, helium is an expensive gas and there is an understandable reluctance for diving operators to use it. Medical advisers must oppose this and emphasize that it is dangerous for men to breathe air below a depth of 50 m or so.

HIGH-PRESSURE NERVOUS SYNDROME

At great depths, breathing oxygen ± helium mixtures, men show various neurological disturbances that are apparently not narcotic but are due to the direct effect of pressures on nerve tissues. This is thought to be so because very similar states can be induced in animals who are ventilated on fluorocarbon liquids containing normal sea-level quantities of oxygen and nitrogen or helium. It is also known that many organic and inorganic processes are disturbed by the applications of high barometric pressures *in vitro*. The high pressures are believed to alter the natural aggregations of water molecules, to increase the ionization of salts, oppose ionic bonding, liquefy gels, and cause various enzymes to fail. It appears to be the major obstacle to ambient-pressure diving much below the edges of the Continental Shelves. At present, men are able to make experimental dives to about 700 m. Various drugs have been investigated as modifiers of the syndrome, but its fundamental cause and protean manifestations suggest this depth will be close to the absolute limit to ambient-pressure diving.

OXYGEN TOXICITY

The hazards of inert gas narcosis, and of decompression illness (see below) could be avoided almost completely if people breathed pure oxygen when they dived. Unfortunately it becomes toxic to the lungs when the alveolar oxygen pressure exceeds half an atmosphere (5 m of sea water) and it becomes toxic to the nervous system when the alveolar, and the arterial, oxygen pressure exceed 2 atm (10 m of sea water). These effects are due to complex chemical interactions, rather than physical solution, and so take time to develop and reverse.

As mentioned elsewhere, respired oxygen is handled by a large number of enzymes and is used in very many ways. Some, such as the production and destruction of neurotransmitters and the synthesis of some steroid hormones, are critical. Increasing the amount of oxygen in simple solution not only affects the balance of some of these processes but also increases the risk of randomly forming the destructive superoxide ion. So, high-pressure oxygen affects body tissues in many ways.

It has two principal actions on the lung. Firstly, it promotes simple absorption atelectasis by replacing the relatively insoluble nitrogen in alveolar spaces. As their servant airways shut off due to transient obstructions, pulmonary blood flow rapidly removes the highly soluble oxygen and CO_2 causing the alveolar spaces to collapse, leading to linear regions of atelectasis that are most obvious in the well-perfused and more readily collapsed basal regions of the lung. Paradoxically, blood leaving the lung is then hypoxic due to admixture with blood perfusing the collapsed spaces.

Secondly, oxygen damages the lung by irritating its endothelial and epithelial surfaces. Some people suggest this is due to the extrapulmonary generation of a noxious agent because the endothelial damage appears first, but it is much more likely to be a direct action of alveolar oxygen on these surfaces. At first there is an exudation of fluid and proliferation of macrophages and an interference with surfactant production. This damage is reversible. If the exposure is prolonged, fibrosis occurs and the lung is permanently scarred.

The time taken for symptoms to appear depends upon the dose. It varies from several hours at half an atmosphere Po_2 to a few hours at 2 atm. Above that pressure, the neurological sequelae overshadow the pulmonary damage that still occurs (Fig. 5).

Oxygen interferes with nervous tissue in a manner that is not yet understood, perhaps because it disrupts many processes rather than one. It manifests itself by epileptiform convulsions that are sometimes, but not always, preceded by aura such as twitching of the face and hands. Any convulsion underwater is potentially fatal and must be avoided. There is a safe latent period, during which oxygen can be breached without any detectable harm to the central nervous system. This time is inversely proportional to depth (i.e. to Po_2). However, the time and threshold level can vary widely in the same individual from day to day. Retention of CO_2 and exertion lower the threshold and shorten the latent period. Like nitrogen narcosis, oxygen toxicity is a preventable hazard in diving. Divers should not breathe oxygen at partial pressures greater than 2 atm except under observation in the decompression chamber. Diving mixtures that are to be breathed for several hours should maintain inspired Po_2 between 0.5 and 1.0 atm. Those that are to be breathed for longer periods should maintain inspired Po_2 between 0.2 and 0.5 atm.

DECOMPRESSION ILLNESS

Oxygen toxicity, nitrogen narcosis, and the high-pressure nervous syndrome set depth limits to diving of 10, 50, and 500 m, respectively, and so are physicochemical obstacles to invading the sea. By contrast, the major medical hazard to diving, decompression sickness, is a physicochemical obstacle on returning from the sea. It occurs because, during any dive, extra inert gas, usually nitrogen or helium, goes into passive solution in the body. On ascent, as the ambient pressure falls, this gas can come out of solution in an uncontrolled way, forming bubbles in the circulation and within tissues. As the ascent continues, these bubbles increase in size and number, blocking blood vessels, and distorting or rupturing cells. On re-descent the bubbles contract and are eventually resorbed. If the first or the subsequent ascent is slow enough, few if any bubbles are formed, the extra gas diffuses into the bloodstream and out of the lungs easily, and the diver reaches the surface unharmed.

Experiments by Haldane at the turn of the century, which have been confirmed subsequently many times, suggest bubble formation occurs whenever ambient pressure falls below about half the total pressure of inert gas in solution. It follows that it is normally safe to ascend from dives to 10 m or less, without hesitation, however long they have endured, and to ascend without stopping, from any deeper dive that has been too brief to take this critical mass of gas on board. For any other dive, return to the surface must be delayed so the ratio of pressure of gas remaining in solution: ambient pressure never exceeds the critical value.

More recent work indicates that the critical value varies from tissue to tissue, and may not reflect a simple ratio of the dissolved nitrogen and ambient pressures, but could be determined by the absolute differences between the two pressures. Because, in general, it is unethical to explore these issues in man, and species differences in susceptibility to decompression illness are very marked, further understanding is most likely to come from accurate epidemiological observations in very large numbers of divers. The development of inexpensive miniature depth–time recorders that can easily be attached to a diver's weight-belt should be very helpful in this regard.

A vast amount of experimental work has been done to determine the safe limits to 'no-stop' diving and the depth–time profiles that have to be followed on returning to the surface after any longer dive. The time-limiting curve for 'no-stop' diving is shown in Fig. 6. It represents the time taken to accumulate 2 atm of dissolved gas in the tissues at the depths shown. The rate of gas accumulation in tissues is determined by the ratio of the solubility of the gas in that tissue to the speed of its blood flow. Because the tissues vary widely in these respects, the body behaves as if it were made up of a series of compartments, the 'fast' ones having short time-constants of inert gas uptake, and the 'slow' ones having long time-constants. The fast tissues such as working muscle dominate the time-course of safe short dives. The slow tissues such as body fat determine the safe ascent rate from long dives. Knowledge of safe practice is tabulated in a series of lengthy decompression schedules, which vary somewhat from one country to another, and are to be found in any textbook of diving medicine. After long (saturation) dives, the ascent is very slow and can take several days.

After relatively brief, shallow descents, divers can return to the surface slowly, stopping for a few minutes at scheduled depths. To do this they normally ascend up a marked shot-line. It is not practical or safe to ascend from deeper or longer dives in this manner, so a submersible recompression chamber is sent to the bottom to collect the diver and return him to the surface in warmth and comfort, or the divers make a limited number of stops in the water and then quickly ascend to the surface and immediately enter a deck-mounted chamber to be recompressed and then decompressed slowly and safely. Usually they are recompressed to 20 m and then given oxygen to breathe intermittently, to accelerate inert gas excretion.

Fig. 5 The pulmonary and central nervous O_2 toxicity versus time curves that are commonly observed (constructed from the data of many workers).

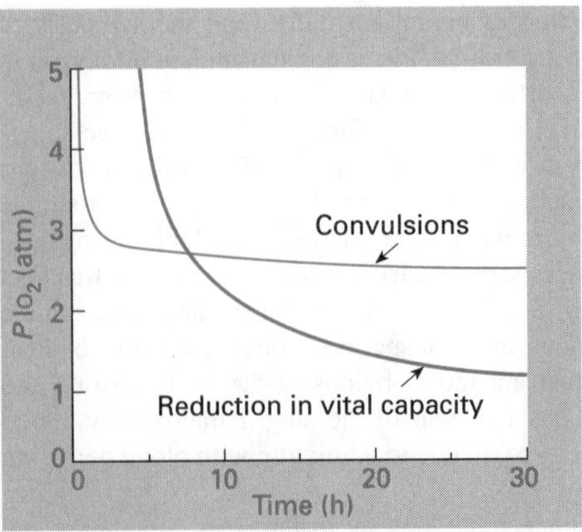

Fig. 6 The 'no-stop' diving curve that determines whether a dive has been shallow and brief enough for the diver to make a free ascent to the surface.

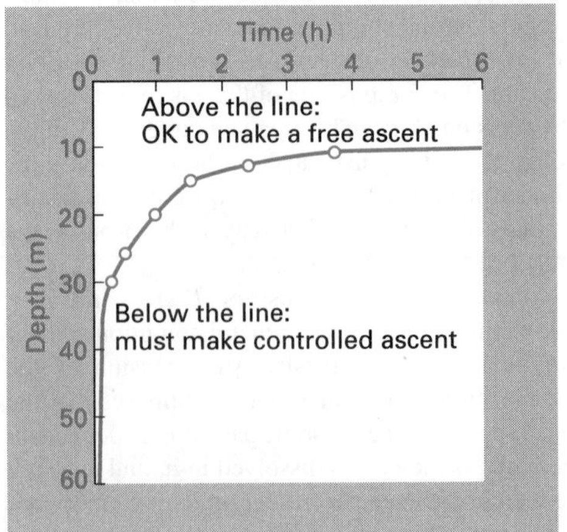

About 1 per cent of dives conducted to authorized schedules, and many badly conducted dives, lead to decompression sickness. This can take two forms, skin irritation or limb pain only (type 1 'bends'), or any other serious manifestation (type 2 'bends'). Skin irritation and mottling alone is treated by oxygen inhalation at the surface and does not require recompression. It is the mildest form of decompression sickness. All other cases should be recompressed as soon as possible. This is the only effective treatment. The object is to reduce the size of existing bubbles and prevent the formation of new ones, before irreversible infarction and oedema have occurred.

About half of all cases involve the central nervous system, most often the lower cervical, the thoracic, or the upper lumbar segments of the spinal cord. Visual disturbances and other cerebral signs are seen often also. Many others involve limb pain, commonly of the shoulders or elbows in divers and of the knees and hips in tunnel workers. A minority of victims experience sudden chest pain, dyspnoea, and cough, believed to be due to bubbles in the pulmonary circulation. Symptoms appear minutes to hours after the end of a dive. Some of them are due to bubble formation directly—others are believed to be secondary to clumping of red cells.

If the symptoms are of limb pain only, the patients are recompressed to 20 m on oxygen. Providing the pain disappears within 10 min of recompression, they are then decompressed over a period of 135 min. If the pain persists, the decompression time is doubled. If there is any evidence of central nervous or chest involvement, at the time of initial diagnosis or subsequently, the patient is immediately put semiprone on the left side, with the buttocks raised, recompressed to 20 m on oxygen and decompressed over at least 4.5 h. Sometimes it is necessary to recompress the patient briefly to 50 m or so to relieve persistent symptoms or signs. Some people give low molecular-weight dextran to combat the clumping of red cells and heparin to reduce any lipaemia from tissue disruption. It is important to emphasize that the only effective treatment is recompression, and that this may still be beneficial even if it cannot be achieved for several hours.

THE PROBLEM OF KEEPING WARM

The general problems of survival in cold water are described in Chapter 8.5.5(c). However, some difficulties are peculiar to divers. They insulate themselves in one of three ways: by cramming as much clothing as possible beneath a supposedly impermeable layer of rubber or canvas sealed at the neck and wrists (a 'dry' suit); by wearing an open-cell foam 'wet' suit that contains air at the surface but immobilizes water freely percolating in; or by wearing a closed-cell suit that consists of gas-filled plastic bubbles. All three suits rely on some gas for insulation and thus are buoyant and compressible. Typically a wet suit will provide some 8 kg of buoyancy, i.e. contain some 8 litres of air. As the diver descends, this gas compresses, making him heavier and colder. The loss of insulation is very noticeable. At depths greater than 50 m it is compounded by the need to breathe helium, which has a high thermal conductivity especially when it is compressed. In fact, the conductivity of helium is so high that gas-filled habitats for saturation diving have to be kept at temperatures close to 30 °C to achieve thermal neutrality. When divers emerge from the habitat they lose heat rapidly through the respiratory tract and through the 'air' filled insulation, which now contains helium. It is often necessary to provide them with personal heating systems (e.g. piped hot water).

ATMOSPHERIC PRESSURE DIVING

In classical diving, men invade the sea breathing gas at ambient pressures which rise linearly with depth. These men are able to deploy most of their sensory and motor skills but are very seriously limited by cold and the chemical consequences of breathing gases at high pressures. Two of these, oxygen toxicity and inert gas narcosis, restrict the choice of breathing mixtures. A third, decompression sickness, greatly reduces the maximum permissible rate of ascent. Divers cannot be launched or recovered when wave heights exceed a few feet, are unable to swim against currents greater than 1½ knots and are usually too cold to work for longer than 90 min. The long times spent in controlled ascent cannot usually be employed profitably, but detain expensive equipment, sometimes in the face of worsening weather. At present, it is difficult to imagine that classical divers will be able to descend much lower than 500 m. This gives them access to the whole of the Continental Shelves but not to the Continental Slopes or the Abyssal Plains beyond.

There are three other ways in which one can explore the sea. First and most safely, one can send down unmanned sensors and manipulators. Almost all of our present knowledge has been obtained in this way. Many of the exploratory devices are dropped at one point as spot samplers to measure local values of particular variables, which they record and transmit from the bottom or on return to the surface. Others can be towed with a fair degree of vertical and lateral control relaying similar information along a cable. Some can be envoyed remotely under sonar or an internally programmed control, storing or transmitting information as they go. As investment pressure rises, more of these will be fitted with manipulators to perform specific tasks.

Unmanned devices do not imperil human life, may be designed to work without a bulky pressure protection, should be able to move freely to and from great depths, and have the important advantage that in need they can be instructed to wait at the bottom indefinitely until surface conditions are favourable for their recovery. Their serious disadvantages are cost, lack of dexterity, and inflexibility of mission purpose. (To get these in perspective, it may be helpful to consider as a parallel the problems of exploring and redeveloping a dry continent, if it could only be done with towed or remote robots operated from night-flying helicopters.) There are bound to be considerable technical improvements in manipulators, sensors, power sources, and programme controls. Similarly, more marine engineering and mining plants will be designed to be built and maintained by telechiric devices. Nevertheless, at present, no one can envisage a time when submarine robots with anything like human capabilities could be constructed for economic sums.

Secondly, men can enter the sea in pressure-resistant vessels that can be towed, powered via a cable, or moved under their own steam. All of the present submersibles are fitted with porthole transparencies, most have additional sensors, and some have primitive manipulators. They can search large areas and some can perform simple tasks. Their present disadvantages are weight, restricted vision and manoeuvrability, bulk, poor manipulator performance, limited operability (most cannot be launched or recovered when wave heights exceed 1 m), high capital and operating costs, and the need for a large and specially equipped surface support vessel.

Thirdly, men can invade the sea in armoured diving suits, a relatively cheap weightless but warm second skin capable of resisting high ambient pressures but putting less restriction on touch, vision, and dexterity than the larger devices. These leave the diver with many of his sensorimotor skills and give him vertical freedom, greater depth range, and very reduced ascent times.

Although such suits were tried and found wanting in the 1930s, they are now easier to make and the need for them has risen greatly. At present they have a working depth limit of about 500 m and are able to ascend and descend freely. The inhabitant remains dry and warm, breathing air at atmospheric pressure throughout. When he surfaces, someone else can descend immediately using the same suit. It is likely that, in the future, much deep-sea diving will be conducted in this way.

THE SELECTION AND MEDICAL CARE OF DIVERS

Divers have a physically demanding job and often must work in sites remote from any medical aid. They must have a high exercise tolerance and be free of any active or latent condition that could erupt while they are away from medical help. In addition, specifically, they must not have any condition that could imperil their own lives or those of their would-be rescuers when they are under water.

In Britain all commercial divers have to pass an annual medical examination conducted by a doctor competent in diving medicine. If the diver is found to be unfit to dive and disagrees with the decision of the examiner he has the right of appeal to an independent tribunal set up by the Health and Safety Executive. The codes of safe diving practice have been summarized in the British 'Health and Safety—Diving Operations at Work Regulations', which took effect in July 1981. These regulations have been nationally and internationally accepted.

In principle, all divers are expected to be physically able and mentally stable people, free of conditions such as epilepsy and ill-controlled diabetes or asthma. They should not be addicted to alcohol or any other drug and they should not have a history, or any other evidence, of obstructive lung disease, ruptured eardrums, or aural surgery. Divers who are generally fit to dive should not be allowed to do so when they have chest, upper airway or ear infections, or when they are overweight (because obesity predisposes to decompression sickness). Neither should they dive while taking any medication that could impair their ability to think clearly or orientate themselves in space correctly.

Unresolved issues

There are several unresolved issues in diving medicine: the nomenclature of the disorders associated with decompression, the management of diving accidents, the role of lung function tests in assessing fitness to dive, the significance of patent foraman ovale in divers, whether people with mild asthma should be allowed to dive, and whether there are any long-term effects of 'safe' diving on the health of divers. These are discussed below.

THE NOMENCLATURE OF THE DISORDERS ASSOCIATED WITH DECOMPRESSION

The two principal hazards of ascent are lung rupture and the evolution of bubbles in blood and tissues (previously known as decompression sickness). On the whole, lung rupture manifests itself within a few minutes of its occurrence, but 'decompression sickness' usually takes several minutes to hours after decompression to become obvious. However, there are exceptions to both rules that can lead to errors in diagnosis and, more importantly, errors in treatment. Many authorities now believe that it is wiser to describe all disorders associated with decompression as decompression illness, defined by the site, acuity, and rate of progress of symptoms before recompression. This system of nomenclature is described in one of the references given at the end of the chapter.

THE MANAGEMENT OF DIVING ACCIDENTS AND EMERGENCIES

Several diving emergencies, for example hypoxia, oxygen toxicity, carbon dioxide poisoning, nitrogen narcosis, hypothermia, various ear, nose, and throat disorders, and underwater blast injury, do not require treatment by recompression, but two of them, acute decompression illness and carbon monoxide poisoning, do. In these two, recompression can be life saving. The Royal Navy's Institute of Naval Medicine at Alverstoke, near Gosport in Hampshire, maintains a 24-h diving medical watch throughout the year (telephone 01705 818888) to provide advice on diagnoses, treatments, and availabilities of recompression chambers. Their advice is also summarized in a freely available report listed at the end of this chapter.

THE ROLE OF LUNG FUNCTION TESTS IN ASSESSING FITNESS TO DIVE

Military and commercial divers are obliged to have annual medical examinations for 'fitness to dive', and sports divers are strongly urged to do likewise. In the past, one of the most stringent requirements of this check-up was that for acceptable spirometry, in particular for an acceptably high forced expiratory volume in 1 s/forced vital capacity (**FEV_1/FVC**) ratio, because of the fear that an obstructed lung was more liable to rupture. It has now become clear that worry is not well founded. The purpose of the medical check is two-fold. Firstly to determine whether the candidate is fit to swim in swift currents and rough waters at remote sites and only secondly to discover whether there is any bar to him or her also diving. In principle anyone who has more than a slightly reduced lung function (FEV_1, FVC, or carbon monoxide transfer) or aerobic capacity will not be fit enough to cope with emergencies in water and they should therefore be advised not to swim except in calm and supervised sites. Diving is often a relaxed affair, but people normally dive in pairs so that in the case of an emergency one diver can get the other out of trouble. At that stage, diving and survival at the surface can be very strenuous indeed. The prime purpose of the medical check is to determine that the candidate is capable of that activity.

THE SIGNIFICANCE OF PATENT FORAMINA OVALES IN DIVERS

On most, possibly almost all, asymptomatic decompressions, many bubbles can be detected in systemic venous bloodstreams. These bubbles are normally trapped in the pulmonary vessels and are resorbed unnoticed. However, about one-quarter of the normal population has a slightly patent foramen ovale, raising the possibility that, in them, some of the systemic venous bubbles might escape through to the left ventricle, bypassing the lung filter, and continuing on to cause cerebrospinal gas embolisms. This thought is reinforced by the observations that as many as 80 per cent of the victims of cerebrospinal gas embolism have patent foramina. However, it is by no means clear whether that is cause or effect. Although systemic venous bubbles are common, arterial gas embolisms are rare. Bubbles have complicated inflammatory interactions with vessel walls, and any significant load arriving in the lung could trigger pulmonary vasoconstriction, raising right heart pressures and opening a previously 'closed' foramen. Present evidence is equivocal and does not appear to justify excluding one-quarter of the population from diving, when gas embolism is a rare event.

SHOULD PEOPLE WITH MILD ASTHMA BE ALLOWED TO DIVE?

It has been the custom to bar asthmatics from diving because of the fear that they were more likely to rupture their lungs on fast ascents. However, very many mild asthmatics are known to have completed very many dives without ill effect. It seems there is a case for relaxing this requirement slightly, but three questions prevail: is the candidate (i) fit enough to cope with a diving emergency, (ii) liable to exercise-induced asthma, and (iii) likely to bronchoconstrict on the inhalation of salt water? Perhaps the most reasonable view at present is to allow a candidate with very mild asthma to dive, providing they can demonstrate a stable and essentially normal spirometry over a 2-month period, they do not have exercise-induced asthma, and they do not constrict abnormally to a saline aerosol.

DOES 'SAFE' DIVING HAVE ANY LONG-TERM EFFECTS ON THE HEALTH OF DIVERS.?

As mentioned earlier most ascents are associated with the appearance of many bubbles in systemic venous streams, but these usually do not cause symptoms, and so such dives are considered to be 'safe'. Decompression tables that have been established experimentally define the boundaries beyond which more than 2 or 3 per cent of divers will experience symptoms of decompression illness. Such dives are 'unsafe'. There is no doubt that the neurological or other sequelae to unsafe dives often fail to resolve completely, but these are regarded as the consequences of unsafe practices. More recently, diving physicians have been asking whether 'safe' dives lead to insiduous, cumulative damage. Although the damage is slight or subclinical, there is definite evidence now that they do. Autopsies on asymptomatic divers with no history of acute decompression illness have revealed their brains and spinal cords contain considerably more microinfarcts than non-diving controls. More importantly, radiographs of the long bones of divers and caisson workers show increasing numbers of aseptic infarcts in a sizeable minority (up to 11 per cent). The incidence is higher in those with a history of decompression illness than those without, but occurs in many with no such history. The infarcts can occur after a single decompression, but their incidence rises with age, depth, and diving intensity. Those in the shafts of bone are asymptomatic, but those at juxta-articular surfaces can be severely disabling. They are more common in caisson workers than divers, but are even seen in professional breath-hold divers, such as the *ama* of Japan, in whom the dissolved gas burden must be light. The aetiology is unknown, but gas embolism is the favoured explanation.

There is also good evidence that commercial diving, especially saturation diving causes the lung's total and vital capacities to expand, its FEV_1:FVC ratio to fall, and its pulmonary capillary blood volume, as judged by carbon monoxide transfer, to fall. The effects are slight but definite and may be cumulative. The expansions in lung volumes are attributed to training effects of breathing compressed gases for long times. The fall in FEV_1:FVC ratio is mainly due to the rise in FVC but there are hints of additional small-airway damage. The fall in pulmonary capillary blood volume appears to be due to transient episodes of hyperoxia during saturation diving procedures, but may also be associated with the influx of bubbles from systemic veins on 'safe' decompressions.

It is also known that commercial divers develop a mild degree of high-tone deafness, currently attributed to the noise of gas flows within their helmets.

Conclusion

Diving is a sometimes very vigorous activity that demands a high degree of mental and physical fitness. It exposes people to several physical and chemical challenges that are reasonably well understood. Because it takes place remote from medical help, there is a strong emphasis on prevention of illness by the following of safe practices. The safe practices have been developed empirically on the non-appearance of symptoms in brief trains of dives. There are now indications that these practices may not be quite as safe as first thought, but the cumulative effects are generally slight.

REFERENCES

Bennett, P.B. and Elliott, D.H. (ed.) (1993). *The physiology and medicine of diving,* (4th edn). Saunders, London.

Bove, A. and Davis, J.C. (ed.) (1992). *Diving medicine,* (2nd edn). Saunders, Philadelphia.

Edmonds, C., Lowry, C., and Pennefather, J. (ed.) (1993). *Diving and subaquatic medicine,* (3rd edn). Butterworth-Heinemann, London.

Elliott, C., Reed, J.W., Cotes, J.E., Robinson, N.G., and King, J. (1990). Narrowing of small lung airways in commercial divers. *European Undersea Biomedical Society,* xx, 197–202.

Francis, T.J.R., and Smith, D. (ed.) (1991). *Describing dysbarism.* Undersea and Hyperbaric Medical Society, Bethesda MD.

Francis, T.J.R., Smith, D.J., and Sykes, J.J.W. (1992). *The prevention and management of diving accidents,* Institute of Naval Medicine Report R92004. Ministry of Defence (Navy), London.

McCallum, R.I. and Harrison, J.A.B. (1993). Dysbaric osteonecrosis: aseptic necrosis of bone. In *The physiology and medicine of diving,* (4th edn), (ed. P.B. Bennet and D.H. Elliott), pp. 563–84. Saunders, London.

Thorsen, E., Reed, J.W., Elliott, C., Golsvik, A., and Hjelle, J.O. (1993). The contribution of hyperoxia to reduced pulmonary function after deep saturation dives. *Journal of Applied Physiology,* **75,** 657–62.

8.5.5(g) Lightning and electric shock

B. A. Pruitt and A. D. Mason

Electrical injury is a phenomenon of modern society whose occurrence rate, though not precisely known, roughly parallels *per capita* use of electric power. In burn centres, the reported frequency of admission for electrical injury ranges from 2 to 8 per cent of admissions, a variation in part dependent upon the inclusion or exclusion of patients with flame injury due to electrical ignition of clothing, with minimal electric injury *per se.* During a recent 10-year period, (1983–1992) 124 or 5.4 per cent of 2316 burn patients admitted to the authors' burn centre had electrical injury; of these, four had been struck by lightning.

Pathophysiology of electrical injury

The accidental inclusion of part of a living body in an electric circuit may produce injury in two ways. The first, which has been called electric shock, may occur at low or high voltage, while the second, thermal injury, occurs principally with higher voltage.

The known determinants of electrical injury include voltage, amperage, type of current, frequency of alternating current, duration of current passage, physical size and configuration of the part involved, and specific points of contact. Unfortunately, the frequencies which are ideal for electric power transmission are within the most dangerous part of the frequency spectrum for the production of both electric shock and thermal injury. Lightning injury is properly viewed as contact with a direct current source at very high voltage and amperage and does not differ in principle from other forms of electrical injury.

Electric shock produces disruption of cyclic bioelectric rhythms in affected organs, e.g., ventricular fibrillation, or induces membrane depolarization, e.g., muscular contraction. The power required to produce such effects is determined by the nature of the current involved and by the precise path of current passage through the body; the effects are strongly dependent upon contact site as well as upon the voltage, power, and frequency of the source.

Thermal injury may be induced either by electrical arcing outside the body or by power dissipation in tissue. High voltage electric arcs develop very high temperatures which are directly injurious to skin and may cause extensive thermal injury by producing ignition of the clothing. Power dissipation (P) in any element of an electric circuit is determined by the potential difference (E) across and current (I) within that element. Those variables define resistance (R):

$$E/I = R$$
$$P = E\,I = E^2/R = I^2\,\mathrm{R}$$

When a part of the body becomes a circuit element, power dissipation within that part produces heat and an increase in temperature. Skin exhibits moderate resistance, especially when dry, but like any insulator, breaks down at sufficient voltage gradient. When this occurs at a contact point, current density and power dissipation reach high levels, producing severe local injury (Fig. 1). In the deeper tissues, current flow is not isotropic, because individual tissues differ in resistance, but except for bone, which has relatively high resistance, these differences are not great. For any specific voltage, power dissipation is greater in tissues of lower resistance and it is a common clinical observation that deep tissues having low resistance are more susceptible to electric injury than those having high resistance. The heat generated within any particular tissue is not confined to that tissue; it is, instead, distributed within the affected part according to the laws of heat flow. Thus, the low resistance soft tissues, contained between an inner core of high resistance bone and an outer shell of high resistance skin, behave as a nearly isotropic volume electric conductor and in any cross-section are nearly uniformly heated by the passage of current. Soft tissue heating parallels current density, which may be approximated as an inverse function of the square of the radius of the body segment in question; heat production per unit volume and rate of temperature increase are greatest in segments of small diameter. The actual temperature achieved is, in turn, a complex function whose principal determinants are current density and the duration of current passage.

Thermal injury of tissue is a function not only of temperature but of duration of exposure to that temperature. At the threshold for injury, which probably lies between 45 and 50°C, injury occurs when exposure is of the order of 100 s; at higher temperatures, the required time decreases exponentially. A block of tissue heated in such a way as to make its temperature uniform throughout and then exposed to a cooler environment cools more rapidly at its periphery than at its core. This suggests that central segments of body parts are more liable to injury following contact with a source of electric power because they sustain longer thermal exposure times; the studies of Hunt *et al.* appear to verify this expectation. Those studies also suggest that duration of current flow is, in a sense, self limiting, since desiccation and carbonization of the points of contact greatly increased the resistance at those points and effectively interrupted current flow at a time inversely proportional to voltage. Other laboratory studies have shown that tissue cross-sectional area and conductivity characteristics result in the greatest current flow occurring in the muscle, fat, skin, and tendon of a limb. In those studies, local arcing and tissue charring did limit the current at voltages below 1000, but at higher voltages such current reduction did not occur. More recent animal studies have confirmed the inverse relationship between current density and cross-sectional area and the direct relationship between current density and severity of tissue damage.

Following such deep tissue injury, occlusion of small nutrient vessels occurs rapidly and tissue ischaemia ensues. In such areas of injury, the patency of larger vessels is often maintained and the observation of bleeding at the time of early debridement does not necessarily imply vascular integrity.

These pathophysiological elements make certain characteristics of electrical injury predictable.

1. Maximal tissue destruction may be expected at points of arcing or of maximal current density, i.e., at contact points and in body segments of small diameter.
2. Extremities are more liable to severe injury than the trunk, and the distal portions of extremities are more liable than the proximal because of current density relationships.
3. Low resistance soft tissues are most liable to thermal injury; one may expect injured muscle to underlie intact skin.
4. Deeper tissues in the path of the current are more liable to injury than overlying peripheral tissues; one may anticipate the occurrence of injured periosseous muscle overlain by uninjured muscle.
5. The true extent of injury is unlikely to be well correlated with the extent of cutaneous burn.

Cell membrane damage may also be caused by the process of electroporation, in which transmembrane potentials of as little as 100 to 500 mV can cause enlargement of pores in cell membranes with associated alteration of function and even cell death. Such changes can apparently occur even when tissue heating is insufficient to cause coagulation necrosis. This process has been implicated as a pathogenic factor in rhabdomyolysis as well as certain otherwise inexplicable neurological signs and symptoms that may persist for prolonged periods after electric injury. Recent laboratory studies by Lee *et al.* have shown that an intravenously administered non-ionic surfactant can partially restore the resistivity of an electropermeabilized muscle. The clinical importance of electroporation and the clinical applicability of surfactant treatment remain undefined.

Fig. 1 The left arm and hand of this patient who made contact with a high voltage line show the typical flexion deformities of the digits and wrist, and charring at the contact site in the first web space and at the sites of arcing at the wrist and antecubital space. Note the more severe damage of the tissues of the hand and distal forearm where the cross-sectional area is relatively small, the darkly discoloured oedematous deeper muscle bulging above the more superficial muscles just proximal to the dorsum of the wrist, and the pale oedematous muscle bulging above the incised fascia in the proximal half of the fasciotomy incision.

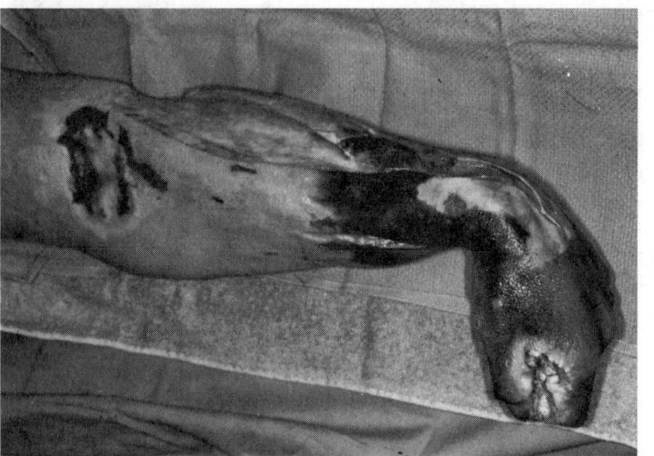

Diagnosis and treatment

The physiological characteristics of high voltage electrical injury are responsible for the differences in clinical presentation and treatment needs between patients sustaining such injury and patients sustaining conventional thermal injury. Significant differences include more frequent cardiopulmonary arrest, greater susceptibility to acute renal failure, frequent need for fasciotomy and early debridement of damaged subfascial tissues, and the occurrence of organ dysfunction of delayed onset.

Cardiopulmonary arrest is much more common in the immediate post-injury period in patients with high voltage electrical or lightning injury than in patients with conventional burns. The arrest may be due to either asystole or fibrillation and must be treated by immediate cardiopulmonary resuscitation. Cardiac arrhythmias can also occur following resuscitation, and patients with such injuries should undergo ECG monitoring for at least 48 h following injury even in the absence of arrhythmias and for 48 h beyond the last ECG evidence of dysrhythmias, if they occur. Hyperkalaemia, which may occur as a consequence of massive tissue destruction, is yet another reason for early post-injury ECG monitoring in patients with high voltage electrical injury, since the serum potassium concentration may reach levels which affect the cardiac conduction system. Hyperkalaemia, depending upon its severity and persistence, should be treated by administration of hypertonic glucose combined with insulin and calcium gluceptate, administration of an ion exchange resin, or performance of haemodialysis.

Two factors conspire to increase the incidence of acute renal failure in patients with high voltage electrical injury. Fluid needs may be underestimated as a result of there being little cutaneous injury, coupled with extensive, but inapparent deep tissue injury. Accordingly, inadequate volumes of resuscitation fluids may be administered and oliguria result. In addition, myoglobin may be liberated from injured muscle and is more likely to precipitate in the renal tubules in the presence of oliguria. Resuscitation fluids should, accordingly, be infused in sufficient volume to obtain an hourly urinary output of 75 to 100 ml in patients who exhibit elevated levels of urinary haemochromogens. If oliguria persists or the haemochromogen level does not promptly diminish despite otherwise adequate resuscitation, a diuretic should be administered to prevent the development of acute renal failure. Although some clinicians advocate the use of a loop diuretic, we prefer the use of mannitol as an osmotic diuretic, and administer 12.5 g (one ampoule) in each litre of intravenous fluid given until the pigment has cleared from the urine. Administration of sodium bicarbonate, acetazolamide, and hypertonic salt solutions to patients with high voltage electrical injury and severe myoglobinuria has been recommended by others. Such treatment is seldom necessary since correction of hypovolaemia returns the blood pH to normal levels and the diuretic effect of the last two agents is, at best, modest in hypovolaemic injured patients. In 25 (20 per cent) of the 124 patients with electrical injury treated recently, haemochromogenuria was evident on admission. Fluid management as described above prevented the development of progressive renal dysfunction and none of the patients developed acute renal failure. It is important to remember that diuretic administration invalidates the hourly urine output as a reliable guide to the adequacy of resuscitation; under these conditions, one must rely upon other haemodynamic criteria to assess the adequacy of resuscitation.

If the electric current has caused injury to tissues beneath the investing fascia of a limb, sufficient oedema may be produced in a muscle compartment to impair nutrient blood flow further or to interrupt flow to distal unburned tissue. Fasciotomy is required in such a situation to prevent further ischaemic damage of unburned tissue by relieving intracompartmental pressure and improving nutrient blood flow. The clinical signs indicating a need for fasciotomy include stony hardness of muscle compartments upon palpation, cyanosis of distal unburned skin, impaired capillary refilling of distal unburned skin or nail beds, and absent or diminished pulsatile flow in distal vessels as assessed by examination with an ultrasonic flowmeter. Although direct intracompartmental pressure measurements have been used in other types of patient to determine the need for fasciotomy, the risk of infection secondary to placing the pressure measurement cannula in burned tissue is great and contraindicates the use of such devices in burned patients. When the indications are present, fasciotomy should be performed as an emergency procedure, using general anaesthesia, as soon as resuscitation has restored haemodynamic stability. When a forearm fasciotomy is performed, the contents of the distal portion of the compartment must be carefully examined, and if the tissues of the carpal tunnel appear to be compromised by oedema, the tunnel should be surgically released as a part of the fasciotomy procedure.

If significant deep tissue injury is suggested by clinical signs but large vessel pulses are intact, arteriography may be helpful in determining the need for operative debridement. Arteriographic evidence of large vessel occlusion secondary to thrombosis may merely confirm clinical findings, but when the arteriogram is performed in the immediate post-injury period, luminal narrowing, irregularity, or 'beading' may be observed in severely injured vessels that will subsequently be occluded by thrombosis. In the absence of other clinical signs of such injury, muscle injury of variable extent may sometimes be indicated by a decrease in the density ('pruning') of muscular nutrient vessels in a limb. The identification of such changes helps to define the level of amputation required to remove muscle which is irreversibly damaged. Some investigators have used a xenon-133 washout technique or technetium-99m pyrophosphate scanning to assess muscle viability following electrical injury. Muscle blood flow of less than 1 ml/min per 100 g of tissue as measured by the xenon-133 washout technique has been equated with non-viable muscle. Both the absence of technetium uptake, interpreted as reflecting avascularity, and increased uptake, interpreted as indicating impairment of blood flow, are considered to be positive results and to mandate excision of muscle. Both of these diagnostic procedures have been evaluated in such a small number of patients as to make it impossible at this time to determine the reliability, accuracy, or clinical usefulness of either. Arteriography, xenon-133 washout studies and technetium-99m pyrophosphate muscle scanning should only be carried out when resuscitation has averted or corrected hypovolaemia and hypotension. Resistivity to 60-Hz current has recently been proposed as a means of assessing the severity of tissue injury due to electricity and identify the necessary extent of debridement. As early as 1 h after electrical injury, resistivity of severely damaged muscle in the hind limb of a dog decreased by 70 per cent, while that of tissue with minimal necrosis decreased by 20 to 40 per cent and that in tissue showing only oedema decreased by 10 to 30 per cent. Longer-term studies will be necessary to determine the sensitivity and specificity of this method.

Fig. 2 The initial level selected for amputation of the limb shown in Fig. 1 reveals the relative pallor of the more severely damaged periosseous tissues in the forearm of this patient. Note the pale muscle belly at 9 o'clock which underlies more darkly coloured viable muscle. The deep tissue damage necessitated revision of the amputation site to a more proximal level.

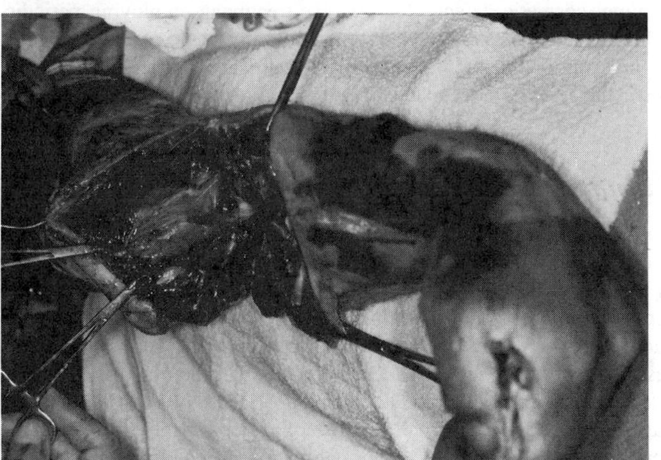

Table 1 *Amputations required in 28 patients with electric injury of upper limb*

Level of amputation	No. of amputations	Mean time of amputation after burn (days)
Shoulder disarticulation	5	2
Above elbow	6	6
Below elbow	9	8
Wrist	5	19
Digit	8	21

Operative exploration of tissue damaged by high voltage electrical injury should be carried out as soon as the patient is haemodynamically stable and should be performed under general anaesthesia. The involved muscle is thoroughly explored, bearing in mind that non-viable deep periosseous muscle can be present beneath more superficial viable muscle (Fig. 2). All necrotic tissue is debrided to reduce the risk of infection and to remove a source of potassium contributing to post-injury hyperkalaemia. Destruction of nerves, tendons, and vessels, or muscle necrosis so extensive as to render a limb useless mandate amputation at a level proximal to the area of tissue necrosis. Such amputations are frequently required in patients with high voltage electrical injury (Table 1). Oedema of the pectoral muscles in patients with high voltage electrical injuries of the upper limb demands exploration of that area and excision of non-viable muscle if it is present. The amputation or exploration wounds are packed open and the patient scheduled for re-examination of the wounds 24 to 48 h later. If, at the time of re-exploration, there is a significant amount of residual necrotic tissue, it is debrided, the wound again packed open, and the patient again scheduled for re-exploration 48 to 72 h later. If at the time of initial or subsequent re-exploration, little or no debridement is necessary, an amputation site may be closed by a 'sausage-type' technique and standard delayed primary closure techniques may be applied to other operative wounds. Since the morphological changes used to assess cell damage due to high voltage electricity are seldom evident within the first 24 h following injury, frozen section microscopy is generally of little help if operation is carried out during the first post-injury day.

The need for repeated debridement of electrically injured tissue and the late rupture of large arteries have been attributed to an injury-specific vasculitis causing progressive vessel occlusion. Angiographic studies in animal models, however, have shown little, if any, progression of vascular injury following electrical injury and no major vessel injury outside the area of tissue destruction. Delayed rupture of large vessels has, in our experience, been associated with desiccation and infection related to debridement and exposure. Recently, Robson *et al.* have correlated increased tissue levels of thromboxane with progressive local necrosis of electrically injured tissue in an animal model and found that the length of injured limb which was salvaged was increased by systemic or topical treatment with antithromboxane agents.

Wang *et al.* have achieved impressive salvage of electrically burned upper limbs by early debridement with vein grafting to replace thrombosed arteries at the wrist level and closure of the wound by a pedicle flap or a microvascular-free flap. Such therapy is indicated only for those patients with sufficient viable tissue to permit useful functional recovery. Delayed local flap coverage and subsequent nerve grafting has also been used to repair a popliteal tissue defect and bridge defects between the sciatic and tibial or sciatic and common peroneal nerves.

Bacterial control is best achieved by the use of Sulfamylon® burn cream in those patients in whom electric injury has damaged only skin and subcutaneous tissue or in those patients with full-thickness burns due to electric ignition of clothing. The active ingredient of this topical chemotherapeutic agent (mafenide acetate) can diffuse into the non-viable tissue and establish an effective antimicrobial concentration at the viable-non-viable tissue interface to limit bacterial proliferation and prevent the development of invasive burn wound sepsis.

Other injuries

The physical characteristics of electrical injury noted previously make visceral damage uncommon, but instances of intestinal perforation, focal gallbladder necrosis, focal pancreatic necrosis, and direct liver injury have been reported. In the case of at least one patient with high voltage electrical injury of the liver, hepatic damage was associated with a coagulopathy. The gastrointestinal tract is rarely directly injured, but is more commonly subject to dysfunction of delayed onset. In one series, three-quarters of patients with high voltage electrical injury showed evidence of gastrointestinal dysfunction within 12 to 18 months of injury and 13 of 45 patients developed cholelithiasis within 2 years.

Neurological deficits indicating either peripheral nerve or spinal cord injury may be evident immediately following injury, or be of delayed onset. A complete neurological examination must be performed on admission and at scheduled intervals thereafter in order to document nerve deficits which occur in patients with high voltage or lightning injury. Peripheral nerve deficits involve motor nerves more commonly than sensory nerves. If peripheral nerve damage is apparent immediately after injury, recovery is rare. Late appearing peripheral nerve deficits may involve nerves far removed from the points of electrical contact and may occur as part of a polyneuritic syndrome with highly variable recovery of function. Immediate post-injury spinal cord deficits are considered to reflect direct neuronal injury, but return of function is more common than in the case of spinal cord deficits of delayed onset, which tend to be permanent. Delayed onset spinal cord deficits are of variable character, ranging from localized nerve deficits with signs of ascending paralysis, transverse myelitis, or an amyotrophic lateral sclerosis-like syndrome to hemiplegia and quadriplegia.

Tetanic contractions of the paraspinus muscles induced by the passage of electric current may produce compression fractures of one or more vertebral bodies. CT scanning is helpful in diagnosing such fractures and assessing the integrity of the neural canal. Vertebral injuries and long bone fractures are not uncommon in electrical powerline workers who fall from a height following electric shock. Radiographs should be obtained as indicated by clinical signs and symptoms to verify or rule out the presence of such fractures.

Cataracts may occur in any patient who has sustained high voltage electrical injury (a 6.2 per cent incidence has been reported in one group of 113 patients), but this complication is most frequent in those patients in whom the contact point has been on the head or neck (Fig. 3). Such cataracts may form during the initial hospital period or may develop as late as 3 or more years after high voltage injury. An ophthalmological examination should be obtained before discharge from hospital as well as at the time of admission and the patient should be informed of the possibility of such sequelae.

House current voltage electrical burns of the mouth may occur when a young child bites an electric cord or sucks on the end of a live extension cord. The injury typically has the pearly white appearance of an avascular full-thickness burn and commonly involves the oral commissure. The frequency of labial artery bleeding (22 per cent in one series) justifies hospital admission of these patients. The timing of debridement appears to exert little influence on morbidity or cosmetic results and what appears initially to be a severe disfiguring lesion often results in a minimal cosmetic defect. Conservative treatment, employing periodic debridement of tissue which is unequivocally necrotic only, permits spontaneous healing with preservation of all viable tissue. Functional or cosmetic defects can be electively repaired later.

Fig. 3 Contact with high voltage source produced extensive full-thickness destruction of scalp and calvarium in this patient. Note charred scalp at margin of defect and exposed cranial suture line. Early obtundation slowly cleared and no long-term neurological sequelae occurred. Bone grafting was needed to repair the calvarial defect several months after the defect was initially closed by split-thickness skin grafting. Bilateral cataracts developed after discharge from hospital.

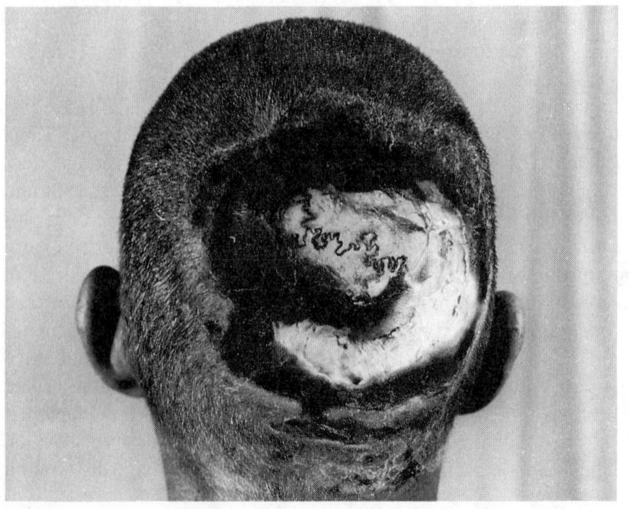

Lightning injury

Cardiopulmonary arrest is particularly common in patients who have been struck by lightning and immediate cardiopulmonary resuscitation is life-saving in such individuals. Recovery of patients who have been reported to be without signs of life for up to 15 or more min following such injury demands the immediate institution of cardiopulmonary resuscitation when such a patient is received in the emergency room. Although evidence of later development of acute myocardial damage has been reported in a small number of patients struck by lightning, persistent or recurrent ECG abnormalities are infrequent.

Neurological sequelae are common following lightning injury and range from coma to isolated nerve deficits and even lower limb paraplegia. These neurological deficits commonly resolve in a matter of hours or, at most, days.

The cutaneous burns present in patients with lightning injury are characteristically superficial and often exhibit an arborescent or spidery splashed-on appearance. Myoglobinuria in such patients is surprisingly uncommon in view of the current flow which occurs during lightning injury. Adequate resuscitation will prevent the development or promptly correct evidence of vasoconstriction and mottling of the skin, which were previously considered to be changes uniquely characteristic of lightning injury. Today, two-thirds of patients who have sustained lightning injuries survive as a result of early institution of cardiopulmonary resuscitation and prompt treatment of the other pathophysiological consequences of such injury.

REFERENCES

Amy, B.W., McManus, W.F., Goodwin, C.W., Jr., and Pruitt, B.A. Jr. (1985). Lightning injury with survival in five patients. *Journal of the American Medical Association*, **253,** 243–5.

Arturson, G. and Hedlund, A. (1984). Primary treatment of 50 patients with high-tension electrical injuries: I. Fluid resuscitation. *Scandinavian Journal of Plastic and Reconstructive Surgery*, **18,** 111–18.

Baxter, C.R. (1970). Present concepts in the management of major electrical injury. *Surgical Clinics of North America*, **50,** 1401–18.

Buchanan, D.L., Erk, Y., and Spira, M. (1983). Electric current arterial injury: a laboratory model. *Plastic and Reconstructive Surgery*, **72,** 199–205.

Burke, J.F., *et al.* (1977). Patterns of high tension electrical injury in children and adolescents and their management. *American Journal of Surgery*, **133,** 492–7.

Chilbert, M., *et al.* (1985). Measure of tissue resistivity in experimental electrical burns. *Journal of Trauma*, **25,** 209–15.

Clayton, J.M., *et al.* (1977). Xenon-133 determination of muscle blood flow in electrical injury. *Journal of Trauma*, **17,** 293–8.

DiVincenti, F.C., Moncrief, J.A., and Pruitt, B.A., Jr. (1969). Electrical injuries: a review of 65 cases. *Journal of Trauma*, **9,** 497–507.

Editorial, Death by lightning. (1977) *Lancet*, **i,** 230.

Fogh-Anderson, P. and Sorensen, B. (1984). Electric oral burns in Danish children with special references to prevention. *Scandinavian Journal of Plastic and Reconstructive Surgery*, **18,** 107–10.

Hunt, J.L., *et al.* (1976). The pathophysiology of acute electric injuries. *Journal of Trauma*, **16,** 335–40.

Hunt, J.L., *et al.* (1974). Vascular lesions in acute electric injuries. *Journal of Trauma*, **14,** 461–73.

Hunt, J.L., Sato, R.M., and Baxter, C.R. (1980). Acute electric burns: current diagnostic and therapeutic approaches to management. *Archives of Surgery*, **115,** 434–8.

Kleiner, J.P. and Wilkin, J.H. (1978). Cardiac effects of lightning stroke. *Journal of the American Medical Association*, **240,** 2757–9.

Layton, T.R., *et al.* (1984). Multiple spine fractures from electric injury. *Journal of Burn Care and Rehabilitation*, **5,** 373–5.

Lazarus, H.M. and Hutto, W. (1982). Electric burns and frostbite: patterns of vascular injury. *Journal of Trauma*, **22,** 581–5.

Lee, R.C., Gottlieb, L.J., and Krizek, T.J. (1992). Pathophysiology and clinical manifestations of tissue injury in electrical trauma. *Advances in Plastic and Reconstructive Surgery*, **8,** 9–16.

Lee, R.C., *et al.* (1992). Surfactant-induced sealing of electropermeabilized skeletal muscle membranes *in vivo. Proceedings of the National Academy of Sciences, USA*, **89,** 4524–8.

Levine, N.S., *et al.* (1975). Spinal cord injury following electrical accidents: case reports. *Journal of Trauma*, **15,** 459–63.

Newsome, T.W., Curreri, P.W., and Eurenius, K. (1972). Visceral injuries: an unusual complication of an electrical burn. *Archives of Surgery*, **105,** 494–7.

Ponten, B., *et al.* (1970). New observations on tissue changes along the pathway of the current in an electrical injury: case report. *Scandinavian Journal of Plastic and Reconstructive Surgery*, **4,** 75–82.

Pruitt, B.A., Jr. (1979). The burn patient: I. Initial care. *Current Problems in Surgery*, **16,** 1–55.

Robson, M.C., Murphy, R.C., and Heggers, J.P. (1984). A new explanation for the progressive tissue loss in electrical injuries. *Plastic and Reconstructive Surgery*, **73,** 431–7.

Saffle, J.R., Crandall, A., and Warden, G.D. (1985). Cataracts: a long-term complication of electrical injury. *Journal of Trauma*, **25,** 17–21.

Sances, A., Jr., *et al.* (1981). Experimental electrical injury studies. *Journal of Trauma*, **21,** 589–97.

Stevenson, J.H. and Zuker, R.M. (1983). Considerations in nerve reconstruction and electric burn injury: case report. *Journal of Burn Care and Rehabilitation*, **4,** 408–10.

Thomson, H.G., Juckes, A.W., and Farmer, A.W. (1965). Electric burns to the mouth in children. *Plastic and Reconstructive Surgery*, **35,** 466–7.

Wang, Z.W., *et al.* (1982). Early surgical treatment of severe electrical injury of bilateral upper extremities: a case report. *Burns*, **9,** 24–9.

Wang, Z.W. and Zoh, W. (1982). Arterial injuries in electrically burned upper limbs and effects of early reconstruction of blood circulation to the wrist. *Burns*, **8,** 379–86.

Zelt, R.G., *et al.* (1986). Experimental high voltage electrical burns: a role of progressive necrosis. *Surgical Forum* **37,** 624–6.

8.5.5(h) Podoconiosis (endemic non-filarial elephantiasis of the lower legs)

A. A. ADISH and E. W. PRICE*

Podoconiosis, formerly known as endemic elephantiasis, is a non-filarial endemic form of elephantiasis of the lower legs. It results from obstruction of the distal superficial lymphatics by soil-borne minerals, rather than by parasites, bacteria, or viruses. The obstructive lymphopathy leads to bilateral but asymmetrical swelling of the feet and lower legs. The disease has been described in the highlands of east and central Africa, and the lowlands of Nigeria, Cameroon, Gabon, Central and south America, Northwestern India, and parts of Indonesia.

Aetiology

The disease is most common among agrarian, barefooted populations in the tropics, is less common in pastoral areas, and absent in infertile and industrial areas. It occurs at an altitude of more than 1500 m, of average temperature of 20°C, and a hot-season rainfall of 1000 mm annually. The areas most affected have reddish-brown volcanic clay soil that is extremely slippery when wet, and very adherent if allowed to dry on the skin.

This soil is characterized by a high proportion of abrasive quartz crystals in fine silts, and of colloidal-sized particles in clays. The predominant silts are amorphous silica and iron oxide, and distorted forms of the aluminosilicate, kaolinite. This combination of soil particles facilitates their penetration through the skin of the feet.

The disease occurs in both sexes, but is more prevalent in men due to excess exposure during farming. The recognition of a familial tendency is reflected in various objections to marrying into an elephantiasis family, and has led to the speculation that there is a congenital inadequacy of the lymphatic system of the lower legs. In acute lymphangitis, streptococci may sometimes be found in the lymph, but the disease can develop without any acute episodes.

Pathology

The abrasive effect of broken crystals of quartz in the soil facilitates the entry of toxic mineral microparticles, such as silica and aluminosilicates (resembling kaolinite), into the dermis of the foot. Careful searching with electron microscopy will demonstrate the presence of silica, aluminium, and iron, either free or within the phagosome of a macrophage (Fig. 1). The effect of these microparticles on the tissue varies from a mild irritation, to a notable pathology.

* Dr. Ernest Price died on 31 January 1990. Much of his second edition chapter has been retained in this edition.

At an early stage, in the dermis collections of lymphocytes related to lymph channels of the superficial lymphatic plexus, and to sweat ducts can be observed. The effect of fibrous thickening of the capsule of the lymph node as well as the subendothelial oedema and collagenosis, interrupts the normal peristalsis of the lymphatic vessels. The development of a fibrous layer across the corticomedullary region of the femoral lymph node acts as a final barrier in cases where the pathology has reached this degree of severity.

Clinical appearances

Three types of disease are described in the early stage. Classification is achieved by clinical observation.

The soft or 'water-bag' type is characterized by lymphoedema. The oedema appears to be mainly subdermal with minimal swelling and fibrotic thickening of the dermis. It is smooth with little hyperkeratotic change. Slight oozing of lymph is common. The skin at this stage can be picked up between the fingers (Fig. 2(a)).

In the hard or 'leathery' type, there is fibrosis of the skin and subcutaneous tissues, which cannot be picked up between the fingers and which do not pit. There is marked hyperkeratosis (Fig. 2(b)).

The 'slipper' type is so-called because the distribution is that of a traditional slipper involving the back of the heel, the borders of the sole and the tips of the toes passing on to the dorsum.

Natural history

The lower legs are progressively involved during the course of several months or years. A burning sensation of the soles and itching over the trunk of the main lymphatic channels is initially confined to one leg. The symptoms occur commonly at night in bed, and are alleviated by uncovering the leg. The occurrence of the monthly menses may initiate symptoms. The pain may be aggravated by excessive alcohol intake or prolonged exertion.

These early symptoms intensify as the permanent swelling develops. Intermittent swelling is first noticed on the dorsum of the foot near the first toe cleft, which then becomes permanent and spreads with or without acute episodes. At the later stage, the swelling may reach the knee, but rarely passes into the thigh. Although both legs are always affected, the disease develops asymmetrically so that swelling of one leg may progress while the other remains quiescent.

In the progressive phase, femoral lymphadenitis and tender swelling of the nodes is a common occurrence, but suppuration is rare. However, the final stage, lymphadenitis or elephantiasis, is established as a permanent condition. Older patients claim that the swelling, size, and extent can decrease with age, but this may be due to the reduced activity in later life.

Fig. 1 Micrograph of femoral lymph node of an elephantiasic person. Note the two macrophages on the left, the upper of which contains a number of clumps of microparticles. Analysis showed that most of these were silica with varying amounts of aluminium, iron, and titanium (× 7200).

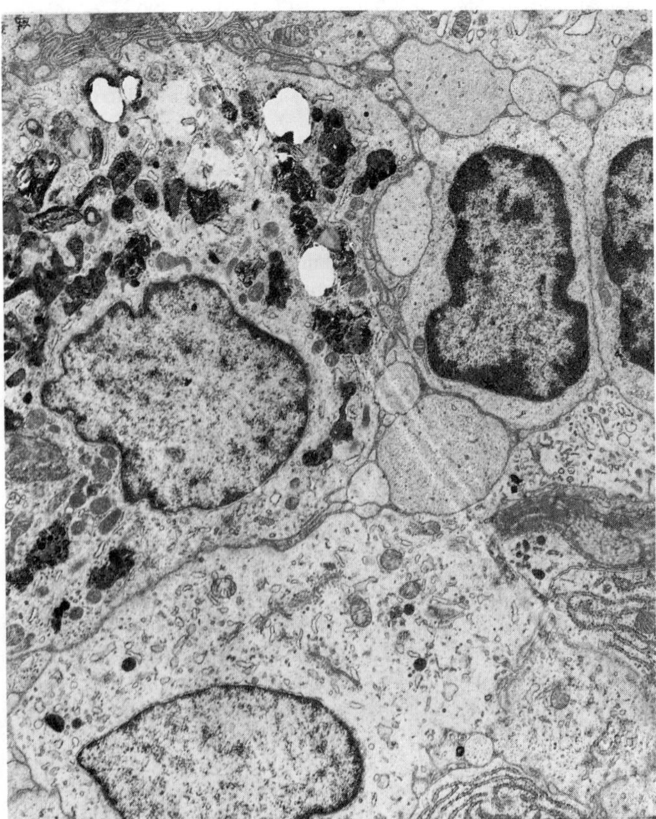

Fig. 2 Clinical types of elephantiasis. (a) The wet or water-bag type. Swelling is readily reduced by compression or elevation. The skin is soft and can be pinched off the bones. (b) The dry or wooden type. Swelling is irreducible by compression or elevation. Note the prominence of hyperkeratosis of the toes with trauma to one toe. Nodulation is frequent.

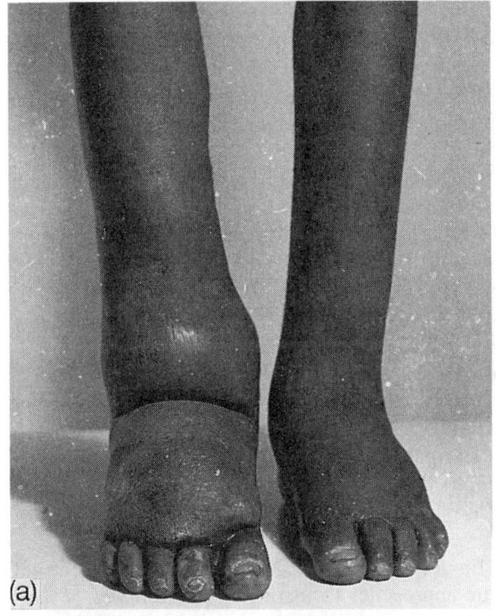

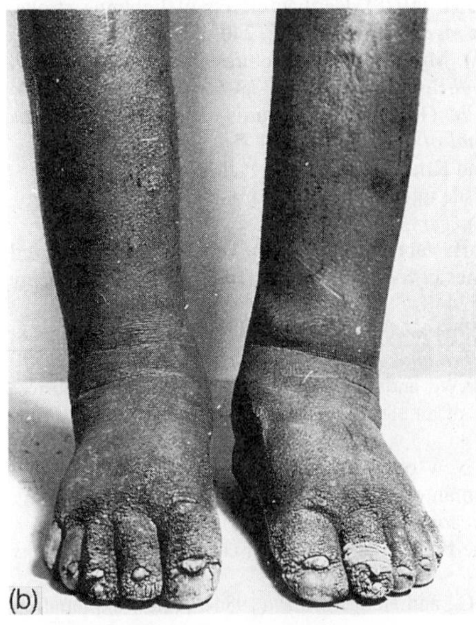

Management

Successful management depends on the understanding and cooperation of patients, and the type of disease. The water-bag type responds better than the leather type. The objectives of management of the disease are:

1. To treat the symptoms. Pain and discomfort can be reduced by an anti-inflammatory analgesic such as aspirin. Persistent itching, which is due to local oedema, will respond to elevation of the limb and elastic stockings.
2. To reduce to a minimum any additional load of minerals in the dermis of the foot. This can be attained by:
   (a) Footwear, with socks and stockings;
   (b) Placing of a mat on the floors of dwellings;
   (c) Changing of residence and/or changing of occupation.
3. To reduce oedema by elevation and compressive bandaging.
4. To reduce fibrogens. Several traditional drugs are used to reduce fibrogens but none is effective in reversing the established fibrosis.

REFERENCES

Kloos, H., Kello, A.B., and Adish, A.A. (1992). Podoconiosis (endemic nonfilarial elephantiasis) in two resettlement schemes in western Ethiopia. *Tropical Doctor*, **22,** 109–12.

Price, E.W. (1984). Environmental factors in the etiology of endemic elephantiasis of the lower legs in tropical Africa. *Tropical and Geographical Medicine*, **36,** 1–5.

Price, E.W. (1984). Non-filarial elephantiasis confirmed as a geochemical disease, and renamed podoconiosis. *Ethiopian Medical Journal*, **26,** 151.

Price, E.W. (1984). Pre-elephantiasic stage of endemic nonfilarial elephantiasis of lower legs ''podoconiosis''. *Tropical Doctor*, **14,** 115–19.

Price, E.W. (1990). *Podoconiosis, non-filarial elephantiasis.* University Press, Oxford.

Tada, M.S., and Marsden, P.D. (1993). Probable podoconiosis in Brasilia. *Revista da Sociedade Brasileira de Medicina Tropical*, **26,** 255.

8.5.5(i) Radiation

R. J. Berry

What kind of radiation?

Radiations are either ionizing or non-ionizing. Ionization involves the forcible ejection of an orbital electron from an atom of matter, creating an ion. When this takes place in a molecule of biological importance, it may lead to biological damage. Non-ionizing radiations may be capable of excitation, but cannot convey sufficient energy to the target molecules to produce this gross structural change.

Ionizing radiations

X-rays

These are electromagnetic waves in the continuous spectrum which includes light and radio waves, but are of very short wavelength. They have no mass and no charge, and are produced in machines by the bombardment of a positively charged anode with a stream of electrons from a heated filament. The energy of the X-rays is determined by the voltage through which the electrons are accelerated, and the penetrating power of the X-rays increases with increasing acceleration voltage. They were first discovered by Röntgen in 1895.

Gamma-rays

These are identical in properties to X-rays but are produced by the spontaneous disintegration of radioactive atoms (see below).

Particle radiations

Unlike X-rays and gamma-rays these have mass, and are produced by the composite parts of atoms such as electrons (beta-particles), protons, or neutrons, or by the nuclei of larger atoms, e.g. helium nuclei (alpha-particles). They may be charged or uncharged. Particulate radiations may come either from the spontaneous disintegration of radioactive atoms or from electrical accelerators, where beams of a wide variety of subatomic particles have been produced.

Sources of radiation

Natural

Cosmic rays

Throughout its evolution humankind has been exposed to cosmic radiation emanating from remote parts of the universe as well as from the sun, which can be regarded as a large thermonuclear reactor. The majority of cosmic rays are very high energy protons and a smaller number of heavier nuclei, mostly alpha-particles. The intensity of exposure of humans to cosmic radiation depends entirely on the altitude at which they are, contributing roughly half of the total external radiation dose from natural sources at sea level but increasing markedly even at high altitudes on land and further still for the crew and passengers of high-flying aircraft. Thus the annual dose from cosmic rays to a person living, for example, in Denver, Colorado at an altitude of around 2000 m is more than twice that for a person living in London. Cosmic rays are energetic and not only irradiate humans on the earth's surface but can also pass through many metres of earth.

Secondary radiations

Secondary radiations are generated in the upper atmosphere and consist largely of gamma-rays and high energy electrons, together with other particles whose ionizing properties are similar to electrons so that their biological effects are also similar. The contribution from secondary irradiation varies with the latitude, being greatest at the poles and lowest at the equator.

Radioactivity

Many of the earth's minerals are naturally radioactive. Atoms are stable only if their nuclei contain an approximately equal number of protons and neutrons and unstable atomic nuclei may undergo spontaneous disintegration. Each element has several isotopes or different forms, with the same number of protons in the nucleus, but differing numbers of neutrons. Many of these isotopes are unstable and are thus radioactive. In body fluids the naturally occurring radioactive isotope of potassium ^{40}K makes the largest contribution to the internal radiation background. In the environment, many naturally occurring materials are radioactive and in the United Kingdom the primary contribution to radiation dose to people comes from radon in the soil. There are wide variations in the natural background of radioactivity throughout the United Kingdom, with some materials such as granite making a significant contribution to the total radiation exposure. In prehistoric times, man evolved from a background in which natural radioactivity levels were far higher than those which obtain today.

Man-made

Among man-made radiations all the types listed above can be produced by machines; X-rays used by doctors are the greatest single man-made source of irradiation of the general population. Nuclear reactors are not only sources of direct radiations (usually absorbed in appropriate shielding) but are also copious producers of radioisotopes. The full consequences of the release of radioisotopes from the 1986 Chernobyl nuclear power plant disaster may not be known for many decades. Finally, and we hope never to be used, nuclear weapons are intense sources of man-made radiation. Except, however, for low-yield 'battlefield' weapons and the 'radiation enhanced' weapons (the so-called 'neutron bomb'), potentially lethal effects of blast and heat occur at greater distances from the point of detonation than do lethal effects from direct radiation.

For both natural and man-made radioactive substances, the qualities of importance are the type of disintegration, the particles or non-particulate radiation produced by the disintegration, the half-life (the time for one-half of the initial activity to have disappeared, half of the remaining activity taking the same time to disappear, etc.) and the initial activity. This is specified in units of disintegrations per second (becquerels) named after the discoverer of radioactivity. The unit which has been used in the past related the number of radioactive disintegrations to the number of disintegrations taking place in 1 g of pure radium, 3.7×10^{10} per second = 1 curie (1 Ci = 3.7×10^{10} Bq, 1 Bq = 2.7×10^{-11} Ci).

Radiation effects

Ionization density

Radiations differ in their effects both qualitatively and quantitatively. X-rays and gamma-rays produce their damage by ejecting orbital electrons from atoms of matter with which they interact. These radiations are sparsely ionizing because the ejected particle is of low mass and limited in its capability for producing damage, so that interactions of many particles are needed to cause major chemical and biological damage. These sparsely ionizing radiations are described as being of low linear energy transfer (low LET) and their effects are dependent upon the rate at which the radiation dose is accumulated, whether protracted in time or fractionated in multiple short bursts. The chemical state of the target molecule can also affect the damage produced by low LET radiations; chemical interactions can cause either potentiation or the radiation damage or protection against it.

Protons, neutrons which eject protons from atoms of matter, and other larger particles are more densely ionizing, and are said to be of high linear energy transfer (high LET). These radiations are less dependent for their effects on the accumulation of multiple damaging events within one target molecule, so that their action is often 'all or none'. They are also less dependent upon the dose rate, dose fractionation, or the chemical state of the target molecule.

Radiation dose

All effects of radiation depend upon the magnitude of the accumulated radiation dose. After a chequered history, beginning with the definition of the röntgen in 1928 (that quantity of radiation which produces in 1 cm^3 of air 1 unit of charge of either sign) absorbed radiation dose is now cited in SI units which have the dimensions of joules (energy) per kilogram (mass of absorbing material). Throughout this section the new units will be given, followed by the old units in parentheses. The basic unit of absorbed radiation dose, 1 J/kg, has been given the eponym 1 gray (1 Gy=100 rad). Conventional SI prefixes are used for multiples and sub-multiples of this unit. To compare the effects of different radiations with the reference standard, which is the effect of sparsely ionizing radiations such as X-rays, the absorbed dose is multiplied by a radiation weighting factor which is selected for the type and energy of the radiation. The value of this factor is determined by the International Commission on Radiological Protection. The product is called equivalent dose, and its unit has the special name of sievert (Sv). Table 1 lists a thousand million-fold range of radiation doses, and their effects upon biological systems.

Total body irradiation of man

As seen in Table 1, the major consequence of radiation exposure is life-shortening, either acutely for doses in excess of 5 to 10 Gy, or due to late effects which may be seen 1 to 40 years after radiation exposure for smaller doses. Clinically important radiation syndromes are as follows.

Table 1 *Effects of total body irradiation*

Equivalent dose (Sv)*	Effect
Sublethal to man	
0.0001	Around 2 weeks' natural background radiation, no detectable effect
0.001 (1 mSv)	Around 6 months' natural background radiation, no detectable effect
0.01	No detectable effect
0.1	Minimal decrease in peripheral lymphocyte count, no clinical effect
1	Mild acute radiation sickness in some individuals (nausea, possible vomiting), no acute deaths, early decrease in peripheral lymphocyte count, decrease in all white blood cells and platelets at 2 to 3 weeks, increase in late risk of leukaemia, solid tumours
Lethal to man	
10	Severe acute radiation sickness, severe vomiting, diarrhoea, death within 30 days of all exposed individuals Severe depression of blood cell and platelet production, damage to gastrointestinal mucosa
100	Immediate severe vomiting, disorientation, coma, death within hours
1000	Death of some micro-organisms, some insects
10 000	Death of most bacteria, some viruses
100 000	Death of all living organisms, denaturation of proteins

*For X-rays and gamma-radiation equivalent dose in Sv is equal to absorbed dose (gray).

Central nervous system syndrome

Above acute exposures of 30 to 100 Gy (3000–10 000 rad) there is a rapid onset of nausea, vomiting which may be severe and repeated, anxiety, disorientation and, within hours, coma and death due to direct radiation effects on central nervous system conduction and to cerebral oedema. There are no definitive pathological signs of damage at autopsy of such individuals.

Gastrointestinal syndrome

Individuals who have received doses in excess of 10 Gy (1000 rad) will also show early onset of nausea and vomiting, usually starting 1 to 2 h after radiation exposure, but often recovering from this by 4 to 6 h. However, they are doomed to die within 4 to 14 days because of radiation damage to the gastrointestinal tract. The convoluted epithelial lining of the small intestine is perhaps the most rapidly renewed tissue in the body; cells born in the intestinal crypts are shed from the tips of villi to the intestinal contents at the end of their normal lifespan approximately 4 to 7 days later. Radiation inhibition of cell division, followed by the reproductive death of the intestinal stem cells results in, first, a shortening of the intestinal villi until the lining of the intestine is as flat as a garden hose. This drastically reduces the surface area available for nutrient and electrolyte diffusion, and results in intractable diarrhoea. Failure of survival of sufficient intestinal stem cells and their proliferation to replace dying intestinal epithelial cells leads to denudation of areas of the bowel, with consequent free access of bowel contents and infection to the blood and leakage of body fluids into the intestinal contents. Dehydration, overwhelming infection, and death follow.

Haemopoietic syndrome

At doses between 1 and 10 Gy (100–1000 rad), although transient nausea and occasional vomiting may be seen in some individuals, the frequency increasing with increasing dose, these early prodromal symptoms disappear rapidly, followed by a period of relative well-being. However, second only to the small bowel, the haemopoietic system is the body tissue which has the most rapid cell turnover. Mature lymphocytes, unlike the majority of body cells, do not need to attempt division before being killed by radiation damage, and undergo rapid interphase cell death within a period of hours. In fact, the change in peripheral lymphocyte count over the first 24 to 48 h after acute radiation exposure can be used as a rough dosimeter for the magnitude of the exposure. As the majority of differentiated peripheral blood cellular elements have normal life-times of 2 to 3 weeks for white cells and platelets, and around 100 days for red cells, no other immediate alterations in blood count are seen. However, haemopoietic stem cells are damaged by radiation, as are cells of other tissues, primarily by the loss of their ability to divide and by their subsequent death on attempting division. Hence, when the normal division stimuli occur there is an initial abortive repopulation of the peripheral blood achieved by 'short cutting' the normal differentiation steps, which further depletes the already damaged haemopoietic stem cell population. By 2 to 3 weeks there is no new input of differentiated, functional white cells and platelets, and the clinical syndrome develops of easy and overwhelming infection due to lack of white cells, and bleeding starting with petechial haemorrhage due to shortage of platelets.

Therapy of acute radiation exposure

It is unlikely that prior warning of radiation exposure would have allowed the ingestion or injection of a radioprotective substance. The only effective, potentially usable radioprotectors so far evolved depend on the production of intracellular hypoxia and/or increasing intracellular-sulphhydryl concentration. Agents such as cysteine, cysteamine, aminoethylisothiouronium (AET), and mercaptoethyl guanidine (MEG) used in near-toxic concentrations have been shown in animal experiments to increase the LD_{50} radiation dose by up to 20 per cent. A thiophosphate compound, *S*-2-(3-aminopropylamino)ethyl phosphorothioic acid, numbered WR 2721, has been evaluated by the United States Army and has achieved similar or greater effectiveness with lower toxicity. However, a more likely scenario is that radiation exposure will occur without prior warning. If large populations have been irradiated even a crude estimation of the radiation dose received will be of importance. Scarce medical resources will have to be devoted only to those patients who have received doses in the LD_{10} to LD_{50} range; those most ill will have been irretrievably lethally irradiated, and the vast majority of those who have received less than LD_{10} radiation dose will recover spontaneously. As the haemopoietic syndrome is life limiting, those patients at highest risk of haemopoietic death will have to be identified by the size of the drop in peripheral blood lymphocyte count over the first 24 to 48 h. A better biological dosimeter but usable for only small numbers of exposed individuals is the number of chromosome aberrations in peripheral blood lymphocytes cultured *in vitro* with phytohaemagglutinin. If facilities exist, venesection and the storing of white cells and platelets against future need is considered by many to be a useful step as well as providing a major early stimulus to proliferation of surviving haemopoietic stem cells. Another useful haemopoietic stimulation is challenge with a strong antigen such as TAB/tetanus toxoid. This is a good public health measure in a disaster situation, and has the advantage of a useful degree of early haemopoietic stimulation.

Following the nuclear reactor accident at Chernobyl and the widespread radioactive contamination from a stolen radioactive source in Goiania, recent experience of management of radiation casualties has been subject to intense scrutiny and a consensus is beginning to emerge. Successes obtained with therapeutic regimes of fluid and electrolyte replacement and platelet transfusion plus appropriate antibiotics have confirmed that infection and haemorrhage are the primary factors causing death from the haemopoietic syndrome. When the number of casualties is sufficiently small, isolation, antimicrobial decontamination of the intestine, systemic antibiotics, transfusion as required of red cells and platelets and supportive measures for empirical treatment of infection have been shown to be highly effective. Current data suggest that the cytokines G-CSF and GM-CSF can accelerate haemopoietic recovery and may be of use in treatment of victims of radiation injury who have received a dose large enough to produce sustained neutropenia but not so large that bone marrow recovery will not occur eventually. The role of bone marrow transplantation is less clear and limited to the few victims whose marrow is unlikely to recover but who have not received lethal damage to the bowel or lungs. Where there is combined injury due to trauma, conventional injuries require normal medical emergency procedures first, as all but the most severe radiation injury is not immediately life-threatening. In particular, wounds should be treated by early definitive surgery in the narrow window of time before radiation-induced suppression of cellular elements necessary for wound healing occurs.

If a major radiation exposure results not from external irradiation but from contamination by radioactive isotopes as after both the Chernobyl reactor accident and the Goiania lost-source incident, information from Health Physics personnel as to the nature of the hazard expected and determination of the initial amount of radioactivity in contaminated casualties is vital—to assess danger to staff as well as patients. If exposure to fallout is expected, a major amount of skin contamination can be avoided by wearing all possible clothing and removing this contaminated clothing once the fallout danger has passed.

First treatment of exposure to radioactive materials by wounding (skin penetration), ingestion, or inhalation may be directed towards removing the radioactive material from the body. Dangerously radioactive material in a wound is treated initially by washing and mechanical scrubbing, and if necessary by adequate surgical excision of the contaminated tissue. Ingestion of radioiodine is treated by giving a single (100–200 mg) dose of stable sodium iodide/iodate so that the amount of the radioisotope which is fixed in the thyroid is minimized. This is most effective if taken before exposure, and only of use within a few hours after exposure. The amount of ^{137}Cs retained in the body can be reduced and its excretion enhanced by treatment with gram quantities of Prussian blue. Ingestion of bone-seeking radionuclides such as ^{90}Sr and actinides such as ^{239}Pu may be treated by administration of chelating agents such as ethylenediamine tetra-acetic acid (EDTA) or diethylenetriamine penta-acetic acid (DTPA) to minimize their deposition in bone. Massive oral doses of stable calcium and parathyroid hormone have also been used with limited success.

Particulate radioactive contamination which has been inhaled may, when the material has particular long-term hazards (e.g. ^{239}Pu), be removed in part by bronchial lavage carried out in centres with appropriate specialist skills.

Late effects of radiation exposure

Leukaemogenesis

Over the period 3 to 10 years after acute radiation exposure there is increased risk of the development of leukaemia, predominantly myeloid leukaemia. The magnitude of risk is proportional to the total radiation dose received. Human experience is based largely on early radiation workers who were exposed unwittingly to large cumulative radiation doses, and the survivors of the Hiroshima and Nagasaki nuclear weapons detonations. However, the first results from the current United Kingdom

National Registry for Radiation Workers have shown a significant connection between the magnitude of occupational radiation exposure and leukaemia incidence although overall this worker population has a lower leukaemia incidence rate than the general public. From such data the dose to double the natural incidence of leukaemia is estimated to lie in the region of a few hundred mGy (a few tens of rads). Leukaemia represents only around 3 per cent of all new malignancies in the United Kingdom, however, and even a relatively large increase in leukaemia incidence may represent a small change in the overall numbers of patients presenting with malignant disease.

Carcinogenesis

Solid tumours are also induced by ionizing radiation exposure, once again increasing in risk as a function of increasing dose, but over periods up to 40 and more years after radiation exposure. The most common sites of radiation-induced tumours are related to the sites in which cancer is most prevalent in the general population. Skin cancer is inevitably high in incidence; other cancers in which increased incidence following radiation exposure has been demonstrated include lung, breast, and bone cancers and lymphomas. A large pool of human experience exists, once again in the early radiation workers, the Hiroshima and Nagasaki survivors, and in specific groups exposed to either inhalation or ingestion of radioactive materials (e.g. uranium miners, radium dial painters) or to the medical use of ionizing radiation for diagnostic or therapeutic purposes (breast cancer in women patients with tuberculosis given a therapeutic artificial pneumothorax, skin and other cancers in patients treated by radiation for ankylosing spondylitis, etc.). For the establishment of general population and occupational exposure limits it is assumed that there is no threshold radiation dose. Age at irradiation is also a factor, with exposure below age 15 probably having about twice the risk per unit dose of subsequent development of malignant disease. Animal and human studies suggest, however, that as the radiation dose increases there is a departure from this inexorable increase in induced malignancy due to the killing by the additional radiation of the transformed cells which presumably would have evolved into a malignant clone. As a guide, on best human data it is suggested that total body exposure of 1cGy (1 rad) gives at most a risk of 1 in 2000 of the development of fatal malignant disease in a particular individual. Thus, uniform exposure of a population of 1 million people to 1cGy may result in the eventual development of about 500 fatal cancers against a background of some 250 000 spontaneous cancer deaths of which some 6000 to 9000 may have resulted from the unavoidable lifelong exposure to natural background radiation.

Radiation damage to the fetus

The developing fetus is particularly susceptible to damage during the period of organogenesis when the loss of reproductive capacity of a cell rest due to evolve into a particular organ may be catastrophic. In particular, irradiation of the fetus during the period 8 to 15 weeks after conception during the period of development of the forebrain may lead to severe mental retardation. The fetus, like the adult, is also subject to an increased risk of the development of leukaemia and solid tumours which is related to the total accumulated radiation dose, but this increased risk per unit dose may be several times greater than for an adult.

Genetic damage

Radiation can produce both dominant lethal events, and recessive changes which are not expressed in the first generation. However, with increasing radiation dose, an increased proportion of those cells in which such transformations have taken place are rendered reproductively inert and cannot pass on their genetic misinformation. Hence, somatic rather than genetic damage is the limiting factor in determining permissible radiation exposure to populations. One study has suggested an association between parental occupational radiation exposure and the risk of development of leukaemia in a child, but this has not been confirmed by other workers.

Controlling human exposure to radiation hazards

ALARA/ALARP

Since the institution of maximum permissible annual radiation exposure levels, pioneered by the International Congress of Radiology in 1928 and intended for radiation workers, progressively more restrictive limits have been imposed for maximum exposure to ionizing radiation not only for those workers but also for the general public. The International Commission on Radiological Protection (ICRP) instituted, in 1977 a new system of radiation protection which was based on three principles.

Justification No practice shall be undertaken involving radiation unless it is likely to bring benefit.

Optimization For any practice involving radiation, the radiation dose used shall be as low as reasonably achievable (ALARA) economic and social considerations being taken into account.

Dose limits No individual shall be exposed to radiation in excess of those limits recommended by the Commission.

In its 1990 recommendations, the Commission has developed this system further by identifying practices, which increase radiation exposures and interventions which reduce them, and by recommending constraints on exposure from individual sources, below dose limits which are now regarded as the level of dose above which the consequences for the individual would be widely regarded as unacceptable. Current dose limits in the United Kingdom are based on the 1977 ICRP recommendations as incorporated into a European Community Directive and given the force of law through regulations made under the Health and Safety at Work, etc. Act, 1974.

DOSE LIMITS TO THE GENERAL PUBLIC

The present average dose to the general public from all sources of radiation is about 2.5 mSv per annum, and the vast majority of this is from natural sources of which exposure to radon gas is the largest and most variable part. By far the largest source of man-made exposure to the general public is from medical uses, as shown in Fig. 1, and of this the

Fig. 1 Sources of radiation exposure to the population of the United Kingdom (reproduced from publication NRPB-R263 of the National Radiological Protection Board with permission).

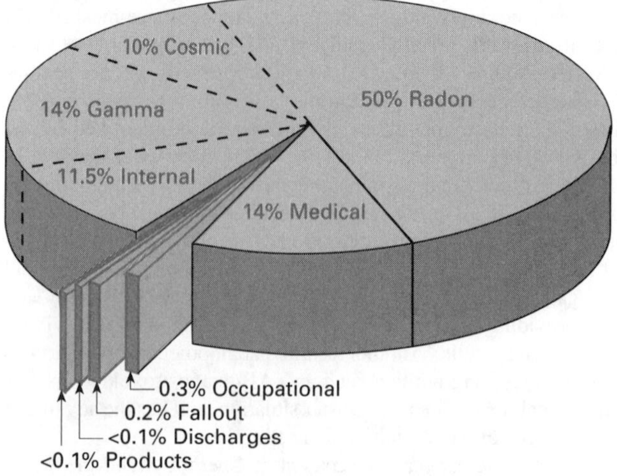

Table 2 *ICRP recommended dose limits (1990)*

	Annual dose limit	
	General public	Radiation workers
Total body exposure (effective dose)	1 mSv, a higher value allowed in special circumstances provided the average over 5 years does not exceed 1 mSv	20 mSv, averaged over defined periods of 5 years and subject to a maximum 50 mSv in any year
Lens of the eye (equivalent dose)	15 mSv	150 mSv
Skin	50 mSv	500 mSv
Hands, feet	-	500 mSv

largest contribution is from diagnostic X-rays. The current legal dose limit for total body exposure for a member of the general public reflects the 1977 recommendations of the ICRP and is 5 mSv, but subject to an average dose limit of 1 mSv per year so that the lifetime whole body equivalent dose to any individual member of the public will not normally exceed 70 mSv. This dose limit is designed to keep at an acceptably low level the stochastic harmful effects of radiation exposure (those all-or-none effects which occur with increasing frequency with increasing dose) and to prevent the occurrence of deterministic harmful effects (for which there is a dose threshold, above which they increase in severity with increasing dose). If only part of the body is irradiated, proportionately higher doses are allowed. The National Radiological Protection Board has recommended that the contribution to dose to the general public from any single source should not exceed 0.5 mSv per year, and all doses should be kept As Low As Reasonably Practicable (ALARP). The 1990 ICRP recommendations are shown in Table 2.

Limits for the inhalation or ingestion of radioactive material depend upon the concentration of those materials in limiting target organs. Thus, the limit for ingestion of radioactive iodine is set by the maximum radiation dose to the thyroid in which it would be concentrated; in fact the limit is set by the concentration in the thyroid of the most susceptible member of the population, a young child.

DOSE LIMITS TO RADIATION WORKERS

The legal dose limit in the United Kingdom currently reflects the European Community Directive implementing the 1977 recommendations of the ICRP, and is 50 mSv per annum to the whole body, with specific limits to individual organs when less than the whole body is irradiated. However, all occupational exposure is subject to demonstration that it is ALARP, and the National Radiological Protection Board has recommended a dose constraint of 15 mSv per year averaged over 5 years with no more than 20 mSv in a single year. The 1990 ICRP recommendations for occupational dose limits are also shown in Table 2. Present regulations of the European Community require that persons be designated radiation workers if there is a likelihood that their annual radiation exposure will exceed one-third of the current dose limits. Volunteers giving informed consent to participate in medical experiments in which radiation is used may not receive a dose greater than the annual dose limit to radiation workers, except in very special circumstances.

EMERGENCY REFERENCE LEVELS

In the event of an unscheduled release of radioactive material into the environment, such as from a nuclear reactor accident, it is necessary to assess the potential radiation dose to the population at risk and then to decide whether appropriate countermeasures should be taken. There are some radiation levels low enough that the risks inherent in taking any action, be it the distribution of stable iodine tablets, or the sheltering or evacuation of a population, may be greater than the risks from the radiation exposure itself. For this reason it is necessary to have emergency reference levels as a planning guide. Emergency reference levels of dose can be translated into initial activities in the air, on pasturage, in drinking water, which would lead to a total body commitment to a dose equal to the emergency reference levels. An incident which produced population doses lower than the emergency reference level would not require specific action, but above this level consideration would be given to intervention such as the destruction of milk, the removal of animals from contaminated pasture, or evacuation of populations. Thus, above a lower bound, there will be a range of action levels up to an upper dose bound above which the introduction of countermeasures is virtually certain. For taking shelter this dose range has been set in the United Kingdom as 3 to 30 mSv, while for more disruptive countermeasures such as evacuation the range is 30 to 300mSV.

Partial body exposure—local radiation effects

When less than the whole body is irradiated, the effect will once again depend on radiation dose, and critically upon what parts of the body are irradiated. Radiation therapy, limited to appropriate parts of the body, has been used to treat malignant disease since Röntgen discovered X-rays in 1895, and there is a considerable literature on the effects of such local irradiation on limiting normal tissues. The radiation effect will also be determined by the fractionation or protraction of the dose in time: the longer the overall time or the larger number of individual radiation exposures, the greater the total dose which can be accumulated before damage is produced. On the skin a single radiation dose in excess of around 8 Gy will cause a transient reddening within a few hours, followed by a more vigorous erythema at 7 to 10 days, its intensity once again depending on total dose accumulated. With increasing radiation dose to the skin, dry or moist desquamation will result, healing by repopulation of the denuded epithelium from surviving basal epithelial cells. For the majority of body tissues the major effect of irradiation is the cessation of division in the stem cells which replenish the differentiated population of the particular tissue. Therefore, radiation effects will be most severe in those tissues in which cell turnover is most rapid. In many organs, although the turnover of parenchymal cells is slow, irradiation damage is produced because of damage to blood vessels resulting in focal ischaemia and often leading to fibrosis. Limiting normal tissues for the clinical radiotherapist in the treatment of cancer include lungs, gastrointestinal tract, kidneys, and central nervous system. Modern radiation therapy uses supervoltage (greater than 1 MV) X-rays or the gamma-rays from ^{60}Co which physically spare the skin. The skin is therefore no longer the limiting normal tissue. Normal tissue tolerance is determined by the induction of fibrosis in subcutaneous connective tissues and in limiting organs within the irradiation volume.

Effects of non-ionizing radiations

Ultraviolet light

Although non-ionizing, ultraviolet light is capable of penetration to at least the basal layer of the skin epithelium, and is specifically absorbed in nucleic acid, including DNA. Because of this it is capable of causing chromosomal damage and cell killing. The clinical development of acute over-exposure to ultraviolet light with early painful erythema followed by dry or moist desquamation is well known in the less pigmented races, but the incidence of skin cancer including melanoma is also highly correlated with exposure to solar ultraviolet light. The intensity of solar ultraviolet radiation increases rapidly with increasing altitude due to the reduced atmospheric scattering and absorption of these light wavelengths. The mechanism of ultraviolet light damage has been relatively well studied; much of this damage is repaired, and individuals deficient in these repair systems such as patients with xeroderma pigmentosum, are exquisitely sensitive to ultraviolet light because of the inability to excise thymine dimers formed by this irradiation in their DNA. Protection against ultraviolet light can be achieved by ingestion of *p*-aminobenzoic acid and a number of sulphonamide antibiotics, and by the use of suitable ultraviolet light absorbing barrier creams.

Radiofrequency electromagnetic waves

The possible hazards to man of exposure to high-intensity radiofrequency electromagnetic waves is more controversial, but individuals chronically exposed to such radiations in high intensity have been reported as developing such conditions as anaemia, alopecia, or psychological disorders. In animal studies, changes in the high spontaneous rate of cancer in particular strains have been reported. The collected publications of the International Radiation Protection Association's Non-ionizing Radiation Committee have now been issued in a single volume and form the most comprehensive bibliography on the subject. The widespread use of radiofrequency 'microwave' ovens for home and restaurant cookery has made their safety a more important question. With the exception of the danger from induction heating, with consequent thermal burn damage, there is no evidence that there is significant risk of danger to the general public from the use of such appliances. The National Radiological Protection Board has recently published a report of an advisory group chaired by Sir Richard Doll which reviewed the evidence and concluded that there is '. . . a tendency for selective publication of results that suggest an increased risk . . .' for leukaemia induction, and that 'In the absence of any unambiguous experimental evidence to suggest that exposure to these electromagnetic fields is likely to be carcinogenic in the broadest sense of the term, the findings to date can be regarded only as sufficient to justify formulating an hypothesis for further investigation.' In the meantime, the National Radiological Protection Board has given advice that acceptable exposures should not result in a rise in body temperature of more than 0.5°C as shown by skin and rectal temperature. Local tissue temperatures should not exceed 38°C for the head, 39°C for the trunk, or 40°C for the limbs. This may be ensured by limiting the mean specific absorption rate in the whole body to 1 W/kg for exposures over 30 min and 2 W/kg for exposures less than 15 min with relaxations to higher levels under specific controlled conditions.

Magnetic fields

With the increasing use of magnetic resonance imaging (MRI) interest has developed in possible hazards to man of exposure to strong and varying magnetic fields. Once again, the biological evidence is largely anecdotal and in part contradictory and mainly involves transient psychological changes. The National Radiological Protection Board has recommended that for static magnetic fields, the individual being imaged should not be exposed to a field greater than 2.5 tesla (T) to the whole or substantial portion of the body. For time varying magnetic fields where the period of magnetic flux density change exceeds 3 ms, exposures should be restricted to root mean square rates of change of less than 20 T/s for all persons. Somewhat higher limits are allowable for rates of change in magnetic flux density when the period of change is less than 10 ms. There is no evidence so far to suggest that the embryo is sensitive to magnetic fields and radiofrequency at the intensities encountered in clinical magnetic resonance imaging, but it is felt to be prudent to exclude pregnant women during the first trimester.

Ultrasound

As with radiofrequency electromagnetic waves, ultrasound can produce local tissue damage by heating, but also by the production of minute bubbles due to cavitation within individual cells. The effects are critically dependent upon the sound frequency, the duty cycle, and the overall length of exposure. For the power levels used conventionally in diagnostic ultrasonography, no significant damage to mammalian cells has been demonstrated, although sophisticated studies of the effect of low-power ultrasound on chromosomes suggest that the margin may not be very wide. The widespread use of medical ultrasound as a non-invasive imaging technique, now with clinical experience of more than 30 years without significant suspicion of induction of fetal abnormalities by diagnostic ultrasound gives reassurance.

REFERENCES

Bond, V.P., Fliedner, T.M., and Archambeau, J.O. (1965). *Mammalian radiation lethality a disturbance in cellular kinetics*. Academic Press, London.

Browne, D., Weiss, J.F., MacVittie, T.J., and Pillar, M.V. (ed.). (1990). *Treatment of Radiation Injuries, Proceedings of the first consensus development conference on the treatment of radiation injuries*. Plenum Press, New York.

Council of the European Communities. (1980). Council directive of 15 July 1980 amending the directives laying down basic safety standards for the health protection of the general public and workers against the dangers of ionizing radiation. *Official Journal of the European Communities*, No. L246, 1-14, 17 September 1980. HMSO, London.

Dennis, J.A., Muirhead, C.R., and Ennis, J.R. (1992). Human health and exposure to electromagnetic radiation. *National Radiological Protection Board Technical Report R-241*. HMSO, London.

Duchene, A.S., Lakey, J.A.R., and Repacholi, M.H. (ed). (1991). IRPA Guidelines on Protection against non-ionizing radiation. *The collected publications of the IRPA non-ionizing radiation Committee*. Pergamon Press, Oxford.

Gardner, M.J., Hall, A.J., Snee, M.P., Downes, S., Powell, C.A., and Terrell, J.D. (1990). Results of a case control study of leukaemia and lymphoma among young people near Sellafield nuclear plant in West Cumbria. *British Medical Journal*, **300,** 429–34.

Hall, E.J. (1973). *Radiobiology for the radiologist*. Harper and Row, Hagerstown, Maryland.

International Commission on Radiological Protection. (1977). Publication 26, Recommendations of the International Commission on Radiological Protection. *Annals of the ICRP*, Vol. 1, no.3. Pergamon Press, Oxford.

International Commission on Radiological Protection. (1991). Publication 60, 1990. Recommendations of the International Commission on Radiological Protection. *Annals of the ICRP*, Vol. 21, no. 1-3. Pergamon Press, Oxford.

Kendall, G.M., *et al.* (1992). Mortality and occupational exposure to radiation: first analysis of the National Registry for Radiation Workers. *British Medical Journal*, **304,** 220–5.

McLaughlin, J.R., King, W.D., Anderson, T.W., Clark, E.A., and Ashmore, J.P. (1993). Paternal radiation exposure and leukaemia in offspring: the Ontario case-control study. *British Medical Journal*, **307,** 959–66.

National Radiological Protection Board. (1990). Board Statement on Emergency Reference Levels. *Documents of the NRPB*, Vol.1 no.4. HMSO, London.

National Radiological Protection Board. (1991). Board Statement on Clinical magnetic resonance diagnostic procedures. *Documents of the NRPB*, Vol.2 no.1. HMSO, London.

National Radiological Protection Board. (1992). Electromagnetic fields and the risk of cancer; report of an advisory group on non-ionising radiation. *Documents of the NRPB*, Vol.3 no.1. HMSO, London.

Otake, M. and Schull, W.J. (1984). *In utero* exposure to A-bomb radiation and mental retardation. *British Journal of Radiology*, **57,** 409–14.

Ross, W.M., Schofield, G.C., Berry, R.J., Lamerton, L.F., and Boag, J.W. (Chairman). (1983). The radiological effects of nuclear war: report of a British Institute of Radiology Working Party. *British Journal of Radiology*, **56,** 147–70.

Urquhart, J.D., *et al.* (1991). Case Control Study of leukaemia and non-Hodgkin's lymphoma in children in Caithness near the Dounreay nuclear installation. *British Medical Journal*, **302,** 687–92.

8.5.5(j) Noise

R. C. Williams

Introduction

Noise is defined in the *Concise Oxford Dictionary* as 'any sound, especially loud or harsh or undesired'. As implied in this definition, there is a subjective element in the perception of sound by the listener as 'noise'. The unpleasant noise for one person may be music to another. It is also possible for a pleasurable sound to have harmful effects. For the purposes of discussion, therefore, the terms 'noise' and 'sound' will be considered synonomous.

The most important effect of noise on man is hearing loss occurring as a consequence of exposure to loud sounds. This effect has been known since the 19th century or earlier. It was appreciated, at least by the beginning of that century, that exposure to naval gunfire could cause deafness, while the first studies on deafness in boilermakers were carried out in 1868 by Toynbee. Since then, studies have been carried out on a wide range of occupational groups confirming the association between occupational noise exposure and hearing loss, the most important of these studies in the United Kingdom being the work by Burns and Robinson in the 1960s. In addition to noise exposure in the workplace, the last 40 years have seen increasing noise exposure in the general community from a variety of sources such as domestic appliances, motor vehicles, and amplified music of all sorts, whether from radios and personal stereos or at discotheques and concerts.

Sound is the perception by the listener of the fluctuations in air pressure produced by a vibrating source. The loudness and character of the sound will depend on the magnitude of the pressure fluctuations and their frequency. In an average healthy young adult, the threshold at which these pressure fluctuations are perceived is 0.00002 pascals (Pa). In noisy manufacturing processes, levels of 2 to 10 Pa are common, whilst the impulse noise from firearms can peak at levels in excess of 1000 Pa. For practical reasons, it is normal to use the logarithmic 'Bel' scale rather than pascals when measuring loudness. The use of such a scale makes it easier to manipulate the wide range of pressure values and corresponds better than a linear scale with the response of the human ear to sound. The unit used is the decibel (dB) which is one-tenth of a 'bel'. The bel scale is a comparative one which requires a reference level, and the one used is the threshold of hearing, 0.00002 Pa.

Since the scale is a logarithmic one, each increase of 3 dB represents a doubling of the energy content. Since, as already stated, the response of the human ear to sound is more logarithmic than linear it therefore requires an increase of 10 dB for a sound to be perceived by the listener as twice as loud.

The number of fluctuations, i.e. cycles per second of the sound pressure wave, constitutes its frequency. The unit of measurement is the hertz (Hz), 1 hertz being one cycle per second. The perception of pitch by the listener is dependent on frequency, the higher the frequency the higher the pitch. The perception of loudness is also affected by frequency. The frequency of any sound will depend on the physical characteristics of the originating source. In practice, it is unusual to have a pure tone and most sounds are made up of a broad spectrum of frequencies of different strengths. It is desirable when measuring sound levels that this is done across the frequency range. This is conventionally done in octave bands, and an example of such an analysis is given in Fig. 1.

In an otologically normal young adult, the ear can perceive sounds in a frequency range from about 25 Hz to about 20 000 Hz (20 kHz). The human ear is most sensitive in the range 500 Hz to 4 kHz, which corresponds to the speech frequencies, vowels being in the range 400 Hz to 2 kHz, and consonants in the range 700 Hz to 4 kHz. There is a rapid fall-off in the sensitivity of the ear in the lower frequencies and a more gradual fall-off in the higher frequencies.

Noise is measured using sound level meters, and all but the most simple instruments have provision for weighting the sensitivity at different frequencies. There are four different scales, the A, B, C, and D scales. The A scale weights the lower frequencies in a similar manner to the response of the human ear, and for this reason is the one most generally used for workplace assessments determining the risk to hearing. It is the normal convention to state the scale when recording the readings, e.g. 90 dB(A). An individual's noise exposure may be expressed as a daily personal noise exposure (Lep,d) or a weekly average of daily personal noise exposure (Lep,w). Formulae are available for calculating both values.

The effect of noise on hearing

The level at which sound becomes harmful to hearing is a matter which continues to be controversial. Susceptibility to hearing loss is subject to normal biological variation, and in any noise-exposed group there will be individuals who may be at increased risk due to disease, toxic agents, or possibly other environmental factors. Current legislation in the United Kingdom, *The Noise At Work Regulations 1989*, which is based on a European Community Directive, specifies 'a first action level of 85 dB(A)'. This should be sufficient to prevent significant hearing loss in otologically normal persons. Within the United Kingdom, the Health and Safety Executive estimated that in 1986 about 1.5 million workers in production industries and construction and around half those in agriculture could be exposed to noise levels above 85 dB(A).

Fig. 1 An analysis of sound levels.

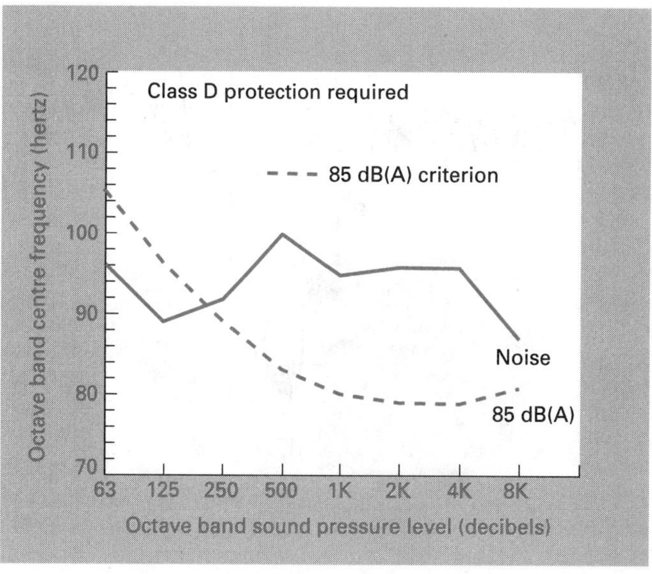

There are four main effects on hearing from noise exposure. These are temporary hearing loss, permanent hearing loss, tinnitus, and recruitment. Initially, exposure to harmful levels of noise causes a temporary loss of hearing, this temporary threshold shift being in the frequency range 4 to 6 kHz. The time taken for recovery is subject to individual variation and the amount of noise exposure; it will usually be complete within 2 weeks of the exposure ceasing.

With continuing noise exposure, the individual will develop a permanent threshold shift, i.e. irreversible hearing loss. The extent of the hearing loss and the rapidity of onset will depend on the susceptibility of the individual and the total noise dose. Again, this hearing loss occurs in the range 4 to 6 kHz. Initially, the lower frequencies are largely unaffected, and there is recovery in the higher frequencies. On audiometric testing, this appears as a characteristic notching of the audiogram, (Fig. 2). With continuing noise exposure, the extent of the loss both increases and extends into the lower frequencies (Fig. 3).

The cause of both the temporary and permanent hearing loss is damage to the hair cells of the cochlea. Permanent hearing loss is due to death of these cells, and is irreversible. The mechanism by which this damage occurs and the reason for the initial loss being greatest at 4 to 6 kHz is unknown. It is known that the hair cells are frequency specific and it is possible the anatomical characteristics of the cochlea make the cells in this frequency band particularly vulnerable to damage.

Tinnitus is a subjective symptom, but is known to occur in association with noise-induced hearing loss. The incidence does not appear related to the severity of the hearing loss. It has been estimated that in 5 to 10 per cent of cases it will be sufficient to cause annoyance and in approximately 1 per cent it will be severe. Some authors have concluded that the incidence is higher for individuals exposed to impulse noise.

Recruitment is a distortion of the perception of sound which occurs in individuals with severe noise-induced hearing loss. It is a response by the damaged cochlea in which sounds well above the threshold of hearing are suddenly heard by the deaf individual at normal or greater than normal loudness. It has a characteristic appearance on the audiogram.

Hearing conservation

The United Kingdom requires every employer, by the Noise Regulations (1990), to 'reduce the risk of damage to the hearing of his employees from exposure to noise to the lowest level reasonably practicable'. A Hearing Conservation Programme should include the following action;

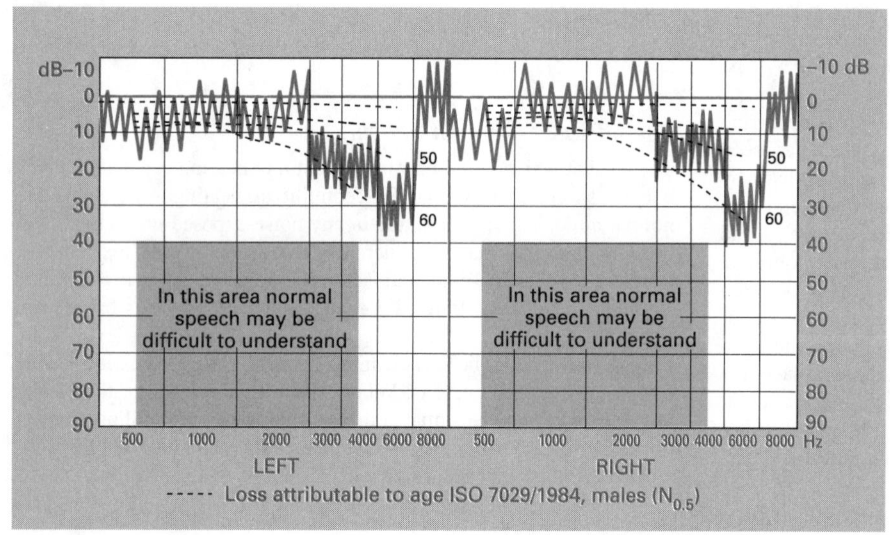

Fig. 2 Hearing loss after continuing noise exposure. Initially the lower frequencies are largely unaffected and there is recovery in the higher frequencies, appearing as a characteristic notching of the audiogram.

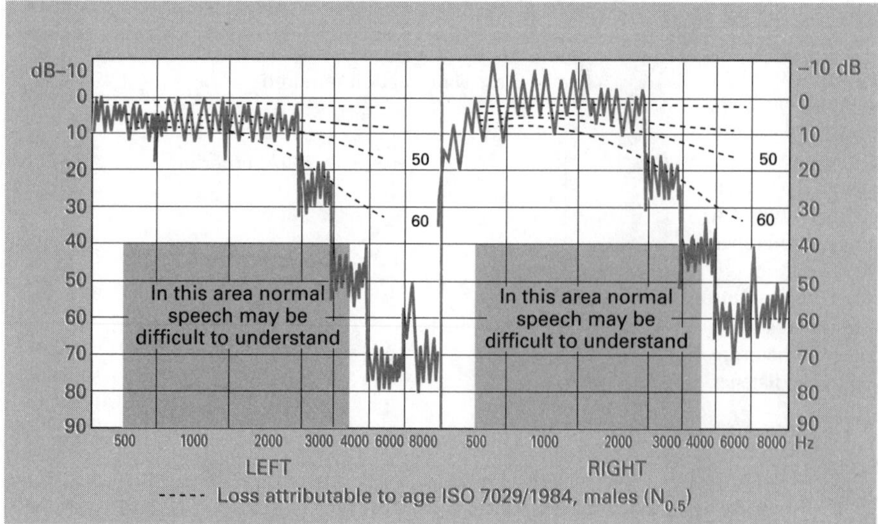

Fig. 3 With continuing noise exposure the extent of the loss increases and extends into the lower frequencies.

an assessment of noise exposure, action to reduce noise levels by engineering means, the provision of hearing protection (Fig. 4), information, instruction, and training for employees on the risk to hearing, and the use of personal protection. Many employers include audiometry screening in the Hearing Conservation Programme, but this is not a legal requirement within the United Kingdom.

Audiometry and the investigation of noise-induced hearing loss

The value of workplace screening audiometry for noise-exposed employees is controversial. Despite criticisms, it is an increasingly used procedure, probably because many employers see it as a protection against claims for noise-induced hearing loss. If the full benefit is to be obtained from such testing, it is essential it is combined with education of employees about the effects of noise and the correct use of hearing protection. There should also be an analysis of the data to assess the effectiveness of the Hearing Conservation Programme and identify at-risk groups. There must be adequate arrangements to ensure the medical follow-up of individuals with abnormal audiograms.

Various classification systems have been proposed for assessing audiometric findings. Within the United Kingdom, there are three main systems in general use. At the workplace, the most commonly used system is probably that suggested in 1987 by the Health and Safety Executive in their discussion document *Audiometry in Industry*. This is based on the sum of the hearing levels at 0.5, 1, and 2 kHz and at 3, 4, and 6 kHZ respectively. A category 1 to 5 is allocated on the basis of this calculation. The United Kingdom Department of Social Security uses a system for assessing disability for industrial injury benefit purposes based on the average at 1, 2, and 3 kHz. The average at 1, 2, and 3 kHz has also been recommended as a basis for assessing hearing disability in guidance published by members of a Working Group on Hearing Disability formed from nominees of the relevant United Kingdom Professional Societies and Associations.

The investigation of individuals for noise-induced hearing loss should include a full history of previous noise exposure, including the provision and use of hearing protection. Enquiry should be made into previous ear disease, ototoxic drug exposure, and any illnesses that could be associated with hearing loss. The individual should be asked about social handicap and the presence of tinnitus. The examination should include otoscopy and audiometry. Full investigation will require the use of an audiometer with facilities for masking and bone conduction testing. It may also be desirable to carry out tympanometry to exclude middle ear disease. In certain circumstances, more sophisticated testing, such as evoked response audiometry, may be required.

Fig. 4 Hearing protection does work but only when worn!

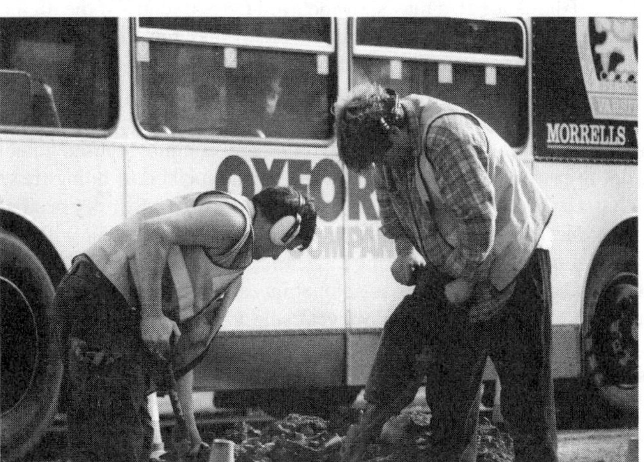

Non-auditory effects of noise

Noise is known to produce a number of other effects on man apart from its effects on hearing. Some of these are mainly of importance in the workplace, but others have an importance in the community as a whole.

In the workplace, loud noise may give rise to difficulties due to interference with the perception of speech. In particular, failure to communicate may give rise to safety hazards. When employees regularly work in loud noise levels, in the long term there will be some adaptation, such as subconscious raising of the voice and lip reading.

A variety of behavioural effects have been attributed to noise. These include annoyance, reduced efficiency, fatigue, and effects on mental health. The fact that noise can cause annoyance is self-evident. The effects of noise on efficiency and fatigue due to noise have been the subject of a number of studies. These have indicated there may be effects, but further work appears necessary. The effects on mental health are difficult to quantify, but there have been some suggestions that there is a greater incidence of psychiatric illness in areas where there are high levels of neighbourhood noise, for example from aircraft.

A number of physiological effects have been attributed to noise, some self-evident such as sleep interference, but also including more specific effects on health, in particular effects on cardiovascular function, especially the blood pressure, and effects on the gastrointestinal system, for example peptic ulcer. The recommended maximum noise level to avoid sleep disturbance is 35 dB(A) averaged over the sleeping period. It has been estimated that 50 per cent of individuals will have sleep disturbance at 50 dB(A). The strongest evidence for an effect on health is for the effect on blood pressure. Several authors have claimed that noise exposure is associated with an increase in blood pressure. Partly because of the difficulties in assessing the effects of noise in isolation from the other causes of hypertension further work is required on this subject.

REFERENCES

Burns, W. and Robinson, D.W., (1970). *Hearing and noise in industry*. HMSO, London.

King, Coles, Lutman, and Robinson. (1992). *Assessment of hearing disability*. Whurr Publishers, London.

Noise at Work. (1989). Noise Guides Nos. 1 and 2. HMSO, London.

Robinson, D.W. (1987). Noise exposure and hearing. A new look at the experimental data. *Health and Safety Executive Report No. 1*. HMSO, London.

8.5.5(k) Vibration

TAR-CHING AW

Definition

Vibration can be defined as the mechanical oscillation of a surface around its reference point. It is measured in terms of:

(a) Frequency (**cycles per second (c.p.s.) or Hertz (Hz)**). The most damaging frequencies are between 25 and 250 Hz;
(b) Magnitude. (m/s^2);
(c) Direction.

Exposure

Exposure to a source of vibration can be transmitted locally usually to the hands and arms, or to the whole body. Occupational exposure and the effects of hand—arm transmitted vibration, differ from that of whole body vibration. Whole body vibration is most likely to affect drivers of tractors, fork-lift trucks, mobile cranes, and helicopters. Hand-arm

Table 1 *Stockholm Scales. Classification of the hand–arm vibration syndrome*

Stage	Grade	Description
1. *Vascular*		
0		No attacks
1	Mild	Occasional attacks affecting only the tips of one or more fingers
2	Moderate	Occasional attacks affecting distal and middle (rarely also proximal) phalanges of one or more fingers
3	Severe	Frequent attacks affecting all phalanges of most fingers
4	Very severe	As in stage 3, with trophic changes in the finger tips
2. *Sensorineural component*		
0_{SN}	Vibration-exposed but no symptoms	
1_{SN}	Intermittent numbness with or without tingling	
2_{SN}	Intermittent or persistent numbness, reduced sensory perception	
3_{SN}	Intermittent or persistent numbness, reduced sensory actile discrimination and/or manipulative dexterity	

vibration exposure occurs in factory workers involved in fettling, chipping, grinding, riveting, swaging, and using drop hammers and hand-held pneumatic hammers, drills, and chisels. It also affects forestry, agricultural, and woodworkers using chain saws, miners drilling rock surfaces, construction and road workers using drills and compactors, and shoe manufacturers using polishing and rotary tools. The pattern of exposure to vibration can be episodic as in the use of a grinding device (e.g. pedestal grinder), random (e.g. in road drilling), and transient (e.g. in the transmission of vibration to a driver when a vehicle hits a pothole in the road). It has been estimated that around 3 per cent of the working population are occupationally exposed to sources of vibration.

Clinical effects

Whole body vibration

Effects include headache, motion sickness, sleep and visual disturbance, urinary and abdominal complaints, and low back pain. In the case of drivers, low back pain may occur as a result of exposure to whole body vibration and poor posture within the vehicle cab. The local effects of hand transmitted vibration have been more extensively studied than whole body vibration, and the rest of this chapter will focus on hand transmitted vibration.

Hand transmitted vibration

Hand–arm transmitted vibration causes secondary Raynaud's phenomenon. This manifests as frequent episodic pallor of the digits, usually on exposure to cold. The condition has also been termed vibration white finger. While the term refers to vascular changes, neurological and musculoskeletal effects are often accompanying features, and may contribute more to the disability experienced. The term 'hand arm vibration syndrome' has been used in preference to vibration white finger, to include the neurological, and musculoskeletal effects. Other suggested terms are vibration induced white finger and hand transmitted vibration syndrome. The latent period between initial exposure and development of symptoms varies with the nature and intensity of exposure. This is usually in the range 5 to 10 years, but may be as little as 1 year.

The vascular effects have been attributed to spasm of the digital vessels, and there is some debate over whether this may be secondary to an effect on the nerve supply to these vessels. The sequence of colour change in the affected digits include pallor, a bluish hue due to cyanosis and redness with spontaneous reversal of the vascular spasm. Exposure to cold precipitates attacks of digital pallor, and patients frequently describe pallor in the morning, or following outdoor activity such as fishing or gardening especially in cold weather. The neurological effects include numbness, reduced temperature perception, loss of manual dexterity, tingling, paraesthesia, and pain. Severe tingling, discomfort, and pain is often described by patients following rapid warming of the hands when the digital blood circulation returns to normal. Inability to distinguish and hold small objects such as coins, and difficulty with manipulating the steering wheel of a car or buttoning up clothes contributes to physical and social disability. Musculoskeletal effects are not as well established, but muscle weakness, exostoses and cysts in the carpal bones, carpal tunnel syndrome, osteoarthritis, and Dupuytren's contracture have been associated with exposure to vibration.

Diagnosis

Diagnosis is based primarily on documentation of relevant and sufficient exposure to vibration and a history consistent with Raynaud's phenomenon. Fingers and thumbs can both be affected. The presence of associated neurological and musculoskeletal features would add support to the diagnosis. Physical examination may show callosities on the hands, loss of touch, pinprick or temperature sensation in the affected digits, muscle weakness, or may show no obvious abnormalities especially in the early stages of the disease. Phalen's sign (tingling sensation in the fingers following flexion of the wrists) and Tinel's sign (sharp tingling along the path of the median nerve on tapping the wrist over the site of the carpal tunnel) are positive if there is associated carpal tunnel syndrome. In rare and very severe cases trophic changes in the finger tips occur leading to gangrene.

Various clinical and special tests have been used in the evaluation of patients with hand arm vibration syndrome. Compression of the nail bed of affected digits for 10 s may show delayed (> 5 s) return of the digital circulation (Lewis–Prusik test). Finger plethysmography allows measurement of changes in finger systolic blood pressure and finger vascular circulation following local cooling. Digital blood pressure measurements using a Doppler device may demonstrate a fall in pressure after cold provocation. Cold provocation tests are commonly used in an attempt to provoke digital pallor. However, the method of doing these tests has not been standardized, and sensitivity is low. Sensory aesthesiometry may detect early loss of tactile perception. Together with the use of a vibrometer for evaluating thresholds of perception of vibration, these tests have found favour as adjunct investigations in cases of hand arm vibration syndrome. In any event, the clinical and occupational history is of greater importance than the results of any of the varied tests available in the diagnosis of hand arm vibration syndrome.

The differential diagnosis should include other causes for Raynaud's phenomenon, or the neurological and musculoskeletal findings. Raynaud's phenomenon may be primary or constitutional (3–4 per cent in men and 10 per cent in women), or secondary to other diseases such as rheumatoid arthritis, lupus erythematosus, scleroderma, other autoimmune disorders, poliomyelitis, syringomyelia, cryoglobulinaemia, occlusive vascular disease, frostbite, and the costoclavicular syndrome. Medications such as ergot, clonidine, and β-blockers, and heavy cigarette smoking may be contributory factors. Occupational exposure to vinyl chloride monomer can cause Raynaud's phenomenon, and n-hexane, carbon disulphide, methyl n-butyl ketone and other occupational neurotoxic agents can produce neurological effects similar to that seen in hand–arm vibration syndrome.

Management, treatment, and prevention.

Vibration induced white finger is a prescribed industrial disease in many countries including the United Kingdom. Workers meeting the criteria for prescription, i.e. having the condition of sufficient severity and working in one of the listed occupations, are entitled to financial benefits. The severity of the disease may be staged according to various schemes.

The Taylor and Pelmear (1975) scale assigns a stage according to the extent and severity of blanching of the digits, and the degree of interference with work and social activities. Four stages for blanching (1–4) are described with a stage 0_T for intermittent tingling, and a stage 0_N for intermittent numbness.

Griffin (1982) and Rigby and Cornish (1984) described a numerical scoring system based on the phalanges affected by blanching. A score of 1 is assigned to the distal phalanges, 2 for the middle, and 3 for the proximal phalanges of the fingers. The proximal phalanx of the thumb is allocated a higher score of 5, and the distal phalanx 4. The total score provides a quantitative basis for assessment of progression of the disease.

In 1987, the Stockholm Workshop scale was proposed to incorporate separate staging for the vascular and sensorineural effects (Table 1). The staging is made separately for each hand. The grade of the disorder is indicated by the stage and the number of affected fingers on each hand; for example, '2L(2)/1R(3)' means two digits at stage 2 in the left hand; and 3 digits at stage one in the right hand.

Depending on the severity of the condition, different medical, occupational hygiene, and management actions can be taken. The action of choice is to eliminate or reduce the source of vibration. Engineering controls may minimize the transmission of vibration from machinery to the body or hands. Specially designed gloves can keep the hands warm and reduce vibration transmission. The patient may be in a position to continue in the job following such action. Where the condition is severe and the source of vibration cannot be eliminated, redeployment away from vibration exposure needs to be considered. In early cases redeployment may arrest or reverse the progression of the symptoms. In severe cases the disease may progress regardless of removal from further exposure to vibration, although there is some suggestion that even in severe cases reversibility can occur. Reversibility is slower in older individuals, and the sensorineural component appears to be slower than the vascular component.

Advice to the patient includes avoidance or reduction of further exposure to vibration, use of appropriate gloves, keeping the body and hands warm, especially in cold weather or when working with cold or pneumatic tools, and cessation of cigarette smoking. Vasodilatory drugs have been used to alleviate symptoms in severe cases. These drugs include tolazoline, inositol, and cyclandelate. Calcium antagonists such as verapamil and nifedipine, angiotensin-converting enzyme inhibitors, prostaglandins, and stanazolol have also been tried. Surgical treatment such as sympathectomy is not recommended for vibration-induced white finger.

A diagnosis of Raynaud's phenomenon should always include detailed inquiry into occupational exposure to vibration. The diagnosis of a case of vibration-induced white finger should be viewed as a sentinel event warranting further investigation of the workplace to assess whether improvements in work practices can be implemented to prevent other cases from occurring.

REFERENCE

Gemne, G. (ed.). (1987). Symptomatology and diagnostic methods in the hand–arm vibration syndrome. *Scandinavian Journal of Work and Environmental Health,* **13,** 271–388.

Tyler, L.E. (ed.). (1993). *FOM Working Party Report on Hand Transmitted Vibration.* Royal College of Physicians, London.

8.5.5(l) Air pollution

J. G. Ayres

Introduction

Concerns about air quality and its effects on health have been expressed for many hundreds of years. The lime burners of the 1300s were blamed for polluting the air and John Evelyn in his famous diary railed against the polluted air of the City of London. The domestic pollution of those years was later compounded by the advent of the Industrial Revolution in the 18th century when the sulphurous emissions from factories were regarded as a necessary evil meaning as it did, jobs and payment for the working population. This grudging acceptance remained until the London Fog Incident of 1952 when, in a space of a week 4000 excess deaths occurred during a particularly severe 'pea souper'. The week was cold, resulting in more coal being burnt in domestic grates and a temperature inversion with a 'blocking' zone of high pressure resulted in accumulation of pollutants at street level. As a result, the Clean Air Act of 1956 was passed which has resulted in a marked reduction in particulate pollution and a lesser reduction in sulphur dioxide levels. This left a feeling in Government that air pollution and its potential health problems had been conquered until in the 1980s it was realized that vehicle emissions were an increasing cause of a different type of air pollution. The pollutants from such emissions, nitrogen dioxide, particulates, and hydrocarbons are potentially harmful in their own right but also act as a substrate for the formation of ozone, the combination of all these pollutants comprising the photochemical pollution (Plate 1) so characteristic of Los Angeles, Athens, and Mexico City.

Although the quality of outdoor air is clearly important, we spend most of our lives indoors and it is now evident that indoor air quality has a role to play in the pathogenesis of lung disease. In the workplace, occupational asthma is an obvious example of an effect of poor indoor air quality (see Section 17.8). Most indoor levels of pollutants are driven by outdoor levels with the exception of nitrogen dioxide which is produced in gas-fired homes, some of the highest personal exposures being recorded near gas cookers. However, the most important indoor pollutant is cigarette smoke, which has a particularly damaging effect on the developing lungs of young children. At present the extent of the health effect(s) of these pollutants, alone or in combination, are a continuing matter for research and debate. Acute effects are often deemed to be small but studies of any health effects of long-term exposure are somewhat lacking.

Measurement of a health effect

The main problem in determining health effects of individual air pollutants is that in real life they are never experienced in isolation. There are multiple potential interactions, not only with other air pollutants, but with other factors such as weather conditions (as seen in the London Fog Incident), levels of airborne allergen, the presence of a respiratory tract infection, exercise, and actively or passively inhaled cigarette smoke. These make determination of specific, pollutant-induced health effects often difficult to unravel.

Point sources of pollution (usually specific factories) are frequently blamed for health effects by the population living nearby. Occasionally, such as has been shown near castor-bean processing factories and steel mills, this can be readily proved but in many cases it is impossible to do so. There are problems in obtaining adequately objective data and

Table 1 *Guideline levels for the air pollutants with respect to human health*

	European Community	World Health Organization
Sulphur dioxide	37–55 p.p.b. (100–150 μg/m^3) (24-h mean) 15–22 p.p.b. (40–60 μg/m^3) (annual mean)	190 p.p.b. (500 μg/m^3) 10 min 135 p.p.b. (350 μg/m^3) 1 h 48 p.p.b. (125 μg/m^3) 24 h 19 p.p.b. (50 μg/m^3) Annual
Sulphur dioxide and smoke Winter smoke	130 μg/m^3 (if smoke < 60, sulphur dioxide 180 μg/m^3) (if smoke >60, sulphur dioxide 130 μg/m^3)	
Annual smoke (98th centile) 250 μg/m^3	(if smoke < 150, sulphur dioxide 350 μg/m^3) (if smoke > 150, sulphur dioxide)	125 μg/m^3 BS (or 120 μg/m^{3}TSP) (24 h mean) (if sulphur dioxide > 125 μg/m^3 (48 p.p.b.))
Smoke		50 μg/m^3 BS (annual mean)
Ozone	50 p.p.b (8-hourly)*	76–100 p.p.b. (150–200 μg/m^3) (1 h mean) 50–60 p.p.b. (100–120 μg/m^3)
Carbon monoxide	None	86 p.p.m. (100 mg/m^3) (not more than 15 min) 50 p.p.m. (60 mg/m^3 (for 30 min))
Lead	2μg/m^3	0.5–1 μg/m^3 (1 year mean)

BS = British Smoke, TSP = total suspended particulates.

*United Kingdom Standard set in 1994.

there are potential sources of confounding in terms of socioeconomic class and cigarette smoking. If hospital admissions (usually respiratory) are increased then an effect is more easily noticed than if the effect is manifest only in terms of symptoms. With diffuse sources of pollution (e.g. vehicle emissions) effects are likely to be noticed because of variable exposures to different sections of the populations either contemporaneously or through variable exposure over time.

There are three main ways whereby a health effect can be assessed: animal studies, challenge studies in humans, and by epidemiological studies. Each have their problems but when determining national ambient air quality standards all available types of data may be taken into consideration. When determining national ambient air quality standards, the aim is to try and define a no observable effect level (NOEL), i.e. the level of a specific pollutant where no health effect can be demonstrated. The rough rule of thumb that has been used is to take as the standard a level one-tenth of the NOEL obtained from human chamber/challenge studies or one-hundredth of the NOEL determined by animal studies. Risk assessment is difficult and very largely arbitrary. Although individual risks are relatively easily measurable in the workplace, when considering ambient airborne pollution individual risk and public health load has been poorly characterized to date.

However, the health effects of outdoor air pollution are considerably less than the risks of active cigarette smoking or the risks of well recognized environmental hazards such as exposure to asbestos. Never the less the true risk to the population of carcinogens from point or diffuse sources of pollution is not clearly quantified.

Outdoor pollution

European Community and World Health Organization guideline levels are summarized in Table 1.

POLYNUCLEAR AROMATIC HYDROCARBONS

These form part of the total hydrocarbons, a wide range of compounds most of which have no known human health effect. When considering total hydrocarbons methane is usually excluded, the remaining hydrocarbons largely comprising alkanes. Because of their association with particulates, total hydrocarbons are usually expressed as parts per billion of carbon. Polynuclear aromatic hydrocarbons are partitioned between the particulate and gas phase, the lower molecular weight molecules being in the gas phase.

The main sources of airborne polycyclic aromatic hydrocarbons are from evaporation of solvents and fuels and from combustion of fuels. Industrial processes and solvent evaporation are responsible for around 50 per cent, road transport for about 25 per cent and gas leaks for 10 per cent of emissions in the United Kingdom. Of these, benzene and, to a lesser extent, benz[*a*]pyrene are known to be carcinogenic. Benzene is present in significant quantities in cigarette smoke and, on average, cigarette smokers take in about 2 mg/day compared with less than 0.2 mg/day for most non-smokers, although passively exposed non-smokers will be exposed to approximately 60 per cent more benzene than non-passive non-smokers. Benzene is a known carcinogen and has been implicated in the development of myeloid leukaemia in adults, although the data for children are more conflicting. Workers exposed to high levels of benzene (e.g. gas works retort house operators, coke oven workers) have higher rates of lung cancer after allowing for cigarette smoking.

LEAD

The effects of occupational exposure to lead and of ingested lead are discussed in Chapters 8.3.6 and 8.5.3(k) respectively. Exposure of the population to lead during the 18th and 19th centuries was probably two to three times greater than at present, the most important source today being the use of lead in petrol. Lead (usually as tetraethyl lead) was introduced as an antiknock agent in petrol but significant reductions in the lead content of leaded petrol in the United Kingdom have occurred over the last 20 years. In 1972 lead content was 0.84 g/l but this had halved by 1981. As a result of European Community legislation in 1986, lead content was reduced to 0.15 g/l which resulted in a 60 per cent reduction in lead emissions. Atmospheric lead levels show a seasonal pattern being approximately double in summer compared with those of winter. An increment in airborne level of 1 μg/m^3 is likely to result in an increase in blood level of 2 μg per cent.

Before 1986, in a very busy, congested city airborne lead levels were around 6 μg/m^3 although a more typical level for a city would be 2 to 3 μg/m^3. Levels fall off quickly with distance from a road and are much lower in suburban (0.5 μg/m^3) and rural (0.1 μg/m^3) areas.

The effect of lead on IQ has been hotly debated. The DHSS Working Party on lead confirmed that children with blood lead levels of greater than 80 μg/dl had impaired IQs and that in any child with a level of between 35 and 80 μg/dl, a source of lead exposure should be sought.

GASEOUS/PARTICULATE POLLUTION

The response by the airways to inhalation of an airborne pollutant is complex. The level and duration of exposure and co-exposure at the same time to another pollutant will affect any response as will the presence of cofactors such as exercise, a concurrent respiratory tract infection, or cigarette smoke. The susceptibility of the individual will also contribute, individuals at the extremes of age, those with greater bronchial responsiveness, and possibly those who are atopic being more likely to be affected. The most susceptible are those with pre-existing chronic lung disease (e.g. asthma, chronic airflow obstruction) and the very young. There is no evidence that individuals with normal lungs will develop asthma if exposed to long-term air pollution although there is good evidence that the prevalence of chronic productive bronchitis is greater in polluted areas, even allowing for cigarette smoking.

Sulphur dioxide (SO_2) and particulates

These are the major constituents of so-called sulphurous air pollution, such as was seen in cities in the United Kingdom before the Clean Air Act. The emissions come from fossil fuel burning (coal and wood) the main emitters being power stations. Small quantities only of sulphur dioxide are emitted from vehicle exhausts, but diesel exhausts expel around 10 times as much particulates as petrol engines. The individual effects of sulphur dioxide and particulates have been difficult to disentangle. Sulphur dioxide causes tracheitis and reduces ciliary function *in vitro*, whilst *in vivo* it can cause bronchoconstriction in exercising asthmatics at levels as low as 0.2 p.p.m., levels which can occasionally be experienced in urban areas today. Non-asthmatic subjects, particularly those who are atopic, will also develop bronchoconstriction with sulphur dioxide on exercise but only at significantly higher exposures. The effect is usually relatively short lived after a single challenge. Many studies worldwide have shown chronic effects of sulphur dioxide on absenteeism, respiratory symptoms, and on prevalence and mortality of chronic bronchitis/chronic airflow obstruction. Acutely, with episodes of sulphur dioxide pollution, transient falls in FEV_1 and peak flow have been seen in asthmatic subjects and increases in hospital admissions have been shown. It is clear from challenge and epidemiological evidence that some individuals are particularly sensitive to the effects of sulphur dioxide. It has been estimated that 25 per cent of asthmatics are sensitive to less than 0.5 p.p.m. of sulphur dioxide while exercising. Recent cross-sectional surveys from France and Poland have suggested that lower levels of FEV_1 and greater respiratory symptoms occur in regions of higher exposure to sulphur dioxide. Earlier British work in postal workers also appeared to show such an effect but is probable that particulate pollution acts either as a confounder or as a cofactor in this situation.

Particulate pollution has usually been measured in the United Kingdom as British Smoke (BS), a measure which assesses the degree of blackening of a filter. This is now being superseded by more accurate measures such as total suspended particulates, which bear a reasonable correlation to BS, and PM10 or PM2.5, particulates less than 10 or 2.5 μm respectively. Recently particulates have been shown to have specific health effects independent of sulphur dioxide. All cause mortality, respiratory mortality, hospital admissions, and respiratory symptoms are significantly correlated to PM10 levels well within WHO guide-lines. In Beijing, long-term particulate exposure causes significant reductions in FEV_1 independent of sulphur dioxide. Particulates also relate more closely to the prevalence of cough and sputum than does sulphur dioxide. Particulates from diesel exhausts are now major contributors to urban particulate levels. Recent work from Japan has shown that diesel exhaust particulates increase an animal's ability to produce allergen specific IgE when challenged, which is a possible explanation for the greater prevalence of hay-fever in urban compared to rural areas in Japan and elsewhere. Particulates and sulphur dioxide, therefore are significantly associated with acute and chronic respiratory disease, independently and in conjunction.

Oxides of nitrogen

The major oxides of nitrogen, nitric oxide (NO), nitrous oxide (N_2O), and nitrogen dioxide (NO_2) are regarded together as NOx. The most important component is nitrogen dioxide, nitric oxide and nitrous oxide having no known deleterious respiratory effects. The major source of nitrogen dioxide is from vehicle emissions, one-third of ambient nitrogen dioxide coming from diesel engines. The highest exposures to ambient nitrogen dioxide for most individuals, however, are seen indoors in gas-fired kitchens, where levels may reach 400 to 500 p.p.b. for short periods. A more usual indoor level is 100 p.p.b. compared to an outdoor urban level of around 30 p.p.b. At 400 p.p.b. ciliary function of isolated human respiratory mucosal cells is impaired. Nitrogen dioxide at very high levels can cause acute pulmonary oedema, but this is only usually seen in the occupational setting (silo filler's disease, Chapter 17.10). The effects of ambient levels of nitrogen dioxide is a matter of much debate and published data are conflicting. An early study showed that 0.1 p.p.m. nitrogen dioxide increased airway responsiveness in exercising asthmatics, but subsequent studies, even up to exposures of 4 p.p.m., showed no effect. A number of epidemiological studies, both cross-sectional and longitudinal (in the short term), have shown significant associations between symptoms and nitrogen dioxide levels, while in Germany the incidence of croup has been shown to relate to levels of nitrogen dioxide. It is reasonable to say that although the evidence for a deleterious direct effect of nitrogen dioxide on human health is conflicting it would be very unwise to rule out such an effect completely. Recently NO_2 has been shown to enhance the bronchoconstrictor response to allergen suggesting a permissive effect of nitrogen dioxide.

Ozone

Ozone is a highly reactive molecule which is formed by the action of ultra-violet light on NOx and hydrocarbon fragments emitted by vehicles. It is formed mostly during the summer months and tends to build up over a prolonged warm spell. Levels are often higher in rural areas downwind from cities as urban nitric oxide neutralizes ozone while the formation of ozone takes a little time as polluted air is taken downwind. It is also probable that ozone enhances the formation of aerosol strong acid, thus significantly affecting the ambient pollutant mix. There is a diurnal variation with peak levels being achieved in late afternoon. In the winter ozone levels are almost unmeasurably low but in summer can exceed hourly values of 100 p.p.b. Rarely in the United Kingdom they will reach 200 p.p.b.

Ozone causes inflammatory changes in the bronchial mucosa at levels as low as 80 p.p.b., at which level changes in vital capacity and FEV_1 can be detected after an exposure of 1 h. Bronchoalveolar lavage after ozone challenge has confirmed recruitment of inflammatory cells at exposures of around 80 p.p.b. Individual responses to challenge with ozone vary widely between normal and asthmatic subjects, but asthmatics appear not to be more sensitive to the effects than normal subjects. It is possible that women are more susceptible. Repetitive exposures seem to produce a lesser response suggesting a latency effect which is difficult to understand in view of the known inflammatory effect of this gas. Summer peaks of ozone and acid have been associated with peaks in hospital admissions for asthma in a number of areas of North America. It has been suggested that a chronic respiratory bronchiolitis found in the lungs of young men dying from non-respiratory causes in Los Angeles (where hourly levels may even reach 300 p.p.b.) is due to chronic ozone exposure but this has been contested. Ozone at levels which do not cause an effect on airway function can cause bronchoconstriction when patients are pre-exposed to usual ambient sulphur dioxide which suggests a potentiating effect of air pollutants, which has great logical appeal. Ozone at 120 p.p.b. has also been shown to enhance the bronchoconstrictor response to inhaled allergen which again reinforces the very likely possibility that current air pollutants exert their effect in a permissive way. This is an area currently under research and is likely to clarify the complex manner in which air pollutants interact with themselves and with other cofactors.

ACID AEROSOLS

Acid air is not to be confused with acid rain although the contributory sources are the same. Acidity in the air is caused by the four major strong acids, sulphuric (formed from sulphur dioxide) nitric (from nitrogen dioxide) and the primary pollutants hydrochloric acid and methane sulphonic acid. Of these it is believed that sulphuric acid is the most important in urban areas, although there are no recent studies to confirm this from the United Kingdom. There are no WHO or European Community levels. Data from the United States Six Cities Study suggest that aerosol strong acid is correlated to the prevalence of cough with sputum but its precise importance in the pathogenesis of lung disease has yet to be determined.

CARBON MONOXIDE

The major source of carbon monoxide for cigarette smokers is, and will remain, cigarette smoke. For non-smokers, including children, there are two main sources, vehicle emissions and passively inhaled cigarette smoke, although indoor cooking can make a significant contribution. Exposures are far greater in tunnels, car parks, garages, and in dense, slow moving traffic. Kerbside levels in towns are of the order of 20 p.p.m. which, with chronic exposure, would produce a carboxyhaemoglobin level of around 3 per cent. WHO guidelines aim to keep blood levels of carboxyhaemoglobin to less than 3 per cent in non-smokers, with recommendations of 86 p.p.m. for 15-min and 50 p.p.m. for 30-min exposures. In non-smokers levels of carboxyhaemoglobin rarely exceed 3 per cent. Carbon monoxide exerts its toxic effect not just by the formation of carboxyhaemoglobin but also because it shifts the oxygen dissociation curve to the left. As a result of these factors, blood levels of around 3.6 per cent will reduce the time to onset of angina on exercise (US Health Effects Institute). The fetuses of smoking mothers may have carboxyhaemoglobin levels up to 2.5 times that of the mother. How the fetus is able to concentrate the carbon monoxide and what the health effects may be to the fetus are unknown.

Source or process specific pollution

Individual factories or other emitters such as power stations or incinerators, are often blamed for perceived high levels of respiratory disease or symptoms in the local population. One problem in determining whether there is a true health effect from a point source is that the complainants are the potential sufferers which introduces a high level of subjectivity into any investigation. Equally, there are many different processes potentially at risk of being regarded as point sources of pollution which may produce well recognized emissions, such as sulphur dioxide or particulates, or may produce process-specific emissions which can be organic or chemical. When considering an investigation into such a source the aim must be to define an increase in respiratory disease or symptoms in the vicinity of the source either with respect to distance from the source or by comparison to a control area. If an effect is demonstrated, attention can turn to the specific emissions involved. It is also essential that prevailing wind direction and details of local topography are considered. Valleys trap pollution and the population downwind of a source will have a higher exposure than the upwind population.

The new United Kingdom Environmental Protection Act has emission guidelines for over 3000 separate processes incorporating a huge number of emissions so that emissions from a suspect source can be viewed with these guidelines in mind (Chapter 17.10).

Sometimes the effect from a point source is very clear. An outbreak of asthma occurring in a community in South Africa in the early 1950s was shown to be due to a change in manufacture in the local castor bean processing factory resulting in the emission of a finer dust. A further change in the process resulted in asthma attacks reducing to the previous very low levels. Similarly, outbreaks of severe asthma occurring in Barcelona in the 1980s were found to occur only on days when soya bean products were being off loaded at the docks into an uncapped silo. Capping of the silo has effectively abolished these epidemic days which were more likely to occur on days of higher ambient nitrogen dioxide, again demonstrating the importance of interaction between different air pollutants. An effect may only be noticed if a factory closes down for a period of time, an unusual occurrence. This occurred with a steel mill in Ohio where respiratory admissions fell when the mill was closed but rose soon after work restarted.

Indoor air pollution

The effect of indoor air quality on health can be considered with respect to the domestic and occupational settings. Domestic exposures are predominantly those of environmental tobacco smoke and nitrogen dioxide, although radon has become a cause for some concern. From the occupational point of view, specific exposures which lead to occupational asthma are dealt with elsewhere (Chapter 17.10) but non-specific problems, such as the 'sick building syndrome' symptom complex will be covered below.

Although we spend the majority of our lives indoors in the United Kingdom (more than 90 per cent of a year) we spend more time outdoors when the weather is good, usually at a time of year when ozone is more likely to be present in significant amounts. We are also more likely to exercise in such conditions. Consequently, personal exposures estimated from indoor/outdoor time activity patterns will give a better idea of time exposure to a specific pollutant/pollutants when trying to estimate a health risk. Individual monitoring would be even better but as yet technology cannot achieve our needs. Nitrogen dioxide is easily measured using passive sampling diffusion tubes, but these can only give weekly exposures and will thus miss out relatively short-lived but high peaks. For exposures over shorter time periods the apparatus required is heavy and expensive.

DOMESTIC EXPOSURES

The most important indoor pollutant is environmental tobacco smoke, health effects from which have been repeatedly confirmed. A smoker of 20 cigarettes a day contributes about 20 $\mu g/m^3$ to 24-h indoor particulate concentrations. Reported particulate levels due to environmental tobacco smoke are variable but in a house containing a number of heavy smokers the 24-h national ambient air quality standard of 260 $\mu g/m^3$ can be exceeded. Various biological markers of environmental tobacco smoke have been assessed, the most consistent being nicotine or cotinine levels in serum, saliva, or urine. Nicotine gives a better indication of recent smoking because of its short half-life while cotinine, with a half-life ranging from 10 to 40 h, is a good indicator of chronic smoking. Neither are present in non-smokers which make them better indicators than carboxyhaemoglobin or serum thiocyanate. Active smokers have salivary cotinine levels of around 300 ng/ml while non-smoking adults have levels of 1.5 ng/ml. In children, those not exposed to environmental tobacco smoke have levels of around 0.2 ng/ml while children whose parents both smoke have levels of around 2.7 ng/ml.

Environmental tobacco smoke has been consistently shown to increase the frequency of respiratory tract infections in children, particularly bronchitis and pneumonia in the first year of life. Hospitalization rates for children in this age group are also increased in those passively exposed. The prevalence of respiratory symptoms are higher in children exposed to environmental tobacco smoke in a dose response manner. An overview of the 11 studies published in this area show an increase in respiratory symptoms from 12.5 per cent in children with two non-smoking parents, to 15.1 per cent in children with one smoking parent, to 18.4 per cent in children whose parents both smoke. Particulate pollution is roughly doubled in homes where two parents smoke compared with those where one only smokes. Environmental tobacco smoke has also been shown to reduce lung function in children. Its irritant effect should not be ignored as this is likely to be the reason most people object to passive smoking. The effect of the irritation *per se* has no known long-term physical effects but the effect on quality of life at home (or work) can be considerable. Patients with asthma find this irritant effect will worsen symptoms.

The most remarkable effect of environmental tobacco smoke is that on the development of lung cancer in passively exposed non-smokers. Two reports in 1981 from Japan and Greece initially established a possible effect. Since then larger and more tightly controlled studies have confirmed a relative risk of around 1.3 of developing lung cancer in those passively exposed. No particular cell type seems to be favoured. Estimates from the United States have suggested that 3000 to 5000 deaths per year from lung cancer can be attributed to passive smoking. All-cause mortality in passive cigarette smokers is increased in both men (relative risk 1.17) and women (relative risk 1.15) allowing for housing, schooling, and marital status.

The role of nitrogen dioxide as a specific cause for increased respiratory disease is less clear. Many studies have been performed, of variable quality, mostly in children. The main problems in determining an effect are the confounding aspects of passive smoking, socioeconomic status, and the presence of asthma in children, and active smoking, occupational exposure, and chronic lung disease in adults. Some, but not all studies were able to take these confounders into consideration. Some studies have shown a doubling of respiratory symptoms in gas-fired homes compared with all electrically-fuelled homes while others have shown no increase. In adults the balance of evidence is against an effect whereas in children there are sufficient positive studies to consider that nitrogen dioxide itself may play a role, although further studies incorporating personal monitoring are needed.

Control of indoor pollution is also contentious. Most attempts are aimed at increasing room ventilation rates which have shown significant improvements in odour levels and occupant satisfaction while air filtration, although attractive, has yet to be shown to be as effective.

Radon-222 is an inert gas, a natural decay product of radium-226, with a half-life of just under 4 days. It decays through four short lived 'radon daughters' to lead-210. Two of the radon daughters, polonium-218 and polonium-214 are alpha-emitters. These cause bronchial mucosal damage when they decay within the lung and inhalation can thus lead to lung cancer in occupationally exposed individuals (predominantly miners, particularly of uranium).

In the 1970s it became clear that radon is invariably present in indoor air and that in some dwellings, levels are unacceptably high. Concentrations of radon are expressed as picocuries (pCi) per litre or as working levels months (WLM) where 1 WLM relates to the amount of emission in a month. In a United States home, average radon concentrations are about 1.5 pCi/l which results in an exposure of about 0.02 WLM monthly, about 0.3 WLM annually, and about 20 WLM over 70 years. The level at which action must be taken in the United Kingdom with regards to a domestic dwelling is 11 pCi/l. The main sources of indoor radon are the rock or soil on which the house is built, building materials used in the construction of the dwelling, natural gas, and water usage. Indoor levels vary considerably and occasionally domestic exposures reach that seen in mines.

There is no doubt that radon in the occupational setting can cause lung cancer and that, in a radon-exposed individual cigarette smoke may increase the dose of alpha-energy to the bronchial mucosa. However, the effect of indoor radon exposure in this regard is more difficult to assess because of methodological problems in determining an effect. There is suggestive data from cross-sectional surveys of an increased lung cancer rate with higher exposures, and modelling has suggested an overall risk of 1.8 to 2-fold but formal longitudinal studies are needed to confirm this.

BUILDING RELATED ILLNESS

In the early 1970s, illnessess or symptom complexes were recognized as being related to occupancy of certain buildings. These conditions can be divided into two general headings, building-related sickness and 'sick building syndrome'.

Building-related sickness

This is defined as an illness arising from exposure to indoor contaminents which causes a distinct, specific, clinical syndrome. These syndromes are either hypersensitivity conditions such as humidifier fever, humidifier lung, or other forms of hypersensitivity pneumonitis, infections such as legionnaire's disease or toxic effects of specific substances such as formaldehyde. Characteristically, symptoms do not disappear on leaving the building and only a small proportion of the occupants are affected. Legionnaire's disease is covered in Chapter 17.7. Other forms of hypersensitivity pneumonitis (e.g. farmer's lung, bird fancier's lung) are dealt with elsewhere but humidifier fever and humidifier lung are specific building related illnesses. Humidifier fever, more commonly seen in the United Kingdom, appears to be a separate entity from humidifier lung, a predominantly American condition, although both are forms of hypersensitivity pneumonitis. The symptoms of both are those of chills, fever, malaise, breathlessness, and myalgia occurring 4 to 12 h after initial exposure. In humidifier fever symptoms are often worse on a Monday which is not usually so in humidifier lung. In both conditions gas transfer and sometimes $P\text{O}_2$ are reduced in the acute phase. The chest radiograph is usually abnormal in humidifier lung with evidence of diffuse, bilateral interstitial shadowing whereas in humidifier fever the radiograph is usually normal. The outlook for the latter is excellent but in humidifier lung, in some cases, pulmonary fibrosis can occur leading to a significant restrictive defect. The pathogenesis in both cases is a hypersensitivity to organic substances from the cooling fluid in the humidifier. In humidifier lung, this is always to thermophilic actinomycetes to which circulating specific antibody can be detected. In humidifier fever the range of allergens is much wider incorporating not only thermophilic actinomycetes but also Gram-negative bacilli, amoebae, and fungi. It is likely that endotoxin plays a part, at least in some cases. Cleaning the contaminated humidifier is effective in dealing with most cases of humidifier fever although in some patients with humidifier lung long-term damage may have ensued.

'Sick (or tight) building' syndrome

'Sick building' syndrome is characterized by an increased prevalence in a particular building of a range of non-specific symptoms typical of mucosal irritation (e.g. sore/dry eyes, sore nose, dry mouth, sore throat) often with lethargy and headaches. Symptoms usually disappear as soon as an affected individual leaves the building and the symptoms will affect more than 20 per cent of the occupants. The first full description of this condition was made in the United Kingdom in 1984 where, in a series of 11 buildings, not necessarily chosen because of complaints from the occupants, the prevalence of typical symptoms was shown to be much higher in non-naturally ventilated compared with naturally ventilated buildings. There does not appear to be a consistent relationship of presence of severity of symptoms to indoor environmental parameters such as temperature, relative humidity, moisture content, carbon monoxide, formaldehyde, or ozone levels. There is some evidence that levels of volatile organic compounds may be involved although their role is likely to be limited. Symptoms are usually reported more often by women than men and by clerical or secretarial staff than managerial or professional staff. It is likely that human factors, such as stress and inability to be able to control the environment, are contributory. It was initially believed that the problem of 'sick building' syndrome was minor but it is now recognized that the financial costs of the condition are substantial. The acceptance of 'sick building' syndrome as an entity has led to the condition playing an important role in new building design. In buildings already affected, modification of the ventilation very often produces significant improvements in symptom severity and frequency. The aim of these design approaches is to reduce symptoms of 'sick building' syndrome so that substantially less than 20 per cent of the occupants are affected.

REFERENCES

Department of Health Advisory Group on the medical aspects of air pollution episodes. (1991). *First report Ozone*. HMSO, London.

Department of Health Advisory Group on the medical aspects of air pollution. (1992). *Second report, sulphur dioxide, particulates, and acid aerosols*. HMSO, London.

Department of Health Advisery Group on the medical aspects of air pollution episodes. (1993). *Third Report. Oxides of nitrogen*. HMSO, London.

Royal College of Physicians. (1970). *Air Pollution and Health*. Pitman, London.

8.5.5(m) Environmental disasters

P. J. Baxter

Over the last two decades at least three million people have been killed by the physical phenomena accompanying natural disasters, and over one billion have suffered adverse health effects or loss of property: 95 per cent of these events occurred in the developing world. Notable technological disasters over the same period, such as the Bhopal incident (India) in 1984, and the reactor fire at Chernobyl (the former USSR) in 1986 have demonstrated the serious hazards posed by modern technology and how the risks may cross international boundaries.

In 1989 the United Nations General Assembly launched a new international initiative proclaiming the 1990s as the International Decade for Natural Disaster Reduction. Technological disasters are not included because the main thrust of the Decade is the application and exploitation of existing scientific and technical knowledge in reducing the effects of natural disasters. Nevertheless interventions in both types of disasters (Table 1) are possible in four definable phases: predisaster planning, preparedness, response, and recovery and reconstruction. Although most health professionals would see their main role in the response phase, for example treating casualties and coping with refugees, major reductions in loss of life will come from advances in diminishing the impact of all phases of disasters. A disaster may be defined as any disruption of the human ecology that exceeds the capacity of the community to function normally. Health workers will only play their full part in disaster reduction when they learn to complement their treatment skills with a multidisciplinary approach to preventive health management that incorporates risk assessment, preparedness, and warning measures. Epidemiology is essential for assisting in the development of preventive measures and for evaluating the health needs after disaster has struck.

Table 1 *Environmental disasters*

Geophysical
Earthquakes
Volcanoes
Weather related
Hurricanes
Tornadoes
Floods
Drought
Technological
Air pollution
Chemical releases
Fires
Nuclear reactor incidents

Natural disasters

Weather-related phenomena

The means already exist accurately to forecast and predict hurricanes and floods using space and hydrological technologies. The most common of natural hazards are floods which affect all nations. Hurricanes, cyclones, and typhoons are severe storms that form over tropical waters, and although their strong winds can reach up to 250 km/h and be very destructive the main damage to life and property is from the flood waves and the accompanying storm surge. Ninety per cent of fatalities are from drowning. Timely evacuation is the key life-saving measure in these events. Tornadoes have a wind velocity of up to 500 km/h and can travel with a width of over 1 km for 300 km over land: they are immensely destructive with most deaths being caused by flying debris. Tornado warnings may be sufficient for some people to take cover in purpose built shelters or the basements of houses.

Earthquakes

This century has witnessed over 1100 devastating earthquakes which have been responsible for 1.53 million recorded deaths. Although about three-quarters of the deaths and injuries in earthquakes are directly due to structural collapse, the actual distribution of the causes of death and the types of injuries incurred in relation to different types of building collapse has not been described. Yet this information, if collected in accordance with an international classification and coding scheme, for example using trauma scores and injury severity scores, would be essential for developing measures to reduce human losses through the design of safer buildings and in devising more advanced rescue techniques and emergency treatment. The dearth of medical data has also limited the development of models for predicting casualty levels. More needs to be known about the determinants of crush syndrome (traumatic rhabdomyolysis) with renal failure in victims whose limbs are trapped for prolonged periods. Crush syndrome was a prominent finding in the disasters in Armenia in 1988 and Mexico City in 1985, but prolonged entrapment is less of a problem in collapses of one-story adobe or wood-framed structures, and there may be other causal or modifying factors such as adverse weather conditions, the effectiveness of emergency medical care, and the time taken to reach hospital.

International initiatives are in progress to devise seismic hazard maps and expert systems in earthquake-prone countries which will provide decision makers with risk management information for long-term planning of land use and to assist with emergency response measures.

Volcanic eruptions

A greater understanding of the devastating hazards of volcanoes emerged following the well-publicized eruption of Mount St Helens (United States) in 1980. Although only about 60 people were killed in the wilderness area surrounding the volcano the explosive destructiveness and the inability to predict this major eruption revealed the serious dangers faced by populations living close to active volcanoes. The most devastating of eruptive phenomena are gravity current flows of debris, namely pyroclastic flows which are often intensely hot and fast moving, and mud flows (lahars) produced by melting ice or heavy rains. Lava flows rarely cause loss of life. The causes of death in pyroclastic flows include heat, asphyxia, burns injuries to the respiratory tract and the skin, and various types of mechanical trauma. Gases may also contribute to loss of life. In 1986 about 1760 people died in a sudden release of a quarter of a million tonnes of carbon dioxide from Lake Nyos, a crater lake in Cameroon. Eruption clouds can contain huge volumes of ash; ash falls can accumulate on the ground and on roofs at rates of over 5 cm/h. At depths greater than 10 cm many weaker buildings may start to collapse, with death and destruction on the scale of major earthquakes. Thus about 300 people died from roof and building collapse in the eruption of Pinatubo in the Philippines in 1991 (Plate 1) despite a massive and successful evacuation from around the volcano. Erupted ash suspended in the air may contain a large proportion of respirable particles (under 10 μm) which may induce asthma and bronchitis in unprotected susceptible people; crystalline silica (quartz) may also pose a potential hazard of silicosis. Ash can incorporate toxic substances such as fluorine, which can kill large numbers of foraging farm animals and endanger human drinking water supplies from surface sources; ground water is also at risk from toxic contamination around the volcano.

Droughts and famine

In contrast, droughts and famine are of slow onset and may affect vast inhabited areas, as in Africa. The socioeconomic factors influencing the vulnerability of populations and the climatological processes that underline drought are presently not well understood and in consequence there has been limited progress in the development of mitigation measures. Famine relief depends primarily on the appropriate provision and distribution of food rather than dramatic medical intervention.

Technological disasters

Major technological hazards may threaten life from explosion (with blast effects) and thermal radiation from fires, as well as discharge into the air which can spread dangerous materials over large areas from point sources. Risk analyses for such eventualities include the development of models for the dispersion of plumes of dense gases and the application of quantified risk assessment methods for predicting plant failure. Such information is being increasingly used to reduce risk in plant or equipment design, in the transport of dangerous substances, and to assist in land use planning for the siting of chemical or nuclear plant, as well as for devising emergency response measures.

Air pollution

Episodes of air pollution severe enough to cause acute increases in mortality in industrialized communities have occurred when adverse meteorological conditions (low winds and temperature inversions) have led to the accumulation of emissions from the combustion of fossil fuels from unabated domestic and industrial sources. Historical examples include the episode in the highly industrialized valley of the Meuse River (Belgium) in 1930, when 63 people died and 6000 fell ill; that in the city of Donora, Pennsylvania, in 1948 when 20 died and 5190 became sick; and that of the classic 'smog' in London (England) in 1952 which was associated with 4000 excess deaths from all causes and in all age groups, but which were mainly ascribed to cardiorespiratory diseases in the elderly. The effects in London were correlated with air levels of sulphur dioxide and particulates, but they are most likely to have been linked to the hydrogen ion concentration and its potential to interfere with the function of cilia in the epithelium of the respiratory tract.

The passing of Clean Air Acts in many countries has virtually eliminated the risk, but the rapid rise in motor traffic is now leading to new air pollution problems. The unburnt hydrocarbons and nitrogen oxides from car exhausts undergo photo-oxidation in sunlight to form ozone which in turn reacts with water to produce hydroxyl radicals. These pollutants will react with moisture to become visible on days of bad pollution as a photochemical smog. Despite much concern over the effects such smog may have in inducing acute respiratory illnesses in cities such as Los Angeles, Athens, and Mexico City, so far devastatingly lethal episodes have not been recorded.

Chemical hazards and fires

The main hazards posed by the chemical industry are large vapour or flammable gas explosions, fire, and toxic releases, but some of the worst chemical disasters have involved the accidental contamination, or deliberate adulteration, of food and alcoholic beverages (Table 2). Incidents involving the chemical contamination of drinking water supplies have also occurred, but major contamination is usually readily detectable through alterations in the water's smell and taste.

Chemicals that are commonly stored or transported under pressure such as chlorine, ammonia, sulphuric acid, hydrogen chloride, phosgene, hydrogen sulphide, and nitrous fumes can also cause accidents. These respiratory irritants are capable of travelling in dangerous concentrations for several kilometres downwind if suddenly released in a chemical plume. They all have the potential to induce bronchospasm, laryngeal oedema, or toxic pulmonary oedema. The medical management of the patient suffering from the pulmonary effects of the inhalation of irritant chemicals and the combustion products of fires is similar.

The world's worst industrial chemical disaster occurred in Bhopal in 1984 when 40 tonnes of methyl isocyanate, a potent respiratory irritant, was released in a few hours and the denser-than-air cloud blew slowly over the town at night. Deaths were caused by pulmonary oedema, and an unknown number of survivors suffered from bronchiolitis obliterans and possibly other organ damage; follow-up studies have been incomplete.

Devastating outbreaks of organic mercury poisoning have occurred as a consequence of methyl mercury being used as a seed dressing for wheat (e.g. Iraq, 1972). Minamata disease arose when methyl mercury was discharged by a chemical plant into Minamata Bay, Japan, where fish, the staple diet of Minamata's citizens, became contaminated with mercury. Victims of methyl and ethyl mercury poisoning suffer neurological damage, such as constriction of visual fields, cerebellar disturbances, dysarthria, and, in offspring of exposed mothers, a cerebral palsy syndrome or impairment of mental development. Polychlorinated biphenyls have accidentally contaminated rice oil during its production in Japan (1967), and again in Taiwan (1979), with similar consequences for those unfortunate enough to consume the oils. The main manifestations were chloracne and dilatation of the meibomian glands, as well as liver abnormalities and hypercholesterolaemia. Teratogenic effects were observed in the children of affected mothers, including developmental and growth abnormalities.

The most puzzling chemical disaster in recent times was the toxic oil syndrome (Spain, 1981) when an outbreak of toxic pneumonia arose from the mass consumption of edible rape-seed oil which had become contaminated by a chemical that remains unidentified to this day. Over 600 people died from the acute pneumonia or from the chronic syndrome (neuropathy, myopathy, sicca syndrome, and scleroderma) that developed in a proportion of the 20 000 people who recovered from the pneumonia. The condition was unique until a remarkably similar disease appeared in 1989 known as eosinophilia myalgia syndrome with prescribed tryptophan.

Whether the chemical is released into the air or into food or drink, special considerations apply to management of the disaster. It is fundamental that the chemical is identified as soon as possible but, as the Bhopal tragedy showed, even if rapid identification is possible knowledge of the chemical's effects in humans may be virtually non-existent. The epidemiological and toxicological means to identify the chemical, and rapidly to document its effects, must be part of the emergency response. Establishing the extent of the exposure in a target population may also be needed, particularly when long-term effects such as carcinogenicity and teratogenicity, are suspected. In prolonged releases into the air, for example in fires, or if the incident has led to ground contamination, urgent decisions on whether or not to evacuate the population

Table 2 *Examples of chemical disasters since 1950*

Year	Country	Location	Type of accident/incident	Chemicals involved	Outcome deaths	Injuries
1950–	Japan	Minamata Bay	Foodstuff contamination (fish)	Methyl mercury	439	2000
1955–9	Turkey		Foodstuff contamination (seed)	Hexachlorobenzene	400	3500
1968	Japan	Kyushu	Foodstuff contamination (oil)	PCBs/PCDFs	0	6400
1971–72	Iraq		Foodstuff contamination (seed)	Methyl mercury	1000s	6071
1974	UK	Flixborough	Plant (explosion)	Cyclohexane	28	89
1975	Italy	Seveso	Plant (runaway reaction)	Dioxin (TCD)/D,2,4,5-T (trichlorophenol)	0	187
1978	Spain	Los Alfaques	Transport accident (explosion)	Propylene	216	200
1979	Taiwan	Yucheng	Foodstuff contamination (oil)	PCBs/PCDFs	0	1900
1981–3	Spain	Madrid	Foodstuff contamination (oil)	As yet uncharacterized	600	20 000
1984	India	Bhopal	Plant (large-scale escape)	Methyl isocyanate	2500	100 000

may be needed. For these and other reasons an expert multidisciplinary team capable of co-ordinating these medical tasks should be on hand to be deployed in major chemical incidents.

Nuclear emergencies

With the ending of the Cold War the greatest risk of nuclear disaster has become the catastrophic failure of a nuclear reactor generating power with the release of volatile and non-volatile fission products into the atmosphere. Exposure to beta- and gamma-radiation from the emissions may result externally through whole-body irradiation from the plume, contamination of skin and clothing, and internally through inhalation and ingestion of contaminated food and water, or absorption through the skin and any wounds. Dosages high enough to cause acute radiation sickness may be received by workers on site, but are unlikely in people living around a nuclear power plant who would be at risk from chronic effects, namely radiation-induced cancer and teratogenic and genetic abnormalities. Estimates of the health risks after reactor accidents are beset with problems of identifying the pathways to humans, and uncertainties over the quantity and composition of the radioactive emissions, and changing assumptions about relationships between dose and effect at low levels of radiation.

The world's first major nuclear accident was the graphite fire in the reactor at Windscale, England, in 1957. The main fission product to be emitted was iodine-131, and a major disaster was averted by the workers who rapidly got the fire under control and by the rapidity of the steps taken to monitor air and food for radioactivity leading to a ban on the consumption of milk from exposed dairy herds. At Three Mile Island, United States, in 1979, a series of mechanical failures and human errors led to a loss of coolant which allowed the fuel to overheat and come near to a core meltdown. Unlike at Windscale the reactor was enclosed in a containment structure, but a disaster would have occurred if the hydrogen bubble above the reactor core had exploded. A negligible amount of radio-iodine was emitted, and the most significant health impact of this incident was probably psychological stress in the local population.

The world's third major reactor accident—and undoubtedly the worst—occurred at Chernobyl, Ukraine, in 1986. Three hundred workers who fought the graphite fire which lasted 10 days suffered radiation sickness, and 32 of them have died. There was no containment building and 150 000 people had to be evacuated from a radius of 30 km affected by surface contamination. A further 600 000 people received significant radiation. As well as iodine-131, the fission products contained the more persistent caesium-137, strontium-90, and plutonium, with the fall-out spreading over large parts of Europe. The total fission products released was estimated at 40 million to 50 million Ci, or over 1000 times that from Windscale. Estimates of increased cancer deaths over the next 70 years following this incident range from 5000 to 40 000. There are now serious concerns about the safety of the rest of Eastern Europe's 58 reactors. In the emergency plans for nuclear accidents a controversial issue is iodine prophylaxis to prevent thyroid cancer from the rapid inhalational uptake of iodine-131 following exposure. The main groups who would benefit from rapid iodine prophylaxis are pregnant and lactating women, neonates, and infants (including breast-fed babies), children, adolescents, and adults such as off-site emergency personnel. There is a hazard to persons with known iodine sensitivity, and patients with hypocomplementaemic vasculitis, and dermatitis herpetiformis. Fatal reactions to iodine administration may occur in those with asymptomatic nodular goitre and latent Graves' disease not under medical care. The administration of stable iodine tablets, which may have to be taken on a repeat daily basis, is now recommended for people in the vicinity of a nuclear accident if exposure to iodine-131 above a previously agreed intervention level is considered likely.

Conclusion

For the main causes of disaster multidisciplinary research involving medicine, science, and engineering will be the key to closing the present wide gaps in our knowledge. Presently the need is often for the dissemination of better technical information and for the education of populations at risk to enable them to develop appropriate emergency preparedness measures, particularly at the local community level. The present era of post-disaster improvisation in natural disasters in developing countries must also give way to well directed and appropriate relief measures. In the devising of innovative mitigation measures health professionals have a leading part to play.

Section 9 *Principles of clinical pharmacology and drug therapy*

9 Principles of clinical pharmacology and drug therapy

J.K. ARONSON AND N.J. WHITE

Clinical pharmacology is the application of scientific principles to understanding the ways in which drugs behave and work in man. It is through such understanding that rational drug therapy can be practised.

The benefit to risk ratio in prescribing

Is your prescription really necessary?
(RICHARD ASHER)

At the heart of every prescribing decision lies an assessment of the benefit to risk ratio. In many cases the doctor will not go through the formal exercise of this calculation, but none the less it will have been made at some time in a general way and it will be the basis, adjusted for the individual case, on which the decision to prescribe is made.

Every time a drug is prescribed, it is with a particular benefit in mind. However, it is also appreciated that there are risks of adverse effects. A doctor who prescribes a drug expects that the potential benefit of the drug will outweigh the potential risks. In some cases he or she will know that that is so. However, in others the benefit/risk ratio may not be known, sometimes because there are insufficient data on which to base a judgement, or because it may be difficult to assess the relative contributions of what appear to be non-comparable risks and benefits.

Take two examples. First, the treatment of pneumococcal pneumonia with penicillin. It is known that the benefit/risk ratio in this case is very high—a cure is likely and adverse effects are usually few and minor. However, if the patient is known to be allergic to penicillin, the risk of a serious adverse effect becomes too great and the benefit/risk ratio drops; in such a case another antibiotic would be used. In this example the benefit/risk ratio is easily determined.

In contrast, consider the treatment with an anticoagulant of a patient with atrial fibrillation and a history of bleeding peptic ulcer. Which outweighs the other: the potential benefit of preventing an embolic stroke by using the anticoagulant, or the potential risk of causing serious gastrointestinal bleeding? These two do not seem to be readily comparable, but a decision has to be made. It may be decided to use the anticoagulant and hope to prevent serious bleeding with a histamine (H_2) antagonist, such as ranitidine, arguing that the degree of morbidity from an embolic stroke is likely to be more serious than that from an acute gastrointestinal bleed, with an approximately equal risk of mortality. However, in an individual case the decision may not be easy.

The benefit/risk ratio of a particular treatment depends on four major factors:

(1) the seriousness of the illness;
(2) the efficacy of the drug;
(3) the seriousness of possible adverse effects;
(4) the risk of possible adverse effects.

If a disease is life threatening, if the drug to be used is highly effective and the only one available, and if the risk of serious adverse effects is negligible, the benefit/risk ratio will be high. At the other end of the spectrum, if the disease is trivial, if the drug is of poor efficacy, with more effective and safer competitors, and if the risk of serious adverse effects is high, the benefit/risk ratio is low. This spectrum is illustrated in Table 1. Most cases will lie somewhere between these two extremes.

To illustrate the principles involved, take the example of phenylbutazone, a highly effective non-steroidal anti-inflammatory drug but with a risk of marrow aplasia of between 1:30 000 and 1:100 000. While there were no other drugs of equal efficacy available, the therapeutic benefit of phenylbutazone was considered great enough to outweigh the relatively high risk of marrow aplasia. However, once other equally effective and safer drugs became available, the risk of its adverse effects was seen to outweigh whatever benefit there was in using it, and its use was restricted.

Note the important features that were considered in making this decision to restrict the use of phenylbutazone. The benefit was considered not in absolute terms but in relation to the severity of the disease and the benefit available from other drugs; while phenylbutazone was more potent therapeutically than other available drugs it was considered highly beneficial, but when equally effective drugs became available its overall benefit was felt to be reduced, despite the fact that the therapeutic effect of the drug itself had not changed during that time. Of course, phenylbutazone is still used today in some cases of severe ankylosing spondylitis that respond poorly to other anti-inflammatory drugs. In those cases the benefit is regarded as outweighing the risk of marrow aplasia.

In order to calculate the benefit/risk ratio the doctor has to know something about each of these four important factors, and an understanding of clinical pharmacology can contribute to the last three. The efficacy of drugs is ideally discovered through double-blind, placebo-controlled clinical trials, although in some cases one may have to rely on the results of trials of less adequate design or even on anecdotal reports. Monitoring for adverse drug reactions will yield information on the types, severity, and risks of adverse reactions (and drug interactions) that may be expected during treatment. Finally, an understanding of the basic clinical pharmacology of a drug (its pharmaceutical properties, its pharmacokinetic properties, its pharmacological actions, and the ways in which those actions are translated into a therapeutic effect) will predict how the benefit/risk ratio will change in particular cases. All these aspects of drug therapy are discussed below.

The therapeutic index of a drug

The therapeutic index of a drug is the ratio of the dose at which adverse effects become important to that at which a therapeutic benefit can be expected. The therapeutic index is not given a numerical value, as precise estimates of these doses are not available and vary from individual to individual. Instead, drugs are divided into two categories, those with high and low therapeutic indices. For example, in the absence of hypersensitivity, penicillins have a high therapeutic index; very large doses can be given without fear of adverse effects. In contrast, digoxin has a low therapeutic index; it takes very little more to cause toxicity than to produce therapeutic benefit. Drugs with a low therapeutic index include the aminoglycoside antibiotics, anticoagulants, anticonvulsants, antihypertensives, some antiparasitic and antiviral agents, cardiac glycosides, cytotoxic take over and immunosuppressant drugs, oral contraceptives, sympathomimetics, and drugs that act on the central nervous system.

The benefit/risk ratio for a particular drug will be more favourable if the drug has a high therapeutic index. If there is a choice between two drugs, each of which has equal efficacy, one would choose the one with the higher therapeutic index.

Table 1 *The factors that affect the benefit to risk ratio*

Seriousness of the indication	Efficacy of the drug	Adverse reactions		Other drugs		Benefit/risk ratio
		Severity	Frequency	Efficacy	Safety	
Life threatening	High	Trivial	Rare	Poor	Poor	Very high
Trivial	Poor	Serious	Frequent	Good	Good	Very low

The principles of clinical pharmacology

Drug therapy can be considered under four headings, the four major processes of clinical pharmacology, each of which is associated with a question about drug therapy. The processes and their associated questions are listed in Table 2 and are illustrated in Fig. 1.

Table 2 *The four processes of clinical pharmacology and the questions with which they are associated in relation to drug therapy*

Process	Question
Pharmaceutical	Is the drug getting into the patient from the appropriate formulation?
Pharmacokinetic	Is the drug getting to its site of action?
Pharmacodynamic	Is the drug producing the required pharmacological effect?
Therapeutic	Is the pharmacological effect being translated into an appropriate therapeutic effect?

The pharmaceutical process

The question associated with the pharmaceutical process is: Is the drug getting into the patient from the appropriate formulation? (In part this question asks about patient compliance, but this is not a pharmaceutical matter and it will be dealt with in a separate section below.)

Pharmaceutical questions in relation to drug therapy are concerned with the nature of the formulation. In most cases there is no need to worry about the formulation of a drug, beyond deciding whether to use the oral or parenteral routes. For example, if you decide to use oral frusemide or bumetanide, the appropriate tablets are prescribed. But sometimes the decision is not so easy. For example, in the United Kingdom there is currently a choice of eight different oral lithium formulations, with differing strengths and absorption characteristics. For glyceryl trinitrate there is a choice of two different types of sublingual formulation, a buccal formulation, and transdermal formulations. To understand the differences it is necessary to understand the concept of systemic availability.

Systemic availability

Systemic availability (commonly known as bioavailability) is a term used to describe the proportion of administered drug that reaches the systemic circulation and is available for distribution to the site of action. It is usually applied in reference to formulations given by the oral route, although it can also refer to other routes of administration, such as intramuscular or transdermal.

- When a drug is given intravenously it all enters the systemic circulation (systemic availability = 100 per cent).
- When a drug is given orally in solution all the drug is immediately available for absorption. The amount of drug that enters the systemic circulation will depend on the extent of absorption and the metabolic effect of the liver as it passes through for the first time (the so-called first-pass effect).
- When a drug is given orally as a tablet or capsule the amount that enters the systemic circulation will also depend on factors intrinsic to the formulation, including the rate of disintegration of the tablet and the rate of dissolution of the drug particles in the intestinal fluid. This may be termed 'pharmaceutical availability'.

When prescribing, doctors depend on the skills of the pharmacist and pharmaceutical chemist in providing formulations of high stability and predictable pharmaceutical availability. When the same drug is available in different formulations, whether from the same or different manufacturers, the doctor may have to decide which to prescribe. This may be particularly important for drugs with a low therapeutic index, for which differences in pharmaceutical availability will have a large impact. For example, if a patient is taking a formulation of low pharmaceutical availability that is producing a good therapeutic effect, switching to a formulation of high availability can cause adverse effects.

Special drug formulations

Most drugs are given orally; oral formulations include elixirs, ordinary (quick-release) tablets and capsules, and modified-release formulations. However, drugs may be given by other routes, including sublingually, buccally, rectally, transdermally, by inhalation, and by injection intravenously, subcutaneously, intramuscularly, or locally.

Sublingual, buccal, and rectal formulations

Drugs that are absorbed through the oral or rectal mucosa enter the venous circulation and pass into the systemic circulation intact, avoiding first-pass metabolism in the liver. For example, sublingual glyceryl trinitrate is effective in doses about 10 times less than those required by the oral route and the effect is rapid. In migraine, nausea and vomiting may impair the absorption of a drug given orally. Ergotamine is most effective when given very early after the start of an attack, and it can be given sublingually, avoiding the oral route. The rectal route can be used for a direct effect on the large bowel (for example, corticosteroids in ulcerative colitis).

Transdermal formulations

Some drugs are well absorbed via the skin, and their transdermal administration via so-called patches allows controlled release of small amounts over a period of hours. Drugs used in this way include glyceryl trinitrate in the long-term treatment of angina pectoris, transdermal hyoscine in the treatment of travel sickness, oestradiol in hormone replacement therapy, and nicotine for stopping smoking.

Inhalations

Inhaled formulations come in several forms, with different intentions. Sodium cromoglycate is formulated as a powder for inhalation, designed to have a local effect on the bronchioles in the treatment and prevention of bronchial asthma. Salbutamol aerosol, on the other hand, is designed to produce bronchodilatation by a metered dose (100 μg) of droplets, whose size (2–5 μm) allows them to penetrate down the bronchial tree to bronchiolar level. About 10 per cent of any drug in an aerosol or other form for inhalation reaches the bronchial tree, the rest being lost in the air, absorbed from the oropharynx, or swallowed. Nebulizers provide continuous administration of aerosolized drugs for short periods of time.

Inhalation can also be used to treat lung infections (e.g. pentamidine for *Pneumocystis carinii* pneumonia).

For migraine, ergotamine can be given by aerosol, with rapid absorption from the tracheobronchial mucosa, avoiding the oral route (for the reasons discussed above under Sublingual).

Subcutaneous, intramuscular, and local injections

Control of the absorption of insulin from the site of subcutaneous injection is achieved by differences in its physical state (for example, crystalline or non-crystalline), in the zinc or protein content, and in the nature and pH of the buffer in which it is suspended. Thus, soluble insulin has a rapid onset and short duration of action (about 6 h), while ultralente insulin, which has large crystals and a high zinc content, has an onset of action at about 7 h and a duration of action of about 36 h.

The absorption of drugs from intramuscular injection sites is sometimes erratic; for phenytoin and diazepam the intramuscular route should be avoided if possible. Intramuscular absorption may be retarded by the use of thick oils, which slow down diffusion of the drug from the site of injection—for example vasopressin tannate in oil in the treatment of diabetes insipidus and fluphenazine decanoate in oil in the treatment of schizophrenia.

Some formulations of anaesthetics for local injection contain adrenaline, which causes vasoconstriction and hence prevents rapid removal of the drug from the site of injection.

Modified-release formulations

Advanced pharmaceutical technology has resulted in oral formulations with novel release mechanisms. These are grouped under the general heading of 'modified-release' formulations, and are usually intended to prolong the duration of action of a drug and to smooth its effects by gradual release during the dosage interval. Examples include formulations of theophylline, nifedipine, diltiazem, lithium, and quinidine. When prescribing these drugs the exact formulation should be specified, as different formulations may provide different systemic availability.

Combination formulations in oral therapy

Combination products for oral use are widely available, but should only be used when the following minimum criteria are met:

- The frequency of administration of the two drugs is the same.
- The fixed doses in the combination product are therapeutically and optimally effective in the majority of cases (i.e. when it is not necessary to alter the dose of one drug independently of the other).

Examples of combination products include:

- Aspirin plus codeine (co-codaprin) or paracetamol plus dihydrocodeine (co-dydramol), pairs of drugs that have different analgesic actions (which summate) and different adverse effects (which do not).
- Levodopa (L-dopa) plus a peripherally-acting dopa decarboxylase inhibitor (benserazide or carbidopa); the peripheral action

Fig. 1 The four processes of clinical pharmacology in relation to drug therapy.

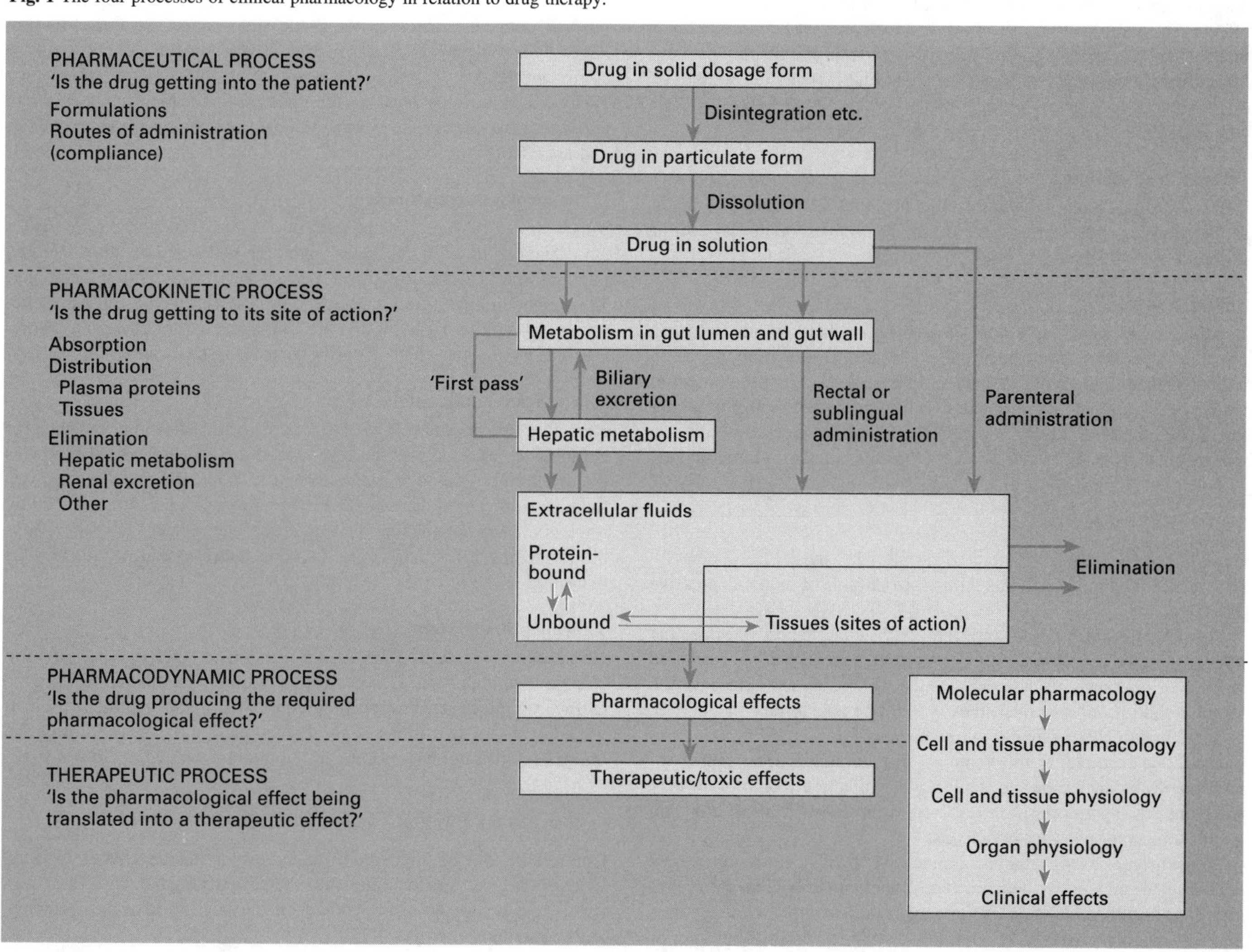

of the decarboxylase inhibitor blocks the peripheral metabolism of L-dopa, which is free to enter the brain, where it is converted to the pharmacologically active product dopamine, producing the therapeutic effect in Parkinson's disease.

- Combined oral contraceptives, which contain an oestrogen and a progestogen.
- The combination of vaccines against diphtheria, tetanus, and pertussis.
- Ferrous sulphate plus folic acid, used in the prevention of anaemia in pregnancy.
- Co-amoxiclav, a combination of amoxycillin and clavulanic acid; the β-lactamase inhibitor, clavulanic acid, prevents the breakdown of amoxycillin by bacterial penicillinase, thus broadening its spectrum.

Patient compliance

Compliance is the extent to which the patient follows a prescribed drug regimen. The extent of non-compliance varies widely, and in different studies has been recorded as low as 10 per cent and as high as 90 per cent. Compliance may be affected by many different factors, including the nature of the treatment, the type of illness, and the behaviour of the patient and doctor.

THE NATURE OF THE TREATMENT

Apart from the cost to the patient (which may be an important factor in some countries), two aspects of the treatment itself are important in determining compliance, the complexity of the regimen and adverse effects. The complexity of the prescribed regimen involves two factors: the frequency of administration (the more often during the day patients have to take a drug the less likely they are to take it) and the number of drugs prescribed (the more drugs prescribed the less likely is overall compliance).

Frequency of administration

When several different tablets (or other formulations) have to be taken at different dosages that involve different numbers of tablets and at different times of the day, compliance suffers.

Adverse effects

If patients experience symptoms that they attribute to adverse drug effects (for example, diarrhoea due to antibiotics or sedation due to anticonvulsants), then, unless they can be persuaded that the potential benefits of treatment outweigh the disadvantages, they will stop taking the medicine. Some patients, notably children, have problems with certain formulations, for example sickly elixirs or large, dry, bitter tablets.

THE TYPE OF ILLNESS

Compliance is likely to be poor in people who are severely mentally disturbed, for example patients with schizophrenia or manic-depressive psychosis.

Physical disability may interfere with compliance, despite the patient's desire to comply. For example, if patients with rheumatoid arthritis or osteoarthritis cannot reach the tablets, or cannot remove the top of a child-proof container, they will not be able to take them.

Sometimes a good response to treatment will discourage further compliance. For example, in the treatment of tuberculosis long courses of multiple drugs are needed to eradicate the infection; compliance may wane once the symptoms have resolved, risking recurrent infection and the emergence of resistant organisms.

Some diseases may promote compliance. Patients with insulin-dependent diabetes may easily become very ill quite quickly if they forget to take their insulin, and that is likely to make them comply, although they may not comply precisely as advised. Patients in whom β-blockers or vasodilators have significantly reduced the frequency of anginal attacks will be conditioned to good compliance.

THE BEHAVIOUR OF THE PATIENT

People tend to forget to take medicines or can't be bothered; they may feel no need for treatment (for example in asymptomatic hypertension); they may be unclear about the prescribing instructions; they may not want to feel dependent or be thought to be dependent on 'drugs'. There may be social or physical reasons why they cannot reach a pharmacist, financial difficulties, or everyday inconveniences in carrying and taking the medication.

THE BEHAVIOUR OF THE DOCTOR

The enthusiasm and confidence with which a treatment is prescribed, and the extent to which these attitudes are transmitted to the patient, may influence not only compliance but also the response to therapy. This is partly related to the placebo effect (see below).

METHODS OF MEASURING COMPLIANCE

Measurement of compliance is important both in everyday practice and in clinical trials. Some methods are listed in Table 3.

Pharmaceutical methods

The fact that patients collect their prescriptions is at least evidence of the first stage of compliance, and can be checked by asking to see the tablets. As a guide to the actual number of tablets that a patient has taken one can count the tablets in the bottle and assume that those missing have been taken. Tablet counting overestimates the extent of compliance.

Recording devices fitted in the caps of medication containers can record the frequency and exact timing of the opening of the container, and are useful in research.

Pharmacokinetic methods

Measurement of some compounds in the plasma or urine may give a good indication of compliance, although it does not allow for the patients who take their treatment only on the day of visiting the doctor. The compound measured may be the drug itself (such as digoxin, phenytoin, or lithium in the plasma, or salicylates in the urine) or a marker (such as riboflavin, which is easily detected in the urine).

Pharmacodynamic methods

Detecting the pharmacological effect of a drug can give evidence of compliance; for example, the response of the heart rate for β-blockers, the prothrombin time for oral anticoagulants, and the reticulocyte count for haematinics. Failure to detect the pharmacological effect of a drug implies non-compliance or inadequate dosage. During long-term antibiotic therapy for urinary tract infection, antibacterial activity can be measured in the urine.

Therapeutic methods

Obviously, if the desired therapeutic effect occurs the question of compliance is unimportant. However, it should be remembered that a good therapeutic outcome may occur irrespective of the treatment used. It would be wrong to attribute a good outcome to the effect of a drug that the patient may not have taken, an important principle in clinical trials.

METHODS OF IMPROVING COMPLIANCE

Compliance may be improved by supervised administration of the drug, by removing barriers to compliance, by simplifying the therapeutic regimen, and by educating the patient on the need to take the medicine, with reminders when possible.

Table 3 *Methods of assessing compliance*

Method	Description	Comments
Tablet counting		
Discrepancy count	The number of tablets dispensed is known, the remaining tablets are counted	The patient is aware of being observed and may dispose of the remaining tablets
Discrepancy estimate	The number of tablets dispensed is known, the patient is asked whether any more are required before the next visit.	The patient is not aware of being closely observed but the count is less accurate
Recording devices		
Medication monitor	A uranium source and photographic film record the regularity with which the drug is removed	Primarily used in research; both methods presuppose that the removal of the drug implied that the drug has been taken
Silicon chip recorder	A silicon-chip recorder is incorporated into the bottle cap and activated whenever the cap is removed	
Detecting substances in plasma, urine, or faeces		
Drug	The concentration of drug is measured directly—for example, plasma phenytoin concentration	Variations may be due to pharmacokinetic differences and not compliance Primarily used in research May be misleading if the drug is taken only on the day of measurement
Inert marker	A compound such as phenobarbitone, riboflavin, or phenol red is incorporated into the drug formulation and can be measured in the urine	
Colour changes	For example, iron colours faeces black, rifampicin turns urine red	
Measuring the pharmacological effect	For example, pupil size with pilocarpine, exercise heart rate with β-adrenoceptor antagonists	

Supervised administration

Administration of a drug by the doctor or nurse ensures compliance. This is possible in hospital or when only occasional administration is required (for example, intramuscular injections of vitamin B_{12}, long-acting depot injections of phenothiazines and thioxanthenes in the treatment of schizophrenia, and supervised twice-weekly antituberculous therapy). Sometimes compliance may be ensured by giving a single dose of a drug at the time of consultation, rather than a short course of tablets (for example, intramuscular antibiotics in the treatment of gonorrhoea). In some cases, compliance may be assured by administration by a relative at home.

Removing barriers to compliance

Compliance may be encouraged by prescribing pleasant-tasting elixirs rather than tablets for children and old people, and by using a drug or formulation that minimizes adverse effects.

Simplification of the therapeutic regimen

The therapeutic regimen can be simplified by reducing both the number of drugs a patient has to take and the frequency of administration. This can sometimes be done with the help of modified-release or combination formulations.

Education and reminders

Educating the patient about why treatment is necessary (for example, the reduction in the risk of tissue damage in treating hypertension or diabetes) is time-consuming but undoubtedly improves compliance. In the treatment of certain infections (for example, in patients with AIDS or tuberculosis and in typhoid carriers) the importance to the community should also be explained.

Even when patients are well motivated, reminders to take the treatment may improve compliance, as it is easy to forget to take medication. A simple *aide-mémoire* consists of the 'calendar pack' used for some medicines, especially oral contraceptives.

Other ways of helping patients include giving them a clearly written list of their current drugs and labelling medicine bottles clearly. Information leaflets may also help in educating and reminding patients about drug therapy.

The pharmacokinetic process

The question associated with the pharmacokinetic process is: Is the drug getting to its site of action? It comprises absorption and systemic availability, distribution, metabolism, and excretion.

Absorption and systemic availability

After oral administration the amount of drug that reaches the systemic circulation depends on its absorption and the extent to which it escapes metabolism in the gastrointestinal tract, the liver, and the lungs. This is called its systemic availability (or bioavailability).

Systemic availability is defined in terms of the amount of administered drug that reaches the systemic circulation intact and the rate at which that happens. The rate of availability depends on pharmaceutical factors (see above) and gastrointestinal absorption, presystemic metabolism being relatively unimportant. On the other hand, the extent of availability depends on both the extent of absorption and the extent of presystemic metabolism.

What is meant by the rate and extent of systemic availability is illustrated in Fig. 2, which shows three curves representing the theoretical plasma concentrations resulting over a period of time after the oral administration of three different formulations of the same dose of the same drug. Each curve contains three features of interest: the peak concentration (C_{max}), the time taken to reach the peak (t_{max}), and the total area under the curve (**AUC**). The C_{max} and t_{max} are measures of the rate of availability, and the total AUC is a measure of its extent. In the three hypothetical cases the rates of availability are clearly different. For formulation I the systemic availability is rapid, perhaps too rapid, leading to potentially toxic plasma concentrations. Formulation II is not so quickly available and plasma concentrations are never in the potentially toxic range. Formulation III is slowly available and plasma concentrations after a single dose are always subtherapeutic. However, in contrast to the rate of availability, the extent of availability of these three formulations, as assessed by the AUC, is the same in each case.

For drugs whose action may depend on the threshold plasma concentration achieved after a single dose (for example, analgesics), such differences may be important. Thus, for the rapid relief of pain a soluble aspirin formulation, giving a curve like formulation II, would be preferable to an enteric-coated formulation, giving a curve like that of formulation III.

A curve of type I can be therapeutically useful if a very fast rate of absorption is needed in order to produce a quick therapeutic effect, for example sublingual glyceryl trinitrate in the relief of an acute attack of angina pectoris, although it is associated with the adverse effect of headache caused by dilatation of extracranial blood vessels.

For drugs whose action is related to a steady-state concentration during multiple dosing, the differences in rate of availability become less important and the chief consideration is the extent.

FACTORS AFFECTING THE RATE OF ABSORPTION

Gastrointestinal motility

Because drug absorption occurs mainly in the upper part of the small intestine, altered gastric emptying will alter the rate. For example, in migraine the rate of absorption of analgesics is reduced because of reduced gastric motility, and the response to oral analgesics may therefore be delayed. This delay can be reduced by giving metoclopramide, which increases the rate of gastric emptying.

When the rate of dissolution of a drug is much longer than the rate of gastric emptying, increased gastrointestinal motility may reduce both the rate and extent of absorption. Thus, enteric-coated formulations may pass through the gut intact, for example when there is severe diarrhoea.

Malabsorption

Although one would expect drug absorption to be impaired in patients with malabsorption, that is not always so. For example, the absorption of propranolol, co-trimoxazole, and cephalexin is increased in patients with coeliac disease, as is the absorption of propranolol in Crohn's disease. Digoxin, however, is less well absorbed from tablets in patients with coeliac disease, radiation-induced enteritis, and other forms of gastrointestinal disease, and thyroxine absorption is impaired in coeliac disease.

Fig. 2 The theoretical plasma concentrations resulting over a period of time after the oral administration of three different formulations of the same dose of the same drug. The profile in each case depends on both the rate and the extent of systemic availability.

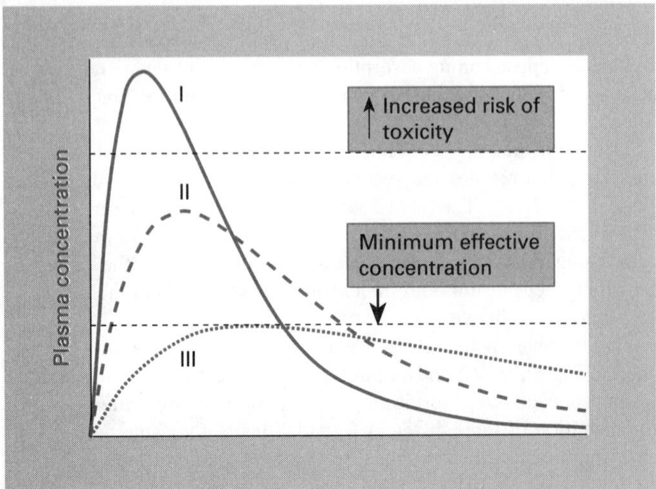

Food

Food may alter the rate and extent of absorption of drugs. For example, eggs impair iron absorption, and milk (and any calcium, aluminium, magnesium, or ferrous salt) impairs tetracycline absorption by the formation of an insoluble chelate. However, effects of this kind are generally of little clinical importance.

First-pass metabolism

First-pass metabolism is metabolism that occurs before the drug enters the systemic circulation. This may happen in the gut lumen (for example, benzylpenicillin and insulin), the gut wall (for example, tyramine, chlorpromazine, and isoprenaline), the liver (the most important), and the lungs (for example, various amines).

There are many examples of drugs that are subject to presystemic metabolism in the liver. For instance, lignocaine is metabolized to two active compounds that have less antiarrhythmic activity than lignocaine itself but are more toxic; propranolol is metabolized to 4-hydroxypropranolol, which is pharmacologically inactive.

When first-pass metabolism results in the formation of compounds with less pharmacological activity than the parent compound there is less efficacy of the drug after oral than intravenous administration. In some cases this may be overcome by using an oral dose greater than that which is effective by the intravenous route. For example, the effective intravenous dose of propranolol is about 5 mg, compared with about 100 mg for oral administration.

In some cases (for example lignocaine and insulin) metabolism is so extensive that it makes oral therapy impossible. However, for some drugs it may be possible to circumvent the liver by giving the drug sublingually, rectally, or transdermally (see above).

Hepatic drug metabolism is discussed in more detail below.

Distribution

PROTEIN BINDING

Many drugs are bound to circulating proteins, usually albumin (acidic drugs), but also globulins (hormones), lipoproteins, and acid glycoproteins (basic drugs). Only non-protein-bound drug can bind to cellular receptors, pass across tissue membranes, and gain access to cellular enzymes, thus being distributed to other body tissues, metabolized, and excreted (for example by the kidney). Thus, changes in protein binding may sometimes cause changes in drug distribution. However, for such changes to be important the drug must be more than 90 per cent bound in the plasma and must not be widely distributed to body tissues. This limits its importance to a few drugs (principally phenytoin and warfarin).

The albumin binding of drugs may be changed in renal impairment (in which the characteristics of albumin binding of drugs are altered by unknown mechanisms), hypoalbuminaemia (drug binding is reduced when the plasma albumin concentration falls below 25 g/l), the last trimester of pregnancy (during which protein binding is reduced partly because of hypoalbuminaemia), and displacement by other drugs.

The binding of drugs to α_1-acid glycoprotein is increased after trauma and surgery, and in inflammatory diseases and infections. For example, the protein binding of quinine is increased in malaria and the binding of lignocaine is increased after myocardial infarction.

TISSUE DISTRIBUTION

The extent of drug distribution to the tissues of the body varies widely. Some drugs are distributed only to the body fluids, while others are bound extensively in tissues. The apparent volume of distribution (see below) gives a mathematical measure of the extent of tissue distribution, but does not give any anatomical or physiological information about that distribution.

The factors that influence the distribution of drugs to different tissues include plasma-protein binding (see above), specific receptor sites in tissues (for example, the binding of cardiac glycosides to Na/K-ATPase in cell membranes throughout the body), regional blood flow (well-perfused organs, such as the heart, kidneys, and liver, tend to accumulate drugs to a greater extent than poorly perfused organs, such as fat and bone), lipid solubility (non-polar drugs, which are relatively lipid-soluble, will distribute more readily to tissues than polar compounds), active transport across cell membranes (for example the adrenergic neurone-blocking drugs), and the effects of other drugs (tricyclic antidepressants inhibit the active transport of the adrenergic neurone-blockers, reducing their access to the site of action in the brain, and thus reducing their efficacy; quinidine reduces the distribution of digoxin by an unknown mechanism).

Some diseases are associated with altered drug distribution, the underlying mechanisms often being obscure. The effects of disease on plasma-protein binding have been mentioned above. Renal failure, apart from its effect on protein binding, may also be associated with a decreased distribution of some drugs (for example, insulin and digoxin). Hyperthyroidism and hypothyroidism respectively increase and reduce the distribution of cardiac glycosides for unknown reasons, resulting in altered plasma digitalis concentrations after a single dose. In cardiac failure the distribution of some antiarrhythmic drugs is reduced (for example, disopyramide and lignocaine). Obesity and malnutrition influence the distribution of drugs that are highly fat soluble (for example, anaesthetics).

Metabolism

Most drug metabolism takes place in the liver, although some occurs elsewhere (for example, suxamethonium in the plasma; insulin and vitamin D in the kidneys; cytosine arabinoside, cyclophosphamide, and other cytotoxic drugs in many cells; and acetylcholine and other neurotransmitters at synapses and within nerves).

Drug metabolism occurs in two phases:

1. Phase I metabolism involves chemical alteration of the basic structure of the drug, for example by oxidation, reduction, or hydrolysis. Oxidation reactions are further subdivided according to whether or not they are effected by the cytochrome-linked mixed function oxidases. Examples of phase I reactions include: the *N*-demethylation of diazepam to desmethyldiazepam, an active metabolite with a long duration of action; the oxidation of theophylline to dimethyluric acid; the oxidation of ethanol to acetaldehyde; the hydrolysis of lignocaine to the toxic metabolites monoethylglycylxylidide and glycylxylidide.
2. Phase II metabolism involves conjugation, for example by sulphation, glucuronidation, methylation, or acetylation. Some drugs are conjugated without prior phase I transformation, while others undergo phase I metabolism before conjugation can take place. The end-products of conjugation are compounds that are more water soluble and therefore more rapidly eliminated by the kidneys. They are usually, although not always, pharmacologically inactive. Examples of phase II reactions include: the glucuronidation of paracetamol; the *N*-acetylation of hydralazine and procainamide; the methylation of desipramine to its active metabolite imipramine. A conjugated product may sometimes be further metabolized. For example, oestrogens are excreted via the bile, deconjugated in the gut by bacteria, and then reabsorbed.

The end-result of drug metabolism is inactivation, although during the process compounds with pharmacological activity may be formed. An inactive compound may be metabolized to an active one; inactive drugs administered for the effects of their active metabolites are called 'pro-drugs'. For example, carfecillin and talampicillin are inactive precursors of carbenicillin and ampicillin respectively, but are much better absorbed than the active drugs. L-Dopa can be regarded as a pro-drug in treating Parkinson's disease because it enters the brain and is metabolized to the active compound dopamine.

The most common type of transformation is metabolism of a pharmacologically active compound to inactive compounds, but sometimes other active compounds are formed first. Examples of parent drugs with active metabolites include diamorphine (which is rapidly metabolized to morphine) and some benzodiazepines (such as diazepam, which is metabolized to desmethyldiazepam, which has a longer duration of action, and to temazepam and oxazepam, which are shorter acting).

Some active compounds are metabolized to toxic compounds. Examples include lignocaine (the accumulation of whose toxic metabolites limits the duration of therapy) and phenytoin (whose main metabolite may inhibit the further metabolism of phenytoin). The normally minor metabolic pathway by which paracetamol is metabolized to a toxic metabolite is enhanced in overdose because the usual detoxifiying pathways are saturated (see Chapter 8.2.1).

The factors that affect hepatic drug metabolism are genetic (see Pharmacogenetics below), other drugs (see Drug interactions below), hepatic blood flow (for drugs with high rates of clearance), liver disease (only important when liver disease is extensive or when there is arteriovenous shunting), and age. The metabolism of some drugs is impaired in old people and in babies under the age of about 6 months, particularly premature babies. In both cases the impairment is due to reduced activity of the hepatic microsomal drug-metabolizing enzymes. For example, in neonatal liver there is a low activity of UDP glucuronyl transferase, which conjugates chloramphenicol; neonates eliminate chloramphenicol slowly, and may suffer peripheral circulatory collapse (the 'grey syndrome') when given it in weight-related doses that are non-toxic to adults.

Excretion

The kidney is the main route whereby drugs are excreted from the body. Other, usually minor, routes include: the lungs (important for paraldehyde); breast milk; sweat, tears, and genital secretions (alarming if the patient is not expecting the orange-red discoloration caused by rifampicin); saliva; and bile. Excretion in bile can lead to the reabsorption of some compounds, for example chloramphenicol (whose inactive metabolites are reactivated by hydrolysis in the gut), oestrogens (which are deconjugated in the gut by bacteria), digitoxin (whose subsequent reabsorption is interrupted by cholestyramine), morphine, rifampicin, and tetracyclines.

Renal excretion of drugs occurs chiefly by three processes (Fig. 3): glomerular filtration, passive tubular reabsorption, and active tubular secretion. Thus, total renal clearance = clearance by filtration + clearance by secretion − retention by reabsorption.

Fig. 3 A diagrammatic representation of a nephron, showing the sites of the three major processes whereby drugs are excreted via the kidney.

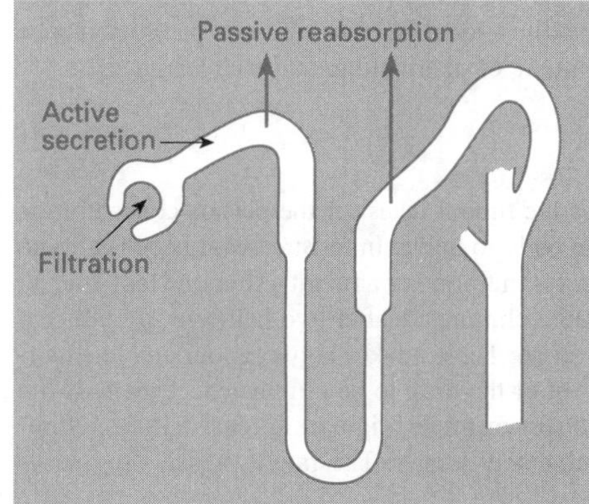

If a drug is mainly metabolized to inactive compounds, renal function will not greatly affect elimination of the active compound. However, if the drug or an active metabolite is excreted unchanged via the kidneys, changes in renal function will influence its elimination.

GLOMERULAR FILTRATION

All drugs are filtered at the renal glomerulus. The extent of filtration is directly proportional to the glomerular filtration rate (**GFR** = 120 ml/min) and to the fraction of unbound drug in the plasma (*fu*). Thus:

$$\text{Rate of clearance by filtration} = fu \times \text{GFR}.$$

If the total renal clearance of a drug is equal to $fu \times$ GFR then it is cleared principally by filtration. It may, of course, also be affected by the other two mechanisms, secretion and reabsorption, but in that case those effects must balance each other. Examples of drugs whose clearance is similar to the GFR (after correction for protein binding) are digoxin, gentamicin, procainamide, methotrexate, and ethambutol. As creatinine is cleared principally by filtration, measurement of the rate of renal clearance of creatinine is useful in estimating the clearance rates of these drugs.

PASSIVE TUBULAR REABSORPTION

Drugs are subject to passive reabsorption by the renal tubules. The elimination of drugs with very low rates of renal clearance (i.e. approaching urine flow rate, or about 1–2 ml/min) will be significantly affected by changes in urine flow rate (because a doubling of flow rate will increase their rate of clearance by 1–2 ml/min, i.e. twofold). However, for weak acids and weak bases the principal factor affecting passive reabsorption is the pH of the renal tubular fluid, because the extent of their ionization (and therefore of their passive reabsorption) depends on the pH when seen in relation to the pK_a of the drug. For example, weak acids with a pK_a below 7.5, such as aspirin, are more highly ionized, and therefore less well reabsorbed, in an alkaline urine. The reverse is true for weak bases with a pK_a greater than 7.5, such as amphetamine, whose reabsorption is reduced, and whose clearance is therefore enhanced, by an acid urine. These principles are sometimes put to use in the treatment of overdose (see Section 8). Renal failure alters passive reabsorption indirectly, by alterations in urine flow rate and pH.

ACTIVE TUBULAR SECRETION

If the renal clearance of a drug is greater than expected by filtration, it is also cleared by active tubular secretion in the proximal tubule. Penicillin is an example. Some drugs inhibit active tubular secretion, and this forms the basis of some drug interactions (see below).

Pharmacokinetic parameters

Formal pharmacokinetics is a rigorous mathematical discipline for describing the way a drug is handled by the body. A full discussion of pharmacokinetics is beyond our scope here, but it is worth discussing three simple and commonly quoted pharmacokinetic parameters: the half-life, the apparent volume of distribution, and the clearance.

HALF-LIFE ($t_{1/2}$)

The half-life of a drug is the time it takes for the plasma concentration or amount of drug in the body to halve. In most cases it is constant, no matter what the starting concentration or amount. After one half-life, 50 per cent of the drug will be eliminated, after two half-lives 75 per cent (50 + 25 per cent), and so on. Thus, it takes between four and five half-lives for about 95 per cent of the drug to be eliminated. If the half-life of the drug is prolonged (for example, digoxin in renal failure), elimination will take proportionately longer. The rate at which drug accumulates in the body during regular multiple dosing is determined by the half-life. Just as it takes four half-lives for 95 per cent of the drug to be eliminated after withdrawal, it takes four half-lives for about 95 per cent of steady state to be reached during regular administration (Fig. 4a and Fig. 5, bottom and middle curves).

The delay in reaching a steady state can be overcome by giving a loading dose. When a drug has a half-life greater than 24 h (for example digoxin, 40 h; digitoxin 7 d; *S*(-)warfarin, 32 h), it takes several days or weeks of regular administration of the same daily dose before the steady-state plasma concentration or amount of drug in the body is reached. Such a delay may be unacceptable if the eventual steady-state plasma concentration is that associated with a therapeutic effect. In such cases a loading dose may be given in order to boost the amount of drug in the body to the required level. This would then be followed by the administration of the regular maintenance dose to maintain the steady state (Fig. 4b and Fig. 5, top curve).

Even when the half-life of a drug is short it may be necessary to give a loading dose if a very rapid effect is required. For example, the half-life of lignocaine is about 1 h; because it would take about 4 h before a steady state was reached a loading dose is usually given, the treatment of cardiac arrhythmias being an urgent matter.

Fig. 4 (a) The theoretical plasma concentrations of a drug over a period of time during its repeated oral administration. With repeated administration there is accumulation to an eventual steady state. (b) If the correct loading dose is given a steady state can be achieved rapidly and then maintained by giving a smaller maintenance dose. In this example, because the drug is being given once every half-life the maintenance dose is half the loading dose.

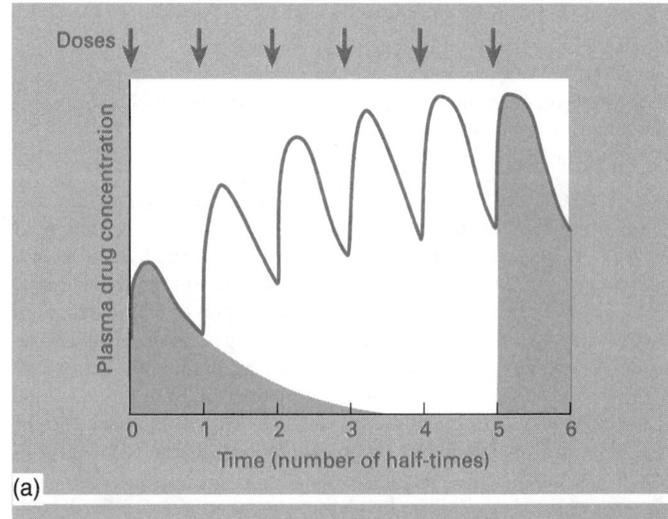

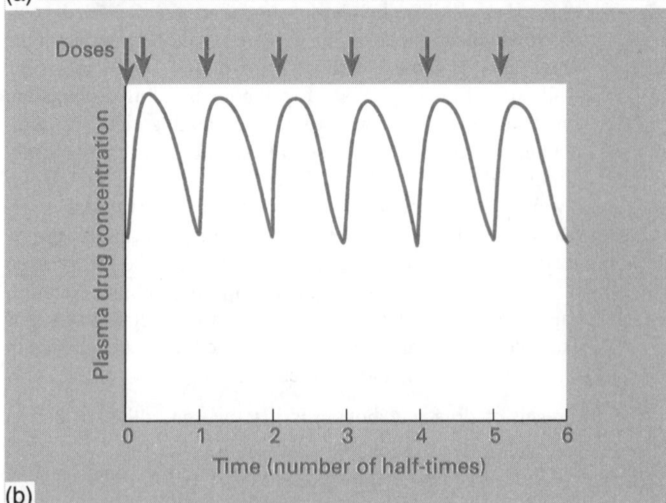

APPARENT VOLUME OF DISTRIBUTION (V)

The apparent volume of distribution is the ratio of the amount of drug in the body to its plasma concentration (V = amount in the body/plasma concentration). The higher the apparent volume the more widely the drug is distributed to the body tissues. For example, warfarin has an apparent volume of distribution of about 0.1 l/kg; its distribution is limited to its site of action and some compartments of body water; in contrast, digoxin has a volume of about 6 l/kg—it is widely distributed to body tissues. Note that the volume of distribution of a drug may be much greater than any actual fluid volume in the body—it is a notional volume that reflects the extent of distribution and should not be interpreted in physiological terms.

To achieve a target plasma concentration it is possible to calculate the loading dose from the relation: V = loading dose/target concentration. The half-life is related to the apparent volume of distribution and the total body clearance: total body clearance × half-life = $\log_e 2$ × volume. Clearance and volume are independent of each other. For example, the rate at which a drug is cleared from the plasma by glomerular filtration is obviously not dependent on the intracellular concentration in the heart. It follows that the half-life must depend on the independent values of clearance and volume. Thus, a change in half-life implies a change in either clearance, or volume, or both.

CLEARANCE (CL)

The clearance of a drug is the fraction of the apparent volume of distribution from which the drug is removed in unit time. It is expressed in units of amount per time (for example ml/min), sometimes corrected for body weight (for example ml/min per kg).

Total body clearance is equal to the sum of the clearances by all routes of elimination, and it is usually subdivided into renal clearance and non-renal clearance (usually assumed to be hepatic). The magnitude of the renal clearance rate of a drug is related to its principal mechanism of renal excretion, as discussed earlier. The plasma concentration at steady state is directly proportional to the clearance rate ($C_{ss} = f \cdot \text{dose}/CL$, where f is the systemic availability). From knowledge of the clearance of a drug it is possible to calculate the appropriate maintenance dose required for a particular plasma concentration. If clearance changes during treatment (for example, because of renal failure), the new maintenance dose can be calculated by comparing the new and old clearance rates ($CL_{old}/CL_{new} = dose_{old}/dose_{new}$).

Fig. 5 Plasma quinine concentrations in cerebral malaria during repeated administration of 5 mg/kg every 8 h (bottom curve), repeated administration of 10 mg/kg every 8 h (middle curve), and repeated administration of 10 mg/kg every 8 h after a loading dose of 20 mg/kg (top curve). (From White, N.J. *et al.* (1983). Quinine loading dose in cerebral malaria. *American Journal of Tropical Medicine and Hygiene,* **32,** 1–5, with permission.)

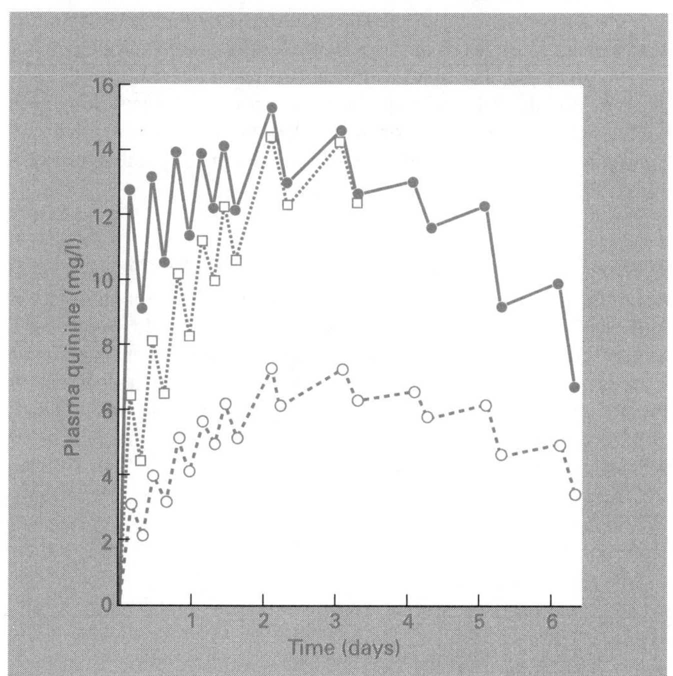

Non-linear kinetics

Although the pharmacokinetics of most drugs are linear, some are not. This means that some aspect of their kinetics becomes saturated in the therapeutic dosage range, so that a linear increase in dosage does not produce a proportionate increase in plasma concentration or effect. This is most clearly seen with phenytoin, whose enzymatic metabolism in the liver becomes saturated at dosages in the therapeutic range; plasma phenytoin concentrations therefore increase non-linearly with dosage (Fig. 6).

The pharmacodynamic process

The question associated with the pharmacodynamic process is: Is the drug producing the required pharmacological effect? It describes all those matters concerned with the pharmacological actions of a drug, whether they be determinants of therapeutic effects or of adverse effects.

Drugs produce their pharmacological effects in many different ways (Table 4). Many of these actions are produced by the stimulation or blockade of a receptor.

Actions via direct effects on receptors

Receptors are proteins situated either in cell membranes or within the cellular cytoplasm. For each type there is a specific group of ligands, drugs or endogenous substances that bind to the receptor and produce pharmacological effects. There are three types of ligands: agonists, antagonists, and partial agonists.

Fig. 6 The relation between daily phenytoin dosage and the associated steady-state plasma phenytoin concentrations in five different patients. Note the large variability in steady-state phenytoin concentrations from patient to patient at any one dosage and the non-linearity of the relation. (After Richens, A. and Dunlop, A. (1975). Serum–phenytoin levels in management of epilepsy. *Lancet,* **ii,** 247–8, with permission © *Lancet.*)

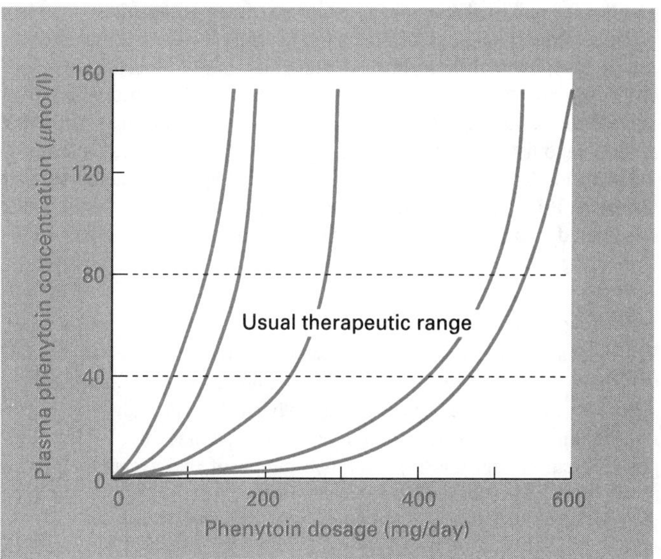

Table 4 *The types of pharmacological actions of drugs*

Actions	Examples
Actions via receptors	
Agonist at a receptor	Morphine
Antagonist at a receptor	Naloxone
Partial agonist at a receptor	Pentazocine
Actions via second messengers	Lithium
Indirect alterations of the effects of endogenous agonists	
Physiological antagonism (insulin)	Glucagon
Increase in endogenous release (monoamines)	Amphetamine
Inhibition of endogenous reuptake (monoamines)	Antidepressants
Inhibition of endogenous metabolism (GABA)	Vigabatrin
Prevention of endogenous release (aldosterone)	ACE inhibitors
Inhibition of transport processes	Diuretics
Actions on enzymes	
Enzyme inhibition	Warfarin
Enzyme activation	Thrombolytic drugs
Enzymatic action	Factor VIII
Other miscellaneous effects	
Chelating agents	Penicillamine
Osmotic diuretics	Mannitol
Volatile general anaesthetics	Halothane
Replacement drugs	Iron salts

Agonists

Ligands that bind to a receptor and produce a response are called agonists. For example, morphine is an agonist at μ-opioid receptors, through which its analgesic action is mediated.

Antagonists

Ligands that prevent an agonist from binding to a receptor and thus prevent its effects are called antagonists (or blockers). However, pure antagonists do not themselves have any pharmacological actions mediated by receptors. For example, naloxone is an opioid-receptor antagonist; when it binds to opioid receptors it prevents or reverses the effects of morphine and other opiates.

Partial agonists

A full agonist is one that is capable of producing a maximal response, when it binds to enough receptors. In contrast, a partial agonist cannot produce the maximal response of which the tissue is capable, even when it binds to the maximum number of available receptors. Thus, above a certain level of binding a partial agonist may bind to receptors without producing any further increase in effect. However, in so doing it may prevent the action of other agonists, and may thus appear to be acting as an antagonist. This mixture of actions is called partial agonism.

For example, pentazocine is a mixed opioid agonist/antagonist at μ-receptors. If it is used in combination with a high dose of a pure agonist it will tend to oppose its action rather than supplement it.

RECEPTOR SUBTYPES

In some cases a receptor may have subtypes, for which certain ligands may have a degree of selectivity. For example, there are at least three subtypes of opioid receptors, μ and δ (both involved in analgesia, gastrointestinal motility, and respiratory depression), and κ (involved in analgesia, sedation, and miosis). The distribution of these receptors varies throughout the nervous system. Most opiates act at μ-receptors, but none is completely selective and they may act at other subtypes.

LONG-TERM EFFECTS OF DRUGS AT RECEPTORS

During long-term therapy the effects of a drug may be altered by adaptive responses, usually accompanied by either increases ('up-regulation') or decreases ('down-regulation') in receptor numbers. Such changes may be responsible for both beneficial and adverse effects of drugs. Examples include:

- The therapeutic response to antidepressants, which may be related to changes in receptors in the brain secondary to the actions of these drugs on neurotransmitter uptake. This explains why the therapeutic response to antidepressants takes a few weeks.
- The way in which the response to L-dopa in Parkinson's disease changes during long-term administration (producing, for example, the 'on-off' effect).
- Withdrawal syndromes, which may occur because long-term changes become unopposed when the drug is withdrawn, for example after the long-term abuse of opiates or the use of benzodiazepines in chronic anxiety.

Actions via direct effects on second messengers

When an agonist stimulates a membrane-bound receptor its effect is produced in one of two ways: either through a so-called second messenger (see Fig. 7) or by changing the activity of an ion channel linked to the receptor. Some drugs may act by affecting second messengers directly. For example, lithium may work by inhibiting phosphatidylinositol turnover at different sites. Theophylline and other xanthines work by inhibiting the breakdown of cyclic AMP.

Actions via indirect alterations of the effects of endogenous agonists

Some drugs indirectly alter the effect of an endogenous agonist rather than acting via a receptor.

Physiological antagonism

Some drugs oppose the physiological effects of others. For example, glucagon is a physiological antagonist of the actions of insulin and can be used to treat hypoglycaemia.

Increase in endogenous release

Some drugs enhance the action of endogenous agonists by increasing their release. For example, amphetamines increase the release of dopamine from nerve endings. Because amphetamines can cause a syndrome similar to schizophrenia, this action has led to the idea that schizophrenia may be related to excess dopamine action in the brain.

Prevention of endogenous release

If a drug prevents the release of an endogenous agonist it will reduce its effects. For example, angiotensin-converting enzyme (ACE) inhibitors prevent the formation of angiotensin II; this prevents the endogenous release of aldosterone, whose effects are thereby reduced, resulting in potassium retention.

Inhibition of endogenous reuptake

Some drugs inhibit the reuptake of endogenous agonists, enhancing their effects. For example, many antidepressants inhibit the reuptake by neurones of certain neurotransmitters, such as noradrenaline and 5-hydroxytryptamine.

Inhibition of endogenous metabolism

Some drugs enhance the effects of endogenous agonists by inhibiting their metabolism. For example, vigabatrin inhibits the metabolism of γ-aminobutyrate (GABA) in the brain, enhancing its actions and suppressing seizures.

Actions via the inhibition of transport processes

Because cations (such as sodium, potassium, and calcium) and other substances (such as organic acids in the kidneys) have so many important roles in the maintenance of normal cellular function, inhibition of their transport is an important type of mechanism of drug action.

Diuretics

Most diuretics act by inhibiting sodium reabsorption in the renal tubules. The loop diuretics frusemide and bumetanide inhibit Na/K/Cl co-transport in the ascending limb of the loop of Henle. The thiazide diuretics inhibit Na/Cl co-transport in the proximal segment of the distal convoluted tubule. The potassium-sparing diuretic amiloride inhibits sodium channels in the distal segment of the distal convoluted tubule.

Calcium antagonists

The calcium antagonists, such as verapamil, diltiazem, and the dihydropyridines (for example, nifedipine), inhibit the transport of calcium via potential-operated calcium channels. The different calcium antagonists have different selectivities for calcium channels in different tissues, and have various actions. For example, verapamil has an antiarrhythmic action in the heart, and nifedipine a vasodilator action on peripheral arterioles.

Drugs acting on potassium channels

Potassium channels in cell membranes control the rate of efflux of potassium from the cells, and this tends to stabilize the cell membrane. Cellular activity will therefore be reduced by drugs that open potassium channels and increased by drugs that close them.

Drugs that open potassium channels include vascular smooth-muscle relaxants, such as minoxidil and hydralazine. Drugs that close them include the sulphonylureas, which increase the release of insulin from pancreatic β-cells, and 3,4-diaminopyridine, which increases the release of acetylcholine at the neuromuscular junction.

Actions via enzyme inhibition

Some drugs act by direct inhibition of enzymes.

Neostigmine

Neostigmine is a reversible cholinesterase inhibitor. It increases the concentration of acetylcholine at the muscle motor end-plate, improving neuromuscular transmission.

Allopurinol

Xanthine and hypoxanthine are oxidized to uric acid by xanthine oxidase; this is inhibited by allopurinol, which therefore reduces the synthesis of uric acid in gout.

Monoamine oxidase (MAO) inhibitors

The monoamine oxidase inhibitors inhibit the metabolism of the monoamines 5-hydroxytryptamine, noradrenaline, and dopamine in the brain, and it is presumably by this action that they produce their antidepressant effect. Just as drugs that act via receptors may be selective for a subtype of a receptor, so MAO inhibitors may be selective for one of the sub-

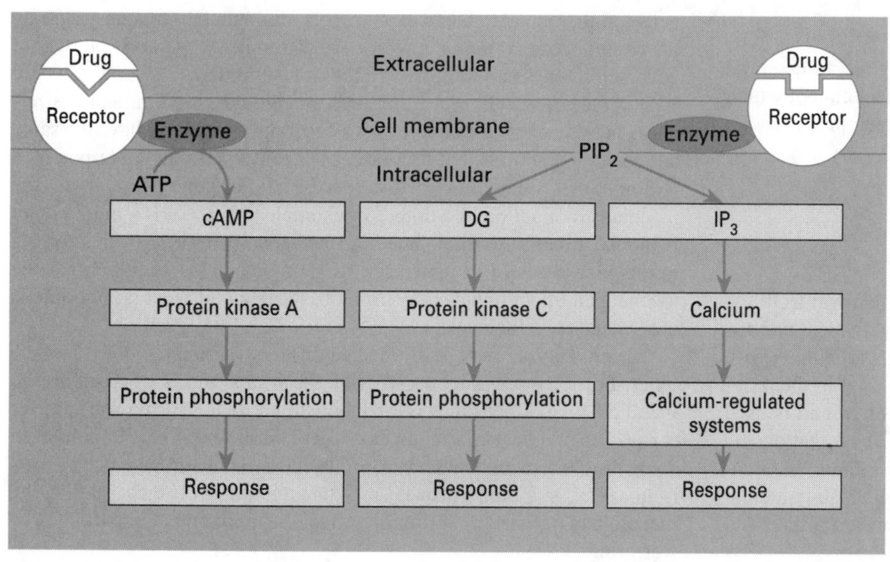

Fig. 7 A schematic representation of the second-messenger systems that mediate the effects of drugs acting at receptors.

types of MAO. For example, selegiline is a selective inhibitor of MAO type B: it inhibits the metabolism of dopamine in the brain and enhances the action of L-dopa in parkinsonism. However, because gut MAO is of type A, selegiline does not produce the 'cheese reaction' (due to tyramine and other amines, see below) that non-selective MAO inhibitors do. In contrast, the antidepressant moclobemide is a selective inhibitor of MAO A; although it inhibits the metabolism of tyramine in the gut it does not inhibit its metabolism by MAO B after absorption.

Cardiac glycosides

The cardiac glycosides act by inhibiting the Na/K pump, changing the disposition of sodium, which secondarily changes calcium disposition within cells.

Other examples

Other drugs that act via enzyme inhibition include warfarin (vitamin K epoxide reductase), aspirin and other non-steroidal anti-inflammatory drugs (the enzymes involved in prostaglandin synthesis), ACE inhibitors, disulfiram (alcohol dehydrogenase), some anticancer drugs, such as cytarabine (DNA polymerase), and some anti-infective agents (bacterial or viral enzymes; for example, trimethoprim inhibits bacterial dihydrofolate reductase, the quinolones inhibit bacterial DNA gyrase, and zidovudine and didanosine inhibit the reverse transcriptase of HIV).

Danazol and stanozolol are examples of drugs that have an indirect inhibitory effect on an enzyme—they stimulate the production of an inhibitor of C1 esterase and are used to treat hereditary angio-oedema, in which there is a deficiency of the inhibitor.

Actions via enzyme activation or direct enzymatic activity

Some drugs activate enzymes or are themselves enzymes.

Drugs that act on the clotting system

The clotting and fibrinolytic factors are enzymes, and certain drugs that act on clotting and fibrinolysis do so by increasing their activity. Heparin acts by activating antithrombin III. The thrombolytic drugs streptokinase, alteplase, and anistreplase are activators of plasminogen.

Enzyme replacement in genetic and acquired enzyme deficiencies

Clotting factor deficiencies can be treated by replacing deficient enzymes of the clotting pathway, for example factor VIII in patients with haemophilia and fresh frozen plasma in warfarin toxicity. Pancreatic enzymes are used in treating malabsorption in patients with chronic pancreatic insufficiency.

Cancer chemotherapy

L-Asparaginase is an enzyme that hydrolyses asparagine, an essential amino acid in the neoplastic cell line, the consequent depletion of which in leukaemic cells may be of therapeutic benefit in some patients with acute lymphoblastic leukaemia.

Actions via other miscellaneous effects

Chelating agents

Drugs that chelate metals can be used to hasten their removal from the body. Calcium sodium edetate (EDTA) chelates many divalent and trivalent metals and is used in the treatment of poisoning, particularly with lead. Dimercaprol chelates some heavy metals and is used in the treatment of mercury poisoning. Desferrioxamine chelates iron and is used in the treatment of iron poisoning and in the iron overload that occurs with repeated blood transfusion (for example, in thalassaemia). Penicillamine chelates copper and is used in the treatment of hepatolenticular degeneration (Wilson's disease); it is also used to chelate cystine and thus prevent renal damage in cystinuria.

Osmotic diuretics

Mannitol is freely filtered at the glomerulus but is reabsorbed to only a small extent by the renal tubules. It therefore increases the concentration of osmotically active particles in the tubular fluid and takes water with it.

Volatile general anaesthetics

General anaesthetics form a diverse group of agents, such as the halogenated hydrocarbons (for example, halothane, methoxyflurane, enflurane, trichloroethylene), and non-halogenated agents (for example, nitrous oxide, ether, and cyclopropane), which produce similar effects on the brain. Their main action is probably on the lipid matrix of the biological membrane, whose biophysical properties they change, resulting in changes in ion fluxes or other functions that are important for neuronal excitability.

Replacement of vitamins and minerals

Some drugs are used simply to replace deficiencies, for example ferrous salts in iron deficiency anaemia and hydroxocobalamin (vitamin B_{12}) in vitamin B_{12} deficiency.

Stereoisomerism and drug action

Stereoisomerism (chirality) of organic compounds is due to asymmetry in one or more of their atoms (usually carbon), resulting in two structures (enantiomers) that cannot be superimposed on each other.

The terminology used to describe chiral compounds is complex, but, in summary, some are called *R* and *S* (from the Latin *rectus* = right and *sinister* = left), others D and L (from the Latin *dexter* = right and *laevus* = left), and yet others *d* and *l*. Examples of drug enantiomers are *R*-warfarin and *S*-warfarin, D-glucose (dextrose) and L-glucose (laevulose), and *d*-propranolol and *l*-propranolol.

Of all synthetic drugs used in clinical practice about 40 per cent are chiral and about 90 per cent of those are marketed in the racemic form (i.e. as an equal mixture of the two enantiomers). Examples include *d,l*-propranolol and *R,S*-warfarin. Naproxen is one of the few examples of a synthetic compound that is marketed as a single enantiomer. In contrast, naturally occurring and semisynthetic compounds are almost all chiral and almost all are marketed as a single isomer. Examples include D-glucose (dextrose) and the naturally occurring amino acids (for example L-dopa).

Enantiomers often have different actions. For example, *l*-propranolol is a β-blocker, while *d*-propranolol has membrane-stabilizing activity like that of local anaesthetics; *l*-sotalol is a β-blocker, while *d*-sotalol has antiarrhythmic effects like those of amiodarone.

Sometimes the difference between enantiomers is a difference between therapeutic and adverse effects, dramatically demonstrated by the example of thalidomide, whose *R*-enantiomer is hypnotic but whose adverse effects seem to be due to the *S*-enantiomer.

In some cases, differences between enantiomers are limited to differences in potency. For example, *S*-warfarin and *R*-warfarin have the same anticoagulant actions, but the former is about five times more potent.

Sometimes enantiomeric differences tell us something about the mechanism of action of a drug. For example, *S*-timolol is a more potent β-blocker than *R*-timolol, but both are equally effective in reducing intraocular pressure in patients with glaucoma. This suggests that the mechanism of action whereby timolol lowers the intraocular pressure is not related to β-blockade.

One enantiomer may be eliminated differently from the body than the other. For example, the half-lives of *S*-warfarin and *R*-warfarin are 32 h and 54 h, and the routes of metabolism are to 7-hydroxywarfarin for *S*-warfarin and to warfarin alcohols for *R*-warfarin. This is important in some drug interactions with warfarin, because some drugs (such as metronidazole, sulphinpyrazone, and phenylbutazone) that inhibit the metabolism of warfarin, primarily affect the more potent enantiomer, *S*-warfarin.

The synthesis of pure enantiomers of synthetic drugs is expensive. However, new techniques may reduce the costs and lead to the emergence of more formulations of pure enantiomers for clinical use.

The therapeutic process

The question associated with the therapeutic process is: Is the pharmacological effect being translated into a therapeutic effect?

Translation of pharmacological effect into therapeutic effect during short-term therapy

The short-term therapeutic and toxic effects of drugs occur as a result of the pharmacological actions we have discussed above. However, the translation of molecular and cellular pharmacological effects into the therapeutic or toxic effect is not a simple process, but one that involves several translational stages at different pharmacological and physiological levels.

Take, for example, the action of salbutamol, a β_2-adrenoceptor agonist, in the treatment of asthma (Fig. 8). Salbutamol stimulates bronchial β_2-adrenoceptors, and so increases the activity of adenylate cyclase; this is its pharmacological effect at the molecular level. The increase in adenylate cyclase activity leads to an increase in the intracellular concentration of cyclic AMP, a pharmacological effect at the cellular level. The increase in cAMP in some way alters the function of bronchial smooth-muscle cells, and results in an inhibition of the release of inflammatory mediators from bronchial mast cells, with effects on cell physiology. All this in turn results in bronchodilatation, an effect on tissue physiology. Bronchodilatation causes improved lung function, an effect on organ physiology. Finally, the patient is able to breathe more easily, the desired clinical effect.

This analysis of the short-term effects of drugs teaches us several things about drug action: how drug action may be modified; how therapeutic and adverse effects may be mediated via different pharmacological effects; the relation between the pharmacological effects of a drug and the rate of onset or duration of its action; and drug/disease interactions.

Fig. 8 The effect of metoclopramide on the absorption of paracetamol. When metoclopramide (10 mg i.v.) was given with paracetamol (1.5 g orally) the rate of paracetamol absorption was increased, as evidenced by a higher and earlier peak paracetamol plasma concentration. (Adapted from Nimmo, J. *et al.* (1973). Pharmacological modification of gastric emptying: effects of propantheline and metoclopramide on paracetamol absorption. *British Medical Journal,* **i**, 587–9, with permission.)

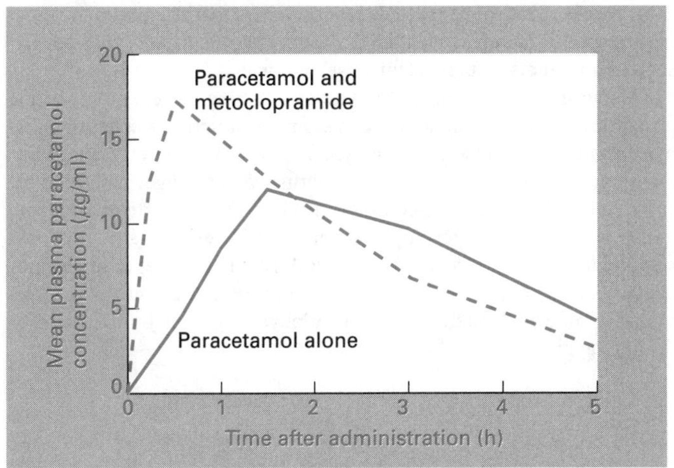

HOW DRUG ACTION MAY BE MODIFIED

There are often ways in which the action of a drug may be beneficially or adversely modified. For example, the action of salbutamol would be expected to be potentiated at the stage at which it alters adenyl cyclase activity by a xanthine derivative, such as theophylline, which increases cellular cAMP concentrations by the inhibition of phosphodiesterase. This turns out to be both a beneficial and an adverse clinical interaction—beneficial because theophylline enhances the therapeutic action of salbutamol, adverse because it also enhances the hypokalaemia that salbutamol may cause by stimulation of Na/K-ATPase.

HOW THERAPEUTIC AND ADVERSE OR OTHER EFFECTS MAY BE MEDIATED VIA DIFFERENT PHARMACOLOGICAL EFFECTS

Some drugs have more than one molecular mechanism of action, and two different therapeutic or adverse effects of a drug may be brought about by two different actions. For example, tetracycline acts as an antibacterial agent by interfering with bacterial protein synthesis, but its therapeutic effect in acne is due to interference with the production of sebum in facial sweat glands.

Alternatively, a therapeutic effect may be brought about by one pharmacological action and an adverse effect by another. For example, the therapeutic effect of salbutamol is brought about by its action on β_2-adrenoceptors, but it causes the unwanted effect of tachycardia by stimulation of β_1-adrenoceptors.

Different therapeutic or adverse effects may be produced by the actions of a single drug on the same or a similar molecular mechanism in different tissues. For example, the inhibition of β_2-adrenoceptors produces bronchoconstriction in the lungs of susceptible individuals and impairs glycogenolysis in the liver.

Peripheral or non-therapeutic effects of drugs can be of clinical importance in several ways. For example, aminoglycoside antibiotics can all cause damage to the middle ear, leading to impaired hearing or loss of balance; these effects are quite separate from the antibiotic activity of these drugs but have to be taken into account when choosing dosage regimens and lead to the requirement of plasma concentration monitoring.

THE RELATION BETWEEN THE PHARMACOLOGICAL EFFECTS OF A DRUG AND THE RATE OF ONSET OR DURATION OF ITS ACTION

The rate of onset of action of a drug is related not only to its pharmacokinetics (i.e. the time it takes for the appropriate amount of drug to build up at the site of action; Fig. 4), but also to the time it takes for the full pharmacodynamic sequence of events to take place. In the case of salbutamol the time between β_2-adrenoceptor stimulation and bronchodilatation (Fig. 8) is of the order of a few minutes. However, for other drugs the sequence of events takes much longer. For example, corticosteroids react with a receptor protein in cellular cytoplasm to form a steroid–receptor complex. This complex enters the cell nucleus, where it binds to chromatin and directs the genetic apparatus to transcribe RNA. This leads, for instance in liver cells, to the production of enzymes involved in gluconeogenesis and amino acid metabolism. Once the steroid has bound to its intracellular receptor it sets off a sequence of reactions that then has its own time-scale, independent of the quantity of steroid, either in the blood or combined with the receptor. The induction of protein synthesis by RNA transcription takes several hours and each new protein has its own biological lifespan. This is why the effect takes hours or days to occur.

Similarly, the duration of action of a drug is related not only to its pharmacokinetics (i.e. the time it takes for the drug to be cleared from the body), but also to the duration of its pharmacological actions. For

Table 5 *The different ways in which adaptation to drug effects may become apparent clinically*

Effect	Example
Therapeutic effects through adaptation	Immunization and vaccination Tricyclic antidepressants
Tolerance—increasing ineffectiveness of therapy:	
Target cell tolerance	Depletion of noradrenaline by ephedrine Change in sulphydryl function by nitrates Opioid tolerance
Physiological homoeostatic mechanisms	Hydralazine (reflex tachycardia) Acetazolamide (acidosis reversing hypokalaemia)
Metabolic autoinduction	Barbiturates, carbamazepine
Withdrawal syndromes:	
Through receptor changes	Opioids, alcohol, benzodiazepines, clonidine, β-blockers
Through physiological adaptation	Corticosteroids
Adverse effects directly due to adaptation	Tardive dyskinesia due to dopamine antagonists

example, aspirin inhibits cyclo-oxygenase by acetylating a serine moiety at the active site of the enzyme. In platelets this leads to inhibition of prostaglandin synthesis for the lifetime of the platelet. Thus, although aspirin is cleared from the body within a few hours, its effect on platelets lasts for days.

DRUG/DISEASE INTERACTIONS

Because of the complex links between the pharmacological effects of a drug and its therapeutic or adverse effects there are many ways in which the pathophysiology of the disease being treated, or of other incidental diseases, can alter the way in which the pharmacological effect is translated into a therapeutic effect.

The use of digoxin in the treatment of cardiac failure is an example of the ways in which drug/disease interactions may influence therapy. Digoxin inhibits the activity of the membrane-bound Na/K pump. This is its pharmacological effect at the molecular level, which causes an increase in the intracellular concentration of sodium, and thereby an alteration in the intracellular disposition of calcium (a pharmacological effect at the cellular level). This in turn leads to an alteration in the action potential of cardiac muscle (a physiological effect at the cellular level), which then causes an increase in the rate of contractility of the myocardial fibres (a physiological effect at the tissue level). There is a consequent increase in cardiac output (a physiological effect at the level of the whole organ).

If this chain of events occurs without interruption the clinical result will be relief of the signs and symptoms of heart failure. However, there are drug/disease interactions that may alter the therapeutic outcome at the different stages in the chain. Thus, potassium depletion enhances the binding of digoxin to the Na/K pump and this increases the extent of inhibition of sodium transport, which can in turn cause digoxin toxicity. In hyperthyroidism there is an alteration in the nature of the interaction between digoxin and the Na/K pump, resulting in resistance to the inhibitory effects of digoxin. Increasing the dose may merely result in digoxin toxicity without ever producing a therapeutic effect. In patients with chronic cor pulmonale, digoxin may inhibit the Na/K pump and may even cause cardiac arrhythmias without ever causing an increase in the rate of myocardial contractility. This may be because of tissue hypoxia and acidosis in cor pulmonale, which may also contribute to an increased risk of digoxin-induced cardiac arrhythmias without therapeutic benefit in patients with acute myocardial infarction. In patients with hypertrophic obstructive cardiomyopathy, although digoxin increases the rate of myocardial contractility, this is not translated into an increase in cardiac output, as there is a fixed obstruction to left ventricular outflow.

This example shows that simply because it is sometimes possible to demonstrate that a drug is having its expected action at a particular pharmacological or physiological level, it cannot automatically be assumed that it will have a consequent therapeutic effect.

Translation of pharmacological effect into therapeutic effect during long-term therapy

Prolonged therapy may bring with it the phenomenon of adaptation to the short-term pharmacological effects of the drug (Table 5). This may have several consequences.

THERAPEUTIC EFFECTS THROUGH ADAPTATION

In immunization, by adapting to an initial immunological challenge, the immune system develops the ability to respond to a subsequent similar challenge, tetanus immunization for example.

Although tricyclic antidepressants very quickly produce inhibition of reuptake of noradrenaline and 5-hydroxytryptamine in the brain, the therapeutic effect of these drugs takes 1 to 2 weeks to become evident. The brain adapts to the increased concentrations of noradrenaline and 5-hydroxytryptamine in the synaptic cleft in certain areas, where the sensitivity of responses to neurotransmitters is decreased by 'down-regulation'; part of this adaptive effect could be the pharmacological action through which these drugs produce their therapeutic effects.

TOLERANCE: INCREASING INEFFECTIVENESS OF THERAPY

Tolerance is a state of decreased responsiveness to a drug, brought about by previous exposure, either to the same drug or to one with similar short-term effects. It may occur in several ways.

Tolerance may develop to the vasoconstricting effects of ephedrine nosedrops, used in the treatment of vasomotor rhinitis, as ephedrine acts by releasing noradrenaline from sympathetic nerve endings and when the noradrenaline is depleted the ephedrine can no longer be effective.

Patients who take long-term glyceryl trinitrate, particularly from transdermal patches, develop tolerance to its effects and may not respond to the acute effects of glyceryl trinitrate. In order to avoid this, patches should not be applied for more than 18 h at a time. This effect probably reflects depletion of tissue sulphydryl groups by oxidation to disulphide groups.

Physiological tolerance by homoeostatic mechanisms

Secondary hyperaldosteronism occurs as a physiological response to sodium loss produced by loop or thiazide diuretics. The enhanced potassium excretion that this causes may be obviated by the use of a potassium-sparing diuretic (for example, amiloride, triamterene, or the aldosterone antagonist spironolactone).

A different type of physiological tolerance occurs in patients given the diuretic acetazolamide. Acetazolamide is a very powerful kaliuretic and can cause severe potassium depletion when it is first given. However, because it inhibits carbonic anhydrase activity in the kidney it causes bicarbonate depletion, and the resulting acidosis causes retention of potassium. Thus, potassium depletion due to acetazolamide lasts only for a few days or weeks.

Metabolic tolerance

Metabolic tolerance results from an increased rate of metabolism of the drug. The most common cause is induction of hepatic microsomal drug-metabolizing enzymes by drugs such as barbiturates, phenytoin, carbamazepine, or griseofulvin. In a particular case, the hepatic inactivation of the carbamazepine is increased after long-term exposure to carbamazepine itself (the phenomenon known as 'autoinduction'), and tolerance occurs spontaneously. Induction of drug metabolism forms the basis of potential adverse drug reactions (see below).

WITHDRAWAL SYNDROMES

A common, though not inevitable, outcome of an adaptive response to long-term drug use is the occurrence of a withdrawal response, which occurs either when the drug is withdrawn or when an antagonist is given, and which usually takes the form of some sort of adverse reaction.

A withdrawal syndrome occurs in opiate addicts when the opiate is withdrawn or when an antagonist, such as naloxone, is given. The symptoms consist of yawning, rhinorrhoea, and sweating, followed by the so-called cold turkey, in which there is shivering and goose flesh. Later, nausea, vomiting, diarrhoea, and hypertension may occur. The acute syndrome subsides within a week, but the addict may have anxiety and sleep disturbances for several weeks or months after. This syndrome can be avoided by introducing increasing doses of methadone as the opiate is withdrawn, as the later withdrawal of methadone, which has a much longer duration of action than morphine, may not result in this syndrome.

Delirium tremens may occur on withdrawal of alcohol from chronic alcoholics. This syndrome consists of disorientation and visual hallucinations.

Withdrawal of benzodiazepines after long-term therapy may result in a disturbance of sleep pattern (rebound insomnia associated with abnormal sleep patterns), agitation, restlessness, and occasionally epileptic convulsions.

There is an increased risk of angina pectoris and myocardial infarction in patients with ischaemic heart disease when β-adrenoceptor antagonists are withdrawn after long-term use. This may be because of an increase in the numbers of cardiac β-adrenoceptors, with increased sensitivity to the β-adrenergic effects of the sympathetic nervous system.

Angina and even myocardial infarction have been reported in munitions workers who have become tolerant of the effects of nitroglycerine (glyceryl trinitrate) and have taken a break from work.

Long-term therapy with corticosteroids suppresses pituitary adrenocorticotrophic hormone (ACTH) secretion, leading to adrenal cortical atrophy. When treatment is suddenly withdrawn, ACTH secretion by the pituitary may take several weeks or months to recover. Because the adrenal cortex has to increase in size again in order to become normally responsive to ACTH the patient is at great risk of an addisonian crisis if stressed.

ADVERSE EFFECTS DIRECTLY DUE TO ADAPTATION

Patients taking neuroleptic drugs (such as chlorpromazine, fluphenazine, and haloperidol) continuously for long periods of time commonly develop abnormal movements (known collectively as tardive dyskinesia). The face, mouth, and tongue are most commonly affected, causing stereotyped sucking and smacking of the lips, lateral jaw movements, and fly catching-like, darting movements of the tongue. Occasionally the dyskinesia may be more widespread and may resemble choreoathetosis. It is thought that the continuous long-term blockade of brain dopamine function with neuroleptic drugs leads to increased sensitivity to the effects of dopamine in certain areas of the brain, perhaps by an increase in dopamine receptor numbers. Tardive dyskinesia may be an expression of such increased sensitivity in extrapyramidal areas of the brain.

Adverse drug reactions

Adverse effects are unwanted effects of drugs, and they may be due to either toxic or side-effects. A toxic effect is an adverse effect that arises through an exaggeration of the pharmacological action that is responsible for the therapeutic effect of the drug (for example, arrhythmias due to digoxin), and is therefore dose related. A side-effect is an adverse effect that arises through some pharmacological action other than that which produces the therapeutic effect (for example, anticholinergic effects of tricyclic antidepressants); such effects may or may not be dose related. The term 'adverse effects' covers all types of unwanted effects.

Incidence

The risks of adverse drug reactions have been variously estimated as follows:

- hospital inpatients: 10 to 20 per cent suffer an adverse reaction;
- deaths in hospital inpatients: 0.24 to 2.9 per cent are due to adverse reactions;
- hospital admissions: 0.3 to 5.0 per cent are due to adverse reactions.

Classification

Adverse drug reactions can be classified into four types (Table 6).

DOSE-RELATED ADVERSE REACTIONS

Dose-related adverse drug reactions are usually due to a pharmacokinetic or pharmacodynamic abnormality producing an exaggeration of a known pharmacological effect of the drug. The pharmacological effect that proves adverse may be the same as that which achieves the therapeutic effect (for example, hypoglycaemia due to insulin), or due to another effect occurring in parallel (for example, the anticholinergic action of tricyclic antidepressants, producing a dry mouth or urinary retention).

Dose-related adverse reactions may occur because of variations in the pharmaceutical, pharmacokinetic, or pharmacodynamic properties of a drug, often due to some disease or pharmacogenetic characteristic of the patient. The following are examples of such mechanisms.

Pharmaceutical variation

Adverse reactions can occur because of the presence of a contaminant, for example pyrogens or even bacteria, in intravenous formulations, if quality control breaks down. If a febrile reaction occurs in a patient being given an infusion, the drip should be taken down and all its components should be sent for bacteriological investigation. The manufacturer should be urgently notified.

Out-of-date formulations may sometimes cause adverse reactions because of degradation products. For example, outdated tetracycline may cause Fanconi's syndrome, because it is degraded to anhydrotetracycline and epiandrotetracycline. The omission of the preservative citric acid from tetracycline formulations has reduced the risk of this effect, but has not removed it completely.

Table 6 *Classification of adverse drug reactions*

Dose-related effects
Pharmaceutical variation
Pharamacokinetic variation:
Pharmacogenetic variation
Hepatic disease
Renal disease
Cardiac disease
Thyroid disease
Drug interactions
Pharmacodynamic variation:
Hepatic disease
Altered fluid and electrolyte balance
Drug interactions
Non-dose-related effects
Immunological reactions
Pseudoallergic reactions
Pharmacogenetic variation
Long-term effects
Adaptive changes
Rebound phenomena
Other long-term effects
Delayed effects
Carcinogenesis
Effects concerned with reproduction:
Impaired fertility
Teratogenesis: adverse effects on the fetus during the early stages of pregnancy
Adverse effects on the fetus during the later stages of pregnancy
Drugs in breast milk

Pharmacokinetic variation

There is a great deal of variation among normal individuals in the rate of elimination of drugs. This variation is most marked for drugs that are cleared by hepatic metabolism and is determined by several factors, which may be genetic, environmental (for example diet, smoking, alcohol), or hepatic (blood flow and intrinsic drug-metabolizing capacity). On top of this normal variation there may occur specific pharmacogenetic or hepatic abnormalities that may be associated with adverse reactions. In addition, renal and cardiac disease can cause alterations in drug pharmacokinetics. Pharmacogenetics is discussed below.

The reserve of the liver parenchyma is large, and adverse reactions due to impaired hepatic metabolism are not common. Nevertheless, in the presence of severe liver disease, care must be taken, particularly with drugs with a low therapeutic index and those subject to extensive first-pass elimination. For example, hepatocellular dysfunction, as in severe hepatitis or advanced cirrhosis, may reduce the clearance of drugs for which the capacity of the liver is limited, phenytoin, theophylline, and warfarin for example. Portosystemic shunting in portal hypertension, associated with cirrhosis, reduces the clearance of drugs normally cleared rapidly by the liver, such as morphine and other narcotic analgesics, propranolol, labetalol, and chlorpromazine.

For drugs that are excreted unchanged by the kidneys or that have active metabolites that are excreted, accumulation will occur in renal failure. Important examples include digoxin, lithium, tetracyclines, aminoglycoside antibiotics, and vancomycin.

Pharmacodynamic variation

There is a great deal of pharmacodynamic variability within the general population, and that variability may be compounded by the effects of disease, as the following examples show.

There are several mechanisms whereby hepatic disease may influence the pharmacodynamic responses to certain drugs. Reduced blood clotting may occur in cirrhosis and acute hepatitis because of reduced production of clotting factors; there is also a bleeding hazard in patients with oesophageal and gastric varices caused by portal hypertension in cirrhosis. Drugs that may impair haemostasis, or that may predispose to bleeding by causing gastric ulceration, should be avoided; these include anticoagulants and non-steroidal anti-inflammatory drugs (for example, aspirin, indomethacin, and ibuprofen).

In patients with hepatic encephalopathy (hepatic coma or precoma), the brain is more sensitive to the effects of drugs with sedative actions. It is therefore wise to avoid opioid and other narcotic analgesics and barbiturates; chlorpromazine dosage should be reduced. Chlormethiazole or short-acting benzodiazepines may be used cautiously as tranquillizers.

Diuretics used for the treatment of ascites and peripheral oedema may precipitate hepatic encephalopathy, particularly if there is too rapid a diuresis.

In hepatic cirrhosis, sodium and water retention may be exacerbated by certain drugs, including indomethacin and phenylbutazone, corticosteroids, and carbamazepine.

The pharmacodynamic effects of some drugs may be altered by changes in fluid and electrolyte balance. For example, the toxic effects of cardiac glycosides are potentiated by both hypokalaemia and hypercalcaemia. The class I antiarrhythmic drugs, such as quinidine, procainamide, and disopyramide, may be more arrhythmogenic if there is hypokalaemia, and this combination causes a particular increase in the risk of polymorphous ventricular tachycardia. Hypocalcaemia prolongs the action of skeletal muscle relaxants such as tubocurarine. Fluid depletion enhances the hypotensive effects of antihypertensive drugs.

NON-DOSE-RELATED ADVERSE REACTIONS

Non-dose-related adverse drug reactions are caused by immunological and pharmacogenetic mechanisms. The features of allergic drug reactions are that there is no relation to the usual pharmacological effects of the drug; there is often a delay between the first exposure to the drug and the occurrence of the subsequent adverse reaction; very small doses of the drug may elicit the reaction once allergy is established; the reaction disappears on withdrawal; and the illness is often recognizable as a form of immunological reaction, for example rash, serum sickness, anaphylaxis, asthma, urticaria, angio-oedema.

Factors associated with an increased risk of allergic drug reactions include a history of allergic disorders (for example, patients with a history of atopic disease and those with hereditary angio-oedema) and HLA status (for example, the risk of nephrotoxicity from penicillamine is increased in patients with the HLA types B8 and DR3 while patients with HLA-DR7 may be protected; the risk of skin reactions with penicillamine is associated with HLA-DRw6, and the risk of thrombocytopenia is associated with HLA-DR4; patients with HLA-DR4 also have a greater risk of the lupus-like syndrome (see below) when it is associated with hydralazine).

Drug allergy and its manifestations are classifiable according to the classification of hypersensitivity reactions, i.e. into four types, types I to IV (see Section 5).

Type I reactions (anaphylaxis; immediate hypersensitivity)

In type I reactions the drug or metabolite interacts with IgE molecules fixed to cells, particularly tissue mast cells and basophil leucocytes. This triggers a process that leads to the release of pharmacological mediators (histamine, 5-hydroxytryptamine, kinins, and arachidonic acid derivatives), which cause the allergic response.

Clinically, type I reactions manifest as urticaria, rhinitis, bronchial asthma, angio-oedema, and anaphylactic shock. Drugs likely to cause anaphylactic shock include penicillins, streptomycin, local anaesthetics, and radio-opaque, iodide-containing, radiographic contrast media.

Type II reactions (cytotoxic reactions)

In type II reactions a circulating antibody of the IgG, IgM, or IgA class interacts with a hapten (drug) combined with a cell membrane constituent (protein), to form a hapten–protein/antigen–antibody complex. Complement is then activated and cell lysis occurs. Most examples are haematological: thrombocytopenia associated with quinidine or quinine ('gin and tonic purpura'), digitoxin, and occasionally rifampicin; 'immune' neutropenia, which can be difficult to distinguish from neutropenia occurring as a direct toxic effect on the bone-marrow, but phenylbutazone, carbimazole, tolbutamide, anticonvulsants, chlorpropamide, and metronidazole have all been incriminated; and the haemolytic anaemias that can also be produced by this mechanism by penicillins, cephalosporins, rifampicin, and quinidine.

Type III reactions (immune-complex reactions)

In type III reactions, antibody (IgG) combines with antigen, that is the hapten–protein complex, in the circulation. The complex thus formed is deposited in the tissues, complement is activated, and damage to capillary endothelium results.

Serum sickness, with fever, arthritis, enlarged lymph nodes, urticaria, and maculopapular rashes, is the typical drug reaction of this type. Penicillins, streptomycin, sulphonamides, and antithyroid drugs may be responsible. Another example of a type III reaction is the acute interstitial nephritis that may be caused by penicillins, some non-steroidal anti-inflammatory drugs, and some diuretics.

Type IV reactions (cell-mediated or delayed hypersensitivity reactions)

In type IV reactions, T lymphocytes are sensitized by a hapten–protein antigenic complex. When the lymphocytes come into contact with the antigen an inflammatory response ensues. Type IV reactions are exemplified by the contact dermatitis caused by local anaesthetic creams, antihistamine creams, and topical antibiotics and antifungal drugs. Skin rashes in response to sulphonamides and thiacetazone are more common in those infected with human immunodeficiency virus.

Pseudoallergic reactions

We include these reactions here for convenience. 'Pseudoallergy' is a term applied to reactions that resemble allergic reactions clinically but for which no immunological basis can be found. For example, asthma and skin rashes caused by aspirin are pseudoallergic reactions. In a proportion of asthmatics, aspirin may trigger an attack of asthma. In cases of extrinsic asthma this may be associated with nasal polyposis and in intrinsic asthma with sinusitis. Aspirin-sensitive asthmatics are often sensitive to other salicylates and to other non-steroidal anti-inflammatory drugs, such as indomethacin and ibuprofen. In addition, about 50 per cent of aspirin-sensitive asthmatics are also sensitive to tartrazine (E102), a yellow dye used as a colouring agent in some drug formulations and foodstuffs.

In some patients the administration of ampicillin or amoxycillin causes a maculopapular erythematous skin rash that resembles the toxic erythema which can occur in penicillin hypersensitivity. However, there is no evidence that the ampicillin rash, as it is called, is immunological in origin. It can be distinguished from true penicillin hypersensitivity by its later onset after the first time of administration (typically 10–14 days compared with 7–10 days in penicillin hypersensitivity, although there is some overlap) and non-recurrence after re-exposure. It is not associated with an increased risk of a serious allergic response to other penicillins, in contrast to penicillin hypersensitivity. An ampicillin rash occurs in about 1 per cent of the normal population, but its incidence is greatly increased in some groups of patients: it occurs almost invariably in patients with some viral infections (for example infectious mononucleosis, cytomegalovirus infection, measles), lymphomas, and leukaemias, and the risk is increased in patients taking allopurinol.

CLINICAL MANIFESTATIONS OF ALLERGIC REACTIONS

The immunological mechanistic approach does not always fit the clinical presentation, in which one is generally faced with some allergic syndrome.

Drug fever as an isolated phenomenon may occur with penicillins, phenytoin, hydralazine, and quinidine. Such fevers are usually of low grade and the patient is generally not very ill. The fever subsides within a few days of stopping the drug. In the case of the penicillins it can sometimes be difficult to distinguish drug fever from a fever that persists because of resistant infection. Fever is also a manifestation of the neuroleptic malignant syndrome, a rare but serious idiosyncratic adverse reaction of unknown cause, in which there is usually a sudden onset of fever, akinesia, rigidity, reduced consciousness, and autonomic disurbances, including tachycardia and hypertension; it can be fatal, and demands emergency treatment by active cooling and intravenous dantrolene.

Rashes of several types may occur, including toxic erythema (due for example to antibiotics, sulphonamides, thiazide diuretics, frusemide, sulphonylureas, and phenylbutazone), urticaria (penicillins, codeine, dextrans, and radiographic contrast media), erythema multiforme (penicillins, sulphonamides, barbiturates, and phenylbutazone), erythema nodosum (sulphonamides and oral contraceptives), cutaneous vasculitis (sulphonamides, phenylbutazone, thiazide diuretics, allopurinol, indomethacin, phenytoin, and alclofenac), exfoliative dermatitis and erythroderma (gold salts, phenylbutazone, isoniazid, and carbamazepine), photosensitivity (amiodarone, sulphonamides, thiazide diuretics, sulphonylureas, tetracyclines, phenothiazines, and nalidixic acid), fixed eruptions (barbiturates, sulphonamides, and tetracyclines), and toxic epidermal necrolysis (Lyell's syndrome) (phenytoin, sulphonamides, gold salts, tetracyclines, allopurinol, and phenylbutazone).

Drugs may produce purpura due to thrombocytopenia (for example, quinine, digitoxin, and rifampicin) or without thrombocytopenia because of capillary damage or fragility (corticosteroids, thiazide diuretics, and meprobamate).

A syndrome mimicking systemic lupus erythematosus, often with joint involvement and generally without renal involvement, may result from treatment with hydralazine, procainamide, phenytoin, or ethosuximide. Although this reaction is conveniently discussed here it is to some extent dose-dependent, as the risk is increased at higher drug doses, and in the cases of hydralazine and procainamide it is more common among slow acetylators.

Thrombocytopenia, neutropenia, haemolytic anaemia, and aplastic anaemia may all occur as adverse drug reactions.

Asthma occurring as a pseudoallergic reaction to aspirin, other non-steroidal anti-inflammatory drugs, and tartrazine has been mentioned above. Other adverse drug reactions in the lung include pneumonitis associated with the lupus-like syndrome (see above), pulmonary eosinophilia, and fibrosing alveolitis.

Jaundice may occur as an allergic response to some drugs through either cholestasis (for example, phenothiazines, erythromycin, and chlorpropamide) or generalized liver damage (for example, halothane, some antituberculous drugs, particularly isoniazid and *p*-aminosalicylic acid, and MAO inhibitors).

LONG-TERM EFFECTS CAUSING ADVERSE REACTIONS

Some adverse effects during long-term therapy are related to both duration of treatment and dose, as follows.

Adaptive changes

These (discussed above) can sometimes form the basis of an adverse reaction. Examples include the development of tolerance to and physical dependence on the narcotic analgesics and the occurrence of tardive dyskinesia in some patients receiving long-term neuroleptic therapy for schizophrenia.

Rebound phenomena

When adaptive changes occur during long-term therapy, sudden withdrawal of the drug may result in rebound reactions. Examples include the typical syndromes that occur after the sudden withdrawal of narcotic analgesics or of alcohol (delirium tremens). Sudden withdrawal of barbiturates may result in restlessness, mental confusion, and convulsions, and a similar syndrome in which anxiety features prominently, may occur after the sudden withdrawal of benzodiazepines. Sleeplessness may also be a feature of the sudden withdrawal of these and a variety of other hypnotic drugs. Sudden withdrawal of some antihypertensive drugs may result in rebound hypertension; this is particularly common with clonidine, which should always be withdrawn slowly. Sudden withdrawal of β-adrenoceptor antagonists may result in rebound tachycardia, which may precipitate myocardial ischaemia.

Sudden withdrawal of corticosteroids can cause acute adrenal insufficiency, and withdrawal of corticosteroids should be very slow after long-term administration.

Reversal of the effects of heparin with protamine sulphate may be associated with rebound hypercoagulability and an increased risk of thromboembolism. However, this risk may have to be taken when there is life-threatening bleeding due to heparin overdosage. In contrast, the withdrawal of oral anticoagulants, such as warfarin, is not accompanied by rebound hypercoagulability.

Other long-term effects

Chloroquine may accumulate in the corneal epithelium (causing a keratopathy) and in the retina (causing a pigmentary retinopathy and blindness). The former occurs in over 90 per cent of patients on long-term therapy, but although the latter is less common it is more serious. The risk increases with daily doses of over 4 mg/kg and in patients also taking probenecid.

Some of the long-term adverse effects of amiodarone are caused by the deposition in the tissues of lipofucsin, including a neuropathy, pulmonary alveolitis, liver damage, microdeposits in the cornea, and skin phototoxicity.

DELAYED EFFECTS CAUSING ADVERSE REACTIONS

Carcinogenesis

The incidence of vaginal adenocarcinoma is increased in the daughters of women who have taken stilboestrol during pregnancy for the treatment of threatened abortion. The extent to which there are changes in the incidences of various tumours in women taking oestrogens, and in particular oral contraceptives, is not settled. However, there is probably an increase in the incidence of uterine endometrial carcinoma in women taking oestrogen replacement therapy for menopausal symptoms, and oral contraceptives increase the incidence of benign liver tumours. Anabolic steroids are associated with an increased risk of liver tumours.

Various anticancer drugs increase the risk of tumours. Examples include the increased risk of bladder cancer in patients taking long-term cyclophosphamide, and of non-lymphocytic leukaemias in patients taking alkylating agents such as melphalan, cyclophosphamide, and chlorambucil. Similarly, patients taking immunosuppressive drug regimens, such as azathioprine with corticosteroids, have a greatly increased risk of developing lymphomas. This has mainly been noted after renal transplantation, but has also been seen in other patients.

Adverse reactions associated with reproduction

Some drugs cause impaired fertility. For example, cytotoxic drugs may cause ovarian failure with amenorrhoea. Reversible impairment of sperm production may be caused by sulphasalazine, nitrofurantoin, MAO inhibitors, and antimalarials, and irreversible impairment by cytotoxic drugs.

Teratogenesis

Teratogenesis occurs when a drug taken during the early stages of pregnancy causes a developmental abnormality in a fetus. The first trimester of pregnancy, and particularly the period from the second to the eighth weeks of gestation, the period of organogenesis, is the most critical, and during this time drugs may cause structural abnormalities. The brain is vulnerable throughout pregnancy.

Table 7 *Some important drugs that may be harmful during early pregnancy*

Drug	Effect
Alcohol	Fetal alcohol syndrome
Androgens	Virilization and multiple congenital defects
Antineoplastic agents	Multiple congenital defects
Carbimazole	Aplasia cutis
Corticosteroids (high dosages)	Cleft palate
Cyproterone	Feminization of male fetus
Diethylstilboestrol	Vaginal adenosis and adenocarcinoma in daughters
Distigmine	Increased uterine tone
Ergotamine	Increased uterine tone
Fibrinolytic drugs	Placental separation
Lithium	Cardiovascular and other malformations
Misoprostol	Increased uterine tone
Phenytoin	Fetal hydantoin syndrome
Tetracyclines	Yellow discoloration of teeth, inhibition of bone growth
Valproate	Neural-tube defects
Vitamin A analogues	Congenital defects
Warfarin	Multiple congenital defects

For a drug to be teratogenic it must first pass across the placenta. The drugs that do this are those that have a low molecular weight, are poorly ionized at physiological pH, and are very fat soluble. The few drugs that do not pass across the placenta illustrate these principles. For example, heparin is ionized and of high molecular weight; tubocurarine is ionized and relatively lipid insoluble; neither crosses the placenta. However, most drugs in the maternal circulation do reach the fetus to some extent.

If a drug is known to be teratogenic in man or animals, then the data sheet will say so. However, if a drug is not known to be teratogenic in man, lack of evidence of teratogenicity in animals cannot be taken as evidence that the drug is not teratogenic in man. Many new drugs are introduced with the advice that they should not be taken during pregnancy, simply for lack of evidence. Some important examples of drugs to avoid during pregnancy are given in Table 7.

Adverse effects on the fetus during the later stages of pregnancy

There are some drugs that are not teratogenic but may have adverse effects on the fetus if given later in pregnancy. Some important drugs that should be avoided or used with care during later pregnancy (and in some cases throughout the whole duration of pregnancy) are listed in Table 8.

What should be done if a woman of childbearing potential is given a drug, and then finds out days or weeks later that she is pregnant? First, it is important to identify the drug and the exact time of exposure to it. If it is a known or a likely teratogen, the relation between the time of exposure and the likely time of conception should be determined. It is sometimes possible to identify the precise date of conception, but if that is not possible one should try to estimate the gestational age by carefully documenting the recent menstrual history and, if necessary, date the pregnancy by ultrasound. If there has been exposure to a known teratogen during the first eight weeks of pregnancy, further investigation may be necessary to identify precise fetal abnormalities. For example, many structural abnormalities can be detected by ultrasound, and neural tube defects may be diagnosed by measurement of serum and amniotic α-

Table 8 *Drugs to be avoided or used with care during later pregnancy*

Drug(s)	Risk to fetus or neonate
Aminoglycoside antibiotics	VIIIth nerve damage
Antithyroid drugs	Goitre and hypothyroidism
Aspirin	Kernicterus, haemorrhage (also maternal)
Benzodiazepines	'Floppy infant syndrome'
Chloramphenicol	Peripheral vascular collapse
Disopyramide	May induce labour
Fibrinolytic drugs	Fetal/maternal haemorrhage
Misoprostol	May induce labour
Narcotic analgesics	Respiratory depression
	Opiate withdrawal syndrome if mother dependent
Nitrofurantoin	Haemolysis
Non-steroidal anti-inflammatory drugs	Closure of the ductus arteriosus
	Delayed and prolonged labour
Pethidine	Respiratory depression
Sulphonamides	Kernicterus
Sulphonylureas	Hypoglycaemia
Tetracyclines	See Table 7
Thiazide diuretics	Thrombocytopenia
Warfarin	Fetal or retroplacental haemorrhage

fetoprotein concentrations. Any decision to advise termination of a pregnancy in such circumstances should be based on a careful consideration of the risk of fetal abnormality from both published information and investigation of the individual case.

Adverse reactions to drugs in breast milk

Some drugs can cause adverse effects in babies after ingestion in breast milk. These include drugs that are so extensively excreted in the milk as to cause dose-related adverse effects in the infant, and drugs that do not necessarily enter the milk in large amounts, but whose adverse effects are not dose related. The latter includes drugs that may cause hypersensitivity reactions (for example, penicillins and sulphonamides), and drugs that are hazardous to babies with glucose 6-phosphate dehydrogenase deficiency (for example, nitrofurantoin and primaquine). Lists of drugs to be avoided can be found in standard reference texts (for example, the *British National Formulary* and the *Physician's Desk Reference*). If there is any doubt about the safety of a drug it is best either to choose another drug or, if the drug must be used, to advise the mother not to breast-feed.

Surveillance methods used in detecting adverse reactions

During the period of clinical trial that a drug undergoes before its general release only the most frequent of adverse reactions will be detected, because so few patients are studied. It is therefore important to have methods for detecting adverse reactions as quickly as possible after marketing, for confirming that the events detected are truly adverse reactions, and for assessing their overall incidence, in order to be able to make some evaluation of the balance of benefit and risk. Some methods of doing this are summarized in Table 9.

Drug interactions

A drug interaction occurs when the effects of one drug (the object drug) are altered by the effects of another drug (the precipitant drug). Usually this results in an adverse drug reaction, but in a few cases a drug interaction may prove beneficial. Interactions form about 7 per cent of all adverse drug reactions; among the few patients who die from adverse drug reactions (about 4 per cent of all deaths) about a third are due to interactions.

Drugs that are likely to precipitate interactions include the following. Drugs that are highly protein bound (aspirin, phenylbutazone, sulphonamides, and trichloracetic acid, a metabolite of chloral hydrate and its congeners), as they are likely to displace object drugs from protein-binding sites. Those that stimulate the metabolism of other drugs, including various anticonvulsants (phenytoin, carbamazepine, and phenobarbitone), rifampicin, dichloralphenazone (because it contains antipyrine), and griseofulvin. Those that inhibit the metabolism of other drugs, including allopurinol, chloramphenicol, cimetidine, metronidazole and other imidazoles (for example, ketoconazole), MAO inhibitors, phenylbutazone and related drugs (for example, azapropazone and sulphinpyrazone), and quinolone antibiotics (for example, ciprofloxacin). Those that affect renal function and alter the renal clearance of object drugs (for example, diuretics, probenecid).

The most likely object drugs in interactions are those that have a steep dose–response curve (i.e. drugs for which a small change in dose results in a relatively large change in therapeutic effect, important in interactions causing decreased efficacy of the object drug), and those that have a low therapeutic index (i.e. drugs for which the dose at which toxic effects start to occur is little more than the therapeutic dose, important in interactions causing toxic effects of the object drug). Drugs that fulfil these criteria include the aminoglycoside antibiotics, anticoagulants, anticonvulsants, antihypertensive drugs, cardiac glycosides, cytotoxic and immunosuppressant drugs, oral contraceptives, and drugs that act on the central nervous system.

Drug interactions can be classified by mechanism. This is done in Table 10, in which some important examples are listed.

Pharmaceutical interactions

Pharmaceutical interactions are physicochemical, either of a drug with an intravenous infusion solution or of two drugs in the same solution. Such interactions result in the loss of activity of the object drug. Pharmaceutical interactions are too numerous to remember in detail, but they can be avoided by adhering to some simple principles. These include giving intravenous drugs by bolus injection if possible or via an infusion burette, by not adding drugs to infusion solutions other than dextrose or saline, and by avoiding mixing drugs in the same infusion solution, unless the mixture is known to be safe (for example, potassium chloride with insulin).

Pharmacokinetic interactions

Pharmacokinetic interactions occur when the absorption, distribution, or elimination (metabolism or excretion) of the object drug is altered by the precipitant drug.

ABSORPTION INTERACTIONS

The absorption of a drug may be altered by another drug, but such effects are rarely of clinical importance. Exceptions include the interactions of cholestyramine with warfarin and digitoxin, whose initial absorption and reabsorption after biliary excretion are reduced, resulting in increased dosage requirements. Oestrogens are metabolized in the liver and some of their metabolites are excreted in the bile, deconjugated by bowel organisms, and reabsorbed. The effect of the combined oral contraceptive can therefore be reduced and pregnancy can result if the bacterial deconjugation of the oestrogen is prevented by a poorly absorbed antibiotic, such as ampicillin.

There are two important examples of beneficial absorption interactions. Metoclopramide increases the rate of gastric emptying and this hastens the absorption of analgesics in the treatment of an acute attack

Table 9 *Some postmarketing surveillance schemes and their advantages and disadvantages*

Scheme	Advantages	Disadvantages
Anecdotal reports	Simple; cheap	Rely on individual vigilance and astuteness; only detect relatively common effects
Voluntary organized reporting	Simple	Under-reporting; reporting bias by 'bandwagon' effect
Intensive event monitoring	Easily organized	Selected population studied for a short time
Cohort studies	Can be prospective; good at detecting effects	Very large numbers required; very expensive
Case-control studies	Excellent for validation and assessment	Will not detect new effects; expensive
Population statistics	Large numbers can be studied	Difficult to coordinate; quality of information may be poor; too coarse
Record linkage	Excellent if comprehensive	Time consuming; expensive; retrospective; relies on accurate records

Table 10 *Mechanisms of drug interactions and some important examples*

Mechanism	Example	Outcome
Physicochemical	Calcium gluconate plus sodium bicarbonate	Precipitation of calcium carbonate in infusion solution
Altered absorption	Reabsorption of oestrogens reduced by antibiotics	Unwanted pregnancy
	Gastric emptying increased by metoclopramide	Increased rate of absorption of simple analgesics
Altered protein binding	Displacement of phenytoin by aspirin	Phenytoin toxicity (transient)
Increased metabolism	Oestrogen metabolism increased by carbamazepine, griseofulvin, phenytoin, rifampicin	Unwanted pregnancy
Reduced metabolism	Warfarin metabolism inhibited by amiodarone, azapropazone, chloramphenicol, cimetidine	Warfarin toxicity
	Theophylline metabolism inhibited by erythromycin	Theophylline toxicity
	Phenytoin metabolism inhibited by isoniazid	Phenytoin toxicity
	Azathioprine metabolism inhibited by allopurinol	Azathioprine toxicity
	Amine metabolism inhibited by MAO inhibitors (includes tyramine in foods and phenylpropanolamine in cold cures)	Acute severe hypertension
Reduced renal elimination	Penicillin/cephalosporin excretion reduced by probenecid	Prolonged duration of antibiotic action
	Lithium excretion reduced by diuretics	Lithium toxicity
	Digoxin excretion reduced by amiodarone, quinidine, verapamil	Digoxin toxicity
Drug effects altered at the same site	Naloxone displaces opioids from opioid receptors	Reversal of opioid toxicity
	Vitamin K competes with warfarin for epoxide reductase	Reversal of the effect of warfarin
	β-Blockers and verapamil	Risk of heart failure or arrhythmias
	Effects of warfarin enhanced by tetracyclines	Warfarin toxicity
	Fibrates and HMGCoA reductase inhibitors	Increased risk of rhabdomyolysis/renal failure
Drug effects altered at different sites	Effects of psychoactive drugs enhanced by alcohol	Increased sedation
	Cytotoxic drugs act at different stages of the cell cycle	Therapeutic potentiation in cancer chemotherapy
Drug effects altered indirectly	Aspirin causes gastric bleeding and reduces platelet aggregation	Increased risk of bleeding with warfarin and impaired haemostasis
	Diuretics cause potassium loss; enhanced effects of antiarrhythmic drugs	Enhanced effects of digoxin (risk of toxicity) (risk of ventricular tachycardia)

of migraine (Fig. 8). Charcoal binds certain drugs in the gut and thus prevents their initial absorption or their reabsorption after biliary excretion or intestinal secretion. This principle is of value in the treatment of self-poisoning with drugs such as phenobarbitone and the tricyclic antidepressants.

PROTEIN-BINDING DISPLACEMENT INTERACTIONS

Displacement of one drug by another from its sites of binding to plasma proteins will cause an increase in the circulating concentration of unbound drug, and thus the potential for an increased effect of the displaced drug. Such interactions are of importance if the object drug is highly protein bound (greater than 90 per cent) and has a low apparent volume of distribution. The important drugs that fulfil these criteria are warfarin, phenytoin, and tolbutamide.

The most common precipitant drugs in protein-binding displacement interactions are sulphonamides, salicylates, and chloral hydrate and some of its congeners (because of their metabolite, trichloracetic acid). In addition, valproate specifically displaces phenytoin.

However, the importance of protein-binding displacement interactions has been exaggerated, and they are often of no clinical importance. The reason is that when drugs such as warfarin, phenytoin, and tolbutamide are displaced their rates of clearance increase in proportion to the degree of displacement. This means that the total concentration of drug in the plasma will fall after displacement, negating the initial effect. Thus, if the patient weathers the initial increase in unbound concentration of the object drug, the interaction will not be of clinical importance.

INTERACTIONS THROUGH INDUCTION OF METABOLISM

Certain drugs increase ('induce') drug metabolism by increasing the amount of endoplasmic reticulum in hepatocytes and by increasing the content of cytochromes P450 and *c* reductase, which catalyse oxidative reactions. Induction of the metabolism of an object drug in this way causes a reduction in its effects (resulting, for example, in epileptic fits while on phenytoin or pregnancy while on an oral contraceptive). Drugs that induce drug metabolism include antipyrine (in dichloralphenazone), barbiturates, carbamazepine, griseofulvin, phenytoin, and rifampicin. The interaction of antipyrine with warfarin is shown in Fig. 9.

INTERACTIONS THROUGH INHIBITION OF METABOLISM

Certain drugs inhibit drug metabolism. Interactions of this type fall into two categories: those in which the precipitant drug is a general inhibitor of oxidative reactions and those in which other specific metabolic pathways are involved.

Important examples of inhibition of drug metabolism by inhibition of oxidative reactions are: inhibition of warfarin metabolism by cimetidine (Fig. 10), metronidazole and other imidazoles, chloramphenicol, norfloxacin and other quinolones, phenylbutazone, azapropazone, and sulphinpyrazone; inhibition of phenytoin metabolism by isoniazid; inhibition of tolbutamide metabolism by phenylbutazone; and inhibition of theophylline metabolism by quinolone and macrolide antibiotics.

The interaction of allopurinol with azathioprine and 6-mercaptopurine is an important example of the effect of inhibition of a specific metabolic pathway. Both 6-mercaptopurine and azathioprine (which is metabolized to 6-mercaptopurine) are metabolized by xanthine oxidase, which is inhibited by allopurinol.

The interaction of MAO inhibitors with dietary tyramine results in severe hypertension, which may be fatal. Inhibition of MAO results in an increase in the noradrenaline content of sympathetic nerve endings. When tyramine is ingested it is normally metabolized by MAO in the gut wall; however, when MAO is inhibited tyramine passes through the gut wall and liver and reaches the systemic circulation. Tyramine releases noradrenaline from its increased stores in nerve endings and a hypertensive crisis results.

EXCRETION INTERACTIONS

Most interactions involving drug excretion occur in the kidneys.

Inhibition of renal tubular secretion

Probenecid inhibits the tubular secretion of penicillins and cephalosporins, prolonging their therapeutic effects. Quinidine, verapamil, and amiodarone inhibit the tubular secretion of digoxin; salicylates inhibit the active secretion of methotrexate; in both cases toxic effects can occur.

Increased renal tubular reabsorption

Diuretics that inhibit renal tubular sodium reabsorption cause compensatory reabsorption of lithium with consequent toxicity (Fig. 11).

Fig. 9 An example of an interaction involving enzyme induction. Dichloralphenazone contains antipyrine, which is a powerful enzyme inducer. It increases the metabolism of warfarin and plasma warfarin concentrations fall. (Adapted from Breckenridge, A. Orme, M. (1971). Clinical implications of enzyme induction. *Annals of the New York Academy of Sciences,* **179,** 421–31, with permission.)

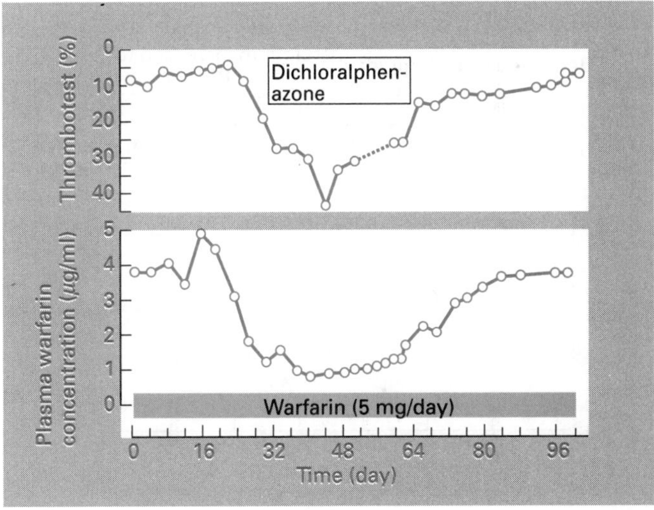

Fig. 10 An example of an interaction involving inhibition of drug oxidation. Plasma warfarin concentrations and the prothrombin time both rose after cimetidine (200 mg three times daily) was introduced in volunteers taking daily maintenance doses of warfarin. (Adapted from Serlin, M.J. *et al.* (1979). Cimetidine: interaction with oral coagulants in man. *Lancet,* **ii,** 317–19, with permission © *Lancet.*)

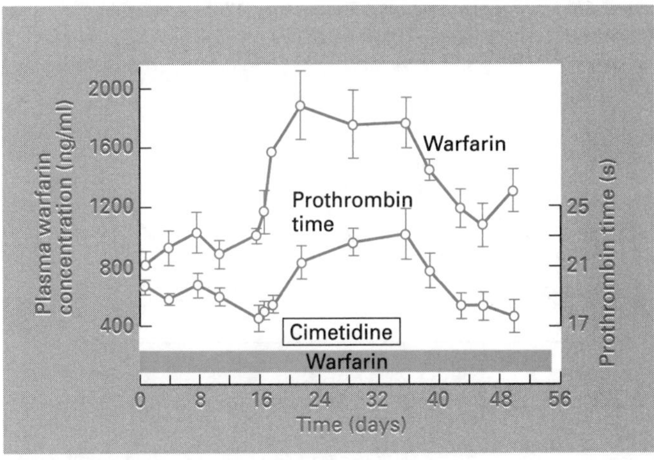

Reduced renal tubular reabsorption

Changing the pH of the urine will alter the reabsorption of drugs that are subject to passive reabsorption. This is put to use in the treatment of overdose with salicylates and amphetamines (by alkalinizing or acidifying the urine, respectively).

Pharmacodynamic interactions

Pharmacodynamic interactions occur when the precipitant drug alters the effect of the object drug at its site of action.

INTERACTIONS AT THE SAME SITE

Direct pharmacodynamic interactions occur when two drugs either act on the same site (antagonism or synergism) or act on two different sites with a similar end-result. Many antagonistic interactions are therapeutically beneficial, including the reversal of the effects of opiates with naloxone and the reversal of the actions of warfarin by vitamin K. In contrast, synergistic interactions are often adverse. The effects of warfarin may be increased or decreased by changes in the affinity of warfarin for vitamin K epoxide reductase (clofibrate, D-thyroxine, anabolic steroids), alterations in the synthesis rate of clotting factors (anabolic steroids), changes in the activity of clotting factors (tetracyclines), or decreased availability of vitamin K secondary to decreased plasma lipids (D-thyroxine, anabolic steroids).

The effects of depolarizing skeletal-muscle relaxants are potentiated by some antibiotics (for example, aminoglycosides, polymixin B, and colistin) and by quinidine and quinine. These interactions are due to the curare-like effects of the precipitant drugs on the motor end-plate of skeletal muscle.

When verapamil and β-adrenoceptor antagonists are used in combination there is an increased risk of cardiac arrhythmias and heart failure.

Fig. 11 An example of an interaction involving inhibition of renal drug excretion. In this case bendrofluazide (5 mg daily) inhibited the renal elimination of lithium, causing an acute increase in plasma lithium concentrations. (Adapted from Chambers, G. *et al.* (1977). Lithium used with a diuretic. *British Medical Journal,* **ii,** 805–6, with permission.)

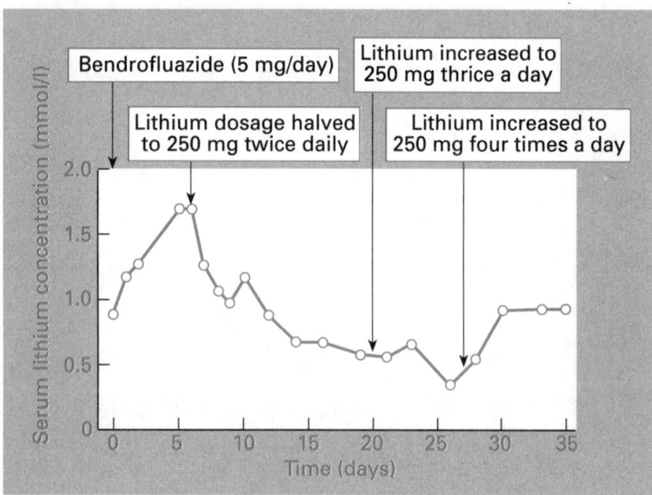

Fig. 12 An example of a pharmacodynamic interaction. Neither doxepin (20 mg three times daily) nor amitriptyline (20 mg three times daily) alone altered the reaction time. Alcohol alone prolonged the reaction time slightly at all times of testing after drug administration (30, 90, and 150 min). However, the combination of alcohol with either doxepin or amitriptyline prolonged the reaction time by much more than one would expect from the separate effects of each component of the combination. (Adapted from Seppala, *et al.* (1975). Effect of tricyclic antidepressants and alcohol in psychomotor skills related to driving. *Clinical Pharmacology and Therapeutics,* **17,** 515–21, with permission.)

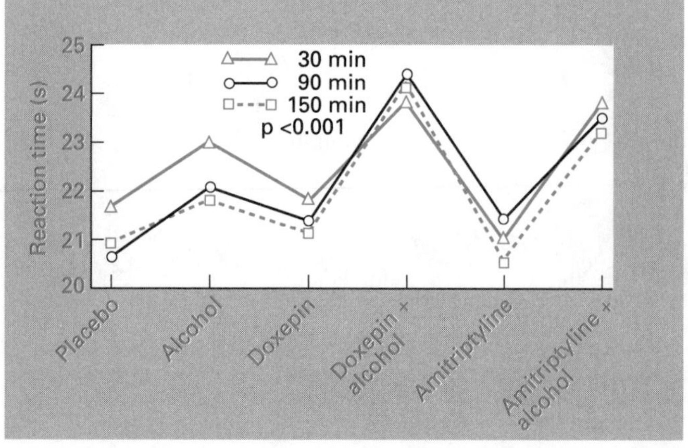

INTERACTIONS AT DIFFERENT SITES

Drugs that have depressant actions on central nervous function may potentiate the effect of each other, whether or not they have effects on the same receptors. The most common example is that of alcohol with any centrally acting drug (Fig. 12).

Other examples include the numerous combinations of cytotoxic drugs used in the treatment of lymphomas and leukaemias, and the use of combinations of antibiotics in the treatment of some infections, even when only one organism is implicated (e.g. in infective endocarditis and tuberculosis). These are beneficial interactions.

INDIRECT PHARMACODYNAMIC INTERACTIONS

In indirect pharmacodynamic interactions a pharmacological, therapeutic, or toxic effect of the precipitant drug in some way alters the therapeutic or toxic effect of the object drug, but the two effects are not themselves related and do not themselves interact.

Warfarin and other anticoagulants may be involved in indirect interactions if platelet aggregation is reduced (for example, by salicylates, dipyridamole, sulphinpyrazone, mefenamic acid, phenylbutazone, and other non-steroidal anti-inflammatory drugs), when there is drug-induced thrombocytopenia, if a drug causes gastrointestinal ulceration (for example, aspirin, phenylbutazone, indomethacin, and other non-steroidal anti-inflammatory drugs), or if a drug causes enhanced fibrinolysis (for example, the biguanides).

Alterations in fluid and electrolyte balance may secondarily alter the effects of some drugs. The effects of cardiac glycosides and the arrhythmogenic effects of some antiarrhythmic drugs (for example, lignocaine, quinidine, procainamide, phenytoin) are increased by potassium depletion (for example, due to potassium-wasting diuretics, corticosteroids, and purgatives).

Pharmacogenetics

Pharmacogenetics is the study of the influence of heredity on the pharmacokinetics of drugs and pharmacodynamic responses to them.

Pharmacokinetic defects

The extent to which an individual metabolizes a drug is, at least in part, genetically determined. For example, monozygotic twins metabolize drugs similarly, while dizygotic twins often do not. For most drugs the variability in metabolism is unimodally distributed. However, for some the distribution is bimodal or trimodal, indicating the existence of separate populations of subjects capable of metabolizing those drugs at discretely different rates. The important pathways of drug metabolism subject to pharmacokinetic variability are acetylation, hydroxylation, and succinylcholine hydrolysis.

ACETYLATION

Acetylation of some drugs is by the hepatic enzyme *N*-acetyltransferase, which has a bimodal distribution. In fast acetylators there is more *N*-acetyltransferase activity, inherited as an autosomal dominant trait, than in slow acetylators, and the difference depends on the amount of hepatic enzyme, rather than a difference in its properties. The ratio of fast:slow acetylators is racially determined, being, for example, 40:60 in Europe, 85:15 in Japan, and 95:5 in the Inuit. Drugs whose acetylation is genetically determined are isoniazid, hydralazine, procainamide, phenelzine, dapsone, and some sulphonamides (for example sulphamethoxypyridazine and sulphapyridine).

Slow acetylators require lower doses of isoniazid and hydralazine than fast acetylators in the treatment of tuberculosis and hypertension, respectively. They are also more likely to develop the lupus erythematosus-like syndrome caused by isoniazid, hydralazine, and procainamide, and the peripheral neuropathy caused by isoniazid (which can be prevented or treated with pyridoxine). The interaction between isoniazid and phenytoin, in which phenytoin metabolism is inhibited by isoniazid, resulting in phenytoin toxicity, occurs more frequently among slow acetylators.

The acetylator status of an individual may be easily assessed by giving a sulphonamide, such as sulphadimidine or sulphapyridine, orally and measuring the relative proportions of acetylated and total sulphonamide in a sample of urine passed 5 to 6 h later.

OXIDATION

Certain varieties of oxidation are bimodally distributed, but, in contrast to acetylation, this is a heterogeneous group of defects, and they are not all uniformly due to decreased amounts of enzyme. Individuals with impaired and normal oxidation are classified as poor and extensive metabolizers, respectively. The main type of defect is the debrisoquine type, an autosomal recessive defect of cytochrome P450 of the type CYP2D6, the gene being located on chromosome 22. It occurs in about 9 per cent of Caucasians, and has a lower prevalence in other racial types.

Drugs besides debrisoquine that are affected include captopril, codeine, flecainide, metoprolol, nortriptyline, perhexiline, phenacetin, phenformin, propafenone, sparteine, and timolol. The dose-related adverse effects of these drugs (for example, lactic acidosis with phenformin, peripheral neuropathy with perhexiline, and central nervous system toxicity with nortriptyline) are more likely in poor hydroxylators. Quinidine inhibits some oxidative reactions and may turn an extensive metabolizer of the debrisoquine type into a poor metabolizer.

The metabolism of mephenytoin is mediated by cytochrome CYP2C, whose activity is bimodally distributed. Poor metabolizers of proguanil (used to prevent malaria) do not convert it to the active form cycloguanil, and may fail to respond to treatment.

Sulphoxidation of penicillamine is polymorphic. Poor sulphoxidation is associated with a fourfold increase in the risk of adverse effects in rheumatoid arthritis. Adverse reactions to gold salts containing a thiol group may also be linked to poor sulphoxidation.

Disease associations with polymorphic metabolism

As some diseases may be related to the effects of environmental chemicals, it is of interest that polymorphic acetylation, hydroxylation, and sulphoxidation have other clinical associations. For example, there may be increased risks of bladder cancer in slow acetylators, of parkinsonism in poor debrisoquine hydroxylators, of bronchogenic carcinoma in extensive debrisoquine hydroxylators, and of primary biliary cirrhosis in poor sulphoxidizers.

SUCCINYLCHOLINE HYDROLYSIS

Succinylcholine is metabolized in the plasma by a non-specific esterase called pseudocholinesterase. Normally this metabolism is fast, the blood is quickly cleared of the drug, and neuromuscular blockade lasts only a few minutes. However, in some individuals the pseudocholinesterase is of abnormal affinity and amount, and does not metabolize the succinylcholine so rapidly, resulting in prolonged neuromuscular blockade. There are three types of abnormalities of pseudocholinesterase, each inherited in autosomal recessive fashion, the dibucaine-resistant, fluoride-resistant, and 'silent' gene types.

In some individuals there is a two- or threefold increase in the concentration of pseudocholinesterase in the plasma, with resistance to the effects of succinylcholine. The prevalence may be as high as 1 in 1000.

Pharmacodynamic defects

Some individuals have biochemical abnormalities that make them peculiarly sensitive or resistant to the effects of certain drugs.

Red-cell enzyme defects (see Section 22)

Unusual drug reactions may occur in individuals whose erythrocytes are deficient in any one of three different but functionally related enzymes, glucose-6-phosphate dehydrogenase, glutathione reductase, and methaemoglobin reductase, which are involved in preventing the oxidation of various cell proteins. If the erythrocyte is exposed to oxidizing agents in these deficiencies, haemolysis occurs, probably because of unopposed oxidation of sulphydryl groups in the cell membrane.

Porphyria (see Section 11)

The hepatic porphyrias, acute intermittent porphyria and porphyria cutanea tarda, are characterized by abnormalities of haem biosynthesis. Certain drugs may precipitate an attack of porphyria.

Malignant hyperthermia

This is a serious, potentially fatal complication of general anaesthesia with halothane, methoxyflurane, and succinylcholine. It occurs in about 1 in 20 000 anaesthetized patients and is inherited in autosomal dominant fashion. It is characterized by an acute rise in body temperature to 40–41°C, muscle stiffness, tachycardia, sweating, cyanosis, and tachypnoea. Creatine kinase activity may rise. Dantrolene, which decreases the amount of calcium released from sarcoplasmic reticulum, is effective, given intravenously in an initial dose of 1 mg/kg, repeated as necessary to a total of 10 mg/kg.

Corticosteroid glaucoma

Intraocular pressure rises during daily use of corticosteroid eyedrops, and the rise is trimodally distributed, 65 per cent, 30 per cent, and 5 per cent of individuals having small, medium, and large increases in pressure, respectively. Those who have a large increase in pressure are at increased risk of glaucoma. Inheritance is autosomal recessive.

Vitamin D-resistant rickets

There are three varieties of rickets in which the disease is resistant to the effects of vitamin D (cholecalciferol), familial hypophosphataemic rickets, vitamin D dependency, and Fanconi's syndrome. They are discussed in Section 12.

Coumarin resistance

Coumarin resistance is a rare defect in which 20 times the usual dose may be required to produce satisfactory anticoagulation. It has autosomal dominant inheritance and the mechanism may be resistance of the vitamin K epoxide reductase to inhibition by warfarin.

Placebos

A placebo (Latin = 'I shall please') was originally a formulation of a pharmacologically inactive compound 'adopted to please rather than to benefit the patient' (OED). However, in its modern usage the term goes further than that. Placebos are of two types, those which contain pharmacologically inactive ingredients, and those which contain some compound with pharmacological activity. Although the former are always knowingly used as placebos by physicians, the latter may be given either in the knowledge that their pharmacological action is not appropriate or in the mistaken belief that it is.

The most common use of the inert placebo is as a dummy for the real treatment in clinical trials, in order to reduce the element of subjective bias. Occasionally, inert placebos, rather than drugs known to have pharmacological activity, are given to patients who are incessantly complaining of some symptom and who are thought to be exaggerating. Pain is the symptom usually involved. If the pain responds to the placebo, then it is often assumed that the patient was making an unnecessary fuss. However, one-third of all people are placebo reactors, that is they will report symptomatic relief of real pain after the administration of an inactive compound, and it would not be surprising if on occasion, and despite real pain appropriate to real pathology, relief was obtained from a placebo. Placebos should not be used in this way.

The issue of a prescription is a common way of ending a patient's visit to the doctor, and not infrequently the doctor will prescribe a compound whose pharmacological action is irrelevant to the case. The doctor may be aware of this, as in the prescription of a vitamin formulation, for example, the patient being informed of the nature of the prescription and being told that it is 'a tonic'. On the other hand, the doctor may misunderstand the proven indications for which a drug has been shown to be effective, for example in the case of a prescription of cimetidine for symptoms of acute 'dyspepsia' in the absence of proven peptic ulceration or oesophagitis.

Some doctors find it difficult to accept that there is no effective treatment for their patient and they feel constrained to try something. There are many examples of pseudotherapy, based on apparently good ideas that do not hold up when examined scientifically, for example the use of cerebral vasodilators in the treatment of senile dementia. Equally, some patients cannot believe that there is not a medicine to cure their disease, and sometimes no amount of talk will persuade them otherwise. Often, in exasperation, the doctor prescribes something that, however tenuously, could be interpreted as being rational treatment, for example the use of diuretics in the treatment of obesity, despite lack of evidence of their long-term efficacy.

If a placebo is to be prescribed, then it should be prescribed with enthusiasm and some show of belief in its efficacy.

Placebos may have adverse effects. If a doctor uses placebos unthinkingly, he or she may ignore the patient's real problem, and that may lead to delayed diagnosis of a treatable condition. Delay in diagnosis, and hence in instituting proper treatment, will be prolonged if the patient initially responds to the placebo. Just as they may relieve real symptoms the use of placebos may be associated with real adverse effects. For example, in a survey of placebo studies, common symptoms were dry mouth (9 per cent), nausea (10 per cent), fatigue (18 per cent), difficulty in concentrating (15 per cent), and headache (25 per cent).

Monitoring drug therapy

Monitoring drug therapy usually involves trying to measure the clinical response directly. If this is difficult, or is not related directly in time to a dose of the drug, another measure of the pharmacological effect may be required. In some cases it may be necessary to resort to measurement of the plasma concentration of the drug.

Monitoring the therapeutic effects of drugs

Some events can be directly monitored in the individual patient, while some are monitored in a population. The latter can be applied to the individual only in terms of a statistical probability derived from the observed population variability. Examples of therapeutic events that can be monitored in the individual include seizure frequency during anticonvulsant drug therapy, muscle power during treatment of myasthenia gravis, the frequency of attacks of angina pectoris, and body weight during diuretic therapy.

Preventive measures in medicine cannot be monitored in the individual and their effects must be gauged by population studies. Examples include the frequency of infections after immunization, the reduction of the risks of hypertension by diuretics, and the prevention of the complications of myocardial infarction by streptokinase and aspirin.

Monitoring the pharmacodynamic effects of drugs

In some circumstances the pharmacological effect of a drug can be carefully measured, followed sequentially, and used as a guide to drug therapy, even though it may not be correlated precisely with the therapeutic effect. Examples include the effect of insulin on the blood glucose concentration in diabetes mellitus, anticoagulants on the prothrombin time, bronchodilators on FEV_1 and peak flow rate in bronchial asthma, and cancer chemotherapy on tumour markers.

Monitoring drug pharmacokinetics (plasma concentration measurement)

This is useful for a few drugs, namely those for which there is difficulty in measuring or interpreting the clinical evidence of therapeutic or toxic effects, for which the relation between dose and plasma concentration is unpredictable, for which there is a good relation between plasma concentration and effect, which have a low therapeutic index, and which are not metabolized to active metabolites. The drugs for which plasma concentration can be useful and which are commonly measured are listed in Table 11.

INDICATIONS FOR MEASURING PLASMA DRUG CONCENTRATIONS

Plasma drug concentrations of the drugs in Table 11 may be measured when individualizing therapy (for example, at the start of therapy when the relation between dose and plasma concentration in the individual is uncertain, when rapid changes in renal function alter the relation between dose and plasma concentration, or when another drug alters the relation between dose and plasma concentration), in the diagnosis of suspected toxicity, and in measuring compliance (see above).

Phenytoin

Plasma concentrations of phenytoin in the toxic range are quite well related to its acute toxic effects, but not to its long-term adverse effects, such as gingival hyperplasia, hirsutism and acne, and folate and vitamin D deficiencies. Steady state takes about 2 weeks of maintenance therapy to occur after a change in dose at low dosages, and the higher the plasma concentration the longer it takes (up to 3 weeks or longer in some patients). For this reason one should not make changes in dosage too frequently. Provided the sample is not taken too soon after a dose (i.e. within 1–2 h), the time of sampling is probably of little importance for phenytoin, as plasma concentrations fluctuate very little during a dosage interval.

Digoxin

Plasma digoxin concentrations correlate well with toxic effects but not with the therapeutic effect within the therapeutic dosage range. The time of blood sampling should be at least 6 h after the previous dose, and 12 h is the best time in patients taking once daily treatment. During regular maintenance dosage without a loading dose, steady state will be reached after about 7 days (normal renal function) to 18 days (functionally anephric). Factors that alter the relation between dose and plasma digitalis concentrations include renal impairment (which reduces the clear-

Table 11 *Usual therapeutic and toxic plasma concentrations of commonly measured drugs*

Drug	Concentration below which a therapeutic effect is unlikely	Concentration above which a toxic effect is more likely
Gentamicin[1]	5 μg/ml (at peak)	12 μg/ml (at peak) 2 μg/ml (at trough)
Digoxin	1.0 nmol/1	3.8 nmol/1
Cyclosporin[2]	80–200 nmol/1	170–300 nmol/1
Lithium	0.4 mmol/1	1.0 mmol/1
Phenytoin	40 μmol/l	80 μmol/1
Theophylline	55 μmol/1	100 μmol/1

[1]Conventional dosage regimens.

[2]Measured in whole blood by specific radioimmunoassay or high-performance liquid chromatography; the actual results depend on the laboratory in which the measurement is made.

ance of digoxin), for example in older people, and drug interactions (see above). Factors that alter the link between the concentrations and effects of digoxin, and make it difficult to interpret the plasma concentration, include potassium depletion (which increases the effect of a given concentration of digitalis on the heart) and thyroid disease (hyperthyroidism causes a decrease in responsiveness and hypothyroidism an increase). Children under 6 months of age have lower plasma digoxin concentrations at a given dose than older children and adults, and they are also more resistant to the pharmacodynamic actions of digitalis; it is not possible clearly to interpret plasma digitalis concentrations in these circumstances. However, plasma concentration measurement is sometimes worth while simply to demonstrate the presence of the drug.

Lithium

Serum lithium concentrations correlate quite well with the therapeutic effect in the range 0.4 to 0.8 mmol/l. At 1.0 to 1.5 mmol/l there is an increase in the incidence of both acute toxicity and long-term adverse effects. Concentrations above 1.5 mmol/l should be avoided. Blood samples should be taken at exactly 12 h after the previous dose, or as near to that as possible. It takes about 3 days for steady state to be reached during regular maintenance therapy, but there is wide variability, and in some patients it may take a week before steady state is reached.

Plasma lithium concentration monitoring is necessary for several reasons. Lithium is nephrotoxic and is excreted by the kidneys; toxicity is thus self-perpetuating because it causes renal damage, further retention of lithium, and further toxicity. Systemic availability varies from individual to individual, is altered by diarrhoea, and varies from formulation to formulation. Changes in sodium balance alter the renal excretion of lithium; for example, renal sodium loss induced by diuretics leads to lithium retention.

Aminoglycoside antibiotics

The same principles apply to all the aminoglycoside antibiotics and we shall illustrate them here with the example of gentamicin. The relation between the plasma concentration of gentamicin and its therapeutic efficacy is complicated by the fact that different organisms have different sensitivities to the antibiotic. The toxic effects of gentamicin on the ears and kidneys are related to the 'peak' concentration (the highest concentration measured after a dose, usually occurring at about 1 h after an intramuscular injection or the start of an intravenous infusion) and the 'trough' concentration (the concentration measured just before the next dose is due).

With standard regimens a peak plasma concentration of 5 to 9 mg/l is generally considered to be necessary, although when gentamicin is used in combination with benzylpenicillin in the treatment of bacterial endocarditis, lower plasma gentamicin concentrations may be effective. Measurement of *in vitro* inhibitory concentrations by the bacteriologist will help to guide therapy. The recommendations for peak and trough concentrations have been based on studies in which several doses of aminoglycosides have been given during the day; with newer regimens involving large single doses once a day, new recommendations will have to be formulated.

Theophylline

Plasma theophylline concentrations correlate well with therapeutic and toxic effects. The time to steady state is usually less than a day, but the half-life varies from patient to patient, because of numerous factors that alter the pharmacokinetics of theophylline, including age, smoking, liver disease, and drug interactions (for example, with the macrolide antibiotics, see Table 10). If the half-life is prolonged, the time to steady state may be as long as 2 to 3 days. Blood samples are best taken just before a dose and should ideally be taken at the same time of day in an individual, because of diurnal variations in trough concentration.

Cyclosporin

Cyclosporin is generally measured in whole blood and the result of the assay may depend on whether the measurement technique is by immunoassay or high-performance liquid chromatography. The time to steady state is about 2 days and samples should be taken just before the next dose is due. Factors that alter the whole blood concentration of cyclosporin without a change in dose include reduced absorption (due to diarrhoea or reduced bile-salt production), reduced metabolism (due to liver disease or inhibition by drugs such as ketoconazole and cimetidine), and increased metabolism (due to enzyme-inducing drugs).

Clinical trials (see also Section 2)

Clinical impressions of the efficacy of a drug can be misleading, partly because of bias on the part of both doctors and patients in favour of the treatment, partly because of the placebo response, and partly because of the selectivity of doctors' memories. The clinical trial is a means whereby the efficacy of a drug may be tested.

Definition

A clinical trial of a drug in a patient has been defined in the United Kingdom Medicines Act of 1968 as an investigation or series of investigations which:

- consists of the administration of one or more medicinal products by, or under the direction of, a doctor or dentist to patients, where
- there is evidence that the products have effects which may be beneficial to the patients, and
- the administration is for the purpose of ascertaining whether, or to what extent, the products have those or any other effects, whether beneficial or harmful (i.e. the assessment of efficacy and risks).

This definition was specifically designed to cover trials of drugs in patients. It could be extended to include, for example, therapeutic procedures (such as a surgical operation) and volunteer trials, in which benefit would not be expected, or indeed required.

The conduct of a clinical trial

The reliability of the conclusions based upon the results of a clinical trial depend entirely upon the care with which the trial is designed, carried out, and analysed.

Aims

The aims of a trial should be formulated before the trial begins. It is generally best to ask one or two specific questions, and to design the trial in order to answer those questions and those questions only. If too many questions are posed in one study, the trial design becomes too complex and organization becomes difficult.

Numbers of subjects (see Section 2)

Control subjects

These are used to eliminate the effect of natural variability of the disease, as proper randomization should produce similar variability among control and study subjects. It is a common misconception that control subjects are necessarily given no treatment or a placebo, but that is not so; if there are ethical problems about withholding therapy the control subjects may be given a treatment that is known to be effective and with which the new treatment will be compared.

If the outcome of the trial can be easily measured, and can be expected to occur within a relatively short period of time, and if the effect of the treatment is reversible, variability can be reduced even further by omitting separate controls and using a 'cross-over' design in which the subject takes one treatment during the first half of the study and the other during the second half.

Randomization

The purpose of randomization is to eliminate bias, for example to avoid recruiting patients who have a particular characteristic to one treatment group and not to the other. If randomization is not done properly, the results of the trial will be invalid. Randomization of a patient to a treatment should not be done until immediately before the treatment begins; once it has occurred the investigator is committed to include that patient's data in the final analysis.

Blindness

Blindness in a trial means that the individual (investigator or patient) does not know what treatment is being given. The purpose of blinding (or 'masking') the investigator is to eliminate bias. The purpose of blinding the patient is to eliminate the differences in responses that can occur because of differences in the patient's expectation of what a particular treatment, or no treatment, may do. The ideal is a double-blind study, one in which both the investigator and the patient are blinded.

Placebos

Placebos (or 'dummies') are used in order to achieve blindness. It is therefore important that placebos should as far as possible be of the same size, shape, colour, texture, weight, taste, and smell as the active formulation.

If two different doses of an active drug are being compared, then any differences in the numbers of tablets to be given must be balanced by placebo tablets. If two different formulations, whether of the same drug or of different drugs, are to be compared, each must be given at the same time as the placebo form of its counterpart (the so-called 'double dummy' technique).

Number of centres

Ideally a clinical trial should be made in one place only, in order to minimize variations in the population and variations in investigators' techniques, and in order to avoid the problems of communication, collection of data, and follow-up. However, because the need for adequate numbers of patients overrides everything else except the elimination of bias, it is often necessary to involve more than one centre.

Criteria for selection or exclusion

Certain groups of individuals are generally excluded from clinical drug trials, unless the trial is designed specifically to study those individuals. These include pregnant women, children, and seriously ill patients. Patients at particular risk of an adverse reaction would also usually be excluded (for example, asthmatic patients in a trial of a β-adrenoceptor antagonist, patients with peptic ulcer in a trial of a non-steroidal anti-inflammatory drug). This principle also applies to the avoidance of drug interactions. Despite difficulties in studying them, one should try not to exclude old patients from drug trials, and it is often worth studying data from old patients separately to try to pick up adverse effects early on, as they are more likely to suffer them. Because poor compliance may reduce the power of a study it is useful to try to identify poor compliers before randomization. This can be done by having a run-in period, during which compliance is specifically studied. Poor compliers may then be excluded before randomization, and this does not introduce bias. A run-in period can also be useful to allow subjects to decide whether or not they want to be included in the study.

Analysis and interpretation

The principles of the analysis of data from clinical trials are outlined in Section 2.

Ethics

This is a very difficult subject, but everyone who is about to be involved in a clinical trial, or whose patients are to be involved in someone else's trial, should be aware of the problems and be prepared to make up his or her own mind about how those problems should be tackled or avoided. The Declaration of Helsinki was formulated by the Eighteenth World Medical Assembly in 1964 to offer guidelines, and there are various other published codes of conduct. International guidelines have recently been prepared by the Council for International Organizations of Medical Science (CIOMS), in collaboration with the World Health Organisation and published as *International Ethical Guidelines for Biomedical Research Involving Human Subjects* (Geneva, 1993).

Consent

It is customary nowadays in almost all cases to seek patients' consent before admitting them to a clinical trial and it is usual to talk in such cases of obtaining the patient's 'informed consent', which consists of two separate processes: giving information and obtaining consent. It is an investigator's duty to inform subjects who are being recruited for trials what the purpose of the trial is, how it will be carried out, and what the important risks will be. It is the duty of the subjects to consider the information given to them and decide whether or not they want to take part in the study, if necessary after consultation with relatives or friends. The investigator should not bring any sort of pressure to bear on the subject, and the decision to take part should be one which the subject has freely taken.

Study design

It is unethical to carry out an improperly designed trial, as it is unethical to subject patients or volunteers to the various hazards and discomforts involved if the trial is too badly designed to yield an answer to one's original question.

The control of ethical problems

Various bodies may exert control of one kind or another on the ethics of a clinical trial. These include the Committee on Safety of Medicines in the United Kingdom and the Food and Drug Administration in the United States (which control the marketing of drugs), ethics committees (institutional review boards) (which scrutinize clinical research proposals and advise whether or not they consider them to be ethical), insurers (who indemnify research workers in case of adverse drug reactions), and the institutions of the law (to which final recourse may be made in the event of disputes).

REFERENCES

This chapter is based on the more detailed text contained in the first section of the *Oxford Textbook of Clinical Pharmacology and Drug*

Therapy (1992), (2nd edn), (D.G. Grahame-Smith and J.K. Aronson) Oxford University Press.

The following are detailed texts on individual subjects.

Pharmacokinetics

Clark, B. and Smith, D.A. (1986). *An introduction to pharmacokinetics,* (2nd edn). Blackwell Scientific, Oxford. A simple introduction to pharmacokinetics without excessive emphasis on mathematics; but you would still have to follow the maths to understand it thoroughly. Contains practical examples.

Gibaldi, M. and Perrier, D. (1982). *Pharmacokinetics,* (2nd edn). Dekker, New York. An excellent text on the mathematics of pharmacokinetics; although it probably contains too much mathematics to be used as an introduction to the subject, much of the text can be read for the purpose of learning principles without needing attention to the mathematics.

Gibson, G.G. and Skett, P. (1986). *Introduction to drug metabolism.* Chapman and Hall, London. Very good introduction to all aspects of drug metabolism. Well referenced.

Rowland, M. and Tozer, T.N. (1989). *Clinical pharmacokinetics. Concepts and applications,* (2nd edn). Lea and Febiger, Philadelphia. An excellent introductory text that needs to be worked through systematically. Covers basic concepts, principles of kinetics as applied to drugs, therapeutic regimens, and individualization of therapy. Well illustrated with practical problems throughout. Light on maths, but appendices deal with some of the practicalities of the mathematical treatment of kinetic data.

Winter, M.E. (1988). *Basic clinical pharmacokinetics,* (2nd edn). Applied Therapeutics, Vancouver. The basic principles of clinical pharmacokinetics outlined, with only essential mathematics. Followed by sections on practical applications for all important drugs, including case studies.

Pharmacological effects of drugs

Bowman, W.C. and Rand, M.J. (1980) *Textbook of pharmacology,* (2nd edn). Blackwell Scientific, Oxford. Excellent reference text covering the basic pharmacology of drugs mostly by organ systems (for example, the blood, the heart) but in some cases by indication (for example, pain, anaesthesia, hypnotics, and sedatives). Six introductory chapters deal with some relevant matters of anatomy, physiology, and biochemistry. The last five chapters deal with the principles of drug action, pharmacokinetics, relevant statistics, 'social' pharmacology, and diet.

Gilman, A.G., Rall, T.W., Nies, A.S., and Taylor, P. (1990) *Goodman and Gilman's The pharmacological basis of therapeutics,* (8th edn). MacMillan, New York. Comprehensive account of basic pharmacology as relevant to therapeutics, arranged by groups of drugs. Useful appendices on prescribing, pharmacokinetic data of individual drugs, and interactions. Very well referenced with both primary and secondary sources.

Adverse effects of drugs

Davies, D.M. (ed.) (1991). *Textbook of adverse drug reactions,* (4th edn). Oxford University Press. Adverse drug reactions classified by organ systems. Introductory chapters deal with history, epidemiology, pathogenesis, detection, and investigation. The final chapter covers medicolegal aspects, and there are four useful appendices (for example 'Effect of drugs on laboratory tests').

Dukes, M.N.G. (ed.) (1992). *Meyler's side effects of drugs,* Vol. 12. Elsevier, Amsterdam. Adverse reactions to drugs discussed under the headings of the individual drugs or groups of drugs, arranged in chapters according to class of drug. Good indexes with separate listings for drugs and diseases.

Dukes, M.N.G./Dukes, M.N.G. and Beeley, L./Dukes, M.N.G. and Aronson J.K./Aronson J.K. and van Boxtel C.J. (ed.) *Side effects of drugs annuals.* Elsevier, Amsterdam. Published annually since 1977. Companion volumes to *Meyler's side effects of drugs (op. cit.),* using the same format, but mostly covering only reports published during the relevant year. A special feature is the 'reviews', in which specific topics are reviewed carefully and distinguished from the rest of the text typographically.

Gross, F.H. and Inman, W.H.W. (ed.) (1977). *Drug monitoring.* Academic Press, London. Proceedings of a symposium on methods of monitoring for adverse drug reactions. Covers virtually every aspect, with references to primary sources.

Drug interactions

Stockley, I. (1991). *Drug interactions,* (2nd edn). Blackwell Scientific, Oxford. Monographs on individual drug interactions arranged in chapters by object drug. Each well-referenced monograph contains a description of the interaction and its mechanism, and an assessment of its importance, with guidance on management. The introductory chapter contains an abbreviated account of basic mechanisms.

Monitoring drug therapy

Aronson, J.K., Hardman, M., and Reynolds D.J.M. (1993). *ABC of monitoring drug therapy.* British Medical Journal, London. Introduction to the principles of monitoring drug therapy by plasma drug concentration measurement. Introductory monographs followed by separate monographs for each important drug.

Clinical trials and statistics

Bland, M. (1987). *An introduction to medical statistics.* Oxford University Press. Good introductory text on statistics with clear examples and relatively little mathematics.

Bradford Hill, A. (1985). *Short textbook of medical statistics,* (2nd edn). Hodder, London. Good introductory text, well oriented towards specific problems (for example, chapters on clinical trials, problems of sampling, collection of statistics). Relatively little mathematics.

Good, C.S. (ed.) (1976). *The principles and practice of clinical trials.* Churchill Livingstone, Edinburgh. Proceedings of a symposium covering the setting up, running, and evaluation of clinical trials. Well illustrated with examples throughout, with references.

Gore, S.M. and Altman, D.G. (1982). *Statistics in practice.* British Medical Association, London. A compilation of articles originally published in the British Medical Journal. Deals in a readable introductory way with a variety of aspects of statistics in clinical practice, particularly in relation to clinical trials. Well referenced.

Pocock, S.J. (1983) *Clinical trials, a practical approach.* Wiley, Chichester. A comprehensive introduction to the design, performance, and analysis of clinical trials, with a short bibliography.

Section 10 *Nutrition*

10.1 Introduction

R. SMITH and W. P. T. JAMES

This introduction gives an overview of nutritional problems and highlights why nutrition is considered so important in both the developed and developing world. Adequate nutrition is essential to life, and many of the conditions mentioned in this book are partly nutritional in origin. The nutritional aspects of some diseases, such as those of the liver, kidney, and pancreas, and of inherited metabolic diseases, are best dealt with in the context of the diseases themselves.

Modern nutrition

It is widely recognized that nutrition is badly taught and that students are ignorant of its theory and practice. This is partly because malnutrition in the developing world is seen wrongly as a single problem of insufficient food whereas the 'malnutrition' of affluent societies is seen to relate principally to overindulgence in food, leading to such problems as obesity. Modern nutrition, however, has now to be understood as the study of a complex metabolic system whereby the body processes not only the nutrients from food but also those many bioactive molecules found in the diet which inhibit or modulate the body's response to such nutrients. Such bioactive molecules include glycoproteins, such as lectins, which are both storage proteins and the natural pesticides of plants. Some, for instance kidney bean lectin, can produce profound intestinal damage unless removed by soaking and adequate cooking before consumption. Others include the flavanoids found in tea and red wine, with marked antioxidant properties, which are being cited as important in preventing coronary heart disease. The phytoestrogens, found for example in soya products, have weak oestrogen effects and alter the sex hormone metabolism of women, perhaps by blocking the activity of the woman's own oestrogens. These phytoestrogens are now being linked to the low breast cancer rates in soya-consuming societies.

As other more subtle effects of nutrients are described, links are becoming apparent between an insufficient intake of nutrients and, for example, poor fetal development, the long-term metabolic programming of adult chronic diseases, and the maintenance of immunological competence in old age. Some nutritionists would now claim that many of the major medical problems of public health importance in all parts of the world have either a nutritional basis or at least an important nutritional contribution. These problems include, in the Third World, blindness and increased childhood morbidity and mortality from vitamin A deficiency, impaired brain development in children and poor work output in adults from iron deficiency anaemia, iodine deficiency disorders which are threatening perhaps a billion children and adults, and subtle deficiencies such as underweight at all ages which enhances the susceptibility to a wide range of communicable diseases.

The basis for many nutritional diseases is multifactorial and involves the cultural aspects of food preparation and social and economic influences, all of which may contribute to an inappropriate diet. These aspects are particularly emphasized in the account of severe malnutrition. Similarly, obesity has many causes, with an interplay between environmental factors and individual variations in susceptibility to weight gain.

With the westernization of the Third World, obesity, maturity-onset diabetes, hypertension, coronary artery disease, and a variety of cancers rapidly emerge. In all these conditions the magnitude of the environmental impact is clear and nutrition is increasingly recognized as the dominant component explaining these different rates of disease. Why particular individuals succumb to a specific disease is a feature of their social conditions, which affect their dietary or exercise patterns and other behaviour, such as smoking, alcohol, and drug use, as well as the interaction of food with genetically controlled metabolic pathways.

Amongst those conditions in which malnutrition is only one aspect of the clinical picture, anorexia nervosa is an example; here nutritional deficiency is associated with complex endocrine and psychological disturbances. In other conditions, such as hypertension and colonic diverticulosis, nutrition is of recognized importance, but the mechanisms and interactions with other factors are elusive and the findings controversial.

Expert committees throughout the world are now increasingly developing policies in an attempt to minimize obesity, diabetes, cardiovascular disease, and cancers through dietary means. A consensus is emerging that diets which are conducive to the prevention of cardiovascular diseases, for example the traditional Mediterranean diet, are also those which minimize the onset of several cancers. How these effects are mediated involves complex studies on nutrient metabolism, clinical studies of the pathophysiological basis of the disease and population surveys to monitor the link between diet and disease. Clinical trials and population intervention studies amplify the basis for considering inappropriate diets as fundamental to the pathogenesis of many of these disorders.

The past four decades have seen appreciable advances in our understanding of the role of the fat- and water-soluble vitamins. Vitamin A for instance, plays a crucial part in controlling the spatial organization of fetal development, vitamin D has a complex role in cellular differentiation as well as calcium homeostasis, and vitamin E modulates the cellular suppression of free-radical induced damage to proteins, fats, and nucleic acids in many different tissues. New knowledge has also emerged on the role of folic acid in cell division and the prevention of neural tube defects, and of pyridoxine in preventing some thrombotic conditions by limiting the development of homocystinaemia. The beneficial impact of vitamin C is increasingly evident in studies on the prevention of oxidative changes in the lens proteins which occur during the development of cataract. Similarly, new roles for selenium in iodine metabolism are now known and the importance of zinc homeostasis in maintaining the thymic proliferation of lymphocytes can now be linked to zinc's control of cell division.

Thus to understand the nutritional basis of a patient's disease requires a knowledge of physiological biochemistry and some molecular biology as well as a perspective of what the patient had actually been eating.

The practical aspect of nutritional assessment requires an understanding of different types of food, their structure, composition, and preparation. These are dealt with generally under the heading of dietetics, details of which will be found in the bibliography. Only a few points will be considered here.

Humans are omnivores, but by necessity many millions of people eat a virtually vegetarian diet. Many forms of edible matter are not used as food for a variety of social, religious, and economic reasons which may bear no relation to their nutritive value. There is usually one food which is the staple diet of a particular culture and this is nearly always vegetable in origin (for instance, wheat, rice, maize, or cassava); another food may be labelled as a prestige component of the diet since it is expensive and therefore usually reserved for special occasions; this is usually meat.

The physical alteration of food by refining or processing can improve or reduce its nutritive value. Thus phytate, which inhibits mineral absorption, may be reduced or the beneficial non-starch polysaccharides (fibre) may be removed by such processes. Foods may be fortified with micronutrients or have added medically undesirable amounts of trans fatty acids, refined sugars, or sodium as salt or monosodium glutamate.

Measuring food intake

Measuring an individual's food intake is not easy. Not only does it fluctuate for social and economic reasons but the control of appetite both in children and adults leads to substantial change in intake from day to day and week to week. It is necessary therefore to measure intake over periods of several days, e.g. a week, to overcome daily fluctuations, but longer monitoring periods are necessary to obtain a consistent picture of usual intakes. Unfortunately, adults often alter their normal behaviour when under study and many reduce their intake and under-report the foods actually consumed as they record details of their diet. This can lead to substantial errors in assessments. Habitual intake may be better assessed by detailed questionnaires about diet with photographs or models of food for estimating portion size. Questionnaires for assessing the relative frequency of consumption of different foods are also used to rank individuals within a population in epidemiological studies, but the method that simply requires a recall of all food eaten in the previous 24 h leads to a consistent underestimation of intake. Given all these difficulties, there is now increasing interest in measuring biochemical markers of intake, e.g. mineral, nitrogen, or vitamin excretion, or blood levels of absorbed nutrients.

Once information is available on the amount of each food eaten, the total nutrients consumed can be estimated by reference to published tables of the average content of each food, these tables often being produced for each country's foods. They need continuous revision as new products are introduced and can give only an approximate estimate of what has actually been consumed.

Measuring food intake does not indicate whether or not an individual is malnourished, since this will depend on the effectiveness of absorption, on the individual's specific needs, and on any metabolic change in utilization. Accurate assessment of the nutritional state of an individual therefore requires direct measurement of his/her size, nutrient stores, metabolism, and functional capacity.

Nutrient requirements

Given the variability between individuals, it is not easy to calculate the amounts of all the nutrients needed to maintain optimum function. In practice national and international expert committees have produced reports that estimate the average nutrient requirement of healthy children of different ages and for adults. This requirement is the minimum needed by the average healthy child or adult to allow for modest or full body nutrient stores or to stimulate a particular metabolic response. Rarely is the value chosen as that needed to produce optimum function. These estimates therefore tend to be somewhat conservative and their derivation is often quite complex.

The reasons why some people have a greater need for nutrients than others are unclear, but presumably include genetic factors. The range of needs in a healthy population can be assessed by a variety of complex techniques, which often include prolonged metabolic balance studies. These assess the intake needed to keep the body's stores, biochemical function, or cellular saturation with a nutrient (such as a vitamin) at a maximum. The criteria of adequacy therefore vary and there can be much debate as to the most appropriate index for specifying a 'healthy' level for the intake of a vitamin or mineral. Requirements will also vary for dietary reasons, for instance intake of other inhibitors of absorption, for physiological reasons, e.g. growth or pregnancy, and for others such as illness. It may be necessary to specify all these before one can obtain a reasonable estimate of the patient's true need. Thus the requirement for the essential amino acid, tyrosine, will be greater in growing children, in convalescing patients depositing new protein, and in pregnant or lactating women. Illness itself may also accelerate amino acid catabolism and require an appreciably higher intake before a new balance between intake and oxidation is achieved.

Examples of increased needs in disease or in people with certain dietary or other habits include the following: an increased need for vitamin A in measles; of vitamin D in people on high cereal diets; of vitamin C in smokers; folate supplements before conception and in early pregnancy, to avoid neural tube defects; zinc supplementation in severe diarrhoea and additional iron in many situations to prevent anaemia, and for optimal development of the infant brain. The United Kingdom Department of Health published revised dietary reference values (DRVs) in 1991. The values were previously known as Recommended Dietary Allowances (RDAs). The term applies to the range of intakes based on an assessment of the distribution of requirements for each nutrient.

Figure 1 provides an illustration of the relationship between these estimated requirements of healthy individuals and the observed nutrient intakes in two populations. In the usual method of calculation, the upper limit of a population's needs is calculated as the mean + 2 SD, since this covers the estimated needs of 97 per cent of the population. This reference nutrient intake (RNI), formerly known as the recommended dietary allowance or RDA, was also considered the 'safe intake'; below this an increasing proportion of the population is at risk of deficiency. Now the European Union estimates have a different nomenclature and the average adult male requirement rather than the population reference intake (PRI; Fig. 1) is proposed for labelling foods. Thus when a portion of breakfast cereal was described as providing 30 per cent of the RDA this meant 30 per cent of the estimated upper limit of the adult male's needs, but will now become 30 per cent of the average healthy males' requirement.

Tables 1 and 2 specify the reference nutrient intakes of vitamins and minerals for healthy people. In Fig. 1, population A is not particularly well fed, since about half the people are eating less than the RNI and are thereby at risk. Those individuals with low constitutional needs for the nutrient being assessed, for example protein, zinc, or vitamin C, will

Fig. 1 Assessing the probability of nutrient deficiency. Note that the average requirement of energy is the value taken to estimate a group's energy needs. This differs from all other nutrients, where an allowance for the 2 SD range of individual need is estimated before specifying the 'safe intake' or 'reference nutrient intake' (RNI). LNRI, lower reference nutrient intake (UK); RNI, reference nutrient intake (UK); PRI, population reference intake (EU).

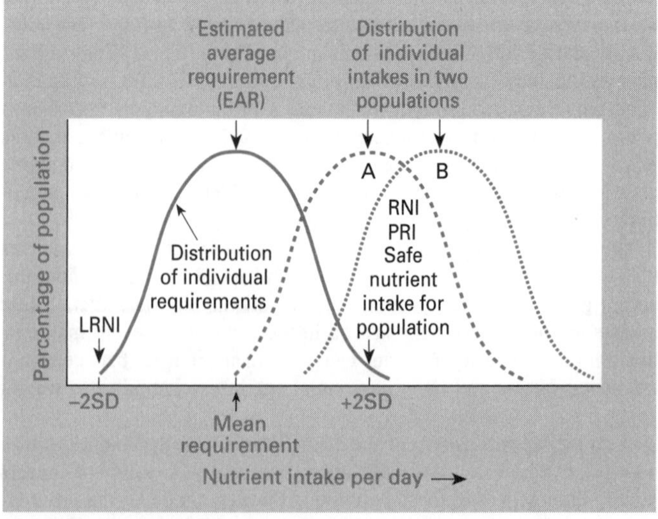

Table 1 *Reference nutrient intakes for vitamins*

Age	Thiamine (mg/day)	Riboflavine (mg/day)	Niacin (nicotinic acid equivalent) (mg/day)	Vitamin B_6 mg/day[d]	Vitamin B_{12} (μg/day)	Folate (μg/day)	Vitamin C (mg/day)	Vitamin A (μg/day)	Vitamin D (μg/day)
0–12 months	0.2–0.3	0.4	3–5	0.2–0.4	0.3–0.4	50	25	350	8.5–7.0
1–10 years	0.5–0.7	0.6–1.0	8–12	0.7–1.0	0.5–1.0	70–150	30	400–500	7–0
Males									
11–50 years	0.9–1.0	1.2–1.3	15–17	1.2–1.4	1.2–1.5	200	35–40	600–700	[b]
Females									
11–50+ years	0.7–0.8	1.1	12–14	1.0–1.2	200	35–40	600	[b]	
Pregnancy	+0.1[c]	+0.3	[a]	[a]	[a]	+100	+10	+100	10
Lactation									
0–4 months	+0.2	+0.5	+2	[a]	+0.5	+60	+30	+350	10
4+ months	+0.2	+0.5	+2	[a]	+0.5	+60	+30	+350	10

[a]No increment.

[b]After age 65 the RNI is 10 μg/day for men and women.

[c]For last trimester only.

[d]Based on protein providing 14.7 per cent of estimated average requirement (EAR) for energy.

Table 2 *Reference nutrient intakes for minerals*

Age	Calcium (mg/day)	Phosphorus[b] (mg/day)	Magnesium (mg/day)	Sodium (mg/day)[c]	Potassium (mg/day)[d]	Chloride[e] (mg/day)	Iron (mg/day)	Zinc (mg/day)	Copper (mg/day)	Selenium (μg/day)	Iodine (μg/day)
0–12 months	525	400	55–80	210–350	800–700	320–500	1.7–7.8	4.0–5.0	0.2–0.3	10–13	50–60
0–10 years	350–550	270–450	85–200	500–1200	800–2000	800–1800	6.9–8.7	5.0–7.0	0.4–7.0	15–30	70–110
Males											
11–50 years	1000–700	775–550	280–300	1600	3100–3500	2500	11.3–8.7	9.0–9.5	0.8–1.2	45–75	130–140
Females											
11–50 years	800–700	625–550	280–270	1600	3100–3500	2500	14.8[f]–8.7	9.0–7.0	0.8–1.2	45–60	130–140
Pregnancy	[a]	[a]	[a]	[a]	[a]	[a]	[a]	[a]	[a]	[a]	[a]
Lactation											
0–4 months	+550	+440	+50	[a]	[a]	[a]	[a]	+6.0	+0.3	+15	[a]
4+ months	+550	+440	+50	[a]	[a]	[a]	[a]	+2.5	+0.3	+15	[a]

[a]No increment.

[b]Phosphorus RNI is set equal to calcium in molar terms.

[c]1 mmol sodium = 23 mg.

[d]1 mmol potassium = 39 mg.

[e]Corresponds to sodium 1 mmol = 35.5 mg.

[f]Insufficient for women with high menstrual losses where the most practical way of meeting iron requirements is to take iron supplements.

remain healthy, but those with a high requirement will be inadequately fed. Since there is no way of knowing this without assessing the individuals concerned, everybody with an intake below the RNI is considered to be at risk. Population B, on the other hand, is rather better off, with about 15 per cent of the population at risk. Many of the intakes proposed in Tables 1 and 2 are based on the concepts depicted in Fig. 1, but often the information on the range of individual need is scanty.

Table 3 gives the RNI for protein. The requirements are based on the report of the FAO/WHO/UNU expert consultation, in which the values were derived on the basis of estimates of the amounts of high-quality egg or milk protein required for nitrogen equilibrium, as measured in nitrogen balance studies. For infants and children, additions were made for growth, and in pregnancy and lactation additions were made to account for the growth of the fetus and to allow adequate breast-milk production. The criteria used were the rate of weight gain or growth, the achievement of a suitably positive nitrogen balance, and the maintenance of a state of well-being.

Energy requirements are different from other nutritional requirements because no allowance can be made for the 2 SD range shown in Fig. 1. If all people were fed to intakes at the highest level, half the group would gain weight because, unlike the case with protein, minerals, or vitamins, there is only a minimal capacity to metabolize excess energy. Recommendations are therefore set as the average of energy requirements for any population group and these are given in Table 4. An estimate of adult energy needs may be made by calculating the likely basal metabolic rate (BMR) for age, weight, and sex as in Table 5. This rate can then be multiplied by a simple factor to allow for varying levels of physical activity as shown in Table 6. For example, the BMR of a 25-year-old male weighing 65 kg would be: $(65 \times 0.063) + 2.896 = 6.99$ MJ/day (from Table 5). If this young man works in an office with only light activity, but is moderately active in his non-working hours, then his average energy requirement would be: $6.99 \times 1.5 = 10.485$ MJ/day (from Table 6). Energy needs decline with age not only because physical activity tends to fall but also because the body loses metabolically active lean tissue, particularly muscle, replacing it with adipose tissue. This change may also result from inactivity.

Table 3 *Reference nutrient intakes for protein*

Age	Reference nutrient intake[a] (g/day)	
0–3 months	12.5[b]	
4–6 months	12.7	
7–9 months	13.7	
10–12 months	14.9	
1–3 years	14.5	
4–6 years	19.7	
7–10 years	28.3	
Males		
11–14 years	42.1	
15–18 years	55.2	
19–50 years	55.5	
50+ years	53.3	
Females:		
11–14 years	41.2	
15–18 years	45.0	
19–50 years	45.0	
50+ years	46.5	
Pregnancy[c]		+6
Lactation[c]		
0–4 months		+11
4+ months		+8

[a]These figures, based on egg and milk protein, assume complete digestibility.

[b]No values for infants 0–3 months are given by WHO. The RNI is calculated from the recommendations of COMA.

[c]To be added to adult requirement through all stages of pregnancy and lactation.

Table 4 *Estimated average requirements (EARs) for energy*

Age	EARs (MJ/day (kcal/day))	
	Males	Females
0–3 months	2.28 (545)	2.16 (515)
4–6 months	2.89 (690)	2.69 (645)
7–9 months	3.44 (825)	3.20 (765)
10–12 months	3.85 (920)	3.61 (865)
1–3 years	5.15 (1230)	4.86 (1165)
4–6 years	7.16 (1715)	6.46 (1545)
7–10 years	8.24 (1970)	7.28 (1740)
11–14 years	9.27 (2220)	7.92 (1845)
15–18 years	11.51 (2755)	8.83 (2110)
19–50 years	10.60 (2550)	8.10 (1940)
51–59 years	10.60 (2550)	8.00 (1900)
60–64 years	9.93 (2380)	7.99 (1900)
65–74 years	9.71 (2330)	7.96 (1900)
75+ years	8.77 (2100)	7.61 (1810)
Pregnancy		+0.80 (200)[a]
Lactation		
1 month		+1.90 (450)
2 months		+2.20 (530)
3 months		+2.40 (570)
4–6 months (Group 1)[b]		+2.00 (480)
4–6 months (Group 2)[c]		+2.40 (570)
> 6 months (Group 1)		+1.00 (240)
> 6 months (Group 2)		+2.30 (550)

[a]Last trimester only.

[b]Exclusive breast-feeding for 3–4 months followed by active weaning.

[c]Breast-feeding primary source of nourishment for 6 months or more. Limited complementary feeds after 3–4 months

Table 5 *Equations for the prediction of basal metabolic rate (Department of Health 1991)*

	Age range (years)	Prediction equation BMR (MJ/day) per kg body weight	95% confidence limits (MJ/day)
Males	10–17	0.074 (wt) + 2.754	± 0.88
	18–29	0.063 (wt) + 2.896	± 1.28
	30–59	0.048 (wt) + 3.653	± 1.40
	60–74	0.0499 (wt) + 2.930	(N/A)
	75+	0.0350 (wt) + 3.434	(N/A)
Females	10–17	0.056 (wt) + 2.898	± 0.94
	18–29	0.062 (wt) + 2.036	± 1.00
	30–59	0.034 (wt) + 3.538	± 0.94
	60–74	0.0386(wt) + 2.875	(N/A)
	75+	0.0410 (wt) + 2.610	(N/A)

N/A, not available.

Table 6 *Basal metabolic rate multiples for light, moderate, and heavy activity*

Non-occupational activity level	Occupational activity level					
	Light		Moderate		Heavy	
	M	F	M	F	M	F
Non-active	1.4	1.4	1.6	1.5	1.7	1.5
Moderatively active	1.5	1.5	1.7	1.6	1.8	1.6
Very active	1.6	1.6	1.8	1.7	1.9	1.7

Long-term nutrient requirements

The concepts and tables set out above deal with the need for a particular quantity of a nutrient to avoid a deficiency state. Excessive intakes are rarely considered a problem, unless very large amounts of vitamins A or D are consumed. For many nutrients adaptive mechanisms in the intestine tend to limit the effects of any dietary excess, e.g. of calcium or iron; water-soluble vitamins are readily excreted in the urine and excess protein intakes can be metabolized readily. Now we recognize that an excess intake of some nutrients, such as saturated fatty acids, may be harmful if ingested for many months or years. The intakes needed to avoid problems that develop from high intakes of substances, such as saturated fatty acids, *trans* fatty acids, sugar, or salt, are even more difficult to quantify than the reference values for vitamins or minerals. Nevertheless, WHO and national committees all now specify the average intake of fat, sugar, salt, and non-starch polysaccharides (formerly known as dietary fibre) that they believe may be conducive to health. Table 7 shows the values given by the United Kingdom Department of Health's *Dietary Reference Values* in 1991 for some of these nutrients. For carbohydrate, fat, and fibre needs the values are expressed as individual minimum and maximum and population averages, rather than the RNI. For a fuller explanation, the reader is referred to the United Kingdom Department of Health's report on Dietary Reference Values (1991).

In many nutritional diseases the patient may be the individual most susceptible to the prevailing pattern of food intake within the community. Only now are we beginning to disentangle the biochemical basis for individual susceptibility to such conditions as ischaemic heart disease, hypertension, and obesity. This new metabolic and molecular understanding is matched by a recognition that particular items in the diet are being ingested in excessive or insufficient amounts. This is a very different view of nutrition from the traditional one which considered nutritional disorders simply as due to protein deficiency or the result

Table 7 *Dietary reference values for fat and carbohydrate for adults as a percentage of daily total energy intake (percentage of food energy)*

	Individual minimum	Population average	Individual maximum
Saturated fatty acids		10 (11)	
cis-Polyunsaturated fatty acids	6 (6.5)	10	
n-3	0.2		
n-6	1.0		
cis-Monosaturated fatty acids		12 (13)	
trans Fatty acids		2 (2)	
Total fatty acids		30 (32.5)	
Total fat		33 (35)	
Non-milk extrinsic sugars	0	10 (11)	
Intrinsic and milk sugars and starch		37 (39)	
Total carbohydrate		47 (50)	
Non-starch polysaccharide	12	18	24

The average percentage contribution to total energy does not total 100 per cent because figures for protein and alcohol are excluded. Protein intakes average 15 per cent of total energy which is above the RNI. It is recognized that many individuals will derive some energy from alcohol, and this has been assumed to average 5 per cent, approximating to current intakes. However, some groups might not drink alcohol, and for some purposes nutrient intakes as a proportion of food energy (without alcohol) might be useful. Therefore average figures are given as percentages both of total energy and, in parentheses, of food energy.

of mineral or vitamin lack. Establishing the ideal nutritional intake of fat, sugar, salt, and non-starch polysaccharide, however, leads to considerable controversy, since the choice of level will have major long-term effects on dietary patterns. These, in turn, have huge economic implications for the food and agriculture industries. Nevertheless, many governments have adopted nutritional advice in an effort to limit the problems of heart disease, hypertension, obesity, and some cancers. These chronic conditions with a nutritional component are dealt with in separate sections of this book.

REFERENCES

Bingham, S.A. (1991). Limitations of the various methods for collecting dietary intake data. *Annals of Nutrition and Metabolism* **35,** 117–27.

Department of Health and Social Security (1980). *Artificial feeds for the young infant.* Report on Health and Social Subjects 18. HMSO, London.

Department of Health (1991). *Dietary Reference Values for food energy and nutrients for the United Kingdom.* Report of the Panel on Dietary Reference Values of the Committee on Medical Aspects of Food Policy, Report on Health and Social Subjects 41. HMSO, London.

Garrow, J. and James, W.P.T. (1993). *Human nutrition and dietetics,* (9th ed). Churchill Livingstone, Edinburgh.

Holland, B., Welch, A.A., Unwin, I.D., Buss, D.H., Paul, A.A., and Southgate, D.A.T. (1991). *McCance and Widdowson's The Composition of Foods.* The Royal Society of Chemistry and MAFF

James, W.P.T. and Schofield, E.C. (1990). *Human energy requirements. A manual for planners and nutritionists.* Oxford University Press.

Secretary of State for Health (1992). *The health of the nation. A strategy for health in England.* HMSO, London.

The Scottish Office (1993). *The Scottish Diet.* Report of a Working Party to the Chief Medical Officer for Scotland. The Scottish Office Home and Health Department, Edinburgh.

World Health Organization (1985). *Energy and protein requirements.* Report of a joint FAO/WHO/UNU Expert Consultation, Technical Report Series 724. World Health Organization, Geneva.

World Health Organization (1988). *Healthy nutrition. Preventing nutrition-related diseases in Europe.* WHO Regional Publications, European Series No. 24, Copenhagen.

World Health Organization (1990). *Diet, nutrition, and the prevention of chronic diseases.* Report of WHO Study Group, Technical Report Series 797. World Health Organization, Geneva.

10.2 Biochemical background

R. SMITH and D. H. WILLIAMSON

Such is the ease with which nutrition usually occurs that it is taken for granted; and only when it is disturbed does this complex physiological process become of clinical interest. At such times it is essential for the physician or surgeon to have some knowledge of the fundamental biochemical processes which underlie normal nutrition, such as the supply and utilization of energy-containing nutrients (upon which life depends), the control of the metabolism of protein, fat, and carbohydrate, and the results of imbalance between fuel supply and demand. It is necessary to know, for example, how metabolic fuels are provided to the tissues; which biochemical changes occur in a patient deprived of food; how an injured person survives; and what are the principles and problems of parenteral feeding. This chapter aims to summarize the relevant biochemical facts of normal human nutrition. It will concern itself exclusively with the metabolism of protein, fat, and carbohydrate and their intermediates. Since much recent knowledge on energy exchange has been derived from studies on obese patients undergoing short or long periods of starvation, the effects of this will also be considered. Further relevant biochemical information will be found in Chapters 10.3 and 11.11.

Production of energy from metabolic fuels

The body requires energy for many functions. These include the synthesis of new tissues, the maintenance of ionic gradients, the processes of secretion and detoxification, the generation of heat, and the performance of exercise and locomotion. To provide this energy the tissues oxidize glucose (from carbohydrate), triacylglycerols, non-esterified fatty acids and ketone bodies (from fat), and amino acids (from protein). These energy-containing substrates or metabolic fuels are provided as a mixture to the tissues in the bloodstream, and their proportional utilization depends on many factors. The oxidation of these fuels is linked to the generation of the high-energy phosphate of adenosine triphosphate (ATP) (Fig. 1) through the tricarboxylic acid (TCA), or citric acid, cycle.

Details of oxidative phosphorylation can be obtained from the references listed at the end of this section. Figure 1 demonstrates the central position of acetyl-CoA whose acetyl group is derived from glucose, fatty acids, ketone bodies, and many amino acids. This carrier molecule brings acetyl units into the TCA cycle. The cyclical oxidation of acetyl-CoA produces 3 moles of $NADH_2$, 1 mole of $FADH_2$, and 2 moles of CO_2 for each mole of acetyl-CoA oxidized. Oxidation of a single glucose molecule can result in the formation of 36 molecules of ATP.

Energy requirements

The normal energy requirements in the adult (which are equal to the energy expenditure) are shown in Chapter 10.1. In the healthy person, energy consumption increases considerably with exercise; fever, surgery, burns, and neoplasms also increase energy demand. Of the total oxygen consumption (which is a convenient measure of aerobic metabolism), more than 90 per cent in the basal state is accounted for by the major organs; approximate figures are: skeletal muscle 30 per cent, abdominal organs 25 per cent, brain 20 per cent, and heart about 11 per cent. During exercise the energy requirements of muscle may increase ten- to fifteen-fold compared with insignificant changes in other organs. Other physiological circumstances increase the energy requirements of other tissues; for instance, that of abdominal organs is increased by eating; and that of a large number of tissues is increased by growth, particularly during infancy or fetal life. In contrast, energy expenditure decreases after middle age.

Some clues about the fuels used to supply this energy may be provided by a comparison between CO_2 production and O_2 consumption (the respiratory quotient), which is 1.0 when carbohydrate is used exclusively as a fuel, and 0.7 for fat. The use of the respiratory quotient to predict the type of fuel being burnt is valid only with certain assumptions and does not provide any information about the proportion of fuel used by different organs.

Fig. 1 The source, production, and utilization of energy from food. The lipids, polysaccharides, and proteins are degraded into their constituents by digestive enzymes. After transport to the tissue cells they are either used for resynthesis (dotted arrows) or mainly converted to acetyl-CoA. The TCA cycle is located in the mitochondria. e^- = electron transport chain. For further explanation see text.

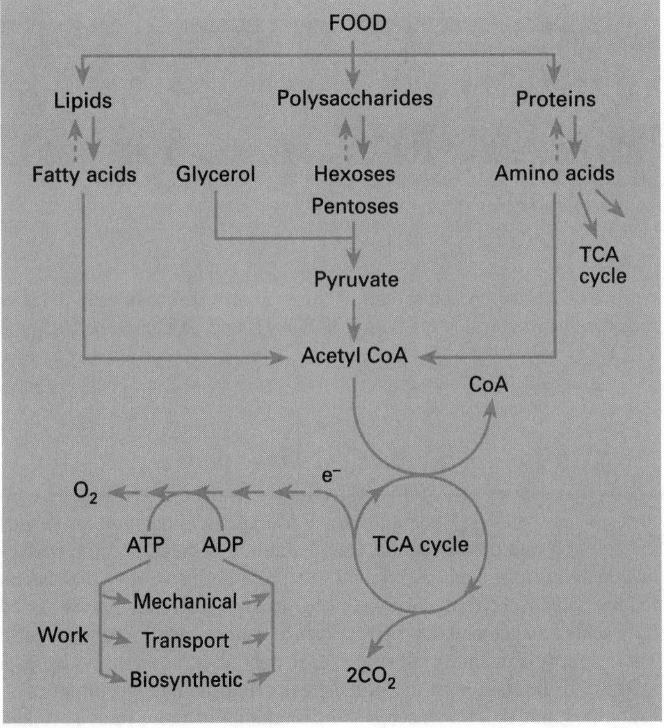

Table 1 *The approximate normal composition of a 70-kg man*

	kg	Percentage of body weight
Water	42	60
Intracellular	28	40
Extracellular	14	20
Solids		
Fat	12.6	18
Protein[a]	11.2	16
Intracellular (muscle)	8.4	12
Extracellular (collagen)	2.8	4
Minerals	3.8	5.4
Carbohydrate	0.4	0.6

[a]The figures for intracellular and extracellular protein are estimates only. The fat content is less than in Fig. 2.

Body composition and metabolic fuels

The available metabolic fuels are related to body composition (Table 1). There are two main protein sites within the body. One of these is extracellular (collagen), located particularly in the bone matrix and skin, and this does not appear to be readily available as a source of fuel. The other is intracellular (striated muscle) which in man is the main source of protein used as of fuel. The amount of adipose tissue varies considerably, and in an obese person may be between 50 and 100 kg above normal. The significance of the differences between muscle and adipose tissue as potential energy sources becomes obvious when it is recalled that muscle protein is associated with about three times its own weight of water and provides 4 kcal/g (about 17 kJ/g) whereas adipose tissue fat is virtually anhydrous, and provides 9 kcal/g (about 38 kJ/g). Thus 100 g of skeletal muscle will yield 100 kcal (420 kJ) whereas 100 g of adipose tissue will yield about 900 kcal (3780 kJ). This means that for a given utilization of energy the weight loss is far less rapid when fat is consumed rather than muscle; that synthesis of fat is by far the most efficient way of storing energy; and that an obese person with an extra 55 kg of adipose tissue has half a million kcal 'in store'. The prime importance of adipose tissue triacylglycerol (triglyceride) as a fuel 'store' is emphasized in Fig. 2. Apart from fat, the only other significant body store of fuel which can be used over a relatively long period is protein, particularly that of skeletal muscle. In starvation, degradation of this tissue for energy purposes is reduced by the selective utilization of fat. In the non-fasting person there are also a number of minor short-term body stores of fuel. These include glycogen, the circulating body pools of free glucose, triacylglycerols, free fatty acids, and amino acids, which are readily used in an overnight fast.

The main metabolic fuels circulate in the plasma as their constituents; protein in the form of amino acids, particularly alanine and glutamine from skeletal muscle; carbohydrate, predominantly as glucose but also (as in exercise) lactate and pyruvate produced in the Cori cycle; and fats as triacylglycerols (chylomicrons, very low density lipoproteins), non-esterified fatty acids, and glycerol. Ketone bodies are formed by partial oxidation of non-esterified fatty acids in the liver.

Fuel supply, utilization, and balance

The supply and utilization of energy-containing substrates is most simply considered with the liver as a transformer between the fuel supply and those tissues that utilize it. Figure 3 shows the main metabolic exchanges, determined by direct cannulation of appropriate vessels, by measurement of isotopically labelled substrate turnover, and by indirect calorimetry in postabsorptive man. After the rapid utilization of short-term fuel stores such as glycogen, the main suppliers of further fuel are fat (in adipose tissue) and protein (in skeletal muscle), and the main utilizers the brain and central nervous system, muscle, abdominal organs, and circulating blood cells.

In a 24-h period the tissues of a normal fasting man will utilize approximately 1800 kcal derived from about 75 g of protein (mainly muscle) and 160 g of triacylglycerol from adipose tissue. Of the 180 g of glucose released from the liver, about 144 g will be totally oxidized by nervous tissue, mainly brain. The remaining 36 g is converted by glycolytic tissues—for example, bone marrow, renal medulla, peripheral nerve, erythrocytes, and to a lesser extent skeletal muscle—to lactate and pyruvate. These metabolites are transported to the liver and kidney and are there resynthesized into glucose. This cycle, the Cori cycle ((2) in Fig. 3), provides a shuttle of carbon which spares gluconeogenesis from protein by limiting the complete oxidation of glucose to carbon dioxide.

Fig. 2 To demonstrate the available metabolic fuels in the normal adult. After the rapid utilization of glycogen, protein and fat are the main fuel 'stores' in fasting. In comparison the energy to be derived from circulating metabolites is insignificant. Note that the scale for the circulating metabolites is 1000 less than for the tissue stores. ECF = extracellular fluid.

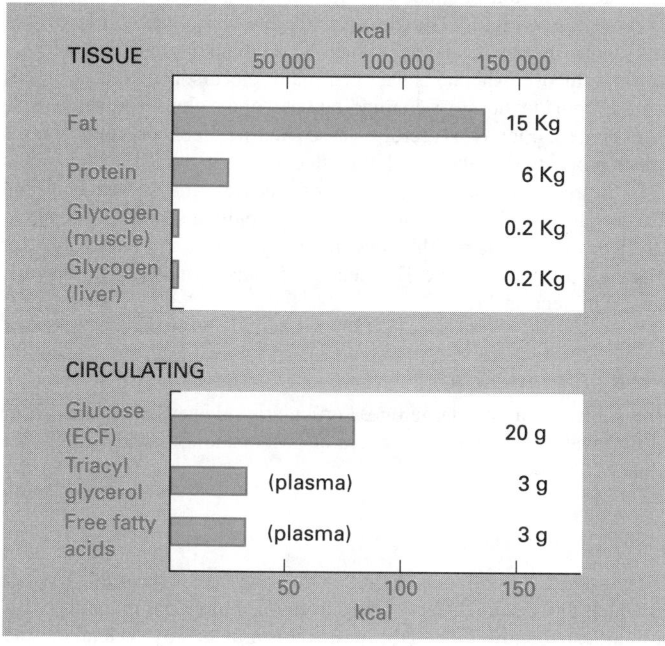

Fig. 3 To demonstrate daily substrate production and utilization (in g) in a post-absorptive 70-kg man consuming 1800 kcal in 24 h. The numbered arrows indicate the direction (but not the extent) of two important cycles: (1) the transfer of glucose from the liver to muscle as part of the glucose-alanine cycle (see Fig. 6), and (2) the production of lactate and pyruvate in the Cori cycle. The dotted arrow indicates the utilization of ketone bodies by nervous tissue (particularly the brain) during starvation.

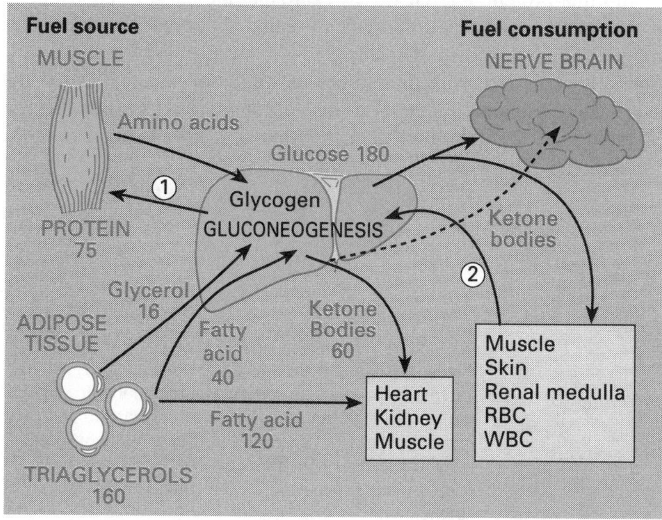

In addition to complete oxidation of glucose (in the brain) and glycolysis (in red cells) in fasting man, the remaining tissues, heart, kidney cortex, skeletal muscle, and other organs use triacylglycerols, fatty acids, or ketone bodies. The liver, which efficiently converts lactate, pyruvate, and the glucogenic amino acids to glucose, requires energy for these processes; again this is derived mainly from fatty acid oxidation.

Figure 3 shows how energy is supplied from the body's own tissues; clearly with exogenous fuel the picture will be more complex, although the mechanisms which control the metabolic pathways will be the same. However, when the food intake and energy requirements are disproportionate, there may be considerable changes in the fuel stores with subsequent alteration in body composition.

The regulation of the balance between fuel supply and its consumption is poorly understood. Normally the intake and utilization of food appear to be closely linked, so that in some adults body weight and composition may remain virtually constant for years. Intake is influenced by appetite and hunger, and probably by other unidentified endocrine or intestinal signals. Many studies on fuel intake in rats are not directly applicable to man, whose larger brain imposes complex controls on eating behaviour and also utilizes a larger proportion of energy. In man the role of the hypothalamus is still debated and the factors which control short and long-term fluctuations in weight remain obscure. These are further considered in relation to obesity (see Chapter 10.5).

Regulation of substrate metabolism

The utilization of a given energy-containing substrate by a tissue depends on many factors; amongst these are its circulating concentration, the blood flow to the tissue, the permeability of the cells and their compartments to the substrate, the mechanism of the entry into the metabolic pathway (initiating enzyme), subsequent intracellular metabolism, and the effects of other substrates and hormones (Table 2).

HORMONES AND METABOLISM (SEE ALSO SECTION 11)

The way in which hormones alter substrate supply are mainly rapid (short-term regulation), but longer-term changes via gene expression do occur. Insulin, glucagon, and the 'stress' hormones (catecholamines, growth hormone, vasopressin) usually have acute effects, although they can also bring about long-term changes in enzyme concentration. The effects of corticosteroids and thyroxine appear to be confined to long-term regulation. The rapid effects of hormones involve either changes in the rate of transport of substrates into the cell or particular cellular compartment or alterations in the activity of key regulatory enzymes. The accepted mechanisms for their action involve:

(1) binding of the hormone to its receptor (usually located on or within the plasma membrane);
(2) generation of a change in concentration of the 'second messenger' (cyclic AMP, cyclic GMP, Ca^{2+} ions); and
(3) interaction of the second messenger with the target enzyme (or transport system).

The target enzyme may not be involved directly in the metabolic process which the particular hormone regulates. In many cases it acts to change the activity of an enzyme (e.g. protein kinase and/or phosphatase) which controls the interconversion of a regulatory enzyme in the metabolic pathway. In this way very small amounts of hormone can bring about large changes in the rate of a metabolic process by a form of enzyme

Table 2 *Summary of regulation of substrate metabolism. A substrate is defined as a substance present in the circulation and capable of being oxidized to yield energy or providing a biosynthetic precursor*

Tissue or compartment	Sites of regulation	Regulators
Vascular	Mixed substrates from diet or stored fuels (blood flow)	Appetite, hormones, substrate–substrate interactions (e.g. Fig. 8)
Cell or organelle membrane	Permeability (passive diffusion or active transport)	Hormones, substrates
Intracellular	Initiating enzyme; other regulatory sites	Hormones, substrates, and other metabolites

cascade (Fig. 4). Impairment of hormone action can occur at any of these stages, by alteration in the number and affinity of the cell-surface receptors, by defects in the generation of the second messenger, or by a deficiency in some other postreceptor event.

By such mechanisms hormones regulate the supply and utilization of metabolic fuels both in health and disease. There is no need to describe their individual effects in detail since much is dealt with in Section 11, but the short-term effects of insulin, glucagon, and catecholamines (Table 3) require mention.

All the actions of insulin are anabolic; protein, glycogen, and fat synthesis and storage are stimulated, and lipolysis and gluconeogenesis inhibited. In contrast, those of catecholamines and glucagon are catabolic. Glucagon exerts its major effect through the liver, increasing glycogen breakdown, gluconeogenesis, and ketogenesis from fatty acids; it also stimulates lipolysis in adipose tissue but has no important effect on muscle. The catecholamines have similar catabolic effects, with muscle as an additional target tissue.

Cortisol is often included as a 'catabolic' hormone, and it may be that its 'permissive' role has been overstressed. It appears to inhibit glucose uptake by peripheral tissues and to increase proteolysis. However, its effects (which are still debated) are delayed rather than immediate.

Finally, it is unwise to deal with the effects of particular hormones in isolation. Just as there are interactions between metabolites, there are also hormone–hormone interactions; for instance glucagon appears to stimulate the production of insulin and growth hormone, whereas catecholamines have the opposite effect.

Carbohydrate metabolism

Although the relative importance of the different metabolic fuels may alter in starvation and other conditions, it is accepted that glucose occupies a central role in whole-body metabolism. This is because it serves as an optimal fuel for so many tissues and an obligatory fuel for brain (except during prolonged starvation or hyperketonaemia), red blood cells, the retina, and the renal medulla.

Glycogen is the storage form of glucose in many tissues, and glucose is liberated from the liver by the action of glucose 6-phosphatase, which is absent in muscle. After an overnight fast about 25 per cent of the 180 g of glucose required daily by a 70-kg man is produced from glycogen. The remainder is formed from lactate and pyruvate, alanine (the main gluconeogenic amino acid), and glycerol (from fat). In postabsorptive man the formation of glucose from lactate represents one part of the Cori cycle (see Fig. 3). Glucose from the liver is converted to pyruvate and lactate in muscle and any which is not oxidized re-enters the liver to form glucose. Alanine is the other major precursor of glucose and its release from the muscle is an important part of the glucose–alanine cycle (see Fig. 6). Finally glycerol released during lipolysis contributes a minor proportion of the circulating glucose.

In the fed state the concentration of glucose remains very constant. This implies that ingested glucose is very rapidly disposed of mainly in the liver, where it is rapidly converted to glycogen and fatty acids (for triacylglycerol secretion). The details of glucose metabolism are discussed in Section 11.

Protein metabolism

The subject is a very large one. Particularly relevant are a knowledge of turnover rate, of the metabolism of different amino acids, and of the glucose–alanine cycle.

PROTEIN TURNOVER

Body protein is continuously broken down and resynthesized. The rate at which this occurs differs widely from one individual to another, and a significant contribution to this turnover is provided by skeletal muscle. Isotope measurements suggest that the whole-body protein breakdown rate (equivalent to the protein synthetic rate) in a young adult is between 3.0 and 3.5 g/kg/day. Measurements of 3-methylhistidine (see below) also suggest that the myofibrillar breakdown rate is about 25 per cent of this. Striated muscle contains sarcoplasmic and myofibrillar protein in approximately equal amounts, and the rate of muscle protein turnover derived from measurements of 3-methylhistidine refers only to that of myofibrillar protein. Even if we disregard the sarcoplasmic contribution to protein turnover, it is important to realize that these measurements imply a daily breakdown of at least 250 g of muscle tissue, since muscle protein is associated with three times its weight of water; if this is not restored by equivalent synthesis, as may occur after operation and injury, the rapid loss of muscle bulk at such a time is readily explained.

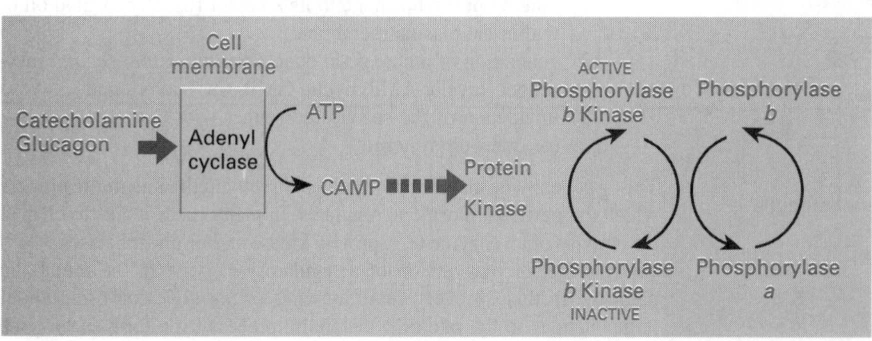

Fig. 4 To demonstrate how a hormone such as adrenaline or glucagon activates a metabolic process in the cell through the adenyl cyclase mechanism and may initiate an enzyme 'cascade'. In this way the eventual metabolic effects of a hormone may be far removed from the initial ones and can be considerably augmented.

Table 3 *Summary of the short-term metabolic effects of some hormones*

Hormone	Target tissues	Effects	Changes in substrate concentration
Insulin	Liver Muscle Adipose tissue Mammary gland	Increases glucose transport (not liver) Increases Glycogen synthesis Protein synthesis Lipogenesis Esterification Decreases Lipolysis Gluconeogenesis	Lowers glucose, fatty acids, ketone bodies, and amino acids
Glucagon	Liver Adipose tissue	Increases Glycogen breakdown Gluconeogenesis Alanine transport (liver) Lipolysis Ketogenesis Decreases Esterification Lipogenesis	Increases glucose, fatty acids, and ketone bodies
Catecholamines	Liver Muscle Adipose tissue	Increase Glycogen breakdown Gluconeogenesis Glycolysis Lipolysis Ketogenesis Decrease Esterification Lipogenesis	Increase glucose, fatty acids, ketone bodies, and lactate

URINE NITROGEN AND 3-METHYLHISTIDINE

The amino groups derived from the metabolism of amino acids in the liver are excreted largely as urea but a significant proportion is also excreted as ammonium ions (Figs 5 and 7). Total urinary nitrogen represents the balance between protein breakdown and synthesis and reflects the re-incorporation of amino acids, liberated into the amino acid pool, into newly formed protein. However, not all amino acids can be re-utilized for synthesis and these include those which have been modified after their incorporation into the peptide chain (i.e. post-translationally modified amino acids) (Fig. 5). 3-Methylhistidine and hydroxyproline provide examples of these; hydroxyproline excretion gives an indication of collagen breakdown rate and 3-methylhistidine that of myofibrillar protein. Both actin and myosin contain 3-methylhistidine derived from post-translational methylation of some histidine residues. In contrast, the sarcoplasmic proteins, which comprise about 50 per cent of the striated muscle, do not contain 3-methylhistidine. 3-Methylhistidine is excreted in the urine and under certain circumstances its rate of excretion can provide an indicator of endogenous muscle protein breakdown, provided that dietary protein is reduced. Since creatinine excretion is an approximate biochemical indicator of muscle mass, the ratio of 3-methylhistidine excretion to that of creatinine can be used to indicate the fractional catabolic rate of skeletal muscle. Measurements have been made in starvation, injury, and various clinical states.

THE BRANCHED-CHAIN AMINO ACIDS

These are leucine, isoleucine, and valine: both their initial and subsequent metabolism is different from those without branched chains (Fig. 5). Thus when they are ingested they largely bypass the liver and are initially metabolized in muscle. This localization in muscle is presumed to have functional significance, and it has been suggested that leucine in particular can stimulate protein synthesis. The way in which it does this is not known, but forms the basis for the attempted therapeutic use of these particular amino acids in nitrogen-losing states.

THE GLUCOSE–ALANINE CYCLE

One pathway that is of particular importance in the exchange of energy is the so-called 'glucose–alanine' cycle (Fig. 6) whereby glucose from the liver is supplied to the peripheral tissues, such as muscle, and alanine is supplied to the liver for deamination. In this way amino groups derived from various amino acids by transamination are transported to the liver in the form of alanine and subsequently disposed of as urea; and the carbon skeletons are used as a source of glucose. Since the proportion of alanine in the amino acids released from muscle is considerably more than that in the amino acids of muscle, it is clear that the released alanine is not entirely derived from muscle protein breakdown. The other major precursors of alanine appear to be glutamate and the branched-chain amino acids. The quantitative importance of this cycle in different conditions and the relative contributions to alanine from different sources remain controversial.

GLUTAMINE

Perhaps the most important amino acid involved in the intertissue transfer of carbon and nitrogen is glutamine. In the fasting state peripheral tissues release alanine and glutamine in approximately equal amounts, but the latter carries two atoms of nitrogen per molecule. The major sites of glutamine utilization are the intestine, the cells of the immune system (as an energy source and nucleotide precursor), and the kidney (as a supply of ammonia for the regulation of acid–base balance). The liver is equipped with the enzymes for synthesizing glutamine (glutamine synthetase) and degrading it (glutaminase), and changes in the activities of these enzymes determine whether the liver extracts or releases glutamine (Fig. 7). The carbon skeleton of glutamine can be used as a gluconeogenic precursor in liver and renal cortex.

Fat metabolism

LIPOLYSIS

In the adipose tissue cell (the adipocyte) stored triacylglycerol is continually broken down to glycerol and non-esterified fatty acids by the action of a hormone-sensitive lipase; the glycerol is eventually used for gluconeogenesis in the liver, and fatty acid may be released to the plasma or be re-esterified within the adipocyte with glycerol-3-phosphate derived from glucose. In the fed state metabolism is directed towards fat storage. During food deprivation or insulin deficiency non-esterified fatty acids are released into the circulation, where they may be used directly as fuel, or converted in the liver to ketone bodies or triacylglycerols for secretion as very low density lipoproteins. Most tissues, apart from red cells and nervous tissue, are capable of using non-esterified fatty acids, and some, such as resting muscle, prefer them to glucose.

KETOGENESIS

There is increasing evidence of the importance of the ketone bodies, acetoacetate and 3-hydroxybutyrate, as tissue fuels, and there are a number of conditions in which their concentration is increased. The control of their production depends on two main steps; the hydrolysis of the fat of adipose tissue by a hormone-sensitive lipase into glycerol and fatty acids; and the metabolism of the long-chain fatty acids into ketone bodies. The former system appears to be largely under the control of insulin, lack of which increases lipolysis. The latter occurs within the liver and is more complex (see Fig. 9). Fatty acids entering the liver may either be re-esterified into triacylglycerols or oxidized. If the rate of fatty acid oxidation is high, there is an increase in the production of ketone bodies; this does not passively follow an increase in the supply of fatty acids but is critically dependent on the activation of the carnitine acyltransferase reaction, itself influenced by the amount of carnitine present, which provides a mechanism to transport long-chain fatty acids into the mitochondria. This process appears to be stimulated by an excess of glucagon relative to that of insulin.

The utilization of ketone bodies as a tissue fuel is particularly important in starvation (see below), where the circulating concentration increases to between 2 and 5 mmol/l, since in this way the breakdown

Fig. 5 A diagram to distinguish the differing metabolic pathways of amino acids and the origin of 3-methylhistidine (3MeH). The glucose–alanine cycle is dealt with in Fig. 6.

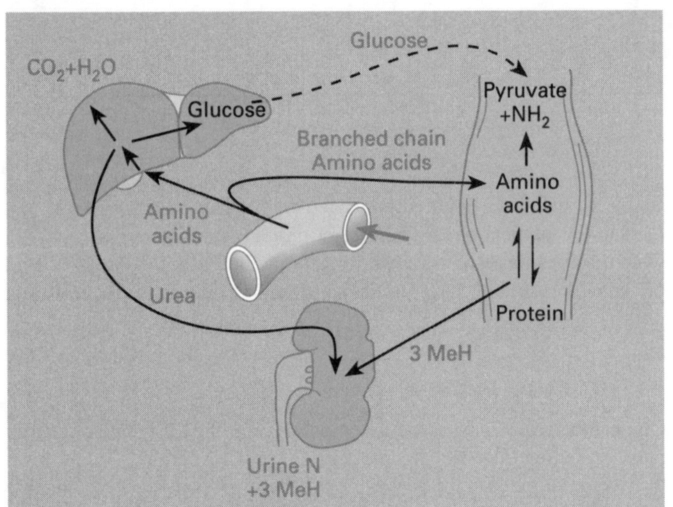

Fig. 7 Co-operation between liver and kidney in acid–base homeostasis. Amino acid oxidation yields ammonium ions and bicarbonate ions which are removed during ureagenesis. In acidosis there is a transfer of NH_4^+ from the liver to the kidney via glutamine (---> →). GLN, glutamine; αKG, α-ketoglutarate.

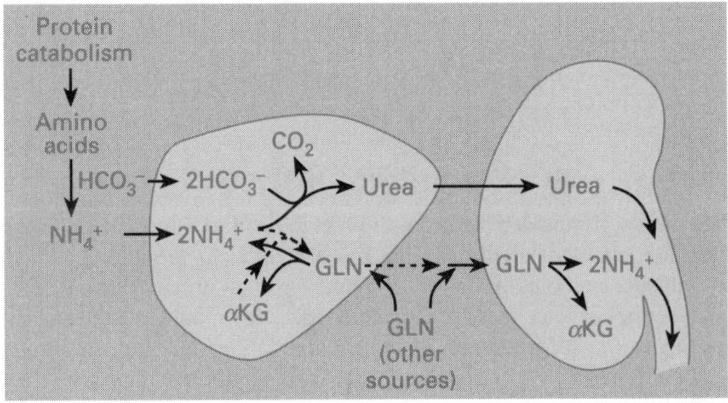

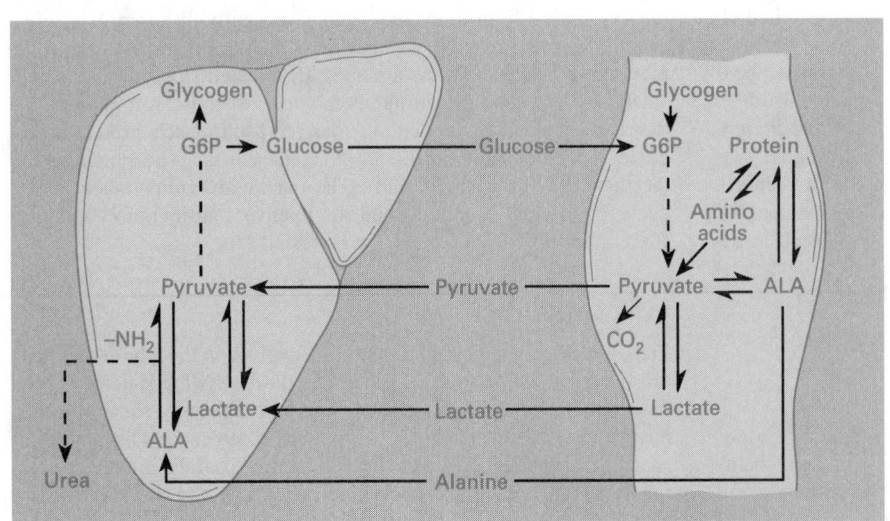

Fig. 6 The glucose–alanine cycle. The sources of alanine within muscle differ according to the state of nutrition. In post-absorptive man alanine (ALA) comes mainly from the transamination of pyruvate derived from glucose. In short-term starvation, alanine is also derived from proteolysis, and pyruvate carbon from partial oxidation of other amino acids. With prolonged starvation less alanine comes from glucose-derived pyruvate and proteolysis is reduced.

of protein for gluconeogenesis is minimized. So far as the brain and central nervous system (which are normally the main consumers of glucose) are concerned, the degree to which ketone bodies are utilized probably depends more on their circulating concentration than on any form of adaptation to starvation, since these tissues already appear to have the necessary enzymes for their metabolism.

TRIACYLGLYCEROLS

Triacylglycerols are transported in the circulation in the form of lipoproteins. Dietary lipid enters the plasma via the lymphatic system as chylomicrons derived from the intestine. Fatty acids synthesized in the liver and esterified to triacylglycerols are secreted as very low density lipoproteins. Both chylomicrons and very low density lipoproteins play an important role in providing fuel for muscle tissue, and fatty acids for milk lipid in the lactating mammary gland. In man, the exact contribution of triacylglycerols as a fuel is not known, but in the rat 50 per cent of the total lipid energy requirement of muscle tissue during starvation is provided by very low density lipoproteins. The other major fate of triacylglycerol is storage in adipose tissue in the fed state. Utilization of triacylglycerols requires their initial conversion to the constituent non-esterified fatty acids and free glycerol in a reaction catalysed by the initiating enzyme, lipoprotein lipase. The latter is active on the luminal surface of capillary endothelial cells.

Fig. 8 To show how one substrate may regulate the use of another. The increasing concentration and availability of non-esterified fatty acids (NEFA) and ketone bodies in starvation decreases the utilization of glucose by muscle. For explanation see text and Randle *et al.* (1988). (−) signifies inhibition.

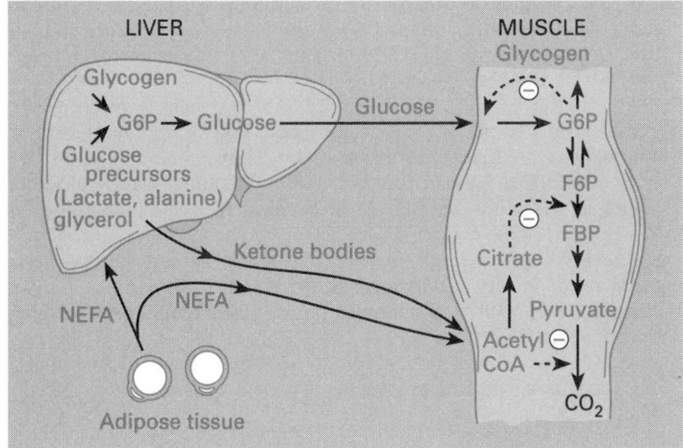

GLUCOSE–LIPID INTERACTIONS

The relationships between utilization of glucose, hepatic carbohydrate status, and lipid metabolism are of considerable nutritional importance. For example, increased availability of blood ketone bodies may reduce the utilization of glucose (Fig. 8). An hepatic link between carbohydrate and lipid metabolism is illustrated in Fig. 9. In order to enter the mitochondrion for subsequent metabolism, fatty acyl-CoA must be converted to the carnitine derivative via the enzyme carnitine acyltransferase (CAT I) located on the outer surface of its inner membrane. On the inner surface, carnitine acyltransferase II (CAT II) then reforms fatty acyl-CoA from the fatty acyl carnitine, with liberation of carnitine. Malonyl-CoA, an intermediate in the pathway of lipogenesis, inhibits CAT I. Glucose derived from glycogen is a major source of carbon for lipogenesis in the liver, and the concentration of malonyl-CoA is directly related to this rate of lipogenesis. Thus an increase in malonyl-CoA will inhibit the further metabolism of fatty acyl-CoA by CAT I and encourage its esterification to triacylglycerols, thus reducing the formation of ketone bodies.

The biochemical effects of starvation

Experimental study of short- and long-term fasting, usually in obese subjects, has shed considerable light on normal metabolic processes and on the way in which the body can adapt to food deprivation. The results obtained from brief fasts have been incorporated in the previous account; in effect they deal with the postabsorptive phase where the small carbohydrate stores, particularly glycogen, have been utilized and energy is provided from protein and fat alone. If the pathways demonstrated during brief fasting persisted during prolonged food deprivation, the loss of protein to provide glucose would be very rapid indeed. However, as mentioned above, the brain can substitute ketone bodies derived from fat for glucose, and with prolonged starvation this occurs progressively. The consequent reduction of protein breakdown is reflected in a fall in urinary nitrogen excretion. As the brain increasingly uses ketone bodies and the liver reduces gluconeogenesis, the kidney produces increased amounts of glucose. This last alteration appears to make the kidney the

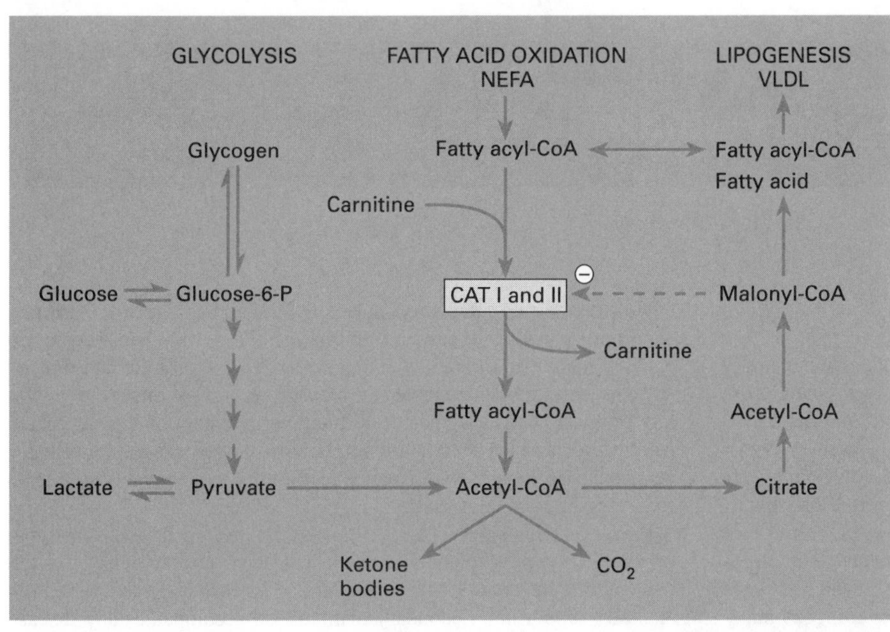

Fig. 9 A scheme of the regulatory links between hepatic carbohydrate status, lipogenesis, and ketogenesis. (−) indicates site of inhibition; CAT I and II indicate carnitine acyl transferase I and II respectively. For explanation see text.

chief gluconeogenetic tissue in prolonged starvation; the glucose is made from deaminated amino acids (mainly glutamine), while the amino groups provide ammonia required to neutralize the keto-acids lost in the urine.

The progressive reduction in gluconeogenesis and protein breakdown does not result from the accompanying fall in insulin levels which would, in contrast, increase gluconeogenesis. It seems likely that proteolysis is reduced by the hyperketonaemia of starvation in two independent ways; first the increasing utilization of ketone bodies, as an alternative fuel to glucose, decreases the requirement of the brain for glucose (derived from protein); and second the direct effect of ketone bodies reduces glucose utilization and alanine release from muscle. This effect can be demonstrated in starving man in whom the infusion of ketone bodies further reduces the already low nitrogen excretion.

In starvation there are only minor changes in the excretion of 3-methylhistidine and hydroxyproline. At the beginning of food deprivation urinary 3-methylhistidine falls to a constant low level as the effect of exogenous protein declines, and the subsequent changes are small. The reported changes in urinary hydroxyproline are variable, but they do suggest that prolonged food deprivation leads to an increase in the breakdown rate of collagen. How much this reflects the use of collagen as a protein source for gluconeogenesis, and how much comes from the skeleton as the result of immobility (especially after surgery, see below) is impossible to say. It does not appear to be due to the effect of acidosis on the skeleton, since it is not affected by the administration of alkali. The combined effects of loss of protein and fat produce considerable changes in body composition, with a reduction of lean body mass in relation to body water. In initial starvation the rapid weight loss is largely due to loss of sodium and water; however, with prolonged starvation body water and extracellular fluid volume decline less than that of lean tissue and sodium is conserved. The continuing breakdown of lean tissues is associated with increased urinary excretion of potassium and zinc, and the eventual fall in the K/N ratio to below 3 (the normal ratio in muscle) is compatible with the breakdown of non-muscular sources of protein such as collagen.

As starvation continues energy requirements also fall. This is partly due to decreasing physical activity; but there is also a fall in the levels of tri-iodothyronine with a subsequent reduction in metabolic rate. The other most important hormonal change is a decrease in insulin secretion.

In summary the fat (and the normal) person when deprived of food switches over to being a ketone-body burner. This spares protein breakdown and allows continued survival. With prolonged starvation the rate of weight loss decreases, fluid is selectively retained, and the metabolic rate falls.

In practice the effects of starvation are rarely as simple as this, since food deprivation usually occurs against a background of injury or infection, or as part of complex picture of protein energy malnutrition.

REFERENCES

Adibi, S.A. (1980). Roles of branched-chain amino acids in metabolic regulations. *Journal of Laboratory and Clinical Medicine*, **95,** 475–84.

Cahill, G.F. (1976). Starvation in man. *Clinics in Endocrinology and Metabolism*, **5,** 397–415.

Elia, M. (1991). The inter-organ flux of substrates in fed and fasted man, as indicated by arterio-venous balance studies. *Nutrition Research Reviews*, **4,** 3–31.

Elia, M., Carter, A., Bacon, S., Winearls, C.G., and Smith, R. (1981). Clinical usefulness of 3-methylhistidine in indicating muscle protein breakdown. *British Medical Journal*, **282,** 351–4.

Garrow, J.S. (1978). *Energy balance and obesity in man*. Elsevier/North Holland Biochemical Press, Amsterdam.

Gibbons, G.F. (1990). Assembly and secretion of hepatic very-low-density lipoprotein. *Biochemistry Journal*, **268,** 1–13.

McGarry, J.D. and Foster, D.W. (1977). Hormonal control of ketogenesis. *Archives of Internal Medicine*, **137,** 495–501.

Newsholme, E.A. and Leech, A.R. (1983) *Biochemistry for the medical sciences*. John Wiley and Sons, Chichester.

Owen, O.E., Tappy, L., Mozzoli, M.A., and Smalley, K.J. (1990). Acute starvation. In *The metabolic and molecular basis of acquired disease*, (ed. R.D. Cohen, B. Lewis, K.G.M.M. Alberti, and A.M. Denman), (1st edn), pp. 550–70. Baillière Tindall, London.

Randle, P.J., Kerbey, A.L., and Espinal, J. (1988). Mechanisms decreasing glucose oxidation in diabetes and starvation: Role of lipid fuels and hormones. *Diabetes/Metabolism Reviews*, **4,** 623–38.

Robinson, A.M. and Williamson, D.H. (1980). Physiological roles of ketone bodies as substrates and signals in mammalian tissues. *Physiological Reviews*, **60,** 143–87.

Snell, K. (1980). Muscle alanine synthesis and hepatic gluconeogenesis. *Biochemical Society Transactions*, **8,** 205–13.

Williamson, D.H. (1984). The regulation of substrate utilization. *Clinical Nutrition*, **2,** 129–36.

Young, V.R. and Munro, H.N. (1978). N^{T}-Methylhistidine (3-methylhistidine) and muscle protein turnover: an overview. *Federation Proceedings*, **37,** 2291–300.

10.3 Severe malnutrition

M.H.N. Golden

Introduction

Nutrition (with genetic constitution) determines the quality and quantity of the substance of the body—the 'soil' in which the 'seeds' of disease germinate; the interaction between the nutritional 'soil' and the aetiological 'seed' will determine the course and cost of many diseases. Nutritional state, with genetic endowment, interacts with aetiological agents in a way which causes, or fails to cause, disease; therefore the role of poor nutrition is important over the whole spectrum of disease. In severe malnutrition there has been a dietary inadequacy sufficient to compromise resistance to disease. Good nutrition leads to health and resistance to disease; poor nutrition leads to ill health and susceptibility to many diseases.

Nutritional state often alters the expression and course of the primary condition as well as its response to treatment. Indeed, it is often accompanying malnutrition that is the major reason for morbidity and mortality, and is the most amenable to treatment. A history of severe weight loss or anorexia is a signal for both active treatment of the associated malnutrition and the modification of treatment regimens for the primary diagnosis. Up to half of all patients admitted to hospital suffer from some degree of malnutrition.

Primary malnutrition is a condition of the dependent and vulnerable who rely on others for nourishment; it is seen most frequently in the young child, the elderly, and particular groups such as prisoners and the mentally subnormal. Secondary malnutrition accompanies any disease which disturbs appetite, digestion, absorption, or utilization of nutrients.

In poor and technologically backward countries malnutrition-associated disease is the major cause of death; it stunts the physical and mental development of the majority of the population. In more advanced societies it accompanies a wide variety of social, psychiatric, medical, and surgical conditions. Slight dementia, grief, physical frailty, deterioration of eyesight, hearing, or teeth, social isolation, and the degenerative diseases combine to make malnutrition common in the elderly.

The term protein energy malnutrition has been used to cover a number of clinical conditions in both adults and children. These include failure to thrive, marasmus, cachexia, phthisis, nutritional dwarfism, kwashiorkor, and nutritional or famine oedema. The large number of terms used reflects emphasis on particular clinical features. Notwithstanding the clinical differences, most of the physiological, biochemical, and body compositional features are common to all varieties of malnutrition, and the principles of classification, investigation, and management are the same for adults and children. The term protein energy malnutrition is best avoided; it carries the false implication that protein and/or energy deficiencies are the direct cause of all the conditions grouped under this rubric. Aetiologically neutral terms such as undernutrition or malnutrition, qualified as necessary, are more appropriate. The term chronic energy deficiency is sometimes used in adults; this is simply a confusing euphemism for thinness.

Nature of nutritional deficiency

If a growing animal is given a diet devoid of iron, there is an initial consumption of stores followed by clinical signs characteristic of iron deficiency: the concentration of iron in the tissues is markedly reduced, but there is no effect on growth or body weight. If such an animal is given a diet devoid of zinc there is an immediate cessation of growth and then loss of weight. After death from zinc deficiency, the concentration of zinc in the major tissues is normal; the animal has died from a nutrient deficiency without any direct evidence of depletion of the nutrient. This may appear confusing. However, in both iron and zinc deficiency the total amount of each within the body is less than normal, but in the case of iron the reduced amount is contained within a normally sized body whereas in the case of zinc the body size has contracted and hence the concentration is maintained. There is clearly a fundamental and distinct difference between these two responses to deprivation of a single nutrient. Most nutrients can be classified into those that give an iron-like (type I) or a zinc-like (type II) response (Table 1). The characteristics of the two types of deficiency are summarized in Table 2.

Type I deficiency

Most physicians consider deficiency in an essential nutrient in terms of a type I deficiency. The classical sequence of events is easily envisaged: the diet is deficient; with the low intake there is a reduction in the tissue concentration; the dependent metabolic pathways are compromised, giving rise to characteristic clinical signs and symptoms. The diagnosis is relatively straightforward and can be achieved by measuring the concentration of the nutrient in a suitable tissue, testing the appropriate metabolic pathway, and demonstrating the effect of replacing the nutrient, *in vitro* or *in vivo,* on a functional system or recognizing specific clinical signs.

Type II deficiency

The position with respect to the type II nutrients is quite different since none of the strategies used to diagnose a type I deficiency are appropriate for a type II deficiency. This gives rise to both conceptual and practical difficulties in the understanding, definition, diagnosis, and treatment of these deficiencies. Much of the controversy surrounding the definition, signs and symptoms, requirements, and diagnosis of type II deficiencies arises from attempts to conceive of type II nutrients as analogous to type I nutrients.

Table 1 *Classification of nutrients according to whether the response to a deficiency is a reduced concentration in the tissues (type I) or a reduced growth rate (type II)*

Type I	Type II
Selenium	Nitrogen
Iodine	Sulphur
Iron	Essential amino acids
Copper	Potassium
Calcium	Sodium
Manganese	Magnesium
Thiamine	Zinc
Riboflavin	Phosphorus
Ascorbic acid	Water
Retinol	
Tocopherol	
Calciferol	
Folic acid	
Cobalamin	
Pyridoxine	

Table 2 *Characteristics of the two types of nutritional deficiency*

Type I	Type II
Tissue level variable	Tissue level fixed
Used in specific pathways	Ubiquitously used
Characteristic physical signs	No characteristic signs
Late or no growth response	Immediate growth response
Stored in body	No body store
Buffered response	Responds to daily input
Not interdependent	Control each other's balance
Little excretory control	Sensitive physiological control

Type II nutrients are the building blocks of tissues which cannot be sustained without the necessary complement of each of these nutrients. A deficiency of any one of them results in catabolism of the tissue and loss of all its components. Resynthesis can only take place in the presence of adequate amounts of all components. Such nutrients can be considered as interdependent, analogous to the requirement for the correct balance of essential amino acids in protein metabolism. They have characteristic ratios that vary over quite a narrow range and are required in the diet in approximately the same ratios as they occur in the body.

An understanding of these particular nutrients is integral to the problem of malnutrition.

1. The response to a deficiency (growth failure with a mild deficiency and weight loss with more profound deficiency) is the same for each type II nutrient. Therefore nutritional growth failure or weight loss *per se* cannot identify which particular nutrient is lacking. Many experiments have been performed in which animals have been fed diets deficient in one or other of these nutrients, and in every case and every species the primary response has been a progressive diminution or cessation of growth followed by weight loss. No other feature has been shown to correspond reproducibly to deficiency, although some endocrine and other physiological adjustments mediate the change from an anabolic to a catabolic state. The response to a prolonged mild deficiency of any of the type II nutrients is stunting, the extent of which is determined by the degree and duration of the deficiency. Acute deficiency leads to tissue loss and wasting in both children and adults. Mild chronic deficiencies are more common than severe acute deficiencies, so that stunting is more common than wasting. About half the world population of children are stunted whereas only 5 to 10 per cent are wasted.

2. A common repertoire of metabolic changes and reductive adaptations takes place in response to any deficiency of type II nutrients. However, because whole tissues are being broken down, or at least there is no net synthesis, all other nutrients which are in excess relative to the deficient nutrient, either from the diet or from catabolized tissue, must be metabolized and excreted; they are not stored in the body. Thus the balance between the various type II nutrients in the diet is important, since a deficiency in any one of them results in a negative balance for all of them. For example if potassium is omitted from a parenteral feeding regimen, the patient will loose nitrogen, zinc, phosphorus, and magnesium; however, type I nutrients such as calcium will not necessarily be in negative balance.
3. If the diet is deficient in any of the type II nutrients mechanisms to conserve that nutrient avidly are activated. Thus it is extremely difficult to demonstrate clinical signs of such a deficiency in the non-growing animal by dietary means alone; usually there must be a coincident pathological loss of the nutrient (for example diarrhoea or renal disease). For this reason the rate of weight gain is the major determinant of the dietary requirement of a type II nutrient. For example children given a diet providing just enough energy for them to maintain body weight, without growing, are able to remain in zinc balance and maintain plasma zinc concentration with an intake of only 1.3 μmol Zn/kg/day. When the same children are gaining weight rapidly, their plasma zinc concentration falls precipitously despite a 10-fold increase in the amount of zinc consumed (14 μmol Zn/kg/day); at this level, the zinc supply limits lean tissue synthesis. No other sign, apart from growth failure and weight loss, is expected from a deficiency of one of these nutrients, unless the deficiency is very profound. There is a corollary which seems to contradict conventional wisdom: a diet which has a sufficiently low concentration of a type II nutrient to give clinical signs other than growth failure will affect the elderly first, then adults, and finally children. This is a consequence of the higher maintenance energy requirement of the child. Thus the protein requirement of a child for maintenance of body weight is about the same as that for an adult (0.6 g/kg/day); however, the maintenance energy requirement for the child is about 400 kJ/kg/day whilst that for the adult is about 160 kJ/kg/day. Hence an adult must have a diet which supplies 6 per cent of the energy as protein to maintain body weight, whereas a child only requires about 2.4 per cent of the energy as protein if he or she is not gaining weight. Therefore type II deficiency in children is expected to cause growth failure only, unless the child has a disease which causes a pathological loss of the nutrient. If a local diet is sufficiently deficient to give rise to other clinical signs, they are seen first in the elderly and last in children. However, there is such a large difference between the concentration which results in growth failure only and that which shows any other feature of deficiency that even where growth failure is common other clinical signs are very rare.
4. As growth rate is the major determinant of the requirement for type II nutrients, a 'catch-up' effect might be expected as a result of restoration of an adequate intake which could be used as a diagnostic test. Unfortunately, this does not necessarily happen. The initial deficiency will result in catabolism and a consequent loss of all the type II nutrients, irrespective of which caused the original problem. Therefore a catch-up response to the supply of only the deficient nutrient will be transient. Normal growth in man is so slow that diagnosis of deficiency in the habitual diet by supplementation is a correspondingly slow and difficult process.
5. One response which seems to be common to a deficiency of each type II nutrient is anorexia which is corrected if the appropriate nutrient is supplied. Such anorexia is related to the relative surfeit of other nutrients, particularly amino acids, which need to be metabolized and excreted to prevent toxicity. Data on specific dietary intake cannot be interpreted without intervention because a large or small intake may be caused by a deficiency of a nutrient which is not being considered. Conceptually, refusal to eat a diet which leads to disordered metabolism makes sense; there is then a metabolic preference for consumption of one's own tissues to satisfy nutritional demands. This strategy may have benefit in the short term by restoring metabolic balance, but in the longer term it leads to severe malnutrition. As growth will be limited by intake of the most deficient nutrient, it is only possible to have an effective 'deficiency' with one type II nutrient at a time—the limiting nutrient. The other nutrients develop a deficit, but this is silent and there is no positive response to any of them. When a dietary supplement is given, which does not contain all the nutrients required for new tissue synthesis, the rate of growth will be determined by the most limiting nutrient in the new diet, not in the original diet or in a supplement alone. Indeed, an incomplete supplement can make a deficiency worse by diluting the original diet.
6. If conventional techniques are used to try to make a diagnosis of deficiency of a specific type II nutrient, the results are likely to mislead. There is little point in performing a muscle biopsy and measuring concentrations because of the effects of the associated loss of whole tissue. If a change in the nutrient concentration is detected in the biopsy, that change is just as likely to be due to deficiency of another type II nutrient or a metabolic alteration unrelated to nutrition as to deficiency of the nutrient of concern. Changes in the concentrations of type II nutrients in tissues can occur as the metabolic state alters. For example, structural to soluble protein ratios affect the essential amino acid concentration of a biopsy; similarly, a reduction in protein synthetic enzymes may lead to loss of zinc from a tissue. Herein lies the difficulty: the responses are not at all specific. Although parvovirus infection may cause anaemia; it would be a foolish person who diagnosed this condition in all those with anaemia; however, transport protein concentrations, for example, are all too often interpreted as signs of dietary protein deficiency in an exactly analogous way.

The type II nutrients have always posed problems to clinicians and nutritionists because of difficulty in diagnosis. Unfortunately, the non-specificity of weight loss and the lack of confirmatory tests of an inadequate intake have led these nutrients to be largely ignored and their importance to be grossly underestimated. As a group, their deficiency is responsible for malnutrition in half the world's children and to unrecognized problems of ill health in many others.

Classification of malnutrition

Any classification system should have the practical use of either identifying those individuals who require intervention or examining the prevalence of malnutrition in a community so that preventive measures can be taken. The system should identify those most at risk, should be simple to apply, and should be accepted internationally.

Children

The most sensitive indicator of malnutrition in childhood is failure to achieve normal growth. Of the many classification systems proposed, three have gained general acceptance. In each of these the size of the child is compared with a 'normal' reference; the reference recommended by the World Health Organization (WHO) is the American NCHS (National Centre for Health Statistics) standard. Other standards have been used, but those derived from elite healthy populations from various countries are all very close to NCHS values.

GOMEZ CLASSIFICATION

The Gomez classification characterizes a child according to its weight relative to that of a normal child of the same age, expressed as a simple percentage. The grades are shown in Table 3. This system is used in public health screening and to evaluate the impact of public health interventions. It has limited clinical use for individuals.

Table 3 *Gomez classification*

Weight for age (% of reference)	$\frac{\text{Weight of subject}}{\text{Weight of normal child of the same age}} \times 100$
90–110	Normal
75–89	Grade I mild malnutrition
60–74	Grade II moderate malnutrition
less than 60	Grade III severe malnutrition

WELLCOME CLASSIFICATION

The Wellcome classification was introduced to overcome the difficulty of misclassification of children with oedema. It groups children according to two criteria: the presence or absence of oedema and, similar to the Gomez system, the weight deficit of the child for its age. The system is shown in Table 4. Each child is assessed for each feature independently so that four possible indices are obtained. An unfortunate result of the introduction of this classification has been the restriction of the definition of kwashiorkor to patients with nutritional oedema alone. Thus the term kwashiorkor is now used with two different meanings: one as a synonym for 'oedematous malnutrition', and the other to denote the clinical syndrome described by Williams where the changes in skin, hair, affect, and fatty liver are also important. Another unfortunate result is that by defining marasmus in terms of a child with a weight for age of less than 60 per cent of the standard, regardless of body habitus, both stunted and wasted children are included in the definition, whereas before it was used to denote only a thin wasted child. It is important to understand clearly how the use of the terms kwashiorkor and marasmus has changed. The Gomez and Wellcome classifications, by using weight for age, fail to differentiate between long-standing failure to grow and acute weight loss.

Table 4 *Wellcome classification of the clinical types of malnutrition*

Weight for age*	No oedema	With oedema
60%–80%	Undernutrition	Kwashiorkor
Less than 60% (~ −4Z)	Marasmus†	Marasmic kswashiorkor

*Percentage of the median NCHS standard

†Includes both wasting and stunting (see Waterlow classification).

WATERLOW CLASSIFICATION

Normal growth is a continuous, balanced, and predictable accretion of tissue that results in a steady increase in both height and weight. An adverse effect which continues for a period of time may result in slowing or cessation of growth. The child is normally proportioned, but as time passes he falls further and further behind other children who are actively growing so that the criteria for severe malnutrition are eventually reached. Because of the shape of the normal growth curve, the younger the child the more rapidly will he fall behind. If a normal child changes growth rate to half normal, he will be twice his present age before he falls below 60 per cent of normal and can be diagnosed as severely malnourished. A child who is exposed to a more severe insult will not only stop growing in height but will also lose weight, becoming underweight for his age much more quickly.

Thus within the group of children who are underweight for their age (Gomez and Wellcome classifications) there are two conceptually different conditions: first, stunted but normally proportioned (nutritional dwarfism); second, of normal height but thin and wasted (the original concept of marasmus). The two conditions can be differentiated by measuring the height as well as the weight and age. Stunting is determined by the height of the child relative to the height of a normal child of the same age (height for age), and wasting as the weight of the child relative to the weight of a normal child of the same height even though the normal child is usually chronologically younger (weight for height). The grades of stunting and wasting are shown in Table 5.

Two methods of expressing the data are in common use. The simplest is to express the weight/height of the child as a percentage of the normal. The second is to express the deficit in terms of multiples of the standard deviation of the normal population of children. The result is called a *Z* score. The *Z* score is much more difficult to calculate, but it is relatively independent of age and expresses stunting and wasting in the same relative units. Clearly, any child who has a *Z* score within ±2 is within the normal range; however, children at the lower end of this range are classified as 'mildly wasted or stunted'. Children who are more than three standard deviations from the normal have severe malnutrition. In children over 6 months of age, a deficit of 5 per cent in height for age or 10 per cent in weight for height is approximately equal to one *Z* score. This system, together within the presence or absence of oedema, anorexia, and complicating illness, is the most useful and appropriate for deciding which individuals require intensive treatment.

Rehabilitation of the wasted child can lead to restoration of lost tissue. However, correction of stunting is more likely to depend on public health measures designed to improve the family circumstances.

MID UPPER ARM CIRCUMFERENCE.

Between the ages of 1 and 5 years there is very little change in the arm circumference of a normal child. Thus this measurement gives a simple anthropometric measure of wasting which is almost independent of age. Table 6 gives an indication of the degree of severity of malnutrition in children with various arm circumferences which can be used for screening in the field.

Adults

BODY MASS INDEX

The assessment of malnutrition in adults is similar to that adopted in the Waterlow classification for children. Stunting in adults usually represents chronic undernutrition in childhood. This may have diagnostic implications but since growth is complete adult stunting is mainly of theoretical interest. It is more useful to define an index of 'thinness'. The most useful measure is the body mass index, defined as weight (in kilograms divided by the square of height (in metres). Table 7 gives values for defining adult grades of malnutrition. The same index is used to define grades of obesity.

Some sick adults cannot stand to have their height measured, and the measurement is not useful in those with kyphosis or scoliosis. Several proxy measures for height can be used in these patients. Although arm span is claimed to be equal to height, this is only valid in those about 1.6 m tall. Clinically, the most useful measurement is the demispan. This is measured as the distance from the middle of the sternal notch to

Table 5 *Waterlow classification*

	Normal	Mild*	Moderate*	Severe*
Weight-for-height deficit (wasting) (%)	90–120† (+2Z to −Z)‡	80–89 (−Z to −2Z)	70–79 (−2Z to −3Z)	<70 (−3Z)
Height-for-age deficit (stunting) (%)	95–110 (+2Z to −Z)	90–94 (−Z to −2Z)	85–89 (−2Z to −3Z)	<85 (−3Z)

*Without oedema. The presence of oedema denotes severe malnutrition (kwashiorkor), even without severe wasting

†Percentage of the median NCHS standard.

‡The Z score is also used to define malnutrition. For weight for age and weight for height, one Z score unit is nearly equal to 10 per cent of the median except in children less than 6 months of age. For height for age one Z score unit is equivalent to 5 per cent of the median.

Table 6 *Mid upper arm circumference in children aged 1 to 5 years*

Circumference	Level of nutrition
>14 cm	Normal
12.5–14 cm	Mild/moderate malnutrition
<12.5 cm	Severe malnutrition

Table 7 *Classification of malnutrition in adults by body mass index (BMI)*

BMI	
>20	Normal
18.5–20	Marginal
17–18.5	Mild malnutrition
16–17	Moderate malnutrition
<16	Severe malnutrition

Table 8 *Classification of adult malnutrition by mid upper arm circumference*

Circumference (cm)	
Male	
≥23	Normal
<23	Malnourished
Female	
≥22	Normal
<22	Malnourished

the tip of the middle finger in the coronal plane. Both sides should be measured; if there is a discrepancy the measurements should be repeated before taking the longest demispan. Height (in metres) in both males and females can then be calculated from the formula

$$\text{height} = 0.73\ (2 \times \text{demispan}) + 0.43.$$

MID UPPER ARM CIRCUMFERENCE.

As with children, the mid upper arm circumference can be used to grade the degree of body wasting in adults. Appropriate cut-off points are given in Table 8.

Clinical features

Severe malnutrition can broadly be divided into three clinical syndromes: marasmus, kwashiorkor, and nutritional dwarfism. In primary malnutrition each of these conditions is associated with poverty, deprivation, and infection; therefore they often coexist in the same individual and the clinical features frequently reflect a mixed picture.

Marasmus

The patient with classical marasmus has obviously lost weight, with prominent ribs, zygoma, and limb joints, gross loss of muscle mass, particularly from the limb girdles (shoulders and buttocks), and almost no subcutaneous fat. The skin, which is thin and atrophic, lies in redundant folds. The pinched look of the face gives the patient an 'old man' look.

Kwashiorkor

The clinical syndrome of kwashiorkor (a word from the Ga language of Ghana signifying the condition that a displaced child develops) was described by Williams in 1933. Typically, a child aged 1 to 2 years with fine friable discoloured hair develops a typical skin rash, oedema, and hepatomegaly. Psychologically he is apathetic when undisturbed and irritable when picked up. Kwashiorkor is an acute illness which develops abruptly. The history of swelling, loss of appetite, and mood change is of a few days only; sometimes there is a history of repeated bouts of swelling but this is uncommon (Fig. 1).

Nutritional dwarfism

On casual observation the nutritional dwarf may appear perfectly normal. It is only when the age of the patient is known that the short stature becomes apparent. However, dental development is less retarded than height, so that the facial shape of these children is inappropriate for their size (Fig. 2).

Oedema

Pitting oedema is the *sine qua non* for making the diagnosis of kwashiorkor. The extent of sodium and water retention in the extracellular fluid is variable. It is commonly 10 to 30 per cent of body weight but may reach 50 per cent in severe cases. The oedema is usually dependent and periorbital. Small accumulations of fluid may be found *post mortem* in the pericardium, pleura, and peritoneum, but large effusions are uncommon; if a serous effusion is present, the possibility of an associated condition such as tuberculosis should always be considered. Adults with kwashiorkor are more likely to have serious effusions. In severe cases the entire body and internal organs are oedematous.

Circulation

The retained sodium and water are not distributed evenly throughout the extracellular compartments. Depletion of the intravascular volume usually accompanies the enormous expansion of the interstitial space. This maldistribution give rise to the anomalous statement that an oedematous patient can be 'dehydrated'. This is semantically incorrect, and the term 'hypovolaemic' should be used to describe these patients. The use of the word 'dehydration' and the attendant concepts have led physicians to treat these patients incorrectly with rehydration solutions. In fact, the hypovolaemia in oedematous patients is a form of toxic shock and should be treated as such.

Hepatomegaly

Hepatomegaly is frequently encountered. The liver may extend to the iliac brim; it is smooth, firm, and not usually tender. The liver enlargement is due to fat accumulation, mainly as triglyceride. Up to half the wet weight of the liver can be due to fat. Indications of liver dysfunction such as petechiae or very slight hyperbilirubinaemia are serious prognostic signs.

Splenomegaly is very unusual in uncomplicated malnutrition: where it occurs it is likely to be associated with particular infections such as malaria, kala azar, or HIV.

Fig. 1 Skin changes of hyperpigmentation with stripping to leave hypopigmentation, most marked on the legs, but also present on the trunk, arms, neck, and face. There is oedema of the legs with obvious wasting in the pectoral region, fullness of the cheeks, and relatively normal hair.

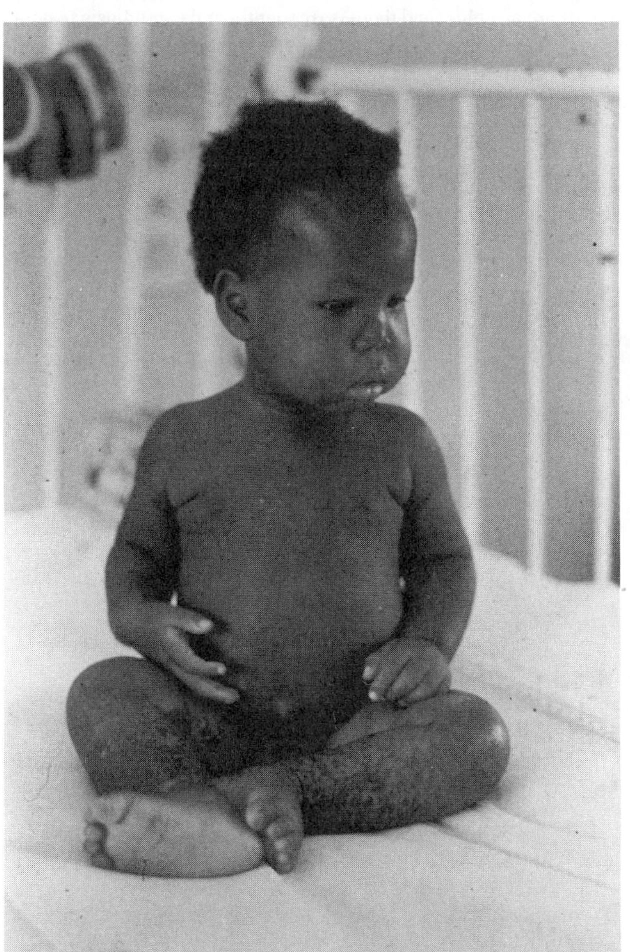

Anorexia

Loss of appetite is a common feature of all forms of severe malnutrition. The most probable underlying causes are infection, type II nutrient deficiency, and liver dysfunction. These patients usually have all three of these underlying causes.

Mood and behaviour

Children have an altered affect. Classically they are apathetic when left alone and cry when they are picked up. The apathy can be very profound, so that the children lie without moving in the position in which they are placed for prolonged periods; they may not try to move or cry during clinical procedures such as venesection. These children are prone to developing bed sores. When they cry, they emit a characteristic monotonous 'bleat' or loud groan rather than a normal 'bawl'. Because of atrophy of the lacrimal glands these children rarely cry with tears.

A series of stereotyped self-stimulating repetitive movements are frequently displayed; this is typical of psychosocial deprivation and absent stimulation. One of the most damaging types of self-stimulating behaviour is rumination. When alone, the child regurgitates the last meal and then re-swallows it; inevitably some is lost. Ruminating children tend to be more alert.

Skin

In kwashiorkor there are a series of sequential changes, the appearance and progression of which are not unlike sunburn. The skin changes usually occur over the course of just a few days. Often the different stages are present simultaneously in different parts of the body. The skin first becomes darker in colour, particularly over pressure areas and places exposed to minor trauma. The superficial dermal layers then dry like thin parchment and split when stretched to reveal pale areas between the cracks—crazy pavement dermatosis (Fig. 3). The dry cracked layer then peals off, leaving extremely thin hypopigmented skin. If it is gently pinched between the fingers numerous small wrinkles appear showing

Fig. 2 Nutritional dwarfism: the normal child on the left is 2 years of age; the child on the right is 8.5 years old.

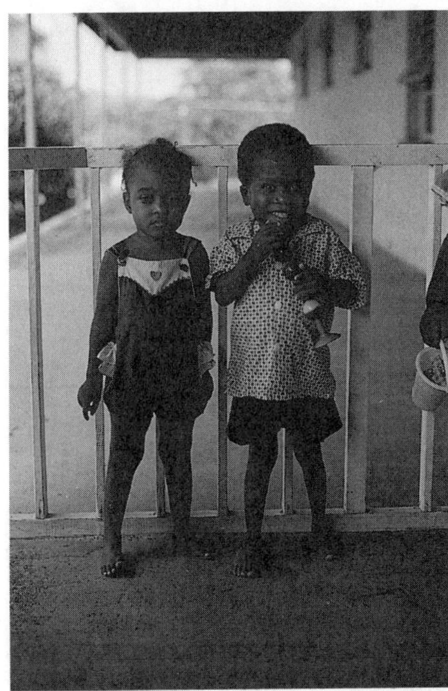

how thin and atrophic the epidermis is. The skin is very friable and ulcerates or macerates, particularly in the flexures, the perineum, and behind the ears (Fig. 4). In severe cases it may appear as if the child has been burnt.

Hair

There is atrophy of the hair roots of the scalp, and the hair can be plucked out easily and painlessly. Some patients go completely bald. The hair itself becomes thin, straight, and 'lifeless'. In patients with naturally curly hair the curls may be lifted up by the new straight hair to give the appearance of trees with straight trunks and a canopy—the 'forest sign'.

The hair may change colour to red, brown, grey, or blond. The reason for this change in colour is unknown. In ambulant patients it appears as if the hair is less resistant than normal to bleaching by the sun. If there are successive bouts of malnutrition interspersed with periods of normal growth the hair may become banded, giving the 'flag sign'. This is very uncommon as affected hair is normally lost after a bout of malnutrition.

Unlike the hair on the scalp, the eyelashes become long and luxuriant. There may also be excessive growth of lanugo hair. In adults pubic and axillary hair is lost and male patients need to shave less frequently.

Cheeks

Fullness of the cheeks, so-called jowls, is commonly associated with oedematous malnutrition. The cause is unknown; it is not due to parotid enlargement. Although there is usually marked parotid atrophy, painless parotid enlargement can occur in some patients, particularly malnourished adults. This seems to be associated with particular geographical locations.

Fig. 3 Oedema and superficial skin stripping in a child with kwashiorkor.

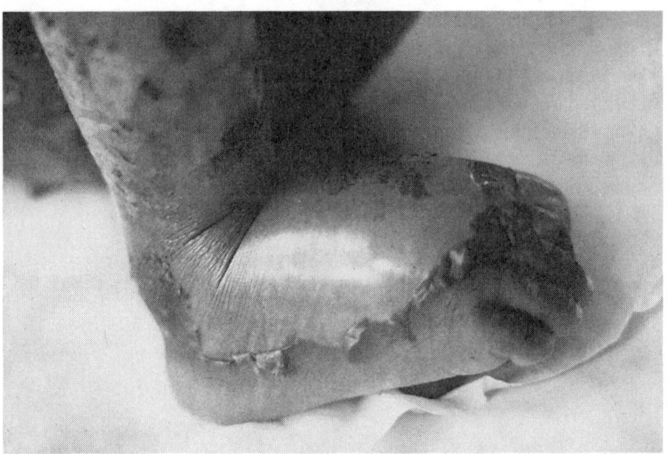

Fig. 4 Open skin lesions on the leg of a child with kwashiorkor.

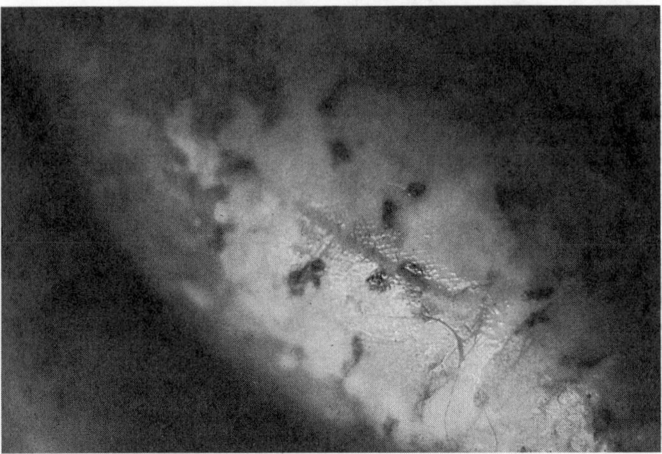

Gynaecomastia

Breast enlargement is not uncommon. It is particularly likely to occur in patients with gross hepatomegaly.

Bone

There is almost always an enlargement of the costochondral junctions giving a 'rickety rosary'. The cause may be related to abnormalities of vitamin D metabolism, or to vitamin C or copper deficiency. Harrison's sulci and other chest deformities from lung infections are quite common. Radiography always reveals marked osteopenia.

Abdominal swelling

The abdomen is usually protuberant (Fig. 5) This is due to gas in the intestine rather than the enlarged liver. Frequently, the abdominal wall is sufficiently thin for peristalsis to be easily visible. Bowel sounds are high pitched and infrequent. In newly admitted patients there is often a succussion splash from the atonic bowel.

Other features

The tympanic membranes are white and thickened (tympanosclerosis). The tonsils are atrophic, and there is frequently oral candidiasis. Angular stomatitis, lingual atrophy, follicular hyperkeratosis, eye signs characteristic of vitamin A deficiency, and other signs of specific type I nutrient deficiencies occur frequently.

Fig. 5 Postmortem appearance of a child who died from kwashiorkor. The enlarged fatty liver (50 per cent triglyceride wet weight), the abundant subcutaneous fat, and the dilated loops of bowel should be noted. In this case the skin appears relatively normal.

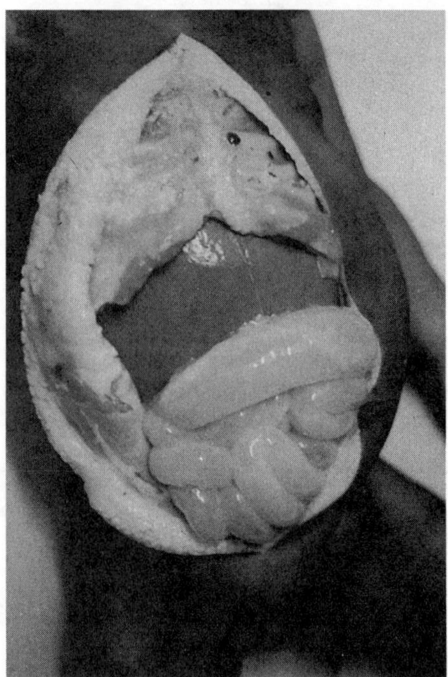

Pathophysiology

The sequence of events that occur in any malnourished individual is illustrated in Fig. 6. Although the defects reinforce each other in a cyclical way, the best starting point is the reduction in dietary intake. This may be due to psychiatric illness, anorexia associated with liver disease, infection, neoplasia, drug intoxication, type II nutrient deficiency, famine or starvation, upper intestinal disease, malabsorption, or other losses of nutrients from the body.

Reduced mass

The first effect of such a reduced intake is a reduction in body mass. This is the most obvious abnormality clinically, and forms the basis for the various anthropometric classifications of malnutrition.

Reduced requirement

As weight is lost absolute nutritional requirements are reduced, partly because of the decreased body mass. This can continue until a new equilibrium is established at a level where the lower intake becomes sufficient to sustain the reduced mass. However, this is not the only mechanism. There is also a relative reduction in requirement so that each gram of body tissue requires less energy. This component of the reduced requirement is very substantial, and is achieved over weeks or months by metabolic adaptation. In rats, the reduction occurs over 5–6 weeks and comprises about one-third of total energy requirement. Prolonged fasting in the obese also gives this magnitude of reduction in basal metabolic rate. Malnourished children gain weight slightly on a diet supplying 400 kJ/kg/day whilst malnourished; when the children are returned to exactly the same diet after recovery they lose weight.

Fig. 6 Schema showing the changes that occur in severe malnutrition.

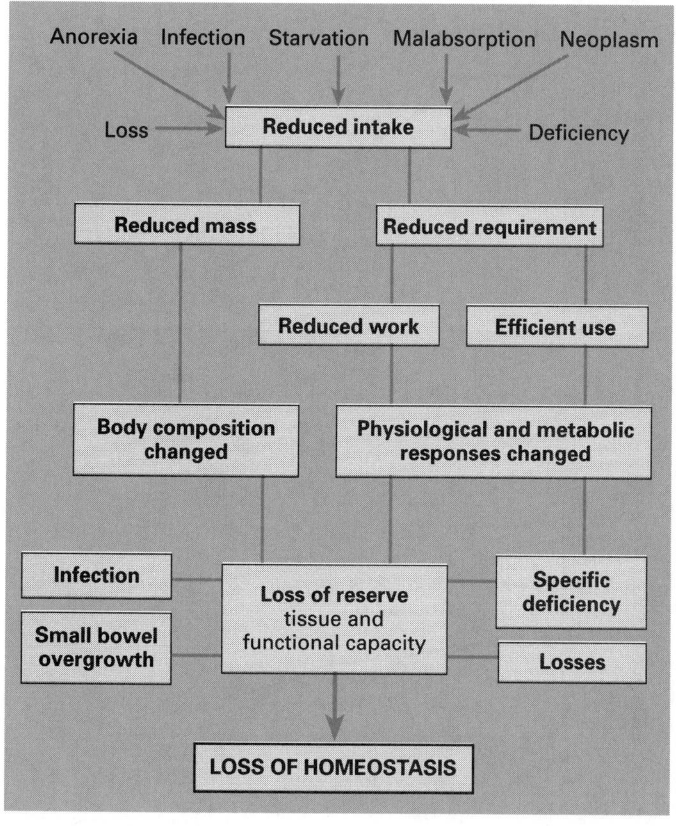

Efficient use

The reduction in relative requirement comes about in two ways. First, ingested food is used more efficiently. For example dynamic measurements show that a much higher proportion of the amino acids released from protein during tissue breakdown are reused to synthesize tissue instead of being oxidized. The physiological mechanisms that conserve nutrients in the body are activated and biochemical pathways involving futile cycles are curtailed. However, food is normally metabolized quite efficiently so that there is a relatively small absolute saving possible from increased efficiency; certainly it cannot account for a 30 per cent reduction in requirement.

Reduced work

By far the most important adaptation is in the actual work performed by the body itself at all levels of organization: the whole body and its organs, tissues, cells, organelles, and enzymatic machinery.

In the well-nourished individual the metabolic capacity far exceeds that usually demanded. Energy is used to maintain this excess capacity or metabolic work. It allows us to cope easily with rapid changes in demand for activity or from imposed stress. Thus we can run at 30 km/h, achieving a cardiac output of 20 l/min, eat 4 MJ of energy with 70 g of protein and 10 g of sodium at one sitting, and then fast for several days without untoward effects. In health, we maintain all the digestive, absorptive, hepatic, and renal capacity to deal with a feast without upsetting our *milieu interieur*. We carry a great deal of physiological redundancy in all our organs. This is why 'non-physiological' stress tests are used to diagnose disordered function at an early stage. Reserves of tissue and functional capacity are energetically expensive to synthesize, replace, and maintain. It is this excess capacity which is sacrificed in malnutrition and is the basis for the reduction in both the functional capacity of the organs and the energy requirements.

Physiological and metabolic changes

Reduction in work by the cells of the body leads to major changes in its physiological and metabolic responses. Indeed, no physiological function has so far been studied in severe undernutrition and found to be 'normal'. Some of the changes are listed in Table 9. Spontaneous physical activity is severely curtailed. The individuals perform no discretionary activity. Children no longer play or explore, and adults sit in a state of suspended animation, only moving when absolutely necessary.

At the other end of the spectrum is a fundamental adaptation—slowing of the sodium pump. Normally, about one-third of basal energy requirements are consumed by this ion pump. Thus this adaptation alone leads to a substantial saving. However, this is at the cost of allowing the intracellular sodium concentration to rise and the intracellular potassium concentration to fall. Of course, the potassium lost from the cell cannot be accommodated in the extracellular fluid and is excreted. Slowing of the sodium pump also leads to a reduction in cellular electrical potential and delay in its restoration; hence there is a reduction in neuromuscular function and muscle rapidly fatigues. Other processes which depend upon a sodium gradient, such as amino acid and glucose transport, have a reduced capacity in malnutrition.

A further third of basal energy requirement is used for the continual cycle of protein synthesis and breakdown in a process known as protein turnover; a considerable saving in energy expenditure is achieved by a reduction of about 40 per cent in the intensity of protein turnover.

There is a reduction in cardiac output due to both a lowered heart rate and a lowered stroke volume. The ventricular function curves (stroke work versus pressure) are altered so that the point of maximum performance occurs at a lower mean pressure; these patients are easily precipitated into heart failure.

Table 9 *Changes in physiological functions in malnourished children*

	Malnourished	Recovered	(MAL-REC)/REC (%)
Metabolic rate (kJ/kg$^{0.75}$/day)	315	417	−24
Sodium pump activity (h^{-1})	3.62	4.94	−27
Intracellular sodium (mmol/kg DS)	169	109	+55
Intracellular potassium (mmol/kg DS)	341	387	−12
Protein synthesis (g/kg/day)	4.0	6.3	−37
Protein breakdown (g/kg/day)	3.7	6.4	−42
Cardiac output (l/min/m^2)	4.77	6.90	−31
Stroke volume (ml/beat/m^2)	44.1	53.0	−22
Circulation time (s)	13.7	10.5	+30
GFR (C_{in} ml/min/m^2)	47.1	92.4	−41
Renal blood flow (C_{pah} ml/min/m^3)	249	321	−22
H^+ excretion after NH_4Cl (μmol/min)	10.4	28.4	−63
Osmolal clearance rate (ml/min)	0.20	0.66	−70
Percentage infused sodium excreted (%)	22.3	48.7	−54
Sodium excreted as a percentage of sodium filtered			
Normal ECF	0.50	1.23	−59
Expanded ECF	0.82	11.07	−93
Response to temperature change	Poikilotherm	Homeotherm	—

DS, dry solids; GFR, glomerular filtration rate; ECF, extracellular fluid volume.

The maximum concentrating and diluting ability of the kidney is severely restricted. There is a very limited capacity to excrete free hydrogen ions, titratable acid, and ammonia in response to an acid load. There is also a specific and severe limitation of the ability to excrete sodium, particularly in response to an expanded extracellular fluid volume. During the early phase of treatment, when the sodium pump is recovering and the excess intracellular sodium is being exported to the extracellular compartment, acute circulatory overload and sudden death can easily occur if the kidney recovers more slowly than the sodium pump.

The motility of the whole intestine is reduced so that transit time in the small intestine is increased. There is a reduction in gastric acid, bile, and pancreatic enzyme production. The cellular enzymes and transport systems for nutrient absorption are compromised and the mucosa becomes flattened; mitotic figures in the crypts become rare. That the defect is one of capacity and not a specific abnormality is demonstrated by the observation that absorption at low rates of presentation (perfusion) is relatively normal, whereas at high rates the digestive and absorptive capacity is overwhelmed.

The malnourished patient becomes poikilothermic. Even a modest reduction to 21 °C or elevation to 33 °C in environmental temperature may lead to hypothermia or pyrexia respectively. It is not unusual for malnourished children in the tropics to develop hypothermia, whereas in temperate climates this condition is commonly in the elderly. Normal individuals increase their oxygen consumption in response to a cool environment in order to maintain body heat by either non-shivering or shivering thermogenesis. Malnourished patients reduce their oxygen consumption in response to a cool environment (Fig. 7); they never shiver.

Marked changes in hormonal balance occur in malnutrition. Growth hormone levels are usually elevated in association with a low insulin concentration and a reduced insulin response to a test meal. Levels of insulin-like growth factors 1 and 2, catecholamine, and glucagon are low. Cortisol levels tend to be high. Levels of both free and bound thyroxine and tri-iodothyronine are low. There are also diminished responses to injected hormones, with down-regulation of most receptors. Although there is glucose intolerance, glucose levels are generally lower than normal. This is partly due to liver dysfunction as the degree of galactose intolerance is similar to the degree of glucose intolerance and there is a marked reduction in gluconeogenesis.

Fig. 7 (a) Response of the body temperature of malnourished children (closed symbols) and recovered children (open symbols) to changes in environmental temperature (squares 33 °C; circles 21 °C); (b) the oxygen consumption upon exposure to a cool environment in malnourished and recovered children. It should be noted that normal children have a higher body temperature and oxygen consumption in a thermoneutral environment.

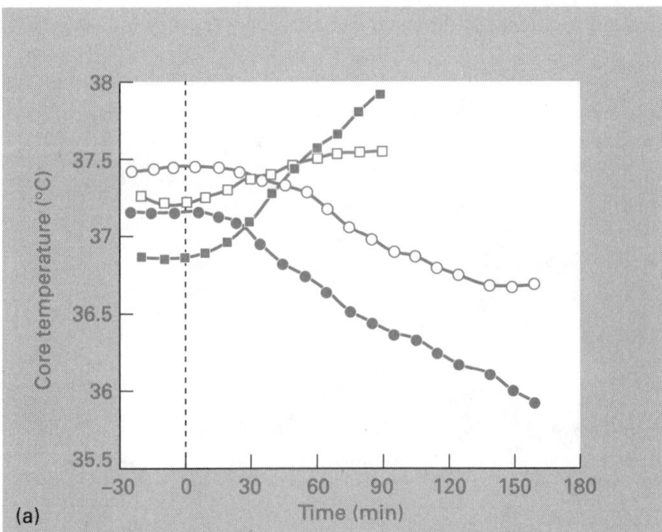

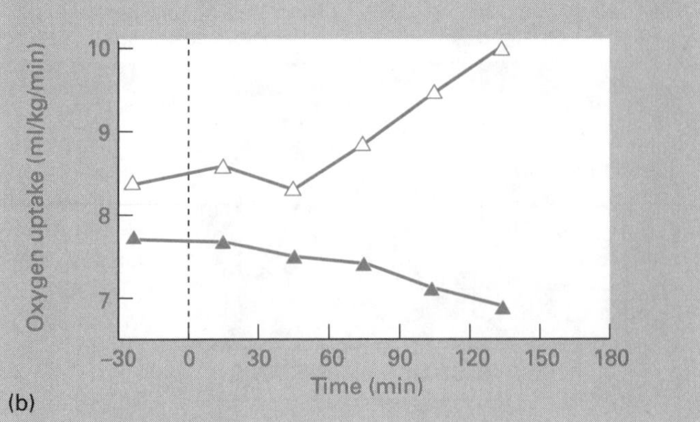

The febrile, acute phase, and inflammatory responses, and the immune system also partake in the reductive adaptation; they are either absent or severely blunted in seriously malnourished patients. Infection is normally recognized by the body's response in terms of fever, leucocytosis, pus formation, tachypnoea, etc.; when these responses do not occur, life-threatening infection may be unrecognized.

Body composition

Changes in body composition occur during malnutrition. Most tissues contribute to the loss of weight, but they do not contribute equally. Subcutaneous fat may virtually disappear and muscle mass is often reduced by more than half. Skin and intestine are also disproportionately affected, whereas the viscera and the central nervous system are relatively well preserved.

The chemical composition of the whole body is altered because of the absolute and relative changes in the size of its organs and as a consequence of the reductive adaptations themselves. Thus the change in activity of the sodium pump invariably leads to increased total body sodium and reduced total body potassium, irrespective of the patient's state of hydration or the serum electrolyte concentrations. When oedema is also present, the malnourished patient has increased extracellular as well as intracellular sodium levels; like the Biblical Lot's wife, these patients become 'pillars of salt'.

The reduction in the metabolic activity of cells leads to a reduction in the levels of enzyme, soluble protein, and RNA complement that are synthesized and maintained by the cell. Most of the trace elements are used to form integral parts of these cellular components. They cannot be retained in the tissues in isolation when the parent proteins are not required. Thus there is a reduction in the tissue concentration of zinc, copper, manganese, and magnesium. The proportionate reduction in each of these components of soft tissue is about the same (Fig. 8). It would be a mistake to measure one component of the tissue and conclude that there is a specific deficiency of that element; the reduction is a consequence of the change in metabolic state. Nevertheless, during reversal of the adaptation the deficits in all these components have to be made good before any weight gain can occur. Iron is an exception. There is an increased concentration of tissue iron in most forms of severe malnutrition, although not in patients with chronic blood loss from, say, intestinal helminthiasis.

Fig. 8 Cellular constituents in malnourished and recovered children. The values are expressed per unit fat free dry weight multiplied by various factors of 10.

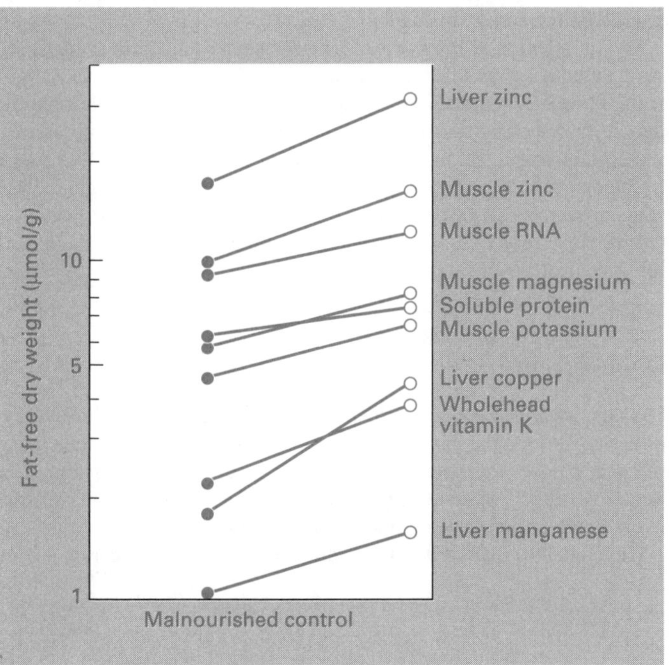

Loss of reserve

The cost of both the reductive adaptations and the reduction in functional tissue mass is to dispense with the reserve capacity to a greater or lesser extent. The malnourished individual has a reduced capacity to respond appropriately to the metabolic, environmental, or infective stresses that do little harm to a well-nourished individual.

Vicious cycles

Superimposed upon the reduced ability to respond to metabolic perturbations and environmental changes are the pathological effects of the stresses themselves. The curtailment of the inflammatory and immune responses results in repeated or, more usually, chronic infections. An atonic gut, achlorhydria, and poor secretion of IgA and bile salts combine to allow normal intestinal flora, both bacteria and fungi, to overgrow the small intestine and stomach. These organisms directly damage the intestine, deconjugate bile salts, and exacerbate any malabsorption. Unless they are suppressed, diarrhoea may worsen when additional food is given. The gas produced and the intestinal stasis is the reason for abdominal swelling in malnutrition; such swelling is characteristic of small bowel overgrowth which should be treated.

The diarrhoea and repeated infections give rise, in turn, to specific nutrient deficiencies, particularly of mineral elements. When the integrity of the skin is breached from the burn-like lesions of severe childhood malnutrition, bedsores, fistulae, and traumatic or surgical lesions which become indolent, blood and serum can be lost in considerable amounts.

The consequences of infections, small bowel overgrowth, malabsorption, nutrient losses, and thermal stress in a patient already adapted to malnutrition is to exacerbate anorexia and further reduce intake. The cycle is now complete. The adaptations are reinforced and physiological function is increasingly compromised. The debilitated patient then reaches a self-perpetuating stage where increasing anorexia and organ dysfunction leads to rapid deterioration and death. Patients often first present *in extremis.*

Loss of homeostasis

As the physiological and tissue reserve is whittled away and the effects of chronic infection and diarrhoea deplete the patient, he or she becomes increasingly 'brittle', like a diabetic patient losing homeostatic control of his blood sugar. However, unlike the diabetic, in the severely malnourished patient it is not just one organ or system which is functionally deranged but all of them. Eventually the patient simply cannot control his *milieu interieur;* everything slows down and stops.

When treatment regimens are planned they must always work within the patient's limited metabolic capacity whilst the reductive adaptations are reversed dietetically. Disequilibrium syndromes can occur during this reversal and lead to sudden unexpected death during early refeeding, even in previously obese patients who have been undergoing a prolonged period of energy restriction.

It is important to note that the classification systems for malnutrition are based almost entirely upon anthropometric criteria (the presence or absence of oedema is the only qualitative criterion), yet illness and death are related to the disordered physiology rather than the precise degree of wasting. There is not necessarily a close correspondence between these two facets of malnutrition. For this reason, clinical signs and features such as anorexia as well as anthropometric criteria, should be used in decisions to admit and treat these patients.

Oedematous malnutrition

Clinically, oedematous malnutrition is unlike other forms of malnutrition in that it is an acute illness. Patients that appear quite well may, over the course of a few days, become extremely irritable, progress through the various stages of skin lesions to give an appearance indistinguishable from burns, develop an enlarging liver, and then suddenly blow up with oedema. When they present they have overall retention of sodium but a low blood pressure and signs of hypovolaemia. In its severe form, the clinical picture is not dissimilar from those of toxic shock syndrome, adult respiratory distress syndrome, multiple organ failure, and so-called sick-cell syndrome. There are also similarities to patients with HIV infection in that there is evidence of profound incompetence of the immune system.

Patients with nutritional oedema, but no wasting or stunting, are metabolically quite different from those with marasmus. They may not show the reductive adaptations characteristic of other forms of severe malnutrition. Other features point to a specific role for infection, cytokines, and free radicals. Thus in oedematous malnutrition, in contrast with marasmus, there is increased excretion of urinary nitrate. Nitrate is the end-product of nitric oxide metabolism and is a measure of the whole-body nitric oxide production rate. The circulating levels and urinary excretion of the leukotrienes are also specifically increased. There is a reduction in cellular glutathione concentration, which is a key intermediate in protection of the body from the effects of free radicals. Measurement of the ratio of NADPH to NADP in cells from these patients show that they have a marked deficit in reducing equivalents. Furthermore, examination of the sulphydryl groups on proteins shows that an unusually large proportion of them are oxidized. Incubation of normal red cells with peroxides *in vitro* reproduces the profile of membrane lipids found in kwashiorkor.

The high intracellular sodium and low potassium concentrations are produced by a different mechanism from the slowing of the sodium pump seen in marasmic patients. The sodium pump is more active than normal in oedematous malnutrition where the cells have an increased complement of $Na^{+}K^{+}$ATPase. In contrast with the marasmic patient, the cell membranes are much more leaky to sodium and potassium; it is this membrane leakiness which leads to the loss of intracellular potassium and increase in intracellular sodium despite the increased activity of the sodium pump. In experiments in which glutathione in normal cells is reduced to the levels seen in oedematous malnutrition, the leakiness of the membrane is reproduced and the same electrolyte abnormalities that are seen in kwashiorkor arise.

In kwashiorkor there is effacement of the podocytes of the glomerulus to resemble minimal-change nephrotic syndrome, but without proteinuria. This is a morphological expression of a change in the surface anionic charge on the cell membranes. The defect can be corrected *in vitro* by perfusion with strongly anionic substances such as heparin. The role played by this change in charge in the formation of oedema is unknown.

Protein synthesis is disrupted in these patients. Electron microscopy of various tissues shows a marked reduction of the protein synthetic machinery. Hepatic export proteins are not made at a sufficient rate to maintain their circulating concentrations. The reduction in lipoprotein synthesis accounts for the large accumulation of triglyceride in the liver.

Most textbooks ascribe kwashiorkor to protein deficiency, but, this concept is now untenable. Protein deficiency does not account for the physiological and biochemical abnormalities; further, experimental protein deficiency does not reproduce the clinical features of kwashiorkor in any species of animal although it does result in stunting and wasting. The oedema can resolve completely on a very low protein diet with no change in plasma albumin level, and in the community no differences have been found in the protein contents of the diets of those who develop kwashiorkor and those who develop marasmus.

How might poverty lead to kwashiorkor? First, poor people live in crowded conditions in a highly contaminated environment and they are susceptible to many severe infections. Indeed, in the tropics epidemics of kwashiorkor follow epidemics of measles. Second, their diets are lacking in many of the type I nutrients that are crucial to protection from free-radical damage, particularly selenium, vitamin E, carotene, vitamin A, vitamin C, riboflavine, thiamine, and nicotinic acid. When an infection stimulates tissue damage, cytokine release, leukotriene synthesis, and free-radical production, these patients lack the machinery needed to protect their liver, skin, and vessels from acute damage. It is this acute damage that produces the syndrome of kwashiorkor.

Investigations

A careful history and examination usually provide most of the information required to treat these patients. The laboratory has a relatively minor role to play, and is used for the identification and characterization of infection and confirmation of type I nutrient deficiencies.

Urine should always be cultured if facilities are available. If there are perineal lesions, urine should be obtained by suprapubic aspiration. Absence of pyuria does not alter the diagnosis of infection in the presence of significant numbers of bacteria in a urethral specimen or any growth at all in a suprapubic specimen.

Tuberculosis is common; its diagnosis presents special difficulties as the Mantoux test is usually negative irrespective of the presence or absence of active disease. Acid-fast bacilli can sometimes be recovered from laryngeal aspirate obtained with a mucus extractor or from gastric washings. The optic fundi should be carefully examined in the dark with mydriasis for characteristic retinal tubercles. The chest radiograph is important and should be scrutinized carefully for small tuberculous lesions.

Infection causes much less shadowing on the chest radiograph than is the case with well-nourished children and may even be absent in the presence of bronchopneumonia. It is important to recognize interstitial lymphocytic pneumonia (HIV associated) because it is specifically treated with steroids which are otherwise contraindicated.

The blood should be examined for malarial parasites, and faeces should be examined for ova and parasites. Testing for sickle-cell disease is important in many communities.

The haematocrit or haemoglobin concentration may be helpful, although anaemia is usually clinically obvious. Changes in haematocrit often give clues to the distribution of fluid between the intravascular and interstitial compartments.

Measurement of plasma constituents is usually unhelpful in management, although thus information can be useful in assessing the prognosis. Plasma concentrations are not necessarily related to whole-body content, particularly for potassium and sodium. Hyponatraemia is frequently found and is a bad prognostic sign.

Therapy should be based on clinical criteria; it should be guided by frequent reappraisal of the direction of clinical progress and does not require laboratory data. Investigations are used for help with diagnosis, not to control treatment.

Management

The aims of treatment are to identify and treat all the life-threatening problems, to feed the patient so that weight is gained at an accelerated rate and 'catches up' with normal, and in children to start to stimulate mental development and to protect the patient from relapse and secure a continued normal development after discharge.

There are two main criteria for admission to residential care:

(1) the presence of anorexia of more than a few days duration.

(2) failure to respond immediately to a trial of outpatient management in the presence of (a) oedema, regardless of weight, or (b) less than 75 per cent weight for height and less than

60 per cent weight for age, or less than 70 per cent weight for height.

Treatment is divided into several phases: an initial acute phase of 1 or 2 days where the immediate threats to life are managed and treatment is initiated, an intermediate phase of about a week during which reversal of the metabolic abnormalities is expected, a rehabilitation phase of 4 to 6 weeks of intense feeding to return the child to a normal body composition, preparation for discharge where long-term outpatient management is initiated, and finally a follow-up phase.

The acute phase

When first admitted the patient needs to be resuscitated; the immediate need is to treat the infections, restore electrolyte balance, and start to reverse the physiological changes without overloading the limited capacity of the heart, kidney, intestine, or liver. The therapeutic implications of the reductive physiological adaptations are given in Table 10.

If the patient has true dehydration, this must be treated with extra fluid. However, patients with severe malnutrition differ from normal subjects in ways that make the diagnosis and treatment of dehydration one of the most difficult aspects of their management. First, signs of dehydration such as sunken eyes, poor skin elasticity, dry mouth, and lack of tears are all unreliable as they are themselves features of malnutrition. The only signs that can be used are those of a compromised circulating volume and an observed loss of fluid. Second, there is far more sodium inside the cells than normal and, if there is oedema, there is also excess extracellular sodium. This is the opposite of a normal person with diarrhoea who has a reduction in whole-body sodium and far less potassium and magnesium than normal in the cells. Third, the patients are very vulnerable to the ill effects of overhydration; fatal heart failure is common during the early stages of treatment. Fourth, there is nearly always some element of 'toxic shock' arising from infections. Thus these patients are quite different from normal subjects with diarrhoea or other types of dehydration. For these reasons, oral rehydration fluids are only given for a short time in limited amounts to restore the circulating volume before feeds are given.

The rehydrating solution used should have a lower sodium content (45 mmol/l) and higher potassium content (40 mmol/l) than is used for normally nourished patients. The oral rehydration solution recommended by the WHO should not be used. Because magnesium, zinc, and phosphorus are also depleted, solutions which contain these ions as well as the major electrolytes are particularly useful. A suitable formula is given in Table 11. Intravenous treatment is dangerous and, if given, needs much closer monitoring than in well-nourished patients.

One of the critical differential diagnoses in the malnourished patient with low tissue perfusion is between dehydration and toxic shock. Toxic shock is perhaps the most difficult complication to treat successfully; it accounts for a large proportion of deaths. In toxic shock, the stress of endotoxaemia is superimposed on the other problems of severe malnutrition. The veins and capillaries dilate, cardiac muscle is weakened, and blood pressure falls. The combined effects of the toxin, the metabolic changes produced by cytokines, and low perfusion of organs leads to increasing shock. Renal perfusion is reduced to a level at which the kidney cannot excrete the end-products of metabolism. The intestine fails to absorb and then secretes fluid; bowel movement diminishes and petechial bleeding occurs throughout the intestine. Liver perfusion is reduced so that gluconeogenesis becomes ineffective and the blood sugar falls. Even the metabolic stress of processing dietary protein can provoke liver failure and high protein diets are dangerous. There is a clouding of consciousness with a progressive decrease of awareness, which results from poor cerebral perfusion, hypoxia, electrolyte disturbance, and hypoglycaemia. The low perfusion of the tissues reduces the metabolic rate to a stage where there is insufficient heat to maintain body temperature.

Incipient toxic shock needs to be recognized in its early stages and its progression prevented. Management depends on the maintenance of cardiac output, the removal of the source of the toxin by treating infection, the prevention of hypoglycaemia and hypothermia, the strict avoidance of any stress such as giving excess fluid or protein, the provision of nutrition, and the correction of deficiencies. If the circulation is compromised, treatment is by cautious plasma expansion.

The principle of dietary management in the acute stage is to give enough to prevent hypoglycaemia and hypothermia, to prevent any further tissue catabolism, and to allow the patient to begin to reassemble cellular enzymes; this must be done within the capacity of the intestine, liver, and other organs. At this stage, not only may the functional capacity be easily exceeded, but deficiencies and nutrient imbalances may be aggravated if too much food is given. It is as important for the patient not to gain new tissue when in this state as it is to prevent the further loss of existing tissue. This is done by strictly controlling the energy intake. Children are given not less than 80 kcal/kg/day and not more than 100 kcal/kg/day; in adults the intake should be 30–40 kcal/kg/day. A child who is given less than 80 kcal/kg/day will continue to use his or her own tissues for food and will deteriorate; a child who is given more than 100 kcal/kg/day may develop a metabolic imbalance.

Because the amount of food that the intestine, liver, and kidney can handle is limited, the diet must be divided into many small portions fed at frequent intervals. The more 'brittle' the patient, the more restricted is his capacity; thus many small feeds must be given at frequent intervals to reach the total desired amount. In the extremely ill patient, the diet is given continuously via a nasogastric drip; intravenous feeding can be used in specialized centres in rich countries but the principles of management are exactly the same with these patients as with children fed orally in the tropics. In the less severely ill patient, food should be divided into hourly, 2-hourly, or 3-hourly portions. It should not be given less frequently than 4-hourly during a complete 24 h period. At this stage the number of feeds that have to be given and the fact that the patients readily develop hypoglycaemia and hypothermia means that they must be fed throughout the night and must have residential care.

The diet should contain every essential nutrient (all the minerals, particularly potassium and magnesium, vitamins, protein, and energy) as the patient needs to repair his tissues; if any one of these is not given in adequate amounts the patient will not recover. However, no nutrient should be present in great excess as this will cause a metabolic stress. The amounts of each nutrient that should be used for treating malnourished patients are given in Table 12. For patients with liver dysfunction, toxic shock, severe anorexia, or oedema a formula with limited amounts of protein and sodium is used—F75 (Table 13); 132 ml/kg/day (5.5 ml/kg/h) of this diet should be given. For other children the diet used during the rapid growth phase (F100) can be given during the acute phase (Table 13).This diet is most easily formulated as a single diet of 1 kcal/ml for use in all phases of treatment; additional water is given in the acute and intermediate phases.

INFECTIONS

Because of the poor inflammatory response, the usual physical signs of infection in the malnourished are unobtrusive or absent; infection expresses itself as apathy, drowsiness, hypothermia, hypoglycaemia, and death. Almost all malnourished children have infections, and many have multiple infections. There is overgrowth of the small intestine with organisms normally present in the colon, and normally commensal organisms, such as *Staphylococcus epidermidis,* become invasive. Infection of the lower respiratory tract, where appropriate samples for culture cannot be easily taken, is particularly common. Infections are frequently the immediate cause of death.

Early effective treatment with antibiotics has an important role in preventing toxic shock, improving the nutritional response to feeding, and preventing mortality. For these reasons blind non-selective wide-spectrum antibiotic treatment is recommended for all patients with severe malnutrition. Some clinicians believe that antibiotics should only

Table 10 *The main physiological changes in severe malnutrition and their implications for management*

Physiological change	Diagnostic and therapeutic implication
Cardiovascular system	
The heart is smaller and thinner than normal. Cardiac output and stroke volume are reduced. Saline infusion leads to greatly increased venous pressure. Overload of the heart readily leads to heart failure. Blood pressure is low. Renal perfusion is reduced. The circulation time is reduced. Plasma volume is usually normal and red-cell volume is reduced	Children are vulnerable to both an increase and decrease in blood volume. Any decrease will further compromise tissue perfusion; an increase can easily produce acute heart failure (increased respiratory rate). If dehydrated give special oral fluid for use in malnutrition (OFUM); do not give intravenous fluid unless in shock. Restrict blood transfusion to 10 ml/kg/day and cover with diuretic. Restrict sodium intake from the diet
Genitourinary system	
Glomerular filtration is reduced. The excretion of acid or of an osmolar load is greatly reduced. Urinary phosphate output is low. Sodium excretion is lower than normal. The kidney is physiologically unresponsive so that an expanded extracellular volume does not lead to increased sodium excretion. Urinary tract infection common	Prevent further tissue breakdown (treat infection and give adequate energy (80–100 kcal/kg/day). Do not give excess protein over and above that needed to restore tissue. Protein should have balanced amino acids (high quality). Avoid salts that can give an acid load (e.g. magnesium chloride, high protein). Make sure that water intake is sufficient
Gastrointestinal system	
The stomach produces much less acid than normal. The motility of the whole intestine is reduced. The pancreas is atrophied and produces a reduced amount of digestive enzymes. The small intestinal mucosa is atrophic with reduced levels of digestive enzymes. Absorption is reduced when a lot of substrate is given either from a high concentration or from large amounts of more dilute solutions.	The digestive and absorptive capacity of the intestine is limited; therefore the patient must be fed frequently with small amounts. If food is malabsrobed the first step is to increase the frequency and reduce the size of each feed (do not dilute the diet and give the same volume). The food is necessary to stimulate the intestine to regrow. There is overgrowth of the intestine with bacteria; this can be treated with antibiotics. Occasionally addition of pancreatic enzymes is useful
Liver	
There is a reduction in the synthesis of all hepatic export proteins. Abnormal metabolites of amino acids are produced. The ability of the liver to take up, metabolize, and excrete toxins is severely limited. The energy production from substrates (such as galactose, fructose) is much slower than normal. Capacity for gluconeogenesis is limited, leading to hypoglycaemia with stress of infection. Biliary secretion is reduced.	The patient should not be given a large meal to metabolize at one time. The amount of protein should be within the capacity of the liver to metabolize it, but sufficient to stimulate synthesis of export proteins. Drugs which depend upon hepatic disposal or are hepatotoxic should be given in reduced doses. Adequate carbohydrate should be given to prevent the necessity for gluconeogenesis
Immune system	
All aspects of immunity are diminished. Lymph glands, tonsils, and the thymus are atrophic. Cell-mediated (T-cell) immunity is particularly depressed. There is very little IgA in secretions. Complement components are low. Phagocytes do not kill ingested bacteria efficiently	Nearly all malnourished children have infections and overgrowth of mucosal surfaces. Blind antibiotic treatment should be given on admission to all children. Treatment will have to continue until the improved nutritional state leads to improvement of the immune system. The children are vulnerable to cross-infection. Acute admissions should be physically separated from recovering chidren.
Inflammatory response	
Tissue damage is not associated with inflammation; white cells do not migrate into areas of damage. The acute phase response is diminished	Signs of infection are often absent even after careful examination. Localized infection like lobar pneumonia is uncommon; generalized infection (bronchopneumonia) is common and may be present with no radiographic or other signs. Raised white-cell count and fever are not necessary. Otitis usually does not give an inflamed or bulging ear. Urinary tract infection is normally symptomless. Hypoglycaemia and hyperthermia are both signs of severe infection
Endocrine	
Insulin is reduced and there is glucose intolerance. IGF-1 is very low, although growth hormone is high. Cortisol is usually high	The endocrine system may not be able to respond appropriately to large meals. Give small frequent meals. Do not give steroids; they are already high.
Temperature regulation	
The children are poikilothermic. Both heat generation in the cold and sweating in the heat are impaired. The children become hypothermic in a cold environment and pyrexial in a hot environment.	Cover the children with clothes and blankets. Keep windows closed at night. Dry children quickly and well after washing and clothe them. Cool fevered children with tepid (not cold) water. Never use alcohol rubs to cool

Physiological change	Diagnostic and therapeutic implication
Cellular function	
The activity of the sodium pump is reduced and the cell membranes are more leaky than normal. This leads to an increase in intracellular sodium and a decrease in intracellular potassium and magnesium. Protein synthesis is reduced	All the children need large doses of potassium and magnesium. Sodium intake should be restricted. During recovery the sodium has to leave the cells and potassium has to enter; this easily leads to cardiac overload and hypokalaemia. Reversal of the electrolyte abnormality should be gradual and should occur after the kidney has recovered. If used at all digoxin doses should be halved
Metabolic rate	
The basal metabolic rate is reduced by about 30%. The energy expenditure due to activity of these children is very low	Internal heat production is limited. Most metabolic processes are sluggish
Body composition	
There is particular atrophy of skin, subcutaneous fat, and muscle. Fat is lost from the orbit. There is atrophy of many glands including the sweat, lachrymal, and salivary glands	Most signs of dehydration are unrealiable: eyes may be sunken with loss of orbital fat. Atrophy leads to folds of skin. Skin, mouth, and eyes are dry owing to gland atrophy. The children have limited reserves of energy. The respiratory muscles are easily exhausted

IGF-1, insulin-like growth factor 1.

Table 11 *Composition of an oral rehydration solution suitable for use in malnourished children (OFUM)*

Component	Concentration per litre
Sodium	45 mmol (45 mEq)
Potassium	40 mmol (40 mEq)
Magnesium	3 mmol (6 mEq)
Glucose	10 g
Sucrose	25 g
Osmolality	291 mOsm
Zinc	300 μmol (19.5 mg)
Copper	45 μmol (2.9 mg)
Selenium	0.6 μmol (47 μg)

be prescribed for clearly defined infection. This approach is only justifiable for senior experienced staff who carefully and personally monitor their patients. Microbiologists often advocate specific treatment of the particular organisms that they manage to isolate and recognize as pathogenic; this can be dangerous in malnourished patients because of the probable presence of multiple organisms, the need to suppress commensals, and failure to sample most of the potential sites of infection.

MEASLES (HERPES AND OTHER SYSTEMIC VIRAL INFECTIONS).

The mortality rate of severely malnourished patients with measles is very high. To reduce the risk of cross-infection from a newly admitted patient who is incubating measles, measles vaccine should be given to all malnourished children on admission. Those with severe malnutrition are often deficient in vitamin A. This is particularly associated with death from measles. However, measles can precipitate severe vitamin A deficiency in patients with reduced stores. As soon as measles is diagnosed, vitamin A should be given to all patients in the ward who have not already received it.

VITAMIN DEFICIENCY

In regions where measles or vitamin A deficiency is known to occur, even if clinical evidence of deficiency is uncommon, vitamin A should

Table 12 *The desirable nutrient intake (per kg body weight) from the diet during the acute and intermediate phases of treatment*

Nutrient		
Water	120–140 ml	120–140 ml
Energy	420 kJ	100 kcal
Protein	1–2 g	1–2 g
Electrolytes		
Sodium	<1.0 mmol	<23 mg
Potassium	>4.0 mmol	>160 mg
Magnesium	>0.6 mmol	>10 mg
Phosphorus	2.0 mmol	60 mg
Calcium	2.0 mmol	80 mg
Trace minerals		
Zinc	30 μmol	2.0 mg
Copper	4.5 μmol	0.3 mg
Selenium	60 nmol	4.7 μg
Iodine	100 nmol	12 μg
Water-soluble vitamins		
Thiamine	70 μg	70 μg
Riboflavin	200 μg	200 μg
Niacin	1000 μg	1000 μg
Pyridoxine	70 μg	70 μg
Cobalamin	100 ng	100 ng
Folic acid	100 μg	100 μg
Ascorbic acid	10 mg	10 mg
Pantothenic acid	300 μg	300 μg
Biotin	10 μg	10 μg
Fat-soluble vitamins		
Retinol	150 μg	150 μg
Calciferol	3 μg	3 μg
Tocopherol	2.2 mg	2.2 mg
Vitamin K	4 μg	4 μg
Lipids		
Total lipid	25–55% energy	
N-6 fatty acids	4.5% energy	
N-3 fatty acids	0.5% energy	

Table 13 *Formula F75 for use in the acute phase and F100 for use in the intermediate and rehabilitation phases of treatment of severely malnourished children*

Ingredient	F75	F100
Dried skim milk	25 g	80 g
Sugar	60g	50 g
Dextrimaltose/rice starch	60 g	–
Vegetable oil	20 g	60 g
Mineral mix	To give the concentrations in Table 12	
Vitamin mix	To give the concentrations in Table 12	
Water	To 1000 ml	To 1000 ml
Energy (kcal/100 ml)	75	100
Protein (% energy)	4.8	11.4
Carbohydrate (% energy)	71	36
Fat (% energy)	25	53
Sodium (mmol/100 ml)	0.6	1.9

be given routinely to all malnourished children on admission in a single dose equivalent to that used to treat vitamin A deficiency.

The patients are usually also deficient in folic acid and should receive 5 mg orally on admission. Many are deficient in riboflavin, ascorbic acid, pyridoxine, thiamine, and the fat-soluble vitamins D, E, and K. Where specific deficiencies are known to be common, the amounts in the diet can be increased, but therapeutic doses should be given to those with clinical signs.

HYPOGLYCAEMIA

All malnourished patients are prone to develop hypoglycaemia which can occur when a patient has not been fed for as short a time as 4 to 6 h. The best way to prevent it is to give more frequent feeds throughout the day and night.

A low body temperature, lethargy, limpness, and clouding of consciousness are usually the only features of hypoglycaemia in malnourished patients, although rigidity, twitching, or convulsions may occur; sweating and pallor, which occur in normal subjects, are unusual. Often the only sign of hypoglycaemia before death is drowsiness. There should be a high index of suspicion of this diagnosis, and if in doubt treatment should be given immediately. If the patient is conscious or can be roused and will drink, glucose in water, sugar in water, or a formula feed by mouth, whichever is most readily available, should be given and the response observed. If the patient is losing consciousness, cannot be roused, or has convulsions, a rapid bolus injection of about 1 ml/kg body weight of sterile 50 per cent glucose should be given intravenously followed by a nasogastric infusion of 10 per cent glucose or sucrose to prevent recurrence. If the intravenous glucose dose cannot be given quickly, about 50 ml of 10 per cent glucose or sucrose in water should be given nasogastrically. When the patient regains consciousness, an oral feed of a milk preparation or glucose in water should be given immediately, followed by frequent oral feeds to prevent recurrence.

HYPOTHERMIA

Hypothermia is a consequence of a low metabolic rate, and frequent feeding is crucial in the management of susceptible patients.

The ideal temperature for the care of malnourished patients is 25 to 30 °C (77–86 °F). Staff, who are active and fully clothed, often find this uncomfortably warm. They do not realize that a room temperature that is comfortable for themselves (20–24 °C) is to cold for malnourished patients, particularly small immobile children. Young infants, those with marasmus, those with large areas of weeping skin, and infected patients are particularly susceptible to hypothermia. Newly admitted patients should not be nursed near windows or in draughts; windows should always be closed at night. If the room feels at all cool, it is too cold for the malnourished patient who should always be properly covered with clothes and blankets. Washing should be kept to a minimum and done during the day, followed by immediate careful drying.

When the rectal temperature is below 35.5 °C (94.9 °F) or the underarm temperature is below 35 °C (95 °F), the patient should be warmed. This is best done by warming the air that is breathed by the patient, for instance by placing a lamp near (but not in contact with) the patient's body or placing warm (not hot) water bottles on the groins and underarms outside the clothes and blankets. Body temperature must be measured every 30 min during rewarming as these patients may rapidly become hyperthermic. All hypothermic patients must also be treated for coincidental hypoglycaemia.

SEVERE ANAEMIA

Blood transfusion is rarely indicated unless anaemia is severe (haemoglobin concentration less than 5 g per 100 ml or haematocrit below 15 per cent). Patients with severe anaemia need a slow blood transfusion of about 10 ml/kg body weight of whole blood or packed cells over a period of about 3 h. If the patient has heart failure, or heart failure is feared as a complication, blood should be given as an exchange transfusion: equal volumes of blood are removed and transfused by taking 2.5 ml/kg before transfusion and then at hourly intervals during the transfusion.

CONGESTIVE HEART FAILURE

This occurs as a complication of overhydration (particularly when intravenous fluids are given), severe anaemia, blood transfusion, plasma transfusion, or with formulae that have a high sodium content. It can also occur during early recovery when the extra food that is given causes sodium to come out of the cells and oedema fluid to be resorbed into the circulation at a faster rate than can be excreted by the kidney. Heart failure may be more common in areas where the diet is low in selenium.

The first important symptom that must be looked for is an increasing respiratory rate; treatment should be started at this stage. However, heart failure has to be differentiated from respiratory infection and toxic shock. They may be difficult to distinguish even after careful examination and consideration of associated signs. In this case the patient must be re-examined at very frequent intervals after any treatment is started so that the diagnosis can be revised if improvement is not rapid. Later signs are respiratory distress, rapid pulse, venous engorgement, cold hands and feet, and a purple discoloration under the fingernails and tongue.

When heart failure is diagnosed, all oral intake and intravenous fluids should be stopped; treatment for heart failure should take precedence over the need for feeding. A loop diuretic (e.g. frusemide 1 mg/kg) given intravenously may be effective, but the renal response may be substantially reduced in very malnourished patients. In such cases venesection (5 ml/kg) is a reasonable emergency approach. The withdrawn blood should be kept sterile in a syringe for retransfusion if the patient's condition deteriorates as a result of this treatment. More often there is an improvement, in which case further venesection is justified, always provided that the total volume of blood removed does not exceed 10 ml/kg. Although this is a very effective treatment in the appropriate circumstances, it should only be used by those with considerable experience. As malnourished patients have a low level of total body potassium and are frequently hypokalaemic, digitalis is rarely used. Trials of agents used in other forms of heart failure, such as angiotensin-converting enzyme inhibitors, have not been conducted in heart failure associated with malnutrition.

When heart failure is due to severe anaemia the treatment is the same, except that 10 ml/kg of red cell concentrate (or whole blood) is transfused in combination with venesection.

Intermediate phase

By the end of the acute phase the patients should have had their dehydration, toxic shock, vitamin A deficiency, and severe anaemia treated, and treatment for infections should have started. The beginning of a return of appetite is the sign that characterizes the intermediate phase of treatment.

Appetite is used as a barometer of progress. Loss of appetite occurs when the patient's metabolic processes cannot cope with the dietary intake. Great care must be taken not to overload the patient at this stage. However, it is necessary to maintain existing tissue whilst the metabolic abnormalities are being corrected and to replace deficiencies. As in the acute phase, the solution to this problem is to provide a source of energy which is marginally above the patients's requirement for maintenance, allowing a small excess for tissue repair. In practice this is achieved by giving not less than 80 and not more than 100 kcal/kg/day. When the patient is taking the diet well the formula can be changed from F75 to F100 (Table 13). The end of the intermediate phase is marked by the return of appetite and hunger. This indicates that the metabolic abnormalities are sufficiently corrected to allow progress to the rehabilitation phase. This usually occurs after 2 to 7 days; some patients with particularly complicated illness may take longer; others, who are hungry initially, can be supplied with high intakes immediately.

There are two ways of reducing the load that is given to the intestine and liver at any one feed. One is to reduce the concentration of the feed whilst keeping the volume constant (e.g. half-strength feeds). This method is not recommended: it either results in the patient receiving insufficient total energy or such large volumes of dilute feed that vomiting occurs. The preferred method is to keep the composition of the diet constant, to reduce the size of each feed, and to give feeds more frequently. This procedure take longer and requires more attendants, but underfeeding already malnourished patients is avoided.

Because these patients may not able to express thirst, their requirement for water may not be met from the formula alone. With such a degree of illness, clinical signs are difficult to interpret. However, extra water can be provided by nasogastric feeding.

MILK INTOLERANCE

Milk intolerance is seldom seen, even among severely malnourished patients; therefore all such patients should be started on a milk-based formula. Intolerance can be diagnosed if there is copious watery diarrhoea which clearly improves when milk intake is reduced and recurs when the patient is challenged with milk a second time. In such cases, milk formulae can be partially or totally substituted by other liquid foods. Milk feeds should be reintroduced and their effects noted before discharging a patient with a confirmed diagnosis of milk intolerance.

Rehabilitation phase

The acute and intermediate phases of treatment together usually take about 7 days, but this period can vary from 2 to 10 days in individual patients. The return of appetite means that infections are under control and that there is no major electrolyte imbalance or deficiency even though the patient's physiological responses are still abnormal and his capacity to eat is limited. If that capacity is exceeded during the early phases of rehabilitation, there will be a corresponding reduction of appetite. At this stage the cellular components needed to absorb and metabolize more food than is necessary for mere maintenance have been resynthesized and there is a capacity to make new tissue. There are still deficits of potassium, magnesium, zinc, and other essential nutrients, and so it is necessary to take in greatly increased amounts of all these components (as well as protein and total calories to allow anabolism. The most important factor determining the rate of recovery is the amount of energy ingested. The principle of this phase is to feed the patient to appetite and actively to encourage eating.

The transition between the intermediate and the rehabilitation phase is achieved simply by increasing the amount of the diet used in the intermediate phase that is dispensed at each feed (by, say, 10 ml per feed) until the patient starts to refuse to finish the feed despite encouragement to take more. Time must be spent with the patient to encourage him to try to finish each feed; the attitude of the attendants is crucial to success. The patient should never be left alone to 'take what he wants'—this is not what is meant by feeding to appetite.

As weight is gained appetite and requirements steadily increase. It is helpful to record weight, intake, and amount refused on a daily chart.

During rehabilitation most children and even adults take between 150 and 220 kcal/kg/day. Children should take a minimum of 130 kcal/kg/day and adults a minimum of 70 kcal/kg/day. The formula should not be discontinued if visible fat appears in the faeces, as a significantly high proportion of fat is still absorbed. However, fat malabsorption is a frequent cause of failure to gain weight at the expected rate. The fat content of the diet should only be decreased if watery diarrhoea is clearly shown to be dependent on dietary fat.

During the first few days of the rehabilitation phase oedematous patients may not gain weight despite an adequate intake because excess fluid is excreted as tissue is produced; in such cases the reduction or disappearance of oedema is clearly seen.

It is appropriate to maintain the patients on the formula until they have achieved a normal weight for height (children) or a body mass index of at least 18 (adults). At this time they usually signal their individual needs by spontaneously reducing their appetites and leaving more of the offered diet uneaten. They then enter the discharge phase of treatment.

With adults the general principles of supplying sufficiently high intakes of energy, protein, and all minerals and vitamins to enable them to gain weight rapidly must still be followed despite the fact that a mixed diet is given. Many normal diets have a low energy density (in the tropics) and have insufficient protein, minerals, and vitamins to sustain rapid rates of growth during catch-up. Further, the mixed diets often contain phytic acid and other chelators which markedly reduce the absorption of some minerals. To counter these effects, a high energy formula should be given between meals composed of the mixed diet. For example if a mixed diet is given three times daily, the formula feed should also be given three times daily to make six 'meals' each day.

Severely malnourished patients have a reduced iron-binding capacity: they are able neither to withhold iron from invading organisms nor to prevent the toxic effects of free iron itself. Iron should not be given during the acute and intermediate phases of treatment, even in the presence of severe anaemia, but should be reserved for the rehabilitation phase. Although iron can be added to the diet, it is preferable to administer it to the patients in the form of a liquid medicine (2 mg/kg/day); this avoids having to use separate diets for the intermediate and rehabilitation phases of treatment.

ASSESSING PROGRESS

Patients should be weighed daily and their weight plotted on a graph. It is useful to indicate weight for height (children) or body mass index (adults) on the graph as the target weight for discharge. Weight gain should be about 5–20 g/kg/day (usually about 10–15 g/kg/day).

EMOTIONAL AND PSYCHOLOGICAL STIMULATION

When patients, particularly children, are in their own homes, they are surrounded by familiar places and people. It is a major psychological trauma for a child to be separated from its mother, family, and surroundings, and to be left alone in a cot. This may be appropriate when a child is acutely sick, but interaction with other children should be actively encouraged during recovery. However, this is often discouraged by hospital staff on the grounds that it increases cross-infection and makes their job more difficult. This attitude, usually from senior staff, is misguided. The best person to be with the child is the mother, and every effort should be made to have her in the ward as much as possible. Malnourished children need affection and tender care from the very start of treatment, and interaction with other children when they become active. This requires patience and understanding by the hospital staff and the child's relatives. When the children have reached the rehabilitation phase, they can be allowed out of their cots for prolonged periods and kept on large play mats with each other. The risk of cross-infection is not increased substantially, and the benefit for the children is much more important than the convenience of the staff.

In hospital, it is not infrequent for 10 or 20 different adults to interact with a patient over the course of a day, each one manipulating but rarely talking to or cuddling the patient. This is not helpful, and is particularly bad if the mother is not staying with the child. Each adult should talk to, smile at, and laugh with the patient affectionately.

Provision of child-oriented care, with affection and tenderness, is insufficient of itself. Severely malnourished children have delayed mental and behavioural development that requires treatment as much as, or more than, their delayed physical development. If such delays persist, they becomes the most serious long-term result of malnutrition. Psychological stimulation through play programmes which start in hospital and continue after discharge can substantially reduce mental retardation.

The austerity of the traditional hospital has no place in the treatment of malnourished children. There should be a large safe fenced area, with mats on the floor, where the children can play. Brightly coloured mobiles should be hung over every cot. Hospital rooms should be brightly coloured with cheerful decorations. Where possible the staff should not wear uniforms, or at least they should have uniforms of similar design to standard maternal dress. Care must be taken to avoid sensory deprivation; the children's faces must not be covered, they must be able to see and hear what is going on around them, and they should not be wrapped or tied to prevent them moving around in the cots. Toys must always be available. The mothers should be taught the importance of play and shown how to make play materials. Toys should be safe, washable, and appropriate for the child's level of development.

In hospital, one person should be in charge of organizing and running a play programme. The play therapist should regularly introduce new activities and play materials which should develop motor and language skills. It is useful to have a curriculum of activities and to play with each child in a structured way for 15 to 30 min each day, in addition to the informal mixing of the children. Mothers should be taught the elements of the curriculum at the appropriate level. It must be emphasized that the family should continue to make toys and play with their children after discharge, and indeed throughout the whole period of development of their child. For this reason, teaching the mother is even more important than teaching the child.

Increased physical activity not only encourages development of the motor skills needed to explore the environment and play effectively but may also enhance growth during nutritional rehabilitation. Passive limb movements and splashing in a warm bath are helpful in immobile children.

Preparation for discharge

There is no sharp dividing line between the end of the rehabilitation phase and the discharge phase. The management of this phase should be started during rehabilitation and completed after discharge. By the time of discharge the child needs to be ready for full integration into the family and community; as this is the environment that led to malnutrition in the first place, the family has to be equipped to prevent recurrence.

A child is usually considered to be ready for discharge when the appropriate weight for height is reached. Although these children are often referred to as 'recovered', this is not usually true. They nearly all have the underlying effects of chronic malnutrition so that they are stunted and have delayed mental development; these defects also require attention. Management of these conditions depends on long-term changes aimed at improving the resources, diet, hygiene, knowledge, and skills of the family as a whole, and not upon care directed at the child alone.

Attaining normal weight for height, of itself, is insufficient reason to discharge a child from daily supervision. One of the problems with traditional hospital management is that anthropometric criteria alone are used for discharge and follow-up is inadequate.

Whenever possible, a home visit by someone who can determine whether adequate care can be provided should guide the decision to discharge. When the patient has been abandoned or the social and economic conditions at the home are hopeless, often because of the absence of a care-giver, appeals should be made for foster homes or other forms of community support.

The patient and care-giver have much to achieve and learn while they are in daily contact with the health staff. Education cannot be left to the last few days before the patient is discharged. Parents or care-givers should be taught about the causes of the patient's malnutrition and how to prevent it in the future, whether the malnourished person is a child or is infirm and elderly. In the case of children, the parents need to know the consequences of malnutrition on future development and the steps that need to be taken, over a considerable time, to reverse any mental impairment and stunting of height, and they need practical instructions on how to feed the child and continue nutritional rehabilitation at home. As these families are the most vulnerable within a community, the opportunity can usefully be taken to give information on child feeding and rearing practices, family planning, personal hygiene, methods of income generation, and sexually transmitted diseases.

Before discharge, children must be vaccinated in accordance with the local health regimen and provision made for booster doses to be given at the appropriate time.

Follow-up after discharge

There should be a plan to follow-up children at regular intervals after discharge. There should also be an efficient strategy for tracing those children that fail to attend follow-up appointments; these are the most vulnerable in society and their parents have not been able to cope. If possible, scheduled follow-up visits should take place at a special clinic for malnourished patients and not at a general clinic. Patients who relapse usually present within 6 months of discharge.

GENERAL CONSIDERATIONS

A child with severe malnutrition may reflect a serious problem in his household; the other children are also at risk. Therefore nutritional and health education is not restricted to avoiding a recurrence of the index case, but should include the prevention or correction of nutritional problems in all the family members, particularly young children, pregnant and lactating women, and the elderly.

The presence of children with severe malnutrition also suggests a high prevalence of malnutrition in that community. Health promotion can include education and promotional programmes for community leaders, local action groups, and the community as a whole. Such programmes focus on the psychological needs of vulnerable groups, the promotion of breast-feeding, appropriate use of weaning foods, nutritional alternatives using traditional foods, personal and environmental hygiene, water management, adequate feeding practices during illness and convalescence, immunization, early treatment of diarrhoea, pneumonia and other diseases, income-generating strategies, and adult literacy classes.

Additional problems with management of malnourished patients

STAFF ATTITUDES

Sometimes a particular patient fails to respond because staff do not believe that their efforts are likely to succeed. Where this exists, the patient's progress is usually poor; this in turn falsely confirms the 'correctness' of the original attitude and efforts are not made for similar patients in the future. This cause of failure to respond is among the most difficult to address, because it is usually based on the experience of long-serving senior staff. The dependence of each patient's well-being and survival on the attitudes of hospital staff should be carefully reviewed.

INFECTIONS

Atypical clinical manifestations of common infections occur in malnourished children. Those that are most commonly overlooked and interfere with a good nutritional response include urinary tract infection, otitis media, tuberculosis, congenital syphilis, cytomegalovirus infection, hepatitis, AIDS, dengue, giardiasis, cryptosporidiosis, and small bowel bacterial overgrowth with secondary malabsorption.

SPECIFIC NUTRIENT DEFICIENCIES

Many specific nutrient deficiencies impair the immune response. They can be the underlying cause of an infection that does not respond as expected to antibiotics. Some patients may have a profound deficiency in one or more specific nutrients that are not adequately replaced by the recommended therapeutic diet and nutrient supplements. Many commercial multivitamin and mineral preparations lack particular nutrients or do not contain sufficient amounts to treat a deficiency; they are generally designed for use as supplements by healthy individuals. Use of such preparations leads to overlooking a deficiency which is assumed to be covered by treatment. The specific deficiencies overlooked most frequently include zinc, magnesium, copper, selenium, folic acid, and vitamin E, although other micronutrients may be involved. Insufficient amounts of potassium and/or magnesium in the diet are common.

PSYCHOLOGICAL PROBLEMS

Nearly all malnourished children have been deprived of psychosocial stimulation. Most fail to thrive, and most develop abnormal modes of self-stimulation such as stereotyped movements.

A severe form of self-stimulation is rumination. Ruminating children regurgitate food from their stomach back to their mouth; much of that food is then lost from the mouth. This usually happens when the children are being ignored, so that rumination is not often observed and its presence is not suspected. Rumination occurs to some extent in up to 10 per cent of malnourished children. Ruminating children usually have a history of vomiting (without diarrhoea), they frequently smell of vomit because of soiling of their clothes and bedclothes, they are unusually alert and suspicious, they do not appear to be distressed by vomiting, they may make stereotyped chewing movements, and they usually take their feeds quite well and yet put on no weight, as if the food has disappeared. Rumination is treated by psychological stimulation until self-stimulation is no longer necessary to achieve gratification. This is best achieved through special attention given by a few staff members with experience and a motherly attitude. They need the skill to show disapproval consistently when the child initiates the vomit-inducing behaviour, without intimidating him, and to encourage other behaviour.

Another cause of failure to thrive is affective deprivation itself, whether as a result of long-term neglect and abuse at home, or because the child feels threatened in the unfamiliar hospital environment. In either case, all those who interact with and care for the child must show affection and give emotional support.

ASSOCIATED PATHOLOGICAL CONDITIONS

Malnutrition accompanies many congenital abnormalities, inborn errors of metabolism, tumours, immunological diseases, and diseases of the major organs. All these conditions occur in areas where primary malnutrition is frequent, just as they do in rich countries. Children with secondary malnutrition will often be misdiagnosed as suffering from primary malnutrition where this condition is prevalent. As the prevalence of primary malnutrition falls, the proportion of malnourished children who have an associated pathology rises. Failure to respond to treatment should lead to investigation of the major organ systems for primary pathology.

HIV INFECTION (ACQUIRED IMMUNODEFICIENCY SYNDROME (AIDS))

Patients with HIV infection are likely to present first with severe malnutrition. In some countries up to half the children presenting with severe malnutrition have HIV infection. It should be particularly suspected in marasmic children with splenomegaly and lymphadenopathy. It is recommended that children infected with HIV should be treated in exactly the same way as malnourished children without the infection. Experience shows that they respond well and gain weight in much the same way as non-infected children.

If severely malnourished patients are tested for HIV, this should be at discharge. A positive HIV test may lead the staff to treat the patient differently (or not at all) and to fail to follow him or her up after discharge. Although HIV testing is needed for epidemiological and prognostic purposes, it is not required or useful for the management of individual cases (except interstitial lymphocytic pneumonia); the result should only be available to the doctor in charge and procedures to maintain this confidentiality should in place.

SPECIFIC DERMATOSIS OF KWASHIORKOR

Spontaneous resolution can be expected with improved nutrition. Atrophy of the skin in the perineum leads to severe napkin dermatitis, particularly in children or the elderly with diarrhoea or incontinence. The perineum should be left exposed to dry without napkins. Application of a barrier such as zinc and castor oil ointment, petroleum jelly, or paraffin gauze dressing (tulle gras) to raw areas helps to relieve pain and prevent infection. Management should be the same as that used for burns. In countries with limited resources the affected areas can be bathed in a dilute solution of 1 per cent potassium permanganate for 10 to 15 min daily; this dries the lesions and inhibits colonizing organisms. The zinc supplement contained in the diet may be insufficient in these patients, as zinc deficiency almost always accompanies severe skin lesions. These patients should always be given systemic antibiotics.

CANDIDIASIS

Most malnourished children have candidiasis. It can be seen as whitish plaques in the mouth; however, even when the mouth is free of lesions, it may occur in the oesophagus, stomach, and rectum, as well as on any damp moist skin. Systemic candidiasis with growth in the respiratory tract and blood can occur in severe malnutrition. Oral nystatin suspension should be given to all patients with candidiasis. In addition, nystatin cream should be applied to any cutaneous lesions. Systemic candidiasis should be treated with ketoconazole.

Drug metabolism in malnourished patients

Changes in the physiology and composition of the malnourished patient will alter the pharmocokinetics of many drugs. There has been very little research on this aspect of either primary malnutrition or even the malnutrition associated with neoplasia or intestinal disease. The response of a patient with 7 per cent of body weight as fat to a fat-soluble drug will be very different from that of a patient with 40 per cent of body weight as fat, and yet this is rarely taken into consideration in prescribing. Poor absorption of drugs from the intestine, disordered hepatic conversion and reduced renal clearance of drugs, increased bacterial deconjugation of drugs excreted in the bile, and alterations in receptors and enzyme targets for drugs each affect their efficacy and potential toxicity. The changes are sufficiently complex for the result of giving a new drug to be unpredictable. These factors should always be considered in the treatment of all malnourished patient and, where available, therapeutic drug monitoring should be used. Clearly, the variables are potentially very important. For example if a patient with malnutrition, secondary to neoplasm, has features of kwashiorkor, is depleted in antioxidant nutrients, and has a low cellular glutathione, giving cytotoxic drugs or radiotherapy may cause irreversible damage.

Conclusion

The problems raised by malnutrition cover the whole spectrum of human experience, from that of the individual to society as a whole, at the medical, social, ethical, moral, and political levels. Malnutrition, particularly amongst children and the elderly, is the most common serious illness in the world today. Lessons learnt from the study and management of malnourished children are relevant to malnourished individuals of all ages and with a wide variety of disorders. A clear understanding of the aetiology and pathogenesis is a prerequisite for designing effective intervention and prevention programmes. The legacy of childhood malnutrition is to be seen in adults who are stunted physically and mentally; it may lay the seeds for many of the chronic diseases of unknown aetiology in adult life.

REFERENCES

Alleyne, G.A.O., Hay, R.W., Picou, D.I.M., Stanfield, J.P., and Whitehead, R.G. (1977). *Protein energy malnutrition.* Edward Arnold, London.

Briend, A. and Golden, M.H. (1993). Treatment of severe child malnutrition in refugee camps. *European Journal of Clinical Nutrition,* **47,** 750–4.

Brooke, O.G. and Salvosa, C.B. (1974). Response of malnourished babies to heat. *Archives of Disease in Childhood,* **49,** 123–7.

Brooke, O.G., Harris, M., and Salvosa, C. (1973). The response of malnourished babies to cold. *Journal of Physiology,* **233,** 75–91.

Golden, M.H. (1982). Trace elements in human nutrition. *Human Nutrition: Clinical Nutrition,* **36,** 185–202.

Golden, M.H. (1985). The consequences of protein deficiency in man and its relationship to the clinical features of kwashiorkor. In: *Nutritional adaptation in man* (ed. K.L. Blaxter and J.C. Waterlow), pp. 169–87. John Libbey, London.

Golden, M.H. (1991). The nature of nutritional deficiency in relation to growth failure and poverty. *Acta Paediatrica Scandanavica,* **374,** 95–110.

Golden, M.H. and Ramdath, D.D. (1987). Free radicals in the pathogenesis of kwashiorkor. *Proceedings of the Nutrition Society,* **46,** 53–68.

Waterlow, J.C. (1992). *Protein-energy malnutrition.* Edward Arnold, London.

10.4 Eating disorders

C. G. Fairburn

Introduction

The term 'eating disorders' is generally used to refer to two closely related psychiatric syndromes, anorexia nervosa and bulimia nervosa. These disorders share many features, and together they are a major source of psychiatric morbidity amongst young women. Anorexia nervosa has long been recognized with particularly good descriptions being published in the 19th century. In contrast, the first series of patients with bulimia nervosa was described as recently as 1979.

Anorexia nervosa

DEFINITION

Three features are required to make a diagnosis of anorexia nervosa. The first is the active maintenance of an unduly low weight: the definition of what constitutes low varies, 15 per cent below the expected weight for the person's age, height, and sex is a widely used figure. The low weight is achieved by a variety of means, including strict dieting or fasting, excessive exercising and, in some, self-induced vomiting. Patients with diabetes mellitus may underuse or omit insulin. Although the low weight may be the most striking feature, the second feature is the most distinctive. This is the presence of certain characteristic attitudes to shape and weight. These are sometimes described as the 'core psychopathology' and they are pathognomonic of anorexia nervosa and bulimia nervosa. Various expressions have been used to describe them, including the 'relentless pursuit of thinness' and a 'morbid fear of fatness'. These concerns are far more intense than the dissatisfaction with shape and weight experienced by many young women today. The third diagnostic feature is amenorrhoea (in postmenarchal females who are not taking an oral contraceptive).

DISTRIBUTION

Anorexia nervosa is largely confined to women aged between 10 and 30 years and to Western countries in which thinness for women is considered attractive. Estimates of the incidence of the disorder range from 0.24 to 14.6 per 100 000 female population per annum, and it seems that the incidence has increased in recent decades. Estimates of the prevalence of the disorder amongst adolescent girls, the group most at risk, range from 0.2 to 1.1 per cent. The disorder is rarely encountered among men (less than 10 per cent of cases are male) and it is also uncommon among non-Caucasians. The social-class distribution seems to be uneven, with there being an overrepresentation of cases from upper socioeconomic groups.

DEVELOPMENT OF THE DISORDER

The onset of anorexia nervosa is usually in adolescence, although prepubertal cases are encountered and occasionally the disorder does not begin until adulthood. Often it starts as normal adolescent dieting which then gets out of control. As the dieting intensifies, weight falls and physiological and psychological features characteristic of semistarvation develop. Additional methods of controlling shape and weight may be adopted at any stage. The characteristic attitudes to shape and weight do not tend to develop until slightly later on.

GENERAL CLINICAL FEATURES

The weight loss is mainly achieved through a severe reduction in food intake. The amount consumed may be very small and some patients fast at times. Typically the range of foods eaten is restricted, with foods viewed as fattening being avoided. Except in long-standing cases, appetite persists and for this reason the term 'anorexia' is not appropriate. Frequent intense exercising is common and adds to the weight loss. Laxative and diuretic misuse and self-induced vomiting may also be practised, particularly by those patients whose control over eating occasionally breaks down. This happens in about one-third of the patients, but the amount eaten is often not truly large.

Accompanying the disturbed eating habits is the so-called body image disturbance. This takes various forms. It may include a perceptual component such that all, or parts, of the body are seen as larger than their true size, and an attitudinal component characterized by an intense dislike of the body or parts of it. Neither feature improves as weight is lost: indeed, both tend to get worse.

Depressed mood, lability of mood, irritability, and anxiety and obsessional symptoms related to eating, are all common features. In more chronic cases there may be hopelessness and thoughts of suicide. There is preoccupation with thoughts about food, eating, shape, and weight, and concentration may be impaired. Outside interests tend to decline as weight is lost and social withdrawal may be marked.

PHYSICAL FEATURES

The physical abnormalities seen in anorexia nervosa have been the subject of much interest. Earlier this century the disorder was mistakenly attributed to pituitary insufficiency, and more recently, and again probably mistakenly, it has been suggested that there might be an underlying primary hypothalamic disorder. The main argument for such a disorder rests upon two observations: first, in small proportion of patients, menstruation ceases prior to weight loss; and secondly, restoration of a healthy weight is not always accompanied by the resumption of regular menstruation. However, it is likely that in both these instances the endocrine disturbance responsible for the menstrual dysfunction is secondary to dieting or overexercising, since both are known to affect menstruation and both often precede the onset of weight loss and persist following weight gain.

Symptoms and signs

Many patients with anorexia nervosa have no physical complaints. However, systematic enquiry often reveals heightened sensitivity to cold and a variety of gastrointestinal symptoms such as constipation, fullness after eating, bloatedness, and vague abdominal pains. Other symptoms encountered include restlessness, lack of energy, low sexual appetite, and early morning wakening. In females who are not taking an oral contraceptive, amenorrhoea is by definition present. Occasionally patients complain of infertility.

On examination, the degree of emaciation may be striking. Growth may be stunted in those with a prepubertal onset and there may be a failure of breast development. Unlike patients with hypopituitarism, axillary and pubic hair is preserved and there is no breast atrophy. A fine downy lanugo hair may be present on the back, arms, and side of face. Typically the skin is dry and the hands and feet are cold. Blood pressure and pulse are low. There may be dependent oedema.

Abnormalities on investigation

Endocrine abnormalities

Many of the abnormalities have been reproduced in studies of the physiological effects of dieting and are reversed by the restoration of healthy eating habits and a normal weight. Luteinizing hormone releasing hormone (LHRH) secretion is impaired, and as a result levels of luteinizing hormone, follicle stimulating hormone and oestradiol are low. There is an immature pattern of luteinizing hormone release. The luteinizing hormone response to LHRH is reduced, but the follicle stimulating hormone response is normal or exaggerated.

Hypothalamic disturbance is also evident in the delayed thyrotropin response to thyrotropin releasing hormone. In addition, there is reduced peripheral conversion of thyroxine to triiodothyronine, and an increased conversion of thyroxine to inactive reverse triiodothyronine. These changes are seen in other chronic illnesses. Thyroxine levels are in the low normal range, whereas triiodothyronine levels are depressed. Clinical evidence of hypothyroidism includes sensitivity to cold, constipation, dry skin, and bradycardia.

Plasma cortisol levels are raised and the normal diurnal variation is lost. These changes are due in part to the increased half-life of cortisol seen in starvation, and in part to a relative increase in cortisol production. Growth hormone levels are also increased, another secondary effect of starvation. Prolactin secretion is normal.

Haematological changes

A normocytic normochromic anaemia is found in a minority of patients and is sometimes attributable to a low intake of iron or folate. Mild neutropenia is common. The erythrocyte sedimentation rate is often low.

Other metabolic abnormalities

Hypercholesterolaemia is frequently present. The mechanism is not understood. Increased serum β-carotene may also be found and reflects increased dietary intake. Life-threatening hypoglycaemia very occasionally occurs and may not present typically due to impaired sympathetic response. Electrolyte disturbance is found in those who vomit frequently or misuse large quantities of laxatives or diuretics.

Other abnormalities

Cranial computed tomography (CT) has revealed enlargement of the cortical sulci and cisternes and dilatation of the ventricles. This appears to be reversible and has been termed 'pseudoatrophy'.

In long-standing cases, osteopenia and osteoporotic fractures are not uncommon and are thought to be secondary to the oestrogen deficiency and low weight. The extent to which the bone loss is reversible has yet to be established.

Delayed gastric emptying and a prolonged gastrointestinal transit time are common and may account for the complaints of fullness after eating, bloatedness, and constipation. Acute gastric dilatation is a rare complication which can be provoked by episodes of overeating or too vigorous attempts at refeeding.

AETIOLOGY

Predisposing factors

Dieting appears to be a general vulnerability factor for both anorexia nervosa and bulimia nervosa. It is a common precursor, and the two disorders are largely confined to countries in which dieting amongst young women is common. However, although many young women diet, few develop an eating disorder. Therefore other aetiological factors must operate. These include a family history of an eating disorder, obesity, and depression. The fact that eating disorders run in families is particularly well established: anorexia nervosa is about eight times more common in the female first-degree relatives of anorectic probands than in the general population. The results of twin studies suggest that this vulnerability may be in part genetic in nature. The personal histories of these patients often include reports of long-standing low self-esteem and extreme perfectionism. The finding that communication between family members is often disturbed is difficult to interpret since it has not been established whether the disturbance predates or follows the onset of the eating disorder.

Maintaining factors

As food intake decreases and weight is lost, there are secondary physical and psychological changes, some of which perpetuate the disorder. For example, delayed gastric emptying will tend to result in fullness even after eating small amounts, and social withdrawal may contribute by isolating the person from his or her peers. Those who have been overweight are understandably pleased with the weight loss and may be complimented on it, and many patients report that exerting strict self-control over their behaviour is rewarding in its own right. Sometimes refusing to eat also has gratifying effects within the family.

ASSESSMENT

Few patients with anorexia nervosa refer themselves for treatment. Usually they are persuaded to seek help by concerned relatives or friends, and as a consequence they attend somewhat reluctantly.

Careful history-taking from both the patient and, if at all possible, from an informant will make the diagnosis clear. It will be evident that the low weight has been achieved through the patient's own efforts and is associated with the characteristic core psychopathology. No physical tests are required to make the diagnosis. Similarly, unless there are positive reasons to suspect another physical condition, no tests are required to exclude other medical disorders. Excluding the presence of coexisting depressive disorder can be difficult, however, since many depressive symptoms are a known consequence of semistarvation. To make this diagnosis it may be necessary to wait until body weight has been restored to a healthy level. It is more straightforward to exclude the possibility that a depressive disorder is the sole diagnosis since the core psychopathology of anorexia nervosa is not present in depression and the weight loss is rarely self-induced.

Some patients present complaining of features associated with anorexia nervosa rather than the disorder itself. For example, they may present with gastrointestinal symptoms, amenorrhoea or infertility, or with depressive or obsessional symptoms. However, once the weight loss has been identified and it has been found to be self-induced, the diagnosis should be clear.

Although physical tests are not required for diagnostic purposes, all patients with anorexia nervosa should have a thorough physical examination and whatever investigations are indicated on the basis of the findings. The electrolytes should be checked of all those who frequently vomit or misuse significant quantities of laxatives or diuretics (see bulimia nervosa).

MANAGEMENT

Patients with anorexia nervosa vary. Some present with short histories and are willing and able to change, while others have an entrenched disorder and resist all attempts to help them.

In principle, there are two aspects to treatment. One is to establish healthy eating habits and a normal weight, and the second is the removal of those factors which have been maintaining the disorder. Both are essential. The returning of eating habits and weight to normal is mainly achieved through a combination of common-sense advice and nutritional counselling. This may be achieved on an inpatient, day-patient, or outpatient basis. Addressing the factors that have been maintaining the eating disorder generally involves the use of more specialized treatments, such as family therapy and cognitive behaviour therapy. Both these treatments require training and are best conducted on an outpatient basis.

Drugs have a limited role. Short-acting minor tranquillizers may occasionally be used to lessen the anxiety some patients experience prior to eating, and if depressive symptoms persist following weight restoration, antidepressant drugs should be prescribed. Tube feeding and intravenous hyperalimentation are rarely indicated.

Occasionally it is appropriate to use drugs to stimulate the resumption of regular menstruation. Most patients whose weight has reached a reasonable level and who are eating healthily restart menstruating within 6 to 12 months. If this does not happen, either clomiphene or luteinizing hormone releasing hormone are usually effective in inducing menstruation. It is not appropriate to use these drugs with patients who are underweight or who are eating abnormally. Instead, their eating disorder should be addressed.

The initial phase of treatment

There are four aspects to this phase of treatment.

Forming a collaborative therapeutic relationship

This is especially important in patients who are reluctant attenders.

Educating the patient

Patients need to learn about the clinical features of anorexia nervosa, the factors relevant to its development and maintenance, and the importance of weight gain. Certain popular books may be recommended.

Agreeing that there is a need for weight gain

A major goal is to establish the need for weight gain. In doing so, it is also important to emphasize that weight restoration is only one part of treatment, albeit a necessary one.

Deciding upon the treatment setting

Most patients with anorexia nervosa may be managed on an outpatient basis. Some need an initial period of day-patient or inpatient treatment followed by outpatient care. Outpatient treatment is not appropriate if the patient's physical health is a cause for concern, or if the patient is depressed and at risk of suicide. Physical indications for admission include: a weight below 70 per cent of the expected weight for the person's age, height, and sex; rapid weight loss; and the presence of medical complications such as massive oedema, severe electrolyte disturbance, and significant intercurrent infection. Under these circumstances admission should be to a general medical ward or a psychiatric unit with good access to general medical help. Partial or full admission to hospital is also indicated if no progress is being made with outpatient care, or if there are no outpatient facilities nearby.

Not infrequently, inpatient treatment is indicated, but the patient does not want to be admitted. Under these circumstances, unless immediate admission to hospital is essential, two options are available: either management on a day-patient basis or a brief trial of outpatient treatment. If the latter option is chosen, patients should be asked to demonstrate that they can gain weight at a reasonable rate (about 1 kg/week). It should be agreed that if they do not succeed, they will come into hospital. A small number of patients refuse admission even though their life is in danger. In such cases compulsory admission to hospital must be seriously considered.

Inpatient treatment

Admission may be to a general or psychiatric hospital. In either case it is a great advantage if the ward staff are experienced in the management of these patients. Weight restoration may be achieved in either setting,but with a psychiatric admission it is easier to make arrangements for the other forms of treatment needed to maximize the maintenance of progress following discharge.

Within a few days of admission, patients should be introduced to the consumption of regular meals and snacks consisting of between 1000 and 1500 kcal/day, and, if possible, by the end of 2 weeks these should be of a normal quantity and composition, consisting of about 2000 kcal/day. However, it is important to note that too rapid refeeding is dangerous since it may result in severe fluid retention, cardiac failure, or acute gastric dilatation. A target weight gain of about 1 kg/week should be set, with the patient and staff monitoring the weight gain each morning. Since between 3000 and 5000 kcal/day are likely to be required to achieve this rate of weight gain, average-sized meals and snacks will not be sufficient. It is the author's view that the best solution is to supplement the patient's diet with energy-rich drinks rather than additional food. Supplements of this type seem preferable to encouraging these patients to overeat, which does little to help establish healthy eating habits and may increase the risk that they develop bulimia nervosa.

The target weight range should be one at which the patient is eating healthily and not dieting, and one at which normal physiological functioning is restored. Once patients enter the target range, the energy-rich drinks should be phased out, leaving them consuming a diet sufficient to maintain their weight. At this stage patients should be given full control over their eating and they should be encouraged to shop, cook, and eat out with friends and family. Unless considerable effort is put into this phase of treatment, the risk of relapse after discharge is considerable.

Other forms of therapy should run concurrently with weight restoration. At first, straightforward support is often best, but once the patient's mental state begins to improve, more specific treatments may be introduced, including family therapy and cognitive behavioural procedures.

With an inpatient regime of this type, body weight is usually restored to a healthy range within 2 to 3 months and the patient discharged 2 to 4 weeks later. The transition from inpatient to outpatient care should be carefully planned.

Day-patient treatment

There is increasing interest in the use of day-patient treatment in place of full admission to hospital for all but the most ill patients. A comprehensive treatment programme can be provided, including supervised eating and weight gain, while patients remain based in their usual social environment. The hope is that day-patient treatment will be found to be associated with a reduced risk of relapse following discharge. This has not yet been established.

Outpatient treatment

This may be the sole form of treatment or it may follow a period of inpatient or day-patient care. Various approaches are used, from simple support and encouragement through to sophisticated forms of individual and family therapy. There has been so little research on the overall management of anorexia nervosa that firm recommendations cannot be made. There is evidence to suggest that family therapy should be used with young patients, and there is interest in using cognitive behavioural techniques with those who are older. (The cognitive behavioural approach is outlined in the section on bulimia nervosa.)

COURSE AND OUTCOME

For some, anorexia nervosa is a relatively benign, self-limiting disorder; for others, about a quarter, it may lead to death or chronic disability. Few consistent predictors of outcome have been identified, the exceptions being a long history and late onset, both of which are associated with a poor prognosis. The presence of a low body weight, bulimic episodes, self-induced vomiting or laxative abuse, and a history of premorbid psychosocial problems also tends to be associated with a poor outcome.

Although at least half the patients recover in terms of their weight and menstrual function, the disturbed attitudes to shape and weight often persist, and eating habits may remain disturbed. Up to a quarter of the patients develop bulimia nervosa. Standardized mortality ratios have been reported between 1.36 and 6.01, the deaths being either a direct result of medical complications or due to suicide. The most recent follow-up studies have obtained lower mortality figures, suggesting that the rate is falling. The outcome in males appears to be essentially the same as that in females.

Bulimia nervosa

DEFINITION

Three features are required to make a diagnosis of bulimia nervosa. The first is the presence of frequent bulimic episodes. By definition, these 'binges' involve the consumption of unusually large amounts of food, given the circumstances, and a sense of loss of control at the time. The second is the use of extreme behaviour to control body shape and weight. This behaviour resembles that used by patients with anorexia nervosa, although self-induced vomiting and laxative or diuretic misuse are much more common. The third feature is the presence of attitudes to shape and weight similar to those found in anorexia nervosa.

There are some patients with anorexia nervosa who have bulimic episodes similar to those of patients with bulimia nervosa and are therefore potentially eligible for both diagnoses. In practice both diagnoses are not given: instead, the diagnosis of anorexia nervosa is given precedence over that of bulimia nervosa.

DISTRIBUTION

People with bulimia nervosa are somewhat older than those with anorexia nervosa, most presenting in their twenties, and they have a broader social class distribution. The disorder is rarely seen in men.

There has been considerable interest in the prevalence of the disorder. Amongst young women in Britain and North America the rate is between 1 and 2 per cent with the great majority of cases not having come to medical attention. Although there are no satisfactory data on the incidence of bulimia nervosa, it seems that the disorder has become more common over the past 25 years. In all countries in which anorexia nervosa is found, there has been a dramatic upsurge in the number of cases of bulimia nervosa: from being viewed as an unusual variant of anorexia nervosa, it is now the most common eating disorder encountered in psychiatric practice (see Fig. 1).

GENERAL CLINICAL FEATURES

There are marked similarities between the clinical features of bulimia nervosa and those of anorexia nervosa. The patients share the same extreme concerns about shape and weight and engage in the same methods of weight control. However, there are two features which distinguish bulimia nervosa from anorexia nervosa: first, the body weight of most patients is in the healthy range; and secondly, there are frequent bulimic episodes. These binges are a source of great shame, they are kept secret

Fig. 1 Rates of referral to an eating disorder centre in Canada (Clarke Institute of Psychiatry and The Toronto General Hospital). (Reprinted with permission from Garner and Fairburn 1988.)

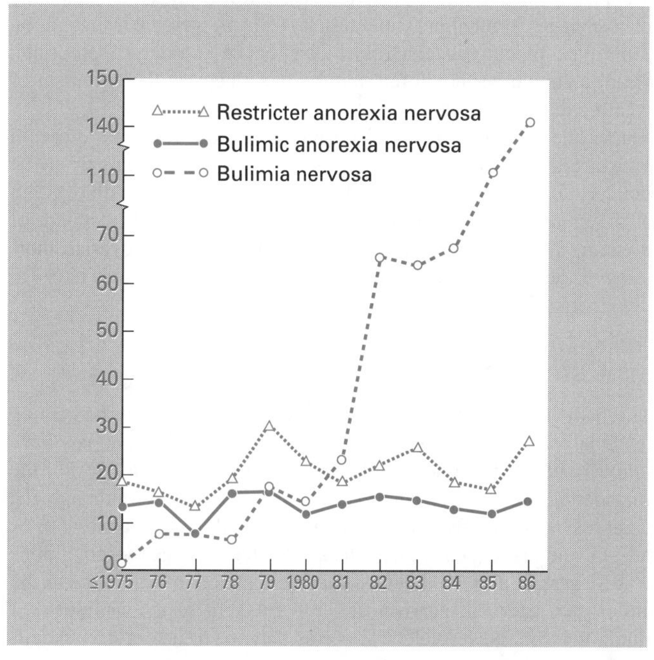

and, in the majority of cases, they are followed by self-induced vomiting or the taking of laxatives. Contrary to the impression given by the popular term 'carbohydrate craving', the proportion of carbohydrate eaten is not remarkable: the distinctive feature is the overall amount of food consumed, on average about 3000 kcal/episode. Some bulimic episodes are extremely large and carry the risk, albeit remote, of acute gastric dilatation or rupture. Between episodes, the patients restrict their food intake in much the same way as patients with anorexia nervosa.

Depressive and anxiety symptoms are also a prominent feature, more so than in anorexia nervosa. A significant minority have problems with alcohol or drugs.

PHYSICAL FEATURES

Symptoms and signs

The majority of patients have few physical complaints. Those most commonly encountered are irregular or absent menstruation, weakness and lethargy, vague abdominal pains, and toothache. On examination, appearance is usually unremarkable. Salivary gland enlargement may be present: typically, this involves the parotids and gives the patient's face a slightly rounded appearance. Sometimes it is associated with a raised serum amylase level, the increase being in the salivary isoenzyme. The underlying pathophysiology is not understood. In those who vomit there may be calluses on the dorsum of the dominant hand (Russell's sign) due to the fingers being used to stimulate the gag reflex. Also, there may be significant erosion of the dental enamel particularly on the lingual surface of the upper front teeth. A minority of patients, particularly those who take large quantities of laxatives or diuretics, have intermittent peripheral or facial oedema.

Abnormalities on investigation

Of most importance is the electrolyte disturbance, which is encountered in about half those who vomit or take laxatives or diuretics. Metabolic alkalosis, hypochloraemia, and hypokalaemia are the most common abnormalities, and they may account for the weakness and tiredness (and on rare occasions hypokalaemic paralysis) experienced by some patients. The overall picture may resemble Bartter's syndrome and has been termed 'pseudo Bartter's syndrome' since it is self-inflicted and usually reversible. Severe electrolyte disturbance is occasionally encountered, particularly low potassium levels, but even when it is long-standing there may be surprisingly few accompanying symptoms. Despite concern about possible cardiac arrhythmias, nephrogenic diabetes insipidus, and the suggestion that chronic hypokalaemia may induce changes in renal proximal tubular cells, aggressive investigation of this type of chronic electrolyte disturbance is rarely appropriate: instead, it should be monitored, but the focus kept on the treatment of the eating disorder itself.

Endocrine abnormalities may be present. These resemble those in anorexia nervosa, but they are not as severe. They are thought to be secondary to the strict dieting and they are probably reversible, given that the menstrual disturbance responds to the successful treatment of the eating disorder. There have been recent reports that ovarian morphology is abnormal in a high proportion of cases. This is also likely to be reversible.

AETIOLOGY

Many patients with bulimia nervosa give a history of disturbed eating stretching back into adolescence, and about one-third of patients have previously fulfilled diagnostic criteria for anorexia nervosa. Most of the remainder started with an anorexia nervosa-like picture, although the weight loss was not of sufficient magnitude to allow the diagnosis to be made. Given this sequence of events and the fact that the two conditions are so similar, it may be assumed that most factors of relevance to the aetiology of anorexia nervosa are also relevant to the aetiology of bulimia nervosa. Nevertheless, it seems that some factors may specifically increase the risk of developing bulimia nervosa rather than anorexia nervosa. These include vulnerability to obesity, affective disorder, and substance abuse, the rates of all three disorders being particularly high amongst the relatives of these patients.

ASSESSMENT

Most people with bulimia nervosa are ashamed of their eating habits and keep them secret for many years. Like those with anorexia nervosa, when they present for help they may complain of features associated with the disorder rather than the disorder itself. For example, they may present with gastrointestinal or gynaecological symptoms, depression, or substance abuse. Under these circumstances making the correct diagnosis may be difficult since there are rarely any clear pointers to the eating disorder.

Those patients who present complaining of the eating disorder are generally referred to psychiatrists, and unlike those with anorexia nervosa, they are usually eager to receive treatment. Assessment is straightforward and the diagnosis can be made with little difficulty. As with anorexia nervosa, no physical tests are needed to make the diagnosis. However, the electrolytes should be checked of all those who frequently vomit or misuse large quantities of laxatives or diuretics.

TREATMENT

The treatment of bulimia nervosa has been the subject of much research. It is clear that the great majority of patients may be managed on an outpatient basis. Treatment in hospital, either partly or fully, is indicated under four unusual circumstances: first, if the patient is either too depressed to be managed as an outpatient or if there is a risk of suicide; secondly, if the patient's physical health is a cause for concern; thirdly, if the patient is in the first trimester of pregnancy, since there is some evidence that the spontaneous abortion rate under these conditions may be high; and fourthly, if the eating disorder proves refractory to outpatient care. If admission to hospital is indicated, it should be brief and serve as a preliminary to outpatient care.

Psychological treatment

The most effective treatment for bulimia nervosa is a specific form of cognitive behaviour therapy. This is a specialized psychological treatment which aims to modify not only the disturbed eating habits but also the disturbed attitudes to shape and weight. It usually involves about 20 sessions over 5 months and results in substantial improvement in all aspects of the psychopathology. The techniques used include the following: the daily self-monitoring of relevant thoughts and behaviour; education about eating, shape, and weight; the use of self-control procedures to help establish a pattern of regular eating; the gradual introduction of avoided foods into the patient's diet; and so-called cognitive restructuring procedures designed to identify and challenge problematic thoughts and attitudes.

Pharmacological treatment

Antidepressant drugs are the only pharmacological treatment to have shown promise. They result in a decline in the frequency of overeating and an improvement in mood, but the effect is not as great as that seen with cognitive behaviour therapy and, more importantly, it is often not maintained. These drugs cannot be recommended as a first-line treatment. Appetite suppressants have no beneficial effect.

Other approaches

Some patients respond to brief educational treatments and self-help manuals probably have a role. For this reason a 'stepped-care' approach to treatment delivery has been proposed in which treatments are provided sequentially according to need. This approach involves a simple treatment being used initially, and moving on to more complex ones only if the patient fails to respond.

COURSE AND OUTCOME

As yet little is known about the course of bulimia nervosa. Some of the cases identified in community surveys appear to be relatively benign in that they are short-lived. In contrast, patients who are referred for treatment often present with long histories and previous unsuccessful attempts at treatment. Most respond well to cognitive behaviour therapy, with the changes being maintained for at least the following 12 months. There have been no studies of long-term outcome. The evidence to date suggests that the disorder tends to 'breed true'; that is, it rarely evolves into anorexia nervosa or any other psychiatric disorder.

PREGNANCY AND CHILDREARING

There is growing concern about the effects of eating disorders on pregnancy and childrearing. This topic has come to the fore with the emergence of bulimia nervosa, since pregnancy does not often occur in the course of anorexia nervosa. In general it seems that eating disorders tend to improve during pregnancy, but the amount of weight gained may be abnormal. The impact on the fetus has yet to be established, although there have been reports of intrauterine growth retardation and low birth weight. Childrearing is influenced in some cases, with there being adverse effects on both infant feeding and growth.

Atypical eating disorders

In addition to anorexia nervosa and bulimia nervosa, various 'atypical eating disorders' are encountered: indeed, they make up over a third of all referrals. They have not been well characterized. Most common are disorders resembling anorexia nervosa or bulimia nervosa but not quite meeting their diagnostic criteria, either because one or more features is absent or because the features are not of sufficient severity, or both. In addition, there are people with eating problems distinct from anorexia nervosa and bulimia nervosa. For example, there are those who vomit when anxious, and people who have difficulty eating or swallowing in public. Both these groups should be classed as having an anxiety disorder and treated accordingly. There is another group of patients who stop eating as a way of bringing attention to themselves. Such people generally have major personality difficulties. In common with those with anxiety disorders, they do not show the attitudes to shape and weight that are characteristic of patients with anorexia nervosa and bulimia nervosa. Their management needs to focus on resolving the problems that brought about their refusal to eat, rather than on the disturbed eating itself.

REFERENCES

Brumberg, J.J. (1988). *Fasting girls*. Harvard, Cambridge. An excellent history of anorexia nervosa

Cooper, P.J. (1993). *Bulimia nervosa: a guide to recovery*. Robinson, London. A self-help manual designed for use as the first step in a stepped-care programme.

Crisp, A.H., Callender, J.S., Halek, C. and Hsu, L.K.G. (1992). Long-term mortality in anorexia nervosa. *British Journal of Psychiatry* **161,** 104–7.

Fairburn, C.G. and Beglin, S.J. (1990). Studies of the epidemiology of bulimia nervosa. *American Journal of Psychiatry* **147,** 401–8.

Fairburn, C.G., Marcus, M.D., and Wilson, G.T. (1993). Cognitive behaviour therapy for binge eating and bulimia nervosa: a comprehensive treatment manual. In *Binge eating: nature, assessment and treatment*, (ed. C.G. Fairburn and G.T. Wilson). Guilford, New York. A detailed description of the most effective form of treatment for bulimia nervosa.

Garner, D.M. and Fairburn, C.G. (1988). Relationship between anorexia nervosa and bulimia nervosa: diagnostic implications. In *Diagnostic issues in anorexia nervosa and bulimia nervosa*, (ed. D.M. Garner and P.E. Garfinkel). Brunner/Mazel, New York.

Garner, D.M. and Garfinkel, P.E. (ed.) (1985). *Handbook of psychotherapy for anorexia nervosa and bulimia nervosa*. Guilford, New York. A collection of chapters describing the various approaches to the treatment of anorexia nervosa and bulimia nervosa.

Goodwin, G.M. (1990). Neuroendocrine function and the biology of the eating disorders. *Human Psychopharmacology* **5,** 249–53.

Hsu, L.K.G. (1990). *Eating disorders*. Guilford, New York. An excellent account of the field.

Lucas, A.R., Beard, C.M., O'Fallon, W.M., and Kurland, L.T. (1991). 50 year trends in the incidence of anorexia nervosa in Rochester, Minnesota: a population-based study. *American Journal of Psychiatry* **148,** 917–22.

Mitchell, J.E., Specker, S.M., and de Zwaan, M. (1991). Comorbidity and medical complications of bulimia nervosa. *Journal of Clinical Psychiatry* **52,** (10, Suppl.), 13–20.

Newman, M.M. and Halmi, K.A. (1988). The endocrinology of anorexia nervosa and bulimia nervosa. *Neurologic Clinics* **6,** 195–212.

Palmer, J.L. (1988). *Anorexia nervosa*, (2nd edn). Penguin, London. A valuable guide for sufferers and their families.

Russell, G.F.M. (1979). Bulimia nervosa: an ominous variant of anorexia nervosa. *Psychological Medicine* **9,** 429–48. The original case series and a classic description of the disorder.

Russell, G.F.M. (1992). Anorexia nervosa of early onset and its impact on puberty. In *Feeding problems and eating disorders in children and adolescents*, (ed. P.J. Cooper and A. Stein)., pp. 85–111. Harwood Academic Publishers, Chur.

Sharp, C.W. and Freeman, C.P.L. (1993). The medical complications of anorexia nervosa. *British Journal of Psychiatry*, **162,** 452–62.

Strober, M. (1991). Family-genetic studies of eating disorders. *Journal of Clinical Psychiatry* **52,** 9–12.

Stunkard, A.J. (1993). A history of binge eating. In *Binge eating: nature, assessment and treatment*, (ed. C.G. Fairburn and G.T. Wilson). Guilford, New York.

10.5 Obesity

J. S. Garrow

Relationship between overweight and mortality and morbidity

DESIRABLE WEIGHT FOR HEIGHT FROM ACTUARIAL DATA

Life insurance companies need to identify those individuals who are at increased risk of dying young, and hence are unprofitable to insure. As early as 1913 the Society of Actuaries published analyses showing that overweight was an important predictor of decreased longevity. At intervals since then the Metropolitan Life insurance agency has published tables of 'desirable weight' for men and women of a given height, the most recent of which was the Build Study 1979. In some publications the range was subdivided according to large, medium, and small frame size, but there is no agreement about how frame size should be mea-

Table 1 *Relationship of life insurance weight (kg) for 'acceptable range', 'overweight', and 'obese' for men and women, and Quetelet's index (QI: kg/m²)*

Height (m)	'Acceptable range' (kg)	QI	'Overweight' (kg)	QI	'Obese' (kg)	QI
Men						
1.6	44–65	17–25	72	28	78	30
1.7	51–73	18–25	80	28	88	30
1.8	58–80	18–25	88	27	96	30
1.9	66–90	18–25	99	27	108	30
Women						
1.5	38–55	17–24	61	27	66	29
1.6	41–59	16–23	65	25	71	28
1.7	45–66	16–23	73	25	79	27
1.8	52–74	16–23	81	25	89	27

sured, nor is there any evidence that this refinement improves the accuracy with which mortality, or total body fat, can be predicted for a person of given age, sex, and height.

There is international consensus that tables showing weight for height can conveniently be replaced by a single index: weight (kg) divided by the square of height (m²). The Belgian astronomer Quetelet observed in 1869 that, among adults of normal body build, weight was proportional to the square of height: in other words W/H^2 was constant. This useful index is therefore called Quetelet's index (QI), but Keys and colleagues in 1972 made a similar observation, and named it body mass index (BMI). In this chapter the QI notation will be used, but BMI can be used interchangeably.

THE EFFECT OF AGE ON DESIRABLE WEIGHT FOR LONGEVITY

Figure 1 shows the general relationship of QI to mortality ratio: the curve is J-shaped, with minimum mortality ratio in the QI range 20 to 25 kg/m². This relationship is similar for both men and women. The nadir of the curve changes with age: between age 20 and 50 years it increases linearly from 20 to 25 kg/m² which, in a person 1.73 m tall, implies an increase from 60 to 75 kg. This does not mean, as has been suggested, that there is a health benefit from a gain of 15 kg during adult life. Several confounding factors operate. First, some people who are very overweight at age 20 will already have died by the age of 50 years. Secondly, the degenerative diseases which are the main cause of excess mortality in obese people take many years to develop, and are therefore more likely to limit life expectancy in a young person than an old one. Thirdly, malignant disease, bowel diseases, and chronic infections tend to cause weight loss and thus increase the mortality ratio in the lower weight ranges. Finally, with increasing age the distribution of fat in the body alters towards a greater proportion intraperitoneally, compared with subcutaneous sites, and this has adverse metabolic consequences, which are discussed below.

Cigarette smoking is also associated with decreased weight and increased mortality, but a large survey by the American Cancer Society has shown that whereas the relation of QI to mortality risk among men or women who smoke 20 cigarettes a day is increased to about 150 per cent of that of non-smokers of the same age, the shape of the curve is little changed (Lew and Garfinkel 1979). It is salutary to advise young smokers who say that they dare not stop for fear of unhealthy weight gain that the health risk of smoking 20 cigarettes a day is similar to that of gaining 20 kg in weight. Since weight gain on stopping smoking is usually far less than 20 kg it is preferable to stop smoking.

OPERATIONAL DEFINITION OF OBESITY IN ADULTS

It is evident from Fig. 1 that obesity can be arbitrarily divided into three grades: a significant effect on longevity begins somewhere in the range 25 to 29.9 kg/m², which is grade I. Above 30 kg/m² the mortality risk is obviously increased (grade II), and above 40 kg/m² the effect on health is severe (grade III). Figure 2 shows bands of weight and height which define these grades: it is a form of presentation which obese patients find easy to understand, and on which it is possible to indicate both their present situation, and also a reasonable target weight which they might profitably try to achieve.

RELATIONSHIP BETWEEN OVERWEIGHT AND FATNESS

Up to this point it has been assumed that overweight is synonymous with excess fatness, but this is not necessarily the case. In 1940 in the United States there was widespread concern because some nationally famous footballers were refused for service as aircrew because they exceeded the weight limits. It fell to Behnke at the naval physiology laboratories to restore national composure by showing that these athletes had a high body density, their excess weight comprising muscle, not fat.

Fig. 1 Mortality ratio in young adults: minimum value is in the range 20–25 kg/m². Values of 30 and 40 kg/m² mark the boundaries between obesity grades I, II, and III.

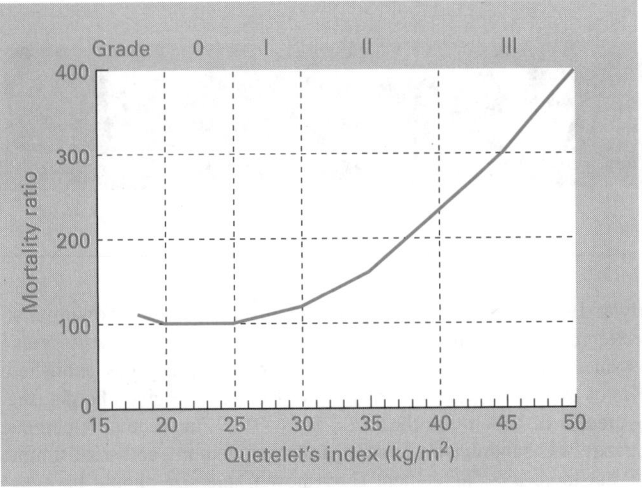

Fig. 2 Weight to height relationship which defines the grades of obesity shown in Fig. 1 (from Garrow 1993).

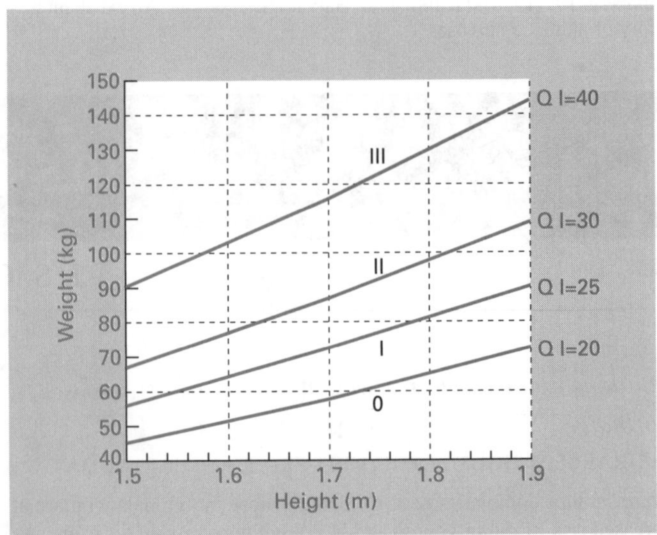

Table 2 *Comparison of the cost, difficulty, and accuracy of methods for measuring total fat (TF), or intra-abdominal fat (IAF) in human subjects*

Method	Cost	Difficulty	Accuracy	
			TF	IAF
Whole-body density	B	A	A	?
Total body water	B	B	B	?
Total body potassium	A	B	B	?
Neutron activation analysis	A	A	B	?
Quetelet's index	E	E	C	?
Skinfolds	E	D	C	D
Electrical impedance	D	D	C[a]	?
Near-infrared reactance	D	E	E	?
Waist/hip circumference	E	E	D	C
CT or NMR imaging	A	A	B	A

A, highest; E, lowest; ?, not specifically measured.

[a]Tetrapolar bioelectrical impedance combined with anthropometry gives a better estimate than either method used alone.

Methods for measuring total body fat

The three classical methods for measuring body fat in living subjects involving measurement of density or water and potassium content, depend on the assumption that body weight is the sum of the weight of fat and the weight of a mixture of non-fat components (called fat-free mass) which has some constant characteristic. This assumption, although necessary, is not quite true. For research purposes, when an accurate estimate of body fat is required, it is preferable to use two or more methods which involve different assumptions about the measurable characteristics of fat-free mass. The advantages and disadvantages of available methods are summarized in Table 2.

Whole-body density

The density of fat in man is 0.90 g/ml, and the fat-free mass is made of a mixture of water (0.993 g/ml), protein (1.34 g/ml), and mineral (3.00 g/ml). If it is assumed that the average density of this mixture is 1.10 g/ml, and whole-body density (d) is measured, then percentage body fat ($F\%$) is given by:

$$F\% = (495/d) - 450.$$

In Table 2 this method is rated most accurate (because the underlying assumption is nearly true, and body weight and volume can be measured very accurately with careful technique) but also most difficult, because the subject must co-operate fully in the measurement of body volume. This is usually done by measuring the volume of water displaced on total immersion, and then subtracting the volume of air in the lungs and airways. Alternatively, a plethysmographic method can be used, which requires immersion up to the neck only.

Total body water

If a known dose of isotopically labelled water is given to a subject and allowed about 3 to 4 h to equilibrate, the final concentration of labelled water in body fluids indicates the weight of total body water (TBW). The isotopes used for labelling are either tritium (the radioactive isotope of hydrogen, ^{3}H), or deuterium (^{2}H), or $^{18}O_2$, which are stable isotopes of hydrogen or oxygen respectively. To measure these with high accuracy it is necessary to use isotope-ratio mass spectrometry, but infrared spectrophotometry can be used with less accuracy (or cost) to measure deuterium. Fat is anhydrous, so if the assumption is made that the fat-free mass (FFM) contains 73 per cent water, then it can be calculated thus:

$$\text{FFM (kg)} = \text{TBW}/0.73$$

and body water can be obtained by subtracting the fat-free mass from body weight. The method is less accurate than measuring density because the assumption that the fat-free mass is 73 per cent water is invalid in people who are very young or very old (in whom the hydration is greater or less, respectively), oedematous, or dehydrated. In very obese patients total body water overestimates fat-free mass, and hence underestimates fat, because adipose tissue contains about 10 per cent extracellular water.

Total body potassium

A naturally occurring long-lived radioactive isotope, ^{40}K, is present at very low concentrations in all potassium, including that in the human body. With very high-sensitivity counters, shielded in massive steel enclosures, it is possible to detect the characteristic γ-radiation coming from ^{40}K and thus calculate total body potassium. Typically, this emission will need to be counted for a period of 15 to 20 min to obtain enough counts to give an estimate of total body potassium (TBK) within an accuracy of 3 per cent. The cost of the equipment is high, as is the cost of staff to maintain it and calibrate it accurately. The average concentration of potassium in the fat-free mass of men is 66 mmol/kg, and in women 60 mmol/kg, so fat-free mass (kg) is given by TBK (mmol)/66 in men and TBK (mmol)/60 in women. The method is of similar accuracy to the estimation of total body water, but is invalid where there is gross disturbance of water or potassium metabolism. It should be noted that in obese people total body potassium underestimates fat-free mass and overestimates fat, because the extracellular water in adipose tissue does not contain significant amounts of potassium. Thus it is not counted as fat-free mass, but (when fat-free mass is subtracted from body weight) contributes to the estimate of fat.

Neutron activation analysis

If a subject is irradiated with neutrons, it is possible to induce measurable short-lived radioactivity in many elements including O, H, N, Ca, P, Na, Cl, and Mg. In principle this gives insight into changes in body composition which do not depend on the assumed constancy of the chemical composition of fat-free mass. However, the method is expensive and involves irradiating the patient and so is not widely available.

Quetelet's index

It is inexpensive and easy to measure the weight and height of a subject but, as noted above, the use of a weight–height index as a measure of fatness will misclassify very muscular individuals as obese. However, for most clinical and epidemiological purposes, Quetelet's index provides a satisfactory measure of obesity in people who are not hypertrophied athletes (in which case it overestimates fatness) or old (in which case it underestimates fatness). Figure 3 shows the relationship between body fat (average of estimates by density, water, and potassium) and weight in 104 women aged between 14 and 60 years, and ranging from 6 to 60 per cent body fat. Differences in fat explain more than 90 per cent of the variation in weight. The regression line has a slope of 1.27, indicating that the excess weight in the obese women is approximately 75 per cent fat and 25 per cent fat-free mass.

Skinfolds

Normally most adipose tissue is in a subcutaneous layer, the thickness of which can be estimated by measuring a skinfold, as illustrated in Fig. 4. Individuals differ in the proportion of fat at different subcutaneous sites, but the sum of skinfolds at biceps, triceps, subscaplar and supra-iliac sites yields an estimate of body fat as shown in Table 3: the error is about 2 kg.

Skinfolds are particularly useful in the estimation of fatness in children, for whom standards are shown in Fig. 5. The method is inexpensive, but requires a skilled observer, and is not applicable to very obese people whose skinfolds would not fit between the jaws of the measuring caliper. Some information is obtained by comparing the subscapular skinfold with limb skinfolds concerning the central distribution of fat, but this is not a reliable method for estimating intra-abdominal fat.

Fig. 3 Relationship between body fat and body weight in 104 women. Body fat was calculated from the mean of estimates by density, water, and potassium in each woman. (From Webster *et al.* 1984.)

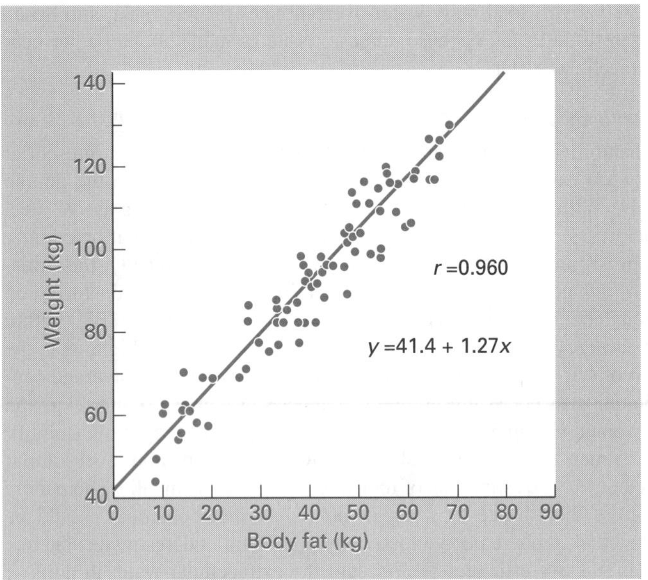

Electrical impedance

Lean tissue is a good conductor of electricity, since it contains an electrolytic solution, whereas fat is not. Measurements of the impedance of the body can be made by passing a small high-frequency current between the hand and foot, but most of the capacity of 'impedance' methods to predict body water and fat-free mass comes from the anthropometric data which are used in the predictive equations. It remains to be seen whether newer multifrequency instruments will provide a significant advance over anthropometric methods.

Near-infrared interactance

The frequency spectrum of light reflected from subcutaneous tissues when illuminated by near-infrared light is modified by the ratio of fat to lean in the underlying tissue. Some inexpensive instruments are commercially available based on this principle, but they have not been shown to be an improvement over anthropometry in the estimation of body fat.

Methods for measuring the distribution of body fat

For reasons discussed below, the health risks associated with obesity relate mainly to that portion of body fat which is within the peritoneal cavity. The following methods yield information about this 'distribution' of body fat.

Waist/hip circumference ratio

Waist circumference is the minimum circumference between the costal margin and iliac crest, measured in the horizontal plane, with the subject

Fig. 4 The measurement of skinfold thicknesses (a) The point at which the skinfold is taken on the arm is measured as half the distance between the acromial and the olecranon processes. A fold of skin and subcutaneous tissue is taken by pinching the tissue between thumb and forefinger as shown and initially placed 2 cm apart. It is essential to maintain the grip with the left hand as shown while the right hand relaxes pressure completely on the handle of the calipers. Above a reading of 20 mm the measurement may decrease despite a firm hold with the left hand. In this case the reading should be taken 2 s after the caliper is applied. The biceps reading is taken in the same plane but at the front of the arm with the hand supinated. The suprailiac measurement is also taken on the left side in the mid-axillary line just above the iliac crest. (Calipers are obtainable from Holtain Ltd, Crosswell, Crymych, Dyfed, UK.) (b) Technique for subcapular measurement.

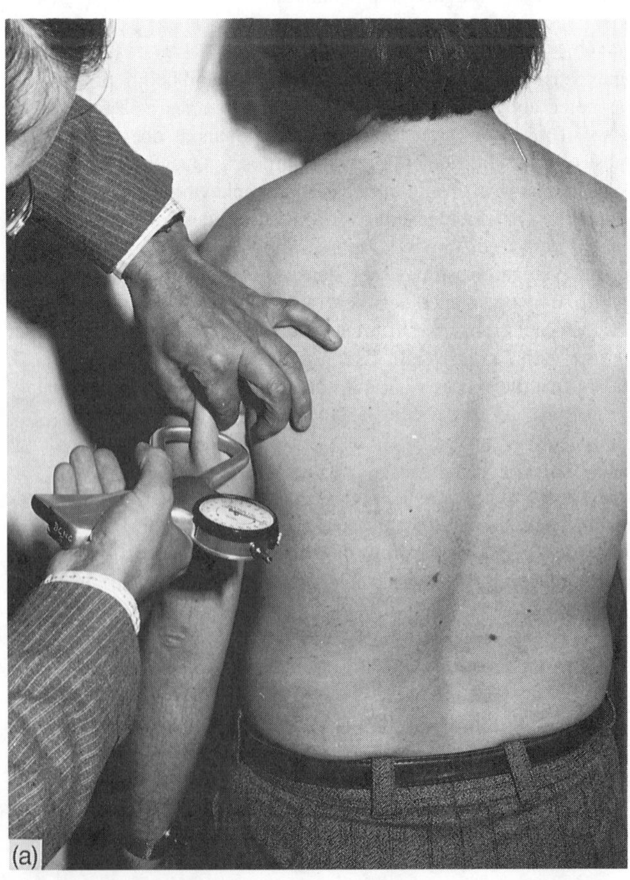

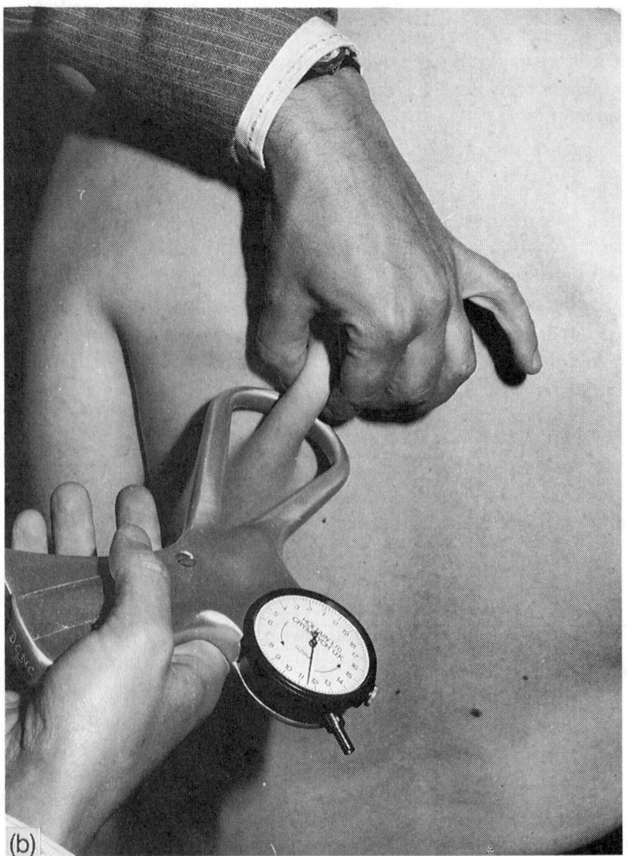

Table 3 *Percentage body fat predicted by the sum of biceps, triceps, subscapular, and suprailiac skinfolds (data of Durnin and Womersley 1974)*

Skinfolds (mm)	Percentage fat							
	Males (age in years)				Females (age in years)			
	17–29	30–39	40–49	50+	16–29	30–39	40–49	50+
15	4.8				10.5			
20	8.1	12.2	12.2	12.6	14.1	17.0	19.8	21.4
25	10.5	14.2	15.0	15.6	16.8	19.4	22.2	24.0
30	12.9	16.2	17.7	18.6	19.5	21.8	24.5	26.6
35	14.7	17.7	19.6	20.8	21.5	23.7	26.4	28.5
40	16.4	19.2	21.4	22.9	23.4	25.5	28.2	30.3
45	17.7	20.4	23.0	24.7	25.0	26.9	29.6	31.9
50	19.0	21.5	24.6	26.5	26.5	28.2	31.0	33.4
55	20.1	22.5	25.9	27.9	27.8	29.4	32.1	34.6
60	21.2	23.5	27.1	29.2	29.1	30.6	33.2	35.7
65	22.2	24.3	28.2	30.4	30.2	31.6	34.1	36.7
70	23.1	25.1	29.3	31.6	31.2	32.5	35.0	37.7
75	24.0	25.9	30.3	32.7	32.2	33.4	35.9	38.7
80	24.8	26.6	31.2	33.8	33.1	34.3	36.7	39.6
85	25.5	27.2	32.1	34.8	34.0	35.1	37.5	40.4
90	26.2	27.8	33.0	35.8	34.8	35.8	38.3	41.2
95	26.9	28.4	33.7	36.6	35.6	36.5	39.0	41.9
100	27.6	29.0	34.4	37.4	36.4	37.2	39.7	42.6
105	28.2	29.6	35.1	38.2	37.1	37.9	40.4	43.3
110	28.8	30.1	35.8	39.0	37.8	38.6	41.0	43.9
115	29.4	30.6	36.4	39.7	38.4	39.1	41.5	44.5
120	30.0	31.1	37.0	40.4	39.0	39.6	42.0	45.1
125	30.5	31.5	37.6	41.1	39.6	40.1	42.5	45.7
130	31.0	31.9	38.2	41.8	40.2	40.6	43.0	46.2
135	31.5	32.3	38.7	42.4	40.8	41.1	43.5	46.7
140	32.0	32.7	39.2	43.0	41.3	41.6	44.0	47.2
145	32.5	33.1	39.7	43.6	41.8	42.1	44.5	47.7
150	32.9	33.5	40.2	44.1	42.3	42.6	45.0	48.2
155	33.3	33.9	40.7	44.6	42.8	43.1	45.4	48.7
160	33.7	34.3	41.2	45.1	43.3	43.6	45.8	49.2
165	34.1	34.6	41.6	45.6	43.7	44.0	46.2	49.6
170	34.5	34.8	42.0	46.1	44.1	44.4	46.6	50.0
175	34.9					44.8	47.0	50.4
180	35.3					45.2	47.4	50.8
185	35.6					45.6	47.8	51.2
190	35.9					45.9	48.2	51.6
195						46.2	48.5	52.0
200						46.5	48.8	52.4
205							49.1	52.7
210							49.4	53.0

standing. Hip circumference is the maximum circumference in the horizontal plane, measured over the buttocks. The ratio of the former to the latter provides an index of the proportion of intra-abdominal fat. The average value for men is about 0.93 with a range of 0.75 to 1.10, and for women 0.83 with a range from 0.70 to 1.00.

Imaging techniques

Images of cross-sections of the body can be obtained by computed tomography, using either X-ray or magnetic resonance techniques. In principle the entire body can be visualized by serial transverse scans, but this is very expensive and time-consuming. In practice, a series of 20 transverse scans provides a very good estimate of the amount and distribution of body fat. This is the gold standard with which less expensive techniques for measuring intraperitoneal fat are compared.

Prevalence of obesity in the United Kingdom and other countries

Surveys of height and weight in a nationally representative sample of adults in the United Kingdom were performed in 1980 and repeated with the same methodology in 1987 and 1991. The data relating to the prevalence of obesity (QI > 30) are summarized in Table 4. In all surveys the prevalence of obesity in both sexes increased between the age of 16 and 50 years, but while in women it continued to increase up to the age of 64, in men it declined. In both sexes and in all age groups the prevalence increased between 1980 and 1987, and between 1987 and 1991.

It is difficult to make valid comparisons between nations, but Table 5 is a compilation of the best available data on the prevalence of obesity in the age group 40 to 60 years in other countries. The values shown in Table 4 indicate that the United Kingdom is fairly typical of north-western Europe: the prevalence is lower in Scandinavian countries and rather higher in The Netherlands, France, and Germany. In Eastern Europe, the former USSR, and in Mediterranean countries the prevalence is higher, especially among women. In every region the prevalence is higher among women than among men.

Aetiology of obesity

CONSIDERATIONS OF ENERGY BALANCE

An obese person has a larger energy store (in the form of fat) than a normal person: typically a person who is 15 kg overweight has 100 000 kcal (25 MJ) more energy stored than a person of normal weight. The laws of thermodynamics tell us that this situation cannot have arisen unless the overweight person had an energy intake which was greater by this amount, or an energy output which was less by this amount, or some combination of these two factors. Medical textbooks, when discussing the aetiology of obesity, offer lists of rare eponymous syndromes, but the statement above applies just as much to patients with the Prader–Willi syndrome as to cases of 'simple' obesity (in the case of the Prader–Willi syndrome the explanation is an excessively large energy intake). It is useful to remember that the genetically determined syndromes associated with obesity in childhood are almost always associated with short stature, and often with mental retardation, whereas obese children without chromosomal abnormalities are almost always tall for their age and are of normal mental development.

Energy intake in obese versus lean persons

Obese people who seek medical help are highly self-selected: invariably they have at some time tried to diet, and have been dissatisfied with the weight loss achieved. The fact that they consult a doctor about their weight usually implies that they believe that the problem must be one of reduced requirements, rather than excessive intake. A diet history tends to confirm this view, since the best a dietitian can do is to calculate the food which the patient recalls (or records) having eaten. Over a week or two this record may be quite accurate, but it is very rarely both accurate and typical of habitual intake. Many studies have shown that when the energy output of obese patients is measured by calorimetry, or by the doubly labelled water technique, the recorded energy intake would have been incapable of maintaining the obese state, so it cannot have been accurate and typical.

Energy output in obese versus lean people

Studies of energy expenditure using the same techniques on groups of lean and obese subjects have shown very consistent results. In both groups, resting metabolic rate accounts for about 70 per cent of total daily energy output (range 62–76 per cent); there is no difference between obese and lean subjects in this respect. However, there is a consistent difference in that the total energy expenditure of the obese

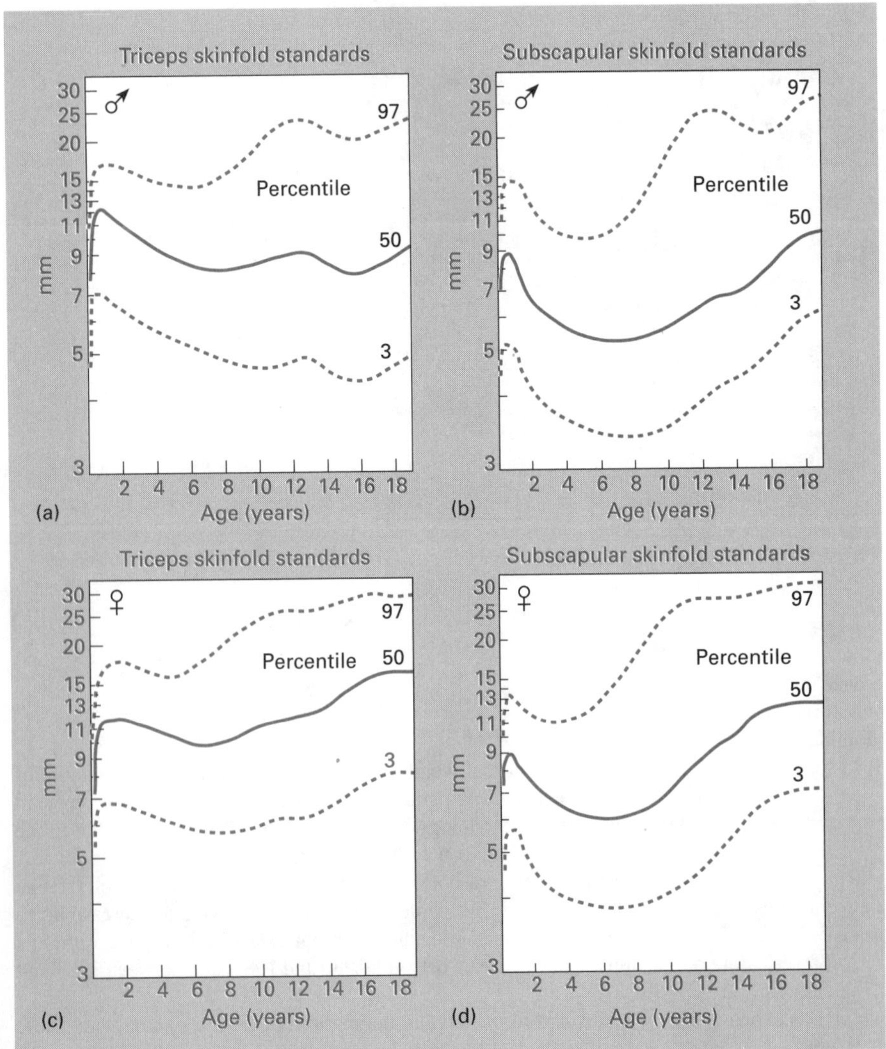

Fig. 5 Standards for triceps and subscapular skinfold thickness in boys and girls. (Redrawn and extracted from *Growth and development chart SEB 45*. Castlemead Publications, Hertford.)

Table 4 *Prevalence (%) of obesity (QI > 30) in a representative sample of men and women between 16 and 64 years in the United Kingdom (data for 1980 from Rosenbaum et al. 1985, for 1987 from Gregory et al. 1990, and for 1991 from White et al. 1994)*

		Age (years)			
		16–24	25–34	35–49	50–64
Men	1980	2.5	4.5	8.0	7.7
	1987	3.0	6.0	11.0	9.0
	1991	5	8	16	18
Women	1980	3.5	4.5	9.9	14.3
	1987	6.0	11.0	10.0	18.0
	1991	6	12	17	23

Table 5 *Prevalence (%) of obesity (QI > 30) among men and women aged 40 to 60 years in Europe and the United States of America*

Area	Men	Women
Northern Europe	10	15
Western Europe	13	16
Mediterranean	16	30
Eastern Europe	18	30
USSR (formerly)	14	44
USA (Caucasian)	15	18
USA (Afro-American)	20	37

group is 124 per cent (range 121 to 128 per cent) of the lean group. The magnitude of the difference between the groups depends on the weight difference: on average, weight differences in women are associated with a difference in daily energy expenditure of about 12 kcal (50 kJ)/kg, and among men of about 15 kcal (63 kJ)/kg. The main determinant of resting metabolic rate (which in turn is the main determinant of total energy expenditure, except in athletes and heavy manual workers) is fat-free mass. Formulae by which resting metabolic rate can be predicted from weight, age, and fat-free mass are given in Table 6.

Mechanisms that maintain energy balance: set-point theory

Maintenance of energy stores is essential for survival in times of famine, to which our ancestors were constantly at risk. Several physiological mechanisms tend to maintain energy balance. Energy intake is to some extent controlled by the sensations of hunger and satiety, but these are readily overridden if there is unlimited supply of varied palatable food. Changes in energy intake also directly affect output: the increase in metabolic rate which occurs during 4 h after a meal is equivalent to about 10 per cent of the ingested energy: this is the metabolic work of assimilating the meal. Energy output increases by about 6 per cent during overfeeding and decreases similarly during underfeeding: the mechanism for this adaptive thermogenesis is not fully understood, but probably involves thyroid and catecholamine metabolism. Finally, weight change causes changes in energy output as described above. These factors combine to buffer large changes in energy balance when the food supply alters.

There is persuasive evidence in laboratory rodents that animals of a particular strain have a set point of weight, to which they tend to return after over- or underfeeding. The evidence for a similar effect in man is very weak.

GENETIC PREDISPOSITION TO OBESITY

It is well known that obesity tends to run in families, but that might imply either genetic or environmental influences, for example obese

Table 6 *Prediction of resting metabolic rate (RMR, kcal/24 h) in adults*

1. From age and weight (W, kg) (data of Schofield 1985)

Age (years)	Men	Women
18–30	RMR = 15.1W + 693	RMR = 14.8W + 488
31–60	RMR = 11.5W + 872	RMR = 8.13W + 846
> 60	RMR = 11.7W + 588	RMR = 9.08W + 660

2. From fat-free mass (FFM, kg), fat mass (FM, kg), and age (A, years) (data of Ravussin *et al.* 1991)

RMR = 13.9FFM + 6.3FM − 4.4A + 941 (men)
RMR = 13.9FFM + 6.3FM − 4.4A + 794 (women)

Table 7 *Percentage of biological (or, in parentheses, adoptive) parents who were overweight or obese, according to the weight class of the adoptee (data of Stunkard et al. 1986)*

Weight class of adoptee	Thin	Medium	Overweight/ obese
Mean QI of adoptee	17.8	23.0	31.4
Percentage of overweight parents			
Mother			
biological	18	35	41
(adoptive)	(34)	(37)	(35)
Father			
biological	35	38	49
(adoptive)	(57)	(53)	(45)

dogs tend to have obese owners, but the effect is clearly not genetic. Table 7 shows the results of a study of the weight status of 540 adult Danish adoptees for whom information was available about the build of both biological and adoptive parents. The weight status of the adoptive mother was not related to that of the adoptee, but that of the biological mother was significantly related. The effect was less marked with the biological father, but (for reasons not understood) there was a significant negative relationship between the weight status of the adoptive father and that of the adoptee. The strongest effect was that thin adoptees rarely had obese biological mothers. In general, adoption studies indicate that about 10 to 30 per cent of variation in obesity is heritable, but the mechanisms are not well understood. Adult offspring of obese parents do not have a significantly reduced metabolic rate compared with the offspring of lean parents.

SOCIAL FACTORS ASSOCIATED WITH OBESITY OR RAPID WEIGHT GAIN

In developed countries there is an inverse relationship between obesity and socioeconomic status, especially among women. Perhaps women of higher social class are influenced by the aphorism ascribed to the Duchess of Windsor, 'No woman can be too rich, or too thin.' The view that obesity in disadvantaged sections of society is caused by a diet of cheap food lacks experimental support: it is true that fruit and fresh vegetables are relatively expensive, and lacking in the diet of poorer people, but food of high energy density, such as meat and cream, are also expensive. The cheapest diet that will provide the daily requirements of nutrients is based mainly on cereals, and is monotonous: both of these characteristics normally lead to undereating, not overeating.

Recent research has indicated the factors associated with rapid weight gain (defined as an increase of > 5 kg in 5 years). In a survey of 12 000 Finnish men and non-pregnant women aged 25–64 years, 15.1

per cent of men and 17.5 per cent of women were in this category. The characteristics in which they differed significantly from the weight-stable members of the population were: a lower level of education, chronic disease, little physical activity at leisure, and heavy alcohol consumption. Weight gain was also observed among those who got married or stopped smoking: these predictors applied both to men and to women.

Mechanisms by which obesity causes disease

A decade ago epidemiologists considered that obesity was not an important cause of disease or mortality, but merely a marker of the true risk factors, such as raised plasma cholesterol, hypertension, and non-insulin-dependent diabetes mellitus. This view was based mainly on multiple regression analyses of the risk factors for total mortality and cardiovascular disease mortality in the Seven Nations Study, which made prospective observations in groups of middle-aged men in the United States, Europe, and Japan. Subsequent research has shown that obesity is not merely a marker, but a cause of these risk factors. Cigarette smoking is an important confounder in this association. Figure 6 indicates causative chains between obesity and some important diseases. The links in these chains are discussed further below.

INSULIN INSENSITIVITY AND ITS CONSEQUENCES

Obese people are insulin resistant and, if their capacity to secrete insulin is limited, very liable to develop non-insulin-dependent diabetes mellitus. The definitive demonstration that the obesity causes the insulin resistance was provided by a study in Vermont by Sims and colleagues. For 6 months they overfed 19 young men who had no personal or family history of obesity or diabetes. At the end of the overfeeding period, when they were in energy balance again, they had increased body weight by 21 per cent, of which 73 per cent was fat. Insulin sensitivity, as measured by oral or intravenous glucose tolerance, decreased significantly and there were coincident increases in fasting levels of insulin and glucose as well as in the insulin response. As weight fell towards the original level these changes reverted to normal. We now know that intra-abdominal fat is especially important in causing insulin insensitivity, since its high lipolytic activity releases high concentrations of free fatty acids into the portal circulation. Insulin insensitivity is the key abnormality in the 'syndrome X' described by Reaven, and is associated with hypertension, high low-density lipoprotein (LDL)-cholesterol, low high-density lipoprotein (HDL)-cholesterol, and an increased risk of atheroma formation. Hypertension is also associated with obesity, and weight reduction has repeatedly been shown to reduce arterial pressure.

METABOLIC EFFECTS OF A LARGE ADIPOSE MASS

Apart from effects mediated by insulin insensitivity, a large adipose mass has three other important effects which predispose to diseases:

Aromatase

This is the enzyme system that converts androgens to oestrogens, and in an obese person there is more aromatase in adipose tissue than in the gonads. This probably accounts for the menstrual problems, polycystic ovaries, and infertility which are often seen in obese women; infertility in obese men; and the excess risk of sex-hormone-sensitive cancers: of the colon, rectum, and prostate in men, and of the endometrium, cervix, ovary, and breast in women.

Cholesterol stores

Such stores in adipose tissue greatly increase the rate of cholesterol excretion in the bile, leading to supersaturation of bile in obese people. This predisposes to the formation of gallstones, cholecystitis, and to gallbladder cancer.

The mechanical load

This load, represented by the excess weight, decreases exercise tolerance and predisposes to inactivity, although there is little evidence that inactivity is an important factor in causing obesity. Inactivity is itself a contributor to insulin insensitivity, and the increased load contributes to

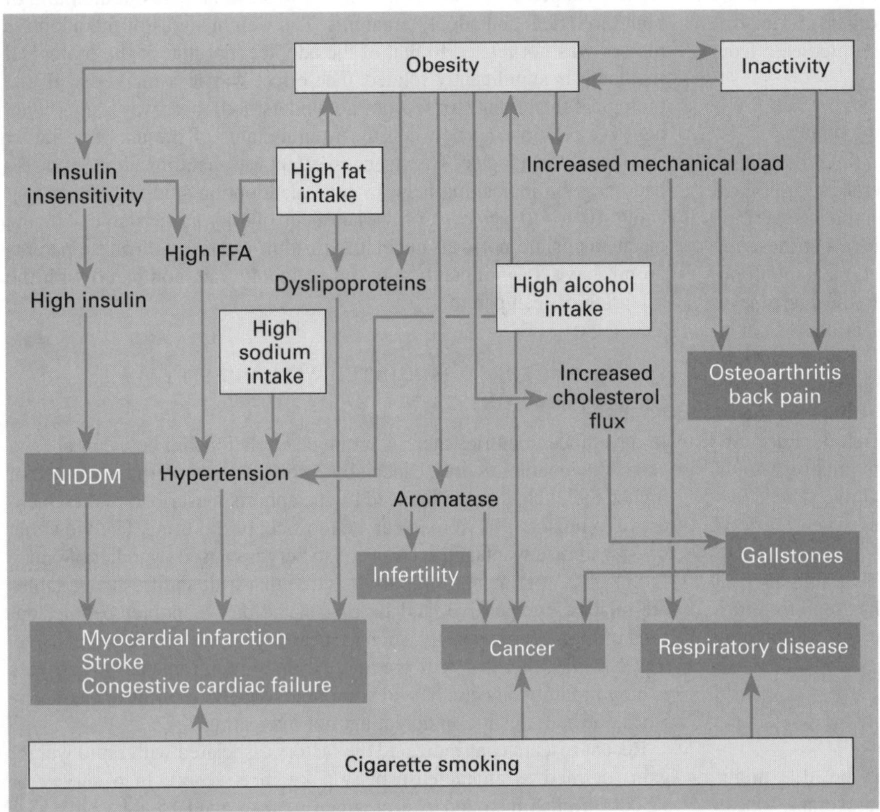

Fig. 6 How obesity causes disease. Important diseases are shown in black boxes, CCF, and alterable lifestyle factors which predispose to these diseases are shown in white boxes; FFA, free fatty acids; NIDDM, non-insulin-dependent diabetes mellitus. (From Garrow 1993.)

osteoarthritis of weight-bearing joints, with a further decrease in exercise tolerance.

CONFOUNDING EFFECTS OF CIGARETTE SMOKING AND ALCOHOL

In view of the widespread effects of obesity on the risks of disease, as illustrated in Fig. 6, it is strange that this association was not seen clearly long ago. In part, the explanation involves the confounding effects of cigarette smoking. For example, there is no clear relationship between QI and risk of fatal stroke, but this is because there is an increased risk in thin smokers and in obese non-smokers, so that if smoking is not taken into account, the relation between QI and death from stroke in non-smokers is obscured.

Alcohol also confounds the assessment of the health risks of obesity. For reasons not understood, alcohol intake is associated with an increased storage of intra-abdominal fat which, as explained above, is particularly important in causing insulin insensitivity.

EFFECTS OF WEIGHT LOSS IN OBESE PEOPLE ON MORTALITY AND MORBIDITY

Life insurance companies have consistently found that obese people who are refused cover at normal premiums, and who subsequently lose weight into the normal range, thereafter have an improved life expectancy. However, this is not totally satisfactory evidence that weight loss reduces the mortality risk in obese people, because those individuals who lose weight in order to enjoy a reduced life insurance premium are self-selected, and probably not typical of all obese people. These people may also have altered other habits affecting health, such as cigarette smoking and physical activity.

Longitudinal surveys have shown that weight loss in the general population is associated with a decrease (and weight gain an increase) in blood pressure, in plasma lipoprotein cholesterol fractions, triglycerides, fasting glucose, post-prandial glucose, uric acid, and in forced vital capacity. However, data on the effect of weight loss on mortality have been equivocal, probably because they did not differentiate between voluntary and involuntary weight loss. In this situation the ideal study design would be one in which obese people were randomly allocated to achieve weight loss, or not, but there are severe ethical and logistic problems in such a design. Not least is the difficulty in obtaining adequate weight loss in the group in whom it is required, and weight stability in the group who expected to maintain their weight.

One argument that has been advanced to suggest that weight loss does not improve the risk of mortality is that, in the United States, the death rate from cardiovascular disease and stroke fell by about 50 per cent between 1972 and 1992, a period in which the prevalence of obesity was increasing. However, although the death rate from cardiovascular disease fell over this period, the attack rate did not; the reduction in death rate seems then to reflect a lower mortality among those who suffered a heart attack or stroke, and not a reduced liability to these disorders.

CLINICAL SIGNIFICANCE OF WEIGHT CYCLING

Surveys in both the United Kingdom and the United States of America have found that individuals who maintain a constant weight over many years have a lower risk of death (particularly from cardiovascular disease) than individuals of the same age, sex, and weight who show large fluctuations in weight. This observation might have several explanations. It may be that the weight cycling is itself injurious to health, since it may imply alternating periods of starvation and overeating, both of which are known to impair insulin sensitivity. It may also be that people who undergo periods of weight loss and regain are manifesting an obsessional personality trait, which is associated with an increased risk of cardiovascular disease. Another explanation is that the weight cycling is associated with some chronic relapsing disease which is the real cause of the excess mortality; or perhaps all these explanations make some contribution. It is unlikely that it will be possible to conduct a trial in which subjects are randomly allocated to cyclical or stable weight programmes, so interpretation of the cause(s) of weight cycling is likely to continue to be inferential. However it is reasonable to conclude that a treatment for obesity which causes weight to be lost and then regained does no good to the patient, and possibly does more harm than not losing weight in the first place.

SOCIAL ISSUES: THE ANTI-DIET MOVEMENT

Weight-loss manoeuvres are the subject of massive attention in the popular media, so the efficacy of new wonder cures is constantly being proclaimed and rebutted by commentators who often have a vested interest. Particularly in the United States, but increasingly in other countries, there is a movement which opposes any attempt to get obese people to lose weight. The argument is based on the belief that dieting causes so much anguish, to so little good effect, that it is ethically unjustified. Of course it is true that many young women who have a QI of less than 25 try unsuccessfully to achieve and maintain an unphysiologically low weight. Their failure to do so still further lowers their self-esteem, and the weight cycling which ensues is probably harmful to health in the way indicated above. However, for people who are obese (QI > 30) the balance of evidence is clearly that treatment of obesity, as set out below, carries much greater potential to do good than harm.

Treatment of obesity

EXPECTATIONS BY PATIENT AND THERAPIST

It is important to appreciate that the relationship between the doctor and an obese patient who requests help with weight loss is unusual. Normally a patient presents with a pain, lump, or other disability, and expects the doctor to make a diagnosis and prescribe a treatment which would not otherwise be available to the patient. This is never the situation with an obese patient. The diagnosis is already known, and almost invariably one or more treatments have been tried, and found wanting. The obese patient therefore comes to the doctor wanting to know why previous treatments failed, and to be given a different treatment which works better.

Doctors also tend to have unrealistic expectations concerning the treatment of obesity. Some assume (wrongly) that all that is required is to send the patient off with a diet sheet. This is stupid: the chance that the patient has never had a diet sheet before is negligible, and the fact that the patient is still obese is evidence that this strategy has failed in the past; there is no reason to suppose it will do any better this time. Others assume (wrongly) that past dietary failure is evidence of some metabolic barrier to weight loss, so the appropriate management is either an extensive trawl through all known hormone assays, or else a sympathetic acknowledgement that the condition is untreatable. The truth lies somewhere between these extremes. Successful treatment of obesity requires patience, motivation, and sound technique on the part of both patient and therapist, but, given these qualities, the chance of a successful outcome is greater than that for many other conditions discussed in this book.

CLINICAL HISTORY RELEVANT TO OBESITY

Table 8 sets out 10 essential questions to which answers are required before starting to advise an obese patient.

1. Target weight

Beware the patient who hopes to reduce from a QI of greater than 30 to one of less than 20 kg/m^2: such a target is very difficult to achieve, and

Table 8 *Ten essential questions to ask an obese patient*

Concerning the patient's target weight
1. What weight do you think you should be?
2. In what way would you benefit if you were (weight given as answer to question 1)?
3. Is your present weight the most you have ever been?
Concerning the patient's perception of dieting
4. Are you on a diet at present?
5. What is the longest time you have kept strictly to a reducing diet?
6. What rate of weight loss do you expect to achieve if you keep to a diet?
7. Do you expect to lose weight without dieting?
Factors which may make dieting more difficult
8. Who does the shopping/cooking at home?
9. What work do you do?
10. Are you on any medication at present?

carries no health benefit if it is achieved. My own practice is to agree to help a patient to achieve QI 25 kg/m^2, but no less.

2. Expected benefit

Some benefits, such as relief from shortness of breath or painful knees, are realistic expectations following weight loss. However, weight loss is no guarantee of social success.

3. Maximum weight

A patient who now weighs 100 kg, but who weighed 130 kg 6 months ago, is far more sophisticated about methods of weight loss than a patient who has never weighed more than 100 kg.

4. Is the patient on a diet now?

If the patient is on a diet, it is necessary to find out what it is, and why the results are unsatisfactory. If the patient is not dieting it is necessary to find out why not. (Question 7 may throw further light on this.)

5. Length of time on diet

If the patient has never kept to a diet for more than a few days it is not surprising that little weight has been lost. It is also not useful to discuss diet plans until something has been done to achieve more prolonged compliance next time.

6. Expected rate of weight loss

The appropriate range of rates of weight loss is shown in Fig. 7: those who are younger, taller, and more overweight may aim for the higher limit, while those who are older, shorter, and less overweight should be satisfied with something near the lower limit. For the first month of dieting the rate of weight loss is more rapid due to the loss of glycogen and the water bound to it. Subsequently the optimum rate of weight loss is 0.5 to 1.0 kg (1–2 lb)/week, which represents an average energy deficit of 500 to 1000 kcal (2–4 MJ)/day. The disadvantages of energy deficits greater than 1000 kcal/day are that there may be excessive loss of lean tissue, it becomes difficult to provide the essential nutrients, it is unnecessarily unpleasant, and there will have to be further large adjustments when the target weight is achieved to find a suitable diet to maintain the new weight. The disadvantages of deficits less than 500 kcal/day are that it takes too long for the subject to reach target weight, unless the initial excess weight was very small.

7. Weight loss without dieting

Usually the patient will realize that restricting energy intake is an inevitable requirement for weight loss. Occasionally, however, a patient comes who believes that modern medicine has developed techniques which escape the thermodynamic imperatives. Unless they are disillusioned on this point no progress will be made.

8. Who cooks/shops?

If the patient buys and cooks the food he/she eats, then, in principle, the patient has control over the diet. In practice, many patients have to eat food prepared by other people, or have to cook for other people. It is not useful to try to advise a change in diet without understanding these constraints.

9. The patient's job

Working differing shifts, or working in a catering environment, may add considerably to the difficulty of dieting.

10. Medication

It is important to consider modifying antihypertensive or hypoglycaemic medication in an obese patient who is going to lose weight. Many other classes of drugs are also relevant: diuretics may cause inexplicable weight changes, psychotropic drugs affect the ability of the patient to achieve the organization and discipline needed for successful dieting, and many obese patients have acquired inappropriate prescriptions for thyroid hormone to treat a presumed low metabolic rate, or bronchodilators to treat their breathlessness.

Having learned something about the patient's perception of an appropriate weight, and the means by which it can be achieved, it is necessary to agree a plan concerning the target weight, the length of time which it is likely to take to achieve this weight (see Fig. 7), and how the target weight, once achieved, can be maintained (see below). It is also important to remember that one of the tasks of the therapist is to restore the patient's self-esteem. It is therefore essential that expectations are realistic; otherwise the enterprise will fail, and this failure will add to the burden of previous failures to lower the patient's self-esteem still further.

Dieting relationship trap

It is remarkable that hostility often arises between obese patients and those who are trying to assist with weight loss. Both parties tend to fall into a 'dieting relationship trap'. The way in which it operates is as follows. Initially the patient comes for advice about losing weight, usually to obtain relief from some of the complications of obesity which have already been mentioned, and is pleased to find a doctor who is willing and able to help with sensible dietary advice. On follow-up visits

Fig. 7 Range of desirable weight loss in obese people. Younger, taller, male, and severely obese patients should aim at the upper line, and older, shorter, female and less overweight patients the lower line. (From Garrow 1993.)

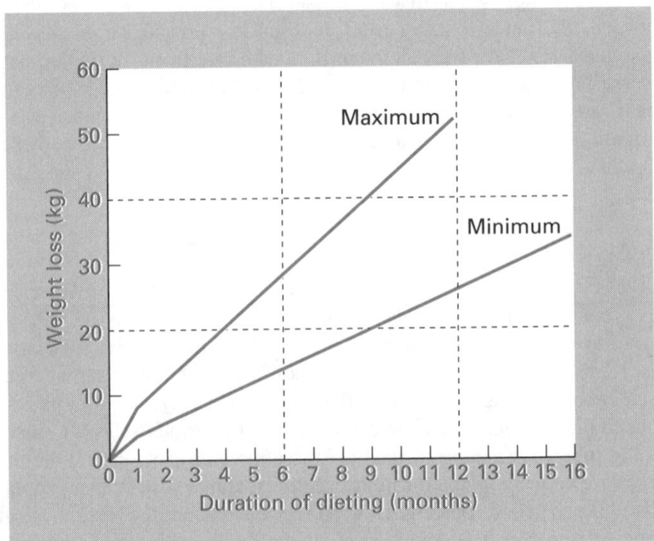

all goes well so long as satisfactory weight loss has been achieved, but the time then comes when the patient returns having not lost weight, or even having regained it. This may precipitate both self-reproach and feelings of unworthiness for any further help, leading to the invitation to the doctor to discharge him or her. Of course, the correct response at this point is to agree with disappointment, to assure the patient that steady weight loss uninterrupted by set-backs is virtually unknown, and to try to identify the factors that precipitated the problem, and how they can best be avoided in the future; above all to provide encouragement, not criticism. The wrong response (into which it is all too easy to slip) is to agree that the patient is wasting the doctor's valuable time, fixing blame for failure on the patient, and so further reducing self-esteem and determination to achieve any further loss of weight.

On the other hand, it is possible to carry sympathy with the patient too far. There is little to be gained from regular monthly meetings between obese patient and doctor at which the lack of any weight loss is noted, the difficulty of dieting is agreed, but nothing is done to increase the chance of success next time.

Matching treatment strategy to degree of obesity

Table 9 shows the treatment strategies which should be considered for different grades of obesity. Unless the history indicates that some other plan should be followed, the first choice for the treatment of an obese patient is a conventional reducing diet. However, finding the best treatment involves trial and error.

Table 9 *Matching treatment strategy of the degree of obesity*

	Grade of obesity			
Treatment	III	II	I	0
Diet				
starvation	No	No	No	No
very-low-calorie	Poss	No	No	No
conventional	Yes(1)	Yes(1)	Yes(1)	No
milk only	Yes(2)	Yes(2)	Poss	No
jaw wiring + waist cord	Yes(3)	Poss	No	No
gastric exclusion surgery	Poss	No	No	No
Drugs				
anorectic	Poss	Poss	No	No
thermogenic	No	No	No	No
Physical training	No	Poss	Yes(2)	Yes
Reassurance	No	No	Poss	Yes

Yes, appropriate treatment, and figure in parentheses indicates order of preference; No, inappropriate; Poss, possible in some circumstances.

Dietary advice

The diet should provide 500 to 1000 kcal/day less than the maintenance energy requirements in order to achieve weight loss at the rate shown in Fig. 7. It must also provide the essential nutrients, so it is logical to seek to restrict those food items which provide energy but little else of nutritional importance, such as sucrose and alcohol. It is also desirable to restrict intake of fat, and particularly saturated fat, partly to reduce the risk of atheromatous heart disease, partly because fat is a concentrated energy source, and partly because there is some evidence that fat has a lower satiating capacity than isoenergetic quantities of carbohydrate or protein. The foods that are not restricted are fruit, vegetables, and whole-grain cereals, since these are important sources of micronutrients and non-starch polysaccharides. It is important that protein intake should be adequate to avoid unnecessary loss of lean tissue, but extremely high protein diets are expensive and have not been shown to be particularly effective or acceptable. Within these guidelines it is possible to construct an infinite variety of nutritionally sound reducing diets which can be adapted to the requirements of individual patients.

It is very difficult to predict which diet will prove most acceptable to a given patient. Presumably the diet that the patient prefers is the one on which obesity developed, so a willingness to change from this is a necessary condition for successful weight loss. Some patients prefer exactly specified diets, whereas others prefer more flexibility. Patients may say that they find dieting difficult because they get hungry, but on closer questioning this may mean that they long for a particular forbidden item of food, such as chocolate. It is not clear whether a small ration of chocolate (in this instance) is helpful or not: people differ. For some patients a monotonous bland diet (such as milk only) is easier to keep to than a varied diet, but for others it is intolerable. A good dietitian will find the best compromise between the diet that will be acceptable and that which will cause the best weight loss.

Frequency and timing of meals

Traditionally, patients are advised to have small, frequent meals, and for a given energy intake this policy seems to decrease hunger over the 24 h compared with a regimen of infrequent larger meals. However, there is no evidence that meal frequency affects total energy output. It is probably useful for patients to establish a formal pattern of eating meals at specified times, since continuous snacking or 'grazing' makes it very difficult to establish any control over total energy intake.

Behaviour therapy

In the past decade psychologists have greatly increased our understanding of dieting behaviour. Most of us eat more or less automatically. If a patient's eating behaviour is to be altered, it is first necessary to become aware of what is being eaten, and the circumstances that tend to trigger inappropriate eating. The mere recording of a food diary is associated with some weight loss in most people, which suggests that we eat less when we are required to pay attention to what we eat, and such a food diary is also useful for the dietitian to assess the patient's habitual diet. There may be recurrent domestic situations which tend to precipitate binge eating; if these can be identified and that situation avoided, the chances of compliance are increased. It is also helpful if other members of the household provide intelligent co-operation with dieting efforts: ignorant nagging or ridicule from other members of the family will defeat all but the most determined dieter.

Weight-loss groups

It is probably useful for the obese patient to have an initial assessment one-to-one with a dietitian, so the necessary information described above can be collected. However, for follow-up sessions there are several advantages in working with groups of about 10 to 15 patients. It is a more efficient use of the dietitian's time to talk to a group of patients than to repeat almost the same message many times to the members of the group individually. Provided that the group is skillfully and sensitively led, patients benefit from being associated with others in a similar situation, and from hearing answers to problems raised by other members of the group. This is particularly true for diffident patients who would not have had the courage to raise the problem themselves. However, group treatment is not a panacea, and may be disastrous if there is a particularly assertive or destructive personality within the group.

Very-low-calorie diets

Commercial diets that provide the recommended daily amounts of micronutrients with minimal energy are attractive to patients wishing to lose weight rapidly. The disadvantage is that the rapid weight loss may signify excessive loss of lean tissue.

Increasing energy output: exercise and drug treatment

Exercise

Physical activity increases energy expenditure, physical fitness, and sensitivity to the action of insulin, all of which are valuable effects for obese people. Although élite athletes can maintain very high levels of energy expenditure for sustained periods, the maximum rate of work of the average non-athlete is about 6 kcal (25 kJ)/min over 1 h. The average resting metabolism is about 1 kcal (4 kJ)/min, so after 1 h the jogger will have used about 360 kcal, while his twin who remained at rest used 60 kcal, so the net cost of an hour's jogging is about 300 kcal. This is probably the upper limit of the increase in energy expenditure which it is realistic to expect overweight people to achieve by exercise. At this level of exercise intensity there is no measurable elevation of metabolic rate when the exercise has stopped. It is often claimed that physical training can selectively increase the fat-free mass of the body, so although the obese person may not experience weight loss, some fat is being replaced by an equal weight of muscle. A recent review of the evidence by Forbes did not find evidence to support this claim. Certainly, obese patients should be encouraged to take exercise within the limitations of their exercise tolerance, and they will benefit in physical fitness by doing so. However, exercise alone is not an effective method for achieving weight loss, nor of significantly altering the proportions of fat and lean issue in the body.

Thermogenic drugs

Thyroxine, given in doses higher than required to match natural production, can reduce weight, but the loss then comprises mainly lean tissue. Recently, there has been intense research to find a drug that will activate energy-wasting reactions in the body without adverse effects. Although several are under development, none has yet proved useful in the treatment of obesity.

Decreasing energy intake: drugs, surgery, jaw wiring

Anorectic drugs

Hunger is a common problem in the dieting patient, so a drug that could abolish or reduce it should be useful. Three types of medication are intended to have this effect. Bulk fillers, such as guar gum, reduce food intake if taken in sufficient quantity, but the discomfort involved in taking quantities that have a significant effect is similar to the discomfort of the hunger which they are designed to relieve, so they are not generally useful. Drugs related to amphetamine have a very significant anorectic effect, but the risks of abuse and psychosis require that the prescription of these drugs is closely controlled. Probably the most widely used anorectic drug is D-fenfluramine, which acts through the serotinergic system in the brain, and is sedative rather than stimulant. Its efficacy was tested in a large, long-term, multicentre study in which the patients were prescribed a conventional energy-restricted diet and a tablet (15 mg D-fenfluramine twice a day or placebo) for 12 months, with monthly assessments (Guy-Grand *et al.* 1989). At 12 months, 37 per cent of the drug group and 45 per cent of those on placebo had withdrawn for various reasons: the mean weight loss among those who completed the trial was 9.82 kg or 7.15 kg, for drug or placebo groups respectively: all the weight loss had occurred in the first 6 months. A 52-week double-blind placebo-controlled randomized trial of fluoxetine (60 mg/day) produced even less favourable results. At the end of the year both patients on drug and placebo had lost only 2 kg. At present the benefits derived from the use of anorectic drugs do not outweigh the disadvantages. Although they decrease hunger in the short term, they cause only a modest increase in weight loss, and do nothing to help with the eventual problem of maintaining weight loss.

Drugs to inhibit digestion and absorption of food from the gut

Several substances will block the action of digestive enzymes *in vitro*, but are not effective in preventing the digestion of a meal when taken orally. If an effective drug is found, it will be difficult to demonstrate its safety for long-term use, since the nutrients that are not absorbed in the small bowel will become available as substrate for anaerobic metabolism by colonic bacteria. This will almost certainly cause flatulence, and may have more serious consequences as the bacteria in the colon adapt to the new energy supply. This class of drugs has not yet been shown to be useful in clinical practice.

Surgical treatment of obesity

This is not an alternative to dieting, but a method for trying to enforce dieting. The minor exception is apronectomy: it is possible for the surgeon to cut away fat hanging in a fold of anterior abdominal wall, but this is really only applicable in severely obese patients, and preferably those who have already lost a considerable amount of their excess fat. Cutting, or sucking, fat from subcutaneous sites is advertised as a cosmetic procedure, but the amount of fat that can be removed is trivial in comparison with the total excess fat in a patient who has medically important obesity. In many cases the cosmetic result from an attempt to remove significant quantities of subcutaneous fat is very unsatisfactory.

Bypass operations

In this class of operations the gut is cut and rejoined to provide a relatively short exposure of the food to the action of digestive enzymes, while the majority of the bowel is short-circuited. The objective is to produce some degree of malabsorption, so that some of the energy in the food is not absorbed, and also so that a large energy intake provokes severe diarrhoea. The weight loss caused by operations of this kind depends more on the aversive consequences if the patient overeats than on failure to absorb what is eaten.

Gastric stapling

In this operation a line of staples closes off all but a small pouch at the fundus, which empties through a small stoma into the main body of the stomach, so only about 50 ml of food can be taken at a time. Typically, patients lose about one-third of their excess weight in the year after operation, but there is then a tendency for weight regain. Weight loss is somewhat greater after the bypass than after the stapling operation, but at the cost of greater metabolic complications, and a greater risk of nutrient deficiencies. Both operations are technically reversible, but weight gain after reversal is rapid and almost universal.

The relative advantages and disadvantages of bypass operations and gastric stapling have been reviewed in a Consensus Statement (1991), the main points of which were:

1. Patients seeking therapy for severe obesity for the first time should be considered for treatment in a non-surgical programme, with integrated components of a dietary regimen, appropriate exercise, and behavioural modification and support.
2. Gastric restrictive or bypass procedures could be considered for the well-informed and motivated patient with acceptable operative risks.
3. Patients who are candidates for surgical procedures should be selected carefully after evaluation by a multidisciplinary team with medical, surgical, psychiatric, and nutritional expertise.
4. The operation should be performed by a surgeon substantially experienced with the appropriate procedures and working in a clinical setting with adequate support for all aspects of management and assessment.
5. Lifetime medical surveillance after surgical therapy is a necessity.

These are views with which experts in the field would agree; the problem in real life is what to do with the severely obese patient who is not well motivated, or is not a good operative risk, or in whom the careful evaluation reveals some other reason why he or she is not ideally suited for surgery. Surgery is often selected because it seems to be the best choice at the time, but this decision may later be regretted by those who inherit the task of lifelong medical supervision.

Gastric balloon

Balloons have been inserted into the stomach to reduce gastric capacity without the hazards associated with abdominal operations in obese people. The results have been disappointing; weight loss is small and not sustained, and the risk of ulcerating the gastric mucosa is significant.

Jaw wiring

It is standard orthodontic practice to wire upper and lower jaws together for treatment of jaw fractures, or when it has been necessary to resect part of the lower jaw. With this procedure the patient can drink, but not chew, and since liquid diets tend to have a low energy density patients often lose weight. Weight loss of about 36 kg in 9 months can be achieved, but not sustained when the wires are removed. The procedure is not justified unless it is combined with some method for helping the patient to maintain the weight loss (see below).

Figure 8 indicates a flow path by which a suitable treatment strategy for a given patient may be identified.

Fig. 8 Flow chart by which an obese patient may be matched to the appropriate treatment strategy.

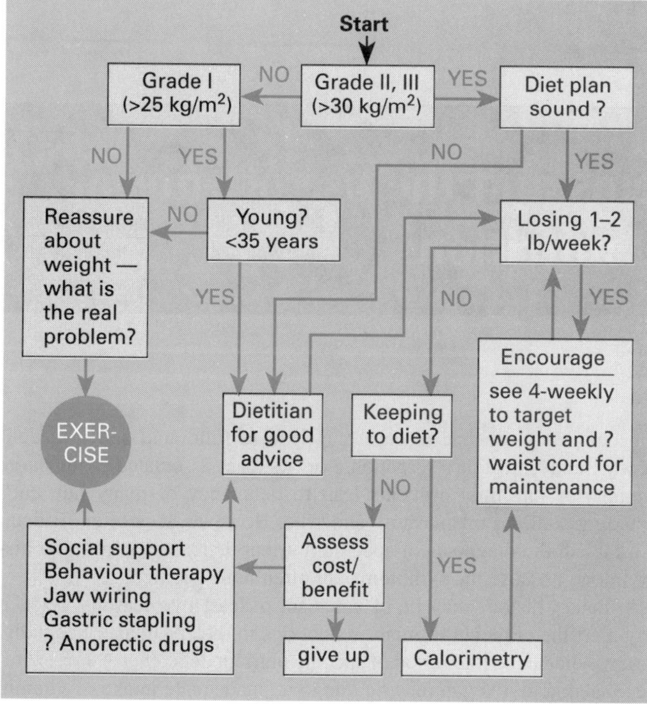

Fig. 9 Change in Quetelet's Index with age in boys. A severely overweight boy aged 5 years can become a normal weight for height 12-year-old by gaining 14 kg (instead of the average 19 kg) over the 7-year interval.

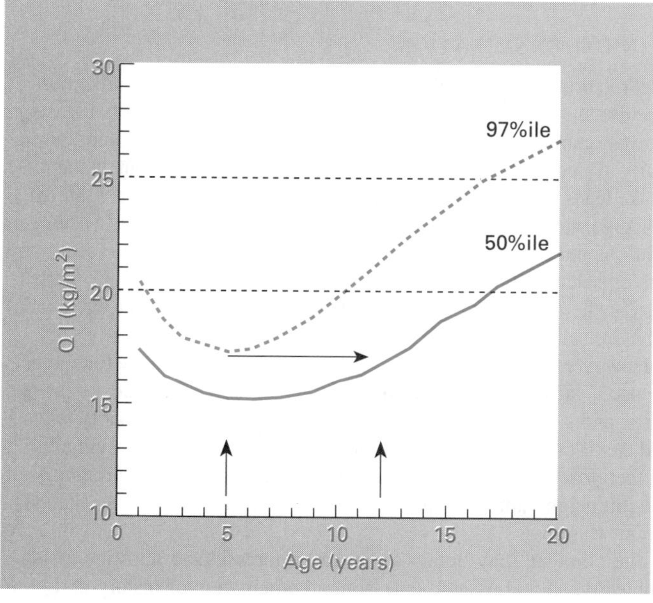

Maintenance of weight loss

If a patient manages to keep to a reducing diet for many months and achieves massive weight loss, it must not be assumed that the weight loss will be automatically maintained when the intense dieting effort is over. On the contrary, it should be assumed that a patient who reduces from, say, 100 kg to 70 kg and then goes back to eating 'normally' (that is, to the diet that previously supported a weight of 100 kg) then that is the weight that will be regained before equilibrium is re-established. We do not know what keeps people of desirable weight at their desirable weight, but whatever this characteristic may be it clearly is not possessed by the formerly obese person.

Most people in affluent countries control their weight, at least in part, by noting unacceptable increases in weight, and altering energy intake (or output) to compensate. To a person who has never been more than 70 kg an increase to 80 kg is a new experience, which will cause some alarm, but this is not true of a person who was previously 100 kg. Previously obese people who have lost weight benefit from a device that warns them of weight gain, which may be a spouse, or flatmate, or a favourite pair of jeans. Alternatively, this monitoring function can be performed by a nylon cord fixed round the waist which becomes tight if excessive weight is gained.

Prevention of obesity

PRIMARY PREVENTION IN CHILDREN

Since about one-third of the adult population in the United Kingdom is already overweight, the opportunities for primary prevention of obesity lie mainly with primary school children. The idea that fatness was determined in infancy by the number of fat cells is no longer tenable: fat babies often do not become fat children, and many fat children were not fat babies. However, fatness at age 13 years is quite a strong predictor of adult fatness, so the optimum time to prevent obesity is in the interval between 5 and 12 years. Figure 9 shows the change in QI among boys aged 1 to 20 years (the curves for girls are similar). Children show a minimum QI at about 5 years of age. At that age a boy on the 50th centile weighs about 19 kg, and will gain another 19 kg by the time he is 12 years old. A boy on the 97th centile at age 5 weighs 24 kg, and if he continues on the 97th centile he will gain another 32 kg by the age of 12 years. However, if the obese boy at age 5 gained only 14 kg in the next 7 years he would then be normal weight for height.

SECONDARY PREVENTION IN ADULTS

The factors that predispose to rapid weight gain in adults have been reviewed above. Unfortunately, adults who are concerned about unwanted weight gain do not get much help from the medical profession until they have become severely obese. It would be better if such people were offered scientifically sound and practical advice about limiting weight gain by means of community slimming clubs, as part of the preventive medicine service.

REFERENCES

Consensus Statement (1991). Gastrointestinal surgery for severe obesity. *NIH Consensus Development Conference, 25–27 March 1991.*

Dore, C., Hesp, R., Wilkins, D. and Garrow, J.S. (1982). Prediction of energy requirements of obese patients after massive weight loss. *Human Nutrition: Clinical Nutrition* **36C,** 41–8.

Durnin, J.V.G.A. and Womersley, J. (1974). Body fat assessed from body density and its estimation from skinfold thickness: measurement on 481 men and women from 16–72 years. *British Journal of Nutrition*, **32,** 77–97.

Forbes, G.B. (1992). Exercise and lean weight: the influence of body weight. *Nutrition Reviews* **50,** 157–61.

Garner, D.M. and Wooley, S.C. (1991). Confronting the failure of behavioral and dietary treatments for obesity. *Clinical Psychology Review* **11,** 729–80.

Garrow, J.S. (1988). *Obesity and related diseases.* Churchill Livingstone, London.

Garrow, J.S. (1992). Treatment of obesity. *Lancet* **340,** 409–13.

Garrow, J.S. (1993). *Human nutrition and dietetics*, Chapter 32. Churchill Livingstone, Edinburgh.

Gregory, J., Foster, K., Tyler, H., and Wiseman, M. (1990). *The dietary and nutritional survey of British adults.* HMSO, London.

Goldstein, D.J., Rampey, A.H., Enas, G.G., Potvin, J.H., Fludzinski, L.A., and Levine, L.R. (1994). Fluoxetine: a randomised clinical trial in the treatment of obesity. *International Journal of Obesity*, **18,** 129–35.

Guy-Grand, B., Apfelbaum, M., Crepaldi, G., Gries, A., Lefebvre, P. and Turner, P. (1989). International trial of long-term dexfenfluramine in obesity. *Lancet* **ii,** 1142–5.

Lew, E.A. and Garfinkel, L. (1979). Variations in mortality by weight among 750,000 men and women. *Journal of Chronic Diseases* **32,** 563–76.

Manson, J.E. *et al.* (1990). A prospective study of obesity and risk of coronary heart disease in women. *New England Journal of Medicine* **322,** 822–9.

Ravussin, E., Zurlo, F., Ferraro, R., and Bogardus, C. (1991). Energy expenditure in man: determinants and risk factors for body weight gain. *Progress in obesity research 1990*, (ed. Y. Oomura), p. 175. Libbey, London.

Rosenbaum, S., Skinner, R.K., Knight, I.B., Garrow, J.S. (1985). A survey of heights and weights of adults in Great Britain. *Annals of Human Biology* **12,** 115–27.

Schofield, C. (1985). An annotated bibliography of source material for basal metabolic rate data. *Human Nutrition: Clinical Nutrition*, **39C** (suppl. 1), 42–91.

Seidell, J.C. (ed.) (1993). *Obesity in Europe: prevalence and public health implications.* WHO, Copenhagen.

Stunkard, A.J., Sorensen, T.I.A., Hanis, C., *et al.* (1986). An adoption study of human obesity. *New England Journal of Medicine*, **314,** 193–8.

Webster, J.D., Hesp, R., and Garrow, J.S. (1984). The composition of excess weight in obese women estimated by body density, total body water and total body potassium. *Human Nutrition: Clinical Nutrition*, **38C,** 299–306.

10.6 Special nutritional problems and the use of enteral and parenteral nutrition

M. Elia

Introduction

Anorexia is a common consequence of disease, and is probably the most important general cause of undernutrition in Western societies. Undernutrition often develops insidiously and its presence may adversely affect clinical outcome in a wide range of conditions. It may increase morbidity following elective surgery and accidental injury; produce non-specific symptoms such as lethargy, depression, and fatigue; reduce tolerance to cytotoxic drugs or radiotherapy, and prolong hospital stay.

New technological advances have made it possible to administer sufficient nutrients to most patient groups at risk of malnutrition, including those with gastrointestinal failure and severe burns, and those who are unconscious. Artificial nutritional support has also extended from hospitals to nursing homes and to the patients' homes to an unprecedented degree. Therefore artificial nutritional support has become an important component of modern clinical medicine.

The response and benefits of nutritional support depend on the severity of the disease, morbidity, and on nutritional status. An assessment of clinical and nutritional status is the first important step towards rationalizing nutritional therapy.

Nutritional assessment

A well-structured history may provide useful information about the likelihood of undernutrition as well as the likelihood of specific nutrient deficiencies. Loss of appetite associated with loss of more than 10 per cent of body weight generally indicates the need for nutritional support. Gastrointestinal disease, especially when associated with vomiting, diarrhoea, or jaundice is likely to lead to malnutrition, but many infective, malignant, or inflammatory diseases also lead to malnutrition. Patients with painful mouth conditions, poorly fitting dentures, and difficulties in swallowing are particularly at risk of developing malnutrition. Alcoholics, the elderly, infirm, and others who do not have regular meals are also at risk.

The clinical history may indicate specific nutrient deficiencies: blood loss leads to iron deficiency; previous gastric surgery to vitamin B_{12} or iron deficiency; coeliac disease may lead to folic acid and iron deficiency; and intestinal resections or fistulae associated with large amounts of intestinal effluents lead to deficiency of many nutrients, including sodium, magnesium, and zinc. However, it is often difficult to establish the diagnosis of specific nutrient deficiencies from the history alone because the symptoms are often non-specific.

A dietary history may be of value for at least two reasons. First, it may alert the clinician to major reductions in dietary intake. Secondly, it may indicate the likelihood of specific nutrient deficiencies. For example, anaemia in a vegan may be due to an inadequate intake of vitamin B_{12}. A diet poor in fruit and vegetables may predispose to vitamin C deficiency and one poor in fish and margarine (which is normally supplemented with vitamin D) may predispose to rickets or osteomalacia, especially in housebound individuals not exposed to sunlight.

CLINICAL EXAMINATION

The relationship of height to weight provides a useful indication of nutritional status. In children an inadequate intake frequently results in growth retardation. Centile charts are useful for this assessment, particularly if sequential measurements are made. In adults an inadequate intake leads to wasting. The body mass index (weight (kg)/height^2 (m^2)) can give some indication of the extent of depletion (Fig. 1), as can skinfold thickness (measured with a caliper), arm circumference, and arm muscle area (calculated from arm circumference and skinfold thickness at the level at which the circumference measurement was made) (Fig. 2).

However, the range of normality is large, and it is possible for subjects to lose a substantial amount of body weight, adipose tissue, or muscle mass, and still exhibit indices that are in the range of normality (Figs 1 and 2), or even above the range of normality (e.g. obese individuals). It is therefore more useful to undertake sequential measurements of weight, height, and other anthropometric measurements rather than single measurements.

The clinician may obtain an overall impression of nutritional status (subjective global assessment) from a combination of history and clinical examination. The examination should include an assessment of

Fig. 1 Ranges of body mass index—weight (kg)/height²(m²). < 17, moderate to severe chronic protein-energy malnutrition (severe if < 15); 17–20, chronic protein energy malnutrition but some normal subjects; 20–25, desirable (some authorities 19–25); 25–30, mildly overweight (grade 1 obesity); 30–40, grade II obesity; > 40, grade III obesity.

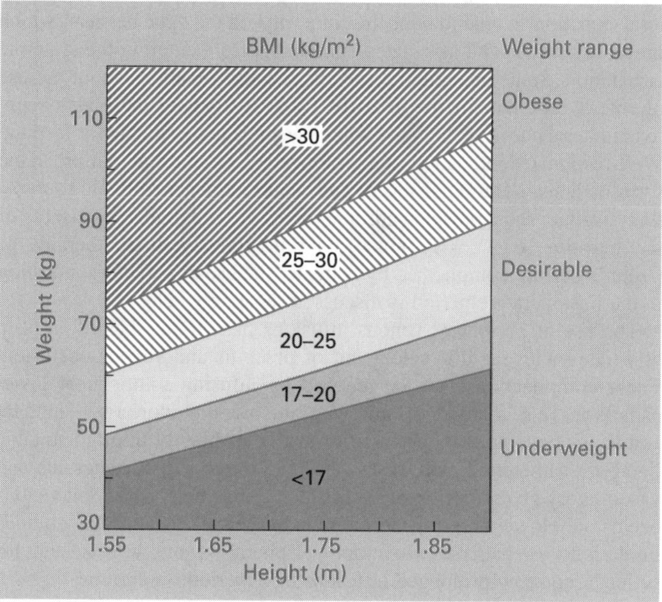

Fig. 2 Percentile curves of triceps skinfold thickness and the estimated mid-upper arm cross-sectional muscle area of American citizens. Based on the US Health and Nutrition Survey (Frisancho 1981, 1984).

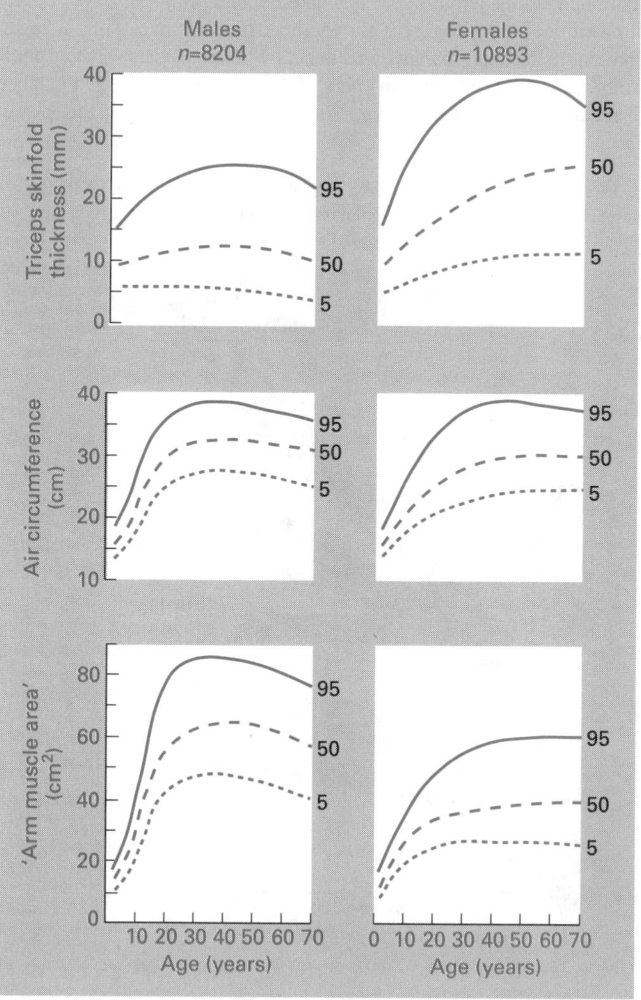

Table 1 *Some signs of specific nutrient deficiencies on examining the limbs and integument*

Nutrient	Sign
Vitamin B_{12}	Anaemia (megaloblastic), atrophic tongue, peripheral neuropathy and subacute combined degeneration of the cord (e.g. absent ankle jerks and upgoing toes)
Folic acid	Anaemia (megaloblastic), atrophic tongue
Vitamin A	Xerophthalmia, hyperkeratosis of the skin
Vitamin C	Easy bruising (positive Hess test)
Vitamin K	Easy bruising (negative Hess test)
Vitamin D	Rickets (swollen wrists, rickety rosary, knock knees), tetany and positive Trousseau's sign (hypocalcaemia), proximal myopathy
Thiamine	Peripheral neuropathy (dry beriberi), oedema (wet beriberi)
Iron	Anaemia (microcytic hypochromic) koilonychia, angular stomatitis, atrophic tongue
Zinc	Bulbous-pustular peristomal and acral dermatitis, loss of hair
Magnesium	Tetany, positive Trousseau's sign
Essential fatty acids	Diffuse scaly dermatitis

muscle wasting, the amount of subcutaneous fat, and presence of oedema and jaundice, but there are many other signs that may be useful, especially on examining the limbs and integument (Table 1). Chelosis or stomatitis may be the result of deficiency of vitamin B complex (but angular stomatitis is common in elderly subjects and may also result from badly fitting dentures); atrophic glossitis may result from folate or vitamin B_{12} deficiency (this may also result from antibiotic therapy); koilonychia may result from severe iron deficiency; tetany may occur in patients with vitamin D deficiency, or hypomagnesaemia; and a rash (acrodermatitis enteropathica) may occur in zinc deficiency. In alcoholics the presence of Wernicke's encephalopathy, Korsakoff's psychosis, and peripheral neuropathy point to the likelihood of thiamine deficiency. Easy bruising may be a sign of scurvy or vitamin K deficiency.

Since the signs and symptoms of many nutrient deficiencies are non-specific, they are often present in a severe form before they can be detected clinically. Usually, deficiencies are present in combinations rather than in isolation.

Preventing and treating malnutrition and the indications for artificial nutritional support

Malnutrition in a variety of clinical conditions has been linked to poor outcome. This, together with the high prevalence of malnutrition reported in some hospitals, has contributed to the recent developments in artificial nutritional support. However, there are many simple things that the clinician can do to improve nutritional state. Nausea may be helped by an antiemetic. A person with dysphagia due to an oesophageal stricture may be helped by the provision of sloppy or liquid meals rather than solid foods. Pain may also cause anorexia, and its relief may improve appetite. Dedicating time to feeding weak and elderly patients may do much to improve nutritional status, or at least prevent the development of malnutrition. This task may be undertaken by nurses, auxiliary staff, or relatives.

When intake is considered inadequate, oral supplements may be tried. If these fail, enteral or parenteral nutrition may have to be used (see below for indications). In some patients it is obvious that artificial nutritional support is necessary from the time of the first consultation. This

Table 2 *Guidelines for the use of enteral nutrition in the adult patient*[a]

1. Clinical settings where artificial enteral nutrition should be a part of routine care
   (a) Protein-energy malnutrition (greater than 10% weight loss) with little or no oral intake for the previous 5 days
   (b) Less than 50% of the required oral nutrient intake for the previous 7–10 days
   (c) Severe dysphasia or swallowing-related difficulties, e.g. head injury, strokes, motor neurone disease
   (d) Major, full-thickness burns
   (e) Massive small bowel resection in combination with parenteral nutrition (in patients with 50–90% small bowel resection, enteral nutrition is given to hasten gut regeneration and return to oral intake)
   (f) Low-output enterocutaneous fistulae (< 500 ml/day)[b] (elemental diets may hasten closure of fistula)
2. Clinical conditions where enteral nutrition would normally be helpful
   (a) Major trauma (see 1(a) and 1(b))
   (b) Radiation therapy (see 1(a) and 1(b))
   (c) Mild chemotherapy (see 1(a) and 1(b))
3. Clinical settings where enteral nutrition is of limited or undetermined value
   (a) Intensive chemotherapy (parenteral nutrition is often indicated)
   (b) Immediate postoperative period or poststress period (especially if an adequate oral intake will be resumed within 5–7 days)
   (c) Acute enteritis
   (d) Less than 10% remaining small intestine (parenteral nutrition is usually indicated)
4. Clinical settings in which enteral nutrition should not be used
   (a) Complete mechanical intestinal obstruction
   (b) Ileus or intestinal hypomotility
   (c) Severe uncontrollable diarrhoea
   (d) High-output fistulae
   (e) Severe acute pancreatitis
   (f) Shock
   (g) Aggressive nutritional support not desired by the patient or legal guardian, and such action being in accordance with hospital policy and existing law
   (h) Prognosis not warranting aggressive nutritional support

[a]Based on the American Society of Parenteral and Enteral Nutrition Board of Directors (ASPEN) (1987).

[b]If the fistula is proximal, the feeding should be distal. If the fistula is distal, sufficient proximal length must be present to allow sufficient absorption. Fistulae due to malignancy, radiation, and distal obstruction are unlikely to close spontaneously.

applies to patients who are unconscious (and likely to remain unconscious for a long period, e.g. following serious head injury), and those who are unable to swallow or have intestinal failure. It also may apply to patients subjected to major surgery, e.g. oesophagogastrectomy, who are routinely prevented from eating for a week or more until the anastomosis has adequately healed, and patients receiving aggressive chemotherapy for haematological malignancies (bone marrow transplantation). These latter patients typically develop severe inflammation of the mucous membranes of the mouth and other parts of the gastrointestinal tract, so that artificial nutritional support (enteral or parenteral nutrition) may be required shortly after the start of treatment. A separate section is dedicated to several of these conditions, but first it is necessary to consider briefly some of the general indications of artificial nutritional support and associated nutritional requirements.

Whenever the gut is available, oral or enteral nutrition should be used because it is simpler, cheaper, and more physiological than parenteral nutrition. In addition, enteral nutrition appears to be better than parenteral nutrition in maintaining the integrity of the 'gut barrier', which prevents bacteria and associated endotoxins from entering the systemic circulation. Some general and specific recommendations about the use of enteral tube feeding are given in Table 2. Some of these also apply to parenteral nutrition, but only when the gut is not available for feeding. Well-recognized indications are prolonged gastrointestinal failure in the form of ileus, peritonitis, severe and recurrent pancreatitis, high intestinal fistulae, short bowel syndrome, or severe inflammatory disease of the intestine, e.g. severe mucositis following cytotoxic therapy, or Crohn's disease complicated by fistulae. The use of parenteral nutrition in the postoperative period is discussed separately below.

The use of peripheral venous infusions of nutrients has often been associated with rapid development of phlebitis and venous occlusion. These complications may be reduced by infusing solutions of lower osmolarity (e.g. a larger volume, less glucose, and more fat—since fat emulsions have an osmolarity close to that of blood), through suitable fine-bore catheters. Small doses of heparin and/or corticosteroids and vasodilatory glycerin trinitrate skin patches may help to prevent venous occlusion. However, peripheral parenteral venous feeding has obvious limitations for patients with poor peripheral venous access, and for patients requiring prolonged infusions of hypertonic solutions.

Nutritional requirements

PROTEIN AND ENERGY

Recommendations about nutrient intake depend on the disease activity and nutritional state. Figure 3 shows the effects of increasing nitrogen intake on the nitrogen balance in subjects who are close to energy equilibrium. Normal individuals in energy balance achieve nitrogen balance at a mean intake of 0.1 g N/kg. The World Health Organization rec-

Fig. 3 Relationship between N intake (1 g N = 6.25 g protein) and N balance in subjects who are receiving sufficient energy to be close to energy balance (see text) (based on Elia 1982; Elwyn 1993).

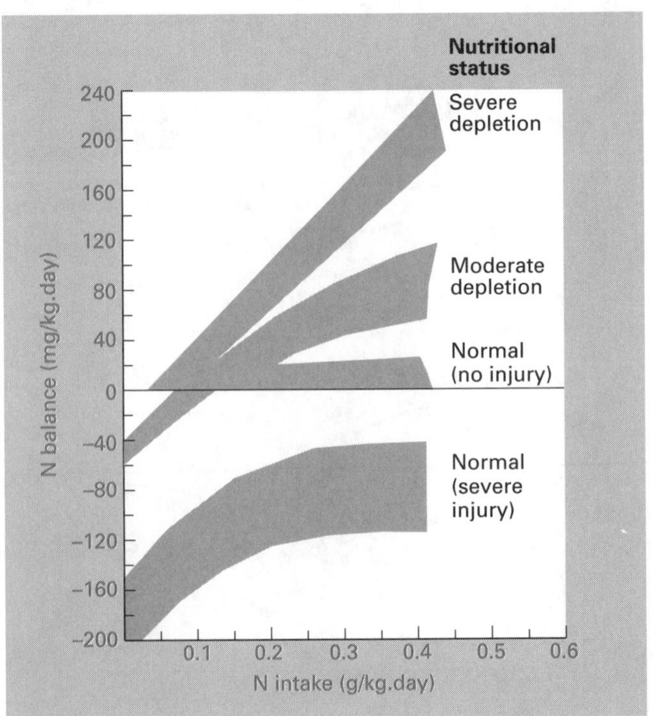

ommends a minimum of 0.12 g N/kg, to take into account the variability between individuals (+ 2 standard deviations). A greater intake produces little improvement in nitrogen balance in normal subjects. In contrast, depleted individuals, particularly those without associated inflammatory or infective disease, continue to achieve a progressively greater positive balance as the nitrogen intake is increased (Fig. 3).

This negative nitrogen balance in catabolic states is due to a combination of the disease itself, which enhances both net muscle proteolysis and liver gluconeogenesis, immobility, and the effect of some drugs such as steroids. The catabolic response is usually greatest within the first few days of injury, but in burned patients it may continue for weeks, albeit to a smaller degree. In normally nourished catabolic patients (e.g. those with sepsis, trauma, burns) who are close to energy balance, an increase in nutritional intake results in improved nutritional balance. However, as Fig. 3 indicates, the curve of N intake v. N balance is shifted downwards (the more severe the injury the greater the catabolism) and to the right. In clinical practice, many patients become malnourished following a severe catabolic injury, so that the response to nutrient intake is intermediate between malnutrition uncomplicated by disease, and severe injury uncomplicated by malnutrition.

From these different responses (Fig. 3) emerge some general and approximate recommendations for nitrogen intake in patients (Fig. 4). The recommended energy intake also varies with the clinical state. In

Fig. 4 Guidelines for estimating the approximate energy and nitrogen (N) requirements (1 g N = 6.25 g protein) for an adult patient receiving artificial nutritional support (based on Elia 1990).

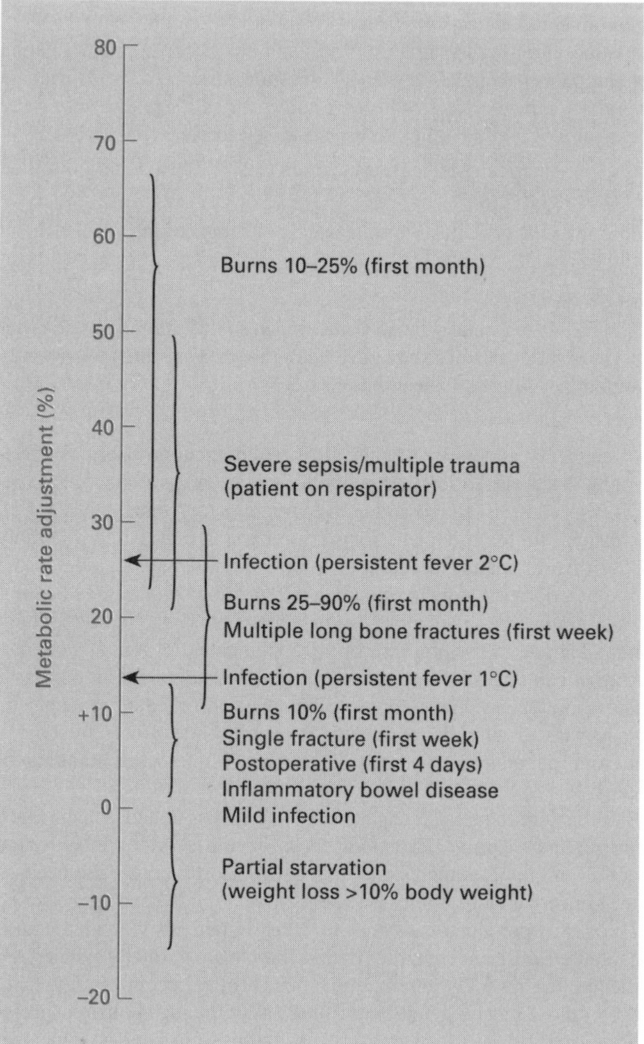

well-nourished individuals who are likely to receive nutritional support for considerable periods of time, it is sensible to aim for energy balance. In the depleted patient, it is desirable to achieve a positive energy balance (as well as a positive nitrogen balance); whereas in obese individuals, loss of adiposity (while limiting the loss of lean tissue) is desirable.

Our concepts about the energy requirement of hospitalized patients have changed considerably over the past 10 to 20 years, so that much less energy is now generally prescribed than previously. This change is due to a combination of factors. One is an over-reaction to the frequent and severe malnutrition which was present before artificial nutritional support became widely practised. Another concerns errors in the interpretation of measurements of metabolic rate. For example, measurements made while patients are receiving large quantities of nutrients will include the thermic effects of the nutrients. Therefore it is incorrect to ascribe any hypermetabolism detected to the disease itself. It is also incorrect to estimate energy requirements for long periods of time based on measurements made over short intervals, especially those obtained during peak hypermetabolism. Furthermore, the effect of pyrexia on energy requirements should not be doubly accounted, as has been done by some professional bodies, since it is already included in the measurement of basal metabolic rate. Another major reason for recommending a lower energy intake than previously stems from change in the clinical management of certain groups of patients. The practice of nursing burned patients in a thermoneutral temperature (26–30 °C or the temperature of minimum resting energy expenditure) and surgically removing necrotic skin tissue, instead of leaving it until it scabs, has contributed to a reduction in energy expenditure.

It is also important to remember that disease is associated with a reduction in physical activity which is often more than sufficient to offset any increase in basal metabolic rate due to disease. Even in ambulatory patients receiving parenteral nutrition in hospital and at home, measurement of total 24-h energy expenditure using tracer techniques has often been found to be 1700 to 2300 kcal/day.

Finally, administration of excess nutrients can increase the likelihood of metabolic complications (e.g. hyperglycaemia, hypermetabolism, increased CO_2 production, and abnormal liver function tests). This, together with recent animal studies suggesting that overfeeding produces a greater mortality in sepsis, has alerted clinicians to the possible dangers of overprescribing nutrients.

Energy requirement may vary substantially with body size, nutritional status, and disease activity. Approximate estimates for requirements are given in Fig. 4. It is thought that most hospitalized adult patients generally require between 1500 and 2500 kcal and between 10 and 15 g N per day. In prescribing artificial feeding it is often possible to approximate the requirements to the contents of three or four standard regimens, to monitor the patient's progress, and to adjust accordingly. It should also be remembered that in some conditions it may be sensible to reduce the intake below normal. For example, the intake of energy can be reduced in the obese, and the intake of protein may be reduced or even temporarily stopped in hepatic encephalopathy. In renal failure it may also be restricted if the aim is to reduce the uraemia and either to avoid dialysis or to increase the interval between dialyses. Fluid restriction in some patients may limit the quantity of nutrients that can be administered. In this case, a compromise between the general clinical needs and nutrient needs is necessary.

FLUID

Usually 1.5 to 3.0 litres of fluid are given to adults receiving enteral or parenteral nutrition, but the intake may vary both above and below this range. Particularly high fluid and electrocyte requirements are necessary in patients with large-output intestinal fistulae. In other situations the fluid allocated to nutritional support is restricted, partly because the patient may already be receiving fluid for other purposes (e.g. infusions of drugs and blood), and partly because the clinical conditions demand it. Low fluid intake may be necessary in oedematous patients, those with renal hepatic or cardiac failure, and patients that have suffered a recent head injury. In this last situation fluid restriction is recommended to limit brain oedema, which can adversely affect the level of consciousness and clinical outcome, but some head-injured subjects may develop diabetes insipidus, when extra fluid is required. Patients with burns also have high fluid requirements. On the other hand, many acute diseases (e.g. various forms of trauma or injury) are associated with impaired renal excretion of water and salt loads, and therefore fluid balance has to be monitored carefully. In the intensive care unit, fluid intake is often modified depending on the results of central venous pressure measurements. Major changes in body weight from one day to the next can also help in the assessment of fluid requirement since these predominantly reflect changes in fluid balance.

MINERALS AND TRACE ELEMENTS

For many adult patients receiving artificial nutritional support, the recommended intake of sodium and potassium intake is often 50 to 100 mmol/day. Chloride intake is usually similar to that of sodium, and phosphate is usually prescribed at a dose of 20 to 40 mmol/day. However, since artificial nutrition is used in a wide range of patients with different disorders, it is not surprising that mineral requirements vary considerably. For example, sodium restriction may be necessary in patients with renal, hepatic, and cardiac failure who are prone to fluid retention. Extra sodium is required in patients with increased loss of gastrointestinal effluents. The additional requirements of sodium and potassium can be predicted from effluent composition as indicated in Table 3. Note that loss of 1 litre of gastrointestinal fluid may more than double the sodium requirements while affecting potassium requirements to a much smaller extent. However, potassium requirements may be increased in patients with excessive renal losses. Potassium requirements may double in patients receiving amphotericin B, which is often given following the use of chemotherapy in bone marrow transplantation. Adequate amounts of potassium and phosphate, which are predominantly intracellular ions, are also necessary during repletion of lean tissue. Indeed, deficiencies of these substances can make the N balance substantially more negative.

The recommended intakes of calcium, magnesium, and many trace elements are quite different for oral/enteral nutrition compared to intravenous nutrition (Table 4). This is because the gut only absorbs a proportion of these nutrients, sometimes less than 10 per cent (e.g. chromium). Prolonged intravenous administration of trace elements at the dose recommended orally may result in toxicity. One of the functions of the gut is to limit the uptake of potentially toxic substances that may be present in excess in the diet or in the gut. The gut is the most important organ regulating the availability of some trace elements into the body, as in the case of iron for which there is little capacity for its disposal by other organs such as the kidney or liver. However, the gut does not appear to be so important in the regulation of fluorine, iodine, or selenium status.

The requirements of trace elements in various diseases are not clearly established, although patients with intestinal fluid losses may have substantial/greater requirements for zinc (Table 4, footnote) and to a lesser extent, chromium. The American Medical Association has recommended that patients on intravenous nutrition may require a fivefold increase in the amount of zinc for every litre of gastrointestinal fluid lost, and a twofold increase in the case of chromium. In contrast, there should be caution about possible toxicities resulting from prolonged intravenous administration of trace elements.

VITAMINS

In contrast to the intravenous recommendations for trace elements, which are generally lower (sometimes severalfold) than those given orally, the reverse is true for vitamins (Table 5). This is partly because the vitamins are generally absorbed to a much greater extent than most trace elements, and partly because their requirement probably increases in many diseases. Although the vitamin requirements in particular diseases, especially infective and active inflammatory ones, are not well established, the requirements for some vitamins may be considerably greater than in health. In addition, some vitamins may degrade during the preparation and storage of parenteral nutrition solutions. For example vitamin A, riboflavin, and vitamin K are photosensitive, and vitamin C may degrade in the presence of trace elements, oxygen, and copper. Thiamine can degrade in the presence of sulphate, which is used as a preservative, and vitamin A palminate may be adsorbed on some plastic storage bags or administration sets. It should be also be remembered that some patients are depleted of vitamins prior to the initiation of therapy.

Manufactured enteral feeds have a long shelf-life and contain trace elements and vitamins. Parenteral feeds have a shorter shelf-life and vitamins and trace elements are often added shortly before use because of the concern about stability (see above). Vitamin K need not be added routinely and particular care must be taken in patients who are on anticoagulants. Sufficient quantities of this vitamin are normally synthesized in the gut, but a weekly intramuscular dose is often recommended, especially in those receiving antibiotics that affect the metabolism of intestinal bacteria. More frequent doses may be given to patients with liver

Table 3 *Approximate electrolyte content of intestinal effluents (mmol/l)*

	Sodium	Potassium	Bicarbonate	Chloride
Gastric	60	15	–	90
Pancreatic	140	5	90	75
Biliary	140	5	35	100
Small intestinal	100	10	25	100
Diarrhoea	60	30	45	45

Table 4 *Recommended daily oral and parenteral intakes of calcium, magnesium, and trace elements in adults*

Mineral or trace element	Oral (mg)[a] Men	Oral (mg)[a] Women	Intravenous (mg)[b]
Calcium	800	800	240–400
Magnesium	350	280	140–290
Iron	10	15	1–2
Zinc	15	12	2.5–4.0[c]
Copper	1.5–3.0	1.5–3.0	0.5–1.5
Iodine	0.15	0.15	0.1–0.2
Manganese	2–5	2–5	0.15–0.8 †
Fluorine	1.5–4.0	1.5–4.0	1–3
Chromium	0.05–0.20	0.05–0.20	0.007–0.013†
Selenium	0.070	0.055	0.03–0.06
Molybdenum	0.075–0.25	0.075–0.25	0.015–0.030

[a]Recommended dietary allowances (National Research Council 1989). The values are for adult males (79 kg) and non-pregnant, non-lactating women (63 kg) aged 25–50 years. Values for those aged > 50 years are generally identical. Some values are indicated as ranges because there is less information on which to base precise recommendations.

[b]Based on American Medical Association (1989), Shenkin and Wretlind (1977), Elia (1990).

[c]Add 2 mg in acute catabolic state and 12–17 mg/l of intestinal effluent lost.

[d]Add 20 μg/l of intestinal fluid lost.

†These doses, especially those at the upper end of the range, are probably overestimates since they have been reported to result consistently in supraphysiological concentrations.

Table 5 *Recommended oral and parenteral intake of vitamins in adults*

Vitamin	Oral (mg)[a] Men	Women	Parenteral (mg)[b]
Water soluble			
Thiamine (B_1)	1.5	1.1	3.0
Riboflavin (B_2)	1.7	1.3	3.6
Niacin (B_5)	19	15	40
Pyridoxine (B_6)	2.0	1.6	4.0
Folate (B_9)	0.2	0.18	0.4
B_{12}	0.002	0.002	0.005
Pantothenic acid (B_3)	(4–7)	4–7	15
Biotin (B_7)	(0.03–0.1)	(0.03–0.1)	0.1
Ascorbic acid (C)	60	60	100
Fat soluble			
Vitamin A[c]	1	0.8	1.0
Vitamin D[d]	0.005	0.005	0.005
Vitamin E[e]	10	8	10
Vitamin K	0.08	0.65	–

[a]Recommended dietary allowances (National Research Council 1989). The values relate to adult males (79 kg) and non-pregnant, non-lactating females (63 kg) aged 25–50 years. Values for those aged > 50 years are similar to those indicated. Some values are indicated as ranges because there is less information on which to base allowances.

[b]Based on American Medical Association (1979).

[c]Retinol equivalents: 1 retinol equivalent = 6 μg β-carotene.

[d]As cholecalciferol: 10 μg cholecalciferol = 400 IU vitamin D.

[e]α-Tocopherol equivalents (TE): 1 mg D-α-tocopherol = 1 αTE.

disease who have a coagulation problem and are at risk of gastrointestinal bleeding. Vitamin B_{12} is also not generally given routinely, but in patients requiring long-term nutritional support, monthly injections can be administered in the same way as they are for patients with pernicious anaemia.

Although the stores of some trace elements and vitamins are large, and deficiencies are not likely to develop for months or possibly years (vitamin A, vitamin D, vitamin B_{12}), it is usual practice to administer a mixture of trace elements and vitamins from the outset of nutritional support, even if this is likely to be for only 1 to 3 weeks. This is because the stores of some vitamins (mainly water-soluble vitamins, e.g. thiamine, riboflavin) are very small. Furthermore, some patients are malnourished at presentation so that the stores of some of the other trace elements or vitamins may already be depleted.

Complications of artificial nutritional support: prevention, treatment, and monitoring

A summary of the complications that may be encountered during parenteral and enteral nutrition is given in Table 6.

PARENTERAL

Mechanical

Complications related to the insertion of a central venous catheter, usually into the subclavian vein, are not common, although pneumothorax may occur in 2 to 3 per cent of cases (the frequency depends on the expertise of the person involved in the procedure). The insertion of the catheter is carried out under aseptic conditions and the position of the catheter tip is confirmed radiologically after insertion. Radiography also helps exclude other complications such as pneumothorax.

Many of the potential problems of parenteral nutrition can be avoided by following appropriate protocols. For example, laying the patient head down while changing feeds and checking the position of locks prevents air embolism, and the use of strict aseptic techniques are essential to prevent catheter-related sepsis (see below).

Occlusion of the catheter may result from reflux of blood into the catheter, but it may also result from coagulation of the feed, especially when all-in-one solutions, which include lipid, are infused. The incidence of catheter blockage depends on the period of catheter use, the diameter of the catheter, and type of catheter (soft polyurethane and Teflon catheters are said to have a lower risk of thrombosis than rigid polyethylene catheters). In patients that have cyclic nocturnal feeding, flushing the catheter with heparin (e.g. 50 U/ml) at the end of feeding reduces the risk of thrombosis. Some recommend routine inclusion of heparin (2–3 U/ml) in the parenteral nutrition solution to prevent both catheter and local venous thrombosis. Several methods may be tried to unblock an occluded catheter. Gentle suction may remove the clot. The clot may be lysed by inserting a solution of urokinase (5000 U/ml) for about 1 h. Alcohol (50 per cent) may be used in a similar way to dissolve lipid-associated occlusions. Insertion of hydrochloric acid (1 M) into the catheter is another potentially effective method.

Infections

Catheter-related infection remains an important complication. Typically the organisms are derived from the skin (e.g. *Staphylococcus aureus*; *Staphylococcus epidermidis*), although a variety of other organisms from the systemic circulation, including Gram-negative organisms and fungi, may seed on to the catheter tip, especially when it is associated with a fibrin clot. Catheter-related sepsis can largely be avoided by the use of aseptic techniques during insertion of the catheter and during the change of feeds, and by avoiding the use of the central venous catheter for purposes other than feeding, such as blood sampling, or administration of drugs and blood.

When catheter-related sepsis is strongly suspected, the catheter should be removed. However, it should be remembered that most episodes of pyrexia are not due to catheter-related sepsis, and the skill of the physician/surgeon in diagnosing alternative causes (e.g. wound infection, pyrexia of trauma, urinary tract infection in patients with urinary catheters, pulmonary embolism) can prevent frequent and unnecessary removal of central venous catheters. Blood cultures taken both from the central venous line and a peripheral vein, and a swab from the catheter entral site, may help to identify the type of organism causing sepsis, and the likelihood that it is related to the catheter.

The procedure of tunnelling the line under the skin, from its site of insertion (typically subclavian vein) to the anterior chest wall, makes dressing and care of the catheter easier, and the location is often more comfortable to the patient. However, there is little evidence that the use of a tunnelling procedure reduces the incidence of catheter-related sepsis.

Multilumen catheters are used in some patients because of the need for multiple uses (sampling and administration of blood, and use for infusion of parenteral solutions including drug therapy). They have the advantages of convenience, especially in patients with limited peripheral venous access. Reports suggest that such catheters probably become infected more frequently than single-lumen catheters which are used solely for parenteral nutrition. This is not surprising because multilumen catheters are more often used for multiple purposes in patients who have more severe disease.

Metabolic complications

Fluid and electrolyte abnormalities are common during parenteral nutrition. This is largely because the underlying condition may result in excess fluid and electrolyte losses (postoperative nasogastric losses, intestinal fistula, etc.) or retention (renal, cardiac, and hepatic failure). Drug therapy may also affect acid–base fluid and electrolyte status. Clinicians involved with the nutritional support of the patient must liaise

Table 6 *Some complications associated with enteral and parenteral nutrition*

	Parenteral	Enteral
Mechanical	Catheter malposition Insertion trauma: pneumothorax, arterial/venous damage (bleeding), branchial plexus injury, chylothorax, cardiac injury, cardiac arrhythmia, fistula	Tube malposition (e.g. placement in trachea) Insertion trauma: nasogastric damage to nasal septum, oesophagus, stomach; perforation (rare); tracheobroncheal fistula (rare) gastrostomy/enterostomy: damage to stomach small bowel; bleeding; peritonitis; leakage, irritation, and infection around the ostomy
	Catheter blockage, kinking, or occlusion Catheter embolus Air embolus	Tube blockage, kinking, or occlusion
	Thrombosis and embolism from catheter tip or vein surrounding catheter	Loss of tube into gastrointestinal tract
Feed/flow related	Substrate overload Glucose: hyperglycaemia and hyperosmolarity (flow related) Fat: infusional hyperlipidaemia Amino acids: hyperammonaemia (infants); uraemia (renal disease)	Diarrhoea or constipation Bloated abdomen and/or cramps Regurgitation/aspiration pneumonia Hyperglycaemia
Infections	Catheter-related sepsis Infected feed/administration set Infection around catheter entry site	Infection of feed or administration set Infection around ostomy
Metabolic	Fluid and electrolyte disturbances Deficiency syndromes, e.g. trace elements, vitamins, essential fatty acids Hyper/hypoglycaemia Substrate overload (see text)	Fluid and electrolyte disturbances Deficiency syndromes (rare with standard feeds in typical patients) Hyper/hypoglycaemia
Organ tissue dysfunction	Abnormal liver function Intestinal atrophy (source of bacterial sepsis) Respiratory distress (excess nutrient administration) Metabolic bone disease	Mainly disease related Aspiration pneumonia may precipitate respiratory distress
Allergic reactions	e.g. to lipid (rare)	Occasionally with some feed constituents (avoided with elemental diets)
Psychological	Anxiety Depression Abnormal self-image Social isolation (home nutrition)	As for parenteral

closely with those involved with other aspects of management. The nutrition team has an important role, partly because it can make the necessary daily adjustments of fluid and electrolytes in the parenteral nutrition solution, and partly because it can make adjustments to other minerals or micronutrients that are not administered routinely to ill patients, for example additions of zinc and magnesium in patients with large persistent intestinal effluent loss. Magnesium deficiency may lead to neuromuscular excitability and tetany. It may also produce hypocalcaemia which is not corrected by calcium administration. Zinc deficiency may impair wound healing and produce dermatitis.

Hyperglycaemia is common in patients receiving parenteral nutrition in hospital. This is largely because glucose intolerance is frequently associated with severe disease. It can be managed by reducing the intake of glucose ($\pm$ increase in lipid intake) or by administering insulin, either as a constant infusion or by intermittent subcutaneous or intramuscular injections, at a dose determined by blood glucose concentrations. Particularly high glucose concentrations may occur if the rate of infusion of nutrients is not adequately regulated. Without the use of an infusion pump the rate of infusion may increase severalfold to cause severe hyperglycaemia, hyperosmolarity, headaches, vomiting, and impaired level of consciousness.

Abnormal liver function tests are frequently observed in patients receiving parenteral nutrition in hospital, for example increased glutamate oxaloacetate transaminase, serum glutamic pyruvic transaminase, and alkaline phosphatase. These are frequently due to the underlying disease (such as sepsis, malignancy, inflammatory bowel disease, pre-existing liver disease) but other factors may be involved: infusion of lipid or excess glucose (leading to hepatic steatosis); bacterial overgrowth in the intestine; and biliary sludge and gallstones. The prolonged absence of oral intake during parenteral nutrition fails to stimulate normal gallbladder contraction and this is probably the major factor responsible for the development of biliary sludge. Detailed investigation of abnormal liver function (biochemical tests, ultrasound scans, and sometimes liver biopsy) may, on occasion, be necessary to discover the underlying pathology.

Phosphate and essential fatty acid deficiencies have both been reported during parenteral nutrition, arising from their lack of inclusion in parenteral nutrition solutions. Phosphate deficiency can cause muscle weakness and impair utilization of protein. It also causes hypercalcaemia and, in the long term, can produce bone disease. Essential fatty acid deficiency produces alopecia, thrombocytopenia, anaemia, and a skin rash as early as 6 weeks after starting intravenous nutritional support without fat. Biochemically, it is diagnosed by an increase in the triene to tetraene ratio (> 0.4) since, in the absence of linoleic acid, oleic acid is metabolized to eicosatrienoic acid. The condition is more likely to develop in patients receiving continuous rather than intermittent parenteral nutrition, because essential fatty acids from the endogenous lipid stores are continually prevented from being released by hyperinsulinaemia. The deficiency syndrome is rapidly reversed by administering an intravenous lipid. Regular application to the skin of oils containing essential fatty acids allows sufficient absorption of fatty acids to treat or prevent this syndrome.

In patients intolerant of lipid (e.g. patients with hyperlipidaemia, some patients with renal or hepatic disease or diabetes) hypertriglyceridaemia results. This may affect the assays of a number of standard biochemical tests, and dilute other plasma constituents (e.g. pseudohyponatraemia). Visual inspection of plasma for lipid several hours after cessation of the lipid infusion can alert the clinician to this problem. Measurement of plasma triglycerides provides a more accurate assessment.

Lipid infusion has been implicated in affecting the function of some organs. For example, hepatic steatosis may cause abnormal liver function tests, and lung deposition in patients with respiratory distress can impair pulmonary function by reducing the permeability of the lung to gases.

Excessive administration of glucose may also have adverse respiratory effects. This is because glucose produces 30 per cent more CO_2/MJ than fat, and an even greater amount of CO_2/MJ when there is net lipogenesis from carbohydrate. Furthermore, excessive administration of glucose increases energy expenditure (dietary-induced thermogenesis) to a greater extent than fat. In patients with impaired pulmonary function this may precipitate respiratory failure, or impair weaning of a patient with respiratory failure from a respirator. However, with the typical amount of glucose infused in most patients this is probably not an important clinical problem. Therefore the use of high-fat regimens generally have little or no advantage over standard or low-fat regimens.

Metabolic bone disease is an occasional problem associated with long-term parenteral nutrition (usually home parenteral nutrition). Several factors may contribute, including corticosteroid therapy, the underlying disease, immobility, and possibly intoxication with aluminium or vitamin D. Excess amino acid intake and heparin have also been implicated. Some studies have reported that the bone histology is not dissimilar to that of osteomalacia, although paradoxically it has been reported that administration of vitamin D can make the condition worse.

Trace element and vitamin deficiencies may occur in patients on long-term parenteral nutrition. Usually this is due to the prescription of insufficient amounts, but excessive losses of intestinal effluents may also be responsible. Deficiencies of several trace elements have been described, for example copper, zinc, iron, selenium, as well as case reports of chromium and molybdenum deficiencies. Several vitamin deficiencies have also been described, including biotin deficiency (eczematous dermatitis, hair loss, depression, anorexia) which is rare under normal circumstances, and night blindness due to vitamin A deficiency.

ENTERAL NUTRITION

The commonest complications associated with enteral feeding in hospitalized patients include nausea or vomiting (10–20 per cent), abnormal bloating and cramps, diarrhoea (5–30 per cent), and constipation (but mainly in long-term feeders at home). Delayed gastric emptying is a feature of many conditions: postoperative abdominal surgery, head injury, severe sepsis, etc. This gastric stasis may lead to accumulation of feed in the stomach, so that eventually the patient develops nausea and vomiting.

In unconscious patients and those with an impaired swallowing reflex, vomiting may lead to aspiration pneumonia, which is one of the most serious complications of enteral nutrition. Gastro-oesophageal regurgitation may also predispose to aspiration pneumonia. Problems associated with poor gastric emptying can be prevented by administering the feed directly into the small intestine. A nasogastric tube may be placed in the small intestine under radiographical control, endoscopically, or during surgery. In those at risk of gastric stasis/regurgitation, gastric pooling can be checked by intermittent aspiration through tubes with a sufficiently wide bore. Continuous infusion of feed into the stomach can prevent the sudden gastric disturbance associated with bolus feeding. The use of an infusion pump to control delivery of feed into the stomach can prevent gastric flooding associated with inadequate manual flow control systems. The use of pharmacological agents, such as metoclopramide or erythromycin, that stimulate gastric emptying may help in susceptible individuals. Erythromycin acts by stimulating the motilin receptor on the smooth muscle of the stomach and small intestine.

Despite the high incidence of diarrhoea in patients receiving enteral-tube feeding in hospital, the mechanism is not entirely understood. However, it is often associated with antibiotic therapy. Lactose intolerance has also been implicated, but most enteral feeds are free of lactose. Rapid delivery of nutrients into the gastrointestinal tract may lead to diarrhoea, especially if the delivery is postpyloric. Here the protective effect of the pylorus in regulating delivery of nutrients into the small intestine is bypassed. A number of other factors have been implicated in causing diarrhoea, including bacterial contamination of enteral diets, an underlying gastrointestinal disease, the use of laxatives, lack of dietary fibre, and neuroendocrine reflexes whereby the administration of feed in the stomach or upper small intestine cause secretion of fluid in the small and large bowel. Diarrhoea may be prevented by taking care not to contaminate the feed with bacteria, controlling the rate of feed infusion, or/and treating the underlying condition. Drugs such as codeine phosphate or loperamide may help to control the symptoms.

Constipation may be a problem in long-term enteral nutrition, particularly in elderly, inactive subjects. Lack of fibre has been implicated, but long-term fibre supplementation studies in such patients are needed to confirm this.

Several metabolic disturbances have been described during enteral feeding: hyperglycaemia in glucose-intolerant subjects; rebound hypoglycaemia after sudden withdrawal of feed; disturbances in plasma potassium, depending on the patient's renal and gastrointestinal function and the potassium content of the feed; hypophosphataemia during refeeding; and abnormalities of liver function which are generally of little clinical significance. The abnormal liver function tests may be due to the underlying disease, drug therapy, or fatty infiltration associated with malnutrition. Refeeding malnourished subjects may produce hypophosphataemia and hypokalaemia as lean tissues containing these electrolytes are accreted.

Trace element deficiencies do not normally occur in patients on long-term enteral feeding but discrepancies have been found between the manufacturers' stated content of some trace elements (copper, zinc, iron, manganese) and the measured content, which was sometimes less than the recommended dietary allowance.

The complications of enteral nutrition at home are similar to those in hospital. Results from a series of 53 patients on home tube-feeding suggest that there are a number of frequent but minor problems of little long-term significance. However, lack of enteral access (due to tube blockage or dislodgement) can be an important problem, because it may lead to dehydration, especially in those with swallowing-related problems who are or prevented from drinking. Flushing of the tubes with water at the end of each feeding period can prevent tube blockage. A blocked tube may be unblocked by flushing it with water in the first instance, followed by a warm solution of sodium bicarbonate or by digesting the coagulated feed with pancreatic enzymes. Coca-Cola® may also be effective in unblocking tubes. If a gastrostomy or enterostomy tube has been dislodged, it is important to replace it quickly because the stoma may rapidly close up and make further access difficult.

Another potentially important problem is regurgitation of feed in patients with impaired gastro-oesophageal function, e.g. elderly people with a hiatus hernia, who have an impaired swallowing reflex. This problem, which can lead to aspiration pneumonia, can be avoided by administering the feed with the upper part of the body elevated to an angle of about 30°, or in those who have a particularly high risk of aspiration it is best to administer the feed directly into the small intestine (jejunostomy feeding).

GENERAL MONITORING OF PATIENTS ON ARTIFICIAL NUTRITIONAL SUPPORT

Careful observations should be made of the patient shortly after the start of enteral or parenteral nutrition, to assess feed tolerance. In patients on parenteral nutrition, urine should be analysed every 4 h to check for glycosuria, and blood glucose should be measured in these patients and others with suspected glucose intolerance. The development of glycosuria in previously stable patients without glycosuria may indicate the development of a complication such as infection before it has been diagnosed clinically. Routine measurements of temperature, pulse, blood pressure, and fluid balance are also essential. Changes in daily weight are the best indices of day-to-day changes in fluid balance. In the longer term, changes in weight usually indicate changes in lean and adipose tissue in response to the support provided.

The frequency with which other investigations are carried out depends on the patient and the underlying condition (also see above). In patients with large losses of gastrointestinal fluids, or those on long-term parenteral nutrition (especially when there is little or no enteral or oral intake), an assessment of trace element and/or vitamin status is often necessary. The catheter site should be inspected regularly as a possible source of infection, and fresh dressings applied as according to standard protocols.

In patients receiving enteral tube feeding, it is important to assess feed tolerance by ensuring that gastric pooling does not occur, especially in those at risk of gastric stasis and those with an impaired swallowing reflex. The development of diarrhoea should lead to a consideration of the possible causes and appropriate action taken (such as adjustment of infusion rate or eradication of specific gastrointestinal pathogens).

Nutritional aspects of specific conditions and situations

The reader is referred to other sections in this book for information on nutritional and fluid and electrolyte aspects of various clinical conditions, e.g. acute and chronic renal failure, malabsorption syndrome, hyperlipidaemia, diabetes mellitus, cystic fibrosis, short bowel syndrome, and enterocutaneous fistulae. Nutritional aspects of a few other conditions, especially those that have gained prominence in recent years, are discussed below.

ACQUIRED IMMUNE DEFICIENCY SYNDROME (AIDS)

AIDS, an increasingly important clinical problem worldwide, has important nutritional consequences. At death, a weight loss of greater than or equal to 20 per cent is common, and in some cases the extent of weight loss may be substantially greater (~40 per cent body weight) and similar to that observed in subjects dying of starvation uncomplicated by disease.

Acute weight loss is usually a consequence of acute infections, whereas more chronic loss is usually associated with an enteropathy. The direct causes of weight loss are multiple. Food intake is usually decreased during acute infections, but during recovery it may be normal or even greater than normal. In advanced disease, decreased food intake is often associated with opportunistic infections in the mouth, pharynx, and oesophagus, which may cause pain and dysphagia. Associated malignancy (Kaposis' sarcoma and non-Hodgkin's lymphoma) may also lead to anorexia. Furthermore, antifungal and antiviral drugs can cause nausea, vomiting, and anorexia, and the use of chemotherapeutic agents for malignancy can produce stomatitis, pharyngitis, and oesophagitis, which can make swallowing painful and distressing. The enteropathy, can be caused by a wide range of pathogens and can lead to steatorrhoea, fluid and electrolyte disturbances, and trace element and vitamin deficiencies. Neurological involvement, which occurs in up to 30 per cent of patients, is also often associated with malnutrition. Dysphagia and coma obviously lead to reduced nutrient intake and malnutrition, and 'dementia', which may affect half the patients with advanced AIDS, may make dietary assessment and management particularly difficult.

Treatment of the underlying condition, such as mouth, throat, and other systemic infections which cause dysphagia, or systemic infections which cause anorexia, can do much to improve nutritional status. There is substantial anabolic potential between acute infective episodes, and the rapid diagnosis and treatment of such infections produce better nutritional results than delayed treatment.

Nutritional assessment should begin at the outset and changes in body weight in relation to the disease process should be closely monitored. Psychological evaluation and social counselling should not be neglected. Anxiety, apathy, and depression are common and may lead to self-neglect, irregular food intake, and deterioration of nutritional status. Support should begin with general nutritional advice about diet, but it may heed to progress to the use of supplements and, occasionally, enteral tube feeding or parenteral nutrition. Enteral nutrition may be used in patients with dysphagia, those with swallowing-related difficulties, those with a decreased level of consciousness, and those with severe weight loss in whom the gastrointestinal tract is functional. Lactose-free feeds and low-fat feeds (with medium-chain triglycerides) are often used in an attempt to improve dietary tolerance, especially in those with an enteropathy. Parenteral nutrition (peripheral or central) may be used when there is intolerance to oral or enteral feeds or in those who develop obstruction. A common indication is in patients with severe diarrhoea (from cryptosporidiosis, for example, or of unknown aetiology) which is resistant to treatment, and which is made worse with enteral feeding.

Surveys have shown that a large proportion of patients with AIDS take supplements of vitamins and trace elements. The clinician should enquire into this practice because, in some cases, ingestion of a large excess of micronutrients may lead to toxicity.

BURNS

Severe burns provide one of the most catabolic and hypermetabolic stimuli to man. The injury response may persist for weeks or months during the period of wound healing. It is not surprising that the nutritional requirements of such patients are greater than for most other catabolic states (see Fig. 3). Nutritional support to metabolically unstable patients (burned or non-burned subjects) can lead to a variety of metabolic complications. Therefore, before aggressive nutritional support is begun, it is important to ensure that some degree of stability is established in haemodynamic and acid–base status.

With minor burns, a normal oral intake, with or without supplements, is all that is required. However, with severe burns, anorexia is frequently severe and prolonged, and artificial nutritional support is usually required.

Feeding through a nasogastric tube is often well tolerated. However, the use of enteral tube feeding may be restricted early after burns because of gastric stasis and occasionally ileus. In most patients gastrointestinal motility improves within 2 to 4 days, so that more nutrients can be administered. Nevertheless, it is important to aspirate the gastric contents intermittently, especially in the early phase after burns, to ensure that there is no gastric pooling. The fluid and electrolyte requirements are often considered in association with nutritional needs, and frequently extra fluid is drunk or given through the enteral feeding tube or intravenous line, to match the increased fluid losses from the skin surface. Some units routinely provide extra micronutrients, but the extent to which vitamin and trace element requirements are increased after burns is poorly defined.

The gastrointestinal tract may not tolerate enteral feeds because of persistent ileus. This may occur in patients with severe burns, and those with other associated problems such as intra-abdominal injuries and sepsis, smoke inhalation, and multiorgan failure resulting in artificial ventilation. In others, the gastrointestinal tract may not tolerate sufficient enteral nutrition to meet the increased requirements of the patient. Therefore some patients need both enteral and parenteral nutrition. The enteral feeding is encouraged because it may maintain gut integrity, prevent bacterial translocation from the gut into the systemic circulation, and speed up the transition from parenteral nutrition to enteral tube feeding and normal oral intake.

HEAD INJURY

Head injury provides another important indication for artificial nutritional support, especially since many patients have an impaired level of consciousness for prolonged periods, which may range from weeks to months.

Head injury frequently coexists with other major injuries, with the result that there is a severe hypermetabolic and catabolic response (for example, the negative N balance may be greater than 20 g N/day in the first week after injury even when a limited intake of nutrients is provided (~800 kcal and 5 g N/day)).

Immobility contributes to the loss of muscle bulk and weight loss can occur very rapidly. One of the major constraints to the use of enteral tube feeding is the delayed gastric emptying, which frequently lasts for more than 10 days after severe head injury. This may be due to the injury alone, but it may also be due to associated abdominal trauma. Using traditional nasogastric feeding techniques in such patients, it is often difficult to provide the full nutritional requirements within 1 to 2 weeks. The impaired level of consciousness and poor or absent swallowing reflex also means that gastric pooling and aspiration are not uncommon. Parenteral nutrition has been used routinely in some centres, which have reported improved nutritional and clinical outcome in comparison with intermittent bolus feeding through a nasogastric tube. However, the use of bolus feeding, especially in patients with severe gastric stasis, was later criticized. More recently, increasing emphasis has been placed on enteral feeding, partly because of its protective effect in preventing mucosal atrophy and bacterial translocation from the gut compared to parenteral nutrition, and partly because parenteral nutrition is associated with a number of potentially serious complications, such as catheter-related sepsis (see above). Therefore, attempts have been made to improve methods of delivering nutrients enterally. This includes the use of pump-assisted delivery and the use of drugs such as metoclopramide and erythromycin, which stimulate gastric emptying. Attempts have also been made to introduce feeds directly into the small intestine, either endoscopically or under radiological control. Bypassing the stomach can allow sufficient delivery of feed to be achieved, but displacement of the tube back into the stomach may occur. Another way of dealing with the problem of gastric stasis is to place jejunostomy tubes, using a laparoscopic percutaneous procedure. Preliminary results of feed tolerance in non-randomized studies of injury are encouraging, but further work is needed.

In patients in whom enteral feeding is not tolerated, for example when there is poor gastric emptying ileus or severe feed-induced diarrhoea, parenteral nutrition is indicated.

TRANSPLANTATION

Artificial nutritional support is required to a varying extent for patients requiring a transplanted organ. With renal transplantation, where the gastrointestinal tract is not affected unless surgical complications occur, it is usual to eat normally shortly after the surgery.

Patients with liver or heart plus lung transplants are usually artificially ventilated in the intensive care unit after transplantation. Artificial nutritional support is often given during this period, especially in those with pre-existing malnutrition or postoperative complications. In those with substantial malnutrition, attempts should be made to improve nutritional status prior to transplantation so that they can cope with the stress of surgery more effectively (see below).

Artificial nutritional support may also be required following treatment with cytotoxic drugs or radiotherapy. In bone marrow transplantation the use of aggressive cytotoxic therapy or radiotherapy may result in inflammation of the mucous membranes of the gastrointestinal tract from mouth to rectum beginning a few days after cytotoxic therapy. Swallowing then becomes painful and diarrhoea a problem. The severity of mucositis may limit the dose of cytotoxic drugs used. A nasogastric tube is often uncomfortable to such patients, and bleeding may occur from friction with the inflamed mucosa, especially in those with thrombocytopenia. Parenteral nutrition is therefore often necessary.

There is much research interest in the use of specific nutrients or bioactive substances to protect the mucosa of the gut from damage by cytotoxic drugs or radiotherapy. Experimental work in animals suggests that glutamine may be particularly effective in this respect. Preliminary evidence in man also suggests that large doses of intravenous glutamine (30–40 g/day) may be beneficial to patients undergoing transplantation, but other work with glutamine supplementation has not been so conclusive. Graft-versus-host reactions complicating marrow or intestinal transplantation may also be accompanied by gastrointestinal symptoms. Severe, prolonged, watery diarrhoea, amounting to several litres a day, presents a serious problem. Parenteral nutrition is usually necessary after intestinal transplantation, partly because the pre-existing bowel disease produces malnutrition (many patients receiving bowel transplants are on long-term parenteral nutrition prior to the transplant), and partly because it is necessary to ensure that sufficient time has been allowed after transplant surgery to ensure that anastomoses have adequately healed, and that mucosal integrity has recovered. Fluid electrolyte and trace elements may need to be given in increased amounts to balance the increased loss associated with gastrointestinal effluents. The protein and energy requirements of patients receiving transplants can be calculated according to the scheme indicated in Fig. 4.

PERIOPERATIVE NUTRITION

Although malnutrition may be present prior to elective surgery, it is most likely postoperatively, especially in those with complications. Many studies have been undertaken to assess whether perioperative nutritional support reduces the complication rate after surgery. They have produced conflicting results, with some suggesting improvements, others no significant effect, and in yet others an increase in infective complications (e.g. catheter-related sepsis) when parenteral nutrition is used. These conflicting results have occurred at least partly because of the multiple other factors that affect the outcome of surgery (age, sex, severity of disease, skill of the surgeon, nursing care, and presence or absence of a nutrition team, and preoperative nutritional status).

The largest multicentre trial of perioperative parenteral nutrition (The Veterans Affairs Total Parenteral Nutrition Co-operative Study Group 1991) involved several hundred patients undergoing elective abdominal and thoracic surgery. The routine administration of parenteral nutrition (from up to 2 weeks before surgery and at least 3 days after surgery) provided no overall benefit. However, in the subgroup of patients who were severely malnourished, perioperative nutritional support decreased the non-infective complications from 42 per cent to between 5 and 23 per cent (depending on the method used to define malnutrition). This and other studies emphasize the importance of patient selection for nutritional support. It is obvious, for instance, that other patient groups, such as those with prolonged ileus, massive bowel resection, fistulae, or recurrent severe pancreatitis, are likely to benefit from parenteral nutrition. Meticulous fluid and electrolyte balance is of major importance (see Table 3) in those with fistulae, with nasogastric aspirates, and those complicated by multiorgan failure.

Patients with prolonged anorexia and intra-abdominal sepsis are also likely to benefit from nutritional support. Parenteral nutrition may be required for long periods, for instance in the patient in whom the fluid output from a fistula gradually decreases in the absence of oral food intake, or after massive intestinal resection (short bowel syndrome) when intestinal adaptation may take weeks or months. In some patients with the short bowel syndrome (< 25 cm small intestine remaining) such support may be required indefinitely.

Home nutritional support

One of the most important recent developments in nutritional support is its use in the community. In 1993 it was estimated that more than 30 per cent of the total artificial nutritional support in Britain (mainly enteral tube feeding) took place in the community, and it is likely that the trend towards more home care will continue to increase. In the United States there are probably more patients receiving enteral tube feeding outside than in hospital. In other countries the trend towards home care has been limited by the lack of an adequate infrastructure and organization, which are necessary to train, discharge, and monitor patients, and to ensure that the feeds and accessories are delivered to the home regularly and reliably.

Artificial nutritional support at home has a number of advantages over treatment in hospital. The patients frequently feel more comfortable in the familiar home environment, where many of them not only care for themselves but also for other family members. Affected adults may frequently go to work and children attend school The treatment of patients at home is cheaper and frees beds for the use of other patients. Treatment at home does involve a major commitment on the part of the patient or carer. It is also associated with potentially serious complications.

INDICATIONS FOR HOME ARTIFICIAL NUTRITION

Home nutritional support is indicated when there is likely to be benefit and the patients or carers are able to perform the necessary tasks to a sufficiently high standard. Whether enteral or parenteral nutrition is used depends on whether the gastrointestinal tract is available for the digestion and absorption of nutrients.

Home parenteral nutrition

Intestinal failure due to Crohn's disease (with or without fistulae), short bowel syndrome, motility disorders (such as scleroderma, and pseudo-obstruction), congenital bowel disease, and radiation enteritis provide important indications. Home parenteral nutrition has also been used in patients with malignancy (usually those with intestinal obstruction) and in patients with AIDS who are unable to tolerate enteral nutrition.

Home enteral tube feeding

The major indications are those associated with swallowing difficulties. These may be obstructive (such as malignancy of the upper gastrointestinal tract) or non-obstructive and due to neurological disorders (for example multiple strokes, Parkinson's disease, motor neurone disease, multiple sclerosis, and primary muscle diseases that affect swallowing). In children, although a neurological disorder of swallowing is an important indication, chronic anorexia leading to failure to thrive is perhaps more common (due to, for example, congenital malformations, severe cystic fibrosis, inborn errors of metabolism, and some gastrointestinal disorders such as Crohn's disease).

AGE DISTRIBUTION

Many reports of home enteral nutrition have noted that 50 per cent or more of the patients are aged over 60 years. This is not too surprising since conditions such as stroke, motor neurone disease, and oesophageal malignancy typically occur in the elderly. Home tube-feeding is also relatively common in children, but it is given less frequently to patients between the ages of 20 and 60 years. This age distribution has particular implications for home care. Many elderly people are unable to care for themselves because of weakness, immobility, arthritis, poor eyesight or hearing, etc., and therefore a carer, usually a family member, has to be identified. Similarly, carers are frequently required for children on home enteral nutrition.

The age distribution of patients on home parenteral nutrition is different, partly because the indication is often Crohn's disease, which occurs predominantly in subjects aged 20 to 50 years.

MANAGEMENT

The principles of artificial nutritional support at home are similar to those in hospital, although special considerations apply to many patients.

Psychological evaluation

The thought that artificial nutritional support may have to be given at home for months or years may cause initial surprise to some patients and they may find it difficult to accept the concept. Nevertheless, given appropriate support, as the patient or carer gains confidence, their fears and anxieties frequently subside. It is always essential to involve family members (or carer) as well as the patient. Contact with patients who are already on home treatment, may do much to reassure. School-age children may also have particular difficulties in coming to terms with this form of therapy, but careful counselling and the use of nocturnal feeding alone, frequently allows them to adjust, attend school, and lead a reasonably normal life.

Training

The training should be supervised only by those experienced in the field. Despite pressure for hospital beds, discharge should not take place until it is clear that the patient is adequately skilled and appropriate arrangements have been made at home.

Patients (or carers of the patients) requiring artificial nutrition at home should learn the basic principles of nutritional support and of asepsis. They should know how to programme the infusion pump that delivers the nutrients, how to add solutions to the feed (if required), how to connect and disconnect the feeds to the catheter/tube, how to change dressings, how to recognize problems associated with feeding, such as a blocked catheter and infection, and how to recognize hyper/hypoglycaemia, measure blood glucose, and screen for glycosuria. Training is often helped by audio-visual aids and written instruction, and reinforced by repeated practice. A trial of home nutritional support over a weekend may be a useful way of assessing the patient's ability to adjust and cope.

Evaluation of the home environment

An assessment of the home environment is essential before discharge. There must be space available for storage of feeds and accessories. A refrigerator is usually necessary for storage of parenteral nutrition solutions and drugs. Modifications to the home can be made to allow routine activities to be carried out more efficiently. A wheelchair or other extra equipment may be very useful for some patients, such as a bed harness for very disabled patients, and adjustable V-shaped boards for children with cystic fibrosis who require physiotherapy and postural drainage of lung secretions.

Financial arrangements

Financial arrangements for home artificial nutrition clearly vary from country to country and in different parts of the same country. A clear statement about finances should be made prior to discharge. In many countries patients and/or carers are entitled to some sort of financial or other support. These should be made known to those entitled to receive them.

Written instructions and follow-up arrangements

Prior to discharge all patients should have written instructions of the routine procedures for home nutritional support and how to recognize and act when complications arise. The patients/carers should also have a telephone number of the appropriate health professional to contact in an emergency, on a 24-h basis.

OUTCOME

The outcome of home nutritional support varies considerably, depending on the underlying condition and the initial selection criteria.

Home parenteral nutrition

The most extensive analysis of outcome of patients on home parenteral nutrition has come from North America (Fig. 5). For a variety of conditions (congenital bowel disease, Crohn's disease, motility disorders of the gut, and radiation enteritis), there is a substantial mortality in the first 2 years (10–30 per cent), but few deaths occur after this period. The mortality is usually due to the underlying condition, although a few deaths arise from the complications of parenteral nutrition. Mortality in patients receiving home parenteral nutrition for AIDS and malignancy has been reported to be high (Fig. 5). For example, in one survey the mortality of AIDS patients receiving parenteral nutrition was as high as 93 per cent in 1 year. This mortality in AIDS and malignancy clearly depends on when nutritional support is started in relation to the stage and severity of the disease. Such a high mortality dictates that such treatment should only be offered to those in whom there is good reason to expect a substantial consequent improvement in the quality of life.

In that context in general, a survey in Britain has revealed that 40 per cent of patients on home parenteral nutrition were independent, able to be fully employed and to look after their families. Fewer than 10 per cent of patients were severely disabled and heavily dependent on others.

Home enteral tube feeding

There is much less information about the outcome of patients receiving home enteral tube feeding. However, in view of the high prevalence of elderly people and the severity of the underlying conditions, a high mortality is to be expected. In one survey an overall mortality of 45 per cent was reported over a period of 2 years. Rates were particularly high for adults who had a malignancy or cerebrovascular disease, as well as for children with major congenital defects. In another community-based study in which enteral tube feeding was given to a group of elderly patients (median age, 76 years) who had suffered from strokes and neurological conditions affecting swallowing, mortality was as high as 50 per cent within the first year. Those with swallowing problems had a better prognosis than those with a stroke. Pneumonia was the most common terminal event.

Fig. 5 Survival of different groups of patients receiving home parenteral nutrition (from Howard *et al.* 1991).

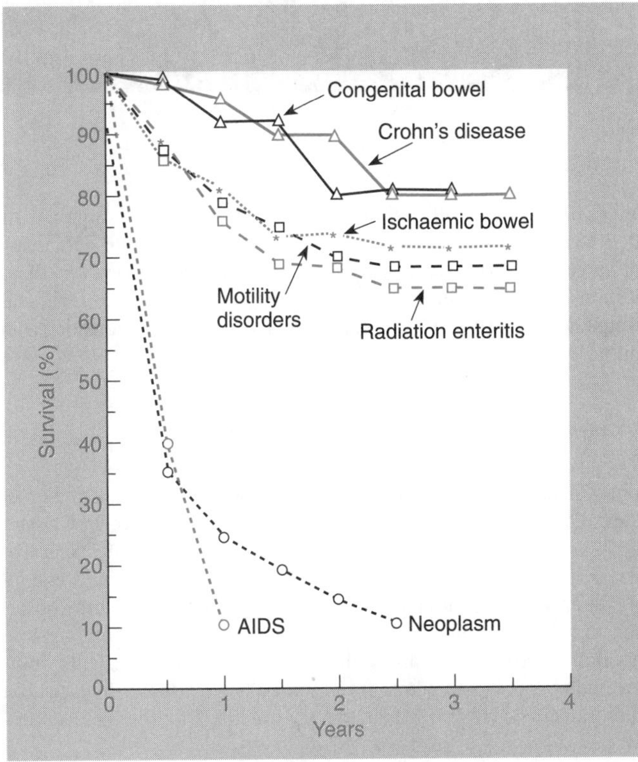

Table 7 *Effect of introducing a nutrition team on the incidence of complications (%) associated with parenteral nutrition*

Percentage with complication	Introduction of team: Before	After	
Catheter-related sepsis	25.0	3.6	Mean of nine studies
Mechanical complications	24.0	6.5	Mean of four studies
Metabolic complications	29.1	12.4	Mean of three studies

From Elia (1993).

Despite the high mortality, many family members feel that the quality of life of affected individuals frequently improves, or does not deteriorate. They appreciate and enjoy being with the affected family member, even in the face of a poor prognosis. In a survey of 70 children receiving home tube feeding, predominantly for failure to thrive, parents reported greater freedom because they did not have to spend so much time trying to feed their children as previously. They also reported that their children were happier and more active than before tube feeding.

MONITORING

Patients on home nutritional support should be seen at regular intervals, at a frequency determined by the needs of the patient or carer and stability of the clinical condition. Nutritional assessment is often based on changes in growth, or body weight (taking into consideration the presence or absence of oedema), but changes in skinfold thicknesses and arm muscle circumference and a variety of biochemical parameters may also be used (for example, urinary creatinine in accurately collected 24-h urine specimens is a reasonable index of muscle mass).

The need for blood counts, urea and electrolytes, and liver function tests varies, depending on the clinical situation. They are more often required for those taking parenteral nutrition. Measurements of trace elements and vitamins are sensible for patients receiving long-term parenteral nutrition, but this may not be necessary for those receiving well-formulated enteral feeds.

ETHICAL CONSIDERATIONS

Legal and ethical considerations about indications, and when to start and terminate home nutritional support, vary from country to country. Furthermore, the law prohibits discontinuation of nutritional support in some states in America but not in others. Particularly difficult ethical issues concern patients with dementia in nursing homes or ordinary homes who stop eating for unknown reasons.

The role of nutrition teams in the management of patients in hospital and at home

Nutritional support is required for a wide range of patients distributed in different wards. A nutrition team, consisting of a clinician, a specialist nurse, dietitian, pharmacist, and possibly others, such as a chemical pathologist and bacteriologist, can advise, supervise, and co-ordinate the management of patients, and maintain high standards of care. It has been shown repeatedly that such teams minimize the incidence of complications associated with nutritional support (see, for example, Table 7 in relation to parenteral nutrition), avoid unnecessary nutritional support, and reduce wastage of feeds. The reduction in the incidence of catheter-related sepsis alone, from a rate of 25 per cent to 3 per cent (Table 7), has substantial economic implications, since one episode of catheter-related sepsis in a British hospital is currently estimated to cost between £1500 and £5000. Nutrition teams also have an important role to play in training patients for home support, providing advice, co-ordinating the supply of feeds and other equipment to the home, and supervising follow-up. In that context, it is regrettable that currently only some 25 to 30 per cent of British hospitals have set up such a team.

REFERENCES

American Medical Association (AMA) (1979). Guidelines for essential trace element preparations for parenteral use. A statement by the nutrition advisory group. *Journal of the American Medical Association* **241,** 2051–4.

American Medical Association Department of Foods and Nutrition (1979). Multivitamin preparations for parenteral use. *Journal of Enteral and Parenteral Nutrition* **3,** 258–62.

ASPEN Board of Directors (1987). Guidelines for the use of enteral nutrition in the adult patient. *Journal of Parenteral and Enteral Nutrition* **11,** 435–9.

Elia, M. (1982). The effects of nitrogen and energy intake on the metabolism of normal, depleted and injured man. Considerations for practical nutritional support. *Clinical Nutrition* **1,** 173–92.

Elia, M. (1990). Artificial nutritional support. *Medicine International* **82,** 3392–6.

Elia, M. (1993). Artificial nutritional support in clinical practice in Britain. *Journal of the Royal College of Physicians* **27,** 1–15.

Elia, M. (1994). Home enteral nutrition: general aspect and a comparison between the United States and Britain. *Nutrition,* **10,** 1–9.

Elwyn, D.H. (1993). Protein and energy requirements: effect of clinical state. *Clinical Nutrition,* **12,** (suppl. 1), S44–S51.

Fischer, J.E. (1991). *Total parenteral nutrition,* (2nd edn). Little, Brown and Company, Boston.

Frisancho, A.R. (1981). New norms of upper limb fat and muscle areas for assessment of nutritional status. *American Journal of Clinical Nutrition* **34,** 2540–5.

Frisancho, A.R. (1984). New standards of weight and body composition by frame size and height for the assessment of nutritional status of adults and the elderly. *American Journal of Clinical Nutrition* **40,** 808–19.

Howard, L., Heaphey, L., Fleming, C.R., Lininger, L. and Steiger, E. (1991). Four years of North American Registry Home Parenteral Nutrition Outcome Data and their implications for patient management. *Journal of Parenteral and Enteral Nutrition* **15,** 384–91.

National Research Council (1989). *Recommended dietary allowances,* (10th ed). National Academic Press, National Academy of Sciences, Washington DC.

Rapp, R.P., Hatton, J., Ott, L., Luer, M. and Young, B. (1993). Specific problems associated with enteral nutrition in patients with head injury. *Clinical Nutrition* **12** (suppl. 1), S70–S74.

Rombeau, J.L. and Caldwell, M.D. (1990). *Enteral and tube feeding,* (2nd edn). W.B. Saunders, Philadelphia.

Shenkin, A. and Wretlind, A. (1977). Complete intravenous nutrition including amino acids, glucose and lipids. In *Nutritional aspects of care in the critically ill,* (ed. J.J. Richards and J.M. Kinney), pp. 345–65. Churchill Livingstone, Edinburgh.

Taylor, S. and Goodinson-McLaren, S. (1992). *Nutritional support: a team approach.* Wolfe Publishing, London.

The Veteran Affairs Total Parenteral Nutrition Co-operative Study Group (1991). Peri-operative total parenteral nutrition in surgical patients. *New England Journal of Medicine* **325,** 525–32.

Wilcock, H., Armstrong, J. and Cottee, S. (1992). Artificial nutrition in a health district with particular reference to tube feeding. *Health Trends* **23,** 93–100.

10.7 Diseases of overnourished societies and the need for dietary change

J. I. Mann

Introduction

A wide range of diseases that are common in affluent societies occur only rarely in developing countries. This observation has been ascribed at least in part to certain aspects of the Western diet. Coronary heart disease, diabetes, obesity, dental caries, osteoporosis, gallstones, functional bowel disease, diverticular disease, appendicitis, haemorrhoids, varicose veins, and certain cancers (most notably colon and breast) are probably the most important. The major incriminating features of the Western diet are energy intake in excess of requirements, excessive quantities of total and saturated fat, insufficient amounts of certain unsaturated fatty acids, excessive amounts of sucrose and other sugars, a deficiency of non-starch polysaccharide (dietary fibre), and inadequate intake of dietary antioxidants (such as the vitamins C and E).

The following paragraphs will summarize the evidence in favour of regarding these conditions as manifestations of malnutrition in affluent societies and will consider the arguments for recommending dietary change. Nutritional deficiencies do occur in affluent societies. These have been reported amongst immigrants and the underprivileged sections of society, especially children,the elderly, and those living on their own. Rickets and iron-deficiency anaemia are amongst the deficiency diseases reported to be increasing in several countries. However, these conditions, other less clinically apparent deficiencies, and the nutritional consequences of excessive intakes of alcohol will not be considered in detail here.

Coronary heart disease

The suggestion that certain dietary practices may be associated with coronary heart disease is based on epidemiological, clinical, and animal studies. The epidemiological and clinical studies discussed in Chapter 15.10.1 provide strong evidence for a deleterious effect of excessive intake of saturated fats (especially myristic acid) and sodium, energy intake in excess of requirements, and inadequate intakes of some unsaturated fatty acids, dietary antioxidants, and perhaps also carbohydrate foods rich in non-starch polysaccharide. Each of these nutrients influences one or more risk factors for coronary heart disease. Intervention studies have shown that when diet is modified to facilitate appropriate changes in these nutrients there is a significant reduction in cardiovascular events, even when the changes are made in middle-aged individuals. The greatest benefit seems to be apparent in those at highest risk, especially when other risk factors related to lifestyle are modified at the same time. While those at the highest personal risk are likely to show the greatest individual benefit from dietary and lifestyle changes, national coronary heart disease rates will only be reduced if changes are made by the population at large. The major purpose of such recommendations would be to reduce the risk of premature morbidity and mortality from coronary heart disease. Large reductions in total mortality and increased life expectancy are unlikely to be seen amongst the first generation making such changes, but the epidemiological data suggest that in succeeding generations, with a greatly reduced lifetime exposure to risk factors related to lifestyle, the greater reduction in cardiovascular events may be reflected in some improvement in overall life expectancy.

Animal studies have provided some confirmatory evidence; several research groups have shown that in monkeys it is possible to induce atheromatous lesions by feeding a diet high in saturated fat. The experimental lesions can be reversed by lipid-lowering measures. The process in animals may differ considerably from that in humans, but such findings do nevertheless provide additional evidence for the role of diet in atherosclerosis. While the evidence suggesting the benefit of dietary change is still questioned by a small number of investigators, it has been sufficient to convince national bodies in those countries with high rates of coronary heart disease to make firm recommendations.

Diabetes mellitus

Diet undoubtedly plays an important aetiological role in non-insulin-dependent diabetes mellitus. As early as 1920 Himsworth suggested that excessive intake of energy, deficiency of dietary carbohydrate, and possibly an excessive intake of fat might increase the risk of diabetes. His conclusions were based on the improved glucose tolerance observed in non-diabetic individuals eating a high carbohydrate compared with a high fat/low carbohydrate diet, the association between high carbohydrate intakes and reduced mortality from diabetes, and the fact that newly diagnosed diabetic patients were found to have a higher intake of total energy (especially energy derived from fatty foods) before the onset of symptoms than non-diabetic controls. Although the findings in his case-control study, and indeed in more recent studies of this kind, are questionable, his conclusions appear to have been confirmed by subsequent epidemiological and clinical studies.

Epidemiological surveys and longitudinal studies in many countries confirm the striking association between increasing degrees of obesity and the risk of developing non-insulin-dependent diabetes mellitus. The association is strongest in those with central (android) obesity and those with a family history of the condition, reflecting the importance of genetic determinants (see also Chapter 11.11). While energy intake in excess of requirements is now universally accepted as an important risk determinant, controversy has raged with regard to the extent to which macronutrient distribution and some micronutrients might be involved in the aetiology of non-insulin-dependent diabetes mellitus. Epidemiological evidence suggests that it is uncommon in people eating a range of 'traditional diets high in fresh fruit, vegetables, and cereals, and therefore high in starches and non-starch polysaccharides and low in fat. Diabetes seems rapidly to assume near-epidemic proportions when traditional lifestyles are exchanged for the Western way of life, particularly when such transitions occur over a short time span. Such changes have been clearly demonstrated in Micronesians, Polynesians, American Indians, and Aboriginal Australians, as well as Chinese and Asian immigrants to Mauritius. A sharp rise in the frequency of non-insulin-dependent diabetes mellitus also emerged from studies of Asian Indian immigrants to Fiji, South Africa, and Britain, and of Chinese in Singapore, Taiwan, and Hong Kong. As lifestyle change starts to occur in China and India, by far the most populous countries in the world, non-insulin-dependent diabetes mellitus may create an enormous public health problem; Zimmet has estimated that there will be 15 million people with diabetes in these two nations by the year 2000. It is not clear which aspects of life-style are involved, and prospective studies in affluent societies have also been unable to identify individual causes. It seems most likely that a combination of factors is responsible. Excess sucrose has largely been exonerated as an important dietary substance likely to provoke diabetes, except perhaps when, alongside a high intake of fat, it contributes towards excessive energy intake. The possible role of chromium and other micronutrient deficiencies in the aetiology remains to be resolved.

Many studies in affluent societies have shown that weight reduction in overweight people and people with diabetes can often result in normal, or near normal, blood glucose levels without the need for oral hypoglycaemic therapy. Furthermore, diets high in soluble forms of non-starch polysaccharides can improve glycaemic control in those with diagnosed diabetes, independent of an effect on body mass. However, in people who are not overweight, sufficient improvement to reduce the need for drug therapy and achieve even near normal blood glucose levels is seen only with extreme dietary change (i.e. diets consisting largely of raw and unprocessed foods and exceptionally low in fat). Intervention studies in people with impaired glucose tolerance suggest that risk of progression to diabetes can be reduced and that this results chiefly from weight loss rather than modification of individual nutrients. Australian aboriginals who have reverted to their traditional lifestyle have shown a marked improvement in several indices of carbohydrate metabolism. However, most intervention studies carried out so far have not continued beyond 2 years, and there is a suggestion that the condition may relapse with time, possibly as a consequence of reverting to previous lifestyle habits. Thus it appears that reducing the level of obesity in the population at large is the single measure most likely to reduce overall rates of non-insulin-dependent diabetes mellitus in high-risk groups.

Although diet is important in the management of insulin-dependent diabetes, nutritional factors have not been detected to contribute to the disease to the same extent as has been the case for non-insulin-dependent diabetes mellitus. Genetic and other environmental factors are believed to be more important. Recent studies have suggested, however, that infants who have been breastfed may have a reduced risk of non-insulin-dependent diabetes mellitus in later life and this observation could be linked with immune mechanisms known to be associated with this condition.

Cancers

Evidence linking the intake of various nutrients to cancer is based on correlation studies (comparison between countries, or over time within a country), studies on migrants, case-control and cohort studies. Animal experiments provide confirmatory evidence, but to date no major intervention trials have been carried out in humans. All the approaches that have been used are fraught with methodological difficulties. In correlation and migrant studies, problems of confounding variables are almost impossible to eliminate; in case-control studies, subjects are asked to recall regular dietary intake before the onset of symptoms; and in cohort studies, dietary assessments, made at a single point in time, provide the estimates of exposure to various nutrients which are related to the subsequent risk of developing cancer. Clearly, such estimates of nutrient intake are not representative of lifetime dietary habits. In a recently published study, mortality from all cancers was significantly lower amongst vegetarians than amongst meat-eaters followed over a prolonged period. This association appeared to be independent of other potentially confounding factors, most notably obesity and cigarette smoking. These findings reinforce the importance of diet in the aetiology of cancer, but since the diet of vegetarians differs from that of meat-eaters in several ways other than the absence of animal protein, it is immensely difficult to disentangle the effects of so many different dietary factors, which are interrelated and may also interact with other lifestyle-related influences. This observation also applies to other stud-

Table 1 *Dietary factors which have been associated with cancers at specific sites*

Cancer site	Related dietary factors: Promoting	Protective
Oesophagus	Alcohol, especially in smokers Certain preserved foods	Several vitamins and minerals
Stomach	Salt-preserved foods	Fresh fruit and vegetables
Colon and rectum	High fat intakes	Vegetables, non-starch polysaccharide
Lung		Green and yellow vegetables
Breast	High energy intake, high fat intakes	
Prostate	High fat intake	

ies. Nevertheless, a number of consistent trends emerge. The foods and nutrients that have been most consistently shown to be related to various cancers are shown in Table 1. A high intake of fat seems to be the most consistent promoting factor, whereas fresh fruit and vegetables appear to protect against several common cancers, and the evidence is generally regarded as sufficient to provide additional justification for advice to reduce intake of fat and increase intake of vegetables and fruit.

Obesity (see also Chapter 10.5)

Of all the conditions associated with overnutrition, obesity is the most obvious. Yet the aetiology of this is still not fully understood. There is no doubt about the increased risk of morbidity and mortality from a wide range of conditions associated with obesity, and surveys in many affluent societies confirm a high and sometimes increasing prevalence. The precise role of nutritional factors remains to be established, but there is clearly no doubt that energy intake in excess of requirements is an essential prerequisite to becoming obese, and in the long term only reduction in energy intake or a substantial increase in output will reduce the proportion of overweight people in the population. It has been suggested that a diet high in fat is more likely to lead to obesity than a high carbohydrate diet of similar energy content because of the low expenditure involved in storing ingested dietary fat. Furthermore, a diet which is high in non-starch polysaccharide may help to reduce obesity by encouraging satiety at a lower level of intake.

Dental caries

Dental caries was exceptionally rare among young people in ancient Britain. Surveys over the past 15 years have suggested that as many as 80 per cent of 5-year-olds require treatment for dental caries and about 10 per cent of all children enter school with more than half their teeth seriously decayed. Some 5 per cent of the adult population in England and Wales and 15 per cent of that in Scotland are edentulous by the age of 30 years. Careful oral hygiene, including the use of fluoride-impregnated toothpaste, fluoridation of the water supply, and perhaps, in future, a vaccine to raise resistance against cariogenic organisms, will decrease the frequency of dental caries, but there are impressive data to suggest a nutritional cause. Amongst the indigenous population of many countries where unrefined foods form the bulk of the diet (e.g. China, Uganda) dental caries once had a very low prevalence. Within a few years of the addition of sugar and other refined foods the frequency showed a rapid increase. A similar change has been shown experimentally in monkeys. In a classical experiment carried out in a Swedish mental hospital, volunteers given toffee apples, chocolate, and caramel in addition to their controlled diet had a thirteenfold greater number of tooth surfaces becoming carious each year, compared with those eating the controlled diet alone. While frequency and timing of intake may be important, and while other dietary factors may also be involved, the overall evidence indicates non-milk extrinsic sugars (see below) as the major dietary component contributing to dental caries.

Osteoporosis

Osteoporosis is now recognized as having reached near-epidemic proportions in many affluent societies. By the age of 65 approximately 20 per cent of women in the United States have suffered from one or more osteoporotic fractures. Lack of physical activity, falling levels of oestrogen, and genetic influences are probably more important than nutrition-related factors in achieving peak bone mass and in the loss of bone mass seen later in life. However, there is a consensus that an adequate intake of dietary calcium, especially by young women early in life, is of value in helping to achieve peak bone mass, and high calcium intakes may help to prevent the loss of cortical bone in some women over 45 years of age (see Section 19).

Constipation and the irritable bowel syndrome

Ninety-nine per cent of a large population sample studied in Britain reported that they defecated at least three times per week. Yet perceived constipation is a frequent complaint. Approximately 3 per cent of all prescriptions written in the National Health Service (in the United Kingdom) are for purgatives and laxatives, at a cost of around £4 000 000, and many times this amount must have been spent in buying these preparations over the counter. In another survey, 6 per cent of people aged between 18 and 80 years described straining when passing stools. No data are available concerning the frequency of passing small stools. There seems little doubt that constipation is uncommon in populations with a high intake of non-starch polysaccharide. In rural Africa stool weights are frequently around 500 g daily, and bowel transit times around 40 h. In Britain stool weights in non-vegetarians are more usually around 100 g (with a very wide range), whereas in vegetarians the average stool weight is over 200 g. Factors other than non-starch polysaccharide might be involved, but the fact that British vegetarians and non-vegetarians with high average daily intakes of non-starch polysaccharide have transit times of less than 75 h and rarely report constipation, whereas those with lower intakes have transit times ranging from 20 to 124 h and frequently complain of constipation, suggests that this dietary component is likely to be particularly relevant. There is no doubt that increasing the non-starch polysaccharide content of the diet (especially that derived from cereals) relieves the symptoms of constipation, an observation now confirmed by controlled clinical trials. There is no direct evidence of a causal link between a diet low in non-starch polysaccharide and the irritable bowel syndrome, but diets rich in non-starch polysaccharide are widely recommended in its treatment and are believed to be of value, even in the absence of formal clinical trials.

Diverticular disease of the colon

The first suggestion that deficiency of non-starch polysaccharides in the diet might be implicated in the aetiology of diverticular disease of the colon came from striking geographical variations in prevalence and the documented increase in disease rates in several European countries since the 1920s. These variations and trends in rates are certainly compatible with a causative link with low non-starch polysaccharide diets, but could also be explained by several alternative dietary and other environmental influences. The best-documented evidence comes from studies of matched patients with and without diverticular disease, from animal experiments, and observations on the effects of treatment with bran. In one study based on diet histories from patients with and without diverticular disease, there was evidence of a lower intake of 'crude fibre' before the onset of symptoms among patients compared with the control subjects. In another study of several hundred volunteers without symptoms, 95 were found to have diverticular disease. Careful dietary histories, which were obtained from all participants, showed that vegetarians, who had a substantially higher non-starch polysaccharide intake than non-vegetarians, were less prone to diverticular disease (12 per cent v. 33 per cent). Moreover non-starch polysaccharide intake was appreciably higher in those without than those with radiological diverticular disease both in vegetarians and non-vegetarians. Animal experiments provide confirmation (for example, rats given a diet low in non-starch polysaccharide have been shown to develop diverticulae, as do rabbits fed with white bread, sugar, and vitamins, and given prostigmine). An increase in non-starch polysaccharide intake is widely recommended to patients with symptomatic diverticular disease, a treatment justified by the findings of some (but not all) controlled clinical trials.

Plausible theories concerning pathogenesis have been suggested; small, hard faeces, undoubtedly features of a diet deficient in non-starch polysaccharide, are associated with narrowing of the colon and the formation of closed segments in which pressure increases. Additional work is then needed by colonic muscles to provide the pressure to move the more solid faeces, producing muscular hypertrophy in addition to the diverticulae at sites of weakness where blood vessels penetrate the muscular coat.

Other diseases

Gallstones, appendicitis, haemorrhoids, varicose veins, and hiatus hernia all occur frequently in developed countries and rarely in developing countries, but the evidence linking these diseases to a nutritional cause is tenuous. Gallstones are undoubtedly associated with obesity. Both gallstones and appendicitis are more common in non-vegetarians than vegetarians and there are some rather indirect data suggesting an association with diets high in sugars and deficient in non-starch polysaccharides. The addition of bran to the diet can make bile less saturated, and experimentally induced gallstones in animals tend to be reduced if foods rich in non-starch polysaccharides are given. Data from the United Kingdom and South Africa taken together provide interesting information concerning appendicitis: appendicitis rates were compared in two matched South African Caucasian groups, the privileged group living in University Halls of Residence and the other living in the establishments for the more indigent where the diets contained more fibre. Annual rates were 7.8 and 1.8 per thousand, respectively. Of course, factors other than diets might explain this, but the similarity in rates to those found in an almost identical study in Bristol (7.6 per thousand in a public school and 0.8 per thousand in an orphanage) are very striking.

The case for dietary change

Many of the conditions listed above are important causes of mortality throughout adult life in Britain and other affluent societies. Non-fatal episodes of illness also account for an enormous drain on resources for health care and profoundly affect society as a whole. Many sets of dietary recommendations for adults have been made, with the hope of reducing the frequency of premature morbidity and mortality from coronary heart disease. Although there is a great deal of evidence to suggest that dietary change will reduce the risk of coronary heart disease, there is a growing realization that recommendations should also take into account other aspects of the relationships between food, nutrients, and health. The earlier focus on macronutrient distribution (percentage energy derived from protein, carbohydrate, and fat) has been extended

Table 2 *Estimated average requirements (EARs) for energy*

	EARs (MJ/day (kcal/day))	
Age	Males	Females
0–3 months	2.28 (545)	2.16 (515)
4–6 months	2.89 (690)	2.69 (645)
7–9 months	3.44 (825)	3.20 (765)
10–12 months	3.85 (920)	3.61 (865)
1–3 years	5.15 (1230)	4.86 (1165)
4–6 years	7.16 (1715)	6.46 (1545)
7–10 years	8.24 (1970)	7.28 (1740)
11–14 years	9.27 (2220)	7.92 (1845)
15–18 years	11.51 (2755)	8.83 (2110)
19–50 years	10.60 (2550)	8.10 (1940)
51–59 years	10.60 (2550)	8.00 (1900)
60–64 years	9.93 (2380)	7.99 (1900)
65–74 years	9.71 (2330)	7.96 (1900)
75+ years	8.77 (2100)	7.61 (1810)
Pregnancy		+0.80[a] (200)
Lactation		
1 month		+1.90 (450)
2 months		+2.20 (530)
3 months		+2.40 (570)
4–6 months (group 1)[b]		+2.00 (480)
4–6 months (group 2)[c]		+2.40 (570)
> 6 months (group 1)[b]		+1.00 (240)
> 6 months (group 2)[c]		+2.30 (550)

[a]Last trimester only.

[b]Active weaning after 4 months.

[c]Breast milk continues to provide the primary source of nourishment for 6 months or more.

Table 3 *Reference nutrient intakes for protein*

Age	Reference nutrient intake[a] (g/day)
0–3 months	12.5
4–6 months	12.7
7–9 months	13.7
10–12 months	14.9
1–3 years	14.5
4–6 years	19.7
7–10 years	28.3
Males	
11–14 years	42.1
15–18 years	55.2
19–50 years	55.5
50+ years	53.3
Females	
11–14 years	41.2
15–18 years	45.0
19–50 years	45.0
50+ years	46.5
Pregnancy[b]	+ 6
Lactation[b]	
0–4 months	+11
4+ months	+ 8

[a]These figures, based on egg and milk protein, assume complete digestibility.

[b]To be added to the adult requirement through all stages of pregnancy and lactation.

Table 4 *Dietary reference values for fat and carbohydrate for adults as a percentage of daily total energy intake (percentage of food energy)*

	Individual minimum	Population average	Individual maximum
Saturated fatty acids		10 (11)	
cis-Polyunsaturated fatty acids		6 (6.5)	10
n-3	0.2		
n-6	1.0		
cis-Monounsaturated acids		12 (13)	
trans Fatty acids		2 (2)	
Total fatty acids		30 (32.5)	
Total fat		33 (35)	
Non-milk extrinsic sugars	0	10 (11)	
Intrinsic and milk sugars and starch		37 (39)	
Total carbohydrate		47 (50)	
Non-starch polysaccharide (g/day)	12	18	24

The average percentage contribution to total energy does not total 100 per cent because figures for protein and alcohol are excluded. Protein intakes average 15 per cent of total energy, which is above the reference nutrient intake. It is recognized that many individuals will derive some energy from alcohol, and this has been assumed to average 5 per cent approximating to current intakes. However, some groups might not drink alcohol and for some purposes nutrient intakes as a proportion of food energy (without alcohol) might be useful. Therefore average figures are given as percentages both of total energy and, in parenthesis, of food energy.

to include recommendations regarding micronutrients, because of the realization that these may also be important in the aetiology and prevention of many chronic diseases, and to ensure that dietary change does not lead to nutritional inadequacies. Indeed, there is increasing evidence that inadequate intakes of some nutrients (to the extent of causing clinical deficiency states) may occur in affluent societies as well as in developing countries, especially amongst new immigrants and, as unemployment increases, amongst the growing number of disadvantaged people. The recently published report on dietary reference values for food energy and nutrients for the United Kingdom represents one of the first attempts to provide comprehensive quantified recommendations concerning all nutrients. Tables 2 to 5 are adapted from this publication.

Tables 2 and 3 give the estimated average requirements for energy and reference nutrient intakes for protein. While these are generally adequate or excessive in most countries, there is evidence that some elderly people do not have sufficient food to achieve adequate intakes of essential micronutrients. It is also important that physical activity is sufficient to enable an adequate intake of total energy and of micronutrients without unacceptable weight gain.

Table 4 shows dietary reference values for fat and carbohydrate for adults expressed as a percentage of total daily energy. The recommended reduction in the population average intake of saturated fatty acids to 10 per cent of total energy (which represents a very considerable reduction from present intakes) is based on the expectation of a reduced risk of coronary heart disease, certain cancers, and obesity and its associated health consequences. Advice regarding polyunsaturated fatty acids includes individual minimum (to prevent deficiency of essential fatty acids) and maximum intakes (to ensure that high intakes do not reduce high-density lipoprotein intakes or increase the risk of gallstones or cancers). The recommended population average intake of 6 per cent polyunsaturated fatty acids represents a modest increase, primarily in the expectation of a reduced risk of coronary heart disease. There are, at present, insufficient data to enable advice to be given regarding the optimal proportions of *n*-6 and *n*-3 polyunsaturated fatty acids. The recommendation is for *cis*-monounsaturated fatty acids to remain unchanged, but if saturated fats are to be reduced, monounsaturated fatty acids would need to be derived from non-animal sources to a greater extent than at present, since saturated and monounsaturated fatty acids occur together in meat. Intake of *trans* fatty acids (found in partially hydrogenated vegetable and fish oils) should not be increased because of adverse effects on lipoproteins. For the first time in such nutritional recommendations advice regarding total fat is based on the sum of fatty acid intake and glycerol, in contrast to the earlier, more arbitrary recommendations which were primarily based on a reduction of total fat. This approach has been adopted on the grounds that the bulk of the scientific evidence relates to advantages and disadvantages of various fatty acids, rather than total fat. Using this technique a reduction in total fat is still required, although the extent of the decrease is not as great as when advice was solely centred around total fat. The evidence for making these recommendations is discussed further in Chapter 15.10.1.

Only about 50 g of carbohydrate daily is required to avoid ketosis, and many populations maintain an adequate nutritional status when carbohydrate provides up to 80 per cent total energy; thus a wide range of intakes is clearly acceptable. However, most Western societies are unaccustomed to a high carbohydrate intake and are reluctant to accept substantial increases in this nutrient. Therefore, a modest increase in total carbohydrate is advised with a limitation on the use of non-milk extrinsic sugars (sucrose and other sugars, apart from those in milk, which are not naturally incorporated into the cellular structure of foods) because of their role in dental caries, especially when consumed frequently. Furthermore, a very high intake of extrinsic sugars (in excess of 30 per cent dietary energy) may be associated with undesirable elevations of plasma glucose, lipids, and insulin. On the other hand, it is considered appropriate (Table 4) that intrinsic sugars (that is, those incorporated into the cellular structure of foods), milk sugars, and starches should provide the balance of dietary energy not provided by protein, fat, and non-milk extrinsic sugars, that is an average of 37 per cent total dietary energy. Foods containing these macronutrients are usually rich in essential micronutrients as well as dietary fibre (non-starch polysaccharide), an increase in which is also recommended because of the convincing evidence for benefit in terms of bowel function and possible benefits regarding a range of diseases of the large intestine, carbohydrate metabolism and insulin and plasma lipids and cardiovascular disease.

Reference nutrient intakes (adequate for most individuals) are provided for vitamins and minerals; selected examples are shown in Table 6. Clinical vitamin deficiencies are uncommon in affluent societies except in at-risk subgroups within populations. For example, immigrants who have migrated from warm to temperate climates may be at risk of vitamin D deficiency, strict vegetarians (who consume no animal or dairy products) may become deficient in vitamin B_{12}, and disadvantaged groups (especially the very young,pregnant and lactating women, and the elderly) may have generally inadequate intakes.

On the other hand inappropriate intakes of certain minerals are fairly common. Excessive intakes of sodium, to such an extent that it probably contributes to hypertension and its consequences, are common throughout the Western world. Targets for reduction may be more important than reference nutrient intakes for sodium. An intake of 140 mmol/day (3.2 g/day), a level currently exceeded in most countries, might be an appropriate maximum. Selenium and iodine are deficient in soils in various parts of the world. Clinical selenium deficiency has only been reported from China, although, with renewed interest in nutrient antioxidants, the role of selenium in the prevention of chronic disease will need to be re-examined in other parts of the world where soils are known to be deficient (e.g. in the South Island of New Zealand). Endemic iodine

Table 5 *Reference nutrient intakes for selected vitamins and minerals*

Age	Vitamin B_{12} μg/day	Folate μg/day	Vitamin A μg/day	Vitamin D μg/day	Calcium mmol/day	Sodium[a] mmol/day	Iron μmol/day	Zinc μmol/day	Selenium μmol/day	Iodine μmol/day
0–3 months	0.3	50	350	8.5	13.1	9	30	60	0.1	0.4
4–6 months	0.3	50	350	8.5	13.1	12	80	60	0.2	0.5
7–9 months	0.4	50	350	7	13.1	14	140	75	0.1	0.5
10–12 months	0.4	50	350	7	13.1	15	140	75	0.1	0.5
1–3 years	0.5	70	400	7	8.8	22	120	75	0.2	0.6
4–6 years	0.8	100	500	–	11.3	30	110	100	0.3	0.8
7–10 years	1.0	150	500	–	13.8	50	160	110	0.4	0.9
Males										
11–14 years	1.2	200	600	–	25.0	70	200	140	0.6	1.0
15–18 years	1.5	200	700	–	25.0	70	200	145	0.9	1.0
19–50 years	1.5	200	700	–	17.5	70	160	145	0.9	1.0
50+ years	1.5	200	700	**	17.5	70	160	145	0.9	1.0
Females										
11–14 years	1.2	200	600	–	20.0	70	260[b]	140	0.6	1.0
15–18 years	1.5	200	600	–	20.0	70	260[b]	110	0.8	1.1
19–50 years	1.5	200	600	–	17.5	70	260[b]	110	0.8	1.1
50+ years	1.5	200	600	**	17.5	70	160	110	0.8	1.1
Pregnancy	*	+100	+100	10	*	*	*	*	*	*
Lactation:										
0–4 months	+0.5	+60	+350	10	+14.3	*	*	+90	+0.2	*
4+ months	+0.5	+60	+350	10	+14.3	*	*	+40	+0.2	*

[a]1 mmol sodium = 23 mg.

[b]Insufficient for women with high menstrual losses where the most practical way of meeting iron requirements is to take iron supplements.

*No increment.

**After 65 years of age the reference nutrient intake is 10 μg/day for men and women.

Table 6 *Food groups and the nutrients they provide*

Food group	Provides
Vegetables and fruits (includes fresh, frozen, canned, and dried)	Carbohydrates: starches and intrinsic sugars Non-starch polysaccharide: soluble and insoluble Vitamins: especially A (yellow and green vegetables), C (dark-green vegetables and most fruits, potatoes), and folate Minerals: magnesium, potassium
Breads and cereals (includes all breads, grains, rice, and pasta)	Protein Carbohydrates, especially starches Non-starch polysaccharide: soluble and insoluble Vitamins: B (except B_{12}), E (wheat germ) Minerals: magnesium, calcium, iron and zinc (whole-grain products)
Milks and dairy products (includes cheese, yoghurt, and ice-cream)	Protein Carbohydrates: milk sugars Fats: higher proportion of saturated fats than polyunsaturated fat or monounsaturated fat Minerals, especially calcium, phosphorus, zinc Vitamins: riboflavin, B_{12}, A
Lean meats, poultry, fish, eggs, nut seeds, and pulses	Protein Fat: both visible and marbled in meat, saturated fat, cholesterol Starches and non-starch polysaccharide: dried beans and peas Vitamins: B_{12}, niacin, thiamine Minerals: iron, zinc, magnesium, copper, potassium, phosphorus, and selenium

A broad indication of the main nutrients supplied by each food group is given. Not all the foods within each group will contain all these nutrients.

deficiency is even more widespread especially in Africa, and clinical deficiency states are largely avoided by the use of iodized salt and sanitizers containing iodine used by the dairy industry. Young women often have insufficient calcium to help achieve peak bone mass, and older women may have an inadequate intake to help prevent an age-related bone loss. Many groups are particularly vulnerable to iron deficiency, due to high physiological requirements (infants and toddlers, adolescents, pregnant women), high losses (menstruating women), or poor absorption (the elderly and people consuming foods high in inhibitors of absorption, such as fibre and tannin in tea).

Table 7 *Food and nutrition guidelines*

1. Eat a variety of foods from each of the four major food groups each day:	
Vegetables and fruits	At least 3 servings of vegetables and 2 servings of fruit each day
Bread and cereals	At least 6 servings each day, including some whole grain
Milk and dairy products	At least 2 servings each day, preferably low fat
Lean meats, poultry, fish, eggs, nuts, or pulses (e.g. dried beans, peas and lentils)	At least 1 serving each day
2. Prepare meals with minimal added fat, especially saturated fat, and salt	
3. Choose prepared foods, drinks, and snacks that are low in fat (especially saturated fat), salt, and sugar	
4. Maintain a healthy body weight by regular physical activity and by healthy eating	
5. If drinking alcohol, do so in moderation	
6. Drink plenty of liquids each day	

Considerable changes in traditional eating patterns are required in order to achieve the recommended changes in distribution of macronutrients. A reduction of high-fat dairy foods, confectionery products, and fatty meats is essential. While these foods are high in saturated fat some are also important sources of calcium, iron, and other essential micronutrients. Education in nutrition is essential in order to ensure that these foods are replaced by others (such as low-fat dairy foods) which will provide sufficient quantities of micronutrients to ensure that deficiencies do not occur, particularly amongst vulnerable groups. Doctors are often asked to give nutritional advice but often lack the information to do so. They and the public require information about food groups and the nutrients they provide (Table 6) as well as appropriate guidelines (Table 7). Dietitians and others trained in nutrition play an invaluable role in providing the public with practical advice to facilitate what are clearly fairly substantial changes from the typical Western diet. Successful implementation of dietary change also requires considerable political motivation. In many Western countries farmers have considerable political influence and in many countries dairy products have government subsidies. Until policies are altered to encourage the consumption of more appropriate food choices, the required changes are unlikely to be adopted by the population as a whole.

REFERENCES

Ahrens, E.H. (1979). Dietary fats and coronary heart disease: Unfinished business. *Lancet* **ii,** 1345–8.

Committee on Medical Aspects of Food Policy (1984). *Diet and cardiovascular disease*. Department of Health and Social Security, no. 28. HMSO, London.

Gear, J., *et al.* (1979). Asymptomatic diverticular disease and intake of dietary fibre. *Lancet* **ii,** 511–14.

Gear, J., Brodribb, A.J., Ware, A., and Mann, J.I. (1981). Fibre and bowel transit times. *British Journal of Nutrition* **45,** 77–82.

Nutrition Taskforce to the Departments of Health (1991). *Food for health*. Department of Health, PO Box 5013, Wellington, New Zealand.

Panel on Dietary Reference Values of the Committee on Medical Aspects of Food Policy (1991). *Report on Health and Social Subjects: 41. Dietary Reference Values for Food Energy and Nutrients for the United Kingdom.* HMSO, London.

Index

Page numbers in **bold** refer to major discussions in the text and include major sections and subsections, but are not necessarily limited to these. Bold page numbers referring to diseases, include discussions on diagnosis, clinical features, pathology and treatment, where relevant.

Page numbers in *italics* refer to pages on which tables are to be found.

vs denotes differential diagnosis or comparisons.

Plates have not been indexed, but are referred to in the text. Biochemical parameters within the tables of Section 33 have not all been indexed individually - readers are advised to seek reference ranges from the appropriate table. Epidemiological data relating to specific countries has only been indexed under the individual countries where major discussions occur. For further information, readers are advised to refer to the epidemiological page reference for the disease in question.

Indexing style/conventions used

Alphabetical order. This index is in letter-by-letter order, whereby hyphens, en-rules and spaces within index headings are ignored in the alphabetization. Terms in brackets are excluded from initial alphabetization eg.

acid(s)
acid-base homeostasis
acidosis
acid phosphatase

Cross-references. Cross-reference terms in *italics* are either general cross-references, or refer to subentry terms within the same main entry (the main entry term is not repeated, in order to save space) i.e. they are not main entry terms.

Index entries have been restricted to two subentry levels. Entries have therefore been reorganised/reworded or relocated where further levels have been required.

eg. *renal failure, acute*, reworded to *acute renal failure*, or *lymphoma, non-Hodgkin's* reworded to *non-Hodgkin's lymphoma.*

Cross-references are inserted to indicate correct keyword term or location of entry.

Some index subentries, particularly those referring to individual pages within a page grouping, have been included more to indicate the extent of the discussion in the text rather than the actual location of the reference.

Abbreviations used in subentries (without explanation):

ACTH	Adrenocorticotrophic hormone (corticotrophin)	hCG	Human chorionic gonadotrophin
AIDS	Acquired immunodeficiency syndrome	HIV	Human immunodeficiency virus
ARDS	Adult respiratory distress syndrome	HPV	Human papilloma virus
CMV	Cytomegalovirus	HTLV	Human T-cell leukaemia virus
COAD	Chronic obstructive airways disease	IL	Interleukin
CPAP	Continous positive airway pressure	LCMV	Lymphocytic choriomeningitis virus
CRF	Corticotrophin releasing hormone (factor)	MAOIs	Monoamine oxidase inhibitors
CT	Computed tomography	MEN	Multiple endocrine neoplasia
DIC	Disseminated intravascular coagulation	MRI	Magnetic resonance imaging
EBV	Epstein-Barr virus	NSAIDs	Non-steroidal anti-inflammatory drugs
ECG	Electrocardiogram/electrocardiography	PAF	Platelet activating factor
EEG	Electroencephalogram/electroencephalography	PEEP	Positive end-expiratory pressure
EMG	Electromyography	PTH	Parathyroid hormone
ERCP	Endoscopic retrograde cholangiopancreatography	RSV	Respiratory syncytial virus
G6PD	Glucose-6-phosphate dehydrogenase	SIADH	Syndrome of inappropriate antidiuretic hormone secretion
GBM	Glomerular basement membrane		
G-CSF	Granulocyte colony-stimulating factor	SLE	Systemic lupus erythematosus
GH	Growth hormone	STDs	Sexually transmitted diseases
GM-CSF	Granulocyte-macrophage colony-stimulating factor	TNF	Tumour necrosis factor
HBV	Hepatitis B virus	TSH	Thyroid stimulating hormone
HCV	Hepatitis C virus		

A

D

E

F

G

H

I

J

M

N

P

Erratum

These entries are missing from the printed index

Q

R

S

T

U

V

W

X

Y

Z